Williams
GYNECOLOGY

Williams GYNECOLOGY

SECOND EDITION

Barbara L. Hoffman, MD
John O. Schorge, MD
Joseph I. Schaffer, MD
Lisa M. Halvorson, MD
Karen D. Bradshaw, MD
F. Gary Cunningham, MD

Department of Obstetrics and Gynecology
University of Texas Southwestern Medical Center at Dallas

Parkland Health and Hospital System
Dallas, Texas

Lewis E. Calver, MS, CMI, FAMI

Biomedical Communications Graduate Program
University of Texas Southwestern Medical Center at Dallas

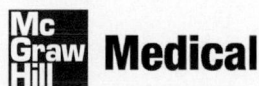

New York   Chicago   San Francisco   Lisbon   London   Madrid   Mexico City
Milan   New Delhi   San Juan   Seoul   Singapore   Sydney   Toronto

Williams Gynecology, Second Edition

Copyright © 2012, 2008 by The McGraw-Hill Companies, Inc. All rights reserved. Printed in China. Except as permitted under the United States copyright Act of 1976, no part of this publication may be reproduced or distributed in any form or by any means, or stored in a data base or retrieval system, without the prior written permission of the publisher.

1 2 3 4 5 6 7 8 9 0 CTP/CTP 17 16 15 14 13 12

ISBN 978-0-07-171672-7
MHID 0-07-171672-6

This book was set in Adobe Garamond by Aptara, Inc.
The editors were Alyssa Fried and Peter J. Boyle.
The production supervisor was Catherine H. Saggese.
Project management was provided by Indu Jawwad, Aptara, Inc.
The designer was Alan Barnett.
The illustration manager was Armen Ovsepyan.
China Translation & Printing, Ltd., was printer and binder.

Library of Congress Cataloging-in-Publication Data

Williams gynecology / [edited by] Barbara L. Hoffman ... [et al.]. –
2nd ed.
    p. ; cm.
Gynecology
Includes bibliographical references and index.
ISBN 978-0-07-171672-7 (hardback : alk. paper)
I. Hoffman, Barbara L.   II. Williams, J. Whitridge (John Whitridge),
1866–1931.   III. Title: Gynecology.
[DNLM: 1. Gynecology.   2. Genital Diseases, Female.
3. Gynecologic
Surgical Procedures. WP 100]
  618.1—dc23
                        2011053203

DEDICATION

This second edition of *Williams Gynecology* is dedicated with great appreciation to Dr. Steven L. Bloom, Chairman of the Department of Obstetrics and Gynecology at the University of Texas Southwestern Medical Center at Dallas. During his tenure as chairman, Steve has been a stalwart supporter of both editions of *Williams Gynecology*. His insight into the needs of authors stems no doubt from his work as one of the editors of our textbook patriarch—*Williams Obstetrics*. As chairman, his vision and leadership have created an environment in which critical evidence-based academic projects can flourish. We have benefited from his effective use of resources, commitment to excellence, and dedication to the advancement of medical education.

CONTENTS

SECTION 1

BENIGN GENERAL GYNECOLOGY

SECTION 2

REPRODUCTIVE ENDOCRINOLOGY, INFERTILITY, AND THE MENOPAUSE

SECTION 3

FEMALE PELVIC MEDICINE AND RECONSTRUCTIVE SURGERY

SECTION 4

GYNECOLOGIC ONCOLOGY

SECTION 5

ASPECTS OF GYNECOLOGIC SURGERY

SECTION 6

ATLAS OF GYNECOLOGIC SURGERY

EDITORS

Barbara L. Hoffman, MD
Associate Professor, Department of Obstetrics and Gynecology
University of Texas Southwestern Medical Center at Dallas

John O. Schorge, MD
Director, Division of Gynecologic Oncology Fellowship
Associate Professor, Department of Obstetrics and Gynecology
Massachusetts General Hospital–Harvard Medical School

Joseph I. Schaffer, MD
Holder, Frank C. Erwin, Jr. Professorship in Obstetrics
    and Gynecology
Director, Division of Gynecology
Director, Division of Female Pelvic Medicine and
    Reconstructive Surgery
Professor, Department of Obstetrics and Gynecology
University of Texas Southwestern Medical Center at Dallas
Chief of Gynecology, Parkland Memorial Hospital, Dallas

Lisa M. Halvorson, MD
Professor, Department of Obstetrics and Gynecology
University of Texas Southwestern Medical Center at Dallas

Karen D. Bradshaw, MD
Holder, Helen J. and Robert S. Strauss and Diana K. and
    Richard C. Strauss Distinguished Chairmanship in
    Women's Health
Director, Lowe Foundation Center for Women's Preventative
    Health Care
Associate Residency Program Director, Department of Obstetrics
    and Gynecology
Professor, Department of Obstetrics and Gynecology
Professor, Department of Surgery
University of Texas Southwestern Medical Center at Dallas

F. Gary Cunningham, MD
Holder, Beatrice and Miguel Elias Distinguished Chair in
    Obstetrics and Gynecology
Professor, Department of Obstetrics and Gynecology
University of Texas Southwestern Medical Center at Dallas

Atlas Art Director

Lewis E. Calver, MS, CMI, FAMI
Chairman, Biomedical Communications Graduate Program
Director, Biomedical Illustration Graduate Studies
Associate Professor, Department of Biomedical Communications
University of Texas Southwestern Medical Center at Dallas

CONTRIBUTORS

Victor E. Beshay, MD
Assistant Professor, Department of Obstetrics and Gynecology
University of Texas Southwestern Medical Center at Dallas
Chapter 10: Endometriosis

Karen D. Bradshaw, MD
Holder, Helen J. and Robert S. Strauss and Diana K. and Richard C.
    Strauss Chairmanship in Women's Health
Director, Lowe Foundation Center for Women's Preventative Health
    Care
Associate Residency Program Director, Department of Obstetrics
    and Gynecology
Professor, Department of Obstetrics and Gynecology
Professor, Department of Surgery
University of Texas Southwestern Medical Center at Dallas
Chapter 13: Psychosocial Issues and Female Sexuality
Chapter 18: Anatomic Disorders
Chapter 21: Menopausal Transition
Chapter 22: The Mature Woman

Anna R. Brandon, PhD, MCS, ABPP
Women's Mood Disorders Center
Department of Psychiatry
University of North Carolina at Chapel Hill School of Medicine
Chapter 13: Psychosocial Issues and Female Sexuality

Bruce R. Carr, MD
Holder, Paul C. MacDonald Distinguished Chair in Obstetrics and
    Gynecology
Director, Division of Reproductive Endocrinology and Infertility
    Fellowship Program
Professor, Department of Obstetrics and Gynecology
University of Texas Southwestern Medical Center at Dallas
Chapter 10: Endometriosis

Kelley S. Carrick, MD
Associate Professor, Department of Pathology
University of Texas Southwestern Medical Center at Dallas
Director of Surgical Pathology Images for Williams Gynecology

Marlene M. Corton, MD
Associate Residency Program Director, Department of Obstetrics
    and Gynecology
Associate Professor, Department of Obstetrics and
    Gynecology
University of Texas Southwestern Medical Center at Dallas
Chapter 25: Anal Incontinence and Functional Anorectal Disorders
Chapter 38: Anatomy

F. Gary Cunningham, MD
Holder, Beatrice and Miguel Elias Distinguished Chair in Obstetrics
    and Gynecology
Professor, Department of Obstetrics and Gynecology
University of Texas Southwestern Medical Center at Dallas
Chapter 5: Contraception and Sterilization
Chapter 6: First-Trimester Abortion
Chapter 38: Anatomy

Kevin J. Doody, MD
Director, Center for Assisted Reproduction, Bedford, TX
Director, In Vitro Fertilization Laboratory at the University of Texas
    Southwestern
Associate Professor, Department of Obstetrics and Gynecology
University of Texas Southwestern Medical Center at Dallas
Chapter 20: Treatment of the Infertile Couple

David M. Euhus, MD
Holder, Marilyn R. Corrigan Distinguished Chair in Breast Cancer
    Surgery
Director of Clinical Cancer Genetics in the Simmons
    Comprehensive Cancer Center
Professor, Department of Surgery
University of Texas Southwestern Medical Center at Dallas
Chapter 12: Breast Disease

Rajiv B. Gala, MD, FACOG
Residency Program Director, Department of Obstetrics and Gynecology
Ochsner Clinic Foundation
Associate Professor of Obstetrics and Gynecology
University of Queensland
Ochsner Clinical School
Chapter 7: Ectopic Pregnancy
Chapter 39: Perioperative Considerations

William F. Griffith, MD
Medical Director, Intermediate Care Center
Director, Vulvology Clinic
Co-Director, Dysplasia Services
Parkland Health and Hospital System, Dallas, Texas
Associate Professor, Department of Obstetrics and Gynecology
University of Texas Southwestern Medical Center at Dallas
Chapter 29: Preinvasive Lesions of the Lower Genital Tract

Lisa M. Halvorson, MD
Professor, Department of Obstetrics and Gynecology
University of Texas Southwestern Medical Center at Dallas
Chapter 6: First-Trimester Abortion
Chapter 15: Reproductive Endocrinology
Chapter 16: Amenorrhea
Chapter 19: Evaluation of the Infertile Couple

Cherine A. Hamid, MD
Assistant Professor, Department of Obstetrics and Gynecology
University of Texas Southwestern Medical Center at Dallas
Chapter 40: Intraoperative Considerations

Alison Brooks Heinzman, MD
Assistant Professor, Department of Obstetrics and Gynecology
University of Texas Southwestern Medical Center at Dallas
Chapter 9: Pelvic Mass

David L. Hemsell, MD
Clinical Professor, Department of Obstetrics and Gynecology
University of Texas Southwestern Medical Center at Dallas
Chapter 3: Gynecologic Infection

Barbara L. Hoffman, MD
Associate Professor, Department of Obstetrics and Gynecology
University of Texas Southwestern Medical Center at Dallas
Chapter 1: Well Woman Care
Chapter 8: Abnormal Uterine Bleeding
Chapter 9: Pelvic Mass
Chapter 11: Pelvic Pain
Chapter 40: Intraoperative Considerations
Chapter 41: Surgeries for Benign Gynecologic Conditions
Chapter 43: Surgeries for Female Pelvic Reconstruction

Siobhan M. Kehoe, MD
Assistant Professor, Department of Obstetrics and Gynecology
University of Texas Southwestern Medical Center at Dallas
Chapter 44: Surgeries for Gynecologic Malignancies

Kimberly A. Kho, MD, MPH
Assistant Professor, Department of Obstetrics and Gynecology
University of Texas Southwestern Medical Center at Dallas
Chapter 42: Minimally Invasive Surgery

Jayanthi S. Lea, MD
Assistant Professor, Department of Obstetrics and Gynecology
University of Texas Southwestern Medical Center at Dallas
Chapter 31: Vulvar Cancer

Eddie H. McCord, MD
Assistant Professor, Department of Obstetrics and Gynecology
University of Texas Southwestern Medical Center at Dallas
Academic Contributor: Benign Gynecology Atlas Art

David Scott Miller, MD, FACOG, FACS
Holder, Dallas Foundation Chair in Gynecologic Oncology
Medical Director of Gynecology Oncology
Parkland Health and Hospital System, Dallas, Texas
Director, Gynecologic Oncology Fellowship Program
Director of Gynecologic Oncology
Professor, Department of Obstetrics and Gynecology
University of Texas Southwestern Medical Center at Dallas
Chapter 33: Endometrial Cancer
Chapter 34: Uterine Sarcoma

Elysia Moschos, MD
Associate Professor, Department of Obstetrics and Gynecology
University of Texas Southwestern Medical Center at Dallas
Chapter 2: Techniques Used for Imaging in Gynecology
Director of Radiologic Images for Williams Gynecology

Phuc D. Nguyen, MD
Former Associate Professor, Department of Radiation Oncology
University of Texas Southwestern Medical Center at Dallas
Chapter 28: Principles of Radiation Therapy

Mary Jane Pearson, MD
Director, Resident Continuity Clinic
Director, Fourth-year Medical Student Programs
Associate Professor, Department of Obstetrics and Gynecology
University of Texas Southwestern Medical Center at Dallas
Chapter 1: Well Woman Care

David D. Rahn, MD
Assistant Professor, Department of Obstetrics and Gynecology
University of Texas Southwestern Medical Center at Dallas
Chapter 23: Urinary Incontinence

Debra L. Richardson, MD, FACOG
Assistant Professor, Department of Obstetrics and Gynecology
University of Texas Southwestern Medical Center at Dallas
Chapter 31: Cervical Cancer
Chapter 32: Vaginal Cancer

David E. Rogers, MD, MBA
Assistant Professor, Department of Obstetrics and Gynecology
University of Texas Southwestern Medical Center at Dallas
Chapter 11: Pelvic Pain

John O. Schorge, MD, FACOG, FACS
Director, Division of Gynecologic Oncology
Associate Professor, Department of Obstetrics and Gynecology
Massachusetts General Hospital – Harvard Medical School
Chapter 27: Principles of Chemotherapy
Chapter 33: Endometrial Cancer
Chapter 34: Uterine Sarcoma
Chapter 35: Epithelial Ovarian Cancer
Chapter 36: Ovarian Germ Cell and Sex-cord-Stromal Tumors
Chapter 37: Gestational Trophoblastic Disease
Chapter 43: Surgeries for Gynecologic Malignancies

Joseph I. Schaffer, MD
Holder, Frank C. Erwin, Jr. Professorship in Obstetrics and Gynecology
Chief of Gynecology
Parkland Health and Hospital System, Dallas, Texas
Director, Division of Gynecology
Director, Division of Female Pelvic Medicine and Reconstructive Surgery
Professor, Department of Obstetrics and Gynecology
University of Texas Southwestern Medical Center at Dallas
Chapter 24: Pelvic Organ Prolapse
Chapter 43: Surgeries for Female Pelvic Reconstruction

Manisha Sharma, MD
Assistant Professor, Department of Obstetrics and Gynecology
University of Texas Southwestern Medical Center at Dallas
Chapter 8: Abnormal Uterine Bleeding

Geetha Shivakumar, MD, MS
Mental Health Trauma Services, Dallas VA Medical Center
Assistant Professor, Department of Psychiatry
University of Texas Southwestern Medical Center at Dallas
Chapter 13: Psychosocial Issues and Female Sexuality

Gretchen S. Stuart, MD, MPHTM
Director, Family Planning Program
Director, Fellowship in Family Planning
Assistant Professor, Department of Obstetrics and Gynecology
University of North Carolina at Chapel Hill
Chapter 5: Contraception and Sterilization

Mayra J. Thompson, MD, FACOG
Associate Professor, Department of Obstetrics and Gynecology
University of Texas Southwestern Medical Center at Dallas
Chapter 42: Minimally Invasive Surgery

Diane M. Twickler, MD, FACR
Holder, Fred Bonte Professorship in Radiology
Vice-Chairman of Academic Affairs
Professor, Department of Radiology
Professor, Department of Obstetrics and Gynecology
University of Texas Southwestern Medical Center at Dallas
Chapter 2: Techniques Used for Imaging in Gynecology
Director of Radiologic Images for Williams Gynecology

Clifford Y. Wai, MD
Director, Fellowship Program in Female Pelvic Medicine and
    Reconstructive Surgery Associate
Professor, Department of Obstetrics and Gynecology
University of Texas Southwestern Medical Center at Dallas
Chapter 23: Urinary Incontinence
Chapter 26: Genitourinary Fistulas and Urethral Diverticulum

Claudia L. Werner, MD
Medical Director of Dysplasia Services
Co-Director Vulvology Clinic
Parkland Health and Hospital System, Dallas, Texas
Associate Professor, Department of Obstetrics and Gynecology
University of Texas Southwestern Medical Center at Dallas
Chapter 29: Preinvasive Lesions of the Lower Genital Tract

Ellen E. Wilson, MD
Director of Pediatric and Adolescent Gynecology Program
Children's Medical Center, Dallas, Texas
Associate Professor, Department of Obstetrics and Gynecology
University of Texas Southwestern Medical Center at Dallas
Chapter 14: Pediatric Gynecology
Chapter 17: Polycystic Ovarian Syndrome and Hyperandrogenism

Larry E. Word, MD
Professor, Department of Obstetrics and Gynecology
University of Texas Southwestern Medical Center at Dallas
Chapter 41: Surgeries for Benign Gynecologic Conditions

ARTISTS

Artist renderings in our surgical atlas were produced by the Chair of the Biomedical Communications Graduate Program and students and faculty within that program.

The world's first degree in medical illustration was awarded by Southwestern Medical School in 1947. Currently, this is one of five accredited medical illustration programs in North America. For those accepted into the program, a Master of Arts degree in Biomedical Communications—Biomedical Illustration is offered by Southwestern School of Health Professions at The University of Texas Southwestern Medical Center at Dallas. The program is two years in length, and a maximum of seven students is now accepted annually.

The program is offered through the Department of Biomedical Communications, and courses are taught by faculty of The University of Texas Southwestern Medical School, Southwestern Graduate School of Biomedical Sciences, and Southwestern School of Health Professions. The program is accredited by the Commission on Accreditation of Allied Health Education Programs and the Association of Medical Illustrators. Mr. Lewis E. Calver has been Program Chairman since 1980.

The program is interdisciplinary. It provides opportunities for development of special knowledge and skills in the application of communication arts and technology to the health sciences. Study of human anatomy, cell biology, neurobiology, and pathology is combined with experience in anatomic, surgical, editorial, and advertising illustration; computer graphics and animation; graphic design; multimedia production; interactive computer-assisted instruction; and instructional design. Additional skills may also be developed in biological illustration, three-dimensional media production, exhibit design, and photography.

Primary Atlas Artists

Lewis E. Calver, MS, CMI, FAMI
Chairman, Biomedical Communications Graduate Program
Director, Biomedical Illustration Graduate Studies
Associate Professor, Department of Biomedical Communications
University of Texas Southwestern Medical Center at Dallas

SangEun Cha
Graduate, Biomedical Communications Graduate Program
University of Texas Southwestern Medical Center at Dallas

Erin Frederikson
Graduate, Biomedical Communications Graduate Program
University of Texas Southwestern Medical Center at Dallas

Alexandra Gordon
Graduate, Biomedical Communications Graduate Program
University of Texas Southwestern Medical Center at Dallas

Jordan Pietz
Graduate, Biomedical Communications Graduate Program
University of Texas Southwestern Medical Center at Dallas

Marie Sena
Graduate, Biomedical Communications Graduate Program
University of Texas Southwestern Medical Center at Dallas

Maya Shoemaker
Graduate, Biomedical Communications Graduate Program
University of Texas Southwestern Medical Center at Dallas

Jennie Swensen
Graduate, Biomedical Communications Graduate Program
University of Texas Southwestern Medical Center at Dallas

Amanda Tomasikiewicz
Graduate, Biomedical Communications Graduate Program
University of Texas Southwestern Medical Center at Dallas

Kristin Yang
Graduate, Biomedical Communications Graduate Program
University of Texas Southwestern Medical Center at Dallas

Contributing Atlas Artists

Katherine Brown
Graduate, Biomedical Communications Graduate Program
University of Texas Southwestern Medical Center at Dallas

T. J. Fels
Graduate, Biomedical Communications Graduate Program
University of Texas Southwestern Medical Center at Dallas

Kimberly Hoggatt-Krumwiede
Associate Professor, Biomedical Communications Graduate Program
University of Texas Southwestern Medical Center at Dallas

Richard P. Howdy, Jr.
Former Instructor, Biomedical Communications Graduate Program
University of Texas Southwestern Medical Center at Dallas

Belinda Klein
Graduate, Biomedical Communications Graduate Program
University of Texas Southwestern Medical Center at Dallas

Anne Matuskowitz
Graduate, Biomedical Communications Graduate Program
University of Texas Southwestern Medical Center at Dallas

Lindsay Oksenberg
Graduate, Biomedical Communications Graduate Program
University of Texas Southwestern Medical Center at Dallas

Kimberly VanExel
Graduate, Biomedical Communications Graduate Program
University of Texas Southwestern Medical Center at Dallas

PREFACE

The first edition of *Williams Obstetrics* was published over a century ago. Since then, the editors of this seminal text have presented a comprehensive and evidenced-based discussion of obstetrics. Patterned after our patriarch, *Williams Gynecology* provides a thorough presentation of gynecology's depth and breadth. In Section 1, general gynecology topics are covered. Sections 2 provides chapters covering reproductive endocrinology and infertility. The developing field of Female Pelvic Medicine and Reconstructive Surgery is presented in Section 3. In Section 4, gynecologic oncology is discussed.

Traditionally, gynecologic information has been offered within the format of either a didactic text or a surgical atlas.

However, because the day-to-day activities of a gynecologist blends these two, so too did we. The initial four sections of our book describe the evaluation and medical treatment of gynecologic problems. The remaining two sections focus on the surgical patient. Section 5 offers detailed anatomy and a discussion of perioperative consideration. Our final section presents an illustrated atlas for the surgical correction of conditions described in Sections 1 through 4. Although discussions of disease evaluation and treatment are evidence based, our text strives to assist the practicing gynecologist and resident. Accordingly, chapters are extensively complemented by illustrations, photographs, diagnostic algorithms, and treatment tables.

ACKNOWLEDGMENTS

During the creation and production of our textbook, we were lucky to have the assistance and support of countless talented professionals both within and outside our department.

First, a task of this size could not be completed without the unwavering support provided by our Department Chairman, Dr. Steven Bloom, and Vice-Chairman, Dr. Barry Schwarz. Their financial and academic endorsement of our efforts has been essential.

Without their academic vision and expert distribution of departmental resources, this undertaking could not have flourished.

In constructing a compilation of this breadth, the expertise of physicians from several departments was needed to add vital, contemporaneous information. We were fortunate to have Dr. Diane Twickler, with joint appointments in the Department of Radiology and Department of Obstetrics and Gynecology, add her insight and knowledge as a specialist in gynecologic radiology. From the Department of Pathology, Dr. Kelley Carrick shared generously from her cadre of outstanding images. She translated her extensive knowledge of gynecologic pathology into concepts relevant for the general gynecologist. Many thanks are extended to Dr. Phuc Nguyen, recently retired from the Department of Radiation Oncology. Dr. Nguyen masterfully explained difficult physics concepts in easy-to-comprehend terms and brought a greatly appreciated enthusiasm to our project. In addition, we are appreciative of the valuable insight and critique provided to this same chapter by Dr. William Hittson. From the Department of Surgery, Dr. David Euhus lent his considerable knowledge of breast disease to contribute both classical and state-of-the-art information to his chapter. His broad research and clinical expertise provided the foundation for his truly comprehensive chapter. From the Department of Psychiatry here at University of Texas Southwestern Medical Center at Dallas and from the University of North Carolina at Chapel Hill School of Medicine, we were lucky to have Drs. Geetha Shivakumar and Anna Brandon, who provided an extensive discussion of psychosocial issues. They expertly distilled a broad topic into a logically organized, practical, and complete presentation. In addition, Dr. Gretchen Stuart, formerly of our department and now a faculty member at the University of North Carolina's Department of Obstetrics and Gynecology, lent her considerable talents in summarizing contraceptive methods and sterilization techniques. Her skillful reorganization of this chapter presents newer trends in contraception counseling. Many warm thanks are extended to Dr. Rajiv Gala, also formerly of our department and now of the Ochsner Clinic. Rajiv masterfully organized and summarized chapters on ectopic pregnancy and perioperative practice. His extensive review of the literature and evidence-based writing shines through both chapters. We thank Dr. Richard Penson, Clinical Director of Medical Gynecologic Oncology at Massachusetts General Hospital. His assistance added significantly to our chapter on chemotherapy fundamentals. Dr. Stephen Heartwell is the Deputy Director of Domestic Programs for the Susan Thompson Buffett Foundation. He served as an important resource for our discussion of first-trimester abortion services.

The beautiful and detailed artwork in our atlas was drawn by the gifted graduate students and Chair of the Biomedical Communications Graduate Program, here at the University of Texas Southwestern Medical Center at Dallas. Graduate students SangEun Cha, Alexandra Gordon, Jennie Swensen, Amanda Tomasikiewicz, and Kristin Yang spent countless hours observing surgical procedures, sketching operative steps, and consulting with surgeons. Their efforts added priceless content to our atlas chapters. We also acknowledge the efforts of our atlas artists from the first edition: Erin Frederikson, Jordan Pietz, Marie Sena, and Maya Shoemaker. Additionally, alumni from the Program provided seminal pieces and include Katherine Brown, Thomas "TJ" Fels, Belinda Klein, Anne Matuskowitz, Lindsay Oksenberg, Constance Tilden, Kimberly VanExel, and faculty member Richard P. Howdy, Jr. Also, Ms. Kimberly Hoggatt-Krumwiede graciously provided several image series to help clarify the steps and missteps of reproductive tract development. Overseeing this monumental task was the Program's Chair, Mr. Lewis Calver. In our first edition, Lew logged tremendous hours sketching art for the urogynecologic section of the atlas. For this edition, he paired his academic talents with Dr. Marlene Corton to create a comprehensive, ageless anatomy chapter. Both of these anatomists committed thankless hours in the cadaver laboratory and in the library to create academically new presentations of female reproductive anatomy. These renderings were crafted and tailored with the gynecologic surgeon in mind to depict important anatomy for these surgeries. Lew also coupled his talents with Drs. Mayra Thompson and Kimberly Kho to create complementary illustrations to their descriptions of minimally invasive procedures. His considerable artistic skills were rivaled only by his dedication to education. Lew added many more hours teaching and advising revisions with his talented students.

Within our own department, the list is too long and the words are too few to convey our heartfelt thanks to all of our department members for their generous contributions. First, Drs. Bruce Carr, David Hemsell, David Miller, and Larry Word, all with well-known and well-established careers, generously contributed their expertise without hesitation. We are indebted to them for their altruism toward our project. From our Gynecology Division, many thanks are extended to Drs. Diane Twickler and Elysia Moschos, who sculpted a clear and detailed summary of traditional and new gynecologic imaging tools. For this edition, these authors updated radiologic images as needed to present ultimate examples of normal anatomy and gynecologic pathology. We were also lucky to have experts in the field of preinvasive lesions of the lower genital tract, Drs. Claudia Werner and William Griffith. They crafted an information-packed, contemporaneous discussion of this topic. In addition, Dr. Griffith has been a steadfast advocate of our project and has extensively added photographic content to many of our chapters. Dr. Eddie McCord worked closely with our medical artist to craft new content for our surgical atlas. His clinical experience and extensive knowledge of anatomy added greatly to the academic value of these illustrations. We were also fortunate to have the expert writing talents of Drs. Mayra Thompson and Kimberly Kho, who provided a clear and evidence-based discussion of minimally invasive surgery. With this second edition, new authors from the gynecology division added their academic expertise to many of the benign gynecology chapters. Our textbook benefitted greatly from the clinical and evidence-based information that Drs. Mary Jane Pearson, Alison Brooks Heinzman, David Rogers, and Manisha Sharma provided in their chapters.

Our Reproductive Endocrinology and Infertility Division also offered a deep bench of talented writers. Dr. Kevin Doody lent his considerable clinical and academic prowess in the treatment of infertility. He penned a chapter that clearly describes the current "state of the art" in this field. Dr. Doody was also a kind benefactor with his spectacular clinical photographs on the topic and contributed these generously to numerous chapters. In addition, Dr. Ellen Wilson brought her wealth of clinical experience to chapters on pediatric gynecology and androgen excess. With her expertise, she crafted chapters that presented practical, prescriptive, and comprehensive discussions of these topics. We are also appreciative of the contributions of a new member to our writing team, Dr. Victor Beshay. Victor teamed with Dr. Bruce Carr to thoroughly yet succinctly summarize the fundamentals of endometriosis.

Dr. Marlene Corton is a skilled urogynecologist and has written extensively on pelvic anatomy. We were thrilled to have her create stunning chapters on anatomy and anal incontinence. Also from the Urogynecology and Female Pelvic Reconstruction Division, Drs. Clifford Wai and David Rahn added expanded content and stellar drawings to our chapter on urinary incontinence. Dr. Wai also masterfully updated his chapter on vesicovaginal fistula and urethral diverticulum. Special thanks are extended to Dr. Ann Word and her contributions to our chapter on pelvic organ prolapse. Her expertise in extracellular matrix remodeling of the female reproductive tract added fundamental content to the discussion of prolapse physiology.

In addition to Drs. Miller and Schorge, the Division of Gynecologic Oncology provided other talented physicians and writers. The topic of vulvar cancer was thoroughly covered by Dr. Jayanthi Lea. Her strengths in clinical practice and resident teaching are evident in her well-organized and evidence-based chapter. We were also thrilled to have Dr. Debra Richardson present comprehensive, clinical discussions of cervical and vaginal cancer in her two chapters. Dr. Siobhan Kehoe lent her surgical expertise to clearly describe and illustrate new laparoscopic and robotic sections to the gynecologic oncology surgical atlas.

Within our text, images add powerful descriptive content to our words. Accordingly, many, many thanks are extended to those who donated surgical and clinical photographs. Of our contributors, many beautiful photographs within our book were taken by Mr. David Gresham, Chief Medical Photographer at the University of Texas Southwestern Medical Center. Dave's eye for detail, shading, and composition allowed even simple objects to shine and be illustrated to their full potential. Since this project's early months, he has been an advocate and valued consultant. Our pathology images were presented at their best thanks to Mr. Mark Smith, a graphics designer here at the University of Texas Southwestern Medical Center. His expertise with micrographs improved the clarity and visual aesthetic of many our microscopic images.

During preparation of this text, we benefited from the expert staff at the University of Texas Southwestern Medical Center at Dallas' South Campus library. As with our first edition, a special "thank you" is extended to Ms. Herldine Radley. Ms. Radley served as priceless asset and expert in library services.

Many of our photographs were taken in the operating rooms at Parkland Hospital. The operative room staff consistently helped us obtain photographs. Moreover, they graciously accommodated our graduate art students as they observed surgeries for their illustration. Special thanks are extended to Ms. Karin Cooper. As is her style, Karin went above and beyond to assist us in securing the photographs that were needed to illustrate many of our chapters. Warm appreciation is similarly given to the operating room staff at University Hospital St. Paul. At St. Paul, our graduate art students were welcomed with open arms by the physicians and OR staff. Students observed, photographed, and queried as skilled surgeons operated. Graciously, Mr. Mack Holmes and Nurse Erlinda Yenchai kindly assisted us in coordinating artists and surgeons. Mr. Moses Walker served as our audiovisual specialist and allowed us to capture spectacular surgical images for our chapters.

In addition, our colleagues in the clinic system and Intermediate Care Center at Parkland Hospital were huge allies in our acquisition of images to illustrate normal and abnormal gynecologic findings. Vera Bell, Sharon Irvin, Mercedes Pineda, and Rebecca Winn, all women's health care nurse practitioners, have been true supporters of our efforts, and we sincerely thank them.

We are truly indebted to our administrative staff, who tirelessly and meticulously typed and organized our content. For this project, we were lucky to have Ms. Connie Utterback serve as our primary administrative assistant. Connie was an integral part of our first edition as well as several editions of *Williams Obstetrics*. She brought her considerable experience, talents, careful attention to detail, and ever-present commitment again to this edition. We are greatly appreciative of her tremendous efforts and unique skills. In addition, Melinda Epstein, Barbara Moore, and Eureka Pinkney added their talents to our undertaking. Ms. Dina Trujillo was a valuable assistant in obtaining needed journal articles. She truly helped to keep our project evidence-based. None of our image and text production would have been possible without the brilliant information technology team in our department. Knowledgeable and responsive, Mr. Charles Richards and Mr. Thomas Ames have supported our project since the first edition. We could not do our job without their expertise.

Williams Gynecology was sculpted into its final form by the talented and dedicated group at McGraw-Hill Publishing, Inc. Ms. Alyssa Fried has brought her considerable intelligence, energetic work ethic, and creativity to our project. Her attention to detail and organizational talents have kept our project on track through an array of potential hurdles with efficiency and style. Our words fall well short in expressing our gratitude. Dr. Anne Sydor has been a steadfast advocate of *Williams Gynecology* since our inaugural edition, and we extend warm thanks for her tremendous support. Ms. Sarah Granlund deserves a crown for her eagle-eyed organization of reams of permissions. Peter Boyle shepherded our book through production. We greatly appreciate his calm and efficient style.

Without the thoughtful, creative efforts of many, our textbook would be a barren wasteland of words. Integral to this process are Armen Ovsepyan and John Williams, at McGraw-Hill, and Alan Barnett of Alan Barnett Design. Special thanks are extended to Mr. Joseph Varghese and Dr. Shetoli Zhimomi at Thomson Digital. They and their artistic team assisted us in revising many of our text images. Their attention to detail and accurate renderings added important academic support to our words. Our text took its final shape under the watchful care of our compositors at Aptara, Inc.

We offer a sincere "thank you" to our residents in training. Their curiosity keeps us energized to find new and effective ways to convey age-old as well as cutting-edge concepts. Their logical questions lead us to holes in our text and thereby always help us to improve our work. We extend special thanks to Dr. Emily Bradbury. Her critique of several of our benign gynecology chapters helped us identify chapter strengths and weaknesses to better serve our readers' needs.

Moreover, the contributors to this text owe a significant debt to the women who have allowed us to participate in their care. The images and clinical expertise presented in this text would not have been possible without their collaborative spirit to help us move medical knowledge forward.

Lastly, we offer an enthusiastic and heartfelt "thank you" to our families and friends. Without their patience, generosity, and encouragement, this task would have been impossible. For them, too many hours with "the book" left them with new responsibilities. And importantly, time away from home left precious family memories unrealized. We sincerely thank you for your love and support.

SECTION 1
BENIGN GENERAL GYNECOLOGY

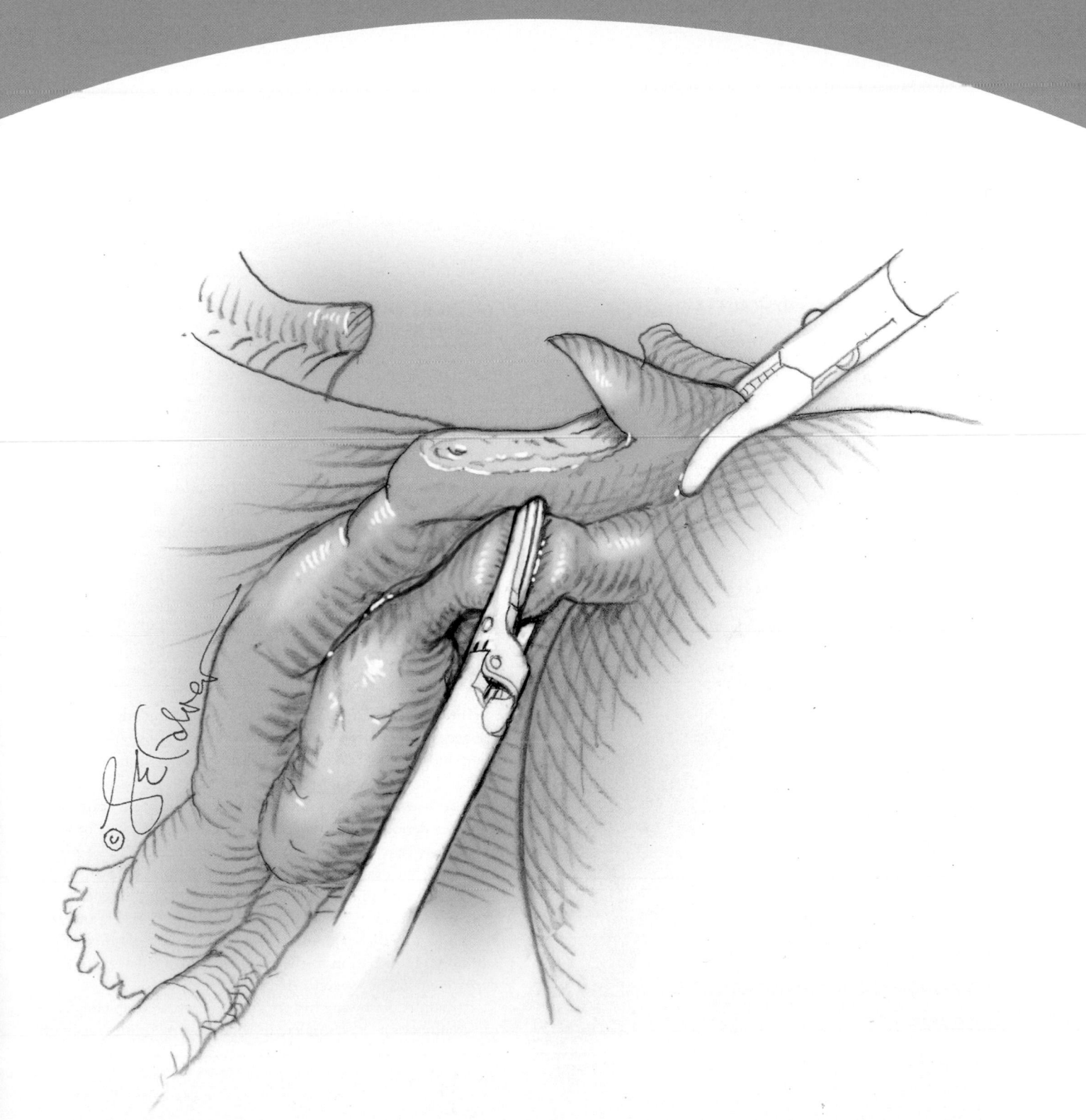

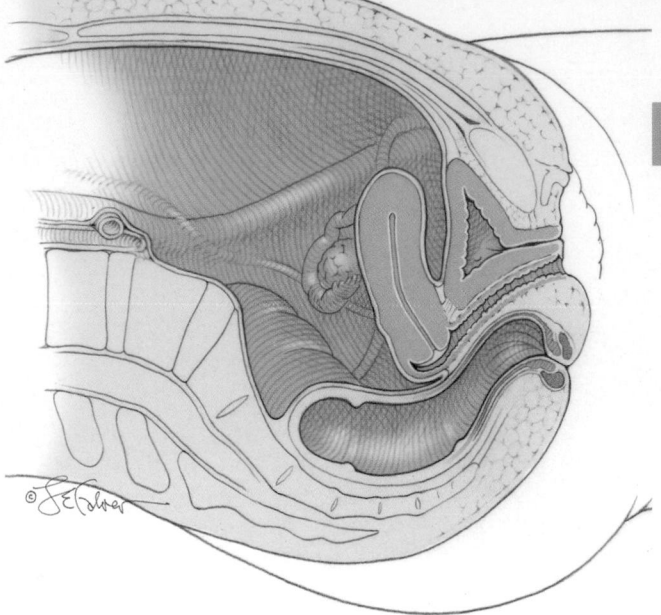

CHAPTER 1

Well Woman Care

MEDICAL HISTORY AND PHYSICAL EXAMINATION

For many women, gynecologists serve as specialist and primary care provider. As such, clinicians are given an opportunity to prevent and treat a wide variety of diseases. The incidence of these may vary greatly depending on the age group treated. Thus, the focus of medical questioning should reflect these changing risks. In addition to questioning regarding specific health complaints, a detailed history, including a thorough family history, can direct appropriate preventive screening.

Various organizations provide guidelines for preventive care and update their recommendations regularly. These include the Centers for Disease Control and Prevention (CDC), the U.S. Preventive Services Task Force (USPSTF), the American Cancer Society, and the American College of Obstetricians and Gynecologists.

The first reproductive health visit is recommended between the ages of 13 and 15 (American College of Obstetricians and Gynecologist, 2011). At this visit, rapport between an adolescent and her gynecologist can be established, the stage of adolescence assessed, and reproductive health care needs addressed. Whether periodic care continues with the gynecologist or with her pediatrician can be discussed at that visit. At this age, an internal pelvic examination is not performed in an asymptomatic adolescent unless otherwise indicated. Specific needs of the adolescent are presented in Chapter 14 (p. 382), and the American College of Obstetricians and Gynecologists offers additional information at their web site: http://www.acog.org/departments/dept_web.cfm?recno=7.

For adults, following historical inventory, a complete physical examination is completed. Many women present with complaints specific to the breast or pelvis. Their evaluation is described next.

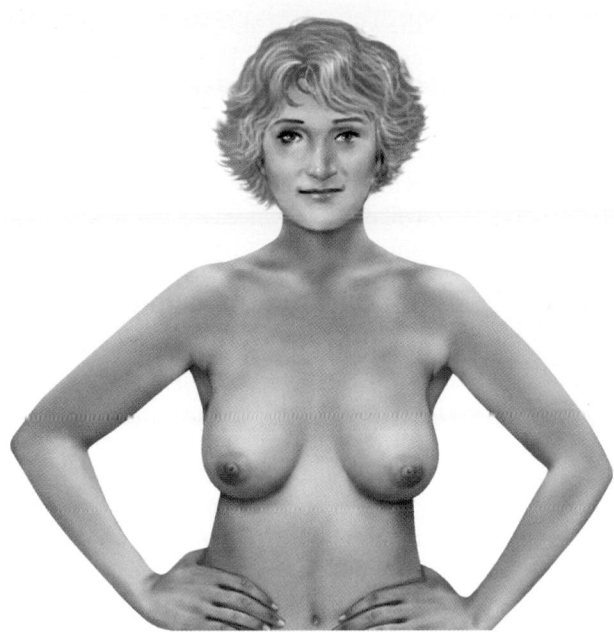

FIGURE 1-1 Drawing depicts visual breast inspection. The patient's gown is dropped briefly to allow inspection. Her hands are pressed against her waist to flex the pectoralis muscles. With the patient leaning slightly forward, breasts are visually inspected to identify for breast contour asymmetry or skin dimpling.

Breast Examination

Self breast examination (SBE) is an examination performed by the patient herself to detect abnormalities. Studies have shown SBE to increase rates of diagnostic testing for ultimately benign breast disease and to be ineffective in lowering breast cancer mortality rates (Kösters, 2008; Thomas, 2002). However, the American College of Obstetricians and Gynecologists (2011a), the American Cancer Society (2011a), and the National Comprehensive Cancer Network (Bevers, 2009) recommend breast self-awareness, which can include self-breast examination (American College of Obstetricians and Gynecologists, 2011a).

In contrast, *clinical breast examination (CBE)* is completed by a clinical health care professional and may identify a small portion of breast malignancies not detected with mammography. Additionally, CBE may identify cancer in young women, who are not typical candidates for mammography (McDonald, 2004). Clinical breast examination can be completed by various methods. However, in an attempt to standardize performance, a committee for the American Cancer Society has described a CBE that includes visual inspection combined with axillary and breast palpation, which is outlined next (Saslow, 2004).

Breast Inspection

Initially, the breasts should be viewed as a woman sits on the table's edge with hands placed at her hips and with pectoralis muscles flexed (Fig. 1-1). Alone, this position enhances asymmetry. Additional arm positions, such as placing arms above the head, do not add vital information. Breast skin is inspected for breast erythema, retraction, scaling, especially over the nipple, and edema, which is termed *peau d'orange* change. Additionally, the breast and axilla are observed for contour symmetry.

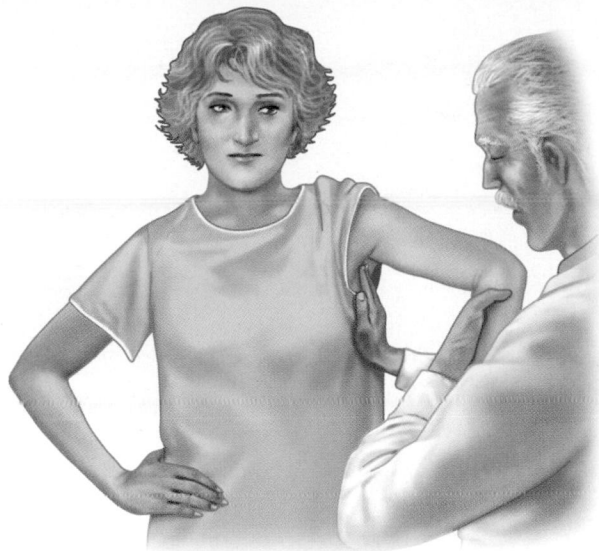

FIGURE 1-2 Drawing depicts one method of axillary lymph node palpation. Finger tips extend to the axillary apex and compress tissue against the chest wall in the rolling fashion shown in Figure 1-4. The patient's arm is supported by the examiner.

Lymph Node Evaluation

Following inspection, axillary, supraclavicular, and infraclavicular lymph nodes are palpated most easily with a woman seated and her arm supported by the examiner (Fig. 1-2). The axilla is bounded by the pectoralis major muscle ventrally and the latissimus dorsi muscle dorsally. Lymph nodes are detected as the examiner's hand glides from high to low in the axilla and momentarily compresses nodes against the lateral chest wall. In a thin patient, one or more normal, mobile lymph nodes less than 1 cm in diameter may commonly be appreciated. The first lymph node to become involved with breast cancer metastasis (the sentinel node) is nearly always located just behind the midportion of the pectoralis major muscle belly.

Breast Palpation

After inspection, breast palpation is completed with a woman supine and with one hand above her head to stretch breast tissue across the chest wall (Fig. 1-3). Examination should include breast tissue bounded by the clavicle, sternal border, inframammary crease, and midaxillary line. Breast palpation within this pentagonal area is approached in a linear fashion. Technique should use the finger pads in a continuous rolling, gliding circular motion (Fig. 1-4). At each palpation point, tissues should be assessed both superficially and deeply (Fig. 1-5). During CBE, intentional attempts at nipple discharge expression are not required unless a *spontaneous* discharge has been described by the patient.

If abnormal breast findings are noted, they are described by their location in the right or left breast, clock position, distance from the areola, and size. Evaluation and treatment of breast and nipple diseases are described more fully in Chapter 12 (p. 333).

During examination, patients are educated that new axillary or breast masses, noncyclic breast pain, spontaneous nipple discharge, nipple inversion, and breast skin changes such

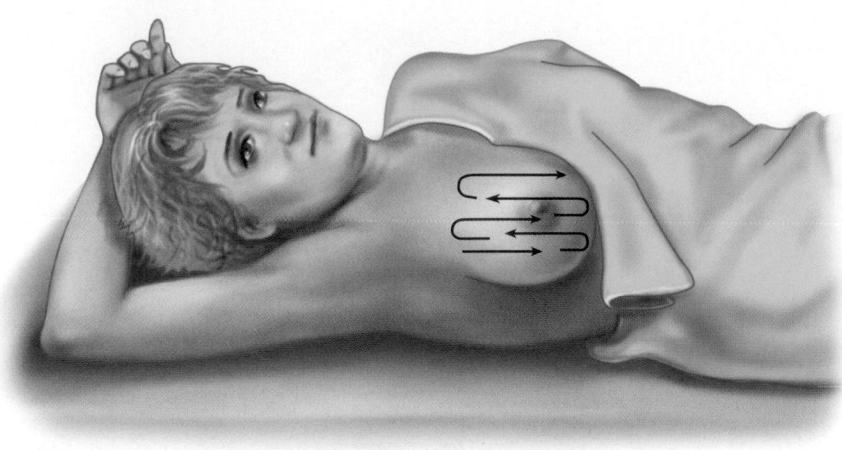

FIGURE 1-3 Drawing depicts recommended patient positioning and direction of palpation during clinical breast examination.

as dimpling, scaling, ulceration, edema, or erythema should be promptly evaluated. Patients who desire to perform SBE should be counseled on its benefits, limitations, and potential harms and instructed to complete SBE the week after menses.

Pelvic Examination

This examination is typically performed with a patient supine, her legs in dorsal lithotomy position, and feet resting in stirrups. The head of the bed is elevated 30 degrees to relax abdominal wall muscles for bimanual examination. A woman should be assured that she may stop or pause the examination at any time. Moreover, each part of the evaluation should be announced or described before its performance.

Inguinal Lymph Nodes and Perineal Inspection

Pelvic cancers and infections may drain to the inguinal lymph nodes, and these should be palpated during examination. Following this, a methodical inspection of the perineum should extend from the mons ventrally, to the genitocrural folds laterally, and to the anus. Infections and neoplasms that involve

the vulva may also involve perianal skin, and this area should be similarly inspected. Some clinicians additionally palpate for Bartholin and paraurethral gland pathology. However, in most cases, patient symptoms and asymmetry in these areas will dictate the need for this specific evaluation.

Speculum Examination

Both metal and plastic specula are available for this examination, each in a variety of sizes to accommodate vaginal length and laxity. The plastic speculum may be equipped with a small light that provides illumination. The metal speculum requires an external light source. Preference between these two types is provider dependent. The vagina and cervix are typically viewed after placement of either a Graves or Pederson speculum (Fig. 1-6). Prior to insertion, a speculum may be warmed with running water or by warming lights mounted within the drawer of the examination table. Additionally, lubrication may add comfort to insertion. Griffith and colleagues (2005) found

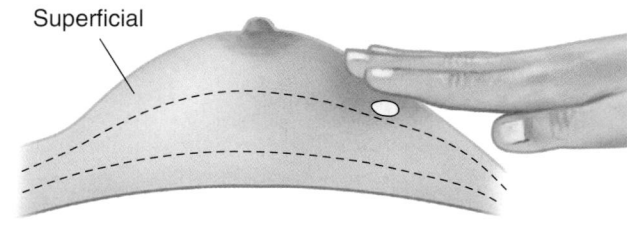

Superficial

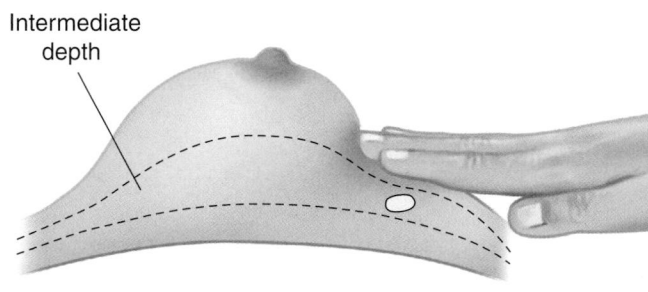

Intermediate depth

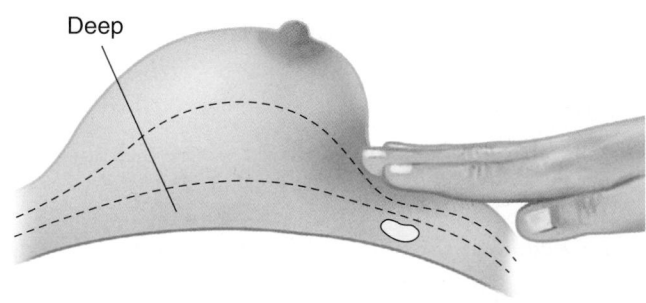

Deep

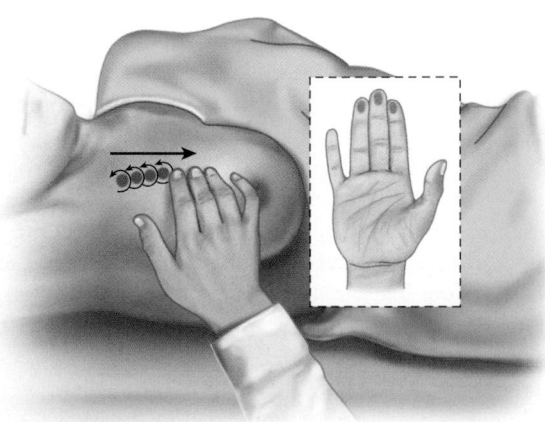

FIGURE 1-4 Drawing depicts recommended palpation technique. The finger pads and a circular rolling motion are used to palpate the entire breast.

FIGURE 1-5 Drawing depicts palpation through several depths at each point along the linear path.

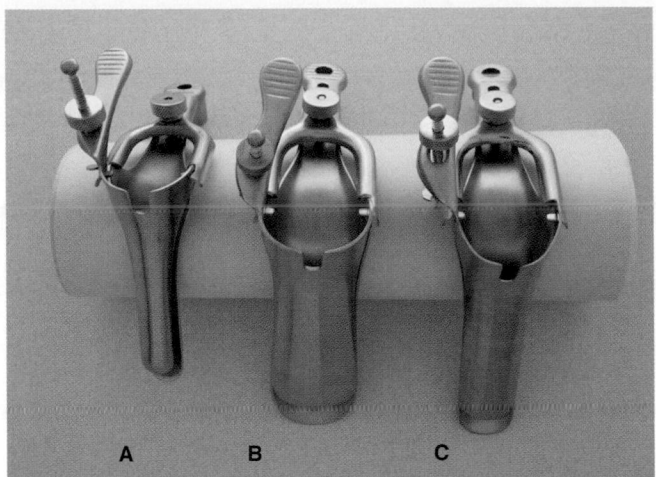

FIGURE 1-6 Photograph displays vaginal specula. **A.** Pediatric Pederson speculum. This may be selected for child, adolescent, or virginal adult examination. **B.** Graves speculum. This may be selected for examination of parous women with relaxed and collapsing vaginal walls. **C.** Pederson speculum. This may be selected for sexually active women with adequate vaginal wall tone. *(Photograph contributed by US Surgitech, Inc.)*

that gel lubricants did not increase unsatisfactory Pap smear cytology rates or decrease *Chlamydia trachomatis* detection rates compared with water lubrication. If gel lubrication is used, a dime-sized aliquot is applied sparingly to the outer surface of the speculum blades.

Prior to insertion, the labia minora are gently separated, and the urethra is identified. Because of urethral sensitivity, the speculum is inserted well below the meatus. Alternatively, prior to speculum placement, an index finger may be placed in the vagina and pressure placed posteriorly. A woman is then encouraged to relax posterior wall muscles to improve comfort with speculum insertion. This practice may prove especially helpful for women undergoing their first examination and for those with infrequent coitus, with dyspareunia, or with heightened anxiety.

With speculum insertion, the vagina commonly contracts, and a woman may note pressure or discomfort. A pause at this point typically is followed by vaginal muscle relaxation. As the speculum bill is completely inserted, it is angled approximately 30 degrees downward to reach the cervix. Commonly, the uterus lies in an anteverted position, and the ectocervix lies apposed against the posterior vaginal wall.

As the speculum is opened, the ectocervix can be identified. Vaginal walls and cervix should be inspected for masses, ulceration, dispigmentation, or unusual discharge. As outlined in Chapter 29 (p. 740), a Pap smear is obtained, and additional swabs for culture or microscopic evaluation may also be collected.

Bimanual Examination

Most often, the bimanual examination is performed after the speculum examination. Some clinicians prefer to complete the bimanual prior to the speculum examination to better identify cervical location before speculum insertion. Either process is appropriate. Uterine and adnexal size, mobility, and tenderness can be assessed during bimanual examination. For women with prior hysterectomy and adnexectomy, bimanual examination is still valuable and can be used to exclude other pelvic pathology.

During this examination, a gloved index and middle finger are inserted together into the vagina until the cervix is reached. For cases of latex allergy, nonlatex gloves should be available. To ease insertion, a water-based lubricant may be initially applied to these gloved fingers. Once the cervix is reached, uterine orientation can be quickly assessed by sweeping the index finger inward along the anterior length of the cervix. In those with an anteverted position, the uterine isthmus is noted to sweep upward, whereas in those with a retroverted position, a soft bladder is palpated. However, in those with a retroverted uterus, if a finger is swept along the cervix's posterior length, the isthmus is felt to sweep downward (Fig. 1-7). With a retroverted uterus, this same finger is continued posteriorly to the fundus and then side-to-side to assess uterine size and tenderness.

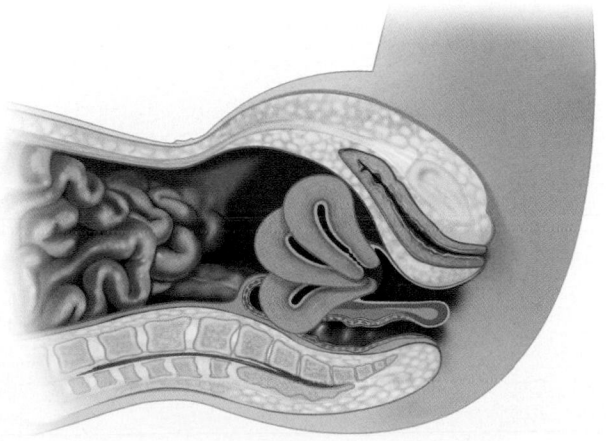
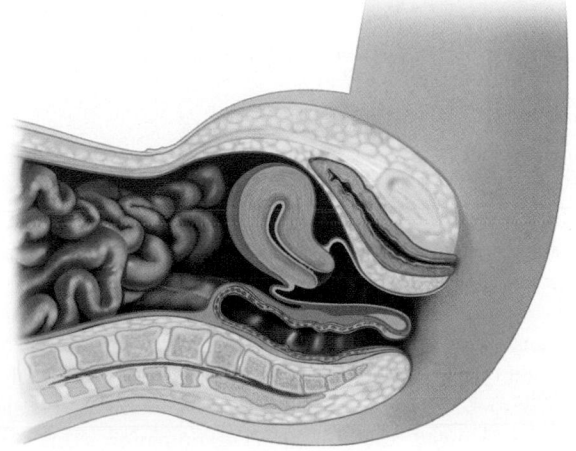

FIGURE 1-7 Drawing depicts uterine positions. **A.** The uterus may be inclined in an anteverted, midplane, or retroverted position. **B.** As shown here, the uterine fundus uterus can be flexed forward, and this is termed anteflexion. Similarly, the fundus may be flexed backward to create a retroflexed uterus.

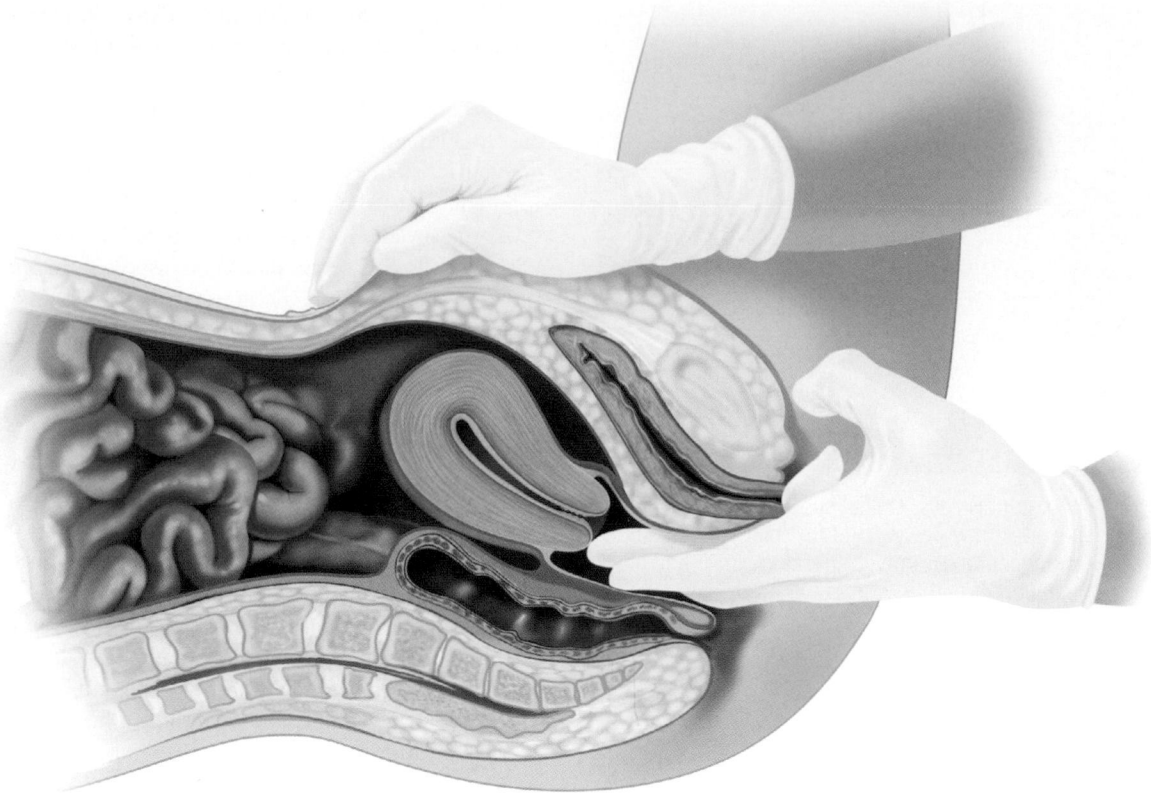

FIGURE 1-8 Drawing depicts bimanual examination. Fingers beneath the cervix lift the uterus toward the anterior abdominal wall. A hand placed on the abdomen detects upward pressure from the uterine fundus. Examination allows assessment of uterine size, mobility, and tenderness.

To determine the size of an anteverted uterus, fingers are placed beneath the cervix, and upward pressure tilts the fundus toward the anterior abdominal wall. A clinician's opposite hand is placed on the abdominal wall to locate the upward fundal pressure (Fig. 1-8).

To assess adnexa, the clinician should use two vaginal fingers to lift the adnexa from the posterior cul-de-sac or ovarian fossa toward the anterior abdominal wall. The adnexa is trapped between these vaginal fingers and the clinician's other hand, which is exerting downward pressure against the lower abdomen. For those with a normal-sized uterus, this abdominal hand is typically best placed just above the inguinal ligament.

Rectovaginal Examination

The decision to perform rectovaginal examination varies among providers. Although some prefer to complete this evaluation on all adults, others elect to perform rectovaginal examination for those with specific indications such as pelvic pain, an identified pelvic mass, or rectal symptoms.

Gloves are changed between bimanual and rectovaginal examinations to avoid contamination of the rectum with potential vaginal pathogens. Also, if fecal occult blood testing is to be done at the time of examination, the glove should be changed after bimanual examination. This minimizes false positive results from contamination by vaginal blood, if present. Initially, an index finger is placed into the vagina and a middle finger into the rectum (Fig. 1-9).

These fingers are swept against one another in a scissoring fashion to assess the rectovaginal septum for scarring or peritoneal studding. The index finger is removed, and the middle finger completes a circular sweep of the rectal vault to exclude masses. If immediate fecal occult blood testing is indicated, it may be performed with a sample from this portion of the examination.

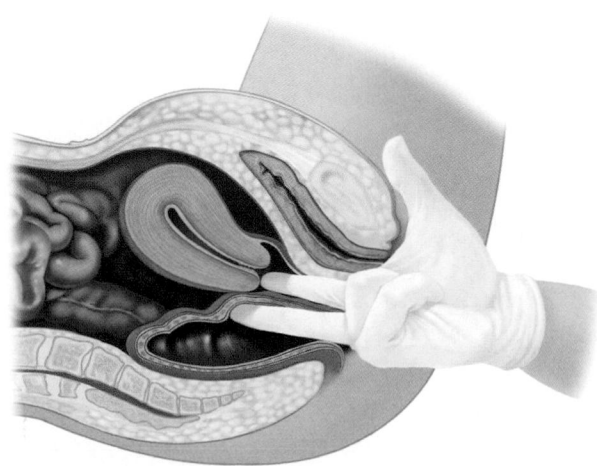

FIGURE 1-9 Drawing depicts rectovaginal examination with assessment of the rectovaginal septum.

PREVENTIVE CARE

As providers of health care for women, gynecologists have an opportunity to evaluate the patient for leading causes of female morbidity and mortality and counsel accordingly. Thus, a familiarity with various screening guidelines is essential. Recommendations by the American College of Obstetricians and Gynecologist (2011c) for primary and preventive care were updated in 2011. Moreover, the U.S. Preventive Services Task Force (2009a) updates its screening guideline recommendations regularly, and this information can be accessed at: http://www.ahrq.gov/clinic/prevenix.htm. These, along with specialty-specific recommendations, can provide valuable information for the clinician who provides preventive care services.

■ Infection Prevention

Vaccination

Although most routine vaccination is completed by adolescence, the need for new or repeat administration of several vaccines should be evaluated in the adult woman. Some are recommended for all adults, whereas others are indicated because of patient comorbidities or occupational exposure risks. For most healthy adults who have completed the indicated childhood and adolescent immunization schedules, those that warrant consideration of additional dosing are diphtheria-tetanus-activated pertussis (Tdap), herpes zoster, and seasonal influenza vaccines. For the human papillomavirus (HPV), two vaccines are now approved by the U.S. Food and Drug Administration (FDA) for females aged 9 to 26 years. Although the ideal recommended age for vaccination is 11 or 12 years, providers should discuss HPV vaccination benefits and offer the vaccine to females aged 13 to 26 (American College of Obstetricians and Gynecologists, 2006a). Screening for HPV vaccine prior to vaccination in those who are already sexually active is not recommended. These vaccines, Gardasil and Cervarix, are discussed in greater detail in Chapter 29 (p. 737).

Table 1-1 summarizes the recommended adult immunization schedule for 2011 and precautions and contraindications for these adult vaccines (Centers for Disease Control and Prevention, 2011). A complete discussion of specific as well as general guidelines can be found at the CDC web site: http://www.cdc.gov/vaccines/recs/schedules/adult-schedule.htm.

Sexually Transmitted Disease Screening

Routine screening for sexually transmitted disease (STD) is not warranted for all women. However, certain testing is recommended for selected groups to decrease morbidity and disease transmission (Table 1-2). In addition, a discussion regarding STD risk factors and regarding STD prevention with barrier condoms and partner selection is recommended for all sexually active adolescents and for adults at increased risk for STDs. These and other infections of the reproductive tract are discussed in Chapter 3 (p. 64).

■ Contraception

For reproductive-aged women, contraceptive needs or plans for pregnancy should be discussed annually. Contraceptive counseling is covered in Chapter 5 (p. 132) but generally should include education on methods and their use, efficacy, side effects, noncontraceptive benefits, and contraindications. However, despite efforts to provide contraception, nearly half of all pregnancies are unintended. Accordingly, a discussion of emergency contraception options is warranted. Additionally, all reproductive-aged women are encouraged to take a 400-μg folic acid supplement daily to prevent fetal neural-tube defects (NTDs) if pregnancy does occur. Women with a previous infant with a NTD should supplement with 4 mg orally each day (American College of Obstetricians and Gynecologists, 2003).

Alternatively, for those desiring pregnancy, topics found in Table 1-3 should be addressed to maximize maternal and fetal health (American College of Obstetricians and Gynecologists, 2005; Jack, 2008).

■ Cancer Screening

For women having periodic health examinations, screening for certain cancers may be indicated for early detection of these malignancies.

Cervical Cancer

Both incidence and mortality rates from cervical cancer in the United States have decreased in the past several decades due to Pap smear screening. The American College of Obstetricians and Gynecologists (2009a) has issued recommendations regarding cervical cytology screening. These are discussed fully in Chapter 29 (p. 742). In brief, either conventional or liquid-based techniques are appropriate, and screening should begin at age 21. Testing is repeated every 2 years for those <30 years. In those ≥30, screening may be stretched to every 3 years for those with no history of cervical intraepithelial neoplasia (CIN) 2 or 3, no immunocompromise, and no diethylstilbestrol exposure in utero. Screening may be discontinued in women aged 65 to 70 with three negative smear results in the preceding 10 years. Moreover, screening may be discontinued following hysterectomy in those with surgery for benign indications and no history of prior high-grade dysplasia.

Endometrial Cancer

For the average-risk woman, routine endometrial cancer screening with biopsy or sonography is not recommended. However, clinicians should educate women, especially those with risk factors, about this cancer's typical symptoms.

Women with multiple family members with colon cancer may have hereditary nonpolyposis colon cancer (HNPCC), also known as Lynch syndrome (Chap. 33, p. 818). For women with known HNPCC or those genetically at high risk for this syndrome, annual screening for endometrial cancer with endometrial biopsy should be offered beginning at age 35 (Smith, 2011).

Ovarian Cancer

Routine screening of asymptomatic women at low risk for ovarian cancer either with cancer antigen 125 (CA125) level measurement or sonography is not recommended (American College of Obstetricians and Gynecologists, 2011d). Currently, annual pelvic examination is the primary prevention tool for these women. However, for women who carry *BRCA1* or

TABLE 1-1. Summary of Recommendations for Adult Immunization

Vaccine Name and Route	Reason to Vaccinate	Vaccine Administration (any vaccine can be given with another)	Contraindications and Precautions[a,b] (mild illness is not a contraindication)
Influenza Trivalent inactivated influenza vaccine (TIV) *Give IM*	• All adults unless contraindicated	• Annually • October and November are ideal months for vaccination • May continue to give TIV and LAIV from December through March	**Precaution** • History of GBS within 6 weeks of previous influenza vaccine
Influenza Live attenuated influenza vaccine (LAIV) *Give intranasally*	• Healthy, nonpregnant persons <50 years		**Contraindication** • Pregnancy • Immunosuppression • Certain serious chronic medical disorders **Precaution** • History of GBS within 6 weeks of previous influenza vaccine • If possible, hold use of "-cyclovir" antivirals[d] for 24 hours before and 14 days after vaccine
Pneumococcal Polysaccharide (PPSV) *Give IM or SC*	• Those ≥65 years • Those with chronic illness, asplenia, or immunosuppression • Smokers; long-term care facility residents	• One-time dose • One-time revaccination is recommended 5 years later for those at highest risk and for those persons ≥65 years if 1st dose was given prior to age 65 and 5 years have elapsed since the 1st dose	
Hepatitis B *Give IM*	• Any adult wishing to obtain Hepatitis B immunity • Household contacts and partners of HBsAg-positive persons; IV drug users; heterosexuals with >1 sex partner; MSM; persons with STDs; recipients of blood replacement products; health care workers; clients and staff at developmental disability institutions or at correctional facilities; travelers to endemic areas[c] • Those with chronic liver disease; ESRD; HIV infection	• Three doses are needed on a 0, 1- to 2-, and 6-month schedule • For the hepatitis A and B combination vaccine, three doses are needed on a 0-, 1-, 6-month schedule	**Precaution** • Pregnancy
Hepatitis A *Give IM*	• Travelers to endemic areas[c] • Chronic liver disease; IV drug use; MSM; receive clotting-factor concentrates • New household contact from endemic area • Anyone wishing to obtain Hepatitis A immunity	• Two doses are needed • The minimum interval between 1st and 2nd doses is 6 months	**Precaution** • Pregnancy

(Continued)

TABLE 1-1. Summary of Recommendations for Adult Immunization *(Continued)*

Vaccine Name and Route	Reason to Vaccinate	Vaccine Administration (any vaccine can be given with another)	Contraindications and Precautions[a,b] (mild illness is not a contraindication)
Td (Tetanus, diphtheria) *Give IM*	• All adults who lack a history of a primary series consisting of at least three doses of tetanus- and diphtheria-containing vaccine • Pregnant women may receive Td vaccination during 2nd or 3rd trimester, if last vaccine >10 years	• For persons who are unvaccinated, complete the primary series with Td (spaced at 0, 1- to 2-month, and 6- to 12-month intervals). One dose of Tdap may be used for one of the three doses • Give Td booster every 10 years after the primary series has been completed.	**Contraindication** • For Tdap only, history of encephalopathy within 7 days following DTP/DTaP **Precaution** • GBS within 6 weeks of receiving a previous dose of tetanus toxoid-containing vaccine • Unstable neurologic condition
Tdap (Tetanus, diphtheria, pertussis) *Give IM*	• 1-time dose as soon as feasible to those listed below who lack prior Tdap vaccine • Postpartum women • Close contact with infants <12 months • Health care personnel	• For adults 19–64 years, a 1-time dose of Tdap is recommended at some point to replace one Td dose	
Varicella *Give SC*	• All adults without evidence of immunity, which is defined as a prior vaccination, previously diagnosed varicella disease, previously diagnosed zoster, U.S.-born before 1980, or laboratory evidence of immunity	• Two doses are needed at 0 and at 1 or 2 months. Even if the second dose is delayed, may still give	**Contraindications** • Pregnancy or possibility of pregnancy within 4 weeks • Immunocompromised persons **Precaution** • Receipt of antibody-containing blood products within last yr • If possible, hold use of "-cyclovir" antivirals[d] for 24 hours before and 14 days after vaccine
Zoster *Give IM*	• Those ≥60 years	• One dose is needed	**Contraindications** • Severe immunosuppression • Pregnancy or possibility of pregnancy within 4 weeks **Precaution** • If possible, hold use of "-cyclovir" antivirals[d] for 24 hours before and 14 days after vaccine
Meningococcal Conjugate vaccine (MCV4) *Give IM* Polysaccharide vaccine (MPSV4) *Give SC*	• Anatomic or function asplenia or terminal complement component deficiencies • Travelers to endemic areas[c] • College freshmen living in dormitories	• One dose is needed • Two-dose series needed at 0 and 2 months for asplenia, complement deficiency, and those with HIV needing vaccination • If age ≤55, use MCV4 • If age ≥56, use MPSV4 • Revaccinate after 5 years with MCV4 if risk persists	**Precaution** • For MCV4 only, history of GBS

(Continued)

TABLE 1-1. Summary of Recommendations for Adult Immunization *(Continued)*

Vaccine Name and Route	Reason to Vaccinate	Vaccine Administration (any vaccine can be given with another)	Contraindications and Precautions[a,b] (mild illness is not a contraindication)
MMR (Measles, mumps, rubella) *Give SC*	• Persons born in 1957 or later should receive at least one dose of MMR if no serologic or clinically documented proof of immunity • Women of childbearing age without acceptable evidence of rubella immunity or vaccination	• One or two doses are needed • Recommend two doses for: postexposure or outbreak setting; college student; healthcare facility worker; international traveler. 4 weeks between doses. • If a pregnant woman is found to be rubella susceptible, administer MMR postpartum	**Contraindications** • Severe immunosuppression • Pregnancy or possibility of pregnancy within 4 weeks **Precaution** • History of thrombocytopenia or thrombocytopenia purpura • Receipt of antibody-containing blood products within last yr
Human Papillomavirus *Give IM*	• All previously unvaccinated females 9–26 years	• Three doses are needed on a 0, 1- to 2-, and 6-month schedule. Use quadrivalent or bivalent vaccine	**Precaution** • In pregnancy, delay until postpartum

[a]Previous anaphylactic reaction to any of a vaccine's components serves as a contraindication for any vaccine.
[b]Moderate to severe illness is a precaution to vaccination.
[c]A list is found at http://wwwnc.cdc.gov/travel/yellowbook/2010/table-of-contents.aspx.
[d]These include acyclovir, famciclovir, valacyclovir.
DTP = diphtheria, tetanus, pertussis vaccine; ESRD = end-stage renal disease; GBS = Guillain-Barré syndrome; HBSAg = hepatitis B surface antigen; IV = intravenous; MSM = men having sex with men; STD = sexually transmitted disease.
Compiled from the Centers for Disease Control and Prevention, 2011, and Fiore, 2010.

BRCA2 gene mutations and who decline prophylactic oophorectomy, these two screening tools may be offered. Those with a strong family history of breast and ovarian cancer may also be viewed to be at higher risk and may be considered for screening. A complete discussion of ovarian cancer screening can be found in Chapter 35 (p. 856).

Breast Cancer

The U.S. Preventive Services Task Force (2009b) has issued new breast cancer screening recommendations regarding CBE, SBE, and breast imaging. As shown in Table 1-4, recommendations of the American College of Obstetricians and Gynecologists (2011a), the American Cancer Society (Smith, 2011), and the USPSTF vary regarding the frequency of screening with breast imaging for women aged 40 to 49 and regarding the use of CBE and SBE. All agree that imaging should be offered to those 50 years and older and that as a woman approaches age 75, breast cancer screening should be individualized. Specifically, patient health status, therapy-associated morbidity, and estimated quality of life gained with cancer treatment should be factored into cancer screening plans for this older age group. A fuller discussion of breast cancer and screening is found in Chapter 12 (p. 347).

Colon Cancer

Colorectal cancer develops in 74,000 women per year in the United States and is the third leading cause of cancer death in women, behind lung and breast cancer (Levin, 2008). Several organizations recommend screening patients at average risk for colorectal cancer beginning at age 50 with any of the methods shown in Table 1-5 (American College of Obstetricians and Gynecologists, 2011b). The preferred method for most is colonoscopy, and the limitations and benefits of each method are noted. Patient adherence to colorectal cancer screening guidelines for women is usually less than 50 percent (Meissner, 2006). Thus, gynecologists can take an active role in counseling patients regarding the importance of appropriate screening.

Fecal occult blood testing (FOBT) is an adequate *annual* screening method when two or three stool samples are self-collected by the patient and the cards returned for analysis. This method relies on a chemical oxidation reaction between the heme moiety of blood and alpha guaiaconic acid, a component of guaiac paper. Heme catalyzes the oxidation of alpha guaiaconic acid by hydrogen peroxide, the active component in the developer. This oxidation reaction yields a blue color (Sanford, 2009). Red meat, raw cauliflower, broccoli, members of the radish family, and melons have similar oxidizing ability and may yield false-positive results. Vitamin C may preemptively react with the reagents and lead to false-negative results. All of these should be eliminated for 3 days before testing. Additionally, women should avoid nonsteroidal antiinflammatory drugs (NSAIDs) 7 days prior to testing to limit risks of gastric irritation and bleeding. These restrictions are cumbersome for some patients and lead to noncompliance with recommended testing.

Alternatively, the fecal immunochemical test (FIT) relies on an immune reaction to human hemoglobin. Similar to FOBT,

TABLE 1-2. Sexually Transmitted Disease Screening Guidelines for Nonpregnant, Sexually Active Asymptomatic Women

Infectious Agent	Recommendations	Risk Factors
Chlamydia trachomatis + *Neisseria gonorrhoeae*	Screen all <25 years Screen those older if risk factors present	New or multiple partners; inconsistent condom use; sex work; current or prior STD
Treponema pallidum	Should screen those with risk factors	Sex work; confinement in adult correction facility; MSM
HIV virus	Should screen all 13–64 years[a] Should screen all 19–64 years[b] Should screen those with risk factors[c]	Multiple partners; injection drug use; sex work; concurrent STD; MSM; transfusion between 1978 and 1985; at-risk partners; initial TB diagnosis
Hepatitis C virus	May screen those with risk factors	Injection drug use; dialysis; partner with hepatitis C; multiple partners; received blood products prior to 1990
Hepatitis B virus	No routine screening	
Herpes simplex virus 2	No routine screening	

[a]Centers for Disease Control and Prevention (2006) recommends screening regardless of risk factors unless the prevalence of undiagnosed HIV infection in the practice is <0.1%. Subsequent annual testing is recommended for those with risk factors.
[b]American College of Obstetricians and Gynecologists (2008) recommends screening regardless of risk factors and screening outside this age range for those at high risk.
[c]U.S. Preventive Services Task Force (2005c) recommends screening for those at increased risk.

HIV = human immunodeficiency virus; MSM = men having sex with men; STD = sexually transmitted disease; TB = tuberculosis.
Compiled from those above and Centers for Disease Control and Prevention, 2010a, and U.S. Preventive Services Task Force, 2004a,b,d; 2005a,b; 2007.

the FIT test is performed for annual screening on two or three patient-collected stool samples but does not require pretesting dietary limitations. Advantages to FIT include greater specificity for human blood and thus fewer false-positive results from dietary meat and vegetables and fewer false-negative results due to vitamin C. All positive test results from FOBT or FIT warrant further evaluation with colonoscopy.

Lastly, screening may be completed with stool DNA (sDNA) testing. This identifies several specific tumor-related DNA mutations in cells shed from colon neoplasms into the bowel contents. This test is currently not widely used, and one significant disadvantage is its high cost relative to other stool screening tests.

It is not uncommon for the gynecologist to perform an FOBT or FIT test on a single stool sample obtained at the time of pelvic examination. However, the single stool sample obtained on digital rectal examination should not be considered a replacement for recommended colorectal cancer screening methods.

Some individuals should be screened more frequently. These include those with a personal history of colorectal cancer or a first-degree relative with colon cancer; those with chronic inflammatory bowel disease; those with prior adenomatous pol-

yps; or those with a known or suspected hereditary colon cancer syndrome such as hereditary nonpolyposis (HNPCC) (Levin, 2008).

Skin Cancer

The increase in skin cancer rates (melanoma and nonmelanoma) in the United States during the past several years has driven interest in regular skin cancer screening. However, the U.S. Preventive Services Task Force (2009a) notes insufficient evidence to recommend whole body screening for skin cancer in the general adult population. In that publication, clinicians are advised to use the "ABCD" system—asymmetry, border irregularity, color, and size (diameter >6 mm) to evaluate skin lesions. The American College of Obstetricians and Gynecologists (2011c) recommends counseling all women about the risks for skin cancer, which include prolonged sun or ultraviolet ray exposure, family or personal history of skin cancer, fair skin, light hair or freckling, immunosuppression, xeroderma pigmentosum, and aging.

■ Osteoporosis

In the United States, approximately 15 percent of women older than 50 years have osteoporosis, and 35 to 50 percent have

TABLE 1-3. Preconceptional Counseling Topics

Condition	Recommendations for Preconceptional Counseling
Abnormal weight	Calculate BMI yearly (see Fig. 1-7, p. 17) *BMI ≥25 kg/m²:* Counsel on diet. Test for diabetes and metabolic syndrome if indicated *BMI ≤18.5 kg/m²:* Assess for eating disorder
Cardiovascular disease	Counsel on cardiac risks during pregnancy. Optimize cardiac function, and offer effective BCM during this time and for those not desiring conception. Discuss warfarin, ACE inhibitor, and ARB teratogenicity, and if possible, switch to less dangerous agent when conception planned. Offer genetic counseling to those with congenital cardiac anomalies
Chronic hypertension	Counsel on specific risks during pregnancy. Assess those with long-standing HTN for ventricular hypertrophy, retinopathy, and renal disease. Counsel women taking ACE inhibitors and ARBs on drug teratogenicity, on effective BCM during use, and on the need to switch agents prior to conception
Asthma	Counsel on asthma risks during pregnancy. Optimize pulmonary function and offer effective BCM during this time
Thrombophilia	Question for personal or family history of thrombotic events or recurrent poor pregnancy outcomes. If found, counsel and screen those contemplating pregnancy. Offer genetic counseling to those with known thrombophilia. Discuss warfarin teratogenicity, offer effective BCM during use, and switch to a less teratogenic agent, if possible, prior to conception
Renal disease	Counsel on specific risks during pregnancy. Optimize blood pressure control and offer effective BCM during this time. Counsel women taking ACE inhibitors and ARBs on their teratogenicity, on effective BCM during use, and on the need to switch agents prior to conception
Gastrointestinal disease	*Inflammatory bowel disease:* Counsel affected women on subfertility risks and risks of adverse pregnancy outcomes. Discuss teratogenicity of MTX and the other immunomodulators, about which less is known, e.g., mycophenolate mofetil, etc. Offer effective BCM during their use and switch agents, if possible, prior to conception
Hepatobiliary disease	*Hepatitis B*: Vaccinate all high-risk women prior to conception (see Table 1-1, pp. 8–10). Counsel chronic carriers on transmission prevention to partners and fetus *Hepatitis C*: Screen high-risk women. Counsel affected women on risks of disease and transmission. Refer for treatment, discuss ramifications of treatment during pregnancy, and offer effective BCM
Hematologic disease	*Sickle-cell disease:* Screen all black women. Counsel those with trait or disease. Test partner if desired *Thalassemias:* Screen women of Southeast Asian or Mediterranean ancestry
Diabetes	Advocate good glucose control, especially in periconceptional period, to decrease known teratogenicity of overt diabetes. Evaluate for retinopathy, nephropathy, hypertension, etc.
Thyroid disease	Screen those with thyroid disease symptoms. Ensure iodine-sufficient diet. Treat overt hyper- or hypothyroidism prior to conception. Counsel on risks to pregnancy outcome
Connective tissue disease	*RA*: Counsel on flare risk after pregnancy. Discuss MTX and leflunomide teratogenicity, as well as possible effects of other immunomodulators. Offer effective BCM during their use and switch agents prior to conception. Halt NSAIDs by 27 weeks' gestation *SLE*: Counsel on risks during pregnancy. Optimize disease and offer effective BCM during this time and for those not desiring conception. Discuss mycophenolate mofetil and cyclophosphamide teratogenicity as well as possible effects of newer immunomodulators. Effective BCM during their use. If possible, switch agents prior to conception
Neurologic and psychiatric disorders	*Depression:* Screen for symptoms of depression. In those affected, counsel on risks of treatment and of untreated illness and high risk of exacerbation during pregnancy and the puerperium *Seizure disorder:* Optimize seizure control using monotherapy if possible

(Continued)

TABLE 1-3. Preconceptional Counseling Topics *(Continued)*

Condition	Recommendations for Preconceptional Counseling
Dermatologic disease	Discuss isotretinoin and etretinate teratogenicity, effective BCM during their use, and need to switch agents prior to conception
Cancer	Counsel on fertility preservation options prior to cancer therapy and on decreased fertility following certain agents. Offer genetic counseling to those with mutation-linked cancers. Evaluate cardiac function in those given cardiotoxic agents, such as adriamycin. Obtain mammography for those given childhood chest radiotherapy. Discuss SERM teratogenicity, effective BCM during their use, and need to switch agents prior to conception. Review chemotherapy and discuss possible teratogenic effects if continued during pregnancy
Infectious diseases	*Asymptomatic bacteruria.* No role for preconceptional screening *Bacterial vaginosis:* No role for preconceptional screening *Influenza:* Vaccinate all women prior to flu season *Malaria:* Counsel to avoid travel to endemic areas during conception. If unable, offer effective BCM during travel or provide chemoprophylaxis for those planning pregnancy *Rubella:* Screen for rubella immunity. If nonimmune, vaccinate and counsel on the need for effective BCM during the subsequent 3 months *Tuberculosis:* Screen high-risk women and treat prior to conception *Tetanus:* Update vaccination, as needed, in all reproductive-aged women *Varicella:* Question regarding immunity. If nonimmune, vaccinate
STDs	*Gonorrhea, syphilis, chlamydial infection:* Screen high-risk women and treat as indicated *HIV:* Screen those 19–64 years and those outside this range if at high risk (see Table 1-2, p. 11). Counsel affected women on risks during pregnancy and on perinatal transmission. Discuss initiation of treatment prior to pregnancy to decrease transmission risk. Offer effective BCM to those not desiring conception *HPV:* Provide Pap smear screening. Vaccinate candidate patients *HSV:* Provide serological screening to asymptomatic women with affected partners. Counsel affected women on risks of perinatal transmission and of preventative measures during the third trimester and labor

ACE = angiotensin-converting enzyme; ARB = angiotensin-receptor blocker; BCM = birth control method; BMI = body mass index; HIV = human immunodeficiency virus; HPV = human papillomavirus; HSV = herpes simplex virus; HTN = hypertension; MTX = methotrexate; NSAID = nonsteroidal antiinflammatory drug; RA = rheumatoid arthritis; SERM = selective estrogen-receptor modulator; SLE = systemic lupus erythematosus; STD = sexually transmitted disease.
Adapted from American College of Obstetricians and Gynecologists, 2008; Fiore, 2010; and Jack, 2008.

osteopenia (Ettinger, 2003). These bone-weakening conditions lead to increased rates of fracture, and bone mass density has been shown to correlate inversely with risks for these fractures. Accordingly, tools that measure bone density such as dual-energy x-ray absorptiometry (DEXA) scanning are used to identify bone loss and predict fracture risk. Table 1-6 lists practice recommendations from the National Osteoporosis Foundation (2010) for postmenopausal patients. Osteoporosis and its prevention and treatment are discussed further in Chapter 21 (p. 563).

■ Obesity
Diagnosis and Risks

In 2007 to 2008, 35 percent of women in the United States were considered obese, and 64 percent were overweight or obese (Flegal, 2010). Body mass index (BMI), although not a direct measure of body fat content, is a valuable tool in assessing a patient's risk for weigh-related medical issues (Table 1-7). Using pounds and inches, BMI is calculated as weight (in pounds), divided by height (in inches) squared, then multiplied by a factor of 703. Using metric measurements, BMI is calculated as weight (in kilograms) divided by height (in meters) squared. An adult BMI calculator can be found at: http://www.cdc.gov/healthyweight/assessing/bmi/adult_bmi/english_bmi_calculator/bmi_calculator.html. For adolescents (and children), BMI is expressed differently. Age and sex are factored, and BMI is calculated as a percentile. A BMI calculator for adolescents can be found at: http://apps.nccd.cdc.gov/dnpabmi/. Table 1-8 reflects the definitions for underweight, overweight, and obesity for adolescents and adults.

In addition to BMI, waist circumference positively correlates with abdominal fat content, which if increased, can serve as a separate comorbid risk. For women, waist circumferences greater than 88 cm (35 inches) are considered increased (National Heart,

TABLE 1-4. Breast Cancer Screening Guidelines

Organization	Screening Mammography	Clinical Breast Examination	Self Breast Examination	Discontinuation of Screening Mammography
American College of Obstetricians and Gynecologists	Age ≥40: annually	Age 20–39: every 1–3 years Age ≥40: annually	Advise breast awareness; consider teaching exam to high-risk patients	Individualize at age 75 and older, consider comorbidities and benefits/risks
American Cancer Society	Age ≥40: annually	Age 20–39: every 1–3 years Age ≥40: annually	Optional for age ≥20	No specific age recommendation; individualize
U.S. Preventive Services Task Force	Age 40–49: no routine screening; can recommend every-2-year screening for selected patients Age 50–74: every 2 years	Inadequate evidence of additional benefit	No	No specific age recommendation; individualize

Compiled from American College of Obstetricians and Gynecologists, 2011a; Smith, 2011; U.S. Preventive Services Task Force, 2009b.

Lung, and Blood Institute, 2000). Waist circumference is measured at the level of the iliac crests at the end of normal expiration. The measuring tape should be snug but not indent the skin.

In addition to the social stigma that often accompanies increased body weight, overweight and obese women are at increased risk for developing hypertension, hypercholesterolemia, type 2 diabetes mellitus, gallbladder disease, knee osteoarthritis, sleep apnea, coronary heart disease (CHD), and certain cancers (Must, 1999; National Task Force on the Prevention and Treatment of Obesity, 2000). Accordingly, treatment of these women is often directed toward weight loss as well as management of other comorbid risk factors (Table 1-9). Gynecologic issues that can be affected by obesity include menstrual patterns, risks for endometrial hyperplasia and endometrial cancer, polycystic ovary syndrome, and choice of contraception. No standard single or panel laboratory test is indicated for the obese patient. Evaluation for comorbidities should be tailored to the patient, taking into consideration her family and social histories. Blood pressure measurement, fasting lipid and glucose screening, and thyroid function testing can all be considered for the obese patient during initial evaluation.

Once a patient is identified as having a BMI outside the desired level, the clinician should assess her readiness for lifestyle change and provide appropriate guidance, support, or referral (Table 1-10). Such tailored counseling may be used not only for weight management but for other behavioral issues, including substance abuse, smoking, and contraception use. Developing a trusting rapport with the patient and helping her move through these stages is important to any type of lasting behavior change (American College of Obstetricians and Gynecologists, 2009b).

Treatment

Lifestyle Changes. Table 1-11 illustrates recommended guidelines to direct therapy for patients identified as overweight or obese (National Heart, Lung, and Blood Institute, 1998). Comorbidities, as defined in Table 1-9, play a significant role in therapy choice. A detailed discussion of dietary weight loss extends beyond this chapter's scope, but several clinician and patient aids can be found at: http://www.nhlbi.nih.gov/guidelines/obesity/prctgd_c.pdf.

In general, for the adult patient, a 10-percent loss within 6 months can be reached in those with BMIs from 27 to 35 with a daily 300- to 500-kcal reduction. In those with higher BMIs, a similar loss can be achieved following a 500- to 1000-kcal reduction. For the adolescent who has a BMI greater than the 85th percentile for age, the clinician must decide whether appropriate counseling can be provided in the office or referral made to a nutritionist. In the adolescent, more than in the adult, the goal may be simply to slow the rate of weight gain to avoid interference with normal growth and development.

TABLE 1-5. Screening Guidelines for the Early Detection of Colorectal Cancer and Adenomas for Average-risk Women Aged 50 years and Older

Tests That Detect Adenomatous Polyps and Cancer[a]		
Test	**Interval**	**Key Issues for Informed Decisions**
Colonoscopy	Every 10 years	Complete bowel prep is required Conscious sedation is used in most centers; patients will miss a day of work and will need a chaperone for transportation from the facility Risks include perforation and bleeding, which are rare but potentially serious; most of the risk is associated with polypectomy
FSIG with insertion to 40 cm or to splenic flexure	Every 5 years	Complete or partial bowel prep is required Sedation usually is not used, so discomfort during the procedure is possible The protective effect of sigmoidoscopy is primarily limited to the portion of the colon examined Patients should understand that positive findings on sigmoidoscopy usually result in a referral for colonoscopy
Double-contrast barium enema (DCBE)	Every 5 years	Complete bowel prep is required If patients have one or more polyps ≥6 mm, colonoscopy will be recommended Risks of DCBE are low; rare cases of perforation have been reported
Computed-tomography colonography (CTC)	Every 5 years	Complete bowel prep is required If patients have one or more polyps ≥6 mm, colonoscopy will be recommended Risks of CTC are low; rare cases of perforation have been reported Extracolonic abnormalities may be identified on CTC that could require further evaluation
Tests That Primarily Detect Cancer[a]		
Test	**Interval**	**Key Issues for Informed Decisions**
gFOBT	Annually	Two to three stool samples collected at home are needed to complete testing; a single sample of stool gathered during a digital exam in the clinical setting is not an acceptable complete stool test
FIT	Annually	Positive tests are associated with an increased risk of colon cancer and advanced neoplasia; colonoscopy should be recommended if the test results are positive If the test is negative, it should be repeated annually Patients should understand that one-time testing is likely to be ineffective
Stool DNA test (sDNA)	Interval uncertain	An adequate stool sample must be obtained and packaged with appropriate preservative agents for shipping to the laboratory The unit cost of the currently available test is significantly higher than other forms of stool testing If the test is positive, colonoscopy will be recommended If the test is negative, the appropriate interval for a repeat test is uncertain

[a]One method from this group is selected.
FIT = fecal immunochemical test; FSIG = flexible sigmoidoscopy; gFOBT = guaiac-based fecal occult blood test.
Adapted from Levin, 2008, with permission; American College of Obstetricians and Gynecologists, 2011b.

CHAPTER 1

TABLE 1-6. General Guidelines for Prevention of Osteoporosis in Postmenopausal Women

Counsel on the risk of osteoporosis and related fractures

Check for secondary causes (Table 21-6, p. 568)

Advise on adequate amounts of calcium (at least 1200 mg per day) and vitamin D (800–1000 IU per day) including supplements if necessary for individuals aged 50 years and older

Recommend regular weight-bearing and muscle-strengthening exercise to reduce the risk of falls and fractures

Advise against tobacco smoking and excessive alcohol intake

In women ≥65 years, recommend bone mineral density testing

In postmenopausal women aged 50–69 years, recommend BMD testing when there is concern based on the risk factor profile (Table 21-7, p. 568)

Recommend BMD testing to those who have had a fracture, to determine degree of disease severity

BMD testing performed in DEXA centers using accepted quality assurance measures is appropriate for monitoring bone loss. For patients on pharmacotherapy, it is typically performed 2 years after initiating therapy and every 2 years thereafter. However, more frequent testing may be warranted in certain clinical situations

BMD = bone mineral density; DEXA = dual-energy x-ray absorptiometry.
Abbreviated from National Osteoporosis Foundation, 2010.

Medications. In addition to diet and exercise, pharmacologic or surgical options may be implemented for selected obese patients. Orlistat (Xenical) is the only FDA-approved agent for obesity. A reversible inhibitor of gastric and pancreatic lipases, orlistat leads to a 30-percent blockage of dietary fat absorption (Henness, 2006). This drug is prescribed as one 120-mg capsule to be taken orally three times daily with meals but is also available over-the-counter in 60-mg capsules (Allī), also taken three times daily. By its mechanism of action, orlistat can create bloating, flatulence, diarrhea, or oily stools, all of which may be limited by a low-fat diet. Associated malabsorption can lead to deficiencies of the fat-soluble vitamins A, D, E, and K, and all patients should receive a daily supplement enriched with these vitamins. Severe liver injury has been reported rarely, and new labeling reflects this risk (Food and Drug Administration, 2010a).

Sibutramine (Meridia) is a centrally acting, selective serotonin- and norepinephrine-reuptake inhibitor that primarily acts as an appetite suppressant. It was voluntarily removed from the U.S. market in 2010 due to concerns for increased cardiovascular adverse events (Food and Drug Administration, 2010b).

Bariatric Surgery. As another adjunct to diet and exercise, bariatric surgery may be selected for those with BMIs ≥40 or with BMIs ≥35 if other comorbid conditions are present (Buchwald, 2005). Of available procedures, two are most commonly performed. *Gastric banding* places an adjustable plastic ring laparoscopically around the stomach to limit food intake. The *Roux-en-Y gastric bypass* creates a small stomach pouch by vertical stapling and limits intake. This smaller stomach is connected directly to the jejunum to bypass the duodenum. This reduces calorie and nutrient absorption. Both surgeries lead to substantial weight loss in individuals with morbid obesity and have been linked with improved comorbid risk factors and decreased mortality rates (Christou, 2004; Sjostrom, 2004). However, surgical complications can be serious and include pulmonary embolism, gastrointestinal leaks at staple or suture lines, stomal obstruction or stenosis, and bleeding (Steinbrook, 2004).

Following bariatric surgery, patients are advised to delay pregnancy for 12 to 18 months. Rapid weight loss during this time poses theoretical risks for intrauterine fetal-growth restriction and nutritional deprivation. However, as weight is lost, fertility rates overall appear to be improved, and risks for pregnancy increase (Merhi, 2009). Accordingly, effective contraception is needed (Centers for Disease Control and Prevention, 2010b). Many contraceptive methods appear to be as effective in women with elevated BMIs as in normal-weight controls. However, the contraceptive patch (OrthoEvra) is less effective in those weighing >90 kg. Use of the subdermal contraceptive rod was not evaluated by the manufacturers in women more than 130 percent of their ideal body weight, and patients should be counseled accordingly. In addition, efficacy of oral contraceptive pills may be impaired in overweight and obese women. Specific to bariatric surgery patients, oral contraception efficacy may be lower in those with bariatric surgery types associated with malabsorption (Society of Family Planning, 2009). Lastly, because of its risk for associated weight gain, depot medroxyprogesterone acetate (DepoProvera) may be an unpopular choice in women trying to lose weight.

Chronic Hypertension

Chronic hypertension is common, and an estimated 39 million American women are hypertensive (American Heart Association, 2010). The risk of hypertension increases with age, and more than 65 percent of those older than 60 years have elevated blood pressures (Ong, 2007; Vasan, 2002). Hypertension is a significant health concern and increases risks of myocardial infarction, stroke, congestive heart failure, renal disease, and peripheral vascular disease. To minimize these effects, gynecologists should be familiar with criteria used to diagnose hypertension. Although many may choose to refer their patients for treatment of

TABLE 1-7. Body Mass Index Tables

BMI	19	20	21	22	23	24	25	26	27	28	29	30	31	32	33	34	35
Height (inches)							**Body Weight (pounds)**										
58	91	96	100	105	110	115	119	124	129	134	138	143	148	153	158	162	167
59	94	99	104	109	114	119	124	128	133	138	143	148	153	158	163	168	173
60	97	102	107	112	118	123	128	133	138	143	148	153	158	163	168	174	179
61	100	106	111	116	122	127	132	137	143	148	153	158	164	169	174	180	185
62	104	109	115	120	126	131	136	142	147	153	158	164	169	175	180	186	191
63	107	113	118	124	130	135	141	146	152	158	163	169	175	180	186	191	197
64	110	116	122	128	134	140	145	151	157	163	169	174	180	186	192	197	204
65	114	120	126	132	138	144	150	156	162	168	174	180	186	192	198	204	210
66	118	124	130	136	142	148	155	161	167	173	179	186	192	198	204	210	216
67	121	127	134	140	146	153	159	166	172	178	185	191	198	204	211	217	223
68	125	131	138	144	151	158	164	171	177	184	190	197	203	210	216	223	230
69	128	135	142	149	155	162	169	176	182	189	196	203	209	216	223	230	236
70	132	139	146	153	160	167	174	181	188	195	202	209	216	222	229	236	243
71	136	143	150	157	165	172	179	186	193	200	208	215	222	229	236	243	250
72	140	147	154	162	169	177	184	191	199	206	213	221	228	235	242	250	258
73	144	151	159	166	174	182	189	197	204	212	219	227	235	242	250	257	265
74	148	155	163	171	179	186	194	202	210	218	225	233	241	249	256	264	272
75	152	160	168	176	184	192	200	208	216	224	232	240	248	256	264	272	279
76	156	164	172	180	189	197	205	213	221	230	238	246	254	263	271	279	287

BMI	36	37	38	39	40	41	42	43	44	45	46	47	48	49	50	51	52	53	54
Height (inches)								**Body Weight (pounds)**											
58	172	177	181	186	191	196	201	205	210	215	220	224	229	234	239	244	248	253	258
59	178	183	188	193	198	203	208	212	217	222	227	232	237	242	247	252	257	262	267
60	184	189	194	199	204	209	215	220	225	230	235	240	245	250	255	261	266	271	276
61	190	195	201	206	211	217	222	227	232	238	243	248	254	259	264	269	275	280	285
62	196	202	207	213	218	224	229	235	240	246	251	256	262	267	273	278	284	289	295
63	203	208	214	220	225	231	237	242	248	254	259	265	270	278	282	287	293	299	304
64	209	215	221	227	232	238	244	250	256	262	267	273	279	285	291	296	302	308	314
65	216	222	228	234	240	246	252	258	264	270	276	282	288	294	300	306	312	318	324
66	223	229	235	241	247	253	260	266	272	278	284	291	297	303	309	315	322	328	334
67	230	236	242	249	255	261	268	274	280	287	293	299	306	312	319	325	331	338	344
68	236	243	249	256	262	269	276	282	289	295	302	308	315	322	328	335	341	348	354
69	243	250	257	263	270	277	284	291	297	304	311	318	324	331	338	345	351	358	365
70	250	257	264	271	278	285	292	299	306	313	320	327	334	341	348	355	362	369	376
71	257	265	272	279	286	293	301	308	315	322	329	338	343	351	358	365	372	379	386
72	265	272	279	287	294	302	309	316	324	331	338	346	353	361	368	375	383	390	397
73	272	280	288	295	302	310	318	325	333	340	348	355	363	371	378	386	393	401	408
74	280	287	295	303	311	319	326	334	342	350	358	365	373	381	389	396	404	412	420
75	287	295	303	311	319	327	335	343	351	359	367	375	383	391	399	407	415	423	431
76	295	304	312	320	328	336	344	353	361	369	377	385	394	402	410	418	426	435	443

TABLE 1-8. Definitions of Abnormal Weight for Adults and Adolescents

Age Group	Underweight	Overweight	Obese
Adolescent	BMI <5th percentile for age	BMI between 85th and 95th percentile for age	BMI >95th percentile for age
Adult	BMI <18.5	BMI 25–29.9	BMI ≥30

TABLE 1-9. Obesity Comorbid Risk Factors

Established coronary heart disease
Other concurrent atherosclerotic disease
   Peripheral vascular disease
   Abdominal aortic aneurysm
   Symptomatic coronary artery disease
Type 2 diabetes mellitus
Sleep apnea
Cigarette smoking
Chronic hypertension
Abnormal lipid levels
   Elevated LDL cholesterol levels
   Elevated triglyceride levels
   Decreased HDL cholesterol levels
Family history of early CHD
Gynecologic abnormalities
   Menorrhagia or metrorrhagia
   Endometrial hyperplasia
   Endometrial cancer
Osteoarthritis
Gallstones

CHD = coronary heart disease; HDL = high-density lipoprotein; LDL = low-density lipoprotein.
Compiled from National Heart, Lung, and Blood Institute, 2000.

TABLE 1-10. Stages of Readiness for Change

Stage of Change	Example of Behavior
Precontemplation	No interest in weight loss; does not perceive a problem
Contemplation	Problem recognition; considering a particular diet
Preparation	Realizes benefits of change; plans changes, e.g., stocks her pantry accordingly
Action	Begins treatment or behavior change
Maintenance	New changes are incorporated into lifestyle

TABLE 1-11. Treatment Recommendations According to BMI

Treatment	BMI 25–26.9	BMI 27–29.9	BMI 30–34.9	BMI 35–39.9	BMI ≥40
Diet, physical activity, behavioral therapy	WCM	WCM	+	+	+
Pharmacotherapy	—	WCM	+	+	+
Surgery	—	—	WCM	WCM	WCM

+ represents the use of indicated treatment regardless of comorbidities; BMI = body mass index; WCM = with comorbidities.
From National Heart, Lung, and Blood Institute, 2000.

TABLE 1-12. Classification and Treatment of Hypertension

Classification	SBP (mm Hg)		DBP (mm Hg)	No Compelling Indication[a]	Those with a Compelling Indication[a]
Normal	<120	*and*	<80	No antihypertensive drug	No antihypertensive drug
Prehypertension	120–139	*or*	80–89	No antihypertensive drug	Drugs for the compelling indication(s)
Stage 1 hypertension	140–159	*or*	90–99	Thiazide-type diuretics for most. May consider ACEIs, ARBs, BBs, CCBs, or combination	Drugs for the compelling indication(s). ACEIs, ARBs, BBs, CCBs as needed
Stage 2 hypertension	≥160	*or*	≥100	Two-drug combination for most, usually thiazide-type diuretic and ACEIs or BB or CCB	Drugs for the compelling indication(s). Add diuretics, ACEIs, ARBs, BBs, CCBs, as needed

[a]Compelling indications include: (1) congestive heart failure, (2) myocardial infarction, (3) diabetes, (4) chronic renal failure, (5) prior stroke. Lifestyle modifications are encouraged for all and include: (1) weight reduction if overweight, (2) alcohol intake limitation, (3) increased aerobic physical activity (30–45 minutes daily), (4) sodium intake reduction (<2.34 g/d), (5) smoking cessation, and (6) Dietary Approaches to Stop Hypertension (DASH) diet (see Table 1–14, p. 20).
ACEI = angiotensin-converting enzyme inhibitor; ARB = angiotensin–receptor blocker; BB = β-blocker; CCB = calcium-channel blocker; DBP = diastolic blood pressure; SBP = systolic blood pressure.
From National Heart, Lung, and Blood Institute, 2003.

hypertension, gynecologists should be aware of target goals and long-term risks associated with this disease.

Diagnosis

Physical Examination. Blood pressures should ideally be taken with a woman seated in a chair with the tested arm resting on a table. An appropriately sized cuff is selected, and the cuff bladder should encircle at least 80 percent of the arm. Hypertension is diagnosed if readings are elevated on at least two separate office visits.

As seen in Table 1-12, categories of hypertension include *prehypertension*, which is diagnosed if readings are in the range 120–139/80–89 mm Hg. This range is important, because women with prehypertension are at significantly increased risk of developing hypertension later (Wang, 2004). Additionally, compared with normal blood pressure readings, prehypertension is associated with greater risks for cardiovascular disease (CVD) (Mainous, 2004).

If hypertension is diagnosed, further examination should exclude underlying causes of hypertension and resultant end-organ disease (Table 1-13). Accordingly, examination should include confirmation of comparable blood pressure in the contralateral arm; optic fundi examination; calculation of BMI and measurement of waist circumference; auscultation for carotid, abdominal, and femoral bruits; thyroid gland palpation; heart and lung auscultation; abdominal examination for renal enlargement and abnormal aortic pulsation; and extremity inspection for edema and pulses.

Laboratory Tests and Other Diagnostic Procedures. Routine laboratory tests recommended before initiating therapy include an electrocardiogram, urinalysis, blood glucose level, hematocrit, lipid profile, thyroid testing, and serum potassium and creatinine measurement. A more extensive search for

TABLE 1-13. Identifiable Causes of Hypertension

Chronic renal disease
Chronic steroid therapy and Cushing syndrome
Coarctation of the aorta
Drug-induced or drug-related
    Nonsteroidal antiinflammatory drugs
    Cocaine and amphetamines
    Sympathomimetics (decongestants, anorectics)
    Combination oral contraceptives
    Adrenal steroids
    Cyclosporine and tacrolimus
    Erythropoietin
    Licorice
    Herbal medicines (ephedra, ma huang)
Pheochromocytoma
Primary aldosteronism
Renovascular disease
Sleep apnea
Thyroid or parathyroid disease

TABLE 1-14. Management of Prehypertension

Strategy	Recommendation	Approximate SBP Reduction	Effect on Incidence or Prevalence of Hypertension
DASH dietary pattern	4–5 fruits/day 4–5 vegetables/day 2–3 low-fat dairy/day <25% fat	3.5 mm Hg	Decreased by 62% (prevalence)
Weight loss	Effective in lowering BP even without attaining normal BMI	1 mm Hg/kg of weight loss	Decreased by 42% (incidence)
Reduced sodium intake	<2400 mg/day	2 mm Hg per 76-mmol/L-per-day decrease	Decreased by 38% (incidence)
Physical activity	Moderate exercise ≥30 minutes most days	3–4 mm Hg	N/A
Moderation of alcohol intake	≤2 oz/day (men) ≤1 oz/day (women)	3.5 mm Hg	N/A

BMI = body mass index; BP = blood pressure; DASH = dietary approaches to stop hypertension; N/A = not available; SBP = systolic blood pressure.
From Svetkey, 2005, with permission.

identifiable causes is not generally indicated unless hypertension is not controlled with initial treatment (Chobanian, 2003).

Treatment

Lifestyle intervention provides an effective means to lower blood pressure and can be used to prevent and treat hypertension (Table 1-14). However, if blood pressure is significantly elevated, or resistant to lifestyle changes alone, or if other comorbid conditions exist, then pharmacologic treatment may be needed to decrease long-term complications. Medications used for treatment are numerous, and an extensive listing can be found in the National Heart, Lung, and Blood Institutes report on hypertension (2003) at: http://www.nhlbi.nih.gov/guidelines/hypertension/express.pdf.

▮ Diabetes Mellitus

Diabetes is common, and approximately 11 million adult women in the United States are diabetic (National Institute of Diabetes and Digestive and Kidney Disease, 2007). The long-term consequences of this endocrine disorder are serious and include coronary heart disease, stroke, peripheral vascular disease, periodontal disease, nephropathy, neuropathy, and retinopathy.

Screening

Currently, the U.S. Preventive Services Task Force (2008) concludes that there is insufficient evidence to recommend routine screening of asymptomatic adults for type 2 diabetes, unless hypertension is coexistent. However, the American

Diabetes Association (2010) recommends that screening be considered at 3-year intervals beginning at age 45, particularly in those with BMIs ≥25. Moreover, testing should be considered at a younger age or completed more often in those who are overweight and have one or more of the other risk factors shown in Table 1-15. Aside from screening, women with overt

TABLE 1-15. Risk Factors for Type 2 Diabetes

Age ≥45 years
Overweight (BMI ≥25)
Family history of diabetes (affected parents or siblings)
Habitual physical inactivity
Race/ethnicity (African-, Hispanic-, Native-, and Asian-Americans, and Pacific Islanders)
Previously identified IFG, IGT, or HbA$_{1c}$ ≥5.7%
History of GDM or delivery of a baby weighing >9 lbs
Hypertension (≥140/90 mm Hg in adults)
HDL cholesterol ≤35 mg/dL and/or triglyceride level ≥250 mg/dL
Polycystic ovary syndrome
Other clinical conditions associated with insulin resistance
History of vascular disease

BMI = body mass index; GDM = gestation diabetes mellitus; HbA$_{1c}$ = hemoglobin A$_{1c}$; HDL = high-density lipoprotein; IFG = impaired fasting glucose; IGT = impaired glucose tolerance.
From American Diabetes Association, 2010.

TABLE 1-16. Diagnostic Criteria for Diabetes Mellitus

HbA_{1c} ≥6.5%. Test should be performed in a laboratory using a method that is NGSP certified
or
FPG ≥126 mg/dL. Fasting is defined as no caloric intake for at least 8 hours
or
2-hours plasma glucose >200 mg/dL during an OGTT. The test should be performed as described by the WHO, using a glucose load containing the equivalent of 75 g anhydrous glucose dissolved in water
or
Symptoms of diabetes plus random plasma glucose concentration ≥200 mg/dL. Classic symptoms of diabetes include polyuria, polydipsia, and unexplained weight loss

Diagnostic Criteria for Impaired Fasting Glucose

FPG: 100–125 mg/dL

Diagnostic Criteria for Impaired Glucose Tolerance

2-hour plasma glucose during 75-g OGTT: 140–199 mg/dL
or
HbA_{1c}: 5.7–6.4%

FPG = fasting plasma glucose; HbA_{1c} = hemoglobin A_{1c}; NGSP = National Glycohemoglobin Standardization Program; OGTT = oral glucose tolerance test; WHO = World Health Organization.
From American Diabetes Association, 2010.

hyperglycemia symptoms such as polyuria, polydipsia, and blurred vision should undergo diagnostic testing for diabetes. Finally, the American College of Obstetricians and Gynecologists (2009c) recommends that all women with gestational diabetes be screened for diabetes 6 to 12 weeks postpartum. If normal, then glycemic status testing is recommended every 3 years.

Diabetes may be diagnosed by different methods, which are shown in Table 1-16. Laboratory measurement of plasma glucose concentration is performed on venous samples, and the above-mentioned values are based on the use of such methods. Elevated values, in the absence of unequivocal hyperglycemia, must be confirmed on a subsequent day by any of these methods. In contrast, capillary blood glucose testing using a blood glucometer is an effective monitoring tool, but is not currently recommended for diagnosing diabetes.

Treatment

For those diagnosed with diabetes, referral to a specialist is indicated. Delayed onset and slower progression of many diabetic complications has been shown to follow control of elevated blood glucose levels (Cleary, 2006; Fioretto, 2006; Martin, 2006). Control can be achieved with diet modification alone or combined with oral hypoglycemic agents or injectable insulin. To lower diabetic morbidity, therapy goals include hemoglobin A_{1c} levels <7 percent, blood pressure readings <130/80 mm Hg, low-density lipoprotein (LDL) levels <100 mg/dL, high-density lipoprotein (HDL) levels >50 mg/dL, triglyceride levels <150 mg/dL, weight loss, and

smoking cessation (National Diabetes Education Program, 2009).

There is an intermediate group whose glucose levels fall below the criteria for diabetes yet are too high to be considered normal. This group is defined as having *impaired fasting glucose* or *impaired glucose tolerance* depending on the test employed (see Table 1-16). These individuals have an increased risk for developing diabetes. To avert or delay diabetes, management of this group includes lifestyle modification to increase physical activity and weight loss, drugs such as metformin, nutritional counseling, and regular diabetes screening (American College of Obstetricians and Gynecologists, 2009c; American Diabetes Association, 2010).

■ Cardiovascular Disease

In 2006, nearly 36 percent of the female population was affected by cardiovascular disease (CVD), and more than 430,000 women died from its complications (American Heart Association, 2010). Guidelines from the American Heart Association encourage surveillance and initial assessment of a woman's risk for CVD (Mosca, 2011). Simplistically, a woman's risk can be calculated by totaling points assigned for smoking, age, lipid levels, and hypertension. An online calculator can be found at: http://hp2010.nhlbihin.net/atpiii/calculator.asp?usertype=prof. Termed the *Framingham 10-year CHD risk score*, point totals are broadly categorized into risk levels as follows: *high risk* (>20-percent risk of CHD), *at risk* (10- to 20-percent 10-year risk), and *optimal risk* (<10-percent risk). Recommendations for CVD are listed in Table 1-17 and are stratified according to these risk levels.

TABLE 1-17. Recommendations for Prevention of Cardiovascular Disease (CVD) in Women

High Risk (>20 percent risk of CVD)	At Risk (10 to 20 percent risk)	Optimal Risk (<10 percent risk)
Strength of Recommendation[a]		
Smoking cessation	Smoking cessation	Physical activity
Physical activity/cardiac rehabilitation	Physical activity	DASH diet
DASH diet	DASH diet	Healthy weight
Healthy weight	Healthy weight	
Blood pressure control	Blood pressure control	
Cholesterol control/therapy (goal <100 mg/dL)	LDL-lowering therapy if ≥190 mg/dL	
β-blocker therapy		
ACE inhibitor or ARB therapy		
Strength of Recommendation[b]		
LDL-lowering therapy (goal <70 mg/dL in very high-risk women)	Aspirin therapy Therapy for other cholesterol or TG elevations	
Glycemic control		
Aspirin/antiplatelet agents		
Omega-3 fatty acids		

ACE = angiotensin-converting enzyme; ARB = angiotensin–receptor blocker; DASH = dietary approach to stop hypertension; LDL = low-density lipoprotein; TG = trigylcerides.
[a]Consistent, good-quality evidence.
[b]Inconsistent or limited-quality evidence.
From Mosca, 2011.

TABLE 1-18. Diagnostic Criteria for Metabolic Syndrome

Any 3 of 5 Criteria Constitute a Diagnosis of Metabolic Syndrome	Categorical Cut Points
Elevated waist circumference[a]	≥102 cm (≥40 inches) in men ≥88 cm (≥35 inches) in women
Elevated TG levels	≥150 mg/dL ***or*** Drug treatment for elevated TG levels[b]
Reduced HDL levels	<40 mg/dL in men <50 mg/dL in women ***or*** Drug treatment for reduced HDL levels[b]
Elevated BP	≥130 mm Hg systolic BP ***or*** ≥85 mm Hg diastolic BP ***or*** Drug treatment for hypertension
Elevated fasting glucose levels	≥100 mg/dL ***or*** Drug treatment for elevated glucose levels

[a]Waist circumference guidelines vary between populations and countries and specific thresholds should be used. Values shown here are for the United States.
[b]Fibrates and nicotinic acid are the most commonly used drugs for elevated TG and reduced HDL. Patients taking these drugs are presumed to have high TG and low HDL levels.
BP = blood pressure; HDL = high-density lipoprotein; TG = triglyceride.
Modified from Alberti, 2009; Grundy, 2005.

Metabolic Syndrome

Diagnosis and Prevalence

This syndrome is a clustering of major cardiovascular disease risk factors (Table 1-18). At present, a single unifying cause of the metabolic syndrome has not been identified, and it may be precipitated by multiple underlying risk factors. Of these, abdominal obesity and insulin resistance appear important (Grundy, 2005). There is current debate surrounding the concept of a metabolic syndrome. However, this syndrome is recognized as a major health risk by the World Health Organization (WHO), American Heart Association, and International Diabetes Federation (Alberti, 2009; Despres, 2006; Grundy, 2006).

This syndrome is common, and approximately 20 to 25 percent of U.S. adults meet diagnostic criteria. Although genders appear equally affected, Mexican Americans show the highest prevalence, and incidence appears to increase in all ethnicities with age (Ford, 2002). The sequelae associated with metabolic syndrome are significant and include an increased risk of type 2 diabetes and mortality from CHD, CVD, and all causes (Lorenzo, 2003; Malik, 2004; Sattar, 2003). Among those with metabolic syndrome, risks are further increased by cigarette smoking and elevated LDL cholesterol levels.

Treatment

Goals of clinical management include reducing risks for clinical atherosclerotic disease and for type 2 diabetes mellitus. Accordingly, primary therapy for metabolic syndrome focuses on lifestyle modification, particularly weight reduction and increased exercise. During evaluation, each metabolic syndrome component should be addressed and treated in accordance with current guidelines. Moreover, drug therapy should follow current guidelines for treatment of each individual component (Eberly, 2006; Grundy, 2006; National Cholesterol Education Program, 2001).

Dyslipidemia

Hypercholesterolemia

Screening and Diagnosis. Data support that LDL cholesterol is the primary atherogenic agent. Although previously believed merely to collect passively within vessel walls, LDL is now felt to be a potent proinflammatory agent and creates the chronic inflammatory response characteristic of atherosclerosis. Logically, elevated levels of total and LDL cholesterol are associated with increased rates of coronary artery disease, ischemic stroke, and other atherosclerotic vascular complications (Horenstein, 2002; Law, 1994).

Preventatively, the National Cholesterol Education Program Adult Treatment Panel III (ATP-III) (2001) recommends that all adults 20 years and older have a serum lipoprotein profile drawn after a 9- to 12-hour fast once every 5 years. This profile includes measurement of total, LDL, HDL and triglyceride concentrations, and Table 1-19 lists interpretation of these levels. However, if other comorbid risks for coronary heart disease are present, then LDL goals are more stringent.

TABLE 1-19. Interpretation of Cholesterol and Triglyceride Levels

Lipoprotein Type (mg/dL)	Interpretation
Total Cholesterol	
<200	Optimal
200–239	Borderline elevated
≥240	Elevated
LDL Cholesterol	
<100	Optimal
100–129	Near optimal
130–159	Borderline elevated
160–189	Elevated
≥190	Very elevated
HDL Cholesterol	
<40	Low
≥60	Elevated
Triglycerides	
<150	Optimal
150–199	Borderline elevated
200–499	Elevated
≥500	Very elevated

HDL = high-density lipoprotein; LDL = low-density lipoprotein.
Compiled from National Cholesterol Education Program, 2001.

Treatment. Lowering LDL levels has been associated with reduced rates of myocardial infarction and ischemic stroke (Goldstein, 2011; Sever, 2003; Thavendiranathan, 2007). Therapy may include lifestyle changes with or without the addition of medication Table 1-20. For those with depressed HDL levels, efforts should be directed toward reaching LDL goals. Additionally, weight management and increased physical activity should be included.

Hypertriglyceridemia

Triglycerides are delivered to tissues by very-low-density lipoprotein (VLDL), which is synthesized and secreted by the liver. This triglyceride-rich lipoprotein is taken up by adipose and muscle, where triglycerides are cleaved from VLDL. Ultimately, a VLDL remnant is created that is atherogenic. For this reason, triglyceride levels can be used as one marker for atherogenic lipoproteins, and high triglyceride levels have been linked to increases in cardiovascular disease (Assmann, 1996; Austin, 1998). Additionally, its clinical importance is underscored by its inclusion in the criteria for the metabolic syndrome (Dunbar, 2005).

Hypertriglyceridemia is diagnosed based on criteria found in Table 1-19. For most with mild or moderate triglyceride elevation, recommendations from ATP-III attempt to lower both LDL and VLDL levels. Alternatively, for those with triglyceride levels greater than 500 mg/dL, treatment goals focus primarily on triglyceride level lowering to prevent pancreatitis.

TABLE 1-20. Oral Lipid Lowering Agents

Drug Class and Agents	Brand Name	Major Indications	Starting Dose	Maximal Dose	Contraindications
HMG CoA reductase inhibitors ("statins")		Elevated LDL			Absolute: Active or chronic liver disease Pregnancy, lactation
Lovastatin	Mevacor, Altocor		20 mg qd	80 mg qd	
Pravastatin	Pravachol		40 mg qhs	80 mg qhs	
Simvastatin	Zocor		20 mg qhs	80 mg qhs	
Fluvastatin	Lescol		20 mg qhs	80 mg qhs	
Atorvastatin	Lipitor		10 mg qhs	80 mg qhs	
Rosuvastatin	Crestor		10 mg qhs	40 mg qhs	
Bile acid sequestrants		Elevated LDL			Absolute: Dysbetalipoproteinemia TG >400 mg/dL
Cholestyramine	Questran		4 g qd	32 g qd	
Colestipol	Colestid		5 g qd	40 g qd	
Colesevelam	Welchol		3750 mg qd	4375 mg qd	
Nicotinic acid		Elevated LDL, low HDL, elevated TG			Absolute: Chronic liver disease Peptic ulcer disease Severe gout
Immediate-release			100 mg tid	1 g tid	
Sustained-release			250 mg bid	1.5 g bid	
Extended-release	Niaspan		500 mg qhs	2 g qhs	
Fibric acid derivatives		Elevated TG, elevated remnants			Absolute: Severe renal or liver disease Gallbladder disease Pregnancy, lactation
Gemfibrozil	Lopid, Gemcor		600 mg bid	600 mg bid	
Fenofibrate	Tricor		145 mg qd	145 mg qd	
Cholesterol absorption inhibitors		Elevated LDL			Relative: Moderate or severe liver disease
Ezetimibe	Zetia		10 mg qd	10 mg qd	
Combination agent		Elevated LDL			Absolute: Liver disease Pregnancy, lactation
Ezetimibe/ simvastatin	Vytorin		10 mg/10 mg qd	10 mg/80 mg qd	
Omega-3 fatty acids	—	Elevated TG	3 g qd	6 g qd	

bid = twice daily; CHD = coronary heart disease; GI = gastrointestinal; HDL = high-density lipoprotein cholesterol; HMG CoA = 3-hydroxy-3methylglutaryl coenzyme A; LDL = low-density lipoprotein cholesterol; TG = triglycerides; qd = daily; qhs = at bedtime; tid = three times daily; WHO = World Health Organization.
Cyclosporine, macrolide antibiotics, various antifungal agents, and cytochrome P450 inhibitors should be used with appropriate caution with fibrates and niacin.
Compiled from National Cholesterol Education Program, 2001, and Rader, 2012.

Stroke

This is the third leading cause of death in the United States. In 2006, approximately 425,000 American women suffered a new or recurrent stroke. Primary prevention is important, because more than 75 percent of strokes are first events (American Heart Association, 2010). Primary care providers should be aware of modifiable risk factors for stroke and treat or refer women for treatment of these factors (Table 1-21).

Exercise

Exercise has known benefits in preventing coronary artery disease, type 2 diabetes, osteoporosis, obesity, depression, insomnia, and breast and colon cancer (Brosse, 2002; Knowler, 2002; Lee, 2003; Vuori, 2001; Youngstedt, 2005). Many of these associations may result from the effects of exercise to lower blood pressure, decrease LDL cholesterol and triglyceride levels, increase HDL cholesterol levels, improve blood sugar control, and reduce weight (Braith, 2006; Pescatello, 2004; Sigal, 2004).

Despite these benefits, based on 2008 U.S. statistics, 64 percent of all women are considered inactive, and only 10 percent exercise more than five times per week (Pleis, 2009). Recommendations from the U.S. Department of Health and Human Services (2008) include moderate-intensity activity such as walking, water aerobics, or yard work for at least

TABLE 1-21. Risk Factors and Treatment Results for Stroke

Risk Factor	Relative Risk	Relative Risk Reduction with Treatment
Hypertension	8	32%
Atrial fibrillation	1.8–2.9	64% with warfarin, 19% with aspirin
Diabetes	1.8–6	No proven effect
Smoking	1.8–2.9	50% at 1 year; baseline risk at 5 years postcessation
Hyperlipidemia	1.8–2.6	16–30%
Carotid stenosis	2.0	50%

Abbreviated from Goldstein, 2011; Smith, 2012.

150 minutes each week or vigorous-intensity activities such as running, swimming laps, or aerobic dancing for 75 minutes each week. Activities should be performed in episodes of at least 10 minutes that are apportioned throughout the week. Additional health benefits are gained with physical activity beyond these amounts.

Although exercise programs have traditionally emphasized dynamic, aerobic lower-extremity exercise, research increasingly suggests that complementary resistance training improves muscular strength and endurance, cardiovascular function, metabolism, coronary risk factors, and psychosocial well-being (Pollock, 2000). Accordingly, government guidelines also encourage biweekly muscle-strengthening activities that involve all the major muscle groups. A fuller listing of general physical activities and their intensity description can be found at the CDC web site: http://www.health.gov/paguidelines/pdf/paguide.pdf.

Thyroid Disease

Dysfunction of the thyroid gland may lead to increased or decreased gland activity. As a result, symptoms of thyroid disease may vary widely, but commonly include changes in weight, temperature tolerances, menstruation, energy level, mood, skin and hair, and gastrointestinal motility. The risk of thyroid disease increases with age, and dysfunction is more common in women. Accordingly, the American Thyroid Association recommends that adults, especially women, be screened for thyroid dysfunction by measurement of a serum thyroid-stimulating hormone (TSH) concentration, beginning at age 35 years and repeated every 5 years thereafter (Ladenson, 2000). The American College of Obstetricians and Gynecologists (2011c) recommends screening initiation at age 50 and a similar 5-year screening interval. Moreover, individuals with clinical manifestations potentially attributable to thyroid dysfunction and those with risk factors for its development may require more frequent testing. People at higher risk for thyroid dysfunction include the elderly, postpartum women, those with prior exposure to high levels of radiation (>20 mGy), and those with Down syndrome. In contrast, the U.S. Preventive Services Task Force (2004c) has found insufficient evidence to recommend for or against routine screening.

Geriatric Screening

In 1996, the Baby Boom generation in the United States, totaling approximately 78 million, began turning 50. Women are living longer, and the current life expectancy for women in the United States is 80 (National Center for Health Statistics, 2010). To describe these individuals, researchers use the categories of *young-old* (ages 65–74), *middle-old* (75–84), and *oldest-old* (85 and older). As a woman moves through these stages, many of her health care needs may not be gynecologic. However, the gynecologist may be the physician contacted by a family member regarding a patient's memory loss or the first physician to notice signs of elder abuse. Accordingly, women's health care providers should be familiar with geriatric screening. Screening for malnutrition, functional status, and cognitive impairment can be included in routine ambulatory screening, whether accomplished by the physician or ancillary staff. Other screening topics include depression, elder abuse, fall risks, sexual dysfunction, urinary incontinence, osteoporosis, cardiovascular disease, and common cancers. These are covered elsewhere in this text, and recommended geriatric preventive care is outlined by the American College of Obstetricians and Gynecologists (2011c).

With screening, questions arise as to when to discontinue routine testing. Many such endpoints have been established by individual specialty organizations. In general, the decision to screen may be modified by the risks associated with the screening test itself, by patient health and comorbidities that might limit evaluation or treatment of a new disease, and by the patient's current estimated life expectancy.

Nutrition

As a woman ages, her body composition changes. Commonly, weight gain starts in her 30s. But as she reaches the geriatric years, weight loss may result secondary to depression, dentition problems, certain medications, neoplasia, or head trauma after a fall. Weight loss may also reflect social issues such as loss of transportation or grief after loss of a loved one. A direct relationship has been shown between weight loss in recently hospitalized elderly patients and mortality in the subsequent

TABLE 1-22. Vulnerable Elders Survey-13 (VES-13)

1. Age _____   **SCORE:** *1 POINT FOR AGE 75–84*
                                             3 POINTS FOR AGE ≥85

2. In general, compared to other people your age, would you say that your health is:

   ☐ Poor,* (*1 POINT*)
   ☐ Fair,* (*1 POINT*)   **SCORE:** *1 POINT FOR FAIR or POOR*
   ☐ Good,
   ☐ Very good, or
   ☐ Excellent

3. How much difficulty, <u>on average</u>, do you have with the following physical activities:

	No difficulty	A little difficulty	Some difficulty	A Lot of difficulty	Unable to do
a. stooping, crouching or kneeling?	☐	☐	☐	☐ *	☐ *
b. liftings or carrying objects as heavy as 10 pounds?	☐	☐	☐	☐ *	☐ *
c. reaching or extending arms above shoulder level?	☐	☐	☐	☐ *	☐ *
d. writing, or handling and grasping small objects?	☐	☐	☐	☐ *	☐ *
e. walking a quarter of a mile?	☐	☐	☐	☐ *	☐ *
f. heavy housework such as scrubbing floors or washing windows?	☐	☐	☐	☐ *	☐ *

SCORE: *I POINT FOR EACH * RESPONSE
IN Q3a THROUGH f. <u>MAXIMUM OF 2 POINTS</u>.*

4. Because of your health or a physical condition, do you have any difficulty:
   a. shopping for personal items (like toilet items or medicines)?
      ☐ YES → Do you get help with shopping?   ☐ YES *   ☐ NO
      ☐ NO
      ☐ DON'T DO → Is that because of your health?   ☐ YES *   ☐ NO
   b. managing money (like keeping track of expenses or paying bills)?
      ☐ YES → Do you get help with managing money?   ☐ YES *   ☐ NO
      ☐ NO
      ☐ DON'T DO → Is that because of your health?   ☐ YES *   ☐ NO
   c. walking across the room? USE OF CANE OR WALKER IS OK.
      ☐ YES → Do you get help with walking?   ☐ YES *   ☐ NO
      ☐ NO
      ☐ DON'T DO → Is that because of your health?   ☐ YES *   ☐ NO
   d. doing light housework (like washing dishes, straightening up, or light cleaning)?
      ☐ YES → Do you get help with light housework?   ☐ YES *   ☐ NO
      ☐ NO
      ☐ DON'T DO → Is that because of your health?   ☐ YES *   ☐ NO
   e. bathing or showering?
      ☐ YES → Do you get help with bathing or showering?   ☐ YES *   ☐ NO
      ☐ NO
      ☐ DON'T DO → Is that because of your health?   ☐ YES *   ☐ NO

SCORE: *4 POINTS FOR ONE OR MORE**

From Saliba, 2001, with permission.

year (Flodin, 2000). Moreover, in elderly women requiring gynecologic surgery, poor nutrition can lead to poor wound healing and delayed recovery. Thus, nutritional assessment is helpful to identify at-risk patients.

An easy to use test, the Mini-Nutritional Assessment Short Form (MNA®-SF), developed by the Nestlé Nutrition Institute, can be used as a screening tool in the ambulatory setting. The short form of MNA uses five questions and the patient's BMI or her calf circumference to assess malnutrition risk (Kaiser, 2009; Rubenstein, 2001; Vellas, 2006). Screening scores <12 points should prompt more detailed assessment with the full MNA form. Both forms are available online at: http://www.mna-elderly.com/mna_forms.html

Functional Status

Functional status refers to a patient's ability to perform both basic and more complex activities for independent living. The basic activities of daily living (ADL) are self-care functions such as grooming and toileting (Katz, 1963). The more complex instrumental activities of daily living (IADL) reflect independent functioning and include checkbook balancing, bill paying, and housekeeping tasks (Lawton, 1969). Declines in such functional status have been linked to increased risks of hospitalization, institutionalization, and death (Walston, 2006). Thus, assessment tools that evaluate ADL and IADL permit early identification, evaluation, and intervention. One of these, the Vulnerable Elders Survey-13 (VES-13), includes questions regarding physical and functional limitations and self-reported health status (Table 1-22). Patients with scores >3 have a fourfold risk of death or functional decline during the subsequent 2 years (Saliba, 2001). This test may be administered by nonclinicians and completed in less than 5 minutes. Tools such as this can help a gynecologist identify patients who appear at risk for functional decline and subsequently refer them for further evaluation if indicated.

Cognitive Function

Dementia is an acquired, chronic condition in which brain cells are destroyed and cognition deteriorates. These changes may present as short- and long-term memory loss, difficulty with problem solving, or inattention to personal hygiene. Although not expert in diagnosis and treatment of cognitive problems, a gynecologist can perform initial screening and provide results that either reassure the patient and her family or prompt more formal evaluation by a geriatrician or neurologist. In the geriatric patient, dementia and depression can be difficult to diagnose separately or as comorbidities. Thus, screening tools for both may be indicated. Those for depression are found in Tables 13-5 and 13-6 (p. 360).

For dementia, the Mini Mental Status Exam, or more recently the Mini-Cog Test, can screen for cognitive impairment in the primary care setting (Borson, 2000, 2006; Folstein, 1975). The Mini-Cog test requires approximately 3 minutes to administer and begins by giving the patient three items to remember early in the interview. Later in the interview, she is asked to recall those three items. For the clock-drawing test, the patient is asked to draw a clock with the hands at a specific time, such as 8:30. A correct clock has numbers 1 through 12

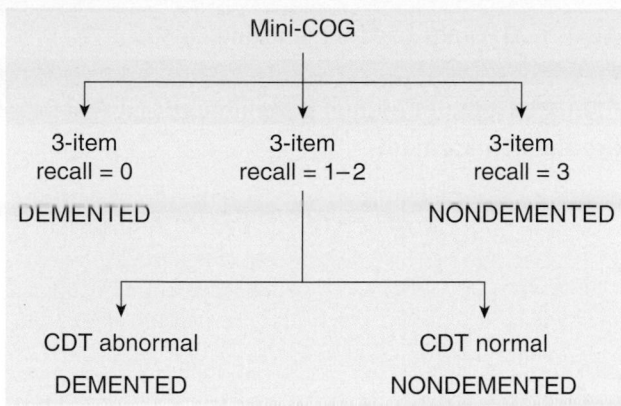

FIGURE 1-10 The Mini-Cog Test. CDT = clock-drawing test. *(From Borson, 2000, with permission.)*

labeled correctly in a clockwise fashion, with two arms (of any length) pointing at the correct numbers for the time requested. It is unlikely that a patient has dementia if the three-item recall test is completed correctly. An algorithm for scoring the Mini-Cog is shown in Figure 1-10. For a Mini-Cog Test suggestive of dementia, referral to an internist, geriatrician, or neurologist, as available to the patient in that community, is indicated.

Mental Health
Depression and Domestic Violence

For women of all ages, these problems are pervasive and account for significant morbidity and mortality. Each is discussed in detail in Chapter 13 (p. 356) and should be routinely screened for at annual visits. For depression, few data support the use of one specific screening method, and simple questions such as "During the past 2 weeks, have you felt down, depressed, or hopeless?" and "Have you felt little interest or pleasure in doing things?" are often effective (Whooley, 1997). These two questions constitute the Personal Health Questionnaire-2 (PHQ2), a validated screening tool for depression (Kroenke, 2003). All positive screening tests should prompt evaluation for depression as outlined in Table 13-5 (p. 360).

For domestic violence, the American College of Obstetricians and Gynecologists (2002) guidelines recommend that physicians routinely ask women direct, specific questions regarding abuse. General introductory statements such as "Because abuse and violence are so common in women's lives, I've begun to ask about it routinely" may be used. Also, the National Domestic Safety Hotline number 1-800-799-SAFE (7233) may be provided to patients (American Medical Association, 1992).

Smoking. Cigarette smoking is the single most preventable cause of death in the United States and has been linked with certain cancers, cardiovascular disease, chronic lung diseases, and stroke. Moreover, specific to gynecology, smoking is linked to diminished fertility, pregnancy complications, and postoperative complications. These are discussed in greater detail in their respective chapters. Yet despite these known effects, in 2003, only 64 percent of U.S. smokers

TABLE 1-23. Drugs Used for Smoking Cessation

Agent	Brand Name	Initial Dosing	Maintenance	Drug Tapering	Therapy Duration
Nicotine Replacement					
Patch[d]	Habitrol Nicoderm CQ	If >10 CPD: a 21-mg patch is reapplied daily weeks 1–6 If <10 CPD: 14-mg patch for weeks 1–6	14-mg patch is used weeks 7–8 ⟶	7-mg patch is used weeks 9–10 7-mg patch is used weeks 7–8	8–12 weeks
Gum[d]	Nicorette 2 mg 4 mg (if ≥25 CPD)	1 piece every 1–2 hour for weeks 1–6 (maximum 24 pieces/d)	1 piece every 2–4 hour for weeks 7–9	1 piece every 4–8 hour for weeks 10–12	12 weeks
Lozenge[b]	Commit 2 mg 4 mg (if smokes <30 min after waking)	1 piece every 1–2 hour for weeks 1–6 (maximum 20 pieces/d)	1 piece every 2–4 hour for weeks 7–9	1 piece every 4–8 hour for weeks 10–12	12 weeks
Inhaler[d]	Nicotrol		6 (average use) to 16 cartridges puffed qd for 12 weeks	Use is then tapered	12–24 weeks
Nasal spray[d]	Nicotrol		1 dose = 1–2 sprays to each nostril per hour (maximum 40 doses/d)	Use is then tapered starting week 9	12–24 weeks
Nicotine Agonists					
Varenicline[c]	Chantix	0.5 mg PO qd for 3 d, then 0.5 mg PO bid for next 4 d	Then 1 mg PO bid		12 weeks
CNS Agents					
Bupropion[c]	Wellbutrin SR Zyban	1–2 weeks prior to cessation: 150 mg PO qd for 3 d	Then 150 mg PO bid		7–12 weeks; may use for 6 months
Nortriptyline[a,d]		25 mg PO qd with gradual increase	75–100 mg PO qd		12 weeks; may use for 6 months
Clonidine[a,c]	Catapres	0.1 mg PO bid, increase by 0.10 mg/d each week as needed	0.15–0.75 mg PO qd		3–10 weeks
	Catapres-TTS	0.1-mg transdermal patch is changed weekly	0.1- to 0.2-mg transdermal patch weekly		

[a]Recommended as second-line agents by U.S. Public Health Service clinical guidelines, 2008.
[b]Has not been evaluated by the Food and Drug Administration (FDA) for pregnancy.
[c]Considered an FDA pregnancy category C drug.
[d]Considered an FDA pregnancy category D drug.
bid = twice daily; CNS = central nervous system; CPD = cigarettes per day; PO = orally; qd = daily.
Compiled from Fiore, 2008.

TABLE 1-24. Medications for Insomnia Approved by the U.S. Food and Drug Administration

Medication	Brand Name	Dose	Indications
Benzodiazepines			
Temazepam	Restoril	7.5–30 mg	For sleep-maintenance insomnia
Estazolam	ProSom	0.5–2 mg	For sleep-maintenance insomnia
Triazolam	Halcion	0.125–0.25 mg	For sleep-onset insomnia
Flurazepam	Dalmane	15–30 mg	For sleep-onset or sleep-maintenance insomnia
Quazepam	Doral	7.5–15 mg	For sleep-onset or sleep-maintenance insomnia
Benzodiazepine-Receptor Agonists			
Eszopiclone	Lunesta	1–3 mg	For sleep-maintenance insomnia
Zolpidem	Ambien	5–10 mg	For sleep-onset insomnia
Zolpidem extended release	Ambien CR	6.25–12.5 mg	For sleep-onset or sleep-maintenance insomnia
Zolipidem (sublingual)	Intermezzo	1.75 mg	For insomnia after middle-of-the-night awakening
Zaleplon	Sonata	5–20 mg	For sleep-onset or sleep-maintenance insomnia
Melatonin-Receptor Agonist			
Ramelteon	Rozerem	8 mg	For sleep-onset insomnia

who had routine examinations were advised by a physician to quit smoking (Torrijos, 2006). The American College of Obstetricians and Gynecologists (2011e) notes that each office visit is an opportunity for intervention. Guidelines from the U.S. Department of Health and Human Services encourage a brief patient intervention that contains five "A's": Ask about tobacco use; Advise cessation; Assess willingness to quit; Assist with medication or treatment referral; Arrange follow-up (Fiore, 2008). Strategies for cessation may include counseling and pharmacotherapy, and both yield increased abstinence rates (Ranney, 2006). Patients can also be referred to the National Cancer Institute's smoking cessation web site: http://www.smokefree.gov. This site provides free, accurate, evidence-based information and professional assistance to help support the immediate and long-term needs of those trying to quit smoking.

Smoking Pharmacotherapy. Nicotine is the key addictive component of tobacco, and it binds to the nicotinic acetylcholine receptor (Coe, 2005; Tapper, 2004). Binding increases central nervous system (CNS) dopamine levels. With smoking cessation, CNS dopamine levels are immediately lowered and cravings follow.

To blunt withdrawal symptoms, several products have been developed. These pharmacologic agents can broadly be divided into: (1) nicotine replacement agents, (2) CNS agents, and (3) nicotine agonists (Table 1-23). Of these, nicotine replacement agents lower nicotine levels gradually, thereby blunting nicotine withdrawal symptoms and increasing the

probability of smoking cessation. Of the CNS agents, bupropion (Zyban, Wellbutrin) is a dopamine-reuptake inhibitor. This drug may maintain central levels of dopamine during cessation and diminish dopamine withdrawal symptoms. Finally, varenicline (Chantix) is a nicotinic acetylcholine-receptor partial agonist. It binds to this receptor to relieve cessation withdrawal symptoms. All of these are effective. Wu and colleagues (2006), however, in their metaanalysis of controlled trials, found higher rates of cessation after 1 year with varenicline.

In 2011, the FDA issued a safety communication regarding the potential small increased risk of certain cardiovascular adverse events in patients with known cardiovascular disease using varenicline. The FDA noted that the drug is effective and that risks should be weighed against the benefits of smoking cessation in a given patient. In addition, the FDA (2009) reported that the use of varenicline or bupropion hydrochloride had been associated with reports of adverse mood or behavior changes. A black box warning describing this is now added to their product labeling.

Substance Abuse. Simple, direct questions regarding use can be brief yet effective tools to identify potential alcohol abuse. A clinician guide for patient evaluation and management is available from the U.S. Department of Health and Human Services (2005) at: http://pubs.niaaa.nih.gov/publications/Practitioner/CliniciansGuide2005/guide.pdf. If usage patterns suggest abuse, then further evaluation or referral is warranted. *Diagnostic and Statistical Manual of Mental*

Disorders, Fourth Edition (DSM-IV-TR) criteria for substance dependence or substance abuse are found in Tables 13-9 and 13-10 (p. 363).

Insomnia

Insomnia is common and its definition includes: (1) difficulty initiating sleep, (2) trouble maintaining sleep, and (3) early waking. Insomnia may be primary or may be secondary to other conditions such as depression, time-zone travel, restless leg syndrome, stimulant use, and sleep apnea (National Institutes of Health, 2005). Accordingly, historical inventory should investigate and treatment should be directed to these and other secondary causes (Becker, 2005).

Treatment of primary insomnia is typically cognitive-behavioral or pharmacologic. Cognitive therapy is aimed at changing patients' beliefs and attitudes regarding sleep. Behavioral therapies are varied and include those that control sleep timing and duration; attempt to improve the bedroom environment; or focus on relaxation or biofeedback techniques (Morgenthaler, 2006; Silber, 2005). Medications may be used to aid sleep, and most agents are of the benzodiazepine family (Table 1-24) (National Institutes of Health, 2005).

REFERENCES

Alberti KG, Eckel RH, Grundy SM, et al: Harmonizing the metabolic syndrome: a joint interim statement of the International Diabetes Federation Task Force on Epidemiology and Prevention; National Heart, Lung, and Blood Institute; American Heart Association; World Heart Federation; International Atherosclerosis Society; and International Association for the Study of Obesity. Circulation 120(16):1640, 2009

American Cancer Society: American Cancer Society Guidelines for the Early Detection of Cancer. 2011. Available at: http://www.cancer.org/Healthy/FindCancerEarly/CancerScreeningGuidelines/american-cancer-society-guidelines-for-the-early-detection-of-cancer. Accessed August 26, 2011

American College of Obstetricians and Gynecologists: Cervical cytology screening. Practice Bulletin No. 109, December 2009a

American College of Obstetricians and Gynecologists: Breast cancer screening. Practice Bulletin No. 122, August 2011a

American College of Obstetricians and Gynecologists: Colonoscopy and colorectal cancer screening strategies. Committee Opinion No. 482, March 2011b

American College of Obstetricians and Gynecologists: Guidelines for Women's Health Care, 2nd ed. Washington, DC, ACOG, 2002

American College of Obstetricians and Gynecologists: Human papillomavirus vaccination. Committee Opinion No. 344, September 2006a

American College of Obstetricians and Gynecologists: Motivational interviewing: a tool for behavior change. Committee Opinion No. 423, January 2009b

American College of Obstetricians and Gynecologists: Neural tube defects. Practice Bulletin No. 44, July 2003

American College of Obstetricians and Gynecologists: Postpartum screening for abnormal glucose tolerance in women who had gestational diabetes mellitus. Committee Opinion No. 435, June 2009c

American College of Obstetricians and Gynecologists: Primary and preventive care: periodic assessments. Committee Opinion No. 483, April 2011c

American College of Obstetricians and Gynecologists: Routine cancer screening. Committee Opinion No. 356, December 2006b

American College of Obstetricians and Gynecologists: Routine human immunodeficiency virus screening. Committee Opinion No. 411, August 2008

American College of Obstetricians and Gynecologists: The importance of preconception care in the continuum of women's health care. Committee Opinion No. 313, September 2005.

American College of Obstetricians and Gynecologists: The role of the obstetrician-gynecologist in the early detection of epithelial ovarian cancer. Committee Opinion No. 477, March 2011d

American College of Obstetricians and Gynecologists: Tobacco use and women's health. Committee Opinion No. 503, September 2011e

American College of Obstetricians and Gynecologists (ACOG) and American College of Allergy, Asthma and Immunology (ACAAI): The use of newer asthma and allergy medications during pregnancy. Ann Allergy Asthma Immunol 84(5):475, 2000

American Diabetes Association: Standards of medical care in diabetes—2010. Diabetes Care 33:S11, 2010

American Heart Association: Heart disease and stroke statistics-2010 update. Available at: http://www.americanheart.org/downloadable/heart/1265665152970DS-3241%20HeartStrokeUpdate_2010.pdf. Accessed August 18, 2010

American Medical Association: Diagnosis and treatment guidelines on domestic violence, 1992. Available at: http://archfami.ama-assn.org/cgi/reprint/1/1/39. Accessed August 17, 2010

Assmann G, Schulte H, von Eckardstein A: Hypertriglyceridemia and elevated lipoprotein(a) are risk factors for major coronary events in middle-aged men. Am J Cardiol 77(14):1179, 1996

Austin MA, Hokanson JE, Edwards KL: Hypertriglyceridemia as a cardiovascular risk factor. Am J Cardiol 81(4A):7B, 1998

Becker PM: Pharmacologic and nonpharmacologic treatments of insomnia. Neurol Clin 23(4):1149, 2005

Bevers TB, Anderson BO, Bonaccio E, et al: NCCN clinical practice guidelines in oncology: breast cancer screening and diagnosis. J Natl Compr Canc Netw 7(10):1060, 2009

Borson S, Scanlan J, Brush M, et al: The Mini-Cog: a cognitive "vital signs" measure for dementia screening in multi-lingual elderly. Int J Geriatr Psychiatry 15:1021, 2000

Borson S, Scanlan J, Watanabe J, et al: Improving identification of cognitive impairment in primary care. Int J Geriatr Psychiatry 21:349, 2006

Braith RW, Stewart KJ: Resistance exercise training: its role in the prevention of cardiovascular disease. Circulation 113(22):2642, 2006

Brosse AL, Sheets ES, Lett HS, et al: Exercise and the treatment of clinical depression in adults: recent findings and future directions. Sports Med 32:741, 2002

Buchwald H: Bariatric surgery for morbid obesity: health implications for patients, health professionals, and third-party payers. J Am Coll Surg 200(4):593, 2005

Centers for Disease Control and Prevention: Recommended adult immunization schedule—United States, 2011. MMWR 60(4):1, 2011

Centers for Disease Control and Prevention: Revised recommendations for HIV testing of adults, adolescents, and pregnant women in health-care settings. MMWR 55(14):1, 2006

Centers for Disease Control and Prevention: Sexually transmitted diseases treatment guidelines, 2010. MMWR 59(12):1, 2010a

Centers for Disease Control and Prevention: U.S. medical eligibility criteria for contraceptive use, 2010. Adapted from the World Health Organization Medical Eligibility Criteria for Contraceptive Use, 4th ed. MMWR Early Release 59 (May 28):1, 2010b

Chobanian AV, Bakris GL, Black HR, et al: The seventh report of the Joint National Committee on Prevention, Detection, Evaluation, and Treatment of High Blood Pressure: the JNC 7 report. JAMA 289(19):2560, 2003

Christou NV, Sampalis JS, Liberman M, et al: Surgery decreases long-term mortality, morbidity, and health care use in morbidly obese patients. Ann Surg 240:416, 2004

Cleary PA, Orchard TJ, Genuth S, et al: The effect of intensive glycemic treatment on coronary artery calcification in type 1 diabetic participants of the Diabetes Control and Complications Trial/Epidemiology of Diabetes Interventions and Complications (DCCT/EDIC) Study. Diabetes 55(12):3556, 2006

Coe JW, Brooks PR, Vetelino MG, et al: Varenicline: an alpha4 beta2 nicotinic receptor partial agonist for smoking cessation. J Med Chem 48(10):3474, 2005

Despres JP, Lemieux I: Abdominal obesity and metabolic syndrome. Nature 444(7121):881, 2006

Dunbar RL, Rader DJ: Demystifying triglycerides: a practical approach for the clinician. Cleve Clin J Med 72(8):661, 2005

Eberly LE, Prineas R, Cohen JD, et al: Metabolic syndrome: risk factor distributing and 18-year mortality in the Multiple Risk Factor Intervention Trial. Diabetes Care 29(1):123, 2006

Ettinger MP: Aging bone and osteoporosis: strategies for preventing fractures in the elderly. Arch Intern Med 163(18):2237, 2003

Fiore AE, Uyeki TM, Broder K, et al: Prevention and control of influenza with vaccines: recommendations of the Advisory Committee on Immunization Practices (ACIP), 2010. MMWR 59(RR-8):1, 2010

Fiore MC, Jaen CR, Baker TB, et al: Treating tobacco use and dependence: 2008 update. Rockville, U.S. Department of Health and Human Services, 2008

Fioretto P, Bruseghin M, Berto I, et al: Renal protection in diabetes: role of glycemic control. J Am Soc Nephrol 17(4 Suppl 2):S86, 2006

Flegal KM, Carroll MD, Ogden CL, et al: Prevalence and trends in obesity among U.S. adults, 1999-2008. JAMA 303(3):235, 2010

Flodin L, Svensson S, Cederholm T: Body mass index as a predictor of 1 year mortality in geriatric patients. Clin Nutr 19(2):121, 2000

Folstein M, Folstein S, McHugh P: "Mini-mental state." A practical method for grading the cognitive state of patients for the clinician. J Psychiatr Res 12:189, 1975

Food and Drug Administration: Chantix (varenicline) may increase the risk of certain cardiovascular adverse events in patients with cardiovascular disease. 2011. Available at: http://www.fda.gov/Drugs/DrugSafety/ucm259161.htm. Accessed August 14, 2011

Food and Drug Administration: Completed safety review of Xenical/Alli (orlistat) and severe liver injury. 2010a. Available at: http://www.fda.gov/Drugs/DrugSafety/PostmarketDrugSafetyInformationforPatientsandProviders/ucm213038.htm. Accessed August 15, 2010

Food and Drug Administration: FDA Requires New Boxed Warnings for the Smoking Cessation Drugs Chantix and Zyban. 2009. Available at: http://www.fda.gov/Drugs/DrugSafety/PostmarketDrugSafetyInformationforPatientsandProviders/DrugSafetyInformationforHeathcareProfessionals/PublicHealthAdvisories/ucm169988.htm. Accessed August 27, 2011

Food and Drug Administration: Meridia (sibutramine hydrochloride) Information. 2010b. Available at :http://www.fda.gov/Drugs/DrugSafety/PostmarketDrugSafetyInformationforPatientsandProviders/ucm191652.htm. Accessed August 26, 2011

Ford ES, Giles WH, Dietz WH: Prevalence of the metabolic syndrome among us adults: findings from the Third National Health and Nutrition Examination Survey. JAMA 287(3):356, 2002

Goldstein LB, Bushnell CD, Adams RJ, et al: Guidelines for the primary prevention of stroke: a guideline for healthcare professionals from the American Heart Association/American Stroke Association. Stroke 42(2):517, 2011

Griffith WF, Stuart GS, Gluck KL, et al: Vaginal speculum lubrication and its effects on cervical cytology and microbiology. Contraception 72(1):60, 2005

Grundy SM: Metabolic syndrome: connecting and reconciling cardiovascular and diabetes worlds. J Am Coll Cardiol 47(6):1093, 2006

Grundy SM, Cleeman JI, Daniels SR, et al: Diagnosis and management of the metabolic syndrome: An American Heart Association/National Heart, Lung, and Blood Institute scientific statement: executive summary. Circulation 112(17):e285, 2005

Hayes SN: Preventing cardiovascular disease in women. Am Fam Physician 74:1331, 2006

Henness S, Perry CM: Orlistat: a review of its use in the management of obesity. Drugs 66(12):1625, 2006

Horenstein RB, Smith DE, Mosca L: Cholesterol predicts stroke mortality in the Women's Pooling Project. Stroke 33(7):1863, 2002

Jack BW, Atrash H, Coonrod DV, et al: The clinical content of preconception care: an overview and preparation of this supplement. Am J Obstet Gynecol 199(6 Suppl 2):S266, 2008

Kahn R, Buse J, Ferrannini E, et al: The metabolic syndrome: time for a critical appraisal: joint statement from the American Diabetes Association and the European Association for the Study of Diabetes. Diabetes Care 28(9):2289, 2005

Kaiser MJ, Bauer JM, Ramsch C, et al: Validation of the Mini Nutritional Assessment short-form (MNA-SF): a practical tool for identification of nutritional status. J Nutr Health Aging 13(9):782, 2009

Katz S, Ford, AB, Moskowitz RW, et al: Studies of illness in the aged. The index of ADL: a standardized measure of biological and psychosocial function. JAMA 185:914, 1963

Knowler WC, Barrett-Connor E, Fowler SE, et al: Reduction in the incidence of type 2 diabetes with lifestyle intervention or metformin. N Engl J Med 346:393, 2002

Kösters JP, Gøtzsche PC: Regular self-examination or clinical examination for early detection of breast cancer. Cochrane Database Syst Rev 3:CD003373, 2008

Kroenke K, Spitzer RL, Williams JB: The Patient Health Questionnaire-2: validity of a two-item depression screener. Med Care 41(11):1284, 2003

Ladenson PW, Singer PA, Ain KB, et al: American Thyroid Association guidelines for detection of thyroid dysfunction. Arch Intern Med 160(11):1573, 2000

Law MR, Wald NJ, Thompson SG: By how much and how quickly does reduction in serum cholesterol concentration lower risk of ischaemic heart disease? BMJ 308(6925):367, 1994

Lawton MP, Brody EM: Assessment of older people: self-monitoring and instrumental activities of daily living. Gerontologist 9:179, 1969

Lee IM: Physical activity and cancer prevention—data from epidemiologic studies. Med Sci Sports Exerc 35(11):1823, 2003

Levin B, Lieberman DA, McFarland B, et al: Screening and surveillance for the early detection of colorectal cancer and adenomatous polyps, 2008: a joint guideline from the American Cancer Society, the U.S. Multi-Society Task Force on Colorectal Cancer, and the American College of Radiology. CA Cancer J Clin 58(3).130, 2008

Lorenzo C, Okoloise M, Williams K, et al: The metabolic syndrome as predictor of type 2 diabetes: the San Antonio heart study. Diabetes Care 26(11):3153, 2003

Mainous AG III, Everett CJ, Liszka H, et al: Prehypertension and mortality in a nationally representative cohort. Am J Cardiol 94(12):1496, 2004

Malik S, Wong ND, Franklin SS, et al: Impact of the metabolic syndrome on mortality from coronary heart disease, cardiovascular disease, and all causes in United States adults. Circulation 110(10):1245, 2004

Martin CL, Albers J, Herman WH, et al: Neuropathy among the diabetes control and complications trial cohort 8 years after trial completion. Diabetes Care 29(2):340, 2006

McDonald S, Saslow D, Alciati MH: Performance and reporting of clinical breast examination: a review of the literature. CA Cancer J Clin 54:345, 2004

Meissner HI, Breen N, Klabunde CN, et al: Patterns of colorectal cancer screening uptake among men and women in the United States. Cancer Epidemiol Biomarkers Prev 15(2):389, 2006

Merhi ZO: Impact of bariatric surgery on female reproduction. Fertil Steril 92(5):1501, 2009

Morgenthaler T, Kramer M, Alessi C, et al: Practice parameters for the psychological and behavioral treatment of insomnia: an update. An American Academy of Sleep Medicine report. Sleep 29(11):1415, 2006

Mosca L, Benjamin EJ, Berra K, et al: Effectiveness-based guidelines for the prevention of cardiovascular disease in women—2011 update: a guideline from the American Heart Association. J Am Coll Cardiol 57(12):1404, 2011

Must A, Spadano J, Coakley EH, et al: The disease burden associated with overweight and obesity. JAMA 282(16):1523, 1999

National Cancer Institute: Breast cancer screening: summary of evidence. 2010. Available at: http://www.cancer.gov/cancertopics/pdq/screening/breast/HealthProfessional/page2#Section_188. Accessed August 12, 2010

National Center for Health Statistics: Health, United States, 2009: with special feature on medical technology. Hyattsville, MD, U.S. Department of Health and Human Services, 2010

National Cholesterol Education Program: Detection, evaluation, and treatment of high blood cholesterol in adults (Adult Treatment Panel III). National Institutes of Health Publication No.01-3670, 2001. Available at: http://www.nhlbi.nih.gov/guidelines/cholesterol/atp3xsum.pdf. Accessed August 12, 2010

National Diabetes Education Program: Guiding principles for diabetes care: for health care providers. National Institutes of Health Publication No.99-4343, 2009. Available at: http://ndep.nih.gov/media/GuidPrin_HC_Eng.pdf. Accessed August 17, 2010

National Heart, Lung, and Blood Institute: Clinical guidelines on the identification, evaluation, and treatment of overweight and obesity in adults. National Institutes of Health Publication No. 98-4083, 1998. Available at: http://www.nhlbi.nih.gov/guidelines/obesity/ob_gdlns.pdf Accessed August 16, 2010

National Heart, Lung, and Blood Institute: The practical guide: identification, evaluation, and treatment of overweight and obesity in adults. National Institutes of Health Publication No. 98-4084, 2000. Available at: http://www.nhlbi.nih.gov/guidelines/obesity/prctgd_c.pdf. Accessed August 16, 2010

National Heart, Lung, and Blood Institute: The seventh report of the Joint National Committee on Prevention, Detection, Evaluation, and Treatment of Hypertension. National Institutes of Health Publication No. 03-5233, 2003. Available at: http://www.nhlbi.nih.gov/guidelines/hypertension/express.pdf. Accessed August 18, 2010

National Institute of Diabetes and Digestive and Kidney Disease: National Diabetes Statistics, 2007. Available at: http://diabetes.niddk.nih.gov/dm/pubs/statistics/index.htm#y_people. Accessed August 18, 2010

National Institutes of Health: NIH state-of-the-science conference statement on manifestations and management of chronic insomnia in adults, NIH Consens State Sci Statements 22(2):1, 2005

National Osteoporosis Foundation: Clinician's guide to prevention and treatment of osteoporosis. Washington, DC, National Osteoporosis Foundation, 2010, p 1

National Task Force on the Prevention and Treatment of Obesity: Overweight, obesity, and health risk. Arch Intern Med 160(7):898, 2000

Nestlé Nutrition Institute: Mini-Nutritional Assessment Short Form (MNA®-SF). 2009. Available at: http://www.mna-elderly.com/forms/mini/mna_mini_english.pdf. Accessed August 17, 2010

Ong KL, Cheung BMY, Man YB, et al: Prevalence, awareness, treatment, and control of hypertension among United States adults 1999-2004. Hypertension 49(1):69, 2007

Pescatello LS, Franklin BA, Fagard R, et al: American College of Sports Medicine position stand. Exercise and hypertension. Med Sci Sports Exerc 36(3):533, 2004

Pleis JR, Lucas JW, Ward BW: Summary health statistics for U.S. adults: National Health Interview Survey, 2008. National Center for Health Statistics. Vital Health Stat 10(242):1, 2009

Pollock ML, Franklin BA, Balady GJ, et al: Resistance exercise in individuals with and without cardiovascular disease: benefits, rationale, safety, and prescription. An advisory from the Committee on Exercise, Rehabilitation, and Prevention, Council on Clinical Cardiology, American Heart Association. Circulation 101(7):828, 2000

Rader DJ, Hobbs HH: Disorders of lipoprotein metabolism. In Longo DL, Kasper DL, Jameson JL, et al (eds): Harrison's Principles of Internal Medicine, 18th ed. New York, McGraw-Hill, 2012

Ranney L, Melvin C, Lux L, et al: Systematic review: smoking cessation intervention strategies for adults and adults in special populations. Ann Intern Med 145(11):845, 2006

Rubenstein LZ, Harker JO, Salva A, et al: Screening for undernutrition in geriatric practice: developing the short-form Mini Nutritional Assessment (MNA-SF). J Geront 56A:M366, 2001

Saliba D, Elliott, M, Rubenstein L, et al: The vulnerable elders' survey: a tool for identifying vulnerable older people in the community. J Am Geriatr Soc 49:1691, 2001

Sanford KW, McPherson RA: Fecal occult blood testing. Clin Lab Med 29(3):523, 2009

Saslow D, Hannan J, Osuch J, et al: Clinical breast examination: practical recommendations for optimizing performance and reporting. CA Cancer J Clin 54:327, 2004

Sattar N, Gaw A, Scherbakova O, et al: Metabolic syndrome with and without C-reactive protein as a predictor of coronary heart disease and diabetes in the West of Scotland Coronary Prevention Study. Circulation 108(4):414, 2003

Sever PS, Dahlof B, Poulter NR, et al: Prevention of coronary and stroke events with atorvastatin in hypertensive patients who have average or lower-than-average cholesterol concentrations, in the Anglo-Scandinavian Cardiac Outcomes Trial—Lipid Lowering Arm (ASCOT-LLA): a multicentre randomised controlled trial. Lancet 361:1149, 2003

Sigal RJ, Kenny GP, Wasserman DH, et al: Physical activity/exercise and type 2 diabetes. Diabetes Care 27(10):2518, 2004

Silber MH: Clinical practice. Chronic insomnia. N Engl J Med 353(8):803, 2005

Sjostrom L, Lindroos AK, Peltonen M, et al: Lifestyle, diabetes, and cardiovascular risk factors 10 years after bariatric surgery. N Engl J Med 351:2683, 2004

Smith RA, Cokkinides V, Brooks D, et al: Cancer Screening in the United States, 2011: a review of current American Cancer Society Guidelines and issues in cancer screening. CA Cancer J Clin 60:99, 2011

Smith WS, English JD, Johnston SC: Cerebrovascular diseases. In Longo DL, Kasper DL, Jameson JL, et al (eds): Harrison's Principles of Internal Medicine, 18th ed. New York, McGraw-Hill, 2012

Society of Family Planning, Higginbotham S: Contraceptive considerations in obese women. Contraception 80(6):583, 2009

Steinbrook R: Surgery for severe obesity. N Engl J Med 350(11):1075, 2004

Svetkey LP: Management of prehypertension. Hypertension 45:1056, 2005

Tapper AR, McKinney SL, Nashmi R, et al: Nicotine activation of alpha4 receptors: sufficient for reward, tolerance, and sensitization. Science 306(5698):1029, 2004

Thavendiranathan P, Bagai A, Brookhart MA, et al: Primary prevention of cardiovascular diseases with statin therapy: a meta-analysis of randomized controlled trials. Arch Intern Med 166:2307, 2006

Thomas DB, Gao DL, Ray RM: Randomized trial of breast self-examination in Shanghai: final results. J Natl Cancer Inst 94(19):1445, 2002

Torrijos RM, Glantz SA: The U.S. Public Health Service "Treating Tobacco Use and Dependence Clinical Practice Guidelines" as a legal standard of care. Tob Control 15(6):447, 2006

U.S. Department of Health and Human Services: Helping patients who drink too much: a clinician's guide, updated 2005 edition. Available at: http://pubs.niaaa.nih.gov/publications/Practitioner/CliniciansGuide2005/guide.pdf. Accessed August 15, 2010

U.S. Department of Health and Human Services: 2008 physical activity guidelines for Americans. Available at: http://www.health.gov/PAGuidelines/pdf/paguide.pdf. Accessed August 15, 2010

U.S. Preventive Services Task Force: Guide to clinical preventive services. 2009a. Available at: http://www.ahrq.gov/clinic/pocketgd09/pocketgd09.pdf. Accessed August 17, 2010

U.S. Preventive Services Task Force: Screening for breast cancer. 2009b. Available at: http://www.ahrq.gov/clinic/uspstf/uspsbrca.htm. Accessed August 12, 2010

U.S. Preventive Services Task Force: Screening for chlamydial infection. 2007. Available at: http://www.ahrq.gov/clinic/uspstf07/chlamydia/chlamydiars.htm. Accessed August 12, 2010

U.S. Preventive Services Task Force: Screening for genital herpes. 2005a. Available at: http://www.uspreventiveservicestaskforce.org/uspstf05/herpes/herpesrs.htm. Accessed August 17, 2010

U.S. Preventive Services Task Force: Screening for gonorrhea. 2005b. Available at: http://www.ahrq.gov/clinic/uspstf/uspsgono.htm. Accessed August 12, 201.

U.S. Preventive Services Task Force: Screening for hepatitis B virus infection. 2004a. Available at: http://www.uspreventiveservicestaskforce.org/3rduspstf/hepbscr/hepbrs.htm. Accessed August 17, 2010

U.S. Preventive Services Task Force: Screening for hepatitis C in adults. 2004b. Available at: http://www.uspreventiveservicestaskforce.org/3rduspstf/hepcscr/hepcrs.htm. Accessed August 17, 2010

U.S. Preventive Services Task Force: Screening for HIV. 2005c. Available at: http://www.ahrq.gov/clinic/uspstf05/hiv/hivrs.htm. Accessed August 12, 2010

U.S. Preventive Services Task Force: Screening for syphilis Infection. 2004d. Available at: http://www.uspreventiveservicestaskforce.org/3rduspstf/syphilis/syphilrs.htm. Accessed August 17, 2010

U.S. Preventive Services Task Force: Screening for thyroid disease, 2004c. Available at: http://www.ahrq.gov/clinic/uspstf/uspsthyr.htm. Accessed February 22, 2007

U.S. Preventive Services Task Force: Screening for type 2 diabetes mellitus in adults. 2008. Available at: http://www.uspreventiveservicestaskforce.org/uspstf08/type2/type2rs.htm. Accessed August 17, 2010

Vasan RS, Beiser A, Seshadri S, et al: Residual lifetime risk for developing hypertension in middle-aged women and men: the Framingham heart study. JAMA 287(8):1003, 2002

Vellas B, Villars H, Abellan G, et al: Overview of MNA® - its history and challenges. J Nutr Health Aging 10:456, 2006

Vuori IM: Dose-response of physical activity and low back pain, osteoarthritis, and osteoporosis. Med Sci Sports Exerc 33(6 Suppl):S551, 2001

Walston J, Hadley EC, Ferrucci L, et al: Research agenda for frailty in older adults: toward a better understanding of physiology and etiology: summary from the American Geriatrics Society/National Institute on Aging Research Conference on Frailty in Older Adults. J Am Geriatr Soc 54(6):991, 2006

Wang Y, Wang QJ: The prevalence of prehypertension and hypertension among U.S. adults according to the new joint national committee guidelines: new challenges of the old problem. Arch Intern Med 164(19):2126, 2004

Whooley MA, Avins AL, Miranda J, et al: Case-finding instruments for depression. Two questions are as good as many. J Gen Intern Med 12(7):439, 1997

Wu P, Wilson K, Dimoulas P, et al: Effectiveness of smoking cessation therapies: a systematic review and meta-analysis. BMC Public Health 6(1):300, 2006

Youngstedt SD: Effects of exercise on sleep. Clin Sports Med 24:355, 2005

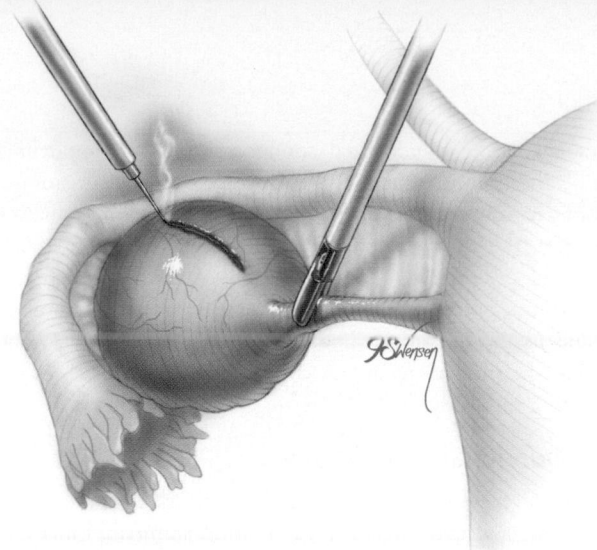

Techniques Used for Imaging in Gynecology

Over the past several decades, a number of technical advances currently allow for superb imaging of female pelvic structures. Modalities include sonography, radiography, computed tomographic (CT) scanning, magnetic resonance (MR) imaging, and less commonly, positron emission tomographic (PET) imaging. Of these, the evolution of sonography has now led to its use in gynecology equivalent to that in obstetrics. Moreover, advances in three-dimensional (3-D) imaging techniques have added such tremendous value to sonographic examination that it rivals the use of CT scanning and MR imaging for evaluation of many gynecologic conditions. MR imaging has been expanded with MR-guided focused ultrasound surgery (MRgFUS) to be used as treatment for uterine leiomyomas.

SONOGRAPHY

Physics

In sonography, the picture displayed on a screen is produced by sound waves reflected back from an imaged structure. Alternating current is applied to a transducer containing piezoelectric crystals, which convert electric energy to high-frequency sound waves. A water-soluble gel applied to the skin or placed within the tip of the transvaginal probe's condom sheath acts as a coupling agent. Sound waves pass through layers of tissue, encounter an interface between tissues of different densities, and are reflected back to the transducer. Converted back into electric energy, they are displayed on a screen. Dense material, such as bone, or a synthetic material, such as an intrauterine device, produces high-velocity reflected waves, also termed *echoes*, which are displayed on a screen as white. Materials such as these are described as *echogenic*. Conversely, fluid is *anechoic,* generates few reflected waves, and appears black on a screen. Middle-density tissues reflect waves to create various shades of gray, and images are described as hypoechoic or hyperechoic relative to tissues immediately adjacent to them. Images are generated so quickly—more than 40 frames/sec—that the picture on the screen appears to move in real-time (Cunningham, 2010d).

Sound reflection is greatest when the difference between the acoustic impedance of two structures is large. This explains why cysts are so well demonstrated with sonography. Strong echoes are produced from the cyst walls, but no echoes arise from fluid

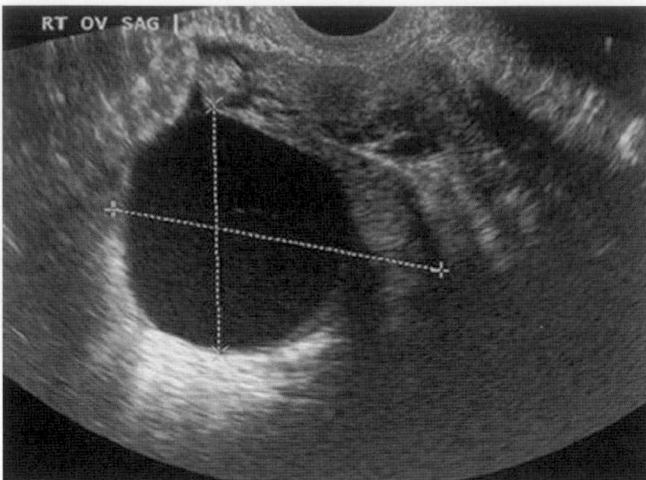

FIGURE 2-1 Transvaginal sonogram of a premenopausal ovary containing a follicular cyst. The cyst fluid appears black or anechoic. Note the white or hyperechoic area under the cyst, a sonographic feature called posterior acoustic enhancement or through-transmission.

within the cyst. As more sound traverses the cyst, more echoes are received from the area behind the cyst, a feature known as *through-transmission* or *acoustic enhancement* (Fig. 2-1). Conversely, with a calcified structure, sound passing through it is minimal and creates a band of reduced echoes beyond it, known as *acoustic shadowing* (Fig. 2-2) (Armstrong, 2001).

Examination Techniques

Guidelines for sonographic examination of the female pelvis have been established by The American Institute of Ultrasound in Medicine (2009). These were developed to serve as standards of quality assurance for patient care and to provide assistance to practitioners performing sonography. Guidelines describe equipment and documentation and may be accessed at http://www.aium.org/publications/guidelines/pelvis.pdf.

All probes should be cleaned after each examination, and vaginal probes should be covered by a protective condom or condom-like sheath before insertion. A female staff member should

always chaperone transvaginal sonography (TVS). Guidelines describe the examination to be performed for each organ and anatomic region in the female pelvis. For instance, in evaluating the uterus, the following should be documented: uterine size, shape, and orientation and description of the endometrium, myometrium, and cervix. A permanent record of the examination and its interpretation should be appropriately labeled and placed in the medical record. A copy is also kept by the facility performing the study.

Transabdominal Sonography

A variety of examination techniques can be used for the sonographic study of the female pelvis. Transabdominal evaluation, using a curved-array 3- to 5-MHz transducer, is still considered the first approach because it provides global identification of all pelvic organs and their spatial relationships to one another (American Institute of Ultrasound in Medicine, 2009). In a non-pregnant patient, a full bladder is usually necessary for adequate visualization, as it pushes the uterus upwards from behind the pubic symphysis and displaces small bowel from the field of view. Moreover, the bladder acts as an *acoustic window*, to improve transmission of ultrasound waves. In patients with large lesions or masses located superior to the bladder dome, the panoramic capabilities provided by transabdominal sonography allow for a more complete disease evaluation (Fleischer, 1997a). Still, assessment of the endometrial cavity is problematic with a transabdominal approach, often necessitating the transvaginal technique.

Transvaginal Sonography

This modality uses higher-frequency (5- to 10-MHz) transducers, which increase sensitivity and spatial image resolution. The probe is positioned in the vaginal fornices, thus the transducer is closer to the region of interest, and there is less beam attenuation in superficial soft tissues. In contrast to transabdominal imaging, the bladder is emptied prior to performing a transvaginal study.

Transrectal and Transperineal Techniques

Transrectal probes or conventional transducers placed over the perineal region are much less commonly employed. They are used for selected indications such as those discussed later in the section on pelvic floor imaging (p. 38).

Harmonic Imaging

This recent modification of sonography is designed to improve tissue visualization and quality by using several frequencies at once from the transmitted ultrasound beam instead of just a single frequency (Armstrong, 2001). Newer probes and post-processing features improve image resolution, particularly at surface interfaces. Also, artifacts that arise from superficial structures such as adipose are reduced.

Focused Ultrasound Therapy

Ultrasound energy during conventional imaging propagates harmlessly through tissue with little energy being absorbed. This energy is deposited as heat but dissipates by the cooling effects of perfusion and conduction. No harmful effects have been recorded at the intensities used for diagnostic purposes in more than 50 years (American Institute of Ultrasound in Medicine, 1991).

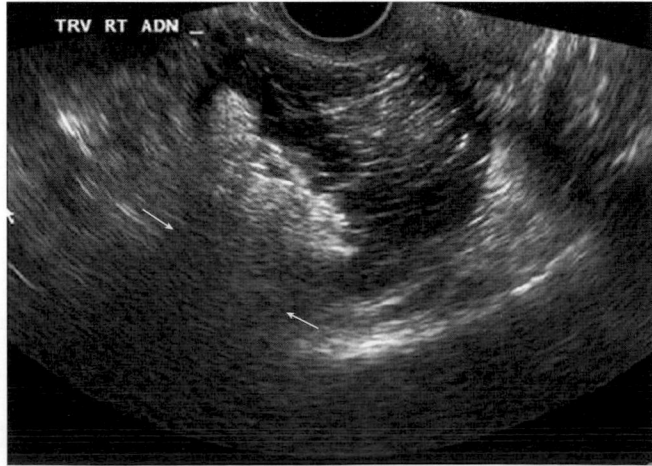

FIGURE 2-2 Transvaginal sonogram of an ovarian teratoma demonstrating posterior acoustic shadowing (*arrows*).

However, if the ultrasound beam carries a high level of energy and is brought to a tight focus, energy carried by the beam is rapidly converted into heat (ter Haar, 1999). When target spot temperatures rise above 55°C, proteins are denatured, cells die, and coagulative necrosis is created (Lele, 1977). In contrast, surrounding tissues are warmed, but not to lethal temperatures.

Doppler Technology

This ultrasound technique can be performed with either transabdominal or transvaginal sonography to determine blood flow through pelvic organs, based on the red blood cell velocity within vessels, especially arteries. The earliest attempt at this technique captured and characterized the spectral waveform of certain vessels identified on a real-time image. Of arterial Doppler spectral waveform parameters, the resistance index and pulsatility index are commonly calculated. These quantitative indices estimate the impedance to red blood cell velocity within the artery and to the organ of interest by expressing the differences between the peak systolic and end-diastolic velocities.

The next application was color Doppler mapping, in which the color-coded pulsed Doppler velocity information is superimposed on the real-time gray-scale image. The color is scaled, such that the brightness of the color is proportional to the velocity of flow. Additionally, color Doppler also provides information regarding the direction of blood flow, and color is assigned to flow direction. Flow approaching the transducer is customarily displayed in red, and flow away from it is shown in blue. Applications of color Doppler in gynecology include evaluation of ovarian masses for torsion or malignancy, improved detection of extrauterine vascularity associated with ectopic pregnancy, and assessment of uterine perfusion in patients with leiomyomas and endometrial disorders.

Power Doppler imaging is a different type of mapping of red blood cell motion. It detects the energy of Doppler signals generated from moving red blood cells by using signal-to-noise characteristics of the vessels compared with surrounding tissues. This modality gives no information regarding blood flow direction, and therefore, data are displayed as a single color, usually yellow. However, power Doppler is more sensitive to low flow velocities, such as in veins and small arteries. The technique may be used to gather additional information regarding disorders of the endometrium.

Saline Infusion Sonography

Also called sonohysterography, saline infusion sonography (SIS) was developed to obtain a more detailed view of the endometrial cavity (Hill, 1997). After voiding, a woman undergoes a comprehensive transvaginal sonographic evaluation. A vaginal speculum is then inserted, the vagina and cervix are swabbed with an antiseptic solution, and a catheter primed with sterile saline is advanced into the cervical canal and past the internal os. We do not routinely use a tenaculum for this. Touching the uterine fundus when advancing the catheter should be avoided as this can induce pain or vasovagal response. It may also shear away endometrium, causing false-positive results. The speculum is carefully removed to avoid dislodging the catheter, the transvaginal probe is reinserted, and sterile saline is injected through the catheter at a rate based

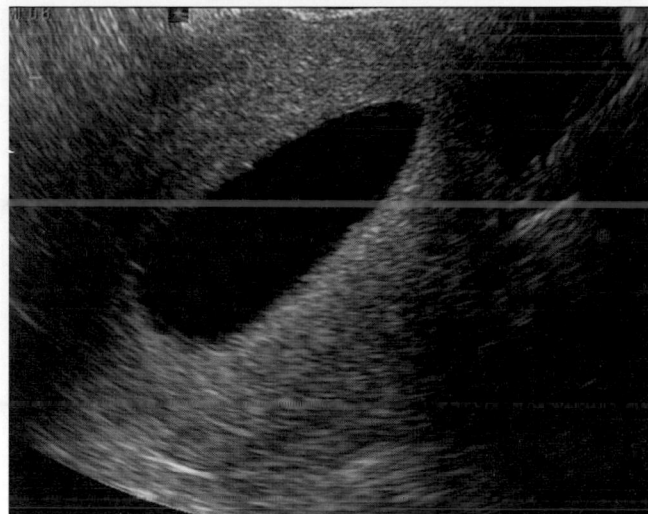

FIGURE 2-3 Saline infusion sonography of a normal endometrial cavity.

on the patient's tolerance. Usually not more than 20 to 40 mL is required to distend the endometrial lumen (Fig. 2-3). During this time, the cavity is observed with TVS. The sonographer scans in the longitudinal plane, imaging from one cornu to the other, and in the transverse plane from the top of the fundus to the cervix. Irregularities of the endometrial surface are well delineated by the anechoic contrast of the saline. At the procedure's conclusion, the catheter is withdrawn under sonographic visualization so that the uterine isthmus and endocervical canal may be evaluated. After removal of the catheter but prior to removal of the transvaginal probe, the upper vagina and vaginal fornices may be evaluated. This technique is referred to as sonovaginography. On average, the entire procedure lasts 5 to 10 minutes.

Many different catheter systems are available, including rigid systems and flexible catheters with and without attached balloons. We use a 7F HSG balloon catheter set (Cooper Surgical), which, by tamponade of the internal cervical os, prevents backflow of the distending medium and provides stable filling and adequate distension. We have found it easy to place and well tolerated (Fig. 2-4). Several distending solutions have been described, including saline, lactated Ringer solution, and 1.5-percent glycine. Sterile saline is inexpensive and provides optimal imaging. Alternatively, the results of two pilot studies investigating the feasibility of a gel-like substance are very promising. The first study used a hydroxyethyl glycerin gel instead of sterile saline for uterine cavity distension (Exalto, 2004). Preliminary results showed excellent distension, stable filling, and no backflow problems. Another study group used a specially designed phase-shifting medium that had a gel-like consistency upon instillation. Its delayed phase shifting properties lead to liquefaction and expulsion once the ultrasound procedure is completed (de Ziegler, 2009). Although technically similar to SIS, as this procedure does not use saline to distend the endometrial cavity, it has been termed "contrast ultrasound." Designed to be markedly simpler than regular SIS, contrast ultrasound does not require a persistent instrument in the uterus or additional infusion during the ultrasound examination. Yet, it provides similar contrast enhancement and images of the uterine cavity comparable with those achieved with SIS. Further study of phase-shifting products is underway.

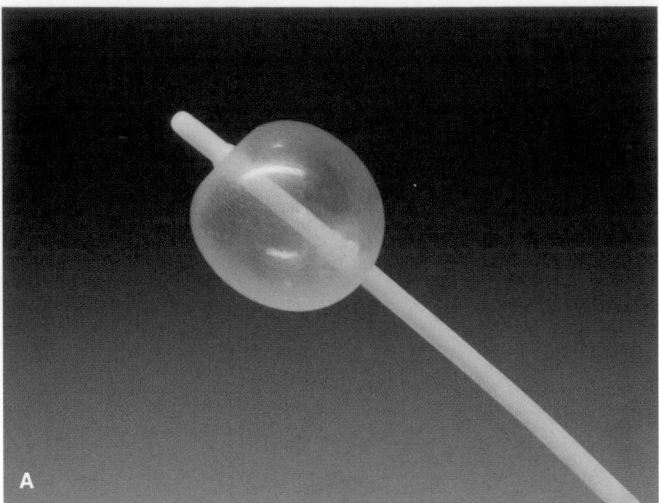

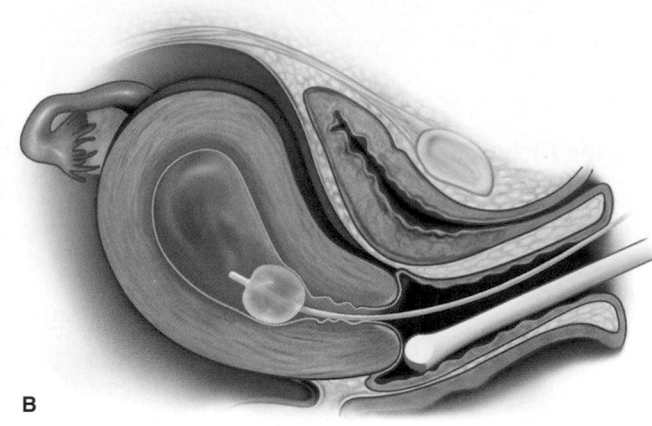

FIGURE 2-4 A. Saline infusion sonography catheter. **B.** Saline infusion sonography.

In the premenopausal woman, SIS is best performed within the first 10 days of the menstrual cycle, and optimally on cycle days 4, 5, or 6 when the lining is thinnest. This timing is recommended to avoid the misinterpretation of menstrual blood clots as intrauterine pathology or conversely, to miss pathology obscured by endometrial growth (Hill, 1997). In addition, such timing should usually preclude pregnancy. For the postmenopausal woman, timing of the procedure is not cycle dependent.

Complications of SIS are minimal, and the risk of infection is less than 1 percent (Bonnamy, 2002). Most recommend prophylactic antibiotics for women with a history of pelvic inflammatory disease and in those who require bacterial endocarditis prophylaxis. Although not evidence based, based on experience in our patient population, we routinely give a single dose of doxycycline, 200 mg orally, following SIS to women with immunocompromise, such as those with diabetes, cancer, or human immunodeficiency virus. We also choose to provide prophylaxis to our infertile patients because of the risk for tubal damage should pelvic infection develop. Pain is usually minimal. It has been our experience that women who have undergone tubal ligation have more discomfort, likely because fluid cannot efflux through the fallopian tubes. A nonsteroidal antiinflammatory drug (NSAID) given 30 minutes prior to the procedure will typically minimize any potential discomfort. Contraindications to SIS include hematometra, pregnancy, active pelvic infection, or obstruction such as with an atrophic or stenotic cervix or vagina. In postmenopausal women with cervical stenosis, we have found the following techniques to be helpful: misoprostol 200 μg orally the evening before and the morning of the procedure; a paracervical block with 1-percent lidocaine without epinephrine; a tenaculum for traction on the cervix; and a sonography-guided sequential cervical dilation with lacrimal duct dilators. Pisal and colleagues (2005) proposed the use of a 20-gauge spinal needle, inserted into the uterine cavity under sonographic guidance, to overcome severe cervical stenosis.

■ Normal Sonographic Findings
Reproductive Tract Organs

In the reproductive years, a normal uterus measures approximately 7.5 × 5.0 × 2.5 cm, but is smaller in the prepubertal,

postmenopausal, or hypoestrogenized woman. Normal uterine stroma returns low-level, uniform echoes. The position of the endometrial and endocervical canals is indicated by linear echogenic stripes, which represent the interfaces between mucus and mucosa (Fig. 2-5). The cervix is best visualized transvaginally with the tip of the probe placed 2 to 3 cm from it. The endocervical canal is a continuation of the endometrial cavity and appears as a thin echogenic line (Fig. 2-6). The vagina is seen as a hypoechoic tubular structure with an echogenic lumen that curves inferiorly over the muscular perineal body at the introitus. The ovaries are ellipsoid. They normally lie in the ovarian fossa with their long axes parallel to the internal iliac vessels and the ureters, which lie posteriorly (Fig. 2-7). Ovarian volume ranges from 4 to 10 cc depending on hormonal status (Cohen, 1990). This volume is calculated using the formula for the volume of an ellipse: $(\pi/6) \times (A \times B \times C)$. In this formula, A, B, and C are the ovarian diameters in centimeters, measured in the three different planes. Ovarian follicles appear as spherical anechoic structures within the ovary and may reach a normal size of 2.5 cm. Normal fallopian tubes are not visible. A small

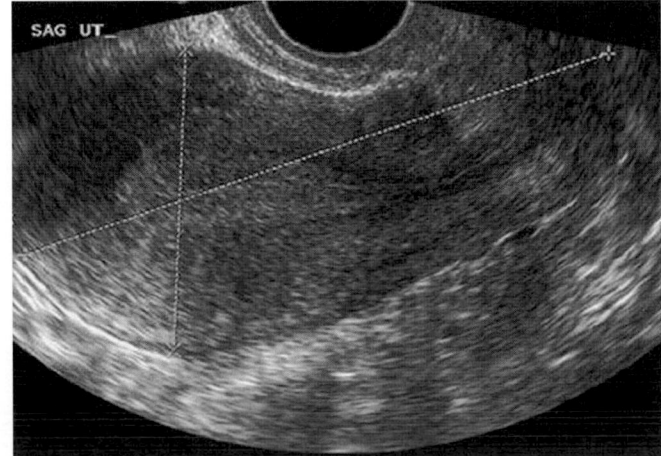

FIGURE 2-5 Transvaginal sonogram in the sagittal plane of an anteverted uterine corpus. Calipers demonstrate measurements of the uterine length (+) and the anterior-posterior dimension (×).

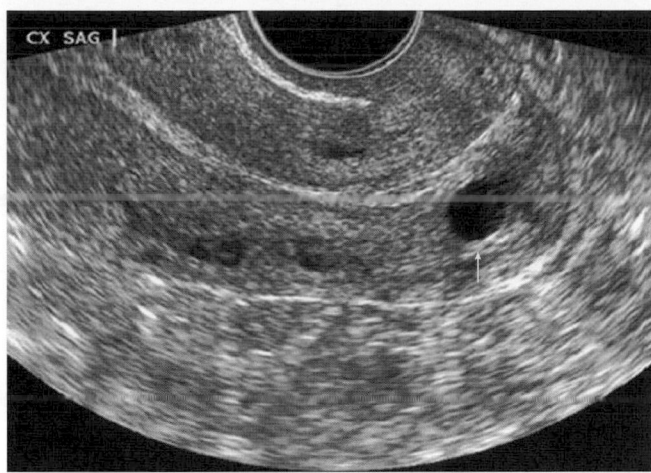

FIGURE 2-6 Transvaginal sonogram in the sagittal plane of a uterine cervix. Arrow points to an endocervical cyst seen posterior to the thin, echogenic endocervical canal.

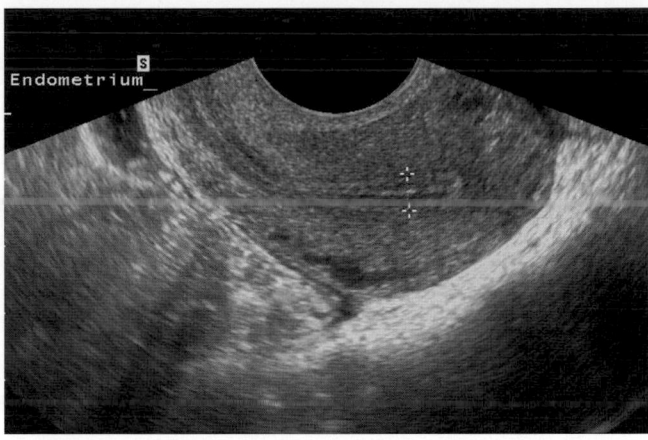

FIGURE 2-8 Transvaginal sonogram in the sagittal plane of a characteristic trilaminar proliferative endometrium. Calipers demonstrate proper measurement of the "double-layer" thickness made of the alternating hyper-hypo-hyperechogenic lines.

amount of fluid in the posterior cul-de-sac is a normal finding and is often seen with ovulation.

Endometrium

Functionally, the endometrium has two main layers: the *stratum basale*, which comprises the densely cellular supporting stroma and varies little with the phase of the menstrual cycle, and the *stratum functionale*, which proliferates during each cycle and partially sloughes at menses. These layers cover the entire cavity.

Sonographic appearances of the endometrium during the menstrual cycle correlate with the phasic changes in its histologic anatomy. During the follicular phase, when the endometrium is under influence of estrogen from ovarian folliculogenesis, the stratum basale appears echogenic due to spectral reflections from the mucus-laden glands. In contrast, the stratum functionale is relatively hypoechoic because of the orderly arrangement of glands that lack secretions. The central opposing surfaces of these two endometrial layers manifest as

a highly reflective, thin midline strip, and the three echogenic lines give the characteristic trilaminar appearance of the proliferative endometrium (Fig. 2-8). Endometrial thickness is measured from the echogenic interface of the anterior basalis layer to the echogenic interface of the posterior basalis layer, thus representing a "double thickness." The hypoechoic halo outside of and adjacent to the endometrium should not be included in the measurement as this is actually the inner compact layer of myometrium. Sonographically, the endometrium should be measured from a sagittal or long-axis image of the uterus in the plane where the central endometrial echo is seen contiguous with the endocervical canal and distinct from the myometrium. Endometrial thickness correlates approximately with the day of the cycle up to day 7 or 8 (Richenberg, 2000).

With ovulation and progesterone production from the corpus luteum during the secretory phase, glandular enlargement and appearance of secretory vacuoles begins. These changes are seen sonographically (Fig. 2-9). During this phase, the endometrium achieves its maximum thickness as the stroma becomes more vascular and edematous.

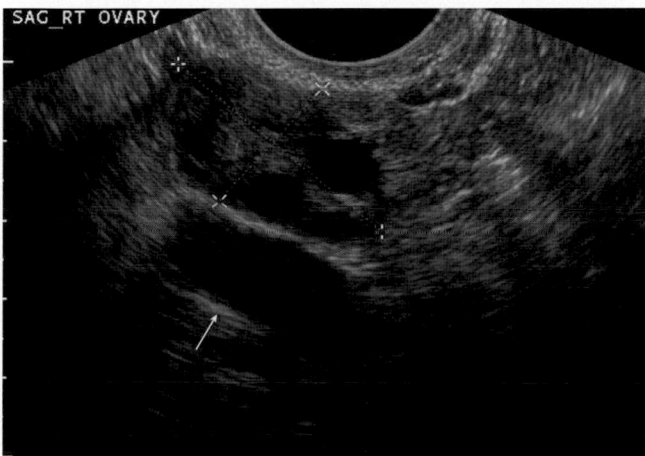

FIGURE 2-7 Transvaginal sonogram in the sagittal plane of a left ovary in a premenopausal woman. The ovary normally lies in the ovarian fossa, anterior to the internal iliac vessels, which are above the arrow.

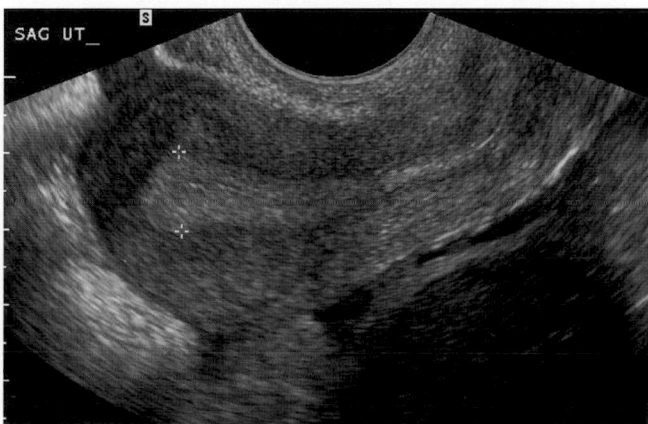

FIGURE 2-9 Transvaginal sonogram in the sagittal plane of a secretory endometrium. The endometrium, which is marked by calipers, has become uniformly echogenic.

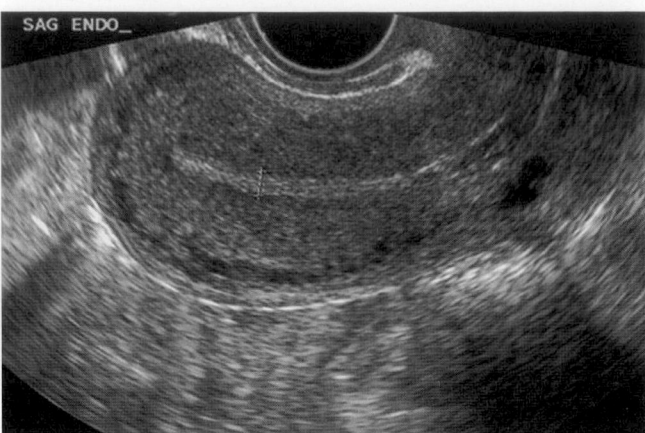

FIGURE 2-10 Transvaginal sonogram in the sagittal plane of a menstrual-phase endometrium, which is marked by calipers.

With menstruation, the endometrium appears as a slightly irregular echogenic interface from sloughed tissue and blood. The thinnest measurements of endometrium are found at conclusion of menses (Fig. 2-10).

With cessation of estrogen stimulation beginning at menopause, the endometrium atrophies, and cyclic sloughing ceases. The postmenopausal endometrium appears thin and uniform (Fig. 2-11).

Pelvic Floor

With the advent of urogynecology as a specialty, sonography is widely used to evaluate pelvic floor anatomy and function. To investigate urethral anatomy, various two-dimensional (2-D) techniques, including transvaginal, transrectal, transperineal, and intraurethral sonography, have been used.

To assess anal sphincter morphology after childbirth, transrectal sonography was the first technique used. This method requires special equipment as well as distension of the anal canal. The technique is of limited value during the immediate postpartum period, and it only provides information regarding

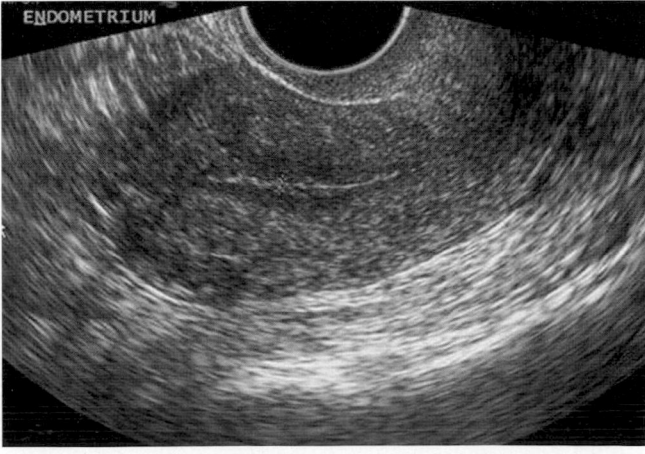

FIGURE 2-11 Transvaginal sonogram in the sagittal plane of an atrophic postmenopausal endometrium.

anal sphincter morphology. Thus, without levator ani muscle assessment, it cannot be used to completely evaluate the posterior compartment (Wisser, 2001). Alternatively, anorectal morphology and the pelvic floor can be assessed with vaginal sonography using a rotating endorectal probe or standard transvaginal probe (Sandridge, 1995; Sultan, 1994). These methods are described further in Chapter 25 (p. 666).

To evaluate the pelvic floor, perineal sonography has been used more recently. The technique requires filling the bladder with approximately 300 mL of saline. With the woman either supine or erect, a 5-MHz curved-array transducer is placed in sagittal orientation to the perineum. This allows real-time imaging of the symphysis pubis, urethra, bladder neck, and bladder. Measurements have been standardized by Schaer and colleagues (1995).

Three-dimensional ultrasound is now increasingly being used to examine pelvic floor anatomy (Coyne, 2008). It has been proposed for imaging paravaginal support, prolapse, and implants used for pelvic floor reconstruction and for antiincontinence surgery. Moreover, this modality allows postprocessing reconstruction of the volume in a coronal plane. This improves visualization of the urethra and the periurethral tissue, which are inaccessible with 2-D ultrasound techniques (Dietz, 2004). Although earlier studies used a transrectal approach to acquire a 3-D volume, technical developments enable abdominal transducers to be used for 3-D translabialtransperineal imaging, which is more acceptable to patients (Dietz, 2007; Huang, 2007; Lee, 2007). Reconstructed tomographic ultrasound imaging, possible with 3-D ultrasound, has been found to be particularly useful in quantifying the degree of levator ani defects in women presenting with symptoms of pelvic floor dysfunction (Dietz, 2007).

■ Clinical Applications

Transvaginal sonography is preferred for evaluation of the normal uterus and adnexa and for diagnosis of gynecologic diseases. These include diagnosis and management of ectopic pregnancy, support for infertility practices, and early detection of ovarian and endometrial cancer.

Transvaginal sonography has few limitations. The only two absolute contraindications are imperforate hymen and patient refusal. A relative contraindication is the patient with a virginal or strictured introitus. These women, however, can usually undergo comfortable examination with proper counseling.

Uterus

Leiomyomas. When visualized with sonography, uterine leiomyomas usually appear as solid, discrete, well-defined masses with a thin hypoechoic periphery (Fig. 2-12). Although most often hypoechogenic in relation to the myometrium, they may also appear hyper- or isoechogenic, especially if degeneration has occurred within the tumor (Lyons, 2000). Shadowing at their lateral borders is common.

For preoperative assessment of women who undergo uterine artery embolization (UAE) for symptomatic leiomyomas, sonography is preferred by most for initial imaging. In these women, 3-D color Doppler sonography can accurately depict tumor vascularity, and in some cases, collateral flow is seen that is not detected by

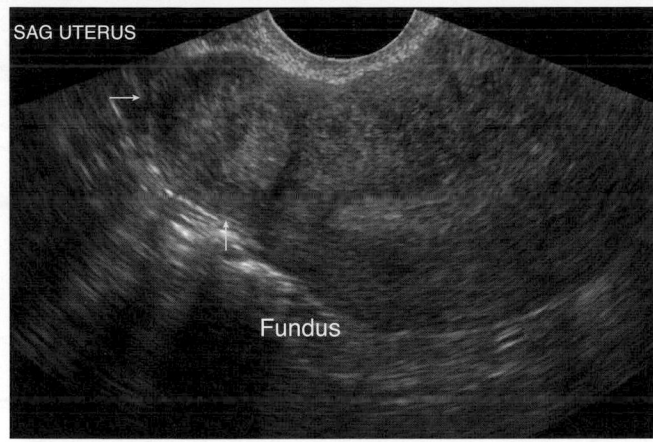

FIGURE 2-12 Transvaginal sonogram of a fundal subserosal leiomyoma (*arrows*).

uterine arteriography (Muniz, 2002). Doppler flow measurements are also useful to predict UAE outcomes, which include shrinkage of the uterus and leiomyomas or embolization failure (McLucas, 2002). In most cases, MR imaging is also performed prior to UAE to add information. Following embolization or gonadotropin-releasing hormone (GnRH) agonist therapy, sonography can also be used to document tumor volume decreases (Fleischer, 2000).

Adenomyosis. Sonographic evaluation of adenomyosis has now become easier and more accurate with the advent of TVS, higher-resolution techniques, and color Doppler capability (Andreotti, 2005). An affected uterus is globular but regular in shape, and the myometrium is asymmetrically thickened with heterogeneous areas (Fig. 2-13). Although a myometrial mass may be present, termed an adenomyoma, it is usually ill defined and does not cause uterine contour changes. Anechoic areas consistent with myometrial cysts are often seen and correspond to dilated endometrial glands (Lyons, 2002). Hypoechoic linear striations are also seen throughout the smooth muscle (Kepkep, 2007). The endometrial-myometrial junction is poorly defined due to heterotopic endometrial tissue extending from the stratum basale.

When evaluated by Doppler sonography, adenomyotic lesions are vascularized, and vessels appear less well-organized than those in the normal myometrium (Atri, 2000; Reinhold, 1999). A recent study by Exacoustos and associates (2011) demonstrated that the coronal view of the uterus obtained by 3-D transvaginal sonography allowed for better visualization and assessment of the myometrial junctional zone, further improving the diagnostic accuracy of sonography for adenomyosis. When specific criteria are used, the ultrasound sensitivity has been reported to approximate 85 percent, and specificity ranges from 50 to 96 percent. Overall accuracy is 68 to 86 percent, which is equivalent to MR imaging (Brosens, 1995; Fedele, 1992; Mark, 1987; Reinhold, 1995; Togashi, 1988, 1989). Magnetic resonance imaging may be helpful in cases that are indeterminate with TVS (p. 55).

Endometrial Abnormalities. Transvaginal sonography is used to accurately evaluate endometrial thickness and appearance, and together with SIS, it plays an important role in managing endometrial disorders. It may be employed to aid in: (1) determining which women should undergo endometrial biopsy, (2) analyzing the endometrium to detect polyps or submucosal leiomyomas, and (3) local assessment of myometrial invasion from endometrial cancer (Fleischer, 1997b).

Transvaginal Sonography. The clinical usefulness of sonography in women with postmenopausal bleeding relies on its ability to accurately measure endometrial thickness (Chap. 8, p. 227). The thickest point along the endometrium from the anterior to posterior endometrial-myometrial junction is measured. In postmenopausal women with endometrial measurements of 4 mm or less, sonographic-pathologic studies have demonstrated that bleeding can be attributed to endometrial atrophy (Ferrazzi, 1996; Goldstein, 1990; Granberg, 1991; Gull, 2000, 2003; Karlsson, 1995). Endometrial hyperplasia, polyps, and carcinoma typically have thicker endometrial measurements.

A number of studies have evaluated the ability of sonography to identify not only thickness but also normal echostructural

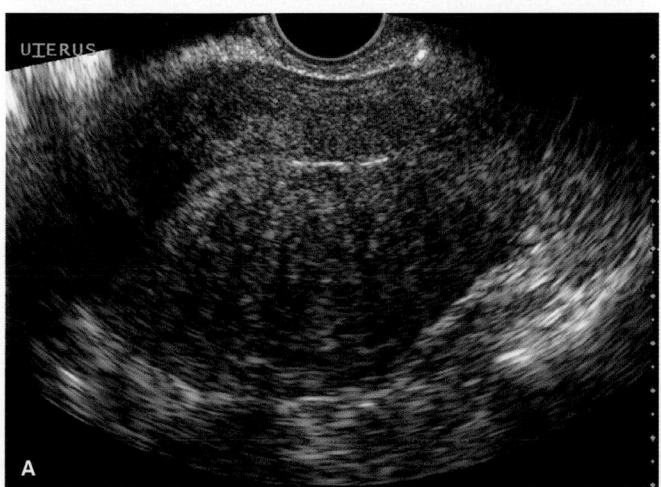

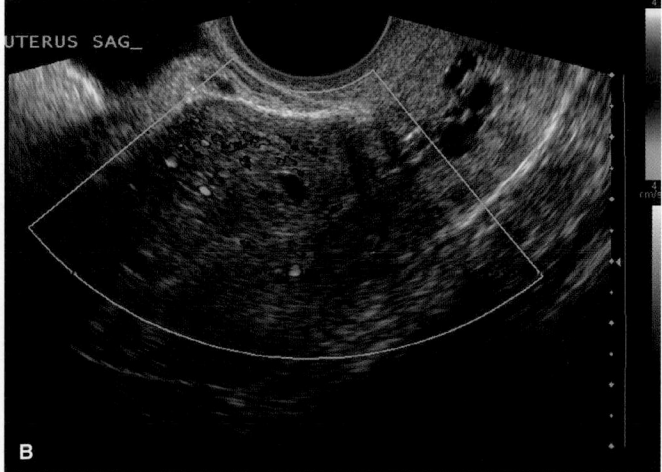

FIGURE 2-13 Adenomyosis. **A.** Transvaginal sonogram in the sagittal plane of a uterus that is globular. The posterior myometrium is asymmetrically thickened, heterogeneous, and exhibits hypoechoic linear striations. **B.** Transvaginal color Doppler evaluation of another case of adenomyosis demonstrates a well-vascularized anterior myometrium and avascular anechoic areas consistent with myometrial cysts. These cysts correspond to dilated endometrial glands.

changes and pathology in the postmenopausal endometrium. Although cystic endometrial changes suggest polyps, homogeneously thickened endometrium suggests hyperplasia, and a heterogeneous structural pattern is suspicious for malignancy, these sonographic findings show much overlap and cannot be used alone (Atri, 1994; Doubilet, 2000; Hulka, 1994; Levine, 1995). Additionally, quantitative color Doppler studies of endometrial vasculature are not informative, because there are no significant differences between resistance and pulsatility indices in benign versus malignant causes of endometrial thickening (Bourne, 1995; Sheth, 1993).

On the other hand, power Doppler assessment of the thickened endometrium appears more promising. Of the few studies that have looked at the qualitative role of transvaginal power Doppler sonography to discriminate between benign and malignant endometrial conditions in women presenting with postmenopausal bleeding and thickened endometrium, investigators found that irregular, branching vessel patterns are good predictors of malignancy (Alcazar, 2003a; Epstein, 2006; Opolskiene, 2007). Some have carried this concept further and evaluated whether quantitative power Doppler ultrasound examination of the endometrium can correctly diagnose endometrial malignancy (Epstein, 2002; Merce, 2007). Indices such as the vascularity index—defined as the vascularized area divided by the endometrial area—can contribute to a correct diagnosis of malignancy in the setting of a thickened endometrium. Regression models, which include power Doppler results to estimate the risk of endometrial cancer, are under development (De Smet, 2006; Mandic, 2006).

Once diagnosed, determining the local extent of endometrial carcinoma is possible using TVS (Ozdemir, 2009; Savelli, 2008). Direct myometrial extension can be assessed, however, false-positive findings may be caused by compression and thinning of the myometrium from large benign lesions. Color Doppler sonography of the myometrial vessels may help to identify invasive endometrial carcinoma. Although useful in evaluating depth of myometrial invasion, sonography is not used to stage endometrial cancer because of its limited ability to evaluate disease beyond the corpus.

Saline Infusion Sonography. In addition to conventional TVS, saline infusion sonography (SIS) has also been used to evaluate the endometrium in various clinical situations (Lindheim, 2003a). These, among others, include abnormal uterine bleeding, clarification of endometrial thickening or other endometrial lesions, visualization of the central endometrial echo when poorly imaged because of uterine position or pathology, evaluation during tamoxifen therapy, and some infertility investigations.

Defining Endometrial Lesions. In further defining endometrial thickening, SIS is the best nonoperative procedure for diagnosing polyps. These lesions are focal and contrast with the diffuse endometrial thickening seen with endometrial hyperplasia. Moreover, polyps and submucosal leiomyomas can often be differentiated based on two findings (Jorizzo, 2001). The first is a difference in echotexture—the leiomyoma is hypoechoic, similar to the myometrium, whereas the polyp is hyperechogenic (Fig. 2-14). Secondly, detection of a strip of endometrium, which overlies the leiomyoma and separates it from the endometrial lumen, differentiates these two (Jorizzo, 2001).

Obviously, SIS cannot be used to differentiate between benign lesions and malignancies with absolute certainty, and any woman with an atypical-appearing or suspicious endoluminal mass requires histologic evaluation to exclude malignancy (Dubinsky, 1999; Fleischer, 1997c; Jorizzo, 1999, 2001). However, SIS can be used to guide directed biopsy of intrauterine pathology (Fig. 2-15) (Dubinsky, 2000; Lindheim, 2003b; Moschos, 2009; Wei, 2006). Limitations primarily involve technical feasibility, such as cervical stenosis or poor visualization due to saline leakage with biopsy instrument insertion. At our institution, saline infusion sonography endometrial sampling (SISES) was prospectively compared with traditional blind endometrial biopsy (EMB) in the diagnosis of benign and malignant endometrial disease in peri- and postmenopausal women with abnormal uterine bleeding. Saline infusion sonography endometrial sampling was superior to EMB in diagnosing endometrial pathology. Specifically, EMB underestimated the incidence of pathology, especially when focal lesions and malignancy were present.

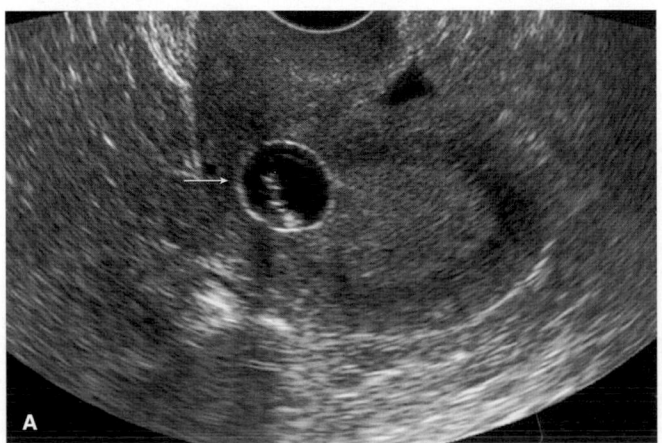
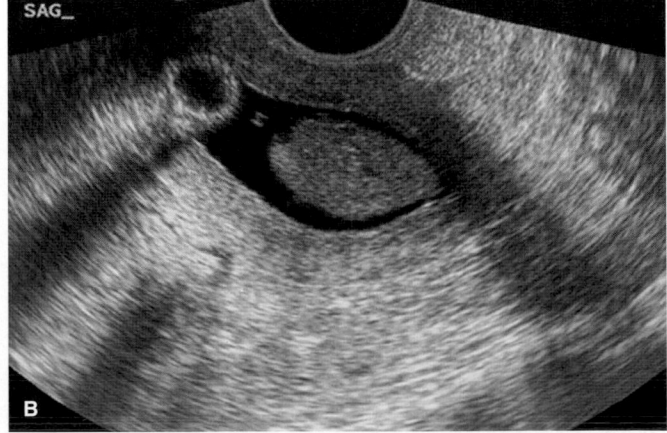

FIGURE 2-14 Endometrial polyp. **A.** Transvaginal sonogram of the endometrium after placement of the saline infusion sonography (SIS) balloon catheter (*arrow*). Note the homogenous-appearing thickened endometrium. **B.** Transvaginal SIS in the same case reveals a hyperechogenic polyp within the endometrial cavity.

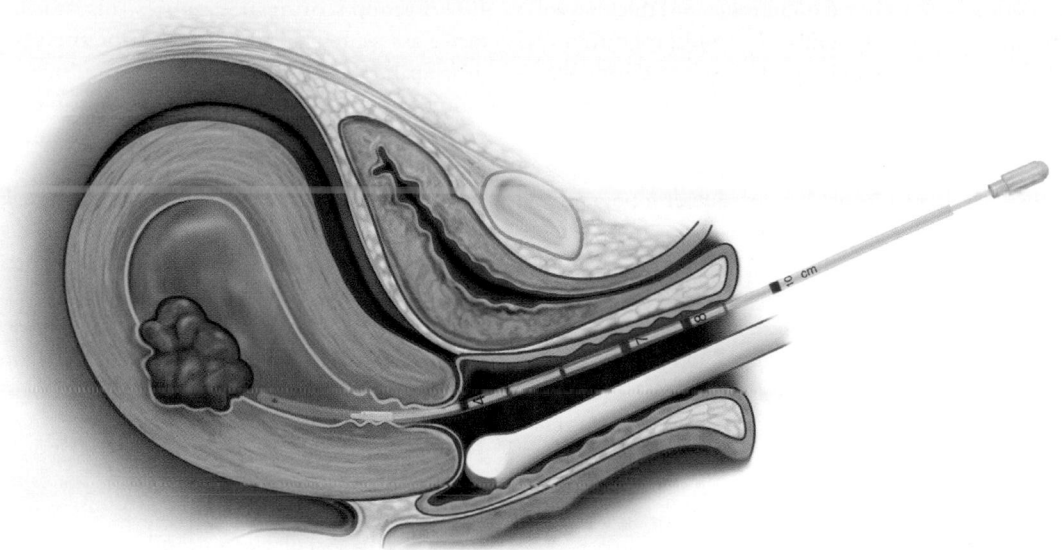

FIGURE 2-15 Saline infusion sonography endometrial sampling (SISES). The cavity is initially distended with saline. Next, an endometrial Pipelle is used to biopsy the endometrium under direct sonographic guidance.

Saline infusion sonography is more accurate than either TVS or hysteroscopy to identify size, location, and depth of myometrial involvement of submucosal leiomyomas (Cicinelli, 1995; Farquhar, 2003; Salim, 2005). This information is useful to predict outcomes and complications of hysteroscopic resection (Bradley, 2000; Emanuel, 1995; Salim, 2005).

Monitoring Tamoxifen Therapy. In women taking tamoxifen, SIS is typically more informative than TVS. Saline infusion sonography helps to delineate hyperplastic conditions in those women with bleeding when taking tamoxifen. Of note, SIS appears to add little value in the asymptomatic woman, and routine sonographic surveillance of asymptomatic women using tamoxifen is not recommended (Bertelli, 2000; Hann, 2001).

Other Uses. Other diagnostic and therapeutic applications of SIS have been described. It is used to locate a "lost" intrauterine device (IUD) and determine whether it is embedded in the myometrium (Bussey, 1996). It has been used to diagnose postabortal remnants, including placenta accreta, and to assess previous cesarean delivery scars in the prediction of future abnormal placentation and in the evaluation of abnormal uterine bleeding (Monteagudo, 2001; Tal, 1997). Coccia and colleagues (2001) used pressure lavage under ultrasound guidance (PLUG) to treat intrauterine adhesions in seven women. This technique uses continuous accumulation of saline for the mechanical disruption of synechiae.

Ovary

Lesion Characterization. Sonography is commonly the initial and often the only imaging procedure performed in the evaluation of pelvic and ovarian masses. Of these, simple cysts are one of the most common, and classic sonographic findings include smooth and regular margins, lack of internal echoes, and increased through-transmission or acoustic enhancement (see Fig. 2-1). Blood-filled cysts, such as hemorrhagic cysts

and endometriomas, have variable appearances because of clot, lysis, and retraction. Internal echoes, septa, mural nodules, solid components, fluid-debris levels, and retracting clot can be seen. Some blood-filled cysts at first may appear solid, with an internal pattern of many small low-level echoes. However, consistent with a cyst, increased through-transmission is present. The sonographic characteristic that has been proven most important for the diagnosis of a hemorrhagic cyst versus an endometrioma is the change over time of the internal structure of the cyst (Fig. 9-17, p. 266) (Derchi, 2001).

With ovarian neoplasms, some sonographic findings may be indicative. For example, a benign serous cystadenoma appears as a cystic mass containing clear fluid with thin internal septations. Mural nodules are infrequent. Mucinous cystadenomas usually are also cystic, and compared with their serous counterparts, they tend to have multiple internal septations, more echogenic fluid, and fluid-debris levels within the cyst. There is no clear boundary between the sonographic appearance of a cystadenoma and a cystadenocarcinoma. However, as a general rule, the greater the amount of solid tissue within the mass, the higher the probability of malignancy. Criteria suggesting cancer are presence of thick septations, multiple papillary projections, solid portions within the mass, and ascites (Table 9-4, p. 264).

Mature cystic teratomas (dermoid cysts) have a classic sonographic appearance (see Fig. 2-2). As described in Chapter 9 (p. 267), these include a markedly hyperechogenic mass with a structure similar to that of surrounding fatty tissue; cystic areas with round echogenic mural nodules; and calcifications, tufts of hair, and fat-fluid levels. These findings reflect the unique tissue contrasts found in these benign tumors.

Malignant Characteristics. Sonography is the best diagnostic technique for preoperative determination of the malignant potential of an ovarian mass (Twickler, 2010). To this end, morphologic scoring systems based on number and thickness of septa, presence and number of papillations, and proportion of solid tissue within the mass have been proposed to standardize the interpretation of findings (DePriest, 1993; Sassone, 1991). When size, morphology, and structure of adnexal masses are combined with color Doppler and spectral analysis of flow signals, the specificity and positive predictive value of sonographic diagnosis is increased (Buy, 1996; Fleischer, 1993; Jain, 1994; Twickler, 1999; Valentin, 1997). In a metaanalysis of 46 studies with 5159 patients, Kinkel and colleagues (2000) reported significantly higher accuracy for combined sonographic techniques compared with that of each individual technique alone. More recently, the International Ovarian Tumor Analysis (IOTA) Group, a collaborative effort that includes nine centers from five European countries, began a prospective, multicenter study from which they developed the most accurate mathematic model to date to calculate the risk of malignancy in an adnexal mass based on sonographic features (Timmerman, 2005).

Neovascularity secondary to angiogenesis within a malignant neoplasm produces a significant increase in color Doppler flow signals. Whereas most benign tumors appear poorly vascularized, most malignant lesions appear well vascularized, with flow signals in both peripheral and central regions—including within septations and solid tumor areas. However, a firm diagnosis based on this alone is not possible. Both avascular malignant tumors and benign hypervascular masses have been reported (Brown, 1994; Kawai, 1992).

Neovascularity within malignancies is made up of abnormal vessels that lack smooth muscle and contain multiple arteriovenous shunts. Consequently, low-impedance flow is expected with such masses as shown in Figure 2-16 (Fleischer, 1993; Kurjak, 1992; Weiner, 1992). Other studies, however, demonstrate significant overlap between values from benign and malignant lesions (Jain, 1994; Levine 1994; Stein, 1994).

Of Doppler parameters, the color content of the tumor probably reflects tumor vascularity better than any other. The overall impression of this vascularity reflects both the number and size of vessels and their functional capacity. The

IOTA group scoring system uses this subjective semiquantitative assessment of flow to describe the vascular features of ovarian masses (Ameye, 2009; Timmerman, 2005). A four-point color score is used to describe tumor blood flow only within septa and solid portions of the mass (Timmerman, 2000).

These observations have led many investigators to evaluate the presence, spatial distribution, and prevalence of flow signals within ovarian masses to distinguish between malignant and benign neoplasms. However, because of overlap of vascular parameters between malignant and benign neoplasms, a firm differential diagnosis based on spectral Doppler evaluation alone is not possible (Valentin, 1997).

Torsion. Although ovarian torsion is a clinical diagnosis, color Doppler evaluation may be helpful. Its sonographic appearance as described in Chapter 9 (p. 271) varies according to the degree of vascular compromise and presence of an adnexal mass. Color Doppler of vessels in the infundibulopelvic ligament may aid the specific diagnosis by demonstrating absent arterial and venous flow. Importantly, the presence of flow does not exclude the diagnosis, but rather central venous signals with tuboovarian torsion are thought to indicate ovarian tissue viability (Fleischer, 1995).

Pelvic Inflammatory Disease

Acute Infection. Although pelvic sonography is commonly performed in women with acute salpingitis, large studies evaluating its sensitivity, specificity, or overall usefulness are lacking (Boardman, 1997; Cacciatore, 1992; Patten, 1990). Sonographic findings vary according to the severity of the disease. In early infection, anatomy may appear normal. With progression, early nonspecific findings include free pelvic fluid, endometrial thickening, endometrial cavity distension by fluid or gas, and indistinct borders of the uterus and ovaries. Enlarged ovaries with increased numbers of small cysts—a "polycystic ovary appearance"—has been shown to correlate with pelvic inflammatory disease (PID). Cacciatore and colleagues (1992) found larger than normal ovarian volumes in women with laparoscopically or endometrial-biopsy-proven PID. They also documented decreasing ovarian size with treatment.

Sonographic findings of the fallopian tubes are the most striking and specific with PID (Fig. 2-17). Although normal tubes are rarely seen unless surrounded by ascites, tubal wall inflammation allows visualization with sonography. As the lumen occludes distally, the tube distends and fills with fluid. Various appearances result (Timor-Tritsch, 1998). The tube may become ovoid or pear shaped, filling with fluid that may be anechoic or echogenic. The tubal wall becomes thickened, measuring ≥5 mm, and incomplete septa are common as the tube folds back upon itself. If the distended tube is viewed in cross section it may demonstrate the *cogwheel sign*, due to thickened endosalpingeal folds (Timor-Tritsch, 1998). Typically, the swollen fallopian tubes extend posteriorly into the cul-de-sac, rather than extending superiorly and anterior to the uterus as large ovarian tumors tend to do. Fluid-debris levels are often visualized in the dilated tubes, and rarely, gas-fluid levels or echogenic bubbles of gas can be seen. Color and power

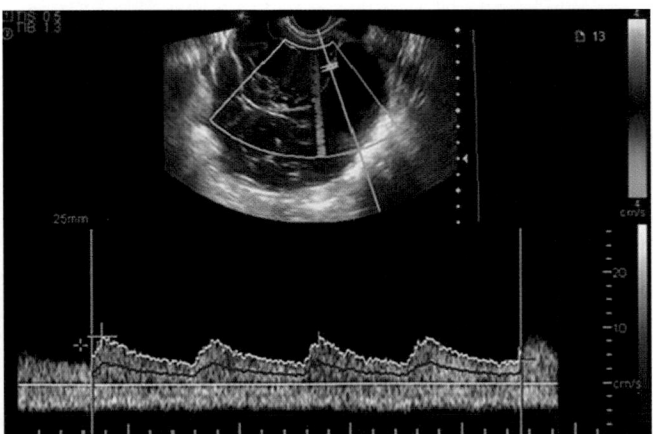

FIGURE 2-16 Complex ovarian mass with irregular cystic areas demonstrating low-impedance [PI = 0.87] flow in a thick septum. This mass was found to be a mucinous cystadenocarcinoma at surgery.

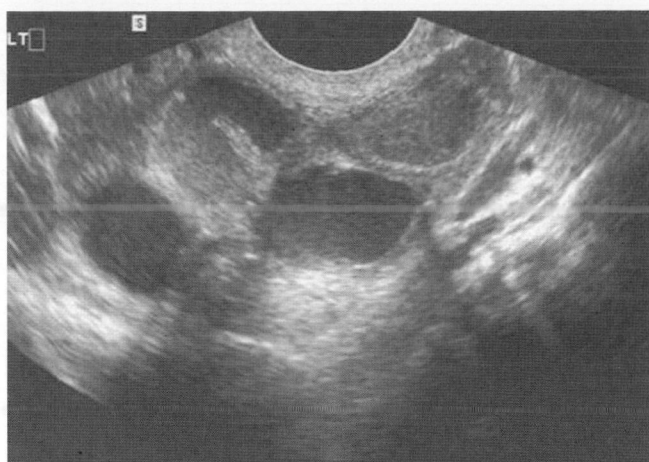

FIGURE 2-17 Transvaginal sonogram in cross-section of an inflamed, dilated tube demonstrating thickened tubal walls, incomplete septa, and echogenic fluid.

Doppler show increased flow from hyperemia in the walls and incomplete septa of the inflamed tubes (Tinkanen, 1993).

Tuboovarian Infection. As the disease progresses, the ovary can become involved. When an ovary adheres to the fallopian tube, but is still visualized, it is called a *tuboovarian complex*. In contrast, a tuboovarian abscess results from a complete breakdown of ovarian and tubal architecture such that the separate structures are no longer identified (Fig. 2-18). If the contralateral side was not affected initially, it may become so. When both tubes are inflamed and occluded, the entire complex typically acquires a U-shape as it fills the cul-de-sac, extending from one adnexal region to the other (Horrow, 2004). The lateral and posterior uterine borders become obscured, and individual tubes and ovaries cannot be distinguished. In women not responding to medical therapy, sonography can be used to guide transvaginal drainage of these lesions (Kaakaji, 2000; Patten, 1990).

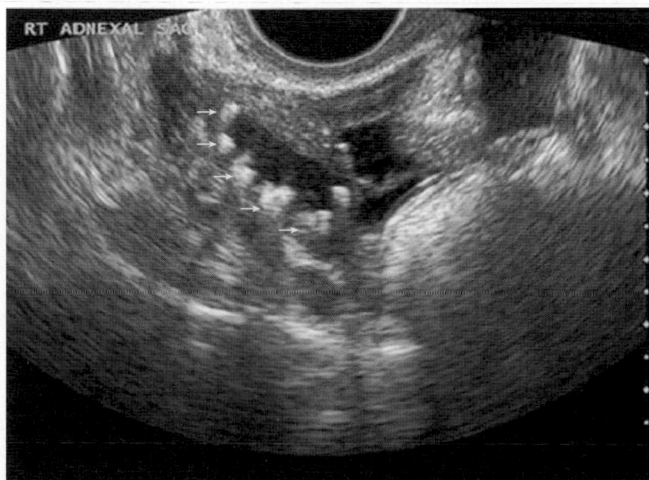

FIGURE 2-18 "Beads on a string" sign. The echogenic mural nodules shown here (*arrows*) within this tuboovarian abscess are thought to represent flattened and fibrotic endosalpingeal folds of the inflamed fallopian tube.

Findings of Prior Infection. Findings of chronic PID include hydrosalpinx. As discussed in Chapter 9 (p. 273), several sonographic findings such as its tubular shape, incomplete septa, and hyperechoic mural nodules can help to distinguish a hydrosalpinx from other cystic adnexal lesions (Fig. 9-26, p. 273). If color flow is detected in a hydrosalpinx, it tends to be less exuberant than flow seen in acute PID. Molander and colleagues (2002) found a higher pulsatility index in patients with a chronic hydrosalpinx (1.5 ± 0.1) than with acute PID (0.84 ± 0.04).

A small number of women with prior PID may have a peritoneal inclusion cyst. These form when ruptured ovarian cyst fluid is trapped around the ovary by adhesions. This diagnosis is suspected if the ovary is surrounded by a loculated fluid collection with thin septations (Horrow, 2002).

Ectopic Pregnancy

Sonography plays a pivotal role in clinical management of suspected ectopic pregnancy. Because a simultaneous uterine and ectopic pregnancy—a heterotopic pregnancy—is rare without assisted reproductive technologies, identification of a uterine pregnancy is the single most important finding for exclusion of an ectopic gestation. Intrauterine pregnancy can be assured if an embryo or if a gestational sac with a double decidual sign is found within the endometrial cavity. All pregnancies can induce an endometrial decidual reaction. However, a double decidual sign, that is, two echogenic external layers encircling the anechoic gestational sac, is caused by the decidua parietalis and decidua capsularis of the developing placenta (Fig. 2-19).

Ectopic pregnancy may present with a large variety of sonographic patterns and locations (Fig. 7-5, p. 204) (Condous, 2007; Moschos, 2008; Valsky, 2008). An extrauterine gestational sac containing an embryo is an unequivocal finding. However, solid and complex adnexal masses in conjunction with an empty uterus and a positive pregnancy test result are frequently encountered. A complex adnexal mass is usually caused by hemorrhage within the ectopic sac or by an ectopic pregnancy that has ruptured into the tube. Complex free fluid or blood clots are often associated (Filly, 1987; Fleischer, 1990; Nyberg, 1987). Placental blood flow within the periphery of the complex adnexal mass–the *ring of fire*–can be seen with transvaginal color Doppler imaging (Fig. 7-7, p. 205). Although this can aid in the diagnosis, this finding can also be seen with a corpus luteum of pregnancy (Pellerito, 1992b).

Intraabdominal Fluid

During routine sonographic evaluation of the pelvis, a small amount of free fluid, as little as 10 mL, is commonly visualized in the posterior cul-de-sac (Khalife, 1998). If free fluid is seen extending to the fundus of the uterus, it is considered to be moderate in amount. Moderate free fluid on transvaginal examination should prompt further evaluation of the paracolic gutters and Morison pouch in the right upper quadrant to assess the extent of the free fluid. Free intraperitoneal fluid is seen in the paracolic gutters and Morison pouch when there is a minimum volume of approximately 500 mL (Abrams, 1999;

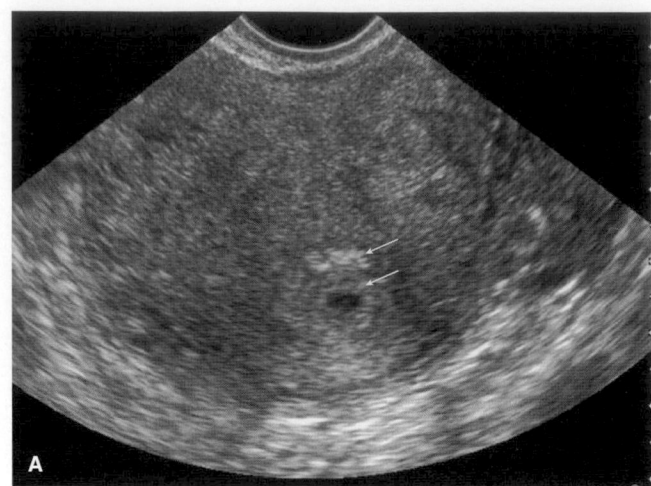
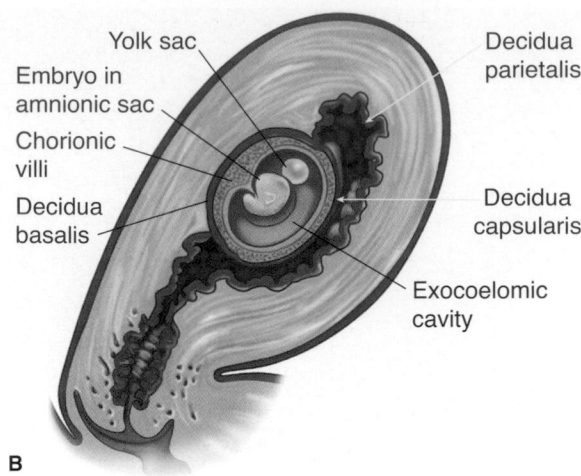

FIGURE 2-19 Transvaginal sonogram and illustration demonstrating a double decidual sign. **A.** Sonogram shows two concentric echogenic layers surrounding the anechoic gestational sac, which are the inner decidua capsularis (*lower arrow*) and the peripheral decidua parietalis (*upper arrow*). **B.** The drawing shows the decidual layers of an early pregnancy. The decidua capsularis and decidua parietalis create the double decidual sign. *(From Cunningham, 2010b, with permission.)*

Branney, 1995; Rodgerson, 2001). Large amounts of anechoic free peritoneal fluid suggest an infectious or inflammatory etiology, such as with ascites. Free fluid that contains low-level echoes or echogenic debris is consistent with hemoperitoneum with clot, such as with a ruptured hemorrhagic cyst or ectopic pregnancy.

The sensitivity of sonography to detect free fluid has led to its increased use in the field of trauma. Focused Assessment with Sonography for Trauma (FAST) is a limited sonographic examination directed solely at identifying free fluid for the diagnosis of intraperitoneal injury. In the context of trauma, free fluid is usually due to hemorrhage. Four specific areas are imaged: perihepatic (right upper quadrant), perisplenic (left upper quadrant), pelvis, and pericardium. FAST has significant advantages over Diagnostic Peritoneal Lavage (DPL) and CT scanning for the evaluation of free intraperitoneal fluid because it is a rapid, noninvasive bedside test. However, there is a significant false-negative rate for the FAST examination (Scalea, 1999). This is in part due to the FAST examination being carried out early in the resuscitation phase when only a small amount of free fluid may have collected in the dependent portions of the peritoneal cavity. In addition, as its use has become more widespread, conflicts have developed regarding credentialing and whether radiologists, emergency physicians, or trauma surgeons should be performing this sonographic technique.

Gestational Trophoblastic Disease

Sonography plays an important role in establishing the diagnosis of hydatidiform mole. A complete hydatidiform mole displays tissue that is interspersed with numerous punctate sonolucencies (Fig. 37-5, p. 902). The appearance varies according to gestational duration and correlates with the size of hydropic villi (Jones, 1975). For example, moles of menstrual age from 8 to 12 weeks typically appear as homogenously echogenic intraluminal tissue, and villi have a maximum diameter of 2 mm. With maturation, vesicles may approximate 10 mm in

diameter, and they are readily seen as sonolucent cystic spaces. These larger villi create a classic transabdominal image termed a "snowstorm" pattern. Fetal tissues and amnionic membranes are absent.

In contrast, features of a partial mole include hydropic placental degeneration and presence of concomitant fetus or fetal parts. Villi are focally swollen and edematous (Fleischer, 2001). Unfortunately, these hydropic villous changes are also seen sonographically in 20 to 40 percent of placentas from nonmolar aborted pregnancies (Reid, 1983). Thus, histologic, genetic, and immunologic analysis of tissue is typically required to differentiate between partial molar and nonmolar pregnancy (Chap. 37, p. 899).

Theca-lutein cysts within the ovary that enlarge under the influence of high serum levels of β-human chorionic gonadotropin (hCG) are also commonly seen with complete molar pregnancies. They are typically bilateral and appear as multiloculated cystic masses that measure between 4 and 8 cm in diameter (Fig. 37-4, p. 901)(Fleischer, 2001).

Sonography with Doppler examination has replaced angiography of the uterus for the detection of invasive disease (Desai, 1991). Sonographically, invasive trophoblastic tissue displays a focal, irregular echogenic region within the myometrium. Doppler sonography can show myometrial implants and their relative aggressiveness by depicting increased and typically turbulent flow to these tumors from the uterine arteries (Long, 1990; Oguz, 2004; Taylor, 1987). Sonography and Doppler analysis may be used to evaluate tumor response to chemotherapy (Hammond, 1980; Maymon, 1996; Ong, 1992; Zhou, 2005). Although, evaluation of the liver and kidney for metastatic disease is usually completed with CT scanning, it may be aided by abdominal sonography (Munyer, 1981).

Infertility

Sonography is employed for four main purposes in the approach to female infertility: (1) identification of abnormal pelvic

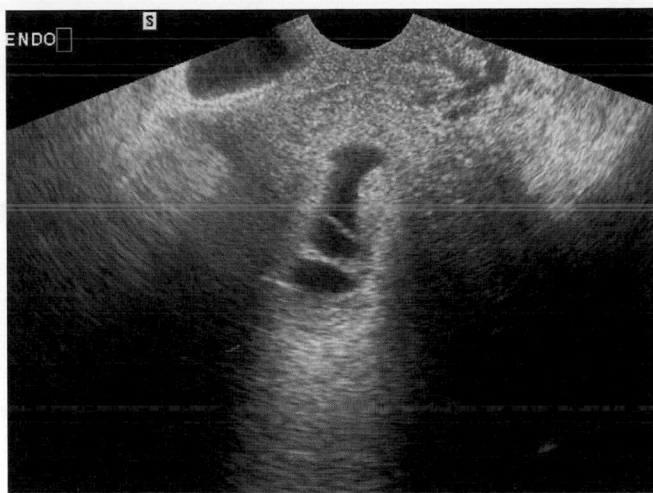

FIGURE 2-20 Asherman syndrome. Transvaginal saline infusion sonography demonstrates echogenic intrauterine synechiae.

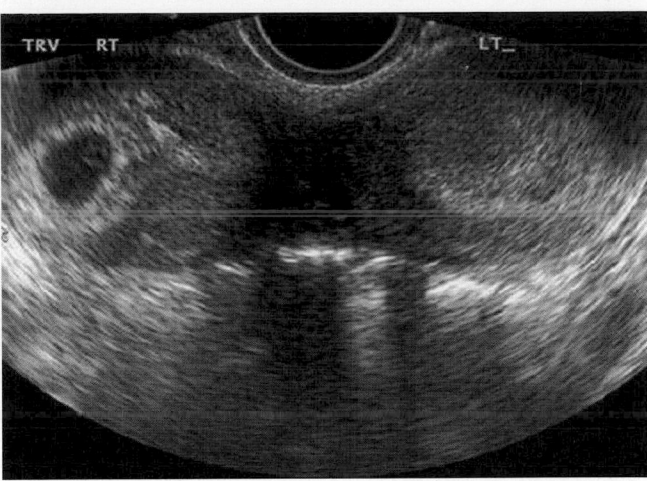

FIGURE 2-21 Uterus didelphys. Transvaginal sonogram in the transverse plane best depicts the two completely separate uterine horns. A gestational sac is evident in the right uterus.

anatomy; (2) detection of pathology causal or contributory to infertility; (3) evaluation of cyclic physiologic uterine and ovarian changes; and (4) surveillance and visual guidance during infertility treatment (Barnhart, 2000; Ekerhovd, 2004; Parsons, 2001).

Sonography can easily demonstrate anatomic uterine defects that may affect both gamete passage and ovum implantation. As discussed, conventional TVS can be used to visualize submucous leiomyomas and polyps, however, relationships of these lesions with the endometrial surface is better seen with SIS (Figs. 8-9 and 9-8, pp. 228 and 253). In those with a history of recurrent abortion, SIS has been used to demonstrate not only müllerian anomalies, but a variety of other uterine cavity defects in up to half of patients (Keltz, 1997). As a screening tool for cavity evaluation in this setting, it appears to be twice as accurate as hysterosalpingography (HSG) and TVS (Soares, 2000). Intrauterine synechiae can be seen as hypoechoic lines disrupting the echogenic endometrium by conventional sonography. These are more definitively seen during SIS as echogenic bands extending from one endometrial surface to the other (Fig. 2-20).

Transvaginal sonography is used initially to detect congenital uterine anomalies that cause infertility or early spontaneous abortion. The addition of 3-D techniques can diagnose congenital abnormalities with a test performance similar to those of HSG, laparoscopy, and MR imaging (Ekerhovd, 2004; Jurkovic, 1995; Salim, 2003). Thereafter, MR imaging is used to characterize and evaluate cases that are complicated or equivocal, especially preoperatively.

A complete duplication anomaly, such as uterus didelphys, can be accurately diagnosed by sonography. In this setting, two separate and divergent uterine horns are seen to have a deep fundal cleft between the two hemiuteri and to have a wide angle between the two endometrial cavities (Fig. 2-21). In contrast, bicornuate and septate uterine anomalies are less confidently differentiated by traditional 2-D transvaginal sonographic techniques. Ideally, the angle between the two endometrial cavities is ≥105° for bicornuate uterus, but ≤75° for septate uterus. Moreover, the fundal shape shows a >1-cm notch

for bicornuate uterus, but a <1-cm notch for septate uterus (Reuter, 1989). Combining TVS findings with SIS provides accuracy up to 90 percent to distinguish the two anomalies. Although MR imaging is frequently employed, 3-D sonography is considered by many to be the best noninvasive method for distinguishing between these uterine anomalies (Fig. 2-22) (Bermejo, 2010; Kupesic, 2001a; Salim, 2003).

A unicornuate uterus without a rudimentary horn is seen as a small, well-formed elliptical uterus that deviates to one side with a single cornu (Salim, 2003). The fundal shape has a concave contour. On 3-D imaging, the unicornuate uterus has the classic "banana" configuration (Fig. 2-23). In 65 percent of cases, however, the unicornuate uterus is associated with a rudimentary

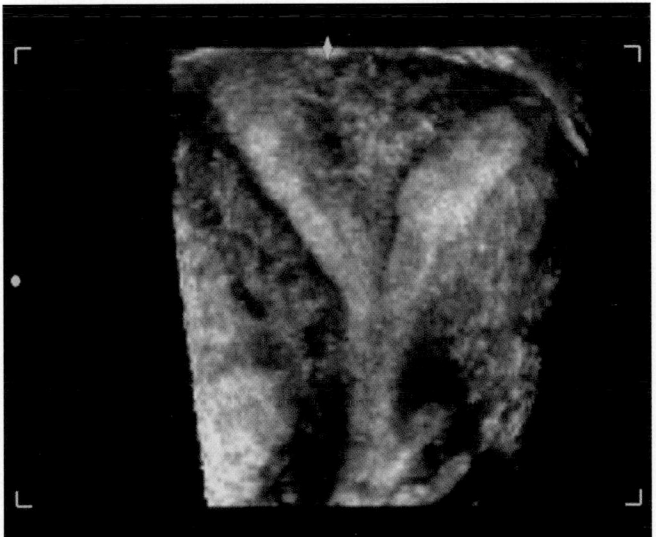

FIGURE 2-22 Septate uterus. The coronal plane of 3-dimensional sonography depicts the normal uterine serosal contour and the narrow angle between the two small endometrial cavities characteristic of a septate uterus. As the septum ends at the uterine isthmus and does not extend into the cervix, this anomaly is properly termed *subseptate*.

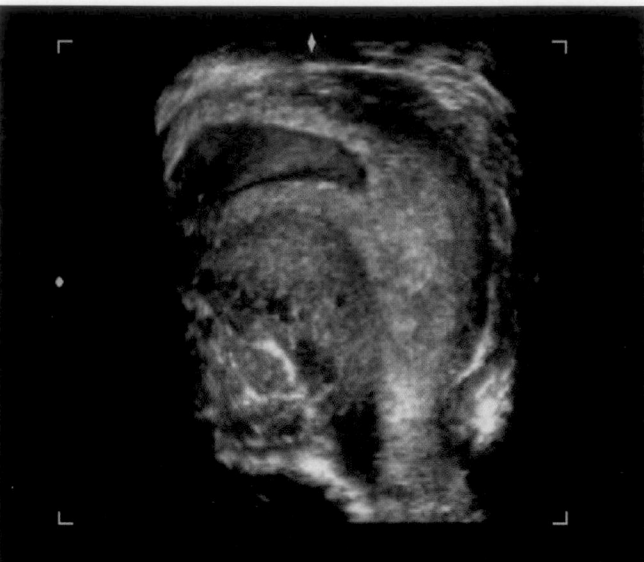

FIGURE 2-23 Unicornuate uterus. The coronal plane of 3-dimensional sonography illustrates the classic "banana" configuration. A gestational sac is seen within the endometrial cavity.

horn, and this is difficult to recognize sonographically (Fig. 18-16, p. 498) (Jayasinghe, 2005). A dilated rudimentary horn is often misdiagnosed as a uterine or adnexal mass (Hall, 1994). Complete evaluation of these cases often requires MR imaging. With most uterine anomalies, especially if unilateral, proper positioning of the kidneys should be documented with transabdominal imaging because of increased rates of associated genitourinary anomalies. Lastly, in women with complex anomalies associated with vaginal agenesis or imperforate hymen, hematocolpos is commonly seen, often with associated hematometra or hematosalpinx (Hall, 1994).

Pelvic endometriosis is another frequent cause of infertility. Sonography is the most common imaging procedure to evaluate suspected endometriosis, although it is mostly used to evaluate endometriotic cysts. Its capability to detect small implants and adhesions is limited. Endometriomas exhibit a variety of sonographic appearances, the most frequent being a pelvic mass with a thick wall and diffuse low-level echoes within the cyst (Fig. 10-6, p. 290). Magnetic resonance imaging is more specific than sonography for identifying endometriomas, and thus, it is indicated in cases with unclear anatomy sonographically (Fig. 10-8, 291).

One of the most powerful uses of sonography in the infertile patient is treatment surveillance. Sonography is used to monitor folliculogenesis in both normal and stimulated cycles. In natural cycles, observation of a developing follicle and prediction of ovulation allow optimal timing for postcoital testing, hCG administration, intercourse, insemination, and ovum collection. At ovulation, the follicle usually disappears, and fluid is observed in the cul-de-sac. At the follicular site, the corpus luteum appears as an irregular oval containing a small quantity of fluid, internal echoes, and a thick wall (Dill-Macky, 2000). In stimulated cycles, sonographic detection of too many follicles allows withholding of hCG induction to prevent ovarian hyperstimulation syndrome. If this develops, sonography is used to grade disease severity through measurements of ovarian size,

detection of ascites, and analysis of renal flow resistances (Fig. 20-4, p. 538) (Barnhart, 2000; Parsons, 2001).

In general, blood flow in the ovulating ovary decreases throughout the menstrual cycle. At ovulation, blood flow velocities dramatically increase in vessels surrounding the corpus luteum because of neovascularization and are seen as low-impedance waveforms. In women undergoing in vitro fertilization (IVF), low ovarian vessel impedance may correlate directly with pregnancy rates (Baber, 1988). Many infertility specialists are now incorporating SIS as a first-line screening tool for uterine evaluation before embryo transfer in women undergoing IVF, ovum donation, and IVF-surrogacy (Gera, 2008; Kim, 1998; Lindheim, 1998; Serafini, 1998; Yauger, 2008). Lastly, sonography can be used to guide interventional maneuvers such as oocyte retrieval and transfer of embryos into the endometrial cavity (Figs. 20-10 and 20-12, p. 546).

Hysterosalpingo-contrast Sonography (Sonosalpingography)

Previously, a fallopian tube could be detected with sonography only when distended by fluid, such as with obstruction. Injection of echogenic contrast material during real-time sonography, called *sonosalpingography, sonohysterosalpingography,* or *hysterosalpingo-contrast sonography* (HyCoSy), is an accurate first-line procedure for the assessment of tubal patency without the need for HSG. Hysterosalpingo-contrast sonography has been shown in many studies to be equivalent to HSG in detecting tubal pathology (Degenhardt, 1996; Heikinen, 1995; Schlief, 1991; Strandell, 1999). It can be performed in an outpatient setting, has good patient acceptance with no risk of x-ray exposure, and can also provide information on uterine cavity and ovarian morphology (Campbell, 1994; Savelli, 2009).

Hysterosalpingo-contrast sonography is done in a manner similar to SIS. Fluid egress from the uterine cavity is blocked by a balloon catheter within the cervical canal. The approximate location of the fallopian tubes as they insert into the uterine cornua is identified with a transvaginal probe. Tubal patency is confirmed by passage of a hyperechoic sonographic contrast medium–Echovist, Albunex, Infoson, air, or sterile saline solution–through the tubes. This gives them a hyperechoic appearance. Color or pulsed Doppler techniques increase the diagnostic accuracy of HyCoSy (Ekerhovd, 2004; Kupesic, 1997). However, a patent tube does not always correlate with a normally functioning tube. Hysterosalpingography may be needed for more accurate delineation of tubal anatomy in selected indications and is still considered a first-line tool in the evaluation of tubal patency in the infertile woman (Cundiff, 1995; Mol, 1996).

Three-Dimensional Sonography

New sonography scanners now allow collection of 3-D data and its representation on a 2-D screen (Kurjak, 2001). This permits a more detailed assessment of the object studied, without restriction of the number and orientation of the scanning planes (Aruh, 1997; Umek, 2002). In gynecology, this tool aids assessment of the uterine cavity, complex ovarian masses, ovarian reserve, uterine anomalies, and interstitial pregnancies (Fig. 2-24) (Izquierdo, 2003).

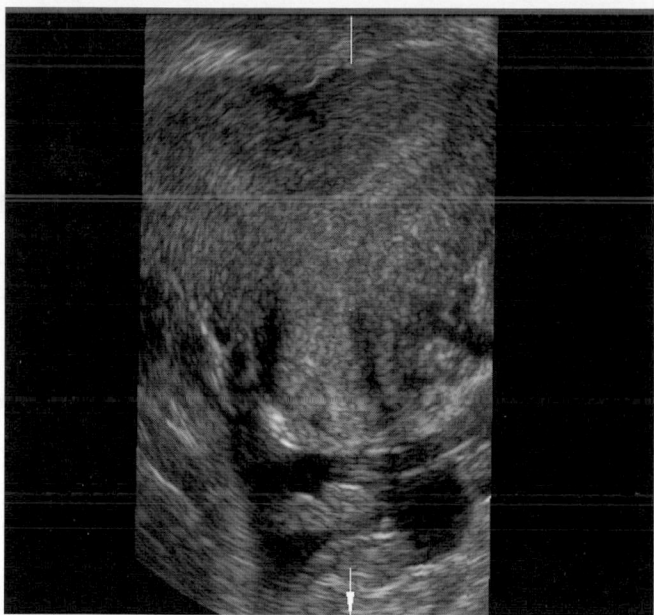

FIGURE 2-24 Arcuate uterus. The coronal plane of 3-dimensional sonography best illustrates this normal uterine variant.

Although conventional SIS or MR imaging is an option to preoperatively map the exact location of leiomyomas in relation to the endometrial cavity and surrounding structures, 3-D sonography and 3-D SIS may also be used (Fig. 19-9, p. 519). This is extremely important in triaging patients for surgery, which depends on knowledge of exact leiomyoma position and extent of endometrial involvement (Sylvestre, 2003; Wamsteker, 1993). These sonography tools may also be used to monitor leiomyoma volume reduction in patients receiving GnRH agonists or following UAE, although MR imaging is more often used following UAE (Chia, 2006).

With 3-D technology, abnormalities of the endometrium and adjacent myometrium, especially focal endometrial thickenings such as polyps, hyperplasia, and cancer, can be better imaged and defined (Andreotti, 2006; Benacerraf, 2008; Bonilla-Musoles, 1997). In their comparative study of 36 women with postmenopausal bleeding, Bonilla-Musoles and associates (1997) compared results from 3-D SIS with findings from TVS, transvaginal SIS, transvaginal color Doppler, and hysteroscopy. Visualization of the uterine cavity and endometrial thickness with 3-D SIS was comparable to hysteroscopy and was better than with the other sonographic techniques. We now routinely implement 3-D imaging for evaluation of an abnormal endometrium during our transvaginal studies and with all SIS procedures. On an investigational front, 3-D sonography with power Doppler angiography (3D-PDA) has been used to discriminate between benign and malignant endometrial disease in women with postmenopausal bleeding and a thickened endometrium (Alcazar, 2009). Three-dimensional power Doppler angiography allows for assessment of endometrial volume, which may more accurately represent the true tissue amount compared with a 2-D measurement of endometrial thickness. Lastly, 3-D power Doppler imaging, enhanced by intravenous contrast, is also being investigated to differentiate

between benign endometrial polyps and endometrial cancer (Lieng, 2008; Song, 2009).

Although traditional TVS will document IUD position adequately in most cases, 3-D sonography offers improved visualization, especially with the levonorgestrel-containing IUD (Bonilla-Musoles, 1996; Lee, 1997; Moschos, 2011). The coronal plane images, which are not possible with 2-D, provide views of both the arms and shaft of the device and the relation of these to the endometrial cavity (Andreotti, 2006; Benacerraf, 2009; Moschos, 2011). Therefore, patients at our institution undergoing gynecologic sonography with IUDs in situ, regardless of the indication for the study, have both a standard 2-D evaluation and a 3-D volume acquisition of the uterus, with reconstruction of the coronal view of the endometrial cavity to establish the type, location, and positioning of the IUD (Fig. 2-25). Another use of 3-D sonography involves transcervical sterilization confirmation. Although the Food and Drug Administration (FDA) still mandates a postprocedural HSG to document proper placement of Essure microinsert coils, 2-D and 3-D TVS has been shown by several investigators to be an acceptable method of confirmation (Fig. 2-26) (Conceptus, 2009; Thiel, 2005).

In detecting malignancies in adnexal masses, most agree that 3-D sonography allows a detailed assessment of the internal structure of ovarian masses (Alcazar, 2003b, 2009; Bonilla-Musoles, 1995; Hata, 1999). Moreover, the addition of color Doppler to 3-D evaluation displays the internal architecture and neovascularization, also characteristic of malignant neoplasms (Kurjak, 2001). However, to date, 3-D power Doppler ultrasound has not shown significantly improved diagnostic accuracy over that of gray-scale and 2-D power Doppler imaging (Geomini, 2007; Jokubkiene, 2007; Sladkevicius, 2007).

A new 3-D technique aimed at differentiating between benign and malignant ovarian masses uses contrast-enhanced TVS for early detection of tumor microvascularity. In studies, patients with complex adnexal masses received a microbubble contrast agent intravenously while undergoing pulse inversion harmonic TVS. Early data show a significant difference in the contrast enhancement kinetic parameters between benign and malignant ovarian masses (Fleischer, 2008, 2009, 2010).

In reproductive medicine, 3-D imaging provides more accurate ovarian volume and follicle counts than measurements estimated from 2-D imaging and is predicted to become the preferred ultrasound technique for infertility ovarian evaluation (Coyne, 2008; Deutch, 2009; Raine-Fenning, 2008). In addition, 3-D ultrasound may also be used to examine endometrial vascularity and determine endometrial receptivity prior to ovarian stimulation (Kupesic, 2001b; Wu, 2003).

Three-dimensional ultrasound is now a commonly used and accurate tool for the assessment of congenital müllerian uterine anomalies (Ghi, 2009; Jurkovic, 1995; Raga, 1996; Salim, 2003). It is as sensitive as hysteroscopy, is as accurate as MR imaging, and provides detailed images of both endometrial cavity shape and external fundal contour (Bermejo, 2010). Thus, müllerian anomalies can be differentiated because the uterine horns and fundal contour can be displayed clearly in

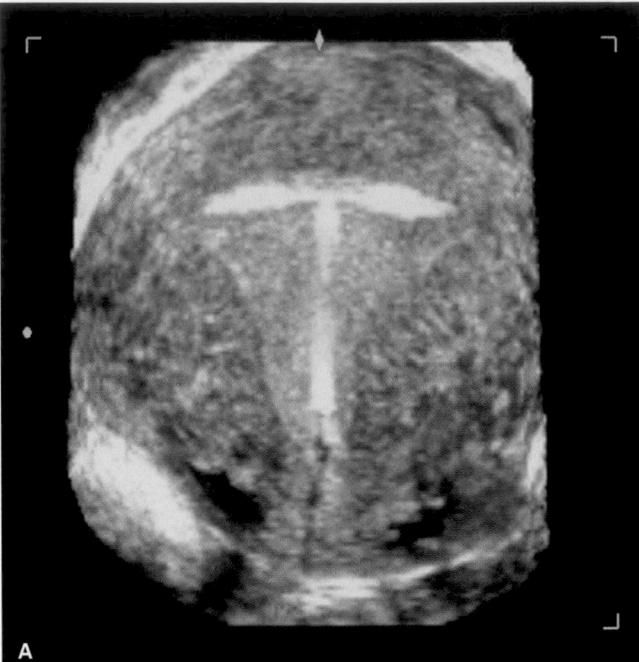

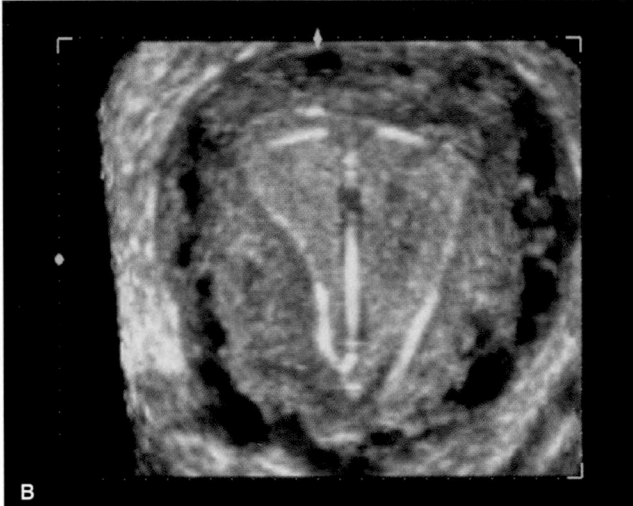

FIGURE 2-25 Intrauterine devices. The coronal planes of 3-dimensional sonography best depict the type and positioning of the Copper T 380A IUD (ParaGard) **(A)** and levonorgestrel-containing IUD (Mirena) **(B)** intrauterine devices within the endometrial cavity.

the same plane (Troiano, 2004). Importantly, 3-D imaging can provide helpful details for preoperative planning and may even help predict the likely outcome of metroplasty (Wu, 1997).

■ Compression Sonography of Lower Extremities

Compression sonography, often combined with color Doppler sonography, is the initial test currently used to detect deep-vein thrombosis (DVT) (Greer, 2003). Sonographic evaluation of leg veins is divided into three parts: (1) the groin and thigh are examined with the patient supine; (2) the popliteal region is examined with the patient lying on her side or sitting; and

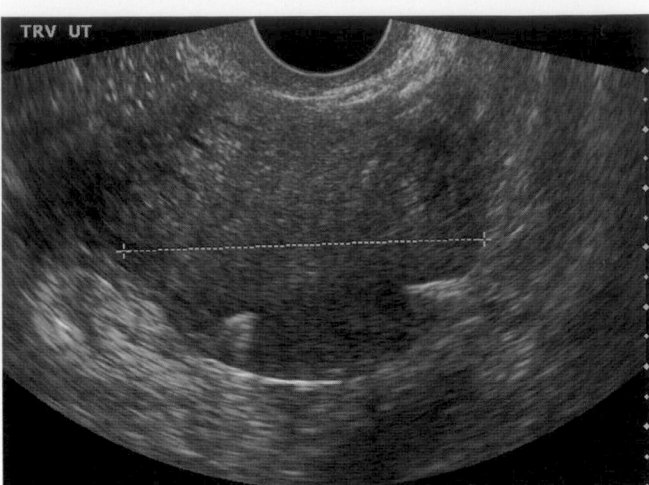

FIGURE 2-26 Essure contraception. Transvaginal sonogram in the transverse plane demonstrates the microinsert coils in the posterior lateral uterus, corresponding to proper placement of the devices in the bilateral cornua.

finally, (3) the calf veins are examined with the patient sitting. Impaired visibility, noncompressibility, and the typical echo pattern of a thrombosed vein confirm the diagnosis (Fig. 2-27) (Andrews, 2005). In symptomatic patients, examination of the femoral, popliteal, and calf trifurcation veins is more than 90-percent sensitive and greater than 99-percent specific for proximal DVT (Davis, 2001; Schellong, 2004). It has a negative predictive value of 98 percent (American College of Obstetricians and Gynecologists, 2000a,b). Moreover, in 220 patients with suspected DVT, Lensing and colleagues (1989) compared compression sonography with contrast venography, the gold standard for DVT detection. They found that both the common femoral and popliteal veins were fully compressible—no thrombosis—in 142 of 143 patients who had a normal venogram (99-percent specific). All 66 patients with proximal vein thrombosis had noncompressible femoral or popliteal veins, or both (100-percent sensitive).

Compression sonography, however, is significantly less reliable for detecting calf vein thromboses (Bates, 2004). However, isolated calf thromboses eventually extend into the proximal veins in up to a fourth of cases. They do so within 1 to 2 weeks of presentation and thus are usually detected by serial sonographic compression examinations (Cunningham, 2010c). The safety of withholding anticoagulation has been established for those patients who have normal serial compression examinations during a week-long surveillance (Birdwell, 1998; Friera, 2002; Heijboer, 1993). Importantly, normal venous sonographic findings do not necessarily exclude pulmonary embolism because the thrombosis may have already embolized, or because it arose from deep pelvic veins, which are inaccessible to sonographic evaluation (Goldhaber, 2004).

RADIOGRAPHY

Plain radiographs are used in gynecologic practice in a manner similar to other medical specialties. Radiographs of the abdomen and pelvis (KUB) are often obtained to assess women

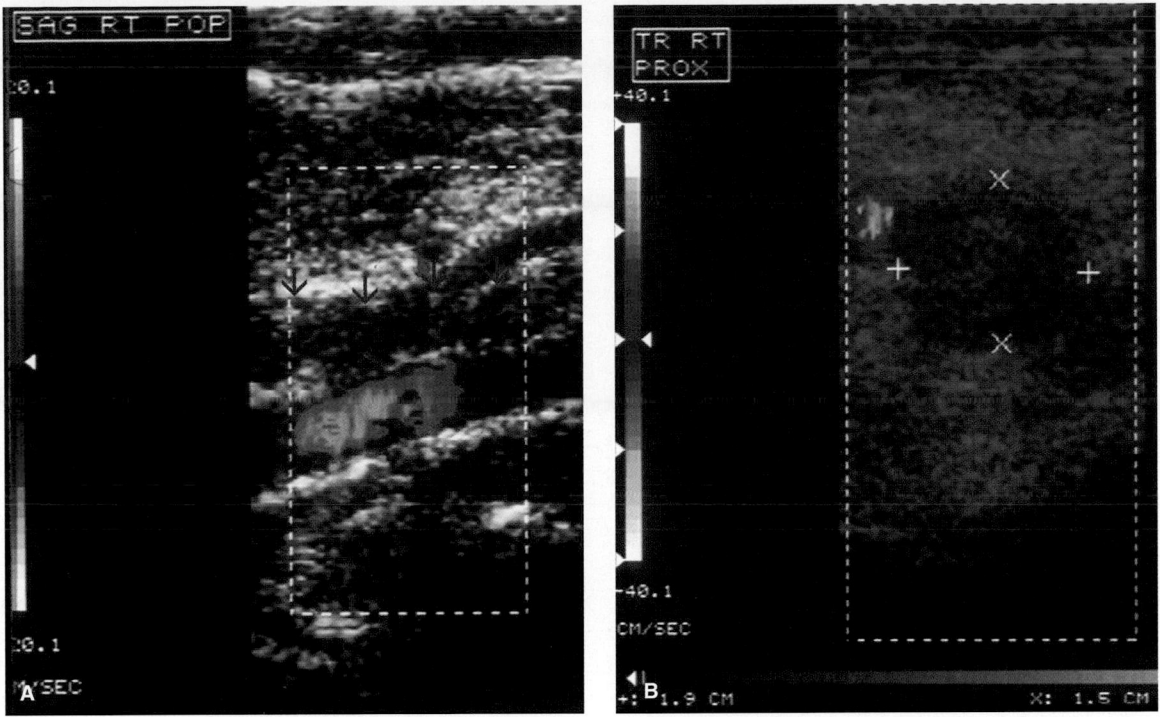

FIGURE 2-27 Sagittal **(A)** and transverse **(B)** images from a lower extremity. Color Doppler ultrasound study in a woman with popliteal vein thrombosis. **A.** Red arrows demarcate the popliteal vein with no flow suggesting clot in the lumen, which sits above the artery demonstrating normal flow as evidenced by the red color map. **B.** The transverse image shows the large size of the vein due to the thrombus (*cursors*), as well as normal flow in the artery, evidenced by the red color map.

with clinically suspected bowel obstruction. This film view can also be used to identify an extrauterine location of a missing IUD. Plain radiographs may also be informative in women with gynecologic malignancies (Soper, 2001). Examples are chest radiographs to screen for pulmonary metastases during malignancy staging, including gestational trophoblastic disease, and for surveillance after initial treatment. As discussed in the next sections, a number of specialized radiographic procedures are especially useful or are specific to evaluation of gynecologic conditions.

Intravenous Pyelography

Excretory urography, also called intravenous pyelography (IVP), is a radiographic study that provides imaging of the urinary tract. In comparison, CT images show more detail of pelvicalyceal and ureteric anatomy but provide less information regarding the renal parenchyma and bladder (Webb, 2001).

After an initial plain radiograph, termed a *scout film*, is used to delineate urinary calculi, then intravenous contrast agent is given. Thereafter, the concentrating function of the proximal tubules renders renal parenchyma radiodense—the *nephrogram phase*—and allows evaluation of renal size, contour, and axis. A radiograph obtained after 5 minutes depicts contrast excreted into the collecting system—the *pyelogram phase*—and the collecting system is evaluated for symmetry and excretion promptness. A final postvoiding radiograph completes the evaluation.

Indications for a preoperative IVP include suspected urinary anomalies in a woman with a coexistent reproductive tract anomaly and confirmation of lower urinary tract patency in

the setting of a compressing pelvic neoplasm. However, many preoperative pyelograms have been replaced with multiphasic CT urography protocols performed on multislice CT scanners (Beyersdorff, 2008). For example, although not a formal part of cervical cancer staging, many clinicians in the United States have substituted CT imaging for IVP in cervical cancer evaluation. CT allows visualization of the cervix, parametria, uterus, adnexa, retroperitoneal lymph nodes, liver, and ureters (International Federation of Obstetricians and Gynecologists, 1998).

As many as 5 to 10 percent of women have an allergic reaction to iodide during IVP, and 1 to 2 percent of these reactions are life threatening. Pretreatment with oral corticosteroids has significantly reduced the incidence of allergic reactions (Lasser, 1987). Nonionic iodinated contrast media agents have a 5- to 30-fold decreased incidence of allergic reactions but are more expensive than traditional ionic contrast media (Mishell, 1997).

There also may be significant nephrotoxicity due to hyperosmolar ionic contrast, which is believed to cause direct tubular insult and ischemic injury. Women with diabetes, renal impairment, and congestive heart failure are at high risk for contrast nephrotoxicity. Low osmotic, nonionic contrast materials are less nephrotoxic and should be considered in special cases such as these (Mishell, 1997).

Voiding Cystourethrography (VCUG) and Positive Pressure Urethrography (PPUG)

These radiographic procedures, discussed in Chapter 26 (p. 687), are used to evaluate the female urethra. However, MR imaging permits superior visualization of urethral abnormalities and is more sensitive than VCUG or PPUG for delineating diverticula with complex structure (Chou, 2008; Daneshgari, 1999; Elsayes, 2006; Neitlich, 1998). For this reason, VCUG is currently more often used to evaluate lower urinary tract trauma, such as fistulas, and patients with prolonged urinary retention. PPUG use has declined due to decreasing numbers of technicians trained to complete the study, difficulty finding appropriate equipment, and the higher sensitivity of MR imaging.

Hysterosalpingography

This radiographic imaging technique is used to evaluate the endocervical canal, the endometrial cavity, and the fallopian tube lumina by injecting radiopaque contrast material through the cervical canal (Chap. 19, p. 516). Used primarily during infertility evaluation, an average HSG study is performed in 10 minutes, involves approximately 90 seconds of fluoroscopic time, and has an average radiation exposure to the ovaries of 1 to 2 rads.

Hysterosalpingography is performed between cycle days 5 and 10. During this time, cessation of menstrual flow minimizes infection and the risk of flushing an ovum from the fallopian tube following ovulation. The test causes cramping, and an NSAID taken 30 minutes prior to the procedure may limit discomfort. An acorn cannula, pediatric Foley catheter, or designated injection catheter is introduced just inside the external cervical os and contrast medium is injected. A paracervical block may be indicated in selected patients, such as those with cervical stenosis. Because rapid injection may cause tubal spasm, slow injection of usually no more than 3 to 4 mL of medium allows a clear outline of the uterine cavity. Generally, only three radiographic views are needed—a preliminary view before injecting contrast, a view showing the fill of the uterine cavity, and the third demonstrating spill of contrast from the tubes into the peritoneal cavity.

There are many variations in the appearance of a normal HSG (Fig. 19-6, p. 517). The endometrial cavity is usually triangular or sometimes T-shaped in the anteroposterior projection. In the lateral view, it is oblong. The contour of the endometrium is usually smooth, but it occasionally has polypoid filling defects that can be isolated or diffuse and can be difficult to distinguish from endometrial polyps or hyperplasia (Lindheim, 2003a). Inadvertent injection of air bubbles introduces artifact. In these instances, SIS is often later obtained for further evaluation of the endometrial cavity.

Contraindications to HSG include acute pelvic infection, active uterine bleeding, pregnancy, and iodine allergy. Complications of HSG are rare but can be serious. The overall risk of acute pelvic infection serious enough to require hospitalization is less than 1 percent, but may be up to 3 percent in women with prior pelvic infection (Stumpf, 1980). In patients with no history of pelvic infection, HSG can be performed without prophylactic antibiotics. If HSG demonstrates dilated fallopian tubes, doxycycline, 100 mg orally twice daily for 3 days, should be given to reduce the incidence of post-HSG PID. In patients with a history of pelvic infection, doxycycline can be administered before the procedure and continued if dilated fallopian tubes are found (American College of Obstetricians and Gynecologists, 2009). Pelvic pain, uterine perforation, and vasovagal reactions may also occur. A number of reactions to the contrast include allergic reactions

and entry into the vascular system with high injection pressures. Embolic phenomena, pelvic peritonitis, and granuloma formation with oil-based contrast agents are rare.

Selective Salpingography

In some cases, it is not possible to distinguish whether tubal blockage seen by HSG is caused by anatomic occlusion or tubal spasm. Hysteroscopic tubal cannulation can further clarify and treat many cases of proximal tubal occlusion as described in Section 42-20 (p. 1176). Alternatively, transcervical selective salpingography and tubal catheterization (SS-TC) under fluoroscopic guidance is another procedure that may be used. It is performed during the follicular phase of the cycle with the catheter forwarded through the cervix and advanced by tactile sensation to the tubal ostium. The position of the catheter is checked fluoroscopically and if satisfactory, water- or oil-soluble contrast is injected. If the obstruction is overcome, the tubal contour is outlined with contrast agent. If the proximal tubal obstruction persists, a guide wire is threaded through the inner cannula of the catheter, advanced toward the obstruction, and gently manipulated to overcome the blockage. The guide wire is then withdrawn, and contrast medium is injected through the catheter to confirm patency. This fluoroscopic tool is effective at diagnosing and treating proximal tubal blockage and is discussed in Chapter 20 (p. 540) (Capitanio, 1991; Das, 2007; Ferraiolo, 1995; Thurmond, 1991; Woolcott, 1995).

Bone Densitometry

Depending on its mineral density, bone absorbs x-rays to different degrees. Because of this, bone density can be evaluated, and most measurements provide site-specific information. However, these studies do not assess either current or past rates of bone remodeling. Thus, sequential density measurements are necessary to assess rates of bone loss over time (Kaplan, 1995). Currently, two common methods are dual energy x-ray absorptiometry (DEXA), which assesses integral bone (cortical and trabecular bone) mineral density in the hip and spine, and quantitative computed tomography (QCT), which evaluates bone mineral in high-turnover trabecular bone.

Of these, DEXA is the best technique for axial osteopenia evaluation (Fig. 21-10, p. 567). It employs two x-ray beams of differing energy levels and accurately measures bone density in the hip and spine—areas most vulnerable to osteoporotic fractures. The spine is commonly scanned between the 1st and 4th lumbar vertebrae. Measurements with DEXA are precise and accurate; radiation dose is low—less than 5 mrem; and patient acceptability is high because the procedure time is usually only 5 to 15 minutes (Jergas, 1993). The reproducibility of DEXA bone mass measurement is excellent to identify a population at high risk for fracture. Although DEXA instruments that measure bone mass at peripheral sites such as the forearm are also available, these may not predict hip fractures as accurately as direct hip measurement. Other advantages include a proven effectiveness in monitoring antifracture treatments and being the standard against which other bone imaging measures are evaluated (Blake, 2007). Disadvantageously, DEXA is a 2-D technique that cannot distinguish between cortical and trabecular bone. In addition, bone spurs, aortic calcifications, and arthritis may falsely elevate reported bone density.

Quantitative computed tomography (QCT) uses either x-rays or gamma rays to provide a cross-sectional view of the vertebral body. As the rate of turnover in trabecular bone is nearly eight times that in cortical bone, this technique can detect early metabolic changes in this highly vulnerable bone type. It provides a volumetric density, which is an advantage in situations in which DEXA may underestimate bone mineral density (Damilakis, 2007). Its precision is excellent but may be reduced with severe osteopenia and kyphosis, increased fat content from obesity or fatty bone marrow in older patients, and by the technical aspects of positioning (Kaplan, 1995; Miller, 1999).

Another technique, that has not yet been validated, is quantitative sonography (QUS) (Pejovic, 1999). This may provide information regarding the structural organization of bone and offers the potential for greater community access to bone mass evaluation (American Association of Endocrinologists, 1996; Philipov, 2000; World Health Organization, 1994). Small portable ultrasound units are available for rapid measurement of heel bone mass in the office, with readings completed in 10 seconds. Quantitative ultrasound is considerably cheaper than DEXA and does not include radiation exposure. However, its utility may be limited to younger patients, ages 35 to 55 years, because older patients' bones often are too compact to allow ultrasound penetration (Pafumi, 2002). Accordingly, QUS analysis of calcaneal bone may be useful to quantify fracture risk as a prescreening tool, to monitor response to treatment, and to identify adverse bone changes associated with disease or medication (Philipov, 2000). However, diagnosis of bone mineral density and osteoporosis by QUS measurements cannot be recommended at the present time (Pocock, 2000).

Considerable progress has been made in the development of MR techniques for assessing osteoporosis. In addition to relaxometry techniques, high-resolution MR imaging, diffusion MR imaging, and in vivo MR spectroscopy may quantify trabecular bone architecture and mineral composition (Damilakis, 2007).

Uterine Artery Embolization

This definitive independent treatment of uterine leiomyomas employs angiography for visualization and embolic occlusion of uterine vasculature. As discussed and illustrated more fully in Chapter 9 (p. 256), blood flow through the uterine arteries is stopped, resulting in preferential leiomyoma ischemia and necrosis.

COMPUTED TOMOGRAPHY

This procedure involves multiple exposures of thin x-ray beams that are translated to 2-D axial images, termed a *slice*, of the particular area of interest. Multiple slices of the target body part are obtained along its length. Multiple-channel helical computed tomography, also called *spiral CT*, allows for continuous acquisition of images in a spiral and the potential for image reformatting in multiple planes. This technique is much faster and permits images to be manipulated for analysis after they have been acquired. Many variables affect radiation dose, especially slice thickness and number of cuts obtained. If a study is performed with contrast, twice as many images will be obtained, and the target-area radiation dose is therefore doubled.

Normal Pelvic Anatomy

The uterus is identified as a homogenous, soft tissue oval or triangular structure situated posterior to the bladder (Fig. 2-28). The uterine walls enhance after intravenous contrast medium. Unlike sonography and MR imaging, the endometrium is not identifiable on CT imaging. The smooth lateral margins of the cervix are well defined because of their contrast against adjacent parametrial fat. There is uniform enhancement of the cervix after intravenous contrast medium administration. The endocervical canal, which can be identified by MR imaging, cannot be distinguished by CT imaging. Images of the vagina and vulva are strongly enhanced by contrast medium (Constant, 1989). Typically, the ovaries are relatively hypodense, variable in appearance and position, and usually situated posterolateral to the uterus (Friedman, 1992).

Computed tomography imaging displays the parametria well and thus is useful for gynecologic malignancies. The parametria contain a large proportion of fatty tissue as well as fibrous tissue, blood vessels, and lymphatics. The cardinal ligaments are seen on axial scans as triangular soft-tissue structures that extend from the lateral borders of the cervix and upper vagina to fuse with the deep fascia covering the levator ani. The round ligaments can be viewed at the upper margin of the parametrium and stretch anterolaterally toward the inguinal ring (Friedman, 1992). The uterosacral ligaments are easily identified on axial and coronal views, passing from the lateral margins of the cervix and vaginal fornices to the sacrum. Finally, the ureter and the uterine arteries can be seen within the broad ligament (Constant, 1989).

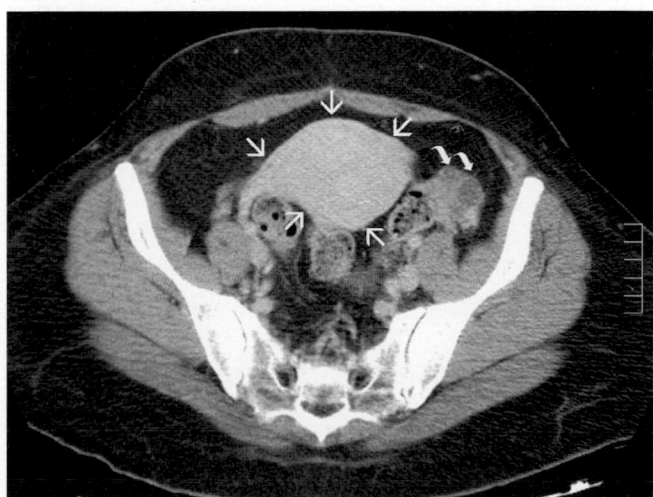

FIGURE 2-28 Computed tomography (CT) of the female pelvis in the axial plane demonstrates the normal uterus (*arrows*) as well as cysts in the left ovary (*curved arrows*).

Imaging Following Gynecologic Surgery

Computed tomography is well suited to diagnose potential complications of hysterectomy and other gynecologic procedures. With regard to ureteral and bladder injuries, CT with intravenous contrast is particularly useful for detecting ureteral obstruction or disruption of the ureter and urinoma formation (Titton, 2003). However, elevated creatinine levels in many of these postoperative patients may preclude its use. Computed tomography cystography is a technique employing retrograde filling of the bladder by gravity drip of 300 to 400 mL of dilute iodinated contrast, followed by helical CT of the bladder with multiplanar reformations (Chan, 2006). This technique is sensitive and specific for the diagnosis of extraperitoneal and intraperitoneal bladder rupture and can also be used to demonstrate fistulas between the bladder and vagina or intestine (Jankowski, 2006; Yu, 2004). Computed tomography is also superior to conventional radiography and barium studies in diagnosing bowel complications, such as small bowel obstruction (Maglinte, 1993). Computed tomography with intravenous and enteral contrast may be more helpful than other imaging modalities in characterizing an abdominal-pelvic fluid collection such as abscess or hematoma (Gjelsteen, 2008).

Gynecologic Malignancy

In most instances, sonography is the preferred initial method of evaluating the female pelvis (Fleischer, 1989; O'Brien, 1984). With pelvic pathology, MR imaging is now often preferable to CT imaging because it does not use radiation and provides excellent views of pelvic structures, in multiple planes (Carr, 2002). For these reasons, literature concerning CT images of benign pelvic disorders is relatively scant.

However, CT imaging is probably the most frequently used imaging technique for the evaluation and surveillance of gynecologic malignancies (Soper, 2001). Oral and rectal contrast allows visualization of the gastrointestinal tract, whereas intravenous contrast enhances blood vessels and viscera. Rapid resolution CT scans have great sensitivity and can be used to detect 2- to 3-mm lesions in the lungs and solid viscera. Scans with contrast yield high-quality information regarding retroperitoneal lymph nodes and ureters. Spiral CT scans record images during arterial, capillary, and venous phases of tissue enhancement during contrast administration, allowing improved imaging of small vessels and tissue interfaces within visceral parenchyma. Whereas sensitivity for intraperitoneal metastases is limited, CT scans can give a useful estimate of bulky metastases, such as in women with advanced ovarian cancer. Disadvantages include radiation exposure, artifacts created by metallic clips or prosthetic joints, and complications related to iodinated intravenous contrast material (Soper, 2001).

POSITRON EMISSION TOMOGRAPHY (PET) IMAGING

This technique uses short-lived radiochemical compounds to serve as tracers for measuring specific metabolic processes suggestive of malignancy or infection (Juweid, 2006). This enables detection of early cancer biochemical anomalies that precede the structural changes identified by other imaging techniques.

As such, PET has become a vital clinical tool, particularly for cancer diagnosis and management. The most common PET radiochemical tracer used clinically is 2-[^{18}F]fluoro-2-deoxy-D-glucose (FDG). This tracer highlights areas of accelerated glycolysis, which is common in neoplastic cells (Goh, 2003).

Data support the use of FDG-PET for imaging gynecologic malignancies. Several studies have demonstrated high sensitivity and specificity of FDG-PET for the initial staging of cervical cancer, especially in patients with no evidence of extrapelvic metastatic disease by MR or CT imaging (Gjelsteen, 2008; Park, 2005). The ability of FDG-PET imaging to assess nodal status in cervical cancer has both prognostic and therapeutic implications. Direct correlation between the extent of lymph node involvement and mortality rates has been shown (Singh, 2003). Prior to lymph node radiation treatment planning, the added anatomic data obtained with PET can be used to guide intensity-modulated radiotherapy (Chap. 28, p. 720). This significantly reduces the amount of radiation delivered to surrounding normal structures (Havrilesky, 2003; Weber, 1995; Wong, 2004).

In addition, FDG-PET scanning can also be used for postsurgical monitoring and surveillance of patients with endometrial and ovarian cancer. Specifically, scanning has been shown to closely correlate with findings at second-look surgery in endometrial and ovarian cancer patients who are in clinical remission (Fig. 2-29) (Belhocine, 2002; Delbeke, 2001; Drieskens, 2003; Iyer, 2010; Kim, 2004; Nanni, 2005; Saga, 2003).

MAGNETIC RESONANCE IMAGING

With this technology, images are constructed based on the radiofrequency signal emitted by hydrogen nuclei after they have been "excited" by radiofrequency pulses in the presence of a strong magnetic field. The radiofrequency signal emitted has characteristics called *relaxation times*. These include the T1-relaxation time (longitudinal) and the T2-relaxation time (transverse).

In a magnetic field, protons will align themselves in the same direction as the field running through the bore of the magnet. If a radiofrequency pulse is applied, these protons are forced out of alignment and rotate in phase with one another. The T1-relaxation is the time it takes for protons to realign with the magnetic field after a radiofrequency pulse is applied. T2-relaxation is the time it takes for the protons to diphase from each other after a radiofrequency pulse is applied.

Because these properties vary among tissues, they are the factors principally responsible for contrast among tissues. The signal intensity of one tissue compared with another, or contrast, can be manipulated by varying the elapsed time between applications of radiofrequency pulses, which is called *repetition time*. Further manipulation of the time between a radiofrequency pulse and sampling the emitted signal is called the *echo delay time*. Sequences with a short repetition time and short echo delay time are called T1-weighted. Sequences with a long repetition time and long echo delay time are regarded as T2-weighted. As examples, the hydrogen molecules in a water-containing area, such as urine in the bladder, have longer relaxation times than those in a solid tissue such as liver. On T1-weighted images, urine in the bladder will appear dark or low signal intensity. On T2-weighted images

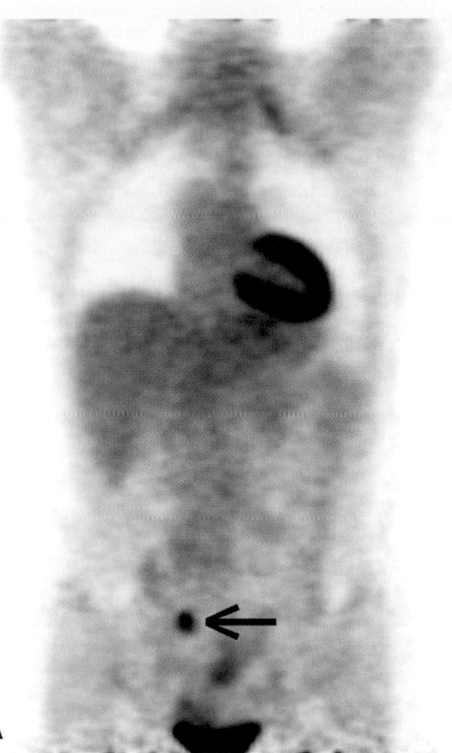

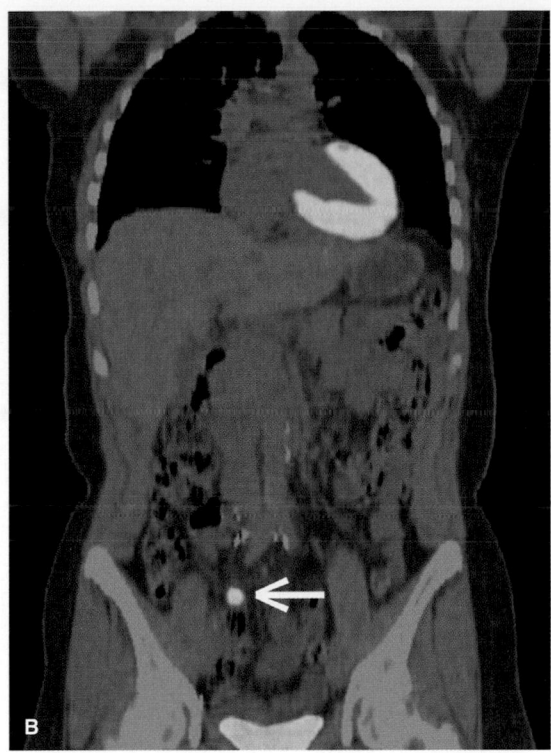

FIGURE 2-29 Positron emission tomography (PET) **(A)** and PET-CT fusion **(B)** images of a woman with recurrence of ovarian cancer. Arrows demarcate abnormal uptake of FDG in the pelvis that represented a 1-cm lymph node. The biopsy of this lymph node revealed recurrent ovarian cancer. *(Images contributed by Dr. Dana Mathews.)*

the same urine will appear bright or high signal intensity. The strength of the magnetic field within the bore of the magnet is measured in tesla (T) (1 tesla = 10,000 gauss).

Technique

The standard imaging technique includes both T1- and T2-weighted sequences, acquired in two planes, usually axial and sagittal. The T1-weighted sequence most clearly delineates organ boundaries and surrounding fat, allows optimal visualization of lymph nodes, and is necessary for tissue and fluid characterization such as hemorrhagic or fat-containing lesions (Nurenberg, 1995). The T2-weighted sequence provides detailed definition of internal organ architecture, such as the zonal anatomy of the uterus and vagina, and aids identification of normal ovaries. T2-weighted images are usually superior in depicting pathologic conditions of the uterus and ovaries.

The multiplanar capability of MR imaging allows a study to be individualized to a specific clinical question. The transverse plane of imaging is routinely acquired in all cases, with additional sequences obtained in either the sagittal or coronal plane. The sagittal plane optimizes visualization of the uterus, whereas the coronal plane is preferred for ovarian evaluation.

Some MR images have better resolution when a paramagnetic contrast agent such as gadolinium diethylenetriamine pentaacetic acid (Gd-DTPA) is given. It is routinely used for evaluation of endometrial and ovarian carcinoma. In the United States, Gd-DTPA is the only contrast material approved for MR imaging. Magnetic resonance contrast changes the local magnetic field in tissues under study. Normal and abnormal

tissues react differently to the contrast, and these differences can be displayed. Side effects are rare, and contrast can be used even if there is a history of allergy to other contrast agents (American College of Radiology, 2004). Magnetic resonance contrast is given in concentrations and doses significantly lower than that used in CT imaging, undergoes renal excretion within 24 hours, and is safe for patients with mildly compromised renal function. However, in their most recent public health advisory on MR contrast, the FDA recommends caution in administering gadolinium-based MR contrast to patients with moderate to end-stage renal disease and consideration of providing hemodialysis immediately after administration of this agent for patients in this category of renal compromise.

Safety

The effects from static magnetic fields and gradient magnetic fields generated with MR imaging have been extensively studied. To date, there are no reported harmful effects, including mutagenic effects, from MR imaging at field strengths used clinically, that is, those less than 2 tesla (American College of Radiology, 1998; Kanal, 2007; Wagner, 1997).

Some, but not all, devices preclude MR imaging. For example, women with intrauterine devices, Essure microinserts, or Filshie clips can be safely imaged. Contraindications, however, include mechanically, electrically, or magnetically activated implants or devices such as internal cardiac pacemakers, neurostimulators, implantable cardiac defibrillators, implantable electronic infusion pumps, cochlear implants, and other such devices. Certain intracranial aneurysm clips and any metallic foreign body in the globe of the eye contraindicate scanning (Cunningham, 2010a).

Use in Gynecology

Sonography is preferred for initial evaluation of suspected gynecologic disease. Magnetic resonance imaging is often used when sonographic findings are equivocal. Common indications include distorted pelvic anatomy, large masses that may be difficult to delineate with sonography, indeterminate cases of adenomyosis, and endometrial disorders in poor surgical candidates (Javitt, 2001). Multiplanar imaging, superior soft-tissue contrast, and large field of view are distinct advantages of MR imaging to assess gynecologic abnormalities (Leung, 2000). A major use of MR imaging is evaluation of pelvic malignancies. Magnetic resonance imaging is also preferable for surveillance in women with cancer because it does not employ ionizing radiation.

Normal Findings

The pelvic organs are generally moderate to low signal intensity on T1-weighted images. T2-weighted images of the menstruating uterus depict a high-signal-intensity endometrium; contiguous low-signal-intensity inner myometrium, which is the junctional zone; and a moderate-signal-intensity outer myometrium (Fig. 2-30) (McCarthy, 1986). The cervix can be distinguished

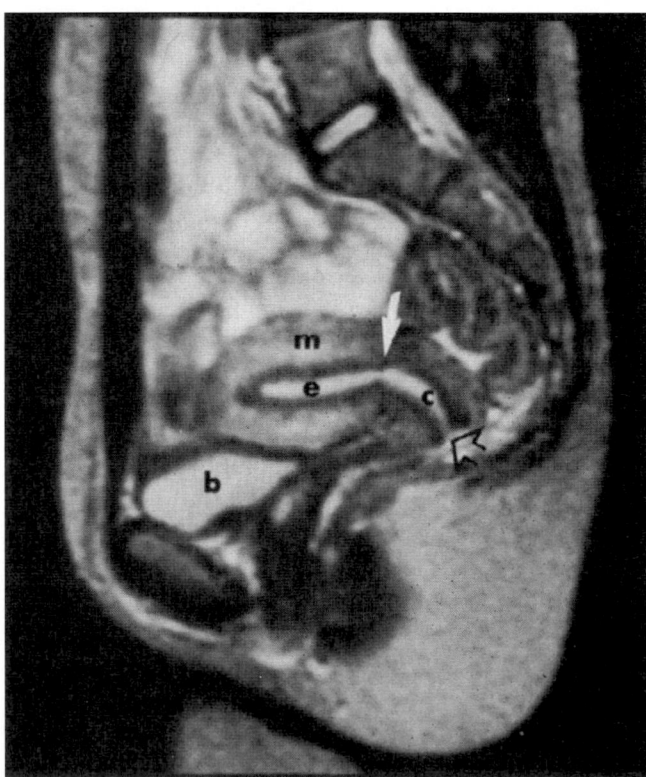

FIGURE 2-30 Sagittal T2-weighted MR image of a normal uterus and cervix. The zonal anatomy of the uterus is depicted, consisting of the endometrium **(e)** and myometrium **(m)**, separated by the dark, low-signal-intensity junctional zone. The cervix **(c)** extends from the level of the internal os (*white arrow*) to the external os (*open arrow*). **b** = bladder.

from the uterine body by its prominent fibrous stroma, which has an overall lower signal intensity. The internal architecture of the cervix is seen on T2-weighted images as central high signal intensity (endocervical glands and mucus) surrounded by low signal intensity (fibrous stroma) and peripheral moderate signal intensity (smooth muscle intermixed with fibrous stroma) (Lee, 1985). T2-weighted images of the vagina depict central high-signal-intensity mucosa and mucus that is surrounded by a low-signal-intensity muscular wall (Hricak, 1988). Ovaries are normally seen on the T2-weighted sequence as moderately high-signal-intensity stroma containing very high-signal-intensity follicles (Dooms, 1986). The fallopian tubes are not typically visualized. Hormonal status influences the MR appearance of all structures and reflects associated physiologic changes.

Magnetic Resonance Imaging in Gynecology

Uterus

Leiomyoma. Magnetic resonance imaging is the most accurate tool for evaluation of leiomyomas (Ascher, 2003). Although TVS remains the initial imaging technique for evaluating women with suspected leiomyomas, false-negative rates may reach 20 percent (Gross, 1983). Its limited field of view, decreased image resolution with increasing patient body fat, and distorted anatomy because of large or multiple leiomyomas are potentially limiting factors (Wolfman, 2006). Leiomyomas less than 2 cm are routinely not identified by TVS, even when symptomatic. Thus, MRI is used when TVS is equivocal or nondiagnostic (Ascher, 2003). Moreover, thorough MR imaging is warranted before UAE and may be used prior to hysteroscopic resection. In addition, the effects of GnRH agonist therapy to shrink leiomyoma volume can be quantified with MR imaging (Lubich, 1991).

As shown in Figure 2-31, leiomyomas have a specific MR appearance and thus can be differentiated from adenomyosis or adenomyoma with 90-percent accuracy (Mark, 1987; Togashi, 1989). This is important when myomectomy is considered, especially in cases with a single large intramural mass. Leiomyomas, even those as small as 0.5 cm, are best seen on T2-weighted images and appear as round, sharply marginated, low-signal-intensity masses relative to the myometrium (Hricak, 1986). Multiplanar views allow for accurate localization as subserosal, intramural, or submucosal. Although not required for management in most cases, the stalk of a prolapsed submucosal leiomyoma can be reliably identified with MR imaging, and its accessibility to hysteroscopic resection can be confirmed. Intramural or subserosal leiomyomas are frequently circumscribed by a high-signal-intensity rim that represents edema from dilated lymphatics and veins. Tumors larger than 3 cm often are heterogeneous because of varying degrees and types of degeneration (Chap. 9, p. 247) (Hricak, 1986; Yamashita, 1993).

As stated earlier, MR imaging is the diagnostic method of choice for preoperative and postprocedural evaluation before UAE (Usadi, 2007). Leiomyoma size, number, and location are critical predictors of procedure success and safety. Moreover, MR imaging depicts these variables more accurately and with less intraobserver variability than sonography (Cura,

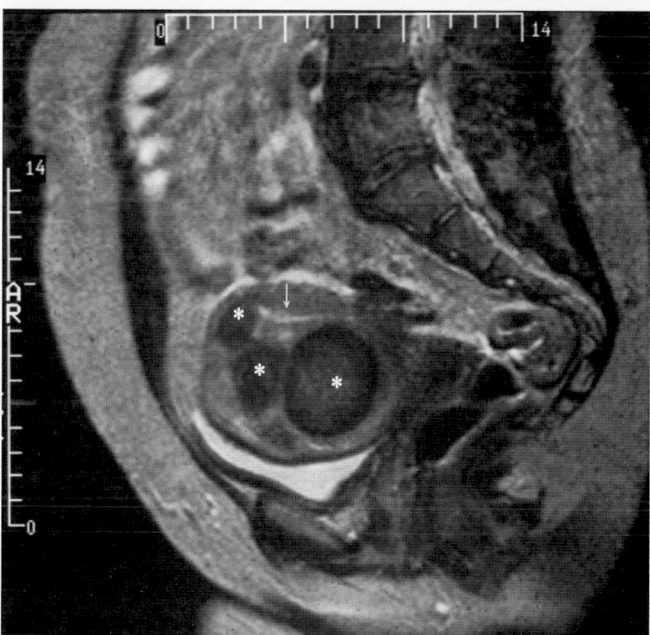

FIGURE 2-31 Sagittal T2-weighted MR image of a uterus demonstrating three leiomyomas. The leiomyomas (*) appear as round, sharply marginated, dark, low-signal-intensity masses in the posterior myometrium. The endometrium is identified as the bright, high-signal-intensity line anterior to the leiomyomas (*arrow*).

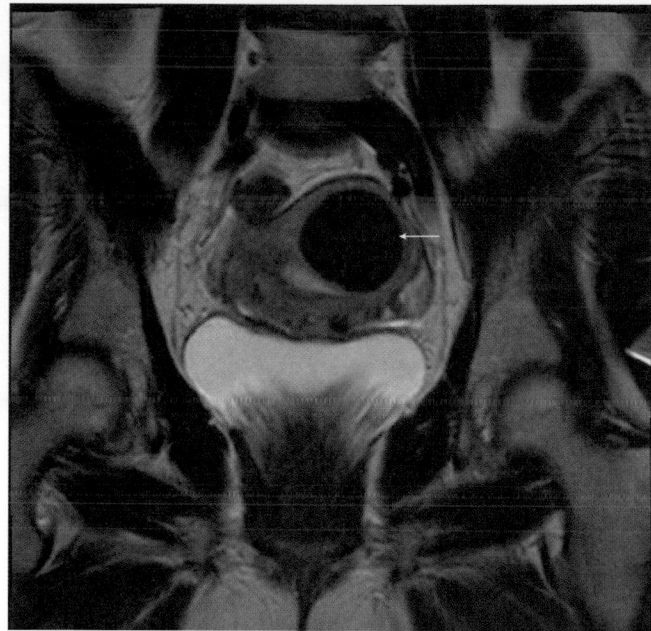

FIGURE 2-32 Coronal T2-weighted MR image of a uterus after uterine artery embolization (UAE). The mural fibroid (*arrow*), having undergone degeneration status post embolization, appears dark and does not enhance after administration of gadolinium contrast. (*Image contributed by Dr. Samuel C. Chao.*)

2006). Hypervascularity, which is seen as a bright signal on T2-weighted images after intravenous gadolinium, correlates with a good response to UAE (Jha, 2000). In contrast, leiomyomas with negligible enhancement and high signal intensity on T1-weighted sequences do not respond to UAE. Contrast MR imaging is also useful for monitoring tumor response after UAE. Successfully embolized leiomyomas demonstrate a decrease in size and no enhancement with contrast, consistent with degeneration (Fig. 2-32) (DeSouza, 1999).

Magnetic resonance imaging guidance of focused ultrasound (MRgFUS) therapy has been used to treat symptomatic leiomyomas (Cline, 1992). Without MR guidance, focused ultrasound therapy is hampered by difficulty in precise beam targeting and in receiving feedback regarding thermal damage. Fortunately, excellent soft-tissue resolution with MR imaging enables precise tissue targeting. Moreover, MR imaging can measure accurate, near real-time thermometry, and thermal damage created by focused ultrasound can be assessed immediately (Hindley, 2004).

A series of high-power ultrasound pulses—sonications—are directed into the leiomyoma, and power is adjusted until an adequate temperature and thermal dose is reached. Pulse duration is generally about 15 seconds, and the interval between pulses, 3 minutes, allows tissues to cool between treatments. The average procedure duration is approximately 3½ hours (Hindley, 2004).

Magnetic resonance imaging guidance of focused ultrasound therapy has been shown to be a safe and feasible minimally invasive alternative for leiomyoma treatment (Chen, 2005; Hesley, 2008; Hudson, 2008; Stewart, 2003). Several studies have demonstrated a relatively rapid improvement in

patient symptoms, a continued decrease in the leiomyoma size over time, a quicker recovery, and few major adverse events in comparison with UAE or myomectomy (Fennessy, 2007; Hindley, 2004; Stewart, 2006, 2007). However, little information is available on costs and long-term results compared with other interventional treatments. Moreover, not all patients are suitable candidates. Obstructions to the energy path such as abdominal wall scars or intraabdominal clips, total uterine size >24 weeks, a desire for future fertility, or general contraindications to MR imaging are limitations. Moreover, leiomyoma characteristics such as size, blood perfusion qualities, or location near adjacent organs may limit feasibility. Other areas of ongoing gynecologic research with this technique include its use in women with symptomatic fibroids desiring future fertility, tumors >10 cm, and adenomyosis (Hesley, 2008).

Adenomyosis. Magnetic resonance imaging has been shown to be equivalent or superior to sonography to diagnose adenomyosis, with a sensitivity of 88 to 93 percent and a specificity of 66 to 91 percent (Ascher, 1994; Reinhold, 1996). The principal advantages of MR imaging over sonography include the reliability of MR to diagnose adenomyosis, particularly focal adenomyomas, in the setting of concomitant pathology such as leiomyomas, and the reproducibility of MR, which allows for accurate treatment monitoring (Reinhold, 1995).

The contrast of adenomyosis to the sharply demarcated, homogeneous MR imaging appearance of leiomyomas is shown in Figure 2-33. Areas of adenomyosis contain internal punctate foci of increased signal on both T1- and T2-weighted images, and they are oval with ill-defined margins (Togashi, 1988, 1989). The high-signal-intensity foci represent ectopic

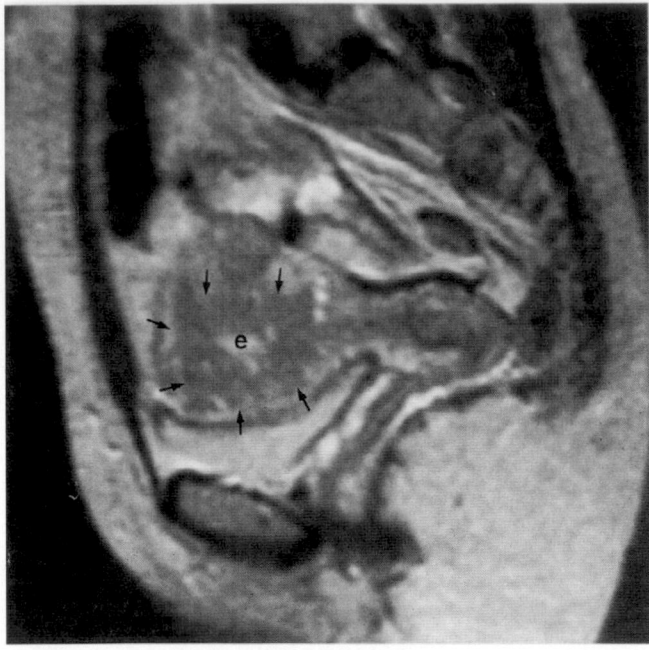

FIGURE 2-33 Sagittal T2-weighted MR image of a uterus with diffuse adenomyosis. Adenomyosis is shown as circumferential thickening of the junctional zone (*arrows*). **e** = endometrium.

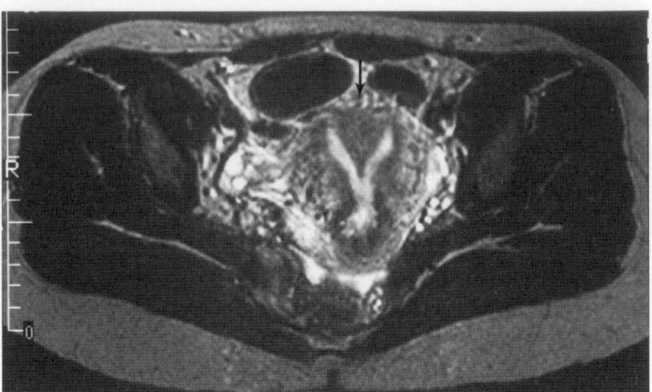

FIGURE 2-34 Transaxial T2-weighted MR image of a septate uterus. A low-signal-intensity fibrous septum (*arrow*) separates the two high-signal-intensity endometrial cavities, and the fundal contour is normal, without indentation.

endometrium and cystically dilated endometrial glands, with or without hemorrhage (Reinhold, 1995, 1996). Diffuse areas of adenomyosis will be evident by thickening of the low-signal-intensity junctional zone (inner myometrium) to ≥12 mm and by linear high-signal-intensity T2-weighted striations radiating out from the endometrial surface. These striations are thought to represent direct invasion of the endometrial basalis layer into the underlying myometrium. Contrast administration does not increase the diagnostic accuracy for adenomyosis (Outwater, 1998).

Congenital Anomalies. As discussed in detail in Chapter 18 (p. 495), müllerian duct anomalies comprise a spectrum of developmental malformations associated with varying degrees of adverse reproductive outcomes. In the past, full evaluation required laparoscopy, laparotomy, HSG, and hysteroscopy. These invasive techniques were largely replaced by MR imaging, which has an accuracy of up to 100 percent (Carrington, 1990; Doyle, 1992; Fielding, 1996; Pellerito, 1992a; Troiano, 2003). As discussed earlier, with advances in 3-D sonography techniques, sonographic evaluation with 3-D image reconstruction, with or without saline infusion, can also be used for diagnosis of müllerian anomalies (Coyne, 2008).

One such example for which MR imaging is particularly adept is differentiation of septate and bicornuate uteri, which is imperative with regard to their clinical implications and surgical treatment. The dividing septum in a bicornuate uterus is composed of myometrium and with MR imaging, is characterized by signal intensity consistent with myometrium. The endometrium of a bicornuate uterus has a normal width and lines two uterine cavities that communicate, as demonstrated by their confluent signal intensity (Carrington, 1990; Fedele, 1989; Pellerito, 1992a). The fundal contour as seen in true coronal sequences is concave. Finally, the

bicornuate uterus typically has a significant fundal notch—larger than 1 cm—between the two horns, and the intercornual distance is greater than 4 cm (Carrington, 1990; Fedele, 1989; Pellerito, 1992a).

The septate uterus is a result of incomplete resorption of the final fibrous septum between the two uterine horns. It is composed of collagen, which has low signal intensity on both T1- and T2-weighted images (Fig. 2-34). The fundal contour of the septate uterus can be convex, flattened, or mildly concave, but the fundal notch is less than 1 cm (Leung, 2000). Also in contrast to the bicornuate uterus, the intercornual distance of the septate uterus is not increased, and thus each uterine cavity is smaller than usual (Carrington, 1990; Forstner, 1994).

Magnetic resonance imaging is also used for more detailed evaluation of a unicornuate uterus and its rudimentary horn. It can determine whether endometrium is contained within the rudimentary horn and whether the horn communicates with the main uterine cavity, a finding of considerable clinical importance (Chap. 18, p. 497) (Leung, 2000). Magnetic resonance imaging can also identify uterine didelphys (Fig. 2-35). Lastly, the superior resolution of MR imaging is also important for planning surgical treatment of cloacal anomalies (Nurenberg, 1995; Pena, 1990).

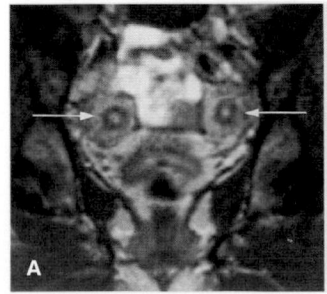
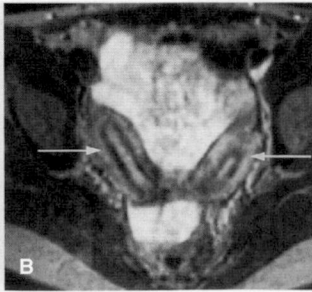

FIGURE 2-35 Uterine didelphys. **A.** Coronal T2-weighted MR image demonstrates two distinct and widely separate endometrial cavities (*arrows*). **B.** Transaxial T2-weighted MR image shows two distinct uterine horns (*arrows*).

Adnexal Masses

Sonography is preferred for initial evaluation of adnexal masses, whereas MR imaging is useful to further characterize adnexal masses whose evaluation by sonography is nondiagnostic or inconclusive (Adusumilli, 2006). Magnetic resonance imaging frequently can provide additional information on soft-tissue composition, for example, differentiating adnexal from pedunculated uterine masses. Magnetic resonance imaging also allows for multiplanar imaging of a larger field of view, which is helpful in defining the origin and extent of pelvic pathology that may be nongynecologic (Foshager, 1996). Because MR imaging does not use ionizing radiation, it may be particularly useful in pregnant women for the characterization of symptomatic or incidentally found adnexal masses with inconclusive sonographic diagnoses (Rajkotia, 2006). Although both sonography and MR imaging are highly sensitive for the detection of adnexal malignancy, MR imaging is slightly more specific (Adusumilli, 2006; Funt, 2002; Jeong, 2000; Sohaib, 2005; Yamashita, 1995).

Endometrial Lesions

Transvaginal sonography and SIS are preferred for characterization of endometrial lesions, such as polyps and endometrial hyperplasia. Magnetic resonance imaging may be helpful when these modalities are nondiagnostic in a patient who is a poor surgical candidate for direct endometrial sampling.

Gynecologic Malignancies

Cervical Cancer. Although not used for screening, MR imaging is excellent for preoperative assessment of gynecologic neoplasms. Its superior soft-tissue contrast resolution and ability to image directly in multiple planes allow evaluation of lymphadenopathy and local tumor extension.

Although CT imaging is typically used for assessment of nodal disease and distant metastases, MR imaging consistently outperforms clinical and CT evaluation of cervical cancer in the assessment of local tumor extension (Choi, 2004; Durfee, 2000; Hricak, 1996, 2007; Narayan, 2003). Current recommendations for MR imaging with cervical cancer include tumor with a transverse diameter >2 cm by physical examination, endocervical or predominately infiltrative tumors that cannot be accurately assessed clinically, and women who are pregnant or have concomitant uterine lesions, such as leiomyomas, that make evaluation difficult (Ascher, 2001; Hricak, 2007). When the extent of parametrial and sidewall invasion is unclear clinically, MR imaging may play an important role in their evaluation (Ascher, 2001). It has a 95- to 98-percent negative-predictive value for parametrial invasion, allowing the absence of parametrial invasion to be determined with confidence (Hricak, 2007; Subak, 1995).

Endometrial Carcinoma. Surgery is currently the most accurate staging method. For the same advantages cited for cervical cancer, MR imaging has recently been gaining acceptance to evaluate endometrial carcinoma (Ascher, 2001). Knowledge of the degree of myometrial and cervical extension affects type of hysterectomy selected, lymph node dissection, and decision to use preoperative intracavitary radiation (Boronow, 1984; Frei, 2000; Larson, 1996). Magnetic resonance imaging has a 92-percent accuracy in staging endometrial cancer, and an 82-percent accuracy in assessing myometrial invasion depth (Hricak, 1987). Therefore, MR imaging is recommended if lymph node metastases are likely, such as from a high-grade tumor; with papillary or clear cell histology; with cervical invasion; or if multifactorial assessment of myometrial, cervical, and lymph node involvement is required (Ascher, 2001).

Ovarian Cancer. Magnetic resonance imaging for ovarian neoplasms is reserved for evaluation when TVS or CT scanning is indeterminate or nondiagnostic. This stems from its increased cost over the other two modalities, decreased availability, and longer imaging and interpretation times (Javitt, 2007; Nurenberg, 1995). Magnetic resonance imaging is particularly useful to assess adnexal mass origin—uterine, ovarian, or nongynecologic—and if ovarian in origin, to determine whether the mass is neoplastic versus nonneoplastic and malignant versus benign (Ascher, 2001). Magnetic resonance imaging is also recommended in pregnant patients and in those with a contraindication to iodinated contrast agents.

Sensitivity of MR imaging for detecting adnexal pathology ranges from 87 to 100 percent and is therefore similar to that of sonography and CT scanning (Siegelman, 1999). The advantages of MR imaging compared with CT scanning in the evaluation of suspected ovarian cancer include its multiplanar capability, its superior contrast resolution, and its increased sensitivity for detecting uterine invasion, extrapelvic peritoneal and lymph node metastases, and tumor extension to omentum, bowel, bone, and vessels (Low, 1995; Tempany, 2000).

Magnetic resonance evaluation of an adnexal mass should include gadolinium-enhanced images to assess tumor vascularity and fat-saturation techniques to differentiate blood from fat in T1-weighted high-signal-intensity lesions (Ascher, 2001). Although histology cannot be diagnosed, findings that are suspicious for malignancy include enhancing solid components, thick septations, nodules, and/or papillary projections.

Urogynecology

Very-fast-sequence MR imaging, termed *dynamic imaging,* allows detailed delineation of the female urethra, levator ani muscles, and surrounding pelvic structures in women with stress urinary incontinence or prolapse of the bladder, uterus, or rectum (Pannu, 2002). Magnetic resonance imaging can be used in the initial evaluation of patients with pelvic organ descent. This may be especially helpful in those who have symptoms of multicompartmental involvement and are being evaluated before a complex pelvic floor reconstruction or in those who have failed previous repairs (Macura, 2006). Grading systems of pelvic organ prolapse and pelvic floor relaxation based on dynamic imaging have been developed (Barbaric, 2001; Fielding, 2000, 2003). Other MR imaging techniques have also been developed for prolapse evaluation. These include upright patient imaging to approximate more normal evacuation positions, placement of various contrast materials into the vagina and rectum to assess vaginal vault prolapse and rectocele, and a suitable replacement for defecography to evaluate prolapse (Bo, 2001; Fielding, 1998; Kelvin, 2000; Lienemann, 2000; Schoenberger, 1998). More recently, MR imaging with

3-D reconstruction has been used to describe levator muscle morphometry in term pregnant nulliparous women to evaluate the effect of pregnancy on the pelvic floor (Boreham, 2005). In the future, improved evaluation of pelvic floor dysfunction with MR imaging can be expected with the routine implementation of upright dynamic imaging in open-configuration MR systems, enhanced visualization of anatomic details achieved with higher magnetic field strength magnets, and standard use of 3-D reconstructions of the pelvic floor (Macura, 2006).

REFERENCES

Abrams BJ, Sukmvanich P, Seibel R, et al: Ultrasound for the detection of intraperitoneal fluid: the role of Trendelenburg position. Am J Emerg Med 17:117, 1999

Adusumilli S, Hussain HK, Caoili EM, et al: MR imaging of sonographically indeterminate adnexal masses. AJR Am J Roentgenol 187:732, 2006

Alcazar JL, Castillo G, Minquez JA, et al: Endometrial blood flow mapping using transvaginal power Doppler sonography in women with postmenopausal bleeding and the thickened endometrium. Ultrasound Obstet Gynecol 21:583, 2003a

Alcazar JL, Galan MJ, Garcia-Manero M, et al: Three-dimensional sonographic morphologic assessment in complex adnexal masses: preliminary experience. J Ultrasound Med 22:249, 2003b

Alcazar JL, Galvan R: Three-dimensional power Doppler ultrasound scanning for the prediction of endometrial cancer in women with postmenopausal bleeding and thickened endometrium. Am J Obstet Gynecol 200:44.e1, 2009

American Association of Endocrinologists: AACE clinical practice guidelines for the prevention and treatment of postmenopausal osteoporosis. Endo Pract 2:157, 1996

American College of Obstetricians and Gynecologists: Antibiotic prophylaxis for gynecologic procedures. Practice Bulletin No. 104, May 2009

American College of Obstetricians and Gynecologists: Prevention of deep vein thrombosis and pulmonary embolism. Practice Bulletin No. 21, October 2000a

American College of Obstetricians and Gynecologists: Thromboembolism in pregnancy. Practice Bulletin No. 19, June 2000b

American College of Radiology: Committee on drugs and contrast media. Manual on contrast media, 5.0 ed. Reston, VA: American College of Radiology Standards, 2004

American College of Radiology: MR safety and sedation. American College of Radiology Standards 457, 1998

American Institute of Ultrasound in Medicine: Guidelines for performance of the ultrasound examination of the female pelvis. 2009. Available at: http://www.aium.org/publications/guidelines/pelvis.pdf. Accessed October 24, 2010

American Institute of Ultrasound in Medicine: Safety considerations for diagnostic ultrasound. AIUM Bioeffects Committee, 1991

Ameye L, Valentin L, Testa AC, et al: A scoring system to differentiate malignant from benign masses in specific ultrasound-based subgroups of adnexal tumors. Ultrasound Obstet Gynecol 33:92, 2009

Andreotti R, Fleischer AC: The sonographic diagnosis of adenomyosis. Ultrasound Q 21:167, 2005

Andreotti RF, Fleischer AC, Mason LE Jr: Three-dimensional sonography of the endometrium and adjacent myometrium: preliminary observations. J Ultrasound Med 25(10):1313, 2006

Andrews E, Jr, Fleischer A: Sonography for deep venous thrombosis: current and future applications. Ultrasound Q 21:213, 2005

Armstrong P, Hawnaur JM, Reznek RH, et al: Imaging techniques. In Armstrong P, Wastie ML (eds): A Concise Textbook of Radiology. London, Arnold, 2001, p 1

Aruh I, Uran B, Demir N: Conservative approach in unruptured cornual pregnancy with a live fetus. Int J Gynecol Obstet 59:43, 1997

Ascher SM, Arnold LL, Patt RH, et al: Adenomyosis: prospective comparison of MR imaging and transvaginal sonography. Radiology 190:803, 1994

Ascher SM, Jha RC, Reinhold C: Benign myometrial conditions: leiomyomas and adenomyosis. Top Magn Reson Imaging 14:281, 2003

Ascher SM, Takahama J, Jha RC: Staging of gynecologic malignancies. Top Magn Reson Imaging 12:105, 2001

Atri M, Nazarnia S, Aldis AE: Transvaginal US appearance of endometrial abnormalities. Radiographics 14:483, 1994

Atri M, Reinhold C, Mehio AR, et al: Adenomyosis: US features with histologic correlation in an in-vitro study. Radiology 215:783, 2000

Baber RJ, McSweeney MB, Gill RW, et al: Transvaginal pulsed Doppler ultrasound assessment of blood flow to the corpus luteum in IVF patients following embryo transfer. Br J Obstet Gynaecol 95:1226, 1988

Barbaric ZL, Marumoto AL, Raz S: Magnetic resonance imaging of the perineum and pelvic floor. Top Magn Reson Imaging 12:83, 2001

Barnhart K, Coutifaris C: The use of ultrasound in the evaluation and treatment of the infertile woman. In Bluth EI, Arger PH, Benson CB, et al (eds): Ultrasound: a practical approach to clinical problems. Stuttgart, Thieme, 2000, p 257

Bates SM, Ginsberg JS: Treatment of deep-vein thrombosis. N Engl J Med 351:268, 2004

Belhocine T, De Barsy C, Hustinx R, et al: Usefulness of (18)F-FDG PET in the posttherapy surveillance of endometrial carcinoma. Eur J Nucl Med Mol Imaging 29:1132, 2002

Benacerraf BR, Shipp TD, Bromley B: Three-dimensional ultrasound detection of abnormally located intrauterine contraceptive devices which are a source of pelvic pain and abnormal bleeding. Ultrasound Obstet Gynecol 34:110, 2009

Benacerraf BR, Shipp TD, Bromley B: Which patients benefit from a 3D reconstructed coronal view of the uterus added to standard routine 2D pelvic sonography? AJR Am J Roentgenol 190(3):626, 2008

Bermejo C, Martinez Ten P, Cantarero R, et al: Three-dimensional ultrasound in the diagnosis of Müllerian duct anomalies and concordance with magnetic resonance imaging. Ultrasound Obstet Gynecol 35:593, 2010

Bertelli G, Valenzano M, Costantini S, et al: Limited value of sonohysterography for endometrial screening in asymptomatic, postmenopausal patients treated with tamoxifen. Gynecol Oncol 78:275, 2000

Beyersdorff D, Zhang J, Schoder H, et al: Bladder cancer: can imaging change patient management? Curr Opin Urol 18:98, 2008

Birdwell BG, Raskob GE, Whitsett TL, et al: The clinical validity of normal compression ultrasonography in outpatients suspected of having deep venous thrombosis. Ann Intern Med 128(1):1, 1998

Blake GM, Fogelman I: Role of dual-energy X-ray absorptiometry in the diagnosis and treatment of osteoporosis. J Clin Densitom 10:102, 2007

Bo K, Lilleas F, Talseth T, et al: Dynamic MRI of the pelvic floor muscles in an upright sitting position. Neurourol Urodyn 20:167, 2001

Boardman LA, Peipert JF, Brody JM, et al: Endovaginal sonography for the diagnosis of upper genital tract infection. Obstet Gynecol 90:54, 1997

Bonilla-Musoles F, Raga F, Osborne NG, et al: Control of intrauterine device insertion with three-dimensional ultrasound: is it the future? J Clin Ultrasound 24:263, 1996

Bonilla-Musoles F, Raga F, Osborne NG, et al: Three-dimensional hysterosonography for the study of endometrial tumors: comparison with conventional transvaginal sonography, hysterosalpingography, and hysteroscopy. Gynecol Oncol 65:245, 1997

Bonilla-Musoles F, Raga F, Osborne NG: Three-dimensional ultrasound evaluation of ovarian masses. Gynecol Oncol 59:129, 1995

Bonnamy L, Marret H, Perrotin F, et al: Sonohysterography: a prospective survey of results and complications in 81 patients. Eur J Obstet Gynecol Reprod Biol 102:42, 2002

Boreham MK, Zaretsky MV, Corton MM, et al: Appearance of the levator ani muscle in pregnancy as assessed by 3-D MRI. Am J Obstet Gynecol 193:2159, 2005

Boronow RC, Morrow CP, Creasman WT, et al: Surgical staging in endometrial cancer: clinical-pathologic findings of a prospective study. Obstet Gynecol 63:825, 1984

Bourne TH: Evaluating the endometrium of postmenopausal women with transvaginal ultrasonography. Ultrasound Obstet Gynecol 6:75, 1995

Bradley LD, Falcone T, Magen AB: Radiographic imaging techniques for the diagnosis of abnormal uterine bleeding. Obstet Gynecol Clin North Am 27:245, 2000

Branney SW, Wolfe RE, Moore EE, et al: Quantitative sensitivity of ultrasound in detecting free intraperitoneal fluid. J Trauma 39:375, 1995

Brosens JJ, de Souza NM, Barker FG, et al: Endovaginal ultrasonography in the diagnosis of adenomyosis uteri: identifying the predictive characteristics. Br J Obstet Gynaecol 102:471, 1995

Brown DL, Frates MC, Laing FC, et al: Ovarian masses: can benign and malignant lesions be differentiated with color and pulsed Doppler US? Radiology 190:333, 1994

Bussey LA, Laing FC: Sonohysterography for detection of a retained laminaria fragment. J Ultrasound Med 15:249, 1996

Buy JN, Ghossain MA, Hugol D, et al: Characterization of adnexal masses: combination of color Doppler and conventional sonography compared with spectral Doppler analysis alone and conventional sonography alone. AJR Am J Roentgenol 166:385, 1996

Cacciatore B, Leminen A, Ingman-Friberg S, et al: Transvaginal sonographic findings in ambulatory patients with suspected pelvic inflammatory disease. Obstet Gynecol 80:912, 1992

Campbell S, Bourne TH, Tan SL, et al: Hysterosalpingocontrast sonography (HyCoSy) and its future role within the investigation of infertility in Europe. Ultrasound Obstet Gynecol 4:245, 1994

Capitanio GL, Ferraiolo A, Croce S, et al: Transcervical selective salpingography: a diagnostic and therapeutic approach to cases of proximal tubal injection failure. Fertil Steril 55:1045, 1991

Carr MW, Grey ML: Magnetic resonance imaging. Am J Nurs 102:26, 2002

Carrington BM, Hricak H, Nuruddin RN, et al: Müllerian duct anomalies: MR imaging evaluation. Radiology 176:715, 1990

Chan DP, Abujudeh HH, Cushing GL Jr, et al: CT cystography with multiplanar reformation for suspected bladder rupture: experience in 234 cases. AJR Am J Roentgenol 187:1296, 2006

Chen S: MRI-guided focused ultrasound treatment of uterine fibroids. Issues Emerg Health Technol 2005, p 1

Chia CC, Huang SC, Chen SS et al: Ultrasonographic evaluation of the change in uterine fibroids induced by treatment with a GnRH analog. Taiwan J Obstet Gynecol 45:124, 2006

Choi SH, Kim SH, Choi HJ, et al: Preoperative magnetic resonance imaging staging of uterine cervical carcinoma: results of prospective study. J Comput Assist Tomogr 28:620, 2004

Chou CP, Levenson RB, Elsayes KM, et al: Imaging of female urethral diverticulum: an update. Radiographics 28(7):1917, 2008

Cicinelli E, Romano F, Anastasio PS, et al: Transabdominal sonohysterography, transvaginal sonography, and hysteroscopy in the evaluation of submucous myomas. Obstet Gynecol 85:42, 1995

Cline HE, Schenck JF, Hynynen K, et al: MR-guided focused ultrasound surgery. J Comput Assist Tomogr 16:956, 1992

Coccia ME, Becattini C, Bracco GL, et al: Pressure lavage under ultrasound guidance: a new approach for outpatient treatment of intrauterine adhesions. Fertil Steril 75:601, 2001

Cohen HL, Tice HM, Mandel FS: Ovarian volumes measured by US: bigger than we think. Radiology 177:189, 1990

Conceptus: Essure. 2009. Available at: http://www.essuremd.com/portals/essuremd/PDFs/TopDownloads/L3002%2009_09%20smaller.pdf. Accessed November 28, 2010

Condous G: Ultrasound diagnosis of ectopic pregnancy. Semin Reprod Med 2:85, 2007

Constant O, Cooke J, Parsons CA: Reformatted computed tomography of the female pelvis: normal anatomy. Br J Obstet Gynaecol 96:1047, 1989

Coyne L, Kannamannadiar J, Raine-Fenning N: 3D ultrasound in gynecology and reproductive medicine. Women's Health 4(5):501, 2008

Cundiff G, Carr BR, Marshburn PB: Infertile couples with a normal hysterosalpingogram. Reproductive outcome and its relationship to clinical and laparoscopic findings. J Reprod Med 40:19, 1995

Cunningham FG, Leveno KL, Bloom SL, et al (eds): General considerations and maternal evaluation. In Williams Obstetrics, 23rd ed. New York, McGraw-Hill, 2010a, p 973

Cunningham FG, Leveno KL, Bloom SL, et al (eds): Implantation, embryogenesis, and placental development. In Williams Obstetrics, 23rd ed. New York, McGraw-Hill, 2010b, p 45

Cunningham FG, Leveno KL, Bloom SL, et al (eds): Thromboembolic disorders. In Williams Obstetrics, 23rd ed. New York, McGraw-Hill, 2010c, p 1020

Cunningham FG, Leveno KL, Bloom SL, et al (eds): Ultrasound and Doppler. In Williams Obstetrics, 23rd ed. New York, McGraw-Hill, 2010d, p 390

Cura M, Cura A, Bugnone A: Role of magnetic resonance imaging in patient selection for uterine artery embolization. Acta Radiol 47:1105, 2006

Damilakis J, Maris T, Karantanas A: An update on the assessment of osteoporosis using radiologic techniques. European Radiology 17:1591, 2007

Daneshgari F, Zimmern PE, Jacomides L: Magnetic resonance imaging detection of symptomatic noncommunicating intraurethral wall diverticula in women. J Urol 161:1259, 1999

Das S, Nardo LG, Seif MW: Proximal tubal disease: the place for tubal cannulation. Reprod Biomed Online 15:383, 2007

Davis JD: Prevention, diagnosis, and treatment of venous thromboembolic complications of gynecologic surgery. Am J Obstet Gynecol 184:759, 2001

Degenhardt F, Jibril S, Eisenhauer B: Hysterosalpingo-contrast-sonography (HyCoSy) for determining tubal patency. Clin Radiology 51:15, 1996

Delbeke D, Martin WH: Positron emission tomography imaging in oncology. Radiol Clin North Am 39:883, 2001

DePriest PD, Shenson D, Fried A, et al: A morphology index based on sonographic findings in ovarian cancer. Gynecol Oncol 51:7, 1993

Desai RK, Desberg LD: Diagnosis of gestational trophoblastic disease: value of endovaginal color flow Doppler sonography. AJR Am J Roentgenol 157:787, 1991

De Smet F, De Brabanter J, Van den Bosch T, et al: New models to predict depth of infiltration in endometrial carcinoma based on transvaginal sonography. Ultrasound Obstet Gynecol 27:664, 2006

DeSouza NM, Williams AD, Larkman DJ, et al: Uterine arterial embolization for leiomyomas: Monitoring of immediate and late perfusion changes with MRI. Proc Int Soc Magn Reson Med 1999, p 1119

Deutch TD, Joergner I, Matson DO, et al: Automated assessment of ovarian follicles using a novel three-dimensional ultrasound software. Fertil Steril 92(5):1562, 2009

de Ziegler D: Contrast ultrasound: a simple-to-use phase-shifting medium offers saline infusion sonography-like images. Fertil Steril 92:369, 2009

Dietz HP: Quantification of major morphological abnormalities of the levator ani. Ultrasound Obstet Gynecol 29:329, 2007

Dietz HP: Ultrasound imaging of the pelvic floor. Part II: three-dimensional or volume imaging. Ultrasound Obstet Gynecol 23:615, 2004

Dill-Macky MJ, Atri M: Ovarian sonography. In Callen PW (eds): Ultrasonography in Obstetrics & Gynecology, 4th ed., Philadelphia, Saunders, 2000, p 857

Dooms GC, Hricak H, Tscholakoff D: Adnexal structures: MR imaging. Radiology 158:639, 1986

Doubilet PM: Vaginal bleeding — postmenopausal. In Bluth EI, Arger PH, Benson CB, et al (eds): Ultrasound: A Practical Approach to Clinical Problems. New York, Thieme, 2000, p 237

Doyle MB: Magnetic resonance imaging in müllerian fusion defects. J Reprod Med 37:33, 1992

Drieskens O, Stroobants S, Gysen M, et al: Positron emission tomography with FDG in the detection of peritoneal and retroperitoneal metastases of ovarian cancer. Gynecol Obstet Invest 55:130, 2003

Dubinsky TJ, Reed S, Mao C, et al: Hysterosonographically guided endometrial biopsy: technical feasibility. AJR Am J Roentgenol 174:1589, 2000

Dubinsky TJ, Stroehlein K, Abu-Ghazzeh Y, et al: Prediction of benign and malignant endometrial disease: hysterosonographic-pathologic correlation. Radiology 210:393, 1999

Durfee SM, Zou KH, Muto MG, et al: The role of magnetic resonance imaging in treatment planning of cervical carcinoma. J Women's Imaging 2:63, 2000

Ekerhovd E, Fried, G, Granberg, S: An ultrasound-based approach to the assessment of infertility, including the evaluation of tubal patency. Best Pract Res Clin Obstet Gynaecol 18(1):13, 2004

Elsayes KM, Mukundan G, Narra VR, et al: Endovaginal magnetic resonance imaging of the female urethra. J Comput Assist Tomogr 30:1, 2006

Emanuel MH, Verdel MJ, Wamsteker K, et al: A prospective comparison of transvaginal ultrasonography and diagnostic hysteroscopy in the evaluation of patients with abnormal uterine bleeding: clinical implications. Am J Obstet Gynecol 172:547, 1995

Epstein E, Skoop L, Isburg PE, et al: An algorithm including results of grayscale and power Doppler ultrasound examination to predict endometrical malignancy in women with postmenopausal bleeding. Ultrasound Obstet Gynecol 20:370, 2002

Epstein E, Valentin L: Gray-scale ultrasound morphology in the presence of absence of intrautrine fluid and vascularity as assesses by color Doppler for discimation between benign and maligant end ometrium in women with postmenopausal bleeding. Ultrasound Obstet Gynecol 28:89, 2006

Exacoustos C, Brienza L, Di Giovanni A, et al: Adenomyosis: three-dimensional sonographic findings of the junctional zone and correlation with histology. Ultrasound Obstet Gynecol 37(4):471, 2011

Exalto N, Stappers C, Emanuel MH, et al: Gel instillation, a new technique for sonohysterography. Hum Reprod 19:I206, 2004

Farquhar C, Ekeroma A, Furness S, et al: A systematic review of transvaginal ultrasonography, sonohysterography and hysteroscopy for the investigation of abnormal uterine bleeding in premenopausal women. Acta Obstet Gynecol Scand 82:493, 2003

Fedele L, Bianchi S, Dorta M, et al: Transvaginal ultrasonography in the diagnosis of diffuse adenomyosis. Fertil Steril 58:94, 1992

Fedele L, Dorta M, Brioschi D, et al: Magnetic resonance evaluation of double uteri. Obstet Gynecol 74(6):844, 1989

Fennessy FM, Tempany CM, McDannold NJ, et al: Uterine leiomyomas: MR imaging-guided focused ultrasound surgery-results of different treatment protocols. Radiology 243:885, 2007

Ferraiolo A, Ferraro F, Remorgida V, et al: Unexpected pregnancies after tubal recanalization failure with selective catheterization. Fertil Steril 63:299, 1995

Ferrazzi E, Torri V, Trio D, et al: Sonographic endometrial thickness: a useful test to predict atrophy in patients with postmenopausal bleeding. An Italian multicenter study. Ultrasound Obstet Gynecol 7:31, 1996

Fielding JR: MR imaging of Müllerian anomalies: impact on therapy. AJR Am J Roentgenol 167:1491, 1996

Fielding JR: MR imaging of pelvic floor relaxation. Radiol Clin North Am 41:747, 2003

Fielding JR, Dumanli H, Schreyer AG, et al: MR-based three-dimensional modeling of the normal pelvic floor in women: quantification of muscle mass. AJR Am J Roentgenol 174:657, 2000

Fielding JR, Griffiths DJ, Versi E, et al: MR imaging of pelvic floor continence mechanisms in the supine and sitting positions. AJR Am J Roentgenol 171:1607, 1998

Filly RA: Ectopic pregnancy: the role of sonography. Radiology 162:661, 1987

Fleischer AC: Gynecologic sonography: instrumentation and techniques. In Fleischer AC, Javitt MC, Jeffrey RB, et al (eds): Clinical Gynecologic Imaging. Lippincott-Raven, 1997a, p 1

Fleischer AC, Cullinan JA, Jones HW: Transvaginal sonography and sonohysterography of endometrial disorders. In Fleischer AC, Javitt MC, Jeffrey RB, Jones HW (eds): Clinical Gynecologic Imaging. Philadelphia, Lippincott-Raven, 1997b, p 150

Fleischer AC, Cullinan JA, Parsons AK: Sonohysterography and sonohysterosalpingography. In Fleischer AC, Javitt MC, Jeffrey RB, et al (eds): Clinical Gynecologic Imaging. Philadelphia, Lippincott-Raven, 1997c, p 315

Fleischer AC, Donnelly EF, Campbell MG, et al: Three-dimensional color Doppler sonography before and after fibroid embolization. J Ultrasound Med 19:701, 2000

Fleischer AC, Gordon AN, Entman SS: Transabdominal and transvaginal sonography of pelvic masses. Ultrasound Med Biol 15:529, 1989

Fleischer AC, Jones HW: Sonography of trophoblastic diseases. In Fleischer AC, Manning FA, Jeanty P, et al (eds): Sonography in Obstetrics & Gynecology, 6th ed. New York, McGraw-Hill, 2001, p 843

Fleischer AC, Lyshchik A, Andreotti RF, et al: Advances in sonographic detection of ovarian cancer: depiction of tumor neovascularity with microbubbles. AJR Am J Roentgenol 194(2):343, 2010

Fleischer AC, Lyshchik A, Jones HW Jr, et al: Contrast-enhanced transvaginal sonography of benign versus malignant ovarian masses: preliminary findings. J Ultrasound Med 27(7):1011, 2008

Fleischer AC, Lyshchik A, Jones HW 3rd, et al: Diagnostic parameters to differentiate benign from malignant ovarian masses with contrast-enhanced transvaginal sonography. J Ultrasound Med 28(10):1273, 2009

Fleischer AC, Pennell RG, McKee MS, et al: Ectopic pregnancy: features at transvaginal sonography. Radiology 174:375, 1990

Fleischer AC, Rodgers WH, Kepple DM, et al: Color Doppler sonography of ovarian masses: a multiparameter analysis. J Ultrasound Med 12:41, 1993

Fleischer AC, Stein SM, Cullinan JA, et al: Color Doppler sonography of adnexal masses. J Ultrasound Med 14:523, 1995

Food and Drug Administration Center for Drug Evaluation and Research. Public health advisory. Update on magnetic resonance imaging (MRI) contrast agents containing gadolinium and nephrogenic fibrosing dermopathy. 2006, Updated 2007. Available at: www.fda.gov/cder/drug/advisory/gadolinium_agents_20061222.htm. Accessed November 28, 2010

Foshager MC, Hood LL, Walsh JW: Masses simulating gynecologic diseases at CT and MR imaging. Radiographics 16:1085, 1996

Forstner R, Hricak H: Congenital malformations of uterus and vagina. Radiology 34:397, 1994

Frei KA, Kinkel K, Bonel HM, et al: Prediction of deep myometrial invasion in patients with endometrial cancer: clinical utility of contrast-enhanced MR imaging-a meta-analysis and Bayesian analysis. Radiology 216:444, 2000

Friedman WN, Rosenfield AT: Computed tomography in obstetrics and gynecology. J Reprod Med 37:3, 1992

Friera A, Gimenez NR, Caballero P, et al: Deep vein thrombosis: can a second sonographic examination be avoided? AJR Am J Roentgenol 178:1001, 2002

Funt SA, Hann LE: Detection and characterization of adnexal masses. Radiol Clin North Am 40:591, 2002

Geomini PM, Coppus SF, Kluivers KB, et al: Is three-dimensional ultrasonography of additional value in the assessment of adnexal masses? Gynecol Oncol 106:153, 2007

Gera PS, Allemand MC, Tatpati LL, et al: Role of saline infusion sonography in uterine evaluation before frozen embryo transfer cycle. Fertil Steril 89:562, 2008

Ghi T, Casadio P, Kuleva M, et al: Accuracy of three-dimensional ultrasound in diagnosis and classification of congenital uterine anomalies. Fertil Steril 92:808, 2009

Gjelsteen A, Ching BH, Meyermann MW, et al: CT, MRI, PET, PET/CT, and ultrasound in the evaluation of obstetric and gynecologic patients. Surg Clin N Am 88:361, 2008

Goh AS, Ng DC: Clinical positron emission tomography imaging—current applications. Ann Acad Med Singapore 32:507, 2003

Goldhaber SZ: Pulmonary embolism. Lancet 363:1295, 2004

Goldstein SR, Nachtigall M, Snyder JR, et al: Endometrial assessment by vaginal ultrasonography before endometrial sampling in patients with postmenopausal bleeding. Am J Obstet Gynecol 163:119, 1990

Granberg S, Wikland M, Karlsson B, et al: Endometrial thickness as measured by endovaginal ultrasonography for identifying endometrial abnormality. Am J Obstet Gynecol 164:47, 1991

Greer IA: Prevention and management of venous thromboembolism in pregnancy. Clin Chest Med 24:123, 2003

Gross BH, Silver TM, Jaffe MH: Sonographic features of uterine leiomyomas: analysis of 41 proven cases. J Ultrasound Med 2:401, 1983

Gull B, Carlsson S, Karlsson B, et al: Transvaginal ultrasonography of the endometrium in women with postmenopausal bleeding: is it always necessary to perform an endometrial biopsy? Am J Obstet Gynecol 182:509, 2000

Gull B, Karlsson B, Milsom I, et al: Can ultrasound replace dilation and curettage? A longitudinal evaluation of postmenopausal bleeding and transvaginal sonographic measurement of the endometrium as predictors of endometrial cancer. Am J Obstet Gynecol 188:401, 2003

Hall DA, Yoder IC: Ultrasound evaluation of the uterus. In Callen PW (ed): Ultrasonography in Obstetrics and Gynecology, 3rd ed. Philadelphia, W.B. Saunders, 1994

Hammond CB, Weed JC, Jr, Currie JL: The role of operation in the current therapy of gestational trophoblastic disease. Am J Obstet Gynecol 136:844, 1980

Hann LE, Gretz EM, Bach AM, et al: Sonohysterography for evaluation of the endometrium in women treated with tamoxifen. AJR Am J Roentgenol 177:337, 2001

Hata T, Yanagihara T, Hayashi K, et al: Three-dimensional ultrasonographic evaluation of ovarian tumours: a preliminary study. Hum Reprod 14:858, 1999

Havrilesky LJ, Wong TZ, Secord AA, et al: The role of PET scanning in the detection of recurrent cervical cancer. Gynecol Oncol 90:186, 2003

Heijboer H, Büller HR, Lensing AW, et al: A comparison of real-time compression ultrasonography with impedance plethysmography for the diagnosis of deep-vein thrombosis in symptomatic outpatients. N Engl J Med 329(19):1365, 1993

Heikinen H, Tekay A, Volpi E, et al: Transvaginal salpingosonography for the assessment of tubal patency in infertile women: methodological and clinical experiences. Fertil Steril 64:293, 1995

Hesley GK, Gorny KR, Henrichsen TL, et al: A clinical review of focused ultrasound ablation with magnetic resonance guidance an option for treating uterine fibroids. Ultrasound Q 24:131, 2008

Hill A: Sonohysterography in the office: instruments and technique. Contemp Obstet Gynecol 42:95, 1997

Hindley J, Gedroyc WM, Regan L, et al: MRI guidance of focused ultrasound therapy of uterine fibroids: early results. AJR Am J Roentgenol 183:1713, 2004

Horrow MM: Ultrasound of pelvic inflammatory disease. Ultrasound Q 20:171, 2004

Horrow MM, Brown KJ: Femscan. Multiloculated pelvic cyst. J Women's Imaging 4:89, 2002

Hricak H, Chang YCF, Thurnher S: Vagina: evaluation with MR imaging. I. Normal anatomy and congenital anomalies. Radiology 169:169, 1988

Hricak H, Gatsonis C, Conkley F, et al: Early invasive cervical cancer: CT and MRI imaging in preoperative evaluation-ACRIN/GOG comparative study of diagnostic performance and interobserver variability. Radiology 245:491, 2007

Hricak H, Powell CB, Yu KK, et al: Invasive cervical carcinoma: Role of MR imaging in pretreatment work-up-cost minimization and diagnostic efficacy analysis. Radiology 198:403, 1996

Hricak H, Stern JL, Fisher MR, et al: Endometrial carcinoma staging by MR imaging. Radiology 162:297, 1987

Hricak H, Tscholakoff D, Heinrichs L, et al: Uterine leiomyomas: correlation of MR histopathologic findings, and symptoms. Radiology 158:385, 1986

Hulka CA, Hall DA, McCarthy K, et al: Endometrial polyps, hyperplasia and carcinoma in postmenopausal women: differentiation with endovaginal sonography. Radiology 191:755, 1994

Huang WC, Yang SH, Yang JM: Three-dimensional transperineal sonographic characteristics of the anal sphincter complex in nulliparous women. Ultrasound Obstet Gynecol 30:210, 2007

Hudson SBA, Stewart, EA: Resonance-guided Focused Ultrasound Surgery. Clin Obstet Gynecol 1:159, 2008

International Federation of Obstetricians and Gynecologists: FIGO annual report on the results of treatment in gynecologic cancer. FIGO 31, 1998

Iyer V, Lee S: MRI, CT and PET/CT for ovarian cancer detection and adnexal lesion characterization. AJR Am J Roentgenol 194:311, 2010

Izquierdo LA, Nicholas C: Three-dimensional transvaginal sonography of interstitial pregnancy. J Clin Ultrasound 31:484, 2003

Jain KA: Prospective evaluation of adnexal masses with endovaginal gray-scale and duplex and color Doppler US: correlation with pathologic findings. Radiology 191:63, 1994

Jankowski JT, Spirnak JP: Current recommendations for imaging in the management of urologic traumas. Urol Clin N Am 33:365, 2006

Javitt MC, Fleischer AC: MRI of the female pelvis: problem solving sonographic uncertainties. In Fleischer AC, Manning FA, Jeanty P, et al (eds): Sonography in Obstetrics & Gynecology, 6th ed. New York, McGraw-Hill, 2001, p 1019

Javitt MC, Fleischer AC, Andreotti RF, et al: Expert panel on women's imaging. Staging and follow-up of ovarian cancer. Reston (VA): Am College of Radiology (ACR) 2007, p 1

Jayasinghe Y, Rane A, Stalewski H, et al: The presentation and early diagnosis of the rudimentary uterine horn. Obstet Gynecol 105(6):1456, 2005

Jeong Y, Outwater EK, Kang HK: Imaging evaluation of ovarian masses. Radiographics 20:144, 2000

Jergas M, Genant HK: Current methods and recent advances in the diagnosis of osteoporosis. Arthritis Rheum 36:1649, 1993

Jha RC, Ascher SM, Imaoka I, et al: Symptomatic fibroleiomyomata: MR imaging of the uterus before and after uterine arterial embolization. Radiology 217:228, 2000

Jokubkiene L, Sladkevicius P, Valentin L: Does three-dimensional power Doppler ultrasound help in discrimination between benign and malignant ovarian masses? Ultrasound Obstet Gynecol 29:215, 2007

Jones W, Lauerson N: Hydatidiform mole with coexistent fetus. Am J Obstet Gynecol 122:267, 1975

Jorizzo JR, Chen MYM, Riccio GJ: Endometrial polyps: sonohysterographic evaluation. AJR Am J Roentgenol 176:617, 2001

Jorizzo JR, Riccio GJ, Chen MYM, et al: Sonohysterography. The next step in the evaluation of the abnormal endometrium. Radiographics 19:S117, 1999

Jurkovic D, Giepel A, Gruboeck K, et al: Three-dimensional ultrasound for the assessment of uterine anatomy and detection of congenital anomalies: a comparison with hysterosalpingography and two-dimensional sonography. Ultrasound Obstet Gynecol 5:233, 1995

Juweid ME, Cheson BD: Positron-emission tomography and assessment of cancer therapy. N Engl J Med 354:496, 2006

Kaakaji Y, Nghiem HV, Nodell C, et al: Sonography of obstetric and gynecologic emergencies. Part II. AJR Am J Roentgenol 174:651, 2000

Kanal E, Barkovich AJ, Bell C, et al: ACR guidance document for safe MR practices: 2007. AJR Am J Roentgenol 188(6):1447, 2007

Kaplan FS: Prevention and management of osteoporosis. Clin Symp 1995, p 47

Karlsson B, Granberg S, Wikland M, et al: Transvaginal ultrasonography of the endometrium in women with postmenopausal bleeding-a Nordic multicenter study. Am J Obstet Gynecol 172:1488, 1995

Kawai M, Kano T, Kikkawa F, et al: Transvaginal Doppler ultrasound with color flow imaging in the diagnosis of ovarian cancer. Obstet Gynecol 79:163, 1992

Keltz MD, Olive DL, Kim AH, et al: Sonohysterography for screening in recurrent pregnancy loss. Fertil Steril 67:670, 1997

Kelvin FM, Maglinte DDT, Hale DS, et al: Female pelvic organ prolapse: a comparison of triphasic dynamic MR imaging and triphasic fluoroscopic cystocolpography. AJR Am J Roentgenol 174:81, 2000

Kepkep K, Tuncay YA, Göynümer G, et al: Transvaginal sonography in the diagnosis of adenomyosis: which findings are most accurate? Ultrasound Obstet Gynecol 3:341, 2007

Khalife S, Falcone T, Hemmings R, et al: Diagnostic accuracy of transvaginal ultrasound in detecting free pelvic fluid. J Reprod Med 43:795, 1998

Kim AH, McKay H, Keltz MD, et al: Sonohysterographic screening before in vitro fertilization. Fertil Steril 69:841, 1998

Kim S, Chung JK, Kang SB, et al: [18F]FDG PET as a substitute for second-look laparotomy in patients with advanced ovarian carcinoma. Eur J Nucl Med Mol Imaging 31:196, 2004

Kinkel K, Hricak H, Lu Y, et al: US characterization of ovarian masses: a meta-analysis. Radiology 217:803, 2000

Kupesic A: Evaluation of Infertile Patients Using Transvaginal Color Doppler and 3-D Imaging. Madrid, Marban, 1997

Kupesic S, Bekavac I, Bjelos D, et al: Assessment of endometrial receptivity by transvaginal color Doppler and three-dimensional power Doppler ultrasonography in patients undergoing in vitro fertilization procedures. J Ultrasound Med 20:125, 2001a

Kupesic S, Kurjak A: Transvaginal color Doppler sonography in the assessment of infertility. In Fleischer AC, Manning FA, Jeanty P, et al (eds): Sonography in Obstetrics & Gynecology, 6th ed. New York, McGraw-Hill, 2001b, p 1078

Kurjak A, Kupesic S: Three-dimensional color power sonography in gynecology. In Fleischer AC, Manning FA, Jeanty P, et al (eds): Sonography in Obstetrics & Gynecology, 6th ed. New York, McGraw-Hill, 2001, p 1225

Kurjak A, Schulman H, Sosic A, et al: Transvaginal ultrasound, color flow, and Doppler waveform of the postmenopausal adnexal mass. Obstet Gynecol 80:917, 1992

Larson DM, Connor GP, Broste SK, et al: Prognostic significance of gross myometrial invasion with endometrial cancer. Obstet Gynecol 88:394, 1996

Lasser EC, Berry CC, Talner LB, et al: Pretreatment with corticosteroids to alleviate reactions to intravenous contrast material. N Engl J Med 317:845, 1987

Lee A, Eppel W, Sam C, et al: Intrauterine device localization by three-dimensional transvaginal sonography. Ultrasound Obstet Gynecol 10:289, 1997

Lee JH, Pretorius DH, Weinstein M, et al: Transperineal three-dimensional ultrasound in evaluating anal sphincter muscles. Ultrasound Obstet Gynecol 30:201, 2007

Lee JKT, Gersell DJ, Balfe DM, et al: The uterus: in vitro MR anatomic correlation of normal and abnormal specimens. Radiology 157:175, 1985

Lele PP, Hazzard DG, Litz ML: Thresholds and mechanisms of ultrasonic damage to "organized" animal tissues. Symposium on Biological Effects and Characterizations of Ultrasound Sources. US Department of Health, Education, and Welfare HEW Publication (FDA) 78-8048:224, 1977

Lensing AWA, Prandoni P, Brandjes D, et al: Detection of deep-vein thrombosis by real-time B-mode ultrasonography. N Engl J Med 320:342, 1989

Leung JWT, Hricak H: Role of magnetic resonance imaging in the evaluation of gynecologic disease. In Callen PW (eds): Ultrasonography in Obstetrics and Gynecology, 4th ed. Philadelphia, W.B. Saunders Company, 2000, p 935

Levine D, Feldstein VA, Babcook CJ, et al: Sonography of ovarian masses: poor sensitivity or resistive index for identifying malignant lesions. AJR Am J Roentgenol 162:1355, 1994

Levine D, Gosink BB, Johnson LA: Change in endometrial thickness in postmenopausal women undergoing hormone replacement therapy. Radiology 197(3):603, 1995

Lienemann A, Anthuber C, Baron A, et al: Diagnosing enteroceles using dynamic magnetic resonance imaging. Dis Colon Rectum 43:205, 2000

Lieng M, Qvigstad E, Dahl GF, et al: Flow differences between endometrial polyps and cancer: a prospective study using intravenous contrast-enhanced transvaginal color flow Doppler and three-dimensional power Doppler ultrasound. Ultrasound Obstet Gynecol 32(7):935, 2008

Lindheim SR, Adsuar N, Kushner DM, et al: Sonohysterography: a valuable tool in evaluating the female pelvis. Obstet Gynecol Surv 58:770, 2003a

Lindheim SR, Morales AJ: Operative ultrasound using an echogenic loop snare for intrauterine pathology. J Am Assoc Gynecol Laparosc 10:107, 2003b

Lindheim SR, Sauer MV: Upper genital-tract screening with hysterosonography in patients receiving donated oocytes. Int J Gynaecol Obstet 60:47, 1998

Long MG, Boulbee JE, Begent RH, et al: Preliminary Doppler studies on the uterine artery and myometrium in trophoblastic tumors requiring chemotherapy. Br J Obstet Gynecol 97:686, 1990

Low RN, Carter WD, Saleh F, et al: Ovarian cancer: comparison of findings with perfluorocarbon-exchanged MR imaging, In-111-CYT-103 immunoscintigraphy, and CT. Radiology 195:391, 1995

Lubich LM, Alderman MG, Ros PR: Magnetic resonance imaging of leiomyomata uteri: Assessing therapy with the gonadotropin-releasing hormone agonist leuprolide. Magn Reson Imaging 9:331, 1991

Lyons EA: Abnormal premenopausal vaginal bleeding: from menarche to menopause. In Bluth EI, Arger PH, Benson CB, et al (eds): Ultrasound: A Practical Approach to Clinical Problems. New York, Thieme, 2000, p 220

Lyons EA: Ultrasound evaluation of bleeding in the non-pregnant patient. Presented at the 102nd Annual Meeting of the American Roentgen Ray Society. Atlanta, Georgia, 2002.

Macura KJ: Magnetic resonance imaging of pelvic floor defects in women. Top Magn Reson Imaging 17:417, 2006

Maglinte DD, Gage SN, Harmon BH, et al: Obstruction of the small intestine: accuracy and role of CT in diagnosis. Radiology 188:61, 1993

Mandic A, Vujkov T, Novakovic P, et al: Clinical-sonographic scoring system in noninvasive diagnosis of endometrial cancer. J BUON 11:197, 2006

Mark AS, Hricak H, Heinrichs LW: Adenomyosis and leiomyoma: differential diagnosis by means of magnetic resonance imaging. Radiology 163:527, 1987

Maymon R, Schneider D, Shulman A, et al: Serial color Doppler flow of uterine vasculature combined with serum b-hCG measurements for improved monitoring of patients with gestational trophoblastic disease. Gynecol Obstet Invest 42:201, 1996

McCarthy S, Tauber C, Gore J: Female pelvic anatomy: MR assessment of variations during the menstrual cycle and with use of oral contraceptives. Radiology 160:119, 1986

McLucas B, Perrella R, Goodwin S, et al: Role of uterine artery Doppler flow in fibroid embolization. J Ultrasound Med 21:113, 2002

Merce LT, Alcazar JL, Lopez C, et al: Clinical references of 3-dimensional sonography and power Doppler angiography for diagnosis of endometrial carcinoma. J Ultrasound Med 26:1279, 2007

Miller PD, Zapalowski C, Kulak CA, et al: Bone densitometry: the best way to detect osteoporosis and to monitor therapy. J Clin Endocrinol Metab 84:1867, 1999

Mishell DR Jr, Stenchever MA, Droegemueller W, et al (eds): Comprehensive Gynecology, 3rd ed. St. Louis, MO, Mosby, 1997, p 691

Mol BW, Swart P, Bossuyt PM, et al: Reproducibility of the interpretation of hysterosalpingography in the diagnosis of tubal pathology. Hum Reprod 11:1204, 1996

Molander P, Sjoberg J, Paavonen J, et al: Transvaginal power Doppler findings in laparoscopically proven acute pelvic inflammatory disease. Ultrasound Obstet Gynecol 17:233, 2002

Monteagudo A, Carreno C, Timor-Tritsch IE: Saline infusion sonohysterography in nonpregnant women with previous cesarean delivery: the "niche" in the scar. J Ultrasound Med 20:1105, 2001

Moschos E, Ashfaq R, McIntire DD, et al: Saline-infusion sonography endometrial sampling compared with endometrial biopsy in diagnosing endometrial pathology. Obstet Gynecol 113:881, 2009

Moschos E, Sreenarasimhaiah S, Twickler DM: First trimester diagnosis of cesarean scar ectopic pregnancies. J Clin Ultrasound 36:504, 2008

Moschos E, Twickler DM: Does the type of intrauterine device affect conspicuity on 2D and 3D ultrasound? AJR Am J Roentgenol 196(6):1439, 2011

Muniz CJ, Fleischer AC, Donnelly EF, et al: Three-dimensional color Doppler sonography and uterine artery arteriography of fibroids: assessment of changes in vascularity before and after embolization. J Ultrasound Med 21:129, 2002

Munyer T, Callen PW, Filly RA, et al: Further observations on the sonographic spectrum of gestational trophoblastic disease. J Clin Ultrasound 9:349, 1981

Nanni C, Rubello D, Farsad M, et al: (18)F-FDG PET/CT in the evaluation of recurrent ovarian cancer: a prospective study on forty-one patients. Eur J Surg Oncol 31:79, 2005

Narayan K, McKenzie A, Fisher R, et al: Estimation of tumor volume in cervical cancer by magnetic resonance imaging. Am J Clin Oncol 26:163, 2003

Neitlich JD, Foster HE, Glickman MG, et al: Detection of urethral diverticula in women: comparison of a high resolution fast spin echo technique with double balloon urethrography. J Urol 159:408, 1998

Nurenberg P, Twickler DM: Magnetic resonance imaging in obstetrics and gynecology. In Cunningham FG, MacDonald PC, Gant NF, et al (eds): Williams Obstetrics, 19th ed. New York, Appleton & Lange, 1995, p 987

Nyberg DA, Mack LA, Jeffrey RB, et al: Endovaginal sonographic evaluation of ectopic pregnancy: prospective study. AJR Am J Roentgenol 149:1181, 1987

O'Brien WF, Buck DR, Nash JD: Evaluation of sonography in the initial assessment of the gynecologic patient. Am J Obstet Gynecol 149:598, 1984

Oguz S, Sargin A, Aytan H, et al: Doppler study of myometrium in invasive gestational trophoblastic disease. Int J Gynecol Cancer 14:972, 2004

Ong MG, Boultbee JE, Langley R, et al: Doppler assessment of the uterine circulation and the clinical behaviour of gestational trophoblastic tumors requiring chemotherapy. Br J Cancer 66:883, 1992

Opolskiene G, Sladkevicius P, Valentin L: Ultrasound assessment of endometrial morphology and vascularity to predict endometrial malignancy in women with postmenopausal bleeding and sonographic endometrial thickness >or= 4.5 mm. Ultrasound Obstet Gynecol 30:332, 2007

Outwater EK, Siegelman ES, Van Deerlin V: Adenomyosis: current concepts and imaging considerations. AJR Am J Roentgenol 170:437, 1998

Ozdemir S, Celik C, Emlik D, et al: Assessment of myometrial invasion in endometrial cancer by transvaginal sonography, Doppler ultrasonography, magnetic resonance imaging and frozen section. Int J Gynecol Cancer 19(6):1085, 2009

Pafumi C, Zizza G, Farina M, et al: Comparison of DEXA and ultrasonometry in the measurement of bone density. Arch Gynecol Obstet 266:152, 2002

Pannu HK: Magnetic resonance imaging of pelvic organ prolapse. Abdom Imaging 27:660, 2002

Park W, Park YJ, Huh SJ, et al: The usefulness of MRI and PET imaging for the detection of parametrial involvement and lymph node metastasis in patients with cervical cancer. Jpn J Clin Oncol 35:260, 2005

Parsons JH, Steer CV: Infertility. In Dewbury K, Meire H, Cosgrove D, et al (eds): Ultrasound Obstetrics and Gynaecology, 2nd ed. London, Churchill Livingstone, 2001, p 99

Patten RM: Pelvic inflammatory disease: endovaginal sonography with laparoscopic correlation. J Ultrasound Med 9:681, 1990

Pejovic T, Olive DL: Contemporary use of bone densitometry. Clin Obstet Gynecol 42:876, 1999

Pellerito JS, McCarthy S, Doyle MB, et al: Diagnosis of uterine anomalies: relative accuracy of MR imaging, endovaginal ultrasound, and hysterosalpingography. Radiology 183:795, 1992a

Pellerito JS, Taylor KJW, Quedens-Case C, et al: Ectopic pregnancy: evaluation with endovaginal color flow imaging. Radiology 183:407, 1992b

Pena A: Atlas of surgical management of anorectal malformations. New York, Springer-Verlag, 1990

Philipov G, Holsman M, Philips PJ: The clinical role of quantitative ultrasound in assessing fracture risk and bone status. Med J Aust 173:208, 2000

Pisal N, Sindos M, O'Riordian J, et al: The use of spinal needle for transcervical saline infusion sonohysterography in presence of cervical stenosis. Acta Obstet Gynecol Scand 84:1019, 2005

Pocock NA, Culton NL, Gilbert GR, et al: Potential roles for quantitative ultrasound in the management of osteoporosis. Med J Aust 173:355, 2000

Raga F, Bonilla-Musoles F, Blanes J, et al: Congenital müllerian anomalies: diagnostic accuracy of three-dimensional ultrasound. Fertil Steril 65:523, 1996

Raine-Fenning N, Jayaprakasan K, Clewes J, et al: SonoAVC: a novel method of automatic volume calculation. Ultrasound Obstet Gynecol 31(6):691, 2008

Rajkotia K, Veeramani M, Katarzyna J: Magnetic resonance imaging of adnexal masses. Top Magn Reson Imag 17:379, 2006

Reid M, McGahan JP, Oi R: Sonographic evaluation of hydatidiform mole and its look-alike. AJR Am J Roentgenol 140:307, 1983

Reinhold C, Atri M, Mehio AR, et al: Diffuse uterine adenomyosis: morphologic criteria and diagnostic accuracy of endovaginal sonography. Radiology 197:609, 1995

Reinhold C, McCarthy S, Bret PM, et al: Diffuse adenomyosis: comparison of endovaginal US and MR imaging with histopathologic correlation. Radiology 199:151, 1996

Reinhold C, Tafazoli F, Mehio AR, et al: Uterine adenomyosis: endovaginal US and MR imaging features with histopathologic correlation. Radiographics 19:S147, 1999

Reuter KL, Daly DC, Cohen SM: Septate versus bicornuate uteri: errors in imaging diagnosis. Radiology 172:749, 1989

Richenberg J, Copperberg P: Ultrasound of the uterus. In Callen PW (ed): Ultrasonography in Obstetrics and Gynecology, 4th ed. Philadelphia, Saunders, 2000, p 814

Rodgerson JD, Heegaard WG, Plummer D, et al: Emergency department right upper quadrant ultrasound is associated with a reduced time to diagnosis and treatment of ruptured ectopic pregnancies. Acad Emerg Med 8(4):331, 2001

Saga T, Higashi T, Ishimori T, et al: Clinical value of FDG-PET in the follow up of postoperative patients with endometrial cancer. Ann Nucl Med 17:197, 2003

Salim R, Lee C, Davies A, et al: A comparative study of three-dimensional saline infusion sonohysterography and diagnostic hysteroscopy for the classification of submucous fibroids. Hum Reprod 20:253, 2005

Salim R, Woelfer B, Backos M, et al: Reproducibility of three-dimensional ultrasound diagnosis of congenital uterine anomalies. Ultrasound Gynecol Obstet 21(6):578, 2003

Sandridge DA, Thorp JM: Vaginal endosonography in the assessment of the anorectum. Obstet Gynecol 86:1007, 1995

Sassone AM, Timor-Tritsch IE, Artner A, et al: Transvaginal sonographic characterization of ovarian disease: evaluation of a new scoring system to predict ovarian malignancy. Obstet Gynecol 78:70, 1991

Savelli L, Ceccarini M, Ludovisi M, et al: Preoperative local staging of endometrial cancer: transvaginal sonography vs. magnetic resonance imaging. Ultrasound Obstet Gynecol 5:560, 2008

Savelli L, Pollastri P, Guerrini M, et al: Tolerability, side effects, and complications of hysterosalpingocontrast sonography (HyCoSy). Fertil Steril 4:1481, 2009

Scalea TM, Rodriquez A, Chiu WC, et al: Focused assessment with sonography for trauma (FAST): results from an international consensus conference. J Trauma 46:466, 1999

Schaer GN, Koechli OR, Schuessler B, et al: Perineal ultrasound for evaluating the bladder neck in urinary stress incontinence. Obstet Gynecol 85:220, 1995

Schellong SM: Complete compression ultrasound for the diagnosis of venous thromboembolism. Curr Opin Pulm Med 10:350, 2004

Schlief R, Deichert U: Hysterosalpingo-contrast sonography of the uterus and fallopian tubes. Results of a clinical trial of a new contrast medium in 120 patients. Radiology 178:213, 1991

Schoenenberger AW, Debatin JF, Guldenschuh I, et al: Dynamic MR defecography with a superconducting, open-configuration MR system. Radiology 206:641, 1998

Serafini P, Nelson J, Batzofin J: IVF-surrogates of donated oocytes. In Sauer MV (ed): Principles of Oocyte and Embryo Donation. New York, Springer-Verlag, 1998, p 313

Sheth S, Hamper UM, Kurman RJ: Thickened endometrium in the postmenopausal woman: sonographic-pathologic correlation. Radiology 187:135, 1993

Siegelman ES, Outwater EK: Tissue characterization in the female pelvis by means of MR imaging. Radiology 212:5, 1999

Singh AK, Grigsby PW, Dehdashti F, et al: FDG-PET lymph node staging and survival of patients with FIGO stage IIIb cervical carcinoma. Int J Radiat Oncol Biol Phys 56:489, 2003

Sladkevicius P, Jokubkiene L, Valentin L: Contribution of morphological assessment of the vessel tree by three-dimensional ultrasound to a correct diagnosis of malignancy in ovarian masses. Ultrasound Obstet Gynecol 30:874, 2007

Soares SR, Barbosa dos Reis MM, Camargos AF: Diagnostic accuracy of sonohysterography, transvaginal sonography, and hysterosalpingography in patients with uterine cavity diseases. Fertil Steril 73:406, 2000

Sohaib SA, Mills TD, Sahdev A, et al: The role of magnetic resonance imaging and ultrasound in patients with adnexal masses. Clin Radiol 60:340, 2005

Song Y, Yang J, Liu Z, et al: Preoperative evaluation of endometrial carcinoma by contrast-enhanced ultrasonography. Br J Obstet Gynaecol 116:294, 2009

Soper JT: Radiographic imaging in gynecologic oncology. Clin Obstet Gynecol 44:485, 2001

Stein SM, Laifer-Narin S, Johnson MB, et al: Differentiation of benign and malignant adnexal masses: relative value of gray-scale, color Doppler and spectral Doppler sonography. AJR Am J Roentgenol 164:381, 1994

Stewart EA, Gedroyc WM, Tempany CMC, et al: Focused ultrasound treatment of uterine fibroid tumors: safety and feasibility of a noninvasive thermoablative technique. Am J Obstet Gynecol 189:48, 2003

Stewart EA, Gostout B, Rabinovici J, et al: Sustained relief of leiomyoma symptoms by using focused ultrasound surgery. Obstet Gynecol 110:279, 2007

Stewart EA, Rabinovici J, Tempany CMC, et al: Clinical outcomes of focused ultrasound surgery for the treatment of uterine fibroids. Fertil Steril 85:22, 2006

Strandell A, Bourne T, Bergh C, et al: The assessment of endometrial pathology and tubal patency: a comparison between the use of ultrasonography and X-ray hysterosalpingography for the investigation of infertility patients. Ultrasound Obstet Gynecol 14:200, 1999

Stumpf PG, March CM: Febrile morbidity following hysterosalpingography: identification of risk factors and recommendations for prophylaxis. Fertil Steril 33:487, 1980

Subak LL, Hricak H, Powell CB, et al: Cervical carcinoma: computed tomography and magnetic resonance imaging for preoperative staging. Obstet Gynecol 86:43, 1995

Sultan AH, Loder PB, Bartram CI: Vaginal endosonography. New approach to image the undisturbed anal sphincter. Dis Colon Rectum 37:1296, 1994

Sylvestre C, Child TJ, Tulandi T, et al: A prospective study to evaluate the efficacy of two- and three-dimensional sonohysterography in women with intrauterine lesions. Fertil Steril 79:1222, 2003

Tal J, Timor-Tritsch IE, Degani S: Accurate diagnosis of postabortal placental remnant by sonohysterography and color Doppler sonographic studies. Gynecol Obstet Invest 43:131, 1997

Taylor KJW, Schwartz PE, Kohorn EI: Gestational trophoblastic neoplasia: diagnosis with Doppler US. Radiology 165:445, 1987

Tempany C, Dou K, Silverman S, et al: Staging of advanced ovarian cancer: comparison of imaging modalities report from the Radiological Diagnostic Oncology Group. Radiology 215:761, 2000

ter Haar G: Therapeutic ultrasound. Eur J Ultrasound 9:3, 1999

Thiel JA, Suchet IB, Lortie K: Confirmation of Essure microinsert tubal coil placement with conventional and volume-contrast imaging three-dimensional ultrasound. Fertil Steril 84(2):504, 2005

Thurmond AS: Selective salpingography and fallopian tube recanalization. AJR Am J Roentgenol 156:33, 1991

Timmerman D, Testa AC, Bourne T, et al: Logistic regression model to distinguish between the benign and malignant adnexal mass before surgery: a multicenter study by the International Ovarian Tumor Analysis Group. J Clin Oncol 23:8794, 2005

Timmerman D, Valentin L, Bourne T, et al: Terms, definitions and measurements to describe the sonographic features of adnexal tumors: a consensus opinion from the International Ovarian Tumor Analysis (IOTA) group. Ultrasound Obstet Gynecol 16:500, 2000

Timor-Tritsch IE, Lerner JP, Monteagudo A, et al: Transvaginal sonographic markers of tubal inflammatory disease. Ultrasound Obstet Gynecol 12:56, 1998

Tinkanen H, Kujansuu E: Doppler ultrasound findings in tubo-ovarian infectious complex. J Clin Ultrasound 21:175, 1993

Titton RL, Gervais DA, Hahn PF, et al: Urine leaks and urinomas: diagnosis and imaging guided intervention. Radiographics 23:1133, 2003

Togashi K, Nishimura K, Itoh K, et al: Adenomyosis: diagnosis with MR imaging. Radiology 166:111, 1988

Togashi K, Ozasa H, Konishi I: Enlarged uterus: differentiation between adenomyosis and leiomyoma with MRI. Radiology 171:531, 1989

Troiano RN: Magnetic resonance imaging of Müllerian duct anomalies of the uterus. Top Magn Reson Imaging 14:269, 2003

Troiano R, McCarthy S: Müllerian duct anomalies: imaging and clinical issues. Radiology 233:19, 2004

Twickler DM, Forte TB, Santos-Ramos R, et al: The Ovarian Tumor Index predicts risk for malignancy. Cancer 86:2280, 1999

Twickler DM, Moschos E: Ultrasound and assessment of ovarian cancer risk. Am J of Roentgenol 194:322, 2010

Umek WH, Laml T, Stutterecker D, et al: The urethra during pelvic floor contraction: observations on three-dimensional ultrasound. Obstet Gynecol 100:796, 2002

Usadi RS, Marshburn PB: The impact of uterine artery embolization on fertility and pregnancy outcome. Curr Opin Obstet Gynecol 19:279, 2007

Valentin L: Gray scale sonography, subjective evaluation of the color Doppler image and measurement of blood flow velocity for distinguishing benign and malignant tumor of suspected adnexal origin. Eur J Obstet Gynecol Reprod Biol 72:63, 1997

Valsky DV, Yagel S: Ectopic pregnancies of unusual location: management dilemmas. Ultrasound Obstet Gynecol 31:245, 2008

Wagner LK, Lester RG, Saldana LR: Exposure of the Pregnant Patient to Diagnostic Radiation, Philadelphia, Medical Physics Publishing, 1997

Wamsteker K, Emanuel MH, de Kruif JH: Transcervical hysteroscopic resection of submucous fibroids for abnormal uterine bleeding: results regarding the degree of intramural extension. Obstet Gynecol 82(5):736, 1993

Webb JAW: Urinary tract: imaging techniques, kidneys and ureters. In Armstrong P, Wastie ML (eds): A Concise Textbook of Radiology. New York, Arnold, 2001, p 189

Weber TM, Sostman HD, Spritzer CE, et al: Cervical carcinoma: determination of recurrent tumor extent versus radiation changes with MR imaging. Radiology 194:135, 1995

Wei AY, Schink JC, Pritts EA, et al: Saline contrast sonohysterography and directed extraction, resection and biopsy of intrauterine pathology using a Uterine Explora curette. Ultrasound Obstet Gynecol 27(2):202, 2006

Weiner Z, Thaler I, Beck D, et al: Differentiating malignant from benign ovarian tumors with transvaginal color flow imaging. Obstet Gynecol 79:159, 1992

Wisser J, Ochsenbein-Imhof N: Sonographic evaluation of the pelvic floor after childbirth. In Fleischer AC, Manning FA, Jeanty P, et al (eds): Sonography in Obstetrics & Gynecology, 6th ed. New York, McGraw-Hill, 2001, p 1195

Wolfman DJ, Ascher SM: Magnetic resonance imaging of benign uterine pathology. Top Magn Reson Imaging 17(6):399, 2006

Wong TZ, Jones EL, Coleman RE: Positron emission tomography with 2-deoxy-2-[18F]fluoro-D-glucose for evaluating local and distant disease in patients with cervical cancer. Mol Imaging Biol 6:55, 2004

Woolcott R, Petchpud A, O'Donnel P, et al: Differential impact on pregnancy rate of selective salpingography, tubal catheterization and wire-guide recanalization in the treatment of proximal fallopian tube obstruction. Hum Reprod 10:1423, 1995

World Health Organization: Assessment of fracture risk and its application to screening for postmenopausal osteoporosis. WHO Reference No. WHO/TSR/843, 1994

Wu HM, Chiang CH, Huang HY, et al: Detection of the subendometrial vascularization flow index by three-dimensional ultrasound may be useful for predicting the pregnancy rate for patients undergoing in vitro fertilization-embryo transfer. Fertil Steril 79:507, 2003

Wu MH, Hsu CC, Huang KE: Detection of congenital müllerian duct anomalies using three-dimensional ultrasound. J Clin Ultrasound 25:487, 1997

Yamashita Y, Torashima M, Hatanaka Y, et al: Adnexal masses: accuracy of characterization with transvaginal US and precontrast and postcontrast MR imaging. Radiology 194:557, 1995

Yamashita Y, Torashima M, Takahashi M: Hyperintense uterine leiomyoma at T2-weighted MR imaging: differentiation with dynamic enhanced MR imaging and clinical implications Radiology 189:721, 1993

Yauger BJ, Feinberg EC, Levens ED, et al: Pre-cycle saline infusion sonography minimizes assisted reproductive technologies cycle cancellation due to endometrial polyps. Fertil Steril 90:1324, 2008

Yu NC, Raman SS, Patel M, et al: Fistulas of the genitourinary tract: a radiologic review. Radiographics 24:1331, 2004

Zhou Q, Lei XY, Xie Q, et al: Sonographic and Doppler imaging in the diagnosis and treatment of gestational trophoblastic disease: a 12-year experience. J Ultrasound Med 24: 15, 2005

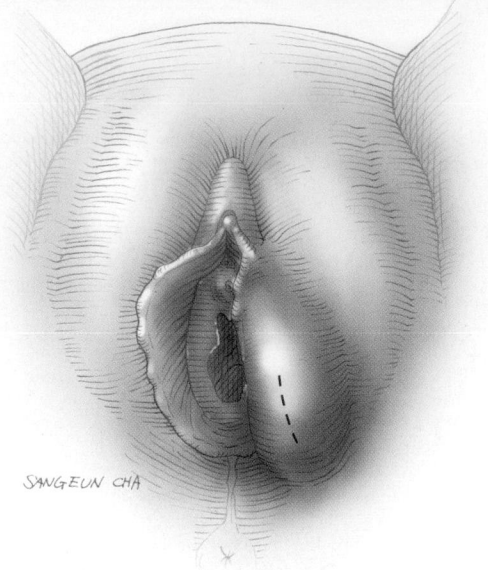

SANGEUN CHA

CHAPTER 3

Gynecologic Infection

NORMAL VAGINAL FLORA

The vaginal flora of a normal, asymptomatic reproductive-aged woman includes multiple aerobic or facultative species as well as obligate anaerobic species (Table 3-1). Of these, anaerobes predominate and outnumber aerobic species approximately 10 to 1 (Bartlett, 1977). These bacteria exist in a symbiotic relationship with the host and are alterable, depending on the microenvironment. They localize where their survival needs are met and have exemption from the infection-preventing destructive capacity of the human host. The function of this vaginal bacterial colonization, however, remains unknown.

Within this vaginal ecosystem, some microorganisms produce substances such as lactic acid and hydrogen peroxide that inhibit nonindigenous organisms (Marrazzo, 2006). Several other antibacterial compounds, termed bacteriocins, provide a similar role and include peptides such as acidocin and lactacin. Moreover, some microbe species have the ability to produce proteinaceous adhesions and attach to vaginal epithelial cells.

For protection from many of these toxic substances, the vagina secretes leukocyte protease inhibitor. This protein protects local tissues against toxic inflammatory products and infection.

Certain bacterial species normally found in vaginal flora have access to the upper reproductive tract. One study of 55 asymptomatic reproductive-aged women found a mean of 4.2 bacterial species recovered from the endocervix, and 2.1 from the endometrial cavity (Hemsell, 1989). Of the species recovered, 17 percent were recovered from the endometrium only, 50 percent were recovered from the endocervix only, and the remainder was recovered from both sites. Also reported is the finding of bacteria in cul-de-sac peritoneal fluid of asymptomatic women undergoing elective tubal sterilization (Spence, 1982). These and other studies show that the female upper reproductive tract is not sterile, but the presence of these bacteria does not indicate active infection. Together, these findings do illustrate the potential for infection following gynecologic surgery and the necessity for antimicrobial prophylaxis (Chap. 39, p. 958). They also explain the potential acceleration of a local acute infection if a pathogen, such as *Neisseria gonorrhoeae,* gains access to the upper tract.

TABLE 3-1. Lower Reproductive Tract Bacterial Flora

Species or Group of Organism

Aerobes
Gram-positive
  Lactobacillus spp.
  Diphtheroids
  Staphylococcus aureus
  Staphylococcus epidermidis
  Group B *Streptococcus*
  Enterococcus faecalis
  Staphylococcus spp.
  Actinomyces israelii
Gram-negative
  Escherichia coli
  Klebsiella spp.
  Proteus spp.
  Enterobacter spp.
  Acinetobacter spp.
  Citrobacter spp.
  Pseudomonas spp.

Anaerobes
Gram-positive cocci
  Peptostreptococcus spp.
  Clostridium spp.
Gram-positive bacilli
  Lactobacillus spp.
  Propionibacterium spp.
  Eubacterium spp.
  Bifidobacterium spp.
Gram-negative
  Prevotella spp.
  Bacteroides spp.
  Bacteroides fragilis group
  Fusobacterium spp.
  Veillonella spp.
Yeast
  Candida albicans and other spp.

Vaginal pH

Typically, the vaginal pH ranges between 4 and 4.5. Although not completely understood, it is believed to result from *Lactobacillus* species' production of lactic acid, fatty acids, and other organic acids. Other bacteria can also contribute organic acids from protein catabolism, and anaerobic bacteria contribute by amino acid fermentation.

Glycogen is present in healthy vaginal mucosa, provides nutrients for many species in the vaginal ecosystem, and is metabolized to lactic acid (Boskey, 2001). Accordingly, as glycogen content within vaginal epithelial cells diminishes after menopause, this decreased substrate for acid production leads to a rise in vaginal pH. Specifically, Caillouette and associates (1997) showed that a vaginal pH of 6.0 to 7.5 in the absence of symptoms was strongly suggestive of menopause. Moreover,

serum follicle-stimulating hormone (FSH) levels and vaginal pH were positively correlated. An inverse relationship, however, was noted between those two and serum estradiol levels.

Altered Flora

Changing any element of this ecology may alter the prevalence of various species. For example, young girls and postmenopausal women not receiving estrogen replacement have a lower prevalence of *Lactobacillus* species compared with that of reproductive-aged women. Devillard and colleagues (2004) reported that hormone replacement therapy restored vaginal lactobacilli populations, which protect against reproductive tract pathogens.

Other events predictably alter lower reproductive tract flora and may lead to patient infection. With the menstrual cycle, transient changes in flora are observed. These are predominantly during the first days of the menstrual cycle and are presumed to be associated with hormonal changes (Keane, 1997). Menstrual fluid also may serve as a nutrient source for several bacterial species, resulting in their overgrowth. What role this plays in the development of upper reproductive tract infection following menstruation is unclear, but an association may be present. For example, women symptomatic with acute gonococcal upper reproductive tract infection characteristically are menstruating or have just completed their menses. The exact role of this timing or of the opening of the cervical canal is unknown. Lastly, treatment with a broad-spectrum antibiotic may result in symptoms attributed to inflammation from *Candida albicans* or other *Candida* spp. by eradicating other species in the flora.

Hysterectomy with removal of the cervix changes lower reproductive tract flora, with or without prophylactic antimicrobial administration. Usually, more anaerobic species are recovered from the vagina postoperatively, with a particular increase in the prevalence of *Bacteroides fragilis*. Of the aerobes, increased prevalence is observed for *Escherichia coli* and *Enterococcus* species. These three species are frequently found in cultures obtained from women who develop pelvic infections following hysterectomy. However, similar increases are also seen in vaginal cultures obtained after hysterectomy in asymptomatic patients (Hemsell, 1988; Ohm, 1975).

Bacterial Vaginosis (BV)

This common, complex, and poorly understood clinical syndrome reflects abnormal vaginal flora. It has been variously named, and former terms include *Haemophilus* vaginitis, *Corynebacterium* vaginitis, *Gardnerella* or anaerobic vaginitis, and nonspecific vaginitis.

For unknown reasons, the vaginal flora's symbiotic relationship shifts to one in which there is overgrowth of anaerobic species including *Gardnerella vaginalis*, *Ureaplasma urealyticum*, *Mobiluncus* species, *Mycoplasma hominis*, and *Prevotella* species. Bacterial vaginosis (BV) is also associated with a significant reduction or absence of the normal hydrogen peroxide-producing *Lactobacillus* species. Whether an altered ecosystem leads to lactobacilli disappearance or whether its disappearance results in the changes observed with BV is unclear.

TABLE 3-2. Bacterial Vaginosis Risk Factors

Oral sex
Douching
Black race
Cigarette smoking
Sex during menses
Intrauterine device
Early age of sexual intercourse
New or multiple sexual partners
Sexual activity with other women

Risk Factors

This condition is not considered by the Centers for Disease Control and Prevention (CDC) (2010b) to be a sexually transmitted disease (STD), and it is seen in women without previous sexual experience. Many risk factors, however, are associated with sexual activity, and an increased risk of acquiring STDs has been reported in affected women (Table 3-2) (Atashili, 2008; Wiesenfeld, 2003). Moreover, a possible role of sexual transmission in the pathogenesis of recurrent BV has been proposed by Bradshaw and colleagues (2006). Successful prevention of BV is limited, but elimination or diminished use of vaginal douches may be beneficial (Brotman, 2008; Klebanoff, 2010).

Diagnosis

Bacterial vaginosis is reported by some to be the most frequent cause of vaginal symptoms resulting in health care visits. Of symptoms, a nonirritating, malodorous vaginal discharge is characteristic, but may not always be present. The vagina is usually not erythematous, and cervical examination reveals no abnormalities.

Clinical diagnostic criteria were first proposed by Amsel and associates (1983) and include: (1) microscopic evaluation of a vaginal-secretion saline preparation, (2) release of volatile amines produced by anaerobic metabolism, and (3) determination of the vaginal pH. First, a saline preparation, also know as a "wet prep," contains a swab-collected sample of discharge mixed with drops of saline on a microscope slide. Clue cells are the most reliable indicators of BV and were originally described by Gardner and Dukes (1955) (Fig. 3-1). These vaginal epithelial cells contain many attached bacteria, which create a poorly defined stippled cellular border. The positive predictive value of this test for the presence of BV is 95 percent.

Adding 10-percent potassium hydroxide (KOH) to a fresh sample of vaginal secretions releases volatile amines that have a fishy odor. This is often colloquially referred to as a "whiff test." The odor is frequently evident even without KOH. Similarly, the alkalinity of seminal fluid and blood are responsible for foul odor complaints after intercourse and with menses. The finding of both clue cells and a positive whiff test result is pathognomonic, even in asymptomatic patients.

Characteristically with BV, the vaginal pH is >4.5, and this results from diminished acid production by bacteria. Similarly, *Trichomonas vaginalis* infection is also associated with anaerobic overgrowth and resultant elaborated amines. Thus, women diagnosed with BV should have no microscopic evidence of trichomoniasis.

The Nugent Score is a system employed for diagnosing BV using microscopic examination of a Gram-stained smear of vaginal discharge. Used primarily in research studies rather than clinical practice, scores are calculated by assessing predominance of three types of bacteria morphology and staining: (1) large gram-positive rods (*Lactobacillus* spp.), (2) small gram-variable rods (*G vaginalis* or *Bacteroides* spp.), and (3) curved gram-variable rods (*Mobiluncus* spp.). A score of 7 to 10 is consistent with BV.

Several gynecologic adverse health outcomes have been observed in women with BV, including vaginitis, endometritis, postabortal endometritis, pelvic inflammatory disease (PID)

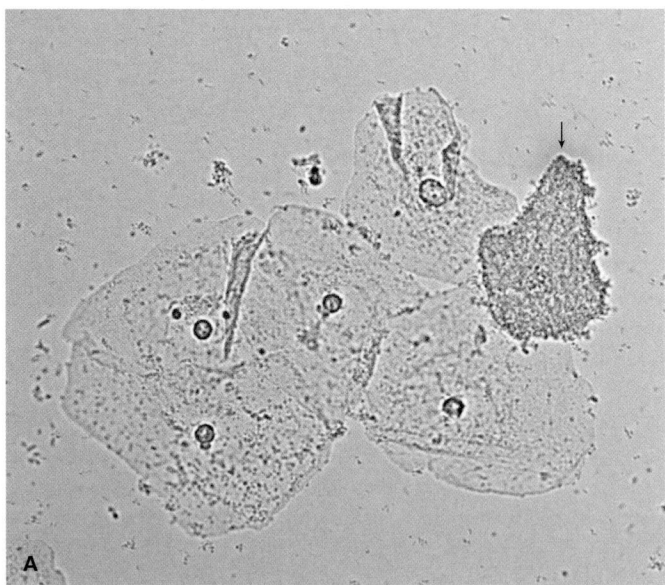 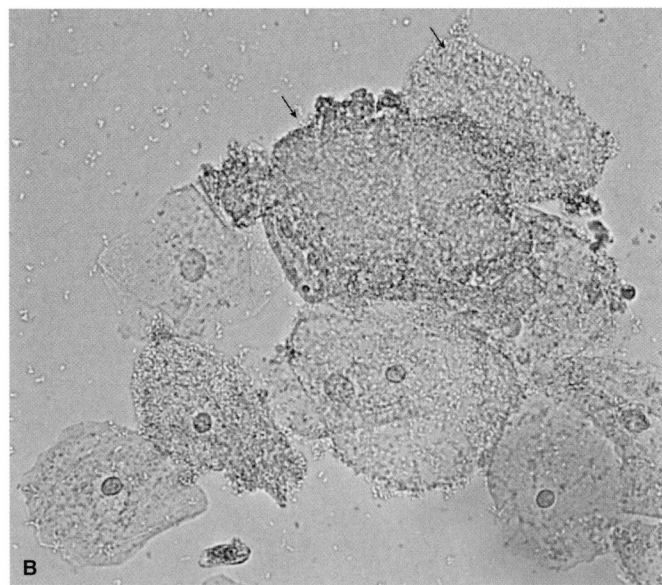

FIGURE 3-1 Photographs of a saline wet preparation reveals clue cells. **A.** Single clue cell (*arrow*) amid normal squamous cells. **B.** Several of these squamous cells are heavily studded with bacteria. Clue cells are covered to the extent that cell borders are blurred and nuclei are not visible (*arrows*). (*Photographs contributed by Dr. Lauri Campagna and Mercedes Pineda, WHNP.*)

TABLE 3-3. Recommended Treatment of Bacterial Vaginosis

Agent	Dosage
Metronidazole (Flagyl)	500 mg orally twice daily for 7 days
Metronidazole gel 0.75% (Metrogel vaginal)	5 g (1 full applicator) intravaginally once daily for 5 days
Clindamycin cream 2% (Cleocin, Clindesse[a])	5 g (1 full applicator) intravaginally at bedtime for 7 days

[a]Drug recalled in 2009 because of manufacturing that did not sufficiently comply with current good manufacturing practices.
Modified from the Centers for Disease Control and Prevention, 2010b.

unassociated with *N gonorrhoeae* or *Chlamydia trachomatis*, and acute pelvic infections following pelvic surgery, especially hysterectomy (Larsson, 1989, 1991, 1992; Soper, 1990).

Treatment

Three regimens have been proposed by the 2010 Centers for Disease Control and Prevention BV working group and are for nonpregnant women (Table 3-3). Alternatives include tinidazole 2 g orally daily for 3 days or clindamycin 300 mg orally twice daily for 7 days. Cure rates with these regimens range from 80 to 90 percent at 1 week, but within 3 months, 30 percent of women have experienced a recurrence of altered flora. At least half have another episode of symptoms associated with this flora change, many of which are correlated with heterosexual contacts (Amsel, 1983; Gardner, 1955; Wilson, 2004). However, treatment of male sexual partners does not benefit women with this recurring condition and is not recommended. Moreover, other forms of therapy such as introduction of lactobacilli, acidifying vaginal gels, and use of probiotics have shown inconsistent effectiveness (Senok, 2009).

ANTIBIOTICS

These drugs are commonly used in gynecology to restore altered flora or treat various infections. The ideal antibiotic is one that exhibits almost complete bioavailability from either oral or parenteral administration, acts promptly to eradicate a diverse variety of aerobic and anaerobic bacteria, fails to induce bacterial resistance, and is nontoxic, nonsensitizing, inexpensive, and easily produced. It does not exist. Despite this, many effective antibiotics are available for the treatment of gynecologic infection.

As a group, antibiotics have been implicated in decreasing the efficacy of oral contraceptives. Fortunately, this has been proven in very few, and these are listed in Table 5-11 (p. 155).

■ Penicillins

Structure

The heart of all penicillins is a β-lactam ring with a side chain and a thiazolidine ring (Fig. 3-2). The β-lactam nucleus provides anti-

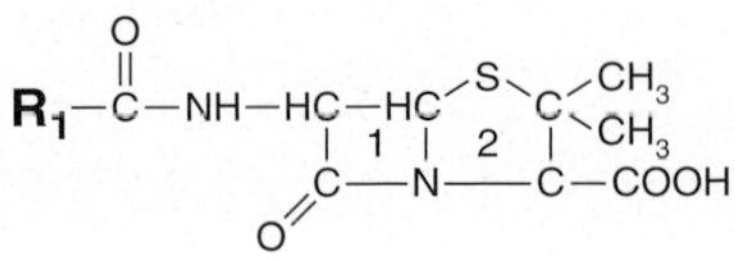

FIGURE 3-2 Basic chemical structure of penicillins. Substitutions at the R_1 position lead to varied antibacterial activity. In this figure, the β-lactam ring is labeled 1, and the thiazolidine ring is numbered 2.

bacterial activity, which is primarily against gram-positive aerobic bacteria. Because of the numerous substitutions at R_1, a variety of antibiotics with altered antibacterial spectra and pharmacologic properties have been synthesized (Table 3-4).

Some bacteria produce an enzyme (β-lactamase) that opens the β-lactam ring and inactivates the drug as a primary bacterial defense mechanism. Clavulanic acid, sulbactam, and tazobactam are inhibitors of β-lactamase and have been combined with several penicillins to enhance the activity spectrum against a broader variety of aerobic and anaerobic bacteria. Additionally, oral probenecid can be prescribed separately for administration with penicillins. This drug lowers the renal-tubular secretion rate of these antibiotics and is used to increase penicillin or cephalosporin plasma levels.

Adverse Reactions

Table 3-5 lists adverse reactions to penicillins (Mayo Clinic, 1991). Up to 10 percent of the general population may manifest an allergic reaction to penicillins. The lowest risk is associated with oral preparations, whereas the highest follows those combined with procaine and given intramuscularly. True anaphylactic (Type I hypersensitivity) reactions are rare, and mortality rates approximate 1 in every 50,000 treatment regimens. If penicillin allergy is noted, yet treatment is still required, desensitization can be performed as described by Wendel and coworkers (1985) and outlined at the CDC web site: http://www.cdc.gov/std/treatment/2006/penicillin-allergy.htm.

Clinical Applications

Excellent tissue penetration is achieved with these agents. Penicillin remains the primary antibiotic for treatment of syphilis, and this family of antibiotics is also useful in treating skin infections and breast cellulitis and breast abscesses. The combination of amoxicillin and clavulanic acid (Augmentin) provides the best oral broad-spectrum antibiotic coverage. Moreover, the ureidopenicillins and those combined with a β-lactamase enzyme inhibitor are effective against acute community-acquired or postoperative pelvic infections. In addition, *Actinomyces israelii* infections, which are an infrequent complication of intrauterine device (IUD) use, are treated with penicillins (American College of Obstetricians and Gynecologists, 2005).

■ Cephalosporins

Structure

Cephalosporins also are β-lactam antimicrobials. Substitutions at the R_1 or R_2 sites of the cephalosporin nucleus significantly

TABLE 3-4. Penicillin Family Classification[a]

Generic (Brand) Name	Route	Dosages Used	Clinical Use of Group	Bacterial Coverage of Group[b]
Natural				
Penicillin G	Oral		Syphilis[c]	*Treponema pallidum*, group A & B
	IV, IM	1–2 million units every 6 hours	Superficial skin cellulitis *Actinomyces* infection	*Streptococcus* spp. & *Enterococcus* spp. Not *Staphylococcus* spp.
				No gram-negative bacteria
Benzathine penicillin G (Bicillin)	IM	2.4 million units		Some anaerobes: *Actinomyces Peptostreptococcus*, & *Clostridium* spp.
Penicillin V (Pen VK)	Oral	250–500 mg every 6 hours		Not *C difficile* or *B fragilis*
Penicillinase-resistant				
Dicloxacillin (Dynapen)	Oral	125–500 mg every 6 hours	Breast cellulitis and breast abscess	Group A & B *Streptococcus* spp. & *Staphylococcus* spp.
Nafcillin sodium (Unipen, Nafcil)	IV	1–2 g every 4–6 hours		Not MRSA or *Enterococcus* spp.
				No gram-negative bacteria
Oxacillin sodium (Prostaphlin)	IV, IM	1–2 g every 4–6 hours		Few anaerobes: *Peptostreptococcus* spp.
Aminopenicillins				
Amoxicillin (Amoxil, Trimox)	Oral	500–1000 mg every 8 hours	Oral treatment of Bartholin or simple vulvar abscess	Group A & B *Streptococcus* spp. & *Enterococcus* spp.
Ampicillin (Omnipen, Principen)	Oral	250–500 mg every 6 hours		Not *Staphylococcus* spp.
	IV	2 g every 6 hours	IV ampicillin: in combination therapy for community-acquired or post-operative pelvic infection[d]	Some gram-negative bacteria: *E coli, P mirabilis, H influenzae, Salmonella* spp., & *Shigella* spp.
Amoxicillin-clavulanic acid (Augmentin)	Oral	500–875 mg every 8–12 hours		Many anaerobes: *Actinomyces, Bacteroides, Peptostreptococcus*, & *Clostridium* spp.
Ampicillin sulbactam (Unasyn)	IV	1.5–3 g every 6 hours	IV Unasyn for community-acquired or postoperative pelvic infection[d]	Not *C difficile*
				Added coverage with Augmentin or Unasyn:
				Many gram-negative bacteria, including *N gonorrhoeae*
				Not *Serratia, Citrobacter, Pseudomonas*, or *Acinetobacter* spp.
Carboxycillins				
Ticarcillin	IV	200–300 mg/kg/d divided and given every 4–6 hours	For community-acquired or postoperative pelvic infection[d] For complicated SSI	Group A & B *Streptococcus* spp. & *Enterococcus* spp. Not *Staphylococcus* spp.
Ticarcillin-clavulanic acid (Timentin)	IV, IM	300 mg/kg/d divided and given every 4 hours		Many gram-negative bacteria, including *N gonorrhoeae* Not *Klebsiella* spp. or *Acinetobacter* spp.
				Few anaerobes: *Clostridium* spp. and *Peptostreptococcus* spp. Not *C difficile*

(Continued)

TABLE 3-4. Penicillin Family Classification[a] *(Continued)*

Generic (Brand) Name	Route	Dosages Used	Clinical Use of Group	Bacterial Coverage of Group[b]
				Added coverage with Timentin: S aureus & S epidermidis Not MRSA Klebsiella spp. & Acinetobacter spp. B fragilis
Uredopenicillins				
Piperacillin (Pipracil)	IV, IM	200–300 mg/kg/d divided and given every 4–6 hours or 3–4 g every 4–6 hours	For community-acquired or postoperative pelvic infection[d]	Group A & B Streptococcus spp. & Enterococcus spp. Not Staphylococcus spp.
Piperacillin-tazobactam (Zosyn)	IV	3.375 mg every 4–6 hours	For complicated SSI	Many gram-negative bacteria, including N gonorrhoeae Not Serratia spp. or Acinetobacter spp.
				Many anaerobes: Actinomyces, Peptostreptococcus, & Clostridium spp. Not C difficile
				Added coverage with Zosyn: S aureus, S epidermidis Not MRSA Serratia spp. & Acinetobacter spp. B fragilis

[a]Penicillins are Food and Drug Administration pregnancy category B drugs.
[b]Purple lettering = gram-positive bacteria; red lettering = gram-negative bacteria; black lettering = anaerobes.
[c]See Table 3-12 for dosages.
[d]See Table 3-31 for dosages.
B fragilis = Bacteroides fragilis; C difficile = Clostridium difficile; E coli = Escherichia coli; H influenzae = Haemophilus influenzae; IM = intramuscular; IV = intravenous; MRSA = methicillin-resistant Staphylococcus aureus; N gonorrhoeae = Neisseria gonorrhoeae; P mirabilis = Proteus mirabilis; S aureus = Staphylococcus aureus; S epidermidis = Staphylococcus epidermidis; SSI = surgical site infection; spp. = species.

alter the spectrum of activity, potency, toxicity, and half-life of these antibiotics (Fig. 3-3). Organization of these qualities has resulted in their division into first-, second-, or third-generation cephalosporins. Although possibly a marketing tool, this classification does allow grouping based on general spectra of activity. Those commonly used by gynecologists are presented in Table 3-6.

Adverse Reactions

Rash and other hypersensitivity reactions are the most common and may develop in up to 3 percent of patients. Cephalosporins are β-lactam antibiotics and if used in those allergic to penicillin, may create the same or accentuated response. Theoretically, this may happen in up to 16 percent of patients (Saxon, 1987). Thus, if an individual developed anaphylaxis with penicillin therapy, cephalosporin administration is contraindicated.

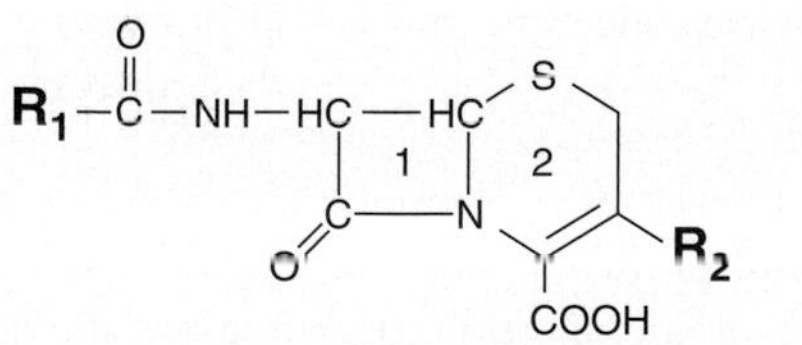

Clinical Applications

First-generation cephalosporins are used primarily for surgical prophylaxis and in the treatment of superficial skin cellulitis. Their activity spectrum is greatest against gram-positive aerobic cocci, with some activity against community-acquired gram-negative rods. However, there is little activity against β-lactamase producing organisms or anaerobic bacteria. Despite this inactivity against many pathogens of pelvic infection that may be acquired during surgery, there is prophylactic efficacy.

Second-generation cephalosporins have enhanced activity against gram-negative aerobic and anaerobic bacteria, with some diminution in effectiveness against aerobic gram-positive cocci. Their primary use is in surgical prophylaxis or for single-agent therapy of major community-acquired or postoperative pelvic infections, including abscess.

Third-generation cephalosporins are effective in treatment of major postoperative pelvic infections, including abscess.

FIGURE 3-3 Basic chemical structure of cephalosporins. Substitutions at R1 and R2 positions lead to varied antibacterial activity.

TABLE 3-5. Penicillin Adverse Reactions

Adverse Reaction	Representative Penicillin
Allergic	
Anaphylaxis	Any penicillin
Urticaria	Any penicillin
Drug fever	Any penicillin
Serum sickness	Penicillin G
Delayed hypersensitivity	Ampicillin
Exfoliative dermatitis	Any penicillin
Neurologic	
Seizure	Penicillin G
Dizziness, paresthesias	Penicillin G procaine
Neuromuscular irritability	Penicillin G
Hematologic	
Hemolytic anemia	Penicillin G
Neutropenia	Oxacillin, piperacillin, penicillin G
Thrombocytopenia	Piperacillin
Platelet dysfunction	Carbenicillin
Renal	
Interstitial nephritis	Any penicillin
Hepatic	
Increased transaminases	Any penicillin
Gastrointestinal	
Nausea, vomiting	Ampicillin
Diarrhea	Ampicillin
Pseudomembranous colitis	Any penicillin
Electrolyte abnormalities	
Sodium overload	Carbenicillin
Hypokalemia	Carbenicillin
Thrombophlebitis	Nafcillin, oxacillin

However, they are used primarily in the treatment of postoperative respiratory tract infections. These agents have documented efficacy as prophylactic agents, but should be reserved for therapy.

Aminoglycosides
Structure and Clinical Applications

This family of compounds includes gentamicin, tobramycin, netilmicin, and amikacin. They differ in antimicrobial activity based on the various amino sugars that form the lateral chains of the central aminoglycoside nucleus. Of the aminoglycosides, gentamicin is primarily selected because of its low cost and clinical efficacy for pathogens recovered from pelvic infections (Table 3-7). For gynecologists, it may be combined with clindamycin with or without ampicillin as a regimen for treatment of serious pelvic infections. Alternatively, gentamicin may be joined with ampicillin and metronidazole. Lastly, it can be used as single-agent therapy for pyelonephritis. Aminoglycoside antibacterial activity is serum/tissue concentration related, and the higher the concentration, the greater the potency.

Adverse Reactions

Aminoglycosides have the potential for significant patient toxicity, which can include ototoxicity, neurotoxicity, and neuromuscular blockade. The inner ear is particularly susceptible to aminoglycosides because of selective accumulation within the hair cells and prolonged half-life within inner ear fluids. Those with vestibular toxicity complain of headaches, nausea, tinnitus, and loss of equilibrium. Cochlear toxicity results in high-frequency hearing loss. If either of these develops, aminoglycoside administration must be stopped promptly. Ototoxicity may be permanent, and risk correlates positively with dose and duration of therapy.

Nephrotoxicity is reversible and may develop in up to 25 percent of patients (Bertino, 1993). Risk factors include older age, renal insufficiency, hypotension, volume depletion, frequent dosing intervals, treatment for 3 or more days, multiple antibiotic administration, or multisystem disease. Toxicity leads to a nonoliguric decrease in creatinine clearance and resultant rise in serum creatinine levels.

Neuromuscular blockade is a rare but potentially life-threatening complication and is dose-related. This family of antibiotics inhibits presynaptic acetylcholine release, blocks acetylcholine receptors, and prevents presynaptic calcium absorption. For this reason, aminoglycoside contraindications include myasthenia gravis or concurrent succinylcholine use. Blockade frequently follows rapid intravenous infusion. For this reason, aminoglycosides are ideally given intravenously over at least 30 minutes. Toxicity is usually detected before respiratory arrest, and at its first signs, intravenous calcium gluconate is administered to reverse this form of aminoglycoside toxicity.

Dosing

Multiple Doses. Aminoglycosides may be parenterally dosed every 8 hours in those with normal renal function. For critically ill patients, an initial dose of between 1.5 and 2 mg/kg for gentamicin, tobramycin, and netilmicin and between 7.5 and 15 mg/kg for amikacin is recommended. Subsequently, maintenance doses are calculated to deliver 3 to 5 mg/kg/d of ideal body weight for the first three aminoglycosides just listed and 15 mg/kg/d for amikacin.

If a patient has decreased renal function, there should be dose reduction or interval lengthening or both. Calculations for these reductions can be found in prescribing information documents at: http://www.drugs.com/pro/gentamicin-sulfate.html and at: http://www.tevausa.com/assets/base/products/pi/Amikacin_PI.pdf. The formula listed below allows one to calculate a rough estimate of creatinine clearance so proper adjustments can be made. This formula is for male patients. The result, multiplied by 0.85, will give a value for female patients.

$$\text{Creatinine clearance (mL/min)} = (140 - \text{age}) \times \text{weight (kg)} \div \text{serum creatinine} \times 72$$

To monitor serum concentration, provide adequate therapeutic levels, and prevent toxicity in patients given multiple daily doses, serum aminoglycoside concentrations should be measured at two points. The first is the peak, drawn either 30 minutes after

TABLE 3-6. Cephalosporin Classification[a]

Generic (Brand) Name	Route	Clinical Use	Bacterial Coverage[b]
First-generation			
Cefadroxil (Duricef)	Oral	Uncomplicated superficial skin cellulitis	Most gram-positive bacteria
Cephalexin (Keflex)	Oral		Not *Enterococcus* spp. or MRSA
Cefazolin (Ancef, Kefzol)	IV	IV for surgical prophylaxis[c]	Few gram-negative bacteria: *E coli, P mirabilis*, & *Klebsiella* spp.
			Not anaerobes
Second-generation			
Cefaclor (Ceclor, Raniclor)	Oral	IV for community-acquired or postoperative pelvic infection[d]	Most gram-positive bacteria
Ceprozil (Cefzil)	Oral		Not *Enterococcus* spp. or MRSA
Cefotetan (Cefotan)	IV, IM		Few gram-negative bacteria: *E coli, P mirabilis, Klebsiella* spp., & *H influenzae*
Cefoxitin (Mefoxin)	IV, IM		
Cefuroxime (Ceftin, Zinacef)	IV, IM		
Cefuroxime axetil (Ceftin, Zinacef)	Oral IV, IM		Few anaerobes: *Peptostreptococcus* spp. & *Clostridium* spp.
			Not *C difficile* or *B fragilis*
Third-generation			
Cefditoren (Spectracef)	Oral	IV forms for postoperative pelvic[d] or respiratory infection	Most gram-positive bacteria
Cefdinir (Omnicef)	Oral		Not *Enterococcus* spp. or MRSA
Cefixime (Suprax)	Oral	Ceftriaxone for STD prophylaxis following sexual assault[e]	Gram-negative bacteria, including *N gonorrhoeae*
Cefpodoxime (Vantin)	Oral		Not *Serratia, Pseudomonas, Morganella*, or *Acinetobacter* spp.
Cefoperazone (Cefobid)	IV, IM		
Cefotaxime (Claforan)	IV, IM		
Ceftazidime (Fortaz, Tazicef)	IV, IM		Few anaerobes: *Peptostreptococcus* spp.
Ceftizoxime (Cefizox)	IV, IM		
Ceftriaxone (Rocephin)	IV, IM		
			Added coverage with IV agents: Most gram-negative bacteria, including *N gonorrhoeae*
			Not *Acinetobacter* spp.
			Anaerobes: *Actinomyces, Clostridium*, & *Peptostreptococcus* spp.
			Not *C difficile* or *Bacteroides* spp.
Fourth-generation			
Cefepime (Maxipime)	IV, IM	For postoperative pelvic infection	Group A & B *Streptococcus* spp., *S aureus*, & *S epidermidis*
			Not MRSA
			Most gram-negative bacteria, including *N gonorrhoeae*
			Few anaerobes: *Peptostreptococcus* spp.

[a]Cephalosporins are Food and Drug Administration pregnancy category B drugs.
[b]Purple lettering = gram-positive bacteria; red lettering = gram-negative bacteria; black lettering = anaerobes.
[c]See Table 39-6 for dosages.
[d]See Table 3-31 for dosages.
[e]See Table 13-16, p. 372, for dosages and complete prophylaxis recommendations following sexual assault. *B fragilis* = *Bacteroides fragilis*; *C difficile* = *Clostridium difficile*; E coli = *Escherichia coli*; H influenzae = *Haemophilus influenzae*; IM = *intramuscular*; IV = *intravenous*; MRSA = methicillin-resistant *Staphylococcus aureus*; N gonorrhoeae = *Neisseria gonorrhoeae*; P mirabilis = *Proteus mirabilis*; S aureus = *Staphylococcus aureus*; S epidermidis = *Staphylococcus epidermidis*; spp. = *species*; STD = sexually transmitted disease.

TABLE 3-7. Other Antibiotics Commonly Used by the Gynecologist

Generic (Brand) Name	Route	Dosages Used	Clinical Use	Bacterial Coverage[a]
Clindamycin[b] (Cleocin)	Oral IV Vaginal Topical	300–600 mg orally every 8 hours 600–900 mg IV every 8 hours 2% vaginal cream 1% skin gel or lotion applied twice daily	Surgical prophylaxis in β-lactam-allergic patients combined with aminoglycoside[e] In combination therapy for community-acquired or postoperative pelvic infection[f] Complicated MRSA infection Vaginal form for BV[g] Topical or oral forms for hidradenitis suppurativa	Gram-positive bacteria, including MRSA Few gram-negative bacteria: *C trachomatis*, some action against *N gonorrhoeae* Anaerobes
Trimethoprim-sulfaoxazole DS[c] (Bactrim DS, Septra DS)	Oral IV	160/800 mg orally every 12 hours 2.5 mg/kg IV every 12 hours	MRSA infection Uncomplicated UTI when *E coli* sensitivity is high[h]	Gram-positive bacteria, including MRSA Some activity against most gram-negative bacteria Not *P mirabilis* or *P aeruginosa* Not anaerobes
Vancomycin[c] (Vancocin)	IV	15–20 mg/kg every 12 hours	In combination, surgical prophylaxis for those with prior MRSA infection[e] Complicated MRSA infection If gram-positive coverage needed in β-lactam allergic patients	Aerobic gram-positive bacteria, including MRSA
Doxycycline[d] (Doryx)	Oral, IV	100 mg twice daily	*C trachomatis* infection, including PID, LGV, granuloma inguinale; syphilis (alternate drug)[i] Orally for hidradenitis suppurativa Uncomplicated MRSA infection Surgical prophylaxis[e]	Gram-positive bacteria, including MRSA Not *Enterococcus* spp. Few gram-negative bacteria: *E coli, Chlamydia* spp., and *Mycoplasma* spp. Few anaerobes: *Clostridium* spp. and *Actinomyces* spp. Not *C difficile* or *Bacteroides* spp.
Gentamicin[d]	IV	Multidose: 2 mg/kg loading dose, then 1.5 mg/kg every 8 hours Single daily dose: 7 mg/kg/d	In combination therapy for community-acquired or postoperative pelvic infection[f] Pyelonephritis[h] Surgical prophylaxis[e]	Not gram-positive bacteria Most gram-negative bacteria Not *N gonorrhoeae* or *Acinetobacter* spp. Not anaerobes

(Continued)

CHAPTER 3

TABLE 3-7. Other Antibiotics Commonly Used by the Gynecologist *(Continued)*

Generic (Brand) Name	Route	Dosages Used	Clinical Use	Bacterial Coverage[a]
Metronizadole[b] (Flagyl)	Oral, IV Vaginal	500 mg orally twice daily for 7 d IV loading dose: 15 mg/kg; maintenance 7.5 mg/kg every 6 hours	In combination therapy for community-acquired or postoperative pelvic infection[f] Vaginal or oral forms for BV[g] Trichomoniasis[j] In combination for PID[k] Surgical prophylaxis[e]	*C difficile* infection Trichomoniasis Bacterial vaginosis pathogens Anaerobes only
Azithromycin[b] (Zithromax)	Oral	1 q daily	*Chlamydia* spp. infection, including: PID, chancroid, and granuloma inguinale[i] STD prophylaxis following sexual assault[l]	Group A and B *Streptococcus* spp. and *S aureus* Not *Enterococcus* spp., MRSA, or *S epidermidis* Not gram-negative bacteria Some anaerobes: *Actinomyces*, *Peptostreptococcus*, and *Clostridium* spp. Not *C difficile* or *B fragilis*

[a]Purple lettering = gram-positive bacteria; red lettering = gram-negative bacteria; black lettering = anaerobes.
[b]Food and Drug Administration pregnancy category B drug.
[c]Food and Drug Administration pregnancy category C drug.
[d]Food and Drug Administration pregnancy category D drug.
[e]See Table 39-6, p. 959, for dosages.
[f]See Table 3-31 for dosages.
[g]See Table 3-3 for dosages.
[h]See Table 3-24 for dosages.
[i]See Table for treatment of specific infection in this chapter for dosages.
[j]See Table 3-18 for dosages.
[k]See Table 3-27 for dosages.
[l]See Table 13-16, p. 372, for dosages and complete prophylaxis recommendations following sexual assault.
B fragilis = *Bacteroides fragilis*; *C trachomatis* = *Chlamydia trachomatis*; *C difficile* = *Clostridium difficile*; *E coli* = *Escherichia coli*; *H influenzae* = *Haemophilus influenzae*; IM = intramuscular; IV = intravenous; LGV = lymphogranuloma venereum; MRSA = methicillin-resistant *Staphylococcus aureus*; *N gonorrhoeae* = *Neisseria gonorrhoeae*; PID = pelvic inflammatory disease; *P mirabilis* = *Proteus mirabilis*; *Pseudomonas aeruginosa* = *P aeruginosa*; *S aureus* = *Staphylococcus aureus*; *Staphylococcus epidermidis* = *S epidermidis*; spp. = species; STD = sexually transmitted disease; UTI = urinary tract infection.

the completion of a 30-minute infusion or 1 hour after an intramuscular injection. These values for gentamicin, tobramycin, and netilmicin should be 4 to 6 µg/mL. For amikacin it should be between 20 and 30 µg/mL. The second blood sample (trough) should be drawn immediately before initiation of the next dose 7.5 or 8 hours later. Trough concentrations should be between 1 and 2 µg/mL for the first three aminoglycosides and 5 to 10 µg/mL for amikacin. These should be repeated if therapy is prolonged (3 to 4 days) or if serum creatinine levels increase. High peak and trough levels are indicators for increased risk of toxicity.

Single Daily Dosing. Increased aminoglycoside concentration enhances antibacterial activity but also toxicity. Once-daily

dosing was evaluated and found to be as or less toxic than multiple daily dosing without sacrificing clinical efficacy (Bertino, 1993). Tulkens and colleagues (1988) reported that once-daily dosing of netilmicin was less toxic than administrations three times daily, without jeopardizing efficacy in the treatment of women with PID. In 1992, Nicolau and associates presented pharmacokinetic data and a nomogram for administering aminoglycosides once daily (Fig. 3-4).

Recommendation for an initial dose, which is 7 mg/kg, is based on the patient's creatinine clearance. For those with a creatinine clearance greater than 60 mL/min, the dosing is every 24 hours. If the clearance is between 40 and 60 mL/min, the recommended dose is every 36 hours. If the

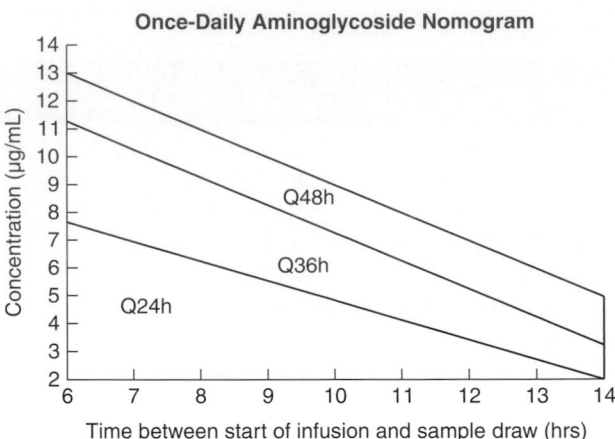

FIGURE 3-4 Once-daily aminoglycoside nomogram.

clearance is less than 40 mL/min, traditional multidosing is recommended.

To use the nomogram presented in Figure 3-4, one obtains a random serum concentration between 8 and 12 hours after the start of the initial dose infusion. One then places that concentration value over the time interval to determine the dosing interval. That applies to gentamicin, tobramycin, and netilmicin. For amikacin, the initial dose is 15 mg/kg, and the resultant concentration at 8 to 12 hours should be divided by 2 and then placed on the nomogram at the dosing interval drawn. With this dosing calculation approach, standard peak and trough levels are unnecessary. A second random sample should be drawn if therapy continues for more than 4 days. Once-daily dosing theoretically is preferable since a higher peak concentration results.

Carbapenems

Structure

The carbapenems are a third class of β-lactam antibiotics that differ from penicillins by substitution of a carbon for a sulfur atom in the five-membered ring and by the addition of a double bond therein (Fig. 3-5). The three antibiotics in this family are imipenem (Primaxin), meropenem (Merrem), and ertapenem (Invanz).

Adverse Reactions

Adverse reactions are comparable to those of the other β-lactam antibiotics. As is true with other β-lactams, if patients have experienced a Type I hypersensitivity reaction to either a penicillin or a cephalosporin, then a carbapenem should not be administered.

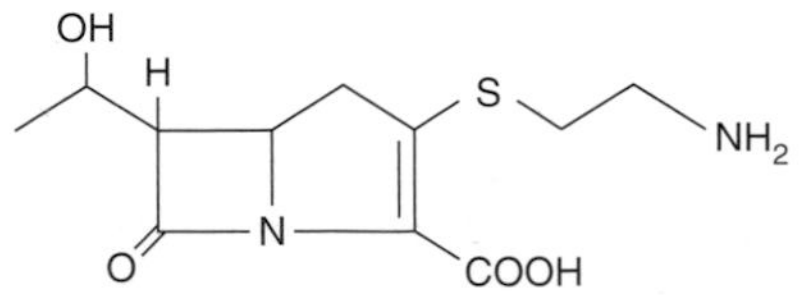

FIGURE 3-5 Basic chemical structure of carbapenems.

Clinical Applications

These antibiotics are designed for polymicrobial bacterial infections, primarily those with resistant aerobic gram-negative bacteria not susceptible to other β-lactam agents. They should be reserved to preserve efficacy by preventing the development of resistance.

Monobactam

The marketed monobactam, Aztreonam, is a synthetic β-lactam. It has a spectrum of activity similar to aminoglycosides, that is, gram-negative aerobic species. Like other β-lactam antibiotics, these compounds inhibit bacterial cell wall synthesis by binding to penicillin-binding proteins or causing cell lysis. It has affinity only for the binding proteins of the gram-negative bacteria and lacks affinity for either gram-positive bacteria or anaerobic organisms. For the gynecologist, aztreonam provides coverage for gram-negative aerobic bacteria, which is usually provided by aminoglycosides, for patients with significantly impaired renal function or aminoglycoside allergy.

Clindamycin

This antibiotic was introduced in the mid-1960s and has been a workhorse in the treatment of serious gynecologic infections. Clindamycin is primarily active against aerobic gram-positive bacteria and anaerobic bacteria, with little activity against aerobic gram-negative bacteria. It is also active against *C trachomatis*. *N gonorrhoeae* is moderately sensitive, and *G vaginalis* is very susceptible to clindamycin. It may be delivered by one of three routes: orally, vaginally (2-percent cream), or intravenously.

The principal application of clindamycin for the gynecologist has been its combination with gentamicin for surgical prophylaxis or for treatment of serious community-acquired or postoperative soft tissue infections or pelvic abscess. Its activity against methicillin-resistant *Staphylococcus aureus* (MRSA) has increased its use in these cases as well as in vulvar abscess. Clindamycin is also used as monotherapy vaginally in the treatment of women with bacterial vaginosis. Moreover, in women with early stages of hidradenitis suppurativa, some patients improve with a long-term topical or oral clindamycin. Because there are parenteral and oral forms of this antibiotic, conversion from the more expensive parenteral therapy to oral therapy can occur early.

Vancomycin

This is a glycopeptide antibiotic that is active only against aerobic gram-positive bacteria. It is primarily used by the gynecologist to treat patients in whom β-lactam therapy is impossible due to a Type I hypersensitivity reaction. Additionally, an oral dose of 120 mg every 6 hours can be given to patients who have developed antibiotic-associated *Clostridium difficile* colitis and who do not respond to oral metronidazole. Lastly, vancomycin is often selected for MRSA infections, which are increasing in incidence.

Adverse Reactions

These are presented in Table 3-8. The most remarkable of these is the "red man" syndrome, which is a dermal reaction

TABLE 3-8. Vancomycin Adverse Effects

Hypersensitivity reactions
Drug fever (rare)
Allergic rash (rare)

Infusion-related side effects
Hypotension
"Red man" syndrome
"Pain and spasm" syndrome

Nephrotoxicity
Rare
Reversible
Enhanced risk with concomitant aminoglycoside
therapy

Neutropenia
Reversible
Develops after prolonged use

Ototoxicity
Hearing loss: often irreversible, rare, associated with
drug levels >30 µg/mL
Enhanced risk with concomitant aminoglycoside
therapy

Thrombophlebitis
Associated with peripheral venous cannulas

developing usually within minutes after initiation of a rapid drug infusion. The reaction, which is a response to histamine release, is an erythematous pruritic rash involving the neck, face, and upper torso. Hypotension also may develop. Intravenous administration over 1 hour or administration of an antihistamine may be protective, if given prior to infusion. Also associated with rapid administration may be painful back and chest muscle spasms.

The most significant of vancomycin's side effects is nephrotoxicity, which is enhanced with aminoglycoside therapy, as is ototoxicity. Both toxicities are associated with high serum concentrations of vancomycin. For that reason, serum peak and trough concentrations are recommended and should range between 20 and 40 µg/mL and 5 and 10 µg/mL, respectively. The initial dose should be 15 mg/kg of ideal body weight.

Metronidazole

This antibiotic was approved by the Food and Drug Administration (FDA) in the early 1960s for the treatment of trichomonal infection and is the principal therapy for this infection. Moreover, it is one of the mainstays of combination antimicrobial therapy given to women with serious postoperative or community-acquired pelvic infections, including pelvic abscess. Since it is active only against obligate anaerobes, metronidazole must be combined with agents effective against gram-positive and gram-negative aerobic bacterial species, such as ampicillin and gentamicin. This antibiotic is also useful in treatment of bacterial vaginosis. It is as effective as vancomycin in the treatment of *C difficile*–associated pseudomembranous colitis.

Tinidazole is another nitroimidazole approved for treatment of trichomoniasis and bacterial vaginosis in nonpregnant adult women. Although more expensive than metronidazole, it may be advantageous for metronidazole-resistant Trichomoniasis (Mammen-Tobin, 2005; Sobel, 2001).

Adverse Reactions

Up to 12 percent of patients taking oral metronidazole may have nausea, and an unpleasant metallic taste has also been described. Patients should abstain from alcohol use to avoid a disulfiram-like effect and emesis. Peripheral neuropathy and convulsive seizures have been reported, are probably dose-related, and are rare.

Fluoroquinolones

This antibiotic class is also known simply as *quinolones*. These have become first-line agents for treating a variety of infections because of their excellent bioavailability with oral administration, tissue penetration, broad-spectrum antibacterial activity, long half-lives, and good safety profile. As with cephalosporins, fluoroquinolones are separated into generations by their development, antibacterial activity, and pharmacokinetic properties (Table 3-9).

Adverse Reactions

Quinolones are contraindicated in children, adolescents, and pregnant and breast-feeding women because they may affect cartilage development. As a family, they are safe, and severe adverse reactions are rare. The side-effect rate ranges from 4 to 8 percent and primarily affects the gastrointestinal (GI) tract following oral administration. Central nervous system symptoms such as headache, confusion, tremors, and seizures have been described, and these develop more frequently in patients with underlying brain disorders.

Clinical Applications

These agents are widely used by gynecologists to treat acute lower urinary tract infections, sexually transmitted diseases, and bacterial intestinal infections. However, they should not be overused. If a less expensive, safer, and equally effective alternative agent is available to treat a given infection, it should be used to preserve fluoroquinolone efficacy.

Tetracyclines

These bacteriostatic antimicrobials are commonly used orally and inhibit bacterial protein synthesis. Doxycycline, tetracycline, and minocycline are active against many gram-positive and gram-negative bacteria, although they are more active against gram-positive species. Susceptible organisms also include several anaerobes, *Chlamydia* and *Mycoplasma* species, and some spirochetes. Accordingly, cervicitis, PID, syphilis, chancroid, lymphogranuloma venereum, and granuloma inguinale respond to these agents. Moreover, tetracyclines are among treatment options for community-acquired skin and soft tissue MRSA infections. Specifically, for these infections, minocycline and doxycycline are superior to tetracycline. Tetracycline is active against *Actinomyces* species and is an alternative for treating actinomycosis. Lastly, these antibiotics bind specific nonmicrobial targets, such as matrix

TABLE 3-9. Selected Quinolone Antibiotics[a]

Generic (Brand) Name	Route	Clinical Use	Bacterial Coverage[b]
Second-generation			
Norfloxacin (Noroxin)	Oral	Acute upper and lower UTI[c]	S aureus
Ciprofloxacin (Cipro)	Oral, IV	Chancroid, granuloma inguinale[d]	Not Enterococcus spp.
Ciprofloxacin extended release (Cipro XR)	Oral	C trachomatis (alternate drug)[e] In combination for surgical prophylaxis[f]	Most gram-negative bacteria Not N gonorrhoeae
Ofloxacin (Floxin)	Oral, IV		Not anaerobes
Third-generation			
Levofloxacin (Levaquin)	Oral, IV	Acute upper and lower UTI[c]	Gram-positive bacteria, including some MRSA activity, also Enterococcus spp.
Moxifloxacin (Avelox)	Oral, IV	C trachomatis (alternate drug)[d]	
Gemifloxacin (Factive)	Oral	In combination for surgical prophylaxis[f]	
			Most gram-negative bacteria Not N gonorrhoeae

[a]Fluoroquinolones are Food and Drug Administration pregnancy category C drugs.
[b]Purple lettering = gram-positive bacteria; red lettering = gram-negative bacteria; black lettering = anaerobes.
[c]See Table 3-24 for dosages.
[d]Ciprofloxacin, see Tables 3-13 and 3-14 for dosages.
[e]Ofloxacin or levofloxacin, see Table 3-20 for dosages.
[f]Ciprofloxacin, ofloxacin, moxifloxacin, see Table 39-6, p. 959, for dosages.
C trachomatis = Chlamydia trachomatis; C difficile = Clostridium difficile; IV = intravenous; MRSA = methicillin-resistant Staphylococcus aureus; N gonorrhoeae = Neisseria gonorrhoeae; S aureus = Staphylococcus aureus; UTI = urinary tract infection.

metalloproteinases (MMPs), and are potent MMP inhibitors. As such, they provide antiinflammatory as well as antimicrobial activity for inflammatory conditions such as acne vulgaris and hidradenitis suppurativa.

Adverse Reactions

With oral administration, tetracyclines can produce direct local GI irritation that manifests as abdominal discomfort, nausea, vomiting, or diarrhea. In teeth and growing bones, tetracyclines readily bind calcium, causing deformity, growth inhibition, or discoloration. Accordingly, tetracyclines are not prescribed for pregnant or nursing women or for children younger than 8 years. Sensitivity to sunlight or ultraviolet light may develop with use. Dizziness, vertigo, nausea, and vomiting may be seen with higher doses. In addition, thrombophlebitis at the intravenous (IV) site frequently follows IV administration. Tetracyclines modify the normal GI flora, which can result in intestinal functional disturbances. Specifically, overgrowth of C difficile may lead to pseudomembranous colitis. As with penicillins and cephalosporins, vaginal flora also may be altered with tetracyclines and lead to Candida species overgrowth and symptomatic vulvovaginitis.

PATHOGENS CAUSING GENITAL ULCER INFECTIONS

Ulceration defines complete loss of the epidermal covering with invasion into the underlying dermis. In contrast, erosion describes partial loss of the epidermis without dermal penetration. These are distinguished by clinical examination. Biopsies are generally not helpful, but these may be if taken from the edge of a new lesion (Fig. 4-2, p. 112). Importantly, biopsy is mandatory if carcinoma is suspected.

Most young sexually active women in the United States who have genital ulcers will have herpes simplex infection, syphilis, or chancroid, but some will have lymphogranuloma venereum or granuloma inguinale. Essentially all are sexually transmitted and are associated with increased risk for human immunodeficiency virus (HIV) transmission. For this reason, HIV and other sexually transmitted disease testing should be offered to such patients. Sexual contacts require examination and treatment, and all involved individuals require reevaluation following treatment.

■ Herpes Simplex Virus Infection

Genital herpes is the most prevalent genital ulcer disease and is a chronic viral infection. The virus enters sensory nerve endings and undergoes retrograde axonal transport to the dorsal root ganglion, where the virus develops lifelong latency. Spontaneous reactivation by various events results in anterograde transport of virus particles/protein to the surface. Here virus is shed, with or without lesion formation. It is postulated that immune mechanisms control latency and reactivation (Cunningham, 2006).

There are two types of herpes simplex virus, HSV-1 and HSV-2. Type 1 HSV is the most frequent cause of oral lesions. Type 2 HSV is found more typically with genital lesions, although both types can cause genital herpes. It is estimated that of American females age 14 to 49 years, 21 percent have suffered a genital HSV-2 infection, and 60 percent of women are seropositive to HSV-1 (Centers for Disease Control and Prevention, 2010a; Xu, 2006).

Most women who have been infected with HSV-2 lack this diagnosis because of mild or unrecognized infections. Infected patients can shed infectious virus while asymptomatic, and most infections are transmitted sexually by patients that are unaware of their infection. Most (65 percent) with active infection are women.

Symptoms

Patient symptoms at initial presentation will depend primarily on whether or not a patient during the current episode has antibody from previous exposure. If a patient has no antibody, the attack rate in an exposed person approaches 70 percent. The mean incubation period is approximately 1 week. Up to 90 percent of those who are symptomatic with their initial infection will have another episode within a year.

The virus infects viable epidermal cells, the response to which is erythema and papule formation. With cell death and cell wall lysis, blisters form. The covering then disrupts, leaving a usually painful ulcer. These lesions develop crusting and heal, but may become secondarily infected. The three stages of lesions are: (1) vesicle with or without pustule formation, which lasts approximately a week; (2) ulceration; and (3) crusting. Virus is predictably shed during the first two phases of an infectious outbreak.

Burning and severe pain accompany initial vesicular lesions. With ulcers, urinary symptoms such as frequency and/or dysuria from direct contact of urine with ulcers may be present (Fig. 3-6). Local swelling may result from vulvar lesions and cause urethral obstruction. Alternatively or additionally, herpetic lesions may involve the vagina, cervix,

bladder, anus, and rectum. Commonly, a woman may have other signs of viremia such as a low-grade fever, malaise, and cephalalgia.

Viral load undoubtedly contributes to the numbers, size, and distribution of lesions. Normal host defense mechanisms inhibit viral growth, and healing starts within 1 to 2 days. Early treatment with an antiviral medication decreases the viral load. Immune-deficient patients are at increased susceptibility and display diminished response and delayed healing.

For a previously uninfected patient, the vesicular, or initial, stage is longer. There is an increased period of new lesion formation and a longer time to healing. Pain persists for the first 7 to 10 days, and lesion healing requires 2 to 3 weeks.

If a patient has had prior exposure to HSV-2, the initial episode is significantly less severe. The duration of pain and tenderness is shorter, and healing time is approximately 2 weeks. Virus is shed usually only during the first week.

Recurrence following HSV-2 infection is common, and almost two thirds of patients have a prodrome prior to lesion onset. Heralding paresthesias are frequently described as pruritus or tingling in the area prior to lesion formation. However, prodromal symptoms may develop without actual lesion formation. Clinical manifestations for women with recurrences are more limited, with only approximately 1 week of symptoms.

Diagnosis

The gold standard for the diagnosis of a herpetic lesion(s) is tissue culture. Specificity is high, but sensitivity is low and declines as lesions heal. In recurrent disease, less than 50 percent of cultures are positive. Polymerase chain reaction (PCR) testing is 1.5 to 4 times more sensitive than culture and will probably replace it. Importantly, a negative culture result does not mean that there is no herpetic infection. Serologic type-specific glycoprotein G-based assays are available to detect antibodies specific to the HSV-specific glycoprotein G2 (HSV-2) and glycoprotein G1 (HSV-1). Assay specificity is ≥96 percent, and the sensitivity of HSV-2 antibody testing ranges from 80 to 98 percent. Although these tests may be used to confirm herpes simplex infection, treatment and additional STD screening may be initiated in clinically obvious cases following physical examination alone.

Treatment

Care Overview. Clinical management is with currently available antiviral therapy. Analgesia with nonsteroidal antiinflammatory drugs or a mild narcotic such as acetaminophen with codeine may be prescribed. In addition, topical anesthetics such as lidocaine ointment may provide relief. Local care to prevent secondary bacterial infection is important.

Patient education is mandatory, and specific topics should include the natural disease history, its sexual transmission, methods to reduce transmission, and obstetric consequences. Acquisition of this infection may have significant psychological impact, and several web sites provide patient information and support. The CDC web site can be accessed at: http://www.cdc.gov/std/Herpes/STDFact-Herpes.htm.

Women with genital herpes should refrain from sexual activity with uninfected partners when prodrome symptoms or

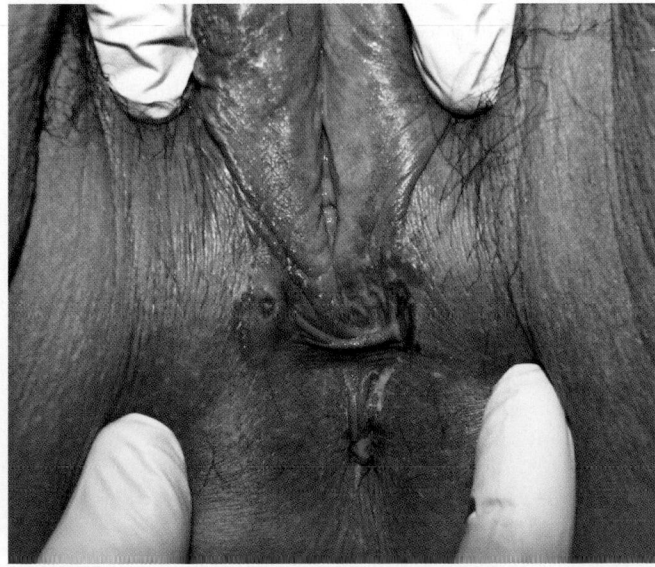

FIGURE 3-6 Genital herpetic ulcers. (*Photograph contributed by Dr. William Griffith.*)

TABLE 3-10. Recommended Oral Medication Regimens for Treatment of Genital Herpes Simplex Infection

First Clinical Episode of Genital Herpes
Acyclovir 400 mg three times daily for 7–10 days
or
Acyclovir 200 mg five times daily for 7–10 days
or
Famciclovir (Famvir) 250 mg three times daily for 7–10 days
or
Valacyclovir (Valtrex) 1 g twice daily for 7–10 days

Episodic Therapy for Recurrent Disease
Acyclovir 400 mg three times daily for 5 days
or
Acyclovir 800 mg twice daily for 5 days
or
Acyclovir 800 mg three times daily for 2 days
or
Famciclovir 125 mg twice daily for 5 days
or
Famciclovir 1 g twice daily for 1 day
or
Valacyclovir 500 mg twice daily for 3 days
or
Valacyclovir 1 g once daily for 5 days

Suppressive Therapy Options
Acyclovir 400 mg twice daily
or
Famciclovir 250 mg twice daily
or
Valacyclovir 0.5 to 1 g once daily

Modified from the Centers for Disease Control and Prevention, 2010b.

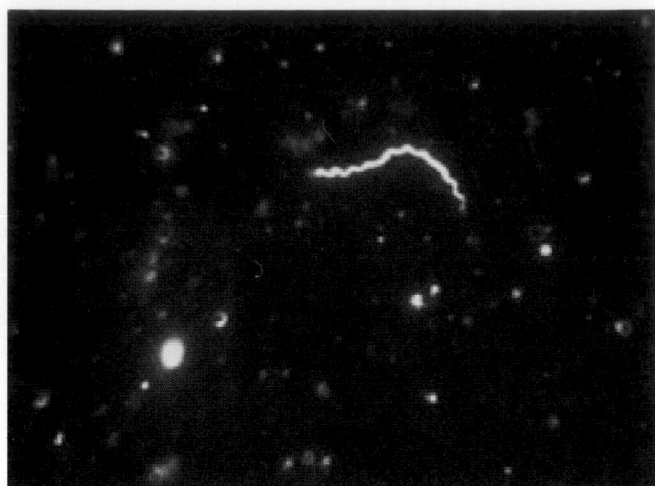

FIGURE 3-7 Microscopic view of Treponema pallidum. With dark-field microscopy, spirochetes appear as motile, bright corkscrews against a black background. *(From Cox, 2003, with permission.)*

80 percent. Safety and efficacy data with acyclovir in such patients for up to 6 years of surveillance are available. Suppressive therapy may eliminate recurrences and decreases sexual transmission of virus by approximately 50 percent (Corey, 2004). Once-daily dosing may result in enhanced compliance and decreased cost.

Syphilis
Pathophysiology

Syphilis is a sexually transmitted infection caused by the spirochete *Treponema pallidum*, which is a slender spiral-shaped organism with tapered ends (Fig. 3-7). Women at highest risk are those from lower socioeconomic groups, adolescents, those with early onset of sexual activity, and those with a large number of lifetime sexual partners. The attack rate for this infection approximates 30 percent. In 2009, more than 44,000 cases of syphilis were reported by state health departments in the United States (Centers for Disease Control and Prevention, 2009).

Primary Syphilis. The natural history of syphilis in untreated patients can be divided into four stages. The hallmark lesion of this infection is termed a *chancre*, in which spirochetes are abundant. Classically, it is an isolated nontender ulcer with raised rounded borders and an uninfected but integrated base. However, it may become secondarily infected and painful. Chancres are commonly found on the cervix, vagina, or vulva, but may also form in the mouth or around the anus (Fig. 3-8). This lesion may develop 10 days to 12 weeks after exposure, with a mean incubation period of 3 weeks. The incubation period is directly related to inoculum size. Without treatment, these lesions spontaneously heal in up to 6 weeks.

Secondary Syphilis. This phase is associated with bacteremia and develops 6 weeks to 6 months after a chancre appears. Its hallmark is a maculopapular rash that may involve the entire body and includes the palms, soles, and mucous membranes (Fig. 3-9). As is true for the chancre, this rash

lesions are present. Latex condom use potentially reduces the risk for herpetic transmission (Martin, 2009; Wald, 2005).

Antiviral Therapy. Currently available antiviral therapy includes acyclovir (Zovirax), famciclovir (Famvir), and valacyclovir (Valtrex). The CDC-recommended oral medications regimens are listed in Table 3-10. Although these agents may hasten healing and decrease symptoms, therapy does not eradicate latent virus or affect future history of recurrent infections.

For women with established HSV-2 infection, therapy may not be necessary if their symptoms are minimal and tolerated by the patient. Episodic therapy for recurrent disease should be initiated at least within 1 day of lesion outbreak or during the prodrome, if it exists. Patients may be given a prescription ahead of time so that medication can be available to begin therapy with prodromal symptoms.

If episodes recur at frequent intervals, a woman may elect daily suppressive therapy, which reduces recurrences by 70 to

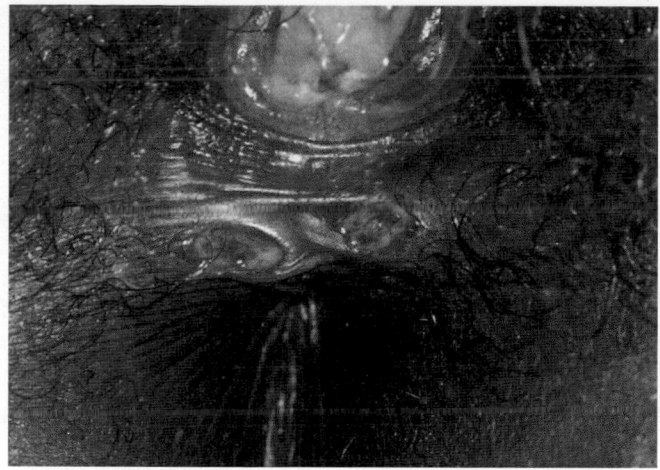

FIGURE 3-8 Vulvar syphilitic chancres on the perineum. *(From Wilkinson, 1995, with permission.)*

actively sheds spirochetes. In warm, moist body areas, this rash may produce broad, pink or gray-white, highly infectious plaques called *condylomata lata* (Fig. 3-10). Because syphilis is a systemic infection, other manifestations may include fever and malaise. Moreover, organ systems such as the kidney, liver, joints, and central nervous system (CNS) (meningitis) may be involved.

Latent Syphilis. During the first year following secondary syphilis without treatment, termed *early latent syphilis*, secondary signs and symptoms may recur. However, lesions associated with these outbreaks are not usually contagious. *Late latent syphilis* is defined as a period greater than 1 year after the initial infection.

Tertiary Syphilis. This phase of untreated syphilis may appear up to 20 years after latency. During this phase, cardiovascular, CNS, and musculoskeletal involvement become apparent. However, cardiovascular and neurosyphilis are half as common in females as in males.

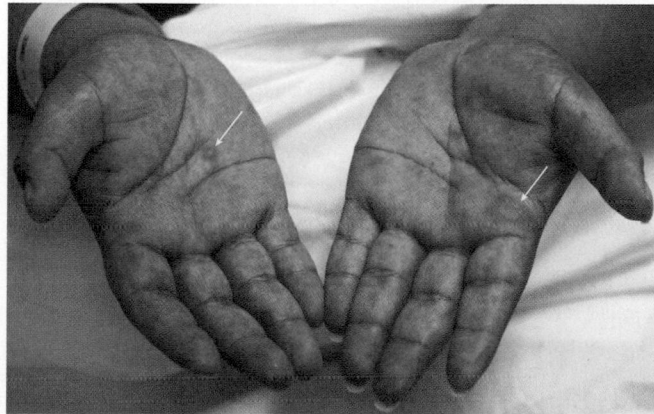

FIGURE 3-9 Photograph of a woman with multiple keratotic papules on her palms *(arrows)*. With secondary syphilis, disseminated papulosquamous eruptions may be seen on the palms, soles, or trunk. *(Photograph contributed by Dr. William Griffith.)*

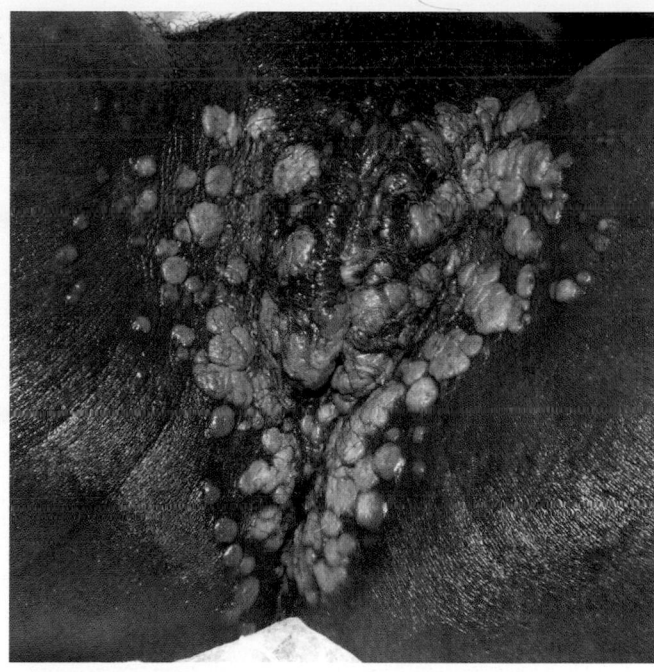

FIGURE 3-10 Photograph of a woman with multiple condyloma lata on her perineum. Soft, flat, moist, pink-tan papules and nodules on the perineum and perianal area are typical of this dermal manifestation of secondary syphilis. *(Photograph contributed by Dr. George Wendel.)*

Diagnosis

Spirochetes are too thin to retain Gram stain. Early syphilis is diagnosed primarily by dark-field examination or direct fluorescent antibody testing of lesion exudate. In the absence of this positive diagnosis, presumptive diagnosis may be reached with serologic tests that are nontreponemal: (1) Venereal Disease Research Laboratory (VDRL) or (2) rapid plasma reagin (RPR) tests (Table 3-11). Alternatively, treponemal-specific tests may be selected: (1) fluorescent treponemal antibody-absorption (FTA-ABS) or (2) *Treponema pallidum* particle agglutination (TP-PA) tests. Clinicians should be familiar with the uses of syphilis serologic tests. *For population screening*, RPR or VDRL testing is appropriate. A positive test result in a woman who has not been treated previously for syphilis or a fourfold titer (two dilutions) increase in a woman previously treated for syphilis should prompt confirmation with treponemal-specific tests. Thus, *for diagnosis confirmation* in a woman with a positive nontreponemal antibody test result or with a suspected clinical diagnosis, FTA-ABS or TP-PA testing should be selected. Finally, *for quantitative measurement* of antibody titers to assess response to treatment, RPR or VDRL tests are typically used.

Following treatment, sequential nontreponemal tests should be performed. During surveillance, the same type test should be used for consistency—either RPR or VDRL. A fourfold titer decrease is required by 6 months after therapy for primary or secondary syphilis or within 12 to 24 months for those with latent syphilis or women with initially high titers (>1:32) (Larsen, 1998). These tests usually become nonreactive after treatment and with time. However, some women may have a persistent low rating, and these patients are described as *serofast*.

TABLE 3-11. Sensitivity of Serodiagnostic Tests in Untreated Syphilis

Test[b]	Mean Percentage Positive (Range) at Indicated Stage of Disease[a]			
	Primary	Secondary	Latent	Tertiary
VDRL, RPR	78 (74–87)	100	95 (88–100)	71 (37–94)
FTA-ABS	84 (70–100)	100	100	96
TP-PA[c]	89	100	100	NA

FTA-ABS = fluorescent treponemal antibody-absorption; NA = not available; RPR = rapid plasma reagin; VDRL = Venereal Disease Research Laboratory; TP-PA = *Treponema pallidum* particle agglutination.
[a]In CDC studies.
[b]The specificity for each of these tests is 94 to 99 percent.
[c]Limited numbers of sera have been evaluated by TP-PA.
From Lukehart, 2007, with permission.

Importantly, women with a reactive treponemal-specific test will more than likely have a positive test for the remainder of their lives, but up to 25 percent may revert to a negative result after several years.

Treatment

Since 1943, penicillin has been the first-line therapeutic agent for this infection, and benzathine penicillin is primarily chosen. Specific recommendations for therapy by the CDC (2010b) are listed in Table 3-12. With treatment, an acute, self-limited febrile response, termed a Jarisch-Herxheimer reaction, may develop within the first 24 hours after treatment of early disease and is associated with headache and myalgia.

As with other STDs, all patients treated for syphilis and their sexual contacts should be tested for other STDs. Patients with evidence of neurologic or cardiac involvement should be treated by an infectious disease specialist. After initial treatment, women should be seen at 6-month intervals for clinical evaluation as well as serologic retesting. A fourfold dilution decrease is anticipated. If this does not occur, a patient either

TABLE 3-12. Recommended Treatment of Syphilis

Primary, secondary, early latent (<1 year) syphilis
Recommended regimen:
  Benzathine penicillin G, 2.4 million units IM once

Alternative oral regimens (penicillin-allergic, nonpregnant women):
  Doxycycline 100 mg orally twice daily for 2 weeks

Late latent, tertiary, and cardiovascular syphilis
Recommended regimen:
  Benzathine penicillin G, 2.4 million units IM weekly times 3 doses

Alternative oral regimen (penicillin-allergic, nonpregnant women):
  Doxycycline 100 mg orally twice daily for 4 weeks

From the Centers for Disease Control and Prevention, 2010b.

has failed treatment or was reinfected and should be reevaluated and retreated. Retreatment recommendations are benzathine penicillin G, 2.4 million units IM weekly for 3 weeks. Thus, if patients with penicillin allergy cannot be followed or if their compliance is questioned, then skin testing, desensitization, and treatment with IM benzathine penicillin is recommended (Wendel, 1985).

Chancroid

This is one of the classic sexually transmitted diseases, but is an uncommon infection in the United States. It appears as local outbreaks predominantly in black and Hispanic males.

It is caused by a nonmotile, nonspore-forming, facultative, gram-negative bacillus, *Haemophilus ducreyi*. Incubation usually spans 3 to 10 days, and host access probably requires a break in the skin or mucous membrane. Chancroid does not cause a systemic reaction, and no prodromal syndrome precedes the appearance of infection.

Symptoms

This disease presents initially as an erythematous papule that becomes pustular and ulcerates within 48 hours. Edges of these painful ulcers are usually irregular with erythematous nonindurated margins. The ulcer bases are usually red and granular and, in contrast to a syphilitic chancre, are typically soft. Lesions are frequently covered with purulent material, and if secondarily infected, a foul odor will result.

The most common locations in women include the fourchette, vestibule, clitoris, and labia. Ulcers on the cervix or vagina may be nontender. Concurrently, approximately half of patients will develop unilateral or bilateral tender inguinal lymphadenopathy. If large and fluctuant, they are termed *buboes*. These may occasionally suppurate and form fistulas, the drainage from which will result in other ulcer formation.

Diagnosis

The diseases most commonly imitating this presentation are syphilis and genital herpes. These may coexist, but uncommonly. Definitive diagnosis requires growth of *H ducreyi* on special media, but sensitivity for culture is less than 80 percent.

TABLE 3-13. Recommended Treatment of Chancroid

Azithromycin (Zithromax) 1 g orally once

or

Ceftriaxone (Rocephin) 250 mg intramuscularly once

or

Ciprofloxacin (Cipro) 500 mg orally twice daily for 3 days

or

Erythromycin base 500 mg orally three times daily for
7 days

Modified from the Centers for Disease Control and
Prevention, 2010b.

TABLE 3-14. Recommended Oral Treatment for
Granuloma Inguinale

Doxycycline (Doryx) 100 mg twice daily for a minimum
of 3 weeks and until lesions have completely healed

or

Azithromycin (Zithromax) 1 g once a week as above

or

Ciprofloxacin (Cipro) 750 mg twice daily as above

or

Erythromycin base 500 mg four times daily as above

or

Trimethoprim-sulfamethoxazole DS (Bactrim DS, Septra
DS) twice daily as above

DS = double strength.
Modified from the Centers for Disease Control and
Prevention, 2010b.

A presumptive diagnosis can be made with identification of gram-negative, nonmotile rods on a Gram stain of lesion contents. Before obtaining either specimen, superficial pus or crusting should be removed with sterile, saline-soaked gauze.

Treatment

The CDC's (2010b) recommended regimens for nonpregnant women are found in Table 3-13. Successful treatment will result in symptomatic improvement within 3 days, and objective evidence of improvement within 1 week. Lymphadenopathy resolves more slowly, and if fluctuant, incision and drainage may be warranted. Those with coexisting HIV infection may require longer therapy courses, and treatment failures are more common. Accordingly, some recommend longer regimens for initial management of known HIV-infected patients.

Granuloma Inguinale

Also known as donovanosis, granuloma inguinale genital ulcerative disease is caused by the intracellular gram-negative bacterium *Calymmatobacterium* (*Klebsiella*) *granulomatis*. This bacterium is encapsulated and has a characteristic appearance in tissue biopsy or cytology specimens (Fig. 3-11). Apparently this disease is only mildly contagious, requires repeated exposures, and has a long incubation period of weeks to months.

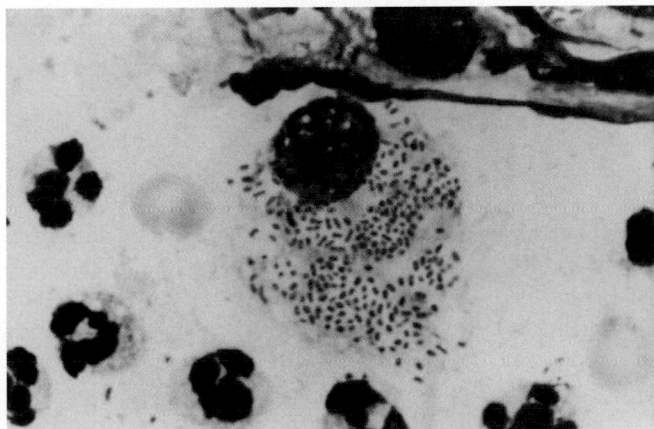

FIGURE 3-11 Photomicrograph of a mononuclear cell containing Donovan bodies. Wright-Giemsa staining creates a "closed safety pin" appearance. (*From Bowden, 2003, with permission.*)

Symptoms

Granuloma inguinale presents as painless inflammatory nodules that progress to highly vascular, beefy red ulcers that bleed easily on contact. If secondarily infected, they may become painful. These ulcers heal by fibrosis, which can result in scarring resembling keloids. Lymph nodes are usually uninvolved, but may become enlarged, and new lesions may appear along these lymphatic drainage channels. Distant lesions have also been reported.

Diagnosis

Diagnosis is confirmed by identification of Donovan bodies during microscopic evaluation of a specimen following Wright-Giemsa staining. Currently, there are no FDA-approved PCR tests for *C granulomatis* DNA.

Treatment

Treatment does stop lesion progression and may be lengthy without formation of granulation tissue in ulcer bases and reepithelialization (Table 3-14). Relapses have been reported up to 18 months after "effective" treatment. A few prospective treatment trials have been published, but these are limited. If successful, improvement will be evident within the first few days of treatment.

Lymphogranuloma Venereum (LGV)

This ulcerative genital disease is caused by *Chlamydia trachomatis* serotypes L1, L2, and L3 and is uncommon in the United States. As is true with other sexually transmitted diseases, this infection is found in lower socioeconomic groups among those with multiple sexual partners.

The chlamydial life cycle is comprised of three stages. Initially, infective particles (elementary bodies) penetrate a host cell. Here they develop into metabolically active reticulate bodies. Binary fission within the cell allows reticulate bodies to transform themselves into multiple elementary bodies. Lastly, these are released by exocytosis.

Symptoms

This infection is commonly divided into three stages as follows: (1) small vesicle or papule, (2) inguinal or femoral lymphadenopathy, and (3) anogenitorectal syndrome. Incubation for this infection ranges from 3 days to 2 weeks. Initial papules heal quickly and without scarring. They appear primarily on the fourchette and posterior vaginal wall up to and including the cervix. Repeated inoculation may result in lesions at multiple sites.

During the second stage, sometimes referred to as the inguinal syndrome, progressive enlargement of inguinal and femoral lymph nodes is observed. Enlarged painful nodes can mat together on either side of the inguinal ligament and create a characteristic "groove sign," which appears in up to one fifth of infected women (Fig. 3-12). In addition, enlarging nodes may rupture through the skin, and chronically draining sinuses may result. Fever may be noted prior to rupture. Commonly, women with LGV develop systemic infection and manifest malaise and fever. Additionally, pneumonitis, arthritis, and hepatitis have been reported with this infection.

In the third stage of LGV, a patient develops rectal pruritus and a mucoid discharge from rectal ulcers. If these become infected, the discharge becomes purulent. This presentation is a result of lymphatic obstruction that follows lymphangitis and that may result in elephantiasis of external genitalia initially and fibrosis of the rectum. Rectal bleeding is common, and a woman may complain of crampy, abdominal pain with abdominal distention, rectal pain, and fever. Peritonitis may follow bowel perforation. Stenosis of the urethra and the vagina has also been reported.

Diagnosis

Lymphogranuloma venereum may be diagnosed following clinical evaluation with exclusion of other etiologies and positive chlamydial testing. A serologic titer that is >1:64 can support the diagnosis. Additionally, lymph node specimens obtained by swab or aspiration may be cultured for *C trachomatis* or tested by immunofluorescence or PCR.

Treatment

The CDC-recommended regimen (2010b) is doxycycline, 100 mg orally twice daily for 21 days. Alternatively, one may use erythromycin base, 500 mg orally four times daily, for the same duration. It is recommended that sexual contacts exposed to a patient within the prior 60 days should be tested for urethral or cervical infection and treated with either standard antichlamydial regimen.

PATHOGENS CAUSING INFECTIOUS VAGINITIS

The term *vaginitis* is the diagnosis given to women who complain of abnormal vaginal discharge with vulvar burning, irritation, or itching. It is one of the most frequent reasons for patient visits to the gynecologist (American College of Obstetricians and Gynecologists, 2008b). The leading causes of symptomatic vaginal discharge are bacterial vaginosis, candidiasis, and trichomoniasis.

Between 7 and 70 percent of women who have vaginal discharge complaints will have no definitive diagnosis (Anderson, 2004). For those in whom identifiable infection is absent, an inflammatory diagnosis and treatment for infection should not be given. In such instances, a woman may seek reassurance, having concern about a recent sexual exposure, and sexually transmitted disease testing may alleviate this.

Importantly, during evaluation, a clinician should obtain a complete history regarding prior vaginal infections and their treatment; duration of symptoms; whether or not the patient has used over-the-counter (OTC) preparations, and if so which type and when; and a complete menstrual and sexual history. The salient features of a menstrual history are outlined in Chapter 8 (p. 222). A sexual history typically include questions regarding age at coitarche, date of most recent sexual activity, number of recent partners, gender of those partners, use of condom barrier protection, method of birth control, prior STD history, and type of sexual activity—anal, oral, or vaginal.

Moreover, a thorough physical examination of the vulva, vagina, and cervix should be performed. Several etiologies may be identified in the office by microscopic examination of the discharge (Table 3-15). First, a saline preparation, described earlier, can be inspected (p. 66). A "KOH-prep" contains a swab-collected sample of discharge mixed with several drops of 10-percent KOH. A whiff test for BV can be completed before placement of the cover slip. KOH leads to osmotic swelling and then lysis of squamous cell membranes. This visually clears the microscopic view and aids identification of fungal buds or hyphae. Finally, vaginal pH analysis may add supportive information. Vaginal pH can be estimated using pH paper test strips. Appropriate readings are obtained by pressing a test strip directly to the upper vaginal wall and resting it there for a few seconds to absorb vaginal fluid. Once the strip is removed, its

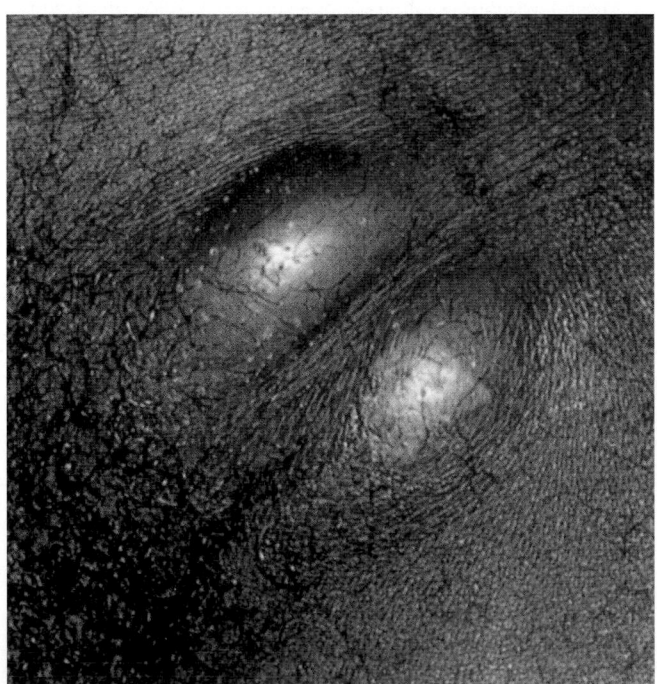

FIGURE 3-12 Photograph of the "groove sign" seen with lymphogranuloma venereum. Enlarged lymph nodes matted together on either side of the inguinal ligament create this characteristic groove. *(From Schachter, 2003, with permission.)*

TABLE 3-15. Summary of Characteristics of Common Vaginal Infections

Category	Physiologic (normal)	Bacterial Vaginosis	Candidiasis	Trichomoniasis	Bacterial (strepto-coccal, staphylococ-cal, *E coli*)
Complaint	None	Bad odor, increased after intercourse and/or menses	Itching, burning, discharge	Frothy discharge, bad odor, dysuria, pruritus, spotting	Thin, watery discharge, pruritus
Discharge	White, clear	Thin, gray or white, adherent, often increased	White "cottage cheese-like"	Green-yellow, frothy, adherent, increased	Purulent
KOH "whiff test"	Absent	Present (fishy)	Absent	May be present	Absent
Vaginal pH	3.8–4.2	>4.5	<4.5	>4.5	>4.5
Microscopic findings	NA	"Clue cells", slight increase in WBCs, clumps of bacteria (saline wet mount)	Hyphae and buds (10-percent KOH solution wet mount)	Trichomonads may be seen moving (saline wet mount)	Many WBCs

E coli = *Escherichia coli*; KOH = potassium hydroxide; NA = not applicable; WBC = white blood cell.

color is determined and matched to color charts on the test strip dispenser. Importantly, blood and semen are alkaline and often will artificially elevate pH. Unfortunately, inexpensive laboratory tests such as these are not as accurate as a clinician would hope (Bornstein, 2001; Landers, 2004).

■ Fungal Infection

This infection is most commonly caused by *Candida albicans*, which can be found in the vaginas of asymptomatic patients and is a commensal of the mouth, rectum, and vagina. Occasionally, other *Candida* species may be involved and include *C tropicalis* and *C glabrata,* among others. Candidiasis is seen more commonly in warmer climates and in obese patients. Additionally, immunosuppression, diabetes mellitus, pregnancy, and recent broad-spectrum antibiotic use predispose women to clinical infection. It can be sexually transmitted, and several studies have reported an association between candidiasis and orogenital sex (Bradshaw, 2005; Geiger, 1996).

Diagnosis

With candidiasis, pruritus, pain, vulvar erythema, and edema with excoriations are common findings (Fig. 3-13). The typical vaginal discharge is described as cottage cheese-like. Vaginal pH is normal (<4.5), and microscopic examination of vaginal discharge with saline or with 10-percent KOH preparations allows yeast identification (Fig. 3-14). *Candida albicans* is dimorphic, with both yeast buds and hyphal forms. It may be present in the vagina as a filamentous fungus (pseudohyphae) or as germinated yeast with mycelia. Vaginal candidal culture is not routinely recommended. However, it may be warranted for those who fail empiric treatment and for women with evidence of infection yet absence of microscopic yeast.

Treatment

The CDC vulvovaginal candidiasis classification (2010b) is presented in Table 3-16. Various treatment formulations that are effective in treating both uncomplicated and complicated infection are presented in Table 3-17. For uncomplicated infection, azoles are extremely effective, but women should be encouraged to return if therapy is unsuccessful.

Women who have four or more candidal infections during a year are classified as having complicated disease, and cultures should be obtained to confirm the diagnosis. Non-*albicans*

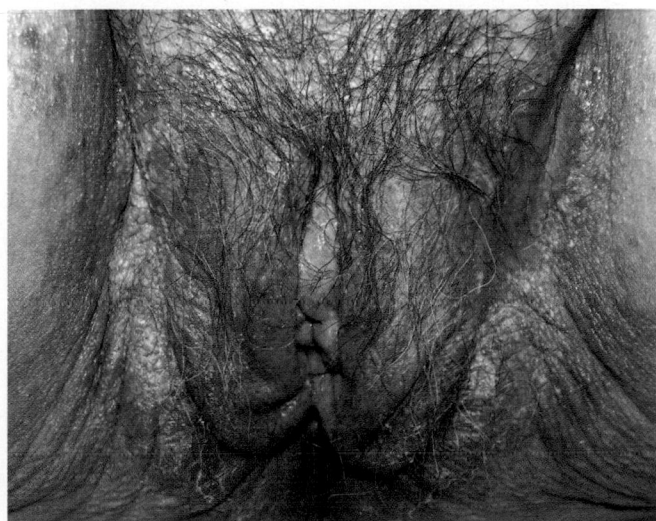

FIGURE 3-13 Thick white discharge, labial erythema, and edema may be seen with candidiasis. *(Photograph contributed by Dr. William Griffith.)*

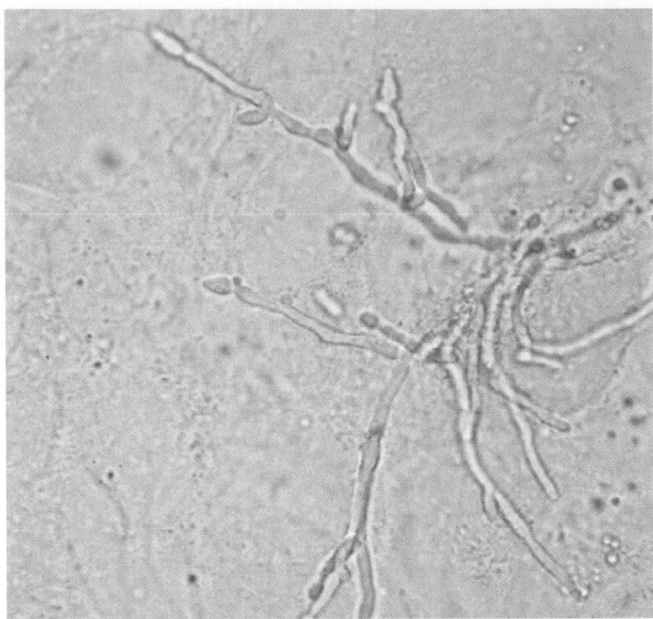

FIGURE 3-14 Photomicrograph of *Candida albicans* in a potassium hydroxide preparation. Serpentine pseudohyphae are seen. *(From Hansfield, 2001, with permission.)*

candidal species are not as responsive to topical azole therapy. Therefore, prolonged local intravaginal therapy regimens and the addition of oral fluconazole (Diflucan), one to three times a week, may be required to achieve clinical cure. Primary treatment for prevention of recurrent infection is oral fluconazole, 100 to 200 mg weekly for 6 months. For non-*albicans* recurrent infection, a 600-mg boric acid gelatin capsule intravaginally daily for 2 weeks has been successful.

TABLE 3-16. Vulvovaginal Candidiasis Classification

Uncomplicated
Sporadic or infrequent
and
Mild to moderate
and
Likely infecting agent is *Candida albicans*
and
Nonimmunocompromised woman

Complicated
Recurrent candidal infection
or
Severe infection
or
Non-*albicans* candidiasis (*C tropicalis, C glabrata*, etc.)
or
Uncontrolled diabetes, immunosuppression, debilitation,
    pregnancy

From the Centers for Disease Control and Prevention, 2010b.

Oral azole therapy has been associated with elevation in liver enzymes. Thus, prolonged oral therapy may not be feasible for that reason or because of interactions with other patient medications such as calcium-channel blockers, warfarin, protease inhibitors, trimetrexate, terfenadine, cyclosporine A, phenytoin, and rifampin. In these cases, local intravaginal therapy once or twice weekly may give a similar clinical response.

Trichomoniasis

Epidemiology

This infection is the most prevalent nonviral STD in the United States (Van der Pol, 2005, 2007). Unlike other STDs, its incidence appears to increase with patient age in some studies. Trichomoniasis is more commonly diagnosed in women because most men are asymptomatic. However, up to 70 percent of male partners of women with vaginal trichomoniasis will have trichomonads in their urinary tract.

This parasite is usually a marker of high-risk sexual behavior, and co-infection with other sexually transmitted pathogens is common, especially *N gonorrhoeae. Trichomonas vaginalis* has predilection for squamous epithelium, and lesions may increase accessibility to other sexually transmitted species. Vertical transmission during birth is possible and may persist for a year.

Diagnosis

Incubation with *T vaginalis* requires 3 days to 4 weeks, and the vagina, urethra, endocervix, and bladder can be infected. No symptoms may be noted in up to one-half of women with trichomoniasis, and such colonization may persist for months or years in some women. However, in those with complaints, vaginal discharge is typically described as foul, thin, and yellow or green. Additionally, dysuria, dyspareunia, vulvar pruritus, and pain may be noted. At times, symptomatology and physical findings are identical to those of acute PID.

With trichomoniasis, the vulva may be erythematous, edematous, and excoriated. The vagina contains the discharge just described, and subepithelial hemorrhages or "strawberry spots" may be seen on the vagina and cervix. Trichomoniasis is typically diagnosed by microscopic identification of parasites in a saline preparation of the discharge. Trichomonads are anteriorly flagellated, and therefore mobile, anaerobic protozoa. They are oval and slightly larger than a white blood cell (WBC) (Fig. 3-15). Trichomonads become less motile with cooling, and slides should be read within 20 minutes. Inspection of a saline preparation is highly specific, yet sensitivity is not as high as hoped (60 to 70 percent). In addition to microscopic findings, vaginal pH is often elevated.

The most sensitive diagnostic technique is culture, which is impractical because special media (Diamond media) is required, and few laboratories are equipped. Moreover, nucleic acid amplification tests (NAATs) for trichomonal DNA are sensitive and specific, but not widely available. Alternatively, the OSOM Trichomonas Rapid Test is an immunochromatographic assay, which has 88-percent sensitivity and 99-percent specificity. It is available for office use, and results are available in 10 minutes (Huppert, 2005, 2007). Trichomonads may also be noted on Pap smear screening, and sensitivity approximates 60 percent (Wiese, 2000). If trichomonads are reported from a

TABLE 3-17. Topical Agents (First-Line Therapy) for the Treatment of Candidiasis

Drug	Brand Name	Formulation	Dosage
Butoconazole	Gynazole-1[a,b]	2% vaginal cream	1 app vaginally for 1 day
	Mycelex-3	2% vaginal cream	1 app vaginally for 3 days
Clotrimazole	Gyne-Lotrimin 7, Mycelex-7	1% vaginal cream	1 app vaginally for 7 days
	Gyne-Lotrimin 3	2% vaginal cream	1 app vaginally for 3 days
	Gyne-Lotrimin 3	200 mg vaginal supp	1 supp daily for 3 days
Clotrimazole Combination Pack	Gyne-Lotrimin 3	200 mg supp + 1% topical cream	1 vaginal supp daily for 3 days. Use cream externally as needed
	Mycelex-7	100 mg supp + 1% topical cream	1 vaginal supp daily for 7 days. Use cream externally as needed
Clotrimazole + Betamethasone	Lotrisone[a]	1% clotrimazole with 0.05% betamethasone cream	Apply cream topically twice daily[c]
Miconazole	Monistat-7	100 mg vaginal supp	1 supp daily for 7 days
	Monistat	2% topical cream	Apply externally as needed
	Monistat-3	4% vaginal cream	1 app vaginally for 3 days
	Monistat-7	2% vaginal cream	1 app vaginally for 7 days
Miconazole Combination Pack	Monistat-3	200 mg vaginal supp + 2% topical cream	1 supp daily for 3 days. Use cream externally twice daily as needed[c]
	Monistat-7	100 mg vaginal supp + 2% topical cream[c]	1 supp daily for 7 days. Use cream externally twice daily as needed[c]
	Monistat Dual Pack	1200 mg vaginal supp + 2% topical cream	1 supp daily for 1 day. Use cream externally twice daily as needed
Terconazole	Terazol 3[a]	80 mg vaginal supp	1 supp daily for 3 days
	Terazol 7[a]	0.4% vaginal cream	1 app vaginally 7 days
	Terazol 3[a]	0.8% vaginal cream	1 app vaginally 3 days
Tioconazole	Monistat-1, Vagistat-1	6.5% vaginal ointment	1 app vaginally, once
Econazole nitrate	Spectrazole	1% topical cream	Apply cream twice daily
Nystatin	Pyolene Nystatin/ Generic	100,000 unit vaginal tablet	1 tablet daily for 14 days (best choice for first-trimester pregnancy)
Nystatin powder	Mycostatin	100,000 units/gram	Apply to vulva twice daily for 14 days
Gentian violet		1% solution	Apply to affected area once

[a]Prescription required.
[b]Drug recalled in 2009 due to manufacturing that did not sufficiently comply with current good manufacturing practices.
[c]Maximum use recommended is 2 weeks.
app = applicatorful; supp = suppository.

PAP smear slide, confirmation by microscopic evaluation of a saline preparation is encouraged prior to treatment.

Women with trichomonal infection should be tested for other sexually transmitted infections. Additionally, sexual contact(s) should be evaluated or referred for evaluation.

Treatment

Oral regimens recommended by the CDC (2010b) are found in Table 3-18. Although each is effective, some report that a 7-day treatment regimen with metronidazole may be more effective in compliant patients. However, compliance may be

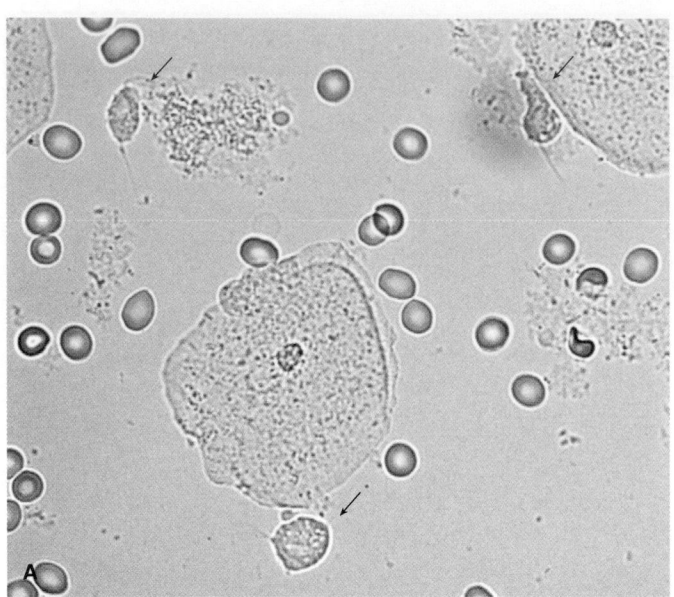

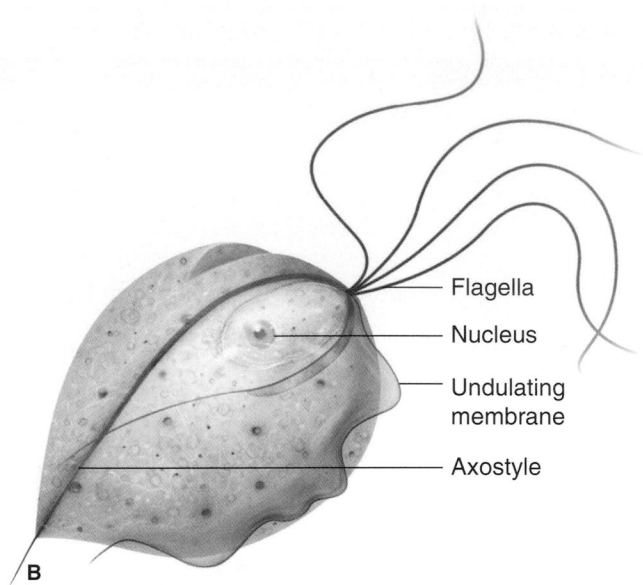

Flagella
Nucleus
Undulating
membrane
Axostyle

FIGURE 3-15 Trichomonads. **A.** Photomicrograph of a vaginal smear saline preparation containing trichomonads (*arrows*). These lie amid larger squamous cells and smaller red blood cells. *(Photograph contributed by Dr. Lauri Campagna and Rebecca Winn, WHNP.)* **B.** Drawing depicts anatomic features of trichomonads. Flagella allow this parasite to be motile.

poor because of longer treatment length and metronidazole side effects. Adverse effects may include a metallic taste and a disulfiram-like reaction (nausea and vomiting) if combined with alcohol. Accordingly, patients should abstain from alcohol during use and for 24 hours following metronidazole therapy and for 72 hours after tinidazole (Tindamax).

Patients who become asymptomatic or who are asymptomatic do not require routine reevaluation. However, recurrence occurs in approximately 30 percent of patients. Condom use may be protective.

There are infrequent patients who have strains that are highly resistant to metronidazole, but these organisms are usually sensitive to tinidazole. Culture and sensitivity should be performed on specimens from patients with frequently recurring infections or from those who do not respond to the initial therapy and who are medication compliant. Oral tinidazole at doses of 500 mg orally three times daily for 7 days or four times daily for 14 days have been effective in curing patients with resistant organisms (Sobel, 2001). For women allergic to the nitroimidazoles, desensitization has been used to allow use of these agents for Trichomoniasis (Helms, 2008).

TABLE 3-18. Recommended Treatment of Trichomoniasis

Primary therapy
Metronidazole (Flagyl) single 2-g dose orally
or
Tinidazole (Tindamax) single 2-g dose orally

Alternative regimen
Metronidazole 500 mg orally twice daily for 7 days

Modified from the Centers for Disease Control and Prevention, 2010b.

PATHOGENS CAUSING SUPPURATIVE CERVICITIS

Neisseria gonorrhoeae

Many women with cervical *N gonorrhoeae* are asymptomatic. For this reason, women at risk should be screened periodically (Table 1-2, p. 11). Risk factors for gonococcal carriage and potential upper reproductive tract infection are: age equal to or less than 25 years, the presence of other sexually transmitted infections, a history of previous gonococcal infection, new or multiple sexual partners, lack of barrier protection, drug use, and commercial sex work. Screening for nonpregnant women at low risk is not recommended (U.S. Preventive Services Task Force, 2005).

Symptoms

Symptomatic lower female reproductive tract gonorrhea may present as vaginitis or cervicitis. Those with cervicitis commonly describe a profuse odorless, nonirritating, and white-to-yellow vaginal discharge. Gonococcus can also infect the Bartholin and Skene glands and the urethra, and it can ascend into the endometrium and fallopian tube to cause upper reproductive tract infection (p. 95).

Diagnosis

Neisseria gonorrhoeae is a gram-negative coccobacillus that invades columnar and transitional epithelial cells, becoming intracellular. For this reason, the vaginal epithelium is not involved.

For gonococcal identification, NAATs are available and have replaced culture in most laboratories. Previously, acceptable specimens were recovered only from the endocervix or urethra. However, newer NAAT collection kits are available for specific collection from the vagina, the endocervix, or urine.

For women without a cervix following hysterectomy, first-void urine samples are collected. For those with a cervix, vaginal-swab specimens are as sensitive and specific as cervical-swab specimens. Cervical samples are acceptable if pelvic examinations are performed, but vaginal-swab specimens are an appropriate sample type even during complete pelvic examination. Urine samples, although acceptable, are least preferred for those with a cervix (Association of Public Health Laboratories, 2009). However, if selected, the initial urine stream, not midstream, should be collected. Of note, these noncultural tests are not FDA-cleared for diagnostic identification of rectal or pharyngeal disease. Thus, cultures should be obtained in those screened at these anatomic sites.

All patients tested for gonorrhea should be tested for other sexually transmitted infections, and sexual contacts should be evaluated and treated or referred for evaluation and treatment. Abstinence should be practiced until therapy is completed and until patients and their treated sexual partners have symptom resolution.

In an effort to prevent and control STDs, guidelines for expedited partner therapy (EPT) have been created by the CDC and supported by the American College of Obstetricians and Gynecologists (2011). EPT is the delivery of a prescription by persons infected with an STD to their sexual partners without clinical assessment of the partners or professional counseling. EPT should ideally not replace traditional strategies, such as standard patient referral, when available. Although acceptable for treatment of heterosexual contacts with gonorrhea or chlamydial infection, data do not support EPT for trichomoniasis or syphilis. Although sanctioned by the CDC, EPT is not legal in several states within the United States. Moreover, the risk of litigation in the event of adverse outcomes may be elevated when a practice has uncertain legal status or is outside formally accepted community practice standards (Centers for Disease Control and Prevention, 2006). The legal status of EPT in each of the 50 states can be found at: http://www.cdc.gov/std/ept/legal/default.htm.

Treatment

Recommendations by the CDC for single-dose therapy of uncomplicated gonococcal infections are outlined in Table 3-19. Importantly, widespread quinolone-resistant gonococci in the United States prompted removal of this antibiotic class from the CDC STD guidelines (2010b). More recently, the CDC (2011) also presented evidence suggesting declining susceptibility to cephalosporins among *N gonorrhoeae* isolates. In response, they issued the recommendation to treat uncomplicated gonococcal infections with single-dose ceftriaxone 250 mg IM combined with azithromycin 2 g orally. Test-of-cure cultures are not necessary, however, reinfection is common. Some recommend retesting 3 months following initial therapy.

■ *Chlamydia trachomatis*

This organism is the second most prevalent of the sexually transmitted disease species recovered in the United States, and its highest prevalence is found in individuals younger than 25 years. Since many with this organism are asymptomatic, annual screening of sexually active women aged ≤25 years and those at risk is recommended (Table 1-2, p. 11).

TABLE 3-19. Recommended Single-dose Treatment of Uncomplicated Gonococcal Infection[a]

Ceftriaxone (Rocephin) 250 mg IM[b]
plus
Azithromycin (Zithromax) 1 g once[b]
or
Doxycycline (Doryx) 100 mg twice daily for 7 days

[a]Test of cure is not recommended routinely for patients with uncomplicated gonorrhea who have been treated with the above recommended regimens. Persons with persistent symptoms of gonococcal infection or whose symptoms recur shortly after treatment should be reevaluated by culture for *N gonorrhoeae*.
[b]Preferred treatment combination.
Modified from the Centers for Disease Control and Prevention, 2011.

Symptoms

This obligate intracellular parasite is dependent on host cells for survival. It causes columnar epithelial infection, and thus, symptoms reflect endocervical glandular infection, with resultant mucopurulent discharge or endocervical secretions. If infected, the endocervical tissue is commonly edematous and hyperemic. Urethritis is another lower genital tract infection that can develop, and dysuria is prominent.

Diagnosis

Microscopic inspection of secretions in a saline preparation typically reveals 20 or more leukocytes per high-power field. More specifically, culture, NAAT, and enzyme-linked immunosorbent assay (ELISA) are available for endocervical specimens. Alternatively, combined gonococcal and chlamydial tests are widely used. As with gonorrhea testing, newer NAAT collection kits permit specific collection from the vagina, the endocervix, or urine. Vaginal-swab specimens are as sensitive and specific as cervical-swab specimens. Cervical samples are acceptable if pelvic examinations are performed, but vaginal-swab specimens are an appropriate sample type even during complete pelvic examination. Urine samples, although acceptable, are least preferred for women with a cervix. However, for women following hysterectomy, first-void urine samples are preferred. Again, these noncultural tests are not FDA-cleared for diagnostic identification of rectal or pharyngeal disease, and culture should be used at these sites. If *C trachomatis* is diagnosed or suspected, then screening for other STDs is indicated.

Treatment

Recommended therapy for *C trachomatis* infection is described in Table 3-20. Azithromycin has the obvious therapeutic compliance advantage of allowing clinicians to observe ingestion at the time of diagnosis. Following treatment, retesting is not

TABLE 3-20. Recommended Oral Treatments of Chlamydial Infection

Primary treatment

Azithromycin (Zithromax) 1 g once
or
Doxycycline (Doryx) 100 mg twice daily for 7 days

Alternative regimens

Erythromycin base 500 mg four times daily for 7 days
or
Erythromycin ethyl succinate 800 mg four times daily for 7 days
or
Ofloxacin 300 mg twice daily for 7 days
or
Levofloxacin (Levaquin) 500 mg once daily for 7 days

Modified from Centers for Disease Control and Prevention, 2010b.

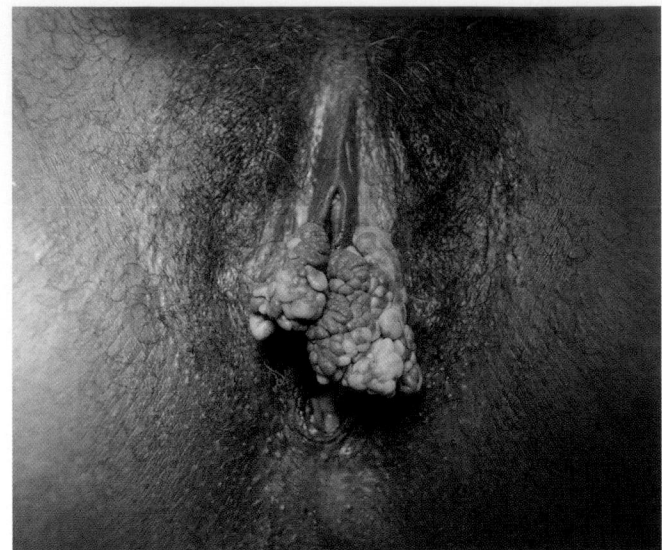

FIGURE 3-16 Photograph of vulvar condyloma acuminata. Multiple exophytic verrucous warts are seen on the labia minora bilaterally.

recommended if symptoms resolve. To prevent further infection, abstinence is recommended until a woman and her partner(s) are treated and are asymptomatic. Sexual partner(s) should be referred for evaluation or examined, counseled, tested, and treated. As with gonorrhea in heterosexual partners, expedited partner therapy is sanctioned by the CDC for selected patients (p. 87).

PATHOGENS CAUSING MASS LESIONS

External Genital Warts

These lesions are created from infection with the human papillomavirus (HPV), and a fuller discussion of the pathophysiology of this virus is found in Chapter 29 (p. 733). Genital warts display differing morphologies, and appearances range from flat papules to the classic verrucous, exophytic lesions, termed condyloma acuminata (Fig. 3-16) (Beutner, 1998). Involved tissues vary, and external genital warts may develop at sites in the lower reproductive tract, urethra, or anus. They are typically diagnosed by clinical inspection, and biopsy is not required unless coexisting neoplasia is suspected (Beutner, 1998; Wiley, 2002). Similarly, HPV serotyping is not required for routine diagnosis.

Treatment

Condyloma acuminata may remain unchanged or spontaneously resolve, and the effect of treatment on future viral transmission is unclear (Centers for Disease Control and Prevention, 2010b). However, many women prefer removal, and lesions can be destroyed with sharp or electrosurgical excision, cryotherapy, or laser ablation. In addition, very large, bulky lesions may be managed with cavitational ultrasonic surgical aspiration (CUSA) (Section 41-28, p. 1087).

Alternatively, topical agents can be applied to resolve lesions through various mechanisms (Table 3-21). Of these, imiquimod cream (Aldara, Zyclara), is a patient-applied, immunomodulatory topical treatment for genital warts. This agent induces macrophages to secrete several cytokines, and of these, interferon-γ is probably the most important. For genital wart clearance, this cytokine stimulates a cell-mediated immune response against HPV (Scheinfeld, 2006). Another topical immune-modulating agent is a 15-percent sinecatechin ointment (Veregen) derived from green-tea leaf extracts. Podophyllin is an antimitotic agent available in a 10- to 25-percent tincture of benzoin solution and disrupts viral activity by inducing local tissue necrosis. A biologically active extract of podophyllin, podofilox, also termed podophyllotoxin, is available in a 0.5-percent solution or gel (Condylox). This can be self-applied by the patient. Alternatively, trichloroacetic acid and bichloroacetic acid are proteolytic agents and are applied serially to warts by clinicians. Intralesional injection of interferon is an effective treatment for warts (Eron, 1986). However, because of its high cost and painful and inconvenient administration, this therapy is not recommended as a primary modality and is best reserved for recalcitrant cases.

Of therapy choices, no data suggest the superiority of one treatment. Thus, in general, treatment should be selected based on clinical circumstances and patient and provider preferences. Importantly, no treatment option, even surgical excision, boasts 100-percent clearance rates. Indeed, clearance rates range from 30 to 80 percent. Accordingly, recurrences are not uncommon following treatment.

Molluscum Contagiosum

The molluscum contagiosum virus is a DNA poxvirus that is transmitted by direct human-to-human contact or by infected

TABLE 3-21. Recommended Treatment of External Genital Warts

Patient-applied:

Podofilox 0.5% solution or gel (Condylox). Patients should apply podofilox solution with a cotton swab, or podofilox gel with a finger, to visible genital warts twice a day for 3 days, followed by 4 days of no therapy. This cycle may be repeated, as necessary, for up to four cycles. The total wart area treated should not exceed 10 cm², and the total volume of podofilox should be limited to 0.5 mL per day.

or

Imiquimod 5% cream (Aldara). Apply imiquimod cream once daily at bedtime, three times a week for up to 16 weeks. 3.75% cream (Zyclara). Apply imiquimod cream once daily at bedtime for up to 8 weeks.
With either cream, the treatment area should be washed with soap and water 6 to 10 hours after the application.

or

Sinecatechin 15% ointment (Veregen). This green tea extract contains catechins and should be applied three times daily (0.5-cm strand to each wart) using a finger to ensure wart coverage. Use is continued until warts are cleared, but not longer than 16 weeks. It should not be washed off, and sexual contact should be avoided when ointment is present.

Provider-administered:

Cryotherapy with liquid nitrogen or cryoprobe. Repeat applications every 1 to 2 weeks.

or

Podophyllin resin 10 to 25 percent in a compound tincture of benzoin. A small amount should be applied to each wart and allowed to air dry. The treatment can be repeated weekly, if necessary. Application should be limited to <0.5 mL of podophyllin or an area of <10 cm² of warts per session. No open lesions or wounds should exist in the area to which treatment is administered. Some specialists suggest thorough washing 1 to 4 hours after application to reduce local irritation.

or

Trichloroacetic acid (TCA) or **Bichloroacetic acid** (BCA) 80 to 90 percent. A small amount should be applied only to the warts and allowed to dry, at which time a white "frosting" develops. This treatment can be repeated weekly if necessary. If an excess amount of acid is applied, the treated area should be powdered with talc, sodium bicarbonate (i.e., baking soda), or liquid soap preparations to remove unreacted acid.

or

Surgical removal either by tangential scissor excision, tangential shave excision, curettage, or electrosurgery.

Alternative regimens:
Intralesional interferon, photodynamic therapy, topical cidofovir.

Modified from the Centers for Disease Control and Prevention, 2010b.

---

fomites. An incubation period of 2 to 7 weeks is typical but can be longer. The host response to viral invasion is papular with central umbilication, giving a characteristic appearance (Fig. 3-17). It may be single or multiple and is commonly seen on the vulva, vagina, thighs, and/or buttocks. Molluscum contagiosum is contagious until lesions resolve.

These lesions are typically diagnosed by visual inspection alone. However, material from a lesion can be collected on a swab, applied to a slide, and submitted to a laboratory for diagnostic staining with Giemsa, Gram, or Wright stains. Molluscum bodies, which are large intracytoplasmic structures, are diagnostic.

Most lesions spontaneously regress within 2 to 3 months. If removal is preferred, lesions may be treated by cryotherapy, electrosurgical needle coagulation, or sharp needle-tip curettage of a lesion's umbilicated center. Alternatively, topical application of agents used in the treatment of genital warts may also be applied effectively to treat molluscum contagiosum (see Table 3-21).

PATHOGENS CAUSING PRURITUS

Scabies

Etiology

Sarcoptes scabiei infect skin and result in an intensely pruritic rash. The mite causing this infection is crab-shaped, and the female digs into the skin and remains there for approximately 30 days, elongating her burrow. Several eggs are laid daily and begin hatching after 3 to 4 days (Fig. 3-18). The baby mites furrow their own burrows, becoming reproductive adults in approximately 10 days. The number of adult mites present on an affected patient averages a dozen, although theoretically there could be hundreds. Mites crawl at a rate of 2.5 centimeters per minute, and sexual transmission is the most likely cause of initial infection, although it can be seen in household contacts.

Diagnosis

A delayed Type IV hypersensitivity reaction to the mites, eggs, and feces develops and results in erythematous papules, vesicles,

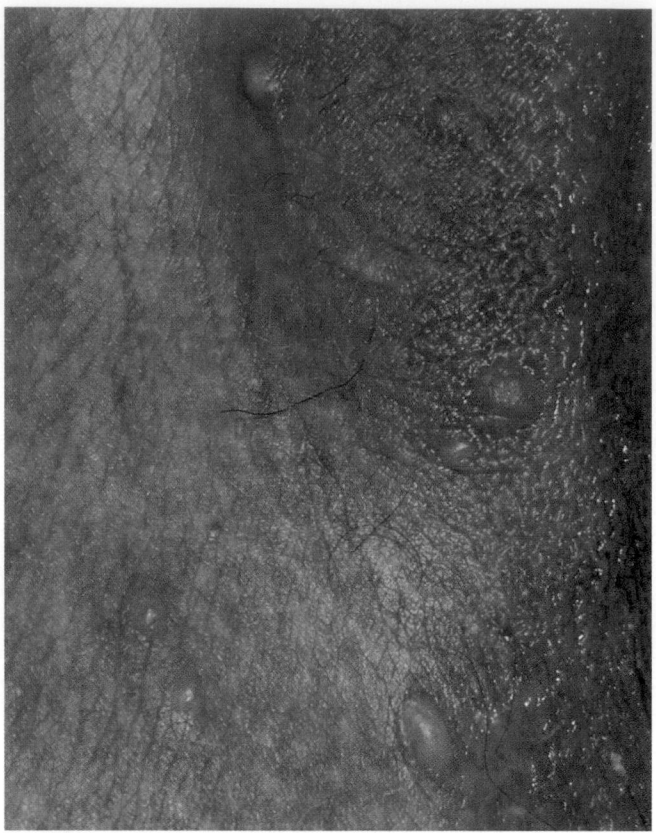

FIGURE 3-17 Photograph of molluscum contagiosum. Flesh-colored, dome-shaped papules with central umbilication are noted.

or nodules in association with skin burrows. Secondary infection, however, may develop and hide these burrows. Most common infection sites include the hands, wrist, elbows, groin, and ankles. Itching is the predominant symptom in these areas.

Burrows are thin elevated tracks in the skin measuring 5 to 10 mm in length. Definitive testing requires scraping across the burrow with a scalpel blade and mixing these fragments in immersion oil on a microscope slide. Identification of mites, eggs, egg fragments, or fecal pellets is diagnostic.

Treatment

Once diagnosed, 1-percent lindane cream (Kwell) is a commonly used agent. A thin layer should be applied from the

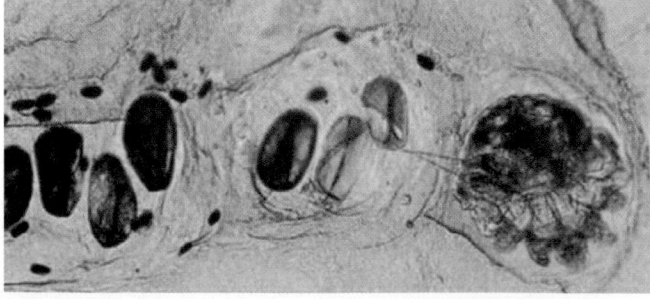

FIGURE 3-18 Photomicrograph of burrow with *Sarcoptes scabiei*. A mite is seen at the end of a burrow (*far right*) with seven eggs and smaller fecal particles. (*From Wolff, 2009, with permission.*)

neck downward with special attention to pruritic areas and the hands, feet, and genital regions. It is recommended that all family members be treated with the exception of pregnant or lactating women and children younger than 2 years. Treatment is effective within 4 hours. Eight to 12 hours after application, a shower or bath should be taken to remove the medication. Only one application is necessary, and bed linens and recently worn clothing should be washed to prevent reinfection.

For pregnant women and young children, 10-percent crotamiton cream or lotion (Eurax) is recommended since it is nontoxic. It should be applied nightly for two nights, and a bath or shower should not be taken for 48 hours. Another treatment regimen is a 5-percent permethrin cream (Elimite), which is effective after a single application. It should be washed off in 8 to 12 hours and is safe in children older than 2 months and in pregnant women.

An antihistamine will help reduce pruritus, which can also be treated with a hydrocortisone-containing cream in adults or with emollients or lubricating agents in infants. If these lesions become infected, antibiotic therapy may be necessary.

Pediculosis

Etiology

Lice are small ectoparasites that measure approximately 1 mm in length (Fig. 3-19). Three species infest humans and include the body louse (*Pediculus humanus*), the crab louse (*Phthirus pubis*), and the head louse (*Pediculus humanus capitis*). Lice attach to the base of human hair with claws that vary in diameter between species. It is this claw's diameter that determines the infestation site. For this reason, the crab louse is found on pubic hair and other hair of similar diameter, such as axillary and facial hair, including eyelashes and eyebrows.

Lice depend on frequent human blood meals, and pubic lice may travel up to 10 centimeters in search of darkness and a new attachment site for blood. They leave voluntarily if the victim becomes febrile or dies, or if there is close contact with another human. Accordingly, pubic lice usually are sexually transmitted, whereas head and body lice may be transmitted by sharing personal objects such as combs, brushes, and clothing.

Symptoms and Diagnosis

The main symptom from louse attachment and biting is pruritus. Scratching results in erythema and inflammation, which increases blood supply to the area. Patients may develop pyoderma and fever if bites become secondarily infected. As is true for mites, the number of lice populating a patient averages a dozen.

Each female adult pubic louse lays approximately four eggs a day, which are glued to the base of hairs. Incubation is approximately 1 month. Their attached eggs, termed nits, can be seen attached to the hair shaft away from the skin line as hair growth progresses (see Fig. 3-19). These nits usually require a magnifying glass for identification. Moreover, suspicious flecks on pubic hair or flecks in clothing can be examined microscopically to see the characteristic louse. Other family members should be evaluated, as should sexual contacts.

Treatment

Pediculicides kill not only adult lice, but also the eggs. A single application is usually effective, but a second application

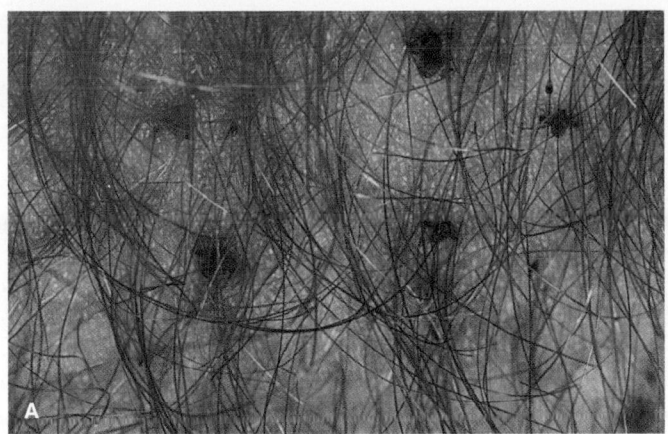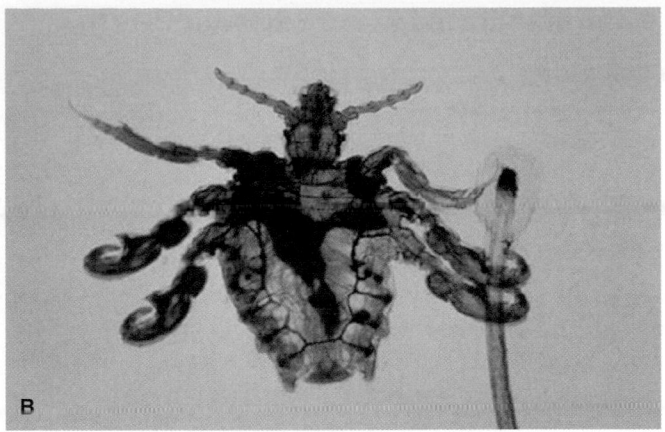

FIGURE 3-19 Phthirus pubis. **A.** Pubic lice are seen attached to hair. In addition, nits are seen as dark dots adhered to pubic hair. *(From Morse, 2003, with permission.)* **B.** Photomicrograph of *Phthirus pubis*. Claw-like legs are ideally suited for clinging to hair shafts. *(From Birnbaum, 2010, with permission.)*

is recommended within 7 to 10 days to kill new hatches. Nonprescription shampoos contain pyrethrins and piperonyl butoxide and should remain on the skin for at least 1 hour. These include brand names such as Rid, Lice-enz, R&C, Pronto, Tegrin LF, and A-200 shampoos.

Alternatively, 1-percent lindane shampoo may also be recommended only for pubic lice treatment. Creams and lotions are reserved for scabies. The treatment is applied to the pubic region for 4 minutes and then rinsed. This compound is percutaneously absorbed through excoriated skin, and seizures have been reported if applied too frequently or not washed off.

Eyelash and eyebrow treatment is problematic. These areas are best treated by applying petrolatum (Vaseline) with a cotton swab at night and washing it off in the morning. Underclothing, bedding, and other infested clothing should be washed and sprayed with Lysol disinfectant. Water temperature greater than 125°F is required to kill lice.

In spite of treatment, pruritus may continue and may be relieved by oral antihistamines, antiinflammatory cream or ointment, or both. The patient should be reevaluated after 1 week to document louse eradication. The sexually transmitted nature of this disease should be discussed, and patients are offered testing for other sexually transmitted infections.

URINARY TRACT INFECTIONS

Symptomatic acute bacterial urinary tract infections (UTIs) are among the most common bacterial infections treated by clinicians. It is estimated that there are more than 8 million office visits per year for these infections in the United States. Cystitis accounts for most of these, whereas more than 100,000 patients are admitted to a hospital annually for acute pyelonephritis treatment. Due to the high incidence of UTI, the Infectious Diseases Society of America has developed guidelines for its treatment (Warren, 1999).

■ Pathogenesis

Because of their pelvic anatomy, women have many more UTIs than men. Bacteria ascending from the colonized urethra enter the bladder and perhaps the kidneys. The short length of the female urethra allows easier access by bacteria to the bladder. Contributing to contamination, the warm moist vulva and rectum are both in close proximity. Similarly, sexual intercourse increases bladder inoculation.

Infections result from the interaction between bacteria and host. Bacterial virulence factors are important, as they enhance colonization and invasion of the lower and upper urinary tract. The principal virulence factors are increased adherence to either vaginal or uroepithelial cells and hemolysin production. The bacterial species most frequently recovered from infected urine culture is *E coli* (Table 3-22).

Once within the bladder, bacteria may ascend within the ureters, enhanced by vesicourethral reflux, into the renal pelvis and cause upper tract infection. Alternatively, the renal parenchyma can be infected by blood-borne organisms, especially during staphylococcal bacteremia. *Mycobacterium tuberculosis* gains access to the kidney through this route and also perhaps by ascension.

TABLE 3-22. Most Common Etiologic Pathogens in Outpatient with Uncomplicated Acute Cystitis

Bacterial Pathogen	Percentage with Pathogen
Gram-negative	
Escherichia coli	50–80
Klebsiella species	6–12
Proteus species	4–6
Enterobacter species	1–6
Morganella species	3–4
Gram-positive	
Enterococcus species	2–12
Coagulase-negative staphylococci (*S saprophyticus*)	5–15
Group B streptococci	2–5

Adapted from Fihn, 2003; Wilson, 2004.

◼ Uncomplicated Acute Bacterial Cystitis

Diagnosis

The most frequent presenting complaints in otherwise healthy, immunocompetent nonpregnant women are dysuria, frequency, urgency, and incontinence.

Studies conducted by the National Institutes of Health (NIH), the Mayo Clinic, and others have shown that most patients can be treated with a short course of antibiotics without examination, urinalysis, or urine culture for an isolated episode of acute uncomplicated bacterial cystitis. It must be emphasized that a patient in this category can always be seen if she prefers. In addition, women should be instructed on clinical changes that warrant further attention such as fever >100.4°C and persistence or recurrence of hematuria, dysuria, and frequency despite treatment.

Women with these exclusions and others require evaluation to exclude other potential causes of their symptoms (Table 3-23). For example, hematuria in a postmenopausal woman may reflect cervical, uterine, or colonic bleeding evident at the time of urination, rather than upper and lower urinary tract infection. Similarly, burning with urination may indicate vulvitis.

◼ Complicated or Recurrent Cystitis

As many as 50 percent of women who suffer an uncomplicated acute bacterial episode of cystitis will have another infection within a year. Up to 5 percent have recurring symptoms soon after treatment. When symptoms develop in such women, the likelihood that a true infection is present is greater than 80 percent.

Diagnosis

Thus, for selected women with complicated or recurrent infections or with persistent or new symptoms during treatment, urinalysis and urine culture are strongly encouraged. For a culture specimen to be informative, it must be accurately collected. A "clean catch" midstream voided urine specimen is usually sufficient. A patient should understand the reasons for and the steps associated with urine specimen collection, which

TABLE 3-23. Exclusions from "Uncomplicated" Cystitis

Persisting symptoms despite >3 days of treatment of urinary tract infection
Symptoms of vaginitis (vaginal discharge/vulvar irritation)
Abdominal and/or pelvic pain, nausea, vomiting
Documented temperature above 38°C (100.4°F)
Recent hospital or nursing home discharge
Documented urologic abnormalities
Recent UTI or urologic surgery
Postmenopausal hematuria
Symptoms >7 days
Immunosuppression
Pregnancy
Diabetes

are designed to prevent contamination by other bacteria from the vulva, vagina, and/or rectum. More than one bacterial species identified in a urine culture usually indicates specimen collection contamination.

Initially, a patient spreads her labia and wipes the periurethral area from front to back with an antiseptic tissue. With labia spread, she begins urinating but does not collect the initial stream. A sample is then collected into a sterile specimen cup. The cup should be handled by the patient in such a way as to avoid contamination. After collection, the urine specimen is delivered promptly to the laboratory and should be plated for culture within 2 hours of collection unless it is refrigerated.

Culture. Urine culture allows accurate identification of an inciting pathogen and susceptibility testing of that pathogen to a variety of antibiotics. Significant bacteriuria is most commonly defined as $\geq 10^5$ bacteria (colony-forming units [cfu]) per milliliter of urine. If urine is collected by either suprapubic aspirate or catheterization, colony counts $\geq 10^2$ cfu/mL are diagnostic. Although a bacterial species may be identified preliminarily, a final urine culture report usually is not available for 48 hours. Thus, empiric treatment is initially begun but modified, as needed, after culture results are available.

Although anaerobic bacteria are part of the vaginal, colonic, and skin flora, they rarely cause UTIs. Hence, urine culture reports do not note anaerobes except in rare instances in which the laboratory has been alerted to and specifically requested to look for an anaerobic species. Fungi can be identified on routine bacteria media and are reported but are rare causes of acute cystitis.

Culture is the gold standard for identifying the etiologic agent of a urinary tract infection, but no laboratory culture techniques help to rapidly identify significant bacteriuria. However, there are rapid tests that give an immediate indication of infection and include microscopy, nitrite testing, and leukocyte esterase testing.

Microscopy. Microscopic examination of a urine specimen allows identification of both pyuria and bacteria. For identification of leukocytes, a specimen should be examined expeditiously because leukocytes deteriorate quickly in urine that has not been appropriately preserved. Standards to define pyuria are inadequate, other than gross counts. Accordingly, the rapid test for leukocyte esterase has become a surrogate for the microscopic WBC count.

Gram staining is a simple, rapid, and sensitive method for detecting a concentration $\geq 10^5$ cfu/mL of a bacterial species. Rapid identification allows appropriate selection of empiric antimicrobial therapy. However, realistically, such testing is typically limited to patients with complicated urinary tract infections or acute pyelonephritis.

Leukocyte Esterase. This test measures esterase enzyme found in urinary leukocytes and enzyme released in poorly preserved specimens. If used alone diagnostically, this test is most beneficial for its high negative predictive value, especially with bacterial colony counts $\geq 10^5$ cfu/mL. If one combines nitrite and leukocyte esterase testing of a clean-catch uncontaminated voided specimen, the specificity of positive tests approaches 100 percent with uropathogen colony counts of $\geq 10^5$ cfu/mL. The negative predictive value is comparable. However, if these specimens have been contaminated with vaginal or colonic bacteria, this test can be falsely positive in the absence of a true uropathogen. *Trichomonas* species also produce esterases. In addition, very concentrated urine or urine with significant proteinuria or glucosuria will decrease the accuracy of this test.

Nitrites. Bacteria metabolically produce nitrites from nitrates. The bacteria in which this is most frequently observed are Enterobacteriaceae, the gram-negative aerobic family of pathogens most commonly responsible for acute UTIs in women. The major drawback of this test is that it does not identify gram-positive pathogens such as staphylococci, streptococci, enterococci, or *Pseudomonas* species. In addition, it ideally requires testing of the first morning urine specimen, because more than 4 hours are required for bacteria to convert nitrates to nitrites at levels that are detectable by the test method. As a single test, the specificity of a positive nitrite test is very high with $\geq 10^5$ cfu/mL of a uropathogen. Its negative predictive value is higher than its positive predictive value.

Treatment

The etiologic pathogens of acute cystitis have progressively changed, as well as their sensitivities to antibiotic regimens. During the past two decades, the frequency of infections caused by group B *Streptococcus* and *Klebsiella* species has increased, whereas *E coli* infection rates have diminished. Also, in many locations, sensitivity patterns in *E coli* warrant a shift in initial empiric treatment from trimethoprim-sulfamethoxazole to a fluoroquinolone for this infection (Table 3-24). If a woman has a sulfa allergy, she can take trimethoprim alone. Treatment courses of any regimen longer than 3 days result in almost twice the number of adverse events, are not more effective in treating uncomplicated cystitis, are more costly, and have higher rates of noncompliance. However, single-dose therapy is less effective than 3-day regimens for this infection. Nitrofurantoin regimens are usually 7 days and are frequently associated with upper GI symptoms.

For significant dysuria, up to 2 days of a bladder analgesic such as phenazopyridine (Pyridium), 200 mg orally up to three times daily, may give significant relief. However, GI upset, yellow-orange stained urine and clothing, and hemolysis in patients with glucose-6-phosphate dehydrogenase (G6PD) deficiency are potential side effects.

Many recurrences develop after intercourse, and low-dose postcoital dosing or continuous 3-day regimens are usually effective at preventing infection recurrence. A woman with two or more episodes of cystitis within 6 months or three infections within a year should be considered for urologic evaluation of her urinary tract.

Asymptomatic Bacteriuria

This is defined as isolation of a specified quantitative count of bacteria in an appropriately collected urine specimen obtained from a person without symptoms or signs referable to urinary

infection (Rubin, 1992). In healthy nonpregnant women, the prevalence of this condition increases with age. It is associated with sexual activity and is more common in diabetics. Moreover, one fourth to one half of elderly women in long-term care facilities have bacteriuria, which is seen primarily in those with chronic neurologic illness and functional impairment.

The Infectious Disease Society of America recommends that nonpregnant premenopausal women not be screened for asymptomatic bacteriuria (Nicolle, 2005). In controlled randomized prospective trials, women randomly given a 1-week course of antibiotic or placebo had similar prevalences of bacteria and incidences of symptomatic infection 1 year after therapy. The same is true for diabetic women, in whom there is evidence of harm with treatment of asymptomatic bacteriuria. Additionally, routine screening is not recommended for older persons living in the community.

Acute Uncomplicated Pyelonephritis
Diagnosis

This infection may be divided into mild (no nausea or vomiting, normal to slightly elevated blood leukocyte count, and normal to low-grade fever) and severe (vomiting, dehydration, evidence of sepsis, high leukocyte count, and fever). Other symptoms may include those of a lower urinary tract infection and varying degrees of back pain and tenderness to percussion over the region of the kidney(s).

Treatment

Traditional therapy for this infection has included hospitalization and intravenous antibiotic treatment for up to 2 weeks. However, studies in young healthy women with normal urinary tracts indicate that 7 to 14 days of oral therapy are sufficient for compliant women with mild infection (see Table 3-24) (Warren, 1999). In one study of more than 50 college women with acute uncomplicated pyelonephritis, resistance to trimethoprim-sulfamethoxazole was 30 percent (Hooton, 1997). Accordingly, an oral fluoroquinolone is recommended treatment unless a pathogen is susceptible to trimethoprim-sulfamethoxazole. At initial diagnosis, clinicians may also administer a parenteral dose prior to starting oral therapy. Alternatively, if a causative organism is gram-positive, then amoxicillin or amoxicillin/clavulanic acid is recommended. Hospitalization is warranted for women who display clinical indications at initial evaluation or fail to improve with outpatient therapy.

PELVIC INFLAMMATORY DISEASE

This is an infection of the upper female reproductive tract organs. Another diagnosis given to this disease is acute salpingitis. Although all may be involved, the reproductive tract organ of importance, with or without abscess formation, is the fallopian tube. Because of difficulty in accurately diagnosing this infection, its true magnitude is unknown. Many women report that they have been treated for PID when they did not

TABLE 3-24. Treatment of Urinary Tract Infection

Infection Category	Antimicrobial Regimen
Uncomplicated cystitis Local *E coli* resistance <20%	Orally for 3 days: Trimethoprim-sulfamethoxazole DS 160/800 mg (Bactrim DS, Septra DS) twice daily *or* Trimethoprim (Bactrim, Septra) 100 mg twice daily *or* Nitrofurantoin macrocrystals (Macrodantin) 50–100 mg four times daily *or* Nitrofurantoin monohydrate macrocrystals (Macrobid) 100 mg twice daily *or* Fosfomycin tromethamine (Monurol) single 3-g dose for only 1 day
Local *E coli* resistance ≥20%	Ciprofloxacin (Cipro) 250 mg twice daily *or* Norfloxacin (Noroxin) 400 mg twice daily *or* Levofloxacin (Levaquin) 250 mg daily
Complicated/recurrent cystitis Postcoital	Same as above unless culture and sensitivity dictate change Orally once: Trimethoprim-sulfamethoxazole SS 80/400 mg 0.5 to 1 tablet *or* Ciprofloxacin 250 mg *or* Levofloxacin 250 mg
Intermittent	Same as uncomplicated acute cystitis, begin with symptom onset
Mild pyelonephritis Gram-negative	Oral 7 to 14 days: Ciprofloxacin 500 mg twice daily *or* Norfloxacin 400 mg twice daily *or* Levofloxacin 250 mg daily
Gram-positive	Amoxicillin-clavulanic acid 875/125 mg (Augmentin) twice daily
Severe pyelonephritis Gram-negative	Intravenous until afebrile 24 to 48 hours, then oral to complete 7–14 days of therapy: Ciprofloxacin 400 mg twice daily *or* Levofloxacin 500 mg daily *or* Cefoxitin (Mefoxin) 2 g every 8 hours with or without aminoglycoside *or* Cefotaxime (Claforan) 1 to 2 g two to four times daily with or without an aminoglycoside
Gram-positive	Ampicillin 3 g every 6 hours *or* Piperacillin-tazobactam 3.375 g (Zosyn) q 6 h *or* Ampicillin-sulbactam 3/1.2 g (Unasyn) q 6 h

DS = double strength; *E coli* = *Escherichia coli*; SS = single strength
Adapted from American College of Obstetricians and Gynecologists, 2008a; Fihn, 2003; and Warren, 1999.

have it, and vice versa. The clinical importance of diagnosing PID is emphasized by its known sequelae, which include tubal-factor infertility, ectopic pregnancy, and chronic pelvic pain. Thus, clinicians should carry a low threshold for diagnosing and treating PID.

Microbiology and Pathogenesis

The exact microbiologic pathogens in the fallopian tube cannot be known for any given patient. Studies have shown that transvaginal culture of the endocervix, endometrium, and cul-de-sac contents reveals different organisms from each site in the same patient. In laparoscopic studies, cervical pathogens and those recovered from the fallopian tube or cul-de-sac are not identical. For that reason, treatment protocols are designed so that most potential pathogens are covered by antibiotic regimens.

Classic salpingitis is associated with and secondary to *N gonorrhoeae* infection, and *C trachomatis* is also commonly recovered (Table 3-25). Another species frequently found is *T vaginalis*. The lower reproductive tract flora in women with PID and in those with bacterial vaginosis is predominately anaerobic species. The microenvironment changes produced by BV may aid ascension of the causative organisms of PID (Soper, 2010). However, Ness and colleagues (2004) and others have shown that bacterial vaginosis is not a risk factor for PID development.

Upper tract infection is believed to be caused by bacteria from the lower reproductive tract that ascend into the upper tract. For this reason, prior tubal ligation may be protective against infection progression in many cases (Levgur, 2000). It is assumed that this ascension is enhanced during menstruation due to loss of endocervical barriers. The gonococcus can cause a direct inflammatory response in the human endocervix, endometrium, and fallopian tube and is one of the true pathogens of human fallopian tube epithelial cells. If normal human fallopian tube cells in cell culture are exposed to potential pathogens such as *E coli*, *B fragilis*, or *Enterococcus faecalis*, no inflammatory response

results. If these bacteria are introduced into a fallopian tube cell culture in which gonococci are present and have caused inflammatory damage, an exaggerated inflammatory response results.

In contrast, intracellular *C trachomatis* does not cause an acute inflammatory response, and little *direct* permanent damage results from chlamydial tubal involvement (Patton, 1983). However, cell-mediated immune mechanisms may be responsible for resulting tissue injury. Specifically, persistent chlamydial antigens can trigger a delayed hypersensitivity reaction with continued tubal scarring and destruction (Toth, 2000).

Lastly, women with pulmonary tuberculosis can develop salpingitis and endometritis. It is assumed that this pathogen is blood-borne, but ascension may still be a possible route. The fallopian tubes also can be infected by direct extension from inflammatory GI disease, especially appendiceal or diverticular abscess rupture.

Diagnosis

Pelvic inflammatory disease can be segregated into "silent" PID and PID. Of these, PID can be further subdivided into acute and chronic.

Silent Pelvic Inflammatory Disease

This condition is thought to result from multiple or continuous low-grade infection in asymptomatic women. Silent PID is not a clinical diagnosis. Rather, it is an ultimate diagnosis given to women with tubal-factor infertility who lack a history compatible with upper tract infection. Many of these patients have antibodies to *C trachomatis* and/or *N gonorrhoeae*. At laparoscopy or laparotomy, these patients may have evidence of prior tubal infection such as adhesions, but for the most part, the fallopian tubes are grossly normal. Internally, however, there are flattened mucosal folds, extensive deciliation of the epithelium, and secretory epithelial cell degeneration (Patton, 1989). Alternatively, hydrosalpinx may be found. Grossly, these fallopian tubes are distended along their entire length. Their distal ends are dilated and clubbed, and fimbria are replaced by or encased by smooth adhesions (Fig. 9-25, p. 273). Sonographically, a hydrosalpinx tends to be anechoic, tubular, serpentine, and often with incomplete septa (Fig. 9-26, p. 273). Lastly, fine adhesions between the liver capsule and anterior abdominal wall may also be evidence of prior silent disease.

Acute Pelvic Inflammatory Disease

Criteria for Diagnosis of Acute Disease. Symptoms characteristically develop during or soon following menstruation. The most recent recommended diagnostic criteria presented by the CDC (2010b) are for sexually active women at risk for STDs who have pelvic or lower abdominal pain, and other etiologies are excluded or unlikely. PID is diagnosed if uterine tenderness, adnexal tenderness, or cervical motion tenderness is present. One or more of the following enhances diagnostic specificity: (1) oral temperature >38.3°C (101.6°F), (2) mucopurulent cervical or vaginal discharge, (3) abundant WBCs on saline microscopy of cervical secretions, (4) elevated erythrocyte sedimentation rate (ESR) or C-reactive protein

---

TABLE 3-25. Pelvic Inflammatory Disease Risk Factors

Douching
Single status
Substance abuse
Multiple sexual partners
Lower socioeconomic status
Recent new sexual partner(s)
Younger age (10 to 19 years)
Other sexually transmitted infections
Sexual partner with urethritis or gonorrhea
Previous diagnosis of pelvic inflammatory disease
Not using mechanical and/or chemical contraceptive barriers
Endocervical testing positive for *Neisseria gonorrhoeae* or *Chlamydia trachomatis*

(CRP), and (5) presence of cervical *N gonorrhoeae* or *C trachomatis*. Thus, a diagnosis of PID is one typically based on clinical findings.

Symptoms and Physical Findings. Presenting symptoms may include lower abdominal and/or pelvic pain, yellow vaginal discharge, menorrhagia, fever, chills, anorexia, nausea, vomiting, diarrhea, dysmenorrhea, and dyspareunia. Patients also may have infective urinary symptoms. Unfortunately, no single symptom is associated with a physical finding that is specific for this diagnosis. Accordingly, other possible sources of acute pelvic pain should be considered (Table 11-1, p. 306).

In women with acute PID, leukorrhea or mucopurulent endocervicitis is common and is diagnosed visually and microscopically. During bimanual pelvic examination, women with acute PID will usually have pelvic organ tenderness. Cervical motion tenderness (CMT) is typically elicited by quickly displacing the cervix laterally with examining vaginal fingers. This reflects pelvic peritonitis and may be considered a vaginal "rebound" test. If a woman has pelvic peritonitis secondary to bacteria and purulent debris that has exuded from the fimbriated end of the fallopian tube, this rapid cervical and peritoneal movement usually causes a marked pain response. Tapping the cul-de-sac with examining finger(s) will give the examiner similar information. This maneuver usually causes a patient significantly less pain because less inflamed peritoneum is involved.

Abdominal peritonitis may be identified by deep probing and quick release of a hand placed on the abdomen—a test for rebound. Alternatively, an examining hand may be positioned with a palm against a woman's midabdomen and gently and quickly moved back and forth (shake). This will identify abdominal peritonitis, often with less patient discomfort.

In women with PID and peritonitis, usually only the lower abdomen is involved. However, inflammation of the liver capsule, which can accompany PID, may lead to right upper quadrant pain, a condition known as Fitz-Hugh-Curtis syndrome. Classically, symptoms of this perihepatitis include sharp, pleuritic right upper quadrant pain that accompanies pelvic pain. The upper abdominal pain may refer to the shoulder or upper arm. With auscultation, a friction rub may be heard along the right anterior costal margin. Importantly, during examination, if all abdominal quadrants are involved, suspicion of a ruptured tuboovarian abscess should be heightened.

Laboratory Testing. In women with lower abdominal pain, tests directed at diagnosing pelvic infection or excluding other pain source are selected. Pregnancy complications can be identified by serum or urine beta-human chorionic gonadotropin testing. A complete blood count (CBC) is selected as a baseline test to exclude hemoperitoneum as the cause of symptoms and identify WBC elevation. In those with significant nausea and vomiting or Fitz-Hugh-Curtis syndrome, liver enzyme values may be normal or mildly elevated. If properly collected, urinalysis findings for infection will be absent. Saline preparation of cervical or vaginal discharge will typically show sheets of leukocytes. In women with suspected acute PID, endocervical testing

for both *N gonorrhoeae* and *C trachomatis* should be performed as described earlier (p. 86). Screening for other STDs should also be incorporated.

Laparoscopy. In Scandinavian countries, women suspected of having acute PID undergo laparoscopy for diagnosis. Tubal serosal hyperemia, tubal wall edema, and purulent exudate issuing from the fimbriated ends of the fallopian tubes, termed *pyosalpinx*, and pooling in the cul-de-sac confirm this diagnosis. Because of this routine practice, Hadgu and coworkers (1986) assembled clinical criteria that preoperatively clinically predicted acute PID and assessed their validity by the absence or presence of disease at laparoscopy. Criteria included: (1) single status, (2) adnexal mass, (3) age younger than 25 years, (4) temperature >38°C, (5) cervical *N gonorrhoeae*, (6) purulent vaginal discharge, and (7) ESR ≥15 mm/h. The preoperative clinical diagnosis of PID was 97-percent accurate if a woman met all seven criteria, allowing avoidance of surgery. However, due to the cost of laparoscopy, antimicrobial therapy based on a clinical diagnosis in patients with historical and physical findings suggestive of acute PID is reasonable.

Sonography. In women with marked abdominal pain and tenderness, appreciation of upper reproductive tract organs during bimanual examination may be limited, and sonography is a primary imaging tool. Normal fallopian tubes are rarely imaged. However, with acute tubal inflammation, the tube swells, its lumen occludes distally, it distends, and its walls and endosalpingeal folds thicken (Fig. 2-17, p. 43). Characteristic findings include: (1) distended, ovoid-shaped tube filled with anechoic or echogenic fluid, (2) fallopian tube wall thickening, (3) incomplete septa, and (4) a "cogwheel" appearance when inflamed tubes are imaged in cross section (Timor-Tritsch, 1998). Sonography may also be used to identify tuboovarian abscess (TOA) or exclude other pathology as the pain source (Molander, 2001). With both pyosalpinx and TOA, color and power Doppler will show increased flow in the walls and septa. If sonography does not lead to a clear diagnosis, computed-tomography (CT) scanning may be indicated (Sam, 2002). In women with right upper quadrant pain suggestive of perihepatitis, chest radiography or upper abdominal sonography may be needed to exclude other pathology.

Endometrial Biopsy. In women suspected of acute PID, some recommend endometrial biopsy to diagnose endometritis. Polymorphonuclear leukocytes on the endometrial surface correlate with acute endometritis, whereas plasma cells in the endometrium are found with chronic endometritis. However, women with uterine leiomyomas or endometrial polyps and no PID frequently also have plasma cells present in the endometrium at endometrial biopsy, as do essentially all women in the lower uterine segment. In the opinion of many, an endometrial biopsy in women with mucopurulent secretions would not provide useful information to alter the diagnosis or therapy (Achilles, 2005).

Tuboovarian Abscess

With infection, the inflamed and suppurative fallopian tube may adhere to the ovary. Sonographically, if both tube and ovary are recognizable, the term *tuboovarian complex* is used. If inflammation proceeds, tissue planes and distinction between the two is lost, and the term *tuboovarian abscess* is applied. Tuboovarian abscesses are typically unilateral and may also involve adjacent structures that include bowel, bladder, and contralateral adnexa. With abscess progression, further structural weakening may lead to abscess rupture and potentially life-threatening peritonitis. Although PID is an important cause of TOA, these may also follow appendicitis, diverticulitis, inflammatory bowel disease, or surgery.

Classically, affected women display signs of PID and a concurrent adnexal or cul-de-sac mass. Sonographically, with TOA, a complex cystic adnexal or cul-de-sac mass with thick irregular walls, areas of mixed echogenicity, septations, and internal echoes from debris are seen (Figs. 2-18, p. 43 and 9-27, p. 274). If the clinical picture is unclear, CT scanning may add information. A thick-walled cystic adnexal mass with internal septations and surrounding inflammatory changes is characteristic (Fig. 3-20). Although not routinely used for TOA imaging, magnetic resonance imaging usually shows a complex pelvic mass with low signal intensity on T1-weighted sequences and heterogeneously high signal intensity on T2-weighted sequences.

Microorganisms frequently cultured include *E coli, Bacteroides* spp., *Peptostreptococcus* spp., and aerobic *Streptococcus* spp. (Landers, 1983). Thus, broad-spectrum antibiotic coverage is selected for initial management of women with unruptured TOA. Most women with TOA will respond to IV antibiotic therapy alone and avoid the need for drainage. Many single-agent regimens have been shown in clinical trial to effectively treat PID complicated by TOAs. These include second- and third-generation cephalosporins (cefoxitin, cefotetan, cefotaxime, ceftizoxime) and certain penicillins (piperacillin, ampicillin/sulbactam, piperacillin/tazobactam). Combination antimicrobial regimens will predictably be more successful. Clindamycin/

gentamicin with or without ampicillin or ampicillin/gentamicin/metronidazole are those most frequently employed. Treatment of a patient with an abscess should include parenteral antimicrobial therapy until the patient has been afebrile for at least 24 hours, preferably 48 to 72 hours.

For those not improved within 2 to 3 days of treatment, prior to attempts at abscess drainage, antimicrobial regimen modification is indicated. Drainage plus antibiotic therapy can be considered as initial treatment for larger abscesses (≥8 cm). For this, drainage can be accomplished with or without surgery. Radiologic drainage is minimally invasive and potentially avoids the higher risks associated with general anesthesia and surgery. In general, pelvic collections can be emptied using transabdominal, transvaginal, transgluteal, or transrectal routes with either CT or sonographic guidance and adequate analgesia. Depending on abscess size and characteristics, contents can be removed with needle aspiration or with catheter placement and short-term drainage. In cases refractory or not amenable to these more conservative measures, exploratory laparoscopy or laparotomy is typically warranted. In those with TOA rupture, emergency surgery is required. Goals of surgery include abscess drainage, excision of necrotic tissues, and peritoneal cavity irrigation.

As is true in all abscesses, drainage is the key to clinical improvement. Although perhaps tempting at laparotomy, removal of the abscess is not necessary unless ovarian parenchyma is involved. This is rare. Electively opening the protective peritoneal and other tissue planes to remove tissues—especially the uterus—in the presence of acute infection does not improve patient outcome compared with percutaneous drainage. As a clinical comparison, infected Bartholin glands are not excised. Rather, they are drained and definitively treated later, when not infected, if necessary.

Infection confined within one organ, such as a pyosalpinx, responds more favorably to antimicrobial therapy because of adequate blood and lymphatic supply. This is true even if attached to an adjacent ovary. However, a cul-de-sac or interloop abscess is more likely to require drainage, because of poor blood and lymphatic supply and a less prompt response to antimicrobial therapy.

Following successful conservative treatment, bilateral adnexal abscesses cannot be equated with guaranteed infertility. In a clinical trial evaluating such patients, 25 percent of women subsequently became pregnant (Hemsell, 1993).

Chronic Pelvic Inflammatory Disease

This diagnosis is given to women who describe a history of acute PID and who have subsequent pelvic pain. Accuracy of this diagnosis clinically is orders of magnitude less than for acute PID. A hydrosalpinx might qualify as a criterion for this diagnosis. Realistically, however, it is a histologic diagnosis (chronic inflammation) made by a pathologist. Thus, the clinical utility of this diagnosis is limited.

Treatment of Pelvic Inflammatory Disease

The most beneficial patient outcomes follow early diagnosis and prompt, appropriate therapy. The primary goal of therapy is to eradicate bacteria, relieve symptoms, and prevent sequelae. Tubal damage or occlusion resulting from infection may lead to

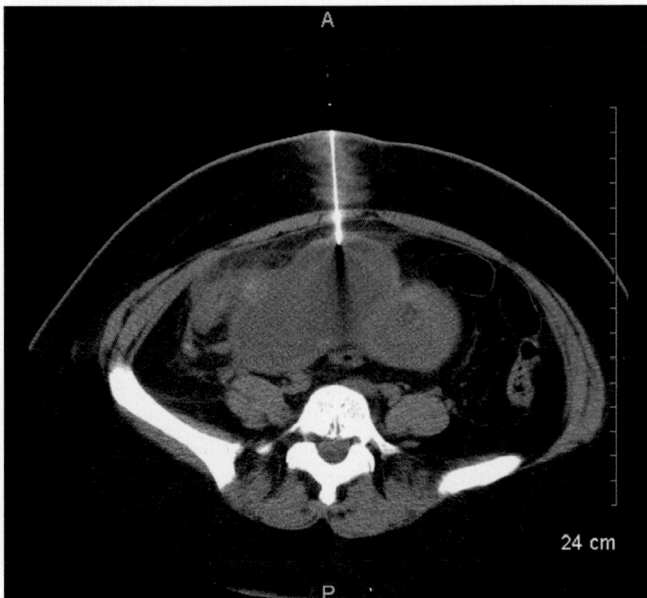

FIGURE 3-20 Computed tomographic (CT) scan of a tuboovarian abscess being drained percutaneous.

TABLE 3-26. Recommended Hospitalization Indications for Parenteral Treatment of Pelvic Inflammatory Disease

Adolescents
Drug addicts
Severe disease
Suspected abscess
Uncertain diagnosis
Generalized peritonitis
Temperature >38.3°C
Failed outpatient therapy
Recent intrauterine instrumentation
White blood cell count >15,000/mm³
Nausea/vomiting precluding oral therapy

TABLE 3-27. Recommended Outpatient Treatment of Pelvic Inflammatory Disease

Ceftriaxone (Rocephin) 250 mg IM once
plus
Doxycycline 100 mg orally twice daily for 14 days
with or without
Metronidazole (Flagyl) 500 mg orally twice daily for 14 days

OR

Cefoxitin (Mefoxin) 2 g IM with 1 g oral probenecid once
plus
Doxycycline 100 mg as above
with or without
Metronidazole as above

OR

Other parenteral third-generation cephalosporin IM given in a single dose[a]
plus
Doxycycline 100 mg as above
with or without
Metronidazole as above

[a]Examples given include ceftizoxime (Cefizox) or cefotaxime (Claforan).
IM = intramuscular.
Modified from the Centers for Disease Control and Prevention, 2010b.

infertility. Rates following one episode approximate 15 percent; two episodes, 35 percent; and three or more episodes, 75 percent (Westrom, 1975). Also, ectopic pregnancy risk is increased 6- to 10-fold and may reach a 10-percent risk for those who conceive. Other sequelae include chronic pelvic pain (15 to 20 percent), recurrent infection (20 to 25 percent), and abscess formation (5 to 15 percent). Unfortunately, women with mild symptoms may remain at home for days or weeks prior to presentation for diagnosis and therapy.

Exactly where a patient should be treated remains controversial. There are proposed criteria that predict better outcome for certain patients with in-hospital parenteral antimicrobial therapy (Table 3-26). However, the high cost of in-hospital treatment prevents routine hospitalization for all women given this diagnosis.

Oral Treatment

In women with a mild to moderate clinical presentation, outpatient treatment and inpatient therapy yield similar results. Clinical treatment with oral therapy is also appropriate for women with HIV infection and PID. These women have the same species recovered compared with non-HIV-infected patients, and response to therapy is similar.

If women have more than moderate disease, they require hospitalization. Dunbar-Jacob and associates (2004) showed that women treated as outpatients took 70 percent of prescribed doses, and for less than 50 percent of their outpatient treatment days. If patients are to be treated as outpatients, an initial parenteral dose may be beneficial. Women treated as outpatients should be reevaluated in approximately 72 hours by phone or in person. If women do not respond to oral therapy within 72 hours, parenteral therapy should be initiated either as an inpatient or as an outpatient if home nursing care is available. This assumes that the diagnosis is confirmed at reevaluation.

Specific treatment recommendations from the CDC are found in Table 3-27. Anaerobes are believed by some to play an important role in upper tract infection and should be treated. Hence, metronidazole may be added to improve anaerobic

coverage. If patients have BV or trichomoniasis, then metronidazole addition is required, although perhaps not for 14 days.

Parenteral Treatment

Any woman who has criteria as outlined in Table 3-26 should be hospitalized for parenteral treatment for at least 24 hours. Following this, if home parenteral treatment is available, this is a reasonable option. Alternatively, if a woman responds clinically and will be appropriately treated by one of the oral regimens in Table 3-27, then she can be discharged on those medications.

Recommendations for parenteral antibiotic treatment of PID are found in Table 3-28. Of these antibiotics, oral and parenteral routes of doxycycline have almost identical bioavailability, but parenteral doxycycline is caustic to veins. Many prospective clinical trials have shown that either of the listed cephalosporins alone, without doxycycline, will result in a clinical cure. For that reason, doxycycline administration could be reserved until the patient can take oral medication. The recommendation is to continue parenteral therapy until 24 hours after the patient clinically improves, and the oral doxycycline should continue to complete 14 days of therapy. Alternatively, if the primary reason for providing doxycycline is to eradicate *C trachomatis*, a 1-g oral dose of azithromycin given while the patient is in the hospital will also achieve that goal.

TABLE 3-28. Recommended Parenteral Treatment of Pelvic Inflammatory Disease

Regimen A

Cefotetan (Cefotan) 2 g IV every 12 hours
or
Cefoxitin (Mefoxin) 2 g IV every 6 hours
plus
Doxycycline 100 mg orally or IV every 12 hours

Regimen B

Clindamycin 900 mg IV every 8 hours
plus
Gentamicin loading dose 2 mg/kg IV or IM followed by a maintenance dose of 1.5 mg/kg every 8 hours. Single daily dosing at 3 to 5 mg/kg per day may be substituted

Alternative Parenteral Regimens

Ampicillin/sulbactam (Unasyn) 3 g IV every 6 hours
plus
Doxycycline 100 mg orally or IV as above

IV = intravenously.
Modified from Centers for Disease Control and Prevention, 2010b.

POSTOPERATIVE INFECTION

Clinical Significance and Risks

Operative site infections continue to account for many hospital-acquired infections. Development of a postoperative infection may result in doubling or even tripling of a predicted hospital stay, resulting in significant patient morbidity and increased health care costs. Risks for postoperative infection are varied (Table 3-29). These include patient and surgical factors, and

TABLE 3-29. Risk Factors for Postoperative Surgical Site Infections

Smoker
Excessive blood loss
Preoperative anemia
Lower socioeconomic status
Immunocompromised patient
Recent operative site surgery
Obesity (abdominal hysterectomy)
Younger age (vaginal hysterectomy)
Older age (abdominal hysterectomy)
Prolonged surgical procedure (>3.5 h)
Foreign body placement (catheter, drain, etc.)
Perioperative HbA1c >7% or CBG >250 in diabetics

CBG = capillary blood glucose; HbA1c = hemoglobin A1c.

preventive strategies are found in Table 39-17 (p. 973). Of these, the degree of wound contamination at the time of surgery plays an important role in these infections.

Because most gynecologic surgical procedures are elective, a gynecologist has time to decrease microbial inoculum. Thus, BV, trichomonal vaginitis, cervicitis, and active urinary tract or respiratory infections ideally are treated and eradicated prior to surgery.

■ Wound Classification

Since 1964, surgical wounds have been classified according to the degree of bacterial contamination of the operative site at the time of surgery. As the number of operative site bacteria (inoculum) increases, so too does the postoperative infection rate.

Clean Wounds

Surgeries that are elective, that are performed for nontraumatic surgical indications, that are without operative site inflammation, and that avoid the respiratory, alimentary, and genitourinary tracts are included in this category. No break occurs in surgical technique. Thus, most laparoscopic and adnexal surgeries are considered to be in this category, and strictly speaking, supracervical hysterectomy could also be added. Without prophylaxis, infection rates range from 1 to 5 percent. Prophylactic antimicrobials do not decrease infection rates following these procedures and are typically not be administered.

Clean Contaminated Wounds

These are surgical wounds in which the respiratory, gastrointestinal, genital, or urinary tract is entered under controlled conditions and without unusual bacterial contamination. Criteria further define that there can be no break in surgical technique. Infection rates range from 5 to 15 percent. This group encompasses most gynecologic procedures including total hysterectomy, cervical conization, and dilatation and curettage (D&C). Of these, hysterectomy is the gynecologic procedure most frequently followed by a surgical site infection. These procedures are usually elective, and hysterectomy requires antimicrobial prophylaxis to reduce postoperative infection rates (Table 39-6, p. 959). (American College of Obstetricians and Gynecologists, 2009).

Contaminated Wounds

Classic cases in this category include open, fresh, accidental wounds; operations with major breaks in sterile technique or gross GI spillage; and incisions in which acute, nonpurulent inflammation is encountered (Mangram, 1999). Infection rates approximate 10 to 25 percent. For this reason, a minimum of 24 hours of perioperative antimicrobial administration is required, and delayed wound closure may be selected. Laparoscopy or laparotomy for acute salpingitis should be included in this category. If abscess is present, these are considered dirty wounds.

Dirty Wounds

These are typically old traumatic wounds or those that involve existing clinical infection or perforated viscera. These operative sites are clinically infected at the time of surgery, and infection rates range from 30 to 100 percent. Accordingly, therapeutic antimicrobial therapy is required.

Surgical Site Infection Classification

In 1992, the CDC provided definitions of hospital-acquired surgical site infections (SSIs). These were modified by Horan and others during the same year. The Joint Commission (JC) currently is emphasizing this morbidity during their hospital accreditation process. Thus, hospitals are more attentive to infection rates and to the rates of individual surgeons. In classifying SSIs, there are two categories, incisional and organ/space (Fig. 3-21). The incisional group is further subdivided into superficial and deep classes. Criteria for each category are detailed in Table 3-30.

Organ/Space

These infections develop in spaces or organs other than that opened by the original incision or manipulated during the surgical procedure. Specific sites include the vaginal cuff, urinary tract, and intraabdominal sites. Of note, vaginal cuff infections are considered in the superficial incisional class and parametritis is classified as a deep incisional infection (Figs. 3-22 and 3-23). In contrast, pelvic infections such as adnexal infection, pelvic abscess, or infected pelvic hematoma fall into the category of organ/space infection (Figs. 3-24 and 3-25).

Diagnosis
Febrile Morbidity

The most frequently used definition for febrile morbidity is an oral temperature of ≥38°C (≥100.4°F) on two or more occasions, 4 or more hours apart, and 24 or more hours following surgery. This condition is seen most frequently after hysterectomy, particularly abdominal hysterectomy; usually is

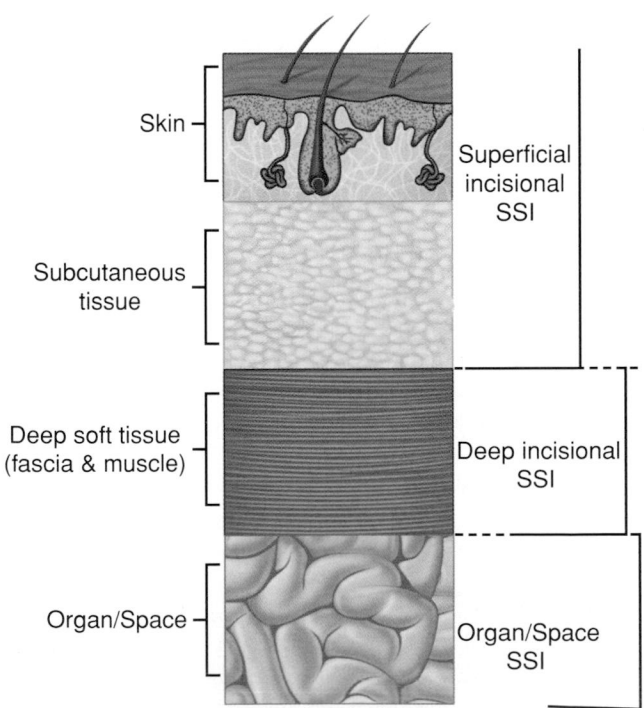

FIGURE 3-21 Anatomy and classification of surgical site infections (SSI). *(Redrawn from Mangram, 1999.)*

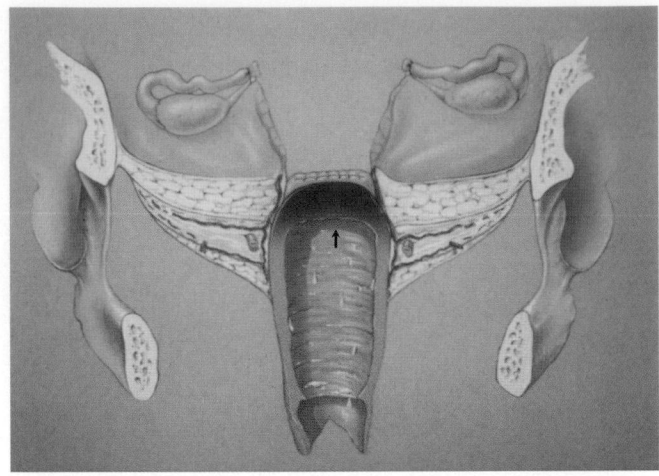

FIGURE 3-22 Vaginal cuff cellulitis. The vaginal surgical margin (*arrow*) is edematous, hyperemic, and tender, and there are purulent secretions in the vagina. Parametria and adnexa are normal during gentle bimanual examination.

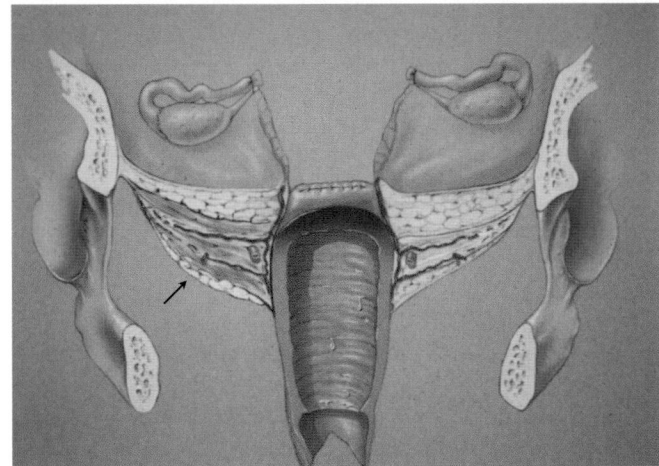

FIGURE 3-23 Pelvic cellulitis in the right parametrium (*arrow*). It is indurated and tender to palpation; no mass is present.

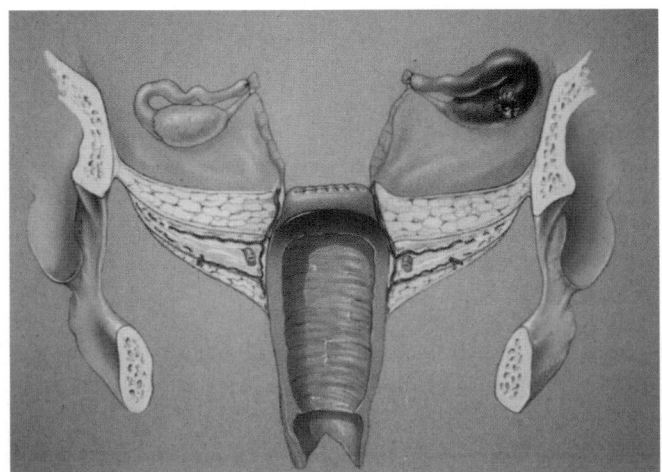

FIGURE 3-24 Adnexal infection after hysterectomy. The parametria are normal. Tenderness without a mass is appreciated in the adnexal area, and its location is dependent on the surgical procedure.

TABLE 3-30. Criteria for Defining Surgical Site Infections

Superficial incisional
Involves only superficial tissues
Develops within 30 days of surgical procedure
Features:
    Purulent drainage or bacteria in culture of tissue or fluid
    Signs or symptoms:
        Tenderness or pain
        Heat or redness
        Localized swelling
        Required opening of superficial incision
    Superficial incision infection diagnosis made by surgeon
Stitch abscesses are not included in this category
Vaginal cuff cellulitis should be included here (see Fig. 3-22)

Deep incisional
Abdominal wall muscle and fascia are involved
Develops within 30 days of surgical procedure
Features:
    Purulent drainage from deep incision, not organ or space component, of surgical site
    Deep incision that spontaneously dehisces or is deliberately opened by a surgeon in a patient who has at least one of
        the following signs or symptoms:
    Temperature $\geq 38°C$ (100.4°F)
    Localized pain or tenderness
    Abscess or other infection found by reoperation, histopathology, or radiology
    Diagnosis made by surgeon
Parametritis (pelvic cellulitis) should be included in this category (see Fig. 3-23)

Organ/space
Develops within 30 days of the surgical procedure
Features:
    Purulent drainage from a drain placed through a stab wound into the organ/space
    Bacteria recovered from tissue or fluid in that organ/space
    Abscess found by reoperation, histopathology, or radiology
    Diagnosis made by surgeon

Modified from Mangram, 1999, with permission.

not associated with other symptoms or signs of infection; and does not require antimicrobial therapy. It has been reported in up to 40 percent of women following abdominal and almost 30 percent of women after vaginal hysterectomy with antimicrobial prophylaxis. It resolves without antibiotic treatment in the absence of other symptoms or signs of infection.

A remote nonsurgical site may also serve as an origin of fever. These may include pulmonary complications, IV site phlebitis, and urinary tract infection. Thus, women who develop recurrent temperature elevation require a thorough history and a careful physical examination by the surgeon, seeking not only surgical but also nonsurgical causes (Chap. 39, p. 971).

Pain

Operative site pain (incisional, lower abdominal, pelvic, and/or lower back) following surgery is normal. Patients who develop an operative site infection report increasing pain in the SSI area, and increasing tenderness is present on physical examination. For most gynecologic patients with pelvic infection, a deep lower abdominal and/or pelvic pain is described. The most common infection sites requiring antimicrobial therapy are the parametria and the vaginal surgical margin. Pelvic abscess or infected pelvic hematoma is least common, and pain is central. Pain associated with abdominal incision infection is localized to the incision.

Physical Examination

Abdominal palpation is an integral part of SSI diagnosis in gynecology. Avoiding an abdominal incision if present, a surgeon slowly, gently, and deeply palpates the lower abdomen over the surgical site following hysterectomy and normally elicits patient discomfort. Tenderness does not mean an acute surgical abdomen or infection. In the immediate postoperative period, this tenderness is expected and decreases quickly.

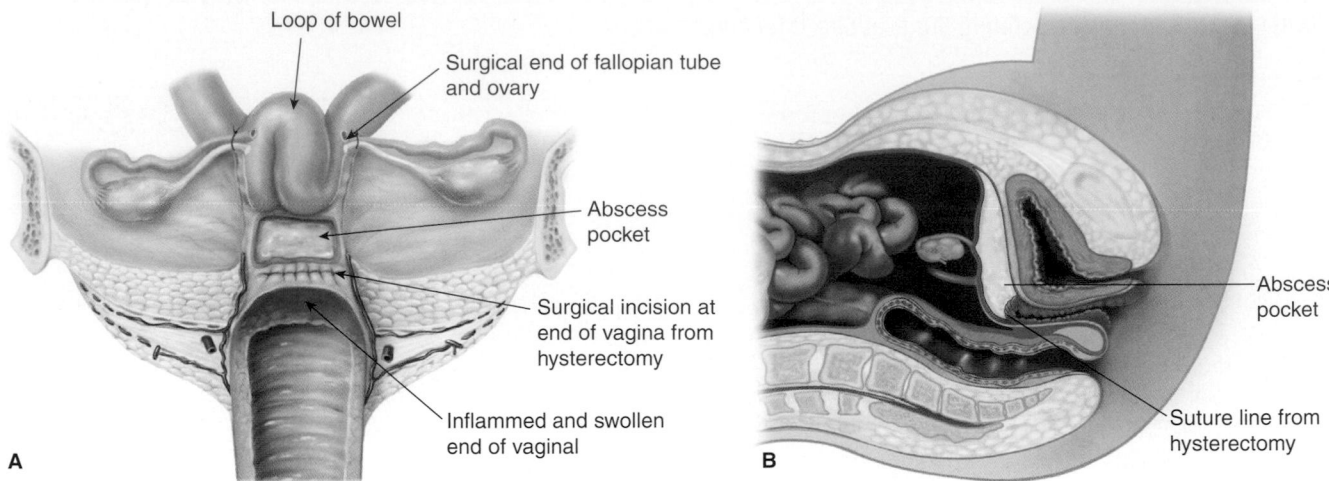

Loop of bowel

Surgical end of fallopian tube and ovary

Abscess pocket

Surgical incision at end of vagina from hysterectomy

Inflammed and swollen end of vaginal

Abscess pocket

Suture line from hysterectomy

A

B

FIGURE 3-25 This is an abscess or infected hematoma that is extraperitoneal and cephalad to the vaginal margins. An adnexal abscess or intraperitoneal abscess should be included, although these are rare. **A.** Coronal view. **B.** Sagittal view.

Women who develop pelvic cellulitis or cuff cellulitis will have increasing tenderness at gentle depression of the lower abdominal wall over the infected area. Tenderness may be bilateral, but more commonly is more marked on one side than the other. Peritoneal signs are not present. Cellulitis, whether it involves the parametria, adnexa, or vaginal cuff, is not associated with a mass.

In the absence of increasing lower abdominal pain and tenderness, a bimanual examination is not necessary for asymptomatic temperature elevation. However, with a combination of fever, increasing tenderness, and new-onset pain, gentle bimanual examination is required to accurately identify the infection site and to exclude or diagnose a mass. Speculum examination usually is not required, and visual findings are similar with or without an existing infection. As is true for routine pelvic examination, most information at bimanual examination is obtained from the vaginal fingers. If a patient is too tender to allow adequate examination, vaginal sonography is indicated. Bowel function is usually not altered by soft tissue cellulitis, but may be by pelvic abscess or infected pelvic hematoma.

Culture

Pelvic infections following hysterectomy are polymicrobial, and for that reason, it is difficult to identify true pathogens. Research has demonstrated that bacteria recovered transvaginally from the pelvis of infected and clinically uninfected women are similar. Accordingly, routine transvaginal culturing of women with cuff or pelvic cellulitis does not add useful information. Moreover, a surgeon should not wait for culture results before starting empiric broad-spectrum antibiotic therapy. However, if initial therapy is partially effective or unsuccessful, then a culture will more predictably identify pathogen(s) since therapy will have eradicated other species. The antibiotic regimen should be changed, and culture results may direct this change. In contrast, abscess or infected hematoma fluid should be cultured since those species are less likely to be vaginal contaminants. The same is true for any fluid or purulent material present in an abdominal incision.

■ Specific Infections
Vaginal Cuff Cellulitis

Essentially all women develop this infection at the vaginal surgical margin after hysterectomy. Normal response to healing is characterized by small-vessel engorgement, which results in erythema and heat. There is vascular stasis with endothelial leakage resulting in interstitial edema, which causes induration. This area is tender, microscopic evaluation of a wet prep reveals numerous WBCs, and purulent discharge is seen in the vagina. This process usually subsides and does not require treatment.

The few women who do require treatment are usually those who present after hospital discharge with mild, but increasing, new-onset lower abdominal pain and have a yellow vaginal discharge. Findings are as above, but the vaginal cuff is more tender than anticipated at this interval from the initial surgical procedure. Oral antimicrobial therapy with a single broad-spectrum agent is appropriate (Table 3-31). A patient should be reevaluated in several days to assess therapeutic efficacy. This may be completed by phone or with an examination if necessary.

Pelvic Cellulitis

This is the most common infection following either vaginal or abdominal hysterectomy. It develops when host humoral and cellular defense mechanisms, combined with preoperative antibiotic prophylaxis, cannot overcome the bacterial inoculum and inflammatory process at the vaginal surgical margin. The inflammatory process spreads into the parametrial region(s), resulting in lower abdominal pain, regional tenderness, and temperature elevation. This usually happens during the late second or third postoperative day. There are no peritoneal signs, and bowel and urinary function are normal. There may be anorexia.

Because patients are discharged on perhaps their first or second postoperative day following vaginal hysterectomy, these patients may be at home before onset of their symptoms, requiring a return visit for evaluation and diagnosis. Hospitalization

TABLE 3-31. Empiric Antimicrobial Regiments for Postgynecologic Surgery Infections

Regimen	Dose
Single-agent intravenous	
Cephalosporin	
Cefoxitin (Mefoxin)	2 g every 6 hours
Cefotetan (Cefotan)	2 g every 12 hours
Cefotaxime (Claforan)	1–2 g every 8 hours
Penicillin ± β-lactamase inhibitor	
Piperacillin	4 g every 6 hours
Piperacillin-tazobactam (Zosyn)	3.375 g every 6 hours
Ampicillin-sulbactam (Unasyn)	3 g every 6 hours
Ticarcillin-clavulanate (Timentin)	3.1 g every 4–6 hours
Carbapenems	
Imipenem-cilastatin (Primaxin)	500 mg every 8 hours
Meropenem (Merrem)	500 mg every 8 hours
Ertapenem (Invanz)	1 g once daily
Combination agent intravenous	
Metronidazole (Flagyl)	Loading dose 15 mg/kg; maintenance 7.5 mg/kg every 6 hours
Ampicillin	2 g every 6 hours
Gentamicin	3–5 mg/kg once daily
or	
Clindamycin	900 mg every 8 hours
Gentamicin	3–5 mg/kg once daily
with or without ampicillin	2 g every 6 hours
Single-agent oral	
Amoxicillin-clavulanate (Augmentin)	875 mg twice daily
Levofloxacin (Levaquin)	500 mg once daily
Clindamycin	300 mg every 6 hours
Metronidazole	500 mg every 6 hours

and treatment with an intravenous broad-spectrum antibiotic regimen is indicated until a patient has been afebrile for 24 to 48 hours, at which time she may be discharged home (see Table 3-31).

Most patients requiring hospitalization for intravenous antibiotic therapy are discharged with a 5- to 7-day oral antimicrobial prescription. Single-agent therapeutic regimens have been shown in prospective randomized trials to be as effective as combination-agent regimens. These infections are polymicrobial, and the regimen selected must have coverage for grampositive and gram-negative aerobic and anaerobic bacteria.

Adnexal Infection

This infection is uncommon and presents almost exactly as does pelvic cellulitis. The difference is in the location of tenderness during bimanual pelvic examination. The cuff and parametrial areas are not usually tender, but the adnexa are areas of tenderness. This infection also may develop after tubal ligation, surgical therapy for ectopic pregnancy, or other adnexal surgery. Empiric antibiotic regimens are identical to those for pelvic cellulitis (see Table 3-31).

Ovarian Abscess

A rare but life-threatening complication following primarily vaginal hysterectomy is ovarian abscess. Presumably, with this infection, surgery is performed in the late proliferative phase of an ovulatory menstrual cycle, and ovaries are in close proximity to the vaginal surgical margin. As expected, physiologic cuff cellulitis develops normally, but when ovulation occurs, bacteria in the area gain access to the ovulation site and the corpus luteum. The corpus luteum normally may become hemorrhagic, and the blood in this functional cyst is a perfect medium for bacterial growth.

Patients in whom this develops have essentially a normal postoperative course until approximately 10 days following surgery. At this time, they experience acute unilateral lower abdominal pain, which then becomes generalized. These symptoms reflect rupture of their abscess and development of generalized abdominal peritonitis. Sepsis commonly follows, and this is a true gynecologic emergency. Immediate exploratory laparotomy is necessary, with preoperative and continued administration of broadspectrum antimicrobials, evacuation of the abscess, and removal of the affected ovary and adjacent fallopian tube if easily accessible. After hospital discharge, oral antibiotics are typically continued for an additional 5 days. This may be variable depending on the clinical setting.

Similarly, women rarely may develop a tuboovarian abscess (usually a pyosalpinx) identical to that seen as an end result of acute PID. This process can be managed medically with intravenous antimicrobials, and surgery is usually not required unless rupture follows. Combination antimicrobial therapy should be continued until a woman has been afebrile for 48 to 72 hours. At this point, IV antibiotics may be replaced by oral agents, which are continued outpatient to complete a 2-week course of therapy. Patients diagnosed with TOA are reevaluated approximately 3 days following hospital discharge and then again 1 and 2 weeks later to document abscess resolution.

Pelvic Abscess/Infected Pelvic Hematoma

Pelvic abscess not involving an adnexal structure is also uncommon. Decades ago, prior to routine administration of antimicrobial prophylaxis, vaginal surgical margins were typically sutured in a fashion to create an open cuff. This method eliminated a closed space between the vagina and peritoneum. If not performed, this space allowed collection of up to 200 mL of blood, serum, and/or lymph between the vaginal margin and the peritoneum following hysterectomy. These fluids provide an excellent milieu for the overgrowth of bacteria inoculated into the adjacent tissues during the surgical procedure. As a result, prior to the initiation of antimicrobial prophylaxis, pelvic infection rates following hysterectomy were as high as 60 percent, and up to 10 percent of these infections were cuff abscesses. However, administration of preoperative prophylactic antibiotics predictability decreases these infection rates following hysterectomy regardless of whether an open or closed cuff is created.

Infected pelvic hematoma may also complicate hysterectomy. In these cases, a postoperative-day-1 hemoglobin is commonly found to be significantly lower in affected women than predicted by intraoperative blood loss. In most instances, reoperation is not required, and fluid or blood product resuscitation, as described in Chapter 40 (p. 1006) suffices. It is this group of women who are at risk for an infected pelvic hematoma.

Women with an infected hematoma will have low-grade temperature elevation (>37.8°C) as their early finding, which is unlike women who develop tissue cellulitis following surgery and whose early symptom of infection is pain and not fever. For this reason, women with an unexplained postoperative hemoglobin decrease should be discharged with instructions to monitor their temperature twice daily for approximately 1 week. They should return for evaluation if their temperature is ≥37.8°C. Pain is a late symptom for these women.

Signs and symptoms of pelvic abscess or infected hematoma are midline, and a mass is discernible centrally. Transvaginal sonography can accurately characterize the dimensions of these (Fig. 3-26). Hospital readmission for therapy is necessary for both. Combination-agent antimicrobial therapy is indicated, and selected regimens should provide gram-positive and gram-negative aerobic and anaerobic coverage. Additionally, opening the vaginal surgical margin, if possible, to allow drainage will aid treatment and accelerate patient response. This can usually be done in a treatment room early, avoiding return to the operating

room. If necessary, these can be drained with sonographic transvaginal guidance or in the operating room. These abscesses or infected hematomas usually remain confined to the extraperitoneal space, and a patient does not usually develop peritonitis. Some patients may develop diarrhea due to the proximity of the rectum, which is usually adjacent to the infected space.

Both infections typically do not present until after a patient is discharged from the hospital. Combination intravenous antibiotics should be administered until a woman has been afebrile 48 to 72 hours. IV antibiotics may then be replaced by oral agents, which are continued outpatient to complete a 2-week course of therapy, if the abscess or hematoma is not drained. If drained, then oral agents continued for 5 to 7 days following IV agents typically are sufficient. Commonly, patients are reevaluated 3 days following hospital discharge and then again 1 and 2 weeks later to document infection resolution.

Abdominal Incision Infection

The superficial and easily accessible location of this infection aids its diagnosis. Although abdominal incision infection may develop alone or with pelvic infection following abdominal hysterectomy, it develops uncommonly after other gynecologic procedures. Unlike pelvic infection, the incidence of this infection is not altered by antimicrobial prophylaxis. Risk factors include obesity, excessive electrosurgical coagulation use, passive drains, and coexistent skin inflammation at the time of surgical incision.

Abdominal incisions are usually the most uncomfortable immediately following gynecologic surgery, but pain decreases daily. Erythema and heat are the first physical signs of this infection, which is usually diagnosed on the fourth or fifth postoperative day—again after discharge from the hospital. A hematoma or seroma may develop in the abdominal wall incision without infection. If these collections are large, opening of the incision and evacuation to prevent infection in those fluids is warranted. Similarly, pus requires incision opening to ensure an intact fascia, as should be done with seromas or hematomas.

Drainage and local care are usually the basis of successful therapy for abdominal incision infection, hematoma, or seroma. Wounds are irrigated with normal saline. Povidone-iodine, iodophor gauze, hydrogen peroxide, and Daiken solution are avoided as they are caustic to healing tissues. However, some recommend their use early but follow with normal saline irrigation. Wet to dry dressings stimulate fibroblastic proliferation and development of healthy granulation tissue. Moistening the dry dressing prior to its removal will ease removal and decrease patient discomfort. At this stage, if infection is absent, then secondary closure can be considered. Wound vacuum-assisted closure devices (Wound VAC) are available for more serious or larger wound areas that are slow to respond (Chap. 39, p. 974).

If there is soft tissue cellulitis adjacent to the incision, antimicrobial therapy is required. If the initial surgery was a clean procedure, then *Staphylococcus* species predominate. Following clean-contaminated or dirty procedures, isolated organisms commonly include gram-negative bacteria—*E coli, P aeruginosa,*

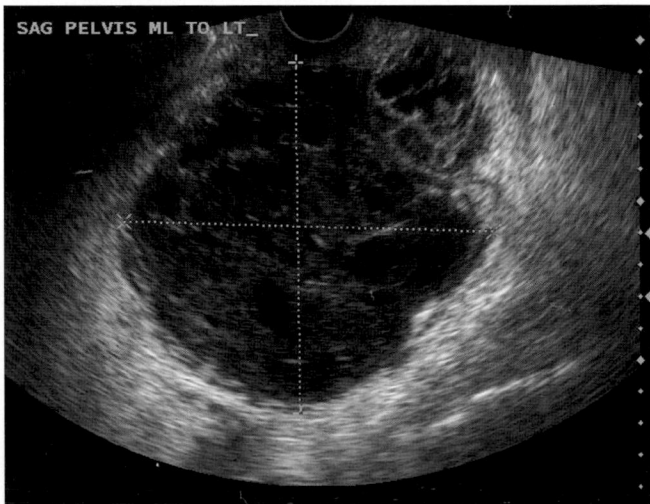

FIGURE 3-26 Transvaginal sonogram of an infected pelvic hematoma following hysterectomy. This 11 × 12 cm collection of blood and clot was drained vaginally in the operative room. *(Image contributed by Dr. Elysia Moschos.)*

and *Enterobacter* species—and gram-positive bacteria, namely, *Staphylococcus* and *Enterococcus* species (Kirby, 2009). Anaerobes are typically not prominent pathogens in these infections but may be present, especially following hysterectomy. Thus, these infections are usually polymicrobial. Antibiotics found in Table 3-31 are suitable regimens. Importantly, the number of infections caused by MRSA has increased dramatically, and coverage for this pathogen should be considered. Suitable antibiotics for MRSA include vancomycin or clindamycin for complicated infections and trimethoprim-sulfamethoxazole, clindamycin, doxycycline, or minocycline for uncomplicated infection. Newer FDA-approved agents against complicated MRSA infections include linezolid (Zyvox), daptomycin (Cubicin), telavancin (Vibativ), quinupristin/dalfopristin (Synercid), and tigecycline (Tygacil). These newer drugs are expensive and may have restricted formulary use to only infectious disease specialists.

Toxic Shock Syndrome

This condition, caused by a toxin (TSS toxin-1) produced by *Staphylococcus aureus*, appears approximately 2 days following surgery or onset of menstruation. Menstrual-associated appearance was initially associated with high-absorbency tampons. The vagina must be colonized by a toxigenic staphylococcal strain, and the patient must lack the specific antibody that can block the superantigen.

The classic nonmenstrual and menstrual toxic shock syndromes have identical clinical symptoms, physical findings, and laboratory results. Women complain of fever, malaise, and diarrhea. In addition to minimal signs of wound infection, if postoperative, a patient has conjunctival and pharyngeal hyperemia without purulence. The tongue is usually reddened, and the skin on the trunk is erythematous but not painful or pruritic. Temperatures are usually above 38.8°C, and orthostatic hypotension or shock may be present. This syndrome results from host cytokines released in response to superantigenic properties of the toxin. The criteria for this diagnosis are presented in Table 3-32.

The wound, if present, should be treated like any other wound. Specifically, it should be cultured to confirm the presence of *S aureus*. However, other cultures (e.g., blood, throat, and cerebrospinal fluid) will be negative. To meet the strict criteria, a woman must have all major and at least three minor criteria. If this is suspected early and if therapy is initiated, the complete syndrome may not develop.

Although treatment with a specific antistaphylococcal antibiotic is required, the hallmark of therapy is entire system support with large volumes of intravenous fluids and electrolytes to replace massive body fluid losses from diarrhea, capillary leakage, and insensible loss. These patients may develop significant edema and are best managed in an intensive care unit. Even with appropriate management, the death rate has been reported to be as high as 5 percent because of subsequent acute respiratory distress syndrome (ARDS), disseminated intravascular coagulopathy (DIC), or hypotension unresponsive to therapy with resultant myocardial failure. This syndrome may also follow gynecologic surgical procedures such as D&C, hysterectomy, urethral suspension, and tubal ligation.

Serologies for Rocky Mountain spotted fever, measles, and leptospirosis must be negative. Viral infection and group A streptococci can cause a similar presentation.

Necrotizing Fasciitis

Although described in the 1870s, it was not named until 1952 by a Parkland Hospital surgeon (Wilson, 1952). It has had various names, including hospital gangrene, acute dermal gangrene, acute streptococcal gangrene, Meleney gangrene, gangrenous erysipelas, and necrotizing erysipelas. Risk factors for this postoperative incision infection are age older than 50 years, arteriosclerotic heart disease, diabetes mellitus, obesity, debilitating disease, smoking, and previous radiation therapy, all of which are associated with decreased tissue perfusion. Also, it has been reported following tubal sterilization, in a suprapubic catheter site after hysterectomy, and even

---

TABLE 3-32. Criteria for Diagnosis of Toxic Shock Syndrome

Major criteria
Hypotension
Orthostatic syncope
Systolic BP <90 mm Hg for adults
Diffuse macular erythroderma
Temperature ≥38.8°C
Late skin desquamation, particularly on the hands, palms, and soles of feet (1 to 2 weeks later)

Minor criteria (organ system involvement)
Gastrointestinal: diarrhea or vomiting
Mucous membranes: oral, pharyngeal, conjunctival, and/or vaginal erythema
Muscular: myalgia or creatinine phosphokinase level greater than twice normal
Renal: BUN and creatinine greater than twice normal or >5 WBCs/HPF in urine, without concurrent UTI
Hematologic: platelet count <100,000 per mm³
Hepatic: SGOT, SGPT, and/or bilirubin levels greater than twice normal
Central nervous system: altered consciousness or disorientation without focal localizing signs

BP = blood pressure; BUN = blood urea nitrogen; HPF = high-powered field; SGOT = serum glutamic oxaloacetic transaminase; SGPT = serum glutamic pyruvic transaminase; UTI = urinary tract infection; WBC = white blood cell.

TABLE 3-33. Criteria for Diagnosis of Necrotizing Fasciitis

Microvascular thrombosis without major vessel occlusion
Extensive necrosis of superficial fascia undermining
    normal skin
Absence of clostridia in wound and/or blood cultures
No muscle involvement
Intensive WBC infiltrate in necrotic subcutaneous tissue
Moderate-to-severe systemic toxic reaction

WBC = white blood cell.

without surgery, especially in vulvar infections of obese diabetic women. Only approximately 20 percent of cases follow surgery, the majority developing after minor injuries or insect bites. Bacteria recovered from women with this infection following surgery are similar to those recovered from any postoperative gynecologic infection site, namely predominantly *E coli*, *E faecalis*, *Bacteroides* spp., *Peptostreptococcus* spp., *S aureus*, groups A and B hemolytic streptococci, and Enterobacteriaceae.

Although this superficial incisional infection begins like any other postoperative infection with pain and erythema, the hallmark for its identification is subcutaneous and superficial fascial necrosis, manifested by excessive tissue edema in adjacent areas (Table 3-33). Blisters or bullae form in tissue that has become avascular and is discolored. There is usually a thin gray transudate. Tissue destruction is far more extensive than is evident by surface examination. The skin will slip over underlying tissue, and if incised, due to the lack of vascularity, there will be no bleeding. Severe systemic toxicity may develop. It is beneficial to get radiographs of the infected area prior to treatment to exclude gas in the tissue produced by *Clostridium perfringens* or other clostridial species. The presence of these bacteria is often associated with myonecrosis.

Although antibiotic administration is required, the cornerstone of treatment is prompt recognition with immediate surgical removal of the devitalized tissue down to tissue that bleeds appropriately. This may result in excision of large areas of tissue, leaving significant disfigurement. However, postponing surgery while waiting for antimicrobial activity will only increase the volume of tissue death. Early fatality rates for patients with this infection approached 80 percent according to Stone and Martin (1972).

Wounds are left open and treated as wound infections as described earlier with local hydrotherapy or a wound VAC. Assistance from a general surgeon for potential grafting is often necessary.

OTHER GYNECOLOGIC INFECTIONS

Vulvar Abscess

These infections develop similarly to other superficial abscesses but have the potential for significant expansion due to the loose areolar tissue in the subcutaneous layers of this area. Risk factors include

diabetes, obesity, perineal shaving, and immunosuppression. Common isolates include *Staphylococcus*, group B *Streptococcus*, and *Enterococcus* species as well as *E coli* and *P mirabilis*. Importantly, Thurman (2008) and Kilpatrick (2010) and their coworkers found MRSA in 40 to 60 percent of cultured vulvar abscesses.

In early stages, surrounding cellulitis may be the most prominent finding, and no abscess is identified. In these cases, sitz baths and oral antibiotics are reasonable treatment. When present, small abscesses may be treated with incision and drainage, abscess packing if indicated, and oral antibiotics to treat surrounding cellulitis. For uncomplicated infection, suitable oral agents will be broad-spectrum and cover MRSA. Trimethoprim-sulfamethoxazole may be used alone. Two-drug therapy with clindamycin or doxycycline combined with a second-generation cephalosporin or with a fluoroquinolone is also a suitable choice, among others. However, for those with immunosuppression or diabetes, hospitalization and IV antibiotic therapy is often warranted due to increased risks for necrotizing fasciitis in these individuals.

Large abscesses typically require admission for drainage under anesthesia. This provides adequate pain control for abscess drainage and for abscess cavity exploration to disrupt loculated areas of pus, as described in Section 41-21 (p. 1068). Suitable IV antimicrobial coverage is broad-spectrum and includes coverage for MRSA (see Table 3-31).

Bartholin Gland Duct Abscess

This infection is managed primarily by drainage (Fig. 3-27). Drainage can typically be complete in an outpatient setting and is described in detail in Section 41-18 (p. 1063).

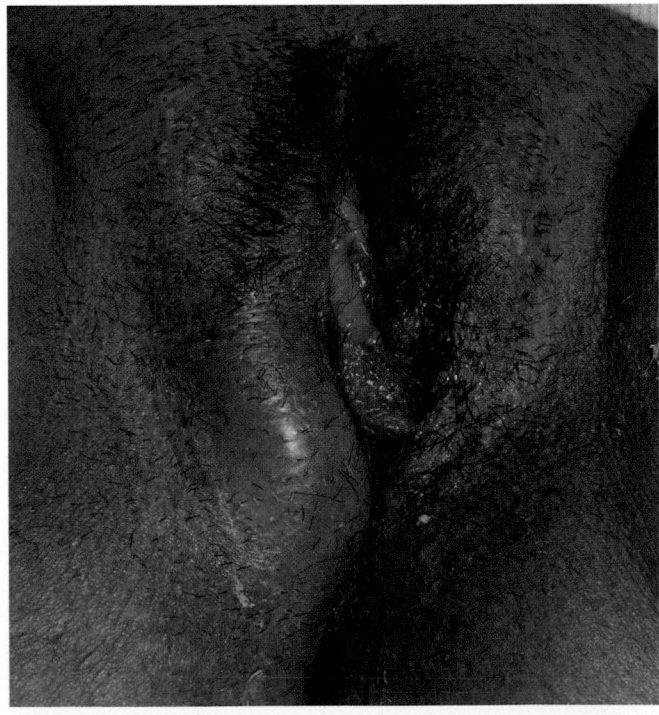

FIGURE 3-27 Photograph of a right Bartholin gland duct abscess.

Antibiotics are commonly added to treat surrounding tissue cellulitis. The most common bacteria isolated from these abscesses include anaerobic *Bacteroides* and *Peptostreptococcus* species and aerobic *E coli*, *S aureus*, and *E faecalis*. Also, *N gonorrhoeae* and *C trachomatis* may be identified (Patil, 2007; Pundir, 2008). Accordingly, polymicrobial coverage is selected, and suitable single agent oral outpatient therapy includes, among others, trimethoprim-sulfamethoxazole, amoxicillin-clavulanate, second-generation cephalosporins, or fluoroquinolones, such as ciprofloxacin. In most cases, abscess cultures are obtained, and screening for sexually transmitted diseases is included.

Actinomyces Infection

Actinomyces israelii is a gram-positive, slow-growing, anaerobic bacterium that rarely leads to infection and abscess. It is found to be part of the indigenous genital flora of healthy women (Persson, 1984). Some have found it more frequently in the vaginal flora of IUD users, and rates of colonization increase with duration of IUD use (Curtis, 1981). Actinomyces are also identified in Pap smears, and Fiorino (1996) cited a 7-percent incidence in IUD users compared with that of less than 1 percent in nonusers. In the absence of symptoms, the incidental finding of *Actinomyces* on cytology is problematic. First, infection is rare, even in those identified to harbor the bacteria. Reviews by Lippes (1999) and Westhoff (2007) suggest that asymptomatic women may retain their IUD and do not require antibiotic treatment. The American College of Obstetricians and Gynecologists (2005) lists four management options for asymptomatic women: (1) expectant management, (2) extended oral antibiotic treatment with the IUD in place, (3) IUD removal, or (4) IUD removal followed by antibiotic treatment. Importantly, if signs or symptoms of infection develop in women who harbor *Actinomyces*, the device should be removed and antimicrobial therapy instituted. Early findings include fever, weight loss, abdominal pain, and abnormal vaginal bleeding or discharge. *Actinomyces* is sensitive to antimicrobials with gram-positive coverage, notably the penicillins.

REFERENCES

Achilles SL, Amortegui AJ, Wiesenfeld HC: Endometrial plasma cells: do they indicate subclinical pelvic inflammatory disease? Sex Transm Dis 32:185, 2005

American College of Obstetricians and Gynecologists: Antibiotic prophylaxis for gynecologic procedures. Practice Bulletin No. 104, May 2009

American College of Obstetricians and Gynecologists: Expedited partner therapy in the management of gonorrhea and Chlamydia by obstetrician-gynecologists. Committee Opinion No. 506, September 2011

American College of Obstetricians and Gynecologists: Intrauterine device. Practice Bulletin No. 59, January 2005

American College of Obstetricians and Gynecologists: Treatment of urinary tract infections in nonpregnant women. Practice Bulletin No. 91, March 2008a

American College of Obstetricians and Gynecologists: Vaginitis. Practice Bulletin No. 72. Obstet Gynecol 107:1195, May 2006, Reaffirmed 2008b

Amsel R, Totten PA, Spiegel CA, et al: Nonspecific vaginitis. Diagnostic criteria and microbial and epidemiologic associations. Am J Med 74:14, 1983

Anderson MR, Klink K, Kohrssen A: Evaluation of vaginal complaints. JAMA 291:1368, 2004

Association of Public Health Laboratories: Laboratory diagnostic testing for *Chlamydia trachomatis* and *Neisseria gonorrhoeae*. Expert Consultation Meeting Summary Report. Atlanta, 2009

Atashili J, Poole C, Ndumbe PM, et al: Bacterial vaginosis and HIV acquisition: a meta-analysis of published studies. AIDS 22(12):1493, 2008

Bartlett JG, Onderdonk AB, Drude E, et al: Quantitative bacteriology of the vaginal flora. J Infect Dis 136(2):271, 1977

Bertino JS Jr., Booker LA, Franck PA, et al: Incidence of and significant risk factors for aminoglycoside-associated nephrotoxicity in patients dosed by using individualized pharmacokinetic monitoring. J Infect Dis 167:173, 1993

Beutner KR, Reitano MV, Richwald GA, et al: External genital warts: report of the American Medical Association Consensus Conference. AMA Expert Panel on External Genital Warts. Clin Infect Dis 27:796, 1998

Birnbaum DM: Microscopic findings. In Knoop KJ, Stack LB, Storrow AB (eds): Atlas of Emergency Medicine, 2nd ed. New York, McGraw-Hill, 2010. Available at: http://www.accessmedicine.com/popup.aspx?aID=6008948&searchStr=pubic lice infestation. Accessed September 29, 2010

Bornstein J, Lakovsky Y, Lavi I, et al: The classic approach to diagnosis of vulvovaginitis: a critical analysis. Infect Dis Obstet Gynecol 9:105, 2001

Boskey ER, Cone RA, Whaley KJ, et al: Origins of vaginal acidity: high D/L lactate ratio is consistent with bacteria being the primary source. Hum Reprod 16(9):1809, 2001

Bowden F: Donovanosis. In Morse S, Ballard RC, Holmes KK, et al (eds): Atlas of Sexually Transmitted Diseases, 3rd ed. Edinburgh, Mosby, 2003, p 103

Bradshaw CS, Morton AN, Garland SM, et al: Higher-risk behavioral practices associated with bacterial vaginosis compared with vaginal candidiasis. Obstet Gynecol 106:105, 2005

Bradshaw CS, Morton AN, Hocking J, et al: High recurrence rates of bacterial vaginosis over the course of 12 months after oral metronidazole therapy and factors associated with recurrence. J Infect Dis 193:1478, 2006

Brotman RM, Klebanoff MA, Nansel TR, et al: A longitudinal study of vaginal douching and bacterial vaginosis—a marginal structural modeling analysis. Am J Epidemiol 168(2):188, 2008

Caillouette JC, Sharp CF, Jr., Zimmerman GJ, et al: Vaginal pH as a marker for bacterial pathogens and menopausal status. Am J Obstet Gynecol 176:1270, 1997

Centers for Disease Control and Prevention: Cephalosporin susceptibility among Neisseria gonorrhoeae isolates—United States, 2000-2010. MMWR 60(26):873, 2011

Centers for Disease Control and Prevention: Expedited partner therapy in the management of sexually transmitted diseases. Atlanta, U.S. Department of Health and Human Services, 2006

Centers for Disease Control and Prevention: Seroprevalence of herpes simplex virus type 2 among persons aged 14-49 years—United States, 2005-2008. MMWR 59(15):456, 2010a

Centers for Disease Control and Prevention: Sexually transmitted disease surveillance, 2009. Atlanta, U.S. Department of Health and Human Services, available at: http://www.cdc.gov/std/stats09/Syphilis.htm. Accessed September 10, 2011

Centers for Disease Control and Prevention: Sexually transmitted diseases treatment guidelines, 2010. MMWR 59(12):1, 2010b

Centers for Disease Control and Prevention: Update to CDC's sexually transmitted diseases treatment guidelines, 2006: fluoroquinolones no longer recommended for treatment of gonococcal infections. MMWR 56(14):332, 2007

Corey L, Wald A, Patel R, et al: Once-daily valacyclovir to reduce the risk of transmission of genital herpes. N Engl J Med 350:11, 2004

Cox D, Liu H, Moreland AA, et al: Syphilis. In Morse S, Ballard RC, Holmes KK, et al (eds): Atlas of Sexually Transmitted Diseases, 3rd ed. Edinburgh, Mosby, 2003, p 42

Cunningham AL, Diefenbach RJ, Miranda-Saksena M, et al: The cycle of human herpes simplex virus infection: virus transport and immune control. J Infect Dis 194(Suppl 1):S11, 2006

Curtis EM, Pine L: Actinomyces in the vaginas of women with and without intrauterine contraceptive devices. Am J Obstet Gynecol 140:880, 1981

Devillard E, Burton JP, Hammond JA, et al: Novel insight into the vaginal microflora in postmenopausal women under hormone replacement therapy as analyzed by PCR-denaturing gradient gel electrophoresis. Eur J Obstet Gynecol Reprod Biol 117:76, 2004

Dunbar-Jacob J, Sereika SM, Foley SM, et al: Adherence to oral therapies in pelvic inflammatory disease. J Womens Health 13:285, 2004

Eron LJ, Judson F, Tucker S, et al: Interferon therapy for condylomata acuminata. N Engl J Med 315:1059, 1986

Fihn SD: Clinical practice: acute uncomplicated urinary tract infection in women. N Engl J Med 349:259, 2003

Fiorino AS: Intrauterine contraceptive device-associated actinomycotic abscess and *Actinomyces* detection on cervical smear. Obstet Gynecol 87:142, 1996

Gardner HL, Dukes CD: *Haemophilus vaginalis* vaginitis: a newly defined specific infection previously classified non-specific vaginitis. Am J Obstet Gynecol 69:962, 1955

Geiger AM, Foxman B: Risk factors for vulvovaginal candidiasis: a case-control study among university students. Epidemiology 7:182, 1996

Hadgu A, Westrom L, Brooks CA, et al: Predicting acute pelvic inflammatory disease: a multivariate analysis. Am J Obstet Gynecol 155:954, 1986

Haefner HK: Current evaluation and management of vulvovaginitis. Clin Obstet Gynecol 42(2):184, 1999

Hansfield HH: Vaginal infections. In Color Atlas and Synopsis of Sexually Transmitted Diseases. New York, McGraw-Hill, 2001, p 169

Helms DJ, Mosure DJ, Metcalf CA, et al: Management of trichomonas vaginalis in women with suspected metronidazole hypersensitivity. Sex Transm Dis 35(5):484, 2008

Hemsell DL, Heard MC, Hemsell PG, et al: Alterations in lower reproductive tract flora after single-dose piperacillin and triple-dose cefoxitin at vaginal and abdominal hysterectomy. Obstet Gynecol 72:875, 1988

Hemsell DL, Hemsell PG, Wendel G Jr, et al: Medical management of severe PID avoiding operations. In Pelvic Inflammatory Disease (PID) Diagnosis and Therapy. Grafelfing, E.R. Weissenbacher, 1993, p 142

Hemsell DL, Obregon VL, Heard MC, et al: Endometrial bacteria in asymptomatic, nonpregnant women. J Reprod Med 34:872, 1989

Hooton TM, Stamm WE: Diagnosis and treatment of uncomplicated urinary tract infection. Infect Dis Clin North Am 11:551, 1997

Huppert JS, Batteiger BE, Braslins P, et al: Use of an immunochromatographic assay for rapid detection of *Trichomonas vaginalis* in vaginal specimens. J Clin Microbiol 43:684, 2005

Huppert JS, Mortensen JE, Reed JL, et al: Rapid antigen testing compares favorably with transcription-mediated amplification assay for the detection of *Trichomonas vaginalis* in young women. Clin Infect Dis 15;45(2):194, 2007

Keane FE, Ison CA, Taylor-Robinson D: A longitudinal study of the vaginal flora over a menstrual cycle. Int J STD AIDS 8:489, 1997

Kilpatrick CC, Alagkiozidis I, Orejuela FJ, et al: Factors complicating surgical management of vulvar abscess. J Reprod Med 55(3-4):139, 2010

Kirby JP, Mazuski JE: Prevention of surgical site infection. Surg Clin North Am 89(2):365, 2009

Klebanoff MA, Nansel TR, Brotman RM, et al: Personal hygienic behaviors and bacterial vaginosis. Sex Transm Dis 37(2):94, 2010

Landers DV, Sweet RL: Tubo-ovarian abscess: contemporary approach to management. Rev Infect Dis 5(5):876, 1983

Landers DV, Wiesenfeld HC, Heine RP, et al: Predictive value of the clinical diagnosis of lower genital tract infection in women. Am J Obstet Gynecol 190:1004, 2004

Larsen SA, Johnson RE: Diagnostic tests. In Larsen SA, Pope V, Johnson RE, et al (eds): Manual of Tests for Syphilis, 9th ed. Washington, DC, Centers for Disease Control and Prevention and American Public Health Association, 1998

Larsson P-G, Bergman B, Försum U, et al: Mobiluncus and clue cells as predictors of pelvic inflammatory disease after first trimester abortion. Acta Obstet Gynecol Scand 68:217, 1989

Larsson P-G, Platz-Christensen J-J, Försum U, et al: Clue cells in predicting infections after abdominal hysterectomy. Obstet Gynecol 77:450, 1991

Larsson P-G, Platz-Christensen J-J, Thejls H, et al: Incidence of pelvic inflammatory disease after first-trimester legal abortion in women with bacterial vaginosis after treatment with metronidazole: a double-blind, randomized study. Am J Obstet Gynecol 166:100, 1992

Levgur M, Duvivier R: Pelvic inflammatory disease after tubal sterilization: a review. Obstet Gynecol Surv 55(1):41, 2000

Lippes J: Pelvic actinomycosis: a review and preliminary look at prevalence. Am J Obstet Gynecol 180:265, 1999

Lukehart SA: Syphilis. In Kasper DL, Braunwald E, Fauci A, et al (eds): Harrison's Internal Medicine Online. Available at: http://www.accessmedicine.com/popup.aspx?aID=2869184. Accessed January 16, 2011

Mammen-Tobin A, Wilson JD: Management of metronidazole-resistant Trichomonas vaginalis–a new approach. Int J STD AIDS 16(7):488, 2005

Mangram AJ, Horan TC, Pearson ML, et al: Guideline for prevention of surgical site infection, 1999. Hospital Infection Control Practices Advisory Committee. Infect Control Hospital Epidemiol 20:250, 1999

Marrazzo JM: A persistent(ly) enigmatic ecological mystery: bacterial vaginosis. J Infect Dis 193:1475, 2006

Martin ET, Krantz E, Gottlieb SL, et al: A pooled analysis of the effect of condoms in preventing HSV-2 acquisition. Arch Intern Med 169(13):1233, 2009

Mayo Clinic: Symposium on Antimicrobial Agents. Mayo Clin Proc 66:931, 1991

Molander P, Sjöberg J, Paavonen J: Transvaginal power Doppler findings in laparoscopically proven acute pelvic inflammatory disease. Ultrasound Obstet Gynecol 17:233, 2001

Morse S, Long J: Infestations. In Morse S, Ballard RC, Holmes KK, et al (eds): Atlas of Sexually Transmitted Diseases, 3rd ed. Edinburgh, Mosby, 2003, p 362

Ness RB, Hillier SL, Kip KE, et al: Bacterial vaginosis and risk of pelvic inflammatory disease. Obstet Gynecol 104:761, 2004

Nicolau D, Quintiliani R, Nightingale CH: Once-daily aminoglycosides. Conn Med 56:561, 1992

Nicolle LE, Bradley S, Colgan R, et al: Infectious Diseases Society of America guidelines for the diagnosis and treatment of asymptomatic bacteriuria in adults. Clin Infect Dis 40:643, 2005

Ohm MJ, Galask RP: The effect of antibiotic prophylaxis on patients undergoing vaginal operations. II. Alterations of microbial flora. Am J Obstet Gynecol 123:597, 1975

Patil S, Sultan AH, Thakar R: Bartholin's cysts and abscesses. J Obstet Gynaecol 27(3):241, 2007

Patton DL, Halbert SA, Kuo CC, et al: Host response to primary *Chlamydia trachomatis* infection of the fallopian tube in pig-tailed monkeys. Fertil Steril 40:829, 1983

Patton DL, Moore DE, Spadoni LR, et al: A comparison of the fallopian tube's response to overt and silent salpingitis. Obstet Gynecol 73:622, 1989

Persson E, Holmberg K: A longitudinal study of Actinomyces israelii in the female genital tract. Acta Obstet Gynecol Scand 63:207, 1984

Pundir J, Auld BJ: A review of the management of diseases of the Bartholin's gland. J Obstet Gynaecol 28(2):161, 2008

Rubin RH, Shapiro ED, Andriole VT, et al: Evaluation of new anti-infective drugs for the treatment of urinary tract infection. Infectious Diseases Society of America and the Food and Drug Administration. Clin Infect Dis 15(Suppl 1):S216, 1992

Sam JW, Jacobs JE, Birnbaum BA: Spectrum of CT findings in acute pyogenic pelvic inflammatory disease. Radiographics 22:1327, 2002

Saxon A, Beall GN, Rohr AS, et al: Immediate hypersensitivity reactions to beta-lactam antibiotics. Ann Intern Med 107:204, 1987

Schachter J, Stephens R: Infections caused by chlamydia trachomatis. In Morse S, Ballard RC, Holmes KK, et al (eds): Atlas of Sexually Transmitted Diseases, 3rd ed. Edinburgh, Mosby, 2003, p 80

Scheinfeld N, Lehman DS: An evidence-based review of medical and surgical treatments of genital warts. Dermatol Online J 12:5, 2006

Senok AC, Verstraelen H, Temmerman M, et al: Probiotics for the treatment of bacterial vaginosis. Cochrane Database Syst Rev 4:CD006289, 2009

Sobel JD, Nyirjesy P, Brown W: Tinidazole therapy for metronidazole-resistant vaginal trichomoniasis. Clin Infect Dis 33:1341, 2001

Soper DE: Pelvic inflammatory disease. Obstet Gynecol 116(2 Pt 1):419, 2010

Soper DE, Bump RC, Hurt WG: Bacterial vaginosis and trichomoniasis vaginitis are risk factors for cuff cellulitis after abdominal hysterectomy. Am J Obstet Gynecol 163:1016, 1990

Spence MR, Blanco LJ, Patel J, et al: A comparative evaluation of vaginal, cervical and peritoneal flora in normal, healthy women: a preliminary report. Sex Transm Dis 9(1):37, 1982

Stone HH, Martin JD Jr: Synergistic necrotizing cellulitis. Ann Surg 175:702, 1972

Thurman AR, Satterfield TM, Soper DE: Methicillin-resistant *Staphylococcus aureus* as a common cause of vulvar abscesses. Obstet Gynecol 112:538, 2008

Timor-Tritsch IE, Lerner JP, Monteagudo A, et al: Transvaginal sonographic markers of tubal inflammatory disease. Ultrasound Obstet Gynecol 12(1):56, 1998

Toth M, Patton DL, Campbell LA, et al: Detection of chlamydial antigenic material in ovarian, prostatic, ectopic pregnancy and semen samples of culture-negative subjects. Am J Reprod Immunol 43(4):218, 2000

Tulkens PM, Clerckx-Braun F, Donnez J: Safety and efficacy of aminoglycosides once-a-day: experimental data and randomized, controlled evaluation in patients suffering from pelvic inflammatory disease. J Drug Dev 1:71, 1988

U.S. Preventive Services Task Force: Screening for gonorrhea: recommendation statement. Ann Family Med 3:263, 2005

Van der Pol B: *Trichomonas vaginalis* infection: the most prevalent nonviral sexually transmitted infection receives the least public health attention. Clin Infect Dis 44:23, 2007

Van der Pol B, Williams JA, Orr DP, et al: Prevalence, incidence, natural history, and response to treatment of *Trichomonas vaginalis* infection among adolescent women. J Infect Dis 192:2039, 2005

Wald A, Langenberg AG, Krantz E, et al: The relationship between condom use and herpes simplex virus acquisition. Ann Intern Med 143(10):707, 2005

Warren JW, Abrutyn E, Hebel JR, et al: Guidelines for antimicrobial treatment of uncomplicated acute bacterial cystitis and acute pyelonephritis in women. Infectious Diseases Society of America (IDSA). Clin Infect Dis 29:745, 1999

Wendel GD Jr, Stark BJ, Jamison RB, et al: Penicillin allergy and desensitization in serious infections during pregnancy. N Engl J Med 312:1229, 1985

Westhoff C: IUDs and colonization or infection with *Actinomyces.* Contraception 75:S48, 2007

Westrom L: Effect of acute pelvic inflammatory disease on fertility. Am J Obstet Gynecol 121:707, 1975

Wiese W, Patel SR, Patel SC, et al: A meta-analysis of the Papanicolaou smear and wet mount for the diagnosis of vaginal trichomoniasis. Am J Med 108(4):301, 2000

Wiesenfeld HC, Hillier SL, Krohn MA, et al: Bacterial vaginosis is a strong predictor of *Neisseria gonorrhoeae* and *Chlamydia trachomatis* infection. Clin Infect Dis 36(5):663, 2003

Wiley DJ, Douglas J, Beutner K, et al: External genital warts: diagnosis, treatment, and prevention. Clin Infect Dis 35(Suppl 2):S210, 2002

Wilkinson EJ, Stone IK: Ulcers. In Atlas of Vulvar Disease. Baltimore, Williams & Wilkins, 1995, p 173

Wilson B: Necrotizing fasciitis. Am Surg 18:416, 1952

Wilson J: Managing recurrent bacterial vaginosis. Sex Transm Infect 80:8, 2004

Wolff K, Johnson RA: Arthropod bites, stings, and cutaneous infections. In Fitzpatrick's Color Atlas and Synopsis of Clinical Dermatology, 6th ed. New York, McGraw-Hill, 2009. Available at: http://www.accessmedicine.com/popup.aspx?aID=5196863&searchStr=scabies. Accessed September 29, 2010

Xu F, Sternberg MR, Kottiri BJ, et al: Trends in herpes simplex virus type 1 and type 2 seroprevalence in the United States. JAMA 296(8):964, 2006

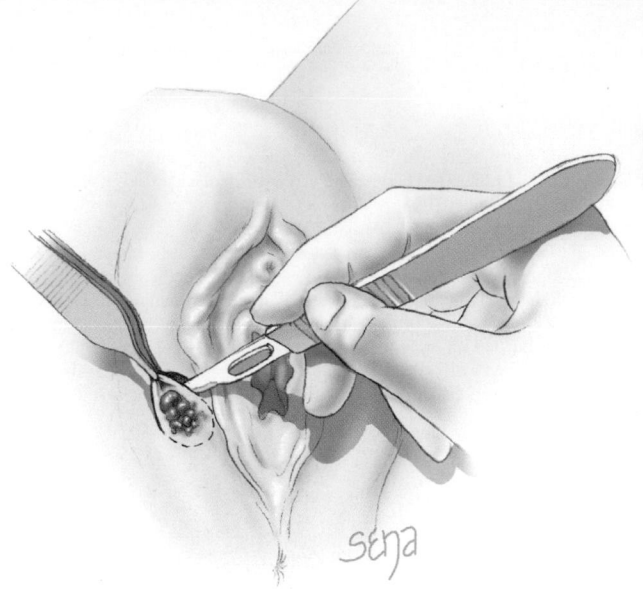

CHAPTER 4

Benign Disorders of the Lower Reproductive Tract

The lower reproductive tract, comprised of the vulva, vagina, and cervix, harbors a wide spectrum of benign and neoplastic diseases. Disorder characteristics often overlap, thus differentiating normal variants, benign diseases, and potentially serious lesions can be challenging. Benign lesions of the lower reproductive tract are common and mastery of their identification and treatment is essential. This chapter highlights the most common conditions encountered.

VULVAR LESIONS

Vulvar skin is more permeable than surrounding tissues because of differences in structure, hydration, occlusion, and susceptibil-

ity to friction (Farage, 2004). As a result, pathology involving the vulva is common, although estimates are difficult because of patient underreporting and clinician misdiagnosis. Lesions may result from infection, trauma, neoplasia, or immune responses. As a result, symptoms may be acute or chronic and may include pain, pruritus, dyspareunia, bleeding, and discharge. Effective therapies are available for most disorders, yet embarrassment and fear may prove significant roadblocks to care for many women.

General Approach to Vulvar Complaints

The initial encounter should include reassurance that the patient's complaints will be investigated thoroughly. Women often minimize and may be uncomfortable with describing their symptoms. Those with chronic conditions may relate protracted histories of assorted diagnoses and treatments by a number of providers and may voice frustration and doubt that relief is possible. These patients should not be promised a cure but rather that every effort will be made to alleviate their symptoms. This may require multiple visits and treatment attempts, and potentially a multidisciplinary approach. A patient-provider partnership in developing a management strategy enhances compliance and satisfaction with care.

Counseling should include discussion of the suspected diagnosis, current treatment plan, and necessary vulvar skin care. Printed materials that explain common conditions, medication use, and skin care are helpful. Patients are often relieved to learn that their complaints and conditions are not unique. Thus, referral to specific national web sites and support groups is usually welcome.

Diagnosis
History

Scheduling adequate time for the initial evaluation is a wise investment, as detailed information is essential. Symptom characterization should include descriptions of duration, location, abnormal sensations, and associated vaginal pruritus or discharge. A thorough medical history should encompass systemic illnesses, medications, and known allergies. Obstetric, sexual, and psychosocial histories and any potentially provocative events around the time of symptom onset often suggest etiologies. Hygiene and sexual practices should be investigated in detail.

Vulvar Pruritus. This is a frequent vulvar symptom of many dermatoses, and the underlying cause is often discoverable during the initial interview. Patients may have been previously diagnosed with psoriasis, eczema, or dermatitis at other body sites. Isolated vulvar pruritus may be associated with initiation of a new medication. Patients may identify foods that provoke or intensify symptoms, and in such cases, a food diary may be helpful. Most often, vulvar pruritus is due to a contact or allergic dermatitis. Common offenders include strongly scented body soaps and laundry products. Excessive washing and use of wash cloths can result in skin drying and mechanical trauma. Washing often becomes more aggressive with pruritus as patients assume their hygiene is lacking. Any of these practices can create an escalating itch-scratch cycle or exacerbate the symptoms of other preexisting dermatoses. Finally, patients frequently use nonprescription remedies for relief of vulvovaginal itching or perceived odor. These products commonly contain multiple known contact allergens, and their use should be discouraged (Table 4-1).

Physical Examination

Examination of the vulva and surrounding skin should be completed using adequate lighting, optimal patient positioning, and magnifying lens or colposcope. Both focal and generalized skin changes are carefully noted, as neoplasia may arise within a field of generalized dermatosis. Abnormal pigmentation, skin texture, nodularity, or vascularity should be evaluated. A small probe such as a cotton swab is used to define the anatomic boundaries of generalized symptoms and to precisely locate focal complaints (Fig. 4-1). A diagram noting vulvar findings and symptoms is useful to assess treatment over time.

Vaginal complaints or vulvar conditions without obvious etiology should prompt vaginal examination. Careful inspection may reveal generalized inflammation or atrophy, abnormal discharge, or focal mucosal lesions such as ulcers. In these cases, saline preparation of secretions for microscopic evaluation ("wet prep"), vaginal pH testing, and aerobic culture should be collected to detect overgrowth of particular bacteria, such as group B *Streptococcus*, or yeast. Finally, a bimanual examination may be performed.

A global skin examination, including the oral mucosa and axillae, may suggest the cause of some vulvar symptoms. Moreover, a focused neurologic examination to evaluate lower extremity sensation and strength as well as perineal sensation and tone may help evaluate vulvar dysesthesias.

TABLE 4-1. Common Vulvar Irritants and Allergens

General Categories	Examples of Specific Agents
Antiseptics	Povidone iodine, hexachlorophene
Body fluids	Semen, feces, urine, saliva
Colored or scented toilet paper	
Condoms	Latex, lubricant, spermicide, thiuram
Contraceptive creams, jellies, foams	Nonoxynol-9, lubricants
Dyes	4-Phenylene diamine
Emollients	Lanolin, jojoba oil, glycerin
Laundry detergents, fabric softeners, and dryer sheets	
Rubber products	Latex, thiuram
Sanitary baby wipes	
Sanitary pads or tampons	
Soaps, bubble bath and salts, shampoos, conditioners	
Topical anesthetics	Benzocaine, lidocaine
Topical antibacterials	Neomycin, bacitracin, polymyxin, framycetin, tea tree oil
Topical corticosteroids	Clobetasol propionate
Topical antifungal creams	Ethylenediamine, sodium metabisulfite

Compiled from American College of Obstetricians and Gynecologists, 2008; Crone, 2000; Fisher, 1973; and Marren, 1992.

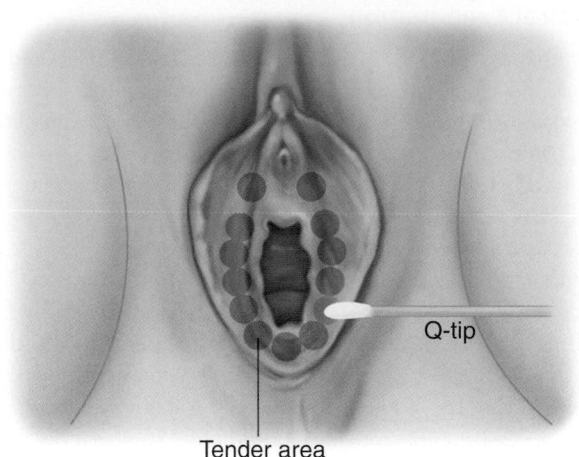

FIGURE 4-1 Pain can be assessed and mapped by systematically touching a cotton-tip applicator to the vulva.

Vulvar Biopsy

Vulvar skin changes are frequently nonspecific and typically will require biopsy for an accurate diagnosis. Biopsy should be strongly considered if the cause of symptoms is not obvious;

focal, hyperpigmented, or exophytic lesions are present; or initial empiric treatment fails. During biopsy, ulcerative lesions are sampled at their edges, and hyperpigmented areas at their thickest region (Mirowski, 2004).

The steps for vulvar biopsy are shown in Figure 4-2. First, the biopsy site is cleaned with an antiseptic agent and infiltrated with a 1- or 2-percent lidocaine solution. Biopsy is performed most easily with a disposable Keyes skin punch. The open, circular blade is designed to remove a core of tissue when gently pressed against the skin and rotated. Keyes punches are available in a variety of diameters, ranging from 2 to 6 mm, and size selection is based on lesion dimensions and whether sampling or excision is the goal. Vulvar skin and lesion thicknesses are variable, and it is important to avoid needless rotation or application of undue pressure on the Keyes punch. Too deep a biopsy will leave a depressed scar. Rotation and pressure should stop when decreased resistance is felt as the dermis is reached. The tissue core is then freed at its base with fine scissors.

Alternatively, a sharp Tischler cervical biopsy instrument may be used for vulvar sampling (Fig. 29-15, p. 750). With this tool, an excessively deep biopsy is avoided by using the side of the instrument to approach the vulvar lesion tangentially and

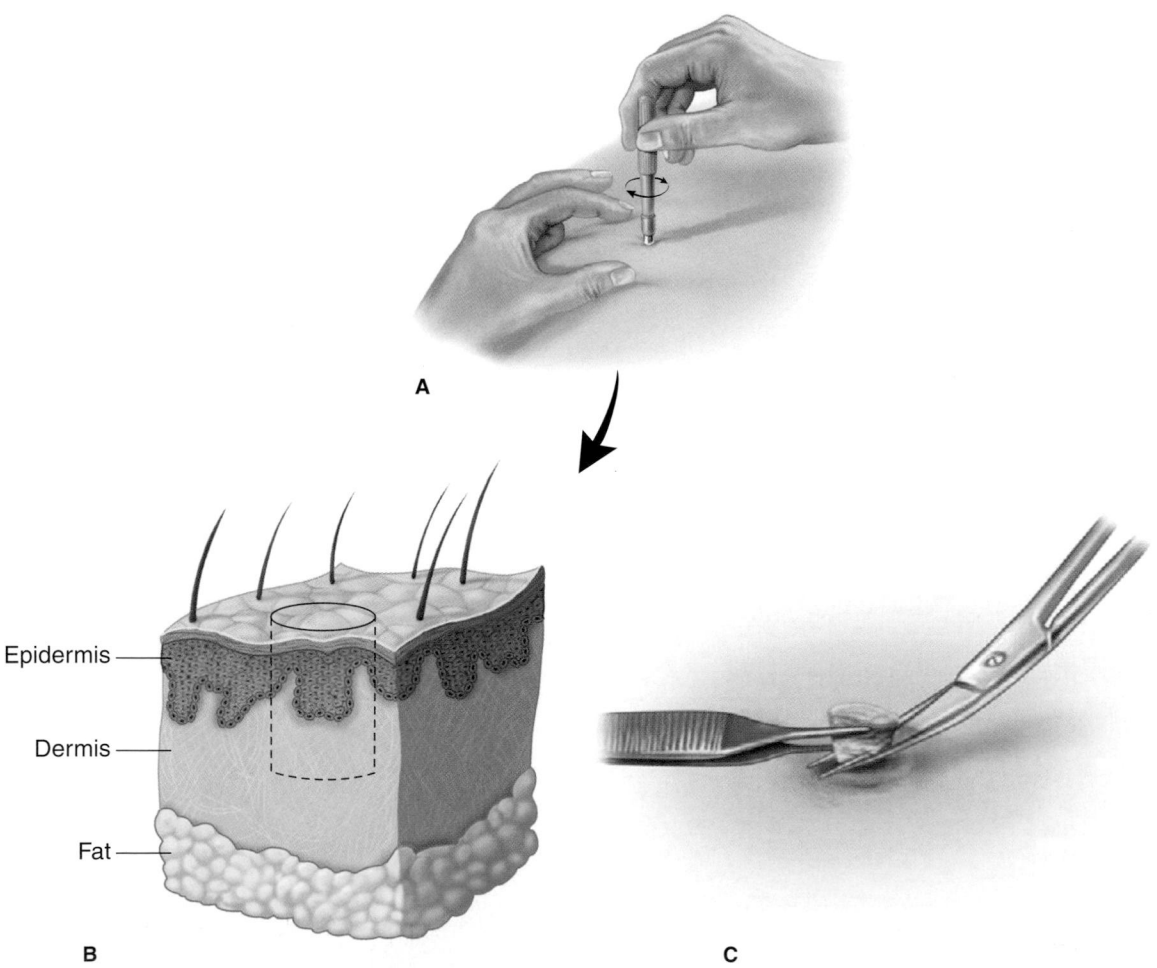

FIGURE 4-2 Vulvar biopsy steps. **A.** A Keyes punch biopsy is placed against the biopsy site. Gentle downward pressure is exerted as the punch is rotated. **B.** A core biopsy is created that extends through the epidermis and partially into the dermis. **C.** Fine forceps are used to elevate the core, while fine scissors incise its base.

by tenting the skin with fine forceps. For raised or pedunculated lesions, a fine scissors may be used. Occasionally, a No. 15-blade scalpel is used for larger focal lesions. Tissue is excised parallel to the natural skinfolds of the vulva to aid healing and minimize scarring.

Following biopsy, bleeding may be controlled with direct pressure, silver nitrate sticks, or Monsel solution. Silver nitrate may leave a permanent discoloration on the skin, which may be upsetting to the patient and confusing at subsequent examinations. If needed, simple interrupted stitches using a fine, absorbable suture provide hemostasis and edge approximation. Nonnarcotic oral analgesics usually suffice to relieve postbiopsy discomfort.

Vulvar Dermatoses

In 2006, the International Society for the Study of Vulvovaginal Disease (ISSVD) adopted the current nomenclature of vulvar dermatoses based on both histopathologic and gross changes (Table 4-2) (Lynch, 2007). For those diseases that may display variable histologic appearances, multiple vulvar biopsies may be required for correct classification.

Lichen Simplex Chronicus

An itch-scratch cycle typically leads to chronic trauma from rubbing and scratching (Lynch, 2004). Early examination reveals excoriations within a background of erythematous skin. With chronic trauma, the skin responds by thickening, termed lichenification. Thus, in long-standing cases, vulvar skin is thick, gray, and leathery with exaggerated skin markings. Skin changes are usually bilateral and symmetric and may extend beyond the labia majora. Intense vulvar pruritus causes functional and psychologic distress, and sleep disruption is common. Potential pruritus triggers include environmental factors (irritation from clothing, heat, sweating), chemical substances contained within hygiene products and topical medications, laundry products, and even food sensitivities (Virgili, 2003). Historical information is typically sufficient to reach the diagnosis.

Treatment involves halting the itch-scratch cycle. First, provocative stimuli should be eliminated. Topical corticosteroid ointments help to reduce inflammation. In addition, lubricants, such as plain petrolatum or vegetable oil, and sitz baths help to restore the skin's barrier function. Oral antihistamine use, trimmed fingernails, and cotton gloves worn at night can help decrease scratching during sleep. If symptoms fail to resolve within 1 to 3 weeks, biopsy is indicated to exclude other pathology. If biopsy is performed, thickening of both the epidermis (acanthosis) and the stratum corneum (hyperkeratosis) is classically found histologically with lichen simplex chronicus.

Lichen Sclerosus

Since the earliest reported cases in the late 1800s, lichen sclerosus has been plagued with confusing terminology. The ISSVD has formally adopted the term *lichen sclerosus* to define

TABLE 4-2. ISSVD Classification of Vulvar Dermatoses: Pathological Subsets and Their Clinical Correlates

Spongiotic pattern
  Atopic dermatitis
  Allergic contact dermatitis
  Irritant contact dermatitis
Acanthotic pattern (formerly squamous cell hyperplasia)
  Psoriasis
  Lichen simplex chronicus
    Primary (idiopathic)
    Secondary (superimposed on lichen sclerosus, lichen planus, etc.)
Lichenoid pattern
  Lichen sclerosus
  Lichen planus
Dermal homogenization/sclerosis pattern
  Lichen sclerosus
Vesiculobullous pattern
  Pemphigoid, cicatricial type
  Liner IgA disease
Acantholytic pattern
  Hailey-Hailey disease
  Darier disease
  Papular genitocrural acantholysis
Granulomatous pattern
  Crohn disease
  Melkersson-Rosenthal syndrome
Vasculopathic pattern
  Aphthous ulcers
  Behçet disease
  Plasma cell vulvitis

ISSVD = International Society for the Study of Vulvovaginal Disease; IgA = immunoglobulin A.

this chronic inflammatory skin condition that predominantly affects the anogenital skin (Moyal-Barracco, 2004b).

Lichen sclerosus classically presents in postmenopausal women, although cases are less commonly found in premenopausal women, children, and men (Fig. 14-9, p. 388). In a referral dermatologic clinic, lichen sclerosus was found in 1:300 to 1:1000 patients with a tendency toward whites (Wallace, 1971). Others estimate an incidence of childhood lichen sclerosus to be 1 in 900 (Powell, 2001).

Pathophysiology. The cause of lichen sclerosus remains unknown, although infectious, hormonal, genetic, and autoimmune etiologies have been suggested. Approximately 20 to 30 percent of patients with lichen sclerosus have other autoimmune disorders, such as Graves disease, type I and II diabetes mellitus, systemic lupus erythematosus, and achlorhydria, with or without pernicious anemia (Bor, 1969; Helm, 1991; Kahana, 1985; Poskitt, 1993). Accordingly, concurrent testing for these disorders is indicated if other suggestive findings are present.

Causation by hormonal disorders has been investigated. Friedrich and Kalra (1984) compared serum androgen and estrogen levels of women with lichen sclerosus with those of age-matched controls. Both dihydrotestosterone (DHT) and androstenedione levels were significantly lower in women with lichen sclerosus, and a reduced local activity of 5α-reductase was implicated. As a result of this study, 2-percent testosterone ointment was widely used in the past to treat lichen sclerosus (Friedrich, 1985; Kaufman, 1974). These results were not replicated in subsequent studies, and testosterone is no longer recommended for treatment of lichen sclerosus (Bornstein, 1998; Cattaneo, 1996; Sideri, 1994).

History. Although some affected women are asymptomatic, most individuals with lichen sclerosus will complain of anogenital symptoms that often worsen at night. Inflammation of local terminal nerve fibers is suspected. Pruritus-induced scratching creates a vicious cycle that may lead to excoriations and thickening of the vulvar skin. Late symptoms can include burning and then dyspareunia due to vulvar skin fragility and architectural changes.

Diagnosis. As mentioned earlier, vulvar and perianal involvement is seen in nearly 85 percent of cases. The typical white, atrophic papules may coalesce into porcelain-white plaques that distort normal anatomy. As a result, labia minora regression, clitoral concealment, urethral obstruction, and introital stenosis may be seen. The skin generally appears thinned and crinkled. Over time a lesion may spread to the perineum and anus and form a "figure-8" or "hourglass" shape (Fig. 4-3) (Clark, 1967). Thickened white plaques or nodularity should prompt biopsy to exclude preinvasive and malignant lesions.

This characteristic clinical picture and histologic confirmation typically lead to the diagnosis. Unfortunately, in long-standing cases, histologic evaluation may be nonspecific, and clinical judgment with close surveillance should guide treatment.

Treatment and Surveillance. Curative options are not available for lichen sclerosus. Thus, treatment goals include symptom control and prevention of anatomic distortion.

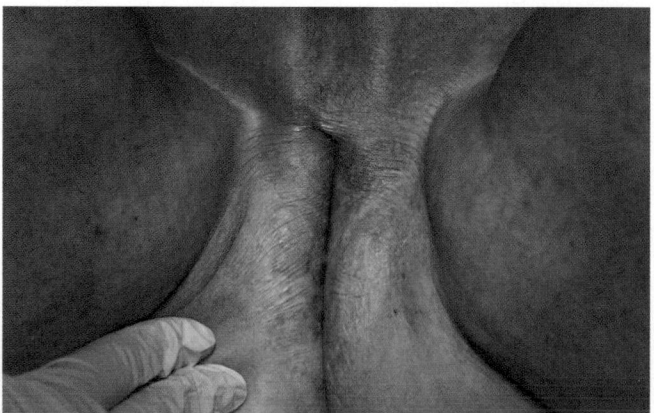

FIGURE 4-3 Vulvar lichen sclerosus. Note the thin and pale vulvar skin and loss of labia minora architecture.

TABLE 4-3. Vulvar Care Recommendations
Avoid using gels, scented bath products, moisturizing wipes, and soaps, as they may contain irritants
Use aqueous creams to clean the vulva
Avoid using a washcloth to clean the vulva
Dab the vulva gently to dry
Avoid wearing tight fitting pants
White cotton underwear is preferred
Avoid washing undergarments in scented or excess detergent. Consider using a multirinse process with cold water to remove any remaining detergent
Consider wearing skirts and wearing no underwear when at home in bed to avoid friction and aid drying

Despite being classified as a nonneoplastic dermatosis, patients with lichen sclerosus have demonstrated an increased risk of vulvar malignancy. Malignant transformation within lichen sclerosus occurs in 4 to 6 percent of patients with stable disease. Histologic cellular atypia may precede a diagnosis of invasive squamous cell carcinoma. Accordingly, lifetime surveillance of women with lichen sclerosus every 6 to 12 months is recommended. Persistently symptomatic, new, or changing lesions should be biopsied (American College of Obstetricians and Gynecologists, 2008; Goolamali, 1974).

Patient Education. As with all vulvar disorders, hygiene recommendations focus on minimizing chemical and mechanical irritation of the skin (Table 4-3). The chronicity of lichen sclerosus and lack of cure elicits an array of emotions. Support groups dedicated to this condition, such as that found at www.lichensclerosus.org, offer needed psychologic support.

Corticosteroids. First-line therapy for lichen sclerosus is an ultrapotent topical corticosteroid preparation such as 0.05-percent clobetasol propionate (Temovate) or 0.05-percent halobetasol propionate (Ultravate). Ointment formulations are preferred by some providers over creams due to their minimal allergenic properties (Table 4-4). Despite theoretic risks of adrenocorticosuppression and iatrogenic Cushing syndrome if used in large doses for extended periods, clobetasol propionate offers effective antiinflammatory, antipruritic, and vasoconstrictive properties (Paslin, 1996).

Initiation of treatment within 2 years of symptom onset usually prevents significant scarring. No treatment scheme is universally accepted for topical corticosteroid use. However, the currently recommended dosing schedule of the British Association of Dermatologists is 0.05-percent clobetasol propionate once nightly for 4 weeks, followed by alternating nights for 4 weeks, and finally tapering to twice weekly for 4 weeks (Neill, 2002). After this initial therapy, recommendations for maintenance therapy vary and range from tapering corticosteroids to "as needed" use to on-going, once- or twice-weekly applications. During initial treatment, some patients may

TABLE 4-4. Topical Medication Guide

Corticosteroid Class	Generic Name	Brand Names and (available forms)	Dosage (apply thin layer)
Low potency	Alclometasone dipropionate 0.05%	Aclovate (cream, ointment)	bid or tid
	Betamethasone valerate 0.01%	Valisone (cream, lotion)	qd or bid
	Fluocinolone acetonide 0.01%	Synalar (solution)	bid or tid
	Hydrocortisone base or acetate 1%, 2.5%	Cortaid or other 1% OTC brands or Hytone, Hycort, or Caldecort 1%, 2.5% (cream, ointment, lotion)	tid or qid
Intermediate potency	Betamethasone valerate 0.1%	Valisone (cream, lotion, ointment)	qd or bid
	Desonide 0.05%	DesOwen (cream, ointment, lotion)	bid or tid
	Fluocinolone acetonide 0.025%	Synalar (cream, ointment)	bid or tid
	Flurandrenolide 0.025%, 0.05%	Cordran (cream, ointment)	bid or tid
	Fluticasone 0.005%, 0.05%	Cutivate 0.005% (ointment), 0.05% (cream)	qd or bid
	Hydrocortisone butyrate 0.1%	Locoid (cream, ointment, solution)	bid or tid
	Hydrocortisone valerate 0.2%	Westcort (cream, ointment)	bid or tid
	Mometasone furoate 0.1%	Elocon (cream, ointment, lotion)	qd
	Prednicarbate 0.1%	Dermatop (cream, ointment)	bid
	Triamcinolone 0.025%, 0.1%	Aristocort, Kenalog (cream, ointment, lotion)	bid
High potency	Amcinonide 0.1%	Cyclocort (cream, ointment, lotion)	bid or tid
	Betamethasone dipropionate 0.05%	Diprolene, Diprosone (cream)	qd or bid
	Desoximetasone 0.05%, 0.25%	Topicort (cream)	bid
	Diflorasone diacetate 0.05%	Maxiflor, Florone (cream)	bid to qid
	Fluocinonide 0.05%	Lidex (cream, gel, ointment)	bid or tid
	Fluocinolone acetonide 0.2%	Synalar-HP (cream)	bid or tid
	Halcinonide 0.1%	Halog (cream, ointment, solution)	qd to tid
	Triamcinolone 0.5%	Aristocort, Kenalog (cream, ointment)	tid or qid
Ultrapotent	Betamethasone dipropionate augmented 0.05%	Diprolene (ointment, gel)	qd or bid
	Clobetasol propionate 0.05%	Temovate (cream, gel, ointment)	bid
	Diflorasone 0.05%	Psorcon (ointment)	bid to qid
	Halobetasol propionate 0.05%	Ultravate (cream, ointment)	bid

bid = twice daily; OTC = over the counter; qd = daily; qid = four times daily; tid = three times daily.

require oral antihistamines or topical 2-percent lidocaine jelly particularly at night to control itching.

Corticosteroids may also be injected into affected areas. One study of eight patients evaluated the efficacy of once-monthly intralesional infiltration of 25 to 30 mg of triamcinolone hexacetonide, equally divided bilaterally, for a total of 3 months. Severity scores decreased in all categories including symptoms, gross appearance, and histopathologic findings (Mazdisnian, 1999).

Other Topical Agents. Estrogen cream is not a primary therapy for lichen sclerosus. However, its addition is indicated for menopausal atrophic changes, labial fusion, and dyspareunia.

Retinoids should be reserved for severe, nonresponsive cases of lichen sclerosus or for patients intolerant of ultrapotent corticosteroids. Topical tretinoin reduces hyperkeratosis, improves dysplastic changes, stimulates collagen and glycosaminoglycan synthesis, and induces local angiogenesis (Eichner, 1992; Kligman, 1986a, 1986b; Varani, 1989). Virgili and colleagues (1995) evaluated the effects of topical 0.025-percent tretinoin (Retin-A, Renova) applied once daily, 5 days a week for 1 year. Complete remission of symptoms was seen in more than 75 percent of women. However, more than one quarter of patients experienced skin irritation, which is common with retinoids.

Tacrolimus (Protopic) and pimecrolimus (Elidel) are topical calcineurin inhibitors that have antiinflammatory and immunomodulating effects. These are indicated for moderate to severe eczema and have shown success in the treatment of lichen sclerosus (Goldstein, 2011; Hengge, 2006). Moreover, these agents compared with topical corticosteroids theoretically lower the risk of skin atrophy, since collagen synthesis is unaffected (Assmann, 2003; Kunstfeld, 2003). However, in the face of Food and Drug Administration (FDA) concerns regarding their link to a variety of cancers, clinicians should exercise caution when prescribing these medications for extended periods (U.S. Food and Drug Administration, 2010).

Photodynamic Therapy. Investigators have evaluated the effects of phototherapy after pretreatment using 5-aminolevulinic acid in one small series of 12 postmenopausal women with advanced lichen sclerosus. Significant reductions in patient symptoms and continued improvement for up to 9 months were noted (Hillemanns, 1999).

Surgery. Surgical intervention should be reserved for significant sequelae and not for primary treatment of uncomplicated lichen sclerosus. For introital stenosis, Rouzier and colleagues (2002) described marked improvements in dyspareunia and quality of sexual intercourse if perineoplasty was performed (Section 41-22, p. 1070). Vaginal dilation and corticosteroids are recommended following most surgical corrections of introital stenosis.

For clitoral adhesions, surgical dissection can be used to free the hood from the glans. Reagglutination can be averted using nightly application of ultrapotent topical corticosteroid ointment (Goldstein, 2007).

Inflammatory Dermatoses

Contact Dermatitis. A primary irritant or allergic substrate can lead to vulvar skin inflammation, termed contact dermatitis (Fig. 4-4). This condition is common, and in unexplained cases of vulvar pruritus and inflammation, irritant contact dermatitis is diagnosed in up to 54 percent of patients (Fischer, 1996).

Irritant contact dermatitis classically presents as immediate burning and stinging upon exposure to an offending agent. In contrast, patients with *allergic contact dermatitis* experience a delayed onset and an intermittent course of pruritus and localized erythema, edema, and vesicles or bullae (Margesson, 2004). A detailed history will aid in differentiating between the two. Inquiry regarding new hygiene routines, personal care products, douches, contraceptive methods, topical medications, or perfumes may help identify the new source of alcohols, antiseptics, or surfactants (see Table 4-1) (Crone, 2000; Fisher, 1973; Marren, 1992).

With allergic contact dermatitis, patch testing may aid in identifying responsible allergen(s). Associated conditions such as candidiasis, psoriasis, seborrheic dermatitis, and squamous cell carcinoma can be excluded through appropriate use of cultures and biopsy.

Treatments for both entities involve elimination of the offending agent, restoration of the natural protective skin barrier, reduction of inflammation, and cessation of scratching (Table 4-5) (Farage, 2004; Margesson, 2004).

Intertrigo. Friction between moist opposed skin surfaces produces this chronic condition. Although most commonly seen

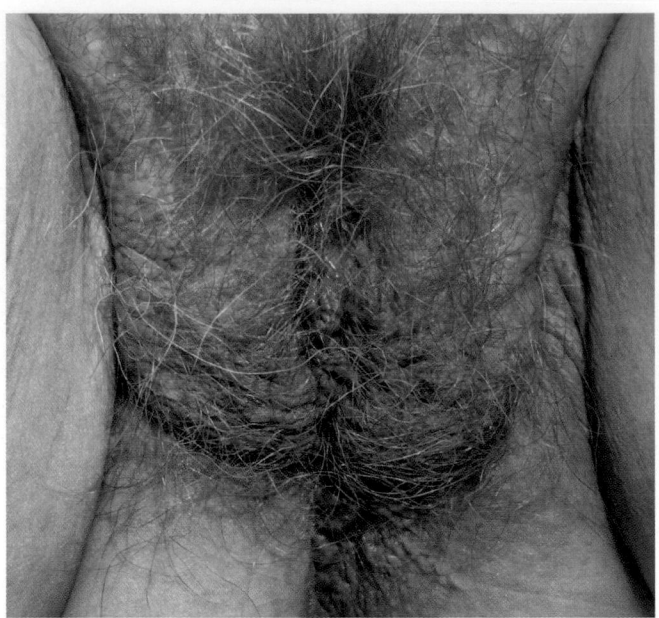

FIGURE 4-4 Vulvar contact dermatitis. Contact sites of the offending agent are seen as symmetric erythema on the vulva.

in the genitocrural folds, skin changes can also be found in the inguinal and intergluteal regions. Superimposed bacterial and fungal infections may complicate the disease process.

The initial erythematous phase, if untreated, can progress to intense inflammation with erosions, exudate, fissuring, maceration, and crusting (Mistiaen, 2004). Symptoms typically include burning and itching. With long-standing intertrigo, hyperpigmentation and verrucous changes may appear.

TABLE 4-5. Treatment of Vulvar Contact Dermatitis

1. Stop offending agents and/or practices
2. Correct vulvar skin barrier function
   a. Sitz bath twice daily with plain water
   b. Apply plain petrolatum
3. Treat any underlying infection
   a. Oral antifungal therapy
   b. Oral antibiotic administration
4. Reduce inflammation
   a. Topical corticosteroids twice daily for 1 to 3 weeks
      i. 0.05% clobatesol propionate ointment
      ii. 0.1% triamcinolone ointment
   b. Systemic corticosteroids for severe irritation
5. Break the itch-scratch cycle
   a. Cool packs (no ice packs, as these may injure skin)
   b. Plain, cold yogurt on a sanitary napkin for 5 to 10 minutes
   c. Consider an SSRI (sertraline [Zoloft] 50 to 100 mg orally once daily) or an antihistamine (hydroxyzine [Vistaril] 25 mg orally three or four times daily)

SSRI = selective serotonin-reuptake inhibitor.
Adapted from Margesson, 2004, with permission.

Treatment entails the use of drying agents such as cornstarch and application of mild topical corticosteroids in the face of inflammation. If skin changes do not respond, then seborrheic dermatitis, psoriasis, atopic dermatitis, pemphigus vegetans, or even scabies should be considered. If superinfection with bacteria or yeast develops, appropriate culture-based therapy is warranted.

To prevent recurrent outbreaks, obese patients are encouraged to lose weight. Other preventative recommendations include wearing light-weight, loose-fitting clothing made of natural fibers (Janniger, 2005).

Atopic Eczema. Classically presenting in the first 5 years of life, atopic dermatitis presents as a severe pruritic dermatitis that follows a chronic, relapsing course. Scaly patches with fissuring are evident on examination. Individuals with atopic eczema may later develop allergic rhinitis and asthma (Spergel, 2003).

Topical corticosteroids and immunomodulators, such as tacrolimus, can be used to control flares (Leung, 2004). In the presence of dry skin, local hydration using emollients and bath oil can offer relief.

Psoriasis. Approximately 1 to 2 percent of the United States' population is affected by psoriasis (Gelfand, 2005). With this condition, thick, red plaques covered with silvery scales are found on extensor limb surfaces. Occasionally, lesions involve the mons pubis or labia (Fig. 4-5). Psoriasis can be exacerbated by nervous stress and menses, with remissions experienced during summer months and pregnancy. Pruritus may be minimal or absent, and this condition is often diagnosed by skin findings alone.

Several treatments are available for psoriasis, and topical corticosteroids are widely used for their rapid efficacy. High-potency corticosteroids are applied to affected areas twice daily for 2 to 4 weeks and then reduced to weekly applications. Diminishing response and skin atrophy are potential disadvantages to long-term use. Recalcitrant cases are best managed by a dermatologist. Vitamin D analogs, such as calcipotriene (Dovonex), although similar in efficacy to potent corticosteroids, are frequently associated with local irritation but avoid skin atrophy (Smith, 2006). Phototherapy offers short-term relief, but long-term treatment plans require a multidisciplinary team approach (Griffiths, 2000). Psoriasis is a T-cell–mediated autoimmune process in which proinflammatory cytokines induce keratinocyte and endothelial cell proliferation. Several FDA-approved immunomodulating biologic agents are available and include infliximab, adalimumab, etanercept, alefacept, and ustekinumab (Smith, 2009).

Lichen Planus

Incidence and Etiology. Lichen planus, an uncommon disease that involves both cutaneous and mucosal surfaces. It equally affects men and women between ages 30 and 60 years (Mann, 1991). Although not completely understood, T-cell autoimmunity directed against basal keratinocytes is thought to underlie its pathogenesis (Goldstein, 2005). Vulvar lichen planus can present as one of three variants: (1) erosive, (2) papulosquamous, or (3) hypertrophic. Of these, erosive lichen planus is the most common vulvovaginal form and the most difficult variant to treat. Lichen planus may be drug-induced, and nonsteroidal antiinflammatory drugs, β-blocking agents, methyldopa, penicillamine, and quinine drugs have been implicated.

Diagnosis. Table 4-6 summarizes the most common imitators of lichen planus. On inspection, papules classically are brightly erythematous or violaceous, flat-topped, shiny polygons most commonly found on the trunk, buccal mucosa, or flexor surfaces of the extremities (Goldstein, 2005; Zellis, 1996). Lacy, white striations (Wickham striae) are frequently found in conjunction with the papules and may also be present on the buccal mucosa (Fig. 4-6). Women typically complain of chronic vaginal discharge with intense vulvovaginal pruritus, burning pain, dyspareunia, and postcoital bleeding. Deep, painful erosions in the posterior vestibule can extend to the labia, resulting in agglutination. With speculum insertion, vulvar skin and vaginal mucosa bleed easily. Erosive lesions can produce adhesions and synechiae, which may lead to vaginal obliteration.

Women with suspected lichen planus require a thorough dermatologic survey looking for extragenital lesions. Nearly one quarter of women with oral lesions will have vulvovaginal involvement, and most with erosive vulvovaginal lichen planus will have oral involvement (Pelisse, 1989). Diagnosis is obtained through biopsy.

Treatment of Vulvar Lichen Planus. Pharmacotherapy remains the first-line treatment for this condition. Additionally, vulvar care recommendations, psychologic support, and discontinuing any medications associated with lichenoid changes should be instituted.

Erosive vulvar lichen planus is treated initially with ultra-potent topical corticosteroid ointments, such as 0.05-percent clobetasol propionate applied daily for up to 3 months, and

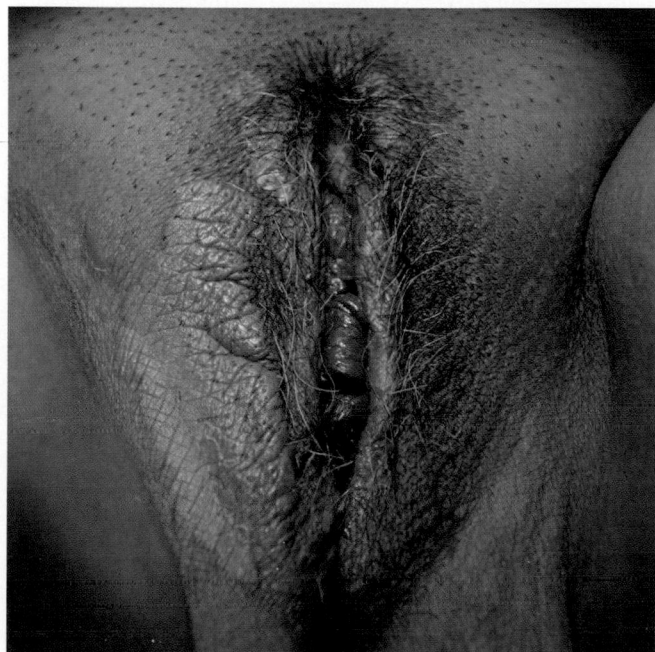

FIGURE 4-5 Psoriasis. Raised plaques are seen on the vulva. *(Photograph contributed by Dr. Saly Thomas.)*

TABLE 4-6. Differential Diagnosis of Lichen Planus

Class of Lichen Planus	Mimicking Condition	Key Features of the Mimicking Condition
Erosive lichen planus	Lichen sclerosus	No vaginal involvement; confirmed by histology
	Pemphigoid vulgaris or benign mucous membrane pemphigoid	Shallow erosive ulcerations with rare vaginal involvement; immunofluorescent histology will confirm (Note: biopsy normal adjacent epithelium)
	Behçet disease	No vaginal involvement; will have ocular involvement; inflammation is perivascular
	Plasma cell vulvitis	Rare; no oral lesions
	Erythema multiforme major/ Stevens-Johnson syndrome	Systemic symptoms
	Desquamative inflammatory vaginitis	Vaginal discharge will have elevated pH, sheets of white cells, and parabasal cells
Papulosquamous lichen planus	Molluscum contagiosum	Biopsy confirmation
	Genital warts	Biopsy confirmation
Hypertrophic lichen planus	Squamous cell carcinoma	Biopsy confirmation

Compiled from Goldstein, 2005; Kaufman, 1974; and Moyal-Barracco, 2004a.

then slowly tapered. Cooper and Wojnarowska (2006) prospectively evaluated the clinical course of 114 women with erosive lichen planus treated with ultrapotent topical corticosteroids. Despite more than 70 percent of women exhibiting good response to twice-daily therapy used for 3 months followed by maintenance therapy, only 9 percent achieved complete remission. Alternatively, these same investigators noted a preparation containing 0.05-percent clobetasol butyrate, 3-percent oxytetracycline, and 100,000 U/g nystatin (Trimovate) to be effective. Although a smaller treatment cohort, more than 90 percent of

women so treated were symptom free following initial treatment.

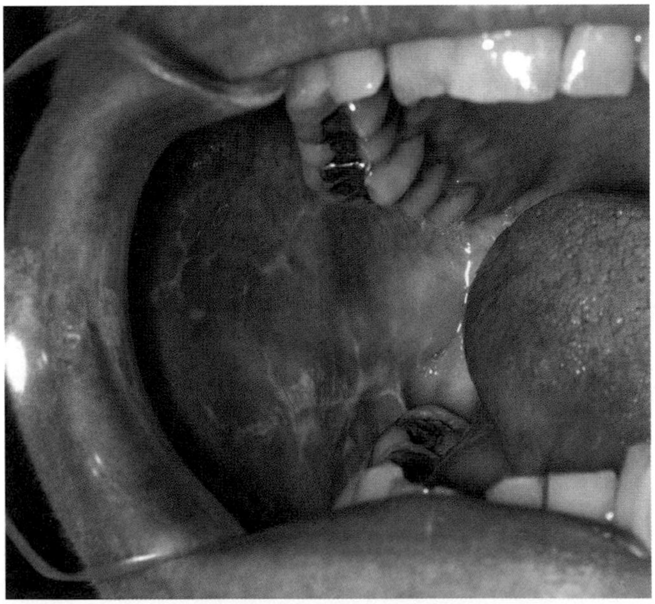

Other agents shown to be beneficial in small case series include systemic corticosteroids, topical tacrolimus ointment, topical cyclosporine, and oral retinoids (Byrd, 2004; Eisen, 1990; Hersle, 1982; Morrison, 2002).

Treatment of Vaginal Lichen Planus. Anderson and colleagues (2002) found that vaginal use of corticosteroid suppositories containing 25 mg of hydrocortisone, commonly prescribed to treat hemorrhoids, was helpful. Specifically, if used twice daily and then tapered to maintain symptom remission, 75 percent of treated women had symptomatic and clinical improvement. For poorly responding patients, compounding pharmacies can provide a 100-mg hydrocortisone suppository. Potent corticosteroids should be prescribed judiciously, as systemic absorption may lead to adrenocorticosuppression (Moyal-Barracco, 2004a). Combining local corticosteroid therapy with vaginal dilator use may help restore coital function in patients with moderate vaginal synechiae. If topical medications fail, systemic treatment with prednisone 40 to 60 mg daily for up to 4 weeks may modulate symptoms (Moyal-Barracco, 2004a). Although no alternative systemic medications have been fully studied, methotrexate, hydroxychloroquine, and mycophenolate mofetil administered by health care providers familiar with their use have been reported effective within a multidisciplinary approach (Eisen, 1993; Frieling, 2003; Lundqvist, 2002). Surgical adhesiolysis is a last resort. Vulvovaginal lichen planus is a chronic, recurrent disease for which symptomatic improvement is possible, but complete control is unlikely.

FIGURE 4-6 Oral lichen planus. Mucosal lesions manifest commonly as lacey, white striations (Wickham striae), although white papules or plaques, erosions, or blisters may also be seen. Oral lesions predominantly affect the buccal mucosa, tongue, and gingiva. (*Photograph contributed by Dr. Edward Ellis.*)

Hidradenitis Suppurativa. This chronic disease is manifest by recurrent papular lesions that may lead to abscess, fistula formation, and scarring predominantly in apocrine gland-bearing skin (Fig. 4-7). In order of frequency, affected areas include the axillae; inguinal, perianal, and perineal skin; inframammary

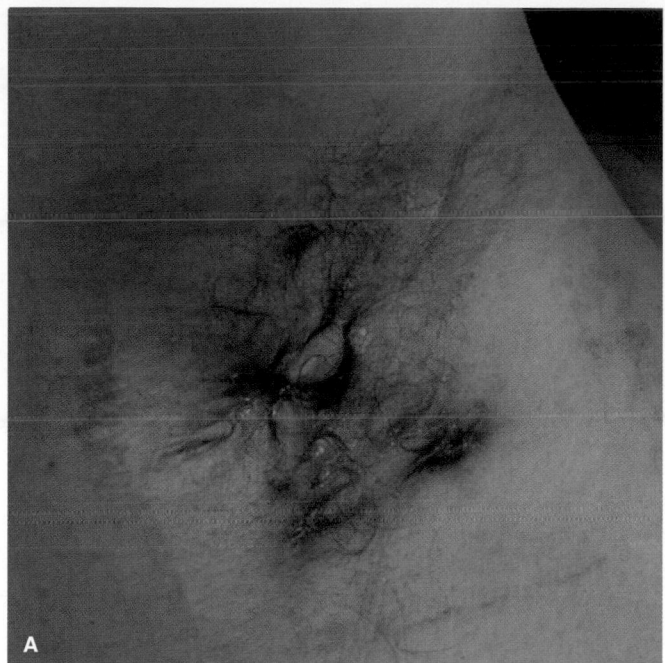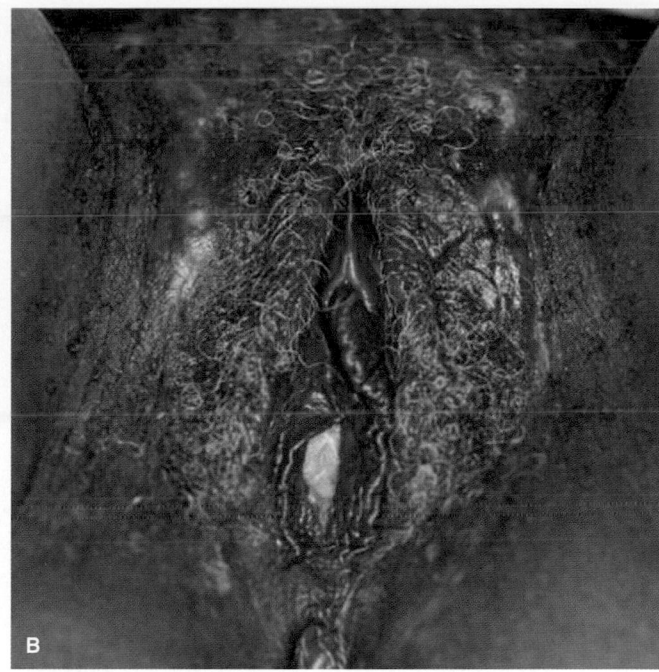

FIGURE 4-7 Hidradenitis suppurativa. **A.** Axilla shows skin puckering created by scarring from prior infection and inflammation. *(From Wolff, 2009, with permission.)* **B.** Mons pubis with multiple draining pustules and thickened scarred skin.

regions; and retroauricular skin. It is characterized by chronic inflammation and obstruction of skin follicles with subsequent subcutaneous abscess formation, skin thickening, and deformity. Abscesses typically form sinus tracts, although polymicrobial superinfection by normal skin flora appears to be independent of the primary disease process (Brook, 1999; Jemec, 1996). The disfigurement and chronic drainage of purulent material can be devastating physically, emotionally, and sexually.

The etiology of hidradenitis suppurativa is unknown. More than one quarter of patients will relate a family history of disease, and an autosomal dominant inheritance pattern has been hypothesized (der Werth, 2000). Although Mortimer and colleagues (1986) found higher plasma concentrations of androgens in women with hidradenitis suppurativa, others have been unable to replicate this finding (Barth, 1996).

Treatment of early cases includes topical or oral antibiotics and warm compresses. Used individually, appropriate long-term oral antibiotics and their dosages include: tetracycline, 500 mg twice daily; erythromycin, 500 mg twice daily; doxycycline, 100 mg twice daily; or minocycline, 100 mg twice daily. Topical 1-percent clindamycin solution applied twice daily may also be effective (Jemec, 1998). More recently, a 10-week course of clindamycin, 300 mg twice daily, plus rifampicin, 600 mg twice daily, has shown efficacy (Gener, 2009).

As reviewed by Rhode and associates (2008), an arsenal of other treatment modalities has been reported with varying efficacy. These include cyproterone acetate (an antiandrogen available in Europe), corticosteroids, isotretinoin, cyclosporine, and infliximab. Nonmedical therapies include laser and phototherapy. Severe, refractory cases may require surgical excision that often involves extensive resection of the vulva and surrounding areas. Plastic surgery techniques are often needed to close these

large defects. Unfortunately, postoperative local recurrences can develop.

Aphthous Ulcers. Nearly 25 percent of women in the second and third decade of life will experience these self-limited mucosal lesions. Classically found on nonkeratinized oral mucosa, aphthous ulcers may also develop on vulvovaginal surfaces. Lesions are painful and can recur every few months.

Although the etiology of aphthous ulcers is unknown, some theorize the origin to be immune-mediated epithelial cell damage (Rogers, 1997). Other described triggers include trauma, infection, hormonal fluctuation, and nutritional deficiencies of B_{12}, folate, iron, or zinc (Torgerson, 2006). Despite the normally self-limited nature of these ulcers, persistent lesions can lead to painful scarring (Rogers, 2003).

High-potency topical corticosteroids can be used at the onset of ulceration. Oral corticosteroids may be used to decrease inflammation in cases resistant to topical corticosteroids. Finally, colchicine, dapsone, and thalidomide have been shown to be effective.

Vulvar Manifestations of Generalized Conditions

Systemic illnesses may initially manifest on the vulvar or vaginal mucosa as bullous, solid, or ulcerative lesions. Examples include systemic lupus erythematosus, erythema multiforme (Stevens-Johnson syndrome), pemphigus, pemphigoid, and sarcoidosis. A thorough history and physical examination usually suffice to link genital lesions with preexisting conditions. However, biopsy of vulvovaginal lesions may provide a new and unexpected diagnosis if the disorder has not yet become evident elsewhere.

Acanthosis Nigricans

This condition is characterized by velvety to warty, brown to black, poorly marginated plaques. These changes are typically found in skin creases, especially on the neck, axillae, and genitocrural folds (Fig. 17-6, p. 467).

Acanthosis nigricans is commonly associated with obesity, diabetes mellitus, and polycystic ovarian syndrome. Thus, if signs or symptoms of these accompany acanthosis nigricans, then appropriate screening is warranted. Common to these three, insulin resistance with compensatory hyperinsulinemia is thought to promote the skin thickening of acanthosis nigricans. Insulin binds to insulin-like growth factor (IGF) receptors and leads to keratinocyte and dermal fibroblast proliferation (Cruz, 1992; Hermanns-Le, 2004). Less commonly, acanthosis nigricans is caused by other insulin-resistance or fibroblast growth-factor disorders (Higgins, 2008).

Treatment of acanthosis nigricans has not been evaluated in randomized trials. However, weight loss can ameliorate insulin resistance, which may lead to lesion improvement. Moreover, in those prescribed metformin for glucose control, improved acanthosis nigricans has been demonstrated (Romo, 2008).

Crohn Disease

Up to one third of women with Crohn disease suffer from anogenital involvement, which typically affects inguinal, genitocrural, and interlabial folds. Such lesions may precede gastrointestinal (GI) symptoms, with edema being the first vulvar manifestation. Subsequent lesions may include characteristic "knife-cut" ulcers, abscesses, as well as fistulas from these lower genital tract lesions to the anus and rectum (Fig. 4-8).

Therapy for gastrointestinal Crohn disease generally benefits external Crohn lesions. Vulvar lesions unrelated to GI disease activity may respond to topical or intralesional corticosteroids or topical metronidazole. Extensive genital surgery often can be avoided or delayed with appropriate vulvar care, nutrition, and close collaboration with a gastroenterologist. In the event

that surgical management is required, excision of the individual fistulous tracts is attempted. Total vulvectomy is reserved for extensive disease. Regardless of management, recurrence is common.

Behçet Disease

This is a rare, chronic, systemic vasculitis that most commonly affects patients in their 20s and 30s and those of Asian or Middle Eastern descent. Behçet disease is characterized by mucocutaneous lesions (ocular, oral, and genital) and associated systemic vasculitis. Oral and genital ulcers appear similar to aphthous ulcers and generally heal within 7 to 10 days. Nevertheless, associated pain can be debilitating. Treatment for these lesions mirrors that of aphthous ulcers.

The exact etiology of Behçet disease remains unknown, although genetic and infectious etiologies are suspected. Vasculitis dominates the disease process, which may involve the brain, GI tract, joints, lungs, and great vessels. Accordingly, in those suspected of Behçet disease, referral to a rheumatologist for additional testing and treatment is recommended.

■ Disorders of Pigmentation

Skin pigmentation should be inspected carefully during each pelvic examination. Benign variations are commonly encountered in clinical practice, especially in women with darker skin. These areas of increased pigment are usually encountered on the labia minora and fourchette. They tend to be bilateral, symmetric, and even in tone and texture. With gentle stretching, the color attenuates evenly. Focal abnormalities should raise suspicion of a premalignant or malignant condition and prompt immediate biopsy to avoid an unnecessary diagnostic delay. As discussed in Chapter 29 (p. 758), high-grade intraepithelial neoplasia and invasive cancer can present as hypo- or hyperpigmented lesions, with or without symptoms. Melanoma is the second most common vulvar malignancy and is discussed in Chapter 31 (p. 803).

Nevus

Acquired nevi commonly develop in adolescence within sun-exposed areas, although vulvar skin is not immune (Krengel, 2005). In contrast, congenital nevi may be found on any skin surface at any age. Pigmented nevi warrant close surveillance as more than half of all melanomas arise from preexisting nevi.

Nevi are classified into three primary groups: junctional, compound, and intradermal. Junctional nevi are less than 1 cm in diameter, flat with minimal surface elevation, and derive from melanocytes within the epidermis. Their color is uniform and lesion margins are well demarcated. This type of nevus is the most likely to become malignant. Compound nevi involve both the dermis and epidermis. Lesions possess regular margins and range in size from 4 to 10 mm. As these lesions age, they may progress into intradermal nevi, which lie completely within the dermis and can become papular or pedunculated.

Vulvar nevi should be biopsied according to guidelines for nevi located elsewhere on the body. Thus, asymmetry, uneven pigmentation, irregular borders, diameter >6 mm, and erosion

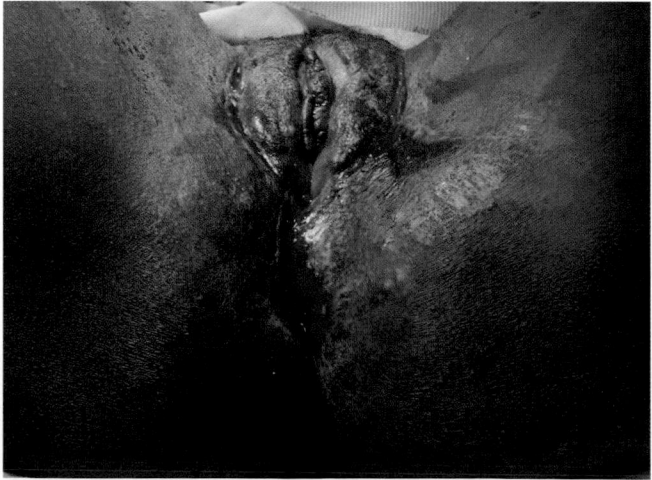

FIGURE 4-8 Vulvar Crohn disease. Knife-cut ulcers in the genitocrural folds and perineum are commonly seen with vulvar Crohn disease. *(Photograph contributed by Dr. F. Gary Cunningham.)*

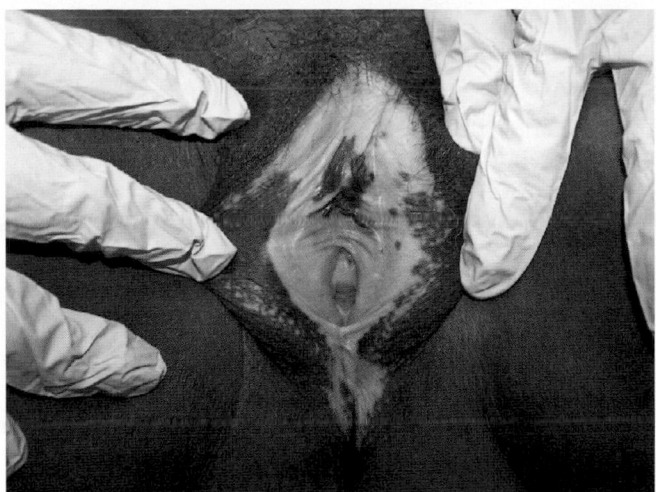

FIGURE 4-9 Vulvar vitiligo.

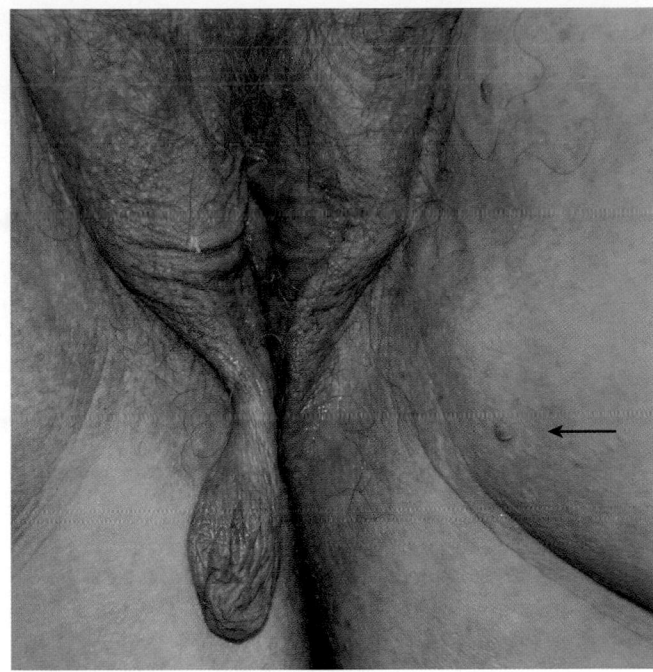

FIGURE 4-10 Vulvar acrocordons (skin tags). Lesions typically are small (*arrow*) and require no intervention. The larger vulvar acrocordon also shown here was excised due to mechanical symptoms from its size.

or fissuring should prompt immediate biopsy. Symptoms of burning or itching should also raise concern. Otherwise inconspicuous nevi warrant a careful descriptive or photographic entry into the medical record and surveillance at least annually until a lesion is deemed stable. Self-examination should be encouraged, and patients should report changes in lesion or symptom status.

Therapy for simple nevi is primarily conservative, with close observation in asymptomatic individuals. As lesions become palpable with subsequent irritation and bleeding, surgical excision serves both a diagnostic and therapeutic role.

Vitiligo

Loss of epidermal melanocytes can result in areas of depigmented skin, termed vitiligo (Fig. 4-9). Global prevalence of this disease averages 0.1 percent, with the incidence peaking in the second decade. No race or ethnicity has greater risks for vitiligo, but the disease may be more disfiguring and distressing for darker-skinned individuals (Grimes, 2005).

Although not fully understood, genetic factors have emerged as the most common cause of vitiligo (Zhang, 2005). Approximately 20 percent of patients have at least one affected first-degree relative. Vitiligo may also share pathogenesis with other autoimmune disorders, such as Hashimoto thyroiditis, Graves disease, diabetes mellitus, rheumatoid arthritis, psoriasis, and vulvar lichen sclerosus (Boissy, 1997).

Most commonly, depigmentation is generalized and symmetric, although distribution may also be acral (limbs, ears), acrofacial, localized, and segmental. We have seen numerous cases of isolated vulvar vitiligo. A number of treatment advances for vitiligo include narrowband ultraviolet (UV) B phototherapy, targeted light therapy, and topical immunomodulators (Grimes, 2005). Most cases are self-limited and explanation of the condition alone is sufficient.

Solid Vulvar Tumors

Most solid vulvar tumors are benign and arise locally. Less commonly, malignant lesions arise on the vulva and are typically

of squamous cell epithelial origin. Rarely, solid vulvar tumors develop as metastatic lesions. Accordingly, many growths warrant biopsy if not obviously identified by visual inspection.

Epidermal and Dermal Lesions

Acrochordon. Commonly known as a skin tag, acrochordons are benign polypoid fibroepithelial lesions. They are most often seen on the neck, axilla, or groin and generally range from 1 to 6 mm in diameter, but can grow much larger (Fig. 4-10). Acrochordons have been linked to diabetes mellitus, and insulin-mediated fibroblast proliferation may explain this relationship (Demir, 2002).

Clinically, an acrochordon is a soft, sessile or pedunculated mass, usually skin colored and devoid of hair. Swelling or ulceration may follow traumatic friction. Surgical removal is recommended for chronic irritation or cosmetic concerns. Smaller lesions, if symptomatic, are easily removed under local anesthesia in an office setting.

Seborrheic Keratosis. Occasionally, vulvar manifestations of seborrheic keratosis may be observed in women with concurrent lesions on the neck, face, or trunk. Sharply circumscribed, slightly raised lesions with a rough, greasy surface are typical. The malignant potential of these slow-growing lesions is minimal, therefore excision is offered only in cases of discomfort.

Keratoacanthoma. These are rapidly growing low-grade malignancies originating in pilosebaceous glands. Lesions begin as firm, round papules that progress to a dome-shaped

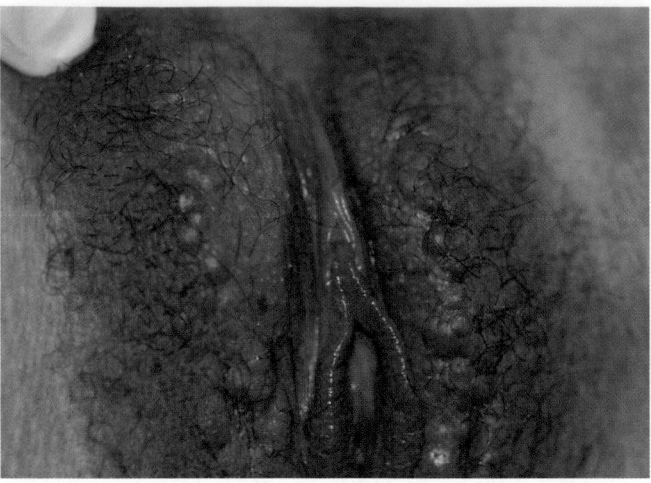

FIGURE 4-11 Vulvar syringoma. Papules are typically arranged in clusters and may extend the length of the labia majora. Syringomas are flesh-colored or yellow and show no anatomic relationship to adjacent pubic hair follicles.

nodule with a central crater. Untreated, the lesion is generally self-limited. However, given its malignant potential and its resemblance to squamous cell carcinoma, surgical excision with a 3- to 5-mm margin is recommended.

Syringoma. These benign eccrine (sweat gland) tumors are found most frequently on the lower eyelid, neck, and face. Rarely, the vulva may be involved bilaterally with multiple 1- to 4-mm firm papules (Fig. 4-11). The clinical appearance of vulvar syringoma is not pathognomonic, thus vulvar punch biopsy will establish the diagnosis and exclude malignancy. Treatment is not required. However, for those with pruritus, mild-potency topical corticosteroids and antihistamines may be helpful. In those with refractory pruritus, surgical excision or lesion ablation may be offered.

Leiomyoma

Vulvar leiomyomas are rare tumors felt to arise either from smooth muscle within the vulva's erectile tissue or from transmigration through the round ligament. Surgical excision to exclude leiomyosarcoma is warranted (Nielsen, 1996).

Fibroma

This rare benign tumor of the vulva arises from deep connective tissues by fibroblast proliferation. Lesions are primarily found on the labia majora and range from 0.6 to 8 cm in diameter. Larger lesions often become pedunculated with a long stalk and may cause pain or dyspareunia. Surgical excision is indicated for symptomatic lesions or if the diagnosis is unclear.

Lipoma

These are large, soft sessile or pedunculated masses composed of mature adipose cells. Similar to fibromas, observation is reasonable in the absence of patient complaints, although symptoms may prompt surgical excision. These lesions lack a fibrous connective tissue capsule. Thus, complete dissection may be complicated by bleeding and require a larger incision.

Ectopic Breast Tissue

Ectopic breast tissue may develop along the theoretical milk lines, which extend bilaterally from the axilla through the breast to the mons pubis (Fig. 4-12). Uncommonly found in the vulva, extramammary breast tissue is hormonally sensitive and may enlarge in response to pregnancy or exogenous hormones. Importantly, these ectopic sites may also develop breast pathologies including fibroadenoma, phyllodes tumor, Paget disease, and invasive adenocarcinoma.

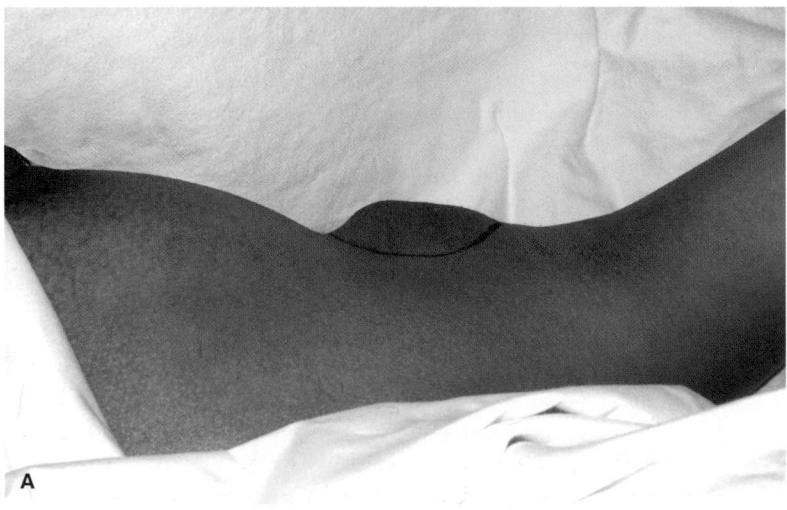
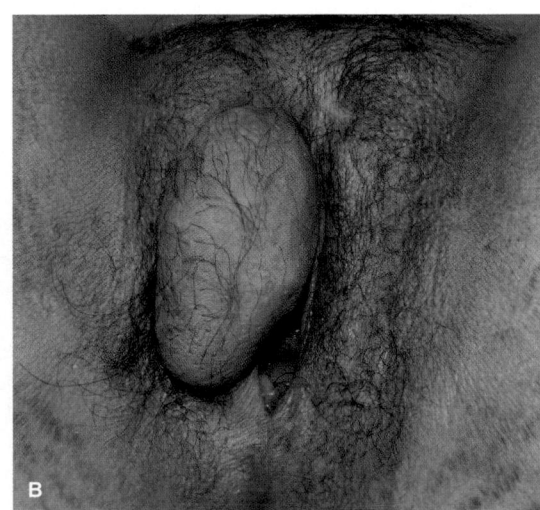

FIGURE 4-12 Ectopic breast tissue in two postpartum patients. **A.** In this patient, axillary ectopic breast tissue required no intervention. Regression followed eventual cessation of breast feeding. **B.** Vulvar ectopic breast tissue. This lesion was excised due to patient discomfort and initially unclear diagnosis. *(Photograph contributed by Dr. Joseph Fitzwater.)*

■ Cystic Vulvar Tumors

Bartholin Gland Duct Cyst and Abscess

Pathophysiology. Mucus produced to moisten the vulva originates in part from the Bartholin glands. Obstruction of this gland's duct is common and may follow infection, trauma, changes in mucus consistency, or congenitally narrowed ducts. However, the underlying cause often is unclear.

In some cases, cyst contents may become infected and lead to abscess formation. These tend to develop in populations with demographic profiles similar to those at high risk for sexually transmitted infections (Aghajanian, 1994). Historically, women with bilateral Bartholin gland duct cysts were assumed to have been infected with *Neisseria gonorrhoeae*. However, studies have demonstrated a wider spectrum of organisms responsible for these cysts and abscesses. Specifically, Tanaka and colleagues (2005) examined 224 patients and isolated approximately two bacterial species per case. In addition, a majority were caused by aerobic bacteria, of which *Escherichia coli* was the most common isolate. Only five cases involved *N gonorrhoeae* or *Chlamydia trachomatis*.

Clinical Findings. Most Bartholin gland duct cysts are small and asymptomatic except for minor discomfort during sexual arousal (Fig. 4-13). With larger or infected cysts, however, patients may complain of severe vulvar pain that precludes walking, sitting, or sexual activity (Fig. 3-27, p. 106).

On physical examination, cysts typically are unilateral, round or ovoid, and fluctuant or tense. If infected, they display surrounding erythema and are tender. The mass is usually located in the inferior labia majora or lower vestibule. Whereas most cysts and abscesses lead to labial asymmetry, smaller cysts may only be detected by palpation. Bartholin abscesses on the verge of spontaneous decompression will exhibit an area of softening, where rupture will most likely occur.

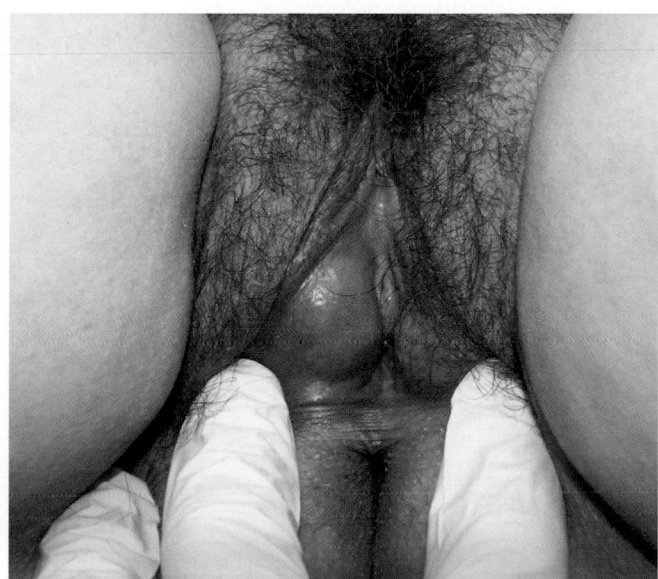

FIGURE 4-13 Bartholin gland duct cyst seen as an asymmetric bulge in the right lower vestibule.

Treatment. Small, asymptomatic Bartholin gland duct cysts require no intervention except exclusion of neoplasia in women older than 40 years. A symptomatic cyst may be managed with one of several techniques. These include incision and drainage (I&D), marsupialization, and Bartholin gland excision, which are described and illustrated in Sections 41-18 through 41-20 (p. 1063). Abscesses are treated with I&D or marsupialization.

Malignancy. After menopause, Bartholin gland duct cysts and abscesses are uncommon and should raise concern for neoplasia. However, carcinoma of the Bartholin gland is rare, and its incidence approximates 0.1 per 100,000 women (Visco, 1996). Most are squamous carcinomas or adenocarcinomas (Copeland, 1986). Given the rarity of these cancers, Bartholin gland excision is typically not indicated. Alternatively, in women older than 40 years, drainage of the cyst and biopsy of suspicious cyst wall sites adequately excludes malignancy (Visco, 1996).

Skene Gland Cyst and Abscess

Ductal occlusion of the Skene gland may lead to cystic enlargement and possible abscess formation. Classically, these lesions can be distinguished during physical examination. Skene gland cysts do not communicate with the urethral lumen and contents are not expressible. Typically, these cysts are located at the distal urethra and often distort the meatus. This is in contrast to most urethral diverticula, which are found most commonly at the mid and proximal urethra.

The etiology remains unknown, although many speculate that infection and trauma are predisposing factors. Main patient symptoms include urinary obstruction, dyspareunia, and pain. The primary treatment of chronic lesions is excision. With acute abscess, either marsupialization or I&D are preferred.

Urethral Diverticulum

The paraurethral glands lie along the inferior urethral wall, and cystic dilatation of one of these glands forms a diverticulum. These sacs often communicate directly with the urethra and bulge into the anterior vaginal wall (Fig. 26-3, p. 683) (Lee, 2005). Although postvoid dribbling is a classic complaint, women may also note pain, dyspareunia, or urinary symptoms. During physical examination, a urethral diverticulum may be palpated as a slight bogginess along the urethral length. Urine or purulent drainage can often be expressed with compression. Urethral diverticula are discussed further in Chapter 26 (p. 683), and their surgical management, which typically involves excision, is illustrated in Section 43-9 (p. 1203).

Epidermoid Cysts

These cysts, also known as *epidermal inclusion cysts* or *sebaceous cysts,* are commonly found on the vulva, and less so in the vagina. Although histologically similar and lined by squamous epithelium, it is unclear if they represent separate entities. Vulvar epidermoid cysts typically form from plugged pilosebaceous units (Fig. 4-14). However, epidermoid cysts can also follow traumatic implantation of epidermal cells into deeper tissues.

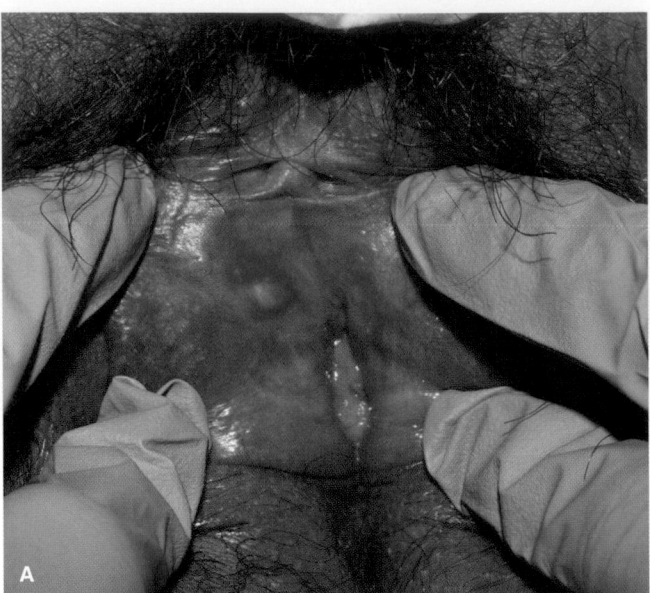
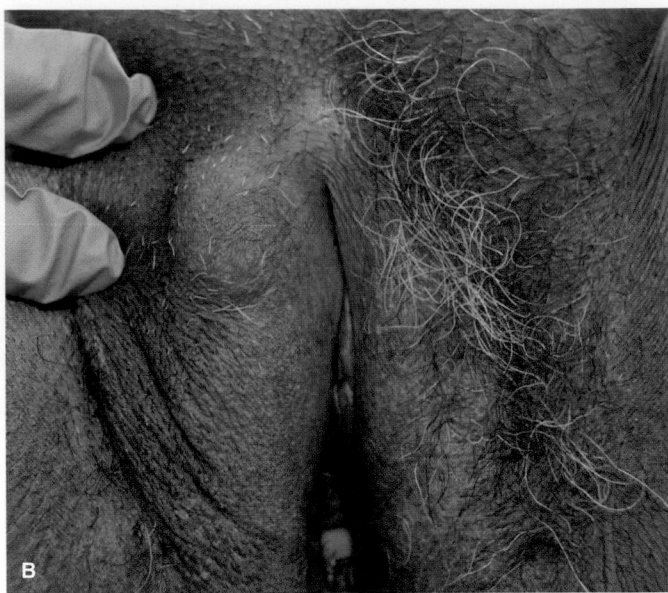

FIGURE 4-14 Epidermal inclusion cysts. **A.** This small lesion on the inner right labia minora required no intervention. **B.** This lesion on the right labia majora was incised and contents expressed due to patient discomfort. It was filled with tan, clay-like material.

Epidermoid cysts are variable in size, typically round or ovoid, and skin colored, yellow, or white. Generally, cysts are filled with viscous, gritty, or caseous foul-smelling material. Epidermoid cysts are generally asymptomatic and require no further evaluation. If symptomatic or secondarily infected, incision and drainage is recommended.

Vulvodynia

In 2003, the ISSVD defined *vulvodynia* as "vulvar discomfort, most often described as burning pain, occurring in the absence of relevant visible findings or a specific, clinically identifiable, neurologic disorder" (Table 4-7) (Moyal-Barracco, 2004b). The term *vestibulitis* was eliminated from ISSVD terminology since inflammatory changes have not been consistently documented. Vulvar pain is described as spontaneous (unprovoked) or triggered by physical pressure (provoked). Provocateurs may include sexual contact, tampon use, or fingertip pressure. Vulvar pain is further categorized as localized or generalized. Like other chronic pain conditions, vulvodynia is enigmatic in its etiology and challenging to treat.

Incidence

Limited studies indicate a prevalence of vulvodynia in the general population of 3 to 11 percent (Lavy, 2007; Reed, 2004). One study estimated that approximately 1 in 50 women will develop vulvodynia each year (Reed, 2008a). Typically, evaluation and management are delayed for years due to patient embarrassment and attempts at self-treatment. Diagnosis and treatment delays, often by multiple providers, are common (Buchan, 2007; Graziottin, 2004; Harlow, 2003). Vulvodynia affects women of all ethnicities over a wide age range that includes preadolescents (Haefner, 2005; Lavy, 2007; Reed, 2008b).

Etiology

Vulvodynia's underlying cause is likely multifactorial and variable among affected individuals. Attempts to identify specific risk factors, such as oral contraceptive pill use or infection (chronic yeast or human papillomavirus), have yielded unconvincing results. Whether predominantly physical or psychosocial factors trigger the pain is controversial, with strong arguments on both sides (Gunter, 2007; Lynch, 2008). Most theories propose that a local injury or noxious stimulus results in maladaptive local and/or central nervous system responses leading to a neuropathic pain syndrome (Chap. 11, p. 306). Interestingly, patients with vulvodynia have an increased prevalence of other chronic pain disorders, including interstitial cystitis, irritable bowel syndrome, fibromyalgia, and temporomandibular pain (Kennedy, 2005; Zolnoun, 2008).

TABLE 4-7. ISSVD Terminology and Classification of Vulvar Pain

A. Vulvar pain related to a specific disorder
  Infectious
  Inflammatory
  Neoplastic
  Neurologic
B. Vulvodynia
  Generalized
  Provoked
  Unprovoked
  Mixed
C. Localized (vestibulodynia, clitorodynia, hemivulvodynia, etc.)
  Provoked
  Unprovoked
  Mixed

ISSVD = International Society for the Study of Vulvovaginal Disease.

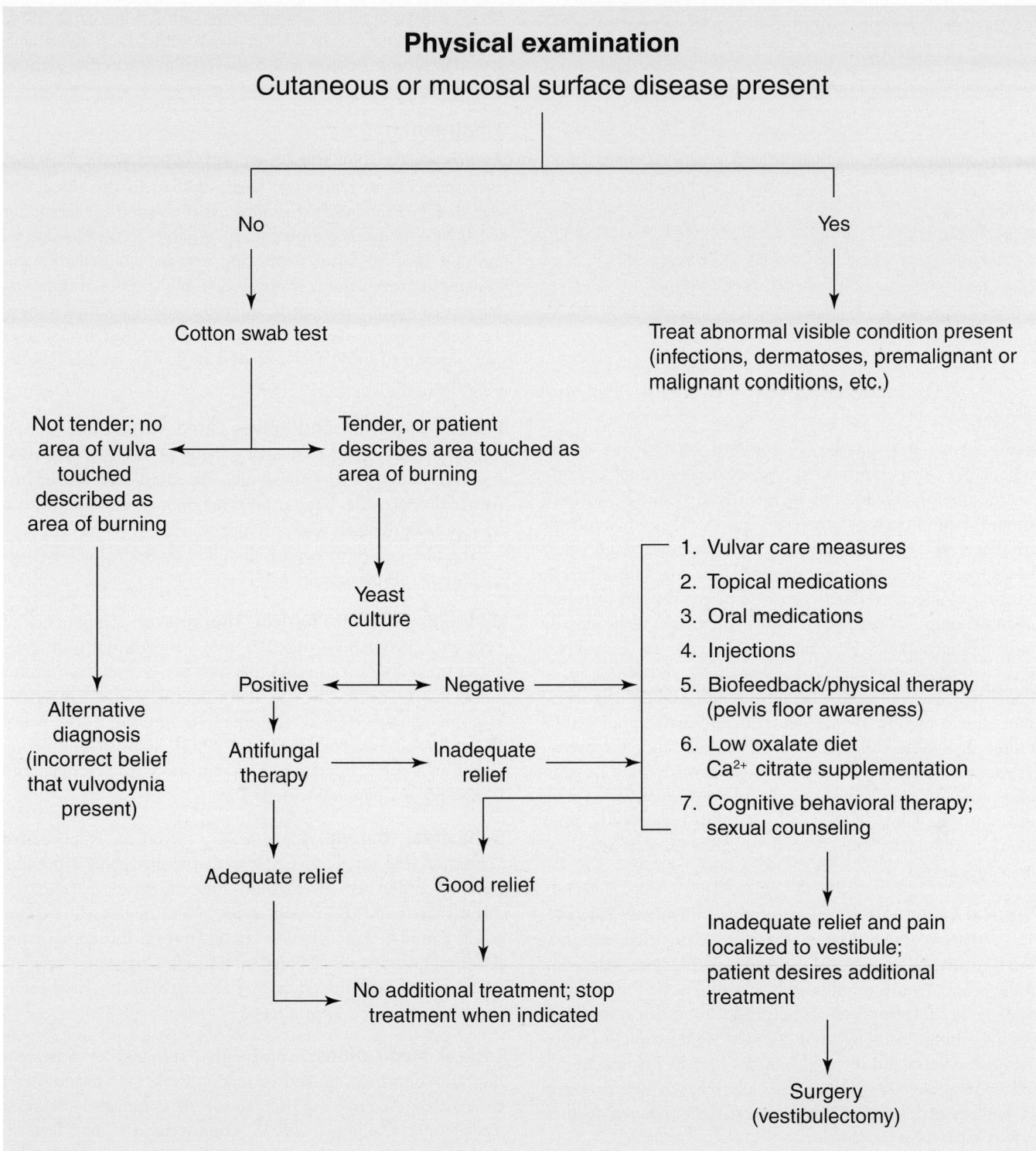

Physical examination

Cutaneous or mucosal surface disease present

No

Yes

Cotton swab test

Treat abnormal visible condition present (infections, dermatoses, premalignant or malignant conditions, etc.)

Not tender; no area of vulva touched described as area of burning

Tender, or patient describes area touched as area of burning

Yeast culture

1. Vulvar care measures
2. Topical medications
3. Oral medications
4. Injections
5. Biofeedback/physical therapy (pelvis floor awareness)
6. Low oxalate diet Ca^{2+} citrate supplementation
7. Cognitive behavioral therapy; sexual counseling

Positive

Negative

Alternative diagnosis (incorrect belief that vulvodynia present)

Antifungal therapy

Inadequate relief

Adequate relief

Good relief

Inadequate relief and pain localized to vestibule; patient desires additional treatment

No additional treatment; stop treatment when indicated

Surgery (vestibulectomy)

FIGURE 4-15 Algorithm for the diagnosis of vulvodynia. *(From Haefner, 2005, with permission.)*

Diagnosis

An evidence-based algorithm for the diagnosis of vulvodynia is provided in Figure 4-15 (Haefner, 2005). Given that vulvodynia is a diagnosis of exclusion, an extensive history is critical to securing the correct diagnosis (Table 4-8) (American College of Obstetricians and Gynecologists, 2006).

History. Vulvodynia refers to vulvar discomfort of at least 3 to 6 months' duration without an identifiable cause. Generalized or localized vulvodynia is described variably as burning, rawness, itching, or cutting pain within affected areas (Bergeron, 2001). Pain may follow a touch stimulus (allodynia) such as tight clothing, undergarments, sexual contact, or pelvic

TABLE 4-8. Questions Appropriate for Investigation of Vulvodynia

When did the pain begin? A precipitating event?
Was the onset gradual or sudden?
Describe the pain and its intensity.
Describe its location. Localized? Generalized?
Aggravating factors? Is it provoked or unprovoked?
Relieving factors?
Prior therapy?
Associated symptoms? Urinary? GI? Dermatologic?
Does pain impact quality of life? Activities?

GI = gastrointestinal.

examination. Sensations may be constant, intermittent, or episodic with exacerbations noted premenstrually (Arnold, 2006).

Questioning should seek to identify frequently associated comorbid conditions or other risk factors. These may include irritable bowel syndrome, interstitial cystitis, psychologic disorders (anxiety, depression, or posttraumatic stress disorder), or a history of infectious diseases such as herpes simplex or zoster. Documentation of past surgical procedures may help identify pudendal nerve injury. A sexual history may reveal clues of past or current abuse, unfavorable coital practices, and contraceptive modalities that could provoke vulvodynia. Additionally, clinicians should inquire about recurrent candidiasis; prior genital trauma, including childbirth-related injuries; and current vulvar care practices. Specifically, questions regarding use of feminine products, panty liners, soaps, and perfumes and type of undergarment fabric worn can be helpful. Importantly, prior therapies should be documented to avoid unnecessary treatment repetition.

Physical Examination. By definition, vulvodynia lacks specific diagnostic physical signs. Therefore, a thorough examination is required to exclude other possible pathologies. Inspection of the external vulva is followed by examination of the vestibular tissue to search for focal, usually mild, erythema at vestibular gland openings. Although not essential, colposcopic investigation of the vulva and directed biopsies may be helpful. Bowen and colleagues (2008) found clinically relevant dermatoses in 61 percent of refractory vulvodynia patients referred to their tertiary care vulvovaginal clinic.

Systematic pain mapping of the vestibule, perineum, and inner thigh is completed and serves as a reference to assess treatment success (see Fig. 4-1). A cotton swab is used to check for allodynia and hyperesthesia. The swab end can first be unwound to form a cotton-fiber wisp. Subsequently, the wooden stick is broken to form a sharp point to retest the same areas. The severity of pain on a 5-point scale should be recorded and followed over time.

Laboratory Testing. No specific laboratory test can diagnose vulvodynia, although a saline "wet prep" of vaginal secretions, vaginal pH testing, and cultures for aerobic bacteria, yeast, and herpes virus can all be helpful in excluding underlying vulvovaginitis (Chap. 3, p. 82). Ulcerative or other focal abnormalities may prompt biopsy and consideration for herpes simplex virus culture.

Treatment

Approximately 1 in 10 women with vulvodynia will experience spontaneous remission (Reed, 2008a). In the absence of well-designed randomized clinical trials, no specific therapy for vulvodynia is deemed superior. In general, a combination of multiple medical forms of therapy may be required to stabilize and improve patient symptoms. In the absence of improvement with medical treatment, surgical excision is a final option. Treatment approaches to vulvodynia are detailed by Haefner and associates (2005) and reviewed by Landry and colleagues (2008).

Patient Education and Vulvar Care. Medical information can be a powerful aid to resolving many of the fears and questions associated with vulvodynia. The National Vulvodynia Association provides patient information and support and can be accessed online at: www.nva.org.

The first step in managing all vulvar disorders includes vulvar care as summarized in Table 4-2.

Biofeedback and Physical Therapy. If components of back pain, pelvic floor muscle spasm, or vaginismus are present, a trained vulvar physical therapist can improve symptoms and coital frequency through use of internal and external massage, myofascial release techniques, acupressure, and pelvic floor muscle retraining (Bergeron, 2002). Steps to completing a thorough pelvic floor muscle examination are described and illustrated in Chapter 11 (p. 313).

Behavioral Therapy. Many believe vulvodynia is more than a psychosexual problem. Compared with the general population, no differences in marital contentment or psychologic distress are found (Bornstein, 1999). Nevertheless, early counseling should include a basic assessment of the intimate partner relationship and of sexual function. Education regarding foreplay, sexual positions, lubrication, and alternatives to vaginal intercourse are offered if appropriate.

Topical Medications. Conservative amounts of 5-percent lidocaine ointment applied to the vestibule 30 minutes prior to sexual intercourse has been shown to significantly decrease dyspareunia (Zolnoun, 2003). Long-term use may lead to healing by minimizing feedback pain amplification. Numerous other topical anesthetic preparations are reported with variable success. However, particular caution should be exercised with benzocaine, which has been associated with increased rates of contact dermatitis.

Eva and colleagues (2003) found decreased estrogen receptor expression in women with vulvodynia. However, topical or intravaginal estrogen therapy has yielded mixed results.

As reported by Boardman and colleagues (2008), topical gabapentin cream is well-tolerated, is effective in the treatment of generalized and localized vulvodynia, and avoids the potential side effects of systemic gabapentin therapy. In their study, 0.5 mL of a 2-, 4-, or 6-percent gabapentin-containing cream was applied three times daily for at least 8 weeks to affected vulvar areas.

Oral Medications. The two major classes of oral medications reported to help vulvodynia are antidepressants and anticonvulsants. Tricyclic antidepressants (TCAs) have become a first-line agent in the treatment of vulvodynia, and reported response rates may reach 47 percent (Munday, 2001). In our experience, amitriptyline started at doses between 5 and 25 mg orally nightly and increased as needed by 10 to 25 mg weekly yields the best results. Final daily doses should not exceed 150 to 200 mg. Importantly, women should remain compliant despite the nearly 4-week lag required to achieve significant pain relief.

Cases resistant to TCAs may be treated with the anticonvulsants gabapentin or carbamazepine (Table 11-5, p. 315) (Ben David, 1999). Oral gabapentin is initiated at a dosage of 100 mg three times daily and gradually increased within 6 to 8 weeks to a maximal daily dose of 3600 mg. Once this dose is reached, pain may be reassessed after 1 to 2 weeks (Haefner, 2005).

Intralesional Injections. In cases of localized vulvodynia, injections using a combination of corticosteroids and local anesthetics have been used (Mandal, 2010; Murina, 2001). Alternatively, the use of botulinum toxin A injections into the levator ani muscles has been reported effective for vulvodynia-related vaginismus (Bertolasi, 2009).

Surgical Therapy. Women with vulvodynia who fail to improve despite aggressive medical therapy are candidates for surgical intervention. Options include local excision of a precise pain locus; complete resection of the vestibule, termed vestibulectomy; or resection of the vestibule and perineum, known as perineoplasty (Section 41-22, p. 1070). Traas and colleagues (2006) reported high success rates with vestibulectomy among women younger than 30 years. Perineoplasty is the most extensive of the three procedures. Its incision extends from just below the urethra to the perineal body, usually terminating above the anal orifice. This procedure may be selected if significant perineal scarring is suspected to contribute to dyspareunia. Overall, improvement rates for appropriately selected patients are high following vulvar excision procedures. However, surgery should be reserved for those with severe localized long-standing vestibular pain who have failed conservative management.

INFECTIOUS LESIONS

Infection is a frequent cause of benign vulvar disease and may involve bacteria, fungi, viruses, or parasites. Ulcerative, proliferative, or suppurative lesions may result, and each is discussed in Chapter 3 (p. 64).

CONGENITAL LESIONS

Structural congenital abnormalities of the lower reproductive tract are uncommon and include those from organ atresia, failure of tissues to regress or to fuse normally, and abnormal hormone signaling. These are discussed in detail in Chapter 18 (p. 481).

VULVOVAGINAL TRAUMA

Hematoma

Given the anatomic location and adipose padding of the adult labia majora, traumatic vulvar and vaginal injuries are rare. Conversely, children lack such well-developed fat pads in the labial area, and activities such as bicycle riding, gymnastics, and bench rails increase their risk of straddle injuries (Virgili, 2000). Less common causes of lower genital tract injury come from coital trauma or assault. A possible sequela of blunt trauma to the relatively vascular vulva is a hematoma.

With a large vulvar hematoma, a general anesthetic may be required for thorough examination of the vulva and vagina. Evaluation can estimate the stability of hematoma size and the integrity of the surrounding bladder, urethra, and rectum. If there is no associated organ injury, the venous nature of most vulvar hematomas makes them candidates for conservative management with cool packs, Foley bladder drainage, and adequate pain control (Propst, 1998).

In general, large vaginal hematomas may require surgical exploration in search of bleeding vessels to secure. An unstable patient may result from retroperitoneal bleeding from a retracted vessel (Gianini, 1991). Postoperatively, a vaginal pack may help tamponade any continued venous leakage.

Laceration

Penetrating trauma accounts for most vaginal injuries. Common causes of trauma include pelvic fracture, forced inanimate objects, coitus, and hydraulic forces such as those experienced with water skiing (Smith, 1996). Atrophic vaginal changes can predispose to injury.

With extensive laceration, examination under anesthesia is often necessary to perform a thorough assessment and to exclude intraperitoneal damage. Moreover, if the peritoneal cavity has been breached, a transabdominal exploration by either laparotomy or laparoscopy is warranted to exclude visceral injury.

Treatment goals include hemostasis and restoration of normal anatomy. Irrigation, debridement, and primary repair are key steps. Uncommonly, infection may require a laceration to be closed by secondary intention. Ultimately, techniques for repairing vulvovaginal trauma are similar to those used for obstetric lacerations.

Sexual Injury

In infants and children, differentiating straddle injury and sexual abuse is often challenging, as injury patterns do not reliably confirm or exclude sexual trauma. Diagnosis requires careful inquiry and correlation of described mechanisms of injury with physical examination findings.

Certain characteristics may serve as alerts for possible sexual abuse. As listed in Table 13-18 (p. 373), these may include genital secretions, concurrent injury at an extragenital site, lack of correlation between history and physical examination, or condyloma acuminata (Dowd, 1994; Emans, 1987). Moreover, injuries to the posterior fourchette; those of the hymeneal area that extend from 3 to 9 o'clock; or vaginal, rectal, or peritoneal perforation should increase suspicion for sexual abuse (Bond, 1995).

In contrast, a unilateral, single, or stellate laceration or bruise in the same shape as the reported blunt object supports a diagnosis of unintentional straddle injury. Lacerations or abrasions of the labia minora, mons pubis, and clitoris that are anterior or lateral to the hymen are typical of this injury.

VAGINAL LESIONS

Foreign Body

Trauma or chronic irritation may be caused by a foreign body placed into the vagina. Females of all ages may be affected, although the objects involved vary by age group. For example, small objects may lodge in a child's vagina during play or self-exploration, whereas an adolescent may complain of being unable to retrieve a forgotten tampon or broken condom. Sexual misadventure or abuse can usually explain the etiology of objects found in adult women. Two items in particular warrant further discussion—the forgotten tampon and vaginal pessary.

Women with a forgotten tampon will typically complain of a foul-smelling vaginal discharge with some associated pruritus, discomfort, or unscheduled bleeding. After further discussion, a history of multiple unsuccessful retrieval attempts may be revealed. In the absence of a leukocytosis, fever, or evidence of an endometritis or salpingitis, simple removal of the tampon is sufficient treatment. Vaginal lavage to cleanse the vagina is not indicated and may actually increase the risk of ascending infection.

Vaginal pessaries are commonly used for the conservative treatment of pelvic organ prolapse or incontinence, and their care is described in Chapter 24 (p. 648). Atrophic vaginal epithelium and inappropriately sized devices increase the risk of ulcerative or erosive complications. Intravaginal estrogen cream for atrophy, monitoring by a health care provider, and periodic removal are helpful to avoid such injuries. Complaints of bloody or foul-smelling discharge should prompt an immediate inspection of the vaginal walls and vault.

Desquamative Inflammatory Vaginitis

This is a rare form of inflammatory vaginitis that occurs primarily in peri- or postmenopausal women. Although the etiology of this vaginitis is unknown, some believe it may represent a variant of erosive vaginal lichen planus (Edwards, 1988). Others note historical triggers such as diarrhea or antibiotic use may precipitate symptoms (Bradford, 2010). Patients typically complain of copious vaginal discharge, introital burning, and dyspareunia, all of which are refractory to common therapies. With examination, a diffuse, exudative, purulent yellow or green discharge and varying degrees of vestibular-vaginal erythema are noted. Microscopy reveals many polymorphonuclear and parabasal cells, but concomitant bacterial or trichomonad forms are absent. The vaginal pH is elevated, and exclusionary test results for gonorrhea and chlamydial infection are negative. Although no randomized

clinical trials are available, Sobel and colleagues (2011) report treatment success with 4 to 5 g of 2-percent clindamycin cream or 10-percent hydrocortisone cream daily intravaginally for 4 to 6 weeks. Whether clindamycin's efficacy is due to its antibacterial action or due to potential antiinflammatory effects is unknown. However, relapse is common.

Diethylstilbestrol-induced Reproductive Tract Abnormalities

In the mid 1900s, diethylstilbestrol (DES), a synthetic nonsteroidal estrogen, was prescribed to women in the United States for a number of pregnancy-related problems. These women's daughters, exposed in utero to DES, show increased rates of vaginal clear cell adenocarcinoma and congenital reproductive tract anomalies (Herbst, 1971). These changes include transverse vaginal septa, circumferential ridges involving the vagina and cervix, and cervical collars of redundant mucosa. Additionally, areas of columnar epithelium within the vaginal squamous mucosa may be found in these women, a condition that is termed *vaginal adenosis*. Vaginal adenosis typically appears red, punctate, and granular. Symptoms include vaginal irritation, discharge, and metrorrhagia, in particular, postcoital bleeding. A fuller discussion of DES-related defects is found in Chapter 18 (p. 502).

Gartner Duct Cyst

These uncommon vaginal cysts develop from remnants of the mesonephric (Wolffian) ducts (Chap. 18, p. 481). They are typically asymptomatic and are usually found within the lateral vaginal wall during routine examination. Symptoms however may include dyspareunia, vaginal pain, and difficulty inserting tampons or other vaginal devices. Examination reveals a tense cyst that is palpable or seen to bulge beneath the lateral vaginal wall. Observation is reasonable in most cases, although marsupialization or excision may be appropriate for symptomatic Gartner duct cysts.

CERVICAL LESIONS

Eversion

The squamocolumnar junction (SCJ) is the border between the columnar epithelium of the endocervix and the squamous epithelium of the ectocervix. As described in Chapter 29 (p. 732), endocervical tissue in some women may migrate outward from the endocervical canal and result in a condition termed eversion or ectropion. As a result, the SCJ lies external to the cervical os. To perform an optimal Pap smear, clinicians must identify and target the SCJ for sampling. Although eversion of the SCJ is a normal finding, asymmetry of the columnar epithelium surrounding the cervical os can mimic an erosive lesion.

Nabothian Cyst

Mucus-secreting columnar cells line the endocervical canal and variable amounts of the ectocervix. During squamous metaplasia,

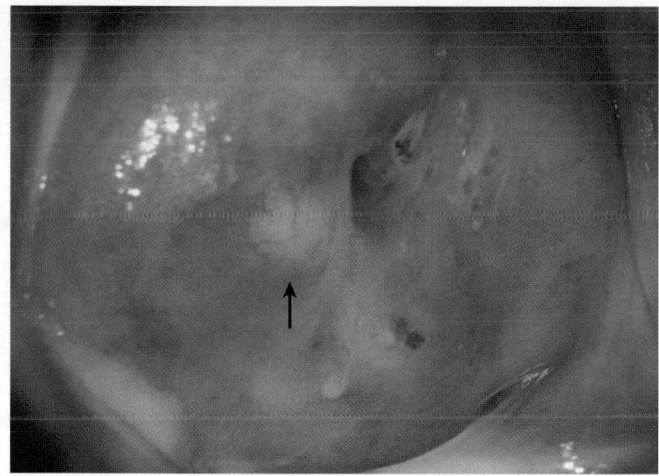

FIGURE 4-16 Cervical nabothian cyst (*arrow*) is seen as a raised, symmetric, smooth, yellow lesion on the ectocervix. Fine, branching blood vessels often course over the surface.

squamous epithelium may cover invaginations of these glandular cells and secretions may accumulate. As this benign process continues, smooth, clear, white or yellow, rounded elevations may form and are visible during routine examination (Fig. 4-16). Nabothian cysts typically warrant no therapy. However, if they grow large enough to make Pap testing or cervical examination difficult, cause symptoms, or need confirmation, they can be opened with a biopsy forceps and drained.

Endocervical Polyp

One of the most common benign neoplasms of the cervix is a hyperplastic projection of the endocervical folds known as an *endocervical polyp* (Fig. 8-14, p. 231). Lesions are usually found during routine cervical surveillance. They are generally asymptomatic but may be associated with leukorrhea or postcoital spotting. Endocervical polyps are rarely malignant, but they are routinely biopsied to remove the entire polyp for pathologic assessment. Additional discussion of management of these lesions is found in Chapter 8 (p. 231).

Cervical Stenosis

Congenital or acquired cervical stenosis commonly involves the internal os. Congenital stenosis is likely due to segmental müllerian hypoplasia. In contrast, postoperative scarring and stenosis of the cervix may result from D&C, cervical conization, loop electrosurgical excision procedure, infection, and neoplasia. Severe atrophic or radiation changes can also be causative.

Symptoms of stenosis in menstruating women include dysmenorrhea, abnormal bleeding, amenorrhea, and infertility. Postmenopausal women are usually asymptomatic until fluid, exudates, or blood accumulates. The terms *hydrometra* (fluid), *pyometra* (pus), or *hematometra* (blood) are used to describe these conditions and are discussed additionally in Chapter 9 (p. 259). An inability to introduce a dilator into the uterine cavity is diagnostic for stenosis. If obstruction is complete, a soft, enlarged uterus is palpable.

Management of cervical stenosis involves dilatation of the cervix with dilators of sequentially increasing diameter. Preoperative misoprostol may aid by softening the cervix Section 42-13 (p. 1157). In postmenopausal women, pretreatment with vaginal estrogen cream for several weeks may assist dilatation. Moreover, sonographic guidance may be useful to avoid uterine perforation, especially in postmenopausal women (Christianson, 2008). Endometrial and endocervical sampling is often indicated in many cases to exclude uterine or cervical malignancy.

Cervical stenosis and its impact on sperm transport and fertility have been poorly studied. As described in Chapter 20 (p. 545), the use of intrauterine insemination (IUI) bypasses the cervix and is a simple and minimally invasive treatment for infertility. IUI is possible for most couples except in cases of severe stenosis.

REFERENCES

Aghajanian A, Bernstein L, Grimes DA: Bartholin's duct abscess and cyst: a case-control study. South Med J 87(1):26, 1994

American College of Obstetricians and Gynecologists: Diagnosis and management of vulvar skin disorders. Practice Bulletin No. 93, May 2008

American College of Obstetricians and Gynecologists: Vulvodynia. Committee Opinion No. 345, October 2006

Anderson M, Kutzner S, Kaufman RH: Treatment of vulvovaginal lichen planus with vaginal hydrocortisone suppositories. Obstet Gynecol 100(2):359, 2002

Arnold LD, Bachmann GA, Rosen R, et al: Vulvodynia: characteristics and associations with comorbidities and quality of life. Obstet Gynecol 107(3): 617, 2006

Assmann T, Becker-Wegerich P, Grewe M, et al: Tacrolimus ointment for the treatment of vulvar lichen sclerosus. J Am Acad Dermatol 48(6):935, 2003

Barth JH, Layton AM, Cunliffe WJ: Endocrine factors in pre- and postmenopausal women with hidradenitis suppurativa. Br J Dermatol 134(6):1057, 1996

Ben David B, Friedman M: Gabapentin therapy for vulvodynia. Anesth Analg 89(6):1459, 1999

Bergeron S, Binik YM, Khalife S, et al: Vulvar vestibulitis syndrome: reliability of diagnosis and evaluation of current diagnostic criteria. Obstet Gynecol 98(1):45, 2001

Bergeron S, Brown C, Lord MJ, et al: Physical therapy for vulvar vestibulitis syndrome: a retrospective study. J Sex Marital Ther 28(3):183, 2002

Bertolasi L, Frasson E, Cappelletti JY, et al: Botulinum neurotoxin type A injections for vaginismus secondary to vulvar vestibulitis syndrome. Obstet Gynecol 114:1008, 2009

Boardman LA, Cooper AS, Blais LR, et al: Topical gabapentin in the treatment of localized and generalized vulvodynia. Obstet Gynecol 112:579, 2008

Boissy RE, Nordlund JJ: Molecular basis of congenital hypopigmentary disorders in humans: a review. Pigment Cell Res 10(1-2):12, 1997

Bond GR, Dowd MD, Landsman I, et al: Unintentional perineal injury in prepubescent girls: a multicenter, prospective report of 56 girls. Pediatrics 95(5):628, 1995

Bor S, Feiwel M, Chanarin I: Vitiligo and its aetiological relationship to organ-specific autoimmune disease. Br J Dermatol 81(2):83, 1969

Bornstein J, Heifetz S, Kellner Y, et al: Clobetasol dipropionate 0.05% versus testosterone propionate 2% topical application for severe vulvar lichen sclerosus. Am J Obstet Gynecol 178(1 Pt 1):80, 1998

Bornstein J, Zarfati D, Goldik Z, et al: Vulvar vestibulitis: physical or psychosexual problem? Obstet Gynecol 93(5 Pt 2):876, 1999

Bowen AR, Vester A, Marsden L, et al: The role of vulvar skin biopsy in the evaluation of chronic vulvar pain. Am J Obstet Gynecol 199(5):467.e-1, 2008

Bradford J, Fischer G: Desquamative inflammatory vaginitis: differential diagnosis and alternate diagnostic criteria. J Low Genit Tract Dis 14(4): 306, 2010

Brook I, Frazier EH: Aerobic and anaerobic microbiology of axillary hidradenitis suppurativa. J Med Microbiol 48(1):103, 1999

Buchan A, Munday P, Ravenhill G, et al: A qualitative study of women with vulvodynia. J Reprod Med 52:15, 2007

Byrd JA, Davis MDP, Rogers RS III: Recalcitrant symptomatic vulvar lichen planus. Arch Dermatol 140(6):715, 2004

Cattaneo A, Carli P, De Marco A, et al: Testosterone maintenance therapy. Effects on vulvar lichen sclerosus treated with clobetasol propionate. J Reprod Med 41(2):99, 1996

Christianson MS, Barker MA, Lindheim SR: Overcoming the challenging cervix: techniques to access the uterine cavity. J Low Genit Tract Dis 12(1):24, 2008

Clark JA, Muller SA: Lichen sclerosus et atrophicus in children. A report of 24 cases. Arch Dermatol 95(5):476, 1967

Copeland LJ, Sneige N, Gershenson DM, et al: Bartholin gland carcinoma. Obstet Gynecol 67(6):794, 1986

Cooper SM, Wojnarowska F: Influence of treatment of erosive lichen planus of the vulva on its prognosis. Arch Dermatol 142(3):289, 2006

Crone AM, Stewart EJ, Wojnarowska F, et al: Aetiological factors in vulvar dermatitis. J Eur Acad Dermatol Venereol 14(3):181, 2000

Cruz PD Jr, Hud JA Jr: Excess insulin binding to insulin-like growth factor receptors: proposed mechanism for acanthosis nigricans. J Invest Dermatol 98(Suppl 6):82S, 1992

Demir S, Demir Y: Acrochordon and impaired carbohydrate metabolism. Acta Diabetol 39(2):57, 2002

der Werth JM, Williams HC: The natural history of hidradenitis suppurativa. J Eur Acad Dermatol Venereol 14(5):389, 2000

Dowd MD, Fitzmaurice L, Knapp JF, et al: The interpretation of urogenital findings in children with straddle injuries. J Pediatr Surg 29(1):7, 1994

Edwards L, Friedrich EG Jr: Desquamative vaginitis: lichen planus in disguise. Obstet Gynecol 71:832, 1988

Eichner R, Kahn M, Capetola RJ, et al: Effects of topical retinoids on cytoskeletal proteins: implications for retinoid effects on epidermal differentiation. J Invest Dermatol 98(2):154, 1992

Eisen D: The therapy of oral lichen planus. Crit Rev Oral Biol Med 4:141, 1993

Eisen D, Ellis CN, Duell EA, et al: Effect of topical cyclosporine rinse on oral lichen planus. A double-blind analysis. N Engl J Med 323(5):290, 1990

Emans SJ, Woods ER, Flagg NT, et al: Genital findings in sexually abused, symptomatic and asymptomatic, girls. Pediatrics 79(5):778, 1987

Eva LJ, MacLean AB, Reid WM, et al: Estrogen receptor expression in vulvar vestibulitis syndrome. Am J Obstet Gynecol 189(2):458, 2003

Farage M, Maibach HI: The vulvar epithelium differs from the skin: implications for cutaneous testing to address topical vulvar exposures. Contact Dermatitis 51(4):201, 2004

Fischer GO: The commonest causes of symptomatic vulvar disease: a dermatologist's perspective. Australas J Dermatol 37(1):12, 1996

Fisher AA: Allergic reaction to feminine hygiene sprays. Arch Dermatol 108(6):801, 1973

Friedrich EG Jr: Vulvar dystrophy. Clin Obstet Gynecol 28(1):178, 1985

Friedrich EG Jr, Kalra PS: Serum levels of sex hormones in vulvar lichen sclerosus, and the effect of topical testosterone. N Engl J Med 310(8):488, 1984

Frieling U, Bonsmann G, Schwarz T, et al: Treatment of severe lichen planus with mycophenolate mofetil. J Am Acad Dermatol 49:1063, 2003

Gelfand JM Stern RS, Nijsten T: The prevalence of psoriasis in African Americans: results from a population-based study. J Am Acad Dermatol 52(1):23, 2005

Gener G, Canoui-Poitrine F, Revuz JE, et al: Combination therapy with clindamycin and rifampicin for hidradenitis suppurativa: a series of 116 consecutive patients. Dermatology 219(2):148, 2009

Gianini GD, Method MW, Christman JE: Traumatic vulvar hematomas. Assessing and treating nonobstetric patients. Postgrad Med 89(4):115, 1991

Goldstein AT, Burrows LJ: Surgical treatment of clitoral phimosis caused by lichen sclerosus. Am J Obstet Gynecol 196(2):126.e-1, 2007

Goldstein AT, Creasey A, Pfau R et al: A double-blind, randomized controlled trial of clobetasol versus pimecrolimus in patients with vulvar lichen sclerosus. J Am Acad Dermatol 64(6):e99, 2011

Goldstein AT, Metz A: Vulvar lichen planus. Clin Obstet Gynecol 48(4):818, 2005

Goolamali SK, Barnes EW, Irvine WJ, et al: Organ-specific antibodies in patients with lichen sclerosus. Br Med J 4(5936):78, 1974

Graziottin A, Brotto LA: Vulvar vestibulitis syndrome: a clinical approach. J Sex Marital Ther 30(3):125, 2004

Griffiths CE, Clark CM, Chalmers RJ, et al: A systematic review of treatments for severe psoriasis. Health Technol Assess 4(40):1, 2000

Grimes PE: New insights and new therapies in vitiligo. JAMA 293(6):730, 2005

Gunter J: Vulvodynia: new thoughts on a devastating condition. Obstet Gynecol Surv 62(12):812, 2007

Haefner HK, Collins ME, Davis GD, et al: The vulvodynia guideline. J Low Genit Tract Dis 9(1):40, 2005

Harlow BL, Stewart EG: A population-based assessment of chronic unexplained vulvar pain: have we underestimated the prevalence of vulvodynia? J Am Med Womens Assoc 58(2):82, 2003

Helm KF, Gibson LE, Muller SA: Lichen sclerosus et atrophicus in children and young adults. Pediatr Dermatol 8(2):97, 1991

Hengge UR, Krause W, Hofmann H, et al: Multicentre, phase II trial on the safety and efficacy of topical tacrolimus ointment for the treatment of lichen sclerosus. Br J Dermatol 155(5):1021, 2006

Herbst AL, Ulfelder H, Poskanzer DC: Adenocarcinoma of the vagina. Association of maternal stilbestrol therapy with tumor appearance in young women. N Engl J Med 284:878, 1971

Hermanns-Le T, Scheen A, Pierard GE: Acanthosis nigricans associated with insulin resistance: pathophysiology and management. Am J Clin Dermatol 5(3):199, 2004

Hersle K, Mobacken H, Sloberg K, et al: Severe oral lichen planus: treatment with an aromatic retinoid (etretinate). Br J Dermatol 106(1):77, 1982

Higgins SP, Freemark M, Prose NS: Acanthosis nigricans: a practical approach to evaluation and management. Dermatol Online J 14(9):2, 2008

Hillemanns P, Untch M, Prove F, et al: Photodynamic therapy of vulvar lichen sclerosus with 5-aminolevulinic acid. Obstet Gynecol 93(1):71, 1999

Janniger CK, Schwartz RA, Szepietowski JC, et al: Intertrigo and common secondary skin infections. Am Fam Physician 72(5):833, 2005

Jemec GB, Faber M, Gutschik E, et al: The bacteriology of hidradenitis suppurativa. Dermatology 193(3):203, 1996

Jemec GB, Wendelboe P: Topical clindamycin versus systemic tetracycline in the treatment of hidradenitis suppurativa. J Am Acad Dermatol 39(6):971, 1998

Kahana M, Levy A, Schewach-Millet M, et al: Appearance of lupus erythematosus in a patient with lichen sclerosus et atrophicus of the elbows. J Am Acad Dermatol 12(1 Pt 1):127, 1985

Kaufman RH, Gardner HL, Brown D Jr, et al: Vulvar dystrophies: an evaluation. Am J Obstet Gynecol 120(3):363, 1974

Kennedy CM, Nygaard IE, Saftlas A, et al: Vulvar disease: a pelvic floor pain disorder? Am J Obstet Gynecol 192:1829, 2005

Kligman AM, Grove GL, Hirose R, et al: Topical tretinoin for photoaged skin. J Am Acad Dermatol 15(4 Pt 2):836, 1986a

Kligman LH: Effects of all-*trans*-retinoic acid on the dermis of hairless mice. J Am Acad Dermatol 15(4 Pt 2):779, 1986b

Krengel S: Nevogenesis—new thoughts regarding a classical problem. Am J Dermatopathol 27(5):456, 2005

Kunstfeld R, Kirnbauer R, Stingl G, et al: Successful treatment of vulvar lichen sclerosus with topical tacrolimus. Arch Dermatol 139(7):850, 2003

Landry T, Bergeron S, Dupuis MJ, et al: The treatment of provoked vestibulodynia. Clin J Pain 24:155, 2008

Lavy RJ, Hynan LS, Haley RW: Prevalence of vulvar pain in an urban, minority population. J Reprod Med 52:59, 2007

Lee JW, Fynes MM: Female urethral diverticula. Best Pract Res Clin Obstet Gynaecol 19 (6):875, 2005

Leung DY, Boguniewicz M, Howell MD, et al: New insights into atopic dermatitis. J Clin Invest 113(5):651, 2004

Lundqvist EN, Wahlin YB, Hofer PA: Methotrexate supplemented with steroid ointments for the treatment of severe erosive lichen ruber. Acta Derm Venereol 82:63, 2002

Lynch PJ: Lichen simplex chronicus (atopic/neurodermatitis) of the anogenital region. Dermatol Ther 17(1):8, 2004

Lynch PJ: Vulvodynia as a somatoform disorder. J Reprod Med 53:390, 2008

Lynch PJ, Moyal-Barracco M, Bogliatto F, et al: 2006 ISSVD classification of vulvar dermatoses: pathological subsets and their clinical correlates. J Reprod Med 52(1):3, 2007

Mandal D, Nunns D, Byrne M, et al: Guidelines for the management of vulvodynia. Br J Dermatol 162(6):1180, 2010

Mann MS, Kaufman RH: Erosive lichen planus of the vulva. Clin Obstet Gynecol 34(3):605, 1991

Margesson LJ: Contact dermatitis of the vulva. Dermatol Ther 17(1):20, 2004

Marren P, Wojnarowska F, Powell S: Allergic contact dermatitis and vulvar dermatoses. Br J Dermatol 126(1):52, 1992

Mazdisnian F, Degregorio F, Mazdisnian F, et al: Intralesional injection of triamcinolone in the treatment of lichen sclerosus. J Reprod Med 44(4):332, 1999

Mirowski GW, Edwards L: Diagnostic and therapeutic procedures. In Edwards L, (ed): Genital Dermatology Atlas. Philadelphia, Lippincott Williams and Wilkins, 2004, p 9

Mistiaen P, Poot E, Hickox S, et al: Preventing and treating intertrigo in the large skin folds of adults: a literature overview. Dermatol Nurs 16(1):43, 2004

Morrison L, Kratochvil FJ III, Gorman A: An open trial of topical tacrolimus for erosive oral lichen planus. J Am Acad Dermatol 47(4):617, 2002

Mortimer PS, Dawber RP, Gales MA: Mediation of hidradenitis suppurativa by androgens. Br Med J (Clin Res Ed) 292(6515):245, 1986

Moyal-Barracco M, Edwards L : Diagnosis and therapy of anogenital lichen planus. Dermatol Ther 17(1):38, 2004a

Moyal-Barracco M, Lynch PJ: 2003 ISSVD terminology and classification of vulvodynia: a historical perspective. J Reprod Med 49(10):772, 2004b

Munday PE: Response to treatment in dysaesthetic vulvodynia. J Obstet Gynaecol 21(6):610, 2001

Murina F, Tassan P, Roberti P, et al: Treatment of vulvar vestibulitis with submucous infiltrations of methylprednisolone and lidocaine. An alternative approach. J Reprod Med 46(8):713, 2001

Neill SM, Tatnall FM, Cox NH: Guidelines for the management of lichen sclerosus. Br J Dermatol 147(4):640, 2002

Nielsen GP, Rosenberg AE, Koerner FC, et al: Smooth-muscle tumors of the vulva. A clinicopathological study of 25 cases and review of the literature. Am J Surg Pathol 20(7):779, 1996

Paslin D: Androgens in the topical treatment of lichen sclerosus. Int J Dermatol 35(4):298, 1996

Pelisse M: The vulvo-vaginal-gingival syndrome. A new form of erosive lichen planus. Int J Dermatol 28(6):381, 1989

Poskitt L, Wojnarowska F: Lichen sclerosus as a cutaneous manifestation of thyroid disease. J Am Acad Dermatol 28(4):665, 1993

Powell J, Wojnarowska F: Childhood vulvar lichen sclerosus: an increasingly common problem. J Am Acad Dermatol 44(5):803, 2001

Propst AM, Thorp JM Jr: Traumatic vulvar hematomas: conservative versus surgical management. South Med J 91(2):144, 1998

Reed BD, Crawford S, Couper M, et al: Pain at the vulvar vestibule: a web-based survey. J Low Genit Tract Dis 8:48, 2004

Reed BD, Haefner HK, Sen A, et al: Vulvodynia incidence and remission rates among adult women. Obstet Gynecol 112:231, 2008a

Reed DR, Cantor LE: Vulvodynia in preadolescent girls. J Low Genit Tract Dis 12(4):257, 2008b

Rhode JM, Burke WM, Cederna PS, et al: Outcomes of surgical management of stage III vulvar hidradenitis suppurativa. J Reprod Med 53:420, 2008

Rogers RS III: Complex aphthosis. Adv Exp Med Biol 528:311, 2003

Rogers RS III: Recurrent aphthous stomatitis: clinical characteristics and associated systemic disorders. Semin Cutan Med Surg 16(4):278, 1997

Romo A, Benavides S: Treatment options in insulin resistance obesity-related acanthosis nigricans. Ann Pharmacother 42(7):1090, 2008

Rouzier R, Haddad B, Deyrolle C, et al: Perineoplasty for the treatment of introital stenosis related to vulvar lichen sclerosus. Am J Obstet Gynecol 186(1):49, 2002

Sideri M, Origoni M, Spinaci L, et al: Topical testosterone in the treatment of vulvar lichen sclerosus. Int J Gynaecol Obstet 46(1):53, 1994

Smith BL: Vaginal laceration caused by water skiing. J Emerg Nurs 22(2):156, 1996

Smith CH, Anstey AV, Barker JN, et al: British Association of Dermatologists' guideline for biologic interventions for psoriasis 2009. Br J Dermatol 161(5):987, 2009

Smith CH, Barker JN: Psoriasis and its management. BMJ 333(7564):380, 2006

Sobel JD, Reichman O, Misra D, et al: Prognosis and Treatment of Desquamative Inflammatory Vaginitis. Obstet Gynecol 117(4):850, 2011

Spergel JM, Paller AS: Atopic dermatitis and the atopic march. J Allergy Clin Immunol 112(Suppl 6):S118, 2003

Tanaka K, Mikamo H, Ninomiya M, et al: Microbiology of Bartholin's gland abscess in Japan. J Clin Microbiol 43(8):4258, 2005

Torgerson RR, Marnach ML, Bruce AJ, et al: Oral and vulvar changes in pregnancy. Clin Dermatol 24(2):122, 2006

Traas MA, Bekkers RL, Dony JM, et al: Surgical treatment for the vulvar vestibulitis syndrome. Obstet Gynecol 107(2 Pt 1):256, 2006

U.S. Food and Drug Administration: Tacrolimus (marketed as Protopic Ointment) Information, 2010. Available at: http://www.fda.gov/Drugs/DrugSafety/PostmarketDrugSafetyInformationforPatientsandProviders/ucm107845.htm. Accessed May 1, 2010

Varani J, Nickoloff BJ, Dixit VM, et al: All-*trans* retinoic acid stimulates growth of adult human keratinocytes cultured in growth factor-deficient medium, inhibits production of thrombospondin and fibronectin, and reduces adhesion. J Invest Dermatol 93(4):449, 1989

Virgili A, Bacilieri S, Corazza M: Evaluation of contact sensitization in vulvar lichen simplex chronicus. A proposal for a battery of selected allergens. J Reprod Med 48(1):33, 2003

Virgili A, Bianchi A, Mollica G, et al: Serious hematoma of the vulva from a bicycle accident. A case report. J Reprod Med 45(8):662, 2000

Virgili A, Corazza M, Bianchi A, et al: Open study of topical 0.025% tretinoin in the treatment of vulvar lichen sclerosus. One year of therapy. J Reprod Med 40(9):614, 1995

Visco AG, Del Priore G: Postmenopausal Bartholin gland enlargement: a hospital-based cancer risk assessment. Obstet Gynecol 87(2):286, 1996

Wallace HJ: Lichen sclerosus et atrophicus. Trans St Johns Hosp Dermatol Soc 57(1):9, 1971

Wolff K, Johnson RA: Disorders of sebaceous and apocrine glands. In Fitzpatrick's Color Atlas & Synopsis of Clinical Dermatology, 6th ed. New York, McGraw-Hill, 2009. Available at: http://www.accessmedicine.com/popup.aspx?aID=5185916. Accessed May 22, 2010

Zellis S, Pincus SH: Treatment of vulvar dermatoses. Semin Dermatol 15(1):71, 1996

Zhang XJ, Chen JJ, Liu JB: The genetic concept of vitiligo. J Dermatol Sci 39(3):137, 2005

Zolnoun DA, Hartmann KE, Steege JF: Overnight 5% lidocaine ointment for treatment of vulvar vestibulitis. Obstet Gynecol 102(1):84, 2003

Zolnoun DA, Rohl J, Moore CG, et al: Overlap between orofacial pain and vulvar vestibulitis syndrome. Clin J Pain 24:187, 2008

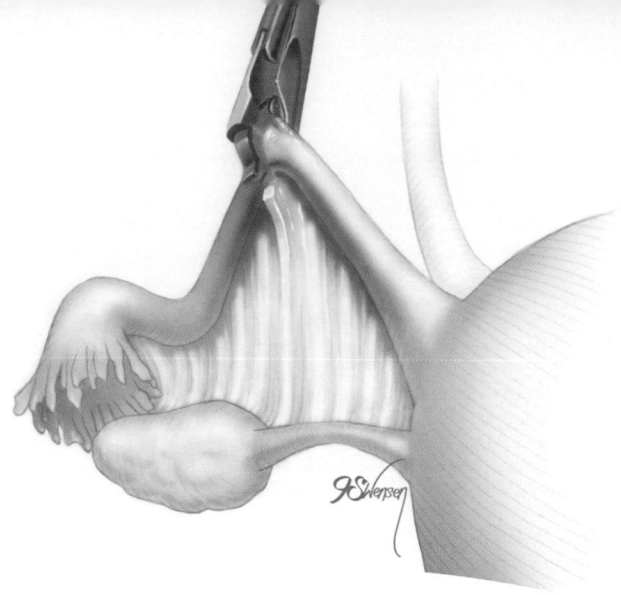

CHAPTER 5

Contraception and Sterilization

Today, an ever-increasing variety of effective methods is available for fertility regulation. Although none is completely without side effects or potential danger, it remains axiomatic that contraception poses fewer risks than pregnancy (Table 5-1). Contraceptive availability is paramount for the care of women as many as half of pregnancies in the United States are unintended. Moreover, in half of these, women were using contraception at the time of conception (Henshaw, 1998). These statistics have prompted a reexamination of contraceptive counseling to prevent unplanned pregnancy (American College of Obstetricians and Gynecologists, 2009b; Grimes, 2009a; Steiner, 2006).

Methods are now grouped according to their effectiveness rather than by type of contraception. *Top-tier* or *first-tier methods* are those that are most effective and are characterized by their ease of use (Fig. 5-1). These methods require only minimal user motivation or intervention and have an unintended pregnancy rate of less than 2 per 100 women during the first year of use (Table 5-2). As expected, these first-tier methods provide the longest duration of contraception after initiation and require the fewest number of return visits. Top-tier methods include intrauterine contraceptive devices, contraceptive implants, and various methods of male and female sterilization. A reduction in unintended pregnancies can be better achieved by increasing the use of these top-tier methods. Thus, although counseling is provided for all contraceptive methods, common misperceptions regarding some of the top-tier methods—especially intrauterine contraception—can also be dispelled (Picardo, 2003).

Second-tier methods include systemic hormonal contraceptives that are available as oral tablets, intramuscular injections, transdermal patches, or transvaginal rings. In sum, their expected failure rate is 3 to 9 percent per 100 users during the first year. This higher rate likely reflects failure to redose at the appropriate interval. Automated reminder systems for these second-tier methods have been repeatedly shown to be ineffective (Halpern, 2006; Hou, 2010).

Third-tier methods include barrier methods for men and women as well as fertility awareness methods such as cycle beads. Their expected failure rate is 10 to 20 percent per 100 users in the first year, however, efficacy increases with

TABLE 5-1. Pregnancy-Related or Method-Related Deaths per 100,000 Fertile Women by Age Group

Method	15–24 Years	25–34 Years	35–44 Years
Pregnancy	5.1	5.5	13.4
Abortion	2.0	1.8	13.4
Intrauterine device	0.2	0.2	0.4
Rhythm, withdrawal	1.3	1.0	1.3
Barrier method	1.0	1.3	2.0
Spermicides	1.8	1.7	2.1
Oral contraceptives	1.1	1.5	1.4
Implants/injectables	0.4	0.6	0.5
Tubal sterilization	1.2	1.1	1.2
Vasectomy	0.1	0.1	0.1

Modified from Harlap, 1991, with permission.

consistent and correct use (American College of Obstetricians and Gynecologists, 2009b).

Fourth-tier methods include spermicidal preparations, which have a failure rate of 21 to 30 percent per 100 first-year users. The withdrawal method is so unpredictable that some have concluded that it does not belong among other contraceptive methods (Doherty, 2009).

MEDICAL ELIGIBILITY CRITERIA

The World Health Organization (2010) has provided evidence-based guidance for the use of all highly effective reversible contraceptive methods by women with various health factors. These guidelines were provided for use by individual countries that then would develop recommendations specific to their circumstances. The Centers for Disease Control and Prevention (2010b, 2011) published *United States Medical Eligibility Criteria (US MEC)* for contraceptive use in the United States. These US MEC guidelines are available and updated regularly at the CDC web site: http://www.cdc.gov/reproductivehealth/UnintendedPregnancy/USMEC.htm. In the US MEC, many

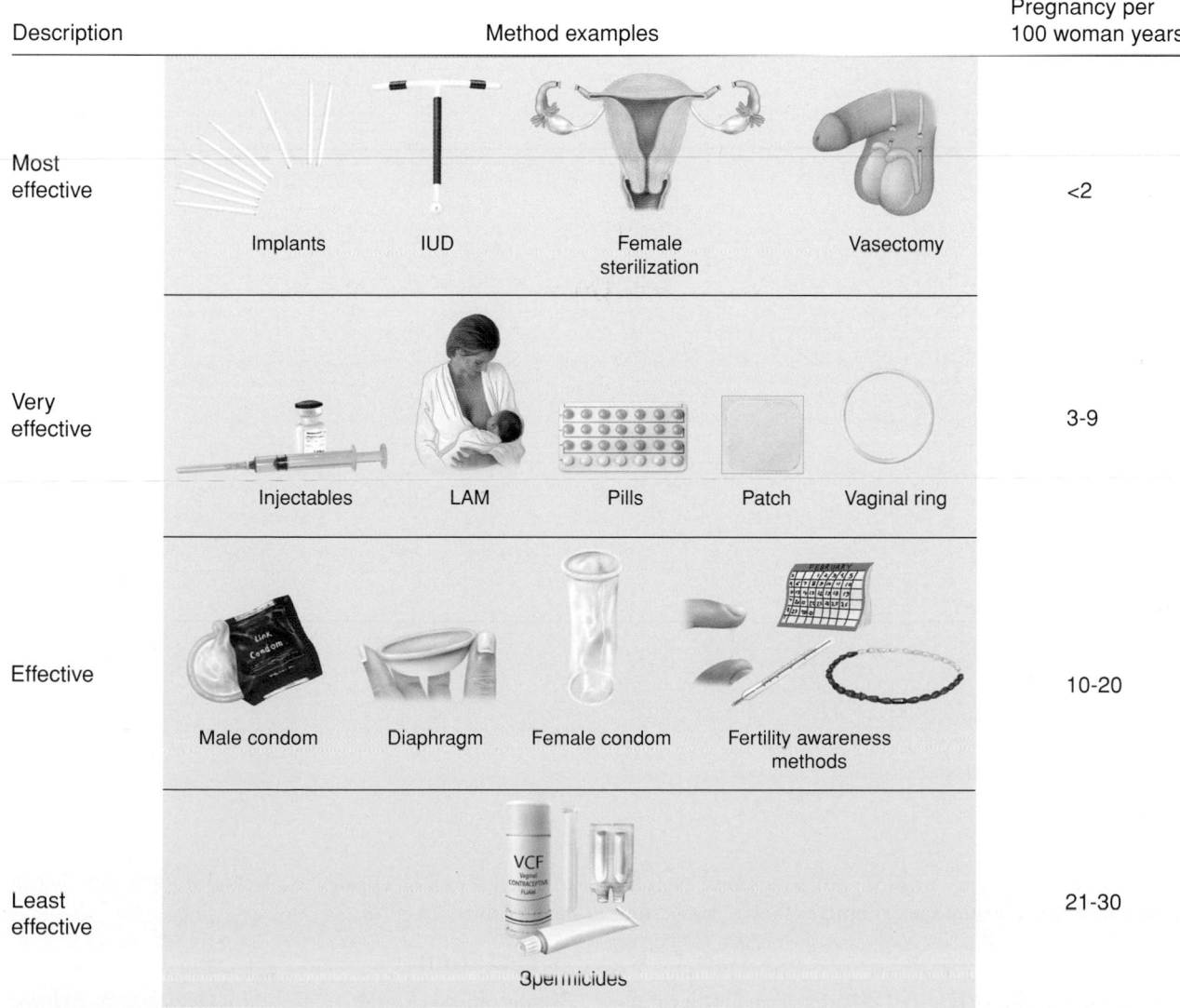

Description	Method examples	Pregnancy per 100 woman years
Most effective	Implants · IUD · Female sterilization · Vasectomy	<2
Very effective	Injectables · LAM · Pills · Patch · Vaginal ring	3-9
Effective	Male condom · Diaphragm · Female condom · Fertility awareness methods	10-20
Least effective	Spermicides	21-30

FIGURE 5-1 Contraceptive effectiveness chart. *(Adapted from World Health Organization, 2007.)*

TABLE 5-2. Percentage of Women Experiencing an Unintended Pregnancy During the First Year of Typical Use and the First Year of Perfect Use of Contraception and the Percentage Continuing Use at the End of the First Year. United States

Method	% of Women Experiencing an Unintended Pregnancy within the First Year of Use		% of Women Continuing Use at 1 Year
	Typical Use	Perfect Use	
No method	85	85	
Spermicides	28	18	42
Fertility awareness-based methods	24		47
Standard Days method		5	
Two Day method		4	
Ovulation method		3	
Symptothermal method		0.4	
Withdrawal	22	4	46
Sponge			36
Parous women	24	20	
Nulliparous women	12	9	
Condom			
Female (fc)	21	5	41
Male	18	2	43
Diaphragm	12	6	57
Combined pill and progestin-only pill	9	0.3	67
Evra patch	9	0.3	67
NuvaRing	9	0.3	67
Depo-Provera	6	0.2	56
Intrauterine contraceptives			
ParaGard (copper T)	0.8	0.6	78
Mirena (LNG)	0.2	0.2	80
Implanon	0.05	0.05	84
Female sterilization	0.5	0.5	100
Male sterilization	0.15	0.10	

Emergency Contraceptives: Emergency contraceptive pills or insertion of a copper intrauterine contraceptive after unprotected intercourse substantially reduces the risk of pregnancy.
Lactational Amenorrhea Method: LAM is a highly effective, *temporary* method of contraception.
LNG-IUS = levonorgestrel intrauterine system.
From Trussell, 2011, with permission.

contraceptive methods are classified into six groups by their similarity: combination oral contraceptive (COC), progestin-only pill (POP), depot medroxyprogesterone acetate (DMPA), implants, levonorgestrel intrauterine device (LNG-IUD), and copper intrauterine device (Cu-IUD). For a given health condition, each of these methods is rated or categorized (1 through 4) to describe its safety profile in a typical woman with that condition (Table 5-3).

Lactation

Among others, lactation is one health factor addressed in the US MEC guidelines. Approximately 20 percent of breast-feeding

TABLE 5-3. Categories within the U.S. Medical Eligibility Criteria

Category	Definition
1	A condition for which there is no restriction for the use of the contraceptive method
2	A condition for which the advantages of using the method generally outweigh the theoretical or proven risks
3	A condition for which the theoretical or proven risks usually outweigh the advantages of using the method
4	A condition that represents an unacceptable health risk if the contraceptive method is used

Centers for Disease Control and Prevention, 2010b.

women will ovulate by 3 months postpartum. Ovulation often precedes menstruation, and these women are at risk for unplanned pregnancy. For women who breast-feed intermittently, effective contraception should begin as if they were not breast-feeding. Moreover, contraception is essential after the first menses unless pregnancy is planned.

Of available methods, copper-containing intrauterine contraception in breast-feeding women has a category 1 or 2 rating, that is, the advantages consistently outweigh the risks. Because progestin-only oral contraceptives have little effect on lactation, they are also preferred by some for use up to 6 months in women who are exclusively breast-feeding. According to the American Academy of Pediatrics and the American College of Obstetricians and Gynecologists (2007), progestin-only contraception may be initiated at 6 weeks postpartum for those exclusively breast-feeding or at 3 weeks if not exclusively. Combination hormone contraception may begin at 6 weeks following delivery, if breast-feeding is well established and the infant's nutritional status is surveilled. This may be initiated as early as 4 weeks after delivery if compliance with later-scheduled postpartum follow-up is a concern and if venous thromboembolism (VTE) risks are absent. The CDC (2011) revised the US MEC guidelines regarding the use of combined hormonal contraception during the puerperium due to the higher risk of VTE during these weeks. The new guidelines are found in Table 5-4.

Concerns regarding hormonal contraceptive use with breast-feeding are based on the theoretical and biologically plausible—but unproven—possibility that systemic progestins may interfere with breast milk production. Importantly, hormonal contraceptives are not purported to harm the quality of breast milk. Minute quantities of the hormones are excreted in breast milk, but no adverse effects on infants have been reported. In their Cochrane review, Truitt and coworkers (2010) summarized the lack of evidence to support a negative impact of hormonal contraception on lactation. Of five studies analyzed, they concluded that all were of poor quality. The one study reporting a negative impact of combination oral contraceptives was significantly limited by a high loss of patient follow-up. They concluded that randomized trials are needed.

Adolescence and Perimenopause

Females at both ends of the reproductive spectrum have unique contraceptive needs, which are discussed in detail in Chapters 14 (p. 396) and 21 (p. 558). With adolescents, since

the mid-1800s, the age of menarche has dropped. Thus, reproductive function is established many years earlier than psychosocial comprehension regarding the consequences of sexual activity. Such early sexual development may result in intermittent spontaneous sexual encounters with a naïve perception of the risks of pregnancy and sexually transmitted infections (Cromer, 1996; Sulak, 1993). Importantly, adolescents have unintended pregnancy rates that approach 85 percent (Finer, 2006). Moreover, adolescent females who do not use a contraceptive at their first sexual encounter are twice as likely to become pregnant during adolescence compared with those who initially use contraception (Abma, 2010). Thus, effective contraception counseling should ideally be provided *before* the onset of sexual activity. In most states, minors have explicit legal authority to consent to contraceptive services, and in many areas, publicly funded clinics provide free contraception to adolescents (Guttmacher Institute, 2011). Moreover, contraception may be provided without a pelvic examination or cervical cancer screening.

In the perimenopause, ovulation becomes irregular and fertility wanes. However, pregnancies do occur, and in women aged ≥40 years, more than one third of all pregnancies are unintended (Finer, 2006). Importantly, pregnancy with advanced maternal age carries an increased risk for pregnancy-related morbidity and mortality. Women in this group may also have coexistent medical problems that may preclude certain methods. Finally, perimenopausal symptoms may be present in this group and may be improved with hormonal methods.

TOP-TIER CONTRACEPTIVE METHODS— MOST EFFECTIVE

Several first-tier methods are available in the United States. These include: (1) a copper-containing intrauterine device, the ParaGard T 380A intrauterine device, (2) a progestin-releasing IUD, the Mirena levonorgestrel-releasing intrauterine system (LNG-IUS), (3) one subdermal implant system, the Implanon single-rod system, and (4) multiple methods of sterilization for men and women.

Intrauterine Contraception

In the past, up to 7 percent of sexually active American women used an intrauterine device (IUD) for contraception. Unnecessary fears and concerns with liability issues caused

TABLE 5-4. U.S. Medical Eligibility Criteria for Use of Various Contraceptive Methods While Breastfeeding

Method	Category[b]	Comments
CHCs		
Breast-feeding		Clinical studies demonstrate conflicting results about effects on milk
<21 days pp	4	volume in women exposed to COCs during lactation; no consistent
21–<30 days pp with risks[a]	3[c]	effect on infant weight has been reported. Adverse health
21–<30 days pp w/o risks	3	outcomes or manifestations of exogenous estrogen in infants
30–42 days pp with risks[a]	3[c]	exposed to CHCs through breast milk have not been demonstrated.
30–42 days pp w/o risks	2	
>42 days pp	2	There is no direct evidence examining the risk for VTE among
		postpartum women using CHCs. VTE risk is elevated during
Non–breast-feeding		pregnancy and postpartum; this risk is most pronounced in the first
<21 days pp	4	weeks after delivery, declining to near baseline levels by 42 days
21–42 days pp with risks[a]	3[c]	postpartum. Use of CHCs, which increases the risk for VTE in healthy
21–42 days pp w/o risks	2	reproductive age women, might pose an additional risk if used
>42 days pp	1	during this time.
DMPA, POPs, Implants		
Breast-feeding		Theoretical concerns that early use may diminish breast milk
<30 days pp	2	production are not supported by evidence. Limited studies
>30 days pp	1	
Non–breast-feeding		Limited evidence suggests no adverse side effects
<30 days pp	1	
>30 days pp	1	
LNG-IUS		
Breast-feeding or not		Theoretical risk of diminished breast milk production. Minimal
<10 minutes pp	2	evidence
10 min to ≤4 weeks pp	2	
≥4 weeks	1	
Puerperal sepsis	4	IUD insertion could worsen condition
Cu-IUC		
Breast-feeding		
<10 minutes pp	1	IUD placement <10 min pp is associated with lower expulsion rates compared with later IUD placement up to >72 hour pp. No comparative data for insertion >72 hour pp
10 min to ≤4 weeks pp	2	At c-section, postplacental placement associated with lower expulsion rate than after vaginal delivery
≥4 weeks	1	No increased risk of infection or perforation associated with pp insertion
Puerperal sepsis	4	IUD insertion could worsen condition

[a]Risk factors include age ≥35 years, previous venous thromboembolism, thrombophilia, immobility, transfusion at delivery, body mass index ≥30, postpartum hemorrhage, postcesarean delivery, preeclampsia, smoking, or peripartum cardiomyopathy.
[b]Category explanation: see Table 5-3.
[c]For women with other risk factors for VTE, these risk factors might increase the classification to a 4.
c-section = cesarean section; CHCs = combination hormonal contraceptives; Cu-IUD = copper-bearing intrauterine device; DMPA = depot medroxyprogesterone acetate; LNG-IUS = levonorgestrel intrauterine system; POPs = progestin-only pills; pp = postpartum.
Adapted from Centers for Disease Control and Prevention, 2010b, 2011.

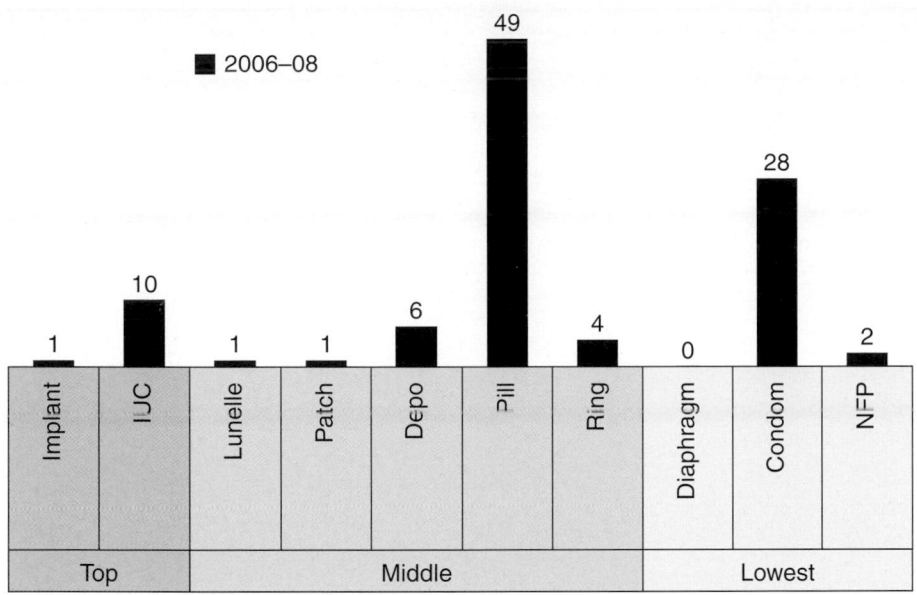

FIGURE 5-2 Chart illustrating rates of contraceptive use by method and by method effectiveness for years 2006–2008 in the United States. *(Data from Mosher, 2010.)*

these highly effective contraceptive methods to become almost obsolete. However, intrauterine contraception (IUC) is once again gaining popularity, and IUC use increased from 2 percent in 2002 to 10 percent in 2008 (Fig. 5-2) (Mosher, 2010). Still, this is much lower compared with worldwide IUC use of 15 percent, and specifically with China—45-percent use and Northern Europe—10-percent use (United Nations, 2007).

Some barriers to IUC use in the United States include cost, politics, and provider failure to offer or encourage use of this highly effective contraceptive method. In an effort to reduce the high proportion of unplanned pregnancies, the American College of Obstetricians and Gynecologists (2007a, 2009b, 2011) encourages use of *long-acting reversible contraceptives (LARC)* for all appropriate candidates, including adolescents. Despite higher up-front costs, the extended span of effective use of IUC results in competitive cost effectiveness compared with other forms of contraception.

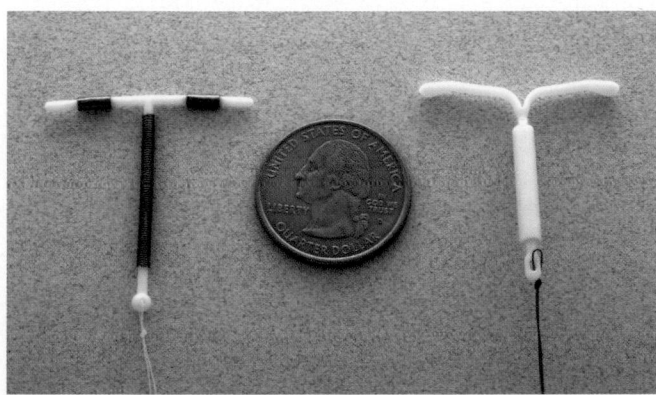

FIGURE 5-3 Intrauterine contraceptive devices available in the United States: Copper-containing ParaGard T 380A (*left*) and levonorgestrel-releasing Mirena (*right*).

Levonorgestrel-Releasing Intrauterine System (LNG-IUS)

Marketed as Mirena, this IUD releases levonorgestrel at a relatively constant rate of 20 mg/day. This small dose mitigates the systemic effects of the progestin. This device is a T-shaped polyethylene structure with the stem encased by a cylinder containing polydimethylsiloxane and levonorgestrel (Fig. 5-3). The cylinder has a permeable membrane that regulates the rate of hormone release. Each device is currently approved for 5 years following insertion, however, evidence supports use for 7 years (Thonneau, 2008).

Mechanism of Action. There are a number of progestin-mediated mechanisms by which LNG-IUS may prevent pregnancy. The progestin renders the endometrium atrophic; it stimulates thick cervical mucus that blocks sperm penetration into the uterus; and it may decrease tubal motility that thereby prevents ovum and sperm union. The progestin may also inhibit ovulation, but this is not consistent (Nilsson, 1984).

Contraindications. Shown in Table 5-5 are the manufacturer's contraindications to use of LNG-IUS. Women who have had a previous ectopic pregnancy may be at increased risk for another because of diminished tubal motility from progestin action. In women with uterine leiomyomas, placement of the LNG-IUS may be problematic if the uterine cavity is distorted. In their metaanalysis, Zapata and associates (2010b) reported the expulsion rate to be approximately 10 percent in women with coexistent leiomyomas. However, they also found that menstrual blood loss in most of these women will be lessened.

Copper-T 380A Intrauterine Device

Marketed as ParaGard, this device is composed of a stem wrapped with 314 mm^2 of fine copper wire, and each arm has a 33-mm^2 copper bracelet—the sum of these is 380 mm^2 of copper. As shown in Figure 5-3, two strings extend from the base of the stem. The Cu-T 380A is approved for 10 years of continuous use, although it has been shown to prevent pregnancy with continuous use for up to 20 years (Bahamondes, 2005).

Mechanism of Action. The intense local inflammatory response induced in the uterus by copper-containing devices leads to lysosomal activation and other inflammatory actions that are spermicidal (Alvarez, 1988; Ortiz, 1987). In the unlikely event that fertilization does occur, the same inflammatory actions are directed against the blastocyst. And finally, the endometrium becomes hostile for implantation.

TABLE 5-5. Manufacturer Contraindications to Use of an Intrauterine Device

ParaGard T 380

ParaGard should not be placed when one or more of the following conditions exist:
1. Pregnancy or suspicion of pregnancy
2. Abnormalities of the uterus resulting in distortion of the uterine cavity
3. Acute pelvic inflammatory disease, or current behavior suggesting a high risk for pelvic inflammatory disease
4. Postpartum endometritis or postabortal endometritis in the past 3 months
5. Known or suspected uterine or cervical malignancy
6. Genital bleeding of unknown etiology
7. Mucopurulent cervicitis
8. Wilson disease
9. Allergy to any component of ParaGard
10. A previously placed IUD that has not been removed

Mirena

Mirena should not be placed when one or more of the following conditions exist:
1. Pregnancy or suspicion of pregnancy
2. Congenital or acquired uterine anomaly if it distorts the uterine cavity
3. Acute pelvic inflammatory disease (PID) or history of, unless there has been a subsequent intrauterine pregnancy
4. Postpartum endometritis or infected abortion in the past 3 months
5. Known or suspected uterine or cervical neoplasia or abnormal Pap smear
6. Genital bleeding of unknown etiology
7. Untreated acute cervicitis or vaginitis or other lower genital tract infections
8. Acute liver disease or liver tumor (benign or malignant)
9. Increased susceptibility to pelvic infection
10. A previously placed IUD that has not been removed
11. Hypersensitivity to any component of Mirena
12. Known or suspected carcinoma of the breast
13. Prior ectopic pregnancy

IUD = intrauterine device.
From Bayer HealthCare, 2009, and Duramed, 2011.

Contraindications. Listed in Table 5-5 are manufacturer's contraindications to use of the Cu-T 380A. In the metaanalysis cited earlier for LNG-IUS use in women with leiomyomas, Zapata and associates (2010b) found no studies relevant to use of copper-containing IUDs in women with significant tumors.

Counseling

During the modern renaissance of IUC, a number of improvements have resulted in safer and more effective methods. That said, there are still some unwanted side effects as well as misconceptions surrounding their use.

Infection. Historically, IUD-associated infections precluded use by young women and those of low parity. Improved device design has mitigated these concerns appreciably. In addition, a number of well-designed studies have shown that sexual behavior and sexually transmitted disease are important risk factors.

With current devices, insertion generally does not increase the risk for pelvic infection. There is no evidence that prophylactic antibiotics are necessary with insertion for women at low risk for sexually transmitted diseases (American College of Obstetricians and Gynecologists, 2009a; Walsh, 1998). Of the less than 1 in 100 women who develop an infection within

20 days of IUD insertion, most usually have a concomitant unrecognized cervical infection. Accordingly, women at higher risk for sexually transmitted lower genital tract infections should be screened either before or at the time of IUD insertion (Centers for Disease Control and Prevention, 2010a; Faúndes, 1998; Grimes, 2000). Alternatively, a small number of pelvic infections are presumed to be caused by intrauterine contamination with normal flora at the time of insertion. Thus, antibiotics selected for treatment of any pelvic infection within the early weeks following IUD insertion should be broad-spectrum to adequately cover all these organisms.

Long-term IUC is not associated with an increased pelvic infection rate in women at low risk for sexually transmitted infections. Indeed, these long-term users have a pelvic infection rate comparable with that of oral contraceptive pill users. Any pelvic infection after 45 to 60 days should be considered sexually transmitted and appropriately treated as described in Chapter 3 (p. 97). For women who develop an infection associated with an IUD, evidence is insufficient to recommend device removal, although this is commonly done. However, close clinical reevaluation is warranted if an IUD remains (Centers for Disease Control and Prevention, 2010b). In women who develop a tuboovarian abscess, the device should be removed immediately after parenteral antibiotic therapy is begun.

Special concerns have arisen for women in whom *Actinomyces* species are identified in the lower genital tract, most commonly during Pap smear cytology reporting. Fiorino (1996) noted a 7-percent incidence in the Pap smears of IUD users compared with a 1-percent incidence in nonusers. Symptomatic pelvic actinomycosis is rare but tends to be indolent and severe.

Currently, in the absence of symptoms, incidental identification of *Actinomyces* species in cytologic specimens has uncertain significance. Treatment options reviewed by the American College of Obstetricians and Gynecologists (2005) include: expectant management, an extended course of antibiotics, IUD removal, or antibiotics plus IUD removal. For women with symptomatic infection, the IUD should be removed and intensive antibiotic therapy given. *Actinomyces* is susceptible to antibiotics with gram-positive coverage, notably the penicillins.

Low Parity and Adolescents.
Nulliparous IUD candidates were previously precluded from IUC use because of fears of pelvic infection and induced sterility. Current studies indicate that the pelvic infection rate is not different from that discussed earlier (Lee, 1998; Society of Family Planning, 2010). Moreover, expulsion rates in nulliparas are similar to those in multiparas. A higher proportion of nulliparas will request removal of the device because of pain or bleeding, but overall, this population reports high levels of satisfaction with IUC. Specifically, after the first year, 75 to 90 percent continue use. Revised labeling now places no restrictions on IUC use based on parity. In addition, for the same reasons, *adolescent* IUD candidates may also appropriately select IUC (American College of Obstetricians and Gynecologists, 2007a).

Human Immunodeficiency Virus (HIV)-Infected Women.
Intrauterine contraception is appropriate for HIV-positive women who are otherwise IUC candidates. Neither device is associated with higher IUD complication rates if used in this population. Moreover, these IUDs do not appear to adversely affect viral shedding or antiretroviral therapy efficacy (American College of Obstetricians and Gynecologists, 2010b).

Postabortal and Postpartum IUD Placement.
An ideal time to improve successful provision of contraception is immediately following abortion or delivery. For women with an induced or spontaneous first- or second-trimester abortion, IUC can be placed immediately after uterine evacuation.

Insertion techniques depend upon uterine size. After first-trimester evacuation, the uterine cavity length seldom exceeds 12 cm. In these instances, the IUD can be placed using the inserter provided in the package. If the uterine cavity is larger, the IUD can be placed using ring forceps with sonographic guidance. In women for whom an IUD is placed immediately after induced abortion, the repeat induced abortion rate is only one third of the rate of women not choosing immediate IUD placement (Goodman, 2008; Heikinheimo, 2008). As perhaps expected, the risk of IUC expulsion is slightly higher when placed immediately after abortion or miscarriage, but the advantages of preventing unplanned pregnancies seem to outweigh this (Bednarek, 2011; Fox, 2011; Grimes, 2010b).

Insertion of an IUD immediately following delivery at or near term has also been studied. Placement by hand or by using an instrument has a similar expulsion rate (Grimes, 2010c). As with postabortion insertion, expulsion rates by 6 months are higher than those in women whose IUD is placed after complete uterine involution. In one study, the expulsion rate in the former group was nearly 25 percent (Chen, 2010). Even in these circumstances, however, immediate placement may be beneficial because in some populations up to 40 percent of women do not return for a postpartum clinic visit (Ogburn, 2005). Finally, postpartum insertion is judged to be category 1 or 2 by the US MEC, that is, its advantages consistently outweigh the risks if puerperal infection is absent (see Table 5-4).

Menstrual Changes.
Commonly, IUC may be associated with changes in menstrual patterns. Women who choose the Cu-T 380A should be informed that increased dysmenorrhea and bleeding with menses may develop. Objectively, these women may have decreased hemoglobin concentrations with this IUD (Hassan, 1999). Treatment with an nonsteroidal antiinflammatory drug (NSAID) will usually diminish the amount of bleeding—even normal amounts—as well as relieve dysmenorrhea. In a Cochrane review that included 15 trials with 2702 women, a number of NSAID formulations found effective included naproxen, ibuprofen, and mefenamic acid (Grimes, 2009b).

With the LNG-IUS, women are counseled to expect irregular spotting for up to 6 months after placement, and thereafter to expect monthly menses to be lighter, or even absent (Bayer HealthCare, 2009). Specifically, the Mirena device is associated with progressive amenorrhea, which is reported by 30 percent of women after 2 years and by 60 percent after 12 years (Ronnerdag, 1999). As in Chapter 8 (p. 238), the LNG-IUS device reduces menstrual blood loss and is an effective treatment for some women with menorrhagia (American College of Obstetricians and Gynecologists, 2006, 2010d). This is often associated with improved dysmenorrhea.

Expulsion.
Approximately 5 percent of women will spontaneously expel their IUD during the first year of use. This is most likely during the first month. Because of this, a woman is instructed to periodically palpate to feel the marker strings protruding from the cervical os. This can be accomplished by either sitting on the edge of a chair or squatting down and then advancing the middle finger into the vagina until the cervix is reached. Following insertion of either IUD, women are reappointed for a visit within several weeks, usually after completion of menses. At this meeting, any side effects are addressed, and IUD placement is confirmed by visualization of the marker strings. Some recommend barrier contraception to ensure contraception during this first month—this may be especially desirable if a device has been expelled previously.

Uterine Perforation.
The uterus may be perforated either with a uterine sound or with an IUD. Perforations may be clinically apparent or silent. Their frequency depends on operator skill and is estimated to be approximately 1 per 1000 insertions (World Health Organization, 1987). In some cases, a partial perforation at insertion is followed by migration of the device completely through the uterine wall. Occasionally, perforation begins spontaneously.

IUD Marker Strings Not Palpable or Visualized
Diagnosis. In some cases, the marker strings may not be palpated or seen with speculum examination. Possibilities include that the device was expelled silently, the device has partially or completely

perforated the uterus, the woman is pregnant and the enlarging uterus has drawn the device upward, or the marker strings are temporarily hidden within the endocervical canal. An IUD should not be considered expelled unless it was seen by the patient.

Initially, an endocervical brush or similar instrument can be used to gently draw the string out of the cervical canal. If unsuccessful, then at least two options are available. After pregnancy has been excluded, the uterine cavity is gently probed using an instrument such as Randall stone forceps or a rod with a hooked end. In some cases, the strings or device will be found with this method. If not successful, at this juncture, or possibly as a first choice, transvaginal sonography (TVS) is performed. As described in Chapter 2 (p. 47), 3-dimensional (3-D) TVS offers improved visualization (Moschos, 2011). As such, patients at Parkland Hospital undergoing gynecologic sonography with IUDs in situ, regardless of the indication for the study, have both a standard 2-D as well as a 3-D evaluation to establish the type, location, and positioning of the IUD (Fig. 2-25, p. 48). If the device is not seen either within the uterine cavity or walls, then an abdominal radiograph, with or without a uterine sound in place, may localize it. Another option includes hysteroscopy (Section 42-14, p. 1162).

Management. These decisions depend upon where the device is located and whether there is a coexistent intrauterine pregnancy. During the interim, a nonpregnant patient should use alternative contraception.

First, a device may penetrate the uterine wall in varying degrees. It should be removed, and this approach varies by IUD location. Devices with a predominantly intrauterine location are typically managed by hysteroscopic IUD removal. In contrast, devices that have nearly completely perforated through the uterine wall are more easily removed laparoscopically.

For women with an intraabdominal IUD, an inert-material device located outside the uterus may cause harm, but not universally. Bowel perforations—both large and small—as well as bowel fistulas have been reported. Once identified laparoscopically, these inert devices can easily be retrieved via laparoscopy or less commonly by colpotomy. Conversely, an extrauterine copper-bearing device induces an intense local inflammatory reaction with adhesions. Thus, they are more firmly adhered, and laparotomy may become necessary (Balci, 2010).

In those with pregnancy and an IUD, early pregnancy identification is important. Up to approximately 14 weeks' gestation, the tail may be visible within the cervix, and if seen, it should be removed. This action reduces subsequent complications such as late abortion, sepsis, and preterm birth (Alvior, 1973). Tatum and colleagues (1976) reported an abortion rate of 54 percent with the device left in place compared with a rate of 25 percent if it was promptly removed. More recently, a study from Israel by Ganer and coworkers (2009) reported pregnancy outcomes from 1988 to 2007 in 292 women who conceived with a copper-containing IUD in place. Outcomes were compared in the two groups of women with and without IUD removal as well as with the general obstetrical population. As shown in Table 5-6, in general, the group of women with an IUD left in place had the worst outcomes. Importantly, however, the

TABLE 5-6. Pregnancy Outcomes in Women Who Conceived with a Copper-Containing IUD in Place

Outcome[a]	IUD in Situ (n = 98)	IUD Removed (n = 194)	No IUD (n = 141,191)	p value
PROM	10.2	7.7	5.7	.021
PTD	18.4	14.4	7.3	<.001
Chorioamnionitis	7.1	4.1	0.7	<.001
FGR	1.0	0.5	1.7	NS
Abruption	4.1	2.1	0.7	<.001
Placenta previa	4.1	0.5	0.5	<.001
Cesarean delivery	32	21	13	<.001
Low birthweight				
<2500 g	11.2	13.4	6.7	<.001
<1500 g	5.1	3.6	1.1	<.001
Perinatal mortality	1.0	1.5	1.2	NS
Malformations	10.2	5.7	5.1	<.041

[a]Outcomes shown as percentages.
FGR = fetal growth restriction; IUD = intrauterine device; NS = not significant; PROM = premature rupture of membranes; PTD = preterm delivery.
Data from Ganer, 2009.

group in whom the IUD was removed still had significantly worse outcomes compared with those of the general population. Of special note, Vessey and associates (1979) had previously reported that fetal malformations were not increased in pregnancies in which the device was left in place. In the Ganer study, it is particularly worrisome that this rate was doubled compared with women in whom the device was removed. There were no chromosomal anomalies identified in fetuses born to women from the two IUD groups, and further distribution was only unusual because there were 12 percent due to skeletal malformations.

Because of these findings, if pregnancy continuation is desired, it is recommended that with early pregnancies the IUD be removed. However, if the tail is not visible, attempts to locate and remove the device may result in pregnancy loss. This risk must be weighed against the risk of leaving the device in place. If removal is attempted, transvaginal sonography can be used. If attempts at removal are followed by evidence for infection, then antimicrobial treatment is begun and is followed by prompt uterine evacuation.

Ectopic Pregnancy. The risk of an associated ectopic pregnancy has been clarified over the past few years. IUC is effective in preventing all pregnancies. Specifically, the contraceptive effect of IUC decreases the absolute number of ectopic pregnancies by half compared with the rate in women who do not use contraception (World Health Organization, 1985, 1987). However, the IUC mechanisms of action are more effective in preventing intrauterine implantation. Thus, if IUC fails, a higher proportion of pregnancies are likely to be ectopic (Furlong, 2002). For this reason, previous ectopic pregnancy is considered a contraindication for use of the LNG-IUS by its manufacturer.

Procedures for Insertion

Before IUD insertion, the Food and Drug Administration (FDA) requires that a woman be given a brochure detailing the side effects and apparent risks from its use. Timing of insertion influences the ease of placement as well as the pregnancy and expulsion rates. When done toward the end of normal menstruation, when the cervix is usually softer and somewhat more dilated, insertion may be easier, and early pregnancy can be excluded. This, however, does not limit insertion to this time. For a woman who is sure she is not pregnant and does not want to be pregnant, insertion may be carried out any time during the menstrual cycle.

Insertion immediately postpartum is more popular in other countries. As discussed on page 139, expulsion and perforation rates are increased, and thus most choose to delay insertion for several weeks. Insertion at 2 weeks is quite satisfactory, and in the Parkland System Family Planning Clinics, insertion is scheduled at 6 weeks postpartum to ensure complete uterine involution. For women who have had an early miscarriage or induced abortion, in the absence of infection, the device may be inserted immediately.

Pain Management

There have been no studies to properly evaluate analgesia for pain associated with insertion. That said, NSAIDs and miso-

prostol are thought to mitigate pain from cervical dilatation and IUC insertion in nulliparous women. However, few studies have adequately evaluated these. Topically applied lidocaine gel may reduce insertion-related pain and warrants further investigation (Allen, 2009).

Technique for Cu-T 380A Insertion

(1) Determine any contraindications, counsel the woman regarding problems associated with device use, and obtain written consent.

(2) Administer an NSAID, with or without codeine, to allay cramps.

(3) Perform a pelvic examination to identify the position and size of the uterus and adnexa. Abnormalities should be evaluated as they may contraindicate the device. Evidence for infection such as a mucopurulent discharge or significant vaginitis should be appropriately treated and resolved before insertion.

(4) The Cu-T 380A should not be loaded into its inserter tube more than 5 minutes before insertion. If longer, the malleable arms tend to retain the "memory" of the inserter and remain bent inward. The IUD arms should lie in the same plane as the flat portion of the blue flange, which is found on the outside of the inserter tube.

(5) Clean the cervical surface with an antiseptic solution, and a tenaculum is placed on the cervical lip. After the uterus is sounded, the blue plastic flange is positioned a distance away from the loaded device tip to reflect this depth.

(6) Pass the inserter tube, with the IUD loaded, into the endometrial cavity. When the blue flange abuts the cervix, insertion stops (Fig. 5-4).

(7) To release the arms, hold the solid white rod steady and withdraw the insertion tube no more than 1 cm. This releases the arms high in the uterine fundus.

(8) While holding the solid white rod steady, gently and carefully move the insertion tube upward toward the top of the uterus, until slight resistance is felt. This will ensure placement of the T at the highest possible position within the uterus.

(9) Hold the insertion tube steady and withdraw the solid white rod.

(10) Gently and slowly withdraw the inserter tube from the cervical canal. Only the marker strings should be visible protruding from the cervix. Trim the threads so that 3 to 4 cm protrude into the vagina. Note the length of the strings in the chart.

(11) If you suspect that the device is not in the correct position, check placement, using sonography if necessary. If it is not positioned completely within the uterus, remove it and replace it with a new device. Do not reinsert an expelled or partially expelled Cu-T 380A.

(12) Remove the tenaculum and observe for bleeding from the tenaculum puncture sites. If there is no bleeding, remove the speculum.

(13) Advise the woman to promptly report any apparent adverse effects.

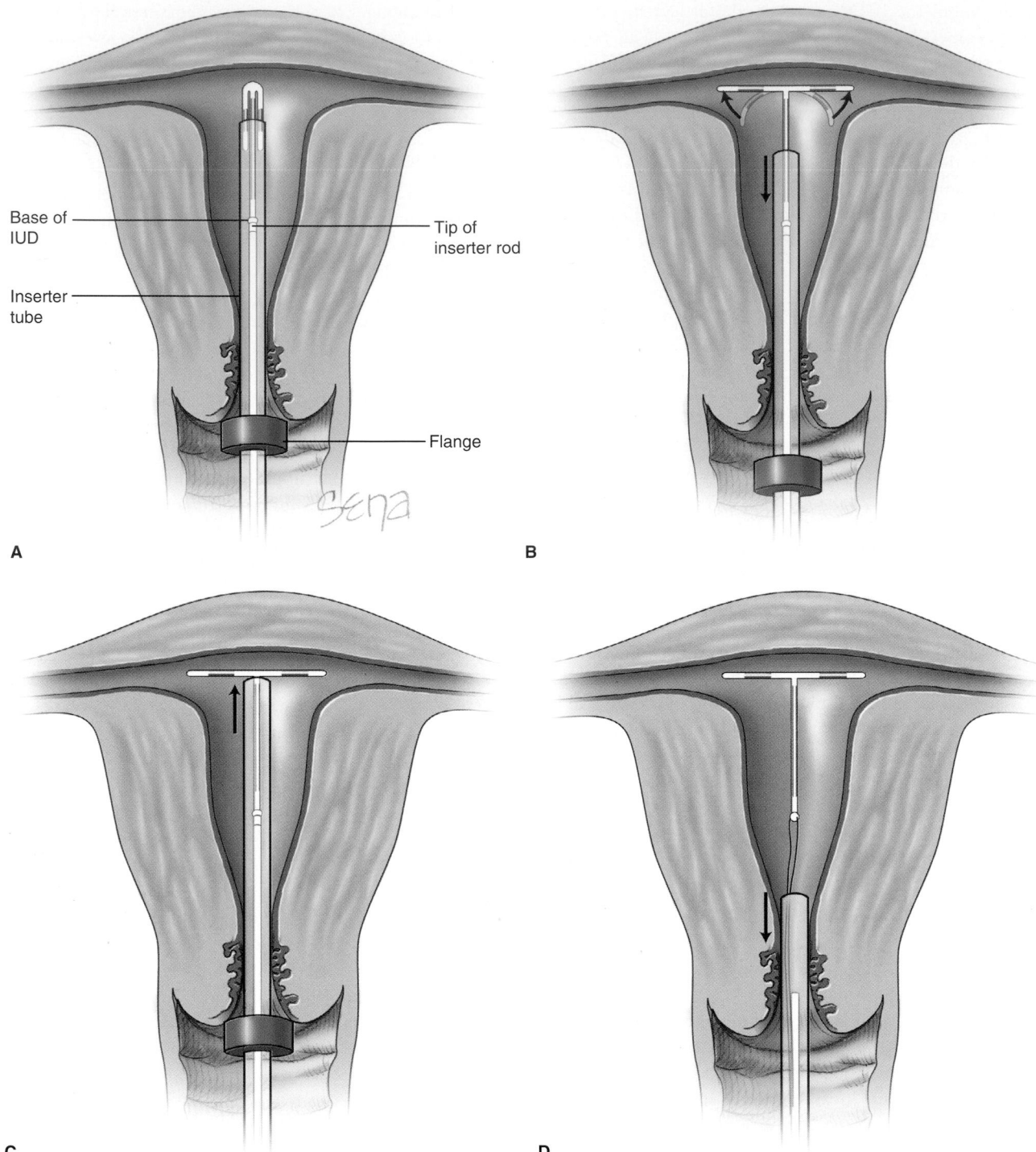

FIGURE 5-4 Insertion of ParaGard T 380A. The uterus is sounded, and the IUD is loaded into its inserter tube not more than 5 minutes before insertion. A blue plastic flange on the outside of the inserter tube is positioned from the IUD tip to reflect the uterine depth. The IUD arms should lie in the same plane as the flat portion of the blue flange. **A.** The inserter tube, with the IUD loaded, is passed into the endometrial cavity. When the blue flange abuts the cervix, insertion stops. **B.** To release the IUD arms, the solid white rod within the inserter tube is held steady while the inserter tube is withdrawn no more than 1 cm. **C.** The inserter tube is then carefully moved upward toward the top of the uterus until slight resistance is felt. **D.** First, the solid white rod and then the inserter tube are withdrawn individually. At completion, only the threads should be visible protruding from the cervix. These are trimmed to allow 3 to 4 cm to extend into the vagina.

Technique for LNG-IUS Insertion

The first five steps are the same as those for the Cu-T 380A just detailed. The technique for LNG-IUS insertion, detailed in the package insert, is now summarized:

(6) Pick up the inserter containing the LNG-IUS and carefully release the threads from behind the slider so that they hang freely.

(7) Ensure that the slider is in the furthermost position away from you—positioned at the top of the handle nearest the device.

(8) While looking at the insertion tube, align the arms of the system horizontally.

(9) Pull on both threads to draw the LNG-IUS into the inserter tube. Note that the knobs at the end of the arms now cover the open end of the inserter (Fig. 5-5).

(10) Fix the threads tightly in the cleft at the end of the handle.

(11) Set the flange to the depth measured by the uterine sound.

(12) To insert the Mirena device, hold the slider firmly in the furthermost position—at the top of the handle. Grasp the cervix with the tenaculum and apply gentle traction to align the cervical canal with the uterine cavity. Gently insert the inserter tube into the cervical canal and advance the inserter tube into the uterus until the flange is situated at a distance 1.5 to 2 cm from the external cervical os. This gives sufficient space for the arms to open within the endometrial cavity. Do not force the inserter.

(13) While holding the inserter steady, release the arms of the device by pulling the slider back until the top of the slider reaches the mark—the raised horizontal line on the handle. Hold this position for 15 to 20 seconds to allow the arms to fully open.

(14) Push the inserter gently into the uterine cavity until its flange touches the cervix. The device should now be in the uterine fundus.

(15) Holding the inserter firmly in position, release the device by pulling the slider down all the way. The threads will be released automatically.

(16) Slowly remove the inserter, cut the marker strings to leave approximately 3 cm visible outside the cervix, and record this length in the patient record.

(17) If there is concern that the IUD is not in the correct position, check placement, using sonography if necessary. Remove the device if it is not positioned completely within the uterus. Do not reinsert a removed system.

■ Progestin Implants

Contraception can be provided by a progestin-containing device that is implanted subdermally and releases the hormone over many years. The devices are coated with a polymer to prevent fibrosis. Several systems have been developed, but only one is available in the United States. The initial implant, the Norplant System (Wyeth), releases levonorgestrel from six silastic rods. It was withdrawn from the U.S. market, and a fund has been established by the manufacturer to ensure access to patients for removal. Supposedly, the silicone-based rods caused ill-defined symptoms that were reversed with removal. Jadelle (Bayer Schering Pharma Oy) has received FDA approval but is not marketed or distributed in the United States (Sivin, 2002). Sino-implant II (Shanghai Dahua Pharmaceutical Co.) is a structurally and pharmacologically similar system to Jadelle. It is manufactured in China and approved for use by several countries in Asia and Africa (Steiner, 2010).

The other implant is the Implanon System (Organon). It is a single-rod subdermal implant containing 68 mg of a progestin—*etonogestrel*—and covered by an ethylene vinyl acetate copolymer. It is discussed next because it is widely available in the United States (Fig. 5-6). Nexplanon (Organon) is the same implant but in a radiopaque form and with an updated insertion device.

Mechanism of Action

The progestin released continuously causes ovulation suppression, increased cervical mucus viscosity, and endometrial atrophic changes (Organon, 2006).

Contraindications

These are similar to those cited for other progestin-containing methods. Specifically, these include pregnancy, thrombosis or thromboembolic disorders, benign or malignant hepatic tumors, active liver disease, undiagnosed abnormal genital bleeding, or breast cancer (Organon, 2006).

Counseling

The etonogestrel subdermal implant will provide contraception for up to 3 years. At this time, the device is removed, and another rod may be placed within the same incision site. Importantly, patients should be counseled that Implanon causes *irregular bleeding* that does not normalize over time. Thus, women who cannot tolerate unpredictable and irregular bleeding should select an alternative method.

Insertion

Implanon is inserted subdermally along the biceps groove of the inner arm and 6 to 8 cm from the elbow. Immediately following insertion, the provider and patient should document that the device is palpable beneath the skin. When Implanon is removed, this superficial location allows in-office extraction of the implant. Through a small incision large enough to admit hemostat tips, the implant is grasped and removed. If desired, a new rod can be placed through this same incision.

If a device is not palpable, it can be imaged with a 10- to 15-MHz sonographic transducer. If this fails to locate the device, magnetic resonance imaging can aid localization (Shulman, 2006). Nexplanon, Norplant, and Jadelle are radiopaque, however, Implanon is not. Thus, radiography is not useful to find this device.

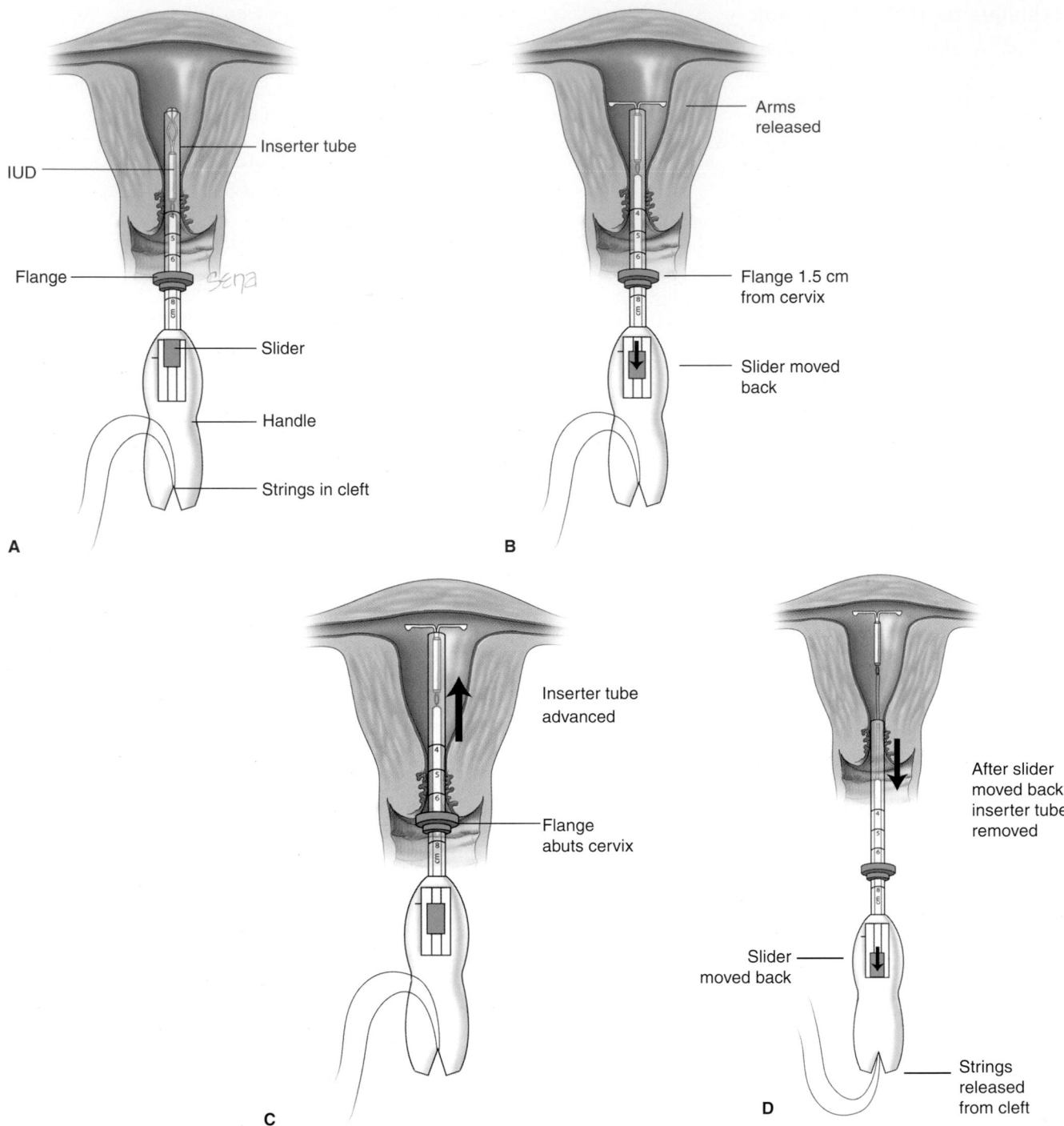

FIGURE 5-5 Insertion of the Mirena intrauterine system. Threads from behind the slider are first released to hang freely. The teal-colored slider found on the handle should be positioned at the top of the handle nearest the device. The IUD arms are oriented horizontally. **A.** As both free threads are pulled outward, the Mirena IUD is drawn into the inserter tube. The threads are then moved upward from below and tightly fixed into the handle's cleft. A flange on the outside of the inserter tube is positioned from the IUD tip to reflect the depth found with uterine sounding. **B.** The inserter tube is gently inserted into the uterus until the flange lies 1.5 to 2 cm from the external cervical os to allow the arms to open. While holding the inserter steady, the IUD arms are released by pulling the slider back to the raised horizontal line on the handle. **C.** The inserter is then gently guided into the uterine cavity until its flange touches the cervix. **D.** The device is released by holding the inserter firmly in position, and pulling the slider back all the way. The threads will be released automatically. The inserter may then be removed. IUD strings are trimmed to leave approximately 3 cm visible outside the cervix.

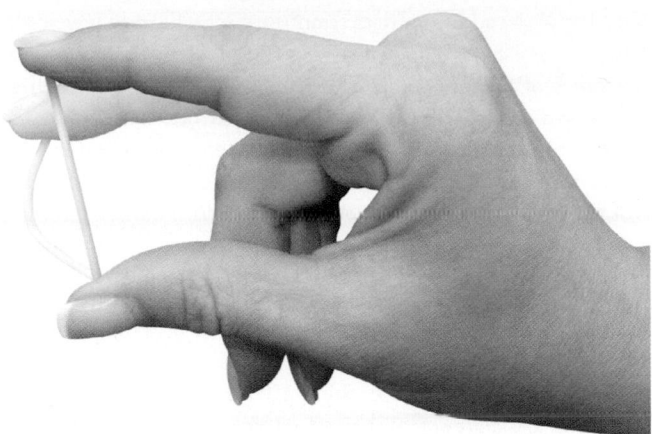

FIGURE 5-6 Implanon System single-rod system. The background image shows rod flexibility. *(Reproduced with permission of N.V. Organon, a subsidiary of Merck & Co, Inc. All rights reserved. Implanon is a registered trademark of N.V. Organon.)*

■ Permanent Contraception—Sterilization

In the United States in 2006, surgical sterilization was the most commonly reported form of contraception in childbearing-aged women. These procedures cannot be tracked accurately because most interval tubal sterilizations and vasectomies are performed in ambulatory surgical centers. However, according to the National Survey of Family Growth, approximately 643,000 female tubal sterilizations are performed annually in the United States (Chan, 2010). The two most commonly employed forms in this country are bilateral tubal ligation—frequently via laparoscopy—and hysteroscopic tubal sterilization. The latter has become popular, and in some settings, it is used in up to half of nonpuerperal female sterilizations (Shavell, 2009).

Over the past 20 years, a number of important multicenter studies regarding sterilization have been performed by investigators of the Collaborative Review of Sterilization (CREST) and the Centers for Disease Control and Prevention. Data from many of these studies are subsequently described.

Female Tubal Sterilization

This is usually accomplished by occlusion or division of the fallopian tubes to prevent ovum passage and thus avoid fertilization. According to the American College of Obstetricians and Gynecologists (2003), 27 percent of couples in the United States select this method. Approximately half of tubal sterilization procedures are performed in conjunction with cesarean delivery or soon after vaginal delivery (MacKay, 2001). Accordingly, this is termed *puerperal sterilization*. The other half of tubal sterilization procedures are done at a time unrelated to recent pregnancy, that is, nonpuerperal tubal sterilization. This is also termed *interval sterilization*. In most instances, nonpuerperal tubal sterilization is accomplished via laparoscopy or hysteroscopy.

Methods for Tubal Interruption.
There are three methods, along with their modifications, that are used for tubal interruption. These include application of a variety of permanent rings or clips to the fallopian tubes; electrocoagulation of a tubal segment; or ligation with suture material, with or without removal of a segment of tube. The steps to these procedures are described in Sections 41-7 (p. 1030) and 42-3 (p. 1123) of the surgical atlas. In a Cochrane review, Nardin and colleagues (2003) concluded that all of these are effective in preventing pregnancy.

Electrocoagulation is used for destruction of a segment of tube and can be accomplished with either unipolar or bipolar current. Although unipolar coagulation has the lowest long-term failure rate, it also has the highest serious complication rate. For this reason, bipolar coagulation is favored by most (American College of Obstetricians and Gynecologists, 2003).

Mechanical methods of tubal occlusion can be accomplished with: (1) a silicone rubber band such as the *Falope Ring* or the *Tubal Ring*, (2) the spring-loaded *Hulka-Clemens Clip*—also known as the *Wolf Clip*, or (3) the silicone-lined titanium *Filshie Clip*. In a randomized trial of 2746 women, Sokal and associates (2000) compared the Tubal Ring and Filshie Clip and reported similar rates of safety and 1-year pregnancy rates of 1.7 per 1000 women. All of these mechanical methods of occlusion have favorable long-term success rate.

Surgical Approaches.
Laparoscopic tubal ligation is the leading method used in this country for nonpuerperal female sterilization (American College of Obstetrics and Gynecologists, 2003). This is frequently done in an ambulatory surgical setting under general anesthesia, and the woman can be discharged several hours later. Alternatively, some choose minilaparotomy using a 3-cm suprapubic incision. This is especially popular in resource-poor countries. With either laparoscopy or minilaparotomy, major morbidity is rare. Minor morbidity, however, was twice as common with minilaparotomy in a study by Kulier and associates (2002). Finally, the peritoneal cavity can also be entered by colpotomy through the posterior vaginal fornix, although this approach is not commonly used.

Counseling.
Indications for this elective procedure include a request for sterilization with clear understanding that this is permanent and irreversible. Each woman should be counseled regarding alternative contraceptive options. Surgical risks are assessed, and occasionally, the procedure may be contraindicated.

Regret.
There will invariably be a number of women who later express regrets about sterilization. From a CREST study, Jamieson and coworkers (2002) reported that by 5 years, 7 percent of women undergoing tubal ligation had regrets. This is not limited to female sterilization, as 6 percent of women whose husbands had undergone vasectomy had similar remorse. The cumulative probability of regret within 14 years of sterilization was 20 percent for women aged 30 or younger at sterilization compared with only 6 percent for those older than 30 years (Hillis, 1999).

Method Failure.
Reasons for interval tubal sterilization failure are not always apparent, but some have been identified. First, surgical error may occur and likely accounts for 30 to 50 percent of cases. Secondly, tubal fistula may complicate occlusion methods. Although usually encountered with

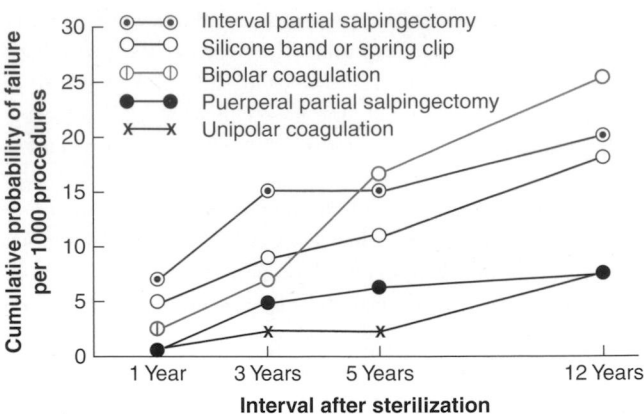

FIGURE 5-7 Data from the U.S. Collaborative Review of Sterilization (CREST) shows the cumulative probability of pregnancy per 1000 procedures by five methods of tubal sterilization. *(Data from Peterson, 1996.)*

electrocoagulation procedures, fistulas are now less likely because an amp meter is used routinely. In some cases, sterilization failure may follow spontaneous reanastomosis of the tubal segments. Equipment failure, such as a defective electric current for electrocoagulation, may be causative. With faulty clips, occlusion is incomplete. Lastly, luteal phase pregnancy may occur and describes the situation in which a woman is already pregnant when the procedure is performed. This can often be avoided by scheduling surgery during the follicular phase of the menstrual cycle and by preoperative human chorionic gonadotropin (hCG) testing.

The overall failure rate reported from the CREST studies was 1.3 percent of 10,685 tubal sterilization surgeries. As shown in Figure 5-7, these rates vary for different procedures. And even with the same operation, failure rates vary. For example, with electrocoagulation, if fewer than three tubal sites are coagulated, the 5-year cumulative pregnancy rate is approximately 12 per 1000 procedures. However, it is only 3 per 1000 if three or more sites are coagulated (Peterson, 1999). The lifetime increased cumulative failure rates over time are supportive that failures after 1 year are not likely due to technical errors. Indeed, Soderstrom (1985) found that most sterilization failures were not preventable.

Ectopic Pregnancy. Pregnancies following tubal sterilization have a high incidence of being ectopically implanted compared with the rate in a general gynecological population. These rates are especially high following electrocoagulation procedures, in which up to 65 percent of pregnancies are ectopic. With failures following other methods—ring, clip, tubal resection—this percentage is only 10 percent (Hendrix, 1999; Peterson, 1999). Importantly, ectopic pregnancy must be excluded when any symptoms of pregnancy develop in a woman who has undergone tubal sterilization.

Menstrual Irregularities. Several studies have evaluated the risk of menorrhagia and intermenstrual bleeding following tubal sterilization, and many have reported no link (DeStefano, 1985;

Shy, 1992). In addition, data from the CREST study have been informative. Peterson and coworkers (2000) compared long-term outcomes of 9514 women who had undergone tubal sterilization with a cohort of 573 women whose partners had undergone vasectomy. Risks for menorrhagia, intermenstrual bleeding, and dysmenorrhea were similar in each group. Perhaps unexpectedly, women who had undergone sterilization had *decreased* duration and volume of menstrual flow, they reported *less* dysmenorrhea, but they had an *increased* incidence of cycle irregularity.

Other Effects. Other long-term effects have also been studied. It is controversial whether risks for subsequent hysterectomy are increased (Pati, 2000). In a CREST surveillance study, Hillis and associates (1997) reported that 17 percent of women undergoing tubal sterilization subsequently had undergone hysterectomy by 14 years. Although they did not compare this incidence with a control cohort, the indications for hysterectomy were similar to those for nonsterilized women who had undergone a hysterectomy.

Women are highly unlikely to develop salpingitis following sterilization (Levgur, 2000). Tubal sterilization appears to have a protective effect against ovarian cancer, but not breast cancer (Westhoff, 2000). The incidence of functional ovarian cysts is increased almost twofold following tubal sterilization (Holt, 2003).

Some psychological sequelae of sterilization were evaluated in a CREST study by Costello and associates (2002). These investigators reported that tubal ligation did not change sexual interest or pleasure in 80 percent of women. In the remaining 20 percent of women who reported a change, 8 of 10 described the changes to be positive.

Tubal Sterilization Reversal. No woman should undergo tubal sterilization believing that subsequent fertility is guaranteed either by surgical reanastomosis or by assisted reproductive techniques. These are technically difficult, expensive, and not always successful. Pregnancy rates vary greatly depending upon age, the amount of tube remaining, and the technology used. Van Voorhis (2000) reviewed a number of reports and found that pregnancy rates varied from 45 to 90 percent with surgical reversals. However, if neosalpingostomy is done for fimbriectomy reversal, the successful pregnancy rate is only 30 percent (Tourgeman, 2001). Of note, pregnancies that result after tubal sterilization reanastomosis are at risk to be ectopic.

Hysterectomy

For a woman with uterine or other pelvic disease for which hysterectomy may be indicated, this may be the ideal form of sterilization.

Transcervical Sterilization

Various methods of sterilization can be completed using a transcervical approach to reach the tubal ostia. Within each ostium, occlusion is achieved by placing either mechanical devices or chemical compounds.

Mechanical Tubal Occlusion. These methods employ insertion of a device into the proximal fallopian tubes via hysteroscopy. Two systems have been approved by the FDA for use in the United States.

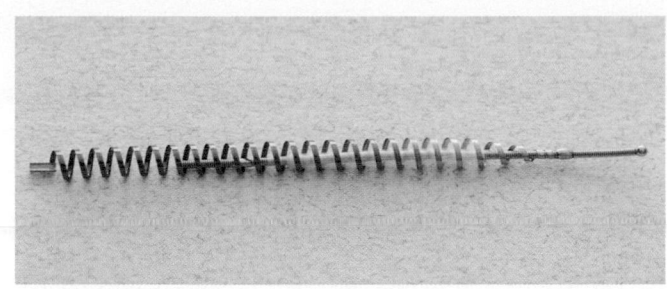

FIGURE 5-8 Microinsert used in the Essure Permanent Birth Control System.

Essure Permanent Birth Control System. The Essure Permanent Birth Control System (Conceptus) was FDA approved in 2002. The device consists of a microinsert made of a stainless steel inner coil that is enclosed in polyester fibers. These fibers are surrounded by an expandable outer coil made of *Nitinol*—a nickel and titanium alloy used in coronary artery stents (Fig. 5-8). Fibroblastic proliferation within the fibers causes tubal occlusion.

Adiana Permanent Contraception. FDA-approved in 2009, Adiana Permanent Contraception (Hologic) is applied by first creating a 60-second radiofrequency thermal injury to the intramural portion of the proximal fallopian tube. This is followed by insertion of a 1.5 × 3.5 mm nonabsorbent silicone elastomer matrix into the tubal lumen. Thermal injury has a depth of 0.5 mm, and during healing, fibroblast growth into the matrix occludes the tubal ostium.

Both systems are installed using similar techniques and are described in Section 42-18 (p. 1172). Analgesia provided by intravenous sedation or paracervical block will successfully alleviate pain (Cooper, 2003). In some women, general anesthesia will be required. Three months following device insertion, hysterosalpingography (HSG) is required to confirm complete occlusion. In some women, occlusion is incomplete at this time, and the study is then repeated at 6 months postoperatively. Until tubal occlusion is established, another method of contraception should be used. Transvaginal sonography has been investigated as an alternative confirmation tool, but currently HSG is required by the FDA (Kerin, 2005; Weston, 2005).

Counseling. By far, the overwhelming advantage of these two methods is that they can be inserted in the office. In addition, the procedure times average less than 20 minutes. Abnormal anatomy may preclude procedure completion. However, in 88 to 95 percent of cases, devices can be successfully placed bilaterally. Once successfully placed, both methods have reported success rates of >95 percent (Castaño, 2010; Gariepy, 2011).

Their biggest drawback is that HSG must be performed at 3 months to verify tubal occlusion

(American College of Obstetricians and Gynecologists, 2010c). At this time, approximately 10 percent of women will be shown to have incomplete occlusion. In fact, the most common reason for pregnancy is from noncompliance with confirmational HSG (Guihai, 2010; Veersema, 2010). Method failure has also been attributed to incorrect HSG interpretation and an established pregnancy prior to the procedure (Levy, 2007).

Chemical Methods of Tubal Occlusion. Agents may be placed into the uterine cavity or tubal ostia to incite an inflammatory response to cause tubal occlusion. A method that has been used worldwide in more than 100,000 women consists of using an IUD-type inserter to place quinacrine pellets into the uterine fundus. It is effective, especially considering its simplicity. Pregnancy rates reported by Sokal and colleagues (2008) were 1 and 12 percent at 1 and 10 years, respectively. Although the World Health Organization recommends against its use because of carcinogenesis concerns, it remains an important method for resource-poor countries (Castaño, 2010; Lippes, 2002).

Male Sterilization

Vasectomy is performed each year in nearly a half million men in the United States (Magnani, 1999). The office procedure is done with local analgesia and usually takes 20 minutes or less to complete. As illustrated in Figure 5-9, a small incision is made in the scrotum, and the lumen of the vas deferens is disrupted to block sperm traveling from the testes. Compared with female tubal sterilization, vasectomy is 30 times less likely to fail and is 20 times less likely to have postoperative complications (Adams, 2009).

Sterility following vasectomy is not immediate nor is its onset reliably predictable. The time until complete expulsion

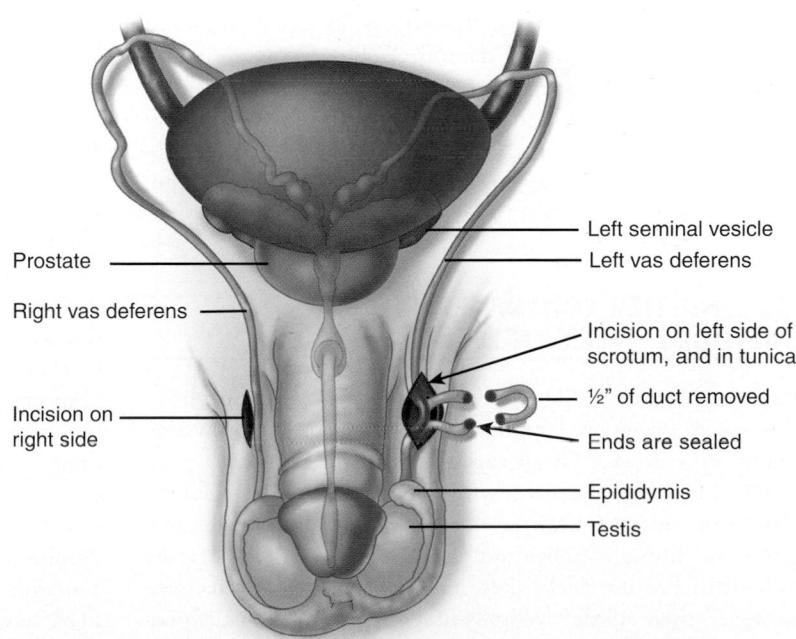

FIGURE 5-9 Schematic showing anatomy and procedure for vasectomy. Within the larger vasectomy incision (*right*), the vas deferens is drawn both as it looks before division (*red*) and after division (*light purple*).

of sperm stored distal to the vas deferens interruption is variable and requires approximately 3 months or 20 ejaculations (American College of Obstetricians and Gynecologists, 2003). Thus, another form of contraception should be used until azoospermia is documented. Although most recommend that semen should be analyzed until two consecutive sperm counts are zero, Bradshaw and coworkers (2001) reported that only one azoospermic semen analysis is sufficient.

Counseling

Method Failure. Sterilization by vasectomy has a failure rate less than 1 percent (Michielsen, 2010). Causes include failure from unprotected intercourse too soon after vasectomy, incomplete occlusion of the vas deferens, or recanalization following suitable separation.

Fertility Restoration. After vasectomy, fertility may be restored either by surgical reanastomosis techniques or by sperm retrieval from the testis. Surgical reversal techniques have evolved since the 1970s and have been reviewed by Kim and Goldstein (2009). Sperm retrieval combined with in vitro fertilization techniques avoids such reversal surgeries and is described in Chapter 20 (p. 546). From their review, Shridharani and Sandlow (2010) concluded that microsurgical reversal is cost effective, but comparative trials with sperm retrieval methods are needed.

Long-Term Effects. Regrets of sterilization were discussed on page 145. Other than these, long-term consequences are rare (Amundsen, 2004). However, because antibodies directed at spermatozoa frequently develop in these men, there were initial concerns these might cause systemic disease. Putative risks were analyzed by Köhler and coworkers (2009) and include cardiovascular disease, immune-complex disorders, psychological changes, male genital cancers, and frontotemporal dementia. Their findings, as well as those of others, are that convincing data are lacking to attribute an increased risk of cardiovascular disease or accelerated atherogenesis to vasectomy (Schwingl, 2000). Moreover, rates of testicular or prostate cancers do not appear increased with this procedure (Cox, 2002; Giovannucci, 1992; Holt, 2008; Köhler, 2009; Lynge, 2002).

SECOND-TIER CONTRACEPTIVE METHODS—VERY EFFECTIVE

Contraceptives considered to be *very effective* are the hormone-containing preparations that include combination oral contraceptives (COCs), progestin-only contraceptive pills (POPs), and contraceptives with estrogens and/or progestins that are made systemically available by injection, transdermal patch, or through application of an intravaginal ring device. When used as intended, these methods are highly effective, however, their efficacy is highly user dependent. Thus, *typical use* considers each woman's compliance with taking a daily pill, changing transdermal patches or rings, or presenting for an injection (see Table 5-2). Such "real world" use significantly diminishes their efficacy, and for women in the United States, these contraceptives have a first-year pregnancy rate of 3 to 9 per 100 users.

■ Combined Hormonal Contraceptives

These are contraceptives that contain an estrogen and a progestin. Combined hormonal contraceptives (CHCs) are available in the United States in three formats—oral contraceptive pills, the transdermal patch, and the intravaginal contraceptive ring. Because of limited data for the transdermal and transvaginal methods relative to that for COCs, their use is usually considered along with those of combined oral contraceptives. For example, *U.S. Medical Eligibility Criteria* shown in Table 5-4 include the patch and ring along with COCs.

Mechanisms of Action

There are multiple contraceptive actions of CHCs. The most important is to inhibit ovulation by suppression of hypothalamic gonadotropin-releasing factors, which prevents pituitary secretion of follicle-stimulating hormone (FSH) and luteinizing hormone (LH). Estrogens suppress FSH release and stabilize the endometrium to prevent metrorrhagia—referred to as *breakthrough bleeding* in this setting. Progestins inhibit ovulation by suppressing LH, they thicken cervical mucus to retard sperm passage, and they render the endometrium unfavorable for implantation. Thus, CHCs have contraceptive effects from both hormones and taken daily for 3 out of every 4 weeks, provide virtually absolute protection against conception.

Pharmacology

Until recently, there were only two estrogens available for use in oral contraceptives in the United States. These were *ethinyl estradiol* and its less commonly used 3-methyl ether, *mestranol.* In 2010, the third estrogen compound—*estradiol valerate*—was approved by the FDA.

Most currently available progestins are *19-nortestosterone* derivatives. However, drospirenone, is a spironolactone analog, and the dose of drospirenone in COCs currently marketed has properties similar to 25 mg of this diuretic (Seeger, 2007). It displays antiandrogenic activity, and its antimineralocorticoid properties may, in theory, cause potassium retention, leading to hyperkalemia. Thus, drospirenone should not be prescribed for those with renal or adrenal insufficiency or with hepatic dysfunction. Moreover, monitoring of serum potassium levels is recommended in the first month for patients chronically treated concomitantly with any drug associated with potassium retention (Bayer Health Care Pharmaceuticals, 2007). Several studies have shown improvement in symptoms for women with premenstrual dysphoric disorder (PMDD) who use the drospirenone-containing COC, Yaz (Lopez, 2009; Yonkers, 2005). The FDA has approved its indications to include treatment of premenstrual syndrome and moderate acne vulgaris for women requesting oral contraception.

Progestins were initially selected for their progestational potency. However, without any scientific basis, they are

TABLE 5-7. Contraindications to the Use of Combination Oral Contraceptives

Pregnancy
Uncontrolled hypertension
Smokers older than 35 years
Diabetes with vascular involvement
Thrombogenic heart arrhythmias
Thrombogenic cardiac valvulopathies
Cerebrovascular or coronary artery disease
Migraines with associated focal neurologic deficits
Thrombophlebitis or thromboembolic disorders
History of deep-vein thrombophlebitis or thrombotic disorders
Undiagnosed abnormal genital bleeding
Known or suspected breast carcinoma
Cholestatic jaundice of pregnancy or jaundice with pill use
Hepatic adenomas or carcinomas, or active liver disease with abnormal liver function
Carcinoma of the endometrium or other known or suspected estrogen-dependent neoplasia

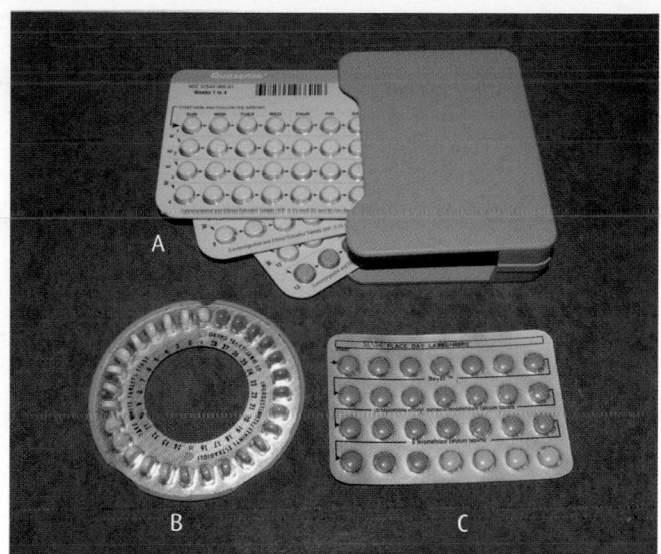

FIGURE 5-10 Various combined oral contraceptive (COC) pills. **A.** Extended-use COCs. Each of the three sequential cards of pills is taken. Placebo pills (*peach*) are found in the bottom card. **B.** 21/7 triphasic COCs. Active pills are taken for 3 weeks and are followed by seven placebo pills (*green*). With triphasic pills, the combination of estrogen and progestin varies with color changes, in this case, from white to blue to dark blue. **C.** 24/4 monophasic COCs. Monophasic pills contain a constant dose of estrogen and progestin throughout the pill pack. With 24/4 dosing regimens, the number of placebo pills is decreased to four.

often compared, marketed, and prescribed based on their presumed estrogenic, antiestrogenic, and androgenic effects (Wallach, 2000). Of note, all progestins lower serum free testosterone levels and thereby limit 5α-reductase, the enzyme necessary to convert testosterone to its active form, dihydrotestosterone. For this reason, progestins can be expected to have salutary effects on androgen-related conditions such as acne.

At the time of their debut over 50 years ago, COCs contained what are now known to be *massive* amounts of both synthetic estrogens and progestins. Because most adverse effects are dose related, side effects of early formulations were much more common compared with those now seen with modern "low-dose" CHCs. For most of the current formulations, the lowest acceptable dose is governed by the ability to prevent unacceptable breakthrough bleeding.

Contraindications

Because of the wide availability of alternate effective contraceptive methods, a number of underlying conditions are considered contraindications to CHC use (Table 5-7).

Combined Oral Contraceptive Pills

Hormone-containing contraceptive pills recently had a celebrated 50th anniversary in this country. These various preparations—used by 12 million women in the United States in 2010—are popularly known by several names. Among others, these include *combination oral contraceptives (COCs), birth control pills (BCPs), oral contraceptives (OCs), oral contraceptive pills (OCPs)*, and most simply, *The Pill*.

Currently, the daily estrogen content in most COCs varies from 20 to 50 μg of ethinyl estradiol, and most pills contain 35 μg or less. Of note, in 2011, the FDA approved the first pill containing only 10 μg of ethinyl estradiol—*Lo*

Loestrin Fe (Warner Chilcott.) With COCs, the progestin dose can be constant throughout the cycle—*monophasic pills*—but the dose frequently is varied—*biphasic and triphasic pills* (Fig. 5-10). In some of these, the estrogen dose is also varied during the cycle. *Combination oral contraceptives* are marketed in almost bewildering variety and are listed in (Table 5-8). There are also generic formulations, and their use has increased. A summary of health benefits associated with combination hormonal contraceptives is found in Table 5-9.

Multiphasic pills were developed in an effort to reduce the amount of total progestin per cycle without sacrificing contraceptive efficacy or cycle control. The reduction is achieved by beginning with a low dose of progestin and increasing it later in the cycle. Theoretically, the lower total dose minimizes the intensity of progestin-induced metabolic changes and adverse side effects. In some of these formulations, the estrogen dose is kept constant, but in others, it is varied. As shown in Table 5-8, in most of these, the estrogen dose is 20 to 40 μg of ethinyl estradiol, whereas in another, estradiol valerate varies from 1- to 3-mg doses. Disadvantages of multiphasic formulations include confusion caused by the multicolored pills—in some brands there are five colors—as well as breakthrough bleeding or spotting, which likely is increased compared with monophasic pills (Woods, 1992).

In a few COCs, inert placebo pills have been replaced by tablets containing iron. These have the suffix Fe added to their name. In addition, Beyaz (Bayer HealthCare) has a

TABLE 5-8. Combination Oral Contraceptive Formulations

Product Name[a]	Estrogen	μg (days)[b]	Progestin	mg (days)
Monophasic Preparations				
20 μg estrogen				
Yaz	EE	20 (24)	Drospirenone	3.00 (24)
Beyaz[c]	EE	20 (24)	Drospirenone	3.00 (24)
Alesse, Aviane, Lutera; Levlite, Lessina, Sronyx	EE	20	Levonorgestrel	0.10
Loestrin 1/20[d], Junel 1/20[d], Microgestin 1/20[d]	EE	20	Norethindrone acetate	1.00
Loestrin 24 Fe[d]	EE	20 (24)	Norethindrone acetate	1.00 (24)
Generesse Fe[d]	EE	25 (24)	Norethindrone	0.80 (24)
30–35 μg estrogen				
Desogen, Ortho-Cept, Apri, Reclipsen, Solia	EE	30	Desogestrel	0.15
Yasmin	EE	30	Drospirenone	3.00
Safyral[c]	EE	30	Drospirenone	3.00
Demulen 1/35, Kelnor, Zovia 1/35	EE	35	Ethynodiol diacetate	1.00
Levlen, Nordette, Levora, Portia, Altavera, Introvale	EE	30	Levonorgestrel	0.15
Lo/Ovral, Cryselle, Low-Ogestrel	EE	30	Norgestrel	0.30
Ovcon-35, Balziva, Zenchent	EE	35	Norethindrone	0.40
Femcon Fe[d]	EE	35	Norethindrone	0.40
Brevicon, Modicon, Necon 0.5/35, Nortrel 0.5/35, Nelova 0.5/35	EE	35	Norethindrone	0.50
Ortho-Novum 1/35, Norinyl 1+35, Necon 1/35, Nortrel 1/35, Norethin 1/35, Nelova 1/35, Cyclafem 1/35	EE	35	Norethindrone	1.00
Loestrin 1.5/30[d], Junel 1.5/30[d], Microgestin 1.5/30[d]	EE	30	Norethindrone acetate	1.50
Ortho-Cyclen, Sprintec, Mononessa, Previfem	EE	35	Norgestimate	0.25
50 μg estrogen				
Ovral, Ogestrel	EE	50	Norgestrel	0.50
Demulen 1/50, Zovia 1/50	EE	50	Ethynodiol diacetate	1.00
Nelova 1/50M	Mes	50	Norethindrone	1.00
Norinyl 1+50; Ortho-Novum 1/50, Necon 1/50	Mes	50	Norethindrone	1.00
Ovcon 50	EE	50	Norethindrone	1.00
Multiphasic Preparations				
10 μg estrogen				
Lo Loestrin Fe[d]	EE	10 (24) 10 (2)	Norethindrone acetate	1.00 (24)
20 μg estrogen				
Mircette, Kariva	EE	20 (21) 0 (2) 10 (5)	Desogestrel	0.15
25 μg estrogen				
Ortho Tri-Cyclen Lo, Tri Lo Sprintec	EE	25	Norgestimate	0.18 (7) 0.215 (7) 0.25 (7)
Cyclessa, Velivet	EE	25	Desogestrel	0.1 (7) 0.125 (7) 0.15 (7)

(Continued)

TABLE 5-8. Combination Oral Contraceptive Formulations *(Continued)*

Product Name[a]	Estrogen	µg (days)[b]	Progestin	mg (days)
Multiphasic Preparations *(Continued)*				
30–35 µg estrogen				
Ortho Tri-Cyclen, Tri-Sprintec, Trinessa, Tri-Previfem	FF	35	Norgestimate	0.18 (7)
				0.215(7)
				0.25 (7)
Tri-Levlen, Triphasil, Trivora, Enpresse, Levonest	EE	30 (6)	Levonorgestrel	0.05 (6)
		40 (5)		0.075 (5)
		30 (10)		0.125 (10)
Estrostep[d], Tri-Legest[d], Tilia Fe	EE	20 (5)	Norethindrone acetate	1.00
		30 (7)		
		35 (9)		
Jenest	EE	35	Norethindrone	0.50 (7)
				1.00 (14)
Ortho-Novum 10/11, Necon 10/11, Nelova 10/11	EE	35	Norethindrone	0.50 (10)
				1.00 (11)
Ortho-Novum 7/7/7, Necon 7/7/7, Nortrel 7/7/7, Cyclafem 7/7/7	EE	35	Norethindrone	0.50 (7)
				0.75 (7)
				1.00 (7)
Tri-Norinyl, Aranelle, Leena	EE	35	Norethindrone	0.50 (7)
				1.00 (9)
				0.50 (5)
Natazia	EV	3 (2)	Dienogest	—
		2 (5)		2.00 (5)
		2 (17)		3.00 (17)
		1 (2)		—
Progestin-Only Preparations				
Ovrette	None		Norgestrel	0.075 (c)
Micronor, Nor-QD, Errin, Camila, Nor-BE, Jolivette, Heather	None		Norethindrone	0.35 (c)
Extended-Cycle Preparations				
20 µg estrogen				
LoSeasonique[e]	EE	20 (84)	Levonorgestrel	0.10 (84)
		10 (7)		
30 µg estrogen				
Seasonale[f], Quasense[f], Jolessa[f]	EE	30 (84)	Levonorgestrel	0.15 (84)
Seasonique[e]	EE	30 (84)	Levonorgestrel	0.15 (84)
		10 (7)		
Continuous Preparation				
Lybrel[g]	EE	20 (28)	Levonorgestrel	0.09

EE = ethinyl estradiol; EV = estradiol valerate; LC = levomefolate calcium; Mes = mestranol.
Numbers in parentheses = number of days at a particular dosage.
(c) = continuous use.
[a]Blue ink denotes original name brand. Black ink denotes subsequent generics.
[b]Administered for 21 days, variations listed in parentheses.
[c]0.451 mg of levomefolate calcium is found in each pill.
[d]Contains or is available in formulas that contain 75-mg doses of ferrous fumarate within the placebo pills.
[e]12 weeks of active pills, 1 week of ethinyl estradiol only.
[f]12 weeks of active pills, 1 week of inert pills.
[g]One pill every day, 365 days each year.
Compiled from U.S. Food and Drug Administration, 2010.

TABLE 5-9. Some Benefits of Combination Estrogen plus Progestin Oral Contraceptives

Increased bone density
Reduced menstrual blood loss and anemia
Decreased risk of ectopic pregnancy
Improved dysmenorrhea from endometriosis
Fewer premenstrual complaints
Decreased risk of endometrial and ovarian cancer
Reduction in various benign breast diseases
Inhibition of hirsutism progression
Improvement of acne
Prevention of atherogenesis
Decreased incidence and severity of acute salpingitis
Decreased activity of rheumatoid arthritis

form of folate—levomefolate calcium—within both its active and placebo pills.

Administration. Ideally, women would begin COCs on the first day of a menstrual cycle, in which case an additional contraceptive method is unnecessary. A more traditional schedule—the *Sunday start*—requires pill initiation on the first Sunday following the onset of menses. If menses begin on a Sunday, then pills are started that day. Lastly, a *quick start* method may be used in which pills are start on any day of the cycle, commonly the day prescribed. This approach improves short-term compliance (Westhoff, 2002, 2007a). Both Sunday start and quick start methods require use of an additional method for 1 week to insure against conception.

To obtain maximum protection and promote regular use, most manufacturers offer dispensers that provide 21 sequential color-coded tablets containing hormones, followed by seven inert tablets of another color (see Fig. 5-10B). Some newer, lower-dose pills regimens continue active hormones for 24 days, followed by 4 inert pills (see Fig. 5-10C). The goal of these 24/4 regimens is to improve the efficacy of very low-dose COCs. Importantly, for maximum contraceptive efficiency, each woman should adopt an effective scheme for assuring daily—or nightly—self-administration.

Missed Pills. During COC use, if one dose is missed, conception is unlikely with higher-dose monophasic estrogen and progestin pills. When this is recognized, taking that day's pill plus the missed pill will minimize breakthrough bleeding. The remainder of the pill pack is completed with one pill taken daily.

If several doses are missed, or if a dose is missed with the lower-dose pills, then the next dose is doubled and an effective barrier technique is added for the subsequent 7 days. The remainder of the pack is completed with one pill taken daily. Alternatively, a new pack can be started with a barrier method as additional contraception for a week. If withdrawal bleeding does not occur during the placebo pills, the pills are continued, but the woman should seek medical attention to exclude pregnancy.

Transdermal System

There is one transdermal system available in the United States—*Ortho Evra patch* (Ortho-McNeil Pharmaceutical). The patch has an inner layer with an adhesive and hormone matrix and an outer water-resistant layer. The patch is applied to the buttocks, upper outer arm, lower abdomen, or upper torso but avoids the breasts. It delivers daily a dose of 150 µg of the progestin, norelgestromin, and 20 µg of ethinyl estradiol. A new patch is applied each week for 3 weeks, followed by a patch-free week to allow for withdrawal bleeding.

In a randomized trial by Audet and associates (2001), the patch was slightly more effective than a low-dose oral contraceptive—1.2 versus 2.2 pregnancies per 100 woman years. Overall, the patch is well tolerated and safe, but dysmenorrhea and breast tenderness were more frequent in the patch group, as was breakthrough bleeding in the first two cycles. Patch replacement was required for either complete—1.8 percent, or partial detachment—2.8 percent. In approximately 3 percent of women, a severe application site reaction precluded further use.

Pooled data suggest that women who weigh 90 kg or more are at increased risk for pregnancy with the patch (Zieman, 2002). Other metabolic and physiologic effects should be those seen with low-dose COCs, with the caveat that accumulated experience is limited. The patch is suitable for women who prefer weekly applications to daily dosing and who meet the other criteria for CHC administration.

Concerns have been raised that CHC delivered by the patch may be associated with an increased risk for venous thromboembolism and other vascular complications. This followed reports that patch use was associated with increased hepatic synthesis of estrogen-sensitive procoagulants compared with COC or vaginal ring use (Jensen, 2008; White, 2006). This is because of different pharmacokinetics attributed to delivery methods. Although peak serum estrogen levels were lower with patch versus COC use, total exposure was greater—a relatively increased net estrogen effect (Kluft, 2008; van den Heuvel, 2005). Despite lack of a convincing clinical association, in 2008, the FDA ordered labeling for the patch to state that users *may* be at increased risk for developing venous thromboembolism. Plaintiff attorneys followed with lawsuits that inevitably curtailed use of the patch method (Phelps, 2009). To date, conclusive evidence for increased morbidity with patch use compared with other CHC use is lacking (Jick, 2006, 2010a,b).

Transvaginal Ring

There is one intravaginal hormonal contraceptive available in the United States—*NuvaRing* (Organon). It is a flexible polymer ring with an outer diameter of 54 mm and an inner diameter of 50 mm (Fig. 5-11). Its core releases a daily dose of 15 µg ethinyl estradiol and 120 µg of the progestin, etonogestrel. These doses very effectively inhibit ovulation, and the failure

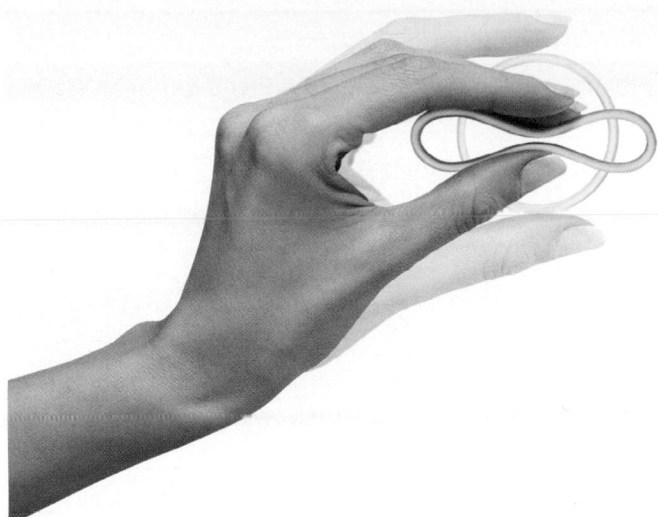

FIGURE 5-11 NuvaRing is an estrogen- and progestin-releasing vaginal contraceptive ring. The background image shows ring flexibility. *(Reproduced with permission of N.V. Organon, a subsidiary of Merck & Co, Inc. All rights reserved. NuvaRing is a registered trademarks of N.V. Organon.)*

rate was reported to be 0.65 pregnancies per 100 woman-years (Mulders, 2001; Roumen, 2001).

Prior to dispensing, the pharmacy must keep rings refrigerated. Once dispensed, their shelf life is 4 months (Burkman, 2002). The ring is initially inserted within 5 days after the onset of menses. It is removed after 3 weeks for one week to allow withdrawal bleeding. After this, a new ring is inserted. Breakthrough bleeding is uncommon. Up to 20 percent of women and 35 percent of men reported being able to feel the ring during intercourse. If bothersome, the ring may be removed for coitus, but it should be replaced within 3 hours.

Intramuscular Administration

The only intramuscular CHC preparation—*Lunelle*—was withdrawn for use in this country by its manufacturer. Each injection contained 25 mg of medroxyprogesterone acetate and 5 mg estradiol cypionate.

Extended Cycle Contraception

The use of CHCs continuously for more than 28 days has become increasingly popular in this country. Their benefits include decreased episodes of cyclic bleeding, fewer menstrual symptoms, and lower costs. Several formulations are available (see Table 5-8). Although these prepackaged cycle formulations are available, extended cycle contraception can also be achieved in other ways. The standard 21- or 28-day COC packs, with the placebo pills discarded, can be used continuously (Lin, 2007). Also, either the transdermal patch or the vaginal ring can be used without the 1-week hormone-free intervals.

Unique Characteristics

A number of factors unique to extended-cycle CHCs are important. Some of these are shared with continuous progestin contraceptive methods such as implants or injections.

The principal change is loss of menstrual normalcy that manifests as less frequent, lighter, and generally unpredictable bleeding episodes. For example, amenorrhea of 6 months or more is reported to affect 8 to 63 percent of extended cycle users. Although considered a benefit by most women, it is far from a guaranteed one. More often, women have fewer bleeding episodes per month. This allows repair of associated anemia in those who had menorrhagia prior to extended-cycle use (Edelman, 2010). But it is also these characteristics that cause some women to be reluctant to use this method, as it may be considered "unnatural" to miss monthly menses. Some are concerned that amenorrhea may be a sign of pregnancy or may affect future fertility. For these, reassurance is given that continuous progestins maintain a healthy endometrium.

Women who use continuous CHC methods report fewer menstrual symptoms that include headaches, fatigue, bloating, and dysmenorrhea compared with women using cyclic contraceptives (Machado, 2010). Moreover, hypothalamic-pituitary-ovarian suppression is greater with continuous use and reduces the possibility of escape ovulation caused by delayed start of a new contraceptive cycle.

Any putative effects of continuous CHC use to cause endometrial cancer would appear to be unfounded. This comes from findings that support a *decreased* risk for endometrial malignancy associated with cyclic CHC use. Thus on a biological basis, it seems reasonable to conclude that this protective effect would also apply to continuous CHC use.

Drug Interactions

Interactions between CHCs and various other medications take two forms. First, hormonal contraceptives may interfere with the actions of some drugs shown in Table 5-10. In contrast, some drugs shown in Table 5-11 may decrease the contraceptive effectiveness of CHCs. Mechanisms for these are multiple and frequently cannot be identified. A major one likely is stimulation or suppression of genes coded for expression of enzymes of the cytochrome oxidase systems.

Pharmacokinetic changes result in decreased serum concentrations of contraceptive steroids. But, the ultimate effect on ovulation suppression is not known as studies are lacking. However, with the information at hand, the effects of these interactions may necessitate that either the dose of contraceptive or that of the other drug be increased or decreased as shown in Tables 5-10 and 5-11 to ensure efficacy.

Special Considerations

Risk of Death. Mortality associated with CHC use is rare in women who are younger than 35 years, have no systemic illness, and do not smoke (see Table 5-1). In an earlier report from a health cooperative, Porter and colleagues (1987) attributed only one death to COCs use for almost 55,000 woman years.

Weight Gain. Excessive weight gain is a concern with use of any hormonal contraceptive. In their most recent Cochrane

TABLE 5-10. Drugs Whose Effectiveness Is Influenced by Combination Oral Contraceptives

Interacting Drug	Evidence	Management of the Interacting Drug
Analgesics		
Acetaminophen	Adequate	Larger dose may be required
Aspirin	Probable	Larger dose may be required
Meperidine	Suspected	Smaller dose may be required
Morphine	Probable	Larger dose may be required
Anticoagulants		
Dicumarol, warfarin	Controversial	
Antidepressants		
Imipramine	Suspected	Decrease dose approximately one third
Anticonvulsant		
Lamotrigine monotherapy	Adequate	Avoid CHCs because anticonvulsant levels are significantly lowered
Tranquilizers		
Diazepam, alprazolam	Suspected	Decrease dose
Temazepam	Possible	May need to increase dose
Other benzodiazepines	Suspected	Observe for increased effect
Antiinflammatories		
Corticosteroids	Adequate	Watch for potentiation of effects, decrease dose accordingly
Bronchodilators		
Aminophylline, theophylline, caffeine	Adequate	Reduce starting dose by one third
Antihypertensives		
Cyclopenthiazide	Adequate	Increase dose
Metoprolol	Suspected	May need to lower dose
Other		
Troleandomycin	Suspected liver damage	Avoid
Cyclosporine	Possible	May use smaller dose
Antiretrovirals	Variable	See manufacturer or other[a]

[a]University of California at San Francisco (UCSF): HIV Insite, 2011.
CHC = combination hormonal contraceptives.
From the Centers for Disease Control and Prevention, 2010b; Gaffield, 2011; Wallach, 2000.

database review of randomized trials, Gallo and associates (2008) again concluded that available evidence was insufficient to determine accurate effects that CHCs might have on weight gain, but that no large effect was obvious.

Obese and Overweight Women. In general, CHCs are highly effective in obese women (Lopez, 2010). However, as with some other drugs, obesity may result in altered pharmacokinetics of some CHC methods. That said, data regarding overweight women are conflicting regarding increased pregnancy risk due to decreased CHC efficacy from lowered bioavailability (Brunner, 2005; Edelman, 2009; Holt, 2002, 2005; Westhoff, 2010). Importantly, in some women, obesity may be synergistic with some of the conditions, described next, that may render CHCs a less optimal contraceptive method.

Combined Hormonal Contraception and Medical Disorders

Interactions of CHCs with some chronic medical disorders may constitute relative or absolute contraindication to CHC use. These are described in the following sections.

Diabetes Mellitus. Higher-dose COCs were associated with insulin antagonistic properties, particularly those mediated by progestins. However, with current low-dose CHCs, these concerns have been mitigated (Speroff, 2001). In healthy women, long-term large prospective studies have found that COCs do not increase the risk for diabetes (Rimm, 1992). Moreover, these agents do not appear to increase the risk for overt diabetes in women with prior gestational diabetes (Kjos, 1998). Lastly, use of these contraceptives is approved for nonsmoking,

TABLE 5-11. Drugs That May Reduce Combined Hormonal Contraceptive Efficacy

Interacting Drug	Evidence
Antituberculous	
Rifampin	Established; reduced efficacy if <50 µg EE pill is used
Antifungals	
Griseofulvin	Strongly suspected
Anticonvulsants and sedatives	
Phenytoin, mephenytoin, phenobarbital, primidone, carbamazepine, ethosuximide, topiramate, oxcarbazepine	Strongly suspected; reduced efficacy if <50 µg EE pill is used; trials lacking
Antibiotics	
Tetracycline, doxycycline	Two small studies find no association
Penicillins	No association documented
Ciprofloxacin	No effect on efficacy of a 30 µg EE + desogestrel pill
Ofloxacin	No effect on efficacy of a 30 µg EE + levonorgestrel pill
Antiretrovirals	Variable effects; see manufacturer or other[a]

[a]University of California at San Francisco (UCSF): HIV Insite, 2011.
EE = ethinyl estradiol.
From the Centers for Disease Control and Prevention, 2010b; Wallach, 2000.

diabetic women who are younger than 35 years and who have no associated vascular disease (American College of Obstetricians and Gynecologists, 2008b).

Cardiovascular Disease. In general, severe cardiovascular disorders limit the use of CHCs, as shown in Table 5-7. For the much more common less severe disorders, however, currently used formulations do not increase associated risks.

Low-dose CHCs do not appreciably increase the absolute risk of clinically significant hypertension (Chasan-Taber, 1996). However, it is common practice for patients to return 8 to 12 weeks following CHC initiation for evaluation of blood pressure and other symptoms. For those with already established chronic hypertension, CHC use is permissible in those with well-controlled otherwise uncomplicated hypertension (American College of Obstetricians and Gynecologists, 2008b). Severe forms of hypertension, especially those with end-organ involvement, usually preclude CHC use.

Women who have had a documented *myocardial infarction* should not be given CHCs. That said, these contraceptives do not increase the de novo risk for myocardial ischemia in nonsmoking women younger than 35 years (Margolis, 2007; Mishell, 2000; World Health Organization Collaborative Study, 1997). Smoking by itself, however, is a potent risk factor for ischemic heart disease, and CHCs used after age 35 years act synergistically to increase this risk.

Cerebrovascular Disorders. Women who have had either an *ischemic* or *hemorrhagic stroke* should not use CHCs. But the incidence of strokes in nonsmoking young women is low,

and use of CHCs does not increase the risk for either type of stroke (World Health Organization Collaborative Study, 1996). This form of vascular disorder is more commonly encountered in those who smoke, have hypertension, or have migraine headaches with visual aura *and* who use CHCs (MacClellan, 2007).

Migraine headaches may be a risk factor for strokes in some young women, and their diagnosis is of some concern in women who plan to use CHCs. In the report by Curtis and coworkers (2002), women using COCs who had *migraine headaches with aura* had a two- to fourfold increased risk for stroke compared with nonusers. Because of this, the World Health Organization (2010) recommends against CHC use in this subset of migraineurs. Alternatively, the American College of Obstetricians and Gynecologists (2008b), because the absolute risk is low, has concluded that CHCs may be considered for young nonsmoking women who have migraine headaches without focal neurologic changes. For many of these women, an intrauterine contraceptive method or a progestin-only pill may be more appropriate (World Health Organization, 2010).

Venous Thromboembolism. From the early history of higher-dose COCs, it was apparent that the risks for *deep-vein thrombosis* and *pulmonary embolism* were significantly increased in women who used these contraceptives (Realini, 1985; Stadel, 1981). These risks were found to be estrogen-dose related and have been appreciably lowered with evolution of low-dose formulations that contain only 20 to 35 µg of ethinyl estradiol (Westhoff, 1998). Of note, a possible increased VTE risk with drosperinone-containing COCs has been shown in two studies, and the FDA has encourage an assessment of benefits and of VTE risks in users of these pills (Food and Drug Administration, 2011; Jick, 2011; Parkin, 2011).

From their review, Mishell and coworkers (2000) concluded that, in general, there was a three- to fourfold increased VTE risk in current COC users, but that this did not persist in former users. However, the risk without contraception is quite low—approximately 1 per 10,000 woman years—and thus the incidence with CHCs is only 3 to 4 per 10,000 woman years. Importantly, these CHC-enhanced risks appear to dissipate rapidly once contraceptive treatment is discontinued. And of equal importance, these risks for venous thrombosis and pulmonary embolism are still lower than those estimated during pregnancy, which has an incidence of 5 to 6 per 10,000 woman years.

Several cofactors increase the incidence of venous thromboembolism in women using estrogen-containing contraceptives or those who are pregnant or postpartum. These include some women with one or more of the many *thrombophilias* that have been described over the past 25 years. Examples include *protein C or S deficiency* or *factor V Leiden mutation* (Chap. 39, p. 960) (Comp, 1996; Mohllajee, 2006). Other factors that increase the risks for thromboembolism are hypertension, obesity, diabetes, smoking, and a sedentary lifestyle (Pomp, 2007, 2008).

Older studies indicated a twofold increased risk for *perioperative thromboembolism* in CHC users (Robinson, 1991). There are no data with the low-dose formulations currently used, and thus, the American College of Obstetricians and Gynecologists (2007b, 2008b) recommends balancing the risks of thromboembolism with those of unintended pregnancy during the 4 to 6 weeks required preoperatively for thrombogenic effects of CHCs to dissipate.

Systemic Lupus Erythematosus. The use of combination hormonal contraception in women with otherwise uncomplicated systemic lupus erythematosus (SLE) has been the "poster child" for evidence-based clinical research. In the past, and with good reason, CHCs were considered to be contraindicated in women with SLE. This was because of their underlying high risk to develop venous and arterial thrombosis along with the thrombogenic effects of older high-dose steroid contraceptive pills. The safety of the low-dose modern COCs in many women with SLE was shown in two randomized trials (Petri, 2005; Sánchez-Guerrero, 2005). Use of CHCs in women with lupus was reviewed by Culwell and colleagues (2009). Importantly, CHCs are not appropriate in women with SLE who have positive testing for antiphospholipid antibodies or have other known contraindications to CHC use.

Seizure Disorders. Approximately 1 million women of reproductive age in the United States are diagnosed with some form of epilepsy. As shown in Tables 5-10 and 5-11, metabolism and clearance of some CHCs are appreciably altered by some, but not all, of the commonly used anticonvulsants. One

mechanism with a number of antiepileptic drugs is potent induction of enzymes of the cytochrome P450 system. This in turn leads to increased metabolism of contraceptive steroids with serum contraceptive steroid levels decreased by as much as half (American College of Obstetricians and Gynecologists, 2008b; Zupanc, 2006).

With few exceptions, these metabolic interactions usually do not result in increased seizure activity. One possible exception is combined use of CHCs and monotherapy with the anticonvulsant lamotrigine. Serum levels of the anticonvulsant are decreased by up to 50 percent, and this may increase the risk for seizures (Gaffield, 2011).

Evidence-based guidelines for use of contraceptives by women with epilepsy are listed in the US MEC (Centers for Disease Control and Prevention, 2010b). Use of CHCs in epileptic women is rated as category 3, that is, theoretical or proven risks usually outweigh the advantages of using the method. They may reduce contraceptive or anticonvulsant effectiveness. Thus, epileptic women using cytochrome P450 enhancing anticonvulsants are counseled regarding alternate contraceptive methods if feasible. If not, a COC containing at least 30 μg of ethinyl estradiol should be used. For those using lamotrigine monotherapy, CHCs are not recommended.

Although they are not CHCs, progestin-only containing preparations are also affected by use of anticonvulsants that induce the cytochrome P450 enzyme system. These result in decreased serum progestin levels, lower rates of effective ovulation suppression, and pose an unacceptable risk of unplanned pregnancy.

Liver Disease. Both estrogens and progestins have known effects on hepatic function. Most commonly seen in pregnancy, cholestasis and cholestatic jaundice are also induced, albeit uncommonly, with CHC use. Because susceptibility is likely due to an inherited gene mutation of bilirubin transport, cholestasis with CHCs is more likely in women affected during a pregnancy. Discontinuing the CHC will result in resolution of symptoms.

There are conflicting reports on whether these cholestatic effects of CHCs increase the risks for subsequent cholelithiasis and cholecystectomy. Any increased risk is likely to be small, and the known effects of increasing parity on gallbladder disease must also be considered.

Regarding women with viral hepatitis or cirrhosis, the World Health Organization has provided recommendations (Kapp, 2009). For women who have active hepatitis, CHCs should not be initiated, but these may be continued in women who experience a flare of their liver disease while already taking CHCs. Use of progestin-only contraception in these women is not restricted. With cirrhosis, mild compensated disease does not limit the use of CHCs. However, in those with severe decompensated disease, all hormonal methods should be avoided.

Neoplastic Diseases. Stimulatory effects of sex steroids on some cancers are a concern. It would appear, however, that overall these hormones do not *cause* cancer (Hannaford, 2007).

A report from the Collaborative Group on Epidemiological Studies of Ovarian Cancer (2008) verified earlier studies that showed a protective effect against endometrial and ovarian cancers (Cancer and Steroid Hormone Study, 1987a,b). This protection decreases as duration from pill discontinuance increases (Tworoger, 2007). Reports concerning possible increased risks for premalignant and malignant changes of the liver, cervix, and breast are conflicting and are presented next.

Hepatic Neoplasia. Some older higher-dose estrogen-containing COCs were linked to risks for hepatic focal nodular hyperplasia and benign hepatic adenomas. Studies done evaluating women taking contemporary low-dose COCs, however, reported no such association (Hannaford, 1997; Heinemann, 1998). Similarly, earlier associations of CHCs with hepatocellular carcinoma have been refuted by the multicenter World Health Organization Study (1989) as well as by Maheshwari and coworkers (2007).

Cervical Dysplasia and Carcinoma. With COC use, there is an increased risk of cervical dysplasia and cervical cancer. These risks increase with duration of use. But, according to the International Collaboration of Epidemiological Studies of Cervical Cancer (2007), if COC use is discontinued, by 10 years, the risk becomes comparable with that of never-users. The reasons for this are speculative and may be related to more frequent human papillomavirus (HPV) exposure because of lesser-used barrier methods. It may also be related to more frequent cytologic screening that COC users may have. Moreover, COCs may increase persistence of HPV infection and HPV oncogene expression (de Villiers, 2003). Importantly, if cervical dysplasia is treated, the recurrence rate is not increased in CHC users.

Breast Cancer. Despite the known stimulatory effects of female sex steroid hormones on breast cancer, it is still unclear whether CHCs have an adverse effect on tumor growth or development. The Collaborative Group on Hormonal Factors in Breast Cancer (1996) analyzed data from studies that included more than 53,000 women with breast cancer and 100,000 nonaffected women. They found a significant 1.24-fold increased risk for current COC users. This risk decreased to 1.16 for those 1 to 4 years after discontinuing COCs and 1.07 for those at 5 to 9 years. The risks were not influenced by age at first use, duration of use, family history of breast cancer, first use prior to pregnancy, or the dose or type of hormone used. This lack of correlation serves to question any causal role of COCs in breast tumorigenesis.

The Collaborative Group investigators also found that COC-associated tumors tended to be to be less aggressive and that cancers were detected at earlier stages. They suggested that the increased cancer diagnosis may have been because of more intensive surveillance among users. In a case-control study—4575 cases and 4682 controls—there was no relationship found with either current or past COC use and breast cancer (Marchbanks, 2002). Finally, women heterozygous for *BRCA1* or *BRCA2* gene mutations have not been shown to have an increased incidence of breast or ovarian cancer with COC use (Brohet, 2007). With regard to benign breast disease, Vessey and Yeates (2007) reported that COC use apparently *lowered* the relative risk.

HIV Infections and Antiretroviral Therapy. Women with HIV infection or acquired immunodeficiency syndrome (AIDS) require special considerations for gynecologic care that are especially important regarding contraceptive use. As outlined by the American College of Obstetricians and Gynecologists (2010b), these women need highly effective contraception that must be compatible with *highly active antiretroviral therapy—HAART*, that places them at low risk for acquiring sexually transmitted infections, and that does not increase their risk of transmitting HIV to their partners.

Although CHCs have been shown safe for use in HIV-positive women, their metabolism may be variably affected by some of the HAART regimens in current use. Details of various HAART regimen interactions with CHCs are available at the University of California, San Francisco HIV InSite web site: http://hivinsite.ucsf.edu/insite?page=ar-00-02.

Other Disorders. In one metaanalysis, Zapata and colleagues (2010a) reported that limited data suggested that COC use did not increase the risk of exacerbation of inflammatory bowel disease. Insufficient data were found in other metaanalyses designed to study contraceptive use in women who had a solid organ transplant or in those who had been diagnosed with peripartum cardiomyopathy (Paulen, 2010; Tepper, 2010).

Progestin-only Contraceptives

Contraceptives that contain only a progestin were developed to obviate the unwanted side effects of estrogens. Progestins can be delivered by a number of mechanisms that include tablets, injections, intrauterine devices (p. 137), and subdermal implants (p. 143).

Progestin-Only Pills

Mechanism of Action. Progestin-only pills—also called *mini-pills*—are taken daily. They do not reliably inhibit ovulation, but instead their effectiveness depends more on cervical mucus alterations and effects on the endometrium. Because the mucus changes do not persist beyond 24 hours, to be maximally effective, a pill should be taken at the same time every day. Their use has not achieved widespread popularity because of a much higher incidence of irregular bleeding and a slightly higher pregnancy rate than that seen with COCs (see Table 5-2).

Progestin-only pills have minimal if any effect on carbohydrate metabolism and coagulation factors. They do not cause or exacerbate hypertension, and thus, they may be ideal for some women at increased risk for other cardiovascular complications. Such women include those with a history of thrombosis or migraine headaches or smokers older than 35 years. The mini-pill is suitable for lactating women because it does not impair milk production. When used in combination with breast-feeding, progestin-only pills are virtually 100-percent effective for up to 6 months (Betrabet, 1987; Shikary, 1987).

Contraindications. Progestin-only pills should not be taken by women with unexplained uterine bleeding, breast cancer, hepatic neoplasms, pregnancy, or active severe liver disease (Janssen-Ortho, 2010).

Counseling. As discussed previously, a major disadvantage of progestin-only tablets is that they must be taken at the same or nearly the same time each day. Importantly, if a progestin-only pill is taken even 4 hours late, an additional form of contraception must be used for the next 48 hours. This may contribute to another major drawback, which is a higher risk for contraceptive failure compared with CHCs. And along with these failures, there is a relative increase in the proportion of ectopic pregnancies (Sivin, 1991). Irregular uterine bleeding is another distinct disadvantage. This may be characterized by amenorrhea, intermenstrual bleeding, or prolonged periods of menorrhagia. As with other progestin-containing methods of contraception, functional ovarian cysts develop with a greater frequency in women using these agents, although they do not usually require intervention (Hidalgo, 2006; Inki, 2002).

The effectiveness of progestin-only tablets is decreased by some medications, which are listed in Tables 5-10 and 5-11. In some cases, women taking these drugs should avoid oral progestin-only preparations.

Injectable Progestins

There are three injectable depot progesterone preparations that are used worldwide. This method is popular in the United States and is used by approximately 6 percent of women choosing a contraceptive. Injectable progestins have mechanisms of action similar to those for oral progestins and include increased cervical mucus viscosity, creation of an endometrium unfavorable for implantation, and unpredictable ovulation suppression.

Injectable preparations include depot medroxyprogesterone acetate (DMPA)—marketed as *Depo-Provera* (Pfizer). A 150-mg dose is given by intramuscular injection every 90 days. A derivative of DMPA is marketed as *depo-subQprovera 104* (Pfizer), and a 104-mg dose is given subcutaneously every 90 days. Because there is slower absorption with subcutaneous injections, the 104-mg dose is equivalent to the 150-mg intramuscular preparation (Jain, 2004). With either method, if the initial dose is given within the first 5 days following menses onset, no back-up contraception is necessary (Haider, 2007). A third injectable depot progestin that is not currently available in the United States is norethindrone ethanthate, which is marketed as *Norgest,* and a 200-mg dose is injected intramuscularly every 2 months.

Injectable progestins have contraceptive efficacy equivalent or better than that of COCs. With perfect use, DMPA has pregnancy rates of 0.3 percent, but typical-use failure rates are as high as 7 percent at 12 months (Kost, 2008; Said, 1986). Depot progesterone does not suppress lactation, and iron-deficiency anemia is less likely in long-term users because of less menstrual bleeding.

Contraindications. Progestin injectables should not be taken by women with pregnancy, unexplained uterine bleeding, breast cancer, active or history of thromboembolic disease, cerebrovascular disease, or significant liver disease (Pfizer, 2010).

Counseling
Bleeding Pattern. Patients interested in DMPA use should be familiar with its potential effects and side effects. First, as is typical of progestin-only contraception, DMPA usually causes *irregular menstrual-type bleeding.* Cromer and coworkers (1994) reported that one fourth of women discontinued its use in the first year because of irregular bleeding. Amenorrhea may develop after extended use, and women should be counseled about this benign effect.

Delayed Return of Fertility Following Cessation. DMPA may also cause prolonged ovulation suppression after injections are stopped. In an earlier study by Gardner and Mishell (1970), one fourth of women did not resume regular menses for up to a year. Accordingly, DMPA may not be the best choice for women who plan to use contraception only briefly before attempting conception.

Bone Density. DMPA causes significantly diminished bone mineral density because of lowered estrogen levels. However, the American College of Obstetricians and Gynecologists (2008a) has concluded that concerns of bone density loss should not prevent or limit use of this contraceptive method.

Bone mineral density loss is most worrisome in long-term users (Scholes, 1999). Moreover, this loss is relevant for adolescents because bone density increases most rapidly from ages 10 to 30 years (Sulak, 1999). Additionally, decreased bone mineral density may be a concern for perimenopausal women, who will shortly be entering the menopause, a time of known accelerated bone loss. These concerns prompted the FDA in 2004 to require a black-box warning that DMPA "should be used as a long-term birth control method—longer than 2 years—only if other birth-control methods are inadequate."

There are some mitigating factors that should be considered regarding this concern. One is that bone loss is greatest during the first and second years of use, and afterwards slows appreciably. Another is that most bone lost during contraceptive use is restored within 5 years after its discontinuance (Clark, 2006; Harel, 2010; Kaunitz, 2006). Finally, there is no evidence that fractures are more common in these women (Lopez, 2009a).

Cancer Risks. Cervical carcinoma in-situ risk is possibly increased with DMPA use, although there are not increased risks for cervical cancer or for hepatic neoplasms with this method (Thomas, 1995). Importantly, the risks for ovarian and endometrial cancers have been shown to be *decreased*

(Earl, 1994; Kaunitz, 1996). In addition, Skegg and colleagues (1995) pooled the results of the New Zealand and World Health Organization case-control studies that included almost 1800 women with breast cancer. Compared with 14,000 controls, DMPA contraceptive use was associated with a twofold cancer risk in the first 5 years of use. However, the overall risk was not increased.

Other Effects. Some women report breast tenderness with DMPA use. Depression has also been reported, but a causal link has not been proven. Finally, although weight gain is often attributed to depot progestins, not all studies have shown this (Bahamondes, 2001; Mainwaring, 1995; Moore, 1995; Taneepanichskul, 1998). Beksinska and coworkers (2010) reported that adolescents who used intramuscular DMPA gained 2.3 kg more weight over 4 to 5 years compared with weight gained by adolescents who used COCs. Subcutaneous DMPA has also been shown to cause modest weight gain in most women (Westhoff, 2007b). Because women who gain weight in the first 6 months of use are more likely to have long-term weight gain, Le and colleagues (2009) suggest that these women may benefit from early counseling.

THIRD-TIER CONTRACEPTIVES— MODERATELY EFFECTIVE

There are two types of contraceptive methods that are considered as moderately effective. One type includes barrier methods, which are designed to prevent functional sperm from reaching and fertilizing the ovum. The other category consists of fertility awareness methods. Perhaps more so than with other contraceptive methods, moderately effective methods have the highest success rates when used by couples who are dedicated to their use.

▪ Barrier Methods

These methods include vaginal diaphragms and male and female condoms. As shown in Table 5-2, the reported pregnancy rate for these methods varies from 2 to 6 percent in the first year of use and is highly dependent on correct and consistent use.

Male Condom

Most condoms are made from latex rubber, and various sizes are manufactured to accommodate anatomy. Less commonly, polyurethane or lamb cecum is used. Condoms provide effective contraception, and their failure rate when used by strongly motivated couples has been as low as 3 or 4 per 100 couple-years of exposure (Vessey, 1982). Generally, and especially in the first year of use, the failure rate is much higher.

A distinct advantage of condoms is that, when used properly, they provide considerable—not absolute—protection against many sexually transmitted infections. Condoms also help to prevent premalignant cervical changes, probably by blocking transmission of the human papillomavirus (HPV) (Winer, 2006).

Counseling. The efficacy of condoms is enhanced appreciably with a reservoir tip. Lubricants should be water based because oil-based products destroy latex condoms and diaphragms (Waldron, 1989). Speroff and Darney (2001) emphasize the following key steps to ensure maximal condom effectiveness:

- It must be used with every coital act.
- It should be in place before contact of the penis with the vagina.
- Withdrawal must occur with the penis still erect.
- The base of the condom must be held during withdrawal.
- Either an intravaginal spermicide or a condom lubricated with spermicide should be employed.

Latex Sensitivity. There are alternative condoms available for latex-sensitive individuals. Condoms made from lamb intestines—*natural skin* or *lambskin condoms*—are effective, but they do not provide protection against sexually transmitted infections. Nonallergenic condoms are made with a synthetic thermoplastic elastomer, such as polyurethane, which is also used in some surgical gloves. These are effective against sexually transmitted infections, but have significantly higher breakage and slippage rates compared with those of latex condoms (Gallo, 2006). In a randomized trial of 901 couples, Steiner and associates (2003) documented breakage and slippage with 8.4 percent of polyurethane condoms compared with only 3.2 percent with latex condoms. They also reported that 6-month typical pregnancy probabilities were 9.0 versus 5.4 percent with polyurethane versus latex condoms, respectively.

Female Condom—Vaginal Pouch

Manufactured by many companies under different names, female condoms prevent pregnancy and sexually transmitted infections. One brand available in the United States is the *FC Female Condom* (Mayer Laboratories)—a polyurethane sheath with a flexible polyurethane ring at each end (Fig. 5-12). The open ring remains outside the vagina, and the closed internal ring is fitted behind the symphysis and beneath the cervix like a diaphragm (Fig. 5-13). It should not be used along with the male condom because together they may slip, tear, or become displaced. In vitro tests have shown the female condom to be impermeable to human immunodeficiency virus, cytomegalovirus, and hepatitis B virus. As shown in Table 5-2, the pregnancy rate is higher than with the male condom.

Diaphragm Combined with Spermicide

The diaphragm consists of a circular rubber dome of various diameters supported by a circumferential metal spring (Fig. 5-14). When used in combination with spermicidal jelly or cream, it can be very effective. The spermicide is applied to the cervical surface centrally in the cup and along the rim. The device is then placed in the vagina so that the cervix, vaginal fornices,

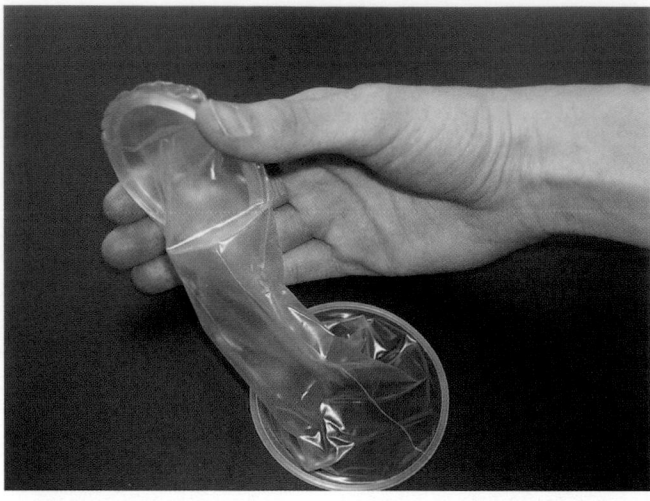

FIGURE 5-12 Female condom. *(Reproduced with permission of The Cervical Barrier Advancement Society and Ibis Reproductive Health.)*

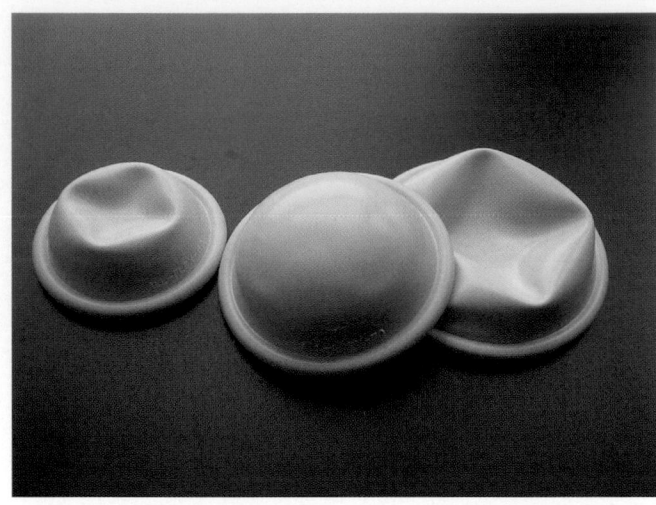

FIGURE 5-14 Group of three diaphragms. *(Reproduced with permission of The Cervical Barrier Advancement Society and Ibis Reproductive Health.)*

and anterior vaginal wall are partitioned effectively from the remainder of the vagina and the penis. At the same time, the centrally placed spermicidal agent is held against the cervix by the diaphragm. When appropriately positioned, the rim is lodged inferiorly deep in the posterior vaginal fornix. Superiorly, the rim lies in close proximity to the inner surface of the symphysis immediately below the urethra (Fig. 5-15). If the diaphragm is too small, it will not remain in place. If too large, it will be uncomfortable when positioned. Because the variables of size and spring flexibility must be specified, the diaphragm is available only by prescription (Allen, 2004).

Because of these reasons regarding proper placement, the diaphragm may not be an effective choice for women with significant pelvic organ prolapse. The malpositioned uterus can cause unstable diaphragm positioning that results in expulsion.

Counseling. The diaphragm and spermicidal agent can be inserted well before intercourse, but if more than 2 hours elapse, additional spermicide should be placed in the upper vagina for maximum protection. Spermicide should also be reapplied before each coital episode. The diaphragm should not be removed for at least 6 hours after intercourse. Because toxic shock syndrome has been described following its use, the diaphragm should not be left in place for longer than 24 hours.

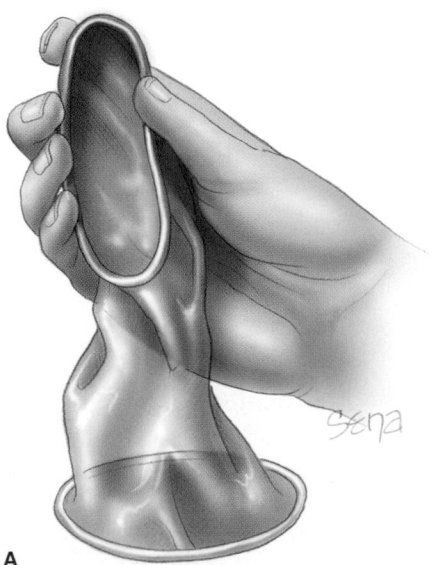

A

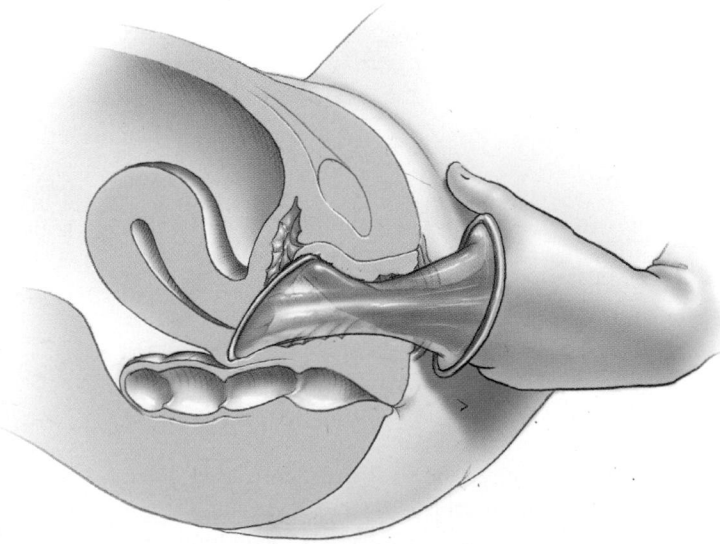

B

FIGURE 5-13 Female Condom insertion and positioning. **A.** The inner ring is squeezed for insertion and is placed similarly to a diaphragm. **B.** The inner ring is pushed inward with an index finger.

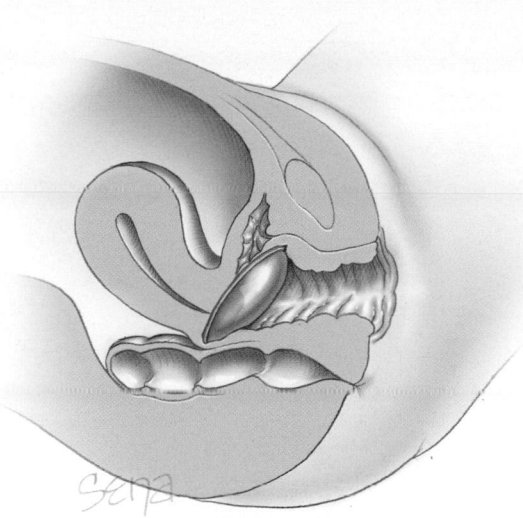

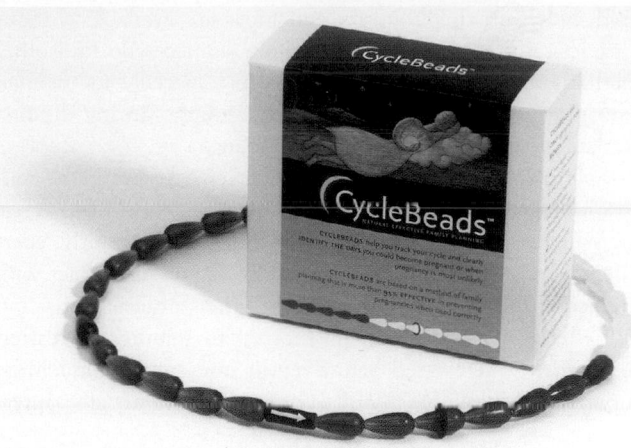

FIGURE 5-16 CycleBeads. *(Reproduced with permission of Cycle Technologies.)*

FIGURE 5-15 A diaphragm in place creates a physical barrier between the vagina and cervix.

FOURTH-TIER CONTRACEPTIVE METHODS—LESS EFFECTIVE

These methods have an extremely high associated failure rate with their use. Fourth-tier methods are comprised of spermicides delivered in various forms, including a barrier sponge.

Proper diaphragm use requires a high level of motivation. Vessey and coworkers (1982) reported a pregnancy rate of only 1.9 to 2.4 per 100 woman-years for motivated users. In a small study, Bounds and colleagues (1995) reported a much higher failure rate of 12.3 per 100 women-years. The unintended pregnancy rate is lower in women older than 35 years compared with younger women.

Diaphragm use has a lower incidence of sexually transmitted infections compared with condom use (Rosenberg, 1992). Conversely, there is a slight increase in the rate of female urinary infections (Cates, 2007).

Spermicides and Microbicides

These contraceptives are marketed variously as creams, jellies, suppositories, film, and aerosol foams (Fig. 5-17). They are

Lea's Shield

This reusable, washable, barrier device is made of silicone and is placed against the cervix. It has only one size, which simplifies the fitting process. The shield protects against pregnancy and sexually transmitted infections. It may be inserted any time prior to intercourse and must be left in place for at least 8 hours thereafter. When used with spermicide, and adjusted for age, the reported 6-month pregnancy rate was 5.6 per 100 users (Mauck, 1996).

Fertility Awareness-Based Methods

This form of contraception is defined by the World Health Organization (2007) as a method that involves identification of the fertile days of the menstrual cycle (Fig. 5-16). The couple may then avoid intercourse or use a barrier method during those days. The comparative efficacy of fertility-based awareness methods remains unknown (Grimes, 2010a). Clearly, proper instruction is critical, and complex charting is involved. These charts, as well as detailed advice, are available from the National Fertility Awareness and Natural Family Planning Service for the United Kingdom at: http://www.fertilityuk.org and from the Natural Family Site at: http://www.bygpub.com/natural.

FIGURE 5-17 Vaginal contraceptive film. The film is first folded in half and then folded up and over the tip of the inserting finger. Once inserted near the cervix, the film will dissolve to provide spermicide.

used widely in this country, and most are available without a prescription. Probable users include women who find other methods unacceptable. They are useful especially for women who need temporary protection, for example, during the first week after starting CHC or while nursing.

Spermicidal agents provide a physical barrier to sperm penetration as well as a chemical spermicidal action. The active ingredient is nonoxynol-9 or octoxynol-9. Importantly, spermicides must be deposited high in the vagina in contact with the cervix shortly before intercourse. Their duration of maximal effectiveness is usually no more than 1 hour. Thereafter, they must be reinserted before repeat intercourse. Douching, if practiced, should be avoided for at least 6 hours after intercourse.

High pregnancy rates are primarily attributable to inconsistent use rather than to method failure. Even if inserted regularly and correctly, however, foam preparations are reported to have a failure rate of 5 to 12 pregnancies per 100 woman-years of use (Trussell, 1990). If pregnancy does occur with use, spermicides are not teratogenic (Briggs, 2002).

Spermicides that primarily contain nonoxynol-9 do not provide protection against sexually transmitted infections. In randomized trials, Roddy and colleagues (1998) compared nonoxynol-9 with and without condom use and found no additional protective effects against chlamydial or HIV infection or gonorrhea. Long-term use of nonoxynol-9 was reported to have minimal effects on vaginal flora (Schreiber, 2006).

Spermicide-Microbicide Combinations

There is currently much interest in combined spermicide-microbicide agents. These have the advantage of being female controlled, and they protect against sexually transmitted infections, including HIV (Weber, 2005). Those in the surfactant class have dual action—they destroy the sperm membrane and they also disrupt the outer envelopes or membranes of viral and bacterial pathogens.

Second-generation microbicides fortify natural defenses by maintaining an acidic pH or maintaining presence of antibodies and enhancing antimicrobial peptides. They also serve to maintain a hostile vaginal environment. Third-generation microbicides work as topical antiretroviral agents. Another possibility is that RNA interference (RNAi) may be used to develop microbicides (Palliser, 2006).

Contraceptive Sponge

The contraceptive sponge *Today* (Allendale Pharmaceuticals) was reintroduced into the United States in 2005. Sold over the counter, it consists of a nonoxynol-9–impregnated polyurethane disc that can be inserted for up to 24 hours prior to intercourse (Fig. 5-18). The disc is moistened and placed directly against the cervix. While in place, it provides contraception regardless of the frequency of coitus. It should remain in place for 6 hours after intercourse. Although perhaps more

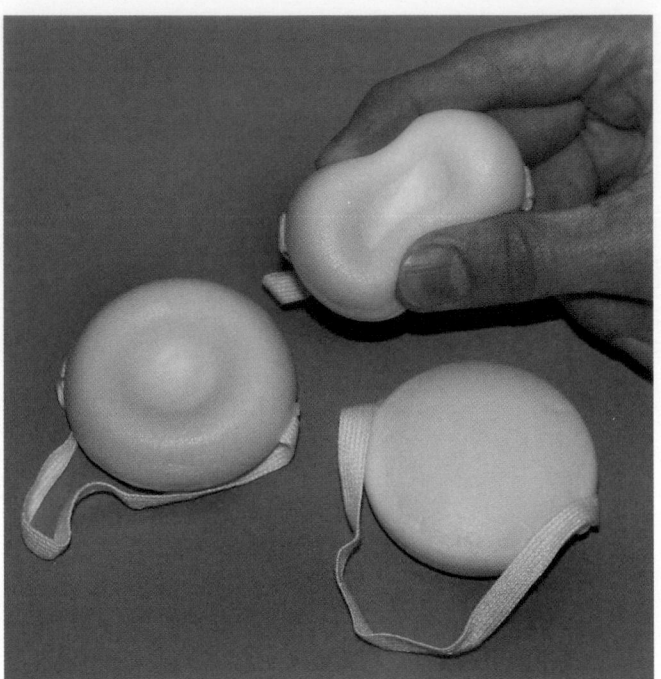

FIGURE 5-18 Today brand vaginal sponge. When in position, the sponge dimple apposes the cervix surface, and the ribbon loop faces outward to allow easy hooking with a finger for removal.

convenient, as shown in Table 5-2, it is less effective than the diaphragm or condom.

EMERGENCY CONTRACEPTION

First popularized by the "morning-after pill" in the 1970s, emergency contraception (EC) has been made widely available in other forms over the past decade. These methods are appropriate for women presenting for contraceptive care following consensual but unprotected sexual intercourse or following sexual assault. There are a number of methods that, if used correctly, will substantially decrease the likelihood of an unwanted pregnancy in these women. According to the American College of Obstetricians and Gynecologists (2010a), methods currently available include sex steroid-containing compounds; antiprogesterone compounds; and the copper-containing IUD (Table 5-12). Importantly, because duration of use is short, women with conditions that might normally contraindicate hormonal forms may be given these for EC.

Information regarding EC is made available to health care providers or patients by a number of 24-hour sources:

- American Congress of Obstetricians and Gynecologists: www.acog.org
- Emergency Contraception Hotline: 1-888-NOT-2-LATE (888-668-2528)
- Emergency Contraception web site: www.not-2-late.com
- Reproductive Health Technologies Project: www.rhtp.org/contraception/emergency/
- Pastillas Anticonceptivas de Emergencia: www.en3dias.org.mx

TABLE 5-12. Methods Available for Use as Emergency Contraception

Method	Formulation	Pills per Dose
Progestin-Only Pill		
Plan B[a]	0.75 mg levonorgestrel	1
Plan B One-Step[b]	1.5 mg levonorgestrel	1
SPRM Pill		
Ella[b]	30 mg ulipristal acetate	1
COC Pills[a,c]		
Ogestrel, Ovral	0.05 mg ethinyl estradiol + 0.5 mg norgestrel	2
Low-Ogestrel, Lo/Ovral, Nordette, Levlen, Levora	0.03 mg ethinyl estradiol + 0.3 mg norgestrel	4
TriLevlen (yellow), Triphasil (yellow), Trivora (pink)	0.03 mg ethinyl estradiol + 0.125 mg levonorgestrel	4
Alesse, Levlite	0.02 mg ethinyl estradiol + 0.1 mg levonorgestrel	5
Copper-Containing IUD		
ParaGard T 380A		

[a]Treatment consists of two doses taken 12 hours apart.
[b]Treatment consists of a single dose taken once.
[c]Use of an antiemetic agent before taking the medication will lessen the risk of nausea, which is a common side effect.
COC = combination oral contraceptive; SPRM = selective progesterone-receptor modulator.

Hormone-Based Emergency Contraception

Mechanisms of Action

Hormonal contraceptives have different mechanisms of action depending on which day of the menstrual cycle intercourse occurs and which day the tablets are given (Croxatto, 2003). One major mode is inhibition or delay of ovulation (Marions, 2004). Other suggested mechanisms include endometrial changes that prevent implantation, interference with sperm transport or penetration, and impairment of corpus luteum function (American College of Obstetricians and Gynecologists, 2010a). There is no evidence that pregnancies that occur despite emergency hormonal contraception are affected. Moreover, emergency hormonal contraception is not a form of medical abortion. Rather, this method prevents ovulation or implantation. It cannot disrupt a zygote that has implanted.

Estrogen-Progestin Combinations

Also known as the *Yuzpe method*, these COC-containing regimens shown in Table 5-12 have been approved by the FDA for use as EC (Yuzpe, 1974). Although more effective the sooner they are taken after unprotected intercourse, pills should be taken within 72 hours of intercourse, but may be given up to 120 hours. Initial dosing is followed 12 hours later by a second dose.

Efficacy is defined by the number of pregnancies observed after treatment divided by the estimated number that would have occurred with no treatment. This *prevented fraction* ranges widely between reports and averages approximately 75 percent with COC regimens (American College of Obstetricians and Gynecologists, 2010a).

Nausea and vomiting are common with COC regimens because of their high estrogen doses (Trussell, 1998a). An oral antiemetic taken at least 1 hour before each dose may reduce these bothersome symptoms. In randomized trials, a 1-hour pretreatment dose of either 50-mg meclizine or 10-mg metoclopramide was found effective (Ragan, 2003; Raymond, 2000). If vomiting occurs within 2 hours of a dose, a replacement dose is given.

Progestin-Only Regimens

A progestin-only method of EC is marketed as *Plan B* and *Plan B One-Step* (Barr Pharmaceuticals). Plan B consists of two tablets, each containing 0.75-mg levonorgestrel. The first dose is taken within 72 hours of unprotected coitus, but may be used up to 120 hours, and the second dose is taken 12 hours later (see Table 5-12). Ngai and associates (2005) also showed that a 24-hour interval between dosing is effective. Plan B One-Step is a single, 1.5-mg levonorgestrel dose, which is taken ideally with 72 hours or up to 120 hours following intercourse.

Most studies, including the multicenter trial by the World Health Organization (von Hertzen, 2002), indicate that the progestin-only regimens are more effective than COC regimens to prevent pregnancy. The American College of Obstetricians and Gynecologists (2010a) cites an approximate 50-percent decreased pregnancy rate with levonorgestrel compared with COCs. Finally, Ellertson and colleagues (2003) reported a 55-percent pregnancy prevention rate even if Plan B was taken as late as 4 to 5 days after unprotected intercourse.

Antiprogestins and Selective Progestin-Receptor Modulators

Compounds have been developed that have contraceptive activity because they prevent progesterone-mediated preparation of the estrogen-primed endometrium for implantation. There are several mechanisms by which antiprogesterone compounds achieve this.

One mechanism of action is by progesterone-receptor modulation, and two compounds are available. First, mifepristone (RU 486)—*Mifeprex* (Danco Laboratories)—is a progesterone antagonist (PA). It either delays ovulation or impairs development of the secretory endometrium. Cheng and colleagues (2008) in their Cochrane review noted that mifepristone in single doses of 25 or 50 mg was superior to other hormonal regimens of EC. Mifepristone also had few side effects. In the United States, mifepristone is not used for EC because of its high cost and because it is not manufactured or marketed in an appropriate dose for EC.

A selective progesterone-receptor modulator (SPRM) was FDA approved in 2010 for postcoital contraception. Ulipristal acetate—*Ella* (Watson)—is taken as a single 30-mg tablet up to 120 hours after unprotected intercourse (Brache, 2010; Russo, 2010; Watson, 2010). Side effects include nausea and prolongation of duration to the next menses.

Copper-Containing Intrauterine Devices

Insertion of a copper-containing IUD is an effective postcoital contraceptive method. Fasoli and coworkers (1989) summarized nine studies that included results from 879 women who chose this as a sole method of postcoital contraception. The only pregnancy reported aborted spontaneously. Trussell and Stewart (1998b) reported that when the IUD was inserted up to 5 days after unprotected coitus, the failure rate was 1 percent. A secondary advantage is that this method also puts in place an effective 10-year method of contraception.

Failure of Emergency Contraception

Every method used for postcoital contraception will have failures. Importantly, these methods generally will not prevent pregnancy resulting from subsequent episodes of intercourse during the same cycle. For these reasons, use of a barrier technique is recommended until the next menses. When menstruation is delayed 3 weeks past its expected onset, the likelihood of pregnancy is increased and appropriate testing is instituted.

REFERENCES

Abma JC, Martinez GM, Copen CE: Teenagers in the United States: sexual activity, contraceptive use, and childbearing, National Survey of Family Growth 2006-2008. National Center for Health Statistics. Vital Health Stat 23(30), 2010

Adams CE, Wald M: Risks and complications of vasectomy. Urol Clin North Am 36(3):331, 2009

Allen RE: Diaphragm fitting. Am Fam Physician 69(1):97, 2004

Allen RH, Bartz D, Grimes DA, et al: Interventions for pain with intrauterine device insertion. Cochrane Database Syst Rev 3:CD007373, 2009

Alvarez F, Brache V, Fernandez E, et al: New insights on the mode of action of intrauterine contraceptive devices in women. Fertil Steril 49(5):768, 1988

Alvior GT Jr: Pregnancy outcome with removal of intrauterine device. Obstet Gynecol 41(6):894, 1973

American Academy of Pediatrics, American College of Obstetricians and Gynecologists: Intrapartum and postpartum care of the mother. In

Lockwood CJ, Lemons JA (eds): Guidelines for Perinatal Care, 6th ed. Washington, DC, AAP/ACOG, 2007, p 169

American College of Obstetricians and Gynecologists: Antibiotic prophylaxis for gynecologic procedures. Practice Bulletin No. 104, May 2009a

American College of Obstetricians and Gynecologists: Benefits and risks of sterilization. Practice Bulletin No. 46, September 2003

American College of Obstetricians and Gynecologists: Clinical management guidelines for obstetrician-gynecologists. Practice Bulletin No. 59, January 2005

American College of Obstetricians and Gynecologists: Depot medroxyprogesterone acetate and bone effects. Committee Opinion No. 415, September 2008a

American College of Obstetricians and Gynecologists: Emergency oral contraception. Practice Bulletin No. 112, May 2010a

American College of Obstetricians and Gynecologists: Gynecologic care for women with human immunodeficiency virus. Practice Bulletin No. 117, December 2010b

American College of Obstetricians and Gynecologists: Hysterosalpingography after tubal sterilization. Committee Opinion No. 458, June 2010c

American College of Obstetricians and Gynecologists: Increasing use of contraceptive implants and intrauterine devices to reduce unintended pregnancy. Committee Opinion No. 450, December 2009b

American College of Obstetricians and Gynecologists: Intrauterine device and adolescents. Committee Opinion No. 392, December 2007a

American College of Obstetricians and Gynecologists: Long-acting reversible contraception: Implants and intrauterine devices. Practice Bulletin No. 121, July 2011

American College of Obstetricians and Gynecologists: Noncontraceptive uses of hormonal contraceptives. Practice Bulletin No. 110, January 2010d

American College of Obstetricians and Gynecologists: Noncontraceptive uses of the levonorgestrel intrauterine system. Committee Opinion No. 337, June 2006

American College of Obstetricians and Gynecologists: Prevention of deep vein thrombosis and pulmonary embolism. Practice Bulletin No. 84, August 2007b

American College of Obstetricians and Gynecologists: Use of hormonal contraception in women with coexisting medical conditions. Practice Bulletin No. 73, June 2006, reaffirmed 2008b

Amundsen GA, Ramakrishnan K: Vasectomy: a "seminal" analysis. South Med J 97:54, 2004

Audet MC, Moreau M, Koltun WD, et al: Evaluation of contraceptive efficacy and cycle control of a transdermal contraceptive patch vs an oral contraceptive: a randomized controlled trial. JAMA 285:2347, 2001

Bahamondes L, Del Castillo S, Tabares G, et al: Comparison of weight increase in users of depot medroxyprogesterone acetate and copper IUD up to 5 years. Contraception, 64(4):223, 2001

Bahamondes L, Faundes A, Sobreira-Lima B, et al: TCu 380A: a reversible permanent contraceptive method in women over 35 years of age. Contraception 72(5):337, 2005

Balci O, Mahmoud AS, Capar M, et al: Diagnosis and management of intra-abdominal, mislocated intrauterine devices. Arch Gynecol Obstet 281(6):1019, 2010

Bayer HealthCare Pharmaceuticals: Mirena (levonorgestrel-releasing intrauterine system): full prescribing information. 2009. Available at: http://www.berlex.com/html/products/pi/Mirena_PI.pdf. Accessed January 15, 2011

Bayer HealthCare Pharmaceuticals: Yasmin, drospirenone and ethinyl estradiol tablets, Physician labeling, 2007. Available at: http://berlex.bayerhealthcare.com/html/products/pi/fhc/Yasmin_PI.pdf. Accessed February 22, 2008

Bednarek PH, Creinin MD, Reeves MF, et al: Immediate versus delayed IUD insertion after uterine aspiration. N Engl J Med 364(23):2208, 2011

Beksinska ME, Smit JA, Kleinschmidt I, et al: Prospective study of weight change in new adolescent users of DMPA, NET-EN, COCs, nonusers and discontinuers of hormonal contraception. Contraception 81(1):30, 2010

Betrabet SS, Shikary ZK, Toddywalla VS, et al: ICMR Task Force Study on hormonal contraception. Transfer of norethindrone (NET) and levonorgestrel (LNG) from a single tablet into the infant's circulation through the mother's milk. Contraception 35:517, 1987

Bounds W, Guillebaud J, Dominik R, et al: The diaphragm with and without spermicide. A randomized, comparative efficacy trial. J Reprod Med 40:764, 1995

Brache V, Cochon L, Jesam C, et al: Immediate pre-ovulatory administration of 30 mg ulipristal acetate significantly delays follicular rupture. Hum Reprod 25(9):2256, 2010

Bradshaw HD, Rosario DJ, James MJ, et al: Review of current practice to establish success after vasectomy. Br J Surg 88:290, 2001

Briggs GG, Freeman RK, Yaffe SJ: Drugs in Pregnancy and Lactation, 6th ed. Baltimore, Williams & Wilkins, 2002

Brohet RM, Goldgar DE, Easton DF, et al: Oral contraceptives and breast cancer risk in the international BRCA 1/2 carrier cohort study: A report from EMBRACE, GENEPSO, GEO-HEBON, and the IBCCS Collaborating Group. J Clin Oncol 25:5327, 2007

Brunner LR, Hogue CJ: The role of body weight in oral contraceptive failure: results from the 1995 national survey of family growth. Ann Epidemiol 15:492, 2005

Burkman RT: Rationale for new contraceptive methods. The Female Patient (Suppl), August 2002

Cancer and Steroid Hormone Study of the Centers for Disease Control and the National Institute of Child Health and Development: Combination oral contraceptive use and the risk of endometrial cancer. JAMA 257:796, 1987a

Cancer and Steroid Hormone Study of the Centers for Disease Control and the National Institute of Child Health and Development: The reduction in risk of ovarian cancer associated with oral-contraceptive use. N Engl J Med 316:650, 1987b

Castaño PM, Adekunle L: Transcervical sterilization. Semin Reprod Med 28(2):103, 2010

Cates W, Raymond EG: Vaginal barriers and spermicides. In Hatcher RA, Trussell J, Nelson AL, et al (eds): Contraceptive Technology, 19th ed. New York, Ardent Media, 2007, p 326

Centers for Disease Control and Prevention: Sexually transmitted diseases treatment guidelines, 2010. MMWR 59(12), 2010a

Centers for Disease Control and Prevention: Update to CDC's U.S. Medical Eligibility Criteria for Contraceptive Use, 2010: revised recommendations for the use of contraceptive methods during the postpartum period. MMWR 60(26):878, 2011

Centers for Disease Control and Prevention: U.S. medical eligibility criteria for contraceptive use, 2010. MMWR 59(4), 2010b

Cha SH, Lee MH, Kim JH, et al: Fertility outcome after tubal anastomosis by laparoscopy and laparotomy. J Am Assoc Gynecol Laparosc 8:348, 2001

Chan LM, Westhoff CL: Tubal sterilization trends in the United States. Fertil Steril 94(1):1, 2010

Chasan-Taber L, Willett WC, Manson JE, et al: Prospective study of oral contraceptives and hypertension among women in the United States. Circulation 94:483, 1996

Chen BA, Reeves MF, Hayes JL, et al: Postplacental or delayed insertion of the levonorgestrel intrauterine device after vaginal delivery: a randomized controlled trial. Obstet Gynecol 116(5):1079, 2010

Cheng L, Gülmezoglu AM, Piaggio GGP, et al: Interventions for emergency contraception. Cochrane Database Syst Rev 2:CD001324, 2008

Clark MK, Sowers M, Levy B, et al: Bone mineral density loss and recovery during 48 months in first-time users of depot medroxyprogesterone acetate. Fertil Steril 86(5):1466, 2006

Collaborative Group on Epidemiological Studies of Ovarian Cancer: Ovarian cancer and oral contraceptives: collaborative reanalysis of data of 45 epidemiological studies including 23,257 women with ovarian cancer and 87,303 controls. Lancet 371:303, 2008

Collaborative Group on Hormonal Factors in Breast Cancer: Breast cancer and hormonal contraceptives: collaborative reanalysis of individual data on 53,297 women with breast cancer and 100,239 women without breast cancer from 54 epidemiological studies. Lancet 347:1713, 1996

Comp PC: Coagulation and thrombosis with OC use: physiology and clinical relevance. Dialogues Contracept 5:1, 1996

Cooper JM, Carignan CS, Cher D, et al: Microinsert nonincisional hysteroscopic sterilization. Obstet Gynecol 102:59, 2003

Costello, C, Hillis S, Marchbanks P, et al: The effect of interval tubal sterilization on sexual interest and pleasure. Obstet Gynecol 100:3, 2002

Cox B, Sneyd MJ, Paul C, et al. Vasectomy and risk of prostate cancer. JAMA 23(287):3110, 2002

Cromer BA, Blair JM, Mahan JD, et al: A prospective comparison of bone density in adolescent girls receiving depot medroxyprogesterone acetate (Depo-Provera), levonorgestrel (Norplant), or oral contraceptives. J Pediatr 129:671, 1996

Cromer BA, Smith RD, Blair JM, et al: A prospective study of adolescents who choose among levonorgestrel implant (Norplant), medroxyprogesterone acetate (Depo-Provera), or the combined oral contraceptive pill as contraception. Pediatrics 94:687, 1994

Croxatto HB, Ortiz ME, Muller AL: Mechanisms of action of emergency contraception. Steroids 68:1095, 2003

Culwell KR, Curtis KM, del Carmen Cravioto M: Safety of contraceptive method use among women with systemic lupus erythematosus: a systematic review. Obstet Gynecol 114(2 Pt 1):341, 2009

Curtis KM, Chrisman CE, Peterson HB: Contraception for women in selected circumstances. Obstet Gynecol 99:1100, 2002

DeStefano F, Perlman JA, Peterson HB, et al: Long term risk of menstrual disturbances after tubal sterilization. Am J Obstet Gynecol 152:835, 1985

de Villiers EM: Relationship between steroid hormone contraceptives and HPV, cervical intraepithelial neoplasia and cervical carcinoma. Int J Cancer 103(6):705, 2003

Doherty IA, Stuart GS: Coitus interruptus is not contraception. Sex Transm Dis 36(12), 2009

Duramed Pharmaceuticals: ParaGard T 380A intrauterine copper contraceptive: prescribing information. Available at: http://www.paragard.com/health_care_professional/global/pdf/Prescribing-Info.pdf. Accessed January 15, 2011

Earl DT, David DJ: Depo-Provera: An injectable contraceptive. Am Fam Physician 49:891, 1994

Edelman A, Gallo MF, Jensen JT, et al: Continuous or extended cycle vs cyclic use of combined hormonal contraceptives for contraception. Cochrane Database Syst Rev 3:CD004695, 2010

Edelman AB, Carlson NE, Cherala G, et al: Impact of obesity on oral contraceptive pharmacokinetics and hypothalamic-pituitary-ovarian activity. Contraception, 80(2):119, 2009

Ellertson C, Evans M, Ferden S, et al: Extending the time limit for starting the Yuzpe regimen of emergency contraception to 120 hours. Obstet Gynecol 101:1168, 2003

Fasoli M, Parazzini F, Cecchetti G, et al: Post-coital contraception: an overview of published studies. Contraception 39:459, 1989

Faúndes A, Telles E, Cristofoletti ML, et al: The risk of inadvertent intrauterine device insertion in women carriers of endocervical Chlamydia trachomatis. Contraception 58(2):105, 1998

Finer LB, Henshaw SK: Disparities in rates of unintended pregnancy in the United States, 1994 and 2001. Perspect Sex Reprod Health 38(2):90, 2006

Fiorino AS: Intrauterine contraceptive device–associated actinomycotic abscess and Actinomyces detection on cervical smear. Obstet Gynecol 87:142, 1996

Food and Drug Administration: Drug safety communication: safety review update on the possible increased risk of blood clots with birth control pills containing drospirenone. 9-26-11. Available at: http://www.fda.gov/Drugs/DrugSafety/ucm273021.htm. Accessed September 27, 2011

Fox MC, Oat-Judge J, Severson K, et al: Immediate placement of intrauterine devices after first and second trimester pregnancy termination. Contraception 83(1):34, 2011

Furlong LA: Ectopic pregnancy risk when contraception fails. J Reprod Med 47:881, 2002

Gaffield ME, Culwell KR, Lee CR: The use of hormonal contraception among women taking anticonvulsant therapy. Contraception 83(1):16, 2011

Gallo MF, Grimes DA, Lopez LM, et al: Non-latex versus latex male condoms for contraception. Cochrane Database Syst Rev 1:CD003550, 2006

Gallo MF, Lopez LM, Grimes DA, et al: Combination contraceptives: effects on weight. Cochrane Database Syst Rev 4:CD003987, 2008

Ganer H, Levy A, Ohel I, et al: Pregnancy outcome in women with an intrauterine contraceptive device. Am J Obstet Gynecol 201:381.e1, 2009

Gardner JM, Mishell DR Jr: Analysis of bleeding patterns and resumption of fertility following discontinuation of a long-acting injectable contraceptive. Fertil Steril 21:286, 1970

Gariepy AM, Creinin MD, Schwarz EB, et al: Reliability of laparoscopic compared with hysteroscopic sterilization at 1 year: a decision analysis. Obstet Gynecol 118(2 Pt 1):273, 2011

Giovannucci E, Tosteson TD, Speizer FE, et al: A long-term study of mortality in men who have undergone vasectomy. N Engl J Med 326:1392, 1992

Goodman S, Henlish SK, Reeves MF, et al: Impact of immediate postabortal insertion of intrauterine contraception on repeat abortion. Contraception 78:143, 2008

Grimes DA: Forgettable contraception. Contraception 80:497, 2009a

Grimes DA: Intrauterine device and upper-genital-tract infection. Lancet 356:1013, 2000

Grimes DA, Gallo MF, Halpern V, et al: Fertility awareness-based methods for contraception. Cochrane Database Syst Rev 1:CD004860, 2010a

Grimes DA, Hubacher D, Lopez LM, et al: Non-steroidal anti-inflammatory drugs for heavy bleeding or pain associated with intrauterine-device use. Cochrane Database Syst Rev 3:CD006034, 2009b

Grimes DA, Lopez LM, Schulz KF, et al: Immediate postabortal insertion of intrauterine devices. Cochrane Database Syst Rev 6:CD001777, 2010b

Grimes DA, Lopez LM, Schulz KF, et al: Immediate post-partum insertion of intrauterine devices. Cochrane Database Syst Rev 5:CD003036, 2010c

Guiahi M, Goldman KN, McElhinney MM, et al: Improving hysterosalpingogram confirmatory test follow-up after Essure hysteroscopic sterilization. Contraception 81(6):520, 2010

Guttmacher Institute: State policies in brief. An overview of minors' consent law. 2011. Available at: http://www.guttmacher.org/statecenter/spibs/spib_OMCL.pdf. Accessed January 14, 2011

Haider S, Darney PD: Injectable contraception. Clin Obstet Gynecol 50(4):898, 2007

Halpern V, Grimes DA, Lopez L, et al: Strategies to improve adherence and acceptability of hormonal methods of contraception. Cochrane Database Syst Rev 1:CD004317, 2006

Hannaford PC, Kay CR, Vessey MP, et al: Combined oral contraceptives and liver disease. Contraception 55:145, 1997

Hannaford PC, Selvaraj S, Elliott AM, et al: Cancer risk among users of oral contraceptives: Cohort data from the Royal College of General Practitioners' oral contraception study. BMJ 335:651, 2007

Harel Z, Johnson CC, Gold MA, et al: Recovery of bone mineral density in adolescents following the use of depot medroxyprogesterone acetate contraceptive injections. Contraception 81(4):281, 2010

Harlap S, Kost K, Forrest JD: Preventing pregnancy, protecting health: a new look at birth control choices in the US. New York, The Alan Guttmacher Institute, 1991

Hassan EO, El-Husseini M, El-Nahal N: The effect of 1-year use of the CuT 380A and oral contraceptive pills on hemoglobin and ferritin levels. Contraception 60(2):101, 1999

Hawkins J, Dube D, Kaplow M, et al: Cost analysis of tubal anastomosis by laparoscopy and by laparotomy. J Am Assoc Gynecol Laparosc 9:120, 2002

Heikinheimo O, Gissler M, Suhonen S: Age, parity history of abortion and contraceptive choices affect the risk of repeat abortion. Contraception 78:149, 2008

Heinemann LA, Weimann A, Gerken G, et al: Modern oral contraceptive use and benign liver tumors: The German Benign Liver Tumor Case-Control Study. Eur J Contracept Reprod Health Care 3:194, 1998

Hendrix NW, Chauhan SP, Morrison JC: Sterilization and its consequences. Obstet Gynecol Surv 54:766, 1999

Henshaw SK: Unintended pregnancy in the United States. Fam Plann Perspect 30:24, 1998

Hidalgo MM, Lisondo C, Juliato CT, et al: Ovarian cysts in users of Implanon and Jadelle subdermal contraceptive implants. Contraception 73(5):532, 2006

Hillis SD, Marchbanks PA, Tylor LR, et al: Poststerilization regret: findings from the United States Collaborative Review of Sterilization. Obstet Gynecol 93:889, 1999

Hillis SD, Marchbanks PA, Tylor LR, et al: Tubal sterilization and long-term risk of hysterectomy: findings from the United States Collaborative Review of Sterilization. Obstet Gynecol 89:609, 1997

Holt SK, Salinas CA, Stanford JL: Vasectomy and the risk of prostate cancer. J Urol 180(6):2565, 2008

Holt VL, Cushing-Haugen KL, Daling JR: Body weight and risk of oral contraceptive failure. Obstet Gynecol 99:820, 2002

Holt VL, Cushing-Haugen KL, Daling JR: Oral contraceptives, tubal sterilization, and functional ovarian cyst risk. Obstet Gynecol 102:252, 2003

Holt VL, Scholes D, Wicklund KG, et al: Body mass index, weight, and oral contraceptive failure risk. Obstet Gynecol 105:46, 2005

Hou MY, Hurwitz S, Kavanagh E: Using daily text-messaging reminders to improve adherence with oral contraceptives. Obstet Gynecol 116:633, 2010

Inki P, Hurskainen R, Palo P, et al: Comparison of ovarian cyst formation in women using the levonorgestrel-releasing intrauterine system vs. hysterectomy. Ultrasound Obstet Gynecol 20(4):381, 2002

International Collaboration of Epidemiological Studies of Cervical Cancer: Cervical cancer and hormonal contraceptives: collaborative reanalysis of individual data for 16,573 women with cervical cancer and 35,509 women without cervical cancer from 24 epidemiological studies. Lancet 370:1609, 2007

Jain J, Dutton C, Nicosia A, et al: Pharmacokinetics, ovulation suppression and return to ovulation following a lower dose subcutaneous formulation of Depo-Provera. Contraception 70(1):11, 2004

Jamieson DJ, Kaufman SC, Costello C, et al: A comparison of women's regret after vasectomy versus tubal sterilization. Obstet Gynecol 99:1073, 2002

Janssen-Ortho: Micronor: product monograph. 2010. Available at: http://www.janssen-ortho.com/JOI/pdf_files/Micronor_E.pdf. Accessed January 10, 2011

Jensen JT, Burke AE, Barnhart KT, et al: Effects of switching from oral to transdermal or transvaginal contraception on markers of thrombosis. Contraception 78(6):451, 2008

Jick SS, Hagberg KW, Hernandez RK, et al: Postmarketing study of ORTHO EVRA* and levonorgestrel oral contraceptives containing hormonal contraceptives with 30 mcg of ethinyl estradiol in relation to nonfatal venous thromboembolism. Contraception 81(1):16, 2010a

Jick SS, Hagberg KW, Kaye JA: ORTHO EVRA and venous thromboembolism: an update. Contraception 81(5):452, 2010b

Jick SS, Hernandez RK: Risk of non-fatal venous thromboembolism in women using oral contraceptives containing drospirenone compared with women using oral contraceptives containing levonorgestrel: case-control study using United States claims data. BMJ 342:d2151, 2011

Jick SS, Kaye JA, Russmann S, et al: Risk of nonfatal venous thromboembolism in women using a contraceptive transdermal patch and oral contraceptives containing norgestimate and 35 μg of ethinyl estradiol. Contraception 73(3):223, 2006

Kapp N, Tilley IB, Curtis KM: The effects of hormonal contraceptive use among women with viral hepatitis or cirrhosis of the liver: a systematic review. Contraception 80(4):381, 2009

Kaunitz AM: Depot medroxyprogesterone acetate contraception and the risk of breast and gynecologic cancer. J Reprod Med 45:419, 1996

Kaunitz AM, Miller PD, Rice VM, et al: Bone mineral density in women aged 25-35 years receiving depot medroxyprogesterone acetate: recovery following discontinuation. Contraception 74(2):90, 2006

Kerin JF, Levy BS: Ultrasound: an effective method for localization of the echogenic Essure sterilization micro-insert: correlation with radiologic evaluations. J Minim Invasive Gynecol 12:50, 2005

Kim HH, Goldstein M: History of vasectomy reversal. Urol Clin North Am 36(3):359, 2009

Kjos SL, Peters RK, Xiang A, et al: Contraception and the risk of type 2 diabetes mellitus in Latina women with prior gestational diabetes mellitus. JAMA 280:533, 1998

Kluft C, Meijer P, LaGuardia KD, et al: Comparison of a transdermal contraceptive patch vs. oral contraceptives on hemostasis variables. Contraception 77(2):77, 2008

Köhler TS, Fazili AA, Brannigan RE: Putative health risks associated with vasectomy. Urol Clin North Am 36(3):337, 2009

Kost K, Singh S, Vaughan B, et al: Estimates of contraceptive failure from the 2002 National Survey of Family Growth. Contraception 77:10, 2008

Kulier R, Boulvain M, Walker D, et al: Minilaparotomy and endoscopic techniques for tubal sterilization. Cochrane Database Syst Rev 3:CD001328, 2002

Le YC, Rahman M, Berenson AB: Early weight gain predicting later weight gain among depot medroxyprogesterone acetate users. Obstet Gynecol 114(2 Pt 1):279, 2009

Lee NC, Rubin GL, Borucki R: The intrauterine device and pelvic inflammatory disease revisited: new results from the Women's Health Study. Obstet Gynecol 72(1):1, 1988

Levgur M, Duvivier R: Pelvic inflammatory disease after tubal sterilization: a review. Obstet Gynecol Surv 55:41, 2000

Levy B, Levie MD, Childers ME: A summary of reported pregnancies after hysteroscopic sterilization. J Minim Invasive Gynecol 2007 14(3):271, 2007

Lin K, Barnhart K: The clinical rationale for menses-free contraception. J Womens Health (Larchmt) 16:1171, 2007

Lippes J: Quinacrine sterilization: the imperative need for clinical trials. Fertil Steril 77:1106, 2002

Lopez LM, Grimes DA, Chen-Mok M, et al: Hormonal contraceptives for contraception in overweight or obese women. Cochrane Database Syst Rev 7:CD008452, 2010

Lopez LM, Grimes DA, Schulz KF, et al: Steroidal contraceptives: effect on bone fractures in women. Cochrane Database Syst Rev 2:CD006033, 2009a

Lopez LM, Kaptein AA, Helmerhorst FM: Oral contraceptives containing drospirenone for premenstrual syndrome. Cochrane Database Syst Rev 2:CD006586, 2009b

Lynge E: Prostate cancer is not increased in men with vasectomy in Denmark. J Urol 168:488, 2002

MacClellan LR, Giles W, Cole J, et al: Probable migraine with visual aura and risk of ischemic stroke: the stroke prevention in young women study. Stroke 38(9):2438, 2007

Machado RB, de Melo NR, Maia H Jr: Bleeding patterns and menstrual-related symptoms with the continuous use of a contraceptive combination of ethinylestradiol and drospirenone: a randomized study. Contraception 81:215, 2010

MacKay AP, Kieke BA, Koonin LM, et al: Tubal sterilization in the United States, 1994-1996. Fam Plann Perspect 33:161, 2001

Magnani RJ, Haws JM, Morgan GT, et al: Vasectomy in the United States, 1991 and 1995. Am J Pub Health 89:92, 1999

Maheshwari S, Sarraj A, Kramer J, et al: Oral contraception and the risk of hepatocellular carcinoma. J Hepatol 47:506, 2007

Mainwaring R, Hales HA, Stevenson K, et al: Metabolic parameters, bleeding, and weight changes in U.S. women using progestin only contraceptives. Contraception 51:149, 1995

Marchbanks PA, McDonald JA, Wilson HG, et al: Oral contraceptives and the risk of breast cancer. N Engl J Med 346:2025, 2002

Margolis KL, Adami HO, Luo J, et al: A prospective study of oral contraceptive use and risk of myocardial infarction among Swedish women. Fertil Steril 88(2):310, 2007

Marions L, Cekan SZ, Bygdeman M, et al: Effect of emergency contraception with levonorgestrel or mifepristone on ovarian function. Contraception 69:373, 2004

Mauck C, Glover LH, Miller E, et al: Lea's Shield: a study of the safety and efficacy of a new vaginal barrier contraceptive used with and without spermicide. Contraception 53:329, 1996

Michielsen D, Beerthuizen R: State-of-the art of non-hormonal methods of contraception: VI. Male sterilization. Eur J Contracept Reprod Health Care 15(2):136, 2010

Mishell DR Jr: Oral contraceptives and cardiovascular events: summary and application of data. Int J Fertil 45:121, 2000

Mohllajee AP, Curtis KM, Martins SL, et al: Does use of hormonal contraceptives among women with thrombogenic mutations increase their risk of venous thromboembolism? A systemic review. Contraception 73:166, 2006

Moore LL, Valuck R, McDougall C, et al: A comparative study of one-year weight gain among users of medroxyprogesterone acetate, levonorgestrel implants, and oral contraceptives. Contraception 52:215, 1995

Moschos E, Twickler DM: Does the type of intrauterine device affect conspicuity on 2D and 3D ultrasound? AJR Am J Roentgenol 196(6):1439, 2011

Mosher WD, Jones J: Use of contraception in the United States: 1982-2008. National Center for Health Statistics. Vital Health Stat 23 (29), 2010

Mulders TM, Dieben T: Use of the novel combined contraceptive vaginal ring NuvaRing for ovulation inhibition. Fertil Steril 75:865, 2001

Nardin JM, Kulier R, Boulvain M: Techniques for the interruption of tubal patency for female sterilisation. Cochrane Database Syst Rev 4:CD003034, 2003

Ngai SW, Fan S, Li S, et al: A randomized trial to compare 24 h versus 12 h double dose regimen of levonorgestrel for emergency contraception. Hum Reprod 20:307, 2005

Nilsson CG, Lahteenmaki P, Luukkainen T: Ovarian function in amenorrheic and menstruating users of a levonorgestrel-releasing intrauterine device. Fertil Steril 41:52, 1984

Ogburn JA, Espey E, Stonehocker J: Barriers to intrauterine device insertion in postpartum women. Contraception 72(6):426, 2005

Organon: Implanon (etonorgestrel implant). Package insert. 2006. Available at: http://www.implanon-usa.com/Authfiles/Images/543_174733.pdf. Accessed January 1, 2011

Ortiz ME, Croxatto HB: The mode of action of IUDs. Contraception 36:37, 1987

Palliser D, Chowdhury D, Wang QY, et al: An siRNA-based microbicide protects mice from lethal herpes simplex virus 2 infection. Nature 439:89, 2006

Parkin L, Sharples K, Hernandez RK, et al: Risk of venous thromboembolism in users of oral contraceptives containing drospirenone or levonorgestrel: nested case-control study based on UK General Practice Research Database. BMJ 342:d2139, 2011

Pati S, Cullins V: Female sterilization: evidence. Obstet Gynecol Clin North Am 27:859, 2000

Paulen ME, Folger SG, Curtis KM, et al: Contraceptive use among solid organ transplant patients: a systematic review. Contraception 82(1):102, 2010

Peterson HB, Jeng G, Folger SG, et al: The risk of menstrual abnormalities after tubal sterilization. N Engl J Med 343:1681, 2000

Peterson HB, Xia Z, Hughes JM, et al: The risk of pregnancy after tubal sterilization: findings from the U.S. Collaborative Review of Sterilization. Am J Obstet Gynecol 174(4):1161, 1996

Peterson HB, Xia Z, Wilcox LS, et al: Pregnancy after tubal sterilization with bipolar electrocoagulation. U.S. Collaborative Review of Sterilization Working Group. Obstet Gynecol 94:163, 1999

Peterson HB, Xia Z, Wilcox LS, et al: Pregnancy after tubal sterilization with silicone rubber band and spring clip application. Obstet Gynecol 97:205, 2001

Petri M, Kim MY, Kalunian, KC, et al: Combined oral contraceptives in women with systemic lupus erythematosus. N Engl J Med 353:2550, 2005

Pfizer: Depo-Provera Full Prescribing Information. 2010. Available at: http://media.pfizer.com/files/products/uspi_depo_provera_contraceptive.pdf. Accessed January 10, 2011

Phelps JY, Kelver ME: Confronting the legal risks of prescribing the contraceptive patch with ongoing litigation. Obstet Gynecol 113(3):712, 2009

Picardo CM, Nichols M, Edelman A, et al: Women's knowledge and sources of information on the risks and benefits of oral contraception. J Am Med Womens Assoc 58:112, 2003

Pomp ER, le Cessie S, Rosendaal FR, et al: Risk of venous thrombosis: obesity and its joint effect with oral contraceptive use and prothrombotic mutations. Br J Haematol 139(2):289, 2007

Pomp ER, Rosendaal FR, Doggen CJ: Smoking increases the risk of venous thrombosis and acts synergistically with oral contraceptive use. Am J Hematol 83:97, 2008

Porter JB, Jick H, Walker AM: Mortality among oral contraceptive users. Obstet Gynecol 70:29, 1987

Ragan RE, Rock RW, Buck HW: Metoclopramide pretreatment attenuates emergency contraceptive-associated nausea. Am J Obstet Gynecol 188:330, 2003

Raymond EG, Creinin MD, Barnhart KT, et al: Meclizine for prevention of nausea associated with use of emergency contraceptive pills: a randomized trial. Obstet Gynecol 95:271, 2000

Realini JP, Goldzieher JW: Oral contraceptives and cardiovascular disease: a critique of the epidemiologic studies. Am J Obstet Gynecol 152:729, 1985

Rimm EB, Manson JE, Stampfer MJ, et al: Oral contraceptive use and the risk of type 2 (non-insulin-dependent) diabetes mellitus in a large prospective study of women. Diabetologia 35:967, 1992

Robinson GE, Burren T, Mackie IJ, et al: Changes in haemostasis after stopping the combined contraceptive pill: Implications for major surgery. BMJ 302:269, 1991

Roddy RE, Zekeng L, Ryan KA, et al: A controlled trial of nonoxynol-9 film to reduce male-to-female transmission of sexually transmitted diseases. N Engl J Med 339:504, 1998

Ronnerdag M, Odlind V: Health effects of long-term use of the intrauterine levonorgestrel-releasing system. Acta Obstet Gynecol Scand 78:716, 1999

Rosenberg MJ, Davidson AJ, Chen JH, et al: Barrier contraceptives and sexually transmitted diseases in women: a comparison of female-dependent methods and condoms. Am J Pub Health 82:669, 1992

Roumen F, Apter D, Mulders TM, et al: Efficacy, tolerability and acceptability of a novel contraceptive vaginal ring releasing etonogestrel and ethinyl estradiol. Hum Reprod 16:469, 2001

Russo JA, Creinin MD: Ulipristal acetate for emergency contraception. Drugs Today (Barc) 46(9):655, 2010

Said S, Omar K, Koetsawang S, et al: A multicentred phase III comparative clinical trial of depot-medroxyprogesterone acetate given three-monthly at doses of 100 mg or 150 mg: 1. Contraceptive efficacy and side effects. World Health Organization Task Force on Long-Acting Systemic Agents for Fertility Regulation. Special Programme of Research, Development and Research Training in Human Reproduction. Contraception 34(3):223, 1986

Sánchez-Guerrero J, Uribe AG, Jiménez-Santana L, et al: A trial of contraceptive methods in women with systemic lupus erythematosus. N Engl J Med 353:2539, 2005

Scholes D, Lacroix AZ, Ott SM, et al: Bone mineral density in women using depot medroxyprogesterone acetate for contraception. Obstet Gynecol 93:233, 1999

Schreiber CA, Meyn LA, Creinin MD, et al: Effects of long-term use of nonoxynol-9 on vaginal flora. Obstet Gynecol 107:136, 2006

Schwingl PJ, Guess HA: Safety and effectiveness of vasectomy. Fertil Steril 73:923, 2000

Seeger JD, Loughlin J, Eng PM, et al: Risk of thromboembolism in women taking ethinylestradiol/drospirenone and other oral contraceptives. Obstet Gynecol 110:587, 2007

Shavell VI, Abdallah ME, Shade GH Jr, et al: Trends in sterilization since the introduction of Essure hysteroscopic sterilization. J Minim Invasive Gynecol 16(1):22, 2009

Shikary ZK, Betrabet SS, Patel ZM, et al: ICMR Task Force Study on hormonal contraception. Transfer of levonorgestrel (LNG) administered through different drug delivery systems from the maternal circulation via breast milk. Contraception 35:477, 1987

Shridharani A, Sandlow JL: Vasectomy reversal versus IVF with sperm retrieval: which is better? Curr Opin Urol 20(6):503, 2010

Shulman LP, Gabriel H: Management and localization strategies for the nonpalpable Implanon rod. Contraception 73(4):325, 2006

Shy KK, Stergachis A, Grothaus LG, et al: Tubal sterilization and risk of subsequent hospital admission for menstrual disorders. Am J Obstet Gynecol 166:1698, 1992

Sivin I: Alternative estimates of ectopic pregnancy risks during contraception. Am J Obstet Gynecol 165:1900, 1991

Sivin I, Nash H, Waldman S: Jadelle levonorgestrel rod implants: a summary of scientific data and lessons learned from programmatic experience. New York, Population Council, 2002

Skegg DCG, Noonan EA, Paul C, et al: Depot medroxyprogesterone acetate and breast cancer. JAMA 273:799, 1995

Society of Family Planning: Use of the Mirena™ LNG-IUS and ParaGard™ CuT380A intrauterine devices in nulliparous women. Contraception 81:367, 2010

Soderstrom RM: Sterilization failures and their causes. Am J Obstet Gynecol 152:395, 1985

Sokal D, Gates D, Amatya R, et al: Two randomized controlled trials comparing the Tubal Ring and Filshie Clip for tubal sterilization. Fertil Steril 74:3, 2000

Sokal DC, Hieu do T, Loan ND, et al: Contraceptive effectiveness of two insertions of quinacrine: results from 10-year follow-up in Vietnam. Contraception 78(1):61, 2008

Speroff L, Darney PD: A Clinical Guide for Contraception, 3rd ed. Philadelphia, Lippincott Williams & Wilkins, 2001, pp 66, 99, 240, 284

Stadel BV: Oral contraceptives and cardiovascular disease. N Engl J Med 305:612, 1981

Steiner M, Lopez M, Grimes D, et al: Sino-implant (II)—a levonorgestrel-releasing two-rod implant: systematic review of the randomized controlled trials. Contraception 81(3):197, 2010

Steiner MJ, Dominik R, Rountree W, et al: Contraceptive effectiveness of a polyurethane condom and a latex condom: a randomized controlled trial. Obstet Gynecol 101:539, 2003

Steiner MJ, Trussell J, Mehta N, et al: Communicating contraceptive effectiveness: a randomized controlled trial to inform a World Health Organization family planning handbook. Am J Obstet Gynecol 195(1):85, 2006

Sulak PJ, Haney AF: Unwanted pregnancies: understanding contraceptive use and benefits in adolescents and older women. Am J Obstet Gynecol 168:2042, 1993

Sulak PJ, Kaunitz AM: Hormonal contraception and bone mineral density. Dialogues Contracept 6:1, 1999

Taneepanichskul S, Reinprayoon D, Khaosaad P: Comparative study of weight change between long-term DMPA and IUD acceptors. Contraception 58:149, 1998

Tatum HJ, Schmidt FH, Jain AK: Management and outcome of pregnancies associated with Copper-T intrauterine contraceptive device. Am J Obstet Gynecol 126:869, 1976

Tepper NK, Paulen ME, Marchbanks PA, et al: Safety of contraceptive use among women with peripartum cardiomyopathy: a systematic review. Contraception 82(1):95, 2010

Thomas DB, Ye Z, Ray RM, et al: Cervical carcinoma in situ and use of Depo-medroxyprogesterone acetate (DMPA). Contraception 51:25, 1995

Thonneau PF, Almont T: Contraceptive efficacy of intrauterine devices. Am J Obstet Gynecol 198(3):248, 2008

Tourgeman DE, Bhaumik M, Cooke GC, et al: Pregnancy rates following fimbriectomy reversal via neosalpingostomy: a 10-year retrospective analysis. Fertil Steril 76:1041, 2001

Truitt ST, Fraser AB, Gallo MF, et al: Combined hormonal versus nonhormonal versus progestin-only contraception in lactation. Cochrane Database Syst Rev 2:CD003988, 2010

Trussell J: Contraceptive efficacy. In Hatcher RA, Trussell J, Nelson AL, et al (eds): Contraceptive Technology, 20th ed. New York, Ardent Media, 2011, p 791

Trussell J, Ellertson C, Stewart F: Emergency contraception. A cost-effective approach to preventing pregnancy. Womens Health Primary Care 1:52, 1998a

Trussell J, Hatcher RA, Cates W Jr, et al: Contraceptive failure in the United States: an update. Stud Fam Plann 21(1):51, 1990

Trussell J, Stewart F: An update on emergency contraception. Dialogues Contracept 5:1, 1998b

Tworoger SS, Fairfield KM, Colditz GA, et al: Association of oral contraceptive use, other contraceptive methods, and infertility with ovarian cancer risk. Am J Epidemiol 166(8):894, 2007

United Nations, Department of Economic and Social Affairs Population Division: World contraceptive use, 2007. Available at: http://www.un.org/esa/population/publications/contraceptive2007/contraceptive2007.htm. Accessed January 11, 2011

University of California at San Francisco: HIV Insite: Database of antiretroviral drug interactions. 2011. Available at: http://hivinsite.ucsf.edu/insite?page=ar-00-02. Accessed January 10, 2011

U.S. Food and Drug Administration: Approved drug products with therapeutic equivalence evaluations. 2010. Available at: http://www.accessdata.fda.gov/scripts/cder/ob/default.cfm. Accessed January 15, 2011

van den Heuvel MW, van Bragt A, Alnabawy AK, et al: Comparison of ethinylestradiol pharmacokinetics in three hormonal contraceptive formulations: the vaginal ring, the transdermal patch and an oral contraceptive. Contraception 72(3):168, 2005

Van Voorhis BJ: Comparison of tubal ligation reversal procedures. Clin Obstet Gynecol 43:641, 2000

Veersema S, Vleugels MPH, Moolenaar LM, et al: Unintended pregnancies after Essure sterilization in the Netherlands. Fertil Steril 93(1):35, 2010

Vessey M, Yeates D: Oral contraceptives and benign breast disease: an update of findings in a large cohort study. Contraception 76(6):418, 2007

Vessey MP, Lawless M, Yeates D: Efficacy of different contraceptive methods. Lancet 1:841, 1982

Vessey MP, Meisler L, Flavel R, et al: Outcome of pregnancy in women using different methods of contraception. Br J Obstet Gynaecol 86:548, 1979

von Hertzen H, Piaggio G, Ding J, et al: Low dose mifepristone and two regimens of levonorgestrel for emergency contraception: a WHO multicentre randomized trial. Lancet 360:1803, 2002

Waldron T: Tests show commonly used substances harm latex condoms. Contracept Tech Update 10:20, 1989

Wallach M, Grimes DA (eds): Modern Oral Contraception. Updates from The Contraception Report. Totowa, NJ, Emron, 2000, pp 26, 90, 194

Walsh T, Grimes D, Frezieres R, et al: Randomized controlled trial of prophylactic antibiotics before insertion of intrauterine devices. Lancet 351:1005, 1998

Watson: Ella prescribing information. 2010. Available at: http://www.accessdata.fda.gov/drugsatfda_docs/label/2010/022474s000lbl.pdf. Accessed January 9, 2011

Weber J, Desai K, Darbyshire J: The development of vaginal microbicides for the prevention of HIV transmission. PLoS Med 2(5):e142, 2005

Westhoff C, Davis A: Tubal sterilization: focus on the U.S. experience. Fertil Steril 73:913, 2000

Westhoff C, Heartwell S, Edwards S, et al: Initiation of oral contraceptive using a quick start compared with a conventional start: a randomized controlled trial. Obstet Gynecol 109:1270, 2007a

Westhoff C, Jain JK, Milsom I, et al: Changes in weight with depot medroxyprogesterone acetate subcutaneous injection 104 mg/0.65 mL. Contraception 75(4):261, 2007b

Westhoff C, Kerns J, Morroni C, et al: Quick start: novel oral contraceptive initiation method. Contraception 66:141, 2002

Westhoff CL: Oral contraceptives and thrombosis: an overview of study methods and recent results. Am J Obstet Gynecol 179:S38, 1998

Westhoff CL, Torgal AH, Mayeda ER, et al: Pharmacokinetics of a combined oral contraceptive in obese and normal-weight women. Contraception, 81(6):474, 2010

Weston G, Bowditch J: Office ultrasound should be the first-line investigation for confirmation of correct ESSURE placement. Aust N Z J Obstet Gynaecol 45:312, 2005

White T, Ozel B, Jain JK, et al: Effects of transdermal and oral contraceptives on estrogen-sensitive hepatic proteins. Contraception 74(4):293, 2006

Winer RL, Hughes JP, Feng Q, et al: Condom use and the risk of genital human papillomavirus infection in young women. N Engl J Med 354:2645, 2006

Woods ER, Grace E, Havens KK, et al: Contraceptive compliance with a levonorgestrel triphasic and a norethindrone monophasic oral contraceptive in adolescent patients. Am J Obstet Gynecol 166:901, 1992

World Health Organization: Combined oral contraceptives and liver cancer. Int J Cancer 43:254, 1989

World Health Organization: Mechanism of action, safety and efficacy of intrauterine devices. Technical Report No. 753, Geneva, Switzerland, WHO, 1987

World Health Organization: Medical Eligibility for Contraceptive Use, 4th ed. Geneva, World Health Organization, 2010

World Health Organization Collaborative Study of Cardiovascular Disease and Steroid Hormone Contraception: Acute myocardial infarction and combined oral contraceptives: results of an international multi-center case-control study. Lancet 349:1202, 1997

World Health Organization Collaborative Study of Cardiovascular Disease and Steroid Hormone Contraception: Ischaemic stroke and combined oral contraceptives: results of an international, multi-center case-control study. Lancet 348:498, 1996

World Health Organization/Department of Reproductive Health and Research (WHO/RHR), Johns Hopkins Bloomberg School of Public Health (SHSPH): Family Planning Handbook for Providers. Baltimore and Geneva, 2007

World Health Organization Special Programme of Research, Development and Research Training in Human Reproduction, Task Force on Intrauterine Devices for Fertility Regulation: A multinational case-control study of ectopic pregnancy. Clin Reprod Fertil 3:131, 1985

Yonkers KA, Brown C, Pearlstein TB, et al: Efficacy of a new low-dose oral contraceptive with drospirenone in premenstrual dysphoric disorder. Obstet Gynecol 106:492, 2005

Yuzpe AA, Thurlow HJ, Ramzy I, et al: Post coital contraception—a pilot study. J Reprod Med 13:53, 1974

Zapata LB, Paulen ME, Cansino C, et al: Contraceptive use among women with inflammatory bowel disease: a systematic review. Contraception 82(1):72, 2010a

Zapata LB, Whiteman MK, Tepper NK, et al: Intrauterine device use among women with uterine fibroids: a systematic review. Contraception 82(1):41, 2010b

Zieman M, Guillebaud J, Weisberg E, et al: Contraceptive efficacy and cycle control with the Ortho Evra™/Evra™ transdermal system: the analysis of pooled data. Fertil Steril 77:S13, 2002

Zupanc M: Antiepileptic drugs and hormonal contraceptives in adolescent women with epilepsy. Neurology 66(Suppl 3):S37, 2006

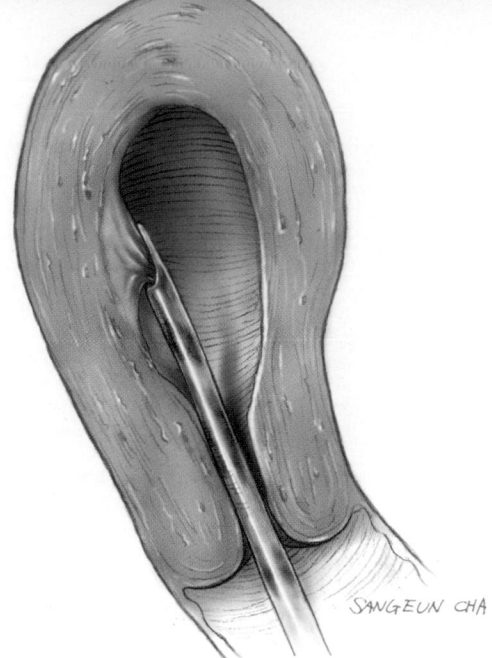

SANGEUN CHA

CHAPTER 6

First-Trimester Abortion

Abortion is the spontaneous or induced termination of pregnancy before fetal viability. Because this definition encompasses deliberate pregnancy terminations, some prefer *miscarriage* to refer to *spontaneous* pregnancy loss. The term *recurrent abortion* is used to describe consecutive pregnancy losses that may have a common cause. The duration of gestation or fetal weight that defines abortion is not consistent between organizations. For example, the National Center for Health Statistics, the Centers for Disease Control and Prevention (CDC), and the World Health Organization all define *abortion* as any pregnancy termination—spontaneous or induced—prior to 20 weeks' gestation or with a fetus born weighing <500 g. These criteria are somewhat self-contradictory because the average weight of a normally developed 20-week fetus is 320 g, whereas a birthweight of 500 g is the mean for 22 to 23 weeks (Moore, 1977). There is even more confusion because definitions vary widely according to state laws.

Technologic development has also resulted in significant evolution leading to current abortion terminology. Transvaginal sonography (TVS) and precise measurement of serum human chorionic gonadotropin (hCG) concentrations allow identification of extremely early pregnancies as well as distinction between intrauterine and ectopic implantations. Their ubiquitous application to everyday practice has spawned a number of other terms. For example, it is now possible to distinguish between a *chemical* and a *clinical* pregnancy. In another example, an ad hoc international consensus group has proposed definitions to clarify outcomes for *pregnancy of unknown location—PUL* (Barnhart, 2011). The goal is early verification of an ectopic pregnancy, which has specific management options. Intrauterine pregnancies are then managed depending on evidence for a living fetus. Those that eventuate in an early spontaneous abortion are also termed *early pregnancy loss* and *early pregnancy failure*.

SPONTANEOUS ABORTION

As just described, spontaneous first-trimester abortion is interchangeably referred to as miscarriage, early pregnancy loss, and early pregnancy failure. Of these, more than 80 percent occur

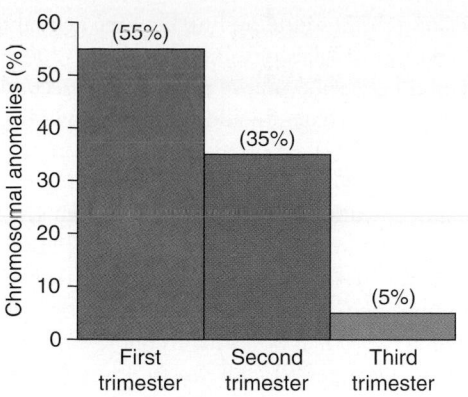

FIGURE 6-1 Frequency of chromosomal anomalies in abortuses and stillbirths during each trimester. Approximate percentages for each group are shown. *(Data from Eiben, 1990; Fantel, 1980; Warburton, 1980.)*

TABLE 6-1. Chromosomal Findings in Early Abortuses

Chromosomal Studies	Reported Incidence Range (Percent)
Normal (euploid)	
46,XY and 46,XX	45 to 55
Abnormal (aneuploid)	
Autosomal trisomy	22 to 32
Monosomy X (45,X)	5 to 20
Triploidy	6 to 8
Tetraploidy	2 to 4
Structural anomaly	2
Double or triple trisomy	0.7 to 2

Data from Eiben, 1990; Kajii, 1980; Simpson, 1980, 2007.

during the first 12 weeks of pregnancy. At this stage, approximately half result from chromosomal anomalies (Fig. 6-1). Of those with a fetus, there is a 1.5 male:female gender ratio (Benirschke, 2000). After 12 weeks, both the abortion rate and the incidence of associated chromosomal anomalies decrease.

During the first 3 months of pregnancy, death of the embryo or fetus nearly always precedes spontaneous expulsion. Early death of the conceptus is usually accompanied by hemorrhage into the decidua basalis, followed by necrosis of adjacent tissues. Thus, the embryofetus detaches, stimulating uterine contractions that result in its expulsion. The intact gestational sac is usually filled with fluid, and a small macerated fetus is found in approximately half of these. In the other half, there is no fetus visible—the so-called *blighted ovum*. Thus, finding the cause of early miscarriage involves ascertaining the cause of fetal death. This is dissimilar from later pregnancy losses in which the fetus usually does not die before expulsion, and thus other explanations are sought.

Incidence

The reported incidence of spontaneous abortion varies with the sensitivity of methods used to identify them. In a meticulous investigation of 221 healthy women studied through 707 menstrual cycles, Wilcox and colleagues (1988) identified pregnancies using precise assays for extremely low serum β-hCG concentrations. They reported that 31 percent of pregnancies were lost *after implantation*. Especially important when considering incidence, two thirds of these early losses were *clinically silent*.

A number of factors are known to influence the clinically apparent miscarriage rate. However, it is not known if these factors play a role in the clinically silent losses. For example, the proportion of clinically apparent miscarriages increases with parity as well as with maternal and paternal age (Gracia, 2005; Kleinhaus, 2006; Warburton, 1964; Wilson, 1986). Their frequency doubles from 12 percent in women before age 20 years to 26 percent in those older than 40. For the same comparison with paternal ages, the frequency of miscarriage increases from 12 to 20 percent. Although it may seem intuitive that these

differences would be similar for clinically silent miscarriages, this has not been studied.

Fetal Factors

Early spontaneous abortions commonly display a developmental abnormality of the zygote, embryo, early fetus, or placenta. Of 1000 miscarriages studied by Hertig and Sheldon (1943), half had a degenerated or absent embryo—the *blighted ovum* described previously. In the other half in which an embryo or fetus was identified, approximately half had a normal 46-chromosomal complement. The remaining pregnancies were aneuploid with any of a variety of abnormal chromosomal numbers such as those shown in Table 6-1.

Aneuploid Abortion

In general, aneuploid fetuses abort earlier than those with a normal chromosomal complement. Kajii (1980) reported that 75 percent of aneuploid fetuses aborted before 8 weeks, but rates of euploid abortions did not peak until approximately 13 weeks. Almost 95 percent of chromosomal abnormalities in aneuploid fetuses are caused by maternal gametogenesis errors. Thus, only 5 percent are due to aberrant paternal chromosomes (Jacobs, 1980).

As shown in Table 6-1, *autosomal trisomy* is the most frequently identified aneuploidy in early miscarriages. Although most trisomies result from *isolated nondisjunction*, balanced structural chromosomal rearrangements are present in one partner in 2 to 4 percent of couples with recurrent miscarriage (American College of Obstetricians and Gynecologists, 2008). Except for chromosome number 1, all other trisomies have been identified, and those with trisomies of number 13, 16, 18, 21, and 22 are most common. Bianco and colleagues (2006) studied almost 47,000 women and reported that a previous miscarriage increased the baseline risk of a subsequent fetal aneuploidy from 1.39 to 1.67 percent. Two or three previous miscarriages increased this risk to 1.84 and 2.18 percent, respectively.

Monosomy X (45,X) is the single most common specific chromosomal abnormality and is also known as *Turner syndrome*.

Most affected fetuses spontaneously abort, but some are live-born phenotypic females (Chap. 18, p. 489). Conversely, *autosomal monosomy* is rare and incompatible with life.

Triploidy is often associated with hydropic placental (molar) degeneration as discussed in detail in Chapter 37 (p. 899). Of hydatidiform moles, partial moles are characteristically triploid. Associated triploid fetuses frequently abort early, and those born later are all grossly malformed. With triploidy in general, advancing maternal and paternal age does not increase the incidence.

Tetraploid fetuses are rarely live born and are most often aborted early in gestation. *Chromosomal structural abnormalities* infrequently cause abortion. Infants with a balanced translocation who are live born usually appear normal as discussed on page 180.

Euploid Abortion

As discussed, chromosomally normal fetuses generally abort later than those with aneuploidy, and their incidence is greatest at 13 weeks (Kajii, 1980). The incidence of euploid abortions increases dramatically after maternal age exceeds 35 years (Stein, 1980).

▪ Maternal Factors

Although there are presumably a large number of causes of euploid abortions, these are poorly enumerated and understood. The well-known influence of maternal age discussed earlier was reviewed by Franz and Husslein (2010). In addition, other implicated causes include various medical and surgical disorders; environmental, nutritional, and lifestyle conditions; immunologically mediated disorders; coagulation abnormalities; and genital developmental abnormalities. Some of these are now discussed, but in no particular order of incidence or importance.

Infections

There are only a few organisms that have been proven to specifically cause abortion. Many infections that cause abortion are systemic and thus infect the fetoplacental unit by blood-borne organisms. Others may infect locally via maternal genitourinary infection or colonization. In actuality, however, infections are an uncommon cause of early abortion (American College of Obstetricians and Gynecologists, 2008). Even insulin-dependent diabetic women, who have an increased a priori abortion risk and who are presumably more susceptible to infections, uncommonly have infection-induced abortions (Simpson, 1996).

Most specific organisms have been found to be unassociated with causing abortions. *Brucella abortus, Campylobacter fetus,* and *Toxoplasma gondii* infections cause abortion in livestock, but not in humans (Feldman, 2010; Hide, 2009; Sauerwein, 1993). It is also likely that there are no abortifacient effects of infections caused by *Listeria monocytogenes, Chlamydia trachomatis,* parvovirus, cytomegalovirus, or herpes simplex virus (Brown, 1997; Feist, 1999; Feldman, 2010; Osser, 1996; Paukku, 1999).

Data concerning the abortifacient effects of some other infections are conflicting. Quinn and coworkers (1983a,b) provided serologic evidence that supports a role for *Mycoplasma hominis* and *Ureaplasma urealyticum.* Conversely, Temmerman and associates (1992) found no link between genital mycoplasmas and abortion. Oakeshott and coworkers (2002) reported an association between *bacterial vaginosis* and second- but not first-trimester miscarriage. In addition, although Temmerman and colleagues (1992) reported an association with human immunodeficiency virus (HIV)-1 infection and abortion, van Benthem and coworkers (2000) found a similar risk for abortion in women before and after they developed HIV infection. Finally, *periodontal disease* is common in pregnant women and has been implicated to cause a host of adverse pregnancy outcomes (Xiong, 2007). Two British cohort studies *suggest* an association between periodontal disease and a two- to fourfold increased risk for miscarriage (Holbrook, 2004; Moore, 2004).

Immunizations

Most routine immunizations can be given safely during pregnancy (Cunningham, 2010d). Fortunately, there is no evidence that active immunization, even with live-virus vaccines, causes miscarriage. One recent example is the pooled analysis of nearly 3600 women given HPV vaccine in early pregnancy (Wacholder, 2010).

Medical Disorders

Increased pregnancy loss associated with diabetes, thyroid disease, and other endocrine disorders is discussed in sections that follow. In general, regarding other acute or chronic diseases, even developing countries report that miscarriages are rarely caused by tuberculosis, malignancies, or other serious conditions.

There are a few specific disorders possibly associated with increased early pregnancy loss. One example is *celiac disease,* which has been reported to cause both male and female infertility as well as recurrent abortions (Sher, 1994). Eating disorders—*anorexia nervosa* and *bulimia nervosa*—are reported to cause subfertility, preterm delivery, and fetal-growth restriction. However, their association with miscarriages is less well studied (Andersen, 2009; Sollid, 2004). *Chronic hypertension* is a common condition associated with increased rates of preeclampsia and fetal-growth restriction, but there are few data concerning early pregnancy loss (August, 2009; Seely, 2011). Perhaps related, Catov and associates (2008) reported an increased risk for fetal-growth restriction in chronically hypertensive women who also had a history of recurrent miscarriages. Another possible link with underlying vascular disease is from the observation that women who have had multiple miscarriages are significantly more likely to have myocardial infarctions later in life (Kharazmi, 2011).

Surgical Disorders and Surgical Procedures During Pregnancy

In general, any putative abortifacient effects of most surgical disorders, like medical disorders discussed earlier, are not well studied. This includes any effects of common surgical procedures performed either before or during pregnancy. One example of extensive interest is pregnancy outcome following *bariatric surgery.* As subsequently discussed on page 173, obesity is an uncontested risk factor for increased miscarriage risk. The unanswered question is whether this risk is mitigated by weight-reduction surgery (Guelinckx, 2009).

Uncomplicated surgical procedures—including abdominal or pelvic surgery—performed during early pregnancy do not appear to increase the risk for abortion (Mazze, 1989). Ovarian tumors or cysts are generally safely resected without causing pregnancy loss. An important exception involves early removal of the corpus luteum or the ovary in which it resides. If performed prior to 10 weeks' gestation, supplemental progesterone should be given. Between 8 and 10 weeks, a single injection of intramuscular 17-hydroxyprogesterone caproate, 150 mg, is given at the time of surgery. If the corpus luteum is excised between 6 to 8 weeks, then two additional 150-mg injections should be given 1 and 2 weeks after the first. Other suitable progesterone replacement regimens include: (1) micronized progesterone (Prometrium) 200 or 300 mg orally once daily, or (2) 8-percent progesterone vaginal gel (Crinone), one premeasured applicator vaginally daily plus micronized progesterone, 100 or 200 mg orally once daily. These are continued until 10 weeks' gestation.

Although *major trauma*—especially abdominal—can cause fetal loss, this is more likely as pregnancy advances. Trauma seldom causes first-trimester miscarriage, and although Parkland Hospital is a busy trauma center, this association is uncommon. Any effects of minor trauma are even more difficult to ascertain.

Radiation and Chemotherapy for Cancer. Therapeutic doses of radiation are undeniably abortifacient, but threshold doses that cause abortion are not precisely known. According to Brent (2009), exposure to <5 rads does not increase the risk for miscarriage.

Female cancer survivors who were treated with abdomino-pelvic radiotherapy may be at increased risk for miscarriage. Wo and Viswanathan (2009) conclude first that fertility may be impaired because of radiation-induced destruction of oocyte reserves leads to premature ovarian failure. Second, radiation damage to the uterus results in reduced volume, impaired distensibility, and vascular and endothelial injury. They reported an associated two- to eightfold increased risk for miscarriages, low-birthweight and growth-restricted infants, preterm delivery, and perinatal mortality in women treated with radiotherapy. Hudson (2010) also summarized effects on subsequent reproduction of radiotherapy, chemotherapy, or both given to treat childhood cancers. They too found an associated increased risk of miscarriage.

Endocrine Abnormalities

Thyroid disorders have long been suspected to cause early pregnancy loss. Severe iodine deficiency—infrequent in developed countries—is associated with excessive miscarriage rates (Castañeda, 2002). In the United States, there are varying degrees of thyroid hormone insufficiency that are common in women. Although overt hypothyroidism is rarely encountered in pregnancy, subclinical hypothyroidism has an incidence of approximately 2 percent (Casey, 2005). It usually is caused by autoimmune *Hashimoto thyroiditis* in which both incidence and severity accrue with age. Despite this common prevalence, any effects of hypothyroidism on early pregnancy loss are still unclear (Krassas, 2010; Negro, 2010). That said, De Vivo (2010) recently reported that subclinical thyroid hormone deficiency may be associated with very early pregnancy loss.

Antithyroid autoantibodies are commonly detected in reproductive-aged women. In two large prenatal screening studies, the prevalence of antibodies to thyroid peroxidase or thyroglobulin was nearly 15 percent (Abbassi-Ghanavati, 2010; Haddow, 2011). Their incidence and concentration are much higher in women with thyroid insufficiency. High serum levels are reported to be associated with an increased incidence of miscarriage even in euthyroid women (Abramson, 2001; Benhadi, 2009; Chen, 2011; Lazarus, 2005). Two prospective studies have confirmed increased miscarriage rates, and preliminary data from one suggests that thyroxine supplementation decreases this risk (Männistö, 2009; Negro, 2006). Effects associated with thyroid disorders in women with *recurrent miscarriage* are considered further on page 186.

Insulin-dependent diabetes has well-known substantively increased risks for spontaneous abortion and major congenital malformations. It can also cause recurrent pregnancy loss and is considered on page 186.

Nutritional Factors

Obesity is associated with subfertility, increases the risk of miscarriage, and results in a host of other adverse pregnancy outcomes (Jarvie, 2010; Satpathy, 2008). Bellver and associates (2010a) studied 6500 women with in vitro fertilization (IVF)-conceived pregnancies and found that pregnancy and live birth rates were reduced progressively for each body mass index (BMI) unit increase. Obesity is also linked to an increased rate of recurrent miscarriage (Lashen, 2004). Finally, and as discussed on page 172, although the risks for many adverse late-pregnancy outcomes are decreased after bariatric surgery, any salutary effects on the miscarriage rate are not clear (Guelinckx, 2009).

Dietary deficiency of any one nutrient or moderate deficiency of all nutrients does not appear to be an important cause of abortion. Extreme cases may be the exception, and *severe hyperemesis gravidarum* may rarely be followed by miscarriage (Maconochie, 2007). And as discussed on page 172, *anorexia* and *bulimia nervosa* are thought to be associated with an increased miscarriage rate (Andersen, 2009). Preconceptional counseling is important because Bulik and colleagues (2010) reported that half of the pregnancies in 62 women with anorexia nervosa were unplanned.

Drug Use and Social Habits

In addition to a list of known teratogenic drugs, various other agents may be associated with an increased risk for miscarriage. Some of those more frequently encountered merit discussion.

According to the CDC (2011b), up to 15 percent of pregnant women admit to *cigarette smoking*. There are well-known adverse effects of smoking on late-pregnancy outcomes, but those for miscarriage are conflicting. Earlier studies linked smoking with a risk for euploid abortion that increased in a linear fashion with the number of cigarettes smoked daily (Armstrong, 1992; Chatenoud, 1998). In a recent questionnaire study, a possible slightly increased risk for miscarriage was found (Gallicchio, 2009). Conversely, a number of other studies do not support this association (Rasch, 2003; Wisborg, 2003). Certainly, it may be intuitive that cigarettes cause early pregnancy loss by a number of mechanisms. One example is magnification of the risk of abnormal placentation as proposed by Catov and associates (2008). They reviewed the Danish National Birth Cohort of more than 81,000 pregnancies and found that smoking was additive to increase the risk of growth-restricted infants in chronically hypertensive mothers.

Alcohol has been well studied for its potent teratogenic and adverse fetal effects. Earlier observations were that both miscarriage and fetal anomaly rates increased with the rates of alcohol abuse during the first 8 weeks of gestation (Armstrong, 1992; Floyd, 1999; Kline, 1980). Such outcomes likely are dose related. For example, Maconochie (2007) observed a significantly increased risk only with regular or heavy alcohol use. Others have reported that low-level alcohol consumption does not significantly increase the risk for abortion (Cavallo, 1995; Kesmodel, 2002).

Caffeine, when consumed "excessively"—not well defined—has been associated with an increased risk for abortion in observational studies. Armstrong (1992) and Cnattingius (2000) reported that consumption of five cups of coffee per day—approximately 500 mg of caffeine—is associated with a slightly increased abortion risk. Klebanoff and associates (1999) reported that women with "extremely elevated" levels of paraxanthine—a caffeine metabolite—had a twofold risk for miscarriage. More recently, two prospective studies were done to study any adverse effects of *moderate* caffeine consumption. Both Savitz (2008) and Weng (2008) reported that consumption of <200 mg of caffeine daily did not increase the miscarriage risk, but one group found a twofold increased risk if >200 mg daily was consumed. Based on all of these findings, the American College of Obstetricians and Gynecologists (2010a) concluded that at this time moderate consumption does not appear to be a major contributor to abortion risk, and that the correlation with high intake is unsettled.

Commonly used *hormonal contraceptives* are not associated with an increased miscarriage rate. Neither are *spermicidal agents.* When *intrauterine devices* fail to prevent pregnancy, however, the risk of abortion, and specifically septic abortion, increases substantively (Ganer, 2009; Moschos, 2011). These and other contraceptive effects are discussed in Chapter 5 (p. 140).

Chemical and Occupational Factors

Some chemicals—for example, benzene—are implicated in causing fetal malformations (Lupo, 2011). Regardless of evidence, it seems prudent to limit exposure of pregnant women to any potentially toxic chemicals. In most cases, however, accurate assessment of any possible relationship between environmental agents and miscarriage is difficult. Some that have been implicated to increase the risk for miscarriage include *arsenic, lead, formaldehyde, benzene,* and *ethylene oxide* (Barlow, 1982). There is mounting evidence for DDT (dichlorodiphenyltrichloroethane) as a cause of miscarriage (Eskenazi, 2009). Use of DDT-containing insecticides had been suspended, but since 2006, its use was again endorsed by the World Health Organization for mosquito control to prevent malaria.

There are a few studies of occupational exposures and abortion risks. Exposure to *video display terminals* and their electromagnetic fields as well as *ultrasound* does not adversely affect miscarriage rates (Schnorr, 1991; Taskinen, 1990). An increased risk of miscarriage has been described for dental assistants exposed to 3 or more hours of *nitrous oxide* per day in offices without gas-scavenging equipment (Boivin, 1997; Rowland, 1995). In their metaanalysis, Dranitsaris and colleagues (2005) found a small incremental risk for spontaneous abortion in women who worked with *cytotoxic antineoplastic chemotherapeutic agents*. In a recent survey, Gallicchio and colleagues (2009) found no increased adverse birth defects in infants born to *cosmetologists*.

Immunological Factors

A number of immune-mediated disorders are associated with early pregnancy loss. A major example is the development of antiphospholipid antibodies directed against binding proteins in plasma (Erkan, 2011). Related to these antibodies, clinical and laboratory findings together provide criteria for the *antiphospholipid antibody syndrome—APS,* which was reviewed by the American College of Obstetricians and Gynecologists (2011a). Because pregnancy loss in these women tends to be repetitive, they are considered with recurrent miscarriage (p. 182).

Inherited Thrombophilias

Complexities of the coagulation cascade include a number of single-gene mutations that affect pro- or anticoagulant proteins. Because these control blood coagulation, any qualitative or quantitative changes in these proteins may increase the risk of either bleeding or arterial and venous thrombosis. Some of the better studied mutations predisposing to thrombosis—collectively termed *thrombophilias*—are caused by mutations of the genes for factor V Leiden, prothrombin, antithrombin, and protein C and protein S.

Soon after their discovery, some thrombophilias were reported to be associated with an increased risk for adverse pregnancy outcomes that included early miscarriage (Scifres, 2008). As the quality of these investigations has improved during the past 10 to 15 years, many of these putative associations have become tenuous (Adelberg, 2002; Carp, 2002; Lockwood, 2010). One major shortcoming is that most large good-quality studies enrolled subjects after the critical period for miscarriage. These well-designed prospective studies, however, have reported no links with later adverse obstetrical outcomes (Dizon-Townsend, 2005; Said, 2010; Silver, 2010). Currently, the American College of Obstetrics and Gynecologists (2011b) is of the opinion that there is not a definitive causal link with these thrombophilias and adverse pregnancy outcomes in general, and abortion in particular. An important caveat is that some thrombophilias may predispose all patients—including pregnant women—to increased risks for thromboembolism.

Genital Tract Anatomic Defects

A number of relatively common genital tract abnormalities—especially those of the uterus—can either prevent pregnancy implantation or disrupt a pregnancy that has implanted.

Of these, congenital anomalies are most commonly implicated, but some acquired anomalies can also cause pregnancy loss. Unless corrected, these defects typically result in repetitive pregnancy losses and thus are considered on page 181.

Paternal Factors

Little is known about paternal factors that may contribute to miscarriage. Certainly, some chromosomal abnormalities in sperm can result in abortion (Carrell, 2003). In a case-control study of more than 92,000 births in the Jerusalem Perinatal Study, Kleinhaus and colleagues (2006) reported that increasing paternal age was significantly associated with an increasing miscarriage rate. The rate was lowest when paternal age was <25 years, and it progressively increased at 5-year intervals and became highest after age 40.

Clinical Classification of Spontaneous Abortion

From a clinical standpoint, abortion can be classified a number of ways. Commonly used subgroups include threatened, inevitable, incomplete, complete, and missed abortion. Septic abortion is when the products of conception, uterus, and other pelvic organs have become infected.

Threatened Abortion

The clinical diagnosis of threatened abortion is presumed when there is a bloody vaginal discharge or bleeding through a closed cervical os. It has long been known that bleeding in early pregnancy is common, and the frequency and associated outcomes were recently quantified by Hasan (2009). Of 4510 women prospectively enrolled early for prenatal care, 27 percent had first-trimester spotting or heavier bleeding, and 43 percent of this group went on to have a miscarriage. As perhaps expected, heavy bleeding increased the risk. In another study, Tongsong (1995) reported that with any amount of bleeding, the risk of miscarriage was substantially lower if there was fetal cardiac activity.

Eddleman and associates (2006) designed an individualized risk assessment model for spontaneous pregnancy loss. They studied 35,000 pregnancies and reported that bleeding during the current pregnancy was by far the most predictive risk factor for pregnancy loss. As shown in Table 6-2, even if miscarriage does not follow early bleeding, the risks for later adverse pregnancy outcomes are increased. In the study by Lykke (2010), nearly 1.8 million deliveries from the Danish National Patient Registry were analyzed. In women with first-trimester vaginal bleeding that did not result in miscarriage, there was a threefold risk for many of the later pregnancy complications listed in Table 6-2.

Some physiologic bleeding near the time of expected menses is painless. With miscarriage, however, bleeding usually begins first, but pain follows a few hours to several days later. Pain may present as low midline cramping; as persistent low backache that is associated with a feeling of pelvic pressure; or as a dull, midline, suprapubic discomfort. Some women have more than one of these. Regardless of clinical presentation, the combination of bleeding and pain predicts a poor prognosis for pregnancy continuation.

TABLE 6-2. Increased Incidence of Some Adverse Outcomes in Women with Threatened Abortion

Maternal	Perinatal
Placenta previa	Preterm ruptured
Placental abruption	membranes
Manual removal of placenta	Preterm birth
Cesarean delivery	Low-birthweight infant
	Fetal-growth restriction
	Perinatal death

From Johns, 2006, Lykke, 2010; Saraswat, 2010; Wijesiriwardana, 2006.

Diagnosis. A woman with an early pregnancy, vaginal bleeding, and pain should be examined. Ectopic pregnancy, ovarian torsion, and the other types of abortion may mimic threatened abortion and should be excluded. To accomplish this, serial quantitative serum β-hCG levels, progesterone levels, and TVS, either alone or in combination, can help ascertain if the fetus is alive and if it is within the uterus. Because none of these tests is 100-percent accurate to confirm fetal death in early gestation, repeat evaluations are often necessary. Data from Barnhart (2004a) shown in Figure 6-2 depict composite serum hCG level disappearance curves in women with bleeding who went on to have an early miscarriage. Serial increasing β-hCG values from women with early pregnancy bleeding who went on to have a normal pregnancy are shown in Figure 6-3. A number of predictive models based on serum hCG levels done 48 hours apart have been described (Chap. 7, p. 203) (Barnhart, 2010; Condous, 2007). Specifically, with a robust uterine pregnancy, serum β-hCG levels should increase at least 53 to 66 percent every 48 hours (Barnhart, 2004a; Kadar, 1982). With serum progesterone levels, concentrations <5 ng/mL suggest a dying pregnancy,

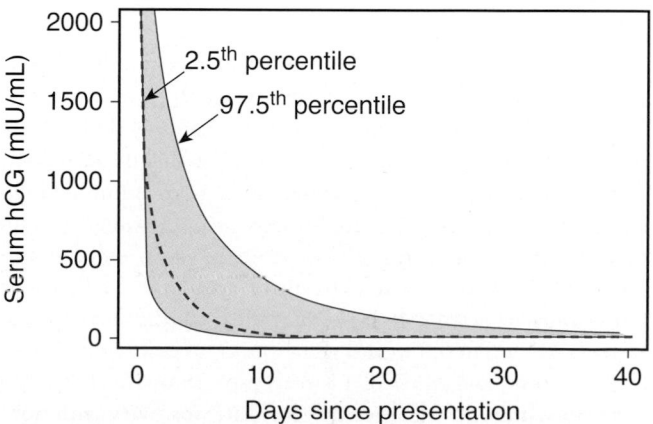

FIGURE 6-2 Composite curve describing decline in serial human chorionic gonadotropin (hCG) values starting at a level of 2000 mIU/mL following early spontaneous miscarriage. The dashed line is the predicted curve based on the summary of data from all women. The colored area within the dashed lines represent the 95-percent confidence intervals. *(Data from Barnhart, 2004a.)*

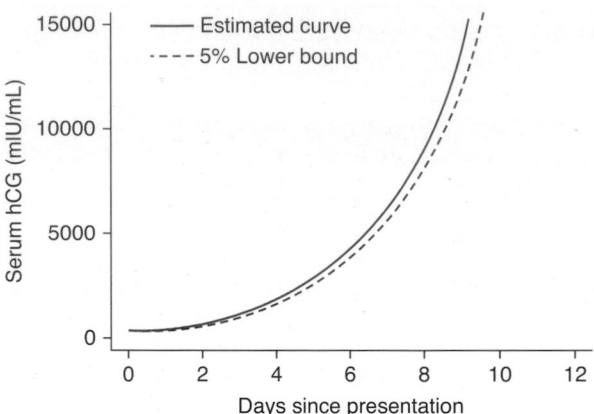

FIGURE 6-3 Composite curve of increasing serum levels of beta-human chorionic gonadotropin (β-hCG) in women with early bleeding and subsequent normal pregnancy *(blue curve)*. Confidence interval of the lower bound of increase is shown by the red line. *(Data from Barnhart, 2004b.)*

whereas values >20 ng/mL support the diagnosis of a healthy pregnancy.

With TVS, the location and viability of gestations can be documented. One of the earliest identified signs is the gestational sac, which is an anechoic fluid collection that represents the exocoelomic cavity (Fig. 2-19, p. 44). With TVS, it can be seen by 4.5 gestational weeks and with maternal serum beta-human chorionic gonadotropin (β-hCG) levels between 1500 and 2000 mIU/mL (Barnhart, 1994; Bree, 1989; Timor-Tritsch, 1988). A word of caution is necessary because a gestational sac may appear similar to other intrauterine fluid accumulations, that is, a pseudogestational sac or pseudosac, as described in Chapter 7 (p. 205).

Differentiating between a gestational sac and a pseudosac early in pregnancy is easier once a yolk sac is seen. Moreover, the American College of Obstetricians and Gynecologists (2009e) advises caution in diagnosing an intrauterine pregnancy in the absence of a definite yolk sac or embryo. The yolk sac is typically seen within a gestational sac at 5.5 weeks' gestation, when a mean sac diameter (MSD) is more than 10 mm. The MSD is reached by summing the three sac diameters and dividing by three. Gestational sacs grow at approximately 1 mm per day. Nyberg and colleagues (1987) suggested that a MSD less than or equal to 0.6 mm/day is evidence for abnormal development.

Soon after appearance of a yolk sac, a 1- to 2-mm embryo adjacent to the yolk sac can be seen at approximately 5 to 6 weeks' gestation (Daya, 1993). Absence of an embryo in a sac with a MSD of 16 to 20 mm or greater is predictive of nonviability (Levi, 1988; Nyberg, 1987). Cardiac activity can be detected at 6 to 6.5 weeks' gestation, at an embryonic length of 1 to 5 mm, and MSD of 13 to 18 mm. Embryos measuring >5 mm without cardiac activity correlate positively with nonviability (Goldstein, 1992; Levi, 1990).

At Parkland Hospital, to ensure that a live uterine pregnancy is not interrupted, we define the threshold of nonviability based on values that are two standard deviations from the mean. Accordingly, anembryonic gestation is diagnosed in cases in which the MSD measures 20 mm and no embryo is seen.

Additionally, nonviability is determined if an embryo measuring 10 mm or more is found but cardiac activity is absent.

Management. With threatened abortion, if bleeding is persistent or heavy, a hematocrit is performed. If blood loss is sufficient to cause significant anemia or hypovolemia, pregnancy evacuation is generally indicated. In these cases in which there is a live fetus, some choose transfusion and further observation.

For women in whom uterine evacuation is not indicated, bed rest is often recommended but has not been shown to improve outcomes. Neither has treatment with a host of medications such as chorionic gonadotropin (Devaseelan, 2010). Acetaminophen-based analgesia will help relieve discomfort.

Anti-D Immunoglobulin. Isoimmunization of D-negative women by D-positive fetal erythrocytes can be prevented with anti-D immunoglobulin. This is recommended by the American College of Obstetricians and Gynecologists (2010b) because without prophylaxis, 2 percent of D-negative women with a spontaneous miscarriage and up to 5 percent of those with an induced abortion will become isoimmunized. Suitable $Rh_0(D)$ immunoglobulin administration options include: (1) 300 µg intramuscularly (IM) for all gestational ages or (2) 50 µg IM for gestations ≤12 weeks but 300 µg IM for gestations ≥13 weeks.

Prophylaxis with a threatened abortion is controversial, and recommendations are limited by the scarcity of evidence-based data (American College of Obstetricians and Gynecologists, 2010b; Hannafin, 2006; Weiss, 2002). Thus, up to 12 weeks' gestation, prophylaxis is optional for women with threatened abortion and a live fetus.

Inevitable Abortion

Obviously, amnionic fluid leaking through a dilated cervix portends almost certain abortion. In these cases, either uterine contractions begin promptly to result in miscarriage, or infection develops. Rarely, a gush of fluid from the uterus during the first half of pregnancy is without serious consequence. The fluid may have collected previously between the amnion and chorion. Because of this, if a sudden discharge of fluid with apparently intact membranes in early pregnancy occurs before pain, fever, or bleeding, then observation is reasonable. If after 48 hours of diminished activity, there has been no additional leakage and there is no bleeding, pain, or fever, then usual activities may be resumed except for any form of vaginal penetration. However, if the gush of fluid is accompanied or followed by continued leakage or by bleeding or pain or fever, then abortion is considered inevitable, and the uterus is emptied.

Incomplete Abortion

When the internal cervical os opens and allows passage of blood and clots, then incomplete abortion is presumed. In these cases, bleeding is caused by partial or total placental detachment, although the fetus or placenta remains in utero or is partially extrude through the dilated os. Before 10 weeks, the fetus and placenta are commonly expelled together, but later they are usually delivered separately. In some women, additional cervical dilatation is necessary before there is spontaneous completion or curettage is performed. Retained placental tissue may simply lie loosely in the cervical canal, thus allowing easy extraction with ring forceps. Suction curettage effectively evacuates the uterus and is described later (p. 189) and is illustrated in Section 41-16 (p. 1059). With miscarriage, removed products of conception should be sent to pathology for standard histologic analysis. With this, products of conception are confirmed, and gestational trophoblastic disease is excluded.

Complete Abortion

In some cases, expulsion of the entire pregnancy is completed before a patient presents for care. A history of heavy bleeding, cramping, and tissue passage is common, and physical examination reveals a closed cervical os. Patients are encouraged to bring in passed tissue. On investigation, tissues indeed may be a complete gestation or erroneously may be blood clots or decidual cast. All pregnancies can induce an endometrial decidual reaction, and sloughing of the decidua can appear as a collapsed sac, that is, a decidual cast. Thus, if a gestational sac is not identified grossly, then sonography is typically performed to differentiate a complete abortion from threatened abortion or ectopic pregnancy. With complete abortion, a thickened endometrium without a gestational sac is seen sonographically. Ectopic pregnancy should always be considered in the differential diagnosis of complete abortion. Condous and colleagues (2005) described 152 women with heavy bleeding who were initially considered to have a completed miscarriage and who had an endometrial thickness <15 mm. Despite these findings, 6 percent of these women were subsequently proven to have an ectopic pregnancy. Thus, unless an intrauterine pregnancy was previously seen sonographically, women with clinical findings suggestive of complete abortion should be surveilled with serial serum hCG measurements, and perhaps sonography, until a diagnosis is established.

Missed Abortion—Early Pregnancy Loss

Current use of the term *missed abortion* requires clarification. Because this was defined many decades before the evolution of current technology, contemporaneous application of the older term is frequently inaccurate. Historically, the term *missed abortion* was used to describe dead products of conception that had usually been retained for weeks or months in a uterus with a closed cervical os. These women usually had early pregnancy findings of amenorrhea, morning sickness, breast changes, and some uterine growth. Because suspected fetal death could not be confirmed, expectant management was the sole option, and spontaneous miscarriage would eventually follow. And because the time of fetal death could not be determined clinically, pregnancy duration, and thus fetal age, was erroneously calculated from the last menses. To elucidate these disparities, Streeter (1930) studied aborted fetuses and observed that the mean interval from death-to-abortion was approximately 6 weeks.

The foregoing historical description of missed abortion must be contrasted with that defined currently with use of serial hormone assays—particularly β-hCG—combined with TVS (Fig. 6-4). There is rapid confirmation of fetal or embryonic death—even in early pregnancies—and many women choose uterine evacuation when the diagnosis is confirmed. Many classify these as a missed abortion, although the term is used interchangeably with *early pregnancy loss*.

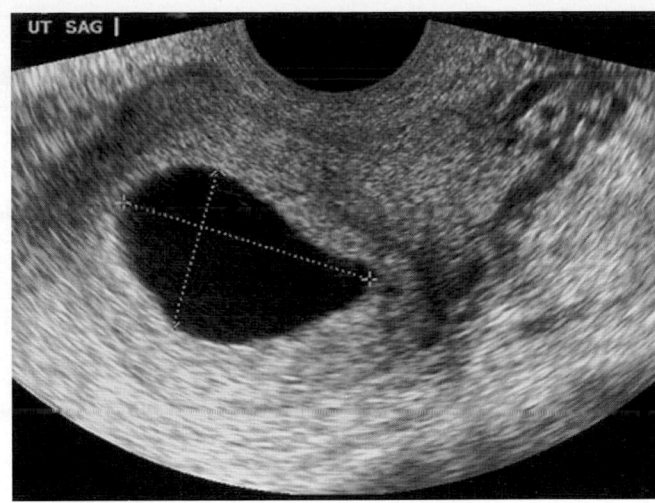

FIGURE 6-4 Transvaginal sonography displays an anembryonic gestation. *(Photograph contributed by Dr. Elysia Moschos.)*

Septic Abortion

Horrific infections and maternal deaths associated with criminal septic abortions have become rare with legalized abortion. Still, women with threatened or incomplete miscarriage can develop infection and sepsis syndrome. Elective abortion, either surgical or medical, is also occasionally complicated by severe and even fatal infections (Barrett, 2002; Ho, 2009). Bacteria that colonize dead conception products initiate maternal infection within the uterus, and infection may extend to cause parametritis, peritonitis, septicemia, and even endocarditis (Vartian, 1991). Particularly worrisome are severe necrotizing infections with toxic-shock syndrome caused by group A streptococcal infections (Daif, 2009).

Treatment of infected abortion or postabortal sepsis includes prompt administration of broad-spectrum antibiotics, and suitable regimens are found in Table 3-31 (p. 103). For women with septic incomplete abortion or for those with retained fragments, intravenous antimicrobial therapy is promptly followed by uterine evacuation. With severe sepsis syndrome, acute respiratory syndrome or disseminated intravascular coagulopathy may develop, and supportive care is essential.

Rare but severe infections with otherwise low-virulence organisms have been described following medical abortions during the past few years. The CDC (2005) reported four deaths associated with medical abortion that was caused by toxic shock syndrome due to *Clostridium sordellii* infection. These infections, as well as similar ones caused by *Clostridium perfringens*, have clinical manifestations that begin within a few days after spontaneous or induced abortion. The hallmark is that these women may be afebrile when first seen with severe endothelial injury, capillary leakage, hemoconcentration, hypotension, and a profound leukocytosis (Cohen, 2007; Fischer, 2005; Ho, 2009). Maternal deaths due to sepsis with these clostridial species are estimated to be 0.58 per 100,000 medical abortions (Meites, 2010).

Antibiotic prophylaxis is recommended following surgical or medical management of spontaneous or induced abortion. The American College of Obstetricians and Gynecologists (2009b)

TABLE 6-3. Randomized Controlled Studies for Management of Early Pregnancy Loss

Study	Inclusion Criteria	No.	Treatment Arms	Outcomes
Blohm (2005)	"Signs of miscarriage"	126	(1) Placebo (2) PGE$_1$, 400 μg vaginally	54% completed at 7 d 81% completed at 7 d; required more analgesia
Nguyen (2005)	Incomplete SAB	149	(1) PGE$_1$, 600 μg orally (2) PGE$_1$, 600 μg orally initially and at 4 hour	60% completed at 3 d 95% at 7 d; 3% curettage
Zhang (2005)	Pregnancy failure[a]	652	(1) PGE$_1$, 800 μg vaginally (2) Vacuum aspiration	71% completed at 3 d; 84% by 8 d; 16% failure 97% successful; 3% failure
Trinder (2006) (MIST Trial)	Incomplete SAB; missed AB	1200	(1) Expectant (2) PGE$_1$, 800 μg vaginally ± 200 mg mifepristone (3) Suction curettage	50% curettage 38% curettage 5% repeat curettage
Dao (2007)	Incomplete SAB	447	(1) PGE$_1$, 600 μg orally (2) Vacuum aspiration	95% completed 100% completed
Shwekerela (2007)	Incomplete SAB	300	(1) PGE$_1$, 600 μg orally (2) Vacuum aspiration	99% completed 100% completed

SAB = spontaneous abortion; PGE$_1$ = prostaglandin E$_1$.
[a]Includes anembryonic gestation, embryonic or fetal death, or incomplete or inevitable SAB.

recommends doxycycline, 100 mg orally 1 hour prior to and then 200 mg orally after a surgical evacuation. At our institution, patients are provided with doxycycline, 100 mg orally twice daily for 10 days. At Planned Parenthood clinics, for medical abortion, doxycycline 100 mg is taken orally daily for 7 days and begins with abortifacient administration (Fjerstad, 2009b).

Management of Spontaneous Abortion

Because death of the conceptus is easily verified by sonography, management can be individualized. In general, any of the three options—expectant, medical, or surgical management—are reasonable unless there is infection or excessive hemorrhage. Results of expectant management of women with suspected first-trimester miscarriage were reported by Luise (2002). Of nearly 1100 women, 81 percent had spontaneous resolution of pregnancy. A major drawback to expectant management, which is also shared by medical treatment, is their association with unpredictable bleeding. Thus, some of these women subsequently require curettage that frequently is unscheduled. Finally, whereas surgical treatment is definitive and predictable, it is invasive and not necessary for all women.

A number of randomized studies have compared these management schemes. These were reviewed by Neilson (2010). A major drawback cited was that between-study comparisons were not completely accurate because of varied inclusion criteria and techniques employed. For example, studies that included women with vaginal bleeding enhanced the success of medical therapy compared with studies that excluded such women

(Creinin, 2006). With these caveats in mind, selected studies reported since 2005 are listed in Table 6-3. These permit some generalizations. First, success is dependent on the type of early pregnancy loss, that is, incomplete versus missed abortion. Second, expectant management of spontaneous incomplete abortion has failure rates as high as 50 percent. Medical therapy with prostaglandin E$_1$ (PGE$_1$) may be related to dose, route, and form—tablet, gel, dissolved—and thus has varying failure rates of 5 to 40 percent. Lastly, curettage results in a quick resolution that is 95- to 100-percent successful.

An important consideration was addressed by Smith (2009), who showed that subsequent pregnancy rates did not differ with the choice of management. Thus, any of several management options can be selected by a woman and her gynecologist with the caveat that prompt medical or surgical completion is warranted when there is dangerous hemorrhage or infection. Dalton (2010) has provided evidence that focused training and education may increase use of office procedures in these cases.

RECURRENT MISCARRIAGE

Terms used to describe repetitive early spontaneous pregnancy losses include *recurrent miscarriage, recurrent spontaneous abortion,* and *recurrent pregnancy loss.* The term *habitual abortion* was used in the past but is generally avoided today. Probably 1 to 2 percent of fertile couples experience recurrent miscarriage, which is classically defined as three or more consecutive losses at ≤20 weeks' gestation or with a fetal weight <500 grams.

Most women with recurrent miscarriage have embryonic or early fetal loss. Recurrent anembryonic miscarriage or those with consecutive losses after 14 weeks are much less common.

Because definitions have varied, it is difficult to compare studies. Terminology differs widely with respect to the number of miscarriages; whether the miscarriages are consecutive or interspersed between viable pregnancies; and whether pregnancies are documented by β-hCG testing, sonographic evaluation, and/or pathologic examination. Moreover, some studies include women with only two instead of three consecutive losses, whereas others include women with three nonconsecutive losses.

At minimum, recurrent miscarriage should be distinguished from sporadic pregnancy loss, which implies that an intervening pregnancy has reached viability with a normal infant. In consideration of this, some investigators distinguish *primary recurrent miscarriage*—no successful pregnancies—from *secondary recurrent miscarriage*—one or more prior live births. Women with one or more intervening normal pregnancies were considered to have a significantly lower recurrent abortion risk. There are, however, recent reports that contradict this presumption.

As shown in Table 6-4, the success rate of a subsequent viable pregnancy decreases as age increases and as the number of consecutive losses increase from two to six. Shown in Table 6-5 are predictive recurrent pregnancy losses with none to three previous miscarriages. In both studies, the risk for subsequent miscarriage is similar following either two or three pregnancies. Findings such as those have led some to recommend evaluation after two miscarriages in couples without prior normal pregnancies and after three pregnancies in those with a prior liveborn (Harger, 1983; Poland, 1977).

The American Society for Reproductive Medicine (2008) has proposed that recurrent pregnancy loss be defined by two or more failed clinical pregnancies confirmed by either sonographic or histopathologic examination. They also recommend that each loss be considered as an impetus for further evaluation

TABLE 6-5. Predicted Miscarriage Rate in Scottish Women with Subsequent Pregnancy According to Number of Prior Miscarriages in More than 150,000 Miscarriages[a]

	Previous Pregnancy Losses			
	0	1	2	3
Pregnancies (n)	143,595	6577	700	115
Subsequent risk for miscarriage	7.0%	13.9%	26.1%	27.8%

[a]Nonconsecutive miscarriages showed the same pattern of risk as consecutive miscarriages.
Data from Bhattacharya, 2010.

and that a thorough evaluation is warranted after three losses. Other considerations include maternal age and the interval between pregnancies. Evaluation and treatment is initiated earlier in couples with concordant subfertility (Reddy, 2007). This practice is further justified by a recent study of more than 1000 women in which women with two pregnancy losses had a prevalence of abnormal test findings similar to that of women with three or more losses (Jaslow, 2010). Remarkably, the chances for a successful pregnancy are more than 50 percent even after five losses in women younger than 45 years (Brigham, 1999).

Etiology

Of the many putative causes of early recurrent abortion, perhaps only three are widely accepted: parental chromosomal abnormalities, antiphospholipid antibody syndrome, and a subset of uterine abnormalities. Other suspected but not proven causes are alloimmunity, endocrinopathies, various infections, and environmental toxins. Moreover, various polymorphisms of gene expression for innumerable inherited factors are likely involved. Eller and colleagues (2011) described polymorphisms that altered vascular endothelial growth factor A (VEGF-A) expression to be more common in women with recurrent miscarriages. Another investigation found that women with exaggerated platelet aggregation were more likely to have recurrent losses (Flood, 2010). The specific type of Th1 and Th2 immune response has also been implicated (Calleja-Agius, 2011). These are only a few examples of genetic research that likely will identify numerous heritable causes of recurrent early pregnancy loss.

Until a few years ago, a variety of inherited thrombophilias were thought to cause recurrent miscarriage. After a number of large studies, however, it appears that these thrombophilias are not associated with a significantly increased risk for pregnancy wastage, including spontaneous miscarriage.

The timing of the losses may provide a clue to their etiology. Genetic factors most frequently result in early embryonic losses, whereas autoimmune or anatomic abnormalities more likely lead to second-trimester losses (Schust, 2002). According to Heuser (2010), for a given individual with idiopathic recurrent pregnancy loss, each miscarriage tends to occur near the same gestational age.

TABLE 6-4. Predicted Success Rate of Subsequent Pregnancy According to Age and Number of Previous Miscarriages in 325 Consecutive Women with Recurrent Miscarriage

Number of Previous Miscarriages at Age (years)	2	3	4	5
	Predicted Success Subsequent Pregnancy (in Percent)			
20	92	90	88	85
25	89	86	82	79
30	84	80	76	71
35	77	73	68	62
40+	69	64	58	52

Data from Brigham, 1999.

Although many causes of recurrent miscarriage parallel those of sporadic miscarriage, the relative incidence differs between the two categories. For example, first-trimester losses in recurrent miscarriage have a significantly lower incidence of genetic abnormalities than are observed in sporadic losses. In one series, the products of conception had a normal karyotype in half of recurrent miscarriages but in only a fourth of sporadic losses (Sullivan, 2004).

Parental Chromosomal Abnormalities

Although these account for only 2 to 4 percent of recurrent losses, karyotypic evaluation of both parents is considered by most to be essential (American College of Obstetricians and Gynecologists, 2008). That said, results from a recent United Kingdom Study raised doubts concerning the cost effectiveness of this practice (Barber, 2010).

A review of 79 studies done more than 25 years ago included data from 8000 couples with two or more miscarriages (Tharapel, 1985). Structural chromosomal anomalies were identified in 3 percent—a fivefold greater incidence than that observed for the general population. Balanced reciprocal translocations accounted for 50 percent of identified abnormalities; Robertsonian translocations for 24 percent; and X chromosome mosaicism such as 47, XXY—*Klinefelter syndrome*—for 12 percent. Inversions and various other anomalies comprised the remainder. The women were twice as likely as the men to harbor the cytogenetic abnormality. The likelihood of a karyotypic abnormality does not differ between consecutive or nonconsecutive pregnancy losses (van den Boogaard, 2010).

Balanced translocations are the most common structural chromosomal abnormality and result in several possible genetic outcomes. These are shown in **Figure 6-5**, and karyotypes may be normal, the same balanced translocation, or an unbalanced translocation. Offspring who inherit the balanced translocation are likely to also experience recurrent miscarriage. The conceptus from an unbalanced translocation will either spontaneously abort or produce an anomalous, frequently stillborn fetus. Thus, a history of second-trimester loss or fetal anomaly should raise the suspicion that one parent may have an abnormal chromosome pattern.

Although the cost effectiveness of karyotyping studies is not universally accepted, some are promoting the use of even more complex and expensive genetic techniques to evaluate these couples. Some of these are genomic hybridization and microarray technology, which can detect chromosomal changes below the threshold of sensitivity for conventional cytogenetic analysis (Rajcan-Separovic, 2010). Currently, we agree with the American College of Obstetricians and Gynecologists (2008) that recurrent miscarriage evaluation should include a standard karyotype of both parents and that more detailed chromosomal evaluation should remain investigational.

Screening Products of Conception

Some recommend that fetal tissue be routinely analyzed for chromosomal abnormalities following a second consecutive miscarriage (Stephenson, 2006). One reason cited is that an abnormal karyotype suggests a sporadic loss and therefore does not predict an increased risk for loss with a subsequent pregnancy.

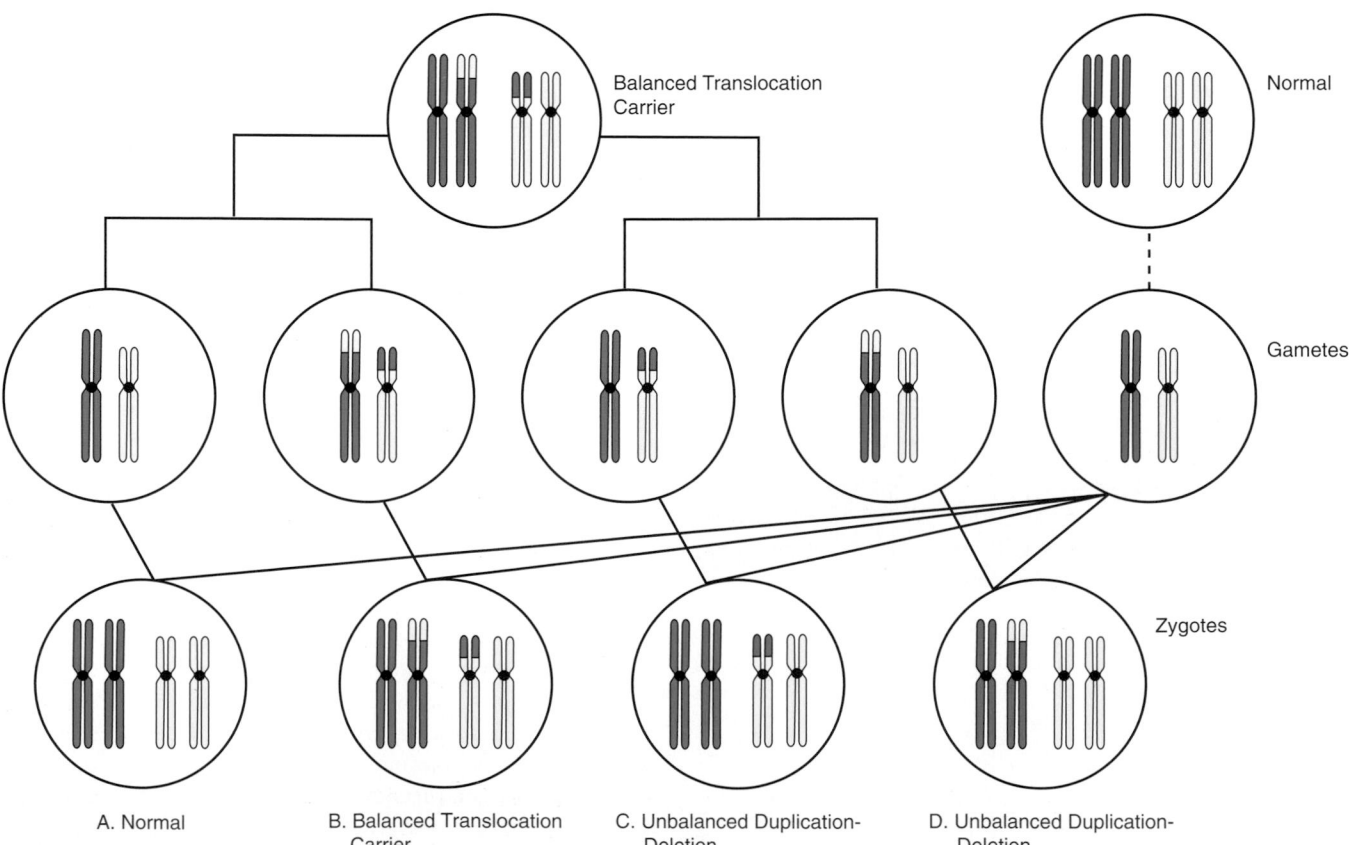

FIGURE 6-5 Gametes produced by a balanced translocation carrier. *(From Cunningham, 2010c.)*

Conversely, an abortus with a normal karyotype might suggest an alternative cause and imply the need for earlier evaluation.

Opponents of such routine karyotyping cite its high cost and possibility of misleading results. This is particularly true if the abnormal cells are derived from a pregnancy with placental mosaicism. Moreover, detection of a 46, XX karyotype may simply reflect contamination with maternal tissues.

In sum, karyotyping of products of conception may not accurately reflect fetal karyotype. Because of the expense and limited information provided, we do not recommend this practice.

Sperm DNA Testing

Increasing attention has been directed to sperm DNA damage and to the presence of reactive oxygen species as an infertility cause. These are discussed further in Chapter 19 (p. 524). It seems reasonable to predict that these abnormalities may also contribute to recurrent pregnancy loss. Carrell and colleagues (2003) have reported a significantly higher rate of both aneuploidy and apoptosis in sperm from the male partner in women with unexplained recurrent miscarriage. Other studies have not supported this finding (Bellver, 2010b). Assays for DNA integrity are not currently integral to recurrent miscarriage evaluation.

Treatment

After thorough genetic counseling, couples with an abnormal karyotype can usually be managed with IVF followed by preimplantation genetic diagnosis (PGD). These techniques are described further in Chapter 20 (p. 548). In one retrospective study of couples with known translocations, PGD was found to increase the rate of successful pregnancy and decrease the length of time to conception (Fischer, 2010). Even so, the prognosis is generally good without intervention for couples with a balanced translocation. Franssen and colleagues (2006) compared two couple cohorts who had experienced at least two miscarriages. There were 278 couples with a balanced translocation and 427 noncarrier couples. In both groups, 85 percent of couples had a healthy child, although the risk for miscarriage was higher in the carrier couples.

Some have recommended that PGD screening be done even in couples with normal karyotypes who have idiopathic recurrent pregnancy loss. This is because of a higher rate of aneuploidy in embryos from women with a history of recurrent miscarriage compared with controls. Results from a large prospective cohort trial, however, found no support for this practice (Platteau, 2005). At this time, the American Society for Reproductive Medicine (2008) does not recommend PGD in couples who are chromosomally normal.

Anatomic Factors

A number of uterine abnormalities have been associated with adverse reproductive outcomes. Although these usually do not affect fertility, some of these anomalies can cause recurrent miscarriage and later pregnancy complications (Reichman, 2010). According to Devi Wold and colleagues (2006), 15 percent of women with three or more consecutive miscarriages will be found to have an acquired or congenital uterine anomaly.

Acquired Abnormalities

Uterine Causes. Pregnancy loss is increased with some acquired uterine abnormalities that include intrauterine synechiae, leiomyoma, and endometrial polyps. Of these, *uterine synechiae*—collectively known as *Asherman syndrome*—usually result from destruction of large areas of endometrium by curettage or ablative procedures. Diagnosis is by hysterosalpingography or saline infusion sonography (Fig. 2-20, p. 45 and Fig. 19-6, p. 517). Katz and colleagues (1996) reviewed 90 women with uterine synechiae who had two or more prior miscarriages. They reported that adhesiolysis decreased the miscarriage rate from 79 to 22 percent, and successful term pregnancies increased from 18 to 69 percent. Other studies have reported similar outcomes with prognosis correlating with disease severity (Al-Inany, 2001; Goldenberg, 1995). Directed hysteroscopic lysis of adhesions is preferable to curettage as discussed and illustrated in Section 42-21 of the atlas (p. 1178).

Uterine leiomyomas are found in a large proportion of adult women and can cause miscarriage, especially if located near the placental implantation site. Of interest, although intramural leiomyomas can alter the expression pattern of a number of endometrial genes, they do not affect expression of genes known to be involved in implantation (Horcajadas, 2008). Common sense suggests that detrimental effects should be greater for submucous compared with intramural leiomyomas, and for large versus small tumors. However, conclusive data are lacking. In a study of women undergoing IVF, pregnancy outcomes were adversely affected by submucous leiomyomas, but not by those that were subserosal or intramural and less than 5 to 7 cm (Jun, 2001; Ramzy, 1998). In contrast, meta-analysis found increased adverse pregnancy outcomes—including miscarriage—following IVF in women with intramural myomas that did not distort the cavity (Sunkara, 2010).

Currently, most agree that consideration be given to excision of submucosal and intracavitary leiomyomas in women with recurrent miscarriage, as discussed in Chapter 9 (p. 251). Ironically, Homer and Saridogan (2010) reviewed outcomes in 227 women after uterine artery embolization for these tumors and found that their risk for miscarriage was *increased*.

Cervical Incompetence. *Incompetent cervix* is a discrete obstetric entity that does not cause first-trimester miscarriage but is associated with an increased risk for second-trimester losses. It usually is manifest by delivery following painless cervical dilatation after 16 to 18 weeks' gestation. Cervical insufficiency may occur following surgical or birth trauma and has also been associated with a molecular defect in collagen synthesis (Dukhovny, 2009). Cervical incompetence is often treated surgically with cervical cerclage placement. Interested readers are referred to Chapter 9 of *Williams Obstetrics*, 23rd edition (Cunningham, 2010a).

Developmental Malformations

Abnormal müllerian duct formation or fusion resulting in congenital uterine anomalies is relatively common. Depending on their variations of anatomy, some may cause increased risks for early miscarriage, whereas others may cause later fetal loss or preterm delivery. Unicornuate, bicornuate, and septate uteri are all associated with increased early miscarriages as well as second-trimester abortions and preterm labor (American College of Obstetricians and Gynecologists, 2008; Reichman, 2010).

Cited prevalence rates for müllerian anomalies vary widely in general populations as well as in women with recurrent miscarriage. This is likely due to differences in the extent of evaluations and the criteria set to define normalcy. Nahum (1998) reviewed 47 studies with more than 573,000 women screened for müllerian uterine malformations. The observed incidence was 1 in 600 in fertile women and 1 in 30 in infertile women for an overall incidence of 1 in 200. The distribution of anomalies and associated loss rates are shown in Table 6-6.

Developmental uterine anomalies are more common in women who have had recurrent pregnancy losses. Salim and colleagues (2003) described nearly 2500 women using 3-dimensional sonography. Anomalies were identified in 24 percent of women with recurrent miscarriage, but in only 5 percent of controls. In a metaanalysis of publications from 1950 to 2007, Saravelos and colleagues (2008) concluded that uterine anomalies are present in approximately 17 percent of patients with recurrent pregnancy loss, 7.3 percent of infertile women, and 6.7 percent of women in the general population.

It has proven difficult to demonstrate that correction of uterine anomalies improves early pregnancy outcome (American College of Obstetricians and Gynecologists, 2008). In one observational study, pregnancy outcomes were reviewed following hysteroscopic metroplasty in 59 women who had a septate uterus and more than two prior miscarriages (Saygili-Yilmaz, 2003). The miscarriage rate decreased from 96 to 10 percent following surgery, and term pregnancies increased from none to 70 percent. In another study from this group, hysteroscopic resection was reported to decrease the incidence of miscarriage from 65 to 15 percent (Saygili-Yilmaz, 2002). Based on these reports and the relative safety of surgical correction, most experts recommend

hysteroscopic resection of a uterine septum in women with recurrent miscarriage, as described in Section 42-19 (p. 1174).

In contrast, surgical repair of a bicornuate uterus requires laparotomy and full-thickness incision of the uterine wall with subsequent risk for uterine dehiscence (Fig. 18-19, p. 500). In these women, surgery is generally not recommended except for women who have had a very high number of pregnancy losses. Additional discussion regarding the incidence, clinical impact, and treatment of congenital anatomic abnormalities can be found in Chapter 18 (p. 481).

Immunologic Factors

Much attention has focused on the immune system playing an important role in recurrent pregnancy loss. Yetman and Kutteh (1996) estimated that 15 percent of more than 1000 women with recurrent miscarriages had recognized immunologic factors. Two primary pathophysiologic models are the *autoimmune theory*—immunity against "self," and the *alloimmune theory*—immunity against antigens from another person.

Autoimmune Factors
Antiphospholipid Antibodies. It had been appreciated that pregnancy wastage is increased in women with systemic lupus erythematosus (Clowse, 2008; Warren, 2004). Subsequently, many women with lupus were identified to have antiphospholipid antibodies—a family of autoantibodies directed against phospholipid-binding plasma proteins (Erkan, 2011). The American College of Obstetricians and Gynecologists (2011a) has reviewed available studies and concludes that positive test results for antiphospholipid antibodies occur in a higher proportion of women with recurrent spontaneous pregnancy loss than in controls. Between 5 and 15 percent of women with recurrent pregnancy loss have clinically significant antibodies compared with only 2 to 5 percent of pregnant controls (Branch, 2010).

When antiphospholipid antibodies are found in conjunction with certain clinical findings, then it is termed the *antiphospholipid antibody syndrome (APS)*. Criteria for the diagnosis of the antiphospholipid antibody syndrome are shown in Table 6-7. These were revised in 2006 by international consensus and have been adopted by the American College of Obstetricians and Gynecologists (2011a). Positive tests are repeated at a minimum of 12 weeks with strict requirements for acceptable laboratory methods and interpretation (Miyakis, 2006). This is the only autoimmune disorder that has been clearly linked to pregnancy wastage. APS can cause recurrent miscarriage, but most cases occur after 10 weeks and are commonly associated with fetal death, preterm delivery, early-onset preeclampsia, and fetal-growth restriction from placental insufficiency and placental thromboses (Clark, 2007a,b).

The mechanisms by which antiphospholipid antibodies result in miscarriage are unclear but can be divided into three general categories—thrombosis, inflammation, and abnormal placentation (Meroni, 2010). *Thrombosis* was initially thought to be due to inhibition of prostacyclin secretion by the vascular endothelium and stimulation of thromboxane A production by platelets. These actions result in vasoconstriction and

TABLE 6-6. Estimated Prevalence of Some Congenital Uterine Malformations and Their Associated Pregnancy Loss Rate

Uterine Anomaly[a]	Proportion (Percent)	SAB Rate (Percent)[b]
Bicornuate	39	40–70
Septate or unicornuate	14–24	34–88
Didelphys	11	40
Arcuate	7	
Hypo- or aplastic	4	

[a]Estimated overall prevalence 1:200 women (Nahum, 1998).
[b]Includes first- and second-trimester losses.
Data from Buttram, 1979; Nahum, 1998; Reddy, 2007; Valli, 2001.

TABLE 6-7. Clinical and Laboratory Criteria for Diagnosis of Antiphospholipid Antibody Syndrome[a]

Clinical Criteria

Obstetric:

One or more unexplained deaths of a morphologically normal fetus at or beyond 10 weeks,

or

Severe preeclampsia or placental insufficiency necessitating delivery before 34 weeks,

or

Three or more unexplained consecutive spontaneous abortions before 10 weeks

Vascular: One or more episodes of arterial, venous, or small vessel thrombosis in any tissue or organ

Laboratory Criteria[b]

Presence of lupus anticoagulant according to guidelines of the International Society on Thrombosis and Hemostasis,

or

Medium or high serum levels of IgG or IgM anticardiolipin antibodies,

or

Anti-β2 glycoprotein-I IgG or IgM antibody

[a]At least one clinical and one laboratory criteria must be present for diagnosis.
[b]These tests must be positive on two or more occasions at least 12 weeks apart.
IgG = immunoglobulin G; IgM = immunoglobulin M.
Modified from Branch, 2010; Erkan, 2011; Miyakis, 2006.

increased in platelet aggregation. More recently, it has been proposed that antiphospholipid antibodies act on trophoblast and endothelial surfaces to inhibit the function of annexin A5, a natural anticoagulant that prevents the activation of factor X and prothrombin (Rand, 2010). Antiphospholipid antibodies may also activate complement to intensify hypercoagulability, which leads to recurrent placental thromboses. *Acute local inflammatory responses* at the placental-maternal interface may also be induced by antiphospholipid antibodies. Finally, *placentation* may be directly affected by these antibodies through impaired decidual expression of integrins and cadherins. This can lead to inhibition of placental proliferation and of syncytial development. This is of particular interest because defective decidual trophoblast invasion—not placental thrombosis—is the most common histologic abnormality identified in APS-related early pregnancy loss (Di Simone, 2007).

Other Autoantibodies. A number of other *antilipid antibody idiotypes* have been described (Bick, 2006). Their measurement is expensive, frequently poorly controlled, and of uncertain relevance in the evaluation of recurrent miscarriage. Results are likewise inconclusive regarding testing for other antibodies including *rheumatoid factor, antinuclear antibodies,* and *antithyroid antibodies.* These latter antibodies are discussed further on page 173. In women with *celiac disease,* an autoimmune disorder due to gluten intolerance, a number of autoantibodies may be found, but their significance to cause miscarriage is unknown. Women with celiac disease are reported to have an increased incidence of pregnancy loss as well as delayed menarche, early menopause, infertility, and fetal-growth restriction (Soni, 2010). Finally, although a polymorphism in the *plasminogen activator inhibitor-1 (PAI-1) gene* reportedly predisposes to miscarriage, other reports have not confirmed this link (Ciacci, 2009; Goodman, 2009).

Treatment of Antiphospholipid Antibody Syndrome. Because of difficulties in its recognition, therapeutic guidelines for APS in women with recurrent miscarriage have been in flux for many years. This is because various treatment regimens were used in studies with variable inclusion criteria, and very few included a placebo arm. A number of studies have compared single-agent or combination therapies using unfractionated heparin, low-molecular-weight heparin, low-dose aspirin, glucocorticoids, or intravenous immunoglobulin (IVIG). As emphasized by Branch and Khamashta (2003), the discrepant reports are confusing, and therapeutic guidelines are blurred.

Many use therapeutic guidelines based on individual indications. For example, treatment during pregnancy is influenced greatly in women with APS who had a previously documented thromboembolism. Other indications include those with APS and a history of recurrent miscarriage, fetal-growth restriction, fetal death, or early-onset preeclampsia, especially if accompanied by HELLP (hemolysis, elevated liver enzyme levels, low platelet count) syndrome (Soh, 2010). For a detailed discussion regarding prophylactic anticoagulation therapy for later-pregnancy and postpartum complications, the reader is referred to Chapter 54 in *Williams Obstetrics*, 23rd edition (Cunningham, 2010b).

Because of the paucity of placebo-controlled trials, attention has been given to heparin and/or aspirin regimens. Ziakas and colleagues (2010) performed a systematic review and meta-analysis of regimens used for treatment of women with APS and recurrent fetal loss (Fig. 6-6). They concluded that the combination of unfractionated heparin and low-dose aspirin significantly benefitted pregnancy outcome in those with first-trimester pregnancy losses. There was no improvement with low-molecular-weight heparin (LMWH) and aspirin combinations. Similar conclusions were reached in a Cochrane Database Review through 2009 (Empson, 2010). The use of LMWH

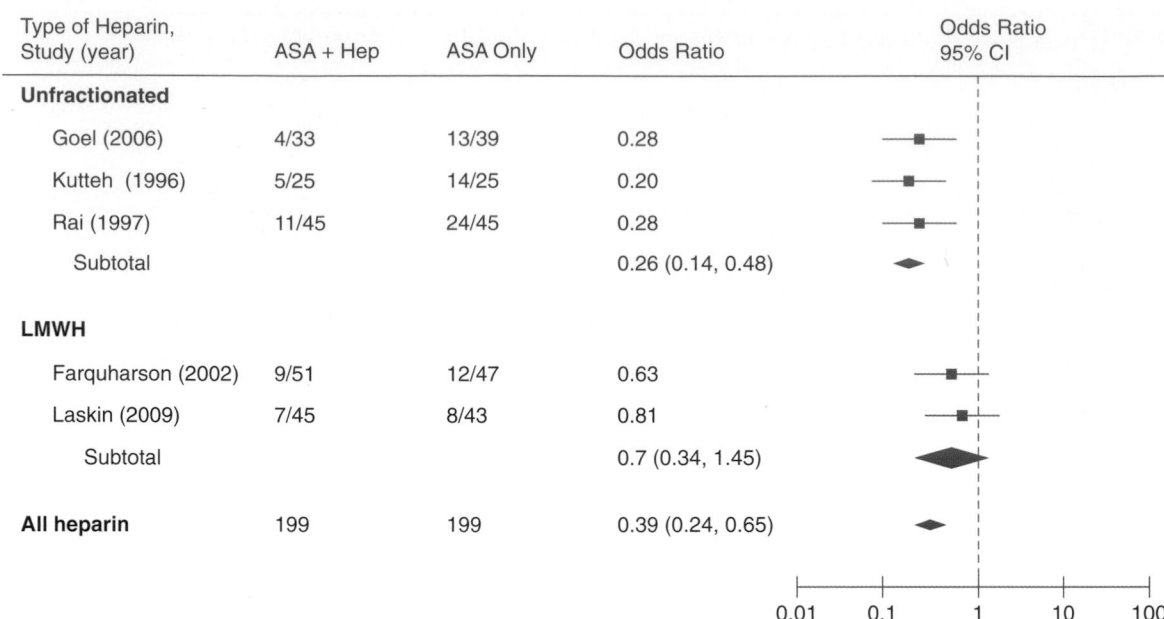

Type of Heparin, Study (year)	ASA + Hep	ASA Only	Odds Ratio	Odds Ratio 95% CI
Unfractionated				
Goel (2006)	4/33	13/39	0.28	
Kutteh (1996)	5/25	14/25	0.20	
Rai (1997)	11/45	24/45	0.28	
Subtotal			0.26 (0.14, 0.48)	
LMWH				
Farquharson (2002)	9/51	12/47	0.63	
Laskin (2009)	7/45	8/43	0.81	
Subtotal			0.7 (0.34, 1.45)	
All heparin	199	199	0.39 (0.24, 0.65)	

FIGURE 6-6 Results of heparin and aspirin given alone or in combination for prevention of first-trimester pregnancy loss in women with antiphospholipid antibody syndrome. ASA = aspirin; CI = confidence interval; Hep = heparin. *(Data from studies cited above and total compilation from Ziakas, 2010.)*

plus aspirin is appealing based on its ease of use and improved safety profile. Until the issue is settled, however, unfractionated heparin is recommended. It may be more effective due to direct inhibition of antiphospholipid antibody binding as well as anticoagulation effects (Franklin, 2003).

Our protocol for treatment of women with APS and recurrent pregnancy loss is similar to that recommended by the American College of Obstetricians and Gynecologists (2011a). Low-dose aspirin—81 mg orally per day—is given along with unfractionated heparin—5000 to 10,000 units subcutaneously daily. Therapy is begun when pregnancy is diagnosed, and it is continued until delivery. Extending treatment for 6 weeks postpartum is considered if there is no history of thrombosis, but definitely recommended for those with a history of thromboembolic events.

Alloimmune Factors

A current and attractive theory suggests that normal pregnancy requires the expression of blocking factors that prevent maternal rejection of paternally derived foreign fetal antigens. The pregnant woman ostensibly will not produce these blocking factors if she shares human leukocyte antigens (HLAs) with the father. Other alloimmune disorders that have been posited to cause recurrent miscarriage include altered natural killer (NK) cell activity and increased lymphocytotoxic antibodies. Berger and associates (2010) found that women with haplotypes caused by various mutations of the HLA-G gene more commonly had recurrent miscarriages compared with normal haplotypes.

Various tests and treatment options have been developed to address this issue. None of these has withstood rigorous scrutiny, and we agree with Reddy (2007) that they are currently considered investigational. Proposed therapies include paternal or third-party leukocyte immunization and IVIG in an attempt to correct the dysregulated response to fetal antigens. Three randomized clinical trials failed to demonstrate any benefit of IVIG or placebo in patients with idiopathic miscarriage (Stephenson, 2010). The American Society for Reproductive Medicine (2006) concluded that IVIG treatment was not effective for recurrent pregnancy loss. Reviews also conclude this to be the case (Ata, 2011; Porter, 2006). Because these treatments have not been adequately tested and are also potentially harmful, we agree with Scott (2003) and others that immunotherapy cannot be recommended at this time.

Empiric Treatment for Unexplained Recurrent Miscarriage

Investigators who conducted some of the early observational studies described similarities between women with recurrent miscarriage ostensibly linked to antiphospholipid antibodies and thrombophilias with women who had otherwise unexplained recurrent pregnancy loss. Because of this, empiric therapy was championed using heparin or aspirin, either alone or in combination. Studies designed to test these regimens were inconclusive because of small numbers (Dolitzky, 2006; Kaandorp, 2009; Rodger, 2008). Subsequently, Kaandorp and colleagues (2010) performed a randomized trial that included 364 Dutch women with at least two unexplained miscarriages. Inclusion criteria included a normal karyotype, no uterine malformations seen with pelvic sonography, no evidence for antiphospholipid antibody syndrome, and a live fetus documented by sonography beginning at 6 weeks' gestation. The women were randomly assigned to be given nadroparin, which is a low-molecular-weight heparin, along with 80 mg of aspirin; aspirin alone; or placebo. As shown in Table 6-8, approximately 65 percent of the entire cohort delivered a live-born infant.

TABLE 6-8. Selected Pregnancy Outcomes from a Randomized Trial of Three Treatment Regimens for Recurrent Miscarriage[a]

| | Treatment Regimen Outcomes (Percent) | | | |
Outcome	Heparin + Aspirin (n=123)	Aspirin (n=120)	Placebo (n=121)	*p* Value
Achieved pregnancy	79	83	85	NS
Live birth	69	62	67	0.52
Miscarriage	22	31	26	0.29
Preeclampsia	2.9	1.6	1.4	0.84
BW <10th percentile	8.7	11.5	7.17	0.69
Preterm delivery	10.1	1.6	4.3	0.11
Congenital malformations	4.3	8.2	2.9	0.39

[a]Parents had normal karyotyping results, and the women included had no uterine malformations noted by sonography, they were antiphospholipid-antibody negative, and a live fetus was documented by sonography beginning at 6 weeks' gestation. No significant differences were noted among the three groups when stratified into ≥24 to <28 wk, ≥28 to <32 wk, and ≥32 to <37 wk groups.
BW = birthweight; NS = not stated.
Data from Kaandorp, 2010.

Importantly, there were no significant differences in pertinent perinatal outcomes—including spontaneous miscarriages—between the three groups. These results clearly argue against the use of these empiric treatments for women with unexplained pregnancy loss.

■ Endocrinologic Factors

Studies evaluating the relationship between recurrent abortion and various endocrinologic abnormalities are inconsistent and have generally been underpowered (American College of Obstetricians and Gynecologists, 2008). According to Arredondo and Noble (2006), 8 to 12 percent of recurrent miscarriages are the result of endocrine factors discussed in the following sections.

Luteal Phase Defect (LPD)

Inadequate development of the endometrium at the time of implantation is termed *luteal phase defect (LPD)*. It is controversial as a cause of miscarriage (Bukulmez, 2004). LPD is generally attributed to insufficient progesterone secretion by the corpus luteum. This may be caused by endocrine dysfunction that prevents normal folliculogenesis and luteal function. These disorders include hyperprolactinemia, thyroid disorders, and polycystic ovarian syndrome.

The gold standard test for LPD is histologic evaluation of a midluteal endometrial biopsy specimen. LPD is diagnosed when histologic dating of the endometrium lags behind menstrual dates by at least 2 days. The formal diagnosis also requires that

two biopsies be out of phase. Unfortunately, such evaluation is invasive and hampered by substantial inter- and intraobserver interpretation variability. More recently, investigators have begun to characterize endometrial markers that are expressed in the periimplantation period. One marker that has been studied is $\alpha v\beta 3$ integrin. At this time, the clinical utility of evaluating for this protein and other markers remains to be proven.

Some suggest that LPD can be diagnosed if the midluteal serum progesterone level is <10 ng/mL. This is unlikely. First, serum progesterone concentrations are highly variable with normal pregnancies. Second, deficient progesterone production may be the consequence rather than the cause of early pregnancy failure (Salem, 1984). Additionally, as many as half of women with histologically defined LPD have a normal serum progesterone level. Progesterone early in pregnancy is secreted by both the corpus luteum and the trophoblast, thus complicating interpretation of the results. Finally, a number of studies have found that serum progesterone measurements are not closely correlated with other markers of endometrial function (Branch, 2010). It may be that determination of endometrial tissue progesterone concentrations will improve the study of LPD. However, at this time, these are not readily available.

Treatment for presumed LPD has included progesterone supplementation, hCG administration to enhance corpus luteum function, or ovulation induction with agents such as clomiphene citrate to generate additional corpora lutea. After their review, Haas and Ramsey (2008) concluded that progesterone treatment during early to midpregnancy does not decrease the risks for miscarriage. Identification and treatment for LPD obviously requires more rigorous evaluation (American College of Obstetricians and Gynecologists, 2008). Although progesterone replacement is controversial for LPD, it is clearly indicated until 8 to 10 weeks in women who have had a corpus luteum removed surgically, such as for an ovarian tumor (p. 173).

Polycystic Ovarian Syndrome (PCOS)

Women with polycystic ovaries have been generally considered to be at an increased risk for miscarriage. However, this association has recently been questioned. There are no reliable data regarding the relative frequency of PCOS in women with recurrent miscarriage compared with normal women. In one study of women with recurrent miscarriage, 8 to 10 percent were identified to have PCOS using the Rotterdam criteria (Chap. 17, p. 460). This frequency of PCOS is similar to that of the general female adult population (Cocksedge, 2009).

A number of mechanisms have been proposed to explain the potential link between PCOS and miscarriage. Current explanations center on the effects on ovarian function caused by elevated serum levels of luteinizing hormone (LH), androgens, or insulin, which are found with PCOS. LH excess may promote infertility by several mechanisms. For example, endometrial LH receptors may be overstimulated by elevated serum LH levels to directly impair implantation. Another possibility is that chronically elevated LH levels adversely affect oocyte development (Homburg, 1998; Watson, 1993). A third mechanism is based on observations that LH induces intraovarian androgen levels, which are known to cause follicular atresia and poor oocyte development (Stanger, 1985; Tulppala, 1993). Thus, if elevated serum LH concentrations indeed cause miscarriage, then its inhibition during a gonadotropin ovulation-induction cycle might decrease the risks for miscarriage. This approach, however, did not improve pregnancy outcome in the controlled trial by Clifford (1996).

Data implicating hyperinsulinemia in pregnancy loss are somewhat stronger. Insulin modulates insulin-like growth factor actions in the ovary, thereby affecting ovarian function. In a retrospective study, pregnancy outcomes were compared in women with PCOS before and after metformin treatment (Glueck, 2002). Metformin (Glucophage) lowers hepatic glucose production and increases insulin sensitivity and thereby lowers insulin levels. These investigators reported that miscarriage rates decreased from 62 to 26 percent when metformin treatment was begun either before or during pregnancy. In a case-control study of 137 infertile women, metformin treatment during pregnancy resulted in decreased risks for miscarriage (Nawaz, 2010). In contrast, however, a systematic review of randomized controlled trials found that there was no improvement in abortion risk with metformin treatment (Palomba, 2009). At this time, routine metformin treatment for women with PCOS solely to treat pregnancy loss, particularly in the absence of insulin resistance, is not recommended.

Diabetes Mellitus

Spontaneous abortion and major congenital malformation rates are both increased in women with insulin-dependent diabetes (Greene, 1999). These risks are clearly related to the degree of metabolic control around the time of conception and in early pregnancy. Importantly, this risk is substantively mitigated with optimal metabolic control. In fact, Mills and colleagues (1988) observed that the miscarriage rate in women with excellent control is similar to that of nondiabetic women. Although diabetes itself is a recognized cause of recurrent miscarriage, diabetic women with recurrent loss may also have levels of insulin resistance greater than diabetic women without miscarriages (Craig, 2002). The causes for this may be similar to those just discussed for women with polycystic ovarian syndrome.

Hypothyroidism

As discussed on page 173, autoimmune thyroid disorders are common in young women. In some of these, antithyroid antibodies are associated with hypothyroidism. But in many, they are indicative of thyroid failure later in life. Both severe iodine deficiency or overt hypothyroidism cause subfertility and increased risk for miscarriage, but effects of subclinical hypothyroidism are less clear. Any effects of thyroid hormone deficiency as a cause of recurrent pregnancy loss have not been studied (Abramson, 2001; Rushworth, 2000). Although obtaining thyroid function tests in symptomatic women is indicated, routine screening for all women with recurrent pregnancy loss is controversial (American College of Obstetricians and Gynecologists, 2008).

Infections

As discussed on page 172, very few infections are firmly associated with early pregnancy loss. It is even less likely that infections would cause recurrent miscarriage because most are sporadic or they stimulate protective maternal antibodies. Routine screening for infection in asymptomatic women is not recommended, nor is empiric antimicrobial therapy (Branch, 2010).

Evaluation and Treatment

Some considerations for evaluation and management of women with recurrent miscarriage are outlined in Table 6-9. Timing and extent of evaluation should be based on maternal age, coexistent infertility, symptoms, and the level of patient anxiety. In our view, after a thorough history and clinical examination, a modicum of testing is done that is directed at likely causes. General testing may include parental karyotyping, uterine cavity evaluation, and testing for antiphospholipid antibody syndrome. There is progressively less support for screening for endocrinologic disorders or thrombophilias. Treatment should always be balanced between the potential morbidity and the strength of the data suggesting likely benefit.

In perhaps half of couples with recurrent miscarriage, a putative cause will emerge. But even for those with no explanatory findings, there can be cautious assurance that the chances of successfully achieving a live birth are reasonably good (Branch, 2010; Reddy, 2007). The results shown previously in Tables 6-4 and 6-5—while age dependent—forecast a reasonable prognosis for a successful subsequent pregnancy even after five recurrent pregnancy losses. Although these couples are anxious to try any treatment, the lack of definitive benefits for many of these should be carefully considered and appropriate counseling offered.

TABLE 6-9. Tests Used for Evaluation of Couples with Recurrent Pregnancy Loss

Etiology	Diagnostic Evaluation	Possible Therapies
Genetic[a]	Karyotype partners	Genetic counseling, donor gametes
Anatomic[a]	Sonohysterography Hysterosalpingogram MR imaging	Septum transection, myomectomy, or adhesiolysis
Immunologic[a]	Lupus anticoagulant Anticardiolipin antibodies Anti-β2 glycoprotein-I antibody	Heparin + aspirin
Endocrinologic[b]	Midluteal progesterone TSH Prolactin Fasting glucose, Hgb A$_{1c}$ Day 3 FSH, estradiol	Progesterone Levothyroxine Dopamine agonist Metformin Counseling
Thrombophilic[b]	Antithrombin deficiency Protein C or S deficiency Factor V Leiden mutation Prothrombin mutation Hyperhomocysteinemia	No proven treatment Folic acid
Toxic	Tobacco, alcohol use Exposure to toxins, chemicals	Eliminate consumption Behavior modification

[a]Testing for these disorders is generally supported by the literature and expert opinion. One or a combination of these tests may be required.
[b]Ongoing controversy regarding testing.
FSH = follicle-stimulating hormone; MR = magnetic resonance; TSH = thyroid-stimulating hormone.
Modified from Kutteh, 2005; Reddy, 2007; and Speroff, 2005.

INDUCED ABORTION

Definitions and Incidence

The term *induced abortion* is defined as the medical or surgical termination of pregnancy before the time of fetal viability. Definitions to describe the incidence include the *abortion ratio,* which is the number of abortions per 1000 live births, and the *abortion rate,* which is the number of these per 1000 women aged 15 to 44 years.

In the United States, abortion statistics may suffer from underreporting. One reason is because clinics inconsistently report medically induced abortions. For example, 827,609 elective abortions were reported to the CDC (2011a) in 2007. In contrast, the Guttmacher Institute (2011) reported that 1.2 million procedures were performed annually from 2005 through 2008.

According to the CDC (2011a), women aged 20 to 29 years accounted for 57 percent of abortions, although the abortion ratios were highest at both extremes of reproductive ages. In 2007, black women had an abortion ratio of 455 compared with 158 per 1000 live births for white women. Procedures were performed during the first 8 weeks in 62 percent of all women, another 29 percent during 9 to 13 weeks, and only 5 percent were done at ≥16 weeks' gestation.

Classification of Induced Abortion

Abortions are performed for various indications that include social, economic, or emotional reasons. Technically, there are no further formal categorizations of induced abortion, but many choose to define them: (1) as indicated or therapeutic or (2) as elective or voluntary.

Therapeutic Abortion

Some medical and surgical disorders that may provide a maternal-health indication for pregnancy termination include recalcitrant cardiac decompensation, pulmonary arterial hypertension, advanced hypertensive vascular disease, diabetes with end-stage organ failure, and some malignancies. Also, many abortions are performed to prevent birth of a fetus with a significant anatomic or mental deformity. The seriousness of fetal deformities is wide ranging, is subjectively variable, and in many cases defies social, legal, or political classification. Finally, in cases of rape or incest, most consider termination indicated.

Elective Abortion

This is usually defined as interruption of pregnancy before fetal viability at patient request for reasons unrelated to maternal or fetal health. These procedures comprise most abortions done today, and approximately one pregnancy is electively terminated for every four live births in the United States (Ventura, 2008). At this rate, Jones and Kavanaugh (2011) estimate that 30 percent of American women will have at least one abortion by age 45. Thus, it is one of the most commonly performed medical procedures (Guttmacher Institute, 2008). The Executive Board of the American College of Obstetricians and Gynecologists (2010c) supports the legal right of women to obtain an abortion prior to fetal viability and considers this a medical matter between a woman and her physician. The Board reaffirmed this opinion in 2010 and emphasized the priority of women's rights to reproductive health-care services over the physician's right to conscientiously refuse to provide such care.

Abortion in the United States

Prior to 1973, abortion was legal in 17 states in this country, however, the process to obtain the procedure varied. This changed in 1973 when the legality of elective abortion was established by the United States Supreme Court in the case of *Roe v. Wade*. The Court defined the extent to which states might regulate abortion:

1. For the stage prior to approximately the end of the first trimester, the abortion decision and the procedure must be left to the medical judgment of the attending physician.
2. For the stage subsequent to approximately the end of the first trimester, the State, in promoting its interest in the health of the mother, may, if it chooses, regulate abortion procedures in ways that are reasonably related to maternal health.
3. For the stage subsequent to viability, the State, in promoting its interest in the potential of human life, if it chooses, may regulate, and even proscribe abortion, except where necessary, in appropriate medical judgment, for the preservation of the life or health of the mother.

Since the 1973 *Roe v. Wade* decision, several other legal decisions merit citation. In 1976, the Congress passed the *Hyde Amendment,* which forbids use of federal funds to provide abortion services except in case of rape, incest, or life-threatening circumstances. In 1992, the Supreme Court reviewed *Planned Parenthood v. Casey* and upheld the fundamental right to abortion, but established that regulations before viability are constitutional as long as they do not impose an "undue burden" on the woman. This decision led to individual state restrictions that limit access to abortion services. Many states have passed legislation that impose counseling requirements, waiting periods, parental consent or notification for minors, facility requirements, funding restrictions, and restrictions on providers allowed to perform the procedures. Another choice-limiting decision was the 2007 Supreme Court decision in which it reviewed *Gonzales v. Carhart* and upheld its Partial-Birth Abortion Ban Act of 2003. This is problematic because there is no medically approved definition of partial-birth abortion according to the Executive Board of The American College of Obstetricians and Gynecologists (2007). The Board goes on to state: "The intervention of legislative bodies into medical decision making is inappropriate, ill advised, and dangerous."

Counseling Before Elective Abortion

There are three basic choices available to a woman considering an abortion: (1) continued pregnancy with its risks and parental responsibilities; (2) continued pregnancy with its risks and responsibilities of arranged adoption; or (3) the choice of abortion with its risks. Knowledgeable and compassionate counselors should objectively describe and provide information regarding these choices so that a woman or couple can make an informed decision (Baker, 2009).

Residency Training in Abortion Techniques

Because of its inherent controversial aspects, abortion training for residents has been both championed and assailed. Among other organizations, the American College of Obstetricians and Gynecologists (2009a) supports abortion training. In 1996, the Accreditation Council for Graduate Medical Education mandated that Obstetrics and Gynecology residency education must include access to experience with induced abortion. In 1999, the *Kenneth J. Ryan Residency Training Program* was established at the University of California at San Francisco to work with residency programs to improve training in abortion and contraception. By 2010, 59 Ryan programs had been started in 28 states and in Canada. These programs provide comprehensive didactics and evidence-based, opt-out clinical training in all methods of medical and surgical uterine evacuation as well as in contraceptive methodology. Other programs, including the one at Parkland Hospital, are less codified, but teach residents technical aspects by management of early missed abortions as well as pregnancy interruption for fetal death, severe fetal anomalies, and life-threatening maternal medical or surgical disorders. Freedman (2010) emphasizes that considerations for abortion training should include social, moral, and ethical aspects.

The American College of Obstetricians and Gynecologists (2010c) respects the need and responsibility of health-care providers to determine their individual positions on induced abortion. It also emphasizes the need to provide standard-of-care counseling and timely referral if providers have individual beliefs that preclude pregnancy termination. At minimum, we agree with Steinauer and colleagues (2005a,b) that any physician trained to care for women must be familiar with various abortion techniques so that complications can be managed or referrals made for suitable care.

Fellowship Training

Programs have been designed for postresidency training in abortion and contraceptive techniques. Formal fellowships in Family Planning are 2-year postgraduate programs that by 2010 were located in 22 departments of obstetrics and gynecology at academic centers across the country. Training includes methods of high-level research and clinical management in all methods of pregnancy prevention and termination.

Techniques for Early Abortion

In the absence of serious maternal medical disorders, abortion procedures do not require hospitalization. With outpatient abortion, capabilities for cardiopulmonary resuscitation and for immediate transfer to a hospital must be available.

TABLE 6-10. Some Techniques Used for First- and Second-Trimester Abortion[a]

Technique	First Trimester	Second Trimester
Surgical	Dilatation and curettage Vacuum aspiration Menstrual aspiration	Dilatation and evacuation (D&E) Dilatation and extraction (D&X) Laparotomy Hysterotomy Hysterectomy

Medical	Prostaglandins E_2, $F_{2\alpha}$, E_1, and analogs
	  Vaginal insertion
	  Parenteral injection
	  Oral ingestion
	Antiprogesterones—RU 486 (mifepristone)
	  and epostane
	Methotrexate—intramuscular and oral
	Various combinations of the above
		Intravenous oxytocin
		Intraamnionic hyperosmotic fluid
		  20-percent saline
		  30-percent urea
		Prostaglandins E_2, $F_{2\alpha}$, E_1, and analogs
		  Intraamnionic injection
		  Extraovular injection[b]
		  Vaginal insertion
		  Parenteral injection
		  Oral ingestion

[a]All procedures are aided by pretreatment using hygroscopic cervical dilators.
[b]Extraovular refers to the potential space between the chorioamnion and decidua.

First- or second-trimester abortion can be performed either medically or surgically by a number of methods that are listed in Table 6-10. Distinctive features of each technique were reviewed by the American College of Obstetricians and Gynecologists (2009c). Results with either surgical or medical methods are comparable with those for spontaneous miscarriage as previously shown in Table 6-3 and now summarized. Both have a high success rate—95 percent with medical and 99 percent with surgical techniques. With medical therapy, surgery is usually avoided as is the need for sedation. However, medical abortion is more time consuming and does not have a predictable outcome. In extreme cases, medical abortion may not be completed for days to a few weeks. Bleeding with medical therapy is usually heavier and unpredictable, and hemorrhage and incomplete abortion are more common with medical versus surgical abortion (Niinimäki, 2009; Robson, 2009). Despite this, medical terminations have lower average costs. Finally, more women who underwent surgical termination had a positive attitude about the procedure compared with those who had a medical abortion.

Techniques for Surgical Abortion

In most cases, preoperative cervical ripening is associated with less pain, a technically easier procedure, and a shorter operative time than if the cervix is not ripened (Kapp, 2010). In either event, termination is done by first dilating the cervix and then evacuating the uterine contents by either sharp or suction curettage or both. These procedures are depicted in Sections 41-15 and 41-16 (p. 1057). Curettage usually requires sedation or analgesia. In addition to intravenously or orally administered sedatives, success has been reported with paracervical lidocaine blockade, with or without other analgesics (Allen, 2009; Cansino, 2009).

Vacuum aspiration is the most commonly used form of suction curettage. It requires a rigid cannula attached to an electric-powered vacuum source. Alternatively, manual vacuum aspiration

is done with a similar cannula that attaches to a handheld syringe for its vacuum source (MacIsaac, 2000; Masch, 2005).

Curettage—either sharp or suction—is recommended before 14 to 15 weeks. The likelihood of complications increases after the first trimester and include perforation, cervical laceration, hemorrhage, incomplete removal of the fetus or placenta, and postoperative infections. Niinimäki and associates (2009) reported results from more than 20,000 Finnish women who had a surgical termination before 63 days. There was a 5.6-percent complication rate. Hemorrhage, incomplete abortion, or infection each comprised one third of complications. A second surgical curettage was necessary in approximately 2 percent. By contrast, 20 percent of more than 22,000 women undergoing a medical termination had such complications as discussed on page 191.

Hygroscopic Dilators. Trauma from mechanical dilatation can be minimized by using devices that slowly dilate the cervix. As shown in Figures 41-16.1 and 41-16.2 (p. 1059), hygroscopic dilators draw water from cervical tissues and expand, gradually dilating the cervix. One such device is derived from various species of *Laminaria* algae that are harvested from the ocean floor. Another is *Dilapan-S,* which is composed of an acrylic-based gel. In a recent Cochrane review, Kapp and associates (2010) found that mechanical dilators decreased the length of first-trimester procedures, but their efficacy was similar to that with medical ripening agents.

Occasionally, a woman who has a hygroscopic dilator placed preparatory to elective abortion will change her mind. Schneider and associates (1991) described this in 21 such cases—7 first- and 14 second-trimester pregnancies. Of the 17 women who chose to continue their pregnancy, there were 14 term deliveries, two preterm deliveries, and one miscarriage 2 weeks later. None suffered infection-related morbidity, including three untreated women with cervical cultures positive for *Chlamydia trachomatis*. In spite of this generally reassuring report, an attitude of irrevocability with regard to dilator placement and abortion seems prudent.

Prostaglandins and Mifepristone. Several pharmaceutical preparations may be used instead of hygroscopic dilators to aid presurgical termination. In the metaanalysis by Kapp (2010) cited earlier, efficacy of these medications was found to be similar to that of hygroscopic dilators. As discussed subsequently, some of these regimens are the same as those used for medically induced abortions. *Misoprostol* (Cytotec), 400 to 600 μg, is administered orally or sublingually or is placed into the posterior vaginal fornix. Of these, Oppegaard and associates (2006) reported that the oral route for misoprostol was unsatisfactory for cervical ripening. Use of misoprostol as an abortifacient is an off-label use of the drug, and patients are counseled accordingly. The progesterone antagonist *mifepristone* (Mifeprex), 200 to 600 μg given orally, is also an effective but expensive cervical-ripening agent. Of other options, *prostaglandins E_2 and $F_{2\alpha}$* have unacceptable side effects compared with misoprostol (Kapp, 2010).

Manual Vacuum Aspiration. This office-based procedure is done using a hand-operated 60-mL syringe and cannula. It is used for surgical treatment of early pregnancy failures as well as elective termination up to 12 weeks' gestation. Masch and Roman (2005) recommend that office-based pregnancy terminations with this method be limited to ≤10 weeks. This is because blood loss increases with procedures between 10 and 12 weeks (Westfall, 1998).

With pregnancies ≤8 weeks, no cervical preparation is often required. After this time, preprocedure treatment is recommended. Paracervical block with or without intravenous sedation is used for anesthesia. With this procedure, a vacuum is created by a syringe that attaches to the cannula. First, the cannula is inserted transcervically into the uterus. The vacuum is then created and produces up to 60 mm Hg suction. Complications are similar to those with the other surgical methods (Goldberg, 2004).

Menstrual Aspiration. Aspiration of the endometrial cavity within 1 to 3 weeks after a missed menstrual period has been referred to as *menstrual extraction, menstrual induction, instant period, traumatic abortion,* and *mini-abortion.* The procedure is done using a flexible 5- or 6-mm Karman cannula and attached syringe. A positive pregnancy test result will eliminate a needless procedure on a nonpregnant woman whose period has been delayed for other reasons. Procedures done this early have unique complications: pregnancy is misdiagnosed, an implanted zygote is missed by the curette, ectopic pregnancy is unrecognized, or infrequently, the uterus is perforated. Even so, Paul and associates (2002) reported a 98-percent success rate in more than 1000 women who underwent this procedure.

To verify placental tissue in the aspirate, MacIsaac and Darney (2000) recommend that the syringe contents be rinsed in a strainer to remove blood. They are then placed in a clear plastic container with saline and examined with back lighting. Placental tissue macroscopically appears soft, fluffy, and feathery. A magnifying lens, colposcope, or microscope can also improve visualization.

Hysterectomy. In women who have significant uterine disease, hysterectomy for abortion may be preferable to either curettage or medical induction.

Medical Abortion

Throughout history, many naturally occurring substances have been used as abortifacients. These remedies generally were ineffective and dangerous. Even today, only a few safe and effective abortifacient drugs are used. According to the American College of Obstetricians and Gynecologists (2009c), outpatient medical abortion is an acceptable alternative to surgical abortion in appropriately selected women at ≤49 days' gestation. Beyond this point, the available data, although less robust, support surgical abortion as the preferable method.

Three medications for early medical abortion have been widely used—either alone or in combination. These are the antiprogestin *mifepristone;* the antimetabolite *methotrexate;* and the prostaglandin *misoprostol.* These agents cause abortion by increasing uterine contractility either by reversing the progesterone-induced inhibition of contractions—mifepristone and methotrexate, or by stimulating the myometrium directly—misoprostol. In addition, mifepristone causes cervical collagen degradation, possibly because of increased expression of matrix metalloproteinase-2 (Clark, 2006). Importantly, methotrexate and misoprostol are teratogens, and their use thus requires a commitment from both the woman and her caregiver to complete the abortion.

A large number and variety of effective dosing schemes are listed in Table 6-11. Misoprostol is used in all three regimens, either following mifepristone or methotrexate administration or given as monotherapy. As discussed on page 178 and previously shown in Table 6-3, any of several regimens used for "early pregnancy loss" are also likely to be successful for elective pregnancy interruption. For elective termination at ≤63 days' gestation, von Hertzen (2009, 2010) and Winikoff (2008) and their associates reported from randomized trials a 92- to 96-percent efficacy with one of the mifepristone/misoprostol regimens given. Fjerstad (2009a) reported similar results from 10 large urban Planned Parenthood clinics. They estimated that buccal misoprostol-oral mifepristone regimens were 87- to 98-percent successful in inducing abortion in women <10 weeks' gestation. With later first-trimester pregnancies, as expected, the success rate is diminished. Dalenda (2010) reported the success rate to be only approximately 80 percent in 122 women at 9 to 12 weeks' gestation.

Contraindications. Most contraindications to medical abortion have evolved from exclusion criteria used in initial clinical trials. Thus, some are relative contraindications, and in addition to specific medication allergies, they have included: an in situ intrauterine device; severe anemia, coagulopathy, or anticoagulant use; and significant medical conditions such as active liver disease, cardiovascular disease, or uncontrolled seizure disorders. Because misoprostol diminishes glucocorticoid activity, women with disorders requiring

TABLE 6-11. Regimens for Medical Termination of Early Pregnancy

Mifepristone/Misoprostol

[a]Mifepristone, 100–600 mg orally followed by:
[b]Misoprostol, 200–600 μg orally or 400–800 μg vaginally, buccally, or sublingually given immediately or up to 72 hours

Methotrexate/Misoprostol

[c]Methotrexate, 50 mg/m^2 intramuscularly or orally followed by:
[d]Misoprostol, 800 μg vaginally in 3–7 days. Repeat if needed 1 week after methotrexate initially given

Misoprostol Alone

[e]800 μg vaginally or sublingually, repeated for up to three doses

[a]Doses of 200 versus 600 mg are similarly effective.
[b]Oral route may be less effective; possibly more side effects, namely, nausea and diarrhea. Sublingual route has more side effects than vaginal route. Shorter intervals (6 hours) with PGE$_1$ given after mifepristone may be less effective than when given >36 hours.
[c]Efficacy similar for routes of administration.
[d]Similar efficacy when given on day 3 versus day 5.
[e]Intervals 3–12 hours given vaginally; 3–4 hours given sublingually.
Data from the American College of Obstetricians and Gynecologists, 2009d; Borgatta, 2001; Coyaji, 2007; Creinin, 2001, 2007; Fekih, 2010; Guest, 2007; Hamoda, 2005; Honkanen, 2004; Jain, 2002; Kulier, 2004; Pymar, 2001; Raghavan, 2009; Schaff, 2000; Shannon, 2006; von Hertzen, 2003, 2007, 2009, 2010; Winikoff, 2008.

glucocorticoid therapy are usually excluded (American College of Obstetricians and Gynecologists, 2009d). In women with renal insufficiency, the methotrexate dose should be modified and given with caution or another regimen administered (Kelly, 2006).

Administration. With the mifepristone/misoprostol regimen, mifepristone treatment is followed by misoprostol given at that same time or up to 72 hours later as shown in Table 6-11. Some prefer that misoprostol be administered on site, after which the woman typically remains for 4 hours. Symptoms are common within 3 hours and included lower abdominal pain, vomiting, diarrhea, fever, and chills/shivering. In the first few hours after misoprostol is given, if the pregnancy appears to have been expelled, an examination is done to confirm expulsion. If the pregnancy has not been expelled, a pelvic examination is performed, and the patient is discharged and appointed to return in 1 to 2 weeks. At this time, if clinical or sonographic evaluation fails to confirm completed abortion, a suction procedure usually is recommended. There are a number of complications, and some may be serious. These included hemorrhage, incomplete abortion, and curettage for hemorrhage, incomplete abortion, or infection (Niinimäki, 2009; von Hertzen, 2010).

In regimens initially employing methotrexate, the misoprostol is given 3 to 7 days later, and women are typically seen at least 24 hours after misoprostol administration. They are next seen approximately 7 days after methotrexate is given, and a sonographic examination is performed. If an intact pregnancy is seen, then another dose of misoprostol is given, and the woman is seen again in 1 week if fetal cardiac activity is present or in 4 weeks if there is no fetal cardiac activity. If abortion

has not occurred by the second visit, it is usually completed by suction curettage.

Bleeding and cramping with medical termination can be significantly worse than symptoms experienced with menses. Adequate analgesia, usually including a narcotic, is provided. The American College of Obstetricians and Gynecologists (2009c) recommends that if there is enough blood to soak two or more pads per hour for at least 2 hours, the woman is instructed to contact her provider to determine whether she needs to be seen.

Unnecessary surgical intervention in women undergoing medical abortion can be avoided if surveillance sonographic results are interpreted appropriately. Specifically, if no gestational sac is present, in the absence of heavy bleeding, intervention in most women is unnecessary. This is true even when, as is common, the uterus contains sonographically evident debris. For postabortal care, however, Clark and colleagues (2010) provided data that routine postprocedure sonographic examination is not necessary. They instead recommend assessment of the clinical course and bimanual pelvic examination.

■ Consequences of Elective Abortion
Maternal Mortality

Legally induced abortion, performed by trained gynecologists, especially when performed during the first 2 months of pregnancy, has a mortality rate of less than 1 per 100,000 procedures (Centers for Disease Control and Prevention, 2011a; Grimes, 2006). In the series from the Finnish Register of almost 43,000 abortions done before 63 days, there was only one procedure-related death (Niinimäki, 2009). The earlier abortion is done, the safer the procedure. The relative risk of procedure-related mortality is estimated to double for each 2 weeks after 8 weeks' gestation. According to Horon (2005), abortion-related deaths are underreported.

Impact on Future Pregnancies

Data relating abortion to subsequent pregnancy outcome are observational, and reports must be interpreted with these limitations in mind. That said, fertility does not appear to be diminished by an elective abortion, except infrequently as a consequence of infection. Similarly, the risks for subsequent ectopic pregnancy are not increased, except possibly in women with preexisting chlamydial infection or in those who develop postabortion infections. It may be reasonable to compare these women with those having a first-trimester miscarriage (Smith, 2009). In those with a first-trimester loss, the 5-year live-birth rate was approximately 80 percent and was similar whether losses were managed expectantly, surgically, or medically.

Some data suggest that induced abortions are associated with increased risks for subsequent adverse pregnancy outcomes. Maconochie (2007) reported that subsequent first-trimester miscarriage was more common in women who had one or more prior elective abortions. From the French EPIPAGE (Etude Epidémiologique sur les Petits Ages Gestationnels) study, Moreau (2005) reported a 1.5-fold increased incidence of very preterm delivery—22 to 32 weeks—in women who had had a prior induced abortion. Shah (2009) performed a systematic review of 37 studies and computed a significantly increased 1.35-fold risk for subsequent low-birthweight and preterm deliveries after one pregnancy termination. These risks increased along with an increased number of procedures. According to Virk (2007), these adverse outcomes are similar in women who had medically versus surgically induced terminations. Multiple abortions using sharp curettage, however, may increase the subsequent risk of placenta previa, whereas vacuum aspiration procedures likely do not (Johnson, 2003).

RESUMPTION OF OVULATION FOLLOWING MISCARRIAGE

Ovulation may resume as early as 2 weeks after an early pregnancy is terminated, whether spontaneous or induced. Lahteenmaki and Luukkainen (1978) detected surges of LH at 16 to 22 days after abortion in 15 of 18 women. Plasma progesterone levels, which had plummeted after the abortion, increased soon after LH surges. These hormonal events agree with histologic changes observed in endometrial biopsies (Boyd, 1972).

These findings are important because postabortion care includes contraception and future pregnancy counseling. Although recommended by some, there appears to be no advantage to delaying conception if this is desired. Love (2010) analyzed the next pregnancy in nearly 31,000 women following a miscarriage and found that those who conceived within 6 months had better pregnancy outcomes than those conceiving later than 6 months after miscarriage.

If pregnancy is to be prevented, effective contraception should be initiated very soon after abortion, and suitable options are presented in Chapter 5 (p. 132). Importantly, there are no gynecological reasons to withhold immediate contraceptive measures should this be chosen (Love, 2010). Hormonal contraceptives can be started at the time of abortion completion. Moreover, IUD insertion immediately following abortion is safe and practical (Bednarek, 2011; Cremer, 2011; Fox, 2011; Grimes, 2010). As expected, the expulsion rate is higher in those with immediate insertion compared with that in women having an IUD inserted at a later visit. However, in populations with poor follow-up compliance, a greater number of IUDs may ultimately be provided to those in whom insertion is immediate.

REFERENCES

Abbassi-Ghanavati M, Casey BM, Spong CY, et al: Pregnancy outcomes in women with thyroid peroxidase antibodies. Obstet Gynecol 116:381, 2010

Abramson J, Stagnaro-Green A: Thyroid antibodies and fetal loss: an evolving story. Thyroid 11:57, 2001

Adelberg AM, Kuller JA: Thrombophilias and recurrent miscarriage. Obstet Gynecol Surv 57:703, 2002

Al–Inany H: Intrauterine adhesions. An update. Acta Obstet Gynecol Scand 80:986, 2001

Allen RH, Fitzmaurice G, Lifford KL, et al: Oral compared with intravenous sedation for first-trimester surgical abortion: a randomized controlled trial. Obstet Gynecol 113(2 pt 1):276, 2009

American College of Obstetricians and Gynecologists: Abortion access and training. Committee Opinion No. 424, January 2009a

American College of Obstetricians and Gynecologists: Abortion policy. College Statement of Policy. January 1993, Reaffirmed July 2007

American College of Obstetricians and Gynecologists: Antibiotic prophylaxis for gynecologic procedures. Practice Bulletin No. 104, May 2009b

American College of Obstetricians and Gynecologists: Antiphospholipid syndrome. Practice Bulletin No. 118, January 2011a

American College of Obstetricians and Gynecologists: Inherited thrombophilias in pregnancy. Practice Bulletin No. 124, September 2011b

American College of Obstetricians and Gynecologists: Management of recurrent early pregnancy loss. Practice Bulletin No. 24, February 2001, Reaffirmed 2008

American College of Obstetricians and Gynecologists: Medical management of abortion. Practice Bulletin No. 67, October 2005, Reaffirmed 2009c

American College of Obstetricians and Gynecologists: Misoprostol for abortion care. Committee Opinion No. 427, February 2009d

American College of Obstetricians and Gynecologists: Moderate caffeine consumption during pregnancy. Committee Opinion No. 462, August 2010a

American College of Obstetricians and Gynecologists: Prevention of Rh D alloimmunization. Practice Bulletin No. 4, May 1999, Reaffirmed 2010b

American College of Obstetricians and Gynecologists: The limits of conscientious refusal in reproductive medicine. Committee Opinion No. 385, November 2007, Reaffirmed December 2010c

American College of Obstetricians and Gynecologists: Ultrasonography in pregnancy. Practice Bulletin No. 101, February 2009e

American Society for Reproductive Medicine: Definitions of infertility and recurrent pregnancy loss. Fertil Steril 90(Suppl 3):S60, 2008

American Society for Reproductive Medicine: Intravenous immunoglobulin (IVIG) and recurrent spontaneous pregnancy loss. Fertil Steril 86(5 Suppl 1): S226, 2006

Andersen AE, Ryan GL: Eating disorders in the obstetric and gynecologic patient population. Obstet Gynecol 114(6):1353, 2009

Armstrong BG, McDonald AD, Sloan M: Cigarette, alcohol, and coffee consumption and spontaneous abortion. Am J Public Health 82:85, 1992

Arredondo F, Noble LS: Endocrinology of recurrent pregnancy loss. Semin Reprod Med 1:33, 2006

Ata B, Tan SL, Shehata F, et al: A systematic review of intravenous immunoglobulin for treatment of unexplained recurrent miscarriage. Fertil Steril 95(3):1080, 2011

August P, Lindheimer MD: Chronic hypertension and pregnancy. In Lindheimer MD, Roberts JM, Cunningham FG (eds): Chesley's Hypertensive Disorders of Pregnancy, 3rd ed. New York, Elsevier, 2009, p 359

Baker A, Beresford T: Informed consent, patient education, and counseling. In Paul M, Lichtenberg ES, Borgatta L, et al (eds): Management of Unintended and Abnormal Pregnancy. West Sussex, UK, Wiley-Blackwell, 2009, p 48

Barber JCK, Cockwell AE, Grant E: Is karyotyping couples experiencing recurrent miscarriage worth the cost? BJOG 117:885, 2010

Barlow S, Sullivan FM: Reproductive Hazards of Industrial Chemicals: An Evaluation of Animal and Human Data. New York, Academic Press, 1982

Barnhart K, Mennuti MT, Benjamin I, et al: Prompt diagnosis of ectopic pregnancy in an emergency department setting. Obstet Gynecol 84(6).1010, 1994

Barnhart K, Sammel MD, Chung K, et al: Decline of serum human chorionic gonadotropin and spontaneous complete abortion: defining the normal curve. Obstet Gynecol 104:975, 2004a

Barnhart K, van Mello NM, Bourne T, et al: Pregnancy of unknown location: a consensus statement of nomenclature, definitions, and outcome. Fertil Steril 95(3):857, 2011

Barnhart KT, Sammel MD, Appleby D, et al: Does a prediction model for pregnancy of unknown location developed in the UK validate on a US population? Hum Reprod 25(10):2434, 2010

Barnhart KT, Sammel MD, Rinaudo PF: Symptomatic patients with an early viable intrauterine pregnancy: hCG curves redefined. Obstet Gynecol 104:50, 2004b

Barrett JP, Whiteside JL, Boardman LA: Fatal clostridial sepsis after spontaneous abortion. Obstet Gynecol 99:899, 2002

Bednarek PH, Creinin MD, Reeves MF: Immediate versus delayed IUD insertion after uterine aspiration. N Engl J Med 364(23):2208, 2011

Bellver J, Ayllón Y, Ferrando M, et al: Female obesity impairs in vitro fertilization outcome without affecting embryo quality. Fertil Steril 93(2):447, 2010a

Bellver J, Meseguer M, Muriel L, et al: Y chromosome microdeletions, sperm DNA fragmentation and sperm oxidative stress as causes of recurrent spontaneous abortion of unknown etiology. Hum Reprod 25(7):1713, 2010b

Benhadi N, Wiersinga WM, Reitsma JB, et al: Higher maternal TSH levels in pregnancy are associated with increased risk for miscarriage, fetal or neonatal death. Eur J Endocrinol 160:985, 2009

Benirschke K, Kaufmann P: Pathology of the Human Placenta, 4th ed. New York, Springer, 2000

Berger DS, Hogge WA, Barmada MM, et al: Comprehensive analysis of HLA-G: implications for recurrent spontaneous abortion. Reprod Sci 17(4):331, 2010

Bhattacharya S, Townend J, Bhattacharya S: Recurrent miscarriage: are three miscarriages one too many? Analysis of a Scottish population-based database of 151,021 pregnancies. Eur J Obstet Gynecol Reprod Biol 150:24, 2010

Bianco K, Caughey AB, Shaffer BL, et al: History of miscarriage and increased incidence of fetal aneuploidy in subsequent pregnancy. Obstet Gynecol 107:1098, 2006

Bick RL, Baker WF Jr: Hereditary and acquired thrombophilia in pregnancy. In Bick RL (ed): Hematological Complications in Obstetrics, Pregnancy, and Gynecology. United Kingdom, Cambridge University Press, 2006, p 122

Blohm F, Fridén BE, Milsom I, et al: A randomized double blind trial comparing misoprostol or placebo in the management of early miscarriage. BJOG 112:1090, 2005

Boivin JF: Risk of spontaneous abortion in women occupationally exposed to anaesthetic gases: a meta-analysis. Occup Environ Med 54:541, 1997

Borgatta L, Burnhill MS, Tyson J, et al: Early medical abortion with methotrexate and misoprostol. Obstet Gynecol 97:11, 2001

Boyd EF Jr, Holmstrom EG: Ovulation following therapeutic abortion. Am J Obstet Gynecol 113:469, 1972

Branch DW, Gibson M, Silver RM: Recurrent miscarriage. N Engl J Med 363:18, 2010

Branch DW, Khamashta MA: Antiphospholipid syndrome: obstetric diagnosis, management, and controversies. Obstet Gynecol 101(6):1333, 2003

Bree RL, Edwards M, Bohm-Velez M, et al: Transvaginal sonography in the evaluation of normal early pregnancy: correlation with HCG level. AJR Am J Roentgenol 153(1):75, 1989

Brent RL: Saving lives and changing family histories: appropriate counseling of pregnant women and men and women of reproductive age, concerning the risk of diagnostic radiation exposures during and before pregnancy. Am J Obstet Gynecol 200(1):4, 2009

Brigham SA, Conlon C, Farquharson RG: A longitudinal study of pregnancy outcome following idiopathic recurrent miscarriage. Hum Reprod 14(11):2868, 1999

Brown ZA, Selke S, Zeh J, et al: The acquisition of herpes simplex virus during pregnancy. N Engl J Med 337:509, 1997

Bukulmez O, Arici A: Luteal phase defect: myth or reality. Obstet Gynecol Clin North Am 31:727, 2004

Bulik CM, Hoffman ER, Von Holle A, et al: Unplanned pregnancy in women with anorexia nervosa. Obstet Gynecol 116:1136, 2010

Buttram VC Jr, Gibbons WE: Müllerian anomalies: a proposed classification (an analysis of 144 cases). Fertil Steril 32(1):40, 1979

Calleja-Agius J, Muttukrishna S, Pizzey AR, et al: Pro- and antiinflammatory cytokines in threatened miscarriages. Am J Obstet Gynecol Feb 23, 2011 [Epub ahead of print]

Cansino C, Edelman A, Burke A, et al: Paracervical block with combined ketorolac and lidocaine in first-trimester surgical abortion: a randomized controlled trial. Obstet Gynecol 114(6):1220, 2009

Carp H, Dolitzky M, Tur Kaspa I, et al: Hereditary thrombophilias are not associated with a decreased live birth rate in women with recurrent miscarriage. Fertil Steril 78:58, 2002

Carrell DT, Wilcox AL, Lowy L, et al: Male chromosomal factors of unexplained recurrent pregnancy loss. Obstet Gynecol 101:1229, 2003

Casey BM, Dashe JS, Wells CE, et al: Subclinical hypothyroidism and pregnancy outcomes. Obstet Gynecol 105(2):239, 2005

Castañeda R, Lechuga D, Ramos RI, et al: Endemic goiter in pregnant women: utility of the simplified classification of thyroid size by palpation and urinary iodine as screening tests. BJOG 109:1366, 2002

Catov JM, Nohr EA, Olsen J, et al: Chronic hypertension related to risk for preterm and term small for gestational age births. Obstet Gynecol 112(2 pt 1):290, 2008

Cavallo F, Russo R, Zotti C, et al: Moderate alcohol consumption and spontaneous abortion. Alcohol 30:195, 1995

Centers for Disease Control and Prevention: Abortion surveillance—United States, 2007. MMWR Surveill Summ 60(1):1, 2011a

Centers for Disease Control and Prevention: Clostridium sordellii toxic shock syndrome after medical abortion with mifepristone and intravaginal misoprostol—United States and Canada, 2001-2005. MMWR 54(29):724, 2005

Centers for Disease Control and Prevention: Tobacco use and pregnancy. Available at: http://www.cdc.gov/reproductivehealth/TobaccoUsePregnancy/index.htm. Accessed March 22, 2011b

Chatenoud L, Parazzini F, Di Cintio E, et al: Paternal and maternal smoking habits before conception and during the first trimester: relation to spontaneous abortion. Ann Epidemiol 8:520, 1998

Chen L, Hu R: Thyroid autoimmunity and miscarriage: a meta-analysis. Clin Endocrinol (Oxf) 74(4):513, 2011

Ciacci C, Tortora R, Scudiero O, et al: Early pregnancy loss in celiac women: the role of genetic markers of thrombophilia. Dig Liver Dis 41:717, 2009

Clark CA, Spitzer KA, Crowther MA, et al: Incidence of postpartum thrombosis and preterm delivery in women with antiphospholipid antibodies and recurrent pregnancy loss. J Rheumatol 34(5):992, 2007a

Clark EAS, Silver RM, Branch DW: Do antiphospholipid antibodies cause preeclampsia and HELLP syndrome? Curr Rheumatol Rep 9:219, 2007b

Clark K, Ji H, Feltovich H et al: Mifepristone-induced cervical ripening: structural, biomechanical, and molecular events. Am J Obstet Gynecol 194:1391, 2006

Clark W, Bracken H, Tanenhaus J, et al: Alternatives to a routine follow-up visit for early medical abortion. Obstet Gynecol 115(2 Pt 1):264, 2010

Clifford K, Rai R, Watson H, et al: Does suppressing luteinizing hormone secretion reduce the miscarriage rate? Results of a randomized controlled trial. BMJ 312:1508, 1996

Clowse ME, Jamison M, Myers E, et al: A national study of the complications of lupus in pregnancy. Am J Obstet Gynecol 199:127.e1, 2008

Cnattingius S, Signorello LB, Anneren G, et al: Caffeine intake and the risk of first-trimester spontaneous abortion. N Engl J Med 343:1839, 2000

Cocksedge KA, Saravelos SH, Metwally M, et al: How common is polycystic ovary syndrome in recurrent miscarriage? Reprod Biomed Online 19(4):572, 2009

Cohen AL, Bhatnagar J, Reagan S, et al: Toxic shock associated with Clostridium sordellii and Clostridium perfringens after medical and spontaneous abortion. Obstet Gynecol 110:1027, 2007

Condous G, Okaro E, Khalid A, Bourne T: Do we need to follow up complete miscarriages with serum human chorionic gonadotrophin levels? BJOG 112:827, 2005

Condous G, Van Calster B, Kirk E, et al: Clinical information does not improve the performance of mathematical models in predicting the outcome of pregnancies of unknown location. Fertil Steril 88(3):572, 2007

Coyaji K, Krishna U, Ambardekar S, et al: Are two doses of misoprostol after mifepristone for early abortion better than one? BJOG 114(3):271, 2007

Craig TB, Ke RW, Kutteh WH: Increased prevalence of insulin resistance in women with a history of recurrent pregnancy loss. Fertil Steril 78:487, 2002

Creinin MD, Huang X, Westhoff C: et al: Factors related to successful misoprostol treatment for early pregnancy failure. Obstet Gynecol 107:901, 2006

Creinin MD, Pymar HC, Schwartz JL: Mifepristone 100 mg in abortion regimens. Obstet Gynecol 98:434, 2001

Creinin MD, Schreiber CA, Bednarek P, et al: Mifepristone and misoprostol administered simultaneously versus 24 hours apart for abortion: a randomized controlled trial. Obstet Gynecol 109(4):885, 2007

Cremer M, Bullard KA, Mosley RM: Immediate vs. delayed post-abortal copper T 380A IUD insertion in cases over 12 weeks of gestation. Contraception 83(6):522, 2011

Cunningham FG, Leveno KL, Bloom SL, et al (eds): Abortion. In Williams Obstetrics, 23rd ed. New York, McGraw-Hill, 2010a, p 215

Cunningham FG, Leveno KL, Bloom SL, et al (eds): Connective-tissue disorders. In Williams Obstetrics, 23rd ed. New York, McGraw-Hill, 2010b, p 1145

Cunningham FG, Leveno KL, Bloom SL, et al (eds): Genetics. In Williams Obstetrics, 23rd ed. New York, McGraw-Hill, 2010c, p 273

Cunningham FG, Leveno KL, Bloom SL, et al (eds): Prenatal care. In Williams Obstetrics, 23rd ed. New York, McGraw-Hill, 2010d, p 207

Daif JL, Levie M, Chudnoff S, et al: Group a Streptococcus causing necrotizing fasciitis and toxic shock syndrome after medical termination of pregnancy. Obstet Gynecol 113(2 Pt 2):504, 2009

Dalenda C, Ines N, Fathia B, et al: Two medical abortion regimens for late first-trimester termination of pregnancy: a prospective randomized trial. Contraception 81(4):323, 2010

Dalton VK, Harris LH, Gold KJ, et al: Provider knowledge, attitudes, and treatment preferences for early pregnancy failure. Am J Obstet Gynecol 202:531.e1, 2010

Dao B, Blum J, Thieba B, et al: Is misoprostol a safe, effective and acceptable alternative to manual vacuum aspiration for postabortion care? Results from a randomized trial in Burkina Faso, West Africa. BJOG 114(11):1368, 2007

Daya S: Accuracy of gestational age estimation by means of fetal crown-rump length measurement. Am Journal Obstet Gynecol 168(3 Pt 1):903, 1993

De Vivo A, Mancuso A, Giacobbe A, et al: Thyroid function in women found to have early pregnancy loss. Thyroid 20(6):633, 2010

Devaseelan P, Fogarty PP, Regan L: Human chorionic gonadotropin for threatened abortion. Cochrane Database Syst Rev 5:DC007422, 2010

Devi Wold AS, Pham N, Arici A: Anatomic factors in recurrent pregnancy loss. Semin Reprod Med 1:25, 2006

Di Simone N, Meroni PL, D'Asta M, et al: Pathogenic role of anti-beta2-glycoprotein I antibodies on human placenta: functional effects related to implantation and roles of heparin. Hum Reprod Update 13(2):189, 2007

Dizon-Townsend D, Miller C, Sibai B, et al: The relationship of the factor V Leiden mutation and pregnancy outcomes for mother and fetus. Obstet Gynecol 106:517, 2005

Dolitzky M, Inbal A, Segal Y, et al: A randomized study of thromboprophylaxis in women with unexplained consecutive recurrent miscarriages. Fertil Steril 86:362, 2006

Dranitsaris G, Johnston M, Poirier S, et al: Are health care providers who work with cancer drugs at an increased risk for toxic events? A systematic review and meta-analysis of the literature. J Oncol Pharm Pract 2:69, 2005

Dukhovny S, Zutshi P, Abbott JF: Recurrent second trimester pregnancy loss: evaluation and management. Curr Opin Endocrinol Diabetes Obes 16:451, 2009

Eddleman K, Sullivan L, Stone J, et al: An individualized risk for spontaneous pregnancy loss: a risk function model. J Soc Gynecol Investig 13:197A, 2006

Eiben B, Bartels I, Bahr-Prosch S, et al: Cytogenetic analysis of 750 spontaneous abortions with the direct-preparation method of chorionic villi and its implications for studying genetic causes of pregnancy wastage. Am J Hum Genet 47:656, 1990

Eller AG, Branch DW, Nelson L, et al: Vascular endothelial growth factor-A gene polymorphisms in women with recurrent pregnancy loss. J Reprod Immunol 88(1):48, 2011

Empson M, Lassere M, Craig J, et al: Prevention of recurrent miscarriage for women with antiphospholipid antibody or lupus anticoagulant. Cochrane Database Syst Rev (2):CD002859, 2005. Edited with no change in conclusions, Issue 1, 2010

Erkan D, Kozora E, Lockshin MD: Cognitive dysfunction and white matter abnormalities in antiphospholipid syndrome. Pathophysiology 18(1):93, 2011

Eskenazi B, Chevrier J, Rosas LG, et al: The Pine River statement: human health consequences of DDT use. Environ Health Perspect 117(9):1359, 2009

Fantel AG, Shepard TH, Vadheim-Roth C, et al: Embryonic and fetal phenotypes: Prevalence and other associated factors in a large study of spontaneous abortion. In Porter IH, Hook EM (eds): Human Embryonic and Fetal Death. New York, Academic Press, 1980, p 71

Farquharson RG, Quenby S, Greaves M: Antiphospholipid syndrome in pregnancy: a randomized, controlled trial of treatment. Obstet Gynecol 100:408, 2002

Feist A, Sydler T, Gebbers JJ, et al: No association of Chlamydia with abortion. J R Soc Med 92:237, 1999

Fekih M, Fathallah K, Ben Regaya L, et al: Sublingual misoprostol for first trimester termination of pregnancy. Int J Gynaecol Obstet 109(1):67, 2010

Feldman DM, Timms D, Borgida AF: Toxoplasmosis, parvovirus, and cytomegalovirus in pregnancy. Clin Lab Med 30(3):709, 2010

Fischer J, Colls P, Esudero T, et al: Preimplantation genetic diagnosis (PGD) improves pregnancy outcome for translocation carriers with a history of recurrent losses. Fertil Steril 94(1):283, 2010

Fischer M, Bhatnagar J, Guarner J, et al: Fatal toxic shock syndrome associated with Clostridium sordellii after medical abortion. N Engl J Med 353:2352, 2005

Fjerstad M, Sivin I, Lichtenberg ES, et al: Effectiveness of medical abortion with mifepristone and buccal misoprostol through 59 gestational days. Contraception 80(3):282, 2009a

Fjerstad M, Trussell, J, Sivin I: Rates of serious infection after changes in regimens for medical abortion. N Engl J Med 361:145, 2009b

Flood K, Peace A, Kent E, et al: Platelet reactivity and pregnancy loss. Am J Obstet Gynecol 203:281.e1, 2010

Floyd RL, Decoufle P, Hungerford DW: Alcohol use prior to pregnancy recognition. Am J Prev Med 17:101, 1999

Fox MC, Oat-Judge J, Severson K: Immediate placement of intrauterine devices after first and second trimester pregnancy termination. Contraception 83(1):34, 2011

Franklin RD, Kutteh WH: Effects of unfractionated and low molecular weight heparin on antiphospholipid antibody binding in vitro. Obstet Gynecol 101:455, 2003

Franssen MTM, Korevaar JC, van der Veen F, et al: Reproductive outcome after chromosome analysis in couples with two or more miscarriages: case-control study. BMJ 332:750, 2006

Franz MB, Husslein PW: Obstetrical management of the older gravida. Womens Health 6(3):463, 2010

Freedman L, Landy U, Steinauer J: Obstetrician-gynecologist experiences with abortion training: physician insights from a qualitative study. Contraception 81(6):525, 2010

Gallicchio L, Miller S, Greene T, et al: Cosmetologists and reproductive outcomes. Obstet Gynecol 113(5):1018, 2009

Ganer H, Levy A, Ohel I, et al: Pregnancy outcome in women with an intrauterine contraceptive device. Am J Obstet Gynecol 201:381.e1, 2009

Glueck CJ, Wang P, Goldenberg N, et al: Pregnancy outcomes among women with polycystic ovary syndrome treated with metformin. Hum Reprod 17:2858, 2002

Goel N, Tuli A, Choudhry R: The role of aspirin versus aspirin and heparin in cases of recurrent abortions with raised anticardiolipin antibodies. Med Sci Monit 12:CR132, 2006

Goldberg AB, Dean G, Kang MS, et al: Manual versus electric vacuum aspiration for early first-trimester abortion: a controlled study of complication rates. Obstet Gynecol 103:101, 2004

Goldenberg M, Sivan E, Sharabi Z, et al: Reproductive outcome following hysteroscopic management of intrauterine septum and adhesions. Hum Reprod 10:2663, 1995

Goldstein SR: Significance of cardiac activity on endovaginal ultrasound in very early embryos. Obstet Gynecol 80(4):670, 1992

Goodman C, Hur J, Goodman CS, et al: Are polymorphisms in the ACE and PAI-1 genes associated with recurrent spontaneous miscarriages? Am J Reprod Immunol 62(6):365, 2009

Gracia CR, Sammel MD, Chittams J, et al: Risk factors for spontaneous abortion in early symptomatic first-trimester pregnancies. Obstet Gynecol 106:993, 2005

Greene MF: Spontaneous abortions and major malformations in women with diabetes mellitus. Semin Reprod Endocrinol 17:127, 1999

Grimes DA: Estimation of pregnancy-related mortality risk by pregnancy outcome, United States, 1991 to 1999. Am J Obstet Gynecol 194:92, 2006

Grimes DA, Lopez LM, Schulz KF, et al: Immediate postabortal insertion of intrauterine devices. Cochrane Database Syst Rev 6:CD001777, 2010

Guelinckx I, Devlieger R, Vansant G: Reproductive outcome after bariatric surgery: a critical review. Hum Reprod Update 15(2):189, 2009

Guest J, Chien PF, Thomson MA, et al: Randomised controlled trial comparing the efficacy of same-day administration of mifepristone and misoprostol for termination of pregnancy with the standard 36 to 48 hour protocol. BJOG 114(2):207, 2007

Guttmacher Institute: State facts about abortion: Texas. September, 2008. Available at: http://www.guttmacher.org/pubs/sfaa/texas.html. Accessed March 23, 2011

Guttmacher Institute: US abortion rate levels off after 30-year decline. Reuters Health Information, January 12, 2011

Haas DM, Ramsey PS: Progesterone for preventing miscarriage. Cochrane Database Syst Rev 2:CD003511, 2008

Haddow JE, McClain MR, Palomaki GE, et al: Thyroperoxidase and thyroglobulin antibodies in early pregnancy and placental abruption. Obstet Gynecol 117:287, 2011

Hamoda H, Ashok PW, Flett GMM, Templeton A: A randomised controlled trial of mifepristone in combination with misoprostol administered sublingually or vaginally for medical abortion up to 13 weeks of gestation. BJOG 112:1102, 2005

Hannafin B, Lovecchio F, Blackburn P: Do Rh-negative women with first trimester spontaneous abortions need Rh immune globulin? Am J Obstet Gynecol 24:487, 2006

Harger JH, Archer DF, Marchese SG, et al: Etiology of recurrent pregnancy losses and outcome of subsequent pregnancies. Obstet Gynecol 62(5):574, 1983

Hasan R, Baird DD, Herring AH, et al: Association between first-trimester vaginal bleeding and miscarriage. Obstet Gynecol 114:860, 2009

Hertig AT, Sheldon WH: Minimal criteria required to prove prima facie case of traumatic abortion or miscarriage: an analysis of 1,000 spontaneous abortions. Ann Surg 117:596, 1943

Heuser C, Dalton J, Macpherson C, et al: Idiopathic recurrent pregnancy loss recurs at similar gestational ages. Am J Obstet Gynecol 203(4):343.e1, 2010

Hide G, Morley EK, Hughes JM, et al: Evidence for high levels of vertical transmission in *Toxoplasma gondii*. Parasitology 136(14):1877, 2009

Ho CS, Bhatnagar J, Cohen AL, et al: Undiagnosed cases of fatal *Clostridium*-associated toxic shock in Californian women of childbearing age. Am J Obstet Gynecol 201:459.e1-7, 2009

Holbrook WJ, Oskarsdottir A, Fridjonsson T, et al: No link between low-grade periodontal disease and preterm birth: a pilot study in a health Caucasian population. Acta Odontol Scand 62:177, 2004

Homburg R: Adverse effects of luteinizing hormone on fertility: fact or fantasy. Baillieres Clin Obstet Gynaecol 12:555, 1998

Homer H, Saridogan E: Uterine artery embolization for fibroids is associated with an increased risk of miscarriage. Fertil Steril 94(1):324, 2010

Honkanen H, Piaggio G, Hertzen H, et al: WHO multinational study of three misoprostol regimens after mifepristone for early medical abortion. BJOG 111(7):715, 2004

Horcajadas JA, Goyri E, Higón MA, et al: Endometrial receptivity and implantation are not affected by the presence of uterine intramural leiomyomas: a clinical and functional genomics analysis. J Clin Endocrinol Metab 93(9):3490, 2008

Horon IL: Underreporting of maternal deaths on death certificates and the magnitude of the problem of maternal mortality. Am J Public Health 95:478, 2005

Hudson MM: Reproductive outcomes for survivors of childhood cancer. Obstet Gynecol 116:1171, 2010

Jacobs PA, Hassold TJ: The origin of chromosomal abnormalities in spontaneous abortion. In Porter IH, Hook EB (eds): Human Embryonic and Fetal Death. New York, Academic Press, 1980, p 289

Jain JK, Harwood B, Meckstroth KR, et al: A prospective randomized, double-blinded, placebo-controlled trial comparing mifepristone and vaginal misoprostol to vaginal misoprostol alone for elective termination of early pregnancy. Hum Reprod 17:1477, 2002

Jarvie E, Ramsay JE: Obstetric management of obesity in pregnancy. Semin Fetal Neonatal Med 15(2):83, 2010

Jaslow CR, Carney JL, Kutteh WH: Diagnostic factors identified in 1020 women with two versus three or more recurrent pregnancy losses. Fertil Steril 93(4):1234, 2010

Johns J, Jauniaux E: Threatened miscarriage as a predictor of obstetric outcome. Obstet Gynecol 107:845, 2006

Johnson LG, Mueller BA, Daling JR: The relationship of placenta previa and history of induced abortion. Int J Gynaecol Obstet 81:191, 2003

Jones RK, Kavanaugh ML: Changes in abortion rates between 2000 and 2008 and lifetime incidence of abortion. Obstet Gynecol 117(6):1358, 2011

Jun SH, Ginsburg ES, Racowsky C, et al: Uterine leiomyomas and their effect on in vitro fertilization outcome: a retrospective study. J Assist Reprod Genet 18:139, 2001

Kaandorp S, Di Nisio M, Goddijn M, et al: Aspiring or anticoagulants for treating recurrent miscarriage in women without antiphospholipid syndrome. Cochrane Database Syst Rev 1:CD004734, 2009

Kaandorp SP, van der Post JAM, Verhoeve HR, et al: Aspirin plus heparin or aspirin alone in women with recurrent miscarriage. N Engl J Med 362:1586, 2010

Kadar N, DeCherney AH, Romero R: Receiver operating characteristic (ROC) curve analysis of the relative efficacy of single and serial chorionic gonadotropin determinations in the early diagnosis of ectopic pregnancy. Fertil Steril 37:542, 1982

Kajii T, Ferrier A, Niikawa N, et al: Anatomic and chromosomal anomalies in 639 spontaneous abortions. Hum Genet 55:87, 1980

Kapp N, Lohr PA, Ngo TD, et al: Cervical preparation for first trimester surgical abortion. Cochrane Database Syst Rev 2:CD007207, 2010

Katz A, Ben-Arie A, Lurie S, et al: Reproductive outcome following hysteroscopic adhesiolysis in Asherman's syndrome. Int J Fertil Menopausal Stud 41:462, 1996

Kelly H, Harvey D, Moll S: A cautionary tale. Fatal outcome of methotrexate therapy given for management of ectopic pregnancy. Obstet Gynecol 107:439, 2006

Kesmodel U, Wisborg K, Olsen SF, et al: Moderate alcohol intake in pregnancy and the risk of spontaneous abortion. Alcohol 37:87, 2002

Kharazmi E, Dossus L, Rohrmann S, et al: Pregnancy loss and risk of cardiovascular disease: a prospective population-based cohort study (EPIC-Heidelberg). Heart 97(1):49, 2011

Klebanoff MA, Levine RJ, DerSimonian R, et al: Maternal serum paraxanthine, a caffeine metabolite, and the risk of spontaneous abortion. N Engl J Med 341:1639, 1999

Kleinhaus K, Perrin M, Friedlander Y, et al: Paternal age and spontaneous abortion. Obstet Gynecol 108:369, 2006

Kline J, Stein ZA, Shrout P, et al: Drinking during pregnancy and spontaneous abortion. Lancet 2:176, 1980

Krassas GE, Poppe K, Glinoer D: Thyroid function and human reproductive health. Endocr Rev 31:702, 2010

Kulier R, Bulmezoglu AM, Hofmeyr GJ, et al: Medical methods for first trimester abortion. Cochrane Database Syst Rev 2:CD002855, 2004

Kutteh WH: Antiphospholipid antibody-associated recurrent pregnancy loss: treatment with heparin and low-dose aspirin is superior to low-dose aspirin alone. Am J Obstet Gynecol 174:1584, 1996

Kutteh WH: Recurrent pregnancy loss. In Carr BR, Blackwell RE, Azziz R (eds): Essential Reproductive Medicine. New York, McGraw-Hill, 2005, p 590

Lahteenmaki P, Luukkainen T: Return of ovarian function after abortion. Clin Endocrinol 2:123, 1978

Lashen H, Fear K, Sturdee DW: Obesity is associated with increased risk of first trimester and recurrent miscarriage: matched case-control study. Hum Reprod 19(7):1644, 2004

Laskin CA, Spitzer KA, Clark CA, et al: Low molecular weight heparin and aspirin for recurrent pregnancy loss: results from the randomized, controlled HepASA Trial. J Rheumatol 36:279, 2009

Lazarus JH: Thyroid disease in pregnancy and childhood. Minerva Endocrinol 30:71, 2005

Levi CS, Lyons EA, Lindsay DJ: Early diagnosis of nonviable pregnancy with endovaginal US. Radiology 167(2):383, 1988

Levi CS, Lyons EA, Zheng XH, et al: Endovaginal US: demonstration of cardiac activity in embryos of less than 5.0 mm in crown-rump length. Radiology 176(1):71, 1990

Lockwood, CJ: Stop screening for inherited thrombophilias in patients with adverse pregnancy outcomes. Contemp OB/GYN 55.5:11, 2010

Love ER, Bhattacharya S, Smith NC, et al: Effect of interpregnancy interval on outcomes of pregnancy after miscarriage: retrospective analysis of hospital episode statistics in Scotland. BMJ 341:c3967, 2010

Luise C, Jermy K, May C, et al: Outcome of expectant management of spontaneous first trimester miscarriage: observational study. BMJ 324:873, 2002

Lupo PJ, Symanski E, Waller DK, et al: Maternal exposure to ambient levels of benzene and neural tube defects among offspring, Texas, 1999-2004. Environ Health Perspect 119:397, 2011

Lykke JA, Dideriksen KL, Lidegaard Ø, et al: First-trimester vaginal bleeding and complications later in pregnancy. Obstet Gynecol 115:935, 2010

MacIsaac L, Darney P: Early surgical abortion: an alternative to and backup for medical abortion. Am J Obstet Gynecol 183:S76, 2000

Maconochie N, Doyle P, Prior S, et al: Risk factors for first trimester miscarriage—results from a UK-population-based case-control study. BJOG 114:170, 2007

Männistö T, Vääräsmäki M, Pouta A, et al: Perinatal outcome of children born to mothers with thyroid dysfunction or antibodies: a prospective population-based cohort study. J Clin Endocrinol Metab 94:772, 2009

Masch RJ, Roman AS: Uterine evacuation in the office. Contemp Obstet Gynecol 51:66-73, 2005

Mazze RI, Källén B: Reproductive outcome after anesthesia and operation during pregnancy: a registry study of 5405 cases. Am J Obstet Gynecol 161:1178, 1989

Meites E, Zane S, Gould C: Fatal *Clostridium sordellii* infections after medical abortions. N Engl J Med 363(14):1382, 2010

Meroni PL, Tedesco F, Locati M, et al: Anti-phospholipid antibody mediated fetal loss: still an open question from a pathogenic point of view. Lupus 19:453, 2010

Miyakis S, Lockshin MD, Atsumi T, et al: International consensus statement on an update of the classification criteria for definite antiphospholipid syndrome (APS). J Thromb Haemost 4:295, 2006

Mills JL, Simpson JL, Driscoll SG, et al: Incidence of spontaneous abortion among normal women and insulin-dependent diabetic women whose pregnancies were identified within 21 days of conception. N Engl J Med 319:1618, 1988

Moore KL: The Developing Human: Clinically Oriented Embryology, 2nd ed. Philadelphia, WB Saunders, 1977

Moore S, Ide M, Coward PY, et al: A prospective study to investigate the relationship between periodontal disease and adverse pregnancy outcome. Br Dent J 197:251, 2004

Moreau C, Kaminski M, Ancel PY, et al: Previous induced abortions and the risk of very preterm delivery: results of the EPIPAGE study. BJOG 112:430, 2005

Moschos E, Twickler DM: Intrauterine devices in early pregnancy: findings on ultrasound and clinical outcomes. Am J Obstet Gynecol 204:427.e1, 2011

Nahum GG: Uterine anomalies. How common are they, and what is their distribution among subtypes? J Reprod Med 43(10):877, 1998

Nawaz FH, Rizvi J: Continuation of metformin reduces early pregnancy loss in obese Pakistani women with polycystic ovarian syndrome. Gynecol Obstet Invest 69(3):184, 2010

Negro R, Formoso G, Mangieri T, et al: Levothyroxine treatment in euthyroid pregnant women with autoimmune thyroid disease: effects on obstetrical complications. J Clin Endocrinol Metab 91(7):2587, 2006

Negro R, Schwartz A, Gismondi R, et al: Universal screening versus case finding for detection and treatment of thyroid hormonal dysfunction during pregnancy. J Clin Endocrinol Metab 95(4):1699, 2010

Neilson JP, Gyte GM, Hickey M, et al: Medical treatments for incomplete miscarriage (less than 24 weeks). Cochrane Database Syst Rev 1:CD007223, 2010

Nguyen NT, Blum J, Durocher J, et al: A randomized controlled study comparing 600 versus 1200 μg oral misoprostol for medical management of incomplete abortion. Contraception 72:438, 2005

Niinimäki M, Pouta A, Bloigu A, et al: Immediate complications after medical compared with surgical termination of pregnancy. Obstet Gynecol 114:795, 2009

Nyberg DA, Mack LA, Laing FC, et al: Distinguishing normal from abnormal gestational sac growth in early pregnancy. J Ultrasound Med 6(1):23, 1987

Oakeshott P, Hay P, Hay S, et al: Association between bacterial vaginosis or chlamydial infection and miscarriage before 16 weeks' gestation: prospective, community based cohort study. BMJ 325:1334, 2002

Oppegaard KS, Qvigstad E, Hesheim BI: Oral versus self-administered vaginal misoprostol at home before surgical termination of pregnancy: a randomized controlled trial. BJOG 113:58, 2006

Osser S, Persson K: Chlamydial antibodies in women who suffer miscarriage. Br J Obstet Gynaecol 103:137, 1996

Palomba S, Falbo A, Orio F Jr, et al: Effect of preconceptional metformin on abortion risk in polycystic ovary syndrome: a systematic review and meta-analysis of randomized controlled trials. Fertil Steril 92(5):1646, 2009

Paukku M, Tulppala M, Puolakkainen M, et al: Lack of association between serum antibodies to Chlamydia trachomatis and a history of recurrent pregnancy loss. Fertil Steril 72:427, 1999

Paul ME, Mitchell CM, Rogers AJ, et al: Early surgical abortion: efficacy and safety. Am J Obstet Gynecol 187:407, 2002

Platteau P, Staessen C, Michiels A, et al: Preimplantation genetic diagnosis for aneuploidy screening in patients with unexplained recurrent miscarriages. Fertil Steril 83(2):393, 2005

Poland B, Miller J, Jones D, et al: Reproductive counseling in patients who have had a spontaneous abortion. Am J Obstet Gynecol 127:685, 1977

Porter TF, LaCoursiere Y, Scott JR: Immunotherapy for recurrent miscarriage. Cochrane Database Syst Rev 2:CD000112, 2006

Pymar HC, Creinin MD, Schwartz JL: Mifepristone followed on the same day by vaginal misoprostol for early abortion. Contraception 64:87, 2001

Quinn PA, Shewchuck AB, Shuber J, et al: Efficacy of antibiotic therapy in preventing spontaneous pregnancy loss among couples colonized with genital mycoplasmas. Am J Obstet Gynecol 145:239, 1983a

Quinn PA, Shewchuck AB, Shuber J, et al: Serologic evidence of Ureaplasma urealyticum infection in women with spontaneous pregnancy loss. Am J Obstet Gynecol 145:245, 1983b

Raghavan S, Comendant R, Digol I, et al: Two-pill regimens of misoprostol after mifepristone medical abortion through 63 days' gestational age: a randomized controlled trial of sublingual and oral misoprostol. Contraception 79(2):84, 2009

Rai R, Cohen H, Dave M: Randomised controlled trial of aspirin and aspirin plus heparin in pregnant women with recurrent miscarriage associated with phospholipid antibodies (or antiphospholipid antibodies). BMJ 314:253, 1997

Rajcan-Separovic E, Diego-Alvarez D, Robinson WP: Identification of copy number variants in miscarriages from couples with idiopathic recurrent pregnancy loss. Hum Reprod 25(11):2913, 2010

Ramzy AM, Sattar M, Amin Y, et al: Uterine myomata and outcome of assisted reproduction. Hum Reprod 13:198, 1998

Rand JH, Wu XX, Quinn AS, et al: The annexin A5-mediated pathogenic mechanism in the antiphospholipid syndrome: role in pregnancy losses and thrombosis. Lupus 19(4):460, 2010

Rasch V: Cigarette, alcohol, and caffeine consumption: risk factors for spontaneous abortion. Acta Obstet Gynecol Scand 82:182, 2003

Reddy UM: Recurrent pregnancy loss: nongenetic causes. Contemp OB Gynecol 52:63, 2007

Reichman DE, Laufer MR: Congenital uterine anomalies affecting reproduction. Best Pract Res Clin Obstet Gynecol 24(2):193, 2010

Robson SC, Kelly T, Howel D, et al: Randomised preference trial of medical versus surgical termination of pregnancy less than 14 weeks' gestation (TOPS). Health Technol Assess 13(53):1, 2009

Rodger MA, Paidas M, McLintock C, et al: Inherited thrombophilia and pregnancy complications revisited. Obstet Gynecol 112:320, 2008

Rowland AS, Baird DD, Shore DL, et al: Nitrous oxide and spontaneous abortion in female dental assistants. Am J Epidemiol 141:531, 1995

Rushworth FH, Backos M, Rai R, et al: Prospective pregnancy outcome in untreated recurrent miscarriages with thyroid autoantibodies. Hum Reprod 15:1637, 2000

Said JM, Higgins JR, Moses EK, et al: Inherited thrombophilia polymorphisms and pregnancy outcomes in nulliparous women. Obstet Gynecol 115(1):5, 2010

Salem HT, Ghaneimah SA, Shaaban MM, et al: Prognostic value of biochemical tests in the assessment of fetal outcome in threatened abortion. Br J Obstet Gynaecol 91:382, 1984

Salim R, Regan L, Woelfer B, et al: A comparative study of the morphology of congenital uterine anomalies in women with and without a history of recurrent first trimester miscarriage. Hum Reprod 18:162, 2003

Saraswat L, Bhattacharya S, Maheshwari A, et al: Maternal and perinatal outcome in women with threatened miscarriage in the first trimester: a systematic review. BJOG 117:245, 2010

Saravelos SH, Cocksedge KA, Li TC: Prevalence and diagnosis of congenital uterine anomalies in women with reproductive failure: a critical appraisal. Hum Reprod Update 14(5):415, 2008

Satpathy HK, Fleming A, Frey D, et al: Maternal obesity and pregnancy. Postgrad Med 120(3):E01, 2008

Sauerwein RW, Bisseling J, Horrevorts AM: Septic abortion associated with Campylobacter fetus subspecies fetus infection: case report and review of the literature. Infection 21:33, 1993

Savitz DA, Chan RL, Herring AH, et al: Caffeine and miscarriage risk. Epidemiology 19:55, 2008

Saygili-Yilmaz E, Yildiz S, Erman-Akar M, et al: Reproductive outcome of septate uterus after hysteroscopic metroplasty. Arch Gynecol Obstet 4:289, 2003

Saygili-Yilmaz ES, Erman-Akar M, Yildiz S, et al: A retrospective study on the reproductive outcome of the septate uterus corrected by hysteroscopic metroplasty. Int J Gynaecol Obstet 1:59, 2002

Schaff EA, Fielding SL, Westhoff C, et al: Vaginal misoprostol administered 1, 2, or 3 days after mifepristone for early medical abortion. A randomized trial. JAMA 284:1948, 2000

Schneider D, Golan A, Langer R, et al: Outcome of continued pregnancies after first and second trimester cervical dilatation by laminaria tents. Obstet Gynecol 78:1121, 1991

Schnorr TM, Grajewski BA, Hornung RW, et al: Video display terminals and the risk of spontaneous abortion. N Engl J Med 324:727, 1991

Schust D, Hill J: Recurrent pregnancy loss. In Berek J (eds): Novak's Gynecology, 13th ed. Philadelphia, Lippincott Williams & Wilkins, 2002

Scifres CM, Macones GA: The utility of thrombophilia testing in pregnant women with thrombosis: fact or fiction? Am J Obstet Gynecol 199:344.e1, 2008

Scott JR: Immunotherapy for recurrent miscarriage. Cochrane Database Syst Rev 2:CD000112, 2003

Seely EW, Ecker J: Clinical practice. Chronic hypertension in pregnancy. N Engl J Med 365(5):439, 2011

Shah PS, Zao J, Knowledge Synthesis Group of Determinants of Preterm/LBW Births: Induced termination of pregnancy and low birthweight and preterm birth: a systematic review and meta-analyses. BJOG 116(11):1425, 2009

Shannon C, Wiebe E, Jacot F: Regimens of misoprostol with mifepristone for early medical abortion: a randomized trial. BJOG 113:621, 2006

Sher KS, Jayanthi V, Probert CS, et al: Infertility, obstetric and gynaecological problems in coeliac sprue. Digest Dis 12:186, 1994

Shwekerela B, Kalumuna R, Kipingili R, et al: Misoprostol for treatment of incomplete abortion at the regional hospital level: results for Tanzania. BJOG 114(11):1363, 2007

Silver RM, Zhao Y, Spong CY, et al: Eunice Shriver National Institute of Child Health and Human Development Maternal-Fetal Medicine Units (NICHD-MFMU) Network. Prothrombin gene G20210A mutation and obstetric complications. Obstet Gynecol 115(1):14, 2010

Simpson JL: Causes of fetal wastage. Clin Obstet Gynecol 50(1):10, 2007

Simpson JL: Genes, chromosomes, and reproductive failure. Fertil Steril 33(2):107, 1980

Simpson JL, Mills JL, Kim H, et al: Infectious processes: an infrequent cause of first trimester spontaneous abortions. Hum Reprod 11:668, 1996

Smith LF, Ewings PD, Guinlan C: Incidence of pregnancy after expectant, medical, or surgical management of spontaneous first trimester miscarriage: long term follow-up of miscarriage treatment (MIST) randomized controlled trial. BMJ 339:b3827, 2009

Soh MC, Nelson-Piercy C: Antiphospholipid antibody syndrome in pregnancy. Expert Rev Obstet Gynecol 5(6):741, 2010

Sollid CP, Wisborg K, Hjort JH, et al: Eating disorder that was diagnosed before pregnancy and pregnancy outcome. Am J Obstet Gynecol 190:206, 2004

Soni S, Badawy SZA: Celiac disease and its effect on human reproduction: a review. J Reprod Med 55:3, 2010

Speroff L, Fritz MA (eds): Recurrent early pregnancy loss. In Clinical Gynecologic Endocrinology and Infertility, 7th ed. Philadelphia, Lippincott, Williams & Wilkins, 2005, p 1093

Stanger JD, Yovich JL: Reduced in-vitro fertilization of human oocytes from patients with raised basal luteinizing hormone levels during the follicular phase. Br J Obstet Gynaecol 92:385, 1985

Stein Z, Kline J, Susser E, et al: Maternal age and spontaneous abortion. In Porter IH, Hook EB (eds): Human Embryonic and Fetal Death. New York, Academic Press, 1980, p 107

Steinauer J, Darney P, Auerbach RD: Should all residents be trained to do abortions? Contemp Obstet Gynecol 51:56, 2005a

Steinauer J, Drey EA, Lewis R, et al: Obstetrics and gynecology resident satisfaction with an integrated, comprehensive abortion rotation. Obstet Gynecol 105:1335, 2005b

Stephenson MD: Management of recurrent early pregnancy loss. J Reprod Med 51:303, 2006

Stephenson MD, Kutteh WH, Purkiss S, et al: Intravenous immunoglobulin and idiopathic secondary recurrent miscarriage: a multicentered randomized placebo-controlled trial. Hum Reprod 25(9):2203, 2010

Streeter GL: Focal deficiencies in fetal tissues and their relation to intra-uterine amputation. Carnegie Institute of Washington, 1930, Publication No. 414, p 5

Sullivan AE, Silver RM, LaCoursiere DY, et al: Recurrent fetal aneuploidy and recurrent miscarriage. Obstet Gynecol 104:784, 2004

Sunkara SK, Khairy M, El-Toukhy T, et al: The effect of intramural fibroids without uterine cavity involvement on the outcome of IVF treatment: a systematic review and meta-analysis. Hum Reprod 25(2):418, 2010

Supreme Court of the United States: Jane Roe et al v Henry Wade, District Attorney of Dallas County. Opinion No. 70-18, January 22, 1973

Supreme Court of the United States: Gonzales, Attorney General v. Carhart, et al. Certiorari to the United States Court of Appeals for the Eighth Circuit. Opinion No. 05–380, April 18, 2007

Supreme Court of the United States: Planned Parenthood v. Casey. Certiorari to the United States Court of Appeals for the Third Circuit. Opinion No. 91-744, June 29, 1992

Taskinen H, Kyyrönen P, Hemminki K: Effects of ultrasound, shortwaves, and physical exertion on pregnancy outcome in physiotherapists. J Epidemiol Community Health 44:196, 1990

Tatum HJ, Schmidt FH, Jain AK: Management and outcome of pregnancies associated with Copper-T intrauterine contraceptive device. Am J Obstet Gynecol 126:869, 1976

Temmerman M, Lopita MI, Sanghvi HC, et al: The role of maternal syphilis, gonorrhoea and HIV-1 infections in spontaneous abortion. Int J STD AIDS 3:418, 1992

Tharapel AT, Tharapel SA, Bannerman RM: Recurrent pregnancy losses and parental chromosome abnormalities: a review. Br J Obstet Gynecol 92:899, 1985

Timor-Tritsch IE, Farine D, Rosen MG: A close look at early embryonic development with the high-frequency transvaginal transducer. Am J Obstet Gynecol 159(3):676, 1988

Tongsong T, Srisomboon J, Wanapirak C, et al: Pregnancy outcome of threatened abortion with demonstrable fetal cardiac activity: a cohort study. J Obstet Gynaecol 21:331, 1995

Trinder J, Brocklehurst P, Porter R, et al: Management of miscarriage: expectant, medical, or surgical? Results of randomized controlled trial (miscarriage treatment (MIST) trial). BMJ 332(7552):1235, 2006

Tulppala M, Stenman UH, Cacciatore B, et al: Polycystic ovaries and levels of gonadotrophins and androgens in recurrent miscarriage: prospective study in 50 women. Br J Obstet Gynaecol 100:348, 1993

Valli E, Zupi E, Marconi D, et al: Hysteroscopic findings in 344 women with recurrent spontaneous abortion. J Am Assoc Gynecol Laparosc 8(3):398, 2001

van Benthem BH, de Vincenzi I, Delmas MD, et al: Pregnancies before and after HIV diagnosis in a European cohort of HIV-infected women. European study on the natural history of HIV infection in women. AIDS 14:2171, 2000

van den Boogaard E, Kaandorp SP, Franssen MT, et al: Consecutive or non-consecutive recurrent miscarriage: is there any difference in carrier status? Hum Reprod 25(6):1411, 2010

Vartian CV, Septimus EJ: Tricuspid valve group B streptococcal endocarditis following elective abortion. Rev Infect Dis 13:997, 1991

Ventura SJ, Abma JC, Mosher WD, et al: Estimated pregnancy rates by outcome for the United States, 1990-2004. Natl Vit Stat Rep 56(15), April 14, 2008

Virk J, Zhang J, Olsen J: Medical abortion and the risk of subsequent adverse pregnancy outcomes. N Engl J Med 16;357(7):648, 2007

von Hertzen H, Honkanen H, Piaggio G, et al: WHO multinational study of three misoprostol regimens after mifepristone for early medical abortion. I: Efficacy. BJOG 110:808, 2003

von Hertzen H, Huong NTM, Piaggio G, et al: Misoprostol dose and route after mifepristone for early medical abortion: a randomized controlled non-inferiority trial. BJOG 117(10):1186, 2010

von Hertzen H, Piaggio G, Huong NT, et al: Efficacy of two intervals and two routes of administration of misoprostol for termination of early pregnancy: a randomised controlled equivalence trial. Lancet 369(9577):1938, 2007

von Hertzen H, Piaggio G, Wojdyla D, et al: Two mifepristone doses and two intervals of misoprostol administration for termination of early pregnancy: a randomized factorial controlled equivalence trial. BJOG 116(3):381, 2009

Wacholder S, Chen BE, Wilcox A, et al: Risk of miscarriage with bivalent vaccine against human papillomavirus (HPV) types 16 and 18: pooled analysis of two randomized controlled trials. BMJ 340:c712, 2010

Warburton D, Fraser FC: Spontaneous abortion risks in man: data from reproductive histories collected in a medical genetics unit. Am J Hum Genet 16:1, 1964

Warburton D, Stein Z, Kline J, et al: Chromosome abnormalities in spontaneous abortion: data from the New York City study. In Porter IH, Hook EB (eds): Human Embryonic and Fetal Death. New York, Academic Press, 1980, p 261

Warren JB, Silver RM: Autoimmune disease in pregnancy: systemic lupus erythematosus and antiphospholipid syndrome. Obstet Gynecol Clin North Am 31:345, 2004

Watson H, Kiddy DS, Hamilton-Fairley D, et al: Hypersecretion of luteinizing hormone and ovarian steroids in women with recurrent early miscarriages. Hum Reprod 8:829, 1993

Weiss J, Malone F, Vidaver J, et al: Threatened abortion: a risk factor for poor pregnancy outcome—a population based screening study (The FASTER Trial). Am J Obstet Gynecol 187:S70, 2002

Weng X, Odouki R, Li DK: Maternal caffeine consumption during pregnancy and the risk of miscarriage: a prospective cohort study. Am J Obstet Gynecol 198:279.e1, 2008

Westfall JM, Sophocles A, Burggraf H, et al: Manual vacuum aspiration for first-trimester abortion. Arch Fam Med 7:559, 1998

Wijesiriwardana A, Bhattacharya S, Shetty A, et al: Obstetric outcome in women with threatened miscarriage in the first trimester. Obstet Gynecol 107:557, 2006

Wilcox AF, Weinberg CR, O'Connor JF, et al: Incidence of early loss of pregnancy. N Engl J Med 319:189, 1988

Wilson RD, Kendrick V, Wittmann BK, et al: Spontaneous abortion and pregnancy outcome after normal first-trimester ultrasound examination. Obstet Gynecol 67:352, 1986

Winikoff B, Dzuba IG, Creinin MD, et al: Two distinct oral routes of misoprostol in mifepristone medical abortion: a randomized controlled trial. Obstet Gynecol 112(6):1303, 2008

Wisborg K, Kesmodel U, Henriksen TB, et al: A prospective study of maternal smoking and spontaneous abortion. Acta Obstet Gynecol Scand 82:936, 2003

Wo JY, Viswanathan AN: Impact of radiotherapy on fertility, pregnancy, and neonatal outcomes in female cancer patients. Int J Radiat Oncol Biol Phys 73(5):1304, 2009

Xiong X, Buekens P, Vastardis S, et al: Periodontal disease and pregnancy outcomes: state-of-the-science. Obstet Gynecol Surv 62(9):605, 2007

Yetman DL, Kutteh WH: Antiphospholipid antibody panels and recurrent pregnancy loss: prevalence of anticardiolipin antibodies compared with other antiphospholipid antibodies. Fertil Steril 66:540, 1996

Zhang J, Gilles JM, Barnhart K, et al: A comparison of medical management with misoprostol and surgical management for early pregnancy failure. N Engl J Med 353:761, 2005

Ziakas PD, Pavlou M, Voulgarelis M: Heparin treatment in antiphospholipid syndrome with recurrent pregnancy loss: a systematic review and meta-analysis. Obstet Gynecol 115(6):1256, 2010

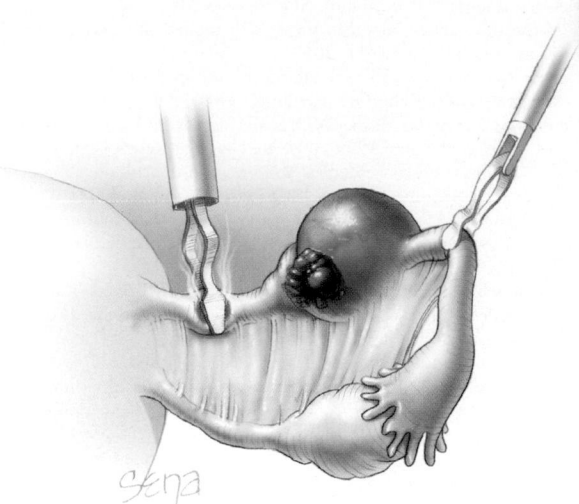

CHAPTER 7

Ectopic Pregnancy

An ectopic or extrauterine pregnancy is one in which the blastocyst implants anywhere other than the endometrial lining of the uterine cavity. As such, they account for 1 to 2 percent of reported pregnancies in the United States (Zane, 2002). With the advent of a sensitive and specific radioimmunoassay for the β-subunit of human chorionic gonadotropin (β-hCG), combined with high-resolution transvaginal sonography (TVS), the initial presentation of a woman with an ectopic pregnancy is seldom as life-threatening as in the past. Nevertheless, ectopic pregnancies remain an important cause of morbidity and mortality in the United States.

CLASSIFICATION

Nearly 95 percent of ectopic pregnancies implant in the fallopian tube. Shown in Figure 7-1 are implantation sites for 1800 surgically treated ectopic pregnancies (Bouyer, 2002). Bilateral ectopic pregnancies are rare, and their estimated prevalence is 1 of every 200,000 pregnancies (al-Awwad, 1999).

EPIDEMIOLOGY

Reported ectopic pregnancy incidence rates are not as reliable as in the past. The dramatic improvements in diagnosis and outpatient treatment protocols render national hospital discharge statistics invalid. According to the Centers for Disease Control and Prevention (1995), the rate of ectopic pregnancy has increased in the United States nearly fourfold from 4.5 per 1000 pregnancies in 1970 to 19.7 per 1000 pregnancies in 1992. This rate is similar to recent estimates by Kaiser Permanente of North California of 20.7 per 1000 pregnancies from 1997 to 2000 (Van Den Eeden, 2005). More recently, Hoover and colleagues (2010) queried a large claims database for women aged 15 to 44 who were privately insured in the United States between 2002 and 2007 and calculated a rate of 6.4 per 1000 pregnancies. However, this reported reduction in ectopic pregnancy rate may not accurately reflect the cases occurring in higher-risk, lower-socioeconomic, uninsured populations.

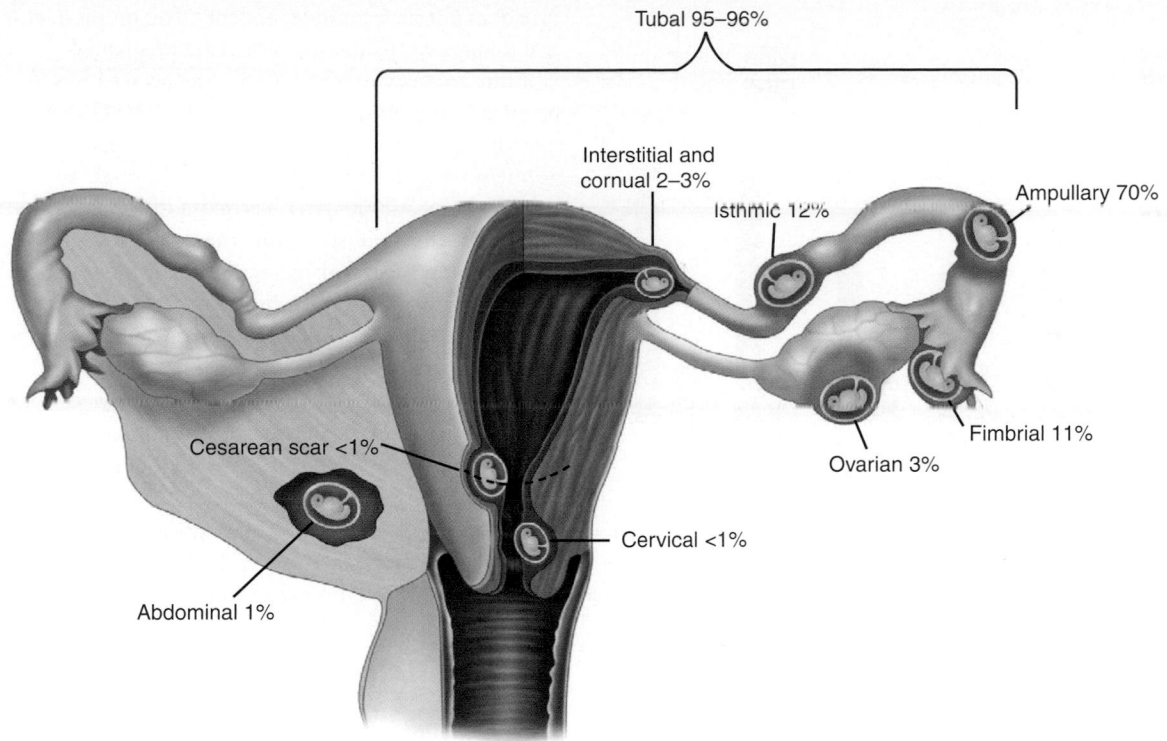

Tubal 95–96%

Interstitial and
cornual 2–3%

Isthmic 12%

Ampullary 70%

Cesarean scar <1%

Fimbrial 11%

Ovarian 3%

Cervical <1%

Abdominal 1%

FIGURE 7-1 Various sites and frequency of ectopic pregnancies. *(From Cunningham, 2010, with permission.)*

A number of factors help to explain the increased incidence of ectopic pregnancies:

1. Greater prevalence of sexually transmitted diseases, specifically chlamydial infections (Rajkhowa, 2000)
2. Diagnostic tools with improved sensitivity
3. Tubal factor infertility, including restoration of tubal patency or documented tubal pathology (Ankum, 1996)
4. Women with delayed childbearing and their accompanied use of assisted reproductive technologies, which carry increased risks of ectopic pregnancy
5. Increased intrauterine device (IUD) use and tubal sterilization, which predispose to ectopic pregnancy with method failure (Mol, 1995).

ECTOPIC PREGNANCY SEQUELAE

Mortality

Ectopic pregnancy remains the leading cause of early pregnancy-related death. Still, current diagnostic and treatment protocols have resulted in a 10-fold decline in the case fatality rate during the past 35 years. The rate in 1970 was 35 deaths per 10,000 ectopic pregnancies compared with 4 per 10,000 in 1989. This was despite the fivefold increase in ectopic pregnancy rates from 17,800 in 1970 to 108,000 in 1992 (Fig. 7-2). Racial disparities affect ectopic pregnancy-related deaths. Nonwhite women had an overall risk of death 3.4 times higher than white women for the 20-year period from 1970 to 1989 (Goldner, 1993). This was so for all age groups as shown in Figure 7-3. Inadequate access to gynecologic and prenatal care may partially explain this trend.

Tubal Rupture

Mortality is directly related to severe hemorrhage from tubal rupture. During the past two decades,

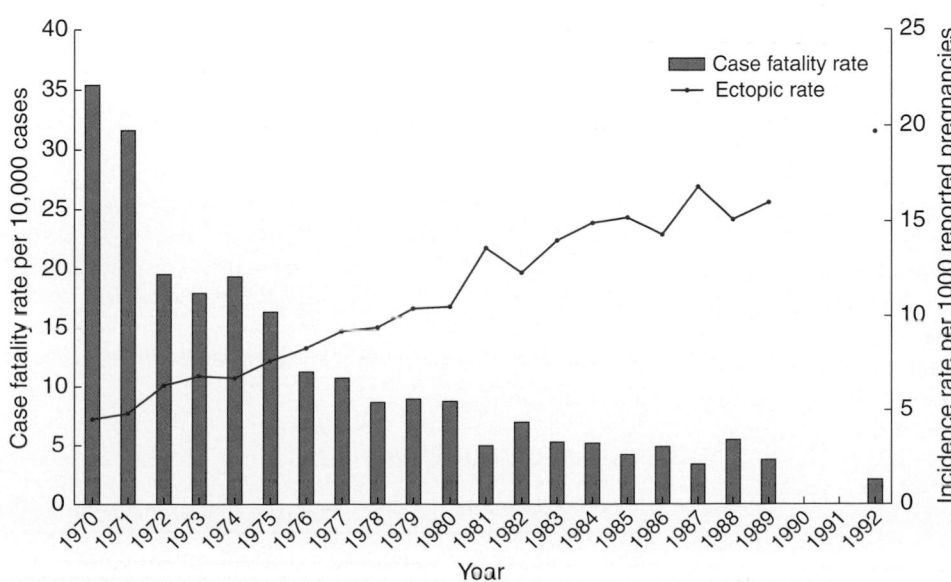

FIGURE 7-2 Case fatality rate and incidence of ectopic pregnancy by year. *(Data from the Centers for Disease Control and Prevention, 1995.)*

SECTION 1

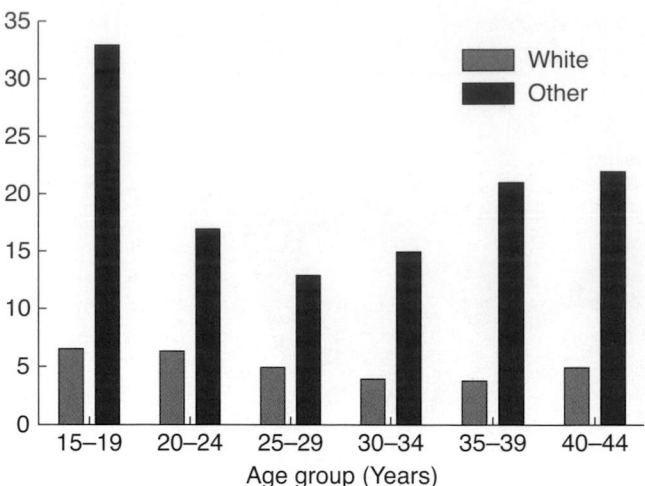

*Per 10,000 ectopic pregnancies.

FIGURE 7-3 Case-fatality rates for ectopic pregnancy by race and age in the United States, 1970–1989. *(From Goldner, 1993, with permission.)*

the rupture rate with ectopic pregnancy ranged from 20 to 35 percent (Job-Spira, 1999; Saxon, 1997). Three risk factors that increase the likelihood of tubal rupture include ovulation induction, serum β-hCG level exceeding 10,000 IU/L when ectopic pregnancy is first suspected, and history of never having used contraception. Appreciation of these risk factors aids a timely diagnosis and prompt surgical intervention. Importantly, minimally invasive treatment options are limited in hemodynamically unstable patients following tubal rupture.

There may be a difference between an "acute" and a "chronic" ectopic pregnancy in regard to risk of tubal rupture. Acute ectopic pregnancies are those with a high serum β-hCG level at presentation and rapid growth leading to an immediate diagnosis. These carry a higher risk of tubal rupture compared with chronic ectopic pregnancies, which demonstrate static or negative serum β-hCG levels (Barnhart, 2003c). Theoretically, an acute ectopic pregnancy has healthy growing trophoblasts that do not result in early bleeding, and women thus present for care later. This is compared with the chronic variety in which minor repeated ruptures or tubal abortion incites an inflammatory response that leads to formation of a pelvic mass. Abnormal trophoblasts die early, and thus lower or negative serum β-hCG levels are found (Brennan, 2000).

Timing of tubal rupture is partially dependent on pregnancy location. As a rule, tubes rupture earlier if implantation is in the isthmic or ampullary portion of the fallopian tube. Later rupture is seen if the ovum implants within the interstitial portion. Rupture is usually spontaneous, but can also be caused by trauma such as that associated from bimanual pelvic examination or coitus.

Tubal Damage

Ultimately, there does not seem to be a direct correlation between tubal damage and long-term prognosis for subsequent pregnancy. Job-Spira and colleagues (1999) reported that rup-

ture does not have an independent effect on the 1-year cumulative frequency of subsequent uterine pregnancy.

Elito and coworkers (2005) prospectively evaluated tubal patency using hysterosalpingography (HSG) after conservative therapy for ectopic pregnancies—either expectant management or systemic methotrexate. Although an initial serum β-hCG level >5000 IU/L carried a 12-fold increased risk of subsequent tubal obstruction, there was no relationship with obstruction and size of the ectopic mass or sonographic landmarks such as tubal ring using color flow Doppler.

Guven and associates (2007) reported a case series of 61 patients with unruptured tubal ectopic pregnancy treated with single or multidose methotrexate. The primary outcome was HSG-proven obstruction rates in the ipsilateral and contralateral fallopian tube. Interestingly, they observed an ipsilateral tubal patency rate of 84 percent in the single-dose group and only 57 percent in the multidose group. They speculated that multidose methotrexate was linked to a higher potential for tubal damage through unclear mechanisms.

RISK FACTORS

An appreciation of risk factors for ectopic pregnancy may lead to a more timely diagnosis. As summarized in Table 7-1, documented tubal pathology, surgery to restore tubal patency, or tubal sterilization carry the highest risks of obstruction and subsequent ectopic pregnancy. A woman with two prior ectopic pregnancies has a 10-fold chance for another (Skjeldestad, 1998).

TABLE 7-1. Risk Factors for Ectopic Pregnancy

Factor	Odds Ratio (95% CI)
Prior ectopic pregnancy	12.5 (7.5, 20.9)
Prior tubal surgery	4.0 (2.6, 6.1)
Smoking >20 cigarettes per day	3.5 (1.4, 8.6)
Prior STD with confirmed PID by laparoscopy and/or positive test for *Chlamydia trachomatis*	3.4 (2.4, 5.0)
Three or more prior spontaneous miscarriages	3.0 (1.3, 6.9)
Age ≥40 years	2.9 (1.4, 6.1)
Prior medical or surgical abortion	2.8 (1.1, 7.2)
Infertility >1 year	2.6 (1.6, 4.2)
Lifelong sexual partners >5	1.6 (1.2, 2.1)
Previous IUD use	1.3 (1.0, 1.8)

IUD = intrauterine device; PID = pelvic inflammatory disease; STD = sexually transmitted disease.
Data from Bouyer, 2003; Buster, 1999.

Smoking, which may be a surrogate marker for sexually transmitted infections, increases the risk of ectopic pregnancy three- to fourfold in women who smoke more than one pack of cigarettes daily (Saraiya, 1998). In addition, there is evidence through animal studies that the fallopian tube is directly affected by cigarette smoke. Smoking alters oocyte cumulus complex pick-up and embryo transport through its effects on ciliary function and smooth muscle contraction (Shaw, 2010; Talbot, 2005).

The use of assisted reproductive technology for sub- or infertile couples has a 0.8-percent incidence of ectopic pregnancy per transfer and 2.2-percent per clinical pregnancy (Coste, 2000). Procedures leading to the highest rates are gamete intrafallopian transfer (3.7 percent), cryopreserved embryo transfer (3.2 percent), and in vitro fertilization (IVF) (2.2 percent) (American Society for Reproductive Medicine and Society for Reproductive Technology, 2002). In women undergoing IVF, the main risk factors for ectopic pregnancy are tubal factor infertility and hydrosalpinges (Strandell, 1999; Van Voorhis, 2006). Moreover, "atypical" implantation—interstitial, abdominal, cervical, ovarian, or heterotopic—is more common following assisted reproductive procedures. A heterotopic pregnancy is an intrauterine pregnancy coexistent with an extrauterine pregnancy.

Women aged 35 to 44 years have a threefold risk of ectopic pregnancy compared with those aged 15 to 25 years (Goldner, 1993). These have been attributed to age-related hormonal changes that alter tubal function (Coste, 2000).

Most forms of contraception lower overall pregnancy rates and thereby lower ectopic pregnancy rates. However, if pregnancy does occur, some methods increase the relative incidence of ectopic pregnancy. For example, a conception with an IUD in place is more often ectopic than a pregnancy with no IUD (Iavazzo, 2008). The levonorgestrel-releasing intrauterine system (LNG-IUS), marketed as Mirena, has a 5-year cumulative pregnancy rate of 0.5 per 100 users, of which half are ectopic (Backman, 2004). Progestin-only contraceptive pills have a slightly increased rate because of their effects to diminish tubal motility. Tubal sterilization can be followed by an ectopic pregnancy. This risk is doubled in women younger than 30 years at the time of sterilization, partially because of age-related fecundity. Tubal bipolar electrosurgical coagulation has failure rates of 32 per 1000 procedures compared with puerperal partial salpingectomy, which has a rate of 1.2 per 1000 procedures (Peterson, 1997).

Prior conservative, pharmacologically induced abortion—but not surgical termination—is associated with an increased risk for ectopic pregnancy (Bouyer, 2003; Tharaux-Deneux, 1998). Antibiotic prophylaxis at the time of abortion may have a protective effect from infection-related inflammatory tubal damage. For example, in a study by Sawaya and colleagues (1996), periprocedure antibiotics decreased the risk of upper genital tract infection by 42 percent.

PATHOPHYSIOLOGY

Histopathology

Lack of a submucosal layer within the fallopian tube provides easy access for the fertilized ovum to burrow through the epithelium and allow implantation within the muscular wall (Fig. 7-4). Moreover, absent resistance allows early trophoblast penetration. As the rapidly proliferating trophoblasts erode the subjacent muscularis layer, maternal blood pours into the spaces within the trophoblastic or the adjacent tissue.

The anatomic location of a tubal pregnancy may predict the extent of damage. Senterman and colleagues (1988) studied histologic samples from 84 isthmic and ampullary pregnancies and reported that half of the ampullary pregnancies were intraluminal, and the muscularis was preserved in 85 percent of these. Conversely, isthmic gestations were found both intra- and extraluminally with greater disruption of the tubal wall.

Inflammation

Acute inflammation has been implicated in the role of tubal damage that predisposes to ectopic pregnancies. Chronic salpingitis and salpingitis isthmica nodosa also have important roles in ectopic pregnancy development (Kutluay, 1994).

Recurrent chlamydial infection causes intraluminal inflammation and subsequent fibrin deposition with tubal scarring (Hillis, 1997). Persistent chlamydial antigens can trigger a delayed hypersensitivity reaction with continued scarring despite negative culture results (Toth, 2000). Whereas endotoxin-producing *Neisseria gonorrhoeae* causes virulent pelvic inflammation that has a rapid clinical onset, chlamydial inflammatory response is chronic and peaks at 7 to 14 days.

There is now compelling evidence that inflammation within the fallopian tube can lead to arrest of the descending embryo while providing a proimplantation signal for embryos within the fallopian tube (Shaw, 2010). Oviduct interstitial cells of Cajal are specialized pacemaker cells responsible for oviduct motility and egg transport. Infections in mice by *Chlamydia muridarum*, which is similar to human *Chlamydia trachomatis*, lead to absent spontaneous pacemaker activity and may offer another explanation for how *Chlamydia* increases ectopic pregnancies in humans (Dixon, 2009).

Another factor involved with oviductal transport of embryos is the cannabinoid receptor (CB1), which is mediated by endocannabinoid signaling. Chronic exposure to nicotine can affect endocannabinoid levels and lead to fallopian tube dysfunction (Horne, 2008).

The increased tubal pregnancy rates in women using assisted reproductive technology has been a conundrum for scientists because the fallopian tube is typically bypassed. Revel and colleagues (2008) sought to establish the relationship between E-cadherin, an adhesion molecule, and tubal ectopic pregnancy implantation sites. They found E-cadherin strongly localized to the tubal embryo implantation site only in women who underwent IVF. This suggests a biologic rather than mechanical factor accounting for the ectopic pregnancies associated with IVF.

CLINICAL MANIFESTATIONS

Symptoms

As women seek care earlier, the ability to diagnose ectopic pregnancy before rupture—even before the onset of symptoms—is not unusual. Despite the classic symptoms of amenorrhea followed by vaginal bleeding and abdominal pain on

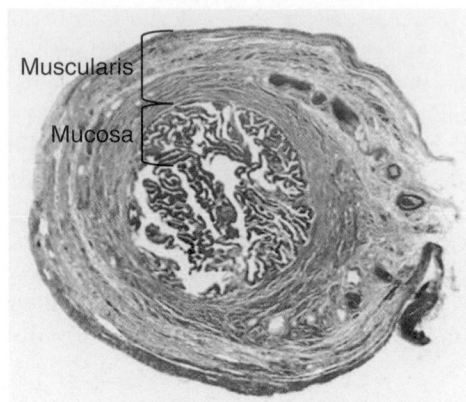

A   Normal fallopian tube

FIGURE 7-4 Photomicrograph of fallopian tubes. **A.** Normal ampullary portion of a fallopian tube at lower magnification. *(Photograph contributed by Dr. Kelley Carrick.)* **B.** Ectopic tubal pregnancy. At higher magnification, chorionic villi *(arrows)* can be seen within the tubal lumen. An area of hemorrhage is seen between the villi and the tubal mucosa. *(Photograph contributed by Dr. Raheela Ashfaq.)*

the affected side, there is no constellation of symptoms that secures the diagnosis with reliability (Dart, 1999). Other pregnancy discomforts such as breast tenderness, nausea, and urinary frequency may accompany more ominous findings. These include shoulder pain worsened by inspiration, which is caused by phrenic nerve irritation from subdiaphragmatic blood, or vasomotor disturbances such as vertigo and syncope from hemorrhagic hypovolemia.

Many women with a small unruptured ectopic pregnancy have unremarkable clinical findings. Nevertheless, the diagnosis should be considered strongly when any of the foregoing symptoms are reported by reproductive-aged women, especially those with risk factors for extrauterine pregnancy.

Rarely, ectopic pregnancies have been the source of abdominal pain in women who previously underwent hysterectomy (Fylstra, 2009). Presumably, postoperative fistulous connections allow sperm to access an ovulated ovum. Possibilities include a non-obliterated cervical stump after supracervical hysterectomy, fistula following vaginal cuff infection, or prolapsed fallopian tube.

■ Clinical Findings

Vital Signs

Although some women have orthostatic findings, normal vital signs are unreliable to exclude a ruptured ectopic pregnancy. Birkhahn and associates (2003) employed the shock index to evaluate the possibility of ruptured ectopic pregnancy. This

index reflects heart rate divided by systolic blood pressure and is used to evaluate trauma patients for hypovolemic or septic shock. The normal range lies between 0.5 and 0.7 for nonpregnant patients. These investigators reported that a shock index of >0.85 increased by 15-fold the likelihood of a ruptured ectopic pregnancy.

Abdominal and pelvic findings are notoriously scant in many women before tubal rupture. With rupture, however, nearly three fourths will have marked tenderness on both abdominal and pelvic examination, and pain is aggravated with cervical manipulation. A pelvic mass, including fullness posterolateral to the uterus, can be palpated in approximately 20 percent of women. Initially, an ectopic pregnancy may feel soft and elastic, whereas extensive hemorrhage produces a firmer consistency. Many times, discomfort precludes palpation of the mass, and limiting examinations may help avert iatrogenic rupture.

DIFFERENTIAL DIAGNOSIS

Symptoms of ectopic pregnancy can mimic multiple entities (Table 7-2). Early pregnancy complications such as threatened or missed abortion or hemorrhagic corpus luteum cyst may be difficult to differentiate (Barnhart, 2003b). Moreover, approximately 20 percent of women with normal pregnancies have early bleeding.

TABLE 7-2. Conditions That Cause Lower Abdominal Pain

Cause	Location	Characteristics	Associated Findings
Pregnancy			
Abortion	Midline or generalized	Crampy, intermittent	(+) UCG; vaginal bleeding
Ectopic	Unilateral or generalized	Crampy, continuous	(+) UCG; vaginal bleeding
Uterus and Cervix			
Endomyometritis ± Cervicitis	Lower abdominal pain	Dull, aching	Vaginal discharge, possible low-grade fever
Endometriosis	Midline	Variable; worse with certain activities and menses	Adnexal mass if endometrioma present
Degenerating leiomyoma	Variable	Sharp or aching	Irregular, enlarged, tender uterus
Adnexal Disease			
Salpingitis	Diffuse	Severe	Moderate to high fever
Tubo-ovarian abscess	Unilateral	Intermittent	Usually high fever
Adnexal torsion	Lower quadrant	Acute, sharp, sudden onset	
Corpus luteum cyst	Unilateral	Aching or sharp	(+/−) UCG
Other			
Appendicitis	Periumbilical, right lower		Anorexia, nausea, vomiting
Diverticulitis	Left lower quadrant	Crampy	Fever, bowel changes
Mesenteric lymphadenitis	Right lower quadrant		
Cystitis	Midline, suprapubic	Acute, spasms	Dysuria, frequency
Renal calculi	Flank, radiating to lower abdomen	Severe, intermittent	Hematuria

UCG = urinary chorionic gonadotropin test result.

A number of nonpregnancy-related disorders can also mimic ectopic pregnancy. In general, a positive test for β-hCG usually excludes these other diagnoses. However, these conditions may exist concurrently with pregnancy—either intrauterine or ectopic.

DIAGNOSIS

Transvaginal sonography and serial serum β-hCG measurements are the most valuable diagnostic aids to confirm clinical suspicions of an ectopic pregnancy.

Laboratory Findings
Serum β-hCG Measurements

Human chorionic gonadotropin is a glycoprotein produced by syncytiotrophoblast and can be detected in serum as early as 8 days after the luteinizing hormone (LH) surge. In normal pregnancies, serum β-hCG levels rise in a log-linear fashion until 60 or 80 days after the last menses, at which time values plateau at approximately 100,000 IU/L. Given an interassay variability of 5 to 10 percent, interpretation of serial values is more reliable when performed by the same laboratory. With a robust uterine pregnancy, serum β-hCG levels should increase at least 53 to 66 percent every 48 hours (Barnhart, 2004; Kadar, 1982). Inadequately rising

serum β-hCG levels indicate only a dying pregnancy, not its location.

Many women present with an unsure last menstrual period, and an educated guess of gestational age is made. In these cases, correlation between the serum β-hCG concentration and TVS findings becomes especially important.

Serum Progesterone Levels

Determination of serum progesterone concentration is used by some to aid ectopic pregnancy diagnosis when serum β-hCG determinations and sonographic findings are inconclusive (Carson, 1993; Stovall, 1992). There is minimal variation in serum progesterone concentration between 5 and 10 weeks' gestation, thus a single value is sufficient. Mol and colleagues (1998) performed a metaanalysis of 22 studies to assess the accuracy of a single serum progesterone level to differentiate ectopic from uterine pregnancy. They found that results were most accurate when approached from the viewpoint of *healthy versus dying pregnancy*. With serum progesterone levels of <5 ng/mL, a dying pregnancy was detected with *near perfect* specificity and with a sensitivity of 60 percent. Conversely, values of >20 ng/mL had a sensitivity of 95 percent with specificity approximating 40 percent to identify a healthy pregnancy. Ultimately, serum progesterone levels can be used to buttress a clinical impression, but *cannot* differentiate between an ectopic and uterine pregnancy.

Hemogram

Ectopic pregnancy can lead to bleeding that may be slight or brisk and that initially may not be clinically evident. Thus, a hemogram is a fast and effective initial screen. The assessment and resuscitation of those with hemorrhage is discussed fully in Chapter 40 (p. 1006).

Sonography

High-resolution sonography has revolutionized the clinical management of women with a suspected ectopic pregnancy. However, routine sonography without a clinical suspicion of ectopic pregnancy does not improve diagnostic and triage efficiency. With TVS, a gestational sac is usually visible between 4½ and 5 weeks, the yolk sac appears between 5 and 6 weeks, and a fetal pole with cardiac activity is first detected at 5½ to 6 weeks. With transabdominal sonography, these structures are visualized slightly later. The sonographic diagnosis of ectopic pregnancy rests on visualization of an adnexal mass separate from the ovary (Fig. 7-5).

When the last menstrual period is unknown, serum β-hCG testing is used to define expected sonographic findings. Each institution must define a β-hCG discriminatory value, that is, the lower limit at which an examiner can reliably visualize pregnancy. At most institutions, this value is a concentration between 1500 and 2000 IU/L. Accurate diagnosis by sonography is three times more likely if the initial β-hCG level is above this value. Technical challenges, such as hemorrhage or leiomyomas, however, can hinder the ability to accurately diagnose an intrauterine gestation even with β-hCG levels above the discriminatory value (Gurel, 2007). The absence of a uterine pregnancy when β-hCG levels are above the discriminatory value suggests an abnormal pregnancy that is an ectopic, an incomplete abortion, or a resolving completed abortion. For example, despite total passage of products of conception with complete abortion, β-hCG testing may still be positive while original β-hCG is metabolized and cleared. Conversely, sonographic findings obtained when β-hCG values lie below the discriminatory value are not diagnostic in nearly two thirds of cases (Barnhart, 1999). In these cases in which neither an intrauterine nor an extrauterine pregnancy is identified, the term *pregnancy of unknown location (PUL)* is used until additional clinical information allows determination of pregnancy location.

Systematic sonographic evaluation is critical to establish the correct diagnosis. Most begin with the endometrial cavity. In pregnancies conceived spontaneously, identification of a uterine pregnancy effectively excludes the possibility of an ectopic implantation. When assisted reproductive technologies are employed, however, careful examination of the tube and ovary is performed even with an intrauterine pregnancy because heterotopic pregnancy rates may be as high as 1 per 100 (Tal, 1996).

An intracavitary fluid collection caused by sloughing of the decidua can create a *pseudogestational sac*, or *pseudosac*. As shown in Figure 7-6, this one-layer collection lies typically in the midline of the uterine cavity. In contrast, a normal gestational sac is eccentrically located (Dashefsky, 1988). Another intracavitary finding is a trilaminar endometrial pattern, which represents two adjacent edematous proliferative-phase endometrial layers

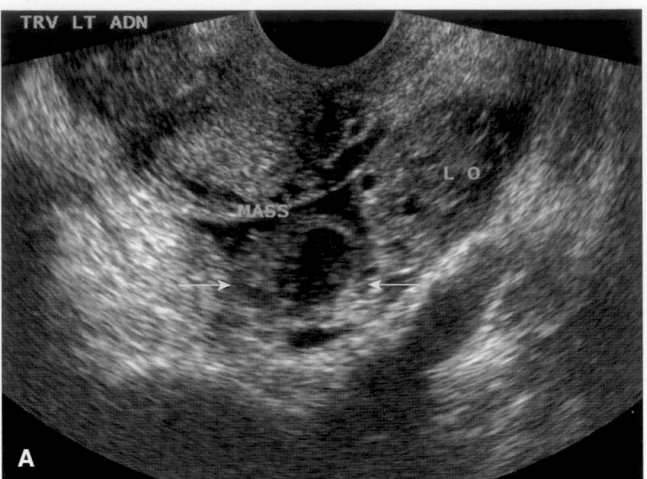

Inhomogeneous mass

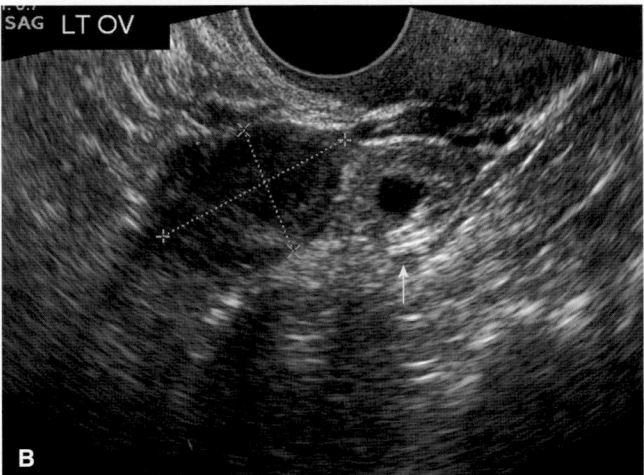

Mass with empty extrauterine sac

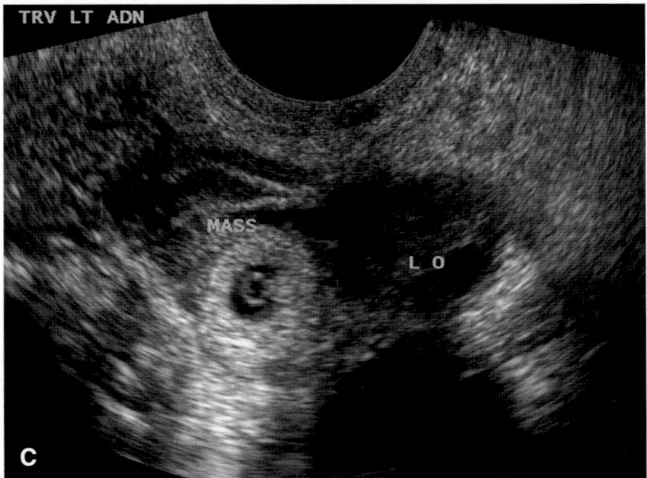

Mass with yolk sac

FIGURE 7-5 Transvaginal sonographic findings with various ectopic pregnancies. For sonographic diagnosis, an ectopic mass should be seen in the adnexa separate from the ovary and may be seen: **(A)** as an inhomogeneous adnexal mass (*yellow arrows*), **(B)** as an empty extrauterine sac with a hyperechoic ring (*arrow*), or **(C)** as a yolk sac and/or fetal pole with or without cardiac activity within an extrauterine sac. LO = left ovary. (*Images contributed by Dr. Elysia Moschos.*)

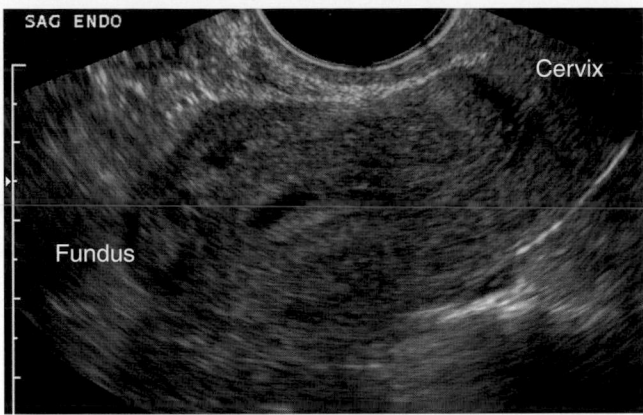

FIGURE 7-6 Transvaginal sonography of a pseudogestational sac within the endometrial cavity. Note its ovoid shape and central location, which are characteristic of these fluid collections. *(Image contributed by Dr. Elysia Moschos.)*

(Fig. 2-8, p. 37) (Lavie, 1996). For the diagnosis of ectopic pregnancy, this finding's specificity is 94 percent but with a sensitivity of only 38 percent (Hammoud, 2005). Endometrial stripe thickness has not been well correlated with ectopic pregnancies. However, Moschos and Twickler (2008) determined that in women with pregnancies of unknown location at presentation, no normal intrauterine pregnancies had a stripe thickness <8 mm.

The fallopian tubes and ovaries are also inspected. Visualization of an extrauterine yolk sac or embryo clearly confirms a tubal pregnancy, although such findings are present in only 15 to 30 percent of cases (Paul, 2000). In some cases, a *halo* or tubal ring surrounded by a thin hypoechoic area caused by subserosal edema can be seen. According to Burry and associates (1993), this has a positive-predictive value of 92 percent and a sensitivity of 95 percent. Brown and associates (1994) conducted a metaanalysis of 10 studies to ascertain the best transvaginal sonographic criteria to diagnose ectopic pregnancy. They reported that the finding of any adnexal mass, other than a simple ovarian cyst, was the most accurate, with a sensitivity of 84 percent, specificity of 99 percent, positive-predictive value of 96 percent, and negative-predictive value of 95 percent. However, not all adnexal masses represent an ectopic pregnancy, and integration of sonographic findings with other clinical information is necessary.

Differentiation of an ectopic pregnancy from a corpus luteum cyst can be challenging. However, Swire and coworkers (2004) observed that the corpus luteum wall is less echogenic compared with both the *halo* and the endometrium. They found that a spongelike, lacelike, or reticular pattern seen within the cyst is classic for hemorrhage (Fig. 9-17, p. 266). Moreover, a corpus luteum is found within the parenchyma of an ovary, whereas an asymmetric ovary should raise suspicion of an ectopic pregnancy (Gurel, 2007). With transvaginal color Doppler imaging, placental blood flow within the periphery of the complex adnexal mass—the *ring of fire*—can be seen (Fig. 7-7). Although this finding can aid ectopic pregnancy diagnosis, it also can be seen with a corpus luteum of pregnancy (Pellerito, 1992). Pulsed-color Doppler sonographic measurements of resistance

indices have been reported to help differentiate between a corpus luteum cyst and ectopic pregnancy, although poor sensitivity limits their utility (Atri, 2003a). Finally, to help characterize a suspicious mass, an examiner can gently palpate an adnexum that is placed between the vaginal probe and the examiner's abdominal hand during real-time scanning. A mass that moves separately from the ovary suggests a tubal pregnancy, whereas a mass that moves synchronously more likely represents a corpus luteum cyst (Levine, 2007).

During sonographic evaluation of the pelvis, free peritoneal fluid suggests intraabdominal bleeding. TVS can detect as little as 50 mL of fluid in the cul-de-sac of Douglas. In addition, transabdominal right-upper-quadrant sonographic evaluation helps assess the extent of hemoperitoneum. Blood in the paracolic gutters and Morison pouch indicates significant hemorrhage. Specifically, free fluid in Morison pouch typically is not seen until a hemoperitoneum reaches 400 to 700 mL (Branney, 1995; Rodgerson, 2001; Rose, 2004). Detection of peritoneal fluid in conjunction with an adnexal mass is highly predictive of ectopic pregnancy (Nyberg, 1991).

Despite technologic advances, the absence of suggestive findings does not exclude an ectopic pregnancy. In addition, TVS has not decreased the prevalence of tubal rupture or need for transfusions at the time of surgery (Atri, 2003b). However, sonography has decreased the need for diagnostic laparoscopy or curettage or both to establish the diagnosis of ectopic pregnancy.

Culdocentesis

With a 16- to 18-gauge spinal needle, the cul-de-sac of Douglas may be entered through the posterior vaginal fornix (Fig. 7-8). The characteristics of the aspirate, in conjunction with clinical findings, may help clarify the diagnosis. Normal-appearing peritoneal fluid is designated as a negative test. If fragments of an old clot or nonclotting blood are found in the aspirate when placed into a dry, clean test tube, then hemoperitoneum is diagnosed. If the aspirated blood clots after it is withdrawn, this

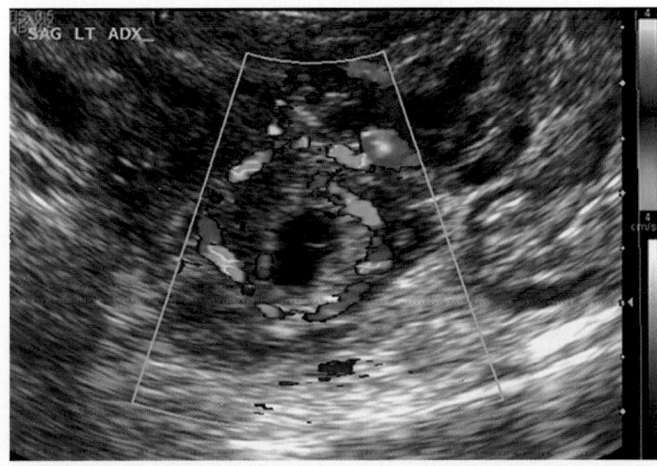

FIGURE 7-7 Color Doppler transvaginal sonography of an ectopic pregnancy. The "ring of fire" reflects placental blood flow around the periphery of the pregnancy. This finding, however, may also be seen with corpus luteum cysts. *(Image contributed by Dr. Elysia Moschos.)*

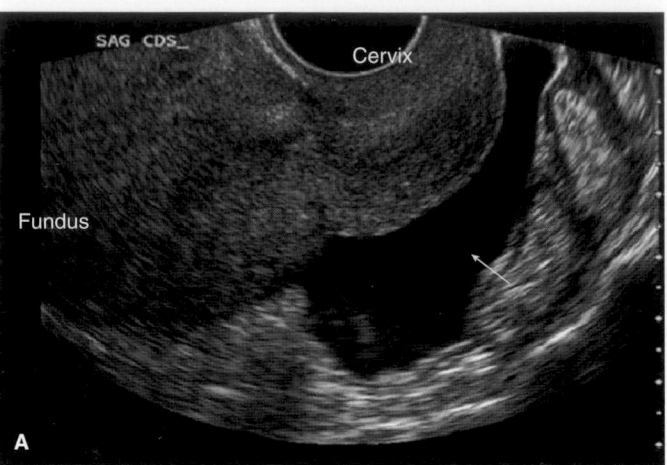
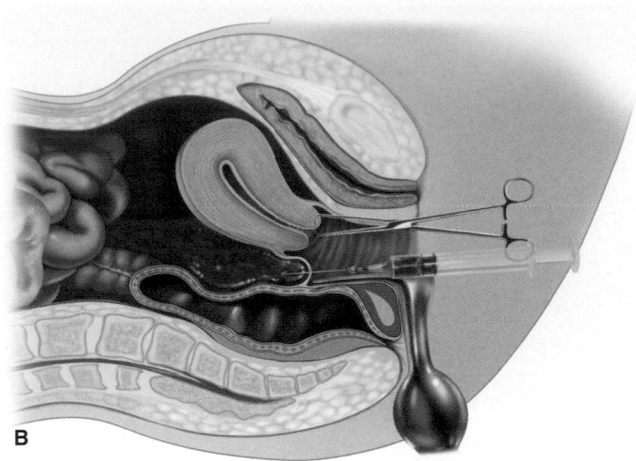

FIGURE 7-8 Techniques to identify intraabdominal bleeding. **A.** Transvaginal sonography of a fluid collection (*arrow*) in the cul-de-sac of Douglas. *(Image contributed by Dr. Elysia Moschos.)* **B.** Culdocentesis. With a 16- to 18-gauge spinal needle attached to a syringe, the cul-de-sac of Douglas is entered through the posterior vaginal fornix as upward traction is applied to the cervix with a tenaculum.

may signify active intraperitoneal bleeding or puncture of an adjacent vessel. If fluid cannot be aspirated, the test can only be interpreted as unsatisfactory. Purulent fluid suggests a number of infection-related causes such as salpingitis or appendicitis. Feculent material may originate from a perforated or ruptured colon or an inadvertent puncture of the rectosigmoid colon.

Historically, culdocentesis was considered an easy bedside test used to diagnose hemoperitoneum. A number of studies have challenged its usefulness, and culdocentesis has been largely replaced by TVS (Glezerman, 1992; Vermesh, 1990). Sonography with findings of echogenic fluid to establish hemoperitoneum is more sensitive and specific than culdocentesis—100 and 100 percent versus 66 and 80 percent, respectively. Also, for most women, sonography is better tolerated.

Endometrial Sampling

There are a number of endometrial changes associated with ectopic pregnancy. These include decidual reaction found in 42 percent of samples, secretory endometrium in 22 percent, and proliferative endometrium in 12 percent, all with an absence of trophoblasts (Lopez, 1994). Many recommend that the absence of trophoblastic tissue be confirmed by curettage before methotrexate treatment is given (Barnhart, 2002; Chung, 2011; Shaunik, 2011). They found that the presumptive diagnosis of ectopic pregnancy is inaccurate in nearly 40 percent of cases without histologic exclusion of a spontaneous pregnancy loss. Nevertheless, the need and method of endometrial sampling must carefully be weighed against the limited risks of methotrexate.

Endometrial biopsy with a Pipelle catheter was studied as an alternative to curettage and found inferior. The sensitivity of obtaining chorionic villi ranged from 30 to 63 percent (Barnhart, 2003b; Ries, 2000). By comparison, frozen section of curettage fragments to identify products of conception is accurate in more than 90 percent of cases (Barak, 2005; Spandorfer, 1996).

Chorionic villi in specimens from women with the diagnosis of spontaneous abortion were identified clinically in only half of cases and by the pathologist in another 30 percent. Thus in

20 percent of women, ectopic pregnancy was still a consideration (Lindahl, 1986).

Novel Serum Markers

A number of small studies have evaluated the utility of novel markers to detect ectopic pregnancy. Of these, vascular endothelial growth factor (VEGF), which is important in placental development, has been investigated alone or in combination (Daniel, 1999; Rausch, 2011). In addition, cancer antigen 125 (CA125), serum creatine kinase, and fetal fibronectin concentrations have been investigated (Ness, 1998; Predanic, 2000). Serum inhibin A levels are significantly lower in women with ectopic pregnancies than in those with normal pregnancies or threatened abortion. This may prove to be a reliable marker in the future (Segal, 2008). Lastly, mass spectrometry-based proteomic techniques have also been used to determine the biochemical blueprint of normal pregnancy and some of its disorders (Shankar, 2005).

SUMMARY OF DIAGNOSTIC EVALUATION

Confirmation by diagnostic laparoscopy remains the gold standard for diagnosis of ectopic pregnancy (Fig. 7-9). That said, with sensitive diagnostic modalities available, ectopic pregnancy can typically be diagnosed prior to surgery, and use of an evidence-based algorithm can assist. After appropriate clinical evaluation, all reproductive-aged women with any suspicion of pregnancy should be tested using a sensitive urine β-hCG assay. Following positive testing, if an intrauterine pregnancy is not confirmed by sonography, if no signs of acute intraabdominal hemorrhage are present, and if an ectopic gestation is suspected, then an evaluation such as the one depicted in Figure 7-10 may be used. Gracia and Barnhart (2001) performed a decision analysis of six diagnostic strategies to evaluate which sequence of tests was most efficient in yielding the fewest missed ectopic pregnancies and interrupted uterine pregnancies. They found the best strategy to include

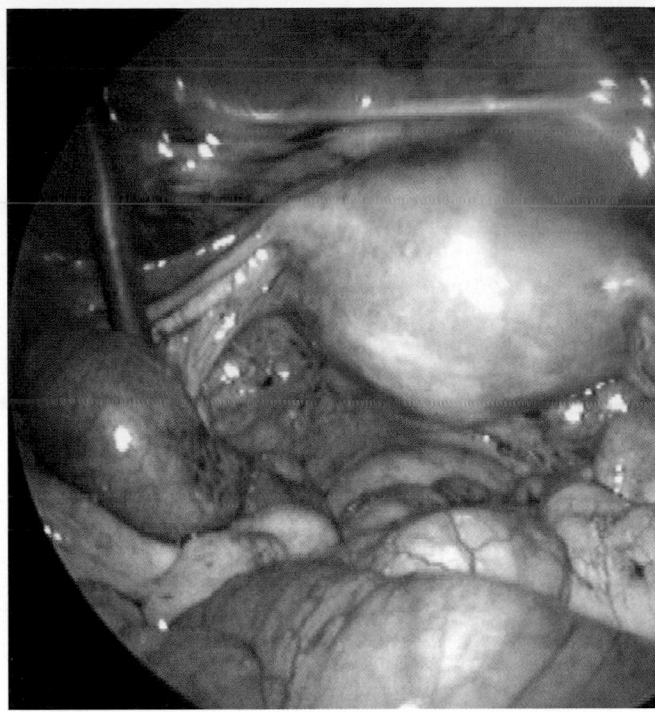

FIGURE 7-9 Laparoscopic photograph of an ectopic pregnancy. A blunt probe elevates a blue, distended left tubal ampulla. *(Photograph contributed by Dr. Kevin Doody.)*

TVS for all women with first-trimester pain or bleeding. If findings are not diagnostic, then serum β-hCG levels are measured. Using this strategy, only 1 percent of all potential uterine pregnancies were interrupted; no ectopic pregnancies were missed; and the average time to diagnosis was 1.46 days. In the event that overall sensitivity of available sonography for detecting uterine pregnancy is less than 93 percent—because of older sonographic equipment, an inexperienced sonographer, patient obesity or discomfort, or distorted anatomy—they recommend initial measurement of serum β-hCG levels and reservation of sonographic examination for those women with levels above the discriminatory zone.

More recently, a scoring system using only patient history and serum β-hCG levels was developed to aid management of pregnancies of unknown location (Barnhart, 2008). Specifically, scores for age, bleeding, serum β-hCG levels, and ectopic and prior miscarriage history were assigned. The sensitivity to intervene for a nonviable gestation was 98 percent, and the specificity to send home a uterine pregnancy was 96 percent. Importantly, the investigators noted that their scoring system should be combined with current strategies to diagnose ectopic pregnancy.

MANAGEMENT

Without intervention, an ectopic tubal pregnancy can lead to tubal abortion, tubal rupture, or spontaneous resolution. *Tubal abortion* is the expulsion of products through the fimbrial end. This tissue can then either regress or reimplant in the abdominal cavity. With reimplantation, bleeding or pain necessitating surgical intervention is a common complication. *Tubal rupture*

is associated with significant intraabdominal hemorrhage. With *spontaneous resolution*, small ectopic pregnancies die and are resorbed without adverse patient effects.

▪ Medical Management

Medical therapy is preferred by most, if feasible. Only methotrexate has been extensively studied as an alternate to surgical therapy (Barnhart, 2009). Other agents that have been used include prostaglandins; the progesterone antagonist mifepristone; traditional Chinese herbal medicines; and potassium chloride or hyperosmolar glucose injected into the ectopic mass (Dengfeng, 2007). The best candidate for medical therapy is a woman who is asymptomatic and motivated and who has resources to be compliant with surveillance. Absolute contraindications for medical therapy with methotrexate include hemodynamic instability, inability to remain compliant with posttherapeutic monitoring, and contraindications to methotrexate itself. With medical therapy, some classic predictors of success include:

1. Initial serum β-hCG level—This is the single best prognostic indicator of treatment success in women given single-dose methotrexate. The prognostic value of the other two predictors may be directly related to their relationship with serum β-hCG concentrations. According to Lipscomb and colleagues (1999), an initial serum value <5000 IU/L was associated with a success rate of 92 percent, whereas an initial concentration >15,000 IU/L had a success rate of 68 percent. In another study, Menon and associates (2007) reported that compared with an initial serum β-hCG level of 2000 to 4999 IU/L, an initial serum β-hCG of 5000 to 9999 IU/L is nearly four times more likely associated with methotrexate therapy failure.

2. Ectopic pregnancy size—There are few data concerning the effect of size on success rates with medical therapy, although many early trials used "large size" as an exclusion criterion. In one study, the success rate with single-dose methotrexate was 93 percent in cases with ectopic masses <3.5 cm, whereas success rates were between 87 and 90 percent when the mass was >3.5 cm (Lipscomb, 1998).

3. Fetal cardiac activity—Identification of cardiac activity sonographically is a relative contraindication to medical therapy, although this is based on limited evidence. Most studies report an increased risk of failure if there is cardiac activity, however, a success rate of 87 percent has been reported (Lipscomb, 1998).

Investigators have evaluated other predictors of treatment failure. Extrauterine yolk sac as a predictor of methotrexate failure has conflicting evidence. A retrospective analysis by Lipscomb and colleagues (2009) found that this sonographic finding added to the risk of single-dose methotrexate failure, but was not an independent predictor. Rapidly rising β-hCG levels both before (>50 percent) and during methotrexate therapy may also portend an increased risk of failure (American Society for Reproductive Medicine, 2008; Dudley, 2004).

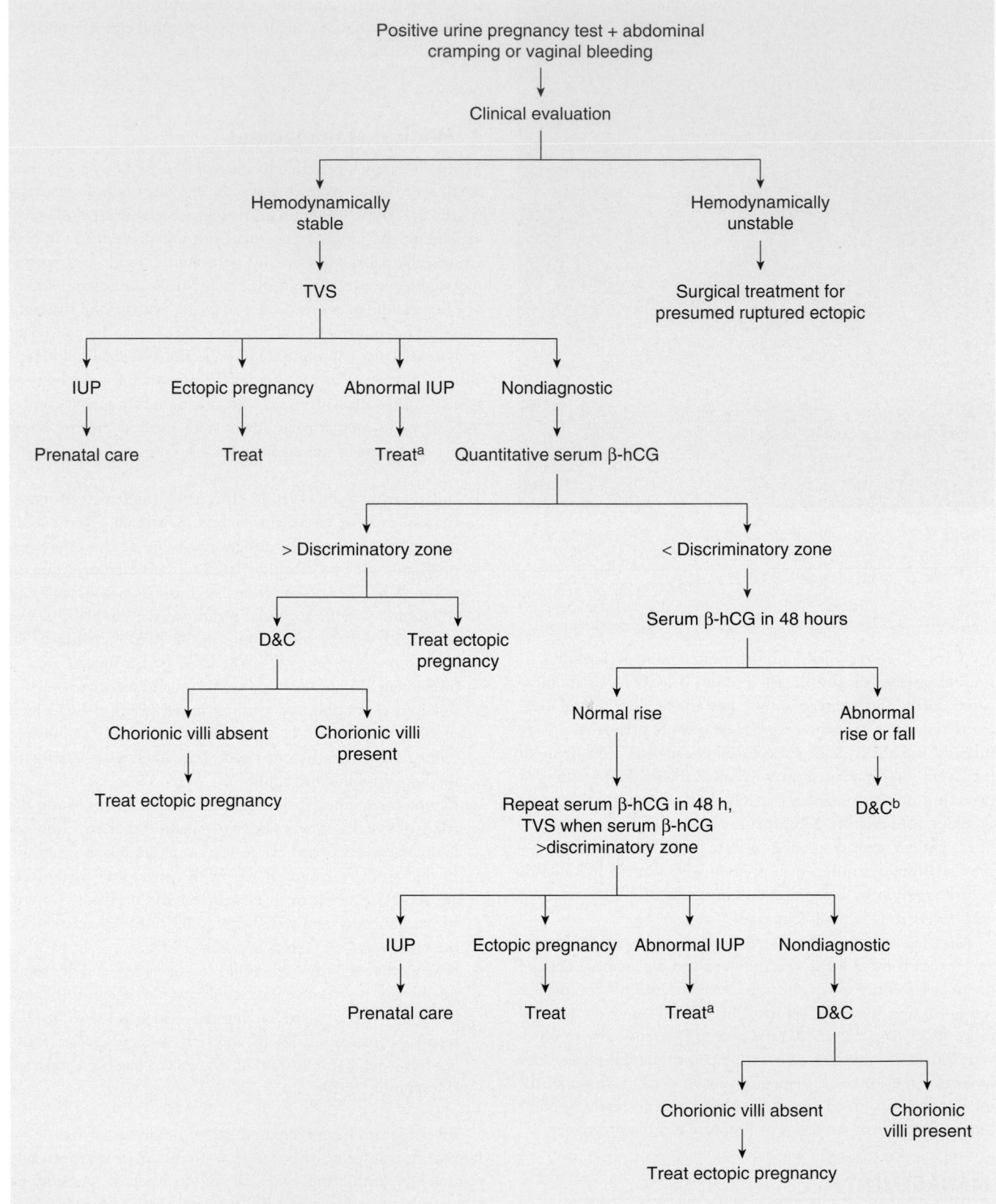

FIGURE 7-10 Algorithm of ectopic pregnancy evaluation.
[a]Abnormal IUPs may be treated by D&C, medical regimens, or expectant management as outlined in Chapter 6, p. 178.
[b]Expectant management may be appropriate in a small select group of women with very low β-hCG levels that are dropping as described on page 212.
β-hCG = β-human chorionic gonadotropin; D&C = dilatation and curettage; IUP = intrauterine pregnancy; TVS = transvaginal sonography.

Methotrexate

This is a folic acid antagonist that competitively inhibits the binding of dihydrofolic acid to the enzyme dihydrofolate reductase. This leads to reduced amounts of purines and thymidylate and thereby an arrest of DNA, RNA, and protein synthesis (Chap. 27, p. 698). It inhibits fast-growing tissue and is used for cancer chemotherapy and for early pregnancy termination. The drug can be given orally, intravenously, or intramuscularly (IM) or can be directly injected into the ectopic pregnancy sac. Currently, parenteral methotrexate administration is used most commonly.

Prior to methotrexate therapy, a complete blood count, serum creatinine and β-hCG levels, liver function tests, and blood type and Rh status should be obtained (American Society for Reproductive Medicine, 2008). Moreover, all except blood typing are repeated prior to additional doses (Lipscomb, 2007). With administration, women should be counseled to avoid the following until treatment is completed: folic acid-containing supplements, which can competitively reduce methotrexate binding to dihydrofolate reductase; nonsteroidal antiinflammatory drugs, which reduce renal blood flow and delay drug excretion; alcohol, which can predispose to concurrent hepatic enzyme elevation; sunlight, which can provoke methotrexate-related dermatitis; and sexual activity, which can rupture the ectopic pregnancy (American College of Obstetricians and Gynecologists, 2008; Chabner, 2006). Importantly, methotrexate is a teratogen, is a Food and Drug Administration pregnancy category X, and can lead to a profound embryopathy (Nurmohamed, 2011; Poggi, 2011).

The most common side effects of methotrexate include stomatitis, conjunctivitis, and transient liver dysfunction, although myelosuppression, mucositis, pulmonary damage, and anaphylactoid reactions have been reported with only one dose of 50 to 100 mg (Isaacs, 1996; Straka, 2004). Side effects are seen in as many as a third of women treated, however, they are usually self-limited. In some cases, leucovorin (folinic acid) is given following treatment to blunt or reverse methotrexate side effects (Table 7-3). Such therapy is termed *leucovorin rescue* (Chap. 27, p. 699).

The single-dose and multidose methotrexate protocols shown in Table 7-3 are associated with overall resolution rates for ectopic pregnancy that approximate 90 percent. To date, Alleyassin and coworkers (2006) have completed the only randomized trial comparing single and multidose administrations. Although the study was underpowered to detect a small difference in success rates, they did observe that 89 percent in the single-dose group and 93 percent in the multidose group were successfully treated. When analyzed from the standpoint of treatment failure, single-dose therapy had a 50-percent higher failure rate compared with multidose therapy (6/54 vs. 4/54). Lipscomb and colleagues (2005) reviewed their institutional experience with methotrexate therapy in 643 consecutively treated patients. They found no significant differences in treatment duration, serum β-hCG levels, or success rates between the multi- and single-dose protocols—95 and 90 percent, respectively. Barnhart and coworkers (2003a) performed a metaanalysis of 26 studies that included 1327 women treated with methotrexate for ectopic pregnancy. Single-dose therapy was more commonly used because of simplicity. It was less expensive, was easily accepted because of less intensive posttherapy monitoring, and did not require leucovorin rescue (Alexander, 1996). The major limitation was that multidose

TABLE 7-3. Medical Treatment Protocols for Ectopic Pregnancy

	Single Dose	Multidose
Dosing	One dose; repeat if necessary	Up to four doses of both drugs until serum β-hCG declines by 15%
Medication Dosage		
Methotrexate	50 mg/m² BSA (day 1)	1 mg/kg, days 1, 3, 5, and 7
Leucovorin	NA	0.1 mg/kg days 2, 4, 6, and 8
Serum β-hCG level	Days 1 (baseline), 4, and 7	Days 0 (baseline), 1, 3, 5, and 7
Indication for additional dose	• If serum β-hCG level does not decline by 15% from day 4 to day 7 • Less than 15% decline during weekly surveillance	If serum β-hCG declines <15%, give additional dose; repeat serum β-hCG in 48 hours and compare with previous value; maximum four doses
Posttherapy surveillance	Weekly until serum β-hCG undetectable	
Methotrexate Contraindications		
Sensitivity to MTX Tubal rupture Breast feeding	Intrauterine pregnancy Hepatic, renal, or hematologic dysfunction	Peptic ulcer disease Active pulmonary disease Evidence of immunodeficiency

BSA = body surface area; β-hCG = β-human chorionic gonadotropin, MTX = methotrexate; NA = not applicable.

treatment had a fivefold greater chance of success than single-dose therapy. Failures included women with tubal rupture, massive intraabdominal hemorrhage, and need for urgent surgery and blood transfusions. Ultimately, most women received between one and four doses of methotrexate. Interestingly, the initial serum β-hCG value was not a valid indicator of how many doses of methotrexate a patient would need for a successful outcome (Nowak-Markwitz, 2009). In the absence of adequately powered randomized trials comparing single- with multidose therapy, we use single-dose methotrexate.

Single-Dose Methotrexate. Intramuscular methotrexate given as a single dose has been the most widely used medical treatment of ectopic pregnancy. Various doses have been studied, and the most popular is the 50 mg/m^2 body surface area (BSA) protocol described by the group from Memphis (Stovall, 1993). In the small randomized trial by Hajenius and colleagues (2000), treatment with 25 mg/m^2 was equally effective as treatment with 50 mg/m^2. BSA can be determined using the nomogram in Figure 27-3 (p. 695) or derived using various internet-based BSA calculators, such as: http://www.globalrph.com/bsa2.htm.

Close monitoring is imperative. A serum β-hCG level is determined prior to methotrexate administration and is repeated on days 4 and 7 following injection. Levels usually continue to rise until day 4. Comparison is then made between day 4 and 7 serum values. If there is a decline by 15 percent or more, then weekly serum β-hCG levels are drawn until they measure <15 IU/L. A decline of less than 15 percent is seen in approximately 20 percent of treated women. In such cases, a second 50 mg/m^2 dose is given, and the protocol is restarted. Approximate time to resolution for all women averages 36 days, but in some, treatment requires 109 days (Lipscomb, 1998).

Others have tried, without success, to develop more convenient serum β-hCG monitoring protocols. Thurman and associates (2010) proposed using a 50-percent drop in values between days 1 and 7 as a predictor of methotrexate success. The protocol had 100-percent sensitivity but only 38- to 58-percent specificity depending on the initial serum β-hCG level. In an attempt to prospectively validate the day-4-to-7 rule while developing a new rule, 69 women receiving methotrexate had serum β-hCG and progesterone levels collected on days 1, 2, 4, 5, and 7. In the end, the original day-4-to-7 guidelines were validated (Kirk, 2007).

During the first few days following methotrexate administration, up to half of women experience abdominal pain that can be controlled with mild analgesics. This *separation pain* presumably results from tubal distension caused by tubal abortion or hematoma formation or both (Stovall, 1993). In some cases, inpatient observation with serial hematocrit determinations and gentle abdominal examinations help assess the need for surgical intervention.

Multidose Methotrexate. The most common regimen is seen in Table 7-3 and consists of up to four doses of parenteral methotrexate, followed by adjunctive doses of leucovorin 24 hours later. Serial serum β-hCG concentrations are obtained. If there is not a 15-percent decline from the previous value—for example, days 0 to 1 or days 1 to 3—an additional methotrexate/leucovorin dose is given, and the serum β-hCG level is repeated 2 days later. A maximum of four doses are given, and weekly serum β-hCG level surveillance continues until values are undetectable.

A hybrid "two dose" protocol has been proposed in an effort to balance the efficacy and convenience of the two most commonly used protocols (Barnhart, 2007). The regimen involves administering 50 mg/m^2 of methotrexate on days 0 and 4 without leucovorin rescue. Although the protocol is still considered experimental, no safety concerns were noted in the 101 patients treated, and the success rate approached 87 percent.

Oral Methotrexate

The bioavailability of oral and parenteral methotrexate is similar (Jundt, 1993). There are only a few trials in which oral methotrexate has been evaluated. Korhonen and colleagues (1996) randomly assigned women with tubal pregnancies without cardiac activity and with serum β-hCG levels <5000 IU/L to be managed expectantly or to receive low-dose oral methotrexate, 2.5 mg daily for 5 days. They found no differences in primary treatment success. Bengtsson and associates (1992) gave 15 mg of methotrexate orally on days 1, 3, and 5 with folinic acid on days 2, 4 and 6. This was successful in 14 of 15 women with a mean resolution time of 24 days.

Mifepristone plus Methotrexate. It seems logical that the addition of 600 mg of mifepristone orally to single-dose methotrexate might improve efficacy and speed resolution of unruptured ectopic pregnancies (Chap. 6, p. 190). In a randomized trial of 212 cases, however, Rozenberg and coworkers (2003) documented no differences in success rates.

Direct Injection into Ectopic Pregnancy

Methotrexate. In efforts to minimize systemic side effects of methotrexate, local injection into the gestational sac under sonographic or laparoscopic guidance has been evaluated. Pharmacokinetic studies with 1 mg/kg of methotrexate injected either into the sac under sonographic guidance or by traditional IM injection showed similar success rates. However, fewer drug-related side effects were seen with local injection (Fernandez, 1995).

Hyperosmolar Glucose. In a small prospective trial, Yeko and colleagues (1995) reported that direct injection of 50-percent glucose into the ectopic mass using laparoscopic guidance was 94-percent successful in women with an unruptured ectopic whose serum β-hCG level was <2500 IU/L. Gjelland and coworkers (1995) reported that treatment success was significantly better in a similar population in which sonographic-rather than laparoscopic-guided injection was used.

Surveillance

Posttherapy monitoring assesses treatment success and screens for signs of persistent ectopic pregnancy. Most medical management protocols have well-defined surveillance schedules. In the absence of symptoms, bimanual examinations are limited to avoid the theoretical risk of manual tubal rupture. Importantly, sonographic monitoring of ectopic mass dimensions can be misleading after serum β-hCG levels have declined to <15 IU/L. Brown and colleagues (1991) described persistent masses to be resolving hematomas rather than persistent trophoblastic tissue. For this reason, posttherapy sonography is reserved for suspected complications such as tubal rupture. Most recommend contraception for 3 to 6 months after successful medical therapy with methotrexate, as this drug may persist in human tissues for up to 8 months after a single dose (Warkany, 1978).

Surgical Management
Laparotomy versus Laparoscopy

There have been at least three prospective studies that compared laparotomy with laparoscopic surgery for ectopic pregnancies (Lundorff, 1991; Murphy, 1992; Vermesh, 1989). Their findings are summarized:

1. There were no significant differences in overall tubal patency determined at second-look laparoscopy. This was despite higher rates of ipsilateral adhesions in the laparotomy group.
2. Each method was followed by a similar number of subsequent uterine pregnancies.
3. There were fewer repeat ectopic pregnancies in women treated laparoscopically, although this was not significant.
4. Laparoscopy resulted in shorter operative times, less blood loss, fewer analgesic requirements, and shorter hospital stays.
5. Laparoscopic surgery was significantly less successful in resolving the tubal pregnancy, however, this was balanced by the just-mentioned benefits of laparoscopy.
6. The costs for laparoscopy were significantly lower than for laparotomy, although some argue that costs are similar when cases converted to laparotomy are considered (Foulk, 1996).

Since completion of these studies, with improvements in laparoscopic equipment and with accrued experience, cases previously managed by laparotomy, such as ruptured tubal or intact interstitial pregnancies, can now be more safely approached using laparoscopy (Sagiv, 2001).

Laparotomy offers a potential advantage to laparoscopy if salpingostomy is planned. A metaanalysis using data from two trials concluded that compared with laparotomic salpingostomy, laparoscopic salpingostomy leads to one case of persistent trophoblastic disease for every 12 women undergoing the laparoscopic approach (Mol, 2008a).

Laparoscopy

To date, there have been no completed randomized trials to guide the choice between conservative—laparoscopic salpingostomy, and definitive—laparoscopic salpingectomy. However, the European Surgery in Ectopic Pregnancy (ESEP) study group is currently assessing this (Mol, 2008b). In an effort to appraise reproductive outcomes after surgical intervention, Becker and coworkers (2011) followed 261 women with and without additional fertility-reducing risk factors who underwent either salpingotomy or salpingectomy. Regardless of surgical choice, subsequent intrauterine pregnancy rates were 92 to 100 percent, respectively, in women without other fertility-reducing risk factors. However, among those with risk factors, intrauterine pregnancy rates were higher with salpingotomy (75 percent) compared with salpingectomy (40 percent).

Salpingectomy

If the contralateral fallopian tube appears normal, then salpingectomy is a reasonable treatment option that avoids the 5 to 8 percent complication rate caused by persistent or recurrent ectopic pregnancy in the same tube (Rulin, 1995).

Many techniques have been described to perform laparoscopic salpingectomy, and a surgical description is found in Section 42-4 (p. 1129). Lim and associates (2007) compared electrosurgical coagulation of the tube and mesosalpinx during laparoscopic salpingectomy with laparoscopic suture-loop (Endoloop) ligation. Endoloop use was associated with significantly shorter operating times (48 vs. 61 minutes) and lower postoperative pain scores.

Salpingostomy

The woman who is hemodynamically stable and strongly desires to preserve fertility is an appropriate candidate for salpingostomy. In addition, serum β-hCG levels may be a factor in patient selection. A retrospective study by Milad and colleagues (1998) found that ectopic resolution rates were lower in women in whom the initial serum β-hCG level was >8000 IU/L. Supportive evidence for this comes from Natale and associates (2003), who reported that serum β-hCG levels >6000 IU/L have a high-risk of implantation into the tubal muscularis.

During salpingostomy, all free and tubal placental tissue should be meticulously removed, especially in cases with tubal rupture. Subsequent intraabdominal implantation of trophoblastic tissue can explain persistent serum β-hCG levels (Bucella, 2009).

Medical versus Surgical Therapy

There are a number of randomized trials that have compared methotrexate treatment with laparoscopic surgery. One multicenter trial compared a multidose methotrexate protocol with laparoscopic salpingostomy and found no differences for tubal preservation and primary treatment success (Hajenius, 1997). However, in this same study group, health-related quality of life factors such as pain, posttherapy depression, and decreased perception of health were significantly impaired after systemic methotrexate compared with laparoscopic salpingostomy (Nieuwkerk, 1998).

There is conflicting evidence when single-dose methotrexate is compared with surgical intervention. In two separate studies, single-dose methotrexate was overall less successful in resolving pregnancy than laparoscopic salpingostomy, although tubal patency and subsequent uterine pregnancy rates were similar between both groups (Fernandez, 1998; Sowter, 2001). Women treated with methotrexate had significantly better physical functioning immediately following therapy, but there were no differences in psychological functioning. Krag Moeller and associates (2009) reported the results from their prospective randomized trial that had a median surveillance period of 8.6 years during which future pregnancy rates were evaluated. Ectopic-resolution success rates were not significantly different between those managed surgically and those treated with methotrexate. Moreover, cumulative spontaneous intrauterine pregnancy rates were not different between the methotrexate group (73 percent) and the surgical group (62 percent).

Based on these studies, we conclude that women who are hemodynamically stable and in whom there is a small tubal diameter, no fetal cardiac activity, and serum β-hCG concentrations <5000 IU/L have similar outcomes with medical or surgical management. Despite lower success rates with medical therapy for women with larger tubal size, higher serum β-hCG levels, and fetal cardiac activity, medical management can be offered to the motivated woman who understands the risks of emergency surgery in the event of treatment failure.

Expectant Management

In select women, some choose close observation in anticipation that there will be spontaneous resorption of an ectopic pregnancy. Intuitively, it is difficult to accurately predict which woman will have an uncomplicated course with such management. Although an initial serum β-hCG concentration has been shown to best predict outcome, the range varies widely. For example, initial values <200 IU/L predict successful spontaneous resolution in 88 to 96 percent of attempts, whereas values >2000 IU/L had success rates of only 20 to 25 percent (Elson, 2004; Trio, 1995). Even with declining values, when the initial β-hCG level exceeded 2000 IU/L, the success rate was only 7 percent (Shalev, 1995). Interestingly, in this study, there was no difference in ipsilateral tubal patency or 1-year fertility rates with either success or failure of expectant management.

Close monitoring is warranted because the risk of tubal rupture persists despite low and declining serum β-hCG levels. An argument could be made that the minimal side effects of methotrexate make it preferable to a potentially prolonged surveillance and associated patient anxiety.

Persistent Ectopic Pregnancy

Incomplete eradication of trophoblastic tissue and its continued growth causes tubal rupture in 3 to 20 percent of women following conservative surgical or medical treatment of ectopic pregnancy (Graczykowski, 1999). Thus, abdominal pain following conservative management should prompt immediate suspicion for persistent trophoblast proliferation.

Following salpingostomy, persistent ectopic pregnancy is more likely with very early pregnancies. Specifically, surgical management is more difficult because pregnancies smaller than 2 cm are harder to visualize and completely remove. To obviate this, Graczykowski and associates (1997) administered a prophylactic dose of 1 mg/m² methotrexate postoperatively, which reduced the incidence of persistent ectopic pregnancy and length of surveillance.

The optimal schedule to identify persistent ectopic pregnancy after surgical therapy has not been determined. Protocols describe serum β-hCG level monitoring from every 3 days to every 2 weeks. Spandorfer and associates (1997) estimated the risk of persistent ectopic pregnancy based on serum β-hCG levels done on the first postoperative day. They observed that if serum β-hCG levels fell by >50 percent compared with presurgical values, then there were no treatment failures within the first 9 days, and thus repeat serum β-hCG determinations 1 week after surgery were appropriate. Conversely, if serum levels fell by <50 percent, then there was a 3.5-fold increased risk of failure within the first week, thus necessitating earlier postoperative evaluation. Importantly, despite low and falling serum β-hCG concentrations, tubal rupture can still occur (Tulandi, 1991).

Currently, standard therapy for persistent ectopic pregnancy is single-dose methotrexate with 50 mg/m² BSA. Although considered, there have been few studies to evaluate low-dose oral methotrexate for this indication.

Anti-D Isoimmunization

If the woman is D negative and her partner has a blood group that is either D positive or unknown, then 300 μg anti-D immune globulin should be given to prevent anti-D isoimmunization.

OVARIAN PREGNANCY

Ectopic implantation of the fertilized egg in the ovary is rare and is diagnosed if four clinical criteria are met. These were outlined by Spiegelberg (1878) and include: (1) the ipsilateral tube is intact and distinct from the ovary; (2) the ectopic pregnancy occupies the ovary; (3) the ectopic pregnancy is connected by the uteroovarian ligament to the uterus; and (4) ovarian tissue can be demonstrated histologically in the placental tissue. A more recent increased incidence in ovarian pregnancy likely is artifactual due to improved imaging modalities. Risk factors are similar to those for tubal pregnancies. In one study, IUD users had a higher proportion of ovarian pregnancies compared with nonusers—5.5 percent versus none (World Health Organization, 1985). Nearly a third of women with an ovarian pregnancy present with hemodynamic instability because of rupture. Diagnosis is based on the classic sonographic description of a cyst with a wide echogenic outer ring on or within the ovary (Comstock, 2005).

INTERSTITIAL PREGNANCY

Interstitial pregnancies implant in the proximal tubal segment that lies within the muscular uterine wall. Swelling lateral to the insertion of the round ligament is the characteristic anatomic finding (Fig. 7-11). Incorrectly, these are sometimes called cornual pregnancies, but this term describes conceptions that develop in the horns of uteri with müllerian anomalies (Lau, 1999; Moawad, 2010). In the past, rupture of interstitial pregnancies usually took place following 8 to 16 weeks of amenorrhea because of the greater distensibility of the

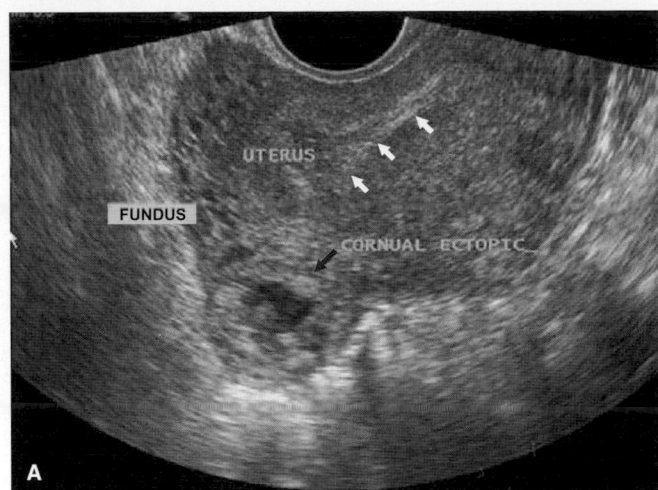 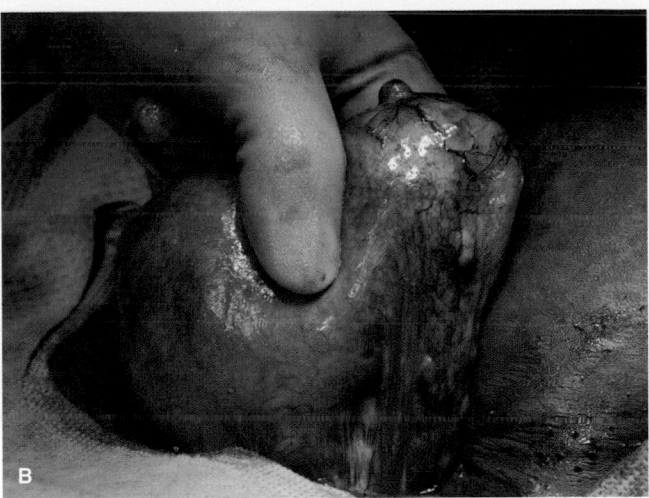

FIGURE 7-11 Interstitial pregnancy. **A.** Transvaginal sonogram, parasagittal view shows an empty uterine cavity and a mass lateral to the uterine fundus. *(Image contributed by Dr. Elysia Moschos.)* **B.** Intraoperative photograph of a uterine fundus and an interstitial pregnancy bulging from the left uterine cornu prior to resection. *(Photograph contributed by Dr. Mario Castellanos.)*

myometrium covering the interstitial segment of fallopian tube. Risk factors are similar to others discussed, although previous ipsilateral salpingectomy is a specific risk factor for interstitial pregnancy (Lau, 1999). Because of the proximity of these pregnancies to the uterine and ovarian arteries, there is a risk of severe hemorrhage, which is associated with mortality rates as high as 2.5 percent (Tulandi, 2004).

Surgical management involves cornual resection either by laparotomy or laparoscopy (Section 41-9, p. 1035). With TVS and serum β-hCG assays, as discussed for suspected tubal pregnancy, interstitial pregnancy can be diagnosed early enough to allow conservative medical therapy (Bernstein, 2001). Given its low incidence, no consensus regarding prediction of success using methotrexate has been established. Jermy and colleagues (2004) reported a 94-percent success with systemic methotrexate using a dose of 50 mg/m² BSA. Their series included four women in whom cardiac activity was verified. Because these women have higher initial serum β-hCG levels at diagnosis, longer surveillance is usually needed. Deruelle and coworkers (2005) advocate postmethotrexate uterine artery embolization to help avert hemorrhage and hopefully hasten ectopic pregnancy resolution.

Hysteroscopic resection of an interstitial pregnancy as well as transcervical suction curettage of interstitial pregnancies have been described. However, long-term results following these techniques are unknown (Sanz, 2002; Zhang, 2004).

Following either medical or conservative surgical management, the risk of uterine rupture with subsequent pregnancies is unclear. Thus, careful observation of these women during pregnancy, along with consideration of elective cesarean delivery, is warranted.

CERVICAL PREGNANCY

The incidence of cervical pregnancy is reported to be between 1 in 8600 and 1 in 12,400 pregnancies (Ushakov, 1997). The incidence appears to be rising because of assisted reproductive technologies, especially IVF and embryo transfer (Ginsburg,

1994; Pattinson, 1994). A risk factor unique to cervical pregnancy is a history of dilation and curettage in a previous pregnancy, seen in nearly 70 percent of cases (Hung, 1996; Pisarska, 1999). Two diagnostic criteria are necessary for cervical pregnancy confirmation: (1) cervical glands are found opposite the placental attachment site, and (2) a portion of or the entire placenta is located below either the entrance of the uterine vessels or the peritoneal reflection on the anterior and posterior uterine surface (Fig. 7-12).

For most hemodynamically stable women with a first-trimester cervical pregnancy, nonsurgical management with systemic methotrexate can be offered and administered as in Table 7-3. Jeng and colleagues (2007) also described 38 cases successfully treated with local methotrexate injection. Resolution and uterine preservation is achieved with methotrexate regimens for gestations <12 weeks in 91 percent of cases (Kung, 1997). In selecting appropriate candidates, Hung and colleagues (1996) noted higher risks of systemic methotrexate treatment failure in those with a gestational age >9 weeks, β-hCG levels >10,000 IU/L, crown-rump length >10 mm, and fetal cardiac activity. For this reason, many induce fetal death with intracardiac or intrathoracic injection of potassium chloride (Jeng, 2007; Verma, 2009). Uterine artery embolization, either before or after methotrexate administration, may be an additional adjunct to limit bleeding complications (Cipullo, 2008; Hirakawa, 2009).

Although conservative management is feasible for many women with cervical pregnancies, surgical intervention may also be selected. Procedures include suction curettage or hysterectomy. Moreover, in those with advanced gestations or with bleeding uncontrolled by conservative methods, hysterectomy is typically required. Importantly, patients should understand the increased risk of urinary tract injury with hysterectomy due to the close proximity of the ureters to the ballooned cervix. Prior to either procedure, uterine artery embolization may be considered to limit intra- and postoperative bleeding (Nakao, 2008; Trambert, 2005). In addition, before curettage, local methotrexate injection into the amnionic sac, ligation of the descending

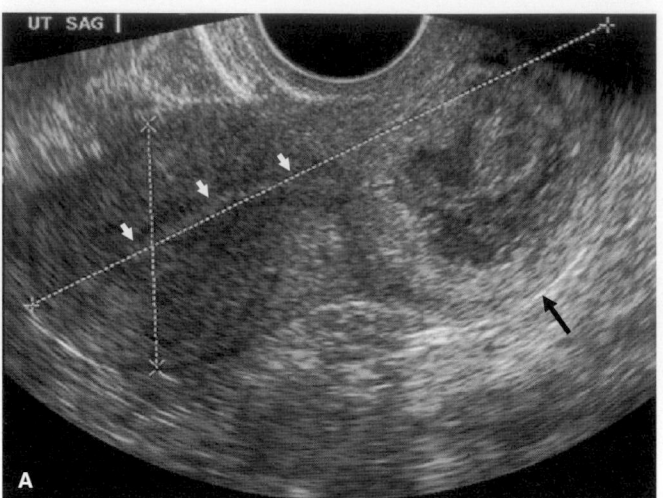

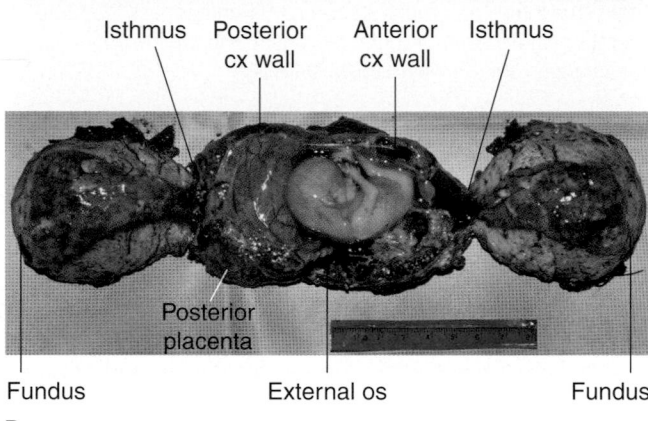

FIGURE 7-12 Cervical pregnancy. **A.** Transvaginal sonography, sagittal view of a cervical pregnancy. Sonographic findings with cervical pregnancy may include: (1) an hourglass uterine shape and ballooned cervical canal; (2) gestational tissue at the level of the cervix (*black arrow*); (3) absent intrauterine gestational tissue (*white arrows*); and (4) a portion of the endocervical canal seen interposed between the gestation and the endometrial canal. *(Image contributed by Dr. Elysia Moschos.)* **B.** Photograph of a hysterectomy specimen containing a cervical ectopic pregnancy. The cervical length was 5–6 cm. *(Photograph contributed by Dr. David Rahn.)*

branches of the uterine arteries, or cerclage placement at the internal os to compress feeding vessels have all been described (Davis, 2008, De La Vega, 2007; Mesogitis, 2005; Trojano, 2009). Following curettage, in the event of hemorrhage, a 26F Foley catheter with a 30-mL balloon can be placed intracervically and inflated to effect hemostasis and to monitor uterine drainage. The balloon remains inflated for 24 to 48 hours and is gradually decompressed over the next few days (Ushakov, 1997). In addition, uterine artery embolization may be considered.

HETEROTOPIC PREGNANCY

A uterine pregnancy in conjunction with an extrauterine pregnancy is termed a heterotopic pregnancy. In the past, incidence estimates were computed to be 1 in 30,000 pregnancies, figuring incidences of dizygotic twinning and ectopic pregnancy of 1 percent each. In pregnancies that result from assisted

reproductive technologies, the rate of heterotopic pregnancies has skyrocketed and may approximate 1 in 100 pregnancies (Habana, 2000). Mechanisms that have been proposed to explain this include hydrostatic forces delivering the embryo into the cornual or tubal area, the tip of the catheter directing transfer toward the tubal ostia, or reflux of uterine secretions leading to retrograde tubal implantation.

When a tubal pregnancy coexists with a uterine pregnancy, potassium chloride can be injected into the tubal pregnancy sac. Methotrexate is contraindicated due to the detrimental effects on the normal pregnancy. Cases of craniofacial, skeletal, cardiopulmonary, and gastrointestinal anomalies have been described even with limited first-trimester methotrexate exposure (Nguyen, 2002).

CESAREAN SCAR PREGNANCY

Implantation within the scar of a previous cesarean delivery through a microscopic tract in the myometrium is uncommon, but carries significant risks of serious maternal morbidity and mortality from massive hemorrhage (Fig. 7-13). The most recent reviews cite the incidence of cesarean scar pregnancy (CSP) to approximate 1 in 2000 pregnancies (Sadeghi, 2010). These microscopic tracts can also stem from other prior uterine surgery—curettage, myomectomy, operative hysteroscopy—and perhaps from manual removal of the placenta (Ash, 2007). Differentiating between a cervicoisthmic pregnancy and a cesarean scar pregnancy can be difficult, and several investigators have described sonographic findings (Jurkovic, 2003; Moschos, 2008). According to Godin (1997), there are four sonographic criteria that should be satisfied for the diagnosis: (1) an empty uterine cavity, (2) an empty cervical canal, (3) a gestational sac in the anterior part of the uterine isthmus, and (4) absence of healthy myometrium between the bladder and gestational sac. Treatment standards are lacking, but options include systemic or locally injected methotrexate, either alone or combined with suction curettage or hysteroscopic removal. Isthmic resection is another method (Michener, 2009; Seow, 2004; Wang, 2009; Yang, 2009). Uterine artery embolization may be used adjunctively to minimize hemorrhage risk (Zhuang, 2009). In most cases the uterus can be preserved, although hysterectomy is also an acceptable and sometimes necessary option (Sadeghi, 2010).

PREVENTION

Ectopic pregnancy is difficult to prevent because few risk factor are modifiable (Butts, 2003). Tubal pathology carries one of the highest risks, and pelvic inflammatory disease plays a major role in tubal adhesions and obstruction. Chlamydial infections constitute nearly half of pelvic inflammatory disease cases, thus efforts have been directed toward screening high-risk populations for asymptomatic infections. These include sexually active women ≤25 years or women with risk factors (Table 1-2, p. 11). Such screening programs in Sweden have demonstrated steady declines in both chlamydial infections and ectopic pregnancy rates, especially in women aged 20 to 24 years (Cates, 1999; Egger, 1998).

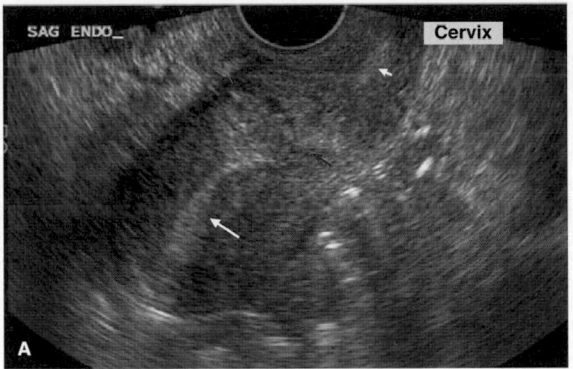

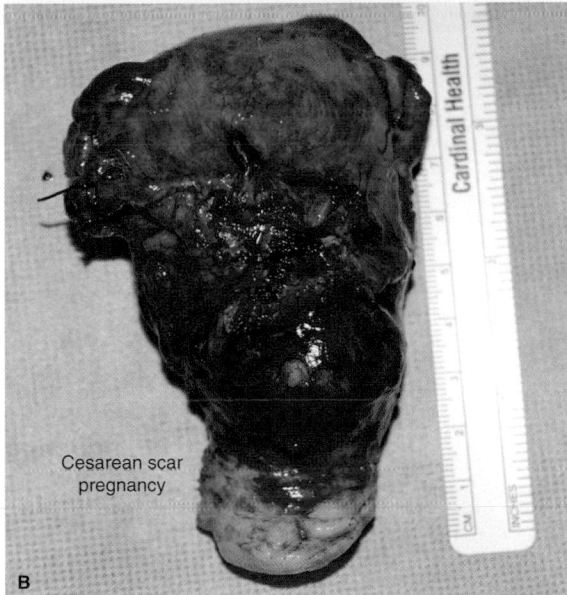

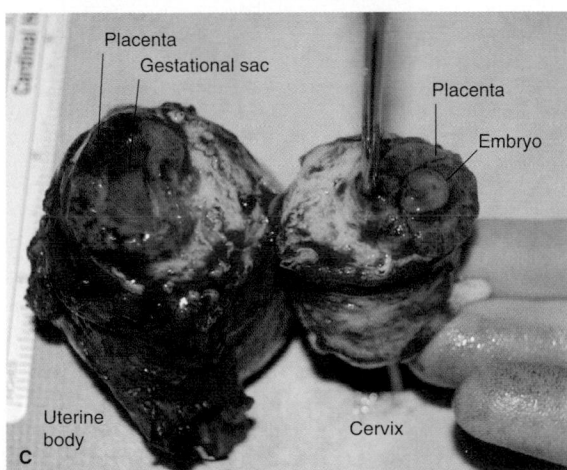

FIGURE 7-13 Cesarean scar pregnancy. **A.** Transvaginal sonogram of a uterus with a cesarean scar pregnancy (CSP) in a sagittal plane. The diagnosis is suggested by sonographic criteria indicative of CSP. First, an empty uterine cavity is identified by a bright hyperechoic endometrial stripe (*long, white arrow*). An empty cervical canal is similarly identified (*short, white arrow*). Lastly, an intrauterine mass is seen in the anterior part of the uterine isthmus (*red arrows*). *(Image contributed by Dr. Elysia Moschos.)* **B.** Hysterectomy specimen containing a cesarean scar pregnancy. **C.** This hysterectomy specimen with a cesarean scar pregnancy is transversely sectioned at the level of the uterine isthmus and through the gestational sac. Only a thin layer of myometrium overlies this pregnancy, which pushes anteriorly through the uterine wall. *(Photograph contributed by Dr. Sunil Balgobin.)*

REFERENCES

al-Awwad MM, al Daham N, Eseet JS: Spontaneous unruptured bilateral ectopic pregnancy: conservative tubal surgery. Obstet Gynecol Surv 54:543, 1999

Alexander JM, Rouse DJ, Varner E, et al: Treatment of the small unruptured ectopic pregnancy: a cost analysis of methotrexate versus laparoscopy. Obstet Gynecol 88:123, 1996

Alleyassin A, Khademi A, Aghahosseini M, et al: Comparison of success rates in the medical management of ectopic pregnancy with single-dose and multiple-dose administration of methotrexate: a prospective, randomized clinical trial. Fertil Steril 85(6):1661, 2006

American College of Obstetricians and Gynecologists: Medical management of ectopic pregnancy. Practice Bulletin No. 94, 2008

American Society for Reproductive Medicine: Medical treatment of ectopic pregnancy. Fertil Steril 90(5 Suppl):S206, 2008

American Society for Reproductive Medicine and Society for Assisted Reproductive Technology: Assisted reproductive technology in the United States: 1999 results generated from the American Society for Reproductive Medicine/Society for Assisted Reproductive Technology Registry. Fertil Steril 78:918, 2002

Ankum WM, Mol BW, Van der Veen F, et al: Risk factors for ectopic pregnancy: a meta-analysis. Fertil Steril 65:1093, 1996

Ash A, Smith A, Maxwell D: Caesarean scar pregnancy. BJOG 114(3):253, 2007

Atri M: Ectopic pregnancy versus corpus luteum cyst revisited: best Doppler predictors. J Ultrasound Med 22:1181, 2003a

Atri M, Valenti DA, Bret PM, et al: Effect of transvaginal sonography on the use of invasive procedures for evaluating patients with a clinical diagnosis of ectopic pregnancy. J Clin Ultrasound 31:1, 2003b

Backman T, Rauramo I, Huhtala S, et al: Pregnancy during the use of levonorgestrel intrauterine system. Am J Obstet Gynecol 190:50, 2004

Barak S, Oettinger M, Perri A, et al: Frozen section examination of endometrial curettings in the diagnosis of ectopic pregnancy. Acta Obstet Gynecol Scand 84:43, 2005

Barnhart K, Hummel AC, Sammel MD, et al: Use of "2-dose" regimen of methotrexate to treat ectopic pregnancy. Fertil Steril 87(2):250, 2007

Barnhart KT: Clinical practice. Ectopic pregnancy. N Engl J Med 361(4):379, 2009

Barnhart KT, Cassanova B, Sammel MD, et al: Prediction of location of a symptomatic early gestation based solely on clinical presentation. Obstet Gynecol 112(6):1319, 2008

Barnhart KT, Fay CA, Suescum M, et al: Clinical factors affecting the accuracy of ultrasonography in symptomatic first-trimester pregnancy. Obstet Gynecol 117(2 Pt 1):299, 2011

Barnhart KT, Gosman G, Ashby R, et al: The medical management of ectopic pregnancy: a meta-analysis comparing "single dose" and "multidose" regimens. Obstet Gynecol 101:778, 2003a

Barnhart KT, Gracia CR, Reindl B, et al: Usefulness of Pipelle endometrial biopsy in the diagnosis of women at risk for ectopic pregnancy. Am J Obstet Gynecol 188:906, 2003b

Barnhart KT, Katz I, Hummel A, et al: Presumed diagnosis of ectopic pregnancy. Obstet Gynecol 100:505, 2002

Barnhart KT, Rinaudo P, Hummel A, et al: Acute and chronic presentation of ectopic pregnancy may be two clinical entities. Fertil Steril 80:1345, 2003c

Barnhart KT, Sammel MD, Rinaudo PF, et al: Symptomatic patients with an early viable intrauterine pregnancy: HCG curves redefined. Obstet Gynecol 104:50, 2004

Barnhart KT, Simhan H, Kamelle SA: Diagnostic accuracy of ultrasound above and below the beta-hCG discriminatory zone. Obstet Gynecol 94:583, 1999

Becker S, Solomayer E, Hornung R, et al: Optimal treatment for patients with ectopic pregnancies and a history of fertility-reducing factors. Arch Gynecol Obstet 283:1, 2011

Bengtsson G, Bryman I, Thorburn J, et al: Low-dose oral methotrexate as second-line therapy for persistent trophoblast after conservative treatment of ectopic pregnancy. Obstet Gynecol 79:589, 1992

Bernstein HB, Thrall MM, Clark WB: Expectant management of intramural ectopic pregnancy. Obstet Gynecol 97:826, 2001

Birkhahn RH, Gaeta TJ, Van Deusen SK, et al: The ability of traditional vital signs and shock index to identify ruptured ectopic pregnancy. Am J Obstet Gynecol 189:1293, 2003

Bouyer J, Coste J, Fernandez H, et al: Sites of ectopic pregnancy: a 10 year population-based study of 1800 cases. Hum Reprod 17:3224, 2002

Bouyer J, Coste J, Shojaei T, et al: Risk factors for ectopic pregnancy: a comprehensive analysis based on a large case-control, population-based study in France. Am J Epidemiol 157:185, 2003

Branney SW, Wolfe RE, Moore EE, et al: Quantitative sensitivity of ultrasound in detecting free intraperitoneal fluid. J Trauma 40(6):1052, 1995

Brennan DF, Kwatra S, Kelly M, et al: Chronic ectopic pregnancy–two cases of acute rupture despite negative beta hCG. J Emerg Med 19(3):249, 2000

Brown DL, Doubilet PM: Transvaginal sonography for diagnosing ectopic pregnancy: positivity criteria and performance characteristics. J Ultrasound Med 13:259, 1994

Brown DL, Felker RE, Stovall TG, et al: Serial endovaginal sonography of ectopic pregnancies treated with methotrexate. Obstet Gynecol 77:406, 1991

Bucella D, Buxant F, Anaf V, et al: Omental trophoblastic implants after surgical management of ectopic pregnancy. Arch Gynecol Obstet 280(1):115, 2009

Burry KA, Thurmond AS, Suby-Long TD, et al: Transvaginal ultrasonographic findings in surgically verified ectopic pregnancy. Am J Obstet Gynecol 168:1796, 1993

Buster JE, Pisarska MD: Medical management of ectopic pregnancy. Clin Obstet Gynecol 42:23, 1999

Butts S, Sammel M, Hummel A, et al: Risk factors and clinical features of recurrent ectopic pregnancy: a case control study. Fertil Steril 80:1340, 2003

Carson SA, Buster JE: Ectopic pregnancy. N Engl J Med 329:1174, 1993

Cates W, Jr.: Chlamydial infections and the risk of ectopic pregnancy. JAMA 281:117, 1999

Centers for Disease Control and Prevention: Ectopic pregnancy—United States, 1990-1992. MMWR Morb Mortal Wkly Rep 44:46, 1995

Chabner BA, Amrein PC, Druker BJ: Antineoplastic agents. In Brunton LL, Lazo JS, Parker KL (eds): Goodman & Gilman's The Pharmacological Basis of Therapeutics, 11th ed. New York, McGraw-Hill, 2006, p 1335

Chung K, Chandavarkar U, Opper N, et al: Reevaluating the role of dilation and curettage in the diagnosis of pregnancy of unknown location. Fertil Steril 96(3):659, 2011

Cipullo L, Cassese S, Fasolino MC et al: Cervical pregnancy: a case series and a review of current clinical practice. Eur J Contracept Reprod Health Care 13(3):313, 2008

Comstock C, Huston K, Lee W: The ultrasonographic appearance of ovarian ectopic pregnancies. Obstet Gynecol 105:42, 2005

Coste J, Fernandez H, Joye N, et al: Role of chromosome abnormalities in ectopic pregnancy. Fertil Steril 74:1259, 2000

Cunningham FG, Leveno KJ, Bloom SL (eds): Ectopic pregnancy. In Williams Obstetrics, 23rd ed. New York, McGraw-Hill, 2010, p 239

Daniel Y, Geva E, Lerner-Geva L, et al: Levels of vascular endothelial growth factor are elevated in patients with ectopic pregnancy: is this a novel marker? Fertil Steril 72:1013, 1999

Dart RG, Kaplan B, Varaklis K: Predictive value of history and physical examination in patients with suspected ectopic pregnancy. Ann Emerg Med 33:283, 1999

Dashefsky SM, Lyons EA, Levi CS, et al: Suspected ectopic pregnancy: endovaginal and transvesical US. Radiology 169:181, 1988

Davis LB, Lathi RB, Milki AA, et al: Transvaginal ligation of the cervical branches of the uterine artery and injection of vasopressin in a cervical pregnancy as an initial step to controlling hemorrhage: a case report. J Reprod Med 53(5):365, 2008

De La Vega GA, Avery C, Nemiroff, et al: Treatment of early cervical pregnancy with cerclage, carboprost, curettage, and balloon tamponade. Obstet Gynecol 109(2 Pt 2):505, 2007

Dengfeng W, Taixiang W, Lina H, et al: Chinese herbal medicines in the treatment of ectopic pregnancy. Cochrane Database Syst Rev CD006224, 2007

Deruelle P, Lucot JP, Lions C, et al: Management of interstitial pregnancy using selective uterine artery embolization. Obstet Gynecol 106:1165, 2005

Dixon RE, Hwang SJ, Hennig GW, et al: Chlamydia infection causes loss of pacemaker cells and inhibits oocyte transport in the mouse oviduct. Biol Reprod 80(4):665, 2009

Dudley PS, Heard MJ, Sangi-Haghpeykar H, et al: Characterizing ectopic pregnancies that rupture despite treatment with methotrexate. Fertil Steril 82(5):1374, 2004

Egger M, Low N, Smith GD, et al: Screening for chlamydial infections and the risk of ectopic pregnancy in a county in Sweden: ecological analysis. BMJ 316:1776, 1998

Elito J, Jr., Han KK, Camano L: Values of beta-human chorionic gonadotropin as a risk factor for tubal obstruction after tubal pregnancy. Acta Obstet Gynecol Scand 84:864, 2005

Elson J, Tailor A, Banerjee S, et al: Expectant management of tubal ectopic pregnancy: prediction of successful outcome using decision tree analysis. Ultrasound Obstet Gynecol 23:552, 2004

Fernandez H, Pauthier S, Doumerc S, et al: Ultrasound-guided injection of methotrexate versus laparoscopic salpingotomy in ectopic pregnancy. Fertil Steril 63:25, 1995

Fernandez H, Yves Vincent SC, Pauthier S, et al: Randomized trial of conservative laparoscopic treatment and methotrexate administration in ectopic pregnancy and subsequent fertility. Hum Reprod 13:3239, 1998

Foulk RA, Steiger RM: Operative management of ectopic pregnancy: a cost analysis. Am J Obstet Gynecol 175:90, 1996

Fylstra DL: Ectopic pregnancy after hysterectomy: a review and insight into etiology and prevention. Fertil Steril 94:431, 2009

Ginsburg ES, Frates MC, Rein MS, et al: Early diagnosis and treatment of cervical pregnancy in an in vitro fertilization program. Fertil Steril 61:966, 1994

Gjelland K, Hordnes K, Tjugum J, et al: Treatment of ectopic pregnancy by local injection of hypertonic glucose: a randomized trial comparing administration guided by transvaginal ultrasound or laparoscopy. Acta Obstet Gynecol Scand 74:629, 1995

Glezerman M, Press F, Carpman M: Culdocentesis is an obsolete diagnostic tool in suspected ectopic pregnancy. Arch Gynecol Obstet 252:5, 1992

Godin PA, Bassil S, Donnez J: An ectopic pregnancy developing in a previous caesarian section scar. Fertil Steril 67:398, 1997

Goldner TE, Lawson HW, Xia Z, et al: Surveillance for ectopic pregnancy—United States, 1970-1989. Morb Mortal Wkly Rep CDC Surveill Summ 42:73, 1993

Gracia CR, Barnhart KT: Diagnosing ectopic pregnancy: decision analysis comparing six strategies. Obstet Gynecol 97:464, 2001

Graczykowski JW, Mishell DR, Jr.: Methotrexate prophylaxis for persistent ectopic pregnancy after conservative treatment by salpingostomy. Obstet Gynecol 89:118, 1997

Graczykowski JW, Seifer DB: Diagnosis of acute and persistent ectopic pregnancy. Clin Obstet Gynecol 42:9, 1999

Gurel S, Sarikaya B, Gurel K, et al: Role of sonography in the diagnosis of ectopic pregnancy. J Clin Ultrasound 35(9):509, 2007

Guven ES, Dilbaz S, Dilbaz B, et al: Comparison of the effect of single-dose and multiple-dose methotrexate therapy on tubal patency. Fertil Steril 88(5):1288, 2007

Habana A, Dokras A, Giraldo JL, et al: Cornual heterotopic pregnancy: contemporary management options. Am J Obstet Gynecol 182:1264, 2000

Hajenius PJ, Engelsbel S, Mol BW, et al: Randomised trial of systemic methotrexate versus laparoscopic salpingostomy in tubal pregnancy. Lancet 350:774, 1997

Hajenius PJ, Mol BW, Bossuyt PM, et al: Interventions for tubal ectopic pregnancy. Cochrane Database Syst Rev CD000324, 2000

Hammoud AO, Hammoud I, Bujold E, et al: The role of sonographic endometrial patterns and endometrial thickness in the differential diagnosis of ectopic pregnancy. Am J Obstet Gynecol 192:1370, 2005

Hillis SD, Owens LM, Marchbanks PA, et al: Recurrent chlamydial infections increase the risks of hospitalization for ectopic pregnancy and pelvic inflammatory disease. Am J Obstet Gynecol 176:103, 1997

Hirakawa M, Tajima T, Yoshimitsu K, et al: Uterine artery embolization along with the administration of methotrexate for cervical ectopic pregnancy: technical and clinical outcomes. AJR Am J Roentgenol 192(6):1601, 2009

Hoover KW, Tao G, Kent CK: Trends in the diagnosis and treatment of ectopic pregnancy in the United States. Obstet Gynecol 115(3):495, 2010

Horne AW, Phillips JA III, Kane N, et al: CB1 expression is attenuated in fallopian tube and decidua of women with ectopic pregnancy. PLoS One 3(12):e3969, 2008

Hung TH, Jeng CJ, Yang YC, et al: Treatment of cervical pregnancy with methotrexate. Int J Gynaecol Obstet 53:243, 1996

Iavazzo C, Salakos N, Vitoratos N: Intrauterine devices and extrauterine pregnancy. A literature review. Clin Exp Obstet Gynecol 35(2):103, 2008

Isaacs JD, Jr., McGehee RP, Cowan BD: Life-threatening neutropenia following methotrexate treatment of ectopic pregnancy: a report of two cases. Obstet Gynecol 88:694, 1996

Jeng CJ, Ko ML, Shen J: Transvaginal ultrasound-guided treatment of cervical pregnancy. Obstet Gynecol 109(5):1076, 2007

Jermy K, Thomas J, Doo A, et al: The conservative management of interstitial pregnancy. BJOG 111:1283, 2004

Job-Spira N, Fernandez H, Bouyer J, et al: Ruptured tubal ectopic pregnancy: risk factors and reproductive outcome: results of a population-based study in France. Am J Obstet Gynecol 180:938, 1999

Jundt JW, Browne BA, Fiocco GP, et al: A comparison of low dose methotrexate bioavailability: oral solution, oral tablet, subcutaneous and intramuscular dosing. J Rheumatol 20:1845, 1993

Jurkovic D, Hillaby K, Woelfer B, et al: First-trimester diagnosis and management of pregnancies implanted into the lower uterine segment cesarean section scar. Ultrasound Obstet Gynecol 21(3):220, 2003

Kadar N, DeCherney AH, Romero R: Receiver operating characteristic (ROC) curve analysis of the relative efficacy of single and serial chorionic gonadotropin determinations in the early diagnosis of ectopic pregnancy. Fertil Steril 37:542, 1982

Kirk E, Condous G, Van Calster B, et al: A validation of the most commonly used protocol to predict the success of single-dose methotrexate in the treatment of ectopic pregnancy. Hum Reprod 22(3):858, 2007

Korhonen J, Stenman UH, Ylostalo P: Low-dose oral methotrexate with expectant management of ectopic pregnancy. Obstet Gynecol 88:775, 1996

Krag Moeller LB, Moeller C, Thomsen SG, et al: Success and spontaneous pregnancy rates following systemic methotrexate versus laparoscopic surgery for tubal pregnancies: a randomized trial. Acta Obstet Gynecol Scand 88(12):1331, 2009

Kung FT, Chang SY, Tsai YC, et al: Subsequent reproduction and obstetric outcome after methotrexate treatment of cervical pregnancy: a review of original literature and international collaborative follow up. Hum Reprod 12:591, 1997

Kutluay L, Vicdan K, Turan C, et al: Tubal histopathology in ectopic pregnancies. Eur J Obstet Gynecol Reprod Biol 57:91, 1994

Lau S, Tulandi T: Conservative medical and surgical management of interstitial ectopic pregnancy. Fertil Steril 72:207, 1999

Lavie O, Boldes R, Neuman M, et al: Ultrasonographic "endometrial three-layer" pattern: a unique finding in ectopic pregnancy. J Clin Ultrasound 24(4):179, 1996

Levine D: Ectopic pregnancy. Radiology 245(2):385, 2007

Lim YH, Ng SP, Ng PH, et al: Laparoscopic salpingectomy in tubal pregnancy: prospective randomized trial using endoloop versus electrocautery. J Obstet Gynaecol Res 33(6):855, 2007

Lindahl B, Ahlgren M: Identification of chorion villi in abortion specimens. Obstet Gynecol 67:79, 1986

Lipscomb GH: Medical therapy for ectopic pregnancy. Semin Reprod Med 25(2):93, 2007

Lipscomb GH, Bran D, McCord ML, et al: Analysis of three hundred fifteen ectopic pregnancies treated with single-dose methotrexate. Am J Obstet Gynecol 178:1354, 1998

Lipscomb GH, Givens VM, Meyer NL, et al: Comparison of multidose and single-dose methotrexate protocols for the treatment of ectopic pregnancy. Am J Obstet Gynecol 192:1844, 2005

Lipscomb GH, Gomez IG, Givens VM, et al: Yolk sac on transvaginal ultrasound as a prognostic indicator in the treatment of ectopic pregnancy with single-dose methotrexate. Am J Obstet Gynecol 200(3):338.e1-4, 2009

Lipscomb GH, McCord ML, Stovall TG, et al: Predictors of success of methotrexate treatment in women with tubal ectopic pregnancies. N Engl J Med 341:1974, 1999

Lopez HB, Micheelsen U, Berendtsen H, et al: Ectopic pregnancy and its associated endometrial changes. Gynecol Obstet Invest 38:104, 1994

Lundorff P, Thorburn J, Hahlin M, et al: Laparoscopic surgery in ectopic pregnancy. A randomized trial versus laparotomy. Acta Obstet Gynecol Scand 70:343, 1991

Menon S, Collins J, Barnhart KT: Establishing a human chorionic gonadotropin cutoff to guide methotrexate treatment of ectopic pregnancy: a systematic review. Fertil Steril 87(3):481, 2007

Mesogitis S, Pilalis A, Daskalakis G, et al: Management of early viable cervical pregnancy. BJOG 112:409, 2005

Michener C, Dickinson JE: Caesarean scar ectopic pregnancy: a single centre case series. Aust N Z J Obstet Gynaecol 49(5):451, 2009

Milad MP, Klein E, Kazer RR: Preoperative serum hCG level and intraoperative failure of laparoscopic linear salpingostomy for ectopic pregnancy. Obstet Gynecol 92:373, 1998

Moawad NS, Mahajan ST, Moniz MH, et al: Current diagnosis and treatment of interstitial pregnancy. Am J Obstet Gynecol 202(1):15, 2010

Mol BW, Ankum WM, Bossuyt PM, et al: Contraception and the risk of ectopic pregnancy: a meta-analysis. Contraception 52:337, 1995

Mol BW, Lijmer JG, Ankum WM, et al: The accuracy of single serum progesterone measurement in the diagnosis of ectopic pregnancy: a meta-analysis. Hum Reprod 13:3220, 1998

Mol F, Mol BW, Ankum WM, et al: Current evidence on surgery, systemic methotrexate and expectant management in the treatment of tubal ectopic pregnancy: a systematic review and meta-analysis. Hum Reprod Update 14(4):309, 2008a

Mol F, Strandell A, Jurkovic D, et al: The ESEP study: salpingostomy versus salpingectomy for tubal ectopic pregnancy, the impact on future fertility: a randomised controlled trial. BMC Womens Health 8:11, 2008b

Moschos E, Sreenarasimhaiah S, Twickler DM: First-trimester diagnosis of cesarean scar ectopic pregnancy. J Clin Ultrasound 36(8):504, 2008

Moschos E, Twickler DM: Endometrial thickness predicts intrauterine pregnancy in patients with pregnancy of unknown location. Ultrasound Obstet Gynecol 32(7):929, 2008

Murphy AA, Nager CW, Wujek JJ, et al: Operative laparoscopy versus laparotomy for the management of ectopic pregnancy: a prospective trial. Fertil Steril 57:1180, 1992

Nakao Y, Yokoyama M, Iwasaka T: Uterine artery embolization followed by dilation and curettage for cervical pregnancy. Obstet Gynecol 111(2 Pt 2):505, 2008

Natale A, Candiani M, Merlo D, et al: Human chorionic gonadotropin level as a predictor of trophoblastic infiltration into the tubal wall in ectopic pregnancy: a blinded study. Fertil Steril 79:981, 2003

Ness RB, McLaughlin MT, Heine RP, et al: Fetal fibronectin as a marker to discriminate between ectopic and intrauterine pregnancies. Am J Obstet Gynecol 179:697, 1998

Nguyen C, Duhl AJ, Escallon CS, et al: Multiple anomalies in a fetus exposed to low-dose methotrexate in the first trimester. Obstet Gynecol 99:599, 2002

Nieuwkerk PT, Hajenius PJ, Ankum WM, et al: Systemic methotrexate therapy versus laparoscopic salpingostomy in patients with tubal pregnancy. Part I. Impact on patients' health-related quality of life. Fertil Steril 70:511, 1998

Nowak-Markwitz E, Michalak M, Olejnik M, et al: Cutoff value of human chorionic gonadotropin in relation to the number of methotrexate cycles in the successful treatment of ectopic pregnancy. Fertil Steril 92(4):1203, 2009

Nurmohamed L, Moretti ME, Schechter T, et al: Importance of timing of gestational exposure to methotrexate for its teratogenic effects when used in setting of misdiagnosis of ectopic pregnancy. Am J Obstet Gynecol Jul 20, 2011 [Epub ahead of print]

Nyberg DA, Hughes MP, Mack LA, et al: Extrauterine findings of ectopic pregnancy of transvaginal US: importance of echogenic fluid. Radiology 178:823, 1991

Paul M, Schaff E, Nichols M: The roles of clinical assessment, human chorionic gonadotropin assays, and ultrasonography in medical abortion practice. Am J Obstet Gynecol 183:S34, 2000

Pattinson HA, Dunphy BC, Wood S, et al: Cervical pregnancy following in vitro fertilization: evacuation after uterine artery embolization with subsequent successful intrauterine pregnancy. Aust N Z J Obstet Gynaecol 34:492, 1994

Pellerito JS, Taylor KJ, Quedens-Case C, et al: Ectopic pregnancy: evaluation with endovaginal color flow imaging. Radiology 193(2):407, 1992

Peterson HB, Xia Z, Hughes JM, et al: The risk of ectopic pregnancy after tubal sterilization. U.S. Collaborative Review of Sterilization Working Group. N Engl J Med 336:762, 1997

Pisarska MD, Carson SA: Incidence and risk factors for ectopic pregnancy. Clin Obstet Gynecol 42:2, 1999

Poggi SH, Ghidini A: Importance of timing of gestational exposure to methotrexate for its teratogenic effects when used in setting of misdiagnosis of ectopic pregnancy. Fertil Steril 96(3):669, 2011

Predanic M: Differentiating tubal abortion from viable ectopic pregnancy with serum CA-125 and beta-human chorionic gonadotropin determinations. Fertil Steril 73:522, 2000

Rajkhowa M, Glass MR, Rutherford AJ, et al: Trends in the incidence of ectopic pregnancy in England and Wales from 1966 to 1996. BJOG 107:369, 2000

Rausch ME, Sammel MD, Takacs P, et al: Development of a Multiple Marker Test for Ectopic Pregnancy. Obstet Gynecol 117(3):573, 2011

Revel A, Ophir I, Koler M, et al: Changing etiology of tubal pregnancy following IVF. Hum Reprod 23(6):1372, 2008

Ries A, Singson P, Bidus M, et al: Use of the endometrial pipelle in the diagnosis of early abnormal gestations. Fertil Steril 74:593, 2000

Rodgerson JD, Heegaard WG, Plummer D, et al: Emergency department right upper quadrant ultrasound is associated with a reduced time to diagnosis and treatment of ruptured ectopic pregnancies. Acad Emerg Med 8(4):331, 2001

Rose JS: Ultrasound in abdominal trauma. Emerg Med Clin North Am 22(3):581, 2004

Rozenberg P, Chevret S, Camus E, et al: Medical treatment of ectopic pregnancies: a randomized clinical trial comparing methotrexate-mifepristone and methotrexate-placebo. Hum Reprod 18:1802, 2003

Rulin MC: Is salpingostomy the surgical treatment of choice for unruptured tubal pregnancy? Obstet Gynecol 86:1010, 1995

Sadeghi H, Rutherford T, Rackow BW: Cesarean scar ectopic pregnancy: case series and review of the literature. Am J Perinatol 27(2):111, 2010

Sagiv R, Debby A, Sadan O, et al: Laparoscopic surgery for extrauterine pregnancy in hemodynamically unstable patients. J Am Assoc Gynecol Laparosc 8:529, 2001

Sanz LE, Verosko J: Hysteroscopic management of cornual ectopic pregnancy. Obstet Gynecol 99:941, 2002

Saraiya M, Berg CJ, Kendrick JS, et al: Cigarette smoking as a risk factor for ectopic pregnancy. Am J Obstet Gynecol 178:493, 1998

Sawaya GF, Grady D, Kerlikowske K, et al: Antibiotics at the time of induced abortion: the case for universal prophylaxis based on a meta-analysis. Obstet Gynecol 87:884, 1996

Saxon D, Falcone T, Mascha EJ, et al: A study of ruptured tubal ectopic pregnancy. Obstet Gynecol 90:46, 1997

Segal S, Gor H, Correa N, et al: Inhibin A: marker for diagnosis of ectopic and early abnormal pregnancies. Reprod Biomed Online 17(6):789, 2008

Senterman M, Jibodh R, Tulandi T: Histopathologic study of ampullary and isthmic tubal ectopic pregnancy. Am J Obstet Gynecol 159:939, 1988

Seow KM, Huang LW, Lin YH: Cesarean scar pregnancy: issues in management. Ultrasound Obstet Gynecol 23(3):247, 2004

Shalev E, Peleg D, Tsabari A, et al: Spontaneous resolution of ectopic tubal pregnancy: natural history. Fertil Steril 63:15, 1995

Shankar R, Gude N, Cullinane F, et al: An emerging role for comprehensive proteome analysis in human pregnancy research. Reproduction 129:685, 2005

Shaunik A, Kulp J, Appleby DH, et al: Utility of dilation and curettage in the diagnosis of pregnancy of unknown location. Am J Obstet Gynecol 204(2):130.e1, 2011

Shaw JL, Dey SK, Critchley HO, et al: Current knowledge of the aetiology of human tubal ectopic pregnancy. Hum Reprod Update 16:432, 2010

Skjeldestad FE, Hadgu A, Eriksson N: Epidemiology of repeat ectopic pregnancy: a population-based prospective cohort study. Obstet Gynecol 91:129, 1998

Sowter M, Farquhar C: Changing face of ectopic pregnancy. Each centre should validate diagnostic algorithms for its own patients. BMJ 315:1312, 1997

Spandorfer SD, Menzin AW, Barnhart KT, et al: Efficacy of frozen-section evaluation of uterine curettings in the diagnosis of ectopic pregnancy. Am J Obstet Gynecol 175:603, 1996

Spandorfer SD, Sawin SW, Benjamin I, et al: Postoperative day 1 serum human chorionic gonadotropin level as a predictor of persistent ectopic pregnancy after conservative surgical management. Fertil Steril 68:430, 1997

Spiegelberg O: Zur Casuistic der Ovarialschwangerschaft. Arch Gynaekol 13:73, 1878

Stovall TG, Ling FW: Single-dose methotrexate: an expanded clinical trial. Am J Obstet Gynecol 168:1759, 1993

Stovall TG, Ling FW, Andersen RN, et al: Improved sensitivity and specificity of a single measurement of serum progesterone over serial quantitative beta-human chorionic gonadotrophin in screening for ectopic pregnancy. Hum Reprod 7:723, 1992

Straka M, Zeringue E, Goldman M: A rare drug reaction to methotrexate after treatment for ectopic pregnancy. Obstet Gynecol 103:1047, 2004

Strandell A, Thorburn J, Hamberger L: Risk factors for ectopic pregnancy in assisted reproduction. Fertil Steril 71:282, 1999

Swire MN, Castro-Aragon I, Levine D: Various sonographic appearances of the hemorrhagic corpus luteum cyst. Ultrasound Q 20:45, 2004

Tal J, Haddad S, Gordon N, et al: Heterotopic pregnancy after ovulation induction and assisted reproductive technologies: a literature review from 1971 to 1993. Fertil Steril 66:1, 1996

Talbot P, Riveles K: Smoking and reproduction: the oviduct as a target of cigarette smoke. Reprod Biol Endocrinol 3:52, 2005

Tharaux-Deneux C, Bouyer J, Job-Spira N, et al: Risk of ectopic pregnancy and previous induced abortion. Am J Public Health 88:401, 1998

Thurman AR, Cornelius M, Korte JE, et al: An alternative monitoring protocol for single-dose methotrexate therapy in ectopic pregnancy. Am J Obstet Gynecol 202(2):139.e1-6, 2010

Toth M, Patton DL, Campbell LA, et al: Detection of chlamydial antigenic material in ovarian, prostatic, ectopic pregnancy and semen samples of culture-negative subjects. Am J Reprod Immunol 43:218, 2000

Trambert JJ, Einstein MH, Banks E, et al: Uterine artery embolization in the management of vaginal bleeding from cervical pregnancy: a case series. J Reprod Med 50:844, 2005

Trio D, Strobelt N, Picciolo C, et al: Prognostic factors for successful expectant management of ectopic pregnancy. Fertil Steril 63:469, 1995

Trojano G, Colafiglio G, Saliani N, et al: Successful management of a cervical twin pregnancy: neoadjuvant systemic methotrexate and prophylactic high cervical cerclage before curettage. Fertil Steril 91(3):935.e17, 2009

Tulandi T, Al Jaroudi D: Interstitial pregnancy: results generated from the Society of Reproductive Surgeons Registry. Obstet Gynecol 103:47, 2004

Tulandi T, Hemmings R, Khalifa F: Rupture of ectopic pregnancy in women with low and declining serum beta-human chorionic gonadotropin concentrations. Fertil Steril 56:786, 1991

Ushakov FB, Elchalal U, Aceman PJ, et al: Cervical pregnancy: past and future. Obstet Gynecol Surv 52:45, 1997

Van Den Eeden SK, Shan J, Bruce C, et al: Ectopic pregnancy rate and treatment utilization in a large managed care organization. Obstet Gynecol 105:1052, 2005

Van Voorhis BJ: Outcomes from assisted reproductive technology. Obstet Gynecol 107:183, 2006

Verma U, Goharkhay N: Conservative management of cervical ectopic pregnancy. Fertil Steril 91(3):671, 2009

Vermesh M, Graczykowski JW, Sauer MV: Reevaluation of the role of culdocentesis in the management of ectopic pregnancy. Am J Obstet Gynecol 162:411, 1990

Vermesh M, Silva PD, Rosen GF, et al: Management of unruptured ectopic gestation by linear salpingostomy: a prospective, randomized clinical trial of laparoscopy versus laparotomy. Obstet Gynecol 73:400, 1989

Wang JH, Xu KH, Lin J, et al: Methotrexate therapy for cesarean section scar pregnancy with and without suction curettage. Fertil Steril 92(4):1208, 2009

Warkany J: Aminopterin and methotrexate: folic acid deficiency. Teratology 17:353, 1978

World Health Organization: A multinational case-control study of ectopic pregnancy. The World Health Organization's Special Programme of Research, Development and Research Training in Human Reproduction: Task Force on Intrauterine Devices for Fertility Regulation. Clin Reprod Fertil 3:131, 1985

Yang Q, Piao S, Wang G, et al: Hysteroscopic surgery of ectopic pregnancy in the cesarean section scar. J Minim Invasive Gynecol 16(4):432, 2009

Yeko TR, Mayer JC, Parsons AK, et al: A prospective series of unruptured ectopic pregnancies treated by tubal injection with hyperosmolar glucose. Obstet Gynecol 85:265, 1995

Zane SB, Kieke BA, Jr., Kendrick JS, et al: Surveillance in a time of changing health care practices: estimating ectopic pregnancy incidence in the United States. Matern Child Health J 6:227, 2002

Zhang X, Liu X, Fan H: Interstitial pregnancy and transcervical curettage. Obstet Gynecol 104(2):1193, 2004

Zhuang Y, Huang L: Uterine artery embolization compared with methotrexate for the management of pregnancy implanted within a cesarean scar. Am J Obstet Gynecol 201(2):152.e1, 2009

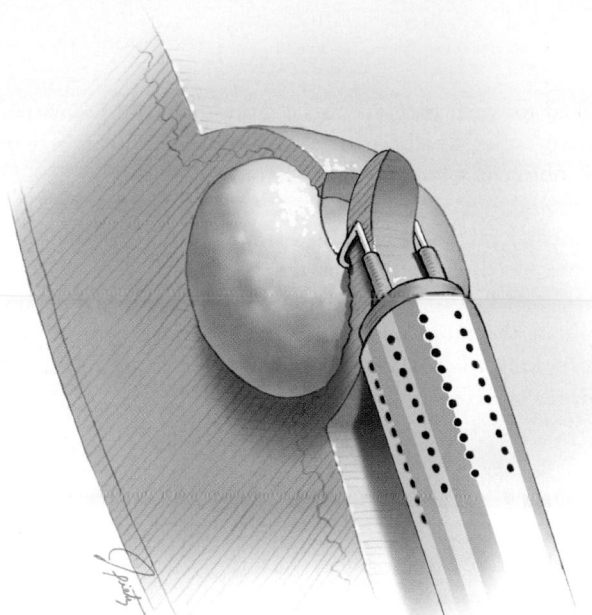

CHAPTER 8

Abnormal Uterine Bleeding

Regular cyclic menstruation results from the choreographed relationship between the endometrium and its regulating factors (Chap. 15, p. 430). Changes in either of these frequently result in abnormal bleeding. Causes of this bleeding include neoplastic growth, hormonal dysfunction, trauma, infection, coagulopathies, and complications of pregnancy (Table 8-1). As a result, abnormal uterine bleeding is a common gynecologic complaint that may affect females of all ages.

DEFINITIONS

Abnormal bleeding may display several patterns. *Menorrhagia* is defined as prolonged or heavy cyclic menstruation. Objectively, menses lasting longer than 7 days or exceeding 80 mL of blood loss are determining values (Hallberg, 1966). *Metrorrhagia* describes intermenstrual bleeding. The term *breakthrough bleeding* is a more informal term for metrorrhagia that accompanies hormone administration. Frequently, women may complain of both patterns, *menometrorrhagia*. In some women, there is diminished flow or shortening of menses, *hypomenorrhea*. Normal menstruation typically occurs every 28 days ± 7 days. Cycles with intervals longer than 35 days describe a state of *oligomenorrhea*. Finally, the term *withdrawal bleeding* refers to the predictable bleeding that results from an abrupt decline in progesterone levels.

Assessing heavy bleeding in a clinical setting has its limitations. For example, several studies have documented the lack of correlation between patient perception of blood loss and objective measurement (Chimbira, 1980c; Fraser, 1984). As a result, methods to objectively assess blood loss have been investigated. Hallberg and associates (1966) describe a technique to extract hemoglobin from sanitary napkins using sodium hydroxide. Hemoglobin is converted to hematin and can be measured spectrophotometrically. The constraints to this approach in a clinical setting are obvious.

Other tools used to estimate menstrual blood loss include hemoglobin and hematocrit evaluation. Hemoglobin concentrations below <12 g/dL increase the chance of identifying women with menorrhagia. A normal level, however, does not exclude menorrhagia, as many women with clinically significant bleeding have normal values.

Another method involves estimating the number and type of pads or tampons used by a woman during menses. Warner and colleagues (2004) found positive correlations between objective menorrhagia and passing clots more than 1 inch in diameter and changing pads more frequently than every

TABLE 8-1. Differential Diagnosis of Abnormal Bleeding

Dysfunctional uterine bleeding
Anovulatory
   Perimenarchal—immature hypothalamic-pituitary-ovarian axis
   Perimenopausal—insensitive ovarian follicles
   Endocrinopathies—see systemic causes
   Drugs—hypothalamic depressants, sex steroids
Ovulatory

Organic lesions
Pregnancy-associated causes—implantation spotting, abortion, ectopic pregnancy, gestational trophoblastic disease, postabortal or postpartum infection
Anatomic uterine lesions
   Neoplasm—leiomyoma, polyp, endometrial hyperplasia, cancer
   Atrophic endometrium
   Infection—sexually transmitted disease, tuberculosis, chronic endometritis
   Mechanical causes—intrauterine device, perforation
   Arteriovenous malformation
   Partial outflow obstruction—congenital müllerian defect, Asherman syndrome
Anatomic nonuterine lesions
   Ovarian lesions—hormone-producing neoplasm
   Fallopian tube lesions—salpingitis, cancer
   Cervical and vaginal lesions—cancer, polyp, infection, atrophic vaginitis, foreign body, trauma

Systemic abnormalities
Exogenous hormone administration—sex steroids, corticosteroids
Coagulopathies
Hepatic failure
Chronic renal failure
Endocrinopathies—hypothyroidism, hyperthyroidism, adrenal disorders, diabetes mellitus, hypothalamic-pituitary disorders, polycystic ovarian syndrome, obesity

Adapted from Leiserowitz, 1996, with permission.

3 hours. Attempts to standardize this type of evaluation have led to development of the pictorial blood assessment chart (PBAC) (Fig. 8-1). With a scoring sheet, patients are asked to record daily the number of sanitary pads or tampons that are lightly, moderately, or completely saturated. Scores are assigned as follows: 1 point for each lightly stained tampon, 5 if moderately saturated, and 10 if completely soaked. Pads are similarly given ascending scores of 1, 5, and 20, respectively. Small clots score 1 point, whereas large clots score 5. Points

are tallied for each menses. Totals more than 100 points per menstrual cycle have been shown to indicate a greater than 80-mL objective blood loss (Higham, 1990; Janssen, 1995; Reid, 2000).

Menstrual calendars are also commonly used to evaluate abnormal bleeding and its patterns (Fig. 8-2). As shown, patients are asked to record dates and quality of blood flow throughout the month. These calendars can be used to aid diagnosis and to document improvement during medical treatment.

INCIDENCE

Abnormal uterine bleeding affects 10 to 30 percent of reproductive-aged women and up to 50 percent of perimenopausal women (Haynes, 1977; Prentice, 2000). Factors that influence the incidence most greatly are age and reproductive status. For example, uterine bleeding is uncommon in prepubertal girls and menopausal women, whereas rates of abnormal bleeding increase significantly in adolescent, perimenopausal, and reproductive-age groups. Familiarity with the most common etiologies of bleeding within these demographics aids diagnosis and treatment.

Childhood

Bleeding prior to menarche should be investigated as an abnormal finding. Initial evaluation should focus on determining the location of the bleeding, because vaginal, rectal, or urethral bleeding can present similarly. In this age group, the vagina, rather than the uterus, is the most common source of bleeding. Vulvovaginitis is the most frequent cause, but dermatologic conditions, neoplastic growths, or trauma by accident, abuse, or foreign body may also be reasons. These are all discussed further in Chapter 14. In addition to vaginal sources, bleeding may also originate from the urethra, secondary to urethral prolapse or infection.

True uterine bleeding usually results from increased estrogen levels. Precocious puberty, accidental exogenous ingestion, or ovarian neoplasms should be considered in these children. Because of the risks associated with these, pelvic examination is requisite to identify the source as vaginal or uterine (Quint, 2001). Thus, adequate evaluation may warrant examination under anesthesia with or without vaginoscopy (Fig. 14-6, p. 386).

Adolescence

In this age group, abnormal uterine bleeding results from anovulation and coagulation defects at disproportionately higher rates compared with older reproductive-aged women (Claessens, 1981; Oral, 2002; Smith, 1998). In contrast, neoplastic growths such as polyps, leiomyomas, and ovarian neoplasms are less frequent. Importantly, pregnancy, sexually transmitted diseases, and sexual abuse should not be ignored in this population.

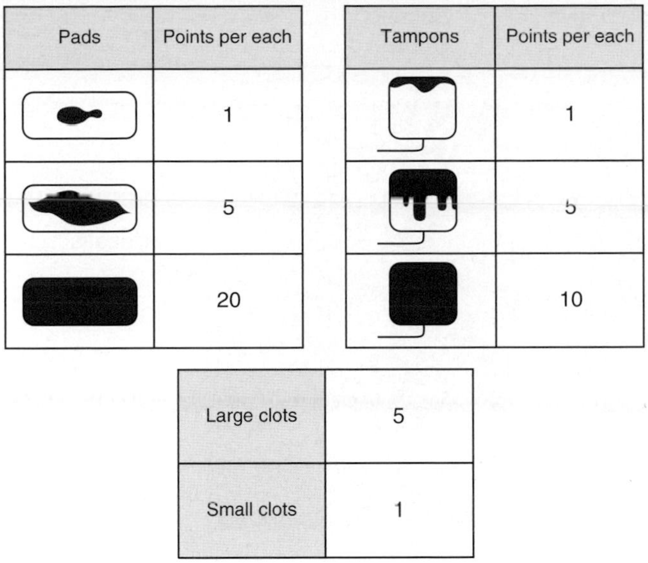

Pads	Points per each
	1
	5
	20

Tampons	Points per each
	1
	5
	10

Large clots	5
Small clots	1

FIGURE 8-1 Scoring for the pictorial bleeding assessment chart. Patients are counseled to evaluate the degree of saturation for each sanitary product used during menstruation. The total number of points are tallied for each menses. Point totals greater than 100 indicate menorrhagia.

Reproductive Age

Menorrhagia is a frequent problem in reproductive-aged women. It is estimated that a woman has a 1 in 20 lifetime chance of consulting her primary physician because of menorrhagia (Bongers, 2004).

Following adolescence, the hypothalamic-pituitary-ovarian axis matures, and anovulatory uterine bleeding is encountered less frequently. With increased sexual activity, rates of bleeding related to pregnancy and sexually transmitted diseases rise. The incidences of leiomyomas and endometrial polyps also increase with age. Accordingly, bleeding from these lesions becomes common in older women within this age group.

Perimenopause

Abnormal uterine bleeding is a frequent clinical problem, accounting for 70 percent of all gynecologic visits by peri- and postmenopausal women. As with perimenarchal girls, anovulatory uterine bleeding from hypothalamic-pituitary-ovarian axis dysfunction becomes a more common finding in this group (Chap. 21, p. 555). In contrast, the incidences of bleeding related to pregnancy and sexually transmitted diseases decrease. With aging, risks of benign and malignant neoplastic growth rise. For example, Seltzer and colleagues (1990) reviewed the charts of 500 perimenopausal women and characterized alterations in their menstrual flow. They found that 18 percent had menorrhagia or metrorrhagia, and a fifth of these were due to premalignant or malignant disease.

Menopause

Bleeding after menopause typically originates from benign disease. Most cases result from atrophy of the endometrium or vagina. Benign endometrial polyps may also cause bleeding in this population.

Even so, malignant neoplasms, especially endometrial carcinoma, are found more frequently in this age group than in others. Less commonly, estrogen-producing ovarian carcinoma may cause endometrial hyperplasia with uterine bleeding. Similarly, ulcerative vulvar, vaginal, or cervical neoplasms may also be sources. And rarely, egress of serosanguinous

Menstrual calendar

Month vs Date	1	2	3	4	5	6	7	8	9	10	11	12	13	14	15	16	17	18	19	20	21	22	23	24	25	26	27	28	29	30	31
January																															
February																														▒	▒
March																															
April																															▒
May																															
June																															▒
July																															
August																															
September																														▒	
October																															
November																														▒	
December																															

Type of bleeding:	Normal:X	Light: /	Heavy: ■	Spotting: S	Provera: P

FIGURE 8-2 Example of a menstrual calendar. Bleeding and its qualities are marked according to the legend at the bottom of the table on the days they occur.

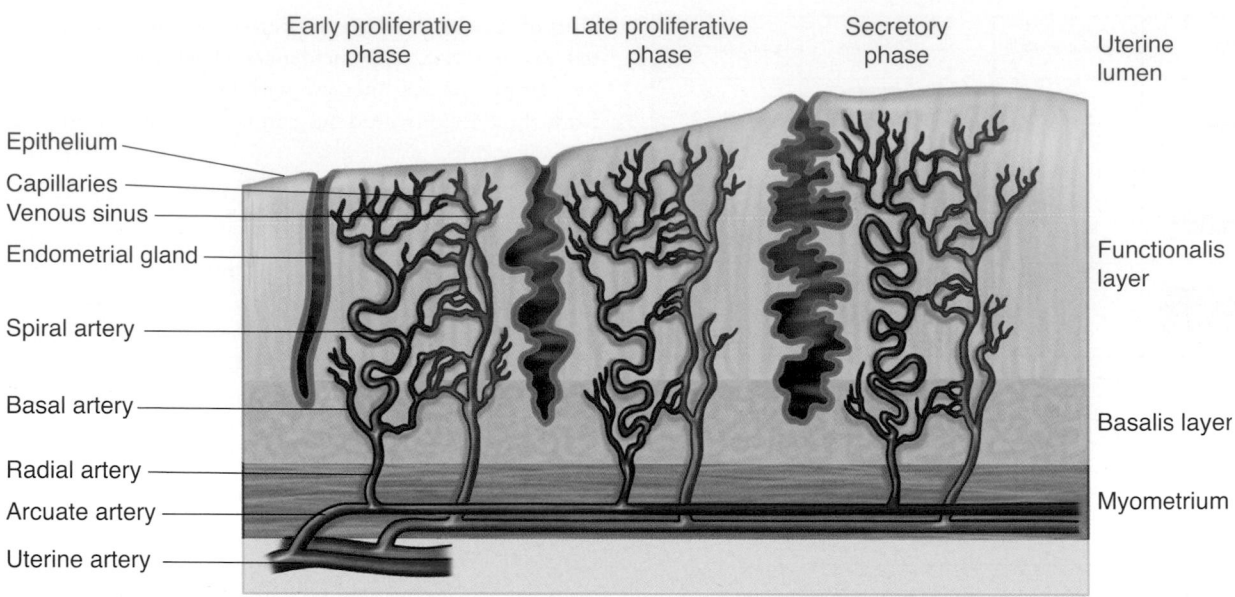

FIGURE 8-3 Drawing of endometrial anatomy as it varies through the menstrual cycle.

discharge from fallopian tube cancers can appear as uterine bleeding.

As with prepubertal females, because bleeding from the rectum, vagina, or urethra may present similarly, clear determination of the bleeding site is critical.

PATHOPHYSIOLOGY

The endometrium consists of two distinct zones, the functionalis layer and the basalis layer (Fig. 8-3). The basalis layer is beneath the functionalis, lies in direct contact with the myometrium, and is less hormonally responsive. The basalis serves as a reservoir for regeneration of the functionalis following menses (Chap. 15, p. 432). In contrast, the functionalis layer lines the uterine cavity, undergoes dramatic change throughout the menstrual cycle, and ultimately sloughs during menstruation. Histologically, the functionalis has a surface epithelium and underlying subepithelial capillary plexus. Also, there are organized stroma and glands in which leukocyte populations are interspersed.

Blood reaches the uterus via the uterine and ovarian arteries. From these, the arcuate arteries are formed and supply the myometrium. These in turn branch into the radial arteries, which extend toward the endometrium at right angles from the arcuate arteries (Fig. 8-4). At the endometrium-myometrium junction, the radial arteries bifurcate to create the basal and spiral arteries. The basal arteries serve the basalis layer of the endometrium and are relatively insensitive to hormonal changes (Abberton, 1999; Hickey, 2000b). The spiral arteries stretch to supply the functionalis layer and end in a subepithelial capillary plexus.

At the end of each menstrual cycle, progesterone levels drop and lead to release of lytic matrix metalloproteinases. These enzymes break down the stroma and vascular architecture of the functionalis layer. Subsequent bleeding and sloughing of

this layer constitute menstruation (Jabbour, 2006). Initially, platelet aggregation and thrombi control blood loss. In addition, the remaining endometrial arteries, under the influence of mediators, vasoconstrict to limit further bleeding (Ferenczy, 2003; Kelly, 2002).

SYMPTOMS

In the initial evaluation of abnormal bleeding, a thorough menstrual history should be collected. Topics typically include age at menarche, date of last menstrual period, and method of birth

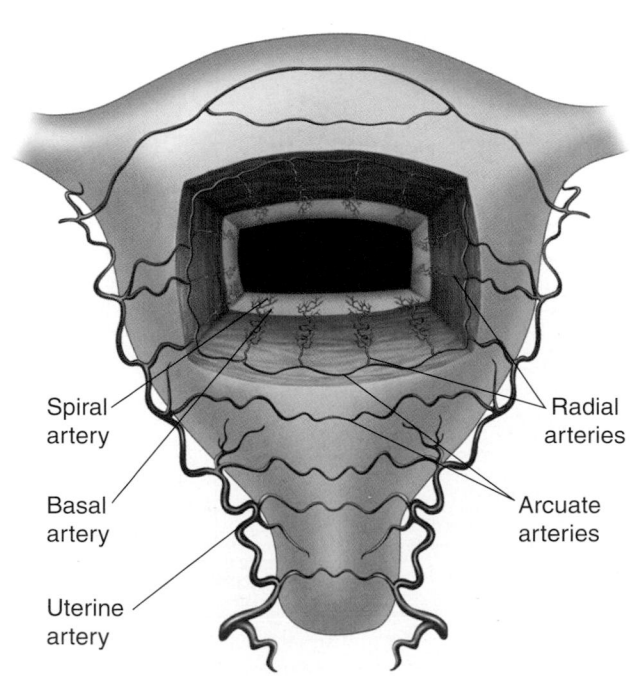

FIGURE 8-4 Uterine blood supply.

control. The timing of her bleeding, bleeding amount, and associated symptoms should also be determined. Disturbances in the regular cycle of endometrial proliferation and sloughing lead to aberrant uterine bleeding. Clinically, various bleeding patterns may result and are described next.

Menorrhagia and Metrorrhagia

These are defined on page 219 and describe abnormalities of bleeding pattern, duration, and flow. Most gynecologic disorders, however, do not consistently display a specific bleeding pattern. Thus, patients may present with menorrhagia or metrorrhagia or both. In most cases, the bleeding pattern in a particular woman is of limited value in diagnosing the underlying cause of bleeding. However, it can be used to assess improvement with treatment.

Postcoital Bleeding

Bleeding following intercourse most commonly develops in women aged 20 to 40 years and in those who are multiparous. No underlying pathology is identified in up to two thirds (Rosenthal, 2001; Selo-Ojeme, 2004). If an identifiable lesion is found, however, it typically is benign (Shalini, 1998). In a review of 248 women with postcoital bleeding, Selo-Ojeme and coworkers (2004) found that a fourth was caused by cervical eversion (Chap. 29, p. 732). Other causes included endocervical polyps, cervicitis, and less commonly, endometrial polyps. In cases of cervicitis, *Chlamydia trachomatis* is a frequent pathogen. Bax and associates (2002) found that the relative risk of chlamydial infection in women with postcoital bleeding was 2.6 times higher than that of a control group without bleeding.

In some women, postcoital bleeding may be from cervical or other genital tract neoplasia. The epithelium associated with cervical intraepithelial neoplasia (CIN) and invasive cancer is thin and friable and readily detaches from the cervix. In women with postcoital bleeding, CIN was found in 7 to 10 percent, invasive cancer in approximately 5 percent, and vaginal or endometrial cancer in less than 1 percent (Sahu, 2007; Selo-Ojeme, 2004; Shalini, 1998). Moreover, some women with postcoital bleeding may have pathologic lesions identified at colposcopic evaluation that had been missed by Pap smear screening (Abu, 2006). Thus, colposcopic examination is considered for women with unexplained postcoital bleeding.

Pelvic Pain

Because of the role of prostaglandins in both menorrhagia and dysmenorrhea, it seems logical that painful cramping would commonly accompany abnormal bleeding (Bieglmayer, 1995; Ylikorkala, 1994). And indeed, dysmenorrhea frequently develops concurrently with abnormal bleeding caused by lesions, infections, and pregnancy complications.

Painful intercourse and noncyclic pain are less frequent in women with abnormal bleeding and usually suggest a structural or infectious source. For example, Lippman and colleagues (2003) reported increased rates of dyspareunia and noncyclic pelvic pain in women with uterine leiomyomas.

DIAGNOSIS

With abnormal uterine bleeding, the diagnostic goal is exclusion of pregnancy or cancer and identification of the underlying pathology to allow optimal treatment. Serum β-hCG testing, sonography (with or without saline infusion), endometrial biopsy, and hysteroscopy are used primarily (Fig. 8-5). In many clinical settings, these tools may be used interchangeably, and modality selection is based on patient variables, available resources, and/or provider training.

Physical Examination

Initially, the site of uterine bleeding must be confirmed because bleeding may also come from the lower reproductive tract, gastrointestinal system, or urinary tract. This is more difficult if there is no active bleeding. In these situations, urinalysis or stool guaiac evaluation may be helpful adjuncts to a thorough physical examination. During examination, specific findings or constellations of findings may suggest an etiology (Table 8-2).

Laboratory Evaluation
β-Human Chorionic Gonadotropin and Hematologic Testing

Miscarriage, ectopic pregnancies, and hydatidiform moles may cause life-threatening hemorrhage. Pregnancy complications are quickly excluded with determination of urine or serum levels of the beta subunit of human chorionic gonadotropin (β-hCG).

Additionally, in women with abnormal uterine bleeding, a complete blood count will identify anemia as well as the degree of blood loss. With chronic loss, erythrocyte indices will reflect a microcytic, hypochromic anemia and show decreases in mean corpuscular volume (MCV), mean corpuscular hemoglobin (MCH), and mean corpuscular hemoglobin concentration (MCHC). Moreover, in women with classic iron-deficiency anemia from chronic blood loss, an elevated platelet count may be seen (Schafer, 2006). In those for whom the cause of anemia is unclear, in those with profound anemia, or in those who fail to improve with oral iron therapy, iron studies may be indicated. Specifically, iron-deficiency anemia produces low serum ferritin and low serum iron levels and an elevated total iron-binding capacity.

Screening for coagulation disorders should be considered in women with menorrhagia and no other obvious cause. This is particularly true for adolescents with menorrhagia. Also, women who convey other personal or family events suggestive of coagulation dysfunction typically warrant screening (American College of Obstetricians and Gynecologists, 2009b). Evaluation includes a complete blood count with platelet count, partial thromboplastin time, and prothrombin

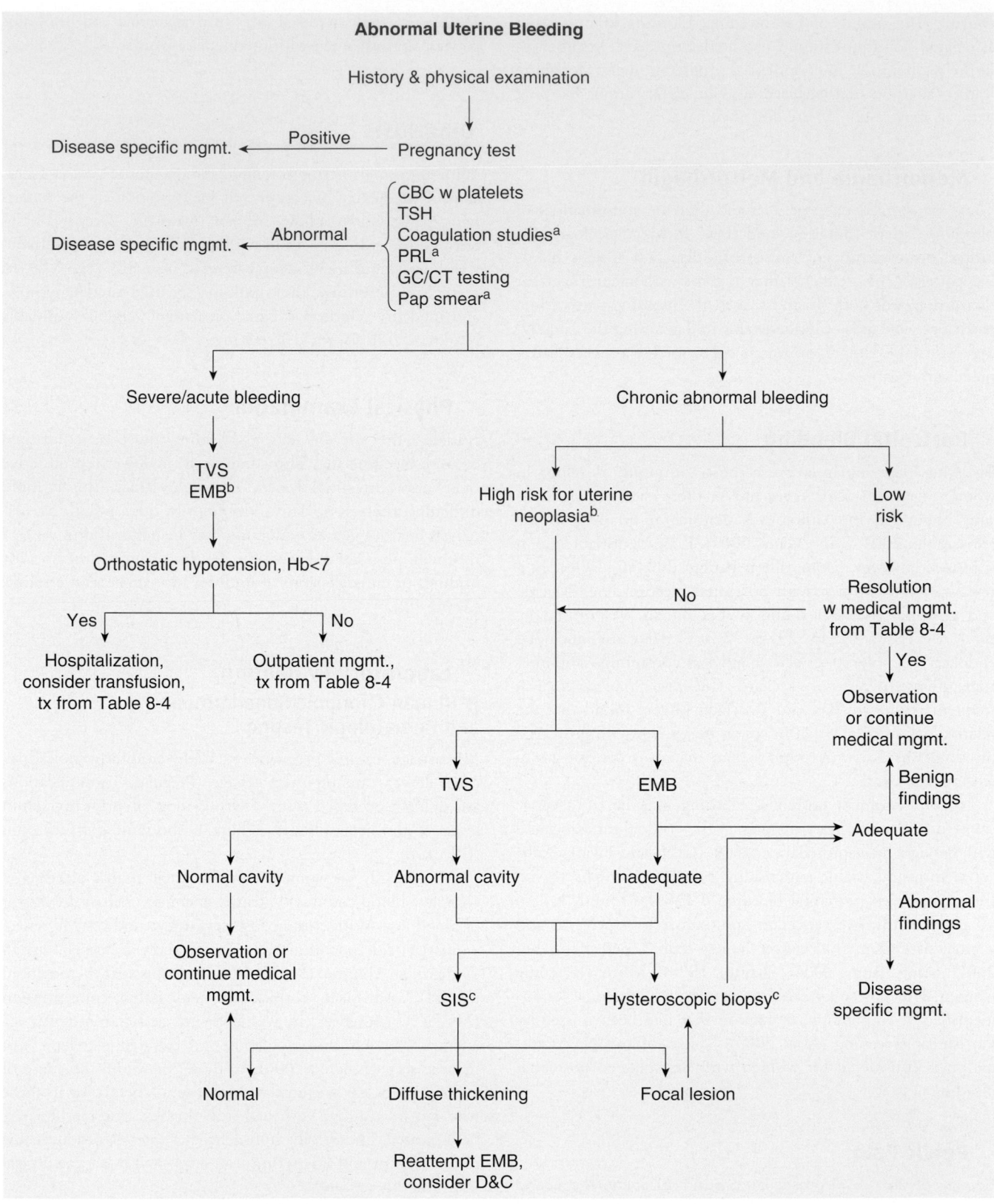

FIGURE 8-5 Diagnostic algorithm to identify endometrial pathology in patients with abnormal uterine bleeding.
[a]Study obtained as indicated by patient history.
[b]Patients with chronic anovulation, obesity, ≥35 years of age, tamoxifen use, or other risks for endometrial cancer.
[c]Both comparable in sensitivity and specificity. Either or both may be selected depending on patient characteristics and physician preference (see p. 228).
CBC = complete blood count; D&C = dilatation and curettage; GC/CT = *Neiserria gonorrhoeae* and *Chlamydia trachomatis;* EMB = endometrial biopsy; Hb = hemoglobin level; PRL = prolactin level; SIS = saline infusion sonography; TSH = thyroid-stimulating hormone level; TVS = transvaginal sonography; tx = treatment.

TABLE 8-2. Clinical Findings Associated with Abnormal Uterine Bleeding

Finding	Bleeding Etiology
Obesity	Anovulatory bleeding Endometrial hyperplasia Endometrial cancer
Signs of PCOS: Acne Hirsutism Obesity Acanthosis nigricans	Anovulatory bleeding Endometrial hyperplasia Endometrial cancer
Hypothyroidism signs: Goiter Weight gain	Anovulatory bleeding
Hyperthyroidism signs: Exophthalmos Weight loss	Unclassified
Increased bruising, gingival bleeding	Coagulopathy
Hyperprolactinemia signs: Galactorrhea Bilateral hemianopsia	Anovulatory bleeding
Longitudinal vaginal septum	Episodic release of trapped menses
Cervicitis	Endometritis
Signs of pregnancy: Cervical bluing Isthmic softening Enlarged uterus	Abortion Ectopic pregnancy Gestational trophoblastic disease
Endocervical mass	Prolapsing leiomyoma or uterine sarcoma Cervical cancer Endocervical polyp
Ectocervical mass	Ectropion Cervical cancer
Enlarged uterus	Pregnancy Leiomyoma Adenomyosis Hematometra Endometrial cancer Uterine sarcoma
Adnexal mass	Ectopic pregnancy Fallopian tube cancer Hormone-producing

PCOS = polycystic ovarian syndrome.

time, and may include special testing for von Willebrand disease (p. 235).

"Wet Prep" Examination and Cervical Cultures

As discussed, cervicitis frequently causes intermenstrual or postcoital spotting (Lindner, 1988). Accordingly, microscopic examination of a saline preparation of cervical secretions or "wet prep" may reveal sheets of neutrophils and red blood cells in women with bleeding caused by cervicitis. In turn, the association between mucopurulent cervicitis and cervical infection with *Chlamydia trachomatis* and *Neisseria gonorrhoeae* is well established (Chap. 3, p. 86) (Marrazzo, 2002). The Centers for Disease Control and Prevention (2006) recommend testing for both when mucopurulent cervicitis is present. Cervicitis secondary to the herpes simplex virus (HSV) may also cause bleeding, and directed cultures may be indicated (Paavonen, 1988). Lastly, trichomoniasis may cause cervicitis and a friable ectocervix.

Cytologic Examination

Both cervical and endometrial cancers can cause abnormal bleeding. Evidence for these tumors can often be found with Pap smear screening.

The most frequent abnormal cytologic results associated with abnormal bleeding involve squamous cell pathology and may reflect cervicitis, intraepithelial neoplasia, or cancer. Less commonly, atypical glandular or endometrial cells may be found. Any of these may suggest the cause of bleeding. Therefore, depending on the cytologic results, colposcopy, endocervical curettage, and/or endometrial biopsy may be indicated. Abnormal cytologic findings and their appropriate evaluation are discussed in Chapter 29 (p. 744).

Endometrial Biopsy

Indications. In women with abnormal bleeding, sampling and histologic evaluation of the endometrium may identify infection or neoplastic lesions such as endometrial hyperplasia or cancer.

Abnormal bleeding is noted in 80 to 90 percent of women with endometrial cancer. The incidence and risk of this cancer increases with age, and three fourths of affected women are postmenopausal. Thus, in postmenopausal patients, the need to exclude cancer intensifies, and endometrial biopsy may be selected for this. In the remaining 25 percent of premenopausal women with endometrial cancer, only 5 percent are younger than 40 years (Peterson, 1968). Most of these younger premenopausal women are obese or have chronic anovulation or both (Rose, 1996). Thus, women in this latter group with abnormal bleeding also warrant exclusion of endometrial cancer. Specifically, the American College of Obstetricians and Gynecologists (2000) recommends endometrial assessment in any woman older than 35 years with abnormal bleeding and also in those younger than 35 years who are suspected of having anovulatory uterine bleeding refractory to medical management.

Sampling Methods. For years, dilatation and curettage (D&C) was used for endometrial sampling. However, because of associated surgical risks, expense, postoperative pain, and need for operative anesthesia, other suitable substitutes were evaluated. In addition, several investigators demonstrated significant rates of incomplete sampling and missed pathology with D&C (Goldstein, 1997; Grimes, 1982; Stock, 1975).

Initial office techniques used metal curettes. Endometrial samples that were removed with these curettes showed significant positive correlation with histologic results obtained from hysterectomy specimens (Ferenczy, 1979; Stovall, 1989). Thus, they were deemed adequate sampling methods. However disadvantages included patient discomfort, cost, and procedure complications such as uterine perforation and infection.

To minimize these, flexible plastic samplers have been evaluated for endometrial biopsy (Figs. 8-6 and 8-7). Advantageously, samples from these catheters have comparable histologic findings with tissues obtained by D&C, hysterectomy, or stiff metal curette (Stovall, 1991). Moreover, they afford greater patient comfort.

Prior to performing endometrial biopsy, pregnancy should be excluded in women of reproductive age. After patient education and consent, a speculum is placed, and the cervix is cleansed with an antibacterial solution, such as povidone-iodine solution. In many cases, a single-tooth tenaculum is needed to stabilize the cervix and permit passage of the Pipelle through the cervical os and into the endometrial cavity. Placing the tenaculum slowly on the anterior cervical can decrease discomfort. Patients also may frequently note cramping with Pipelle insertion. The Pipelle is directed toward the fundus until resistance is met. Markings on the device allow measurement of uterine depth, and this value should be recorded in the procedure note. The Pipelle stilette is then retracted to create suction within the cylinder. Several times, the hollow tube is withdrawn to the level of the internal cervical os and advanced back to the fundus. The device is gently turned during its advance and retraction to allow thorough sampling of all endometrial surfaces. Uncommonly, a vagal response may follow Pipelle insertion. In this instance, the procedure is terminated, and patient support is provided.

Despite its advantages, there are limitations to endometrial sampling with the Pipelle device. First, a tissue sample that is inadequate for histologic evaluation or an inability to pass the catheter into the endometrial cavity is encountered

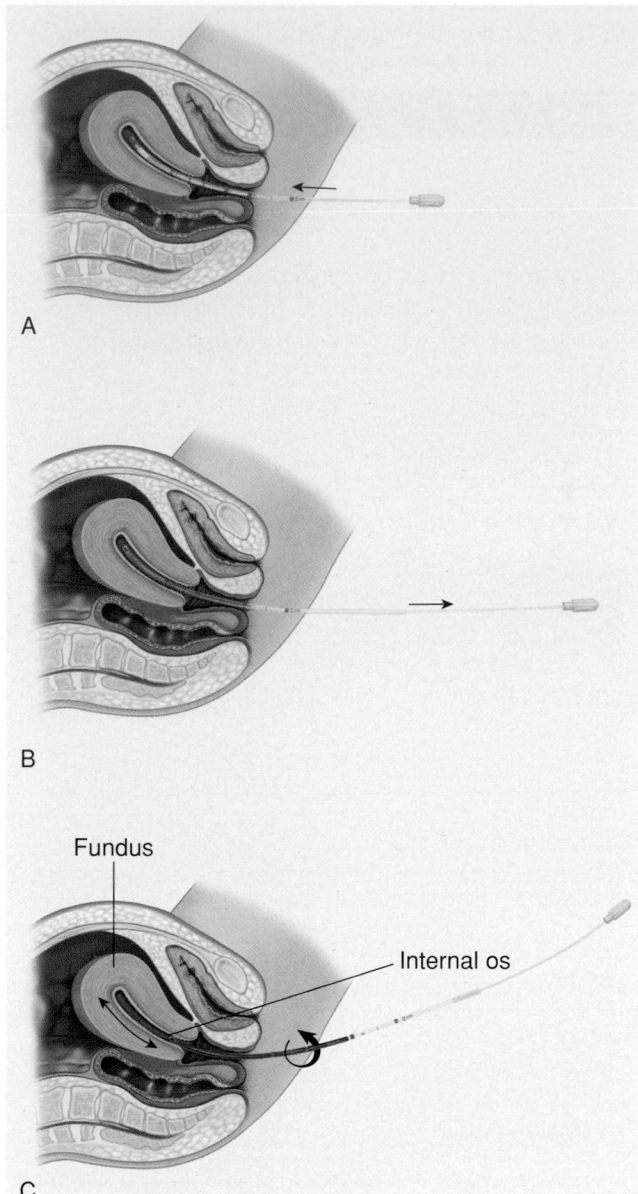

FIGURE 8-6 Steps of endometrial biopsy. **A.** During biopsy, the Pipelle is inserted through the cervical os and directed to the uterine fundus. Markings on the device permit assessment of uterine depth. **B.** The stilette of the Pipelle is retracted to create suction within the cylinder. **C.** Several times, the pipelle is withdrawn to the level of the internal cervical os and advanced back to the fundus. The Pipelle is gently turned during its advance and retraction to allow thorough sampling of all endometrial surfaces.

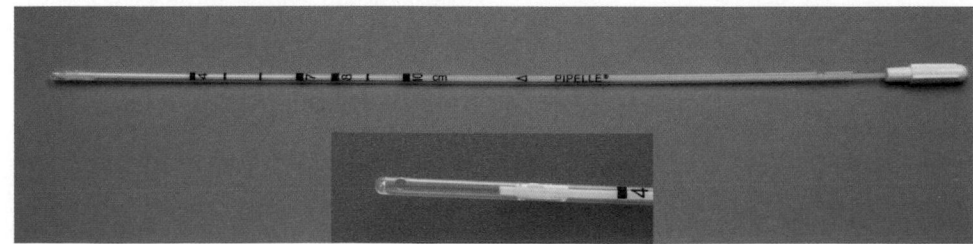

FIGURE 8-7 Photograph of a Pipelle endometrial sampling device. Note the fluted opening *(inset)* at the end of the device, which draws endometrial tissue up into the narrow cylinder.

in up to 28 percent of biopsy attempts (Smith-Bindman, 1998). Cervical stenosis and large submucous leiomyomas are common causes of obstruction. An incomplete evaluation necessitates further investigation with D&C, transvaginal sonography with or without saline infusion, or diagnostic hysteroscopy (Emanuel, 1995). Second, endometrial biopsy has a cancer-detection failure rate of 0.9 percent. Thus, a positive histologic result is accurate to diagnose cancer, but a negative result does not definitively exclude it. Therefore, if an endometrial biopsy with normal tissue is obtained, but abnormal bleeding continues despite conservative treatment, or if the suspicion of endometrial cancer is high, then further diagnostic efforts are warranted (Clark, 2002; Hatasaka, 2005). Finally, endometrial sampling is associated with a greater percentage of false-negative results if the pathology is focal, such as with endometrial polyps. In a study of 639 women evaluated by diagnostic office hysteroscopy and endometrial biopsy, Svirsky and colleagues (2008) found that the sensitivity of endometrial sampling for detection of endometrial polyps and submucosal fibroids was only 8.4 and 1.4 percent, respectively. Because of these limitations with endometrial sampling, investigators have evaluated the use of sonography, hysteroscopy, or both to replace or complement endometrial sampling.

Sonography
Transvaginal Sonography (TVS)

With improved resolution, this technology is chosen by many instead of endometrial biopsy as a first-line tool to assess abnormal bleeding. Advantageously, it allows assessment of both the myometrium and the endometrium. Thus, if abnormal bleeding stems from myometrial pathology such as leiomyomas, sonography offers anatomic information that is not afforded by hysteroscopy or endometrial biopsy. In addition, TVS compared with these other two typically offers greater patient comfort and suitable detection of endometrial hyperplasia and cancer (Ferrazzi, 1996; Karlsson, 1995; Van den Bosch, 2008).

When the endometrium is imaged in a sagittal view, opposed endometrial surfaces appear as a hyperechoic *endometrial stripe* down the center of the uterine body (Fig. 8-8 and Fig. 2-8, p. 37). In postmenopausal women, this endometrial thickness has been correlated with endometrial cancer risk. Although endometrial thickness varies among patients, ranges have been established. Granberg and coworkers (1991) found thickness measurements of 3.4 ± 1.2 mm in postmenopausal women with an atrophic endometrium, 9.7 ± 2.5 mm in those with endometrial hyperplasia, and 18.2 ± 6.2 mm in those with endometrial cancer. Subsequently, a number of investigations have similarly focused on endometrial thickness as it relates to the risk of endometrial hyperplasia and cancer in postmenopausal women. Sensitivities of 95 to 97 percent have been reported using a measurement of ≤4 mm for exclusion of endometrial cancer. This guideline can be employed whether or not a patient is taking hormone replacement therapy (Bakour, 1999; Karlsson, 1995; Tsuda, 1997). Women with endometrial thicknesses >4 mm typically require additional evaluation with saline infusion sonography (SIS), hysteroscopy, or endometrial biopsy (American College of Obstetricians and Gynecologists, 2009a).

Similarly, researchers have attempted to create endometrial thickness guidelines for premenopausal women. Merz and colleagues (1996) found that the normal endometrial thickness in premenopausal women did not exceed 4 mm on day 4 of the menstrual cycle, nor did it measure more than 8 mm by day 8. However, endometrial thicknesses can vary considerably among premenopausal women, and suggested evidence-based abnormal thresholds range from ≥4 mm to >16 mm (Breitkopf, 2004; Goldstein, 1997; Shi, 2008). Thus, consensus for endometrial thickness guidelines has not been established for this group. At our institution, no additional evaluation is recommended for a normal-appearing endometrium measuring ≤10 mm in a premenopausal female experiencing abnormal uterine bleeding if she has no other risk factors to prompt further testing. Risk factors for endometrial carcinoma include extended abnormal uterine bleeding, chronic anovulation, diabetes, obesity, hypertension, and tamoxifen use (Hatasaka, 2005).

Qualities other than endometrial thickness are also considered because textural changes may indicate pathology. For example, punctate cystic areas within the endometrium may indicate a polyp (p. 230). Conversely, hypoechoic masses that distort the endometrium and originate from the inner layer of myometrium most commonly are submucous fibroids. Although there are no specific sonographic findings that are characteristic of endometrial cancer, some findings have been linked with greater frequency (Fig. 33-4, p. 821). For example, intermingled hypo- and hyperechoic areas within the endometrium may indicate malignancy. Endometrial cavity fluid

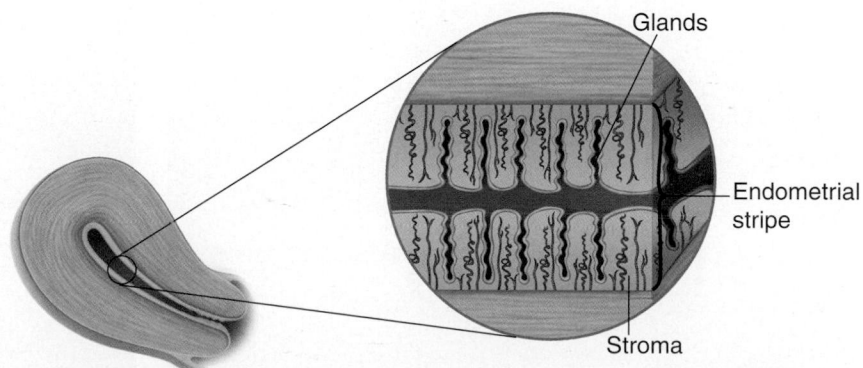

FIGURE 8-8 The sonographic endometrial stripe in a sagittal plane represents the thickness created by the apposed anterior and posterior endometrium. In premenopausal women, stripe thickness will vary during the menstrual cycle as the endometrium gradually thickens and then is sloughed.

collections and an irregular endometrial-myometrial junction have also been implicated. Thus, with these findings, even with a normal endometrial stripe width in postmenopausal patients, endometrial biopsy or hysteroscopy with biopsy should be considered to exclude malignancy (Dubinsky, 2004; Krissi, 1998; Sheikh, 2000).

Although the use of these criteria can safely reduce endometrial biopsies for many patients, others consider false-negative rates as too high with this strategy for evaluation of postmenopausal women (Timmermans, 2010). Some advocate hysteroscopy with direct biopsy or D&C to evaluate postmenopausal bleeding (Litta, 2005; Tabor, 2002). In other patient populations, the 4-mm guideline may also be inappropriate. For example, van Doorn and coworkers (2004) reported decreased diagnostic accuracy in diabetic or obese women, and they recommend consideration of endometrial sampling.

A major limitation of TVS is its higher false-negative rate in diagnosing focal intrauterine pathology. This results in part from the physical inability of TVS to clearly assess the endometrium when there is concurrent uterine pathology such as leiomyomas or polyps. In these cases, saline infusion sonography or hysteroscopy may be informative.

Saline Infusion Sonography (SIS)

This simple, minimally invasive, and effective sonographic procedure can be used to visually evaluate the myometrium, endometrium, and endometrial cavity. To perform SIS, a small catheter is threaded through the cervical os and into the endometrial cavity (Chap. 2, p. 35). Through this catheter, sterile saline is infused, and the uterus is distended. Sonography is then performed using a traditional transvaginal technique. SIS is contraindicated in women who are pregnant or who could be pregnant, or who have a pelvic infection or unexplained pelvic tenderness (American College of Obstetricians and Gynecologists, 2008).

Also known as *sonohysterography*, this method allows visualization of common masses associated with abnormal uterine bleeding such as endometrial polyps, submucous leiomyomas, and intracavitary blood clots. These masses frequently create nondescript distortion or thickening of the endometrial lining when imaged with TVS. Thus, compared with TVS, SIS typically permits superior detection of intracavitary masses and differentiation of lesions as being endometrial, submucous, or intramural (Fig. 8-9) (Pasrija, 2004; Ryu, 2004). In addition, Moschos and colleagues (2009) describe a method of sonographically guided Pipelle endometrial biopsy during SIS (Fig. 2-15, p. 41). Although not yet widely used, this technique enables directed histologic sampling of endometrial pathology and has proved superior to blind endometrial biopsy in providing a diagnosis for abnormal bleeding in peri- and postmenopausal women.

SIS has also been compared with hysteroscopy to detect uterine cavitary focal lesions. De Kroon and coworkers (2003) performed a metaanalysis of 24 studies and reported SIS to equal the diagnostic accuracy of hysteroscopy. Importantly, neither hysteroscopy nor SIS can reliably discriminate between benign and malignant focal lesions. Thus, because of the malignant potential of many focal lesions, biopsy or excision of most structural lesions, when identified, is recommended for those with risk factors. For this, operative hysteroscopy is typically used.

SIS does have disadvantages. First, it is cycle dependent and best performed in the proliferative phase of the cycle to minimize false negative and false positive results. For example, focal lesions may be concealed in a thick, secretory endometrium. Also, the amount of endometrial tissue that can develop during the normal secretory phase can be mistaken for a small polyp or focal hyperplasia (Goldstein, 2004). In addition, SIS usually causes more patient discomfort than TVS, and approximately 5 percent of examinations cannot be completed because of cervical stenosis or patient discomfort. As expected, stenosis is more prevalent in postmenopausal

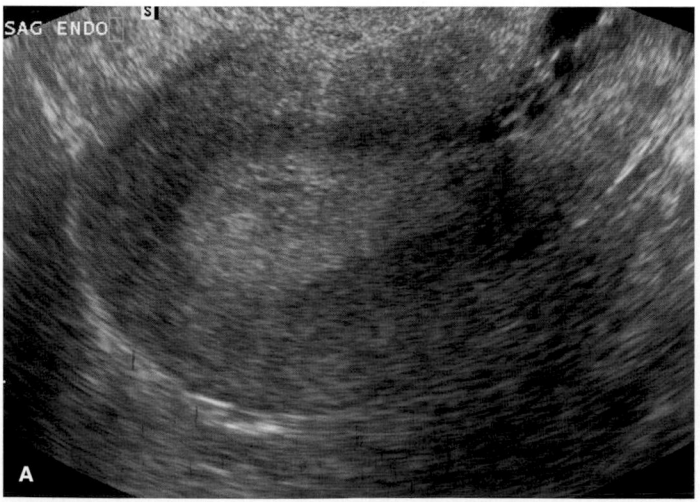
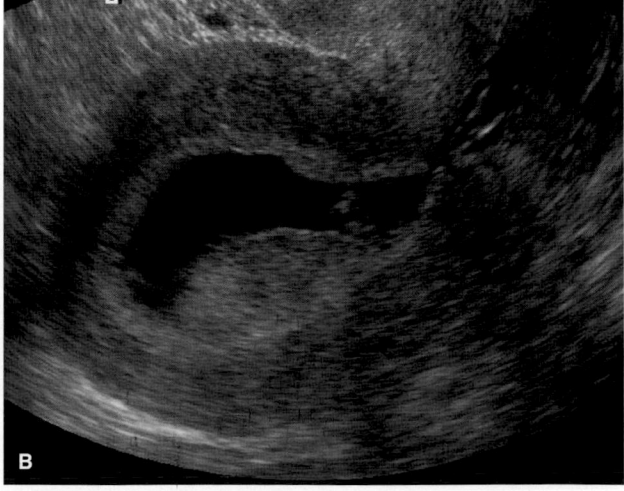

FIGURE 8-9 Transvaginal sonography of the uterus in the sagittal plane. **A.** The endometrium is thickened in this postmenopausal patient. **B.** Saline infusion sonography reveals a posterior endometrial mass and further delineates its size and qualities. *(Images contributed by Dr. Elysia Moschos.)*

women (de Kroon, 2003). This rate of incompletion mirrors that of diagnostic hysteroscopy.

Although accurate for identifying focal lesions, SIS may not add to the value of TVS in evaluating diffuse lesions such as hyperplasia and cancer. Therefore, in postmenopausal women with abnormal bleeding, and in whom the exclusion of cancer is more relevant than evaluating focal intracavitary lesions, use of SIS alone as an initial diagnostic tool may not have advantages over TVS.

Transvaginal Color Doppler Sonography (TV-CDS)

This technique has been evaluated to identify and differentiate endometrial pathology in the context of uterine bleeding (Alcazar, 2003, 2004; Jakab, 2005). In one study, Fleischer and colleagues (2003) used TV-CDS to distinguish submucous leiomyomas and endometrial polyps. They reported that endometrial polyps usually had only one arterial feeding vessel (Fig. 8-10). In contrast, submucous leiomyomas generally received blood flow from several vessels arising from the inner myometrium.

Three-dimensional sonography and 3-D SIS have been evaluated, but their contribution to the evaluation of abnormal uterine bleeding is yet undefined (Chap. 2, p. 46) (Clark, 2004).

Hysteroscopy

This procedure involves inserting an optic endoscope, usually 3 to 5 mm in diameter, into the endometrial cavity and is explained in detail in Section 42-13 (p. 1157). The uterine cavity is then distended with saline or another medium for visualization (Fig. 8-11). In addition to inspection, biopsy of the endometrium allows histologic diagnosis of visually abnormal areas and has been shown to be a safe and accurate means to identify pathology. In fact, for many studies done to investi-

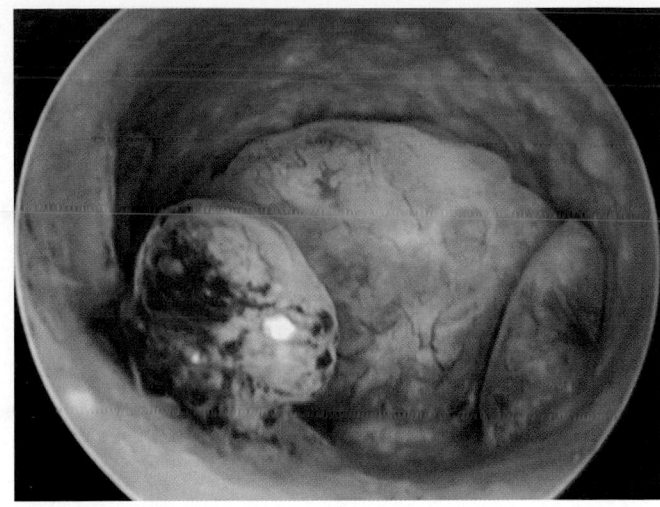

FIGURE 8-11 Hysteroscopy demonstrating endometrial polyps. *(Photograph contributed by Dr. Catherine Chappell.)*

gate the accuracy of TVS or SIS for evaluation of intracavitary uterine pathology, hysteroscopy is used as the "gold standard" for comparison.

The main advantage of hysteroscopy is to detect intracavitary lesions such as leiomyomas and polyps that might be missed using transvaginal sonography or endometrial sampling (Tahir, 1999). Some have advocated hysteroscopy as the primary tool for the diagnosis of abnormal uterine bleeding. Although it is accurate for identifying endometrial cancer, it is less accurate for endometrial hyperplasia. Thus, some recommend endometrial biopsy or endometrial curettage in conjunction with hysteroscopy (Ben-Yehuda, 1998; Clark, 2002).

There are other limitations to hysteroscopy. Cervical stenosis sometimes will block successful introduction of the endoscope, and heavy bleeding may limit an adequate examination (Beukenholdo, 2003). Hysteroscopy is more expensive and technically challenging than TVS or SIS. Although office hysteroscopy can be painful, use of a 3.5-mm minihysteroscope instead of the conventional 5-mm endoscope significantly decreases patient discomfort (Cicinelli, 2003). Associated infection and uterine perforation have been reported, but fortunately, their incidences are low (Bradley, 2002; Vercellini, 1997).

There is concern that peritoneal seeding with malignant cells may take place during hysteroscopy in some women subsequently diagnosed with endometrial cancer (Bradley, 2004; Zerbe, 2000). Accordingly, caution is advised with hysteroscopy in women at high risk for endometrial cancer (Oehler, 2003). Although there may be a risk of peritoneal contamination by cancer cells with hysteroscopy, patient prognosis overall does not appear to be worsened if this occurs (Polyzos, 2010; Revel, 2004).

Summary of Diagnostic Procedures

There is no one clear sequence to the use of endometrial biopsy, TVS, SIS, and hysteroscopy when evaluating abnormal uterine

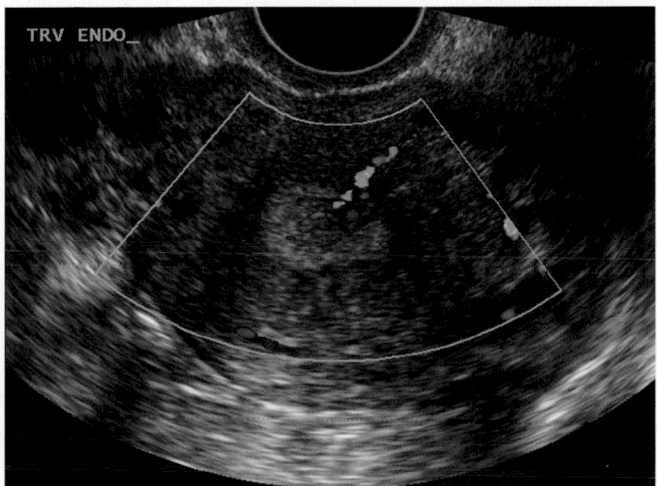

FIGURE 8-10 TV-CDS of an endometrial polyp. Color flow feature identifies a single feeder vessel, which is characteristic of a polyp. *(Image contributed by Dr. Elysia Moschos.)*

bleeding. None of these will distinguish all anatomic lesions with high sensitivity and specificity. That said, TVS for several reasons is a logical first step. It is well tolerated, cost effective, and requires relatively minimal technical skill. Additionally, it has the advantage of reliably determining whether a lesion is diffuse or focal and myometrial or endometrial. Once anatomic lesions have been identified, subsequent evaluation requires individualization. If endometrial hyperplasia or cancer is suspected, then endometrial biopsy may offer advantages. Alternatively, possible focal lesions may be best investigated with either hysteroscopy or SIS. Ultimately, the goal of diagnostic evaluation is to identify and treat pathology and specifically to exclude endometrial carcinoma. Thus, selection of appropriate tests depends upon their accuracy in characterizing the most likely anatomic lesions.

ETIOLOGY AND MANAGEMENT OPTIONS

As described earlier, uterine bleeding may result from structural abnormalities, hormonal changes, coagulopathies, infection, neoplasia, or complications of pregnancy. The risks and incidences of these etiologies change significantly with age and reproductive status. In approximately half of cases, no organic pathology is identified, and dysfunctional uterine bleeding is diagnosed, that is, a diagnosis of exclusion (Rees, 1987).

Pregnancy Associated

Abnormal bleeding during early pregnancy is encountered in 15 to 20 percent of pregnancies (Everett, 1997; Weiss, 2004). Although frequently no reason is found to account for bleeding, it may reflect early abortion, ectopic pregnancy, cervical infection, hydatidiform mole, cervical eversion, or polyp. Detailed discussions of bleeding associated with pregnancy and hydatidiform mole are found in Chapters 6, 7, and 37.

Structural Abnormalities
Pathology Associated with Uterine Enlargement

Structural abnormalities are frequent causes of abnormal bleeding, and of these, leiomyomas by far are the most common. The impact of these tumors in clinical gynecology cannot be understated. Other less frequent structural causes of bleeding include adenomyosis, hematometra, and hypertrophic myometrium. A detailed discussion of all these disorders and their treatment is presented in Chapter 9.

Endometrial Polyps

These soft, fleshy intrauterine growths are comprised of endometrial glands and fibrotic stroma and are covered by a surface epithelium (Fig. 8-12). Polyps are common, and their prevalence in the general population approximates 8 percent (Dreisler, 2009a). However, in those with abnormal bleeding, rates range from 10 to 30 percent (Bakour, 2000; Goldstein, 1997). Intact polyps may be single or multiple, may measure from a few millimeters to several centimeters, and may be sessile or pedunculated (Kim, 2004). Estrogen and progesterone have been implicated in their growth. These hormones elongate

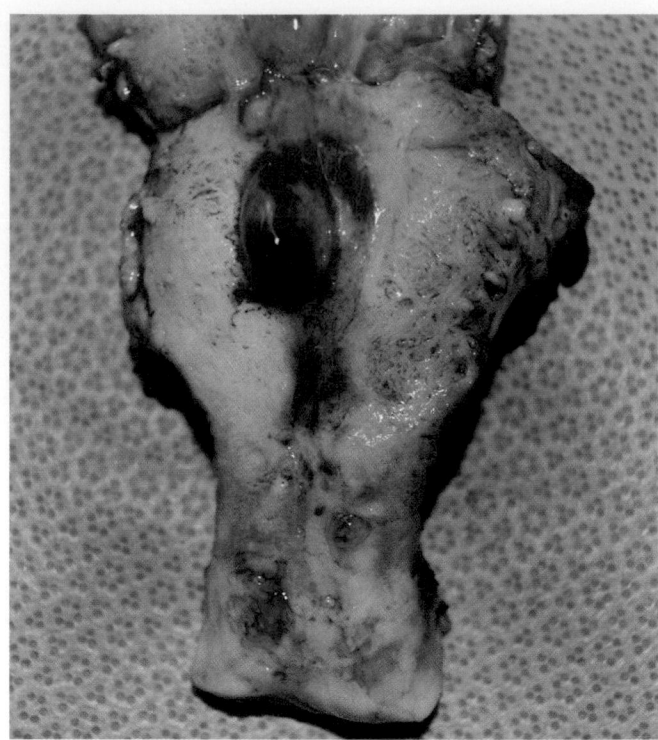

FIGURE 8-12 Single endometrial polyp found within the endometrial cavity of a hysterectomy specimen.

endometrial glands, stromal tissue, and spiral arteries, leading to creation of the characteristic polypoid appearance (Jakab, 2005).

Patient risk factors include increasing age, obesity, and tamoxifen use (Dibi, 2009; Reslova, 1999). Although some studies suggest an association between hormone replacement therapy and polyp formation, others do not (Bakour, 2002; Dreisler, 2009a; Maia, 2004; Oguz, 2005). Use of oral contraceptive pills appears to be protective (Dreisler, 2009b). In addition, for women taking tamoxifen, use of the contraceptive levonorgestrel-releasing intrauterine system (LNG-IUS) lowers rates of endometrial polyp formation (Chan, 2007; Chin, 2009; Gardner, 2009).

More than 70 percent of women with endometrial polyps will complain of menorrhagia or metrorrhagia (Preutthipan, 2005; Reslova, 1999). Specifically, stromal congestion within the polyp is thought to cause venous stasis with apical necrosis and bleeding (Jakab, 2005). Although bleeding is a common symptom, with the introduction of transvaginal sonography, a large number of women with asymptomatic polyps have also been identified during imaging for other indications (Goldstein, 2002).

Infertility has been linked indirectly with endometrial polyps. For example, small studies have shown increased pregnancy rates and fewer early pregnancy losses in infertile women following hysteroscopic excision (Pérez-Medina, 2005; Preutthipan, 2005; Varasteh, 1999). Although the exact mechanisms related to infertility are unknown, several causes have been suggested. Metalloproteinases associated with implantation and cytokines that impact embryo development have been implicated. Both are found in greater amount in polyps than normal surrounding uterine tissue (Inagaki, 2003). Alternatively, polyps found near the tubal ostia may hinder ostium function and block

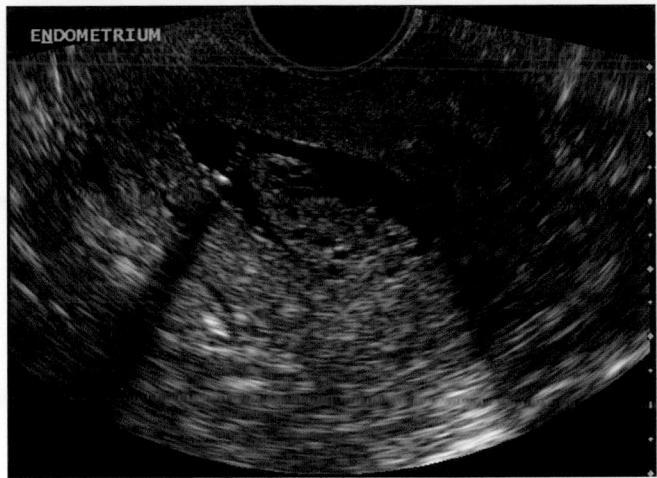

FIGURE 8-13 Saline infusion sonography of an endometrial polyp. Small, sonolucent areas within this endometrial mass represent cystic areas commonly found within theses polyps. *(Image contributed by Dr. Elysia Moschos.)*

sperm migration (Shokeir, 2004; Yanaihara, 2008). For these reasons, many advocate polyp removal in infertile women.

The main diagnostic tools for evaluation of endometrial polyps include transvaginal sonography, saline infusion sonography, and hysteroscopy. Although endometrial biopsy may identify polyps, it has decreased sensitivity for detecting focal lesions compared with these other modalities.

In premenopausal women, TVS is best performed prior to day 10 of the cycle to lower the risk of false-positive findings. With TVS, an endometrial polyp may appear as a nonspecific endometrial thickening or as a round or elongated focal mass within the endometrial cavity. Sonolucent cystic spaces, which correspond to dilated endometrial glands, may be seen within some polyps (Fig. 8-13) (Nalaboff, 2001). Transvaginal sonography may be augmented with color Doppler. Visualization of a single feeding vessel is typical of endometrial polyps as is shown in Figure 8-10 (Fleischer, 2003).

Saline infusion sonography and hysteroscopy are both accurate in identifying endometrial polyps (Nanda, 2002; Soares, 2000). With SIS, polyps appear as echogenic, smooth, intracavitary masses with either broad bases or thin stalks and are outlined by fluid (see Fig. 8-9B) (Jorizzo, 2001). Hysteroscopy identifies nearly all cases of endometrial polyps (see Fig. 8-11). The main advantage of hysteroscopy is the ability to identify and remove the polyp concurrently.

The Pap smear is an ineffective tool to identify polyps. However, it occasionally incidentally leads to their identification. For example, 5 percent of postmenopausal women with benign endometrial cells identified on Pap smear were found to have endometrial polyps (Karim, 2002; Wu, 2001). Moreover, in postmenopausal women with atypical glandular cells of undetermined significance (AGUS), endometrial polyps were the most common underlying pathology found (Obenson, 2000).

Most polyps are benign, and premalignant or malignant transformation develops in only 4 to 5 percent (Baiocchi, 2009; Golan, 2010; Wang, 2010). Thus, operative hysteroscopic pol-

ypectomy is recommended for symptomatic women or those with risk factors for malignant transformation (Machtinger, 2005; Savelli, 2003). These risks include postmenopausal status, age >60 years, polyp size greater than 1.5 cm, and tamoxifen use (Baiocchi, 2009; Ferrazzi, 2009; Golan, 2010). During hysteroscopic polypectomy, background sampling of the endometrium should be considered in those with endometrial cancer risk factors (Rahimi, 2009).

For asymptomatic women with polyps but without risk factors for malignant transformation, management may be more conservative. Some advocate removal of all endometrial polyps because premalignant and malignant transformation has been identified in even asymptomatic premenopausal women (Golan, 2010). However, the risk for transformation in these patients with small lesions is low, and many of these polyps spontaneously resolve or slough (Ben-Arie, 2004; DeWaay, 2002).

Endocervical Polyps

These lesions represent overgrowths of benign endocervical stroma covered by epithelium. Also called cervical polyps, they typically appear as single, red, smooth elongated masses extending from the endocervical canal (Fig. 8-14). Polyps vary in size and range from several millimeters to 2 or 3 centimeters. These common growths are found more frequently in multiparas and rarely in prepubertal females. Endocervical polyps are typically asymptomatic, but they can cause metrorrhagia, postcoital bleeding, and symptomatic vaginal discharge. Many endocervical polyps are identified by visual inspection during pelvic examination. In other instances, Pap smear findings of atypical glandular cells of undetermined significance (AGUS) may prompt investigation and lead to identification of endocervical polyps higher in the endocervical canal (Burja, 1999; Obenson, 2000).

Endocervical polyps are typically benign, and premalignant or malignant transformation develops in less than 1 percent

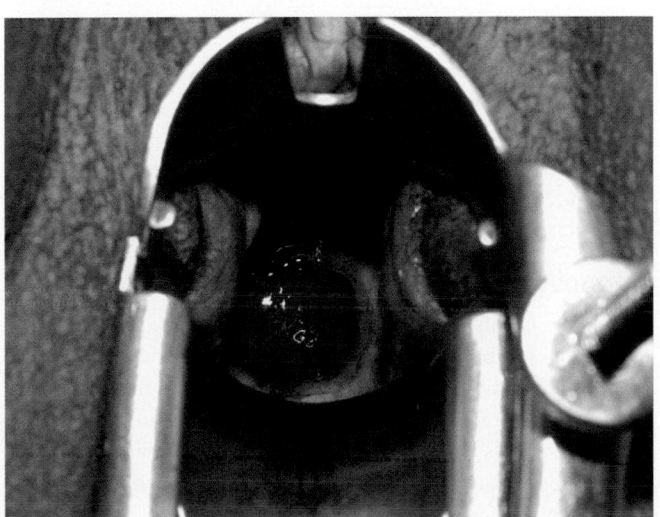

FIGURE 8-14 Photograph of an endocervical polyp. These are soft, fleshy pedunculated growths that extend from the endocervical canal. *(Photograph contributed by Dr. Claudia Werner.)*

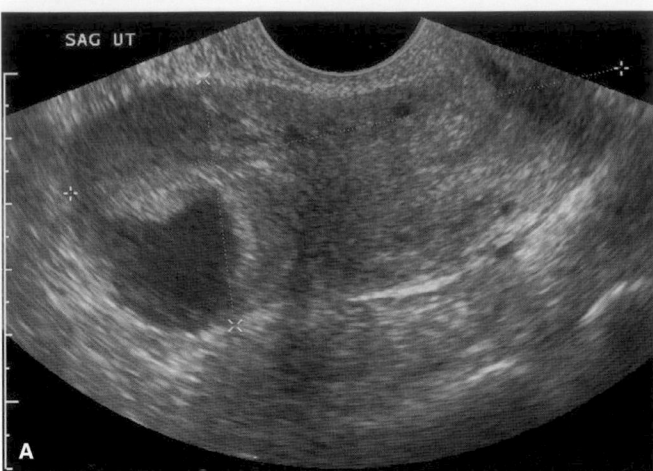 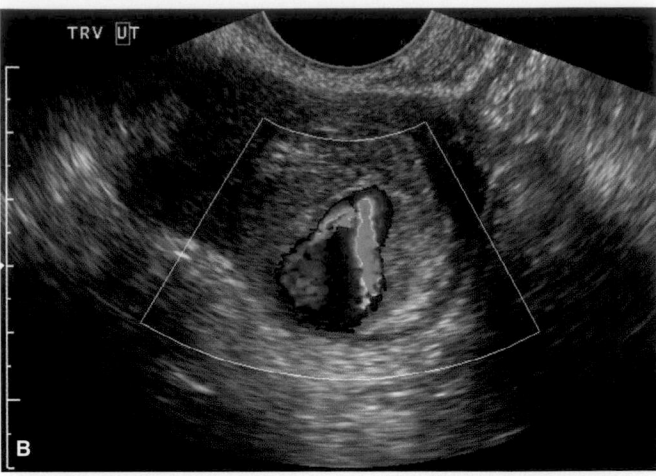

FIGURE 8-15 Transvaginal sonography of an arteriovenous malformation (AVM). **A.** Sagittal image of the uterus with an irregular-shaped anechoic space *(calipers)* within the posterior fundal myometrium. **B.** Color Doppler evaluation of this area in the transverse plane demonstrates the classic mosaic color pattern of an AVM. *(Images contributed by Dr. Elysia Moschos.)*

(Buyukbayrak, 2011; Chin, 2008; Schnatz, 2009). However, cervical cancer can present as polypoid masses and can mimic these benign lesions. Accordingly, most recommend removal and histologic evaluation of all polyps. However, several studies have stratified affected patients by age, symptoms, and cytology and found no preinvasive disease or cancer in polyps of young, asymptomatic women with concurrent normal Pap smear cytology (MacKenzie, 2009; Younis, 2010).

If the stalk is slender, endocervical polyps are removed by grasping the polyp with a ring or polyp forceps. The polyp is twisted repeatedly about the base of its stalk to strangulate its feeding vessels. With repeated twisting the base will narrow and avulse. Monsel solution (ferric subsulfate) can be applied with direct pressure to the resulting stalk stub to complete hemostasis. Infrequently, a thick-pedicle polyp may warrant surgical excision if heavier bleeding or significant pain is anticipated. Patients should be counseled that polyp recurrence rates range from 6 to 15 percent (Berzolla, 2007; Younis, 2010).

Müllerian Defects

Congenital structural lesions of the reproductive tract may at times cause chronic intermenstrual bleeding superimposed upon normal menstrual cycling. In most of these women, sequestered sites have a patent outflow that captures menstrual flow and then releases it slowly to create episodic bleeding (Fig. 18-14, p. 495) (Hatasaka, 2005).

Arteriovenous Malformation (AVM)

These consist of a mixture of arterial, venous, and small capillary-like channels with fistulous connections. Uterine AVMs may be congenital or acquired, and vessel sizes may vary considerably (Majmudar, 1998). Acquired AVMs are usually single, large vessels that form after trauma from cesarean delivery or D&C or that develop concurrently with cervical or endometrial cancer, with gestational trophoblastic disease, or with intrauterine device use (Ghosh, 1986). Uterine AVMs are rare and more frequently involve the corpus, but may also be found in the cervix (Lowenstein, 2004).

Affected patients often present with menorrhagia or menometrorrhagia after a miscarriage, curettage, or other intracavitary uterine surgery. Heavy uterine bleeding without associated cervical trauma or uterine perforation may be presenting signs. Symptoms can develop slowly or appear suddenly and with life-threatening bleeding (Timmerman, 2003).

In some cases, AVMs are first visualized with sonography because of its ready availability and widespread use. Sonographic characteristics are nonspecific and may include hypoechoic tubular structures within the myometrium (Fig. 8-15). Color Doppler ultrasound may provide a more specific image with large-caliber vessels and blood flow reversals. Angiography is used to confirm the diagnosis of AVMs and may be concurrently therapeutic when performed with embolization (Cura, 2009). Computed tomographic (CT) scanning with contrast, magnetic resonance (MR) imaging, saline infusion sonography, and hysteroscopy have also been used to image these (Lowenstein, 2004; Timmerman, 2003).

Arteriovenous malformations have been treated traditionally by hysterectomy. However, less invasive approaches have also been used. These include arterial embolization or surgical coagulation of the AVM feeding vessels (Corusic, 2009; Ghosh, 1986; Majmudar, 1998; Yokomine, 2009).

■ External Sources

Intrauterine Device (IUD)

Copper-Containing Intrauterine Device. These intrauterine devices have long been associated with menorrhagia and metrorrhagia (Bilian, 2002; Milsom, 1995). Several explanations for this bleeding have been suggested. At the cellular level, unbalanced ratios of prostaglandins and thromboxane have been proposed as a potential source of IUD-induced menorrhagia (Zhang, 1992). This gains credence in that clinical studies have shown bleeding improvement with prostaglandin inhibitors such as nonsteroidal antiinflammatory drugs (NSAIDs) (Roy, 1981).

At the tissue level, endometrial vascularity, congestion, and degeneration are increased in IUD users. These changes result in interstitial hemorrhage, which may lead to metrorrhagia (Shaw, 1979a,b). At the organ level, some have suggested that IUD rotation, embedding, or perforation may cause excessive bleeding. There have been studies that support as well as refute this (Faundes, 1997; Pizarro, 1989).

Following exclusion of pregnancy, infection, or gross structural pathology, patients with IUD-related bleeding may initially be managed with an empiric trial of NSAIDs. Persistent or refractory bleeding, however, may reflect other gynecologic pathology. These patients should be managed similarly to other women with the initial complaint of abnormal uterine bleeding. However, sonographic evaluation may be limited by IUD shadowing. Endometrial biopsy with small catheters can be performed without removal of the device (Grimes, 2007).

Levonorgestrel-Releasing Intrauterine System. This system, marketed as Mirena, can lead to abnormal uterine bleeding in some users. The cause of bleeding is not clear, but down-regulation of estrogen and progesterone receptors, increased local leukocyte populations, and alterations of endometrial vascular morphology, hemostasis, and endometrial repair have all been proposed (Oliveira-Ribeiro, 2004; Rhoton-Vlasak, 2005).

The endometrial effects of progestins are thought to predominate, and evidence is accruing that low-dose progestins increase endometrial vascular fragility (Hickey, 2000a, 2002; Roopa, 2003). The LNG-IUS is associated with development of superficial, thin-walled vessels with increased diameters. Combined with endometrial surface irregularity, these may cause the breakthrough bleeding often seen. As the endometrium becomes atrophic, these vascular abnormalities gradually resolve at a time thought to coincide clinically with progestin-induced amenorrhea (McGavigan, 2003).

Bleeding associated with the LNG-IUS may be managed similarly to that with the copper-containing IUD, and NSAIDs serve as first-line treatment. Patients can be reassured that most patients experience a decline in menstrual flow and are typically satisfied with its use after 3 months (Irvine, 1999).

Progestin-only Contraception

Bleeding disturbances are common not only with the LNG-IUS as just described, but also with other progestin-only methods of birth control. This bleeding is characteristically irregular and light, but may also be frequent and prolonged.

Combination Hormonal Contraception

Bleeding associated with combination oral contraceptive pills (COCs) is common. As many as 30 to 50 percent of women experience abnormal uterine bleeding in the first month that COCs are initiated (Nelson, 2011). The presumed source of this bleeding stems from endometrial atrophy that is induced by the progestin component of COCs. During this process, spiral arterioles do not characteristically coil, and they become thinner and more sinusoidal. In addition, venules become dilated and prone to thrombosis. This often leads to local tissue infarction and is thought to be the cause of breakthrough bleeding (Deligdisch, 2000; Ober, 1977).

Fortunately, the incidence of bleeding decreases significantly with time. For example, Rosenburg and Long (1992) found that after 6 months of COC use, only approximately 10 percent of patients experienced breakthrough bleeding. Accordingly, during the early months of pill use, only counseling and reassurance are typically required (Schrager, 2002). If bleeding persists, selecting a different COC formulation may be required (Chap. 5, p. 150). If bleeding continues despite pill changes, other pathology should be considered.

Hormone Replacement Therapy (HRT)

Irregular spotting or bleeding is a well-known side effect of hormone replacement therapy and is a frequent reason for discontinuation (Chap. 22, p. 585) (Reynolds, 2002). Bleeding may develop both in women using continuous (daily) therapy and in those taking cyclic (sequential) replacement, but is less likely during the first year in those using a cyclic regimen (Furness, 2009). Intrauterine pathology has been shown to be four times more frequent in patients with continued abnormal bleeding after 6 months of HRT use, as well as in those who have abnormal bleeding after achieving initial amenorrhea. Thus, evaluation of bleeding is recommended for this patient subset (Leung, 2003).

Tamoxifen

This selective estrogen-receptor modulator (SERM) is used as an adjunct for treatment of estrogen-receptor–positive breast cancer. Although it diminishes estrogen action in breast tissue, it stimulates proliferation in the endometrium. Tamoxifen use has been linked to hyperplasia, polyps, and carcinoma of the endometrium and to uterine sarcomas (Cohen, 2004).

Screening women who use tamoxifen but who do not have abnormal bleeding has not proved effective. Specifically, protocols that use sonography or endometrial biopsy to efficiently identify endometrial cancer in asymptomatic users have failed (Barakat, 2000; Love, 1999). Thus, unless a patient has been identified to be at higher risk for endometrial cancer, a woman using tamoxifen should undergo evaluation for endometrial cancer only if symptoms of bleeding develop (American College of Obstetricians and Gynecologists, 2006).

Infection

In addition to cervicitis, abnormal bleeding can also be caused by chronic endometritis. This diagnosis is confirmed by the finding of plasma cells within an endometrial biopsy specimen. Chronic endometritis was found by Greenwood and Moran (1981) in up to 10 percent of endometrial biopsies performed for abnormal bleeding. Chronic endometritis typically develops insidiously. Although bleeding is a common complaint with endometritis, women may also describe vaginal discharge and lower abdominal pain.

Chronic endometritis has been linked to infectious disease. Specifically, *Neisseria gonorrhoeae*, *Chlamydia trachomatis*, agents of bacterial vaginosis, and *Mycoplasma* species have each been implicated in causing this low-grade endometrial inflammation (Crum, 2006; Gilmore, 2007; Haggerty, 2009). Abnormal uterine bleeding from endometritis may be observed in those with acute as well as subclinical or silent pelvic inflammatory disease (PID) (Ness, 2004; Wiesenfeld, 2002). In one study,

Wiesenfeld and coworkers (2002) found subclinical PID and endometritis in 27 percent of women with *C trachomatis,* in 26 percent of women infected with *N gonorrhoeae,* and in 15 percent of those with bacterial vaginosis. Accordingly, obtaining cultures for these two pathogens is reasonable in sexually active patients. However, in some patients, infection does not seem to play a role, and the histopathologic findings derive solely from inflammatory changes. For example, chronic endometritis may be associated with structural lesions such as endometrial polyps or submucous leiomyomas, or it may follow events such as abortion or pregnancy. Thus, deciding whether or not treat with antibiotics can be challenging, but empiric treatment with an antibiotic course has been shown to improve symptoms in women with chronic endometritis (Eckert, 2004). At our instivtution, patients are typically given a course of doxycycline, 100 mg orally twice daily for 10 days. For bleeding associated with PID, treatment follows that outlined in Table 3-27 (p. 98).

■ Systemic Causes

Renal Disease

Severe renal dysfunction is frequently accompanied by endocrine disturbances that often result in hypoestrogenism, amenorrhea, and infertility (Matuszkiewicz-Rowińska, 2004). In a study of 100 women with chronic renal failure undergoing dialysis, Cochrane and Regan (1997) reported that 80 percent of those menstruating complained of menorrhagia. This is also of concern because bleeding may worsen the chronic anemia associated with renal failure. The mechanism behind these abnormalities is not clear, but hypothalamic dysregulation of gonadotropin secretion is suspected (Bry-Gauillard, 1999).

Treatment of abnormal bleeding due to chronic renal insufficiency is problematic. NSAIDs are contraindicated, because they cause renal artery vasoconstriction with adverse effects on glomerular function. Administration of cyclical progestins is typically unhelpful. Instead, Cochrane and Regan (1997) suggest high-dose medroxyprogesterone acetate to create endometrial atrophy and amenorrhea. They also reported that most women with renal insufficiency respond to low-dose COCs, which offer the additional benefit of improved cycle control. However, in women with severe hypertension or systemic lupus erythematosus, these may be contraindicated. Fong and Singh (1999) have reported success with the LNG-IUS in renal transplant patients with menorrhagia secondary to uterine leiomyomas.

If patients with renal failure and severe menorrhagia cannot take or do not respond to medical therapy, then surgical treatments are considered. Jeong and coworkers (2004) found endometrial ablation to be successful, and 87 percent of women showed diminished bleeding. In some women, however, hysterectomy is required. Minimally invasive surgical hysterectomy approaches have been described in the setting of renal failure and are effective (Jeong, 2004; Kuzel, 2009; Raff, 2008).

Liver Disease

Depending on its severity, liver dysfunction can lead to menstrual abnormalities (Stellon, 1986). In studies evaluating menstruation in women with end-stage liver disease before transplantation, menstrual dysfunction is reported by 60 percent

(de Koning, 1990; Mass, 1996). The underlying mechanism for bleeding is not clear, but as in renal failure, hypothalamic-pituitary-ovarian axis dysfunction has been implicated. The liver serves a primary role in the metabolism and excretion of sex hormones, and liver dysfunction is associated with high levels of circulating estrogen. This, in turn, may lead to the inappropriately low serum luteinizing-hormone and follicle-stimulating hormone levels seen in these women (Bell, 1995; Cundy, 1991).

Hemostatic dysfunction may also contribute to abnormal bleeding. With the exception of von Willebrand factor, all of the coagulation proteins and most of their inhibitors are synthesized in the liver. In addition, thrombocytopenia is common in women with portal hypertension and splenomegaly.

Evidencd-based studies directing the treatment of menorrhagia in women with liver disease are lacking. As outlined by the World Health Organization (Kapp, 2009a,b), hormonal therapy may be inappropriate for some affected women. Specifically, in those with chronic viral hepatitis or with mild compensated cirrhosis, hormonal contraceptive use is not restricted. In those with active hepatitis or a flare of their chronic viral disease, initiation of progestin-only contraception is reasonable, whereas estrogen-containing products are avoided. In those with severe, decompensated cirrhosis, all hormonal contraception should be avoided.

Thyroid Disease

Both hyperthyroidism and hypothyroidism can cause menstrual disturbances ranging from amenorrhea to menorrhagia (Koutras, 1997). In many women, these menstrual abnormalities antedate other clinical findings of thyroid disease (Joshi, 1993). Thus, in most women with abnormal uterine bleeding, measurement of serum TSH levels is recommended.

With hyperthyroidism, hypomenorrhea and amenorrhea are more frequent complaints, and menorrhagia is noted in only approximately 5 percent. With severe overt hypothyroidism, women commonly present with anovulation, amenorrhea, and anovulatory dysfunctional uterine bleeding (p. 236). These women may also display defects in hemostasis. This may be due to decreased coagulation factor levels that have been identified in some hypothyroid patients. With either hypo- or hyperthyroidism, treatment of the underlying thyroid disorder usually corrects uterine bleeding abnormalities (Krassas, 1999; Wilansky, 1989).

Coagulopathy

Many coagulation defects that lead to menorrhagia can be broadly categorized as either: (1) dysfunction of platelet adherence or (2) defects in platelet plug stabilization. First, during initial stages of hemostasis, platelets adhere to breaks in a vessel wall by the binding of their receptors to exposed collagen. This bridging is dependent on von Willebrand factor (vWF), a plasma protein. Once bound, platelets are activated and release a potent agonist of their aggregation, thromboxane. Thus, low platelet number, defects in vWF quality or quantity, platelet receptor defects, or thromboxane inhibitors may all lead to poor platelet adherence and menorrhagia. Second, the coagulation cascade leads to fibrin formation, which stabilizes aggregated platelets. Defects in the clotting factors that comprise these cascades may also predispose to abnormal bleeding (Ewenstein, 1996).

In general, coagulopathies are infrequent causes of gynecologic bleeding. However, in the subset of women with menorrhagia and normal anatomy, the incidence is significantly higher (Kadir, 1998; Philipp, 2005). Moreover, a history of easy bruising, bleeding complications with surgery or obstetric delivery, recurrent hemorrhagic cysts, epistaxis, and gastrointestinal bleeding or a family history of bleeding disorders should raise concern for coagulopathy. In addition, the American College of Obstetricians and Gynecologists (2001) has also recommended specifically testing for von Willebrand disease in adolescents with severe menorrhagia and in women with significant menorrhagia without another identifiable cause, and consideration of testing prior to hysterectomy in those with severe uterine bleeding.

Laboratory screening for coagulopathies includes a complete blood count (CBC) with platelets, prothrombin time (PT), and partial thromboplastin time (PTT). Bleeding time has not been shown to be specific or sensitive and thus is not routinely recommended. More commonly identified coagulopathies include von Willebrand disease (vWD), thrombocytopenia, and disorders of platelet function. Deficiencies of factors VIII and IX (hemophilia A and B) and other factor deficiencies are uncommon. Specific screening for each is discussed subsequently.

Thrombocytopenia or Platelet Dysfunction.

As described, platelets are an integral part of thrombus formation, and low counts may lead to abnormal bleeding. Thrombocytopenia may be broadly categorized as resulting from disorders that increase platelet destruction, decrease platelet production, or increase platelet sequestration.

Alternatively, normal platelet counts may be found, but platelet dysfunction and thus their poor aggregation may be the underlying defect. First, prolonged use of thromboxane inhibitors such as NSAIDs and aspirin may lead to platelet dysfunction. These drugs are commonly taken by women with abnormal bleeding due to its close association with dysmenorrhea. Accordingly, patients should be asked about chronic use of these drugs. Much less often, primary genetic defects in platelet receptors lead to platelet dysfunction and abnormal bleeding.

As a group, evidenced-based data directing the treatment of platelet-associated menorrhagia are limited (Levens, 2007; Martin-Johnston, 2008). With the exception of NSAIDs, options for treatment include those described later for dysfunctional uterine bleeding.

Von Willebrand Disease.

Von Willebrand factor (vWF) is a glycoprotein synthesized in endothelial cells and megakaryocytes and is integral to platelet adherence at sites of endothelial injury. It also prevents clearance of factor VIII, which is rapidly depleted without vWF and becomes clinically deficient (McGrath, 2010). Diminished amount or decreased function of vWF characterizes the several variants of von Willebrand disease (Table 8-3). Von Willebrand disease is an inherited bleeding disorder, and autosomal dominant and recessive patterns of transmission exist.

The disorder is more common in white than in African-American women, and the prevalence of von Willebrand disease approximates 1 percent in the general population (Miller, 2003; Nichols, 2008). However, in women with abnormal bleeding and normal pelvic anatomy, the rate of von Willebrand disease was found to be 13 percent (Shankar, 2004). Affected individuals commonly complain of menorrhagia, and rates of 60 to 70 percent have been noted (Kadir, 1998, 1999; Lak, 2000). Heavy menstruation typically begins with menarche in these patients.

In screening for coagulopathy, women with von Willebrand disease may display a prolonged PTT. Specific tests include measurement of von Willebrand-ristocetin cofactor activity, von Willebrand factor antigen concentration, and factor VIII activity (James, 2009b). Of note, factor VIII and vWF levels reach a nadir during menses and are relatively increased in women using COCs. However, testing should not be rescheduled nor COCs halted to complete patient evaluation (James, 2009a). Consultation with a hematologist is recommended because the diagnosis of von Willebrand disease, especially in its mild form, can be difficult.

Treatments for women with menorrhagia and von Willebrand disease include hormonal contraception, desmopressin, plasma concentrates, antifibrinolytics, or surgery. Combination oral contraceptive pills are often used as first-line treatment and have been noted to arrest uterine hemorrhage in

TABLE 8-3. vWD Classification and Laboratory Values

Condition	Description	vWf:RCo (IU/dL)	vWf:Ag (IU/dL)	FVIII activity
Type 1	Partial quantitative vWF deficiency	<30	<30	↓ or Normal
Type 2	Qualitative vWF deficiency	<30	<30–200	↓ or Normal
Type 3	Virtually complete vWF deficiency	<3	<3	↓↓↓ (<10 IU/dL)
Normal		50–200	50–200	Normal

FVIII = coagulation factor VIII; vWD = von Willebrand disease; vWF = von Willebrand factor; vWF:Ag = von Willebrand factor antigen; vWF:RCo = von Willebrand factor: risocetin cofactor activity.
Adapted from Nichols, 2009.

88 percent of affected women (Foster, 1995). Also, Kingman and coworkers (2004) reported that the LNG-IUS effectively decreased blood loss and induced amenorrhea in 56 percent of 16 women with inherited bleeding disorders. Extended-cycle COC use or depot medroxyprogesterone acetate are other options for menorrhagia in these women (American College of Obstetricians and Gynecologists, 2009b). Additional treatment may also include the antifibrinolytic drugs aminocaproic acid and tranexamic acid. These agents inhibit conversion of plasminogen to plasmin and thereby diminish fibrinolysis and stabilize formed clots (Nichols, 2008). Importantly, agents that prevent platelet adhesion, such as aspirin or NSAIDs, should be avoided in affected individuals.

In those no longer desiring fertility, surgical intervention may be considered. Preliminary success has been found with endometrial ablation for women with von Willebrand disease-related menorrhagia, but long-term success rates are lower than in those without a bleeding disorder (Rubin, 2004). Dilatation and curettage is not effective long-term to control bleeding in affected women and may worsen blood loss (James, 2009a). Hysterectomy is curative, although rates of bleeding complications from hysterectomy in women with von Willebrand disease are higher than those in unaffected women (James, 2009c). In preparation for surgical procedures, preoperative consultation with a hematologist is recommended to coordinate preoperative desmopressin or factor concentrate administration (American College of Obstetricians and Gynecologists, 2009b).

For severe bleeding, both vWF and factor VIII are replaced by administration of the plasma-derived concentrates, Humate-P or Alphanate. Factor replacement is combined with desmopressin. This vasopressin analog promotes release of vWF from endothelial cells and is available in intravenous, subcutaneous, and intranasal forms (Federici, 2008; Lee, 2005). Desmopressin side effects include flushing, transient blood pressure changes, and headache, but these rarely limit use. However, because of its antidiuretic properties, monitoring for hyponatremia is warranted if multiple doses or shorter dosing intervals are used (Rodeghiero, 2008). A comprehensive list of management and dosing guidelines for various clinical situations for those with vWD is available from The National Heart, Lung, and Blood Institute at: http://www.nhlbi.nih.gov/guidelines/vwd.

Coagulation Cascade Factor Deficiencies. These coagulopathies usually manifests as a prolonged prothrombin time or activated partial thromboplastin time (aPTT). As with von Willebrand disease, affected women may present with menorrhagia. Hemophilia A and B are inherited X-linked deficiencies of factor VIII and IX, respectively. Women carriers of the gene, however, can have decreased levels of factor VIII or IX. In some cases, factor levels are low enough to cause mild hemophilia, which may manifest as abnormal bleeding (Mannucci, 2001; Siegel, 2005).

Other coagulation factor deficiencies are usually inherited as autosomal recessive traits and are rare. This group includes dysfibrinogenemia, hypofibrinogenemia, prothrombin deficiency, and deficiency of factors V, VII, X, XI, and XIII. Menorrhagia has been reported in as many as 50 percent of affected women (Lukes, 2005). Treatment of these disorders is by factor replace-

ment (Mannucci, 2004). Menorrhagia can be addressed similarly to von Willebrand disease.

Anticoagulation Therapy. Although this treatment confers a risk of major bleeding events, minor bleeding problems such as menstrual irregularities are also often encountered. Initially, coagulation studies including PT, PTT, and platelet count should be obtained as bleeding may be related to excess anticoagulant activity. Patients should also be queried regarding recent dosage changes. Physical examination is completed, and imaging and endometrial sampling are performed as indicated.

Management can be challenging, as many traditional treatment options carry increased risks in these women. Long-term administration of estrogen-containing agents to manipulate the endometrium is contraindicated in those at risk for thromboembolism. Moreover, surgical interventions are associated with increased rates of intra- and postoperative bleeding or thromboembolic complications. The LNG-IUS has been found to be an effective treatment for menorrhagia in many of these women (Pisoni, 2006; Vilos, 2009). If a surgical approach is desired, endometrial ablation can be considered. If hysterectomy is required, anticoagulation can be reversed prior to surgery as described in Chapter 39 (p. 954).

Dysfunctional Uterine Bleeding

Once the just-described organic causes of abnormal uterine bleeding have been excluded, the term *dysfunctional uterine bleeding (DUB)* is used. Up to half of women with abnormal bleeding will have DUB (Hickey, 2000b). The term is further categorized as *anovulatory DUB* or *ovulatory DUB*. Eighty to 90 percent of DUB is associated with anovulation. With this form, bleeding episodes are irregular and amenorrhea, metrorrhagia, and menorrhagia are common. For example, many women with anovulation may be amenorrheic for weeks to months followed by irregular, prolonged, and heavy bleeding. The other 10 to 20 percent of DUB cases are described as ovulatory DUB. Ovulation occurs with normal cyclicity, and menorrhagia is thought to originate from defects in the bleeding control mechanisms of menstruation.

Pathophysiology

Anovulatory DUB. If ovulation does not occur, no progesterone is produced, and a proliferative endometrium persists. At the tissue level, a chronic proliferative endometrium is typically associated with stromal breakdown, decreased spiral arteriole density, and dilated and unstable venous capillaries (Singh, 2005). Because endometrial vessels become markedly dilated, bleeding can be severe. At the cellular level, the availability of arachidonic acid is reduced, and prostaglandin production is impaired. For these reasons, bleeding associated with anovulation is thought to result from alterations in endometrial vascular structure and prostaglandin concentration and from an increased endometrial responsiveness to vasodilating prostaglandins (Hickey, 2000b, 2003).

Ovulatory DUB. This form of DUB is thought to stem predominately from vascular dilatation alone. For example, women with ovulatory bleeding lose blood at rates three times faster than women with normal menses, but the number of spiral arterioles is not increased (Abberton, 1999). Thus in women with ovulatory DUB, it is thought that the vessels supplying the endometrium have decreased vascular tone and therefore increased rates of blood loss due to vasodilatation (Rogers, 2003). A number of causes that provoke this change in vascular tone have been suggested, and prostaglandins have been strongly implicated.

Treatment

Medical treatment of dysfunctional uterine bleeding includes NSAIDs, COCs, progestins, androgens, and agonists of gonadotropin-releasing hormone (GnRH). The use of tranexamic acid (antifibrinolytic agent) was approved by the U.S. Food and Drug Administration (FDA) for the treatment of menorrhagia in 2009. Etamsylate has also been described, but this agent is not commonly used in the United States.

Nonsteroidal Antiinflammatory Drugs. These medicines are effective and well-tolerated oral agents commonly used for the treatment of DUB (Table 8-4). The rationale for their use stems from the suspected role of prostaglandins in the pathogenesis of DUB. A number of investigators have documented the effectiveness of NSAIDs in decreasing DUB-related menorrhagia (Makarainen, 1986b; Marchini, 1995). Among NSAIDs, there are no differences in clinical efficacy, although responses to a particular agent may vary among individuals (Lethaby, 2007).

Women lose 90 percent of menstrual blood volume during the first 3 days of menses (Haynes, 1977). Accordingly, NSAIDs are most effective if used with the onset of menses or just prior to its onset and continued throughout its duration. Therefore, one advantage to NSAIDs is that they are taken only during menstruation. Another advantage is that commonly associated dysmenorrhea also improves with NSAIDs.

The so-called conventional NSAIDs nonspecifically inhibit both cyclooxygenase-1 (COX-1), an enzyme critical to normal platelet function, and COX-2, which mediates inflammatory response mechanisms. Conventional NSAIDs are effective analgesics, but their use with bleeding may not be ideal considering their inhibitory effects on platelet function. Another class of NSAIDs inhibits only COX-2, and these COX-2 inhibitors do not interfere with platelet aggregation and hemostasis (Leese, 2000). However, long-term use of COX-2 inhibitors has been linked with increased rates of myocardial infarction, stroke, and heart failure (Farkouh, 2009; Solomon, 2006). Moreover, data showing an advantage in menorrhagia control with COX-2 inhibitors compared with conventional NSAIDs are lacking.

Oral Progestins. With anovulation, the resulting unopposed estrogen stimulation causes proliferation of the endometrium and erratic bleeding. Progestins halt endometrial growth and allow for an organized sloughing following their withdrawal (Saarikoski, 1990). Thus, progestin treatment of women with

TABLE 8-4. Medical Treatment of Menorrhagia[a,b]

Acute Treatment[c]

Premarin	25 mg IV q4h for up to three doses	DeVore, 1982
Premarin	2.5 mg pill q6h	DeVore, 1982
COCs	1 pill tid for up to 7 days (then taper)	Munro, 2006

Chronic Treatment

NSAID

Mefenamic acid	500 mg tid for 5 days, beginning with menses	Bonnar, 1996
Naproxen	550 mg on first day of menses, then 275 mg daily	Hall, 1987
Ibuprofen	600 mg daily throughout menses	Makarainen, 1986a
Flurbiprofen	100 mg bid for 5 days, beginning with menses	Andersch, 1988
Meclofenamate	100 mg tid for 3 days, beginning with menses	Vargyas, 1987

Other classes

COCs	One pill daily	Agarwal, 2001
Tranexamic acid	650 mg pill: 2 pills tid for 5 days, beginning with menses	Lukes, 2010
Norethindrone	5 mg tid days 5 through 26 of cycle (ovulatory DUB)	Irvine, 1998
	5 mg tid days 15 through 26 of cycle (anovulatory DUB)	Higham, 1993
Danazol	100 mg or 200 mg daily throughout cycle	Chimbira, 1980b
GnRH agonists	3.75 mg IM each month (maximum 6 months of use)	Shamonki, 2000
LNG-IUS	Intrauterine placement	Reid, 2005

[a]All agents are administered orally except high-dose Premarin, GnRH agonists, and LNG-IUS.
[b]All anemic patients should also initiate oral iron supplementation.
[c]Antiemetics may be required to control nausea and vomiting with these high-dose estrogen-containing regimens.
bid = twice daily; COCs = combination oral contraceptive pills; DUB = dysfunctional uterine bleeding; GnRH = gonadotropin-releasing hormone; IM = intramuscularly; IV = intravenously; LNG-IUS = levonorgestrel-containing intrauterine system; NSAID = nonsteroidal antiinflammatory drug; qid = four times daily; tid = three times daily.

anovulatory DUB is usually successful. Of the progestins, either norethindrone—also known as norethisterone—or medroxyprogesterone acetate may be used. Norethindrone, 5 mg, is given orally two or three times daily, or medroxyprogesterone acetate 10 mg is taken orally once daily. This is followed by withdrawal bleeding 3 to 5 days after completion of a 10-day course. Importantly, patients should be educated that menses will begin *after* rather than *during* their progesterone course. For long-term menstrual regulation, these same dosages are taken during days 16 through 25 following the first day of the most recent menstrual flow (Fraser, 1990).

In contrast, ovulatory DUB is not due to a progestin deficiency but rather results from altered prostaglandin synthesis or disruption of hemostasis. As expected, ovulatory menorrhagia is relatively unresponsive to cyclic administration of oral progestins (Cameron, 1987, 1990; Preston, 1995; Singh, 2005). Despite this, women with ovulatory DUB may respond to longer treatment schedules. Norethindrone, 5 mg, or medroxyprogesterone acetate, 10 mg, each given orally three times daily for days 5 to 26 of each menstrual cycle, have proved effective (Fraser, 1990; Irvine, 1998). Unfortunately, prolonged use of high-dose progestins is often associated with side effects such as mood changes, weight gain, bloating, headaches, and atherogenic changes in the lipid profile (Lethaby, 2008). For these reasons, they are considered unacceptable by many women for near-daily long-term use.

Combination Oral Contraceptive Pills.

Evidence suggests that these hormonal agents effectively treat DUB, and when used long term, reduce flow by 40 to 70 percent (Agarwal, 2001; Fraser, 1991). Advantages to COC use include the additional benefits of reducing dysmenorrhea and providing contraception. Their presumed method of action is endometrial atrophy. There may also be diminished prostaglandin synthesis and decreased endometrial fibrinolysis (Irvine, 1999).

In addition to chronic use for the treatment of dysfunctional uterine bleeding, COCs can be used acutely to manage menorrhagia. Pills containing at least 30 μg of ethinyl estradiol should be prescribed, and a complete list of COC formulations is found in Table 5-8 (p. 150). If bleeding is significant, the regimen begins with one pill every 8 hours until the bleeding has stopped or markedly diminished for at least 24 hours. An antiemetic may be needed to control nausea. For most women, bleeding will diminish within 24 to 48 hours. After bleeding has slowed, the COC dosage is decreased to one pill every 12 hours for the next 3 to 7 days. A once-a-day dosage is then continued for 21 days to be followed by withdrawal menses. This type of dose-diminishing regimen is colloquially known as a "COC taper." Effective modification of this regimen may include less frequent dosing or smaller doses. Following this taper, COCs may be stopped or continued long-term for cycle control (Munro, 2006).

Estrogen.

High-dose estrogen therapy may be useful in controlling acute, heavy bleeding. Conjugated equine estrogens (Premarin) are administered orally at dosages up to 10 mg daily, given in four divided doses. Similarly, the drug can be given intravenously in 25-mg doses every 4 hours for up to three doses (DeVore, 1982). Once bleeding has slowed, patients can be transitioned to an oral taper using COCs.

Gonadotropin-Releasing Hormone Agonists.

The profound hypoestrogenic state created by these agents induces endometrial atrophy and amenorrhea in most women. Side effects, however, may be dramatic and include those typical for the menopause. In addition, associated bone loss precludes their long-term use, and treatment is typically limited to 6 months. This family of drugs, however, may be helpful in the short term to induce amenorrhea and allow women to rebuild their red blood cell mass. From this group, leuprolide acetate (Lupron) is used at our institution. Depending on the degree of anemia and other associated factors, a 3.75-mg dose, given each month, or an 11.25-mg dose, given every 3-months, is administered intramuscularly.

Levonorgestrel Releasing Intrauterine System.

Intrauterine devices were initially developed for contraceptive purposes. However, the addition of progestins to inert intrauterine devices was found to decrease expulsion rates, improve contraceptive efficacy, and in some cases, lessen menorrhagia. The LNG-IUS device was designed to take advantage of these attributes and has been shown to reduce menstrual loss by 74 to 97 percent after 3 months' use (Singh, 2005; Stewart, 2001). The LNG-IUS can be used in most women, including adolescents, as a first-line treatment. Contraindications are found in Table 5-5 (p. 138). It is particularly useful for reproductive-aged women with menorrhagia who wish to retain fertility.

Several investigations have compared the LNG-IUS with medical therapy, with endometrial ablation, or with hysterectomy. First, compared with mefenamic acid given during menses or with oral progesterone given 21 days each cycle, the LNG-IUS proved more effective in decreasing blood loss (Irvine, 1998; Lethaby, 2005; Reid, 2005). If compared with endometrial ablation, the LNG-IUS appears to have similar therapeutic effects up to 2 years after treatment (Kaunitz, 2009). Finally, Hurskainen and associates (2001, 2004), in their randomized controlled trial of 236 women, showed that when assigned either to LNG-IUS or hysterectomy as a treatment for menorrhagia, after 1 year and again after 5 years, the two treatments were associated with equal improvements in health status, quality of life, and psychosocial well-being. However, 42 percent of those assigned to the LNG-IUS eventually underwent hysterectomy.

Androgens (Danazol and Gestrinone).

Danazol is a derivative of the synthetic steroid 17α-ethinyl testosterone. The net effect of danazol creates a hypoestrogenic and hyperandrogenic environment, which induces endometrial atrophy. As a result, menstrual loss is reduced by approximately half, and it may even induce amenorrhea in some women (Beaumont, 2002; Chimbira, 1980a; Higham, 1993).

For heavy menstrual bleeding, suggested dosing is 100 to 200 mg taken daily (Chimbira, 1980b). Unfortunately, this agent has significant androgenic side effects that include weight gain, oily skin, and acne. Thus, danazol is usually reserved as a second-line drug for short-term use prior to surgery (Bongers, 2004).

Gestrinone is derived synthetically from a 19-nortestosterone steroid nucleus. Its mechanism of action, side effects, and indications for the treatment of menorrhagia are similar to those of danazol. The recommended dose for the treatment of menorrhagia is 2.5 mg daily every 3 to 4 days. The drug is used in the United Kingdom and other countries, but is not approved for use in the United States.

Tranexamic Acid. This is an antifibrinolytic drug and exerts its effects by reversibly blocking lysine binding sites on plasminogen. Decreased plasmin levels follow. As a result of lower plasmin levels, fibrinolytic activity within endometrial vessels is diminished, fibrin is not broken down, and thereby bleeding is prevented.

In women with DUB, fibrinolytic activity within the endometrium is increased compared with that of women with normal menses (Gleeson, 1994). Clinically, tranexamic acid has been shown effective to reduce bleeding in women with DUB-related menorrhagia (Kriplani, 2006; Lethaby, 2000). In addition, it requires administration only during menstruation and has few minor reported side effects that are predominantly gastrointestinal and dose-dependent. The recommended dose is two 650-mg tablets orally taken three times daily for a maximum of 5 days during menstruation (Lukes, 2010).

Although used in other parts of the world for many years, tranexamic acid (Lysteda) was only approved by the U.S. FDA to treat menorrhagia in 2009. The drug has no effect on other blood coagulation parameters such as platelet count, activated partial thromboplastin time, and prothrombin time (Wellington, 2003). However, its use in the United States had previously been limited by concern that increased systemic thrombotic activity may lead to increased rates of thromboembolism. Contraindications to tranexamic acid include a history of or an intrinsic risk for thromboembolic disease. In addition, strong caution is recommended in concurrently prescribing hormonal contraceptives that also increase thromboembolic risk.

Etamsylate (Ethamsylate). This hemostatic agent is the diethylammonium salt of dihydroxy-2,5-benzenesulfonate. It has been in clinical use for more than 30 years, but its mechanism of action is still not completely understood. Also spelled *ethamsylate*, this agent is suspected to act in early hemostasis by increasing platelet adhesiveness and aggregation (Hernandez, 2004). Its effectiveness varies in randomized trials, and ranges from no reduction in flow to a 50-percent decrease (Bonnar, 1996; Chamberlain, 1991). In this country, etamsylate does not have a clinical role in the treatment of menorrhagia (Irvine, 1999).

Iron Therapy. Women with abnormal uterine bleeding may become anemic. Thus, patient care typically is directed toward bleeding abatement and oral iron replacement. Ferrous salts vary in their content of elemental iron. Thus, equivalent common replacement regimens include ferrous sulfate, 325 mg three times daily, or ferrous fumarate, 200 mg three times daily (Adamson, 2008). The presence of acid in the duodenum improves iron solubility and absorption. Accordingly, iron should be taken between meals or at bedtime. Epigastric discomfort and constipation are common side effects. These may be countered with dose reductions, use of enteric-coated iron tablets, and/or higher-fiber diets (Alleyne, 2008).

Uterine Artery Embolization. This procedure is most commonly used to treat menorrhagia secondary to uterine leiomyomas (Chap. 9, p. 256). Rarely, in those not responding to conservative measures, this intervention may be considered for dysfunctional uterine bleeding in women with excessive acute blood loss or with coagulopathic disorders or in those who refuse blood products (Salazar, 2009).

Surgery. For many women, conservative medical management may either be unsuccessful or associated with significant side effects. Surgical management of menorrhagia may include hysterectomy and procedures to destroy the endometrium.

Dilatation and Curettage (D&C). Curettage is rarely used for long-term treatment because its effects are only temporary. In the occasional woman, D&C is performed to arrest severe bleeding refractory to high-dose estrogen administration (American College of Obstetricians and Gynecologists, 2000; Stabinsky, 1999).

Endometrial Destructive Procedures. Although medical therapy is generally used first, more than half of women with menorrhagia undergo hysterectomy within 5 years of referral to a gynecologist. In at least a third of these, an anatomically normal uterus is removed (Coulter, 1991; Roy, 2004). As alternatives to hysterectomy, less invasive procedures have been devised that either destroy or resect the endometrium and lead to amenorrhea in a manner similar to Asherman syndrome (Chap. 16, p. 444).

Currently acceptable procedures for endometrial resection or ablation employ laser, radiofrequency, electrical, or thermal energies (Oehler, 2003). These methods are described and illustrated in detail in Section 42-17 (p. 1169). They are considered as either first- or second-generation techniques according to their temporal introduction into use and their need for hysteroscopic guidance. A number of studies that compared first- and second-generation techniques have shown them equally effective (Gervaise, 1999; Meyer, 1998).

After resection or ablation, 70 to 80 percent of women experience significantly decreased flow, and 15 to 35 percent of these develop amenorrhea. Increasing treatment failures due to endometrial regeneration accrue with time following the procedure. For example, in a long-term surveillance of 301 women following ablation, Martyn and coworkers (1998) reported that the cumulative failure rate increased from 13 percent at 2 years to 27 percent at 5 years. In these women, the amenorrhea rate remained relatively constant at approximately 40 percent. Vilos (2004) noted that subsequent hysterectomy approximated 12 percent by 5 years following ablation.

Although success rates for treatment of heavy bleeding are not as high as with hysterectomy, patient satisfaction rates are surprisingly comparable. Moreover, resection and ablation procedures have significantly lower complication rates when compared with hysterectomy.

Following ablation, later evaluation of the endometrium for recurrent abnormal bleeding can be challenging. Uterine cavity anatomy is often distorted by synechiae and uterine wall agglutination. The failure rate of endometrial sampling has been reported to be as high as 33 percent. Moreover, endometrial stripe evaluation by transvaginal sonography or hysteroscopic examination may be limited (Ahonkallio, 2009). Accordingly,

TABLE 8-5. Considerations with Endometrial Ablation

Contraindications
Pregnancy
Acute pelvic infection
Endometrial hyperplasia or genital tract cancer
Women wishing to preserve their fertility
Postmenopausal women
Expectation of amenorrhea
Intrauterine device in place

Concerns
Women at high risk for endometrial cancer[a]
Large or distorted endometrial cavity[b]
Prior uterine surgery: classical cesarean delivery,
    transmural myomectomy[c]

[a]Risks include obesity, chronic anovulation, tamoxifen use, unopposed estrogen use, and diabetes mellitus.
[b]Each device has specific cavity-size limitations.
[c]May be associated with increased risk of damage to surrounding tissue.

endometrial ablation is not routinely recommended for patients at high risk for endometrial cancer (American Society for Reproductive Medicine, 2008). Other contraindications are listed in Table 8-5.

Hysterectomy. Removal of the uterus is the most effective treatment for bleeding, and overall patient satisfaction rates approximate 85 percent. Moreover, subjective improvement of dysmenorrhea and premenstrual symptoms has also been reported following hysterectomy (Aberdeen Endometrial Ablation Trials Group, 1999; Mousa, 2001). Disadvantages to hysterectomy include more frequent and severe intraoperative and postoperative complications compared with either conservative medical or ablative surgical procedures. Operating time, hospitalization, recovery times, and costs are also greater. The procedure is discussed in detail in Section 41-12 (p. 1020).

REFERENCES

Abberton KM, Healy DL, Rogers PAW: Smooth muscle alpha actin and myosin heavy chain expression in the vascular smooth muscle cells surrounding human endometrial arterioles. Hum Reprod 14:3095, 1999

Aberdeen Endometrial Ablation Trials Group: A randomised trial of endometrial ablation versus hysterectomy for the treatment of dysfunctional uterine bleeding: outcome at four years. Aberdeen Endometrial Ablation Trials Group. Br J Obstet Gynaecol 106:360, 1999

Abu J, Davies Q, Ireland D: Should women with postcoital bleeding be referred for colposcopy? J Obstet Gynaecol 26(1):45, 2006

Adamson JW: Iron deficiency and other hypoproliferative anemias. In Fauci AS, Braunwald E, Kasper DL, et al (eds): Harrison's Principles of Internal Medicine, 17th ed. New York, McGraw-Hill, 2008, p 632

Agarwal N, Kriplani A: Medical management of dysfunctional uterine bleeding. Int J Gynecol Obstet 75:199, 2001

Ahonkallio SJ, Liakka AK, Martikainen HK, et al: Feasibility of endometrial assessment after thermal ablation. Eur J Obstet Gynecol Reprod Biol 147(1):69, 2009

Alcazar JL, Castillo G, Minguez JA, et al: Endometrial blood flow mapping using transvaginal power Doppler sonography in women with postmenopausal bleeding and thickened endometrium. Ultrasound Obstet Gynecol 21:583, 2003

Alcazar JL, Galan MJ, Minguez JA, et al: Transvaginal color Doppler sonography versus sonohysterography in the diagnosis of endometrial polyps. J Ultrasound Med 23:743, 2004

Alleyne M, Horne MK, Miller JL: Individualized treatment for iron-deficiency anemia in adults. Am J Med 121(11):943, 2008

American College of Obstetricians and Gynecologists: Management of anovulatory bleeding. Practice Bulletin No. 14, March 2000

American College of Obstetricians and Gynecologists: Sonohysterography. Technology Assessment No. 5, December 2008

American College of Obstetricians and Gynecologists: Tamoxifen and uterine cancer. Committee Opinion No. 336, June 2006

American College of Obstetricians and Gynecologists: The role of transvaginal sonography in the evaluation of postmenopausal bleeding. Committee Opinion No. 426, February, 2009a

American College of Obstetricians and Gynecologists: Von Willebrand's disease in gynecologic practice. Committee Opinion No. 263, December 2001

American College of Obstetricians and Gynecologists: Von Willebrand disease in women. Committee Opinion No. 451, December 2009b

American Society for Reproductive Medicine: Indications and options for endometrial ablation. Fertil Steril 90(5 Suppl):S236, 2008

Andersch B, Milsom I, Rybo G: An objective evaluation of flurbiprofen and tranexamic acid in the treatment of idiopathic menorrhagia. Acta Obstet Gynecol Scand 67:645, 1988

Baiocchi G, Manci N, Pazzaglia M, et al: Malignancy in endometrial polyps: a 12-year experience. Am J Obstet Gynecol 201(5):462.e1, 2009

Bakour SH, Dwarakanath LS, Khan KS, et al: The diagnostic accuracy of ultrasound scan in predicting endometrial hyperplasia and cancer in postmenopausal bleeding. Acta Obstet Gynecol Scand 78:447, 1999

Bakour SH, Gupta JK, Khan KS: Risk factors associated with endometrial polyps in abnormal uterine bleeding. Int J Gynecol Obstet 76(2):165, 2002

Bakour SH, Khan KS, Gupta JK: The risk of premalignant and malignant pathology in endometrial polyps. Acta Obstet Gynecol Scand 79:317, 2000

Barakat RR, Gilewski TA, Almadrones L, et al: Effect of adjuvant tamoxifen on the endometrium in women with breast cancer: a prospective study using office endometrial biopsy. J Clin Oncol 18:3459, 2000

Bax CJ, Oostvogel PM, Mutsaers JA, et al: Clinical characteristics of *Chlamydia trachomatis* infections in a general outpatient department of obstetrics and gynaecology in the Netherlands. Sex Transm Infect 78:E6, 2002

Beaumont H, Augood C, Duckitt K, et al: Danazol for heavy menstrual bleeding. Cochrane Database Syst Rev 2:CD001017, 2002

Bell H, Raknerud N, Falch JA, et al: Inappropriately low levels of gonadotrophins in amenorrhoeic women with alcoholic and non-alcoholic cirrhosis. Eur J Endocrinol 132:444, 1995

Ben-Arie A, Goldchmit C, Laviv Y, et al: The malignant potential of endometrial polyps. Eur J Obstet Gynecol Reprod Biol 115:206, 2004

Ben-Yehuda OM, Kim YB, Leuchter RS: Does hysteroscopy improve upon the sensitivity of dilatation and curettage in the diagnosis of endometrial hyperplasia or carcinoma? Gynecol Oncol 68:4, 1998

Berzolla CE, Schnatz PF, O'Sullivan DM, et al: Dysplasia and malignancy in endocervical polyps. J Womens Health 16(9):1317, 2007

Beukenholdt R, Guerrero K: An audit of a specialist registrar-run outpatient diagnostic hysteroscopy service in a district general hospital. J Obstet Gynaecol 23:294, 2003

Bieglmayer C, Hofer G, Kainz C, et al: Concentrations of various arachidonic acid metabolites in menstrual fluid are associated with menstrual pain and are influenced by hormonal contraceptives. Gynecol Endocrinol 9:307, 1995

Bilian X: Intrauterine devices. Best Pract Res Clin Obstet Gynaecol 16:155, 2002

Bongers MY, Mol BWJ, Brolmann HAM: Current treatment of dysfunctional uterine bleeding. Maturitas 47:159, 2004

Bonnar J, Sheppard BL: Treatment of menorrhagia during menstruation: randomised controlled trial of ethamsylate, mefenamic acid, and tranexamic acid. BMJ 313:579, 1996

Bradley LD: Complications in hysteroscopy: prevention, treatment and legal risk. Curr Opin Obstet Gynecol 14 (4):409, 2002

Bradley WH, Boente MP, Brooker D, et al: Hysteroscopy and cytology in endometrial cancer. Obstet Gynecol 104(5 Pt 1):1030, 2004

Breitkopf DM, Frederickson RA, Snyder RR: Detection of benign endometrial masses by endometrial stripe measurement in premenopausal women. Obstet Gynecol 104(1):2004

Bry-Gauillard H, Touraine P, Mamzer-Bruneel MF, et al: Complete regression of a major hyperprolactinaemia after renal transplantation. Nephrol Dial Transplant 14:466, 1999

Burja IT, Thompson SK, Sawyer WL Jr, et al: Atypical glandular cells of undetermined significance on cervical smears. A study with cytohistologic correlation. Acta Cytol 43:351, 1999

Buyukbayrak EE, Karsidag AYK, Kars B, et al: Cervical polyps: evaluation of routine removal and need for accompanying D&C. Arch Gynecol Obstet 283:581, 2011

Cameron IT, Haining R, Lumsden MA, et al: The effects of mefenamic acid and norethisterone on measured menstrual blood loss. Obstet Gynecol 76(1):85, 1990

Cameron IT, Leask R, Kelly RW, et al: The effects of danazol, mefenamic acid, norethisterone and a progesterone-impregnated coil on endometrial prostaglandin concentrations in women with menorrhagia. Prostaglandins 34:99, 1987

Centers for Disease Control and Prevention: Sexually transmitted diseases treatment guidelines—2006. MMWR 55:2006

Chamberlain G, Freeman R, Price F, et al: A comparative study of ethamsylate and mefenamic acid in dysfunctional uterine bleeding. Br J Obstet Gynaecol 98:707, 1991

Chan SS, Tam WH, Yeo W, et al: A randomised controlled trial of prophylactic levonorgestrel intrauterine system in tamoxifen-treated women. BJOG 114(12):1510, 2007

Chimbira TH, Anderson AB, Cope E, et al: Effect of danazol on serum gonadotrophins and steroid hormone concentrations in women with menorrhagia. Br J Obstet Gynaecol 87:330, 1980a

Chimbira TH, Anderson AB, Naish C, et al: Reduction of menstrual blood loss by danazol in unexplained menorrhagia: lack of effect of placebo. Br J Obstet Gynaecol 87:1152, 1980b

Chimbira TH, Anderson AB, Turnbull A: Relation between measured menstrual blood loss and patient's subjective assessment of loss, duration of bleeding, number of sanitary towels used, uterine weight and endometrial surface area. Br J Obstet Gynaecol 87:603, 1980c

Chin J, Konje JC, Hickey M: Levonorgestrel intrauterine system for endometrial protection in women with breast cancer on adjuvant tamoxifen. Cochrane Database Syst Rev 4:CD007245, 2009

Chin N, Platt AB, Nuovo GJ: Squamous intraepithelial lesions arising in benign endocervical polyps: a report of 9 cases with correlation to the Pap smears, HPV analysis, and immunoprofile. Int J Gynecol Pathol 27(4):582, 2008

Cicinelli E, Parisi C, Galantino P, et al: Reliability, feasibility, and safety of minihysteroscopy with a vaginoscopic approach: experience with 6,000 cases. Fertil Steril 80(1):199, 2003

Claessens EA, Cowell CA: Acute adolescent menorrhagia. Am J Obstet Gynecol 139:277, 1981

Clark TJ: Outpatient hysteroscopy and ultrasonography in the management of endometrial disease. Curr Opin Obstet Gynecol 16:305, 2004

Clark TJ, Voit D, Gupta JK, et al: Accuracy of hysteroscopy in the diagnosis of endometrial cancer and hyperplasia: a systematic quantitative review. JAMA 288:1610, 2002

Cochrane R, Regan L: Undetected gynaecological disorders in women with renal disease. Hum Reprod 12:667, 1997

Cohen I: Endometrial pathologies associated with postmenopausal tamoxifen treatment. Gynecol Oncol 94:256, 2004

Corusic A, Barisic D, Lovric H, et al: Successful laparoscopic bipolar coagulation of a large arteriovenous malformation due to invasive trophoblastic disease: a case report. J Minim Invasive Gynecol 16(3):368, 2009

Coulter A, Bradlow J, Agass M, et al: Outcomes of referrals to gynaecology outpatient clinics for menstrual problems: an audit of general practice records. Br J Obstet Gynaecol 98:789, 1991

Crum CP, Lee KR (eds): Diagnostic Gynecologic and Obstetric Pathology. Philadelphia, Elsevier, 2006, p 466

Cundy TF, Butler J, Pope RM, et al: Amenorrhoea in women with non-alcoholic chronic liver disease. Gut 32:202, 1991

Cura M, Martinez N, Cura A, et al: Arteriovenous malformations of the uterus. Acta Radiol 50(7):823, 2009

de Koning ND, Haagsma EB: Normalization of menstrual pattern after liver transplantation: consequences for contraception. Digestion 46:239, 1990

de Kroon CD, de Bock GH, Dieben SW, et al: Saline contrast hysterosonography in abnormal uterine bleeding: a systematic review and meta-analysis. BJOG 110:938, 2003

Deligdisch L: Hormonal pathology of the endometrium. Mod Pathol 13:285, 2000

DeVore GR, Owens O, Kase N: Use of intravenous Premarin in the treatment of dysfunctional uterine bleeding—a double-blind randomized control study. Obstet Gynecol 59:285, 1982

DeWaay DJ, Syrop CH, Nygaard IE, et al: Natural history of uterine polyps and leiomyomata. Obstet Gynecol 100:3, 2002

Dibi RP, Zettler CG, Pessini SA, et al: Tamoxifen use and endometrial lesions: hysteroscopic, histological, and immunohistochemical findings in postmenopausal women with breast cancer. Menopause 16(2):293, 2009

Dreisler E, Sorensen SS, Ibsen PH, et al: Prevalence of endometrial polyps and abnormal uterine bleeding in a Danish population aged 20-74 years. Ultrasound Obstet Gynecol 33(1):102, 2009a

Dreisler E, Sorensen SS, Lose G: Endometrial polyps and associated factors in Danish women aged 36-74 years. Am J Obstet Gynecol 200(2):147.e1, 2009b

Dubinsky TJ: Value of sonography in the diagnosis of abnormal vaginal bleeding. J Clin Ultrasound 32:348, 2004

Eckert LO, Thwin SS, Hillier SL, et al: The antimicrobial treatment of subacute endometritis: a proof of concept study. Am J Obstet Gynecol 190:305, 2004

Emanuel MH, Verdel MJ, Wamsteker K, et al: A prospective comparison of transvaginal ultrasonography and diagnostic hysteroscopy in the evaluation of patients with abnormal uterine bleeding: clinical implications. Am J Obstet Gynecol 172:547, 1995

Everett C: Incidence and outcome of bleeding before the 20th week of pregnancy: prospective study from general practice. BMJ 315:32, 1997

Ewenstein BM: The pathophysiology of bleeding disorders presenting as abnormal uterine bleeding. Am J Obstet Gynecol 175(3 Pt 2):770, 1996

Farkouh ME, Greenberg BP: An evidence-based review of the cardiovascular risks of nonsteroidal anti-inflammatory drugs. Am J Cardiol 103(9):1227, 2009

Faundes D, Bahamondes L, Faundes A, et al: No relationship between the IUD position evaluated by ultrasound and complaints of bleeding and pain. Contraception 56:43, 1997

Federici AB: The use of desmopressin in von Willebrand disease: the experience of the first 30 years (1977-2007). Haemophilia 14 (Suppl 1):5, 2008

Ferenczy A: Pathophysiology of endometrial bleeding. Maturitas 45(1):1, 2003

Ferenczy A, Shore M, Guralnick M, et al: The Kevorkian curette. An appraisal of its effectiveness in endometrial evaluation. Obstet Gynecol 54:262, 1979

Ferrazzi E, Torri V, Trio D, et al: Sonographic endometrial thickness: a useful test to predict atrophy in patients with postmenopausal bleeding. An Italian multicenter study. Ultrasound Obstet Gynecol 7(5):315, 1996

Ferrazzi E, Zupi E, Leone FP, et al: How often are endometrial polyps malignant in asymptomatic postmenopausal women? A multicenter study. Am J Obstet Gynecol 200(3):235.e1, 2009

Fleischer AC, Shappell HW: Color Doppler sonohysterography of endometrial polyps and submucosal fibroids. J Ultrasound Med 22:601, 2003

Fong YF, Singh K: Effect of the levonorgestrel-releasing intrauterine system on uterine myomas in a renal transplant patient. Contraception 60(1):51, 1999

Foster PA: The reproductive health of women with von Willebrand disease unresponsive to DDAVP: results of an international survey. On behalf of the Subcommittee on von Willebrand Factor of the Scientific and Standardization Committee of the ISTH. Thromb Haemost 74(2):784, 1995

Fraser IS: Treatment of ovulatory and anovulatory dysfunctional uterine bleeding with oral progestogens. Aust N Z J Obstet Gynaecol 30(4):353, 1990

Fraser IS, McCarron G: Randomized trial of 2 hormonal and 2 prostaglandin-inhibiting agents in women with a complaint of menorrhagia. Aust N Z J Obstet Gynaecol 31:66, 1991

Fraser IS, McCarron G, Markham R: A preliminary study of factors influencing perception of menstrual blood loss volume. Am J Obstet Gynecol 149:788, 1984

Furness S, Roberts, H, Marjoribanks J, et al: Hormone replacement therapy in postmenopausal women and risk of endometrial hyperplasia. Cochrane Database Syst Rev 2:CD000402, 2009

Gardner FJ, Konje JC, Bell SC, et al: Prevention of tamoxifen induced endometrial polyps using a levonorgestrel releasing intrauterine system long-term follow-up of a randomised control trial. Gynecol Oncol 114(3):452, 2009

Gervaise A, Fernandez H, Capella-Allouc S, et al: Thermal balloon ablation versus endometrial resection for the treatment of abnormal uterine bleeding. Hum Reprod 14:2743, 1999

Ghosh TK: Arteriovenous malformation of the uterus and pelvis. Obstet Gynecol 68:40S, 1986

Gilmore H, Fleischhacker D, Hecht JL: Diagnosis of chronic endometritis in biopsies with stromal breakdown. Hum Pathol 28(4):581, 2007

Gleeson NC: Cyclic changes in endometrial tissue plasminogen activator and plasminogen activator inhibitor type 1 in women with normal menstruation and essential menorrhagia. Am J Obstet Gynecol 171:178, 1994

Golan A, Cohen-Sahar B, Keidar R, et al: Endometrial Polyps: Symptomatology, menopausal status and malignancy. Gynecol Obstet Invest 70(2):107, 2010

Goldstein SR: Menorrhagia and abnormal bleeding before the menopause. Best Pract Res Clin Obstet Gynaecol 18:59, 2004

Goldstein SR, Monteagudo A, Popiolek D, et al: Evaluation of endometrial polyps. Am J Obstet Gynecol 186:669, 2002

Goldstein SR, Zeltser I, Horan CK, et al: Ultrasonography-based triage for perimenopausal patients with abnormal uterine bleeding. Am J Obstet Gynecol 177(1):102, 1997

Granberg S, Wikland M, Karlsson B, et al: Endometrial thickness as measured by endovaginal ultrasonography for identifying endometrial abnormality. Am J Obstet Gynecol 164:47, 1991

Greenwood SM, Moran JJ: Chronic endometritis: morphologic and clinical observations. Obstet Gynecol 58:176, 1981

Grimes D: Intrauterine devices (IUDs). In Hatcher RA, Trussell J, Nelson AL (eds): Contraceptive Technology. New York, Ardent Media, 2007, p 123

Grimes DA: Diagnostic dilation and curettage: a reappraisal. Am J Obstet Gynecol 142:1, 1982

Haggerty CL, Totten PA, Ferris M, et al: Clinical characteristics of bacterial vaginosis among women testing positive for fastidious bacteria. Sex Transm Infect 85(4):242, 2009

Hall P, Maclachlan N, Thorn N, et al: Control of menorrhagia by the cyclo-oxygenase inhibitors naproxen sodium and mefenamic acid. Br J Obstet Gynaecol 94:554, 1987

Hallberg L, Hogdahl AM, Nilsson L, et al: Menstrual blood los——a population study. Variation at different ages and attempts to define normality. Acta Obstet Gynecol Scand 45:320, 1966

Hatasaka H: The evaluation of abnormal uterine bleeding. Clin Obstet Gynecol 48:258, 2005

Haynes PJ, Hodgson H, Anderson AB, et al: Measurement of menstrual blood loss in patients complaining of menorrhagia. Br J Obstet Gynaecol 84:763, 1977

Hernandez MR, Alvarez-Guerra M, Escolar G, et al: The hemostatic agent ethamsylate promotes platelet/leukocyte aggregate formation in a model of vascular injury. Fundam Clin Pharmacol 18:423, 2004

Hickey M, Dwarte D, Fraser IS: Superficial endometrial vascular fragility in Norplant users and in women with ovulatory dysfunctional uterine bleeding. Hum Reprod 15:1509, 2000a

Hickey M, Fraser I: Human uterine vascular structures in normal and diseased states. Microsc Res Tech 60:377, 2003

Hickey M, Fraser IS: Clinical implications of disturbances of uterine vascular morphology and function. Baillier's Best Pract Res Clin Obstet Gynaecol 14:937, 2000b

Hickey M, Fraser IS: Surface vascularization and endometrial appearance in women with menorrhagia or using levonorgestrel contraceptive implants. Implications for the mechanisms of breakthrough bleeding. Hum Reprod 17:2428, 2002

Higham JM, O'Brien PM, Shaw RW: Assessment of menstrual blood loss using a pictorial chart. Br J Obstet Gynaecol 97:734, 1990

Higham JM, Shaw RW: A comparative study of danazol, a regimen of decreasing doses of danazol, and norethindrone in the treatment of objectively proven unexplained menorrhagia. Am J Obstet Gynecol 169:1134, 1993

Hurskainen R, Teperi J, Rissanen P, et al: Clinical outcomes and costs with the levonorgestrel-releasing intrauterine system or hysterectomy for treatment of menorrhagia: randomized trial 5-year follow-up. JAMA 291:1456, 2004

Hurskainen R, Teperi J, Rissanen P, et al: Quality of life and cost-effectiveness of levonorgestrel-releasing intrauterine system versus hysterectomy for treatment of menorrhagia: a randomized trial. Lancet 357(9252):273, 2001

Inagaki N, Ung L, Otani T, et al: Uterine cavity matrix metalloproteinases and cytokines in patients with leiomyoma, adenomyosis or endometrial polyp. Eur J Obstet Gynecol Reprod Biol 111:197, 2003

Irvine GA, Cameron IT: Medical management of dysfunctional uterine bleeding. Best Pract Res Clin Obstet Gynaecol 13:189, 1999

Irvine GA, Campbell-Brown MB, Lumsden MA, et al: Randomised comparative trial of the levonorgestrel intrauterine system and norethisterone for treatment of idiopathic menorrhagia. BJOG 105:592, 1998

Jabbour HN, Kelly RW, Fraser HM, et al: Endocrine regulation of menstruation. Endocr Rev 27(1):17, 2006

Jakab A, Ovari L, Juhasz B, et al: Detection of feeding artery improves the ultrasound diagnosis of endometrial polyps in asymptomatic patients. Eur J Obstet Gynecol Reprod Biol 119:103, 2005

James AH, Kouides PA, Abdul-Kadir R, et al: Von Willebrand disease and other bleeding disorders in women: consensus on diagnosis and management from an international expert panel. Am J Obstet Gynecol 201(1):12.e1, 2009a

James AH, Manco-Johnson MJ, Yawn BP, et al: Von Willebrand disease: key points from the 2008 National Heart, Lung, and Blood Institute guidelines. Obstet Gynecol 114(3):674, 2009b

James AH, Myers ER, Cook C, et al: Complications of hysterectomy in women with von Willebrand disease. Haemophilia 15(4):926, 2009c

Janssen CA, Scholten PC, Heintz AP: A simple visual assessment technique to discriminate between menorrhagia and normal menstrual blood loss. Obstet Gynecol 85:977, 1995

Jeong KA, Park KH, Chung DJ, et al: Hysteroscopic endometrial ablation as a treatment for abnormal uterine bleeding in patients with renal transplants. J Am Assoc Gynecol Laparosc 11(2):252, 2004

Jorizzo JR, Chen MYM, Riccio GJ: Endometrial polyps: sonohysterographic evaluation. AJR Am J Roentgenol 176:617, 2001

Joshi JV, Bhandarkar SD, Chadha M, et al: Menstrual irregularities and lactation failure may precede thyroid dysfunction or goitre. J Postgrad Med 39:137, 1993

Kadir RA, Economides DL, Sabin CA, et al: Assessment of menstrual blood loss and gynaecological problems in patients with inherited bleeding disorders. Haemophilia 5:40, 1999

Kadir RA, Economides DL, Sabin CA, et al: Frequency of inherited bleeding disorders in women with menorrhagia. Lancet 351:485, 1998

Kapp N: WHO provider brief on hormonal contraception and liver disease. Contraception 80(4):325, 2009a

Kapp N, Tilley IB, Curtis KM: The effects of hormonal contraceptive use among women with viral hepatitis or cirrhosis of the liver: a systematic review. Contraception 80(4):381, 2009b

Karim BO, Burroughs FH, Rosenthal DL, et al: Endometrial-type cells in cervico-vaginal smears: clinical significance and cytopathologic correlates. Diagn Cytopathol 26:123, 2002

Karlsson B, Granberg S, Wikland M, et al: Transvaginal ultrasonography of the endometrium in women with postmenopausal bleeding—a Nordic multi-center study. Am J Obstet Gynecol 172:1488, 1995

Kaunitz AM, Meredith S, Inki P, et al: Levonorgestrel-releasing intrauterine system and endometrial ablation in heavy menstrual bleeding: a systematic review and meta-analysis. Obstet Gynecol 113:1104, 2009

Kelly RW, King AE, Critchley HO: Inflammatory mediators and endometrial function–focus on the perivascular cell. J Reprod Immunol 57:81, 2002

Kim KR, Peng R, Ro JY, et al: A diagnostically useful histopathologic feature of endometrial polyp: the long axis of endometrial glands arranged parallel to surface epithelium. Am J Surg Pathol 28:1057, 2004

Kingman CE, Kadir RA, Lee CA, et al: The use of levonorgestrel- releasing intrauterine system for treatment of menorrhagia in women with inherited bleeding disorders. BJOG 111(12):1425, 2004

Koutras DA: Disturbances of menstruation in thyroid disease. Ann NY Acad Sci 816:280, 1997

Krassas GE, Pontikides N, Kaltsas T, et al: Disturbances of menstruation in hypothyroidism. Clin Endocrinol 50:655, 1999

Kriplani A, Kulshrestha V, Agarwal N, et al: Role of tranexamic acid in management of dysfunctional uterine bleeding in comparison with medroxyprogesterone acetate. J Obstet Gynaecol 26(7):673, 2006

Krissi H, Bar-Hava I, Orvieto R, et al: Endometrial carcinoma in a post-menopausal woman with atrophic endometrium and intra-cavitary fluid: a case report. Eur J Obstet Gynecol Reprod Biol 77:245, 1998

Kuzel D, Toth D, Cindr J, et al: Minimally invasive and hysteroscopic diagnosis and treatment of patients after organ transplantation. J Obstet Gynaecol Res 35(2):339, 2009

Lak M, Peyvandi F, Mannucci PM: Clinical manifestations and complications of childbirth and replacement therapy in 385 Iranian patients with type 3 von Willebrand disease. Br J Haematol 111:1236, 2000

Lee CA, Abdul-Kadir R: Von Willebrand disease and women's health. Semin Hematol 42:42, 2005

Leese PT, Hubbard RC, Karim A, et al: Effects of celecoxib, a novel cyclooxygenase-2 inhibitor, on platelet function in healthy adults: a randomized, controlled trial. J Clin Pharmacol 40:124, 2000

Leiserowitz GS, Graves R: Abnormal uterine bleeding. In Steven CS, Sullivan ND, Tilton P (eds): Manual of Outpatient Gynecology. Boston, Little, Brown, 1996, p 83

Lethaby A, Augood C, Duckitt K: Nonsteroidal anti-inflammatory drugs for heavy menstrual bleeding. Cochrane Database Syst Rev 4:CD000400, 2007

Lethaby A, Cooke I, Rees MC: Progesterone or progestogen-releasing intrauterine systems for heavy menstrual bleeding. Cochrane Database Syst Rev 4:CD002126, 2005

Lethaby A, Farquhar C, Cooke I: Antifibrinolytics for heavy menstrual bleeding. Cochrane Database Syst Rev 4:CD000249, 2000

Lethaby A, Irvine G, Cameron I: Cyclical progestogens for heavy menstrual bleeding. Cochrane Database Syst Rev 1:CD001016, 2008

Leung PL, Tam WH, Kong WS, et al: Intrauterine pathology in women with abnormal uterine bleeding taking hormone replacement therapy. J Am Assoc Gynecol Laparosc 10(2):260, 2003

Levens ED, Scheinberg P, DeCherney AH: Severe menorrhagia associated with thrombocytopenia. Obstet Gynecol 110(4):913, 2007

Lindner LE, Geerling S, Nettum JA, et al: Clinical characteristics of women with chlamydial cervicitis. J Reprod Med 33:684, 1988

Lippman SA, Warner M, Samuels S, et al: Uterine fibroids and gynecologic pain symptoms in a population-based study. Fertil Steril 80:1488, 2003

Litta P, Merlin F, Saccardi C, et al: Role of hysteroscopy with endometrial biopsy to rule out endometrial cancer in postmenopausal women with abnormal uterine bleeding. Maturitas 50:117, 2005

Love CD, Muir BB, Scrimgeour JB, et al: Investigation of endometrial abnormalities in asymptomatic women treated with tamoxifen and an evaluation of the role of endometrial screening. J Clin Oncol 17:2050, 1999

Lowenstein L, Solt I, Deutsch M, et al: A life-threatening event: uterine cervical arteriovenous malformation. Obstet Gynecol 103:1073, 2004

Lukes AS, Kadir RA, Peyvandi F, et al: Disorders of hemostasis and excessive menstrual bleeding: prevalence and clinical impact. Fertil Steril 84:1338, 2005

Lukes AS, Moore KA, Muse KN: Tranexamic Acid Treatment for Heavy Menstrual Bleeding. Obstet Gynecol 116(4):865, 2010

Machtinger R, Korach J, Padoa A, et al: Transvaginal ultrasound and diagnostic hysteroscopy as a predictor of endometrial polyps: risk factors for premalignancy and malignancy. Int J Gynecol Cancer 15:325, 2005

MacKenzie IZ, Naish C, Rees CM, et al: Why remove all cervical polyps and examine them histologically? BJOG 116(8):1127, 2009

Maia H Jr, Maltez A, Studard E, et al: Effect of previous hormone replacement therapy on endometrial polyps during menopause. Gynecol Endocrinol 18:299, 2004

Majmudar B, Ghanee N, Horowitz IR, et al: Uterine arteriovenous malformation necessitating hysterectomy with bilateral salpingo-oophorectomy in a young pregnant patient. Arch Pathol Lab Med 122:842, 1998

Makarainen L, Ylikorkala O: Ibuprofen prevents IUCD-induced increases in menstrual blood loss. Br J Obstet Gynaecol 93:285, 1986a

Makarainen L, Ylikorkala O: Primary and myoma-associated menorrhagia: role of prostaglandins and effects of ibuprofen. Br J Obstet Gynaecol 93:974, 1986b

Mannucci PM, Duga S, Peyvandi F: Recessively inherited coagulation disorders. Blood 104:1243, 2004

Mannucci PM, Tuddenham EGD: The hemophilias—from royal genes to gene therapy. N Engl J Med 344:1773, 2001

Marchini M, Tozzi L, Bakshi R, et al: Comparative efficacy of diclofenac dispersible 50 mg and ibuprofen 400 mg in patients with primary dysmenorrhea. A randomized, double-blind, within-patient, placebo-controlled study. Int J Clin Pharmacol Ther 33:491, 1995

Marrazzo JM, Handsfield HH, Whittington WL: Predicting chlamydial and gonococcal cervical infection: implications for management of cervicitis. Obstet Gynecol 100:579, 2002

Martin-Johnston MK, Okoji OY, Armstrong A: Therapeutic amenorrhea in patients at risk for thrombocytopenia. Obstet Gynecol Surv 63(6):395, 2008

Martyn P, Allan B: Long-term follow-up of endometrial ablation. J Am Assoc Gynecol Laparosc 5:115, 1998

Mass K, Quint EH, Punch MR, et al: Gynecological and reproductive function after liver transplantation. Transplantation 62:476, 1996

Matuszkiewicz-Rowińska J, Skorzewska K, Radowicki S, et al: Endometrial morphology and pituitary-gonadal axis dysfunction in women of reproductive age undergoing chronic haemodialysis—a multicentre study. Nephrol Dial Transplant 19:2074, 2004

McGavigan CJ, Dockery P, Metaxa-Mariatou V, et al: Hormonally mediated disturbance of angiogenesis in the human endometrium after exposure to intrauterine levonorgestrel. Hum Reprod 18:77, 2003

McGrath RT, McRae E, Smith OP, et al: Platelet von Willebrand factor—structure, function and biological importance. Br J Haematol 148(6):834, 2010

Merz E, Miric-Tesanic D, Bahlmann F, et al: Sonographic size of uterus and ovaries in pre- and postmenopausal women. Ultrasound Obstet Gynecol 7(1):38, 1996

Meyer WR, Walsh BW, Grainger DA, et al: Thermal balloon and rollerball ablation to treat menorrhagia: a multicenter comparison. Obstet Gynecol 92:98, 1998

Miller CH, Haff E, Platt SJ, et al: Measurement of von Willebrand factor activity: relative effects of ABO blood type and race. J Thromb Haemost 1:2191, 2003

Milsom I, Andersson K, Jonasson K, et al: The influence of the Gyne-T 380S IUD on menstrual blood loss and iron status. Contraception 52:175, 1995

Moschos E, Ashfaq R, McIntire DD, et al: Saline-infusion sonography endometrial sampling compared with endometrial biopsy in diagnosing endometrial pathology. Obstet Gynecol 113(4):881, 2009

Mousa HA, Abou El Senoun GM, Mahmood TA: Medium-term clinical outcome of women with menorrhagia treated by rollerball endometrial ablation versus abdominal hysterectomy with conservation of at least one ovary. Acta Obstet Gynecol Scand 80:442, 2001

Munro MG, Mainor N, Basu R, et al: Oral medroxyprogesterone acetate and combination oral contraceptives for acute uterine bleeding: a randomized controlled trial. Obstet Gynecol 108(4):924, 2006

Nalaboff KM, Pellerito JS, Ben Levi E: Imaging the endometrium: disease and normal variants. Radiographics 21:1409, 2001

Nanda S, Chadha N, Sen J, et al: Transvaginal sonography and saline infusion sonohysterography in the evaluation of abnormal uterine bleeding. Aust N Z J Obstet Gynaecol 42:530, 2002

Nelson AL, Cwiak C: Combined oral contraceptives. In Hatcher RA, Trussell J, Nelson AL (eds): Contraceptive Technology, 20th ed. New York, Ardent Media, 2011, 313

Ness RB, Brunham RC, Shen C, et al: Associations among human leukocyte antigen (HLA) class II DQ variants, bacterial sexually transmitted diseases, endometritis, and fertility among women with clinical pelvic inflammatory disease. Sex Transm Dis 31:301, 2004

Nichols WL, Hultin MB, James AH, et al: Von Willebrand disease (VWD): evidence-based diagnosis and management guidelines, the National Heart, Lung, and Blood Institute (NHLBI) Expert Panel report (USA). Haemophilia 14(2):171, 2008

Nichols WL, Rick ME, Ortel TL, et al: Clinical and laboratory diagnosis of von Willebrand disease: a synopsis of the 2008 NHLBI/NIH guidelines. Am J Hematol 84(6):366, 2009

Obenson K, Abreo F, Grafton WD: Cytohistologic correlation between AGUS and biopsy-detected lesions in postmenopausal women. Acta Cytol 44:41, 2000

Ober WB: Effects of oral and intrauterine administration of contraceptives on the uterus. Hum Pathol 8:513, 1977

Oehler MK, Rees MC: Menorrhagia: an update. Acta Obstet Gynecol Scand 82:405, 2003

Oguz S, Sargin A, Kelekci S, et al: The role of hormone replacement therapy in endometrial polyp formation. Maturitas 50(3):231, 2005

Oliveira-Ribeiro M, Petta CA, De Angelo Andrade LAL, et al: Correlation between endometrial histology, microvascular density and calibre, matrix metalloproteinase-3 and bleeding pattern in women using a levonorgestrel-releasing intrauterine system. Hum Reprod 19:1778, 2004

Oral E, Cagdas A, Gezer A, et al: Hematological abnormalities in adolescent menorrhagia. Arch Gynecol Obstet 266:72, 2002

Paavonen J, Stevens CE, Wolner-Hanssen P, et al: Colposcopic manifestations of cervical and vaginal infections. Obstet Gynecol Surv 43:373, 1988

Pasrija S, Trivedi SS, Narula MK: Prospective study of saline infusion sonohysterography in evaluation of perimenopausal and postmenopausal women with abnormal uterine bleeding. J Obstet Gynaecol Res 30:27, 2004

Pérez-Medina T, Bajo-Arenas J, Salazar F, et al: Endometrial polyps and their implication in the pregnancy rates of patients undergoing intrauterine insemination: a prospective randomised study. Hum Reprod 20:1632, 2005

Peterson EP: Endometrial carcinoma in young women. A clinical profile. Obstet Gynecol 31:702, 1968

Philipp CS, Faiz A, Dowling N, et al: Age and the prevalence of bleeding disorders in women with menorrhagia. Obstet Gynecol 105:61, 2005

Pisoni CN, Cuadrado MJ, Khamashta MA, et al: Treatment of menorrhagia associated with oral anticoagulation: efficacy and safety of the levonorgestrel releasing intrauterine device (Mirena coil). Lupus, 15(12):877, 2006

Pizarro E, Schoenstedt G, Mehech G, et al: Uterine cavity and the location of IUDs following administration of meclofenamic acid to menorrhagic women. A pilot study. Contraception 40:413, 1989

Polyzos NP, Mauri D, Tsioras S, et al: Intraperitoneal dissemination of endometrial cancer cells after hysteroscopy: a systematic review and meta-analysis. Int J Gynecol Cancer 20(2):261, 2010

Prentice A: When does heavy flow merit treatment? Practitioner 244:174, 2000

Preston JT, Cameron IT, Adams EJ, et al: Comparative study of tranexamic acid and norethisterone in the treatment of ovulatory menorrhagia. Br J Obstet Gynaecol 102:401, 1995

Preutthipan S, Herabutya Y: Hysteroscopic polypectomy in 240 premenopausal and postmenopausal women. Fertil Steril 83:705, 2005

Quint EH, Perlman SE: Premenarchal vaginal bleeding. J Pediatr Adolesc Gynecol 14:135, 2001

Raff GJ, Kasper KM, Hollinger EF Jr, et al: Laparoscopic hysterectomy in patients with prior renal transplantation. J Minim Invasive Gynecol 15(2):223, 2008

Rahimi S, Marani C, Renzi C, et al: Endometrial polyps and the risk of atypical hyperplasia on biopsies of unremarkable endometrium: a study on 694 patients with benign endometrial polyps. Int J Gynecol Pathol 28(6):522, 2009

Rees M: Menorrhagia. Br Med J (Clin Res Ed) 294:759, 1987

Reid PC, Coker A, Coltart R: Assessment of menstrual blood loss using a pictorial chart: a validation study. BJOG 107:320, 2000

Reid PC, Virtanen-Kari S: Randomised comparative trial of the levonorgestrel intrauterine system and mefenamic acid for the treatment of idiopathic menorrhagia: a multiple analysis using total menstrual fluid loss, menstrual blood loss and pictorial blood loss measurements. BJOG 112:1121, 2005

Reslova T, Tosner J, Resl M, et al: Endometrial polyps. A clinical study of 245 cases. Arch Gynecol Obstet 262:133, 1999

Revel A, Tsafrir A, Anteby SO, et al: Does hysteroscopy produce intraperitoneal spread of endometrial cancer cells? Obstet Gynecol Surv 59:280, 2004

Reynolds RF, Obermeyer CM, Walker AM, et al: The role of treatment intentions and concerns about side effects in women's decision to discontinue postmenopausal hormone therapy. Maturitas 43:183, 2002

Rhoton-Vlasak A, Chegini N, Hardt N, et al: Histological characteristics and altered expression of interleukins (IL) IL-13 and IL-15 in endometria of levonorgestrel users with different uterine bleeding patterns. Fertil Steril 83:659, 2005

Rodeghiero F: Management of menorrhagia in women with inherited bleeding disorders: general principles and use of desmopressin. Haemophilia 14 (Suppl 1):21, 2008

Rogers PA, Abberton KM: Endometrial arteriogenesis: vascular smooth muscle cell proliferation and differentiation during the menstrual cycle and changes associated with endometrial bleeding disorders. Microsc Res Tech 60:412, 2003

Roopa BA, Loganath A, Singh K: The effect of a levonorgestrel-releasing intra-uterine system on angiogenic growth factors in the endometrium. Hum Reprod 18:1809, 2003

Rose PG: Endometrial carcinoma. N Engl J Med 335:640, 1996

Rosenberg MJ, Long SC: Oral contraceptives and cycle control: A critical review of the literature. Adv Contracept 8:35, 1992

Rosenthal AN, Panoskaltsis T, Smith T, et al: The frequency of significant pathology in women attending a general gynaecological service for postcoital bleeding. BJOG 108:103, 2001

Roy S, Shaw ST Jr: Role of prostaglandins in IUD-associated uterine bleeding–effect of a prostaglandin synthetase inhibitor (ibuprofen). Obstet Gynecol 58:101, 1981

Roy SN, Bhattacharya S: Benefits and risks of pharmacological agents used for the treatment of menorrhagia. Drug Saf 27:75, 2004

Rubin G, Wortman M, Kouides PA: Endometrial ablation for von Willebrand disease-related menorrhagia—experience with seven cases. Haemophilia 10:477, 2004

Ryu JA, Kim B, Lee J, et al: Comparison of transvaginal ultrasonography with hysterosonography as a screening method in patients with abnormal uterine bleeding. Korean J Radiol 5:39, 2004

Saarikoski S, Yliskoski M, Penttila I: Sequential use of norethisterone and natural progesterone in pre-menopausal bleeding disorders. Maturitas 12:89, 1990

Sahu B, Latheef R, Aboel Magd S: Prevalence of pathology in women attending colposcopy for postcoital bleeding with negative cytology. Arch Gynecol Obstet 276(5):471, 2007

Salazar GM, Petrozza JC, Walker TG: Transcatheter endovascular techniques for management of obstetrical and gynecologic emergencies. Tech Vasc Interv Radiol 12(2):139, 2009

Savelli L, De Iaco P, Santini D, et al: Histopathologic features and risk factors for benignity, hyperplasia, and cancer in endometrial polyps. Am J Obstet Gynecol 188:927, 2003

Schafer AI: Essential thrombocythemia and thrombocytosis. In Lichtman MA, Beutler E, Kipps TJ, et al (eds): Williams Hematology, 7th ed., New York, McGraw-Hill, 2006

Schnatz PF, Ricci S, O'Sullivan DM: Cervical polyps in postmenopausal women: is there a difference in risk? Menopause 16(3):524, 2009

Schrager S: Abnormal uterine bleeding associated with hormonal contraception. Am Fam Physician 65:2073, 2002

Selo-Ojeme DO, Dayoub N, Patel A, et al: A clinico-pathological study of postcoital bleeding. Arch Gynecol Obstet 270:34, 2004

Seltzer VL, Benjamin F, Deutsch S: Perimenopausal bleeding patterns and pathologic findings. J Am Med Womens Assoc 45:132, 1990

Shalini R, Amita S, Neera MA: How alarming is post-coital bleeding–a cytologic, colposcopic and histopathologic evaluation. Gynecol Obstet Invest 45:205, 1998

Shamonki MI, Ziegler WF, Badger GJ, et al: Prediction of endometrial ablation success according to perioperative findings. Am J Obstet Gynecol 182:1005, 2000

Shankar M, Lee CA, Sabin CA, et al: von Willebrand disease in women with menorrhagia: a systematic review. BJOG 111:734, 2004

Shaw ST Jr, Macaulay LK, Hohman WR: Morphological studies on IUD-induced metrorrhagia. I. Endometrial changes and clinical correlations. Contraception 19(1):47, 1979a

Shaw ST Jr, Macaulay LK, Hohman WR: Vessel density in endometrium of women with and without intrauterine contraceptive devices: a morphometric evaluation. Am J Obstet Gynecol 135:202, 1979b

Sheikh M, Sawhney S, Khurana A, et al: Alteration of sonographic texture of the endometrium in post-menopausal bleeding. A guide to further management. Acta Obstet Gynecol Scand 79:1006, 2000

Shi AA, Lee SL: Radiological reasoning: algorithmic workup of abnormal vaginal bleeding with endovaginal sonography and sonohysterography. AJR Am J Roentgenol 191(6 Suppl):S68, 2008

Shokeir TA, Shalan HM, El Shafei MM: Significance of endometrial polyps detected hysteroscopically in eumenorrheic infertile women. J Obstet Gynaecol Res 30:84, 2004

Siegel JE: Abnormalities of hemostasis and abnormal uterine bleeding. Clin Obstet Gynecol 48:284, 2005

Singh RH, Blumenthal P: Hormonal management of abnormal uterine bleeding. Clin Obstet Gynecol 48:337, 2005

Smith YR, Quint EH, Hertzberg RB: Menorrhagia in adolescents requiring hospitalization. J Pediat Adolesc Gynecol 11:13, 1998

Smith-Bindman R, Kerlikowske K, Feldstein VA, et al: Endovaginal ultrasound to exclude endometrial cancer and other endometrial abnormalities. JAMA 280:1510, 1998

Soares SR, dos Reis MMBB, Camargos AF: Diagnostic accuracy of sonohysterography, transvaginal sonography, and hysterosalpingography in patients with uterine cavity diseases. Fertil Steril 73:406, 2000

Solomon SD, Pfeffer MA, McMurray JJ, et al: Effect of celecoxib on cardiovascular events and blood pressure in two trials for the prevention of colorectal adenomas. Circulation 114:1028, 2006

Stabinsky SA, Einstein M, Breen JL: Modern treatments of menorrhagia attributable to dysfunctional uterine bleeding. Obstet Gynecol Surv 54:61, 1999

Stellon AJ, Williams R: Increased incidence of menstrual abnormalities and hysterectomy preceding primary biliary cirrhosis. Br Med J (Clin Res Ed) 293:297, 1986

Stewart A, Cummins C, Gold L, et al: The effectiveness of the levonorgestrel-releasing intrauterine system in menorrhagia: a systematic review. Br J Obstet Gynaecol 108:74, 2001

Stock RJ, Kanbour A: Prehysterectomy curettage. Obstet Gynecol 45:537, 1975

Stovall TG, Ling FW, Morgan PL: A prospective, randomized comparison of the Pipelle endometrial sampling device with the Novak curette. Am J Obstet Gynecol 165:1287, 1991

Stovall TG, Solomon SK, Ling FW: Endometrial sampling prior to hysterectomy. Obstet Gynecol 73:405, 1989

Svirsky R, Smorgick N, Rozowski U, et al: Can we rely on blind endometrial biopsy for detection of focal intrauterine pathology? Am J Obstet Gynecol 199(2):115.e1, 2008

Tabor A, Watt HC, Wald NJ: Endometrial thickness as a test for endometrial cancer in women with postmenopausal vaginal bleeding. Obstet Gynecol 99:663, 2002

Tahir MM, Bigrigg MA, Browning JJ, et al: A randomised controlled trial comparing transvaginal ultrasound, outpatient hysteroscopy and endometrial biopsy with inpatient hysteroscopy and curettage. Br J Obstet Gynaecol 106:1259, 1999

Timmerman D, Wauters J, Van Calenbergh S, et al: Color Doppler imaging is a valuable tool for the diagnosis and management of uterine vascular malformations. Ultrasound Obstet Gynecol 21:570, 2003

Timmermans A, Opmeer BC, Khan KS, et al: Endometrial thickness measurement for detecting endometrial cancer in women with postmenopausal bleeding: a systematic review and meta-analysis. Obstet Gynecol 116(1):160, 2010

Tsuda H, Kawabata M, Kawabata K, et al: Improvement of diagnostic accuracy of transvaginal ultrasound for identification of endometrial malignancies by using cutoff level of endometrial thickness based on length of time since menopause. Gynecol Oncol 64:35, 1997

Van den Bosch T, Verguts J, Daemen A, et al: Pain experienced during transvaginal ultrasound, saline contrast sonohysterography, hysteroscopy and office sampling: a comparative study. Ultrasound Obstet Gynecol 31(3):346, 2008

Van Doorn LC, Dijkhuizen FP, Kruitwagen RF, et al: Accuracy of transvaginal ultrasonography in diabetic or obese women with postmenopausal bleeding. Obstet Gynecol 104:571, 2004

Varasteh NN, Neuwirth RS, Levin B, et al: Pregnancy rates after hysteroscopic polypectomy and myomectomy in infertile women. Obstet Gynecol 94:168, 1999

Vargyas JM, Campeau JD, Mishell DR Jr: Treatment of menorrhagia with meclofenamate sodium. Am J Obstet Gynecol 157:944, 1987

Vercellini P, Cortesi I, Oldani S, et al: The role of transvaginal ultrasonography and outpatient diagnostic hysteroscopy in the evaluation of patients with menorrhagia. Hum Reprod 12(8):1768, 1997

Vilos GA: Hysteroscopic and nonhysteroscopic endometrial ablation. Obstet Gynecol Clin North Am 31:687, 2004

Vilos GA, Tureanu V, Garcia M, et al: The levonorgestrel intrauterine system is an effective treatment in women with abnormal uterine bleeding and anticoagulant therapy. J Minim Invasive Gynecol 16(4):480, 2009

Wang JH, Zhao J, Lin J: Opportunities and risk factors for premalignant and malignant transformation of endometrial polyps: management strategies. J Minim Invasive Gynecol 17(1):53, 2010

Warner PE, Critchley HO, Lumsden MA, et al: Menorrhagia I: measured blood loss, clinical features, and outcome in women with heavy periods: a survey with follow-up data. Am J Obstet Gynecol 190:1216, 2004

Weiss JL, Malone FD, Vidaver J, et al: Threatened abortion: a risk factor for poor pregnancy outcome, a population-based screening study. Am J Obstet Gynecol 190:745, 2004

Wellington K, Wagstaff AJ: Tranexamic acid: a review of its use in the management of menorrhagia. Drugs 63:1417, 2003

Wiesenfeld HC, Hillier SL, Krohn MA, et al: Lower genital tract infection and endometritis: insight into subclinical pelvic inflammatory disease. Obstet Gynecol 100:456, 2002

Wilansky DL, Greisman B: Early hypothyroidism in patients with menorrhagia. Am J Obstet Gynecol 160:673, 1989

Wu HH, Schuetz MJ III, Cramer H: Significance of benign endometrial cells in Pap smears from postmenopausal women. J Reprod Med 46:795, 2001

Yanaihara A, Yorimitsu T, Motoyama H: Location of endometrial polyp and pregnancy rate in infertility patients. Fertil Steril 90(1):180, 2008

Ylikorkala O: Prostaglandin synthesis inhibitors in menorrhagia, intrauterine contraceptive device-induced side effects and endometriosis. Pharmacol Toxicol 75(Suppl 2):86, 1994

Yokomine D, Yoshinaga M, Baba Y, et al: Successful management of uterine arteriovenous malformation by ligation of feeding artery after unsuccessful uterine artery embolization. J Obstet Gynaecol Res 35(1):183, 2009

Younis MTS, Iram S, Anwar B, et al: Women with asymptomatic cervical polyps may not need to see a gynaecologist or have them removed: An observational retrospective study of 1126 cases. Eur J Obstet Gynecol Reprod Biol 150(2):190, 2010

Zerbe MJ, Zhang J, Bristow RE, et al: Retrograde seeding of malignant cells during hysteroscopy in presumed early endometrial cancer. Gynecol Oncol 79(1):55, 2000

Zhang JY, Luo LL: [Intrauterine device-induced menorrhagia and endometrial content of prostacyclins]. [Chinese]. Chung-Hua Fu Chan Ko Tsa Chih [Chinese J Obstet Gynecol] 27:167, 1992

CHAPTER 8

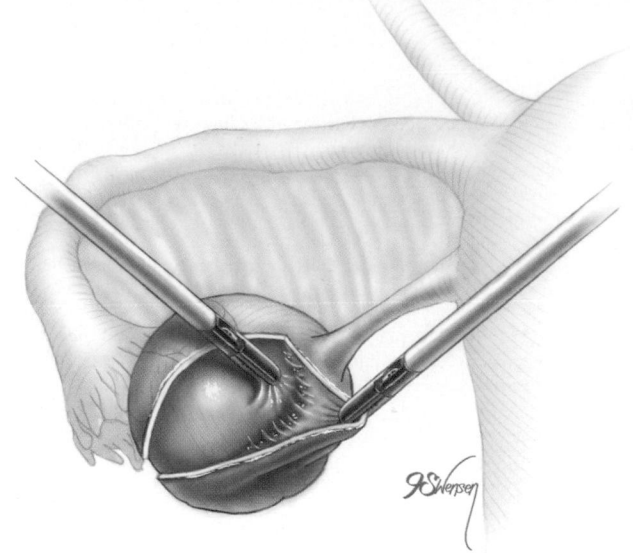

Pelvic masses are common clinical findings and may involve the reproductive organs or nongynecologic structures. They may be identified in asymptomatic women during routine pelvic examination or may cause symptoms. Typical complaints include pain, pressure sensations, dysmenorrhea, or abnormal uterine bleeding. Although most pelvic masses are acquired lesions, a few arise as congenital anomalies. In the evaluation of pelvic masses, laboratory tests are typically uninformative, but levels of serum β-human chorionic gonadotropin (hCG)

or tumor markers may be helpful. Initially, imaging with sonography is preferred, but computed tomography (CT) or magnetic resonance (MR) imaging may be useful when the nature of the mass is still uncertain. The treatment of pelvic masses varies with patient symptoms, age, and risk factors. Although medical management is possible for many pelvic masses, for others, surgical treatment offers the highest success rates.

DEMOGRAPHIC FACTORS

Age has the greatest influence in evaluation of a pelvic mass. Pathology varies greatly with age, and neoplasms are more prevalent in older women.

Prepubertal Girls

Most gynecologic pelvic masses in this age group involve the ovary. Even during childhood, the ovaries are typically active, and many of these masses are functional cysts (de Silva, 2004; Deligeoroglou, 2004). Neoplastic lesions usually are benign germ cell tumors, and mature cystic teratomas (dermoid cysts) are the most common (Brown, 1993; Islam, 2008). Malignant ovarian tumors in children and adolescents are rare and account for only 0.9 percent of all malignancies in this age group (Young, 1975). As discussed in Chapter 14 (p. 389), asymptomatic simple cysts may initially be considered functional and observed. For those that are complex or persistent, additional surgical evaluation is typically indicated. Laparoscopy and in many cases, ovarian cystectomy, rather than oophorectomy, are appropriate approaches in this population.

Adolescents

For the most part, the incidence and type of ovarian pathology found in adolescents are similar to those in prepubertal girls. In addition to functional ovarian cysts, with the onset of reproductive function, pelvic masses in adolescents may also include endometriomas and the sequelae of pelvic inflammatory disease and pregnancy. Gynecologic masses present a special diagnostic challenge in children and adolescents, because benign neoplasms greatly outnumber malignant ones, and their clinical signs and symptoms are often nonspecific.

Reproductive-Aged Women

A number of genital tract disorders cause pelvic masses in adult women. Uterine enlargement due to pregnancy, functional ovarian cysts, and leiomyoma are among the most common. Endometrioma, mature cystic teratoma, acute or chronic tubo-ovarian abscess, and ectopic pregnancies are other frequent causes. Most pelvic masses in this age group are benign, but malignancy rates typically increase with age.

Postmenopausal Women

With the cessation of ovulation and reproductive function, the causes of pelvic mass also change. Simple ovarian cysts and leiomyomas are still a common source. Although menopause typically results in atrophy of leiomyomas, uterine enlargement can still be noted in many women. Importantly, malignancy is a more frequent cause of pelvic masses in this demographic group. Uterine tumors, including adenocarcinoma and sarcoma, can cause associated uterine enlargement. In addition, ovarian cancer accounts for nearly 3 percent of new cancers among all women, with an estimated 21,990 new cases expected in the United States in 2011 (American Cancer Society, 2011).

UTERUS

Uterine enlargement is common and most frequently is the result of pregnancy or leiomyomas. Less often, enlargement is from adenomyosis, hematometra, or an adherent adnexal mass.

Leiomyomas

Leiomyomas are benign smooth muscle neoplasms that typically originate from the myometrium. They are often referred to as *uterine myomas*, and because their considerable collagen content creates a fibrous consistency, they are incorrectly called *fibroids*. Their incidence among women is generally cited as 20 to 25 percent, but has been shown to be as high as 70 to 80 percent in studies using histologic or sonographic examination (Buttram, 1981; Cramer, 1990; Day Baird, 2003). Moreover, the documented value varies depending on age and race of the study population (Day Baird, 2003).

In many women, leiomyomas are clinically insignificant. Conversely, their number, size, or location within the uterus can provoke a variety of symptoms. Taken together, these symptoms constitute an important segment of gynecologic practice. For example, of all inpatient hospitalizations for gynecologic problems from 1998 to 2005, uterine leiomyomas were the most common diagnosis and comprised 27 percent of gynecologic admissions (Whiteman, 2010).

Pathology

Grossly, leiomyomas are round, pearly white, firm, rubbery tumors that on cut-surface display a whorled pattern (Fig. 9-1). A typically involved uterus contains 6 to 7 tumors of varying size (Cramer, 1990). Leiomyomas possess a distinct autonomy from their surrounding myometrium because of a thin, outer connective tissue layer. This clinically important cleavage plane allows leiomyomas to be easily "shelled out" of the uterus during surgery. Histologically, leiomyomas contain elongated smooth muscle cells aggregated in bundles. Mitotic activity, however, is rare and is a key point in their differentiation from leiomyosarcoma.

The typical appearance of leiomyomas may change if normal muscle tissue is replaced with various degenerative substances following hemorrhage and necrosis. This process is collectively termed *degeneration*, and the replacement substances dictate the naming of these degenerative types. Forms include hyaline, calcific, cystic, myxoid, carneous or red, and fatty. These gross changes should be recognized as normal variants by both surgeon and pathologist.

Necrosis and degeneration develops frequently in leiomyomas because of the limited blood supply within these tumors. Leiomyomas have a lower arterial density compared with the surrounding normal myometrium (Fig. 9-2). Moreover, their lack of vascular organization leaves some tumors vulnerable to hypoperfusion and ischemia (Farrer-Brown, 1970; Forssman, 1976). As discussed later, acute pain may accompany degeneration.

Cytogenetics

Each leiomyoma is derived from a single progenitor myocyte. Thus, multiple tumors within the same uterus each show independent cytogenetic origins (Mashal, 1994; Townsend, 1970). The primary mutation initiating tumorigenesis is unknown, but identifiable karyotypic defects are found in approximately 40 percent of leiomyomas (Rein, 1998; Xing, 1997). A number of unique defects involving chromosomes 6, 7, 12, and 14 and less commonly X, 1, 3, 10, 13 have been identified to correlate with rates and direction of tumor growth (Brosens, 1998; Hodge, 2007). It is anticipated that further characterization of the specific functions of these karyotypic changes will help to define the important steps in leiomyoma development.

Estrogen Effects

Uterine leiomyomas are estrogen- and progesterone-sensitive tumors (Table 9-1). Consequently, they develop during the reproductive years. After menopause, leiomyomas generally shrink, and new tumor development is infrequent. Thus, it seems that many risk or protective factors depend on circumstances that chronically alter estrogen or progesterone levels or both. This concept is integral in understanding many of the risk factors associated with leiomyoma development and growth and in formulating treatment plans. Sex steroid hormones likely mediate their effect by stimulating or inhibiting transcription and production of cellular growth factors.

Leiomyomas themselves create a hyperestrogenic environment, which appears requisite for their growth and maintenance. First, compared with normal myometrium, leiomyoma

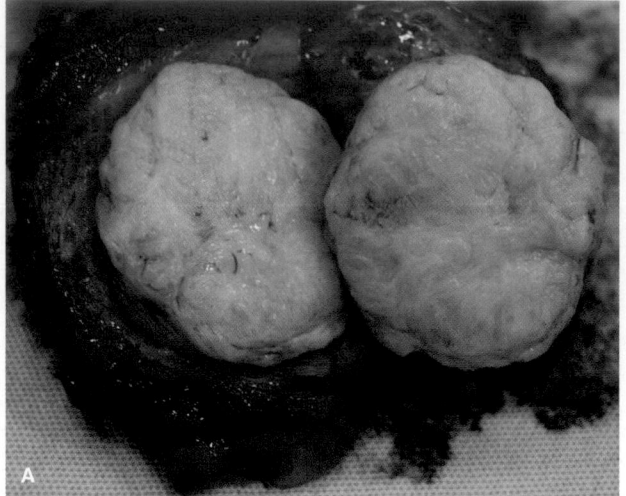

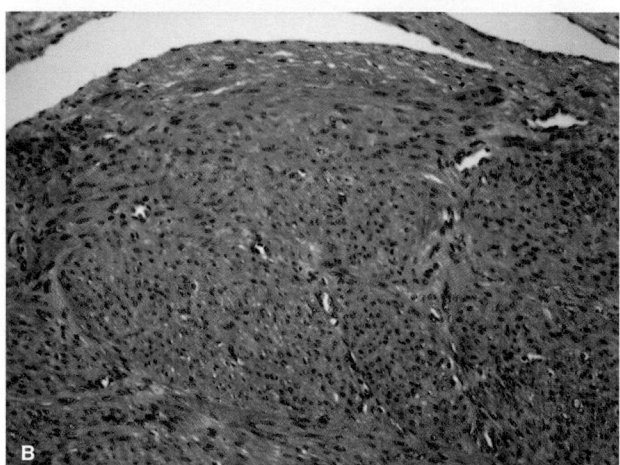

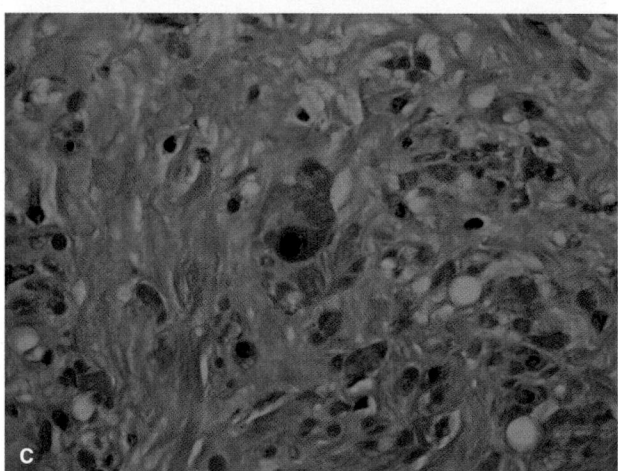

FIGURE 9-1 A. This bisected, off-white, whorled leiomyoma, which is distinct from the surrounding myometrium in this bisected uterine fundus, is a typical leiomyoma example. **B.** Histologically, leiomyomas contain interlacing, elongated smooth muscle cells with eosinophilic cytoplasm. Smooth muscle cells are more tightly packed within leiomyomas compared with those of the surrounding myometrium and give these tumors a more cellular appearance microscopically. **C.** The appearance of leiomyomas may vary depending on the degree and type of degeneration present. With hyaline degeneration, abundant pink glassy hyaline is interspersed between smooth muscle cells. *(Photographs B and C contributed by Dr. Raheela Ashfaq.)*

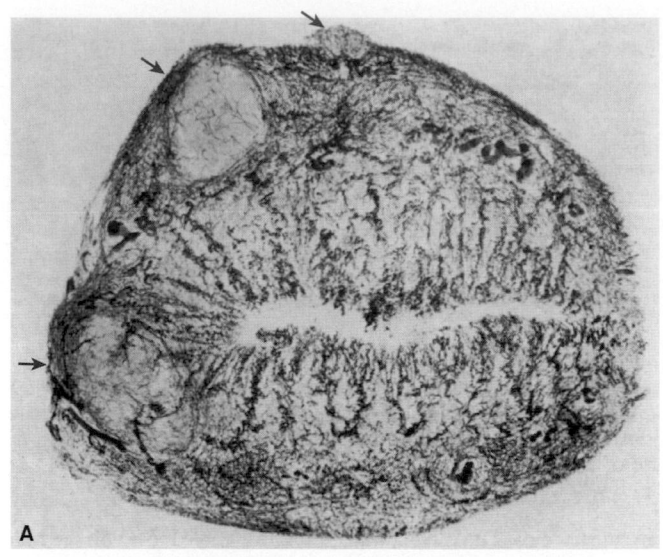

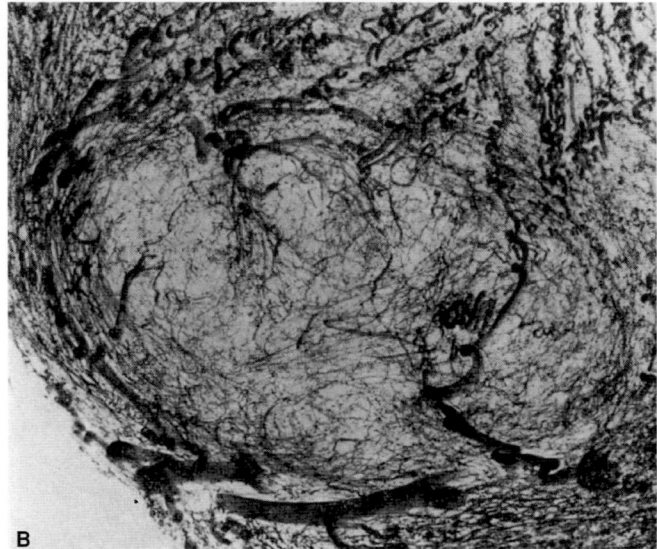

FIGURE 9-2 A. A transverse slice of uterus following arterial injection of a radiopaque medium shows the arterial supply in a subserosal and two intramural leiomyomas (*arrows*). **B.** Higher magnification of the arterial supply in the lower of the two intramural leiomyomas. Vessels are seen as thick, irregular black lines encircling and leading into the leiomyoma. *(From Farrer-Brown, 1970, with permission.)*

cells contain a greater density of estrogen receptors, which results in greater estradiol binding. Second, these tumors convert less estradiol to the weaker estrone (Englund, 1998; Otubu, 1982; Yamamoto, 1993). A third mechanism described by Bulun and colleagues (1994) involves higher levels of cytochrome P450 aromatase in leiomyomas compared with normal myocytes. This specific cytochrome isoform catalyzes the conversion of androgens to estrogen in a number of tissues (Chap. 15, p. 403).

There are a number of conditions associated with sustained estrogen exposure that encourage leiomyoma formation. For example, the increased years of persistent estrogen production found with early menarche and with an increased body mass index (BMI) are each linked with a greater risk of leiomyomas (Marshall, 1998; Wise, 2005). Obese women produce more

TABLE 9-1. Relationships of Patients Factors, Leiomyoma Risk, and Steroid Hormones

Factor	Effect on Risk	Potential Reason
Early menarche	Increased	Increased years of estrogen exposure
Elevated BMI	Increased	Increased conversion of androgens to estrogens
Affected family member	Increased	Genetic differences in hormone production or metabolism
African-American race	Increased	Genetic differences in hormone production or metabolism
PCOS	Increased	Unopposed estrogen secondary to anovulation
Postmenopausal	Decreased	Hypoestrogenism
Increased parity	Decreased	Break in chronic estrogen exposure; uterine remodeling during postpartum involution
Combination oral contraceptives	Decreased or null	Exposure to estrogen opposed by progesterone
Cigarette smoking	Decreased	Decreased serum estrogen levels

BMI = body mass index; PCOS = polycystic ovarian syndrome.

estrogens from increased adipose conversion of androgens to estrogen and also display decreased hepatic production of sex hormone binding globulin (Glass, 1989). Also, those with polycystic ovarian syndrome (PCOS) have a higher risk, which is thought secondary to the sustained estrogen exposure that accompanies chronic anovulation (Wise, 2007).

In premenopausal women, estrogen and progesterone hormone treatment probably has no inductive effect on leiomyoma formation. With few exceptions, oral contraceptive combination pills either lower or have no effect on this risk (Chiaffarino, 1999; Parazzini, 1992; Ross, 1986).

Studies evaluating the effects of hormone replacement therapy, however, do show a small increased risk of leiomyoma development (Polatti, 2000; Reed, 2004). In women with existing tumors, Palomba and associates (2002) evaluated the relationship between leiomyoma growth and differing doses of medroxyprogesterone acetate (MPA) in hormone replacement therapy. Because higher doses of MPA were associated with leiomyoma growth, they recommended using the lowest possible dose of MPA in these patients.

Finally, smoking alters estrogen metabolism and lowers physiologically active serum estrogen levels (Daniel, 1992; Michnovicz, 1986). This may explain why women who smoke generally have a lower risk for leiomyoma formation (Parazzini, 1992).

Progestin Effects

The role of progesterone in leiomyomas is less clear, and indeed both stimulatory and inhibitory effects have been reported. For example, exogenous progestins have been shown to limit leiomyoma growth in clinical trials (Goldzieher, 1966; Tiltman, 1985). Similarly, epidemiologic studies link depot medroxyprogesterone use with a lower incidence of leiomyoma development (Lumbiganon, 1996).

In contrast, other studies report a stimulatory influence of progestins on leiomyoma growth. For example, the antiprogestin RU486 induces atrophy in most leiomyomas (Murphy, 1993). Moreover, in women treated with gonadotropin-releasing hormone (GnRH) agonists, leiomyomas typically decrease in size. However, if progestins are given simultaneously, there may be *increased* leiomyoma growth (Carr, 1993; Friedman, 1994). More recent research suggests that progesterone is the *primary* mitogen for tumor growth and that estrogen's role is to upregulate progesterone receptors (Ishikawa, 2010).

Risk Factors

During the reproductive years, the incidence of this tumor increases with age. In a study by Day Baird and associates (2003), the cumulative incidence by age 50 years was nearly 70 percent in white and more than 80 percent in African-American women. Sporadic case reports such as the one by Perkins and colleagues (2009) document their rarity in teenagers. Lower rates of leiomyomas are linked with pregnancy, and women giving birth at an early age, those with higher parity, and those with a more recent pregnancy all display lower incidences of leiomyoma formation (Wise, 2004). This association has been theorized to result from uterine remodeling that occurs during postpartum uterine involution (Parker, 2007).

Leiomyomas are more common in African-American women compared with white, Asian, or Hispanic women. Few studies have been done to ascertain these ethnic differences, but in African-American women, some investigators have found significantly higher aromatase mRNA levels within their leiomyomas or higher prevalences of estrogen-receptor gene polymorphisms that predispose to leiomyomas (Al-Hendy, 2006; Ishikawa, 2009). Heredity likely plays a role in susceptibility to the initial mutation involved with leiomyoma development. For example, family and twin studies have shown the risk of leiomyoma formation to be approximately two times greater in women with affected first-degree relatives (Sato, 2002; Vikhlyaeva, 1995).

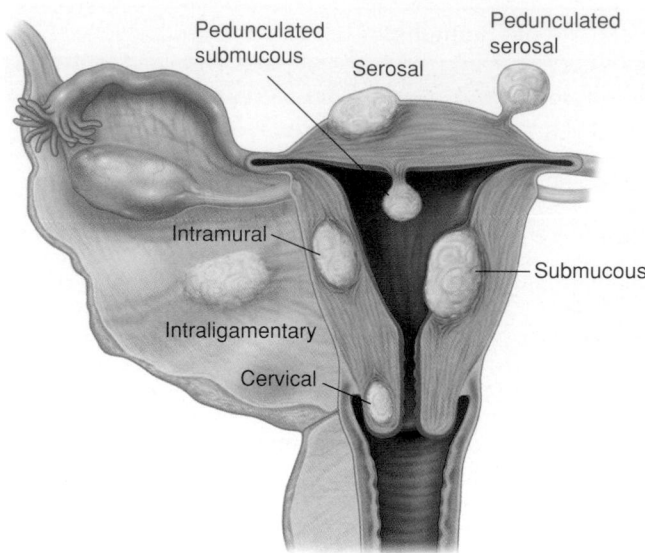

FIGURE 9-3 Leiomyomas can be categorized as shown. However, the borders of most leiomyomas overlap these distinct regions.

Classification of Uterine Leiomyoma

Leiomyomas are classified based on their location and direction of growth (Fig. 9-3). *Subserosal leiomyomas* originate from myocytes adjacent to the uterine serosa, and their growth is directed outward. When these are attached only by a stalk to their progenitor myometrium, they are called *pedunculated leiomyomas*. *Parasitic leiomyomas* are subserosal variants that attach themselves to nearby pelvic structures from which they derive vascular support, and then may or may not detach from the parent myometrium. *Intramural leiomyomas* are those with growth centered within the uterine walls. Finally, *submucous leiomyomas* are proximate to the endometrium and grow toward and bulge into the endometrial cavity. For endoscopic resection evaluation, submucous leiomyomas are further classified by their depth of involvement. The European Society of Hysteroscopy defines leiomyomas as follows: type 0, if the mass is located entirely within the uterine cavity; type I, if less than 50 percent is located within the myometrium; and type II, if greater than 50 percent of the mass is surrounded by myometrium (Wamsteker, 1993). Only about 0.4 percent of leiomyomas develop in the cervix (Tiltman, 1998). Leiomyomas have also been found less commonly in the ovary, fallopian tube, broad ligament, vagina, and vulva.

Leiomyomatosis. Extrauterine smooth muscle tumors, which are benign yet infiltrative, may develop in women with concurrent uterine leiomyomas and are termed leiomyomatosis. In such cases, the diagnosis of malignant metastasis from a leiomyosarcoma must be excluded.

Intravenous leiomyomatosis is a rare, benign smooth muscle tumor that invades and extends serpiginously into the uterine and other pelvic veins, the vena cava, and even the cardiac chambers. Although histologically benign and usually amenable to resection, the tumor can be fatal as a consequence of venous obstruction or cardiac involvement (Uchida, 2004; Worley, 2009; Zhang, 2010).

Benign metastasizing leiomyomas derive from morphologically benign uterine leiomyomas that disseminate hematogenously. Lesions have been found in the lungs, gastrointestinal tract, spine, and brain (Alessi, 2003). Classically, these are found in women who have a recent or distant history of pelvic surgery (Zaloudek, 2002).

Disseminated peritoneal leiomyomatosis appears as multiple small nodules on the peritoneal surfaces of the abdominal cavity or the abdominal organs or both. They are usually found in women of reproductive age, and 70 percent are associated with pregnancy or combination oral contraceptives (Robboy, 2000).

More recently, case reports describe multiple small peritoneal leiomyomas found following laparoscopic myomectomy or hysterectomy. These cases have been described as parasitic leiomyomas or as disseminated peritoneal leiomyomatosis. Morcellation and implantation of tumor remnants following initial surgery have been implicated (Kho, 2009; Miyake, 2009; Paul, 2006; Sinha, 2007).

Treatments for these benign conditions may involve hysterectomy with oophorectomy, tumor debulking, and more recently, use of GnRH agonists, aromatase inhibitors, selective estrogen-receptor modulators, or chemotherapy (Bodner, 2002; Lin, 2009; Rivera, 2004).

Symptoms

Most women with leiomyomas are asymptomatic. However, symptomatic patients typically complain of bleeding, pain, pressure sensation, or infertility. In general, the larger the leiomyoma, the greater the likelihood of symptoms (Cramer, 1990). Although most symptoms are chronic, acute pain may accompany a degenerating leiomyoma or tumor prolapse from the uterus. Acute distress may also follow rare complications such as torsion of a subserosal pedunculated leiomyoma, acute urinary retention, deep-vein thromboembolism, or intraperitoneal hemorrhage (Gupta, 2009).

Bleeding. This is the most common symptom and usually presents as menorrhagia (Olufowobi, 2004). The pathophysiology underlying this bleeding may relate to dilatation of venules. Bulky tumors are thought to exert pressure and impinge on the uterine venous system, which causes venous dilatation within the myometrium and endometrium (Figs. 9-4 and 9-5). For this reason, intramural and subserosal tumors have been shown to have the same propensity to cause menorrhagia as submucous ones (Wegienka, 2003).

Dysregulation of local vasoactive growth factors is also thought to promote vasodilatation. When engorged venules are disrupted at the time of menstrual sloughing, bleeding from these markedly dilated venules overwhelms the usual hemostatic mechanisms (Stewart, 1996).

Pelvic Discomfort and Dysmenorrhea. A sufficiently enlarged uterus can cause pressure sensation, urinary frequency, incontinence, or constipation. Rarely, leiomyomas extend laterally to compress the ureter and lead to obstruction and hydronephrosis. Although dysmenorrhea is common, in a population-based cross-sectional study, Lippman and coworkers (2003) reported that women with leiomyomas more fre-

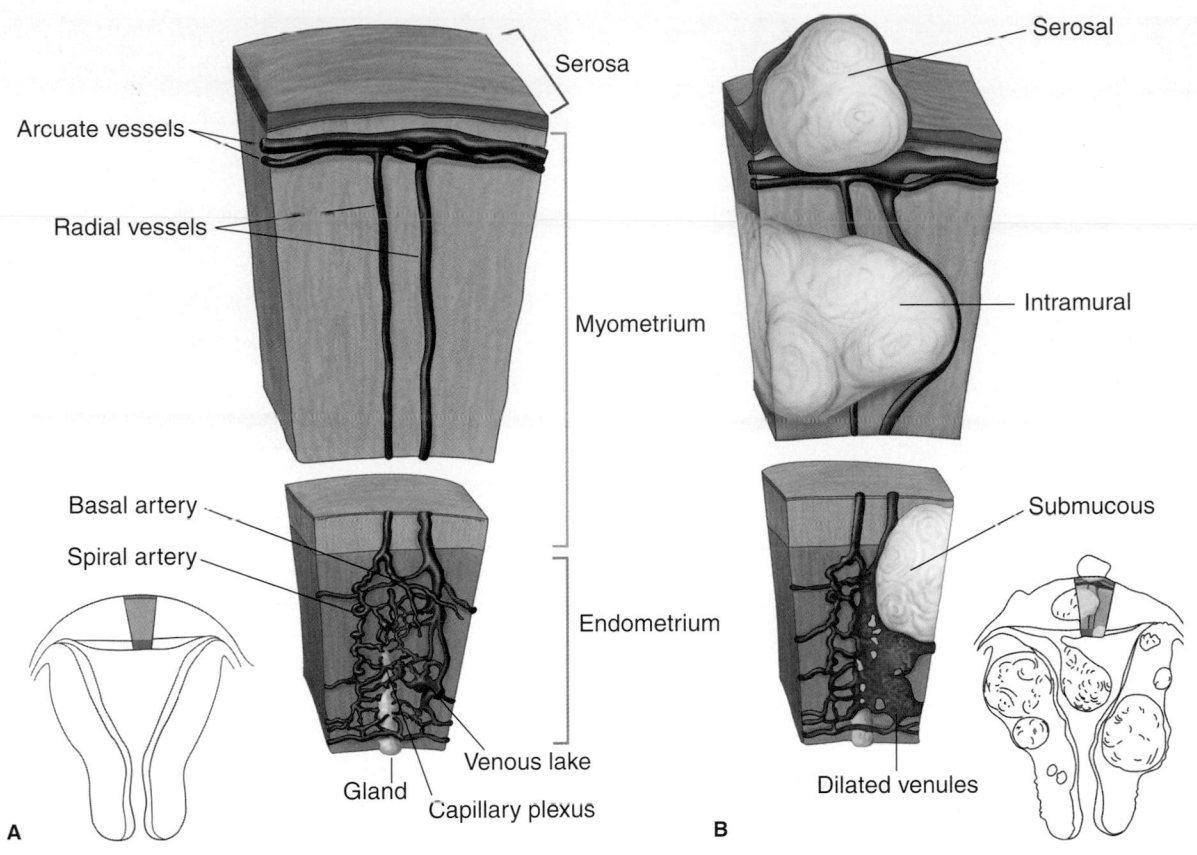

FIGURE 9-4 One mechanism by which leiomyomas cause menorrhagia. For both images, the inset shows the area from which the large uterine wedge in the main image was taken. **A.** Normal uterine vasculature. **B.** At any level within the myometrium, leiomyomas can compress adjacent veins and thereby cause dilatation of distal endometrial venules. With menstrual shedding of the endometrium, these venules are disrupted. Typical endometrial hemostatic mechanisms are unable to completely control bleeding from these dilated vessels, and menorrhagia results. *(Redrawn from Buttram, 1981.)*

quently had dyspareunia or noncyclical pelvic pain than dysmenorrhea.

Acute Pelvic Pain. This is a less frequent complaint with leiomyomas, but is most often seen with a degenerating or prolapsing leiomyoma. As described earlier, leiomyomas may degenerate, and such tissue necrosis can be associated with acute pain, fever, and leukocytosis. This constellation may mimic other causes of acute pelvic pain. Sonography is typically performed to help identify a cause, and usually a nondescript leiomyoma is found. Computed tomography may also be obtained, especially if clear interpretation of pelvic anatomy is obscured by multiple large leiomyomas or if appendicitis is a considered diagnosis. Treatment of a degenerating leiomyoma is nonsurgical and includes analgesics and antipyretics as needed. However, broad-spectrum antibiotics are often administered as differentiating between leiomyoma degeneration and endometritis may often be difficult. In most cases, symptoms improve within 24 to 48 hours.

Women with prolapse of a tumor from the endometrial cavity will typically present with complaints of cramping or acute pain as the tumor stretches and passes through the endocervical canal. Associated bleeding or serosanguineous discharge is common. Visual inspection is usually diagnostic, although sonography is often performed to evaluate the size and number of coexisting uterine leiomyomas and exclude other possible

sources of pain (Fig. 9-6). In leiomyomas not immediately removed, preoperative biopsy may be indicated because some cases of uterine sarcoma or cervical cancer can appear similar. Surgical treatment involves severing the leiomyoma from its stalk and is described in detail in Section 41-11 (p. 1043).

Infertility and Pregnancy Wastage. Although the mechanisms are not clear, leiomyomas can be associated with infertility. It is estimated that 2 to 3 percent of infertility cases are due solely to leiomyomas (Buttram, 1981; Kupesic, 2002). Their putative effects include occlusion of tubal ostia and disruption of the normal uterine contractions that propel sperm or ova. Distortion of the endometrial cavity may also diminish implantation and sperm transport. Importantly, leiomyomas are associated with endometrial inflammation and vascular changes that may disrupt implantation (Brosens, 2003; Farhi, 1995; American Society for Reproductive Medicine, 2006).

There is a stronger association of subfertility with submucous leiomyomas than with tumors located elsewhere. Improved pregnancy rates following hysteroscopic resection have provided most of the indirect evidence for this link (Vercellini, 1999). In one study, Garcia and Tureck (1984) reported pregnancy rates approaching 50 percent following myomectomy in women with submucous leiomyomas as their sole source of infertility.

The relationship between subfertility and intramural and subserosal leiomyomas that do not distort the endometrial

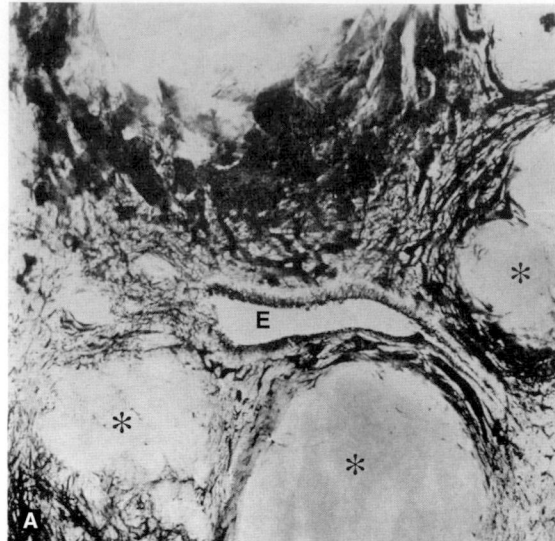

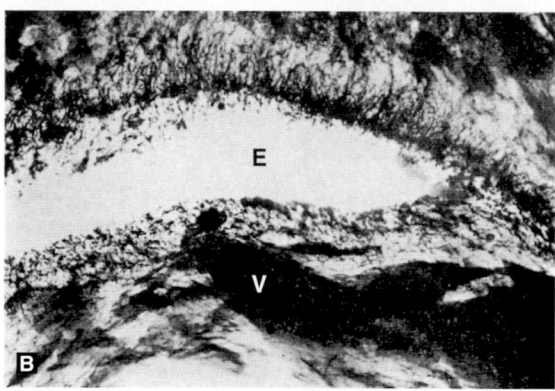

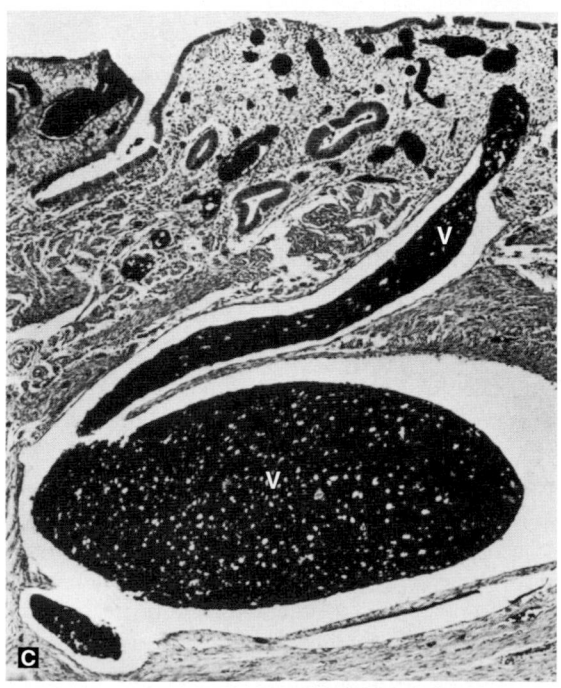

FIGURE 9-5 Micrographs of uterine vasculature following venous injection of a radiopaque medium. **A.** Dilated venous plexuses are seen as a black network. Note the multiple leiomyomas (*asterisks*) and endometrial cavity (*E*). **B.** Higher magnification shows black dilated venules in the base of the endometrium. **C.** A dilated endometrial venule communicates with an enlarged vessel in the inner myometrium. *(From Farrer-Brown, 1970, 1971, with permission.)*

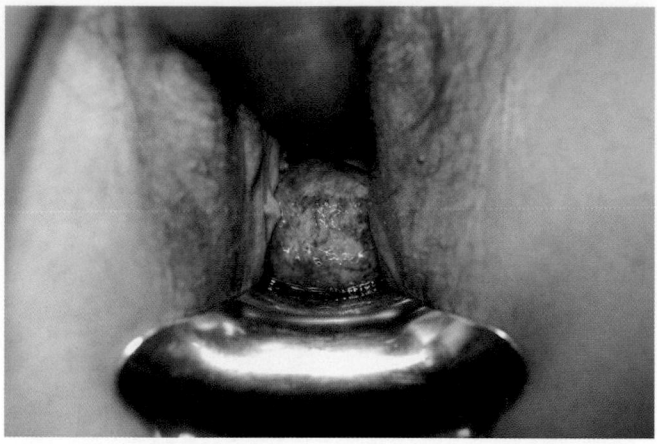

FIGURE 9-6 Preoperative photograph of the perineum show vaginal retractors placed along the upper and lower vaginal walls. With this retraction, a round, hyperemic leiomyoma is seen. The tumor and its elongated stalk prolapsed from the uterine cavity, through the cervix, and into the vagina. *(Photograph contributed by Dr. David Rogers.)*

cavity is more tenuous. A number of investigators have reported equally good in vitro fertilization (IVF) success rates in women with and without leiomyomas that did not distort the endometrial cavity (Farhi, 1995; Oliveira, 2004). Others, however, have reported adverse fertility effects from intramural and subserosal leiomyomas (Hart, 2001; Marchionni, 2004). Importantly, the strength of this evidence must be weighed against the morbidity associated with intramural myomectomy (Klatsky, 2008).

Both uterine leiomyoma and spontaneous miscarriage are common, and an association between these has not been shown convincingly. Benson and associates (2001) showed that pregnancy loss rates increased with increasing number of leiomyomas but was unaffected by tumor size or location. Other indirect evidence comes from studies that cite significantly lower spontaneous abortion rates following resection (Campo, 2003; Vercellini, 1999).

Other Clinical Manifestations. Rarely, women with leiomyomas may develop *myomatous erythrocytosis syndrome*. This may result from excessive erythropoietin production by the kidneys or by the leiomyomas themselves (Vlasveld, 2008; Yokoyama, 2003). In either case, red cell mass returns to normal following hysterectomy.

Leiomyomas occasionally may cause *pseudo-Meigs syndrome*. Traditionally, Meigs syndrome consists of ascites and pleural effusions that accompany benign ovarian fibromas. However, any pelvic tumor including large, cystic leiomyomas or other benign ovarian cysts can cause this. The presumed etiology stems from discordancy between the arterial supply and the venous and lymphatic drainage from the leiomyomas. Resolution of ascites and hydrothorax follows hysterectomy.

Diagnosis

Leiomyomas are often detected by pelvic examination with findings of uterine enlargement, irregular contour, or both. In reproductive-aged women, uterine enlargement should prompt determination of a urine or serum β-hCG level.

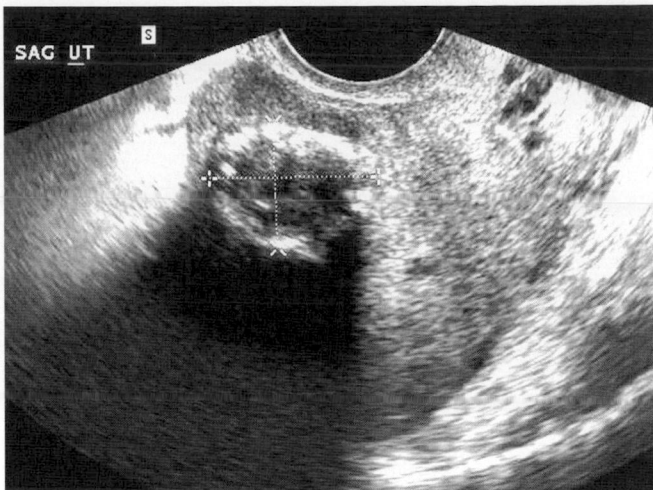

FIGURE 9-7 Transvaginal sonogram of an intramural leiomyoma with a calcified border. *(Image contributed by Dr. Elysia Moschos.)*

Imaging.

Sonography is initially done to define pelvic anatomy (Chap. 2, p. 38). The sonographic appearances of leiomyomas vary from hypo- to hyperechoic depending on the ratio of smooth muscle to connective tissue and whether there is degeneration. Calcification and cystic degeneration create the most sonographically distinctive changes (Fig. 9-7). Calcifications appear hyperechoic and commonly rim the tumor or are randomly scattered throughout the mass (Kurtz, 1979). Cystic or myxoid degeneration typically fills the leiomyoma with multiple, smooth-walled, round, irregularly sized but generally small hypoechoic areas.

If menorrhagia, dysmenorrhea, or infertility accompanies a pelvic mass, then the endometrial cavity may be evaluated for submucous leiomyomas, endometrial polyps, congenital anomalies, or synechiae. As describe in detail in Chapter 8 (p. 228), if the endometrium is thick or irregular, then saline infusion sonography (SIS) or hysteroscopy may provide additional infor-

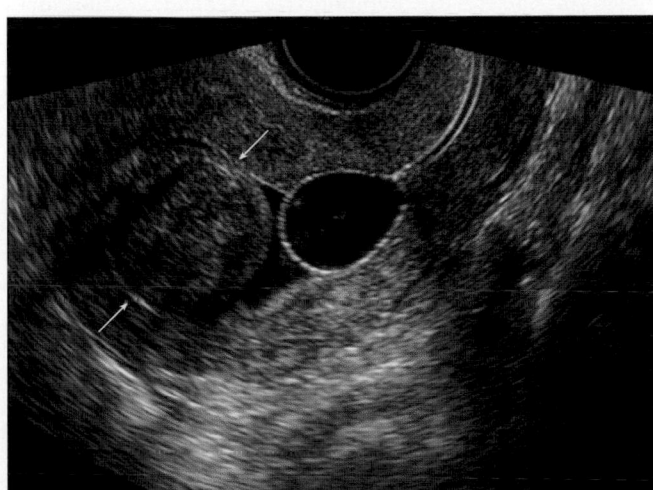

FIGURE 9-8 Submucous leiomyoma (*yellow arrows*) is clearly outlined during saline infusion sonography (SIS). The SIS catheter balloon is seen in the lower uterine cavity (*red arrow*). *(Image contributed by Dr. Elysia Moschos.)*

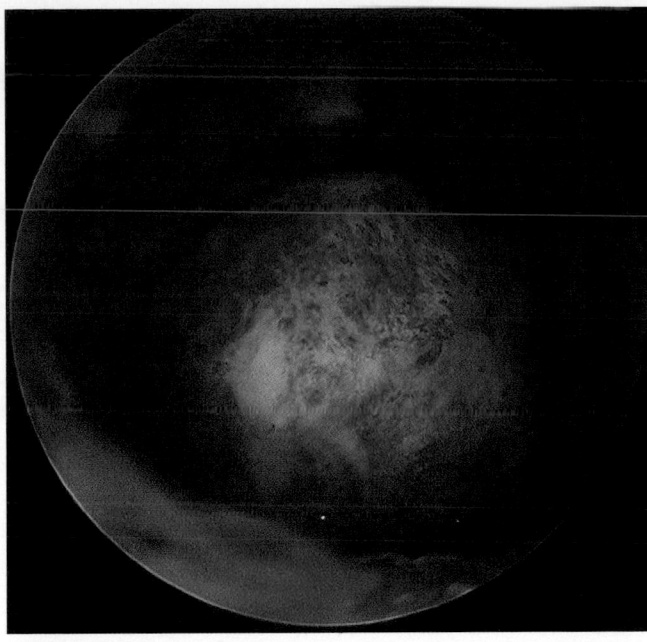

FIGURE 9-9 Hysteroscopic photograph of a submucous leiomyoma prior to resection. *(Photograph contributed by Dr. Karen Bradshaw.)*

mation (Figs. 9-8 and 9-9). For the infertile woman, hysterosalpingography (HSG) may be used during initial evaluation to define endometrial pathology as well as tubal patency. Weinraub and associates (1996) reported use of 3-dimensional SIS. However, any clear advantage over 2-dimensional SIS or hysteroscopy has not been demonstrated (de Kroon, 2004).

Leiomyomas have characteristic vascular patterns that can be identified by color flow Doppler. A peripheral rim of vascularity from which a few vessels arise to penetrate into the center of the tumor is traditionally seen. Doppler imaging can be used to differentiate an extrauterine leiomyoma from other pelvic masses or a submucous leiomyoma from an endometrial polyp or adenomyosis (Chap. 2, p. 35) (Fleischer, 2003).

Magnetic resonance imaging may be required when imaging is limited by body habitus or distorted anatomy. This tool allows more accurate assessment of the size, number, and location of leiomyomas, which may help identify appropriate patients for alternatives to hysterectomy such as myomectomy or uterine artery embolization (p. 256) (Zawin, 1990). Importantly, for a dominant fundal uterine mass, MR imaging can also aid differentiation of a fundal leiomyoma, which is a suitable myomectomy indication, from adenomyosis, which is an unsuitable indication for this procedure.

Management

Observation. Regardless of their size, asymptomatic leiomyomas usually can be observed and surveilled during annual pelvic examination (American College of Obstetricians and Gynecologists, 2001). However, assessment of the adnexa may be hindered by uterine size or contour, and adequate uterine and adnexal assessment may be limited by patient obesity. In these cases, some may choose to add annual sonographic surveillance (Cantuaria, 1998; Guarnaccia, 2001).

TABLE 9-2. Indications for the Medical Treatment of Uterine Leiomyoma

Agent	NSAIDs	COCs	DMPA	LNG-IUS	GnRH Agonist
Symptom					
Dysmenorrhea	+	+	+	+	+
Menorrhagia	−	+	+	+	+
Dyspareunia	−	−	−	−	+
Pelvic pressure	−	−	−	−	+
Infertility	−	−	−	−	+

COCs = combination oral contraceptive pills; DMPA = depot medroxyprogesterone acetate; GnRH = gonadotropin-releasing hormone; LNG-IUS = levonorgestrel-releasing intrauterine system (Mirena); NSAIDs = nonsteroidal antiinflammatory drugs.

Leiomyomas in general are slow-growing. A longitudinal sonography-based study showed the average diameter growth to be only 0.5 cm/yr, although diameter growth greater than 3 cm/yr has been observed (DeWaay, 2002). Moreover, growth rates of leiomyomas within the same patient will vary widely, and some tumors will even spontaneously regress (Peddada, 2008). Therefore, predicting leiomyoma growth or symptom onset is difficult, and watchful waiting may be the best option for an individual asymptomatic patient.

In the past, most preferred surgical removal of a large, asymptomatic leiomyomatous uterus because of concerns regarding cancer risks and increased operative morbidity if left to grow larger. These concerns have been disproven, and thus, otherwise asymptomatic women with large leiomyomas can also be managed expectantly (Parker, 1994; Stovall, 1994). In addition, most infertile women with uterine leiomyomas are initially managed expectantly. For those with symptomatic tumors, surgery should be timed closely to planned pregnancy, if possible, to limit the risk of tumor recurrence.

Drug Therapy. In some women with symptomatic leiomyomas, medical therapy may be preferred (Table 9-2). In addition, because leiomyomas typically regress postmenopausally, some women choose medical treatment to relieve symptoms in anticipation of menopause. In others, medical therapy such as GnRH agonists is used as an adjunct to surgery.

Nonsteroidal Antiinflammatory Drugs (NSAIDs). Women with dysmenorrhea have higher endometrial levels of prostaglandins $F_{2\alpha}$ and E_2 than asymptomatic women (Willman, 1976; Ylikorkala, 1978). Accordingly, treatment of dysmenorrhea and menorrhagia associated with leiomyomas is based on the role of prostaglandins as mediators of these symptoms. A number of NSAIDs have proved effective for dysmenorrhea, yet there is not one considered to be superior (Table 10-2, p. 285).

Prostaglandins are also associated with menorrhagia. That said, benefits of NSAIDs for leiomyoma-related bleeding are less clear. The few studies done have had conflicting results (Anteby, 1985; Mäkäräinen, 1986; Ylikorkala, 1986). Available data do not support their use as sole agents for leiomyoma-related menorrhagia.

Hormonal Therapy. Both combination oral contraceptive pills (COCs) and progestins have been used to induce endometrial atrophy and decrease prostaglandin production in women with leiomyomas. Friedman and Thomas (1995) studied 87 women with leiomyomas and reported that those taking low-dose COCs had significantly shorter menses and no evidence of uterine enlargement. Orsini and colleagues (2002) reported similar results. Although the data supporting its use is not robust, the levonorgestrel-releasing intrauterine system (LNG-IUS) has also been shown to improve menorrhagia in women with leiomyoma-related bleeding (Grigorieva, 2003; Kaunitz, 2007; Magalhães, 2007). Importantly, leiomyomas that distort the endometrial cavity preclude LNG-IUS use (Bayer, 2009). Compared with women without leiomyomas, those with tumors experience higher IUD-expulsion rates.

Based on the above studies, steroid contraceptives are a reasonable treatment option for menstrual-related leiomyoma symptoms. However, because of the unpredictable effects of progestins on leiomyoma growth, the American College of Obstetricians and Gynecologists (2008) recommends close monitoring of leiomyoma and uterine size. In contrast, the American Society for Reproductive Medicine (2006) does not recommend either progestins or combination COCs for leiomyoma-related symptoms.

Androgens. Both danazol and gestrinone have been found to shrink leiomyoma volume and improve bleeding symptoms (Coutinho, 1989; De Leo, 1999). Unfortunately, their prominent side effects, which include acne and hirsutism, preclude their use as first-line agents (Chap. 10, p. 294).

GnRH Agonists. These compounds are synthetic derivatives of the GnRH decapeptide. Amino-acid substitution makes them resistant to degradation, thereby increasing their half-life and prolonging receptor binding. They are inactive if taken orally, but intramuscular, subcutaneous, and intranasal preparations are available. Leuprolide acetate (Lupron Depot) is approved by the U.S. Food and Drug Administration (FDA) for leiomyoma treatment and is available in a 3.75-mg monthly dose or 11.25-mg 3-month dose, both given intramuscularly (IM). Less frequently used GnRH agonists include goserelin (Zoladex) administered as a 3.6-mg monthly or 10.8-mg 3-month subcutaneous depot implant; triptorelin (Trelstar) given as a 3.75-mg monthly IM injection; and nafarelin (Synarel) used in a 200-mg twice-daily nasal spray regimen. These later three are not specifically FDA-approved for leiomyoma treatment, but off-label use with these has been shown effective.

GnRH agonists shrink leiomyomas by targeting the growth effects of estrogen and progesterone. Initially, these agonists stimulate receptors on pituitary gonadotropes to cause a supraphysiological release of both luteinizing hormone (LH) and follicle-stimulating hormone (FSH). Also called a *flare*, this phase typically lasts 1 week. With their long-term action, however, agonists downregulate receptors in gonadotropes, thus creating desensitization to further GnRH stimulation. Correspondingly, decreased gonadotropin secretion leads to suppressed estrogen and progesterone levels 1 to 2 weeks after initial GnRH agonist administration (Broekmans, 1996). Another possible mechanism is that leiomyomas themselves may contain GnRH receptors, and agonists may directly decrease leiomyoma size (Chegini, 1996; Wiznitzer, 1988).

Results with GnRH agonist treatment include dramatic decreases in uterine and leiomyoma volume. Most women experience a mean decrease in uterine volume of 40 to 50 percent, and most of this occurs during the first 3 months of therapy. Clinical benefits of reduced leiomyoma volumes include pain relief and diminished menorrhagia, usually amenorrhea. During this time, anemic women are given oral iron therapy to rebuild their red cell mass and increase iron stores (Filicori, 1983; Friedman, 1990). Most recommend treatment for a total of 3 to 6 months. Following GnRH agonist discontinuance, normal menses resume in 4 to 10 weeks. Unfortunately, leiomyomas then regrow, and uterine volumes regain pretreatment sizes within 3 to 4 months (Friedman, 1990). Despite regrowth, Schlaff and coworkers (1989) reported symptom relief for approximately 1 year in half of women given GnRH agonists.

GnRH agonists have significant costs, risks, and side effects. Side effects result from the profound drop in serum estrogen levels and have been reported to occur in up to 95 percent of women treated with this method (Letterie, 1989). Side effects include vasomotor symptoms, libido changes, vaginal epithelium dryness, and accompanying dyspareunia. Despite these, less than 10 percent of patients terminate treatment secondary to side effects (Parker, 2007). Importantly, 6 months of agonist therapy can result in a 6-percent loss in trabecular bone, not all of which may be recouped following discontinuation (Scharla, 1990). As a result, these agents alone are not recommended for longer than 6 months' use.

To obviate the severity of these side effects, several medications have been added to GnRH agonist treatment. The goal of this *add-back therapy* is to counter side effects—most importantly, vasomotor effects and bone loss—without mitigating the effects on uterine and leiomyoma volume decrease. This is possible because the estrogen level required to improve vasomotor symptoms and minimize bone loss is below the estrogen threshold that would restimulate leiomyoma growth. Mizutani and coworkers (1998) found that GnRH agonists suppress leiomyoma cell proliferation and induce cell apoptosis by the fourth week of GnRH agonist therapy. They proposed that add-back therapy be withheld until after this time. Because of these and other observations, add-back therapy is typically begun 1 to 3 months following GnRH agonist initiation.

Add-back therapy traditionally includes estrogen combined with a progestin, and those studied have generally been low-dose preparations equivalent to menopausal hormonal therapy. An oral regimen of medroxyprogesterone acetate (MPA), 10 mg (days 16–25), combined with equine estrogen, 0.625 mg (days 1–25), or an oral continuous daily regimen of MPA 2.5 mg and equine estrogen 0.625 mg may be used.

Add-back therapy with selective estrogen-receptor modulators (SERMs), such as tibolone and raloxifene, has also been shown to prevent bone loss. Advantages of SERMs include the ability to begin them concurrently with GnRH agonist treatment without negating the agonist effects of leiomyoma shrinkage. Unfortunately, a high percentage of women complain of vasomotor symptoms while taking SERMs (Palomba, 1998, 2004).

Because of the limitations of GnRH agonist therapy, the American College of Obstetricians and Gynecologists (2008) recommends that it should not be used longer than 6 months without add-back therapy. The American Society for Reproductive Medicine (2006) states that GnRH agonist treatment with add-back therapy may be considered for longer than a 6-month, yet finite, duration in those anticipating menopause, but not for younger affected women.

Preoperatively, GnRH agonists offer several advantages. Their use decreases menorrhagia and may allow correction of anemia. Decreased uterine size as a result of treatment may allow a less complicated or extensive surgical procedure. For example, hysterectomy or myomectomy may be performed through a smaller laparotomy incision or by vaginal hysterectomy, laparoscopy, or hysteroscopy (Crosignani, 1996; Mencaglia, 1993; Stovall, 1994). A fuller discussion of preoperative GnRH agonist use for leiomyomas can be found in Section 41-10 (p. 1039).

GnRH Antagonists. Two agents in this class, cetrorelix and ganirelix, are currently FDA-approved for infertility use in women undergoing controlled ovarian hyperstimulation. These have also been studied for treatment of leiomyomas (Engel, 2007; Flierman, 2005). Their profound hypoestrogenic effects are similar to those of GnRH agonists, but they avoid the initial gonadotropin flare and have a more rapid onset of action. Daily subcutaneous injections induce leiomyoma shrinkage comparable to that with GnRH agonists (Gonzalez-Barcena, 1997; Kettel, 1993). The limitation of these drugs is that they are daily injectables, and a depot form of cetrorelix did not provide adequate or consistent suppression of estrogen production or leiomyoma growth (Felberbaum, 1998).

Antiprogestins. Physiologically, progesterone binds to either progesterone receptor A (PR-A) or B (PR-B). Of these, PR-A is found in leiomyomas in greater amounts than PR-B (Viville, 1997). Specific agents can competitively bind these receptors and are classified as *antiprogestins* if they universally prompt antagonist effects, or as *selective progesterone-receptor modulators (SPRMs)* if they exert antiprogesterone effects in some tissues but progestational effects in others (Spitz, 2009). Although none are currently available clinically for this indication, several trials support their efficacy for leiomyoma treatment.

Mifepristone, also known as RU486, is an antiprogestin that has been used for treatment of leiomyomas. Mifepristone diminishes leiomyoma volume by approximately half. Various doses have been used and include 2.5, 5, 10, or 50 mg given daily over 12 weeks (Eisinger, 2003, 2009; Murphy, 1993). Steinauer and colleagues (2004) reported that mifepristone was effective in improving symptoms. Of those treated, 91 percent developed amenorrhea, 75 percent reported improved pain relief, and 70 percent had fewer pressure symptoms. In a comparison of leuprolide acetate treatment and mifepristone therapy, Reinsch and associates (1994) showed comparable decreases in uterine volume, yet mifepristone was better tolerated.

Mifepristone therapy, however, has several drawbacks. Approximately 40 percent of treated women complain of vasomotor symptoms. In addition, its antiprogestational effects expose the endometrium to unopposed estrogen. The spectrum of endometrial findings is a topic of research and range from simple endometrial hyperplasia to a new category described as *PRM-associated endometrial changes* (Mutter, 2008). Moreover, mifepristone (Mifeprex) is currently FDA-approved solely for early pregnancy termination. It is only manufactured as 200-mg tablets, a dose well above that needed for leiomyoma therapy. Ulipristal (CDB-2914) is another antiprogestin that is structurally similar to mifepristone and has shown clinical promise as well (Levens, 2008).

In addition to antiprogestins, use of SPRMs for leiomyoma treatment has gained interest. One such SPRM, asoprisnil, was shown to suppress uterine bleeding, shrink leiomyoma volume, yet avoid estrogen-deficiency symptoms and breakthrough bleeding (Chwalisz, 2005, 2007; Williams, 2007). However, some subjects receiving asoprisnil developed endometrial changes during a phase III extension trial, and dosing was prematurely halted for all subjects (U.S. National Institutes of Health Clinical Trials, 2008).

Uterine Artery Embolization (UAE).

UAE is an angiographic interventional procedure that delivers polyvinyl alcohol (PVA) microspheres or other synthetic particulate emboli into both uterine arteries. Uterine blood flow is thereby obstructed, producing ischemia and necrosis. Because vessels serving leiomyomas have a larger caliber, these microspheres are preferentially directed to the tumors, sparing the surrounding myometrium.

During UAE, an angiographic catheter is placed in either femoral artery and advanced under fluoroscopic guidance to sequentially catheterize both uterine arteries (Figs. 9-10 and 9-11). Failure to embolize both uterine arteries allows existing collateral circulation between the two uterine arteries to sustain leiomyoma blood flow and is associated with significantly lower success rates (Bratby, 2008).

UAE is a management option for women with uterine leiomyomas who have significant symptoms despite medical management and who might otherwise be considered a candidate for hysterectomy or myomectomy. Due to pregnancy complications following UAE, this procedure is typically not considered for

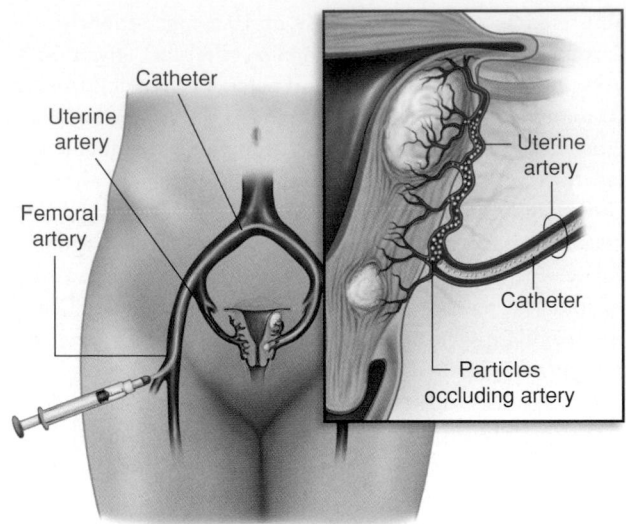

FIGURE 9-10 Diagram of uterine artery embolization (UAE).

women who have not completed childbearing (Hovsepian, 2009; Stokes, 2010). Other patient limitations are listed in Table 9-3. In addition, not all leiomyomas are suitable. Specifically, pedunculated submucous or subserosal tumors are excluded, because of concerns for tumor necrosis and subsequent sloughing.

Prior to UAE, a woman should have a thorough evaluation by her gynecologist (American College of Obstetricians and Gynecologists, 2004). Patients should have a current Pap smear, negative testing for *Neisseria gonorrhoeae* and *Chlamydia trachomatis*, and saline "wet prep" results that are clear of infection. Endometrial biopsy should be completed in those with endometrial cancer risk factors. Complete blood count, creatine level, prothrombin time, and partial thromboplastin time should also be obtained (Andrews, 2009; Bradley, 2009).

Following UAE, pain typically requires a 24- to 48-hour hospital admission for management. For subsequent pain control, most patients can usually be prescribed NSAIDs and have a rapid return to daily activities (Edwards, 2007). However, as a result of leiomyoma necrosis, approximately 10 percent of patients develop significant postprocedural symptoms and require hospital readmission. The *postembolization syndrome* usually lasts 2 to 7 days and is classically marked by pelvic pain and cramping, nausea and vomiting, low-grade fever, and malaise. White blood cell count elevation is common and seen in approximately 20 percent of cases (Ganguli, 2008). Intensity of these symptoms varies, and pain management strategies include oral, intravenous, epidural, or patient-controlled analgesia regimens.

Ultimately, embolization is effective for leiomyoma-related symptoms. Several randomized controlled trials have shown high rates of patient satisfaction and symptom improvement (Dutton, 2007; Edwards, 2007; Goodwin, 2008; Hehenkamp, 2008). Compared with hysterectomy, UAE is associated with shorter hospitalization, reduced 24-hour pain scores, and earlier return to daily activities. UAE also compares favorably with myomectomy for symptom relief (Goodwin, 2006; Siskin, 2006). However, many patients do not achieve adequate improvement, and long-term surveillance reveals that approximately 25 percent of UAE-treated patients will require an additional

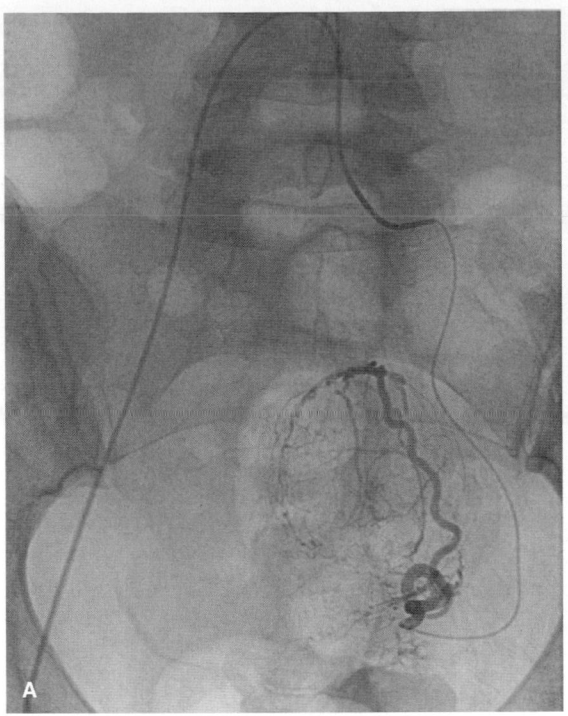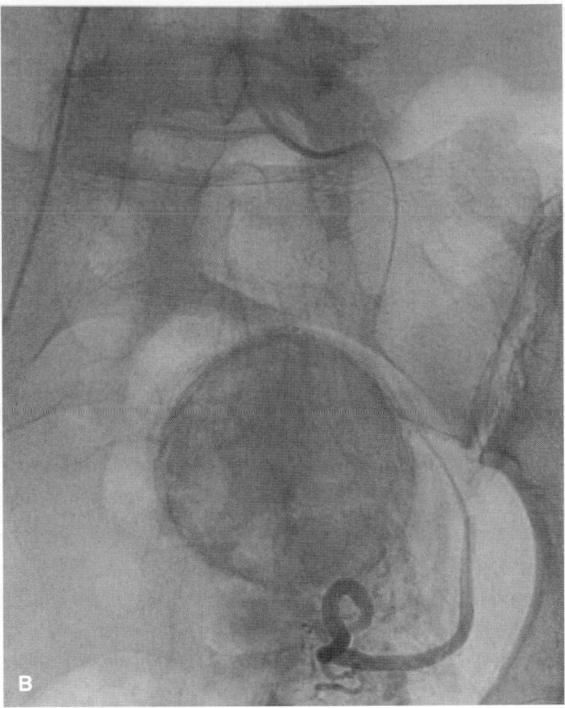

FIGURE 9-11 Fluoroscopic images obtained during uterine artery embolization (UAE). **A.** Before embolization, the leiomyoma can be identified by its numerous, hypertrophied, tortuous arteries wrapping around its periphery and extending within it. **B.** After embolization, most of the blood vessels are occluded by particles and appear truncated. Leiomyomas are again easily visualized and appear dark and smudged as the contrast/particle mixture stagnates within the tumor. *(Images contributed by Dr. Samuel C. Chao.)*

TABLE 9-3. UAE Absolute and Relative Contraindications

Absolute
Pregnancy
Active uterine or adnexal infection
Suspected reproductive tract malignancy[a]

Relative	**Reason**
Coagulopathy	Bleeding complications
Renal impairment	Renal effects of contrast
Desire for future fertility	Pregnancy complications
Uterine size >20–24 weeks	Difficult to embolize
Prior salpingectomy or salpingo-oophorectomy	Altered arterial anatomy
Prior pelvic radiation	Altered arterial anatomy
Concurrent GnRH agonist use	Hinders embolization
Pedunculated: subserosal or submucous leiomyoma	Necrosis causes detachment
Large hydrosalpinx	Increased infection risk
Severe contrast allergy	Allergic reaction risk

[a]May be used palliatively or as an adjunct to surgery.
GnRH = gonadotropin-releasing hormone; UAE = uterine artery embolization.
Compiled from American College of Obstetricians and Gynecologists, 2008; American Society of Reproductive Medicine, 2006; Hovsepian, 2009; Stokes, 2010.

---

subsequent procedure (Dutton, 2007; Goodwin, 2008; Kooij, 2010).

There are a number of complications associated with UAE. Leiomyoma tissue passage is common and likely is seen only with leiomyomas that have contact with the endometrial surface. Necrotic leiomyomas that pass into the vagina usually can be removed in the office. Those that do not pass spontaneously from the uterine cavity or that remain firmly attached to the uterine wall may require dilatation and evacuation (Spies, 2002). Groin hematoma and prolonged vaginal discharge are other frequent complications (Volkers, 2006). Transient amenorrhea, which lasts at most a few menstrual cycles, is also commonly seen following UAE and can be associated with transiently increased FSH levels (Hovsepian, 2006; Tropeano, 2010). Permanent amenorrhea, however, develops occasionally, and more commonly in older patients (Hehenkamp, 2007). This likely results from concurrent embolization of the ovaries via the anastomosis between the uterine and ovarian arteries. Rarely, embolization may also involve and incite necrosis of surrounding tissues such as the uterus, adnexa, bladder, and soft tissues.

A number of complications have been identified in women during pregnancy subsequent to UAE. Although the number of evaluable pregnancies is small, consistent complications include increased rates of miscarriage, postpartum hemorrhage, and cesarean delivery (Homer, 2010). Other complications noted by some, but not all studies, include higher rates of preterm delivery, fetal malpresentation, fetal-growth restriction, and abnormal placentation (Goldberg, 2004; Pron, 2005; Walker, 2006).

Magnetic Resonance Imaging-Guided Focused Ultra-sound (MRgFUS). Preliminary studies indicate that this therapy is a safe and feasible, minimally invasive alternative for leiomyoma treatment. In 2004, the FDA approved the device for this procedure (Stewart, 2003). As discussed in Chapter 2 (p. 55), this technique focuses ultrasound energy to a degree that heats targeted leiomyomas to incite necrosis during 2- to 3-hour treatment sessions. Advantageously, it is noninvasive, is performed with conscious sedation, and is associated with rapid recovery and return to daily activities. However, studies have shown that 28 percent of women seek alternative treatments for their symptoms by 12 months following MRgFUS (Fennessy, 2007; Stewart, 2006). Moreover, not all patients are suitable candidates. Contraindications include obstructions to the energy path such as abdominal wall scars or intraabdominal clips, total uterine size >24 weeks, a desire for future fertility, or contraindications to MR imaging. Moreover, leiomyoma characteristics such as size, blood perfusion qualities, and location near adjacent tissues may limit feasibility (Hesley, 2008). Although few major adverse events have been documented, long-term data regarding the duration of symptom relief are limited (Stewart, 2007).

Surgical Management

Bleeding and pain symptoms may improve in many women using medical treatment or radiologic interventions. However, for many, surgery for leiomyomas is necessary and includes hysterectomy, myomectomy, and myolysis.

Hysterectomy. Removal of the uterus is the definitive and most common surgical treatment for leiomyomas. Hysterectomy for leiomyomas can be performed vaginally, abdominally, or laparoscopically. Approximately, 600,000 hysterectomies are performed annually in the United States. Although the most common indication is leiomyomas, the percentage performed for this indication has trended downward from 44 percent in 2000 to 38 percent in 2004 (Whiteman, 2008). In a study of 418 women undergoing hysterectomy for benign gynecologic conditions, Carlson and coworkers (1994) found that hysterectomy for women with symptomatic leiomyomas resulted in satisfaction rates greater than 90 percent. There were marked improvements in pelvic pain, urinary symptoms, fatigue, psychological symptoms, and sexual dysfunction.

Removal of the ovaries is not required. The decision to perform oophorectomy at the time of hysterectomy factors age and cancer risk, among others, and is discussed fully in Section 41-12 (p. 1045). Other considerations prior to hysterectomy include uterine size and preoperative hematocrit. In some cases, preoperative GnRH agonist use may provide advantages.

Myomectomy. Resection of tumors is an option for symptomatic women who desire future childbearing or for those who decline hysterectomy. This can be performed laparoscopically, hysteroscopically, or via laparotomy incision, and each is described in detail in the surgical atlas. Myomectomy usually improves pain, infertility, or bleeding. For example, menorrhagia improves in approximately 70 to 80 percent of patients following tumor removal (Buttram, 1981; Olufowobi, 2004).

Myomectomy Versus Hysterectomy. Historically, hysterectomy has been recommended for women not seeking pregnancy. Many believed that myomectomy, compared with hysterectomy, carried a greater risk for perioperative morbidity. As experience accrued, myomectomy has been shown to be effective and to carry perioperative risks comparable with hysterectomy. In a number of reports, blood loss, intraoperative injuries, and febrile morbidity were similar (Iverson, 1996; Sawin, 2000).

Disadvantageously, postoperative intraabdominal adhesions and leiomyoma recurrence are more common after myomectomy compared with hysterectomy (Stricker, 1994). Recurrence rates following myomectomy range from 40 to 50 percent (Acien, 1996; Fedele, 1995). New leiomyoma development appears diminished in women who become pregnant following myomectomy, perhaps because of protective effects of increasing parity (Candiani, 1991).

Laparoscopic Myomectomy. Laparoscopic leiomyoma resection may be performed with successful outcomes (Hurst, 2005; Mais, 1996). In one study, Seracchioli and coworkers (2000) reviewed results of 131 women following myomectomy for at least one large leiomyoma. They reported equivalent pregnancy rates with fewer transfusions, shorter hospital stays, and less febrile morbidity in women undergoing laparoscopic resection compared with laparotomy. Moreover, laparoscopic myomectomy appears to incite less adhesion formation than does laparotomy (Bulletti, 1996; Dubuisson, 2000; Takeuchi, 2002).

Limitations to a laparoscopic approach, however, include uterine size and laparoscopic surgical skills, especially suturing techniques. Most advocate a multilayer suture closure of leiomyoma beds following enucleation to mirror that with abdominal myomectomy (Agdi, 2010; Glasser, 2008; Parker, 2006). In addition, several investigators have recommended limiting resection to those tumors less than 8 to 10 cm because of increased hemorrhage and operating time with larger tumors (Dubuisson, 2001; Takeuchi, 2003).

Hysteroscopy. Hysteroscopic resection of submucous leiomyomas has long-term effectiveness of 60 to 90 percent for the treatment of menorrhagia (Derman, 1991; Emanuel, 1999; Hallez, 1995). Hysteroscopic leiomyoma resection also improves fertility rates, especially when tumors are the sole cause of infertility (Fernandez, 2001; Vercellini, 1999). In their review, Donnez and Jadoul (2002) calculated an overall pregnancy rate of 45 percent following hysteroscopic tumor resection in women with leiomyoma as their sole identified source of infertility.

Endometrial Ablation. There are several tissue-destructive modalities that can ablate the endometrium, and they are discussed in detail in Section 42-17 (p. 1169). These techniques are effective for women with dysfunctional uterine bleeding, but when used as a sole technique for leiomyoma-related bleeding, the failure rate approaches 40 percent (Goldfarb, 1999; Yin, 1998). The use of this technique is also limited by the size and location of the leiomyoma. In some cases, ablation is used as an adjunct following hysteroscopic leiomyoma resection in women with menorrhagia.

Investigational Approaches. A number of techniques are available to induce leiomyoma necrosis and shrinkage. These include mono- or bipolar electrosurgery, laser vaporization, or cryotherapy. All of these techniques are used laparoscopically and consume a great deal of operating room time, incite variable degrees of necrosis within the leiomyoma and surrounding normal myometrium, and produce significant postoperative pain. Data regarding long-term symptom relief, recurrence rates, and effects on fertility and pregnancy are lacking (Agdi, 2008; Levy, 2008).

Methods to occlude the uterine artery have also been investigated. These include laparoscopic bilateral artery ligation and an approach that places transvaginal clamps temporarily across the uterine arteries (Hald, 2009; Holub, 2008; Vilos, 2010). Until clinical trials are done, all of the methods described here are currently considered experimental (Sharp, 2006).

Hematometra
Pathogenesis

In this condition, menstrual outflow obstruction traps blood and distends the uterus and at times, the proximal cervix. Many cases of hematometra develop at menarche if menstrual flow is obstructed by congenital anomalies (Chap. 18, p. 492). In this setting, a distended vagina, termed *hematocolpos,* is also commonly associated, and distended fallopian tubes, called *hematosalpinx,* may be seen. A number of acquired abnormalities such as scarring and neoplasms can also obstruct menstrual flow. For example, hematometra may follow radiation treatment, prolonged hypoestrogenism with atrophy, or surgeries of the endometrial cavity or endocervical canal. Similarly, it may develop in those with Asherman syndrome or with malignancies of the uterus or cervix.

Diagnosis

Women with hematometra classically complain of cyclic, midline pain. But they can also present with vague complaints such as low back pain and pelvic fullness. With total obstruction, there is amenorrhea. Partial obstruction causes pain accompanied by scant dark bleeding that may have a foul odor and may not be cyclic. If uterine distension is significant, compression by the large uterus can even result in urinary retention or constipation. If secondary infection and pyometra develop, fever and leukocytosis may be noted. Findings on pelvic examination include an enlarged, soft, or even cystic midline uterine corpus that may be tender to palpation. Clinical findings may mimic early pregnancy, leiomyoma cystic degeneration, leiomyosarcoma, and gestational trophoblastic disease. Thus, urine or serum β-hCG assay may be helpful. Importantly, in cases in which the underlying cause is unclear, endocervical and endometrial biopsy is helpful to exclude malignancy.

Sonography is the principal diagnostic tool. Imaging shows a smooth, symmetric hypoechoic enlargement of the uterine cavity (Fig. 9-12). Low-level internal echoes may variably be present (Wu, 1999). A hematosalpinx is seen less commonly

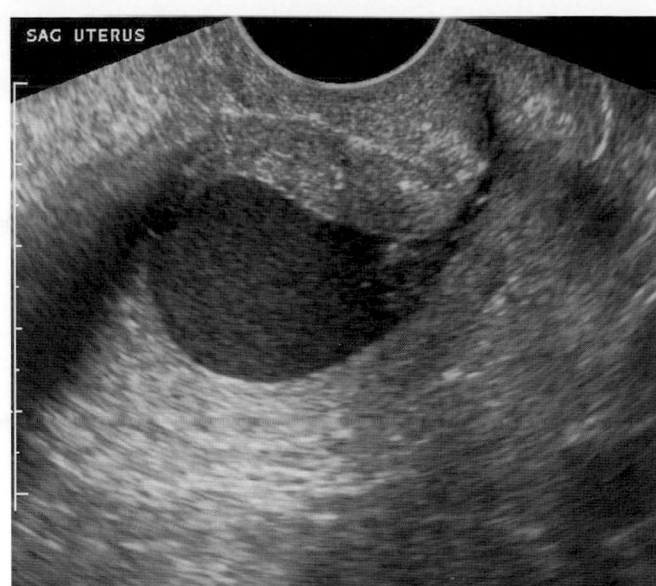

FIGURE 9-12 Sonographic transvaginal sagittal image of hematometra. The uterine walls and proximal cervix are dilated by retained blood, which appears hypoechoic. *(Image contributed by Dr. Elysia Moschos.)*

and is identified as hypoechoic tubular distensions lateral to the uterus (Sailer, 1979). MR imaging can also be used to help determine the exact location of the obstruction and may provide a more complete anatomic evaluation.

Treatment

For most cases of hematometra, relief of the obstruction and evacuation of blood are the goals. Cervical dilatation usually relieves the accumulation (Borten, 1984). Some have described hysteroscopy following dilatation to access blood pockets and to lyse adhesions (Cooper, 2000). Congenital abnormalities may require more extensive procedures to correct the obstruction (Chap. 18, p. 492).

Adenomyosis

Adenomyosis is characterized by uterine enlargement caused by ectopic rests of endometrium—both glands and stroma—located deep within the myometrium. These rests may be scattered throughout the myometrium—*diffuse adenomyosis,* or they may form a circumscribed nodular focal collection—*focal adenomyosis.* Although either form may be suspected clinically, the diagnosis is usually based on histologic findings in surgical specimens. Accordingly, reported incidences in hysterectomy specimens vary depending on the histologic criteria as well as the degree of sectioning, but range from 20 to 60 percent (Bird, 1972; Parazzini, 1997).

Pathophysiology

Anatomy. On gross examination, there typically is global uterine enlargement, but this rarely exceeds that of a 12-week pregnancy. The surface contour is smooth and regular and generalized softening and reddish myometrial discoloration is common. The grossly cut uterine surface typically appears spongy with focal areas of hemorrhage (Fig. 9-13).

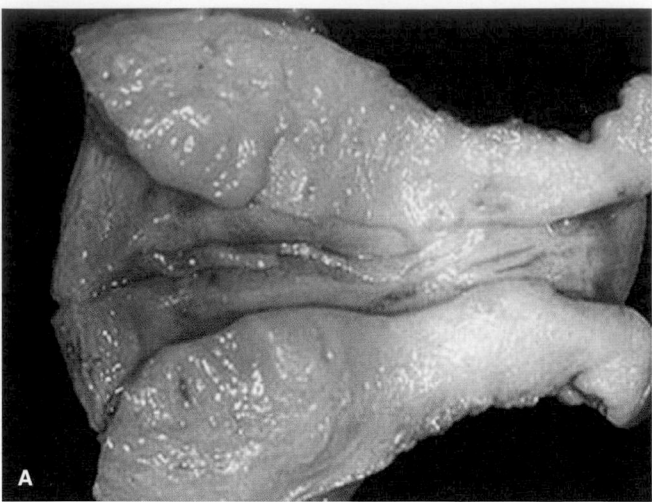
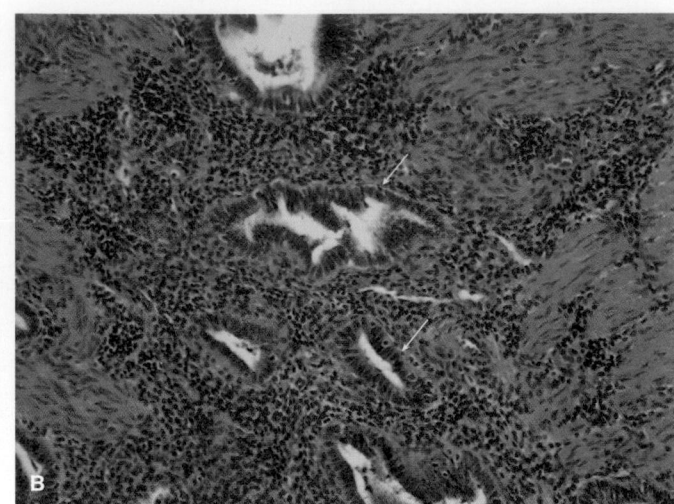

FIGURE 9-13 Adenomyosis. **A.** Gross bivalved uterine specimen. Note the spongy texture of this uterus with adenomyosis. **B.** Microscopically benign endometrial glands (*arrows*) and stroma infiltrate deeply into the myometrium. *(Photographs contributed by Dr. Raheela Ashfaq.)*

The ectopic foci of glands and stroma that are found in the myometrium in adenomyosis originate from the basalis layer of the endometrium. Because cells from the basalis layer do not undergo the typical proliferative and secretory changes during the menstrual cycle, hemorrhage within these foci is minimal.

Pathogenesis. The most widely held theory regarding adenomyosis development describes the downward invagination of the endometrial basalis layer into the myometrium. The endometrial-myometrial interface is unique from most mucosal-muscular interfaces in that it lacks an intervening submucosa. Accordingly, even in normal uteri, the endometrium commonly invades the myometrium superficially.

Mechanisms that incite deep myometrial invasion are unknown, but in some cases, there is myometrial weakness caused by prior pregnancy or surgery, or by decreased immunologic activity at the endometrial-myometrial interface (Ferenczy, 1998; Levgur, 2000). Estrogen and progesterone likely play a role in its development and maintenance. For example, adenomyosis develops during the reproductive years and regresses after menopause. Regardless of the permissive cause, cell migration and invasion proceed.

An alternative theory is that adenomyosis is caused by metaplasia of pluripotent müllerian tissue.

Risk Factors

Parity and age are significant risk factors for adenomyosis. Specifically, nearly 90 percent of cases are in parous women, and nearly 80 percent develop in women in their 40s and 50s (Lee, 1984).

Adenomyosis is associated with other pathologies that are affected by cytochrome P450 aromatase expression and higher tissue estrogen levels. These include leiomyomas, endometriosis, and endometrial cancer (Azziz, 1989). As discussed in Chapter 10, however, endometriosis has markedly different epidemiologic characteristics and is thought to arise from another mechanism. Oral contraceptives are not associated with

adenomyosis, however, adenomyosis is found more commonly in women taking the selective estrogen-receptor modulator, tamoxifen (Cohen, 1997; Parazzini, 1997). Other identified potential risk factors are history of chronic endometritis, abortion, uterine trauma from childbirth, and hyperestrogenism.

Symptoms

Approximately one third of women with adenomyosis have symptoms. Their severity correlates with increasing number of ectopic foci and extent of invasion (Levgur, 2000; Nishida, 1991; Sammour, 2002). Menorrhagia and dysmenorrhea are common. Menorrhagia possibly results from increased and abnormal vascularization of the endometrial lining. Dysmenorrhea is thought to be caused by increased prostaglandin production found in adenomyotic tissues compared with that in normal myometrium (Koike, 1992). Perhaps 10 percent of women with adenomyosis complain of dyspareunia. Because adenomyosis typically develops in older parous women in their 40s and 50s, infertility is not a frequent complaint (Nikkanen, 1980).

Diagnosis

Cancer Antigen 125 (CA125). For many years, the diagnosis of adenomyosis in most cases has been made retrospectively following pathologic evaluation of a hysterectomy specimen. Serum levels of the tumor marker CA125 have been evaluated as a diagnostic tool but have not proved to be helpful. Although CA125 levels are typically elevated in women with adenomyosis, they may also be elevated in those with leiomyomas, endometriosis, pelvic infection, and pelvic malignancies (Menon, 1999).

Sonography. Transabdominal sonography does not consistently identify the often subtle myometrial changes of adenomyosis, thus imaging with TVS is preferred, and MR imaging may be complementary (Bazot, 2001; Reinhold, 1998).

In the hands of experienced sonographers, findings of diffuse adenomyosis may include: (1) anterior or posterior myometrial

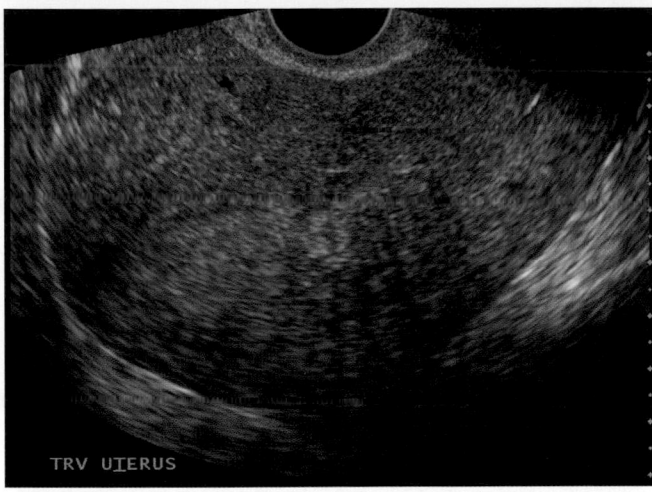

FIGURE 9-14 Sonographic transvaginal sagittal image of adeno-myosis. *(Image contributed by Dr. Elysia Moschos.)*

wall appearing thicker than its counterpart, (2) myometrial texture heterogeneity, (3) small myometrial hypoechoic cysts, representing cystic glands within ectopic endometrial foci, (4) striated projections extending from the endometrium into the myometrium, and (5) ill-defined endometrial echo (Fig. 9-14) (Reinhold, 1999).

Focal adenomyosis appears as discrete hypoechoic nodules that may sometimes be differentiated from leiomyomas by their poorly defined margins, elliptical rather than globular shape, minimal mass effect on surrounding tissues, lack of calcifications, and presence of anechoic cysts of varying diameter (Fedele, 1992; Reinhold, 1998).

Because these findings are often subtle, operator experience influences diagnostic accuracy more than with most other pelvic pathology. Moreover, the presence of other concurrent uterine disease such as leiomyomas or endometrial cancer also limits accuracy. In these settings, MR imaging has proved highly accurate for diagnosis (Fig. 2-33, p. 56).

Management

Medical Treatment. The main objective of treatment is relief from pain and bleeding. Conservative therapy for symptomatic adenomyosis is similar to that for primary menorrhagia or dysmenorrhea (Chap. 8, p. 237). First, NSAIDs are often given (Fraser, 1986; Marjoribanks, 2003). Combination oral contraceptives and progestin-only regimens can be used to induce endometrial atrophy and decrease endometrial prostaglandin production to improve dysmenorrhea and menorrhagia. The levonorgestrel-releasing intrauterine system, marketed as Mirena, has also been shown effective for treatment of adenomyosis-related bleeding (Bragheto, 2007; Sheng, 2009).

Because adenomyosis and endometriosis share endometrial origins, some have used GnRH agonists or danazol in a fashion similar to the treatment of endometriosis. There have been no clinical trials, however, to study these practices.

Interventional Treatment. Hysterectomy is the definitive treatment and as with other conditions, the type of surgical procedure depends on uterine size and associated uterine or abdominopelvic pathology.

Endometrial ablation or resection using hysteroscopy has been used to successfully treat dysmenorrhea and menorrhagia caused by adenomyosis (Molnar, 1997; Wortman, 2000). However, complete eradication of deep adenomyosis is problematic, and residual disease is responsible for a significant number of treatment failures. Because of this, McCausland and McCausland (1996) recommended preoperative sonography or MR imaging to identify deep lesions and to thereby improve patient selection. Another caveat is that any injury to the endometrial lining, including ablation, may be the initiating insult that activates endometrial tissue to grow into the myometrium, thus *causing* adenomyosis.

Uterine artery embolization (p. 256) has also been used to relieve symptoms for some women. However, success rates vary widely, ranging from 25 to 85 percent, and approximately 50 percent of patients still require eventual hysterectomy (Jha, 2003; Kim, 2007; Lohle, 2007; Stokes, 2010; Toh, 2003).

Myometrial Hypertrophy

In some women, especially those with high parity, there is global enlargement of the uterus but no associated underlying identifiable pathology found in hysterectomy specimens (Fraser, 1987). Also known as gravid hypertrophy, this condition results from myometrial fiber enlargement and not hyperplasia or interstitial fibrosis (Traiman, 1996). One definition includes uterine weights exceeding 120 g for nulliparas and 210 g for multiparas (Zaloudek, 2002). Symptoms are uncommon but may include menstrual irregularities, and of these, menorrhagia is the most frequent complaint.

Uterine or Cervical Diverticula

These rare ballooned sacculations communicate with and extend out from the endometrial cavity or endocervical canal. Many develop after cesarean delivery and are thought to arise at sites of uterine dehiscence. Others are thought to be congenital anomalies developing from a localized duplication of the distal müllerian duct on one side (Engel, 1984). The diverticulum may serve as a passive repository for menstrual flow, with intermittent expulsion of blood producing pain and intermenstrual bleeding. In addition, these saccules may become secondarily infected (Umezaki, 2004).

Transvaginal sonography (TVS) or saline infusion sonography are typically used to evaluate women with these symptoms. Hysterosalpingography, hysteroscopy, and MR imaging have been used to show communication to the endometrium (Erickson, 1999). Treatment includes excision of the diverticulum or hysterectomy.

OVARY

Ovarian masses are a frequent finding in general gynecology. Of these masses, most are cystic, and functional ovarian cysts

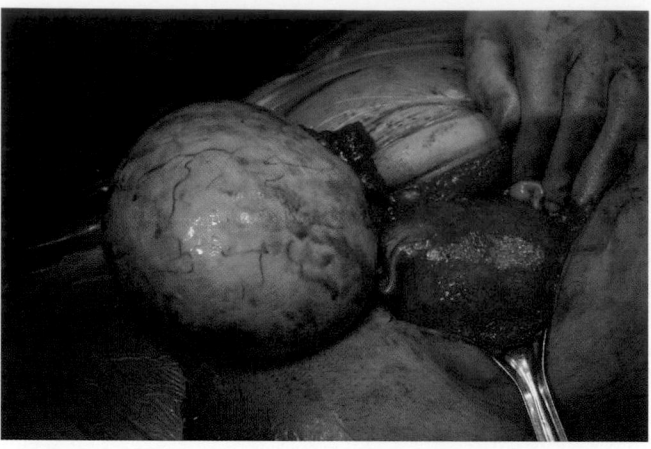

FIGURE 9-15 Intraoperative photograph of a large benign mucinous cystadenoma. The fimbriated end of the fallopian tube is seen above the ovary, and the uterus lies to the right.

comprise a large portion. Neoplasms constitute most of the remainder, and the majority of these are benign (Fig. 9-15). However, despite continuous improvement in diagnostic methods, it is often impossible to clinically differentiate between benign and malignant conditions. Thus, management must balance concerns of performing an operation for an innocent lesion with the risk of not removing an ovarian malignancy.

Ovarian Cystic Masses as a Group

Histologically, ovarian cystic masses are often divided into those derived from neoplastic growth, *ovarian cystic neoplasms*, and those created by disruption of normal ovulation, *functional ovarian cysts*. Differentiation of these is not always clinically apparent using either imaging tools or tumor markers. Accordingly, ovarian cysts are often managed as a single composite clinical entity.

These cysts often require excision because of symptoms or the possibility of cancer, and consequently, their economic impact is significant. In their review of U.S. inpatient hospitalization for 2010, Whiteman and colleagues (2010) reported that approximately 7 percent of gynecologic admissions were for benign ovarian cysts.

Pathogenesis

The incidence of ovarian cysts varies only slightly with patient demographics and ranges from 5 to 15 percent (Dorum, 2005; Millar, 1993; Porcu, 1994). The exact mechanisms leading to cyst formation are unclear. Angiogenesis is an essential component of both the follicular and luteal phases of the ovarian cycle. It also participates in various pathologic ovarian processes, including follicular cyst formation, polycystic ovarian syndrome, ovarian hyperstimulation syndrome, and benign and malignant ovarian neoplasms. There is evidence that vascular endothelial growth factor (VEGF) serves as a major mediator of angiogenesis and specifically as it factors into the development of ovarian neoplasms (Gómez-Raposo, 2009). Accordingly, monoclonal antibodies that target VEGF have proved effective in the treatment of many ovarian cancers (Kumaran, 2009).

Symptoms

Most women with ovarian cysts are asymptomatic. If symptoms develop, pain and vague pressure sensations are common. Cyclic pain with menstruation may indicate endometriosis with an associated endometrioma. Intermittent pain may reflect early torsion, whereas acute severe pain may indicate torsion with resulting ovarian ischemia. Other causes of acute pain include cyst rupture or tuboovarian abscess. In contrast, vague pressure or achiness may be the only symptom and can result from stretching of the ovarian capsule. In advanced ovarian malignancies, women complain of increased abdominal girth and early satiety from ascites or from an enlarged ovary.

In some women, evidence of hormonal disruption may be found. For example, excess estrogen production from granulosa cell stimulation may disrupt normal menstruation or initiate bleeding, even in prepubertal or postmenopausal patients. Similarly, virilization may result from increased androgens produced by theca cell stimulation.

Diagnosis

Many ovarian cysts are asymptomatic and found incidentally on routine pelvic examination or during imaging studies for another indication. Findings may vary, but typically masses are mobile, cystic, nontender, and found lateral to the uterus.

Human Chorionic Gonadotropin. In the evaluation of adnexal pathology, serum β-hCG testing provides valuable information. Detection of serum β-hCG may indicate ectopic pregnancy or a corpus luteum of pregnancy. Less commonly, β-hCG can also serve as a tumor marker in defining ovarian neoplasm.

Tumor Markers. Tumor markers are typically proteins that are produced by tumor cells or by the body in response to tumor cells. Several such markers have been used to identify ovarian malignancies.

Cancer antigen 125 is an antigenic determinant on a high-molecular-weight glycoprotein produced by mesothelial cells that line the peritoneal, pleural, and pericardial cavities. It is used as a tumor marker because serum levels are often elevated in women with epithelial ovarian cancer. Unfortunately, CA125 is not a tumor-specific antigen, and it is elevated in up to 1 percent of healthy controls. It may also be elevated in women with nonmalignant disease such as leiomyomas, endometriosis, and salpingitis. Despite these limitations, serum CA125 determinations may be helpful and are often used in the evaluation of ovarian cysts. Serum alpha-fetoprotein (AFP) levels may be elevated in those rare patients with a yolk sac tumor or embryonal cell carcinoma. Increased serum levels of β-hCG may indicate an ovarian choriocarcinoma, a mixed germ cell tumor, or embryonal cell carcinoma. Inhibins A and B are markers for granulosa cell tumors. Lastly, lactate dehydrogenase (LDH) levels may be increased in those with dysgerminoma, whereas elevated carcinoembryonic antigen (CEA) and cancer antigen 19-9 (CA19-9) levels arise from secretions of mucinous epithelial ovarian carcinomas.

Imaging. Both transvaginal sonography (TVS) and transabdominal sonography (TAS) are excellent methods, and cyst size is the main determinant in selecting between the two. For lesions confined to the true pelvis, TVS has superior resolution, whereas TAS is more useful for large tumors (Marret, 2001). Characteristic findings for specific types of ovarian cysts have been described and have also been defined to discriminate malignant from benign lesions (Table 9-4) (Granberg, 1989; Minaretzis, 1994; Okugawa, 2001).

Traditional gray-scale sonography may also be augmented with color flow Doppler. Transvaginal color Doppler sonography (TV-CDS) may add information regarding the nature of the lesion, its malignant potential, and the presence of torsion (Emoto, 1997; Rosado, 1992; Wu, 1994). However, for assessing simple ovarian cysts and the risk of malignancy, TV-CDS typically provides no significant advantage compared with conventional TVS (Vuento, 1995).

Use of MR imaging for ovarian cyst evaluation has been investigated. Its added value compared with sonography is limited in most clinical settings. However, MR imaging may clarify situations in which anatomy or patient habitus complicates sonographic imaging (Outwater, 1996).

Management

Observation. Most ovarian cysts are functional, and most spontaneously regress within 6 months of identification. High-dose oral contraceptive pills have been used by some to hasten functional cyst resolution. However, several investigators have found no additional benefit to this adjunctive therapy (American College of Obstetricians and Gynecologists, 2010; Grimes, 2009; Turan, 1994).

The risk of ovarian malignancy increases with age. Despite this, for postmenopausal women with a simple ovarian cyst, expectant management may also be reasonable. A number of investigators have confirmed the safety of this approach when several criteria are met: (1) sonographic evidence of a thin-walled, unilocular cyst, (2) cyst diameter less than 5 cm, (3) no cyst enlargement during surveillance, and (4) normal serum CA125 level (Menon, 1999; Nardo, 2003). Moreover, the American College of Obstetricians and Gynecologists (2007) notes that simple cysts up to 10 cm in diameter by sonographic evaluation may safely be followed even in postmenopausal women.

Surgical Excision. Despite efforts by researchers to classify lesions by radiologic and serologic means, there is considerable morphologic similarity among cyst types and between those that are malignant and benign. Accordingly, for many cases, surgical excision of the cyst serves as the definitive diagnostic tool.

Cystectomy Versus Oophorectomy. Of these, cystectomy offers the advantage of ovarian preservation, but at the risk of cyst rupture and tumor spill. With ovarian cancer, such spill and subsequent malignant seeding can worsen patient prognosis. Thus, the decision for one surgical technique in preference over the other is influenced by lesion size, patient age, and intraoperative findings. For example, in premenopausal women, smaller lesions generally require only cystectomy with preserva-

tion of reproductive function. Larger lesions may necessitate oophorectomy because of increased risks of cyst rupture during enucleation, difficulty in reconstructing ovarian anatomy following large cyst removal, and the greater risk of malignancy in these bigger cysts. However, in postmenopausal women, oophorectomy is preferred because the risk for cancer is higher and benefits to ovarian salvage are limited (Okugawa, 2001).

Clinical findings of malignancy at the time of surgery will dictate further actions. Multiple small lesions studding the peritoneal surface, ascites, and exophytic growths extending from the ovarian capsule should prompt appropriate surgical staging and treatment for ovarian cancer as discussed in Chapters 35 and 36 (p. 868).

Laparoscopy. The surgical approach for cyst excision is also dictated by clinical factors. Laparoscopy has many advantages, but it generally has been underused for management of ovarian cysts. Concerns of increased rates of cyst rupture and tumor spill have caused many to avoid this modality. That said, many investigators have documented the safety of laparoscopic cystectomy and oophorectomy (Lin, 1995; Mais, 1995; Yuen, 1997).

Minilaparotomy. For small or moderately sized cysts, laparotomy incisions can usually be minimized. As a result, most who undergo minilaparotomy can be discharged the day of surgery (Berger, 1994; Flynn, 1999). Although minilaparotomy typically offers shorter operative times, lower rates of cyst rupture, and greater cost savings compared with laparoscopy, this approach can limit a surgeon's ability to lyse adhesions and inspect peritoneal surfaces for signs of ovarian malignancy.

Laparotomy. Women with a greater potential for malignancy are best managed by laparotomy with a midline vertical incision. This provides a surgical field large enough for oophorectomy or cyst enucleation without tumor rupture and for surgical staging if malignancy is found. In those with a low risk of malignancy and a smaller cyst, laparotomy through a low transverse incision may be appropriate.

Cyst Aspiration. Historically, there has been hesitation to aspirate ovarian cysts because of possible intraperitoneal seeding by early-stage ovarian cancer. Moreover, nondiagnostic, false-positive, and false-negative results are common (Dejmek, 2003; Martinez-Onsurbe, 2001; Moran, 1993). For these reasons, rare indications exist for this procedure alone.

Role of the Generalist. Ovarian cysts frequently require surgical treatment. Most of these lesions are benign and typically are removed by general gynecologists. When malignancy is present, however, formal cancer staging should accompany excision. Studies support that optimal surgical resection and proper staging performed by gynecologic oncologists during the primary operation for ovarian cancers are major factors in long-term survival. Thus, women with pelvic masses and preoperative findings suspicious for malignancy are generally referred. The American College of Obstetricians and Gynecologists (2011) and Society of Gynecologic Oncologists have jointly presented guidelines regarding clinical criteria that should prompt referral to a gynecologic oncologist (Table 9-5). If one or more criteria

TABLE 9-4. Recommended Management of Asymptomatic Ovarian Masses Found with Imaging

Type of Ovarian Mass	Recommendation
Cysts with Benign Qualities	
Simple Cyst	Simple cysts, regardless of patient age, are almost certainly benign
Premenopausal	
≤3 cm diameter	Normal anatomic finding
≤5 cm diameter	No additional treatment required
>5 but ≤7 cm diameter[a]	TVS repeated in 6–12 weeks to document resolution; if persistent, then yearly TVS[b]
>7 cm diameter[a]	MRI or surgical evaluation
Postmenopausal	
≤1 cm diameter	Normal anatomic finding
≤5 cm diameter[a]	CA125 measurement; if normal level, then TVS repeated in 6–12 weeks; if persistent cyst, then yearly TVS[b]
>7 cm diameter[a]	MRI or surgical evaluation
Hemorrhagic Cyst[c]	
Premenopausal	
≤3 cm diameter corpus luteum	Normal anatomic finding
≤5 cm diameter	No additional treatment required
>5 but ≤7 cm diameter	TVS repeated in 6–12 weeks; if persistent, then consider MRI or surgical evaluation
Early postmenopausal[d] Any size	CA125 measurement; if normal, then TVS repeated in 6–12 weeks; if persistent cyst, then consider MRI or surgical evaluation
Late postmenopausal[d] Any size	Surgical evaluation
Endometrioma	TVS repeated in 6–12 weeks; if persistent, then yearly TVS[b]
Mature cystic teratoma (dermoid cyst)	If not surgically removed[e], then yearly TVS[b]
Hydrosalpinx	May be observed as clinically indicated
Peritoneal inclusion cyst	May be observed as clinically indicated
Cysts with Indeterminate, but Probably Benign, Qualities	
Indeterminate for: hemorrhagic cyst, mature cystic teratoma, endometrioma	
Premenopausal	TVS repeated in 6–12 weeks; if persistent cyst, then consider surgical evaluation or MRI
Postmenopausal	Consider surgical evaluation
Thin-walled cyst with single thin septation or focal cyst wall calcification	Same as for simple cyst described above
Multiple thin septations (<3 mm)	Consider surgical evaluation
Nodule (non-hyperechoic) without flow	Consider surgical evaluation or MRI
Cysts with Qualities Suggesting Malignancy	
Thick (>3 mm) irregular septations	Consider surgical evaluation
Nodule with blood flow	Consider surgical evaluation

[a]The American College of Obstetricians and Gynecologists (ACOG) (2007) recommends a threshold up to 10 cm for simple cysts in all age groups.
[b]Shorter time interval may be selected for surveillance as clinically indicated.
[c]Color Doppler as an adjunct is recommended to exclude solid components.
[d]All postmenopausal women with an adnexal mass should undergo breast examination, digital rectal examination, and mammography, if not already performed in the last year due to the high rate of metastasis from other primary tumors to the ovary.
[e]Some studies have found that stable small dermoid cysts may be observed in premenopausal women.
CA125 = cancer antigen 125; MRI = magnetic resonance imaging; TVS = transvaginal sonography.
Adapted from American College of Obstetricians and Gynecologists, 2007; Levine, 2010.

TABLE 9-5. Guidelines for Referral of Newly Diagnosed Pelvic Mass to Gynecologic Oncologist

Premenopausal woman (<50 years)
Very elevated CA125 level
Ascites
Evidence of abdominal or distant metastasis
(by examination or imaging study)

Postmenopausal woman (≥50 years)
Elevated CA125 level
Ascites
Nodular or fixed pelvic mass
Evidence of abdominal or distant metastasis
(by examination or imaging study)

Compiled from the American College of Obstetricians and Gynecologists and Society of Gynecologic Oncologists, 2011.

from this list or other suspicious findings are identified, referral is recommended (Im, 2005).

Another potential tool to assist in appropriate referral is the OVA1 test. Described further in Chapter 35 (p. 861), this test is a serum screen for five biomarkers. It can be used to aid the triage of women already determined to require surgery for ovarian pathology.

Functional Ovarian Cysts

These are common, originate from ovarian follicles, and are created by hormonal dysfunction during ovulation. They are subcategorized as either *follicular cysts* or *corpus luteum cysts* based on both their pathogenesis and histologic qualities. They are not neoplasms and derive mass from accumulation of intrafollicular fluids rather than cellular proliferation. Hormonal dysfunction prior to ovulation results in expansion of the follicular antrum with serous fluid and formation of a follicular cyst. In contrast, following ovulation, excessive hemorrhage may fill the corpus luteum, creating a corpus luteum cyst. Although these cysts generally have similar symptoms and management, they differ in the potential hormones produced as well as histologic appearance.

Risk Factors

Smoking. Several epidemiologic studies have linked smoking with functional cyst development (Holt, 2005; Wyshak, 1988). Although the exact mechanism(s) by which cigarette smoking exerts its affect is unknown, changes in gonadotropin secretion and ovarian function are suspected (Michnovicz, 1986; Zumoff, 1990).

Contraception. High-dose oral hormonal contraceptives suppress ovarian activity and protect against cyst development (Ory, 1974). Subsequent studies, however, have shown only modest protective effects from low-dose monophasic or low-dose triphasic contraceptives (Chiaffarino, 1998; Holt, 2003). The American College of Obstetricians and Gynecologists

(2010) does not support the use of COCs for cyst prevention or treatment.

In contrast, there is an increased incidence of follicular cysts reported with many progestin-only contraceptives. Recall that continuous, low-dose progestins do not completely suppress ovarian function. As a result, dominant follicles may develop in response to gonadotropin secretion, yet the normal ovulatory process is frequently disrupted, and follicular cysts develop. In clinical studies, cystic masses were found on bimanual pelvic examination in 2 to 9 percent of women using the progestin-only implants (Brache, 2002). Similarly, levonorgestrel-containing intrauterine devices have been associated with the development of functional ovarian cysts (Inki, 2002).

Tamoxifen. Women treated with tamoxifen for breast cancer—either pre- or postmenopausal—have an increased risk for ovarian cyst formation. Most studies report rates of 15 to 30 percent compared with 7 percent cited for the general postmenopausal population (Cohen, 2003; Mourits, 1999). Premenopausal women are disparately affected, and from 30 to 80 percent develop cysts (Mourits, 1999; Shushan, 1996).

Most of these are believed to be functional cysts, but the exact mechanism by which tamoxifen stimulates their formation is unknown. Fortunately, most resolve with time whether tamoxifen treatment is continued or discontinued (Lindahl, 1997; Shushan, 1996). If small simple cysts are found, these women should undergo sonographic surveillance. However, if clinical signs of malignancy are present, then surgical exploration is indicated, and tamoxifen use is discontinued.

Diagnosis and Treatment

Functional cysts are managed similarly to other cystic ovarian lesions. Consequently, sonography is the imaging tool of choice for evaluation. Typically, follicular cysts are completely rounded anechoic lesions with thin, regular walls (Fig. 9-16).

Conversely, corpus luteum cysts are termed "great imitators" because of their varied sonographic characteristics

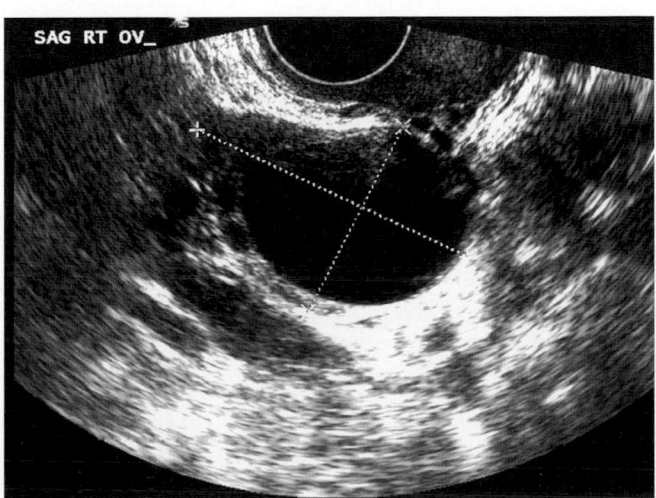

FIGURE 9-16 Sonographic transvaginal sagittal image of an ovary containing a follicular cyst. Note the smooth walls and lack of internal echoes. *(Image contributed by Dr. Elysia Moschos.)*

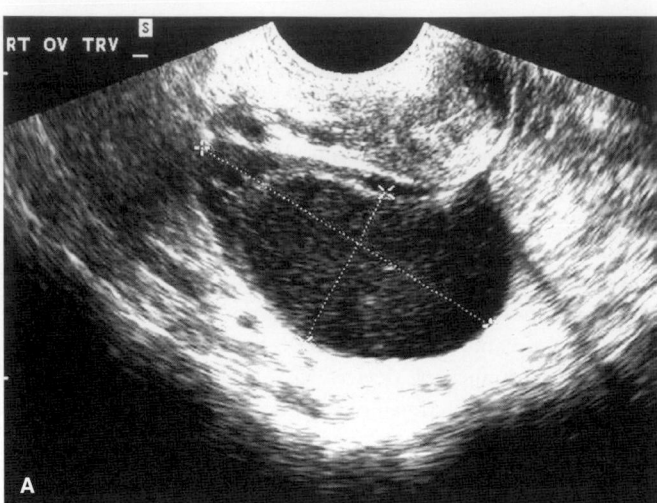
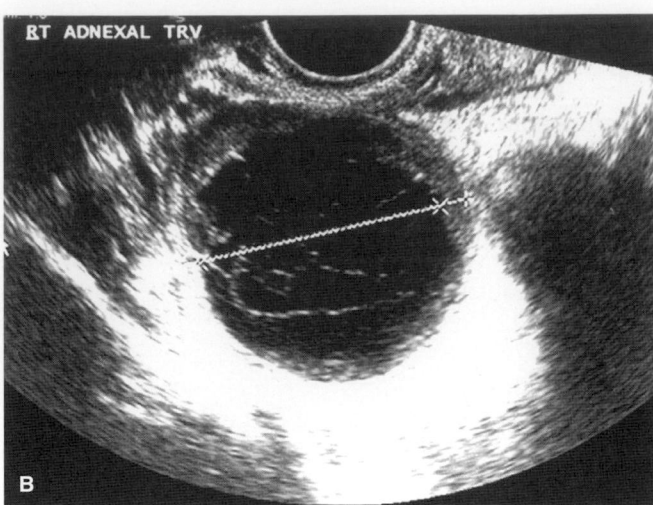

FIGURE 9-17 Sonographic transvaginal transverse images of two hemorrhagic corpus luteum cysts. **A.** Diffuse low-level echoes, which are commonly associated with hemorrhage, are seen throughout this smooth-walled cyst. **B.** Reticular interfaces are another commonly demonstrated sonographic finding within a resolving hemorrhagic cyst. *(Images contributed by Dr. Elysia Moschos.)*

(Fig. 9-17). Immediately following hemorrhage into its cavity, the cyst generally appears echogenic and mimics a solid mass. With evolution of the clot, a lacy reticular pattern develops. As the clot hemolyzes, a distinct line often forms between the serum and retracting clot. With further retraction, the clot may appear as an intramural nodule. Imaging with transvaginal color Doppler typically displays a brightly colored ring because of the increased vascularity surrounding the cyst (Swire, 2004; Yoffe, 1991). This *ring of fire* is also common to ectopic pregnancies (Fig. 7-7 p. 205).

If asymptomatic, women with findings of functional ovarian cyst may be observed. However, surgical evaluation is often required for persistent cysts.

Theca Lutein Cysts

These are an uncommon type of follicular cyst, characterized by luteinization and hypertrophy of their theca interna layer. Bilateral, multiple smooth-walled cysts form and range in size from 1 to 4 cm in diameter (Russell, 2009). This condition is termed *hyperreactio lutealis*, and the cysts are thought to result from stimulation by elevated (LH) or β-hCG levels. Commonly associated conditions include gestational trophoblastic disease, multifetal gestation, diabetes, fetal hydrops, and ovarian hyperstimulation during assisted reproductive techniques (Fig. 37-4, p. 901). These cysts typically resolve spontaneously following removal of the stimulating hormone source. Torsion may complicate this condition and is treated as described on page 270.

Benign Neoplastic Ovarian Cysts

These benign lesions, in combination with functional ovarian cysts, comprise most ovarian masses. Ovarian neoplasms can be distinguished histologically and are grouped as epithelial-stromal tumors, germ cell tumors, sex cord-stromal tumors,

and others shown in Table 9-6 depending on their cell type of origin. Of benign ovarian neoplasms, serous and mucinous cystadenomas and mature cystic teratoma are by far the most common (Pantoja, 1975b).

Benign Serous and Mucinous Tumors

These are members of the surface epithelial-stromal neoplasia group. *Benign serous tumors* are typically thin-walled, unilocular cysts filled with serous fluid and are lined by cells similar to those lining the fallopian tube. They are bilateral in up to 20 percent of cases. *Benign mucinous tumors* are typically thicker-walled, mucoid-containing tumors that may be small, but can often attain large diameters. They may be uni- or multilocular and are lined by a single columnar layer whose cells contain abundant mucin (Fig. 9-18) (Prat, 2009).

In categorizing tumors within the epithelial-stromal family, benign tumors are designated as *adenomas*; malignant tumors, as *carcinomas*; and those with exuberant cellular proliferation without invasive behavior as *low malignant potential* (Chen, 2003). The prefix *cyst-* describes predominantly cystic neoplasms. In most epithelial-stromal tumors, the epithelial component dominates. Thus, a benign cystic ovarian mass with a tubal-like epithelium is termed serous cystadenoma. In those in which ovarian stroma is prominent, the suffix *–fibroma* is used. Thus, *serous cystadenomafibroma* describes a benign, mainly cystic tumor of the ovarian epithelial-stromal tumor group in which solid stromal components are also prominent (Prat, 2009).

Ovarian Teratoma

These belong to the germ cell family of ovarian neoplasms. Teratomas arise from a single germ cell, and therefore, may contain any of the three germ layers—ectoderm, mesoderm, or endoderm. These layers typically form tissues that are foreign

TABLE 9-6. World Health Organization Histologic Classification of Ovarian Tumors

Surface epithelial-stromal tumors
  Serous tumors
  Mucinous tumors
  Endometrioid tumors
  Clear cell tumors
  Transitional cell tumors: Brenner tumor, transitional cell carcinoma (non-Brenner type)
  Squamous cell tumors
  Mixed epithelial tumors
  Undifferentiated carcinoma

Sex cord-stromal tumors
  Granulosa-stromal cell tumors: granulosa cell tumors, thecoma-fibroma group
  Sertoli-stromal cell tumors
  Sex cord tumor with annular tubules
  Gynandroblastoma
  Unclassified
  Steroid (lipid) cell tumors: stromal luteoma, Leydig cell tumor, unclassified

Germ cell tumors
  Dysgerminoma
  Yolk sac tumors (endodermal sinus tumors)
  Embryonal carcinoma
  Polyembryoma
  Choriocarcinoma
  Teratomas: immature, mature, monodermal, mixed germ cell

Others
  Gonadoblastoma
  Germ cell sex cord-stromal tumor of nongonadoblastoma type
  Tumors of rete ovarii
  Mesothelial tumors
  Tumors of uncertain origin, miscellaneous tumors
  Gestational trophoblastic diseases
  Soft tissue tumors not specific to ovary
  Malignant lymphomas, leukemias, plasmacytomas
  Unclassified tumors
  Secondary (metastatic) tumors
  Tumorlike lesions

Adapted from Chen, 2003; Scully, 1999.

to the ovary and that have a disorganized structure. As a result, teratomas usually contain a haphazard collection of tissues such as hair, fat, bone, and teeth. Aptly, their name derives from the Greek word *teras*, meaning monster. The term "dermoid" was later coined to describe these tumors, because of the prevalence of dermal elements in these cysts (Pantoja, 1975b).

Teratomas are classified as:

Immature teratoma—This neoplasm is malignant. Immature tissues from one, two, or all three germ cell layers are found and frequently coexist with mature elements.

Mature teratoma—This benign tumor contains mature forms of the three germ cell layers, and subcategories include:

(1) Mature cystic teratomas develop into cystic structures and may be known by several names, including *mature cystic teratoma, benign cystic teratoma,* and *dermoid cyst.*
(2) Mature solid teratoma has elements formed within a solid mass.
(3) Fetiform teratomas or homunculus forms a doll-shape and contains a solid arrangement of the germ cell layers that displays considerably normal spatial differentiation.

Monodermal teratoma—This benign tumor is composed either solely or predominantly of only one highly specialized tissue type. Of the monodermal teratomas, those composed dominantly of thyroid tissue are termed *struma ovarii.*

Mature Cystic Teratoma. These common tumors comprise approximately 10 to 25 percent of all ovarian neoplasms and 60 percent of all benign ovarian neoplasms (Katsube, 1982; Koonings, 1989; Peterson, 1955).

Pathology. These cystic tumors are typically slow growing, and most measure between 5 and 10 cm (Comerci, 1994; Pantoja, 1975a). They are bilateral in approximately 10 percent of cases (Caruso, 1971; Katsube, 1982; Peterson, 1955). When sectioned, most cysts appear unilocular and typically contain one area of localized growth, which protrudes into the cystic cavity. Alternatively designated as *Rokitansky protuberance, dermoid plug, dermoid process, dermoid mamilla,* or *embryonal rudiment,* this protuberance may occasionally be absent or multiple.

Microscopically, endodermal or mesodermal derivatives may be found, but ectodermal elements usually predominate. The cyst is typically lined with keratinized squamous epithelium and contains abundant sebaceous and sweat glands. Hair and fatty secretions are commonly found within (Fig. 9-19). The Rokitansky protuberance is usually the site where the most varied tissue types are found and is also a common location of malignant transformation.

Malignant transformation develops in only 1 to 3 percent of cases, typically in women older than 40. These cancers comprise only 1 percent of all ovarian malignancies (Kelley, 1961; Koonings, 1989; Peterson, 1957). Because of the preponderance of squamous epithelium lining these cysts, it seems logical that squamous cell carcinoma comprises 80 percent of malignant cases.

Tumor Origin. The diverse tissues found within teratomas are thought not to arise by fertilization of the egg by sperm. Instead, they are theorized to develop from genetic material contained within a single oocyte. As a result, almost all mature cystic teratomas have a 46, XX karyotype (Eppig, 1977; Linder, 1975). Complete embryonic development from asexual

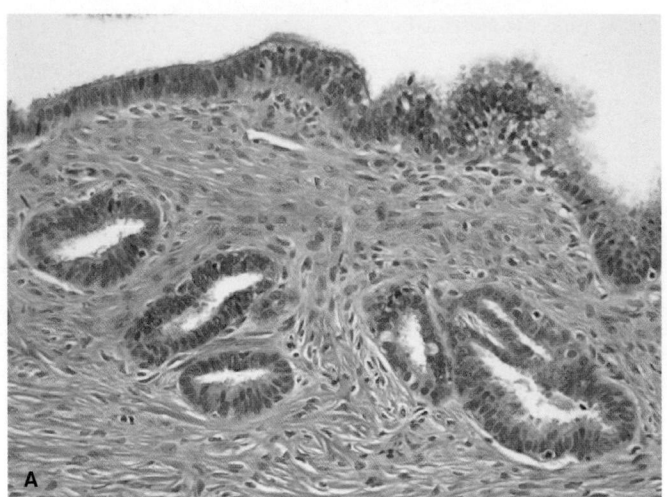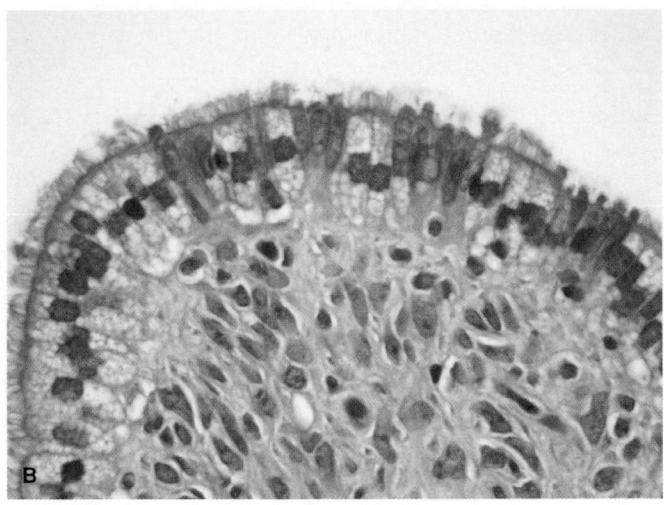

Serous cystadenoma

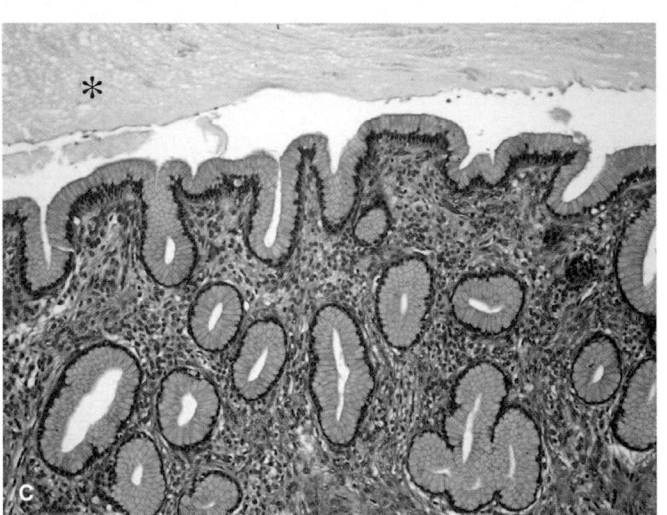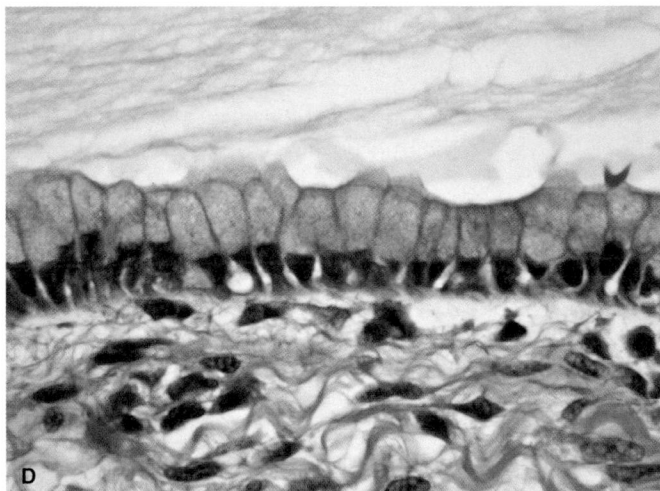

Mucinous cystadenoma

FIGURE 9-18 Serous **(A,B)** and mucinous **(C,D)** cystadenomas. **A.** This simple cyst has a fibrous wall and is lined by a single layer of benign, columnar tubal-type epithelium with cilia. The epithelium may also be simple cuboidal or attenuated and flattened. **B.** High-power view of its ciliated, tubal-type lining. **C.** Mucinous cystadenomas are typically multiloculated cysts lined by a single layer of benign mucin-containing epithelium. Mucinous fluid is secreted by the epithelium and contained within the cystic mass. In this image, it appears as amorphous material above the epithelium and is stained pink (*asterisk*). **D.** High-power view of simple columnar, mucin-containing epithelium. (*Photographs contributed by Dr. Kelley Carrick.*)

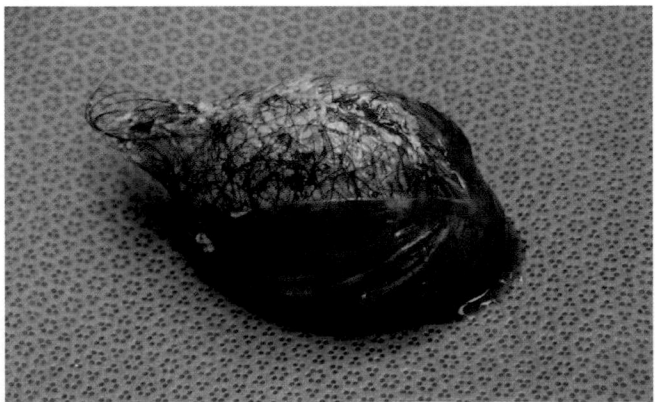

FIGURE 9-19 Photograph of a sectioned mature cystic teratoma following cystectomy. Abundant hair and sebum, characteristic of these neoplasms, is evident.

reproduction—*parthenogenesis*—is found in lower phylogenetic organisms. In mammals, the process falls well short of normal embryogenesis, but some embryonic tissue development does occur.

Complications. Almost 15 percent of mature cystic teratomas undergo torsion, but cyst rupture is rare. Presumably, their thick cyst wall resists rupture compared with other ovarian neoplasms. If cysts do rupture, acute peritonitis is common, and Fielder and associates (1996) attributed peritonitis to the sebum and hair contents of these cysts. They showed the benefits of intraoperative lavage to prevent peritonitis and adhesion formation. Alternatively, chronic leakage of teratoma contents can lead to a granulomatous peritonitis that may often initially be visually misinterpreted as widespread malignancy (Phupong, 2004).

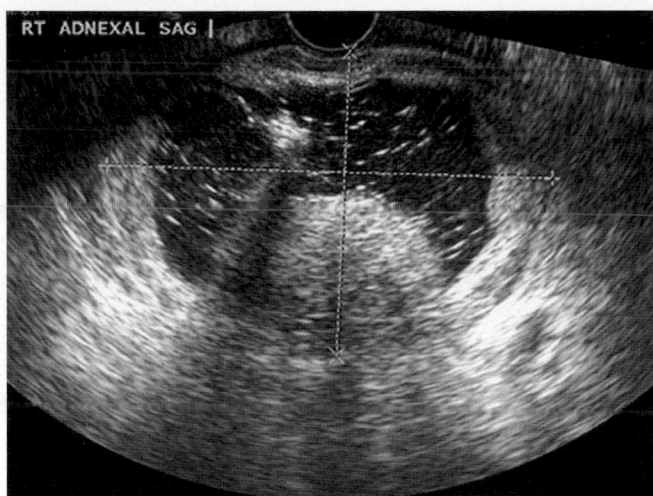

FIGURE 9-20 Sonogram revealing characteristics of mature cystic teratoma. *(Image contributed by Dr. Elysia Moschos.)*

Diagnosis. Symptoms from mature cystic teratomas are similar to those of other ovarian cysts. As a result, sonography is the main imaging tool used in their identification (Fig. 9-20). Mature cystic teratomas—more so than most ovarian tumors—display a number of characteristic sonographic features:

(1) Tip of the iceberg—This sign is created by amorphous echogenic interfaces of fat, hair, and tissues in the foreground that shadow and thus obscure structures behind them (Guttman, 1977).

(2) Fat-fluid or hair-fluid levels—A distinct linear demarcation can be seen when free serous fluid interfaces with sebum alone or sebum mixed with hair.

(3) Hair—This frequent component of mature cystic teratomas, when intermixed with sebum, forms accentuated lines and dots that represent hair in longitudinal and transverse planes (Bronshtein, 1991).

(4) Rokitansky protuberance—This mural nodule found in most mature teratomas has a characteristic sonographic appearance. The typically rounded protuberance ranges in size from 1 to 4 cm, is predominantly hyperechoic, and creates an acute angle with the cyst wall.

Although these findings are frequently seen in mature cystic teratomas, they may also be found in other ovarian cysts. For example, Patel and associates (1998) reported modest positive-predictive values for these findings individually. However, they described values of 100 percent when two or more were found within a given lesion.

Treatment. For most women with mature cystic teratoma, surgical excision provides a definitive diagnosis, affords relief of symptoms, and prevents complications of torsion, rupture, and malignant degeneration. In the past, most recommended that the opposite ovary be explored because of the high frequency of bilateral lesions. Surgeons commonly bivalved, wedged, or biopsied grossly normal contralateral ovaries. With accurate sonographic imaging, these procedures are no longer indicated with a normal appearing contralateral ovary (Comerci, 1994).

Although most of these masses are surgically removed, a few studies have supported surveillance only for cysts measuring <6 cm in premenopausal women, especially those desiring future fertility (Alcázar, 2005; Caspi, 1997; Hoo, 2010). These studies document slow tumor growth that averages less than 2 mm/yr. If the mass is not removed, sonography is recommended every 6 to 12 months initially (Levine, 2010),

■ Solid Ovarian Tumors

Completely solid ovarian masses typically are benign. That said, these masses should still be removed because of the inability to exclude malignancy in these tumors. Ovarian tumors that may present as a solid masses include: sex cord-stromal tumors, Krukenberg tumor, ovarian leiomyoma and leiomyosarcoma, carcinoid, primary lymphoma, and transition cell tumors, also called Brenner tumors (Fig. 9-21).

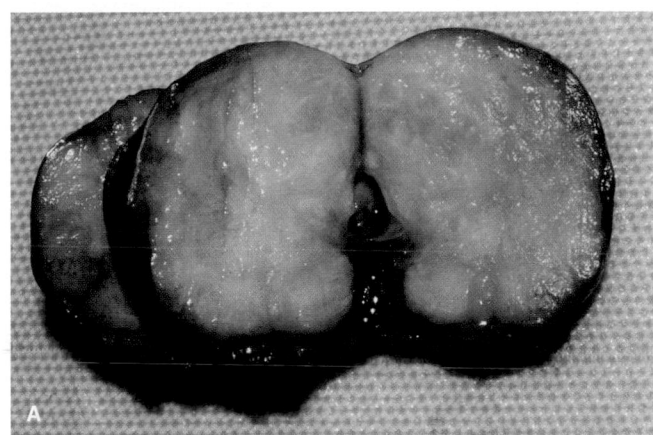

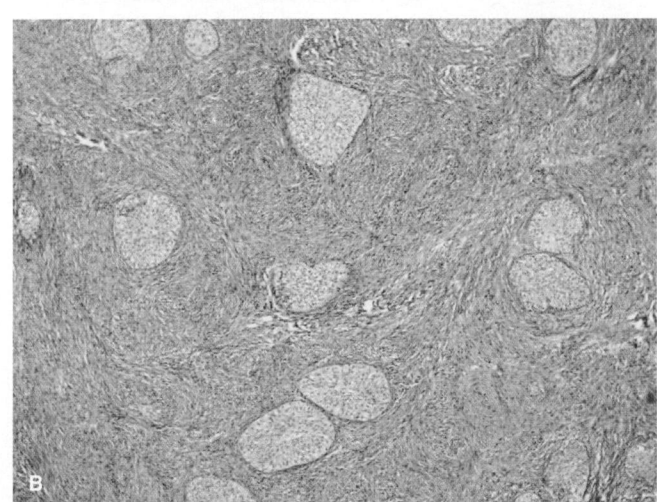

FIGURE 9-21 Photographs of a Brenner tumor following oophorectomy. **A.** A well-circumscribed, tan to yellow, rubbery mass with a smooth to slightly bosselated cut surface is characteristic of these tumors. During preparation of this specimen for histologic assessment, ink (in this case, black) was applied to the external surface of the mass to allow identification of inner and outer surfaces during microscopic evaluation. **B.** Typical of these tumors, sharply demarcated nests of transitional-type epithelial cells are found within a densely fibrous stroma. These epithelial cells have prominent cell borders, pale to lightly eosinophilic cytoplasm, and oval nuclei, without atypia or mitotic activity. *(Photograph contributed by Dr. Jason Mull.)*

Ovarian Remnant Syndrome

Persistent functional ovarian tissue following incomplete oophorectomy can present as a pelvic mass if ovarian pathology develops. They most commonly cause pain and are discussed in detail in Chapter 11 (p. 317) (Mahdavi, 2004). Dense adhesive disease at the time of oophorectomy is the greatest risk factor, and women with a history of pelvic inflammatory disease, endometriosis, or prior pelvic surgery are more commonly affected (Nezhat, 2005).

TORSION OF ADNEXAL MASSES

Torsion involves the twisting of adnexal components. Most commonly, the ovary and fallopian tube rotate as a single entity around the broad ligament. Infrequently, an ovary may alone turn about its mesovarium, and rarely a fallopian tube twists alone about the mesosalpinx (Lee, 1967). Torsion may occur with normal adnexa, but in 50 to 80 percent of cases unilateral ovarian masses are identified (Nichols, 1985; Warner, 1985).

Incidence

Adnexal torsion accounts for 3 percent of gynecologic emergencies. Although most common during the reproductive years, postmenopausal women may also be affected (Hibbard, 1985). A disproportionate number of cases of adnexal torsion develop during pregnancy, and these compose 20 to 25 percent of all torsion cases.

Pathophysiology

Adnexal masses with increased mobility have greater torsion rates. Congenitally long uteroovarian ligaments create excessively mobile mesovaria or fallopian tubes and may increase the risk in even normal adnexa (Bellah, 1989; Graif, 1988). Similarly, pathologically enlarged ovaries with a diameter >6 cm will typically rise from the true pelvis. Without these bony confines, mobility and risk of torsion are increased. Accordingly, the highest rates of torsion are found in adnexal masses from 6 to 10 cm (Houry, 2001). Torsion of the adnexa more commonly involves the right adnexa, likely due to limited mobility of the left ovary caused by the sigmoid colon (Hasiakos, 2008).

Two key points assist in initially maintaining blood flow to the involved adnexal structures despite twisting of their vascular pedicles. First, adnexa are supplied from the respective adnexal branches of both the uterine and ovarian vessels. During torsion, one of these, but not the other, may be involved. Second, although low-pressure veins draining the adnexa are compressed by the twisting pedicle, high-pressure arteries initially resist compression. As a result of this continued inflow but arrested egress of blood, the adnexa become congested and edematous, but do not infarct. Because of this, it is reasonable to conservatively manage cases of early torsion at the time of surgery. With continued stromal swelling, however, arteries may become compressed, leading to adnexal infarction and necrosis and necessitating adnexectomy.

Anatomy

Grossly, a torsed adnexa is enlarged and often appears hemorrhagic (Fig. 9-22). On cut surface and microscopically, the ovarian tissue may be edematous, hemorrhagic, or necrotic.

Symptoms and Physical Findings

Classically, the woman with adnexal torsion complains of sharp lower abdominal pain with sudden onset that worsens intermittently over several hours. The pain usually is localized to the involved side, with radiation to the flank, groin, or thigh. Low-grade fever suggests adnexal necrosis. Nausea and vomiting frequently accompany the pain.

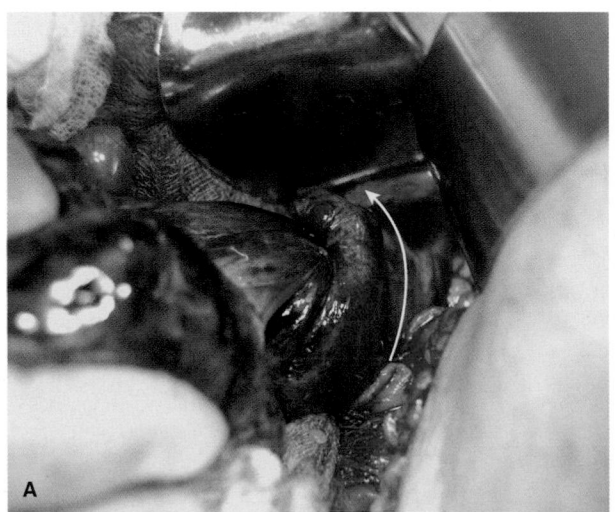
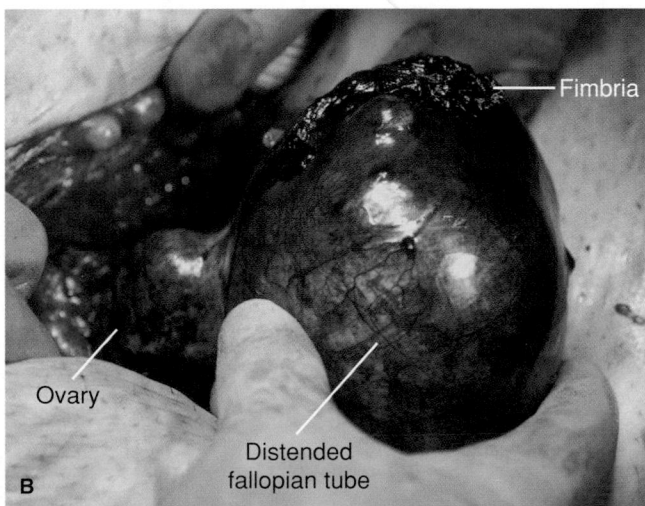

FIGURE 9-22 Intraoperative photographs of adnexal torsion. **A.** Twisting of the infundibulopelvic ligament leads to strangulation of ovarian vessels within it. **B.** A cyanotic ovary and fallopian tube result and are shown here. Hemorrhage into the tubal walls created this massively dilated fallopian tube. Dusky fimbria are seen at the end of the tube. *(Photographs contributed by Dr. Jason Harn.)*

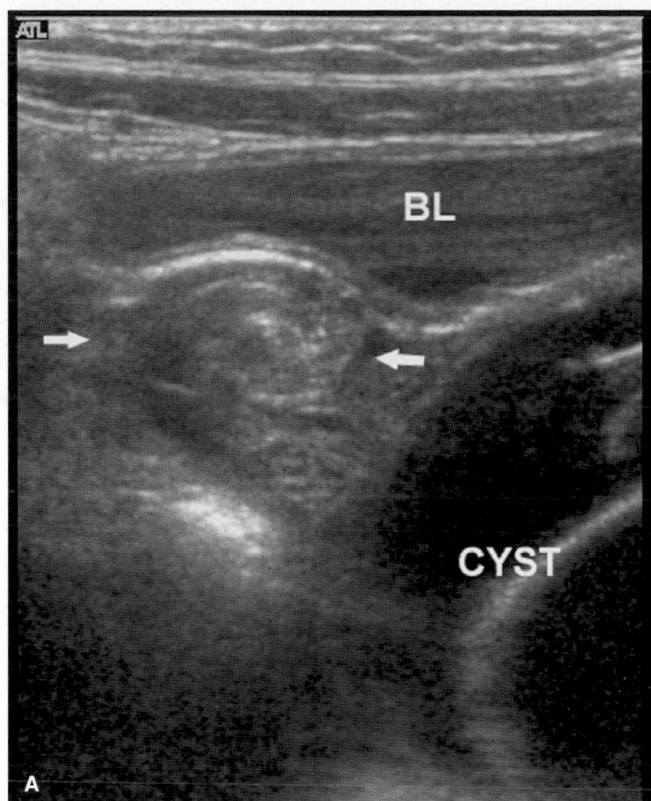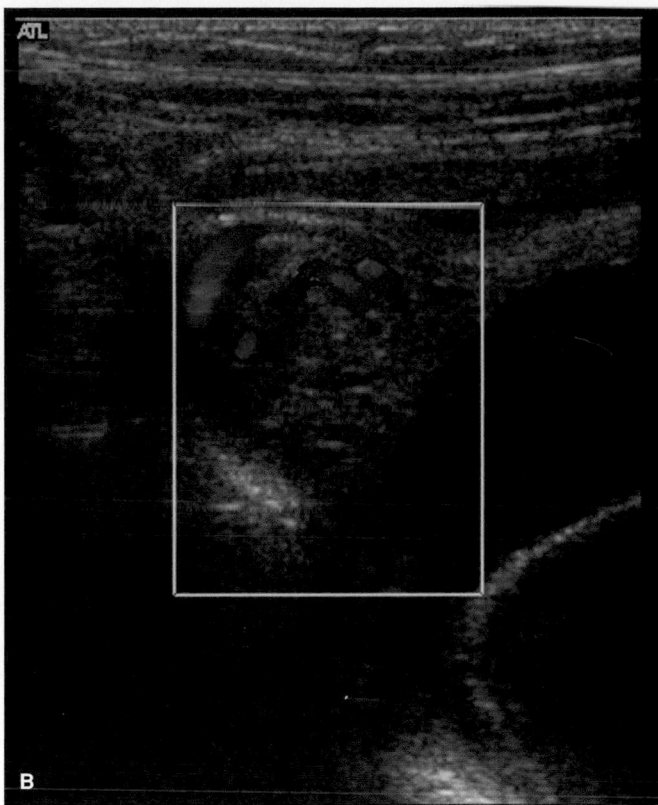

FIGURE 9-23 Whirlpool sign of ovarian torsion seen with transvaginal sonography. **A.** Conventional transabdominal sonography. White arrows point to torsion of ovarian vessels. BL = bladder. **B.** Transvaginal color Doppler shows twisting of the vessels. *(Vijayaraghavan, 2004, with permission.)*

Lack of clear physical findings can add to the difficulty in reaching this diagnosis. An adnexal mass may not be palpable, and during early its stages, significant tenderness or discomfort may not be elicited during examination.

Diagnosis
Imaging

Sonography plays an essential role in evaluation. Sonographic findings, however, can vary widely depending on the degree of vascular compromise, the characteristics of any associated intraovarian or intratubal mass, and the presence or absence of adnexal hemorrhage. Sonographically, torsion may mimic ectopic pregnancy, tuboovarian abscess, hemorrhagic ovarian cyst, and endometrioma. Accordingly, rates of correct sonographic diagnosis range from 50 to 75 percent (Graif, 1984; Helvie, 1989).

Despite these limitations, specific findings associated with ovarian torsion have been described. First, the presence of multiple follicles rimming an enlarged ovary has a reported detection rate of 64 percent (Farrell, 1982; Graif, 1988). This finding reflects the ovarian congestion and edema described earlier. As shown in Figure 9-23, the twisted pedicle may also appear as a bull's-eye target, whirlpool, or snail shell, that is, a rounded hyperechoic structure with multiple, inner, concentric hypoechoic broad rings (Vijayaraghavan, 2004).

Transvaginal color Doppler sonography (TV-CDS) may add significant information for clinical evaluation. In many affected women, disruption of normal adnexal blood flow can be seen (Albayram, 2001). However in some cases, incomplete or intermittent torsion may at times display using TV-CDS both venous and arterial flow with varied and confusing findings. Thus, disruption of vascular flow is highly suggestive of torsion, but torsion should not be excluded on the basis of a normal Doppler study alone, especially in the setting of suggestive signs and symptoms (Bar-On, 2010).

Computed tomography or MR imaging may be helpful in complicated cases or in those with ambiguous clinical presentation such as seen with incomplete or chronic torsion (Rha, 2002).

Management

Salvage of the involved adnexa, resection of any associated cyst or tumor, and possible oophoropexy are goals of treatment. Findings of adnexal necrosis or rupture with hemorrhage, however, may necessitate removal of adnexal structures.

Torsion may be evaluated by laparoscopy or laparotomy. Previously, adnexectomy was usually done to avoid possible thrombus release upon detorsion and subsequent embolism. Evidence does not support this. McGovern and coworkers (1999) reviewed nearly 1000 cases of torsion and found the rare occurrence of pulmonary embolism in only 0.2 percent. In fact, these cases of embolism were associated with adnexal excision and were not linked to conservative untwisting of the pedicle.

In a study of 94 women with adnexal torsion, Zweizig and associates (1993) reported no increased morbidity in women undergoing initial untwisting of the adnexa compared with those undergoing adnexectomy.

For these reasons, detorsion of the adnexa is generally recommended. Within minutes following detorsion, congestion is relieved, and ovarian volume and cyanosis typically diminish. For many, absence of these changes may prompt adnexal removal. A persistently black-bluish ovary, however, is not pathognomonic for necrosis, and the ovary may still recover. Cohen and associates (1999) reviewed 54 cases in which adnexa were preserved regardless of their appearance following detorsion. They reported functional integrity and successful subsequent pregnancy in almost 95 percent. Bider and colleagues (1991) observed no increased postoperative infection morbidity in cases similarly managed. Because necrosis may still occur, conservative management requires postoperative vigilance for fever, leukocytosis, and peritoneal signs.

Following detorsion, there is no consensus as to the management of the adnexa. As conservative management has evolved, the incidence of repeated torsion will likely increase. Specific ovarian lesions should be excised. Cystectomy in an ischemic, edematous ovary, however, may technically be difficult. Therefore, some authors recommend later cystectomy, if still present 6 to 8 weeks after primary intervention (Rody, 2002). Unilateral or bilateral oophoropexy has been described to minimize the risk of repeat ipsilateral torsion or contralateral adnexal torsion, especially in the pediatric population (Djavadian, 2004; Germain, 1996). Varying techniques in case reports and case series have been described to secure the ovary. These include shortening of the uteroovarian ligament with a running stitch through the ligament or suturing of either the ovary or the uteroovarian ligament to the posterior aspect of the uterus, the lateral pelvic wall, or the round ligament (Fuchs, 2010; Weitzman, 2008).

Management during pregnancy does not differ. However, if the corpus luteum is removed before 10 weeks' gestation, progestational support is recommended until 10 weeks' gestation to maintain the pregnancy. Suitable regimens include: (1) micronized progesterone (Prometrium) 200 or 300 mg orally once daily; (2) 8-percent progesterone vaginal gel (Crinone) one premeasured applicator vaginally daily plus micronized progesterone 100 or 200 mg orally once daily; or (3) intramuscular 17-hydroxyprogesterone caproate (Delalutin), 150 mg. If between 8 and 10 weeks, then only one injection is required immediately after surgery. If the corpus luteum is excised between 6 to 8 weeks, then two additional doses should be given 1 and 2 weeks after the first.

PARAOVARIAN MASSES

Paratubal/Paraovarian Cysts

Most of these cysts are not neoplastic, but are either distended remnants of the paramesonephric duct or mesothelial inclusion cysts. The most common paramesonephric cyst is the *hydatid of Morgagni,* which is pedunculated and typically dangles from one of the fimbria (**Fig. 9-24**). Extremes of size

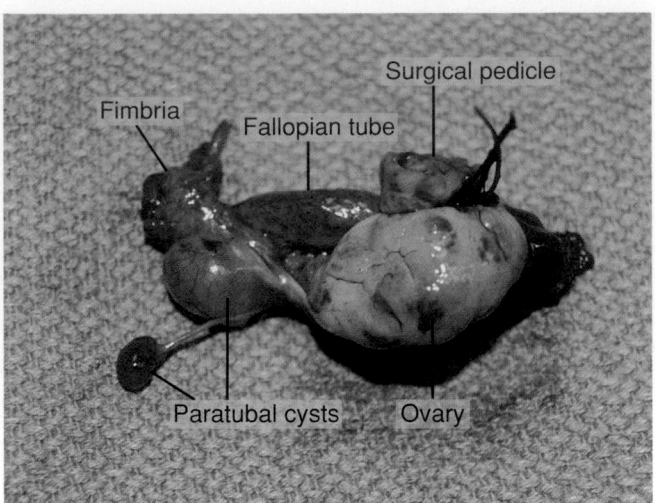

FIGURE 9-24 Surgical specimen containing fallopian tube, ovary, and paratubal cysts. The pedunculated and thin-walled nature of these cysts is typical.

have been noted, but most measure less than 3 cm (Genadry, 1977). The reported incidence of paraovarian cysts varies, but one autopsy series cited a rate of approximately 5 percent of adnexal cysts (Dorum, 2005). Neoplastic paraovarian cysts are rare, and histologically resemble tumors of ovarian origin. They are usually cystadenomas or cystadenofibromas and are rarely of borderline potential or malignant (Honore, 1980; Korbin, 1998).

Cysts are most commonly identified in asymptomatic women at the time of surgery or sonography for other gynecologic problems. If symptoms develop, they mimic those of other ovarian pathology, such as abdominal or pelvic pain. They are infrequently associated with complications such as hemorrhage, rupture, or torsion (Genadry, 1977).

Transvaginal sonography is often used as a primary evaluation tool for symptomatic woman, and most of these cysts have thin, smooth walls, and anechoic centers. Sonography, however, has limitations in differentiating between paraovarian and ovarian pathology (Athey, 1985; Barloon, 1996). Moreover, MR imaging is poor in differentiating between ovarian and paraovarian cysts (Ghossain, 2005). Thus, many women are managed similarly to those with the diagnosis of ovarian cyst. When surgically managed, cystectomy or less frequently, drainage and fulguration of the cyst wall are performed. When noted as an incidental intraoperative finding, these cysts are generally excised, although this is not an evidence-based practice.

Paraovarian Solid Tumors

Leiomyomas are the most common solid paraovarian mass with pathophysiology identical to those within the myometrium. Infrequently, congenital anomalies such as an accessory or supernumerary ovary, rudimentary uterine horn, or pelvic kidney may present as a pelvic mass with or without symptoms. One rare solid paraovarian tumor arises as a remnant of the

Wolffian duct and has been termed the *female adnexal tumor of probable Wolffian origin*. Other rare malignant paraovarian solid tumors include sarcomas, lymphoma, adenocarcinoma, pheochromocytoma, and choriocarcinoma.

Most paraovarian solid tumors are asymptomatic and identified on routine pelvic examination. Occasionally, there is unilateral pelvic and abdominal pain. Sonography and MR imaging are used to visualize these masses, although accurate differentiation between benign and malignant lesions is typically not possible. Thus, most solid masses are surgically removed.

FALLOPIAN TUBE PATHOLOGY

The bulk of tubal pathologies involve ectopic pregnancy or the sequelae of pelvic inflammatory disease (PID). Fallopian tube neoplasms are rare.

■ Hydrosalpinx

This chronic swelling of the fallopian tube is commonly a long-term result of PID. Accordingly, risk factors are the same as those for PID. Grossly, the fine fimbria and tubal ostia are obliterated and replaced by a smooth, clubbed end (Fig. 9-25). The ballooned, thin walls of the elongated tube are whitish and translucent, and the tube is typically distended with a clear serous fluid. Depending on the degree and location of the ipsilateral ovary, the hydrosalpinx may be adhered to it.

Hydrosalpinx may be found in asymptomatic women during pelvic examination or sonography done for other indications. Some women note infertility or chronic pelvic pain. The differential diagnosis mimics that for other cystic pelvic lesions discussed on p. 262. In general, no laboratory test is helpful,

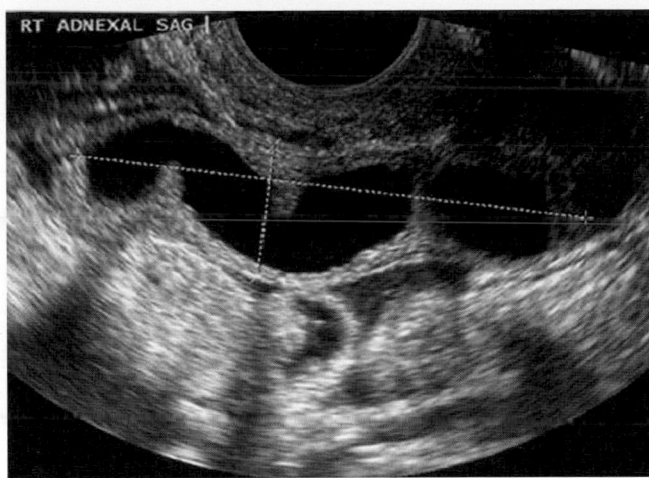

FIGURE 9-26 Transvaginal sonogram of hydrosalpinx. Incomplete septa, which are folds of the dilated tube, are seen within this fusiform, fluid-filled structure. *(Image contributed by Dr. Elysia Moschos.)*

and serum CA125 level testing for presumed ovarian malignancy is typically negative.

Sonography has low sensitivity for detection of hydrosalpinges during infertility evaluation. However, in women with sonographic findings, there is usually a thin-walled, hypoechoic cystic fusiform structure with incomplete septa (Fig. 9-26). In some, multiple hyperechoic mural nodules measuring 2 to 3 mm arch around the inner circumference of the tube to create the *beads on a string* sign (Fig. 2-18, p. 43). These nodules represent fibrotic endosalpingeal folds.

Management varies depending on the conviction of diagnosis, desire for future fertility, and associated symptoms. In asymptomatic women who have completed childbearing, and in whom the sonographic evidence supports the diagnosis of hydrosalpinx, expectant management is typical. In those with pelvic pain, infertility, or in whom the diagnosis is uncertain, diagnostic laparoscopy is typically preferred.

For women not wishing to preserve fertility, laparoscopic treatment may include lysis of adhesions and salpingectomy. Conversely, in women who desire fertility, surgical intervention depends on the degree of tubal damage. As the degree of tubal distortion increases, fertility rates decrease (Schlaff, 1990). In women with mild tubal disease, laparoscopic neosalpingostomy has resulted in 80-percent pregnancy rates and is a reasonable approach (Fig. 20-7, p. 541). In those women with severe disease, IVF may offer a greater chance at fertility.

Of note, women with a hydrosalpinx who undergo IVF have approximately half the pregnancy rate of other women (American Society for Reproductive Medicine, 2004). One theoretical explanation is that the hydrosalpinx fluid bathes the endometrial cavity with toxic fluid that contains bacteriologic agents, debris, lymphocytes, cytokines, lymphokines, and prostaglandins. This is suggested to lower blastocyst implantation rates (Johnson, 2004; Strandell, 2002). This is supported by studies showing improved subsequent pregnancy, implantation, and live birth rates following resection of hydrosalpinges

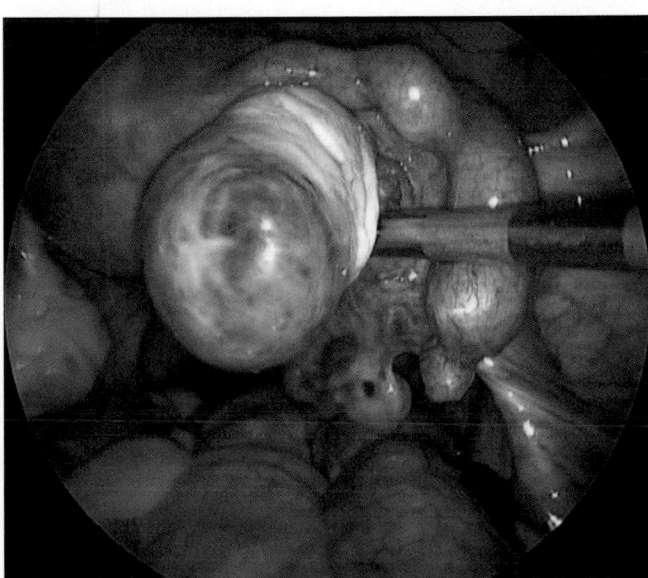

FIGURE 9-25 Laparoscopic photograph of a hydrosalpinx. Note the thin-walled ballooned fallopian tube and its clubbed end stretching from the uterine cornua and draping behind the blunt probe. A typical corpus luteum cyst is seen at the distal end of the ovary. *(Photograph contributed by Dr. Karen Bradshaw.)*

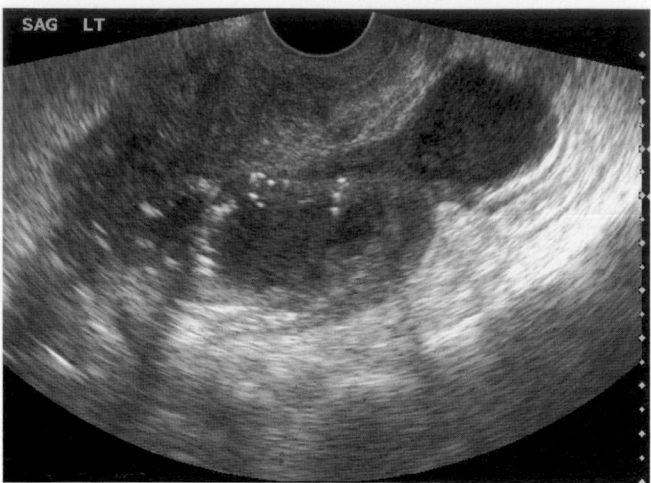

FIGURE 9-27 Sonographic transvaginal sagittal image of a tuboovarian complex. *(Image contributed by Dr. Elysia Moschos.)*

prior to IVF (Dechaud, 1998; Johnson, 2004; Strandell, 1999). For all of these reasons, the American Society for Reproductive Medicine (2004) recommends such surgery prior to IVF.

Benign Neoplasms

These are rare in the fallopian tube. The most common benign tumor is the mesothelioma, which is found in less than 1 percent of hysterectomy specimens (Pauerstein, 1968). Previously termed adenomatoid tumors, these 1- to 2-cm, well-circumscribed solid nodules arise in the tubal wall (Salazar, 1972). Tubal leiomyomas are uncommon and derive from the smooth muscle of the muscularis, from the broad ligament, or from vessels in either location. Additionally, hemangioma, lipoma, chondroma, adenofibroma, cystadenofibroma, angiomyolipoma, and neural tumors may rarely develop.

Tuboovarian Abscess

This is an inflammatory mass involving the fallopian tube, ovary, and often surrounding structures. If an ovary adheres to the fallopian tube, but is still visualized, it is called a *tuboovarian complex*. In contrast, a *tuboovarian abscess* results from a complete breakdown of ovarian and tubal architecture such that the separate structures are no longer identified. Either is usually a consequence of PID, although occasionally diverticulitis or pelvic malignancy may be the generative source. These women usually present with lower abdominal pain, fever, and leukocytosis, and with unilateral or bilateral adnexal masses. Sonography is typically diagnostic. Normal adnexal anatomy, either unilaterally or bilaterally, is obliterated and replaced with a cystic or multiseptated mass that contains multiple internal echoes (Fig. 9-27). Also, in this setting, CT imaging performed with both IV and oral contrast may provide improved sensitivity, although at higher cost. Treatment consists of broad-spectrum antibiotics, analgesia, and antipyretics. Large isolated abscesses may benefit from percutaneous drainage. Rarely, surgery with hysterectomy and adnexectomy is required, but is reserved for cases refractory to conservative measures. Abscess rupture causes severe pain and progressive peritonitis and is a surgical emergency. These abscesses and their management are more fully discussed in Chapter 3 (p. 96).

REFERENCES

Acien P, Quereda F: Abdominal myomectomy: results of a simple operative technique. Fertil Steril 65(1):41, 1996

Agdi M, Tulandi T: Endoscopic management of uterine fibroids. Best Pract Res Clin Obstet Gynaecol 22(4):707, 2008

Agdi M, Tulandi T: Minimally invasive approach for myomectomy. Semin Reprod Med 28(3):228, 2010

Albayram F, Hamper UM: Ovarian and adnexal torsion: spectrum of sonographic findings with pathologic correlation. J Ultrasound Med 20(10):1083, 2001

Alcázar JL, Castillo G, Jurado M, et al: Is expectant management of sonographically benign adnexal cysts an option in selected asymptomatic premenopausal women? Hum Reprod 20(11):3231, 2005

Alessi G, Lemmerling M, Vereecken L, et al: Benign metastasizing leiomyoma to skull base and spine: a report of two cases. Clin Neurol Neurosurg 105(3):170, 2003

Al-Hendy A, Salama SA: Ethnic distribution of estrogen receptor-alpha polymorphism is associated with a higher prevalence of uterine leiomyomas in black Americans. Fertil Steril 86(3):686, 2006

American Cancer Society: Cancer facts and figures 2011. Atlanta, American Cancer Society, 2011

American College of Obstetricians and Gynecologists: Alternatives to hysterectomy in the management of leiomyomas. Practice Bulletin No. 96, August 2008

American College of Obstetricians and Gynecologists: Management of adnexal masses. Practice Bulletin No. 83, 2007

American College of Obstetricians and Gynecologists: Noncontraceptive uses of hormonal contraceptives. Practice Bulletin No. 110, 2010

American College of Obstetricians and Gynecologists: Surgical alternatives to hysterectomy in the management of leiomyomas. Practice Bulletin No. 16, 2001

American College of Obstetricians and Gynecologists: The role of the generalist obstetrician-gynecologist in the early detection of ovarian cancer. Committee Opinion No. 477, December 2011

American College of Obstetricians and Gynecologists: Uterine artery embolization. Committee Opinion No. 293, February 2004

American Society for Reproductive Medicine: Myomas and reproductive function. Fertil Steril 86(5 Suppl 1):S194, 2006

American Society for Reproductive Medicine: Salpingectomy for hydrosalpinx prior to in vitro fertilization. Fertil Steril 82(Suppl 1):117, 2004

Andrews RT, Spies JB, Sacks D, et al: Patient care and uterine artery embolization for leiomyomata. J Vasc Interv Radiol 20(7 Suppl)S307, 2009

Anteby SO, Yarkoni S, Ever Hadani P: The effect of a prostaglandin synthetase inhibitor, indomethacin, on excessive uterine bleeding. Clin Exp Obstet Gynecol 12(3-4):60, 1985

Athey PA, Cooper NB: Sonographic features of parovarian cysts. AJR Am J Roentgenol 144(1):83, 1985

Azziz R: Adenomyosis: current perspectives. Obstet Gynecol Clin North Am 16(1):221, 1989

Barloon TJ, Brown BP, Abu-Yousef MM, et al: Paraovarian and paratubal cysts: preoperative diagnosis using transabdominal and transvaginal sonography. J Clin Ultrasound 24(3):117, 1996

Bar-On S, Mashiach R, Stockheim D, et al: Emergency laparoscopy for suspected ovarian torsion: are we too hasty to operate? Fertil Steril 93(6):2012, 2010

Bayer HealthCare Pharmaceuticals: Mirena (levonorgestrel-releasing intrauterine system). Highlights of prescribing information, 2009. Available at: http://berlex.bayerhealthcare.com/html/products/pi/Mirena_PI.pdf. Accessed July 8, 2010

Bazot M, Cortez A, Darai E, et al: Ultrasonography compared with magnetic resonance imaging for the diagnosis of adenomyosis: correlation with histopathology. Hum Reprod 16(11):2427, 2001

Bellah RD, Griscom NT: Torsion of normal uterine adnexa before menarche: CT appearance. AJR Am J Roentgenol 152(1):123, 1989

Benson CB, Chow JS, Chang-Lee W, et al: Outcome of pregnancies in women with uterine leiomyomas identified by sonography in the first trimester. J Clin Ultrasound 29(5):261, 2001

Berger GS: Outpatient pelvic laparotomy. J Reprod Med 39(8):569, 1994

Bider D, Mashiach S, Dulitzky M, et al: Clinical, surgical and pathologic findings of adnexal torsion in pregnant and nonpregnant women. Surg Gynecol Obstet 173(5):363, 1991

Bird CC, McElin TW, Manalo-Estrella P: The elusive adenomyosis of the uterus—revisited. Am J Obstet Gynecol 112(5):583, 1972

Bodner K, Bodner-Adler B, Wierrani F, et al: Intravenous leiomyomatosis of the uterus. Anticancer Res 22(3):1881, 2002

Borten M, Friedman EA: Drainage of postabortion hematometra by Foley catheter. Am J Obstet Gynecol 149(8):908, 1984

Brache V, Faundes A, Alvarez F, et al: Nonmenstrual adverse events during use of implantable contraceptives for women: data from clinical trials. Contraception 65(1):63, 2002

Bradley LD: Uterine fibroid embolization: a viable alternative to hysterectomy. Am J Obstet Gynecol 201(2):127, 2009

Bragheto AM, Caserta N, Bahamondes L, et al: Effectiveness of the levonorgestrel-releasing intrauterine system in the treatment of adenomyosis diagnosed and monitored by magnetic resonance imaging. Contraception 76(3):195, 2007

Bratby MJ, Hussain FF, Walker WJ: Outcomes after unilateral uterine artery embolization: a retrospective review. Cardiovasc Intervent Radiol 31(2):254, 2008

Broekmans FJ: GnRH agonists and uterine leiomyomas. Human Reprod 11(Suppl 3):3, 1996

Bronshtein M, Yoffe N, Brandes JM, et al: Hair as a sonographic marker of ovarian teratomas: improved identification using transvaginal sonography and simulation model. J Clin Ultrasound 19(6):351, 1991

Brosens I, Deprest J, Dal Cin P, et al: Clinical significance of cytogenetic abnormalities in uterine myomas. Fertil Steril 69(2):232, 1998

Brosens J, Campo R, Gordts S, et al: Submucous and outer myometrium leiomyomas are two distinct clinical entities. Fertil Steril 79(6):1452, 2003

Brown MF, Hebra A, McGeehin K, et al: Ovarian masses in children: a review of 91 cases of malignant and benign masses. J Pediatr Surg 28(7):930, 1993

Bulletti C, Polli V, Negrini V, et al: Adhesion formation after laparoscopic myomectomy. J Am Assoc Gynecol Laparosc 3(4):533, 1996

Bulun SE, Simpson ER, Word RA: Expression of the CYP19 gene and its product aromatase cytochrome P450 in human uterine leiomyoma tissues and cells in culture. J Clin Endocrinol Metab 78(3):736, 1994

Buttram VC Jr, Reiter RC: Uterine leiomyomata: etiology, symptomatology, and management. Fertil Steril 36(4):433, 1981

Campo S, Campo V, Gambadauro P: Reproductive outcome before and after laparoscopic or abdominal myomectomy for subserous or intramural myomas. Eur J Obstet Gynecol Reprod Biol 110(2):215, 2003

Candiani GB, Fedele L, Parazzini F, et al: Risk of recurrence after myomectomy. Br J Obstet Gynaecol 98(4):385, 1991

Cantuaria GH, Angioli R, Frost L, et al: Comparison of bimanual examination with ultrasound examination with ultrasound examination before hysterectomy for uterine leiomyoma. Obstet Gynecol 92(1):109, 1998

Carlson KJ, Miller BA, Fowler FJ Jr: The Maine Women's Health Study: II. Outcomes of nonsurgical management of leiomyomas, abnormal bleeding, and chronic pelvic pain. Obstet Gynecol 83(4):566, 1994

Carr BR, Marshburn PB, Weatherall PT, et al: An evaluation of the effect of gonadotropin-releasing hormone analogs and medroxyprogesterone acetate on uterine leiomyomata volume by magnetic resonance imaging: a prospective, randomized, double blind, placebo-controlled, crossover trial. J Clin Endocrinol Metab 76(5):1217, 1993

Caruso PA, Marsh MR, Minkowitz S, et al: An intense clinicopathologic study of 305 teratomas of the ovary. Cancer 27(2):343, 1971

Caspi B, Appelman Z, Rabinerson D, et al: The growth pattern of ovarian dermoid cysts: a prospective study in premenopausal and postmenopausal women. Fertil Steril 68(3):501, 1997

Chegini N, Rong H, Dou Q, et al: Gonadotropin-releasing hormone (GnRH) and GnRH receptor gene expression in human myometrium and leiomyomata and the direct action of GnRH analogs on myometrial smooth muscle cells and interaction with ovarian steroids in vitro. J Clin Endocrinol Metab 81(9):3215, 1996

Chen VW, Ruiz B, Killeen JL, et al: Pathology and classification of ovarian tumors. Cancer 97(S10):2631, 2003

Chiaffarino F, Parazzini F, La Vecchia C, et al: Oral contraceptive use and benign gynecologic conditions. A review. Contraception 57(1):11, 1998

Chiaffarino F, Parazzini F, La Vecchia C, et al: Use of oral contraceptives and uterine fibroids: results from a case-control study. Br J Obstet Gynaecol 106(8):857, 1999

Chwalisz K, Larsen L, Mattia-Goldberg C, et al: A randomized, controlled trial of asoprisnil, a novel selective progesterone receptor modulator, in women with uterine leiomyomata. Fertil Steril 87(6):1399, 2007

Chwalisz K, Perez MC, Demanno D, et al: Selective progesterone receptor modulator development and use in the treatment of leiomyomata and endometriosis. Endocr Rev 26(3):423, 2005

Cohen I, Beyth Y, Shapira J, et al: High frequency of adenomyosis in postmenopausal breast cancer patients treated with tamoxifen. Gynecol Obstet Invest 44(3):200, 1997

Cohen I, Potlog-Nahari C, Shapira J, et al: Simple ovarian cysts in postmenopausal patients with breast carcinoma treated with tamoxifen: long-term follow-up. Radiology 227(3):844, 2003

Cohen SB, Oelsner G, Seidman DS, et al: Laparoscopic detorsion allows sparing of the twisted ischemic adnexa. J Am Assoc Gynecol Laparosc 6(2):139, 1999

Comerci JT Jr, Licciardi F, Bergh PA, et al: Mature cystic teratoma: a clinicopathologic evaluation of 517 cases and review of the literature. Obstet Gynecol 84(1):22, 1994

Cooper JM, Brady RM: Late complications of operative hysteroscopy. Obstet Gynecol Clin North Am 27(2):367, 2000

Coutinho EM, Gonçalves MT: Long-term treatment of leiomyomas with gestrinone. Fertil Steril 51(6):939, 1989

Cramer SF, Patel A: The frequency of uterine leiomyomas. Am J Clin Pathol 94(4):435, 1990

Crosignani PG, Vercellini P, Meschia M, et al: GnRH agonists before surgery for uterine leiomyomas. A review. J Reprod Med 41(6):415, 1996

Daniel M, Martin AD, Faiman C: Sex hormones and adipose tissue distribution in premenopausal cigarette smokers. Int J Obes Relat Metab Disord 16(4):245, 1992

Day Baird D, Dunson DB, Hill MC, et al: High cumulative incidence of uterine leiomyoma in black and white women: ultrasound evidence. Am J Obstet Gynecol 188(1):100, 2003

de Kroon CD, Louwe LA, Trimbos JB, et al: The clinical value of 3-dimensional saline infusion sonography in addition to 2-dimensional saline infusion sonography in women with abnormal uterine bleeding: work in progress. J Ultrasound Med 23(11):1433, 2004

De Leo V, la Marca A, Morgante G: Short-term treatment of uterine fibromyomas with danazol. Gynecol Obstet Invest 47(4):258, 1999

de Silva KS, Kanumakala S, Grover SR, et al: Ovarian lesions in children and adolescents—an 11-year review. J Pediatr Endocrinol 17(7):951, 2004

Dechaud H, Daures JP, Arnal F, et al: Does previous salpingectomy improve implantation and pregnancy rates in patients with severe tubal factor infertility who are undergoing in vitro fertilization? A pilot prospective randomized study. Fertil Steril 69(6):1020, 1998

Dejmek A: Fine needle aspiration cytology of an ovarian luteinized follicular cyst mimicking a granulosa cell tumor. A case report. Acta Cytol 47(6):1059, 2003

Deligeoroglou E, Eleftheriades M, Shiadoes V, et al: Ovarian masses during adolescence: clinical, ultrasonographic and pathologic findings, serum tumor markers and endocrinological profile. Gynecol Endocrinol 19(1):1, 2004

Derman SG, Rehnstrom J, Neuwirth RS: The long-term effectiveness of hysteroscopic treatment of menorrhagia and leiomyomas. Obstet Gynecol 77(4):591, 1991

DeWaay DJ, Syrop CH, Nygaard IE, et al: Natural history of uterine polyps and leiomyomata. Obstet Gynecol 100(1):3, 2002

Djavadian D, Braendle W, Jaenicke F: Laparoscopic oophoropexy for the treatment of recurrent torsion of the adnexa in pregnancy: case report and review. Fertil Steril 82(4):933, 2004

Donnez J, Jadoul P: What are the implications of myomas on fertility? A need for a debate? Human Reproduction 17(6):1424, 2002

Dorum A, Blom GP, Ekerhovd E, et al: Prevalence and histologic diagnosis of adnexal cysts in postmenopausal women: an autopsy study. Am J Obstet Gynecol 192(1):48, 2005

Dubuisson JB, Fauconnier A, Babaki-Fard K, et al: Laparoscopic myomectomy: a current view. Hum Reprod Update 6(6):588, 2000

Dubuisson JB, Fauconnier A, Fourchotte V, et al: Laparoscopic myomectomy: predicting the risk of conversion to an open procedure. Hum Reprod 16(8):1726, 2001

Dutton S, Hirst A, McPherson K, et al: A UK multicentre retrospective cohort study comparing hysterectomy and uterine artery embolization for the treatment of symptomatic uterine fibroids (HOPEFUL study): main results on medium-term safety and efficacy. BJOG 114(1):1340, 2007

Edwards RD, Moss JG, Lumsden MA, et al: Uterine-artery embolization versus surgery for symptomatic uterine fibroids. N Engl J Med 356(4):360, 2007

Eisinger SH, Fiscella J, Bonfiglio T, et al: Open-label study of ultra low-dose mifepristone for the treatment of uterine leiomyomata. Eur J Obstet Gynecol Reprod Biol 146(2):215, 2009

Eisinger SH, Meldrum S, Fiscella K, et al: Low-dose mifepristone for uterine leiomyomata. Obstet Gynecol 101(2):243, 2003

Emanuel MH, Wamsteker K, Hart AA, et al: Long-term results of hysteroscopic myomectomy for abnormal uterine bleeding. Obstet Gynecol 93(5 Pt 1):743, 1999

Emoto M, Iwasaki H, Mimura K, et al: Differences in the angiogenesis of benign and malignant ovarian tumors, demonstrated by analyses of color

Doppler ultrasound, immunohistochemistry, and microvessel density. Cancer 80(5):899, 1997

Engel G, Rushovich AM: True uterine diverticulum. A partial mullerian duct duplication? Arch Pathol Lab Med 108(9):734, 1984

Engel JB, Audebert A, Frydman R, et al: Presurgical short term treatment of uterine fibroids with different doses of cetrorelix acetate: a double-blind, placebo-controlled multicenter study. Eur J Obstet Gynecol Reprod Biol 134(2):225, 2007

Englund K, Blanck A, Gustavsson I, et al: Sex steroid receptors in human myometrium and fibroids: changes during the menstrual cycle and gonadotropin-releasing hormone treatment. J Clin Endocrinol Metab 83(11):4092, 1998

Eppig JJ, Kozak LP, Eicher EM, et al: Ovarian teratomas in mice are derived from oocytes that have completed the first meiotic division. Nature 269(5628):517, 1977

Erickson SS, Van Voorhis BJ: Intermenstrual bleeding secondary to cesarean scar diverticuli: report of three cases. Obstet Gynecol 93(5 Pt 2):802, 1999

Farhi J, Ashkenazi J, Feldberg D, et al: Effect of uterine leiomyomata on the results of in-vitro fertilization treatment. Hum Reprod 10(10):2576, 1995

Farrell TP, Boal DK, Teele RL, et al: Acute torsion of normal uterine adnexa in children: sonographic demonstration. AJR Am J Roentgenol 139(6):1223, 1982

Farrer-Brown G, Beilby JO, Tarbit MH: The vascular patterns in myomatous uteri. J Obstet Gynaecol Br Commonw 77(11):967, 1970

Farrer-Brown G, Beilby JO, Tarbit MH: Venous changes in the endometrium of myomatous uteri. Obstet Gynecol 38(5):743, 1971

Fedele L, Bianchi S, Dorta M, et al: Transvaginal ultrasonography in the diagnosis of diffuse adenomyosis. Fertil Steril 58(1):94, 1992

Fedele L, Parazzini F, Luchini L, et al: Recurrence of fibroids after myomectomy: a transvaginal ultrasonographic study. Hum Reprod 10(7):1795, 1995

Felberbaum RE, Germer U, Ludwig M, et al: Treatment of uterine fibroids with a slow-release formulation of the gonadotrophin releasing hormone antagonist cetrorelix. Hum Reprod 13(6):1660, 1998

Fennessy FM, Tempany CM, McDannold NJ, et al: Uterine leiomyomatas: MR imaging-guided focused ultrasound surgery—results of different treatment protocols. Radiology 243(3):885, 2007

Ferenczy A: Pathophysiology of adenomyosis. Hum Reprod Update 4(4):312, 1998

Fernandez H, Sefrioui O, Virelizier C, et al: Hysteroscopic resection of submucosal myomas in patients with infertility. Hum Reprod 16(7):1489, 2001

Fielder EP, Guzick DS, Guido R, et al: Adhesion formation from release of dermoid contents in the peritoneal cavity and effect of copious lavage: a prospective, randomized, blinded, controlled study in a rabbit model. Fertil Steril 65(4):852, 1996

Filicori M, Hall DA, Loughlin JS, et al: A conservative approach to the management of uterine leiomyoma: pituitary desensitization by a luteinizing hormone-releasing hormone analogue. Am J Obstet Gynecol 147(6):726, 1983

Fleischer AC, Shappell HW: Color Doppler sonohysterography of endometrial polyps and submucosal fibroids. J Ultrasound Med 22(6):601, 2003

Flierman PA, Oberyé JJ, van der Hulst VP, et al: Rapid reduction of leiomyoma volume during treatment with the GnRH antagonist ganirelix. BJOG 112(5):638, 2005

Flynn MK, Niloff JM: Outpatient minilaparotomy for ovarian cysts. J Reprod Med 44(5):399, 1999

Forssman L: Distribution of blood flow in myomatous uteri as measured by locally injected 133Xenon. Acta Obstet Gynecol Scand 55(2):101, 1976

Fraser IS: Menorrhagia due to myometrial hypertrophy: treatment with tamoxifen. Obstet Gynecol 70(3 Pt 2):505, 1987

Fraser IS, McCarron G, Markham R, et al: Measured menstrual blood loss in women with menorrhagia associated with pelvic disease or coagulation disorder. Obstet Gynecol 68(5):630, 1986

Friedman AJ, Daly M, Juneau-Norcross M, et al: Long-term medical therapy for leiomyomata uteri: a prospective, randomized study of leuprolide acetate depot plus either oestrogen-progestin or progestin "add-back" for 2 years. Hum Reprod 9(9):1618, 1994

Friedman AJ, Lobel SM, Rein MS, et al: Efficacy and safety considerations in women with uterine leiomyomas treated with gonadotropin-releasing hormone agonists: the estrogen threshold hypothesis. Am J Obstet Gynecol 163(4 Pt 1):1114, 1990

Friedman AJ, Thomas PP: Does low-dose combination oral contraceptive use affect uterine size or menstrual flow in premenopausal women with leiomyomas? Obstet Gynecol 85(4):631, 1995

Fuchs N, Smorgick N, Tovbin Y, et al: Oophoropexy to prevent adnexal torsion: how, when, and for whom? J Minim Invasive Gynecol 17(2):205, 2010

Ganguli S, Faintuch S, Salazar GM, et al: Postembolization syndrome: changes in white blood cell counts immediately after uterine artery embolization. J Vasc Interv Radiol 19(3):443, 2008

Garcia CR, Tureck RW: Submucosal leiomyomas and infertility. Fertil Steril 42(1):16, 1984

Genadry R, Parmley T, Woodruff JD: The origin and clinical behavior of the parovarian tumor. Am J Obstet Gynecol 129(8):873, 1977

Germain M, Rarick T, Robins E: Management of intermittent ovarian torsion by laparoscopic oophoropexy. Obstet Gynecol 88(4 Pt 2):715, 1996

Ghossain MA, Braidy CG, Kanso HN, et al: Extraovarian cystadenomas: ultrasound and MR findings in 7 cases. J Comput Assist Tomogr 29(1):74, 2005

Glass AR: Endocrine aspects of obesity. Med Clin North Am 73(1):139, 1989

Glasser MH: Minimally invasive approaches to myomectomy. In Nezhat C, Nezhat F, Nezhat C (eds): Nezhat's Operative Gynecologic Laparoscopy and Hysteroscopy. New York, Cambridge University Press, 2008, p 319

Goldberg J, Pereira L, Berghella V, et al: Pregnancy outcomes after treatment for fibromyomata: uterine artery embolization versus laparoscopic myomectomy. Am J Obstet Gynecol 191(1):18, 2004

Goldfarb HA: Combining myoma coagulation with endometrial ablation/resection reduces subsequent surgery rates. JSLS 3(4):253, 1999

Goldzieher JW, Maqueo M, Ricaud L, et al: Induction of degenerative changes in uterine myomas by high-dosage progestin therapy. Am J Obstet Gynecol 96(8):1078, 1966

Gómez-Raposo C, Mendiola M, Barriuso J, et al: Angiogenesis and ovarian cancer. Clin Transl Oncol 11(9):564, 2009

Gonzalez-Barcena D, Alvarez RB, Ochoa EP, et al: Treatment of uterine leiomyomas with luteinizing hormone-releasing hormone antagonist cetrorelix. Hum Reprod 12(9):2028, 1997

Goodwin SC, Bradley LD, Lipman JC, et al: Uterine artery embolization versus myomectomy: a multicenter comparative study. Fertil Steril 85(1):14, 2006

Goodwin SC, Spies JB, Worthington-Kirsch R, et al: Uterine artery embolization for treatment of leiomyomata: long-term outcomes from the FIBROID Registry. Obstet Gynecol 111(1):22, 2008

Graif M, Itzchak Y: Sonographic evaluation of ovarian torsion in childhood and adolescence. AJR Am J Roentgenol 150(3):647, 1988

Graif M, Shalev J, Strauss S, et al: Torsion of the ovary: sonographic features. AJR Am J Roentgenol 143(6):1331, 1984

Granberg S, Wikland M, Jansson I: Macroscopic characterization of ovarian tumors and the relation to the histological diagnosis: criteria to be used for ultrasound evaluation. Gynecol Oncol 35(2):139, 1989

Grigorieva V, Chen-Mok M, Tarasova M, et al: Use of a levonorgestrel-releasing intrauterine system to treat bleeding related to uterine leiomyomas. Fertil Steril 79(5):1194, 2003

Grimes DA, Jones LB, Lopez LM, et al: Oral contraceptives for functional ovarian cysts. Cochrane Database Syst Rev 2:CD006134, 2009

Guarnaccia MM, Rein MS: Traditional surgical approaches to uterine fibroids: abdominal myomectomy and hysterectomy. Clin Obstet Gynecology 44(2):385, 2001

Gupta S, Manyonda IT: Acute complications of fibroids. Best Pract Res Clin Obstet Gynaecol 23(5):609, 2009

Guttman PH Jr: In search of the elusive benign cystic ovarian teratoma: application of the ultrasound "tip of the iceberg" sign. J Clin Ultrasound 5(6):403, 1977

Hald K, Noreng HJ, Istre O, et al: Uterine artery embolization versus laparoscopic occlusion of uterine arteries for leiomyomas: long-term results of a randomized comparative trial. J Vasc Interv Radio 20(10):1303, 2009

Hallez JP: Single-stage total hysteroscopic myomectomies: indications, techniques, and results. Fertil Steril 63(4):703, 1995

Hart R, Khalaf Y, Yeong CT, et al: A prospective controlled study of the effect of intramural uterine fibroids on the outcome of assisted conception. Hum Reprod 16(11):2411, 2001

Hasiakos D, Papakonstantinou K, Kontoravdis A, et al: Adnexal torsion during pregnancy: report of four cases and review of the literature. J Obstet Gynaecol Res 34(4 Pt 2):683, 2008

Hehenkamp WJ, Volkers NA, Birnie E, et al: Symptomatic uterine fibroids: treatment with uterine artery embolization or hysterectomy—results from the randomized clinical Embolisation versus Hysterectomy (EMMY) trial. Radiology 246(3):823, 2008

Hehenkamp WJ, Volkers NA, Broekmans FJ, et al: Loss of ovarian reserve after uterine artery embolization: a randomized comparison with hysterectomy. Hum Reprod 22(7):1996, 2007

Helvie MA, Silver TM: Ovarian torsion: sonographic evaluation. J Clin Ultrasound 17(5):327, 1989

Hesley GK, Gorny KR, Henrichsen TL, et al: A clinical review of focused ultrasound ablation with magnetic resonance guidelines: an option for treating uterine fibroids. Ultrasound Q 24(2):131, 2008

Hibbard LT: Adnexal torsion. Am J Obstet Gynecol 152(4):456, 1985

Hodge JC, Morton CC: Genetic heterogeneity among uterine leiomyomata: insights into malignant progression. Hum Mol Genet 16(1):r7, 2007

Holt VL, Cushing-Haugen KL, Daling JR: Oral contraceptives, tubal sterilization, and functional ovarian cyst risk. Obstet Gynecol 102(2):252, 2003

Holt VL, Cushing-Haugen KL, Daling JR: Risk of functional ovarian cyst: effects of smoking and marijuana use according to body mass index. Am J Epidemiol 161(6):520, 2005

Holub Z, Mara M, Kuzel D, et al: Pregnancy outcomes after uterine artery occlusion: prospective multicentric study. Fertil Steril 90(5):1886, 2008

Homer J, Saridogan E: Uterine artery embolization for fibroids is associated with an increased risk of miscarriage. Fertil Steril 94(1):324, 2010

Honore LH, O'Hara KE: Serous papillary neoplasms arising in paramesonephric parovarian cysts. A report of eight cases. Acta Obstet Gynecol Scand 59(6):525, 1980

Hoo W, Yazebek J, Holland T, et al: Expectant management of ultrasonically diagnosed ovarian dermoid cysts: is it possible to predict the outcome? Ultrasound Obstet Gynecol 36(2):235, 2010

Houry D, Abbott JT: Ovarian torsion: a fifteen-year review. Ann Emerg Med 38(2):156, 2001

Hovsepian DM, Ratts VS, Rodriquez M, et al: A prospective comparison of the impact of uterine artery embolization, myomectomy, and hysterectomy on ovarian function. J Vasc Interv Radiol 17(7):1111, 2006

Hovsepian DM, Siskin GP, Bonn J, et al: Quality improvement guidelines for uterine artery embolization for symptomatic leiomyomata. J Vasc Interv Radiol 20(7 Suppl):S193, 2009

Hurst BS, Matthews ML, Marshburn PB: Laparoscopic myomectomy for symptomatic uterine myomas. Fertil Steril 83(1):1, 2005

Im SS, Gordon AN, Buttin BM, et al: Validation of referral guidelines for women with pelvic masses. Obstet Gynecol 105(1):35, 2005

Inki P, Hurskainen R, Palo P, et al: Comparison of ovarian cyst formation in women using the levonorgestrel-releasing intrauterine system vs. hysterectomy. Ultrasound Obstet Gynecol 20(4):381, 2002

Ishikawa H, Ishi K, Serna VA, et al: Progesterone is essential for maintenance and growth of uterine leiomyomata. Endocrinology 151(6):2433, 2010

Ishikawa H, Reierstad S, Demura M, et al: High aromatase expression in uterine leiomyoma tissue of African-American women. J Clin Endocrinol Metab 94(5):1752, 2009

Islam S, Yamout SZ, Gosche JR: Management and outcomes of ovarian masses in children and adolescents. Am Surg 74(11):1062, 2008

Iverson RE Jr, Chelmow D, Strohbehn K, et al: Relative morbidity of abdominal hysterectomy and myomectomy for management of uterine leiomyomas. Obstet Gynecol 88(3):415, 1996

Jha RC, Takahama J, Imaoka I, et al: Adenomyosis: MRI of the uterus treated with uterine artery embolization. AJR Am J Roentgenol 181(3):851, 2003

Johnson NP, Mak W, Sowter MC: Surgical treatment for tubal disease in women due to undergo in vitro fertilisation. Cochrane Database Syst Rev 3:CD002125, 2004

Katsube Y, Berg JW, Silverberg SG: Epidemiologic pathology of ovarian tumors: a histopathologic review of primary ovarian neoplasms diagnosed in the Denver Standard Metropolitan Statistical Area, 1 July-31 December 1969 and 1 July-31 December 1979. Int J Gynecol Pathol 1(1):3, 1982

Kaunitz AM: Progestin-releasing intrauterine systems and leiomyoma. Contraception 75(Suppl):S130, 2007

Kelley RR, Scully RE: Cancer developing in dermoid cysts of the ovary. A report of 8 cases, including a carcinoid and a leiomyosarcoma. Cancer 14:989, 1961

Kettel LM, Murphy AA, Morales AJ, et al: Rapid regression of uterine leiomyomas in response to daily administration of gonadotropin-releasing hormone antagonist. Fertil Steril 60(4):642, 1993

Kho KA, Nezhat C: Parasitic myomas. Obstet Gynecol 114(3):611, 2009

Kim MD, Kim S, Kim NK, et al: Long-term results of uterine artery embolization for symptomatic adenomyosis. AJR Am J Roentgenol 188:176, 2007

Klatsky PC, Tran ND, Caughey AB, et al: Fibroids and reproductive outcomes: a systematic literature review from conception to delivery. Am J Obstet Gynecol 198(4):357, 2008

Koike H, Egawa H, Ohtsuka T, et al: Correlation between dysmenorrheic severity and prostaglandin production in women with endometriosis. Prostaglandins Leukot Essent Fatty Acids 46(2):133, 1992

Kooij SM, Hehenkamp WJ, Wolkers NA, et al: Uterine artery embolization vs hysterectomy in the treatment of symptomatic uterine fibroids: 5-year outcome from the randomized EMMY trial. Am J Obstet Gynecol 203:105.e1, 2010

Koonings PP, Campbell K, Mishell DR Jr, et al: Relative frequency of primary ovarian neoplasms: a 10-year review. Obstet Gynecol 74(6):921, 1989

Korbin CD, Brown DL, Welch WR: Paraovarian cystadenomas and cystadenofibromas: sonographic characteristics in 14 cases. Radiology 208(2):459, 1998

Kumaran GC, Jayson GC, Clamp AR: Antiangiogenic drugs in ovarian cancer. Br J Cancer 100(1):1, 2009

Kupesic S, Kurjak A, Skenderovic S, et al: Screening for uterine abnormalities by three-dimensional ultrasound improves perinatal outcome. J Perinat Med 30(1):9, 2002

Kurtz AB, Rubin CS, Kramer FL, et al: Ultrasound evaluation of the posterior pelvic compartment. Radiology 132(3):677, 1979

Lee NC, Dicker RC, Rubin GL, et al: Confirmation of the preoperative diagnoses for hysterectomy. Am J Obstet Gynecol 150(3):283, 1984

Lee RA, Welch JS: Torsion of the uterine adnexa. Am J Obstet Gynecol 97(7):974, 1967

Letterie GS, Coddington CC, Winkel CA, et al: Efficacy of a gonadotropin-releasing hormone agonist in the treatment of uterine leiomyomata: long-term follow-up. Fertil Steril 51(6):951, 1989

Levens ED, Potlog-Nahari C, Armstrong AY, et al: CDB-2914 for uterine leiomyomata treatment: a randomized controlled trial. Obstet Gynecol 111(5):1129, 2008

Levgur M, Abadi MA, Tucker A: Adenomyosis: symptoms, histology, and pregnancy terminations. Obstet Gynecol 95(5):688, 2000

Levine D, Brown DL, Andreotti RF, et al: Management of asymptomatic ovarian and other adnexal cysts imaged at US: Society of Radiologists in Ultrasound Consensus Conference Statement. Radiology 256(3):943, 2010

Levy BS: Modern management of uterine fibroids. Acta Obstet Gynaecol Scand 87(8):812, 2008

Lin P, Falcone T, Tulandi T: Excision of ovarian dermoid cyst by laparoscopy and by laparotomy. Am J Obstet Gynecol 173(3 Pt 1):769, 1995

Lin YC, Wei LH, Shun CT, et al: Disseminated peritoneal leiomyomatosis responds to systemic chemotherapy. Oncology 76(1):55, 2009

Lindahl B, Andolf E, Ingvar C, et al: Endometrial thickness and ovarian cysts as measured by ultrasound in asymptomatic postmenopausal breast cancer patients on various adjuvant treatments including tamoxifen. Anticancer Res 17(5B):3821, 1997

Linder D, McCaw BK, Hecht F: Parthenogenic origin of benign ovarian teratomas. N Engl J Med 292(2):63, 1975

Lippman SA, Warner M, Samuels S, et al: Uterine fibroids and gynecologic pain symptoms in a population-based study. Fertil Steril 80(6):1488, 2003

Lohle PN, De Vries J, Klazen CA, et al: Uterine artery embolization for symptomatic adenomyosis with or without uterine leiomyomas with the use of calibrated tris-acryl gelatin microspheres: midterm clinical and MR imaging follow-up. J Vasc Interv Radiol 18(7):835, 2007

Lumbiganon P, Rugpao S, Phandhu-fung S, et al: Protective effect of depot-medroxyprogesterone acetate on surgically treated uterine leiomyomas: a multicentre case-control study. Br J Obstet Gynaecol 103(9):909, 1996

Magalhães J, Aldrighi JM, de Lima GR: Uterine volume and menstrual patterns in users of the levonorgestrel-releasing intrauterine system with idiopathic menorrhagia or menorrhagia due to leiomyomas. Contraception 75(3):193, 2007

Mahdavi A, Berker B, Nezhat C, et al: Laparoscopic management of ovarian remnant. Obstet Gynecol Clin North Am 31(3):593, 2004

Mais V, Ajossa S, Guerriero S, et al: Laparoscopic versus abdominal myomectomy: a prospective, randomized trial to evaluate benefits in early outcome. Am J Obstet Gynecol 174(2):654, 1996

Mais V, Ajossa S, Piras B, et al: Treatment of nonendometriotic benign adnexal cysts: a randomized comparison of laparoscopy and laparotomy. Obstet Gynecol 86(5):770, 1995

Mäkäräinen L, Ylikorkala O: Primary and myoma-associated menorrhagia: role of prostaglandins and effects of ibuprofen. Br J Obstet Gynaecol 93(9):974, 1986

Marchionni M, Fambrini M, Zambelli V, et al: Reproductive performance before and after abdominal myomectomy: a retrospective analysis. Fertil Steril 82(1):154, 2004

Marjoribanks J, Proctor ML, Farquhar C: Nonsteroidal anti-inflammatory drugs for primary dysmenorrhoea. Cochrane Database Syst Rev 4:CD001751, 2003

Marret H: [Doppler ultrasonography in the diagnosis of ovarian cysts: indications, pertinence and diagnostic criteria]. [French]. J Gynecol Obstet Biol Reprod (Paris) 30(1 Suppl):S20, 2001

Marshall LM, Spiegelman D, Manson JE, et al: Risk of uterine leiomyomata among premenopausal women in relation to body size and cigarette smoking. Epidemiology 9(5):511, 1998

Martinez-Onsurbe P, Ruiz VA, Sanz Anquela JM, et al: Aspiration cytology of 147 adnexal cysts with histologic correlation. Acta Cytol 45(6):941, 2001

Mashal RD, Fejzo ML, Friedman AJ, et al: Analysis of androgen receptor DNA reveals the independent clonal origins of uterine leiomyomata and the secondary nature of cytogenetic aberrations in the development of leiomyomata. Genes Chromosomes Cancer 11(1):1, 1994

McCausland AM, McCausland VM: Depth of endometrial penetration in adenomyosis helps determine outcome of rollerball ablation. Am J Obstet Gynecol 174(6):1786, 1996

McGovern PG, Noah R, Koenigsberg R, et al: Adnexal torsion and pulmonary embolism: case report and review of the literature. Obstet Gynecol Surv 54(9):601, 1999

Mencaglia L, Tantini C: GnRH agonist analogs and hysteroscopic resection of myomas. Int J Gynaecol Obstet 43(3):285, 1993

Menon U, Talaat A, Jeyarajah AR, et al: Ultrasound assessment of ovarian cancer risk in postmenopausal women with CA125 elevation. Br J Cancer 80(10):1644, 1999

Michnovicz JJ, Hershcopf RJ, Naganuma H, et al: Increased 2-hydroxylation of estradiol as a possible mechanism for the anti-estrogenic effect of cigarette smoking. N Engl J Med 315(21):1305, 1986

Millar DM, Blake JM, Stringer DA, et al: Prepubertal ovarian cyst formation: 5 years' experience. Obstet Gynecol 81(3):434, 1993

Minaretzis D, Tsionou C, Tziortziotis D, et al: Ovarian tumors: prediction of the probability of malignancy by using patient's age and tumor morphologic features with a logistic model. Gynecol Obstet Invest 38(2):140, 1994

Miyake T, Enomoto T, Ueda Y, et al: A case of disseminated peritoneal leiomyomatosis developing after laparoscopic-assisted myomectomy. Gynecol Obstet Invest 67(2):96, 2009

Mizutani T, Sugihara A, Nakamuro K, et al: Suppression of cell proliferation and induction of apoptosis in uterine leiomyoma by gonadotropin-releasing hormone agonist (leuprolide acetate). J Clin Endocrinol Metab 83(4):1253, 1998

Molnar BG, Baumann R, Magos AL: Does endometrial resection help dysmenorrhea? Acta Obstet Gynecol Scand 76(3):261, 1997

Moran O, Menczer J, Ben Baruch G, et al: Cytologic examination of ovarian cyst fluid for the distinction between benign and malignant tumors. Obstet Gynecol 82(3):444, 1993

Mourits MJ, de Vries EG, Willemse PH, et al: Ovarian cysts in women receiving tamoxifen for breast cancer. Br J Cancer 79(11-12):1761, 1999

Murphy AA, Kettel LM, Morales AJ, et al: Regression of uterine leiomyomata in response to the antiprogesterone RU 486. J Clin Endocrinol Metab 76(2):513, 1993

Mutter GL, Bergeron C, Deligdisch L, et al: The spectrum of endometrial pathology induced by progesterone receptor modulators. Mod Pathol 21(5):591, 2008

Nardo LG, Kroon ND, Reginald PW: Persistent unilocular ovarian cysts in a general population of postmenopausal women: is there a place for expectant management? Obstet Gynecol 102(3):589, 2003

Nezhat C, Kearney S, Malik S, et al: Laparoscopic management of ovarian remnant. Fertil Steril 83(4):973, 2005

Nichols DH, Julian PJ: Torsion of the adnexa. Clin Obstet Gynecol 28(2):375, 1985

Nikkanen V, Punnonen R: Clinical significance of adenomyosis. Ann Chir Gynaecol 69(6):278, 1980

Nishida M: Relationship between the onset of dysmenorrhea and histologic findings in adenomyosis. Am J Obstet Gynecol 165(1):229, 1991

Okugawa K, Hirakawa T, Fukushima K, et al: Relationship between age, histological type, and size of ovarian tumors. Int J Gynaecol Obstet 74(1):45, 2001

Oliveira FG, Abdelmassih VG, Diamond MP, et al: Impact of subserosal and intramural uterine fibroids that do not distort the endometrial cavity on the outcome of in vitro fertilization-intracytoplasmic sperm injection. Fertil Steril 81(3):582, 2004

Olufowobi O, Sharif K, Papaionnou S, et al: Are the anticipated benefits of myomectomy achieved in women of reproductive age? A 5-year review of the results at a UK tertiary hospital. J Obstet Gynaecol 24(4):434, 2004

Orsini G, Laricchia L, Fanelli M: [Low-dose combination oral contraceptives use in women with uterine leiomyomas]. [Italian]. Minerva Ginecol 54(3):253, 2002

Ory H: Functional ovarian cysts and oral contraceptives. Negative association confirmed surgically. A cooperative study. J AM Med Assoc 228(1):68, 1974

Otubu JA, Buttram VC, Besch NF, et al: Unconjugated steroids in leiomyomas and tumor-bearing myometrium. Am J Obstet Gynecol 143(2):130, 1982

Outwater EK, Mitchell DG: Normal ovaries and functional cysts: MR appearance. Radiology 198(2):397, 1996

Palomba S, Affinito P, Tommaselli GA, et al: A clinical trial of the effects of tibolone administered with gonadotropin-releasing hormone analogues for the treatment of uterine leiomyomata. Fertil Steril 70(1):111, 1998

Palomba S, Orio F Jr, Russo T, et al: Gonadotropin-releasing hormone agonist with or without raloxifene: effects on cognition, mood, and quality of life. Fertil Steril 82(2):480, 2004

Palomba S, Sena T, Morelli M, et al: Effect of different doses of progestin on uterine leiomyomas in postmenopausal women. Eur J Obstet Gynecol Reprod Biol 102(2):199, 2002

Pantoja E, Noy MA, Axtmayer RW, et al: Ovarian dermoids and their complications. Comprehensive historical review. Obstet Gynecol Surv 30(1):1, 1975a

Pantoja E, Rodriguez-Ibanez I, Axtmayer RW, et al: Complications of dermoid tumors of the ovary. Obstet Gynecol 45(1):89, 1975b

Parazzini F, Negri E, La Vecchia C, et al: Oral contraceptive use and risk of uterine fibroids. Obstet Gynecol 79(3):430, 1992

Parazzini F, Vercellini P, Panazza S, et al: Risk factors for adenomyosis. Hum Reprod 12(6):1275, 1997

Parker WH: Etiology, symptomatology, and diagnosis of uterine myomas. Fertil Steril 87(4):725, 2007

Parker WH: Laparoscopic myomectomy and abdominal myomectomy. Clin Obstet Gynecol 49(4):789, 2006

Parker WH, Fu YS, Berek JS: Uterine sarcoma in patients operated on for presumed leiomyoma and rapidly growing leiomyoma. Obstet Gynecol 83(3):414, 1994

Patel MD, Feldstein VA, Lipson SD, et al: Cystic teratomas of the ovary: diagnostic value of sonography. AJR Am J Roentgenol 171(4):1061, 1998

Pauerstein CJ, Woodruff JD, Quinton SW: Development patterns in "adenomatoid lesions" of the fallopian tube. Am J Obstet Gynecol 100(7):1000, 1968

Paul PG, Koshy AK: Multiple peritoneal parasitic myomas after laparoscopic myomectomy and morcellation. Fertile Steril 85(2):492, 2006

Peddada SD, Laughlin SK, Miner, K, et al: Growth of uterine leiomyomata among premenopausal black and white women. Proc Natl Acad Sci USA 105(50):19887, 2008

Perkins JD, Hines RR, Prior DS: Uterine leiomyoma in an adolescent female. J Natl Med Assoc 101(6):611, 2009

Peterson WF: Malignant degeneration of benign cystic teratomas of the ovary; a collective review of the literature. Obstet Gynecol Surv 12(6):793, 1957

Peterson WF, Prevost EC, Edmunds FT, et al: Benign cystic teratomas of the ovary; a clinico-statistical study of 1,007 cases with a review of the literature. Am J Obstet Gynecol 70(2):368, 1955

Phupong V, Sueblinvong T, Triratanachat S: Ovarian teratoma with diffused peritoneal reactions mimicking advanced ovarian malignancy. Arch Gynecol Obstet 270(3):189, 2004

Polatti F, Viazzo F, Colleoni R, et al: Uterine myoma in postmenopause: a comparison between two therapeutic schedules of HRT. Maturitas 37(1):27, 2000

Porcu E, Venturoli S, Dal Prato L, et al: Frequency and treatment of ovarian cysts in adolescence. Arch Gynecol Obstet 255(2):69, 1994

Prat J: Ovarian serous and mucinous epithelial-stromal tumors. In Robboy SJ, Mutter GL, Prat J, et al (eds): Robboy's Pathology of the Female Reproductive Tract, 2nd ed. Churchill Livingstone Elsevier, 2009, p 611

Pron G, Mocarski E, Bennett J, et al: Pregnancy after uterine artery embolization for leiomyomata: the Ontario multicenter trial. Obstet Gynecol 105(1):67, 2005

Reed SD, Cushing-Haugen KL, Daling JR, et al: Postmenopausal estrogen and progestogen therapy and the risk of uterine leiomyomas. Menopause 11(2):214, 2004

Rein MS, Powell WL, Walters FC, et al: Cytogenetic abnormalities in uterine myomas are associated with myoma size. Mol Hum Reprod 4(1):83, 1998

Reinhold C, Tafazoli F, Mehio A, et al: Uterine adenomyosis: endovaginal US and MR imaging features with histopathologic correlation. Radiographics 19:S147-60, 1999

Reinhold C, Tafazoli F, Wang L: Imaging features of adenomyosis. Hum Reprod Update 4(4):337, 1998

Reinsch RC, Murphy AA, Morales AJ, et al: The effects of RU 486 and leuprolide acetate on uterine artery blood flow in the fibroid uterus: a prospective, randomized study. Am J Obstet Gynecol 170(6):1623; 1994

Rha SE, Byun JY, Jung SE, et al: CT and MR imaging features of adnexal torsion. Radiographics 22(2):283, 2002

Rivera JA, Christopoulos S, Small D, et al: Hormonal manipulation of benign metastasizing leiomyomas: report of two cases and review of the literature. J Clin Endocrinol Metab 89(7):3183, 2004

Robboy SJ, Bentley RC, Butnor K, et al: Pathology and pathophysiology of uterine smooth-muscle tumors. Environ Health Perspect 108 (Suppl 5):779, 2000

Rody A, Jackisch C, Klockenbusch W, et al: The conservative management of adnexal torsion—a case-report and review of the literature. Eur J Obstet Gynecol Reprod Biol 101(1):83, 2002

Rosado WM Jr, Trambert MA, Gosink BB, et al: Adnexal torsion: diagnosis by using Doppler sonography. AJR Am J Roentgenol 159(6):1251, 1992

Ross RK, Pike MC, Vessey MP, et al: Risk factors for uterine fibroids: reduced risk associated with oral contraceptives. Br Med J Clin Res Ed 293(6543):359, 1986

Russell P, Robboy SJ: Ovarian cysts, tumor-like, iatrogenic and miscellaneous conditions. In Robboy SJ, Mutter GL, Prat J, et al (eds): Robboy's Pathology of the Female Reproductive Tract, 2nd ed. Churchill Livingstone Elsevier, 2009, p 577

Sailer JF: Hematometra and hematocolpos: ultrasound findings. AJR Am J Roentgenol 132(6):1010, 1979

Salazar H, Kanbour A, Burgess F: Ultrastructure and observations on the histogenesis of mesotheliomas, "adenomatoid tumors," of the female genital tract. Cancer 29(1):141, 1972

Sammour A, Pirwany I, Usubutun A, et al: Correlations between extent and spread of adenomyosis and clinical symptoms. Gynecol Obstet Invest 54(4): 213, 2002

Sato F, Mori M, Nishi M, et al: Familial aggregation of uterine myomas in Japanese women. J Epidemiol 12(3):249, 2002

Sawin SW, Pilevsky ND, Berlin JA, et al: Comparability of perioperative morbidity between abdominal myomectomy and hysterectomy for women with uterine leiomyomas. Am J Obstet Gynecol 183(6):1448, 2000

Scharla SH, Minne HW, Waibel-Treber S, et al: Bone mass reduction after estrogen deprivation by long-acting gonadotropin-releasing hormone agonists and its relation to pretreatment serum concentrations of 1,25-dihydroxyvitamin D_3. J Clin Endocrinol Metab 70(4):1055, 1990

Schlaff WD, Hassiakos DK, Damewood MD, et al: Neosalpingostomy for distal tubal obstruction: prognostic factors and impact of surgical technique. Fertil Steril 54(6):984, 1990

Schlaff WD, Zerhouni EA, Huth JA, et al: A placebo-controlled trial of a depot gonadotropin-releasing hormone analogue (leuprolide) in the treatment of uterine leiomyomata. Obstet Gynecol 74(6):856, 1989

Scully R, Sobin L: Histological Typing of Ovarian Tumours, Vol 9. New York, Springer Berlin, 1999

Seracchioli R, Rossi S, Govoni F, et al: Fertility and obstetric outcome after laparoscopic myomectomy of large myomata: a randomized comparison with abdominal myomectomy. Hum Reprod 15(12):2663, 2000

Sharp HT: Assessment of new technology in the treatment of idiopathic menorrhagia and uterine leiomyomata. Obstet Gynecol 108(4):990, 2006

Sheng J, Zhang WY, Zhang JP, et al: The LNG-IUS study on adenomyosis: a 3-year follow-up study on the efficacy and side effects of the use of levonorgestrel intrauterine system for the treatment of dysmenorrhea associated with adenomyosis. Contraception 79(3):189, 2009

Shushan A, Peretz T, Uziely B, et al: Ovarian cysts in premenopausal and postmenopausal tamoxifen-treated women with breast cancer. Am J Obstet Gynecol 174(1 Pt 1):141, 1996

Sinha R, Sundaram M, Mahajan C, et al: Multiple leiomyomas after laparoscopic hysterectomy: report of two cases. J Minim Invasiv Gynecol 14(1): 123, 2007

Siskin GP, Shlansky-Goldberg RD, Goodwin SC, et al: A prospective multicenter comparative study between myomectomy and uterine artery embolization with polyvinyl alcohol microspheres: long-term clinical outcomes in patients with symptomatic uterine fibroids. J Vasc Interv Radiol 17(8):1287, 2006

Spies JB, Spector A, Roth AR, et al: Complications after uterine artery embolization for leiomyomas. Obstet Gynecol 100(5 Pt 1):873, 2002

Spitz IM: Clinical utility of progesterone receptor modulators and their effect on the endometrium. Curr Opin Obstet Gynecol 21(4):318, 2009

Steinauer J, Pritts EA, Jackson R, et al: Systematic review of mifepristone for the treatment of uterine leiomyomata. Obstet Gynecol 103(6):1331, 2004

Stewart EA, Gedroyc WM, Tempany CM, et al: Focused ultrasound treatment of uterine fibroid tumors: safety and feasibility of a noninvasive thermoablative technique. Am J Obstet Gynecol 189(1):48, 2003

Stewart EA, Gostout B, Rabinovici J, et al: Sustained relief of leiomyoma symptoms by using focused ultrasound surgery. Obstet Gynecol 110(2 pt 1):279, 2007

Stewart EA, Nowak RA: Leiomyoma-related bleeding: a classic hypothesis updated for the molecular era. Hum Reprod Update 2(4):295, 1996

Stewart EA, Rabinovici JU, Tempany CM, et al: Clinical outcomes of focused ultrasound surgery for the treatment of uterine fibroids. Fertil Steril 85(1): 22, 2006

Stokes LS, Wallace MJ, Godwin RB, et al: Quality improvement guidelines for uterine artery embolization for symptomatic leiomyomas. J Vasc Interv Radiol 21:1153, 2010

Stovall TG, Summit RL Jr, Washburn SA, et al: Gonadotropin-releasing hormone agonist use before hysterectomy. Am J Obstet Gynecol 170(6):1744; 1994

Strandell A, Lindhard A: Why does hydrosalpinx reduce fertility? The importance of hydrosalpinx fluid. Hum Reprod 17(5):1141, 2002

Strandell A, Lindhard A, Waldenstrom U, et al: Hydrosalpinx and IVF outcome: a prospective, randomized multicentre trial in Scandinavia on salpingectomy prior to IVF. Hum Reprod 14(11):2762, 1999

Stricker B, Blanco J, Fox HE: The gynecologic contribution to intestinal obstruction in females. J Am Coll Surg 178(6):617, 1994

Swire MN, Castro-Aragon I, Levine D: Various sonographic appearances of the hemorrhagic corpus luteum cyst. Ultrasound Q 20(2):45, 2004

Takeuchi H, Kinoshita K: Evaluation of adhesion formation after laparoscopic myomectomy by systematic second-look microlaparoscopy. J Am Assoc Gynecol Laparosc 9(4):442, 2002

Takeuchi H, Kuwatsuru R: The indications, surgical techniques, and limitations of laparoscopic myomectomy. J Soc Laparoendosc Surg 7(2):89, 2003

Tiltman AJ: Leiomyomas of the uterine cervix: a study of frequency. Int J Gynecol Pathol 17(3):231, 1998

Tiltman AJ: The effect of progestins on the mitotic activity of uterine fibromyomas. Int J Gynecol Pathol 4(2):89, 1985

Toh CH, Wu CH, Tsay PK, et al: Uterine artery embolization for symptomatic uterine leiomyoma and adenomyosis. J Formos Med Assoc 102(10):701, 2003

Townsend DE, Sparkes RS, Baluda MC, et al: Unicellular histogenesis of uterine leiomyomas as determined by electrophoresis by glucose-6-phosphate dehydrogenase. Am J Obstet Gynecol 107(8):1168, 1970

Traiman P, Saldiva P, Haiashi A, et al: Criteria for the diagnosis of diffuse uterine myohypertrophy. Int J Gynaecol Obstet 54(1):31, 1996

Tropeano G, Di Stasi C, Amoroso S, et al: Long-term effects of uterine fibroid embolization on ovarian reserve: a prospective cohort study. Fertil Steril 94(6):2296, 2010

Turan C, Zorlu CG, Ugur M, et al: Expectant management of functional ovarian cysts: an alternative to hormonal therapy. Int J Gynaecol Obstet 47(3):257, 1994

Uchida H, Hattori Y, Nakada K, et al: Successful one-stage radical removal of intravenous leiomyomatosis extending to the right ventricle. Obstet Gynecol 103(5 Pt 2):1068, 2004

Umezaki I, Takagi K, Aiba M, et al: Uterine cervical diverticulum resembling a degenerated leiomyoma. Obstet Gynecol 103(5 Pt 2):1130, 2004

U.S. National Institutes of Health Clinical Trials: Study to evaluate the safety of asoprisnil in the treatment of uterine fibroids. May, 2008. Available online through ClinicalTrialsFeeds.org at: http://clinicaltrials.gov/ct2/show/NCT00156208. Accessed July 3, 2010

Vercellini P, Zaina B, Yaylayan L, et al: Hysteroscopic myomectomy: long-term effects on menstrual pattern and fertility. Obstet Gynecol 94(3):341, 1999

Vijayaraghavan SB: Sonographic whirlpool sign in ovarian torsion. J Ultrasound Med 23(12):1643, 2004

Vikhlyaeva EM, Khodzhaeva ZS, Fantschenko ND: Familial predisposition to uterine leiomyomas. Int J Gynaecol Obstet 51(2):127, 1995

Vilos GA, Vilos EC, Abu-Rafea B, et al: Transvaginal Doppler-guided uterine artery occlusion for the treatment of symptomatic fibroids: summary results from two pilot studies. J Obstet Gynaecol Can 32(2):149, 2010

Viville B, Charnock-Jones DS, Sharkey AM, et al: Distribution of the A and B forms of the progesterone receptor messenger ribonucleic acid and protein in uterine leiomyomata and adjacent myometrium. Hum Reprod 12(4):815, 1997

Vlasveld LT, de Wit CW, Vermeij RA, et al: Myomatous erythrocytosis syndrome: further proof for the pathogenic role of erythropoietin. Neth J Med 66(7):283, 2008

Volkers NA, Hehenkamp WJ, Birnie E, et al: Uterine artery embolization in the treatment of symptomatic uterine fibroid tumors (EMMY trial): periprocedural results and complications. J Vasc Interv Radiol 17(3):471, 2006

Vuento MH, Pirhonen JP, Makinen JI, et al: Evaluation of ovarian findings in asymptomatic postmenopausal women with color Doppler ultrasound. Cancer 76(7):1214, 1995

Walker WJ, McDowell SJ: Pregnancy after uterine artery embolization for leiomyomata: a series of 56 completed pregnancies. Am J Obstet Gynecol 195(5):1266, 2006

Wamsteker K, Emanuel MH, de Kruif JH: Transcervical hysteroscopic resection of submucous fibroids for abnormal uterine bleeding: results regarding the degree of intramural extension. Obstet Gynecol 82(5):736, 1993

Warner MA, Fleischer AC, Edell SL, et al: Uterine adnexal torsion: sonographic findings. Radiology 154(3):773, 1985

Wegienka G, Baird DD, Hertz-Picciotto I, et al: Self-reported heavy bleeding associated with uterine leiomyomata. Obstet Gynecol 101(3):431, 2003

Weinraub Z, Maymon R, Shulman A, et al: Three-dimensional saline contrast hysterosonography and surface rendering of uterine cavity pathology. Ultrasound Obstet Gynecol 8(4):277, 1996

Weitzman VN, DiLuigi AJ, Maier DB, et al: Prevention of recurrent adnexal torsion. Fertil Steril 90(5):2018.e1, 2008

Whiteman MK, Hillis SD, Jamieson DJ, et al: Inpatient hysterectomy surveillance in the United States, 2000-2004. Am J Obstet Gynecol 198(1):34. e1, 2008

Whiteman MK, Kuklina E, Jamieson DJ, et al: Inpatient hospitalization for gynecologic disorders in the United States. Am J Obstet Gynecol 202(6).541.e1, 2010

Williams AR, Critchley HO, Osei J, et al: The effects of the selective progesterone receptor modulator asoprisnil on the morphology of uterine tissues after 3 months treatment in patients with symptomatic uterine leiomyomata. Hum Reprod 22(6):1696, 2007

Willman EA, Collins WP, Clayton SG: Studies in the involvement of prostaglandins in uterine symptomatology and pathology. Br J Obstet Gynaecol 83(5):337, 1976

Wise LA, Palmer JR, Harlow BL, et al: Reproductive factors, hormonal contraception, and risk of uterine leiomyomata in African-American women: a prospective study. Am J Epidemiol 159(2):113, 2004

Wise LA, Palmer JR, Spiegelman D, et al: Influence of body size and body fat distribution on risk of uterine leiomyomata in U.S. black women. Epidemiology 16(3):346, 2005

Wise LA, Palmer JR, Stewart EA, et al: Polycystic ovary syndrome and risk of uterine leiomyomata. Fertil Steril 87(5):1108, 2007

Wiznitzer A, Marbach M, Hazum E, et al: Gonadotropin-releasing hormone specific binding sites in uterine leiomyomata. Biochem Biophys Res Commun 152(3):1326, 1988

Worley MJ Jr, Aelion A, Caputo TA, et al: Intravenous leiomyomatosis with intracardiac extension: a single-institution experience. Am J Obstet Gynecol 201(6):574.e1, 2009

Wortman M, Daggett A: Hysteroscopic endomyometrial resection. J Soc Laparoendosc Surg 4(3):197, 2000

Wu CC, Lee CN, Chen TM, et al: Incremental angiogenesis assessed by color Doppler ultrasound in the tumorigenesis of ovarian neoplasms. Cancer 73(4):1251, 1994

Wu MP, Wu CC, Chang FM, et al: Endometrial carcinoma presenting as hematometra mimicking a large pelvic cyst. J Clin Ultrasound 27(9):541, 1999

Wyshak G, Frisch RE, Albright TE, et al: Smoking and cysts of the ovary. Int J Fertil 33(6):398, 1988

Xing YP, Powell WL, Morton CC: The del(7q) subgroup in uterine leiomyomata: genetic and biologic characteristics. Further evidence for the secondary nature of cytogenetic abnormalities in the pathobiology of uterine leiomyomata. Cancer Genet Cytogenet 98(1):69, 1997

Yamamoto T, Noguchi T, Tamura T, et al: Evidence for estrogen synthesis in adenomyotic tissues. Am J Obstet Gynecol 169(3):734, 1993

Yin CS, Wei RY, Chao TC, et al: Hysteroscopic endometrial ablation without endometrial preparation. Int J Gynaecol Obstet 62(2):167, 1998

Ylikorkala O, Dawood MY: New concepts in dysmenorrhea. Am J Obstet Gynecol 130(7):833, 1978

Ylikorkala O, Pekonen F: Naproxen reduces idiopathic but not fibromyoma-induced menorrhagia. Obstet Gynecol 68(1):10, 1986

Yoffe N, Bronshtein M, Brandes J, et al: Hemorrhagic ovarian cyst detection by transvaginal sonography: the great imitator. Gynecol Endocrinol 5(2):123, 1991

Yokoyama Y, Shinohara A, Hirokawa M, et al: Erythrocytosis due to an erythropoietin-producing large uterine leiomyoma. Gynecol Obstet Invest 56(4):179, 2003

Young JL Jr, Miller RW: Incidence of malignant tumors in U. S. children. J Pediatr 86(2):254, 1975

Yuen PM, Yu KM, Yip SK, et al: A randomized prospective study of laparoscopy and laparotomy in the management of benign ovarian masses. Am J Obstet Gynecol 177(1):109, 1997

Zaloudek C, Hendrickson M: Mesenchymal tumors of the uterus. In Kurman RJ (eds): Blaustein's Pathology of the Female Genital Tract. New York, Springer, 2002, p 577

Zawin M, McCarthy S, Scoutt LM, et al: High-field MRI and US evaluation of the pelvis in women with leiomyomas. Magn Reson Imaging 8(4):371, 1990

Zhang C, Miao Q, Liu X, et al: Intravenous leiomyomatosis with intracardiac extension. Ann Thorac Surg 89(5):1641, 2010

Zumoff B, Miller L, Levit CD, et al: The effect of smoking on serum progesterone, estradiol, and luteinizing hormone levels over a menstrual cycle in normal women. Steroids 55(11):507, 199

Zweizig S, Perron J, Grubb D, et al: Conservative management of adnexal torsion. Am J Obstet Gynecol 168(6 Pt 1):1791, 1993

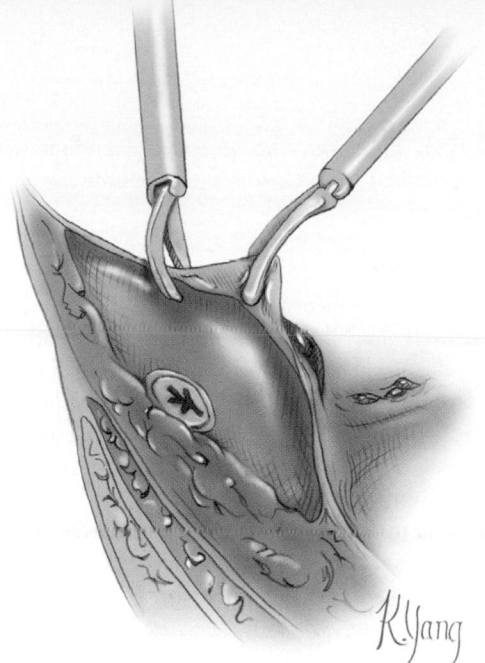

Endometriosis

Endometriosis is a common benign gynecologic disorder defined as the presence of endometrial glands and stroma outside of the normal location. First identified in the mid-19th century, endometriosis is most commonly found on the pelvic peritoneum but may also be found on the ovaries, rectovaginal septum, and ureter, and rarely in the bladder, pericardium, and pleura (Comiter, 2002; Giudice, 2004; Von Rokitansky, 1860). Endometriosis is a hormonally dependent disease and as a result is chiefly found in reproductive-aged women. Women with endometriosis may be asymptomatic, subfertile, or suffer varying degrees of pelvic pain. Endometrial tissue located within the myometrium is termed adenomyosis, or sometimes referred to as endometriosis in situ, and is discussed in greater detail in Chapter 9 (p. 259).

INCIDENCE

The incidence of endometriosis is difficult to quantify, as women with the disease are often asymptomatic, and imaging modalities have low sensitivities for diagnosis. The primary method of diagnosis is laparoscopy, with or without biopsy for histologic diagnosis (Kennedy, 2005; Marchino, 2005b). Using this standard, investigators have reported the annual incidence of surgically diagnosed endometriosis to be 1.6 cases per 1000 women aged between 15 and 49 years (Houston, 1987). In asymptomatic women, the prevalence of endometriosis ranges from 2 to 22 percent, depending on the population studied (Eskenazi, 1997; Mahmood, 1991; Moen, 1997). However, because of its link with infertility and pelvic pain, endometriosis is notably more prevalent in subpopulations of women with these complaints. In infertile women, the prevalence has been reported to be between 20 and 50 percent and in those with pelvic pain, between 40 and 50 percent (Balasch, 1996; Eskenazi, 2001; Meuleman, 2009).

PATHOPHYSIOLOGY

Etiology

Although the definitive cause of endometriosis remains unknown, several theories with supporting evidence have been described.

Retrograde Menstruation

The earliest and most widely accepted theory describes retrograde menstruation through the fallopian tubes and subsequent dissemination of endometrial tissue within the peritoneal cavity (Sampson, 1927). Refluxed endometrial fragments adhere to and invade the peritoneal mesothelium and develop a blood supply, which leads to continued implant survival and growth (Giudice, 2004).

First proposed in the 1920s, this theory has gained support with the findings of greater volumes of refluxed blood and endometrial tissue in the pelves of women with endometriosis (Halme, 1984). Uterine hyperperistalsis and dysperistalsis have been noted in women with endometriosis and resulted in subsequent increased endometrial reflux (Leyendecker, 2004). Additionally, D'Hooghe (1997) demonstrated that surgical obliteration of the cervical outflow tract in baboons leads to the induction of endometriosis. Women with amenorrhea due to outflow tract obstruction similarly have a high incidence of endometriosis, which is often relieved by correction of the obstruction (Sanfilippo, 1986).

Lymphatic or Vascular Spread

Evidence also supports the concept of endometriosis originating from aberrant lymphatic or vascular spread of endometrial tissue (Ueki, 1991). Findings of endometriosis in unusual locations, such as the perineum or groin, bolster this theory (Mitchell, 1991; Pollack, 1990). The retroperitoneal region has abundant lymphatic circulation. Thus, cases in which no peritoneal implants are found, but solely isolated retroperitoneal lesions are noted, suggest lymphatic spread (Moore, 1988). Additionally, the tendency of endometrial adenocarcinoma to spread via the lymphatic route indicates the ease with which endometrium can be transported by this method (McMeekin, 2003). Although this theory remains attractive, few studies have experimentally evaluated this form of endometriosis transmission.

Coelomic Metaplasia

The theory of coelomic metaplasia suggests that the parietal peritoneum is a pluripotential tissue that can undergo metaplastic transformation to tissue histologically indistinguishable from normal endometrium. Because the ovary and the progenitor of the endometrium, the müllerian ducts, are both derived from coelomic epithelium, metaplasia may explain the development of ovarian endometriosis. In addition, the theory has been extended to include the peritoneum because of the proliferative and differentiation potential of the peritoneal mesothelium. This theory is attractive in instances of endometriosis in the absence of menstruation, such as in premenarchal and postmenopausal women, and in males treated with estrogen and orchiectomy for prostatic carcinoma (Dictor, 1988; Pinkert, 1979). However, the absence of endometriosis in other tissues derived from coelomic epithelium argues against this theory.

Induction Theory

Finally, the induction theory proposes that some hormonal or biologic factor(s) may induce the differentiation of undifferentiated cells into endometrial tissue (Vinatier, 2001). These substances may be exogenous or released directly from the endometrium (Bontis, 1997). In vitro studies have demonstrated the potential for ovarian surface epithelium, in response to estrogens, to undergo transformation to form endometriotic lesions (Matsuura, 1999). Although many putative factors have been identified, their propensity to cause endometriosis in some women but not in others demonstrates the still-unidentified etiology of this disease.

Hormonal Dependence

Estrogen has been definitively established as having a causative role in the development of endometriosis (Gurates, 2003). Although most estrogen in women is produced directly by the ovaries, numerous peripheral tissues are also known to create estrogens through aromatization of ovarian and adrenal androgens. Endometriotic implants have been shown to express aromatase and 17β-hydroxysteroid dehydrogenase type 1, the enzymes responsible for conversion of androstenedione to estrone and of estrone to estradiol, respectively. Implants, however, are deficient in 17β-hydroxysteroid dehydrogenase type 2, which inactivates estrogen (Kitawaki, 1997; Zeitoun, 1998). This enzymatic combination ensures that implants will be exposed to an estrogenic environment. Furthermore, the locally produced estrogens within endometriotic lesions may exert their biologic effect within the same tissue or cell in which they are produced, a process referred to as *intracrinology*.

In contrast, normal endometrium does not express aromatase and has elevated levels of 17β-hydroxysteroid dehydrogenase type 2 in response to progesterone (Satyaswaroop, 1982). As a result, progesterone antagonizes the estrogen effects in normal endometrium during the luteal phase of the menstrual cycle. Endometriosis, however, manifests a relative progesterone-resistant state, which prevents attenuation of the estrogen stimulation in this tissue (Attia, 2000).

Prostaglandin E_2 (PGE_2) is the most potent inducer of aromatase activity in endometrial stromal cells, acting through the prostaglandin EP_2 receptor subtype (Noble, 1997; Zeitoun, 1999). Estradiol produced in response to the increased aromatase activity subsequently augments PGE_2 production by stimulating the cyclooxygenase type 2 (COX-2) enzyme in uterine endothelial cells (Fig. 10-1) (Bulun, 2002; Gurates, 2003). This creates a positive feedback loop and potentiates the estrogenic effects on proliferation of endometriosis. This concept of locally produced estrogens and intracrine estrogen action in endometriosis serves as the basis for aromatase inhibitor use. These agents diminish aromatase activity in cases of endometriosis that are refractory to standard therapy.

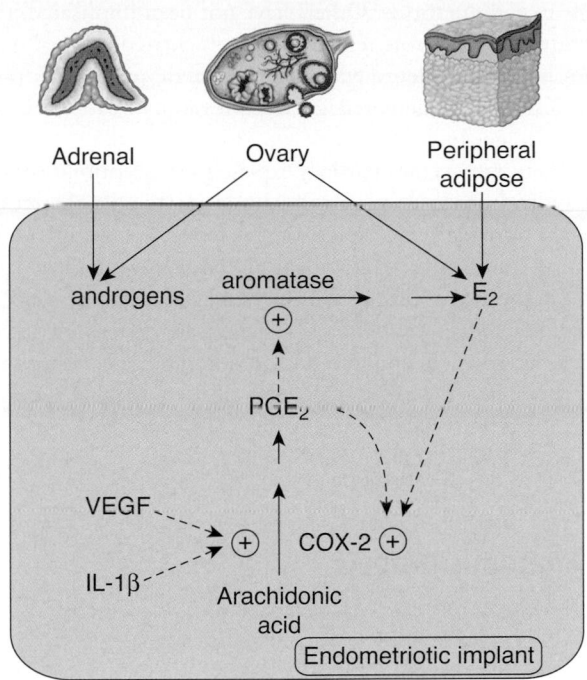

FIGURE 10-1 Activation of COX-2 in endometrial stromal cells results in upregulation of PGE_2, a potent stimulator of aromatase in endometrial stromal cells. Aromatase activity results in intracellular aromatization of androgens to increase intracellular estradiol via a paracrine mechanism. *(Redrawn from Gurates, 2003.)*

Role of the Immune System

Although most women experience retrograde menstruation, which may play a role in the seeding and establishment of implants, few develop endometriosis. Menstrual tissue and endometrium that are refluxed into the peritoneal cavity are usually cleared by immune cells such as macrophages, natural killer (NK) cells, and lymphocytes. For this reason, immune system dysfunction is one likely mechanism for the genesis of endometriosis in the presence of retrograde menstruation (Seli, 2003). Impaired cellular and humoral immunity and altered growth factor and cytokine signaling have each been identified in endometriotic tissues.

Macrophages act as scavenger cells in various tissues, and increased numbers have been found in the peritoneal cavities of women with endometriosis (Haney, 1981; Olive, 1985b). This increased population might logically act to suppress endometrial proliferation. However, macrophages in these women instead have a stimulatory effect on endometriotic tissue. In one study, circulating monocytes obtained from women with endometriosis enhanced the in vitro proliferation of cultured endometrial cells, whereas monocytes from women without endometriosis had the opposite effect (Braun, 1994). Therefore, it appears that impaired function, and not population size, of macrophages allows endometriotic tissue proliferation.

Natural killer cells are immune cells that have cytotoxic activity against foreign cells. Although the number of NK cells is unaltered in the peritoneal fluid of women with endometriosis, decreased NK cell cytotoxicity against endometrium has been demonstrated (Ho, 1995; Wilson, 1994). Specifically, the peritoneal fluid from women with endometriosis has been found to suppress NK cell activity, suggesting that soluble factors may play a role in NK cell suppression (Oosterlynck, 1993).

Cellular immunity may also be disordered in women with endometriosis, and T lymphocytes are implicated. For example, in women with endometriosis compared with unaffected women, total lymphocyte numbers or helper/suppressor subpopulation ratios do not differ in peripheral blood, but peritoneal fluid lymphocyte numbers are increased (Steele, 1984). Also, the cytotoxic activity of T lymphocytes against autologous endometrium in affected women is impaired (Gleicher, 1984).

Humoral immunity has also been shown to be altered in affected women and is suggested to play a role in the development of endometriosis. Endometrial antibodies of the IgG class are more frequently detected in the sera of women with endometriosis (Odukoya, 1995). One study also identified IgG and IgA autoantibodies against endometrial and ovarian tissues in the sera and in cervical and vaginal secretions of affected women (Mathur, 1982). These results suggest that endometriosis may be, in part, an autoimmune disease. This may explain some of the factors influencing lower pregnancy and in vitro fertilization (IVF) implantation rates in women with endometriosis (Dmowski, 1995).

Cytokines are small, soluble immune factors involved in paracrine and autocrine signaling of other immune cells. Numerous cytokines, especially interleukins, have been implicated in the pathogenesis of endometriosis. Increased levels of interleukin-1β (IL-1β) have been identified in the endometrial fluid of those with endometriosis (Mori, 1991). Moreover, IL-6 levels are increased in endometrial stromal cells of affected women (Tseng, 1996). Accordingly, IL-6 serum levels greater than 2 pg/mL and tumor necrosis factor-α (TNF-α) peritoneal fluid levels more than 15 pg/mL may be used to discriminate between those with or without endometriosis (Bedaiwy, 2002). Similarly, IL-8 peritoneal fluid levels are elevated in affected individuals and stimulate proliferation of endometrial stromal cells (Arici, 1996, 1998; Ryan, 1995). Testing for these factors is mainly a research tool and not clinically used for endometriosis diagnosis.

Other noninterleukin cytokines and growth factors are associated with the pathogenesis of endometriosis. For example, both monocyte chemoattractant protein-1 (MCP-1) and RANTES (regulated on activation, normal T-cell expressed and secreted) are chemoattractant for monocytes. Levels of these cytokines are increased in the peritoneal fluid of those with endometriosis and positively correlate with disease severity (Arici, 1997; Khorram, 1993). In addition, vascular endothelial growth factor (VEGF) is an angiogenic growth factor, which is upregulated by estradiol in endometrial stromal cells and peritoneal fluid macrophages. Levels of this factor are increased in the peritoneal fluid of affected women (McLaren, 1996). Although the exact role of these cytokines is not clear, perturbations in their expression and activity further support an immunologic role in the pathogenesis of endometriosis.

RISK FACTORS

Familial Clustering

There is evidence of a familial inheritance pattern for endometriosis. Although no apparent Mendelian genetics inheritance pattern has been identified, the increased incidence in first-degree relatives suggests a polygenic/multifactorial inheritance pattern. For example, in a genetic study of women with endometriosis, Simpson and colleagues (1980) noted that 5.9 percent of female siblings and 8.1 percent of the mothers of affected women had endometriosis, compared with 1 percent of the husband's female first-degree relatives. Further research has revealed that women with endometriosis and an affected first-degree relative were more likely to have severe endometriosis (61 percent) than women without an affected first-degree relative (24 percent) (Malinak, 1980). Moreover, Stefansson and associates (2002), in their analysis of a large population-based study in Iceland, demonstrated a higher kinship coefficient in women with endometriosis compared with matched controls. In this study, the risk ratios were 5.2 for sisters and 1.56 for cousins. Studies have also demonstrated concordance for endometriosis in monozygotic twin-pairs, suggesting a familial/genetic basis (Hadfield, 1997; Treloar, 1999).

Genetic Mutations and Polymorphisms

The rates of familial clustering just noted suggest polygenic inheritance, and several candidate genes have been investigated. The largest study to date, examining more than 1000 affected sister-pair families, has identified a region on chromosome 10q26 that demonstrates significant linkage in these sisters affected with endometriosis (Treloar, 2005). This study also revealed a smaller linkage on chromosome 20p13. Two candidate genes within or near this locus have been identified. One such gene is *EMX2*, which encodes a transcription factor necessary for reproductive tract development. It has been shown to be aberrantly expressed in the endometrium of women with endometriosis (Daftary, 2004). The second gene is *PTEN*, a tumor suppressor gene implicated in the malignant transformation of ovarian endometriosis (Bischoff, 2000). Studies are currently underway to further determine the role of these genes in endometriosis.

Microarray technology has been used to analyze differences in gene expression in eutopic endometrium (endometrium found normally lining the endometrial cavity) from women without endometriosis compared with that from women with endometriosis (Kao, 2003). Researchers found that several genes were regulated differently in the eutopic endometrium in women with endometriosis. These include those coding for interleukin 15, glycodelin, Dickkopf-1, semaphorin E, aromatase, progesterone receptor, and various angiogenic factors. Some of these genes have previously been shown to play a role in endometriosis. Others have not been implicated until recently, and their role remains to be elucidated. Several other genes have been identified, through genetic mutations, polymorphisms, or differential gene expression, to be associated with endometriosis.

Genetic factors may partially explain the susceptibility of certain individuals to develop endometriosis. Genetic aberrations may also provide some explanation as to the reason endometriosis may lead to the development of endometrioid adenocarcinoma in the ovary. The mechanism of malignant transformation is not clear but is thought to be genetically determined. Loss of heterozygosity in endometriotic lesions and of certain tumor suppressor genes such as *p53*, as well as numerical chromosome aberrations have been described (Korner, 2006; Sainz de la Cuesta, 1996, 2004).

Anatomic Defects

Reproductive outflow tract obstruction can predispose to development of endometriosis, likely through exacerbation of retrograde menstruation (Breech, 1999). Accordingly, endometriosis has been identified in women with noncommunicating uterine horn, imperforate hymen, and transverse vaginal septum (Chap. 18, p. 492) (Schattman, 1995). Because of this association, diagnostic laparoscopy to identify and treat endometriosis is suggested at the time of corrective surgery for many of these anomalies. Repair of such anatomic defects is thought to decrease the risk of developing endometriosis (Joki-Erkkila, 2003; Rock, 1982).

Environmental Toxins

Numerous studies have suggested that exposure to environmental toxins may play a role in the development of endometriosis. The toxins most commonly implicated are 2,3,7,8-tetrachlorodibenzo-*p*-dioxin (TCDD) and other dioxin-like compounds (Rier, 2003). In binding, TCDD activates the aryl hydrocarbon receptor. This receptor functions as a basic transcription factor and similar to the steroid hormone receptor family of proteins, leads to the transcription of various genes. As a result, TCDD and other dioxin-like compounds may stimulate endometriosis through increases in interleukin levels, activation of cytochrome P450 enzymes such as aromatase, and alterations in tissue remodeling. Moreover, TCDD in conjunction with estrogen appears to stimulate endometriosis formation, and TCDD appears to block the progesterone-induced regression of endometriosis (Rier, 2003).

In the environment, TCDD and dioxin-like compounds are waste by-products of industrial processing. Ingestion of contaminated foods or accidental contact is the most common method of exposure. Although endometriosis and TCDD were initially linked in primates, human studies also note a higher prevalence of endometriosis in women with high breast milk dioxin concentrations (Koninckx, 1994; Rier, 1993). In addition, subsequent studies have demonstrated higher serum dioxin levels in infertile women with endometriosis compared with those in infertile controls (Mayani, 1997).

CLASSIFICATION AND LOCATION OF ENDOMETRIOSIS

Classification System

The primary method of endometriosis diagnosis is visualization of endometriotic lesions by laparoscopy, with or without biopsy for histologic confirmation. Since the extent of endometriosis can vary widely between individuals, attempts have been made to develop a standardized classification to objectively assess the extent of endometriosis. Following several revisions since 1979, the current American Society for Reproductive Medicine (ASRM) classification system (1997) allows description of disease extent, differentiation between superficial and invasive disease, better correlation of surgical findings with clinical outcomes, and description of endometriotic lesion morphology as white, red, or black. Some biochemical activities within implants and possibly disease prognosis can be predicted by implant morphology (Vernon, 1986). However, this system has limitations and is not a good predictor of pregnancy following treatment and does not correlate well with symptoms of pain (American College of Obstetricians and Gynecologists, 1999). In this system, endometriosis is classified as stage I (minimal), stage II (mild), stage III (moderate), and stage IV (severe) (Fig. 10-2). This newest classification does not include certain endometriosis locations, such as bowel, in staging of the disease.

Anatomic Sites

Endometriosis may develop anywhere within the pelvis and on other extrapelvic peritoneal surfaces. Most commonly, endometriosis is found in the dependent areas of the pelvis. The ovary, pelvic peritoneum, anterior and posterior cul-de-sacs, and uterosacral ligaments are frequently involved (Fig. 10-3). Additionally, the rectovaginal septum, ureter, and rarely

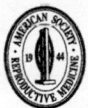

AMERICAN SOCIETY FOR REPRODUCTIVE MEDICINE REVISED CLASSIFICATION OF ENDOMETRIOSIS

Patient's Name _____ Date _____

Stage I (Minimal) - 1-5
Stage II (Mild) - 6-15
Stage III (Moderate) - 16-40
Stage IV (Severe) - >40
Total _____

Laparoscopy _____ Laparotomy _____ Photography _____
Recommended Treatment _____

Prognosis _____

	ENDOMETRIOSIS	<1cm	1-3cm	>3cm
PERITONEUM	Superficial	1	2	4
	Deep	2	4	6
OVARY	R Superficial	1	2	4
	Deep	4	16	20
	L Superficial	1	2	4
	Deep	4	16	20

	POSTERIOR CULDESAC OBLITERATION	Partial		Complete
		4		40

	ADHESIONS	<1/3 Enclosure	1/3-2/3 Enclosure	>2/3 Enclosure
OVARY	R Filmy	1	2	4
	Dense	4	8	16
	L Filmy	1	2	4
	Dense	4	8	16
TUBE	R Filmy	1	2	4
	Dense	4*	8*	16
	L Filmy	1	2	4
	Dense	4*	8*	16

*If the fimbriated end of the fallopian tube is completely enclosed, change the point assignment to 16.

Denote appearance of superficial implant types as red [(R), red, red-pink, flamelike, vesicular blobs, clear vesicles], white [(W), opacifications, peritoneal defects, yellow-brown], or black [(B) black, hemosiderin deposits, blue]. Denote percent of total described as R____%, W____% and B____%. Total should equal 100%.

Additional Endometriosis: _____   Associated Pathology: _____

To Be Used with Normal Tubes and Ovaries   To Be Used with Abnormal Tubes and/or Ovaries

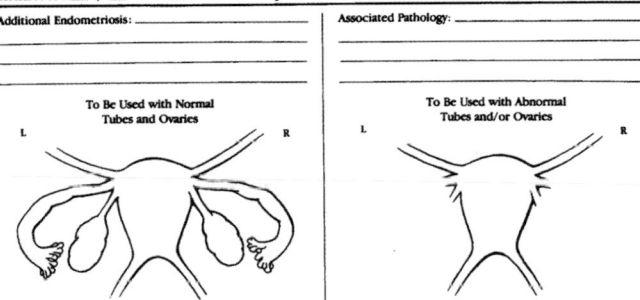

FIGURE 10-2 American Society for Reproductive Medicine Revised Classification of Endometriosis. *(From the American Society for Reproductive Medicine, 1997, with permission.)*

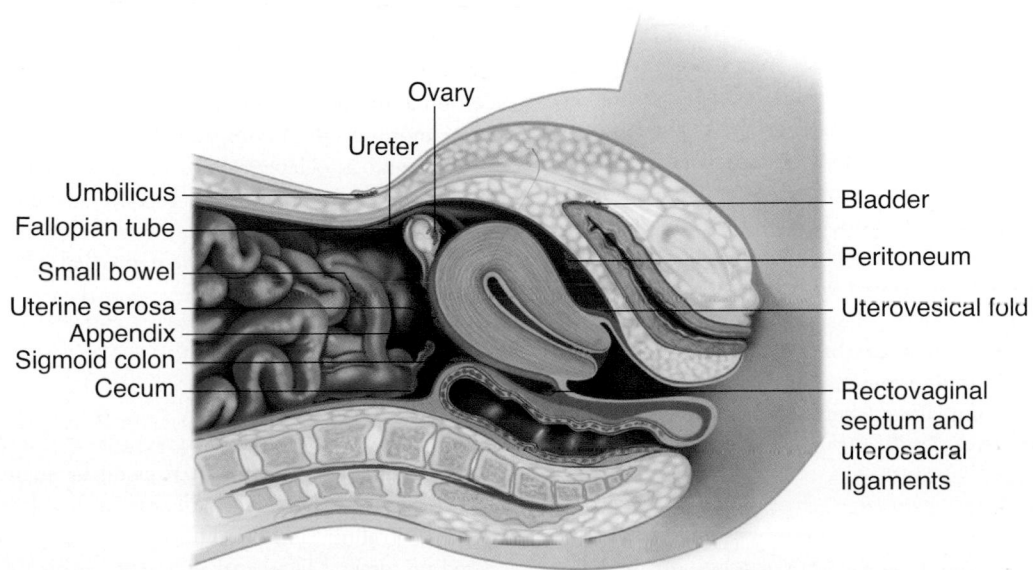

Umbilicus
Fallopian tube
Small bowel
Uterine serosa
Appendix
Sigmoid colon
Cecum

Ureter
Ovary

Bladder
Peritoneum
Uterovesical fold

Rectovaginal septum and uterosacral ligaments

FIGURE 10-3 Possible locations of endometriosis within the abdomen and pelvis.

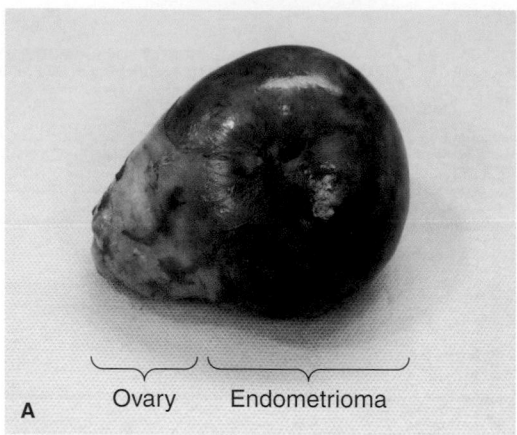
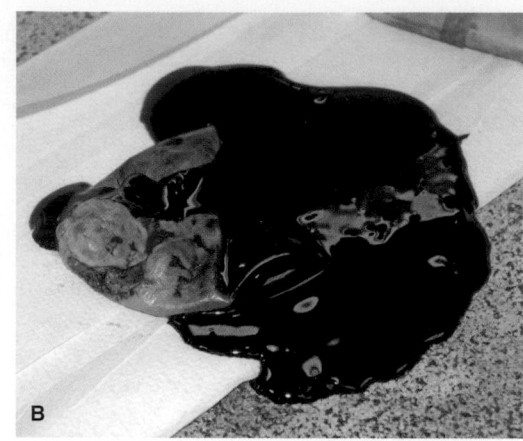

FIGURE 10-4 Photographs of an endometrioma. **A.** Surgical specimen of an ovary containing an endometrioma. **B.** Upon opening the endometrioma, chocolate-like fluid is seen. *(Photographs contributed by Dr. Roxanne Pero.)*

the bladder, pericardium, surgical scars, and pleura may be affected. One pathologic review revealed that endometriosis has been identified on all organs except the spleen (Markham, 1989). Rare sites of endometriosis may present with atypical cyclic symptoms. For example, women with urinary tract endometriosis may describe cyclic irritative voiding symptoms and hematuria; those with rectosigmoid involvement may note cyclic rectal bleeding; and pleural lesions have been associated with menstrual pneumothorax or hemoptysis (Price, 1996; Roberts, 2003; Ryu, 2007; Sciume, 2004).

Ovarian endometriomas are a common manifestation of endometriosis (Fig. 10-4). These smooth-walled, dark-brown ovarian cysts are filled with a chocolate-appearing fluid and may be unilocular or when larger, multilocular. Ovarian endometriomas are thought to form through invagination of ovarian cortex and subsequent incorporation of menstrual debris that had been adherent to the ovarian surface (Hughesdon, 1957). Another theory has suggested that endometriomas develop as a result of coelomic metaplasia of invaginated epithelial inclusions (Nisolle, 1997).

PATIENT SYMPTOMS

Although women with endometriosis may be asymptomatic, symptoms are common and typically include chronic pelvic pain and infertility. Some researchers have suggested that certain early menstrual changes may be associated with endometriosis. In a case-control trial of 512 Australian women, a history of dysmenorrhea was associated with subsequent diagnosis of endometriosis, whereas menarche after age 14 years was strongly and inversely associated with endometriosis (Treloar, 2010). The current ASRM classification of endometriosis, which describes the extent of disease bulk, poorly predicts symptoms. Thus clinically, women with extensive disease (stage IV) may note few complaints, whereas those with minimal disease (stage I) may have significant pain or subfertility or both.

Pain

Endometriosis is a common cause of pelvic pain, which in affected women can vary greatly and may be cyclic or chronic

(Mathias, 1996). The underlying cause of this pain is unclear, but proinflammatory cytokines and prostaglandins released by endometriotic implants into the peritoneal fluid may be one source (Giudice, 2004). Additionally, evidence suggests that pain from endometriosis correlates with depth of invasion and that the site of pain may indicate lesion location (Chapron, 2003; Koninckx, 1991). Endometriosis pain may result from neuronal invasion of endometriotic implants that subsequently develop a sensory and sympathetic nerve supply, which may undergo central sensitization (Chap. 11, p. 305) (Berkley, 2005). This leads to persistent hyperexcitability of the neurons and subsequent persistent pain, despite surgical excision. Hyperinnervation of intestinal deep infiltrating endometriosis may explain why this lesion type causes severe pain (Wang, 2009). Whatever the cause, clinically, women with endometriosis experience different manifestations of pain.

Dysmenorrhea

Cyclic pain with menstruation is noted commonly in women with endometriosis. Typically, endometriosis-associated dysmenorrhea precedes menses by 24 to 48 hours and is less responsive to nonsteroidal antiinflammatory drugs (NSAIDs) and combination oral contraceptives (COCs). This pain is thought to be more severe in comparison with primary dysmenorrhea. Cramer and associates (1986) demonstrated a positive correlation between dysmenorrhea severity and endometriosis risk. Furthermore, deeply infiltrating endometriosis, that is, disease that extends >5 mm under the peritoneal surface, also appears to positively correlate with dysmenorrhea severity (Chapron, 2003).

Dyspareunia

Endometriosis-associated dyspareunia is most often related to rectovaginal septum or uterosacral ligament disease and is less commonly associated with ovarian involvement (Murphy, 2002; Vercellini, 1996b). During intercourse, tension on diseased uterosacral ligaments may trigger this pain (Fauconnier, 2002). Although some women with endometriosis may describe a history of dyspareunia since coitarche, endometriosis-associated dyspareunia is suspected if pain develops after years of pain-free intercourse (Ferrero, 2005). The degree of discomfort, however, appears to be independent of disease severity (Fedele, 1992).

Dysuria

Although less frequent symptoms of endometriosis, painful urination and cyclic urinary frequency and urgency may be noted in affected women. Endometriosis may be suspected if these symptoms are concurrent with negative urine culture results (Vercellini, 1996a). If hematuria or significant bladder symptoms are noted, cystoscopy may be performed for further evaluation and diagnosis confirmation.

Defecatory Pain

Painful defecation develops less commonly than the other types of pelvic pain and typically reflects rectosigmoid involvement with endometriotic implants (Azzena, 1998). Symptoms may be chronic or cyclic, and they may be associated with constipation, diarrhea, or cyclic hematochezia (Remorgida, 2007).

Noncyclic Pain

Chronic pelvic pain is the most common symptom associated with endometriosis. Approximately 40 to 60 percent of women with chronic pelvic pain are found to have endometriosis at the time of laparoscopy (Eskenazi, 1997). Some studies have demonstrated a correlation of pain severity with advanced stage disease, whereas other studies have not (Fedele, 1992; Muzii, 1997).

The focus of chronic pain may vary. If the rectovaginal septum or uterosacral ligaments are involved with disease, pain may radiate to the rectum or lower back. Alternatively, pain radiating down the leg and causing cyclic sciatica may reflect posterior peritoneal endometriosis or direct sciatic nerve involvement (Possover, 2007; Vercellini, 2003b; Vilos, 2002).

Some individuals complaining of abdominal pain have abdominal wall endometriosis. In some cases, endometriomas developed in the abdominal scar after surgical procedures such as uterine surgery or cesarean delivery, whereas others are unrelated to prior surgery and develop spontaneously (Fig. 10-5) (Papavramidis, 2009; Steck, 1966).

▮ Infertility

The incidence of endometriosis in women with subfertility is 20 to 30 percent (Waller, 1993). In addition, although wide variability is reported, patients with infertility appear to have a greater incidence of endometriosis than fertile controls (13 to 33 percent versus 4 to 8 percent) (D'Hooghe, 2003; Strathy, 1982). Furthermore, Matorras and colleagues (2001) noted an increased prevalence of more severe stages of endometriosis in women with infertility. Adhesions that are caused by endometriosis may impair normal oocyte pick-up and transport by the fallopian tube. Beyond mechanical impairment of ovulation

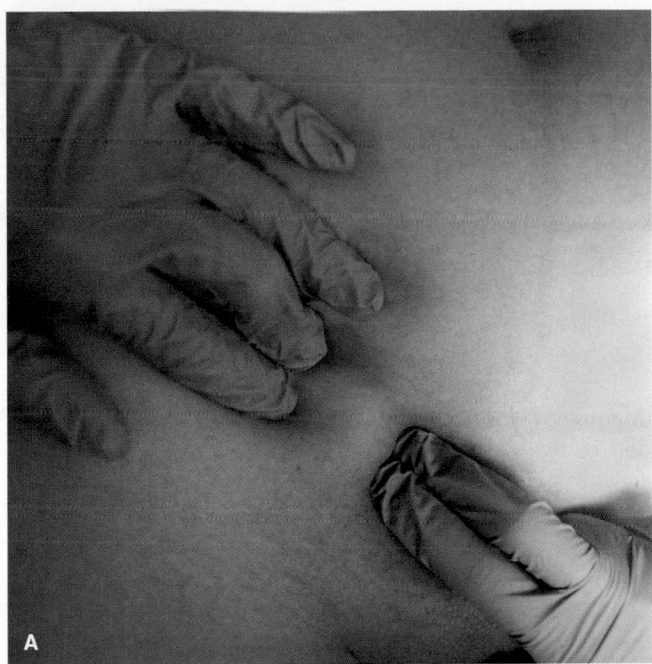

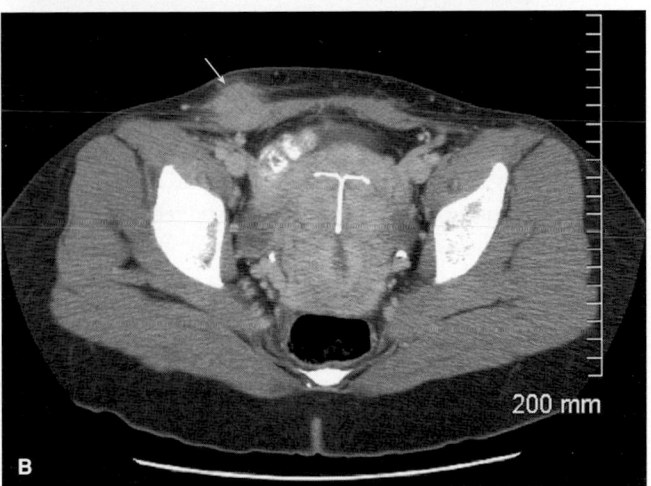

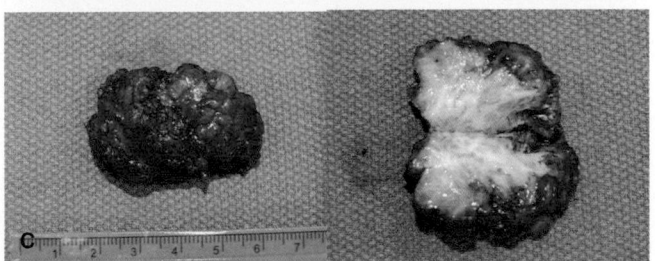

FIGURE 10-5 Endometriosis within a Pfannenstiel incision scar. **A.** Preoperative photograph delineates the borders of the mass. **B.** Computed tomography imaging shows a subcutaneous mass extending down to the anterior abdominal wall fascia (*arrow*). **C.** Excised mass (*left*). Bivalving the mass (*right*) reveals white fibrous scarring within yellow subcutaneous fat. Pathologic evaluation confirmed endometriosis. (*Photographs contributed by Dr. Christi Capet.*)

and fertilization, more subtle defects also appear to be involved in the pathogenesis of infertility in women with endometriosis. Such defects include perturbations in ovarian and immune function as well as implantation.

Minimal or Mild Disease

Although evidence suggests that severe forms of endometriosis are associated with infertility, support for an association and causation of infertility by milder forms of endometriosis is less abundant (D'Hooghe, 1996; Schenken, 1980). Primate studies have shown that surgically induced endometriosis resulted in a 35-percent pregnancy rate in animals with minimal endometriosis, a 12-percent rate in those with advanced endometriosis, and no pregnancies if ovarian adhesions were present. These rates compared poorly with a 42-percent pregnancy rate in control animals (Schenken, 1984).

Human studies demonstrating a causation of subfertility by minimal or mild endometriosis are lacking, but an association is suggested by the differing prevalence of endometriosis between infertile patients and fertile women. For example, evaluating women with minimal disease, Rodriguez-Escudero and colleagues (1988) reported that women with minimal endometriosis had a monthly fecundity rate of 6 percent and a 12-month cumulative pregnancy rate of 47 percent. Although this is much lower than that of normal fertile women, participation bias likely exists in such studies. Furthermore, a prospective cohort study demonstrated that women with minimal or mild endometriosis had a fecundity similar to that of those with unexplained infertility. Well-designed, prospective randomized controlled trials have found conflicting evidence as to whether surgical treatment of minimal or mild endometriosis improves fecundity rates and cumulative pregnancy rates in these women. One of these studies demonstrated improved fertility, but a trial with fewer women noted no improvement (Marcoux, 1997; Parazzini, 1999).

Moderate or Severe Disease

In moderate to severe endometriosis (stage III to IV), tubal and ovarian architecture are often distorted. As a result, impaired fertility would be expected. Unfortunately, few studies report fecundity rates in women with severe endometriosis. One investigation comparing mild, moderate, and severe endometriosis revealed a monthly fecundity rate of 8.7 percent in those with mild disease, 3.2 percent with moderate disease, and no pregnancies with severe disease (Olive, 1985a). There are no well-designed studies examining the effectiveness of surgical therapy in patients with severe endometriosis, but cumulative pregnancy rates have reached 30 percent after surgical excision (Adamson, 1993; Osuga, 2002). This rate appears to be greater than that of women who undergo expectant management.

Folliculogenesis and Embryogenesis Effects

Some researchers have suggested that folliculogenesis is impaired in women with endometriosis. The development and quality of embryos in women with endometriosis undergoing IVF were compared with those of embryos originating from women with tubal factor infertility (Pellicer, 1995). There were significantly fewer blastomeres per embryo and a significantly greater rate of embryonic developmental arrest in the endometriosis group. This suggests a possible decreased develop-mental competence of oocytes originating from the ovaries of women with endometriosis. Another investigation found that oocyte number may be decreased in women with endometriosis (Suzuki, 2005). In addition, researchers have attempted to determine if the follicular environment is different in women with endometriosis. However, studies demonstrating qualitative and quantitative changes in steroidogenesis have found conflicting results (Garrido, 2002; Harlow, 1996; Pellicer, 1998). Apoptosis is another attractive theory for decreased oocyte competence in women with endometriosis, but well-designed studies are lacking.

Endometrial Changes

Abnormalities in endometrial development in women with endometriosis support the possibility that implantation defects may be responsible for subfertility associated with endometriosis. For example, abnormalities in gene expression are found in the eutopic endometrium from women with endometriosis compared with women without endometriosis (Kao, 2003). Specifically, deficient $\alpha v \beta 3$ integrin expression in the periimplantation endometrium of women with endometriosis has been demonstrated, and this may be associated with decreased uterine receptivity (Lessey, 1994). The role of apoptosis on periimplantation endometrium is another area of study still largely unexplored.

Other Factors

Abnormalities in inflammation and cytokine activity in women with endometriosis may play a role in endometriosis-associated infertility. Sperm function may be altered in women with endometriosis, and sperm may undergo increased phagocytosis by macrophages in affected women (Haney, 1981; Muscato, 1982). Moreover, sperm binding to the zona pellucida appears to be adversely changed (Qiao, 1998). However, investigations of the effects of endometriosis on sperm motility and the acrosome reaction reveal conflicting results (Bielfeld, 1993; Curtis, 1993; Tasdemir, 1995).

Intestinal and Ureteral Obstruction

Endometriosis may involve the small bowel, cecum, appendix, or rectosigmoid colon and lead to intestinal obstruction in some cases (Cameron, 1995; Varras, 2002; Wickramasekera, 1999). Endometriosis of the gastrointestinal tract is usually confined to the subserosa and muscularis propria. However, more severe cases may involve the bowel wall transmurally and create a clinical and radiologic picture consistent with malignancy (Decker, 2004). Accurate preoperative diagnosis and management are difficult due to the atypical presentation. Laparoscopy typically provides the definitive diagnosis. Treatment is often surgical, with resection and primary anastomosis of the affected intestinal segment. In women without obstructing symptoms, however, conservative management with hormonal therapy may be considered.

In a large series by Antonelli and coworkers (2006), the prevalence of urinary tract endometriosis was 2.6 percent. In this series of 31 patients, 12 had bladder endometriosis, 15 had ureteral endometriosis, and four had both ureteral and bladder involvement. Urinary tract endometriosis may present variably, including frequency, urgency, and ureteral obstruction progressing eventually to loss of kidney function (Douglas, 2004). Treatment is either medical or surgical. Surgical treatment generally employs resection techniques and is usually tailored to relieve ureteral obstruction.

DIAGNOSIS

◼ Physical Examination

Visual Inspection

For the most part, endometriosis is a disease confined to the pelvis. Accordingly, abnormalities during visual inspection are often lacking. Some exceptions include endometriosis within an episiotomy scar or surgical scar, most often within a Pfannenstiel incision (Koger, 1993; Zhu, 2002). Rarely, endometriosis may develop spontaneously within the perineum or perianal region (Watanabe, 2003).

Speculum Examination

Examination of the vagina and cervix often reveals no signs of endometriosis. Occasionally, blue or red powder-burn lesions may be seen on the cervix or the posterior fornix of the vagina. These lesions may be tender or bleed with contact. One study found that speculum examination displayed endometriosis in 14 percent of patients diagnosed with deeply infiltrating endometriosis (Chapron, 2002).

Bimanual Examination

Pelvic organ palpation may reveal anatomic abnormalities suggestive of endometriosis. Uterosacral ligament nodularity and tenderness may reflect active disease or scarring along the ligament. An enlarged, cystic adnexal mass may represent an ovarian endometrioma, which may be mobile or adhered to other pelvic structures. Bimanual examination may reveal a retroverted, fixed, tender uterus, or a firm, fixed posterior cul-de-sac. However, examination is generally inaccurate in assessing the extent of endometriosis, especially if the lesions are extragenital.

Although pelvic organ palpation may assist diagnosis, the sensitivity and specificity of focal pelvic tenderness in detecting endometriosis displays wide variation and ranges from 36 to 90 percent and 32 to 92 percent, respectively (Chapron, 2002; Eskenazi, 2001; Koninckx, 1996; Ripps, 1992). For example, Chapron and coworkers (2002) palpated a painful nodule in 43 percent of patients with deeply infiltrating endometriosis. In another study of 91 women with chronic pelvic pain and surgically confirmed endometriosis, the bimanual examination was normal 47 percent of the time (Nezhat, 1994). Pelvic nodularities secondary to endometriosis may be more easily detected by bimanual examination during menses (Koninckx, 1996).

◼ Laboratory Testing

Laboratory investigations are often undertaken to exclude other causes of pelvic pain (Table 10-1). Initially, a complete blood

TABLE 10-1. Differential Diagnosis of Endometriosis

Gynecologic
Pelvic inflammatory disease
   Tuboovarian abscess
   Salpingitis
   Endometritis
Hemorrhagic ovarian cyst
Ovarian torsion
Primary dysmenorrhea
Degenerating leiomyoma
Ectopic pregnancy
Other pregnancy complications

Nongynecologic
Interstitial cystitis
Chronic urinary tract infection
Renal calculi
Inflammatory bowel disease
Irritable bowel syndrome
Diverticulitis
Mesenteric lymphadenitis
Musculoskeletal disorders

count (CBC), serum or urine human chorionic gonadotropin assay, urinalysis and urine cultures, vaginal cultures, and cervical swabs may be obtained to exclude infections or pregnancy complications.

Serum CA125

Numerous serum markers have been studied as possible adjuncts in the diagnosis of endometriosis. No serum marker has been studied in greater detail than CA125 (cancer antigen 125). Found as an antigenic determinant on a glycoprotein, CA125 has been identified in several adult tissues such as fallopian tube epithelium, the endometrium, the endocervix, the pleura, and the peritoneum. As discussed in Chapter 35 (p. 856), this marker is used in ovarian cancer evaluation and surveillance. Recognized by monoclonal antibody assays, elevated CA125 levels have been shown to positively correlate with endometriosis severity (Hornstein, 1995a). Unfortunately, although demonstrating adequate specificity, the assay has poor sensitivity in detecting mild endometriosis. A metaanalysis of studies evaluating CA125 in the diagnosis of endometriosis revealed a sensitivity of only 28 percent and a specificity of 90 percent (Mol, 1998). This marker appeared to be a better test in diagnosing stage III and IV endometriosis. Although the role of this test in clinical practice is uncertain, it may be useful in the presence of a sonographically detected ovarian cyst suggestive of an endometrioma.

Other Serum Markers

Cancer antigen 19-9 (CA 19-9), another antigenic glycoprotein, is a serum marker that has also been shown to positively correlate with endometriosis severity (Harada, 2002).

Serum placental protein 14 (PP14; glycodelin-A) was initially shown to have adequate sensitivity (59 percent), but this has not been confirmed by other studies (Telimaa, 1989). Interleukin-6 (IL-6) serum levels above 2 pg/mL (90-percent sensitivity and 67-percent specificity) and tumor necrosis factor-α peritoneal fluid levels above 15 pg/mL (100-percent sensitivity and 89-percent specificity) may be used to discriminate between those with or without endometriosis (Bedaiwy, 2002). Several other serum markers have been studied, with limited diagnostic accuracy (Bedaiwy, 2004). As mentioned earlier, most of these tests are rarely used outside of research settings.

Diagnostic Imaging

Sonography

Both transabdominal and transvaginal (TVS) sonographic approaches have been used extensively in the diagnosis of endometriosis. TVS is the mainstay in evaluating symptoms associated with endometriosis. It is accurate in detecting endometriomas and aids exclusion of other causes of pelvic pain. However, imaging of superficial endometriosis or endometriotic adhesions is inadequate. Small endometriotic plaques or nodules may occasionally be seen, but these findings are inconsistent (Carbognin, 2004).

More recently, sonovaginography, a technique involving vaginal saline instillation to more accurately localize rectovaginal endometriosis, and transrectal sonography have assisted in the diagnosis and evaluation of endometriosis, especially endometriosis on bowel (Brosens, 2003; Menada, 2008). Transvaginal sonography appears to be as effective as a transrectal approach in identifying posterior pelvic endometriosis. However, the transrectal approach may delineate rectal involvement more accurately and may be more appropriate when planning surgery (Bazot, 2003).

Endometriomas can be diagnosed by TVS with adequate sensitivity in most settings if they are 20 mm in diameter or greater. Specifically, sensitivity and specificity of TVS to diagnose endometriomas range from 64 to 90 percent and from 22 to 100 percent, respectively (Moore, 2002). Endometriomas classically present as cystic structures with low-level internal echoes (Fig. 10-6). However, true to their nickname, "the great mimicker," they can also demonstrate other sonographic features such as thick septations, thickened walls, and echogenic wall foci (Athey, 1989; Patel, 1999). Color Doppler transvaginal sonography often demonstrates pericystic, but not intracystic, flow (Carbognin, 2004).

Computed Tomographic (CT) Scanning

This modality has been suggested for the diagnosis and evaluation of the extent of bowel endometriosis. Biscaldi and colleagues (2007) described the use of multislice CT scanning combined with colon distension by water enteroclysis to determine the presence and depth of bowel endometriotic lesions. This technique had a sensitivity of 98.7 percent and a specificity of 100 percent in identifying women with bowel endometriosis (Fig. 10-7).

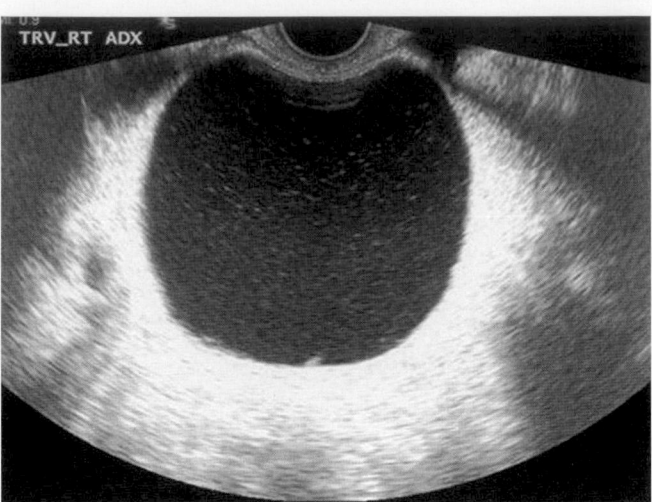

FIGURE 10-6 Transvaginal sonogram demonstrating ovarian endometrioma. A cyst with diffuse internal low-level echoes is seen. *(Image contributed by Dr. Elysia Moschos.)*

Magnetic Resonance Imaging

This modality has been increasingly used as a noninvasive method for endometriosis diagnosis. Small nodules may be recognized as high-signal-intensity lesions on T1-weighted sequences, and plaque lesions have a similar appearance, with a

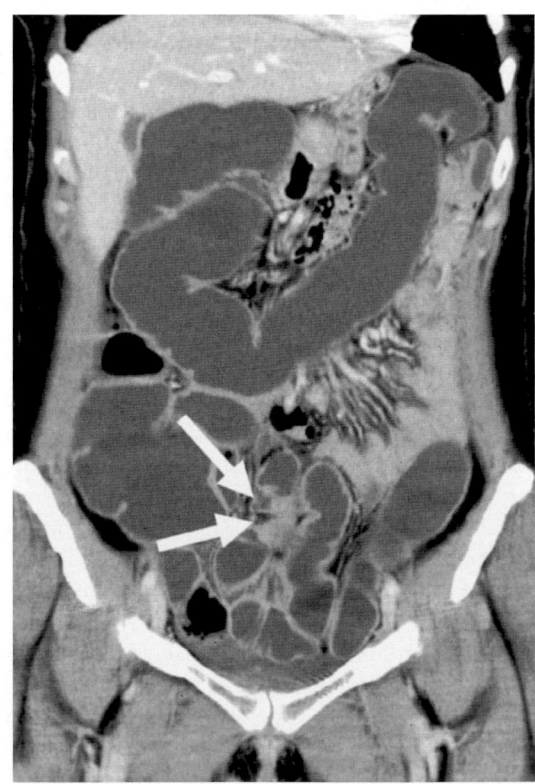

FIGURE 10-7 Coronal section during multislice CT-enteroclysis. The arrow indicates an endometriotic nodule located on the sigmoid colon that does not penetrate the muscularis propria. *(From Biscaldi, 2007, with permission.)*

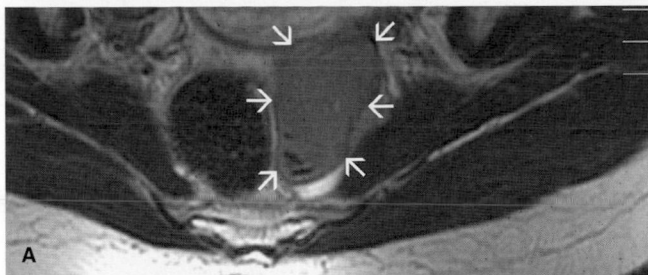

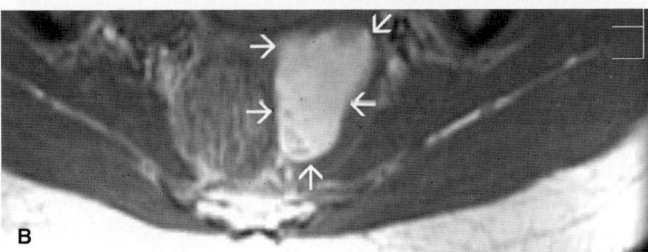

FIGURE 10-8 Magnetic resonance images of an endometrioma (*arrows*) just lateral to the rectum. **A.** Consistent with subacute blood, low-intensity-signals are found on T2-weighted sequences. **B.** High-intensity-signals are seen on T1-weighted sequences. (*Images contributed by Dr. Diane Twickler.*)

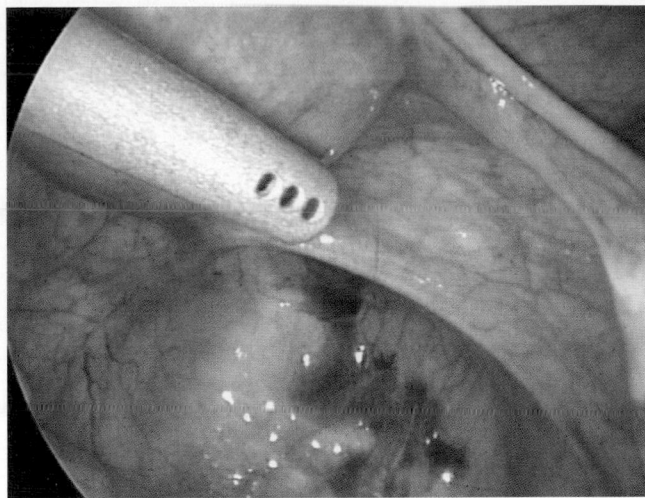

FIGURE 10-9 A red and white endometriotic lesion seen on the pelvic peritoneum during laparoscopy. (*Photograph contributed by Dr. Karen Bradshaw.*)

variable signal on T2-weighted sequences (Carbognin, 2004). An endometrioma appears as a high-signal-intensity mass on T1-weighted sequences, with a tendency toward low intensity in T2-weighted sequences (Fig. 10-8). Adhesions usually have a low signal intensity and obscure organ interfaces (Choudhary, 2009).

Diagnostic Laparoscopy

This tool is the primary method used for diagnosing endometriosis (Kennedy, 2005). Laparoscopic findings are variable and may include discrete endometriotic lesions, endometrioma, and adhesion formation.

The pelvic organs and pelvic peritoneum are typical locations for endometriosis. Lesions are variable colors, which may include red (red, red-pink, or clear), white (white or yellow-brown), and black (black or black-blue) (Fig. 10-9). Dark lesions are pigmented by hemosiderin deposition from trapped menstrual debris. White and red lesions most commonly correlate with the histologic findings of endometriosis (Jansen, 1986). In addition to color differences, endometriotic lesions may differ morphologically. They can appear as smooth blebs on peritoneal surfaces, as holes or defects within the peritoneum, or as flat stellate lesions whose points are formed by surrounding scar tissue. Endometriotic lesions may be superficial or may deeply invade the peritoneum or pelvic organs. Although these characteristics may allow endometriosis to be diagnosed with accuracy, pain symptoms correlate poorly with laparoscopic findings (Kennedy, 2005).

Laparoscopic visualization of ovarian endometriomas has a sensitivity and specificity of 97 percent and 95 percent, respectively (Vercellini, 1991). Because of this, ovarian biopsy is rarely required for diagnosis.

Pathologic Analysis

Although current guidelines do not require biopsy and histologic evaluation for the diagnosis of endometriosis, some suggest that relying solely on laparoscopic findings in the absence of histologic confirmation often results in overdiagnosis (American Society for Reproductive Medicine, 1997). Specifically, the greatest discordance between laparoscopic and histologic findings is noted in scarred lesions (Marchino, 2005a; Walter, 2001). Histologic diagnosis requires both endometrial glands and stroma found outside the uterine cavity (Fig. 10-10). Additionally, hemosiderin deposition and fibromuscular metaplasia are frequently noted (Murphy, 2002). The gross appearance of endometriotic lesions often suggests certain microscopic findings. For example, if examined microscopically, red lesions are frequently vascularized, whereas white lesions more often display fibrosis and few vessels (Nisolle, 1997).

TREATMENT

Diagnosis and treatment of endometriosis depends on a woman's specific symptoms, symptom severity, location of endometriotic lesions, goals for treatment, and desire to conserve future fertility. As shown in Figure 10-11, determining whether a patient is seeking treatment for infertility or pain is essential, as therapy for these two is different (Olive, 2001). If infertility is the presenting symptom, then fertility-preserving treatment without ovulation suppression will be required. In contrast, if the patient has severe, recalcitrant pain and has completed childbearing, definitive surgery may be warranted.

Expectant Management

For many women, symptoms will preclude them from choosing expectant management. However, for those with mild symptoms

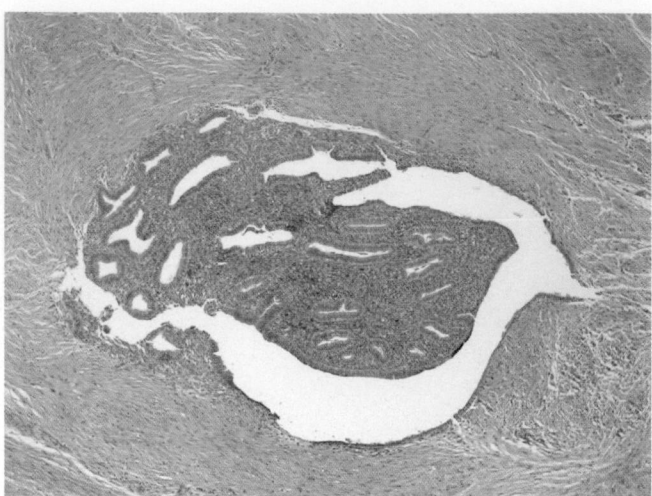

FIGURE 10-10 Endometriosis. This focus of endometrial glands and stroma was identified in the abdominal wall at the lateral aspect of a prior cesarean delivery Pfannenstiel incision. *(Photograph contributed by Dr. Kelley Carrick.)*

or for asymptomatic women diagnosed incidentally, expectant management may be appropriate. For example, Sutton and associates (1997) expectantly managed patients initially diagnosed by laparoscopy with minimal to moderate endometriosis. At second-look laparoscopy after 1 year, 29 percent of women had disease regression, 42 percent remained unchanged, and 29 percent had disease progression. Other investigators have shown similar rates of disease regression with expectant management (Thomas, 1987). However, studies evaluating infertile women have demonstrated lower fecundity rates after expectant management than following surgical treatment (Marcoux, 1997; Milingos, 2002). These studies are confined to patients with minimal to moderate endometriosis, and there are no well-designed trials examining the effect of expectant management on severe endometriosis.

Medical Treatment of Pain
Nonsteroidal Antiinflammatory Drugs

These agents nonselectively inhibit the cyclooxygenase isoenzymes 1 and 2 (COX-1 and COX-2), and within this group, the selective COX-2 inhibitors specifically inhibit the COX-2 isoenzyme. Both these enzymes are responsible for the synthesis of prostaglandins involved in the pain and inflammation associated with endometriosis. For example, endometriotic tissue has been shown to express COX-2 at greater levels than eutopic endometrium (Cho, 2010; Ota, 2001). Therefore, therapy aimed at lowering these prostaglandin levels may play a role in alleviating endometriosis-associated pain.

NSAIDs are often first-line therapy in women with primary dysmenorrhea or pelvic pain prior to laparoscopic confirmation of endometriosis, and in women with minimal or mild pain symptoms associated with known endometriosis. Although animal models have demonstrated disease regression with NSAID treatment, few studies have critically evaluated their effective-

ness in disease regression in surgically confirmed endometriosis (Efstathiou, 2005). However, evidence exists for their efficacy in patients with dysmenorrhea and pelvic pain (Table 10-2) (Nasir, 2004). Due to the cardiovascular risks with long-term use of selective COX-2 inhibitors, these medications should be used at the lowest possible dose and for the shortest duration necessary (Jones, 2005).

Combination Oral Contraceptives

These agents have been a mainstay for the treatment of pain associated with endometriosis. Although no randomized controlled trials have compared COCs with placebo, abundant observational evidence supports the role of COCs in the relief of endometriosis-related pain (Harada, 2008; Vercellini, 1993; Vessey, 1993). These drugs appear to act by inhibiting gonadotropin release, decreasing menstrual flow, and decidualizing implants. In addition, COCs have been shown to reduce nerve fiber density and nerve growth factor expression in endometriotic lesions (Tokushige, 2009). COCs also have the added benefit of contraception, suppression of ovulation, and other noncontraceptive benefits (Chap. 5, p. 152).

COCs can be used conventionally in a cyclic regimen or may be used continuously, without a break for withdrawal menses. The continuous regimen may be preferable for its decreased frequency of painful menses in women who fail to achieve adequate relief with cyclic COC therapy (Vercellini, 2003c; Wiegratz, 2004). Traditionally, monophasic COCs have been used in endometriosis treatment, but no evidence supports their clinical superiority to multiphasic COCs. Additionally, low-dose COCs (containing 20 µg ethinyl estradiol) have not proved superior to conventional-dose COCs for the treatment of endometriosis and may lead to higher rates of abnormal bleeding (Gallo, 2005).

Progestins

Progestational agents have long been used in the treatment of endometriosis. Progestins are known to antagonize estrogenic effects on the endometrium, causing initial decidualization and subsequent endometrial atrophy. Similar to COCs, progestins have been shown to reduce nerve fiber density and nerve growth factor expression in endometriotic lesions (Tokushige, 2009). Progestins may be administered for endometriosis treatment in numerous ways and include oral progestins, depot medroxyprogesterone acetate (DMPA) (Depo-Provera), a levonorgestrel-releasing intrauterine device (IUD), and the newer selective progesterone-receptor modulators (SPRMs).

One well-designed, randomized controlled trial compared the effect of oral medroxyprogesterone acetate (MPA) 100 mg daily given for 6 months and placebo. At second-look laparoscopy, partial or total resolution of peritoneal implants was noted in 60 percent of progestin-treated women compared with 18 percent of the placebo group. Furthermore, pelvic pain and defecatory pain were significantly reduced (Telimaa, 1987). Side effects of high-dose MPA included acne, edema, weight

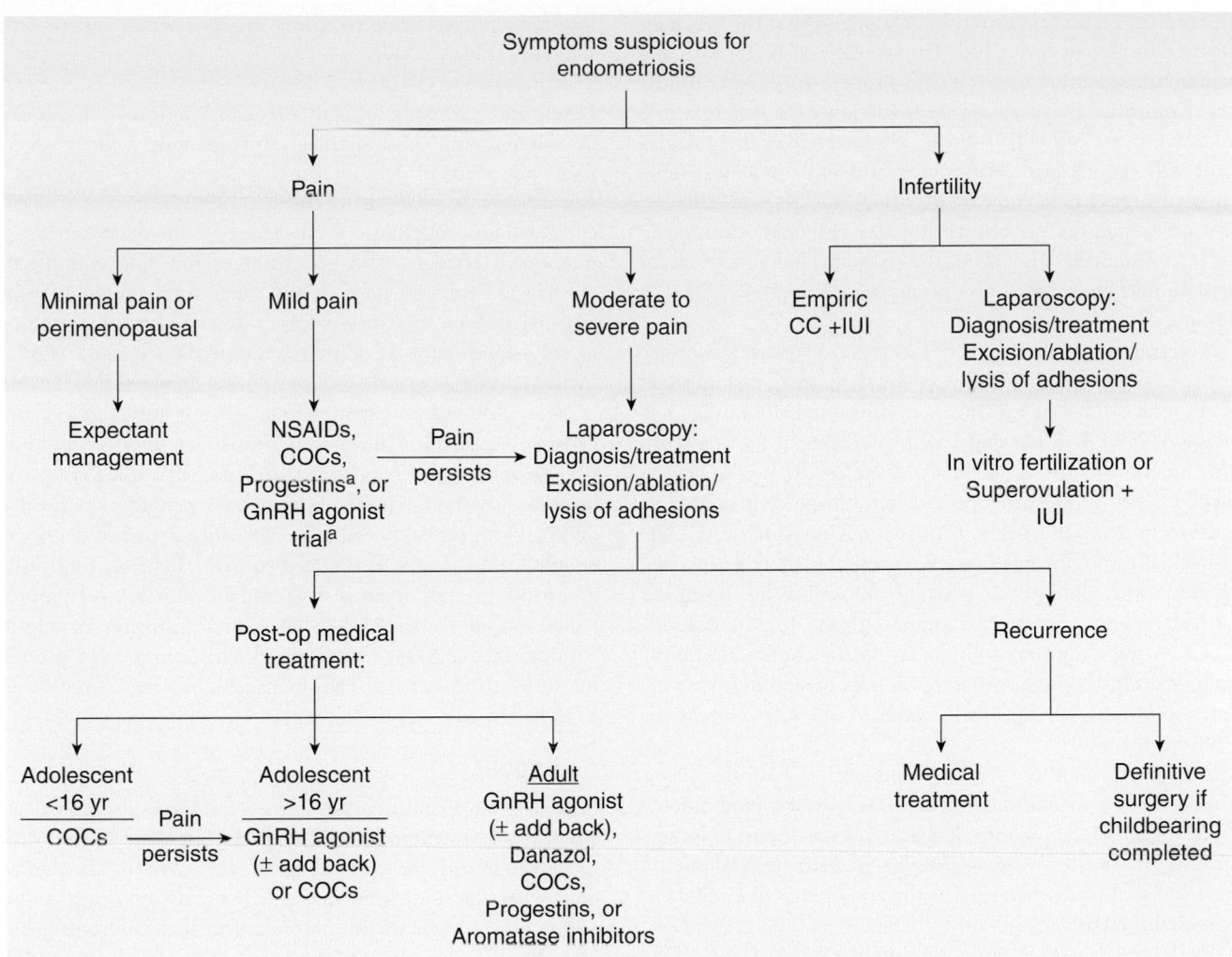

FIGURE 10-11 Diagnostic and treatment algorithm for women with presumptive or proven endometriosis. CC = clomiphene citrate (Clomid); COCs = combination oral contraceptive pills; GnRH = gonadotropin-releasing hormone; IUI = intrauterine insemination; NSAIDs = nonsteroidal antiinflammatory drugs. ªAgents not recommended for adolescents younger than 16 years.

gain, and irregular menstrual bleeding. In practice, MPA is prescribed in oral dosages ranging from 20 to 100 mg daily. Alternatively, MPA may be given intramuscularly in depot form in a dosage of 150 mg every 3 months. In depot form, MPA may delay resumption of normal menses and ovulation

and should not be used in women contemplating imminent pregnancy.

In 2004, the U.S. FDA issued a "black box warning" in the Depo-Provera package insert to highlight that prolonged use may result in bone density loss, that this loss is

TABLE 10-2. Commonly Used Oral Nonsteroidal Antiinflammatory Drugs (NSAIDs) in the Treatment of Endometriosis-Associated Dysmenorrhea

Generic Name	Trade Name	Dosage	Adverse Effects
Ibuprofen	Motrin, Advil, Nuprin	400 mg every 4–6 hours	Nausea; epigastric pain; anorexia; constipation; gastrointestinal bleeding
Naproxen	Naprosyn, Aleve	500 mg initially, then 250 mg every 6–8 hours	Same as above
Naproxen sodium	Anaprox	550 mg initially, then 275 mg every 6–8 hours	Same as above
Mefenamic acid	Ponstel	500 mg initially, then 250 mg every 6 hours, starting with menses and continued for 3 days	Same as above
Ketoprofen	Orudis, Oruvail	50 mg every 6–8 hours	Same as above

greater with increasing duration of use, and that the loss may not be completely reversible. The warning also states that a woman should limit use of Depo-Provera to 2 years unless other contraceptive methods are inadequate for her. It is still unknown if use of DMPA during adolescence or early adulthood will reduce peak bone mass and will increase osteoporotic fracture risks later in life. Bone density surveillance with dual energy x-ray absorptiometry (DEXA) scanning is not recommended. Therefore, the risks and benefits of treatment should be weighed if contemplating long-term DMPA therapy.

Norethindrone acetate (NETA) is a 19-nortestosterone synthetic progestin that has been used to treat endometriosis. In one study, investigators administered an initial oral dosage of NETA, 5 mg daily, with increases of 2.5 mg daily until amenorrhea or a maximal dosage of 20 mg daily was reached. They found an approximately 90-percent reduction in dysmenorrhea and pelvic pain (Muneyyirci-Delale, 1998). Additionally, NETA has been shown to be effective in conjunction with long-term gonadotropin-releasing hormone (GnRH) agonist therapy for endometriosis. In this fashion, NETA, 5 mg daily oral administration, in conjunction with prolonged GnRH agonist therapy, results in significant symptom resolution while protecting against bone loss (Hornstein, 1998; Surrey, 2002).

Dienogest, another synthetic progestin, has also been studied for use in endometriosis. In a 12-week randomized, double-blind, placebo-controlled study, it was found to be significantly more effective than placebo for reducing endometriosis-associated pain when used orally at a dosage of 2 mg daily (Strowitzki, 2010).

The levonorgestrel-releasing intrauterine system (LNG-IUS) (Mirena) has traditionally been used for contraception and dysfunctional uterine bleeding (Chap. 5, p. 137). However, the LNG-IUS has also been used for the treatment of endometriosis. This IUD delivers levonorgestrel directly to the endometrium and is effective for up to 5 years. An observational trial revealed symptomatic improvement in patients with endometriosis using the LNG-IUS, with symptom improvement continuing up to 30 months (Lockhat, 2005). The continuation rate at 3 years, however, was only 56 percent, mostly due to intolerable bleeding, persistent pain, and weight gain. A randomized controlled trial comparing LNG-IUS with GnRH agonist therapy showed equivalent improvement in pain symptoms, without the concomitant hypoestrogenism that accompanies GnRH agonist treatment (Petta, 2005). Accordingly, these findings make the LNG-IUS an attractive option in treating women with endometriosis. However, in patients with bowel endometriosis, the levonorgestrel IUD may not be effective in symptom control (Hinterholzer, 2007).

Progesterone Antagonists and Selective Progesterone-Receptor Modulators

A new and novel option in the treatment of endometriosis has been the use of progesterone antagonists (PAs) and selective progesterone-receptor modulators (SPRMs). PAs bind to and inactivate progesterone receptors. In contrast, SPRMS, depending on their individual pharmacologic profile, may activate or inactivate progesterone receptors variably within different tissue types (Elger, 2000).

Mifepristone (RU486; Mifeprex) is a PA and is currently FDA-approved solely for early pregnancy termination. Studied in women with endometriosis, mifepristone reduced pelvic pain and extent of endometriosis, when used for 6 months at oral dosages of 50 mg daily (Kettel, 1996). However, as a side effect, its antiprogestational effects expose the endometrium to unopposed estrogen. The spectrum of resulting endometrial changes is a topic of research and range from simple endometrial hyperplasia to a new category described as progesterone-receptor-modulator–associated endometrial changes (PAEC) (Mutter, 2008).

Most SPRMs are experimental and not available for clinical use. Asoprisnil (J867) is a SPRM that induces endometrial atrophy and amenorrhea. In Phase II studies, asoprisnil improved dysmenorrhea and pelvic pain symptoms (Chwalisz, 2005). However, some subjects receiving asoprisnil developed endometrial changes during a phase III extension trial, using asoprisnil to treat leiomyomas, and dosing was prematurely halted for all subjects (U.S. National Institutes of Health Clinical Trials, 2008). These novel agents may hold promise for future treatment of endometriosis, but are currently not FDA approved.

Androgens

Prior to the availability of newer medications, androgens played a bigger role in endometriosis treatment. In fact, the first medication approved for endometriosis treatment in the United States was the androgen danazol. This class of drugs is now falling out of favor mainly secondary to their androgenic side effects.

Danazol is a synthetic androgen that is an isoxazole derivative of 17-α-ethinyl testosterone. The predominant mechanism of action appears to be suppression of the midcycle luteinizing hormone (LH) surge and thereby to create a chronic anovulatory state (Floyd, 1980). Danazol occupies receptor sites on sex hormone-binding globulin (SHBG) to increase serum free testosterone levels and also binds directly to androgen and progesterone receptors. As a result, danazol creates a hypoestrogenic, hyperandrogenic state that induces endometrial atrophy in endometriotic implants (Fedele, 1990). Danazol at dosages of 200 mg given orally three times daily proved superior to placebo for the reduction of endometriotic implants and pelvic pain symptoms after 6 months of therapy (Telimaa, 1987). The recommended dosage of danazol is 600 to 800 mg orally daily. Unfortunately, significant androgenic side effects develop at this dosage and include acne, hot flashes, hirsutism, adverse serum lipid profiles, voice deepening (possibly irreversible), elevation of liver enzyme levels, and mood changes. Moreover, due to possible teratogenicity, this medication should be taken in conjunction with effective contraception. Because of this adverse side-effect profile, danazol is prescribed less frequently, and if administered, its duration should be limited.

Gestrinone (ethylnorgestrienone; R2323) is an antiprogestational agent prescribed in Europe for endometriosis treatment. Although it has antiprogestational, antiestrogenic, and androgenic effects, it predominantly induces a progesterone withdrawal effect and decreases the number of estrogen and progesterone receptors. Endocrinologic changes during therapy with gestrinone show that basal concentrations of gonadotropin levels remain unchanged, estradiol concentrations vary, and free testosterone levels increase, with concomitant androgenic side effects (Forbes, 1993). Gestrinone equals the effectiveness of danazol and of GnRH agonists for relief of endometriosis-related pain (Prentice, 2000a). Furthermore, during 6 months of treatment, gestrinone was not associated with the bone density loss commonly seen with GnRH agonist use and was more effective in persistently decreasing moderate to severe pelvic pain (Gestrinone Italian Study Group, 1996). Unfortunately, gestrinone appears to lower high-density lipoprotein (HDL) levels. Gestrinone is administered orally, 2.5 to 10 mg weekly, with divided doses given daily or three times weekly.

GnRH Agonists

Endogenous pulsatile release of GnRH leads to pulsatile secretory activity of the gonadotropes within the anterior pituitary. This pulsatile release results in pituitary release of gonadotropins, with subsequent ovarian steroidogenesis and ovulation. Continuous, nonpulsatile GnRH administration, however, results in pituitary desensitization and subsequent loss of ovarian steroidogenesis (Rabin, 1980). These features allow pharmacologic use of GnRH agonists for the treatment of endometriosis. With loss of ovarian estradiol production, the hypoestrogenic environment removes the stimulation normally provided to the endometriotic implants and creates a pseudomenopausal state during treatment. In addition to their direct effect on estrogen production, GnRH agonists have also been shown to reduce COX-2 levels in patients with endometriosis, providing another mechanism for endometriosis treatment (Kim, 2009).

GnRH agonists are inactive if taken orally, but intramuscular, subcutaneous, and intranasal preparations are available. Leuprolide acetate (Lupron Depot) is available in a 3.75-mg monthly dose or an 11.25-mg 3-month dose, both given intramuscularly (IM). Less frequently used GnRH agonists include goserelin (Zoladex) administered as a 3.6-mg monthly or a 10.8-mg 3-month subcutaneous depot implant; triptorelin (Trelstar) given as a 3.75-mg monthly IM injection; and nafarelin (Synarel) used in a 200-mg twice-daily nasal spray regimen. All of these except triptorelin carry specific FDA approval for endometriosis treatment.

Pain Improvement. GnRH agonists may be used empirically prior to laparoscopy in women with chronic pelvic pain and clinical suspicion of endometriosis. In a study by Ling (1999), after 3 months of GnRH agonist treatment, pain scores significantly declined compared with those after placebo. Subsequent laparoscopy revealed that 93 percent of these women had surgically diagnosed endometriosis. Accordingly, many suggest that in similar patients, depot leuprolide acetate may be used empirically in lieu of laparoscopy for satisfactory symptom improvement. Empiric GnRH agonist can also be used for the diagnosis of endometriosis in older adolescent patients. The American College of Obstetricians and Gynecologists (2005), in their committee opinion on endometriosis in the adolescent, recommend the use of empiric GnRH agonist in patients older than 18 years if their pain persists after NSAIDs and COCs. If pain improves after a GnRH agonist trial, then a diagnosis of endometriosis can be made. An empiric trial is not routinely offered to patients younger than 18 years because the effects of these GnRH agonists on bone formation and long-term bone density have not been adequately studied.

In those with *surgically confirmed* endometriosis, numerous studies have demonstrated the effectiveness of GnRH agonist therapy to improve pain symptoms. For example, in their randomized controlled trial, Dlugi and coworkers (1990) compared depot leuprolide acetate with placebo and found significant decreases in pelvic pain severity with GnRH agonist therapy. Similar findings were obtained comparing buserelin, another GnRH agonist, with expectant management during a 6-month period (Fedele, 1993). The GnRH agonists seem to provide greater relief when administered for 6 months compared with 3 months (Hornstein, 1995b).

In trials with other drugs for the treatment of endometriosis, GnRH agonists compared favorably. Vercellini and associates (1993) found equal degrees of pain improvement during their comparison of GnRH agonist therapy with a low-dose cyclic COC regimen. However, dyspareunia was less in the GnRH agonist-treated group. In addition, a metaanalysis revealed that GnRH agonists were equally effective in improving pain scores and decreasing endometriotic implants compared with danazol (Prentice, 2000b).

Add-Back Therapy. Concerns regarding the long-term effects of prolonged hypoestrogenism preclude extended treatment with GnRH agonists. Hypoestrogenic symptoms include hot flushes, insomnia, reduced libido, vaginal dryness, and headaches. Of particular concern is the effect of hypoestrogenism on bone mineral density (BMD). Both spine and hip BMD decrease at 3 and 6 months of GnRH agonist therapy, with only partial recovery at 12 to 15 months after treatment (Orwoll, 1994). Because of the increased risk of osteoporosis, therapy is usually limited to the shortest possible duration—usually no greater than 6 months.

Estrogen may be added to GnRH agonist therapy to counteract bone loss and is termed *add-back therapy* (Fig. 10-12) (Carr, 1995). With the addition of such hormonal add-back therapy, a GnRH agonist may occasionally be used longer than 6 months. Barbieri (1992) suggested that tissues have varied sensitivity to estrogen, and that a concentration of estrogen that will partially prevent bone loss may not stimulate endometrial growth. Thus, the goal of add-back is to supply enough estrogen to minimize GnRH agonist side effects while still maintaining a hypoestrogenic state sufficient to suppress endometriosis. This "estrogen threshold" has not been established, but is thought to approximate 30 to 40 pg/mL of estradiol. Therefore, the addition of a small amount of hormones as add-back may alleviate side effects while maintaining therapeutic efficacy.

SECTION 1

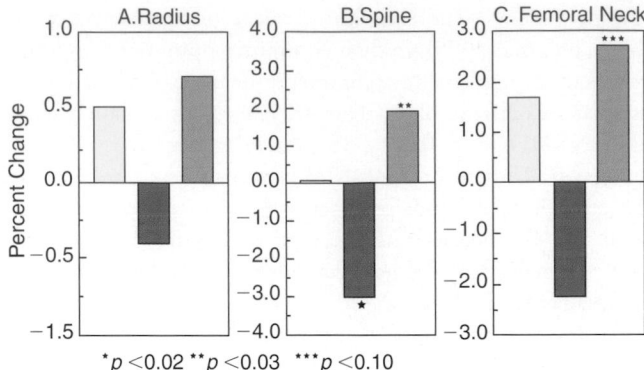

$*p < 0.02 \quad **p < 0.03 \quad ***p < 0.10$

FIGURE 10-12 Changes in bone mineral density in the radius, spine and femoral neck in women treated for 6 months with COCs (*yellow bar*), GnRH agonist (*blue bar*), or GnRH agonist plus COCs (*green bar*). *(From Carr, 1995.)*

Add-back can be accomplished with the use of norethindrone acetate, 5 mg orally given daily, with or without conjugated equine estrogen (Premarin) 0.625 mg orally daily for 12 months. This regimen has been shown to provide extended pain relief beyond the duration of treatment and to preserve bone density (Surrey, 2002). Other regimens have used transdermal estradiol 25 µg with daily 5 mg oral MPA and showed that GnRH remained effective in reducing endometriosis pain (Edmonds, 1996). In addition, traditional COCs may be used effectively as add-back. The extent of bone loss has been evaluated with add-back therapy, and although bone loss was noted in all patients undergoing GnRH agonist treatment, the extent of loss was lower in the add-back group (Edmonds, 1994; Zupi, 2004).

Add-back therapy can be initiated either immediately with the GnRH agonist or after 3 to 6 months of agonist therapy. However, several studies have shown that little benefit is gained in deferring add-back therapy and that patients who receive add-back concurrently with agonist therapy have reduced bone loss (Al-Azemi, 2009; Kiesel, 1996).

GnRH Antagonists

GnRH antagonists are another category of GnRH analogs capable of suppressing gonadotropin production. Unlike GnRH agonists, GnRH antagonists do not produce an initial release or *flare* of gonadotropins, and thus, suppression of gonadotropins and sex steroid hormones is immediate.

GnRH antagonists are mainly used for suppression of premature ovulation in IVF cycles and have not been well studied for endometriosis treatment. Nonetheless, some researchers have evaluated GnRH antagonist therapy for endometriosis using the rat model, and have found them to be effective in causing disease regression (Altintas, 2008; Jones, 1987; Sharpe, 1990). Küpker and colleagues (2002) studied the effect of the antagonist cetrorelix in 15 endometriosis patients. They administered subcutaneous injections of cetrorelix at a dosage of 3 mg weekly for 8 weeks. Patients were symptom free during treatment, and estrogen-withdrawal symptoms did not occur. The most common side effect was vaginal bleeding. Second-look laparoscopy showed disease regression in 60 percent of study

participants. The GnRH antagonists hold promise for endometriosis treatment, although long-term depot forms are not currently available. They seem to be better tolerated and may not require add-back therapy. Currently, nonpeptide orally bioactive GnRH antagonists are under development, and some have been studied for endometriosis. At this stage, more studies are still needed prior to full clinical use of these agents.

Aromatase Inhibitors

As previously mentioned, endometrial tissue locally produces aromatase, the enzyme responsible for estrogen synthesis. In endometriotic tissue, estrogen may be produced locally through aromatization of circulating androgens. This may be the reason for postmenopausal endometriosis and for intractable symptoms in some women despite treatment. The aromatase inhibitor anastrozole (Arimidex) was first used for endometriosis treatment in a woman with postmenopausal endometriosis after total hysterectomy and bilateral salpingo-oophorectomy (Takayama, 1998). The patient experienced significant pain relief, significant endometriotic lesion size reduction, and a 6-percent reduction in lumbar spine BMD after 9 months of treatment. Subsequently, further study has examined aromatase inhibitors in conjunction with low-dose, continuous COC add-back therapy for 6 months. This small Phase II trial using anastrozole revealed a significant pain reduction in 14 of 15 women with previously intractable pain from endometriosis (Amsterdam, 2005). Aromatase inhibitors have hypoestrogenic side-effect profiles that are similar to those of GnRH agonists, but hold promise in severe, refractory cases of endometriosis. Additional study is needed to establish the efficacy of such regimens (American College of Obstetricians and Gynecologists, 2008).

Other Medications

Other medical therapies have been attempted to control endometriosis symptoms. Two potentially promising agents are simvastatin and rosiglitazone. Simvastatin (Zocor) is an HMG-CoA reductase inhibitor used to lower cholesterol levels. It also exerts an inhibitory effect on endometriosis development in a mouse model and inhibits human endometriotic stromal cell proliferation in tissues from women with endometriosis (Bruner-Tran, 2009; Nasu, 2009).

Rosiglitazone (Avandia) is an insulin sensitizer used to treat diabetes. In addition, its binding to special receptors leads to immunomodulation, decreased aromatase activity, and in turn, decreased endometriosis burden in animal models (Aytan, 2007; Lebovic, 2007). In women with endometriosis receiving rosiglitazone, pain symptoms were noted to improve (Moravek, 2009). Further randomized trials are necessary prior to using these agents clinically.

Surgical Treatment of Endometriosis-Related Pain

Lesion Removal and Adhesiolysis

Because the primary method for diagnosis of endometriosis is laparoscopy, surgical treatment of endometriosis at the time of diagnosis is an attractive option. Numerous studies have examined removal of endometriotic lesions, through either excision or ablation. Unfortunately, many of these studies are uncontrolled or retrospective. However, a single randomized controlled trial compared laparoscopic ablation of endometriotic lesions plus laparoscopic uterine nerve ablation with diagnostic laparoscopy performed alone. In the ablation group, 63 percent of women attained significant symptom relief compared with 23 percent in the expectant management group. Unfortunately, recurrence is common following surgical excision. Jones (2001) demonstrated pain recurrence in 74 percent of patients at a mean time of 73 months following surgery. The median time for recurrence was 20 months.

The optimal method of endometriotic implant ablation for maximal symptom relief is controversial. Laser ablation does not appear to be more effective than conventional electrosurgical ablation of endometriosis (Blackwell, 1991). A randomized controlled trial comparing ablation with excision of endometriotic lesions in women with stage I or II endometriosis revealed similar reductions in pain scores at 6 months (Wright, 2005). For deeply infiltrative endometriosis, some authors have advocated radical surgical excision, although well-designed trials are lacking (Chapron, 2004).

Adhesiolysis is postulated to effectively treat pain symptoms in women with endometriosis by restoring normal anatomy. Unfortunately, most studies are poorly designed and retrospective. As a result, a definitive link between adhesions and pelvic pain is unclear (Hammoud, 2004). For example, one randomized controlled trial demonstrated no overall pain relief from adhesiolysis compared with expectant management (Peters, 1992). However, within this study, one woman with severe, dense vascularized bowel adhesions experienced pain relief following adhesiolysis.

Endometrioma Resection

Endometriomas are often treated surgically, as ovarian masses often prompt surgical investigation. Historically, endometriomas have been treated by total ovarian cystectomy or by aspiration coupled with ablation of the cyst capsule. One randomized controlled trial compared cystectomy with surgical drainage and bipolar coagulation of the endometrioma's inner lining (Beretta, 1998). Cystectomy led to lower rates of pelvic pain compared with drainage and coagulation (10 percent versus 53 percent). Additionally, cumulative pregnancy rates were higher following cystectomy during 24-month surveillance (67 percent versus 24 percent). Endometriomas may recur. Liu and coworkers (2007) found an approximately 15 percent recurrence rate at 2 years following initial surgery.

It is also important to note that women who undergo endometrioma excision may subsequently have a reduction in ovarian reserve (Almog, 2010; Ragni, 2006; Somigliana, 2003). This reduction in ovarian reserve may later prove detrimental to future fertility. Accordingly, in women who are asymptomatic and who have small cysts that display classic findings of an endometrioma, surveillance is an option. Following initial diagnosis, repeat TVS is recommended 6 to 12 weeks later to exclude hemorrhagic cyst. Endometriomas may then be sonographically surveilled in asymptomatic women yearly, or sooner at the clinician's discretion (American College of Obstetricians and Gynecologists, 2007; Levine, 2010). If surgery is indicated, to minimize loss in ovarian function, the endometrioma should be resected with removal of minimal normal ovarian tissue. In addition, limiting use of electrosurgical coagulation is one technique to avoid ovarian damage.

Presacral Neurectomy

For some women, transection of presacral nerves lying within the interiliac triangle may provide relief of chronic pelvic pain (Chap. 11, p. 316). Results from a randomized controlled trial revealed significantly greater pain relief at 12 months postoperatively in women treated with presacral neurectomy (PSN) and endometriotic excision compared with that from endometriotic excision alone (86 percent versus 57 percent) (Zullo, 2003). However, all of these women had midline pain. An earlier metaanalysis demonstrated a significant decrease in pelvic pain after PSN compared with that following more conservative procedures, but only in those with midline pain (Wilson, 2000). Neurectomy may be performed laparoscopically, but it is technically challenging. For these reasons, PSN is used in a limited manner and not recommended routinely for management of endometriosis-related pain.

Laparoscopic Uterine Nerve Ablation

There is no evidence that laparoscopic uterine nerve ablation (LUNA) is effective in treating endometriosis-related pain (Vercellini, 2003a). In a randomized controlled trial of 487 women with chronic pelvic pain lasting longer than 6 months, with or without minimal endometriosis, LUNA did not improve pain, dysmenorrhea, dyspareunia, or quality-of-life scores compared with laparoscopy without pelvic denervation (Daniels, 2009).

Abdominal versus Laparoscopic Approach

All of the surgical procedures just listed can be approached either through laparotomy or laparoscopy. Operative laparoscopy has been used for treatment of ovarian endometriomas for more than 20 years, and strong evidence supports laparoscopy over laparotomy in managing benign ovarian masses (Mais, 1995; Reich, 1986; Yuen, 1997). Unfortunately, a large number of endometriomas are still treated by laparotomy, with 50 percent of physicians surveyed in the United Kingdom still treating endometriomas in this manner (Jones, 2002). Although laparoscopic treatment of endometrioma carries an associated 5-percent risk for conversion to laparotomy, laparoscopy should be the primary procedure of choice because of its efficacy and low rates of postoperative morbidity (Canis, 2003).

Studies also demonstrate the effectiveness and low morbidity rates in laparoscopic excision of endometriotic implants. Also, laparoscopic presacral neurectomy appears to be as effective as laparotomy (Nezhat, 1992; Redwine, 1991). Adhesiolysis should be performed by laparoscopy when safe, and laparoscopy leads to less de novo adhesion formation than laparotomy (Gutt, 2004).

Hysterectomy with Bilateral Salpingo-oophorectomy

This procedure is the definitive and most effective therapy for women with endometriosis who do not wish to retain their reproductive function. Women who forego bilateral oophorectomy during hysterectomy for endometriosis have a sixfold greater risk of recurrent chronic pelvic pain and an eightfold greater risk of requiring additional surgery compared with women who undergo concomitant bilateral oophorectomy (Namnoum, 1995). For this reason, hysterectomy alone has no role in the treatment of chronic pelvic pain secondary to endometriosis.

Despite its effectiveness in endometriosis treatment, limitations of hysterectomy with bilateral salpingo-oophorectomy include surgical risks, pain recurrence, and hypoestrogenism effects. Of women who undergo hysterectomy and bilateral salpingo-oophorectomy for chronic pelvic pain, 10 percent have recurrent symptoms and 3.7 percent required additional pelvic surgery. Accordingly, a consensus conference recommendation from an expert panel of gynecologists in the United States stated that hysterectomy with bilateral salpingo-oophorectomy should be reserved for women with symptomatic endometriosis who have completed childbearing and recognize the risk of premature hypoestrogenism, including possible osteoporosis and decreased libido (Gambone, 2002).

Approach to Hysterectomy with Oophorectomy. There is no single correct procedure for hysterectomy and bilateral salpingo-oophorectomy for patients with endometriosis, and surgery may be completed laparoscopically, abdominally, or vaginally. However, adhesions and distorted anatomy secondary to endometriosis often makes a laparoscopic or vaginal approach difficult. In addition, the need to remove ovaries may make a vaginal approach less feasible. Accordingly, the choice of procedure will depend on equipment availability, operator experience, and extent of disease.

Postoperative Hormone Replacement. In response to concerns of increased cardiovascular disease and breast cancer risks with postmenopausal hormone therapy (HT) use, efforts have been directed to minimize indiscriminant HT use (Anderson, 2004; Rossouw, 2002). Women with endometriosis who undergo hysterectomy with oophorectomy, however, represent a subset of menopausal women who may be better candidates for HT than women with natural menopause. First, women with surgical menopause are usually younger and would likely benefit from replacement of estrogen that is lost by removal of functional ovaries. Estrogen replacement should be considered in women with an early surgical menopause to prevent hypoestrogenic side effects such as hot flashes, osteoporosis, or decreased libido. Although evidence is lacking, some suggest treatment in these women continue until the time of expected natural menopause.

Although unopposed estrogen may be used in postmenopausal women in the absence of a uterus, disease recurrence has been reported with this therapy in women with severe endometriosis first treated with hysterectomy and oophorectomy (Taylor, 1999). Symptoms required repeat surgery and did not recur with combined estrogen and progestin regimens. Additionally, cases of endometrial carcinoma have been reported in women with endometriosis treated with unopposed estrogen after hysterectomy and oophorectomy (Reimnitz,

1988; Soliman, 2004). This is rare and may arise from incompletely resected pelvic endometriosis. Therefore, adding a progestin to estrogen replacement therapy may be considered in women with severe endometriosis treated surgically.

The optimal timing for hormone replacement initiation following hysterectomy with oophorectomy is unclear (American College of Obstetricians and Gynecologist, 1999). Some have advocated a 6-week delay to allow hormonal ablation of residual disease. However, the evidence to support a recommendation is limited. One small study showed no significant differences in postoperative recurrent pain rates whether hormones were initiated immediately after surgery or delayed (Hickman, 1998).

Treatment of Endometriosis-Related Infertility

Medical therapy used for treatment of endometriosis-related pain has not been shown to be effective in increasing fecundity in women with endometriosis (Hughes, 2003). Surgical ablation has been suggested to be beneficial for women with infertility and minimal to mild endometriosis, although the effect was minimal (Marcoux, 1997). Other researchers did not appreciate a fertility benefit to surgical ablation for mild to moderate endometriosis (Parazzini, 1999). Moderate to severe endometriosis may be treated with surgery to restore normal anatomy and tubal function. However, well-designed trials examining the role of surgery for subfertility in women with severe endometriosis are lacking. Alternatively, patients with endometriosis and infertility are candidates for fertility treatments such as controlled ovarian hyperstimulation, intrauterine insemination, and IVF (Chap. 20, p. 545).

REFERENCES

Adamson GD, Hurd SJ, Pasta DJ, et al: Laparoscopic endometriosis treatment: is it better? Fertil Steril 59:35, 1993

Al-Azemi M, Jones G, Sirkeci F, et al: Immediate and delayed add-back hormonal replacement therapy during ultra long GnRH agonist treatment of chronic cyclical pelvic pain. BJOG 116:1646, 2009

Almog B, Sheizaf B, Shalom-Paz E, et al: Effects of excision of ovarian endometrioma on the antral follicle count and collected oocytes for in vitro fertilization. Fertil Steril 94(6):2340, 2010

Altintas D, Kokcu A, Tosun M, et al: Comparison of the effects of cetrorelix, a GnRH antagonist, and leuprolide, a GnRH agonist, on experimental endometriosis. J Obstet Gynaecol Res 34:1014, 2008

American College of Obstetricians and Gynecologists: Aromatase inhibitors in gynecology. Committee Opinion No. 412, August 2008

American College of Obstetricians and Gynecologists: Endometriosis in adolescents. Committee Opinion No. 310, April 2005

American College of Obstetricians and Gynecologists: Management of adnexal masses. Practice Bulletin No. 83, July 2007

American College of Obstetricians and Gynecologists: Medical management of endometriosis. Practice Bulletin No. 11, December 1999

American Society for Reproductive Medicine: Revised American Society for Reproductive Medicine classification of endometriosis: 1996. Fertil Steril 67:817, 1997

Amsterdam LL, Gentry W, Jobanputra S, et al: Anastrozole and oral contraceptives: a novel treatment for endometriosis. Fertil Steril 84:300, 2005

Anderson GL, Limacher M, Assaf AR, et al: Effects of conjugated equine estrogen in postmenopausal women with hysterectomy: the Women's Health Initiative randomized controlled trial. JAMA 291:1701, 2004

Antonelli A, Simeone C, Zani D, et al: Clinical aspects and surgical treatment of urinary tract endometriosis: our experience with 31 cases. Eur Urol 49:1093, 2006

Arici A, Oral E, Attar E, et al: Monocyte chemotactic protein-1 concentration in peritoneal fluid of women with endometriosis and its modulation of expression in mesothelial cells. Fertil Steril 67:1065, 1997

Arici A, Seli E, Zeyneloglu HB, et al: Interleukin-8 induces proliferation of endometrial stromal cells: a potential autocrine growth factor. J Clin Endocrinol Metab 83:1201, 1998

Arici A, Tazuke SI, Attar E, et al: Interleukin-8 concentration in peritoneal fluid of patients with endometriosis and modulation of interleukin-8 expression in human mesothelial cells. Mol Hum Reprod 2.40, 1996

Athey PA, Diment DD: The spectrum of sonographic findings in endometriomas. J Ultrasound Med 8:487, 1989

Attia GR, Zeitoun K, Edwards D, et al: Progesterone receptor isoform A but not B is expressed in endometriosis. J Clin Endocrinol Metab 85:2897, 2000

Aytan H, Caliskan AC, Demirturk F, et al: Peroxisome proliferator-activated receptor-gamma agonist rosiglitazone reduces the size of experimental endometriosis in the rat model. Aust N Z J Obstet Gynecol 47(4):321, 2007

Azzena A, Litta P, Ferrara A, et al: Rectosigmoid endometriosis: diagnosis and surgical management. Clin Exp Obstet Gynecol 25:94, 1998

Balasch J, Creus M, Fabregues F, et al: Visible and non-visible endometriosis at laparoscopy in fertile and infertile women and in patients with chronic pelvic pain: a prospective study. Hum Reprod 11:387, 1996

Barbieri RL: Hormone treatment of endometriosis: the estrogen threshold hypothesis. Am J Obstet Gynecol 166:740, 1992

Bazot M, Detchev R, Cortez A, et al: Transvaginal sonography and rectal endoscopic sonography for the assessment of pelvic endometriosis: a preliminary comparison. Hum Reprod 18:1686, 2003

Bedaiwy MA, Falcone T: Laboratory testing for endometriosis. Clin Chim Acta 340:41, 2004

Bedaiwy MA, Falcone T, Sharma RK, et al: Prediction of endometriosis with serum and peritoneal fluid markers: a prospective controlled trial. Hum Reprod 17:426, 2002

Beretta P, Franchi M, Ghezzi F, et al: Randomized clinical trial of two laparoscopic treatments of endometriomas: cystectomy versus drainage and coagulation. Fertil Steril 70:1176, 1998

Berkley KJ, Rapkin AJ, Papka RE: The pains of endometriosis. Science 308:1587, 2005

Bielfeld P, Graf M, Jeyendran RS, et al: Effects of peritoneal fluids from patients with endometriosis on capacitated spermatozoa. Fertil Steril 60:893, 1993

Biscaldi E, Ferrero S, Fulcheri E, et al: Multislice CT enteroclysis in the diagnosis of bowel endometriosis. Eur Radiol 17:211, 2007

Bischoff FZ, Simpson JL: Heritability and molecular genetic studies of endometriosis. Hum Reprod Update 6:37, 2000

Blackwell RE: Applications of laser surgery in gynecology. Hype or high tech? Surg Clin North Am 71:1005, 1991

Bontis JN, Vavilis DT: Etiopathology of endometriosis. Ann N Y Acad Sci 816:305, 1997

Braun DP, Muriana A, Gebel H, et al: Monocyte-mediated enhancement of endometrial cell proliferation in women with endometriosis. Fertil Steril 61:78, 1994

Breech LL, Laufer MR: Obstructive anomalies of the female reproductive tract. J Reprod Med 44:233, 1999

Brosens I, Puttemans P, Campo R, et al: Non-invasive methods of diagnosis of endometriosis. Curr Opin Obstet Gynecol 15:519, 2003

Bruner-Tran KL, Osteen KG, Duleba AJ: Simvastatin protects against the development of endometriosis in a nude mouse model. J Clin Endocrinol Metab 94:2489, 2009

Bulun SE, Yang S, Fang Z, et al: Estrogen production and metabolism in endometriosis. Ann N Y Acad Sci 955:75, 2002

Cameron IC, Rogers S, Collins MC, et al: Intestinal endometriosis: presentation, investigation, and surgical management. Int J Colorectal Dis 10:83, 1995

Canis M, Mage G, Wattiez A, et al: The ovarian endometrioma: why is it so poorly managed? Laparoscopic treatment of large ovarian endometrioma: why such a long learning curve? Hum Reprod 18:5, 2003

Carbognin G, Guarise A, Minelli L, et al: Pelvic endometriosis: US and MRI features. Abdom Imaging 29:609, 2004

Carr BR, Breslau NA, Givens C, et al: Oral contraceptive pills, gonadotropin-releasing hormone agonists, or use in combination for treatment of hirsutism: a clinical research center study. J Clin Endocrinol Metab 80:1169, 1995

Chapron C, Chopin N, Borghese B, et al: Surgical management of deeply infiltrating endometriosis: an update. Ann NY Acad Sci 1034:326, 2004

Chapron C, Dubuisson JB, Pansini V, et al: Routine clinical examination is not sufficient for diagnosing and locating deeply infiltrating endometriosis. J Am Assoc Gynecol Laparosc 9;115, 2002

Chapron C, Fauconnier A, Dubuisson JB, et al: Deep infiltrating endometriosis: relation between severity of dysmenorrhoea and extent of disease. Hum Reprod 18:760, 2003

Cho S, Park SH, Choi YS, et al: Expression of cyclooxygenase-2 in eutopic endometrium and ovarian endometriotic tissue in women with severe endometriosis. Gynecol Obstet Invest 69:93, 2010

Choudhary S, Fasih N, Papadatos D, et al: Unusual imaging appearances of endometriosis. AJR Am J Roentgenol 192:1632, 2009

Chwalisz K, Perez MC, Demanno D, et al: Selective progesterone receptor modulator development and use in the treatment of leiomyomata and endometriosis. Endocr Rev 26:423, 2005

Comiter CV: Endometriosis of the urinary tract. Urol Clin North Am 29:625, 2002

Cramer DW, Wilson E, Stillman RJ, et al: The relation of endometriosis to menstrual characteristics, smoking, and exercise. JAMA 255:1904, 1986

Curtis P, Lindsay P, Jackson AE, et al: Adverse effects on sperm movement characteristics in women with minimal and mild endometriosis. Br J Obstet Gynaecol 100:165, 1993

D'Hooghe TM: Clinical relevance of the baboon as a model for the study of endometriosis. Fertil Steril 68:613, 1997

D'Hooghe TM, Bambra CS, Raeymaekers BM, et al: The cycle pregnancy rate is normal in baboons with stage I endometriosis but decreased in primates with stage II and stage III-IV disease. Fertil Steril 66:809, 1996

D'Hooghe TM, Debrock S, Hill JA, et al: Endometriosis and subfertility: is the relationship resolved? Semin Reprod Med 21:243, 2003

Daftary GS, Taylor HS: EMX2 gene expression in the female reproductive tract and aberrant expression in the endometrium of patients with endometriosis. J Clin Endocrinol Metab 89:2390, 2004

Daniels J, Gray R, Hills RK, et al: Laparoscopic uterosacral nerve ablation for alleviating chronic pelvic pain: a randomized controlled trial. JAMA 302:955, 2009

Decker D, Konig J, Wardelmann E, et al: Terminal ileitis with sealed perforation—a rare complication of intestinal endometriosis: case report and short review of the literature. Arch Gynecol Obstet 269:294, 2004

Dictor M, Nelson CE, Uvelius B: Priapism in a patient with endometrioid prostatic carcinoma. A case report. Urol Int 43:245, 1988

Dlugi AM, Miller JD, Knittle J: Lupron depot (leuprolide acetate for depot suspension) in the treatment of endometriosis: a randomized, placebo-controlled, double-blind study. Lupron Study Group. Fertil Steril 54:419, 1990

Dmowski WP, Rana N, Michalowska J, et al: The effect of endometriosis, its stage and activity, and of autoantibodies on in vitro fertilization and embryo transfer success rates. Fertil Steril 63:555, 1995

Douglas C, Rotimi O. Extragenital endometriosis: a clinicopathological review of a Glasgow hospital experience with case illustrations. J Obstet Gynaecol 24:804, 2004

Edmonds DK: Add-back therapy in the treatment of endometriosis: the European experience. Br J Obstet Gynaecol 103(Suppl 14):10, 1996

Edmonds DK, Howell R: Can hormone replacement therapy be used during medical therapy of endometriosis? Br J Obstet Gynaecol 101 (Suppl 10):24, 1994

Efstathiou JA, Sampson DA, Levine Z, et al: Nonsteroidal antiinflammatory drugs differentially suppress endometriosis in a murine model. Fertil Steril 83:171, 2005

Elger W, Bartley J, Schneider B, et al: Endocrine pharmacological characterization of progesterone antagonists and progesterone receptor modulators with respect to PR-agonistic and antagonistic activity. Steroids 65:713, 2000

Eskenazi B, Warner ML: Epidemiology of endometriosis. Obstet Gynecol Clin North Am 24:235, 1997

Eskenazi B, Warner M, Bonsignore L, et al: Validation study of nonsurgical diagnosis of endometriosis. Fertil Steril 76:929, 2001

Fauconnier A, Chapron C, Dubuisson JB, et al: Relation between pain symptoms and the anatomic location of deep infiltrating endometriosis. Fertil Steril 78:719, 2002

Fedele L, Bianchi S, Bocciolone L, et al: Buserelin acetate in the treatment of pelvic pain associated with minimal and mild endometriosis: a controlled study. Fertil Steril 59:516, 1993

Fedele L, Bianchi S, Bocciolone L, et al: Pain symptoms associated with endometriosis. Obstet Gynecol 79:767, 1992

Fedele L, Marchini M, Bianchi S, et al: Endometrial patterns during danazol and buserelin therapy for endometriosis: comparative structural and ultrastructural study. Obstet Gynecol 76:79, 1990

Ferrero S, Esposito F, Abbamonte LH, et al: Quality of sex life in women with endometriosis and deep dyspareunia. Fertil Steril 83:573, 2005

Floyd WS: Danazol: endocrine and endometrial effects. Int J Fertil 25:75, 1980

Forbes KL, Thomas FJ: Tissue and endocrine responses to gestrinone and danazol in the treatment of endometriosis. Reprod Fertil Dev 5:103, 1993

Gallo MF, Nanda K, Grimes DA, et al: 20 mcg versus >20 mcg estrogen combined oral contraceptives for contraception. Cochrane Database Syst Rev 2:CD003989, 2005

Gambone JC, Mittman BS, Munro MG, et al: Consensus statement for the management of chronic pelvic pain and endometriosis: proceedings of an expert-panel consensus process. Fertil Steril 78:961, 2002

Garrido N, Krussel JS, Remohi J, et al: Expression and function of 3beta hydroxysteroid dehydrogenase (3beta HSD) type II and corticosteroid binding globulin (CBG) in granulosa cells from ovaries of women with and without endometriosis. J Assist Reprod Genet 19:24, 2002

Gestrinone Italian Study Group: Gestrinone versus a gonadotropin-releasing hormone agonist for the treatment of pelvic pain associated with endometriosis: a multicenter, randomized, double-blind study. Gestrinone Italian Study Group. Fertil Steril 66:911, 1996

Giudice LC, Kao LC: Endometriosis. Lancet 364:1789, 2004

Gleicher N, Dmowski WP, Siegel I, et al: Lymphocyte subsets in endometriosis. Obstet Gynecol 63:463, 1984

Gurates B, Bulun SE: Endometriosis: the ultimate hormonal disease. Semin Reprod Med 21:125, 2003

Gutt CN, Oniu T, Schemmer P, et al: Fewer adhesions induced by laparoscopic surgery? Surg Endosc 18:898, 2004

Hadfield RM, Mardon HJ, Barlow DH, et al: Endometriosis in monozygotic twins. Fertil Steril 68:941, 1997

Halme J, Hammond MG, Hulka JF, et al: Retrograde menstruation in healthy women and in patients with endometriosis. Obstet Gynecol 64:151, 1984

Hammoud A, Gago LA, Diamond MP: Adhesions in patients with chronic pelvic pain: a role for adhesiolysis? Fertil Steril 82:1483, 2004

Haney AF, Muscato JJ, Weinberg JB: Peritoneal fluid cell populations in infertility patients. Fertil Steril 35:696, 1981

Harada T, Kubota T, Aso T: Usefulness of CA19-9 versus CA125 for the diagnosis of endometriosis. Fertil Steril 78:733, 2002

Harada T, Momoeda M, Taketani Y, et al: Low-dose oral contraceptive pill for dysmenorrhea associated with endometriosis: a placebo-controlled, double-blind, randomized trial. Fertil Steril 90:1583, 2008

Harlow CR, Cahill DJ, Maile LA, et al: Reduced preovulatory granulosa cell steroidogenesis in women with endometriosis. J Clin Endocrinol Metab 81:426, 1996

Hickman TN, Namnoum AB, Hinton EL, et al: Timing of estrogen replacement therapy following hysterectomy with oophorectomy for endometriosis. Obstet Gynecol 91(5 Pt 1):673, 1998

Hinterholzer S, Riss D, Brustmann H: Symptomatic large bowel endometriosis in a woman with a hormonal intrauterine device: a case report. J Reprod Med 52:1055, 2007

Ho HN, Chao KH, Chen HF, et al: Peritoneal natural killer cytotoxicity and CD25+ CD3+ lymphocyte subpopulation are decreased in women with stage III-IV endometriosis. Hum Reprod 10:2671, 1995

Hornstein MD, Harlow BL, Thomas PP, et al: Use of a new CA 125 assay in the diagnosis of endometriosis. Hum Reprod 10:932, 1995a

Hornstein MD, Surrey ES, Weisberg GW, et al: Leuprolide acetate depot and hormonal add-back in endometriosis: a 12-month study. Lupron Add-Back Study Group. Obstet Gynecol 91:16, 1998

Hornstein MD, Yuzpe AA, Burry KA, et al: Prospective randomized double-blind trial of 3 versus 6 months of nafarelin therapy for endometriosis associated pelvic pain. Fertil Steril 63:955, 1995b

Houston DE, Noller KL, Melton LJ III, et al: Incidence of pelvic endometriosis in Rochester, Minnesota, 1970–1979. Am J Epidemiol 125:959, 1987

Hughes E, Fedorkow D, Collins J, et al: Ovulation suppression for endometriosis. Cochrane Database Syst Rev 3:CD000155, 2003

Hughesdon PE: The structure of endometrial cysts of the ovary. J Obstet Gynaecol Br Emp 64:481, 1957

Jansen RP, Russell P: Nonpigmented endometriosis: clinical, laparoscopic, and pathologic definition. Am J Obstet Gynecol 155:1154, 1986

Joki-Erkkila MM, Heinonen PK: Presenting and long-term clinical implications and fecundity in females with obstructing vaginal malformations. J Pediatr Adolesc Gynecol 16:307, 2003

Jones KD, Fan A, Sutton CJ: The ovarian endometrioma: why is it so poorly managed? Indicators from an anonymous survey. Hum Reprod 17:845, 2002

Jones KD, Haines P, Sutton CJ: Long-term follow-up of a controlled trial of laser laparoscopy for pelvic pain. JSLS 5:111, 2001

Jones RC: The effect of a luteinizing hormone-releasing hormone antagonist on experimental endometriosis in the rat. Acta Endocrinol (Copenh) 114:379, 1987

Jones SC: Relative thromboembolic risks associated with COX-2 inhibitors. Ann Pharmacother 39:1249, 2005

Kao LC, Germeyer A, Tulac S, et al: Expression profiling of endometrium from women with endometriosis reveals candidate genes for disease-based implantation failure and infertility. Endocrinology 144:2870, 2003

Kennedy S, Bergqvist A, Chapron C, et al: ESHRE guideline for the diagnosis and treatment of endometriosis. Hum Reprod 20:2698, 2005

Kettel LM, Murphy AA, Morales AJ, et al: Treatment of endometriosis with the antiprogesterone mifepristone (RU486). Fertil Steril 65:23, 1996

Khorram O, Taylor RN, Ryan IP, et al: Peritoneal fluid concentrations of the cytokine RANTES correlate with the severity of endometriosis. Am J Obstet Gynecol 169:1545, 1993

Kiesel L, Schweppe KW, Sillem M, et al: Should add-back therapy for endometriosis be deferred for optimal results? Br J Obstet Gynaecol 103(Suppl 14):15, 1996

Kim YA, Kim MR, Lee JH, et al: Gonadotropin-releasing hormone agonist reduces aromatase cytochrome P450 and cyclooxygenase-2 in ovarian endometrioma and eutopic endometrium of patients with endometriosis. Gynecol Obstet Invest 68:73, 2009

Kitawaki J, Noguchi T, Amatsu T, et al: Expression of aromatase cytochrome P450 protein and messenger ribonucleic acid in human endometriotic and adenomyotic tissues but not in normal endometrium. Biol Reprod 57:514, 1997

Koger KE, Shatney CH, Hodge K, et al: Surgical scar endometrioma. Surg Gynecol Obstet 177:243, 1993

Koninckx PR, Braet P, Kennedy SH, et al: Dioxin pollution and endometriosis in Belgium. Hum Reprod, 9:1001, 1994

Koninckx PR, Meuleman C, Demeyere S, et al: Suggestive evidence that pelvic endometriosis is a progressive disease, whereas deeply infiltrating endometriosis is associated with pelvic pain. Fertil Steril 55:759, 1991

Koninckx PR, Meuleman C, Oosterlynck D, et al: Diagnosis of deep endometriosis by clinical examination during menstruation and plasma CA-125 concentration. Fertil Steril 65:280, 1996

Korner M, Burckhardt E, Mazzucchelli L: Higher frequency of chromosomal aberrations in ovarian endometriosis compared to extragonadal endometriosis: a possible link to endometrioid adenocarcinoma. Mod Pathol 19:1615, 2006

Küpker W, Felberbaum RE, Krapp M, et al: Use of GnRH antagonists in the treatment of endometriosis. Reprod Biomed Online 5:12, 2002

Lebovic DI, Mwenda JM, Chai DC, et al: PPAR-gamma receptor ligand induces regression of endometrial explants in baboons: a prospective, randomized, placebo-and drug-controlled study. Fertil Steril 88(4 Suppl):1108, 2007

Lessey BA, Castelbaum AJ, Sawin SW, et al: Aberrant integrin expression in the endometrium of women with endometriosis. J Clin Endocrinol Metab 79:643, 1994

Levine D, Brown DL, Andreotti RF, et al: Management of asymptomatic ovarian and other adnexal cysts imaged at US: Society of Radiologists in Ultrasound Consensus Conference Statement. Radiology 256(3):943, 2010

Leyendecker G, Kunz G, Herbertz M, et al: Uterine peristaltic activity and the development of endometriosis. Ann N Y Acad Sci 1034:338, 2004

Ling FW: Randomized controlled trial of depot leuprolide in patients with chronic pelvic pain and clinically suspected endometriosis. Obstet Gynecol 93:51, 1999

Liu X, Yuan L, Shen F, et al: Patterns of and risk factors for recurrence in women with ovarian endometriomas. Obstet Gynecol 109(6):1411, 2007

Lockhat FB, Emembolu JO, et al: The efficacy, side-effects and continuation rates in women with symptomatic endometriosis undergoing treatment with an intra-uterine administered progestogen (levonorgestrel): a 3 year follow-up. Obstet Gynecol Surv 60:443, 2005

Mahmood TA, Templeton A: Prevalence and genesis of endometriosis. Hum Reprod 6:544, 1991

Mais V, Ajossa S, Piras B, et al: Treatment of nonendometriotic benign adnexal cysts: a randomized comparison of laparoscopy and laparotomy. Obstet Gynecol 86:770, 1995

Malinak LR, Buttram VC Jr, Elias S, et al: Heritage aspects of endometriosis. II. Clinical characteristics of familial endometriosis. Am J Obstet Gynecol 137:332, 1980

Marchino GL, Gennarelli G, Enria R, et al: Diagnosis of pelvic endometriosis with use of macroscopic versus histologic findings. Fertil Steril 84:12, 2005a

Marchino GL, Gennarelli G, Enria R, et al: Laparoscopic visualization with histologic confirmation represents the best available option to date in the diagnosis of endometriosis. Fertil Steril 84:38, 2005b

Marcoux S, Maheux R, Berube S: Laparoscopic surgery in infertile women with minimal or mild endometriosis. Canadian Collaborative Group on Endometriosis. N Engl J Med 337:217, 1997

Markham SM, Carpenter SE, et al: Extrapelvic endometriosis. Obstet Gynecol Clin North Am 16:193, 1989

Mathias SD, Kuppermann M, Liberman RF, et al: Chronic pelvic pain: prevalence, health-related quality of life, and economic correlates. Obstet Gynecol 87:321, 1996

Mathur S, Peress MR, Williamson HO, et al: Autoimmunity to endometrium and ovary in endometriosis. Clin Exp Immunol 50:259, 1982

Matorras R, Rodriguez F, Pijoan JI, et al: Women who are not exposed to spermatozoa and infertile women have similar rates of stage I endometriosis. Fertil Steril 76:923, 2001

Matsuura K, Ohtake H, Katabuchi H, et al: Coelomic metaplasia theory of endometriosis: evidence from in vivo studies and an in vitro experimental model. Gynecol Obstet Invest 47(Suppl 1):18, 1999

Mayani A, Barel S, Soback S, et al: Dioxin concentrations in women with endometriosis. Hum Reprod 12:373, 1997

McLaren J, Prentice A, Charnock-Jones DS, et al: Vascular endothelial growth factor is produced by peritoneal fluid macrophages in endometriosis and is regulated by ovarian steroids. J Clin Invest 98:482, 1996

McMeekin DS, Tillmanns T: Endometrial cancer: treatment of nodal metastases. Curr Treat Options Oncol 4:121, 2003

Menada MV, Remorgida V, Abbamonte LH, et al: Transvaginal ultrasonography combined with water-contrast in the rectum in the diagnosis of rectovaginal endometriosis infiltrating the bowel. Fertil Steril 89:699, 2008

Meuleman C, Vandenabeele B, Fieuws S, et al: High prevalence of endometriosis in infertile women with normal ovulation and normospermic partners. Fertil Steril 92:68, 2009

Milingos S, Mavrommatis C, Elsheikh A, et al: Fecundity of infertile women with minimal or mild endometriosis. A clinical study. Arch Gynecol Obstet 267:37, 2002

Mitchell AO, Hoffman AP, Swartz SE, et al: An unusual occurrence of endometriosis in the right groin: a case report and review of the literature. Mil Med 156:633, 1991

Moen MH, Schei B: Epidemiology of endometriosis in a Norwegian county. Acta Obstet Gynecol Scand 76:559, 1997

Mol BW, Bayram N, Lijmer JG, et al: The performance of CA-125 measurement in the detection of endometriosis: a meta-analysis. Fertil Steril 70:1101, 1998

Moore J, Copley S, Morris J, et al: A systematic review of the accuracy of ultrasound in the diagnosis of endometriosis. Ultrasound Obstet Gynecol 20:630, 2002

Moore JG, Binstock MA, et al: The clinical implications of retroperitoneal endometriosis. Am J Obstet Gynecol 158:1291, 1988

Moravek MB, Ward EA, Lebovic DI: Thiazolidinediones as therapy for endometriosis: a case series. Gynecol Obstet Invest 68:167, 2009

Mori H, Sawairi M, Nakagawa M, et al: Peritoneal fluid interleukin-1 beta and tumor necrosis factor in patients with benign gynecologic disease. Am J Reprod Immunol 26:62, 1991

Muneyyirci-Delale O, Karacan M: Effect of norethindrone acetate in the treatment of symptomatic endometriosis. Int J Fertil Womens Med 43:24, 1998

Murphy AA: Clinical aspects of endometriosis. Ann N Y Acad Sci 955:1, 2002

Muscato JJ, Haney AF, Weinberg JB: Sperm phagocytosis by human peritoneal macrophages: a possible cause of infertility in endometriosis. Am J Obstet Gynecol 144:503, 1982

Mutter GL, Bergeron C, Deligdisch L, et al: The spectrum of endometrial pathology induced by progesterone receptor modulators. Mod Pathol 21(5):591, 2008

Muzii L, Marana R, Pedulla S, et al: Correlation between endometriosis-associated dysmenorrhea and the presence of typical or atypical lesions. Fertil Steril 68:19, 1997

Namnoum AB, Hickman TN, Goodman SB, et al: Incidence of symptom recurrence after hysterectomy for endometriosis. Fertil Steril 64:898, 1995

Nasir L, Bope ET: Management of pelvic pain from dysmenorrhea or endometriosis. J Am Board Fam Pract 17(Suppl):S43, 2004

Nasu K, Yuge A, Tsuno A, et al: Simvastatin inhibits the proliferation and the contractility of human endometriotic stromal cells: a promising agent for the treatment of endometriosis. Fertil Steril 92:2097, 2009

Nezhat C, Nezhat F: A simplified method of laparoscopic presacral neurectomy for the treatment of central pelvic pain due to endometriosis. Br J Obstet Gynaecol 99:659, 1992

Nezhat C, Santolaya J, Nezhat FR: Comparison of transvaginal sonography and bimanual pelvic examination in patients with laparoscopically confirmed endometriosis. J Am Assoc Gynecol Laparosc 1:127, 1994

Nisolle M, Donnez J: Peritoneal endometriosis, ovarian endometriosis, and adenomyotic nodules of the rectovaginal septum are three different entities. Fertil Steril 68:585, 1997

Noble LS, Takayama K, Zeitoun KM, et al: Prostaglandin E2 stimulates aromatase expression in endometriosis-derived stromal cells. J Clin Endocrinol Metab 82:600, 1997

Odukoya OA, Wheatcroft N, Weetman AP, et al: The prevalence of endometrial immunoglobulin G antibodies in patients with endometriosis. Hum Reprod 10:1214, 1995

Olive DL, Pritts EA: Treatment of endometriosis. N Engl J Med 345:266, 2001

Olive DL, Stohs GF, Metzger DA, et al: Expectant management and hydrotubations in the treatment of endometriosis-associated infertility. Fertil Steril 44:35, 1985a

Olive DL, Weinberg JB, Haney AF: Peritoneal macrophages and infertility: the association between cell number and pelvic pathology. Fertil Steril 44:772, 1985b

Oosterlynck DJ, Meuleman C, Waer M, et al: Immunosuppressive activity of peritoneal fluid in women with endometriosis. Obstet Gynecol 82:206, 1993

Orwoll ES, Yuzpe AA, Burry KA, et al: Nafarelin therapy in endometriosis: long-term effects on bone mineral density. Am J Obstet Gynecol 171:1221, 1994

Osuga Y, Koga K, Tsutsumi O, et al: Role of laparoscopy in the treatment of endometriosis-associated infertility. Gynecol Obstet Invest 53(Suppl 1):33, 2002

Ota H, Igarashi S, Sasaki M, et al: Distribution of cyclooxygenase-2 in eutopic and ectopic endometrium in endometriosis and adenomyosis. Hum Reprod 16:561, 2001

Papavramidis TS, Sapalidis K, Michalopoulos N, et al: Spontaneous abdominal wall endometriosis: a case report. Acta Chir Belg 109:778, 2009

Parazzini F: Ablation of lesions or no treatment in minimal-mild endometriosis in infertile women: a randomized trial. Gruppo Italiano per lo Studio dell'Endometriosi. Hum Reprod 14:1332, 1999

Patel MD, Feldstein VA, Chen DC, et al: Endometriomas: diagnostic performance of US. Radiology 210:739, 1999

Pellicer A, Oliveira N, Ruiz A, et al: Exploring the mechanism(s) of endometriosis-related infertility: an analysis of embryo development and implantation in assisted reproduction. Hum Reprod 10(Suppl 2):91, 1995

Pellicer A, Valbuena D, Bauset C, et al: The follicular endocrine environment in stimulated cycles of women with endometriosis: steroid levels and embryo quality. Fertil Steril 69:1135, 1998

Peters AA, Trimbos-Kemper GC, Admiraal C, et al: A randomized clinical trial on the benefit of adhesiolysis in patients with intraperitoneal adhesions and chronic pelvic pain. Br J Obstet Gynaecol 99:59, 1992

Petta CA, Ferriani RA, Abrao MS, et al: Randomized clinical trial of a levonorgestrel-releasing intrauterine system and a depot GnRH analogue for the treatment of chronic pelvic pain in women with endometriosis. Hum Reprod 20:1993, 2005

Pinkert TC, Catlow CE, Straus R: Endometriosis of the urinary bladder in a man with prostatic carcinoma. Cancer 43:1562, 1979

Pollack R, Gordon PH, Ferenczy A, et al: Perineal endometriosis. A case report. J Reprod Med 35:109, 1990

Possover M, Chiantera V: Isolated infiltrative endometriosis of the sciatic nerve: a report of three patients. Fertil Steril 87(2):417.e17, 2007

Prentice A, Deary AJ, Bland E: Progestagens and anti-progestagens for pain associated with endometriosis. Cochrane Database Syst Rev 2:CD002122, 2000a

Prentice A, Deary AJ, Goldbeck-Wood S, et al: Gonadotrophin-releasing hormone analogues for pain associated with endometriosis. Cochrane Database Syst Rev 2:CD000346, 2000b

Price DT, Maloney KE, Ibrahim GK, et al: Vesical endometriosis: report of two cases and review of the literature. Urology 48:639, 1996

Qiao J, Yeung WS, Yao YQ, et al: The effects of follicular fluid from patients with different indications for IVF treatment on the binding of human spermatozoa to the zona pellucida. Hum Reprod 13:128, 1998

Rabin D, McNeil LW: Pituitary and gonadal desensitization after continuous luteinizing hormone-releasing hormone infusion in normal females. J Clin Endocrinol Metab 51:873, 1980

Ragni G, Somigliana E, Benedetti F, et al: Damage to ovarian reserve associated with laparoscopic excision of endometriomas: a quantitative rather than a qualitative injury. Am J Obstet Gynecol 193:1908, 2005

Redwine DB: Conservative laparoscopic excision of endometriosis by sharp dissection: life table analysis of reoperation and persistent or recurrent disease. Fertil Steril 56:628, 1991

Reich H, McGlynn F: Treatment of ovarian endometriomas using laparoscopic surgical techniques. J Reprod Med 31:577, 1986

Reimnitz C, Brand E, Nieberg RK, et al: Malignancy arising in endometriosis associated with unopposed estrogen replacement. Obstet Gynecol 71:444, 1988

Remorgida V, Ferrero S, Fulcheri E, et al: Bowel endometriosis: presentation, diagnosis, and treatment. Obstet Gynecol Surv 62(7):461, 2007

Rier S, Foster WG: Environmental dioxins and endometriosis. Semin Reprod Med 21: 145, 2003

Rier SE, Martin DC, Bowman RE, et al: Endometriosis in rhesus monkeys (Macaca mulatta) following chronic exposure to 2,3,7,8-tetrachlorodibenzo-p-dioxin. Fundam Appl Toxicol 21:433, 1993

Ripps BA, Martin DC: Correlation of focal pelvic tenderness with implant dimension and stage of endometriosis. J Reprod Med 37:620, 1992

Roberts LM, Redan J, Reich H: Extraperitoneal endometriosis with catamenial pneumothoraces: a review of the literature. JSLS 7:371, 2003

Rock JA, Zacur HA, Dlugi AM, et al: Pregnancy success following surgical correction of imperforate hymen and complete transverse vaginal septum. Obstet Gynecol 59:448, 1982

Rodriguez-Escudero FJ, Neyro JL, Corcostegui B, et al: Does minimal endometriosis reduce fecundity? Fertil Steril 50:522, 1988

Rossouw JE, Anderson GL, Prentice RL, et al: Risks and benefits of estrogen plus progestin in healthy postmenopausal women: principal results From the Women's Health Initiative randomized controlled trial. JAMA 288:321, 2002

Ryan IP, Tseng JF, Schriock ED, et al: Interleukin-8 concentrations are elevated in peritoneal fluid of women with endometriosis. Fertil Steril 63:929, 1995

Ryu JS, Song ES, Lee KH, et al: Natural history and therapeutic implications of patients with catamenial hemoptysis. Resp Med 101(5):1032, 2007

Sainz de la Cuesta R, Eichhorn JH, Rice LW, et al: Histologic transformation of benign endometriosis to early epithelial ovarian cancer. Gynecol Oncol 60:238, 1996

Sainz de la Cuesta R, Izquierdo M, Canamero M, et al: Increased prevalence of p53 overexpression from typical endometriosis to atypical endometriosis and ovarian cancer associated with endometriosis. Eur J Obstet Gynecol Reprod Biol 113:87, 2004

Sampson JA: Peritoneal endometriosis due to menstrual dissemination of endometrial tissue into the peritoneal cavity. Am J Obstet Gynecol 14:442, 1927

Sanfilippo JS, Wakim NG, Schikler KN, et al: Endometriosis in association with uterine anomaly. Am J Obstet Gynecol 154:39, 1986

Satyaswaroop PG, Wartell DJ, Mortel R: Distribution of progesterone receptor, estradiol dehydrogenase, and 20 alpha-dihydroprogesterone dehydrogenase activities in human endometrial glands and stroma: progestin induction of steroid dehydrogenase activities in vitro is restricted to the glandular epithelium. Endocrinology 111:743, 1982

Schattman GL, Grifo JA, Birnbaum S: Laparoscopic resection of a noncommunicating rudimentary uterine horn. A case report. J Reprod Med 40:219, 1995

Schenken RS, Asch RH: Surgical induction of endometriosis in the rabbit: effects on fertility and concentrations of peritoneal fluid prostaglandins. Fertil Steril 34:581, 1980

Schenken RS, Asch RH, Williams RF, et al: Etiology of infertility in monkeys with endometriosis: luteinized unruptured follicles, luteal phase defects, pelvic adhesions, and spontaneous abortions. Fertil Steril 41:122, 1984

Sciume C, Geraci G, Pisello F, et al: [Intestinal endometriosis: an obscure cause of cyclic rectal bleeding]. Ann Ital Chir 75:379, 2004

Seli E, Arici A: Endometriosis: interaction of immune and endocrine systems. Semin Reprod Med 21:135, 2003

Sharpe KL, Bertero MC, Vernon MW: Rapid regression of endometriosis by a new gonadotropin-releasing hormone antagonist in rats with surgically induced disease. Prog Clin Biol Res 323:449, 1990

Simpson JL, Elias S, Malinak LR, et al: Heritable aspects of endometriosis. I. Genetic studies. Am J Obstet Gynecol 137:327, 1980

Soliman NF, Evans AJ: Malignancy arising in residual endometriosis following hysterectomy and hormone replacement therapy. J Br Menopause Soc 10:123, 2004

Somigliana E, Ragni G, Benedetti F, et al: Does laparoscopic excision of endometriotic ovarian cysts significantly affect ovarian reserve? Insights from IVF cycles. Hum Reprod 18:2450, 2003

Steck WD, Helwig EB: Cutaneous endometriosis. Clin Obstet Gynecol 9:373, 1966

Steele RW, Dmowski WP, Marmer DJ: Immunologic aspects of human endometriosis. Am J Reprod Immunol 6:33, 1984

Stefansson H, Geirsson RT, Steinthorsdottir V, et al: Genetic factors contribute to the risk of developing endometriosis. Hum Reprod 17:555, 2002

Strathy JH, Molgaard CA, Coulam CB, et al: Endometriosis and infertility: a laparoscopic study of endometriosis among fertile and infertile women. Fertil Steril 38:667, 1982

Strowitzki T, Faustmann T, Gerlinger C, et al: Dienogest in the treatment of endometriosis-associated pelvic pain: a 12-week, randomized, double-blind, placebo-controlled study. Eur J Obstet Gynecol Reprod Biol 151(2):193, 2010

Surrey ES, Hornstein MD: Prolonged GnRH agonist and add-back therapy for symptomatic endometriosis: long-term follow-up. Obstet Gynecol 99:709, 2002

Sutton CJ, Pooley AS, Ewen SP, et al: Follow-up report on a randomized controlled trial of laser laparoscopy in the treatment of pelvic pain associated with minimal to moderate endometriosis. Fertil Steril 68:1070, 1997

Suzuki T, Izumi S, Matsubayashi H, et al: Impact of ovarian endometrioma on oocytes and pregnancy outcome in in vitro fertilization. Fertil Steril 83:908, 2005

Takayama K, Zeitoun K, Gunby RT, et al: Treatment of severe postmenopausal endometriosis with an aromatase inhibitor. Fertil Steril 69:709, 1998

Tasdemir M, Tasdemir I, Kodama H, et al: Effect of peritoneal fluid from infertile women with endometriosis on ionophore-stimulated acrosome loss. Hum Reprod 10:2419, 1995

Taylor M, Bowen-Simpkins P, Barrington J: Complications of unopposed oestrogen following radical surgery for endometriosis. J Obstet Gynaecol 19:647, 1999

Telimaa S, Kauppila A, Ronnberg L, et al: Elevated serum levels of endometrial secretory protein PP14 in patients with advanced endometriosis. Suppression by treatment with danazol and high-dose medroxyprogesterone acetate. Am J Obstet Gynecol 161:866, 1989

Telimaa S, Puolakka J, Ronnberg L, et al: Placebo-controlled comparison of danazol and high-dose medroxyprogesterone acetate in the treatment of endometriosis. Gynecol Endocrinol 1:13, 1987

Thomas EJ, Cooke ID: Successful treatment of asymptomatic endometriosis: does it benefit infertile women? Br Med J (Clin Res Ed) 294:1117, 1987

Tokushige N, Markham R, Russell P, et al: Effect of progestogens and combined oral contraceptives on nerve fibers in peritoneal endometriosis. Fertil Steril 92:1234, 2009

Treloar SA, Bell TA, Nagle CM, et al: Early menstrual characteristics associated with subsequent diagnosis of endometriosis. Am J Obstet Gynecol 202:534, 2010

Treloar SA, O'Connor DT, O'Connor VM, et al: Genetic influences on endometriosis in an Australian twin sample. Fertil Steril 71:701, 1999

Treloar SA, Wicks J, Nyholt DR, et al: Genomewide linkage study in 1,176 affected sister pair families identifies a significant susceptibility locus for endometriosis on chromosome 10q26. Am J Hum Genet 77:365, 2005

Tseng JF, Ryan IP, Milam TD, et al: Interleukin-6 secretion in vitro is upregulated in ectopic and eutopic endometrial stromal cells from women with endometriosis. J Clin Endocrinol Metab 81:1118, 1996

Ueki M: Histologic study of endometriosis and examination of lymphatic drainage in and from the uterus. Am J Obstet Gynecol 165:201, 1991

U.S. National Institutes of Health Clinical Trials: Study to evaluate the safety of asoprisnil in the treatment of uterine fibroids. May, 2008. Available online through ClinicalTrialsFeeds.org at: http://clinicaltrials.gov/ct2/show/NCT00156208. Accessed July 3, 2010

Varras M, Kostopanagiotou E, Katis K, et al: Endometriosis causing extensive intestinal obstruction simulating carcinoma of the sigmoid colon: a case report and review of the literature. Eur J Gynaecol Oncol 23:353, 2002

Vercellini P, Aimi G, Busacca M, et al: Laparoscopic uterosacral ligament resection for dysmenorrhea associated with endometriosis: results of a randomized, controlled trial. Fertil Steril 80:310, 2003a

Vercellini P, Chapron C, Fedele L, et al: Evidence for asymmetric distribution of sciatic nerve endometriosis. Obstet Gynecol 102:383, 2003b

Vercellini P, Frontino G, De Giorgi O, et al: Continuous use of an oral contraceptive for endometriosis-associated recurrent dysmenorrhea that does not respond to a cyclic pill regimen. Fertil Steril 80:560, 2003c

Vercellini P, Meschia M, De Giorgi O, et al: Bladder detrusor endometriosis: clinical and pathogenetic implications. J Urol 155:84, 1996a

Vercellini P, Trespidi L, Colombo A, et al: A gonadotropin-releasing hormone agonist versus a low-dose oral contraceptive for pelvic pain associated with endometriosis. Fertil Steril 60:75, 1993

Vercellini P, Trespidi L, De Giorgi O, et al: Endometriosis and pelvic pain: relation to disease stage and localization. Fertil Steril 65:299, 1996b

Vercellini P, Vendola N, Bocciolone L, et al: Reliability of the visual diagnosis of ovarian endometriosis. Fertil Steril 56:1198, 1991

Vernon MW, Beard JS, Graves K, et al: Classification of endometriotic implants by morphologic appearance and capacity to synthesize prostaglandin F. Fertil Steril 46:801, 1986

Vessey MP, Villard-Mackintosh L, Painter R: Epidemiology of endometriosis in women attending family planning clinics. BMJ 306:182, 1993

Vilos GA, Vilos AW, Haebe JJ: Laparoscopic findings, management, histopathology, and outcome of 25 women with cyclic leg pain. J Am Assoc Gynecol Laparosc 9:145, 2002

Vinatier D, Orazi G, Cosson M, et al: Theories of endometriosis. Eur J Obstet Gynecol Reprod Biol 96:21, 2001

Von Rokitansky C: Ueber Uterusdrusen-neubuildung in Uterus and Ovarilsarcomen. Z Ges Aerzte Wein 37:577, 1860

Waller KG, Lindsay P, Curtis P, et al: The prevalence of endometriosis in women with infertile partners. Eur J Obstet Gynecol Reprod Biol 48:135, 1993

Walter AJ, Hentz JG, Magtibay PM, et al: Endometriosis: correlation between histologic and visual findings at laparoscopy. Am J Obstet Gynecol 184:1407, 2001

Wang G, Tokushige N, Russell P, et al: Hyperinnervation in intestinal deep infiltrating endometriosis. J Minim Invasive Gynecol 16:713, 2009

Watanabe M, Kamiyama G, Yamazaki K, et al: Anal endosonography in the diagnosis and management of perianal endometriosis: report of a case. Surg Today 33:630, 2003

Wickramasekera D, Hay DJ, Fayz M: Acute small bowel obstruction due to ileal endometriosis: a case report and literature review. J R Coll Surg Edinb 44:59, 1999

Wiegratz I, Kuhl H: Long-cycle treatment with oral contraceptives. Drugs 64:2447, 2004

Wilson ML, Farquhar CM, Sinclair OJ, et al: Surgical interruption of pelvic nerve pathways for primary and secondary dysmenorrhoea. Cochrane Database Syst Rev 2:CD001896, 2000

Wilson TJ, Hertzog PJ, Angus D, et al: Decreased natural killer cell activity in endometriosis patients: relationship to disease pathogenesis. Fertil Steril 62:1086, 1994

Wright J, Lotfallah H, Jones K, et al: A randomized trial of excision versus ablation for mild endometriosis. Fertil Steril 83:1830, 2005

Yuen PM, Yu KM, Yip SK, et al: A randomized prospective study of laparoscopy and laparotomy in the management of benign ovarian masses. Am J Obstet Gynecol 177:109, 1997

Zeitoun KM, Bulun SE: Aromatase: a key molecule in the pathophysiology of endometriosis and a therapeutic target. Fertil Steril 72:961, 1999

Zeitoun K, Takayama K, Sasano H, et al: Deficient 17 beta-hydroxysteroid dehydrogenase type 2 expression in endometriosis: failure to metabolize 17 beta-estradiol. J Clin Endocrinol Metab 83:4474, 1998

Zhu L, Wong F, Lang JH: Perineal endometriosis after vaginal delivery—clinical experience with 10 patients. Aust N Z J Obstet Gynaecol 42:565, 2002

Zullo F, Palomba S, Zupi E, et al: Effectiveness of presacral neurectomy in women with severe dysmenorrhea caused by endometriosis who were treated with laparoscopic conservative surgery: a 1-year prospective randomized double-blind controlled trial. Am J Obstet Gynecol 189:5, 2003

Zupi E, Marconi D, Sbracia M, et al: Add-back therapy in the treatment of endometriosis-associated pain. Fertil Steril 82:1303, 2004

CHAPTER 11

Pelvic Pain

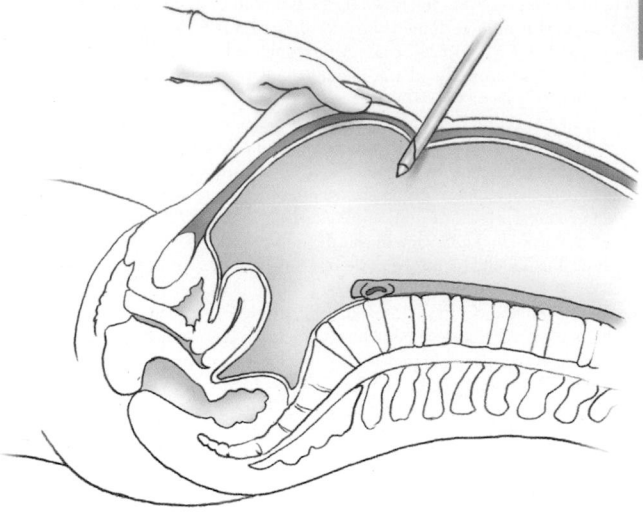

Pain in the lower abdomen and pelvis is one of the most common patient complaints. In addition to the human costs of illness and distress, the economic results can be measured in billions of dollars from medical charges as well as lost wages and productivity. Accurate diagnosis and treatment offers an opportunity to minimize this toll.

Pain is subjective and often ambiguous, and thus, difficult to diagnose and treat. Therefore, clinicians should understand the mechanisms underlying human pain perception, which involves complex physical, biochemical, emotional, and social interactions. Providers are obligated to search for organic sources of pain, but equally important, they should avoid overtreatment for an illness or injury that is minor or short lived.

PAIN PATHOPHYSIOLOGY

Pain is a protective mechanism meant to warn of an immediate threat and to prompt withdrawal from noxious stimuli. Pain is usually followed by an emotional response and inevitable behavioral consequences. These are often as important as the pain itself. Merely the threat of pain may elicit responses even in the absence of actual injury.

When categorized, pain may be considered *somatic* or *visceral* depending on the type of afferent nerve fibers involved. Additionally, pain is described by the physiologic steps that produce it and can be defined as *inflammatory* or *neuropathic* (Kehlet, 2006). Both categorizations are helpful in diagnosing the underlying sources of pain and selecting effective treatment.

Somatic Pain

Somatic pain stems from nerve afferents of the somatic nervous system, which innervates the parietal peritoneum, skin, muscles, and subcutaneous tissues (Fig. 23-3, p. 611). Somatic pain is typically sharp and localized. It is found on either the right or left within dermatomes that correspond to the innervation of involved tissues (Fig. 11-1).

Visceral Pain

Visceral pain stems from afferent fibers of the autonomic nervous system, which transmits information from the viscera and visceral peritoneum. Noxious stimuli typically include stretching, distension, ischemia, necrosis, or spasm of abdominal organs. The visceral afferent fibers that transfer these stimuli are sparse. Thus, the resulting diffuse sensory input leads to pain that is often described as a generalized, dull ache.

Visceral pain often localizes to the midline because visceral innervation of abdominal organs is usually bilateral (Flasar, 2006). Also, visceral afferents follow a segmental distribution,

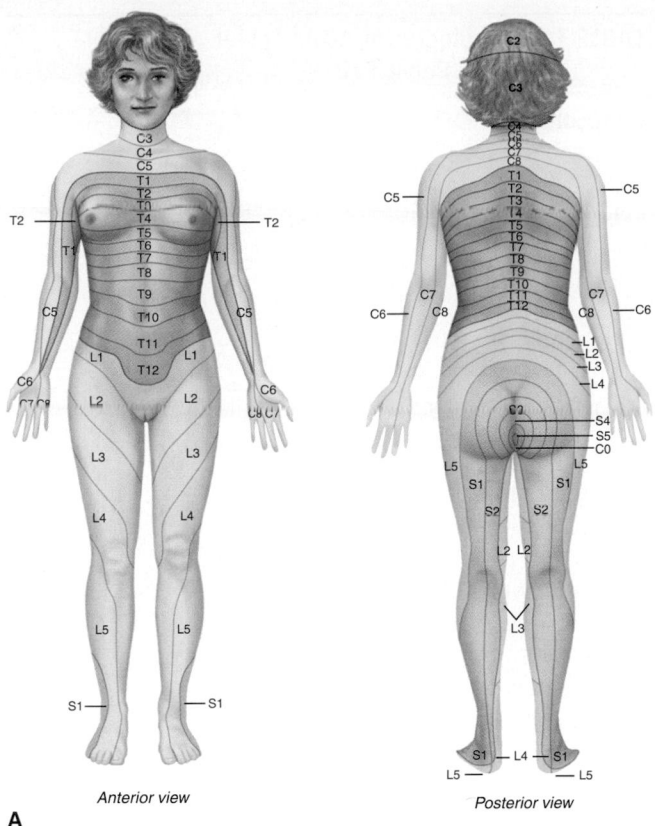

Anterior view

Posterior view

A

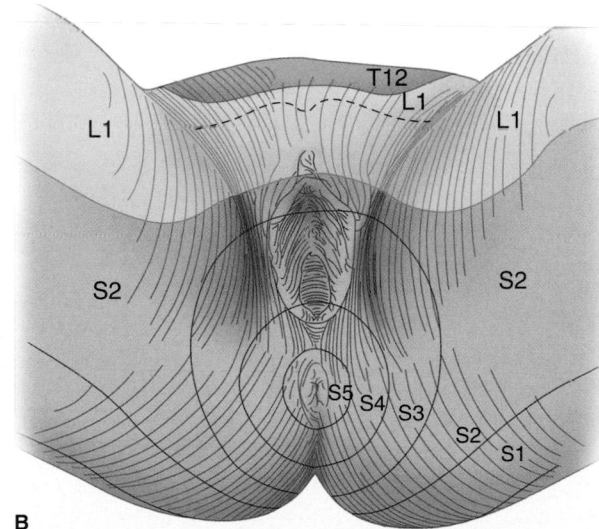

B

FIGURE 11-1 Dermatome maps. A dermatome is an area of skin supplied by a single spinal nerve. **A.** Body dermatomes. **B.** Perineal dermatomes. *(Redrawn from Rogers, 2000, with permission.)*

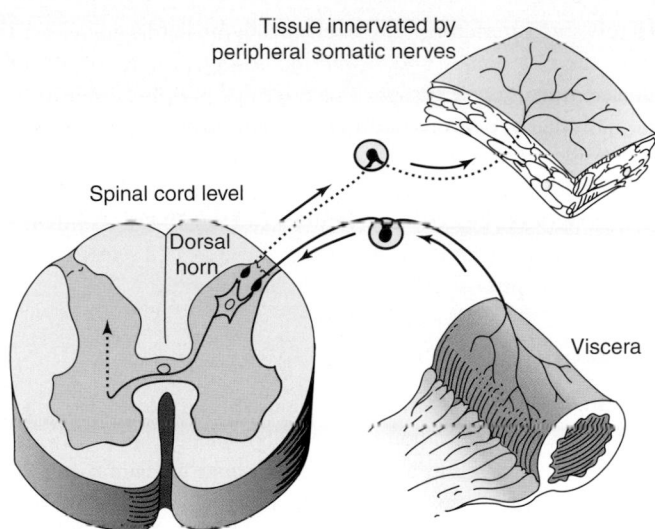

FIGURE 11-2 Viscerosomatic convergence. Pain impulses originating from an organ may impact dorsal horn neurons that are synapsing concurrently with peripheral somatic nerves. These impulses may then be perceived by the brain as coming from a peripheral somatic source such as muscle or skin rather than the diseased viscera. *(Redrawn from Perry, 2000, with permission.)*

Visceral afferent fibers are poorly myelinated, and action potentials may easily spread from them to adjacent somatic nerves. As a result, visceral pain may at times be referred to dermatomes that correspond to these adjacent somatic nerve fibers (Giamberardino, 2003). In addition, both peripheral somatic and visceral nerves often synapse in the spinal cord at the same dorsal horn neurons. These neurons, in turn, relay sensory information to the brain. The cortex recognizes the signal as coming from the same dermatome regardless of its visceral or somatic nerve origin. This phenomenon, termed *viscerosomatic convergence*, may lead to difficulty in a patient distinguishing internal organ pain from abdominal wall or pelvic floor pain (Fig. 11-2) (Perry, 2003).

Inflammatory Pain

With acute pain, noxious stimuli such as a knife cut, burn, or crush injury activate sensory pain receptors, more formally termed nociceptors. Action potentials travel from the periphery to dorsal horn neurons in the spinal cord. Here, reflex arcs may lead to immediate muscle contraction, which removes and protects the body from harm. Additionally, within the spinal cord, sensory information is augmented or dampened and may then be transmitted to the brain. In the cortex, it is recognized as pain (Janicki, 2003). After an acute stimulus is eliminated, activity of the nociceptor quickly diminishes.

If tissues are injured, then inflammation typically follows. Body fluids, along with inflammatory proteins and cells, are called to the injury site to limit tissue damage. Because cells and most inflammatory proteins are too large to cross normal endothelium, vasodilation and increased capillary permeability are required features of this response. Chemical mediators of this process are prostaglandins released from the damaged tissue and cytokines, which are produced in white blood cells and endothelial cells. Cytokines include interleukins, tissue necrosis

and visceral pain is typically localized by the brain's sensory cortex to an approximate spinal cord level that is determined by the embryologic origin of the involved organ. For example, pathology in midgut organs, such as the small bowel, appendix, and caecum, cause perceived periumbilical pain. In contrast, disease in hindgut organs, such as the colon and intraperitoneal portions of the genitourinary tract, cause midline pain in the suprapubic or hypogastric area (Gallagher, 2004).

factors, and interferons. These sensitizing mediators are released into affected tissues and lower the conduction threshold of nociceptors in these tissues. This is termed peripheral sensitization. Similarly, neurons within the spinal cord display increased excitability, termed central sensitization. As a result, within inflamed tissues, the perception of pain is increased relative to the strength of the external stimulus (Kehlet, 2006). As inflammation decreases and healing ensues, the increased sensitivity to stimuli and thus the perception of pain subsides.

Neuropathic Pain

In some individuals, sustained noxious stimuli can lead to persistent central sensitization and to a permanent loss of neuronal inhibition. As a result, a decreased threshold to painful stimuli remains despite resolution of the inciting stimuli (Butrick, 2003). This persistence characterizes neuropathic pain, which is felt to underlie many chronic pain syndromes. The concept of neuropathic pain helps explain in part why many with chronic pain have discomfort disproportionately greater to the amount of coexistent disease found. During central sensitization, neurons within spinal cord levels above or below those initially affected may eventually become involved. This phenomenon results in chronic pain that may be referred across several spinal cord levels.

Thus, in assessing patients with chronic pain, a clinician may find an ongoing inflammatory condition. In these cases, inflammatory pain dominates, and treatment is directed at resolving the underlying inflammatory condition. However, for many, evaluation may reveal no or minimal current pathology. In these cases, pain is neuropathic, and treatment thus focuses on management of pain symptoms.

ACUTE PAIN

Acute lower abdominal pain and pelvic pain are common complaints. The definition varies based on duration, but in general, discomfort is present less than 7 days. The sources of acute lower abdominal and pelvic pain are extensive, and a thorough history and physical examination can aid in narrowing the list (Table 11-1).

Diagnosis

A timely and accurate diagnosis is the goal and ensures the best medical outcome and prognosis for the patient. Accordingly, one should attempt to obtain a patient's history while performing the initial physical examination element, that of observing the patient. Her general appearance and specific physical and emotional attributes are noted. Although history and examination are described separately here, in the clinical setting they should be performed almost simultaneously for optimal results.

History

In addition to a thorough medical and surgical history, a verbal description of the pain and its associated factors is essential. For example, duration can be informative, and pain with abrupt onset may be more often associated with organ torsion, rup-

---

TABLE 11-1. Etiologies of Acute Lower Abdominal and Pelvic Pain

Gynecologic
Dysmenorrhea
Incomplete or complete abortion
Pelvic inflammatory disease
Ovarian torsion
Ectopic pregnancy
Tuboovarian abscess
Mittelschmerz
Ovarian mass
Prolapsing leiomyoma
Outflow tract obstruction

Gastrointestinal
Gastroenteritis
Colitis
Irritable bowel disease
Appendicitis
Diverticulitis
Inflammatory bowel disease
Constipation
Small bowel obstruction
Mesenteric ischemia
Gastrointestinal malignancy

Urologic
Cystitis
Pyelonephritis
Urinary tract stone
Perinephric abscess

Musculoskeletal
Hernia
Peritonitis
Abdominal wall trauma

Miscellaneous
Diabetic ketoacidosis
Herpes zoster
Opiate withdrawal
Hypercalcemia
Sickle cell crisis
Vasculitis
Abdominal aortic aneurysm rupture
Abdominal aortic aneurysm dissection
Porphyria
Heavy metal toxicity

---

ture, or ischemia. The nature of pain may add value. Patients with acute pathology involving pelvic viscera may describe *visceral pain* that is midline, diffuse, dull, achy, or cramping. They may repeatedly shift or roll to one side to find a comfortable position. One example is the diffuse midline periumbilical pain of early appendicitis.

The underlying pelvic pathology may extend from the viscera to cause inflammation of its adjacent parietal peritoneum.

In these cases, sharp *somatic pain* is found, which is localized, often unilateral, and focused to a specific corresponding dermatome. Again using appendicitis as an example, the classic migration of pain to the site of peritoneal irritation in the right lower quadrant illustrates acute somatic pain. In other instances, sharp, localized pain may not originate from the parietal peritoneum, but from pathology in specific muscles or in isolated areas of skin or subcutaneous tissues. In either instance, with somatic pain, patients classically rest motionless to avoid movement of the affected peritoneum, muscle, or skin.

Colicky pain may reflect bowel obstructed by adhesion, neoplasia, stool, or hernia. It may also result from increased bowel peristalsis in those with irritable or inflammatory bowel disease or infectious gastroenteritis. Alternatively, colic may follow forceful uterine contractions with the passage of products of conception, prolapsing submucous leiomyomas, or endometrial polyps. In addition, stones in the lower urinary tract may cause spasms of pain as they are passed.

Associated symptoms may also direct diagnosis. For example, absence of dysuria, hematuria, frequency, or urgency will exclude urinary pathology in most instances. Gynecologic causes are often associated with vaginal bleeding, vaginal discharge, dyspareunia, or amenorrhea. Alternatively, exclusion of diarrhea, constipation, or gastrointestinal (GI) bleeding lowers the probability of GI disease.

Vomiting complaints, however, are less informative, although the temporal relationship of vomiting to the pain may be helpful. In the acute surgical abdomen, if vomiting occurs, it usually follows as a response to pain and results from vagal stimulation. This vomiting is typically severe and develops without nausea. For example, nausea and vomiting have been found in approximately 75 percent of adnexal torsion cases (Descargues, 2001; Huchon, 2010). Therefore, the acute onset of unilateral pain that is severe and associated with a tender adnexal mass in a patient with nausea and vomiting should alert one to the increased probability of adnexal torsion. Conversely, if vomiting is noted prior to the onset of pain, a surgical abdomen is less likely (Miller, 2006).

In general, well-localized pain or tenderness, persisting for longer than 6 hours and unrelieved by analgesics, has an increased likelihood of acute peritoneal pathology.

Physical Examination

General Appearance.
Initial examination begins with observation of a patient while obtaining her history. A woman's general appearance, including facial expression, diaphoresis, pallor, and degree of agitation, often indicates the urgency of the clinical problem.

Vital Signs.
Elevated temperature, tachycardia, and hypotension should prompt an expedited evaluation, as the risk for intraabdominal pathology increases with their presence. Constant, low-grade fever is common in inflammatory conditions such as diverticulitis and appendicitis, and higher temperatures may be seen with pelvic inflammatory disease (PID), advanced peritonitis, or pyelonephritis.

Pulse and blood pressure evaluation should assess orthostatic changes if intravascular hypovolemia is suspected. A pulse increase of 30 beats per minute or a systolic blood pressure drop of 20 mm Hg or both, between lying and standing after 1 minute, is often reflective of hypovolemia. If noted, establishment of intravenous access and rehydration may be required prior to completion of the examination. However, certain neurologic disorders and medications, such as tricyclic antidepressants or antihypertensives, may also produce similar orthostatic blood pressure changes.

Abdominal Examination.
Visual inspection of the abdomen focuses on prior surgical scars, which may increase the possibility of bowel obstruction from postoperative adhesions or incisional hernia. Additionally, abdominal distension may be seen with bowel obstruction, perforation, or ascites. After inspection, auscultation of the abdomen may identify hyperactive or high-pitched bowel sounds characteristic of bowel obstruction. Hypoactive sounds, however, provide less diagnostic information.

Palpation of the abdomen should systematically explore each abdominal quadrant and begin away from the area of indicated pain. Peritoneal irritation is suggested by rebound tenderness or by abdominal rigidity due to involuntary guarding or reflex spasm of the abdominal muscles.

Pelvic Examination.
In general, pelvic examination should be performed in reproductive-aged women, as gynecologic pathology and complications of pregnancy are a common cause of pain in this age group. The decision to proceed with this examination in geriatric and pediatric patients may be based on clinical information.

Of findings, purulent vaginal discharge or cervicitis may reflect PID (Chap. 3, p. 93). Vaginal bleeding may stem from pregnancy complications, benign or malignant reproductive tract neoplasia, or acute vaginal trauma. Pregnancy, leiomyomas, and adenomyosis are common causes of uterine enlargement, and the former two may also create uterine softening. Cervical motion tenderness indicates peritoneal irritation and may be seen with PID, appendicitis, diverticulitis, and intraabdominal bleeding. A tender adnexal mass may reflect ectopic pregnancy, tuboovarian abscess, or ovarian cyst with torsion, hemorrhage, or rupture. Alternatively, a tender mass may be an abscess of nongynecologic origin such as one involving the appendix or colon diverticulum. Rectal examination can add information regarding the source and size of pelvic masses as well as the possibility of colorectal pathologies. Stool guaiac testing for occult blood, although less sensitive when not performed serially, is still warranted in many patients (Rockey, 2005). Those with complaints of rectal bleeding, painful defecation, or significant bowel habit changes are examples.

In emergency room settings, women with acute pain may experience waits between their initial assessment and subsequent testing. For these patients, recent literature supports early administration of analgesia. Fears that analgesia will mask patient symptoms and hinder accurate diagnosis have not been supported (McHale, 2001; Pace, 1996). Thus, barring significant hypotension or drug allergy, morphine sulfate may be administered judiciously in these situations.

Laboratory Testing

Despite benefits from a thorough history and physical examination, the sensitivity of these two in diagnosing the cause of abdominal pain is low (Gerhardt, 2005). Thus, laboratory and diagnostic testing are typically required. In women with acute abdominal pain, complications of pregnancy are common. Thus, either urine or serum β-hCG testing is recommended in those of reproductive age without a history of hysterectomy. Complete blood count (CBC) can aid in assessment of hemorrhage, both uterine and intraabdominal, and assess the possibility of infection. Urinalysis may be used to evaluate possible urolithiasis or cystitis. In addition, microscopic evaluation and culture of vaginal discharge can add support to clinically suspected cases of PID.

Radiologic Imaging

Sonography. In women with acute pelvic pain, several imaging options are available. However, transvaginal and transabdominal pelvic sonography are preferred modalities if an obstetric or gynecologic cause is suspected (Andreotti, 2009). Sonography provides a high sensitivity for detection of structural pelvic pathology. It is widely available, can usually be obtained quickly, requires little patient preparation, is relatively noninvasive, and avoids ionizing radiation. Disadvantageously, examination quality is affected by the skill and experience of the sonographer (Angle, 2010).

In most cases, the transvaginal approach offers superior resolution of the reproductive organs (Chap. 2, p. 38). Transabdominal sonography may still be necessary if the uterus or adnexal structures are significantly enlarged or if they lie beyond the transvaginal probe's field of view. Color Doppler imaging during sonography permits evaluation of the vascular characteristics of pelvic structures. In women with acute pain, the addition of Doppler studies is particularly useful if adnexal torsion or ectopic pregnancy is suspected (Twickler, 2010). Perforation of the uterine wall by an intrauterine device (IUD) and hematometra caused by menstrual outflow obstruction from müllerian agenesis anomalies are less common causes of acute pain. For determining IUD location, imaging müllerian abnormalities, and other indications, 3-dimensional (3-D) sonography has become invaluable (Bermejo, 2010; Moschos, 2011).

Conventional Radiography. Although the sensitivity is low for most gynecologic conditions, plain film radiographs may still useful when obstruction or perforation of the bowel is suspected (Leschka, 2007). Dilated loops of small bowel, air-fluid levels, the presence or absence of gas in the colon, or the finding of free air under the diaphragm are all significant findings when attempting to differentiate between a gynecologic and GI cause for acute pain.

Computed Tomography. Computed tomography (CT) and, more recently, multidetector computed tomography (MDCT) have been increasingly used to evaluate acute abdominal pain in adults. CT offers a global examination that can identify numerous abdominal and pelvic conditions, often with a high level of confidence (Hsu, 2005). Compared with other imaging tools, it has superior performance in identifying GI and urinary tract causes of acute pelvic and lower abdominal pain (Andreotti, 2009). Noncontrasted renal colic CT has largely replaced the conventional intravenous pyelogram looking for ureteral obstruction. The combination of both oral and intravenous contrast is preferred in the evaluation of GI abnormalities such as appendicitis.

CT has several advantages in addition to its high sensitivity for most nongynecologic disorders. It can be performed quickly; is not perturbed by gas, bone, or obesity; and is not operator-dependent. Disadvantages include the occasional lack of availability, high cost, inability to use contrast media in patients who are allergic or have renal dysfunction, and exposure to low levels of ionizing radiation (Leschka, 2007).

Currently, there is considerable ongoing debate regarding the safety and possible overuse of CT. Of major concern is the potential increase in cancer risk directly attributable to ionizing radiation, which is estimated to be even higher in younger patients and women (Einstein, 2007). Radiation doses from CT scans are generally considered to be 100 to 500 times those from conventional radiography (Smith-Bindman, 2010). Investigators in a large multicenter analysis found that the median effective radiation dose from a multiphase abdomen and pelvic CT scan was 31 mSv, and this correlates with a lifetime attributable risk of four cancers per 1000 patients (Smith-Bindman, 2009). By way of comparison, health care workers at risk of repeated radiation exposure are generally limited to 100 mSv over 5 years with a maximum of 50 mSv allowed in any given year (Fazel, 2009).

In the acute clinical setting, the benefits of CT imaging frequently outweigh these risks. One analysis conducted in the Netherlands found that the rate of false positive diagnoses of appendicitis among adults decreased from 24 to 3 percent from 1996 to 2006. They noted that this decrease correlated with the increased rate of CT use during the same interval (Raman, 2008). Appendiceal perforation rates also decreased from 18 to 5 percent. Considering that the false positive diagnosis of appendicitis in women has been found to be as high as 42 percent, this certainly represents improvement in clinical outcomes.

Magnetic Resonance (MR) Imaging. If available, MR imaging is becoming an important tool for women with acute pelvic pain if initial sonography is nondiagnostic. Common reasons for noninformative sonographic evaluations include patient obesity and pelvic anatomy distortion secondary to large leiomyomas, müllerian anomalies, or exophytic tumor growth.

As a first-line tool, MR imaging is often selected for pregnant patients, for whom ionizing radiation exposure should be limited. However, for most acute disorders, it provides little advantage over 3-D sonography or CT (Bermejo, 2010; Brown, 2005). Lack of availability can be a disadvantage after hours, on weekends, or in smaller hospitals and emergency departments (Brown, 2005).

Laparoscopy

Operative laparoscopy is the primary treatment for suspected appendicitis, adnexal torsion, or some ectopic pregnancies and for cases of ruptured ovarian cyst associated with symptomatic hemorrhage. Moreover, diagnostic laparoscopy may be useful if no pathology can be identified by conventional diagnostics. However, in stable patients with acute abdominal pain, noninvasive testing is typically fully exhausted before considering this approach (Sauerland, 2006).

Decision to Operate. The decision to perform a surgical procedure in the clinical setting of acute pelvic pain is not always an easy one. If the patient is clinically stable, the decision can be made in a timely manner, with appropriate evaluation and consultation. In a less stable patient with signs of peritoneal irritation, possible hemoperitoneum, organ torsion, shock, and/or impending sepsis, the decision to operate should be made

decisively unless there are overwhelming clinical contraindications to immediate surgery.

CHRONIC PAIN

Persistent pain may be visceral, somatic, or mixed in origin. As a result, it may take several forms in women and include: dysmenorrhea, dyspareunia, vulvodynia, chronic pelvic pain (CPP), musculoskeletal pain, intestinal cramping, or dysuria. The list of pathologies that may underlie these chronic pain symptoms is extensive and includes both psychological and organic disorders (Table 11-2). Moreover, pathology in one

TABLE 11-2. Sources of Chronic Pelvic Pain in Women

Gynecologic	Musculoskeletal
Endometriosis	Hernias
Adenomyosis	Muscular strain
Leiomyomas	Faulty posture
Intraabdominal adhesions	Myofascial pain
Ovarian mass	Levator ani syndrome
Adnexal mass	Fibromyositis
Reproductive tract cancer	Degenerative joint disease
Pelvic organ prolapse	Lumbar vertebrae compression
Pelvic muscle trigger points	Disk herniation or rupture
Intrauterine contraceptive device	Coccydynia
Endometrial or endocervical polyps	Spondylosis
Chronic ectopic pregnancy	
Ovarian retention syndrome	**Neurologic**
Ovarian remnant syndrome	Neurologic dysfunction
Postoperative peritoneal cysts	Abdominal cutaneous nerve entrapment
Chronic PID	Neuralgia of iliohypogastric, ilioinguinal, lateral femoral
Chronic endometritis	cutaneous, and/or genitofemoral nerves
Outflow tract obstruction	Pudendal neuralgia
Broad ligament herniation	Piriformis syndrome
Pelvic congestion syndrome	Spinal cord or sacral nerve tumor
Urologic	**Miscellaneous**
Chronic urinary tract infection	Psychiatric disorders
Detrusor dyssynergia	Physical or sexual abuse
Interstitial cystitis	Shingles
Radiation cystitis	
Urinary tract stone	
Urinary tract cancer	
Urethral diverticulum	
Gastrointestinal	
Irritable bowel syndrome	
Constipation	
Diverticular disease	
Colitis	
Inflammatory bowel disease	
GI tract cancer	
Celiac disease	
Chronic intermittent bowel obstruction	

GI = gastrointestinal; PID = pelvic inflammatory disease.

organ can commonly lead to dysfunction in adjacent systems. As a result, a woman with chronic pain may have more than one cause of pain and overlapping symptoms. Thus, a comprehensive evaluation of multiple organ systems and psychological state is essential for complete treatment.

Chronic Pelvic Pain

Chronic pelvic pain is a common gynecologic problem, and Mathias and colleagues (1996) estimated its prevalence in reproductive-aged women to be 15 percent. There is no universally accepted definition of chronic pelvic pain. However, many investigators distinguish it from dysmenorrhea and dyspareunia and define it as: (1) noncyclic pain that persists for 6 or more months; (2) pain that localizes to the anatomic pelvis, to the anterior abdominal wall at or below the umbilicus, or to the lumbosacral back or buttocks; and (3) pain that is of sufficient severity to cause functional disability or lead to medical intervention (American College of Obstetricians and Gynecologists, 2008).

Etiology

Causes of chronic pelvic pain fall within a broad spectrum, but endometriosis, symptomatic leiomyomas, and irritable bowel syndrome are commonly diagnosed. Importantly, endometriosis is a frequent cause of CPP, but it typically is also associated with cyclic symptoms. Diagnosis and treatment of pain related to this condition are discussed fully in Chapter 10 (p. 289). Evaluation and management of chronic pain secondary to leiomyomas is described in Chapter 9 (p. 250).

The pathophysiology of CPP is unclear in many patients and may have a significant association with neuropathic pain, described earlier (p. 306). Chronic pelvic pain shows increased association with irritable bowel syndrome, interstitial cystitis, and vulvodynia. These are also considered by many to be chronic visceral pain syndromes stemming from neuropathic pain (Janicki, 2003).

Diagnosis

History. More than with many other gynecologic complaints, a detailed history and physical examination are integral to diagnosis. A pelvic pain questionnaire can be used initially to obtain information. One example is available from the International Pelvic Pain Society and may be accessed at: http://www.pelvicpain.org/resources/handpform.aspx. Additionally, a body silhouette diagram can be provided to patients for them to mark specific sites of pain. One example is the McGill Pain Questionnaire and Short Form (MPQ, MPQ-SF), which combines a list of pain descriptors with a body map for patients to mark sites of pain. This can be accessed at http://www.npcrc.org/usr_doc/adhoc/painsymptom/McGill%20Pain%20Inventory.pdf (Melzack, 1987). At minimum, the series of questions found in Table 11-3 may provide valuable information.

In addition to questionnaires, pain scales can improve pain assessment, and several types are available (Herr, 2004). Of

TABLE 11-3. Questions Relevant to Chronic Pelvic Pain
What is the pain's quality, severity, and location?
When and how did your pain start, and how has it changed?
What makes your pain better or worse?
Other symptoms or health problems?
Do you have frequency, urgency, or bloody urine?
Do you have nausea or vomiting, diarrhea, constipation, or rectal bleeding?
Do you have pain with your periods?
Did your pain start initially as menstrual cramps?
Have you had surgery? What was the reason?
How many pregnancies have you had?
How did you deliver? Was there an episiotomy?
Current and prior birth control?
Prior sexually transmitted disease or pelvic infection?
Pain with deep penetration during intercourse?
Are you depressed or anxious?
Treated for mental illness in the past?
Have you been or are you now being abused physically or sexually?
Prior evaluations or treatments for your pain?
Have any previous treatments helped?
What medications are you taking now?
How has the pain affected your quality of life?
What do you believe or fear is causing your pain?

these, the Visual Analog Scale, Numerical Rating Scale, and the Verbal Descriptor Scale are shown in Figure 11-3.

Obstetric History. Pregnancy and delivery can be traumatic to neuromuscular structures and have been linked with pelvic organ prolapse, pelvic floor muscle myofascial pain syndromes, and symphyseal or sacroiliac joint pain. Paterson

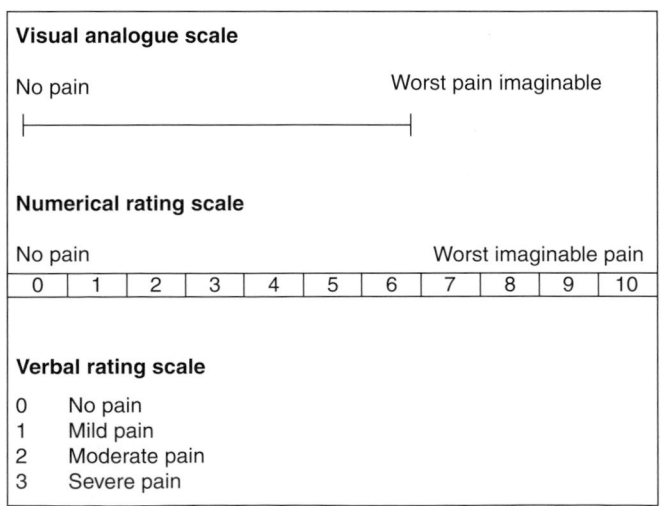

FIGURE 11-3 Rating scales for pain. The visual analogue, numerical, and verbal rating scales are shown.

(2009) reported that 9 percent of postpartum patients continue to experience genital and/or pelvic pain for more than 1 year after delivery. In addition, injury to the ilioinguinal or iliohypogastric nerves during Pfannenstiel incision for cesarean delivery may lead to lower abdominal wall pain even years after the initial injury (Whiteside, 2003). Following delivery, recurrent, cyclic pain and swelling in the vicinity of a cesarean incision or within an episiotomy suggests endometriosis within the scar itself (Fig. 10-5, p. 287). Alternatively, in a nulliparous woman with infertility, pain may stem from endometriosis, pelvic adhesions, or chronic pelvic inflammatory disease.

Surgical History. Prior abdominal surgery increases a woman's risk for pelvic adhesions, especially if infection, bleeding, or large areas of denuded peritoneal surfaces were involved. Adhesions were found in 40 percent of patients who underwent laparoscopy for chronic pelvic pain suspected to be of gynecologic origin (Sharma, 2011). The incidence of adhesions increases with the number of prior surgeries (Dubuisson, 2010). Lastly, certain disorders persist or commonly recur, and thus information regarding prior surgeries for endometriosis, adhesive disease, or malignancy should be sought.

Psychosocial History. There is a significant association between chronic pelvic pain and physical, emotional, or sexual abuse (American College of Obstetricians and Gynecologists, 2011; Jamieson, 1997; Lampe, 2000). A metaanalysis by Paras and associates (2009) demonstrated that sexual abuse is associated with an increased lifetime diagnosis rate of functional bowel disorders, fibromyalgia, psychogenic seizure disorder, and chronic pelvic pain. Additionally, for some women, chronic pain is an acceptable means to cope with social stresses. For these reasons, patients should be questioned regarding domestic violence and satisfaction with family relationships. Furthermore, an inventory of depressive symptoms is essential, as depression may cause or result from chronic pelvic pain (Table 13-5, p. 360).

Physical Examination. The etiology of chronic pain is varied, and information gathered from physical examination can often clarify the source and direct further testing. In a woman with chronic pain, even routine examination may be extremely painful. For example, in those with neuropathic pain, mere light touch may elicit pain. Therefore, examination should proceed slowly to allow relaxation between each step. Moreover, the patient should be reassured that she may ask for the examination to be halted at any time.

Terms used to describe examination findings include *allodynia* and *hyperesthesia,* among others. Allodynia is a painful response to a normally innocuous stimulus, such as a cotton swab. Hyperalgesia is an extreme response to a painful stimulus.

Stance and Gait. Women with intraperitoneal pathology may compensate with changes in posture. Such adjustments can create secondary musculoskeletal sources of pain (p. 324). Alternatively, musculoskeletal structures may be the site of referred pain from these organs (Table 11-4). Thus, careful observation of a woman's posture and gait is integral in the evaluation of chronic pelvic pain.

Initially, a woman is examined while standing. Posture should be evaluated anteriorly, posteriorly, and laterally. Posterior, inspection for scoliosis and horizontal stability of the shoulders, gluteal folds, and knee creases is performed. Asymmetry may reflect musculoskeletal disorders.

Lateral visual examination may reveal lordosis and concomitant kyphosis. This combination has been noted in some women with CPP and termed *typical pelvic pain posture* (TPPP) (Fig. 11-4) (Baker, 1993). Also, abnormal tilt of the pelvic bones can be assessed by simultaneously placing an open palm on each side between the posterior superior iliac spine (PSIS)

TABLE 11-4. Musculoskeletal Origins of Chronic Pelvic Pain

Structure	Innervation	Referred Pain Sites
Hip	T12–S1	Lower abdomen; anterior medial thigh; knee
Lumbar ligaments, facets/discs	T12–S1	Low back; posterior thigh and calf; lower abdomen; lateral trunk; buttock
Sacroiliac joints	L4–S3	Posterior thigh; buttock; pelvic floor
Abdominal muscles	T5–L1	Abdomen; anteromedial thigh; sternum
Pelvic and back muscles		
Iliopsoas	L1–L4	Lateral trunk; lower abdomen; low back; anterior thigh
Piriformis	L5–S3	Low back; buttock; pelvic floor
Pubococcygeus	S1–L4	Pelvic floor; vagina; rectum; buttock
Obturator internal/external	L3–S2	Pelvic floor; buttock; anterior thigh
Quadratus lumborum	T12–L3	Anterior lateral trunk; anterior thigh; lower abdomen

Modified from Baker, 1993, with permission.

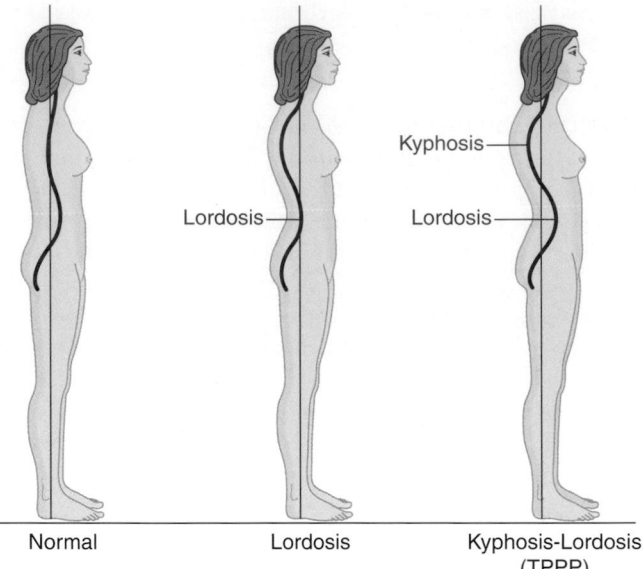

FIGURE 11-4 Concurrent lordosis and kyphosis are common postural changes associated with chronic pelvic pain. TPPP = typical pelvic pain posture. *(Redrawn from Howard, 2000, with permission.)*

and anterior superior iliac spine (ASIS). Normally, the ASIS lies one-quarter inch below the level of the PSIS, and greater distances may suggest abnormal tilt. Pelvic tilt may be associated with hip osteoarthritis and other orthopedic problems (Labelle, 2005; Yoshimoto, 2005).

Anterior inspection should focus on symmetry of the ASISs, umbilicus, and weight bearing. If one leg is dominant in weight bearing, the nonbearing leg is often externally rotated and slightly flexed at the knee. In addition to carriage, the anterior abdominal wall and inguinal areas should be inspected for hernias. Direct and indirect inguinal hernias and femoral hernias are often noted only when the woman is standing. Hernias that involve the anterior abdominal wall and pelvic floor are most commonly associated with CPP. Less frequently, *sciatic hernia,* which is herniation of peritoneum and peritoneal contents through the greater sciatic foramen, and *obturator hernia,* which is that through the obturator canal, have also been rarely described as sources of pain (Chang, 2005; Miklos, 1998; Moreno-Egea, 2006; Servant, 1998). Inspection of the perineum and vulva with the patient standing may identify varicosities. These are often asymptomatic or may cause superficial discomfort. Such varicosities may also coexist with internal pelvic varicosities. These internal varicosities can create a deep pelvic ache and are the underlying cause of pelvic congestion syndrome (p. 317).

Any observed limitation in mobility may also be informative. A patient should be asked to bend forward at the waist. Limitation in forward flexion may reflect primary orthopedic disease or adaptive shortening of back extensor muscles. This shortening is seen frequently in women with chronic pain and TPPP (Fig. 11-5). In such cases, patients are unable to create a normal convex curve with this motion.

Muscle weakness may also indicate orthopedic disease. A Trendelenburg test, in which a patient is asked to balance on one foot, can indicate dysfunction of hip abductor muscles or hip joint. With a positive test, when a woman elevates a leg by flexing the hip, the ipsilateral iliac crest droops.

Gait may also be evaluated by having the patient walk across the room. An *antalgic gait,* known as a limp, refers to a posture or gait that minimizes weight bearing on a lower limb or joint and indicates a higher probability of musculoskeletal pain.

Supine. The anterior abdominal wall should be evaluated for abdominal scars. These may be sites of hernia or nerve entrapment or may indicate a risk for intraabdominal adhesive disease. Auscultation for bowel sounds and bruits should follow. Increased bowel activity may reflect irritable or inflammatory bowel diseases. Bruits should prompt investigation for vascular pathology.

While supine, a woman is asked to demonstrate with one finger the point of maximal pain and then encircle the total surrounding area of involvement. Superficial palpation of the anterior abdominal wall by a clinician may reveal sites of tenderness or knotted muscle that may reflect nerve entrapment or myofascial pain syndrome (p. 324). Moreover, pain with elevation of the head and shoulders while tensing the abdominal wall muscles, *Carnett sign,* is typical of anterior abdominal wall pathology. Conversely, if the source of pain originates from inside the abdominal cavity, discomfort usually decreases with such elevation (Thomson, 1991). Moreover, Valsalva maneuver during head and shoulder elevation may display diastasis of the rectus abdominis muscle or hernias. Diastasis recti can be differentiated in most cases from a ventral hernia. With diastasis, the borders of the rectus abdominis muscle can be palpated bilaterally along the entire length of the protrusion. Deep palpation of the lower abdomen may identify pathology originating from pelvic viscera. Dullness to percussion or a shifting fluid wave may reflect ascites.

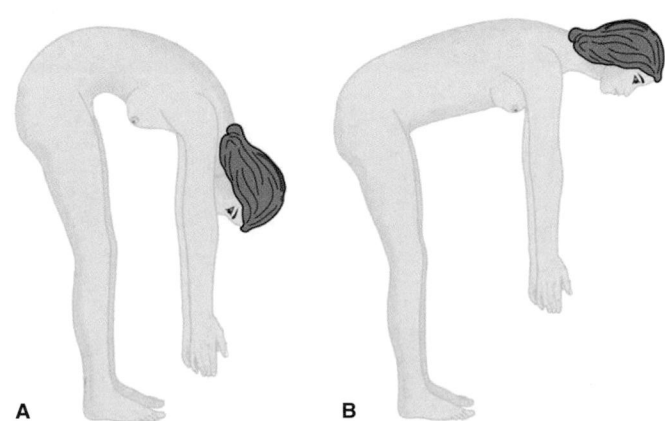

FIGURE 11-5 Mobility testing. **A.** Normal flexion of the lower back. **B.** Limited flexion may be seen in those with orthopedic disease or in those with chronic pelvic pain. *(From Baker, 1998, with permission.)*

Tests of mobility may give additional information. In most cases, a woman can elevate her leg 80 degrees from the horizontal toward her head, termed a *straight leg test*. Pain with leg elevation may be seen with lumbar disc, hip joint, or myofascial pain syndromes. Additionally, symphyseal pain with this test may indicate laxity in the symphysis pubis or pelvic girdle. Both the obturator and iliopsoas tests may indicate myofascial pain syndromes involving these muscles or disorders of the hip joint. With the obturator test, a supine patient brings one knee into 90 degrees of flexion while the foot remains planted. The ankle is immobilized, and the knee is gently pulled laterally and then medially to assess for tenderness. With the iliopsoas test, a supine woman attempts to flex each hip separately against resistance from the examiner's hand. If pain is described with flexion, the test result is positive.

Sitting. A patient's posture in the sitting position should be inspected. Myofascial pain syndromes involving pelvic floor muscles often lead patients to shift weight to one buttock or to sit toward a chair's front edge.

Lithotomy. Pelvic examination should begin with inspection of the vulva for generalized changes and localized lesions as outlined in Chapter 4 (p. 111). Specifically, erythema may reflect vulvitis or chronic fungal infection. Alternatively, thinning of vulvar skin may result from lichen sclerosus or atrophic changes. The vestibular area should be carefully inspected next. One or more focal areas of redness involving the vestibular gland openings, associated with exquisite tenderness to palpation, indicate vulvar vestibulitis.

After inspection, systematic pressure point palpation of the vulva is completed with a small cotton swab to map areas of pain (Fig. 4-1, p. 112). Palpation of the vagina ideally begins with one finger, which is gradually inserted 3 to 4 cm. Systematic sweeping pressure against the pelvic floor muscles along their length may identify isolated knots of taut muscle in those with myofascial pain syndrome of the pelvic floor. Typically, the pubococcygeus, iliococcygeus, and obturator internus muscles can be reached with a vaginal finger (Fig. 11-6). Additionally, tenderness of the urethra and bladder are potential indicators of urethral diverticulum or interstitial cystitis, respectively. Pain with deep palpation of the vaginal fornices may be seen with endometriosis, and cervical motion tenderness may be noted with acute and chronic PID. If pain follows gentle movement of the coccyx, then articular disease of the coccyx, termed *coccydynia,* is suspected.

Assessment of the uterus may reveal an enlarged uterus, often with an irregular contour, due to leiomyomas. Globular enlargement with softening is more typical of adenomyosis. Immobility of the uterus may follow scarring from endometriosis, PID, malignancy, or adhesive disease from prior surgeries. Evaluation of the adnexa may reveal tenderness or mass. Such lateral tenderness may reflect endometriosis, diverticular disease, or pelvic congestion syndrome.

Rectal examination and rectovaginal palpation of the rectovaginal septum should be included. Palpation of hard stool or hemorrhoids may indicate GI disorders, whereas nodularity of the rectovaginal septum may be found with endometriosis or neoplasia. Myofascial tenderness involving the puborectalis and coccygeus muscles may be noted by sweeping the index finger with pressure across these muscles (see Fig. 11-6). Lastly, stool testing for occult blood may be performed during digital rectal examination at the initial visit. Alternatively, home test kits for occult blood are available at most pharmacies and at many physicians' offices.

Testing
Laboratory Evaluation. For women with chronic pelvic pain, diagnostic testing may add valuable information. Results from urinalysis and urine culture may indicate urinary tract stones, urinary tract malignancy, or recurrent infection as sources of pain. Thyroid disease can affect physiologic functioning and may be found in those with bowel or bladder symptoms. Thus, serum thyroid-stimulating hormone (TSH) levels are commonly assayed. Diabetes can lead to neuropathy, and screening may be completed with urinalysis or serum evaluation.

Radiologic Imaging and Endoscopy. These modalities may be informative, and of these, transvaginal sonography is widely used by gynecologists to evaluate chronic pelvic pain. Sonography of the pelvic organs may reveal endometriomas, leiomyomas, ovarian cysts, dilated pelvic veins, and other structural lesions. However, despite its applicability for many gynecologic disorders, sonography has poor sensitivity in identifying endometriotic implants or most adhesions. Similarly, CT or MR imaging may be used, but often adds little additional information to that obtained with sonography.

In those with bowel symptoms, barium enema may indicate internal or external obstructive lesions, malignancy, and diverticular or inflammatory bowel disease. However, flexible sigmoidoscopy and colonoscopy may offer more information because colonic mucosa can be directly inspected and biopsied if necessary. In those in whom pelvic congestion syndrome is suspected, the use of transvaginal color Doppler ultrasound, CT, and MR imaging have all been reported, however, pelvic venography is considered the primary tool. This technique requires cannulation of the femoral vein to access the internal iliac vessels for contrast injection (p. 318).

Cystoscopy, laparoscopy, flexible sigmoidoscopy, and colonoscopy may each be employed, and patient symptoms will dictate their use. In those with symptoms of chronic pain and urinary symptoms, cystoscopy is typically advised. If GI complaints are dominant, then flexible sigmoidoscopy or colonoscopy may be warranted. For many women with no obvious cause of their CPP, laparoscopy is often performed. Approximately 40 percent of all gynecologic laparoscopies are performed for this indication (Howard, 1993). Importantly, intraoperative explanations for CPP are commonly found in those with normal preoperative examinations (Cunanan, 1983; Kang, 2007). Laparoscopy allows direct identification and in many cases, treatment of intraabdominal pathology. Therefore, laparoscopy is considered by many to be the gold standard for evaluation of chronic pelvic pain (Sharma, 2011).

One laparoscopic approach to CPP is performed under local anesthesia with the patient conscious and available for questioning regarding sites of pain (Howard, 2000; Swanton, 2006). Termed *conscious pain mapping,* this technique has resulted

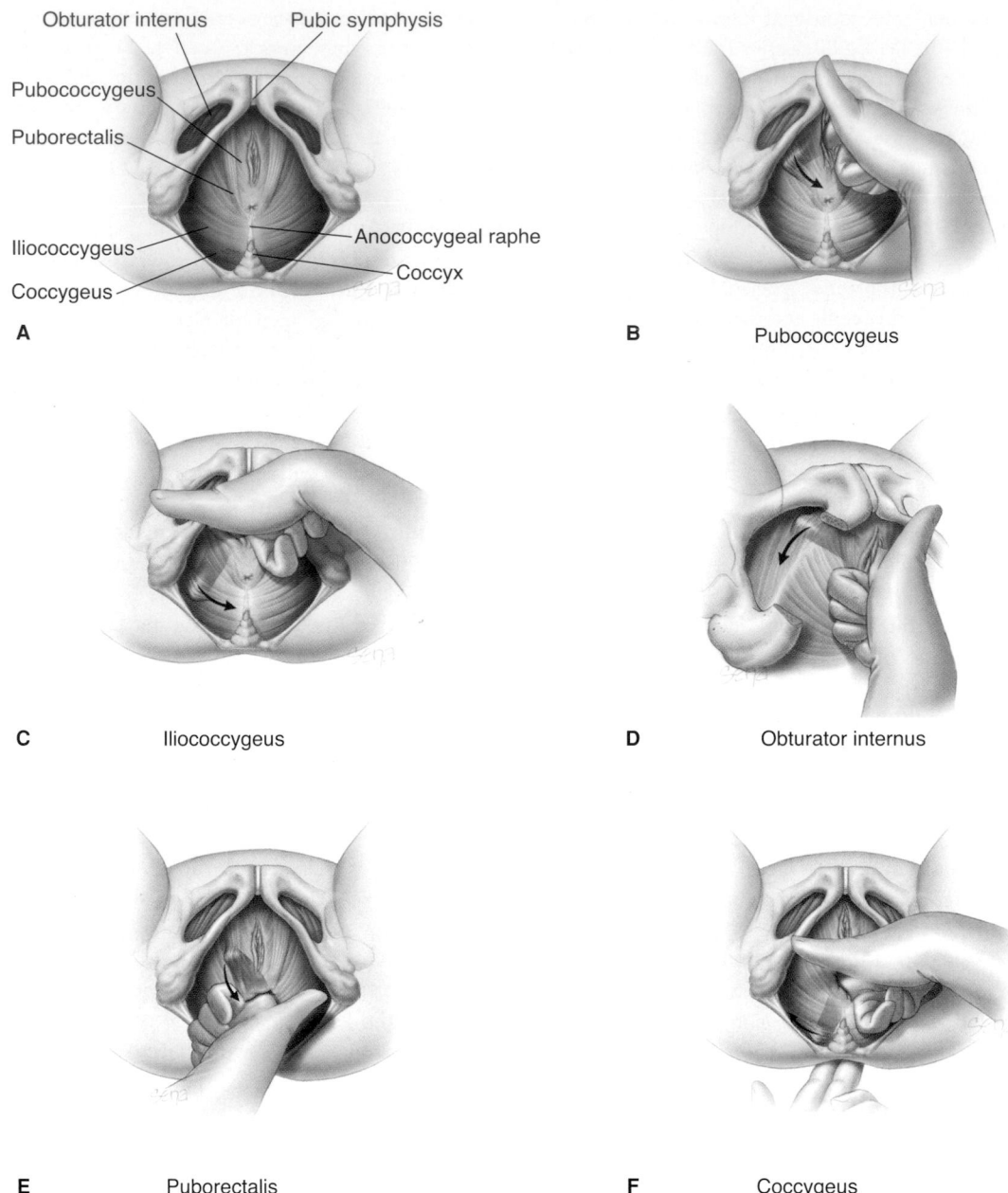

FIGURE 11-6 Pelvic floor muscle examination. *(Images contributed by Ms. Marie Sena.)*

in more targeted treatment and improved postoperative pain scores. However, its clinical use to date has been limited.

Treatment

In many women with CPP, an identifying source is found, and treatment is dictated by the diagnosis. However, in other cases, pathology may not be identified, and treatment is directed toward dominant symptoms.

Analgesics. Treatment of pain typically begins with oral analgesics such as acetaminophen or nonsteroidal antiinflammatory drugs (NSAIDs) (Table 10-2, p. 293). Acetaminophen is a widely used and effective analgesic despite having no significant antiinflammatory properties. Alternatively, NSAIDs are particularly helpful if inflammatory states underlie the pain.

If satisfactory relief is not achieved, then a mild opioid such as codeine, propoxyphene, or hydrocodone may be added to this regimen (Table 39-12, p. 965). Opioids are most effective and least addictive if given on a scheduled basis and at doses that adequately relieve pain. If pain persists, stronger opioids such as morphine, methadone, fentanyl, oxycodone, and hydromorphone can replace milder ones. Close and regular surveillance is essential (Gunter, 2003). An alternative to classic opioids is tramadol hydrochloride, which in addition to its mild central opioid effect also inhibits serotonin and norepinephrine reuptake.

Hormonal Suppression. Endometriosis is a common disorder found in women with CPP and is estrogen-dependent. Thus, hormonal suppression may be considered, especially in those with coexistent dysmenorrhea or dyspareunia and who lack dominant bladder or bowel symptoms. As discussed in Chapter 10 (p. 292), combination oral contraceptives, progestins, gonadotropin-releasing hormone (GnRH) agonists, and certain androgens have proved effective.

Antidepressants and Anticonvulsants. For many, CPP represents neuropathic pain, and therapy has been extrapolated from treatment of such pain in other disorders. Tricyclic antidepressants have repeatedly been shown to reduce neuropathic pain independent of their antidepressant effects (Saarto, 2005). Moreover, antidepressants are a logical choice, as clinically significant depression is commonly comorbid with pain. Amitriptyline (Elavil) and its metabolite nortriptyline (Pamelor) have the best documented efficacy in the treatment of neuropathic and nonneuropathic pain syndromes (Table 11-5) (Bryson, 1996). Selective serotonin-reuptake inhibitors do not

TABLE 11-5. Antidepressants and Antiepileptic Drugs Used in Chronic Pain Syndromes

Drug (Brand name)	Dosage	Side Effects
Antidepressants		
Tricyclic antidepressants		Dry mouth, constipation, urinary retention, sedation, weight gain
Amitriptyline (Elavil)[a] Imipramine (Tofranil)[a]	For both, 10–25 mg at bedtime; increase by 10–25 mg per week up to 75–150 mg at bedtime or a therapeutic drug level	Tertiary amines have greater anticholinergic side effects
Desipramine (Norpramin)[a] Nortriptyline (Pamelor)[a]	For both, 25 mg in the morning or at bedtime; increase by 25 mg per week up to 150 mg per day or a therapeutic drug level	Secondary amines have fewer anticholinergic side effects
Selective Serotonin-Reuptake Inhibitors		
Fluoxetine (Prozac)[a] Paroxetine (Paxil)[a]	For both, 10–20 mg per day; up to 80 mg per day for fibromyalgia	Nausea, sedation, decreased libido, sexual dysfunction, headache, weight gain
Novel Antidepressants		
Bupropion (Wellbutrin)[a]	100 mg per day; increase by 100 mg per week up to 200 mg twice daily (400 mg per day)	Anxiety, insomnia or sedation, weight loss, seizures (at dosages above 450 mg per day)
Venlafaxine (Effexor)[a]	37.5 mg per day; increase by 37.5 mg per week up to 300 mg per day	Headache, nausea, sweating, sedation, hypertension, seizures Serotoninergic properties in dosages below 150 mg per day; mixed serotoninergic and noradrenergic properties in dosages above 150 mg per day
Antiepileptic Drugs		
First-generation agents		
Carbamazepine (Tegretol)	200 mg per day; increase by 200 mg per week up to 400 mg three times daily (1200 mg per day)	Dizziness, diplopia, nausea, aplastic anemia
Phenytoin (Dilantin)[a]	100 mg at bedtime; increase weekly up to 500 mg at bedtime	Blood dyscrasias, hepatotoxicity
Second-generation agents		
Gabapentin (Neurontin)	100–300 mg at bedtime; increase by 100 mg every 3 days up to 1800 to 3600 mg per day taken in divided doses three times daily	Drowsiness, dizziness, fatigue, nausea, sedation, weight gain
Pregabalin (Lyrica)	150 mg at bedtime for diabetic neuropathy; 300 mg twice daily for postherpetic neuralgia	Drowsiness, dizziness, fatigue, nausea, sedation, weight gain
Lamotrigine (Lamictal)[a]	50 mg per day; increase by 50 mg every 2 weeks up to 400 mg per day	Dizziness, constipation, nausea; rarely, life-threatening rashes

[a]Not approved by the U.S. Food and Drug Administration for treatment of neuropathic pain.
Abbreviated from Maizels, 2005, with permission.

appear to be as effective as tricyclic antidepressants (Gilron, 2006).

In addition to antidepressants, anticonvulsants have also been used effectively in treatment of CPP. Of these, gabapentin and carbamazepine are most commonly used to reduce neuropathic pain (Wiffen, 2005a,b).

Polypharmacy. Combining drugs with different sites or mechanisms of action may often improve pain. For example, an NSAID and an opioid may be partnered, especially in conditions in which inflammation is dominant. If muscle spasm underlies pain, then pairing a tranquilizer or a muscle relaxant with an opioid or with an NSAID may improve results (Howard, 2003).

Surgery

Neurolysis. Nerve destruction, termed *neurolysis,* involves nerve transection or injection of a neurotoxic chemical. Nerve transection cuts a specific peripheral nerve or may be performed on an entire nerve plexus.

Presacral neurectomy (PSN) describes interruption of somatic pain fibers from the uterus that course within the superior hypogastric plexus (Fig. 38-13, p. 929). This procedure is performed by incising the pelvic peritoneum over the sacrum and then identifying and transecting the sacral nerve plexus. In women so treated, approximately 75 percent note a greater than 50 percent decline in pain (American College of Obstetricians and Gynecologists, 2008).

However, presacral neurectomy is technically challenging and requires familiarity with operating in the presacral space. Surgery has been associated with long-term constipation and urinary retention postoperatively. Infrequently, life-threatening hemorrhage may be encountered from the middle sacral vessels, which run in the presacral space.

Alternatively, laparoscopic uterine nerve ablation (LUNA) involves the destruction of the uterine nerve fibers that pass to the uterus with the uterosacral ligament. During LUNA, most surgeons destroy approximately 2 cm of uterosacral ligament near its attachment to the uterus (Lifford, 2002). Based on pelvic innervation, these surgeries are indicated only for treatment of centrally located pelvic pain and have been performed to treat refractory endometriosis-related CPP and dysmenorrhea. However, in one trial, almost 500 women with CPP were randomly assigned to laparoscopy and intraoperative treatment of identified pathology or to a combination of laparoscopy, treatment, and LUNA. The addition of LUNA did not improve pain scores (Daniels, 2009). Moreover, comparisons of LUNA and presacral neurectomy show significantly greater long-term pain relief with presacral neurectomy (Proctor, 2005).

Hysterectomy. When thorough evaluation excludes an organic cause and conservative medical therapy has failed, a total hysterectomy and bilateral salpingo-oophorectomy is considered definitive management. For many women with CPP, hysterectomy is effective in resolving pain and improving quality of life (Kjerulff, 2000; Stovall, 1990). However, for others, hysterectomy may fail to relieve CPP. This result may follow more commonly in those who are younger than 30 years, those who have mental illness, or those with no identifiable pelvic

pathology (Gunter, 2003). Almost 40 percent of women with no identified pelvic pathology will have persistent pain after hysterectomy (Hillis, 1995).

Specific Causes of Chronic Pelvic Pain

As noted earlier, endometriosis and leiomyomas are common causes of CPP and are discussed in detail in Chapters 9 and 10. Additional potential gynecologic sources of chronic pain include pelvic adhesive disease, ovarian remnant syndrome, and pelvic congestion syndrome.

Pelvic Adhesions. Adhesions are fibrous connections between opposing organ surfaces or between an organ and abdominal wall, at sites where there should be no connection. They vary in vascularity and thickness. Adnexal adhesions may be classified according to a system developed by the American Society for Reproductive Medicine (Table 11-6) (American Fertility Society, 1988).

Adhesions are common, and in laparoscopies performed for CPP, they are found in approximately one quarter of cases (Howard, 1993). However, not all adhesive disease creates pain. For example, Thornton and associates (1997) found no relationship between pelvic pain and women with intraabdominal adhesions.

Pathophysiology. The relationship between chronic pelvic pain and adhesions is incompletely understood. In those with CPP, intraperitoneal adhesions are believed to cause pain when they distort normal anatomy or when movement stretches the peritoneum or organ serosa. This theory is supported by studies using conscious pain mapping. Filmy adhesions that allowed significant movement between two structures had

TABLE 11-6. Adnexal Adhesion Scoring System				
Adhesions		**<1/3 Enclosure**	**1/3 to 2/3 Enclosure**	**>2/3 Enclosure**
Ovary R	Filmy	1	2	4
	Dense	4	8	16
L	Filmy	1	2	4
	Dense	4	8	16
Tube R	Filmy	1	2	4
	Dense	4[a]	8[a]	16
L	Filmy	1	2	4
	Dense	4[a]	8[a]	16

[a]If the fimbriated end of the fallopian tube is completely enclosed, change the point assignment to 16.
Scores 0 to 5 reflect minimal disease; those from 6 to 10 indicate mild disease; those from 11 to 20 signify moderate disease; and those from 21 to 32 reflect severe disease.
L = left; R = right.
From The American Fertility Society, 1988, with permission.

the highest association with pain, whereas adhesions that prohibited movement had the lowest pain scores. Moreover, adhesions that had a relationship to the peritoneum had a high association with pain (Demco, 2004). Sensory nerve fibers have been identified histologically, ultrastructurally, and immunohistochemically in human peritoneal adhesions obtained at laparotomy, lending additional support to these theories (Suleiman, 2001).

Diagnosis. Risks for adhesions include prior surgery, prior intraabdominal infection, and endometriosis. Less commonly, inflammation from radiation, chemical irritation, or foreign-body reaction may be causes. Pain is typically aggravated by sudden movement, intercourse, or other specific activities.

Laparoscopy is the primary tool used to diagnose adhesions. In general, sonography lacks sensitivity. However, Guerriero and coworkers (1997) noted a positive correlation with ovarian adhesions if the ovarian surface borders appeared blurred. Also, adhesions were suspected if the ovary appeared immediately adjacent to the uterus and if this position persisted despite manipulation of these organs with the sonography transducer.

Treatment. Surgical lysis is often used to treat pain symptoms, and a number of observational studies have shown pain improvement (Fayez, 1994; Steege, 1991; Sutton, 1990). However, two randomized studies comparing adhesion lysis with expectant management found no difference in pain scores after 1 year (Peters, 1992; Swank, 2003). Others who support the continued judicious use of adhesiolysis in the treatment of pelvic pain question the statistical methods used in these studies (Roman, 2009). When performed, adhesiolysis is associated with a significant risk of adhesiogenesis, especially in cases involving endometriosis (Parker, 2005). Thus, the decision to lyse adhesions should be individualized, and if lysis is performed, steps should be taken to minimize reformation (Hammoud, 2004). Gentle tissue handling, adequate hemostasis, and adhesion barriers have all been shown to be helpful (American Society for Reproductive Medicine, 2008).

Ovarian Remnant Syndrome and Ovarian Retention Syndrome.

Following oophorectomy, remnants of an excised ovary may create symptoms that are termed *ovarian remnant syndrome*. Distinction is made between this syndrome and ovarian retention syndrome, also known as residual ovary syndrome. *Ovarian retention syndrome* involves symptoms stemming from an ovary intentionally left at the time of previous gynecologic surgery (El Minawi, 1999). Although differentiated by the amount of ovarian tissue involved, both syndromes have nearly identical symptoms and are diagnosed and treated similarly.

Although an uncommon cause of CPP, women with symptomatic ovarian remnants most typically complain of chronic or cyclic pain or dyspareunia. The onset of symptoms is variable and may begin years following surgery (Nezhat, 2005).

Women with these syndromes may have a pelvic mass palpable on bimanual examination (Orford, 1996). Sonography is informative in many cases. In those with ovarian remnants, ovaries may be identified in some cases by a thin rim of ovarian cortex surrounding a coexistent ovarian cyst (Fleischer, 1998).

Indeterminate cases may require CT or MR imaging. In cases where ureteral compression is suspected, intravenous pyelography may be warranted. Laboratory testing, specifically follicle-stimulating hormone (FSH) levels in reproductive-aged women with a history of a bilateral oophorectomy, may be helpful. Levels in premenopausal range are suggestive of retained functioning ovarian tissue (Magtibay, 2005).

Although medical treatment has included hormonal manipulation to suppress functioning tissue, surgical excision is required in many symptomatic cases (Lafferty, 1996). Because the ureter is commonly intimately involved with adhesions encasing a remnant, laparotomy is warranted in many cases. However, in those with advanced laparoscopic skills, successful outcomes can be achieved (Nezhat, 2000, 2005).

Pelvic Congestion Syndrome.

Retrograde blood flow through incompetent valves can often create tortuous, congested ovarian or pelvic veins. Chronic pelvic ache, pressure, and heaviness may result and is termed *pelvic congestion syndrome* (Beard, 1988).

Pathophysiology. Currently, it is not clear whether congestion results from mechanical dilatation, ovarian hormonal dysfunction, or both. Higher rates of ovarian varicosities and pelvic congestion syndrome are noted in parous women. A mechanical theory describes a dramatic increase in pelvic vein diameter during late pregnancy that leads to ovarian vein valve incompetence and pelvic varicosities. Additionally, estrogen has been implicated in pelvic congestion syndrome in that estrogen acts as a venous dilator. Moreover, pelvic congestion syndrome resolves following menopause, and antiestrogenic medical therapy has been shown to be effective in these cases (Farquhar, 1989; Gangar, 1993). Most likely, both factors play roles. The cause of pain with pelvic congestion remains unclear, but increased dilatation, concomitant stasis, and release of local nociceptive mediators have been suggested (Giacchetto, 1989; Soysal, 2001).

Diagnosis. Affected women may describe pelvic ache or heaviness that may worsen premenstrually, after prolonged sitting or standing, or following intercourse. During bimanual examination, tenderness at the junction of the outer and middle thirds of a line drawn between the symphysis and anterior superior iliac spine or direct ovarian tenderness may be found. In addition, varicosities in the thigh, buttocks, perineum, or vagina may be associated (Venbrux, 1999).

The left ovarian venous plexus drains into the left ovarian vein, which empties into the left renal vein. The right ovarian vein generally drains directly into the inferior vena cava. Both ovarian veins may have numerous trunks (Fig. 11-7). Pelvic venography of this vascular anatomy is a primary diagnostic tool in women suspected of pelvic congestion syndrome, and embolization can be concurrently performed in identified candidates. Alternatively, CT, MR imaging, sonography, and diagnostic laparoscopy can identify varicosities. However, because these modalities are performed while a woman is prone, some varicosities decompress in this position and may be missed (Park, 2004; Umeoka, 2004).

Treatment. Treatments for pelvic congestion syndrome have included chronic progestin or GnRH agonist administration,

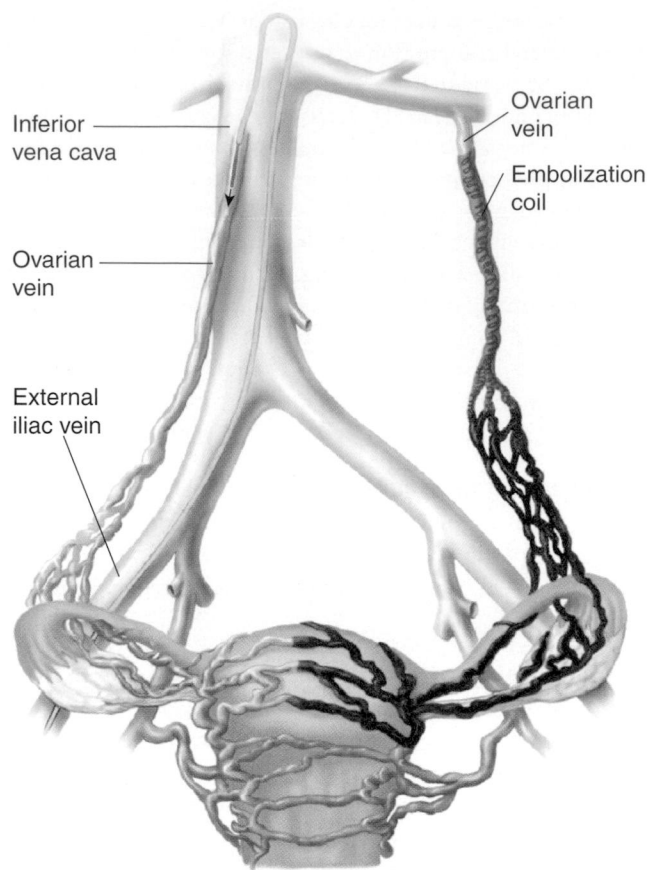

Inferior
vena cava

Ovarian
vein

Embolization
coil

Ovarian
vein

External
iliac vein

FIGURE 11-7 On the image's right, pelvic varices have already been treated with sclerosant and coils in the left ovarian vein. On the image's left, a guiding catheter is threaded into the right ovarian vein to perform ovarian venography and embolization. *(From Kim, 2006, with permission.)*

ovarian vein embolization or ligation, and hysterectomy with bilateral salpingo-oophorectomy (BSO), although none is definitive. For example, Beard and colleagues (1991) found that almost one third of women had some residual pain following total hysterectomy with BSO for this condition.

Embolization appears to afford effective treatment, and percentages of women with pain improvement range from 65 to 95 percent (Kim, 2006; Maleux, 2000; Venbrux, 2002). Ovarian vein sclerotherapy provided symptomatic relief at 1 year in 17 of 20 patients who were treated (Tropeano, 2008). Chung and coworkers (2003) compared embolization against hysterectomy and oophorectomy and found embolization more effective. Long-term studies on its effects past 1 year, however, are lacking.

Alternatively, medical treatment with GnRH agonists or with medroxyprogesterone acetate, 30 mg orally daily, has been shown to be effective for some women with pelvic congestion syndrome, although symptoms typically recur after medication is discontinued (Reginald, 1989).

Dysmenorrhea

Cyclic pain with menstruation is common and accompanies most menses (Balbi, 2000; Weissman, 2004). This pain is classically described as cramping and is often accompanied by low backache, nausea and vomiting, headache, or diarrhea.

The term *primary dysmenorrhea* describes cyclic menstrual pain without an identifiable associated pathology, whereas *secondary dysmenorrhea* frequently complicates endometriosis, leiomyomas, PID, adenomyosis, endometrial polyps, and menstrual outlet obstruction. For this reason, secondary dysmenorrhea may be associated with other gynecologic symptoms, such as dyspareunia, dysuria, abnormal bleeding, or infertility.

Compared with secondary dysmenorrhea, primary dysmenorrhea more commonly begins shortly after menarche. Pain characteristics, however, typically fail to differentiate between the two types, and primary dysmenorrhea is usually diagnosed following exclusion of known associated causes.

Risks for Primary Dysmenorrhea

When other factors are removed, primary dysmenorrhea equally affects women regardless of race and socioeconomic status. However, increased pain duration or severity is positively associated with earlier age at menarche, long menstrual periods, smoking, and increased body mass index (BMI). In contrast, parity appears to improve symptoms (Harlow, 1996; Sundell, 1990).

Pathophysiology

During endometrial sloughing, endometrial cells release prostaglandins as menstruation begins. Prostaglandins stimulate myometrial contractions and incite ischemia. Women with more severe dysmenorrhea have higher levels of prostaglandins in menstrual fluid, and these levels are highest during the first 2 days of menstruation. Prostaglandins are also implicated in secondary dysmenorrhea. However, anatomic mechanisms can also be identified, depending on the type of accompanying pelvic disease.

Diagnosis

In women with menstrual cramps and no other associated findings or symptoms, no additional evaluation may be initially required once pregnancy is excluded, and empiric therapy may be prescribed (Proctor, 2006). In women at risk for PID, cultures for *Chlamydia trachomatis* and *Neisseria gonorrhoeae* are indicated. Moreover, if pelvic evaluation is incomplete due to body habitus, then transvaginal sonography may be informative to exclude structural pelvic pathology.

Treatment

Nonsteroidal Antiinflammatory Drugs. Because prostaglandins have been implicated in the genesis of dysmenorrhea, administration of NSAIDs is logical, and studies support their use (Marjoribanks, 2003; Zhang, 1998). These drugs and their dosages are found in Table 10-2 (p. 293).

Steroid Hormone Contraception. Combination hormone birth control methods are believed to improve dysmenorrhea by lowering prostaglandin production, and observational studies of combination oral contraceptives (COCs) have noted improved dysmenorrhea in users (Brill, 1991; Gauthier, 1992; Hendrix, 2002; Milsom, 1990). In addition, extended or continuous administration of COCs may be useful in women with pain not controlled with traditional pill use (Chap. 5, p. 153) (Sulak, 1997).

Progestin-only contraceptives are also used to effectively treat dysmenorrhea. The levonorgestrel-releasing intrauterine system (LNG-IUS), depot medroxyprogesterone acetate injection, and progestin-releasing implanted rods have been shown to be effective in improving dysmenorrhea (Chap. 5, pp. 137 and 157) (Baldaszti, 2003; Varma, 2006).

Gonadotropin-Releasing Hormone Agonists and Androgens. The estrogen-lowering effects of these agents lead to endometrial atrophy and diminished prostaglandin production. Although gonadotropin-releasing hormone agonists and androgens such as danazol have been shown to be effective in treating dysmenorrhea, their substantial side effects preclude their routine and long-term use. A fuller discussion and list of dosages for these agents and their side effects can be found in Chapter 9 (p. 254).

Complementary and Alternative Medicine. Diet changes, herbal medicine, and physical treatments have each been sparsely evaluated in the treatment of dysmenorrhea. Oral vitamins E and B_1 (thiamine), magnesium, fish oil, low-fat diet, and the herb Toki-shakuyaku-san have all been shown to improve dysmenorrhea. However, evidence derives from small and typically nonrandomized trials (Barnard, 2000; Gokhale, 1996; Harel, 1996; Wilson, 2001; Ziaei, 2001). Additionally, data are limited but positive toward the use of exercise, topical heat, acupuncture, and transcutaneous electrical nerve stimulation (TENS) (Akin, 2001, 2004; Fugh-Berman, 2003; Golub, 1968; Helms, 1987; Kaplan, 1994).

Surgery. Cases of dysmenorrhea refractory to conservative management are unusual, and in such instances, surgery may be indicated. Hysterectomy is effective in treating dysmenorrhea, but may be unwanted in those desiring future fertility. For these women, presacral neurectomy or LUNA may be indicated.

Dyspareunia

Dyspareunia is a frequent gynecologic complaint. In reproductive-aged U.S. women, the 12-month prevalence is 15 to 20 percent (Glatt, 1990; Laumann, 1999). Painful intercourse may be associated with vulvar, visceral, musculoskeletal, neurogenic, or psychosomatic disorders. Moreover, coexistent etiologies may lead to similar symptoms. For example, women with vulvodynia have been shown in many cases to have coexistent pelvic floor muscle spasm, both of which may cause dyspareunia (Reissing, 2005). Because of the frequent association between dyspareunia and CPP and frequent overlap of etiologies, physical examination and diagnostic testing often follow that for women with CPP (p. 311).

Dyspareunia may be subclassified as *insertional,* that is, pain with vaginal entry, or *deep,* which is associated with deep thrusting. Of insertional dyspareunia cases, vulvodynia, vulvitis, and poor lubrication comprise the majority. Of deep dyspareunia cases, endometriosis, pelvic adhesions, and bulky leiomyomas are frequent causes. In many women, both insertional and deep dyspareunia may be present.

Additional terms include *primary dyspareunia,* which describes the onset of painful intercourse coincident with coitarche, and *secondary dyspareunia,* which is painful intercourse after a period of pain-free sexual activity. Sexual abuse, female genital mutilation, and congenital anomalies most frequently lead to primary dyspareunia, whereas sources of secondary dyspareunia are more varied. Lastly, dyspareunia should be clarified as *generalized,* occurring in all episodes of intercourse, or as *situational,* associated with only specific partners or sexual positions.

Diagnosis

History taking in women with dyspareunia should include questions regarding associated symptoms such as vaginal discharge, vulvar pain, dysmenorrhea, CPP, or scant lubrication. Onset of symptoms and their temporal association with obstetric delivery, pelvic surgery, or sexual abuse is often informative. In addition, dyspareunia may be found in those who breast feed, presumably because of hypoestrogenism-derived vaginal atrophy seen with lactation (Buhling, 2006; Signorello, 2001). Psychosocial topics such as relationship satisfaction or depression should also be covered.

Inspection of the vulva should mirror that for chronic pain. In particular, generalized erythema, episiotomy scars, or atrophy is sought. Erythema may indicate contact or allergic dermatitis or infection, particularly fungal infection. Accordingly, a historical inventory of potential skin irritants, a saline slide preparation, vaginal pH testing, and vaginal cultures are performed. Specifically, a vaginal fungal culture may be required in some cases. This is because several noncandidal species may be difficult to detect if microscopic analysis is solely used (Edwards, 2003; Haefner, 2005).

Some, but not all, have found a positive correlation between degree of pelvic organ prolapse and dyspareunia (Burrows, 2004; Ellerkmann, 2001). If noted, its degree should be assessed with pelvic organ prolapse evaluation (POP-Q) (Chap. 24, p. 636).

Physical examination should evaluate the distal, mid-, and proximal vagina. Evaluation may first begin with palpation of the Bartholin and periurethral glands. Additionally, cotton-swab testing is used to map painful areas (Fig. 4-1, p. 112). Next, insertion of a single digit into the distal vagina may elicit *vaginismus,* that is, reflex contraction of the muscles associated with distal vaginal penetration (Basson, 2000). This contraction response is normal, but prolonged spasm of the bulbocavernosus, pubococcygeus, piriformis, and obturator internus muscles may cause pain. In some cases, spasm may be a conditioned response to a current or former physical pain (Bachmann, 1998).

With deeper digital examination, midvaginal pain may be triggered. This may be seen with interstitial cystitis, congenital anomalies, or following radiation therapy or pelvic reconstructive surgeries.

Deep dyspareunia is more commonly caused by disorders that also cause CPP. Focal points of this examination are discussed on page 311. Similarly, diagnostic testing for deep dyspareunia in great part mirrors that for CPP. Urine and vaginal cultures may indicate infection, and radiologic imaging may reveal structural visceral disease.

Treatment

Resolution of dyspareunia is highly dependent on the underlying cause. For those with vaginismus, structured desensitization is effective. Patients gradually gain control with comfortably inserting dilators of increasing size into the introitus. Concurrent psychological counseling in such cases is often warranted. Poor lubrication may be countered with education directed toward adequate arousal techniques and use of external lubricants.

Surgery may be indicated for structural pathologies and may include ablation of endometriosis, lysis of adhesions, and restoration of normal anatomy. For those with dyspareunia related to a retroverted uterine position, uterine suspension has been shown in small studies to be effective (Perry, 2005).

Dysuria

Evaluation of dysuria begins with a careful pelvic inspection to exclude vaginitis, vulvar lesions, and urethral diverticulum. A voiding diary can be informative, and for those with associated dyspareunia, a sexual history should be obtained. The most common cause of dysuria is infection, and urinalysis and urine culture are therefore initial tests. Similarly, *N gonorrhoeae, C trachomatis,* and herpes simplex virus infections should be excluded. For those with chronic dysuria, urodynamic studies may help to identify those with detrusor overactivity, significantly decreased compliance, or bladder outlet obstruction (Chap. 23, p. 621). Cystoscopy is used to identify the hallmark mucosal findings of interstitial cystitis and exclude neoplastic growths or stones (Irwin, 2005). Adjunctively, sonography or laparoscopy may be indicated to exclude structural pelvic pathology or endometriosis.

Interstitial Cystitis/Painful Bladder Syndrome

This chronic inflammatory disorder of the bladder is typified by symptoms of frequency, urgency, and pelvic pain (Bogart, 2007). With interstitial cystitis (IC), this triad is found in combination with characteristic mucosal changes and reduced bladder capacity (Hanno, 1994). Cystoscopically, *Hunner ulcers* are reddish-brown mucosal lesions with small vessels radiating toward a central scar and are found in approximately 10 percent of cases (Fig. 11-8) (Messing, 1978; Nigro, 1997). The other more common finding is *glomerulations,* which are small petechiae or submucosal hemorrhages. In addition to cases with classic IC findings, *painful bladder syndrome* describes chronic IC symptoms in those who lack cystoscopic findings of IC or other bladder pathology (Abrams, 2002).

Prevalence. The prevalence of IC in the United States is variable and cited at 30 to 60 per 100,000 (Curhan, 1999; Jones, 1997). It is diagnosed more commonly in women, in Caucasians, in smokers, and in those in their 40s (Kennedy, 2006; Propert, 2000). There is a strong association between IC and endometriosis. The two conditions share similar symptoms, and many patients evaluated for chronic pelvic pain have been found to have either one or both conditions (Butrick, 2007; Paulson, 2007). In addition, IC is associated with irri-

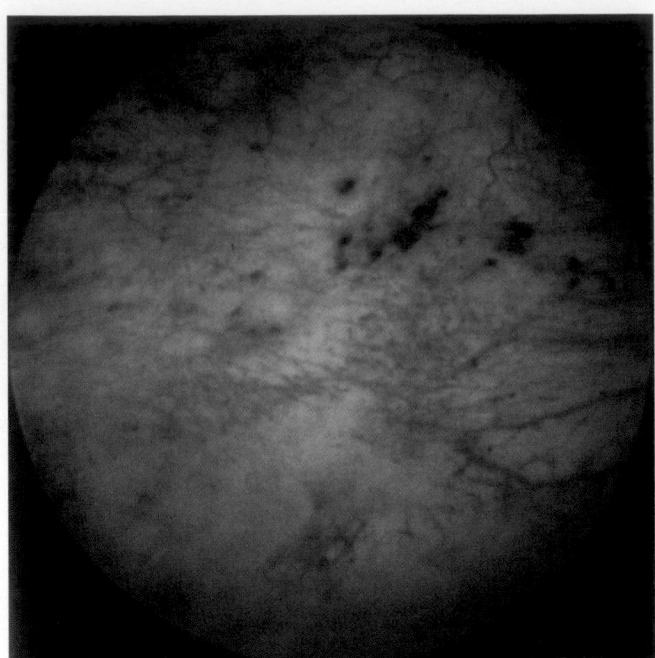

FIGURE 11-8 Cystoscopic photograph displays Hunner ulcers. *(From Reuter, 1987, with permission.)*

table bowel syndrome, generalized pain disorders, fibromyalgia, pelvic floor dysfunction, and depression (Aaron, 2000; Clauw, 1997; Novi, 2005; Peters, 2007).

Pathophysiology. The exact cause of IC is unknown, and current theories include increased mucosal permeability or mast cell activation (Sant, 2007; Warren, 2002). Glycosaminoglycans are an important component of the mucin layer that covers and protects the bladder urothelium. One theory explains that IC symptoms originate from a defect in the protective bladder glycosaminoglycan component. This leads to increased bladder mucosa permeability (Parsons, 2003).

Diagnosis. Koziol (1994) reported symptoms in a series of IC sufferers and found frequency, urgency, and pelvic pain to be most common. Frequency occurs both in the day and night, and voiding events average 16 times per day but can reach 40 times daily. Pain is described as vaginal, suprapubic, or lower abdominal and often worsens during the week before menstruation. It is commonly exacerbated by spicy foods; by alcoholic, acidic, carbonated, or caffeinated beverages; and by coitus, stress, or exercise. Pain is often relieved with voiding, but typically recurs as the bladder refills. Additionally, women commonly describe dyspareunia (Metts, 2001).

Many other conditions can produce symptoms similar to those of IC, and most urologists have therefore regarded IC as being a diagnosis of exclusion. Accordingly, urine culture is obtained, and patients suspected of having IC typically undergo cystoscopy. Bladder biopsy is not required to diagnose IC, but biopsies are often performed to exclude other bladder pathology such as cancer. Urodynamic testing is recommended in those with urgency. In women with IC, both bladder capacity and compliance are decreased.

Treatment. Interstitial cystitis is a chronic disorder with exacerbations and remissions. There is no universally accepted therapy, and for some, expectant management is appropriate. Of therapies, dietary restriction of acidic foods or drinks, oral pentosan polysulfate sodium (Elmiron), oral amitriptyline or antihistamines, intravesical instillation of agents such as heparin or dimethyl sulfoxide (DMSO), or hydrodistension of the bladder are among the more commonly used (Rovner, 2000). The Interstitial Cystitis Association serves as an important resource to patients and clinicians for therapy options and can be accessed at: http://www.ichelp.org.

GASTROINTESTINAL DISEASE

In a significant number of cases, GI disease is found as an underlying cause of chronic pelvic pain. Gastrointestinal causes may be organic or functional (see Table 11-2). Thus, initial screening may follow that for CPP. However, symptoms such as fever, GI bleeding, weight loss, anemia, and abdominal mass should prompt a stronger search for organic pathology. Investigations may include sigmoidoscopy or colonoscopy to exclude inflammation, diverticula, or tumors. For those with diarrhea, stool examination for leukocytes or for ova and parasites may be indicated. Moreover, serologic testing for celiac disease may be valuable. When indicated, sonography may aid in distinguishing gastrointestinal from gynecologic pathology.

Colonic Diverticular Disease

Colon diverticula are small defects in the muscular layer of the colon through which colonic mucosa and submucosa herniate. Diverticular disease of the colon is common in both men and women. It develops in approximately 10 percent of adults younger than 40 years and in greater than 50 percent of those 80 years and older. The sigmoid and descending colon are typically affected.

Chronic symptoms of diverticular disease include abdominal pain that localizes to the left lower quadrant, obstipation, and rectal fullness. More seriously, diverticula may cause acute or chronic GI bleeding or may become infected. Infection may be difficult to distinguish clinically from PID or tuboovarian abscess. In these cases, CT is the recommended imaging technique and has a sensitivity for diagnosis greater than 90 percent and a specificity approaching 100 percent (Ambrosetti, 1997).

Chronic diverticular disease is usually treated with a high-fiber diet and long-term suppressive therapy with antibiotics. With acute severe infection, hospitalization, parenteral antibiotics, surgical or percutaneous abscess drainage, or partial colectomy may be required. Suspected rupture of a diverticular abscess with peritonitis is an indication for immediate surgical exploration (Jacobs, 2007).

Celiac Disease

This is an inherited autoimmune intolerance to gluten, which is a component of wheat, barley, or rye. In affected individuals, ingestion of gluten creates an immune-mediated reaction that damages the small intestine mucosa and leads to varying degrees of malabsorption. Celiac disease is common, and its incidence in the general population approaches 1 percent (Green, 2007). Its incidence is suspected to be even higher if those with GI symptoms are screened. There is a gender bias to the disease, and two to three times as many women as men are affected (Green, 2005).

The most common presenting symptoms are abdominal pain and diarrhea. Other findings include weight loss, osteopenia, and fatigue from anemia; all of which stem from malabsorption. In addition, celiac disease has been associated with infertility, although the mechanism is not understood. Celiac disease should be suspected in those with characteristic findings and in those with a family history of the disorder.

Diagnosis requires both duodenal biopsy and a positive response to a gluten-free diet. However, a significant number of patients presenting with abdominal pain and diarrhea do not have celiac disease. Accordingly, many physicians will screen with noninvasive serologic tests to avoid unnecessary biopsy. Of available diagnostic tests, serologic screening for IgA antiendomysial antibodies and IgA antitissue transglutaminase antibodies is accurate more than 90 percent of the time (van der Windt, 2010).

Functional Bowel Disorders

Also known as *functional gastrointestinal disorders* (FGIDs), this group of functional disorders has symptoms attributable to the lower GI tract and includes those listed in Table 11-7. In defining these chronic conditions, symptoms must have begun more than 6 months previously and have occurred more than 3 days a month during the last 3 months (Longstreth, 2006). The diagnosis always presumes the absence of a structural or biochemical explanation for symptoms (Thompson, 1999).

Irritable Bowel Syndrome

Definition and Incidence. This functional bowel disorder is defined as abdominal pain that improves with defecation and is associated with a change in bowel habits. Subtypes are divided by the predominant stool pattern and include constipative, diarrheal, and mixed stool categories. Although defining criteria are listed in Table 11-7, other symptoms that may support the diagnosis include abnormal stool frequency (fewer than three bowel movements per week or more than three per day), abnormal stool form, straining, urgency, passing mucus, and bloating (Longstreth, 2006).

Irritable bowel syndrome (IBS) is common, and its prevalence in the general population is estimated to be near 10 percent. The prevalences of diarrhea-predominant and constipation-predominant IBS are equivalent (Saito, 2002).

Pathophysiology. With IBS, neural, hormonal, genetic, environmental, and psychosocial factors are variably involved

TABLE 11-7. Functional Gastrointestinal (GI) Disorders

Functional Bowel Disorders

Irritable bowel syndrome (IBS)	Recurrent abdominal pain or discomfort at least 3 days per month in the last 3 months associated with 2 or more of the following: (1) improved with defecation; (2) onset associated with a change in stooling frequency; (3) onset associated with a change in stool form
Functional abdominal bloating	Must include *both* of the following: (1) recurrent feeling of bloating or visible distension at least 3 days/month in 3 months; (2) insufficient criteria for a diagnosis of functional dyspepsia, IBS, or other functional GI disorder
Functional constipation	Must include *two or more* of the following: (1) straining during at least 25% of defecations; (2) lumpy or hard stools in at least 25% of defecations; (3) sensation of incomplete evacuation for at least 25% of defecations; (4) sensation of anorectal obstruction/blockage for at least 25% of defecations; (5) manual maneuvers to aid at least 25% of defecations; (6) fewer than three defecations per week Loose stools are rarely present without the use of laxatives There are insufficient criteria for IBS
Functional diarrhea	Loose or watery stools without pain, occurring in at least 75% of stools
Unspecified functional bowel disorder	Bowel symptoms not attributable to an organic etiology that do not meet criteria for the previously defined categories

Functional Abdominal Pain

Functional abdominal pain	At least 6 months of: (1) continuous or nearly continuous abdominal pain; and (2) no or only occasional relation of pain with physiologic events (e.g., eating, defecation, or menses); (3) some loss of daily functioning; (4) pain is not feigned (e.g., malingering); (5) insufficient criteria for other functional gastrointestinal disorders that would explain the abdominal pain
Unspecified functional abdominal pain	

Adapted from Longstreth, 2006, and Thompson, 1999.

(Drossman, 2002). The primary pathophysiologic mechanism of IBS, however, is thought to involve dysregulation in interactions between the central nervous system (CNS) and enteric nervous system (ENS). Such brain-gut dysfunction may eventually cause alterations of GI mucosal immune response, intestinal motility and permeability, and visceral sensitivity. In turn, these produce abdominal pain and altered bowel function (Harris, 2006; Mayer, 2008). Specifically, serotonin (5-hydroxytryptamine, 5-HT) is involved with regulating intestinal motility, visceral sensitivity, and gut secretion and is thought to play an important role in IBS (Atkinson, 2006; Gershon, 2005).

Diagnosis. Organic diseases such as those in Table 11-2 are excluded prior to the diagnosis of IBS. However, for young patients who have typical IBS symptoms and no symptoms of organic disease, few tests are required. Testing is individualized, and factors that typically prompt greater testing include older patient age, longer duration and greater severity of symptoms, absent psychosocial factors, presence of organic disease symptoms, and family history of GI disease.

Treatment

Diet. Traditionally, therapy to increase daily fiber intake has been employed. Although dietary fiber is effective in treating constipation, it has not been shown to be effective for diarrhea-dominant cases of IBS or for IBS-associated pain (Quartero, 2005). Management of food intolerances can be another potentially valuable treatment adjunct (Alpers, 2006).

Medications. In general, drug therapy is directed toward dominant symptoms. For those with constipation-dominant IBS, commercial fiber analogs may help if increased dietary fiber is unsuccessful (Table 11-8) (Ramkumar, 2005). In addition, stimulation of the serotonin receptor subtype 5-hydroxytryptamine-4 (5-HT$_4$) increases colonic transit time and inhibits visceral sensitivity. Specifically, tegaserod (Zelnorm), a partial 5-HT$_4$-receptor agonist, increases colonic motility and has been effective in relief of constipation-predominant IBS (Layer, 2005; Tack, 2005). However, in 2007, Novartis suspended U.S. sales of Zelnorm in compliance with a request by the Food and Drug Administration (FDA). An increased incidence of cardiovascular events in those using this

TABLE 11-8. Agents Used to Treat Irritable Bowel Syndrome (IBS)

Symptom	Drug	Oral Dosage
Diarrhea	Loperamide	2–4 mg when necessary; maximum 12 g/d
	Cholestyramine resin	4 g with meals
Constipation	Psyllium husk	3.4 g bid with meals, then adjust
	Methylcellulose	2 g bid with meals, then adjust
	Calcium polycarbophil	1 g qd to qid
	Lactulose syrup	10–20 g bid
	70% sorbitol	15 mL bid
	Polyethylene glycol 3350	17 g in 8 oz. water qd
	Magnesium hydroxide	2–4 tbsp qd
Abdominal pain	Tricyclic antidepressants	Start at 25–50 mg hs, then adjust
	Selective serotonin-reuptake inhibitors	Begin with a small dose and increase as needed

bid = twice daily; hs = at bedtime; qd = daily; qid = four times daily.
Modified from Longstreth, 2006, with permission.

agent prompted the FDA's action. It is available now only for special cases (U.S. Food and Drug Administration, 2010).

For those with diarrhea-dominant symptoms, loperamide (Imodium) or diphenoxylate (Lomotil) are effective in slowing bowel motility. As substances stay longer in the intestine, more water is absorbed from fecal matter. Thus, for those with severe diarrhea, alosetron (Lotronex), a selective serotonin 5-HT₃-receptor antagonist, interacts with receptors of enteric nervous system neurons to slow bowel motility. Use of this drug decreases pain, urgency, and stool frequency (Camilleri, 2000; Chey, 2004; Ford, 2009). However, due to cases of ischemic colitis associated with its use, alosetron is now strictly regulated and available only through an FDA prescribing program (Chang, 2006; U.S. Food and Drug Administration, 2009).

For patients with pain secondary to bowel spasm, antispasmodic agents decrease intestinal smooth muscle activity and are thought to decrease abdominal discomfort. Agents available in the United States include dicyclomine (Bentyl) and hyoscyamine (Levsin). In general, these agents are safe, are inexpensive, and have been shown to be effective (Quartero, 2005). However, evidence-based data supporting their use are few, and anticholinergic side effects of these agents often limit their long-term use (Schoenfeld, 2005).

Tricyclic antidepressants may help patients with IBS both by an anticholinergic effect on the gut and by mood-modifying action. Tricyclic antidepressants may slow intestinal transit time and have been shown to be effective in treatment of diarrhea-dominant IBS (Hadley, 2005). Alternatively, another class of antidepressant, the selective serotonin-reuptake inhibitors (SSRIs), has been shown in small studies to be useful for irritable bowel syndrome (Tabas, 2004; Vahedi, 2005).

Psychological Therapy. Psychological or behavioral treatments may help some patients. Of these, cognitive-behavioral therapy and hypnotherapy have been shown to be effective (Drossman, 2003; Gonsalkorale, 2003; Payne, 1995).

MUSCULOSKELETAL ETIOLOGIES

Clinical syndromes involving the muscles, nerves, and skeletal system of the lower abdomen and pelvis are frequently encountered but often overlooked by gynecologists in our never-ending quest to identify visceral sources of chronic pelvic pain.

Abdominal Wall Hernia

Defects in anterior abdominal wall or femoral fascia can lead to herniation of bowel or other intraabdominal contents through these rents. Such herniation can cause pain. Moreover, if the blood supply of herniated contents is compromised acutely, then bowel obstruction or bowel ischemia can necessitate prompt surgical intervention.

Hernias may develop at sites of inherent anatomic weakness, and common types in women include ventral, umbilical, and incisional hernias. Indirect inguinal, direct inguinal, and femoral hernias are types less commonly found in females. Spigelian hernias are rare. As shown in Figure 11-9, ventral hernias are caused by fascial defects typically occurring in the midline. Umbilical hernias are those involving defects of the umbilical ring. Indirect inguinal hernias are those in which abdominal contents herniate through the internal inguinal ring and into the inguinal canal. As shown in Figure 11-10, contents may then exit the external inguinal ring. In contrast, contents of a direct inguinal hernia bulge through a fascial defect within Hesselbach triangle. This triangle is bordered by the inguinal ligament, the inferior epigastric vessels, and the lateral border of the rectus abdominis muscle. Spigelian hernias can occur anywhere along the lateral border of the rectus abdominis. However, the most frequent location is at the level of the arcuate line.

Conditions that increase intraabdominal pressure such as pregnancy, ascites, peritoneal dialysis, and chronic cough are known hernia risk factors. Congenital or acquired anatomic

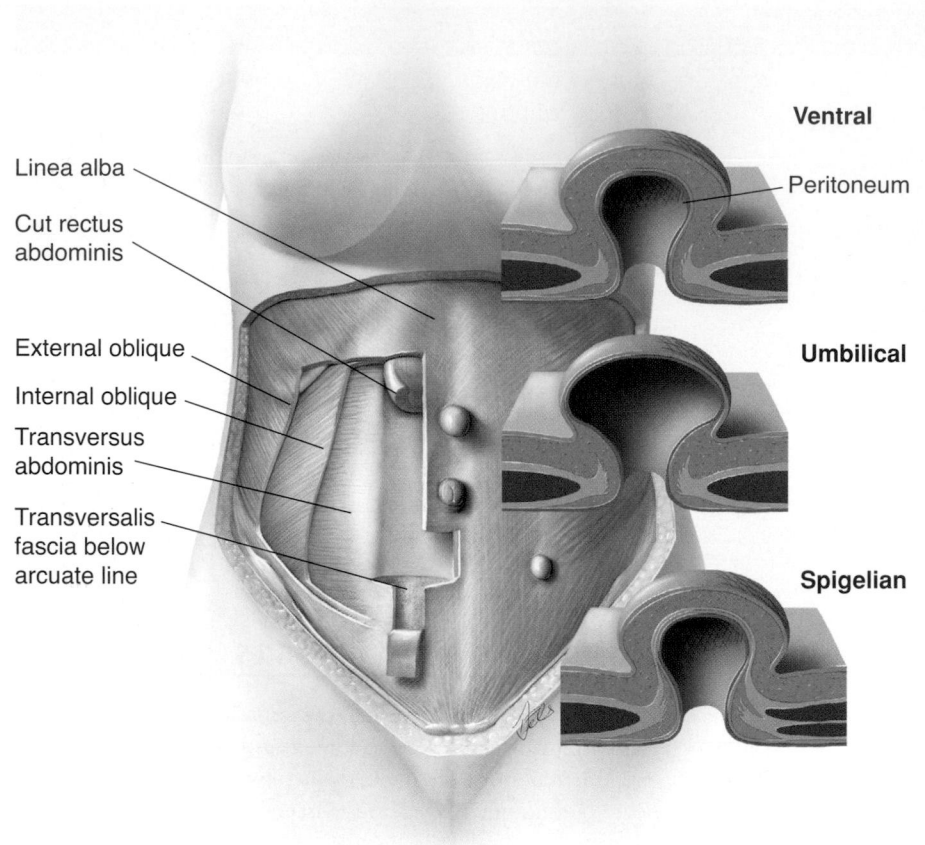

Linea alba
Cut rectus abdominis
External oblique
Internal oblique
Transversus abdominis
Transversalis fascia below arcuate line

Ventral
Peritoneum
Umbilical
Spigelian

A hyperirritable area within a muscle can lead to persistently contracted fibers and cause pain, weakness, or autonomic reactions (Simons, 1999). The primary reactive area within the muscle is termed a *trigger point (TrP)* and is identified as a palpable taut, ropy band. These myofascial trigger points can affect any muscle, and those involving muscles of the anterior abdominal wall, pelvic floor, and pelvic girdle can be sources of chronic pelvic pain. For this reason, the American College of Obstetricians and Gynecologists (1997) recommends an assessment of the musculoskeletal system prior to laparoscopy or hysterectomy for CPP.

Pathophysiology

Trigger points are thought to form as the end of a metabolic crisis within a muscle. Dysfunction of a neuromuscular endplate can lead to sustained acetylcholine release, persistent depolarization, sarcomere shortening, and creation of a taut muscle band. Affected fibers compress capillaries and decrease local blood flow. The resulting ischemia leads to release of substances that activate peripheral nerve nociceptors and in turn cause pain (McPartland, 2004).

A persistent barrage of nociceptive signals from TrPs may eventually lead to central sensitization and the potential for neuropathic pain (p. 306). Signals may spread segmentally within the spinal cord to cause localized or referred pain (Gerwin, 2005). Trigger points can also initiate somatovisceral responses such as vomiting, diarrhea, and bladder spasm, which may add confusion to the diagnosis.

Incidence and Risk Factors

The incidence of myofascial disease is unknown. However, in an evaluation of 500 patients with chronic pelvic pain, Carter (1998) found 7 percent of patients primarily had trigger points as a source of their pain. Moreover, of nearly 1000 women evaluated for CPP, 22 percent were found to have significant tenderness of the levator ani muscles, and 14 percent were found to have significant tenderness of the piriformis muscles (Gomel, 2007). Prevalence appears to be greatest in those between 30 and 50 years of age. Risk factors are varied, although many trigger points can be traced to a prior specific trauma such as a sporting injury or to chronic biomechanical overload of a muscle (Sharp, 2003). Accordingly, in evaluating patients with chronic pain and suspected myofascial pain syndrome, a detailed inventory of sporting injuries, traumatic injuries, obstetric deliveries, surgeries, and work activities is essential.

FIGURE 11-9 Hernias that may involve the anterior abdominal wall include ventral, umbilical, or much less commonly, Spigelian. *(Image contributed by Mr. T. J. Fels.)*

weakness or connective tissue disorders are also associated. Because of the potential risks associated with organ herniation and strangulation, hernias are typically repaired once identified. Small ventral, umbilical, or incisional hernias may be repaired by gynecologic surgeons. In these cases, the hernia sac is excised and fascia reapproximated. Patients with larger hernias, which usually require mesh placement, or hernias in the inguinal area are typically referred to a general surgeon.

Myofascial Pain Syndrome

Many musculoskeletal conditions can lead to CPP and are listed in Table 11-2. In addition to these, chronic visceral inflammatory conditions such as endometriosis, interstitial cystitis, or IBS may lead to pathologic changes in nearby muscles and/or nerves. In turn, these changes can be the genesis of myofascial pain syndromes of the abdominal wall or pelvic floor. Knowledge and awareness of these complex associations allows a physician to more effectively address all the components leading to pain, rather than narrowly focusing on an isolated visceral disorder. As a result, a patient is less likely to suffer misdiagnosis and inappropriate treatment. Instead, appropriate referral for physical therapy or pain management can be initiated.

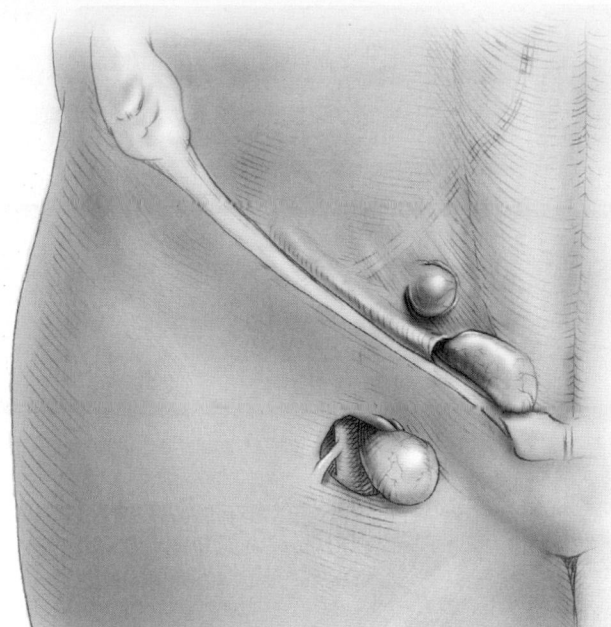

FIGURE 11-10 Indirect and direct inguinal hernias and femoral hernia. A direct hernia is cause by a fascial defect within Hesselbach triangle. An indirect hernia forms from intraabdominal contents exiting through the inguinal canal. Femoral hernias form from contents exiting through the femoral ring. *(Image contributed by Ms. Kristin Yang.)*

Diagnosis

Marking by the patient of painful sites on a body silhouette diagram can be an informative first step. Involvement of specific muscles will often give characteristic patterns. Patients typically describe the pain as aggravated by specific movement or activity and relieved by certain positions. Cold, damp exposure generally worsens the pain. Pressure on a trigger point causes pain and produces effects on a target area or *referral zone*. This specific and reproducible area of referral rarely coincides with dermatologic or neuronal distribution and is the feature that differentiates myofascial pain syndromes from fibromyalgia (Lavelle, 2007).

Muscle examination may be completed by flat palpation, pincer palpation, or deep palpation depending on muscle location. Flat palpation uses fingertips to roll over superficial muscles, which are only accessible at the surface (Fig. 11-11). This technique is commonly used to assess the anterior abdominal wall muscles. In those muscles with greater accessibility, pincer palpation grasps the muscle belly between the thumb and fingers. With any of the palpation techniques, spot tenderness and taut muscle bands can often be appreciated in those with myofascial pain syndrome. Classically, the involved muscle displays weakness and restricted stretch. Additionally, TrP pressure may also elicit a local muscle twitch response or reproduce a patient's referred pain or both.

Muscle Groups

Anterior Abdominal Wall Trigger Points.
The muscles of the rectus abdominis, the obliques, and transversus abdominis muscles may all develop TrPs that lead to chronic pain. Associated somatovisceral pelvic symptoms from these

muscles may include diarrhea or urinary frequency, urgency, or retention.

Within the rectus abdominis muscle, painful TrPs are frequently found along the linea semilunaris, which is the term for this muscle's lateral margin (Suleiman, 2001). Additional TrP sites in the rectus abdominis muscle commonly develop at the muscle's insertion into the pubic bone and also below the umbilicus. Within the external oblique muscle, trigger points

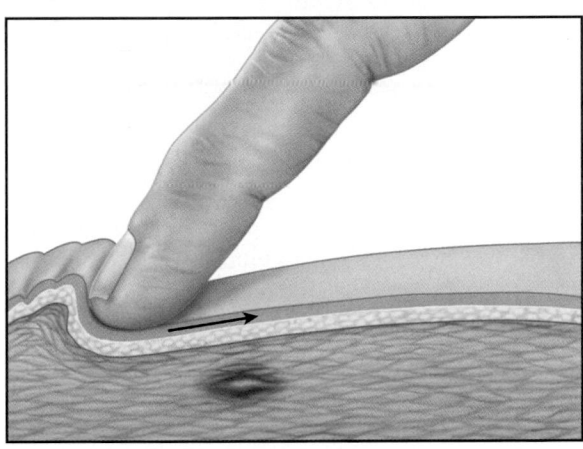

A

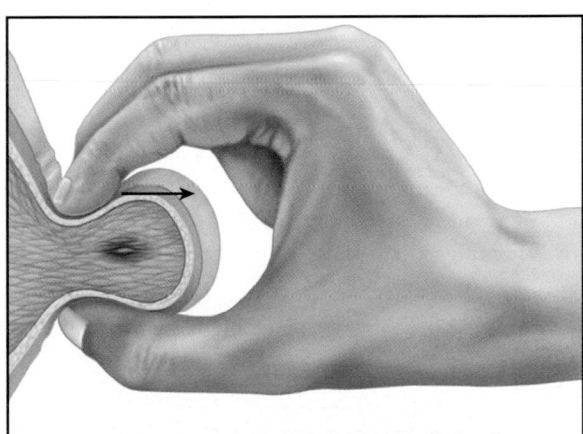

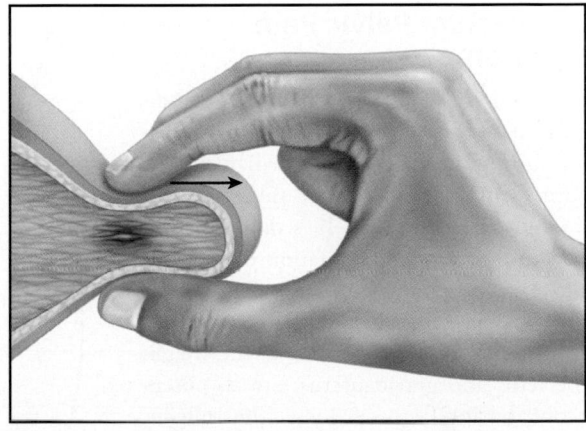

B

FIGURE 11-11 Techniques for trigger point palpation. **A.** With flat palpation, fingertips stroke across the muscle surface. **B.** With pincer palpation. The muscle is grasped and palpation for trigger points is completed as the muscle slips through the fingers.

frequently involve its lateral attachment to the anterior iliac crest, and pain usually refers to the pubic bone.

Pelvic Muscle Trigger Points.

After examination of the anterior abdominal wall, muscles of the pelvis should be evaluated. Following careful inspection of the external genitalia, vaginal examination should proceed slowly and cautiously with the index finger only and initially without a palpating abdominal hand. Muscles within the pelvis include the levator ani, coccygeus, obturator internus, and deep transverse perineal and piriformis muscles. These are assessed for painful spasm or trigger points (see Fig. 11-6) (Vercellini, 2009). Trigger points involving these muscles and anal sphincter muscles are frequently associated with poorly localized pain that may be described as involving the coccyx, hip, or back (Figs. 11-12 and 11-13). Dyspareunia is common.

Pain stemming from TrPs involving the levator ani muscles has had a variety of names including *levator ani spasm syndrome* and *coccydynia*. Currently, *levator ani syndrome* is the preferred term. Coccydynia is reserved for coccygeal pain originating from skeletal trauma to the coccyx.

Treatment

The goal of treatment is inactivation of trigger points, which then allows stretching and release of taut muscle bands. Therapies are varied and include, among others: TrP release maneuvers, biofeedback, TrP dry needling or injection, and local heat. Pharmacologic agents such as NSAIDs, other analgesics, muscle relaxants, or tranquilizers are also employed.

■ Peripartum Pelvic Pain Syndrome

Also known as pelvic girdle pain, this condition is characterized by persistent pain that begins during pregnancy or immediately postpartum. Pain is prominent around the sacroiliac joints and symphysis. It is thought to be related to injury or inflammation of the ligaments in the pelvis and/or lower spine. Muscle weakness, postural adjustments of pregnancy, and hormonal changes, as well as the weight of the fetus and gravid uterus, are all potential contributing factors (Mens, 1996). Pelvic girdle pain is common. Significant pain is estimated to afflict approximately 20 percent of pregnant women and 7 percent of those during the 3 months following delivery (Albert, 2002; Wu, 2004). Diagnosis is usu-

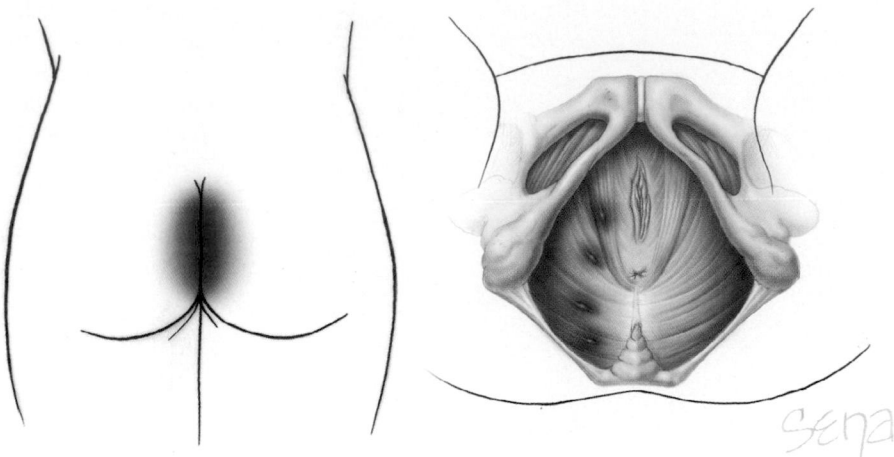

FIGURE 11-12 Pattern of referred pain (*red shading in the left image*) created by trigger points in the levator ani and coccygeus muscles (*right image*). *(Images contributed by Ms. Marie Sena.)*

ally clinical and based on findings during specific orthopedic joint manipulation tests. These are used to recreate or provoke the pain. Treatment includes physical therapy, exercise, and analgesics typically used for CPP, as described earlier (p. 314) (Vermani, 2010; Vleeming, 2008).

NEUROLOGIC ETIOLOGIES

Nerve compression can lead to chronic pelvic pain and may involve nerves of the anterior abdominal wall or those within the pelvis.

■ Anterior Abdominal Wall Nerve Entrapment Syndromes

As discussed, anterior abdominal wall pain is frequently mistaken for visceral pain. Common neurologic causes include entrapment of the anterior cutaneous branches of the intercostal

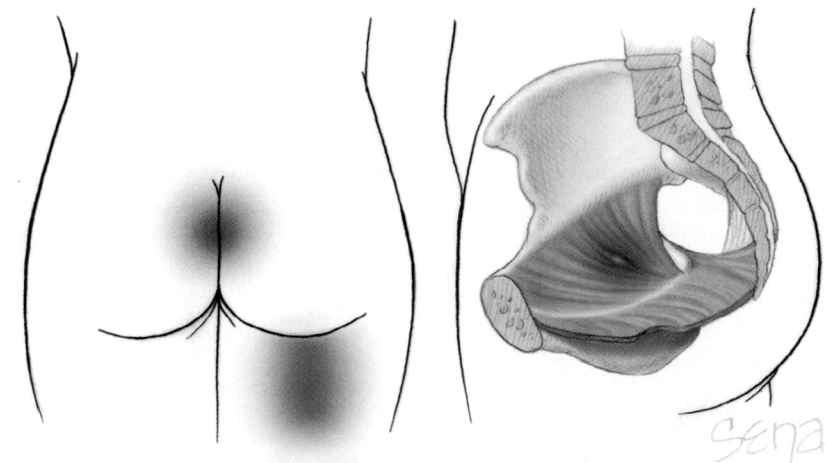

FIGURE 11-13 An extensive pattern of referred pain (*red shading in the left image*) can be created by trigger points in the obturator internus muscle (*right image*). *(Images contributed by Ms. Marie Sena.)*

nerves or compression of branches of the ilioinguinal, iliohypogastric, genitofemoral, and lateral femoral cutaneous nerves (Greenbaum, 1994).

Pathophysiology

Peripheral nerves can be compressed either within narrow anatomic canals or rings or beneath tight ligaments, fibrous bands, or sutures. Thus, common sites of compression for a given nerve are often predictable based on their anatomy. For example, each anterior cutaneous branch of an intercostal nerve traverses anteriorly through the rectus abdominis muscle. Each branch and its corresponding vessels travels through a fibrous ring found within the lateral aspect of rectus abdominis muscle (Fig. 11-14). On crossing the anterior rectus sheath, each branch divides and then courses within the subcutaneous tissues. Fat surrounding the neurovascular bundle appears to pad the enclosed structures within the fibrous ring (Srinivasan, 2002). However, if this bundle receives excessive intra- or extraabdominal pressure, compression of the bundle against the fibrous ring can cause nerve ischemia and pain (Applegate, 1997).

Alternatively, nerve entrapment, injury, or neuroma formation may involve branches of the ilioinguinal, iliohypogastric, lateral femoral cutaneous, or genitofemoral nerves (Chap. 40, p. 983). Involvement may follow inguinal hernia repair, low transverse abdominal incisions, and lower abdominal laparoscopic trocar placement. Hypoesthesia is the more common finding with these injuries, but pain may variably develop within months of surgery or after several years.

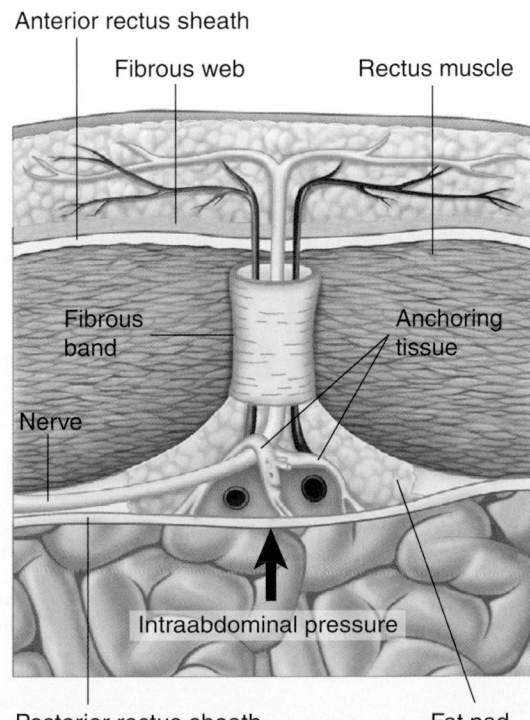

Anterior rectus sheath

Fibrous web   Rectus muscle

Fibrous band   Anchoring tissue

Nerve

Intraabdominal pressure

Posterior rectus sheath   Fat pad

FIGURE 11-14 Drawing displays nerve entrapment of the anterior cutaneous branches of one of the intercostal nerves. The nerve is compressed as it traverses the rectus abdominis muscle within a fibrous sheath. *(Redrawn from Greenbaum, 1994, with permission.)*

Diagnosis and Treatment

Criteria for diagnosing nerve entrapment are clinical and include: (1) pain aggravated by patient movement or light skin pinching over the affected area and (2) pain improvement following local anesthetic injection. In general, electromyography is not useful because it lacks adequate sensitivity (Knockaert, 1996).

In most cases, pain will improve with local injection of anesthetic agents with or without corticosteroids. One- or 2-percent lidocaine and a 40-mg/mL concentration of triamcinolone can be combined in a 1:1 ratio. Less than half a milliliter is injected at each pain site. Additional treatments may include oral analgesics, biofeedback, and gabapentin. If conservative options fail to bring sufficient relief, neurolysis with injection of 5- to 6-percent absolute alcohol or phenol or surgical neurectomy may be required (Madura, 2005; Suleiman, 2001).

Pudendal Neuralgia
Pathophysiology

Neuralgia is sharp, severe, shooting pain that follows the path of the involved nerve. Nerve entrapment of the pudendal nerve may cause this type of pain in the perineum. Pudendal neuralgia is rare, usually develops after age 30, and is characterized by pain in the sensory distribution of the pudendal nerve. The three branches of this nerve are the perineal nerve, the inferior rectal nerve, and the dorsal nerve to the clitoris (Fig. 38-28, p. 944). Thus, pain can involve the vagina, vulva, mons veneris, clitoris, labia, perineum, buttocks, inner leg, or anorectal areas and is frequently usually unilateral. In affected individuals, allodynia and hyperesthesia may be extreme to the point of disability. The pain is frequently aggravated by sitting, relieved by standing or sitting on a toilet seat, and may increase during the day.

In addition to an extensive sensory distribution, the pudendal nerve supplies motor innervation to the external anal sphincter muscle and to much of the pelvic diaphragm, including the levator ani (Stav, 2009). Disturbance of the pudendal nerve can create loss of motor function in the external anal sphincter and thereby, fecal incontinence. In one study of patients evaluated for fecal incontinence, 56 percent demonstrated a pudendal neuropathy. In 67 percent of these patients, the neuropathy was unilateral (Gooneratne, 2007). Fecal incontinence is more fully discussed in Chapter 25 (p. 659).

Diagnosis and Treatment

The diagnosis of pudendal neuralgia is clinical, and no one test or combination of tests is pathognomonic for this condition. That said, clinical suspicion may be supported by objective testing. This may include neurophysiologic testing such as pudendal nerve motor latency and electromyography (EMG), both described in Chapter 25 (p. 668). Rarely, CT or MR imaging may be informative, although these may be performed to exclude other pathology.

Treatment may involve physical therapy; behavioral modification; medications such as gabapentin or tricyclic antidepressants; pudendal nerve blockade, with or without corticosteroids; and surgical nerve decompression. Lastly, pudendal nerve stimulation has demonstrated beneficial effects on pelvic floor functional impairments and pain (Carmel, 2010; Spinelli, 2005). However, limited data exist regarding this modality.

Piriformis Syndrome
Pathophysiology

Compression of the sciatic nerve by the piriformis muscle may lead to buttock or low back pain in the distribution of the sciatic nerve (Broadhurst, 2004; Fishman, 2002). This is termed the *piriformis syndrome.* Proposed mechanisms for compression include contracture or spasm of the piriformis muscle from trauma, overuse and muscle hypertrophy, and congenital variations in which the sciatic nerve or its divisions pass through this muscle (Hopayian, 2010).

Despite being first described more than 60 years ago, this condition remains controversial regarding its existence as a true clinical entity. That said, Fishman and associates (2002) estimate the piriformis syndrome to be responsible for 6 to 8 percent of cases of low back pain and sciatica in the United States each year.

Diagnosis and Treatment

Symptoms include pain and tenderness involving the buttocks, with or without radiation into the posterior thigh. Pain is worse with activity, prolonged sitting, walking, and internal rotation of the hip (Kirschner, 2009). Dyspareunia has a common but variable association and has been demonstrated in 13 to 100 percent of cases (Hopayian, 2010).

Diagnosis of the piriformis syndrome is clinical and based on findings during specific orthopedic joint manipulation tests. Nerve conduction and EMG are typically nondiagnostic. Uncommonly, MR imaging may be helpful by identifying a swollen or enlarged piriformis muscle or anatomic variation in the muscle (Petchprapa, 2010). Treatment is conservative and includes physical therapy, NSAIDs, muscle relaxants, or neuropathic pain agents such as gabapentin, nortriptyline, or carbamazepine. Therapeutic injections of local anesthetics, with or without corticosteroids, or of botulinum toxin may be used. Surgery is reserved for refractory cases.

REFERENCES

Aaron LA, Burke MM, Buchwald D: Overlapping conditions among patients with chronic fatigue syndrome, fibromyalgia, and temporomandibular disorder. Arch Intern Med 160:221, 2000

Abrams P, Cardozo L, Fall M, et al: The standardisation of terminology of lower urinary tract function: report from the Standardisation Subcommittee of the International Continence Society. Neurourol Urodyn 21:167, 2002

Akin M, Price W, Rodriguez G Jr, et al: Continuous, low-level, topical heat wrap therapy as compared to acetaminophen for primary dysmenorrhea. J Reprod Med 49:739, 2004

Akin MD, Weingand KW, Hengehold DA, et al: Continuous low-level topical heat in the treatment of dysmenorrhea. Obstet Gynecol 97:343, 2001

Albert HB, Godskesen M, Westergaard JG: Incidence of four syndromes of pregnancy-related pelvic joint pain. Spine 27(24):2831, 2002

Alpers DH: Diet and irritable bowel syndrome. Curr Opin Gastroenterol 22:136, 2006

Ambrosetti P, Grossholz M, Becker C, et al: Computed tomography in acute left colonic diverticulitis. Br J Surg 84:532, 1997

American College of Obstetricians and Gynecologists: Adult manifestations of childhood sexual abuse. Committee Opinion No. 498, August 2011

American College of Obstetricians and Gynecologists: Chronic pelvic pain. Practice Bulletin No. 51, March 2004, Reaffirmed May 2008

American College of Obstetricians and Gynecologists: Hysterectomy, abdominal or vaginal for chronic pelvic pain. Criteria Set No. 29, November 1997

American Fertility Society: The American Fertility Society classifications of adnexal adhesions, distal tubal occlusion, tubal occlusion secondary to tubal ligation, tubal pregnancies, mullerian anomalies and intrauterine adhesions. Fertil Steril 49:944, 1988

American Society for Reproductive Medicine, Society of Reproductive Surgeons: Pathogenesis, consequences, and control of peritoneal adhesions in gynecologic surgery. Fertil Steril 90(5 Suppl):S144, 2008

Andreotti RF, Lee SI, Choy G, et al: ACR appropriateness criteria on acute pelvic pain in the reproductive age group. JACR J Am Coll Radiol 6(4):235, 2009

Angle RH, Ackerman SJ, Irshad A: Practical imaging of acute pelvic pain in premenopausal women. Contemp Diagn Radiol 33(1):1, 2010

Applegate WV, Buckwalter NR: Microanatomy of the structures contributing to abdominal cutaneous nerve entrapment syndrome. J Am Board Fam Pract 10:329, 1997

Atkinson W, Lockhart S, Whorwell PJ, et al: Altered 5-hydroxytryptamine signaling in patients with constipation- and diarrhea-predominant irritable bowel syndrome. Gastroenterology 130(1):34, 2006

Bachmann GA, Phillips NA: Sexual dysfunction. In Steege JF, Metzger DA, Levy BS (eds): Chronic Pelvic Pain: An Integrated Approach. Philadelphia, WB Saunders, 1998, p 77

Baker PK: Musculoskeletal origins of chronic pelvic pain. Diagnosis and treatment. Obstet Gynecol Clin North Am 20:719, 1993

Baker PK: Musculoskeletal problems. In Steege JF, Metzger DA, Levy BS (eds): Chronic Pelvic Pain: An Integrated Approach. Philadelphia, WB Saunders, 1998, p 232

Balbi C, Musone R, Menditto A, et al: Influence of menstrual factors and dietary habits on menstrual pain in adolescence age. Eur J Obstet Gynecol Reprod Biol 91:143, 2000

Baldaszti E, Wimmer-Puchinger B, Loschke K: Acceptability of the long-term contraceptive levonorgestrel-releasing intrauterine system (Mirena): a 3-year follow-up study. Contraception 67:87, 2003

Barnard ND, Scialli AR, Hurlock D, et al: Diet and sex-hormone binding globulin, dysmenorrhea, and premenstrual symptoms. Obstet Gynecol 95:245, 2000

Basson R, Berman J, Burnett A, et al: Report of the international consensus development conference on female sexual dysfunction: definitions and classifications. J Urol 163:888, 2000

Beard RW, Kennedy RG, Gangar KF, et al: Bilateral oophorectomy and hysterectomy in the treatment of intractable pelvic pain associated with pelvic congestion. Br J Obstet Gynaecol 98:988, 1991

Beard RW, Reginald PW, Wadsworth J: Clinical features of women with chronic lower abdominal pain and pelvic congestion. Br J Obstet Gynaecol 95:153, 1988

Bermejo C, Martínez Ten P, Cantarero R, et al: Three-dimensional ultrasound in the diagnosis of müllerian duct anomalies and concordance with magnetic resonance imaging. Ultrasound Obstet Gynecol 35(5):593, 2010

Bogart LM, Berry SH, Clemens JQ: Symptoms of interstitial cystitis, painful bladder syndrome and similar diseases in women: a systematic review. J Urol 177(2):450, 2007

Brill K, Norpoth T, Schnitker J, et al: Clinical experience with a modern low-dose oral contraceptive in almost 100,000 users. Contraception 43:101, 1991

Broadhurst NA, Simmons DN, Bond MJ: Piriformis syndrome: correlation of muscle morphology with symptoms and signs. Arch Phys Med Rehabil 85(12):2036, 2004

Brown MA, Sirlin CB: Female pelvis. Magn Reson Imaging Clin North Am 13(2):381, 2005

Bryson HM, Wilde MI: Amitriptyline. A review of its pharmacological properties and therapeutic use in chronic pain states. Drugs Aging 8:459, 1996

Buhling KJ, Schmidt S, Robinson JN, et al: Rate of dyspareunia after delivery in primiparae according to mode of delivery. Eur J Obstet Gynecol Reprod Biol 124:42, 2006

Burrows LJ, Meyn LA, Walters MD, et al: Pelvic symptoms in women with pelvic organ prolapse. Obstet Gynaecol 104(5 Pt 1):982, 2004

Butrick CW: Interstitial cystitis and chronic pelvic pain: new insights in neuropathology, diagnosis, and treatment. Clin Obstet Gynaecol 46:811, 2003

Butrick CW: Patients with chronic pelvic pain: endometriosis or interstitial cystitis/painful bladder syndrome? J Soc Laparoendosc Surg 11(2):182, 2007

Camilleri M, Northcutt AR, Kong S, et al: Efficacy and safety of alosetron in women with irritable bowel syndrome: a randomised, placebo-controlled trial. Lancet 355:1035, 2000

Carmel M, Lebel M, Tu le M: Pudendal nerve neuromodulation with neurophysiology guidance: a potential treatment option for refractory chronic pelvi-perineal pain. Int Urogynecol J Pelvic Floor Dysfunct 21(5):613, 2010

Carter JE: Surgical treatment for chronic pelvic pain. JSLS 2:129, 1998

Chang L, Chey WD, Harris L, et al: Incidence of ischemic colitis and serious complications of constipation among patients using alosetron: systematic review of clinical trials and post-marketing surveillance data. Am J Gastroenterol 101(5):1069, 2006

Chang SS, Shan YS, Lin YJ, et al: A review of obturator hernia and a proposed algorithm for its diagnosis and treatment. World J Surg 29:450, 2005

Chey WD, Chey WY, Heath AT, et al: Long-term safety and efficacy of alosetron in women with severe diarrhea-predominant irritable bowel syndrome. Am J Gastroenterol 99:2195, 2004

Chung MH, Huh CY: Comparison of treatments for pelvic congestion syndrome. Tohoku J Exp Med 201:131, 2003

Clauw DJ, Schmidt M, Radulovic D, et al: The relationship between fibromyalgia and interstitial cystitis. J Psychiatr Res 31:125, 1997

Cunanan RG Jr, Courey NG, Lippes J: Laparoscopic findings in patients with pelvic pain. Am J Obstet Gynecol 146:589, 1983

Curhan GC, Speizer FE, Hunter DJ, et al: Epidemiology of interstitial cystitis: a population based study. J Urol 161:549, 1999

Daniels J, Gray R, Hills RK, et al: Laparoscopic uterosacral nerve ablation for alleviating chronic pelvic pain: a randomized controlled trial. JAMA 302(9):955, 2009

Demco L: Pain mapping of adhesions. J Am Assoc Gynecol Laparosc 11:181, 2004

Descargues G, Tinlot-Mauger F, Gravier A, et al: Adnexal torsion: a report on forty-five cases. Eur J Obstet Gynecol Reprod Biol 98:91, 2001

Drossman DA, Camilleri M, Mayer EA, et al: AGA technical review on irritable bowel syndrome. Gastroenterology 123:2108, 2002

Drossman DA, Toner BB, Whitehead WE, et al: Cognitive-behavioral therapy versus education and desipramine versus placebo for moderate to severe functional bowel disorders. Gastroenterology 125:19, 2003

Dubuisson J, Botchorishvili R, Perrette S, et al: Incidence of intraabdominal adhesions in a continuous series of 1000 laparoscopic procedures. Am J Obstet Gynecol 203(2):111.e1, 2010

Edwards L: New concepts in vulvodynia. Am J Obstet Gynecol 189(3, Suppl 1):S24, 2003

Einstein AJ, Henzlova MJ, Rajagopalan S: Estimating risk of cancer associated with radiation exposure from 64-slice computed tomography coronary angiography. JAMA 298(3):317, 2007

El Minawi AM, Howard FM: Operative laparoscopic treatment of ovarian retention syndrome. J Am Assoc Gynecol Laparosc 6:297, 1999

Ellerkmann RM, Cundiff GW, Melick CF, et al: Correlation of symptoms with location and severity of pelvic organ prolapse. Am J Obstet Gynecol 185:1332, 2001

Farquhar CM, Rogers V, Franks S, et al: A randomized controlled trial of medroxyprogesterone acetate and psychotherapy for the treatment of pelvic congestion. Br J Obstet Gynaecol 96:1153, 1989

Fayez JA, Clark RR: Operative laparoscopy for the treatment of localized chronic pelvic-abdominal pain caused by postoperative adhesions. J Gynecol Surg 10:79, 1994

Fazel R, Krumholz HM, Wang Y, et al: Exposure to low-dose ionizing radiation from medical imaging procedures. N Engl J Med 361(9):849, 2009

Fishman LM, Dombi GW, Michaelsen C, et al: Piriformis syndrome: diagnosis, treatment and outcome—a ten-year study. Arch Phys Med Rehabil 83:295, 2002

Flasar MH, Goldberg E: Acute abdominal pain. Med Clin North Am 90:481, 2006

Fleischer AC, Tait D, Mayo J, et al: Sonographic features of ovarian remnants. J Ultrasound Med 17:551, 1998

Ford AC, Brandt LJ, Young C, et al: Efficacy of 5-HT₃ antagonists and 5-HT₄ agonists in irritable bowel syndrome: systematic review and meta-analysis. Am J Gastroenterol 104(7):1831, 2009

Fugh-Berman A, Kronenberg F: Complementary and alternative medicine (CAM) in reproductive-age women: a review of randomized controlled trials. Reprod Toxicol 17:137, 2003

Gallagher EJ: Acute abdominal pain. In Tintinalli JE, Kelen GD, Stapczynski JS, et al (eds): Tintinalli's Emergency Medicine: A Comprehensive Study Guide. New York, McGraw-Hill, 2004

Gangar KF, Stones RW, Saunders D, et al: An alternative to hysterectomy? GnRH analogue combined with hormone replacement therapy. Br J Obstet Gynaecol 100:360, 1993

Gauthier A, Upmalis D, Dain MP: Clinical evaluation of a new triphasic oral contraceptive: norgestimate and ethinyl estradiol. Acta Obstet Gynecol Scand (Suppl 156):27, 1992

Gerhardt RT, Nelson BK, Keenan S, et al: Derivation of a clinical guideline for the assessment of nonspecific abdominal pain: the Guideline for Abdominal Pain in the ED Setting (GAPEDS) Phase 1 Study. Am J Emerg Med 23:709, 2005

Gershon MD: Nerves, reflexes, and the enteric nervous system: pathogenesis of the irritable bowel syndrome. J Clin Gastroenterol 39(4 Suppl 3):S184, 2005

Gerwin RD: A review of myofascial pain and fibromyalgia—factors that promote their persistence. Acupunct Med 23:121, 2005

Giacchetto C, Catizone F, Cotroneo GB, et al: Radiologic anatomy of the genital venous system in female patients with varicocele. Surg Gynecol Obstet 169:403, 1989

Giamberardino MA: Referred muscle pain/hyperalgesia and central sensitisation. J Rehab Med (41 Suppl):85, 2003

Gilron I, Watson CP, Cahill CM, et al: Neuropathic pain: a practical guide for the clinician. Can Med Assoc J 175:265, 2006

Glatt AE, Zinner SH, McCormack WM: The prevalence of dyspareunia. Obstet Gynecol 75:433, 1990

Gokhale LB: Curative treatment of primary (spasmodic) dysmenorrhoea. Indian J Med Res 103:227, 1996

Golub LJ, Menduke H, Lang WR: Exercise and dysmenorrhea in young teenagers: a 3-year study. Obstet Gynecol 32:508, 1968

Gomel V: Chronic pelvic pain: a challenge. J Minim Invasive Gynecol 14(4):521, 2007

Gonsalkorale WM, Miller V, Afzal A, et al: Long term benefits of hypnotherapy for irritable bowel syndrome. Gut 52:1623, 2003

Gooneratne ML, Scott SM, Lunniss PJ: Unilateral pudendal neuropathy is common in patients with fecal incontinence. Dis Colon Rectum 50(4):449, 2007

Green PH: The many faces of celiac disease: clinical presentation of celiac disease in the adult population. Gastroenterology 128(4 Suppl):S74, 2005

Green PHR, Cellier C: Celiac disease. N Engl J Med 357(17):1731, 2007

Greenbaum DS, Greenbaum RB, Joseph JG, et al: Chronic abdominal wall pain. Diagnostic validity and costs. Dig Dis Sci 39:1935, 1994

Guerriero S, Ajossa S, Lai MP, et al: Transvaginal ultrasonography in the diagnosis of pelvic adhesions. Hum Reprod 12:2649, 1997

Gunter J: Chronic pelvic pain: an integrated approach to diagnosis and treatment. Obstet Gynecol Surv 58:615, 2003

Hadley SK, Gaarder SM: Treatment of irritable bowel syndrome. Am Fam Physician 72:2501, 2005

Haefner HK, Collins ME, Davis GD, et al: The vulvodynia guideline. J Lower Gen Tract Dis 9:40, 2005

Hammoud A, Gago LA, Diamond MP: Adhesions in patients with chronic pelvic pain: a role for adhesiolysis? Fertil Steril 82:1483, 2004

Hanno PM: Diagnosis of interstitial cystitis. Urol Clin North Am 21:63, 1994

Harel Z, Biro FM, Kottenhahn RK, et al: Supplementation with omega-3 polyunsaturated fatty acids in the management of dysmenorrhea in adolescents. Am J Obstet Gynecol 174:1335, 1996

Harlow SD, Park M: A longitudinal study of risk factors for the occurrence, duration and severity of menstrual cramps in a cohort of college women. Br J Obstet Gynaecol 103:1134, 1996

Harris LA, Chang L: Irritable bowel syndrome: new and emerging therapies. Curr Opin Gastroenterol 22:128, 2006

Helms JM: Acupuncture for the management of primary dysmenorrhea. Obstet Gynaecol 69:51, 1987

Hendrix SL, Alexander NJ: Primary dysmenorrhea treatment with a desogestrel-containing low-dose oral contraceptive. Contraception 66:393, 2002

Herr KA, Spratt K, Mobily PR, et al: Pain intensity assessment in older adults: use of experimental pain to compare psychometric properties and usability of selected pain scales with younger adults. Clin J Pain 20:207, 2004

Hillis SD, Marchbanks PA, Peterson HB: The effectiveness of hysterectomy for chronic pelvic pain. Obstet Gynaecol 86:941, 1995

Hopayian K, Song F, Riera R, et al: The clinical features of the piriformis syndrome: a systematic review. Eur Spine J 19(12):2095, 2010

Howard FM: Chronic pelvic pain. Obstet Gynecol 101:594, 2003

Howard FM: The role of laparoscopy in chronic pelvic pain: promise and pitfalls. Obstet Gynecol Surv 48:357, 1993

Howard FM, El Minawi AM, Sanchez RA: Conscious pain mapping by laparoscopy in women with chronic pelvic pain. Obstet Gynaecol 96:934, 2000

Hsu CT, Rosioreanu A, Friedman RM, et al: Computed tomography imaging of the acute female pelvis. Contemp Diagn Radiol 28(18):1, 2005

Huchon C, Fauconnier A: Adnexal torsion: a literature review. Eur J Obstet Gynecol 150(1):8, 2010

Irwin P, Samsudin A: Reinvestigation of patients with a diagnosis of interstitial cystitis: common things are sometimes common. J Urol 174:584, 2005

Jacobs D: Diverticulitis. N Engl J Med 357(20):2057, 2007

Jamieson DJ, Steege JF: The association of sexual abuse with pelvic pain complaints in a primary care population. Am J Obstet Gynaecol 177:1408, 1997

Janicki TI: Chronic pelvic pain as a form of complex regional pain syndrome. Clin Obstet Gynaecol 46:797, 2003

Jones CA, Nyberg L: Epidemiology of interstitial cystitis. Urology 49(5A Suppl):2, 1997

Kang SB, Chung HH, Lee HP, et al: Impact of diagnostic laparoscopy on the management of chronic pelvic pain. Surg Endosc 21(6):916, 2007

Kaplan B, Peled Y, Pardo J, et al: Transcutaneous electrical nerve stimulation (TENS) as a relief for dysmenorrhea. Clin Exp Obstet Gynaecol 21:87, 1994

Kehlet H, Jensen TS, Woolf CJ: Persistent postsurgical pain: risk factors and prevention. Lancet 367:1618, 2006

Kennedy CM, Bradley CS, Galask RP, et al: Risk factors for painful bladder syndrome in women seeking gynecologic care. Int Urogynecol J 17:73, 2006

Kim HS, Malhotra AD, Rowe PC, et al: Embolotherapy for pelvic congestion syndrome: long-term results. J Vasc Intervent Radiol 17:289, 2006

Kirschner JS, Foye PM, Cole JL: Piriformis syndrome, diagnosis and treatment. Muscle Nerve 40(1):10, 2009

Kjerulff KH, Rhodes JC, Langenberg PW, et al: Patient satisfaction with results of hysterectomy. Am J Obstet Gynecol 183:1440, 2000

Knockaert DC, Boonen AL, Bruyninckx FL, et al: Electromyographic findings in ilioinguinal-iliohypogastric nerve entrapment syndrome. Acta Clin Belg 51:156, 1996

Koziol JA: Epidemiology of interstitial cystitis. Urol Clin North Am 21:7, 1994

Labelle H, Roussouly P, Berthonnaud E, et al: The importance of spino-pelvic balance in L5-S1 developmental spondylolisthesis: a review of pertinent radiologic measurements. Spine 30(6 Suppl):S27, 2005

Lafferty HW, Angioli R, Rudolph J, et al: Ovarian remnant syndrome: experience at Jackson Memorial Hospital, University of Miami, 1985 through 1993. Am J Obstet Gynaecol 174:641, 1996

Lampe A, Solder E, Ennemoser A, et al: Chronic pelvic pain and previous sexual abuse. Obstet Gynaecol 96:929, 2000

Laumann EO, Paik A, Rosen RC: Sexual dysfunction in the United States: prevalence and predictors. JAMA 281:537, 1999

Lavelle ED, Lavelle W, Smith HS: Myofascial trigger points. Med Clin North Am 91(2):229, 2007

Layer P, Keller J, Mueller-Lissner S, et al: Tegaserod: long-term treatment for irritable bowel syndrome patients with constipation in primary care. Digestion 71:238, 2005

Leschka S, Alkadhi H, Wildermuth S, et al: Acute abdominal pain: diagnostic strategies. In Marincek B, Dondelinger RF (eds): Emergency Radiology. New York, Springer, 2007, p 411

Lifford KL, Barbieri RL: Diagnosis and management of chronic pelvic pain. Urol Clin North Am 29:637, 2002

Longstreth GF, Thompson WG, Chey WD, et al: Functional bowel disorders. Gastroenterology 130:1480, 2006

Madura JA, Madura JA, Copper CM, et al: Inguinal neurectomy for inguinal nerve entrapment: an experience with 100 patients. Am J Surg 189:283, 2005

Magtibay PM, Nyholm JL, Hernandez JL, et al: Ovarian remnant syndrome. Am J Obstet Gynecol 193:2062, 2005

Maizels M, McCarberg B: Antidepressants and antiepileptic drugs for chronic non-cancer pain. Am Fam Physician 71:483, 2005

Maleux G, Stockx L, Wilms G, et al: Ovarian vein embolization for the treatment of pelvic congestion syndrome: long-term technical and clinical results. J Vasc Intervent Radiol 11:859, 2000

Marjoribanks J, Proctor ML, Farquhar C: Nonsteroidal anti-inflammatory drugs for primary dysmenorrhoea. Cochrane Database Syst Rev 4:CD001751, 2003

Mathias SD, Kuppermann M, Liberman RF, et al: Chronic pelvic pain: prevalence, health-related quality of life, and economic correlates. Obstet Gynecol 87:321, 1996

Mayer E: Irritable bowel syndrome. N Engl J Med 358(16):1692, 2008

McHale PM, LoVecchio F: Narcotic analgesia in the acute abdomen—a review of prospective trials. Eur J Emerg Med 8:131, 2001

McPartland JM: Travell trigger points—molecular and osteopathic perspectives. J Am Osteopath Assoc 104:244, 2004

Melzack R: The short-form McGill Pain Questionnaire. Pain 30(2):191, 1987

Mens JM, Vleeming A, Stoeckart R, et al: Understanding peripartum pelvic pain: implications of a patient survey. Spine 21(11):1363, 1996

Messing EM, Stamey TA: Interstitial cystitis: early diagnosis, pathology, and treatment. Urology 12:381, 1978

Metts JF: Interstitial cystitis: urgency and frequency syndrome. Am Fam Physician 64:1199, 2001

Miklos JR, O'Reilly MJ, Saye WB: Sciatic hernia as a cause of chronic pelvic pain in women. Obstet Gynaecol 91:998, 1998

Miller SK, Alpert PT: Assessment and differential diagnosis of abdominal pain. Nurse Pract 31:38, 2006

Milsom I, Sundell G, Andersch B: The influence of different combined oral contraceptives on the prevalence and severity of dysmenorrhea. Contraception 42:497, 1990

Moreno-Egea A, La Calle MC, Torralba-Martinez JA, et al: Obturator hernia as a cause of chronic pain after inguinal hernioplasty: elective management using tomography and ambulatory total extraperitoneal laparoscopy. Surg Laparosc Endosc Percutan Tech 16:54, 2006

Moschos E, Twickler DM: Does the type of intrauterine device affect conspicuity on 2D and 3D ultrasound? AJR Am J Roentgenol 196(6):1439, 2011

Nezhat C, Kearney S, Malik S, et al: Laparoscopic management of ovarian remnant. Fertil Steril 83:973, 2005

Nezhat CH, Seidman DS, Nezhat FR, et al: Ovarian remnant syndrome after laparoscopic oophorectomy. Fertil Steril 74:1024, 2000

Nigro DA, Wein AJ, Foy M, et al: Associations among cystoscopic and urodynamic findings for women enrolled in the Interstitial Cystitis Data Base (ICDB) Study. Urology 49(5A Suppl):86, 1997

Novi JM, Jeronis S, Srinivas S, et al: Risk of irritable bowel syndrome and depression in women with interstitial cystitis: a case-control study. J Urol 174:937, 2005

Orford VP, Kuhn RJ: Management of ovarian remnant syndrome. Aust N Z J Obstet Gynaecol 36:468, 1996

Pace S, Burke TF: Intravenous morphine for early pain relief in patients with acute abdominal pain. Acad Emerg Med 3:1086, 1996

Paras ML, Murad MH, Chen LP, et al: Sexual abuse and lifetime diagnosis of somatic disorders: a systematic review and meta-analysis. JAMA 302(5):550, 2009

Park SJ, Lim JW, Ko YT, et al: Diagnosis of pelvic congestion syndrome using transabdominal and transvaginal sonography. Am J Roentgenol 182:683, 2004

Parker JD, Sinaii N, Segars JH, et al: Adhesion formation after laparoscopic excision of endometriosis and lysis of adhesions. Fertil Steril 84:1457, 2005

Parsons CL: Prostatitis, interstitial cystitis, chronic pelvic pain, and urethral syndrome share a common pathophysiology: lower urinary dysfunctional epithelium and potassium recycling. Urology 62:976, 2003

Paterson LQ, Davis SN, Khalifé S, et al: Persistent genital and pelvic pain after childbirth. J Sex Med 6(1):215, 2009

Paulson JD, Delgado M: Relationship between interstitial cystitis and endometriosis in patients with chronic pelvic pain. J Soc Laparoendosc Surg 11(2):175, 2007

Payne A, Blanchard EB: Controlled comparison of cognitive therapy and self-help support groups in the treatment of irritable bowel syndrome. J Consult Clin Psychol 63:779, 1995

Perry CP: Peripheral neuropathies and pelvic pain: diagnosis and management. Clin Obstet Gynaecol 46:789, 2003

Perry CP, Presthus J, Nieves A: Laparoscopic uterine suspension for pain relief: a multicenter study. J Reprod Med 50:567, 2005

Petchprapa CN, Rosenberg ZS, Sconfienza LM, et al: MR imaging of entrapment neuropathies of the lower extremity. Part 1. The pelvis and hip. Radiographics 30(4):983, 2010

Peters AAW, Trimbos-Kemper GCM, Admiraal C, et al: A randomized clinical trial on the benefit of adhesiolysis in patients with intraperitoneal adhesions and chronic pelvic pain. Br J Obstet Gynaecol 99:59, 1992

Peters KM, Carrico DJ, Kalinowski SE, et al: Prevalence of pelvic floor dysfunction in patients with interstitial cystitis. Urology. 70(1):16, 2007

Proctor M, Farquhar C: Diagnosis and management of dysmenorrhoea. BMJ 332:1134, 2006

Proctor ML, Latthe PM, Farquhar CM, et al: Surgical interruption of pelvic nerve pathways for primary and secondary dysmenorrhoea. Cochrane Database Syst Rev 4:CD001896, 2005

Propert KJ, Schaeffer AJ, Brensinger CM, et al: A prospective study of interstitial cystitis: results of longitudinal follow-up of the interstitial cystitis data base cohort. The Interstitial Cystitis Data Base Study Group. J Urol 163:1434, 2000

Quartero AO, Meineche-Schmidt V, Muris J, et al: Bulking agents, antispasmodic and antidepressant medication for the treatment of irritable bowel syndrome. Cochrane Database Syst Rev 2:CD003460, 2005

Raman SS, Osuagwu FC, Kadell B, et al: Effect of CT on false positive diagnosis of appendicitis and perforation. N Engl J Med 358(9):972, 2008

Ramkumar D, Rao SSC: Efficacy and safety of traditional medical therapies for chronic constipation: systematic review. Am J Gastroenterol 100:936, 2005

Reginald PW, Adams J, Franks S, et al: Medroxyprogesterone acetate in the treatment of pelvic pain due to venous congestion. Br J Obstet Gynaecol 96:1148, 1989

Reissing ED, Brown C, Lord MJ, et al: Pelvic floor muscle functioning in women with vulvar vestibulitis syndrome. J Psychosom Obstet Gynecol 26:107, 2005

Reuter HJ: Bladder. In Atlas of Urologic Endoscopy Diagnosis and Treatment. New York, Thieme Medical Publishers, 1987, p 85

Rockey DC: Occult gastrointestinal bleeding. Gastroenterol Clin North Am 34:699, 2005

Rogers RM Jr: Basic pelvic neuroanatomy. In Steege JF, Metzger DA, Levy BS (eds): Chronic Pelvic Pain: An Integrated Approach. Philadelphia, WB Saunders, 1998, p. 46

Roman H, Hulsey TF, Marpeau L, et al: Why laparoscopic adhesiolysis should not be the victim of a single randomized clinical trial. Am J Obstet Gynecol 200(2):136.e1, 2009

Rovner E, Propert KJ, Brensinger C, et al: Treatments used in women with interstitial cystitis: the Interstitial Cystitis Data Base (ICDB) study experience. The Interstitial Cystitis Data Base Study Group. Urology 56:940, 2000

Saarto T, Wiffen PJ: Antidepressants for neuropathic pain. Cochrane Database Syst Rev 3:CD005454, 2005

Saito YA, Schoenfeld P, Locke GR, III: The epidemiology of irritable bowel syndrome in North America: a systematic review. Am J Gastroenterol 97:1910, 2002

Sant GR, Kempuraj D, Marchand JE, et al: The mast cell in interstitial cystitis: role in pathophysiology and pathogenesis. Urology 69(4 Suppl):34, 2007

Sauerland S, Agresta F, Bergamaschi R, et al: Laparoscopy for abdominal emergencies: evidence-based guidelines of the European Association for Endoscopic Surgery. Surg Endosc 20:14, 2006

Schoenfeld P: Efficacy of current drug therapies in irritable bowel syndrome: what works and does not work. Gastroenterol Clin North Am 34:319, 2005

Servant CT: An unusual cause of sciatica. A case report. Spine 23:2134, 1998

Sharma D, Dahiya K, Duhan N, et al: Diagnostic laparoscopy in chronic pelvic pain. Arch Gynecol Obstet 283(2):295, 2011

Sharp HT: Myofascial pain syndrome of the abdominal wall for the busy clinician. Clin Obstet Gynaecol 46:783, 2003

Signorello LB, Harlow BL, Chekos AK, et al: Postpartum sexual functioning and its relationship to perineal trauma: a retrospective cohort study of primiparous women. Am J Obstet Gynecol 184:881, 2001

Simons DG, Travell JG: Travell and Simons' Myofascial Pain and Dysfunction: the Trigger Point Manual, 2nd ed. Baltimore, Williams & Wilkins, 1999

Smith-Bindman R: Is computed tomography safe? N Engl J Med 363(1):1, 2010

Smith-Bindman R, Lipson J, Marcus R, et al: Radiation dose associated with common computed tomography examinations and the associated lifetime attributable risk of cancer. Arch Intern Med 169(22):2078, 2009

Soysal ME, Soysal S, Vicdan K, et al: A randomized controlled trial of goserelin and medroxyprogesterone acetate in the treatment of pelvic congestion. Hum Reprod 16:931, 2001

Spinelli M, Malaguti S, Giardiello G, et al: A new minimally invasive procedure for pudendal nerve stimulation to treat neurogenic bladder: description of the method and preliminary data. Neurourol Urodyn 24(4):305, 2005

Srinivasan R, Greenbaum DS: Chronic abdominal wall pain: a frequently overlooked problem. Practical approach to diagnosis and management. Am J Gastroenterol 97:824, 2002

Stav K, Dwyer P, Roberts F, et al: Pudendal neuralgia fact or fiction? Obstet Gynecol Surv 64(3):190, 2009

Steege JF, Stout AL: Resolution of chronic pelvic pain after laparoscopic lysis of adhesions. Am J Obstet Gynecol 165:278, 1991

Stovall TG, Ling FW, Crawford DA: Hysterectomy for chronic pelvic pain of presumed uterine etiology. Obstet Gynecol 75:676, 1990

Sulak PJ, Cressman BE, Waldrop E, et al: Extending the duration of active oral contraceptive pills to manage hormone withdrawal symptoms. Obstet Gynecol 89:179, 1997

Suleiman S, Johnston DE: The abdominal wall: an overlooked source of pain. Am Fam Physician 64:431, 2001

Sundell G, Milsom I, Andersch B: Factors influencing the prevalence and severity of dysmenorrhoea in young women. Br J Obstet Gynaecol 7:588, 1990

Sutton C, MacDonald R: Laser laparoscopic adhesiolysis. J Gynecol Surg 6:155, 1990

Swank DJ, Swank-Bordewijk SCG, Hop WCJ, et al: Laparoscopic adhesiolysis in patients with chronic abdominal pain: a blinded randomised controlled multi-centre trial. Lancet 361:1247, 2003

Swanton A, Iyer L, Reginald PW: Diagnosis, treatment and follow up of women undergoing conscious pain mapping for chronic pelvic pain: a prospective cohort study. BJOG 113:792, 2006

Tabas G, Beaves M, Wang J, et al: Paroxetine to treat irritable bowel syndrome not responding to high-fiber diet: a double-blind, placebo-controlled trial. Am J Gastroenterol 99:914, 2004

Tack J, Muller-Lissner S, Bytzer P, et al: A randomised controlled trial assessing the efficacy and safety of repeated tegaserod therapy in women with irritable bowel syndrome with constipation. Gut 54:1707, 2005

Thompson WG, Longstreth GF, Drossman DA, et al: Functional bowel disorders and functional abdominal pain. Gut 45(Suppl 2):II43, 1999

Thomson WH, Dawes RF, Carter SS: Abdominal wall tenderness: a useful sign in chronic abdominal pain. Br J Surg 78:223, 1991

Thornton JG, Morley S, Lilleyman J, et al: The relationship between laparoscopic disease, pelvic pain and infertility; an unbiased assessment. Eur J Obstet Gynaecol Reprod Biol 74:57, 1997

Tropeano G, Di Stasi C, Amoroso S, et al: Ovarian vein incompetence: a potential cause of chronic pelvic pain in women. Eur J Obstet Gynecol Reprod Biol 139(2):215, 2008

Twickler DM, Moschos E: Ultrasound and assessment of ovarian cancer risk. AJR Am J Roentgenol 194(2):322, 2010

Umeoka S, Koyama T, Togashi K, et al: Vascular dilatation in the pelvis: identification with CT and MR imaging. Radiographics 24:193, 2004

U.S. Food and Drug Administration: Lotronex (alosetron hydrochloride) information. 2009. Available at: http://www.fda.gov/Drugs/DrugSafety/PostmarketDrugSafetyInformationforPatientsandProviders/ucm110450.htm. Accessed October 8, 2010

U.S. Food and Drug Administration: Zelnorm (tegaserod maleate) Information. 2010. Available at: http://www.fda.gov/Drugs/DrugSafety/PostmarketDrugSafetyInformationforPatientsandProviders/ucm103223.htm. Accessed October 8, 2010

Vahedi H, Merat S, Rashidioon A, et al: The effect of fluoxetine in patients with pain and constipation-predominant irritable bowel syndrome: a double-blind randomized-controlled study. Aliment Pharmacol Ther 22:381, 2005

Van der Windt DA, Jellema P, Mulder CJ, et al: Diagnostic testing for celiac disease among patients with abdominal symptoms: a systematic review. JAMA 303(17):1738, 2010

Varma R, Sinha D, Gupta JK: Non-contraceptive uses of levonorgestrel-releasing hormone system (LNG-IUS)—a systematic enquiry and overview. Eur J Obstet Gynecol Reprod Biol 125:9, 2006

Venbrux AC, Chang AH, Kim HS, et al: Pelvic congestion syndrome (pelvic venous incompetence): impact of ovarian and internal iliac vein embolotherapy on menstrual cycle and chronic pelvic pain. J Vasc Intervent Radiol 13:171, 2002

Venbrux AC, Lambert DL: Embolization of the ovarian veins as a treatment for patients with chronic pelvic pain caused by pelvic venous incompetence (pelvic congestion syndrome). Curr Opin Obstet Gynecol 11:395, 1999

Vercellini P, Somigliana E, Viganò P, et al: Chronic pelvic pain in women: etiology, pathogenesis and diagnostic approach. Gynecol Endocrinol 25(3):149, 2009

Vermani E, Mittal R, Weeks A: Pelvic girdle pain and low back pain in pregnancy: a review. Pain Pract 10(1):60, 2010

Vleeming A, Albert HB, Ostgaard HC, et al: European guidelines for the diagnosis and treatment of pelvic girdle pain. Eur Spine J 17(6):794, 2008

Warren JW, Keay SK: Interstitial cystitis. Curr Opin Urol 12:69, 2002

Weissman AM, Hartz AJ, Hansen MD, et al: The natural history of primary dysmenorrhoea: a longitudinal study. BJOG 111:345, 2004

Whiteside JL, Barber MD, Walters MD, et al: Anatomy of ilioinguinal and iliohypogastric nerves in relation to trocar placement and low transverse incisions. Am J Obstet Gynaecol 189:1574, 2003

Wiffen PJ, McQuay HJ, Edwards JE, et al: Gabapentin for acute and chronic pain. Cochrane Database Syst Rev 3:CD005452, 2005a

Wiffen PJ, McQuay HJ, Moore RA: Carbamazepine for acute and chronic pain. Cochrane Database Syst Rev 3:CD005451, 2005b

Wilson ML, Murphy PA: Herbal and dietary therapies for primary and secondary dysmenorrhoea. Cochrane Database Syst Rev 3:CD002124, 2001

Wu WH, Meijer OG, Uegaki K, et al: Pregnancy-related pelvic girdle pain (PPP), I: terminology, clinical presentation, and prevalence. Eur Spine J 13(7):575, 2004

Yoshimoto H, Sato S, Masuda T, et al: Spinopelvic alignment in patients with osteoarthrosis of the hip: a radiographic comparison to patients with low back pain. Spine 30:1650, 2005

Zhang WY, Li Wan PA: Efficacy of minor analgesics in primary dysmenorrhoea: a systematic review. Br J Obstet Gynaecol 105:780, 1998

Ziaei S, Faghihzadeh S, Sohrabvand F, et al: A randomised placebo-controlled trial to determine the effect of vitamin E in treatment of primary dysmenorrhoea. BJOG 108:1181, 2001

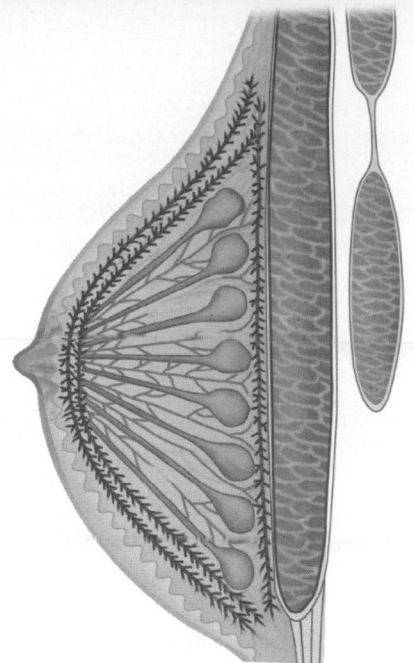

Breast disease in women encompasses a spectrum of benign and malignant disorders, which present most commonly as breast pain, nipple discharge, or palpable mass. The specific causes of these symptoms vary with patient age. Benign dis orders predominate in young premenopausal women, whereas malignancy rates increase with advancing age. Evaluation of breast disorders usually requires the combination of a careful history, physical examination, imaging, and when indicated, biopsy.

ANATOMY

Ductal System

The glandular portion of the breast is comprised of 12 to 15 independent ductal systems that each drain approximately 40 lobules (Fig. 12-1). Each lobule consists of 10 to 100 milk-producing acini that drain into small terminal ducts (Parks, 1959). Terminal ducts drain into larger collecting ducts that merge into even larger ducts, which exhibit a saccular dilation just below the nipple called a lactiferous sinus (Fig. 12-2).

In general, only six to eight openings are visible on the nipple surface. These drain the dominant ductal systems, which account for approximately 80 percent of the breast's glandular volume (Going, 2004). Minor ducts either terminate just below the nipple surface or open on the areola near the base of the nipple. The areola itself contains numerous lubricating sebaceous glands, called Montgomery glands, which are often visible as punctate prominences.

In addition to epithelial structures, the breast is composed of varying proportions of collagenous stroma and fat. The distribution and abundance of these stromal components accounts for a breast's consistency when palpated and for its imaging characteristics.

Lymphatic Drainage

Afferent lymphatic drainage of the breast is provided by dermal, subdermal, interlobar, and prepectoral systems (Fig. 12-3) (Grant, 1953). Each of these may be viewed as a lattice of valveless channels that interconnect with every other system and that ultimately drain into one or two axillary lymph nodes

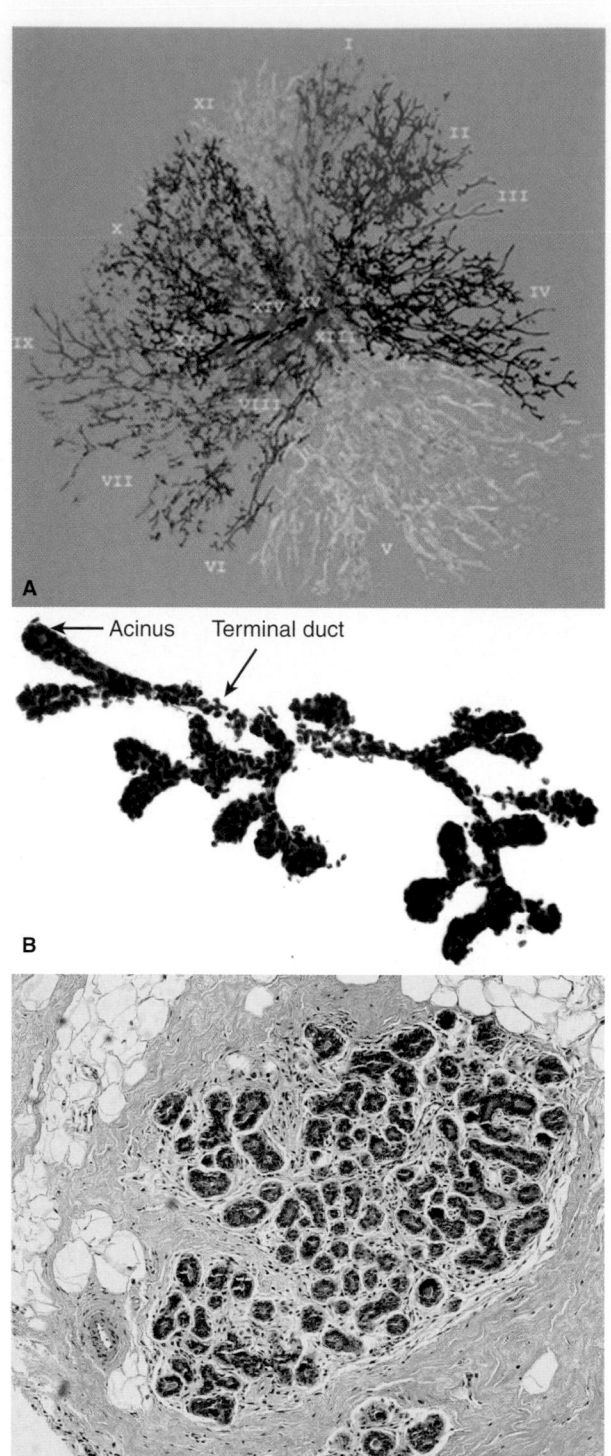

FIGURE 12-1 A. Ductal anatomy of the breast. *(From Going, 2004, with permission.)* **B.** Terminal duct-acinar structure from a fine-needle aspiration biopsy. **C.** Histology of a normal lobule.

(the sentinel nodes). Because all of these systems are interconnected, the breast drains as a unit, and injection of colloidal dyes in any part of the breast at any level will result in accumulation of dye in the same one or two axillary sentinel lymph nodes. The axillary lymph nodes receive most of the lymphatic drainage of the breast, and consequently are the nodes most frequently involved with breast cancer metastases (Hultborn, 1955). However, there are also alternate drainage pathways that do not appear to interconnect with other networks and that drain directly into internal mammary, supraclavicular, contralateral axillary, or abdominal lymph node basins.

DEVELOPMENT AND PHYSIOLOGY

During fetal development, the primordial breast arises from the basal layer of the epidermis. Before puberty, the breast is a rudimentary bud comprised of a few branching ducts capped with alveolar buds, end buds, or small lobules (Osin, 1998). At puberty, usually between the ages of 10 and 13 years, ovarian estrogen and progesterone cooperate to direct organized communication between breast epithelial cells and mesenchymal cells, resulting in extensive branching of the ductal system and development of lobules (Ismail, 2003). Specific disorders of this development are discussed in Chapter 14 (p. 390). Final differentiation of the breast is mediated by progesterone and prolactin and is not completed until the first full-term pregnancy (Grimm, 2002; Ismail, 2003).

During the reproductive years, terminal ducts near the acini and the acini themselves are most sensitive to ovarian hormones and prolactin. Most forms of benign and malignant breast disease arise in these terminal duct-acinar structures. Breast epithelial cells proliferate during the luteal phase of the menstrual cycle when estrogen and progesterone levels are increased, and then undergo programmed cell death at the end of the luteal phase, when levels of these hormones decline (Anderson, 1982; Soderqvist, 1997). This effect is mediated by paracrine signaling induced by estrogen receptor activation and is associated with an increase in the water content of the extracellular matrix (Stoeckelhuber, 2002). This is often recognized as breast fullness and tenderness the week preceding menses.

At menopause, when ovarian estrogen production ceases, breast lobules involute, and the collagenous stroma is replaced by fat. Because estrogen receptor expression is negatively regulated by estrogen, there is an increase in estrogen receptor expression after menopause (Khan, 1997). Despite a decline in ovarian estrogen production, postmenopausal women continue to produce estrogen through the action of the enzyme aromatase, which converts adrenal androgens to estrogen (Bulun, 1994). Aromatase is found in fat, muscle, and breast tissue.

EVALUATION OF A BREAST LUMP

It is not possible to distinguish benign from malignant or cystic from solid breast masses by clinical examination. However, findings from clinical examination, interpreted in conjunction with imaging and pathology (the triple test), contribute significantly to management decisions (Hermansen, 1987).

Physical Examination

The breast is comma shaped, and the comma's tail corresponds to the axillary tail of Spence. This extension can be large, especially during pregnancy and lactation, and is frequently mistaken for an axillary mass.

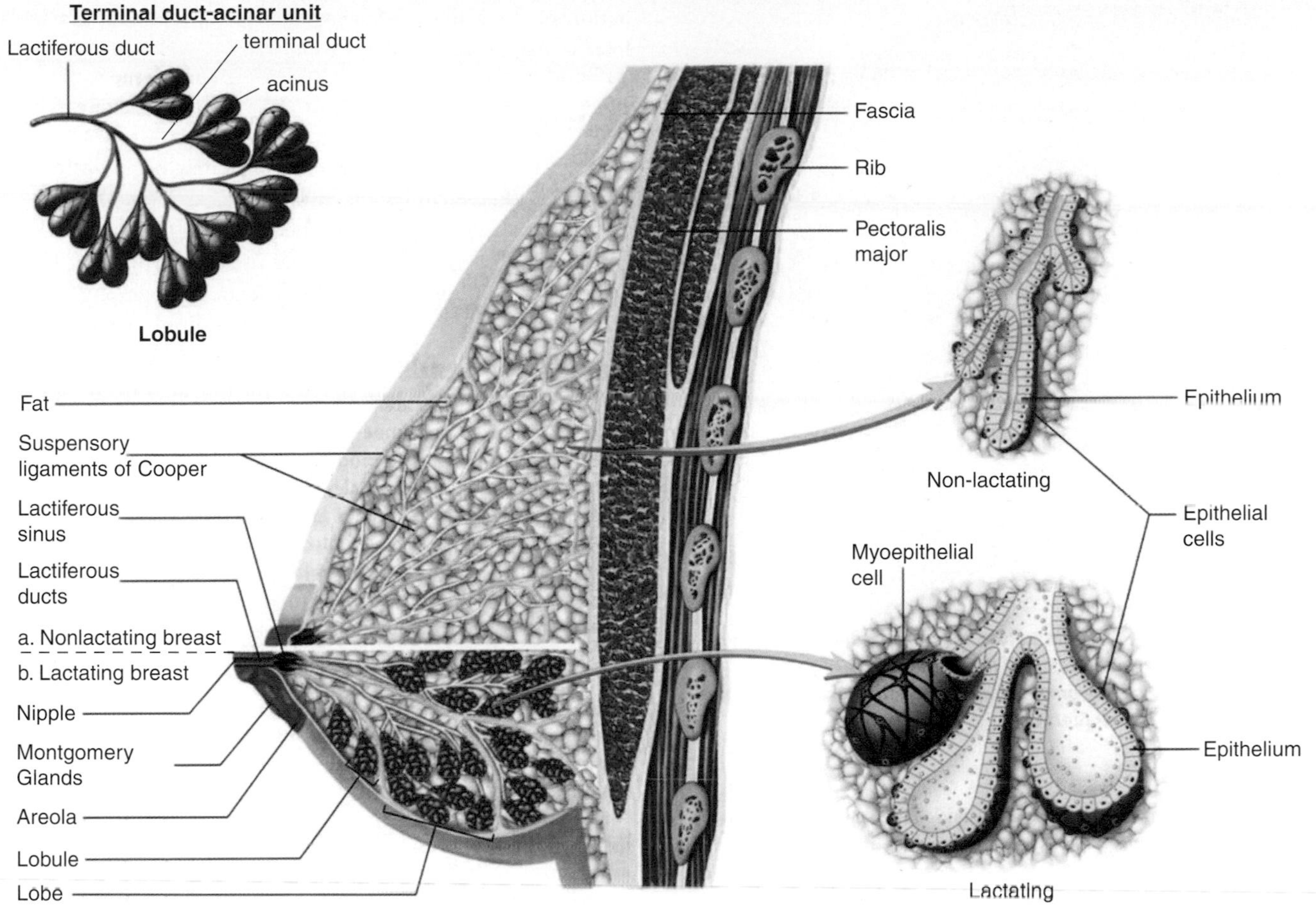

Terminal duct-acinar unit
Lactiferous duct
terminal duct
acinus
Lobule
Fascia
Rib
Pectoralis major
Fat
Suspensory ligaments of Cooper
Lactiferous sinus
Lactiferous ducts
a. Nonlactating breast
b. Lactating breast
Nipple
Montgomery Glands
Areola
Lobule
Lobe
Epithelium
Non-lactating
Epithelial cells
Myoepithelial cell
Epithelium
Lactating

FIGURE 12-2 Breast anatomy. *(From Seeley, 2006, with permission.)*

Clinical examination of the breast begins with inspection of the breast to determine whether there is dimpling, nipple retraction, or skin changes. This examination is described further in Chapter 1 (p. 3). The presence and character of expressible nipple discharge is recorded. In addition, the location of a mass is specifically documented according to its clock position and then measured along the long axis using a ruler or caliper (Fig. 12-4). The distance from the center of the nipple to the center of the mass is specified. Since many health care providers are typically involved in the evaluation and management of the same breast mass, the most useful entry in the clinical record will define the location and size of the mass (e.g., right

Subclavicular nodes
Superior
Internal mammary nodes
External mammary nodes
To axillary nodes of opposite side
Sappey
Lateral
Medial
Circumareolar
Inferior
A
Right breast
Subclavius muscle
Axillary vein
Apical nodes
I Transmuscular or transpectoral lymphatic paths
I
Rotter's node (Interpectoral node)
Pectoralis minor
II
II Retromuscular or retropectoral lymphatic path
Pectoralis major
B

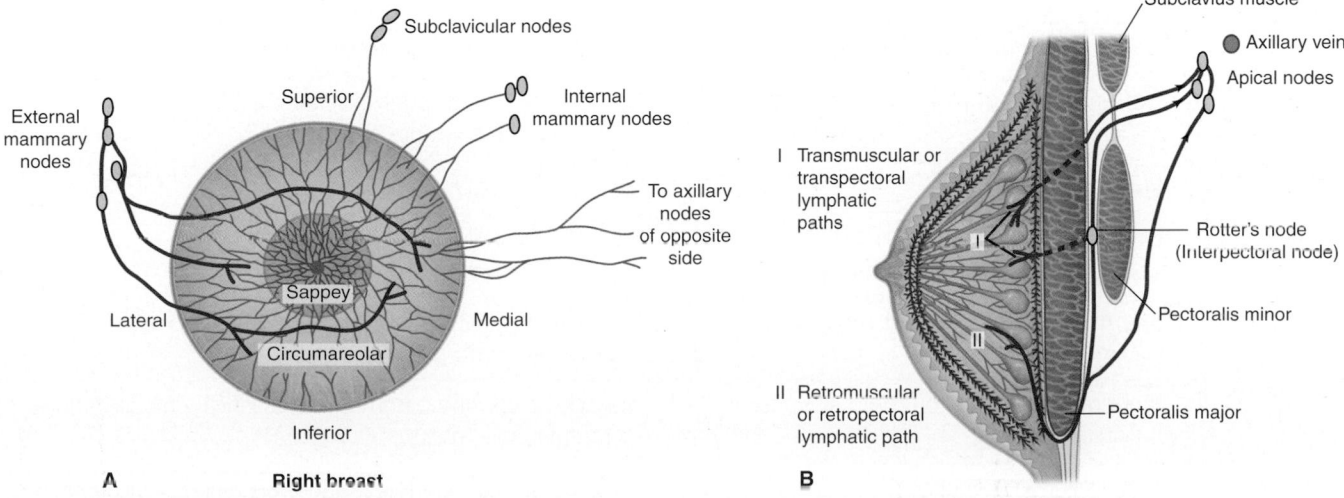

FIGURE 12-3 Lymphatic drainage of the breast. **A.** Accessory drainage pathways. **B.** Classic axillary drainage pathways. *(From Grant, 1953, with permission.)*

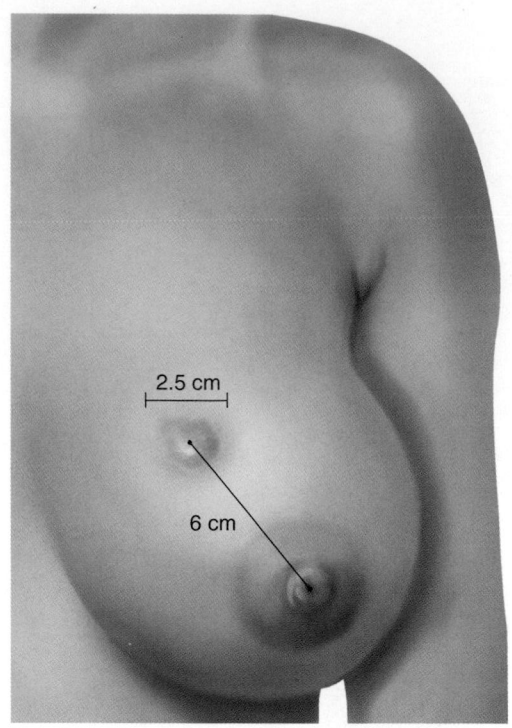

FIGURE 12-4 Recording the location of a breast mass as "Left breast, 2.5-cm mass, 10:00, 6 cm FN." FN = from the nipple.

breast, 2-cm mass, 3:00, 4 cm from the nipple). Although clinical examination alone can never exclude malignancy, noting that a mass has benign features such as smoothness, roundness, and mobility will factor into the ultimate decision to excise or observe a lesion. Evaluation should also include careful exami-

nation of the axillae, infraclavicular fossa, and supraclavicular fossa (Chap. 1, p. 3).

Diagnostic Imaging

Diagnostic imaging of a suspected mass may begin with mammography that includes magnification, extra compression, or extra views beyond the usual medial lateral oblique and cranial caudal views that are typically used for screening. Unlike screening mammography, diagnostic mammography may be appropriate for women of any age. In addition, sonography is invaluable for determining whether a mass is cystic or solid and is a component of most diagnostic imaging algorithms. Certain features of solid masses, such as irregular margins, internal echoes, or a width-to-height ratio <1.7, may suggest malignancy (Stavros, 1995).

Breast Imaging Reporting and Data System

Diagnostic imaging results should be summarized according to the Breast Imaging Reporting and Data System (BI-RADS) classification (Table 12-1) (D'Orsi, 1998). Lesions that are graded BI-RADS 5 are highly suggestive of malignancy, and ≥95 percent of these are ultimately proven to be cancerous. Decreasing numerical grades are associated with diminishing probability of malignancy.

Breast Biopsy

Evaluation of a solid breast mass is completed by needle biopsy. These biopsies should be performed after an imaging test or a minimum of 2 weeks prior to an imaging test, as resulting

TABLE 12-1. Breast Imaging Reporting and Data System (BI-RADS)

BI-RADS Category	Description	Examples
0	Additional views or sonography required	Focal asymmetry, microcalcifications, or a mass identified on a screening mammogram
1	No abnormalities identified	Normal fat and fibroglandular tissue
2	Not entirely normal, but definitely benign	Fat necrosis from a prior excision, stable biopsy-proven fibroadenoma, stable cyst
3	Probably benign	Circumscribed mass that has been followed for <2 years
4A	Low suspicion for malignancy, but intervention required	Probable fibroadenoma, complicated cyst
4B	Intermediate suspicion for malignancy, intervention required	Partially indistinctly marginated mass otherwise consistent with a fibroadenoma
4C	Moderate suspicion, but not classic for carcinoma	New cluster of fine pleomorphic calcifications, ill-defined irregular solid mass
5	Almost certainly malignant	Spiculated mass, fine linear and branching calcifications
6	Biopsy-proven carcinoma	Biopsy-proven carcinoma

TABLE 12-2. Performance Characteristics of the Concordant Triple Test[a]

Citation	Number	Sensitivity	Specificity	Positive Predictive Value	Negative Predictive Value	Accuracy
Hermansen, 1987	458	1.00	0.74	0.64	1.00	0.82
Kreuzer, 1976	240	0.99	0.99	0.99	0.99	0.99
Kaufman, 1994	159	1.00	0.98	0.98	1.00	0.99
Hardy, 1990	116	0.98	0.53	0.68	0.97	0.76
Thomas, 2002	108	0.98	1.00	1.00	0.98	0.99
Butler, 1990	86	1.00	0.52	0.97	1.00	0.98
Du Toit, 1992	73	1.00	1.00	1.00	1.00	1.00

[a]Cytologic diagnoses of "definitively malignant" and "suspicious for malignancy" are considered positive. The triple test includes clinical examination, imaging, and needle biopsy. Only cases that were malignant by all three tests or benign by all three tests are included in the calculations.

tissue trauma can produce image artifacts that simulate malignancy (Sickles, 1983). Options include fine-needle aspiration (FNA) biopsy or core-needle biopsy (Boerner, 1999). The trend in recent years has been to prefer core-needle biopsy (Tabbara, 2000). Although FNA takes less time to perform and is less expensive than core-needle biopsy, it is less likely to provide a specific diagnosis and has a higher insufficient sample rate (Shannon, 2001). Fine-needle aspiration retrieves clusters of epithelial cells that may be interpreted as benign or malignant, but cannot reliably differentiate between benign proliferative lesions and fibroepithelial neoplasms or between ductal carcinoma in situ and invasive cancer (Boerner, 1999; Ringberg, 2001).

In contrast, core-needle biopsy is performed using an automated device that takes one core at a time or is completed using a vacuum-assisted device that, once initially positioned, delivers multiple cores. Needle biopsy of solid masses is generally preferred prior to excision, as the results of the biopsy contribute significantly to surgical planning (Cox, 1995).

Triple Test

The combination of clinical examination, imaging, and needle biopsy is called the *triple test*. When all three assessments suggest a benign lesion or all three suggest a breast cancer, the triple test is said to be concordant. A concordant benign triple test is >99-percent accurate, and breast lumps in this category can be followed by clinical examination alone at 6-month intervals (Table 12-2). If any of the three assessments suggests malignancy, the lump should be excised regardless of results from the other two. It is always appropriate to offer excision of a fully evaluated breast lump, even after a benign concordant triple test, as breast lumps can be a source of significant anxiety.

Cysts

Most breast cysts arise from apocrine metaplasia of lobular acini. They are generally lined by a single layer of epithelium

that ranges from flattened to columnar. From one autopsy series that included 725 women, investigators reported microcysts in 58 percent and cysts >1 cm in 21 percent (Davies, 1964). The incidence of breast cysts peaks between 40 and 50 years, and the lifetime incidence of palpable breast cysts is estimated to be 7 percent (Haagensen, 1986b).

Breast cysts are diagnosed and classified by sonographic examination. There are three types of cysts: simple, complicated, and complex (Berg, 2003). Simple cysts are sonolucent, have a smooth margin, and show enhanced through-transmission (Fig. 12-5). These lesions do not require special management or monitoring, but they may be aspirated if painful. Recurrent cysts can be reimaged and reaspirated, but recurrent symptomatic cysts are best managed by excision.

Complicated cysts show internal echoes during sonography and can sometimes be indistinguishable from solid masses. Internal echoes are usually caused by proteinaceous debris, but all complicated cysts should be aspirated. The aspirated material may be submitted for culture if it is purulent, or for cytology if there are worrisome clinical or imaging features. If the sonographic abnormality does not resolve completely with aspiration, a core-needle biopsy is usually performed.

Complex cysts show septa or intracystic masses during sonographic evaluation. An intracystic mass usually represents a papilloma, but medullary carcinoma, papillary carcinoma, and some infiltrating ductal carcinomas can present as complex cysts. Although some have advocated core-needle biopsy for the evaluation of complex cysts, this procedure can decompress a cyst, making it difficult to localize at the time of surgery. Additionally, papillary lesions diagnosed by needle biopsy will require excision. Thus, it seems reasonable to recommend excision of all complex cysts.

Fibroadenoma

Fibroadenomas represent a focal developmental abnormality of a breast lobule and as such are not true neoplasms.

Definitive diagnosis

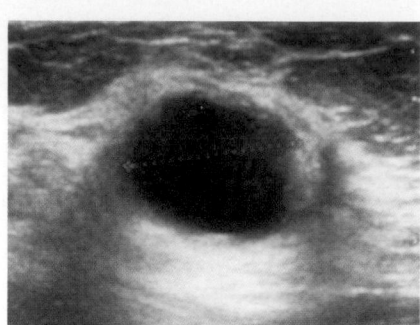

Simple cyst

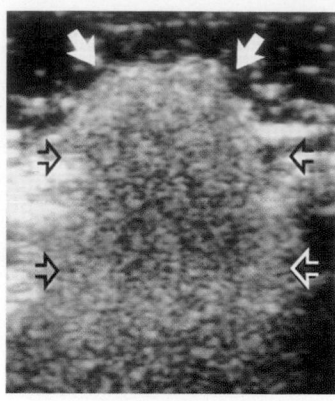

Silicone

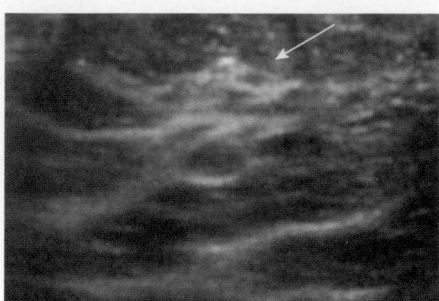

Fibroglandular ridge

Requires needle biopsy

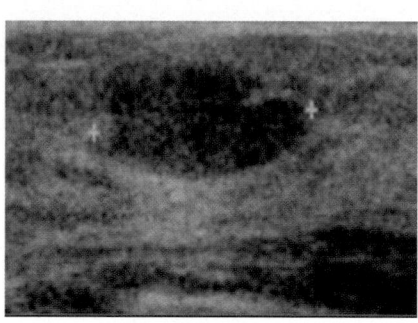

Solid - benign

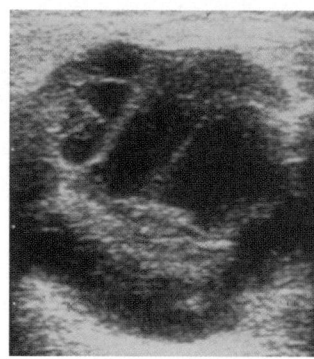

Complex cyst

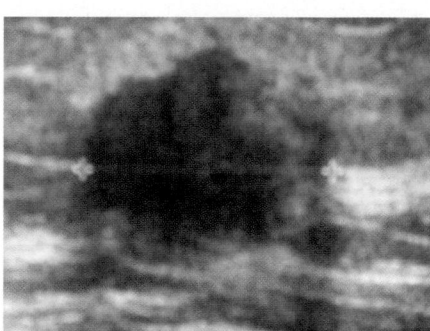

Suspicious

FIGURE 12-5 Sonographic appearance of palpable breast masses.

Histologically, fibroadenomas are comprised of glandular and cystic epithelial structures surrounded by a cellular stroma. Fibroadenomas account for 7 to 13 percent of breast clinic visits and had a prevalence of 9 percent in one autopsy series (Dent, 1988; Franyz, 1951). They often present in adolescence, are recognized most frequently in premenopausal women, and usually spontaneously involute at menopause.

Fibroadenomas classified as benign concordant by the triple test can be safely followed without excision. Because some fibroadenomas may grow large, and because benign phyllodes tumors are often indistinguishable from fibroadenomas by imaging and needle biopsy, a fibroadenoma that is growing should be excised.

Phyllodes Tumors

Histologically, phyllodes tumors are similar to fibroadenomas in that epithelial-lined spaces are surrounded by cellular stroma. However, with phyllodes tumors, the stromal cells are monoclonal and neoplastic. Phyllodes tumors are classified as benign, intermediate, or malignant, based on the degree of stromal cell atypia, number of mitoses, tumor margin characteristics, and abundance of stromal cells (Oberman, 1965). Phyllodes tumors account for less than 1 percent of breast neoplasms, and the median age at diagnosis is 40 years (Haagensen, 1986a; Reinfuss, 1996).

Malignant phyllodes tumors can metastasize to distant organs, with lung being the primary site. Chest radiographs or chest computed-tomography (CT) scanning are appropriate staging tests for malignant cases. Phyllodes tumors rarely metastasize to lymph nodes, thus axillary staging is not required unless there are clinically involved nodes (Chaney, 2000).

Treatment consists of wide local excision with a minimum 1-cm margin. Mastectomy may be required to achieve this margin, as the median tumor size at presentation is 5 cm. Local recurrence rates for completely excised tumors range from 8 percent for benign lesions to 36 percent for malignant lesions (Barth, 1999).

NIPPLE DISCHARGE

Fluid can be expressed from the nipple ducts of at least 40 percent of premenopausal women, 55 percent of parous women, and 74 percent of women who have lactated within 2 years (Wrensch, 1990). The fluid generally issues from more than one duct and may range from milky white to dark green or brown. Green coloration is related to the content of cholesterol diepoxides and is not suggestive of underlying infection or malignancy (Petrakis, 1988).

Multiduct discharges that are elicited only following manual expression are considered physiologic and do not require

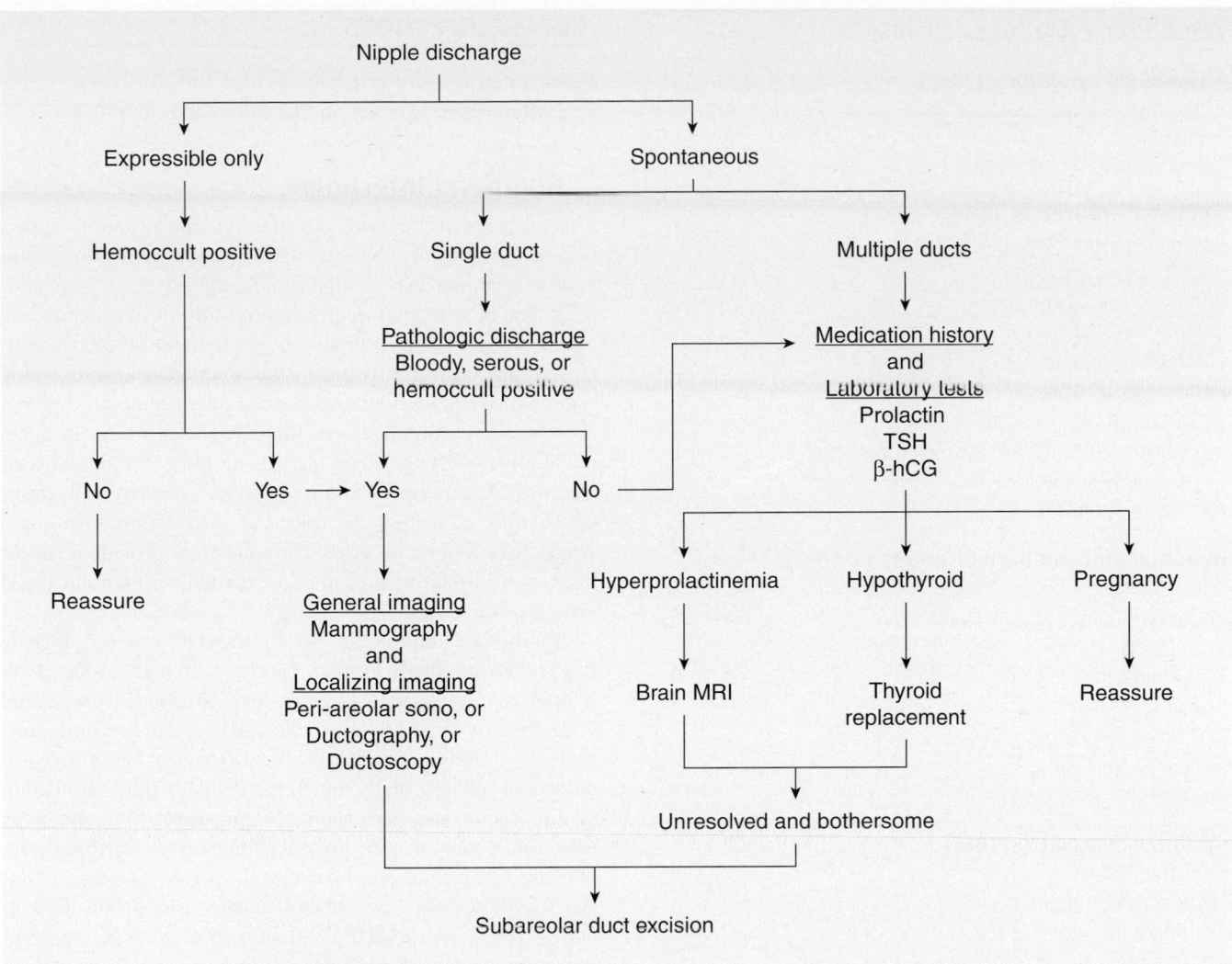

FIGURE 12-6 Diagnostic algorithm to evaluate nipple discharge. hCG = human chorionic gonadotropin; MRI = magnetic resonance imaging; TSH = thyroid-stimulating hormone.

additional evaluation. However, spontaneous discharges should be considered pathologic and merit evaluation (Fig. 12-6). Spontaneous milky nipple discharge, also called galactorrhea, may result from a variety of causes (Tables 12-3 and 12-4). Pregnancy is another frequent cause of new-onset spontaneous discharge, and a bloody multiduct discharge during pregnancy is not uncommon.

Pathologic nipple discharge is defined as a spontaneous single-duct discharge that is serous or bloody. The rate of underlying malignancy ranges from approximately 2 percent for young women with no associated findings on imaging or physical examination to 20 percent for older women with associated findings (Cabioglu, 2003; Lau, 2005). Most pathologic nipple discharges are caused by benign intraductal papillomas, which are simple milk duct polyps (Urban, 1978). They arise in the major milk ducts, generally within 2 cm of the nipple, and contain a velvety papillary epithelium on a central fibrovascular stalk.

Evaluation of a pathologic nipple discharge begins with breast examination. Careful evaluation can frequently locate a trigger point on the areolar edge that elicits the discharge when

pressed. Occult-blood testing and microscopic examination of the discharge can provide additional information. A glass slide that has been touched to the discharge and immediately fixed in 95-percent alcohol may be used for cytologic assessment. Nipple fluid samples are acellular in 25 percent of cases and thus cannot exclude an underlying malignancy (Papanicolaou, 1958). However, malignant cells, if found, are highly correlated with an underlying cancer (Gupta, 2004).

Following these examinations, diagnostic mammography and an assessment of the subareolar ducts by ductography, mammary ductoscopy, or sonography is indicated. Diagnostic mammography is usually negative, but may occasionally identify an underlying ductal carcinoma in situ (DCIS). Mammary ductography, also known as galactography, requires cannulating the affected duct, injecting radiocontrast, and then performing mammography (Fig. 12-7). In contrast, ductoscopy involves dilation and cannulation of the discharging breast duct, followed by passage of an endoscope measuring only 0.6 to 1.2 mm in diameter.

An evaluation of the subareolar ducts, as just described, is required to localize an intraductal lesion for subsequent

TABLE 12-3. Causes of Galactorrhea

Physiologic conditions (14%)
Pregnancy and postpartum state
Breast stimulation
"Witch's milk" in neonates

Neoplastic processes (18%)
Pituitary adenoma (prolactinoma)
Bronchogenic carcinoma
Renal adenocarcinoma
Lymphoma
Craniopharyngioma
Hydatidiform mole
Hypernephroma
Mixed growth hormone-secreting and prolactin-
   secreting tumors
Null-cell adenoma

Hypothalamic-pituitary disorders (<10%)
Craniopharyngioma and other tumors
Infiltrative conditions
Sarcoidosis
Tuberculosis
Schistosomiasis
Pituitary-stalk resection
Multiple sclerosis
Empty-sella syndrome

Systemic diseases (<10%)
Hypothyroidism
Chronic renal failure
Cushing disease
Acromegaly

Medications and herbs (20%)

Chest wall irritation (<10%)
Irritating clothes or ill-fitting brassieres
Herpes zoster
Atopic dermatitis
Burns
Breast surgery
Spinal cord injury or surgery
Spinal cord tumor
Esophagitis
Esophageal reflux

Idiopathic (35%)
Hyperprolactinemia
Euprolactinemia

From Pena, 2001, with permission.

excision. However, pathologic nipple discharge is *definitively* diagnosed and treated by subareolar duct excision, which is also known as microductectomy (Locker, 1988). Subareolar duct excision can also be used to treat bothersome multiduct discharges not associated with prolactinoma.

BREAST INFECTIONS

Breast infections are generally divided into puerperal, which develop during pregnancy and lactation, and nonpuerperal.

Puerperal Infections

This infection of the breast is characterized by a warm, tender, diffuse erythema of the breast with systemic signs of infection such as fever, malaise, myalgias, and leukocytosis. It is successfully treated with oral or intravenous antibiotics, depending on the severity, but may also progress to form deep parenchymal abscesses that require surgical drainage. Sonographic examination is highly sensitive for identifying underlying abscesses if mastitis does not improve rapidly with antibiotics. Women with puerperal mastitis should continue to breast feed or breast pump during treatment to prevent milk stasis, which may contribute to infection progression (Thomsen, 1983). Cracked or excoriated nipples may provide a source of entry for bacteria and should be treated with lanolin-based lotions or ointments.

Appropriate antibiotics for puerperal mastitis include those covering staphylococcal species, although group A & B *Streptococcus*, *Corynebacterium*, and *Bacteroides* species and *Escherichia coli* may also less frequently be isolated. Commonly, cephalexin (Keflex) or dicloxacillin (Dynapen), each given at dosages of 500 mg orally four times daily, or the combination of amoxicillin and clavulanate (Augmentin), 500 mg orally three times daily, may be prescribed for 7 days. Erythromycin, 500 mg orally four times daily, will provide adequate coverage for those with a penicillin allergy. Methicillin-resistant *Staphylococcus aureus* (MRSA) has become a more prevalent community-acquired pathogen causing mastitis in pregnancy and the puerperium (Laibl, 2005; Stafford, 2008). If MRSA is suspected or if a patient fails to improve on an initial regimen, then trimethoprim-sulfamethoxazole double strength (Bactrim DS, Septra DS), one or two tablets orally twice daily, or clindamycin, 300 mg orally three times daily, is a suitable choice. In ill patients with extensive infection, hospitalization and intravenous (IV) antibiotics are typically required. In these complicated cases, MRSA coverage may be prudent, and clindamycin, 600 mg IV every 8 hours, or vancomycin, 1 g IV every 12 hours, can be administered. Intravenous antibiotics are typically given until the woman is afebrile for 24 to 48 hours. Oral antibiotics are then continued to complete a 7- to 10-day course.

Focal mastitis may result from an infected galactocele. A tender mass will usually be palpable at the site of skin erythema. Needle aspiration of the galactocele and antibiotics are frequently all that is required, but recurrence or progression may mandate surgical drainage.

Nonpuerperal Infections
Cellulitis

Uncomplicated cellulitis in a nonirradiated breast and in a nonpuerperal setting is uncommon. Accordingly, its occurrence should prompt imaging and biopsies to exclude inflammatory breast cancer.

TABLE 12-4. Medications and Herbs Associated with Galactorrhea

Antidepressants and anxiolytics
Alprazolam (Xanax)
Buspirone (BuSpar)
Monoamine oxidase inhibitors
    Moclobemide (Manerlx; available in Canada)
Selective serotonin-reuptake inhibitors
    Citalopram (Celexa)
    Fluoxetine (Prozac)
    Paroxetine (Paxil)
    Sertraline (Zoloft)
Tricyclic antidepressants

Antihypertensives
Atenolol (Tenormin)
Methyldopa (Aldomet)
Reserpine (Serpasil)
Verapamil (Calan)

Antipsychotics

Histamine H$_2$-receptor blockers
Cimetidine (Tagamet)
Famotidine (Pepcid)
Ranitidine (Zantac)

Hormones
Conjugated estrogen and medroxyprogesterone
    (Premphase, Prempro)
Medroxyprogesterone contraceptive injections
    (Depo-Provera)
Combination hormonal contraception

Phenothiazines
Chlorpromazine (Thorazine)
Prochlorperazine (Compazine)

Other drugs
Amphetamines
Anesthetics
Arginine
Cannabis
Cisapride (Propulsid)
Cyclobenzaprine (Flexeril)
Danazol (Danocrine)
Dihydroergotamine (DHE 45)
Domperidone
Isoniazid
Metoclopramide (Reglan)
Octreotide (Sandostatin)
Opiates
Rimantadine (Flumadine)
Sumatriptan (Imitrex)
Valproic acid (Depakene)

Herbs
Anise
Blessed thistle
Fennel
Fenugreek seed
Marshmallow
Nettle
Red clover
Red raspberry

From Pena, 2001, with permission.

Abscess

Nonpuerperal breast abscesses are generally classified as peripheral or subareolar. Peripheral abscesses usually are skin infections such as folliculitis or infection of epidermal inclusion cysts or Montgomery glands. These abscesses are all adequately treated by drainage and the antibiotics discussed in the previous section.

In contrast, subareolar abscesses arise from keratin-plugged milk ducts directly behind the nipple. The abscess itself usually presents under the areola, and fistulous communications between multiple abscesses are common. Simple drainage is

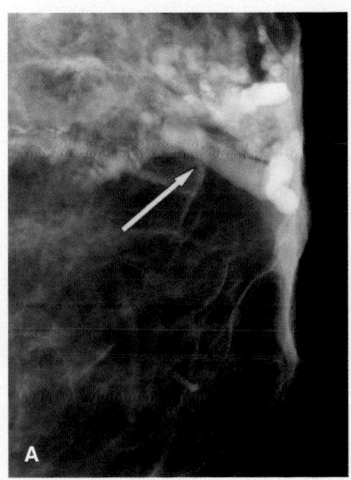
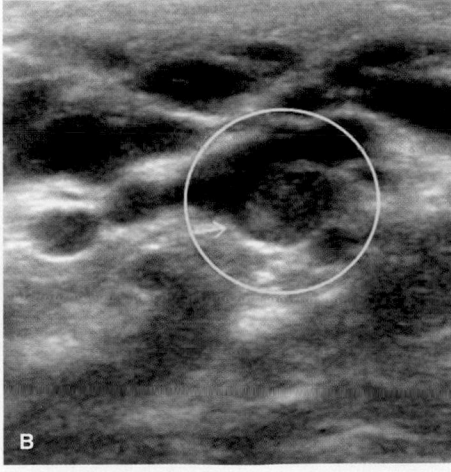

FIGURE 12-7 Imaging for a pathologic nipple discharge. **A.** Ductography shows dilated ducts and a filling defect (*arrow*). **D.** Periareolar sonogram with an intraductal mass, which is seen within the yellow circle.

associated with a recurrence rate of nearly 40 percent, thus effective treatment requires subareolar duct excision and complete removal of sinus tracts. In general, surgical drainage of nonpuerperal breast abscesses should always be accompanied by biopsy of the abscess wall, as breast cancer occasionally presents as an abscess (Benson, 1989; Watt-Boolsen, 1987).

MASTALGIA

Breast pain is common, and the prevalence is higher for women nearing menopause than for younger women (Euhus, 1997; Maddox, 1989). The precise etiology of mastalgia is unknown, but it is likely related to estrogen- and progesterone-mediated changes in interstitial water content, and therefore in interstitial pressure.

Mastalgia is generally classified as cyclic or noncyclic. Noncyclic mastalgia is often focal and shows no relationship to the menstrual cycle. Although focal mastalgia is frequently caused by a simple cyst, breast cancer occasionally presents as focal breast pain. Therefore, this complaint is evaluated by careful clinical examination, targeted imaging, and needle biopsy of any palpable or imaging abnormalities.

In contrast, cyclic mastalgia is usually bilateral, diffuse, and most severe during the late luteal phase of the menstrual cycle

(Gateley, 1990). It remits with the onset of menstruation. Cyclic mastalgia requires no specific evaluation and is generally managed symptomatically with nonsteroidal antiinflammatory agents (Fig. 12-8). A variety of other treatments have been proposed including bromocriptine, vitamin E, or oil of evening primrose. However, outcomes are no better than placebo in the best randomized clinical trials, except for bromocriptine in the subset of women with elevated prolactin levels (Kumar, 1989; Mansel, 1990). For the most severe cases, several agents are effective when administered during the last 2 weeks of the menstrual cycle. These include: (1) danazol, 200 mg orally daily; (2) the selective estrogen-receptor modifier toremifene (Fareston), 20 mg orally daily; or (3) tamoxifen (Nolvadex), 20 mg orally daily. Pregnancy must first be excluded and then avoided if these medications are used.

BENIGN PROLIFERATIVE BREAST DISEASE

Fibrocystic Change

The primary tissue components of the breast are fat, fibrous stroma, and epithelial structures. The hormonally responsive component is the epithelium, but considerable paracrine communication exists between the epithelium and stroma. Hormonal stimulation may result in dilated fluid-filled lobular

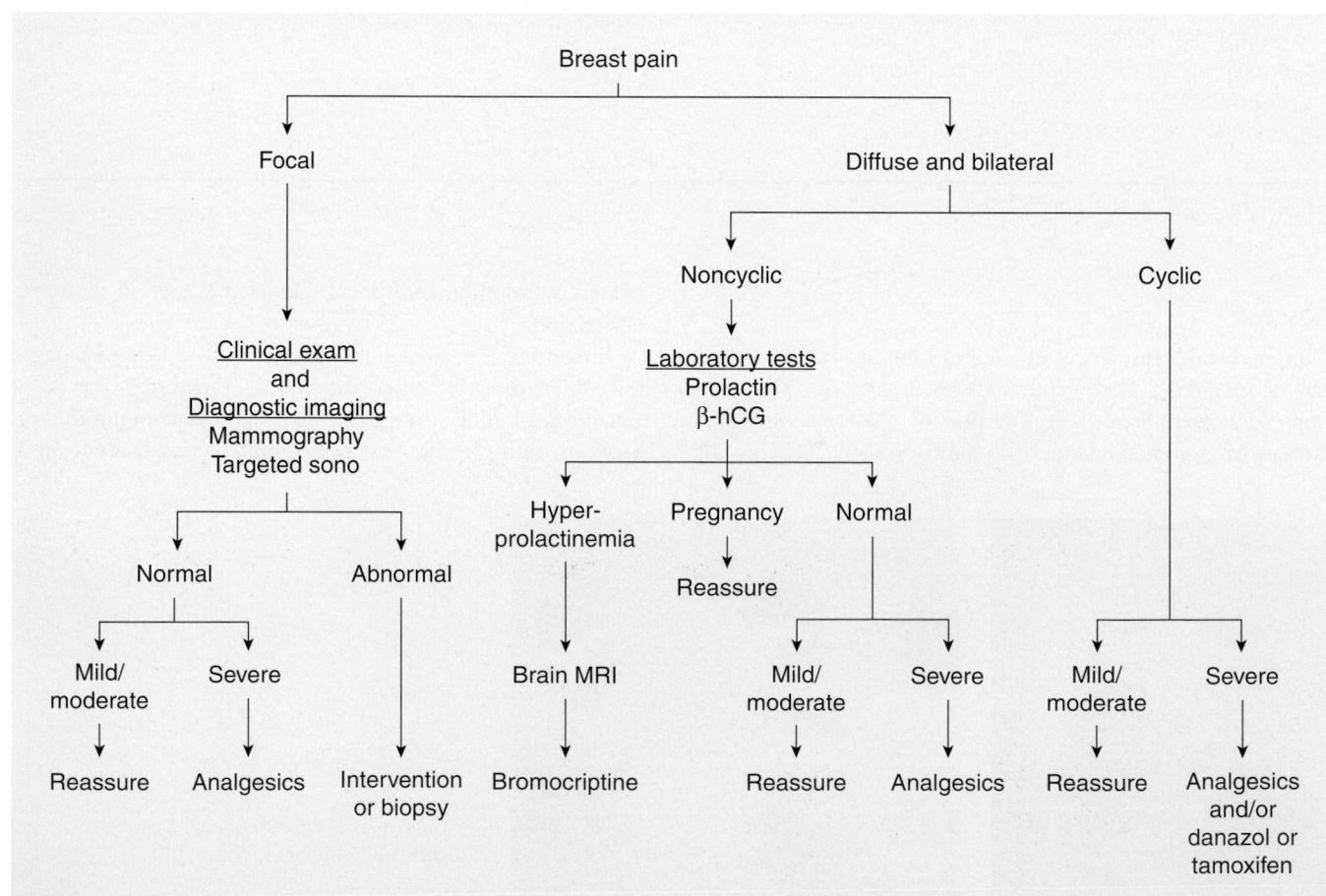

FIGURE 12-8 Diagnostic algorithm to evaluate mastalgia. Oil of evening primrose or vitamin E is frequently used for mild/moderate pain, but the effects are no better than placebo. hCG = human chorionic gonadotropin; MRI = magnetic resonance imaging.

acini interpreted as microcysts on histologic sections and is usually accompanied by relative stromal abundance. This is commonly referred to as fibrocystic change. Depending on the particular pattern of epithelial structures and associated stroma, a breast may appear mammographically dense, feel nodular to palpation, or both. Fibrocystic change is generally classified as proliferative or nonproliferative according to the epithelial features of the process.

Ductal and Lobular Hyperplasia

For the most part, proliferative changes develop in the terminal ducts and acini of the lobules. These structures are usually lined by an inner layer of cuboidal luminal epithelial cells and an outer layer of myoepithelial cells. Proliferation of the luminal epithelial cells results in terminal ducts or acini with several layers of cells, which is referred to as ductal or lobular hyperplasia, respectively. As this process progresses, the terminal ducts or acini become packed with cells, which begin to show nuclear atypia. This condition is referred to as atypical ductal hyperplasia (ADH) or atypical lobular hyperplasia (ALH), respectively. As more and more terminal ducts or acini become involved, the condition is recognized as ductal carcinoma in situ (DCIS) or lobular carcinoma in situ (LCIS), depending on whether the cells are arising from the ducts or acini, respectively (Fig. 12-9) (Ringberg, 2001). In general, women with typical epithelial hyperplasia have a relative risk for breast cancer of about 1.5, whereas women with atypical hyperplasia have a relative risk of approximately 4.5 (Dupont, 1993; Sneige, 2002).

These traditional histologic designations are gradually being replaced by a standardized scoring system that reflects the risk for subsequent breast cancer. Based on the cell of origin, extent, and grade, the proposed categories include ductal intraepithelial neoplasia (DIN) low risk, 1, 2, and 3, and lobular intraepithelial neoplasia (LIN) 1, 2, or 3 (Bratthauer, 2002; Tavassoli, 2005).

LOBULAR CARCINOMA IN SITU

Lobular carcinoma in situ is not associated with any specific mammographic or palpable features and thus is only diagnosed incidentally. Classic LCIS has not traditionally been viewed as a direct precursor of breast cancer, but rather as a marker of increased breast cancer risk. This is because subsequent breast cancers develop with nearly the same frequency in both breasts (Chuba, 2005). The risk of subsequent breast cancer is approximately 1 percent per year but is modified upward by early age at diagnosis, family history of breast cancer, and extensive disease (Bodian, 1996).

Lobular carcinoma in situ tends to be multifocal and bilateral. Therefore, local excision with clear margins is frequently not possible and not necessary. Accordingly, management options include enhanced surveillance, chemoprevention, or bilateral prophylactic mastectomy. Surveillance may include twice-yearly clinical examinations and mammography alternating with screening magnetic resonance (MR) imaging. There are no data yet to show that screening MR imaging reduces breast cancer mortality rates among women with LCIS, but the infiltrating lobular cancers that can develop are frequently mammographically occult. Five years of tamoxifen has been shown to reduce breast cancer incidence by 56 percent in women with LCIS (Fisher, 1998). The selective estrogen-receptor modulator raloxifene (Evista) may be an option for postmenopausal women (Vogel, 2006). Most women with LCIS do not opt for bilateral prophylactic mastectomy. However, for women with LCIS and a family history of breast cancer or for women who are continuing to require multiple biopsies, it is often a welcome solution.

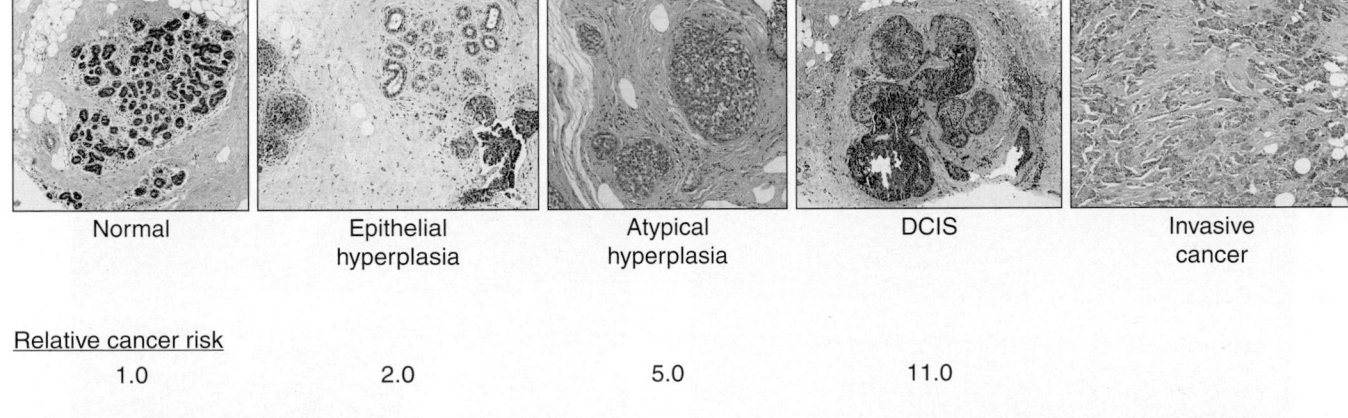

| Normal | Epithelial hyperplasia | Atypical hyperplasia | DCIS | Invasive cancer |

Relative cancer risk

| 1.0 | 2.0 | 5.0 | 11.0 | |

Tumor suppressor gene methylation

Allelic imbalances

Oncogene amplification

FIGURE 12-9 Histologic progression from normal breast tissue to cancer. DCIS = ductal carcinoma in situ.

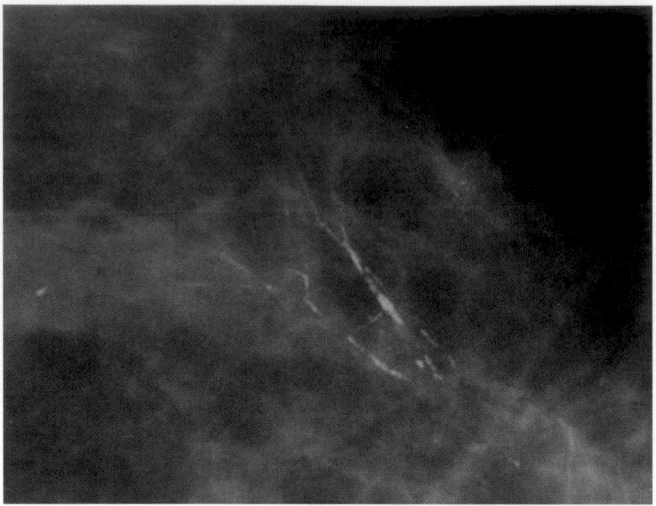

FIGURE 12-10 Linear and branching calcifications associated with ductal carcinoma in situ. *(Image contributed by Dr. Phil Evans.)*

DUCTAL CARCINOMA IN SITU

Ductal carcinoma in situ can be understood as a condition in which cancer cells fill portions of a mammary ductal system without invading beyond the duct's basement membrane (Ringberg, 2001). Although DCIS cells have accumulated many of the DNA changes common to invasive breast cancer, they lack certain critical changes that would permit them to persist outside of the duct (Aubele, 2002). Ductal carcinoma in situ is currently classified as stage 0 breast cancer.

The incidence of DCIS in the United States has increased in parallel with that of invasive breast cancer during the past two decades. But, similar to invasive breast cancer, the incidence has plateaued during the past several years (Virnig, 2010). Ductal carcinoma in situ currently accounts for 25 to 30 percent of all breast cancers in the United States. It is most commonly diagnosed by screening mammography as it is frequently associated with pleomorphic, linear, or branching calcifications (Fig. 12-10).

Ductal carcinoma in situ is classified by morphologic type, the presence or absence of comedonecrosis, and nuclear grade. The common morphologic types include cribriform, solid, micropapillary, and comedo (Fig. 12-11). Comedonecrosis appears as a necrotic eosinophilic core down the center of a duct packed with cancer cells. Of all of the classifying variables, nuclear grade is the most predictive for associated invasive cancer, for extent of disease, and for recurrence after treatment (Ringberg, 2001).

Incompletely treated DCIS may recur locally, and 50 percent of recurrences are associated with fully developed invasive breast

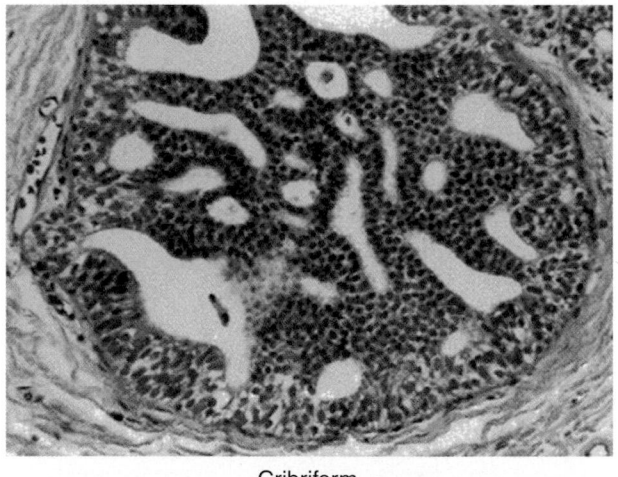

Cribriform

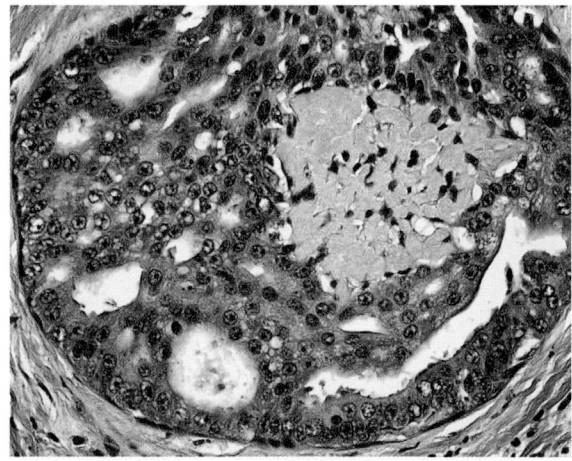

Comedo

Solid

Micropapillary

FIGURE 12-11 Morphologic types of ductal carcinoma in situ (DCIS).

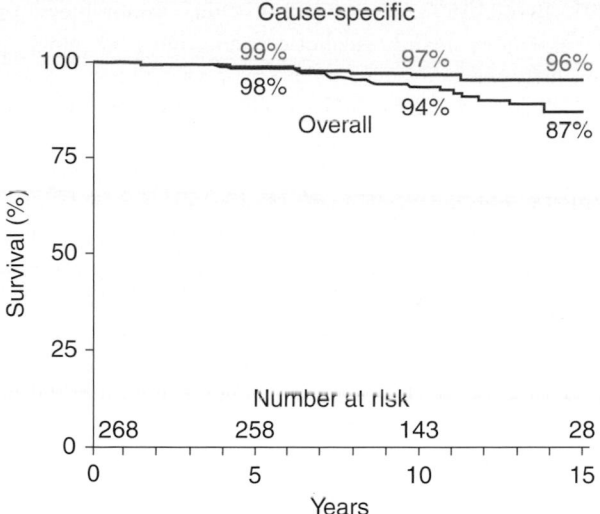

FIGURE 12-12 Cause-specific and overall survival for ductal carcinoma in situ. *(From Solin, 1996, with permission.)*

cancer. The principal treatment of DCIS is wide excision with a negative margin. This may require mastectomy if DCIS is extensive or if there are other contraindications to breast conservation. When breast conservation is possible, postoperative breast irradiation will reduce the local recurrence rate from 18 percent to 9 percent and is considered standard adjuvant treatment (Fisher, 1993). For those treated with breast conservation and radiation, the breast cancer-specific survival rate is 96 percent (Fig. 12-12) (Solin, 1996). Axillary staging is generally not included in the management of DCIS, although some have advocated sentinel node biopsy for large, high-grade DCIS diagnosed by needle biopsy and treated by lumpectomy, as occult invasive cancer is diagnosed in 10 percent (Wilkie, 2005). Sentinel lymph node (SLN) biopsy in conjunction with mastectomy is less controversial, as it is not possible to go back and perform SLN biopsy if an occult invasive cancer is diagnosed in this setting.

Five years of tamoxifen is recommended for estrogen-receptor-positive DCIS treated by breast conservation (Fisher, 1999). Although tamoxifen is not associated with a statistically significant improvement in overall survival rates, it does significantly reduce the incidence of ipsilateral invasive cancer and also reduces the risk of contralateral breast cancer.

■ Paget Disease of the Nipple

This type of DCIS presents as a focal eczematous rash of the nipple (Fig. 12-13). Ductal carcinoma cells, responding to chemoattractants secreted by cells in the dermis, migrate to the surface of the nipple, inducing skin breakdown (Schelfhout, 2000). The condition is easily diagnosed histologically following excision of the affected nipple tip after nipple-areolar blockade using local anesthetic. Evaluation should also include careful clinical examination, as an associated mass is identified in approximately 60 percent of cases (Ashikari, 1970). Among those with no palpable abnormalities, mammography will show suspicious densities or calcifications in 21 percent (Ikeda, 1993). An underlying DCIS is identified in about two thirds of cases, and an invasive cancer in approximately one third (Ashikari, 1970).

Treatment includes wide excision with negative margins. Breast conservation, which requires central breast resection including the nipple-areolar complex and all identifiable underlying disease, is followed by postoperative breast irradiation (Bijker, 2001). Axillary staging by sentinel node biopsy is not required unless an invasive component is identified or total mastectomy is performed.

BREAST CANCER RISK FACTORS

The most profound breast cancer risk factor is female gender. In addition, the incidence of breast cancer, as for most other cancers, increases with advancing age. Other significant risk factors are related to reproductive variables, benign proliferative breast disease, and family history of breast or ovarian cancer.

■ Reproductive Factors
Ovulatory Cycles

Ovulatory menstrual cycles exert stress on the breast epithelium by inducing proliferation in the late luteal phase. If conception does not occur, proliferation is followed by programmed cell death (Anderson, 1982; Soderqvist, 1997). Early age at menarche is associated with earlier onset of ovulatory cycles and increased breast cancer risk (den Tonkelaar, 1996; Vihko, 1986). Conversely, early menopause, whether it is natural or surgical, is associated with a reduced breast cancer risk (Kvale, 1988). Indeed, the lifetime number of ovulatory cycles is linearly related

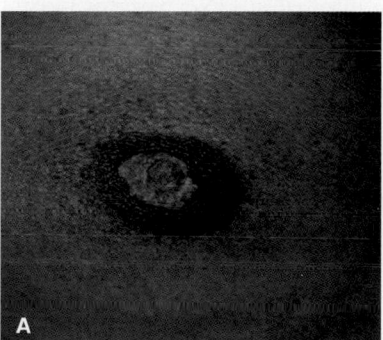 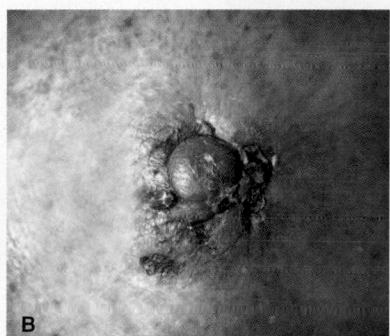 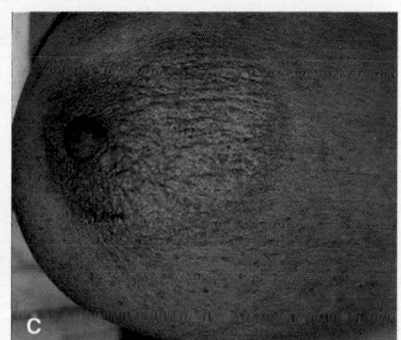

FIGURE 12-13 A. and **B.** Paget disease of the nipple. **C.** Benign reactive dermatitis. *(Photographs contributed by Dr. Marilyn Leitch.)*

to breast cancer risk (Clavel-Chapelon, 2002). Pregnancy generates very high levels of circulating estradiol, which is associated with a transient increase in short-term risk. But pregnancy also provides relief from ovarian cycling. Consequently, increasing parity is associated with a reduced lifetime risk.

Pregnancy

The breast is unique among all human organs in that it exists as a primordium for a decade or more before entering a highly proliferative state at menarche, and then does not fully mature until the first live birth. Immature breast epithelium is more susceptible to carcinogens than postlactational epithelium (Russo, 1996). Therefore, the longer a first live birth is delayed, the greater the breast cancer risk. Relative to nulliparity, first live births before the age of 28 years are associated with reduced breast cancer risk, whereas those thereafter are associated with increased risk (Gail, 1989). Both early age at first live birth and greater numbers of live births are associated with reduced breast cancer risk (Layde, 1989; MacMahon, 1970; Pathak, 1986; Pike, 1983).

Benign Proliferative Breast Disease and Family History

As discussed earlier, benign proliferative breast disease is a marker of breast cancer risk, with relative risks ranging from 1.5 to 4.5 depending on whether epithelial cells are atypical or not (Dupont, 1993). A family history of breast cancer may also indicate an increased breast cancer risk, particularly with affected first-degree relatives (parents, siblings, or offspring), an early age at diagnosis, or bilateral breast cancer (Claus, 1994; Colditz, 1993).

Other Factors

Increased mammographic density is emerging as an important breast cancer risk factor. The incidence of breast cancer among women with almost entirely dense breasts is three- to sixfold greater than that of women with almost entirely fatty breasts, a relative risk approaching that conferred by a diagnosis of atypical ductal hyperplasia (Fig. 12-14) (Barlow, 2006; Boyd,

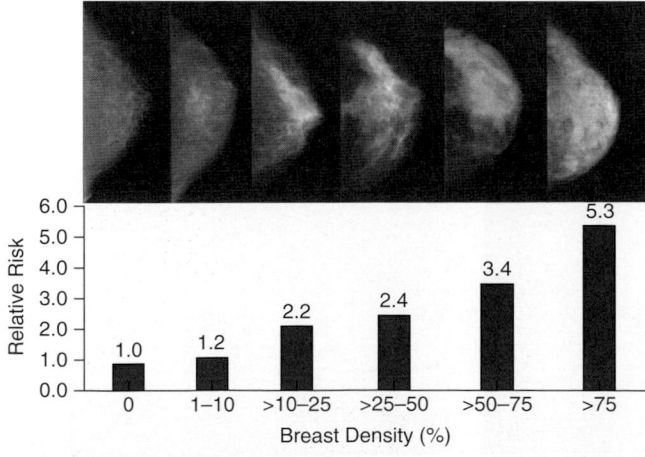

FIGURE 12-14 Relative risk of breast cancer increases with increasing mammographic breast density. *(From Santen, 2005, with permission.)*

1995; Byrne, 1995; Ursin, 2003). Other minor breast cancer risk factors include alcohol consumption (>2 ounces per day), increased body mass index (for postmenopausal women only), increased height, and current use of combined estrogen-progestin hormone replacement therapy (Friedenreich, 2001; Lahmann, 2004; Macinnis, 2004; Smith-Warner, 1998; Writing Group for the Women's Health Initiative Investigators, 2002). Use of estrogen-only hormone replacement therapy does not appear to be associated with an increased breast cancer risk (LaCroix, 2011; The Women's Health Initiative Steering Committee, 2004). In general, all of these risk factors are more prevalent in developed countries than in less developed countries. Consequently, breast cancer is more common in industrialized cultures (Parkin, 2001).

Gail Model

Gail (1989) evaluated more than a dozen potential breast cancer risk factors in a population of women undergoing screening mammography. Of these, age, age at menarche, age at first live birth, number of breast biopsies, and number of first-degree relatives with breast cancer emerged as the most important factors. The Gail model is a mathematical tool for calculating breast cancer risk based on these risk factors and has been independently validated (Costantino, 1999; Rockhill, 2001). A risk calculator is available to physicians through the National Cancer Institute website at http://www.cancer.gov/bcrisktool/. However, shortcomings of the model include an inability to predict which women in a large group will actually develop breast cancer, failure to account for other risk factors (such as LCIS), and failure to adequately address family history factors. Although newer models, such as the Tyrer-Cuzick model, combine genetic risk factors with the established Gail factors and also include parity, age at menopause, height, body mass index, and history of LCIS or atypical ductal hyperplasia, no other model has been independently validated as extensively as the Gail model (Tyrer, 2004). A recent modification of the Gail model includes a factor for mammographic density (Chen, 2006).

Breast Cancer Genetics

Nearly 30 percent of breast cancers have some familial component, but fewer than 10 percent are caused by inherited mutations in major breast cancer susceptibility genes (Antoniou, 2006; Lichtenstein, 2000). These genes operate in an autosomal dominant fashion and are involved in DNA repair or in controlling the cell cycle so that DNA can be repaired before the cell divides.

Family histories that suggest inherited susceptibility include early-onset breast cancer (<50 years), bilateral breast cancer, male breast cancer, multiple affected relatives in one generation, breast cancer in multiple generations, development of cancers that are known to be associated with a particular syndrome, and two or more cancers in one relative, especially if they develop at an early age. CancerGene is a widely used computer program for estimating gene mutation probabilities based on family history information and is available at: http://www4.utsouthwestern.edu/breasthealth/cagene. When possible, genetic testing is a powerful tool for determining who in the family is truly at high risk.

Inherited Breast-Ovarian Cancer Syndrome

This syndrome accounts for 5 to 7 percent of breast cancers (Malone, 2000). Approximately 45 percent of individuals with this syndrome carry a *BRCA1* gene mutation, and 35 percent have a *BRCA2* mutation. Twenty percent of families with inherited breast-ovarian cancer syndrome test negative for *BRCA1* and *BRCA2* gene mutations, suggesting that other genes remain to be identified.

Hallmarks of the BRCA1 form include early age at breast cancer diagnosis (median 44 years); high-grade, estrogen and progesterone receptor–negative breast cancers; and associated ovarian cancer (Foulkes, 2004). The lifetime risk for breast cancer ranges from 35 to 80 percent, and for ovarian cancer 16 to 57 percent (Easton, 1995; Ford, 1994, 1998). Individuals who have developed both breast and ovarian cancer have an 86-percent probability of carrying a BRCA gene mutation (Cvelbar, 2005).

Women with *BRCA2* gene mutations develop breast cancer at about the same age as women with sporadic breast cancer, thus age at diagnosis is not usually a good criterion for recognizing this syndrome. Ovarian cancer is an associated cancer, but develops less frequently than it does in BRCA1 families. Males with *BRCA2* mutations develop breast cancer at approximately the same frequency as females without mutations, and 4 to 40 percent of male breast cancers are related to *BRCA2* mutations (Friedman, 1997; Thorlacius, 1996). Other associated cancers are listed in Table 12-5. Early premenopausal bilateral oophorectomy significantly reduces the incidence of both breast and ovarian cancer in women with inherited breast-ovarian cancer syndrome and is discussed further in Chapter 35 (p. 857) (Domchek, 2010; Kauf, 2002; Rebbeck, 2002).

Other recognized gene syndromes are associated with increased breast cancer risk (see Table 12-5). Their associated mutations affect genes involved with DNA repair, growth factor signaling, and cell-cell interactions. It is increasingly recognized that mutations in these genes, although rare, can cause predisposition syndromes that are very similar to those caused by *BRCA1* and *BRCA2* mutations.

Treatment options for breast cancers that arise in the context of an inherited predisposition syndrome are the same as for sporadic breast cancers. However, many of these women choose bilateral mastectomy, as the risk of an ipsilateral second primary breast cancer in a preserved breast can be as high as 3 to 4 percent annually, and the risk of a contralateral breast cancer is similar (Haffty, 2002; Seynaevea, 2004). Breast conservation is, however, an acceptable option for a highly motivated and well-informed patient (Pierce, 2010; Robson, 1999).

BREAST CANCER SCREENING

Screening Mammography

This radiographic test is currently the best and most thoroughly validated breast cancer screening test available. It has been evaluated in eight large randomized trials, the most recent of which was conducted in Canada in the 1980s (Begg, 2002). Controversies surrounding the benefits of screening

TABLE 12-5. Genetic Syndromes Associated with an Increased Risk of Breast Cancer

Syndrome Name	Genetic Mutation	Associated Disorders
Inherited breast-ovarian cancer	BRCA1 BRCA2	Cancers of the breast, ovary, pancreas, stomach, biliary system, and prostate and melanoma; male breast cancer for BRCA2
Li-Fraumeni	p53	Sarcoma, leukemia, melanoma and cancers of the breast, brain, adrenal cortex, pancreas, lung, cervix, and prostate
Cowden	PTEN	Breast: adenosis, fibrosis, hamartoma, fibroadenoma, and cancer (male and female); thyroid disease; ileum and colon hamartomatous polyps; facial tricholemmomas; macrocephaly; and oral papillomatosis
Peutz-Jegher	LKB1	Gastrointestinal hamartomatous polyps; cancers of the breast, small bowel, colon/rectum, pancreas, ovary, endometrium, cervix, lung, and testicle; and oral melanin pigmentation
p16^{INK4a} and p14^{ARF}	p16^{INK4a} p14^{ARF}	Leukemia/lymphoma, melanoma and cancers of the breast, pancreas, cervix, gallbladder, lung, larynx, prostate, liver, and intestine
Ataxia telangiectasia mutated	ATM	Lymphoma, leukemia, and breast cancer; cerebellar ataxia; telangiectasias; vitiligo; and café-au-lait spots
CHK2	CHK2	Sarcoma, leukemia, melanoma and cancers of the brain, adrenal cortex, pancreas, lung, cervix, and prostate; male and female breast cancer

p16^{INK4a} and p14^{ARF} may also be known as dysplastic nevus syndromes.
Data compiled from Borg, 2000; Concannon, 2002; The Breast Cancer Linkage Consortium, 1999; The CHEK2-Breast Cancer Consortium, 2002; Evans, 1997; Lim, 2003; and Schrager, 1998.

SECTION 1

mammography largely center on the impact of the test on breast cancer-specific and overall mortality rates. However, at this time, it is generally accepted that for women aged 50 to 69 years, screening mammography reduces breast cancer mortality rates. Considerable uncertainty remains for women between the ages of 40 and 49, but several influential organizations including the American Cancer Society, the American College of Obstetricians and Gynecologists (2011a), and the American College of Radiology have recommended that yearly screening mammography begin at age 40 (Lee, 2010; Smith, 2011). Recent improvements in screening mammography including digital mammography and computer-assisted diagnosis have improved the sensitivity of the test for some subgroups, challenging the contemporary relevance of older screening trials (Pisano, 2005).

It is important to recognize that most women with screen-detected abnormalities (~95 percent) do not have breast cancer, although the true-positive rate increases with increasing age (Feig, 2000). In addition, up to 25 percent of women diagnosed with breast cancer will have had a normal mammogram in the preceding 12 to 24 months.

Screening Sonography

This modality identifies mammographically occult breast cancer in less than 1 percent of women. However, in one large study, this translated into a 42-percent increase in screen-detected cancers (Gordon, 2002; Kolb, 2002). Screening sonography, however, is time consuming to perform, and the accuracy is highly dependent on the operator.

Screening Magnetic Resonance Imaging

This screening option has recently been evaluated among genetically high-risk women. It is particularly attractive in this group of women, who develop breast cancer at a rate of 2 percent per year between the ages of 25 and 50, a time during which mammography sensitivity is reduced by dense breast tissue. In general, MR imaging shows higher sensitivity and specificity than mammography, but the test has been criticized for its expense and high false-positive rate (Leach, 2005; Stoutjesdijk, 2001; Tilanus-Linthorst, 2000; Warner, 2001). Nevertheless, for 100 women with a strong family history of breast cancer and a negative mammogram, nine abnormal MR imaging scans would be expected, and three of these would represent mammographically occult breast cancer.

Breast MR imaging requires specially trained radiologists and specialized equipment (a breast coil and a high-resolution magnet). It is performed with and without intravenous gadolinium contrast (Orel, 2001). Areas of suspicious enhancement identified by MR imaging are evaluated by targeted sonographic examination and biopsied under sonographic guidance. If a lesion is not visible during sonography, then MR imaging-guided core biopsy is performed.

Other Radiologic Tools

Other screening modalities in the developmental stage include breast tomosynthesis, sestamibi scanning,

electrical impedance scanning, and thermography (Dobbins, 2003; Martin, 2002; Parisky, 2003; Sampalis, 2002). Of these, breast tomosynthesis warrants special mention, as it is likely to be adopted into the clinic in the near future. Tomosynthesis is a digital approach that obtains multiple images as the x-ray source and collector are rotated around the breast. Image slices are then reconstructed by a computer. This approach enhances calcifications and densities that would normally be obscured by intervening dense tissue.

Screening Physical Examination

The value of a screening clinical breast examination (CBE) performed by health care providers should not be neglected (Jatoi, 2003). Four of the large randomized mammography trials collected information on CBE and found that 44 to 74 percent of the breast cancers were detected by this approach. Sensitivity and specificity were higher for CBE than mammography among young women. The American College of Obstetricians and Gynecologists (2011b) recommends CBE during a woman's routine periodic assessment for those 19 years and older.

Enthusiasm for breast self-examination (BSE) has diminished subsequent to publication of a very large randomized trial performed in Shanghai, China, that found no improvement in mortality rates (Thomas, 2002). Although there is less interest in promoting systematic breast self-examination, it seems reasonable to encourage women to remain breast-aware. The American College of Obstetricians and Gynecologists (2011a) notes that BSE has the potential to detect palpable breast masses and can be recommended.

INVASIVE BREAST CANCER

In the United States, breast cancer is the most common cancer in women and the second most common cause of cancer-related mortality (second to lung) (Siegel, 2011). Although the incidence of breast cancer increased steadily in the United States through the 1980s and 1990s, it has leveled at approximately 125 cases per year per 100,000 and is declining for some ethnicities (Fig. 12-15).

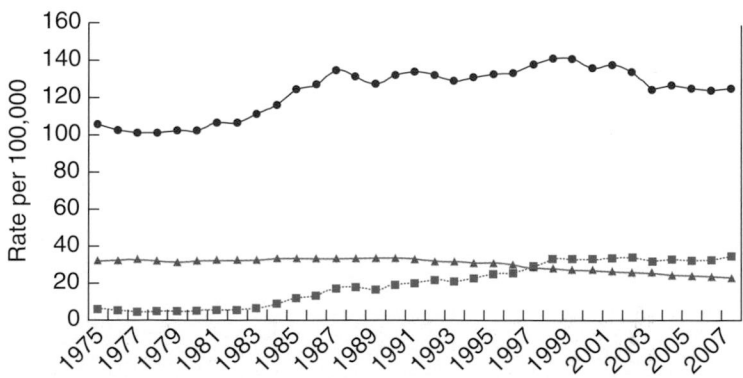

FIGURE 12-15 Trends in breast cancer incidence and mortality in the United States. Curve of decreasing breast cancer rates in United States. ● = incidence of invasive breast cancer; ■ = incidence in situ; ▲ = mortality rate. *(Data from Altekruse, 2010.)*

Tumor Characteristics

Primary cancers of the breast comprise 97 percent of malignancies affecting the breast, whereas 3 percent represent metastases from other sites. The most common of these, in descending order, are the contralateral breast, lymphoma, lung, and melanoma (Georgiannos, 2001). Cancers of mammary epithelial structures account for most of primary breast cancer. Infiltrating ductal carcinoma is the most common form of invasive breast cancer (~80 percent), and infiltrating lobular carcinoma is the second most common (~15 percent). Other malignancies such as phyllodes tumors, sarcoma, and lymphoma comprise the remainder.

Apart from stage, the primary tumor characteristics that most influence prognosis and treatment decisions are hormone receptor status, nuclear grade, and Her-2/neu expression (Bast, 2001). Approximately two thirds of breast cancers are estrogen and progesterone receptor positive. This feature is generally associated with a better prognosis and more treatment options.

Her-2/neu is a membrane tyrosine kinase that cooperates with other Her-family receptors to generate proliferation and survival signals in breast cancer cells. Approximately 25 percent of breast cancers have increased expression of Her-2/neu (Masood, 2005). These cancers are usually sensitive to the humanized monoclonal antibody trastuzumab (Herceptin), which represents the first in a new class of targeted therapies (Plosker, 2006).

Gene expression profiling has been used to classify individual tumors. It is anticipated that in the future, individualized therapies will be selected based on the pattern of nuclear and growth factor receptors that are active in a given tumor (Habel, 2006; van de Vijver, 2002).

Breast Cancer Staging

Careful breast cancer staging is essential for predicting outcome, planning treatment, and comparing treatment effects in clinical trials. Each patient is assigned both a clinical and a pathologic stage. The clinical stage is based on examination and radiographic findings, whereas a pathologic stage is based on actual tumor measurements and pathologic assessments of lymph nodes after primary surgery. Surgical staging of breast cancer is based on the TNM system, which includes primary tumor size (T), regional lymph node involvement (N), and presence of distant metastases (M) (Table 12-6). For patients with a clinically and sonographically negative axilla, sentinel lymph node biopsy has largely replaced complete axillary dissection for nodal staging (Giuliano, 1995; Lyman, 2005). Alternatively, axillary metastases may be diagnosed preoperatively by sonography-guided needle biopsy in 18 percent of patients with clinically negative axillae (Sapino, 2003).

The most common metastatic site of breast cancer is the bone, and practice varies with respect to screening for metastatic disease. However, common screening modalities include CT of the chest, abdomen, and pelvis combined with bone scintigraphy or combined whole body positron emission tomography and CT (PET/CT) (Chap. 2, p. 52) (Kumar, 2005). Bone scintigraphy is usually recommended in patients assessed by PET/CT, as PET/CT can miss osteolytic bone metastases.

Breast Cancer Treatment

Breast cancer is best treated in a multidisciplinary environment that includes surgeons, medical oncologists, and radiation oncologists. Surgery and radiation therapy are aimed at eliminating all local or regional tumor in a way that maximizes cosmetics and minimizes the risk of local or regional recurrence. There is some evidence that these local modalities reduce the risk of subsequent metastases and therefore impact survival (Early Breast Cancer Trialists Collaborative Group, 2005).

TABLE 12-6. Breast Cancer Surgical Staging

T Stage		Stage Grouping			
Tis	In situ	0	Tis	N0	M0
T1	≤2 cm	I	T1	N0	M0
T2	>2 cm but ≤5 cm	IIA	T0	N1	M0
T3	>5 cm		T1	N1	M0
T4	Involvement of skin or chest wall or inflammatory cancer		T2	N0	M0
			T2	N1	M0
		IIB	T3	N0	M0
N Stage		IIIA	T0	N2	M0
N0	No lymph node involvement		T1	N2	M0
N1	1–3 nodes		T2	N2	M0
N2	4–9 nodes		T3	N1	M0
N3	≥10 nodes or any infraclavicular nodes		T3	N2	M0
		IIIB	T4	N0	M0
M Stage			T4	N1	M0
M0	No distant metastases		T4	N2	M0
M1	Distant metastases	IIIC	Any T	N3	M0
		IV	Any T	Any N	M1

However, a significant proportion of patients with apparently localized disease have tumor cells detectable in their blood or bone marrow at diagnosis, making systemic treatment with chemotherapy, hormone manipulation, or targeted therapies the primary approach for reducing the risk of metastases and death (Euhus, 2005).

Surgery

Although Halstead (1894) revolutionized the treatment of breast cancer by demonstrating improved outcome for patients treated with radical mastectomy, results from recent randomized clinical trials have appropriately fostered a trend towards less aggressive surgery. Specifically, it has been thoroughly documented that lumpectomy with postoperative radiation therapy results in the same breast cancer-specific survival rate as total mastectomy (Fisher, 2002a,b). During surgery, more extensive axillary lymph node dissection is indicated for patients with a positive sentinel node finding or with axillary disease diagnosed by needle biopsy (Lyman, 2005). This procedure results in lymphedema in 15 to 50 percent of women, depending on how it is measured (Morrell, 2005). It is also associated with persistent shoulder or arm symptoms in up to 70 percent (Kuehn, 2000). Following lumpectomy, whole breast irradiation is the standard, although preliminary data for accelerated partial breast irradiation are encouraging (Jeruss, 2006; Zannis, 2005).

Chemotherapy

In the past, adjuvant chemotherapy was reserved for patients with nodal metastases and in these cases, was always given after definitive surgery. However, randomized prospective trials have shown that adjuvant chemotherapy improves survival rates for high-risk node-negative patients as well (Fisher, 2004; National Institutes of Health, 2000). More and more, however, the decision for chemotherapy is influenced by specific measures of tumor biology.

If used, adjuvant chemotherapy is usually administered after primary surgery but before radiation therapy. Neoadjuvant chemotherapy is given prior to definitive surgery and is gaining popularity. Neoadjuvant chemotherapy permits assessment of a given tumor's sensitivity to the selected agents, and the tumor shrinkage that often results permits less aggressive surgery.

Modern breast cancer chemotherapy usually includes an anthracycline such as doxorubicin (Adriamycin), in conjunction with cyclophosphamide (Cytoxan) (Trudeau, 2005). Taxanes may replace anthracyclines in the near future, as they are less toxic and are associated with equivalent or superior outcomes (Nabholtz, 2005). Chemotherapeutic agents are described more fully in Chapter 27 (p. 692).

Hormonal Therapy and Targeted Therapies

Adjuvant hormonal therapy is used for estrogen-receptor-positive tumors. In pre- or postmenopausal women, one option is the selective estrogen-receptor modulator tamoxifen. As discussed in Chapter 27 (p. 705), important side effects of tamoxifen include menopausal symptoms, increased risks of thromboembolic events, and higher rates of endometrial polyps and endometrial cancer. Although this cancer risk is increased, surveillance of the endometrium with routine transvaginal sonography or endometrial biopsy is not recommended. Endometrial evaluation is reserved for those with abnormal bleeding and follows that outlined in Chapter 8 (p. 225).

In postmenopausal women, aromatase inhibitors may be used, and Food and Drug Administration (FDA)-approved agents include anastrozole (Arimidex), letrozole (Femara), and exemestane (Aromasin) (Jaiyesimi, 1995; Kudachadkar, 2005). In postmenopausal women, most circulating estradiol is derived from the peripheral conversion of androgens by the enzyme aromatase. Administration of aromatase inhibitors reduces circulating estradiol to nearly undetectable levels in these women. The addition of an aromatase inhibitor after tamoxifen is associated with a 23- to 39-percent improvement in disease-free survival rates and a nearly 50-percent reduction in contralateral breast cancer rates (Geisler, 2006).

Unlike tamoxifen, aromatase inhibitors are associated with greater rates of bone loss and fractures. For this reason, annual bone mineral density testing is recommended for those taking aromatase inhibitors. For women with mild or moderate bone loss, exercise and supplementation with vitamin D and calcium are encouraged. Bisphosphonates are recommended for severe loss, and a fuller discussion of these drugs is found in Chapter 22 (p. 593) (Hilner, 2003).

Bisphosphonates, such as zoledronic acid (Zometa), are indicated for the treatment of bone metastases, and ample evidence supports their use to prevent cancer-treatment-induced bone loss. There is currently considerable interest in determining whether bisphosphonate use in the adjuvant setting can reduce the risk of bone metastases. Several trials are currently ongoing.

Therapies that target specific biological pathways are becoming available. Trastuzumab is a humanized monoclonal antibody that is very effective against Her-2/neu overexpressing tumors. In addition, bevacizumab (Avastin), a vascular endothelial growth factor (VEGF) antagonist, is finding a place in the clinic (Gonzalez-Angulo, 2006; Rugo, 2004). In addition, dozens of other antibodies and small molecules that target growth factors and receptor tyrosine kinases or their intermediaries are currently being evaluated in clinical trials (Kaklamani, 2004). These biologic agents are described more fully in Chapter 27 (p. 706).

■ Surveillance

Long-term surveillance of breast cancer patients after treatment includes periodic history and physical examination, both general and directed at eliciting signs or symptoms of recurrence. Women who elected breast conservation should be aware that the remaining breast tissue requires surveillance indefinitely, as ipsilateral second primary breast cancers develop at a rate of approximately 1 percent per year and contralateral breast cancers at approximately 0.7 percent per year (Fatouros, 2005; Fisher, 1984; Gao, 2003). Laboratory and imaging tests are obtained to further evaluate specific signs or symptoms. The use of screening tests other than mammography to identify asymptomatic recurrences is not recommended (Emens, 2003; Khatcheressian, 2006).

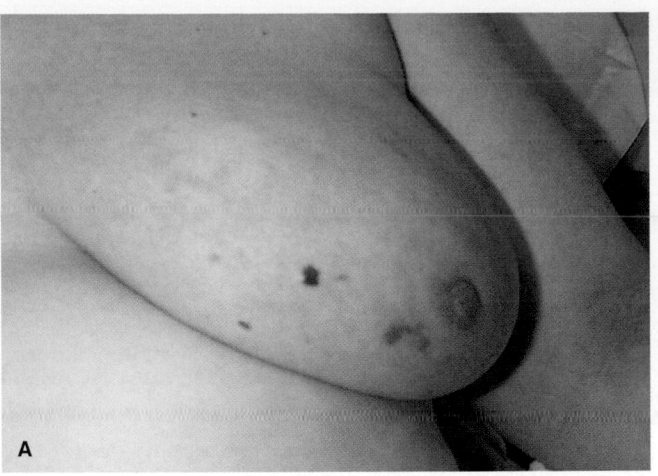 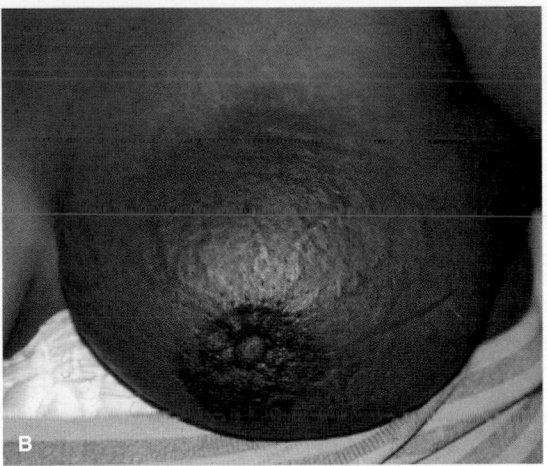

FIGURE 12-16 Photographs of inflammatory breast cancer. **A.** Subtle erythematous blush and edema in inflammatory breast cancer. **B.** Classic inflammatory breast cancer. *(Photographs contributed by Dr. Marilyn Leitch.)*

Inflammatory Breast Cancer

Inflammatory breast cancer accounts for 1 to 5 percent of breast cancers (Chang, 1998; Dawood, 2010). This cancer presents with skin changes that can range from a faint red blush to a flaming-red rash associated with skin edema (peau d'orange change) (Fig. 12-16). It is distinguished from a neglected advanced primary breast cancer by its rapid onset and progression within just a few weeks. The cancer spreads rapidly throughout the entire breast and creates diffuse induration. As a result, the breast may enlarge to two to three times its original volume within weeks (Taylor, 1938).

Although mastitis or even congestive heart failure can produce a similar clinical appearance, inflammatory breast cancer must be definitively excluded. This always includes diagnostic mammography and punch biopsy of the skin. However, it also may require multiple biopsies and additional imaging tests such as MR imaging or sestamibi scanning. Treatment begins with induction chemotherapy, which is followed by modified radical mastectomy (total mastectomy and axillary dissection) and then postoperative chest wall irradiation with or without additional chemotherapy (Cariati, 2005). The 5-year survival rate is 30 to 55 percent, which is significantly worse than for neglected advanced primary breast cancer (Brenner, 2002; Harris, 2003).

BREAST CANCER PREVENTION

Obesity and a sedentary lifestyle are two modifiable risk factors that should be addressed in high- and lower-risk women. Although some studies have reported a reduced breast cancer risk among women consuming five or more servings a day of fresh fruits and vegetables, prospective studies have not convincingly linked any single dietary practice to breast cancer incidence (Gandini, 2000; Meskens, 2005). Regular physical activity is consistently associated with reduced breast cancer risk in case-control and cohort studies (Lee, 2003).

Women at high risk for breast cancer have three main options. (1) enhanced surveillance, (2) chemoprevention, or (3) prophylactic surgery. Enhanced surveillance usually consists of clinical examination every 6 months, alternating mammography with breast MR imaging or screening sonography. Enhanced surveillance can begin 10 years before the earliest age of breast cancer diagnosis in a family.

The U.S. FDA has approved tamoxifen for breast cancer chemoprevention in pre- or postmenopausal women 35 years or older with a 5-year Gail model risk ≥1.7 percent. Five years of tamoxifen is associated with a 49-percent reduction in breast cancer incidence, including both invasive breast cancer and DCIS (Fisher, 1998). However, tamoxifen is associated with an increased incidence of endometrial cancer in postmenopausal women and an increased risk of thromboembolic disease including deep-vein thrombosis, pulmonary embolism, and stroke.

Raloxifene is another selective estrogen-receptor modulator that reduces the incidence of invasive breast cancer to the same extent as tamoxifen, but it does not reduce the risk of DCIS to the same extent (Vogel, 2006). Raloxifene has been associated with a lower risk of endometrial cancer and thromboembolic complications than tamoxifen. Raloxifene has not been evaluated in premenopausal women, although tamoxifen has.

Prophylactic surgery is usually reserved for women at very high risk for breast cancer. This includes women with inherited mutations in breast cancer predisposition genes and some women with LCIS, particularly if it is extensive or associated with a family history of breast cancer. Bilateral prophylactic oophorectomy performed in premenopausal women with BRCA gene mutations has been shown to reduce the risk of breast cancer by 50 percent and the risk of ovarian cancer by more than 90 percent (Eisen, 2005; Kauf, 2002; Rebbeck, 2002). Early surgical menopause is often accompanied by estrogen withdrawal symptoms, which can significantly impact quality of life. Hormone replacement therapy in this setting does not appear to diminish the breast cancer risk-reducing benefits of oophorectomy (Rebbeck, 2005).

Bilateral prophylactic mastectomy is usually performed as a skin sparing procedure with immediate reconstruction. Bilateral prophylactic mastectomy reduces breast cancer risk by more than 90 percent, but it is currently unclear whether overall or breast cancer-specific survival rates are increased (Hartmann, 2001; Lostumbo, 2004; McDonnell, 2001; Peralta, 2000). Breast cancers may develop after prophylactic mastectomy if there is residual breast tissue (usually in the upper outer quadrant or axillary tail). They may also develop in the skin of a mastectomy flap.

REFERENCES

Altekruse SF, Kosary CL, Krapcho M, et al (eds): SEER Cancer Statistics Review, 1975-2007. Bethesda, National Cancer Institute, 2010. Available at: http://seer.cancer.gov/csr/1975_2007/. Accessed September 14, 2010

American College of Obstetricians and Gynecologists: Breast cancer screening. Practice Bulletin No. 122, August 2011a

American College of Obstetricians and Gynecologists: Primary and preventive care: periodic assessments. Committee Opinion No. 483, April 2011b

Anderson TJ, Ferguson DP, Raab G: Cell turnover within "resting" human breast: influence of parity, contraceptive pill, age and laterality. Br J Cancer 46:276, 1982

Antoniou AC, Easton DF: Models of genetic susceptibility to breast cancer. Oncogene 25:5898, 2006

Ashikari R, Park K, Huvos AG, et al: Paget's disease of the breast. Cancer 26:680, 1970

Aubele M, Werner M, Hofler H: Genetic alterations in presumptive precursor lesions of breast carcinomas. Anal Cell Pathol 24:69, 2002

Barlow W, White E, Ballard-Barbash R, et al: Prospective breast cancer risk prediction model for women undergoing screening mammography. J Natl Cancer Inst 98:1204, 2006

Barth RJ: Histologic features predict local recurrence after breast conserving therapy of phyllodes tumors. Breast Cancer Res Treat 57:291, 1999

Bast RC, Ravdin P, Hayes DF, et al: 2000 update of recommendations for the use of tumor markers in breast and colorectal cancer: Clinical Practice Guidelines of the American Society of Clinical Oncology. J Clin Oncol 19:1865, 2001

Begg CB: The mammography controversy. Oncologist 7:174, 2002

Benson EA: Management of breast abscesses. World J Surg 13:753, 1989

Berg WA, Campassi CI, Loffe OB: Cystic lesions of the breast: sonographic-pathologic correlation. Radiology 227:183, 2003

Bijker N, Rutgers EJ, Duchateau L, et al: Breast-conserving therapy for Paget disease of the nipple: a prospective European Organization for Research and Treatment of Cancer study of 61 patients. Cancer 91:472, 2001

Bodian CA, Perzin KH, Lattes R: Lobular neoplasia. Long term risk of breast cancer and relation to other factors. Cancer 78:1024, 1996

Boerner S, Fornage BD, Singletary E, et al: Ultrasound-guided fine-needle aspiration (FNA) of nonpalpable breast lesions. Cancer (Cancer Cytopathol) 87:19, 1999

Borg A, Sandberg T, Nilsson K, et al. High frequency of multiple melanomas and breast and pancreas carcinomas in CDKN2A mutation-positive melanoma families. J Natl Cancer Inst 92:1260, 2000

Boyd NF, Byng JW, Jong RA, et al: Quantitative classification of mammographic densities and breast cancer risk: results from the Canadian National Breast Screening Study. J Natl Cancer Inst 87:670, 1995

Bratthauer GL, Tavassoli FA: Lobular intraepithelial neoplasia: previously unexplored aspects assessed in 775 cases and their clinical implications. Virchows Archiv 440:134, 2002

Brenner B, Siris N, Rakowsky E, et al: Prediction of outcome in locally advanced breast cancer by post-chemotherapy nodal status and baseline serum tumour markers. Br J Cancer 87:1404, 2002

Bulun SE, Simpson ER: Competitive RT-CR analysis indicates levels of aromatase cytochrome P450 transcripts in adipose tissue of buttocks, thighs, and abdomen of women increase with advancing age. J Clin Endocrinol Metab 78:428, 1994

Butler JA, Vargas HI, Worthen N, et al: Accuracy of combined clinical-mammographic-cytologic diagnosis of dominant breast masses. Arch Surg 125:893, 1990

Byrne C, Schairer C, Wolfe J, et al: Mammographic features and breast cancer risk: effects with time, age, and menopause status. J Natl Cancer Inst 87:1622, 1995

Cabioglu N, Hunt KK, Singletary S, et al: Surgical decision making and factors determining a diagnosis of breast carcinoma in women presenting with nipple discharge. J Am Coll Surg 196:354, 2003

Cariati M, Bennett-Britton TM, Pinder SE, et al: "Inflammatory" breast cancer. Surg Oncol 14:133, 2005

Chaney AW, Pollack A, Mcneese MD, et al: Primary treatment of cystosarcoma phyllodes of the breast. Cancer 89:1502, 2000

Chang S, Parker SL, Pham T, et al: Inflammatory breast carcinoma incidence and survival. The surveillance, epidemiology, and end results program of the National Cancer Institute, 1975–1992. Cancer 82:2366, 1998

Chen J, Pee D, Ayyagari R, et al: Projecting absolute invasive breast cancer risk in white women with a model that includes mammographic density. J Natl Cancer Inst 98:1215, 2006

Chuba PJ, Hamre MR, Yap J, et al: Bilateral risk for subsequent breast cancer after lobular carcinoma-in-situ: analysis of surveillance, epidemiology, and end results data. J Clin Oncol 23:5534, 2005

Claus EB, Risch N, Thompson WD: Autosomal dominant inheritance of early-onset breast cancer. Implications for risk prediction. Cancer 73:643, 1994

Clavel-Chapelon F, Group EN: Cumulative number of menstrual cycles and breast cancer risk: results from the E3N cohort study of French women. Cancer Causes Control 13:831, 2002

Colditz GA, Willett WC, Hunter DJ, et al: Family history, age and risk of breast cancer. Prospective data from the Nurses Health Study. JAMA 270:1563, 1993

Concannon P: ATM heterozygosity and cancer risk. Nat Genet 32:89, 2002

Costantino JP, Gail MH, Pee D, et al: Validation studies for models projecting the risk of invasive and total breast cancer incidence. J Natl Cancer Inst 91:1541, 1999

Cox CE, Reintgen DS, Nicosia SV, et al: Analysis of residual cancer after diagnostic breast biopsy: an argument for fine-needle aspiration cytology. Ann Surg Oncol 2:201, 1995

Cvelbar M, Ursic-Vrscaj M, Rakar S: Risk factors and prognostic factors in patients with double primary cancer: epithelial ovarian cancer and breast cancer. Eur J Gynaecol Oncol 26:59, 2005

Dawood S: Biology and management of inflammatory breast cancer. Expert Rev Anticancer Ther 10(2):209, 2010

Domchek SM, Friebel TM, Singer CF, et al: Association of risk-reducing surgery in BRCA1 or BRCA2 mutation carriers with cancer risk and mortality. JAMA 304(9):967, 2010

D'Orsi CJ, Bassett LW, Feig SA, et al: Illustrated Breast Imaging Reporting and Data System: illustrated BI-RADS, 3rd ed. Reston, VA, American College of Radiology, 1998

Davies HH, Simons M, Davis JB: Cystic disease of the breast. Relationship to carcinoma. Cancer 17:757, 1964

den Tonkelaar I, de Waard F: Regularity and length of menstrual cycles in women aged 41–46 in relation to breast cancer risk: results from the DOM-project. Breast Cancer Res Treat 38:253, 1996

Dent DM, Macking EA, Wilkie W: Benign breast disease clinical classification and disease distribution. Br J Clin Pract 42(Suppl 56):69, 1988

Dobbins JT, Godfrey DJ: Digital x-ray tomosynthesis: current state of the art and clinical potential. Phys Med Biol 48:R65, 2003

Du Toit RS, Grobler SP, Brink C, et al: The role of mammography to evaluate palpable breast tumors. S Afr Med J 30:15, 1992

Dupont WD, Parl FF, Hartman WH, et al: Breast cancer risk associated with proliferative breast disease and atypical hyperplasia. Cancer 71:1258, 1993

Early Breast Cancer Trialists Collaborative Group (EBCTG): Effects of radiotherapy and of differences in the extent of surgery for early breast cancer on local recurrence and 15-year survival: an overview of the randomized trials. Lancet 366:2087, 2005

Easton DF, Ford D, Bishop T, et al: Breast and ovarian cancer incidence in BRCA1-mutation carriers. Am J Hum Genet 56:265, 1995

Eisen A, Lubinski J, Klijn J, et al: Breast cancer risk following bilateral oophorectomy in BRCA1 and BRCA2 mutation carriers: an international case-control study. J Clin Oncol 23:7491, 2005

Emens LA, Davidson NE: The follow-up of breast cancer. Semin Oncol 30:338, 2003

Euhus DM: Clinical relevance of circulating tumor cells in the management of breast cancer. Biol Ther Breast Cancer 6:6, 2005

Euhus DM, Uyehara C: Influence of parenteral progesterones on the prevalence and severity of mastalgia in premenopausal women. A multi-institutional cross-sectional study. J Am Coll Surg 184:596, 1997

Evans SC, Lozano G: The Li-Fraumeni syndrome: an inherited susceptibility to cancer. Mol Med Today 3:390, 1997

Fatouros M, Roukos DH, Arampatzis I, et al: Factors increasing local recurrence in breast-conserving surgery. Expert Rev Anticancer Ther 5:737, 2005

Feig SA: Age-related accuracy of screening mammography: how should it be measured? Radiology 214:633, 2000

Fisher B, Anderson S, Bryant J, et al: Twenty-year follow-up of a randomized trial comparing total mastectomy, lumpectomy, and lumpectomy plus irradiation for the treatment of invasive breast cancer. N Engl J Med 347:1233, 2002a

Fisher B, Costantino J, Redmond C, et al: Lumpectomy compared with lumpectomy and radiation therapy for the treatment of intraductal breast cancer. N Engl J Med 328:1581, 1993

Fisher B, Costantino JP, Wickerham DL, et al: Tamoxifen for prevention of breast cancer: report of the National Surgical Adjuvant Breast and Bowel Project P-1 Study. J Natl Cancer Inst 90:1371, 1998

Fisher B, Dignam J, Wolmark N, et al: Tamoxifen in treatment of intraductal breast cancer: National Surgical Adjuvant Breast and Bowel Project B-24 randomised controlled trial. Lancet 353:1993, 1999

Fisher B, Jeong JH, Anderson S, et al: Twenty-year follow-up of a randomized trial comparing radical mastectomy, total mastectomy, and total mastectomy followed by irradiation. N Engl J Med 347:567, 2002b

Fisher ER, Fisher B, Sass R, et al: Pathologic findings from the National Surgical Adjuvant Breast Project (Protocol No. 4): XI. Bilateral breast cancer. Cancer 54:3002, 1984

Fisher ER, Land SR, Fisher B, et al: Pathologic findings from the National Surgical Adjuvant Breast and Bowel Project. Twelve-year observations concerning lobular carcinoma in situ. Cancer 100:238, 2004

Ford D, Easton DF, Bishop DT, et al: Risks of cancer in BRCA-1 mutation carriers. Lancet 343:692, 1994

Ford D, Easton DF, Stratton M, et al: Genetic heterogeneity and penetrance analysis of the BRCA1 and BRCA2 genes in breast cancer families. Am J Hum Genet 62:676, 1998

Foulkes WD, Metcalfe K, Sun P, et al: Estrogen receptor status in BRCA1- and BRCA2-related breast cancer: the influence of age, grade, and histological type. Clin Cancer Res 10:2029, 2004

Franyz VK, Pickern JW, Melcher GW, et al: Incidence of chronic cystic disease in so-called normal breast: a study based on 225 post-mortem examinations. Cancer 4:762, 1951

Friedenreich CM: Review of anthropometric factors and breast cancer risk. Eur J Cancer Prev 10:15, 2001

Friedman LS, Gayther SA, Kurosaki T, et al: Mutation analysis of BRCA1 and BRCA2 in a male breast cancer population. Am J Hum Genet 60:313, 1997

Gail MH, Brinton LA, Byar DP, et al: Projecting individualized probabilities of developing breast cancer for white females who are being examined annually. J Natl Cancer Inst 81:1879, 1989

Gandini S, Merzenich H, Robertson C, et al: Meta-analysis of studies on breast cancer risk and diet: the role of fruit and vegetable consumption and the intake of associated micronutrients. Eur J Cancer 36:636, 2000

Gao X, Fisher SG, Emami B: Risk of second primary cancer in the contralateral breast in women treated for early-stage breast cancer: a population-based study. Int J Radiat Oncol Biol Phys 56:1038, 2003

Gateley CA, Mansel RE: Management of cyclic breast pain. Br J Hosp Med 43:330, 1990

Geisler J, Lonning PE: Aromatase inhibitors as adjuvant treatment of breast cancer. Crit Rev Oncol Hematol 57:53, 2006

Georgiannos SN, Chin J, Goode AW, et al: Secondary neoplasms of the breast: a survey of the 20th century. Cancer 92:2259, 2001

Giuliano AE, Dale PS, Turner RR, et al: Improved axillary staging of breast cancer with sentinel lymphadenectomy. Ann Surg 222:394, 1995

Going JJ, Moffat DF: Escaping from Flatland: clinical and biological aspects of human mammary duct anatomy in three dimensions. J Pathol 203:538, 2004

Gonzalez-Angulo AM, Hortobagyi GN, Esteva FJ: Adjuvant therapy with trastuzumab for HER-2/neu-positive breast cancer. Oncologist 11:857, 2006

Gordon PB: Ultrasound for breast cancer screening and staging. Radiol Clin North Am 40:431, 2002

Grant RN, Tabah EJ, Adair FE: The surgical significance of the subareolar lymph plexus in cancer of the breast. Surgery 33:71, 1953

Grimm SL, Seagroves TN, Kabotyanski EB, et al: Disruption of steroid and prolactin receptor pattern in the mammary gland correlates with a block in lobuloalveolar development. Mol Endocrinol 16:2675, 2002

Gupta RK, Gaskell D, Dowle CS, et al: The role of nipple discharge cytology in the diagnosis of breast disease: a study of 1948 nipple discharge smears from 1530 patients. Cytopathology 15:326, 2004

Haagensen CD: Cystosarcoma phyllodes. In Diseases of the Breast. Philadelphia, WB Saunders, 1986a, p 284

Haagensen CD: Gross cystic disease. In Diseases of the Breast. Philadelphia, WB Saunders, 1986b, p 250

Habel LA, Shak S, Jacobs MK, et al: A population-based study of tumor gene expression and risk of breast cancer death among lymph node-negative patients. Breast Cancer Res 8:R25, 2006

Haffty BG, Harrold E, Khan AJ, et al: Outcome of conservatively managed early-onset breast cancer by BRCA1/2 status. Lancet 359:1471, 2002

Halstead W: The results of operations for cure of cancer of the breast performed at Johns Hopkins Hospital. Johns Hopkins Hosp Bull 4:497, 1894

Hardy JR, Powles TJ, Judson I, et al: How many tests are required in the diagnosis of palpable breast abnormalities? Clin Oncol 2:148, 1990

Harris EE, Schultz D, Bertsch H, et al: Ten-year outcome after combined modality therapy for inflammatory breast cancer. Int J Radiat Oncol Biol Phys 55:1200, 2003

Hartmann LC, Sellers TA, Schaid DJ, et al: Efficacy of bilateral prophylactic mastectomy in BRCA1 and BRCA2 gene mutation carriers. J Natl Cancer Inst 93:1633, 2001

Hermansen C, Skovgaard Poulsen H, Jensen J, et al: Diagnostic reliability of combined physical examination, mammography, and fine-needle puncture ("triple-test") in breast tumors. A prospective study. Cancer 60:1866, 1987

Hilner BE, Ingle JN, Chlebowski RT, et al: American Society of Clinical Oncology 2003 update on role of bisphosphonates and bone disease in women with breast cancer. J Clin Oncol 21(21):4042, 2003

Hultborn KA, Larsen LG, Raghnult I: The lymph drainage from the breast to the axillary and parasternal lymph nodes: studies with the aid of colloidal Au 198. Acta Radiol 45:52, 1955

Ikeda DM, Helvie MA, Frank TS, et al: Paget's disease of the nipple: radiologic-pathologic correlation. Radiology 189:89, 1993

Ismail PM, Amato P, Soyal SM, et al: Progesterone involvement in breast development and tumorigenesis—as revealed by progesterone receptor "knockout" and "knockin" mouse models. Steroids 68:779, 2003

Jaiyesimi IA, Buzdar AU, Decker DA, et al: Use of tamoxifen for breast cancer: twenty-eight years later. J Clin Oncol 13:513, 1995

Jatoi I: Screening clinical breast exam. Surg Clin North Am 83:789, 2003

Jeruss JS, Vicini FA, Beitsch PD, et al: Initial outcomes for patients treated on the American Society of Breast Surgeons MammoSite clinical trial for ductal carcinoma-in-situ of the breast. Ann Surg Oncol 13:967, 2006

Kaklamani V, O'Regan RM: New targeted therapies in breast cancer. Semin Oncol 31(2 Suppl 4):20, 2004

Kauf ND, Satagopan JM, Robson ME, et al: Risk-reducing salpingo-oophorectomy in women with a BRCA1 or BRCA2 mutation. N Engl J Med 346:1609, 2002

Kaufman Z, Shpitz B, Shapiro M, et al: Triple approach in the diagnosis of dominant breast masses: combined physical examination, mammography, and fine-needle aspiration. J Surg Oncol 56:254, 1994

Khan SA, Rogers MA, Khurana KK, et al: Estrogen receptor expression in benign breast epithelium and breast cancer risk. J Natl Cancer Inst 89:37, 1997

Khatcheressian JL, Wolff AC, Smith TJ, et al: American Society of Clinical Oncology 2006 Update of the Breast Cancer Follow-Up and Management Guidelines in the Adjuvant Setting. J Clin Oncol 24:1, 2006

Kolb TM, Lichy J, Newhouse JH: Comparison of the performance of screening mammography, physical examination, and breast US and evaluation of factors that influence them: an analysis of 27,825 patient evaluations. Radiology 225:165, 2002

Kreuzer G, Boquoi E: Aspiration biopsy, cytology, mammography and clinical exploration: a modern set up in diagnosis of tumors of the breast. Acta Cytol 20:319, 1976

Kudachadkar R, O'Regan RM: Aromatase inhibitors as adjuvant therapy for postmenopausal patients with early stage breast cancer. CA Cancer J Clin 55:145, 2005

Kuehn T, Klauss W, Darsow M, et al: Long-term morbidity following axillary dissection in breast cancer patients—clinical assessment, significance for life quality and the impact of demographic, oncologic and therapeutic factors. Breast Cancer Res Treat 64:275, 2000

Kumar R, Nadig MR, Chauhan A: Positron emission tomography: clinical applications in oncology. Part 1. Expert Rev Anticancer Ther 5:1079, 2005

Kumar S, Mansel RE, Scanlon F: Altered responses of prolactin, luteinizing hormone and follicle stimulating hormone secretion to thyrotropin releasing hormone/gonadotropin releasing hormone stimulation in cyclical mastalgia. Br J Surg 71:870, 1989

Kvale G, Heuch I: Menstrual factors and breast cancer risk. Cancer 62: 1625, 1988

LaCroix AZ, Chlebowski RT, Manson JE: Health outcomes after stopping conjugated equine estrogens among postmenopausal women with prior hysterectomy. JAMA 305(13):1305, 2011

Lahmann PH, Hoffmann K, Allen N, et al: Body size and breast cancer risk: findings from the European Prospective Investigation into Cancer and Nutrition (EPIC). Int J Cancer 111:762, 2004

Laibl VR, Sheffield JS, Roberts S, et al: Clinical presentation of community-acquired methicillin-resistant Staphylococcus aureus in pregnancy. Obstet Gynecol 106(3):461, 2005

Lau S, Küchenmeister, I, Stachs A, et al: Pathological nipple discharge: surgery is imperative in postmenopausal women. Ann Surg Oncol 12:246, 2005

Layde PM, Webster LA, Baughman LA, et al: The independent associations of parity, age at first full term pregnancy, and duration of breastfeeding with the risk of breast cancer. Cancer and Steroid Hormone Study Group. J Clin Epidemiol 42:963, 1989

Leach MO, Boggis CR, Dixon AK, et al: Screening with magnetic resonance imaging and mammography of a UK population at high familial risk of breast cancer: a prospective multicentre cohort study (MARIBS). Lancet 365:1769, 2005

Lee CH, Dershaw DD, Kopans D, et al: Breast cancer screening with imaging: recommendations from the Society of Breast Imaging and the ACR on the use of mammography, breast MRI, breast ultrasound, and other technologies for the detection of clinically occult breast cancer. J Am Coll Radiol 7(1):18, 2010

Lee IM: Physical activity and cancer prevention—data from epidemiologic studies. Med Sci Sports Exerc 35:1823, 2003

Lichtenstein P, Holm NV, Verkasalo PK, et al: Environmental and heritable factors in the causation of cancer—analyses of cohorts of twins from Sweden, Denmark, and Finland. N Engl J Med 343:78, 2000

Lim W, Hearle N, Shah B, et al: Further observations on LKB1/STK11 status and cancer risk in Peutz-Jeghers syndrome. Br J Cancer 89:308, 2003

Locker AP, Galea MH, Ellis IO, et al: Microdochectomy for single-duct discharge from the nipple. Br J Surg 75:700, 1988

Lostumbo L, Carbine N, Wallace J, et al: Prophylactic mastectomy for the prevention of breast cancer. Cochrane Database Syst Rev 4:CD002748, 2004

Lyman GH, Giuliano AE, Somerfield MR, et al: American Society of Clinical Oncology Guideline recommendations for sentinel lymph node biopsy in early-stage breast cancer. J Clin Oncol 23:7703, 2005

MacInnis RJ, English DR, Gertig DM, et al: Body size and composition and risk of postmenopausal breast cancer. Cancer Epidemiol Biomarkers Prev 13:2117, 2004

MacMahon B, Cole P, Lin TM, et al: Age at first birth and breast cancer risk. Bull World Health Organ 43:209, 1970

Maddox PR, Mansel RE: Management of breast pain and nodularity. World J Surg 13:699, 1989

Malone KE, Daling JR, Neal C, et al: Frequency of BRCA1/BRCA2 mutations in a population-based sample of young breast carcinoma cases. Cancer 88:1393, 2000

Mansel RE, Dogliotti L: European multicenter trial of bromocriptine in cyclical mastalgia. Lancet 335:190, 1990

Martin G, Martin R, Brieva MJ, et al: Electrical impedance scanning in breast cancer imaging: correlation with mammographic and histologic diagnosis. Eur Radiol 12:1471, 2002

Masood S: Prognostic/predictive factors in breast cancer. Clin Lab Med 25:809, 2005

McDonnell SK, Schaid DJ, Myers JL, et al: Efficacy of contralateral prophylactic mastectomy in women with a personal and family history of breast cancer. J Clin Oncol 19: 3938, 2001

Meskens FL, Szabo E: Diet and cancer: the disconnect between epidemiology and randomized clinical trials. Cancer Epidemiol Biomarkers Prev 14:1366, 2005

Morrell RM, Halyard MY, Schild SE, et al: Breast cancer-related lymphedema. Mayo Clin Proc 80:1480, 2005

Nabholtz JM, Gligorov J: Docetaxel in the treatment of breast cancer: current experience and future prospects. Expert Rev Anticancer Ther 5:613, 2005

National Institutes of Health: Adjuvant therapy for breast cancer. NIH Consensus Statement, National Institutes of Health. Available at: http://consensus.nih.gov/2000/2000AdjuvantTherapyBreastCancer114PDF.pdf. Accessed January 20, 2007

Oberman HA: Cystosarcoma phyllodes: a clinicopathologic study of hypercellular periductal neoplasms of the breast. Cancer 28:697, 1965

Orel SG, Schnall MD: MR imaging of the breast for the detection, diagnosis, and staging of breast cancer. Radiology 220:13, 2001

Osin PP, Anbazhagan R, Bartkova J, et al: Breast development gives insights into breast disease. Histopathology 33:275, 1998

Papanicolaou GN, Holmquist DG, Bader GM, et al: Exfoliative cytology in the human mammary gland and its value in the diagnosis of breast cancer and other diseases of the breast. Cancer 11:377, 1958

Parisky YR, Sardi A, Hamm R, et al: Efficacy of computerized infrared imaging analysis to evaluate mammographically suspicious lesions. Am J Roentgenol 180:263, 2003

Parkin DM: Global cancer statistics in the year. Lancet Oncol 2:533, 2001

Parks AG: The micro-anatomy of the breast. Ann R Coll Surg Engl 25:235, 1959

Pathak DR, Speizer FE, Willett WC, et al: Parity and breast cancer risk: possible effect on age at diagnosis. Int J Cancer 37:21, 1986

Pena KS, Rosenfeld JA: Evaluation and treatment of galactorrhea. Am Fam Physician 63:1763, 2001

Peralta E, Ellenhorn J, Wagman L, et al: Contralateral prophylactic mastectomy improves the outcome of selected patients undergoing mastectomy for breast cancer. Am J Surg 180:439, 2000

Petrakis NL, Miike R, King EB, et al: Association of breast fluid coloration with age, ethnicity and cigarette smoking. Breast Cancer Res Treat 11:255, 1988

Pierce LJ, Phillips KA, Griffith KA, et al: Local therapy in BRCA1 and BRCA2 mutation carriers with operable breast cancer: comparison of breast conservation and mastectomy. Breast Cancer Res Treat 121(2):389, 2010

Pike MC, Krailo MD, Henderson BE, et al: "Hormonal" risk factors, "breast tissue age" and the age-incidence of breast cancer. Nature 303:767, 1983

Pisano ED, Gatsonis C, Hendrick E, et al: Diagnostic performance of digital versus film mammography for breast-cancer screening. N Engl J Med 353:1773, 2005

Plosker GL, Keam SJ: Trastuzumab: a review of its use in the management of HER2-positive metastatic and early-stage breast cancer. Drugs 66:449, 2006

Rebbeck T, Friebel T, Wagner T, et al. Effect of short-term hormone replacement therapy on breast cancer risk reduction after bilateral prophylactic oophorectomy in BRCA 1 and BRCA 2 mutation carriers: the PROSE Study Group. J Clin Oncol 23:7804, 2005

Rebbeck TR, Lynch HT, Neuhausen SL, et al: Prophylactic oophorectomy in carriers of BRCA1 and BRCA2 mutations. N Engl J Med 346:1616, 2002

Reinfuss M, Mitus J, Duda K, et al: The treatment and prognosis of patients with phyllodes tumor of the breast: an analysis of 170 cases. Cancer 77:910, 1996

Ringberg A, Anagnostaki L, Anderson H, et al: Cell biological factors in ductal carcinoma in situ (DCIS) of the breast—relationship to ipsilateral local recurrence and histopathological characteristics. Eur J Cancer 37:1514, 2001

Robson M, Levin D, Federici M, et al: Breast conservation therapy for invasive breast cancer in Ashkenazi women with BRCA gene founder mutations. J Natl Cancer Inst 91:2112, 1999

Rockhill B, Spiegelman D, Byrne C, et al: Validation of the Gail et al model of breast cancer risk prediction and implications for chemoprevention. J Natl Cancer Inst 93:358, 2001

Rugo HS: Bevacizumab in the treatment of breast cancer: rationale and current data. Oncologist 9(Suppl):143, 2004

Russo IH, Russo J: Mammary gland neoplasia in long-term rodent studies. Environ Health Perspect 104:938, 1996

Sampalis FS, Denis R, Picard D, et al: International prospective evaluation of scintimammography with 99m technetium sestamibi. Am J Surg 185:544, 2002

Santen RJ, Mansel R: Benign breast disorders. N Engl J Med 353:275, 2005

Sapino A, Cassoni P, Zanon E, et al: Ultrasonographically-guided fine-needle aspiration of axillary lymph nodes: role in breast cancer management. Br J Cancer 88:702, 2003

Schelfhout VR, Coene ED, Delaey B, et al: Pathogenesis of Paget's disease: epidermal heregulin-alpha, motility factor, and the HER receptor family. J Natl Cancer Inst 92:622, 2000

Schrager CA, Schneider D, Gruener AC, et al: Clinical and pathological features of breast disease in Cowden's syndrome: an underrecognized syndrome with an increased risk of breast cancer. Hum Pathol 29:47, 1998

Seeley RR, Stephens TD, Tate P: Reproductive system. In Anatomy and Physiology, 7th ed. New York, McGraw-Hill, 2006, p 1058

Seynaevea C, Verhooga LC, van de Boscha LM, et al: Ipsilateral breast tumour recurrence in hereditary breast cancer following breast-conserving therapy. Eur J Cancer 40:1150, 2004

Shannon J, Douglas-Jones AG, Dallimore NS: Conversion to core biopsy in preoperative diagnosis of breast lesions: is it justified by results? J Clin Pathol 54:762, 2001

Sickles EA, Klein DL, Goodson WH, et al: Mammography after needle aspiration of palpable breast masses. Am J Surg 145:395, 1983

Siegel R, Ward E, Brawley O: Cancer statistics, 2011: the impact of eliminating socioeconomic and racial disparities on premature cancer deaths. CA Cancer J Clin 61(4):212, 2011

Smith RA, Cokkinides V, Brooks D, et al: Cancer screening in the United States, 2011: a review of current American Cancer Society Guidelines and issues in cancer screening. CA Cancer J Clin 61(1):8, 2011

Smith-Warner SA, Spiegelman D, Yaun SS, et al: Alcohol and breast cancer in women: a pooled analysis of cohort studies. JAMA 279:535, 1998

Sneige N, Wang J, Baker BA, et al: Clinical, histopathologic, and biologic features of pleomorphic lobular (ductal-lobular) carcinoma in situ of the breast: a report of 24 cases. Mod Pathol 15:1044, 2002

Soderqvist G, Isaksson E, von Schoultz B, et al: Proliferation of breast epithelial cells in healthy women during the menstrual cycle. Am J Obstet Gynecol 176:123, 1997

Solin LJ, Kurtz J, Fourquet A, et al: Fifteen-year results of breast-conserving surgery and breast irradiation for the treatment of ductal carcinoma in situ of the breast. J Clin Oncol 14:754, 1996

Stafford I, Hernandez J, Laibl V, et al: Community-acquired methicillin-resistant *Staphylococcus aureus* among patients with puerperal mastitis requiring hospitalization. Obstet Gynecol 112(3):533, 2008

Stavros AT, Thickman D, Rapp CL, et al: Solid breast nodules: use of sonography to distinguish between benign and malignant lesions. Radiology 196:123, 1995

Stoeckelhuber M, Stumpf P, Hoefter EA, et al: Proteoglycan-collagen associations in the non-lactating human breast connective tissue during the menstrual cycle. Histochem Cell Biol 118:221, 2002

Stoutjesdijk MJ, Boetes C, Jager GJ, et al: Magnetic resonance imaging and mammography in women with a hereditary risk of breast cancer. J Natl Cancer Inst 93:1095, 2001

Tabbara SO, Frost AR, Stoler MH, et al: Changing trends in breast fine-needle aspiration: results of the Papanicolaou Society of Cytopathology Survey. Diagn Cytopathol 22:126, 2000

Tavassoli FA: Breast pathology: rationale for adopting the ductal intraepithelial neoplasia (DIN) classification. Nature Clin Pract Oncol 2:116, 2005

Taylor G, Meltzer A: Inflammatory carcinoma of the breast. Am J Cancer 33:33, 1938

The Breast Cancer Linkage Consortium: Cancer risks in BRCA2 mutation carriers. J Natl Cancer Inst 91:1310, 1999

The CHEK2-Breast Cancer Consortium: Low-penetrance susceptibility to breast cancer due to CHEK2*1100delC in noncarriers of BRCA1 or BRCA2 mutations. Nat Genet 31:55, 2002

The Women's Health Initiative Steering Committee: Effects of conjugated equine estrogen in postmenopausal women with hysterectomy: The Women's Health Initiative randomized controlled trial. JAMA 291:1701, 2004

Thomas DB, Gao DL, Ray RM, et al: Randomized trial of breast self-examination in Shanghai: final results. J Natl Cancer Inst 94:1445, 2002

Thomsen AC, Hansen KB, Moller BR: Leukocyte counts and microbiological cultivation in the diagnosis of puerperal mastitis. Am J Obstet Gynecol 146:938, 1983

Thorlacius S, Olafsdottir G, Tryggvadottir L, et al: A single BRCA2 mutation in male and female breast cancer families from Iceland with varied cancer phenotypes. Nat Genet 13:117, 1996

Tilanus-Linthorst MM, Obdeijn IM, Bartels KC, et al: First experiences in screening women at high risk for breast cancer with MR imaging. Breast Cancer Res Treat 63:53, 2000

Trudeau M, Charbonneau F, Gelmon K, et al: Selection of adjuvant chemotherapy for treatment of node-positive breast cancer. Lancet Oncol 6:886, 2005

Tyrer J, Duffy SW, Cuzick J: A breast cancer prediction model incorporating familial and personal risk factors. Stat Med 23:1111, 2004

Urban J, Egeli R: Non-lactational nipple discharge. CA Cancer J Clin 283:3, 1978

Ursin G, Ma H, Wu AH, et al: Mammographic density and breast cancer in three ethnic groups. Cancer Epidemiol Biomarkers Prev 12:332, 2003

van de Vijver MJ, He YD, van't Veer L, et al: A gene expression signature as a predictor of survival in breast cancer. N Engl J Med 347:1999, 2002

Vihko RK, Apter DL: The epidemiology and endocrinology of the menarche in relation to breast cancer. Cancer Surv 5:561, 1986

Virnig BA, Tuttle TM, Shamliyan T, et al: Ductal carcinoma in situ of the breast: a systematic review of incidence, treatment, and outcomes. J Natl Cancer Inst 102(3):170, 2010

Vogel VG, Costantino JP, Wickerham DL, et al: Effects of tamoxifen vs raloxifene on the risk of developing invasive breast cancer and other disease outcomes. The NSABP Study of Tamoxifen and Raloxifene (STAR) P-2 Trial. JAMA 295:2727, 2006

Warner E, Plewes DB, Shumak RS, et al: Comparison of breast magnetic resonance imaging, mammography, and ultrasound for surveillance of women at high risk for hereditary breast cancer. J Clin Oncol 19:3524, 2001

Watt-Boolsen S, Rasmussen NR, Blichert-Toft M: Primary periareolar abscess in the non-lactating breast: risk of recurrence. Am J Surg 155:571, 1987

Wilkie C, White L, Dupont E, et al: An update of sentinel lymph node mapping in patients with ductal carcinoma in situ. Am J Surg 190:563, 2005

Wrensch WR, Petrakis NL, Gruenke LD, et al: Factors associated with obtaining nipple aspirate fluid: analysis of 1428 women and literature review. Breast Cancer Res Treat 15:39, 1990

Writing Group for the Women's Health Initiative Investigators: Risks and benefits of estrogen plus progestin in healthy post-menopausal women: principal results from the Women's Health Initiative randomized controlled trial. JAMA 288:321, 2002

Zannis V, Beitsch P, Vicini F, et al: Descriptions and outcomes of insertion techniques of a breast brachytherapy balloon catheter in 1403 patients enrolled in the American Society of Breast Surgeons MammoSite breast brachytherapy registry trial. Am J Surg 190:530, 2005

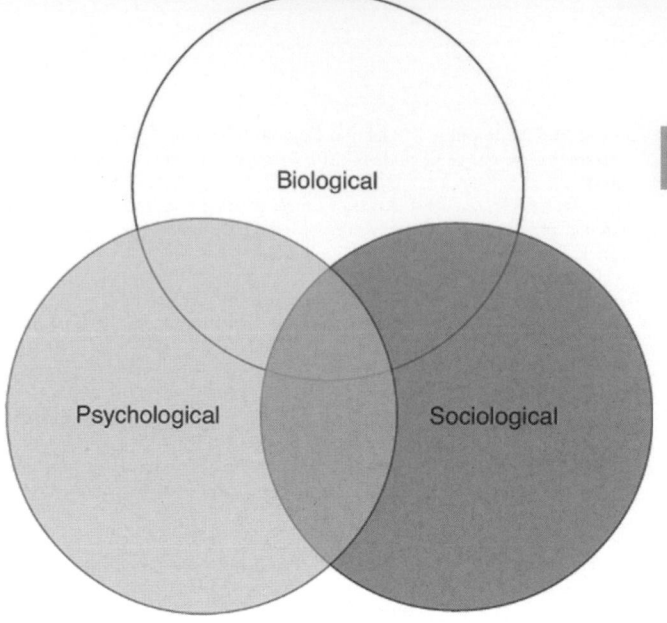

More than 30 years ago, psychiatrist George Engel (1977) coined a word to describe a developing paradigm for patient care, the "biopsychosocial model." The model encouraged formulating treatments that considered the mind and body of a patient as two intertwining systems influenced by yet a third system—society.

Twenty years before this paradigm, Erik Erikson (1963) created a model that describes psychological maturation across the life span. Combining these two models yields a dimensional perspective helpful for the evaluation, diagnosis, and treatment of any patient (Table 13-1).

Not only do women use more health care services in general than men in the United States, but more women approach their physicians with psychiatric complaints, and more women have comorbid illness than men (Andrade, 2003; Burt, 2005; Kessler, 1994). Coupled with the "almost universal recognition" that primary care is where most patients with psychiatric illness are first seen, obstetricians and gynecologists will often be the first to evaluate a woman in psychiatric distress (Goldberg, 2003). A clinical interview such as one presented in Table 13-2 can guide assessment and includes all three domains from the biopsychosocial model.

COMMON PSYCHIATRIC PRESENTATIONS

Mood, anxiety, and alcohol or substance use disorders are three families of psychiatric disorders commonly seen and often are comorbid with reproductive disorders (American Psychiatric Association, 2000a). Each family is characterized by a predominant feature, and each disorder within that family is identified by specific symptoms of that feature. These three groups are defined by specific criteria described by the *Diagnostic and Statistical Manual of Mental Disorders, Fourth Edition, Text Revision* (DSM-IV-TR), published by the American Psychiatric Association (2000a). The DSM-IV-TR is currently being updated, with the DSM-V expected in 2013 and described at http://www.dsm5.org/Pages/Default.aspx. Material in this chapter is based upon the DSM-IV.

Mood Disorders

The spectrum of mood disorders is divided into depressive disorders (major depressive disorder, dysthymic disorder,

TABLE 13-1. Biopsychosocial Development

	Adolescence: 11–18 yrs	Early Adulthood: 18–34 yrs	Middle Adulthood: 35–60 yrs	Late Adulthood: 61 yrs–death
Biologic	Pubertal hormonal changes Reproductive organ development Physical growth spurts Menarche Initiation of sexual activity	Hormonal activity Sexual activity Pregnancy	Hormonal changes Menopausal transition	Postmenopausal risks Age-related illness
Psychological	Identity construction Family functioning Peer relations Academic achievement	Role transitions Partner selection Motherhood Divorce Career choices and success Economic status	Marital status Late childbearing or "empty nest" Caring for aging parents Grandparenthood Career success and/or change Economic stability	Widowhood/ divorce Remarriage Losses Extended family and friends Retirement Economic security
Social	School Home Neighborhood Church	College Workplace Home Neighborhood Church	Home Workplace Neighborhood Church Community	Home Neighborhood Church Community World-at-large

and depressive disorder not otherwise specified); the bipolar disorders (bipolar I, bipolar II, cyclothymic disorder, and bipolar disorder not otherwise specified); and two etiologic disorders (mood disorder due to a general medical condition and substance-induced mood disorder) (Table 13-3). Individuals with bipolar disorders demonstrate episodes both of depression and of mania, which are described in Table 13-4.

Mood Disorder Prevalence

The lifetime prevalence for mood disorders in the general U.S. population is approximately 20 percent (Kessler, 2005). Depression is the second leading cause of disability in women, and females are 1.5 times more likely to suffer from a major depressive episode than men (National Institute of Mental Health, 2010). Women also commonly have one or more comorbid psychiatric disorders, most commonly anxiety disorder and/or substance use disorder.

Diagnosis of Mood Disorders

Self-report questionnaires are often used to identify individuals who require further psychiatric evaluation (screening measures) and gauge the frequency and intensity of depressive symptoms (severity measures). The Quick Inventory of Depressive Symptomatology-Self Report (QIDS-SR) is one such tool easily implemented for clinical use (Tables 13-5 and 13-6) (Rush, 2003). By patient report, this questionnaire assesses the symptom severity required by DSM-IV criteria to diagnose major depressive disorder. Further information regarding this

instrument and its translation into 30 languages are available at www.ids qids.org.

Anxiety Disorders

Anxiety disorders have the highest prevalence rates in the United States. Lifetime prevalence rates approximate 30 percent, and women are 1.6 times more likely to be diagnosed than men (Kessler, 2005). For women, the key transitions of menarche, pregnancy, and menopause may cause anxious feelings because of the perceived irreversible life changes that they may herald (Bibring, 1959). Criteria established in the DSM-IV may provide guidelines to help distinguish anxiety disorder from normally expected worries (Tables 13-7 and 13-8).

Alcohol and Substance Disorders

In the United States, the lifetime prevalence for alcohol and substance disorders approximates 15 percent. This diagnosis is twice as likely in males, although rates in women are increasing (Kessler, 2005). Indicators of substance misuse are found in Tables 13-9 and 13-10. Often these disorders coexist with depression and anxiety. An in-depth discussion of these issues is beyond this chapter's scope, but additional information regarding alcohol and other commonly abused substances, including prescription medications, is available at www.nida.nih.gov.

TABLE 13-2. Psychiatric Assessment of Women: Clinically Significant Considerations

Component	Consideration
History of present illness and past psychiatric history	Characterize symptoms in relation to: 1. A specific phase of the menstrual cycle 2. Use of hormonal contraception 3. Pregnancy 4. Postpartum period 5. Breast feeding or weaning 6. Abortion 7. Infertility treatment 8. Hysterectomy 9. Menopausal transition
Medications	Exogenous hormones and all over-the-counter medications and supplements
Dietary assessment	Ritualistic or restrictive eating patterns, binging, self-induced vomiting, and use of diet pills, laxatives, emetics, and diuretics
Alcohol and drug use	Covert use, especially of prescription medications
Family psychiatric history	History of premenstrual dysphoric disorders and postpartum mood disorders
Medical history	Autoimmune illnesses (e.g., lupus, thyroiditis, or fibromyalgia) that may present with psychiatric symptoms History of sexually transmitted disease that may affect current sexual functioning and childbearing capacity
Menstrual history	Pregnancy, menstruation-related symptoms Perimenopausal symptoms
Social and developmental history	Sexual preference, relationship styles, level of satisfaction with current relationships Tendency to take on certain role in relationships (e.g., caregiver, nurturer, or dependent or helpless role) Current or past sexual, physical, or emotional abuse
Socioeconomic status	Level of economic support and ability to meet ongoing financial needs If patient is a single mother, inquire about child support

Adapted from Burt, 2005, with permission.

EATING DISORDERS

Eating disorders are classified by DSM-IV as anorexia nervosa (AN), bulimia nervosa (BN), and eating disorder not otherwise specified (Tables 13-11 and 13-12). The core symptoms of both anorexia and bulimia are preoccupation with weight gain and excessive self-evaluation of weight and body shape. These disorders are 10 to 20 times more common in females than in males, particularly in those aged 15 to 24 years (Mitchell, 2006). During adolescence, an estimated 4 percent of girls have some form of eating disorder, and approximately 0.3 percent suffer from anorexia nervosa. Anorexia usually begins early in adolescence and peaks at ages 17 to 18 years. Bulimia nervosa is more prevalent than anorexia but typically has a later onset (Hoek, 1998, 2006).

Pathophysiology

The exact etiology of eating disorders is unknown. However, evidence suggests that there is a strong familial aggregation for eating disorders (Stein, 1999). In the restricting type of AN, the concordance rate among monozygotic twins has been shown to approximate 66 percent, and for dizygotic twins—10 percent (Treasure, 1989).

Various biologic factors have been implicated in the development of eating disorders. Abnormalities in neuropeptides, neurotransmitters, and hypothalamic-pituitary-adrenal and hypothalamic-pituitary-gonadal axes are reported (Stoving, 1999, 2001). In addition, psychological and psychodynamic factors related to an absence of autonomy are thought to influence obsessive preoccupations (Fassino, 2007). Although eating

TABLE 13-3. Diagnostic Criteria for a Major Depressive Episode

A. **≥5 criteria present during the same 2-week period or a change from previous functioning.**
At least one of these:
Depressed mood most of the day, nearly every day (can be irritability in kids)
Markedly diminished interest or pleasure in most activities, most of the day, most days
The balance of 5 from these:
Significant weight loss/gain, change in appetite, or failure to make expected gains
Insomnia or hypersomnia nearly every day
Psychomotor agitation or retardation nearly every day, *observable by others*
Fatigue or loss of energy nearly every day
Feelings of worthlessness or excessive or inappropriate guilt nearly every day
Diminished ability to think or concentrate or indecisiveness
Recurrent thoughts of death, recurrent suicidal ideation, plans, or attempt
B. The symptoms do not meet the criteria for a Mixed Episode
C. Symptoms cause significant distress or impairment in functioning
D. Symptoms are not due to a substance or a general medical condition
E. Symptoms not better accounted for by bereavement ≥2 months or marked

Specifiers:
Mild, Moderate, or Severe with or without Psychotic Features
Chronic
With Catatonic Features
With Melancholic Features
With Atypical Features
With Postpartum Onset

Adapted from American Psychiatric Association, 2000a, with permission.

TABLE 13-4. Diagnostic Criteria for Manic Episodes

Criteria for manic episodes
A. Distinct period of abnormally and persistently elevated, expansive, or irritable mood, lasting at least 1 week
B. During the period of mood disturbance, ≥3 of the following symptoms have persisted to a significant degree:
Inflated self-esteem or grandiosity
Decreased need for sleep
More talkative than usual
Flight of ideas or experiences racing thoughts
Distractibility
Increase in activity or psychomotor agitation
Excessive involvement in pleasurable or risky activities with high potential for negative or painful consequences
C. The criteria for a major depressive episode are not fulfilled
D. The patient is markedly impaired occupationally or socially, is psychotic, or needs to be hospitalized to prevent harm to self or others
E. The symptoms are not due to the direct physiologic effects of a substance or a general medical condition

Criteria for a hypomanic episode
A. A distinct period of persistently elevated, expansive, or irritable mood, lasting throughout at least 4 days, that is clearly abnormal from the usual mood
B. During the period of mood disturbance, ≥3 of the above symptoms (same as for mania) have persisted to a significant degree
C. The episode is associated with an unequivocal change in functioning that is uncharacteristic of the person when not symptomatic
D. The disturbance in mood and the change in functioning are observable by others
E. The episode is not severe enough to cause marked impairment in social or occupational functioning or to necessitate hospitalization, and there are no psychotic features
F. The symptoms are not due to the direct physiologic effects of a substance or a general medical condition

Adapted from American Psychiatric Association, 2000a, with permission.

TABLE 13-5. The Quick Inventory of Depressive Symptomatology (16-Item) (Self-Report) (QIDS-SR$_{16}$)

Name or ID: _____   Date: _____

CHECK THE ONE RESPONSE TO EACH ITEM THAT BEST DESCRIBES YOU FOR THE PAST SEVEN DAYS.

During the past seven days...

1. Falling Asleep:
- ☐ 0 I never take longer than 30 minutes to fall asleep.
- ☐ 1 I take at least 30 minutes to fall asleep, less than half the time.
- ☐ 2 I take at least 30 minutes to fall asleep, more than half the time.
- ☐ 3 I take more than 60 minutes to fall asleep, more than half the time.

2. Sleep During the Night:
- ☐ 0 I do not wake up at night.
- ☐ 1 I have a restless, light sleep with a few brief awakenings each night.
- ☐ 2 I wake up at least once a night, but I go back to sleep easily.
- ☐ 3 I awaken more than once a night and stay awake for 20 minutes or more, more than half the time.

3. Waking Up Too Early:
- ☐ 0 Most of the time, I awaken no more than 30 minutes before I need to get up.
- ☐ 1 More than half the time, I awaken more than 30 minutes before I need to get up.
- ☐ 2 I almost always awaken at least one hour or so before I need to, but I go back to sleep eventually.
- ☐ 3 I awaken at least one hour before I need to, and can't go back to sleep.

4. Sleeping Too Much:
- ☐ 0 I sleep no longer than 7–8 hours/night, without napping during the day.
- ☐ 1 I sleep no longer than 10 hours in a 24-hour period including naps.
- ☐ 2 I sleep no longer than 12 hours in a 24-hour period including naps.
- ☐ 3 I sleep longer than 12 hours in a 24-hour period including naps.

During the past seven days...

5. Feeling Sad:
- ☐ 0 I do not feel sad.
- ☐ 1 I feel sad less than half the time.
- ☐ 2 I feel sad more than half the time.
- ☐ 3 I feel sad nearly all of the time.

Please complete either 6 or 7 (not both)

6. Decreased Appetite:
- ☐ 0 There is no change in my usual appetite.
- ☐ 1 I eat somewhat less often or lesser amounts of food than usual.
- ☐ 2 I eat much less than usual and only with personal effort.
- ☐ 3 I rarely eat within a 24-hour period, and only with extreme personal effort or when others persuade me to eat.

-OR-

7. Increased Appetite:
- ☐ 0 There is no change from my usual appetite.
- ☐ 1 I feel a need to eat more frequently than usual.
- ☐ 2 I regularly eat more often and/or greater amounts of food than usual.
- ☐ 3 I feel driven to overeat both at mealtime and between meals.

Please complete either 8 or 9 (not both)

8. Decreased Weight (Within the Last Two Weeks):
- ☐ 0 I have not had a change in my weight.
- ☐ 1 I feel as if I have had a slight weight loss.
- ☐ 2 I have lost 2 pounds or more.
- ☐ 3 I have lost 5 pounds or more.

-OR-

9. Increased Weight (Within the Last Two Weeks):
- ☐ 0 I have not had a change in my weight.
- ☐ 1 I feel as if I have had a slight weight gain.
- ☐ 2 I have gained 2 pounds or more.
- ☐ 3 I have gained 5 pounds or more.

disorders are believed to be a western cultural phenomenon, rates of eating disorders are also increasing in nonwestern cultures (Fichter, 2004).

▮ Diagnosis

Anorexia Nervosa

This disorder is divided into two subtypes: (1) a restricting type and (2) a bulimic type, which is distinct from bulimia nervosa. Symptoms begin in the form of unique eating habits that become more and more restrictive. Advanced symptoms may include extreme food intake restriction and excessive exercise.

Up to 50 percent of anorectics also show bulimic behavior, and these types may alternate during the course of anorexic illness. Bulimic-type anorectics have been found to engage in two distinct behavior patterns, those who binge and purge and those who solely purge.

Individuals with anorexia commonly defend their eating behaviors upon confrontation and rarely recognize their illness. They increasingly isolate themselves socially as their disorder progresses. Multiple somatic complaints such as gastrointestinal symptoms and cold intolerance are common. In the disorder's later stages, weight loss becomes more apparent, and medical complications may prompt patients to seek help. These

TABLE 13-5. The Quick Inventory of Depressive Symptomatology (16-Item) (Self-Report) (QIDS-SR$_{16}$) *(Continued)*

During the past seven days...

10. Concentration/Decision-Making:
- ☐ 0 There is no change in my usual capacity to concentrate or make decisions.
- ☐ 1 I occasionally feel indecisive or find that my attention wanders.
- ☐ 2 Most of the time, I struggle to focus my attention or to make decisions.
- ☐ 3 I cannot concentrate well enough to read or cannot make even minor decisions.

11. View of Myself:
- ☐ 0 I see myself as equally worthwhile and deserving as other people.
- ☐ 1 I am more self-blaming than usual.
- ☐ 2 I largely believe that I cause problems for others.
- ☐ 3 I think almost constantly about major and minor defects in myself.

12. Thoughts of Death or Suicide:
- ☐ 0 I do not think of suicide or death.
- ☐ 1 I feel that life is empty or wonder if it's worth living.
- ☐ 2 I think of suicide or death several times a week for several minutes.
- ☐ 3 I think of suicide or death several times a day in some detail, or I have made specific plans for suicide or have actually tried to take my life.

13. General Interest:
- ☐ 0 There is no change from usual in how interested I am in other people or activities.
- ☐ 1 I notice that I am less interested in people or activities.
- ☐ 2 I find I have interest in only one or two of my formerly pursued activities.
- ☐ 3 I have virtually no interest in formerly pursued activities.

During the past seven days...

14. Energy Level:
- ☐ 0 There is no change in my usual level of energy.
- ☐ 1 I get tired more easily than usual.
- ☐ 2 I have to make a big effort to start or finish my usual daily activities (for example, shopping, homework, cooking, or going to work).
- ☐ 3 I really cannot carry out most of my usual daily activities because I just don't have the energy.

15. Feeling Slowed Down:
- ☐ 0 I think, speak, and move at my usual rate of speed.
- ☐ 1 I find that my thinking is slowed down or my voice sounds dull or flat.
- ☐ 2 It takes me several seconds to respond to most questions, and I'm sure my thinking is slowed.
- ☐ 3 I am often unable to respond to questions without extreme effort.

16. Feeling Restless:
- ☐ 0 I do not feel restless.
- ☐ 1 I'm often fidgety, wringing my hands, or need to shift how I am sitting.
- ☐ 2 I have impulses to move about and am quite restless.
- ☐ 3 At times, I am unable to stay seated and need to pace around.

From Rush, 2003, with permission.

TABLE 13-6. Quick Inventory of Depressive Symptomatology-Self Report (QIDS-SR$_{16}$) Scoring Instructions

1. Enter the highest score on any one of the four sleep items (items 1 to 4)
   Enter the highest score on any one of the four weight items (items 6 to 9)
   Enter the highest score on either of the two psychomotor items (items 15 and 16)
2. There will be one score for each of the nine Major Depressive Disorder symptom domains
3. Add the scores of the nine items (sleep, weight, psychomotor changes, depressed mood, decreased interest, fatigue, guilt, concentration, and suicidal ideation) to obtain the total score; total scores range from 0 to 27
4. 0–5: no depressive symptoms; 6–10: mild symptoms; 11–15: moderate symptoms; 16–20: severe symptoms; 21–27: very severe symptoms

From Rush, 2003.

TABLE 13-7. Anxiety Disorders

Panic attack
Agoraphobia
Specific phobia
Social phobia
Obsessive-compulsive disorder
Posttraumatic stress disorder
Acute stress disorder
Generalized anxiety disorder
Anxiety disorder due to a general medical condition
Substance-induced anxiety disorder
Anxiety disorder not otherwise specified

Adapted from American Psychiatric Association, 2000a, with permission.

individuals often present with dental problems, general nutritional deficiency, electrolyte abnormalities (hypokalemia and alkalosis), and decreased thyroid function. Electrocardiogram changes such as QT prolongation (bradycardia) and inversion or flattened T-waves may be noted. Rare complications include gastric dilation, arrhythmias, seizure, and death.

Bulimia Nervosa

This disorder is identified by periods of uncontrolled eating of high-calorie foods (binges), followed by self-induced vomiting (purging). Moreover, bulimic women may often misuse laxatives or diuretics. Unlike anorexia, those with bulimia often recognize their maladaptive behaviors.

Most bulimics have normal weights, although their weight may fluctuate. Thus, physical findings may be more subtle. One of the most characteristic signs is knuckle calluses found on the dorsum of the dominant hand. Termed *Russell sign*, calluses form in response to repetitive contact with acidic stomach contents during purging (Strumia, 2005).

Comorbidity of Eating Disorders

Anorexia nervosa and bulimia nervosa are complex disorders, affecting both psychological and physical systems (Klump, 2009). These eating disorders often are accompanied by comorbid depression and anxiety symptoms. Rates of mood symptoms approximate 50 percent, and anxiety symptoms, 60 percent (Braun, 1994). Simple phobia and obsessive-compulsive behaviors may also coexist. In many cases, patients with anorexia appear to have rigid, perfectionistic personalities and have low sexual interest. Patients with bulimia often display sexual conflicts, problems with intimacy, and impulsive suicidal tendencies (American Psychiatric Association, 2000b).

Prognosis of Eating Disorders

Data concerning the long-term physical and psychological prognosis of women with eating disorders is limited. Most may symptomatically improve with aging. However, complete recovery from anorexia nervosa is rare, and many continue to have distorted body perceptions and peculiar eating habits. Overall, the prognosis for bulimia is better than that for anorexia.

Treatment of Eating Disorders

Treatment of eating disorders involves a multidisciplinary approach. The American Psychiatric Association practice guidelines for eating disorders include: (1) nutritional rehabilitation, (2) psychosocial treatment that includes individual and family therapies, and (3) pharmacotherapeutic treatment of concurrent psychiatric symptoms (American Psychiatric Association, 2000b). Online resources for information and support are provided by the National Eating Disorder Association (www.edap.org) and Academy for Eating Disorders (www.aedweb.org). Health care providers should also be aware of

TABLE 13-8. Diagnostic Criteria for Generalized Anxiety Disorder

A. Excessive anxiety and worry occurring more days than not for at least 6 months, about a number of events or activities
B. The person finds it difficult to control the worry
C. The anxiety and worry are associated with three or more of the following six symptoms:
   1. Restlessness or feeling keyed up or on edge
   2. Being easily fatigued
   3. Difficulty concentrating or mind going blank
   4. Irritability
   5. Muscle tension
   6. Sleep disturbance
D. The focus of the anxiety and worry is not confined to features of another psychiatric disorder (e.g. worry about having a panic attack [Panic Disorder]; being embarrassed in public [Social Phobia]; gaining weight [Anorexia Nervosa])
E. The anxiety, worry, or physical symptoms cause clinically significant distress or impairment in social, occupational, or other important areas of functioning
F. The disturbance is not due to the direct physiologic effects of a substance or a general medical condition and does not occur exclusively during a mood disorder or a psychotic disorder

Adapted from American Psychiatric Association, 2000a, with permission.

TABLE 13-9. Diagnostic Criteria for Substance Dependence

A maladaptive pattern of substance use, leading to clinically significant impairment or distress, as manifested by three or more of the following, occurring at any time in the same 12-month period:
(1) Tolerance, defined by either:
  (a) a need for markedly increased amounts of the substance
  (b) markedly diminished effect with continued use of the same amount of the substance
(2) Withdrawal, manifested by:
  (a) characteristic withdrawal syndrome for the substance
  (b) the same or a closely related substance is taken to relieve or avoid withdrawal symptoms
(3) The substance is often taken in larger amounts or over a longer period than is intended
(4) There is a persistent desire or unsuccessful efforts to cut down or control substance use
(5) A great deal of time is spent in activities necessary to obtain the substance, use the substance, or recover from its effects
(6) Important social, occupational, or recreational activities are given up or reduced because of substance use
(7) Substance use is continued despite knowledge of having a persistent or recurrent physical or psychological problem that is likely to have been caused or exacerbated by the substance

Adapted from American Psychiatric Association, 2000a, with permission.

TABLE 13-10. Diagnostic Criteria for Substance Abuse

A. A maladaptive pattern of substance use leading to clinically significant impairment or distress, as manifested by one or more of the following, occurring within a 12-month period:
  (1) Recurrent substance use resulting in a failure to fulfill major role obligations at work, school, or home
  (2) Recurrent substance use in situations in which it is physically hazardous
  (3) Recurrent substance-related legal problems
  (4) Continued substance use despite having persistent or recurrent social or interpersonal problems caused or exacerbated by the effects of the substance
B. The symptoms have never met the criteria for Substance Dependence for this class of substance

Adapted from American Psychiatric Association, 2000a, with permission.

TABLE 13-11. Diagnostic Criteria for Anorexia Nervosa

A. Refusal to maintain body weight at or above a minimally normal weight for age and height (less than 85% of that expected)
B. Intense fear of gaining weight or becoming fat, even though underweight
C. Disturbance in the way in which one's body weight or shape is experienced, undue influence of body weight or shape on self-evaluation, or denial of the seriousness of the current low weight
D. In postmenarcheal females, amenorrhea

Restricting Type: No binge-eating or purging behaviors

Binge-Eating/Purging Type: Binge-eating and self-induced vomiting, or the misuse of laxatives, diuretics, or enemas

Adapted from American Psychiatric Association, 2000a, with permission.

TABLE 13-12. Diagnostic Criteria for Bulimia Nervosa

A. Recurrent episodes of binge eating:
1. Eating, in a discrete period of time, an amount of food definitely larger than most people would eat in a similar period of time under similar circumstances
2. A sense of lack of control over eating during the episode
B. Recurrent inappropriate compensatory behavior to prevent weight gain, such as self-induced vomiting; misuse of laxatives, diuretics, enemas, or other medications; fasting; or excessive exercise
C. Binge eating and inappropriate compensatory behaviors both occur, on average, at least twice a week for 3 months
D. Self-evaluation is unduly influenced by body shape and weight
E. The disturbance does not occur exclusively during episodes of Anorexia Nervosa

Purging Type: Regularly engaging in purging behaviors

Nonpurging Type: Compensatory behaviors are inappropriate, such as fasting or excessive exercise, but do not include vomiting or the misuse of laxatives

Adapted from American Psychiatric Association, 2000a, with permission.

pro-eating-disorder web sites, which may enable anorexic behaviors (Norris, 2006).

PREMENSTRUAL DISORDERS

Frequently, women of reproductive age experience symptoms during the late luteal phase of their menstrual cycle, and collectively these complaints are termed *premenstrual syndrome (PMS)* or *premenstrual tension (PMT)*. Nearly 300 different symptoms have been reported and typically include both psychiatric and physical complaints (Table 13-13) (Endicott, 2006; Halbreich, 2003a). For most women, these symptoms are self-limited. However, approximately 15 percent report moderate to severe symptoms that cause some impairment or require special consideration (Wittchen, 2002).

Premenstrual dysphoric disorder (PMDD) and *premenstrual dysphoria (PMD)* are independent clinical conditions that are identified by an accompanying psychosocial or functional impairment (Yonkers, 2008). PMDD carries significant functional impairment, and diagnosis should be reserved for those who meet the strict DSM-IV criteria (American Psychiatric Association, 2000a). In practice, however, the diagnosis of PMDD is often confused with PMD, particularly if a woman's complaints match some PMDD criteria. The prevalence of true PMDD in the general female population is considered 3 to 8 percent (Wittchen, 2002).

Pathophysiology of Premenstrual Syndrome

The exact causes of premenstrual disorders are unknown, although several different biologic factors have been suggested. Of these, estrogen, progesterone, and the neurotransmitters gamma amino butyric acid (GABA) and serotonin are frequently studied (Halbreich, 2003b).

Sex Steroids

Premenstrual syndrome is cyclic. Symptoms begin following ovulation and resolve with menses. They are less common in women with surgical oophorectomy or drug-induced ovarian hypofunction such as with gonadotropin-releasing hormone (GnRH) agonists. Moreover, women with anovulatory cycles rarely report PMS symptoms. For these reasons, PMS pathophysiology research has focused on the sex steroids estrogen and progesterone.

Central Nervous System Interaction. Estrogen and progesterone are neuroactive steroids and influence the central nervous system (CNS) neurotransmitters: serotonin, noradrenaline, and GABA. The predominant action of estrogen is neuronal excitability, whereas progestins are inhibitory (Halbreich, 2003b).

Specifically, PMS is believed, in part, to be associated with neuroactive progesterone metabolites. Of these, allopregnanolone is a potent modulator of GABA receptors, and its effects mirror those of low-dose benzodiazepines, barbiturates, and alcohol. However, the negative mood symptoms in women with PMDD may be caused by a paradoxical effect of allopregnanolone mediated via the GABA receptor (Backstrom, 2003, 2011). Wang and colleagues (1996) noted fluctuations in allopregnanolone across the various menstrual cycle phases. These changes were implicated with PMS symptom severity. However, this finding has not been consistently replicated by others (Rapkin, 1997; Schmidt, 1994; Sundstrom, 1998).

Serotonin

Evidence also supports a role for serotonergic system dysregulation in PMS pathophysiology. Decreased serotonergic activity has been noted in the luteal phase. Moreover, trials of serotonergic treatments have shown symptom reduction in women with PMS (Cohen, 2004; Halbreich, 2002a; Yonkers, 1996).

Renin-Angiotensin-Aldosterone System

Sex steroids also interact with the renin-angiotensin-aldosterone system (RAAS) to alter electrolyte and fluid balance. The antimineralocorticoid properties of progesterone and possible estrogen activation of the RAAS system may explain PMS symptoms of bloating and weight gain.

TABLE 13-13. Endicott Daily Record of Problem Severity

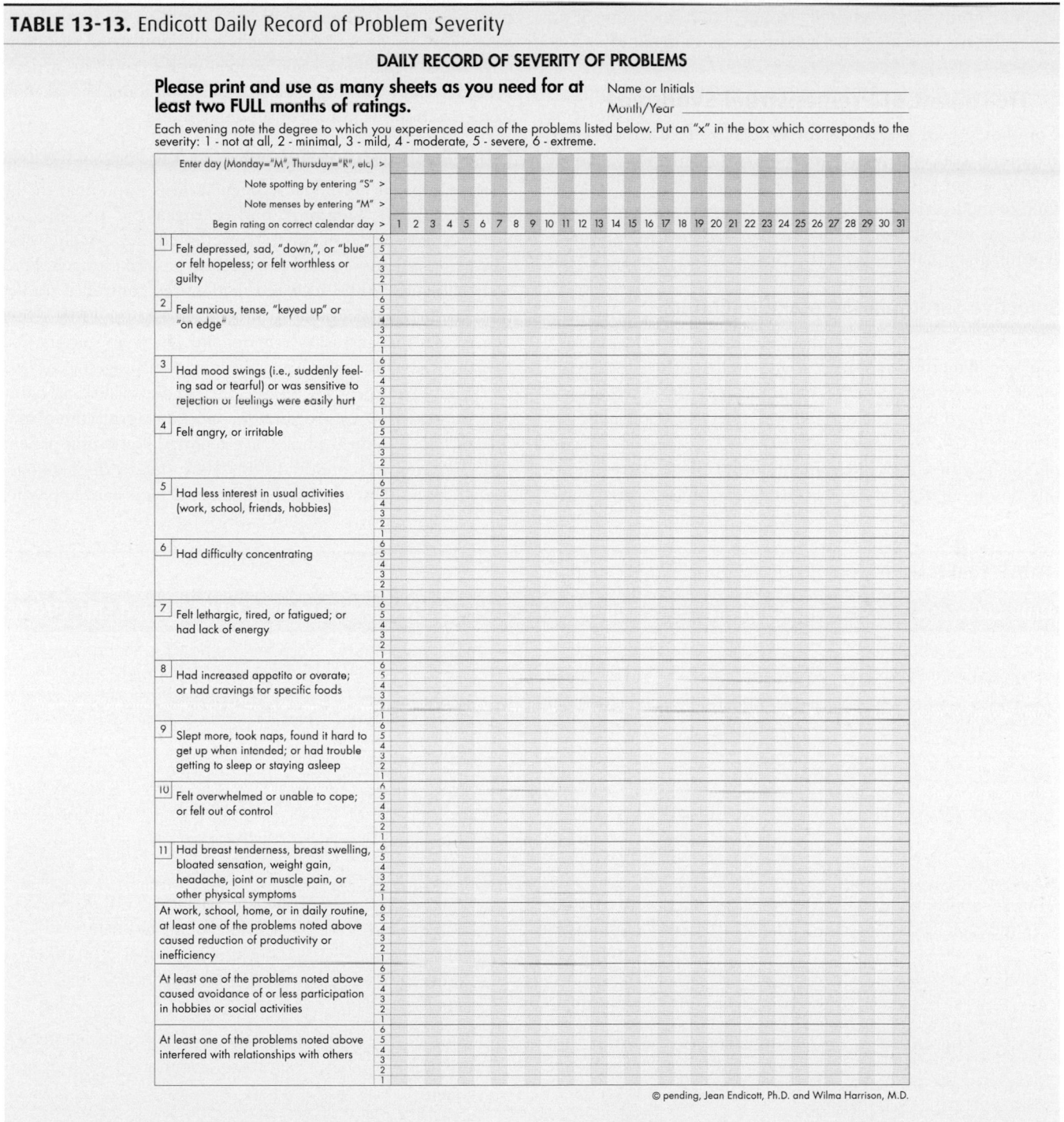

DAILY RECORD OF SEVERITY OF PROBLEMS

Please print and use as many sheets as you need for at least two FULL months of ratings.

Name or Initials _____

Month/Year _____

Each evening note the degree to which you experienced each of the problems listed below. Put an "x" in the box which corresponds to the severity: 1 - not at all, 2 - minimal, 3 - mild, 4 - moderate, 5 - severe, 6 - extreme.

Enter day (Monday="M", Thursday="R", etc) >
Note spotting by entering "S" >
Note menses by entering "M" >
Begin rating on correct calendar day > 1 2 3 4 5 6 7 8 9 10 11 12 13 14 15 16 17 18 19 20 21 22 23 24 25 26 27 28 29 30 31

1. Felt depressed, sad, "down,", or "blue" or felt hopeless; or felt worthless or guilty
2. Felt anxious, tense, "keyed up" or "on edge"
3. Had mood swings (i.e., suddenly feeling sad or tearful) or was sensitive to rejection or feelings were easily hurt
4. Felt angry, or irritable
5. Had less interest in usual activities (work, school, friends, hobbies)
6. Had difficulty concentrating
7. Felt lethargic, tired, or fatigued; or had lack of energy
8. Had increased appetite or overate; or had cravings for specific foods
9. Slept more, took naps, found it hard to get up when intended; or had trouble getting to sleep or staying asleep
10. Felt overwhelmed or unable to cope; or felt out of control
11. Had breast tenderness, breast swelling, bloated sensation, weight gain, headache, joint or muscle pain, or other physical symptoms

At work, school, home, or in daily routine, at least one of the problems noted above caused reduction of productivity or inefficiency

At least one of the problems noted above caused avoidance of or less participation in hobbies or social activities

At least one of the problems noted above interfered with relationships with others

© pending, Jean Endicott, Ph.D. and Wilma Harrison, M.D.

■ Diagnosis of Premenstrual Syndrome

Women with PMS usually present with complaints from multiple systems, and these symptoms display temporal association with the menstrual cycle luteal phase (see Table 13-13). Symptoms must begin at least 5 days (American College of Obstetricians and Gynecologists [ACOG] criteria, 2000) or 1 week (DSM-IV) before menses and remit within 4 days (ACOG criteria) or a few days (DSM-IV) after menses onset. Evaluation of women complaining of PMS symptoms includes prospective daily symptom rating for at least two or three menstrual cycles.

In certain instances, PMS symptoms may be an exacerbation of underlying primary psychiatric condition(s). Thus, during evaluation, other common psychiatric conditions such as depression, dysthymia, and anxiety disorders should be excluded. Additionally, other medical conditions that have a multisystem presentation should be considered. These include hypothyroidism, systemic lupus erythematosus, endometriosis, anemia, fibromyalgia, chronic fatigue syndrome, fibrocystic breast disease, irritable bowel syndrome, and migraine.

Treatment of Premenstrual Syndrome

Commonly used treatments for PMS have focused on either symptom reduction or modification of underlying hormonal dysregulation. Clinicians may consider treatment options for mild to moderate cases. However, if treatment fails or if symptoms are severe, then psychiatric referral may be indicated (Cunningham, 2009).

Selective Serotonin-Reuptake Inhibitors

Most psychotropic medications are effective in reducing psychologic symptom severity. Several well-controlled trials of selective serotonin-reuptake inhibitors (SSRIs) have shown these drugs to be efficacious and well tolerated (Cohen, 2002; Halbreich, 2002b; Yonkers, 1996, 1997). Standard dosages of SSRIs with either intermittent (luteal phase) or continuous dosing strategy are now considered primary therapy for

psychological symptoms of PMS (Table 13-14). In addition, short-term use of anxiolytics such as alprazolam or buspirone offer added benefits to some women with prominent anxiety. However, in prescribing anxiolytics, caution should be taken in women with prior history of substance abuse.

Estrogen and Progesterone

Because gonadal hormonal dysregulation is implicated in the genesis of PMS symptoms, both estrogen and progesterone therapies have been evaluated. However, efficacy is highly variable with progesterone and to some extent with estrogen. Ford and colleagues (2009) reviewed randomized controlled studies that assessed progesterone treatment efficacy for PMS. Only two studies met inclusion criteria, and reviewers summarized that the trials did not prove or disprove that progesterone was an effective treatment for PMS. Other studies evaluating estrogen, progesterone, or progesterone-blocking agent administration during the luteal phase have reported worsening patient PMS symptoms (Schmidt, 1998). Thus, due to the heterogeneous actions of estrogen and progesterone, it is hard to predict

TABLE 13-14. List of Common Psychotropic Medications

Drug Class	Indication	Examples[a]	Brand Name	Commonly Reported Side Effects
Selective serotonin-reuptake inhibitors (SSRIs)	Depressive, anxiety, and premenstrual disorders	Fluoxetine[c] Citalopram[c] Escitalopram[c] Sertraline[c] Paroxetine[d] Fluvoxamine[c]	Prozac, Sarafem Celexa Lexapro Zoloft Paxil Luvox	Nausea, headache, insomnia, diarrhea, dry mouth, sexual dysfunction
Serotonin noradrenergic-reuptake inhibitors (SNRIs)	Depressive, anxiety, and premenstrual disorders	Venlafaxine XR[c] Duloxetine[c]	Effexor Cymbalta	Dry mouth, anxiety, agitation, dizziness, somnolence, constipation
Tricyclic and tetracyclic antidepressants	Depressive and anxiety disorders	Desipramine[c] Nortriptyline[d] Amitriptyline[c] Doxepin[c] Maprotiline[b]	Norpramin Pamelor, Aventyl Elavil Sinequan Ludiomil	Drowsiness, dry mouth, dizziness, blurred vision, confusion, constipation, urinary retention and frequency
Benzodiazepines	Anxiety disorders	Alprazolam[d] Clonazepam[d] Diazepam[d]	Xanax Klonopin Valium	Drowsiness, ataxia, sleep changes, impaired memory, hypotension
Others	Depressive and anxiety disorders	Nefazodone[c] Trazodone[c] Bupropion SR, XL[c]	Serzone Desyrel Wellbutrin	Headache, dry mouth, orthostatic hypotension, somnolence
	Anxiety disorders	Buspirone[b] Hydroxyzine[c]	Buspar Vistaril, Atarax	Dizziness, drowsiness, headache
	Sleep agents	Zaleplon[c] Zolpidem[c] Ramelteon[c] Eszopiclone[c]	Sonata Ambien Rozerem Lunesta	Headache, somnolence, amnesia, fatigue

[a]Superscript reflects Food and Drug Administration pregnancy category.
SR = sustained release; XR/XL = extended release.

who would likely benefit from exogenous treatment with these hormones.

In addition, data are limited in support of combination oral contraceptive (COC) pills for this indication. However, certain COCs (Yaz, Beyaz) containing the spironolactone-like progestin drospirenone show evidence of therapeutic benefits for PMS symptoms and are Food and Drug Administration (FDA) indicated for treatment of PMDD (Chap. 5, p. 148) (Rapkin, 2008).

Other Agents

Prostaglandin inhibitors such as ibuprofen and naproxen offer benefits through their antiinflammatory effects and alleviate cramping and headaches associated with PMS (Table 10-2, p. 293). Diuretics such as spironolactone or combined hydrochlorothiazide and triamterene (Dyazide) may be prescribed to alleviate fluid retention and leg edema. Monitoring for potential side effects such as orthostatic hypotension and hypokalemia is critical, since these can be severe.

GnRH agonists and synthetic androgens, such as danazol, alleviate symptoms by suppressing ovulation. However, their substantial side effects should be weighed against the potential benefits in women with premenstrual disorders (Chap. 10, p. 294). Diet can aggravate PMS, and foods and beverages high in sugar and caffeine may worsen symptoms (Johnson, 1995). In contrast, vitamins such as pyridoxine (vitamin B_6) and vitamin E may offer added benefits. Pyridoxine is a cofactor to tryptophan hydroxylase, which is the key enzyme in serotonin synthesis (Wyatt, 1999). The recommended dose of pyridoxine is 50 to 100 mg/day, but doses exceeding 100 mg/day are avoided to prevent pyridoxine toxicity. In smaller trials, minerals such as calcium and magnesium have shown benefits. Magnesium in combination with vitamin B_6 appears to reduce anxiety-related premenstrual symptoms (De Souza, 2000). Calcium benefits are possibly through relief of calcium-deficiency symptoms such as muscle cramps (Thys-Jacobs, 2000).

PREGNANCY AND POSTPARTUM DISORDERS

Although pregnancy was previously viewed as protective against depression, not only do some women experience the first onset of depression during this time, but this is also a period of vulnerability for relapse of psychiatric disorders (Cohen, 2006a). Treatment is critical, as suicide is a leading cause of maternal death in developed countries (Lindahl, 2005). Etiologic studies have been inconclusive, but both hormonal changes and psychosocial stressors are implicated in the onset and maintenance of symptoms (Bloch, 2006; Boyce, 2005). Accordingly, it has been suggested that health professionals thoroughly assess psychiatric and psychosocial history to enable early identification, prevention, and treatment of perinatal depression (Moses-Kolko, 2004).

For the most part, psychiatric disorders during pregnancy have a course and presentation similar to those same disorders in nonpregnant women. For this reason, there are no distinct diagnostic criteria for psychiatric disorders experienced during pregnancy and the puerperium. However, flagging episodes

that occur in relation to childbirth may be beneficial, and thus a specifier of "postpartum onset" is often included in the diagnosis.

Mood Disorders in the Perinatal Period
Depression During Pregnancy
Risks for Depression in Pregnancy. The prevalence of depression during pregnancy has been estimated to be highest (11 percent) in the first trimester and to fall to 8.5 percent in the second and third trimesters. Studies specifically investigating depression during pregnancy have found associations with life stress, previous episodes of depression, poor social support (particularly from the partner), and maternal anxiety (Lancaster, 2010).

Diagnosis of Depression in the Perinatal Period. The Edinburgh Postnatal Depression Scale (EPDS) is a screening measure specifically developed to identify and assess the severity of depressive symptoms during pregnancy and the puerperium (Cox, 1987). Unlike screening measures that include symptoms also characteristic of pregnancy itself (appetite, weight change, sleep disturbance, and fatigue), the EPDS inquires about neurovegetative symptoms that are more specific to depression. Available in a number of languages, the EPDS is an efficient way for a clinician to identify patients who are at risk for being depressed during both pregnancy and puerperium. It is available through the American Academy of Pediatrics at http://www.aap.org/sections/scan/practicingsafety/Toolkit_Resources/Module2/EPDS.pdf. At this time, the American College of Obstetricians and Gynecologists (2010) notes that evidence is insufficient evidence to currently recommend universal screening.

Treatment of Depression in Pregnancy. No antidepressant has been approved by the U.S. FDA during pregnancy (Kornstein, 2001). The FDA classifies most SSRIs as category C drugs. However, concerns regarding increased rates of congenital cardiac malformations with first-trimester paroxetine (Paxil) exposure led the manufacturer to change its pregnancy category from C to D (GlaxoSmithKline, 2008). Also, the American College of Obstetricians and Gynecologists (2008) recommends that paroxetine use be avoided in women who are either pregnant or planning pregnancy. Moreover, fetal echocardiography should be considered for women with early pregnancy paroxetine exposure. However, because of the large number of fetal outcomes analyzed, the American College of Obstetricians and Gynecologists (2008) concludes that the absolute risk of any birth defect is small and that SSRIs are not major teratogens.

Two types of neonatal effects have been described following SSRI use in pregnancy, and the U.S. FDA (2006a,b) has issued Public Health Advisories regarding these. First, a neonatal behavioral syndrome, termed *serotonin syndrome*, is characterized by transient jitteriness, increased muscle tone, feeding or digestive disturbances, irritability, and respiratory distress. More seriously, persistent pulmonary hypertension in the newborn (PPHN) has also been associated with SSRI use during pregnancy. Fortunately, the absolute risk among exposed infants is small—6 to 12 per 1000. A fuller discussion of these and other psychiatric medications and pregnancy can be found in Chapter 14 of Williams Obstetrics, 23rd edition (Cunningham, 2010). Online resources regarding teratogenicity include Reprotox at: www.reprotox.org and TERIS at:http://depts.washington.edu/terisweb.

On balance, women who discontinue antidepressant medication during pregnancy relapse into depression significantly more frequently than women who maintain their pharmacologic treatment (Cohen, 2006a). In addition, suicide remains a significant cause of pregnancy-associated death. The American College of Obstetricians and Gynecologists (2008) stresses that the potential risks of SSRI use in pregnancy must be considered in the context of the risk of depression relapse if their administration is discontinued. Thus, treatment with these medications during pregnancy should be individualized. To support clinicians in weighing these risks and benefits, the American Psychiatric Association (APA) and American College of Obstetricians and Gynecologists (2008) have published guidelines for the management of depression during pregnancy (Field, 2006; Shadigian, 2005; Wisner, 2000; Yonkers, 2009).

Nonpharmacologic and complementary approaches have also been used as potential treatment options during pregnancy. These include omega fatty acid supplementation, acupuncture, massage, sleep cycle manipulation, cognitive behavioral therapy, and interpersonal psychotherapy (Brandon, 2011; Carter, 2005; Manber, 2004; Parry, 2000; Spinelli, 2003). The published guidelines of APA and ACOG suggest that psychotherapy, in particular, is a practical first-line approach for mild to moderate depression (Yonkers, 2009).

Depression in the Postpartum

Risks. Depression after childbirth has largely been divided into three categories: postpartum blues, postpartum depression, and postpartum psychosis. The strongest predictors of postpartum depression include prior history of depression or anxiety, family history of psychiatric illness, poor marital relationship, low levels of social support, and stressful life events in the previous 12 months (Boyce, 2005; Sayil, 2007).

Classification

Postpartum Blues. This transient state of heightened emotional reactivity can develop in up to 50 percent of postpartum patients. The onset is 2 to 14 days after childbirth, and its duration is less than 2 weeks (Gaynes, 2005). Blues generally require no intervention. Rest and social support contribute significantly to remission. However, postpartum blues do constitute a significant risk factor for subsequent depression during the puerperium.

Postpartum Depression. According to the DSM-IV, postpartum depression refers to the diagnosis of major depressive disorder within 4 weeks after childbirth. However, in research and most clinical settings, any depression developing within 12 months following childbirth is considered to have postpartum onset. With this definition, the prevalence of postpartum depression approximates 15 percent in postpartum women (Gaynes, 2005).

Postpartum depression warrants careful assessment by a mental health professional, as treatment should be initiated immediately to minimize impaired caregiving. Infants of depressed mothers have exhibited cognitive, temperamental, and developmental differences compared with infants of nondepressed mothers (Kaplan, 2009; Newport, 2002). SSRIs are usually first-line agents, although caution is necessary in breast-feeding mothers. In addition, a number of psychosocial interventions have demonstrated efficacy in treating postpartum depression. Of these, the most significant effects have been achieved with interpersonal therapy and cognitive behavioral therapy (Clark, 2003; Dennis, 2005). Additionally, Postpartum Support International is an excellent resource of information for both clinicians and patients. Information can be obtained at www.postpartum.net and the MedEd PPD web site at http://mededppd.org/default2.asp.

Postpartum Psychosis. This condition develops in less than 2 percent of new mothers, and its onset is generally within 2 weeks of childbirth (Gaynes, 2005). The risk for this severe form of depression is increased for women who have had prior mood disorders. Particularly, prior postpartum psychosis increases by 30 to 50 percent a woman's risk with subsequent deliveries (American Psychiatric Association, 2000a). Evaluation and antipsychotic pharmacologic treatment are essential for these women. Hospitalization is often indicated until the safety of mother and infant is assured.

Other Psychiatric Disorders in the Perinatal Period

Clinicians most often focus on mood disorders during the perinatal period. However, other psychiatric illnesses such as anxiety disorders, bipolar disorders, and schizophrenia may also be present. Of these, bipolar disorders and schizophrenia are serious, recurrent psychiatric illnesses that require pharmacologic treatment. Treatment planning is critical with such patients, and decisions should always be made in collaboration with a psychiatric professional. A careful balance must be struck between minimizing medication risk to the fetus and maternal risk from untreated or undertreated disease.

Perinatal Loss

Perinatal loss did not become a subject of professional research until the 1970s. Although many studies have focused on identifying factors that modify grieving styles, a few have focused on interventions with families after perinatal loss. Study results show that health care providers are most helpful if they speak directly, use understandable language, and share information that might provide parents a sense of control over their situation and might address their fears. Additional time with health professionals and a perception of being a priority is also important to parents (DiMarco, 2001).

Since grief is individual, no generalizations can be made concerning clinical treatment in such situations. Thus, a clinician must ask a patient what she needs and wants. Couples therapy may be helpful if mother and father find it difficult to grieve congruently. Family therapy may be indicated if other children need support to process the loss and their parents' grief. Interventions include openness to expressions of grief, assessment of readiness for another pregnancy, and referral of couples to resources such as hospital support groups and internet sites such as that sponsored by the Hygeia Foundation at: http://www.hygeia.org.

MENOPAUSAL TRANSITION AND MENOPAUSE

Risks for Psychiatric Disorders During Menopausal Transition

Menopausal transition has long been investigated as a vulnerable period for emergence of mood symptoms. Anxiety, irritable mood, and sleep problems are more likely to develop in perimenopausal women than in premenopausal women (Brandon, 2008; Bromberger, 2001; Freeman, 2006). Moreover, recent data suggest that rates of new-onset depression during menopausal transition are nearly twice that of premenopausal rates (Cohen, 2006b). This risk persists even after adjusting for sleep disturbances and vasomotor symptoms.

Other possible risks for depression and anxiety are a prior history of depression, severe premenstrual distress, hot flashes, and disrupted sleep. Demographic predictors of increased risk during the menopausal period are lower educational status, African-American ethnicity, unemployment, and major life stressors (Bromberger, 2001; Freeman, 2006; Maartens, 2002). Moreover, psychosocial issues include a woman's recognition that her reproductive years are ending and that her children will leave to establish their own lives. Developmentally, many women are transitioning from being focused on family to finding other avenues to invest time and energy.

Mood vulnerability during menopausal transition is believed to follow erratic physiologic fluctuations in reproductive hormones. Detailed discussion of these hormones as they relate to mood changes during this transition is found in Chapter 21 (p. 572).

Evaluation During Menopausal Transition

Women with psychological symptoms warrant a comprehensive psychosocial inventory and risk factor assessment. Importantly, since medical conditions may concurrently develop during this transition, evaluation should exclude these before symptoms are considered psychosomatic. Specifically, thyroid function should be evaluated.

Treatment of Mood Symptoms During Menopausal Transition

The approach to treating mood symptoms involves both pharmacotherapy and psychotherapy (Brandon, 2008). Recommended psychotropic medications are SSRIs and selective noradrenergic-reuptake inhibitors (SNRIs). These agents are good options for women who do not wish to use hormone therapy. Additional benefits include alleviation of vasomotor symptoms and sleep disturbance (Chap. 22, p. 588).

Studies suggest that short-term administration of estrogen is an option for perimenopausal women with depressive symptoms (Soares, 2001). However, this benefit should be weighed against safety concerns raised in the Women's Health Initiative (WHI) Study and others (Chap. 22, p. 583). The psychotropic role of estrogen-progesterone preparations in postmenopausal women remains unclear.

LATE LIFE

According to estimates by the U.S. Census Bureau, the number of elderly people in the United States will significantly increase during the next decades as the "Baby Boomer" generation ages. By 2030, nearly 20 percent of the population will be older than 65 years (He, 2005). Psychosocial issues addressed are significantly different for these women. Stressors may include diminished mental and physical function as well as loss of partner, family, or friends. Erikson identified the task of this final developmental stage of life as one of consolidation and integration. In this model, women retrospectively examine their lives. They may manage their last years with integrity and with satisfaction in a life well lived, or may suffer despair, feeling that all was in vain.

Mental Disorders in the Elderly

According to the 2000 U.S. Census, functionally impairing mental disorders affected 11 percent of adults aged 65 to 74 and 10 percent of those older than 74 (He, 2005). Of these disorders, depression, anxiety, late-onset psychotic and paranoid disorders, and alcoholism are those most likely to be observed in a clinical practice (Zarit, 1998). However, the prevalence of depression is generally thought to be lower in postmenopausal women compared with that in reproductive-aged women. Moreover, most studies suggest that the gender gap between rates of depression closes in late life. As in the general population, anxiety is the most common psychiatric disorder in the elderly (Zarit, 1998).

Evaluation of Psychiatric Disorders in Late Life

If a psychiatric disorder is suspected, careful evaluation is required to exclude underlying medical causes for these changes. For example, depression may be a comorbid disorder with or an early symptom of Alzheimer and Parkinson disease (Polidori, 2001). Alternatively, depression, anxiety, and psychosis may also result from single medications or drug combinations.

Specific screening questionnaires for depression have been developed for the elderly such as the Geriatric Depression Scale (Brink, 1982). This screening tool is available in various languages at http://www.stanford.edu/~yesavage/GDS.html. In addition, neuropsychologic evaluation is helpful to discriminate between mood symptoms and cognitive impairment. A fuller discussion and examples of cognitive screening tests are found in Chapter 1 (p. 27).

Treatment of Psychiatric Disorders in Late Life

Recognizing the natural decline in serotonin levels with aging, many gerontologists prescribe SSRIs for their patients. However, communication between all treating physicians to coordinate medications and minimize interactions is particularly important for elderly patients.

Psychosocial treatments are often helpful for the patient and where applicable, her caregivers. Cognitive behavioral therapy and interpersonal therapy have both been found effective with the elderly. Moreover, family therapy can be of great value to those struggling with end-of-life issues, functional impairments, multiple losses, and caregiver burden. Social workers are also of tremendous value if a patient and family need to locate additional resources for care.

A metaanalysis of 89 treatment studies for depression in older adults found that pharmacotherapy and psychotherapy achieved comparable results in treatment of depression. In contrast, an analysis of 32 treatment studies for anxiety found pharmacotherapy slightly more effective than psychotherapy (Pinquart, 2006, 2007). Thus, treatment planning may be individualized and should assess patient preference, contraindications, and treatment access (Pinquart, 2006).

ADDITIONAL DISORDERS THAT PRESENT ACROSS THE LIFE SPAN

Somatoform Disorders

Recurrent, multiple, often unexplained physical symptoms are hallmark features of somatoform disorders. These disorders are common, and their estimated prevalence in general clinical practice is 16 percent (de Waal, 2004). Their prevalence may be even higher in specialty clinics such as pain management clinics.

Somatoform disorders are complex and poorly understood. However, symptoms cause significant distress and/or impairment in various domains of an affected individual's life. Moreover, one in four somatoform patients suffer from comorbid anxiety and depressive symptoms. Thus, a multidisciplinary approach is often required to effectively manage these women's symptoms.

SEXUAL ASSAULT

Sexual assault is a crime of violence, often motivated by aggression and rage, with the assailant using sexual contact as a weapon for power and control. Sexual assault can include a range of coercive behaviors ranging from kissing, fondling, and molestation to rape or attempted rape. Linden (1999) defines sexual assault as "an event that occurred without the victim's consent, involved the use of force or the threat of force, and involved actual or attempted penetration of the victim's vagina, mouth, or rectum."

According to recent statistics, one in six to one in three women will be raped during her lifetime (Anderson, 2009; Luce, 2010). Up to 39 percent of these women have been found to be sexually assaulted more than once (Kilpatrick, 1992). Many rapes are unreported, because of a victim's feelings of shame and guilt. Based on survey data, Resnick (2000) reported that only 54 percent of victims actually reported the crime of being sexually assaulted.

Well-known sequelae of rape include isolation, depression, anxiety, somatic symptoms, suicide attempts, and posttraumatic stress disorder (PTSD). The experience has a strong effect on the victim's subsequent health and thus is a major public health issue. Importantly, in caring for sexual assault victims, clinicians should be familiar with the complex array of reactions (emotional and physical), common injuries, and elements of proper evaluation and treatment of these patients. Immediate management of a woman who has been sexually assaulted should address three areas: legal, medical, and psychosocial. Care is coordinated among law enforcement officers, medical personnel, and psychosocial support staff. It is critical that the survivor be assured that she is safe and not to blame for the assault (Luce, 2010).

Common Physical Findings with Sexual Assault

Initial evaluation of a sexual assault victim should concentrate on identifying serious or life-threatening injuries. Although 70 percent of rape victims were found to sustain no obvious physical injuries, 24 percent sustained minor injuries, and up to 5 percent sustained major nongenital injuries. The most common nongenital injuries in these victims include bruises, cuts, scratches, and swelling (81 percent); internal injuries and unconsciousness (11 percent); and knife or gunshot wounds (2 percent) (Sommers, 2001). Although death is rare (0.1 percent sustain fatal injuries), the fear of death during an assault is one of the most intense reactions (Deming, 1983; Marchbanks, 1990).

Once life-threatening injuries are excluded by the provider, a patient should be moved to a quiet, private setting for further evaluation. A systematic, thorough, but compassionate approach to obtaining a history and collecting evidence is essential for appropriate patient treatment and for future prosecution of her assailant (American College of Obstetricians and Gynecologists, 2011c).

Rape Examination/Legal Documentation

Although valid evidence may be collected up to 5 days after sexual assault, immediate examination increases the opportunity to obtain valuable physical evidence (Table 13-15). Consent is obtained prior to physical and genital examination and evidence collection. This step helps to reestablish a victim's sense of control and is crucial for entry of evidence in a court of law (Plaut, 2004). Providers should emphasize that vital information may be lost if evidence is not collected early and that evidence collection does not commit a victim to pressing criminal charges (Linden, 1999). Moreover, a patient should be counseled that she may terminate an examination if it is too emotionally or physically painful.

Most states have standardized kits known as "rape kits" for evidence collection. First, clothing is collected as a patient

TABLE 13-15. Important Elements of Physical Examination and Evidence Collection Following Sexual Assault

Physical Examination

General appearance

Affect/emotional status

Complete examination of head, body, and extremities; record injuries on body diagram

Pelvic examination, with colposcopy if available, to exclude lower reproductive tract trauma

Elements of Evidence Collection

Swabs and smears of involved orifices and skin surfaces

Oral, saline "swish and collect" sample if oral sex coerced

Fingernail scrapings from the patient, if the victim scratched the assailant's skin or clothing

Clothing collected in labeled paper bags

Head hair combings; then head hairs cut or pulled from patient for comparison

Pubic hair combings; then pubic hair cut or pulled from patient for comparison

Blood sample for patient blood typing for comparison with assailant's type

undresses on a white sheet and is placed in properly labeled bags. Any debris, such as hair, fibers, mud, or leaves, should also be collected. Documentation of all physical injuries is critical, and objective evidence of trauma (even minor) is associated with increased chances of successful prosecution. Evidence gathering includes a sample of the patient's saliva and swabs of all involved orifices or skin surfaces. If the patient had scratched the assailant in defense, then fingernail scrapings should be collected. A thorough pelvic examination with evidence collection is essential, even if there are no complaints of genital pain. Up to one third of victims can have traumatic genital injuries without symptoms. Common patterns of genital injury include tears of the posterior fourchette and fossa, labial abrasions, and hymenal bruising. Significant genital injuries are more common in postmenopausal or prepubertal victims (Jones, 2009). Colposcopy should be used, if available, as this technique increases detection of more subtle injuries to the cervix and vagina. Lenahan and coworkers (1998) reported that colposcopy increased genital trauma recognition from 6 percent to 53 percent. Using a colposcope in combination with toluidine blue enhancement, Slaughter and colleagues (1997) documented an injury rate as high as 94 percent in sexually assaulted women examined within 48 hours. In addition, a Wood lamp may aid identification of semen on the skin, which then should be collected with moistened cotton swabs. A blood sample is collected for typing, to differentiate the blood type of the victim from that of the assailant. After evidence is collected, it is signed, sealed, and locked in a secure place to ensure that legal evidence procedures are maintained (Rambow, 1992). *Chain of evidence* is a legal concept that describes an unbroken chain of protection, from origin of collection to court, for a sample or exhibit (Lowe, 2009).

Treatment Following Sexual Assault

Pregnancy Prevention

Medication prophylaxis to prevent pregnancy and common sexually transmitted diseases is provided to women following sexual assault. The risk of rape-related pregnancy approximates 5 percent per rape among reproductive-aged victims (Holmes, 1996). Most of these pregnancies, unfortunately, occur in adolescents, often the victims of incest, who never report the incident nor receive medical attention. Because of variation in a woman's menstrual cycle, pregnancy prophylaxis, also termed *emergency contraception*, should be offered to all victims (Table 5-12, p. 163). Prophylaxis can be administered for up to 72 hours after rape, but is most effective in the first 24 hours (Table 13-16). Some studies indicate that prophylaxis may be effective for up to 5 days following penile penetration.

A negative pregnancy test to exclude a preexisting pregnancy should be confirmed before administering emergency contraceptive methods. Side effects of estrogen/progestin combinations (Yuzpe method) include nausea (in up to 50 percent of patients), vomiting (in up to 20 percent), breast tenderness, and heavier menstrual period. With use of levonorgestrel (Plan B), the risk of nausea is reduced to 23 percent and vomiting to 6 percent (Arowojolu, 2002). An oral antiemetic, such as phenergan 25 mg, can be prescribed 30 minutes prior to administration to decrease nausea.

Patients should be informed that the timing of their next menses may be altered following this prophylaxis. Although current regimens are 74 to 89 percent effective, women should be counseled to return if their next menses is more than 1 to 2 weeks late (Task Force on Postovulatory Methods of Fertility Regulation, 1998; Trussell, 1996; Yuzpe, 1982).

Sexually Transmitted Disease Prevention

The risk of acquiring a sexually transmitted disease (STD) after rape has been estimated. The risk of developing trichomoniasis is approximately 12 percent; bacterial vaginosis, 12 percent; gonorrhea, 4 percent to 12 percent; chlamydial infection, 2 to 14 percent; syphilis, 5 percent; and human immunodeficiency virus (HIV) infection, <1 percent (Jenny, 1990; Katz, 1997; Schwarcz, 1990). However, these risks are difficult to predict and vary by geographic location, type of assault, assailant, severity of trauma at the site of a potential exposure, and presence of preexisting infections. General recommendations describe antibiotic prophylaxis for gonorrhea, trichomoniasis, and chlamydial infection and vaccination for hepatitis B virus (see Table 13-16).

The fear of contracting HIV after sexual assault is common in survivors and is often the primary concern following rape (Baker, 1990). However, postexposure prophylaxis (PEP) against HIV remains controversial, given the low risk of transmission after a single sexual assault (Gostin, 1994). The per-contact risk of HIV transmission from an HIV-positive person with receptive penile-anal exposure is estimated to be 0.5 to 3.2 percent and with receptive penile-vaginal exposure, 0.05 to 0.15 percent (Wieczorek, 2010). Although rare, HIV transmission associated with receptive oral intercourse has been reported. Experts recommend offering PEP to candidates who are at a higher risk of being exposed to HIV and who are

TABLE 13-16. Pregnancy and Sexually Transmitted Disease Prevention Following Sexual Assault

Testing
Pregnancy test (urine or serum)
Serum hepatitis B surface antigen (HBsAg) assay
Serum Venereal Disease Research Laboratory (VDRL) test
Cultures for *Neisseria gonorrhoeae* and *Chlamydia trachomatis* from each penetrated site
Microscopic evaluation of vaginal discharge saline prep
If HIV PEP is planned, then CBC, serum liver function tests, and serum creatinine level

Treatment
Plan B: levonorgestrel 0.75 mg, one pill orally every 12 hours for two doses **or** other methods (see Table 5-12, p. 163)
Ceftriaxone 250 mg intramuscularly, single dose
Azithromycin 1 g orally, single dose
Metronidazole 2 g orally, single dose

Optional Treatment
Hepatitis B vaccination (see Table 1-1, p. 11).
Oral HIV PEP for 4 weeks[a,b]:
   Zidovudine 300 mg/lamivudine 150 mg (Combivir) one pill twice daily; **or**
   Tenofovir 300 mg/emtricitabine 200 mg (Truvada) one pill once daily; **or**
   Ritonavir 50 mg/lopinavir 200 mg (Kaletra) two pills twice daily plus
     tenofovir 300 mg/emtricitabine 200 mg (Truvada) one once daily

[a]Abbreviated from Lanovitz, 2009.
[b]Additional regimens found in CDC guidelines (Smith, 2005).
CBC = complete blood count; HIV = human immunodeficiency virus; PEP = postexposure prophylaxis.

willing to complete the full course of medications and comply with surveillance testing. The risks and side effects of these medications and need for close monitoring should be discussed with patients (Wieczorek, 2010). Nausea is a common side effect with PEP. Thus, a prescription for an antiemetic such as phenergan, to be used as needed, can be considered (Table 39-10, p. 963). PEP should begin within 72 hours, if indicated (Table 13-17). For sexual assault patients presenting outside of this time frame, information should be provided regarding follow-up HIV antibody testing and referral options.

Psychological Response to Sexual Assault

Survivors of sexual assault may display an array of reactions that commonly include anxiety, agitation, crying, or a quiet, calm, and distant affect. Burgess and Holmstrom (1974) first characterized the "rape trauma syndrome." They described two response phases to the trauma of sexual assault: (1) the acute disorganization phase, lasting several weeks, and (2) the reorganization phase, lasting from several weeks to years. During the acute phase, common initial emotional reactions include shock and disbelief, fear, shame, self-blame, humiliation, anger, isolation, grief, and loss of control. Somatic reactions may be common (p. 370). During the reorganization phase, feelings of vulnerability, despair, guilt, and shame may continue. Symptoms may include nonspecific anxiety, somatic complaints, or depression.

Subsequent Care Following Sexual Assault

Survivors should be referred to local rape crisis centers and encouraged to visit within 1 to 2 days. Victims of sexual assault have been shown to experience numerous negative effects on their lives. These may include resource disruption (e.g., unemployment, divorce), deterioration in interpersonal functioning, elevated risk of suicide, and an increased use of medical services (Kelleher, 2009). Thus, ongoing counseling and support is vital.

All sexual assault victims should receive medical evaluation at 1 to 2 weeks. If STD prophylaxis was declined, then cultures are repeated. Surveillance blood testing for HIV and syphilis (rapid plasma reagin [RPR]) should be performed at 6 weeks, 3 months, and 6 months if initial test results are negative. Remaining hepatitis vaccinations are administered during visits, if needed.

CHILD SEXUAL ABUSE

Sexual abuse is defined as a child engaged in sexual activities that he or she cannot comprehend, for which he or she is developmentally unprepared and cannot give consent, and/or that violate societal laws or social taboos (Kellogg, 2005). Such abuse is not uncommon in the United States. Thus, indicators that should prompt evaluation include: (1) statements by the child or family of abuse, (2) genital or anal injury without concordant history of unintentional trauma, (3) semen or pregnancy identified, or (4) sexually transmitted disease diagnosed beyond the incubation period of vertical (natal mother-to-child) transmission (Bechtel, 2010). Determining whether genital findings in children are normal variants or indicative of assault can be

TABLE 13-17. HIV PEP after Sexual Assault

Assess for risk of HIV infection in the assailant
Determine characteristics of the assault that may increase the risk of HIV transmission (i.e., mucosal trauma and bleeding)
Consider consulting an HIV specialist or the National Clinicians' Postexposure Prophylaxis Hotline: 888-448-4911
Discuss low seroconversion rates in a risk-targeted approach and highlight the toxicity of routine antiretroviral PEP
If the patient starts PEP, schedule follow-up within 7 days
If prescribing PEP, obtain CBC, serum liver function tests, and serum creatinine level
Check HIV serology at baseline, 6 weeks, and then at 3 and 6 months

CBC = complete blood count; HIV = human immunodeficiency virus; PEP = postexposure prophylaxis.
Adapted from the Centers for Disease Control and Prevention, 2010.

difficult, and these have been categorized according to their likelihood of associated sexual abuse. An exhaustive list of normal and indeterminate signs has been compiled by Adams and colleagues (2007, 2008), and those considered diagnostic are listed in Table 13-18. A provider completing the examination should have formal training in the evaluation of suspected child sexual abuse, including didactic learning and practical experience. A list of local specialist providers can be found on the American Academy of Pediatrics Section on Child Abuse and Neglect web site at: http://www.aap.org/sections/childabuseneglect. Importantly, acute injuries associated with child sexual abuse heal and resolve rapidly. Thus, examination should be completed as soon as sexual assault is suspected (McCann, 2007).

In girls evaluated for STDs during sexual abuse examination, the prevalence of STDs is low (Girardet, 2009a). Thus, the decision to obtain specimens from a child is individualized. Situations that typically prompt testing include: (1) if STD signs or complaints are identified; (2) if the suspected assailant has or is at high risk for an STD; (3) if another child or adult in the household has an STD; (4) if a patient or parent requests testing; or (5) if evidence of genital, oral, or anal penetration or ejaculation is found (Centers for Disease Control and Prevention, 2010).

Recommended testing includes: cultures for *Neisseria gonorrhoeae* from the pharynx, anus, and vagina; cultures for *Chlamydia trachomatis* from the anus and vagina; and wet mount evaluation of a vaginal swab specimen for *Trichomonas vaginalis* infection and bacterial vaginosis. Decisions regarding serologic testing for *Treponema pallidum*, HIV, and hepatitis B virus are individualized. Swab specimens from the vagina, rather than endocervical specimens, are recommended for prepubertal girls. Moreover, the Centers for Disease Control and Prevention (CDC) (2010) advocate *N gonorrhoeae* and *C trachomatis* culture rather than evaluation with nucleic acid amplification tests (NAATs).

The general concept that sexually transmissible infections found beyond the neonatal period are evidence of sexual abuse has exceptions. For example, perinatally acquired *C trachomatis* infection has, in some cases, persisted up to age 3 years in girls. Genital warts have been diagnosed in children who have no other evidence of sexual abuse. Finally, most hepatitis B virus (HBV) infections in children result from household exposure to those with chronic HBV infection (Centers for Disease Control and Prevention, 2010).

STD prophylaxis for children who have been sexually abused is generally not recommended due to lower rates of associated

TABLE 13-18. Findings Diagnostic of Sexual Contact in Suspected Child Sexual Abuse

Acute genital or perianal lacerations or extensive bruising[a]
Perianal or fourchette scarring[a]
An area between 4 and 8 o'clock on the rim of the hymen where it appears to have been torn through to, or nearly to, the base
Positive genital, anal, or pharyngeal culture for *Neisseria gonorrhoeae*[b]
Confirmed diagnosis of syphilis[b]
Positive culture or saline prep for *Trichomonas vaginalis* in a child older than 1 year
Positive genital or anal culture for *Chlamydia trachomatis* in a child older than 3 years
Positive serology for HIV[b]
Pregnancy
Sperm identified in specimens taken directly from a child's body

[a]If other medical conditions such as Crohn disease, coagulopathy, or labial adhesion are not explanatory for findings.
[b]If perinatal transmission, transmission from blood products, and needle contamination have been excluded.
HIV = human immunodeficiency virus.
Adapted from Adams, 2007, 2008.

infection and a greater guarantee of scheduled follow-up. However, if the clinical setting dictates or if test results are positive for infection, antibiotics may be provided. *For those weighing less than 45 kg*, treatment for gonorrhea includes a 125-mg single dose of ceftriaxone (Rocephin) intramuscularly (IM). For chlamydial infection, oral erythromycin 50 mg/kg/d in four divided doses for 14 days is given. *For children above 45 kg*, a single dose of ceftriaxone 250 mg IM plus a single 1-g oral dose of azithromycin will treat gonorrhea. For chlamydial infection, a single 1-g oral dose of azithromycin or doxycycline (for those older than 8 years) 100 mg twice daily for 7 days can be prescribed (Centers for Disease Control and Prevention, 2010, 2011; Woods, 2005). Rates of HIV transmission following sexual abuse are very low in children, and compliance with PEP regimens, once prescribed, is poor (Girardet, 2009b). However, antiretroviral treatment is well tolerated by children, and PEP can be offered based on the clinical setting. If antiretroviral PEP is considered, it should be initiated, similar to other prophylaxis, within the first 72 hours, and the CDC (2010) recommends consulting professionals who specialize in care of HIV-infected children.

In addition to treatment of physical trauma, psychosocial evaluation should be a part of care. Importantly, childhood sexual abuse can have long-term psychological and/or gynecologic sequelae (American College of Obstetricians and Gynecologists, 2011a).

INTIMATE PARTNER VIOLENCE

Definition

Intimate partner violence (IPV) refers to harm inflicted by one intimate partner to the other, with the intention of causing pain or controlling the other's behavior. Women account for 89 percent of IPV cases reported among couples (Chambliss, 2008). The terms IPV, *domestic violence (DV), gender-based violence,* or *violence against women* encompass a multitude of abuses directed at women and girls. The United Nation Declaration on the Elimination of Violence Against Women (1993) defines violence as acts that cause, or have the potential to cause, harm. Introduction of the term "gender based" emphasizes that the act is rooted in inequality between women and men (Krantz, 2005).

Violence against women varies and includes battering, sexual assault, incest, and elder abuse (Burge, 1997; Straka, 2006). Most victims know their assailant and have been assaulted more than once. The average length of victimization before presentation to health care providers or the police is 4 years for abused women (Tjaden, 2000).

Intimate Partner Violence Statistics

The CDC's National Center for Injury Prevention and Control (2000) estimates that nearly 5.3 million incidents of IPV occur each year among U.S. women aged 18 years and older. These incidents result in nearly 2 million injuries and 1400 deaths nationwide every year (Wilson, 2006). Three studies conducted in family practice settings found that the lifetime prevalence of husband-to-wife violence (slapping or worse) ranged from 36 percent to 44 percent (Elliott, 1995; Hamberger, 1992;

Pence, 1993). Many deaths due to IPV may go unrecognized as death certificate data are notoriously inaccurate. Deaths from other causes, such as suicide or substance abuse, may not be recognized as having IPV as the underlying cause.

Risk Factors

Race

Whites and African-Americans have higher rates of IPV than Hispanics. IPV during pregnancy is more frequent, more severe, and has a higher risk of homicide among white women than either African-American or Hispanic females.

Young Adulthood

Younger women are at greater risk for IPV than are older women (Chambliss, 2008). Peters and colleagues (2002) analyzed data from 5298 domestic violence reports. They found that women aged 16 to 24 years are at greatest risk for IPV, a risk that is more than twice that for women aged 25 to 34 years. Rates of IPV decrease throughout women's reproductive years and reach a nadir in those aged 65 or older.

Substance Abuse

Alcohol and substance abuse continue to play a large role in IPV both for perpetrators and for their victims. Victims develop substance abuse problems as they attempt to medicate their physical and emotional pain. Most women with posttraumatic stress disorder and substance use have histories of physical or sexual abuse. Kyriacou (1999) reported that 45 percent of men and 20 percent of women have been drinking when IPV occurs.

Prior Exposure to Violence

Hotaling and Sugarman (1986) found only one consistent risk marker of being an abused wife. Witnessing violence as a child was a significant risk factor reported in 11 of 15 studies.

Intimate Partner Violence During Pregnancy

Women should be screened for IPV perinatally. Seven to 20 percent of pregnant women may be victims, and homicide is reported as the leading cause of death during pregnancy. Most cases result from partner abuse (Gazmararian, 1996; Shadigian, 2005). Therefore, screening for IPV is an important component of prenatal care. The Antenatal Psychosocial Health Assessment (ALPHA) is a questionnaire that evaluates psychosocial health during pregnancy and contains sections that screen for domestic violence. This screening tool can be found at http://www.dfcm.utoronto.ca/Assets/DFCM+Digital+Assets/ALPHA_Guide_english.pdf.

Domestic Violence in Late Life

The social and medical problems of elder abuse are escalating with an increasing senior population. Currently, an estimated 2 million older adults are mistreated annually, and 84 percent of cases are unreported (Jayawardena, 2006). Elder abuse is divided into seven categories by The National Center on Elder Abuse: physical, emotional, and sexual abuse, financial exploitation, neglect, self-neglect, and miscellaneous (Tatara, 1997). Of these, neglect is the most prevalent form, occurs most often in the home, and is perpetrated most frequently by family members. Identified risk factors are caregiver stress, patient cognitive impairment, need for assistance with daily life activities, conflicted family relationships, and poor social support.

Diagnosis

Women who have been assaulted are far more likely to seek help from their medical provider than from legal personnel, mental health professionals, or victim advocates. Victims of violence have an unusually high rate of medical use for years after the assault and may present with psychiatric and somatic complaints to their primary care provider (Koss, 1992). Although some clinicians may feel awkward asking patients, researchers agree that *the single most important thing a physician can do for a battered woman is to ask about violence* (Linden, 1999). Additionally, health care providers should ask about IPV if they identify symptoms or behaviors that may be associated with victimization (Burge, 1997). These may include bruising, unexplained injuries, depression or anxiety, alcohol or drug abuse, unexplained chronic pain, isolation, inability to cope, limited access to care, noncompliance, husbands with extremely controlling behaviors or intense jealousy, or husbands with substance abuse.

The American Congress of Obstetricians and Gynecologists (2010) recommends that physicians screen all patients for IPV at routine gynecologic visits, family planning visits, the first prenatal visit, at least once per trimester, and at the postpartum visit. Screening can be conducted by making the following statement and asking three simple questions. "Because violence is so common in many women's lives and because there is help available for women being abused, I now ask every patient about domestic violence:

1. Within the past year—or since you have been pregnant—have you been hit, slapped, kicked, or otherwise physically hurt by someone?
2. Are you in a relationship with a person who threatens or physically hurts you?
3. Has anyone forced you to have sexual activities that made you feel uncomfortable?"

Management of Intimate Partner Violence
Patient Validation and Referral

If a patient discloses IPV, a clinician should validate and normalize a patient's perspective. Patients should be counseled that many women have assault experiences, that most are afraid to confide these, that memories about the experience can be painful, and that concern about future assaults is a reasonable fear. Following disclosure, a clinician should express concern for the woman's safety and health and convey a willingness to discuss relationship issues at any time. Moreover, information describing community resources should be offered. The National Domestic Violence Hotline (1-800-799-SAFE [7233]) is a nonprofit telephone referral service, with access to more than 5000 women's shelters nationally. Resources are also available on their web site at: http://www.ndvh.org/.

Documentation

Battery is a crime, yet few states specifically require reporting of IPV. A small number of states require mandatory arrest of batterers, and a few jurisdictions aggressively pursue cases of IPV. Accordingly, clinicians should know their state laws to properly and adequately inform their patients. In addition, providers should thoroughly document physical findings of violence. Such data may be required if criminal charges are pursued.

FEMALE SEXUALITY

Sexuality may be one of the most complex and yet basic components of human behavior. Expressions of sexuality and intimacy remain important throughout life. A woman's expression of her sexuality is unique to her and is likely to change over time. Pleasure or anhedonia from sex can also have a considerable impact on overall quality of life (Wylie, 2009). Sexuality encompasses sexual identity, sexual function, and sexual relationships. Although basic sexual drive is biologic, its expression is determined by a variety of psychological, social, environmental, spiritual, and learned factors. Thus, sexual satisfaction, for women, is often less dependent on the physical components of sex than on the quality of the relationship and the context in which sexual behavior is undertaken.

Biologic Cycle

In describing the sexual response cycle, several investigators have assumed that sexual responses follow a predictable and linear sequence of events from excitement to resolution. The number of stages within this response cycle varies, and those containing from two to four stages have been described (Fig. 13-1). The traditional view of the sexual response cycle describes progression through discrete sequential stages of desire, arousal, orgasm, and resolution. However, it is now recognized that these phases

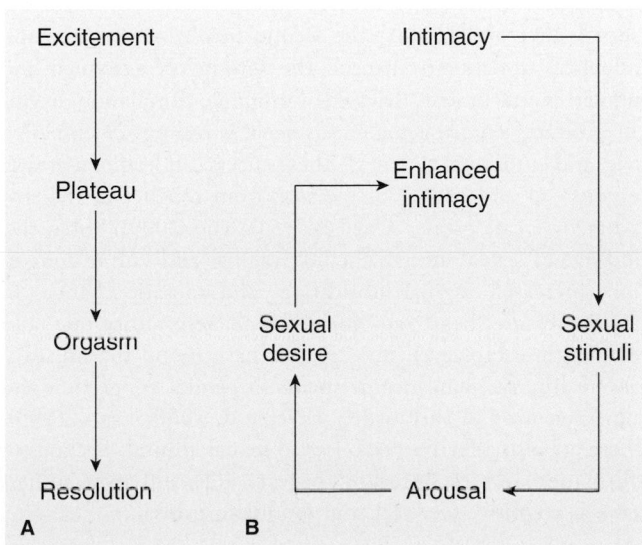

FIGURE 13-1 Models of female sexual response. Model **(A)** adapted from Masters, 1966. Model **(B)** adapted from Basson, 2000.

overlap and that their sequence may vary (Basson, 2006; Rosen, 2008). In more recent models, the woman begins in a state that is desire neutral. If she experiences adequate emotional intimacy from her partner, she may seek or be receptive to sexual stimuli. Receptivity to sexual stimuli allows the woman to move from sexual neutrality to arousal. If the mind continues to process the stimuli to further arousal, desire will encourage the woman to move forward to sexual satisfaction and orgasm. This positive outcome fosters intimacy and reinforces sexual motivation.

Drive/Desire

The basis of desire and perceived arousal in women is poorly understood, but it appears to involve interactions among multiple neurotransmitters, sex hormones, and environment. Early in the female sexual response cycle, erotic stimulation is associated with a desire, also termed *libido*, for sexual interaction. Libido varies and is considered to be the cerebral component of sexuality.

Several other factors have been closely linked to women's sexual satisfaction and libido. Based on survey data, these include stable past and current mental health, positive emotional well-being and self-image, rewarding past sexual experiences, positive feelings for her partner, and positive expectations for the relationship (Bancroft, 2003; Dennerstein, 2005; Laumann, 2005).

Arousal

A woman's sexual arousal is complex and correlates positively with the sexual stimulus and its emotional context. This subconscious reflex is organized by the autonomic nervous system and processed in the limbic system in response to mental or physical stimuli that are recognized as sexual. In 1998, Fisher described the emotion/motivation system, whereby basic emotions are seen to arise from distinct systems of neural activity. She proposed that humans have three primary motivation circuits or systems and that these brain systems have evolved to direct behavior. The first involves androgens and influences lust (sexual drive and libido). The second involves dopamine and influences attraction (romance). The third involves oxytocin and influences attachment. Released after nipple stimulation, oxytocin produces entactogenic effects such as feelings of empathy, love, and emotional closeness. These effects can lead to a greater response to and feeling of pleasure from touch and thereby, indirectly create greater sexual desire (Wylie, 2009). Subjective findings of sexual arousal include vaginal and vulvar congestion, increased vaginal lubrication, and somatic changes in blood pressure, heart rate, muscle tone, respiratory rate, and temperature. However, investigators have found that in sexually healthy women, measurements of genital congestion and subjective arousal vary widely (Everaerd, 2000; Laan, 1995). There are also affective responses to sexual arousal. Feelings of affirmation and joy or feelings of fear, guilt, and awkwardness serve as cognitive feedback and modulate arousal.

Clitoral Changes with Arousal

In the basal state, clitoral corporal and vaginal smooth muscles are tonically contracted. After sexual stimulation, neurogenic and endothelial release of nitric oxide leads to clitoral cavernosa artery relaxation. Arterial inflow follows and creates increased clitoral intracavernosal pressure and clitoral engorgement (Cellek, 1998). Extrusion of the glans clitoris and enhanced sensitivity results.

Vaginal and Vulvar Changes with Arousal

In the basal state, the vaginal epithelium reabsorbs sodium from the submucosal capillary plasma transudate. However, after sexual stimulation, several neurotransmitters, including nitric oxide and vasoactive intestinal peptide, are released. These modulate vaginal vascular and nonvascular smooth muscle relaxation (Palle, 1990). A dramatic increase in submucosal capillary flow follows and overwhelms sodium reabsorption. As a result, 3 to 5 mL of vaginal transudate is produced, and this enhanced lubrication is essential for pleasurable coitus. Vaginal smooth-muscle relaxation increases vaginal length and luminal diameter, especially in the distal two thirds of the vagina.

Release

Masters and Johnson (1966) proposed that orgasmic release is a reflex-like response that follows once a plateau of excitement has been reached or exceeded. The physiologic and behavioral indices of orgasm involve the whole body–facial grimaces, generalized myotonia, carpopedal spasms, and contractions of the gluteal and abdominal muscles. For women, orgasm is also marked by rhythmic contractions of the uterus, the vaginal barrel, and the rectal sphincter. These gradually diminish in intensity, duration, and regularity following orgasm. The subjective experience of orgasm includes feeling of intense pleasure with a peaking and rapid, exhilarating release. These sensations are reported to be singular, regardless of the manner in which orgasm is achieved (Newcomb, 1983). Women are unique in their ability to be multiorgasmic, that is, capable of a series of distinguishable orgasmic responses without a lowering of excitement between them.

Resolution

After orgasm, the anatomic and physiologic changes of excitement reverse. In women, genital vasocongestion diminishes, and the vagina shortens and narrows. A filmy sheet of perspiration covers the body, and elevated heart and respiration rates gradually return to normal. If orgasm has occurred, there is concomitant psychologic and physical relaxation. If orgasm does not occur, a similar physiologic process occurs, but at a slower rate.

Normal Variations in the Physiologic Response

Sexual function and variations in the physiologic response may be affected by many biologic and psychologic aspects of reproduction and the life cycle.

Pregnancy and Sexuality

During pregnancy, sexual function may change, and a reduction in sexual desire and coital frequency is typical (Hyde,

1996). These changes may stem from fears of causing fetal harm during intercourse or orgasm. In addition, fatigue, physical discomfort, or feeling less physically attractive are other reasons.

Women who suffer recurrent miscarriage, infertility, or undergo therapeutic abortion, and even those during a normal puerperium, will have alterations in their physiologic and psychologic sexual response. Hyde (1996) found that women who are breast feeding report less sexual activity and less satisfaction that those who were not breast feeding. The study failed to demonstrate marked differences according to the method of delivery, although women who had cesarean delivery were more likely to resume intercourse 4 weeks postpartum than women who had delivered vaginally. In the puerperium, the combination of a new baby, fatigue, hormonal changes, and a healing episiotomy scar may contribute to diminished frequency and enjoyment of sexual intercourse (Srivastava, 2008). However, at 12 to 18 months after childbirth, Klein and associates (2009) found no significant difference in sexual function between women who delivered vaginally without episiotomy, deep perineal laceration, or operative vaginal delivery by forceps or vacuum and women who underwent elective cesarean delivery.

Sexuality During Menopausal Transition

The baseline data from the Study of Women's Health Across the Nation (SWAN) addressed sexual behavior in 3262 women aged 42 to 52 years who were either premenopausal or in early menopausal transition. Evidence suggests that in early menopausal transition, there were few changes in sexual practices or function (Cain, 2003). However, in late menopausal transition or with oophorectomy in younger women, the decline in estrogen, and possibly androgen, levels can interfere with physiologic response (Avis, 2000; Gast, 2009). Masters and Johnson (1966) described a delay in clitoral reaction time, delayed or absent vaginal lubrication, decreased vaginal congestion, and reduced duration of contractions with orgasm. Moreover, loss of estrogen diminishes genital blood flow, vaginal lubrication, and vaginal tissue structural integrity (Freedman, 2002; Pauls, 2005). Sarrel and associates (1990) correlated improved libido and orgasm with estrogen replacement in postmenopausal women. Others have shown improvement in vaginal lubrication, blood flow, and vaginal compliance in menopausal women using systemic estrogen replacement (Berman, 1999; Semmens, 1982). Gast and colleagues (2009) showed that women receiving low-dose conjugated estrogens had a significant improvement in dyspareunia, sexual experience, and quality of life, although this did not translate into increased coital activity.

Sexuality in Late Life

With aging, sexuality continues to play an important role in the maintenance of physical and mental health. Klausmann (2002) and Dennerstein (2001) both suggest that even many years after menopause, an increase in desire and interest is consistently reported with a new relationship. The opportunity for sexual activity in the form of intercourse, however, is often dependent on partner issues. Both partner availability and partner health

begin to shape the frequency with which this form of sexual activity occurs. As erectile dysfunction in men increases with aging and women live longer than men, the "partner gap" becomes a major cause of sexual dissatisfaction for older women (Srivastava, 2008). Of older women, 40 to 47 percent masturbate.

In general, sexual activity declines with increasing age. Activity is reported in 30 to 78 percent of 60-year-old women, in 11 to 74 percent of those older than 70 years, and in 8 to 43 percent of 80-year-old women (Morley, 2003). Few data describe sexual function in those older than 80. However, as the "Baby Boomer" cohort, which is a more sexually open group than prior generations, continues to age, there may be greater desire to maintain this quality of life (Morley, 1992).

SEXUAL DISORDERS

Psychiatric sexual dysfunction is characterized by painful intercourse or disturbances in desire, arousal, orgasm, or resolution that cause marked distress and relationship difficulty (Table 13-19). Sexual dysfunction stemming from dyspareunia may also originate from gynecologic disease and is discussed more fully in Chapter 11 (p. 319).

Incidence

Although many studies have investigated female sexual dysfunction, prevalence rates are difficult to establish due to differing criteria and measures of sexual functioning. However, one literature review estimated that 64 percent of women experience low or no sexual desire, 35 percent have difficulty achieving orgasm, and 26 percent experience sexual pain (Hayes, 2006). Most difficulties last less than 6 months, but one third may persist longer.

Risk Factors

Psychosocial risk factors for sexual dysfunction include comorbid psychologic disorders, negative emotions, maladaptive cognitions (such as inaccurate expectations), cultural factors, lack of education regarding sexual functioning, couple distress, and absent physical attraction (Bach, 2001). Of these, psychiatric disorders such as depression and anxiety are frequently comorbid with sexual disorders. Thus, for most patients who suffer from sexual dysfunction, evaluations should not stop with an organic explanation (Bach, 2001).

Evaluation of Sexual Dysfunction

A thorough sexual history includes recording the patient's medical, surgical, social, and psychiatric history (American College of Obstetricians and Gynecologists, 2011b). In accordance with the biopsychosocial approach, diagnosis of sexual disorders begins by judging if dysfunction is caused exclusively by a general medical condition, drug abuse, medication (e.g., antidepressants often disrupt sexual response), or toxin exposure. Subsequently, evaluation for a primary psychiatric disorder should follow. Assessment typically inventories a woman's ethnic, cultural, religious, and social backgrounds and includes

TABLE 13-19. Sexual Function Disorders

Hypoactive Sexual Desire Disorder
Persistently or recurrently deficient or absent sexual fantasies and desire for sexual activity, taking into account factors such as age and the context of the person's life

Sexual Aversion Disorder
Persistent or recurrent extreme aversion to and avoidance of all genital sexual contact with a sexual partner

Female Sexual Arousal Disorder
Persistent or recurrent inability to attain or maintain until completion of sexual activity an adequate lubrication-swelling response of sexual excitement

Female Orgasmic Disorder
Persistent or recurrent delay in, or absence of, orgasm following a normal excitement phase taking into account factors such as age, sexual experience, and the adequacy of sexual stimulation she receives

Dyspareunia
Recurrent or persistent genital pain associated with sexual intercourse (not caused exclusively by vaginismus or lack of lubrication)

Vaginismus
Recurrent or persistent involuntary spasm of the musculature of the lower third of the vagina that interferes with sexual intercourse

In all the Above Disorders
The disturbance causes marked distress or interpersonal difficulty
Sexual dysfunction is not better accounted for by another psychiatric disorder and is not due exclusively to the direct physiologic effects of a substance or a general medical condition

Types: Lifelong vs. acquired; generalized vs. situational; due to psychological factors vs. due to combined factors

Adapted from American Psychiatric Association, 2000a, with permission.

a frank discussion regarding her current sexual partner(s) and sexual expectations. Clinical assessment should incorporate the patient's age, sexual experience, and symptom frequency and chronicity and should determine whether a woman perceives her symptoms as distressing or impairing (American Psychiatric Association, 2000a). Importantly, a woman should be asked if the sexual difficulty has always been present or has developed only within a certain time and if it persists across all situations or only appears in certain circumstances. Finally, referral to a psychiatrist or psychologist may be indicated for a thorough psychiatric interview.

Treatment of Sexual Dysfunction

Multidisciplinary treatment is ideal for patients with sexual dysfunction. A team would typically include the referring physician, gynecologist, psychologist, and a nurse-specialist. For organic disorders, it may be necessary to include specialists in urology, gastroenterology, and anesthesiology. Psychological approaches usually include some combination of sexual education, communication enhancement, identification of emotional and cultural factors, cognitive-behavioral therapy, and couples therapy.

REFERENCES

Adams JA: Guidelines for medical care of children evaluated for suspected sexual abuse: an update for 2008. Curr Opin Obstet Gynecol 20:435, 2008

Adams JA, Kaplan RA, Starling SP, et al: Guidelines for medical care of children who may have been sexually abused. J Pediatr Adolesc Gynecol 20:163, 2007

American College of Obstetricians and Gynecologists: Adult manifestations of childhood sexual abuse. Committee Opinion No. 498, August, 2011a

American College of Obstetricians and Gynecologists: Female sexual dysfunction. Practice Bulletin No. 119, April 2011b

American College of Obstetricians and Gynecologists: Premenstrual syndrome. Practice Bulletin No. 15, April 2000

American College of Obstetricians and Gynecologists: Screening for depression during and after pregnancy. Committee Opinion No. 453, February 2010

American College of Obstetricians and Gynecologists: Sexual assault. Committee Opinion No. 499, August 2011c

American College of Obstetricians and Gynecologists: Use of psychiatric medications during pregnancy and lactation. Practice Bulletin No. 92, April 2008

American Congress of Obstetricians and Gynecologists: Screening tools—domestic violence. 2010. Available at: http://www.acog.org/departments/dept_notice.cfm?recno=17&bulletin=585. Accessed August 23, 2010

American Psychiatric Association: Diagnostic and Statistical Manual of Mental Disorders, Fourth Edition, Text Revision. Washington, DC, American Psychiatric Association, 2000a

American Psychiatric Association: Practice Guideline for the Treatment of Patients with Eating Disorders, 2nd ed. In Practice Guidelines for the Treatment of Psychiatric Disorders, Compendium 2000. Washington, DC, American Psychiatric Association, 2000b

Anderson SL, Parker BJ, Bourguignon CM: Predictors of genital injury after nonconsensual intercourse. Adv Emerg Nurs J 31(3):236, 2009

Andrade L, Caraveo-Anduaga JJ, Berglund P, et al: The epidemiology of major depressive episodes: results from the International Consortium of Psychiatric Epidemiology (ICPE) Surveys. Int J Methods Psychiatr Res 12(1):3, 2003

Arowojolu AO, Okewole IA, Adekunle AO: Comparative evaluation of the effectiveness and safety of two regimens of levonorgestrel for emergency contraception in Nigerians. Contraception 66(4):269, 2002

Avis NE, Stellato R, Crawford S, et al: Is there an association between menopause status and sexual functioning? Menopause 7(5):297, 2000

Bach AK, Wincze JP, Barlow DH: Sexual Dysfunction. New York, Guilford Press, 2001

Backstrom T, Andersson A, Andree L, et al: Pathogenesis in menstrual cycle-linked CNS disorders. Ann NY Acad Sci 1007(1):42, 2003

Bäckström T, Haage D, Löfgren M, et al: Paradoxical effects of GABA-A modulators may explain sex steroid induced negative mood symptoms in some persons. Neuroscience 191:46, 2011

Baker TC, Burgess AW, Brickman E, et al: Rape victims' concern about possible exposure to HIV infection. J Interpers Violence 549, 1990

Bancroft J, Loftus J, Long JS: Distress about sex: a national survey of women in heterosexual relationships. Arch Sex Behav 32(3):193, 2003

Basson R: Clinical practice. Sexual desire and arousal disorders in women. N Engl J Med 354(14):1497, 2006

Basson R: The female sexual response: a different model. J Sex Marital Ther 26(1):51, 2000

Bechtel, K: Sexual abuse and sexually transmitted infection in children and adolescents. Curr Opin Pediatr 22:94, 2010

Berman JR, Berman LA, Werbin TJ, et al: Clinical evaluation of female sexual function: effects of age and estrogen status on subjective and physiologic sexual responses. Int J Impot Res 11(Suppl 1):S31, 1999

Bibring GL: Some considerations of the psychological processes in pregnancy. Psychoanal Study Child 14:113, 1959

Bloch M, Rotenberg N, Koren D, et al: Risk factors for early postpartum depressive symptoms. Gen Hosp Psychiatry 28(1):3, 2006

Boyce P, Hickey A: Psychosocial risk factors to major depression after childbirth. Soc Psychiatry Psychiatr Epidemiol 40(8):605, 2005

Brandon AR, Freeman MP: When She Says "No" to Medication: Psychotherapy for Antepartum Depression. Curr Psychiatry Rep Aug 30, 2011 [Epub ahead of print]

Brandon AR, Shivakumar G, Freeman MP : Perimenopausal depression. Curr Psychiatr 7(10):38, 2008

Braun DL, Sunday SR, Halmi KA: Psychiatric comorbidity in patients with eating disorders. Psychol Med 24(4):859, 1994

Brink TL, Yesavage JA, Lum O, et al: Screening tests for geriatric depression. Clin Gerontol 1(1):37, 1982

Bromberger JT, Meyer PM, Kravitz HM, et al: Psychologic distress and natural menopause: a multiethnic community study. Am J Public Health 91(9):1435, 2001

Burge SK: Violence against women. Prim Care 24(1):67, 1997

Burgess AW, Holmstrom LL: Rape trauma syndrome. Am J Psychiatry 131(9):981, 1974

Burt VK, Hendrick VC: Clinical Manual of Women's Mental Health. Washington, DC, American Psychiatric Publishing, 2005, p 6

Cain VS, Johannes CB, Avis NE, et al: Sexual functioning and practices in a multi-ethnic study of midlife women: baseline results from SWAN. J Sex Res 40(3):266, 2003

Carter FA, Carter JD, Luty SE, et al: Screening and treatment for depression during pregnancy: a cautionary note. Aust N Z J Psych 39:255, 2005

Cellek S, Moncada S: Nitrergic neurotransmission mediates the non-adrenergic non-cholinergic responses in the clitoral corpus cavernosum of the rabbit. Br J Pharmacol 125(8):1627, 1998

Centers for Disease Control and Prevention: Cephalosporin susceptibility among Neisseria gonorrhoeae isolates—United States, 2000–2010. MMWR 60(26):873, 2011

Centers for Disease Control and Prevention: Full report of the prevalence, incidence, and consequences of violence against women. 2000. Available at: http://www.ncjrs.gov/pdffiles1/nij/183781.pdf. Accessed August 23, 2010

Centers for Disease Control and Prevention: Sexually transmitted diseases treatment guidelines, 2010. MMWR 59(12):1, 2010

Chambliss LR: Intimate partner violence and its implication for pregnancy. Clin Obstet Gynecol 51(2):385, 2008

Clark R, Tluczek A, Wenzel A: Psychotherapy for postpartum depression: a preliminary report. Am J Orthopsychiatry 73(4):441, 2003

Cohen LS, Altshuler LL, Harlow BL, et al: Relapse of major depression during pregnancy in women who maintain or discontinue antidepressant treatment. JAMA 295(5):499, 2006a

Cohen LS, Miner C, Brown EW, et al: Premenstrual daily fluoxetine for premenstrual dysphoric disorder: a placebo-controlled, clinical trial using computerized diaries. Obstet Gynecol 100(3):435, 2002

Cohen LS, Soares CN, Lyster A, et al: Efficacy and tolerability of premenstrual use of venlafaxine (flexible dose) in the treatment of premenstrual dysphoric disorder. J Clin Psychopharmacol 24(5):540, 2004

Cohen LS, Soares CN, Vitonis AF, et al: Risk for new onset of depression during the menopausal transition: the Harvard study of moods and cycles. Arch Gen Psychiatry 63(4):385, 2006b

Cox J, Holden J, Sagovsky R: Detection of postnatal depression: Development of the 10-item Edinburgh postnatal depression scale. Br J Psychiatry 150:782, 1987

Cunningham FG, Leveno KL, Bloom SL, et al (eds): Teratology and medications that affect the fetus. In Williams Obstetrics, 23rd ed. New York, McGraw-Hill, 2010

Cunningham J, Yonkers KA, O'Brien S, et al: Update on research and treatment of premenstrual dysphoric disorder. Harv Rev Psychiatry 17(2):120, 2009

De Souza MC, Walker AF, Robinson PA, et al: A synergistic effect of a daily supplement for 1 month of 200 mg magnesium plus 50 mg vitamin B_6 for the relief of anxiety-related premenstrual symptoms: a randomized, double-blind, crossover study. J Womens Health Gend Based Med 9(2):131, 2000

de Waal MW, Arnold IA, Eekhof A, et al: Somatoform disorders in general practice: prevalence, functional impairment and comorbidity with anxiety and depressive disorders. Br J Psychiatry 184:470, 2004

Deming JE, Mittleman RE, Wetli CV: Forensic science aspects of fatal sexual assaults on women. J Forensic Sci 28(3):572, 1983

Dennerstein L, Dudley E, Burger H: Are changes in sexual functioning during midlife due to aging or menopause? Fertil Steril 76(3):456, 2001

Dennerstein L, Lehert P, Burger H, et al: Sexuality. Am J Med 118(12, Suppl 2):59, 2005

Dennis CL: Psychosocial and psychological interventions for prevention of postnatal depression: systematic review. BMJ 331(7507):1, 2005

DiMarco MA, Menke EM, McNamara T: Evaluating a support group for perinatal loss. MCN Am J Matern Child Nurs 26(3):135, 2001

Elliott BA, Johnson MM: Domestic violence in a primary care setting. Patterns and prevalence. Arch Fam Med 4(2):113, 1995

Endicott J, Nee J, Harrison W: Daily record of severity of problems (DRSP): reliability and validity. Arch Womens Ment Health 9(1):41, 2006

Engel GL: The need for a new medical model: a challenge for biomedicine. Science 196(4286):129, 1977

Erikson EH: Childhood and Society, 2nd ed. New York, Norton, 1963

Everaerd W, Laan E, Both S, et al: Female Sexuality. New York, Wiley, 2000

Fassino S, Daga GA, Pierò A, et al: Psychological factors affecting eating disorders. Adv Psychosom Med 28:141, 2007

Fichter MM, Xepapadakos F, Quadflieg N, et al: A comparative study of psychopathology in Greek adolescents in Germany and in Greece in 1980 and 1998—18 years apart. Eur Arch Psychiatry Clin Neurosci 254(1):27, 2004

Field T, Hernandez-Reif M, Diego M: Risk factors and stress variables that differentiate depressed from nondepressed pregnant women. Infant Behav Dev 29(2):169, 2006

Fisher HE: Lust, attraction, and attachment in mammalian reproduction. Hum Nat 9:23, 1998

Ford O, Lethaby A, Roberts H, et al: Progesterone for premenstrual syndrome. Cochrane Database Syst Rev 2:CD003415, 2009

Freedman MA: Female sexual dysfunction. Int J Fertil Womens Med 47(1):18, 2002

Freeman EW, Sammel MD, Lin H, et al: Associations of hormones and menopausal status with depressed mood in women with no history of depression. Arch Gen Psychiatry 63(4):375, 2006

Gast MJ, Freedman MA, Vieweg AJ, et al: A randomized study of low-dose conjugated estrogens on sexual function and quality of life in postmenopausal women. Menopause 16(2):247, 2009

Gaynes BN, Gavin N, Meltzer-Brody S, et al: Perinatal depression: prevalence, screening accuracy, and screening outcomes. Evid Rep Technol Assess(Summ) 119:1, 2005

Gazmararian JA, Lazorick S, Spitz AM, et al: Prevalence of violence against pregnant women. JAMA 275(24):1915, 1996

Girardet RG, Lahoti S, Howard LA, et al: Epidemiology of sexually transmitted infections in suspected child victims of sexual assault. Pediatrics 124(1):79. 2009a

Girardet RG, Lemme S, Biason TA, et al: HIV post-exposure prophylaxis in children and adolescents presenting for reported sexual assault. Child Abuse Negl 33:173, 2009b

GlaxoSmithKline: Paxil (paroxetine hydrochloride) prescribing information, January 2008. Available at: http://us.gsk.com/products/assets/us_paxil.pdf. Accessed July 25, 2010

Goldberg G: Psychiatry and primary care. World Psychiatry 2(3):153, 2003

Gostin LO, Lazzarini Z, Alexander D, et al: HIV testing, counseling, and prophylaxis after sexual assault. JAMA 271(18):1436, 1994

Halbreich U: The etiology, biology, and evolving pathology of premenstrual syndromes. Psychoneuroendocrinology 28(Suppl 3):55, 2003a

Halbreich U: The pathophysiologic background for current treatments of premenstrual syndromes. Curr Psychiatr Rep 4(6):429, 2002a

Halbreich U, Bergeron R, Yonkers KA, et al: Efficacy of intermittent, luteal phase sertraline treatment of premenstrual dysphoric disorder. Obstet Gynecol 100(6):1219, 2002b

Halbreich U, Borenstein J, Pearlstein T, et al: The prevalence, impairment, impact, and burden of premenstrual dysphoric disorder (PMS/PMDD). Psychoneuroendocrinology 28(Suppl 3):1, 2003b

Hamberger LK, Saunders DG, Hovey M: Prevalence of domestic violence in community practice and rate of physician inquiry. Fam Med 24(4):283, 1992

Hayes RD, Bennett CM, Fairley CK, et al: What can prevalence studies tell us about female sexual difficulty and dysfunction? J Sex Med 3(4):589, 2006

He W, Sengupta M, Velkoff VA, et al: 65+ in the United States: 2005. Available at: http://www.census.gov/prod/2006pubs/p23-209.pdf. Accessed August 23, 2010

Hoek HW: Incidence, prevalence and mortality of anorexia nervosa and other eating disorders. Curr Opin Psychiatry 19(4):389, 2006

Hoek HW, van Furth EF: [Anorexia nervosa and bulimia nervosa: I. Diagnosis and treatment]. Ned Tijdschr Geneeskd 142(33):1859, 1998

Holmes MM, Resnick HS, Kilpatrick DG, et al: Rape-related pregnancy: estimates and descriptive characteristics from a national sample of women. Am J Obstet Gynecol 175(2):320, 1996

Hotaling GT, Sugarman DB: An analysis of risk markers in husband to wife violence: the current state of knowledge. Violence Vict 1(2):101, 1986

Hyde JS, DeLamater JD, Plant EA, et al: Sexuality during pregnancy and the year postpartum. J Sex Res 33:143, 1996

Jayawardena KM, Liao S: Elder abuse at end of life. J Palliat Med 9(1):127, 2006

Jenny C, Hooton TM, Bowers A, et al: Sexually transmitted diseases in victims of rape. N Engl J Med 322(11):713, 1990

Johnson SR: Menstruation. In O'Hara MW, Reiter RC, Johnson SR, et al (eds): Psychological Aspects of Women's Reproductive Health. New York, Springer, 1995

Jones JS, Rossman L, Diegel R, et al: Sexual assault in postmenopausal women: epidemiology and patterns of genital injury. Am J Emerg Med 27(8):922, 2009

Kaplan PS, Burgess AP, Sliter JK, et al: Maternal sensitivity and the learning-promoting effects of depressed and nondepressed mothers' infant-directed speech. Infancy 14(2):143, 2009

Katz MH, Gerberding JL: Postexposure treatment of people exposed to the human immunodeficiency virus through sexual contact or injection-drug use. N Engl J Med 336(15):1097, 1997

Kelleher C, McGilloway S: "Nobody ever chooses this . . .": a qualitative study of service providers working in the sexual violence sector—key issues and challenges. Health Soc Care Community 17(3):295, 2009

Kellogg N: The evaluation of sexual abuse in children. Pediatrics 116:506, 2005

Kessler RC, Berglund P, Demler O, et al: Lifetime prevalence and age-of-onset distributions of DSM-IV disorders in the National Comorbidity Survey Replication. Arch Gen Psychiatry 62(6):593, 2005

Kessler RC, McGonagle KA, Zhao S, et al: Lifetime and 12-month prevalence of DSM-III-R psychiatric disorders in the United States. Results from the National Comorbidity Survey. Arch Gen Psychiatry 51(1):8, 1994

Kilpatrick DG, Edmunds C, Seymour A: Rape in America: a report to the nation. Arlington, VA, National Center for Victims of Crime; Charleston, SC, Medical University of South Carolina, National Crime Victim Research and Treatment Center, 1992

Klausmann D: Sexual motivation and the duration of the relationship. Arch Sex Behav 31:275, 2002

Klein K, Worda C, Leipold H, et al: Does the mode of delivery influence sexual function after childbirth? J Womens Health (Larchmt) 18(8):1227, 2009

Klump KL, Bulik CM, Kaye WK, et al: Academy for eating disorders position paper: eating disorders are serious mental illnesses. Int J Eat Disord 42(2):97, 2009

Kornstein SG: The evaluation and management of depression in women across the life span. J Clin Psychiatry 62(Supp l24):11, 2001

Koss MP, Heslet L: Somatic consequences of violence against women. Arch Fam Med 1(1):53, 1992

Krantz G, Garcia-Moreno C: Violence against women. J Epidemiol Community Health 59(10):818, 2005

Kyriacou DN, Anglin D, Taliaferro E, et al: Risk factors for injury to women from domestic violence against women. N Engl J Med 341(25):1892, 1999

Laan E, Everaerd W, van der Velde J, et al: Determinants of subjective experience of sexual arousal in women: feedback from genital arousal and erotic stimulus content. Psychophysiology 32(5):444, 1995

Lancaster CA, Gold KJ, Flynn HA, et al: Risk factors for depressive symptoms during pregnancy: a systematic review. Am J Obstet Gynecol 202(1):5, 2010

Landovitz RJ, Currier JS: Clinical practice. Postexposure prophylaxis for HIV infection. N Engl J Med 361(18):1768, 2009

Laumann EO, Nicolosi A, Glasser DB, et al: Sexual problems among women and men aged 40-80 y: prevalence and correlates identified in the global study of sexual attitudes and behaviors. Int J Impot Res 17(1):39, 2005

Lenahan LC, Ernst A, Johnson B: Colposcopy in evaluation of the adult sexual assault victim. Am J Emerg Med 16(2):183, 1998

Lindahl V, Pearson JL, Colpe L: Prevalence of suicidality during pregnancy and the postpartum. Arch Womens Ment Health 8(2):77, 2005

Linden JA: Sexual assault. Emerg Med Clin North Am 17 (3):685, 1999

Lowe SM, Rahman N, Forster G: Chain of evidence in sexual assault cases. Int J STD AIDS 20(11):799, 2009

Luce H, Schrager S, Gilchrist V: Sexual assault of women. Am Fam Physician 81(4):489, 2010

Maartens LWF, Knottnerus JA, Pop VJ: Menopausal transition and increased depressive symptomatology: a community based prospective study. Maturitas 42(3):195, 2002

Manber R, Schnyer RN, Allen JJB, et al: Acupuncture: a promising treatment for depression during pregnancy. J Affect Disord 83(1):89, 2004

Marchbanks PA, Lui KJ, Mercy JA: Risk of injury from resisting rape. Am J Epidemiol 132(3):540, 1990

Masters EH, Johnson VE: Human Sexual Response. Boston, Little, Brown, 1966

McCann J, Miyamoto S, Boyle C, et al: Healing of nonhymenal genital injuries in prepubertal and adolescent girls: a descriptive study. Pediatrics 120:1000, 2007

Mitchell AM, Bulik CM: Eating disorders and women's health: an update. J Midwifery Womens Health 51(3):193, 2006

Moore T, Parrish H, Black BP: Interconception care for couples after perinatal loss: a comprehensive review of the literature. J Perinat Neonatal Nurs 25(1):44, 2011

Morley JE: Sexual function and the aging woman. Ann Intern Med 307, 1992

Morley JE, Kaiser FE: Female sexuality. Med Clin North Am 87(5):1077, 2003

Moses-Kolko EL, Roth EK: Antepartum and postpartum depression: healthy mom, healthy baby. J Am Med Womens Assoc 59(3):181, 2004

National Institute of Mental Health: The numbers count: mental disorders in America. 2010. Available at: http://www.nimh.nih.gov/publicat/numbers.cfm. Accessed August 23, 2010

Newcomb MD, Bentler PM: Dimensions of subjective female orgasmic responsiveness. J Pers Soc Psychol 44(4):862, 1983

Newport DJ, Wilcox MM, Stowe ZN: Maternal depression: a child's first adverse life event. Semin Clin Neuropsychiatry 7(2):113, 2002

Norris ML, Boydell KM, Pinhas L, et al: Ana and the Internet: a review of pro-anorexia websites. Int J Eat Disord 39(6):443, 2006

Palle C, Bredkjaer HE, Ottesen B, et al: Vasoactive intestinal polypeptide and human vaginal blood flow: comparison between transvaginal and intravenous administration. Clin Exp Pharmacol Physiol 17(1):61, 1990

Parry B, Curran ML, Stuenkel CA, et al: Can critically timed sleep deprivation be useful in pregnancy and postpartum depression? J Affect Disord 60:201, 2000

Pauls RN, Kleeman SD, Karram MM: Female sexual dysfunction: principles of diagnosis and therapy. Obstet Gynecol Surv 60(3):196, 2005

Pence E, Paymar M: Education groups for men who batter: the Duluth Model. New York, Springer, 1993

Peters J, Shackelford TK, Buss DM: Understanding domestic violence against women: using evolutionary psychology to extend the feminist functional analysis. Violence Vict 17 (2):255, 2002

Pinquart M, Duberstein PR: Treatment of anxiety disorders in older adults: a meta-analytic comparison of behavioral and pharmacological interventions. Am J Geriatr Psychiatry 15(8):639, 2007

Pinquart M, Duberstein PR, Lyness JM: Treatments for later-Life depressive conditions: a meta-analytic comparison of pharmacotherapy and psychotherapy. Am J Psychiatry 163(9):1493, 2006

Plaut SM, Graziottin A, Heaton PW: Sexual Dysfunction. Oxford, UK, Health Press Limited, 2004

Polidori MC, Menculini G, Senin U, et al: Dementia, depression and parkinsonism: a frequent association in the elderly. J Alzheimer Dis 3(6):553, 2001

Rambow B, Adkinson C, Frost TH, et al: Female sexual assault: medical and legal implications. Ann Emerg Med 21:717, 1992

Rapkin AJ: YAZ in the treatment of premenstrual dysphoric disorder. J Reprod Med 53(9 Suppl):729, 2008

Rapkin AJ, Morgan M, Goldman L, et al: Progesterone metabolite allopregnanolone in women with premenstrual syndrome. Obstet Gynecol 90(5):709, 1997

Resnick H, Acierno R, Holmes M, et al: Emergency evaluation and intervention with female victims of rape and other violence. J Clin Psychol 56(10):1317, 2000

Rosen RC, Bachmann GA: Sexual well-being, happiness, and satisfaction, in women: the case for a new conceptual paradigm. J Sex Marital Ther 34(4):291, 2008

Rush AJ, Trivedi MH, Ibrahim HM, et al: The 16-item quick inventory of depressive symptomatology (QIDS), clinician rating (QIDS-C), and self-report (QIDS-SR): a psychometric evaluation in patients with chronic major depression. Biol Psychiatry 54(5):573, 2003

Sarrel PM: Sexuality and menopause. Obstet Gynecol 75(4 Suppl):26S, 1990

Sayil M, Gure A, Uçanok Z: First time mothers' anxiety and depressive symptoms across the transition to motherhood: associations with maternal and environmental characteristics. Women Health 44(3):61, 2007

Schmidt PJ, Nieman LK, Danaceau MA, et al: Differential behavioral effects of gonadal steroids in women with and in those without premenstrual syndrome. N Engl J Med 338(4):209, 1998

Schmidt PJ, Purdy RH, Moore PH Jr, et al: Circulating levels of anxiolytic steroids in the luteal phase in women with premenstrual syndrome and in control subjects. J Clin Endocrinol Metab 79(5):1256, 1994

Schwarcz SK, Whittington WL: Sexual assault and sexually transmitted diseases: detection and management in adults and children. Rev Infect Dis 12 (S6):682, 1990

Semmens JP, Wagner G: Estrogen deprivation and vaginal function in postmenopausal women. JAMA 248(4):445, 1982

Shadigian E, Bauer ST: Pregnancy-associated death: a qualitative systematic review of homicide and suicide. Obstet Gynecol Surv 60(3):183, 2005

Slaughter L, Brown CR, Crowley S, et al: Patterns of genital injury in female sexual assault victims. Am J Obstet Gynecol 176(3):609, 1997

Smith DK, Grohskopf LA, Black RJ, et al: Antiretroviral postexposure prophylaxis after sexual, injection-drug use, or other nonoccupational exposure to HIV in the United States: recommendations from the U.S. Department of Health and Human Services. MMWR 54(2):1, 2005

Soares CN, Almeida OP, Joffe H: Efficacy of estradiol for the treatment of depressive disorders in perimenopausal women: a double-blind, randomized, placebo-controlled trial. Arch Gen Psychiatry 58(6):529, 2001

Sommers MS, Schafer J, Zink T, et al: Injury patterns in women resulting from assault. Trauma Violence Abuse 2(3):240, 2001

Spinelli M, Endicott J: Controlled clinical trial of interpersonal psychotherapy versus parenting education for depressed pregnant women. Am J Psychiatry 160(3):555, 2003

Srivastava R, Thakar R, Sultan A: Female sexual dysfunction in obstetrics and gynecology. Obstet Gynecol Surv 63(8):527, 2008

Stein D, Kaye WH: Familial aggregation of eating disorders: results from a controlled family study of bulimia nervosa. Int J Eat Disord 26(2):211, 1999

Stoving RK, Hangaard J, Hagen C: Update on endocrine disturbances in anorexia nervosa. J Pediatr Endocrinol 14(5):459, 2001

Stoving RK, Hangaard J, Hansen-Nord M, et al: A review of endocrine changes in anorexia nervosa. J Psychiatr Res 33(2):139, 1999

Straka SM, Montminy L: Responding to the needs of older women experiencing domestic violence. Violence Against Women 12(3):251, 2006

Strumia R: Dermatologic signs in patients with eating disorders. Am J Clin Dermatol 6(3):165, 2005

Sundstrom I, Backstrom T: Citalopram increases pregnanolone sensitivity in patients with premenstrual syndrome: an open trial. Psychoneuroendocrinology 23(1):73, 1998

Task Force on Postovulatory Methods of Fertility Regulation: Randomised controlled trial of levonorgestrel versus the Yuzpe regimen of combined oral contraceptives for emergency contraception. Lancet 352(9126):428, 1998

Tatara T, Kuzmekus LB: Summaries of statistical data on elder abuse in domestic settings for FY95 and FY 96. National Center on Elder Abuse, Elder Abuse Information Series No. 2, Washington, DC, 1997

Thys-Jacobs S: Micronutrients and the premenstrual syndrome: the case for calcium. J Am Coll Nutr 19(2):220, 2000

Tjaden P, Thoennes N: Extent, nature, and consequences of intimate partner violence: findings from the national Violence Against Women Survey. National Institute of Justice Centers for Disease Control and Prevention, 2000

Treasure J, Holland AJ: Genetic vulnerability to eating disorders: evidence from twin and family studies. In Remschmidt H (ed): Child and Youth Psychiatry: European Perspectives. New York, Hogrefe and Hubert, 1989, p 59

Trussell J, Ellertson C, Stewart F: The effectiveness of the Yuzpe regimen of emergency contraception. Fam Plann Perspect 28 (2):58, 1996

United Nations General Assembly (UNGA): Declaration on the elimination of violence against women. United Nations General Assembly (UNGA) 1993. Available at: http://www.un.org/documents/ga/res/48/a48r104.htm. Accessed August 23, 2010

U.S. Food and Drug Administration: Public Health Advisory—Combined use of 5-hydroxytryptamine receptor agonists (Triptans), selective serotonin reuptake inhibitors (SSRIs) or selective serotonin/norepinephrine reuptake inhibitors (SNRIs) may result in life-threatening serotonin syndrome, 2006a. Available at: http://www.fda.gov/Drugs/DrugSafety/PublicHealthAdvisories/ucm124349.htm. Accessed July 25, 2010

U.S. Food and Drug Administration: Public Health Advisory: Treatment challenges of depression in pregnancy and the possibility of persistent pulmonary hypertension in newborns, 2006b. Available at: http://www.fda.gov/Drugs/DrugSafety/PublicHealthAdvisories/ucm124348.htm. Accessed July 25, 2010

Wang M, Seippel L, Purdy RH, et al: Relationship between symptom severity and steroid variation in women with premenstrual syndrome: study on serum pregnenolone, pregnenolone sulfate, 5 alpha-pregnane-3,20-dione and 3 alpha-hydroxy-5 alpha-pregnan-20-one. J Clin Endocrinol Metab 81(3):1076, 1996

Wieczorek K: A forensic nursing protocol for initiating human immunodeficiency virus post-exposure prophylaxis following sexual assault. J Forensic Nurs 6(1):29, 2010

Wilson JS, Websdale N: Domestic violence fatality review teams: an interprofessional model to reduce deaths. J Interprof Care 20(5):535, 2006

Wisner KL, Zarin DA, Holmboe ES, et al: Risk-benefit decision making for treatment of depression during pregnancy. Am J Psychiatry 157(12):1933, 2000

Wittchen HU, Becker E, Lieb R, et al: Prevalence, incidence and stability of premenstrual dysphoric disorder in the community. Psychol Med 32(1):119, 2002

Woods CR: Sexually transmitted diseases in prepubertal children: mechanisms of transmission, evaluation of sexually abused children, and exclusion of chronic perinatal viral infections. Semin Pediatr Infect Dis 16(4):317, 2005

Wyatt KM, Dimmock PW, Jones PW, et al: Efficacy of vitamin B-6 in the treatment of premenstrual syndrome: systematic review. Br Med J 318:1375, 1999

Wylie K, Mimoun S: Sexual response models in women. Maturitas 63(2):112, 2009

Yonkers KA, Halbreich U, Freeman E, et al: Sertraline in the treatment of premenstrual dysphoric disorder. Psychopharmacol Bull 32(1):41, 1996

Yonkers KA, Halbreich U, Freeman E, et al: Symptomatic improvement of premenstrual dysphoric disorder with sertraline treatment. A randomized controlled trial. Sertraline Premenstrual Dysphoric Collaborative Study Group. JAMA 278(12):983, 1997

Yonkers KA, O'Brien PM, Eriksson E: Premenstrual syndrome. Lancet 371(9619):1200, 2008

Yonkers KA, Wisner KL, Stewart DE, et al: The management of depression during pregnancy: a report from the American Psychiatric Association and the American College of Obstetricians and Gynecologists. Gen Hosp Psychiatry 31(5):403, 2009

Yuzpe AA, Smith RP, Rademaker AW: A multicenter clinical investigation employing ethinyl estradiol combined with dl-norgestrel as postcoital contraceptive agent. Fertil Steril 37(4):508, 1982

Zarit SH, Zarit JM: Mental Disorders in Older Adults: Fundamentals of Assessment and Treatment. New York, Guilford Press, 1998

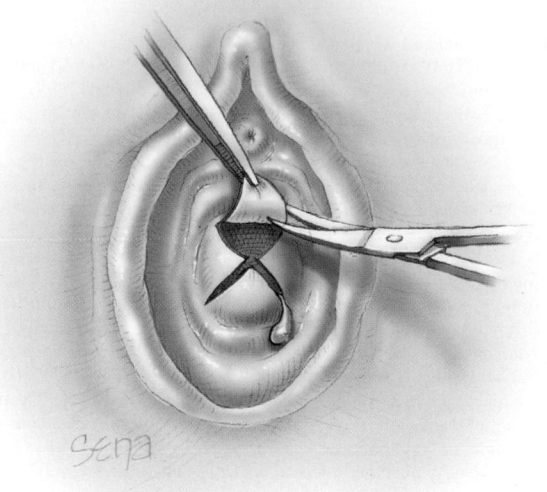

Pediatric gynecology is a unique subspecialty that encompasses knowledge from various specialties including general pediatrics, gynecology, reproductive endocrinology, as well as pediatric endocrinology and pediatric urology. Treatment of a particular patient may thus require the collaboration of clinicians from one or more of these fields.

Gynecologic disorders in children can differ greatly from those encountered in the adult female. Even the simple physical examination of the genitalia differs significantly. Thus, a thorough understanding of such differences can aid in clarifying and diagnosing the variety of gynecologic abnormalities seen in this age group.

PHYSIOLOGY AND ANATOMY

Hypothalamic-Pituitary-Ovarian (HPO) Axis

A carefully orchestrated cascade of events unfolds in the neuroendocrine system and regulates development of the female reproductive system.

In utero, gonadotropin-releasing hormone (GnRH) neurons develop in the olfactory placode. These neurons migrate through the forebrain to the arcuate nucleus of the hypothalamus by 11 weeks' gestation (Fig. 16-5, p. 447). They form axons that extend to the median eminence and to the capillary plexus of the pituitary portal system (Fig. 15-11, p. 414) (Ronnekliev, 1990; Schwanzel-Fukuda, 1989; Silverman, 1987). Gonadotropin-releasing hormone, a decapeptide, is influenced by higher cortical centers and is released from these neurons in a pulsatile fashion into the pituitary portal plexus. As a result, by midgestation, the GnRH "pulse generator" stimulates secretion of gonadotropins, that is, follicle-stimulating hormone (FSH) and luteinizing hormone (LH), from the anterior pituitary. In turn, the pulsatile release of gonadotropins stimulates ovarian synthesis and release of gonadal steroid hormones. Concurrently, accelerated germ cell division and follicular development begins, resulting in the creation of 6 to 7 million oocytes by 5 months' gestation. By late gestation, gonadal steroids exert a negative feedback upon secretion of both the pituitary gonadotropins and hypothalamic GnRH. During this time, oocyte number decreases through a process of gene-related apoptosis to reach a level of 1 to 2 million by birth (Vaskivuo, 2001).

At birth, FSH and LH concentrations rise abruptly in response to the fall in placental estrogen levels and are highest in the first 3 months of life (Fig. 14-1). This transient rise in gonadotropin levels is followed by an increase in gonadal steroid concentrations, which is thought to explain instances of neonatal breast budding, minor bleeding from endometrial

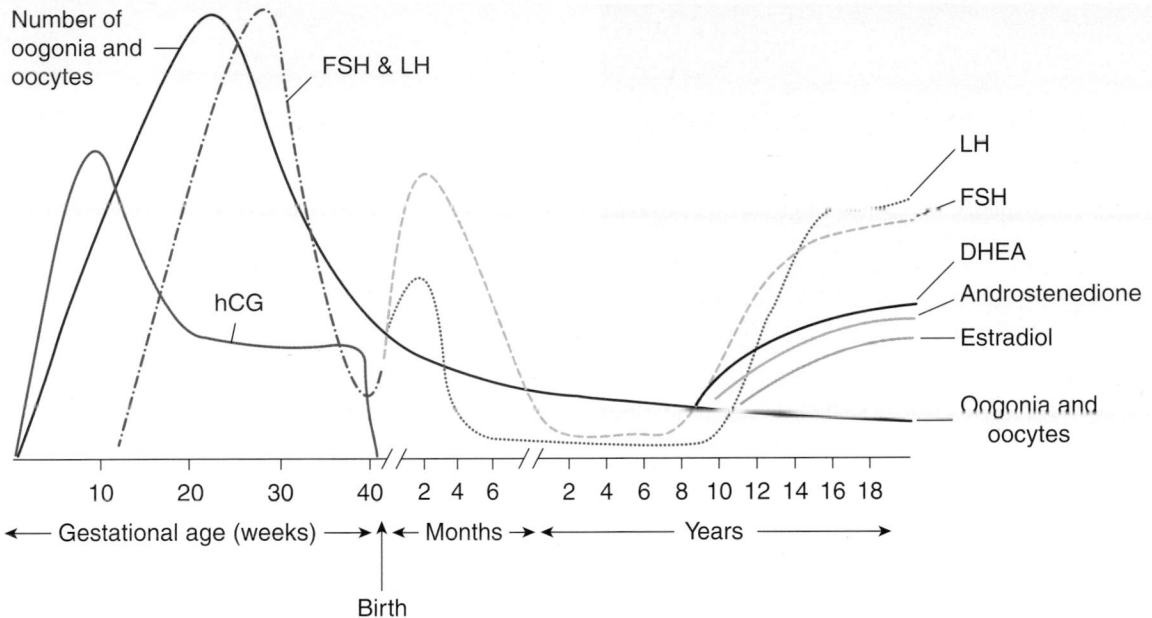

FIGURE 14-1 Variation in oocyte number and hormone levels during prenatal and postnatal periods. (DHEA = dehydroepiandrosterone; FSH = follicle-stimulating hormone; hCG = human chorionic gonadotropin; LH = luteinizing hormone.) *(Adapted from Speroff, 2005, with permission.)*

shedding, and short-lived ovarian cysts. Following these initial months, gonadotropin levels gradually decline to reach prepubertal levels by age 1 to 4 years.

The childhood years are thus characterized by low plasma levels of FSH, LH, and estradiol. Estradiol levels typically measure <10 pg/mL, and LH values are <0.3 mIU/mL. Both may be assessed if precocious development is suspected (Neely, 1995; Resende, 2007; Sathasivam, 2010). During childhood, ovaries undergo active follicular growth and oocyte atresia. As a result of this attrition, by puberty, only 300,000 to 500,000 oocytes remain (Speroff, 2005).

■ Anatomy

Pelvic anatomy also changes during pediatric development. In the neonate, sonographically, the uterus measures approximately 3.5 cm in length and 1.5 cm in width. Because the cervix is larger than the fundus, the neonatal uterus is typically spade-shaped (Nussbaum, 1986; Ratani, 2004). An echogenic central endometrial stripe is common and reflects the transiently elevated gonadal steroid levels described earlier. Fluid is seen within the endometrial cavity in 25 percent of female newborns. Ovarian volume measures ≤1 cm³, and small cysts are frequently found (Cohen, 1993; Garel, 2001).

During childhood, the uterus measures 2.5 to 4 cm and is tubular as a result of the cervix and fundus being now equal size (Fig. 14-2). The ovaries increase in size as childhood progresses, and volumes range from 2 to 4 cm³ (Ziereisen, 2005).

■ Pubertal Changes

Puberty marks the normal physiologic transition from childhood to sexual and reproductive maturity. Each landmark of hormonal and anatomic change during this time represents a spectrum of what is considered "normal."

With puberty, primary sexual characteristics of the hypothalamus, pituitary, and ovaries initially undergo an intricate maturation process. This maturation leads to the complex development of secondary sexual characteristics involving the breast, sexual hair, and genitalia, in addition to a limited acceleration in body growth.

Marshall and Tanner (1969) recorded breast and pubic hair development in 192 English schoolgirls and created the *Tanner stages* to describe pubertal development (Fig. 14-3). Initial pubertal changes occur between ages 8 and 13 years in most North American females (Tanner, 1985). Changes before or after are categorized as either precocious puberty or delayed puberty and warrant evaluation. In most girls, breast budding, termed *thelarche,* is the first physical sign of puberty and begins at approximately age 10 years (Aksglaede, 2009; Biro, 2006; Rosenfield, 2009). In a minority, pubic hair growth, known as *pubarche,* develops first. Following breast and pubic hair growth, adolescents, during a 3-year span from ages 10.5 to 13.5 years, undergo an accelerated increase in height, termed a *growth spurt*. Since these original population studies, U.S. girls have trended to start thelarche and menarche earlier. Differences in onset timing are also related to race and higher body mass index (Euling, 2008; Rosenfield, 2009). For example, the mean age of menarche in white girls is 12.7 years and 6 months earlier, or 12.1, in black girls (Tanner, 1973).

GYNECOLOGIC EXAMINATION

An adolescent who has reached the age of 18 may consent to medical examination and treatment. Prior to this age, a minor child must have the consent of a parent or legal guardian (except in emergency) for examination and treatment.

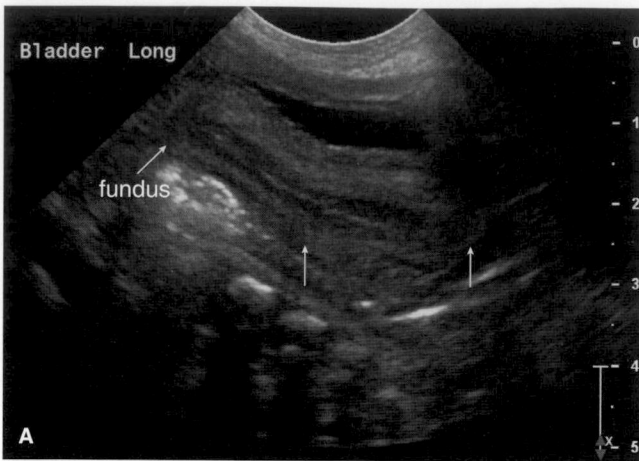

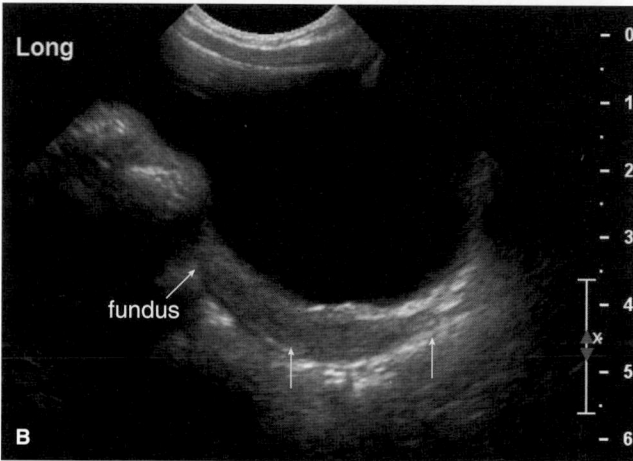

FIGURE 14-2 Transabdominal pelvic sonograms. **A.** Normal neonatal uterus. Midline longitudinal sonogram of the pelvis in this 3-day-old newborn demonstrates the uterus posterior to the bladder. Yellow arrows mark the fundus, isthmus, and cervix, respectively. The anteroposterior (AP) diameter of the cervix is greater than that of the fundus and creates a spade-shaped uterus. Due to the effect of maternal and placental hormones, a central echogenic endometrial cavity stripe is clearly visible. **B.** Normal prepubertal uterus. Midline longitudinal sonogram of the pelvis in this 3-year-old girl demonstrates the uterus posterior to the bladder. Yellow arrows mark the fundus, isthmus, and cervix, respectively. The uterus is homogeneously hypoechoic. The AP diameter of the cervix is equal to that of the fundus, and this gives the uterus a tubular shape. *(Images contributed by Dr. Neil Fernandes.)*

A routine yearly examination of a child by her pediatrician will generally include a brief examination of the breasts and external genitalia. Congenital anomalies, if visible externally—such as imperforate hymen, may be identified during such examination. Alternatively, if parent or child has a specific complaint regarding vulvovaginal pain, rash, bleeding, discharge, or lesions, a gynecologic examination is directed toward the area of concern.

Importantly, a parent or guardian should be present at the examination. This allows the child to understand that the examination is sanctioned. Moreover, clinicians can

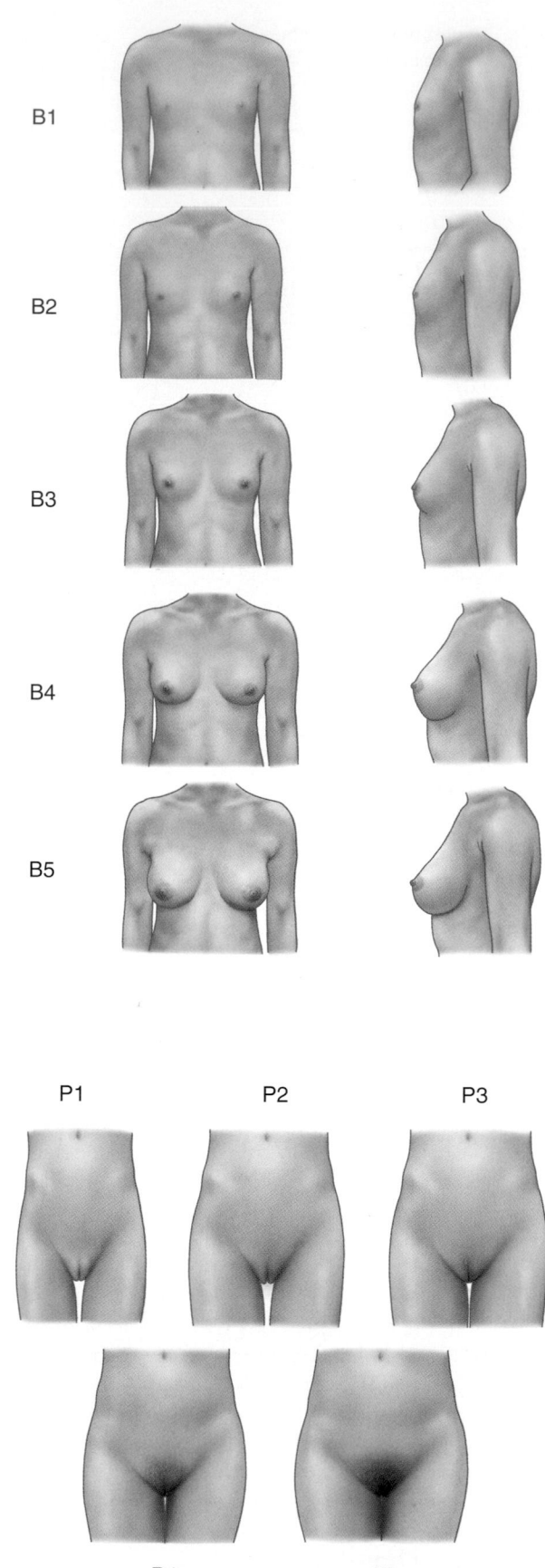

FIGURE 14-3 The Tanner stages of female breast and pubic hair development.

use this opportunity to inform a parent about findings and potential treatment. This may also be an opportune time to emphasize points regarding inappropriate genital touching by others and the importance of parental notification if this occurs. In mid-to-late adolescence, however, a patient may prefer, for privacy reasons, not to be examined with a parent present.

"Child-friendly" objects in the examination room such as posters, books, toys, and pictures and distracting conversation can ease fears and significantly aid in examination of the young female. Similarly, using an anatomically appropriate doll to explain the examination and having the child repeat the procedure on the doll may decrease anxiety.

The examination begins with a less-threatening approach of checking the ears, throat, heart, and lungs. Breasts are inspected. The external genital examination is best performed with the child in a frog-leg or knee-chest position to improve visualization. Occasionally, the patient may feel more comfortable sitting in a parent's lap. Sitting on a chair or examination table, the parent allows the child's legs to straddle the parent's thighs (Fig. 14-4).

Once the child is optimally positioned, each labium may be gently held with a thumb and forefinger and pulled toward the examiner and laterally. In this manner, the introitus, hymen, and lower portion of the vagina are inspected (Fig. 14-5). An internal examination is rarely necessary unless a foreign body, tumor, or vaginal bleeding is suspected. This evaluation is best accomplished under general anesthesia in an ambulatory care center. Vaginoscopy may be performed using a hysteroscope or cystoscope to provide illumination as well as irrigation (Baldwin, 1995; Pokorny, 1997). During vaginoscopy, normal

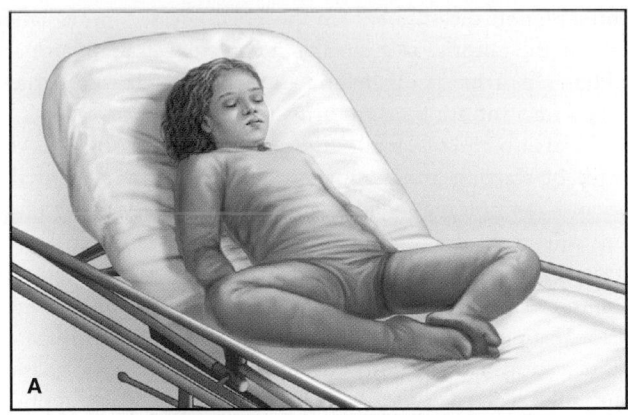

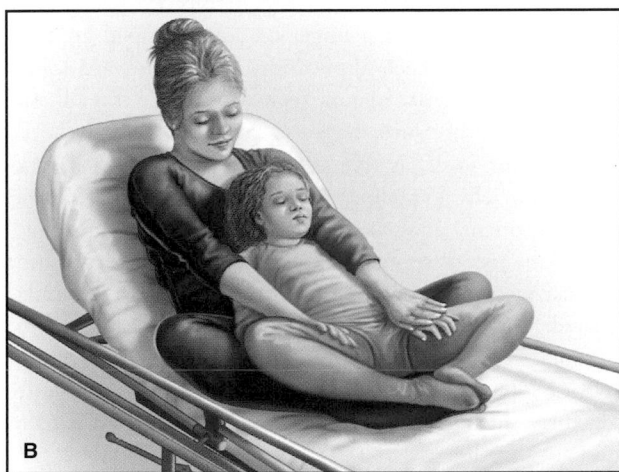

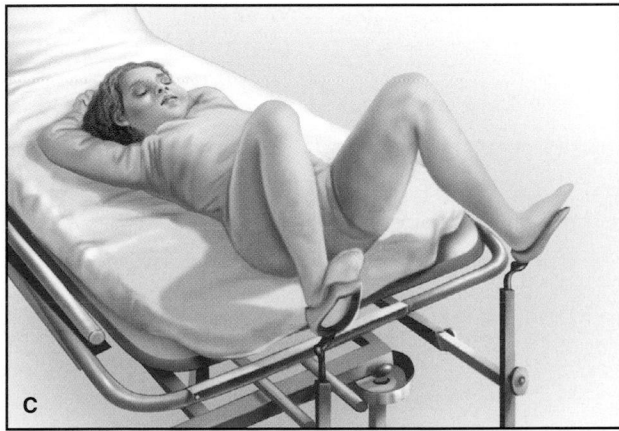

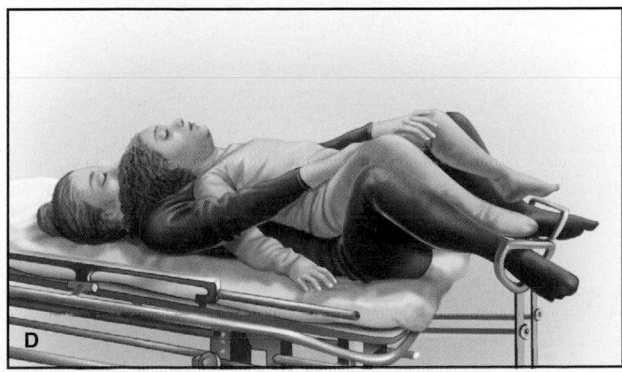

FIGURE 14-4 Positions for examination of the pediatric patient **(A–D)**.

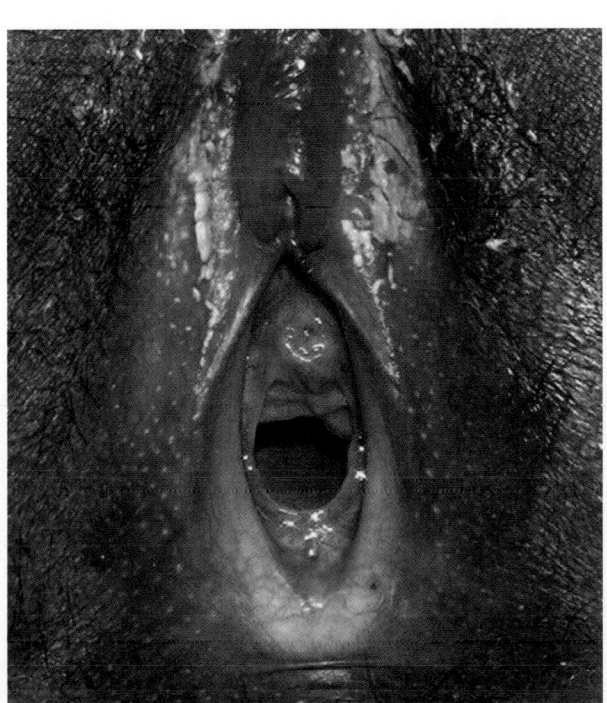

FIGURE 14-5 Photograph of normal prepubertal genitalia.

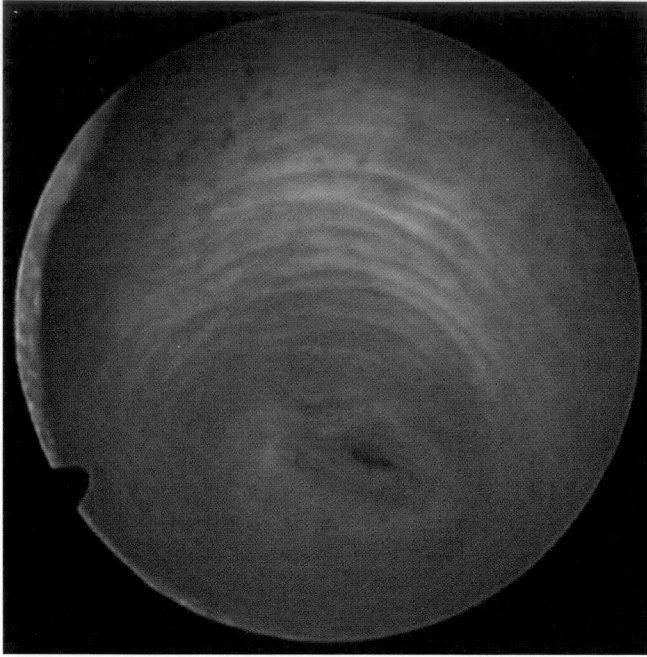

FIGURE 14-6 Photograph taken during vaginoscopy in an 8-year-old female. Typical for prepubertal girls, the cervix is almost flush with the proximal vagina.

saline is used as the distension medium (Fig. 14-6). The labia majora are manually approximated to occlude the vagina and achieve vaginal distension.

PROBLEMS IN PEDIATRIC GYNECOLOGY

Labial Adhesion

Adhesion between the labia minora begins as a small posterior midline fusion, which is usually asymptomatic. This fusion may remain an isolated minor finding or may progress toward the clitoris to completely close the vaginal orifice. Also termed *labial agglutination*, this adhesion develops in 1 to 5 percent of prepubertal girls and in approximately 10 percent of female infants within the first year of life (Berenson, 1992; Christensen, 1971).

The cause of labial adhesion is unknown, although hypoestrogenism is implicated. This fusion typically develops in a low-estrogen environment—it is seen in infants and young girls and tends to undergo spontaneous resolution at puberty (Jenkinson, 1984). Additionally, erosion of the vulvar epithelium is thought to underlie some cases of labial adhesion. For example, adhesion has been found in association with vulvar irritation such as with lichen sclerosus, with herpes simplex viral infection, and with vulvar trauma following sexual abuse (Berkowitz, 1987).

The diagnosis is made by visual inspection of the vulva. The labia majora appear normal, whereas the labia minora are fused with a distinct thin line of demarcation or *raphe* between them (Fig. 14-7). Extensive agglutination may leave only a

ventral pinhole meatus between the labia. Located immediately beneath the clitoris, this small opening may lead to urinary dribbling as urine pools behind the adhesion. In these cases, urinary tract infection or urethritis may develop.

The treatment of labial adhesion varies according to the degree of scarring and symptoms. In many instances, if the patient is asymptomatic, no treatment is necessary as the adhesion will typically resolve spontaneously with the rise of estrogen levels at puberty. Extensive adhesion with urinary symptoms, however, will require treatment with an estrogen cream. Estradiol (Estrace) cream or alternatively, conjugated equine estrogen (Premarin) cream may be applied to the fine, thin raphe twice daily for 2 weeks, followed by daily applications for an additional 2 weeks. A generous pea-sized amount of cream is placed with a finger or cotton-tipped applicator to the raphe. With each application, gentle outward traction is exerted on the labia majora to help separate the adhesion. Similarly, light pressure may also be applied with the cotton applicator itself, as tolerated. After adhesion separation, a petroleum jelly (Vaseline) or vitamins A and D ointment (A&D ointment) may be applied nightly for 6 months to decrease the risk of recurrence. If the adhesion reforms during the subsequent months or years, the process may be similarly repeated. Occasionally, with overuse of estrogen cream, local irritation, vulvar pigmentation, and minor breast budding may develop, at which time, topical treatment is discontinued. These side effects are reversible once treatment is halted. Alternatively, the use of 0.05-percent betamethasone cream applied twice daily for 4 to 6 weeks has been reported as successful treatment (Mayoglou, 2009; Meyers, 2006).

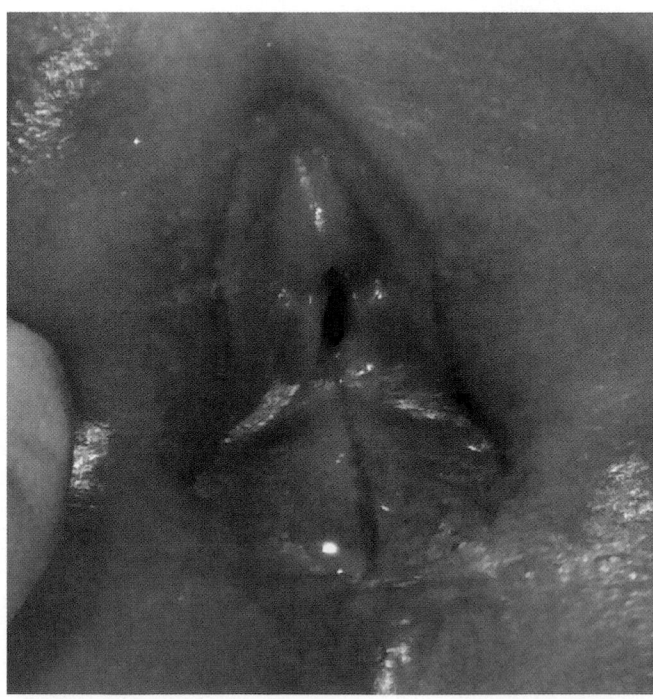

FIGURE 14-7 Labial adhesion. Labia minora are agglutinated in the midline. *(Photograph contributed by Dr. Mary Jane Pearson.)*

Manual separation of labial adhesion in an outpatient setting without analgesia is not generally advised as significant pain may result. In addition, recurrence is much more common. However, if the adhesion persists despite consistent use of estrogen cream as described earlier, labia minora separation may be attempted several minutes after applying 5-percent lidocaine ointment to the adhesion raphe.

If separation is not easily accomplished or tolerated by the child, surgical separation is recommended in an operating room under general anesthesia as an outpatient procedure. Division of the fused labia, also termed *introitoplasty*, involves a midline incision with light cautery and should not require suturing. To prevent repeated agglutination after surgery, an estrogen cream should be applied nightly for 2 weeks. This is followed by an emollient cream nightly for at least 6 months.

Congenital Anatomic Anomalies

Several anatomic and müllerian abnormalities present in early adolescence as obstructions to menstrual outflow. Described in Chapter 18, those most commonly seen include imperforate hymen, transverse vaginal septum, cervical and vaginal agenesis with an intact uterus, and the OHVIRA syndrome (obstructed hemivagina with ipsilateral renal agenesis) (Han, 2010; Reddy, 2009; Smith, 2007). These are often diagnosed in an adolescent with primary amenorrhea and cyclic pain. An adolescent with OHIVRA will present with menses that become increasingly painful over 6 to 9 months.

Vulvitis
Allergic and Contact Dermatitis

Inflammation of the vulva may develop in isolation or in association with vaginitis. In such cases, prepubertal girls may complain of vulvar discomfort and itching. Although the underlying pathophysiology of allergic and contact dermatitis varies, the clinical appearance is usually similar. In affected females, vesicles or papules form on bright-red, edematous skin (Fig. 14-8). However, in chronic cases, scaling, skin fissuring, and lichenification may be noted. In response, a detailed history should be directed to the level of hygiene, degree of continence, and exposure to potential skin irritants. Frequently, children may develop diaper dermatitis as a result of urine and stool exposure. Corrective measures include attempts to keep the skin dry by more frequent diaper changes or by application of emollient creams, such as Vaseline or A&D ointment, to create a moisture barrier.

Significant pruritus may develop from contact or allergic vulvitis. Typical offending agents include bubble baths and soaps, laundry detergents, fabric softeners and dryer sheets, bleach, and perfumed or colored toilet paper (Table 4-1, p. 112). Topical creams, lotions, and ointments used to soothe an area may also be an irritant to some children. For most, removing the offending agent and encouraging once- or twice-daily sitz baths is sufficient. These baths consist of placing two tablespoons of baking soda in warm water and soaking for 20 minutes. If itching is severe, an oral medication may be prescribed such as hydroxyzine hydrochloride (Atarax) 2 mg/kg/d

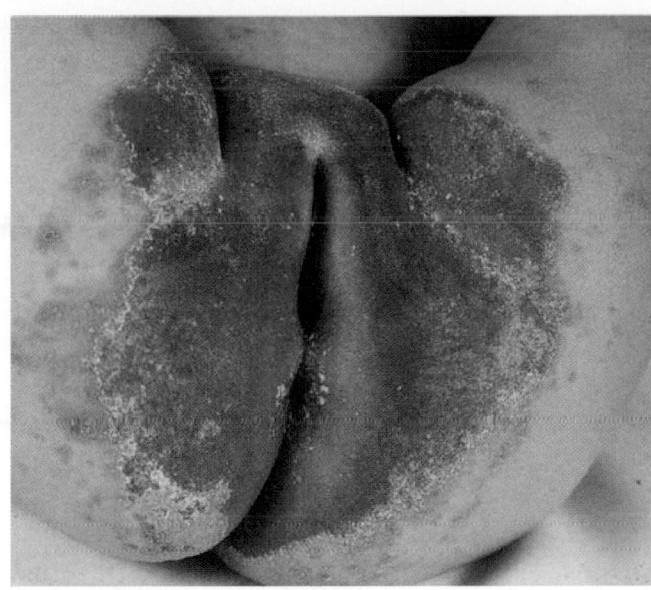

FIGURE 14-8 Diaper rash dermatitis and secondary candidiasis in a girl receiving antibiotic therapy. *(From Wolff, 2005, with permission.)*

divided in four doses, or application of a 2.5-percent topical hydrocortisone ointment twice daily for 1 week.

Lichen Sclerosus

Vulvitis may also be caused by lichen sclerosus. With this, the vulva displays hypopigmentation; atrophic, parchment-like skin; and occasional fissuring. Lesions are usually symmetrical and may form an "hourglass" appearance around the vulva and perianal areas (Fig. 14-9). Occasionally, the vulva may develop dark purple vulvar ecchymoses, which may bleed.

Similar to labial adhesion, lichen sclerosus can develop concurrently with hypoestrogenism or with inflammation. Lichen sclerosus is found more commonly in the postmenopausal years and can be associated with vulvar malignancy. In contrast, this association is not found in affected pediatric patients. The exact pathophysiology is unknown, although twin and cohort studies suggest a genetic role (Meyrick Thomas, 1986; Sherman, 2010).

Patients may complain of intense itching, discomfort, bleeding, excoriations, and dysuria. Diagnosis typically relies on visual inspection. However, rarely, a vulvar biopsy may be indicated if the classic skin changes are absent.

Treatment consists of topical corticosteroid cream such as 2.5-percent hydrocortisone, applied nightly to the vulva for 6 weeks. If improvement is noted, the dose may be lowered to 1-percent hydrocortisone and continued for 4 to 6 weeks. Thereafter, strict attention to hygiene and the use of petroleum-based ointments is recommended. Severe cases will require a more potent corticosteroid such as 0.05-percent clobetasol propionate (Temovate), applied twice daily for 2 weeks. This initial dosing is followed by an individualized regimen, which slowly tapers the dose to a once-weekly bedtime application. The long-term prognosis for childhood lichen sclerosus is unclear. Although some cases resolve at puberty, small case series suggest that as many as 75 percent of affected children have disease that

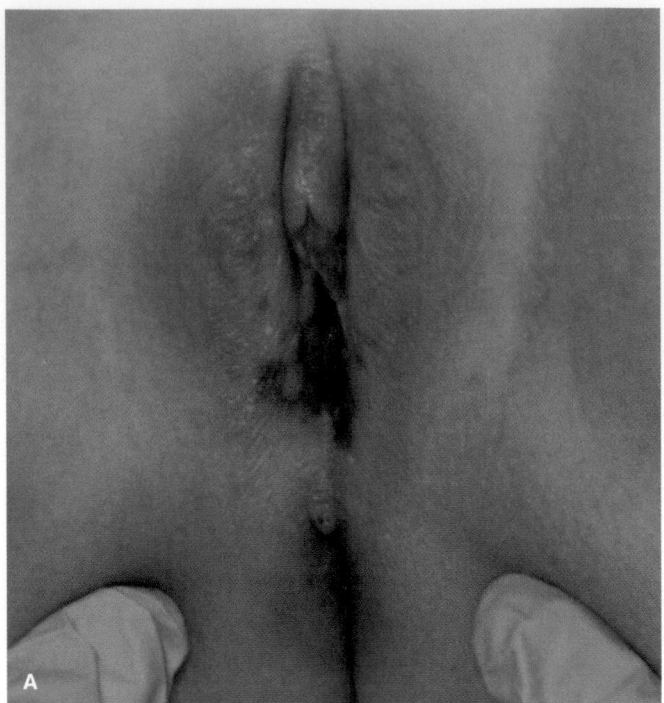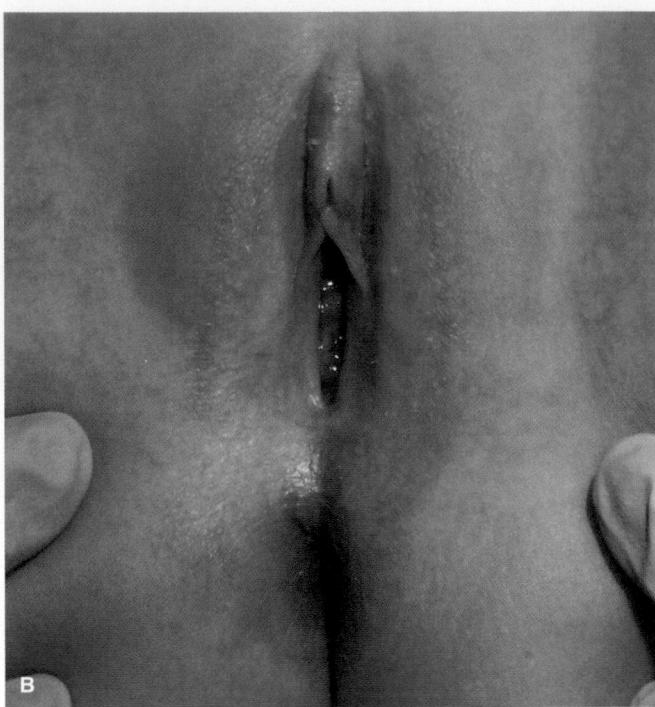

FIGURE 14-9 Photographs of lichen sclerosus before and after treatment. **A.** Findings include thin, parchment-like skin on the labia majora, ecchymoses on the labia minora and majora, and mild disease on the perianal skin. Involvement of both the vulva and perianal skin gives a figure-of-eight shape to affected areas. **B.** Skin texture and ecchymoses improved following treatment. *(Photographs contributed by Dr. Mary Jane Pearson.)*

persists or recurs following puberty (Berth-Jones, 1991; Powell, 2002; Smith, 2009).

Infection

Some common infectious organisms that may cause prepubertal vulvitis include group A beta-hemolytic streptococcus, *Candida* species, and pinworms. Group A beta-hemolytic streptococcus may present with a bright "beefy" red appearance of the vulva and introitus. The child may elicit symptoms of dysuria, vulvar pain, pruritus, or bleeding. In most cases, vulvovaginal culture and clinical setting typically lead to diagnosis. Group A beta-hemolytic streptococcus may be treated with an oral first-generation penicillin or cephalosporin or other appropriate antibiotic for 2 to 4 weeks.

Candidiasis is rarely seen in nonestrogenized prepubertal girls. It more often develops during the first year of life, after a course of antibiotics, or in females with juvenile diabetes or an immunocompromised condition. Diagnosis is assisted by the visual inspection of a reddened, raised rash with well-demarcated borders and occasional satellite lesions. Microscopic examination of a vaginal sample prepared with 10-percent potassium hydroxide (KOH) will help identify hyphae (Fig. 3-14, p. 84). Treatment consists of twice-daily vulvar application of antifungal creams such as clotrimazole, miconazole, or butoconazole for 10 to 14 days or until the rash is cleared.

Enterobius vermicularis, also known as *pinworm*, can be a source of intense vulvar itching, particularly at night. Nocturnal pruritus results from an intestinal infection with these 1-cm-long, threadlike white worms that often exit the anus at night (Pierce, 1992; Zeiguer, 1993). Inspecting this area with a flashlight at night when the child is asleep, parents may identify worms perianally. The "Scotch-tape test" entails pressing a piece of cellophane tape to the perianal area in the morning, affixing the tape to a slide, and visualizing eggs with microscopy. Treatment consists of mebendazole (Vermox), 100 mg orally in a single dose and repeated after 1 week.

Physiologic Discharge

Physiologic discharge is often seen transiently in the newborn as a result of exposure to maternal estrogen in utero. This usually appears as a clear to white mucous discharge. Also in the first few days after birth, the endometrium may undergo transient shedding, and a bloody discharge is seen.

Vulvovaginitis

This is one of the most common gynecologic problems of prepubertal girls. Three fourths of vulvovaginitis cases in this age group are nonspecific, with culture results yielding "normal flora." Alternatively, several infectious agents, discussed subsequently, may be identified.

Nonspecific Vulvovaginitis

Several months after birth, as estrogen levels wane, the vulvovaginal epithelium becomes thin and atrophic. As a result of this change, the vulva and vagina are more susceptible to irritants and infections until puberty.

TABLE 14-1. Causes of Vulvovaginitis in Children

Poor vulvar hygiene
Inadequate front-to-back wiping after bowel movements
Lack of labial fat pads and labial hair
Short distance from the anus to the vagina
Nonestrogenized vulvovaginal epithelium
Foreign body insertion into the vagina
Chemical irritants such as soaps, bubble baths, shampoos
Coexistent eczema or seborrhea
Chronic disease and altered immune status
Sexual abuse

Many visits to the pediatric gynecologist involve vulvovaginal complaints. The pathogenesis is not well defined, but known instigating factors that can lead to nonspecific vulvovaginitis are included in Table 14-1. Symptoms include itching, vulvar redness, discharge, dysuria, and odor. Most children and those adolescents who are not sexually active tolerate speculum examination poorly. But a vaginal swab for bacterial culture is typically comfortably obtained. In cases of nonspecific vulvovaginitis, cultures typically only isolate normal vaginal flora. Culture results that reveal bowel flora suggest contamination with fecal aerobes.

Treatment is directed toward correction of the underlying cause. Itching and inflammation may be relieved with the use of a low-dose topical corticosteroid (hydrocortisone, 1 or 2.5 percent). Occasionally, severe itching can lead to a secondary bacterial infection that requires oral antibiotic treatment. Antibiotics commonly used include amoxicillin, an amoxicillin plus clavulanic acid combination, or a similar cephalosporin given during a 7- to 10-day course.

Infectious Vulvovaginitis

Infectious vulvovaginitis often presents with a malodorous, yellow or green purulent discharge, and vaginal cultures are routinely obtained in these cases. The respiratory pathogen group A beta-hemolytic streptococcus is the most common specific infectious agent found in prepubertal females and is isolated from 7 to 20 percent of girls with vulvovaginitis (Pierce, 1992; Piippo, 2000). Treatment of group A beta-hemolytic streptococcus consists of amoxicillin, 40 mg/kg, taken orally three times daily for 10 days. Less frequently, other respiratory pathogens found include *Haemophilus influenzae, Staphylococcus aureus,* and *Streptococcus pneumoniae.* Enteric pathogens such as *Shigella* and *Yersinia* species may also be found by culture of vaginal discharge. Classically, *Shigella* species incite a mucopurulent bloody discharge, which typically follows diarrhea caused by the same organism. Treatment is with oral trimethoprim-sulfamethoxazole (TMP-SMZ), 6 to 10 mg/kg/d, divided and given every 12 hours (Bogaerts, 1992).

As discussed in Chapter 13, sexual abuse may result in infections including those caused by *Neisseria gonorrhoeae, Chlamydia trachomatis,* herpes simplex virus (HSV), *Trichomonas vaginalis,* and human papillomavirus (HPV) (Fig. 14-10). The clinical presentation of each mirrors the infectious findings in adults.

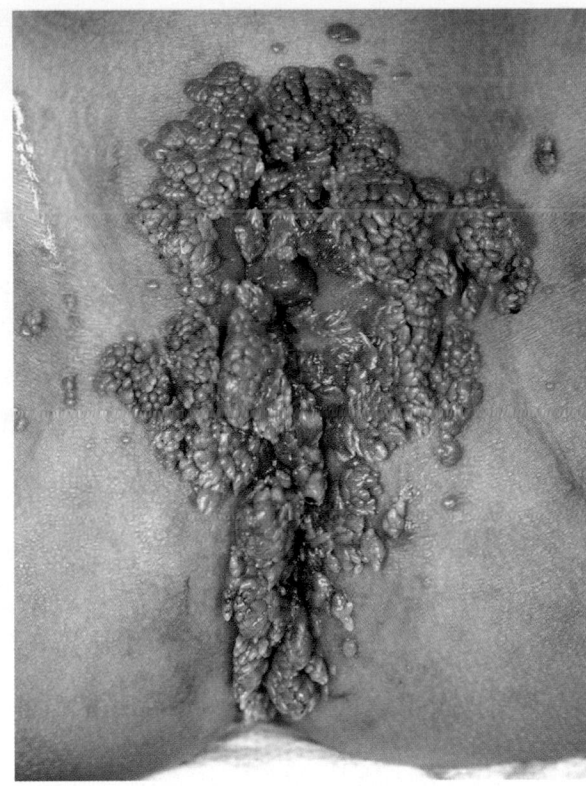

FIGURE 14-10 Vulvar condyloma in a prepubertal girl.

Although some of these may result from vertical transmission, child protective services should be notified of any child suspected to be the victim of sexual abuse (Chap. 13, p. 372).

Genital Trauma

The prepubertal vulva is less protected from blunt injury due to the lack of labial fat pads (Fig. 14-11). In addition, children are more physically active, thereby increasing the risk of trauma. Fortunately, most injuries to the vulva are blunt, minor, and accidental. Sharp-object penetration, however, may cause more serious injury to the vulvovaginal area. Sexual or physical abuse should be also considered in many cases of genital trauma. Management of vulvovaginal trauma is discussed in greater detail in Chapter 4 (p. 127).

Ovarian Tumors

Ovarian masses, typically cysts, are common in childhood. They may be found prenatally during maternal sonographic evaluation, as well as during the prepubertal years and adolescence. Although most are benign, approximately 1 percent of all malignant tumors in this age group are of ovarian origin (Breen, 1977, 1981).

Fetal and Neonatal Ovarian Cysts

Almost all ovarian masses in this age group are cystic and are typically identified incidentally on maternal sonographic examination. Although the true incidence of fetal ovarian cysts is not known, some cystic development has been reported in 30 to 70 percent of fetuses (Brandt, 1991; Lindeque, 1988). Most cysts result

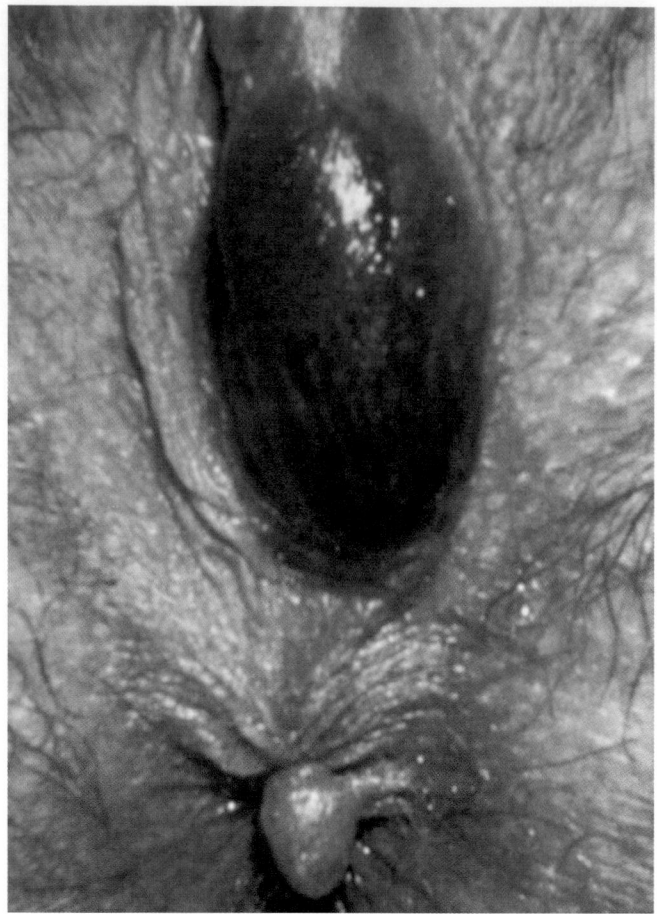

FIGURE 14-11 Straddle injury of the vulva with hematoma formation. *(From the North American Society for Pediatric and Adolescent Gynecology, 2001, with permission.)*

may be discovered incidentally during abdominal examination or during sonographic examination for some other indication. Enlarging cysts may cause an increased abdominal girth or chronic pain. Hormone-secreting cysts may lead to isosexual or heterosexual precocious puberty, and thus evaluation for signs of early pubertal development is indicated. Moreover, rupture, hemorrhage, or torsion may precipitate acute abdominal pain, similar to that seen in adults (Chap. 9, p. 270).

In the older adolescent and adult, transvaginal sonography is the preferred tool to evaluate ovarian tumors. However, a prepubertal child will not tolerate examination with a transvaginal probe. Therefore, in this age group, transabdominal pelvic sonography is most frequently used. Computed tomography is helpful if a mature cystic teratoma (dermoid cyst) is suspected, as fat is better appreciated with this modality. Although magnetic resonance (MR) imaging is preferred for evaluation of congenital müllerian anomalies, it is less helpful than pelvic sonography for ovarian mass determination. The most common complex cysts found in childhood and adolescence are germ cell tumors, specifically benign mature cystic teratoma (Panteli, 2009). Rarely, tumors may be malignant germ cell tumors or epithelial ovarian tumors (Schultz, 2006; Tapper, 1983).

As with those of the fetal and neonatal periods, small simple ovarian cysts without septation or internal echoes may be monitored with serial sonographic examination. Most less than 5 cm will resolve within 1 to 4 months (Thind, 1989). Persistent or enlarging cysts warrant surgical intervention, and laparoscopy is the preferred method. Optimal management includes fertility-sparing ovarian cystectomy with preservation of normal ovarian tissue.

Following puberty, ovarian cysts in adolescents, as in adults, are a frequent finding. Management mirrors that of adnexal masses found in adults as described in Chapter 9 (p. 262).

Breast Development and Disease

At puberty, under the influence of ovarian hormones, the breast bud grows rapidly. The epithelial sprouts of the mammary gland branch further and become separated by increasing deposition of fat.

Newborns may have some minor breast budding due to transplacental passage of maternal hormones in utero. Similarly, newborn breasts may produce *witches' milk*, which is a bilateral white nipple discharge, also as a result of maternal hormone stimulation. Both effects are transient, and most often diminish during several weeks to months.

Breast development, termed *thelarche*, begins in most girls between the ages of 8 and 13 years. Thelarche prior to age 8 or lack of breast development by age 13 is considered abnormal and should be investigated (p. 391).

Breast Examination

This evaluation begins in the newborn period and extends through the prepubertal and adolescent years as abnormalities can develop in any age group. Assessment includes inspection for accessory nipples, infection, lipoma, fibroadenoma, and premature thelarche.

from maternal hormonal stimulation in utero. They are typically unilateral, asymptomatic, and tend to regress spontaneously by 4 months after birth, whether they are simple or complex.

During the neonatal period and infancy, ovarian cysts may also develop. These result from the postnatal gonadotropin surge seen with the withdrawal of maternal hormones after birth. Most cysts are simple, asymptomatic, and tend to regress within several months.

The risk of malignancy in fetal and neonatal ovarian cysts is low, although rupture, intracystic hemorrhage, visceral compression, and torsion followed by autoamputation of the ovary or adnexa may be seen. For uncomplicated fetal or neonatal cysts measuring less than 5 cm in diameter, appropriate management is observation and sonographic examination every 4 to 6 weeks (Bagolan, 2002; Murray, 1995; Nussbaum, 1988; Spence, 1992). For simple cysts measuring greater than 5 cm, percutaneous cyst aspiration may be considered to prevent torsion (Bryant, 2004; Salkala, 1991). Large complex ovarian cysts that do not regress postnatally require surgical excision.

Prepubertal Ovarian Masses

As in the newborn, most ovarian masses in children are cystic, and presenting symptoms are varied. Asymptomatic cysts

Polythelia

Accessory nipples, also termed *polythelia*, are common and noted in 1 percent of patients. Most frequently, a small areola and nipple are found along the embryonic milk line, which extends from the axilla to the groin bilaterally. Accessory nipples are usually asymptomatic, and excision is not required. Rarely, however, they may contain glandular tissue that can lead to pain, nipple discharge, or development of fibroadenomas (Aughsteen, 2000; Oshida, 2003).

Premature Thelarche

Thelarche may begin before age 8 in some girls and is most commonly seen in girls aged less than 2 years (Fig. 14-12). This early breast maturation is termed *premature thelarche*. It differs from precocious puberty in that it is benign, self-limited, and develops in isolation, without other signs of pubertal development. Premature thelarche is suspected when minimal breast tissue growth or nipple maturation is noted during surveillance, but the patient's height falls within established percentile curves. Monitoring body growth and breast changes alone may suffice, but in those with increased height or weight or with other pubertal changes, additional testing for precocious puberty is warranted. Accordingly, analysis of the patient's growth curve and Tanner stage, a radiographic bone age study, and gonadotropin measurement may be indicated (p. 393).

To explain bone age, as children develop, their bones change in size and shape. These changes can be seen radiographically and can be correlated with chronologic age. Thus, the radiographic "bone age" is the average age at which children in general reach a particular stage of bone maturation. Girls with early estrogen excess from precocious puberty show growth-rate acceleration, rapid bone age advancement, early cessation of growth, and eventual short stature. Bone age can be determined at many skeletal sites, and the left hand and wrist are by far the most commonly used.

Premature thelarche is suggested if the bone age is synchronous and falls within 1 year of chronologic age. However, if the bone age is advanced by 2 or more years, puberty has begun and evaluation of precocious puberty is indicated. In those with isolated premature thelarche, serum estradiol levels may be slightly elevated, and this is seen more commonly in very low-birthweight infants (Escobar, 1976; Ilicki, 1984; Klein, 1999; Nelson, 1983). In addition, serum gonadotropin levels are low. In most cases, premature breast development regresses or stabilizes, and treatment consists of reassurance with careful surveillance for other signs of precocious puberty.

Breast Asymmetry

Asymmetrical breast growth may be seen often during early breast development stages in adolescent girls aged 13 to 14 years. A thorough examination should be performed to check for a breast mass such as a fibroadenoma or cyst. If no mass is identified, then yearly breast examinations are performed to determine the extent and persistence of asymmetry.

The etiology of breast asymmetry is not known, although there have been cases of sports injuries or surgical trauma occurring during early breast development that may have led to asymmetry (Goyal, 2003; Jansen, 2002). Moreover, a strong association with asymmetry and tuberous breast formation has been noted (DeLuca-Pytell, 2005).

In most cases, asymmetry will resolve by the completion of breast maturity (Templeman, 2000). Therefore, a decision toward surgical intervention involving augmentation or reduction mammoplasty is not made until full breast growth is attained. Until that time, adolescents may be fitted with padded bras or even prosthetic inserts to ensure symmetry when fully clothed. Although most adolescents with minor breast asymmetry choose not to undergo surgical intervention, others may elect to visit with a plastic surgeon to discuss options, particularly if the asymmetry is pronounced.

Breast Hypertrophy

Rarely, adolescents develop extremely large breasts without concurrent large breast masses. Breast hypertrophy can be symptomatic, and complaints may include back pain, shoulder discomfort from bra-strap pressure, kyphosis, and psychologic distress. These young women will often seek reduction mammoplasty, but surgery should be delayed until breast growth is completed, as determined by serial breast measurements, typically between the ages of 15 to 18 years.

Tuberous Breasts

With normal breast development, growth on the breast's ventral surface projects the areola forward, and peripheral growth enlarges the breast base. In some adolescents, the fascia is densely adhered to the underlying muscle and fails to be separated from

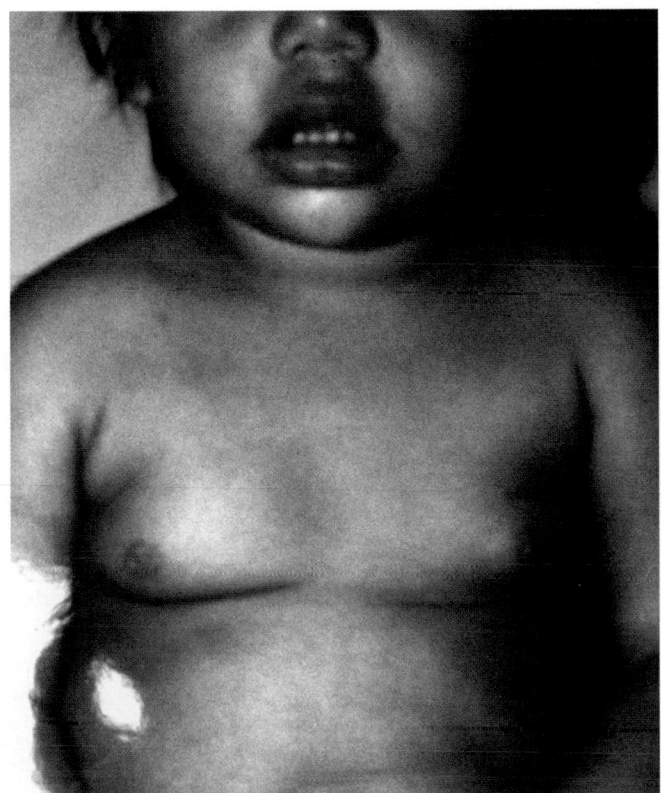

FIGURE 14-12 Premature thelarche. *(From the North American Society for Pediatric and Adolescent Gynecology, 2001, with permission.)*

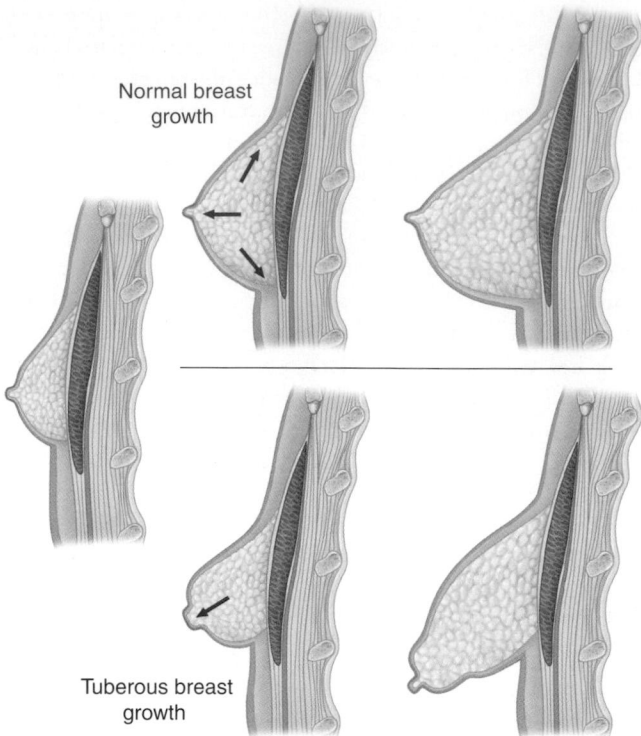

Normal breast growth

Tuberous breast growth

FIGURE 14-13 Comparison of normal and tuberous breast development. *(Redrawn from Grolleau, 1999, with permission.)*

its muscular layer by laterally expanding breast tissue (Fig. 14-13). This restricts peripheral expansion of the breast base, and breast growth is directed forward. These are termed *tuberous breasts.* This appearance can also follow exogenous hormone replacement that may be prescribed to girls with a lack of breast development from genetic, metabolic, or endocrine conditions. To avoid tuberous development in this setting, hormone replacement is initiated at small dosages and gradually increased over time. For example, conjugated equine estrogen (Premarin), 0.3 mg, may be given orally each day for 6 months, followed by incremental dose increases every 6 months, through doses 0.625 mg and 0.9 mg, to finally reach 1.25 mg daily. Medroxyprogesterone acetate (Provera), 10 mg, is given orally each day for 12 days of the month to prompt withdrawal periods. Once estrogen dosing has reached 1.25 mg daily, the patient may alternatively be placed on a low-dose oral contraceptive pill instead.

Lack of Breast Development

Congenital absence of breast glandular tissue, termed *amastia*, is rare. More commonly, a lack of breast development results from low estrogen levels caused by constitutionally delayed puberty, debilitating chronic disease, radiation or chemotherapy, genetic disorders such as gonadal dysgenesis, or extremes of physical activity such ballet or endurance sport. Treatment is based on the etiology. For example, once a competitive athlete completes her career, breast development may begin spontaneously without hormonal treatment. In contrast, to prompt breast development and prevent osteoporosis, patients with gonadal dysgenesis will require some form of hormonal replacement, such as that described earlier for the prevention of tuberous breasts.

Nipple Discharge

Nipple discharge may present in varied colors, which may indicate their etiology. For example, milky discharge typifies galactorrhea; cloudy, yellow, or light-green liquid may indicate infection; greenish-brown discharge is commonly associated with ductal ectasia; whereas a serosanguineous nipple fluid may reflect an intraductal papilloma or rarely cancer. In general, the pathophysiology and management of these discharges mirrors that of the adult female (Chap. 12, p. 338).

Breast Cysts

When an adolescent presents with a complaint of a breast lump, the findings are often consistent with fibrocystic changes. These are characterized by patchy or diffuse, bandlike thickenings or lumps. Sonography may aid in distinguishing between a cystic and solid mass and in defining cyst qualities (Garcia, 2000). In contrast, mammography has a limited role in the evaluation of child and adolescent breast tissue due to high breast tissue density. Mammography has limited sensitivity and specificity in young developing breasts, and their normally dense breast tissue yields high rates of false-negative results (Williams, 1986).

Actual breast cysts are found on occasion and will usually resolve spontaneously over a few weeks to months. If a cyst is large, persistent, or symptomatic, a fine-needle aspiration may be performed using local analgesia in an office setting.

Breast Masses

Most breast masses in children and adolescents are benign and may include normal but asymmetric breast bud development; fibroadenoma; fibrocyst; lymph node; or abscess. The most common breast mass identified in adolescence is the fibroadenoma, which accounts for 68 to 94 percent of all masses (Daniel, 1968; Goldstein, 1982). Fortunately, breast cancer in pediatric populations is rare, and cancer complicated less than 1 percent of breast masses identified in this group (Gutierrez, 2008; Neinstein, 1994). However, primary breast cancer may develop more frequently in pediatric patients with a history of prior radiation, especially treatment directed to the chest wall. Additionally, metastatic disease is considered in those with a history of malignancy.

Following identification of a breast mass on physical examination in a young female, sonography is the primary imaging method. Magnetic resonance imaging is not routinely recommended because of its high cost and limited availability.

Treatment of breast masses includes observation, needle biopsy, and surgical excision. Observation may be appropriate for small asymptomatic lesions considered to be fibroadenomas. Alternatively, in many cases, a tissue diagnosis with a minimally invasive procedure such as fine-needle aspiration is indicated. Additionally, sonography-guided core needle biopsy is another percutaneous option. In any mass not surgically excised, clinical surveillance is recommended to ensure stability of the mass (Weinstein, 2003). Masses that are symptomatic, large, or enlarging are preferably excised using local analgesia or general anesthesia in an ambulatory surgical center.

Mastitis is rare in the pediatric population, and its incidence displays a bimodal distribution—in the neonatal period and

TABLE 14-2. Causes of Vaginal Bleeding in Children

Foreign body
Genital tumors
Urethral prolapse
Lichen sclerosus
Vulvovaginitis
Condyloma acuminata
Trauma
Precocious puberty
Exogenous hormone usage

in children older than 10 years. The etiology in these cases is unclear, but the association with breast enlargement during these two periods has been implicated. *Staphylococcus aureus* is the most common isolate, and abscess develops more commonly than in the adult (Faden, 2005; Stricker, 2006). In adolescents, infections may be also associated with lactation and pregnancy, trauma related to sexual foreplay, shaving periareolar hair, and nipple piercing (Templeman, 2000; Tweeten, 1998). Infections are treated with antibiotics and occasional drainage if an abscess has formed (Chap. 12, p. 340).

Vaginal Bleeding

Neonates may present with vaginal bleeding during the first week of life due to the withdrawal of maternal estrogen at birth. Bleeding typically resolves after a few days. Prepubertal bleeding in a child, however, merits careful evaluation (Table 14-2). Most instances of vaginal bleeding in the prepubertal girl are due to local causes and can be elucidated with a simple history and physical examination. Occasionally, an examination under anesthesia with saline vaginoscopy is required for diagnosis, particularly if a foreign body is in the upper vagina.

Precocious Puberty

Early pubertal development may be seen in both sexes, but females are much more commonly affected, with a sex ratio of 23:1 (Bridges, 1994). For girls, precocious puberty has historically been defined as the development of breast or pubic hair in those younger than 8 years. However, Herman-Giddens and colleagues (1997) noted that girls in the United States overall are undergoing normal pubertal development at younger ages than previously reported. In addition, racial differences exist. Puberty begins earliest in black girls, followed by Hispanic and white girls. Accordingly, to limit the proportion of girls requiring unneeded evaluation for precocious puberty, some have suggested lowering the age for evaluation of precocious puberty (Herman-Giddens, 1997; Kaplowitz, 1999).

Premature pubertal development may result from various causes. These have been categorized based on pathogenesis and include central precocious puberty, peripheral precocious puberty, heterosexual precocious puberty, and temporal variation of normal puberty. Most girls evaluated for precocious puberty are found to have normal pubertal development that has merely begun prior to standard temporal milestones and does not stem from underlying pathology. However, because many of the underlying etiologies of precocious puberty carry significant sequelae, girls with early pubertal development should be fully evaluated when identified.

Central Precocious Puberty (Gonadotropin Dependent)

Early activation of the hypothalamic-pituitary-ovarian axis leads to GnRH secretion, increased gonadotropin formation, and in turn, increased gonadal steroid levels. Often termed *true precocious puberty*, central precocious puberty is rare and affects 1 in 5000 to 10,000 individuals in the general population (Partsch, 2002). The most common cause of central precocious puberty is idiopathic, however, central nervous systems lesions must be excluded (Table 14-3).

Symptoms of central precocious puberty are similar to those of normal puberty—with breast development, pubic hair growth, growth spurt, and eventual menses—however, at an earlier age. As outlined in Table 14-4, testing includes a left hand and wrist bone age radiographic measurement. In affected girls, advanced skeletal maturation is seen. In addition, serum FSH, LH, and estradiol levels are elevated for chronologic age and typically lie in the pubertal range. Early in the process, however, FSH and LH levels may only be elevated in the evenings, and a GnRH stimulation test can be helpful. During GnRH stimulation, GnRH (3.5 µg/kg; not to exceed 100 µg) is infused intravenously, and gonadotropin levels are measured before and at sequential intervals after infusion. Central precocious puberty is confirmed by a rise in serum LH levels following infusion. In contrast, lack of LH and FSH level elevation after infusing GnRH suggests peripheral precocious puberty. In those with elevated gonadotropin levels, computed tomography and MR imaging of the central nervous system may identify a cerebral abnormality associated with central precocious puberty.

Treatment goals focus on preventing short adult height and limiting the psychologic effects of early pubertal development. Epiphyseal fusion is an estrogen-dependent process. Accordingly, girls with precocious puberty are at risk for early growth-plate closure and short stature in adulthood. Treatment consists of a GnRH agonist, which serves to downregulate pituitary gonadotropes and inhibit FSH and LH release. Estrogen levels drop, and often there is a marked regression of breast and uterine size. If therapy is instituted after menses have begun, they will cease. Timing for the discontinuation of GnRH therapy and reinitiation of pubertal development is determined by the primary therapy goals: maximizing height, synchronizing puberty with peers, and allaying psychological distress. From a review of several studies, the mean age at treatment discontinuation was approximately 11 years (Carel, 2009).

Peripheral Precocious Puberty (Gonadotropin Independent)

Less commonly, elevated estrogen levels may originate from a peripheral source, such as an ovarian cyst. Termed peripheral precocious puberty, this category is characterized by lack of

TABLE 14-3. Etiologies of Precocious Puberty

Central (GnRH dependent)
Idiopathic[a]
Central nervous system (CNS) tumors:
   Astrocytomas, adenomas, gliomas, germinomas
Congenital anomaly:
   Hamartomas, hydrocephalus, arachnoid or suprasellar
      cysts, septooptic dysplasia, empty sella syndrome
CNS infection
Head trauma
Ischemia
Iatrogenic: Radiation, chemotherapy, surgical
Adoption from underdeveloped to developed country

Peripheral (GnRH independent)
Estrogen- or testosterone-producing tumors:
   Adrenal/ovarian carcinoma or adenoma
   Ovarian germ cell tumor: granulosa cell tumor,
      theca cell tumor, Leydig cell tumor
Gonadotropin- or hCG-producing tumors:
   Choriocarcinoma, dysgerminoma, teratoma,
      gonadoblastoma
   Hepatoblastoma, chorioepithelioma
Congenital adrenal hyperplasia:
   21-hydroxylase deficiency, 11-hydroxylase
      deficiency
Exogenous exposure to androgen or estrogen
McCune-Albright syndrome
Ovarian follicular cysts
Primary hypothyroidism
Aromatase excess syndrome
Glucocorticoid resistance

[a]The most common cause of precocious puberty is idiopathic.
CNS = central nervous system; GnRH = gonadotropin-releasing hormone; hCG = human chorionic gonadotropin.
Compiled from Muir, 2006; Nathan, 2005.

TABLE 14-4. Evaluation of Precocious Puberty

For girls presenting with signs of estrogen excess:
   Radiographic bone age
   Serum FSH, LH, estradiol, TSH levels
   Pelvic sonography
   MRI of the CNS with contrast medium

For girls presenting with signs of virilization:
   Radiographic bone age
   Serum FSH, LH, estradiol levels
   Serum DHEAS, testosterone levels
   Serum 17α-hydroxyprogesterone level
   Serum androstenedione level
   Serum 11-deoxycortisol level

A GnRH stimulation test may help differentiate premature thelarche from true central and peripheral precocious puberty.

CNS = central nervous system; DHEAS = dehydroepiandrosterone sulfate; FSH = follicle-stimulating hormone; GnRH = gonadotropin-releasing hormone; LH = luteinizing hormone; MRI = magnetic resonance imaging; TSH = thyroid-stimulating hormone.

GnRH pulsatile release, low levels of pituitary gonadotropins, yet increased serum estrogen concentrations.

Although the originating source is variable, the most common cause is a granulosa cell tumor, accounting for more than 60 percent of cases (Emans, 1998). Other types of ovarian cysts, adrenal disorders, iatrogenic disorders, and primary hypothyroidism are additional causes (see Table 14-3). McCune-Albright syndrome is characterized by polyostotic fibrous dysplasia, irregular café-au-lait spots, and endocrinopathies. Precocious puberty is a frequent finding and results from estrogen production in the ovarian cysts that are common in these girls.

In girls with peripheral precocious puberty, estrogen levels are characteristically elevated, whereas serum levels of LH and FSH are low. Bone age determination shows advanced aging, and GnRH stimulation shows no elevation in serum LH levels.

Treatment of peripheral precocious puberty consists of eliminating the estrogen. For those with exogenous exposure, elimination of the estrogen source, such as hormonal pills or creams, is sufficient. An estrogen-secreting ovarian or adrenal tumor will require surgical excision, and hypothyroidism is treated with thyroid hormone replacement.

Heterosexual Precocious Puberty

Androgen excess with signs of virilization is rare in childhood (Chap. 17, p. 469). Termed *heterosexual precocious puberty*, this condition is most commonly caused by increased androgen secretion from the adrenal gland or ovary. Causes include androgen-secreting ovarian or adrenal tumors, congenital adrenal hyperplasia, Cushing syndrome, and exposure to exogenous androgens. Treatment is directed at correction of the underlying etiology.

Variations of Normal Puberty

Although standardized age guidelines accurately reflect the timing of pubertal development in most girls, others begin development early. Premature thelarche, premature adrenarche, and premature menarche describe the premature pubertal development of breast tissue, pubic hair, and menses, respectively. Each develops in isolation and without other evidence of pubertal development.

As described earlier (p. 391), *premature thelarche* is a diagnosis of exclusion, and evaluation for precocious puberty in these girls reveals bone ages consistent with chronologic age. Normal FSH and LH levels, normal or slightly elevated estradiol levels, normal pelvic sonographic examination, and normal growth are noted. Treatment consists of careful surveillance and reassurance that the remainder of pubertal development will progress at a normal age. *Adrenarche* is the onset of dehydroepiandrosterone (DHEA) and DHEA sulfate (DHEAS) production from the adrenal zona reticularis, which can be detected at around 6 years. The phenotypic result of adrenarche is the development of axillary and pubic hair, termed *pubarche,* which begins in girls at approximately age 8 years (Auchus, 2004). *Premature adrenarche* is defined therefore as the growth of pubic hair prior to age 8, but other signs of estrogenization or virilization are absent. Most girls will have an increased level of DHEAS, which suggests that the adrenal gland is maturing prematurely (Korth-Schultz, 1976). Some girls with premature adrenarche are found to develop polycystic ovarian syndrome in adolescence (Ibanez, 1993; Miller, 1996). Others are found to have a partial deficiency of 21 hydroxylase. Therefore, girls with premature adrenarche should be screened for precocious puberty. Treatment of premature adrenarche includes reassurance and monitoring at 3- to 6-month intervals for other signs of puberty.

Uterine bleeding that occurs once for several days or monthly, without other signs of puberty is termed *premature menarche.* This condition is rare, and other sources of bleeding should be considered and excluded first.

Delayed Puberty

Puberty is considered delayed if no secondary sexual characteristics are noted by age 13, which is more than two standard deviations from the mean age, or if menses have not commenced by age 16 (Table 14-5). Delayed puberty affects 3 percent of adolescents. Causes include chronic anovulation, constitutional delay, anatomic abnormalities, hypergonadotropic hypogonadism, and hypogonadotropic hypogonadism. With the exception of constitutional delay, these other abnormalities are discussed in greater detail in Chapters 16 and 18.

Constitutional delay is the most common, and these adolescents have a lack of both secondary sexual characteristics and pubertal growth spurt by age 13 years (Albanese, 1995; Ghali, 1994; Malasanoa, 1997). The probable cause is a delay in reactivation of the GnRH pulse generator (Layman, 1994). Patients may be started on low-dose estrogen until puberty progresses, at which point estrogen may be discontinued. During low-dose estrogen treatment, it is not necessary to introduce progesterone withdrawal because in early puberty there is a similar long period of unopposed estrogen prior to ovulatory cycles.

Sexuality
Gender Identity

Many couples choose to learn the gender of their baby before delivery, whereas others choose to wait until the birth. Typically, girls are "raised as girls" and boys, "raised as boys." Gender-appropriate clothes and behaviors, as determined by the local community, are adopted by the child and reinforced by parental approval. Behaviors in conflict with gender are generally discouraged. However, young children will often explore various behaviors, both masculine and feminine, which comprise the variety of normal experiences in the process of sex-role socialization (Maccoby, 1974; Mischel, 1970; Serbin, 1980).

TABLE 14-5. Causes of Delayed Puberty

Constitutional (physiologic delay)[a]
Chronic anovulation (polycystic ovarian syndrome)
Anatomic
   Imperforate hymen
   Transverse vaginal septum
   Vaginal and/or cervical agenesis
   Müllerian agenesis
Androgen insensitivity syndrome (testicular feminization)
Hypergonadotropic hypogonadism
   Gonadal dysgenesis (Turner syndrome)
   Pure gonadal dysgenesis (46,XX or 46,XY)
   Premature ovarian failure
      Idiopathic
      Resistant ovary syndrome
      Autoimmune oophoritis
      Chemotherapy
      Radiation
      17α-Hydroxylase deficiency
      Aromatase deficiency
      Galactosemia
Hypogonadotropic hypogonadism
   Central nervous system etiologies
      Tumors (i.e., craniopharyngioma)
      Infection
      Trauma
      Chronic disease (i.e., celiac disease or Crohn disease)
      GnRH deficiency (Kallman syndrome)
      Isolated gonadotropin deficiency
      Hypothyroidism
      Hyperprolactinoma
   Adrenal
      Congenital adrenal hyperplasia
      Cushing syndrome
      Addison disease
   Psychosocial
      Eating disorders
      Excessive exercise
      Stress, depression

[a]The most common cause of delayed puberty is constitutional delay. GnRH = gonadotropin-releasing hormone.

The task of determining sexual assignment becomes more challenging in cases of ambiguous genitalia in the newborn. Initially, the possibility of life-threatening disease such as congenital adrenal hyperplasia should be investigated. As described in Chapter 18, gender assignment may be difficult and best delayed until test results identify genetic gender and the underlying problem.

The final gender assignment in such cases is termed the *sex of rearing* and reflects the pattern of gender behavior to be emphasized. The final determination for the sex of rearing is based not only on the individual's karyotype but also on the functional capacity of the external genitalia. For example,

SECTION 1

TABLE 14-6. Percentages of Sexually Active Adolescents in the United States According to School Grade

Grade	Ever Had Intercourse	Currently Active	≥4 Lifetime Partners
9	29.3	21.6	6.3
10	39.6	29.3	7.6
11	52.5	41.5	12.9
12	65.0	53.1	19.1

Summarized from Eaton, 2010.

boys born with congenital absence of the penis, a rare disorder, are usually raised as females after bilateral orchidectomy and reconstruction of the scrotum to have the appearance of labia. If parental attitudes towards the assigned gender are consistent, most children assume the sex of rearing regardless of their genotype.

Adolescent Perceptions of Sexual Activity

Adolescent sexuality develops during a period of rapid change that provides opportunities for adolescents to experience both risk-taking and health-promoting behaviors. Data from two large surveys of U.S. adolescents reveal that the percentage of those who become sexually active increases steadily after age 13 (Table 14-6) (Abma, 2010; Eaton, 2010).

Research suggests that adolescents view health care providers as an important resource for information and education regarding healthy sexual development. However, many parents and educators oppose sexuality education because of concerns that providing such information will encourage the onset of intercourse, termed *coitarche*, and will increase the frequency of intercourse. On the contrary, several studies have found that such education will actually delay the onset and frequency of sexual activity, increase contraceptive use, and reduce the rate of unprotected intercourse (Kirby, 1999, 2001). A national survey in 1999 noted that 75 percent of adolescents attending grades 7 through 12 in public secondary schools reported that they received classes in sexuality education (Hoff, 2000). A large percentage wanted more information on specific topics such as contraception, sexually transmitted diseases (STDs), condom use, and emotional issues.

Oral sex is now a more commonplace practice among adolescents. The National Survey of Family Growth in 2005 reported that one in four adolescents aged 15 to 19 years who had not had sexual intercourse reported practicing oral sex with an opposite partner. Of those adolescents who practiced sexual intercourse, 83 percent of females and 88 percent of males stated they had engaged in oral sex (Mosher, 2005). Adolescents may see oral sex as an alternative way to maintain their "technical virginity," prevent pregnancy, or avoid STDs, or they may perceive it as a step on the way to engaging in sexual intercourse with a dating partner.

Sexual activity and partner violence appear to have a frequent association in adolescent populations (Chap. 13, p. 374). For example, Kaestle and Halpern (2005) noted that violent victimization was more likely to occur in romantic relationships that included sexual intercourse (37 percent) compared with those that did not (19 percent). Abma and colleagues (2010) reported that among females with coitarche before age 20, 7 percent described their first intercourse as nonvoluntary.

Contraception

Despite the availability of a wide range of contraceptive options, nearly one half of pregnancies in the United States are unintended (Finer, 2006). Of adolescents, more than 20 percent do not use contraception at first intercourse, and there is a median delay of 22 months before seeking prescription methods after the sexual debut (Finer, 1998).

Recent trends in contraceptive technology include effective methods that enhance patient compliance. Discussed in Chapter 5, these new methods include the contraceptive patch, vaginal ring, levonorgestrel-releasing intrauterine system, extended-use oral contraceptive pills, and subdermal etonogestrel-releasing implant. The most commonly used contraceptive by adolescents is the combination oral contraceptive (COC) pill. Data from the National Survey on Family Growth for 2006 to 2008 revealed that of females using birth control, 30 percent used COC pills; 10 percent used other hormonal methods; and 54 percent used condoms solely or as part of a dual method (Abma, 2010). Intrauterine devices, both copper- and progestin-containing, are available options for adolescents who meet IUD criteria (American College of Obstetricians and Gynecologists, 2007, 2009). The levonorgestrel-releasing intrauterine system (LNG-IUS) (Mirena) is worldwide becoming an accepted, safe contraceptive choice of nulliparas, including adolescents (Yen, 2010). One study of 179 adolescents found an 85-percent continuation rate after 1 year with the LNG-IUS (Paterson, 2009).

The role of the clinician caring for sexually active adolescents is twofold—prevention of unintended pregnancy and protection against sexually transmitted diseases. Ideally, counseling should begin prior to the onset of sexual activity. This discussion should also include education on the use of emergency contraception.

Adolescents commonly express concerns about contraceptive services, and these include necessity of a concurrent pelvic examination, short- and long-term contraceptive side effects, and confidentiality. Adolescents should be informed that a pelvic examination is not necessary when a contraceptive is prescribed. Many adolescents have misperceptions about contraception, including beliefs that it may cause infertility or birth defects, and such concerns may be important topics during contraceptive counseling (Clark, 2001).

According to guidelines from the American College of Obstetricians and Gynecologist (2009), Pap smear screening should not begin until age 21 regardless of sexual activity. HIV-positive status is an exception, and full guideline recommendations are described in Chapter 29 (p. 742). Sexually active adolescents should be counseled and screened for gonorrhea and chlamydial infection (U.S. Preventive Services Task Force, 2005, 2007). For these, as described in Chapter 3, simple vaginal swabs are accurate if specific nucleic acid amplification tests (NAATs) are used. Also, urine samples for NAATs are acceptable, although not the preferred sample (Association of Public Health Laboratories, 2009). Other STDs should be screened as clinically indicated.

Information on HPV vaccination can also be offered. Two HPV vaccines, Cervarix (GlaxoSmithKline) and Gardasil (Merck), are approved by the Food and Drug Administration for females aged 9 through 26 years. The Centers for Disease Control and Prevention (2009) recommend a series of three doses for girls, beginning with a first injection at age 11 or 12 years. A second dose is administered 1 to 2 months later, and a third dose is given 6 months after the initial one. These vaccines are discussed further in Chapter 29 (p. 737).

For these types of services, the Supreme Court has ruled that minors have the right to the availability of contraceptives (*Carry v. Population Services International*, 431 U.S. 678 1977). Moreover, current law dictates that all states provide consent to adolescents for treatment of "medically emancipated" conditions such as contraception, STDs, pregnancy, substance abuse, and mental health. These are legally designated medical situations for which an adolescent may receive care without the permission or knowledge of a parent or legal guardian (Akinbami, 2003).

REFERENCES

Abma JC, Martinez GM, Copen CE: Teenagers in the United States: Sexual activity, contraceptive use, and childbearing, National Survey of Family Growth 2006-2008. National Center for Health Statistics. Vital Health Stat 23:30, 2010

Akinbami LJ, Gandhi H, Cheng TL: Availability of adolescent health services and confidentiality in primary care practices. Pediatrics 111:394, 2003

Aksglaede L, Sørensen K, Petersen JH, et al: Recent decline in age at breast development: the Copenhagen Puberty Study. Pediatrics 123(5):e932, 2009

Albanese A, Stanhope R: Investigation of delayed puberty. Clin Endocrinol 43:105, 1995

American College of Obstetricians and Gynecologists: Increasing use of contraceptive implants and intrauterine devices to reduce unintended pregnancy. Committee Opinion No. 450, December 2009

American College of Obstetricians and Gynecologists: Intrauterine device and adolescents. Committee Opinion No. 392, December 2007

Association of Public Health Laboratories: Laboratory diagnostic testing for *Chlamydia trachomatis* and *Neisseria gonorrhoeae*. Expert Consultation Meeting Summary Report. Atlanta, GA, 2009

Auchus RJ, Rainey WE: Adrenarche—physiology, biochemistry and human disease. Clin Endocrinol 60(3):288, 2004

Aughsteen AA, Almasad JK, Al-Muhtaseb MH: Fibroadenoma of the supernumerary breast of the axilla. Saudi Med J 21:587, 2000

Bagolan P, Giorlandino C, Nahom A, et al: The management of fetal ovarian cysts. J Pediatr Surg 37:25, 2002

Baldwin DD, Landa HM: Common problems in pediatric gynecology. Urol Clin North Am 22:161, 1995

Berenson AB, Heger AH, Hayes JM, et al: Appearance of the hymen in prepubertal girls. Pediatrics 89:3878, 1992

Berkowitz CD, Elvik SL, Logan MK: Labial fusion in prepubescent girls: a marker for sexual abuse? Am J Obstet Gynecol 156(1):16, 1987

Berth-Jones J, Graham-Brown RA, Burns DA: Lichen sclerosus et atrophicus—a review of 15 cases in young girls. Clin Exp Dermatol 16(1):14, 1991

Biro FM, Huang B, Crawford PB, et al: Pubertal correlates in black and white girls. J Pediatr 148(2):234, 2006

Bogaerts J, Lepage P, De Clercq A, et al: *Shigella* and gonococcal vulvovaginitis in prepubertal central African girls. Pediatr Infect Dis J 11:890, 1992

Brandt ML, Luks FI, Filiatrault D, et al: Surgical indications in antenatally diagnosed ovarian cysts. J Pediatr Surg 26:276, 1991

Breen JL, Bonamo JF, Maxson WS: Genital tract tumors in children. Pediatr Clin North Am 28:355, 1981

Breen JL, Maxson WS: Ovarian tumors in children and adolescents. Clin Obstet Gynecol 20:607, 1977

Bridges NA, Christopher JA, Hindmarsh PC, et al: Sexual precocity: sex incidence and aetiology. Arch Dis Child 70:116, 1994

Bryant AE, Laufer MR: Fetal ovarian cysts: incidence, diagnosis and management. J Reprod Med 49:329, 2004

Carel JC, Eugster EA, Rogol A, et al: Consensus statement on the use of gonadotropin-releasing hormone analogs in children. Pediatrics 123:e752, 2009

Centers for Disease Control and Prevention: Vaccines and preventable diseases: HPV vaccine—questions and answers. 2009. Available at: http://ww.cdc.gov/vaccines/vpd-vac/hpv/vac-faqs.htm. Accessed June 27, 2010

Christensen EH, Oster J: Adhesions of labia minora (synechia vulvae) in childhood: a review and report of fourteen cases. Acta Paediatr Scand 60:709, 1971

Clark LR: Will the pill make me sterile? Addressing reproductive health concerns and strategies to improve adherence to hormonal contraceptive regimens in adolescent girls. J Pediatr Adolesc Gynecol 4(4):151, 2001

Cohen HL, Shapiro M, Mandel F, et al: Normal ovaries in neonates and infants: a sonographic study of 77 patients 1 day to 24 months old. AJR Am J Roentgenol 160:583, 1993

Daniel WA Jr, Mathews MD: Tumors of the breast in adolescent females. Pediatrics 41:743, 1968

DeLuca-Pytell DM, Piazza RC, Holding JC, et al. The incidence of tuberous breast deformity in asymmetric and symmetric mammoplasty patients. Plast Reconstruct Surg 116(7):1894, 2005

Eaton DK, Kann L, Kinchen S, et al: Youth risk behavior surveillance—United States, 2009. MMWR Surveill Summ 59(5):1, 2010

Emans S, Laufer M, Goldstein D: Pediatric and Adolescent Gynecology, 5th ed. Philadelphia: Lippincott Williams & Wilkins, 2005, pp 127, 159

Escobar ME, Rivarola MA, Bergada C: Plasma concentration of oestradiol-17beta in premature thelarche and in different types of sexual precocity. Acta Endocrinol 81:351, 1976

Euling SY, Herman-Giddens ME, Lee PA, et al: Examination of U.S. puberty-timing data from 1940 to 1994 for secular trends: panel findings. Pediatrics 121:S172, 2008

Faden H: Mastitis in children from birth to 17 years. Pediatr Infect Dis J 24(12):1113, 2005

Finer LB, Henshaw SK: Disparities in rates of unintended pregnancy in the United States, 1994 and 2001. Perspect Sex Reprod Health 38(2):90, 2006

Finer LB, Zabin LS: Does the timing of the first family planning visit still matter? Fam Plann Perspect 30(1):30, 1998

Garcia CJ, Espinoza A, Dinamarca V, et al: Breast US in children and adolescents. Radiographics 20:1605, 2000

Garel L, Dubois J, Grignon A, et al: US of the pediatric female pelvis: a clinical perspective. Radiographics 21(6):1393, 2001

Ghali K, Rosenfield RL: Disorders of pubertal development: too early, too much, too late, or too little. Adolesc Med 5:19, 1994

Goldstein DP, Miler V: Breast masses in adolescent females. Clin Pediatr 21:17, 1982

Goyal A, Mansel RE: Iatrogenic injury to the breast bud causing breast hypoplasia. Postgrad Med J 79(930):235, 2003

Grolleau JL, Lanfrey E, Lavigne B, et al: Breast base anomalies: treatment strategy for tuberous breasts, minor deformities, and asymmetry. Plast Reconstruct Surg 104(7):2040, 1999

Gutierrez JC, Housri N, Koniaris LG et al: Malignant breast cancer in children: a review of 75 patients. J Surg Res 147(2):182, 2008

Han B, Herndon CN, Rosen MP, et al: Uterine didelphys associated with obstructed hemivagina and ipsilateral renal anomaly (OHVIRA) syndrome. Radiology Case Reports [Online] 5:327, 2010

Herman-Giddens ME, Slora EJ, Wasserman RC, et al: Secondary sexual characteristics and menses in young girls seen in office practice: a study from the Pediatric Research in Office Settings network. Pediatrics 99:505, 1997

Hoff T, Greene L, McIntosh M, et al: Sex Education in America: a View from Inside the Nation's Classrooms. Menlo Park CA: Henry J. Kaiser Family Foundation, 2000

Ibanez L, Potau N, Virdis R, et al: Postpubertal outcome in girls diagnosed of premature pubarche during childhood: increased frequency of functional ovarian hyperandrogenism. J Clin Endocrinol Metab 76:1599, 1993

Ilicki A, Prager LR, Kauli R, et al: Premature thelarche—natural history and sex hormone secretion in 68 girls. Acta Paediatr Scand 73:756, 1984

Jansen DA, Spencer SR, Leveque JE: Premenarchal athletic injury to the breast bud as the cause for asymmetry: prevention and treatment. Breast J 8:108, 2002

Jenkinson SD, MacKinnon AE: Spontaneous separation of fused labia minora in prepubertal girls. Br Med J (Clin Res Ed) 289:160, 1984

Kaestle CE, Halpern CT: Sexual intercourse precedes partner violence in adolescent romantic relationships. J Adolesc Health 36(5):386, 2005

Kaplowitz PB, Oberfield SE: Reexamination of the age limit for defining when puberty is precocious in girls in the United States. Implications for evaluation and treatment. Drug and Therapeutics and Executive Committees of the Lawson Wilkins Pediatric Endocrine Society. Pediatrics 104:936, 1999

Kirby D: Emerging answers: research findings on programs to reduce teenage pregnancy. The National Campaign to Prevent Teen Pregnancy, Washington, DC, 2001

Kirby D: Reducing adolescent pregnancy: approaches that work. Contemp Pediatr 16:83, 1999

Klein KO, Mericq V, Brown-Dawson JM, et al: Estrogen levels in girls with premature thelarche compared with normal prepubertal girls as determined by an ultrasensitive recombinant cell bioassay. J Pediatr 134:190, 1999

Korth-Schultz S, Levine LS, New M: Dehydroepiandrosterone sulfate (DS) levels, a rapid test for abnormal adrenal androgen secretion. J Clin Endocrinol Metab 42:1005, 1976

Layman LC, Reindollar RH: Diagnosis and treatment of pubertal disorders. Adolesc Med 5:37, 1994

Lindeque BG, du Toit JP, Muller LM, et al: Ultrasonographic criteria for the conservative management of antenatally diagnosed fetal ovarian cysts. J Reprod Med 33:196, 1988

Maccoby EE, Jacklin CN: The Psychology of Sex Differences. Stanford, CA: Stanford University Press, 1974

Malasanoa TH: Sexual development of the fetus and pubertal child. Clin Obstet Gynecol 40:153, 1997

Marshall WA, Tanner JM: Variations in pattern of pubertal changes in girls. Arch Dis Child 44(235):291, 1969

Mayoglou L, Dulabon L, Martin-Alguacil N, et al: Success of treatment modalities for labial fusion: a retrospective evaluation of topical and surgical treatments. J Pediatr Adolesc Gynecol 22(4):247, 2009

Meyers JB, Sorenson CM, Wisner BP, et al: Betamethasone cream for the treatment of pre-pubertal labial adhesions. J Pediatr Adolesc Gynecol 19(6):401, 2006

Meyrick Thomas RH, Kennedy CT: The development of lichen sclerosus et atrophicus in monozygotic twin girls. Br J Dermatol 114:337, 1986

Miller DP, Emans SJ, Kohane I: A follow-up study of adolescent girls with a history of premature pubarche. J Adolesc Health 18(4):301, 1996

Mischel W: Sex-typing and socialization. In Mussen PH (ed): Carmichaels Manual of Child Psychology, 3rd ed., Vol 11. New York, Wiley, 1970, pp 3-72

Mosher WD, Chandra A, Jones J: Sexual behavior and selected health measures: men and women 15-44 years of age, United States, 2002. Adv Data, 362:1, 2005

Muir A: Precocious puberty. Pediatr Rev 27:373, 2006

Murray S, London S: Management of ovarian cysts in neonates, children, and adolescents. Adolesc Pediatr Gynecol 8:64, 1995

Nathan BM, Palmert MR: Regulation and disorders of pubertal timing. Endocrinol Metab Clin North Am 34(3):617, 2005

Neely EK, Hintz RL, Wilson DM, et al: Normal ranges for immuno- chemiluminometric gonadotropin assays. J Pediatr 124(1):40, 1995

Neinstein LA: Review of breast masses in adolescents. Adolesc Pediatr Gynecol 7:119, 1994

Nelson KG: Premature thelarche in children born prematurely. J Pediatr 103:756, 1983

North American Society for Pediatric and Adolescent Gynecology: The PediGYN teaching slide set. Philadelphia, 2001, slides 31, 84

Nussbaum A, Sanders R, Jones M: Neonatal uterine morphology as seen on real-time US. Radiology 160:641, 1986

Nussbaum AR, Sanders RC, Hartman DS, et al: Neonatal ovarian cysts: sonographic-pathologic correlation. Radiology 168:817, 1988

Oshida K, Miyauchi M, Yamamoto N, et al: Phyllodes tumor arising in ectopic breast tissue of the axilla. Breast Cancer 10:82, 2003

Panteli C, Curry J, Kiely E, et al: Ovarian germ cell tumours: a 17-year study in a single unit. Eur J Pediatr Surg 19(2):96, 2009

Partsch CJ, Heger S, Sippell WG: Management and outcome of central precocious puberty. Clin Endocrinol 56(2):129, 2003

Paterson H, Ashton J, Harrison-Woolrych M: A nationwide cohort study of the use of the levonorgestrel intrauterine device in New Zealand adolescents. Contraception 79(6):433, 2009

Pierce AM, Hart CA: Vulvovaginitis: causes and management. Arch Dis Child 67:509, 1992

Piippo S, Lenko H, Vuento R: Vulvar symptoms in paediatric and adolescent patients. Acta Paediatr 89:431, 2000

Pokorny S: Pediatric & adolescent gynecology. Compr Ther 23:337, 1997

Powell J, Wojnarowska F: Childhood vulvar lichen sclerosus. The course after puberty. J Reprod Med 47(9):706, 2002

Ratani RS, Cohen HL, Fiore E: Pediatric gynecologic ultrasound. Ultrasound Q 20:127, 2004

Reddy J, Schantz-Dunn J, Laufer MR: Obstructed hemivagina, uterine didelphys and ipsilateral renal anomaly (OHVIRA) syndrome: an unusual presentation. J Pediatr Adolesc Gynecol 22(2):e52, 2009

Resende EA, Lara BH, Reis JD, et al: Assessment of basal and gonadotropin-releasing hormone-stimulated gonadotropins by immunochemiluminometric and immunofluorometric assays in normal children. J Clin Endocrinol Metab 92(4):1424, 2007

Ronnekliev OK, Resko JA: Ontogeny of gonadotropin-releasing hormone-containing neurons in early fetal development of the rhesus macaques. Endocrinology 126:498, 1990

Rosenfield RL, Lipton RB, Drum ML: Thelarche, pubarche, and menarche attainment in children with normal and elevated body mass index. Pediatrics 123:84, 2009

Salkala E, Leon Z, Rouse G: Management of antenatally diagnosed fetal ovarian cysts. Obstet Gynecol Surv 46:407, 1991

Sathasivam A, Garibaldi L, Shapiro S, et al: Leuprolide stimulation testing for the evaluation of early female sexual maturation. Clin Endocrinol (Oxf) 73(3):375, 2010

Schultz KA, Ness KK, Nagarajan R, et al: Adnexal masses in infancy and childhood. Clin Obstet Gynecol 49(3):464, 2006

Schwanzel-Fukuda M, Pfaff DW: Origin of luteinizing hormone-releasing hormone neurons. Nature 338:161, 1989

Serbin LA: Sex-role socialization: a field in transition. In Lahey BB, Kazdin AE (eds): Advances in Clinical Child Psychology, Vol 3. New York, Plenum, 1980, p 41

Sherman V, McPherson T, Baldo M, et al: The high rate of familial lichen sclerosus suggests a genetic contribution: an observational cohort study. J Eur Acad Dermatol Venereol 24(9):1031, 2010

Silverman A-J, Jhamandas J, Renaud LP: Localization of luteinizing hormone-releasing hormone (LHRH) neurons that project to the median eminence. J Neurosci 7:2312, 1987

Smith NA, Laufer MR: Obstructed hemivagina and ipsilateral renal anomaly (OHVIRA) syndrome: management and follow-up. Fertil Steril 87(4):918, 2007

Smith SD, Fischer G: Childhood onset vulvar lichen sclerosus does not resolve at puberty: a prospective case series. Pediatr Dermatol 26(6):725, 2009

Spence JEH, Domingo M, Pike C: The resolution of fetal and neonatal ovarian cysts. Adolesc Pediatr Gynecol 5:27, 1992

Speroff L, Fritz M: Clinical gynecologic endocrinology and infertility, 7th ed. Baltimore, Lippincott Williams & Wilkins, 2005, p 362

Stricker T, Navratil F, Forster I, et al: Nonpuerperal mastitis in adolescents. J Pediatr 148(2):278, 2006

Tanner JM: Trend toward earlier menarche in Long, Oslo, Copenhagen, the Netherlands and Hungary. Nature 243:95, 1973

Tanner JM, Davies PWS: Clinical longitudinal standards for height and height velocity for North American children. J Pediatr 107:317, 1985

Tapper D, Lack EE: Teratomas in infancy and childhood. A 54-year experience at the Children's Hospital Medical Center. Ann Surg 198(6):398, 1983

Templeman C, Hertweck SP: Breast disorders in the pediatric and adolescent patient. Obstet Gynecol Clin North Am 27(1):19, 2000

Thind CR, Carty HM, Pilling DW: The role of ultrasound in the management of ovarian masses in children. Clin Radiol 40:180, 1989

Tweeten SS, Rickman LS: Infectious complications of body piercing. Clin Infect Dis 26(3):735, 1998

U.S. Preventive Services Task Force: Screening for chlamydial infection. 2007. Available at: http://www.ahrq.gov/clinic/uspst/uspschlm.htm. Accessed June 8, 2010

U.S. Preventive Services Task Force: Screening for gonorrhea. 2005. Available at: http://www.ahrq.gov/clinic/uspst/uspsgono.htm. Accessed June 8, 2010

Vaskivuo TE, Anttonen M, Herva R, et al: Survival of human ovarian follicles from fetal to adult life: apoptosis, apoptosis-related proteins, and transcription factor GATA-4. J Clin Endocrinol Metab 86:3421, 2001

Weinstein SP, Conant EF: Eleven-year-old with breast mass. Pediatr Case Rev 3(2):91, 2003

Williams SM, Kaplan PA, Peterson JC, et al: Mammography in women under age 30: is there clinical benefit? Radiology 161:49, 1986

Wolff K, Johnson RA, Suurmond D: Cutaneous fungal infections. In Fitzpatrick's Color Atlas & Synopsis of Clinical Dermatology, 5th ed. Online. New York, McGraw-Hill. Available at: http://www.accessmedicine.com/content.aspx?aID=757192&searchStr=diaper+rash#757192. Accessed January 20, 2007

Yen S, Saah T, Adams Hillard PJ: IUDs and adolescents—an under-utilized opportunity for pregnancy prevention. J Pediatr Adolesc Gynecol 23(3):123, 2010

Zeiguer NJ, Muchinik GR, Geulfand L, et al: Vulvovaginitis in Argentinian children: evaluation of determinant pathogens. J Pediatr Adolesc Gynecol 6:25, 1993

Ziereisen F, Guissard G, Damry N, et al: Sonographic imaging of the paediatric female pelvis. Eur Radiol 15:1296, 2005

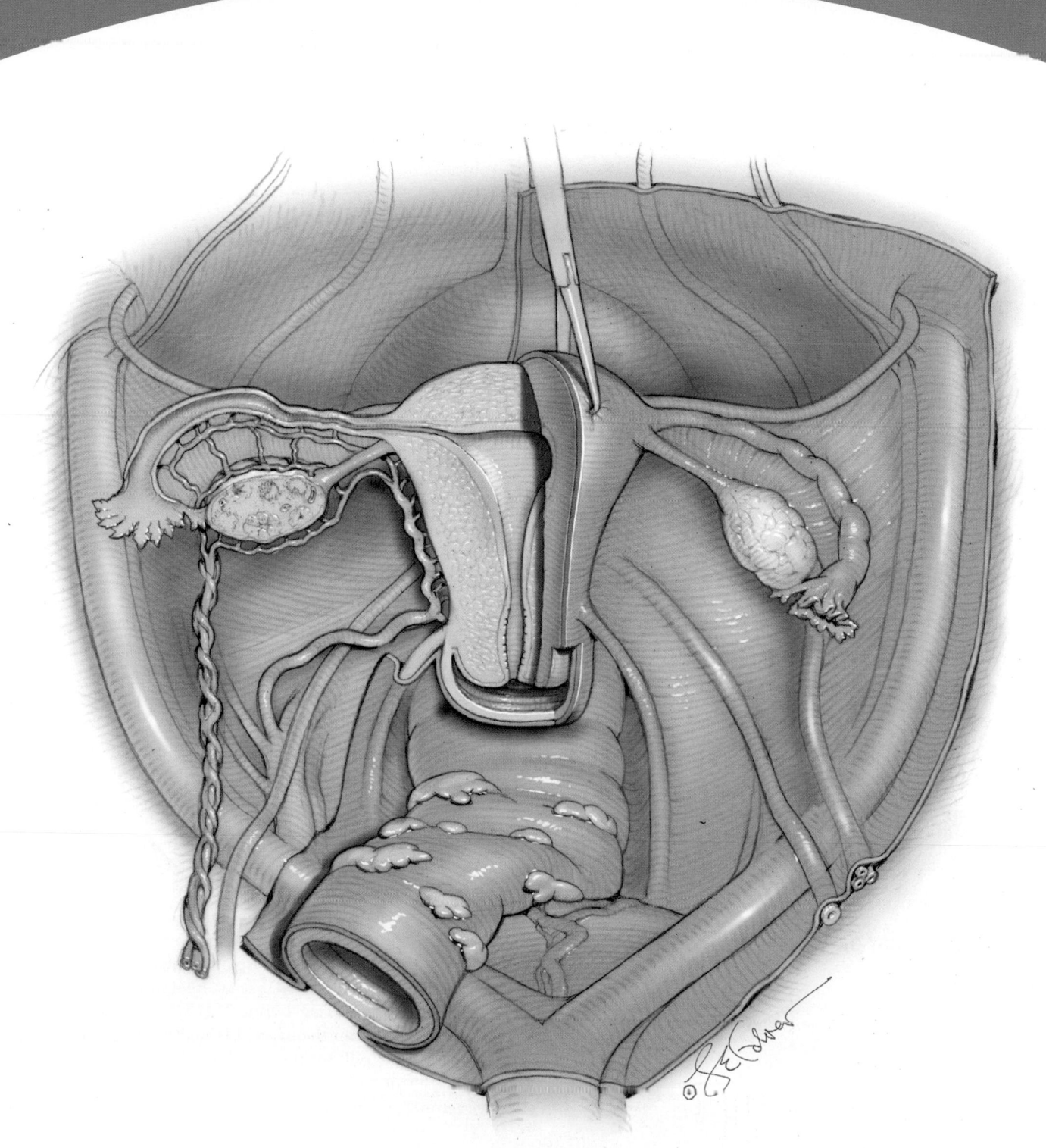

Reproductive Endocrinology

Reproductive endocrinology is the study of hormones and neuroendocrine factors that are produced by and/or affect reproductive tissues. These tissues include the hypothalamus, anterior pituitary gland, ovary, endometrium, and placenta. A hormone is classically described as a cell product that is secreted into the peripheral circulation and that exerts its effects in distant target tissues (Fig. 15-1). This is termed *endocrine secretion*. Additional forms of cell-to-cell communication exist and are critical for reproductive physiology. *Paracrine* communication, common within the ovary, refers to chemical signaling between neighboring cells. *Autocrine* communication occurs when a cell releases substances that influence its own function. Production of a substance within a cell that affects that cell before secretion is termed an *intracrine* effect.

Neurotransmitters, in classic neural pathways, cross a small extracellular space called a synaptic junction and bind to dendrites of a second neuron (Fig. 15-2). Alternatively, these factors are secreted into the vascular system and are transported to other tissues where they exert their effects in a process termed *neuroendocrine secretion* or *neuroendocrine signaling*. An example of neuroendocrine signaling is gonadotropin-releasing hormone (GnRH) secretion into the portal vasculature with effects on the gonadotropes within the anterior pituitary gland.

In overview, normal reproductive function requires precise quantitative and temporal regulation of the hypothalamic-pituitary-ovarian axis (Fig. 15-3). Within the hypothalamus, specific nuclei release GnRH in pulses. This decapeptide binds to surface receptors on the gonadotrope subpopulation of the anterior pituitary gland. In response, gonadotropes secrete glycoprotein gonadotropins, that is, luteinizing hormone (LH) and follicle-stimulating hormone (FSH), into the peripheral circulation. Within the ovary, LH and FSH bind to the theca and granulosa cells to stimulate folliculogenesis as well as ovarian production of an array of steroid hormones (estrogens, progesterone, and androgens), gonadal peptides (activin, inhibin,

Endocrine action

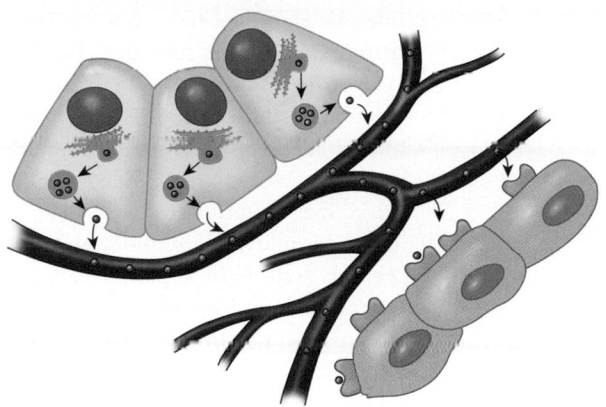

Paracrine action   Autocrine action

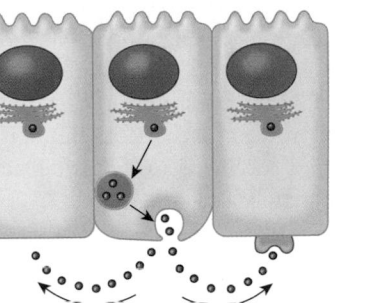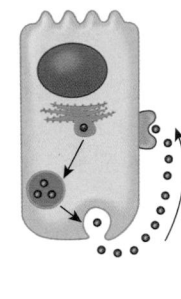

FIGURE 15-1 Drawing depicts different types of hormone communication. Endocrine: hormones travel through the circulation to reach their target cells. Paracrine: hormones diffuse through the extracellular space to reach their target cells, which are neighboring cells. Autocrine: hormones feed back on the cell of origin, without entering the circulation.

Neurotransmitter secretion (e.g, dopamine)

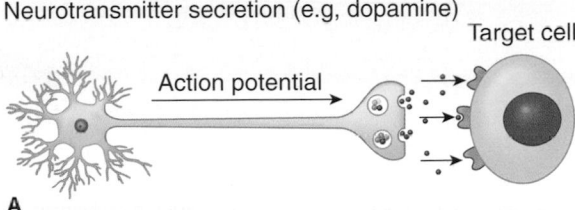

A

Neurohormone secretion (e.g, GnRH)

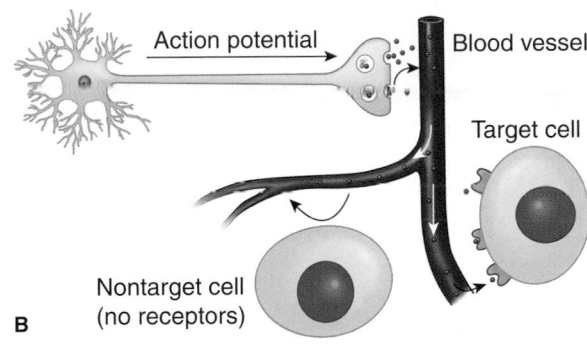

B

FIGURE 15-2 Drawing illustrates types of neurotransmitter secretion. **A.** Classic neurotransmitter release and binding. Transmission of an action potential down a neural axon leads to release of neurotransmitters, which travel across a synaptic cleft to reach their target cell. **B.** Neurohormonal secretion. An action potential leads to release of neurotransmitters. In this instance, neurotransmitters enter into and travel through the circulation to reach their target organ.

and follistatin), and growth factors. Among other functions, these ovarian-derived factors feed back to the hypothalamus and pituitary gland to inhibit, or at the midcycle surge, to augment GnRH and gonadotropin secretion. The ovarian steroids are also critical for preparing the endometrium for implantation of the embryo if pregnancy ensues.

HORMONE BIOSYNTHESIS AND MECHANISM OF ACTION

Hormones can be broadly classified as either steroids or peptides, each with their own mode of biosynthesis and mechanism of action. The receptors for these hormones can be divided into two groups: (1) those present on the cell surface, which in general interact with hormones that are water soluble, namely peptides, and (2) those that are primarily intracellular and interact with lipophilic hormones such as steroids. Hormones are normally present in serum and tissues in very low concentrations. Therefore, receptors must have both high affinity and high specificity for their ligand to produce the correct biologic response.

Peptide Hormones in Reproduction
Luteinizing Hormone, Follicle-Stimulating Hormone, and Human Chorionic Gonadotropin

Structurally, LH and FSH are heterodimers that contain a common α-subunit linked to either an LHβ or FSHβ subunit, respectively. The glycoprotein α-subunit also interacts with the thyroid-stimulating hormone β-subunit to form thyroid-stimulating hormone (TSH) and with the human chorionic gonadotropin β-subunit to form human chorionic gonadotropin (hCG). The similarity of these hormones can have clinical sequelae. For example, molar pregnancies frequently produce very high levels of hCG, which can bind to TSH receptors, producing hyperthyroidism. Importantly, with any of these peptide hormones, only the dimers possess biologic activity. Although the subunits can be found in their unassociated form in the circulation, these "free" subunits are not known to have physiologic significance.

The LH and hCG β-subunits are encoded by two separate genes within a gene grouping called the LH/CG cluster. The amino acid sequence of the human LH and CG β-subunits demonstrates approximately 80-percent similarity, however, the hCG β-subunit contains an additional 24-amino-acid extension on the carboxy terminus. The presence of these additional amino acids has allowed the development of highly specific assays for LH and hCG.

Female Reproductive Axis

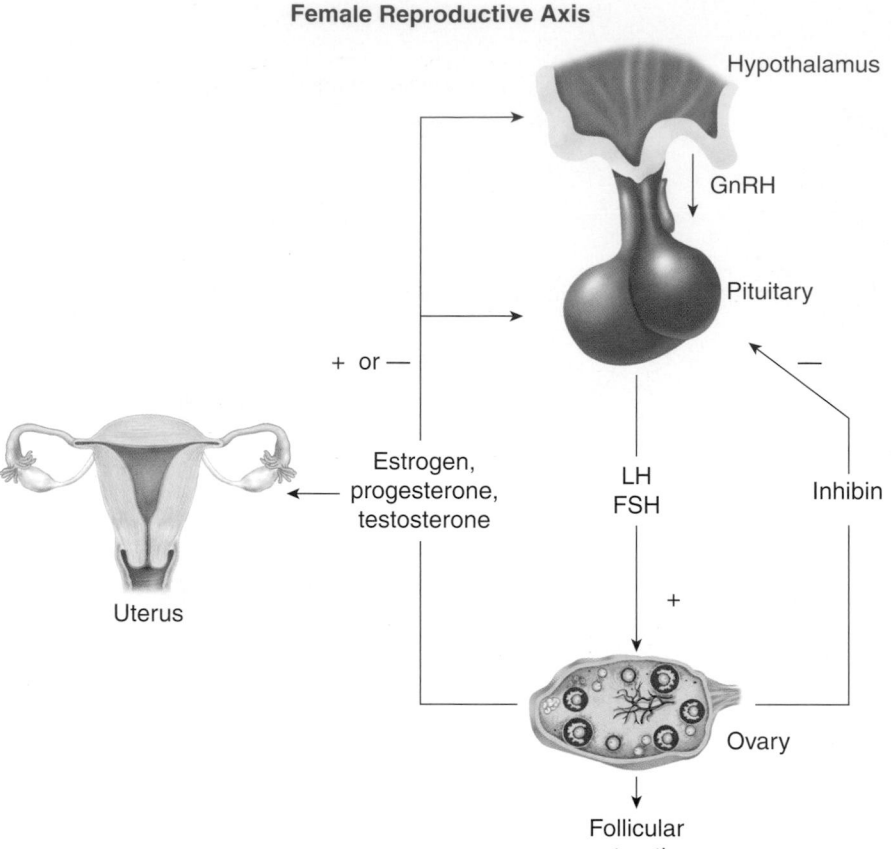

FIGURE 15-3 Diagram depicts positive and negative feedback loops seen with the hypothalamic-pituitary-ovarian axis. Pulsatile release of gonadotropin-releasing hormone (GnRH) leads to release of luteinizing hormone (LH) and follicle-stimulating hormone (FSH) from the anterior pituitary. Effects of LH and FSH result in follicle maturation, ovulation, and production of the sex steroid hormones (estrogen, progesterone, and testosterone). Rising serum levels of these hormones exert negative feedback inhibition on GnRH and gonadotropin release. Sex-steroid hormones vary in their effects on the endometrium and myometrium as discussed in the text. Inhibin, produced in the ovary, has a negative effect on gonadotropin release.

Activin, Inhibin, and Follistatin

Three polypeptide factors—*inhibin*, *activin*, and *follistatin*—were initially isolated from follicular fluid based on their selective effects on FSH biosynthesis and secretion (de Kretser, 2002). As suggested by their names, inhibin decreases and activin stimulates gonadotrope function. Follistatin suppresses FSHβ gene expression, most likely by binding to and thereby preventing the interaction of activin with its receptor (Besecke, 1997). Subsequent studies have indicated that these peptides also affect biosynthesis of LH and the GnRH receptor, although these responses are less robust (Kaiser, 1997).

Inhibin and activin are closely related peptides. Inhibin consists of an α-subunit (unrelated to the LH glycoprotein α-subunit) linked by a disulfide bridge to one of two highly homologous β-subunits to form inhibin A ($\alpha\beta_A$) or inhibin B ($\alpha\beta_B$). Activin is composed of homodimers ($\beta_A\beta_A$, $\beta_B\beta_B$) or heterodimers ($\beta_A\beta_B$) of the same β-subunits as inhibin (Dye, 1992). More recently, a number of additional β-subunit isoforms have been identified. In contrast, follistatin is structurally unrelated to either inhibin or activin.

Although originally isolated from follicular fluid, these "gonadal" peptides are expressed by a wide variety of reproductive tissues in which they provide diverse, tissue-specific functions (Meunier, 1988). The messenger ribonucleic acids (mRNAs) that encode the inhibin/activin subunits, follistatin, and the activin receptor have been detected in the pituitary, ovary, testes, and placenta as well as in the brain, adrenal, liver, kidney, and bone marrow (Kaiser, 1992; Muttukrishna, 2004). Activins have recently been shown to negatively impact female germ cell survival during development and germ cell activation during folliculogenesis (Ding, 2010; Liu, 2010). Of these peptides, inhibin is currently believed to be most critical for the feedback regulation of gonadotropin gene expression. In contrast, activin and follistatin effects on gonadotrope function most likely occur through the action of locally released peptides acting as autocrine/paracrine factors.

Steroid Hormones in Reproduction
Classification

Sex steroids are divided into three groups based on the number of carbon atoms that they contain. Each carbon in this structure is assigned a number identifier, and each ring is assigned a letter (Fig. 15-4). The 21-carbon series includes progestins as well as glucocorticoids and mineralocorticoids. Androgens contain 19 carbons, whereas estrogens have 18.

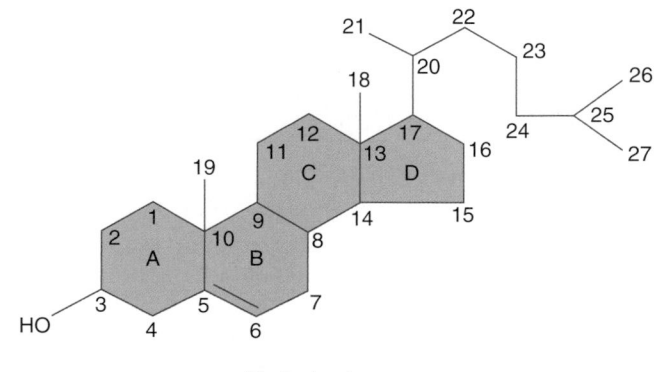

Cholesterol

FIGURE 15-4 Diagram displays the chemical structure of cholesterol, which is the common precursor in sex-steroid biosynthesis. All sex steroids contain the basic cyclopentanephenanthrene molecule, which consists of three 6-carbon rings and one 5-carbon ring.

Steroids are given scientific names according to a generally accepted convention in which functional groups below the plane of the molecule are preceded by the α symbol and those above the plane of the molecule are indicated by a β symbol. A Δ symbol indicates a double bond. Those steroids with a double bond between carbon atoms 5 and 6 are called Δ^5 steroids (pregnenolone, 17-hydroxypregnenolone, and dehydroepiandrosterone), whereas those with a double bond between carbons 4 and 5 are termed Δ^4 steroids (progesterone, 17-hydroxyprogesterone, androstenedione, testosterone, mineralocorticoids, and glucocorticoids).

Steroidogenesis

Sex steroid hormones are synthesized in the gonads, adrenal gland, and placenta. Cholesterol is the primary building block in steroidogenesis, and all steroid-producing tissues, except the placenta, are capable of synthesizing cholesterol from the two-carbon precursor, acetate. Steroid hormone production, which involves at least 17 enzymes, primarily occurs in the abundant smooth endoplasmic reticulum found in steroidogenic cells (Mason, 2002).

Steroidogenic enzymes catalyze four basic modifications of the steroid structure: (1) side-chain cleavage (desmolase reaction), (2) conversion of hydroxyl groups to ketones (dehydrogenase reactions), (3) addition of a hydroxyl group (hydroxylation reaction), and (4) removal or addition of hydrogen to create or reduce a double bond (Table 15-1). The steroid biosynthesis pathway is shown in simplified form in Figure 15-5. This

TABLE 15-1. Steroidogenic Enzymes		
Enzyme	**Cellular Location**	**Reactions**
P450scc	Mitochondria	Cholesterol side chain cleavage
P450c11	Mitochondria	11-Hydroxylase 18-Hydroxylase 19-Methyloxidase
P450c17	Endoplasmic reticulum	17-Hydroxylase 17,20-Lyase
P450c21	Endoplasmic reticulum	21-Hydroxylase
P450arom	Endoplasmic reticulum	Aromatase

pathway is identical in all steroidogenic tissues, but the distribution of products synthesized by each tissue is determined by the presence of requisite enzymes. For example, the ovary is deficient in 21-hydroxylase and 11β-hydroxylase and therefore is unable to produce corticosteroids. Of note, it is becoming increasingly clear that many steroidogenic enzymes exist as multiple isoforms with different precursor preferences and directional activities. As a result, specific steroids may be produced via multiple pathways in addition to the classic pathway shown in Figure 15-5 (Auchus, 2009).

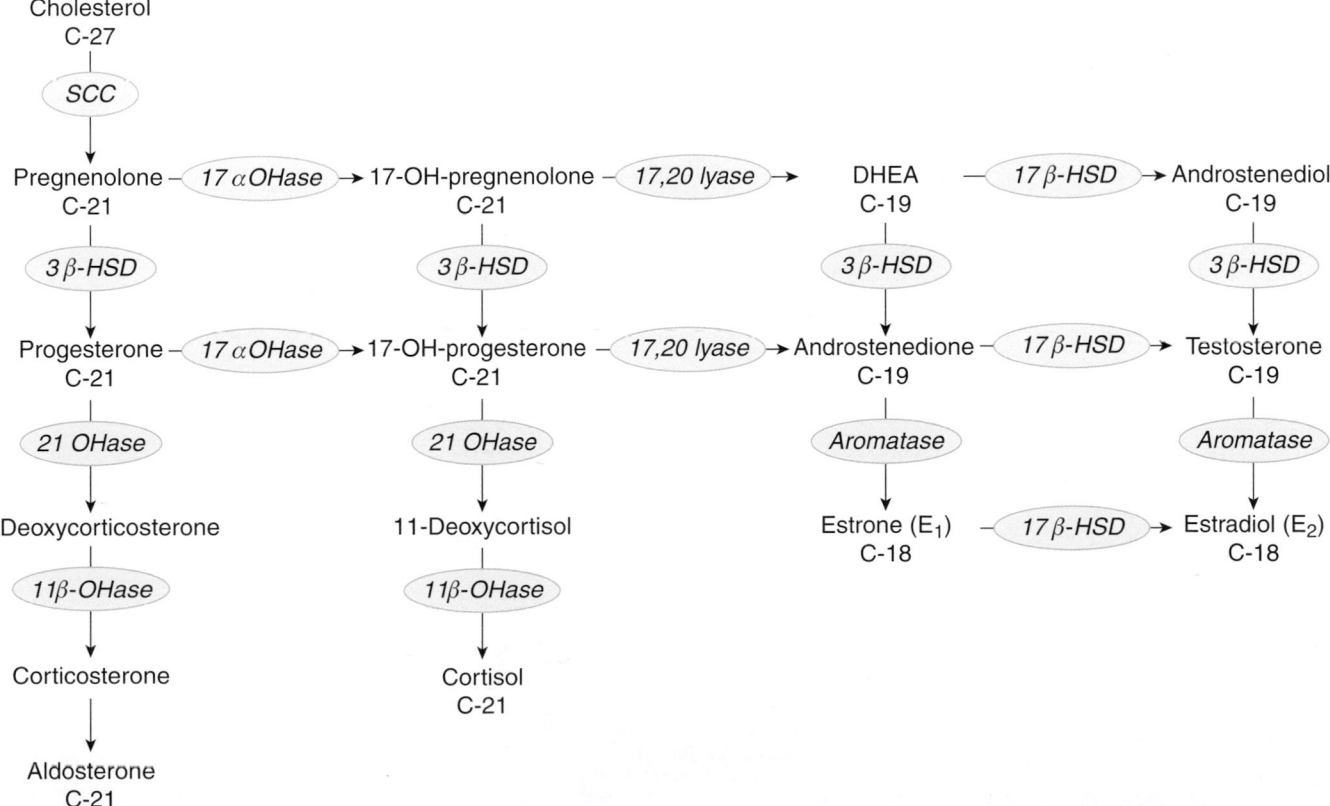

FIGURE 15-5 Diagram depicts steps in the steroidogenesis pathway. Enzymes are found within the blue ovals. The C-18, C-19, or C-21 designation beneath the sex steroid reflects the number of carbon atoms it contains. 3β-HSD = 3β-hydroxysteroid dehydrogenase; 11β-OHase = 11β-hydroxylase; 17αOHase = 17α-hydroxylase; 17β-HSD = 17β-hydroxysteroid dehydrogenase; 21OHase = 21-hydroxylase; DHEA = dehydroepiandrosterone; SCC = side-chain cleavage enzyme.

Steroid Metabolism

Steroids are metabolized mainly in the liver and to a lesser extent in the kidney and intestinal mucosa. Hydroxylation of estradiol results in production of estrone or catechol estrogens. These estrogens are then conjugated to glucuronides or sulfates to form water-soluble compounds for excretion in the urine. Accordingly, administration of certain pharmacologic steroid hormones may be contraindicated in those with active liver or renal disease.

Steroid Synthesis in the Adrenal Gland

The adult fetal gland is composed of three zones. Each of these zones expresses a different complement of steroidogenic enzymes and as a result, synthesizes different products. The zona glomerulosa lacks 17α-hydroxylase activity but contains large amounts of aldosterone synthase (P450aldo) and therefore produces mineralocorticoids. The zona fasciculata and zona reticularis, both of which express the 17α-hydroxylase gene, synthesize glucocorticoids and androgens, respectively.

Derivation of Circulating Estrogens and Androgens in the Female

Circulating estrogens in the reproductive-aged female are a mixture of both estradiol and the less potent estrone. Although a small amount of estriol is produced through peripheral conversion in the nonpregnant female, estriol production is primarily limited to production by the placenta during pregnancy.

Estradiol is the primary estrogen produced by the ovary during reproductive years. Levels are derived both from direct synthesis in developing follicles and through conversion of estrone. Estrone is secreted directly by the ovary and can also be converted from androstenedione in the periphery. Androgens are converted to estrogens in many tissues, but conversion primarily occurs secondary to aromatase activity in the skin and adipose tissue.

Of the androgens, the ovary produces primarily androstenedione and dehydroepiandrosterone (DHEA) with smaller amounts of testosterone. Although the adrenal cortex primarily produces mineralocorticoids and glucocorticoids, it also contributes to approximately one half of the daily production of androstenedione and DHEA and essentially all of the sulfated form of DHEA (DHEAS). Twenty-five percent of circulating testosterone is secreted by the ovary, 25 percent is secreted by the adrenal gland, and the remaining 50 percent is produced by peripheral conversion of androstenedione to testosterone (Fig. 15-6) (Silva, 1987).

Steroid Hormone Transport in the Circulation

Most steroids in the peripheral circulation are bound to carrier proteins, either specific proteins such as sex hormone-binding globulin (SHBG), thyroid-binding globulin, or corticosteroid-binding globulin, or to nonspecific proteins such as albumin. Only 1 to 2 percent of androgens and estrogens are unbound or free.

Only the unbound steroid fraction is believed to be biologically active, although albumin's low affinity for sex steroids may allow steroids bound to this protein to exert some effects. The amount of free hormone is in equilibrium with the amount

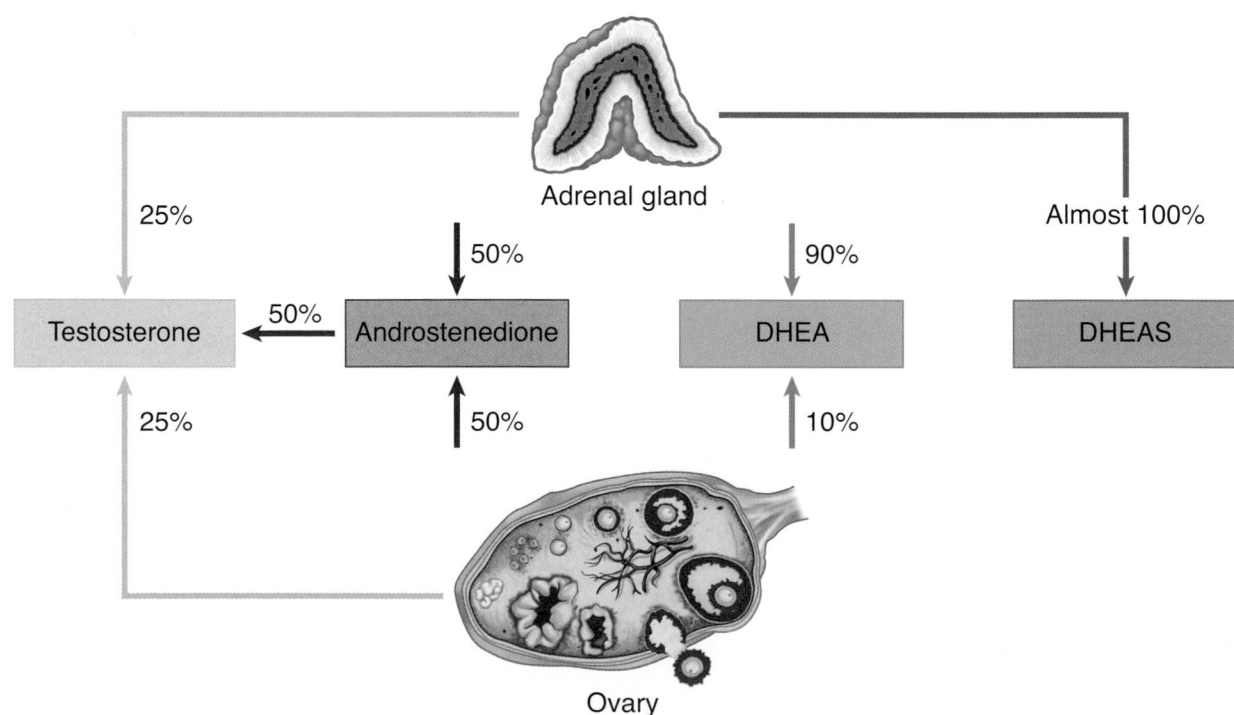

FIGURE 15-6 Diagram depicts the approximate contribution of the adrenal glands and ovaries to levels of androgens, dehydroepiandrosterone (DHEA), and DHEA sulfate (DHEAS).

bound. As a result, small changes in carrier protein expression can produce substantial alterations in steroid effect.

Sex hormone-binding globulin (SHBG) circulates as a homodimer that binds a single steroid molecule. This binding protein is primarily synthesized in the liver, although it has also been detected in other tissues such as the brain, placenta, endometrium, and testes (Hammond, 1989, 1996). SHBG levels are increased by hyperthyroidism, pregnancy, and estrogen administration. In contrast, androgens, progestins, growth hormone (GH), insulin, and corticoids decrease SHBG levels. An increase in weight, particularly central body fat, can significantly blunt SHBG expression and thereby increase free hormone levels.

Note that unbound hormone can be technically difficult to measure and results should be interpreted with caution. Free testosterone levels are the most commonly ordered free steroid hormone tests. The most accurate assays require dialysis of the sample and are performed by a limited number of commercial laboratories. The more available calculated free levels are relatively inaccurate. Unlike thyroid hormone measurements, the measurement of free testosterone is rarely necessary for clinical diagnosis in the female. For example, measurement of testosterone levels in patients with presumed polycystic ovarian syndrome (PCOS) is important for eliminating the presence of an androgen-producing tumor. Normal or high-normal levels of total testosterone are consistent with the diagnosis of PCOS. Because testosterone decreases SHBG levels, patients with normal total testosterone levels, but with clinical evidence of hyperandrogenism (hirsutism and/or acne), invariably have either increased free testosterone levels or increased sensitivity of the hair follicle and sebaceous glands. In most cases, the measurement of free testosterone levels is unlikely to add more information than total testosterone levels.

Steroidogenesis and Clinical Disorders

Congenital Adrenal Hyperplasia. Typically due to a 21-hydroxylase deficiency, classic congenital adrenal hyperplasia (CAH) is one of the most common autosomal recessive metabolic diseases. It is estimated to occur in 1:10,000 to 1:15,000 births (Trakakis, 2010). Although CAH has been reported in a wide range of ethnic groups, it is most common in the Ashkenazi Jewish population. Alternatively, deficiencies in 11β-hydroxylase activity account for 5 to 8 percent of CAH cases.

Patients with CAH exhibit a broad range of clinical phenotypes depending on the extent of enzymatic deficiency. On one extreme, gene conversions and large deletions result in severe enzyme deficiency and present as salt-wasting CAH in the neonate. For example, in the more common form of CAH, a block at the 21-hydroxylase step results in markedly reduced levels of aldosterone and cortisol. The back-up of precursors shifts steroidogenesis toward the androgen pathway. Therefore, females with CAH will present with female pseudohermaphroditism (female karyotype with masculinized external genitalia) (Chap. 18, p. 489). Unless corticosteroid replacement is provided, these children will die in the neonatal period. A less severe mutation may lead to so-called simple

virilizing CAH. As its name suggests, this condition is notable for sufficient corticosteroid production but increased androgen levels.

In a nonclassic form of CAH, also known as late-onset or adult-onset CAH, hyperandrogenemia does not present until puberty. The incidence of nonclassic disease has been estimated at 1:1000 births. At puberty, activation of the adrenal axis increases steroidogenesis, unmasking a mild 21-hydroxylase activity deficiency. Levels of adrenocorticotropin hormone (ACTH) may increase due to the lack of negative feedback by cortisol, further exacerbating androgen production. These patients often present with hirsutism, acne, and anovulation. Thus, late-onset CAH may mimic PCOS.

Diagnostically, serum 17α-hydroxyprogesterone (17-OHP) levels provide a sensitive screen for the presence of CAH (Chap. 17, p. 471). Levels should be measured during the follicular phase to avoid false positives from 17-OHP secretion by the corpus luteum.

Synthesis of Estrogens from Androgens. Aromatization of C19 androgens by P450arom (aromatase; CYP19) yields C18 estrogens containing a phenolic ring (see Fig. 15-5). In addition to the ovary, aromatase is expressed in significant levels in adipose tissue, skin, and brain (Boon, 2010). Clinically important, sufficient estrogen can be derived from peripheral aromatization to produce endometrial bleeding in postmenopausal women, especially those who are overweight or obese.

5α-Reductase Types 1 and 2. The 5α-reductase enzyme exists in two forms, each encoded by a separate gene. The type 1 enzyme is found in the liver, kidneys, skin, and brain. In contrast, the type 2 enzyme is predominantly expressed in the male genitalia (Russell, 1994). 5α-reductase converts testosterone to a more potent androgen, 5α-dihydrotestosterone (DHT). Because DHT promotes transformation of vellus hair to terminal hair, medications that antagonize 5α-reductase are often effective in the treatment of hirsutism (Stout, 2010).

RECEPTOR STRUCTURE AND FUNCTION

Steroid hormones and peptide factors differ in their specific DNA interaction, yet both ultimately lead to DNA transcription and protein production. In the nucleus, steroid-bound receptors bind to DNA-regulatory elements within target-gene promoter regions. In the case of peptide factors, sequential phosphorylation ultimately activates proteins bound to gene promoter sequences. Following gene activation, the enzyme ribonucleic acid (RNA) polymerase transcribes the information into mRNA, which carries the coded information into the cytoplasmic compartment of cells. There, the information is translated by ribosomes into proteins.

■ G-Protein Coupled Receptors
Intracellular Signaling Systems

G-protein coupled receptors are a large family of cell-membrane associated receptors that bind peptide factors. These receptors consist of a hydrophilic extracellular domain, an intracellular domain, and a hydrophobic transmembrane domain that spans the cell membrane seven times. When bound to hormone, these receptors undergo a conformational change, activate intracellular signaling pathways, and through a series of phosphorylation events, ultimately modulate transcription of multiple genes within the target cell.

Gonadotropin-Releasing Hormone Receptor

The GnRH receptor (GnRH-R) is a member of the G-protein coupled receptor superfamily. Expression of GnRH-R has been identified in the ovary, testes, hypothalamus, prostate, breast, and placenta (Yu, 2011). Gonadotropin-releasing hormone itself may be expressed in the pituitary, gonads, and placenta (Kim, 2007). Although data are still preliminary, GnRH and its receptor may form an autocrine/paracrine regulatory network in reproductive tissues in addition to the classic neuroendocrine hypothalamic-pituitary system.

To add further complexity, it is now known that humans express two forms of GnRH as well as two forms of the receptor (Cheng, 2005). The GnRH II receptor likely is more widely expressed than the classic GnRH I receptor. GnRH II peptide may also have a different expression pattern than GnRH I (Neill, 2002). Significant future work will be required to determine the overlapping and divergent functions of these new proteins.

Gonadotropin Receptors

Both LH and hCG bind to a single G-protein coupled receptor known as the LH/CG receptor. Relative to LH, hCG has a slightly higher affinity for the receptor and has a longer half-life. In contrast, FSH binds to a unique G-protein coupled receptor.

Within the ovary, the LH/CG receptor is expressed on thecal cells, interstitial cells, and luteal cells. In the granulosa cells of preantral follicles, LH/CG receptor mRNA is nearly undetectable. Expression of this receptor is markedly induced during follicular maturation, with high levels observed in differentiated granulosa cells. LH/CG receptors have been identified in the human endometrium, myometrium, fallopian tubes, and brain (Camp, 1991). The function of the LH/CG ligand-receptor system is unknown for these other tissues. In contrast, FSH receptor expression appears to be restricted to the granulosa cells of the ovary and the Sertoli cells of the testis.

■ Steroid Hormone Receptors
Classification of Steroid Receptor Superfamily Members

Despite their structural similarities, estrogens, progestins, androgens, mineralocorticoids, and glucocorticoids all interact with unique receptors known as nuclear hormone receptors. The nuclear receptor superfamily consists of three receptor groups: (1) those that bind steroidal ligands, (2) those that have affinity for nonsteroidal ligands, and (3) those with no known ligand.

In the first group, receptors are gene transcription factors with known steroidal ligands, such as estrogen, progesterone, and androgens. The second group contains nonsteroid ligand-activated receptors such as thyroid hormone and retinoic acid receptors. Lastly, orphan receptors comprise the largest component of the nuclear receptor superfamily. By definition, these receptors do not have an identified ligand and are believed to be constitutively active, although their activity may be altered by posttranslational modifications such as phosphorylation.

Modular Structure of the Steroid Receptor Superfamily

Free steroids diffuse into cells and combine with specific receptors (Fig. 15-7A). Subsequently, steroid receptors enhance or repress gene transcription through interactions with specific DNA sequences, called hormone responsive elements, in the promoter region of target genes (Klinge, 2001). Members of this receptor superfamily exhibit a modular structure of distinct domains as depicted in (Fig. 15-8). Each of these regions provides activities required for full receptor function.

In general, nuclear receptors have two regions that are critical for gene activation, termed activation function 1 and activation function 2 (AF1 and AF2). AF1 is located in the A/B domain and is usually ligand independent. AF2 is in the ligand-binding domain (E) and is often hormone-dependent. The highly conserved DNA-binding region (C) consists of "zinc fingers," so called because the presence of zinc introduces a loop in the amino acid sequence, creating a structure that inserts into the DNA helix.

Estrogen, Progesterone, and Androgen Receptors

Receptors for estrogen are localized to the nucleus. In contrast, progesterone receptors (PRs), androgen receptors (AR), and those for mineralocorticoids and glucocorticoids are cytoplasmic in the absence of ligand. Ligand binding to these latter receptors allows translocation to the nucleus.

Two isoforms of estrogen receptors, ERα and ERβ, have been cloned and are encoded by separate genes. These receptors are differentially expressed in tissues and appear to subserve distinct functions (Fig. 15-9) (Kuiper, 1997). For example, both ERα and ERβ are required for normal ovarian function. However, mice lacking ERα are anovulatory and accumulate cystic follicles, whereas the ovaries of ERβ-null mice are normal histologically despite impaired ovulation (Couse, 2000).

The progesterone receptor also exists in at least two isoforms. Encoded from a single gene, PRA and PRB are identical except for an additional 164 amino acids at the amino terminus (Conneely, 2002). A third PR isoform, designated PRC, differs from the other two in its DNA-binding domain and has been postulated to act as a progestin inhibitor (Wei, 1996). As with the estrogen receptors, the PR isoforms are not interchangeable. For example, PRA is required for normal ovarian and uterine functions but is expendable in the breast (Lydon, 1996). Of note, estrogen is a key stimulator of PR expression. As a result, PR expression is generally very low in hypoestrogenic states.

Only one form of the androgen receptor has been identified. This receptor contains the classic steroid receptor structure. Mutations in this receptor are responsible for androgen

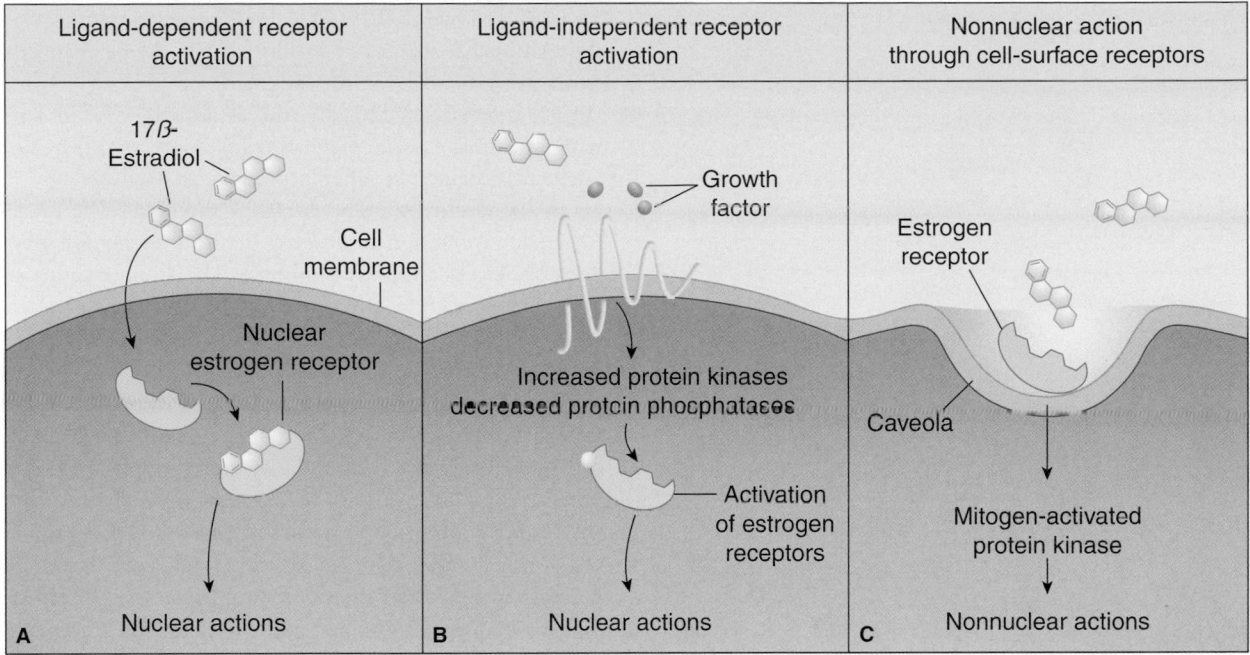

FIGURE 15-7 Estrogen-receptor ligand-dependent and ligand-independent activation. **A.** Classically, the estrogen receptor can be activated by estrogen. Unbound hormone is free to bind with empty steroid receptors found either in the cytoplasm or more commonly, in the cell's nucleus. Hormone-bound receptors then bind to specific DNA promoter sequences. This binding typically leads to DNA transcription and eventually to specific protein synthesis. **B.** The estrogen receptor can also be activated independently of estrogen. Growth factors can increase the activity of protein kinases that phosphorylate different sites on the receptor molecule. This unbound, yet activated, receptor will then exert transcriptional effects. **C.** Nonnuclear estrogen-signaling pathways can also produce effects. Cell-membrane estrogen receptors are located in invaginations called caveolae. Estrogen binding to these estrogen receptors is linked to the mitogen-activated protein kinase pathway and results in a rapid, nonnuclear effect. *(From Gruber, 2002, with permission.)*

insensitivity syndrome (AIS) in 46,XY patients characterized by lack of sexual hair, lack of a uterus and fallopian tubes, a vaginal pouch, and intraabdominal testes (Chap. 18, p. 489) (Brinkmann, 2001).

ESTROGEN RECEPTOR

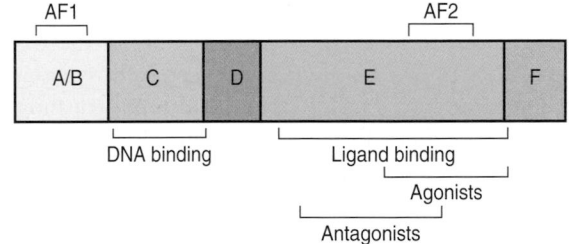

PROGESTERONE RECEPTOR

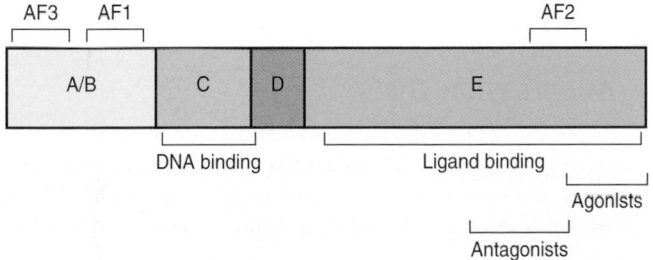

FIGURE 15-8 Drawing depicts the concept of functional domains within estrogen and progesterone receptors. Note distinct sites for ligand and DNA binding. *(From O'Malley, 1999, with permission.)*

Nongenomic Actions of Steroids

Recent studies have introduced the concept that a subset of steroids, including estrogens and progestins, may alter cell function via nongenomic effects, that is, independent of the classic nuclear hormone receptors (see Fig. 15-7C). These nongenomic effects occur rapidly and may be mediated via cell-surface receptors (Moore, 1999). Pharmacologic agents under development specifically target these nongenomic effects to allow more precise therapy for steroid-sensitive disorders.

Receptor Expression and Desensitization

Many factors modulate the cellular response to sex steroids and peptide factors. Of these, the number of receptors within a cell or on the cell membrane is critical for attaining a maximal hormonal response. Importantly, the number of receptors on a cell can be modified at multiple levels of gene expression, from gene transcription through receptor protein degradation.

Hormonally induced negative regulation of receptors is termed *homologous downregulation* or *desensitization*. Desensitization provides a mechanism for limiting the duration of a hormonal response by decreasing the sensitivity of a cell to a constant level of hormone upon prolonged exposure.

Within the reproductive system, the process of desensitization is best understood for the GnRH receptor and is used clinically to produce a hypoestrogenic state. Pharmacologic agonists of GnRH, such as leuprolide acetate (Lupron), initially stimulate receptors on pituitary gonadotropes to cause

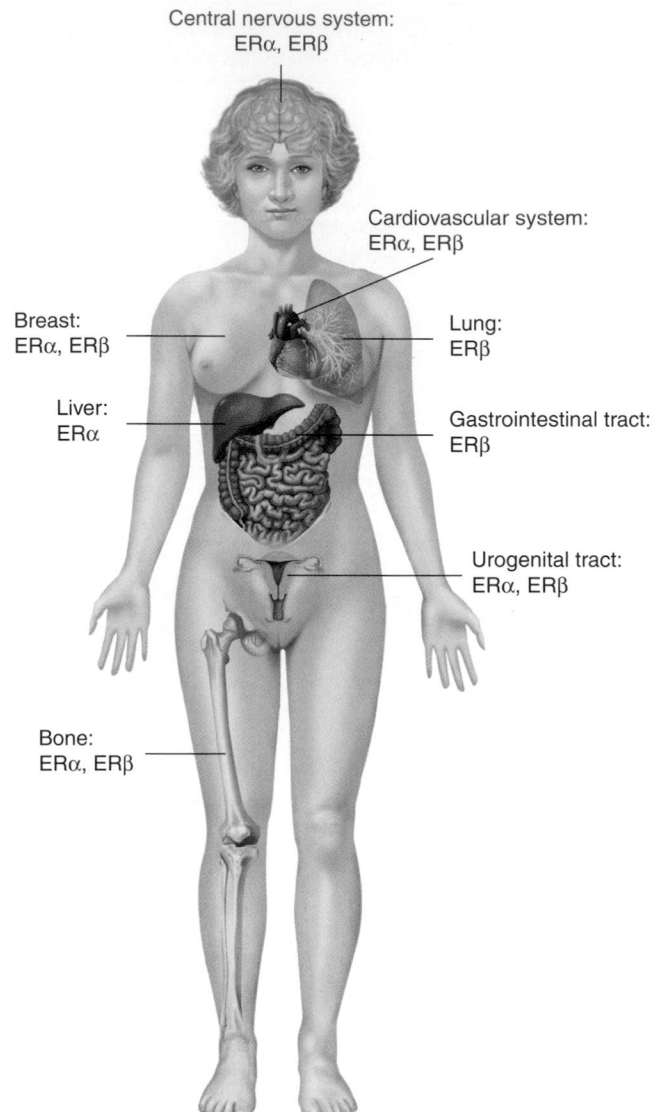

Central nervous system:
ERα, ERβ

Cardiovascular system:
ERα, ERβ

Breast:
ERα, ERβ

Lung:
ERβ

Liver:
ERα

Gastrointestinal tract:
ERβ

Urogenital tract:
ERα, ERβ

Bone:
ERα, ERβ

FIGURE 15-9 Distribution of specific estrogen receptors within certain organs. ERα = estrogen receptor alpha; ERβ = estrogen receptor beta.

a supraphysiologic release of both LH and FSH. With their long-term action, however, agonists downregulate receptors in gonadotropes, thus creating desensitization to further GnRH stimulation. Correspondingly, decreased gonadotropin secretion leads to suppressed estrogen and progesterone levels 1 to 2 weeks after initial GnRH agonist administration.

IMMUNOASSAYS FOR PEPTIDE AND STEROID HORMONES

Immunoassays

These have been developed for essentially all polypeptide, steroid, and thyroid hormones. Immunoassays are remarkably sensitive and in most cases, are easily automated. For many hormones, the concentration is reported as international units per volume rather than as a mass per volume (Table 15-2). It is critical to know which reference standard is used by a specific assay as results may differ significantly. Reference preparations

are produced by the World Health Organization (WHO) or by the National Institutes of Health (NIH). More than 20 standards are available for measurement of LH, FSH, prolactin (PRL), and hCG. Clinically, this issue may arise in a patient with a possible ectopic pregnancy in which serial β-hCG levels are being obtained at different health care facilities.

The possibility of a "hook effect" should also be considered in the interpretation of results. In the presence of very high hormone levels, antibody binding will be saturated and can give a falsely low reading.

In addition, the amount of immunoreactive hormone present in a sample does not necessarily correlate with the biologic activity of that hormone. For example, PRL exists in multiple isoforms, many of which are immunologically detectable, but not biologically active. Similarly, alternate glycosylation patterns of the gonadotropins at different times of the reproductive life span are believed to alter their biologic activity.

"Normal ranges" should also be interpreted with care as a stated normal range is often broad. The hormone level of an individual may double and the level may still lie within a normal range, although the result is actually abnormal for that individual. In the context of the pituitary gland and its target endocrine glands, it may be adequate to measure the pituitary hormone alone. However, interpretation of the result may be clarified by the addition of the target hormone level. For example, in many laboratories, an abnormal TSH value will lead to "reflex" testing for thyroid hormone levels. Low levels of both members of a stimulating-hormone and target-gland hormone pair indicate an abnormality in either hypothalamic or pituitary function (Table 15-3). High levels of a target-gland hormone coupled with low levels of its stimulating pituitary hormone suggest autonomous secretion by the target organ such as occurs in the hyperthyroidism of Graves disease.

Stimulation Tests

These tests may be used when hypofunction of an endocrine organ is suspected. These tests use a known endogenous stimulating hormone to assess the reserve capacity of the tissue of interest. The trophic hormone used may be a hypothalamic releasing factor such as GnRH or thyrotropin-releasing hormone (TRH). Alternatively, a substitute pituitary hormone, such as hCG as a substitute for LH or cosyntropin (Cortrosyn) for ACTH may be used. The ability of the target gland to respond is measured by an increase in the appropriate hormone's plasma level. One example, the "GnRH stim" test, may be useful in evaluation of abnormal pubertal development and is described in Chapter 14 (p. 393). Unfortunately, clinical-grade GnRH is often unavailable.

Suppression Tests

These tests may be performed when endocrine hyperfunction is suspected. For example, a "dexamethasone suppression test" may be given to a patient with suspected hypercortisolism (Cushing disease or syndrome). Described in full in Chapter 17 (p. 472), this test gauges the ability of dexamethasone to inhibit ACTH secretion and thus cortisol production by the adrenal. The failure of glucocorticoid treatment to suppress cortisol production would be consistent with primary hyperadrenalism.

TABLE 15-2. Reference Ranges for Selected Reproductive Steroids in Adult Human Serum

Steroid	Subjects	Reference Values
Androstenedione	Men	2.8–7.3 nmol/L
	Women	3.1–12.2 nmol/L
Testosterone	Men	6.9–34.7 nmol/L
	Women	0.7–2.8 nmol/L
Dihydrotestosterone	Men	1.0–3.10 nmol/L
	Women	0.07–.086 nmol/L
Dehydroepiandrosterone	Men/Women	5.5–24.3 nmol/L
Dehydroepiandrosterone sulfonate	Men/Women	2.5–10.4 µmol/L
Progesterone	Men	<0.3–1.3 nmol/L
	Women	
	Follicular	0.3–3.0 nmol/L
	Luteal	19.0–45.0 nmol/L
Estradiol	Men	<37–210 pmol/L
	Women	
	Follicular	<37–360 pmol/L
	Luteal	625–2830 pmol/L
	Midcycle	699–1250 pmol/L
	Postmenopausal	<37–140 pmol/L
Estrone	Men	37–250 pmol/L
	Women	
	Follicular	110–400 pmol/L
	Luteal	310–660 pmol/L
	Postmenopausal	22–230 pmol/L
Estrone sulfonate	Men	600–2500 pmol/L
	Women	
	Follicular	700–3600 pmol/L
	Luteal	1100–7300 pmol/L
	Postmenopausal	130–1200 pmol/L

From O'Malley, 1999, with permission.

ESTROGENS AND PROGESTINS IN CLINICAL PRACTICE

A multitude of both estrogen and progesterone preparations are available for use in clinical practice. Each of these medications differs in its biologic efficacy, and clinicians should understand the reasons behind some of these differences.

Estrogens

Classic estrogens are 18-carbon steroid compounds containing a phenolic ring (Fig. 15-10). This group contains the natural estrogens—estradiol, estrone, estriol, conjugated equine estrogens (CEE), and their derivatives. The predominant synthetic C-18 estrogen is ethinyl estradiol, the estrogen present in combination oral contraceptives. Synthetic nonsteroidal estrogens include diethylstilbestrol (DES) and selective estrogen-receptor modulators

(SERMs) such as tamoxifen and clomiphene citrate. Despite their variation from the classic steroid ring shape, these nonsteroidal estrogens are still able to bind to the estrogen receptor.

Of the natural estrogens, 17β-estradiol is the most potent followed by estrone and then estriol. In comparing some

TABLE 15-3. Classification of Functional Amenorrhea

Description	LH/FSH	Estrogen
*Hyper*gonadotropic *Hypo*gonadism	High	Low
*Hypo*gonadotropic *Hypo*gonadism	Low	Low

FSH = follicle-stimulating hormone; LH = luteinizing hormone.

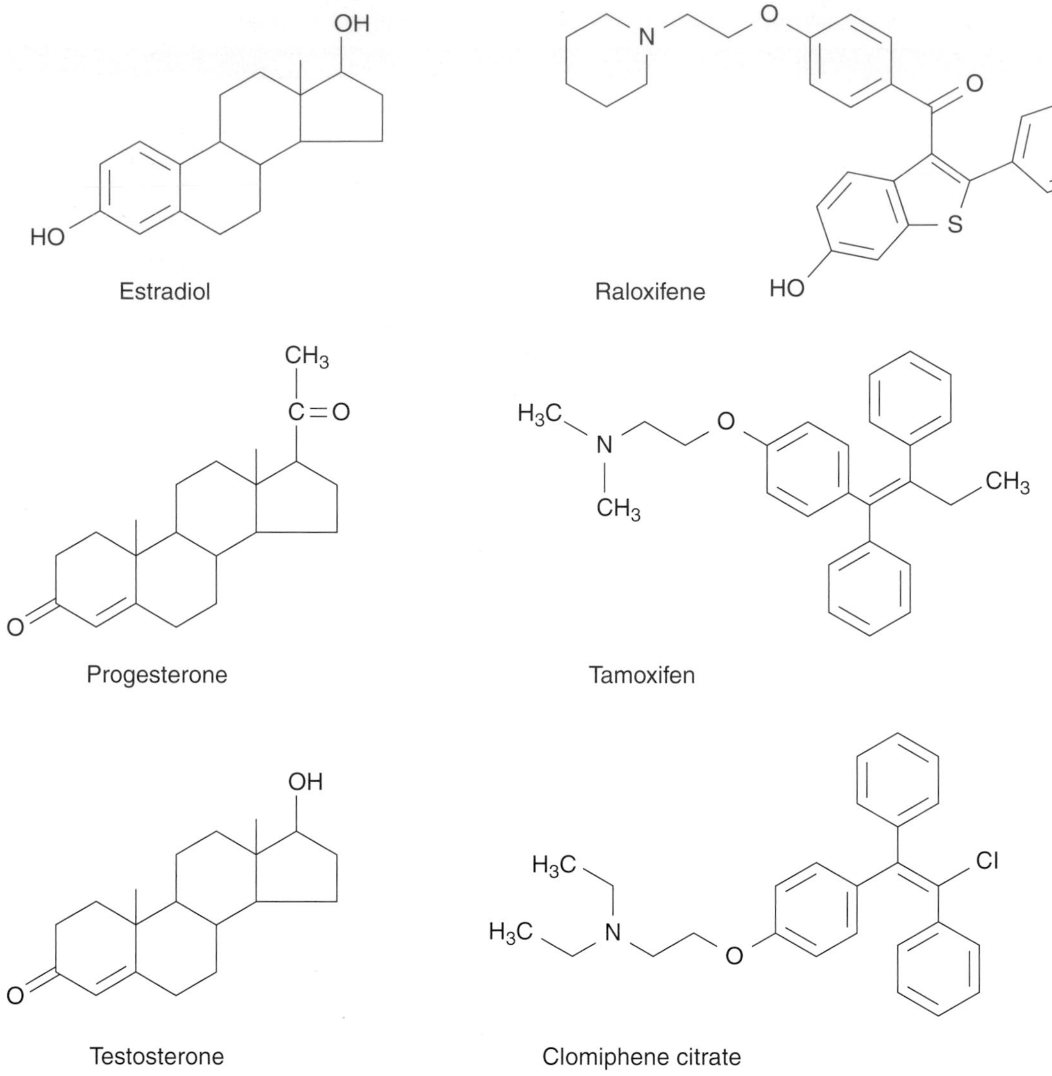

FIGURE 15-10 Chemical structure of important sex steroids and selective estrogen-receptor modulators.

pharmacologically used estrogens, ethinyl estradiol has been estimated to be approximately 100 to 1000 times more potent on a per weight basis than either micronized estradiol or CEE in terms of increasing sex hormone-binding globulin levels, which is one marker of estrogen potency (Kuhl, 2005; Mashchak, 1982).

Progestogens

Although there is no formal rule, progestogens are commonly categorized as natural progesterone and as synthetic progestogens called progestins. Only progesterone can maintain human pregnancy. Synthetic progestins can be classified as derivatives of either 19-norprogesterone or 19-nortestosterone (Kuhl, 2005). Of the 19-norprogesterones, the most commonly used are medroxyprogesterone acetate and megestrol acetate.

Most progestins used in contraceptives are derived from 19-nortestosterone. These are commonly described as first generation (norethindrone), second generation (levonorgestrel, norgestrel), or third generation (desogestrel, norgestimate). Each generation has been designed to have progressively less androgenic effect. The fourth-generation progestin, drospirenone,

is unique in that it is derived from spironolactone. Although it has no androgenic activity, drospirenone has an affinity for the mineralocorticoid receptor approximately five times that of aldosterone. This explains its diuretic action.

Selective Steroid-Receptor Modulators

As indicated by their names, these synthetic compounds bind to their target receptors and exert tissue-specific effects, acting as agonists in some tissues and antagonists in others (Table 15-4). The best known of these are the selective estrogen-receptor modulators (SERMs) (Haskell, 2003). The divergent effects of the SERMs can be attributed to many factors at the molecular level. Each SERM binds to an estrogen receptor to generate a unique molecular confirmation, which in turn affects the interaction of the complex with transcriptional cofactors and gene promoter regions. The response will also be modified by the relative expression of ERα and ERβ receptors in the target tissue (see Fig. 15-9).

The hormonal milieu may also be important in determining the agonist–antagonist profile of a specific SERM. For example,

TABLE 15-4. Estrogenic Agonist or Antagonist Effects of Tamoxifen, Raloxifene, and Estradiol

Drug	Breast	Bone	Lipids	Uterus
Tamoxifen	Antagonist	Agonist	Agonist	Agonist
Raloxifene	Antagonist	Agonist	Agonist	Antagonist
Estradiol	Agonist	Agonist	Agonist	Agonist

a SERM may act as an estrogen agonist in a low-estrogen state, such as menopause, but as a competitive antagonist in a patient with high circulating levels of the potent estrogen estradiol. The unique pharmacologic profiles of these compounds expand their therapeutic utility.

More recently, selective progesterone-receptor modulators (SPRMs) have been developed in the hope of improving emergency contraception efficacy and expanding treatment options for disorders including leiomyomas and endometriosis (Chap. 5, p. 163 and Chap. 9, p. 255) (Chwalisz, 2005). Selective androgen-receptor modulators (SARMs) are also under investigation for the treatment of osteopenia and decreased libido in women. Ideally, these will avoid the virilizing effects of testosterone treatment (Negro-Vilar, 1999).

As indicated by the preceding discussion, the agonist–antagonist effect of a steroid hormone is inextricably related to the clinical tissue of interest. Although this concept is most frequently discussed in terms of selective steroid modulators, in fact, all steroid hormones within a class exert differences in their pattern of action across tissues. As a result, when a steroid is chosen for treatment, each clinical endpoint should be considered individually.

Steroid Hormone Potency

The efficacy of estrogen and progesterone treatments is altered by a large number of factors such as: (1) receptor binding affinity, (2) formulation, (3) route of administration, (4) metabolism, and (5) affinity for binding globulins. First, even small chemical modifications can substantially impact the biologic effects of steroid preparations. For example, the progestins in clinical use all exert progestogenic effects, but may also act as weak androgens, antiandrogens, glucocorticoids, or antimineralocorticoids. These differences are likely explained by variations in binding affinity for the relevant steroid receptor (Table 15-5).

Second, estrogens and progestins can be administered as oral, transdermal, vaginal, or intramuscular preparations, among others. The choice of carrier molecule impacts hormone bioavailability. For example, although crystalline progesterone is poorly absorbed via the intestine, dispersion of the progesterone into small particles (micronization) markedly increases surface area and uptake.

Third, oral medications pass through the intestine and the liver prior to systemic dissemination. As these tissues are sites for steroid metabolism, oral medications and their levels may be significantly altered prior to reaching their target organs. As an example, the bioavailability of orally administered micronized progesterone is less than 10 percent and compares poorly with the estimated 50- to 70-percent bioavailability for norethindrone and 100 percent for levonorgestrel. This difference is due to a high level of "first pass" metabolism of micronized progesterone (Stanczyk, 2002). As another example, the half-life of ethinyl estradiol is greatly extended relative to that of unconjugated estradiol by the presence of the ethinyl group, which impairs metabolism.

TABLE 15-5. Relative Binding Affinities of Steroid Receptors and Serum Binding Globulins to Progestogens

Progestogen	PR	AR	ER	GR	MR	SHBG	CBG
Progesterone	50	0	0	10	100	0	36
Medroxyprogesterone acetate	115	5	0	29	160	0	0
Levonorgestrel	150	45	0	1	75	50	0
Etonogestrel	150	20	0	14	0	15	0
Norgestimate	15	0	0	1	0	0	0
Dienogest	5	10	0	1	0	0	0
Drospirenone	35	65	0	6	230	0	0

AR = androgen receptor; CBG = corticoid-binding globulin; ER = estrogen receptor; GR = glucocorticoid receptor; MR = mineralocorticoid receptor; PR = progesterone receptor; SHBG = sex hormone-binding globulin.
Abbreviated from Wiegratz, 2004, with permission.

TABLE 15-6. Relative Potency of Various Estrogens Concerning Clinical and Metabolic Parameters[a]

Estrogen	Suppression of		Increase Serum Levels of			
	Hot Flashes	FSH	HDL	SHBG	CBG	Angiotensinogen
Estradiol-17β	100	100	100	100	100	
Estriol	30	20				
CEE	120	110	150	300	150	500
Ethinyl estradiol	12,000	12,000	40,000	50,000	60,000	35,000

[a]The values are estimated on a weight basis.
CBG = corticoid-binding globulin; CEE = conjugated equine estrogens; FSH = follicle-stimulating hormone;
HDL = high-density lipoprotein; SHBG = sex hormone-binding globulin.
Abbreviated from Kuhl, 2005, with permission.

Absorption and metabolism rates may differ between individuals due to inherited or acquired differences in liver, intestinal, and renal function (Kuhl, 2005). Local metabolism will also impact steroid efficacy and can include conversion between steroids (for example, androgens to estrogens by aromatase) or within a steroid type (for example, estradiol to the weaker estrone). Diet, alcohol consumption, cigarette smoking, exercise, and stress have all been postulated to alter steroid metabolism. The presence of thyroid disease also affects drug metabolism rates.

Lastly, steroid potency depends on affinity for the various carrier proteins produced by the liver. Only unbound hormone and to a much lesser extent, the amount bound to albumin or cortisol-binding protein (CBG) is functionally active. Steroid bound to sex hormone-binding globulin is considered to be inactive. Approximately 38 percent of estradiol is bound to SHBG, 60 percent is bound to albumin, and the remainder is free. In contrast, ethinyl estradiol is bound nearly exclusively to albumin, and this increases its bioavailability (Barnes, 2007). As shown in Table 15-5, significant differences in carrier binding are also observed for progestogens (Wiegratz, 2004).

Importantly, hormonal status affects expression of carrier proteins. Specifically, estrogens and thyroid hormone stimulate and androgens blunt serum SHBG levels. To add further complexity, it is now believed that target cells can secrete SHBG, which then acts locally as a membrane receptor to stimulate cyclic adenosine monophosphate (cAMP) intracellular signaling pathways (Rosner, 2010).

Additional Steroid Assays

As previously described, immunoassays for gonadal steroids are widely available (p. 408). However, these assays do not provide any insight into the biologic activity of these hormones. Two additional types of assays provide additional information: (1) in vitro receptor-binding assays and (2) bioassays. Of these, receptor-binding assays can determine the affinity of a hormone for a specific receptor, but do not provide any insight into the functional impact of this interaction.

With bioassays, a limited number of studies have evaluated the efficacy of estrogens in women using clinical, endocrinologic, and metabolic parameters (Table 15-6) (Kuhl, 2005). As seen in animal studies, different preparations vary markedly in their potency. Of note, estrogens also demonstrate differences in terms of their tissue specificity. For example, 17β-estradiol and CEE suppress pituitary FSH to a similar extent, whereas CEE is a more potent stimulator of liver SHBG production.

REPRODUCTIVE NEUROENDOCRINOLOGY

Neurotransmitters

The list of known neurotransmitters continues to expand as our understanding of their anatomic distribution, mode of regulation, and mechanism of action increases. Neurotransmitters can be classified as: (1) biogenic amines (dopamine, epinephrine, norepinephrine, serotonin, histamine), (2) neuropeptides, (3) acetylcholine, (4) excitatory amino neurotransmitters (glutamate, glycine, aspartic acid), (5) the inhibitory amino acid gamma amino butyric acid (GABA), (6) gaseous transmitters (nitric oxide, carbon monoxide), and (7) miscellaneous factors (cytokines, growth factors).

Neuropeptides in Reproduction

Over 50 neuropeptides have been described that influence behavior, pain perception, memory, appetite, thirst, temperature, homeostasis, and sleep. Clinically important neuropeptides include the endogenous opiates, kisspeptin, neuropeptide Y (NPY), galanin, and pituitary adenylate cyclase-activating peptide.

Endogenous Opiates

Depending on the precursor peptide from which they are derived, these neuropeptides can be categorized into three classes—endorphins, enkephalins, and dynorphins. Of these, endorphins (endogenous morphines) are cleavage products of the proopiomelanocortin (POMC) gene, which also yields ACTH and α-melanocyte stimulating hormone (α-MSH)

(Howlett, 1986; Taylor, 1997). The endorphins serve a wide range of physiologic functions including the regulation of temperature, cardiovascular and respiratory systems, pain perception, mood, and reproduction.

Proopiomelanocortin is produced in highest concentration in the anterior pituitary gland, but is also expressed in the brain, sympathetic nervous system, gonads, placenta, gastrointestinal tract, and lungs. The primary peptide synthesized from this pathway depends on the tissue source. For example, the predominant products in the brain are the opiates, whereas pituitary biosynthesis results principally in ACTH production.

Central opioidergic neurons are important mediators of the anterior and posterior pituitary gland. Administration of morphine or its analogs causes release of growth hormone and PRL and inhibition of gonadotropins and TSH release (Grossman, 1983; Houben, 1994). In addition, functional hypothalamic amenorrhea due to eating disorders, intensive exercise, and stress is correlated with an increase in endogenous opiates (Chap. 16, p. 449). Elevated PRL levels also increase opioid levels in the hypothalamus. This may provide a mechanism, in addition to increased dopamine levels, for the suppression of GnRH pulsatility that occurs with hyperprolactinemia (Khoury, 1987; Petraglia, 1985).

Kisspeptin

The past 5 years has seen a rapid advance in our understanding of the critical role that hypothalamic kisspeptin neurons play in sexual differentiation, puberty initiation, and adult reproductive function. Kisspeptin neurons send processes to GnRH neurons, allowing direct control of GnRH secretion. Interestingly, one group of kisspeptin neurons may mediate negative steroid feedback, whereas another is responsible for the positive feedback observed before ovulation (Lehman, 2010; Pineda, 2010).

Ever more complex interactions are being characterized between kisspeptin neurons and factors that are known to be important links between energy homeostasis and reproductive function. In a number of cases, kisspeptin neuronal activity both regulates the function of other neural networks and is reciprocally regulated by those same systems. Examples include neurons that express neuropeptide Y, galanin, or POMC (Fu, 2010). The adipose-derived factor leptin has also been shown to regulate kisspeptin expression (Chap. 16, p. 449).

Neuropeptide Y and Galanin

Neurons expressing NPY or galanin are located throughout the hypothalamus and project to kisspeptin neurons, to GnRH neurons, and to other areas of the central nervous system with roles in reproductive function. NPY and galanin secretion vary in response to changes in energy level as seen in anorexia or conversely, obesity. Both of these neuropeptides have been shown to alter GnRH pulsatility and to potentiate GnRH-induced gonadotrope secretion (Lawrence, 2011; Peters, 2009).

Pituitary Adenylate Cyclase-Activating Peptide

Pituitary adenylate cyclase-activating peptide (PACAP) was first isolated from the hypothalamic arcuate nucleus in sheep (Anderson, 1996). As suggested by its name, PACAP binds to receptors present in the pituitary and stimulates gonadotropin secretion, albeit more weakly than GnRH. It has been determined that gonadotropes themselves secrete PACAP, suggesting an autocrine–paracrine role for this hormone. PACAP modulates GnRH-receptor expression and conversely, GnRH alters PACAP-receptor expression on the gonadotrope cell surface. Furthermore, pituitary PACAP gene expression is markedly increased by GnRH (Grafer, 2009). Thus, these two important neuropeptides are functionally linked at the level of the anterior pituitary.

THE HYPOTHALAMIC-PITUITARY AXIS

Anatomy

The hypothalamus is the source of many important neurotransmitters studied in reproductive function, and consists of nuclei located at the base of the brain, just superior to the optic chiasm. Pituitary function is primarily influenced by neurons located within the arcuate, ventromedial, dorsomedial, and paraventricular nuclei of the hypothalamus (Fig. 15-11).

Neurons within the hypothalamus form synaptic connections with other neurons throughout the central nervous system (CNS). In addition, a subset of the hypothalamic neurons project to the median eminence. In the median eminence, a dense network of capillaries arises from the superior hypophyseal arteries. These capillaries drain into portal vessels that traverse the pituitary stalk and then form a capillary network within the anterior pituitary gland (adenohypophysis). The primary direction of this hypophyseal portal system is from hypothalamus to pituitary, however, retrograde flow also exists. This creates an ultrashort feedback loop between the pituitary gland and hypothalamic neurons. The hypothalamus is thus a critical locus for integration of information from the environment, nervous system, and multiple other organ systems.

Anterior Pituitary Hormones

Intimately connected to the hypothalamus, the anterior pituitary gland contains five hormone-producing cell types: (1) gonadotropes (which produce LH and FSH), (2) lactotropes (PRL), (3) somatotropes (GH), (4) thyrotropes (TSH), and (5) adrenocorticotropes (ACTH). Of these, gonadotropes comprise approximately 10 to 15 percent of all hormonally active cells in the anterior pituitary (Childs, 1983).

With the exception of PRL, which is under tonic inhibition, pituitary hormones are stimulated by hypothalamic neuroendocrine secretion. Although initially felt to be under separate control, it now is known that both of the gonadotropins, LH and FSH, are regulated by a single releasing peptide, called gonadotropin-releasing hormone, which acts on the anterior pituitary's gonadotrope subpopulation. Most gonadotropes contain secretory granules that contain both LH and FSH, although a significant number of cells are monohormonal, that is, secrete only LH or only FSH.

Of the other pituitary-releasing hormones, corticotropin releasing hormone (CRH) stimulates biosynthesis and secretion of ACTH by the pituitary adrenocorticotropes. Thyrotropin-releasing hormone (TRH) increases secretion by

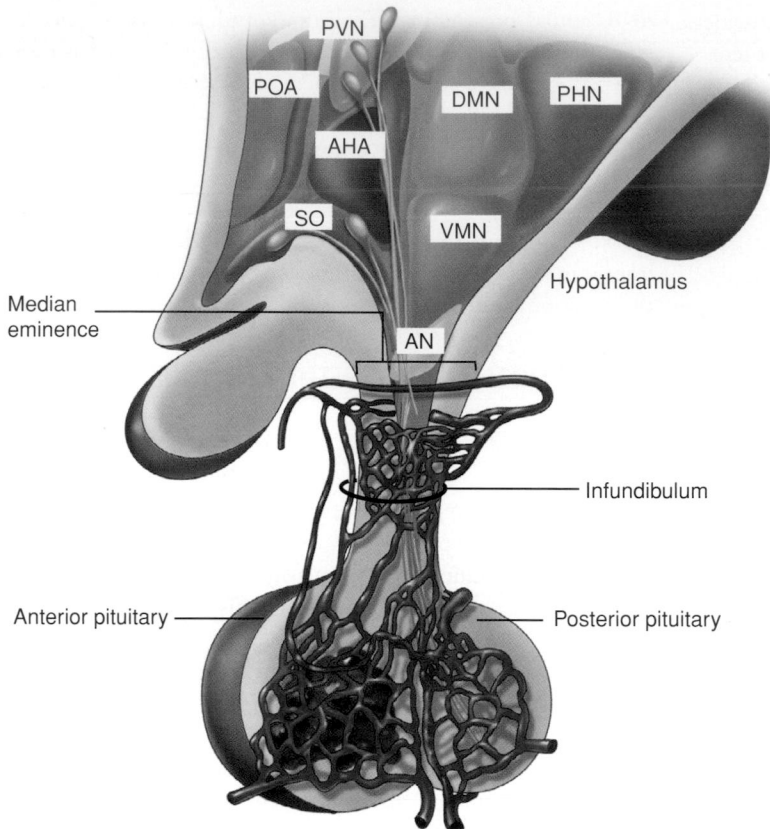

FIGURE 15-11 Diagram depicts a sagittal section through the hypothalamus and pituitary gland with rostral structures to the left and caudal ones to the right. The hypothalamus is anatomically and functionally linked with the anterior pituitary by the portal system of blood supply. The posterior pituitary contains the axon terminals of neurons arising in the supraoptic (SO) nucleus and paraventricular nucleus (PVN) of the hypothalamus. AHA = anterior hypothalamic area; AN = arcuate nucleus; DMN = dorsomedial nucleus; PHN = posterior hypothalamic nucleus; POA = preoptic area; VMN = ventromedial nucleus. *(From Cunningham, 2010b, with permission.)*

the thyrotropes of TSH, also known as *thyrotropin*. Various hypothalamic secretagogues regulate expression of somatotrope-derived growth hormone (GH). Lastly, PRL expression is primarily under inhibitory regulation by dopamine. As a consequence of these regulatory mechanisms, damage to the pituitary stalk results in hypopituitarism for LH, FSH, GH,

ACTH, and TSH, but an associated increase in PRL secretion.

Hypothalamic Releasing Peptides

These peptides have characteristics that are important for both their biologic function and clinical use. First, they are small peptides with short half-lives of a few minutes due to their rapid degradation. Secondly, hypothalamic releasing peptides are released in minute quantities and are highly diluted in the peripheral circulation. Therefore, biologically active concentrations of these factors are locally restricted to the anterior pituitary gland. Clinically, the extremely low concentrations of these hormones render them essentially undetectable in serum. Thus, levels of their corresponding pituitary factors are measured as surrogate markers.

Gonadotropin-Releasing Hormone

Isolated in the early 1970s, GnRH is a decapeptide with a half-life of less than 10 minutes. Pharmacologic amino acid changes can markedly extend its half-life and change its biologic activity from an agonist to an antagonist (Fig. 15-12) (Redding, 1973). Most information concerning GnRH and the GnRH receptor is based on studies of a single isoform of each. Recently, however, additional molecular forms of GnRH and its receptor have been identified (p. 406).

Migration of the Gonadotropin-Releasing Hormone Neurons. Many hypothalamic neurons arise within the central nervous system, but GnRH-containing neurons have a unique embryologic origin. Specifically, progenitor GnRH neurons originate in the medial olfactory placode and migrate along the vomeronasal nerve into the hypothalamus (Fig. 16-5, p. 447). A series of soluble factors regulate GnRH neuronal migration at specific locations along their migratory route. These factors include secreted signaling molecules such as GABA, adhesion

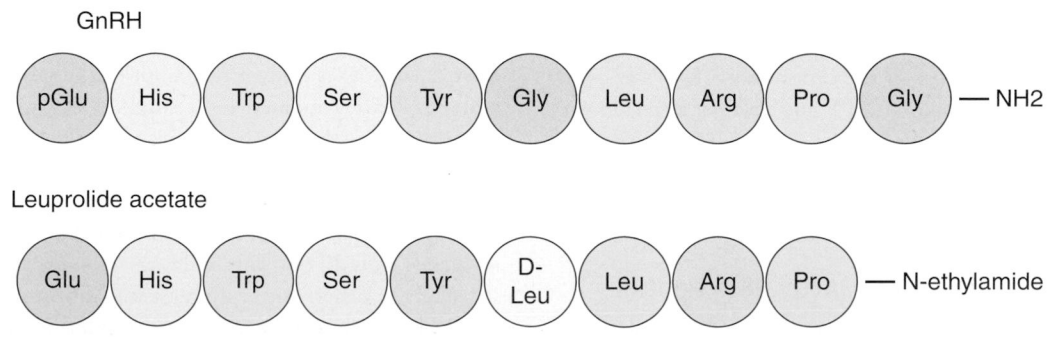

FIGURE 15-12 Schematic drawing shows the similar amino acid composition of the decapeptide gonadotropin-releasing hormone (GnRH) and of its synthetic agonist leuprolide acetate.

molecules, and growth factors (Tobet, 2006; Wierman, 2004). Failure of normal migration may result from a variety of genetic defects in these signalling molecules and can lead to Kallmann syndrome, which is discussed in greater detail in Chapter 16 (p. 447).

In primates, GnRH cell bodies are primarily located within the arcuate nucleus. From these neuronal cell bodies, GnRH is axonally transported along the tuberoinfundibular tract to the median eminence. Gonadotropin-releasing hormone (GnRH) is then secreted into the portal system that drains directly to the anterior pituitary gland and stimulates gonadotropin biosynthesis and secretion. The number of GnRH neurons in the adult is strikingly low, with only a few thousand cells dispersed within the arcuate nucleus.

The olfactory origin of GnRH neurons and nasal epithelial cells suggest a link between reproduction and olfactory signals. Compounds released by one individual that affect other members of the same species are known as *pheromones*. Pheromones obtained from the axillary secretions of women in the late follicular phase accelerate the LH surge and shorten menstrual cycles of women exposed to these chemicals. Secretions from women in the luteal phase have the opposite effects. Thus, pheromones may be one mechanism by which women who are together frequently often exhibit synchronous menstrual cycles (Stern, 1998).

A subset of GnRH neurons sends projections into other areas of the central nervous system, including the limbic system. These projections are not required for gonadotropin secretion, but may play a role in modulation of reproductive behavior (Nakai, 1978; Silverman, 1987).

Pulsatile Gonadotropin-Releasing Hormone Secretion.

In elegant experiments, Knobil (1974) demonstrated that pulsatile delivery of GnRH to the pituitary gonadotropes was required to achieve sustained gonadotropin secretion in a primate model. As shown in Figure 15-13, continuous infusion with GnRH rapidly decreased both LH and FSH secretion, an effect that is easily reversed with a return to pulsatile stimulation. This characteristic is exploited clinically by administration of long-acting GnRH agonists to treat steroid-dependent conditions such as endometriosis, leiomyomas, breast cancer, and

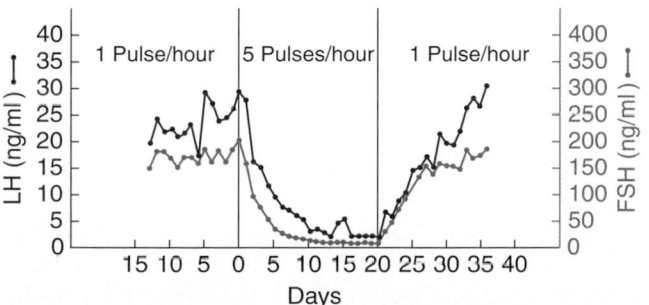

FIGURE 15-13 Graph shows changes in luteinizing hormone (LH) and follicle-stimulating hormone (FSH) levels with variation in gonadotropin-releasing hormone (GnRH) pulsatile release. *(From Knobil, 1980, with permission.)*

prostate cancer. Such agonists disrupt pulsatile GnRH release, lead to depressed gonadotropin release, and in turn result in lowered serum ovarian sex steroid levels.

Pulsatile release of GnRH is more frequent but of lower amplitude during the follicular phase compared with the luteal phase. More rapid pulse frequencies preferentially stimulate LH, whereas slower frequencies favor FSH secretion (Wildt, 1981). Therefore, changes in GnRH pulse frequency affect the absolute levels as well as the ratio of LH to FSH release.

Pulsatile activity is currently believed to be an intrinsic property of GnRH neurons. Other hormones and neurotransmitters thus provide modulatory effects (Clayton, 1981; Yen, 1985). In animal models, estrogen increases GnRH pulse frequency and therefore leads to an increase in LH levels relative to FSH levels. In contrast, progesterone decreases GnRH pulsatility. As less frequent GnRH pulses preferentially stimulate FSH over LH secretion, the increase in progesterone during the luteal phase may explain the preferential stimulation of FSH observed toward the end of this phase. This rise in FSH is critical for the initiation of follicular recruitment.

Opioid Peptides and Gonadotropin-Releasing Hormone. Opioid tone in the brain plays a central role in menstrual cyclicity by suppressing the hypothalamic release of GnRH (Funabashi, 1994). Estrogen promotes endorphin secretion, and this is increased further with the addition of progesterone (Cetel, 1985). Thus, endorphin levels increase during the follicular phase, peak during the luteal phase, and drop markedly during menses. This pattern suggests that opioid tone acts along with progesterone to decrease GnRH pulse frequency in the luteal phase relative to the follicular phase. For reasons that are not fully understood, a release from opioid suppression of GnRH occurs at the time of ovulation (King, 1984).

For many years, it was thought that GnRH neurons did not express estrogen receptors, and therefore, estrogen feedback at the hypothalamus must occur via effects on hypothalamic neurons with synaptic connections to the GnRH neurons. However, it is now known that GnRH neurons express the estrogen receptor ERβ. Progesterone receptors have not been identified in GnRH-expressing neurons. Therefore, it is currently believed that the ovarian steroids affect GnRH neuronal activity via direct and indirect mechanisms, with opioids acting as a critical intermediary for negative feedback.

◼ Other Hypothalamic-Pituitary Axes
Dopamine and Prolactin

The most important neurotransmitters in reproductive neuroendocrinology are the three monoamines—dopamine, norepinephrine, and serotonin. Dopamine-containing fibers that regulate pituitary function arise chiefly in the hypothalamic arcuate nucleus and project to the median eminence where dopamine enters the portal vessels. Dopamine present in hypophyseal portal vessel blood is of sufficient concentration

TABLE 15-7. Hypothalamic-Pituitary Products and Their End Organs

Hypothalamus	Pituitary	End Organ
GnRH	LH/FSH	Gonads
Dopamine	PRL	Breast
TRH	TSH	Thyroid
CRH	ACTH	Adrenal
GHRH	GH	Somatic

ACTH = adrenocorticotropin hormone; CRH = corticotropin-releasing hormone; FSH = follicle-stimulating hormone; GH = growth hormone; GHRH = growth hormone–releasing hormone; GnRH = gonadotropin-releasing hormone; LH = luteinizing hormone; PRL = prolactin; TRH = thyrotropin-releasing hormone; TSH = thyroid-stimulating hormone.

to inhibit PRL release, and dopamine is the principal prolactin inhibitory factor (PIF) (Table 15-7). In contrast, prolactin-releasing factors, although less potent, include TRH, vasopressin, vasoactive intestinal peptide (VIP), endogenous opioids, and acetylcholine.

There are five forms of the dopamine receptor divided into two groups, D_1 and D_2. Cells in the anterior pituitary gland primarily express the D_2 subtypes. The medical treatment of prolactinomas has been improved in terms of both effectiveness and patient tolerance by the development of the D_2-specific ligands. For example, the dopamine agonist cabergoline is a D_2-specific ligand, whereas bromocriptine is nonspecific.

Thyrotropin-Releasing Hormone

As indicated by its name, thyrotropin-releasing hormone (TRH) stimulates secretion of thyroid-stimulating hormone (TSH) from the anterior pituitary gland's thyrotrope subpopulation. Of note, TRH is also a potent prolactin-releasing factor and results in a clinical link between hypothyroidism and secondary hyperprolactinemia (Fig. 16-8, p. 452) (Krieger, 1980).

Thyroid-stimulating hormone binds to specific receptors on the plasma cell membrane of thyroid cells, stimulating the biosynthesis of thyroid hormones through an increase in thyroid gland size and vascularity. Thyroid hormone exerts negative feedback on TRH and TSH releasing cells.

Corticotropin-Releasing Hormone

This is the primary hypothalamic factor that stimulates synthesis and secretion of ACTH. Consisting of 41 amino acid residues, corticotropin-releasing hormone (CRH) is distributed in multiple locations within the hypothalamus and other CNS areas. Release of CRH is stimulated by catecholaminergic input from other brain pathways and inhibited by endogenous opioids.

Corticotropin-releasing hormone binds to a family of CRH receptors and stimulates ACTH biosynthesis and secretion. In turn, ACTH stimulates glucocorticoid production by the adrenal's zona fasciculata and androgen production by its zona reticularis. Corticotropin-releasing hormone secretion is under negative-feedback regulation by circulating cortisol produced in the adrenal gland. In contrast, mineralocorticoid production by the zona glomerulosa is primarily regulated via the renin-angiotensin system. As a result, abnormalities in the CRH–ACTH pathway do not result in electrolyte disturbances.

Central CRH pathways are believed to mediate many stress responses (Sutton, 1982). Clinically, in women with hypothalamic amenorrhea, CRH levels have been found to be elevated. Increased levels of CRH inhibit hypothalamic GnRH secretion by direct action as well as by augmenting central opioid concentrations (Fig. 16-7, p. 449). This functional pathway may explain the association between hypercortisolism and menstrual abnormalities.

Growth Hormone–Releasing Hormone

Growth hormone secretion by pituitary somatotropes is primarily regulated through stimulation by hypothalamic growth hormone-releasing hormone (GHRH) and inhibition by somatostatin. Expression of GHRH is limited to the hypothalamus with the exception of placental and immune cells, which also secrete this hormone. In contrast, somatostatin is widely distributed in the CNS as well as in the placenta, pancreas, and gastrointestinal tract.

As with GnRH, GHRH depends on pulsatile secretion to exert a physiologic effect. Exercise, stress, sleep, and hypoglycemia stimulate GH release, whereas free fatty acids and other factors related to adiposity blunt growth hormone release. Estrogen, testosterone, and thyroid hormone also play a role in increased GH secretion.

Growth hormone stimulates skeletal and muscle growth, regulates lipolysis, and promotes the cellular uptake of amino acids. This hormone induces insulin resistance and therefore, GH excess may be associated with new-onset diabetes mellitus. Most of the growth effects of GH are mediated via the insulin-like growth factors, IGF-I and IGF-II. These growth factors are produced in high quantities in the liver for release into the circulation. Many of the target tissues also synthesize IGFs where they exert local effects. Within the ovary, IGF-I modulates steroid action during folliculogenesis. This factor also acts to suppress GH secretion. Circulating IGF-I and IGF-II are bound to binding proteins, which modulate IGF action at target tissues. In terms of mediating growth factor activity, regulating expression of these binding proteins may be as important as regulation of the IGFs themselves in modulating growth factor activity.

Posterior Pituitary Gland

Unlike the anterior pituitary gland, the posterior pituitary (neurohypophysis) consists of the axon terminals of magnocellular neurons arising in the supraoptic and paraventricular nuclei of the hypothalamus (see Fig. 15-11). These neurons synthesize the nine-amino-acid cyclic peptides oxytocin and arginine vasopressin. Precursors for these peptides are produced in the neuronal cell body and transported down the axon in secretory granules. During transport, precursors are cleaved into mature peptides and a carrier protein—neurophysin (Verbalis, 1983). Activation of these neurons generates an axon potential that results in calcium influx and secretion of granule contents into the perivascular space. These secreted peptides then enter adjacent blood vessels for transport throughout the peripheral circulation.

Oxytocin

Oxytocin has significant roles in both parturition and lactation (Kiss, 2005). It is currently believed that this peptide does not play a role in labor initiation as serum oxytocin levels are constant until the expulsive portion of labor (Fisher, 1983). Nevertheless, an increase in myometrial and decidual oxytocin-receptor expression has been noted near term, primarily due to an increase in estrogen levels.

It is well documented that oxytocin is the primary mediator of myometrial contractility once labor has been initiated. Cervical and vaginal stimulation results in an acute release of oxytocin from the posterior pituitary in a process known as the *Ferguson reflex*. Clinically, oxytocin's ability to induce uterine contractions is exploited to induce or augment labor.

Vaginal distension, such as occurs with coitus, also increases oxytocin release. Based on this observation, it has been suggested that oxytocin may be responsible for the rhythmic uterine and tubal contractions that aid sperm delivery to the oocyte. Oxytocin may also play a role in orgasm and ejaculation.

The anterior pituitary hormone prolactin is critical for milk production in breast alveoli. The glandular cells of the alveoli are surrounded by a mesh of myoepithelial cells. Suckling triggers nerve impulses from mechanoreceptors in the nipple and areola that increase hypothalamic neuronal activity. Axon terminals passing to the posterior pituitary gland release oxytocin, which causes the myoepithelial cells to contract and thereby express milk from the alveoli into the ducts and sinuses (Crowley, 1992). Other conditioned stimuli, such as the sight, sound, or smell of a baby or sexual arousal, will have similar effects. Inhibition of milk let-down can follow stress, fear, embarrassment, or distraction. Therefore, women are encouraged to find a relaxing, private environment when breast feeding.

Oxytocin expression has been detected in multiple tissues in addition to the posterior pituitary gland, including the anterior pituitary, placenta, fallopian tubes, and gonads, with high expression in the corpus luteum (Williams, 1990). Its function in these tissues has yet to be elucidated.

ABNORMALITIES IN THE HYPOTHALAMIC-PITUITARY AXIS

Abnormalities in the hypothalamic-pituitary axis result in hypogonadotropic hypogonadism and can be categorized as either developmental or acquired. Developmental lesions due to inherited genetic defects include Kallmann syndrome and idiopathic hypogonadotropic hypogonadism. Acquired abnormalities include functional disorders (eating disorders, excessive exercise, stress) and hypothalamic-pituitary lesions due to tumor, infiltrative diseases, infarction, surgery, or radiation therapy. Information regarding functional hypothalamic disorders and other causes of hypogonadotropic hypogonadism

can be found in Chapter 16 (p. 447). Hyperprolactinemia and pituitary adenomas will be discussed in the following sections.

Hyperprolactinemia
Etiology of Hyperprolactinemia

Elevated circulating prolactin levels can be caused by a variety of physiologic activities including pregnancy, sleep, eating, and coitus. Increased prolactin levels, which in general can lead to galactorrhea, may also be observed following chest wall stimulation such as occurs with suckling, breast examination, chest wall surgery, herpes zoster infection, or nipple piercing (Table 12-3, p. 340). Prolactin is primarily regulated by tonic dopamine inhibition of secretion. Prolactin secretion is increased by serotonin, norepinephrine, opioids, estrogen, and TRH. Therefore, medications that block dopamine-receptor action (phenothiazines) or deplete catecholamine levels (monoamine oxidase inhibitors) may increase PRL levels (Table 12-4, p. 341). Moreover, hyperprolactinemia may be caused by tumor, radiation, or infiltrative diseases such as sarcoid and tuberculosis, which damage the pituitary stalk and prevent dopamine-mediated inhibition of PRL secretion.

Primary hypothyroidism is also associated with mild elevations in serum PRL levels (Van Gaal, 1981). Specifically, low-circulating thyroid hormone levels produce a reflex increase in hypothalamic TRH levels due to loss of feedback inhibition. Thyrotropin-releasing hormone can bind directly to anterior pituitary lactotropes and stimulate PRL production (Haisenleder, 1992). As a rule, thyroid function tests should be measured when confirming a diagnosis of hyperprolactinemia as a patient may require thyroid replacement rather than further evaluation for pituitary adenoma.

Prolactin-secreting adenomas, also termed prolactinomas, are the most common pituitary adenoma and the most common adenomas to be diagnosed by gynecologists. Most affected women present with microadenomas and signs of PRL excess such as galactorrhea and amenorrhea (Davis, 2004).

Diagnosis of Hyperprolactinemia

Serum Prolactin Levels. Hyperprolactinemia is, by definition, present in any patient with an elevated serum PRL level. Optimally, PRL levels are drawn in the morning, that is, at the time of the PRL nadir. Prior to testing, breast examination is avoided to prevent false-positive results. If a mildly elevated PRL level is found, sampling should be repeated because PRL levels vary throughout the day. Moreover, many factors including the stress of venipuncture may produce false elevations.

Normal PRL levels are typically less than 20 ng/mL in nonpregnant women, although the upper limit of normal varies by assay. Importantly, PRL levels rise nearly 10-fold during pregnancy and make detection of a prolactinoma difficult at this time. Occasionally, the reported prolactin value will be falsely low due to a "hook effect" present in the assay (Frieze, 2002). That is, the presence of very high levels of endogenous hormone oversaturate the test antibodies and thereby prevent required binding between a patient's PRL and the labeled assay PRL. This problem is overcome with dilution of a patient's

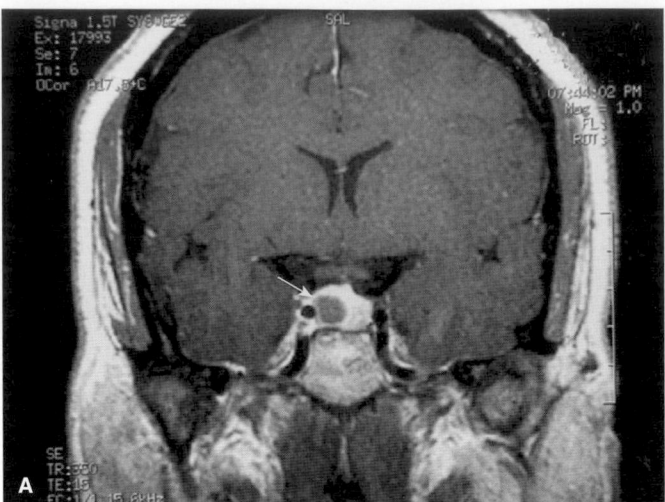
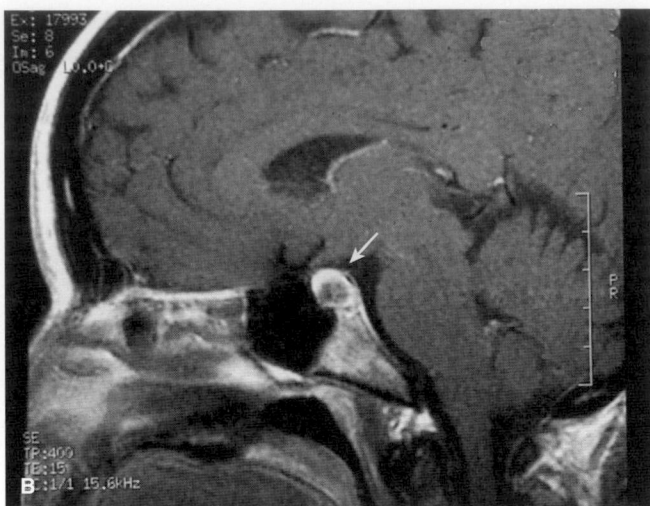

FIGURE 15-14 Magnetic resonance image of a pituitary microadenoma (*arrow*). **A.** Coronal image. **B.** Sagittal image.

sample. Importantly, a mismatch between the adenoma size noted on magnetic resonance (MR) imaging and the degree of PRL level elevation should alert a clinician to either the possibility of an incorrect assay result or the likelihood that the macroadenoma is actually not primarily PRL secreting. Macroadenomas of any cell type may damage the pituitary stalk and prevent transfer of hypothalamic dopamine to the lactotropes.

Conversely, a patient may rarely have an elevated PRL level on assay despite a lack of clinical features of hyperprolactinemia. The hyperprolactinemia in these patients is thought to be secondary to alternate forms of PRL, including the so-called big or macroprolactin, which contains multimers of native PRL. Macroprolactin is not physiologically active but may be detected by PRL assays (Fahie-Wilson, 2005).

Radiologic Imaging. Magnetic resonance imaging is advisable for all patients with confirmed hyperprolactinemia. Some experts advocate limiting imaging to women with a PRL level exceeding 100 ng/mL as lower levels are most likely due to small microadenomas (Fig. 15-14). Although this is undoubtedly a safe approach in most women, mildly elevated PRL levels also may be due to pituitary stalk compression by a nonprolactin-secreting macroadenoma or a craniopharyngioma, which are diagnoses with severe potential consequences.

The availability of sensitive neuroimaging techniques now affords earlier diagnosis and intervention. In the past, pituitary adenomas were identified using a coned-down view of the sella turcica during standard head radiography. Although computed tomography (CT) scanning provides useful information on tumor size, bony artifacts may limit interpretation. Therefore, MR imaging, using both T1- and T2-weighted images, has become the preferred radiologic approach due to its high sensitivity and excellent spatial resolution (Ruscalleda, 2005). Frequently, MR imaging is performed with and without gadolinium infusion for maximum definition of tumor size and extension.

Hyperprolactinemia and Amenorrhea

The primary mechanism by which hyperprolactinemia results in amenorrhea is believed to be due to a reflex increase in

central dopamine (Fig. 16-8, p. 452). Stimulation of the dopaminergic receptors on the GnRH neurons alters GnRH pulsatility, thereby disrupting folliculogenesis. As dopamine receptors have also been identified in the ovaries, detrimental effects on folliculogenesis may also play a role. Additional mechanisms undoubtedly exist in view of the complexity of the interactions between the various hormones, peptides, and neurotransmitters that influence hypothalamic function.

Pituitary Adenomas
Classification of Adenomas

Pituitary adenomas are the most common cause of acquired pituitary dysfunction and comprise approximately 10 percent of all intracranial tumors. Clinically, symptoms of galactorrhea, menstrual disturbances, or infertility may lead to its diagnosis. Most tumors are benign, and only an estimated 0.1 percent of adenomas develop into frank carcinoma with metastasis (Kaltsas, 2005). Nevertheless, pituitary adenomas may cause striking abnormalities in both endocrine and nervous system function (Table 15-8).

Pituitary adenomas were historically classified as eosinophilic, basophilic, or chromophobic according to their hematoxylin and eosin staining characteristics. Tumors are now classified by their hormonal expression pattern as determined by immunohistochemistry (Fig. 15-15). Adenomas are further grouped by size into microadenomas (<10 mm in diameter) and macroadenomas (>10 mm in diameter).

Most adenomas secrete PRL, however, adenomas may secrete any of the pituitary hormones either as a single hormone (monohormonal adenoma) or in combinations (multihormonal adenoma). In the past, a subset of tumors was considered nonsecreting. However, with more sensitive assays, most have been determined to secrete the common α-subunit or the gonadotropin β-subunits and therefore are gonadotrope-derived. Rarely, both α- and β-subunits are secreted as functional dimeric hormone.

TABLE 15-8. Clinical Features of Pituitary Adenomas

Adenoma Cell Origin	Hormone Product	Clinical Syndrome	Reproductive Effects	Testing	Typical Results	Treatment
Lactotrope	PRL	Hypogonadism, galactorrhea	Disrupts GnRH pulsatility	Serum PRL level	Elevated	Surgical excision; dopamine agonist; see Fig. 15-16
Gonadotrope	FSH, LH, subunits	Silent or hypogonadism; less commonly, gonadotropin excess or panhypopituitarism	Disrupts GnRH pulsatility	Serum gonadotropin α-subunit	Elevated	Surgical excision
Somatotrope	GH	Acromegaly/gigantism, menstrual irregularity	Disrupts GnRH pulsatility, ovarian steroidogenesis, LH receptor synthesis, and inhibin secretion	IGF-I level, 100-g glucose suppression test	Elevated No GH suppression	Surgical excision; somatostatin agonists: octreotide or lanreotide
Corticotrope	ACTH	Cushing syndrome, amenorrhea	Disrupts GnRH pulsatility	24-hr urine collection with free cortisol measurement	Elevated serum ACTH and urinary cortisol levels	Surgical excision; ketoconazole blunts adrenal steroidogenesis
				CRH stimulation test	Elevated serum ACTH and cortisol levels	
				BIPSS	ACTH levels in BIPSS sample higher than in serum	
Thyrotrope	TSH	Thyrotoxicosis, menstrual abnormalities	Increases SHBG; Increases conversion of androgens to estrogens	Serum TSH, T_3, and T_4 levels	All elevated	Surgical excision, PTU or tapazole preoperatively to normalize thyroid levels, β-blockers to control associated tachycardia

ACTH = adrenocorticotropin hormone; BIPSS = bilateral inferior petrosal sinus sampling; CRH = corticotropin-releasing hormone; FSH = follicle-stimulating hormone; GH = growth hormone; GnRH = gonadotropin releasing hormone; IGF — insulin-like growth factor; LH = luteinizing hormone; PRL = prolactin; PTU = propylthiouracil; SHBG = sex hormone-binding globulin; TSH = thyroid-stimulating hormone. T_3 = triiodothyronine; T_4 = thyroxine.

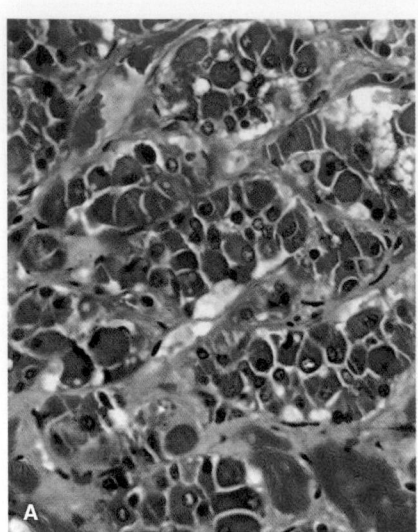 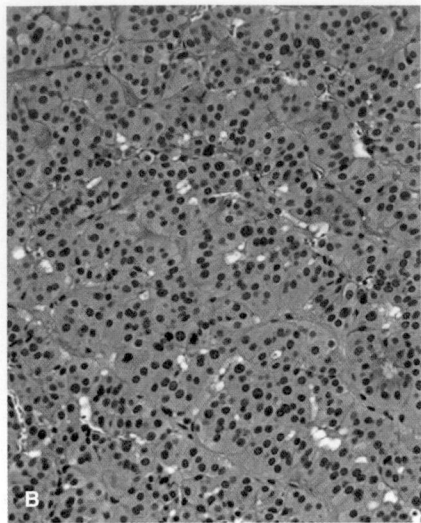 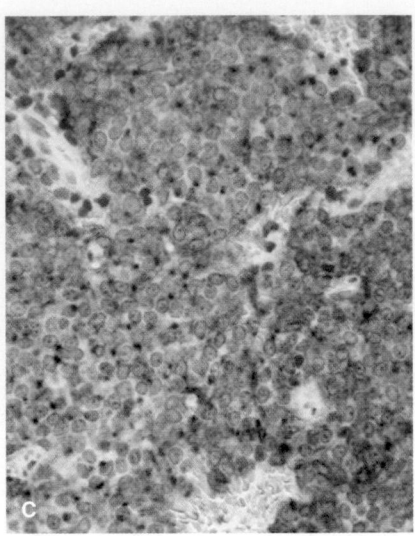

FIGURE 15-15 Photomicrographs from the anterior pituitary gland. **A.** Normal anterior pituitary gland. Secretory cells of the various types are arranged in small clusters between sinusoidal capillaries (H&E, 200×). **B.** Pituitary adenoma. In contrast to normal anterior pituitary gland, adenomas are composed of highly monomorphic cells. Note the absence of small clusters and sinusoids (H&E, 100×). **C.** Prolactin-secreting adenoma. Immunohistochemistry demonstrates expression of prolactin by many of the neoplastic cells. The dot-like pattern is characteristic of many prolactin-producing adenomas (HRP/DAB, 100×). *(Photographs contributed by Dr. Jack Raisanen.)*

Pituitary Adenoma Symptoms

Endocrinopathy. Pituitary adenomas may cause symptoms via excess hormone secretion and lead to clinical conditions such as hyperprolactinemia, acromegaly, or Cushing disease. Alternatively, adenomas may result in hormone deficiency due to damage of other pituitary cell types or of the pituitary stalk by an expanding adenoma or following treatment of the primary lesion.

As might be predicted, pituitary microadenomas are typically diagnosed during evaluation of an endocrinopathy, whereas macroadenomas frequently come to medical attention when a patient presents with symptoms from invasion of surrounding structures. The anterior pituitary gland neighbors both the optic chiasm and cavernous sinuses. Disruption of the optic chiasm by suprasellar growth of the pituitary mass may present as bitemporal hemianopsia in which patients have loss of the outer portion of the right and left visual fields. The cavernous sinuses are a paired collection of thin-walled veins located on either side of the sella turcica. Pituitary tumor compression can lead to cavernous sinus syndrome, which consists of a constellation of symptoms including headache, visual disturbances, and cranial nerve palsies, specifically cranial nerves III, IV, and VI.

Reproductive Effects of Pituitary Adenomas. Any pituitary mass or infiltrate can present as an abnormality in reproductive function that may include delayed puberty, anovulation, oligomenorrhea, and infertility. The exact mechanisms linking adenomas to menstrual dysfunction are not well understood for many adenoma subtypes, with the exception of prolactinomas. Macroadenomas likely affect reproductive function either by compressing the pituitary stalk with resultant hyperprolactinemia or less commonly, by directly compressing gonadotropes.

Pregnancy and Pituitary Adenomas. The pituitary gland enlarges during pregnancy, primarily due to hypertrophy and hyperplasia of the lactotropes in response to elevated serum estrogen levels. Although there is a risk of tumor enlargement during pregnancy, clinical experience has shown that the risk is small, particularly for microadenomas (Molitch, 2010). However, because significant expansion may lead to headaches or compression of the optic chiasm and blindness, visual field testing should be considered every trimester for women with macroadenomas. Although therapy is likely to be safe, most experts advise that dopamine agonist therapy be discontinued during pregnancy (Webster, 1996).

Pituitary Apoplexy. Spontaneous hemorrhage into a pituitary adenoma, termed *pituitary apoplexy*, is a rare life-threatening medical emergency. Apoplexy may lead to severe hypoglycemia, hypotension, CNS hemorrhage, and death. Signs and symptoms include acute visual changes, severe headache, neck stiffness, hypotension, loss of consciousness, and coma. These symptoms result from:(1) leakage of blood and necrotic material into the subarachnoid space, (2) acute hypopituitarism, and (3) development of a rapidly expanding hemorrhagic intrasellar mass that compresses the optic chiasm, cranial nerves, or hypothalamus and internal carotid arteries.

Treatment of Hyperprolactinemia and Pituitary Adenomas

Medical

Dopamine agonists may be considered in any patient with hyperprolactinemia in whom a large non-prolactin producing tumor or other cause of hyperprolactinemia has been excluded. In this situation, it is likely that the patient has an undetectable microadenoma, although the incidence of this occurrence is decreasing with the advent of highly sensitive magnetic resonance (MR) imaging.

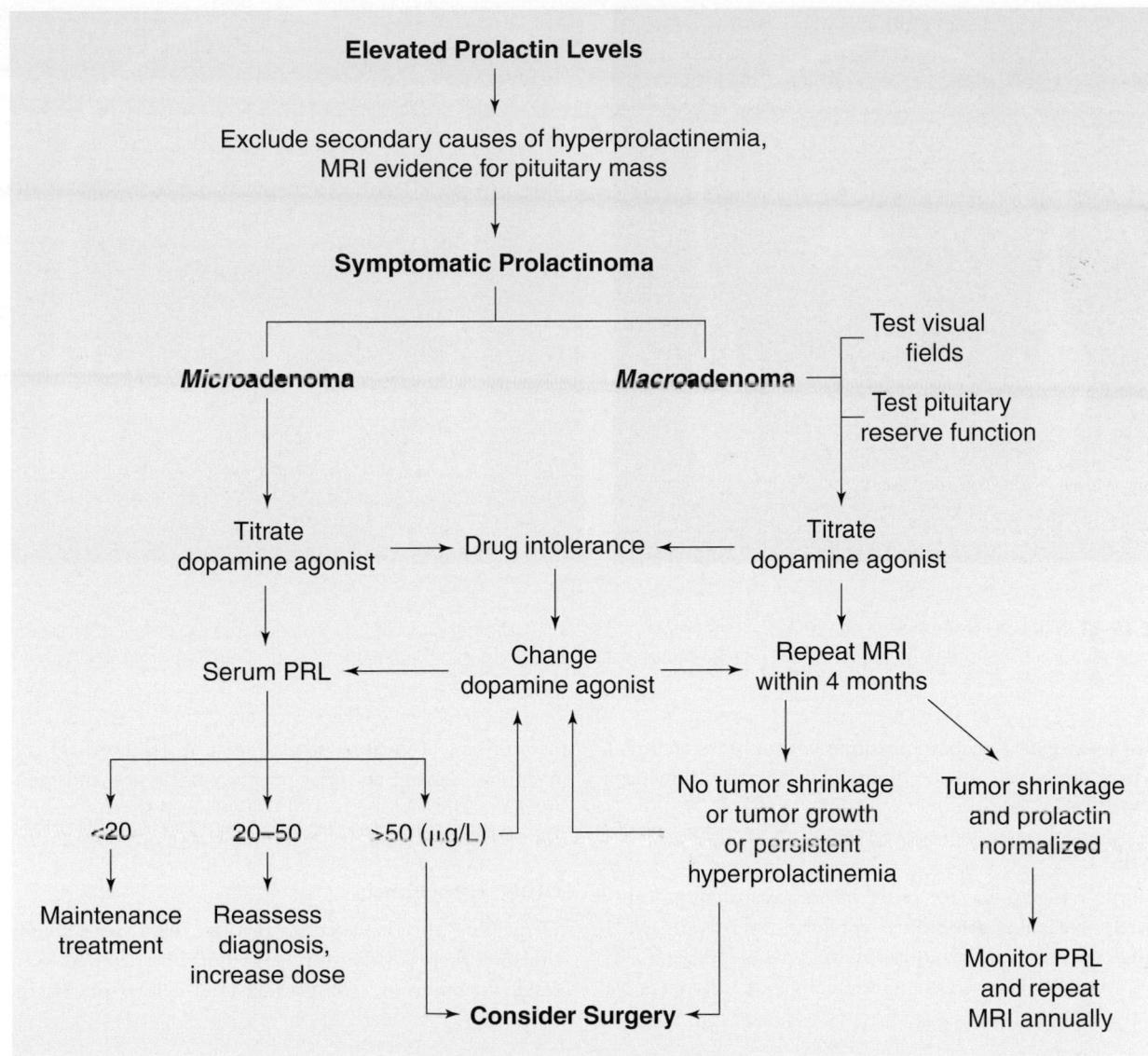

Elevated Prolactin Levels

Exclude secondary causes of hyperprolactinemia,
MRI evidence for pituitary mass

Symptomatic Prolactinoma

*Micro*adenoma   *Macro*adenoma — Test visual fields

Test pituitary reserve function

Titrate dopamine agonist → Drug intolerance ← Titrate dopamine agonist

Serum PRL ← Change dopamine agonist → Repeat MRI within 4 months

<20   20–50   >50 (μg/L)   No tumor shrinkage or tumor growth or persistent hyperprolactinemia   Tumor shrinkage and prolactin normalized

Maintenance treatment   Reassess diagnosis, increase dose   **Consider Surgery**   Monitor PRL and repeat MRI annually

FIGURE 15-16 Algorithm describing the evaluation and treatment of pituitary prolactinomas. MRI = magnetic resonance imaging; PRL = prolactin. *(From Melmed, 2008, with permission.)*

Most pituitary tumors grow slowly, and many cease growth after attainment of a certain size. Thus, asymptomatic patients with a microprolactinoma may be managed conservatively with serial MR imaging and serum PRL levels every 1 to 2 years as the risk of progression to a macroadenoma is less than 10 percent (Schlechte, 1989). These women should be followed for even mild changes in menstrual cyclicity as they are at risk for developing hypoestrogenism and resultant risk for osteopenia or osteoporosis (Klibanski, 1980).

When tumors of any size are associated with symptoms of amenorrhea or galactorrhea, therapy should be considered (Fig. 15-16). Neurosurgical evaluation is mandatory when visual field defects or severe headaches are present. In general, first-line treatment is medical for both micro- and macroadenomas. Specifically, women should receive a dopamine agonist such as the nonspecific dopamine-receptor agonist bromocriptine (Parlodel) or the dopamine-receptor type 2 agonist cabergoline (Dostinex).

These dopamine agonists decrease PRL secretion and shrink tumor size (Molitch, 2001). However, bromocriptine treatment is associated with a number of common side effects, including headache, postural hypotension, blurred vision, drowsiness, and leg cramps. Most of these are attributable to activation of type 1 dopamine receptors. Due to its receptor specificity, cabergoline treatment is generally better tolerated than bromocriptine. Cabergoline also has a longer half-life than bromocriptine, allowing once- or twice-weekly dosing compared with the multiple daily doses that may be required for bromocriptine. Typical initial cabergoline dosages are 0.25 mg orally twice weekly. Cabergoline has been found to be more effective than bromocriptine in normalizing PRL levels (Di Sarno, 2001; Webster, 1994). Nevertheless, cabergoline can be prohibitively expensive. Most patients can tolerate bromocriptine if started at a low dose—½ tab or 0.125 mg—each night to minimize associated nausea and dizziness. This dose can be slowly increased to three times

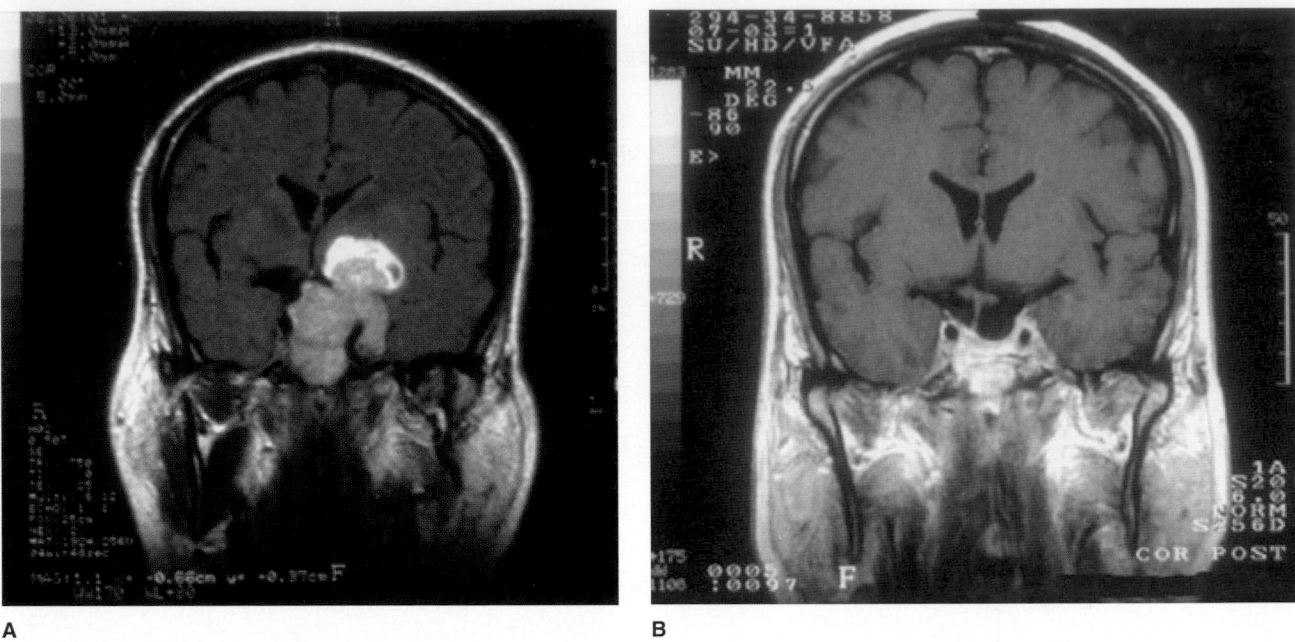

FIGURE 15-17 Magnetic resonance image of a pituitary before and after surgical resection of a macroadenoma. **A.** Preoperative coronal image reveals tumor measuring greater than 10 mm. **B.** Postoperative coronal image of the same patient following tumor excision.

daily as tolerated. Reliable measurement of posttreatment serum prolactin levels can be obtained 1 month following a steady medication dose.

Surgical

Neurosurgery is required for refractory tumors or those causing acutely worsening symptoms. The pituitary is approached through a transsphenoidal route whenever possible (Fig. 15-17). Complications of surgery, although rare, include intraoperative

hemorrhage, a cerebrospinal fluid leak (rhinorrhea), diabetes insipidus, damage to other pituitary cell types, and meningitis (Arafah, 1986; Molitch, 1999). Radiation therapy may be used for patients with surgically nonresectable or persistent tumors.

Other Treatments

Depending on the success of these approaches, additional therapies such as radiation therapy may be required to manage residual symptoms. The gamma knife allows precise focus of

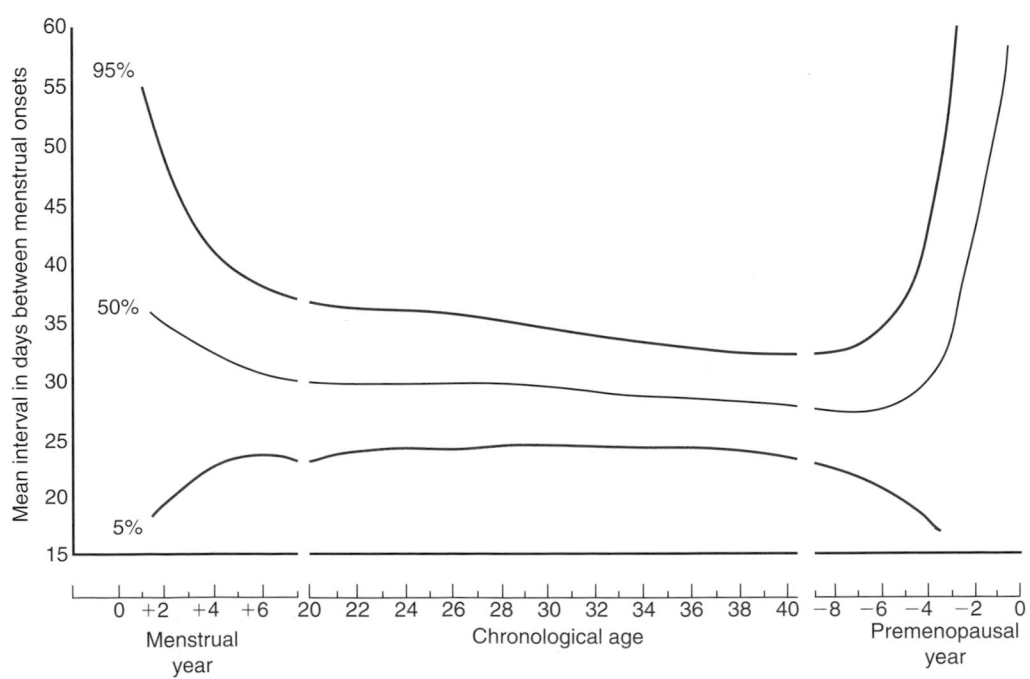

FIGURE 15-18 Graphic depiction of menstrual cycle length variation with age. *(Data from Treloar, 1967.)*

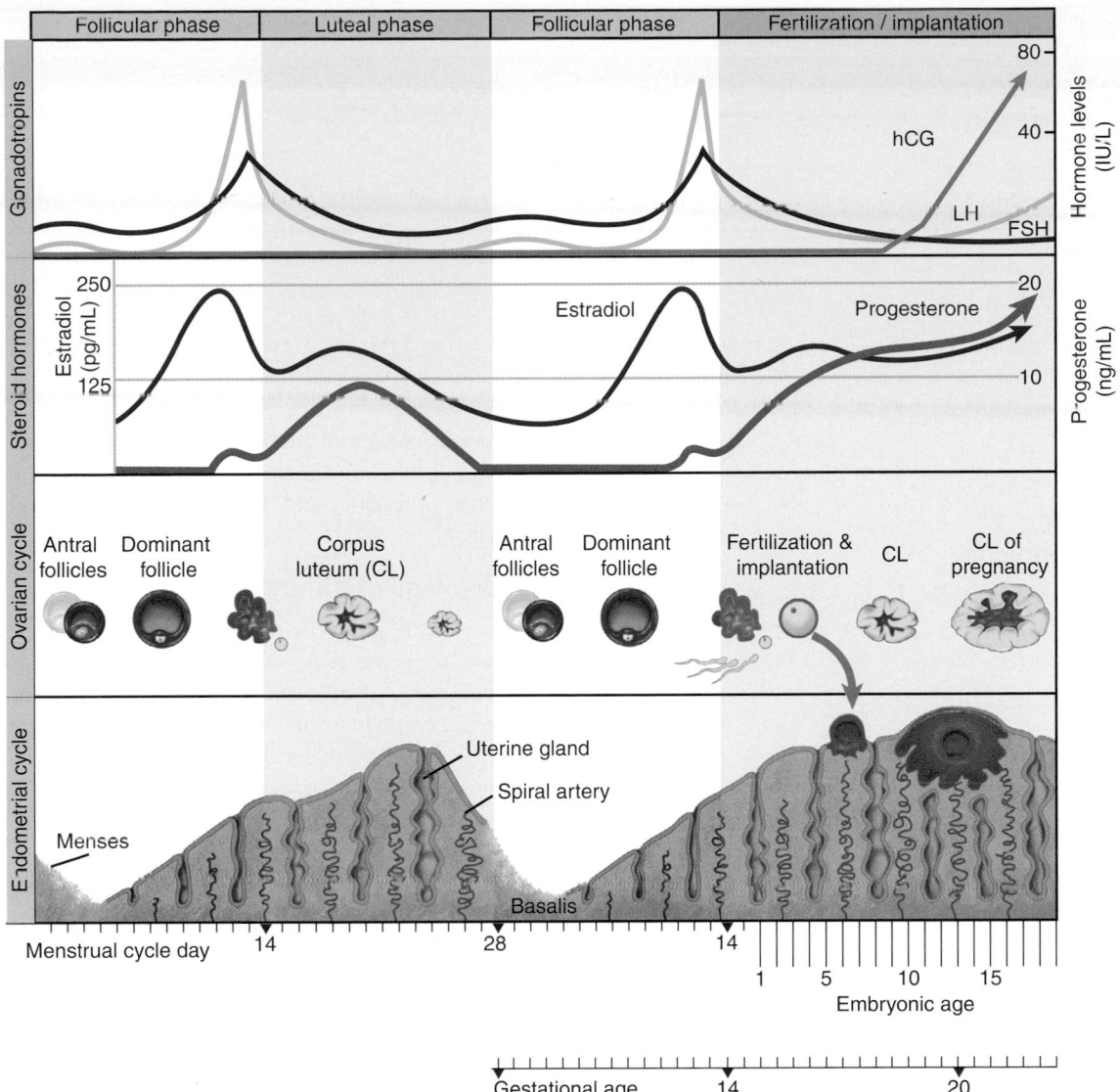

FIGURE 15-19 Gonadotropin control of the ovarian and endometrial cycles. The ovarian-endometrial cycle has been structured as a 28-day cycle. The follicular phase (days 1 to 14) is characterized by rising levels of estrogen, thickening of the endometrium, and selection of the dominant "ovulatory" follicle. During the luteal phase (days 15 to 28), the corpus luteum (CL) produces estrogen and progesterone, which prepare the endometrium for implantation. If implantation occurs, the developing blastocyst will begin to produce human chorionic gonadotropin (hCG) and rescue the corpus luteum, thus maintaining progesterone production. FSH = follicle-stimulating hormone; LH = luteinizing hormone. *(From Cunningham, 2010a, with permission.)*

the radiation beam, significantly decreasing local tissue damage and improving patient tolerance. Gene therapy has been proposed as a treatment for pituitary tumors. Possibilities include the introduction of genes that encode growth-inhibiting factors by retroviral infection. Additional studies are needed to determine whether this approach will be safe and efficacious (Seilicovich, 2005).

MENSTRUAL CYCLE

The "typical" menstrual cycle is defined as 28 ± 7 days with menstrual flow lasting 4 ± 2 days and an average blood loss of 20 to 60 mL. By convention, the first day of vaginal bleeding is considered day 1 of the menstrual cycle. Menstrual

cycle intervals vary among women and often for an individual woman at different times of her reproductive life (Fig. 15-18). In a study of more than 2700 women, menstrual cycle intervals were found to be most irregular in the 2 years following menarche and the 3 years preceding menopause (Treloar, 1967). Specifically, a trend toward shorter intervals is common during early menopausal transition, but is followed by interval lengthening in later transition. The menstrual cycle is least variable between the ages of 20 and 40 years.

When viewed from a perspective of ovarian function, the menstrual cycle can be defined as a preovulatory follicular phase and postovulatory luteal phase (Fig. 15-19). Corresponding phases in the endometrium are termed the proliferative and secretory phases (Table 15-9). For most women,

TABLE 15-9. Menstrual Cycle Characteristics

	Menstrual Phases		
Cycle day	1–5	6–14	15–28
Ovarian phase	Early follicular	Follicular	Luteal
Endometrial phase	Menstrual	Proliferative	Secretory
Estrogen/progesterone	Low levels	Estrogen	Progesterone

the luteal phase of the menstrual cycle is stable, lasting 13 to 14 days. Thus, variations in normal cycle length generally result from variations in the duration of the follicular phase (Ferin, 1974).

The Ovary
Ovarian Morphology

The adult human ovary is oval with a length of 2 to 5 cm, a width of 1.5 to 3 cm, and a thickness of 0.5 to 1.5 cm. During the reproductive years, the ovary weighs between 5 and 10 g. It is comprised of three parts: an outer cortical region, which contains both the germinal epithelium and the follicles; a medullary region, which consists of connective tissue, myoid-like contractile cells, and interstitial cells; and a hilum, which contains blood vessels, lymphatics, and nerves that enter the ovary (Fig. 15-20).

Ovaries have two interrelated functions: the generation of mature oocytes and the production of steroid and peptide hormones that create an environment in which fertilization and subsequent implantation in the endometrium can occur. Endocrine functions of the ovary correlate closely to the morphologic appearance and disappearance of follicles and corpus luteum.

Embryology of the Ovary

The ovary develops from three major cellular sources: (1) primordial germ cells, which arise from the endoderm of the yolk sac and differentiate into the primary oogonia; (2) coelomic epithelial cells, which develop into granulosa cells; and (3) mesenchymal cells from the gonadal ridge, which become the ovarian stroma. Additional information regarding gonadal differentiation can be found in Chapter 18 (p. 482).

OVARY

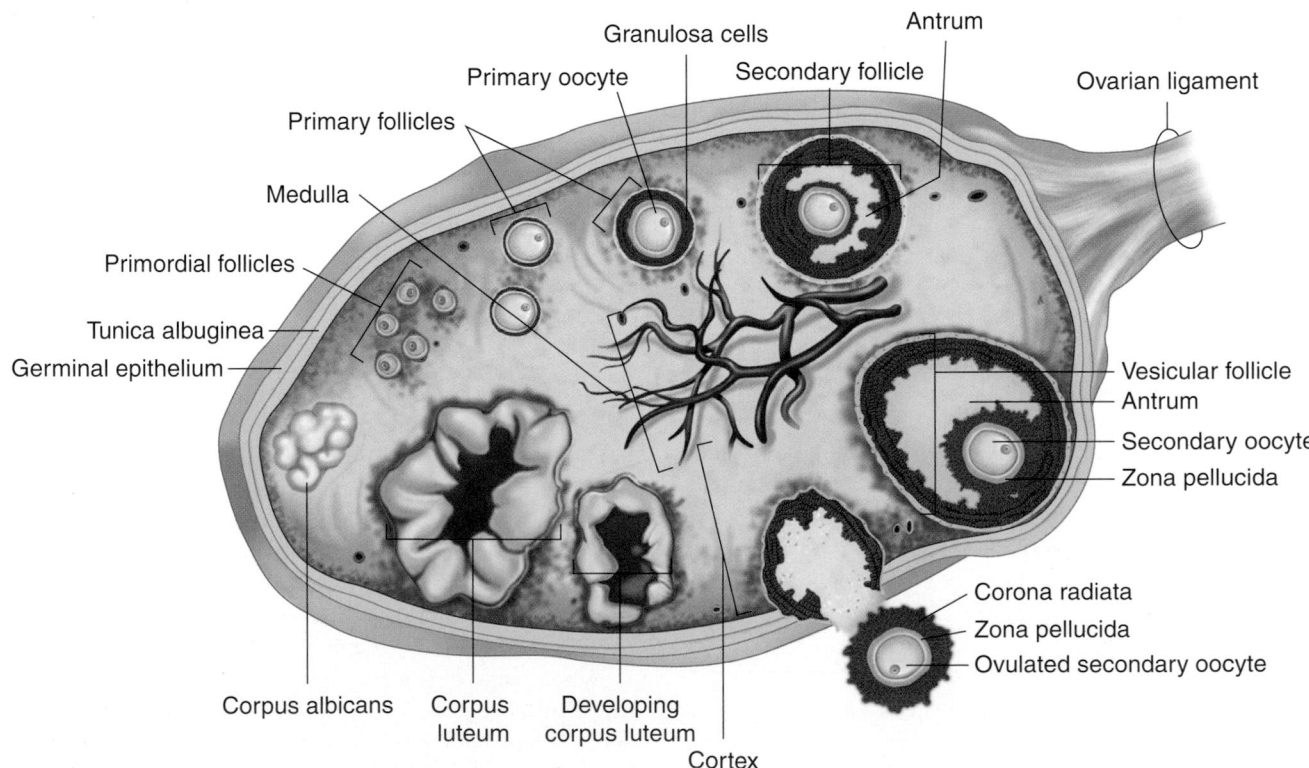

FIGURE 15-20 Drawing depicts ovarian anatomy and various sequential steps of follicular development.

Primordial germ cells can be identified in the yolk sac as early as the third week of gestation (Baker, 1963). These cells begin their migration into the gonadal ridge during the sixth week of gestation and generate the primary sex cords. It is not possible to distinguish the ovary from the testes by histologic criteria until approximately 10 to 11 weeks of fetal life.

After the primordial cells reach the gonad, they continue to multiply through successive mitotic divisions. Starting at 12 weeks' gestation, a subset of oogonia will enter meiosis to become primary oocytes (Baker, 1967). Primary oocytes are surrounded by a single layer of flattened granulosa cells, creating a primordial follicle.

Oocyte Loss with Aging

All oogonia either develop into primary oocytes or become atretic. Based on our current understanding of ovarian function, additional oocytes cannot be generated postnatally. This differs markedly from the male situation in which sperm are produced continuously throughout adulthood. Recent studies have suggested that ovarian stem cells may be able to generate mature oocytes, however, this field of investigation is currently highly controversial (Notarianni, 2011).

The maximal number of oogonia is achieved at the 20th week of gestation, at which time 6 to 7 million oogonia are present in the ovary (Baker, 1963). Approximately 1 to 2 million oogonia are present at birth. Fewer than 400,000 are present at the initiation of puberty, of which fewer than 500 are destined to ovulate (Peters, 1978). Therefore, most germ cells are lost through atresia (Hsueh, 1996).

There is now strong evidence that follicular atresia is not a passive, necrotic process, but rather a precisely controlled active process, namely apoptosis, which is under hormonal control. Apoptosis begins in utero and continues throughout reproductive life.

Meiotic Division During Oocyte Maturation

As previously mentioned, primary oogonia enter meiosis in utero to become primary oocytes. These oocytes are arrested in development at prophase I during the first meiotic division. Meiotic division resumes at ovulation in response to the LH surge. Once again, the process is arrested, this time in the second meiotic metaphase. The arrest of meiosis prior to ovulation is believed to be due to production of an oocyte maturation inhibitor (OMI) by the granulosa cells (Tsafriri, 1982). Meiosis is completed only if fertilization occurs (Fig. 15-21).

Completion of the first meiotic division within the oocyte results in production of a polar body, which contains chromosomal material but minimal cytoplasm. With completion of meiosis following fertilization, a second polar body is extruded. The maternal nucleus, called a pronucleus, fuses with the paternal pronucleus to generate a preembryo with a 46,XX or 46,XY karyotype.

Stromal Cells

Ovarian stroma contains interstitial cells, connective tissue cells, and contractile cells. Of these, connective tissue cells provide structural support to the ovary. Interstitial cells sur-

rounding a developing follicle differentiate into theca cells. Under gonadotropin stimulation, these cells increase in size and develop lipid stores, characteristic of steroid-producing cells (Saxena, 1972).

Another group of interstitial cells is present in the ovarian hilum and therefore are known as hilus cells. These cells closely resemble testicular Leydig cells, and hyperplasia or neoplastic changes in hilar cells may result in virilization from excess testosterone secretion. The normal role of these cells is unknown, but their intimate association with blood vessels and neurons suggest that they may convey systemic signals to the remainder of the ovary (Upadhyay, 1982).

Ovarian Hormone Production
Ovarian Steroidogenesis

The normal functioning ovary synthesizes and secretes the sex-steroid hormones—estrogens, androgens, and progesterone in a precisely controlled pattern determined, in part, by the pituitary gonadotropins, FSH and LH. The most important secretory products of ovarian steroid biosynthesis are progesterone and estradiol. However, the ovary also secretes quantities of estrone, androstenedione, testosterone, and 17α-hydroxyprogesterone. Sex-steroid hormones play an important role in the menstrual cycle by preparing the uterus for implantation of a fertilized ovum. If implantation does not occur, ovarian steroidogenesis declines, the endometrium degenerates, and menstruation ensues.

Two-Cell Theory of Ovarian Steroidogenesis. Ovarian estrogen biosynthesis requires the combined action of two gonadotropins (LH and FSH) on two cell types (theca and granulosa cells). First proposed by Falck in 1959, this concept is known as the two-cell theory of ovarian steroidogenesis (Fig. 15-22) (Peters, 1980). Until the late antral stage of follicular development, LH-receptor expression is limited to the thecal compartment, and FSH-receptor expression is limited to the granulosa cells.

Theca cells express all of the enzymes needed to produce androstenedione. This includes high levels of CYP17 gene expression, whose enzyme product catalyzes 17-hydroxylation—the rate-limiting step in the conversion of progesterones to androgens (Sasano, 1989). This enzyme is absent in the granulosa cells, so they are incapable of producing the precursor needed to produce estrogens. Granulosa cells therefore rely on the theca cells as their primary source for estrogen precursors.

In response to LH stimulation, theca cells synthesize the androgens androstenedione and testosterone. These androgens are secreted into the extracellular fluid and diffuse across the basement membrane to the granulosa cells to provide precursors for estrogen production. In contrast to theca cells, granulosa cells express high levels of aromatase activity in response to FSH stimulation. Thus, these cells efficiently convert androgens to estrogens, primarily the potent estrogen estradiol. In sum, ovarian steroidogenesis is dependent on the effects of LH and FSH acting independently on the theca cells and granulosa cells, respectively.

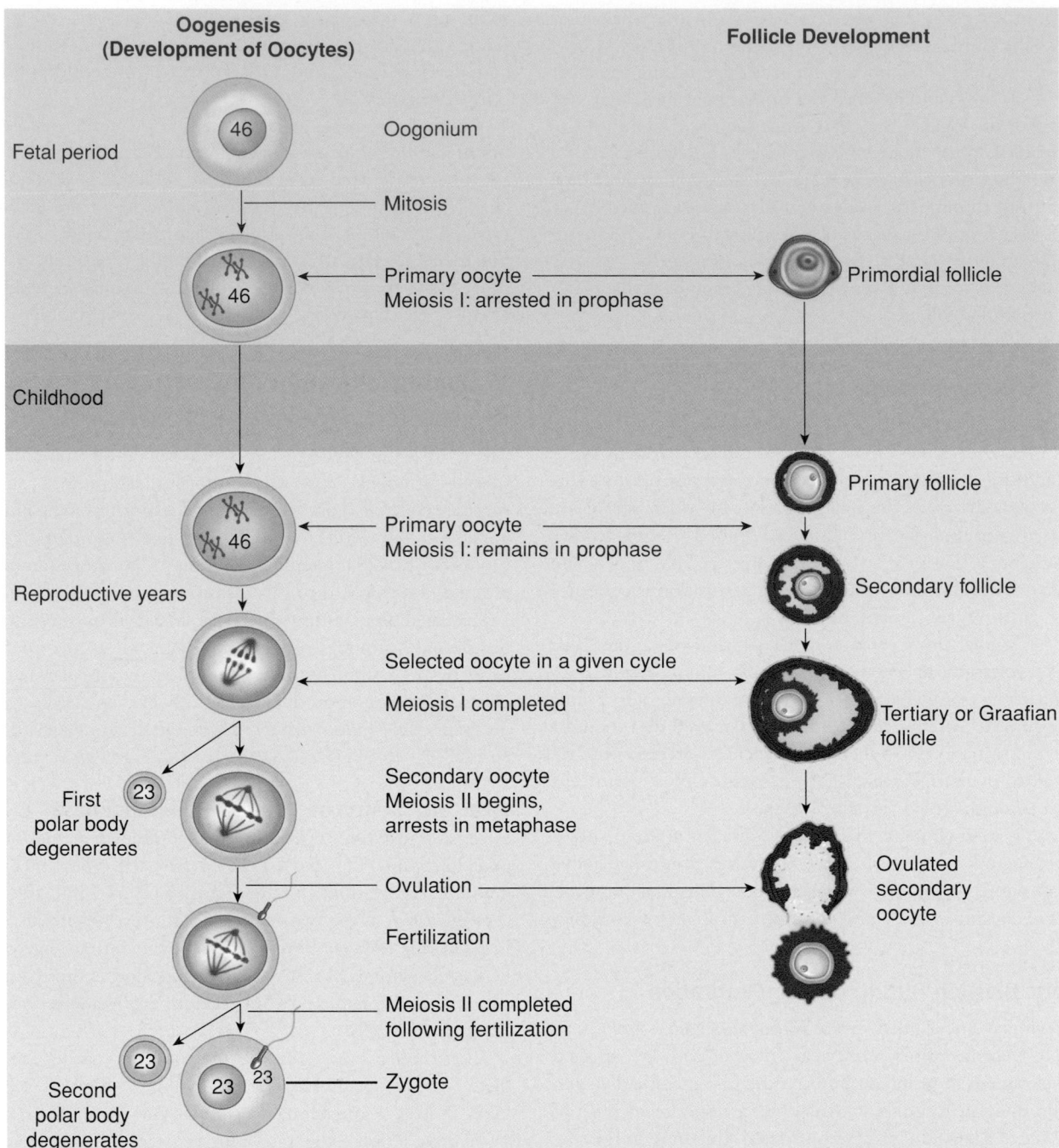

FIGURE 15-21 Drawing illustrates the steps of oocyte development and corresponding follicular maturation. In the fetal period, once the primordial germ cells arrive in the gonad, they differentiate into oogonia. Mitotic division of oogonia increases the population. Many oogonia further differentiate into primary oocytes, which begin meiosis. However, the process arrests during prophase. A primary oocyte with its surrounding epithelial cells is called a primordial follicle. In childhood, primary oocytes remain suspended in prophase I. Beginning in puberty and extending through the reproductive years, several primordial follicles mature each month into primary follicles. A few of these continue development to secondary follicles. One or two secondary follicles progress to a tertiary or Graafian follicle stage. At this stage, the first meiotic division completes to produce a haploid secondary oocyte and a polar body. During this process, cytoplasm is conserved by the secondary oocyte. Consequently, the polar body is disproportionately small. The secondary oocyte halts meiosis at its second metaphase. One of the secondary oocytes is then released at ovulation. If the oocyte is fertilized, completion of the second meiotic division follows. If fertilization fails to occur, then the oocyte degenerates prior to completion of the second meiotic division.

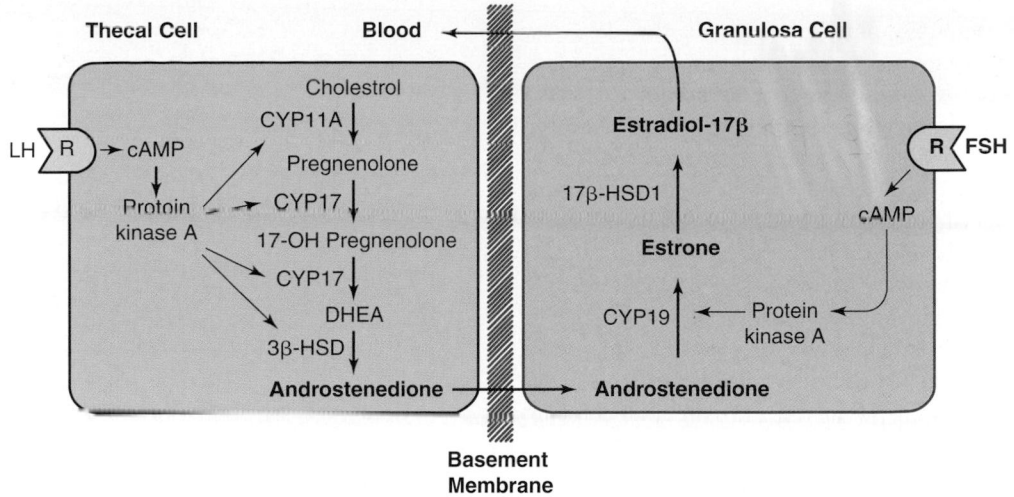

FIGURE 15-22 Diagram illustrates the two-cell theory of ovarian follicular steroidogenesis. Theca cells contain large numbers of luteinizing hormone (LH) receptors. Binding of LH to these receptors leads to cyclic AMP activation and synthesis of androstenedione from cholesterol. Androstenedione diffuses across the basement membrane of theca cells to enter granulosa cells of the ovary. Here, under the activation of follicle-stimulating hormone (FSH), androstenedione is converted by the enzyme aromatase to estrone and estradiol. cAMP = cyclic adenosine monophosphate; CYP11A = cholesterol side-chain cleavage enzyme; CYP17 = 17α-hydroxylase; CYP19 = aromatase; DHEA = dehydroepiandrosterone; 3β-HSD = 3β-hydroxysteroid dehydrogenase; 17β-HSD1 = 17β-hydroxysteroid dehydrogenase; R = receptor. *(Redrawn from Carr, 2005, with permission.)*

Steroidogenesis across the Life Span

Childhood. The human ovary has the capacity to produce estrogens by 8 weeks' gestation, however, a minimal amount of steroid is actually synthesized at any time during fetal development (Miller, 1988).

Circulating levels of the gonadotropins LH and FSH vary markedly at different ages of a woman's life. During the second trimester of fetal development, the plasma levels of gonadotropins rise to levels similar to those observed in menopause (Faiman, 1976). The fetal hypothalamic-pituitary axis continues to mature during the second trimester of pregnancy, becoming more sensitive to the high circulating levels of estrogen and progesterone secreted by the placenta (Kaplan, 1976; Yen, 1986). In response to the high levels of these steroids, fetal gonadotropins fall to low levels prior to birth. After delivery, gonadotropin levels rise abruptly in the neonate due to separation from the placenta and subsequent freedom from inhibition by placental steroids (Winter, 1976).

The elevated levels of gonadotropins in the newborn persist for the first few months of life, declining to low levels in early childhood (Winter, 1976). There may be multiple etiologies for the low gonadotropin levels during this period of life. The hypothalamic-pituitary axis has been found to have increased sensitivity to negative feedback, even by the low circulating levels of gonadal steroids at this stage (Yen, 1986). There is growing

evidence that there is an intrinsic role of the central nervous system in maintaining low gonadotropin levels. In support of this mechanism, low levels of LH and FSH are found in children with gonadal dysgenesis (Conte, 1975).

Puberty. One of the first signs of puberty is a sleep-associated increase in LH secretion (Fig. 15-23). Over time, increased

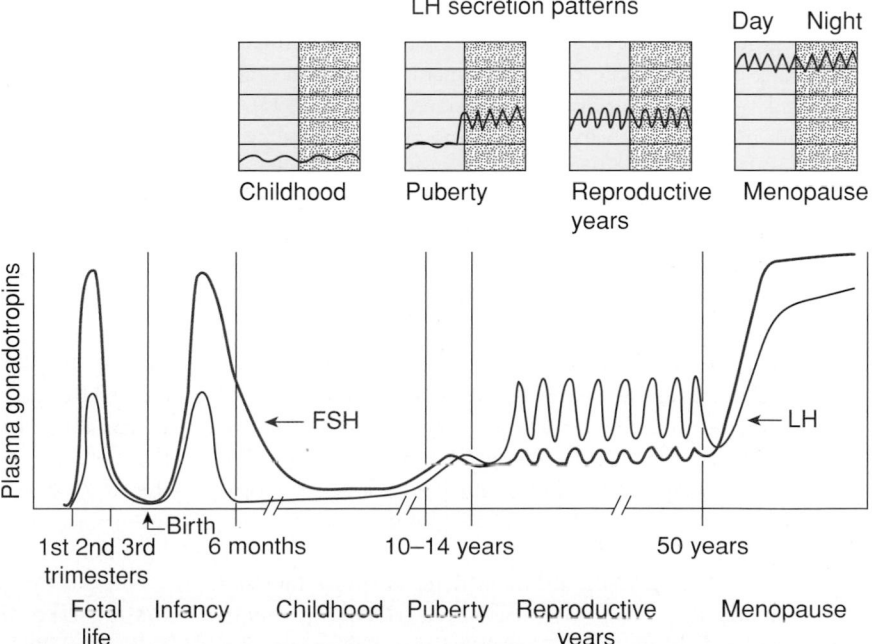

FIGURE 15-23 The upper diagram illustrates variations in luteinizing hormone (LH) secretion during the day and night during different life stages. The lower diagram depicts LH and follicle-stimulating hormone (FSH) level variations during different life stages in the female. *(Redrawn from Carr, 1998, with permission.)*

gonadotropin secretion is noted throughout the day. An increased FSH to LH ratio is typical in the premenarchal girl and postmenopausal woman. During the reproductive years, LH exceeds FSH levels, inverting this ratio.

Increased gonadotropin levels stimulate ovarian estradiol production. The rise in estrogen levels results in the growth spurt, maturation of the female internal and external genitalia, and development of a female habitus including breast enlargement (thelarche). Activation of the pituitary-adrenal axis results in an increase in adrenal androgen production and the associated development of axillary and pubic hair (adrenarche or pubarche). Increased gonadotropin levels ultimately lead to ovulation and subsequent menses, with the timing of the first menstrual period defining menarche. This developmental process takes approximately 3 to 4 years and is discussed further in Chapter 14 (p. 382).

Menopause. The postmenopausal ovary contains only a few follicles. As a result, plasma estrogen and inhibin levels decrease markedly after cessation of ovulatory cycles. Through loss of this negative feedback, LH and FSH levels are strikingly elevated in postmenopausal women. Elevated LH levels can stimulate production of C_{19} steroids (mainly androstenedione) in ovarian stromal cells. This ovarian-derived androstenedione as well as adrenal androgens can be converted by peripheral tissues to estrone, the principal estrogen in the plasma of postmenopausal women. The major site for the conversion of androstenedione to estrone is adipose tissue. Peripheral conversion of circulating androstenedione to estrone is directly correlated to body weight. For a given body weight, conversion is higher in postmenopausal women than in premenopausal women. These low circulating estrogen levels are usually inadequate to protect against bone loss.

Gonadal Peptides and the Menstrual Cycle

Activin-Inhibin-Follistatin System. Ovaries synthesize and secrete a group of peptide factors—inhibin, activin, and follistatin. Circulating inhibin is believed to be primarily gonadal in origin as serum levels drop abruptly after castration (Demura, 1993).

Serum inhibin levels vary widely across the menstrual cycle (Groome, 1996; McLachlan, 1987). During the early follicular phase, FSH stimulates the secretion of inhibin B by the granulosa cells (Buckler, 1989) (Fig. 15-24). However, increasing levels of circulating inhibin B blunt FSH secretion later in the follicular phase. During the luteal phase, regulation of inhibin production comes under the control of LH and switches from inhibin B to inhibin A (McLachlan, 1989). Inhibin B levels peak during the midluteal phase, decrease with the loss of luteal function, and remain low during the luteal-follicular transition and early follicular phase. The inverse relationship between circulating inhibin levels and FSH secretion is consistent with a negative-feedback role for inhibin in regulating FSH secretion.

Serum levels of activin, although detectable, are low and remain stable across the menstrual cycle (Demura, 1993). Follistatin levels likewise are unchanged across the reproductive cycle. Furthermore, circulating follistatin levels are similar in GnRH-deficient and postmenopausal women as well as in women after oophorectomy (Kettel, 1996; Khoury, 1995). These data strongly suggest that circulating follistatin is not

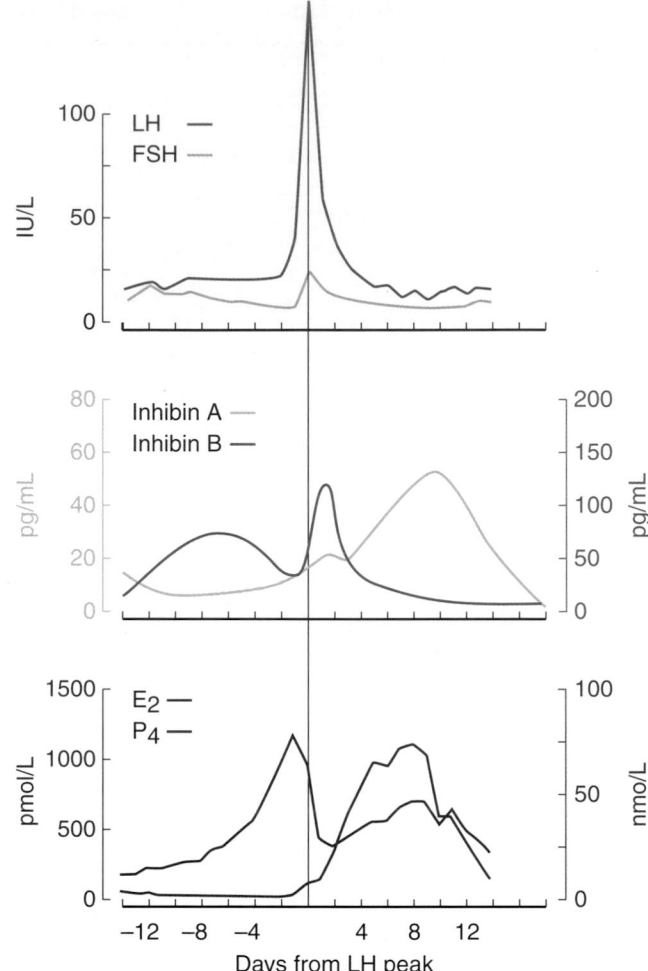

FIGURE 15-24 Graphs display gonadotropin, inhibin, and sex-steroid level changes during a normal menstrual cycle. In the first graph, peaking of luteinizing hormone (LH) (*purple line*) and follicle-stimulating hormone (FSH) (*pink line*) levels is displayed. In the middle graph, changing levels of inhibin A and inhibin B levels are shown. Note that inhibin B levels (*green line*) peak temporally near the midcycle surge in the LH level, whereas maximal elevation of inhibin A (*orange line*) occurs several days following this peak. In the third graph, elevations in estradiol levels (*red line*) are noted prior to the surge in LH levels and in the midluteal phase. Progesterone levels (*blue line*) peak in the midluteal phase. E_2 = estradiol; P_4 = progesterone.

derived from the ovary, although its source remains unknown. Essentially all of the follistatin is bound by activin throughout the menstrual cycle (McConnell, 1998). Therefore, although the ovary does make both activin and follistatin, these factors appear to act locally rather than modulate gonadotrope function.

Insulin-Like Growth Factor. The relative roles of IGF-I and IGF-II in mediating ovarian function may differ across species, but current data suggest that IGF-II is more important in the human (el Roeiy, 1993). Gonadotropins stimulate IGF-II production in theca cells, granulosa cells, and luteinized granulosa cells. Receptors for IGF are expressed on the theca and granulosa cells, supporting an autocrine/paracrine action in the follicle (Hernandez, 1992). Follicle-stimulating hormone also mediates expression of IGF-binding proteins. This system, although complex, allows additional fine-tuning of intrafollicular activity (Adashi, 1991; Thierry van Dessel, 1996).

Follicular Development

Follicular development begins with primordial follicles that were generated during fetal life (see Fig. 15-20). These follicles consist of an oocyte arrested in the first meiotic division surrounded by a single layer of flattened granulosa cells. These follicles are separated from the stroma by a thin basement membrane. Preovulatory follicles are avascular. As a result, they are critically dependent on diffusion and on the later development of gap junctions for obtaining nutrients and clearing metabolic waste. Diffusion also allows passage of steroid precursors from the thecal to the granulosa cell layer.

Primary Follicle

In the next stage of development, the granulosa cells become cuboidal and increase in number to form a pseudostratified layer. The follicle is now termed a primary follicle. Intercellular gap junctions develop between adjacent granulosa cells and between granulosa cells and the developing oocyte (Albertini, 1974). These connections allow the passage of nutrients, ions, and regulatory factors between cells. Gap junctions also allow cells without gonadotropin receptors to receive signals from cells with receptor expression (Fletcher, 1985). As a result, hormone-mediated effects can be transmitted throughout the follicle.

During this stage, the oocyte begins secretion of an acellular coat known as the zona pellucida. The human zona pellucida contains at least three proteins, named ZP1, ZP2, and ZP3. In current physiologic models, receptors on the acrosome head of the sperm recognize ZP3. This interaction results in release of acrosomal contents, penetration of the zona pellucida, and fertilization of the egg. Although the precise mechanism may differ between species, enzymes released from the acrosome induce alterations in ZP2 resulting in hardening of the coat. This process prevents fertilization of the oocyte by more than one sperm (Nixon, 2007).

Secondary Follicle

Development of a secondary, or preantral, follicle includes final growth of the oocyte and a further increase in granulosa cell number. The stroma differentiates into the theca interna and the theca externa, which abuts the surrounding stroma (Eppig, 1979).

Tertiary Follicle

With ongoing development, follicular fluid begins to collect between the granulosa cells, ultimately producing a fluid-filled space known as the antrum. The follicle is now termed a tertiary, or antral, follicle. Further accumulation of antral fluid results in a rapid increase in follicular size and development of a preovulatory, or Graafian, follicle.

Granulosa cells in the antral follicle are histologically and functionally divided into two groups. The granulosa cells surrounding the oocyte form the cumulus oophorus, whereas the granulosa cells surrounding the antrum are known as mural granulosa cells.

Antral fluid consists of a plasma filtrate and factors secreted by the granulosa cells. These locally produced factors, which include estrogen and growth factors, are present in substantially higher concentrations in follicular fluid than in the circulation and are likely critical for successful follicular maturation (Asimakopoulos, 2006; Silva, 2009).

Gonadotropins and Follicular Development

Early stages of development (up to the secondary follicle) do not require gonadotropin stimulation and thus are said to be "gonadotropin-independent." Final follicular maturation requires the presence of adequate amounts of circulating LH and FSH and is therefore said to be "gonadotropin-dependent" (Butt, 1970). Of note, data are beginning to accumulate which suggest that progression from gonadotropin-independent to -dependent stages is not as discrete as previously believed.

Concept of a Selection Window

Follicular development is a multistep process, which proceeds over at least 3 months and culminates in ovulation from a single follicle. Each month, a group of follicles known as a cohort begins a phase of semisynchronous growth. The size of this cohort appears to be proportional to the number of inactive primordial follicles within the ovaries and has been estimated at 3 to 11 follicles per ovary in young women (Gougeon, 1994; Hodgen, 1982; Pache, 1990).

It is important to emphasize that the ovulatory follicle is recruited from a cohort that began development two to three cycles prior to the ovulatory cycle. During this time, most follicles will die as they will not be at an appropriate stage of development during the selection window.

During the luteal-follicular transition, a small increase in FSH levels is responsible for selection of the single dominant follicle that will ultimately ovulate (Schipper, 1998). As previously described, theca cells produce androgens and granulosa cells generate estrogens. Estrogen levels increase with increased follicular size, enhance the effects of FSH on granulosa cells, and create a feed-forward action on follicles that produce estrogens.

It has also been suggested that the intrafollicular levels of members of the insulin-like growth factor family (IGFs) may synergize with FSH to help select the dominant follicle. Additional studies have demonstrated elevated levels of vascular endothelial growth factor (VEGF) around the follicle that will be selected. This follicle would presumably be exposed to higher levels of circulating factors such as FSH.

Granulosa cells also produce inhibin B, which passes from the follicle into the plasma and specifically inhibits the release of FSH, but not of LH, by the anterior pituitary. The combined production of estradiol and inhibin B by the dominant follicle results in the decline of follicular-phase FSH levels and may be responsible at least in part for the failure of the other follicles to reach preovulatory status during any one cycle.

Estrogen-Dominant Follicular Microenvironment

Ongoing follicular maturation requires the successful conversion from an "androgen-dominant" microenvironment to an "estrogen-dominant" microenvironment. At low concentrations, androgens stimulate aromatization and contribute to estrogen production. However, intrafollicular androgen levels will rise if aromatization in the granulosa cells lags behind androgen production by the thecal layer. At higher concentrations, androgens are converted to the more potent 5α-androgens, such as dihydrotestosterone. These androgens inhibit aromatase activity, cannot be aromatized to estrogens, and inhibit FSH induction of LH-receptor expression on the granulosa cells (Hillier, 1980; Jia, 1985; McNatty, 1979b).

This model predicts that follicles that lack adequate FSH receptor and granulosa cell number will remain primarily androgenic and will therefore become atretic. In support of this model, an increased androgen-to-estrogen ratio is found in the follicular fluid of atretic follicles, and a number of studies have demonstrated that high estrogen levels prevent apoptosis.

Insulin-like growth factor also has apoptosis-suppressing activity and is produced by granulosa cells. This action of IGF-I is suppressed by certain IGF-binding proteins that are present in the follicular fluid of atretic follicles. The action of FSH to prevent atresia may therefore result, in part, from its ability to stimulate IGF-I synthesis and suppress the synthesis of the IGF-binding proteins.

Phases of the Menstrual Cycle

Follicular Phase

During the end of a previous cycle, estrogen, progesterone, and inhibin levels decrease abruptly with a corresponding increase in circulating FSH levels (see Fig. 15-24) (Hodgen, 1982). As just described, this increase in FSH level is responsible for recruitment of the cohort of follicles that contains the follicle destined for ovulation. Despite general belief, sonographic studies in women have demonstrated that ovulation does not alternate sides, but occurs randomly from either ovary (Baird, 1987).

In women with waning ovarian function, the FSH level at this time of the cycle is elevated relative to that of younger women, presumably due to a loss of ovarian inhibin production in the previous luteal phase. As a result, measurement of an early follicular or cycle day 3 FSH and estradiol levels are frequently obtained in infertility clinics. The accelerated increase in serum FSH levels results in more robust recruitment of follicles and may explain both the shortened follicular phase observed in these older reproductive-aged women and the increased incidence of spontaneous twinning.

During the midfollicular phase, follicles produce increased amounts of estrogen and inhibin, resulting in a decline in FSH levels through negative feedback. This drop in FSH levels is believed to contribute to selection of the follicle destined to ovulate, termed the *dominant follicle*. Based on this theory, remaining follicles express decreased numbers of FSH receptors and therefore are unable to respond adequately to declining FSH levels. Also of note, the ovary expresses the potent angiogenic factor VEGF. Follicles that will undergo atresia have a limited blood supply, presumably due to decreased VEGF expression, which effectively decreases delivery of circulating factors to these follicles (Ravindranath, 1992).

During most of follicular development, granulosa cell responses to FSH stimulation include an increase in granulosa cell number, an increase in aromatase expression, and in the presence of estradiol, expression of LH receptors on the granulosa cells. With the development of LH-receptor expression during the late follicular phase, granulosa cells begin to produce small amounts of progesterone. This progesterone decreases granulosa cell proliferation, thereby slowing follicular growth (Chaffkin, 1992). Progesterone is primarily responsible for generating the FSH surge (Erickson, 1979; McNatty, 1979a). Progesterone also augments the positive feedback of estrogen as discussed in the following section (Couzinet, 1992). This latter effect may explain the occasional induction of ovulation in anovulatory amenorrheic women when given progesterone to induce menses.

Ovulation and the Luteinizing Hormone Surge

Ovulation, the process by which the oocyte-cumulus is released from the follicle, has been compared with an inflammatory response. As such, products induced by these signaling cascades include gene products that rupture the follicle and remodel the follicular remnant into a corpus luteum.

Toward the end of the follicular phase, estradiol levels increase dramatically. For reasons that are not completely understood, with this rapid increase, estradiol is no longer inhibitory and instead develops positive feedback effects at both the hypothalamus and anterior pituitary gland to generate the LH surge. Estradiol concentrations of 200 pg/mL for 50 hours are necessary to initiate a gonadotropin surge (Young, 1976).

The LH surge acts rapidly on both the granulosa and theca cells of the preovulatory follicle to terminate the genes involved in follicular expression while at the same time turning on the expression of genes required for ovulation and luteinization. In addition, the LH surge initiates the reentry of the oocyte into meiosis, expansion of the cumulus oophorus, synthesis of prostaglandins, and luteinization of granulosa cells. The mean duration of the LH surge is 48 hours, and ovulation occurs approximately 36 to 40 hours after the onset of the LH surge (Hoff, 1983; Lemarchand-Beraud, 1982). Abrupt termination of the surge is postulated to be due to acutely increasing steroid and inhibin secretion by the corpus luteum.

The granulosa cells surrounding the oocyte differ from mural granulosa cells in that they do not express LH receptors or synthesize progesterone. Cumulus oophorus granulosa cells develop tight gap junctions between themselves and with the oocyte. The cumulus mass that accompanies the ovulating oocyte is believed to be important for providing a rough surface and increased size to improve oocyte "pick-up" by the tubal fimbria.

Discordant oocyte maturation and luteinization is prevented by the action of locally produced factors, including oocyte maturation inhibitor (OMI) and luteinization inhibitor. Endothelin-1 has been proposed to be the luteinization inhibitor, whereas the identity of the OMI is under active investigation (Tedeschi, 1992). Intrafollicular activin may also help to prevent premature luteinization as it suppresses progesterone production by granulosa cells (Li, 1992).

Recently, members of an epidermal growth factor-like family, that is, amphiregulin, epiregulin, and beta-cellulin, were found to substitute for both the morphologic and biochemical events triggered by LH, including both expansion of the cumulus and maturation of the oocyte. Thus, these growth factors are part of the downstream cascade that begins with LH binding to its receptor and ends with ovulation.

Based on sonographic surveillance, extrusion of the oocyte only lasts a few minutes (Knobil, 1994). The exact mechanism of this expulsion is poorly defined but is not due to an increase in follicular pressure (Espey, 1974). The presence of proteolytic enzymes in the follicle, including plasmin and collagenase, suggest that these enzymes are responsible for follicular wall thinning (Beers, 1975). The preovulatory gonadotropin surge stimulates expression of tissue plasminogen activator by the granulosa and theca cells. The surge also decreases expression of plasminogen inhibitor, resulting in a marked increase in plasminogen activity (Piquette, 1993).

Prostaglandins also reach a peak concentration in follicular fluid during the preovulatory gonadotropin surge (Lumsden, 1986). Prostaglandins may stimulate smooth muscle contraction in the ovary, thereby contributing to ovulation (Yoshimura, 1987). Women undergoing infertility treatment are advised to avoid prostaglandin synthetase inhibitors in the preovulatory period to avoid luteinized unruptured follicle syndrome (LUFS) (Priddy, 1990; Smith, 1996). The incidence of LUFS has been estimated at 4.5 percent in cycling women. However, significant controversy exists as to whether LUFS should be considered pathologic or simply a sporadic event (Kerin, 1983).

Luteal Phase

Following ovulation, the remaining follicular cells differentiate into the corpus luteum, literally *yellow body* (Corner, 1956). This process, which requires LH stimulation, includes both morphologic and functional changes known as luteinization. The granulosa and theca cells proliferate and undergo hypertrophy to form granulosa-lutein cells and smaller theca-lutein cells, respectively (Patton, 1991). The conversion of a granulosa cell into a large luteal cell is a dramatic example of cellular differentiation.

During corpus luteum formation, the basement membrane that separates granulosa cells from theca cells degenerates and allows vascularization of previously avascular granulosa cells. Capillary invasion begins 2 days after ovulation, reaching the center of the corpus luteum by the fourth day. This increase in perfusion provides these luteal cells with access to circulating low-density lipoprotein (LDL), which is used to provide precursor cholesterol for steroid biosynthesis. This marked increase in blood supply can have clinical implications as pain from a hemorrhagic corpus luteum cyst is a relatively frequent presentation to emergency rooms.

As might be predicted by its name, steroidogenesis in the corpus luteum is under the primary control of luteinizing hormone from the anterior pituitary gland. Based on its steroidogenic products, the luteal phase is considered progesterone dominant, in contrast to the estrogen dominance of the follicular phase. Increased vascularization, cellular hypertrophy, and an increased number of intracellular organelles transform the corpus luteum into the most active steroidogenic tissue in the body. Maximal levels of progesterone production are observed in the midluteal phase and have been estimated at an impressive 40 mg of progesterone per day. Ovulation can be safely assumed to have occurred if the progesterone level exceeds 3 ng/mL on cycle day 21. A progesterone level greater than 10 to 15 ng/mL generally indicates adequate luteal function and no need for progesterone supplementation.

Although progesterone is the most abundant ovarian steroid during the luteal phase, estradiol is also produced in significant quantities. Estradiol levels drop transiently immediately after the LH surge. This decrease may explain the midcycle spotting noticed by some women. The reason for this decrease is not known, but it may result from a direct inhibition of granulosa cell growth by increasing progesterone levels (Hoff, 1983). The decline in estradiol levels is followed by a steady increase to reach a maximum during the midluteal phase.

The corpus luteum also produces large quantities of the polypeptide inhibin A. This coincides with a decrease in circulating FSH levels in the luteal phase. If inhibin A levels decline at the end of the luteal phase, FSH levels rise once more to begin selection of a oocyte cohort for the next menstrual cycle.

Gonadotropins and Luteal Function. Normal hormonal function of the corpus luteum depends on adequate serum LH levels, the presence of LH receptors on the luteal cells, and a sufficient number of luteal cells (Vande Wiele, 1970). As a result, it is critical that LH receptor expression on the granulosa cells was appropriately induced during the prior follicular phase. In support of the importance of this hormone for survival of the corpus luteum, it has been demonstrated that blunted serum LH concentrations are correlated with a shortened luteal phase.

Luteal function is further influenced by gonadotropin levels during the preceding follicular phase. A reduction in LH or FSH secretion is correlated with poor luteal function (McNeely, 1988; Stouffer, 1980). Presumably, a lack of FSH leads to a decrease in the total number of granulosa cells. Furthermore, luteal cells in these suboptimal cycles will have a decreased number of FSH-induced LH receptors and thus will be less responsive to LH stimulation.

Luteolysis. If pregnancy does not occur, the corpus luteum regresses through a process called luteolysis. The mechanism for luteolysis is poorly understood, but luteal regression is presumed to be tightly regulated and luteal cycle length varies minimally. Following luteolysis, the blood supply to the corpus luteum diminishes, progesterone and estrogen secretion drop precipitously, and the luteal cells undergo apoptosis and become fibrotic. This creates the *corpus albicans* (white body).

If pregnancy occurs, hCG produced by the early gestation "rescues" the corpus luteum from atresia by binding to and activating the LH receptor on luteal cells. Human CG stimulation of corpus luteum steroidogenesis maintains endometrial stability until placental steroid production is adequate to

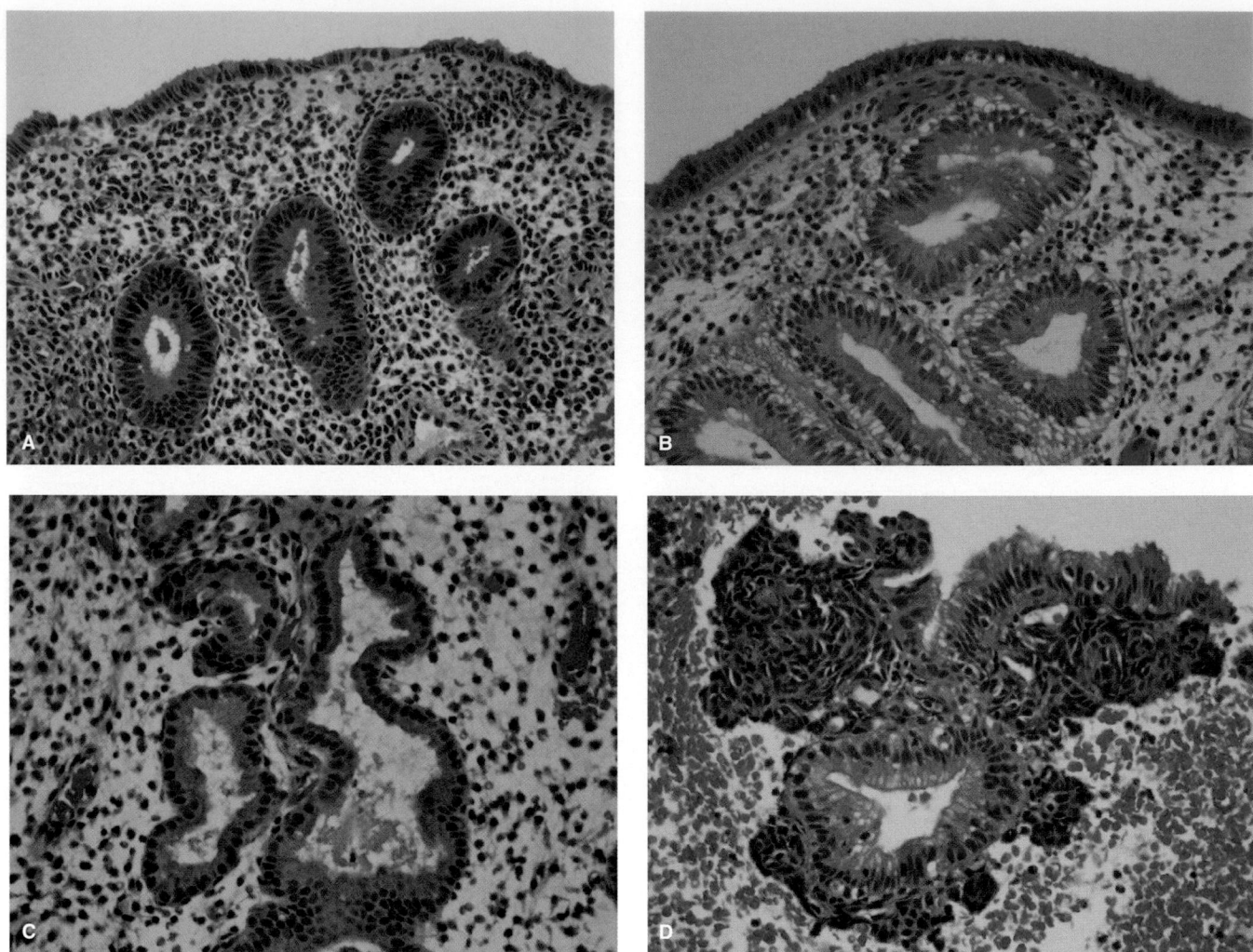

FIGURE 15-25 Photomicrograph illustrating endometrial changes during the menstrual cycle. **A.** Proliferative phase: straight to slightly coiled, tubular glands are lined by pseudostratified columnar epithelium with scattered mitoses. **B.** Early secretory phase: coiled glands with a slightly widened diameter are lined by simple columnar epithelium with clear subnuclear vacuoles. **C.** Late secretory phase: serrated, dilated glands with intraluminal secretion are lined by short columnar cells. **D.** Menstrual phase: fragmented endometrium with condensed stroma and glands with secretory vacuoles are seen in a background of blood. *(Photographs contributed by Dr. Kelley Carrick.)*

assume this function late in the first trimester. For this reason, surgical removal of the corpus luteum during pregnancy should be followed by progesterone replacement as outline in Chapter 9 (p. 272) until approximately 10 weeks' gestation.

ENDOMETRIUM

Histology across the Menstrual Cycle

The endometrium consists of two layers: the *basalis layer,* which lies against the myometrium, and the *functionalis layer,* which is apposed to the uterine lumen (Fig. 8-3, p. 222). The basalis layer, which does not change significantly across the menstrual cycle, is critical for regeneration of the endometrium following menstrual sloughing. The functionalis layer of the endometrium can be further divided into the superficial and thin, *stratum compactum,* which consists of gland necks and dense

stroma. The underlying *stratum spongiosum* contains glands and large amounts of loosely organized stroma and interstitial tissue.

After menstruation, the endometrium is 1 to 2 mm thick. Under the influence of estrogen, the glandular and stromal cells of the functionalis layer proliferate rapidly following menses (Fig. 15-25). This period of rapid growth, termed the *proliferative phase*, corresponds to the ovary's follicular phase. As this phase progresses, glands become more tortuous and cells lining the glandular lumen undergo pseudostratification. The stroma remains compact. Endometrial thickness is approximately 12 mm at the time of the LH surge and does not increase significantly thereafter.

Following ovulation, the endometrium transforms into a secretory tissue. The period during and after transformation is defined as the *secretory phase* of the endometrium and correlates to the ovary's *luteal phase* of the menstrual cycle. Glycogen-rich subnuclear vacuoles appear in cells lining the glands. Under further stimulation by progesterone, these vacuoles move from the glandular cells' base toward their lumen and expel their contents. This secretory process peaks on approximately postovulatory day 6, coinciding with the day of implantation. Throughout the luteal phase, glands become increasingly tortuous, and the stroma becomes more edematous. In addition, spiral arteries that feed the endometrium increase their number and coiling.

If a blastocyst does not implant, then the corpus luteum is not maintained by placental hCG, progesterone levels drop, and endometrial glands begin to collapse. Polymorphonuclear leukocytes and monocytes from nearby vasculature infiltrate the endometrium. The spiral arteries constrict leading to local ischemia, and lysosomes release proteolytic enzymes that accelerate tissue destruction. Prostaglandins (PGs), particularly prostaglandin $F_{2\alpha}$, are present in the endometrium and likely contribute to arteriolar vasospasm. Prostaglandin $F_{2\alpha}$ also induces myometrial contractions, which may aid in expelling the endometrial tissue.

The entire endometrial functionalis layer is thought to exfoliate with menstruation, leaving only the basalis layer to provide cells for endometrial regeneration. However, in a number of reports, investigators have found large variations in the amount of tissue shed from different levels of the endometrium. Following menstruation, reepithelialization of the desquamated endometrium is believed to be initiated within 2 to 3 days after the onset of menses and to be completed within 48 hours.

Regulation of Endometrial Function
Tissue Degradation and Hemorrhage

Within the endometrium, a large number of proteins maintain a delicate balance between tissue integrity and the localized tissue destruction required for menstrual sloughing or for trophoblast invasion during implantation. Genes encoding these tissue proteins are believed to be regulated by cytokines, growth factors, and steroid hormones, although the details of this regulation are still incomplete.

Of these tissue proteins, tissue factor is a membrane-associated protein that activates the coagulation cascade on contact with blood. In addition, urokinase and tissue plasminogen activator (TPA) are both fibrinolytic, increasing the conversion of plasminogen to plasmin and activating tissue breakdown. TPA activity is blocked by plasminogen activator inhibitor 1, also present in the endometrial stroma (Lockwood, 1993; Schatz, 1995). Importantly, matrix metalloproteinases (MMPs) are a family of enzymes with overlapping substrate specificities for collagens and other extracellular matrix components. The compositions of the MMPs vary within the different endometrial tissues and during the menstrual cycle. Endogenous MMP inhibitors, called tissue inhibitors of matrix metalloproteinases, are also increased premenstrually and limit MMP degradative activity.

Vasoconstriction and Myometrial Contractility

Effective menstruation depends on appropriately timed endometrial vasoconstriction and myometrial contraction. Vasoconstriction produces ischemia, which leads to endome-trial damage and subsequent menstrual sloughing. Within the endometrium, epithelial and stromal cells secrete endothelin-1, a member of a family of potent vasoconstrictors. Enkephalinase, which degrades endothelins, is expressed at its highest levels in the midsecretory endometrium (Head, 1993). However, in the late luteal phase, drops in serum progesterone levels lead to a loss of enkephalinase expression. This permits increased endothelin activity, which in turn provides a physiologic system inclined toward vasoconstriction.

In concert with endometrial sloughing, myometrial contractions control blood loss by compressing endometrial vasculature and help to expel menstrual discharge. A fall in serum progesterone decreases an enzyme that degrades prostaglandins. This allows increasing $PGF_{2\alpha}$ activity in the myometrium and triggers myometrial contractions (Casey, 1980).

Estrogens and Progestins

The expression of estrogen receptors and progesterone receptors in the endometrium is highly regulated across the menstrual cycle. This regulation of steroid receptor number provides an additional mechanism for controlling steroid effects on endometrial development and function.

Estrogen receptors are expressed in the nuclei of epithelial, stromal, and myometrial cells, and a peak concentration is seen during the proliferative phase. However, during the luteal phase, rising progesterone levels decrease estrogen receptor expression (Lessey, 1988).

Endometrial progesterone receptors peak at midcycle in response to rising estrogen levels. By midluteal phase, progesterone receptor expression in the endometrium is nearly absent, although expression remains strong in the stromal compartment (Lessey, 1988; Press, 1988).

The proliferation and differentiation of the uterine epithelium is under the control of estradiol, progesterone, and various growth factors. The importance of estrogens for endometrial development is emphasized by the documented increase in endometrial hyperplasia in women receiving unopposed estrogen therapy. Estrogen exerts its effects directly, through interaction with estrogen receptors and through induction of various growth factors including IGF-1, transforming growth factor α, and epidermal growth factor (Beato, 1989; Dickson, 1987). The effects of progesterone on endometrial growth vary among endometrial layers. Progesterone is clearly critical for the conversion of the functionalis layer from a proliferative to a secretory pattern. Moreover, progesterone also appears to promote cellular proliferation in the basalis layer.

Growth Factors and Cell Adhesion Molecules

A large number of growth factors and associated receptors have been identified in the endometrium (Table 15-10). Each of these factors has its own pattern of expression, and this complexity has made it difficult to determine which of the factors is most critical for endometrial function (Ohlsson, 1989; Sharkey, 1995).

In addition to growth factors, cell adhesion molecules found within the endometrium play an important role in endometrial function. These molecules fall into four classes: the integrins,

TABLE 15-10. Endometrial Growth Factors and Their Function

Growth Factors	Suggested Function	Production Site
Transforming growth factor-β (TGF-β) family	Regulates extracellular matrix organization through regulation of TIMPs and PAI-1	Epithelial and stromal cells
Epidermal growth factor (EGF)	Stimulates stromal cell differentiation, regulates endometrial cell expression of integrins	Stromal and glandular cells
Insulin-like growth factors (IGF-I and IGF-II)	Promotes mitosis and differentiation in the endometrium	Endometrium, ovary, trophoblasts
IGF binding protein-1 (IGFBP-1)	Modulates trophoblast invasion	Decidualized stromal cells
Platelet-derived growth factor (PDGF)	Promotes angiogenesis, stimulates stromal cell proliferation	Stromal cells, activated platelets
Vascular endothelial growth factor (VEGF)	Modulates angiogenesis and vascular permeability	Glandular cells
Tumor necrosis factor-β (TNF-β)	Promotes mitogenic, angiogenic, inflammatory, and immunomodulatory effects	Endometrium, trophoblasts
Macrophage colony-stimulating factor (MCSF)	Stimulates monocyte maturation, regulates mature macrophage cell function	Endometrium, decidua, placenta
Leukemia inhibitory factor (LIF)	Promotes blastocyst implantation	Endometrium, blastocyst, placenta

PAI-1 = plasminogen activator inhibitor-1; TIMP = tissue inhibitor of matrix metalloproteinase.

the cadherins, the selectins, and members of the immuno-globulin superfamily. Each has been implicated in endometrial regeneration and embryo implantation.

Implantation Window

In the human, the embryo enters the uterine cavity 2 to 3 days after fertilization with implantation beginning approximately 4 days later (Fig. 15-26). Studies in humans and animal models have demonstrated that normal implantation and embryonic development require synchronous development of the endometrium and the embryo (Pope, 1988). The human blastocyst may have less stringent requirements for implantation than other species as ectopic implantation occurs relatively frequently.

Uterine receptivity can be defined as the temporal window of endometrial maturation during which trophectoderm attaches to the endometrial epithelial cells with subsequent invasion into the endometrial stroma. Based on a number of studies, the window of implantation in the human is relatively broad, extending from day 20 through day 24 of the menstrual cycle. Precise determination of this temporal window is critical since only those factors expressed during this time act as direct functional mediators of uterine receptivity.

Several investigators have attempted to correlate biochemical markers and ultrastructural features of the endometrium with the presence of uterine receptivity. Endometrial maturation is associated with loss of both surface microvilli and ciliated cells as well as the development of cellular protrusions, called *pinopods*, on the apical surface of the endometrium. Specifically, the presence of pinopods is considered to be an important morphologic marker of peri-implantation endometrium. Pinopod formation is known to be highly progesterone dependent (Yoshinaga, 1989).

A wide variety of factors are believed to be important for uterine receptivity, including cell adhesion molecules—integrins, selectins, cadherins, and mucins—as well as immunoglobulins and cytokines. Integrins have been a particularly well-studied factor in this regard (Casals, 2010). However, to date, no single integrin molecule has been determined to be the critical marker for identification of the implantation window (Achache, 2006).

Endometrial Dating and Luteal Phase Defect. In a classic study, Noyes and colleagues (1950) described a system for correlating the endometrial histologic appearance with menstrual cycle phase. With their system, a discrepancy of more than 2 days, termed a *luteal phase defect*, was linked to implantation failure and early pregnancy loss (Olive, 1991). Endometrial biopsy for this purpose has been used for infertility evaluation. Its current limited role is discussed further in Chapter 19 (p. 513).

ENDOCRINOLOGY OF PREGNANCY

Extensive endocrine changes occur in the maternal circulation during pregnancy because of altered maternal physiology as

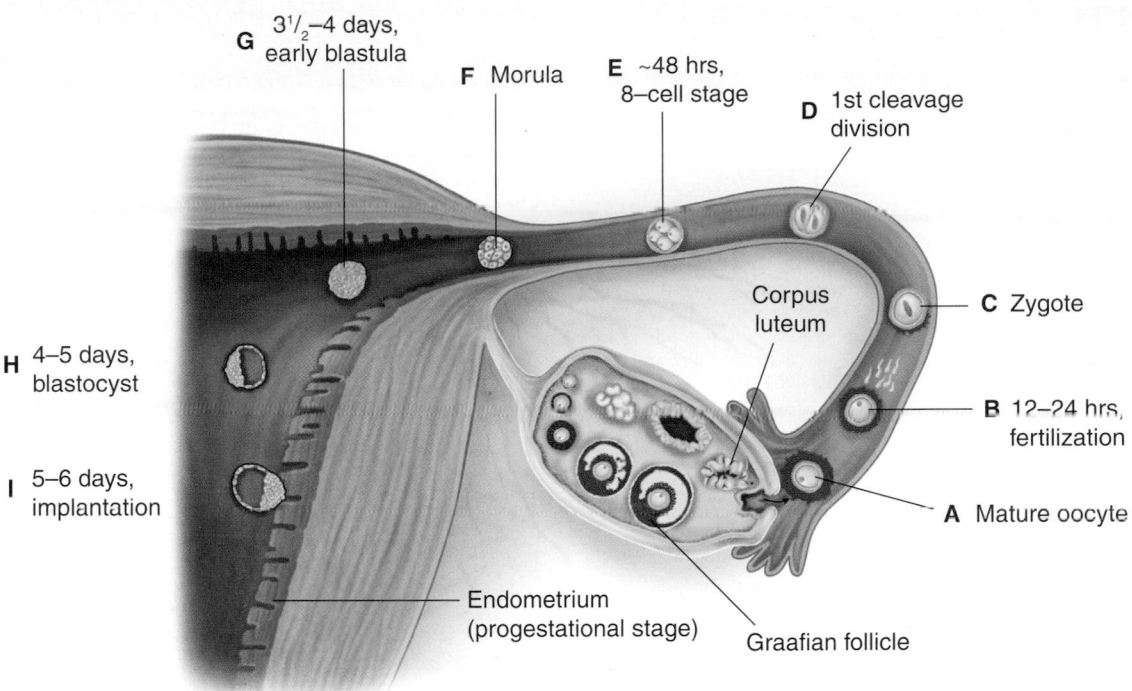

G 3½–4 days, early blastula

F Morula

E ~48 hrs, 8–cell stage

D 1st cleavage division

Corpus luteum

C Zygote

H 4–5 days, blastocyst

B 12–24 hrs, fertilization

I 5–6 days, implantation

A Mature oocyte

Endometrium (progestational stage)

Graafian follicle

FIGURE 15-26 Illustration depicts key points of conception: ovulation, fertilization, zygote transport through the fallopian tube, and implantation.

well as contributions by the placenta and fetus. A more detailed discussion of these changes can be found in *Williams Obstetrics*, 23rd edition (Cunningham, 2010a).

Human Chorionic Gonadotropin

Human chorionic gonadotropin is produced by the placental syncytiotrophoblast and can be detected in serum as early as 7 to 9 days after the LH surge. In early pregnancy, hCG levels increase rapidly, doubling approximately every 2 days. Levels of this peptide hormone peak at approximately 100,000 mIU/mL during the first trimester of pregnancy. This is followed by a relatively sharp decrease in the early second trimester and maintenance at lower levels throughout the remainder of pregnancy.

Human CG binds to LH/CG receptors on corpus luteum cells and stimulates steroidogenesis in the ovary. To maintain endometrial integrity and uterine quiescence, hCG levels are critical for corpus luteum steroid production during early pregnancy before the placenta attains adequate steroidogenic capability. The transfer in production of estrogens and progesterone from the ovary to the placenta is often called the "luteal-placental shift."

As the placenta is the primary source for hCG production, measurement of plasma hCG levels has proved to be an effective screening tool for pregnancies with altered placental mass or function. Relatively elevated levels of hCG are observed in association with multifetal gestation or a fetus with Down syndrome. Lower hCG levels are observed in cases of poor placentation such as occurs in ectopic pregnancy or spontane-

ous miscarriage. Serial hCG measurements can be very helpful to monitor these latter conditions as the doubling time is relatively reliable.

Markedly abnormal elevations in hCG levels are most often observed in the presence of gestational trophoblastic disease, including hydatidiform mole and choriocarcinoma (Chap. 37, p. 898). As noted previously, hCG and TSH share a common α-subunit and related β-subunits. Due to this structural similarity, hCG can bind to and activate TSH-receptors in the thyroid gland. This explains the association of molar pregnancy with hyperthyroidism.

Human CG can also be a useful tumor marker for nontrophoblastic neoplasias. Ectopic (nonplacental) production of hCG, either the intact dimer or the β-subunit, is frequently associated with germ cell tumors and has been reported for a variety of tumors arising from the mucosal epithelium of the cervix, bladder, lung, and nasopharynx (Chap. 36, p. 880). It has been postulated that hCG inhibits apoptosis in these tumors, thereby allowing rapid growth (Iles, 2007).

Placental Steroids
Luteal-Placental Shift

The corpus luteum is the major source of sex steroid production in early pregnancy. Surgical removal of the corpus luteum will result in miscarriage before the switch to placental steroid production. Thus, in such cases, postoperative progesterone supplementation is required to maintain early pregnancies, and replacement regimens are discussed in Chapter 9 (272).

REFERENCES

Achache H, Revel A: Endometrial receptivity markers, the journey to successful embryo implantation. Hum Reprod Update 12:731, 2006

Adashi EY, Resnick CE, Hurwitz A, et al: Ovarian granulosa cell-derived insulin-like growth factor binding proteins: modulatory role of follicle-stimulating hormone. Endocrinology 128:754, 1991

Albertini DF, Anderson E: The appearance and structure of intercellular connections during the ontogeny of the rabbit ovarian follicle with particular reference to gap junctions. J Cell Biol 63:234, 1974

Anderson ST, Sawangjaroen K, Curlewis JD: Pituitary adenylate cyclase-activating polypeptide acts within the medial basal hypothalamus to inhibit prolactin and luteinizing hormone secretion. Endocrinology 137:3424, 1996

Arafah BM, Brodkey JS, Pearson OH: Gradual recovery of lactotroph responsiveness to dynamic stimulation following surgical removal of prolactinomas: long-term follow-up studies. Metabolism 35:905, 1986

Asimakopoulos B, Koster F, Felberbaum R, et al: Cytokine and hormonal profile in blood serum and follicular fluids during ovarian stimulation with the multidose antagonist or the long agonist protocol. Hum Reprod 21:3091, 2006

Auchus RJ: Non-traditional metabolic pathways of adrenal steroids. Rev Endocr Metab Disord 10:27, 2009

Baird DT: A model for follicular selection and ovulation: lessons from superovulation. J Steroid Biochem 27:15, 1987

Baker TG: A quantitative and cytological study of germ cells in human ovaries. Proc R Soc Lond B Biol Sci 158:417, 1963

Baker TG, Franchi LL: The fine structure of oogonia and oocytes in human ovaries. J Cell Sci 2:213, 1967

Barnes RR, Levrant SG: Pharmacology of estrogens. In Treatment of the Postmenopausal Woman. New York, Columbia University Press, 2007, p 767

Beato M: Gene regulation by steroid hormones. Cell 56:335, 1989

Beers WH: Follicular plasminogen and plasminogen activator and the effect of plasmin on ovarian follicle wall. Cell 6:379, 1975

Besecke LM, Guendner MJ, Sluss PA, et al: Pituitary follistatin regulates activin-mediated production of follicle-stimulating hormone during the rat estrous cycle. Endocrinology 138:2841, 1997

Boon WC, Chow JD, Simpson ER: The multiple roles of estrogens and the enzyme aromatase. Prog Brain Res 181:209, 2010

Brinkmann AO: Molecular basis of androgen insensitivity. Mol Cell Endocrinol 179 (1-2):105, 2001

Buckler HM, Healy DL, Burger HG: Purified FSH stimulates production of inhibin by the human ovary. J Endocrinol 122:279, 1989

Butt WR, Crooke AC, Ryle M, et al: Gonadotrophins and ovarian development; proceedings of the two Workshop Meetings on the Chemistry of the Human Gonadotrophins and on the Development of the Ovary in Infancy. Birmingham, 1969. Edinburgh, E & S Livingstone, 1970

Camp TA, Rahal JO, Mayo KE: Cellular localization and hormonal regulation of follicle-stimulating hormone and luteinizing hormone receptor messenger RNAs in the rat ovary. Mol Endocrinol 5:1405, 1991

Carr BR: The ovary. In Carr BR, Blackwell RE (eds): Textbook of Reproductive Medicine, 2nd ed. Stamford, Appleton Lange, 1998, p 210

Carr BR: The ovary and the normal menstrual cycle. In Carr BR, Blackwell RE, Azziz R (eds): Essential Reproductive Medicine. New York, McGraw-Hill, 2005, p 79

Casals G, Ordi J, Creus M, et al: Osteopontin and αvß3 integrin as markers of endometrial receptivity: the effect of different hormone therapies. Reprod Biomed Online 21:349, 2010

Casey ML, Hemsell DL, MacDonald PC, et al: NAD+-dependent 15-hydroxyprostaglandin dehydrogenase activity in human endometrium. Prostaglandins 19:115, 1980

Cetel NS, Quigley ME, Yen SS: Naloxone-induced prolactin secretion in women: evidence against a direct prolactin stimulatory effect of endogenous opioids. J Clin Endocrinol Metab 60:191, 1985

Chaffkin LM, Luciano AA, Peluso JJ: Progesterone as an autocrine/paracrine regulator of human granulosa cell proliferation. J Clin Endocrinol Metab 75:1404, 1992

Cheng CK, Leung PC: Molecular biology of gonadotropin-releasing hormone (GnRH)-I, GnRH-II, and their receptors in humans. Endocr Rev 26:283, 2005

Childs GV, Hyde C, Naor Z, et al: Heterogeneous luteinizing hormone and follicle-stimulating hormone storage patterns in subtypes of gonadotropes separated by centrifugal elutriation. Endocrinology 113:2120, 1983

Chwalisz K, Perez MC, Demanno D, et al: Selective progesterone receptor modulator development and use in the treatment of leiomyomata and endometriosis. Endocr Rev 26:423, 2005

Clayton RN, Catt KJ: Gonadotropin-releasing hormone receptors: characterization, physiological regulation, and relationship to reproductive function. Endocr Rev 2:186, 1981

Conneely OM, Mulac-Jericevic B, DeMayo F, et al: Reproductive functions of progesterone receptors. Recent Prog Horm Res 57:339, 2002

Conte FA, Grumbach MM, Kaplan SL: A diphasic pattern of gonadotropin secretion in patients with the syndrome of gonadal dysgenesis. J Clin Endocrinol Metab 40:670, 1975

Corner GW Jr: The histological dating of the human corpus luteum of menstruation. Am J Anat 98:377, 1956

Couse JF, Curtis HS, Korach KS: Receptor null mice reveal contrasting roles for estrogen receptor alpha and beta in reproductive tissues. J Steroid Biochem Mol Biol 74:287, 2000

Couzinet B, Brailly S, Bouchard P, et al: Progesterone stimulates luteinizing hormone secretion by acting directly on the pituitary. J Clin Endocrinol Metab 74:374, 1992

Crowley WR, Armstrong WE: Neurochemical regulation of oxytocin secretion in lactation. Endocr Rev 13:33, 1992

Cunningham FG, Leveno KJ, Bloom SL, et al (eds): Implantation, embryogenesis, and placental development. In Williams Obstetrics, 23rd ed. New York, McGraw-Hill, 2010a, pp 37, 62

Cunningham FG, Leveno KJ, Bloom SL, et al (eds): Parturition. In Williams Obstetrics, 23rd ed. New York, McGraw-Hill, 2010b, p 159

Davis JR: Prolactin and reproductive medicine. Curr Opin Obstet Gynecol 16:331, 2004

de Kretser DM, Hedger MP, Loveland KL, et al: Inhibins, activins, and follistatin in reproduction. Hum Reprod Update 8:529, 2002

Demura R, Suzuki T, Tajima S, et al: Human plasma free activin and inhibin levels during the menstrual cycle. J Clin Endocrinol Metab 76:1080, 1993

Dickson RB, Lippman ME: Estrogenic regulation of growth and polypeptide growth factor secretion in human breast carcinoma. Endocr Rev 8:29, 1987

Ding CC, Thong KJ, Krishna A, et al: Activin A inhibits activation of human primordial follicles in vitro. J Assist Reprod Genet 27:141, 2010

Di Sarno A, Landi ML, Cappabianca P, et al: Resistance to cabergoline as compared with bromocriptine in hyperprolactinemia: prevalence, clinical definition, and therapeutic strategy. J Clin Endocrinol Metab 86:5256, 2001

Dye RB, Rabinovici J, Jaffe RB: Inhibin and activin in reproductive biology. Obstet Gynecol Surv 47:173, 1992

el Roeiy A, Chen X, Roberts VJ, et al: Expression of insulin-like growth factor-I (IGF-I) and IGF-II and the IGF-I, IGF-II, and insulin receptor genes and localization of the gene products in the human ovary. J Clin Endocrinol Metab 77:1411, 1993

Eppig JJ: A comparison between oocyte growth in coculture with granulosa cells and oocytes with granulosa cell-oocyte junctional contact maintained in vitro. J Exp Zool 209:345, 1979

Erickson GF, Wang C, Hsueh AJ: FSH induction of functional LH receptors in granulosa cells cultured in a chemically defined medium. Nature 279:336, 1979

Espey LL: Ovarian proteolytic enzymes and ovulation. Biol Reprod 10:216, 1974

Fahie-Wilson MN, John R, Ellis AR: Macroprolactin; high molecular mass forms of circulating prolactin. Ann Clin Biochem 42:175, 2005

Faiman C, Winter JS, Reyes FI: Patterns of gonadotrophins and gonadal steroids throughout life. Clin Obstet Gynaecol 3:467, 1976

Ferin M, International Institute for the Study of Human Reproduction: Biorhythms and Human Reproduction; a conference sponsored by the International Institute for the Study of Human Reproduction. New York, Wiley, 1974

Fisher DA: Maternal-fetal neurohypophyseal system. Clin Perinatol 10:695, 1983

Fletcher WH, Greenan JR: Receptor mediated action without receptor occupancy. Endocrinology 116:1660, 1985

Frieze TW, Mong DP, Koops MK: "Hook effect" in prolactinomas: case report and review of literature. Endocr Pract 8:296, 2002

Fu LY, van den Pol AN: Kisspeptin directly excites anorexigenic proopiomelanocortin neurons but inhibits orexigenic neuropeptide Y cells by an indirect synaptic mechanism. J Neurosci 30:10205, 2010

Funabashi T, Brooks PJ, Weesner GD, et al: Luteinizing hormone-releasing hormone receptor messenger ribonucleic acid expression in the rat pituitary during lactation and the estrous cycle. J Neuroendocrinol 6:261, 1994

Gougeon A, Ecochard R, Thalabard JC: Age-related changes of the population of human ovarian follicles: increase in the disappearance rate of non-growing and early-growing follicles in aging women. Biol Reprod 50:653, 1994

Grafer CM, Thomas R, Lambrakos L, et al: GnRH stimulates expression of PACAP in the pituitary gonadotropes via both the PKA and PKC signaling systems. Mol Endocrinol 23:1022, 2009

Groome NP, Illingworth PJ, O'Brien M, et al: Measurement of dimeric inhibin B throughout the human menstrual cycle. J Clin Endocrinol Metab 81:1401, 1996

Grossman A: Brain opiates and neuroendocrine function. Clin Endocrinol Metab 12:725, 1983

Gruber CJ, Tschugguel W, Schneeberger C, al: Production and actions of estrogens. N Engl J Med 346(5):340, 2002

Haisenleder DJ, Ortolano GA, Dalkin AC, et al: Differential actions of thyrotropin (TSH)-releasing hormone pulses in the expression of prolactin and TSH subunit messenger ribonucleic acid in rat pituitary cells in vitro. Endocrinology 130:2917, 1992

Hammond GL, Bocchinfuso WP: Sex hormone-binding globulin: gene organization and structure/function analyses. Horm Res 45:197, 1996

Hammond GL, Underhill DA, Rykse HM, et al: The human sex hormone-binding globulin gene contains exons for androgen-binding protein and two other testicular messenger RNAs. Mol Endocrinol 3:1869, 1989

Haskell SG: Selective estrogen receptor modulators. South Med J 96:469, 2003

Head JR, MacDonald PC, Casey ML: Cellular localization of membrane metalloendopeptidase (enkephalinase) in human endometrium during the ovarian cycle. J Clin Endocrinol Metab 76:769, 1993

Hernandez ER, Hurwitz A, Vera A, et al: Expression of the genes encoding the insulin-like growth factors and their receptors in the human ovary. J Clin Endocrinol Metab 74:419, 1992

Hillier SG, van den Boogaard AM, Reichert LE Jr, et al: Intraovarian sex steroid hormone interactions and the regulation of follicular maturation: aromatization of androgens by human granulosa cells in vitro. J Clin Endocrinol Metab 50:640, 1980

Hodgen GD: The dominant ovarian follicle. Fertil Steril 38:281, 1982

Hoff JD, Quigley ME, Yen SS: Hormonal dynamics at midcycle: a reevaluation. J Clin Endocrinol Metab 57:792, 1983

Houben H, Denef C: Bioactive peptides in anterior pituitary cells. Peptides 15:547, 1994

Howlett TA, Rees LH: Endogenous opioid peptides and hypothalamo-pituitary function. Annu Rev Physiol 48:527, 1986

Hsueh AJ, Eisenhauer K, Chun SY, et al: Gonadal cell apoptosis. Recent Prog Horm Res 51:433, 1996

Iles RK: Ectopic hCGbeta expression by epithelial cancer: malignant behaviour, metastasis and inhibition of tumor cell apoptosis. Mol Cell Endocrinol 260:264, 2007

Jia XC, Kessel B, Welsh TH Jr, et al: Androgen inhibition of follicle-stimulating hormone-stimulated luteinizing hormone receptor formation in cultured rat granulosa cells. Endocrinol 117:13, 1985

Kaiser UB, Conn PM, Chin WW: Studies of gonadotropin-releasing hormone (GnRH) action using GnRH receptor-expressing pituitary cell lines. Endocr Rev 18:46, 1997

Kaiser UB, Lee BL, Carroll RS, et al: Follistatin gene expression in the pituitary: localization in gonadotropes and folliculostellate cells in diestrous rats. Endocrinology 130:3048, 1992

Kaltsas GA, Nomikos P, Kontogeorgos G, et al: Clinical review: diagnosis and management of pituitary carcinomas. J Clin Endocrinol Metab 90:3089, 2005

Kaplan SL, Grumbach MM, Aubert ML: The ontogenesis of pituitary hormones and hypothalamic factors in the human fetus: maturation of central nervous system regulation of anterior pituitary function. Recent Prog Horm Res 32:161, 1976

Kerin JF, Kirby C, Morris D, et al: Incidence of the luteinized unruptured follicle phenomenon in cycling women. Fertil Steril 40:620, 1983

Kettel LM, DePaolo LV, Morales AJ, et al: Circulating levels of follistatin from puberty to menopause. Fertil Steril 65:472, 1996

Khoury RH, Wang QF, Crowley WF Jr, et al: Serum follistatin levels in women: evidence against an endocrine function of ovarian follistatin. J Clin Endocrinol Metab 80:1361, 1995

Khoury SA, Reame NE, Kelch RP, et al: Diurnal patterns of pulsatile luteinizing hormone secretion in hypothalamic amenorrhea: reproducibility and responses to opiate blockade and an alpha 2-adrenergic agonist. J Clin Endocrinol Metab 64:755, 1987

Kim HH, Mui KL, Nikrodhanond AA, et al: Regulation of gonadotropin-releasing hormone in nonhypothalamic tissues. Semin Reprod Med 25:326, 2007

King JC, Anthony EL: LHRH neurons and their projections in humans and other mammals: species comparisons. Peptides 5(Suppl 1).195, 1984

Kiss A, Mikkelsen JD: Oxytocin—anatomy and functional assignments: a minireview. Endocr Regul 39:97, 2005

Klibanski A, Neer RM, Beitins IZ, et al: Decreased bone density in hyperprolactinemic women. N Engl J Med 303:1311, 1980

Klinge CM: Estrogen receptor interaction with estrogen response elements. Nucleic Acids Res 29:2905, 2001

Knobil E: On the control of gonadotropin secretion in the rhesus monkey. Recent Prog Horm Res 30:1, 1974

Knobil E: The neuroendocrine control of the menstrual cycle. Recent Prog Horm Res 36:53, 1980

Knobil E: The Physiology of Reproduction. New York, Raven Press, 1994

Krieger DT: Neuroendocrinology, the Interrelationships of the Body's Two Major Integrative Systems in Normal Physiology and in Clinical Disease. Sunderland, MA, Sinauer Associates, 1980

Kuhl H: Pharmacology of estrogens and progestogens: influence of different routes of administration. Climacteric 8(Suppl 1):3, 2005

Kuiper GG, Carlsson B, Grandien K, et al: Comparison of the ligand binding specificity and transcript tissue distribution of estrogen receptors alpha and beta. Endocrinology 138:863, 1997

Lawrence C, Fraley GS: Galanin-like peptide (GALP) is a hypothalamic regulator of energy homeostasis and reproduction. Front Neuroendocrinol 32:1, 2011

Lehman MN, Coolen LM, Goodman RL: Minireview: kisspeptin/neurokinin B/dynorphin (KNDy) cells of the arcuate nucleus: a central node in the control of gonadotropin-releasing hormone secretion. Endocrinology 151:3479, 2010

Lemarchand-Beraud T, Zufferey MM, Reymond M, et al: Maturation of the hypothalamo-pituitary-ovarian axis in adolescent girls. J Clin Endocrinol Metab 54:241, 1982

Lessey BA, Killam AP, Metzger DA, et al: Immunohistochemical analysis of human uterine estrogen and progesterone receptors throughout the menstrual cycle. J Clin Endocrinol Metab 67:334, 1988

Li W, Yuen BH, Leung PC: Inhibition of progestin accumulation by activin-A in human granulosa cells. J Clin Endocrinol Metab 75:285, 1992

Liu CF, Parker K, Yao HH: WNT4/beta-catenin pathway maintains female germ cell survival by inhibiting activin betaB in the mouse fetal ovary. PLoS One 5:e10382, 2010

Lockwood CJ, Nemerson Y, Krikun G, et al: Steroid-modulated stromal cell tissue factor expression: a model for the regulation of endometrial hemostasis and menstruation. J Clin Endocrinol Metab 77:1014, 1993

Lumsden MA, Kelly RW, Templeton AA, et al: Changes in the concentration of prostaglandins in preovulatory human follicles after administration of hCG. J Reprod Fertil 77:119, 1986

Lydon JP, DeMayo FJ, Conneely OM, et al: Reproductive phenotypes of the progesterone receptor null mutant mouse. J Steroid Biochem Mol Biol 56(1-6 Spec No):67, 1996

Mashchak CA, Lobo Ra, Dozono-Takano R, et al: Comparison of pharmacodynamic properties of various estrogen formulations. Am J Obstet Gynecol 144:511, 1982

Mason JI: Genetics of Steroid Biosynthesis and Function. New York, Taylor & Francis, 2002

McConnell DS, Wang Q, Sluss PM, et al: A two-site chemiluminescent assay for activin-free follistatin reveals that most follistatin circulating in men and normal cycling women is in an activin-bound state. J Clin Endocrinol Metab 83:851, 1998

McLachlan RI, Cohen NL, Vale WW, et al: The importance of luteinizing hormone in the control of inhibin and progesterone secretion by the human corpus luteum. J Clin Endocrinol Metab 68:1078, 1989

McLachlan RI, Robertson DM, Healy DL, et al: Circulating immunoreactive inhibin levels during the normal human menstrual cycle. J Clin Endocrinol Metab 65:954, 1987

McNatty KP, Makris A, DeGrazia C, et al: The production of progesterone, androgens, and estrogens by granulosa cells, thecal tissue, and stromal tissue from human ovaries in vitro. J Clin Endocrinol Metab 49:687, 1979a

McNatty KP, Makris A, Reinhold VN, et al: Metabolism of androstenedione by human ovarian tissues in vitro with particular reference to reductase and aromatase activity. Steroids 34:429, 1979b

McNeely MJ, Soules MR: The diagnosis of luteal phase deficiency: a critical review. Fertil Steril 50:1, 1988

Melmed S, Jameson JL: Disorders of the anterior pituitary and hypothalamus. In Kasper DL, Braunwald E, Fauci AS, et al (eds): Harrison's Principles of Internal Medicine, 17th ed. New York, McGraw-Hill, 2008, p 2206

Meunier H, Rivier C, Evans RM, et al: Gonadal and extragonadal expression of inhibin alpha, beta A, and beta B subunits in various tissues predicts diverse functions. Proc Natl Acad Sci U S A 85:247, 1988

Miller WL: Molecular biology of steroid hormone synthesis. Endocr Rev 9:295, 1988

Molitch ME: Disorders of prolactin secretion. Endocrinol Metab Clin North Am 30:585, 2001

Molitch ME: Management of prolactinomas during pregnancy. J Reprod Med 44(Suppl 12).1121, 1999

Molitch ME: Prolactinomas and pregnancy. Clin Endocrinol (Oxf) 73:147, 2010

Moore FL, Evans SJ: Steroid hormones use non-genomic mechanisms to control brain functions and behaviors: a review of evidence. Brain Behav Evol 54:41, 1999

Muttukrishna S, Tannetta D, Groome N, et al: Activin and follistatin in female reproduction. Mol Cell Endocrinol 225:45, 2004

Nakai Y, Plant TM, Hess DL, et al: On the sites of the negative and positive feedback actions of estradiol in the control of gonadotropin secretion in the rhesus monkey. Endocrinology 102:1008, 1978

Negro-Vilar A: Selective androgen receptor modulators (SARMs):a novel approach to androgen therapy for the new millennium. J Clin Endocrinol Metab 84:3459, 1999

Neill JD: GnRH and GnRH receptor genes in the human genome. Endocrinology 143:737, 2002

Nixon B, Aitken RJ, McLaughlin EA: New insights into the molecular mechanisms of sperm-egg interaction. Cell Mol Life Sci 64:1805, 2007

Notarianni E: Reinterpretation of evidence advanced for neo-oogenesis in mammals, in terms of a finite oocyte reserve. J Ovarian Res 4:1, 2011

Noyes RW, Hertig AT, Rock J: Dating the endometrial biopsy. Fertil Steril 1:3, 1950

Ohlsson R: Growth factors, protooncogenes and human placental development. Cell Differ Dev 28:1, 1989

Olive DL: The prevalence and epidemiology of luteal-phase deficiency in normal and infertile women. Clin Obstet Gynecol 34:157, 1991

O'Malley BW, Strott CA: Steroid hormones: metabolism and mechanism of action. In Yen SS, Jaffe RB, Barbieri RL (eds): Reproductive Endocrinology, 4th ed. Philadelphia, Saunders, 1999, p 128

Pache TD, Wladimiroff JW, de Jong FH, et al: Growth patterns of nondominant ovarian follicles during the normal menstrual cycle. Fertil Steril 54:638, 1990

Patton PE, Stouffer RL: Current understanding of the corpus luteum in women and nonhuman primates. Clin Obstet Gynecol 34:127, 1991

Peters EE, Towler KL, Mason DR, et al: Effects of galanin and leptin on gonadotropin-releasing hormone-stimulated luteinizing hormone release from the pituitary. Neuroendocrinology 89:18, 2009

Peters H, Byskov AG, Grinsted J: Follicular growth in fetal and prepubertal ovaries of humans and other primates. Clin Endocrinol Metab 7:469, 1978

Peters H, Joint A: The Ovary: A Correlation of Structure and Function in Mammals. Berkeley, University of California Press, 1980

Petraglia F, D'Ambrogio G, Comitini G, et al: Impairment of opioid control of luteinizing hormone secretion in menstrual disorders. Fertil Steril 43:534, 1985

Pineda R, Aguilar E, Pinilla L, et al: Physiological roles of the kisspeptin/GPR54 system in the neuroendocrine control of reproduction. Prog Brain Res 181:55, 2010

Piquette GN, Crabtree ME, el Danasouri I, et al: Regulation of plasminogen activator inhibitor-1 and -2 messenger ribonucleic acid levels in human cumulus and granulosa-luteal cells. J Clin Endocrinol Metab 76:518, 1993

Pope WF: Uterine asynchrony: a cause of embryonic loss. Biol Reprod 39:999, 1988

Press MF, Udove JA, Greene GL: Progesterone receptor distribution in the human endometrium. Analysis using monoclonal antibodies to the human progesterone receptor. Am J Pathol 131:112, 1988

Priddy AR, Killick SR, Elstein M, et al: The effect of prostaglandin synthetase inhibitors on human preovulatory follicular fluid prostaglandin, thromboxane, and leukotriene concentrations. J Clin Endocrinol Metab 71:235, 1990

Ravindranath N, Little-Ihrig L, Phillips HS, et al: Vascular endothelial growth factor messenger ribonucleic acid expression in the primate ovary. Endocrinology 131:254, 1992

Redding TW, Kastin AJ, Gonzales-Barcena D, et al: The half-life, metabolism and excretion of tritiated luteinizing hormone-releasing hormone (LH-RH) in man. J Clin Endocrinol Metab 37:626, 1973

Rosner W, Hryb DJ, Kahn SM, et al: Interactions of sex hormone-binding globulin with target cells. Mol Cell Endocrinol 316:79, 2010

Ruscalleda J: Imaging of parasellar lesions. Eur Radiol 15:549, 2005

Russell DW, Wilson JD: Steroid 5 alpha-reductase: two genes/two enzymes. Annu Rev Biochem 63:25, 1994

Sasano H, Okamoto M, Mason JI, et al: Immunolocalization of aromatase, 17 alpha-hydroxylase and side-chain-cleavage cytochromes P-450 in the human ovary. J Reprod Fertil 85:163, 1989

Saxena BB, Beling CG, Gandy HM, et al: Gonadotropins. New York, Wiley-Interscience, 1972

Schatz F, Aigner S, Papp C, et al: Plasminogen activator activity during decidualization of human endometrial stromal cells is regulated by plasminogen activator inhibitor 1. J Clin Endocrinol Metab 80:2504, 1995

Schipper I, Hop WC, Fauser BC: The follicle-stimulating hormone (FSH) threshold/window concept examined by different interventions with exogenous FSH during the follicular phase of the normal menstrual cycle: duration, rather than magnitude, of FSH increase affects follicle development. J Clin Endocrinol Metab 83:1292, 1998

Schlechte J, Dolan K, Sherman B, et al: The natural history of untreated hyperprolactinemia: a prospective analysis. J Clin Endocrinol Metab 68:412, 1989

Seilicovich A, Pisera D, Sciascia SA, et al: Gene therapy for pituitary tumors. Curr Gene Ther 5:559, 2005

Sharkey AM, Dellow K, Blayney M, et al: Stage-specific expression of cytokine and receptor messenger ribonucleic acids in human preimplantation embryos. Biol Reprod 53:974, 1995

Silva JR, Figueiredo JR, van den Hurk R: Involvement of growth hormone (GH) and insulin-like growth factor (IGF) system in ovarian folliculogenesis. Theriogenology 71:1193, 2009

Silva PD, Gentzschein EE, Lobo RA: Androstenedione may be a more important precursor of tissue dihydrotestosterone than testosterone in women. Fertil Steril 48:419, 1987

Silverman AJ, Jhamandas J, Renaud LP: Localization of luteinizing hormone-releasing hormone (LHRH) neurons that project to the median eminence. J Neurosci 7:2312, 1987

Smith G, Roberts R, Hall C, et al: Reversible ovulatory failure associated with the development of luteinized unruptured follicles in women with inflammatory arthritis taking non-steroidal anti-inflammatory drugs. Br J Rheumatol 35:458, 1996

Stanczyk FZ: Pharmacokinetics and potency of progestins used for hormone replacement therapy and contraception. Rev Endocr Metab Disord 3:211, 2002

Stern K, McClintock MK: Regulation of ovulation by human pheromones. Nature 392:177, 1998

Stouffer RL, Hodgen GD: Induction of luteal phase defects in rhesus monkeys by follicular fluid administration at the onset of the menstrual cycle. J Clin Endocrinol Metab 51:669, 1980

Stout SM, Stumpf JL: Finasteride treatment of hair loss in women. Ann Pharmacother 44:1090, 2010

Sutton RE, Koob GF, Le Moal M, et al: Corticotropin releasing factor produces behavioural activation in rats. Nature 297:331, 1982

Taylor HS, Vanden Heuvel GB, Igarashi P: A conserved Hox axis in the mouse and human female reproductive system: late establishment and persistent adult expression of the Hoxa cluster genes. Biol Reprod 57:1338, 1997

Tedeschi C, Hazum E, Kokia E, et al: Endothelin-1 as a luteinization inhibitor: inhibition of rat granulosa cell progesterone accumulation via selective modulation of key steroidogenic steps affecting both progesterone formation and degradation. Endocrinology 131:2476, 1992

Thierry van Dessel HJ, Chandrasekher Y, Yap OW, et al: Serum and follicular fluid levels of insulin-like growth factor I (IGF-I), IGF-II, and IGF-binding protein-1 and -3 during the normal menstrual cycle. J Clin Endocrinol Metab 81:1224, 1996

Tobet SA, Schwarting GA: Minireview: recent progress in gonadotropin-releasing hormone neuronal migration. Endocrinology 147:1159, 2006

Trakakis E, Basios G, Trompoukis P, et al: An update to 21-hydroxylase deficient congenital adrenal hyperplasia. Gynecol Endocrinol 26:63, 2010

Treloar AE, Boynton RE, Behn BG, et al: Variation of the human menstrual cycle through reproductive life. Int J Fertil 12(1 Pt 2):77, 1967

Tsafriri A, Dekel N, Bar-Ami S: The role of oocyte maturation inhibitor in follicular regulation of oocyte maturation. J Reprod Fertil 64:541, 1982

Upadhyay S, Zamboni L: Ectopic germ cells: natural model for the study of germ cell sexual differentiation. Proc Natl Acad Sci U S A 79:6584, 1982

Van Gaal L, Abs R, De Leeuw I, et al: Hypothyroidism and prolactin. Eur J Obstet Gynecol Reprod Biol 12:315, 1981

Vande Wiele RL, Bogumil J, Dyrenfurth I, et al: Mechanisms regulating the menstrual cycle in women. Recent Prog Horm Res 26:63, 1970

Verbalis JG, Robinson AG: Characterization of neurophysin-vasopressin prohormones in human posterior pituitary tissue. J Clin Endocrinol Metab 57:115, 1983

Webster J: A comparative review of the tolerability profiles of dopamine agonists in the treatment of hyperprolactinaemia and inhibition of lactation. Drug Saf 14:228, 1996

Webster J, Piscitelli G, Polli A, et al: A comparison of cabergoline and bromocriptine in the treatment of hyperprolactinemic amenorrhea. Cabergoline Comparative Study Group. N Engl J Med 331:904, 1994

Wei LL, Hawkins P, Baker C, et al: An amino-terminal truncated progesterone receptor isoform, PRc, enhances progestin-induced transcriptional activity. Mol Endocrinol 10:1379, 1996

Wiegratz I, Kuhl H: Progestogen therapies: differences in clinical effects? Trends Endocrinol Metab 15:277, 2004

Wierman ME, Pawlowski JE, Allen MP, et al: Molecular mechanisms of gonadotropin-releasing hormone neuronal migration. Trends Endocrinol Metab 15:96, 2004

Wildt L, Hausler A, Marshall G, et al: Frequency and amplitude of gonadotropin-releasing hormone stimulation and gonadotropin secretion in the rhesus monkey. Endocrinology 109:376, 1981

Williams CL, Nishihara M, Thalabard JC, et al: Duration and frequency of multiunit electrical activity associated with the hypothalamic gonadotropin releasing hormone pulse generator in the rhesus monkey: differential effects of morphine. Neuroendocrinology 52:225, 1990

Winter JS, Hughes IA, Reyes FI, et al: Pituitary-gonadal relations in infancy: 2. Patterns of serum gonadal steroid concentrations in man from birth to two years of age. J Clin Endocrinol Metab 42:679, 1976

Yen SS, Quigley ME, Reid RL, et al: Neuroendocrinology of opioid peptides and their role in the control of gonadotropin and prolactin secretion. Am J Obstet Gynecol 152:485, 1985

Yen SSC, Jaffe RB: Reproductive Endocrinology: Physiology, Pathophysiology, and Clinical Management. Philadelphia, Saunders, 1986

Yoshimura Y, Wallach EE: Studies of the mechanism(s) of mammalian ovulation. Fertil Steril 47:22, 1987

Yoshinaga K, Serono Symposia USA: Blastocyst Implantation. Boston, Adams, 1989

Young JR, Jaffe RB: Strength-duration characteristics of estrogen effects on gonadotropin response to gonadotropin-releasing hormone in women. II. Effects of varying concentrations of estradiol. J Clin Endocrinol Metab 42:432, 1976

Yu B, Ruman J, Christman G: The role of peripheral gonadotropin-releasing hormone receptors in female reproduction. Fertil Steril 95:465, 2011

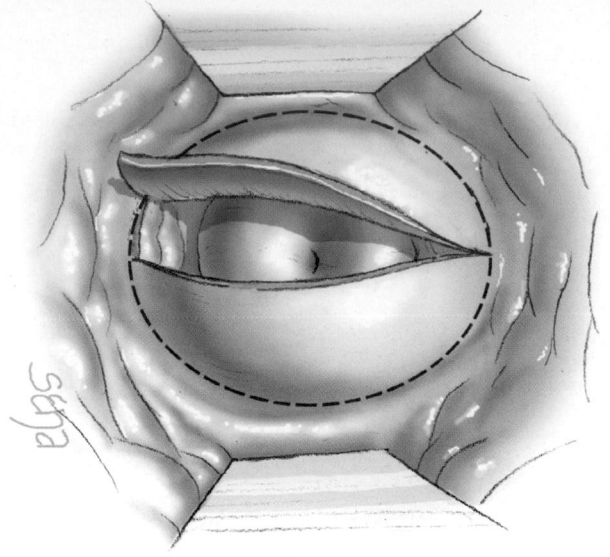

CHAPTER 16

Amenorrhea

Evaluation and management of a patient with amenorrhea is common in gynecology, and the prevalence of pathologic amenorrhea ranges from 3 to 4 percent in reproductive-aged populations (Bachmann, 1982; Pettersson, 1973). Amenorrhea is diagnosed in a female: (1) who has not menstruated by age 14 years and who lacks other evidence of pubertal development; (2) who has not menstruated by age 16, even in the presence of other pubertal signs; or (3) who has previously menstruated but has been without menses for a time equivalent to a total of three previous cycles or 6 months. Although amenorrhea has classically been defined as primary (no prior menses) or secondary (cessation of menses), this distinction may lead to diagnostic error and should be avoided.

In some circumstances, evaluation reasonably may be initiated despite the absence of these strict criteria. Examples include a patient with the stigmata of Turner syndrome, obvious virilization, or a history of uterine curettage. An evaluation for delayed puberty should also be considered before the ages just listed if the patient or her parents are concerned.

Although the list of possible etiologies is extensive, most causes will fall into a limited number of categories (Tables 16-1 and 16-2). Of course, amenorrhea is a normal state prior to puberty, during pregnancy and lactation, and following the menopause.

NORMAL MENSTRUAL CYCLE

A differential diagnosis for amenorrhea can be developed based on requirements for normal menses. Generation of a cyclic, controlled pattern of uterine bleeding requires precise temporal and quantitative regulation of a number of reproductive hormones (Chap. 15, p. 423).

First, the hypothalamic-pituitary-ovarian axis must be functional. The hypothalamus releases pulses of gonadotropin-releasing hormone (GnRH) into the portal circulation at defined frequencies and amplitude. Gonadotropin-releasing hormone stimulates the synthesis and secretion of the gonadotropins, luteinizing hormone (LH) and follicle-stimulating hormone (FSH), by the gonadotrope cells of the anterior pituitary gland. These gonadotropins enter the peripheral circulation and act on the ovary to stimulate both follicular development and ovarian hormone production. These ovarian hormones include the steroid hormones (estrogen, progesterone, and androgens), as well as the peptide hormone inhibin. As suggested by its name, inhibin blocks FSH synthesis and secretion. Gonadal steroids are typically inhibitory at both the pituitary and the hypothalamus. However, development of a mature follicle results

TABLE 16-1. Primary Amenorrhea: Frequency of Etiologies

Presentation	Frequency (%)
Hypergonadotropic hypogonadism	43
45,X and variants	27
46,XX	14
46,XY	2
Eugonadism	30
Müllerian agenesis	15
Vaginal septum	3
Imperforate hymen	1
AIS	1
PCOS	7
CAH	1
Cushing and thyroid disease	2
Low FSH without breast development	27
Constitutional delay	14
GnRH deficiency	5
Other CNS disease	1
Pituitary disease	5
Eating disorders, stress, excess exercise	2

AIS = androgen insensitivity syndrome; CAH = congenital adrenal hyperplasia; CNS = central nervous system; FSH = follicle-stimulating hormone; GnRH = gonadotropin-releasing hormone; PCOS = polycystic ovarian syndrome.
Adapted from Reindollar, 1981, with permission.

TABLE 16-2. Secondary Amenorrhea: Frequency of Etiologies[a]

Etiology	Frequency (%)
Low or normal FSH level: various	67.5
Eating disorders, stress, excess exercise	15.5
Nonspecific hypothalamic	18
Chronic anovulation (PCOS)	28
Hypothyroidism	1.5
Cushing syndrome	1
Pituitary tumor/empty sella	2
Sheehan syndrome	1.5
High FSH level: gonadal failure	10.5
46,XX	10
Abnormal karyotype	0.5
High prolactin level	13
Anatomic	7
Asherman syndrome	7
Hyperandrogenic states	2
Late-onset CAH	0.5
Ovarian tumor	1
Undiagnosed	0.5

[a]Excluding pregnancy diagnoses.
CAH = congenital adrenal hyperplasia; FSH = follicle-stimulating hormone; PCOS = polycystic ovarian syndrome.
Adapted from Reindollar, 1986, with permission.

in a rapid rise in estrogen levels. These levels act positively at the pituitary to generate a midcycle surge in LH release. The mechanism by which this previously negative estrogen feedback switches to positive feedback is unknown. In addition to LH release, circulating estrogens stimulate the development of a thickened, proliferative endometrial lining.

Following ovulation, LH stimulates luteinization of the follicular granulosa cells and surrounding theca cells to form the corpus luteum. The corpus luteum continues to produce estrogen, but also secretes high levels of progesterone. Progesterone converts the endometrium to a secretory pattern. If pregnancy occurs, the corpus luteum is "rescued" by human chorionic gonadotropin (hCG) secreted from early syncytiotrophoblast. hCG is similar structurally to LH and assumes the role of corpus luteum support during early pregnancy. If pregnancy does not occur, then progesterone and estrogen secretion ceases, the corpus luteum regresses, and endometrial sloughing ensues. The pattern of this "progesterone withdrawal bleed" will vary in duration and blood loss among women, but should be relatively constant across cycles for each individual.

Amenorrhea may follow disruption of this choreographed communication. However, menses may be absent even in the presence of normal cyclic hormonal changes due to the presence of anatomic abnormalities. The endometrium must be able to respond normally to hormonal stimulation, and the cervix, vagina, and introitus must be present and patent.

CLASSIFICATION SYSTEM

Numerous classification systems for the diagnosis of amenorrhea have been developed, and all have their strengths and weaknesses. One useful scheme is outlined in Table 16-3. This system divides the causes of amenorrhea into anatomic versus hormonal etiologies with further division into inherited versus acquired disorders.

As described earlier, normal menses require adequate ovarian production of steroid hormones. Decreased ovarian function (hypogonadism) may result either from a lack of stimulation by the gonadotropins (*hypo*gonadotropic hypogonadism) or from primary failure of the ovary (*hyper*gonadotropic hypogonadism) (Table 16-4). A number of disorders are associated with relatively normal LH and FSH levels (*eu*gonadotropic), however, there is loss of appropriate cyclicity. A classic example within this category is polycystic ovarian syndrome as discussed further on page 451.

ANATOMIC DISORDERS

Anatomic abnormalities that may present as amenorrhea can broadly be viewed as either inherited or acquired disorders of the outflow tract (uterus, cervix, vagina, and introitus).

TABLE 16-3. Classification Scheme for Amenorrhea

Anatomic

Inherited
- Müllerian agenesis (partial or complete)
- Vaginal septum
- Cervical atresia
- Imperforate hymen
- Labial fusion

Acquired
- Intrauterine synechiae (Asherman syndrome)
- Cervical stenosis

Hormonal/Endocrinologic

Hypergonadotropic Hypogonadism (POF)
Inherited
- Chromosomal (gonadal dysgenesis)
- Single-gene disorders

Acquired
- Infectious
- Autoimmune
- Iatrogenic
- Environmental
- Idiopathic

Hypogonadotropic Hypogonadism
Disorders of the hypothalamus = hypothalamic amenorrhea
Inherited
- Idiopathic hypogonadotropic hypogonadism (IHH)
- Kallmann syndrome

Acquired
- Hypothalamic amenorrhea ("functional")
  - Eating disorders
  - Excessive exercise
  - Stress
- Destructive processes
  - Tumor
  - Radiation
  - Trauma
  - Infection
  - Infiltrative disease
- Pseudocyesis

Eugonadotropic Amenorrhea
Inherited
- Polycystic ovarian syndrome
- Adult-onset congenital adrenal hyperplasia
- Ovarian tumors (steroid producing)

Acquired
- Hyperprolactinemia
- Thyroid disease
- Cushing syndrome
- Acromegaly

Hypogonadotropic Hypogonadism (cont'd)
Disorders of the anterior pituitary gland
Inherited
- Pituitary hypoplasia

Acquired
- Adenoma
  - Prolactinoma
- Destructive processes
  - Macroadenoma
  - Metastases
  - Radiation
  - Trauma
  - Infarction (Sheehan syndrome)
  - Infiltrative disease

Chronic disease
- End-stage kidney disease
- Liver disease
- Malignancy
- Acquired immunodeficiency syndrome (AIDS)
- Malabsorption syndromes

TABLE 16-4. Categories of Amenorrhea Based on Gonadotropin and Estrogen Levels

Type of Hypogonadism	LH/FSH	Estrogen	Primary Defect
Hypergonadotropic	High	Low	Ovary
Hypogonadotropic	Low	Low	Hypothalamus/pituitary
Eugonadotropic	Normal[a]	Normal[a]	Varied

[a]Generally in normal range, but lack cyclicity.
FSH = follicle-stimulating hormone; LH = luteinizing hormone.

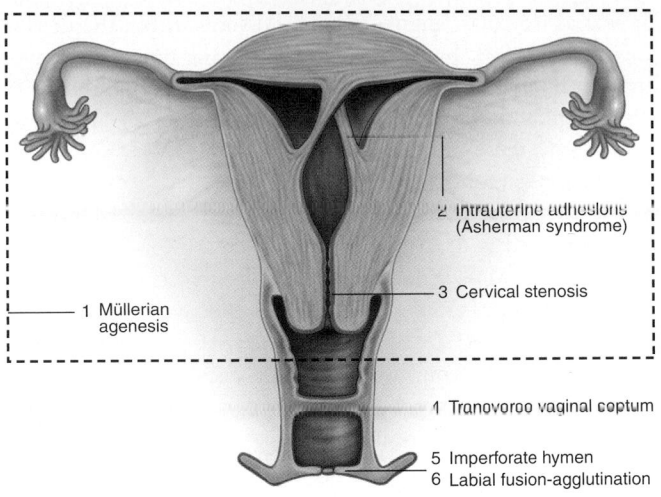

FIGURE 16-1 Drawing demonstrating anatomic defects that may lead to amenorrhea.

- 2 Intrauterine adhesions (Asherman syndrome)
- 3 Cervical stenosis
- 1 Müllerian agenesis
- 4 Transverse vaginal septum
- 5 Imperforate hymen
- 6 Labial fusion-agglutination

TABLE 16-5. Comparison of Müllerian Agenesis and Androgen Insensitivity Syndrome

Presentation	Müllerian Agenesis	Androgen Insensitivity
Inheritance pattern	Sporadic	X-linked recessive
Karyotype	46,XX	46,XY
Breast development	Yes	Yes
Axillary and pubic hair	Yes	No
Uterus	No	No
Gonad	Ovary	Testis
Testosterone	Female levels	Male levels
Associated anomalies	Yes	No

Inherited

These are a frequent cause of amenorrhea in adolescents, and pelvic anatomy is abnormal in approximately 15 percent of women with primary amenorrhea (The Practice Committee of the American Society for Reproductive Medicine, 2006). Figure 16-1 depicts the range of anatomic defects that may present with amenorrhea. These are additionally discussed in Chapter 18 (p. 492).

Distal Outflow Tract Obstruction

Amenorrhea will be observed in the presence of an imperforate hymen (1 in 2000 women), a transverse vaginal septum (1 in 70,000 women), or isolated atresia of the vagina (Banerjee, 1999; Parazzini, 1990; Reid, 2000). Patients with these anomalies have a 46,XX karyotype, female secondary sexual characteristics, and normal ovarian function. Therefore, the amount of uterine bleeding is normal, but its normal path for egress is obstructed or absent. These patients may note moliminal symptoms, such as breast tenderness, food cravings, and mood changes, which are attributable to elevated progesterone levels. In addition, accumulation of menstrual blood behind an obstruction frequently results in cyclic abdominal pain. In women with outflow tract obstruction, an increase in retrograde menstruation may lead to development of endometriosis with associated complications such as chronic pain and infertility. Also, although structurally normal, labia in some girls may be severely agglutinated and can lead to obstruction and amenorrhea. Most cases are treated early with topical estrogen and/or manual separation as described in Chapter 14 (p. 386). Thus, outflow obstruction in most of these cases is avoided.

Müllerian Defects

During embryonic development, the müllerian ducts give rise to the upper vagina, cervix, uterine corpus, and fallopian tubes. Müllerian agenesis may be partial or complete. Accordingly, amenorrhea may result from outflow obstruction or from a lack of endometrium in cases involving uterine agenesis. In complete müllerian agenesis, often called Mayer-Rokitansky-Kuster-Hauser syndrome, patients fail to develop any müllerian structures, and examination reveals only a vaginal dimple. In a report from Finland, approximately 1 in 5000 newborn females were identified with this disorder. Thus, it ranks second only to gonadal dysgenesis as a cause of primary amenorrhea (Aittomaki, 2001; Reindollar, 1981).

The presentation of complete müllerian agenesis may be confused with complete androgen insensitivity syndrome. In the latter condition, the patient has a 46,XY karyotype and functioning testes. However, underlying androgen receptor mutations prevent normal testosterone binding, normal male ductal system development, and virilization. These two syndromes are compared in Table 16-5. More information about these disorders can be found in Chapter 18 (p. 481).

Acquired

Other abnormalities of the uterus that cause amenorrhea include cervical stenosis and extensive intrauterine adhesions.

Cervical Stenosis

Postoperative scarring and stenosis of the cervix may follow dilatation and curettage (D&C), cervical conization, loop electrosurgical excision procedures, infection, and neoplasia. Severe atrophic or radiation changes can also be causative.

Stenosis most commonly involves the internal os, and symptoms in menstruating women include amenorrhea, abnormal bleeding, dysmenorrhea, and infertility. Postmenopausal women are usually asymptomatic until fluid, exudates, or blood accumulates. The terms *hydrometra* (fluid), *pyometra* (pus), or *hematometra* (blood) are used to describe these conditions and are discussed additionally in Chapter 9 (p. 259). An inability to introduce a dilator into the uterine cavity is diagnostic. If obstruction is complete, a soft, enlarged uterus is palpable. Management of cervical stenosis involves dilatation of the cervix and exclusion of neoplasia in indicated cases as described in Chapter 4 (p. 129).

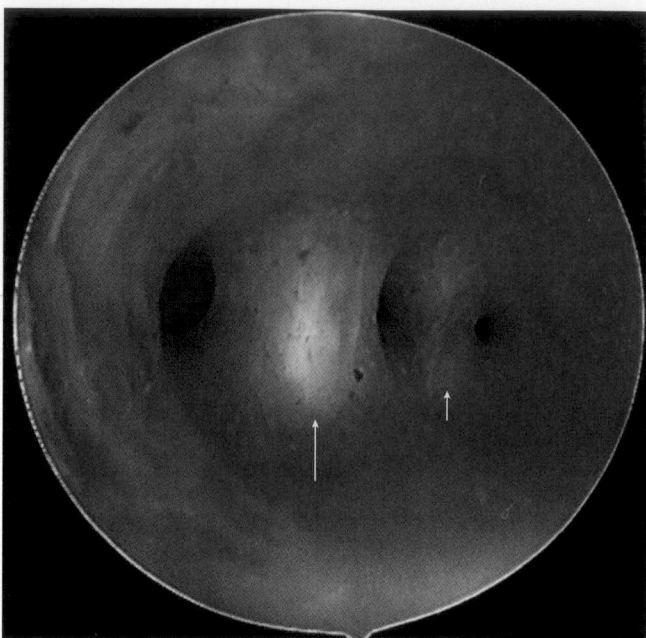

FIGURE 16-2 Hysteroscopic photograph displays intrauterine adhesions (*arrows*) found with Asherman syndrome. *(Photograph contributed by Dr. Ellen Wilson.)*

Intrauterine Adhesions (Asherman Syndrome)

Also known as uterine synechiae and when symptomatic, as Asherman syndrome, the spectrum of scarring includes filmy adhesions, dense bands, or complete obliteration of the uterine cavity (Fig. 16-2). The endometrium is divided into a functionalis layer, which lines the endometrial cavity, and a basalis layer, which regenerates the functionalis layer after each menstrual cycle. Destruction of the basalis endometrium prevents endometrial thickening in response to ovarian steroids. Therefore, no tissue is produced nor subsequently sloughed when steroid hormone levels fall at the end of the luteal phase.

Amenorrhea may be observed with extensive intrauterine scarring. In less severe cases, patients may present with hypomenorrhea or with recurrent pregnancy loss due to failure of normal placentation. In their evaluation of 292 women with intrauterine adhesions, Schenker and Margalioth (1982) noted delivery of term pregnancies in only 30 percent of 165 pregnancies. The remaining pregnancies either were spontaneously aborted (40 percent) or delivered prematurely.

Endometrial damage may follow vigorous curettage, usually in association with postpartum hemorrhage, miscarriage, or elective abortion complicated by infection. In a series of 1856 women with Asherman syndrome, 88 percent followed postabortal or postpartum uterine curettage (Schenker, 1982). Damage may also result from other uterine surgery, including metroplasty, myomectomy, or cesarean delivery, or from infection related to an intrauterine device. Although rare in the United States, tuberculous endometritis is a relatively common cause of Asherman syndrome in developing countries (Buttram, 1977; Klein, 1973; Sharma, 2009).

When intrauterine adhesions are suspected, hysterosalpingography is indicated. Intrauterine adhesions characteristically appear as irregular, angulated filling defects within the uterine cavity (Fig. 19-6, p. 517). At times, uterine polyps, leiomyomas, air bubbles, and blood clots may masquerade as adhesions. Transvaginal sonography or saline infusion sonography may help clarify these difficult cases (Fig. 2-20, p. 45), but definitive diagnosis requires hysteroscopy.

Hysteroscopic lysis of adhesions is the preferred surgical treatment and is described in Section 42-21 (p. 1178). Prior to the commonplace use of operative hysteroscopy, dilatation and curettage was employed. Although effective in lysing intrauterine adhesions, D&C unfortunately also injured normal endometrium. In contrast, the direct inspection afforded by hysteroscopy allows precise division of adhesion bands and clear documentation of the location and degree of adhesions and the results of the operative repair. As with uterine septum resection, laparoscopy may be a necessary adjunct to guide excision in severe cases to reduce risks of uterine perforation and intraperitoneal injury. Rates of success vary depending on the presenting symptoms, but a summary of the literature by Yu and coworkers (2008) showed a 74-percent pregnancy rate after hysteroscopic lysis in women who wanted to have a child, and of those, an 80-percent live birth rate. However, if only patients with severe disease are evaluated, pregnancy rates range from only 20 to 45 percent, and live births rates approximate only 30 percent (Fedele, 2006).

ENDOCRINE DISORDERS

Hypergonadotropic Hypogonadism (Premature Ovarian Failure)

The term *hypergonadotropic hypogonadism* refers to any process in which: (1) ovarian function is decreased or absent (hypogonadism) and (2) due to the lack of negative feedback, the gonadotropins LH and FSH have increased serum levels (hypergonadotropic). This category of disorders implies primary dysfunction at the level of the ovary, rather than centrally at the hypothalamus or pituitary. This process can also be termed *premature menopause* or *premature ovarian failure* (POF), with a current trend toward the term *primary ovarian insufficiency* (POI). The latter two terms are preferable as they better describe the pathophysiology of this condition.

Premature ovarian failure is defined as loss of oocytes and the surrounding support cells prior to age 40 years. The diagnosis is determined by two serum FSH levels greater than 40 mIU/mL obtained at least 1 month apart. This definition distinguishes POF from the physiologic loss of ovarian function, which occurs with normal menopause. The incidence of premature ovarian failure has been estimated at 1 in 1000 women less than 30 years and 1 in 100 women less than 40 years (Coulam, 1986). A careful evaluation is mandatory. Nevertheless, in most cases, the etiology of POF is not determined.

Heritable Disorders

Chromosomal Defects. Gonadal dysgenesis is the most frequent cause of POF. In this disorder, a normal complement of germ cells is present in the early fetal ovary. However, oocytes undergo accelerated atresia, and the ovary is replaced by a

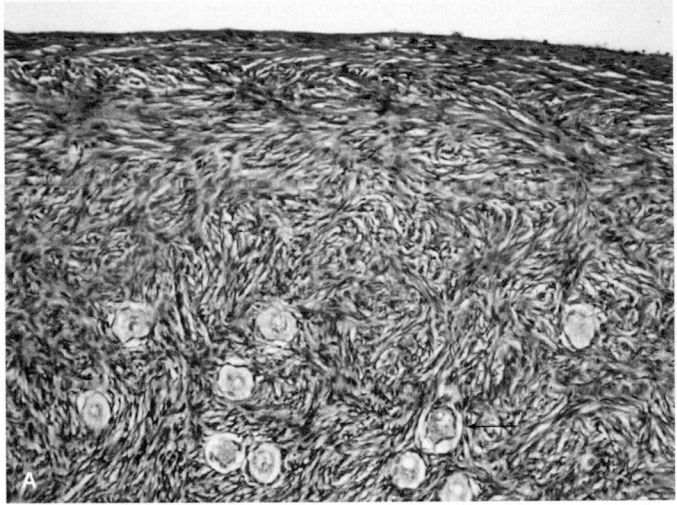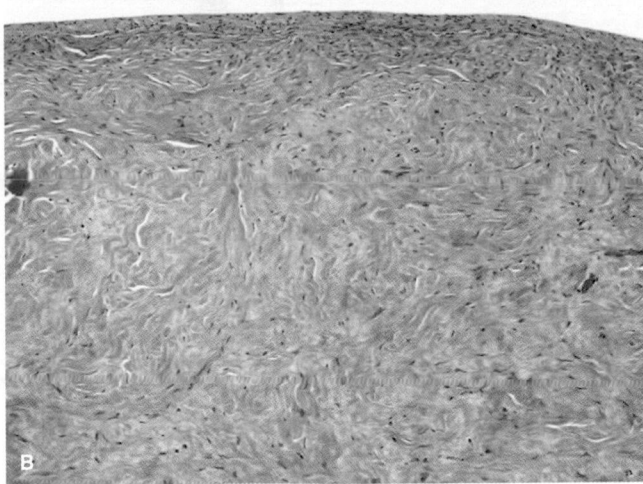

FIGURE 16-3 Photomicrographs of histologic samples. **A.** Normal premenopausal ovarian cortex with multiple primordial follicles. *(Photograph contributed by Dr. Kelley Carrick.)* **B.** Ovary from a woman with gonadal dysgenesis. Streak ovary showing ovarian-type stroma with no primordial follicles. *(Photograph contributed by Dr. Raheela Ashfaq.)*

fibrous streak—termed a streak gonad (Figs. 16-3 and 16-4) (Simpson, 1975; Singh, 1966). Individuals with gonadal dysgenesis may present with a variety of clinical features and can be divided into two broad groups based on whether the patient's karyotype is normal or abnormal (Schlessinger, 2002).

Deletion of genetic material from an X chromosome accounts for approximately two thirds of gonadal dysgenesis patients (Devi, 1998; Tho, 1981). These individuals are said to have Turner syndrome. A 45,X karyotype is found in approximately half of these patients, most of whom have associated somatic defects including short stature, webbed neck, low hairline, shield-shaped chest, and cardiovascular defects (Turner, 1972). Characteristics of the Turner phenotype are listed in Table 16-6.

The remaining patients with gonadal dysgenesis and identifiable abnormalities of the X chromosome have chromosomal mosaicism with or without associated structural abnormalities of the X chromosome. In these cases, the most common form of mosaicism is a 45,X/46,XX karyotype (Tho, 1981). Short stature and somatic abnormalities are most closely linked to deletions in the short arm of the X chromosome (Xp). In contrast, patients with deletion of the long arm of the X chromosome frequently have normal stature or may even have a eunuchoid body type. The low levels of estrogens in these patients result in delayed closure of the epiphyses of the long bones, resulting in long arms and legs relative to the torso. This appearance is termed a *eunuchoid habitus* (Baughman, 1968; Hsu, 1970).

Approximately 90 percent of individuals with gonadal dysgenesis due to loss of X genetic material never menstruate. The

TABLE 16-6. Characteristic Findings in Women with Turner Syndrome

Height 142–147 cm
Micrognathia
Epicanthal folds
Low-set ears
Sensorineural hearing loss
Otitis media leading to conductive loss
High-arched palate
Webbing of the neck
Chest square and shield-like
Lack of breast development
Areolae widely spaced
Coarctation of the aorta
Short fourth metacarpal
Cubitus valgus
Renal abnormalities
Autoimmune disorders
Autoimmune thyroiditis
Diabetes mellitus

FIGURE 16-4 Photograph taken of a streak gonad (*dotted line*) during laparoscopy. Fallopian tube fimbria are grasped by a laparoscopic instrument. *(Photograph contributed by Dr. Victor Beshay.)*

Fallopian tube

IP ligament

remaining 10 percent have sufficient residual follicles to experience menses and rarely, may achieve pregnancy. However, the menstrual and reproductive lives of such individuals are invariably brief (Kaneko, 1990; Simpson, 1975; Tho, 1981).

In some cases of gonadal dysgenesis, chromosomal mosaicism may also include the presence of a Y chromosome, such as 45,X/46,XY. Thus, chromosomal analysis should be performed in all cases of amenorrhea associated with premature ovarian failure, particularly before age 30. The presence of a Y chromosome cannot be determined clinically as only a few patients will demonstrate signs of androgen excess. A streak gonad should be removed if Y chromosomal material is present, as nearly 25 percent of these patients will develop a malignant germ cell tumor (Chap. 36, p. 882) (Manuel, 1976; Simpson, 1975; Troche, 1986).

The remaining one third of patients with gonadal dysgenesis will have a normal karyotype (46,XX or 46,XY) and are said to have "pure" gonadal dysgenesis. Patients with a 46,XY genotype and gonadal dysgenesis (Swyer syndrome) are phenotypically female due to the lack of secretion of testosterone and antimüllerian hormone (AMH) by the dysgenetic testes. The etiology of the gonadal failure in both genetically male and female patients is poorly understood but is likely due to single gene defects or destruction of gonadal tissue in utero, perhaps by infection or toxins (Wilson, 1992).

Specific Genetic Defects. In addition to the chromosomal abnormalities just described, patients may experience POF due to single gene mutations. Recent studies have demonstrated a significant relationship between fragile X syndrome and premature ovarian failure. This syndrome is caused by a triple repeat sequence mutation in the X-linked *FMR1* (fragile X mental retardation) gene. The fully expanded mutation (>200 CGG repeats) is the most common known inherited genetic cause of mental retardation and of autism. The expanded sequence is hypermethylated, resulting in silencing of gene expression. Males with the so-called premutation (50 to 200 CGG repeats) are at risk for fragile-X associated tremor/ataxia syndrome (FXTAS). Although the mechanism is unclear, it has been observed that females with the premutation have a 13- to 26-percent risk of developing POF. It is estimated that 0.8 to 7.5 percent of sporadic POF and 13 percent of familial POF is due to premutations in this gene. The prevalence of premutations in women approximates 1 in 129 to 1 in 300 (Wittenberger, 2007).

Less common gene mutations include mutation in the *CYP17* gene. This results in decreased 17 alpha-hydroxylase and 17,20-lyase activity, thereby preventing the production of cortisol, androgens, and estrogens (Fig. 15-5, p. 403). These patients have sexual infantilism and primary amenorrhea due to absent estrogen secretion. *Sexual infantilism* describes patients with a lack of breast development, lack of pubic and axillary hair, and a small uterus. Mutations in the *CYP17* gene also lead to increased adrenocorticotropin hormone (ACTH) secretion, thereby stimulating mineralocorticoid secretion. This, in turn, leads to the development of hypokalemia and hypertension (Goldsmith, 1967).

Mutations in the LH and FSH receptors have also been reported. These mutations prevent normal response to circulating gonadotropins, a condition termed *resistant ovary syndrome* (Aittomaki, 1995).

Although frequently cited, galactosemia is a rare cause of POF. Classic galactosemia affects 1 in 30,000 to 1 in 60,000 live births. Inherited as an autosomal-recessive disorder, this condition leads to abnormal galactose metabolism due to a deficiency of galactose-1-phosphate uridyl transferase, encoded by the *GALT* gene (Rubio-Gozalbo, 2010). Galactose metabolites are believed to have a direct toxic effect on many cell types, including germ cells. Potential complications include neonatal death, ataxic neurologic disease, cognitive disabilities, and cataracts. Primary or premature ovarian failure will develop in almost 85 percent of females if left untreated. Treatment is lifelong dietary restriction of galactose, which is present in milk-based foods. Galactosemia is frequently diagnosed during newborn screening programs or pediatric evaluation for associated growth and developmental impairment and long before a patient would present to a gynecologist (Kaufman, 1981; Levy, 1984; Robinson, 1984).

Acquired Abnormalities

Hypergonadotropic hypogonadism can be acquired via infection, autoimmune disease, medical treatments, or other causes. Infectious causes of POF are rare and poorly understood, with mumps oophoritis the most frequently reported (Morrison, 1975).

Autoimmune disorders are estimated to account for 40 percent of POF cases (Hoek, 1997; LaBarbera, 1988). Ovarian failure may be one component of autoimmune pituitary polyglandular failure and accompanied by hypothyroidism and adrenal insufficiency, or it may follow other autoimmune disorders such as systemic lupus erythematosus. POF has also been associated with myasthenia gravis, idiopathic thrombocytopenic purpura, rheumatoid arthritis, vitiligo, and autoimmune hemolytic anemia (de Moraes, 1972; Jones, 1969; Kim, 1974). Although a number of antiovarian antibodies have been characterized, there is currently no validated serum antibody marker to assist in the diagnosis of autoimmune POF (The Practice Committee of the American Society for Reproductive Medicine, 2006). Therefore, lacking a firm diagnosis, all women with POF should be evaluated for the presence of autoimmune disorders (p. 456).

Iatrogenic ovarian failure is a relatively common presentation. This group includes patients who have undergone surgical removal of the ovaries due to recurrent ovarian cysts, endometriosis, or severe pelvic inflammatory disease. A patient may experience amenorrhea following pelvic radiation for malignancies, such as Hodgkin disease. Preventively, ovaries may be surgically repositioned (oophoropexy), if possible, out of the anticipated radiation field prior to therapy (Terenziani, 2009; Williams, 1999).

Ovarian failure may also follow chemotherapy for treatment of malignancies or severe autoimmune diseases. Alkylating agents are believed to be particularly damaging to ovarian function. To minimize the resulting oocyte depletion, a number of investigators advocate the use of GnRH agonists or antagonists concurrent with or prior to therapy (Blumenfeld, 1999; Pereyra, 2001; Somers, 2005).

A number of mechanisms by which GnRH analogs exert their protective effects have been proposed. These medications decrease ovarian blood flow, and thereby decrease exposure of the ovaries to chemotherapeutic agents (Blumenfeld, 2003).

Dividing cells are known to be more sensitive than cells at rest to the cytotoxic effects of chemotherapeutic agents. Therefore, it has also been suggested that pituitary-gonadal axis inhibition may protect the germinal epithelium by inhibiting oogenesis. Alternatively, as GnRH receptors have been identified in the ovary, GnRH analogs may act directly in the ovary to decrease granulosa cell metabolism (Peng, 1994). However, this explanation is not totally satisfactory, as the early stages of oogenesis occur independently of gonadotropin stimulation.

It should be emphasized that the efficacy of GnRH analog treatment remains highly controversial. Recent advances in oocyte and ovarian tissue cryopreservation make it likely that the removal of oocytes prior to treatment will become the preferred approach.

The chance of developing ovarian failure is correlated with increasing radiation and chemotherapeutic dose. Permanent ovarian failure almost invariable results from a dose of more than 8 Gy (800 rads) applied directly to the ovary (Ash, 1980). Patient age is also a significant factor. Younger patients are less likely to develop failure and more likely to regain ovarian function over time (Gradishar, 1989; Wallace, 1989).

A wide variety of environmental toxins have a clear detrimental effect on follicular health. These include cigarette smoking, heavy metals, solvents, pesticides, and industrial chemicals (Jick, 1977; Mlynarcikova, 2005; Sharara, 1998).

Hypogonadotropic Hypogonadism

The term *hypogonadotropic hypogonadism* implies that the primary abnormality lies in the hypothalamic-pituitary axis. A decrease in gonadotropin stimulation of the ovaries leads to loss of ovarian folliculogenesis. Generally in these patients, LH and FSH levels, although low, will still be in the detectable range (<5 mIU/mL). However, levels may be undetectable in patients with complete absence of hypothalamic stimulation, such as occurs in Kallmann syndrome. In addition, absent pituitary function due to abnormal development or severe pituitary damage may lead to similarly low levels. Thus, the group of hypogonadotropic hypogonadism disorders may be viewed as a continuum with perturbations leading to luteal dysfunction, oligomenorrhea, and in the most severe presentation, amenorrhea.

Disorders of the Hypothalamus

Inherited Abnormalities of the Hypothalamus.

Inherited hypothalamic abnormalities primarily consist of those patients with idiopathic hypogonadotropic hypogonadism (IHH). Of these patients, a subset have associated defects in the ability to smell (hyposmia or anosmia) and are said to have Kallmann syndrome. This syndrome can be inherited as an X-linked, an autosomal dominant, or an autosomal recessive disorder (Cadman, 2007; Layman, 1999; Waldstreicher, 1996). The X-linked form was the first to be characterized and follows mutation in the *KAL1* gene on the short arm of the X chromosome. Expressed during fetal development, this gene encodes an adhesion protein named anosmin-1. As this protein is critical for normal migration of both GnRH and olfactory neurons, loss of normal anosmin-1 expression results in both reproductive and olfactory deficits (Fig. 16-5) (Franco, 1991; Soussi-Yanicostas, 1996). Based on postmortem analyses, Kallmann patients have a normal complement of GnRH neurons, however, these neurons fail to migrate and remain near the nasal epithelium

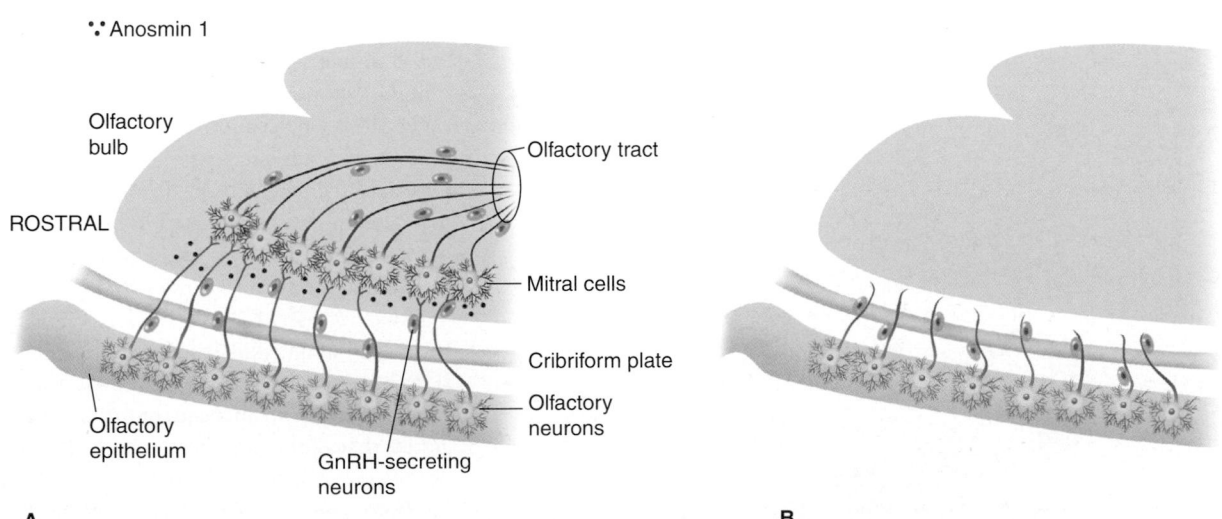

FIGURE 16-5 Drawing depicts normal GnRH neuron migration and the pathogenesis of Kallmann syndrome. **A.** During normal development, olfactory neurons arising in the olfactory epithelium extend their axons through the cribriform plate of the ethmoid bone to reach the olfactory bulb. Here, these axons synapse with dendrites of mitral cells, whose axons form the olfactory tract. Mitral cells secrete anosmin-1, which is the protein product of the *KAL1* gene. This protein is necessary to direct the olfactory axons to their correct location in the olfactory bulb. The GnRH-secreting neurons use this axonal path to migrate from the olfactory placode to the hypothalamus. **B.** Patients with Kallmann syndrome due to a *KAL1* mutation lack anosmin-1 expression. As a result, the axons of the olfactory neurons cannot interact properly with mitral cells, and their migration ends between the cribriform plate and olfactory bulb. As GnRH neuronal migration is dependent on this axonal pathway, GnRH migration likewise ends at this location, resulting in the migration defect found in Kallman syndrome. *(Redrawn from Rugarli, 1993.)*

(Quinton, 1997). As a result, locally secreted GnRH is unable to stimulate gonadotropin secretion by the anterior pituitary gland. Marked decreases in ovarian estrogen production result in a lack of breast development or menstrual cycles.

Kallmann syndrome is also associated with midline facial anomalies such as cleft palate, unilateral renal agenesis, cerebellar ataxia, epilepsy, neurosensory hearing loss, and synkinesis (mirror movements of the hands) (Winters, 1992; Zenaty, 2006). Kallmann syndrome can be distinguished from IHH by olfactory testing. This can be done easily in the office with strong odorants such as ground coffee or perfume. Interestingly, many of these patients are unaware of their deficit.

Over the past 10 years, an array of autosomal genes have been identified that contribute to normal development, migration, and secretion by GnRH neurons (Fig. 16-6). Mutations in a number of these genes have been described in patients with hypothalamic amenorrhea. As a result, the percentage of patients in whom this disorder need be considered idiopathic is gradually decreasing. Of note, mutation in the *CHD7* gene may cause either normosmic IHH or Kallmann syndrome, thereby blurring the distinction between these disorders.

Acquired Hypothalamic Dysfunction
Functional Disorders or Hypothalamic Amenorrhea.
Inherited hypothalamic abnormalities are much less common than acquired deficiencies. Most commonly, gonadotropin deficiency leading to chronic anovulation is believed to arise from functional disorders of the hypothalamus or higher brain centers. Also called "hypothalamic amenorrhea," this diagnosis encompasses three main categories: eating disorders, excessive exercise, and stress. From a teleologic perspective, amenorrhea in time of starvation or extreme stress can be seen as a mechanism to prevent pregnancy at a time in which resources are suboptimal for raising a child.

Each woman appears to have her own hypothalamic "setpoint" or sensitivity to environmental factors. For example, individual women can tolerate markedly different amounts of stress without developing amenorrhea.

Eating Disorders. The eating disorders anorexia nervosa and bulimia can both result in amenorrhea. Anorexia nervosa is associated with severe caloric restriction, weight loss, self-induced vomiting, excess use of laxatives, and compulsive exercise (Chap. 13, p. 358). Weight loss is generally less severe in bulimic women, who eat in binges and then purge.

Hypothalamic dysfunction is severe in anorexia and may affect other hypothalamic-pituitary axes in addition to the reproductive axis. Amenorrhea in anorexia nervosa can precede, follow, or appear coincidentally with weight loss. In addition, even with return to normal weight, not all women with anorexia will regain normal menstrual function.

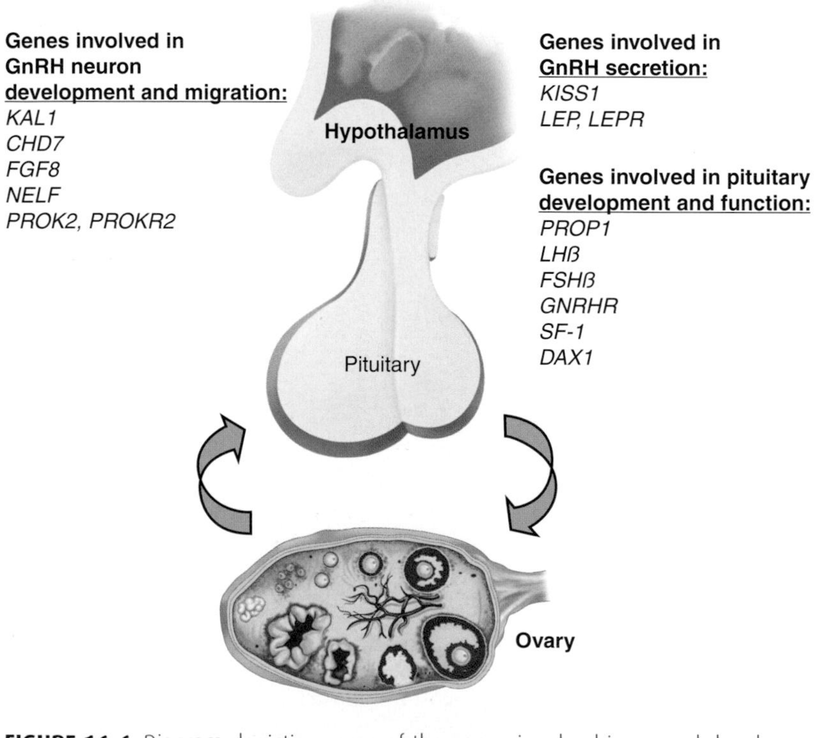

Exercise-Induced Amenorrhea. Exercise-induced amenorrhea is most common in women whose exercise regimen is associated with significant loss of fat, including ballet, gymnastics, and long-distance running (De Souza, 1991; Frisch, 1980). In those women who continue to menstruate, cycles are notable for their variability in cycle interval and length due to reduced hormonal function, including shortened luteal phases (De Souza, 1998). Puberty may be delayed in girls who begin training before menarche (Frisch, 1981).

In 1970, Frisch and Revelle proposed the concept that an adolescent girl needed to achieve a critical body weight to begin menstruating. This mass was initially postulated to be approximately 48 kilograms and was subsequently refined to a minimal body mass index (BMI) approaching the normal of ≥ 19. BMI is calculated as: $BMI = weight(kg)/[\text{square of height } (m^2)]$ (Frisch, 1974a,b). Figure 1-7 (p. 17) displays a BMI nomogram. Subsequent studies have suggested that, although there is a clear correlation between body fat and reproductive function (at both ends of the weight spectrum), overall energy balance better predicts the onset and maintenance of menstrual cycles (Billewicz, 1976; Johnston, 1975). For example, many elite athletes regain menstrual cyclicity following a decrease in exercise intensity prior to any change in weight (Abraham, 1982).

Stress-Induced Amenorrhea. Stress-induced amenorrhea may be associated with clearly

Genes involved in GnRH neuron development and migration:
KAL1
CHD7
FGF8
NELF
PROK2, PROKR2

Hypothalamus

Genes involved in GnRH secretion:
KISS1
LEP, LEPR

Genes involved in pituitary development and function:
PROP1
LHβ
FSHβ
GNRHR
SF-1
DAX1

Pituitary

Ovary

FIGURE 16-6 Diagram depicting some of the genes involved in normal development and function of the hypothalamic-pituitary-ovarian axis. Identified mutations in these genes now explain some forms of hypogonadotropic hypogonadism that were previously considered idiopathic. *(Adapted from Achermann, 2001, and Bianco, 2009.)*

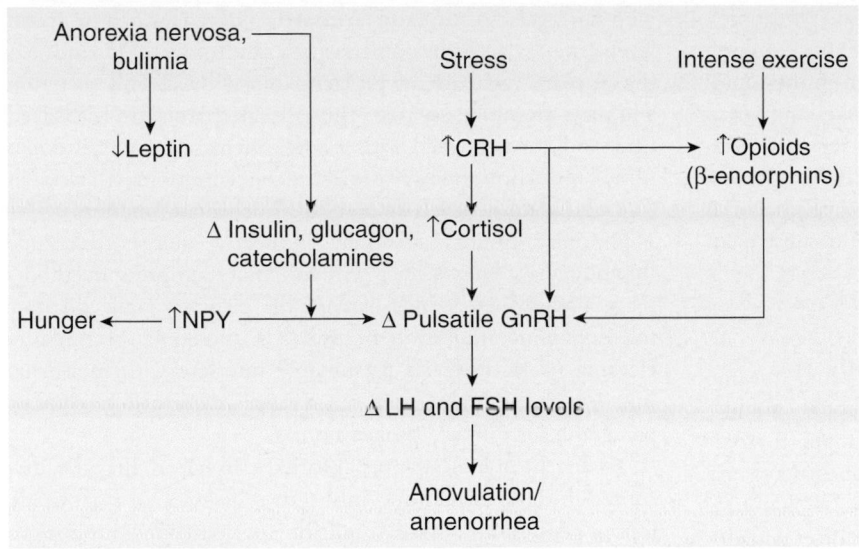

FIGURE 16-7 Diagram depicting a simplified model for the development of amenorrhea in women with eating disorders, high stress levels, or rigorous exercise. CRH = corticotropin-releasing hormone; FSH = follicle-stimulating hormone; GnRH = gonadotropin-releasing hormone; LH = luteinizing hormone; NPY = neuropeptide Y.

traumatic life events, such as death of a family member or divorce. Nevertheless, less severe life events and even positive events may be associated with stress. For example, stress-related amenorrhea is frequently associated with leaving for college, test taking, or wedding planning.

Eating disorders, exercise, and stress may alter menstrual function through overlapping mechanisms. This observation may be in part because these problems are often not found in isolation. For example, women with eating disorders frequently exercise excessively and are undoubtedly under stress as they attempt to control their eating patterns.

Pathophysiology of Functional Hypothalamic Amenorrhea. Figure 16-7 depicts a simplified model for the development of amenorrhea in these patients. It must be emphasized that each cause of functional hypothalamic amenorrhea may act via one or all of these pathways. Furthermore, in many cases, the factors known to impact reproductive function are likely acting indirectly on GnRH neurons by various neuronal subtypes with synaptic connections to GnRH neurons.

Exercise in particular has been associated with an increase in levels of endogenous opioids (β-endorphins), producing the so-called runner's high. Opioids alter GnRH pulsatility as demonstrated by treatment of humans and animal models with antiopiates, such as naloxone.

As part of the stress response, each of these conditions may lead to an increase in corticotropin-releasing hormone (CRH) release by the hypothalamus, which in turn results in cortisol secretion by the adrenal gland. CRH alters the pattern of pulsatile GnRH secretion, whereas cortisol may act directly or indirectly to disrupt GnRH neuronal function.

Eating disorders are thought to impact ovulatory function through a number of hormonal factors, including insulin, glucagon, and leptin. First identified in 1994, leptin is a 167-amino acid protein encoded by the *ob* gene and produced in white adipose tissue (Zhang, 1994). Leptin receptors have been identified in the central nervous system and a wide range of peripheral tissues (Chen, 1996; Lee, 1996; Tartaglia, 1995).

Primarily produced in adipose tissue, leptin provides an important link between energy balance and reproduction, albeit one of many mechanisms (Schneider, 2004). Patients with anorexia nervosa have been found to have low circulating leptin levels (Mantzoros, 1997). Conversely, mutation of the human leptin gene results in morbid obesity, diabetes mellitus, and hypogonadism. This trio can be successfully reversed with recombinant human leptin (Licinio, 2004). This has led to the concept of leptin as a "satiety factor." It has been hypothesized that a decrease in leptin production due to weight loss could secondarily stimulate neuropeptide Y, which is known to stimulate hunger and alter GnRH pulsatility. Leptin likely acts through a wide variety of additional neurotransmitters and neuropeptides, including the β-endorphins, and α-melanocyte-stimulating hormone (Tartaglia, 1995).

Pseudocyesis. Although rare, the diagnosis of pseudocyesis should be considered in any woman presenting with amenorrhea and pregnancy symptoms. Pseudocyesis exemplifies the ability of the mind to control physiologic processes. Approximately 550 cases of pseudocyesis have been reported in the medical literature in women ranging from ages 6 to 79 years. These patients fervently believe that they are pregnant and subsequently demonstrate a number of pregnancy signs and symptoms, including amenorrhea.

Endocrine evaluation in a limited number of patients has failed to demonstrate a consistent pattern of hormonal derangements. Alterations in LH pulse frequency concurrent with elevated serum androgen levels may explain amenorrhea. Elevated serum prolactin levels and resultant galactorrhea have been noted in a subset of patients. Growth hormone secretion appears to be blunted.

A common link in these patients is a history of severe grief, such as recent miscarriage or infant death. Psychiatric treatment is generally required to treat the associated depression, which is often exacerbated when the patient is informed that she is not pregnant (Bray, 1991; Starkman, 1985; Whelan, 1990).

Anatomic Destruction. Any process that destroys the hypothalamus can impair GnRH secretion and lead to the development of hypogonadotropic hypogonadism and amenorrhea. Due to the complex interaction of input to the GnRH neurons, these abnormalities do not need to directly impact the GnRH neurons but may operate indirectly by altering activity of modulatory neurons.

The tumors most often associated with amenorrhea include craniopharyngiomas, germinomas, endodermal sinus tumors, eosinophilic granuloma (Hand-Schuller-Christian syndrome), and gliomas, as well as metastatic lesions. The most common of these tumors, craniopharyngiomas, are located in the suprasellar region and frequently present with headaches and visual changes. Impaired GnRH secretion has been reported with infections, such as tuberculosis, and with infiltrative diseases, such as sarcoidosis. Trauma or radiation to the hypothalamus can also result in hypothalamic dysfunction and subsequent amenorrhea.

Disorders of the Anterior Pituitary Gland

The anterior pituitary gland consists of gonadotropes (producing LH and FSH), lactotropes (prolactin), thyrotropes (thyroid-stimulating hormone), corticotropes (adrenocorticotropin hormone), and somatotropes (growth hormone) (Chap. 15, p. 413). Although various disorders may directly affect gonadotropes, many causes of pituitary-derived amenorrhea may also follow abnormalities in other pituitary cell types, which in turn alter gonadotrope function.

Inherited Abnormalities of the Pituitary Gland. Our
understanding of the genetic mechanisms that regulate normal pituitary development and function is rapidly advancing. An increasing number of cohorts have been described with combined pituitary hormone deficiency and central facial and/or neurologic defects due to a failure of midline fusion, a condition known as septo-optic dysplasia. Many of these patients have a mutation in the *PROP1* gene (Cadman, 2007; Layman, 1999). Second, mutations in genes that encode the LH or FSH β-subunits or the GnRH receptor have also been identified as rare causes of hypogonadotropic hypogonadism. Hypothalamic and pituitary dysfunction with associated gonadal dysgenesis and adrenal hypoplasia has been well described in patients with mutations in the nuclear hormone receptors steroidogenic factor-1 (SF-1, NR5A1) and DAX1 (NR0B1) (Beranova, 2001; Layman, 1997, 1998; Matthews, 1993; Weiss, 1992). Most recently, attention has focused on kisspeptin-1 and its receptor, G-protein-coupled receptor 54 (GPR54). Mutations in this receptor result in delayed puberty and hypogonadotropic hypogonadism, demonstrating that this ligand-receptor system is a critical stimulus of GnRH secretion (Pallais, 2006; Seminara, 2006).

Acquired Pituitary Dysfunction. Most pituitary dysfunction is acquired after menarche and therefore presents with normal pubertal development followed by secondary amenorrhea. Nevertheless, in rare cases, these disorders may begin prior to puberty, resulting in delayed pubertal development and primary amenorrhea (Howlett, 1989).

Pituitary adenomas are the most common cause of acquired pituitary dysfunction and are discussed in detail in Chapter 15 (p. 418). The most common adenomas secrete prolactin. However, excessive secretion of any pituitary-derived hormone can result in amenorrhea.

Increased serum prolactin levels are found in as many as one tenth of amenorrheic women, and more than half of women with both galactorrhea and amenorrhea have elevated prolactin levels (the "galactorrhea-amenorrhea syndrome"). Dopamine is the primary regulator of prolactin biosynthesis and secretion and plays an inhibitory role. Thus, elevated prolactin levels feed back and are associated with a reflex increase in central dopamine production to lower prolactin concentrations. This rise in central dopamine levels alters GnRH neuronal function.

Pituitary tumors also may indirectly alter gonadotrope function via a mass effect. Growth may compress neighboring gonadotropes or may damage the pituitary stalk, disrupting dopamine inhibition of prolactin secretion. Secondarily elevated prolactin levels presumably interfere with menstrual function through the same mechanisms described in the last paragraph for primary prolactinomas.

As in the hypothalamus, pituitary function may be disrupted by inflammation, infiltrative disease, or metastatic lesions. Although a rare condition, peripartum lymphocytic hypophysitis can be a dangerous cause of pituitary failure. Infiltrative diseases include sarcoidosis and hemochromatosis. In addition, loss of anterior pituitary function may be observed following surgical or radiation treatment of pituitary adenomas.

Sheehan syndrome refers to panhypopituitarism. It classically follows massive postpartum hemorrhage and associated hypotension. Abrupt, severe hypotension leads to pituitary ischemia and necrosis (Kelestimur, 2003). In its most severe form, these patients develop shock due to pituitary apoplexy. Pituitary apoplexy is characterized by a sudden onset of headache, nausea, visual deficits, and hormonal dysfunction due to acute hemorrhage or infarction within the pituitary. In less severe forms, loss of gonadotrope activity in the pituitary leads to anovulation and subsequent amenorrhea. Damage to the other pituitary cell types may present as failure to lactate, loss of sexual and axillary hair, and manifestation of hypothyroidism and adrenal insufficiency symptoms. The pituitary cell types are differentially sensitive to damage. For this reason, prolactin secretion deficiency is the most common, followed by loss of gonadotropin and growth hormone release, loss of ACTH production, and least commonly, by decreases in thyroid-stimulating hormone (TSH) secretion (Veldhuis, 1980).

Other Causes of Hypogonadotropic Hypogonadism

Hypogonadotropic amenorrhea may be observed in a wide variety of chronic diseases including end-stage kidney disease, liver disease, malignancies, acquired immunodeficiency syndrome, and malabsorption syndromes. The mechanisms by which these disorders result in menstrual dysfunction are poorly understood. End-stage kidney disease is known to be associated with an increase in prolactin as well as altered serum leptin levels, both of which may disrupt normal GnRH pulsatility (Ghazizadeh, 2007). Of patients with nonalcoholic chronic liver disease, the cause of the low gonadotropin levels has not been elucidated and in fact, is only observed in a subset of amenorrheic patients (Cundy, 1991). Patients with malabsorption due to celiac disease have been reported to have delayed menarche, secondary amenorrhea, and early menopause, which have been attributed to deficiencies in trace elements, such as zinc and selenium. These are required for normal gonadotropin biosynthesis and secretion (Özgör, 2010). Chronic diseases may also produce amenorrhea through common mechanisms, such as stress and nutritional deficiencies.

■ Eugonadotropic Amenorrhea

A number of disorders that produce amenorrhea are not associated with significantly abnormal gonadotropin levels. In these women, chronic sex-steroid secretion interferes with the normal feedback between the ovary and the hypothalamic-pituitary axis. Lack of cyclicity interferes with normal oocyte maturation and ovulation, and menstruation fails to occur.

Due to relatively normal gonadotropin levels, these patients will secrete estrogen and therefore can also be said to have *chronic anovulation with estrogen present*. This is in contrast to the patients with ovarian failure or hypothalamic-pituitary failure in which estrogen is absent. This distinction may be useful during evaluation and treatment.

Polycystic Ovarian Syndrome (PCOS)

This syndrome is by far the most common cause of chronic anovulation with estrogen present and is discussed fully in Chapter 17 (p. 460). Patients with PCOS may have a wide variety of menstrual presentations. First, complete amenorrhea may follow anovulation. Without ovulation, progesterone is lacking, and an absent progesterone withdrawal fails to prompt menses. In some women with PCOS, however, amenorrhea may be attributable to the ability of androgens, which are elevated in PCOS patients, to atrophy the endometrium. Alternatively, menometrorrhagia may be noted and results from unopposed estrogen stimulation of the endometrium. Within this unstable, thickened proliferative-phase endometrium, episodic stromal breakdown and shedding leads to irregular bleeding. Vessels may be abnormally large in anovulatory endometria, and bleeding may be severe. Lastly, women with PCOS may complete occasional ovulatory cycles, and normal withdrawal menses occur.

Polycystic ovarian syndrome can be appropriately characterized as an inherited form of eugonadotropic amenorrhea. Although a specific gene defect has not been identified, an increased incidence of PCOS is found in the mothers and sisters of affected individuals.

Adult-Onset Congenital Adrenal Hyperplasia

This condition closely mimics the presentation of PCOS with hyperandrogenism and irregular menstrual cycles. Most commonly, adult-onset congenital adrenal hyperplasia (CAH), also termed late-onset CAH, is due to a mutation in the *CYP21* gene, which encodes the 21-hydroxylase enzyme. With a mild mutation, patients are asymptomatic until adrenarche with its associated requirement for increased adrenal steroidogenesis. Patients with CAH are unable to convert an adequate percent-

age of progesterone to cortisol and aldosterone, thus shunting progesterone precursors to toward the androgen pathway (Fig. 15-5, p. 403). As in PCOS, elevated androgen levels blunt oocyte maturation and thereby result in anovulation and amenorrhea.

Ovarian Tumor

Although uncommon, chronic anovulation with estrogen present can also be observed with ovarian tumors producing either estrogens or androgens. Examples of these tumors include granulosa cell tumors, thecal cell tumors, and mature cystic teratomas.

Hyperprolactinemia and Hypothyroidism

As discussed earlier, hyperprolactinemia can be categorized as a cause of pituitary hypogonadotropic hypogonadism. Of note, however, many of these patients may have relatively normal gonadotropin levels, although as a group, their estrogen levels will be mildly depressed. Significantly elevated serum prolactin levels are almost always due to the presence of a pituitary mass, such as a prolactin-secreting adenoma. Nevertheless, when obtaining a history, it is important to remember that many medications and herbs have been associated with galactorrhea and may be predicted to disrupt menstrual cyclicity (Table 12-4, p. 341). The antipsychotic group of medications is perhaps the most commonly encountered in this clinical setting.

Thyroid disease is also a relatively common cause of oligoamenorrhea associated with gonadotropins in the normal range. Classically, hypothyroidism is stated to cause amenorrhea, whereas hyperthyroidism is implicated in menorrhagia (Chap. 8, p. 234). Although less common, hyperthyroidism may also be encountered in the amenorrheic patient.

A mechanism by which hyperprolactinemia and hypothyroidism may lead to amenorrhea is outlined in Figure 16-8. In this model, a primary decrease in circulating thyroid hormone levels leads to a compensatory increase in hypothalamic thyrotropin-releasing hormone (TRH). As part of the thyroid axis, TRH increases TSH by the thyrotropes in the pituitary gland. In addition, TRH also binds to the pituitary lactotropes, increasing prolactin secretion.

An increase in circulating prolactin results in a compensatory increase in central dopamine, the primary inhibitor of prolactin secretion. The increase in central dopamine levels alters GnRH secretion, thereby disrupting normal cyclic gonadotropin secretion and preventing ovulation. Note that this increase in prolactin may be primary, for example from a prolactinoma, or may be secondary due to an elevation in TRH levels. In secondary hyperprolactinemia, prolactin levels are generally less than 100 ng/mL.

There are undoubtedly other mechanisms by which thyroid disease and elevated prolactin levels disturb menstrual function, but these are poorly understood at present. For example, thyroid receptors are found in most cell types. Also, thyroid hormone increases sex hormone-binding globulin levels, altering the levels of unbound, and thereby active, ovarian steroids. In

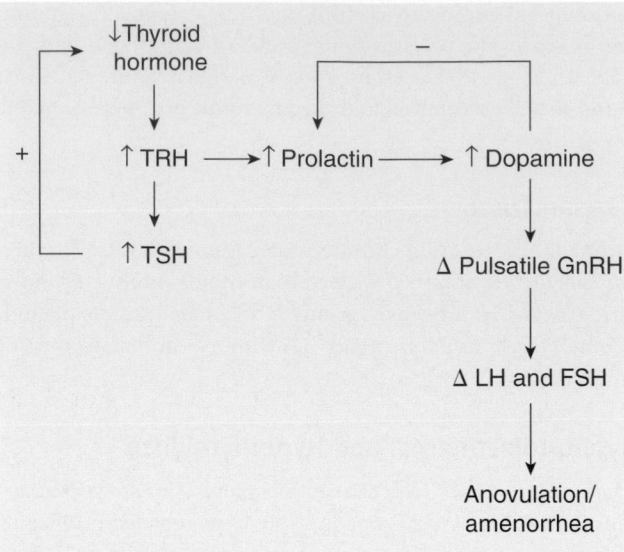

FIGURE 16-8 Diagram depicting a simplified model for the development of amenorrhea in women with hyperprolactinemia or hypothyroidism. FSH = follicle-stimulating hormone; GnRH = gonadotropin-releasing hormone; LH = luteinizing hormone; TRH = thyrotropin-releasing hormone; TSH = thyroid-stimulating hormone.

addition, prolactin receptors have been identified in the ovary and in the endometrium.

EVALUATION

History

An algorithm for approaching the patient with amenorrhea is presented in Figure 16-9. The evaluation of menstrual abnormalities should start with questions regarding pubertal development. Did the patient experience normal puberty in terms of onset and progression as outlined in Chapter 14 (p. 383)? Did she ever achieve regular menstrual cyclicity? The cycle interval, duration, and amount of menstrual flow should be characterized. It is important to determine when a change in this pattern was noted and whether the change was sudden or gradual. Did the development of amenorrhea correlate with pelvic infection, surgery, radiation therapy, chemotherapy, or other illnesses?

A surgical history should focus on prior pelvic surgery, particularly intrauterine surgery including dilatation and curettage. Complications associated with this surgery, particularly infection, should be sought.

A focused review of symptoms can also be helpful. For example, new-onset headaches or visual changes may suggest a tumor of the central nervous system or pituitary gland. Pituitary tumors may impinge on the optic chiasm, resulting in bitemporal hemianopsia, that is, the loss of both right and left outer visual fields. Bilateral breast discharge is consistent with the diagnosis of hyperprolactinemia. The presence of thyroid disease may be associated with heat or cold intolerance, weight changes, and sleep abnormalities. Hot flashes

and vaginal dryness suggest hypergonadotropic hypogonadism, that is, premature ovarian failure. Hirsutism and acne are frequently seen with PCOS or with adult-onset CAH. Cyclic pelvic pain would suggest a reproductive tract outlet obstruction.

Important questions regarding family history include premature cessation of menses or a history of autoimmune disease, including thyroid disease, which would suggest an increased risk for POF. A history of irregular menses, infertility, or signs of excess androgen production may be noted in those with PCOS. Sudden neonatal death may have occurred in family members carrying mutations in the *CYP21* gene responsible for CAH.

The social history should investigate exposure to environmental toxins, including cigarettes. Any medications should be noted, especially those that increase prolactin levels, such as antipsychotics.

Physical Examination

General appearance can be helpful in the evaluation of amenorrhea. A low BMI, perhaps in conjunction with tooth enamel erosion from recurrent vomiting, is highly suggestive of an eating disorder. Signs of Turner syndrome should be evaluated, including the presence of short stature and other stigmata such as webbed neck or shield-shaped chest. Midline facial defects, such as cleft palate, are consistent with a developmental defect of the hypothalamus or anterior pituitary gland. Hypertension in a prepubertal girl would be consistent with mutation in the *CYP17* gene and shunting of the steroidogenic pathway toward aldosterone.

Visual field defects, particularly bitemporal hemianopsia, may indicate a pituitary gland or central nervous system tumor. Skin should be inspected for acanthosis nigricans, hirsutism, or acne, which may indicate PCOS or other causes of hyperinsulinemia and/or hyperandrogenism. The presence of supraclavicular fat and abdominal striae with hypertension may be noted in those with Cushing syndrome. Hypothyroidism may present with an abnormally enlarged thyroid gland, delayed reflexes, and bradycardia. During breast examination, bilateral galactorrhea implies the presence of hyperprolactinemia. A more complete discussion of the evaluation and treatment of galactorrhea can be found in Chapter 12 (p. 338).

Examination of the genitalia should start by noting hair pattern. A sparse or absent female hair pattern may be due to either lack of adrenarche or androgen insensitivity syndrome. Conversely, elevated androgen levels will result in a male pattern of genital hair growth. In contrast to the triangular pattern of hair in females, male pubic hair extends to the umbilicus, forming a triangle, or male escutcheon. Markedly elevated levels of androgens may also produce signs of virilization, most noticeably clitoromegaly (Figs. 17-2, p. 464, and 17-10, p. 471). These women may also note voice deepening and male pattern balding.

Evidence of estrogen production includes a pink, moist vagina and cervical mucus. A vaginal smear will demonstrate mostly superficial epithelial cells (Fig. 21-11, p. 576).

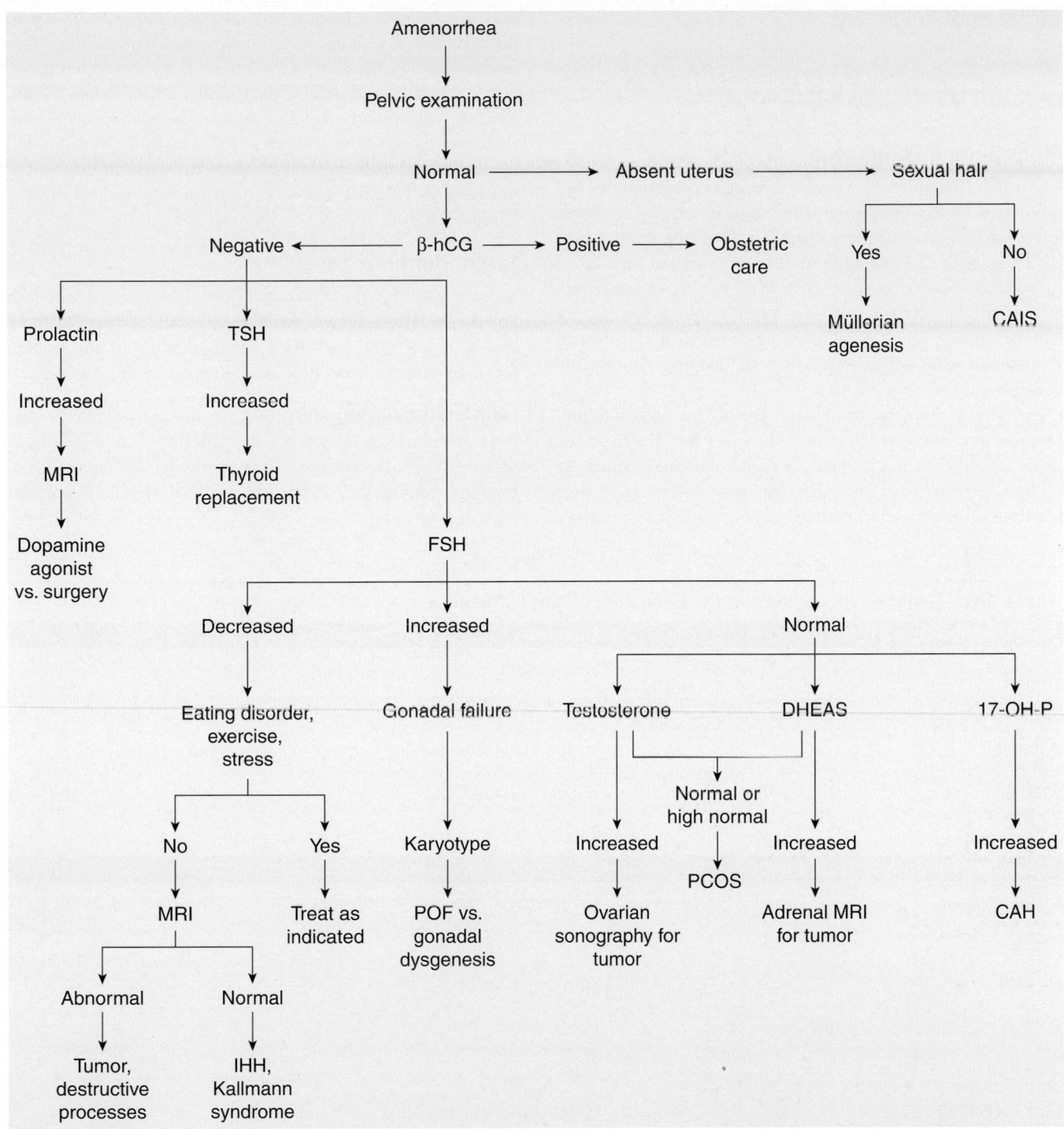

FIGURE 16-9 Diagnostic algorithm to evaluate amenorrhea. AIS = androgen insensitivity syndrome; CAH = congenital adrenal hyperplasia; CAIS = complete androgen insensitivity syndrome; DHEAS = dehydroepiandrosterone sulfate; FSH = follicle-stimulating hormone; hCG = human chorionic gonadotropin; IHH = idiopathic hypogonadotropic hypogonadism; MRI = magnetic resonance imaging; 17-OH-P = 17-hydroxyprogesterone; PCOS = polycystic ovarian syndrome; POF = premature ovarian failure; TSH = thyroid-stimulating hormone.

Determination of müllerian anomalies by physical examination is described in Chapter 18 (p. 495). Rectal and digital vaginal examination may help identify a uterus above an obstruction at the level of the introitus or in the vagina. The presence of hematocolpos suggests normal ovarian and endometrial function.

Laboratory and Radiologic Testing

The differential diagnosis of amenorrhea is extensive, but evaluation of most women is relatively straightforward. As for all disorders, testing may be modified by patient history and physical examination.

Exclusion of Pregnancy

All reproductive-aged women with amenorrhea should be assumed pregnant until proven otherwise. Therefore, urinary or serum β-hCG level measurement is prudent.

Progesterone Withdrawal

Classically, patients are given exogenous progesterone and monitored for a progesterone withdrawal bleed, which follows a few days after completion of progesterone (the progesterone challenge test). If bleeding ensues, then a woman is assumed to produce estrogen and to have a developed endometrium and patent outflow tract. If bleeding does not follow, then a patient is given estrogen followed by progesterone treatment. If a woman again fails to bleed, then an anatomic abnormality is diagnosed.

A number of factors can lead to an incorrect test interpretation. First, estrogen levels may fluctuate both in hypothalamic amenorrhea and in the early stages of ovarian failure. As a result, patients with these disorders may have at least some bleeding after progesterone withdrawal. Specifically, menses may be observed after progesterone administration in up to 40 percent of women with hypothalamic amenorrhea due to stress, weight loss, or exercise and in up to 50 percent of women with ovarian failure (Nakamura, 1996; Rebar, 1990). Second, women with high androgen levels, such as occurs with PCOS and CAH, may have an atrophic endometrium and fail to bleed. Up to 20 percent of women in whom estrogen is present will fail to bleed following progesterone withdrawal (Rarick, 1990).

Serum Hormone Levels

As suggested by the Practice Committee of the American Society for Reproductive Medicine (2006), it may be more reasonable to begin with hormonal evaluation in any woman found to have a normal pelvic examination (Table 16-7).

Follicle-Stimulating Hormone. A normal FSH level suggests an anatomic defect or eugonadotropic hypogonadism, such as PCOS. In contrast, a low level suggests hypothalamic-pituitary dysfunction, and an elevated FSH level is consistent with ovarian failure.

TABLE 16-7. Tests Commonly Used in the Evaluation of Amenorrhea

Primary Laboratory Tests	Diagnosis
β-hCG	Pregnancy
FSH	Hypogonadotropic versus hypergonadotropic hypogonadism[a]
Estradiol	Hypogonadotropic versus hypergonadotropic hypogonadism
Prolactin	Hyperprolactinemia
TSH	Thyroid disease (hypothyroidism)
Secondary Laboratory Tests	
Testosterone	PCOS and exclude ovarian tumor
DHEAS	Exclude adrenal tumor
17-OH-P	Late-onset CAH
2-hour glucose tolerance test	PCOS
Fasting lipid panel	PCOS
Autoimmune testing	Premature ovarian failure
Karyotype	Premature ovarian failure <35 years
Radiologic Evaluation	
Sonography	PCOS or to determine presence of uterus
HSG or saline infusion sonography	Müllerian anomaly or intrauterine synechiae
Magnetic resonance imaging	Müllerian anomaly or hypothalamic-pituitary disease

[a]Hypogonadotropic hypogonadism includes functional causes of hypothalamic amenorrhea (excessive exercise, eating disorders, and stress). Hypergonadotropic hypogonadism refers primarily to premature ovarian failure.
CAH = congenital adrenal hyperplasia; DHEAS = dehydroepiandrosterone sulfate; FSH = follicle-stimulating hormone; hCG = human chorionic gonadotropin; HSG = hysterosalpingography; 17-OH-P = 17-hydroxyprogesterone; PCOS = polycystic ovarian syndrome; TSH = thyroid-stimulating hormone.

Patients with PCOS, hyperprolactinemia, or thyroid disease would be expected to have normal FSH levels. Although many patients with PCOS have elevated LH-to-FSH level ratios >2, testing for this relationship is unnecessary as a normal ratio does not exclude this diagnosis.

If an FSH value is low, it may be helpful to repeat this measurement with the addition of an LH level to confirm hypogonadotropic hypogonadism. Additional testing may include a GnRH stimulation test. Although a number of different protocols have been employed, one common approach has been intravenous injection of 100 µg of GnRH as a bolus, followed by LH and FSH measurement at 0, 15, 30, 45, and 60 minutes. Although both LH and FSH levels will be blunted, FSH levels will be high relative to LH ratios in patients with hypogonadotropic hypogonadism or delayed puberty (Job, 1977; Yen, 1973). However, clinicians may be unable to perform this test due to a lack of consistently available clinical-grade GnRH.

An elevated FSH level strongly suggests the presence of hypergonadotropic hypogonadism (premature ovarian failure). This diagnosis requires two FSH levels >40 mIU/mL obtained at least 1 month apart. At least two elevated values are required because the course of POF may fluctuate over time. This fluctuation likely explains the occasional pregnancy that has been reported in these women. Patients should keep a menstrual calendar while testing is completed, as bleeding 2 weeks following an elevated serum FSH level may simply indicate that the sample was obtained during a gonadotropin surge.

As adjuncts to FSH testing, ancillary markers that will increase the sensitivity and specificity of ovarian reserve testing have been investigated. Many clinicians obtain measurements for estradiol in addition to FSH, although this has not been consistently shown to increase diagnostic accuracy. Attention has turned more recently to the use of circulating antimüllerian hormone (AMH) levels (Chap. 19, p. 515) (Li, 2011). The granulosa cells of preantral and small antral follicles produce large amounts of AMH, but production decreases as follicles mature and become FSH-dependent. The role of AMH in the adult ovary is poorly understood. It may contribute to the entry rate of primordial follicles into the developing follicular cohort or may play a role in dominant follicle selection. AMH levels are directly proportional to the number of early developing follicles and provide a useful measure of follicle number. In contrast to FSH and estradiol, AMH levels are relatively constant across the menstrual cycle, increasing the usefulness of this test (Broekmans, 2008). In addition to AMH, measurement of an alternative granulosa cell product, inhibin B, has been suggested. However, more recent studies suggest that inhibin levels do not adequately predict the degree of follicular dysfunction (Knauff, 2009).

Prolactin and Thyroid-Stimulating Hormone. These hormone levels should be tested in most patients with amenorrhea, as prolactin-secreting adenomas and thyroid disease are relatively common and require specific treatment. Furthermore, hypothyroidism may secondarily lead to elevated prolactin levels as shown in Figure 16-8. Because of this close relationship between thyroid disease and prolactin levels, both hormones should be measured simultaneously. Treatment for hypothyroidism will also normalize prolactin levels. If a TSH level is elevated, an unbound thyroxine (free T_4) level is drawn to confirm clinical hypothyroidism.

Testosterone. Serum levels of this hormone should be measured in any woman with suspected PCOS or with clinical signs of androgen excess. Hormonal evaluation should include measurement of serum total testosterone levels. Measurement of free testosterone levels is generally unwarranted as these assays are more expensive and more variable. Mild elevations in testosterone levels are consistent with the diagnosis of PCOS. However, values exceeding 200 ng/dL may suggest the presence of an ovarian tumor and should be evaluated with pelvic sonography.

Dehydroepiandrosterone Sulfate (DHEAS). Secretion of this hormone is essentially limited to the adrenal gland. High normal levels or even very mild elevations are consistent with PCOS. Adrenal adenomas may produce circulating DHEAS levels above 700 µg/dL and warrant investigation with magnetic resonance (MR) imaging or computed tomography (CT) scanning of the adrenals. Measurement of 17-hydroxyprogesterone (17-OH-P) aims to identify patients with adult-onset CAH. However, confirmation of this diagnosis can be difficult due to the overlap in values among normal patients and heterozygote and homozygote carriers of mutations in the 21 hydroxylase (*CYP21A2*) gene. Accordingly, adrenal stimulation with ACTH (Cortrosyn), termed the ACTH stimulation test or colloquially the *cort stim test,* may be required (Chap. 17, p. 471).

Radiologic Evaluation

Any patient with hypogonadotropic hypogonadism should be assumed to have an anatomic abnormality until proven otherwise by imaging of the brain and pituitary gland with MR imaging or CT scanning. Thus, functional hypothalamic amenorrhea due to stress, exercise, or eating disorder is a diagnosis of exclusion. Imaging is highly sensitive for identification of destructive disorders such as tumors or infiltrative diseases of the hypothalamus or pituitary. Patients with Kallmann syndrome frequently demonstrate defects in the development of the olfactory bulbs and sulci of the rhinencephalon (Klingmuller, 1987).

Other Serum Testing

If an eating disorder is suspected, an immediate assessment of serum electrolytes is warranted as imbalances can be life-threatening. An electrocardiogram should also be considered in those patients perceived to have more severe disease. A reverse tri-iodothyronine (rT_3) level is often elevated in patients with functional hypothalamic amenorrhea.

Women with PCOS should be screened for insulin resistance and lipid abnormalities. These are commonly found in affected patients and increase the risks for diabetes and cardiovascular disease (Chap. 17, p. 472). Although no consensus exists, it is probably prudent to repeat these tests every few years.

Chromosomal Analysis

Patients with gonadal dysgenesis, such as Turner syndrome, should be considered for karyotyping. Classic teaching suggests that this test is unnecessary after age 30. However, consideration should be given to testing patients up to age 35, as a rare individual with mosaicism may retain functional oocytes and thus sustain cyclic menses longer than expected. As previously indicated, a Y cell line requires bilateral oophorectomy because of the increased risk for ovarian tumors. Due to the close association between stature and abnormalities in the X chromosome, many specialists advise karyotyping all women with premature ovarian failure who are shorter than 60 inches (Saenger, 2001). Chromosomal studies should also be considered in any woman with a familial history of premature ovarian failure.

Specific Disorders

Premature Ovarian Failure. Many patients with POF will not have a clear etiology for their disorder. Presumption of an autoimmune disorder is probably wise, based on their potential long-term consequences. Although testing for these disorders varies widely among experts, a list of associated autoimmune disorders is shown in Table 16-8.

Anatomic Disorders. These can be evaluated with a number of modalities depending on the suspected etiology. A sonographic examination is frequently useful as a first screen in those with a grossly normal uterus (Figs. 2-21 through 2-24, p. 45). Hysterosalpingography (HSG) or saline infusion sonography (SIS) is excellent for the detection of intrauterine synechiae or developmental anomalies (Figs. 2-20, p. 45, 19-6, p. 517, and 19-8, p. 519). Magnetic resonance imaging is frequently used for delineation of anatomic structures, such as a noncommunicating or hypoplastic uterine horn.

Müllerian dysgenesis may be associated with various malformations in other organ systems. With complete müllerian agenesis, approximately one third of individuals will have urinary tract abnormalities including an ectopic kidney, unilateral renal agenesis, horseshoe kidney, or abnormal collecting ducts. Skeletal anomalies, generally of the spine, may be present in up to 12 percent of these patients (Fore, 1975; Griffin, 1976). Renal sonography and radiographs of the lower spine are indicated in these women. The incidence of associated abnormalities differs among the types of müllerian dysgenesis. Abnormalities are most common with complete agenesis or duplication anomalies, such as bicornuate uterus or uterine didelphys. They are less common with disorders of resorption, such as uterine septum (Fedele, 1990; Letterie, 1988; Reinhold, 1997).

TREATMENT

The treatment of amenorrhea depends on the etiology as well as the aims of a patient, such as a desire to treat hirsutism or become pregnant.

Anatomic abnormalities will require surgical correction, if possible, and are discussed in Chapter 18 (p. 481). Hypothyroidism should be treated with thyroid replacement, and a suggested dosage of levothyroxine is 1.6 µg/kg of body weight per day (Baskin, 2002). For most, a reasonable starting dose is 50 to 100 µg of levothyroxine orally daily. TSH response is slow, and levels should be rechecked 6 to 8 weeks following initiation. A TSH level in the lower range of normal is the therapeutic goal. If needed, a dose may be increased in an increment of 12.5 or 25 µg (Jameson, 2008). Women with hyperprolactinemia should receive a dopamine agonist, such as bromocriptine or cabergoline. Macroadenomas may require surgery if secondary deficits such as visual changes are observed. Both medical and surgical specifics of pituitary disease treatment are described in Chapter 15 (p. 421).

Estrogen Replacement

This therapy should be instituted in essentially every patient with hypogonadism to avoid osteoporosis. As in postmenopausal women, bone loss is accelerated in the first few years following estrogen deprivation. Therefore, treatment should be instituted quickly. Women with a uterus also require continuous or intermittent progesterone administration to protect against endometrial hyperplasia or cancer (Chap. 22, p. 585). There is no consensus, however, on an optimal regimen in these patients. Some experts recommend that women in their 20s should receive higher doses of estrogen than is routinely given to postmenopausal women, as this is a time of ongoing bone deposition. Frequently, it is easiest to prescribe combination oral contraceptive (COC) pills. Younger women may prefer this treatment as their friends may also use these pills, and in their minds, hormone replacement therapy may be associated with aging. Additionally, there is also no consensus on the duration of treatment in this patient population. For most individuals, continuation until approximately age 50, the usual age of menopause, seems reasonable.

TABLE 16-8. Evaluation of Premature Ovarian Failure due to Presumptive Autoimmune Disease

Test(s)	Target Organ
Free T$_4$, TSH	Thyroid
Calcium, phosphorus, albumin	Parathyroid
ACTH	Adrenal
Fasting glucose, HbA1c	Islet cells
CBC	Red blood cells (hemolytic anemia or pernicious anemia)
Platelets	Idiopathic thrombocytopenia

ACTH = adrenocorticotropin hormone; CBC = complete blood count; HbA1c = hemoglobin A1c; TSH = thyroid-stimulating hormone; T$_4$ = thyroxine.

Patients who have eating disorders or who exercise excessively will require behavior modification. In a patient with an eating disorder, psychiatric intervention is imperative due to the significant morbidity and mortality associated with this diagnosis (Chap. 13, p. 358) (American Psychiatric Association, 2000). Elite athletes may choose not to alter their exercise regimens and will therefore require estrogen treatment.

Polycystic Ovarian Syndrome

Treatment of affected women may include cyclic progesterone treatment or COCs or other forms of estrogen-progesterone treatment (Chap. 17, p. 474). Insulin-sensitizing agents such as metformin may be indicated in those with diabetes mellitus. In those with hyperandrogenism due to PCOS, combination oral contraceptives and/or spironolactone are often warranted.

Women with adult-onset CAH can be treated with low-dose corticosteroids to partially block ACTH stimulation of adrenal function and thereby decrease overproduction of adrenal androgens.

Infertility

Alternative approaches may be required in a patient who desires conception and many of these are discussed more fully in Chapter 20 (p. 529). Adequate treatment of hyperprolactinemia and thyroid disease will result in ovulation and in normal fertility for most women. If clearly linked to infertility, anatomic abnormalities should be surgically corrected whenever possible. However, depending on the type and severity of the abnormality, a surrogate to carry a gestation may be needed. Premature ovarian failure cannot be reversed, and these individuals can be offered in vitro fertilization using a donor oocyte to conceive. Women with hypogonadotropic hypogonadism, assuming that behavior modification is not successful, should be referred to an infertility specialist for treatment with pulsatile GnRH or with gonadotropins. Most patients will receive gonadotropin therapy because pulsatile GnRH is more complex to administer, and GnRH is not reliably available. Women with PCOS will frequently ovulate following treatment with the selective estrogen-receptor modulator clomiphene citrate. Clomiphene citrate is believed to act by transient inhibition of estrogen feedback at the hypothalamus and pituitary gland. This treatment, however, is not effective in those with hypogonadotropic hypogonadism, as they lack significant levels of circulating estrogen.

Patient Education

Finally, as in all medical conditions, patients should be adequately counseled regarding their diagnosis, the long-term implications of their diagnosis, and treatment options. Many women are under the mistaken impression that it is dangerous not to have a menstrual period. They should be reassured that this, in and of itself, is not a concern. On the other hand, all women with an intact endometrium should understand the risks of unopposed estrogen action, whether the estrogen is exogenous, such as through hormone therapy, or endogenous, such as in PCOS. Clinicians should counsel hypoestrogenic women about the importance of estrogen replacement to protect against bone loss. As described in Chapter 22 (p. 585), estrogen may have additional benefits, which should also be explained. In addition, even if not raised by the patient, the potential for future childbearing should be discussed.

REFERENCES

Abraham SF, Beumont PJ, Fraser IS, et al: Body weight, exercise and menstrual status among ballet dancers in training. Br J Obstet Gynaecol 89(7):507, 1982

Achermann JC, Weiss J, Eun-Jig L, et al: Inherited disorders of the gonadotropin hormones. Mol Cell Endocrinol 179:89, 2001

Aittomaki K, Eroila H, Kajanoja P: A population-based study of the incidence of müllerian aplasia in Finland. Fertil Steril 76(3):624, 2001

Aittomaki K, Lucena JL, Pakarinen P, et al: Mutation in the follicle-stimulating hormone receptor gene causes hereditary hypergonadotropic ovarian failure. Cell 82(6):959, 1995

American Fertility Society: The American Fertility Society classifications for adnexal adhesions, distal tubal occlusion, tubal occlusion secondary to tubal ligations, tubal pregnancies, müllerian anomalies, and intrauterine adhesions. Fertil Steril 49:944, 1988

American Psychiatric Association: Practice guideline for the treatment of patients with eating disorders (revision). American Psychiatric Association Work Group on Eating Disorders. Am J Psychiatry 157(1 Suppl):1, 2000

Ash P: The influence of radiation on fertility in man. Br J Radiol 53(628):271, 1980

Bachmann GA, Kemmann E: Prevalence of oligomenorrhea and amenorrhea in a college population. Am J Obstet Gynecol 144(1):98, 1982

Banerjee N, Kriplani A, Takkar D: Rare delivery complication caused by an undiagnosed uterine septum. Aust N Z J Obstet Gynaecol 39(1):113, 1999

Baskin HJ, Cobin RH, Duick DS, et al: American Association of Clinical Endocrinologists medical guidelines for clinical practice for the evaluation and treatment of hyperthyroidism and hypothyroidism. Endocr Pract 8(6):457, 2002

Baughman FA Jr, Vander Kolk KJ, Mann JD, et al: Two cases of primary amenorrhea with deletion of the long arm of the X chromosome (46, XXq-). Am J Obstet Gynecol 102(8):1065, 1968

Beranova M, Oliveira LM, Bedecarrats GY, et al: Prevalence, phenotypic spectrum, and modes of inheritance of gonadotropin-releasing hormone receptor mutations in idiopathic hypogonadotropic hypogonadism. J Clin Endocrinol Metab 86(4):1580, 2001

Bianco SDC, Kaiser UB: The genetic and molecular basis of idiopathic hypogonadotropic hypogonadism. Nat Rev Endocrinol 5:569, 2009

Billewicz WZ, Fellowes HM, Hytten CA: Comments on the critical metabolic mass and the age of menarche. Ann Hum Biol 3(1):51, 1976

Blumenfeld Z: Gynaecologic concerns for young women exposed to gonadotoxic chemotherapy. Curr Opin Obstet Gynecol 15(5):359, 2003

Blumenfeld Z, Avivi I, Ritter M, et al: Preservation of fertility and ovarian function and minimizing chemotherapy-induced gonadotoxicity in young women. J Soc Gynecol Investig 6(5):229, 1999

Bray MA, Muneyyirci-Delale O, Kofinas GD, et al: Circadian, ultradian, and episodic gonadotropin and prolactin secretion in human pseudocyesis. Acta Endocrinol (Copenh) 124(5):501, 1991

Broekmans FJ, Visser JA, Laven JSE, et al: Anti-müllerian hormone and ovarian dysfunction. Trends Endocrinol Metab 19(9):340, 2008

Buttram VC Jr, Turati G: Uterine synechiae: variations in severity and some conditions which may be conducive to severe adhesions. Int J Fertil 22(2):98, 1977

Cadman SM, Kim SH, Hu Y, et al: Molecular pathogenesis of Kallmann's syndrome. Horm Res 67(5):231, 2007

Chen H, Charlat O, Tartaglia LA, et al: Evidence that the diabetes gene encodes the leptin receptor: identification of a mutation in the leptin receptor gene in db/db mice. Cell 84(3):491, 1996

Christianson MS, Barker MA, Lindheim SR: Overcoming the challenging cervix: techniques to access the uterine cavity. J Low Genit Tract Dis 12(1):24, 2008

Coulam CB, Adamson SC, Annegers JF: Incidence of premature ovarian failure. Obstet Gynecol 67(4):604, 1986

Cundy TF, Butler J, Pope RM, et al: Amenorrhoea in women with non-alcoholic chronic liver disease. Gut 32(2):202, 1991

de Moraes RM, Blizzard RM, Garcia-Bunuel R, et al: Autoimmunity and ovarian failure. Am J Obstet Gynecol 112(5):693, 1972

De Souza MJ, Metzger DA: Reproductive dysfunction in amenorrheic athletes and anorexic patients: a review. Med Sci Sports Exerc 23(9):995, 1991

De Souza MJ, Miller BE, Loucks AB, et al: High frequency of luteal phase deficiency and anovulation in recreational women runners: blunted elevation in follicle-stimulating hormone observed during luteal-follicular transition. J Clin Endocrinol Metab 83(12):4220, 1998

Devi AS, Metzger DA, Luciano AA, et al: 45,X/46,XX mosaicism in patients with idiopathic premature ovarian failure. Fertil Steril 70(1):89, 1998

Fedele L, Bianchi S, Frontino G: Septums and synechiae: approaches to surgical correction. Clin Obstet Gynecol 49(4):767, 2006

Fedele L, Dorta M, Brioschi D, et al: Magnetic resonance imaging in Mayer-Rokitansky-Kuster-Hauser syndrome. Obstet Gynecol 76(4):593, 1990

Fore SR, Hammond CB, Parker RT, et al: Urologic and genital anomalies in patients with congenital absence of the vagina. Obstet Gynecol 46(4):410, 1975

Franco B, Guioli S, Pragliola A, et al: A gene deleted in Kallmann's syndrome shares homology with neural cell adhesion and axonal path-finding molecules. Nature 353(6344):529, 1991

Frisch RE: A method of prediction of age of menarche from height and weight at ages 9 through 13 years. Pediatrics 53(3):384, 1974a

Frisch RE, Gotz-Welbergen AV, McArthur JW, et al: Delayed menarche and amenorrhea of college athletes in relation to age of onset of training. JAMA 246(14):1559, 1981

Frisch RE, McArthur JW: Menstrual cycles: fatness as a determinant of minimum weight for height necessary for their maintenance or onset. Science 185(4155):949, 1974b

Frisch RE, Revelle R: Height and weight at menarche and a hypothesis of critical body weights and adolescent events. Science 169(943):397, 1970

Frisch RE, Wyshak G, Vincent L: Delayed menarche and amenorrhea in ballet dancers. N Engl J Med 303(1):17, 1980

Ghazizadeh S, Lessan-Pezeshkii M: Reproduction in women with end-stage renal disease and effect of kidney transplantation. Iran J Kidney Dis 1(1):12, 2007

Goldsmith O, Solomon DH, Horton R: Hypogonadism and mineralocorticoid excess. The 17-hydroxylase deficiency syndrome. N Engl J Med 277(13):673, 1967

Gradishar WJ, Schilsky RL: Ovarian function following radiation and chemotherapy for cancer. Semin Oncol 16(5):425, 1989

Griffin JE, Edwards C, Madden JD, et al: Congenital absence of the vagina. The Mayer-Rokitansky-Kuster-Hauser syndrome. Ann Intern Med 85(2):224, 1976

Hoek A, Schoemaker J, Drexhage HA: Premature ovarian failure and ovarian autoimmunity. Endocr Rev 18(1):107, 1997

Howlett TA, Wass JA, Grossman A, et al: Prolactinomas presenting as primary amenorrhoea and delayed or arrested puberty: response to medical therapy. Clin Endocrinol (Oxf) 30(2):131, 1989

Hsu LY, Hirschhorn K: Genetic and clinical considerations of long-arm deletion of the X chromosome. Pediatrics 45(4):656, 1970

Jameson JL, Weetman AP: Disorders of the thyroid gland. In Fauci AS, Braunwald E, Kasper DL, et al (eds): Harrison's Principles of Internal Medicine, 17th ed. New York, McGraw-Hill, 2008, p 2232

Jick H, Porter J: Relation between smoking and age of natural menopause. Report from the Boston Collaborative Drug Surveillance Program, Boston University Medical Center. Lancet 1(8026):1354, 1977

Job JC, Chaussain JL, Garnier PE: The use of luteinizing hormone-releasing hormone in pediatric patients. Horm Res 8(3):171, 1977

Johnston FE, Roche AF, Schell LM, et al: Critical weight at menarche. Critique of a hypothesis. Am J Dis Child 129(1):19, 1975

Jones GS, Moraes-Ruehsen M: A new syndrome of amenorrhae in association with hypergonadotropism and apparently normal ovarian follicular apparatus. Am J Obstet Gynecol 104(4):597, 1969

Kaneko N, Kawagoe S, Hiroi M: Turner's syndrome—review of the literature with reference to a successful pregnancy outcome. Gynecol Obstet Invest 29(2):81, 1990

Kaufman FR, Kogut MD, Donnell GN, et al: Hypergonadotropic hypogonadism in female patients with galactosemia. N Engl J Med 304(17):994, 1981

Kelestimur F: Sheehan's syndrome. Pituitary 6(4):181, 2003

Kim MH: "Gonadotropin-resistant ovaries" syndrome in association with secondary amenorrhea. Am J Obstet Gynecol 120(2):257, 1974

Klein SM, Garcia CR: Asherman's syndrome: a critique and current review. Fertil Steril 24(9):722, 1973

Klingmuller D, Dewes W, Krahe T, et al: Magnetic resonance imaging of the brain in patients with anosmia and hypothalamic hypogonadism (Kallmann's syndrome). J Clin Endocrinol Metab 65(3):581, 1987

Knauff EAH, Eijemans MJC, Lambalk CB, et al: Anti-Müllerian hormone, inhibin B, and antral follicle count in young women with ovarian failure. J Clin Endocrinol Metab 94:786, 2009

LaBarbera AR, Miller MM, Ober C, et al: Autoimmune etiology in premature ovarian failure. Am J Reprod Immunol Microbiol 16(3):115, 1988

Layman LC: Genetics of human hypogonadotropic hypogonadism. Am J Med Genet 89(4):240, 1999

Layman LC, Cohen DP, Jin M, et al: Mutations in gonadotropin-releasing hormone receptor gene cause hypogonadotropic hypogonadism. Nat Genet 18(1):14, 1998

Layman LC, Lee EJ, Peak DB, et al: Delayed puberty and hypogonadism caused by mutations in the follicle-stimulating hormone beta-subunit gene. N Engl J Med 337(9):607, 1997

Lee GH, Proenca R, Montez JM, et al: Abnormal splicing of the leptin receptor in diabetic mice. Nature 379(6566):632, 1996

Letterie GS, Wilson J, Miyazawa K: Magnetic resonance imaging of müllerian tract abnormalities. Fertil Steril 50(2):365, 1988

Levy HL, Driscoll SG, Porensky RS, et al: Ovarian failure in galactosemia. N Engl J Med 310(1):50, 1984

Li HW, Anderson RA, Yeung WS, et al: Evaluation of serum antimullerian hormone and inhibin B concentrations in the differential diagnosis of secondary oligoamenorrhea. Fertil Steril 96(3):774, 2011

Licinio J, Caglayan S, Ozata M, et al: Phenotypic effects of leptin replacement on morbid obesity, diabetes mellitus, hypogonadism, and behavior in leptin-deficient adults. Proc Natl Acad Sci USA 101(13):4531, 2004

Mantzoros C, Flier JS, Lesem MD, et al: Cerebrospinal fluid leptin in anorexia nervosa: correlation with nutritional status and potential role in resistance to weight gain. J Clin Endocrinol Metab 82(6):1845, 1997

Manuel M, Katayama PK, Jones HW, Jr.: The age of occurrence of gonadal tumors in intersex patients with a Y chromosome. Am J Obstet Gynecol 124(3):293, 1976

Matthews CH, Borgato S, Beck-Peccoz P, et al: Primary amenorrhoea and infertility due to a mutation in the beta-subunit of follicle-stimulating hormone. Nat Genet 5(1):83, 1993

Mlynarcikova A, Fickova M, Scsukova S: Ovarian intrafollicular processes as a target for cigarette smoke components and selected environmental reproductive disruptors. Endocr Regul 39(1):21, 2005

Morrison JC, Givens JR, Wiser WL, et al: Mumps oophoritis: a cause of premature menopause. Fertil Steril 26(7):655, 1975

Nakamura S, Douchi T, Oki T, et al: Relationship between sonographic endometrial thickness and progestin-induced withdrawal bleeding. Obstet Gynecol 87(5 Pt 1):722, 1996

Özgör B, Selimoğlu MA: Coeliac disease and reproductive disorders. Scand J Gastroenterol 45(4):395, 2010

Pallais JC, Bo-Abbas Y, Pitteloud N, et al: Neuroendocrine, gonadal, placental, and obstetric phenotypes in patients with IHH and mutations in the G-protein coupled receptor, GPR54. Mol Cell Endocrinol 254-255:70, 2006

Parazzini F, Cecchetti G: The frequency of imperforate hymen in northern Italy. Int J Epidemiol 19(3):763, 1990

Peng C, Fan NC, Ligier M, et al: Expression and regulation of gonadotropin-releasing hormone (GnRH) and GnRH receptor messenger ribonucleic acids in human granulosa-luteal cells. Endocrinology 135(5):1740, 1994

Pereyra PB, Mendez Ribas JM, Milone G, et al: Use of GnRH analogs for functional protection of the ovary and preservation of fertility during cancer treatment in adolescents: a preliminary report. Gynecol Oncol 81(3):391, 2001

Pettersson F, Fries H, Nillius SJ: Epidemiology of secondary amenorrhea. I. Incidence and prevalence rates. Am J Obstet Gynecol 117(1):80, 1973

The Practice Committee of the American Society for Reproductive Medicine: Current evaluation of amenorrhea. Fertil Steril 86(Supp 5S):148, 2006

Quinton R, Hasan W, Grant W, et al: Gonadotropin-releasing hormone immunoreactivity in the nasal epithelia of adults with Kallmann's syndrome and isolated hypogonadotropic hypogonadism and in the early midtrimester human fetus. J Clin Endocrinol Metab 82(1):309, 1997

Rarick LD, Shangold MM, Ahmed SW: Cervical mucus and serum estradiol as predictors of response to progestin challenge. Fertil Steril 54(2):353, 1990

Rebar RW, Connolly HV: Clinical features of young women with hypergonadotropic amenorrhea. Fertil Steril 53(5):804, 1990

Reid RL: Amenorrhea. In Copeland LJ (ed): Textbook of Gynecology. Philadelphia, Saunders, 2000

Reindollar RH, Byrd JR, McDonough PG: Delayed sexual development: a study of 252 patients. Am J Obstet Gynecol 140(4):371, 1981

Reindollar RH, Novak M, Tho SP, et al: Adult-onset amenorrhea: a study of 262 patients. Am J Obstet Gynecol 155(3):531, 1986

Reinhold C, Hricak H, Forstner R, et al: Primary amenorrhea: evaluation with MR imaging. Radiology 203(2):383, 1997

Robinson AC, Dockeray CJ, Cullen MJ, et al: Hypergonadotrophic hypogonadism in classical galactosaemia: evidence for defective oogenesis. Case report. Br J Obstet Gynaecol 91(2):199, 1984

Rubio-Gozalbo ME, Gubbels CS, Bakker JA, et al: Gonadal function in male and female patients with classic galactosemia. Human Reprod Update 16(2):177, 2010

Rugarli E, Ballabio A: Kallmann syndrome. From genetics to neurobiology. JAMA 270(22):2713, 1993

Saenger P, Albertsson Wikland K, Conway GS, et al: Recommendations for the diagnosis and management of Turner syndrome. J Clin Endocrinol Metab 86(7):3061, 2001

Schenker JG, Margalioth EJ: Intrauterine adhesions: an updated appraisal. Fertil Steril 37(5):593, 1982

Schlessinger D, Herrera L, Crisponi L, et al: Genes and translocations involved in POF. Am J Med Genet 111(3):328, 2002

Schneider JE: Energy balance and reproduction. Physiol Behav 81(2):289, 2004

Seminara SB: Mechanisms of disease: the first kiss-a crucial role for kisspeptin-1 and its receptor, G-protein-coupled receptor 54, in puberty and reproduction. Nat Clin Pract Endocrinol Metab 2(6):328, 2006

Sharara FI, Seifer DB, Flaws JA: Environmental toxicants and female reproduction. Fertil Steril 70(4):613, 1998

Sharma JB, Roy KK, Pushparaj M, et al: Hysteroscopic findings in women with primary and secondary infertility due to genital tuberculosis. Int J Gynaecol Obstet 104(1):49, 2009

Simpson JL: Gonadal dysgenesis and abnormalities of the human sex chromosomes: current status of phenotypic-karyotypic correlations. Birth Defects Orig Artic Ser 11(4):23, 1975

Singh RP, Carr DH: The anatomy and histology of XO human embryos and fetuses. Anat Rec 155(3):369, 1966

Somers EC, Marder W, Christman GM, et al: Use of a gonadotropin-releasing hormone analog for protection against premature ovarian failure during cyclophosphamide therapy in women with severe lupus. Arthritis Rheum 52(9):2761, 2005

Soussi-Yanicostas N, Hardelin JP, Arroyo-Jimenez MM, et al: Initial characterization of anosmin-1, a putative extracellular matrix protein synthesized by definite neuronal cell populations in the central nervous system. J Cell Sci 109(Pt 7)1749, 1996

Starkman MN, Marshall JC, La Ferla J, et al: Pseudocyesis: psychologic and neuroendocrine interrelationships. Psychosom Med 47(1):46, 1985

Tartaglia LA, Dembski M, Weng X, et al: Identification and expression cloning of a leptin receptor, OB-R. Cell 83(7):1263, 1995

Terenziani M, Piva L, Meazza C, et al: Oophoropexy: a relevant role in preservation of ovarian function and pelvic irradiation. Fertil Steril 91(3):935.e15, 2009

Tho PT, McDonough PG: Gonadal dysgenesis and its variants. Pediatr Clin North Am 28(2):309, 1981

Troche V, Hernandez E: Neoplasia arising in dysgenetic gonads. Obstet Gynecol Surv 41(2):74, 1986

Turner H: Classic pages in obstetrics and gynecology by Henry H. Turner. A syndrome of infantilism, congenital webbed neck, and cubitus valgus. Endocrinology, vol. 23, pp. 566-574, 1938. Am J Obstet Gynecol 113(2):279, 1972

Veldhuis JD, Hammond JM: Endocrine function after spontaneous infarction of the human pituitary: report, review, and reappraisal. Endocr Rev 1(1):100, 1980

Waldstreicher J, Seminara SB, Jameson JL, et al: The genetic and clinical heterogeneity of gonadotropin-releasing hormone deficiency in the human. J Clin Endocrinol Metab 81(12):4388, 1996

Wallace WH, Shalet SM, Crowne EC, et al: Ovarian failure following abdominal irradiation in childhood: natural history and prognosis. Clin Oncol (R Coll Radiol) 1(2):75, 1989

Weiss J, Axelrod L, Whitcomb RW, et al: Hypogonadism caused by a single amino acid substitution in the beta subunit of luteinizing hormone. N Engl J Med 326(3):179, 1992

Whelan CI, Stewart DE: Pseudocyesis—a review and report of six cases. Int J Psychiatry Med 20(1):97, 1990

Williams RS, Littell RD, Mendenhall NP: Laparoscopic oophoropexy and ovarian function in the treatment of Hodgkin disease. Cancer 86(10):2138, 1999

Wilson EE, Vuitch F, Carr BR: Laparoscopic removal of dysgenetic gonads containing a gonadoblastoma in a patient with Swyer syndrome. Obstet Gynecol 79(5):842, 1992

Winters SJ: Expanding the differential diagnosis of male hypogonadism. N Engl J Med 326(3):193, 1992

Wittenberger MD, Hagerman RJ, Sherman SL, et al: The FMR1 premutation and reproduction. Fertil Steril 87(3):456, 2007

Yen SS, Rebar R, VandenBerg G, et al: Hypothalamic amenorrhea and hypogonadotropinism: responses to synthetic LRF. J Clin Endocrinol Metab 36(5):811, 1973

Yu D, Wong YM, Cheong Y, et al: Asherman syndrome—one century later. Fertil Steril 89(4):759, 2008

Zenaty D, Breton's P, Lambe C, et al: Paediatric phenotype of Kallmann syndrome due to mutations of fibroblast growth factor receptor 1 (FGFR1). Mol Cell Endocrinol 254-255:78, 2006

Zhang Y, Proenca R, Maffei M, et al: Positional cloning of the mouse obese gene and its human homologue. Nature 372(6505):425, 1994

CHAPTER 16

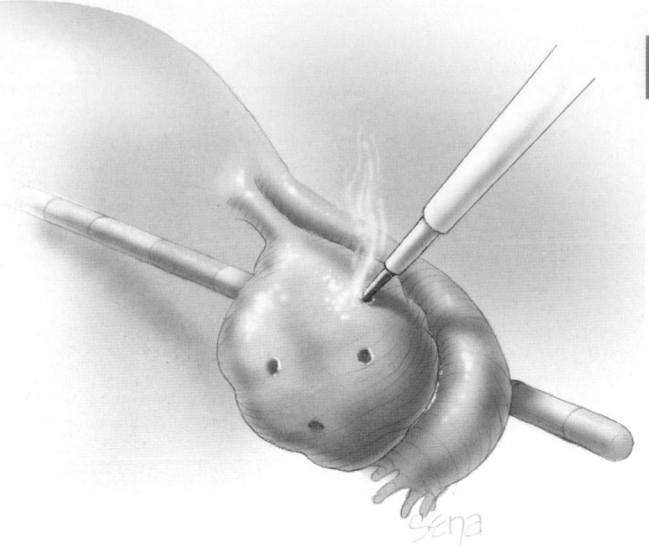

CHAPTER 17

Polycystic Ovarian Syndrome and Hyperandrogenism

Polycystic ovarian syndrome (PCOS) is a common endocrinopathy typified by oligoovulation or anovulation, signs of androgen excess, and multiple small ovarian cysts. These signs and symptoms may vary widely between women as well as within individuals over time. As a result, women with PCOS may first present to various medical specialists, including gynecologists, internists, endocrinologists, or dermatologists. Thus, a familiarity with PCOS is essential for physicians in each of these specialties.

INCIDENCE

Polycystic ovarian syndrome is the most common endocrine disorder of reproductive-aged women and affects approximately 4 to 12 percent (Asunción, 2000; Diamanti-Kandarakis, 1999; Farah, 1999; Knochenhauer, 1998). Although symptoms of androgen excess may vary among ethnicities, PCOS appears to equally affect all races and nationalities.

DEFINITION

Polycystic Ovarian Syndrome

In 2003 in Rotterdam, The Netherlands, a consensus meeting between the European Society of Human Reproduction and Embryology and the American Society for Reproductive Medicine (ESHRE/ASRM)—The Rotterdam ESHRE/ASRM-Sponsored PCOS Consensus Workshop Group, 2004—redefined PCOS (Table 17-1). Affected individuals must have two of the following three criteria: (1) oligo- and/or anovulation, (2) hyperandrogenism (clinical and/or biochemical), and (3) polycystic ovaries identified sonographically. However, because other etiologies, such as congenital adrenal hyperplasia, androgen-secreting tumors, and hyperprolactinemia, may also lead to oligoovulation and/or androgen excess, these must be excluded. Thus, PCOS is at present a diagnosis of exclusion.

The Rotterdam criteria constitute a broader spectrum than that formerly put forward by the National Institutes of Health (NIH) Conference in 1990 (Zawadzki, 1990). The latter defined PCOS by ovulatory dysfunction plus clinical hyperandrogenism and/or hyperandrogenemia without regard to ovarian sonographic appearance. Controversy exists as to which definition is more appropriate, and many investigators still use the NIH 1990 criteria as a basis to define PCOS in their population studies (Chang, 2005).

TABLE 17-1. Definition of Polycystic Ovarian Syndrome

ESHRE/ASRM (Rotterdam) 2003
To include two out of three of the following:
1. Oligo- or anovulation
2. Clinical and/or biochemical signs of hyperandrogenism
3. Polycystic ovaries (with exclusion of related disorders)

NIH (1990)
To include both of the following:
1. Oligo-ovulation
2. Hyperandrogenism and/or hyperandrogenemia (with exclusion of related disorders)

AE-PCOS (2009)
1. Hyperandrogenism: hirsutism and/or hyperandrogenemia
   and
2. Ovarian dysfunction: Oligo-anovulation and/or polycystic ovaries
   and
3. Exclusion of other androgen-excess or related disorders

AE-PCOS = Androgen Excess and PCOS Society;
ASRM = American Society for Reproductive Medicine;
ESHRE = European Society of Human Reproduction and Embryology; NIH = National Institutes of Health;
PCOS = polycystic ovarian syndrome.
From Azziz, 2009; The Rotterdam ESHRE/ASRM-Sponsored PCOS Consensus Workshop Group, 2004; Zawadzki, 1990.

Lastly, a third organization—The Androgen Excess and PCOS Society (AE-PCOS)—has also defined criteria for PCOS (Azziz, 2009). As is shown in Table 17-1, these criteria are similar to those outlined in Rotterdam.

Ovarian Hyperthecosis and HAIRAN Syndrome

Often considered a more severe form of PCOS, ovarian hyperthecosis is a rare condition characterized by nests of luteinized theca cells distributed throughout the ovarian stroma. Affected women exhibit severe hyperandrogenism and may occasionally display frank virilization signs such as clitoromegaly, temporal balding, and deepening of the voice (Culiner, 1949). In addition, a much greater degree of insulin resistance and acanthosis nigricans is typically is found (Nagamani, 1986).

The hyperandrogenic-insulin resistant-acanthosis nigricans (HAIRAN) syndrome is uncommon and consists of marked hyperandrogenism, severe insulin resistance, and acanthosis nigricans (Barbieri, 1994). The etiology of this disorder is unclear, and HAIRAN syndrome may represent either a variant of PCOS or a distinct genetic syndrome. Both ovarian hyperthecosis and HAIRAN are exaggerated phenotypes of PCOS, and their treatment mirrors that for PCOS described later in the chapter.

ETIOLOGY

The underlying cause of PCOS is unknown. However, a genetic basis that is both multifactorial and polygenic is suspected, as there is a well-documented aggregation of the syndrome within families (Franks, 1997). Specifically, an increased prevalence has been noted between affected individuals and their sisters (32 to 66 percent) and mothers (24 to 52 percent) (Govind, 1999; Kahsar-Miller, 2001; Yildiz, 2003). Some have suggested an autosomal dominant inheritance with expression in both females and males. For example, first-degree male relatives of women with PCOS have been shown to have significantly higher rates of elevated circulating dehydroepiandrosterone sulfate (DHEAS) levels, early balding, and insulin resistance compared with control males (Legro, 2000, 2002).

Identification of candidate genes linked to PCOS has been a major research focus, given the large potential benefit for both diagnosis and management of this disorder. In general, putative genes include those involved in androgen synthesis and those associated with insulin resistance. Clinical and in vitro studies of human ovarian theca cells have suggested dysregulation of the *CYP11a* gene in patients with PCOS. This gene encodes the cholesterol side-chain cleavage enzyme, which is the enzyme that performs the rate-limiting step in steroid biosynthesis (Fig. 15-5, p. 403). Evidence also suggests upregulation of other enzymes in the androgen biosynthetic pathway (Franks, 2006). In addition, the insulin receptor gene on chromosome 19p13.2 may be involved (Urbanek, 2005). Further investigation, however, is needed to determine the roles of these gene products in the pathogenesis of PCOS.

PATHOPHYSIOLOGY

Gonadotropins

Anovulation in women with PCOS is characterized by inappropriate gonadotropin secretion (Fig. 17-1). Specifically, alterations in gonadotropin-releasing hormone (GnRH) pulsatility lead to preferential production of luteinizing hormone (LH) compared with follicle-stimulating hormone (FSH) (Hayes, 1998; Waldstreicher, 1988). It is currently unknown whether hypothalamic dysfunction is a primary cause of PCOS or is secondary to abnormal steroid feedback. In either case, serum LH levels rise, and increased levels are observed clinically in approximately 50 percent of affected women (Balen, 2002; van Santbrink, 1997). Similarly, luteinizing hormone:follicle-stimulating hormone (LH:FSH) ratios are elevated and rise above 2:1 in approximately 60 percent of patients (Rebar, 1976).

Insulin Resistance

Women with PCOS also display greater degrees of insulin resistance and compensatory hyperinsulinemia than nonaffected women. Insulin resistance is defined as a reduced glucose-uptake response to a given amount of insulin. The mechanism of this decreased insulin sensitivity appears to

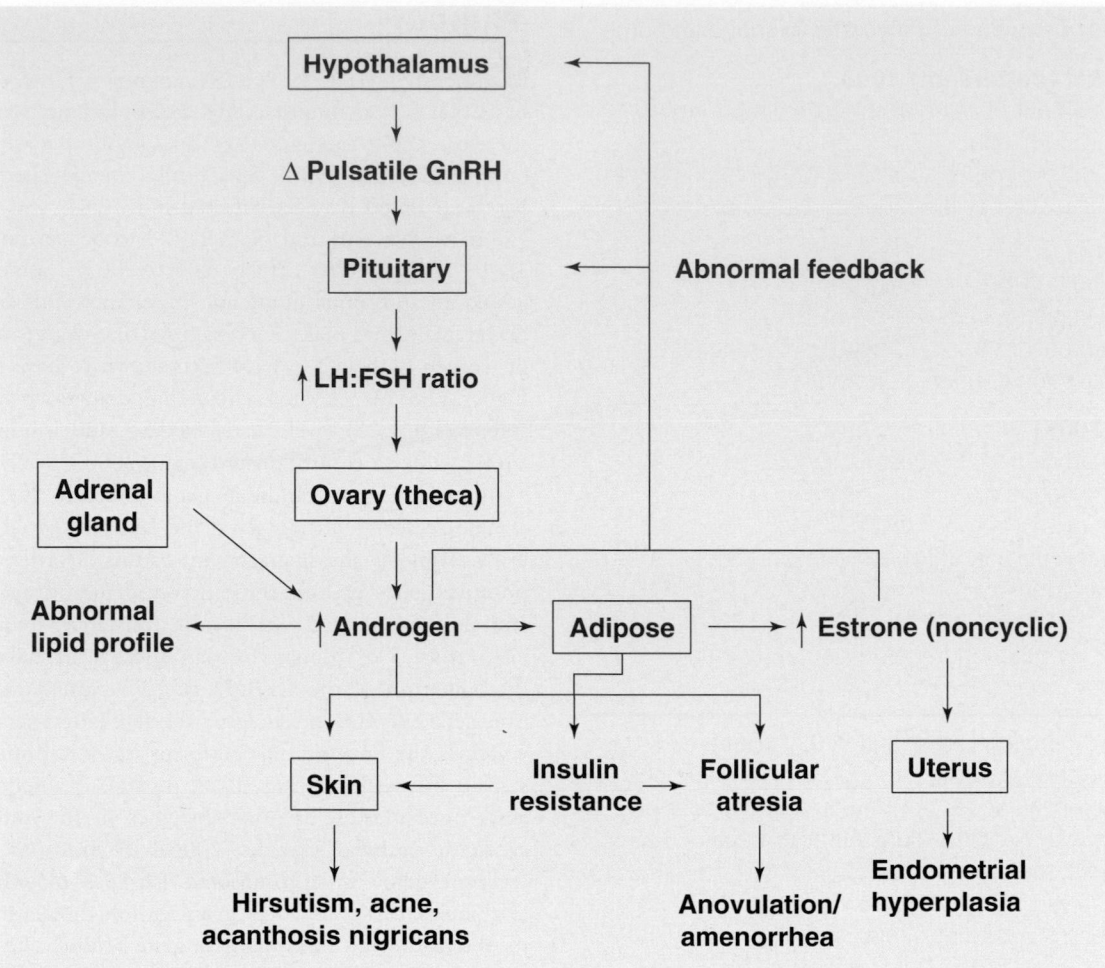

FIGURE 17-1 Model for the initiation and maintenance of polycystic ovarian syndrome (PCOS). Alterations in pulsatile gonadotropin-releasing hormone (GnRH) release may lead to a relative increase in luteinizing hormone (LH) versus follicle-stimulating hormone (FSH) biosynthesis and secretion. LH stimulates ovarian androgen production, while the relative paucity of FSH prevents adequate stimulation of aromatase activity within the granulosa cells, thereby decreasing androgen conversion to the potent estrogen estradiol.

Increased intrafollicular androgen levels result in follicular atresia. Increased circulating androgen levels contribute to abnormalities in patient lipid profiles and the development of hirsutism and acne. Increased circulating androgens can also be derived from the adrenal gland.

Elevated serum androgens (primarily androstenedione) are converted in the periphery to estrogens (primarily estrone). As conversion occurs primarily in the stromal cells of adipose tissue, estrogen production will be augmented in obese PCOS patients. This conversion results in chronic feedback at the hypothalamus and pituitary gland, in contrast to the normal fluctuations in feedback observed in the presence of a growing follicle and rapidly changing levels of estradiol. Unopposed estrogen stimulation of the endometrium may lead to endometrial hyperplasia.

Insulin resistance due to genetic abnormalities and/or increased adipose tissue contributes to follicular atresia in the ovaries as well as the development of acanthosis nigricans in the skin.

Lack of follicular development results in anovulation and subsequent oligo- or amenorrhea.

Note that this syndrome may develop from primary dysfunction of any one of a number of organ systems. For example, elevated ovarian androgen production may be due to an intrinsic abnormality in enzymatic function and/or abnormal hypothalamic-pituitary stimulation with LH and FSH.

The common denominator is development of a self-perpetuating noncyclic hormonal pattern.

be due to a postbinding abnormality in insulin-receptor-mediated signal transduction (Dunaif, 1997). Both lean and obese women with PCOS are found to be more insulin resistant than nonaffected weight-matched controls (Dunaif, 1989, 1992).

Insulin resistance has been associated with an increase in several disorders including type 2 diabetes mellitus (DM), hypertension, dyslipidemia, and cardiovascular disease. Therefore, PCOS is not simply a disorder of short-term consequences such as irregular periods and hirsutism, but also one of long-term health sequelae (Table 17-2).

Androgens

Both insulin and LH stimulate androgen production by the ovarian theca cell (Dunaif, 1992). As a result, affected ovaries

TABLE 17-2. Consequences of Polycystic Ovarian
Syndrome

Short-term consequences
Obesity
Infertility
Irregular menses
Abnormal lipid levels
Hirsutism/acne/androgenic alopecia
Glucose intolerance/acanthosis nigricans

Long-term consequences
Diabetes mellitus
Endometrial cancer
Cardiovascular disease

---

secrete elevated levels of testosterone and androstenedione. Specifically, elevated free testosterone levels are noted in 70 to 80 percent of women with PCOS, and 25 to 65 percent exhibit elevated levels of DHEAS (Moran, 1994, 1999; O'Driscoll, 1994). In turn, elevated androstenedione levels contribute to an increase in estrone levels through peripheral conversion of androgens to estrogens by aromatase.

Sex Hormone-Binding Globulin

Women with PCOS display decreased levels of sex hormone-binding globulin (SHBG). This glycoprotein, produced in the liver, binds most sex steroids. Only approximately 1 percent of these steroids are unbound and thus free and bioavailable. The synthesis of SHBG is suppressed by insulin as well as androgens, corticoids, progestins, and growth hormone (Bergh, 1993). Because of suppressed SHBG production, less circulating androgen is bound and thus more remains available to bind with end-organ receptors. It is for this reason that some women with PCOS will have total testosterone levels in the normal range, but will be clinically hyperandrogenic due to elevated free testosterone levels.

In addition to hyperandrogenism, low SHBG levels have also been linked to impaired glucose control and a risk for developing type 2 DM (Ding, 2009). The mechanism of this association is not fully understood and may reflect a role for SHBG in glucose homeostasis. Moreover, in several small studies, a relationship has been found between lower plasma SHBG levels in first-trimester pregnancies and subsequent gestational diabetes (Smirnakis, 2007; Thadhani, 2003). Specific to PCOS, Veltman-Verhulst and colleagues (2010) evaluated SHBG levels in women with PCOS and found a similar association with low SHBG levels and subsequent development of gestational diabetes mellitus.

Anovulation

Although androgen levels are typically elevated in women with PCOS, progesterone levels are low due to anovulation. The precise mechanism leading to anovulation is unclear, but hypersecretion of LH has been implicated in menstrual irregularity.

In addition, anovulation may result from insulin resistance, as a substantial number of anovulatory patients with PCOS may resume ovulatory cycles when treated with metformin, an insulin sensitizer (Nestler, 1998). It has been suggested that oligoovulatory women with PCOS exhibit a milder phenotype of ovarian dysfunction than anovulatory PCOS patients and have a more favorable response to ovulation induction agents (Burgers, 2010).

Finally, the large antral follicle cohort seen in PCOS may contribute to anovulation. Some patients who have undergone ovarian wedge resection or laparoscopic ovarian drilling have found significant improvement in their menstrual regularity. One study demonstrated that 67 percent of PCOS patients developed regular menses following such surgery compared with only 8 percent prior to surgery (Amer, 2002).

SIGNS AND SYMPTOMS

In women with PCOS, complaints stem from varied endocrine effects and may include menstrual irregularities, infertility, manifestations of androgen excess, or other endocrine dysfunction. Symptoms classically become apparent within a few years of puberty.

Menstrual Dysfunction

Menstrual dysfunction in women with PCOS may range from amenorrhea to oligomenorrhea to episodic menometrorrhagia with anemia. In many women with PCOS, amenorrhea and oligomenorrhea result from anovulation. In this setting, failed ovulation precludes progesterone production and then also progesterone withdrawal to trigger menses. Alternatively, amenorrhea may result from elevated androgen levels in those with PCOS. Specifically, androgens may counteract estrogen to produce an atrophic endometrium. It is therefore not uncommon to observe amenorrhea and a thin endometrial stripe in PCOS patients with elevated androgen levels.

In contrast to amenorrhea, women with PCOS may have heavy and unpredictable bleeding. In these women, progesterone is not produced due to anovulation, and chronic estrogen exposure results. This produces constant mitogenic stimulation of the endometrium. The instability of the thickened endometrium results in an unpredictable bleeding pattern.

Characteristically, oligomenorrhea (fewer than eight menstrual periods in 1 year) or amenorrhea (absence of menses for 3 or more consecutive months) with PCOS begins with menarche. Approximately 50 percent of *all* postmenarchal girls have irregular periods for up to 2 years due to immaturity of the hypothalamic-pituitary-ovarian axis. However, in girls with PCOS, monthly ovulatory menstrual cycles are not established by midadolescence, and they typically continue to have irregular cycles.

Lastly, some evidence suggests that PCOS patients with prior irregular cycle intervals may develop regular cycle patterns as they age. A decreasing antral follicle cohort as women enter their 30s and 40s may lead to a concurrent decrease in androgen production (Elting, 2000).

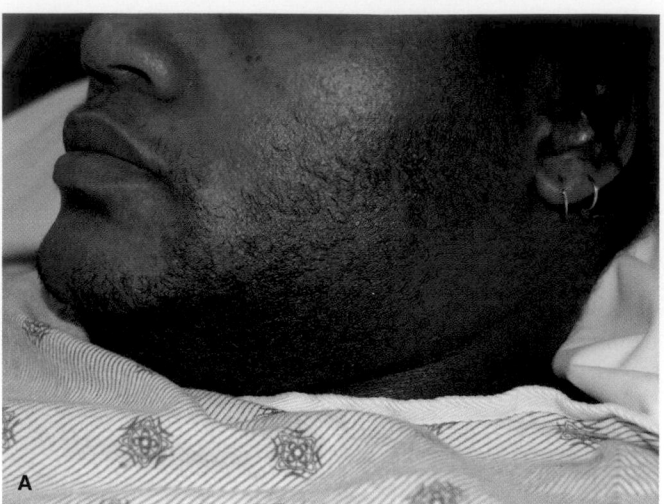 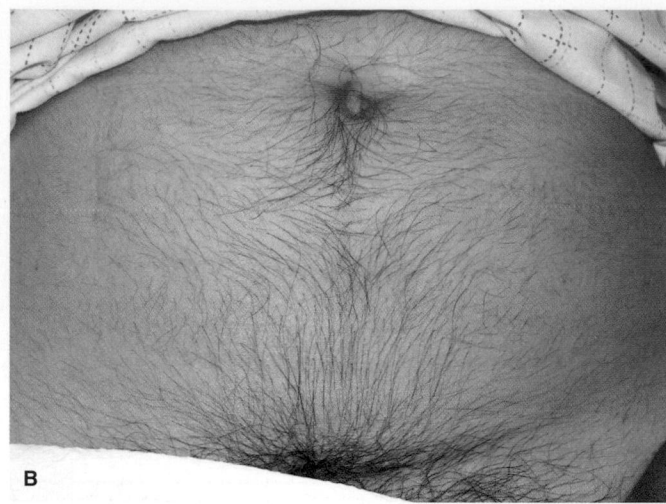

FIGURE 17-2 Photographs of hirsutism. **A.** Facial hirsutism. *(Photograph contributed by Dr. Tamara Chao.)* **B.** Male pattern escutcheon.

Hyperandrogenism

This condition is typically manifested clinically by hirsutism, acne, and/or androgenic alopecia. In contrast, signs of virilization such as increased muscle mass, decreased breast size, deepening of the voice, and clitoromegaly are not typical of PCOS. Virilization reflects higher androgen levels and should prompt investigation for an androgen-producing tumor of the ovary or the adrenal gland.

Hirsutism

In a female, hirsutism is defined as coarse, dark, terminal hairs distributed in a male pattern (Fig. 17-2). Hirsutism should be distinguished from hypertrichosis, which is a generalized increase in lanugo, that is, the soft, lightly pigmented hair associated with some medications and malignancies. Polycystic ovarian syndrome accounts for 70 to 80 percent of cases of hirsutism. Idiopathic hirsutism is the second most frequent cause (Azziz, 2003).

Women with PCOS typically report hirsutism beginning in late adolescence or the early 20s. Additionally, a variety of drugs may also lead to hirsutism, and their use should be investigated (Table 17-3).

Pathophysiology of Hirsutism. Elevated androgen levels play a major role in determining the type and distribution of hair (Archer, 2004). Within a hair follicle, testosterone is converted by the enzyme 5α-reductase to dihydrotestosterone (DHT). Although both testosterone and DHT convert short, soft vellus hair to coarse terminal hair, DHT is markedly more effective than testosterone (Fig. 17-3). Conversion is irreversible, and only hairs in androgen-sensitive areas are changed in this manner to terminal hairs. As a result, the most common areas affected with excess hair growth in women with PCOS include the upper lip, chin, sideburns, chest, and linea alba of the lower abdomen. Specifically, *escutcheon* is the term used to describe the hair pattern of the lower abdomen. In women, a triangular pattern overlies the mons pubis, whereas in men it also extends up the linea alba to form a diamond shape.

Ferriman-Gallwey Scoring System. To quantify the degree of hirsutism for research purposes, the Ferriman-Gallwey scoring system was developed in 1961 and later modified in 1981 (Ferriman, 1961; Hatch, 1981). Within the modified system, abnormal hair distribution is assessed in nine body areas and scored from 0 to 4 (Fig. 17-4). Increasing numeric scores correspond to greater hair density within a given area. Many investigators define hirsutism as a score of 8 or greater using the modified version.

This system is cumbersome and therefore is not used frequently in clinical settings. A simplified version that assesses only three body areas has been investigated (Cook, 2011). Nevertheless, scoring may be useful for following treatment

TABLE 17-3. Medications That May Cause Hirsutism and/or Hypertrichosis

Drug	Brand Name
Hirsutism	
Anabolic steroids	
Danazol	Danocrine
Metoclopramide	Reglan
Methyldopa	Aldomet
Phenothiazines	
Progestins	
Reserpine	Serpasil
Testosterone	
Hypertrichosis	
Cyclosporine	Sandimmune
Diazoxide	Hyperstat
Hydrocortisone	
Minoxidil	Rogaine
Penicillamine	Cuprimine
Phenytoin	Dilantin
Psoralens	Oxsoralen
Streptomycin	

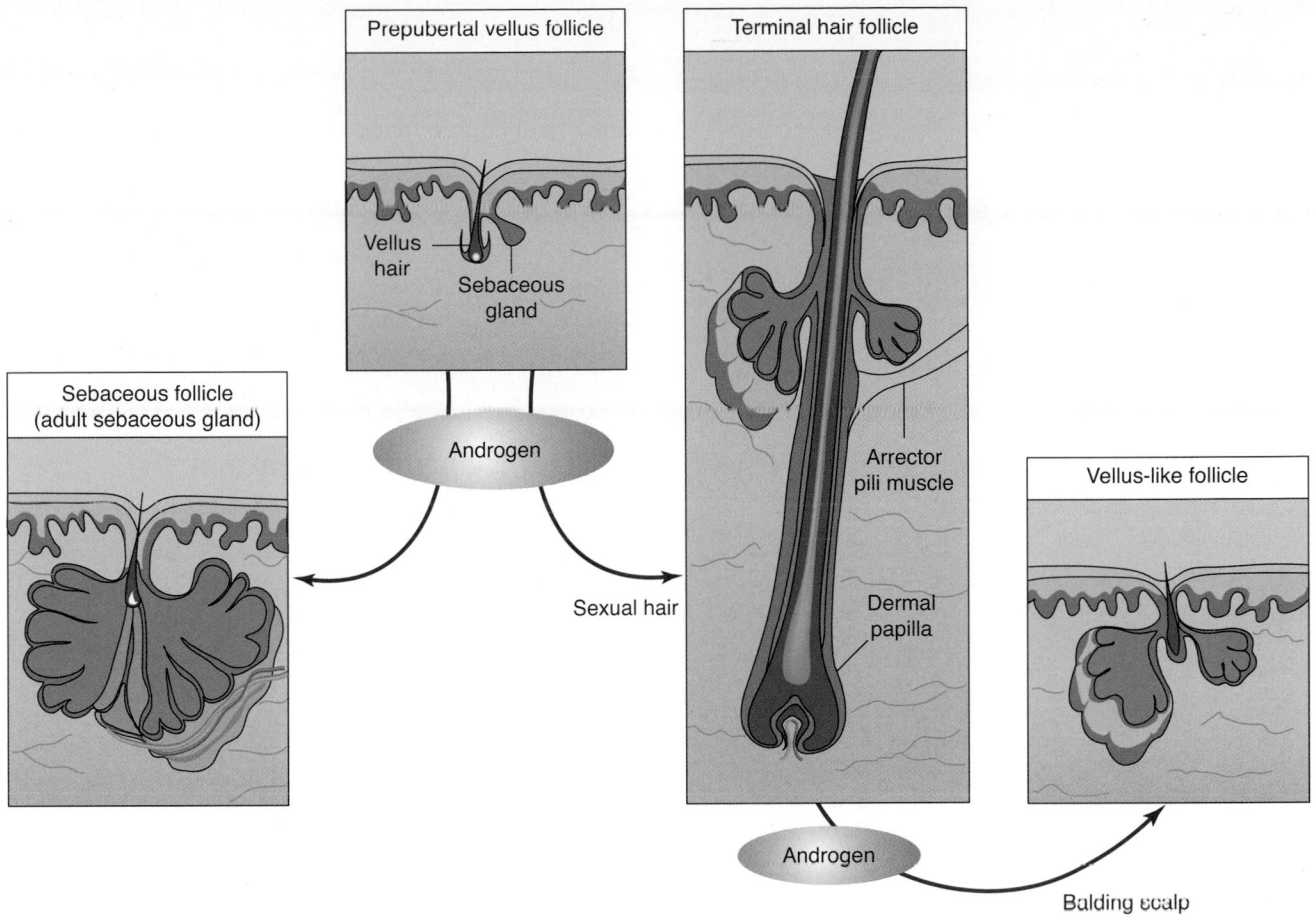

FIGURE 17-3 Androgenic effects on the pilosebaceous unit. In some hair-bearing areas, androgens stimulate sebaceous glands, and increased sebum may lead to acne. In other areas, vellus follicles respond to androgens and are converted to terminal follicles, leading to hirsutism. Under the influence of androgens, terminal hairs that were not previously dependent on androgens revert to a vellus form and balding results. *(Redrawn from, 2005, with permission.)*

responses in individual patients. Alternatively, many specialists choose to classify hirsutism more generally as mild, moderate, or severe depending on the location and density of hair growth.

Ethnicity. The concentration of hair follicles per unit area does not differ between men and women, however, racial and ethnic differences do exist. Individuals of Mediterranean descent have a higher concentration of hair follicles than northern Europeans, and a much higher concentration than Asians (Speroff, 1999). For this reason, Asians with PCOS are much less likely to present with overt hirsutism than other ethnic groups. Additionally, there is also a strong familial tendency for the development of hirsutism, due to genetic differences in target tissue sensitivity to androgens and in the activity of 5α-reductase.

Acne

Acne vulgaris is a frequent clinical finding in adolescents. However, acne that is particularly persistent or of late onset should suggest PCOS (Homburg, 2004). The prevalence of acne in women with PCOS is unknown, although one study found that 50 percent of adolescents with PCOS have moderate acne (Dramusic, 1997). In addition, an elevation of androgen

levels has been reported in 80 percent of women with severe acne, 50 percent with moderate acne, and 33 percent with mild acne (Bunker, 1989). Women with moderate to severe acne have an increased prevalence (52 to 83 percent) of polycystic ovaries identified during sonographic examination (Betti, 1990; Bunker, 1989; Jebraili, 1994).

Pathogenesis of Acne. The pathogenesis of acne vulgaris involves four factors: blockage of the follicular opening by hyperkeratosis, sebum overproduction, proliferation of commensal *Propionibacterium acnes,* and inflammation (Purdy, 2006). In women with androgen excess, overstimulation of androgen receptors in the pilosebaceous unit results in increased sebum production that eventually leads to inflammation and comedone formation (see Fig. 17-3). Inflammation leads to the main long-term side effect of acne—scarring. Accordingly, treatment is directed at minimizing inflammation, decreasing keratin production, lowering colonization of *P acnes,* and reducing androgen levels to diminish sebum production (Moghetti, 2006).

As in the hair follicle, testosterone is converted within sebaceous glands to its more active metabolite, DHT, by 5α-reductase. 5α-reductase has two isoenzymes, type 1 and type 2. Of these, type 1 isoenzyme predominates in sebaceous

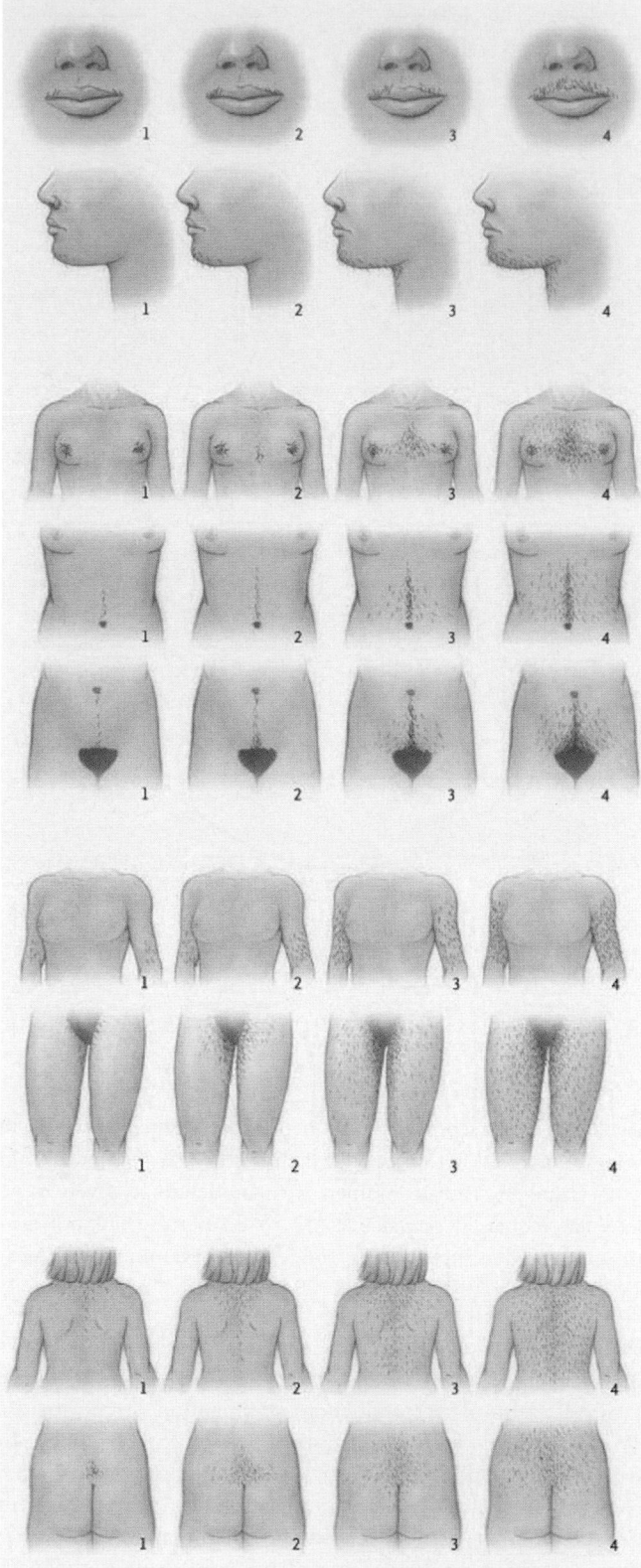

FIGURE 17-4 Depiction of the modified Ferriman-Gallwey system for scoring hirsutism.

glands. In skin types prone to acne, such as the face, the activity of type 1 isoenzyme is greater and implies that more DHT is being produced in these sebaceous glands (Thiboutot, 2004).

Alopecia

Female androgenic alopecia is a less common finding in women with PCOS. Hair loss progresses slowly and is characterized either by diffuse thinning at the crown with preservation of the frontal hairline or by bitemporal recession (Cela, 2003). Its pathogenesis involves an excess of 5α-reductase activity in the hair follicle leading to a rise in DHT levels. In addition, there is an increased expression of androgen receptors in these individuals (Chen, 2002).

Alopecia, however, may reflect other serious disease. For this reason, affected women should also be evaluated to exclude thyroid dysfunction, anemia, or other chronic illness.

Other Endocrine Dysfunction
Insulin Resistance

Although not well characterized, the association between insulin resistance, hyperandrogenism, and PCOS has long been recognized. The precise incidence of insulin resistance in women with PCOS has been difficult to discern due to lack of a simple method for determining insulin sensitivity in an office setting. Although obesity is known to exacerbate insulin resistance, one classic study demonstrated that both lean and obese women with PCOS have increased rates of insulin resistance and type 2 DM compared with weight-matched controls without PCOS (Fig. 17-5) (Dunaif, 1989, 1992).

Acanthosis Nigricans. This skin condition is characterized by thickened, gray-brown velvety plaques seen in flexure areas such as the back of the neck, the axillae, the crease beneath the breast, the waist, and the groin (Fig. 17-6) (Panidis, 1995). Thought to be a cutaneous marker of insulin resistance, acanthosis nigricans may be found in individuals with or without PCOS. Insulin resistance leads to hyperinsulinemia, which is believed to stimulate keratinocyte and dermal fibroblast growth, producing the characteristic skin changes (Cruz, 1992). Acanthosis nigricans is more often found in obese women with PCOS (50 percent incidence) than those with PCOS and normal weight (5 to 10 percent). Rarely, it is seen with genetic syndromes or malignancy of the gastrointestinal tract, such as adenocarcinoma of the stomach or pancreas (Torley, 2002).

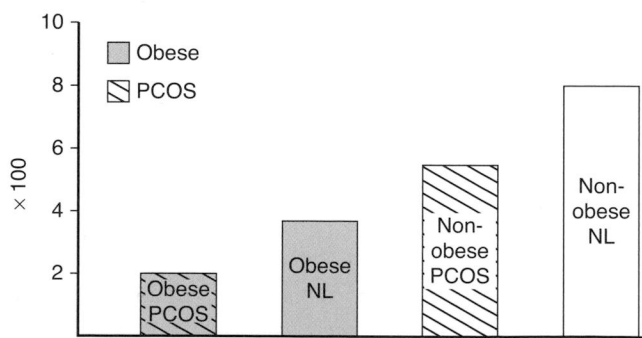

FIGURE 17-5 Insulin sensitivity is decreased in obese women with polycystic ovarian syndrome. NL = normal (those without PCOS); PCOS = polycystic ovarian syndrome. *(Adapted from Dunaif, 1989, with permission.)*

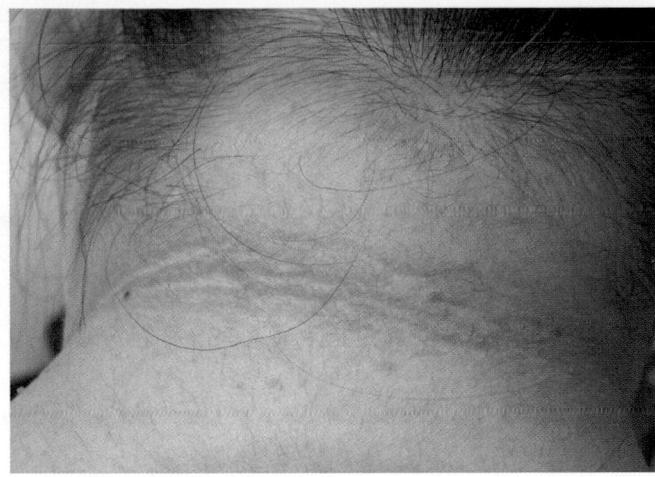

FIGURE 17-6 Photograph shows acanthosis nigricans on the back of the neck.

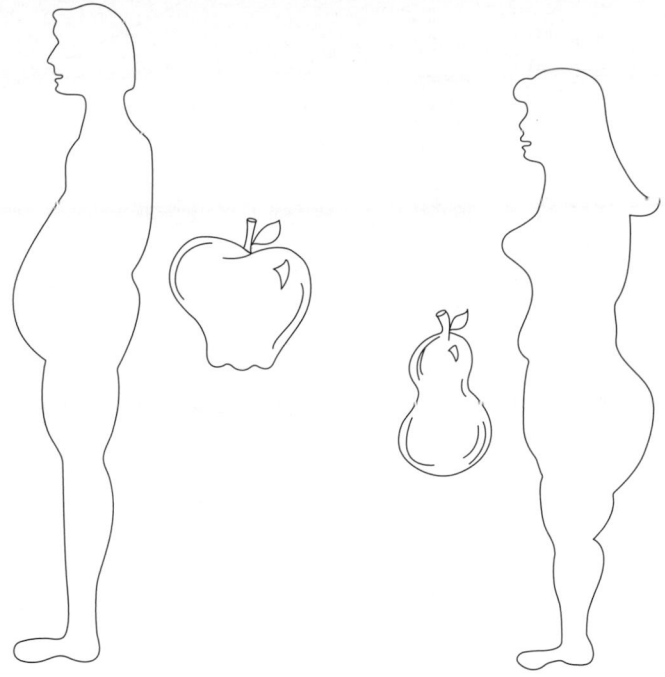

FIGURE 17-7 Obesity may present with a central distribution of body fat, also described in lay terms as an "apple-shaped" pattern. Alternatively, fat may predominate in the hips and buttocks in what is often termed a "pear-shaped" distribution.

When acanthosis nigricans is associated with malignancy, the onset is usually more abrupt, and skin involvement is more extensive (Moore, 2008).

Impaired Glucose Tolerance and Type 2 Diabetes Mellitus. Women with PCOS are at increased risk for impaired glucose tolerance (IGT) and type 2 DM. Based on oral glucose tolerance testing of obese women with PCOS, the prevalence of IGT and DM is approximately 30 percent and 7 percent, respectively (Legro, 1999). Similar findings were reported in a group of obese adolescents with PCOS (Palmert, 2002). Even after adjusting for body mass index (BMI), women with PCOS remained more likely to have DM (Lo, 2006). Specifically, β cell dysfunction that is independent of obesity has been reported in patients with PCOS (Dunaif, 1996a).

Dyslipidemia

The classic atherogenic lipoprotein profile seen in PCOS is characterized by elevated low-density lipoprotein (LDL) and triglyceride levels and total cholesterol:high-density lipoprotein (HDL) ratios, and by depressed HDL levels (Banaszewska, 2006). Independent of total cholesterol levels, these changes may increase the risk of cardiovascular disease in women with PCOS. The prevalence of dyslipidemia in PCOS approaches 70 percent (Legro, 2001; Rocha, 2011; Talbott, 1998).

Obesity

Compared with age-matched controls, women with PCOS are more likely to be obese, as reflected by elevated BMIs and waist:hip ratios (Talbott, 1995). This ratio reflects an android or central pattern of obesity, which itself is an independent risk factor for cardiovascular disease (Fig. 17-7) (Nishizawa, 2002). This pattern of increased waist circumference and thick subcapsular skinfolds has also been predictive of insulin resistance (Lee, 2010).

As noted earlier, insulin resistance is believed to play a large role in the pathogenesis of PCOS and is often exacerbated by obesity (Dunaif, 1989). Affected women show a high waist-to-hip ratios, enlarged adipocytes, reduced serum adiponectin levels, and lower lipoprotein lipase activity (Mannerås-Holm, 2011). Thus, obesity can have a synergistic effect on PCOS and can worsen ovulatory dysfunction, hyperandrogenism, and the appearance of acanthosis nigricans.

Obstructive Sleep Apnea

Obstructive sleep apnea is more common in women with PCOS and is likely related to central obesity and insulin resistance (Fogel, 2001; Vgontzas, 2001). However, some research has determined that the risk of sleep apnea is 30- to 40-fold higher in women with PCOS compared with weight-matched controls. This evidence points towards a link between obstructive sleep apnea and the metabolic and hormonal abnormalities associated with PCOS. There may be two subtypes of PCOS, that is, PCOS with or without obstructive sleep apnea. PCOS women with this condition may be at much higher risk for DM and cardiovascular disease than women with PCOS who do not have obstructive sleep apnea (Nitsche, 2010).

Metabolic Syndrome and Cardiovascular Disease

This syndrome is characterized by insulin resistance, obesity, atherogenic dyslipidemia, and hypertension. The metabolic syndrome is associated with an increased risk of cardiovascular disease (CVD) and type 2 DM (Chap. 1, p. 21) (Schneider, 2006). The prevalence of metabolic syndrome is reported to be approximately 45 percent in women with PCOS compared with 4 percent in age-adjusted controls (Fig. 17-8) (Dokras, 2005). Polycystic ovarian syndrome shares several

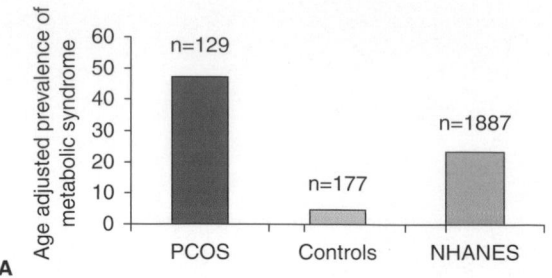

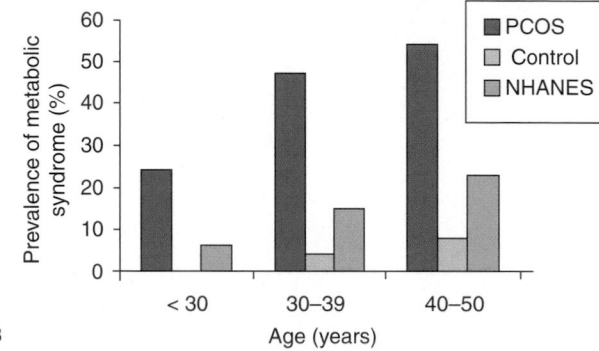

FIGURE 17-8 A. Women with polycystic ovarian syndrome (PCOS) have an increased risk of metabolic syndrome compared with age-adjusted controls and with women from NHANES III. **B.** In women with PCOS, the risk of metabolic syndrome begins earlier than in controls or those from NHANES III. The Third National Health and Nutrition Survey (NHANES III) collected data from a representative sample of the noninstitutionalized civilian U.S. population from 1988 through 1994 (Ford, 2002). *(From Dokras, 2005, with permission.)*

endocrine features with the metabolic syndrome, although definitive evidence for an increased incidence of CVD in women with PCOS is lacking (Legro, 1999; Rebuffe-Scrive, 1989; Talbott, 1998). However, in a small group of women with PCOS, Dahlgren and colleagues (1992) predicted a relative risk of myocardial infarction of 7.4. Another 10-year surveillance study showed an odds ratio of 5.91 for CVD in overweight Caucasian women with PCOS (Talbott, 1995). Thus, evidence suggests that women with PCOS should have CVD factors identified and treated (Table 1-17, p. 22) (Mosca, 2011).

In addition to components of the metabolic syndrome, other markers of subclinical disease link PCOS and CVD. Women with PCOS have been found to have a greater incidence of left ventricular diastolic dysfunction and increased internal and external carotid artery stiffness (Lakhani, 2000; Tiras, 1999). Moreover, in affected women, several studies have found greater endothelial dysfunction, which is described as an early event in the evolution of atherosclerosis (Diamanti-Kandarakis, 1999; Orio, 2004; Paradisi, 2003; Tarkun, 2004).

Endometrial Neoplasia

In women with PCOS, a threefold increased risk of endometrial cancer has been reported. Endometrial hyperplasia and endometrial cancer are long-term risks of chronic anovulation,

and neoplastic changes in the endometrium are felt to arise from chronic unopposed estrogen (Chap. 33, p. 817) (Coulam, 1983). Moreover, the effects of hyperandrogenism and hyperinsulinemia to lower SHBG levels and increase circulating estrogen levels may add to this risk.

Few women who develop endometrial cancer are younger than 40 years, and most of these premenopausal women are obese or have chronic anovulation or both (Peterson, 1968; Rose, 1996). Thus, the American College of Obstetricians and Gynecologists (2000) recommends endometrial assessment in any woman older than 35 years with abnormal bleeding, and in those younger than 35 years who are suspected of having anovulatory uterine bleeding refractory to medical management (Chap. 8, p. 225).

Infertility

Infertility or subfertility is a frequent complaint in women with PCOS and results from anovulatory cycles. Moreover, in women with infertility secondary to anovulation, PCOS is the most common cause and accounts for 80 to 90 percent of cases (Adams, 1986; Hull, 1987). Infertility evaluation and treatment in women with PCOS is described in more detail in Chapter 20 (p. 530).

Pregnancy Loss

Women with PCOS who become pregnant are known to experience an increased rate (30 to 50 percent) of early miscarriage compared with a baseline rate of approximately 15 percent in the general population (Homburg, 1998b; Regan, 1990; Sagle, 1988). The etiology of early miscarriage in women with PCOS is unclear. Initially, retrospective and observational studies showed an association between LH hypersecretion and miscarriage (Homburg, 1998a; Howles, 1987). However, one prospective study showed that lowering LH levels with GnRH agonists failed to show a benefit from this therapy (Clifford, 1997).

Others have suggested that insulin resistance is related to miscarriage in these women. To lower loss rates, an insulin level lowering drug, metformin (Glucophage), has been investigated. Metformin, a biguanide, lowers serum insulin levels by reducing hepatic glucose production and increasing the sensitivity of liver, muscle, fat, and other tissues to the uptake and effects of insulin.

Several retrospective studies have indicated that women with PCOS taking metformin during pregnancy have a lower incidence of miscarriage (Glueck, 2001; Jakubowicz, 2002). In addition, a prospective study demonstrated a lower miscarriage rate for women conceiving while taking metformin compared with those using clomiphene citrate (Palomba, 2005). However, a metaanalysis of 17 studies failed to show an effect of metformin administration on miscarriage risk in women with PCOS (Palomba, 2009). Until further randomized controlled trials are performed studying the effects of metformin (a category B drug) on pregnancy outcome, the use of this medication in gestation for miscarriage prevention is not recommended.

Complications in Pregnancy

Several pregnancy and neonatal complications have been associated with PCOS. One large metaanalysis found women with PCOS to have a two- to threefold higher risk of gestational diabetes, pregnancy-induced hypertension, preterm birth, and perinatal mortality, unrelated to multifetal gestations (Boomsma, 2006). Metformin has been studied as a tool to mitigate these complications. However, investigators in one study found that metformin treatment during pregnancy did not reduce rates of these complications (Vanky, 2010).

Many women with PCOS require the use of ovulation induction medications or in vitro fertilization to conceive. These practices substantially increase the risk of multifetal gestations, which are associated with increased rates of maternal and neonatal complications (Chap. 20, p. 538).

Psychologic Health

Women with PCOS may present with various psychosocial problems such as anxiety, depression, low self-esteem, reduced quality of life, and negative body image (Deeks,

2010; Himelein, 2006). If depression is suspected, a screening tool such as the one found in Table 13-5 (p. 360) may be implemented.

DIAGNOSIS

Polycystic ovarian syndrome is often referred to as a diagnosis of exclusion. Thus, routine exclusion of other potentially serious disorders that may clinically appear similar to PCOS is warranted (Table 17-4). For women who present with complaints of hirsutism, the algorithm in Figure 17-9 can be used.

Thyroid-Stimulating Hormone and Prolactin

Thyroid disease may frequently lead to menstrual dysfunction similar to that seen in women with PCOS (Chap. 8, p. 234). Accordingly, a serum TSH level is typically measured during evaluation.

Similarly, hyperprolactinemia is a well-known cause of menstrual irregularities and occasionally amenorrhea. Elevated

---

TABLE 17-4. Differential Diagnoses of Ovulatory Dysfunction and Hyperandrogenism

	Laboratory Testing	Indicative Results[a]
Causes of oligo- or anovulation		
PCOS	Total T level	Usually increased
	DHEAS level	May be mildly increased
	LH:FSH ratio	Typically >2:1
Hyperthyroidism	TSH level	Decreased
Hypothyroidism	TSH level	Increased
Hyperprolactinemia	PRL level	Increased
Hypogonadotropic hypogonadism	FSH, LH, E_2 levels	All decreased
POF	FSH, LH levels	Increased
	E_2 levels	Decreased
Causes of hyperandrogenism		
PCOS		
Late-onset CAH	17-OH-P level	>200 ng/dL
Androgen-secreting ovarian tumor	Total T level	>200 ng/dL
Androgen-secreting adrenal tumor	DHEAS level	>700 µg/dL
Cushing syndrome	Cortisol level	Increased
Exogenous androgen use	Toxicology screen	Increased
Summary of testing in those suspected of PCOS		
Serum levels of FSH, LH, TSH, Total T, PRL, DHEAS, 17-OH-P		
2hr-GTT		
Lipid profile		
Measurement of BMI, waist circumference, BP		

[a]Based on reference laboratory ranges of normal.
BMI = body mass index; BP = blood pressure; CAH = congenital adrenal hyperplasia; DHEAS = dehydroepiandrosterone sulfate; E_2 = estradiol; FSH = follicle-stimulating hormone; GTT = glucose tolerance test; LH = luteinizing hormone; 17-OH-P = 17-hydroxyprogesterone; PCOS = polycystic ovarian syndrome; POF = premature ovarian failure; PRL = prolactin; T = testosterone; TSH = thyroid-stimulating hormone.

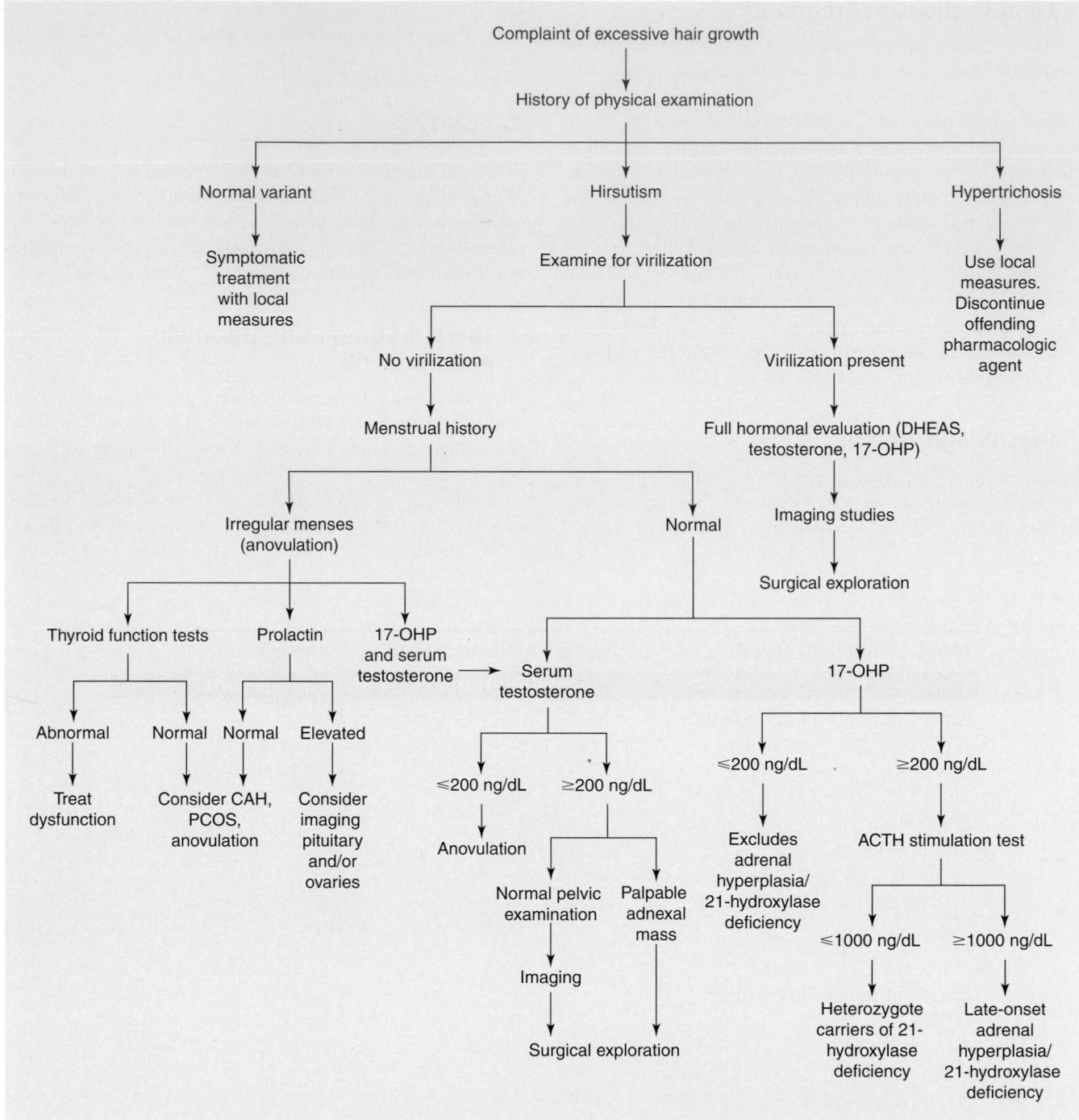

FIGURE 17-9 Algorithm for diagnosis of polycystic ovarian syndrome. ACTH = adrenocorticotropin hormone; CAH = congenital adrenal hyperplasia; DHEAS = dehydroepiandrosterone sulfate; PCOS = polycystic ovarian syndrome; 17-OHP = 17-hydroxyprogesterone. *(From Hunter, 2003, with permission.)*

prolactin levels lead to anovulation through inhibition of GnRH pulsatile secretion from the hypothalamus. A list of potential causes of hyperprolactinemia and treatments are found in Chapter 15 (p. 417).

Testosterone

Tumors of the ovary or adrenal are a rare but serious cause of androgen excess. A variety of ovarian neoplasms, both benign and malignant, may produce testosterone and lead to viriliza-

tion. Among others, these include the sex cord-stromal tumors (Chap. 36, p. 879). Importantly, women with an abrupt onset, typically within several months, or sudden worsening of virilizing signs should prompt concern for a hormone-producing ovarian or adrenal tumor. Symptoms may include deepening of the voice, frontal balding, severe acne or hirsutism or both, increased muscle mass, and clitoromegaly (Table 17-5 and Fig. 17-10).

Diagnostically, serum testosterone levels may be used to exclude ovarian tumors. Free testosterone levels are more

TABLE 17-5. Clinical Features of Virilization

Acne
Hirsutism
Amenorrhea
Clitoromegaly
Androgenic alopecia
Decreased breast size
Deepening of the voice
Increased muscle mass

sensitive than total testosterone levels as an indicator of hyperandrogenism. However, although improving, current free testosterone assays lack a uniform laboratory standard (Miller, 2004). For this reason, total testosterone levels remain the best approach for excluding a tumor. Threshold values beyond 200 ng/dL of total testosterone warrant evaluation for an ovarian lesion (Derksen, 1994).

Pelvic sonography is the preferred method to exclude an ovarian neoplasm in a female with very high androgen levels. Alternatively, computed tomography (CT) or magnetic resonance (MR) imaging may also be used in this setting.

Dehydroepiandrosterone Sulfate

Dehydroepiandrosterone sulfate is produced essentially exclusively by the adrenal gland. Therefore, serum DHEAS levels above 700 µg/dL are highly suggestive for the presence of an adrenal neoplasm. Adrenal imaging with abdominal CT or MR

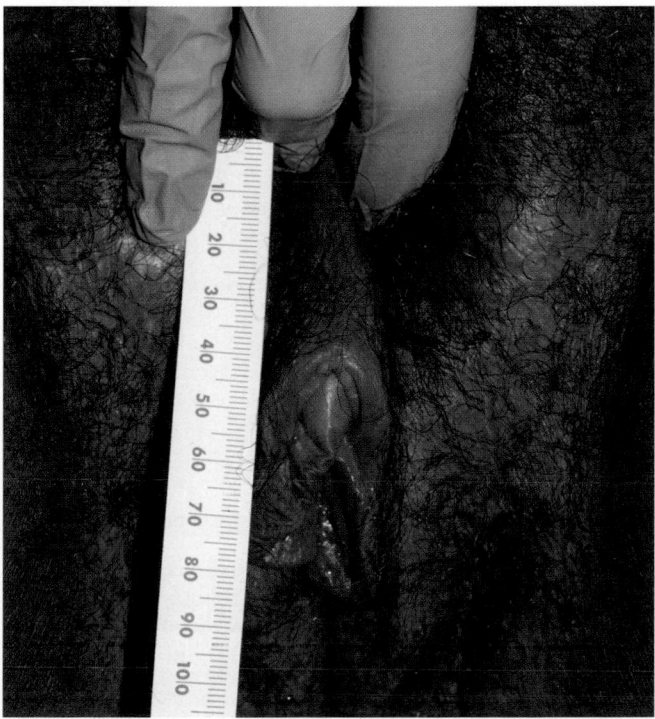

FIGURE 17-10 Virilization manifest by clitoromegaly. The normal adult clitoris is generally 1 to 1.5 cm long and 0.5 cm wide in the nonerect state. *(Photograph contributed by Dr. Ben Li.)*

imaging is indicated for any patient with DHEAS levels that exceed this value.

Gonadotropins

During evaluation of amenorrhea, FSH and LH levels are typically measured to exclude premature ovarian failure and hypogonadotropic hypogonadism (see Table 17-4). Past this, however, LH and FSH levels have little additive value to the diagnosis of PCOS. Although classically LH levels measure at least twofold higher than FSH levels, this is not found in all women with PCOS. Specifically, one third of women with PCOS have circulating LH levels in the normal range, a finding more common in obese patients (Arroyo, 1997; Taylor, 1997). Moreover, serum LH levels are affected by sample timing within a menstrual cycle, use of oral contraceptive pills, and BMI.

17α-Hydroxyprogesterone

The term *congenital adrenal hyperplasia* (CAH) describes several autosomal recessive disorders that result from complete or partial deficiency of an enzyme involved in cortisol and aldosterone synthesis, usually 21-hydroxylase or less frequently 11-hydroxylase (Fig. 15-5, p. 403). Symptoms of CAH and their severity are varied. It may present in the neonate with ambiguous genitalia and life-threatening hypotension (Chap. 18, p. 488). Alternatively, symptoms may be milder and delayed until adolescence or adulthood.

In this late-onset form of CAH, the enzyme deficiency leads to a relative cortisol deficiency. In response, adrenocorticotropic hormone (ACTH) levels are increased to normalize cortisol production. Adrenal hyperplasia and elevated androgens results as a consequence of this accommodation. Thus, symptoms of late-onset CAH reflect accumulation of precursor C_{19} steroid hormones. These precursors are converted to dehydroepiandrosterone, androstenedione, and testosterone. Thus, signs of virilization predominate.

With late-onset CAH, the most commonly affected enzyme is 21-hydroxylase, and deficiency leads to accumulation of its substrate, 17-hydroxyprogesterone. Serum values are drawn in the morning from a fasting patient. Threshold values of 17-hydroxyprogesterone that measure more than 200 ng/dL should prompt an ACTH stimulation test. With this test, synthetic ACTH, 250 µg, is injected intravenously, and a serum 17-hydroxyprogesterone level is measured 1 hour later.

To explain this test, the ACTH given during testing stimulates uptake of cholesterol and synthesis of pregnenolone. If 21-hydroxylase activity is ineffective, steroid precursors up to and including progesterone, 17-hydroxypregnenolone, and especially 17-hydroxyprogesterone accumulate in the adrenal cortex and in circulating blood. Thus, in affected individuals, serum levels of 17-hydroxyprogesterone can reach many times their normal concentrations. Levels above 1000 ng/dL are indicative of late-onset CAH.

Cortisol

Cushing syndrome results from prolonged exposure to elevated levels of either endogenous or exogenous glucocorticoids. Of these, the syndrome is most frequently caused by administration of exogenous glucocorticoids. Alternatively, the term *Cushing disease* is reserved for cases of Cushing syndrome in which the constellation of symptoms stem from increased secretion of ACTH by a pituitary tumor. Individuals with Cushing syndrome may present with many symptoms suggestive of PCOS such as menstrual dysfunction, acne or hirsutism, truncal obesity, dyslipidemia, and glucose intolerance. Classically, moon facies and abdominal purple striae are also noted. Cushing syndrome is rare. Accordingly, routine screening in all women with oligomenorrhea is not indicated. However, in those with moon facies, abdominal striae, central fat distribution, proximal muscle weakness, and easy bruising, screening should be strongly considered (Nieman, 2008).

Initial laboratory testing is directed at confirming excessive glucocorticoid production. Analysis of a 24-hour urine collection for urinary free cortisol excretion is the preferred initial test. Normal values are less than 90 μg per 24 hours, and those in excess of 300 μg per day are considered diagnostic for Cushing syndrome (Kirk, 2000; Meier, 1997). Alternatively, a dexamethasone suppression test may be selected to avoid the difficulty of obtaining a 24-hour urine collection in some women. This, however, has a higher false-positive rate. With the suppression test, 1 mg of dexamethasone is taken orally at 11 PM, and a plasma cortisol level is measured at 8 AM the following morning. In women with a normally functioning feedback loop, administration of the corticosteroid dexamethasone should lower ACTH secretion and thus diminish adrenal cortex production of cortisol. Normal testing values are below 5 μg/dL (Crapo, 1979). However, if a woman has an exogenous or an ectopic endogenous source of cortisol, then cortisol levels during suppression testing will remain elevated. Treatment of Cushing syndrome depends on the underlying source of excess glucocorticosteroids.

Measurements of Insulin Resistance and Dyslipidemia

Many women with PCOS have insulin resistance and compensatory hyperinsulinemia. Although the consensus meeting in Rotterdam suggested that tests of insulin resistance are *not* required to diagnose or treat PCOS, these tests are often used to evaluate glucose metabolism and impaired insulin secretion in these women (The Rotterdam ESHRE/ASRM-Sponsored PCOS Consensus Workshop Group, 2004).

The gold standard for evaluating insulin resistance has been the hyperinsulinemic euglycemic clamp. Unfortunately, this test as well as the intravenous glucose tolerance test (IV GTT) requires an intravenous line and frequent sampling, are labor and time intensive, and are not practical in a clinical setting. Accordingly, other less sensitive surrogate markers that evaluate insulin resistance are used and include: (1) 2-hour glucose tolerance test (2-hr GTT), (2) fasting serum insulin level, (3) homeostasis model assessment of insulin resistance (HOMA IR), (4) quantitative insulin sensitivity check (QUICKI), and (5) calculation of serum glucose:insulin ratios.

Of these, a 2-hr GTT is frequently used to exclude IGT and type 2 DM. This test is particularly important in obese PCOS patients who are at higher risk for both (Table 17-6). Over time, women with PCOS demonstrate a worsening of IGT, with a reported conversion rate of approximately 2 percent per year to type 2 DM. Importantly, measurements of fasting glucose and glycohemoglobin levels will not detect early worsening of insulin resistance and glucose intolerance. This affirms the importance of periodic assessment of glucose tolerance with a 2-hr GTT in this population (Legro, 1999, 2005). In their position statement, the AE-PCOS (Salley, 2007) recommends 2-hr GTT testing for individuals with PCOS. Those with normal glucose tolerance are rescreened at least once every 2 years or more frequently if additional risks exist. Those with impaired glucose tolerance are tested annually. As an alternative, Hurd and associates (2011) found HbA1c testing to also be a suitable screen for DM. Normal and abnormal test result ranges are found in Table 1-16 (p. 21).

In addition to assessment of insulin resistance, a fasting lipid profile is used to evaluate dyslipidemia. Evaluation and treatment of dyslipidemia is further described in Chapter 1 (p. 23).

Endometrial Biopsy

An endometrial biopsy is recommended in women older than age 35 with abnormal bleeding and in younger women with anovulatory bleeding refractory to hormonal treatment. Steps of this procedure are found in Chapter 8 (p. 225).

Sonography

Histologically, a polycystic ovary (PCO) displays increases in volume, number of ripening and atretic follicles, cortical stromal thickness, and number of hilar cell nests

TABLE 17-6. Diagnosis of Impaired Glucose Tolerance and Diabetes Mellitus

	Normal Range	Impaired Glucose Tolerance	Diabetes Mellitus
Fasting blood glucose level	<100 mg/dL	100–125 mg/dL	≥126 mg/dL
2-hr GTT	<140 mg/dL	140–199 mg/dL	≥200 mg/dL

2-hr GTT = 2-hour oral glucose tolerance test.
From American Diabetes Association, 2010.

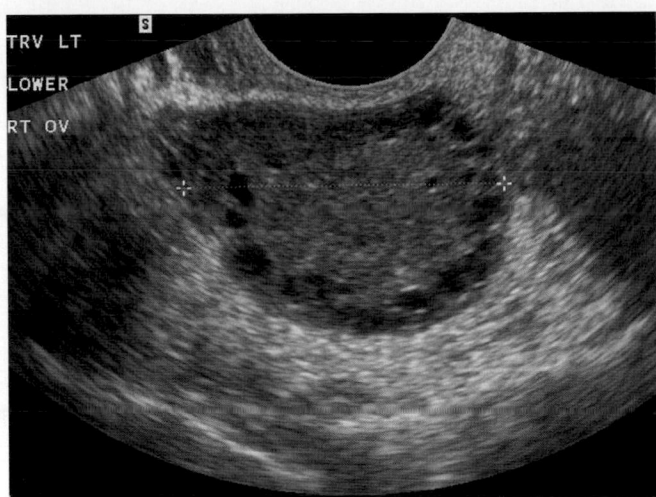

FIGURE 17-11 Transvaginal sonography displays multiple small hypoechoic cysts. *(Image contributed by Dr. Elysia Moschos.)*

(Hughesdon, 1982). Many of these tissue changes can be seen sonographically, and pelvic sonography is commonly used to evaluate the ovaries in women with suspected PCOS. Sonography is particularly important for women with PCOS seeking fertility and in women with signs of virilization. A high-definition transvaginal approach is superior and has a higher detection rate of PCO than the transabdominal route. However, a transabdominal route is preferred for virginal adolescents.

Sonographic criteria for polycystic ovaries from the 2003 Rotterdam conference include ≥12 small cysts (2 to 9 mm in diameter) or an increased ovarian volume (>10 mL) or both (Fig. 17-11). Often there is an increased amount of stroma relative to the number of follicles (Balen, 2003). Only one ovary with these findings is sufficient to define PCOS. However, criteria do not apply to women taking combination oral contraceptive pills (The Rotterdam ESHRE/ASRM-Sponsored PCOS Consensus Workshop Group, 2004).

In contrast, other findings are not valuable diagnostically. For example, the typical "black pearl necklace" appearance, in which follicles are distributed just underneath the capsule in a row, and the perceived increase in stromal echogenicity have been eliminated as diagnostic criteria. Moreover, a polycystic ovary should not be confused with a multicystic ovary, which is normal size, contains six or more follicles without peripheral displacement, and lacks an increase in central stromal volume.

Remarkably, studies using sonography have shown that at least 23 percent of young women have ovaries that exhibit PCO morphology, yet many of these women have no other symptoms of PCOS (Clayton, 1992; Polson, 1988). In addition, a polycystic appearance of the ovaries can often be found in other conditions of androgen excess, such as congenital adrenal hyperplasia, Cushing syndrome, and exogenous use of androgenic medications. For this reason, PCO morphology found during sonographic examination is not used solely to make the diagnosis of PCOS.

Diagnosis of PCOS in Adolescence

Several independent *prepubertal* risk factors for PCOS have been identified. These include above average or low birthweight for gestational age, premature adrenarche, atypical sexual precocity, and obesity with acanthosis nigricans (Rosenfield, 2007). That said, diagnosing PCOS in adolescence is difficult due to the fact that adolescents frequently have irregular menses for 2 to 4 years after menarche, and acne is common. Moreover, in adolescence, transabdominal rather than transvaginal pelvic sonography is generally performed, and image resolution is poorer. In adolescents with incomplete criteria for a firm diagnosis of PCOS, careful surveillance is warranted as they may be diagnosed at a later time (Carmina, 2010).

TREATMENT

The choice of treatment for each symptom of PCOS depends on a woman's goals and the severity of endocrine dysfunction. Thus, anovulatory women desiring pregnancy will undergo significantly different treatment than adolescents with menstrual irregularity and acne. Patients often seek treatment for a singular complaint and may see various specialists from dermatologists, nutritionists, aestheticians, and endocrinologists prior to evaluation by a gynecologist.

Observation

Women with PCOS who have fairly regular cycle intervals (8 to 12 menses per year) and have mild hyperandrogenism may choose not to be treated. In these women, however, periodic screening for dyslipidemia and diabetes mellitus is prudent.

Weight Loss

For obese women with PCOS, lifestyle changes focused on diet and exercise are paramount to treatment at each stage of life. Even a modest amount of weight loss (5 percent of body weight) can result in restoration of normal ovulatory cycles in some women. This improvement results from reductions in insulin and androgen levels, the latter mediated through increases in SHBG levels (Huber-Buchholz, 1999; Kiddy, 1992; Pasquali, 1989).

The optimal diet that best improves insulin sensitivity is not known. Diets high in carbohydrates increase insulin secretion rates, whereas diets high in protein and fat lower those rates (Bass, 1993; Nuttall, 1985). However, very-high-protein diets are concerning with respect to stresses on kidney function. Moreover, they afford only short-term weight loss initially with lesser benefits over time (Legro, 1999; Skov, 1999). Thus, it appears that a well-balanced hypocaloric diet offers the most benefit in treating obese women with PCOS.

Exercise

Exercise is known to have a beneficial effect in treating patients with type 2 DM (Nestler, 1998). The most dramatic effect of lifestyle intervention was published in 2002 as the Diabetes Prevention Program. Women and men at risk for diabetes were asked to lose at least 7 percent of their weight and to exercise for 150 minutes each week. This group had a twofold greater benefit in delaying the onset of diabetes compared with a group given metformin alone. Both groups fared better than a placebo group (Knowler, 2002). Few studies, however, have looked specifically at the effect of exercise on insulin action and reproductive function in women with PCOS (Jaatinen, 1993; Nybacka, 2011). In addition to DM, women with PCOS may have comorbid risk factors for CVD. In patients with PCOS, exercise has been shown to improve cardiovascular capacity (Vigorito, 2007).

■ Treatment of Oligoovulation and Anovulation

Women with oligoovulation or anovulation typically have fewer than eight menses per year, often skip menses for several months at a time, or simply have amenorrhea. Flow may be scanty or may be very long and heavy, resulting in anemia.

Combination Oral Contraceptive Pills

A first-line treatment for menstrual irregularities is combination oral contraceptive pills (COCs), which will induce regular menstrual cycles. In addition, COCs reduce androgen levels. Specifically, COCs suppress gonadotropin release, which results in decreased ovarian androgen production. Moreover, the estrogen component increases SHBG levels. Lastly, the progestin component antagonizes the endometrial proliferative effect of estrogen, thus reducing risks of endometrial hyperplasia due to unopposed estrogen.

Theoretically, COCs that contain progestins with fewer androgenic properties are preferred. Such progestins include norethindrone; a third-generation progestin, such as norgestimate or desogestrel; or the newer progestin drospirenone. However, no COC pill has shown superiority compared with another in reducing hirsutism (Sobbrio, 1990). Alternative combination hormonal contraceptive options include the contraceptive patch and vaginal ring (Chap. 5, p. 152).

In initiating therapy, if a woman's last menses was more than 4 weeks prior, a pregnancy test is indicated. If negative, progesterone is given to produce a withdrawal bleed prior to COC initiation. Typical regimens include: medroxyprogesterone acetate (MPA) (Provera), 10 mg orally daily for 10 days; MPA, 10 mg orally twice daily for 5 days; or micronized progesterone (Prometrium), 200 mg orally daily for 10 days. Patients are counseled that bleeding is expected to begin after completion of the progestin course.

Cyclic Progestogens

In patients who are not candidates for combination hormonal contraception, progesterone withdrawal is recommended every 1 to 3 months. Examples of regimens used include: MPA, 5 to 10 mg orally daily day for 12 days, or micronized progesterone, 200 mg orally each evening for 12 days. Patients should be counseled that intermittent progestins will not reduce symptoms of acne or hirsutism, nor will they provide contraception.

Insulin Sensitizing Agents

Although the use of insulin sensitizers in PCOS has not been approved by the Food and Drug Administration (FDA), they have been found to be increasingly beneficial for both metabolic and gynecologic issues. Of these agents, metformin is the most commonly prescribed, particularly in women with impaired glucose tolerance and insulin resistance. This drug improves peripheral insulin sensitivity by reducing hepatic glucose production and increasing target tissue sensitivity to insulin. Metformin decreases androgen levels in both lean and obese women, leading to increased rates of spontaneous ovulation (Batukan, 2001; Essah, 2006; Haas, 2003).

A number of studies have demonstrated that up to 40 percent of anovulatory women with PCOS will ovulate, and many will achieve pregnancy with metformin alone (Fleming, 2002; Neveu, 2007). Metformin is a category B drug and is safe to use as an ovulatory induction agent. As such, it may be used alone or in concert with other medications such as clomiphene citrate (Chap. 20, p. 533). Specifically, metformin has been shown to increase the ovulatory response to clomiphene citrate in patients who were previously clomiphene resistant (Nestler, 1998). Despite these positive findings regarding metformin and ovulation induction, in a randomized prospective study of 626 women, Legro and colleagues (2007) found higher live-birth rates with clomiphene citrate alone (22 percent) than with metformin alone (7 percent).

A rare adverse side effect of metformin is lactic acidosis, which is almost exclusively found in patients with renal insufficiency, liver disease, or congestive heart failure. More common side effects are gastrointestinal, and these can be minimized by starting at a low dose and gradually increasing the dose over several weeks to an optimal level. In clinical studies, 1500 to 2000 mg in divided doses daily with meals is typically used.

The thiazolidinediones, also known as glitazones, are another class of medications used for patients with diabetes mellitus and include rosiglitazone (Avandia) and pioglitazone (Actos). These agents bind to insulin receptors on cells throughout the body, causing them to become more responsive to insulin and thereby lowering serum glucose and insulin levels. Similar to metformin, rosiglitazone and pioglitazone have been shown to improve ovulation in some patients (Azziz, 2001; Dunaif, 1996b; Ehrmann, 1997). However, the glitazones are category C drugs and thus should be used as ovulation induction agents in rare cases and discontinued once pregnancy is achieved.

■ Hirsutism

In the treatment of hirsutism, a primary goal is lowering androgen levels to halt further conversion of vellus hairs to terminal ones. However, medical therapies will not eliminate abnormal hair growth already present. Moreover, treatments may require 6 to 12 months before clinical improvement is apparent. For this reason, clinicians should be familiar with temporary hair removal methods that may be used in the interim. Permanent cosmetic therapies may then be implemented once medications have reached maximal therapeutic effect.

Combination Oral Contraceptives

As described earlier, COCs are effective in establishing regular menses and lowering ovarian androgen production. As an additional effect, the estrogen component of these pills leads to increased SHBG levels. With higher SHBG levels, a greater amount of free testosterone is bound and thus becomes biologically unavailable at the hair follicle.

Gonadotropin-Releasing Hormone Agonists

As described in Chapter 9 (p. 255), GnRH agonists effectively lower gonadotropin levels over time and in turn subsequently lower androgen levels. Despite their effectiveness in treating hirsutism, administration of these agents is not a preferred long-term treatment method due to associated bone loss, high cost, and menopausal side effects.

Eflornithine Hydrochloride

This antimetabolite topical cream is applied twice daily to areas of facial hirsutism and is an irreversible inhibitor of ornithine decarboxylase. This enzyme is necessary for hair follicle cell division and function, and its inhibition results in slower hair growth. It does not permanently remove hair, and thus women are required to continue routine methods of hair removal while using this medicine.

Clinical results from eflornithine hydrochloride (Vaniqa) may require 4 to 8 weeks of use. However, clinical trials have shown that approximately one third of patients have marked improvement after 24 weeks of eflornithine use compared with placebo, and 58 percent showed some overall improvement in hirsutism scores (Balfour, 2001).

Androgen-Receptor Antagonists

Antiandrogens are competitive inhibitors of androgen binding to the androgen receptor. Although these agents are effective in the treatment of hirsutism, they carry a risk for several side effects. Metrorrhagia may frequently develop. In addition, as antiandrogens, these drugs bear a theoretical risk of pseudohermaphroditism in male fetuses of women using such medications in early pregnancy. Accordingly, these drugs are commonly used in conjunction with oral contraceptive pills, which prompt regular menses and provide effective contraception.

None of the antiandrogen agents are approved by the FDA for treatment of hyperandrogenism and thus are used off-label. Spironolactone (Aldactone), in a dosage of 50 to 100 mg orally twice daily, is the primary antiandrogen used currently in the United States. In addition to its antiandrogen effects, this drug also affects hair conversion from vellous to terminal by its direct inhibition of 5α-reductase. Spironolactone is also a potassium-sparing diuretic. As such, it should not be prescribed for chronic use in combination with agents that can also raise blood potassium levels, such as potassium supplements, angiotensin-converting enzyme (ACE) inhibitors, nonsteroidal antiinflammatory drugs such as indomethacin, or other potassium-sparing diuretics.

In Europe, Canada, and Mexico, the preferred antiandrogen is cyproterone acetate, usually marketed in an oral contraceptive pill. However, this agent is not approved by the FDA (Van der Spuy, 2003). Flutamide is another nonsteroidal antiandrogen marketed for the treatment of prostate cancer, but is rarely used for hirsutism due to its potential hepatotoxicity.

5α-Reductase Inhibitors

Conversion of testosterone to DHT may be effectively decreased by the 5α-reductase inhibitor finasteride. This drug is available as a 5-mg tablet for prostate cancer (Proscar) and a 1-mg tablet for the treatment of male alopecia (Propecia). Most studies have used 5-mg daily doses and have found finasteride to be modestly effective in the treatment of hirsutism (Fruzzetti, 1994; Moghetti, 1994)

Side effects are low with finasteride, although decreased libido has been noted. However, as with other antiandrogens, the risk of male fetal teratogenicity is present, and effective contraception must be used concurrently.

Hair Removal

Hirsutism is often treated by mechanical means, and these include both depilation and epilation techniques. In addition to hair removal, lightening hair color with bleach is an additional cosmetic option.

Depilation. Depilation describes hair removal above the skin surface. Shaving is the most common form and does not exacerbate hirsutism, contrary to the myth that it will increase hair follicle density. Alternatively, topical chemical depilatories are also effective. Available in gel, cream, lotion, aerosol, and roll-on forms, these agents contain calcium thioglycolate. This agent breaks disulfide bonds between hair protein chains, causing hair to break down and separate easily from the skin surface.

Epilation

Mechanical Removal. In contrast to depilation, epilation removes the entire hair shaft and root and includes techniques such as plucking, waxing, threading, electrolysis, and laser treatment. Threading, also known as *khite* in Arabic, is a fast method for removing entire hairs and is commonly used in the Middle East and India. Hairs are snared within an outstretched strand of twisted cotton thread and pulled out.

Thermal Destruction. Although waxing and plucking allow effective temporary hair removal, permanent epilation may be achieved with thermal destruction of the hair follicle. Electrolysis, performed by a trained individual, involves placement of a fine electrode and passage of electric current to destroy individual follicles. It requires repetitive treatments over several weeks to months, can be painful, and may result in scarring.

Alternatively, laser therapy uses specific laser wavelengths to permanently destroy follicles. During this process, termed *selective photothermolysis,* only target tissues absorb laser light and are heated. Surrounding tissues fail to absorb the selective wavelength and receive minimal thermal damage. For this reason, light skinned women with dark hairs are better candidates for laser treatment due to the selective wavelength absorption by their hair.

TABLE 17-7. Algorithm of Acne Treatment

	First-Line Therapy	Therapy Alternatives for Female Patients	Maintenance Therapy
Mild			
Comedonal	T. retinoid	Salicylic acid	T. retinoid ± BPO or BPO/AB
Papular/Pustular	T. retinoid + BPO or BPO/AB		
Moderate			
Papular/pustular	T. retinoid + oral antibiotic + BPO or BPO/AB	COCs + T. retinoid ± BPO or BPO/AB	T. retinoid ± BPO or BPO/AB
Nodular	T. retinoid + oral antibiotic ± BPO or BPO/AB	COCs + T. retinoid ± BPO or BPO/AB	
Severe nodular	Oral isotretinoin	COCs + oral antibiotic + T. retinoid ± BPO or BPO/AB	T. retinoid ± BPO or BPO/AB

AB = topical antibiotic; BPO = benzoyl peroxide; BPO/AB = benzoyl peroxide and topical antibiotic combination agent; COCs = combination oral contraceptives; T. retinoid = topical retinoid. See Table 17-8 for specific agents. Modified from Zaenglein, 2006, with permission.

Advantageously, laser treatment can cover a wider surface area than electrolysis and therefore requires fewer treatments. It causes less pain, but is expensive and can result in dyspigmentation.

Prior to any epilation technique, topical anesthetics may be prescribed. Specifically, a topical cream combination of 2.5-percent lidocaine and 2.5-percent prilocaine (EMLA cream 5%) can be applied as a thick layer that remains for 2 hours under an occlusive dressing and is removed just prior to epilation. Recommended adult dosing is 1.5 to 2 g for each 10 cm² area of skin treated.

Acne

One part of acne treatment is similar to that for hirsutism and involves lowering of androgen levels. Therapy may include: (1) combination oral contraceptive pills; (2) antiandrogens such as spironolactone or flutamide, which inhibit binding of androgen to its receptor; or (3) 5α-reductase inhibitors such as finasteride. In addition to lowering androgen levels, other therapies may be added. For this reason, women with moderate to severe acne may benefit from consultation with a dermatologist (Table 17-7).

Topical Retinoids

Derived from vitamin A, topical retinoids regulate the follicular keratinocyte and normalize its desquamation. In addition, this group of agents also has direct antiinflammatory properties and thereby targets two factors linked to acne vulgaris (Zaenglein, 2006). The most commonly used agent with retinoid activity is tretinoin (Table 17-8). Adapalene and tazarotene have also been shown to be effective (Gold, 2006; Leyden, 2006). Initially, a pea-sized dab sufficient to cover the entire face is applied every third night and progressively increased as tolerated to nightly application (Krowchuk, 2005). Tretinoin may cause a transient worsening of acne during the first weeks of treatment.

Concerning teratogenicity, tretinoin and adapalene are category C drugs and thus are not recommended for use during pregnancy or breastfeeding. However, epidemiologic studies currently do not support a link between topical retinoids and birth defects (Jick, 1993; Loureiro, 2005). Tazarotene is category X and similarly is not used during these times or without highly effective contraception.

Topical Benzoyl Peroxide

Benzoyl peroxide is an excellent antimicrobial and antiinflammatory agent. It is the active ingredient in many over-the-counter products used for acne. Some prescription products also combine benzoyl peroxide with antibiotics such as clindamycin or erythromycin (see Table 17-8).

Topical and Systemic Antibiotics

Topical antibiotics typically include erythromycin and clindamycin, whereas oral antibiotics most often used for acne include doxycycline, minocycline, and erythromycin. Oral antibiotics are more effective than topical therapies, but can have a variety of side effects such as sun sensitivity and gastrointestinal upset.

Isotretinoin

Oral isotretinoin (Accutane) is an analog of vitamin A that is highly effective for the treatment of severe recalcitrant acne. Despite its efficacy, oral isotretinoin is teratogenic if taken during the first trimester of pregnancy. Malformations typically involve the cranium, face, heart, central nervous system, and thymus. Therefore, isotretinoin administration should be limited to women using a highly effective method of contraception.

TABLE 17-8. Topical Acne Medications

Drug	Formulation (Brand Name)	Strength (%)
Retinoids		
Tretinoin	Cream (Retin A)	0.025, 0.05, 0.1
	Cream (Renova)	0.02, 0.05
	Gel (Retin A)	0.01, 0.025
	Gel (Atralin)	0.05
	Solution (Retin A)	0.05
	Microsphere gel (Retin-A Micro)	0.04, 0.1
	Polymerized cream or gel (Avita)	0.025
Adapalene	Cream, gel, solution, or lotion (Differin)	0.1
Tazarotene	Cream or gel (Tazorac, Avage)	0.05, 0.1[a]
BPO/antibiotic combined agent		
BPO/erythromycin	Gel (Acanya)	2.5/1.2
	Gel (Benzaclin, Duac)	5/1
BPO/clindamycin	Gel (Benzamycin)	5/3
Retinoid/antibiotic combined agent		
Tretinoin/clindamycin	Gel (Ziana, Veltin)	0.025/1.2

[a]Indicated for psoriasis.
BPO = benzoyl peroxide.

Acanthosis Nigricans

Optimal treatment for acanthosis nigricans should be directed towards decreasing insulin resistance and hyperinsulinemia (Field, 1961). Specifically, a few studies have shown an improvement in acanthosis nigricans with insulin sensitizers (Walling, 2003). Other methods, including topical antibiotics, topical and systemic retinoids, keratolytics, and topical corticosteroids have been tried with limited success (Schwartz, 1994).

Surgical Therapy

Although ovarian wedge resection is now rarely performed, laparoscopic ovarian drilling has been shown to restore ovulation in a significant number of women with PCOS who were found to be resistant to clomiphene citrate (Section 42-8, p. 1139) (Hendriks, 2007). Rarely, oophorectomy is a viable option for women not seeking fertility who exhibit signs and symptoms of ovarian hyperthecosis and accompanying severe hyperandrogenism.

REFERENCES

Adams J, Polson DW, Franks S: Prevalence of polycystic ovaries in women with anovulation and idiopathic hirsutism. Br Med J (Clin Res) 293:355, 1986

Amer SA, Gopalan V, Li TC, et al: Long term follow-up of patients with polycystic ovarian syndrome after laparoscopic ovarian drilling: clinical outcome. Hum Reprod 17:2035, 2002

American College of Obstetricians and Gynecologists: Management of anovulatory bleeding. Practice Bulletin No. 14, March 2000

American Diabetes Association: Standards of medical care in diabetes—2010, Diabetes Care 33:S11, 2010

Archer JS, Chang RJ: Hirsutism and acne in polycystic ovary syndrome. Best Pract Res Clin Obstet Gynecol 18:737, 2004

Arroyo A, Laughlin GA, Morales AJ, et al: Inappropriate gonadotropin secretion in polycystic ovary syndrome: influence of adiposity. J Clin Endocrinol Metab 82:3728, 1997

Asunción M, Calvo RM, San Millán JL, et al: A prospective study of the polycystic ovary syndrome in unselected Caucasian women from Spain. J Clin Endocrinol Metab 85:2434, 2000

Azziz R: The evaluation and management of hirsutism. Obstet Gynecol 101:995, 2003

Azziz R, Carmina E, Dewailly D, et al: The Androgen Excess and PCOS Society criteria for the polycystic ovary syndrome: the complete task force report. Fertil Steril 91:456, 2009

Azziz R, Ehrmann D, Legro RS, et al: Troglitazone improves ovulation and hirsutism in the polycystic ovary syndrome: a multicenter, double blind, placebo-controlled trial. J Clin Endocrinol Metab 86:1626, 2001

Balen A, Michelmore K: What is polycystic ovary syndrome? Are national reviews important? Hum Reprod 17:2219, 2002

Balen AH, Laven JS, Tan SL, et al: Ultrasound assessment of the polycystic ovary: international consensus definitions. Hum Reprod Update 9:505, 2003

Balfour JA, McClellan K: Topical eflornithine. Am J Clin Dermatol 2:197, 2001

Banaszewska B, Duleba A, Spaczynski R: Lipids in polycystic ovary syndrome: role of hyperinsulinemia and effects of metformin. Am J Obstet Gynecol 194:1266, 2006

Barbieri RL: Hyperandrogenism, insulin resistance and acanthosis nigricans. 10 years of progress. J Reprod Med 39:327, 1994

Bass KM, Newschaffer CJ, Klag MJ, et al: Plasma lipoprotein levels as predictor of cardiovascular death in women. Arch Intern Med 153:2209, 1993

Batukan C, Baysal B: Metformin improves ovulation and pregnancy rates in patients with polycystic ovary syndrome. Arch Gynecol Obstet 265:124, 2001

Bergh C, Carlsson B, Olsson JH, et al: Regulation of androgen production in cultured human thecal cells by insulin-like growth factor I and insulin. Fertil Steril 59:323, 1993

Betti R, Bencini PL, Lodi A, et al: Incidence of polycystic ovaries in patients with late onset or persistent acne: hormonal reports. Dermatologica 181:109, 1990

Boomsma CM, Eijkemans MJC, Hughes EG: A meta-analysis of pregnancy outcomes in women with polycystic ovary syndrome. Hum Reprod Update 12:673, 2006

Bunker CB, Newton JA, Kilborn J, et al: Most women with acne have polycystic ovaries. Br J Dermatol 121:675, 1989

Burgers JA, Fong SL, Louwers YV, et al: Oligoovulatory and anovulatory cycles in women with polycystic ovary syndrome (PCOS): what's the difference? J Clin Endocrinol Metab 95(12):E485, 2010

Carmina E, Oberfield SE, Lobo RA: The diagnosis of polycystic ovary syndrome in adolescents. Am J Obstet Gynecol 203(3):201.e1, 2010

Cela E, Robertson C, Rush K, et al: Prevalence of polycystic ovaries in women with androgenic alopecia. Eur J Endocrinol 149:439, 2003

Chang WY, Knochenhauer ES, Bartolucci AA, et al: Phenotypic spectrum of polycystic ovary syndrome: clinical and biochemical characterization of the three major clinical subgroups. Fertil Steril 83:1717, 2005

Chen W, Thiboutot D, Zouboulis CC: Cutaneous androgen metabolism: basic research and clinical perspectives. J Invest Dermatol 119:992, 2002

Clayton R, Ogden V, Hodgkinson J, et al: How common are polycystic ovaries in normal women and what is their significance for the fertility of the population? Clin Endocrinol 37:127, 1992

Clifford K, Rai R, Regan L: Future pregnancy outcome in unexplained recurrent first trimester miscarriage. Hum Reprod 12:387, 1997

Cook H, Brennan K, Azziz R: Reanalyzing the modified Ferriman-Gallwey score: is there a simpler method for assessing the extent of hirsutism? Fertil Steril Sept 15, 2011 [Epub ahead of print]

Coulam CB, Annegers JF, Kranz JS: Chronic anovulation syndrome and associated neoplasia. Obstet Gynecol 61:403, 1983

Crapo L: Cushing's syndrome: a review of diagnostic tests. Metab Clin Exp 28:955, 1979

Cruz PD Jr, Hud JA Jr: Excess insulin binding to insulin-like growth factor receptors: proposed mechanism for acanthosis nigricans. J Invest Dermatol 98(Suppl):82S, 1992

Culiner A, Shippel S: Virilism and theca-cell hyperplasia of the ovary: a syndrome. BJOG 56:439, 1949

Dahlgren E, Janson PO, Johansson S, et al: Polycystic ovary syndrome and risk for myocardial infarction. Evaluated from a risk factor model based on a prospective population study of women. Acta Obstet Gynecol Scand 71:599, 1992

Deeks AA, Gibson-Helm ME, Teede HJ: Anxiety and depression in polycystic ovary syndrome: a comprehensive investigation. Fertil Steril 93(7):2421, 2010

Derksen J, Nagesser SK, Meinders AE, et al: Identification of virilizing adrenal tumors in hirsute women. N Engl J Med 331:968, 1994

Diamanti-Kandarakis E, Kouli CR, Bergiele AT, et al: A survey of the polycystic ovary syndrome in the Greek island of Lesbos: hormonal and metabolic profile. J Clin Endocrinol Metab 84:4006, 1999

Ding EL, Song Y, Manson JE, et al: Sex hormone-binding globulin and risk of type 2 diabetes in women and men. N Engl J Med 361(12):1152, 2009

Dokras A, Bochner M, Hollinrake E: Screening women with polycystic ovary syndrome for metabolic syndrome. Obstet Gynecol 106:131, 2005

Dramusic V, Rajan U, Wong YC, et al: Adolescent polycystic ovary syndrome. Ann NY Acad Sci 816:194, 1997

Dunaif A: Insulin resistance and the polycystic ovary syndrome: mechanisms and implication for pathogenesis. Endocrine Rev 18:774, 1997

Dunaif A, Finegood DT: Beta-cell dysfunction independent of obesity and glucose intolerance in the polycystic ovary syndrome. J Clin Endocrinol Metab 81:942, 1996a

Dunaif A, Scott D, Finegood D, et al: The insulin-sensitizing agent troglitazone improves metabolic and reproductive abnormalities in the polycystic ovary syndrome. J Clin Endocrinol Metab 81:3299, 1996b

Dunaif A, Segal KR, Futterweit W, et al: Profound peripheral insulin resistance, independent of obesity, in polycystic ovary syndrome. Diabetes 38:1165, 1989

Dunaif A, Segal KR, Shelley DR, et al: Evidence for distinctive and intrinsic defects in insulin action in polycystic ovary syndrome. Diabetes 41:1257, 1992

Ehrmann DA, Schneider DJ, Burton E, et al: Troglitazone improves defects in insulin action, insulin secretion, ovarian steroidogenesis, and fibrinolysis in women with polycystic ovary syndrome. J Clin Endocrinol Metab 82:2108, 1997

Elting MW, Korsen TJM, Rekers-Mombarg LTM: Women with polycystic ovary syndrome gain regular menstrual cycles when aging. Hum Reprod 15, 24, 2000

Essah PA, Apridonidze T, Iuorno MJ, et al: Effects of short-term and long-term metformin treatment on menstrual cyclicity in women with polycystic ovary syndrome. Fertil Steril 86:230, 2006

Farah L, Lazenby AJ, Boots LR, et al: Prevalence of polycystic ovary syndrome in women seeking treatment from community electrologists (Alabama Professional Electrology Association Study Group). J Reprod Med 44:870, 1999

Ferriman D, Gallwey JD: Clinical assessment of body hair growth in women. J Clin Endocrinol Metab 21:1440, 1961

Field JB, Johnson P, Herring B: Insulin-resistant diabetes associated with increased endogenous plasma insulin followed by complete remission. J Clin Invest 40:1672, 1961

Fleming R, Hopkinson ZE, Wallace AM, et al: Ovarian function and metabolic factors in women with oligomenorrhea treated with metformin in a randomized double blind placebo-controlled trial. J Clin Endocrinol Metab 87:569, 2002

Fogel RB, Malhotra A, Pillar G, et al: Increased prevalence of obstructive sleep apnea syndrome in obese women with polycystic ovary syndrome. J Clin Endocrinol Metab 86:1175, 2001

Ford ES, Giles WH, Dietz WH: Prevalence of metabolic syndrome among US adults: findings from the third National Health and Nutrition Examination Survey. JAMA 287:356, 2002

Franks S: Candidate genes in women with polycystic ovary syndrome. Fertil Steril 86 (Suppl 1):S15, 2006

Franks S, Gharani N, Waterworth D, et al: The genetic basis of polycystic ovary syndrome. Hum Reprod 12:2641, 1997

Fruzzetti F, de Lorenzo D, Parrini D, et al: Effects of finasteride, a 5 alpha-reductase inhibitor, on circulating androgens and gonadotropin secretion in hirsute women. J Clin Endocrinol Metab 79(3):831, 1994

Glueck CJ, Phillips H, Cameron D, et al: Continuing metformin throughout pregnancy in women with polycystic ovary syndrome appears to safely reduce first-trimester spontaneous abortion: a pilot study. Fertil Steril 75:46, 2001

Gold LS: The MORE trial: effectiveness of adapalene gel 0.1% in real-world dermatology practices. Cutis 78(1 Suppl):12, 2006

Govind A, Obhrai MS, Clayton RN: Polycystic ovaries are inherited as an autosomal dominant trait: analysis of 29 polycystic ovary syndrome and 10 control families. J Clin Endocrinol Metab 84:38, 1999

Haas DA, Carr BR, Attia GR: Effects of metformin on body mass index, menstrual cyclicity, and ovulation induction in women with polycystic ovary syndrome. Fertil Steril 79:469, 2003

Hatch R, Rosenfield RL, Kim MH, et al: Hirsutism: implications, etiology, and management. Am J Obstet Gynecol 140:815, 1981

Hayes FJ, Taylor AE, Martin KA, et al: Use of a gonadotropin-releasing hormone antagonist as a physiologic probe in polycystic ovary syndrome: assessment of neuroendocrine and androgen dynamics. J Clin Endocrinol Metab 83:2243, 1998

Hendriks ML, Ket JC, Hompes PG, et al: Why does ovarian surgery in PCOS help? Insight into the endocrine implications of ovarian surgery for ovulation induction in polycystic ovary syndrome. Hum Reprod Update 13(3):249, 2007

Himelein MJ, Thatcher SS: Polycystic ovary syndrome and mental health: a review. Obstet Gynecol Surv 61(11):723, 2006

Homburg R: Adverse effects of luteinizing hormone on fertility: fact or fantasy. Baillieres Clin Obstet Gynaecol 12(4):555, 1998a

Homburg R, Armar NA, Eshel A, et al: Influence of serum luteinising hormone concentrations on ovulation, conception, and early pregnancy loss in polycystic ovary syndrome. BMJ 297(6655):1024, 1998b

Homburg R, Lambalk CB: Polycystic ovary syndrome in adolescence—a therapeutic conundrum. Hum Reprod 19:1039, 2004

Howles CM, Macnamee MC, Edwards RG: Follicular development and early function of conception and non-conceptional cycles after human in vitro fertilization: endocrine correlates. Hum Reprod 2:17, 1987

Huber-Buchholz MM, Carey DG, Norman RJ: Restoration of reproductive potential by lifestyle modification in obese polycystic ovary syndrome: role of insulin sensitivity and luteinizing hormone. J Clin Endocrinol Metab 84:1470, 1999

Hughesdon PE: Morphology and morphogenesis of the Stein-Leventhal ovary and of so-called "hyperthecosis." Obstet Gynecol Surv 37:59, 1982

Hull MG: Epidemiology of infertility and polycystic ovarian disease: endocrinological and demographic studies. Gynaecol Endocrinol 1:235, 1987

Hurd WW, Abdel-Rahman MY, Ismail SA, et al: Comparison of diabetes mellitus and insulin resistance screening methods for women with polycystic ovary syndrome. Fertil Steril 96(4):1043, 2011

Jaatinen TA, Anttila L, Erkkola R, et al: Hormonal responses to physical exercise in patients with polycystic ovarian syndrome. Fertil Steril 60:262, 1993

Jakubowicz DJ, Iuorno MJ, Jakubowicz S, et al: Effects of metformin on early pregnancy loss in the polycystic ovary syndrome. J Clin Endocrinol Metab 87:524, 2002

Jebraili R, Kaur S, Kanwar AJ, et al: Hormone profile & polycystic ovaries in acne vulgaris. Indian J Med Res 100:73, 1994

Jick SS, Terris BZ, Jick H: First trimester topical tretinoin and congenital disorders. Lancet 341:1181, 1993

Kahsar-Miller MD, Nixon C, Boots LR, et al: Prevalence of polycystic ovary syndrome (PCOS) in first-degree relatives of patients with PCOS. Fertil Steril 75:53, 2001

Kiddy DS, Hamilton-Fairley D, Bush A, et al: Improvement in endocrine and ovarian function during dietary treatment of obese women with polycystic ovary syndrome. Clin Endocrinol (Oxf) 36:105, 1992

Kirk LF Jr, Hash RB, Katner HP, et al: Cushing's disease: clinical manifestations and diagnostic evaluation. Am Fam Physician 62:1119, 1133, 2000

Knochenhauer ES, Key TJ, Kahsar-Miller M, et al: Prevalence of the polycystic ovary syndrome in unselected black and white women of the southeastern United States: a prospective study. J Clin Endocrinol Metab 83:3078, 1998

Knowler WC, Barrett-Connor E, Fowler SE, et al: Diabetes Prevention Program Research Group. Reduction in the incidence of type 2 diabetes with lifestyle intervention or metformin. N Engl J Med 346:393, 2002

Krowchuk DP: Managing adolescent acne: a guide for pediatricians. Pediatr Rev 26:250, 2005

Lakhani K, Constantinovici N, Purcell WM, et al: Internal carotid artery haemodynamics in women with polycystic ovaries. Clin Sci (Lond) 98:661, 2000

Lee JK, Wu CK, Lin LY, et al: Insulin resistance in the middle-aged women with "tigerish back and bearish waist". Diabetes Res Clin Pract 90(3):e85, 2010

Legro RS: Is there a male phenotype in polycystic ovary syndrome families? J Pediatr Endocrinol Metab 13(Suppl 5):1307, 2000

Legro RS, Barnhart HX, Schlaff WD, et al: Clomiphene, metformin, or both for infertility in the polycystic ovary syndrome. N Engl J Med 356(6):551, 2007

Legro RS, Gnatuk CL, Kunselman AR, et al: Changes in glucose tolerance over time in women with polycystic ovary syndrome: a controlled study. J Clin Endocrinol Metab 90:3236, 2005

Legro RS, Kunselman AR, Demers L, et al: Elevated dehydroepiandrosterone sulfate levels as the reproductive phenotype in the brothers of women with polycystic ovary syndrome. J Clin Endocrinol Metab 87:2134, 2002

Legro RS, Kunselman AR, Dodson WC, et al: Prevalence and predictors of risk for type 2 diabetes mellitus and impaired glucose tolerance in polycystic ovary syndrome: a prospective, controlled study in 254 affected women. J Clin Endocrinol Metab 84:165, 1999

Legro RS, Kunselman AR, Dunaif A: Prevalence and predictors of dyslipidemia in women with polycystic ovary syndrome. Am J Med 111:607, 2001

Leyden J, Thiboutot DM, Shalita AR, et al: Comparison of tazarotene and minocycline maintenance therapies in acne vulgaris: a multicenter, double-blind, randomized, parallel-group study. Arch Dermatol 142:605, 2006

Lo JC, Feigenbaum SL, Yang J, et al: Epidemiology and adverse cardiovascular risk profile of diagnosed polycystic ovary syndrome. J Clin Endocrinol Metab 91(4):1357, 2006

Loureiro KD, Kao KK, Jones KL, et al: Minor malformations characteristics of the retinoic acid embryopathy and other birth outcomes in children of women exposed to topical tretinoin during early pregnancy. Am J Med Genet A 136:117, 2005

Mannerås-Holm L, Leonhardt H, Kullberg J, et al: Adipose tissue has aberrant morphology and function in PCOS: enlarged adipocytes and low serum adiponectin, but not circulating sex steroids, are strongly associated with insulin resistance. J Clin Endocrinol Metab 96(2):E304, 2011

Meier CA, Biller BM: Clinical and biochemical evaluation of Cushing's syndrome. Endocrinol Metab Clin North Am 26:741, 1997

Miller KK, Rosner W, Lee H, et al: Measurement of free testosterone in normal women and women with androgen deficiency: comparison of methods. J Clin Endocrinol Metab 89:525, 2004

Moghetti P, Castello R, Magnani CM, et al: Clinical and hormonal effects of the 5 alpha-reductase inhibitor finasteride in idiopathic hirsutism. J Clin Endocrinol Metab 79:1115, 1994

Moghetti P, Toscano V: Treatment of hirsutism and acne in hyperandrogenism. Best Pract Res Clin Endocrinol Metab 20:221, 2006

Moore RL, Devere TS: Epidermal manifestations of internal malignancy. Dermatol Clin 26(1):17, 2008

Moran C, Knochenhauer E, Boots LR, et al: Adrenal androgen excess in hyperandrogenism: relation to age and body mass. Fertil Steril 71:671, 1999

Moran C, Tapia MC, Hernandez E, et al: Etiological review of hirsutism in 250 patients. Arch Med Res 25:311, 1994

Mosca L, Benjamin EJ, Berra K, et al: Effectiveness-based guidelines for the prevention of cardiovascular disease in women—2011 update: a guideline from the American Heart Association. J Am Coll Cardiol 57(12):1404, 2011

Nagamani M, Dinh TV, Kelver ME: Hyperinsulinemia in hyperthecosis of the ovaries. Am J Obstet Gynecol 154:384, 1986

Nestler JE, Jakubowicz DJ, Evans WS, et al: Effects of metformin on spontaneous and clomiphene-induced ovulation in the polycystic ovary syndrome. N Engl J Med 338:1876, 1998

Neveu N, Granger L, St Michel P, et al: Comparison of clomiphene citrate, metformin, or the combination of both for first-line ovulation induction and achievement of pregnancy in 154 women with polycystic ovary syndrome. Fertil Steril 87(1):113, 2007

Nieman LK, Biller BM, Findling JW, et al: The diagnosis of Cushing's syndrome: an Endocrine Society Clinical Practice Guideline. J Clin Endocrinol Metab 93(5):1526, 2008

Nishizawa H, Shimomura I, Kishida K, et al: Androgens decrease plasma adiponectin, an insulin-sensitizing adipocyte-derived protein. Diabetes 51:2734, 2002

Nitsche K, Ehrmann DA: Obstructive sleep apnea and metabolic dysfunction in polycystic ovary syndrome. Best Pract Res Clin Endocrinol Metab 24(5):717, 2010

Nuttall FQ, Gannon MC, Wald JL, et al: Plasma glucose and insulin profiles in normal subjects ingesting diets of varying carbohydrate, fat, and protein content. J Am Coll Nutr 4:437, 1985

Nybacka A, Carlström K, Ståhle A, et al: Randomized comparison of the influence of dietary management and/or physical exercise on ovarian function and metabolic parameters in overweight women with polycystic ovary syndrome. Fertil Steril Sept 28, 2011 [Epub ahead of print]

O'Driscoll JB, Mamtora H, Higginson J, et al: A prospective study of the prevalence of clearcut endocrine disorders and polycystic ovaries in 350 patients presenting with hirsutism or androgenic alopecia. Clin Endocrinol 41:231, 1994

Orio F, Palomba S, Cascella T, et al: Early impairment of endothelial structure and function in young normal-weight women with polycystic ovary syndrome. J Clin Endocrinol Metab 89:4588, 2004

Palmert MR, Gordon CM, Kartashov AI, et al: Screening for abnormal glucose tolerance in adolescents with polycystic ovary syndrome. J Clin Endocrinol Metab 87(3):1017, 2002

Palomba S, Falbo A, Orio F Jr, et al: Effect of preconceptional metformin on abortion risk in polycystic ovary syndrome: a systematic review and meta-analysis of randomized controlled trials. Fertil Steril 92(5):1646, 2009

Palomba S, Orio F, Falo A, et al: Prospective parallel randomized, double-blind, double dummy controlled clinical trial comparing clomiphene citrate and metformin as the first-line treatment for ovulation induction in nonobese anovulatory women with polycystic ovary syndrome. J Clin Endocrinol Metab 90:4068, 2005

Panidis D, Skiadopoulos S, Rousso D, et al: Association of acanthosis nigricans with insulin resistance in patients with polycystic ovary syndrome. Br J Dermatol 132:936, 1995

Paradisi G, Steinberg HO, Shepard MK, et al: Troglitazone therapy improves endothelial function to near normal levels in women with polycystic ovary syndrome. J Clin Endocrinol Metab 88:576, 2003

Pasquali R, Antenucci D, Casimirri F, et al: Clinical and hormonal characteristics of obese amenorrheic hyperandrogenic women before and after weight loss. J Clin Endocrinol Metab 68:173, 1989

Peterson EP: Endometrial carcinoma in young women. A clinical profile. Obstet Gynecol 31:702, 1968

Polson DW, Adams J, Wadsworth J, et al: Polycystic ovaries—a common finding in normal women. Lancet 1:870, 1988

Purdy S, de Berker D: Acne. BMJ 333:949, 2006

Rebar R, Judd HL, Yen SS, et al: Characterization of the inappropriate gonadotropin secretion in polycystic ovary syndrome. J Clin Invest 57:1320, 1976

Rebuffe-Scrive M, Cullberg G, Lundberg PA, et al: Anthropometric variables and metabolism in polycystic ovarian disease. Horm Metab Res 21:391, 1989

Regan L, Owen EJ, Jacobs HS: Hypersecretion of luteinising hormone, infertility, and miscarriage. Lancet 336:1141, 1990

Rocha MP, Marcondes JA, Barcellos CR, et al: Dyslipidemia in women with polycystic ovary syndrome: incidence, pattern and predictors. Gynecol Endocrinol 27(10):814, 2011

Rose PG: Endometrial carcinoma. N Engl J Med 335:640, 1996

Rosenfield RL: Clinical review: identifying children at risk for polycystic ovary syndrome. J Clin Endocrinol Metab 92(3):787, 2007

Rosenfield RL: Hirsutism. N Engl J Med 353:2578, 2005

Sagle M, Bishop K, Ridley N, et al: Recurrent early miscarriage and polycystic ovaries. BMJ 297:1027, 1988

Salley KES, Wickham EP, Cheang KI, et al: Glucose intolerance in polycystic ovary syndrome. A position statement of the Androgen Excess Society. J Clin Endocrinol Metab 92:4546, 2007

Schneider JG, Tompkins C, Blumenthal RS, et al: The metabolic syndrome in women. Cardiol Rev 14:286, 2006

Schwartz RA: Acanthosis nigricans. J Am Acad Dermatol 31:1, 1994

Skov AR, Toubro S, Bulow J, et al: Changes in renal function during weight loss induced by high vs. low-protein low-fat diets in overweight subjects. Int J Obes 23:1170, 1999

Smirnakis KV, Plati A, Wolf M, et al: Predicting gestational diabetes: choosing the optimal early serum marker. Am J Obstet Gynecol 196(4):410.e1, 2007

Sobbrio GA, Granata A, D'Arrigo F, et al: Treatment of hirsutism related to micropolycystic ovary syndrome (MPCO) with two low-dose oestrogen oral contraceptives: a comparative randomized evaluation. Acta Eur Fertil 21:139, 1990

Speroff L, Glass RH, Kase NG: Hirsutism. In Speroff L, Glass RH, Kase NG, (eds): Clinical Gynecologic Endocrinology and Infertility, 6th ed. Baltimore, Williams & Wilkins, 1999, p 523

Talbott E, Clerici A, Berga SL, et al: Adverse lipid and coronary heart disease risk profiles in young women with polycystic ovary syndrome: results of a case-controlled study. J Clin Epidemiol 51:415, 1998

Talbott E, Guzick D, Clerici A, et al: Coronary heart disease risk factors in women with polycystic ovary syndrome. Arterioscler Thromb Vasc Biol 15:821, 1995

Tarkun I, Arslan BC, Canturk Z, et al: Endothelial dysfunction in young women with polycystic ovary syndrome: relationship with insulin resistance and low-grade chronic inflammation. J Clin Endocrinol Metab 89:5592, 2004

Taylor AE, McCourt B, Martin KA, et al: Determinants of abnormal gonadotropin secretion in clinically defined women with polycystic ovary syndrome. J Clin Endocrinol Metab 82:2248, 1997

Thadhani R, Wolf M, Hsu-Blatman K, et al: First-trimester sex hormone binding globulin and subsequent gestational diabetes mellitus. Am J Obstet Gynecol 189(10):171, 2003

The Rotterdam ESHRE/ASRM-Sponsored PCOS Consensus Workshop Group: Revised 2003 consensus on diagnostic criteria and long-term health risks related to polycystic ovary syndrome (PCOS). Hum Reprod 19:41, 2004

Thiboutot D: Acne: hormonal concepts and therapy. Clin Dermatol 22:419, 2004

Tiras MB, Yalcin R, Noyan V, et al: Alterations in cardiac flow parameters in patients with polycystic ovarian syndrome. Hum Reprod 14:1949, 1999

Torley D, Bellus GA, Munro CS: Genes, growth factors and acanthosis nigricans. Br J Dermatol 147:1096, 2002

Urbanek M, Woodroffe A, Ewens KG, et al: Candidate gene region for polycystic ovary syndrome (PCOS) on chromosome 19p 13.2. J Clin Endocrinol Metab 90:6623, 2005

Van der Spuy ZM, le Roux PA: Cyproterone acetate for hirsutism. Cochrane Database Syst Rev 4:CD001125, 2003

van Santbrink EJ, Hop WC, Fauser BC: Classification of normogonadotropin infertility: polycystic ovaries diagnosed by ultrasound versus endocrine characteristics of PCOS. Fertil Steril 67:452, 1997

Vanky E, Stridsklev S, Heimstad R, et al: Metformin versus placebo from first trimester to delivery in polycystic ovary syndrome: a randomized, controlled multicenter study. J Clin Endocrinol Metab 95(12):E448, 2010

Veltman-Verhulst SM, van Haeften TW, Eijkemans MJ, et al: Sex hormone-binding globulin concentrations before conception as a predictor for gestational diabetes in women with polycystic ovary syndrome. Hum Reprod (12):3123, 2010

Vgontzas AN, Legro RS, Bixler EO, et al: Polycystic ovary syndrome is associated with obstructive sleep apnea and daytime sleepiness: role of insulin resistance. J Clin Endocrinol Metab 86:517, 2001

Vigorito C, Giallauria F, Palomba S, et al: Beneficial effects of a three-month structured exercise training program on cardiopulmonary functional capacity in young women with polycystic ovary syndrome. J Clin Endocrinol Metab 92(4):1379, 2007

Waldstreicher J, Santoro NF, Hall HJE, et al: Hyperfunction of the hypothalamic-pituitary axis in women with polycystic ovarian disease: indirect evidence of partial gonadotroph desensitization. J Clin Endocrinol Metab 66:165, 1988

Walling HW, Messingham M, Myers LM, et al: Improvement of acanthosis nigricans on isotretinoin and metformin. J Drugs Dermatol 2:677, 2003

Yildiz BO, Yarali H, Oguz H, et al: Glucose intolerance, insulin resistance, and hyperandrogenemia in first degree relatives of women with polycystic ovary syndrome. J Clin Endocrinol Metab 88:2031, 2003

Zaenglein AL, Thiboutot DM: Expert committee recommendations for acne management. Pediatrics 118:1188, 2006

Zawadzki JK, Dunaif A: Diagnostic criteria for polycystic ovary syndrome: towards a rational approach. In Dunaif A, Givens JR, Haseltine F, et al (eds): Polycystic Ovary Syndrome. Boston, Blackwell Scientific, 1990, p 377

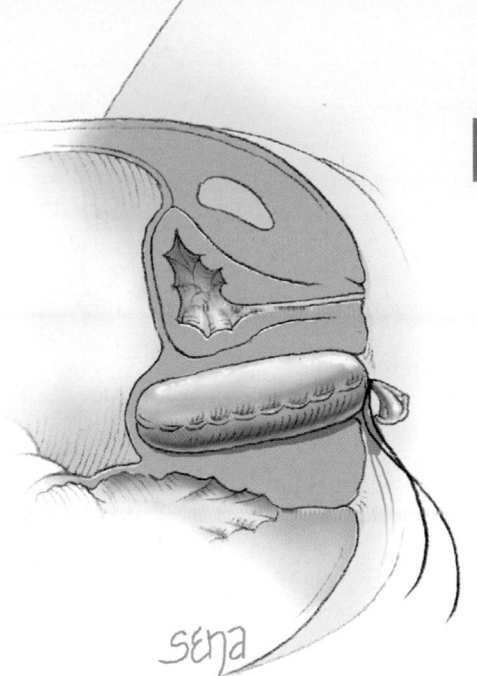

CHAPTER 18

Anatomic Disorders

Congenital anatomic disorders of the female reproductive tract occur frequently and may result from genetic mutation, developmental arrest, abnormal hormonal exposure, or exposure to environmental insults that exert their effects at critical stages of embryonic development. Disorders range from congenital absence of the vagina and uterus, to lateral or vertical fusion defects of the müllerian ducts, to external genitalia that are ambiguous in sexual differentiation. Anatomic defects of the urinary tract are commonly found in these patients due to the concurrent embryonic development of the reproductive and urinary tracts.

NORMAL EMBRYOLOGY

Overview

An understanding of the complex embryology of the female reproductive system often aids in clarifying the structure of malformations and their association with other genitourinary anomalies (Shatzkes, 1991; Yin, 2005). Like most organ systems, the female urogenital tract develops from multiple cell types that undergo important spatial growth and differentiation. Development occurs during relatively narrow time windows and is governed by time-linked patterns of gene expression (Park, 2005). Some of the molecular mechanisms underlying this process have recently been uncovered with modern molecular genetics and are discussed later.

The urogenital tract is functionally divided into the urinary system and genital system. The urinary organs include the kidneys, ureters, bladder, and urethra. The reproductive organs consist of the gonads, ductal system, and external genitalia.

Both the urinary and genital systems develop from intermediate mesoderm, which extends along the entire embryo length. During initial embryo folding, a longitudinal ridge of this intermediate mesoderm develops along each side of the primitive abdominal aorta and is called the urogenital ridge (Fig. 18-1). Primordial germ cells first appear in the outer ectodermal layer of the embryo. At approximately 40 days of gestation, these germ cells migrate along the hindgut to the urogenital ridge (Fig. 18-1B). This ridge then divides into the nephrogenic and genital ridges.

At approximately 60 days of gestation, the nephrogenic ridges develop into the mesonephric kidneys (mesonephros) and paired mesonephric ducts, also termed Wolffian ducts (Figs. 18-1B and Fig. 18-2A). These mesonephric ducts connect the mesonephric

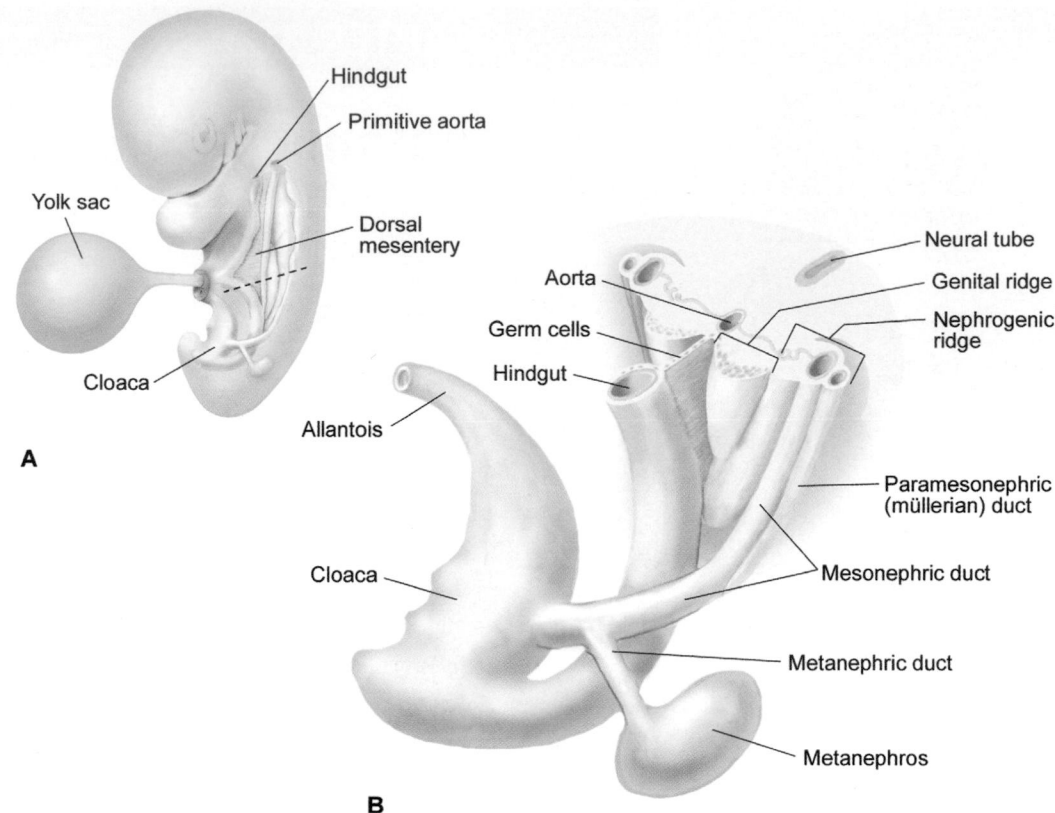

FIGURE 18-1 Early development of the embryonic genitourinary tract. **A.** In the developing embryo, the urogenital ridge forms from coelomic mesenchyme lateral to the primitive aorta. **B.** Cross section through the embryo shows division of the urogenital ridges into the genital ridge (future gonad) and nephrogenic ridge, which contains the mesonephros and mesonephric (Wolffian) ducts. The metanephros is the primitive kidney and is connected by the mesonephric ducts to the cloaca. Primordial germ cells migrate along the dorsal mesentery of the hindgut to reach the genital ridge. Paramesonephic (müllerian) ducts develop lateral to the mesonephric ducts. *(Images contributed by Kim Hoggatt-Krumwiede, MA.)*

kidneys (destined for resorption) to the cloaca, which is a common opening into which the embryonic urinary, genital, and alimentary tracts join (Fig. 18-2B). Recall that evolution of the renal system passes sequentially through the pronephric and mesonephric stages to reach the permanent metanephric system. The ureteric bud arises from the mesonephric duct at approximately the fifth week of fetal life. It lengthens to become the metanephric duct (ureter) and induces differentiation of the metanephros, which will eventually become the final functional kidney.

The paired paramesonephric ducts, also termed the müllerian ducts, develop from an invagination of the coelomic epithelium at approximately the sixth week and grow alongside the mesonephric ducts (Figs. 18-1B and 18-2B). The caudal portions of the müllerian ducts approximate one another in the midline and end behind the cloaca (Fig. 18-2C). The cloaca is divided by formation of the urorectal septum by the seventh week and is separated to create the rectum and the urogenital sinus (Fig. 18-2D). The urogenital sinus is considered in three parts: (1) the cephalad or vesicle portion, which will form the urinary bladder; (2) the middle or pelvic portion, which creates the female urethra; and (3) the caudal or phallic part, which will give rise to the distal vagina and to the greater vestibular (Bartholin), urethral, and paraurethral (Skene) glands. During differentiation of the urinary bladder,

the caudal portion of the mesonephric ducts is incorporated into the trigone portion of the bladder wall. Consequently, the caudal portion of the metanephric ducts (ureters) penetrates the bladder with distinct and separate orifices (Fig. 18-2D).

The close association between the mesonephric (Wolffian) and paramesonephric (müllerian) ducts has important clinical relevance because developmental insult to either system is often associated with anomalies that involve the kidney, ureter, and reproductive tract. For example, Kenney and colleagues (1984) showed that up to 50 percent of females with uterovaginal malformations have associated urinary tract anomalies.

Gonadal Differentiation

Mammalian sex is determined genetically. Individuals with X and Y chromosomes normally develop as males, whereas those with two X chromosomes develop as females. Before 7 weeks of embryonic development, embryos of male or female sex are indistinguishable (Table 18-1).

During this indeterminate time, the genital ridge begins as coelomic epithelium with underlying mesenchyme. The epithelium proliferates, and cords of epithelium invaginate into the mesenchyme to create primitive sex cords. In both 46,XX and

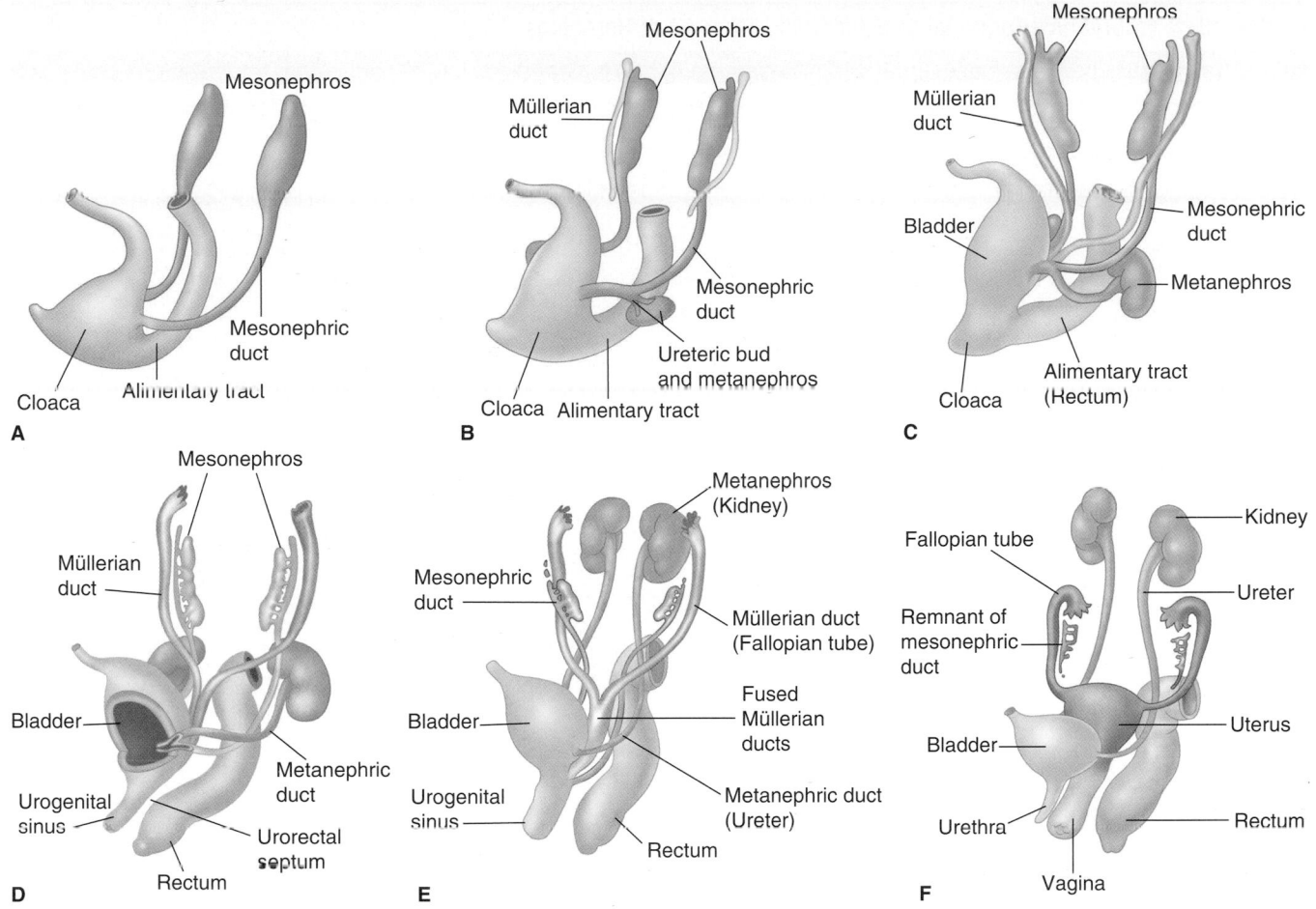

FIGURE 18-2 Embryonic development of the female genitourinary tract. *(Redrawn from Shatzkes, 1991.)*

46,XY embryos, the primordial germ cells are first identified as large polyhedral cells in the yolk sac. As noted earlier, these germ cells migrate by amoeboid motion along the hindgut dorsal mesentery to populate the undifferentiated genital ridge. Thus, the major cellular components of the early genital ridge include primordial germ cells and somatic cells.

At this point, the presence or absence of gonadal determinant genes determines fetal gender development (Fig. 18-3) (Taylor, 2000). Sexual differentiation is dependent upon the genetic sex that is determined at fertilization of the X-bearing oocyte by either an X- or Y-chromosome bearing sperm. In humans, the gene, named *the sex-determining region of the Y (SRY)*, is the testis-determining factor. In the presence of *SRY*, gonads develop as testes. Other important gonadal developmental genes include *SF1, SOX9, WT1, WNT4*, and *DAX1* (Viger, 2005).

In males, cells in the medullary region of the primitive sex cords differentiate into Sertoli cells, and these cells organize to form the testicular cords (Fig. 18-3A). Testicular cords are identifiable at 6 weeks and consist of these Sertoli cells and tightly packed germ cells. Early in the second trimester, the cords develop a lumen and become seminiferous tubules. Development of a testis-specific vasculature is crucial for normal testicular development (Ross, 2005).

The developing Sertoli cells begin to secrete antimüllerian hormone (AMH) (also called müllerian inhibitory substance—MIS) during developmental weeks 7 to 8. This gonadal hormone causes regression of the ipsilateral paramesonephric (müllerian duct) system, and this involution is completed by 9 to 10 weeks' gestation (Marshall, 1978). AMH also controls the rapid gubernacular growth necessary for the transabdominal descent of the testis. Serum AMH levels remain elevated in boys during childhood and then decline at puberty to the low levels seen in adult men. In contrast, girls have undetectable AMH levels until puberty, when serum levels become measurable. Clinically, AMH levels can be used to measure ovarian reserve and to predict the success of controlled ovarian hyperstimulation during assisted reproduction (Chap. 19, p. 515).

In the testes, Leydig cells arise from the original mesenchyme of the gonadal ridge and lie between the testicular cords. Their differentiation begins approximately 1 week after Sertoli cell development. The Leydig cells begin to secrete testosterone by 8 weeks' gestation. At weeks 15 to 18, testosterone production peaks as a result of stimulation of the testes by human chorionic gonadotropin (hCG). Testosterone acts in a paracrine manner on the ipsilateral mesonephric (Wolffian) duct to promote virilization of the duct into the epididymis, vas deferens, seminal vesicle, and ejaculatory duct. The androgens testosterone and

TABLE 18-1. Embryonic Urogenital Structures and Their Adult Homologs

Indifferent Structure	Female	Male
Genital ridge	Ovary	Testis
Primordial germ cells	Ova	Spermatozoa
Sex cords	Granulosa cells	Seminiferous tubules, Sertoli cells
Gubernaculum	Uteroovarian and round ligaments	Gubernaculum testis
Mesonephric tubules	Epoophoron, paroophoron	Efferent ductules, paradidymis
Mesonephric ducts	Gartner duct	Epididymis, ductus deferens, seminal vesicle, and ejaculatory duct
Paramesonephric ducts	Uterus Fallopian tubes Upper vagina	Prostatic utricle Appendix of testis
Urogenital sinus	Bladder Urethra Vagina Urethral and paraurethral glands Greater (Bartholin) and lesser vestibular glands	Bladder Urethra Prostatic utricle Prostate glands Bulbourethral glands
Genital tubercle	Clitoris	Glans penis
Urogenital folds	Labia minora	Floor of penile urethra
Labioscrotal swellings	Labia majora	Scrotum

dihydrotestosterone are essential for male phenotype development. These androgens control differentiation and growth of the internal and external genitalia and also prime male differentiation of the brain.

In the female embryo, without the influence of the *SRY* gene, the bipotential gonad develops into the ovary. Compared with testicular development, ovarian differentiation is delayed by approximately 2 weeks. Development is first characterized by the absence of testicular cords in the gonad. The primitive sex cords degenerate, and the mesothelium of the genital ridge forms secondary sex cords (Fig. 18-3B). These secondary cords become the granulosa cells that band together to form the follicular structures that surround the germ cells. Oocytes and the surrounding granulosa cells begin communication when the resting primordial follicles are stimulated to grow under the influence of follicle-stimulating hormone (FSH) at puberty. The medullary portion of the gonad regresses and forms the rete ovarii within the ovarian hilum.

Germ cells that carry two X chromosomes undergo mitosis during their initial migration to the female genital ridge. They reach a peak number of 6 to 7 million by 20 weeks' gestation. At this time, the fetal ovary demonstrates mature organization, with the presence of stroma and primordial follicles containing oocytes. During the third trimester, oocytes begin meiosis but arrest during meiosis I until the oocyte undergoes ovulation after menarche. Atresia of the oocytes starts in utero, leading to a reduced number of germ cells at birth (Fig. 14-1, p. 383).

■ Ductal System Development

Sexual differentiation of the reproductive ducts begins in week 7 due to the influence of gonadal hormones (testosterone and AMH) and other factors on the mesonephric (Wolffian) and paramesonephric (müllerian) ducts.

In the female, the lack of AMH allows müllerian ducts to persist. These ducts grow caudally along with the mesonephric ducts. During their elongation, both duct systems become enclosed in peritoneal folds that later give rise to the broad ligaments of the uterus (Fig. 18-4). At approximately 10 weeks' gestation and during their caudal migration, the two distal portions of the müllerian ducts approach each other in the midline and fuse even before they reach the urogenital sinus. The fused ducts form a tube called the uterovaginal canal. This tube then inserts into the urogenital sinus at Müller tubercle (Fig. 18-2E).

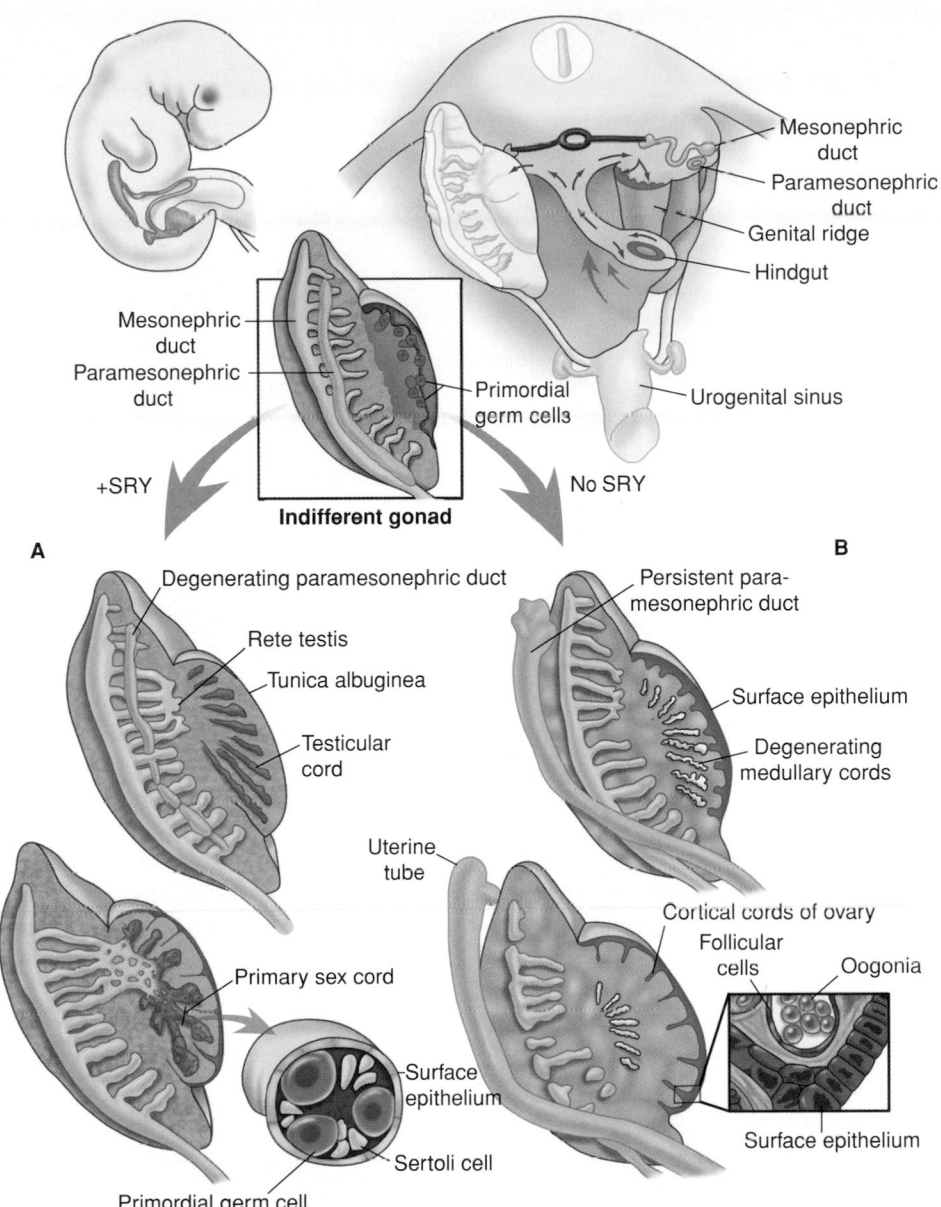

FIGURE 18-3 Development of the gonads and ductal systems in male **(A)** and female **(B)** embryos. *(From Cunningham, 2010, with permission.)*

By 12 weeks, the uterine corpus and cervix differentiate, and the uterine wall thickens. Initially, the upper pole of the uterus contains a thick midline septum that undergoes dissolution to create the uterine cavity. Dissolution of the uterine septum is usually completed by 20 weeks. The unfused cephalad portions of the müllerian ducts become the fallopian tubes (Fig. 18-2F). Any failure of lateral fusion of the two müllerian ducts or failure to reabsorb the septum between them results in separate uterine horns or some degree of persistent midline uterine septum.

Most investigators suggest that the vagina develops under the influence of the müllerian ducts and estrogenic stimulation. The vagina forms partly from the müllerian ducts and partly from the urogenital sinus (Masse, 2009). Specifically, the upper vagina derives from the fused müllerian ducts. The distal vagina develops from the bilateral sinovaginal bulbs, which are cranial evagination of the urogenital sinus.

During vaginal development, the müllerian ducts reach the urogenital sinus at Müller tubercle (Fig. 18-5A). Here, cells in the sinovaginal bulbs proliferate cranially to lengthen the vagina and create a solid vaginal plate (Fig. 18-5B). During the second trimester, these cells desquamate, allowing full canalization of the vaginal lumen (Fig. 18-5C). The hymen is the partition that remains to a varying degree between the dilated, canalized, fused sinovaginal bulbs and the urogenital sinus (Fig. 18-5B,C). The hymen usually becomes perforated shortly before or after birth. An imperforate hymen represents persistence of this membrane.

External Genitalia

Early development of the external genitalia is similar in both sexes. By 6 weeks' gestation, three external protuberances have

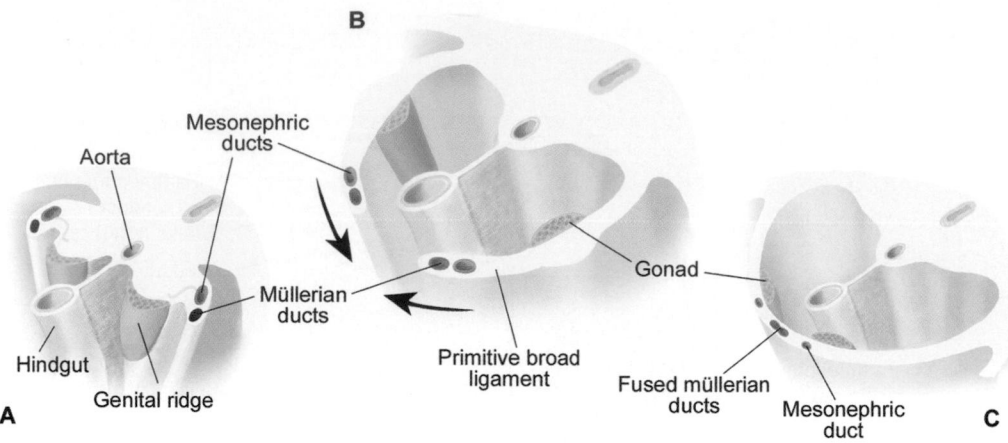

FIGURE 18-4 Development of the broad ligaments. **A.** The müllerian ducts initially lie lateral to the developing gonad. **B.** The müllerian ducts then move medially. **C.** In the midline, the müllerian ducts fuse, and the developing ovaries come to lie laterally. The mesonephric duct ultimately degenerates, but remnants may be found in the mesovarium and broad ligaments. *(Images contributed by Kim Hoggatt-Krumwiede, MA.)*

developed surrounding the cloacal membrane. These are the left and right genital swellings, which meet ventrally to form the third protuberance, the genital tubercle (Fig. 18-6A). The genital swellings become the labioscrotal folds. The urogenital sinus extends onto the surface of the enlarging genital tubercle to form the urethral groove, which is flanked on either side by the urethral folds, which lie within the labioscrotal folds. By week 7 of gestation, the urogenital membrane ruptures, exposing the cavity of the urogenital sinus to amnionic fluid. The genital tubercle elongates to form the phallus in males and the clitoris in females.

It is not until week 12 of gestation that one is able to visually differentiate between male and female external

genitalia (Fig. 18-7). In the male fetus, dihydrotestosterone (DHT), formed locally by the 5-α reduction of testosterone, prompts the anogenital distance to lengthen, the phallus to enlarge, the labioscrotal folds to fuse and form the scrotum, and subsequently, the urethral folds to merge and enclose the penile urethra (Fig. 18-6B). In the female fetus, in the absence of DHT, the anogenital distance does not lengthen, and the labioscrotal and urethral folds do not fuse (Fig. 18-6C). The genital tubercle bends caudally to become the clitoris, and the urogenital sinus becomes the vestibule of the vagina. The labioscrotal folds create the labia majora, whereas the urethral folds persist as the labia minora.

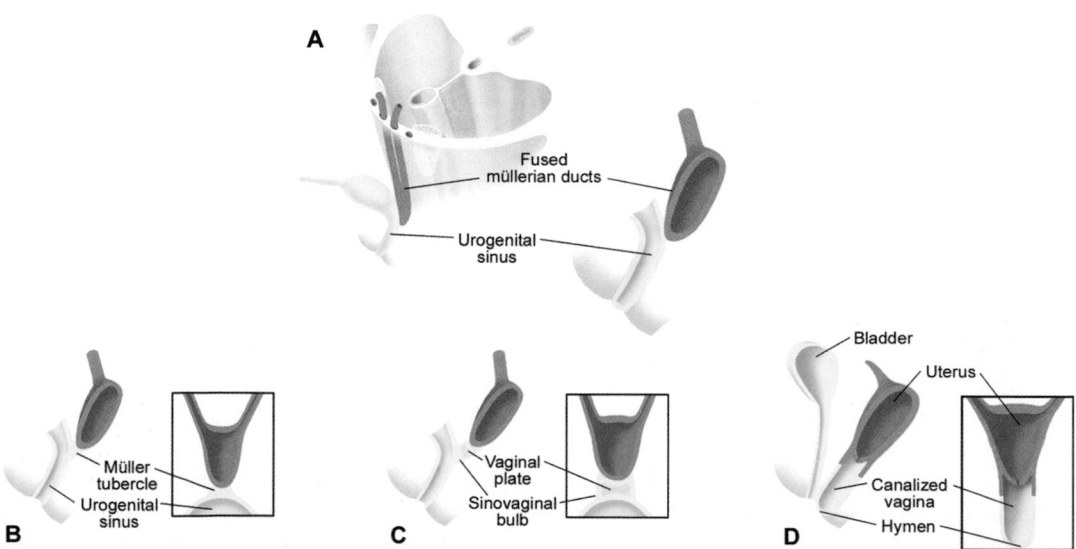

FIGURE 18-5 Development of the lower female reproductive tract. **A.** The fused müllerian ducts join the urogenital sinus at Müller tubercle. **B.** From the urogenital sinus, the sinovaginal bulbs evaginate and proliferate cranially to create the vaginal plate **(C)**. **D.** Lengthening of the vaginal plate and canalization leads to development of the lower vagina. The upper vagina develops from the caudal end of the fused müllerian ducts. *(Images contributed by Kim Hoggatt-Krumwiede, MA.)*

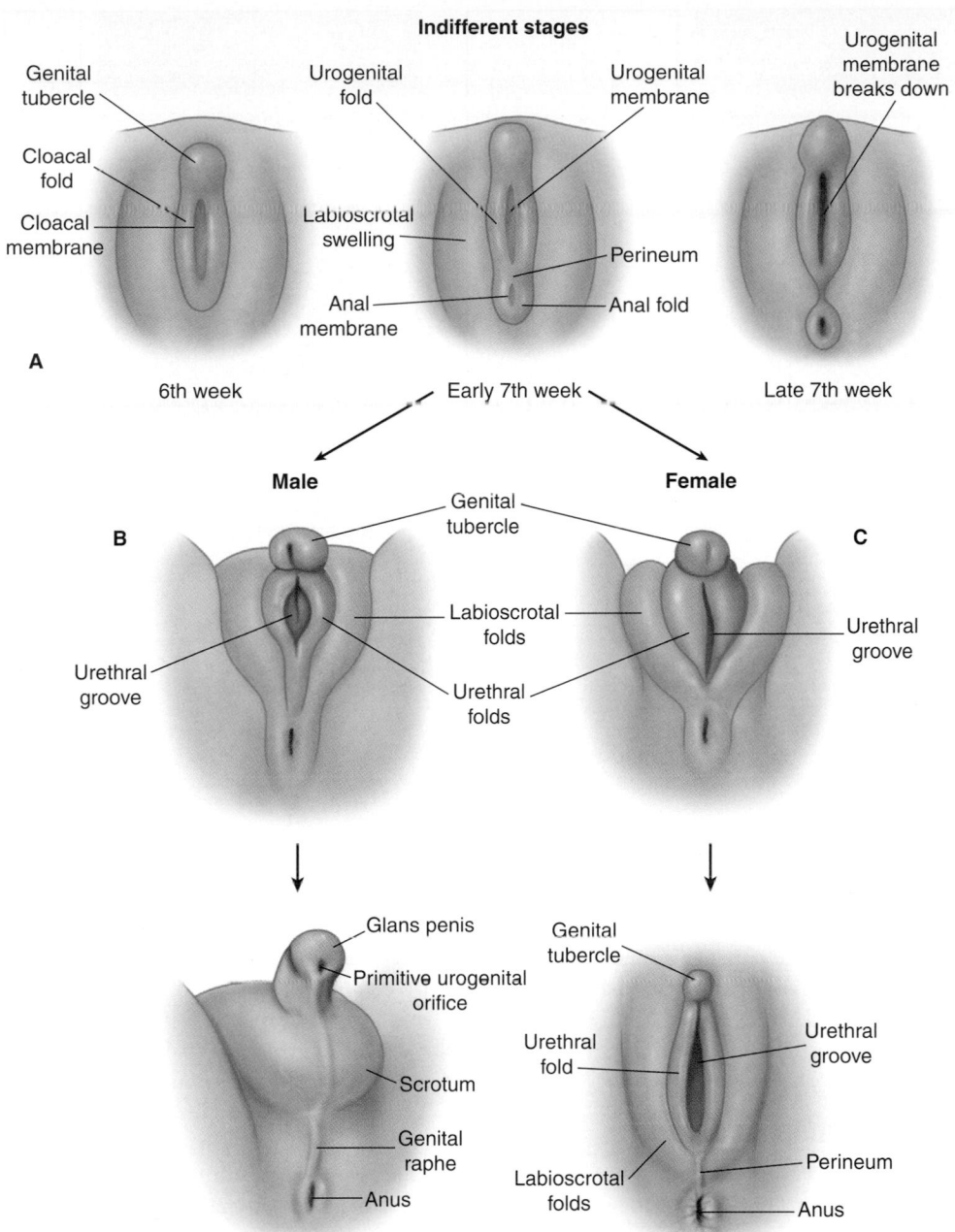

FIGURE 18-6 Development of the external genitalia. **A.** Indifferent stage. **B.** Virilization of external genitalia. **C.** Feminization.

Genetic Influences on Development

The pathways regulating female sexual differentiation have remained incompletely defined, but *WNT4*, *WT1*, *SF1*, and *DAX1* genes are important for normal development (MacLaughlin, 2004). For example, Vainio and colleagues (1999) showed that mice with a WNT4 mutation lack a vagina and uterus but retained testosterone-producing cells in the ovaries. Biason-Lauber and colleagues (2008) describe a human phenotype for WNT4 deficiency. Affected individual have müllerian agenesis as well as signs of ovarian hyperandrogenism, due to an abundance of Leydig cells in the ovaries.

Hox genes are regulators that encode highly conserved transcription factors. These factors control aspects of mor-

phogenesis and cell differentiation during normal embryonic development. Vertebrate Hox genes in groups 9–13 play a role in determining positional identity along the axis of the developing paramesonephric duct. *HoxA9* is one such gene that is expressed at high levels in areas destined to become the fallopian tube (Park, 2005). *HoxA10* and *11* are expressed in the developing and adult uterus. *HoxA11* is expressed in primordia of the lower uterine segment and cervix, whereas *HoxA13* is expressed in the ectocervix and upper vagina. No *HoxA12* has been described (Du, 2004). These and other ovarian determinant genes play an active role in gonadal and reproductive tract morphogenesis, but mechanisms are yet to be elucidated fully (MacLaughlin, 2004; Taylor, 2000).

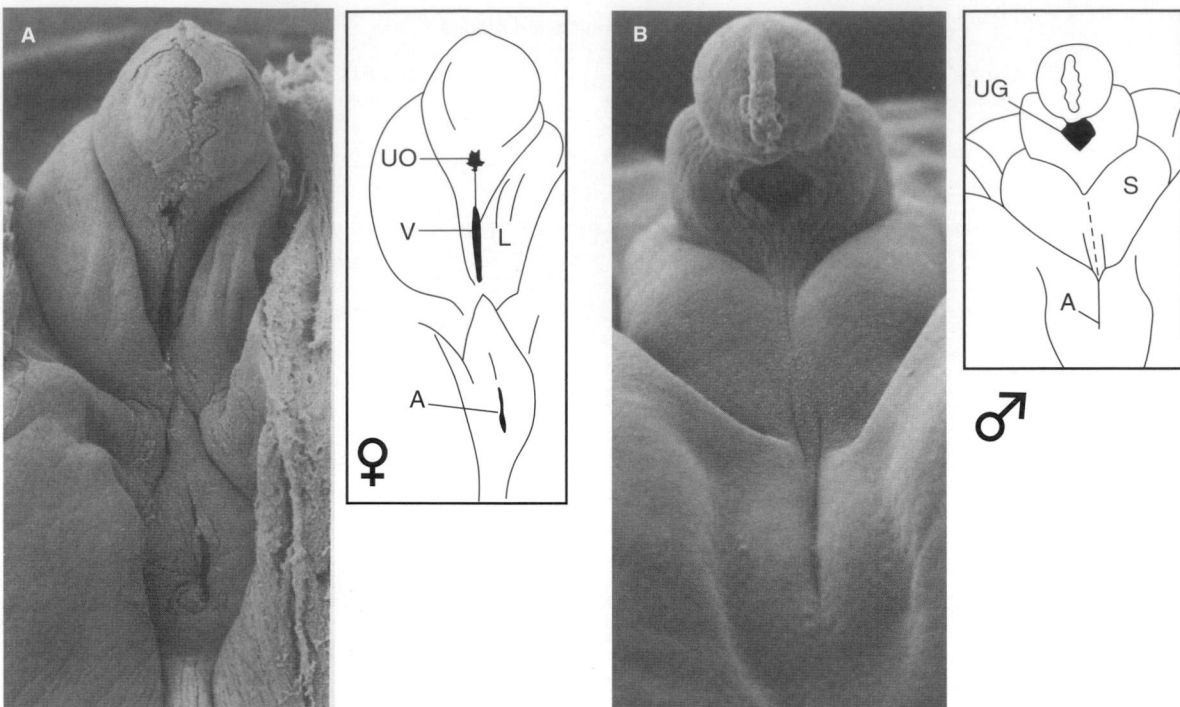

FIGURE 18-7 Scanning electron micrographs of external genitalia. **A.** 11-week female fetus. **B.** 10-week male fetus. A = anus; L = labia majora; S = scrotal fold; UG = urethral groove; UO = urethral orifice; V = vagina. *(From O'Rahilly, 2001, with permission.)*

DISORDERS OF SEX DEVELOPMENT

Disorders of sex development (DSD) are congenital conditions in which chromosomal, gonadal, or anatomic sexual development is atypical. These can be classified broadly into three categories according to gonadal histology (Table 18-2).

Female Pseudohermaphroditism (Category I)

Discordance between gonadal sex (46,XX) and the phenotypic appearance of external genitalia (masculinized) results from excessive fetal androgen exposure. In affected individuals, the ovaries and female internal ductal structures such as the uterus, cervix, and upper vagina are present. Accordingly, all patients with female pseudohermaphroditism are potentially fertile. The external genitalia, however, are virilized to a varying degree depending on the amount and timing of androgen exposure. As a result, virilization may range from modest clitoromegaly

TABLE 18-2. Classification of Ambiguous Genitalia

Category I	Female pseudohermaphroditism
Category II	Male pseudohermaphroditism
Category III	Disorders of genetic or gonadal development
	A. Gonadal dygenesis
	B. True hermaphroditism
	C. Embryonic testicular regression

to more extreme posterior labial fusion and development of a phallus with a penile urethra. Degrees of virilization can be described by the Prader score, which ranges from 0 for a normal-appearing female to 5 for a normal, virilized male.

Excessive androgen exposure may stem from adrenal abnormalities or nonadrenal sources. Fetal congenital adrenal hyperplasia due to the deficiency of 21-hydroxylase enzyme (CYP21) is the most common cause of female pseudohermaphroditism, with an incidence approximating one in 14,000 live births (White, 2000). In many cases, congenital adrenal hyperplasia can be diagnosed antenatally, and early maternal dexamethasone therapy can ameliorate the masculine phenotype (MacLaughlin, 2004). In addition, fetal 11β-hydroxylase (CYP11B) and 3β-hydroxysteroid dehydrogenase deficiencies can also lead to androgen excess and ambiguous genitalia (Fig. 15-5, p. 403).

Nonadrenal causes include maternal exposure to drugs such as testosterone, danazol, norethindrone, and other androgen derivatives. Maternal virilizing ovarian tumors, such as luteoma of pregnancy and Sertoli-Leydig cell tumor, or virilizing adrenal tumors may be other sources. Fortunately, these neoplasms infrequently cause fetal virilization because of the tremendous ability of the placental synciotrophoblast to convert C_{19} steroids (androstenedione and testosterone) to estradiol via the enzyme aromatase (Cunningham, 2010).

The three embryonic structures that are commonly affected by elevated androgen levels are the clitoris, labioscrotal folds, and urogenital sinus. Accordingly, successful reconstructive surgery in affected individuals should correct these structural abnormalities to ensure a good cosmetic result and adequate sexual function. To allow future fertility, vaginal adequacy is critical. Thus, the objectives of feminizing genitoplasty are to decrease enlarged clitoral size while maintaining vascularity and sensory innervations, to reduce and feminize the labioscrotal folds, and most importantly, to address the urogenital sinus, which usually involves creating a separate vaginal introitus in the perineum (Hensle, 2002).

Male Pseudohermaphroditism (Category II)

Insufficient androgen exposure of a fetus destined to be a male leads to male pseudohermaphroditism. The karyotype is 46,XY and testes are present. The uterus is generally absent as a result of normal embryonic AMH production by the Sertoli cells. These patients are most often sterile from abnormal spermatogenesis and have a small inadequate phallus for sexual function.

The etiology of male pseudohermaphroditism may involve: (1) enzyme defects in the biosynthesis of testosterone, (2) peripheral enzyme defects, or (3) abnormalities in the androgen receptor. First, within the testes, five enzyme defects have been associated with impaired testosterone production and include deficiencies of cholesterol side-chain cleavage enzyme (P450scc); 3β-hydroxysteroid dehydrogenase; 17α-hydroxylase; 17,20-desmolase (P450c17a); and 17β-hydroxysteroid dehydrogenase (Fig. 15-5, p. 403). The latter two enzyme deficiencies can also cause congenital adrenal hyperplasia. Secondly, peripherally, a defect in the 5-α reductase enzyme leads to impaired conversion of testosterone to DHT, the active androgen in peripheral tissues.

Finally, the androgen receptor may be defective and result in androgen-insensitivity syndrome (AIS). The estimated incidence of AIS ranges between one in 13,000 to 41,000 live births (Bangsboll, 1992; Blackless, 2000). The gene for the androgen receptor is found on the long arm of the X chromosome. Mutations may result in production of a nonfunctional receptor that will not bind androgen or may lead to receptors that bind androgen but are unable to effect full transcriptional activation. As a result, there may be complete resistance to androgens and no genital ambiguity (external genitalia appear as normal female). Alternatively, an incomplete form is associated with varying degrees of virilization and genital ambiguity. Milder forms of AIS have been described in men with severe male factor infertility and poor virilization. Testosterone therapy via patch or injection may be needed for continued masculine response.

Patients with complete androgen-insensitivity syndrome (CAIS) appear as phenotypically normal females at birth. They often present at puberty with primary amenorrhea and scant or absent pubic and axillary hair. These girls develop breasts during pubertal maturation due to abundant androgen-to-estrogen conversion. In affected individuals, external genitalia appear normal; scant or absent pubic hair is noted; the vagina is shortened; no cervix is seen; and the uterus and fallopian tubes are absent. Testes may be palpable in the labia or inguinal area or may be found intraabdominally. Laboratory evaluation demonstrates elevated luteinizing hormone (LH) levels, nor-

mal or slightly elevated male testosterone levels, and a 46,XY karyotype.

In CAIS patients, surgical excision of the testes after puberty is recommended to decrease the associated risk of germ cell tumors, which may be as high as 20 to 30 percent (Chap. 36, p. 882) (Chavhan, 2008). Additionally, estrogen should be replaced to reach physiologic levels, and a functional vagina is created either by dilation or surgical vaginoplasty. Examples of adequate hormonal replacement include 0.05 to 0.1 mg of estradiol transdermally; 0.5 to 1 mg of oral estradiol; or 0.625 to 1.25 mg of oral conjugated estrogen. Adequate replacement in these patients is important to maintain breast development and bone mass and to provide relief from vasomotor symptoms.

"Women" with CAIS were never virilized in utero or postnatally due to their total inability to respond to androgens. They have a female gender identity. In affected individuals, sexual function may be normal, whereas others may complain of sexual difficulties (Lewis, 1986; Minto, 2003; Vague, 1983; Wisniewski, 2000). Most common are sexual infrequency and vaginal penetration difficulty, as is seen sometimes with müllerian agenesis. Treatment with estrogen cream and dilators may lead to vaginal dilation and satisfactory intercourse. In others, vaginal reconstruction, as discussed in Section 41-25 (p. 1075), may be offered.

Disorders of Genetic or Gonadal Development (Category III)

Several conditions, such as gonadal dysgenesis, true hermaphroditism, and embryonic testicular regression, may all lead to the development of ambiguous or infantile genitalia.

Gonadal Dysgenesis

Abnormal development of the gonads, that is, *gonadal dysgenesis*, results most often from nondisjunction of parental chromosomes and leads to streak gonads. In affected patients, gonadal failure is indicated by elevated gonadotropin levels.

In 50 to 60 percent of patients with gonadal dysgenesis, the karyotype is 45,X, and this condition is called Turner syndrome. The classic stigmata of Turner syndrome are shown in (Fig. 18-8). Of these, cubitus valgus is an elbow deformity that deviates the forearm greater than 15 degrees when the arm is extended at the side. Associated problems include cardiac anomalies (especially coarctation of the aorta), renal anomalies, hearing impairment, otitis media and mastoiditis, and an increased incidence of hypertension, achlorhydria, diabetes mellitus, and Hashimoto thyroiditis. This syndrome may be recognized in childhood. However, some patients are not diagnosed until adolescence, when they present with short stature, prepubertal female genitalia, and primary amenorrhea. The uterus and vagina are normal and capable of responding to exogenous hormones.

Other patients with gonadal dysgenesis have a mosaic karyotype (e.g., 46,XX/45,X) or a structural abnormality of the second X chromosome. They may exhibit some or all of the signs of Turner syndrome. Patients with mosaicism are more likely to have some pubertal maturation.

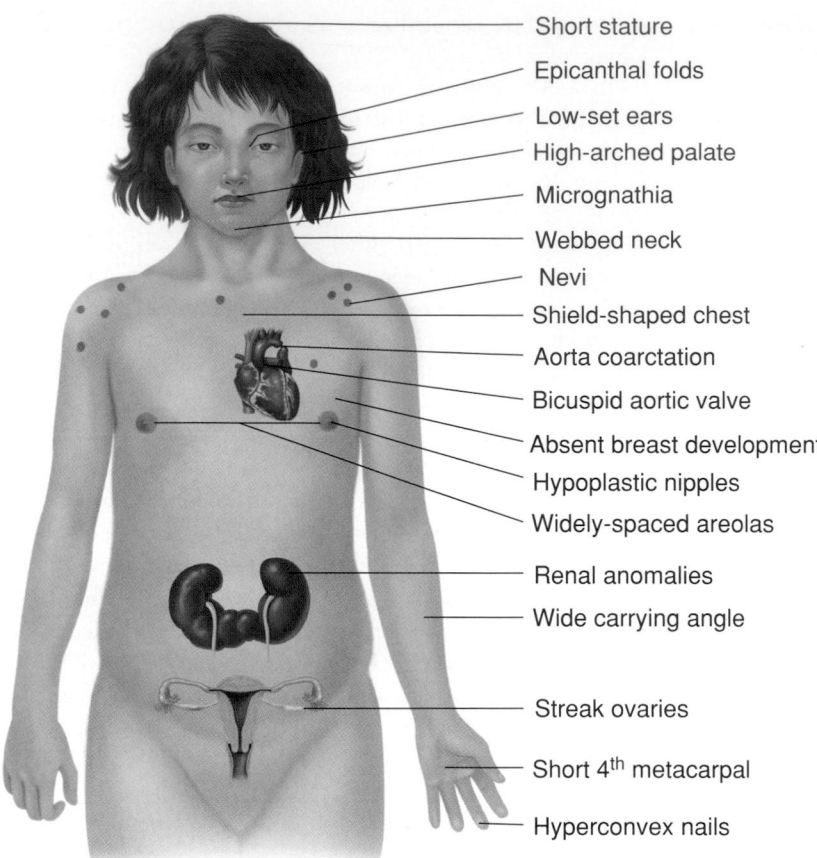

Short stature
Epicanthal folds
Low-set ears
High-arched palate
Micrognathia
Webbed neck
Nevi
Shield-shaped chest
Aorta coarctation
Bicuspid aortic valve
Absent breast development
Hypoplastic nipples
Widely-spaced areolas
Renal anomalies
Wide carrying angle
Streak ovaries
Short 4th metacarpal
Hyperconvex nails

FIGURE 18-8 Characteristic physical findings that may be found in women with Turner syndrome.

The term *pure gonadal dysgenesis* includes patients with normal stature and the gonadal abnormality of Turner syndrome. The karyotype may be 46,XY or 46,XX. In XY patients (Swyer syndrome), the absent testis results from the lack of SRY or other testis-determining factors on the Y chromosome. These streak gonads fail to produce androgens or AMH. Patients appear as normal prepubertal females and have a normal müllerian system due to absent AMH. Because of the Y chromosome, these patients are at increased risk of gonadal tumors and thus require gonad removal. In those with pure gonadal dysgenesis and a 46,XX karyotype, the defect in gonadal development has not been clarified.

All types of gonadal dysgenesis typically require hormone treatment to effect breast development. Our protocol uses estradiol, 0.25 mg orally each day for approximately 6 months beginning near age 12 or at the time of diagnosis. The estradiol dose is sequentially increased every 6 months through daily doses of 0.5 mg, 0.75 mg, 1 mg, and then 2 mg. We colloquially term this the "start low and go slow" protocol. Progesterone is begun after approximately 1 year of unopposed estrogen treatment. Each month, micronized progesterone, 200 mg orally nightly, is given for 12 nights and then stopped to permit withdrawal bleeding. This method mimics normal pubertal hormonal stimulation of breast tissue. The patient is then maintained on 2 mg of oral estradiol and monthly withdrawal to progesterone. Alternatively, a low-dose

combination oral contraceptive would also be acceptable maintenance.

True Hermaphroditism

With this condition, affected individuals have both ovarian and testicular gonadal tissue. The most common karyotype in true hermaphrodites is 46,XX, followed by 46,XX/46,XY. The phenotype of a 46,XX true hermaphrodite includes a unilateral ovotestis with a contralateral ovary or testis, or bilateral ovotestes. The gonadal location varies from abdominal to inguinal to scrotal. The nature of the internal ductal system depends on the ipsilateral gonad and its degree of differentiation. The amount of AMH and testosterone present determines the degree to which the internal ductal system is masculinized or feminized. External genitalia are usually ambiguous and undermasculinized due to an inadequate amount of testosterone.

In *46,XX sex-reversed males,* male sexual differentiation occurs in the presence of a 46,XX karyotype. In this condition, varying lengths of DNA from the Y chromosome are translocated to the X chromosome during meiosis. The *SRY* gene is abnormally translocated to the X chromosome in approximately 60 percent of 46,XX sex-reversed males (Kolon, 1998; Schweikert, 1982). In individuals without SRY translocation, it is likely that other downstream Y, X, or autosomal testis-determining factor genes are present or activated. SRY guides the gonad to develop along testicular lines, and testicular hormone function is near normal. Production of AMH prompts müllerian system regression, and androgens promote development of the Wolffian system and external genitalia masculinization. Spermatogenesis, however, is absent due to a lack of certain genes on the long arm of the Y chromosome. These individuals are not usually diagnosed until puberty or during an infertility evaluation. Semen analysis reveals azoospermia. The testes are usually small and may be cryptorchid. The penis may be small, and hypospadias is present in approximately 10 percent.

Embryonic Testicular Regression

Individuals with this condition may or may not produce AMH, and therefore the uterus may be present or absent. Similarly, the karyotype may or may not be abnormal, that is, 46,XY/45,X (mixed gonadal dysgenesis); 46,XX (true hermaphroditism); or 46,XY (embryonic testicular regression). There is variable androgen secretion among these disorders, and thus phenotypic presentations may be diverse.

Klinefelter's syndrome (47,XXY) occurs in one in 500 births or 1 to 2 percent of all males. These individuals tend to be tall, undervirilized males with gynecomastia and small, firm testes. They have significantly reduced fertility due to hypogonadism and are at increased risk for germ cell tumors, osteoporosis, and breast cancer.

Gender Assignment

At birth, gender assignment to the normal newborn usually involves a simple assessment of the external genitalia and a straightforward joyful declaration of male or female by the obstetrician. Delivery of a newborn with a disorder of sex development is a potential medical emergency and presents a serious psychosocial, diagnostic, medical and possibly surgical challenge for a multispecialty medical team. Ambiguous external genitalia in a newborn can create possible long-lasting psychosexual and social ramifications for the individual and family. Ideally, as soon as the neonate with ambiguous genitalia is stable, parents should be able to hold the child, if possible. The newborn should be referred to as "your baby." The obstetrician should explain that the genitalia are incompletely formed and should emphasize the seriousness of the situation and the need for rapid consultation and laboratory testing (Fig. 18-9). Other suggested terms to use while discussing ambiguous development include "phallus," "gonads," "folds" to reference underdeveloped labia or scrotum and "urogenital sinus" to describe the vagina or urethra. Relevant neonatal physical examination should evaluate: (1) ability to palpate gonads in the labioscrotal or inguinal regions, (2) ability to palpate uterus during rectal examination, (3) phallus size, (3) genitalia pigmentation, and (4) presence of other syndromic features. The newborn's metabolic condition should be assessed, as hyperkalemia, hyponatremia, and hypoglycemia may be indicative of congenital adrenal hyperplasia. The mother should be examined for signs of hyperandrogenism (Thyen, 2006). In addition, pediatric endocrinologists and reproductive endocrinologists should be consulted as soon as possible. During education of the family, the need for accurate determination of gender and sex of rearing should be emphasized. Discussions should include the need for hormonal stimulation at puberty and potential later surgical reconstruction.

DEFECTS OF THE BLADDER AND PERINEUM

Bladder exstrophy follows failure of the cloacal membrane to be reinforced by an ingrowth of mesoderm. The bilaminar cloacal membrane lies at the caudal end of the germinal disc and forms the infraumbilical abdominal wall. Normally, an ingrowth of mesoderm between the ectodermal and endodermal layers of the cloacal membrane leads to formation of the lower abdominal musculature and the pelvic bones. Without reinforcement, the cloacal membrane may prematurely rupture. Depending on the extent of the infraumbilical defect and the stage of development at which it ruptures, bladder exstrophy, cloacal exstrophy, or epispadias results (Gearhart, 1992).

The incidence of bladder exstrophy has been estimated to range between 1 in 10,000 and 1 in 50,000 (Lattimer, 1966; Rickham, 1960). This anomaly displays a predilection for males, and the male-to-female ratio approximates 2:1.

Exstrophy is characterized by an exposed bladder lying outside the abdomen. Associated findings commonly include abnormal external genitalia and a widened symphysis pubis, caused by the outward rotation of the innominate bones. Stanton (1974) noted that 43 percent of 70 females with bladder exstrophy had associated reproductive tract anomalies. The urethra and vagina are typically short, and the vaginal orifice is frequently stenotic and displaced anteriorly. The clitoris is duplicated or bifid, and the labia, mons pubis, and clitoris are divergent. The uterus, fallopian tubes, and ovaries are typically normal except for occasional müllerian duct fusion defects.

Reconstruction of the female genitalia presents a less complex problem than that in the male. Surgical closure of the exstrophy is currently performed in the first 3 years of life as a staged surgical procedure (Damario, 1994; Dees, 1949). Vaginal dilatation or vaginoplasty may be required to allow satisfactory intercourse in mature females (Jones, 1973). Long term, the defective pelvic floor may predispose women to uterine prolapse (Gearhart, 1992).

DEFECTS OF THE CLITORIS

Congenital abnormalities of the clitoris are unusual, but they include clitoral duplication, female phallic urethra, or clitoromegaly. Clitoral duplication, also known as bifid clitoris, usually develops in association with bladder exstrophy, described previously, or with epispadias. The disorder is rare, and the incidence approximates one in 480,000 females (Elder, 1992).

In those with epispadias but without bladder exstrophy, visibly apparent anomalies include a widened, patulous urethra; absent or bifid clitoris; nonfused labial folds (majora and minora); and flattened mons pubis. Vertebral abnormalities and diastases of the pubic symphysis are also commonly associated.

Another clitoral anomaly is the female phallic urethra and is found in association with the persistent cloaca (Sotolongo, 1983). The phallic urethra opens at the tip of the clitoris. This anomaly affects 4 to 8 percent of girls with persistent cloaca and has been described in association with embryonic exposure to cocaine (Karlin, 1989).

Clitoromegaly noted at birth is suggestive of fetal female exposure to excessive androgens. Clitoromegaly is defined as a clitoral index >10 mm^2. This index is determined by the glans length times the width. Moreover, early androgen exposure in females may lead to fusion of the labioscrotal folds and findings of a single perineal opening, the urogenital sinus. Labia are rugated and scrotumlike. A gonad found in the groin or labia majora, however, should raise the concern of male pseudohermaphroditism.

Frequently in premature neonates, the clitoris may appear large, but it does not change size and appears to regress as the infant grows. Other causes of newborn clitoromegaly include breech presentation with vulvar swelling, chronic severe vulvovaginitis, and neurofibromatosis (Dershwitz, 1984; Greer, 1981).

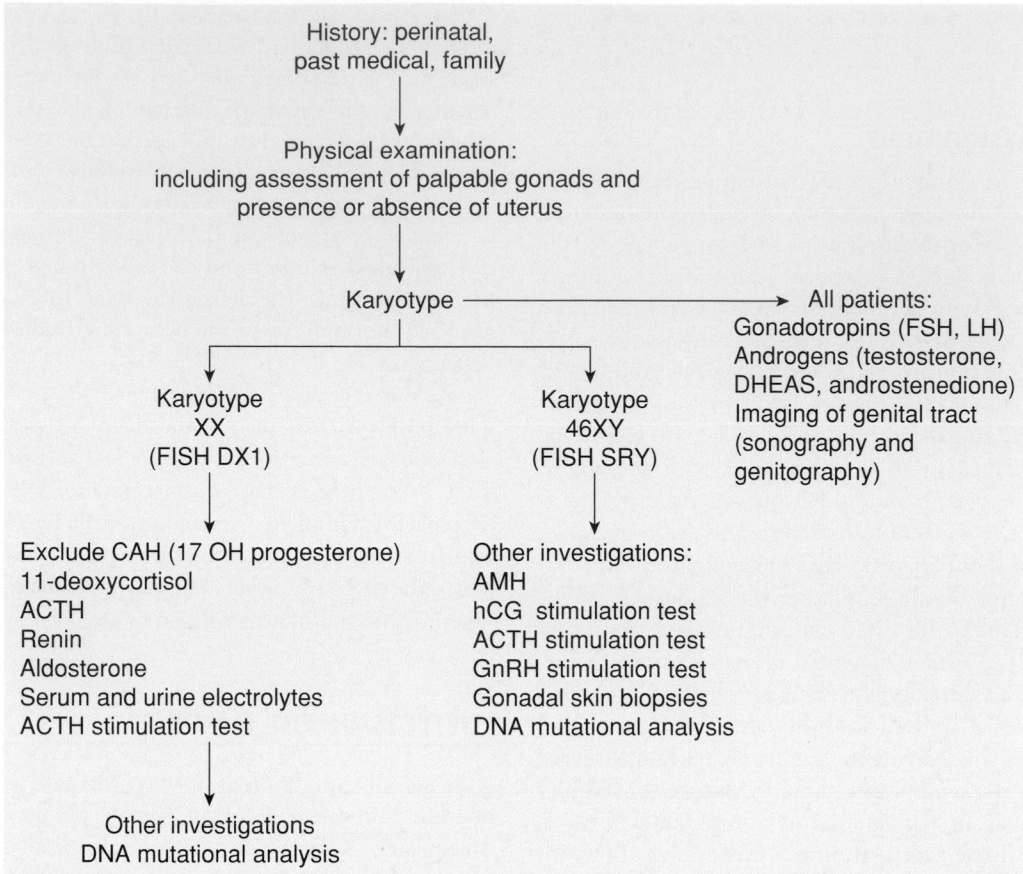

FIGURE 18-9 One algorithm for investigating disorders of sexual development. Genitography is a fluoroscopic study in which contrast is flushed retrograde into the urogenital sinus orifice to potentially highlight the urethra, bladder, and vagina. ACTH = adrenocorticotropic hormone; AMH = antimüllerian hormone; CAH = congenital adrenal hyperplasia; DHEAS = dehydroepiandrosterone sulfate; FISH = fluorescent in situ hybridization; FSH = follicle-stimulating hormone; GnRH = gonadotropin-releasing hormone; hCG = human chorionic gonadotropin; LH = luteinizing hormone. *(Adapted from Allen, 2009, with permission.)*

HYMENEAL DEFECTS

The hymen is the membranous vestige of the junction between the sinovaginal bulbs and the urogenital sinus (see Fig. 18-4). It generally becomes perforate during fetal life to establish a connection between the vaginal lumen and the perineum. A variety of hymeneal abnormalities include imperforate, microperforate, annular, septate, cribriform (sievelike), naviculate (boat-like), or septate types (Fig. 18-10) (Breech, 1999). Imperforate hymen follows failure of the inferior end of the vaginal plate to canalize, and its incidence approximates 1 in 1000 to 2000 females (Parazzini, 1990). Although typically sporadic, imperforate hymen in multiple family members has been reported (Lim, 2003; Stelling, 2000; Usta, 1993).

If the hymen is imperforate, blood from endometrial sloughing or mucus accumulates in the vagina. During the neonatal period, significant amounts of mucus can be secreted secondary to maternal estradiol stimulation. The newborn may have a bulging, translucent yellow-gray mass at the vaginal introitus. This condition is termed hydro/mucocolpos. Most cases are asymptomatic and resolve as the mucus is reabsorbed and estrogen levels decrease. However, large hydro/mucocolpos may

cause respiratory distress or may obstruct the ureters, resulting in hydronephrosis (Breech, 2009).

After menarche, adolescents with imperforate hymen present with trapped menstrual blood behind the hymen, which creates a bluish bulge at the introitus (Fig. 18-11). With cyclic menstruation, the vaginal canal greatly distends, and the cervix may dilate and allow formation of a hematometra and hematosalpinx. Cyclic pain, amenorrhea, abdominal pain mimicking acute abdomen, and difficulty with urination or defecation may be presenting symptoms (Bakos, 1999). Moreover, retrograde menstruation may lead to the development of endometriosis. Other obstructive reproductive tract anomalies that are located more cephalad, such as transverse vaginal septum, may present similarly.

Patients with microperforate, cribriform, or septate hymen will typically complain of menstrual irregularities or difficulty with tampon placement or intercourse. Imperforate or microperforate hymen may be corrected when diagnosed and is illustrated in Section 41-17 (p. 1062). Breech and Laufer (1999) advocate repair when estrogen is present to improve tissue healing, either in infancy or after thelarche, but before menarche. This timing avoids the formation of hematocolpos and possible

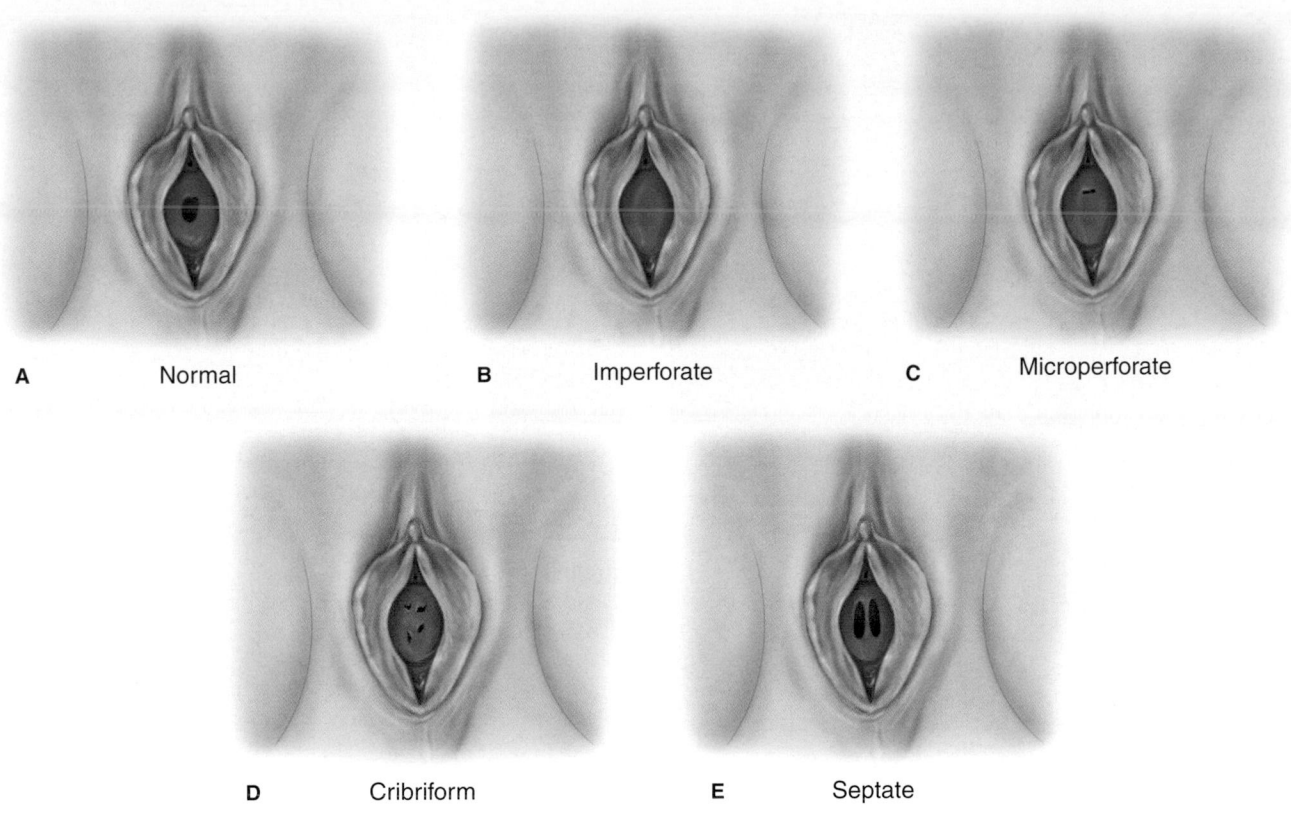

| A | Normal | B | Imperforate | C | Microperforate |

| D | Cribriform | E | Septate |

FIGURE 18-10 Types of hymens.

hematometra. Laparoscopy may be performed concurrently with hymenectomy to exclude endometriosis. Importantly, clinicians should avoid needle aspiration of a hematocolpos for diagnosis or treatment. Aspiration may seed the retained blood with bacteria and increase infection risks. Moreover, recurrent hematocolpos secondary to inadequate drainage is common following needle aspiration alone.

Hymeneal cysts in the newborn must be differentiated from an imperforate hymen with hydro/mucocolpos (Nazir, 2006). These cysts typically have an opening and may regress spontaneously (Berkman, 2004). They may also be treated by incision and drainage. Simple puncture of these without anesthesia has also been successfully performed.

TRANSVERSE VAGINAL SEPTUM

Transverse vaginal septa are believed to arise from failed müllerian duct fusion or failed canalization of the vaginal plate (Fig. 18-12). The anomaly is uncommon, and Banerjee (1998) reported an incidence of 1 in 70,000 females. A septum may be obstructive, with mucus or menstrual blood accumulation, or nonobstructive, with mucus and blood egress.

Transverse vaginal septum can develop at any level within the vagina but is more common in the upper portion. This corresponds to the junction between the vaginal plate and the caudal end of the fused müllerian ducts (see Fig. 18-5). Rock (1982) found that 46 percent of septa were located in the upper vagina,

35 percent in the middle, and 19 percent in the lower vagina. The thickness of the septum may vary, and thicker septa tend to lie nearer the cervix. Typically, a septum is thin (average thickness of 1 cm), but Rock (1982) reported septal thicknesses up to 5 to 6 cm.

In neonates and infants, obstructive transverse vaginal septum has been associated with fluid and mucus collection in the upper vagina. The resulting mass may be large enough to compress abdominal or pelvic organs. In addition, pyomucocolpos, pyometra, and pyosalpinges may develop from ascension of vaginal or perineal bacteria through small perforations within a septum (Breech, 1999). In contrast to other müllerian duct defects, transverse vaginal septum is associated with few urologic abnormalities.

Patients with transverse vaginal septum usually present with symptoms similar to those of imperforate hymen. The diagnosis is suspected when an abdominal or pelvic mass is palpated or when a foreshortened vagina and inability to identify the cervix is encountered. Diagnosis is confirmed by either sonography or magnetic resonance (MR) imaging. Magnetic resonance imaging is most helpful prior to surgery to determine the septal thickness and depth (Fig. 18-13). In addition, MR imaging may identify whether a cervix is present, and thereby allow differentiation of a high vaginal septum from cervical agenesis.

Surgical repair technique is dependent upon septal thickness, and skin grafts may occasionally be necessary to cover the defect left by excision of very thick septa. Smaller septa

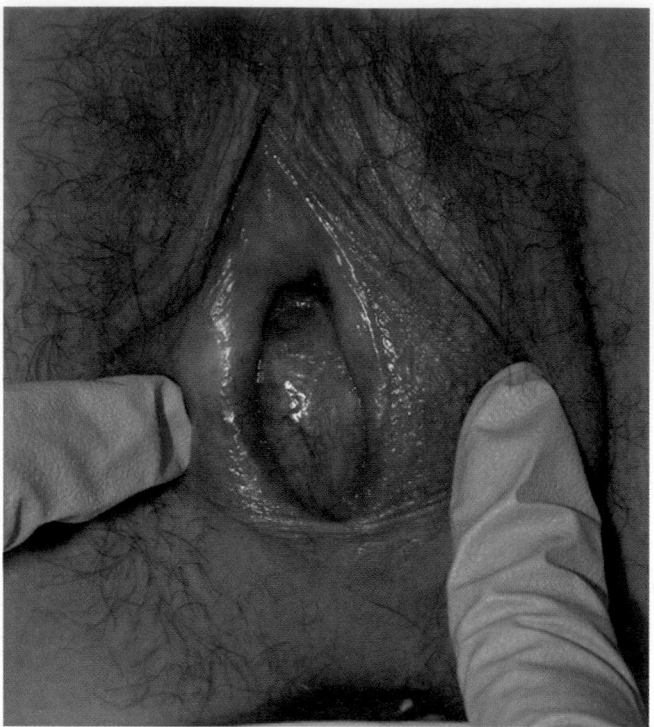

FIGURE 18-11 Photograph of imperforate hymen. *(Photograph contributed by Dr. Ellen Wilson.)*

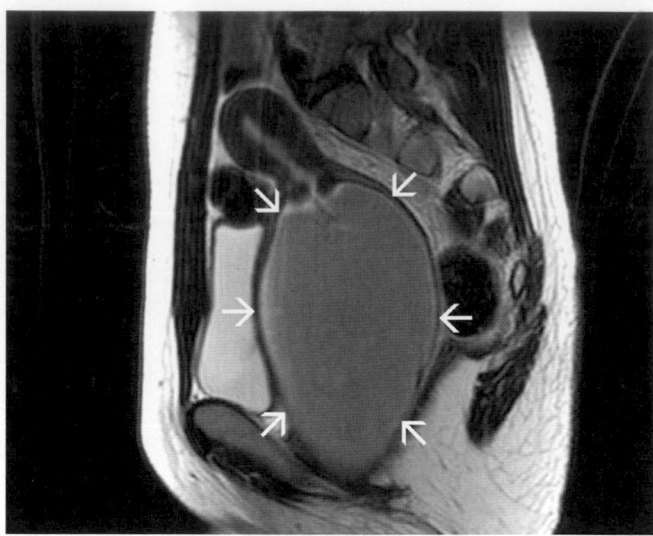

FIGURE 18-13 Magnetic resonance image of complete low transverse septum with obstruction. Marked hematocolpos is identified *(arrows)* in this 13-year-old female. The relatively low signal intensity on the T2-weighted images is consistent with subacute blood. The uterus is seen above the hematocolpos. *(Image contributed by Dr. Doug Sims.)*

may be removed by excision followed by end-to-end anastomosis of the upper and lower vagina (Section 41-24, p. 1073). Alternative to excision with end-to-end anastomosis, Garcia (1967) reported a Z-plasty technique that may minimize scar formation. Sanfilippo (1986) recommends laparoscopy concurrently with transverse vaginal septum excision because of the high rate of endometriosis due to retrograde menstruation from outflow tract obstruction.

LONGITUDINAL VAGINAL SEPTUM

A longitudinal vaginal septum results from defective lateral fusion and incomplete reabsorption of the caudal portion of the müllerian ducts. These septa may be partial or extend the complete vaginal length. Longitudinal septa are generally seen with partial or complete duplication of the cervix and uterus. They may also accompany anorectal malformations (Breech, 2009). Of affected women, up to 20 percent may have renal abnormalities.

Affected individuals complain of difficulty with intercourse. Vaginal bleeding may occur despite placement of a tampon, because the tampon is placed in only one of the duplicated vaginas. The nonobstructed form can be managed conservatively unless dyspareunia develops. However, an obstructive variety of longitudinal vaginal septum can develop (Fig. 18-14). Typically, the patient presents in adolescence with normal menarche, but reports worsening, monthly unilateral vaginal and pelvic pain from outflow obstruction (Carlson, 1992). During examination, a patent vagina and cervix is noted, but a unilateral vaginal and pelvic mass can be palpated. Obstructed hemivagina is almost universally associated with ipsilateral renal agenesis. Together obstructed hemivagina with ipsilateral renal agenesis has been labeled OHVIRA syndrome.

Surgical correction consists of wide excision of the obstructing septum, taking precautions to avoid the urethra/bladder and rectum. During excision, sonographic guidance can be useful to identify the distended upper vagina (Breech, 2009). Joki-Erkkila and Heinonen (2003) followed 26 females after surgical repair of obstructive outflow tract anomalies. They found a high rate of vaginal stricture requiring reoperation,

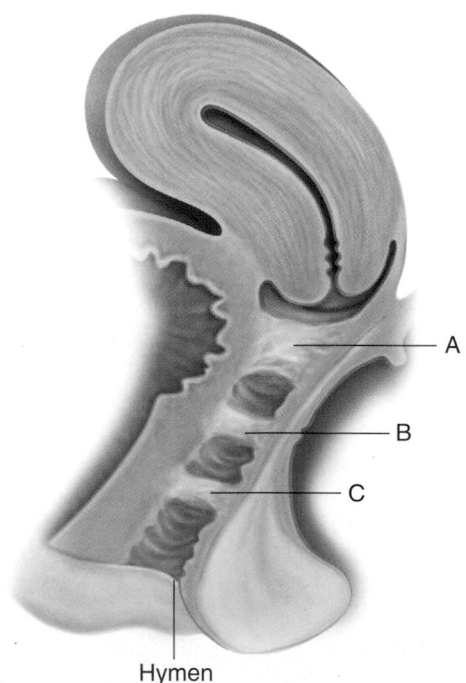

A

B

C

Hymen

FIGURE 18-12 Potential locations of transverse vaginal septa. *(Redrawn from Rock, 1982.)*

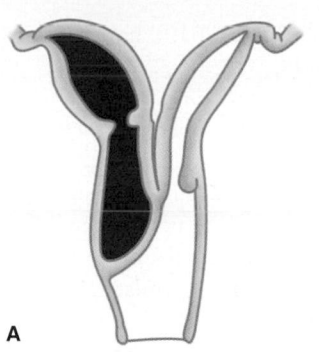 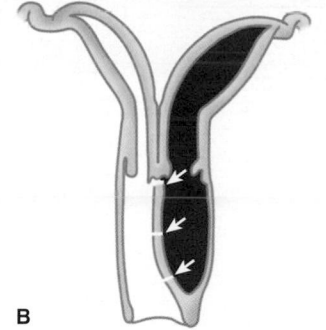 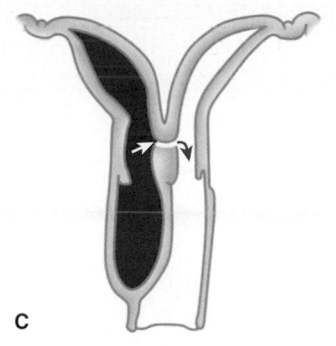

FIGURE 18-14 Uterine didelphys with obstructed hemivagina. **A.** Complete obstruction. **B.** Partial vaginal communication. **C.** Partial uterine communication. *(Adapted from Rock, 1980.)*

as well as dysfunctional uterine bleeding, dyspareunia, and dysmenorrhea.

CONGENITAL VAGINAL CYSTS

Although in each sex the müllerian or Wolffian ducts marked for degeneration do regress, vestigial remnants can be found and may become clinically apparent. Mesonephric (Wolffian) remnants may give rise to Gartner duct cysts. Clinically important müllerian remnants are typically found as vaginal cysts.

As a whole, vaginal cysts are reported in approximately 1 in 200 females (Hwang, 2009). Remnant cysts are typically located in the anterolateral wall of the vagina, although they may be found at various locations along its length. Most are asymptomatic, benign, measure 1 to 7 cm in diameter, and do not require surgical excision. Deppisch (1975) described 25 cases of symptomatic vaginal cysts and reported a wide range of symptoms. These included dyspareunia, vaginal pain, difficulty with tampon use, urinary symptoms, and palpable mass. If these cysts become infected and intervention is required during the acute phase, cyst marsupialization is preferred.

Occasionally, a remnant cyst may cause chronic symptoms that warrant excision. Pelvic magnetic resonance (MR) imaging can be helpful prior to surgery to determine the extent of the cyst and its anatomic relationship to the ureter or bladder base (Hwang, 2009). Of note, complete vaginal cyst excision may be more difficult than anticipated, as some may extend up into the broad ligament and anatomically approximate the distal course of the ureter.

MÜLLERIAN ANOMALIES

Anomalies of the uterus may be congenital or acquired and typically present with menstrual abnormalities, pelvic pain, infertility, or pregnancy wastage. The true incidence of congenital müllerian anomalies, of which uterine malformations constitute the majority, is unknown. Most cases are diagnosed during evaluation for obstetric or gynecologic problems, but in the absence of symptoms, most anomalies remain undiagnosed. Because nearly 57 percent of women with uterine defects have successful fertility and pregnancy, the true incidence of congenital müllerian defects may be significantly understated. Simon

and colleagues (1991) found uterine anomalies in 3 percent of 679 fertile women undergoing laparoscopic tubal sterilization. Nahum (1998) found that the prevalence of uterine anomalies in the general population was 1 in 201 women or 0.5 percent.

Anatomic uterine defects have long been recognized as a cause of obstetric complications. Recurrent pregnancy loss, preterm labor, abnormal fetal presentation, and prematurity constitute the major reproductive problems encountered. Cunningham and colleagues (2010) provide a full discussion of specific müllerian defects and their obstetric importance. Müllerian defects are also associated with renal anomalies in 30 to 50 percent of cases, and defects include renal agenesis, severe renal hypoplasia, and ectopic or duplicate ureters (Sharara, 1998).

Various classification schemes for female reproductive tract anomalies exist, but the most commonly used system was proposed by Buttram and Gibbons (1979) and adapted by the American Society for Reproductive Medicine (American Fertility Society, 1988) (Table 18-3). Within this system, six categories organize similar embryonic developmental defects. Moreover, Acien (2009) and Rock (2010) have described types of uterovaginal and cervical malformations that do not adapt to the usual classification systems. Such anomalies should be described and drawn in detail in a patient's medical record for future reference.

Segmental Müllerian Hypoplasia or Agenesis

Some form of müllerian aplasia, hypoplasia, or agenesis affects one in every 4000 to 10,000 females and is a common cause of primary amenorrhea (American College of Obstetricians and Gynecologists, 2006). Uterine agenesis follows failed development of the lower portion of the müllerian ducts and usually leads to absence of the uterus, cervix, and upper part of the vagina (Patton, 1994). Variants may display absence of the upper vagina but presence of the uterus. Normal ovaries are found, and affected individuals otherwise develop as phenotypically normal females and present with primary amenorrhea.

Vaginal Atresia

Females with vaginal atresia lack the lower portion of the vagina, but otherwise have normal external genitalia (Fig. 18-15A). Embryologically, the urogenital sinus fails to contribute its

TABLE 18-3. Classification of Müllerian Anomalies

I. Segmental müllerian hypoplasia or agenesis
   a. Vaginal
   b. Cervical
   c. Uterine
   d. Tubal
   e. Combined
II. Unicornuate uterus
   a. Rudimentary horn with cavity, communicating to unicornuate uterus
   b. Rudimentary horn with cavity, not communicating to unicornuate uterus
   c. Rudimentary horn with no cavity
   d. Unicornuate uterus without a rudimentary horn
III. Uterine didelphys
IV. Bicornuate uterus
   a. Complete bifurcation (bicollis)
   b. Partial bifurcation (unicollis)
V. Septate uterus
   a. Complete septation
   b. Partial septation
VI. Arcuate uterus
VII. Diethylstilbestrol-related anomalies

From the American Fertility Society, 1988, with permission.

expected caudal portion of the vagina (Simpson, 1999). As a result, the lower portion of the vagina, usually one fifth to one third of the total length, is replaced by 2 to 3 cm of fibrous tissue. In some individuals, however, vaginal atresia may extend to near the cervix.

Since most affected women have normal external genitalia and upper reproductive tract organs, vaginal atresia does not often become apparent until menarche. Adolescents generally present shortly after physiologic menarche with cyclic pelvic pain due to hematocolpos or hematometra. On physical examination, breasts, pubic hair distribution, perineum, and hymeneal ring are normal. But beyond the hymeneal ring, only a vaginal dimple or small pouch is found. A rectoabdominal examination confirms the presence of midline organs. Additionally, sonographic or MR imaging will display upper reproductive tract organs. Of these, MR imaging is the most accurate diagnostic tool, as the length of the atresia, the amount of upper vaginal dilatation, and the presence or absence of a cervix can be identified. Identification of the cervix in such cases distinguishes vaginal atresia from müllerian agenesis. Laparoscopy, however, is often necessary when anatomy cannot be fully evaluated with radiographic studies. Treatment follows that for müllerian agenesis.

Cervical Agenesis

Because of the common müllerian source, women with congenital absence of the cervix typically also lack the upper vagina. The uterus, however, usually develops normally (Fig. 18-15C).

In addition to agenesis, Rock (2010) has described various forms of cervical dysgenesis.

Women with cervical agenesis initially present similarly to patients with other reproductive tract obstructive anomalies, that is, with primary amenorrhea and cyclic abdominal or pelvic pain. If a functional endometrium is present, a patient may have a distended uterus, and endometriosis may have developed secondary to retrograde menstrual flow. A single midline uterine fundus is the norm, although bilateral hemiuteri have also been described (Dillon, 1979).

Radiographic studies, sonography, and MR imaging are helpful in evaluating anatomy. If imaging demonstrates an obstructed uterus, hysterectomy has been recommended by some (Rock, 1984). In contrast, Niver (1980) and others report creation of an epithelialized endocervical tract and vagina. However, significant morbidity, including infection, recurrent obstruction requiring hysterectomy, and death due to sepsis has been reported with establishment of such a vaginal-uterine connection (Casey, 1997; Rock, 2010). Alternatively, conservative management with GnRH antagonists or agonists or with combination oral contraceptive pills may be used to suppress retrograde menses and possible endometriosis until a patient is ready for reproduction options (Doyle, 2009). Thus, the uterus may be retained for possible reproductive potential. Thijssen and associates (1990) reported a successful pregnancy using zygote intrafallopian tube transfer in a patient with cervical agenesis. Gestational surrogacy offers another viable option for these women.

Müllerian Agenesis

Congenital absence of both the uterus and vagina is termed müllerian aplasia, müllerian agenesis, or Mayer-Rokitansky-Kuster-Hauser syndrome (American College of Obstetricians and Gynecologists, 2006). In classic müllerian agenesis, patients have a shallow vaginal pouch, only measuring 1 to 2 inches deep. In addition, the uterus, cervix, and upper part of the vagina are absent. Typically, a portion of the distal fallopian tubes are present. Also, normal ovaries are expected, given their separate embryonic source. Most patients with müllerian agenesis have only small rudimentary müllerian bulbs without endometrial activity. However, in 2 to 7 percent of women with this condition, active endometrium develops and patients typically present with cyclic abdominal pain (American College of Obstetricians and Gynecologists, 2002). Surgical excision of symptomatic rudimentary bulbs is required. With müllerian agenesis, traditional conception is impossible, but pregnancy may be achieved using the combination of oocyte retrieval, in vitro fertilization, and gestational surrogacy.

Evaluation for associated congenital renal or other skeletal anomalies is essential in individuals with müllerian hypoplasia or agenesis. Approximately 15 to 36 percent of women with uterine agenesis also have defects of the urinary system, and 12 percent may have scoliosis. Recently a syndrome known as MURCS (müllerian duct aplasia, renal aplasia, cervicothoracic somite dysplasia) has been described (Oppelt, 2006). Other skeletal malformations observed include spina bifida, sacralization (partial fusion to the sacrum) of L5, lumbarization (nonfusion of the first and second sacral segments) of the sacral bone,

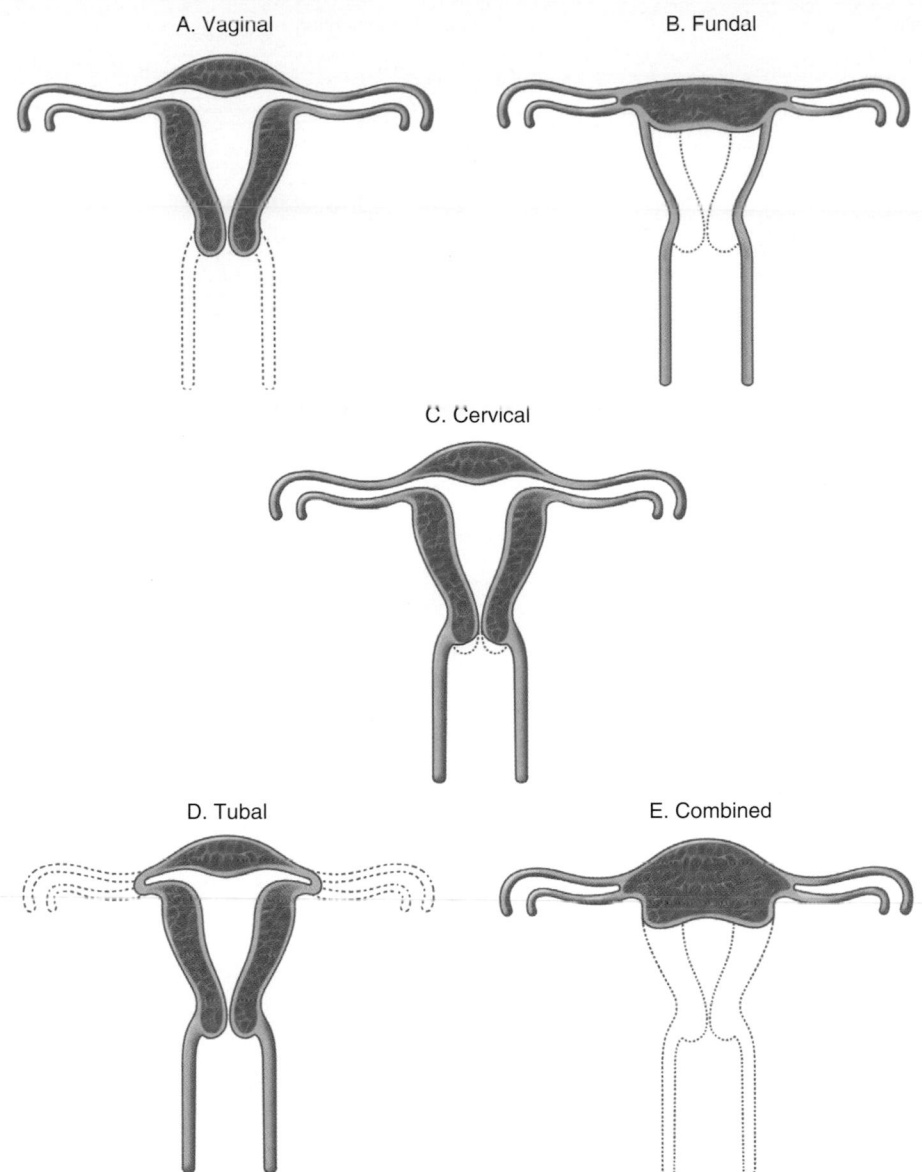

A. Vaginal   B. Fundal

C. Cervical

D. Tubal   E. Combined

FIGURE 18-15 Class I müllerian anomalies include types of segmental müllerian agenesis shown here as well as complete agenesis of müllerian structures.

repeated coitus. Overall, vaginal dilatation techniques are successful in forming a functional vagina in as many as 90 percent of cases (Croak, 2003; Roberts, 2001).

Surgical procedures are seen by many as a more immediate solution to creation of a neovagina, and several methods have been reported. The method used most commonly by gynecologists is the McIndoe vaginoplasty (McIndoe, 1950). As illustrated in Section 41-25 (p. 1075), a canal is created within the connective tissue between the bladder and rectum. A split-thickness skin graft obtained from the patient's buttocks or thigh is then used to line the neovagina. Strickland (1993) has reported excellent function and patient satisfaction. Modifications of the McIndoe procedure include the use of other materials to line the neovagina.

All of these methods require a commitment to scheduled postoperative dilatation to avoid significant vaginal stricture (Breech, 1999). Accordingly, these procedures should be considered only if the patient is mature and willing to adhere to a postoperative regimen of regular intercourse or manual dilatation with dilators.

To avoid these postoperative requirements, pediatric surgeons more frequently use a segment of bowel to create the vagina. These colpoplasties most commonly use sigmoidal or ileal segments and require laparotomy and bowel anastomosis. Many patients complain of a persistent vaginal discharge from the gastrointestinal mucosa. Kapoor (2006) reported on 14 such sigmoid vaginoplasties and noted good cosmetic results and no cases of colitis, stenosis, or excessive mucus.

In contrast, the Vecchietti procedure uses an initial abdominal surgery to create an apparatus for passive vaginal dilatation. A sphere, attached to two wires, is placed in the vaginal dimple. The wires are guided through the potential neovaginal space to exit on the anterior abdominal wall. The wires are places on continuous tension, which is increased periodically to stretch the blind vaginal pouch (Vecchietti, 1965).

Unicornuate Uterus

Failure of one müllerian duct to develop and elongate results in a unicornuate uterus (Fig. 18-16). This anomaly is common, and Zanetti (1978) found an incidence of 14 percent in a series of 1160 uterine anomalies. With unicornuate uterus, a functional uterus, normal cervix, and normal round ligament and fallopian tube are found on one side. On the contralateral side,

and malformations of the cervical vertebrae. Cardiac malformations and neurologic disturbances appear to play a lesser role and include ventricular septal defects and unilateral hearing problems. Fifty to 60 percent of women with müllerian agenesis have secondary malformations and thus should be regarded as having a complex multiorgan and multisystem syndrome.

Treatment. One treatment goal for most of these women is creation of a functional vagina. This may be accomplished conservatively or surgically. There are several conservative approaches, and each attempts to progressively invaginate the vaginal dimple to create a canal of adequate size. Graduated hard glass dilators were initially recommended by Frank (1938). Ingram (1981) modified the Frank method by affixing the dilators to a bicycle seat mounted upon a stool. This affords patients hand mobility for other activities during the 30 min to 2 h spent each day for passive dilation (American College of Obstetricians and Gynecologists, 2002). A vagina may also be created with

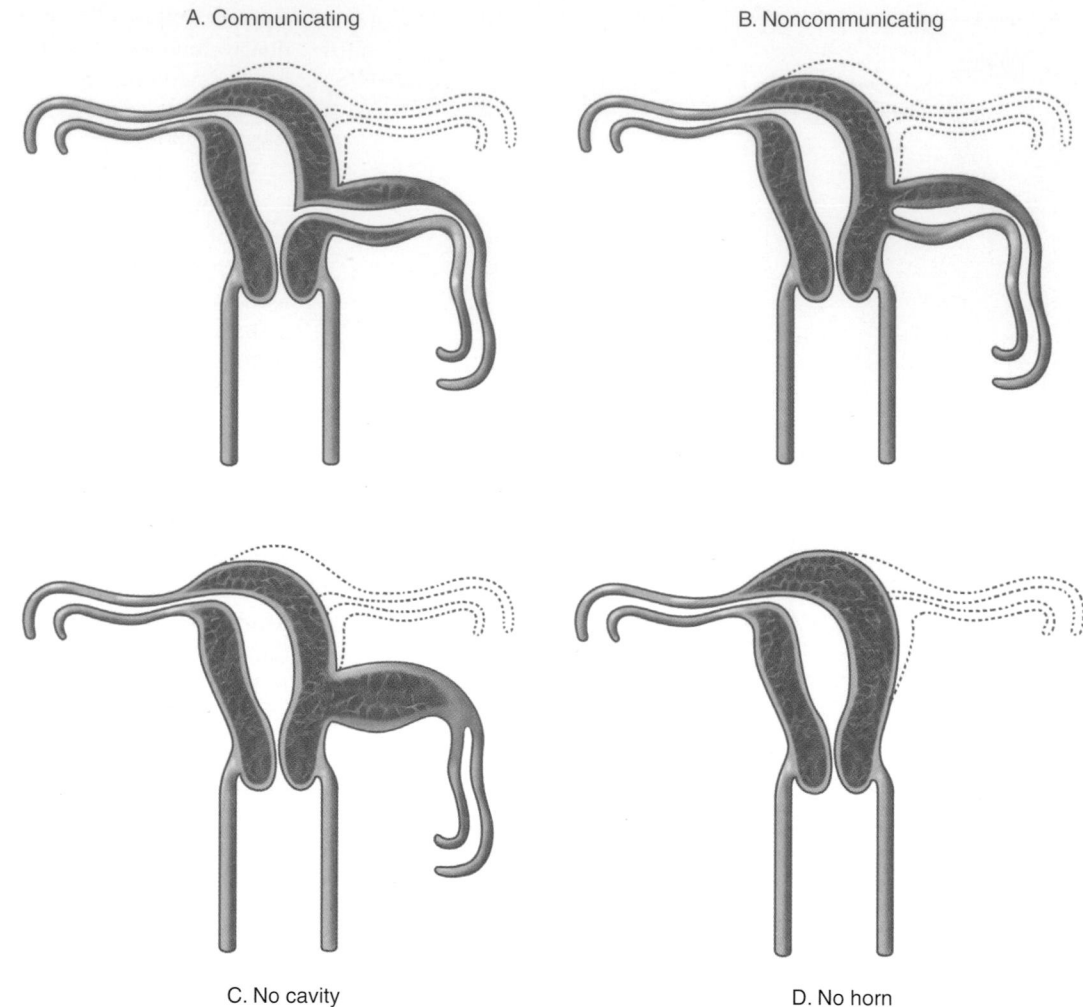

A. Communicating

B. Noncommunicating

C. No cavity

D. No horn

FIGURE 18-16 Class II müllerian anomalies include forms of unicornuate uterus. Types vary depending on whether a rudimentary horn is present, whether the horn is communicating or noncommunicating, and whether it contains a cavity and functional endometrium. (*From Cunningham, 2010, with permission.*)

müllerian structures develop abnormally, and agenesis or more frequently a rudimentary uterine horn is identified. A rudimentary horn may communicate or more commonly not communicate with the unicornuate uterus. In addition, the endometrial cavity of the rudimentary horn may be obliterated or may contain some functioning endometrium. Active endometrium in a noncommunicating horn will eventually be symptomatic with cyclic unilateral pain (Rackow, 2007).

Women with a unicornuate uterus have an increased incidence of infertility, endometriosis, and dysmenorrhea (Fedele, 1987, 1994; Heinonen, 1983). On physical examination, the uterus is often markedly deviated. Hysterosalpingography, combined with sonography or MR imaging, is a key study during evaluation. Typically, hysterosalpingography (HSG) films show a deviated banana-shaped cavity with a single fallopian tube. Rudimentary development of a uterine horn in association with a unicornuate uterus is best confirmed by sonography. This modality is sufficiently accurate and may be more reliable than laparoscopy in determining whether rudimentary structures contain endometrial tissue. Three-dimensional transvaginal sonography has also been used reliably to diagnose and classify müllerian anomalies

(Raga, 1996). In addition, renal sonography is performed, as 40 percent of women with a unicornuate uterus also have some degree of renal agenesis, usually ipsilateral to the anomalous side (Rackow, 2007).

Women with unicornuate uterus have impaired pregnancy outcomes. A review of studies reveals a spontaneous abortion rate of 36 percent, a preterm delivery rate of 16 percent, and a live birth rate of 54 percent (Rackow, 2007). Obstetric complications, such as breech presentation, fetal growth restriction, dysfunctional labor, and cesarean delivery, are also more common (Acien, 1993).

The pathogenesis of pregnancy loss associated with unicornuate uterus is incompletely understood, but reduced uterine capacity or anomalous distribution of the uterine artery has been suggested (Burchell, 1978). Moreover, cervical incompetence may contribute to the risk for premature delivery and late-trimester abortion. Accordingly, a unicornuate uterus should be suspected in any woman with a history of pregnancy loss, premature delivery, or abnormal fetal lie.

No current surgeries are available to enlarge the unicornuate uterus cavity. Some obstetricians recommend prophylactic cervical cerclage, but adequate trials assessing outcome are lacking. Selection of a gestational surrogate may circumvent these anatomic limitations. Other patients, however, seem to carry their pregnancies longer with each subsequent gestation and may eventually reach fetal viability prior to labor.

Pregnancy may also occur in the rudimentary horn. In noncommunicating horns, this is thought to result from the intraabdominal transit of sperm from the contralateral fallopian tube. Pregnancy is associated with a high rate of uterine rupture, typically prior to 20 weeks (Rolen, 1966). Because of the high maternal morbidity secondary to intraperitoneal hemorrhage, excision of a cavitary rudimentary horn is indicated whenever it is identified (Heinonen, 1997; Nahum, 2002). To that end, Dicker (1998) has reported the laparoscopic removal of rudimentary horn pregnancy.

If the rudimentary horn is obliterated, removal is not routinely recommended. Salpingectomy or salpingo-oophorectomy on the side with the rudimentary horn, however, has been suggested to prevent ectopic pregnancy in women with a unicornuate uterus, although the ectopic pregnancy risk is low.

Uterine Didelphys

A didelphic uterus results from failed fusion of the paired müllerian ducts. This anomaly is characterized by two separated uterine horns, each with an endometrial cavity and uterine cervix (Fig. 18-17). A longitudinal vaginal septum runs between the two cervices in most cases. Heinonen (1984) reported that all 26 women with uterine didelphys in his series had a longitudinal vaginal septum. Occasionally, one hemivagina is obstructed by an oblique or transverse vaginal septum (see Fig. 18-14) (Hinckley, 2003).

Uterine didelphys should be suspected if a longitudinal vaginal septum or if two separate cervices are discovered. HSG is recommended to confirm the diagnosis and exclude communication between the uteri.

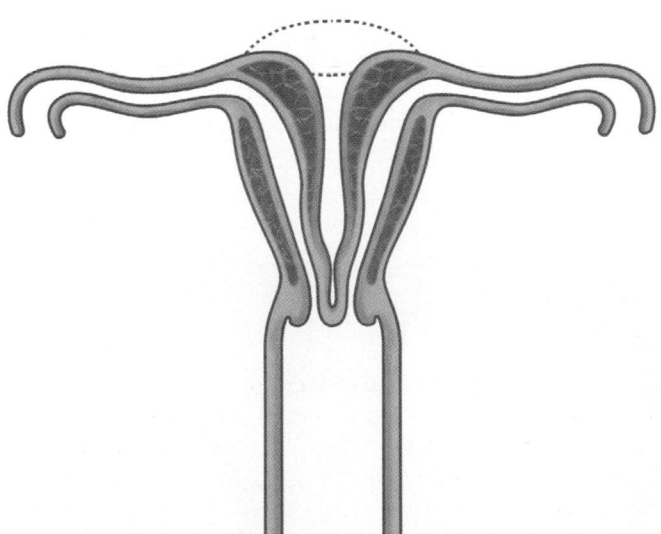

FIGURE 18-17 Class III müllerian anomaly is uterine didelphys. Two distinct uterine cavities and two cervices are found. Although not shown here, most cases also have a longitudinal vaginal septum in the upper vagina. *(From Cunningham, 2010, with permission.)*

Pregnancies develop in one of the two horns, and of the major uterine malformations, the didelphic uterus has the best reproductive prognosis. Compared with the unicornuate uterus, although the potential for uterine growth and capacity appears similar, the uterine didelphys probably has an improved blood supply through collateral connections between the two horns. Alternatively, improved fetal survival may be secondary to earlier diagnosis, which favors earlier and more intensive prenatal care (Patton, 1994). Heinonen (2000) followed 36 women with uterus didelphys long term and found that 34 of 36 women (94 percent) who wanted to conceive had at least one pregnancy, and they produced 71 pregnancies. Of these pregnancies, 21 percent were spontaneously aborted and 2 percent were ectopic. The rate for fetal survival was 75 percent; for prematurity, 24 percent; for fetal growth restriction, 11 percent; for perinatal mortality, 5 percent; and for cesarean delivery, 84 percent. In this series, pregnancy located more commonly (76 percent) in the right horn than in the left. Because the spontaneous abortion rate mirrors that of women with normal uterine cavities, surgical procedures in response to pregnancy loss are rarely indicated. Thus, surgery should be reserved for highly selected patients in whom repeated late-trimester losses or premature delivery has occurred with no other apparent etiology.

Bicornuate Uterus

This anomaly is caused by incomplete fusion of the müllerian ducts. It is characterized by two separate but communicating endometrial cavities and a single uterine cervix. Failed fusion may extend to the cervix, resulting in a complete bicornuate uterus, or may be partial, causing a milder abnormality (Fig. 18-18). Women with a bicornuate uterus can expect reasonable success—approximately 60 percent—in delivering a living child. As with many uterine anomalies, premature delivery is a substantial obstetric risk. Heinonen and colleagues (1982) reported a 28-percent abortion rate and a 20-percent incidence of premature labor in women with a partial bicornuate uterus. Women with a complete bicornuate uterus had a 66-percent incidence of preterm delivery and a lower fetal survival rate.

Hysterosalpingography is the initial diagnostic step. Classically, the uterine horns show a marked divergence, but various morphologic findings are possible. Because HSG may not accurately distinguish a bicornuate from a septate uterus, additional testing is necessary. Sonography has been used successfully to differentiate the two and their distinction is described in Chapter 2 (p. 56). Malini (1984) reviewed 50 cases of uterine anomalies and compared sonographic findings with those obtained by HSG and laparoscopy. Sonography was confirmatory or diagnostic of the suspected anomaly in most cases (88 percent). Moreover, the diagnostic accuracy of sonography may be improved when coupled with HSG. Reuter and coworkers (1989) reported a diagnostic accuracy of 90 percent when the two techniques were used. A potentially more accurate method uses MR imaging. Pellerito (1992) evaluated uterine anomalies by MR imaging and correctly identified all of 24 bicornuate uteri. Although fundal

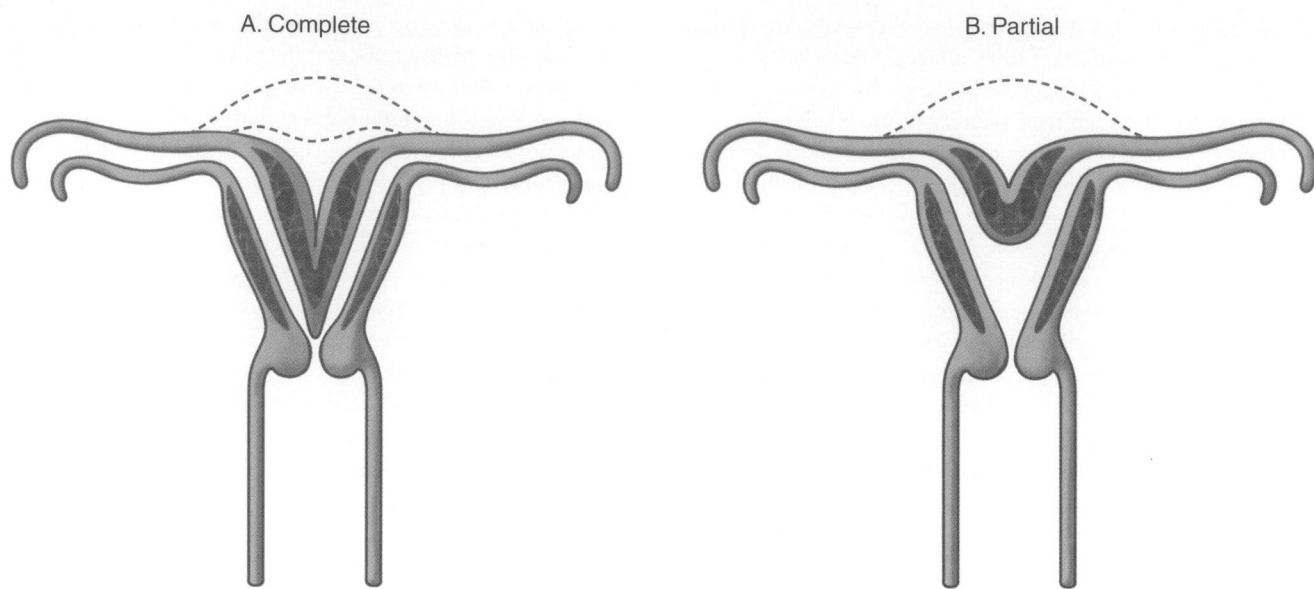

FIGURE 18-18 Class IV müllerian anomalies are forms of bicornuate uterus. Incomplete fusion of the midline müllerian ducts during embryogenesis partially or completely divides the endometrial cavity into two longitudinal halves.

contour and septal conformation can be accurately visualized by MR imaging, its high cost precludes its use in all cases. Thus, sonography and HSG seem acceptable imaging techniques in the initial investigation. When the presumptive diagnosis is a septate uterus, laparoscopy is indicated for a definitive diagnosis and before hysteroscopic resection of the septum is initiated.

Surgical reconstruction of the bicornuate uterus has been advocated in women with multiple spontaneous abortions and in whom no other causative factors are identified. Strassman (1952) described the surgical technique that unified equal-sized endometrial cavities (Fig. 18-19). Reproductive outcome after unification generally has been good. In 289 women, preoperative pregnancy loss was more than 70 percent. Following surgery, more than 85 percent of pregnancies ended in delivery of a viable infant. The actual benefit of metroplasty for a bicornuate uterus, however, has not been tested in a controlled clinical series. As in surgery for uterine didelphys, metroplasty should be reserved for women in whom recurrent pregnancy loss occurs with no other identifiable cause.

Septate Uterus

Following fusion of the müllerian ducts, failure of their medial segments to regress can create a permanent septum within the uterine cavity. Its contours can vary widely and depends on the amount of persistent midline tissue. The septum can project minimally from the uterine fundus or can extend completely to the cervical os (Fig. 18-20). Moreover, septa can develop segmentally, resulting in partial communications of the partitioned uterus (Patton, 1994). The histologic structure of septa ranges from fibrous to fibromuscular.

The true incidence of these anomalies is not known because they are usually only detected in women with obstetric complications. Although this defect does not predispose to increase rates of preterm labor or cesarean delivery, septate uterus is associated with a marked increase in spontaneous abortion rates

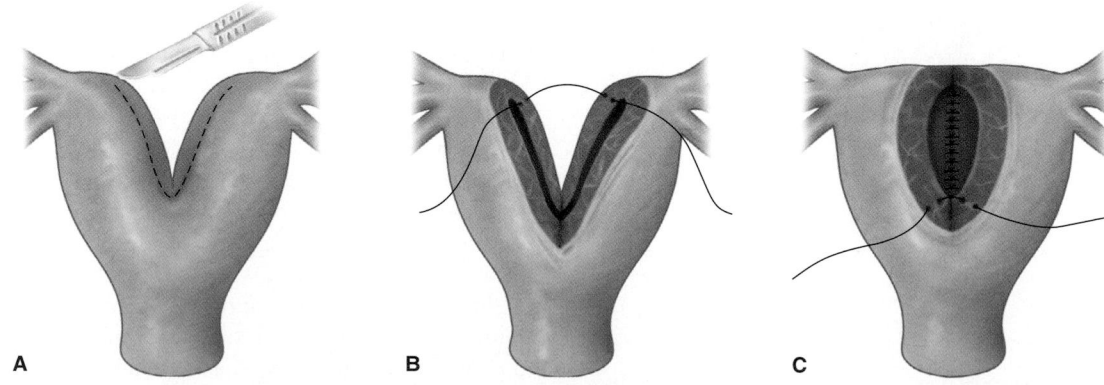

FIGURE 18-19 Strassman metroplasty is one of several techniques of bicornuate uterus repair. **A.** Excision of intervening uterine wall. **B.** Reapproximation of posterior uterine wall with a layer of myometrial sutures. **C.** Shown here, reapproximation of the anterior wall is closed similarly. Following placement of myometrial sutures, a layer of subserosal sutures is placed in the anterior and posterior walls.

A. Complete   B. Partial

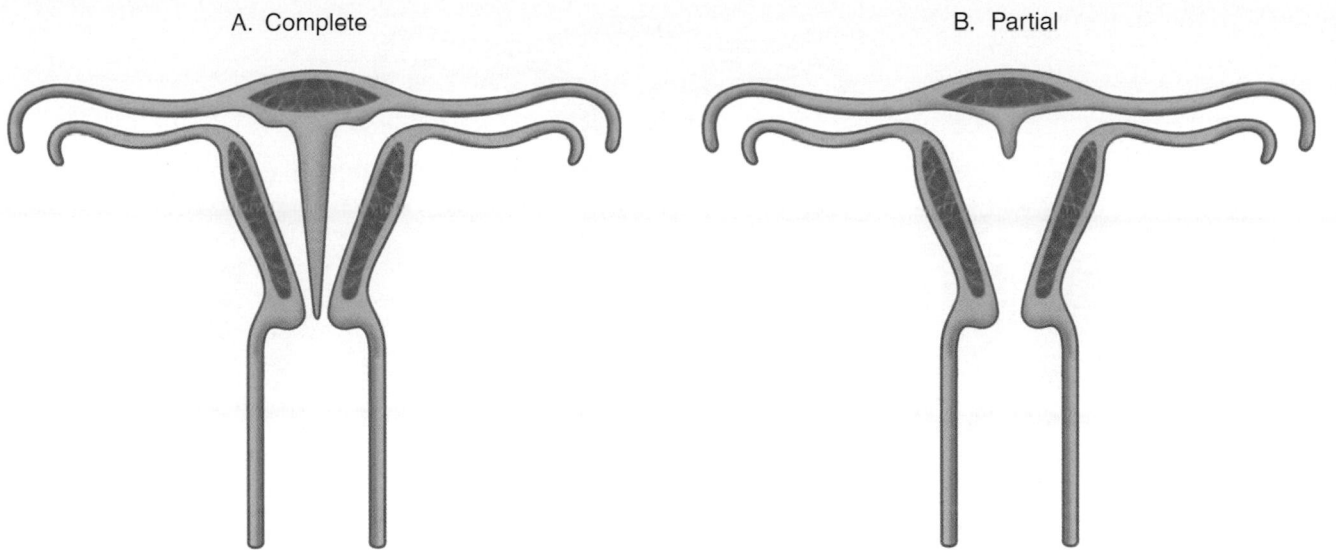

FIGURE 18-20 Class V müllerian anomalies include forms of septate uterus. The fibrous or fibromuscular septum may extend partially into the uterine cavity or may extend the entire length.

(Heinonen, 2006). Woelfer and colleagues (2001) reported a first-trimester spontaneous abortion rate for septate uterus of 42 percent. Moreover, early pregnancy loss is significantly more common with a septate than with a bicornuate uterus (Proctor, 2003).

This extraordinarily high pregnancy wastage likely results from partial or complete implantation on a largely avascular septum, from distortion of the uterine cavity, and from associated cervical or endometrial abnormalities. Based on operative experience for septal defects, the blood supply to the fibromuscular septum appears markedly reduced compared with normal myometrium. In addition to spontaneous abortion, septate uterus may infrequently cause fetal malformation, and Heinonen (1999) described three newborns with a limb-reduction defect born to women with septate uterus.

Diagnosis of the septate uterus follows guidelines established for the bicornuate uterus and includes HSG and sonography. Historically, abdominal metroplasty for septate uterus was shown to decrease fetal wastage and ultimately improve fetal survival (Blum, 1977; Rock, 1977). Two main disadvantages to metroplasty include the requirement of cesarean delivery to prevent uterine rupture and the high rate of postoperative pelvic adhesion formation and subsequent infertility.

Currently, hysteroscopic septum resection is an effective and safe alternative to treat women with septate uterus (Section 42-19, p. 1174). Typically, operative hysteroscopy is combined with laparoscopic surveillance to reduce the risk of uterine perforation. After the initial case reports by Chervenak and Neuwirth (1981), many investigators have confirmed satisfactory live birth rates with the procedure (Daly, 1983; DeCherney, 1983; Israel, 1984). In a retrospective review, Fayez (1986) evaluated reproductive outcome in women who had either an abdominal metroplasty or hysteroscopic septoplasty. They noted an 87-percent live birth rate in the hysteroscopic group compared with a 70-percent rate in the abdominal group. Similarly, Daly and associates

(1989) reported impressive results after hysteroscopic surgery. Proponents of hysteroscopic resection describe reduced rates of pelvic adhesions, shortened postoperative convalescence, lowered operative morbidity, and avoidance of mandatory cesarean delivery (Patton, 1994).

Arcuate Uterus

An arcuate uterus displays only mild deviation from normal uterine development. Anatomic hallmarks include a slight midline septum within a broad fundus, sometimes with minimal fundal cavity indentation (Fig. 18-21). Most clinicians report no worsening of reproductive outcomes. Conversely, Woelfer and colleagues (2001) found excessive second-trimester losses and preterm labor. Surgical resection is indicated only if excessive rates of pregnancy loss are encountered and other etiologies for recurrent spontaneous abortion have been excluded.

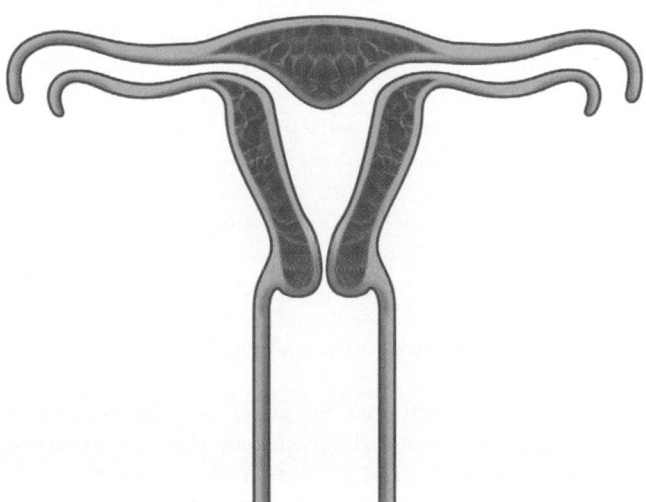

FIGURE 18-21 Class VI müllerian anomaly is arcuate uterus. *(From Cunningham, 2010, with permission.)*

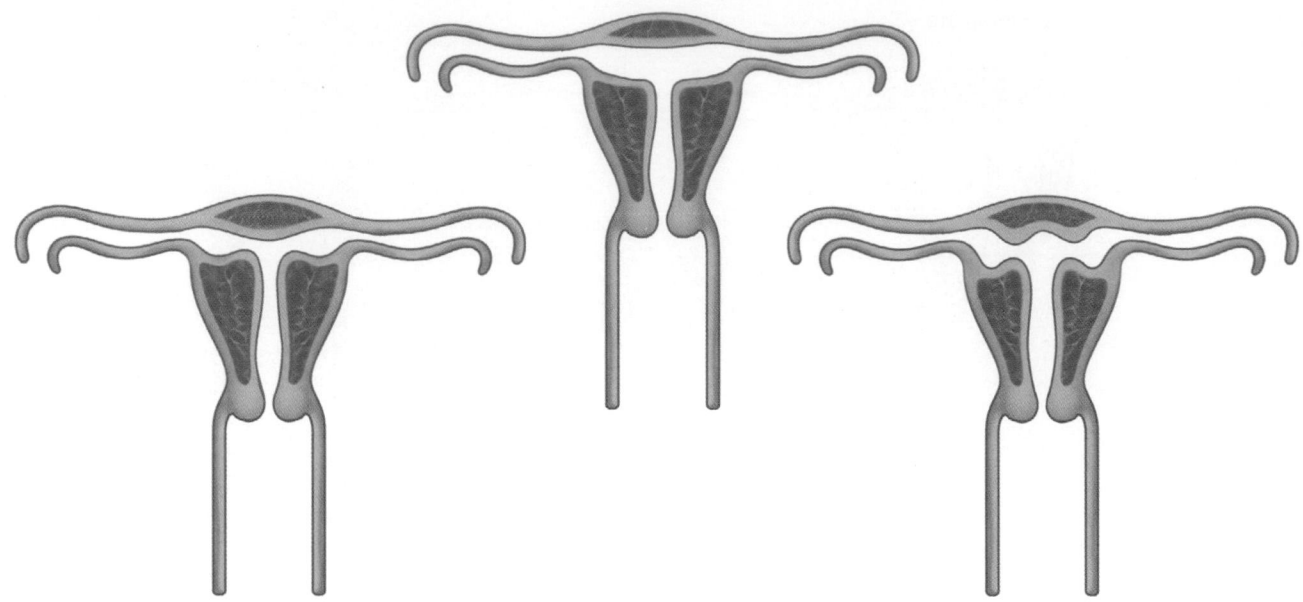

FIGURE 18-22 Class VII diethylstilbestrol-induced uterine anomalies.

Diethylstilbestrol-Induced Reproductive Tract Abnormalities

Diethylstilbestrol (DES), a synthetic nonsteroidal estrogen, was prescribed to an estimated 3 million pregnant women in the United States from the late 1940s through the early 1960s. Early reports claimed the drug was useful in treating abortion, preeclampsia, diabetes, hot flashes, and preterm labor (Masse, 2009). It was unfortunately ineffective for these indications. Almost 20 years later, Herbst and coworkers (1971) found that DES exposure in utero was linked to the development of a "T shaped" uterus and an increased incidence of clear cell adenocarcinomas of the vagina and cervix. The risk of this vaginal malignancy approximates 1 in 1000 exposed daughters. Daughters also have increased risks of developing vaginal and cervical intraepithelial neoplasia, suggesting that DES exposure could affect gene regulation (Herbst, 2000). DES has also been shown to suppress the *WNT4* gene and alter Hox gene expression in mice müllerian ducts. This provides a plausible molecular mechanism for the uterine abnormalities, vaginal adenosis, and rarely, carcinoma observed in exposed patients (Masse, 2009).

During normal development, the vagina is originally lined by a glandular epithelium derived from the müllerian ducts. By the end of the second trimester, this layer is replaced by squamous epithelium extending up from the urogenital sinus. Failure of the squamous epithelium to completely line the vagina is termed adenosis. Although variable, it typically appears red, punctate, and granular. Common symptoms include vaginal irritation, discharge, and metrorrhagia, in particular postcoital bleeding. Moreover, adenosis is associated with vaginal clear cell adenocarcinoma.

Genitourinary malformations following DES exposure in utero have also been noted and include those of the cervix, vagina, uterine cavity, and fallopian tubes. Transverse septa, circumferential ridges involving the vagina and cervix, and cervical collars ("cockscomb cervix") have been found. Women with cervicovaginal abnormalities are more likely to have uterine anomalies, such as smaller uterine cavities, shortened upper uterine segments, and "T-shaped" and irregular cavities (Fig. 18-22) (Barranger, 2002). Fallopian tube abnormalities include shortened and narrowed dimensions and absent fimbria. Hysterosalpingography remains the primary imaging tool for identification of these anomalies.

Males exposed to DES in utero also have structural abnormalities. Cryptorchidism, testicular hypoplasia, microphallus, and hypospadias have been reported (Hernandez-Dias, 2002). Moreover, Klip and colleagues (2002) provided evidence of a transgeneration effect, in which male fetuses conceived by daughters of DES-exposed women have increased rates of hypospadias.

Women exposed to DES, in general, have impaired conception rates (Goldberg, 1999; Palmer, 2001; Senekjian, 1988). Reduced fertility in these women is poorly understood but is associated with cervical hypoplasia and atresia. Of those who do conceive, the incidence of spontaneous pregnancy loss, ectopic pregnancy, and preterm delivery are increased, again particularly in those with associated structural abnormalities (Goldberg, 1999; Hoover, 2011).

FALLOPIAN TUBE ANOMALIES

The fallopian tubes develop from the unpaired distal ends of the müllerian ducts. Congenital anomalies of the fallopian tube include accessory ostia, complete or segmental absence of the fallopian tube, and several embryonic cystic remnants (Woodruff, 1969). The remnants of the mesonephric duct in the female include a few blind tubules in the mesovarium, the *epoophoron,* and similar ones adjacent to the uterus, collectively called the *paroophoron* (Fig. 18-2F) (Moore, 2008). The epoophoron or paroophoron may develop into clinically identifiable cysts. Remnants of the müllerian duct may also be found along its embryologic course. The most common is a small, blind cystic structure attached by a pedicle to the distal end of the fallopian tube, the hydatid of Morgagni (Fig. 9-24, p. 272) (Zheng, 2009).

Paratubal cysts are frequent incidental discoveries during gynecologic operations for other abnormalities or are found on sonographic examination. They may be of mesonephric, mesothelial, or paramesonephric origin. Most of these cysts are asymptomatic and slow growing and are discovered during the third and fourth decades of life.

In utero exposure to DES has been associated with various tubal abnormalities. Short, tortuous tubes or ones with shriveled fimbria and small ostia have been linked to infertility (DeCherney, 1981).

OVARIAN ANOMALIES

A *supernumerary ovary* is an ectopic ovary that has no connection with the broad, uteroovarian, or infundibulopelvic ligaments (Wharton, 1959). This rare gynecologic anomaly may be located in the pelvis, retroperitoneum, paraaortic area, colonic mesentery, or omentum. Aberrant migration of part of the gonadal ridge after incorporation of germ cells describes one theory (Printz, 1973).

In contrast, the term *accessory ovary* describes excess ovarian tissue nearby and connected to a normally placed ovary. Wharton (1959) estimated that both accessory ovary and supernumerary ovary were rare. Moreover, 3 of 4 patients with supernumerary ovary and 5 of 19 patients with accessory ovary had additional congenital defects, most frequently abnormalities of the genitourinary tract.

An absent ovary, with or without an associated tube, may result from congenital agenesis or from ovarian torsion with necrosis and reabsorption (Eustace, 1992; James, 1970). The incidence has been suggested to be approximately 1 in 11,240 women (Sivanesaratnam, 1986).

REFERENCES

Acien P: Reproductive performance of women with uterine malformations. Hum Reprod 8(1):122, 1993

Acien P, Acien M, Sanchez-Ferrer ML: Müllerian anomalies "without a classification": from the didelphys-unicollis uterus to the bicervical uterus with or without septate vagina. Fertil Steril 91(6):2369, 2009

Allen L: Disorders of sexual development. Obstet Gynecol Clin North Am 36(1):25, 2009

American College of Obstetricians and Gynecologists: Nonsurgical diagnosis and management of vaginal agenesis. Committee Opinion No. 274, July 2002

American College of Obstetricians and Gynecologists: Vaginal agenesis: diagnosis, management, and routine care. Committee Opinion No. 355, December 2006

American Fertility Society: The American Fertility Society classifications of adnexal adhesions, distal tubal occlusion, tubal occlusion secondary to tubal ligation, tubal pregnancies, müllerian anomalies and intrauterine adhesions. Fertil Steril 49(6):944, 1988

Bakos O, Berglund L: Imperforate hymen and ruptured hematosalpinx: a case report with a review of the literature. J Adolesc Health 24(3):226, 1999

Banerjee R, Laufer MR: Reproductive disorders associated with pelvic pain. Semin Pediatr Surg 7(1):52, 1998

Bangsboll S, Qvist I, Lebech PE, et al: Testicular feminization syndrome and associated gonadal tumors in Denmark. Acta Obstet Gynecol Scand 71(1):63, 1992

Barranger E, Gervaise A, Doumerc S, et al: Reproductive performance after hysteroscopic metroplasty in the hypoplastic uterus: a study of 29 cases. BJOG 109(12):1331, 2002

Berkman DS, McHugh MT, Shapiro E: The other interlabial mass: hymenal cyst. J Urol 171(5):1914, 2004

Biason-Lauber A, Konrad D: WNT4 and sex development. Sex Dev 2(4–5):210, 2008

Blackless M, Charuvastra A, Derryck A, et al: How sexually dimorphic are we? Review and synthesis. Am J Hum Biol 12(2):151, 2000

Blum M: Prevention of spontaneous abortion by cervical suture of the malformed uterus. Int Surg 62(4):213, 1977

Breech LL, Laufer MR: Müllerian anomalies. Obstet Gynecol Clin North Am 36(1):47, 2009

Breech LL, Laufer MR: Obstructive anomalies of the female reproductive tract. J Reprod Med 44(3):233, 1999

Burchell RC, Creed F, Rasoulpour M, et al: Vascular anatomy of the human uterus and pregnancy wastage. Br J Obstet Gynaecol 85(9):698, 1978

Buttram VC Jr, Gibbons WE: Müllerian anomalies: a proposed classification. (An analysis of 144 cases.) Fertil Steril 32(1):40, 1979

Carlson RL, Garmel GM: Didelphic uterus and unilaterally imperforate double vagina as an unusual presentation of right lower-quadrant abdominal pain. Ann Emerg Med 21(8):1006, 1992

Casey AC, Laufer MR: Cervical agenesis: septic death after surgery. Obstet Gynecol 90(4 Pt 2):706, 1997

Chavhan GB, Parra DA, Oudjhane K, et al: Imaging of ambiguous genitalia: classification and diagnostic approach. Radiographics 28(7):1891, 2008

Chervenak FA, Neuwirth RS: Hysteroscopic resection of the uterine septum. Am J Obstet Gynecol 141(3):351, 1981

Croak AJ, Gebhart JB, Klingele CJ, et al: Therapeutic strategies for vaginal müllerian agenesis. J Reprod Med 48(6):395, 2003

Cunningham FG, Leveno KJ, Bloom SL (eds): Reproductive tract abnormalities. In Williams Obstetrics, 23rd ed. New York, McGraw-Hill, 2010, p 894

Daly DC, Maier D, Soto-Albors C: Hysteroscopic metroplasty: six years' experience. Obstet Gynecol 73(2):201, 1989

Daly DC, Walters CA, Soto-Albors CE, et al: Hysteroscopic metroplasty: surgical technique and obstetric outcome. Fertil Steril 39(5):623, 1983

Damario MA, Carpenter SE, Jones HW Jr, et al: Reconstruction of the external genitalia in females with bladder exstrophy. Int J Gynaecol Obstet 44:245, 1994

DeCherney AH, Cholst I, Naftolin F: Structure and function of the fallopian tubes following exposure to diethylstilbestrol (DES) during gestation. Fertil Steril 36(6):741, 1981

DeCherney A, Polan ML: Hysteroscopic management of intrauterine lesions and intractable uterine bleeding. Obstet Gynecol 61(3):392, 1983

Dees JE: Congenital epispadias with incontinence. J Urol 62(4):513, 1949

Deppisch LM: Cysts of the vagina: Classification and clinical correlations. Obstet Gynecol 45(6):632, 1975

Dershwitz RA, Levitsky LL, Feingold M: Picture of the month. Vulvovaginitis: a cause of clitorimegaly. Am J Dis Child 138(9):887, 1984

Dicker D, Nitke S, Shoenfeld A, et al: Laparoscopic management of rudimentary horn pregnancy. Hum Reprod 13(9):2643, 1998

Dillon WP, Mudaliar NA, Wingate MB: Congenital atresia of the cervix. Obstet Gynecol 54(1):126, 1979

Doyle JO, Laufer MR: Mayer-Rokitansky-Kuster-Hauser (MRKH) syndrome with a single septate uterus: a novel anomaly and description of treatment options. Fertil Steril 92(1):391, 2009

Du H, Taylor HS: Molecular regulation of müllerian development by Hox genes. Ann NY Acad Sci 1034:152, 2004

Elder J: Congenital anomalies of the genitalia. In Walsh PC, Retik AB, Stamey TA, et al (eds): Campbell's Urology. Philadelphia, WB Saunders, 1992, p 1920

Eustace DL: Congenital absence of fallopian tube and ovary. Eur J Obstet Gynecol Reprod Biol 46(2-3):157, 1992

Fayez JA: Comparison between abdominal and hysteroscopic metroplasty. Obstet Gynecol 68(3):399, 1986

Fedele L, Bianchi S, Marchini M, et al: Ovulation induction in the treatment of primary infertility associated with unicornuate uterus: report of five cases. Hum Reprod 9(12):2311, 1994

Fedele L, Zamberletti D, Vercellini P, et al: Reproductive performance of women with unicornuate uterus. Fertil Steril 47(3):416, 1987

Frank RT: The formation of an artificial vagina without an operation. Am J Obstet Gynecol 141:910, 1938

Garcia RF: Z-plasty for correction of congenital transverse vaginal septum. Am J Obstet Gynecol 99(8):1164, 1967

Gearhart JP, Jeffs RD: Exstrophy of the bladder, epispadias, and other bladder anomalies. In Walsh PC, Retik AB, Stamey TA, et al (eds): Campbell's Urology. Philadelphia, WB Saunders, 1992, p 1772

Goldberg JM, Falcone T: Effect of diethylstilbestrol on reproductive function. Fertil Steril 72(1):1, 1999

Greer DM Jr, Pederson WC: Pseudo-masculinization of the phallus. Plast Reconstr Surg 68(5):787, 1981

Heinonen PK: Clinical implications of the didelphic uterus: long-term follow-up of 49 cases. Eur J Obstet Gynecol Reprod Biol 91(2):183, 2000

Heinonen PK: Clinical implications of the unicornuate uterus with rudimentary horn. Int J Gynaecol Obstet 21(2):145, 1983

Heinonen PK: Complete septate uterus with longitudinal vaginal septum. Fertil Steril 85(3):700, 2006

Heinonen PK: Limb anomalies among offspring of women with a septate uterus: a report of three cases. Early Hum Dev 56(2-3):179, 1999

Heinonen PK: Unicornuate uterus and rudimentary horn. Fertil Steril 68(2):224, 1997

Heinonen PK: Uterus didelphys: a report of 26 cases. Eur J Obstet Gynecol Reprod Biol 17(5):345, 1984

Heinonen PK, Saarikoski S, Pystynen P: Reproductive performance of women with uterine anomalies. An evaluation of 182 cases. Acta Obstet Gynecol Scand 61(2):157, 1982

Hensle TW, Bingham J: Feminizing genitoplasty. Adv Exp Med Biol 511:251, 2002

Herbst AL: Behavior of estrogen-associated female genital tract cancer and its relation to neoplasia following intrauterine exposure to diethylstilbestrol (DES). Gynecol Oncol 76(2):147, 2000

Herbst AL, Ulfelder H, Poskanzer DC: Adenocarcinoma of the vagina. Association of maternal stilbestrol therapy with tumor appearance in young women. N Engl J Med 284(15):878, 1971

Hernandez-Diaz S: Iatrogenic legacy from diethylstilbestrol exposure. Lancet 359(9312):1081, 2002

Hinckley MD, Milki AA: Management of uterus didelphys, obstructed hemivagina and ipsilateral renal agenesis. A case report. J Reprod Med 48(8):649, 2003

Hoover RN, Hyer M, Pfeiffer RM, et al: Adverse health outcomes in women exposed in utero to diethylstilbestrol. N Engl J Med 365(14):1304, 2011

Hwang JH, Oh MJ, Lee NW, et al: Multiple vaginal müllerian cysts: a case report and review of literature. Arch Gynecol Obstet 280(1):137, 2009

Ingram JM: The bicycle seat stool in the treatment of vaginal agenesis and stenosis: a preliminary report. Am J Obstet Gynecol 140(8):867, 1981

Israel R, March CM: Hysteroscopic incision of the septate uterus. Am J Obstet Gynecol 149(1):66, 1984

James DF, Barber HR, Graber EA: Torsion of normal uterine adnexa in children. Report of three cases. Obstet Gynecol 35(2):226, 1970

Joki-Erkkila MM, Heinonen PK: Presenting and long-term clinical implications and fecundity in females with obstructing vaginal malformations. J Pediatr Adolesc Gynecol 16(5):307, 2003

Jones HW Jr: An anomaly of the external genitalia in female patients with exstrophy of the bladder. Am J Obstet Gynecol 117(6):748, 1973

Kapoor R, Sharma DK, Singh KJ, et al: Sigmoid vaginoplasty: long-term results. Urology 67(6):1212, 2006

Karlin G, Brock W, Rich M, et al: Persistent cloaca and phallic urethra. J Urol 142(4):1056, 1989

Kenney PJ, Spirt BA, Leeson MD: Genitourinary anomalies: radiologic-anatomic correlations. RadioGraphics 4:233, 1984

Klip H, Verloop J, van Gool JD, et al: Hypospadias in sons of women exposed to diethylstilbestrol in utero: a cohort study. Lancet 359(9312):1102, 2002

Kolon TF, Ferrer FA, McKenna PH: Clinical and molecular analysis of XX sex reversed patients. J Urol 160(3 Pt 2):1169, 1998

Lattimer JK, Smith MJ: Exstrophy closure: a follow up on 70 cases. J Urol 95(3):356, 1966

Lewis VG, Money J: Sexological theory, H-Y antigen, chromosomes, gonads, and cyclicity: two syndromes compared. Arch Sex Behav 15(6):467, 1986

Lim YH, Ng SP, Jamil MA: Imperforate hymen: report of an unusual familial occurrence. J Obstet Gynaecol Res 29(6):399, 2003

MacLaughlin DT, Donahoe PK: Sex determination and differentiation. N Engl J Med 350(4):367, 2004

Malini S, Valdes C, Malinak LR: Sonographic diagnosis and classification of anomalies of the female genital tract. J Ultrasound Med 3(9):397, 1984

Marshall FF: Embryology of the lower genitourinary tract. Urol Clin North Am 5(1):3, 1978

Masse J, Watrin T, Laurent A, et al: The developing female genital tract: from genetics to epigenetics. Int J Dev Biol 53(2-3):411, 2009

McIndoe A: The treatment of congenital absence and obliterative conditions of the vagina. Br J Plast Surg 2(4):254, 1950

Minto CL, Liao KL, Conway GS, et al: Sexual function in women with complete androgen insensitivity syndrome. Fertil Steril 80(1):157, 2003

Moore KL, Persaud TVN: The urogenital system. In The Developing Human. Philadelphia, Saunders, 2008, p 243

Nahum GG: Rudimentary uterine horn pregnancy. The 20th-century worldwide experience of 588 cases. J Reprod Med 47(2):151, 2002

Nahum GG: Uterine anomalies. How common are they, and what is their distribution among subtypes? J Reprod Med 43(10):877, 1998

Nazir Z, Rizvi RM, Qureshi RN, et al: Congenital vaginal obstructions: varied presentation and outcome. Pediatr Surg Int 22(9):749, 2006

Niver DH, Barrette G, Jewelewicz R: Congenital atresia of the uterine cervix and vagina: three cases. Fertil Steril 33(1):25, 1980

Oppelt P, Renner SP, Kellermann A, et al: Clinical aspects of Mayer-Rokitansky-Kuster-Hauser syndrome: recommendations for clinical diagnosis and staging. Hum Reprod 21(3):792, 2006

O'Rahilly R, Muller F: Human Embryology and Teratology, 3rd ed. New York, Wiley Liss, 2001, p 340

Palmer JR, Hatch EE, Rao RS, et al: Infertility among women exposed prenatally to diethylstilbestrol. Am J Epidemiol 154(4):316, 2001

Parazzini F, Cecchetti G: The frequency of imperforate hymen in northern Italy. Int J Epidemiol 19(3):763, 1990

Park SY, Jameson JL: Minireview: transcriptional regulation of gonadal development and differentiation. Endocrinology 146(3):1035, 2005

Patton PE: Anatomic uterine defects. Clin Obstet Gynecol 37(3):705, 1994

Pellerito JS, McCarthy SM, Doyle MB, et al: Diagnosis of uterine anomalies: relative accuracy of MR imaging, endovaginal sonography, and hysterosalpingography. Radiology 183(3):795, 1992

Printz JL, Choate JW, Townes PL, et al: The embryology of supernumerary ovaries. Obstet Gynecol 41(2):246, 1973

Proctor JA, Haney AF: Recurrent first trimester pregnancy loss is associated with uterine septum but not with bicornuate uterus. Fertil Steril 80(5):1212, 2003

Rackow BW, Arici A: Reproductive performance of women with müllerian anomalies. Curr Opin Obstet Gynecol 19(3):229, 2007

Raga F, Bonilla-Musoles F, Blanes J, et al: Congenital müllerian anomalies: diagnostic accuracy of three-dimensional ultrasound. Fertil Steril 65(3):523, 1996

Reuter KL, Daly DC, Cohen SM: Septate versus bicornuate uteri: errors in imaging diagnosis. Radiology 172(3):749, 1989

Rickham PP: Vesicointestinal fissure. Arch Dis Child 35:967, 1960

Roberts CP, Haber MJ, Rock JA: Vaginal creation for müllerian agenesis. Am J Obstet Gynecol 185(6):1349, 2001

Rock JA, Jones HW Jr: The clinical management of the double uterus. Fertil Steril 28(8):798, 1977

Rock JA, Jones HW Jr: The double uterus associated with an obstructed hemivagina and ipsilateral renal agenesis. Am J Obstet Gynecol 138(3):339, 1980

Rock JA, Roberts CP, Jones HW Jr: Congenital anomalies of the uterine cervix: lessons from 30 cases managed clinically by a common protocol. Fertil Steril 94(5):1858, 2010

Rock JA, Schlaff WD, Zacur HA, et al: The clinical management of congenital absence of the uterine cervix. Int J Gynaecol Obstet 22(3):231, 1984

Rock JA, Zacur HA, Dlugi AM, et al: Pregnancy success following surgical correction of imperforate hymen and complete transverse vaginal septum. Obstet Gynecol 59(4):448, 1982

Rolen AC, Choquette AJ, Semmens JP: Rudimentary uterine horn: obstetric and gynecologic implications. Obstet Gynecol 27(6):806, 1966

Ross AJ, Capel B: Signaling at the crossroads of gonad development. Trends Endocrinol Metab 16(1):19, 2005

Sanfilippo JS, Wakim NG, Schikler KN, et al: Endometriosis in association with uterine anomaly. Am J Obstet Gynecol 154(1):39, 1986

Schweikert HU, Weissbach L, Leyendecker G, et al: Clinical, endocrinological, and cytological characterization of two 46,XX males. J Clin Endocrinol Metab 54(4):745, 1982

Senekjian EK, Potkul RK, Frey K, et al: Infertility among daughters either exposed or not exposed to diethylstilbestrol. Am J Obstet Gynecol 158(3 Pt 1):493, 1988

Sharara FI: Complete uterine septum with cervical duplication, longitudinal vaginal septum and duplication of a renal collecting system. A case report. J Reprod Med 43(12):1055, 1998

Shatzkes DR, Haller JO, Velcek FT: Imaging of uterovaginal anomalies in the pediatric patient. Urol Radiol 13(1):58, 1991

Simon C, Martinez L, Pardo F, et al: Müllerian defects in women with normal reproductive outcome. Fertil Steril 56(6):1192, 1991

Simpson JL: Genetics of the female reproductive ducts. Am J Med Genet 89(4):224, 1999

Sivanesaratnam V: Unexplained unilateral absence of ovary and fallopian tube. Eur J Obstet Gynecol Reprod Biol 22(1-2):103, 1986

Sotolongo JR Jr, Gribetz ME, Saphir RL, et al: Female phallic urethra and persistent cloaca. J Urol 130(6):1186, 1983

Stanton SL: Gynecologic complications of epispadias and bladder exstrophy. Am J Obstet Gynecol 119(6):749, 1974

Stelling JR, Gray MR, Davis AJ, et al: Dominant transmission of imperforate hymen. Fertil Steril 74(6):1241, 2000

Strassman E: Plastic unification of double uterus. Am J Obstet Gynecol 64(1):25, 1952

Strickland JL, Cameron WJ, Krantz KE: Long-term satisfaction of adults undergoing McIndoe vaginoplasty as adolescents. Adolesc Pediatr Gynecol 6:135, 1993

Taylor HS: The role of HOX genes in the development and function of the female reproductive tract. Semin Reprod Med 18(1):81, 2000

Thijssen RF, Hollanders JM, Willemsen WN, et al: Successful pregnancy after ZIFT in a patient with congenital cervical atresia. Obstet Gynecol 76(5 Pt 2):902, 1990

Thyen U, Lanz K, Holterhus PM, et al: Epidemiology and initial management of ambiguous genitalia at birth in Germany. Horm Res 66(4):195, 2006

Usta IM, Awwad JT, Usta JA, et al: Imperforate hymen: report of an unusual familial occurrence. Obstet Gynecol 82(4 Pt 2 Suppl):655, 1993

Vague J: Testicular feminization syndrome. An experimental model for the study of hormone action on sexual behavior. Horm Res 18(1-3):62, 1983

Vainio S, Heikkilä M, Kispert A, et al: Female development in mammals is regulated by Wnt-4 signalling. Nature 397(6718):405, 1999

Vecchietti G: [Creation of an artificial vagina in Rokitansky-Kuster-Hauser syndrome]. Attual Ostet Ginecol 11(2):131, 1965

Viger RS, Silversides DW, Tremblay JJ: New insights into the regulation of mammalian sex determination and male sex differentiation. Vitam Horm 70:387, 2005

Wharton LR: Two cases of supernumerary ovary and one of accessory ovary, with an analysis of previously reported cases. Am J Obstet Gynecol 78:1101, 1959

White PC, Speiser PW: Congenital adrenal hyperplasia due to 21-hydroxylase deficiency. Endocr Rev 21(3):245, 2000

Wisniewski AB, Migeon CJ, Meyer-Bahlburg HF, et al: Complete androgen insensitivity syndrome: long-term medical, surgical, and psychosexual outcome. J Clin Endocrinol Metab 85(8):2664, 2000

Woelfer B, Salim R, Banerjee S, et al: Reproductive outcomes in women with congenital uterine anomalies detected by three-dimensional ultrasound screening. Obstet Gynecol 98(6):1099, 2001

Woodruff JC, Pauersteine CJ: The fallopian tube: structure, function, pathology and management. Baltimore, Williams & Wilkins, 1969, p 18

Yin Y, Ma L: Development of the mammalian female reproductive tract. J Biochem 137(6):677, 2005

Zanetti E, Ferrari LR, Rossi G: Classification and radiographic features of uterine malformations: hysterosalpingographic study. Br J Radiol 51(603):161, 1978

Zheng W, Robboy SJ: Fallopian tube. In Robboy SJ, Mutter GL, Prat J (eds): Robboy's Pathology of the Female Reproductive Tract. London, Churchill Livingstone, 2009, p 509

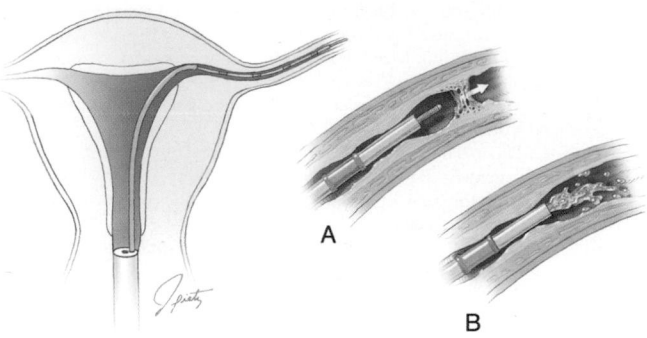

Evaluation of the Infertile Couple

Infertility is defined as the inability to conceive after 1 year of unprotected intercourse of reasonable frequency. It can be subdivided into *primary infertility*, that is, no prior pregnancies, and *secondary infertility*, referring to infertility following at least one prior conception.

Conversely, fecundability is the ability to conceive, and data from large population studies show that a monthly probability of conceiving is 20 to 25 percent. In those attempting conception, approximately 50 percent of women will be pregnant at 3 months, 75 percent will be pregnant at 6 months, and more than 85 percent will be pregnant by 1 year (Fig. 19-1) (Guttmacher, 1956; Mosher, 1991).

Infertility is a common condition, affecting 10 to 15 percent of reproductive-aged couples. Of note, even without treatment, approximately half of women will conceive in the second year of attempting. Although the prevalence of infertility is believed to have remained relatively stable during the past 40 years, the demand for infertility evaluation and treatment has increased (Chandra, 2010). With the well-publicized advances in infertility treatment, patients now have greater hope that medical intervention will help them achieve their goal.

Most couples are more correctly considered to be *subfertile,* rather than infertile, as they will ultimately conceive if given enough time. This concept of subfertility can be reassuring to couples. However, there are obvious exceptions, such as the woman with bilaterally obstructed fallopian tubes or the azoospermic male.

It is generally agreed that an infertility evaluation should be considered in any couple that has failed to conceive in 1 year. There are a number of clinical scenarios, however, in which evaluation should be considered sooner. For example, to delay evaluation in an anovulatory woman or a woman with a history of severe pelvic inflammatory disease (PID) may not be appropriate. Furthermore, fecundability is highly age related, thus evaluation at 6 months should be performed in women older than 40 years who desire conception, and according to some experts, in women older than 35. As a part of infertility evaluation, the patient should be prepared for an anticipated pregnancy. A comprehensive list of preconceptional topics is found in Table 1-3 (p. 12).

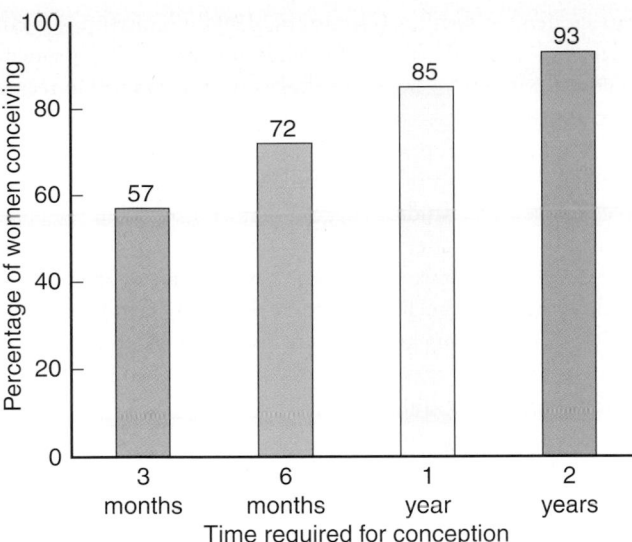

FIGURE 19-1 Time required for conception.

ETIOLOGY OF INFERTILITY

Successful pregnancy requires a complex sequence of events including ovulation, ovum pick-up by a fallopian tube, fertilization, transport of a fertilized ovum into the uterus, and implantation into a receptive uterine cavity. With male infertility, sperm of adequate number and quality must be deposited at the cervix near the time of ovulation. Remembering these critical events can help direct a clinician to develop an appropriate evaluation and treatment strategy.

In general, infertility can be attributed to the female partner one third of the time, the male partner one third of the time, and both partners in the remaining one third. This approximation emphasizes the importance of evaluating both members of the couple before instituting therapy. Estimates of the incidence of various causes of infertility are shown in Table 19-1 (Abma, 1997; American Society for Reproductive Medicine, 2006a).

It should be strongly urged that both partners be present for the initial consultation. A visit to a health care provider for infertility evaluation provides an excellent opportunity for educating a couple regarding the normal process of conception. Many myths surround the ability to conceive, such as the importance of coital position and the need to remain horizontal following ejaculation. These myths can add undue stress to an already stressful situation and should be dispelled.

Couples should be educated regarding the concept of a fertile window for conception. The chance of conception is increased

TABLE 19-1. Etiology of Infertility

Male	25%
Ovulatory	27%
Tubal/uterine	22%
Other	9%
Unexplained	17%

from the 5 days preceding ovulation through the day of ovulation (Wilcox, 1995). If the male partner has normal semen characteristics, a couple should have daily intercourse during this period to maximize the chance of conception. Although sperm concentrations will drop with increasing coital frequency, this decrease is generally too small to negatively impact the chance of fertilization (Stanford, 2002). Couples should also be reminded to avoid oil-based lubricants, which are harmful to sperm.

MEDICAL HISTORY

The Female History
Gynecologic

As with any medical condition, a thorough history and physical examination is critical (American Society for Reproductive Medicine, 2000). For the female partner, questions should include a complete gynecologic history. Specifically, questions regarding menstruation (frequency, duration, recent change in interval or duration, hot flashes, and dysmenorrhea), prior contraceptive use, and duration of infertility should be asked. Also pertinent is a history of recurrent ovarian cysts, endometriosis, leiomyomas, sexually transmitted diseases, or PID. Because prior conception indicates ovulation and a patent fallopian tube in the patient's past, this history should be sought. A prolonged time to conception may suggest subfertility and may increase the chance of determining an etiology in a couple. Pregnancy complications such as miscarriage, preterm delivery, retained placenta, postpartum dilatation and curettage, chorioamnionitis, or fetal anomalies should be noted. A history of abnormal Pap smears may be pertinent, particularly if a woman underwent cervical conization, which could lower cervical mucus quality and alter cervical canal anatomy. When gathering a medical history, a coital history, including frequency and timing of intercourse, should be obtained. Symptoms such as dyspareunia may point to endometriosis and a need for earlier laparoscopic evaluation of the female partner.

Medical

The medical history should be aimed at eliciting symptoms of hyperprolactinemia or thyroid disease. Symptoms of androgen excess such as acne or hirsutism may point to polycystic ovarian syndrome (PCOS) or much less commonly, congenital adrenal hyperplasia. Prior chemotherapy or pelvic irradiation may suggest ovarian failure.

Surgical

The surgical history should focus on pelvic and abdominal surgeries. Surgical treatment of ruptured appendicitis or diverticulitis should raise suspicion for pelvic adhesive disease or tubal obstruction or both. Prior uterine surgery can be associated with intrauterine adhesions.

Medications

Questions regarding medications should be include over-the-counter medications, such as nonsteroidal antiinflammatory drugs, that may adversely affect ovulation. In most instances, use of herbal remedies should be discouraged. Women should

TABLE 19-2. Effects of Obesity and Environmental Factors on Fertility

Factor	Impact on Fertility
Obesity (BMI >35)	2-fold increase TTC
Underweight (BMI <19)	4-fold increase TTC
Smoking	60% increase RR
Alcohol (>2/day)	60% increase RR
Illicit drugs	70% increase RR
Toxins	40% increase RR
Caffeine (>250 mg/day)	45% decrease fecundability

BMI = body mass index; RR = relative risk of infertility; TTC = time to conception.
Abbreviated from American Society for Reproductive Medicine, 2008a, with permission.

be encouraged to take a daily vitamin with at least 400 µg of folic acid to decrease the chance of neural-tube defects. In those with a previously affected child, 4 g should be taken orally daily (American College of Obstetricians and Gynecologists, 2003).

Social

A social history should focus on lifestyle and environmental factors such as eating habits and exposure to toxins. Abnormalities in gonadotropin-releasing hormone (GnRH) and gonadotropin secretion are clearly related to body mass indices >25 or <17 (Table 1-7, p. 17) (Grodstein, 1994a). Although difficult to achieve, even modest weight reduction in overweight women is correlated with normalized menstrual cycles and subsequent pregnancies (Table 19-2).

Accumulating data also suggest that cigarette smoking lowers fertility in both women and men (Hughes, 1996; Hull, 2000; Kunzle, 2003; Laurent, 1992). The prevalence of infertility is higher and the time to conception is longer in women who smoke, or even those exposed passively to cigarette smoke. Toxins in the smoke can accelerate follicular depletion and increase genetic mutations in gametes or early embryos (Sharara, 1994; Shideler, 1989). Admittedly, current data do not prove causation, but only correlation, between smoking and infertility or adverse pregnancy outcomes. Nevertheless, an estimated 25 percent of women in the reproductive age group smoke, and the desire for pregnancy can be a powerful motivator toward cessation (Augood, 1998). Table 1-23 (p. 28) contains a list of agents approved by the Food and Drug Administration for smoking cessation.

Alcohol consumption should also be limited. Heavy alcohol intake decreases fertility in women and has been associated with a decrease in sperm counts and increase in sexual dysfunction in men (Klonoff-Cohen, 2003; Nagy, 1986). A standardized alcoholic drink is typically defined as 12 ounces of beer, 5 ounces of wine, or 1.5 ounces of hard alcohol. Based on a number of studies, five to eight drinks per week negatively

impacts female fertility (Grodstein, 1994b; Tolstrup, 2003). As alcohol is also detrimental to early pregnancy, it is prudent to advise patients to avoid alcohol consumption while trying to conceive.

Caffeine consumption has also been linked to decreased fecundability. A cup of coffee contains approximately 115 mg of caffeine. Most studies suggest that consumption of more than 250 mg of caffeine daily by the female partner is associated with a modest, but statistically significant, decrease in fertility and increase in time to conception. Caffeine intake greater than 500 mg per day has also been demonstrated to increase recurrent miscarriage rates (Bolumar, 1997; Caan, 1998; Cnattingius, 2000).

Illicit drugs may also impact fecundability. Marijuana suppresses the hypothalamic-pituitary-gonadal axis in both men and women, and cocaine can impair spermatogenesis (Bracken, 1990; Smith, 1987a). Although uncommon, fecundability is reduced with occupational exposure to the dry cleaning fluid perchloroethylene and to toluene used in the printing business. Heavy metals and pesticides should also be avoided, as they may both decrease fertility rates and increase the risk of recurrent miscarriage (Orejuela, 1998).

Ethnicity

The ethnic background of both partners is important for determining the need for preconceptional testing, such as screening for sickle cell anemia in African-Americans, for Tay-Sachs disease and other disorders in Ashkenazi Jews, and for cystic fibrosis in patients of northern European descent (American College of Obstetricians and Gynecologists, 2005, 2007, 2009). A family history of infertility, recurrent miscarriage, or fetal anomalies may also point to a genetic etiology. Although the inheritance pattern is complex, data suggest that both PCOS and endometriosis occur in familial clusters. For example, a woman carries an estimated sevenfold increased risk of endometriosis over the general population if a single first-degree family member has the disease (Moen, 1993).

The Male History

The male partner should be questioned regarding pubertal development and difficulties with sexual function. Erectile dysfunction, particularly in conjunction with decreased beard growth, may suggest decreased testosterone levels. Ejaculatory dysfunction should also be evaluated, including investigation of developmental anomalies such as hypospadias, which could result in suboptimal semen deposition (Benson, 1997).

Sexually transmitted diseases or frequent genitourinary infections, including epididymitis or prostatitis, may result in obstruction of the vas deferens. Mumps in an adult can lead to testicular inflammation and damage to the spermatogenic stem cells (Beard, 1977). Moreover, a history of cryptorchidism, testicular torsion, or testicular trauma may suggest abnormal spermatogenesis (Anderson, 1990; Bartsch, 1980; Sigman, 1997; Tas, 1996). Compared with fertile males, males with a history of unilateral or bilateral cryptorchidism (failure of testes to descend) have fertility rates of 80 percent and 50 percent, respectively (Lee, 1993). The reason for poor semen characteristics in

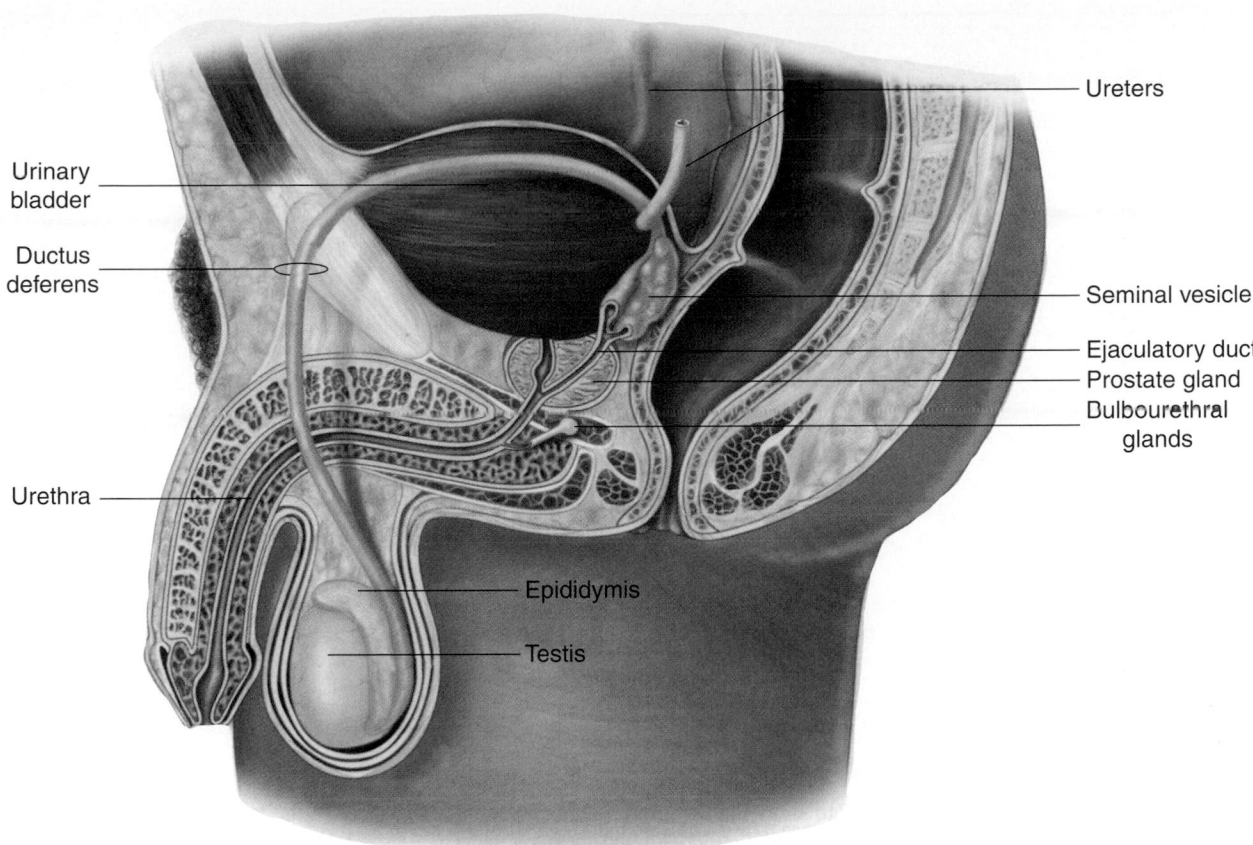

FIGURE 19-2 Male genitalia. *(From McKinley, 2006, with permission.)*

these patients is unclear. The relatively warm intraabdominal temperature may cause permanent damage to the stem cells. Alternatively, genetic abnormalities that led to the abnormal location of the testes may also affect sperm production.

A history of varicocele should also be obtained. A varicocele consists of dilated veins of the pampiniform plexus of the spermatic cords that drain the testes (Figs. 19-2 and 19-3). Varicoceles are believed to raise scrotal temperature, however, the negative

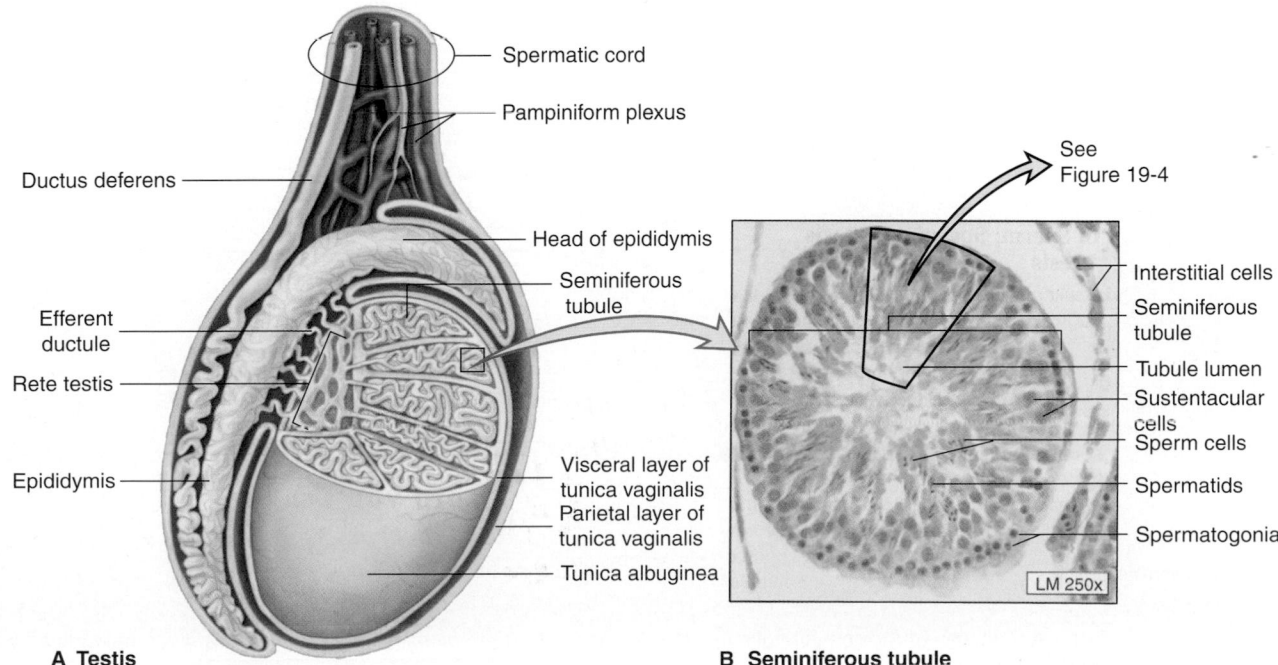

FIGURE 19-3 Male testis. **A.** Gross anatomy of a testis. **B.** Cutaway of the testis reveals the microscopic structure of a seminiferous tubule. *(From McKinley, 2006, with permission.)*

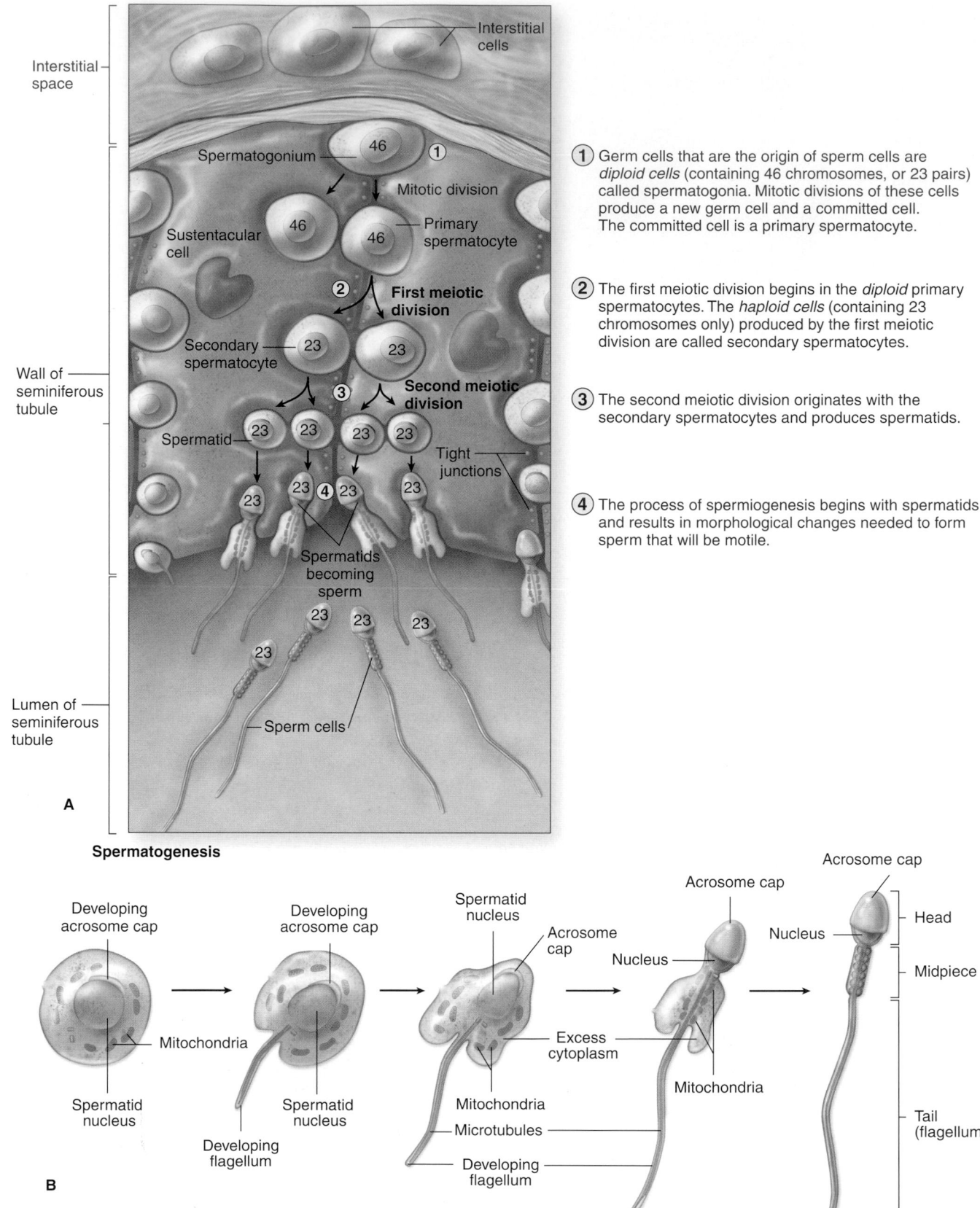

1 Germ cells that are the origin of sperm cells are *diploid cells* (containing 46 chromosomes, or 23 pairs) called spermatogonia. Mitotic divisions of these cells produce a new germ cell and a committed cell. The committed cell is a primary spermatocyte.

2 The first meiotic division begins in the *diploid* primary spermatocytes. The *haploid cells* (containing 23 chromosomes only) produced by the first meiotic division are called secondary spermatocytes.

3 The second meiotic division originates with the secondary spermatocytes and produces spermatids.

4 The process of spermiogenesis begins with spermatids and results in morphological changes needed to form sperm that will be motile.

FIGURE 19-4 Male testis. **A.** Cutaway of the seminiferous tubule from Figure 19-3 shows the mitotic and meiotic divisions involved with spermatogenesis. **B.** Structural changes required during spermiogenesis. *(From McKinley, 2006, with permission.)*

affects of varicoceles on fertility are controversial (Chehval, 1992; Jarow, 2001; World Health Organization, 1992). Although 30 to 40 percent of men seen in infertility clinics are diagnosed with a varicocele, nearly 20 percent of men in the general population are similarly affected. Although there has been substantial disagreement on the benefits gained from varicocele repair, metaanalyses suggest that varicocele repair improves fertility (American Society for Reproductive Medicine, 2008b; Schlesinger, 1994; Steckel, 1993). If a varicocele is suspected, it should be evaluated by a urologist, preferably one with a specific interest in infertility.

Spermatogenesis, from stem cell to mature sperm, within the epididymis, takes nearly 90 days (Fig. 19-4). Therefore, any detrimental event in the prior 3 months can adversely affect semen characteristics (Hinrichsen, 1980; Rowley, 1970). Spermatogenesis is optimal at temperatures slightly below body temperature, hence the location of the testes outside of the pelvis. Illness with high fevers or chronic hot tub use can temporarily impair sperm quality. There is no definitive evidence that boxer underwear is advantageous (Tas, 1996).

The medical portion of the male history should focus on prior treatment with chemotherapy or local radiation therapy that may damage the spermatogonial stem cells. Hypertension, diabetes mellitus, and neurologic disorders may be associated with erectile dysfunction or retrograde ejaculation. Several medications are known to worsen semen parameters and include cimetidine, erythromycin, gentamicin, tetracycline, and spironolactone (Sigman, 1997). As described previously, cigarettes, alcohol, illicit drugs, and environmental toxins all adversely affect semen parameters (Muthusami, 2005; Ramlau-Hansen, 2007). The increasing use of anabolic steroids also decreases sperm production by suppressing the production of intratesticular testosterone (Gazvani, 1997). Although the effects of many medications are reversible, anabolic steroid abuse may lead to lasting or even permanent damage to testicular function.

PHYSICAL EXAMINATION

Examination of the Female Patient

A physical examination may provide many clues to the cause of infertility. Vital signs, height, and weight should be recorded.

A particularly short stature may reflect a genetic condition such as Turner syndrome. Hirsutism, alopecia, or acne indicates the need to measure androgen levels. Acanthosis nigricans is consistent with insulin resistance associated with PCOS or much less commonly, Cushing syndrome. Galactorrhea is often indicative of hyperprolactinemia. Additionally, thyroid abnormalities should be noted. Many of these diagnoses and their management are discussed in greater detail in other chapters (Table 19-3).

A pelvic examination may be particularly informative. Inability to place a speculum through the introitus may raise doubts about coital frequency. The vagina should be moist and rugated, and the cervix should have a reasonable amount of mucus. Both indicate adequate estrogen production. An enlarged or irregularly shaped uterus may reflect leiomyomas, whereas a fixed uterus suggests pelvic scarring due to endometriosis or prior pelvic infection. Uterosacral nodularity or ovarian masses may additionally implicate endometriosis.

All women should have a normal Pap smear result within the year preceding treatment. Negative cultures for *Neisseria gonorrhoeae* and *Chlamydia trachomatis* should be obtained to ensure that cervical manipulation during evaluation and treatment does not cause an ascending infection. The breast examination must be normal, and when indicated by age or family history, a mammogram should be obtained prior to initiating hormonal treatment.

Examination of the Male Patient

Most gynecologists will not feel comfortable performing a complete physical examination of the male. Nevertheless, parts of this evaluation are relatively easy to perform, and a gynecologist at minimum should understand the primary focus of the examination. As signs of testosterone production, normal secondary sexual characteristics such as beard growth, axillary and pubic hair, and perhaps male pattern balding should be present. Gynecomastia or eunuchoid habitus may suggest Klinefelter syndrome (47,XXY karyotype) (De Braekeleer, 1991).

The penile urethra should be at the tip of the glans for proper semen deposition in the vagina. Testicular length

TABLE 19-3. Chapters with Relevant Information about Infertility

Etiology	Diagnosis	Chapter Title	Chapter Number
Ovulatory dysfunction	PCOS	PCOS and hyperandrogenism	Chapter 17
	Hypothalamic-pituitary	Amenorrhea	Chapter 16
	Age-related	Menopausal transition	Chapter 21
	POF	Amenorrhea	Chapter 16
Tubal disease	PID	Gynecologic infection	Chapter 3
Uterine abnormalities	Congenital	Anatomic disorders	Chapter 18
	Leiomyomas	Pelvic mass	Chapter 9
	Asherman syndrome	Amenorrhea	Chapter 16
Other	Endometriosis	Endometriosis	Chapter 10

PCOS = polycystic ovarian disease; POF = premature ovarian failure; PID = pelvic inflammatory disease.

should be at least 4 cm with a minimal testicular volume of 20 mL (Charny, 1960; Hadziselimovic, 2006). Small testes are unlikely to be producing normal sperm numbers. A testicular mass may indicate testicular cancer, which can present as infertility. The epididymis should be soft and nontender to exclude chronic infection. Epididymal fullness may suggest vas deferens obstruction. The prostate should be smooth, nontender, and normal size. Additionally, the pampiniform plexus of veins should be palpated for varicocele (Jarow, 2001). Importantly, both vas deferens should be palpable. Congenital bilateral absence of the vas deferens is associated with mutation in the gene responsible for cystic fibrosis (Anguiano, 1992).

EVALUATION FOR SPECIFIC CAUSES OF INFERTILITY

The infertility evaluation can be conceptually simplified into confirmation of: (1) ovulation, (2) normal female reproductive tract anatomy, and (3) normal semen characteristics. The specifics regarding evaluation of each of these categories will be detailed in the following sections and are shown in Table 19-4.

■ Etiology of Infertility in the Female
Ovulatory Dysfunction

Ovulation may be perturbed by abnormalities within the hypothalamus, anterior pituitary, or ovaries. Hypothalamic disorders may be acquired or inherited. Acquired disorders include those due to lifestyle, for example, excessive exercise, eating disorders, or stress. Alternatively, dysfunction or improper migration of

the hypothalamic gonadotropin-releasing hormone neurons may be inherited, such as that which occurs in idiopathic hypothalamic hypogonadism (IHH) or in Kallmann syndrome. Thyroid disease and hyperprolactinemia may also contribute to menstrual disturbances. A full discussion of disorders that result in menstrual disturbances is found in Chapter 16 (p. 440).

Menstrual Pattern. A patient's menstrual history is an excellent predictor of regular ovulation. A woman with cyclic menses at an interval of 25 to 35 days and duration of bleeding of 3 to 7 days is most likely ovulating. Although these numbers vary widely, each woman will have her own normal pattern. Therefore, these figures should not significantly vary across cycles for an individual woman.

Probable ovulation is also suggested by *mittelschmerz*, which is midcycle pelvic pain associated with ovulation, or by moliminal symptoms such as breast tenderness, acne, food cravings, and mood changes. Ovulatory cycles are more likely to be associated with dysmenorrhea, although severe dysmenorrhea may suggest endometriosis.

Basal Body Temperature. Basal body temperature (BBT) charting has long been used to identify ovulation. This test requires that a woman's morning oral temperature be graphically charted (Fig. 19-5). Oral temperatures are usually 97.0° to 98.0°F during the follicular phase. A postovulatory rise in progesterone levels increases basal temperature by approximately 0.4° to 0.8°F. This *biphasic* temperature pattern is strongly predictive of ovulation (Bates, 1990). Nevertheless, although this test has the advantage of being inexpensive, it is insensitive in many women. Furthermore, for a couple wishing to conceive, the temperature increase follows ovulation, and therefore the

TABLE 19-4. Infertility Testing

Etiology	Evaluation
Ovulatory dysfunction	Serum midluteal progesterone level Ovulation predictor kit Early follicular FSH ± estradiol level (ovarian reserve) ± Antimüllerian hormone (AMH) level ± Serum measurements (TSH, prolactin, androgens) ± Ovarian sonography (antral follicle count) ± Basal body temperature chart ± Endometrial biopsy (luteal phase defect)
Tubal/pelvic disease	Hysterosalpingography Laparoscopy with chromotubation
Uterine factors	Hysterosalpingography Transvaginal sonography Saline infusion sonography Magnetic resonance imaging Hysteroscopy Laparoscopy
Cervical factor	± Postcoital test
Male factor	Semen analysis

FSH = follicle-stimulating hormone; TSH = thyroid-stimulating hormone.

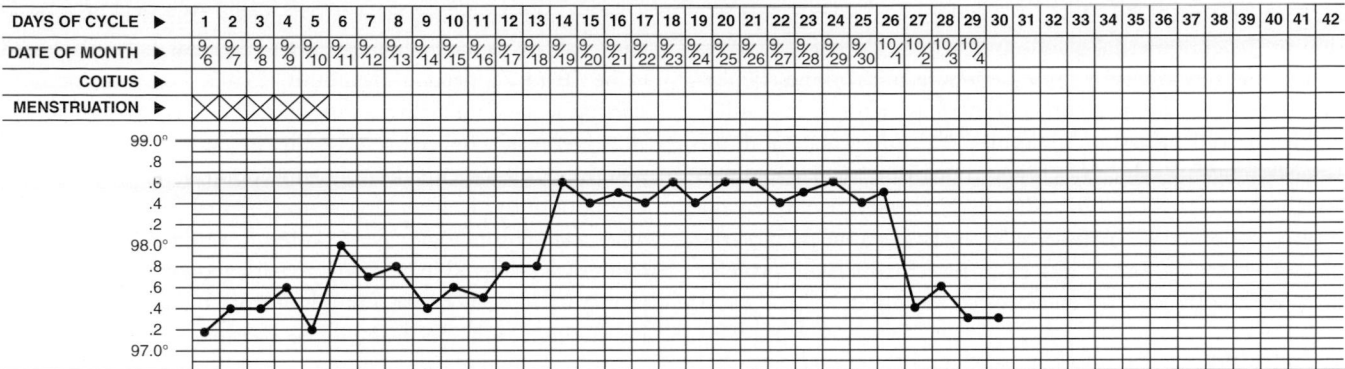

FIGURE 19-5 Biphasic pattern seen on this basal body temperature chart suggests ovulation. *(From Chang, 2005, with permission).*

window of maximal fertility has been missed (Grinsted, 1989; Luciano, 1990; Moghissi, 1992). Although this test may be useful for a couple first attempting to conceive, it has generally fallen out of favor as an infertility diagnostic tool.

Ovulation Predictor Kits. A number of additional tests for ovulation have been developed. Urinary ovulation predictor kits are widely available in pharmacies. These kits, which measure the concentration of urinary luteinizing hormone (LH) by colorimetric assay, have become relatively easy to use and provide clear instructions regarding interpretation.

In general, a woman should begin testing 2 to 3 days prior to the predicted LH surge, and testing should be continued daily. There is no clear consensus regarding the optimal time of day to test. Some infertility specialists suggest that the concentrated first morning void is a logical testing time. Others are concerned that this sample may provide a false-positive result, and they suggest testing the second morning urine. Other clinicians reason that the serum LH peak occurs in the morning and that the greatest likelihood of detecting a urinary peak would be in the late afternoon or evening. Timing is probably not critical as long as the test is performed daily, as the LH surge spans only 48 to 50 hours. In most instances, ovulation will occur the day following the urinary LH peak (Luciano, 1990; Miller, 1996).

If equivocal results are obtained, the test can be repeated in 12 hours. In one study, urine LH surge assays were estimated to have 100-percent sensitivity and 96-percent accuracy, although this is undoubtedly an overestimate of typical-use results (Grinsted, 1989; Guermandi, 2001).

Serum Progesterone. Ovulation can also be tested by measuring midluteal phase serum progesterone levels. In a classic 28-day cycle, serum is obtained on cycle day number 21 following the first day of menstrual bleeding, or 7 days following ovulation. Levels during the follicular phase are generally <2 ng/mL. Values above 4 to 6 ng/mL are highly correlated with ovulation and progesterone production by the corpus luteum (Guermandi, 2001). Progesterone is secreted as pulses, and therefore a single measurement is not indicative of overall production during the luteal phase. As a result, an absolute threshold for acceptable progesterone levels has not been clearly established.

Nevertheless, Hull and colleagues (1982) have reported that a midluteal progesterone concentration of greater than 9.4 ng/mL is predictive of higher pregnancy rates than those observed in patients with progesterone levels less than 10 ng/mL.

Many clinicians choose to empirically treat any patient with a progesterone level below this value with natural progesterone. Although this approach is unlikely to be harmful, the utility of this management is unproven. Accordingly, the midluteal progesterone level is best regarded as an excellent measure for the occurrence of ovulation, but not an absolute indicator of adequate luteal function.

Endometrial Biopsy. Adequate progesterone levels are required for endometrial preparation prior to implantation. Luteal phase defect (LPD) occurs when suboptimal progesterone production results in inadequate endometrial development. Thus, it was proposed that an endometrial biopsy would reflect both corpus luteum function and endometrial response, and thereby provide more clinically relevant information than a serum progesterone level alone. Noyes and associates (1975) described a sequence of histologic events in the endometrium in the periovulatory, luteal, and early menstrual stages. These investigators defined LPD as a lag in the histologic appearance of the endometrium of greater than 2 days relative to the actual day of the cycle determined retrospectively. This discrepancy in dating is termed an *out-of-phase biopsy*. Classically, an endometrial biopsy is obtained as close to the impending menstrual cycle as possible based on previous cycle length and more recently, on the timing of the LH surge.

Unfortunately, the utility of this test is severely hampered by high intraobserver and interobserver variability (Balasch, 1992; Scott, 1993). The estimated frequency of LPD in the infertile population has ranged widely, but is generally agreed to be between 5 and 10 percent. Nevertheless, a finding of an out-of-phase biopsy occurs nearly as frequently in fertile as in infertile women, with a large overlap in incidence between the two groups (Aksel, 1980; Balasch, 1992; Davis, 1989; Scott, 1993). This observation has led many experts to conclude that LPD may not exist as a clinical entity. Certainly in its current form, the endometrial biopsy has little predictive value. For all of these reasons, this test is no longer considered a routine part of the infertility evaluation.

It is interesting to note that impressive advances are being made in our understanding of the timing of protein expression in the endometrial glands and stroma. Potential markers for uterine receptivity include osteopontin, cytokines (leukemia inhibitory factor, colony-stimulating factor-1, and interleukin-1), cell adhesion molecules (the integrins), and the L-selectin ligand, which has been proposed to mediate embryo attachment (Carson, 2002; Kao, 2003; Lessey, 1998). In the future, endometrial biopsies may again become part of the diagnostic evaluation if expression patterns of these proteins prove to be predictive of endometrial receptivity.

Sonography. Serial ovarian sonographic evaluations can demonstrate the development of a mature antral follicle and its subsequent collapse during ovulation. This approach is time consuming, and ovulation can be missed. However, sonography is an excellent approach for supporting the diagnosis of PCOS (Chap. 17, p. 472).

Female Aging and Ovulatory Dysfunction

Epidemiology. There is a clear inverse relationship between female age and fertility (Table 19-5) (American Society for Reproductive Medicine, 2006a). A classic study was performed in the Hutterites, a community that eschews contraception. After ages 34, 40, and 45, the incidence of infertility was 11 percent, 33 percent, and 87 percent, respectively. The average age at last pregnancy was 40.9 years (Tietze, 1957). Another interesting study evaluated cumulative pregnancy rates in women using donor insemination. In women younger than 31 years, 74 percent achieved pregnancy within 1 year. These rates fell to 62 percent for women between 31 and 35 years, and further declined to 54 percent in women older than 35 (Treloar, 1998).

Physiology. Age-related infertility is most closely linked to the loss of viable oocytes. At midgestation, a normal human female fetus has approximately 7 million oocytes, which will decrease to between 1 and 2 million by birth (Fig. 14-1, p. 383). Ongoing atresia of nondominant follicles proceeds throughout a woman's reproductive life span. Approximately 300,000 follicles are present at puberty, and <1000 follicles at the onset of menopause. Thus, even before a female reaches menarche, she has lost most of her eggs.

As a woman ages, risks of genetic abnormalities and mitochondrial deletions in the remaining oocytes are substantially increased (Keefe, 1995; Pellestor, 2003). These factors result

in decreased pregnancy rates and increased miscarriage rates in both spontaneous and stimulated cycles. The overall miscarriage risk in women older than 40 years has been estimated to be 50 to 75 percent (Maroulis, 1991). For these reasons, starting at age 35, fertility testing should be strongly considered after failure to conceive for 1 year, or perhaps even after six months, in all patients desiring conception.

Importantly, ovarian reserve can be lost for many reasons other than chronologic age. As a result, testing should also be seriously considered in any woman with an unexplained change in menstrual cyclicity or a family history of early menopause. Furthermore, evaluation should be considered in heavy smokers or in women with a history of ovarian surgery, chemotherapy, or pelvic irradiation.

An array of serum and sonographic tests has been developed to evaluate a patient's likelihood of conception, and a number of these are described subsequently. The optimal combination of tests is under ongoing revision. Currently, measurement of early follicular follicle-stimulating hormone (FSH) and estradiol levels is probably the most cost-effective approach for the general practitioner. In general, testing for thyroid disease and hyperprolactinemia also seems prudent as these disorders may be associated with ovulatory defects that may be mild and difficult to ascertain by history.

Follicle-Stimulating Hormone. Measurement of serum FSH levels in the early follicular phase is a simple and sensitive predictor of ovarian reserve (Toner, 1991). With declining ovarian function, the granulosa cells and luteal cells secrete less inhibin, a peptide hormone that is responsible for inhibiting FSH secretion by the anterior pituitary gonadotropes (Chap. 15, p. 402). With loss of luteal inhibin, FSH levels rise in the early follicular phase. Measurement of serum FSH levels is classically performed on cycle day number 3 following the onset of menses, the so-called "cycle day 3" FSH level. However, it is reasonable to test between days 2 and 4. A value >10 mIU/mL indicates significant loss of ovarian reserve and should prompt a more rapid evaluation and more intensive treatment. In a large study evaluating in vitro fertilization (IVF) cycles, a day-3 FSH level exceeding 15 mIU/mL was predictive of significantly lower pregnancy rates (Muasher, 1988; Scott, 1995; Toner, 1991).

Estradiol. Many clinicians also measure serum estradiol levels simultaneously (Buyalos, 1997; Licciardi, 1995). Addition of an estradiol measurement may decrease the incidence of false-negative results of FSH values alone. Somewhat paradoxically, despite the overall depletion of ovarian follicles, estrogen levels in older women will be elevated early in the cycle due to increased stimulation of ovarian steroidogenesis by elevated FSH levels. A cycle-day-3 estradiol level of >80 pg/mL is considered abnormal. It should be noted that reference levels for estradiol and FSH can vary between laboratories. Therefore, clinicians should become familiar with their own laboratory's normal values.

Inhibin B. Attempts to identify additional markers of ovarian reserve have included measurement of the granulosa cell product inhibin B. Inhibin B increases during the follicular phase, leading to progressive inhibition of FSH secretion by the

TABLE 19-5. Female Aging and Infertility

Female Age (years)	Infertility
20–29	8.0%
30–34	14.6%
35–39	21.9%
40–44	28.7%

pituitary gland. As with FSH and estradiol, inhibin B must be measured early in the follicular phase due to large fluctuations in serum levels across the cycle. Although initially promising, inhibin B levels have not been shown to add substantially to the information gained from FSH testing, and therefore, this test is falling out of favor.

Antimüllerian Hormone. Antimüllerian hormone (AMH) is the most recent circulating factor to be analyzed as a predictor of ovarian reserve (La Marca, 2009). As suggested by its name, AMH is expressed by the fetal testes during male differentiation to prevent development of the müllerian system (fallopian tubes, uterus, and upper vagina). AMH is also expressed by the granulosa cells of small preantral follicles, with limited expression in larger follicles. This observation suggests that AMH plays a role in recruitment of a dominant follicle. Measurement of AMH levels has an advantage over FSH and inhibin testing, as expression is independent of cycle stage. Furthermore, AMH levels may drop prior to observable changes in FSH or estradiol levels, providing an earlier marker of waning ovarian function. Recent studies suggest that AMH levels correlate with ovarian primordial follicle number more strongly than FSH or inhibin levels (Hansen, 2011). Interestingly, AMH levels are increased two- to threefold in women with PCOS compared with normally cycling women. This observation is consistent with the multiple early follicles found in these patients.

Clomiphene Citrate Challenge Test. The clomiphene citrate challenge test (CCCT) is believed to be a more sensitive indicator of diminished ovarian reserve than measurement of "unstimulated" hormone levels (Navot, 1987). Clomiphene citrate (Clomid) is a nonsteroidal estrogen-receptor modulator. Although the exact mechanism is not fully understood, clomiphene is believed to block the negative-feedback inhibition of endogenous estrogens on FSH secretion (Fig. 20-1, p. 533). With the test, a woman takes 100 mg of clomiphene citrate daily orally on cycle day numbers 5 through 9. Estradiol and FSH levels are measured on day 3, and an FSH level is measured on day 10. Follicle-stimulating hormone elevations at either time point are indicative of diminished ovarian reserve.

In general, a simple day-3 FSH level measurement is probably adequate as an initial screen. However, consideration should be given to performing a CCCT in women with a borderline FSH level or in those older than 40.

Antral Follicle Count. Sonographic evaluation of the follicular phase antral follicle count (AFC) is commonly used in infertility practice as a reliable predictor for subsequent response to ovulation induction (Frattarelli, 2000; Maseelall, 2009). The number of small antral follicles reflects the size of the resting follicular pool. Antral follicles between 2 and 10 mm are counted in both ovaries. The total AFC is usually between 10 and 20 in a reproductive-aged woman. A count less than 10 predicts poor response to gonadotropin stimulation.

Testing Interpretation. Abnormal test results from any of the preceding methods correlate with a poorer prognosis for achieving pregnancy whatever the woman's age. Referral to an infertility specialist is advisable in these patients. Conversely, a normal test does not negate the impact of a woman's age on her fertility status. This information may be useful in counseling a couple regarding prognosis. Poor results in an older woman can supply an impetus either to attempt donor oocyte IVF or to pursue alternatives such as adoption. Borderline results in a younger woman may suggest a need for more intensive treatment.

Tubal and Pelvic Factors

Symptoms such as chronic pelvic pain or dysmenorrhea may suggest tubal obstruction or pelvic adhesions or both. Adhesions can prevent normal tubal movement, ovum pickup, and transport of the fertilized egg into the uterus. A wide variety of etiologies may contribute to tubal disease, including pelvic infection, endometriosis, and prior pelvic surgery.

A history of PID is highly suspicious for pelvic adhesions or damage to the fallopian tubes. Tubal infertility has been estimated to follow in 12 percent, 23 percent, and 54 percent of women following one, two, or three cases of PID, respectively (Lalos, 1988). Nevertheless, an absent PID history is not overly reassuring, as nearly one half of patients who are found to have tubal damage have no clinical history of antecedent disease (Rosenfeld, 1983).

Approximately one third to one fourth of all infertile women in developed countries are diagnosed with tubal disease (Serafini, 1989; World Health Organization, 2007). In the United States, the most common causes of tubal disease are infection with *C trachomatis* or *N gonorrhoeae* (Chap. 3, p. 93). In contrast, in developing countries, genital tuberculosis may account for 3 to 5 percent of infertility cases (Aliyu, 2004; Nezar, 2009). As a result, this diagnosis should be considered in immigrant populations from countries with endemic infection. In these cases, tubal damage and endometrial adhesions are underlying causes. Genital tuberculosis typically follows hematogenous seeding of the reproductive tract from an extragenital primary infection. The likelihood of a return to fertility after antitubercular treatment is low, and IVF with embryo transfer remains the most reliable approach (Aliyu, 2004).

Within implants of endometriosis, inflammation and chronic bleeding can also lead to fallopian tube obstruction or development of severe pelvic adhesions. In addition, a history of ectopic pregnancy, even if treated medically with methotrexate, implies the likelihood of significant tubal damage. Residual adhesions are common after even the most meticulous pelvic surgery. This is particularly true in cases with pelvic inflammation due to blood, infection, or irritation caused by mature cystic teratoma (dermoid) contents.

Salpingitis isthmica nodosa is an inflammatory condition of the fallopian tube, characterized by nodular thickening of its isthmic portion. Histologically, smooth muscle proliferation and diverticula of tubal epithelium contribute to this thickening. This uncommon condition is typically bilateral and progressive and leads ultimately to tubal occlusion and infertility (Saracoglu, 1992). Fertility options include those for proximal tubal occlusion as discussed in Chapter 20 (p. 540). In addition, the risk of ectopic pregnancy is increased with salpingitis isthmica nodosa.

Testing for tubal patency can be performed by hysterosalpingography (HSG) or by chromotubation during laparoscopy. Chapter 2 (p. 50) contains an additional discussion of HSG performance. Regarding treatment, fimbrioplasty may be considered in cases of distal tubal obstruction without significant hydrosalpinx. Attempts may also be made to correct proximal obstruction with balloon tuboplasty via hysteroscopy. However, with the advent of successful pregnancy rates using IVF, tubal surgery rates are decreasing. All of these options are described fully in Chapter 20.

Uterine Abnormalities

Congenital Anomalies. Uterine anomalies can be either inherited or acquired. Common inherited anomalies include uterine septum, bicornuate uterus, unicornuate uterus, and uterine didelphys. With the possible exception of a large uterine septum, the impact of these anomalies on conception has been difficult to verify, although a subset are clearly associated with pregnancy complications. A uterine septum can now be removed relatively simply and safely with hysteroscopy as described in Section 42-19 (p. 1174). Most infertility specialists will proceed with surgery if this anomaly is identified.

Diethylstilbestrol. In utero exposure to this synthetic estrogen has been linked to malformations of uterine development in addition to an increased risk for vaginal adenosis. More information on this topic can be found in Chapter 18 (p. 502). The classic uterine appearance is a small, T-shaped uterus. Fortunately, this problem is seen progressively less frequently in infertility clinics as this drug is no longer used and most affected women are leaving reproductive age (Goldberg, 1999).

Acquired Abnormalities. Acquired anomalies include intrauterine polyps, leiomyomas, and Asherman syndrome.

Endometrial Polyps. These soft fleshy growths are estimated to be present in 3 to 5 percent of infertile women (Farhi, 1995; Soares, 2000). The prevalence is higher in women with symptoms, such as intermenstrual or postcoital bleeding (Chap. 8, p. 230). Although these complaints typically prompt hysteroscopic removal, most data have not clearly demonstrated an indication for removing polyps in otherwise asymptomatic women (Ben-Arie, 2004; DeWaay, 2002). Of note, however, one study has suggested that removal of even small polyps (under 1 cm) may improve pregnancy rates following intrauterine insemination (Perez-Medina, 2005).

Leiomyomas. These benign smooth muscle tumors may also prevent normal implantation, depending on their size and location (Pritts, 2001). Certainly, it is reasonable to assume that leiomyomas that obstruct a fallopian tube, distort the uterine cavity, or fill the uterine cavity would be detrimental to implantation. The endometrium overlying these tumors is less vascular and the surrounding myometrium exhibits dysfunctional contractility, both of which may contribute to decreased rates of successful pregnancy. It seems equally reasonable to postulate that a subserosal leiomyoma would not adversely affect pregnancy.

Farhi and colleagues (1995) studied the effects of uterine leiomyomas on IVF success rates. In 28 women with a normal uterine cavity, the pregnancy rate was 30 percent per embryo transfer. In 18 women with an abnormal cavity, the pregnancy rate was only 9 percent per transfer. Although this suggests that removal of submucous leiomyomas should improve fecundability, there are no randomized, prospective trials to confirm this conclusion.

Appropriate intervention is even more ambiguous in the patient with intramural leiomyomas that do not abut the endometrium (Stovall, 1998). Thus far, it has not been possible to develop an algorithm based on number, volume, or location of these tumors that accurately predicts the need to remove them, either to improve implantation rates or to decrease pregnancy complications such as miscarriage, placental abruption, or preterm labor. Nevertheless, many experts will consider surgical removal of a leiomyoma greater than 5 cm or multiple smaller tumors in this size range. Importantly, surgical benefits should be weighed against postoperative complications that lower subsequent fertility. These include creation of Asherman syndrome following the removal of large submucosal leiomyomas, formation of pelvic adhesions, or the need for cesarean delivery if the full myometrial thickness is transected.

Asherman Syndrome. The presence of intrauterine adhesions, also called *synechiae*, is termed *Asherman syndrome*. This diagnosis is discussed in detail in Chapter 16 (p. 444). Asherman syndrome occurs most frequently in women with a history of uterine dilation and curettage, particularly in the context of infection and pregnancy (Schenker, 1996). The clinical history will often include an acute postsurgical decrease in menstrual bleeding or even amenorrhea. A woman with an intrauterine device (IUD) complicated by infection or a woman with genital tuberculosis is also at high risk for intrauterine adhesions. Treatment of Asherman syndrome involves hysteroscopic lysis of the adhesions as described in Section 42-21 (p. 1178). Although dilation and curettage has been used, hysteroscopy provides more precise control with less secondary scarring. Electrosurgical coagulation is rarely required, as the bands in most cases are composed of connective tissue with poor blood supply.

Radiologic and Surgical Approaches for Evaluation of Pelvic Structures

There are several approaches for evaluating pelvic anatomy: (1) hysterosalpingography, (2) transvaginal sonography with or without saline instillation, (3) 3-D transvaginal sonography, (4) hysteroscopy, (5) laparoscopy, and (6) pelvic imaging by magnetic resonance (MR) imaging. As shown in Table 19-6, each has its own advantages and disadvantages.

Hysterosalpingography. This radiographic tool can be useful for evaluating the shape and size of the uterine cavity, in addition to defining tubal status. Hysterosalpingography is generally performed on cycle day numbers 5 through 10. At this time, there should be minimal intrauterine clotting that could block tubal outflow or give the false impression of an intrauterine abnormality. Furthermore, a woman should not have ovulated and possibly conceived. For this test, iodinated contrast medium is infused through a catheter placed into the

TABLE 19-6. Advantages and Disadvantages of Various Methods for Evaluating Pelvic Anatomy

	Tubal Patency	Uterine Cavity	Developmental Defects	Endometriosis or PAD	Ovaries
HSG	+	+	−	+/−	−
TVS	−	+/−	+/−	−	+
3-D TVS	−	+	+	−	+
SIS	−	+	+/−	−	+
MR imaging	−	+	+	−	+
Hysteroscopy	−	+	+ (with laparoscopy)	−	−
Laparoscopy	+	−	+ (with hysteroscopy)	+	+

HSG = hysterosalpingography; MR = magnetic resonance; PAD = pelvic adhesive disease; SIS = saline-infusion sonography; TVS = transvaginal sonography.

uterus. Under fluoroscopy, dye is followed as it fills the uterine cavity, then the tubal lumen, and finally spills out of the tubal fimbria into the pelvic cavity (Fig. 19-6).

Tubal Disease. In a large metaanalysis, HSG was demonstrated to have 65-percent sensitivity and 83-percent specificity for tubal obstruction (Swart, 1995). Tubal contractions, particularly cornual spasm, can give the incorrect impression of proximal fallopian tube obstruction (a false-positive result). Much less commonly reported is a scenario in which a false-negative result is obtained when the fallopian tube is seen as patent by HSG, although subsequently it is determined to be

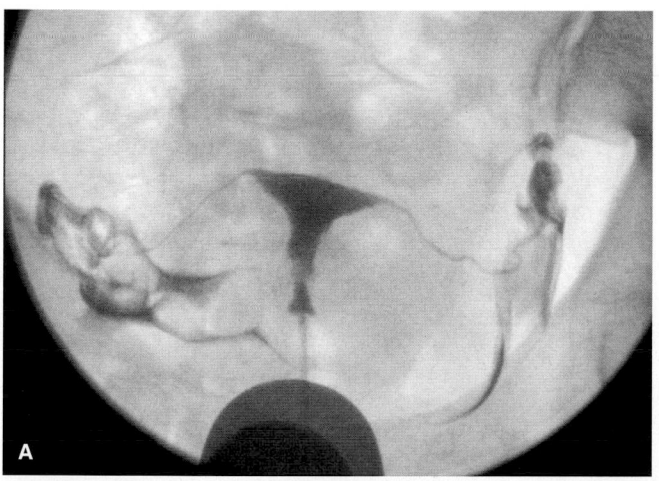

Normal

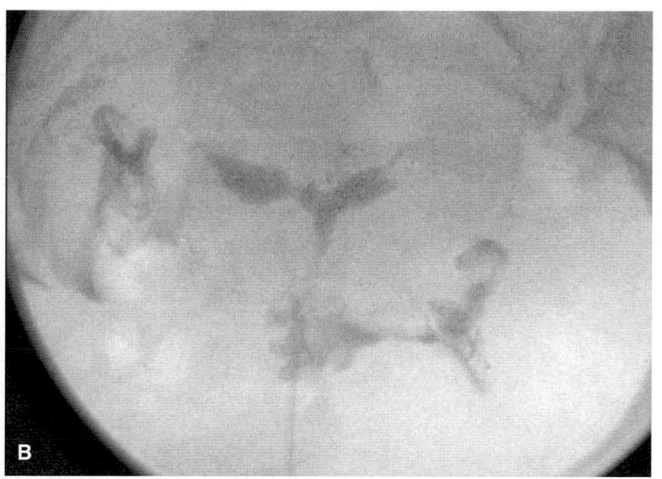

Asherman syndrome

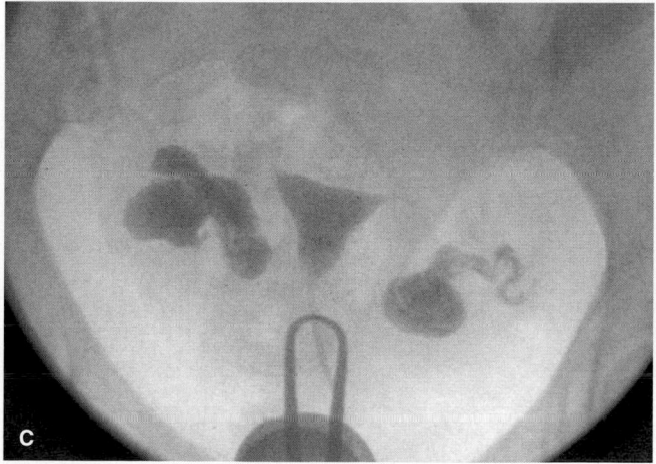

Bilateral hydrosalpinges

FIGURE 19-6 Hysterosalpingogram findings. These images are digitally reversed, causing the radiopaque contrast to appear black against a radiolucent background. **A.** Normal hysterosalpingogram. Radiopaque dye fills the uterine cavity and spills from both fallopian tubes into the peritoneal cavity. The dye catheter is seen directly beneath the endometrial contour. **B.** Asherman syndrome. Contrast dye fills a small and irregularly shaped endometrial cavity, often described as having a "moth-eaten" appearance. **C.** Bilateral hydrosalpinges. Note the marked tubal dilation and lack of spill of contrast medium at the fimbrial ends. *(Images contributed by Dr. Kevin Doody.)*

blocked. Many causes of tubal disease affect both tubes, and therefore, unilateral disease is unusual. Unilateral obstruction with a normal contralateral tube is most likely due to the dye following the path of least resistance during the HSG procedure. However, laparoscopy with chromotubation should be considered prior to treatment to confirm a final diagnosis.

Hysterosalpingography is not reliable in detecting peritubal or pelvic adhesions, although loculations of dye around the tubes may be suggestive. Thus, HSG is an excellent predictor of tubal patency, but is less effective at predicting normal tubal function or the presence of pelvic adhesions. Pregnancy rates have been reported to be increased following HSG and have been suggested to result from flushing of intratubal debris. However, these reports followed evaluation with oil-based dyes rather than water-based dyes, which are currently preferred.

Uterine Pathology. Hysterosalpingography also provides analysis of the contour of the intrauterine cavity. A polyp, leiomyoma, or adhesion within the cavity will block dye diffusion, resulting in an intrauterine "defect" in dye opacity on the radiograph (Fig. 19-7). Although false positives may be obtained due to blood clots, mucus plugs, or shearing of the endometrium during placement of the intrauterine catheter, HSG has been shown to accurately identify intrauterine pathology. In one study of more than 300 women in which hysteroscopy was used as the gold standard, HSG was determined to be 98-percent sensitive and 35-percent specific, with a positive predictive value of 70 percent and a negative predictive value of 8 percent. Most misdiagnoses were due to an inability to distinguish polyps from submucous leiomyomas. This is a minimal problem, as these patients will undergo further evaluation and treatment in either case (Preutthipan, 2003; Randolph, 1986). Although other studies have not provided such impressive results, it is clear that HSG is a powerful tool for evaluation of the uterine cavity.

Hysterosalpingography can also define developmental uterine anomalies (Fig. 19-8). A Y-shaped uterus identified during HSG may represent either a uterine septum or a bicornuate uterus. In these cases, the external contour of the uterine

fundus must be evaluated using MR imaging, high-resolution sonography, 3-dimensional (3-D) sonography, or laparoscopy. A smooth fundal contour is consistent with a diagnosis of uterine septum. This is an important distinction, as a septum is often resected, but a bicornuate uterus is generally not treated. In general, uterine anomalies do not cause infertility, but may be associated with miscarriage or later fetal loss, creating a management dilemma. Accordingly, it may be reasonable to surgically treat some uterine anomalies in an effort to improve pregnancy outcome. However, a couple must be carefully counseled that conception itself is unlikely to be affected. A further discussion of the fertility effects of congenital anomalies is found in Chapter 18.

Sonography. Transvaginal pelvic sonography may be helpful in determining uterine anatomy, particularly during the luteal phase, when the thickened endometrium acts as contrast to the myometrium. Although 3-D sonography machines are not yet widely available, their development is advancing the discriminatory abilities of sonography (Fig. 19-9).

The infusion of saline into the endometrial cavity during sonography performed in the follicular phase provides another approach for achieving contrast between the cavity and uterine walls. This procedure has many names including hysterosonography, sonohysterography, or saline infusion sonography (SIS). Details of this procedure are described in Chapter 2 (p. 35). Saline infusion sonography has been reported to have a sensitivity of 75 percent and specificity of more than 90 percent for detecting endometrial defects. It has an acceptable positive predictive value of 50 percent and an excellent negative predictive value of 95 percent, which greatly exceeds the negative predictive value of HSG (Soares, 2000). Moreover, SIS may be more sensitive than HSG in determining whether a cavitary defect is a pedunculated leiomyoma or a polyp (Figs. 8-9 and 8-10, p. 229). Perhaps more importantly, SIS can help determine what portion of a submucous leiomyoma is within the cavity, as only those with less than a 50-percent intramural component are approached for hysteroscopic resection.

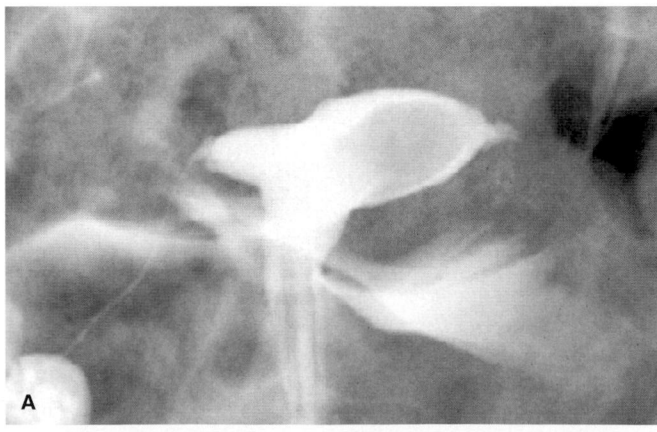

Submucous leiomyoma

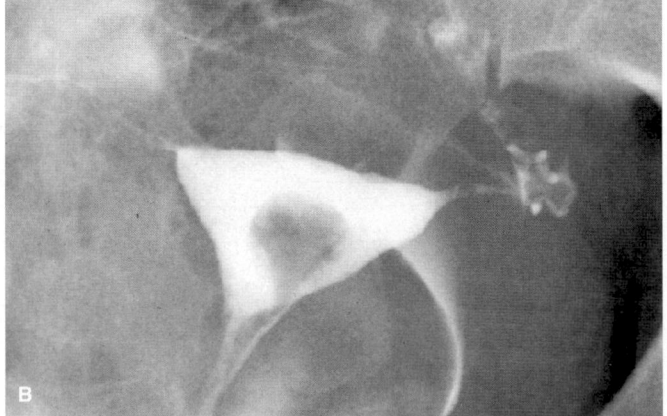

Endometrial polyp

FIGURE 19-7 Appearance of leiomyoma and endometrial polyps on hysterosalpingogram (HSG). **A.** A broad-based filling defect is formed during HSG by a submucous leiomyoma. Note distortion of the left cornu by this mass. **B.** A more irregular filling defect is created by an endometrial polyp. Note that polyps generally have a less substantial attachment to the myometrium. *(Images contributed by Dr. Diane Twickler.)*

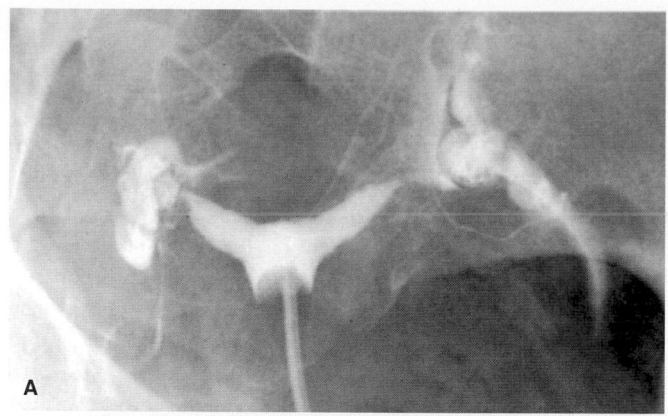

Bicornuate uterus

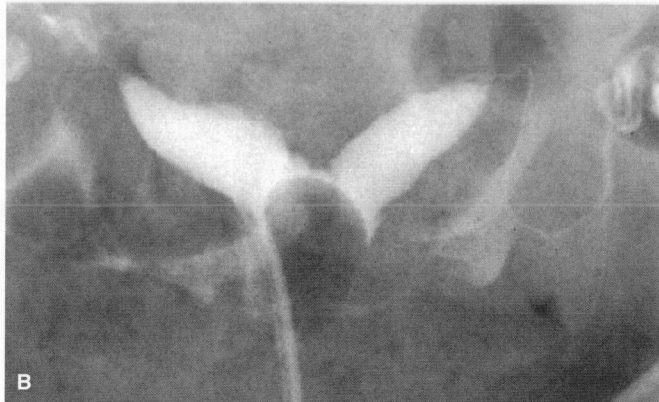

Septate uterus

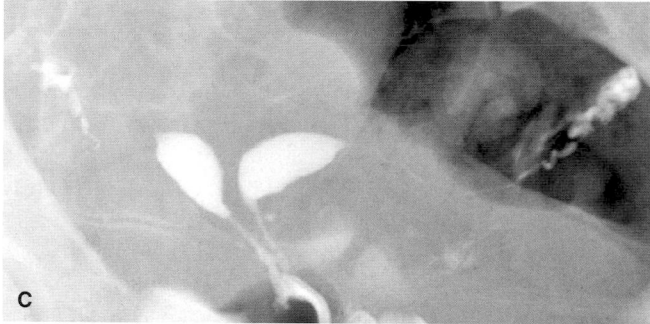

Uterine didelphys

FIGURE 19-8 Hysterosalpingograms show müllerian developmental anomalies. **A.** Bicornuate uterus, due to a failure of müllerian duct fusion, produces a fundal defect with wide-spaced uterine horns. **B.** Septate uterus is due to a failure of resorption. This moderate septum displaces the radiopaque dye to the level of the radiolucent injector balloon. **C.** Uterine didelphys consisting of two completely separate müllerian systems including duplication of the cervix. *(Images contributed by Dr. Diane Twickler.)*

The primary limitation of SIS is that it does not provide information regarding the fallopian tubes, although rapid loss of saline into the pelvis is certainly consistent with at least unilateral patency. Saline infusion sonography is generally less painful than HSG and does not require radiation exposure. Therefore, it is the preferred method if information about tubal patency is not required, such as in patients who are known to require IVF.

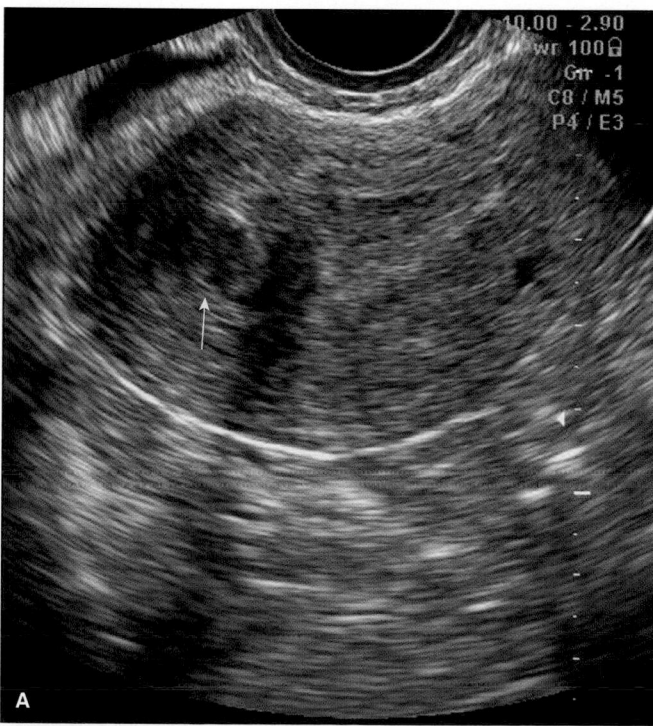

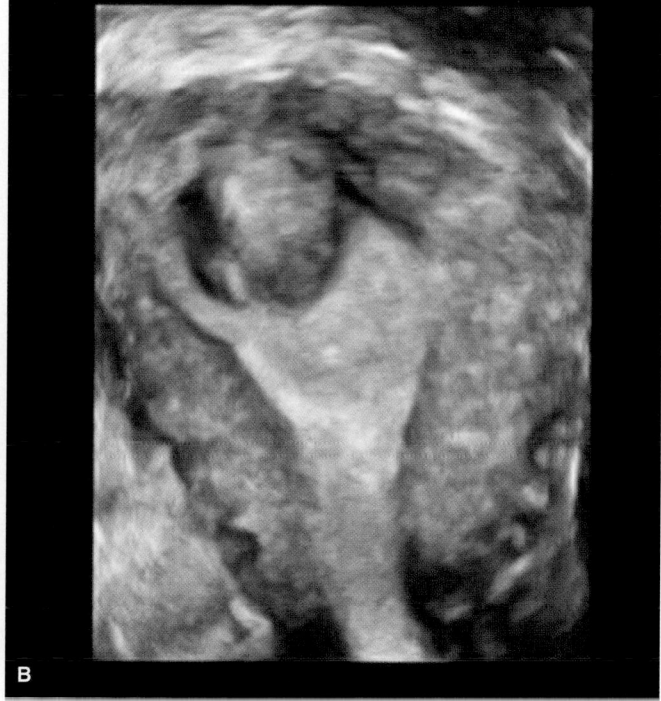

FIGURE 19-9 Sonograms display the same submucous leiomyoma. **A.** Transvaginal sonography. **B.** 3-D sonography. *(Images contributed by Dr. Victor Beshay.)*

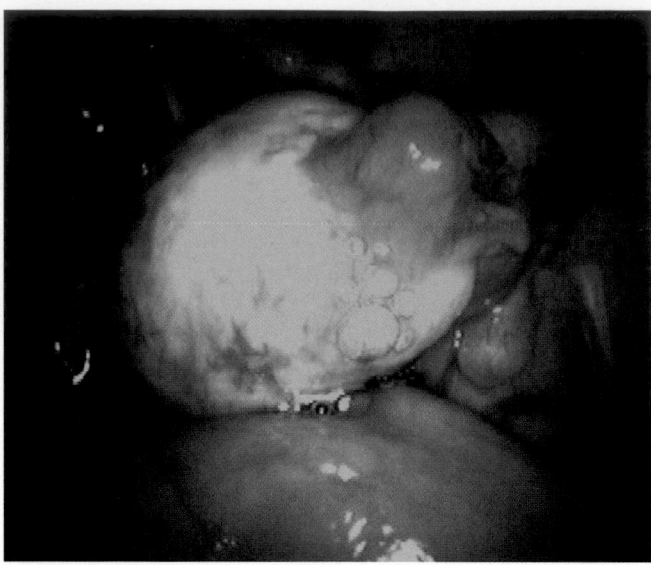

FIGURE 19-10 Chromotubation seen at laparoscopy. Note the spill of blue dye from the fimbriated end of the fallopian tube onto the ovarian surface. *(Image contributed by Dr. Kevin Doody.)*

Laparoscopy. Direct inspection provides the most accurate assessment of pelvic pathology, and laparoscopy is the gold standard approach. Chromotubation may be performed, in which a dilute dye is injected through an acorn cannula placed against the cervix or through a balloon catheter positioned within the uterine cavity (Figs. 42-1.7 and 42-1.8, p. 1102). Tubal spill is evaluated through the laparoscope (Fig. 19-10). Indigo carmine dye is preferable to methylene blue, as the methylene blue rarely may induce acute methemoglobinemia, particularly in patients with glucose-6-phosphate dehydrogenase deficiency. One 5-mL vial of indigo carmine is mixed with 50 to 100 mL of sterile saline for injection through the cervical cannula. Laparoscopy allows both diagnosis and immediate surgical treatment of abnormalities such as endometriosis or pelvic adhesions. Laparoscopic ablation of endometriotic lesions or adhesions may increase subsequent pregnancy rates (Chap. 10, p. 287).

As laparoscopy is an invasive procedure, it is not advocated in place of HSG as part of the initial infertility evaluation. Exceptions include women with a history or symptoms suggestive of endometriosis or prior pelvic inflammation. However, even in these women, a preliminary HSG may be informative (De Hondt, 2005).

If laparoscopy is clearly indicated, then hysteroscopy can also be performed to evaluate the uterine cavity while the patient is under anesthesia. Moreover, in operative hysteroscopic cases, laparoscopy can help direct surgery and avoid perforation, for example, during septal incision.

Laparoscopy also may be considered in patients who fail to conceive with clomiphene citrate or gonadotropin ovulation induction. If pelvic disease is found and treated, progression to IVF may be avoided. With improvements in IVF success rates, this latter argument is becoming less justifiable, as the cost of surgery well exceeds the cost of an IVF cycle.

Hysteroscopy. Endoscopic evaluation of the intrauterine cavity is the primary method for defining intrauterine abnormalities. Hysteroscopy can be performed in an office or operating room. With improved instrumentation, the ability to concurrently diagnose and treat abnormalities in the office is increasing. However, substantially more extensive hysteroscopic surgery is possible in the operating room. A fuller discussion of hysteroscopy and its indications is found in Section 42-13 (p. 1157).

Cervical Factors

The cervical glands secrete mucus that is normally thick and impervious to sperm and ascending infections. High estrogen levels at midcycle change the characteristics of this mucus, and it becomes thin and stretchy. Estrogen-primed cervical mucus filters out nonsperm components of semen and forms channels that help direct sperm into the uterus (Fig. 19-11). Midcycle mucus also creates a reservoir for sperm. This allows ongoing release during the next 24 to 72 hours and extends the potential time for fertilization (Katz, 1997).

Abnormalities in mucus production are most frequently observed in women who have undergone cryosurgery, cervical conization, or a loop electrosurgical excision procedure (LEEP) for treatment of an abnormal Pap smear. Cervical infection may also negatively impact mucus quality, although the data in this area have been controversial. Implicated agents include *C trachomatis*, *N gonorrhoeae*, *Ureaplasma urealyticum*, and *Mycoplasma hominis* (Cimino, 1993). Although there may be no advantage in terms of mucus quality, obtaining cultures for *C trachomatis* and *N gonorrhoeae* seems prudent to avoid causing ascending infection during HSG or intrauterine inseminations.

Postcoital Test. Also known as the Sims-Huhner test, this test can be performed to evaluate cervical mucus (Oei, 1995a,b). A couple is requested to have intercourse on the day of ovulation. The woman is seen in the office within a few hours, and a sample of the cervical mucus is obtained from the cervical os with forceps or by aspiration. In the presence of high estrogen levels, the mucus should be copious and relatively clear. Mucus should be able to be stretched to >5 cm after being placed between two glass slides. These qualities are summarized by the term *spinnbarkeit*. At least five motile sperm per high-power field should be visible under the microscope, although some authorities feel that a single, forward-moving sperm is adequate. There should be a minimal number of other cell types, such as inflammatory cells. When dried, the mucus should form a ferning pattern. This is crystallization of an increased salt concentration in the mucus, which is prompted by increased preovulatory estrogen levels (see Fig. 19-11A).

The most common reason for an abnormal test is improper timing. If mucus is scanty and thick, often termed *hostile*, then sperm motility evaluation is futile, and the test should be repeated.

Despite the preceding discussion, the utility of the postcoital test is probably negligible in most circumstances. There is limited consensus on the definition of a normal test, and the predictive value for conception is poor (Oei, 1995b). Moreover, various approaches to improve an abnormal postcoital test have not convincingly increased pregnancy rates. In a prospective, randomized controlled trial, a normal postcoital test did not predict increased cumulative pregnancy rates (Oei, 1998).

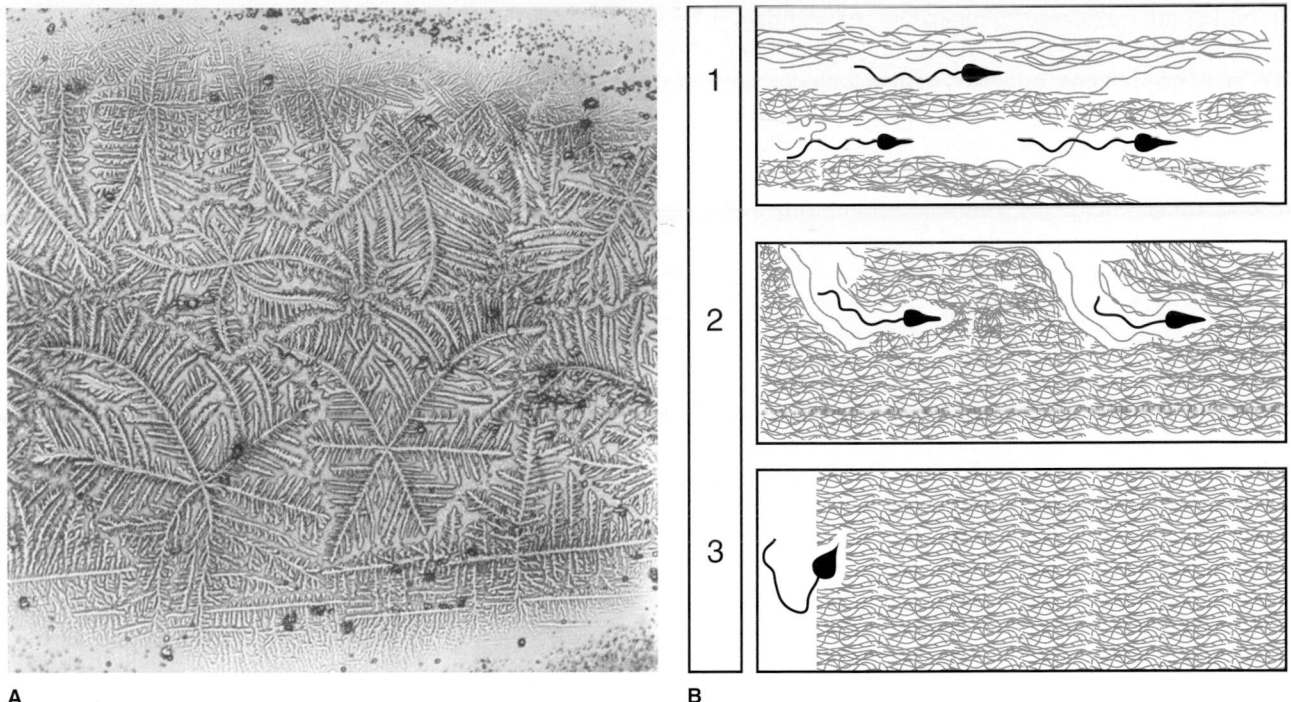

FIGURE 19-11 A. A ferning pattern is seen when periovulatory cervical mucus is spread and dried on a microscope slide. *(Photograph contributed by Dr. James C. Glenn.)* **B.** Examples of postcoital test slides. **Slide 1:** Columns within adequate cervical mucus help direct sperm into the uterine cavity. In patients with increasingly thick hostile mucus (**slides 2 & 3**), sperm display decreased motility.

Many infertility specialists recommend literally bypassing the cervix with intrauterine insemination (IUI) in any woman with a history of cervical surgery, especially if she has noted a decrease in midcycle mucus production. The remaining utility of the postcoital test is for couples who will not consider intrauterine insemination or do not have intrauterine insemination readily available. It may also be useful in regions of the world in which more specific testing cannot be obtained, as a postcoital test will provide basic information regarding mucus production, appropriate intercourse practices, and presence of motile sperm.

Etiology of Infertility in the Male

Causes of male infertility can roughly be categorized as abnormalities of sperm production, abnormalities of sperm function, and obstruction of the ductal outflow tract.

Normal Spermatogenesis

During evaluation of a male infertility patient, the basics of male reproductive physiology should be understood. Analogous to the ovary, testes have two functions: the generation of mature germ cells (sperm) and the production of male hormones, primarily testosterone. The seminiferous tubules contain developing sperm and support cells called *Sertoli cells* or *sustentacular cells* (see Fig. 19-4). The Sertoli cells form tight junctions that produce a blood-testis barrier. This avascular space within the seminiferous tubules protects sperm from antibodies and toxins, but also makes these cells dependent on diffusion for oxygen, nutrients, and metabolic precursors. Located between the seminiferous tubules are Leydig cells, also called *interstitial*

cells, which are responsible for steroid hormone production. In simplistic terms, Leydig cells are similar to the thecal cells of the ovary.

Unlike the ovary, testes contain stem cells that allow ongoing production of mature germ cells throughout a male's life. In a fertile male, approximately 100 to 200 million sperm are produced each day (Sigman, 1997). The process begins with a diploid (46,XY) spermatogonial cell, which grows and becomes a primary spermatocyte. The first meiotic division produces two secondary spermatocytes, and completion of meiosis results in four mature sperm with a haploid (23,X or 23,Y) karyotype. During this developmental process, most sperm cytoplasm is lost, mitochondria that provide energy are positioned in the sperm midpiece, and sperm flagella develop.

Production of sperm requires approximately 70 days to complete. An additional 12 to 21 days is needed for sperm to be transported into the epididymis. Here, they further mature and develop motility (Heller, 1963; Hinrichsen, 1980; Rowley, 1970). Importantly, due to this prolonged developmental period, the results of a semen analysis reflect events during the past 3 months, not a single point in time.

To fertilize an oocyte, human sperm must undergo a process known as *capacitation*. Capacitation results in sperm hyperactivation (an extreme increase in movement) as well as the ability of sperm to release acrosomal contents, which allow penetration of the zona pellucida.

Normal spermatogenesis is dependent on high local levels of testosterone. Luteinizing hormone from the anterior pituitary gland stimulates production of testosterone by the Leydig cells in the interstitium of the testes. Follicle-stimulating hormone increases LH receptors on the Leydig cells, thus indirectly contributing to testosterone production. In addition, FSH increases production of sex hormone-binding globulin, also called androgen-binding protein. Androgen-binding protein binds testosterone and maintains high concentrations of this hormone in the seminiferous tubules (Sigman, 1997).

In addition to hormone levels, testicular volume often reflects spermatogenesis, and a normal volume is between 15 and 25 mL. Most this volume is provided by the seminiferous tubules. Thus, decreased testicular volume is a strong indicator of abnormal spermatogenesis.

Spermatogenesis is directed by genes on the Y chromosome. There are also important contributions by autosomal genes, which continue to be elucidated. Therefore, genetic abnormalities may also adversely affect this process, as discussed later in this chapter.

Male fertility likely decreases modestly with age. A number of studies have demonstrated that pregnancy rates decrease and time to conception increases as male age increases. Studies of semen parameters across age have suggested that sperm concentration is maintained, however, sperm motility and morphology progressively worsen (Levitas, 2007). The clinical significance of this change is unclear (Kidd, 2001). In short, although advancing male age may have an impact on fertility, it is probably insignificant compared with aging changes in women.

Semen Analysis

This is a core test in evaluation of male fertility status. For this test, the male is asked to refrain from ejaculation for 2 to 3 days, and a specimen is collected by masturbation into a sterile cup. If masturbation is not an option, then a couple can use specially designed silastic condoms without lubricants. Importantly, the sample should arrive in the laboratory within an hour of ejaculation to allow for optimal analysis.

The sample undergoes liquefaction, that is, thinning of the seminal fluid, due to enzymes from the liquid contribution of the prostate gland. This process takes 5 to 20 minutes and allows more accurate evaluation of the sperm contained in the seminal fluid. Ideally, two semen samples separated by at least a month should be analyzed. In practice, frequently only a single sample is analyzed if parameters are normal.

The reference values for the semen analysis are shown in Table 19-7 (World Health Organization, 1999). A clinician should remember a number of critical aspects with regard to this test. First, semen characteristics will vary across time in a single individual. Second, semen analysis results, particularly morphologic interpretation, will differ between laboratories. Therefore, reference ranges for the laboratory being used should be known. Note that the concept of "reference" range is more appropriate than "normal" range. Although total motile sperm count correlates with fertility, not all males with "normal" semen parameters display normal fertility (Guzick, 2001). The lack of absolute predictive value for this test is likely due to the fact that it does not provide information regarding sperm function, that is, the ultimate ability to fertilize an oocyte.

Most semen analysis reports will indicate semen volume, pH, and presence or absence of fructose. Nearly 80 percent of semen volume comes from the seminal vesicles. Seminal fluid

TABLE 19-7. Semen Analysis

Volume	>1.5 mL[a]
Count	>20 million/mL[a]
Motility	>50%[a]
Morphology	>30%[b]
	>14%[a] (Kruger)[c]
WBCs	<1 million/mL[a]
Round cells	<5 million/mL[a]

WBCs = white blood cells.
[a]From World Health Organization, 1999, with permission.
[b]From World Health Organization, 1992, with permission.
[c]From Kruger, 1988, with permission.

is alkaline and is thought to protect sperm from acidity present in prostatic secretions and in the vagina. Seminal fluid also provides fructose as an energy source for sperm. An acidic pH or lack of fructose suggests a seminal vesicle or ejaculatory duct problem.

Semen Volume. Low semen volume is often simply due to incomplete specimen collection or short abstinence interval. However, it may indicate partial obstruction of the vas deferens (ductus deferens) or retrograde ejaculation. Partial or complete vas deferens obstruction may be caused by infection, tumor, prior testicular or inguinal surgery, or trauma. Retrograde ejaculation follows failed closure of the bladder neck during ejaculation and allows seminal fluid to flow backward into the bladder. Retrograde ejaculation should be suspected in men with diabetes mellitus, spinal cord damage, or a history of prostate or other retroperitoneal surgery that may have damaged nerves (Hershlag, 1991). Medications, particularly β-blockers, may contribute to this problem. A postejaculatory urinalysis can detect sperm in the bladder and confirm the diagnosis. If urine is properly alkalinized, these sperm are viable and can be retrieved to achieve pregnancy.

Sperm Count. A male partner may have normal sperm counts, *oligospermia* (low counts), or *azoospermia* (no sperm). Oligospermia is defined as a concentration of fewer than 20 million sperm per milliliter, and counts less than 5 million per milliliter are considered severe.

The prevalence of azoospermia is approximately 1 percent of all men. Azoospermia may be due to obstruction in the outflow tract, termed obstructive azoospermia, such as that which occurs with congenital absence of the vas deferens, severe infection, or vasectomy. Azoospermia may also follow testicular failure (non-obstructive azoospermia). In the latter case, careful centrifugation and analysis may identify a small number of motile sperm adequate for IVF use. Alternatively, this latter group may have viable sperm obtainable through either epididymal aspiration or testicular biopsy. Endocrine and genetic evaluation is indicated for men with abnormal sperm counts, as will be described later.

Sperm Motility. Decreased sperm motility is termed *asthenospermia*. Some laboratories will distinguish between rapid (grade 3 to 4), slow (grade 2), and nonprogressive (grade 0 to 1) movement. Total progressive motility is the percentage of sperm exhibiting forward movement (grades 2 to 4). Asthenospermia has been attributed to prolonged abstinence, antisperm antibodies, genital tract infections, or varicocele.

The hypoosmotic swelling test can help to differentiate between dead and nonmotile sperm. Unlike dead sperm, living sperm can maintain an osmotic gradient. Thus, when mixed with a hypoosmotic solution, living nonmotile sperm with normal membrane function will swell and coil as fluid is absorbed (Casper, 1996). Once identified, these viable sperm may be used for intracytoplasmic sperm injection.

Sperm Morphology. Abnormal sperm morphology is termed *teratospermia*. Many laboratories use the original classification, in which normal morphology is characterized by more than 50 percent of sperm exhibiting normal shape. More recently, Kruger and colleagues (1988) have developed strict criteria for defining normal morphology. Their studies defined a more detailed characterization of normal sperm morphology, which showed improved correlation with fertilization rates during IVF cycles. Their criteria require careful analysis of the shape and size of the sperm head, the relative size of the acrosome in proportion to the head, and characteristics of the tail, including length, coiling, or the presence of two tails (Fig. 19-12). Fertilization rates are highest with normal morphology percentages greater than 14 percent. Significantly decreased fertilization rates are seen when normal morphology percentages falls below 4 percent.

Round cells in a sperm sample may represent either leukocytes or immature sperm. White blood cells (WBCs) can be distinguished from immature sperm using a variety of techniques, including a myeloperoxidase stain for WBCs (Wolff, 1995). True leukocytospermia is defined as greater than 1 million WBCs per milliliter and may indicate chronic epididymitis or prostatitis. In this scenario, many andrologists consider empiric antibiotic treatment prior to obtaining a repeat semen analysis. A common protocol would include doxycycline at a dosage of 100 mg orally twice daily for 2 weeks. Alternative approaches include culture of any expressible discharge or of the semen sample.

Unless a general obstetrician-gynecologist has developed a particular interest and expertise in the area of infertility, repeated abnormal semen analyses are an indication for referral to an infertility specialist. Although the partner may be referred directly to a urologist, it may be more reasonable to refer the couple to a reproductive endocrinologist, as the female will also require evaluation. Treatment is likely to be more complex in these couples and will typically be directed to both partners. The reproductive specialist can determine the need for further referral of the male partner to a urologist for investigation of genetic, anatomic, hormonal, or infectious abnormalities.

Antisperm Antibodies

Although these antibodies may be detected in as many as 10 percent of men, controversy exists regarding the negative

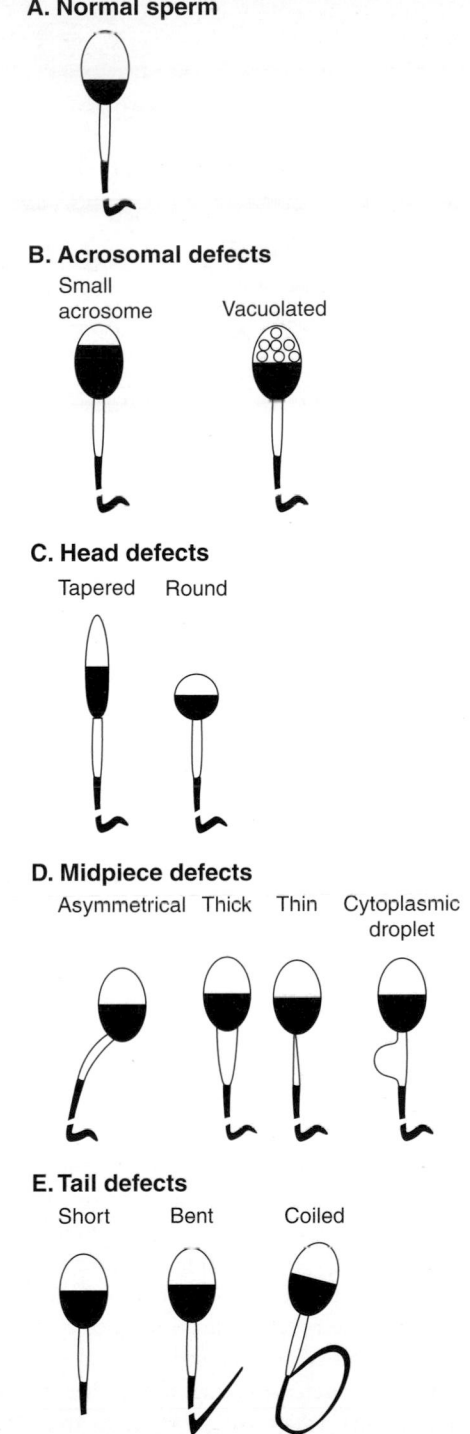

FIGURE 19-12 Some types of abnormally formed spermatozoa.

fertility effects of antisperm antibodies found in semen. These antibodies may be particularly prevalent following vasectomy, testicular torsion, testicular biopsy, or other clinical situations in which the blood-testis barrier is breached (Turek, 1994). It is currently felt that only IgG or IgA, bound to the sperm head or midpiece, are critical for decreasing fertilization capacity.

The most commonly employed assay contains immunobeads, which are mixed with the sperm preparation. These

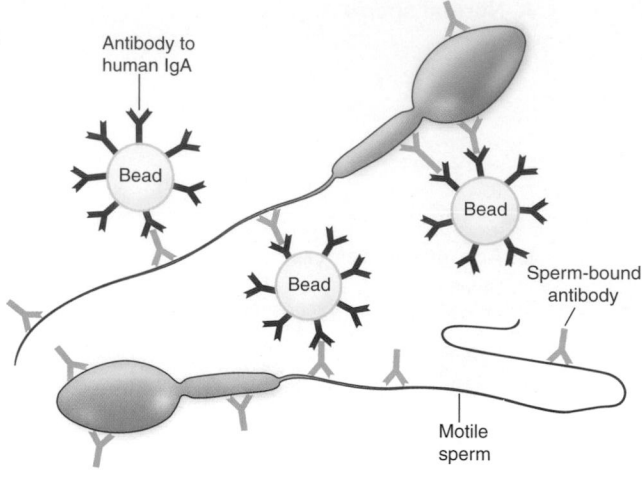

The immunobead reaction

FIGURE 19-13 Immunoreactive beads bind to antibodies that are bound to sperm.

beads will bind to antibodies present in a sperm sample. This mixture can be visualized under a standard microscope. With affected individuals, beads bind to antibodies that have bound to sperm (Fig. 19-13). Treatment historically included corticosteroids, but it is unclear that this approach improves fertility. Moreover, significant side effects, including aseptic necrosis of the hip, have been reported in treated patients.

Current data suggest that antisperm antibodies do not need to be tested routinely as part of an infertility evaluation unless the male partner has a clear risk factor for these antibodies. An exception would be those patients who will undergo IVF. In an affected antibody-positive population, fertilization rates are improved using intracytoplasmic sperm injection.

DNA Fragmentation

During the past 10 years, interest has increased regarding elevated sperm DNA fragmentation as a cause of male factor infertility (Sakkas, 2010; Zini, 2009). Although some degree of DNA damage is likely repaired during embryogenesis, the location and extent of damage may negatively affect fertilization rates and increase miscarriage rates. Increased levels of DNA damage are associated with advanced paternal age and external factors such as cigarette smoking, chemotherapy, radiation, environmental toxins, varicocele, and genital tract infections. Studies have observed increased levels of reactive oxygen species in sperm samples with abnormal DNA fragmentation rates. In response to this observation, it has been proposed that dietary supplementation with the antioxidants vitamin C and vitamin E may be beneficial. However, data are currently lacking regarding the efficacy of this approach.

A wide array of assays is currently available to analyze for DNA integrity and include the Sperm Chromatin Structure Assay (SCSA) and the terminal deoxynucleotidyl transferase-mediated dUTP nick-end labeling (TUNEL) assay. The SCSA is based on the increased susceptibility of DNA with single-strand or double-strand breaks to denature in weak acid. The TUNEL assay exploits the ability of labeled nucleotides to inter-

calate into DNA breaks for subsequent measurement. These tests are currently hampered by a lack of consensus regarding appropriate threshold values and by conflicting data regarding their ability to predict successful pregnancy. As a result, this testing is likely beyond the scope of the generalist at this point. Nevertheless, the concept that sperm DNA integrity can be adversely affected through multiple mechanisms provides useful insight into a previously underappreciated cause of male infertility.

Assays of Sperm Function

A wide variety of assays to test sperm function have been developed during the past few decades. The predictive significance of these assays is questionable, as they are based on highly nonphysiologic conditions, and results vary widely from infertility center to infertility center. Most are no longer used or are used only intermittently by infertility specialists. These tests are briefly described to provide more complete information to the general practitioner. However, they should not be considered part of a basic infertility evaluation.

Mannose Fluorescence Assay. The sperm's ability to recognize the zona pellucida of an oocyte is dependent on a number of proteins and sugars on the zona surface, including the sugar mannose. Acrosomal mannose-ligand receptor activity has been shown to correlate with IVF pregnancy rates (Benoff, 1993).

For this receptor assay, mannose residues in bovine serum albumin are modified so that they release fluorescence. A capacitated sperm sample from a patient is mixed with this fluorescent preparation. In a parallel experiment, sperm from a known fertile donor is mixed with the same fluorescent preparation in a separate dish. The patient's binding pattern is compared with the pattern obtained with the fertile male sample.

Hemizona Assay. The hemizona assay is a technique for analyzing the sperm's ability to bind to the zona pellucida. Human oocytes are bisected (to prevent fertilization) and are mixed either with the partner's sperm or with fertile donor sperm. The hemizona index is calculated by dividing the number of patient sperm bound by the number of control sperm bound and multiplying by 100 (Burkman, 1988).

Sperm Penetration Assay. The sperm penetration assay is performed by mixing capacitated human sperm with hamster oocytes. The zona pellucida typically prevents cross-species sperm binding and must first be removed from these test oocytes. The number of oocytes that are penetrated by sperm is calculated. The presumption is that more oocytes will be penetrated by sperm from fertile men than by sperm from infertile men (Smith, 1987b).

Acrosomal Reaction. Penetration of an oocyte requires that sperm undergo an acrosomal reaction, during which the enzymatic contents of the acrosome are released on interaction with the oocyte membrane. Various methods can be used to induce the acrosomal reaction in a patient's sperm sample. The percentage of sperm that undergoes the reaction is compared with that of a fertile male's control sample (Sigman, 1997).

Hormonal Evaluation of the Male

Hormonal testing in the male is analogous to endocrine testing in an anovulatory female. Essentially, abnormalities may be due to central defects in hypothalamic-pituitary function or to defects within the testes. Most urologists will defer testing unless a sperm concentration is less than 10 million/mL. Testing will include measurements of serum FSH and testosterone levels.

Low FSH and low testosterone levels are consistent with hypothalamic dysfunction, such as idiopathic hypogonadotropic hypogonadism or Kallmann syndrome (Chap. 16, p. 447). In these patients, sperm production may be achieved with gonadotropin treatment. Although frequently successful, at least 6 months may be required for detection of sperm production.

Elevated FSH and low testosterone levels provide evidence of testicular failure, and most men with oligospermia fall into this category. In this patient group, it is important to determine, based on testosterone levels, whether testosterone replacement is indicated. Normal spermatogenesis requires high levels of intratesticular testosterone, which cannot be achieved with exogenous testosterone. Furthermore, many of these men will lack spermatogonial stem cells. Therefore, testosterone replacement will not rescue sperm production. In fact, replacement will decrease gonadotropin stimulation of remaining testicular function through negative feedback at the hypothalamus and pituitary. Unless the couple has chosen to use donor sperm, testosterone replacement should be deferred during fertility treatment. However, replacement will provide other benefits, such as improved libido and sexual function, maintenance of muscle mass and bone density, and a general sense of well-being.

Additional hormonal testing may be included as part of an evaluation of the infertile male. Elevated serum prolactin levels and thyroid dysfunction impact spermatogenesis and are the most likely endocrinopathies to be detected (Sharlip, 2002; Sigman, 1997).

Genetic Testing of the Male

Genetic abnormalities are a relatively common cause of abnormal semen characteristics. Approximately 15 percent of azoospermic men and 5 percent of severely oligospermic men will have an abnormal karyotype. Although genetic abnormalities cannot be corrected, they may have implications for the health of the patient or his offspring. Therefore, karyotyping should be pursued when indicated by poor semen analysis results. The lower limit in sperm concentration for such testing varies between practitioners but lies between 3 and 10 million sperm per milliliter.

Klinefelter syndrome (47,XXY) will be a frequent finding. Klinefelter syndrome is observed in approximately 1 in 500 men in the general population and accounts for 1 to 2 percent of male infertility. Classically, these men are tall, are undervirilized, and have gynecomastia and small, firm testes (De Braekeleer, 1991). As the phenotype varies widely, lack of these characteristics should not preclude chromosomal evaluation. Conversely, a clinician should strongly consider obtaining karyotype testing in any male with these characteristics.

Autosomal abnormalities will also be found in a subset of men with severe oligospermia.

A patient with severely decreased sperm counts and a normal karyotype should be offered testing for microdeletion of the Y chromosome. Up to 15 percent of men with severe oligospermia or azoospermia will have small deletions in the region of the Y chromosome, termed the *azoospermia factor (AZF) region*. If the deletion is within the AZFa or AZFb subregions, then it is unlikely that viable sperm can be recovered for use in IVF. Most men with an AZFc deletion will have viable sperm at biopsy. However, these deletions should be presumed to be inherited by their offspring. The clinical significance of microdeletions in the recently identified AZFd region is unknown, as these patients have apparently normal spermatogenesis (Hopps, 2003; Kent-First, 1999; Pryor, 1997).

Patients may decline testing for microdeletion of the Y chromosome for various reasons. Beyond infertility, no known health risks are associated with these deletions. Many couples with azoospermia will chose to use donor sperm, and thus identification of this mutation may not be pertinent. Other couples reason that if the husband is able to have a child despite this deletion, there is no significant disadvantage if the abnormality is transmitted to any offspring.

Obstructive azoospermia may be due to congenital bilateral absence of the vas deferens (CBAVD). Approximately 70 to 85 percent of men with CBAVD will be found to have mutations in the cystic fibrosis transmembrane conductance regulator gene (*CFTR* gene), although not all will have clinical cystic fibrosis (Oates, 1994; Ratbi, 2007). Conversely, essentially all men with clinical cystic fibrosis will have CBAVD. Fortunately, testicular function in these men is usually normal, and adequate sperm may be obtained by epididymal aspiration to achieve pregnancy through IVF. Careful genetic counseling and testing of the female partner for carrier status is critical in these situations.

Testicular Biopsy

Evaluation of a severely oligospermic or azoospermic male may include either open or percutaneous testicular biopsy to determine whether viable sperm are present in the seminiferous tubules (Sharlip, 2002). For example, even men with testicular failure diagnosed by elevated serum FSH levels may have adequate sperm on biopsy for use in intracytoplasmic sperm injection. The biopsy specimen can be cryopreserved for future extraction of sperm during an IVF cycle. However, freshly biopsied specimens are generally felt to provide higher success rates. Thus, the biopsy may have diagnostic, prognostic, and therapeutic value.

CONCLUSION

Figure 19-14 provides an algorithm for the evaluation of an infertile couple. Details will vary between practitioners and will be affected by patient presentation. In general, the female partner should have some form of testing to confirm ovulation and should undergo HSG, whereas the male partner should have semen analysis performed. In older women, evaluation of an early follicular FSH level is essential to ensure adequate follicular reserves. A subset of couples will decline HSG and

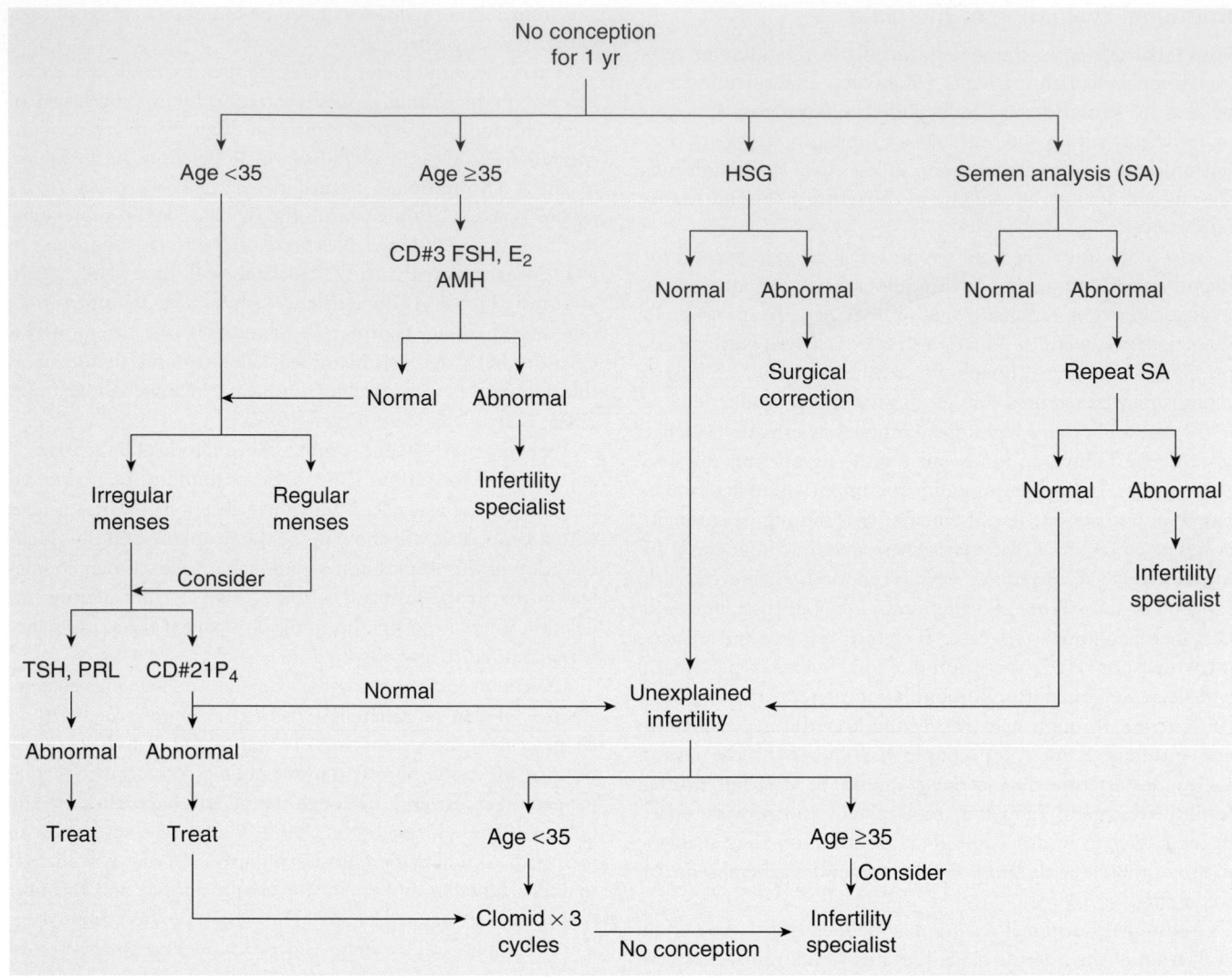

FIGURE 19-14 Diagnostic algorithm for evaluation of the infertile couple. AMH = antimüllerian hormone; CD#3 = cycle day 3; CD#21 = cycle day 21; E_2 = estradiol; FSH = follicle-stimulating hormone; HSG = hysterosalpingography; P_4 = progesterone; PRL = prolactin; SA = semen analysis; TSH = thyroid-stimulating hormone.

semen analysis if the woman has a clear ovulatory defect. These couples should be reminded that there is a relatively high incidence of couples having two abnormalities, one of which would be missed by this approach. These patients may be treated, but should be strongly encouraged to complete the evaluation if they do not conceive within a few months. Options for treatment are discussed in Chapter 20.

REFERENCES

Abma J, Chandra A, Mosher W, et al: Fertility, family planning, and women's health: new data from the 1995 National Survey of Family Growth. Vital Health Stat 23:1, 1997

Aksel S: Sporadic and recurrent luteal phase defects in cyclic women: comparison with normal cycles. Fertil Steril 33:372, 1980

Aliyu MH, Aliyu SH, Salihu HM: Female genital tuberculosis: a global review. Int J Fertil Womens Med 49:123, 2004

American College of Obstetricians and Gynecologists: Hemoglobinopathies in pregnancy. Practice Bulletin No. 78, January 2007

American College of Obstetricians and Gynecologists: Neural tube defects. Practice Bulletin No. 44, July 2003

American College of Obstetricians and Gynecologists: Prenatal and preconceptional carrier screening for genetic diseases in individuals of Eastern European Jewish descent. Committee Opinion No. 442, October 2009

American College of Obstetricians and Gynecologists: Update on carrier screening for cystic fibrosis. Committee Opinion No. 325, December 2005

American Society for Reproductive Medicine: Aging and fertility in women. Fertil Steril 86(Suppl 4):S248, 2006a

American Society for Reproductive Medicine: Effectiveness and treatment for unexplained infertility. Fertil Steril 86(5, Suppl 1):S111, 2006b

American Society for Reproductive Medicine: Optimal evaluation of the infertile female. Fertil Steril 82(Suppl 1):S169, 2000

American Society for Reproductive Medicine: Optimizing natural fertility. Fertil Steril 90(Suppl 3):S1, 2008a

American Society for Reproductive Medicine: Report on varicocele and fertility. Fertil Steril 90(Suppl):S247, 2008b

Anderson J, Williamson R: Fertility after torsion of the spermatic cord. Br J Urol 65:225, 1990

Anguiano A, Oates R, Amos J, et al: Congenital bilateral absence of the vas deferens. A primarily genital form of cystic fibrosis. JAMA 267:1794, 1992

Augood C, Duckitt K, Templeton A: Smoking and female infertility: a systematic review and meta-analysis. Hum Reprod 13:1532, 1998

Balasch J, Fabregues F, Creus M, et al: The usefulness of endometrial biopsy for luteal phase evaluation in infertility. Hum Reprod 7:973, 1992

Bartsch G, Frank S, Marberger H, et al: Testicular torsion: late results with special regard to fertility and endocrine function. J Urol 124:375, 1980

Bates G, Garza D, Garza M: Clinical manifestations of hormonal changes in the menstrual cycle. Obstet Gynecol Clin North Am 17:299, 1990

Beard C, Benson R Jr, Kelalis P, et al: The incidence and outcome of mumps orchitis in Rochester, Minnesota, 1935 to 1974. Mayo Clin Proc 52:3, 1977

Ben-Arie A, Goldchmit C, Laviv Y, et al: The malignant potential of endometrial polyps. Eur J Obstet Gynecol Reprod Biol 115:206, 2004

Benoff S, Cooper G, Hurley I, et al: Human sperm fertilizing potential in vitro is correlated with differential expression of a head-specific mannose-ligand receptor. Fertil Steril 59:854, 1993

Benson GS: Erection, Emission, and Ejaculation: Physiologic Mechanism, 3rd ed. St. Louis, MO, Mosby, 1997

Bolumar F, Olsen J, Rebagliato M, et al: Caffeine intake and delayed conception: a European multicenter study on infertility and subfecundity. European Study Group on Infertility Subfecundity. Am J Epidemiol 145:324, 1997

Bracken M, Eskenazi B, Sachse K, et al: Association of cocaine use with sperm concentration, motility, and morphology. Fertil Steril 53:315, 1990

Burkman L, Coddington C, Franken D, et al: The hemizona assay (HZA): development of a diagnostic test for the binding of human spermatozoa to the human hemizona pellucida to predict fertilization potential. Fertil Steril 49:688, 1988

Buyalos R, Daneshmand S, Brzechffa P: Basal estradiol and follicle-stimulating hormone predict fecundity in women of advanced reproductive age undergoing ovulation induction therapy. Fertil Steril 68:272, 1997

Caan B, Quesenberry C Jr, Coates A: Differences in fertility associated with caffeinated beverage consumption. Am J Public Health 88:270, 1998

Carson D, Lagow E, Thathiah A, et al: Changes in gene expression during the early to mid-luteal (receptive phase) transition in human endometrium detected by high-density microarray screening. Mol Hum Reprod 8:871, 2002

Casper R, Meriano J, Jarvi K, et al: The hypo-osmotic swelling test for selection of viable sperm for intracytoplasmic sperm injection in men with complete asthenozoospermia. Fertil Steril 65:972, 1996

Chandra A, Stephen EH: Infertility service use among U.S. women: 1995 and 2002. Fertil Steril 93(3):725, 2010

Chang WY, Agarwal SK, Azziz R: Diagnostic evaluation and treatment of the infertile couple. In Carr BR, Blackwell RE, Azziz R (eds): Essential Reproductive Medicine. New York, McGraw-Hill, 2005, p 366

Charny C: The spermatogenic potential of the undescended testis before and after treatment. J Urol 38:697, 1960

Chehval M, Purcell M: Deterioration of semen parameters over time in men with untreated varicocele: evidence of progressive testicular damage. Fertil Steril 57:174, 1992

Cimino C, Borruso A, Napoli P, et al: Evaluation of the importance of Chlamydia t. and/or Mycoplasma h. and/or Ureaplasma u. genital infections and of antisperm antibodies in couples affected by muco-semen incompatibility and in couples with unexplained infertility. Acta Eur Fertil 24:13, 1993

Cnattingius S, Signorello L, Anneren G, et al: Caffeine intake and the risk of first-trimester spontaneous abortion. N Engl J Med 343:1839, 2000

Daudin M, Bieth E, Bujan L, et al: Congenital bilateral absence of the vas deferens: clinical characteristics, biological parameters, cystic fibrosis transmembrane conductance regulator gene mutations, and implications for genetic counseling. Fertil Steril 74:1164, 2000

Davis O, Berkeley A, Naus G, et al: The incidence of luteal phase defect in normal, fertile women, determined by serial endometrial biopsies. Fertil Steril 51:582, 1989

De Braekeleer M, Dao T: Cytogenetic studies in male infertility: a review. Hum Reprod 6:245, 1991

De Hondt A, Peeraer K, Meuleman C, et al: Endometriosis and subfertility treatment: a review. Minerva Ginecol 57:257, 2005

DeWaay DJ, Syrop CH, Nygaard IE, et al: Natural history of uterine polyps and leiomyomata. Obstet Gynecol 100:3, 2002

Farhi J, Ashkenazi J, Feldberg D, et al: Effect of uterine leiomyomata on the results of in-vitro fertilization treatment. Hum Reprod 10:2576, 1995

Frattarelli J, Lauria-Costab D, Miller B, et al: Basal antral follicle number and mean ovarian diameter predict cycle cancellation and ovarian responsiveness in assisted reproductive technology cycles. Fertil Steril 74:512, 2000

Gazvani M, Buckett W, Luckas M, et al: Conservative management of azoospermia following steroid abuse. Hum Reprod 12:1706, 1997

Goldberg J, Falcone T: Effect of diethylstilbestrol on reproductive function. Fertil Steril 72:1, 1999

Grinsted J, Jacobsen J, Grinsted L, et al: Prediction of ovulation. Fertil Steril 52:388, 1989

Grodstein F, Goldman M, Cramer D: Body mass index and ovulatory infertility. Epidemiology 5:247, 1994a

Grodstein F, Goldman M, Cramer D: Infertility in women and moderate alcohol use. Am J Public Health 84:1429, 1994b

Guermandi E, Vegetti W, Bianchi M, et al: Reliability of ovulation tests in infertile women. Obstet Gynecol 97:92, 2001

Guttmacher A: Factors affecting normal expectancy of conception. JAMA 161:855, 1956

Guzick D, Overstreet J, Factor-Litvak P, et al: Sperm morphology, motility, and concentration in fertile and infertile men. N Engl J Med 345:1388, 2001

Hadziselimovic F: Early successful orchidopexy does not prevent from developing azoospermia. Int Braz J Urol 32(5):570, 2006

Hansen KR, Hodnett GM, Knowlton N, et al: Correlation of ovarian reserve tests with histologically determined primordial follicle number. Fertil Steril 95(1):170, 2011

Heller C, Clermont Y: Spermatogenesis in man: an estimate of its duration. Science 140:184, 1963

Hershlag A, Schiff S, DeCherney A: Retrograde ejaculation. Hum Reprod 6:255, 1991

Hinrichsen M, Blaquier J: Evidence supporting the existence of sperm maturation in the human epididymis. J Reprod Fertil 60:291, 1980

Hopps CV, Mielnik A, Goldstein M, et al: Detection of sperm in men with Y chromosome microdeletions of the AZFa, AZFb, and AZFc regions. Hum Reprod 18(8):1660, 2003

Hughes E, Brennan B: Does cigarette smoking impair natural or assisted fecundity? Fertil Steril 66:679, 1996

Hull MG, Savage P, Bromham DR, et al: The value of a single serum progesterone measurement in the midluteal phase: a criterion of a potentially fertile cycle ("ovulation") derived from treated and untreated conception cycles. Fertil Steril 37(3):355, 1982

Hull MG, North K, Taylor H, et al: Delayed conception and active and passive smoking. The Avon Longitudinal Study of Pregnancy and Childhood Study Team. Fertil Steril 74:725, 2000

Jarow J: Effects of varicocele on male fertility. Hum Reprod Update 7:59, 2001

Kao L, Germeyer A, Tulac S, et al: Expression profiling of endometrium from women with endometriosis reveals candidate genes for disease-based implantation failure and infertility. Endocrinology 144:2870, 2003

Katz D, Slade D, Nakajima S: Analysis of pre-ovulatory changes in cervical mucus hydration and sperm penetrability. Adv Contracept 13:143, 1997

Keefe D, Niven-Fairchild T, Powell S, et al: Mitochondrial deoxyribonucleic acid deletions in oocytes and reproductive aging in women. Fertil Steril 64:577, 1995

Kent-First M, Muallem A, Shultz J, et al: Defining regions of the Y-chromosome responsible for male infertility and identification of a fourth AZF region (AZFd) by Y-chromosome microdeletion detection. Mol Reprod Dev 53:27, 1999

Kidd S, Eskenazi B, Wyrobek A: Effects of male age on semen quality and fertility: a review of the literature. Fertil Steril 75:237, 2001

Klonoff-Cohen H, Lam-Kruglick P, Gonzalez C: Effects of maternal and paternal alcohol consumption on the success rates of in vitro fertilization and gamete intrafallopian transfer. Fertil Steril 79:330, 2003

Kruger T, Acosta A, Simmons K, et al: Predictive value of abnormal sperm morphology in in vitro fertilization. Fertil Steril 49:112, 1988

Kunzle R, Mueller M, Hanggi W, et al: Semen quality of male smokers and nonsmokers in infertile couples. Fertil Steril 79:287, 2003

Lalos O: Risk factors for tubal infertility among infertile and fertile women. Eur J Obstet Gynecol Reprod Biol 29:129, 1988

La Marca A, Broekmans FJ, Volpe A, et al: Anti-Mullerian hormone (AMH): what do we still need to know? Hum Reprod 24(9):2264, 2009

Laurent S, Thompson S, Addy C, et al: An epidemiologic study of smoking and primary infertility in women. Fertil Steril 57:565, 1992

Lee P: Fertility in cryptorchidism: does treatment make a difference? Endocrinol Metab Clin North Texas 22:479 1993

Lessey B: Endometrial integrins and the establishment of uterine receptivity. Hum Reprod 13(Suppl 3):247, 1998

Levitas E, Lunenfeld E, Weisz N, et al: Relationship between age and semen parameters in men with normal sperm concentration: analysis of 6022 semen samples. Andrologia 39(2):45, 2007

Licciardi F, Liu H, Rosenwaks Z: Day 3 estradiol serum concentrations as prognosticators of ovarian stimulation response and pregnancy outcome in patients undergoing in vitro fertilization. Fertil Steril 64:991, 1995

Luciano A, Peluso J, Koch E, et al: Temporal relationship and reliability of the clinical, hormonal, and ultrasonographic indices of ovulation in infertile women. Obstet Gynecol 75(3 Pt 1):412, 1990

Maroulis G: Effect of aging on fertility and pregnancy. Semin Reprod Endocrinol 9:165, 1991

Maseelall PB, Hernandez-Rey AE, Oh C, et al: Antral follicle count is a significant predictor of livebirth in in vitro fertilization cycles. Fertil Steril 91 (4 Suppl):1393, 2009

McKinley M, O'Loughlin VD: Reproductive System in Human Anatomy. New York, McGraw-Hill, 2006, p 873

Miller P, Soules M: The usefulness of a urinary LH kit for ovulation prediction during menstrual cycles of normal women. Obstet Gynecol 87:13, 1996

Moen M, Magnus P: The familial risk of endometriosis. Acta Obstet Gynecol Scand 72:560, 1993

Moghissi K: Ovulation detection. Endocrinol Metab Clin North Am 21:39, 1992

Mosher W, Pratt W: Fecundity and infertility in the United States: incidence and trends. Fertil Steril 56:192, 1991

Muasher S, Oehninger S, Simonetti S, et al: The value of basal and/or stimulated serum gonadotropin levels in prediction of stimulation response and in vitro fertilization outcome. Fertil Steril 50:298, 1988

Muthusami KR, Chinnaswamy P: Effect of chronic alcoholism on male fertility hormones and semen quality. Fertil Steril 84(4):919, 2005

Nagy F, Pendergrass P, Bowen D, et al: A comparative study of cytological and physiological parameters of semen obtained from alcoholics and non-alcoholics. Alcohol Alcohol 21:17, 1986

Navot D, Rosenwaks Z, Margalioth E: Prognostic assessment of female fecundity. Lancet 2:645, 1987

Nezar M, Goda H, El-Negery M, et al: Genital tract tuberculosis among fertile women: an old problem revisited. Arch Gynecol Obstet 280(5):787, 2009

Nikolaou D, Templeton A: Early ovarian ageing: a hypothesis. Detection and clinical relevance. Hum Reprod 18:1137, 2003

Noyes R, Hertig A, Rock J: Dating the endometrial biopsy. Am J Obstet Gynecol 122:262, 1975

Oates R, Amos J: The genetic basis of congenital bilateral absence of the vas deferens and cystic fibrosis. J Androl 15:1, 1994

Oei SG, Helmerhorst FM, Bloemenkamp KW: Effectiveness of the postcoital test: randomised controlled trial. BMJ 317(7157):502, 1998

Oei S, Helmerhorst F, Keirse M: When is the post-coital test normal? A critical appraisal. Hum Reprod 10:1711, 1995a

Oei S, Keirse M, Bloemenkamp K, et al: European postcoital tests: opinions and practice. Br J Obstet Gynaecol 102:621, 1995b

Orejuela F, Lipshultz LL: Effects of working environment on male reproductive health. Contemp Urol 10:86, 1998

Pellestor F, Andreo B, Arnal F, et al: Maternal aging and chromosomal abnormalities: new data drawn from in vitro unfertilized human oocytes. Hum Genet 112:195, 2003

Perez-Medina T, Bajo-Arenas J, Salazar F, et al: Endometrial polyps and their implication in the pregnancy rates of patients undergoing intrauterine insemination: a prospective, randomized study. Hum Reprod 20:1632, 2005

Preutthipan S, Linasmita V: A prospective comparative study between hysterosalpingography and hysteroscopy in the detection of intrauterine pathology in patients with infertility. J Obstet Gynaecol Res 29:33, 2003

Pritts E: Fibroids and infertility: a systematic review of the evidence. Obstet Gynecol Surv 56:483, 2001

Pryor J, Kent-First M, Muallem A, et al: Microdeletions in the Y chromosome of infertile men. N Engl J Med 336:534, 1997

Ramlau-Hansen CH, Thulstrup AM, Aggerholm AS, et al: Is smoking a risk factor for decreased semen quality? A cross-sectional analysis. Human Reproduction 22(1):188, 2007

Randolph J Jr, Ying Y, Maier D, et al: Comparison of real-time ultrasonography, hysterosalpingography, and laparoscopy/hysteroscopy in the evaluation of uterine abnormalities and tubal patency. Fertil Steril 46:828, 1986

Ratbi I, Legendre M, Niel F, et al: Detection of cystic fibrosis transmembrane conductance regulator (CFTR) gene rearrangements enriches the mutation spectrum in congenital bilateral absence of the vas deferens and impacts on genetic counseling. Hum Reprod 22(5):1285, 2007

Rosenfeld DL, Scholl G, Bronson R, et al: Unsuspected chronic pelvic inflammatory disease in the infertile female. Fertil Steril 39:44, 1983

Rowley M, Teshima F, Heller C: Duration of transit of spermatozoa through the human male ductular system. Fertil Steril 21:390, 1970

Sakkas D, Alvarez JG: Sperm DNA fragmentation: mechanisms of origin, impact on reproductive outcome, and analysis. Fertil Steril 93(4):1027, 2010

Saracoglu OF, Mungan T, Tanzer F: Pelvic tuberculosis. Int J Gynaecol Obstet 37:115, 1992

Schenker J: Etiology of and therapeutic approach to synechia uteri. Eur J Obstet Gynecol Reprod Biol 65:109, 1996

Schlesinger M, Wilets I, Nagler H: Treatment outcome after varicocelectomy. A critical analysis. Urol Clin North Am 21:517, 1994

Scott RT Jr, Hofmann GE: Prognostic assessment of ovarian reserve. Fertil Steril 63:1, 1995

Scott R, Snyder R, Bagnall J, et al: Evaluation of the impact of intraobserver variability on endometrial dating and the diagnosis of luteal phase defects. Fertil Steril 60:652, 1993

Serafini P, Batzofin J: Diagnosis of female infertility. A comprehensive approach. J Reprod Med 34(1):29, 1989

Sharara F, Beatse S, Leonardi M, et al: Cigarette smoking accelerates the development of diminished ovarian reserve as evidenced by the clomiphene citrate challenge test. Fertil Steril 62:257, 1994

Sharlip I, Jarow J, Belker A, et al: Best practice policies for male infertility. Fertil Steril 77:873, 2002

Shideler S, DeVane G, Kalra P, et al: Ovarian-pituitary hormone interactions during the perimenopause. Maturitas 11:331, 1989

Sigman M, Jarow J: Endocrine evaluation of infertile men. Urology 50:659, 1997

Smith C, Asch R: Drug abuse and reproduction. Fertil Steril 48:355, 1987a

Smith R, Johnson A, Lamb D, et al: Functional tests of spermatozoa. Sperm penetration assay. Urol Clin North Am 14:451, 1987b

Soares S, Barbosa dos Reis M, Camargos A: Diagnostic accuracy of sonohysterography, transvaginal sonography, and hysterosalpingography in patients with uterine cavity diseases. Fertil Steril 73:406, 2000

Stanford J, White G, Hatasaka H: Timing intercourse to achieve pregnancy: current evidence. Obstet Gynecol 100:1333, 2002

Steckel J, Dicker A, Goldstein M: Relationship between varicocele size and response to varicocelectomy. J Urol 149:769, 1993

Stovall D, Parrish S, Van Voorhis B, et al: Uterine leiomyomas reduce the efficacy of assisted reproduction cycles: results of a matched follow-up study. Hum Reprod 13:192, 1998

Swart P, Mol B, van der Veen F, et al: The accuracy of hysterosalpingography in the diagnosis of tubal pathology: a meta-analysis. Fertil Steril 64:486, 1995

Tas S, Lauwerys R, Lison D: Occupational hazards for the male reproductive system. Crit Rev Toxicol 26:261, 1996

te Velde E, Pearson P: The variability of female reproductive ageing. Hum Reprod Update 8:141, 2002

Tietze C: Reproductive span and rate of reproduction among Hutterite women. Fertil Steril 8:89, 1957

Tolstrup J, Kjaer S, Holst C, et al: Alcohol use as predictor for infertility in a representative population of Danish women. Acta Obstet Gynecol Scand 82:744, 2003

Toner J, Philput C, Jones G, et al: Basal follicle-stimulating hormone level is a better predictor of in vitro fertilization performance than age. Fertil Steril 55:784, 1991

Treloar S, Do K, Martin N: Genetic influences on the age at menopause. Lancet 352:1084, 1998

Turek PJ, Lipshultz LI: Immunologic infertility. Urol Clin North Am 21(3):447, 1994

Wilcox A, Weinberg C, Baird D: Timing of sexual intercourse in relation to ovulation. Effects on the probability of conception, survival of the pregnancy, and sex of the baby. N Engl J Med 333:1517, 1995

Wolff H: The biologic significance of white blood cells in semen. Fertil Steril 63:1143, 1995

World Health Organization: Laboratory Manual for the Examination of Human Semen and Sperm-Cervical Mucus Interaction. Cambridge University Press, 1999

World Health Organization: The influence of varicocele on parameters of fertility in a large group of men presenting to infertility clinics. Fertil Steril 57(6):1289, 1992

World Health Organization: Women and sexually transmitted infections. 2007. Available at: http://www.who.int/mediacentre/factsheets/fs110/en/. Accessed August 21, 2010

Zini A, Sigman M: Are tests of sperm DNA damage clinically useful? Pros and cons. J Androl 30:219, 2009

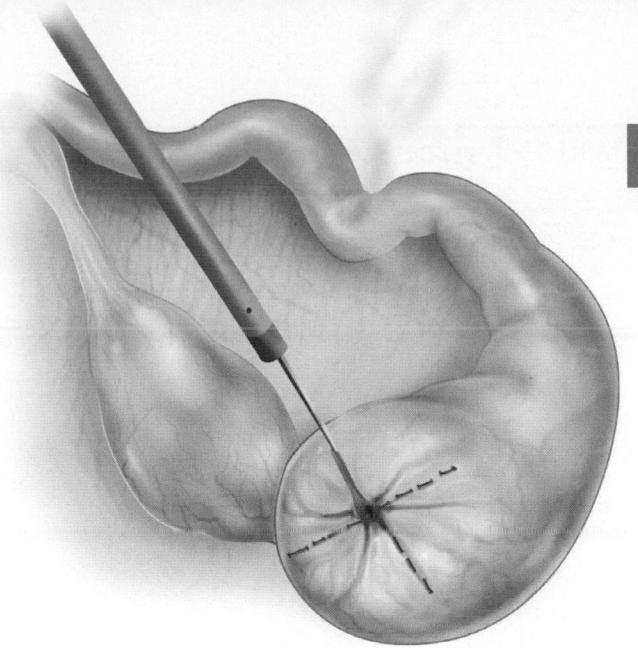

CHAPTER 20

Treatment of the Infertile Couple

Infertility results from diseases of the reproductive system that impair the body's ability to perform basic reproductive function. It is defined as the failure to achieve a successful pregnancy after 12 months or more of regular unprotected intercourse (American Society for Reproductive Medicine, 2008a). Ten to 15 percent of the reproductive-aged population is infertile, and men and women are equally affected.

Infertility treatment is a complex process influenced by numerous factors. Important considerations include duration of infertility, a couple's age (especially the female's), and diag-

nosed cause. Additionally, the level of distress experienced by a couple should be taken into account.

In general, a first step involves identification of a primary cause and contributing factors, and treatment is aimed at their direct correction. Most couples are treated with conventional therapies such as medication or surgery. In many cases, therapy can begin without a complete evaluation, especially if a cause is obvious. However, if pregnancy does not quickly follow, then more thorough testing is required.

In contrast, evaluation commonly may not yield a satisfactory explanation or may identify causes that are not amenable to direct correction. For such cases, recent advances in assisted reproduction have provided effective treatments. These approaches, however, are not without disadvantages. For example, in vitro fertilization (IVF) has been linked with higher rates of some fetal and maternal complications. Appropriate treatments may also pose ethical dilemmas for couples or their physician. For example, selective reduction of a multifetal pregnancy may improve survival chances for some fetuses but at the cost of others. Lastly, infertility treatment can be a financial burden, a significant source of emotional stress, or both.

An infertility specialist should not dictate treatment, but should offer and explain therapy options, which may include expectant management or even adoption.

LIFESTYLE THERAPIES

Environmental Factors

Increasing information suggests that some male and female infertility may result from environmental contaminants or toxins (Giudice, 2006). Endocrine-disrupting chemicals such as dioxins and polychlorinated biphenyls, as well as agricultural pesticides and herbicides, phthalates (used in making plastic materials), lead, and bisphenol A (used in the manufacture of polycarbonate plastic and resins), have been shown to be reproductive toxicants (Hauser, 2008; Mendola, 2008).

Although direct links to infertility in humans are not conclusive, clinicians should counsel patients that environmental exposures to toxic substances should be avoided if possible. Currently, these cautions should be discussed carefully to avoid alarm.

▪ Smoking

At least one fifth of reproductive-aged men and women in the United States smoke cigarettes (Centers for Disease Control and Prevention, 2011). Several comprehensive reviews have summarized cumulative data on cigarette smoking and female fecundity, and all support the conclusion that smoking has an adverse effect (American Society for Reproductive Medicine, 2008d). Moreover, smoking's negative effects on female fecundity do not appear to be overcome by assisted reproductive technologies (ART). A 5-year prospective study of 221 couples found that the risk of failing to conceive with ART was more than doubled in smokers. Each year that a woman had smoked was associated with a 9-percent increase in the risk of unsuccessful ART cycles (Klonoff-Cohen, 2001).

The effect of smoking on male fertility is more difficult to discern. Although smokers often have reduced sperm concentrations and motility comparatively, these often remain within the normal range.

Smoking is associated with an increased miscarriage rate in both natural and assisted conception cycles. The mechanism for this has not been elucidated, but the vasoconstrictive and antimetabolic properties of some components of cigarette smoke such as nicotine, carbon dioxide, and cyanide may lead to placental insufficiency.

Specifically, smoking has been linked to higher rates of abruption, fetal-growth restriction, and preterm labor (Cunningham, 2010). In addition, smoking in pregnant women is associated with an increased risk of trisomy 21 that results from maternal meiotic nondisjunction (Yang, 1999). For these reasons, smoking should be discouraged for both male and female partners planning pregnancy.

Many women are unaware of the effects of smoking on fertility, and education is an important first step toward cessation (Table 20-1). If behavioral approaches fail, use of medical adjuncts such as nicotine replacement therapy, bupropion (Zyban), or varenicline (Chantix) may prove effective (Table 1-23, p. 28). Nicotine preparations are designated as category D. Bupropion and varenicline are nonnicotine Food and Drug Administration (FDA)-approved agents and carry a category C designation (Fiore, 2008). Although studies of these agents in pregnant women have been limited, ideally, pharmacologic smoking cessation therapies are best used prior to conception.

▪ Alcohol

Alcohol consumption is widespread and increasing in many countries. It is well known that chronic alcohol abuse during pregnancy may lead to fetal alcohol syndrome, but the impact on fertility has been less well studied. Retrospective investigations have generally found that moderate alcohol intake in women has no significant effect on fertility, whereas a high intake has been associated with

TABLE 20-1. Women's Awareness of Health Risks Associated with Smoking

Smoking Risk	Women Aware of Risk
Respiratory disease	99%
Heart disease	96%
Pregnancy complications	91%
Spontaneous abortion	39%
Ectopic pregnancy	27%
Infertility	22%
Early menopause	18%

Abbreviated from Roth, 2001, with permission.

reduced fecundability. However, one prospective study of Danish couples attempting pregnancy demonstrated a decreased fecundability even among women with a weekly alcohol intake of five or fewer drinks (Jensen, 1998). This finding needs further corroboration, but it seems reasonable to encourage women to avoid alcohol when they are trying to become pregnant.

▪ Caffeine

Caffeine is one of the most widely used pharmacologically active substances in the world. Studies have suggested that a positive dose–response relationship between caffeine and impaired fertility does exist. Hassan and Killick (2004) determined that women who consumed seven or more cups of coffee or tea per day were 1.5 times more likely to be subfertile. Accordingly, recommendations of caffeine intake moderation in infertile women seem prudent.

▪ Weight Optimization
Obese Women

Ovarian function is dependent on weight. Low body-fat content is associated with hypothalamic hypogonadism. In contrast, central body fat is associated with insulin resistance and contributes to ovarian dysfunction in many women with polycystic ovarian syndrome (PCOS). Lifestyle modification in overweight infertile women with PCOS leads to a reduction of central fat and improved insulin sensitivity, decreased hyperandrogenemia, lowered luteinizing hormone (LH) concentrations, and restoration of normal fertility in many cases (Hoeger, 2001; Kiddy, 1992). Even a 5 to 10 percent reduction in body weight has been shown to be successful in these women (Table 20-2) (Kiddy, 1992; Pasquali, 1989). Apart from diet, exercise can also improve insulin sensitivity. Weight loss and exercise are inexpensive and should be recommended as first-line management of obese women with PCOS.

Although pharmacologic options can effectively treat anovulation if weight cannot be lost, it should be noted that obesity is a significant risk factor for obstetric and perinatal

TABLE 20-2. Efficacy of Lifestyle Intervention in Anovulatory Infertile Women

Parameter	Completed, $n = 67$ (Mean ± SD or %)	Drop-Out, $n = 20$ (Mean ± SD or %)
BMI, basal	37.4 ± 6.9	35.9 ± 4.1
PCOS status	79%	72%
Anovulatory at baseline	81%	75%
Change in BMI	−3.7 ± 1.6	−0.4 ± 1.4[a]
Resumed spontaneous ovulation	90%	None
Pregnancies (cumulative: spontaneous or assisted reproductive technologies)	77%	None

The original cohort included 87 infertile obese women, most of whom had PCOS, and treatment consisted of a long-term lifestyle intervention program, including physical activity and hypocaloric diet. Those who completed were compared with those who dropped out.
[a]$p < .05$
BMI = body mass index; PCOS = polycystic ovarian syndrome.
From Pasquali, 2006, with permission.

complications. Some maternal risks include higher rates of gestational diabetes, cesarean delivery, preeclampsia, unexplained stillbirth, and surgical wound infection. Obesity also has been associated with an increased risk of birth defects (American Society for Reproductive Medicine, 2008b). Therefore, strong consideration should be given to delaying treatments in morbidly obese women until their body mass index (BMI) can be reduced below 40. This is especially true if treatments involve surgical risks or risk of multifetal gestation.

Weight-loss options are discussed in Chapter 1 (p. 13). If bariatric surgery is selected, conception should be delayed for 12 to 18 months (American College of Obstetricians and Gynecologists, 2005). This is because rapid weight loss during this time poses theoretical risks for intrauterine fetal-growth restriction and nutritional deprivation.

Underweight Women

Although obesity is more commonly encountered, undernutrition can also be a problem. The reproductive axis is closely linked to nutritional status, and inhibitory pathways suppress ovulation in subjects with significant weight loss (Table 20-3 and Fig. 16-7, p. 449). Anorexia nervosa and bulimia nervosa affect up to 5 percent of reproductive-aged women and may cause amenorrhea, infertility, and in those who do conceive, an increased likelihood of miscarriage. Fortunately, recovery may follow minimal acquisition of weight because energy balance has a more important effect than body fat mass.

▪ Exercise

Physical activity has been demonstrated to have numerous health benefits. The relationship between exercise and fertility, however, is not straightforward. Competitive female athletes often experience amenorrhea, irregular cycles or luteal dysfunction, and infertility. This may be related not specifically to physical activity itself, but rather to low body-fat content or physical stress associated with competition.

At this time, insufficient data exist to support or discourage physical activity in infertile women in the absence of documented ovarian dysfunction associated with obesity or low body weight.

▪ Nutrition

In the absence of obesity or significant undernutrition, the role of diet in infertility is unclear. High-protein diets and gluten intolerance (celiac disease) have been investigated as underlying causes in women. However, study sizes have been small, and conflicting results found (Collin, 1996; Jackson, 2008; Meloni, 1999). In men, dietary antioxidants have been proposed as a potential way to improve male reproductive outcomes by reducing oxidative damage in sperm DNA (Ross, 2010). Although promising, large well-designed studies to guide clinical use are needed (Patel, 2008). Additionally, the nutritional supplement, carnitine, had been often touted as a potential benefit for male infertility. This finding, however, has not been confirmed by a randomized, prospective trial (Sigman, 2006).

Despite a lack of conclusive benefits of nutritional supplements or diet modification in infertile couples, it does seem reasonable to recommend daily multivitamin supplementation to both. Folic acid is contained in most multivitamins, and daily doses of 400 μg orally are recommended for women attempting pregnancy to reduce the incidence of neural-tube defects in their fetuses (American College of Obstetricians and Gynecologists, 2003).

▪ Stress Management

Stress has been implicated in reproductive failure. Although severe stress can result in anovulation, less significant stress

TABLE 20-3. Relation of Comorbid Mental Disorders to Amenorrhea at Baseline and 10- to 15-year Follow Up Among 173 Women with Bulimia Nervosa

Lifetime Mental Disorder	Current Amenorrhea				Amenorrhea Over 10- to 15-Year Follow-Up			
	Total	Rate		Analysis	Total	Rate		Analysis
	n	n	%	p	n	n	%	p
Anorexia nervosa				<.02				<.001
Present	59	16	27.1		50	43	86.0	
Subthreshold	23	4	17.4		19	9	47.4	
Absent	78	7	9.0		74	19	25.7	
Mood disorder				<.03				<.07
Present	104	10	9.6		92	51	55.4	
Absent	55	16	29.1		51	20	39.2	
Anxiety disorder				<.16				<.68
Present	48	5	10.4		42	22	52.4	
Absent	112	22	19.6		101	49	48.5	

From Crow, 2002, with permission.

may also play a role, but a mechanism has yet to be defined. Patients with higher stress levels have been found to have lower pregnancy rates when undergoing IVF treatments (Thiering, 1993). Accordingly, consideration should be given to screening all infertile couples for evidence of anxiety or depression. Although pharmacologic management of stress is not typically recommended during infertility treatments, a "mind/body" approach that combines psychological counseling and meditation may be considered for those patients manifesting high levels of anxiety (Domar, 1990).

CORRECTION OF AN IDENTIFIED CAUSE

Correction of Ovarian Dysfunction

Hyperprolactinemia

Prolactin is a pituitary hormone that plays an important role in a variety of reproductive functions, and elevated levels are commonly encountered in clinical endocrinology practice. If hyperprolactinemia is found, then physiologic, pharmacologic, or other secondary causes of hormone hypersecretion should be sought (Tables 12-3 and 12-4, p. 340). In the absence of hypothyroidism or a pharmacologic cause of hyperprolactinemia, imaging studies should be performed to identify microadenoma or macroadenoma of the pituitary gland.

Dopamine agonists are the primary treatment of hyperprolactinemia (Chap. 15, p. 420). Surgical therapies should only be considered with prolactin-secreting adenomas resistant to medical therapy.

When conception does occurs, because the risk of tumor expansion is low during pregnancy, dopamine-agonist therapy is typically stopped. However, if symptomatic tumor enlargement develops, a dopamine agonist may be reinstituted (Molitch, 1999, 2010).

Hypothyroidism

Thyroid disorders are prevalent in reproductive-aged individuals and affect women four to five times more frequently than men. Clinical hypothyroidism is associated with changes in cycle length and amount of bleeding. Specifically, oligomenorrhea and amenorrhea are frequent findings. Although ovulation and conception can still occur in those with mild hypothyroidism, treatment with thyroxine usually restores a normal menstrual pattern and enhances fertility (Chap. 16, p. 456).

Subclinical hypothyroidism may also be associated with ovarian dysfunction (Strickland, 1990). Lincoln and associates (1999) found a 2-percent incidence of elevated thyroid-stimulating hormone (TSH) levels in 704 asymptomatic women seeking evaluation for infertility. In those with elevated TSH levels and associated ovarian dysfunction, correction of hypothyroidism led to pregnancy in 64 percent of patients. In addition to a possible effect on fertility, subclinical hypothyroidism may also adversely affect pregnancy outcomes.

Ovulation Induction

Ovarian dysfunction is the most common indication for the use of medications to induce ovulation. These agents can also be used in ovulatory women to increase the likelihood of pregnancy in couples with other causes of infertility or unexplained infertility. Use of these medications to promote follicular development and prompt ovulation is called *superovulation* or *ovulation enhancement*. If these agents are administered solely to stimulate follicles, and egg harvesting is completed by ART, then the term *controlled ovarian hyperstimulation* is used. In contrast, we prefer the term *ovulation induction* to describe treatment with medications to stimulate normal ovulation in women with ovarian dysfunction.

Frequent causes of ovarian dysfunction include PCOS and diminished ovarian reserve. Less often, central (hypothalamic or

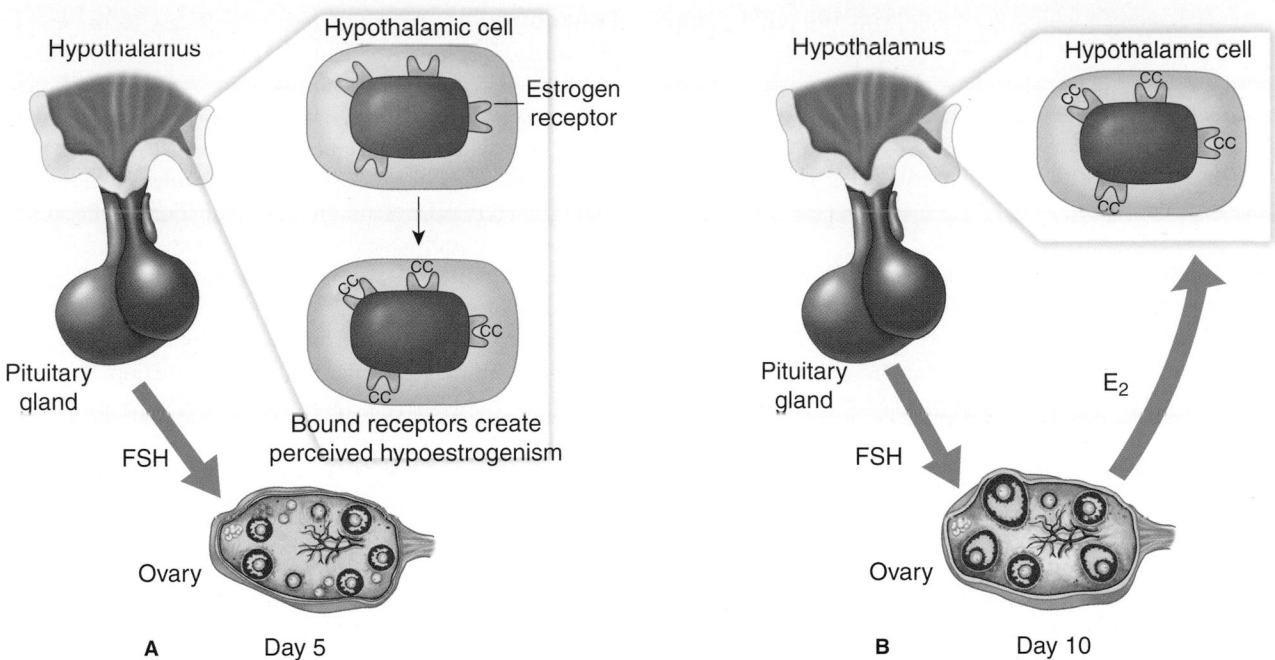

FIGURE 20-1 Effect of clomiphene citrate (CC) administration. **A.** Clomiphene binds to the estrogen receptor in the pituitary and hypothalamus. This causes an effective reduction in hypothalamic estrogen receptor number. Because of this reduced receptor number, the hypothalamus and pituitary are effectively blinded to true circulating estrogen levels, and perceived hypoestrogenism results. As a result, estrogen's negative feedback is interrupted centrally, and follicle-stimulating hormone (FSH) secretion increases from the anterior pituitary. This leads to maturation of multiple follicles. **B.** By the late follicular phase, because of clomiphene citrate's long retention within tissues, estrogen receptor depletion continues centrally. As a result, increased estradiol (E_2) secretion from the ovary is not capable of exerting normal negative feedback on FSH release. This leads to a growth of multiple dominant follicles and multiple ovulations.

pituitary) disorders or thyroid dysfunction can result in infertility. Rarely, ovarian tumors or adrenal abnormalities lead to abnormal ovarian function. Treatment of ovarian dysfunction should be based on the identified cause as well as the results of any prior attempted therapy.

Clomiphene Citrate

Pharmacologic Effects. Clomiphene citrate (CC) is the initial treatment for most anovulatory infertile women. Chemically similar to tamoxifen, CC is a nonsteroidal triphenylethylene derivative that demonstrates both estrogen agonist and antagonist properties (Fig. 15-10, p. 410). Antagonist properties predominate except at very low estrogen levels. As a result, negative feedback that is normally produced by estrogen in the hypothalamus is reduced (Fig. 20-1). Gonadotropin-releasing hormone (GnRH) secretion is altered and stimulates pituitary gonadotropin release. The resulting increase in follicle-stimulating hormone (FSH) levels, in turn, drives ovarian follicular activity.

Tamoxifen has also been used successfully for ovulation induction. However, it is not approved by the FDA for this indication and has not been demonstrated to have significant advantage compared with CC.

Administration. Clomiphene citrate is administered orally, typically starting on the third to fifth day after the onset of spontaneous or progestin-induced menses. Ovulation rates, conception rates, and pregnancy outcome are similar regardless whether treatment begins on cycle day 2, 3, 4, or 5. Prior to

therapy, sonography is advisable to exclude signs of significant spontaneous follicular maturation or residual follicular cysts. In general at our institution, clomiphene can be administered if no follicle is >20 mm and the endometrium is less than 5 mm. A pregnancy test is also indicated after spontaneous menses. Although not a proven teratogen, CC is classified as category X by the FDA and thus is contraindicated in suspected or documented pregnancy.

The dose required to achieve ovulation correlates with body weight. However, there is no reliable way to accurately predict which dose will be required in an individual woman (Lobo, 1982). Consequently, CC is titrated empirically to establish the lowest effective dose for each patient. Treatment typically begins with a single 50-mg tablet taken daily orally for 5 consecutive days. Doses are increased by a 50-mg increment in each subsequent cycle until ovulation is induced. The dose of clomiphene citrate should not be increased if normal ovulation is confirmed. Thus, lack of pregnancy alone does not justify an increase in dose. The effective dose of CC ranges from 50 mg/day to 250 mg/day, although doses in excess of 100 mg/day are not approved by the FDA. Some studies have suggested that adjunctive therapy with glucocorticoids may benefit some patients not responsive to CC alone (Elnashar, 2006; Parsanezhad, 2002). The precise mechanism is unclear, although several direct and indirect actions of dexamethasone have been suggested. This therapy may be empiric or individualized based on elevated dehydroepiandrosterone sulfate (DHEAS) levels.

In general, women failing to ovulate with 100 mg/day dosing or failing to conceive following 3 to 6 months of ovulatory response to CC should be considered candidates for alternative treatments. In a retrospective study including 428 women who received CC for ovulation induction, 84.5 percent of pregnancies achieved with treatment occurred during the first three ovulatory cycles (Gysler, 1982).

Insulin-Sensitizing Agents.

Although PCOS appears to be a heterogeneous disorder, many women with this condition exhibit insulin resistance (Chap. 17, p. 461). Insulin resistance leads to compensatory hyperinsulinemia and dyslipidemia. Given the strong evidence that hyperinsulinemia plays a pivotal pathogenic role in development of PCOS, it is reasonable to assume that interventions that reduce circulating insulin levels in women with PCOS may restore normal reproductive endocrine function. As discussed, weight loss, nutrition, and exercise have clearly led to reduced hyperinsulinemia, resolution of hyperandrogenism, and in many cases, resumption of ovulatory function in overweight women with PCOS. However, women may be poorly compliant, and weight loss is rarely maintained over time.

Insulin-sensitizing agents show promise in the treatment of PCOS. When administered to insulin-resistant patients, these compounds act to increase target tissue responsiveness to insulin, thereby reducing the body's need for compensatory hyperinsulinemia (Antonucci, 1998). Current insulin sensitizing agents include the biguanides and thiazolidinediones (Chap. 17, p. 474).

Studies suggest that metformin (Glucophage), given with meals 500 mg orally three times daily or 850 mg twice daily and administered to women with PCOS, increased the frequency of spontaneous ovulation, menstrual cyclicity, and ovulatory response to CC (Nestler, 1998; Palomba, 2005; Vandermolen, 2001). In contrast, a large, prospective, randomized, multicenter trial does not support the hypothesis that metformin, either alone or in combination with CC, improves the live-birth rate in women with PCOS (Legro, 2007).

Gonadotropins.

Clomiphene citrate is easy to use and leads to ovulation in most patients (Hammond, 1983). However, pregnancy rates are disappointing and approximate 50 percent or less (Raj, 1977; Zarate, 1971). Lower than expected pregnancy rates with CC have been attributed to its long half-life and peripheral antiestrogenic effects, mainly on the endometrium and cervical mucus. In such individuals, who are often classified as "clomiphene resistant," the next step is traditionally the administration of exogenous gonadotropin preparations via injections, instead of CC.

As with CC, the goal of ovulation induction with gonadotropins is simply to normalize ovarian function. Ideally, the dose used should be the minimum required to cause normal development of a single dominant follicle. Because the response to gonadotropins can vary greatly from individual to individual and even from cycle to cycle, intensive monitoring is required to adjust dosage and timing of ovulation.

Gonadotropin preparations vary in terms of their source (urinary or recombinant) and by the presence or absence of LH activity (Table 20-4). Traditional urinary-derived human menopausal gonadotropin (hMG) preparations are extracted and purified from the urine of postmenopausal women, and their active components are both FSH and LH. These preparations also contain human chorionic gonadotropin (hCG), which is mainly derived from pituitary secretion of hCG in postmenopausal women. LH and hCG can both bind to the same receptor (luteinizing hormone/chorionic gonadotropin receptor [LHCGR]). In purified hMG, hCG is the primary source of the LH activity, although significant LH is also present in the older, non-highly purified hMG products (Filicori, 2002). Highly purified urinary preparations allow for administration via subcutaneous route with minimal or no reaction at the injection site. Alternatives to hMG include highly purified urinary gonadotropin preparations and purified recombinant FSH.

Both LH and FSH activity are required for normal ovarian steroidogenesis and follicular development. In many cases, pure FSH preparations can be used because of adequate endogenous LH production. However, for ovulation induction in

---

TABLE 20-4. Gonadotropin Preparations Used for Ovulation Induction

Name	Product Type	FSH Activity	LH Activity	hCG Activity
Bravelle Fertinex[a]	Vial	Highly purified urinary	Minimal	Minimal
Follistim Gonal-f	Pen or vial	Highly purified recombinant	None	None
Menopur	Vial	Highly purified urinary	Minimal	Highly purified urinary
Repronex Pergonal[a] Humagon[a]	Vial	Urinary	Urinary	Urinary

FSH = follicle-stimulating hormone; hCG = human chorionic gonadotropin; LH = luteinizing hormone.
[a]No longer available.

patients with hypogonadotropic amenorrhea, LH activity must be provided from an exogenous source. Options include hMG, recombinant LH, and low-dose (diluted) urinary or recombinant hCG. Ovulation induction in women with PCOS can be performed either with FSH-only containing products because of endogenous LH or with those containing both LH and FSH activity. At present, data do not support the superiority of one preparation over another.

Gonadotropin development will likely continue. A long-acting FSH is commercially available in Europe and is being tested in the United States. This recombinant molecule was created by adding a DNA sequence to the human FSH gene. This extra sequence (naturally present on the beta subunit of hCG) allows for more glycosylation and hence a prolonged clearance. Low-molecular-weight molecules (nonproteins) are also in the early stages of clinical development. Advantages of these nontraditional gonadotropins include oral delivery.

Most clinicians begin ovulation induction attempts at a low gonadotropin dosage of 50 to 75 IU/day. This is gradually increased if no ovarian response (as assessed by serum estradiol measurements) is noted after several days (Fig. 20-2). This is referred to as a "step-up" protocol. A "step-down" protocol can also be used with the advantage of a decreased duration of stimulation. However, the risk of excessive ovarian response, such as multiple follicle development or ovarian hyperstimulation syndrome, may be increased with this method. With either approach, if a patient fails to conceive, subsequent cycles may be started at higher doses based on prior response.

In general, results of gonadotropin stimulation in women with PCOS are less successful than those in patients with hypogonadotropic amenorrhea (Balen, 1994). Women with PCOS have ovaries highly sensitive to gonadotropin stimulation. They have a higher risk of excessive ovarian response and of multifetal pregnancy than those with normal ovaries (Farhi, 1996).

Aromatase Inhibitors.
Gonadotropins are associated with more effective ovulation induction and higher pregnancy rates than CC. However, gonadotropins are expensive and carry higher risks for ovarian hyperstimulation syndrome and multifetal gestation. Accordingly, aromatase inhibitors have been investigated as ovulation inducing agents (Fig. 20-3). These were originally developed for breast cancer treatment and effectively inhibit *aromatase*, a cytochrome P450 hemoprotein that catalyzes the rate-limiting step in estrogen production. Aromatase inhibitors are orally administered, easy to use, relatively inexpensive, and associated with typically minor side effects.

The most widely used aromatase inhibitor to induce ovulation in anovulatory and ovulatory infertile women is letrozole (Femara). Compared with CC, its use is associated with a thicker endometrium and a trend toward higher pregnancy rates following ovulation induction. When used in combination with gonadotropins, letrozole leads to lower gonadotropin requirements and pregnancy rates comparable to those for gonadotropin treatment alone (Carper, 2003; Mitwally, 2004). The typical dosage used is 2.5 mg to 5 mg orally daily for 5 days.

Data suggesting that letrozole use for infertility treatment might be associated with a higher risk of congenital cardiac and bone malformations in the newborn are contradictory (Biljan, 2005; Tulandi, 2006). However, in 2005, the manufacturer issued a statement to physicians worldwide advising that letrozole use in premenopausal women, specifically its use for ovulation induction, is contraindicated (Fontana, 2005). As a result, it is not likely that letrozole will gain widespread acceptance for ovulation induction in the near future. Well-designed randomized prospective trials confirming safety are needed.

A second aromatase inhibitor, anastrozole (Arimidex), is of the same compound class as letrozole and has also been approved for treatment of women with breast cancer. At this time, no concerns have been raised regarding its teratogenicity. Experience with anastrozole in ovulation induction at this time is limited, however, and ideal dosage requirements are currently unknown.

Complications of Fertility Drugs
Ovarian Hyperstimulation Syndrome. Ovarian hyperstimulation syndrome (OHSS) is a clinical symptom complex associated with ovarian enlargement resulting from exogenous gonadotropin therapy. Symptoms may include abdominal pain and distension, ascites, gastrointestinal problems, respiratory compromise, oliguria, hemoconcentration, and thromboembolism. These symptoms may develop during ovulation induction or in early pregnancies that were conceived through exogenous ovarian stimulation.

Pathophysiology. The etiology of OHSS is complex, but hCG, either exogenous or endogenous (derived from a resulting pregnancy), is believed to be an early contributing factor. Development of OHSS involves increased vascular permeability and loss of fluid, protein, and electrolytes into the peritoneal cavity, which leads to hemoconcentration. Increased capillary permeability is felt to result from vasoactive substances produced by the corpus luteum. Vascular endothelial growth factor (VEGF) is believed to play a major role, and angiotensin II may also be involved. Hypercoagulability may be related to hyperviscosity following hemoconcentration. Alternatively, it may be secondary to the high estrogen levels present, and these high levels can increase coagulation factors. Predisposing factors for OHSS include multifollicular ovaries such as with PCOS, young age, high estradiol levels during ovulation induction, and pregnancy.

Diagnosis and Treatment. Abdominal pain is prominent and caused by ovarian enlargement together with accumulation of peritoneal fluid. Although sonographic examination of women with OHSS usually reveals enlarged ovaries with numerous follicular cysts and ascites, OHSS is a clinical diagnosis (Fig. 20-4). Several different classification schemes have been proposed to categorize the severity of this syndrome (Table 20-5).

Treatment of OHSS is generally supportive. Paracentesis is typically performed transvaginally as an outpatient and can ameliorate abdominal discomfort and relieve respiratory distress. Reaccumulation of ascites may prompt additional paracenteses or rarely placement of a percutaneous "pigtail" catheter

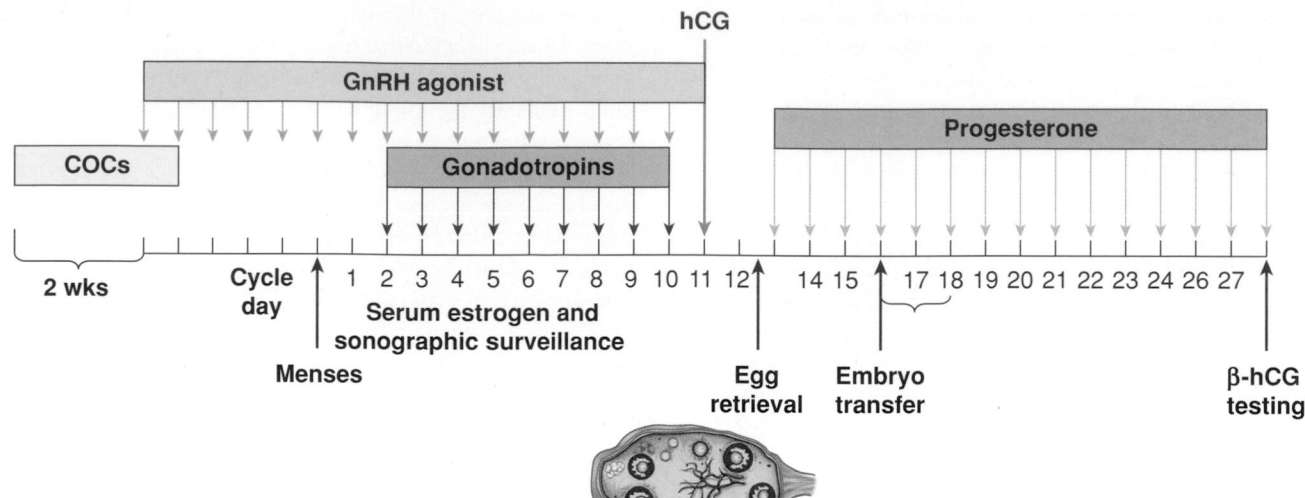

A

≥ 3 follicles at ≥ 17 mm

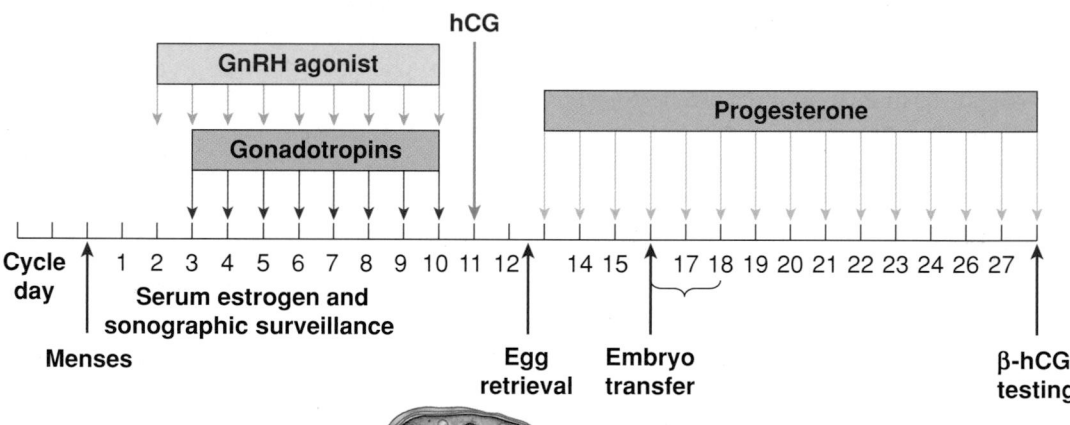

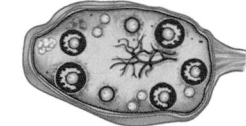

B

≥ 3 follicles at ≥ 17 mm

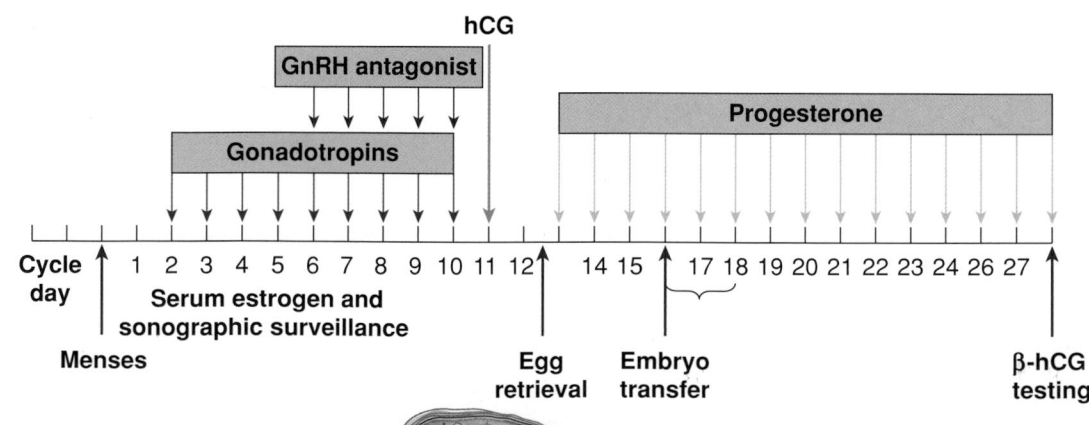

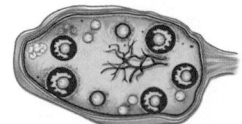

C

≥ 3 follicles at ≥ 17 mm

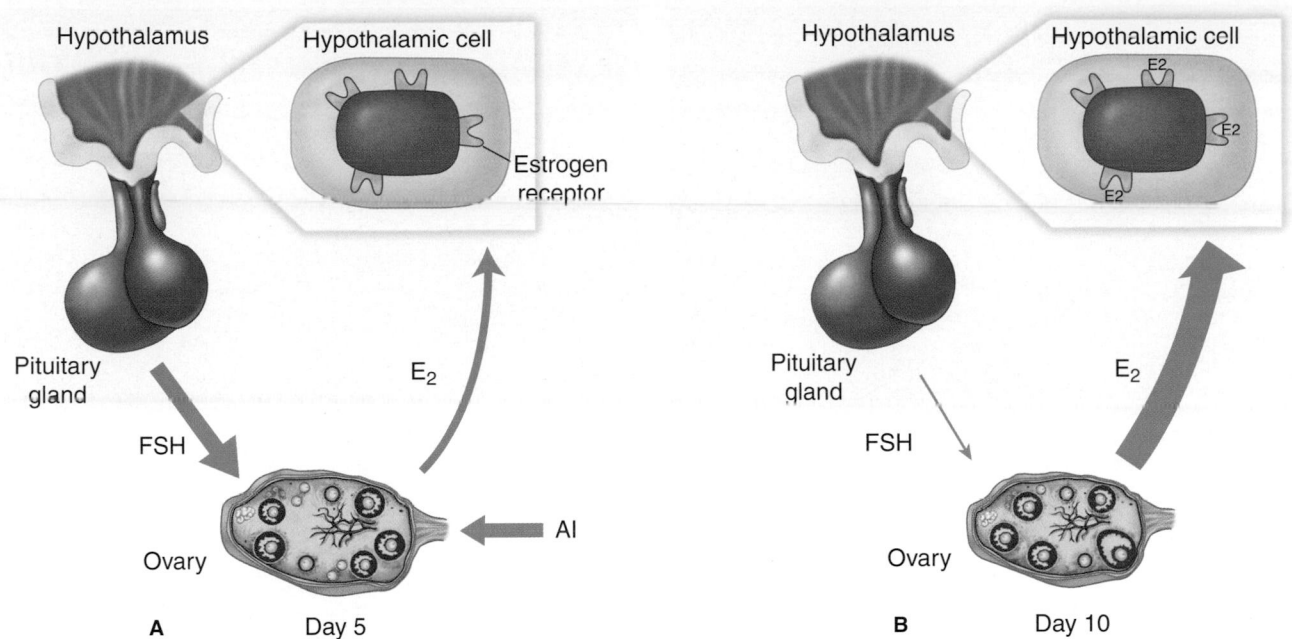

FIGURE 20-3 Effect of aromatase inhibitor (AI) administration. **A.** Administration suppresses ovarian estradiol (E_2) secretion and reduces estrogen negative feedback at the pituitary and hypothalamus. As a result, increased follicle-stimulating hormone (FSH) secretion from the anterior pituitary stimulates growth of multiple ovarian follicles. **B.** Later in the follicular phase, the effect of the aromatase inhibitor is reduced, and E_2 levels increase as a result of follicular growth. Because aromatase inhibitors do not affect estrogen receptors centrally, the increased E_2 levels result in normal central negative feedback on FSH secretion. Follicles smaller than the dominant follicle undergo atresia, with resultant monofollicular ovulation in most cases.

for continuous drainage. Untreated hypovolemia can lead to renal, hepatic, or pulmonary end-organ failure. Thus, fluid balance must be maintained by replacement with an isotonic fluid such as normal saline. Monitoring of electrolytes is critical. Because of hypercoagulability in these women, prophylaxis for thromboembolism should be strongly considered with severe OHSS (Table 39-9, p. 962).

Prevention. Strategies to avoid OHSS during exogenous ovulation induction include decreasing follicular stimulation (a decreased FSH dose), "coasting" (withholding FSH administration for 1 or more days prior to the hCG trigger injection), prophylactic treatment with volume expanders, and substitution of hCG for FSH during the final days of ovarian stimulation. With this last strategy, low-dose hCG administration

---

FIGURE 20-2 Drug protocols for ovulation induction.
A. Downregulation gonadotropin-releasing hormone (GnRH) agonist protocol. This is also known as the *long protocol*. In this diagram, the long protocol is combined with combination oral contraceptive (COC) pill pretreatment.

With the long protocol, GnRH agonists are begun typically 7 days prior to gonadotropins. GnRH agonists suppress endogenous pituitary release of gonadotropins. This minimizes the risk of a premature luteinizing hormone (LH) surge and thus premature ovulation. During all protocols, serial serum estrogen levels and sonographic surveillance of follicular development accompany gonadotropin administration. Human chorionic gonadotropin (hCG) serves as a surrogate for LH and is administered to trigger ovulation when sonography shows three or more follicles measuring at least 17 mm. Eggs are retrieved 36 hours later. Embryos are transferred back to the uterus 3–5 days following retrieval. Progesterone supplementation, with either vaginal preparations or intramuscular injection, follows during the luteal phase to support the endometrium.

The goal of COC pretreatment is to prevent ovarian cyst formation. One of the major drawbacks of GnRH agonist therapy is the induction of initial transient gonadotropin release or *flare*, which may lead to ovarian cyst formation. Functional ovarian cysts can prolong the duration of pituitary suppression required prior to gonadotropin initiation and may also exert a detrimental effect on follicular development because of their steroid production. Moreover, COC pretreatment may improve induction results by providing an entire cohort of follicles synchronized at the same developmental stage that will reach maturity at the same time once stimulated by gonadotropins.
B. GnRH flare protocol. This is also known as the *short protocol*. GnRH agonists initially bind gonadotropes and stimulate follicle-stimulating hormone (FSH) and LH release. This initial flare of gonadotropes stimulates follicular development. Following this initial surge of gonadotropins, the GnRH agonist causes receptor downregulation and an ultimately hypogonadotropic state. Gonadotropin injections begin 2 days later to continue follicular growth. As with the long protocol, continued GnRH agonist therapy prevents premature ovulation.
C. GnRH antagonist protocol. As with GnRH agonists, these agents are combined with gonadotropins to prevent premature LH surge and ovulation. This protocol attempts to minimize risk of ovarian hyperstimulation syndrome (OHSS) and GnRH side effects, such as hot flashes, headaches, bleeding, and mood changes.

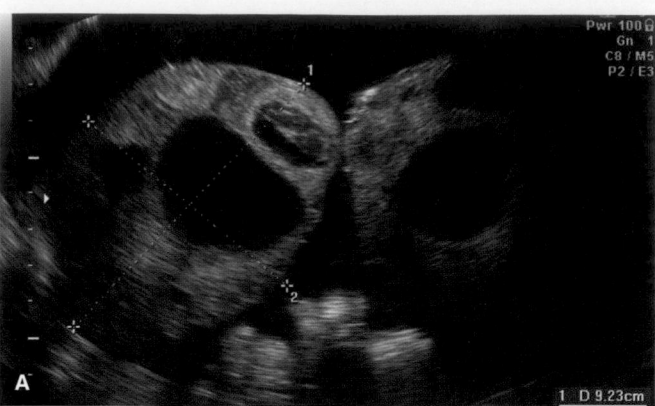 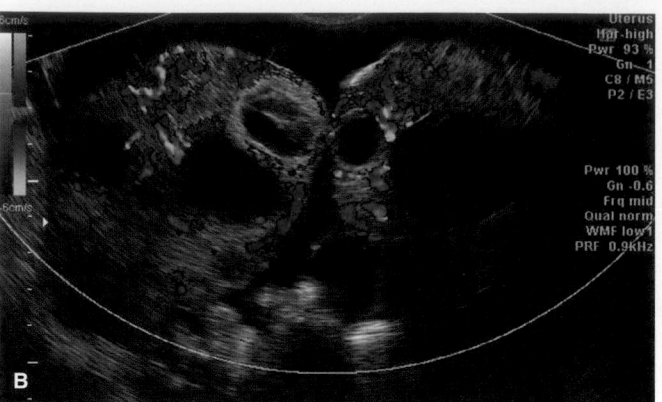

FIGURE 20-4 A. Transvaginal sonogram of ovaries with multiple large cysts secondary to ovarian hyperstimulation syndrome. Ovaries are enlarged and meet in the midline. Ascites surrounds these enlarged ovaries. **B.** Color Doppler transvaginal sonography is often performed to exclude ovarian torsion in these patients.

can support maturation of larger ovarian follicles, but has been postulated to directly or indirectly increase atresia rates of small antral follicles and thereby lower rates of OHSS.

If concern of OHSS is present during induction, then the hCG trigger can be withheld, resulting in cycle cancellation. Alternatively, a single dose of GnRH agonist such as leuprolide acetate (Lupron) can be used in place of hCG. This results in an endogenous LH surge, which can bring about the final stages of follicle and oocyte maturation without significant risk of OHSS. Prevention of pregnancy does not completely eliminate the risk of OHSS but certainly serves to limit the duration of the symptoms. Thus, an additional option in ART cycles is to freeze all embryos and forgo embryo transfer that cycle.

Multifetal Gestation. From 1980 through 1997, the number of twin births rose by more than 50 percent, and the number of higher-order multifetal births increased by more than 400 percent (Fig. 20-5) (Martin, 1999). In an analysis of data from these years, the Centers for Disease Control and Prevention (2000) estimated that approximately 20 percent of triplets and higher-order multifetal births were attributable to spontaneous events; 40 percent were related to ovulation inducing drugs

without ART; and 40 percent resulted from ART. However, further analysis of the same data indicates that the overwhelming majority of all multifetal births results from spontaneously conceived twin gestations and that only approximately 10 percent result from IVF and related procedures.

Complications. Higher-order multifetal pregnancy is an adverse outcome of infertility treatment. In general, increased fetal number leads to greater risk of perinatal and maternal morbidity and mortality. Prematurity leads to most adverse events in these cases, but fetal-growth restriction and discordance may also be factors.

Monozygotic gestation rates are also increased in ovulation induction and ART, and these pregnancies are associated with greater fetal risks. These include a three- to fivefold higher perinatal mortality rate compared with that of dizygotic twins. Moreover, monozygotic twins have a 30-percent risk of twin-twin transfusion syndrome (TTTS). This condition results from abnormal flow through deep vascular anastomoses within the shared placenta. TTTS is associated with a greater risk of severe neurologic damage and accounts for a significant portion of increased perinatal mortality rates. Additionally, congenital anomalies are increased two- to threefold in monozygotic twins versus singleton neonates, with an estimated incidence of 10 percent. Initially, extended embryo culture and zona manipulation were postulated to increase the risk of monozygosity. More recently, well-designed prospective trials have refuted this contention (Papanikolaou, 2010).

Management. Patients with higher-order multifetal gestations are faced with options of continuing their pregnancy with all the risks previously described, terminating the entire pregnancy, or selecting multifetal pregnancy reduction (MFPR). MFPR reduces the number of fetuses to decrease the risk of maternal and perinatal morbidity and mortality. Although MFPR decreases the risks associated with preterm delivery, it often creates profound ethical dilemmas. Moreover, multifetal reduction lowers, but does not eliminate, the risk of fetal-growth restriction in remaining fetuses. With MFPR, pregnancy loss and prematurity are primary risks. However, current data

---

TABLE 20-5. Classification and Staging of Ovarian Hyperstimulation Syndrome

Grade 1: Abdominal distension/discomfort
Grade 2: Grade 1 plus nausea and vomiting or diarrhea
Ovaries enlarged 5–12 cm
Grade 3: Sonographic evidence of ascites
Grade 4: Clinical evidence of ascites or hydrothorax or difficulty breathing
Grade 5: All of the above plus decreased blood volume, hemoconcentration, diminished renal perfusion and function, and coagulation abnormalities

From Whelan, 2000, with permission.

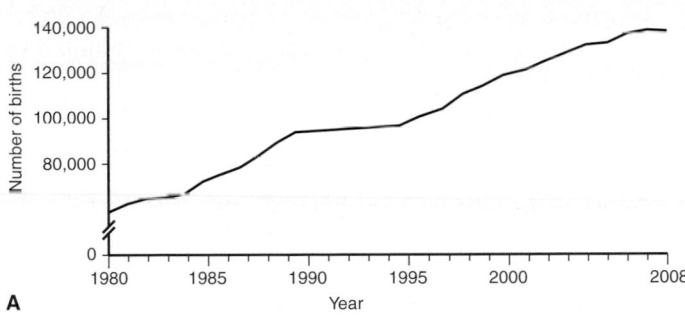

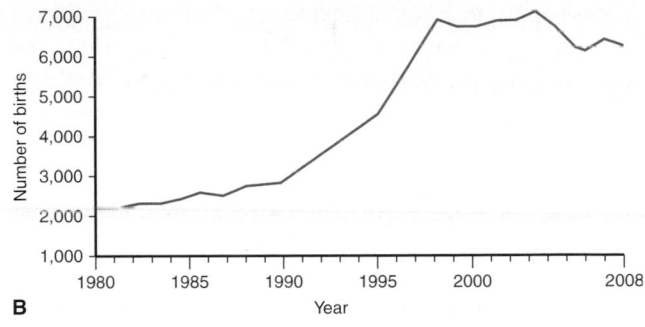

FIGURE 20-5 Trends in frequency of multifetal gestations. **A.** Number of twin births in the United States from 1980 to 2008. **B.** Number of triplet and higher order multifetal births in the United States for the same time period. *(Data from Martin, 2010.)*

suggest that such complications have decreased as experience with the procedure has grown (Evans, 2008).

Prevention. Several issues in infertility care contribute to the increased incidence of higher-order multifetal pregnancies. An infertile couple's sense of urgency may lead to a preference for more aggressive strategies involving gonadotropin treatment or for more embryos to be transferred in IVF cycles. Clinicians may feel competitive pressures to achieve higher pregnancy rates and may be inclined to turn to superovulation or IVF earlier in treatment or to transfer a greater number of embryos.

There have been efforts to lower the rates of multifetal gestation in patients undergoing ovulation induction or superovulation by using serum estradiol limits and arbitrary sonographic criteria of follicular size. These, however, have been ineffective. In a multicenter randomized clinical trial involving 1255 ovulation induction cycles, hCG was withheld if the estradiol concentration rose above 3000 pg/mL or if more than six follicles greater than 18 millimeters in diameter were present (Guzick, 1999). Despite these limits on hCG administration, the multifetal gestation rate was still 30 percent. Although sonography and serum estradiol monitoring have not reduced the incidence of multifetal gestation or OHSS, the risk of multifetal pregnancy does correlate with the magnitude of follicular response as indicated by follicle number and serum estradiol levels. However, there is no consensus among centers regarding specific sonographic criteria or estradiol levels beyond which hCG should not be administered.

When the likelihood of multifetal gestation is felt to be excessive, IVF can be undertaken to reduce the risk. Because the number of embryos transferred can be strictly controlled, this strategy can minimize the risk of higher-order multifetal gestations. Guidelines set forth by the American Society for Reproductive Medicine and the Society for Assisted Reproductive Technology (2009) have led to a significant reduction in triplet (and higher) gestations (Table 20-6).

Ovarian Drilling

Surgical ovarian wedge resection was the first established treatment for anovulatory PCOS patients. It was largely abandoned because of postsurgical adhesion formation, which converted endocrinologic subfertility to mechanical subfertility (Adashi, 1981; Buttram, 1975; Stein, 1939). As a result, it was replaced by medical ovulation induction with CC and gonadotropins (Franks, 1985). However, medical ovulation induction, as discussed earlier, has limitations. Accordingly, surgical therapy using laparoscopic techniques and termed *laparoscopic ovarian drilling* is an alternative for women resistant to medical therapies.

During laparoscopic ovarian drilling, electrosurgical coagulation, laser vaporization, or harmonic scalpel may be used to create multiple perforations into the ovarian surface and stroma (Section 42-8, p. 1139). In many uncontrolled observational studies, drilling has led to temporary, higher rates of spontaneous postoperative ovulation and conception or to improved medical ovulation induction (Armar, 1990, 1993; Farhi, 1995; Greenblatt, 1987; Kovacs, 1991).

The mechanism of action with laparoscopic ovarian drilling is thought to be similar to that with ovarian wedge resection. Both procedures may destroy ovarian androgen-producing tissue and thereby reduce peripheral conversion of androgens to estrogens. Specifically, a fall in serum levels of androgens

TABLE 20-6. Recommended Limits on the Numbers of Embryos to Transfer

	Age			
Prognosis	<35 years	35–37 years	38–40 years	41–42 years
Cleavage-stage embryos[a]				
Favorable[b]	1–2	2	3	5
All others	2	3	4	5
Blastocysts[a]				
Favorable[b]	1	2	3	3
All others	2	2	3	3

[a]Justification for transferring one additional embryo more than the recommended limit should be clearly documented in the patient's medical record.
[b]Favorable = first cycle of in vitro fertilization (IVF), good embryo quality, excess embryos available for cryopreservation, or previous successful IVF cycle.
American Society for Reproductive Medicine and Society for Assisted Reproductive Technology, 2009, with permission.

and LH and an increase in FSH levels have been demonstrated after ovarian drilling (Armar, 1990; Greenblatt, 1987). The endocrine changes following surgery are thought to convert the adverse androgen-dominant intrafollicular environment to an estrogenic one and to restore the hormonal environment to normal by correcting disturbances of ovarian-pituitary feedback (Aakvaag, 1985; Balen, 1993). Thus, both local and systemic effects are thought to promote follicular recruitment and maturation and subsequent ovulation.

Risks of ovarian drilling include postoperative adhesion formation as well as the other risks of laparoscopic surgery (Section 42-1, p. 1095). Additionally, theoretical risks of diminished ovarian reserve and premature ovarian failure remain to be well investigated. As surgery is more invasive, ovarian drilling is generally not offered prior to consideration of medical therapies.

Correction of Diminished Ovarian Reserve

Ovarian dysfunction may result from ovarian failure or from a diminished ovarian reserve, either of which may follow normal aging, disease, or surgical castration. Even if a woman is spontaneously menstruating, a basal (day 2 or 3) FSH level above 15 IU/L predicts that medical therapies, including exogenous gonadotropins, will be of little benefit. For these women, the option of using donor eggs should be considered (p. 546). Expectant management may also be considered, although the likelihood of pregnancy is low.

Correction of Anatomic Abnormalities

Anatomic distortions of the female reproductive tract are a major cause of infertility and may prevent ovum entry into the fallopian tube; impair transport of ova, sperm, or embryos; or interfere with implantation. The three primary types of anatomic abnormalities include tubal factors, peritoneal factors, and uterine factors. Each has differing effects and therefore may require different therapies.

Tubal Factors

Tubal occlusion can arise from congenital abnormality, infection, or iatrogenic causes. Additionally, a small subset of tubal infertility is idiopathic. Not only the cause of tubal damage but also the nature of an anatomic abnormality is important. For example, proximal tubal occlusion, distal tubal occlusion, and tubal absence differ markedly in their treatment.

Proximal tubal occlusion describes obstruction proximal to the fimbria and may develop at the tubal ostium, isthmus, or ampulla. Specifically, *midtubal occlusion* is considered a subset of proximal occlusion. Proximal tubal occlusion may be secondary to tubal resection, luminal obliteration, or simply plugging with mucus or debris. In contrast, *distal tubal occlusion* describes obstruction at the tube's fimbria. It typically results from prior pelvic infection and may be associated with concomitant adnexal adhesions.

Tubal Cannulation. Proximal tubal occlusion is often amenable to direct techniques. If diagnosed at the time of hysterosalpingography (HSG), consideration should be given to performing concurrent selective salpingography. A catheter is placed such that it wedges within the tubal ostium. This allows significant hydrostatic pressure to be applied to the tube. Such pressure will likely overcome most instances of tubal spasm or plugging by mucus or debris. If tubal patency cannot be reestablished, an inner catheter with guide wire is used to cannulate the tube. In most instances, this creates patency in isolated, short segmental areas of scarring. Scarring of a longer segment or luminal obliteration, however, is not amenable to correction with tubal cannulation. In these women, surgical segmental resection with reanastomosis or IVF may be considered.

Tubal Reconstruction. Tubal obstruction that is not amenable to treatment with selective salpingography has traditionally been treated surgically. Options include hysteroscopic cannulation, surgical reanastomosis, and neosalpingostomy. Although there have been considerable increases in the success rates of ART, reproductive surgery remains an important option or complement to ART for many couples.

Proximal Tubal Obstruction. Some types of tubal blockage have a much better prognosis with surgical therapy than others. For example, hysteroscopic cannulation of fallopian tubes can treat some types of proximal obstruction in a fashion similar to selective salpingography. Described in Section 42-20 (p. 1176), hysteroscopic cannulation is best performed with concurrent laparoscopy to verify distal tubal patency.

Proximal obstruction not amenable to cannulation techniques can be treated with segmental resection and reanastomosis (Fig. 20-6). In most cases, this can be done as an outpatient procedure through a minilaparotomy incision. However, obstruction extending medially into the interstitial portion of the tube is more technically challenging to repair and more prone to obstruction postoperatively. Therefore, proximal occlusion extending to the interstitial segment that cannot be treated with cannulation is best treated in most instances with IVF.

Proximal and midtubal occlusion that results from prior sterilization can be treated with either tubal reanastomosis or IVF. From a patient perspective, outpatient tubal reanastomosis avoids ovarian stimulation and increased risk for multifetal gestation and provides an ability to conceive normally. In general, although the monthly probability of pregnancy following tubal reversal is likely lower than that for age-matched controls without prior sterilization, the cumulative chance of pregnancy is high. However, IVF should be strongly considered if other fertility factors are present or the type of sterilization performed does not permit reconstruction. For example, in cases of sterilization completed by fimbriectomy, neosalpingostomy can be corrective. However, the probability of pregnancy is lower, and IVF should be considered.

The "reversibility" of sterilization can generally be determined by review of the operative report and pathology report if the procedure involved segmental resection. If operative records are unavailable or suggest that reanastomosis may not be feasible, laparoscopy is performed prior to laparotomy to assess chances of surgical success.

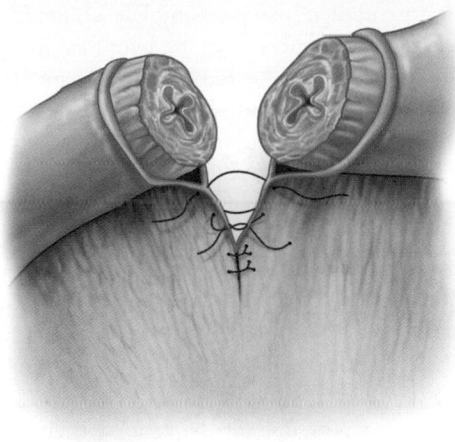

A

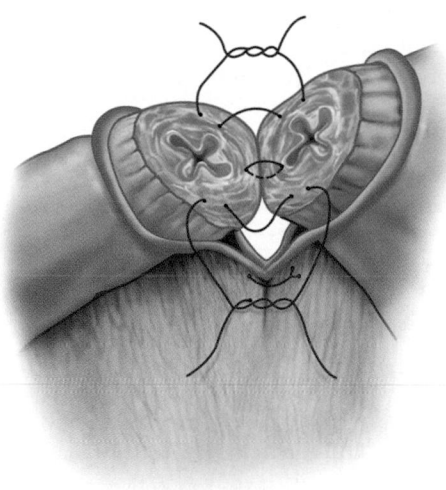

B

FIGURE 20-6 Surgical reanastomosis of fallopian tube segments. The scarred portion of the tube is sharply excised until nonfibrotic tubal tissues are reached. **A.** The mesosalpinx is reapproximated with interrupted stitches using 6-0 delayed-absorbable suture. **B.** The tubal muscularis is reapproximated with single stitches in each quadrant using 7-0 delayed-absorbable suture. Tubal serosa is closed with interrupted or running 6-0 delayed-absorbable suture.

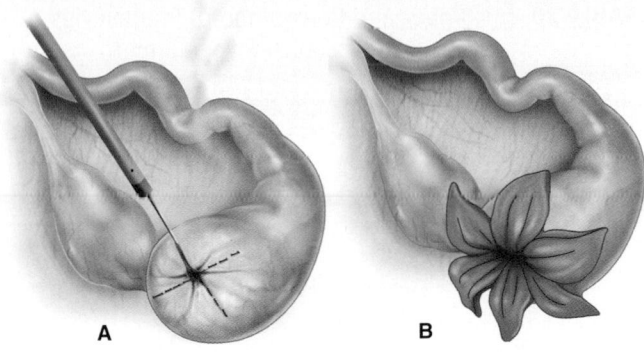

A   **B**

FIGURE 20-7 Neosalpingostomy. **A.** The distal end of the clubbed fallopian tube is opened sharply or with electric or laser energy. **B.** The endosalpinx is everted using Cuff or Bruhat technique.

Outpatient reversal of sterilization is most commonly done by minilaparotomy. Incision size typically varies from 3 to 6 cm depending on a patient's weight and anatomy. Some surgeons are able to complete some of these procedures by laparoscopy. Robotic control may be helpful for this but may increase operating time and expense.

Distal Tubal Obstruction. Following pelvic inflammatory disorders, normal fimbrial anatomy may be destroyed or fimbria may be encased by concomitant adnexal adhesions. In these cases, neosalpingostomy can be performed at minilaparotomy or laparoscopy (Fig. 20-7). However, women desiring neosalpingostomy for treatment of distal occlusion should be counseled that the risk of ectopic pregnancy is high, the likelihood of pregnancy is 50 percent or lower, and postoperative reocclusion is common (Bayrak, 2006). Moreover, hydrosalpinges

that are dilated more than 3 cm in diameter, that are associated with significant adnexal adhesions, or that display an obviously attenuated endosalpinx (fallopian tube mucosa) yield a poor prognosis. These tubes are best treated by salpingectomy. As described in Chapter 9 (p. 273), if both tubes are affected, bilateral salpingectomy is recommended prior to proceeding with IVF (American Society for Reproductive Medicine, 2008e).

Uterine Factors

Three types of uterine factors have been implicated in infertility and include leiomyomas, endometrial polyps, and intrauterine adhesions. Mechanisms of infertility with these factors have not been clearly elucidated. However, the end result is decreased endometrial receptivity and reduced likelihood of embryo implantation.

Leiomyomas. Leiomyomas are common benign tumors of the uterus and have been associated with infertility in some women. Retrospective studies have suggested a benefit from surgically removing these tumors to increase efficacy of both natural and assisted conception (Griffiths, 2006).

There are no randomized controlled trials to clearly demonstrate that myomectomy improves fertility. However, in view of the many retrospective observational studies that suggest this, it is reasonable to offer myomectomy to infertile women if tumors are large or impinge on the endometrial cavity. Myomectomy can be performed using hysteroscopy or laparoscopy or via laparotomy, and selection of the approach is discussed in Chapter 9 (p. 258). Currently, no studies validate one method compared with another in terms of efficacy. Therefore, clinical judgment should determine the most appropriate technique from the standpoint of safety, restoration of normal uterine anatomy, and speed of recovery.

Endometrial Polyps. These soft, fleshy endometrial growths are commonly diagnosed during evaluation of infertility. Several studies have suggested good pregnancy rates following polypectomy, although the mechanism by which polyps may impair fertility has not been established. The requirement to

TABLE 20-7. Number and Percentage of Pregnancies after Hysteroscopic Polypectomy (n = 204)

	Polypectomy n = 101 (%)	Control n = 103 (%)	p-value
Subsequent pregnancy	64 (63.4)	29 (28.2)	<0.001

RR 2.1 (95% CI 1.5–2.9).
From Pérez-Medina, 2005, with permission.

remove even small polyps in infertile women has been previously debated. However, a prospective trial of 204 women with polyps and with an additionally diagnosed cervical factor, male factor, or unexplained infertility appears to give some clear guidance.

In this trial, women were randomized to one of two groups prior to treatment with intrauterine insemination (IUI) (Pérez-Medina, 2005). The first group underwent polypectomy. The second underwent only hysteroscopic biopsy of the polyp to obtain histologic confirmation. All patients were managed expectantly for three cycles prior to proceeding with up to four cycles of IUI. The pregnancy rate in the polypectomy group was more than twice as high regardless of polyp size (Table 20-7). These data suggest that endometrial polyps can significantly impair outcome of infertility treatment. Thus, it would seem prudent to perform hysteroscopic polypectomy in all infertile patients if a polyp is identified (Section 42-15, p. 1164).

Intrauterine Adhesions. Adhesions within the endometrial cavity, also called *synechiae*, can range from asymptomatic small bands to complete or near-complete obliteration of the endometrial cavity. If amenorrhea or hypomenorrhea results, the condition is termed *Asherman syndrome* (Chap. 16, p. 444).

Treatment involves surgical adhesiolysis to restore normal uterine cavity size and configuration. Dilatation and curettage (D&C) and abdominal approaches have previously been used. However, with the advantages of hysteroscopy, the role of these other techniques has been minimized.

Hysteroscopic adhesion resection may range from simple lysis of a small band to extensive adhesiolysis of dense intrauterine adhesions using scissors, electrosurgical cutting, or laser energy (Section 42-21, p. 1178). However, women whose uterine fundus is completely obscured and those with a markedly narrowed, fibrotic cavity present the greatest therapeutic challenge. Several techniques have been described for these difficult cases, but outcome is far worse than in patients with small band adhesions. In those women with severe Asherman syndrome that is not amenable to reconstructive surgery, gestational carrier surrogacy is a valuable option (p. 546).

Peritoneal Disease

Endometriosis and pelvic adhesions are two types of peritoneal disease that frequently contribute to infertility and that may develop independently or concurrently.

Endometriosis. This condition and its effects on infertility are extensively discussed in Chapter 10 (p. 287). In women with minimal or mild disease, evidence supporting lesion ablation is limited, and use of empiric general fertility-boosting procedures such as ART or superovulation combined with IUI or ART is reasonable. These treatments have been validated to increase fecundity in women with stage I and II disease (Table 20-8) (Guzick, 1999).

TABLE 20-8. Cycle Fecundity in Women with Stage I or II Endometriosis, According to Treatment

Group	Unexplained Infertility	Endometriosis-Associated Infertility			
Treatment	Guzick[a]	Deaton[a]	Chaffin[a]	Fedele[a]	Kemmann[a]
No treatment or intracervical insemination	0.02	0.033	—	0.045	0.028
IUI	0.05[b]	—	—	—	—
Clomiphene	—	—	—	—	0.066
Clomiphene/IUI	—	0.095[b]	—	—	—
Gonadotropins	0.04[b]	—	0.066	—	0.073[b]
Gonadotropins/IUI	0.09[b]	—	0.129[b]	0.15[b]	—
IVF	—	—	—	—	0.222[b]

[a]And their colleagues.
[b]p <.05 for treatment vs. no treatment.
IUI = intrauterine insemination; IVF = in vitro fertilization.
From American Society for Reproductive Medicine, 2006b, with permission.

Moderate and severe endometriosis results in distortion of anatomic relationships of reproductive organs. In many cases, surgical treatment may improve anatomy, and pregnancy may result (American Society for Reproductive Medicine, 2006b). Unfortunately, advanced disease may prevent adequate restoration of pelvic anatomy. Therefore, a surgeon's operative findings and anticipated surgical results should guide postoperative strategy. If satisfactory surgical outcome is achieved, it is reasonable to attempt pregnancy for 6 to 12 months prior to considering other options such as IVF. It should be remembered that endometriosis in some cases may recur quickly, and unnecessary delay in attempting pregnancy postoperatively is not advised.

Several studies suggest that in women with advanced endometriosis, long-term treatment with GnRH agonists before initiation of a cycle may improve fecundity (Dicker, 1992; Surrey, 2002). At the present time, however, this treatment strategy is not universally accepted.

If endometriomas are noted, surgical options include cyst drainage, drainage followed by cyst wall ablation, or cyst excision. All three procedures can be performed laparoscopically in nearly all circumstances given adequate surgeon experience. Simple drainage minimizes ovarian destruction, but commonly results in rapid cyst recurrence. One histologic study demonstrated that a mean of 60 percent of the cyst wall (range of 10 to 98 percent) was lined by endometrium to a depth of 0.6 mm (Muzii, 2007). Therefore, drainage and ablation may not destroy all endometrium to this depth. Thus, this approach is also associated with significant risk of cyst recurrence as well as thermal damage to the ovary. For these reasons, laparoscopic excision of the cyst wall by a stripping technique should be considered optimal treatment for most endometriomas (Section 42-6, p. 1133). Hart and coworkers (2008) compared ablative surgery and cyst excision and noted more favorable results for diminished pain, cyst recurrence, and spontaneous pregnancy with excision. However, excision is inevitably accompanied by removal of normal ovarian tissue and often leads to decreased ovarian volume and diminished ovarian reserve (Almog, 2010; Exacoustos, 2004; Ragni, 2005).

Pelvic Adhesions. Pelvic adhesions may result from endometriosis, prior surgery, or pelvic infection and often vary in their density and vascularity. Adhesions may impair fertility by distorting adnexal anatomy and by interfering with gamete and embryo transport, even in the absence of tubal disease.

Surgical lysis may restore pelvic anatomy in some cases, but adhesions may recur, especially if they are dense and vascular. Adherence to microsurgical principles and minimally invasive surgery may help decrease adhesion formation. Although numerous adjuvants, such as adhesion barriers, have been used to reduce the risk of postoperative adhesion formation, currently none have been validated to improve fecundity (American Society for Reproductive Medicine, 2006a, 2008f).

Among infertile women with adnexal adhesions, pregnancy rates after adhesiolysis are 32 percent at 12 months and 45 percent at 24 months of surveillance. These rates can be compared with 11 percent at 12 months and 16 percent at 24 months in those left untreated (Tulandi, 1990). As with

severe endometriosis, clinical judgment regarding operative findings and results of surgery should guide the strategy postoperatively. IVF is the best option for those with a poor prognosis for restoration of normal anatomy.

Correction of Cervical Abnormalities

In response to follicular estradiol production, the cervix should produce abundant thin mucus. If present, this mucus acts as a conduit and functional reservoir for sperm (Fig. 19-11B, p. 521). Accordingly, inadequate cervical mucus impairs sperm transport to the upper female reproductive tract.

Causes of abnormal or deficient mucus include infection, prior cervical surgery, use of antiestrogens (e.g., clomiphene citrate) for ovulation induction, and sperm antibodies. However, many women with decreased or hostile mucus have no history of predisposing factors.

Examination of cervical mucus may reveal gross evidence of chronic cervicitis that deserves treatment. Doxycycline, 100 mg orally twice daily for 10 days, is an appropriate therapy. In those with decreased mucus volume, treatments include short-term supplementation with exogenous estrogen, such as ethinyl estradiol, and the use of the mucolytic expectorant guaifenesin. However, the value of estrogen and guaifenesin has not been confirmed. Moreover, exogenous estrogens could have a negative effect on follicular development and ovarian function.

For these reason, most clinicians treat noninfectious, suspected cervical mucus abnormalities with IUI. Although this approach also has not been validated with randomized prospective trials, the theoretical basis for this approach seems sound (Helmerhorst, 2005). Additionally, IUI has been demonstrated to be effective for treatment of unexplained infertility. As a result, many clinicians forgo cervical mucus testing and proceed directly with IUI treatments in the absence of tubal disease (Fig. 20-8).

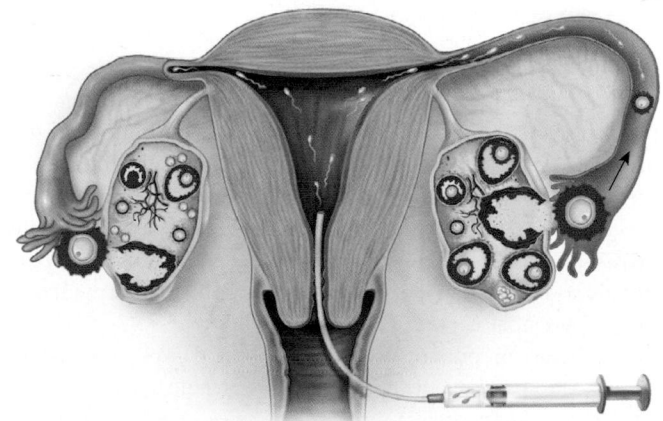

FIGURE 20-8 Intrauterine insemination (IUI). Prior to IUI, partner or donor sperm is washed and concentrated. IUI is usually combined with superovulation, and signs of impending ovulation are monitored with transvaginal sonography. At the time of suspected ovulation, a long, thin catheter is threaded through the cervical os and into the endometrial cavity. A syringe containing the sperm concentrate is attached to the catheter's distal end, and the sperm sample is injected into the endometrial cavity.

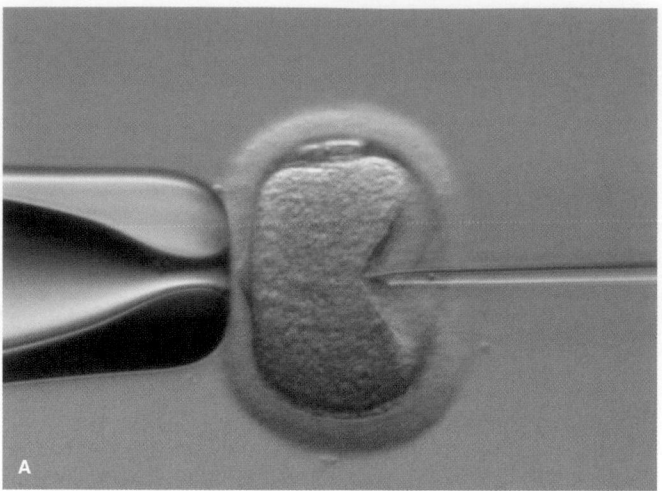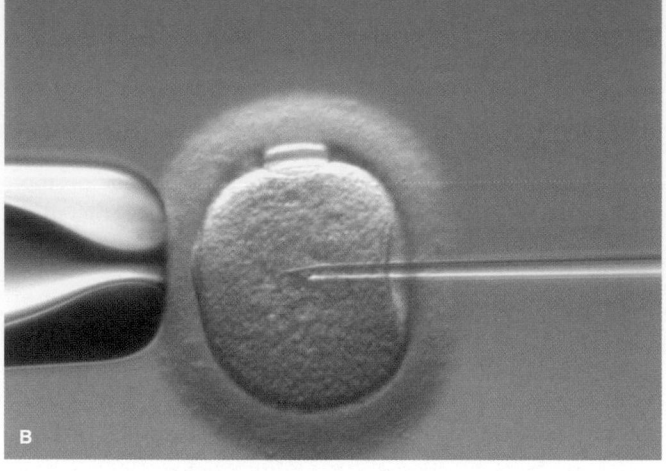

FIGURE 20-9 Photomicrographs of intracytoplasmic sperm injection.

Correction of Male Infertility

Male infertility has varied causes and may include abnormalities of semen volume such as *aspermia* and *hypospermia* or of sperm number such as *azoospermia* and *oligospermia*. Additionally, motility may be limited, termed *asthenospermia*, or sperm structure may be abnormal, *teratozoospermia*. Accordingly, therapy should be planned only after thorough evaluation (Chap. 19, p. 521).

In the absence of identifiable correctable cause, it is appropriate to offer IUI or ART as treatment options. The choice of whether to proceed initially with IUI therapies as opposed to the more intensive and expensive ART treatments is dependent on several factors. These include duration of infertility, age of the female, and history of prior treatments. If ART is considered for male factor, intracytoplasmic sperm injection (ICSI) is typically selected rather than traditional IVF (Fig. 20-9).

Aspermia

This condition is characterized by a complete lack of semen and results from failure to ejaculate. The physiology of ejaculation includes emission of sperm with accessory gland fluid into the urethra, simultaneous closure of the urethral sphincters, and forceful ejaculation of semen through the urethra. Emission and closure of the bladder neck are primarily alpha-adrenergically mediated thoracolumbar sympathetic reflex events with supraspinal modulation. Ejaculation is a sacral spinal reflex mediated by the pudendal nerve.

Anejaculation or anorgasmia is not a rare complaint and may be related to psychogenic factors, organic erectile dysfunction, or impaired parasympathetic sacral spinal reflex. Appropriate treatments depend on the cause and may include psychologic counseling or erectile dysfunction treatment with sildenafil citrate (Viagra) or other similar medication. Vibratory stimulation may also be effective in some instances. Electroejaculation is an invasive procedure and is generally used for men with spinal cord injuries who are unresponsive to the therapies just described.

Men who always achieve orgasm but never experience prograde ejaculation or have a greatly reduced prograde volume typically have retrograde ejaculation. Therefore, administration of oral pseudoephedrine or other alpha-adrenergic agent to aid bladder neck closure is warranted. However, for many, pharmacologic methods are ineffective, and IUI may be performed using sperm processed from a voided urine specimen collected after ejaculation.

A minority of men who achieve orgasm, but not prograde ejaculation, have failure of emission. Treatment with sympathomimetic agents may be attempted in these individuals as well, although pharmacologic therapies have generally met with limited success. Alternatively, testicular or epididymal extraction of sperm via aspiration or biopsy may be used in cases refractory to medication. As with electroejaculation, this technique recovers a limited number of viable sperm and is best suited for use with ICSI.

Hypospermia

Hypospermia or low semen volume (<2 mL) impairs transport of sperm into cervical mucus and may be associated with decreased sperm density or motility. Retrograde ejaculation may underlie this condition, and treatment follows that described for aspermia.

Alternatively, hypospermia may follow partial or complete ejaculatory duct obstruction. In these cases, transurethral resection of the narrowed portion of the ejaculatory duct has resulted in marked improvement in semen parameters, and pregnancies have been achieved. However, couples should be counseled that postoperative complete obstruction of the ejaculatory ducts is not rare. Thus, consideration should be given to cryopreservation of sperm prior to surgical attempts in those individuals with partial obstruction.

Azoospermia

Characterized by the total absence of sperm in semen, azoospermia may result from obstruction in the male reproductive tract or from nonobstructive causes.

Obstructive azoospermia, especially resulting from prior vasectomy or ejaculatory duct obstruction, may be amenable to surgical treatment. However, congenital absence of the vas deferens (CBAVD) is a common cause of azoospermia and unfortunately, is not treatable surgically. In such candidates, testicular sperm extraction (TESE) may be performed in conjunction with ICSI. CBAVD is associated with cystic fibrosis, and thus, antepartum screening of both partners is considered.

Nonobstructive azoospermia may be caused by a karyotypic abnormality such as Klinefelter syndrome (47,XXY) or balanced translocation, by deletion of a small portion of the Y chromosome, by testicular failure, or by unexplained causes. In many cases, TESE may be combined effectively with ICSI in those with Klinefelter syndrome and Y microdeletion of the AZFc region. However, in men with Y microdeletion in the AZFa or AZFb region, this ART combination has been ineffective (Choi, 2004).

Oligospermia

Oligospermia is diagnosed if fewer than 20 million sperm are present per milliliter of semen. Causes are varied and include hormonal, genetic, environmental (including medications), and unexplained causes. Also, an obstructive cause, especially ejaculatory duct obstruction, should be considered if oligospermia is seen in conjunction with low semen volume. If severe oligospermia (<5 to 10 million sperm per milliliter) is noted, an evaluation similar to that for azoospermia is warranted.

Oligospermia in the absence of decreased sperm motility not uncommonly reflects hypogonadotropic hypogonadism. In general, hypogonadotropic hypogonadism is best treated with FSH and hCG administered to the male. Alternatively, clomiphene citrate and aromatase inhibitors, although not FDA-approved treatment for this indication, may be considered in some instances for males, especially if obesity and elevated serum estradiol levels are present. Spermatogenesis is a long process lasting approximately 100 days, and several months may be required to identify significant improvements in sperm density with either treatment.

Environmental factors such as excessive exposure to high temperatures should be investigated. Drug and medication history should also be obtained. If an environmental factor is identified, correction may improve sperm numbers.

Asthenospermia

Asthenospermia or decreased sperm motility may be seen alone or in combination with oligospermia or other abnormal semen parameters. In general, asthenospermia does not respond to directed treatments. Expectant management may be considered, especially if the duration of infertility is short and maternal age is less than 35 years. For treatment, IUI and ICSI are preferred, although IUI is generally not successful in severe cases (Centola, 1997). If fewer than 1 million motile sperm are available for insemination following semen processing, or the couple has experienced >5 years of infertility, then ICSI should be considered as initial therapy (Ludwig, 2005).

Teratozoospermia

Teratozoospermia or abnormal sperm morphology is most often seen in conjunction with oligospermia, asthenospermia,

and oligoasthenospermia. Directed treatments for teratozoospermia are not available, and therapy options include IUI and ART. Because teratozoospermia may commonly be accompanied by sperm function defects that may impair fertilization, ICSI should be considered if ART is selected.

Varicocele

This results from dilatation of the pampiniform plexus of the spermatic vein and is usually left-sided (Fig. 19-3, p. 509). Traditional treatment is surgical ligation of the internal spermatic vein. With ligation, several surgical techniques have been employed, but inguinal ligation or subinguinal ligation are the most frequently performed. More recently, interventional radiographic techniques that selectively catheterize and embolize the internal spermatic vein with sclerosing solutions, tissue adhesives, or detachable balloons or coils have been used as alternatives. Despite the widespread application of varicocele treatments, there is insufficient evidence to conclude that treatment of a clinical varicocele in couples with male subfertility improves the likelihood of conception (Evers, 2003). The American Society for Reproductive Medicine (2008c) notes that repair may be appropriate for selected couples.

UNEXPLAINED INFERTILITY

Unexplained infertility may represent one of the most common infertility diagnoses with a reported prevalence of up to 30 percent (Dodson, 1987). The diagnosis of unexplained infertility is highly subjective and depends on the diagnostic tests performed or omitted and on their level of quality. Paradoxically, a diagnosis of unexplained infertility, therefore, will be more often reached if the evaluation is incomplete or of poor quality (Gleicher, 2006). Nevertheless, by definition, a diagnosis of unexplained infertility cannot be directly treated. Expectant management may be considered especially with infertility of short duration and with relatively young maternal age. However, if treatment is desired, then IUI, superovulation, and ART are empiric appropriate interventions to consider.

INTRAUTERINE INSEMINATION

This technique uses a thin flexible catheter to place a prepared semen sample into the uterine cavity. First, motile, morphologically normal spermatozoa are separated from dead sperm, leukocytes, and seminal plasma. This highly motile fraction is then inserted transcervically near the anticipated time of ovulation. Intrauterine insemination can be performed with or without superovulation and is appropriate therapy for treatment of cervical factors, mild and moderate male factors, and unexplained infertility.

If performed for cervical factors, IUI timed by urine LH surge is an initial strategy that achieves reasonable pregnancy rates of up to 11 percent per cycle (Steures, 2004). Although this rate is lower than that seen with superovulation combined with IUI, the side effects and costs of superovulation are avoided.

In contrast, for unexplained infertility and for male factors, IUI is most commonly performed in conjunction with superovulation. A combination of clomiphene citrate and IUI was evaluated by Deaton and colleagues (1990) in a randomized trial. In this study, the treatment group had a significantly higher pregnancy rate (9.5 percent) compared with controls (3.3 percent). Gonadotropin treatment (FSH or hMG) alone has been shown to increase the likelihood of pregnancy, but the benefit is markedly improved with the addition of IUI.

ASSISTED REPRODUCTIVE TECHNOLOGIES

The term *assisted reproductive technologies* describes clinical and laboratory techniques used to achieve pregnancy in infertile couples for whom direct corrections of underlying causes are not feasible. In principle, IUI meets this definition. By convention, however, ART procedures are those that at some point require extraction and isolation of an oocyte. These techniques include, but are not limited to, in vitro fertilization, intracytoplasmic sperm injection, egg donation, gestational carrier surrogacy, gamete intrafallopian transfer (GIFT), and zygote intrafallopian transfer (ZIFT). Additional ART associated techniques include egg and embryo cryopreservation, testicular sperm extraction, in vitro maturation of oocytes (IVM), and preimplantation genetic diagnosis (PGD).

In Vitro Fertilization

During IVF, mature oocytes from stimulated ovaries are retrieved transvaginally with sonographic guidance (Fig. 20-10). Sperm and ova are then combined in vitro to prompt fertilization (Fig. 20-11). If successful, viable embryos are transferred transcervically into the endometrial cavity using sonographic guidance (Fig. 20-12).

Similar to IUI, substantial benefit is achieved using controlled ovarian hyperstimulation prior to egg retrieval. Many

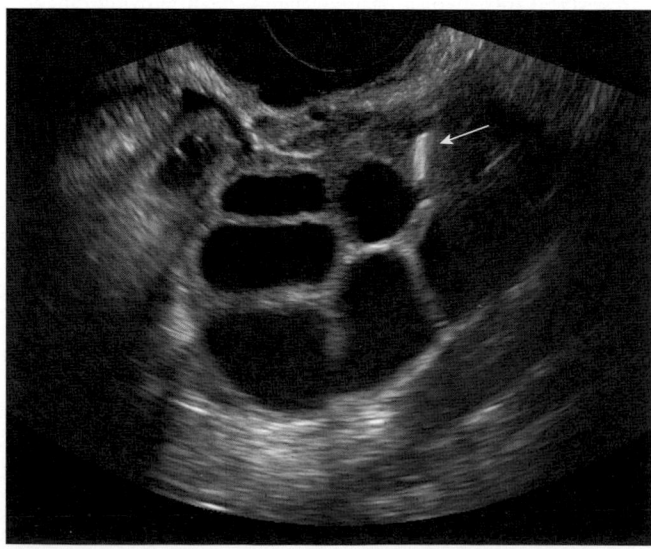

FIGURE 20-10 Transabdominal sonogram demonstrates transvaginal oocyte retrieval. The needle is seen in the upper right portion of the image as a hyperechoic line (*arrow*) entering a mature follicle.

ova are genetically or functionally abnormal. Thus, exposure of several ova to sperm results in an increased chance of a healthy embryo. Most often, a GnRH agonist is used in conjunction with gonadotropins (FSH or hMG). These agonists prevent the possibility of spontaneous LH surge and ovulation prior to egg retrieval. Optimally, 10 to 20 ova are harvested, and from these, one healthy embryo is ideally transferred back to the uterus.

Unfortunately, methods to determine embryo health are imperfect. Therefore, to maximize the probability of pregnancy, more than one embryo is typically transferred, thus resulting in increased risk of multifetal gestation.

More recently, advances in culture conditions permit embryos to be cultured to the blastocyst stage. This allows transfer of fewer embryos, yet maintains high pregnancy rates (Langley, 2001).

As discussed earlier, hydrosalpinges should be removed or tubal interruption performed prior to proceeding with IVF to increase implantation rates and decrease the risk of miscarriage.

Intracytoplasmic Sperm Injection

This variation on IVF is most applicable to male factor infertility. During the micromanipulation technique of ICSI, cumulus cells surrounding an ovum are enzymatically digested, and a single sperm is directly injected through the zona pellucida and oocyte cell membrane. Pregnancy rates with ICSI are comparable with those achieved with IVF for other causes of infertility.

For azoospermic men, ICSI has made pregnancy in their partners possible. In these cases, sperm are mechanically extracted from the testis or epididymis.

Gestational Carrier Surrogacy

This variation on IVF places a fertilized egg into the uterus of a surrogate, rather than into the "intended mother." Indications are varied, and this approach may be appropriate for women with uncorrectable uterine factors, for those in whom pregnancy would pose significant health risks, and for those with repetitive unexplained miscarriage.

Gestational carrier surrogacy has legal and psychosocial issues. In most states, a surrogate is the legal parent and therefore, adoption must be completed after birth to give the intended mother her parental rights. However, a few states have adopted specific laws that extend protection to the intended parents.

Egg Donation

Egg donation may be employed in cases of infertility associated with ovarian failure or diminished ovarian reserve. Additionally, this technique may also be used to achieve pregnancy in fertile women when offspring would be at risk for maternally transmitted genetic disease. Egg donors may be known to the recipient couple or more commonly, are anonymous young women recruited by an agency or IVF center.

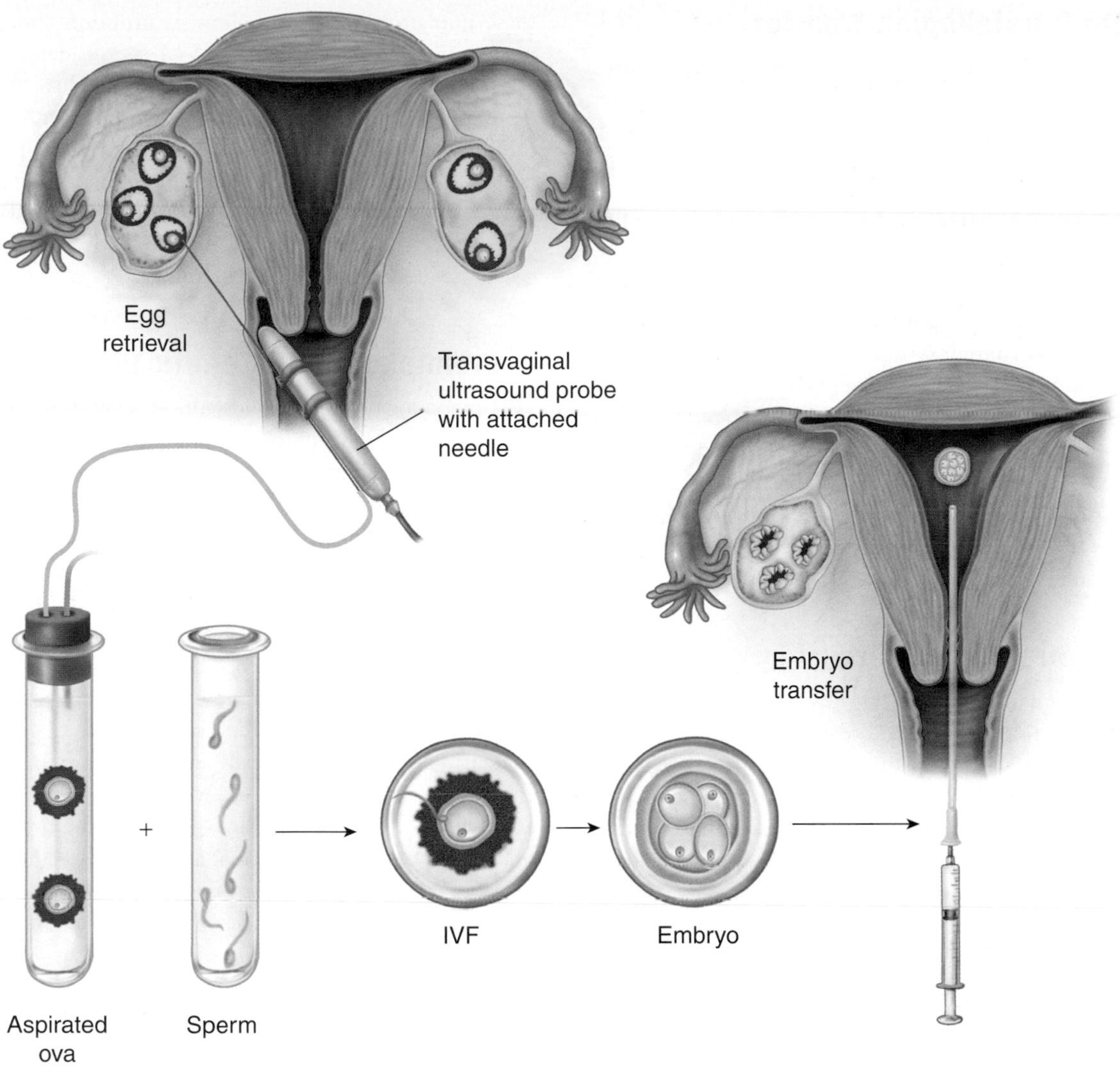

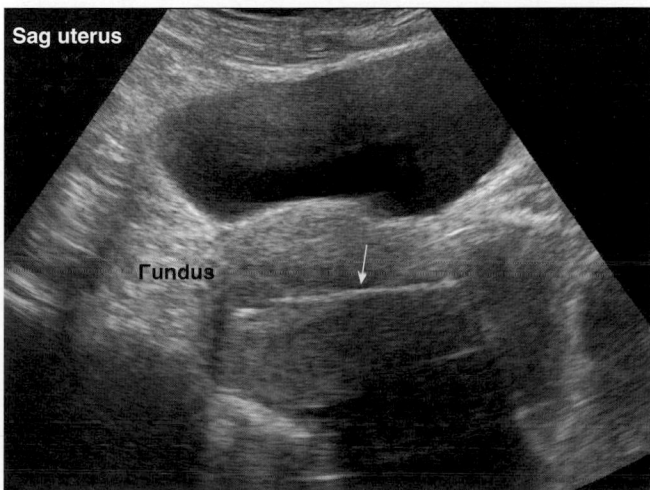

Egg retrieval

Transvaginal ultrasound probe with attached needle

Embryo transfer

Aspirated ova

Sperm

IVF

Embryo

FIGURE 20-11 In vitro fertilization (IVF). Controlled ovarian hyperstimulation is achieved with one of the protocols displayed in Figure 20-2, and follicle maturation is monitored over several days sonographically. Near ovulation, a transvaginal approach under sonographic guidance is used to harvest eggs from the ovaries. These oocytes are fertilized in vitro, and fertilized eggs develop to the blastocyst stage. Blastocysts are then drawn up into a syringe and delivered into the endometrial cavity under sonographic guidance.

Sag uterus

Fundus

FIGURE 20-12 Embryo transfer performed using abdominal sonographic guidance for proper placement. Catheter (*arrow*) is seen within the endometrial cavity.

At present, highest success rates require use of "fresh" or noncryopreserved oocytes. For this reason, an egg donation cycle requires synchronization of the recipient's endometrium with egg development in the donor.

To accomplish this, the egg donor completes one of the superovulation protocols outlined in Figure 20-2. Concurrently, if a recipient is not menopausal, GnRH agonists are used to suppress gonadotropin production in the receiving woman. This allows a scheduled priming of her endometrium with estrogen and progesterone. Following gonadotropin suppression, exogenous estrogen is given to the recipient. This estrogen administration begins just prior to the start of gonadotropin administration to the egg donor. After a donor receives hCG to allow the final stages of follicle and egg maturation, the recipient begins progesterone to prepare her endometrium. In the recipient, estrogen and progesterone are typically continued until late in the first trimester when placental production of these hormones is deemed to be adequate.

Gamete Intrafallopian Transfer

This technique is similar to IVF in that egg retrieval is performed after controlled ovarian hyperstimulation. Unlike IVF, however, fertilization and early embryo development do not take place in the laboratory. Eggs and sperm are placed via catheter through the fimbria and deposited directly into the oviduct. This transfer of gametes is most commonly performed at laparoscopy. Like IUI, GIFT is most applicable for unexplained infertility and should not be considered for tubal factor causes of infertility.

This technique was most popular in the late 1980s and early 1990s. However, as laboratory techniques have improved, IVF has largely replaced GIFT. In general, GIFT is more invasive, provides less diagnostic information, and requires transfer of more than two eggs for optimal pregnancy chances, which increases the risk of higher-order multifetal gestation. Thus, the major indication for GIFT at present is to avoid the religious or ethical concerns that some patients may have with fertilization taking place outside the body.

Zygote Intrafallopian Transfer

This technique is a variant of IVF with similarities to GIFT. Zygote transfer is not performed directly into the uterine cavity, but rather into the fallopian tube at laparoscopy. If the transfer is completed after a zygote has begun to divide, the procedure is more accurately termed tubal embryo transfer (TET). Although a normal fallopian tube may provide a superior environment for the early-stage embryo, this advantage has been lessened with improvements in laboratory culture methods. Accordingly, ZIFT currently should be considered most appropriately in the rare case in which transcervical transfer during IVF is technically not feasible.

Embryo Cryopreservation

With IVF, many eggs are retrieved to yield ultimately one to three healthy embryos for transfer. This frequently leads to extra embryos. Successful freezing and thawing of embryos has been possible for two decades. Moreover, advances in cryoprotectants and techniques have allowed improved survival rates of embryos frozen at a variety of developmental stages. With cryopreservation, these supernumerary embryos can yield pregnancies later, obviating the need for ovarian stimulation and egg retrieval.

Oocyte Cryopreservation

Significant technical challenges have been encountered with cryopreservation of unfertilized eggs. At this time, oocyte cryopreservation is still considered by most to be experimental, and long-term outcomes are unknown. This technique, however, is proving useful in attempting to preserve the fertility potential of women facing gonadotoxic chemotherapy. As success improves, oocyte cryopreservation may assist women desiring to delay childbearing and will likely lead to expansion of egg donation programs.

In Vitro Maturation

This technique has been used to achieve pregnancy by aspirating antral follicles from unstimulated ovaries and culturing these immature oocytes to allow resumption and completion of meiosis in vitro. Currently, IVM is considered experimental, and long-term outcomes are unknown. This technique may be useful in patients with PCOS in whom stimulation poses a significant risk of OHSS. Additionally, it is possible that refinement and evolution of this technique may make possible maturation of ova from preantral follicles. This could potentially allow preservation of fertility potential for women in whom gonadotoxic chemotherapy is required.

Preimplantation Genetic Diagnosis

This laboratory technique identifies genetic abnormalities in eggs or embryos prior to their transfer. Thus, risk for transmission of hereditable disease is a well-established indication for preimplantation genetic diagnosis (PGD). Other proposed indications include recurrent miscarriage, advanced maternal age, and multiple failed IVF cycles. Preimplantation genetic diagnosis is currently not considered an experimental procedure, and implementation of newly developed methods for genetic analysis will likely continue to broaden its application (Society for Assisted Reproductive Technology and American Society for Reproductive Medicine, 2008).

During this technique, cells are removed from a developing embryo. Multiple options exist with regard to timing of biopsy and source of genetic material. Biopsy of the first and second polar body has the advantage of avoiding cell removal from the developing embryo. However, two separate micromanipulation procedures are required, and genetic abnormalities of paternal origin are not detected. Biopsy of cleavage-stage embryos (6- to 8-cell stage) allows evaluation of both maternal and paternal contribution to the genome (Fig. 20-13). However, biopsy at this stage may only partially reflect the embryo's genetic makeup if mitotic nondisjunction has occurred and embryonic mosaicism has been created. In addition, biopsied normal embryos have a significantly decreased implantation rate. Most recently, biopsy of the trophectoderm at the blastocyst stage has been suggested to hold several advantages (Fig. 20-14). The trophectoderm is the layer from which the trophoblasts and thus the placenta develop. Biopsy from this layer allows evaluation of several (5 to 7) cells while avoiding removal of fetal cells. Unfortunately, biopsy of embryos at this late stage may require embryo cryopreservation following biopsy if genetic analysis cannot be performed rapidly.

Initially, multicolor fluorescent in situ hybridization (FISH) was employed to test single cells for structural aberrations and/or aneuploidy. This method limits the number of chromosomes that can be analyzed and has largely been replaced by more sophisticated procedures that allow for determination of the full embryonic karyotype. These newer techniques include comparative genomic hybridization (CGH) and automated quantitative real-time polymerase chain reaction (qPCR). Additionally, different microarray technologies are available including single-nucleotide polymorphism (microarray SNP) and microarray CGH (Fig. 20-15). To analyze single cells for disease-specific DNA mutations (e.g., cystic fibrosis or sickle cell disease) different strategies are used requiring linkage analysis or DNA sequencing. More recently, SNP microarrays have

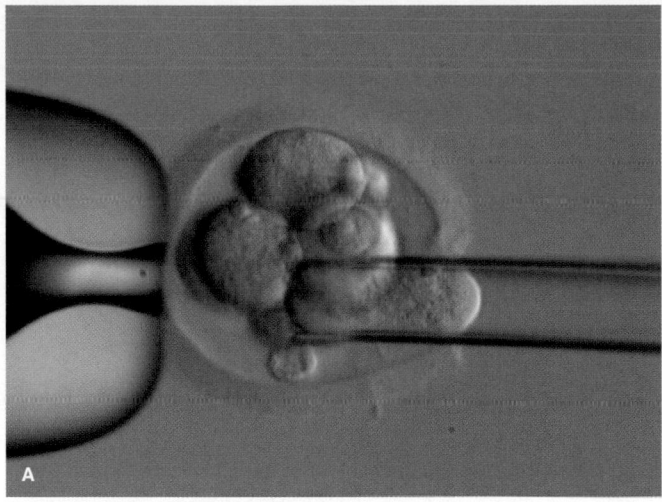 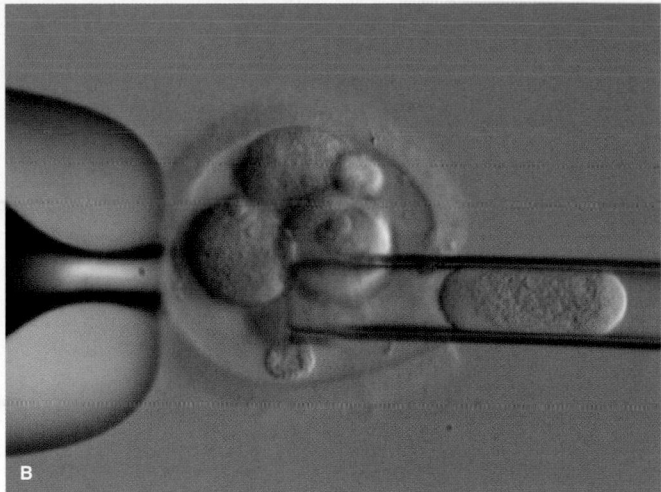

FIGURE 20-13 Photomicrographs of embryo biopsy.

now been validated for simultaneous testing of aneuploidy and translocations as well as single gene defects.

The PGD strategies and technologies continue to evolve rapidly. This evolution has been characterized by increasing validation of accuracy and decreasing expense. It has been suggested that in the near future, PGD might be applied more broadly to couples undergoing IVF that are not known to be at increased risk for genetically abnormal offspring. This routine application of PGD may allow for more accurate embryo assessment and may facilitate a desired shift to elective single embryo transfer (eSET) thus decreasing the risk of multiple gestation. A decrease in miscarriage risk may be an added benefit. Studies are currently underway to test these hypotheses.

◼ Complications of Assisted Reproductive Technologies

Assisted reproductive technologies in most cases lead to successful delivery of healthy singleton pregnancies. However, there are complications of pregnancy that may develop more fre-

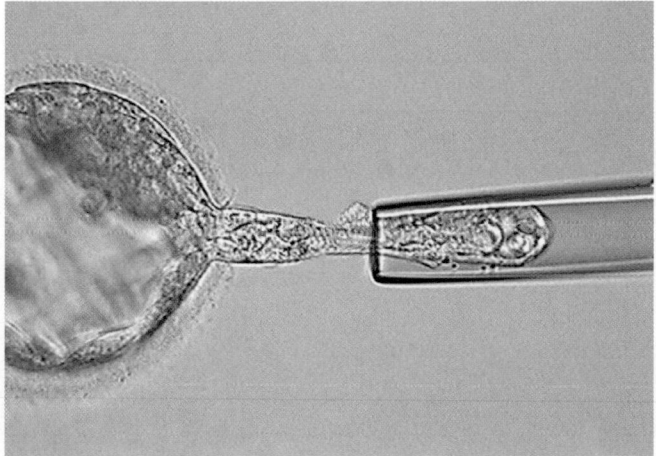

FIGURE 20-14 Photomicrograph of trophectoderm biopsy. The trophectoderm is distinct from the embryonic inner cell mass and gives rise to trophoblastic cells.

quently in those conceived using ART. Of maternal risks, preeclampsia, placenta previa, and placental abruption are more common in IVF-conceived pregnancies (Table 20-9). Of fetal risks, multifetal gestation, discussed earlier, is the most common. In addition, perinatal mortality, preterm delivery, low birthweight, and fetal-growth restriction have been implicated in IVF singleton gestations. These trends persist even following adjustment for age and parity (Reddy, 2007). Other studies, however, have not confirmed this increase in risk (Fujii, 2010). Additionally, congenital anomalies and epigenetic issues are concerns (Table 20-10).

Discussions regarding the risks for congenital anomalies began shortly after the initial success of IVF and intensified following the use of ICSI. Specifically, studies do suggest a higher incidence of congenital anomalies in infants conceived with ovulation induction, IUI, or IVF compared with those from the general population (El-Chaar, 2009; Reddy, 2007). Interpretation of most published studies, however, is complex. For example, the patient population undergoing IVF is very different from the general obstetric population with respect to age and other factors. If data are adjusted for maternal age or duration of subfertility, the risk of congenital anomalies does not appear to be increased with ART (Shevell, 2005; Zhu, 2006). This implies that much of the risk is intrinsic to the infertile couple and not related to the procedure itself.

An increase in the risk of epigenetic issues has also been reported. Although these conditions appear to be rare, their importance cannot be overstated. For review, each autosomal gene is represented by two copies, or alleles, and one copy is inherited from each parent. For most genes, both alleles are expressed simultaneously. However, approximately 150 human genes are *imprinted*, and with these genes, only one of the alleles is expressed. Imprinted genes are under control of an imprinting center that directs embryogenesis and viability. Alteration of the cellular environment can interfere with this regulation and may follow gamete manipulation or inadequate in vitro culture conditions. As a result, accelerated embryo growth, birth complications, placental abnormalities, and polyhydramnios have been observed in nonhuman mammalian ART pregnancies.

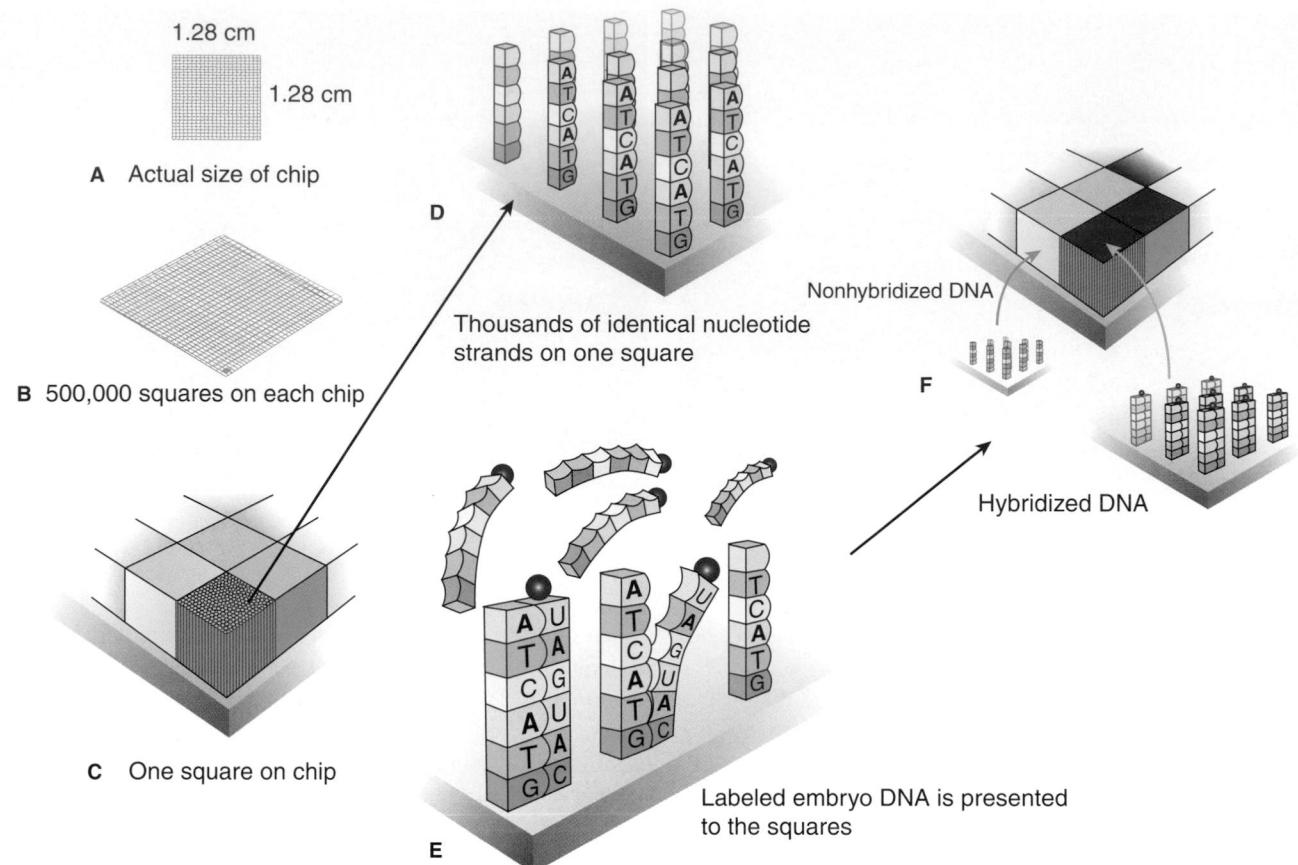

1.28 cm

1.28 cm

A Actual size of chip

B 500,000 squares on each chip

C One square on chip

D Thousands of identical nucleotide strands on one square

E Labeled embryo DNA is presented to the squares

F Nonhybridized DNA

Hybridized DNA

FIGURE 20-15 Preimplantation genetic evaluation using microarray technology. **A.** Actual microarray chip size. **B.** Each chip contains thousands of squares. **C** & **D.** Each square contains thousands of identical oligonucleotides attached to the square surface, and each square is unique in its nucleotide content. **E.** During genetic analysis, a mixture containing tagged DNA from the embryo is presented to the chip. Complementary DNA sequences bind. **F.** If a laser is shined on the chip, DNA sequences that have bound glow. This signals a matching sequence.

In humans, imprinted genes may contribute to behavior and language development, alcohol dependency, schizophrenia, and bipolar affective disorders. Imprinting may also increase risks for obesity, for cardiovascular disease, and for childhood and adult cancers. Of imprinting disorders, only rates of the rare Beckwith-Wiedemann syndrome have currently been suggested to be increased in human ART. Additionally, causation has not been conclusively proved. However, in view of these increased risks, it is reasonable to consider more intensive prenatal assessment in pregnancies conceived by IVF.

Studies assessing cognitive development after ART have for the most part been reassuring, although conflicting studies do exist. Many studies are suboptimal due to small sample size, choice of comparison group, and confounding and mediating

TABLE 20-9. Potential Risks in Singleton IVF-Conceived Pregnancies

	Absolute Risk (%) in IVF-Conceived Pregnancies	Relative Risk (vs. Non–IVF-Conceived Pregnancies)
Preeclampsia	10.3%	1.6 (1.2–2.0)
Placenta previa	2.4%	2.9 (1.5–5.4)
Placental abruption	2.2%	2.4 (1.1–5.2)
Gestational diabetes	6.8%	2.0 (1.4–3.0)
Cesarean delivery[a]	26.7%	2.1 (1.7–2.6)

[a]Please note that most experts believe the rate of cesarean delivery to be well above the 26.7% rate quoted here.
IVF = in vitro fertilization.
From Society for Assisted Reproductive Technology, 2009, with permission.

TABLE 20-10. Potential Risks in Singleton IVF Pregnancies

	Absolute Risk (%) in IVF Pregnancies	Relative Risk (vs. Non-IVF Pregnancies)
Preterm birth	11.5	2.0 (1.7–2.2)
Low birthweight (<2500 g)	9.5	1.8 (1.4–2.2)
Very low birthweight (<1500 g)	2.5	2.7 (2.3–3.1)
Small for gestational age	14.6	1.6 (1.3–2.0)
NICU admission	17.8	1.6 (1.3–2.0)
Stillbirth	1.2	2.6 (1.8–3.6)
Neonatal mortality	0.6	2.0 (1.2–3.4)
Cerebral palsy	0.4	2.8 (1.3–5.8)
Genetic risks		
Imprinting disorder	0.03	17.8 (1.8–432.9)
Major birth defect	4.3	1.5 (1.3–1.8)
Chromosomal abnormalities (after ICSI):		
of a sex chromosome	0.6	3.0
of another chromosome	0.4	5.7

IVF = in vitro fertilization; NICU = neonatal intensive care unit.
From Society for Assisted Reproductive Technology, 2009, with permission.

factors (Carson, 2010). Fortunately, currently available data suggest that there are no differences between the psychomotor development of preschool children conceived by IVF and that of naturally conceived children. Similarly, the socioemotional development of children conceived by IVF appears comparable with that of naturally conceived children (Ludwig, 2006).

CONCLUSION

The treatment of infertility should be initiated only after a thorough investigation as outlined in Chapter 19. The initial focus should be to identify lifestyle or environmental issues that may contribute to or cause the reproductive impairment. Obesity, inadequate nutrition, and associated stress should not be overlooked. In general, it is desirable to correct any identifiable contributors to subfertility. In many cases, no obvious cause can be detected. In other couples, the cause(s) may be identifiable, but not amenable to directed corrective therapies. In these circumstances, generalized fertility-boosting strategies may be recommended. These treatments include intrauterine insemination (with or without superovulation) and ART. It is important to recognize that superovulation and ART are not without risks, and couples should be appropriately counseled. Additionally, these techniques may involve third parties (egg, sperm, or embryo donors, or gestational carriers). These procedures are associated with unique psychosocial, legal, and ethical considerations. Emerging technologies such as preimplantation genetic testing bring additional ethical issues that must be confronted and resolved by both patient and practitioner.

REFERENCES

Aakvaag A: Hormonal response to electrocautery of the ovary in patients with polycystic ovarian disease. Br J Obstet Gynaecol 92:1258, 1985

Adashi EY, Rock JA, Guzick D, et al: Fertility following bilateral ovarian wedge resection: a critical analysis of 90 consecutive cases of the polycystic ovary syndrome. Fertil Steril 36:30, 1981

Almog B, Sheizaf B, Shalom-Paz E, et al: Effects of excision of ovarian endometrioma on the antral follicle count and collected oocytes for in vitro fertilization. Fertil Steril 94(6):2340, 2010

American College of Obstetricians and Gynecologists: Neural tube defects. Practice Bulletin No. 44, July 2003

American College of Obstetricians and Gynecologists: Obesity in pregnancy. Committee Opinion No. 315, September 2005

American Society for Reproductive Medicine: Control and prevention of peritoneal adhesions in gynecologic surgery. Fertil Steril 86(Suppl 4):S1, 2006a

American Society for Reproductive Medicine: Definitions of infertility and recurrent pregnancy loss. Fertil Steril 90(3 Suppl):S60, 2008a

American Society for Reproductive Medicine: Endometriosis and infertility. Fertil Steril 86(5 Suppl 1):S156, 2006b

American Society for Reproductive Medicine: Obesity and reproduction: an educational bulletin. Fertil Steril 90(5 Suppl):S21, 2008b

American Society for Reproductive Medicine: Report on varicocele and infertility. Fertil Steril 90(3 Suppl):S247, 2008c

American Society for Reproductive Medicine: Smoking and infertility. Fertil Steril 90(5 Suppl):S254, 2008d

American Society for Reproductive Medicine, Society for Assisted Reproductive Technology: Guidelines on number of embryos transferred. Fertil Steril 92(5):1518, 2009

American Society for Reproductive Medicine, Society of Reproductive Surgeons: Salpingectomy for hydrosalpinx prior to in vitro fertilization. Fertil Steril 90(Suppl 5):S66, 2008e

American Society for Reproductive Medicine, Society of Reproductive Surgeons: Pathogenesis, consequences, and control of peritoneal adhesions in gynecologic surgery. Fertil Steril 90(5 Suppl):S144, 2008f

Antonucci T, Whitcomb R, McLain R, et al: Impaired glucose tolerance is normalized by treatment with the thiazolidinedione troglitazone. Diabetes Care 20:188, 1998

Armar N, McGarrigle H, Honour J, et al: Laparoscopic ovarian diathermy in the management of anovulatory infertility in women with polycystic ovaries: endocrine changes and clinical outcomes. Fertil Steril 53:45, 1990

Armar NA, Lachelin GC: Laparoscopic ovarian diathermy: an effective treatment for anti-oestrogen resistant anovulatory infertility in women with the polycystic ovary syndrome. Br J Obstet Gynecol 100(2):P161, 1993

Balen A, Braat D, West C, et al: Cumulative conception and livebirth rates after the treatment of anovulatory infertility: safety and efficacy of ovulation induction. Hum Reprod 9:1563, 1994

Balen A, Tan SL, Jacobs H, et al: Hypersecretion of luteinising hormone. A significant cause of infertility and miscarriage. Br J Obstet Gynaecol 100:1082, 1993

Bayrak A, Harp D, Saadat P, et al: Recurrence of hydrosalpinges after cuff neosalpingostomy in a poor prognosis population. J Assist Reprod Genet 23:285, 2006

Biljan MM, Hemmings R, Brassard N, et al: The outcome of 150 babies following the treatment with letrozole or letrozole and gonadotropins. Fertil Steril 84(Suppl 1):S95, 2005

Buttram VC, Vaquero C: Post-ovarian wedge resection adhesive disease. Fertil Steril 26:874, 1975

Carson C, Kurinczuk JJ, Sacker A, et al: Cognitive development following ART: effect of choice of comparison group, confounding and mediating factors. Hum Reprod 25(1):244, 2010

Casper RF: Letrozole: ovulation or superovulation? Fertil Steril 80:1335, 2003

Centers for Disease Control and Prevention: Vital signs: current cigarette smoking among adults aged ≥18 years—United States, 2005-2010. MMWR 60(35):1207, 2011

Centers for Disease Control and Prevention: Contribution of assisted reproductive technology and ovulation-inducing drugs to triplet and higher-order multiple births—United States, 1980–1997. MMWR 49:535, 2000

Centola GM: Successful treatment of severe oligozoospermia with sperm washing and intrauterine insemination. J Androl 18:448, 1997

Choi JM, Chung P, Veeck L, et al: AZF microdeletions of the Y chromosome and in vitro fertilization outcome. Fertil Steril 81:337, 2004

Collin P, Vilska S, Heinonen PK, et al: Infertility and coeliac disease. Gut 39(3):382, 1996

Crow SJ, Thuras P, Keel PK, et al: Long-term menstrual and reproductive function in patients with bulimia nervosa. Am J Psychiatry 159:1048, 2002

Cunningham FG, Leveno KL, Bloom SL, et al (eds): Teratology and medications that affect the fetus. In Williams Obstetrics, 23rd ed, New York, McGraw-Hill, 2010, p 329

Deaton J, Gibson M, Blackmer K, et al: A randomized, controlled trial of clomiphene citrate and intrauterine insemination in couples with unexplained infertility or surgically corrected endometriosis. Fertil Steril 54:1083, 1990

Dicker D, Goldman JA, Levy T, et al: The impact of long-term gonadotropin-releasing hormone analogue treatment on preclinical abortions in patients with severe endometriosis undergoing in vitro fertilization-embryo transfer. Fertil Steril 57:597, 1992

Dodson WC, Whitesides DB, Hughes CL, et al: Superovulation with intrauterine insemination in the treatment of infertility: a possible alternative to gamete intrafallopian transfer and in vitro fertilization. Fertil Steril 48:441, 1987

Domar AD, Seibel MM, Benson H, et al: The mind/body program for infertility: a new behavioral treatment approach for women with infertility. Fertil Steril 54: 1183, 1990

El-Chaar D, Yang Q, Gao J, et al: Risk of birth defects increased in pregnancies conceived by assisted human reproduction. Fertil Steril 92(5):1557, 2009

Elnashar A, Abdelmageed E, Fayed M, et al: Clomiphene citrate and dexamethazone in treatment of clomiphene citrate-resistant polycystic ovary syndrome: a prospective placebo-controlled study. Hum Reprod 21(7):1805, 2006

Evans MI, Britt DW: Fetal reduction 2008. Curr Opin Obstet Gynecol 20(4): 386, 2008

Evers JL, Collins JA: Assessment of efficacy of varicocele repair for male subfertility: a systematic review. Lancet 361(9372):1849, 2003

Exacoustos C, Zupi E, Amadio A, et al: Laparoscopic removal of endometriomas: sonographic evaluation of residual functioning ovarian tissue. Am J Obstet Gynecol 191(1):68, 2004

Farhi J, Soule S, Jacobs HS, et al: Effect of laparoscopic ovarian electrocautery on ovarian response and outcome of treatment with gonadotropins in clomiphene citrate-resistant patients with polycystic syndrome. Fertil Steril 64:930, 1995

Farhi J, West C, Patel A, et al: Treatment of anovulatory infertility: the problem of multiple pregnancy. Hum Reprod 11:429, 1996

Filicori M, Cognigni GE, Taraborrelli S, et al: Modulation of folliculogenesis and steroidogenesis in women by graded menotropin administration. Hum Reprod 17:2009, 2002

Fiore MC, Jaén CR, Baker TB, et al: Treating tobacco use and dependence: 2008 update. Clinical Practice Guideline. Rockville, MD, U.S. Department of Health and Human Services, Public Health Service, 2008

Fontana PG, Leclerc JM: Contraindication of Femara (letrozole) in premenopausal women. 2005. Available at: www.hc-sc.gc.ca/dhp-mps/alt_formats/hpfb-dgpsa/pdf/medeff/femara_hpc-cps-eng.pdf. Accessed October 15, 2010

Franks S, Adams J, Mason H, et al: Ovulation disorders in women with polycystic ovary syndrome. Clin Obstet Gynecol 12:605, 1985

Fujii M, Matsuoka R, Bergel E, et al: Perinatal risk in singleton pregnancies after in vitro fertilization. Fertil Steril 94(6):2113, 2010

Giudice LC: Infertility and the environment: the medical context. Semin Reprod Med 24:129, 2006

Gleicher N, Barad D: Unexplained infertility: does it really exist? Hum Reprod 21:1951, 2006

Greenblatt E, Casper RF: Endocrine changes after laparoscopic ovarian cautery in polycystic ovarian syndrome. Am J Obstet Gynecol 156:279, 1987

Griffiths A, D'Angelo A, Amso N, et al: Surgical treatment of fibroids for subfertility. Cochrane Database Syst Rev 3:CD003857, 2006

Guzick DS, Carson SA, Coutifaris C, et al: Efficacy of superovulation and intrauterine insemination in the treatment of infertility. N Engl J Med 340:177, 1999

Gysler M, March CM, Mishell DR Jr, et al: A decade's experience with an individualized clomiphene treatment regime including its effect on the postcoital test. Fertil Steril 37:161, 1982

Hammond M, Halme J, Talbert L, et al: Factors affecting the pregnancy rate in clomiphene citrate induction of ovulation. Obstet Gynecol 62:196, 1983

Hart RJ, Hickey M, Maouris P, et al: Excisional surgery versus ablative surgery for ovarian endometriomata. Cochrane Database Syst Rev 2:CD004992, 2008

Hassan MA, Killick SR: Negative lifestyle is associated with a significant reduction in fecundity. Fertil Steril 81:384, 2004

Hauser R, Sokol R: Science linking environmental contaminant exposures with fertility and reproductive health impacts in the adult male. Fertil Steril 89(2 Suppl):e59, 2008

Helmerhorst FM, Van Vliet HAAM, Gornas T, et al: Intra-uterine insemination versus timed intercourse for cervical hostility in subfertile couples. Cochrane Database Syst Rev 4:CD002809, 2005

Hoeger K: Obesity and weight loss in polycystic ovary syndrome. Obstet Gynecol Clin North Am 28:85, 2001

Jackson JE, Rosen M, McLean T, et al: Prevalence of celiac disease in a cohort of women with unexplained infertility. Fertil Steril 89(4):1002, 2008

Jensen TK, Hjollund NH, Henriksen TB, et al: Does moderate alcohol consumption affect fertility? Follow up study among couples planning first pregnancy. BMJ 317:505, 1998

Kiddy DS, Hamilton-Fairly D, Bush A, et al: Improvement in endocrine and ovarian function during dietary treatment of obese women with polycystic ovary syndrome. Clin Endocrinol (Oxf) 36:105, 1992

Klonoff-Cohen H, Natarajan L, Marrs R, et al: Effects of female and male smoking on success rates of IVF and gamete intra-Fallopian transfer. Hum Reprod 16:1389, 2001

Kovacs G, Buckler H, Bangah M, et al: Treatment of anovulation due to polycystic ovarian syndrome by laparoscopic ovarian electrocautery. Br J Obstet Gynaecol 98:30, 1991

Langley MT, Marek DM, Gardner DK, et al: Extended embryo culture in human assisted reproduction treatments. Hum Reprod 16:902, 2001

Legro RS, Barnhart HX, Schlaff WD, et al: Clomiphene, metformin or both for infertility in polycystic ovary syndrome. N Engl J Med 356(6):551, 2007

Lincoln SR, Ke RW, Kutteh WH: Screening for hypothyroidism in infertile women. J Reprod Med 44:455, 1999

Lobo RA, Gysler M, March CM, et al: Clinical and laboratory predictors of clomiphene response. Fertil Steril 37:168, 1982

Ludwig AK, Diedrich K, Ludwig M, et al: The process of decision making in reproductive medicine. Semin Reprod Med 23(4):348, 2005

Ludwig AK, Sutcliffe AG, Diedrich K, et al: Post-neonatal health and development of children born after assisted reproduction: a systematic review of controlled studies. Eur J Obstet Gynecol Reprod Biol 127(1):3, 2006

Martin JA, Hamilton BE, Sutton PD, et al: Births: final data for 2008. Natl Vital Stat Rep 59:1, 2010

Martin JA, Park MM: Trends in twin and triplet births: 1980–97. Natl Vital Stat Rep 47:1, 1999

Meloni GF, Desole S, Vargiu N, et al: The prevalence of celiac disease in infertility. Hum Reprod 14:2759, 1999

Mendola P, Messer LC, Rappazzo K: Science linking environmental contaminant exposures with fertility and reproductive health impacts in the adult female. Fertil Steril 89(2 Suppl):e81, 2008

Mirwally MF, Casper RF: Aromatase inhibition reduces the dose of gonadotropin required for controlled ovarian hyperstimulation. J Soc Gynecol Invest 11:406, 2004

Molitch ME: Management of prolactinomas during pregnancy. J Reprod Med 44:1121, 1999

Molitch ME: Prolactinomas and pregnancy. Clin Endocrinol (Oxf) 73:147, 2010

Muzii L, Bianchi A, Bellati F, et al: Histologic analysis of endometriomas: what the surgeon needs to know. Fertil Steril 87(2):362, 2007

Nestler JE, Jakubowicz DJ, Evans WS, et al: Effects of metformin on spontaneous and clomiphene-induced ovulation in the polycystic ovary syndrome. N Engl J Med 338:1876, 1998

Palomba S, Orio F, Falbo A, et al: Prospective parallel randomized, double blind, double-dummy controlled clinical trial comparing clomiphene citrate and metformin as the first-line treatment for ovulation induction in nonobese anovulatory women with polycystic ovary syndrome. J Clin Endocrinol Metab 90:4068, 2005

Papanikolaou EG, Fatemi H, Venetis C, et al: Monozygotic twinning is not increased after single blastocyst transfer compared with single cleavage-stage embryo transfer. Fertil Steril 93(2):592, 2010

Parsanezhad ME, Alborzi S, Motazedian S, et al: Use of dexamethasone and clomiphene citrate in the treatment of clomiphene citrate-resistant patients with polycystic ovary syndrome and normal dehydroepiandrosterone sulfate levels: a prospective, double-blind, placebo-controlled trial. Fertil Steril 78(5):1001, 2002

Pasquali R, Antenucci D, Casmirri F, et al: Clinical and hormonal characteristics of obese amenorrheic hyperandrogenic women before and after weight loss. J Clin Endocrinol Metab 68:173, 1989

Pasquali R, Gambineri A, Pagotto U: The impact of obesity on reproduction in women with polycystic ovary syndrome. BJOG 113:1148, 2006

Patel SR, Sigman M: Antioxidant therapy in male infertility. Urol Clin North Am 35(2):319, 2008

Pérez-Medina T, Bajo-Arenas J, Salazar F, et al: Endometrial polyps and their implication in the pregnancy rates of patients undergoing intrauterine insemination: a prospective, randomized study. Hum Reprod 20:1632, 2005

Ragni G, Somigliana E, Benedetti F, et al: Damage to ovarian reserve associated with laparoscopic excision of endometriomas: a quantitative rather than a qualitative injury. Am J Obstet Gynecol 193(6):1908, 2005

Raj S, Thompson I, Berger M, et al: Clinical aspects of polycystic ovary syndrome. Obstet Gynecol 49(5):552, 1977

Reddy UM, Wapner RJ, Rebar RW, et al: Infertility, assisted reproductive technology, and adverse pregnancy outcomes: executive summary of a National Institute of Child Health and Human Development workshop. Obstet Gynecol 109(4):967, 2007

Ross C, Morriss A, Khairy M, et al: A systematic review of the effect of oral antioxidants on male infertility. Reprod Biomed Online 20(6):711, 2010

Roth L, Taylor HS: Risks of smoking to reproductive health: assessment of women's knowledge. Am J Obstet Gynecol 184:934, 2001

Shevell T, Malone FD, Vidaver J, et al: Assisted reproductive technology and pregnancy outcome. Obstet Gynecol 106(5 Pt 1):1039, 2005

Sigman M, Glass S, Campagnone J, et al: Carnitine for the treatment of idiopathic asthenospermia: a randomized, double-blind, placebo-controlled trial. Fertil Steril 85(5):1409, 2006

Society for Assisted Reproductive Technology: Informed consent for assisted reproduction: in vitro fertilization, intracytoplasmic sperm injection, assisted hatching, embryo cryopreservation. pp 20, 22, 2009. Available at: http://www.sart.org/. Accessed August 26, 2011

Society for Assisted Reproductive Technology, American Society for Reproductive Medicine: Preimplantation genetic testing: a Practice Committee opinion. Fertil Steril 90(5 Suppl):S136, 2008

Stein IF, Cohen MR: Surgical treatment of bilateral polycystic ovaries. Am J Obstet Gynecol 38:465, 1939

Steures P, van der Steeg JW, Verhoeve HR, et al: Does ovarian hyperstimulation in intrauterine insemination for cervical factor subfertility improve pregnancy rates? Hum Reprod 19:2263, 2004

Strickland DM, Whitted WA, Wians FH Jr: Screening infertile women for subclinical hypothyroidism. Am J Obstet Gynecol 163(1 Pt 1):262, 1990

Surrey ES, Silverberg KM, Surrey MW: Effect of prolonged gonadotropin-releasing hormone agonist therapy on the outcome of in vitro fertilization-embryo transfer in patients with endometriosis. Fertil Steril 78:699, 2002

Thiering P, Beaurepaire J, Jones M, et al: Mood state as a predictor of treatment outcome after in vitro fertilization/embryo transfer technology (IVF/ET). J Psychosom Res 37:481, 1993

Tulandi T, Collins JA, Burrows E, et al: Treatment-dependent and treatment-independent pregnancy among women with periadnexal adhesions. Am J Obstet Gynecol 162:354, 1990

Tulandi T, Martin J, Al-Fadhli R, et al: Congenital malformations among 911 newborns conceived after infertility treatment with letrozole or clomiphene citrate. Fertil Steril 85:1761, 2006

Vandermolen DT, Ratts VS, Evans WS, et al: Metformin increases the ovulatory rate and pregnancy rate from clomiphene citrate in patients with polycystic ovary syndrome who are resistant to clomiphene citrate alone. Fertil Steril 75:310, 2001

Whelan JG III, Vlahos NF: The ovarian hyperstimulation syndrome. Fertil Steril 73:883, 2000

Yang Q, Sherman SL, Hassold TJ, et al: Risk factors for trisomy 21: maternal cigarette smoking and oral contraceptive use in a population-based case-control study. Genet Med 1:80, 1999

Zarate A, Herdmandez-Ayup S, Rios-Montiel A: Treatment of anovulation in the Stein-Leventhal syndrome. Analysis of ninety cases. Fertil Steril 22:188, 1971

Zhu JL, Basso O, Obel C, et al: Infertility, infertility treatment, and congenital malformations: Danish national birth cohort. BMJ 333(7570):679, 2006

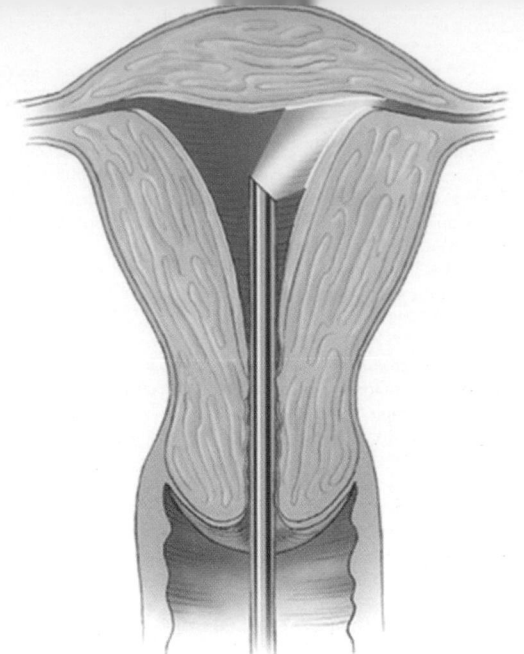

The menopausal transition is a progressive endocrinologic continuum that takes reproductive-aged women from regular, cyclic, and predictable menses that are characteristic of ovulatory cycles, to a final menstrual period associated with ovarian senescence. With improvements in medical treatment and increased focus on preventive health care, average life expectancy has increased. As a result, most women can now expect to live at least one third of their lives in the postmenopause. Specifically, in the 2010 United States census, nearly 42 million women were aged 55 years and older (U.S. Census Bureau, 2011). Importantly, menopausal transition and the years of life spent in the postmenopausal state bring with them issues related to both quality of life and disease prevention and management (Lund, 2008).

DEFINITIONS

The term *menopause* refers to a point in time that follows 1 year after the cessation of menstruation. The *postmenopause* describes those years following this point. The average age of women experiencing their final menstrual period is 51.5 years, but cessation of menses due to ovarian failure may occur at any age. *Premature ovarian failure* refers to cessation of menses before age 40 and is associated with an elevated follicle-stimulating hormone (FSH) level (Chap. 16, p. 444). The older terms *perimenopause* or *climacteric* generally refer to the time period in the late reproductive years, usually late 40s to early 50s. Characteristically, it begins with menstrual cycle irregularity and extends to 1 year after permanent cessation of menses. The more correct terminology for this time is *menopausal transition*. This transition typically develops over a span of 4 to 7 years, and the average age at its onset is 47 years (Burger, 2008; McKinlay, 1992).

The first standardized classification guidelines for female reproductive aging were proposed in 2001 at the Stages of Reproductive Aging workshop (STRAW) (Fig. 21-1). The purpose of the STRAW report was to clarify the stages and

Final Menstrual Period (FMP)

Stages:	−5	−4	−3	−2	−1	0	+1	+2
Terminology:	Reproductive			Menopausal Transition			Postmenopause	
	Early	Peak	Late	Early	Late*		Early*	Late
				Perimenopause				
Duration of Stage:	Variable			Variable		ⓐ 1 yr	ⓑ 4 yrs	Until demise
Menstrual Cycles:	Variable to regular	Regular		Variable cycle length (>7 days different from normal)	≥2 Skipped cycles and an interval of amenorrhea (≥60 days)	Amen × 12 mos	None	
Endocrine:	Normal FSH		↑ FSH	↑ FSH			↑ FSH	

*Stages most likely to be characterized by vasomotor symptoms   ↑ = elevated

FIGURE 21-1 The stages of reproductive aging. Amen = Amenorrhea; FSH = follicle-stimulating hormone level. *(Redrawn from Soules, 2001, with permission).*

nomenclature of normal female reproductive aging. These staging criteria are intended to be guidelines rather than strictly applied diagnoses. Every stage may not occur in a given individual, and if they do occur, they may not progress in the exact sequence provided (Hale, 2009). The group concluded that because the terms *perimenopause* and *climacteric* are not used consistently, they should be used only with patients and in the lay press and not in scientific papers. The term *menopausal transition* is the preferred term (Soules, 2001).

The STRAW report divides reproductive and postreproductive life into several stages. The anchor for the staging system is the final menstrual period (FMP), and the age range and duration of each stage varies. Five stages precede and two stages follow the FMP. Stage −5 refers to the early reproductive period, stage −4 to the reproductive peak, and stage −3 to the late reproductive period. Stage −2 refers to the early menopausal transition and stage −1 to the late menopausal transition. Stage +1a refers to the first year after the FMP, stage +1b refers to years 2 to 5 postmenopause, and stage +2 refers to the ensuing later postmenopausal years.

In the early menopausal transition (stage −2), a woman's menstrual cycles remain regular, but the interval between cycles may be altered by 7 or more days. Typically, cycle lengths become shorter. Compared with younger women, FSH levels are elevated, and serum estrogen levels may be increased in the early follicular phase. Normal ovulatory cycles may be interspersed with anovulatory cycles during this transition, and conception can occur unexpectedly. The late menopausal transition (stage −1) is characterized by two or more skipped menses and at least one intermenstrual interval of 60 days or more due to longer and longer duration of anovulation (Soules, 2001).

All of the preceding definitions are currently the best description of a woman's transit through menopause, but these will certainly be subject to modification in the future.

INFLUENTIAL FACTORS

A number of environmental, genetic, and surgical influences may speed ovarian aging. For example, smoking advances the age of menopause by approximately 2 years (Gold, 2001; Wallace, 1979). In addition, chemotherapy, pelvic radiation, ovarian surgery, and hysterectomy may also lead to an earlier age of menopause. During the menopausal transition, more erratic fluctuations in female reproductive hormones can lead to an array of physical and psychological symptoms as outlined in Table 21-1 (Bachmann, 2001; Dennerstein, 1993).

PHYSIOLOGIC CHANGES

Hypothalamus-Pituitary-Ovarian Axis Changes

During the reproductive life of a woman, gonadotropin-releasing hormone (GnRH) is released in a pulsatile fashion by the arcuate nucleus of the medial basal hypothalamus. It binds to GnRH receptors on the pituitary gonadotropes to stimulate cyclic release of the gonadotropins—luteinizing hormone (LH) and FSH. These gonadotropins, in turn, stimulate the production of the ovarian sex steroids estrogen and progesterone and the peptide hormone inhibin. During the reproductive years, estrogen and progesterone exert positive and negative feedback on pituitary gonadotropin production and on the amplitude and frequency of GnRH release. Produced in the granulosa cells, inhibin exerts important negative feedback influence over FSH secretion from the pituitary. This tightly regulated endocrine system leads to ovulatory menstrual cycles that are regular and predictable.

The transition from ovulatory cycles to menopause typically begins in the late 40s and in early menopausal transition

TABLE 21-1. Symptoms Associated with Menopausal Transition

Changes in menstrual patterns
Shorter cycles are typical (by 2–7 days)
Longer cycles are possible
Irregular bleeding (heavier, lighter, with spotting)

Vasomotor symptoms
Hot flashes
Night sweats
Sleep disturbances

Psychological and mental disturbances
Worsening premenstrual syndrome
Depression
Irritability
Mood swings
Loss of concentration
Poor memory

Sexual dysfunction
Vaginal dryness
Decreased libido
Painful intercourse

Somatic symptoms
Headache
Dizziness
Palpitations
Breast pain and enlargement
Joint aches and back pain

Other symptoms
Urinary incontinence
Dry, itchy skin
Weight gain

(stage −2). Levels of FSH rise slightly and lead to an increased ovarian follicular response. This, in turn, creates overall higher estrogen levels (Jain, 2005; Klein, 1996). This rise in FSH levels is attributed to a decrease in ovarian inhibin secretion, rather than to a decrease in estradiol production. As described earlier, inhibin regulates FSH through negative feedback, and decreased inhibin levels lead to elevated levels of FSH. In perimenopausal women, estradiol production fluctuates with these changing FSH levels and can reach higher concentration than those observed in women younger than 35. Estradiol levels generally do not decrease significantly until late in the menopausal transition. Despite continuing regular cyclic menstruation, progesterone levels during the early menopausal transition are lower than in women of mid-reproductive age (Santoro, 2004). Testosterone levels do not vary appreciably during menopausal transition.

In late menopausal transition, women exhibit impaired folliculogenesis and an increasing incidence of anovulation compared with mid-reproductive-aged women. Also, during this time, ovarian follicles undergo an accelerated rate of loss until eventually the supply of follicles is depleted. These changes, including the increase in FSH levels, reflect the reduced quality

and capability of aging follicles to secrete inhibin (Reyes, 1977; Santoro, 1996).

Antimüllerian hormone (AMH) is a glycoprotein secreted by the granulosa cells of secondary and preantral follicles. Circulating concentrations remain relatively stable across the menstrual cycle in reproductive-aged women and correlate with the number of early antral follicles. As such, data suggest that AMH can be used as a marker of ovarian reserve (Kwee, 2008; La Marca, 2010). Levels of AMH decrease markedly and progressively across the menopausal transition (Hale, 2007).

With ovarian failure in the menopause (stage +1b), ovarian steroid hormone release ceases, and the negative-feedback loop is opened. Subsequently, GnRH is released at maximal frequency and amplitude. As a result, circulating FSH and LH levels rise up to fourfold higher than in the reproductive years (Klein, 1996).

Among these hormonal changes within the hypothalamic-pituitary-ovarian axis, few show variation distinct enough to be use as serum markers of menopausal transition. As discussed later, the diagnosis of menopausal transition is mainly based on historical information. In the postmenopause, however, because of the just-described marked rise in FSH levels, this gonadotropin becomes a more reliable marker.

Ovarian Changes

Ovarian senescence is a process that has been shown to actually begin in utero within the embryonic ovary due to programmed oocyte atresia (Fig. 14-1, p. 383). From birth onward, primordial follicles are continuously being activated, mature partially, and then regress. This follicular activation continues in a constant pattern that is independent of pituitary stimulation.

Evidence, however, suggests that this regular activation of follicles is accelerated during late reproductive life. A more rapid depletion of ovarian follicles starts in the late 30s and early 40s and continues until a point at which the menopausal ovary is virtually devoid of follicles (Figs. 21-2 and 21-3). For example, Richardson and colleagues (1987) performed a quantitative histologic study of the endometrium and ovaries from 17 women aged 44 to 55 years who were in menopausal transition. These were coupled with a single hormonal measurement and a reproductive history from each of these women who subsequently underwent oophorectomy and hysterectomy for uterine leiomyomas or menorrhagia. The six women who reported regular cycles had an average of 1700 follicles in the selected ovary compared with an average of 180 follicles in the ovaries of those who reported irregular cycles.

An average woman may experience approximately 400 ovulatory events during her reproductive lifetime. This represents a very small percentage of the 6 to 7 million oocytes present at the 20th week of gestation, or even the 400,000 oocytes present at birth. The process of atresia of the nondominant cohort of follicles, largely independent of menstrual cyclicity, is the prime event that leads to the eventual loss of ovarian activity and menopause.

Adrenal Steroid Changes

Dehydroepiandrosterone sulfate (DHEAS) is produced almost exclusively in the adrenal gland. With advancing age, adrenal

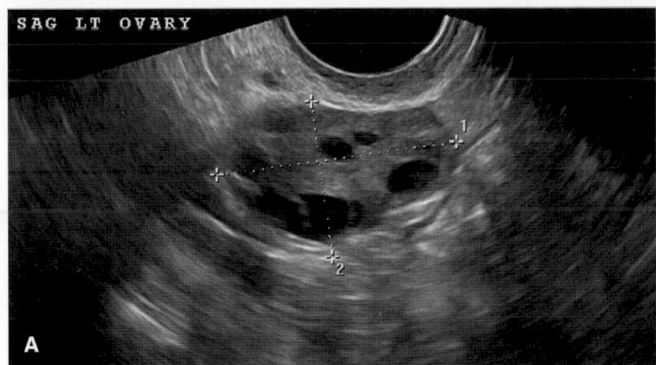

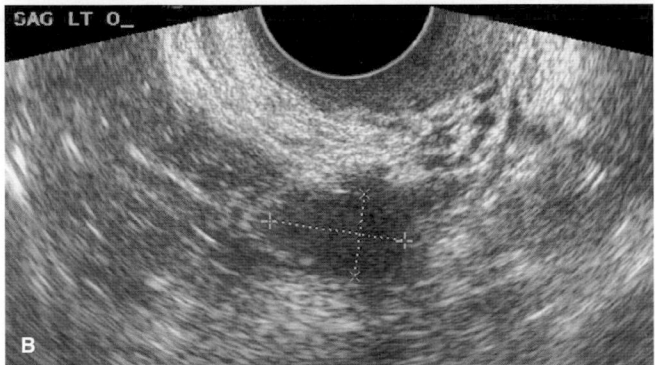

FIGURE 21-2 Transvaginal sonographic images of pre- and post-menopausal ovaries, which are marked by calipers. **A.** In general, premenopausal ovaries have greater volume and contain follicles, which are seen as multiple, small, anechoic smooth-walled cysts. **B.** In comparison, postmenopausal ovaries have smaller volume and are characteristically devoid of follicular structures. *(Images contributed by Dr. Elysia Moschos.)*

production of DHEAS declines. Adrenal hormone levels have been studied in aging women by Labrie (1997) and Burger (2000), each with their colleagues. They found that in women aged 20 to 30 years, DHEAS concentrations peaked during these years, with an average of 6.2 micromoles, and then decreased steadily. In women 70 to 80 years, DHEAS levels were diminished by 74 percent to 1.6 micromoles. Other adrenal hormones decrease with aging as well. Androstenedione peaks at ages 20 to 30 years and then decreases to 62 percent of this peak level in women aged 50 to 60 years. Pregnenolone diminishes by 45 percent from reproductive life to menopause. The ovary contributes to the production of these hormones during the reproductive years, but after menopause, only the adrenal gland continues this hormone synthesis.

Burger and associates (2000) prospectively studied 172 women during the menopausal transition as a part of the Melbourne Women's Midlife Health Project. In their longitudinal analysis of hormone levels in these patients, no relationship between a woman's final menstrual period and the decline in DHEAS level was noted. Advancing age, regardless of menopausal status, determined DHEAS level decline.

■ Sex Hormone-Binding Globulin Level Changes

The principal sex steroids—estradiol and testosterone—circulate in the blood bound to a glycoprotein carrier produced in the liver, known as sex hormone-binding globulin (SHBG). Production of SHBG declines after the menopause and may lead to increased levels of free or unbound estrogen and testosterone.

Reproductive age ovary

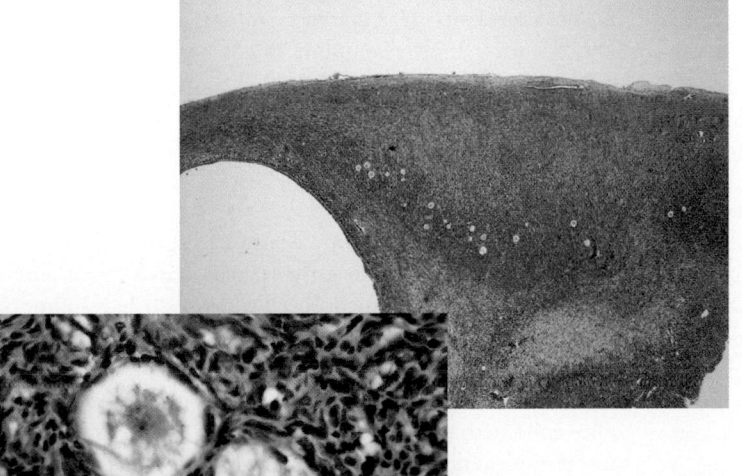

Primordial follicles

Menopausal ovary

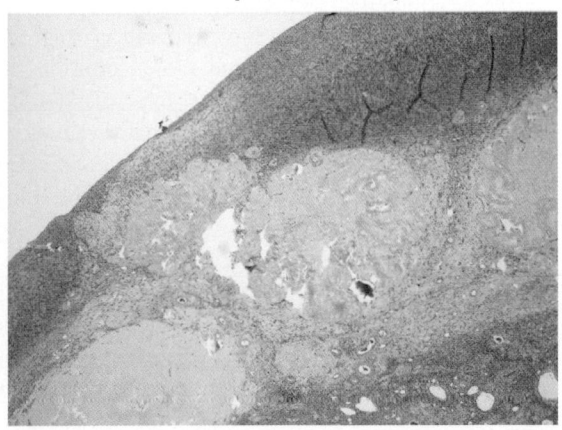

FIGURE 21-3 Microscopic differences between a reproductive-age and menopausal ovary. **A.** Reproductive-age ovary. Note preponderance of primordial follicles. **B.** High-power image of primordial follicles. **C.** The menopausal ovary shows abundance of atretic follicles and persistent pale pink corpora albicans. *(Photographs contributed by Dr. Raheela Ashfaq.)*

Endometrial Changes

Microscopic changes in the endometrium directly reflect the level of systemic estrogen and progesterone and thus may change dramatically depending on the phase of menopausal transition. During early menopausal transition, the endometrium may reflect ovulatory cycles, which are prevalent during this time. During the later stage of menopausal transition, anovulation is common, and the endometrium will display estrogen's effect when unopposed by progesterone. Accordingly, proliferative changes or disordered proliferative changes are frequently findings on pathologic examination of endometrial biopsy (EMB) samples. After menopause, the endometrium becomes atrophic due to lack of estrogen stimulation (Fig. 21-4).

Menstrual Disturbances

Abnormal uterine bleeding is common during the menopausal transition. Treloar and coworkers (1981) found that menses were irregular in more than one half of all women studied during menopausal transition. Because the time interval surrounding menopause is characterized by relatively high, acyclic estrogen levels and relatively low progesterone production, women in the menopausal transition are at increased risk for developing endometrial hyperplasia or carcinoma. However, in all women, regardless of menopausal status, the etiology of abnormal bleeding should be determined as outlined in Chapter 8 (p. 223). Anovulation is the most common cause of erratic bleeding during the transition, although endometrial hyperplasia and carcinoma, estrogen-sensitive neoplasms such as endometrial polyps and uterine leiomyomas, and pregnancy-related events should always be considered.

Endometrial cancer is suspected in any woman in menopausal transition with abnormal uterine bleeding. The overall incidence of endometrial cancer is approximately 0.1 percent of women in this group per year, but in women with abnormal uterine bleeding, the risk increases to 10 percent (Lidor, 1986). Malignant precursors of endometrial cancer such as complex endometrial hyperplasia become more common during the menopausal transition. Endometrial hyperplasia and neoplasia are traditionally diagnosed from histologic evaluation of endometrial specimens. Thus, sampling of the endometrium is an important part of the evaluation of abnormal bleeding.

Although endometrial neoplasia is the greatest concern during this time, EMB frequently reveals a nonneoplastic endometrium displaying estrogen effects unopposed by progesterone. In premenopausal women, this results from anovulation. In postmenopausal women, unopposed estrogen may be derived from extragonadal endogenous estrogen production, which may result from increased aromatization of androgen to estrogen due to obesity. In addition, decreased SHBG levels lead to increased levels of free and therefore bioavailable, estrogen (Moen, 2004). Unopposed estrogen administration can also account for these effects in postmenopausal women.

Evaluation of Abnormal Bleeding

Sonography. Evaluation of the endometrium by transvaginal sonography is currently the imaging method of choice in the diagnostic evaluation of abnormal uterine bleeding. In postmenopausal women, an endometrial thickness of ≤4 mm has a 99-percent negative predictive value in excluding endometrial carcinoma. A thickness >4 mm is a nonspecific finding (American College of Obstetricians and Gynecologists, 2009). Endometrial biopsy is advised in any postmenopausal women with abnormal bleeding and endometrial thickness >4 mm.

In premenopausal women, evidence is lacking regarding the application of this criterion. However, a biopsy is typically indicated in premenopausal women ≥35 years. Moreover, in those younger than 35, if a clinical history suggests long-term unopposed estrogen exposure, a biopsy is prudent even if the endometrial thickness is "normal" (4 to 10 mm).

Saline infusion sonography (SIS) improves the characterization of endometrial thickening and the detection and description of endometrial lesions. Moreover, Moschos and colleagues (2009) described the usefulness of SIS-EMB. With this, focal areas of endometrium may be biopsied with an endometrial Pipelle under sonographic guidance during SIS (Fig. 2-15, p. 41).

Endometrial Biopsy. The diagnostic approach to a woman in menopausal transition with abnormal bleeding has evolved over the past century from operating room dilatation and curettage (D&C), to outpatient vacuum-suction curettage, to eventually the Pipelle plastic catheter (Fig. 8-6, p. 444) (Goldstein, 2010; Stovall, 1991). Importantly, although the risk of pregnancy is diminished during menopausal transition, pregnancy should be excluded prior to uterine biopsy.

Fewer than 10 percent of postmenopausal women cannot be adequately evaluated by office biopsy. Inability to enter the uterine cavity is the most common reason for failure. In such instances, pretreatment with the prostaglandin E_1 analog misoprostol (Cytotec), 200 or 400 μg vaginally or 400 μg orally the night before biopsy, may be helpful. Misoprostol softens the cervix and typically allows passage of a Pipelle through a stenotic os. This may avert the need for forceful dilatation in the office or D&C in the operating room. Side effects of misoprostol may include nausea, diarrhea, uterine cramping, and uterine bleeding.

If adequate Pipelle sampling is not possible and histologic endometrial evaluation is indicated, then outpatient D&C may be performed (Section 41-15, p. 1057). In many cases, D&C may be coupled with hysteroscopy, which adds accuracy to identification of focal lesions.

Hysteroscopy. Hysteroscopy is also useful to evaluate abnormal uterine bleeding. It allows for evaluation of focal intrauterine lesions and targeted biopsy of specific lesions such as submucous leiomyomas, endometrial polyps, or focal areas of endometrial hyperplasia or endometrial cancer (Section 42-13, p. 1157). Patients with a stenotic cervical os that does not allow an in-office endometrial biopsy to be performed can be pretreated with misoprostol, as described earlier, to ease cervical dilation and help reduce the risk of uterine perforation during hysteroscopy.

Fertility Potential

Contraception

Many women in their late 40s do not consider themselves fertile. Accordingly, many will stop contraception use but will still have occasional ovulatory cycles. Pregnancies do occur in this

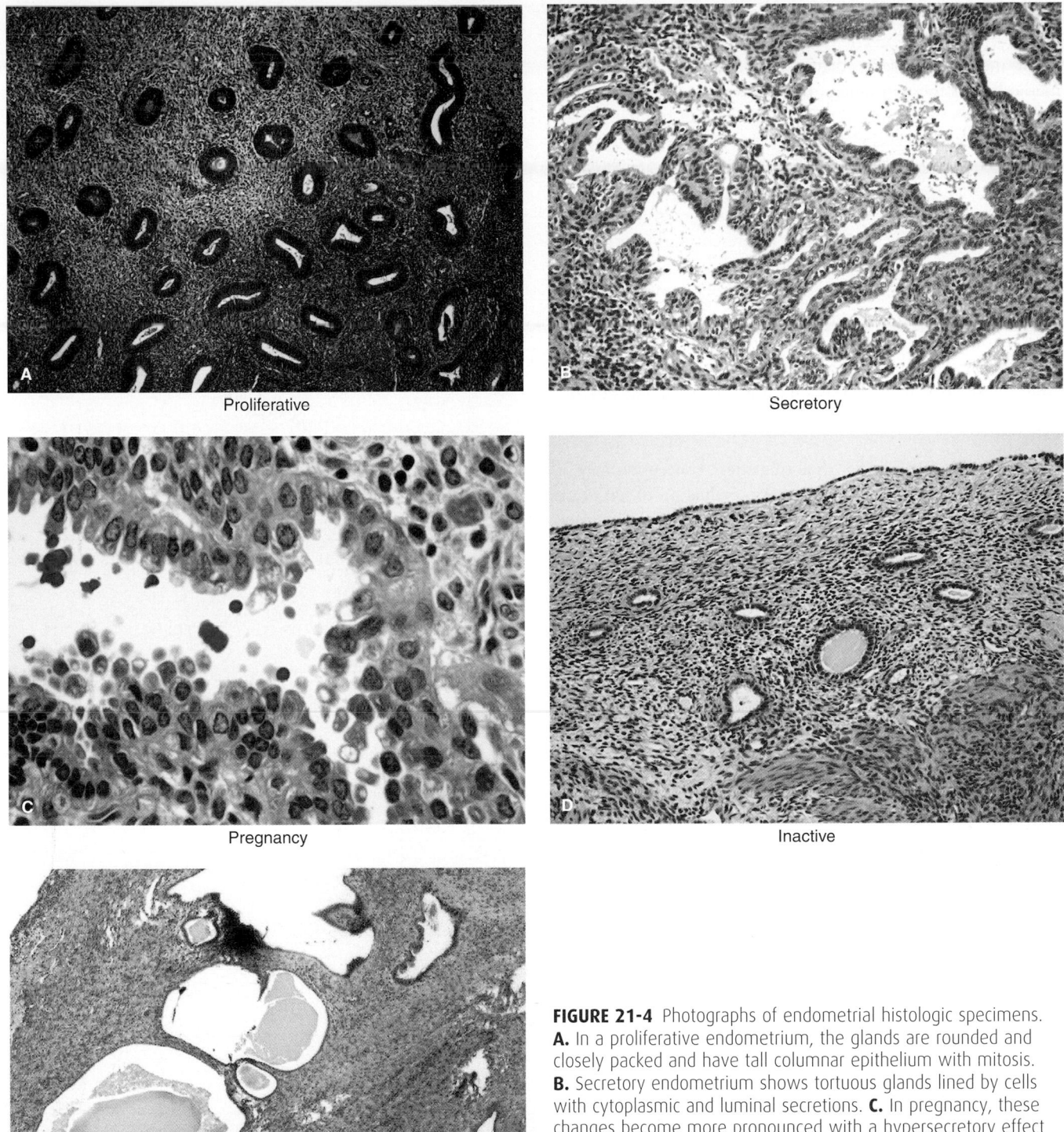

Proliferative

Secretory

Pregnancy

Inactive

Atrophic

FIGURE 21-4 Photographs of endometrial histologic specimens. **A.** In a proliferative endometrium, the glands are rounded and closely packed and have tall columnar epithelium with mitosis. **B.** Secretory endometrium shows tortuous glands lined by cells with cytoplasmic and luminal secretions. **C.** In pregnancy, these changes become more pronounced with a hypersecretory effect demonstrated by cell clearing and cytoplasmic blebs. **D.** Inactive endometrial tissue shows only scattered, inactive nonproliferating glands in the basalis. **E.** With endometrial atrophy, cystic changes can occur. *(Photographs contributed by Dr. Raheela Ashfaq.)*

age group, and in women aged ≥40 years, more than one third of all pregnancies are unintended (Finer, 2006). Importantly, pregnancy with advanced maternal age carries an increased risk for pregnancy-related morbidity and mortality. In selecting appropriate contraception for these women, several points should be considered. First, as described later, postmenopausal women display an increased rate of bone loss compared with

reproductive-aged women. Thus, depot medroxyprogesterone acetate (DMPA), which is associated with bone density loss with prolonged use, may not be a first-line choice for some women in menopausal transition. The American College of Obstetricians and Gynecologists (2008), however, has concluded that concerns of bone density loss should not prevent or limit use of this contraceptive method (Chap. 5, p. 158).

In addition to the normal physiologic changes of menopausal transition, women in this group may also have coexistent medical problems that preclude certain contraceptive methods. For these instances, the Centers for Disease Control and Prevention (2010) has created guidelines to aid the safe selection of contraception for women with certain health conditions. These U.S. Medical Eligibility Criteria are available online at: http://www.cdc.gov/mmwr/pdf/rr/rr59e0528.pdf. Lastly, symptoms related to physiologic changes of menopausal transition, such as hot flashes, may be present in this group and may be improved with hormonal methods.

Contraception can be discontinued by all women at the age of 55 years. No spontaneous pregnancies above that age have been reported. Some women may still have menstrual bleeding above this age, but ovulation is extremely rare and any oocytes are likely to be of poor quality and not viable (Gebbie, 2010).

Infertility

For women entering menopausal transition, conception may be difficult. For those desiring pregnancy, evaluation of fertility is often accelerated. In addition, infertility treatment may require assisted reproductive technologies, described in Chapter 20 (p. 529). Advanced maternal age during pregnancy is associated with increased risks. Among others, these include miscarriage, chromosomal abnormalities, cesarean delivery, gestational diabetes, pregnancy-induced hypertension, and stillbirth (Montan, 2007; Schoen, 2009). Accordingly, women entertaining conception would benefit from counseling on these risks.

◼ Central Thermoregulation Changes
Incidence

Of the many symptoms of menopause that may affect quality of life, the most common are symptoms related to thermoregulation. These vasomotor symptoms may be described as *hot flashes*, *hot flushes*, and *night sweats*. Kronenberg (1990) tabulated all of the published epidemiologic studies and determined that vasomotor symptoms developed in 11 to 60 percent of menstruating women during the transition. In the Massachusetts Women's Health Study, the incidence of hot flashes increased from 10 percent during the premenopausal period to approximately 50 percent after cessation of menses (McKinlay, 1992). Hot flashes begin an average of 2 years before the FMP, and 85 percent of women who experience them will continue to experience them for more than 1 year. Of these women, 25 to 50 percent will have hot flashes for 5 years, and >15 percent may experience them for >15 years (Kronenberg, 1990). Longitudinal studies have shown that hot flashes are associated with low exercise levels, smoking, high FSH and low estradiol levels, increasing body mass, ethnicity, socioeconomic status, and a history of premenstrual dysphoric disorder (PMDD) or depression (Gold, 2006; Guthrie, 2005).

Vasomotor Symptoms

Thermoregulatory and cardiovascular changes that accompany a hot flash have been well documented. An individual hot flash generally lasts 1 to 5 minutes, and skin temperatures rise because of peripheral vasodilation (Kronenberg, 1990).

This change is particularly marked in the fingers and toes, where skin temperature can increase 10 to 15°C. Most women sense a sudden wave of heat that spreads over the body, particularly on the upper body and face. Sweating begins primarily on the upper body, and it corresponds closely in time with an increase in skin conductance (Fig. 21-5). Sweating has been observed in women during 90 percent of hot flashes (Freedman, 2001).

Increases in both awake and sleep systolic blood pressure are noted with hot flashes (Gerber, 2007). In addition, heart rate increases 7 to 15 beats per minute at approximately the same time as peripheral vasodilatation and sweating. Heart rate and

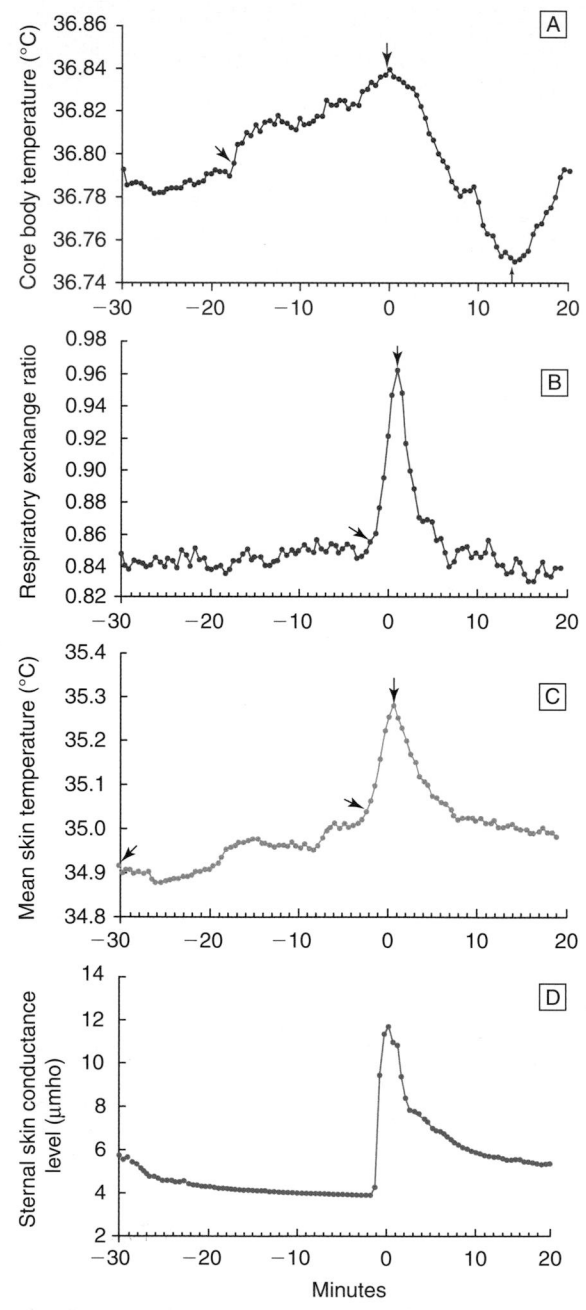

FIGURE 21-5 Physiologic changes (means) during a hot flash. **A.** Core body temperature. **B.** Respiratory exchange ratio. **C.** Skin temperature. **D.** Sternal skin conductance. Time 0 is the beginning of the sternal skin conductance response. *(Redrawn from Freedman, 1998, with permission.)*

skin blood flow usually peak within 3 minutes of the onset of the hot flash. Simultaneously with sweating and peripheral vasodilation, the metabolic rate also significantly rises. Hot flashes may also be accompanied by palpitations, anxiety, irritability, and panic.

Five to 9 minutes after a hot flash begins, core temperature decreases 0.1 to 0.9°C due to heat loss from perspiration and increased peripheral vasodilation (Molnar, 1981). If the heat loss and sweating are significant, a woman may experience chills. Skin temperature gradually returns to normal, sometimes taking 30 minutes or longer.

Pathophysiology of Vasomotor Symptoms

Despite the prevalence and impact of hot flashes, the pathophysiology of vasomotor symptoms is not clearly understood (Bachmann, 2005). Some dysfunction of central thermoregulatory centers in the hypothalamus is likely the cause of this common symptom. The medial preoptic area of the hypothalamus contains the thermoregulatory nucleus responsible for regulating perspiration and vasodilatation, which is the primary mechanism of heat loss in humans. If exposed to temperature changes, this nucleus activates these heat dissipation mechanisms. These maintain core body temperature in a regulated normal range, called the *thermoregulatory zone.*

Estrogens. Certainly, estrogens play a vital role in the development of hot flashes (Fig. 21-6). Although there is no clear correlation between the two, estrogen withdrawal or rapid fluctuation in levels, rather than low estrogen concentration, is suspected (Erlik, 1982; Overlie, 2002). This hypothesis is supported by the fact that women with gonadal dysgenesis (Turner syndrome), who lack normal estrogen levels, do not experience hot flashes unless first exposed to estrogen and then withdrawn from treatment.

Neurotransmitters. Although estrogen withdrawal clearly has a significant impact on hot flash development, recent research has demonstrated that other factors are involved (Bachmann, 2005). For example, Freedman (1998, 2001) hypothesized that changes in neurotransmitter levels may contribute to hot flashes. Altered neurotransmitter concentrations may create a narrow thermoregulatory zone and a lowered sweating threshold. Thus, even subtle changes in core body temperature may trigger heat loss mechanisms. The changes in levels of β-endorphins and other neurotransmitters affect the thermoregulatory center in the hypothalamus and make some women more prone to hot flashes (Pinkerton, 2009).

Norepinephrine. This is thought to be the primary neurotransmitter responsible for lowering the thermoregulatory set point and triggering the heat loss mechanisms associated with hot flashes (Rapkin, 2007). Plasma levels of norepinephrine metabolites are increased before and during hot flashes. Moreover, studies have shown that norepinephrine injections can increase core body temperature and induce a heat loss response (Freedman, 1990). Conversely, medications that decrease norepinephrine levels may reduce vasomotor symptoms (Laufer, 1982).

Estrogens are known to modulate adrenergic receptors in many tissues. Freedman (2001) suggested that hypothalamic

α_2-adrenergic receptors are decreased by menopause-related decreases in estrogen levels. They showed that a decline in presynaptic α_2-adrenergic receptors leads to increased norepinephrine levels, thereby causing vasomotor symptoms.

Serotonin. Also known as 5-hydroxytryptamine (5-HT), serotonin is likely to be another neurotransmitter that is involved in the pathophysiology of hot flashes (Slopien, 2003). Estrogen level fluctuations may increase the sensitivity of the hypothalamic serotonin 5-HT2A receptor. Specifically, estrogen withdrawal is associated with a decreased blood serotonin level, which is followed by upregulation of serotonin receptors in the hypothalamus. Activation of specific serotonin receptors has been shown to mediate heat loss (Gonzales, 1993). However, the role of serotonin in central regulatory pathways is complex because binding at some serotonin receptors can exert negative feedback on other serotonin receptor types (Bachmann, 2005). Therefore, the effect of a change in serotonin activity depends on the type of receptor activated.

In sum, these and other studies suggest that reductions and significant fluctuations in estradiol levels lead to a decline in inhibitory presynaptic α_2-adrenergic receptors and an increase in hypothalamic norepinephrine and serotonin release. Norepinephrine and serotonin lower the set point in the thermoregulatory nucleus and allow heat loss mechanisms to be triggered by subtle changes in core body temperature.

Sleep Dysfunction and Fatigue

Sleep disruption is a common complaint of women with hot flashes. Women may awake several times during the night and may be drenched in sweat. Disturbed sleep can lead to fatigue, irritability, depressive symptoms, cognitive dysfunction, and impaired daily functioning.

The relationship between hot flashes and impaired sleep has been studied (Table 21-2). Hollander and associates (2001) studied a cohort of late reproductive-aged women and found that women with a greater incidence of hot flashes were more likely to report poor sleep than were women with fewer vasomotor symptoms. Kravitz and colleagues (2003) found that the prevalence of sleep disturbance ranges from 32 to 40 percent in the early menopausal transition and from 38 to 46 percent in the late menopausal transition.

Many women begin to have prolonged feelings of fatigue, exhaustion, and lack of energy during menopausal transition. Fatigue may be related to night sweats and difficulty sleeping or an independent risk factor that is yet to be identified. Commonsense education for patients during menopausal transition may prove valuable (Table 21-3).

Risk Factors for Vasomotor Symptoms

Several risk factors have been associated with an increased probability of hot flashes. These include surgical menopause, race/ethnicity, body mass, and smoking. Surgical menopause is associated with a 90-percent probability of hot flashes during the first year after oophorectomy, and symptoms can be more abrupt and severe than those associated with natural menopause. Research has also demonstrated that the prevalence of vasomotor symptoms varies among racial and

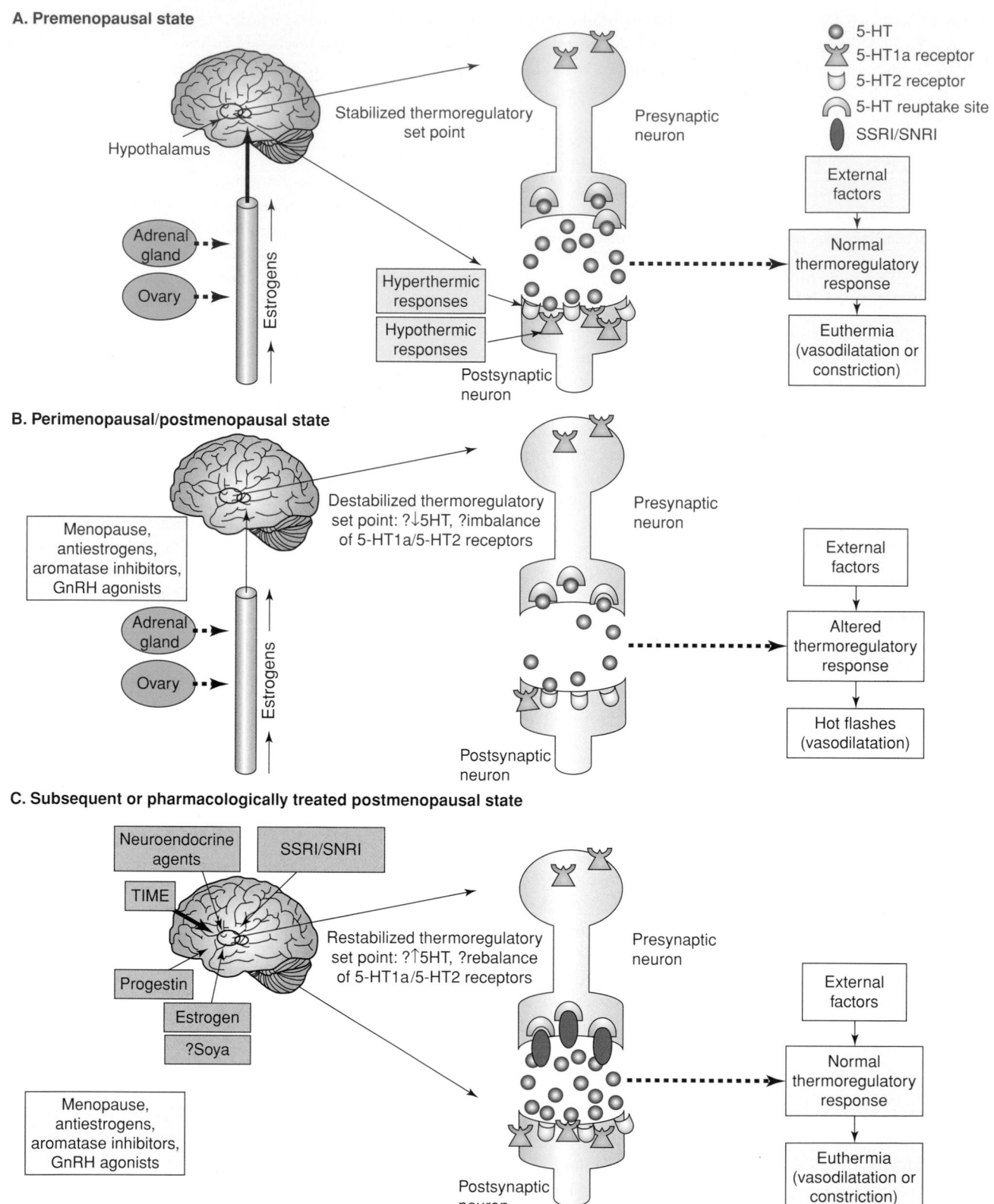

FIGURE 21-6 Diagram of the interactions between sex steroid hormones and serotonin in the central nervous system (CNS) and their effects on thermoregulatory response. A symbol legend is in the upper right corner. Serotonin (5-HT) receptors are those for the neurotransmitter serotonin. **A.** Estrogen stabilizes the CNS thermoregulatory set point and leads to a normal thermoregulatory response. **B.** During menopausal transition, decreased estrogen levels lead to instability of the set point and an altered response to external thermal stimuli. **C.** Gradually over time, the set point becomes stable again. Alternatively, pharmacologic intervention with exogenous estrogen or selective serotonin-reuptake inhibitors (SSRIs) may also stabilize the set point. 5-HT = 5-hydroxytryptamine; GnRH = gonadotropin-releasing hormone; SNRI = selective norepinephrine reuptake inhibitor. *(Redrawn from Stearns, 2002, with permission.)*

TABLE 21-2. Insomnia by Severity of Hot Flashes and Menopausal Symptoms

	Insomnia Symptoms ≥ 6 mo					
Variable	DIS	DMS	NRS	At Least One Symptom	GSD	DSM-IV Insomnia Diagnosis
Hot flashes (%)						
None (n = 673)	7.7	30.5	6.8	12.9	36.0	10.5
Mild (n = 172)	11.6	47.1	15.1	15.1	52.9	23.3
Moderate (n = 89)	19.1	56.2	25.8	28.1	66.3	30.3
Severe (n = 48)	35.4[a]	68.8[a]	35.4[a]	52.1[a]	81.3[a]	43.8[a]
Menopausal status (%)						
Premenopause (n = 562)	9.4	30.2[a]	9.3	15.3	36.5	13.0
Perimenopause (n = 219)	16.0	49.8	20.1[a]	23.3	56.6[a]	26.0
Postmenopause (n = 201)	9.0	44.8	8.0	12.9	50.7	14.4

[a]$p < .001$

DIS = difficulty initiating sleep; DMS = difficulty maintaining sleep; DSM-IV = *Diagnostic and Statistical Manual of Mental Disorders, Fourth Edition*; GSD = global sleep dissatisfaction; NRS = nonrestorative sleep.
From Ohayon, 2006, with permission.

ethnic groups. Hot flashes appear to be more common in African-American than in white women and are more common among white than among Asian women (Gold, 2001; Kuh, 1997).

The impact of body mass on hot flash frequency is not clear. Some investigators have reported that thinner women are more likely to experience hot flashes, whereas others have found that heavier women are more commonly affected (Erlik, 1982; Thurston, 2008; Wilbur, 1998). Other risk factors include early menopause, low circulating levels of estradiol, a sedentary lifestyle, smoking, and use of selective estrogen-receptor modulators (SERMs) (Bachmann, 2005). In addition, women exposed to high ambient temperatures may experience more frequent and severe hot flashes. Randolph (2005) found that the incidence of hot flashes in climates of 31°C may be four times as great as that in climates of 19°C. A thorough discussion of treatment options for hot flashes is found in Chapter 22 (p. 585).

Bone Metabolism and Structural Changes

Normal bone is a dynamic, living tissue that is in a continuous process of destruction and rebuilding. This bone remodeling, also described as *bone turnover*, allows adaptation to mechanical changes in weight bearing and other physical activities.

Bone Remodeling Physiology

The skeleton consists of two bone types (Fig. 21-7). Cortical bone is the bone of the peripheral skeleton (arms and legs) and accounts for 80 percent of total bone weight. Trabecular bone is the bone of the axial skeleton, which includes the spinal column, pelvis, hip, and proximal femur. The process of bone remodeling involves a constant resorption of bone, carried out by multinucleated giant cells known as *osteoclasts*, which mature originally from blood monocytes. A concurrent process of bone formation is completed by *osteoblasts*, which are a specialized tissue fibroblast (Fig. 21-8).

The osteoclast is the only bone-resorbing cell. Activated osteoclasts secrete hydrochloric acid and collagen degrading enzymes

TABLE 21-3. Fatigue Prevention Instructions

Obtain adequate sleep every night
Exercise regularly to reduce stress
Avoid long work hours and maintain your personal schedule
If stress is environmental, take vacations, switch jobs, or approach your company or family to help resolve sources of your stress
Limit intake of alcohol, drugs, and nicotine
Eat a healthy and well-balanced diet
Drink adequate amounts water (8 to 10 glasses) during the early part of the day
Consider seeing a specialist in menopausal medicine

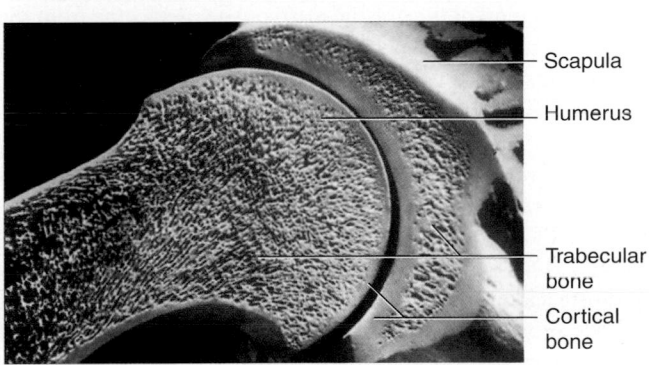

FIGURE 21-7 Photograph of bone with trabecular and cortical bone labeled. *(From Saladin, 2005, with permission.)*

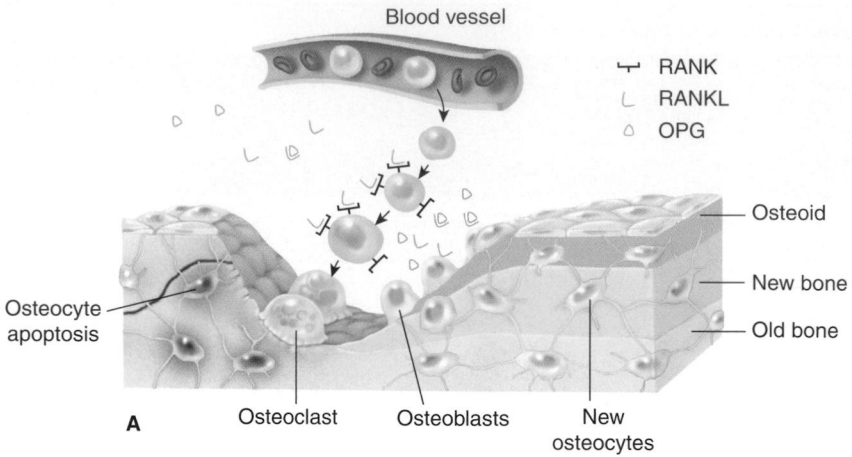

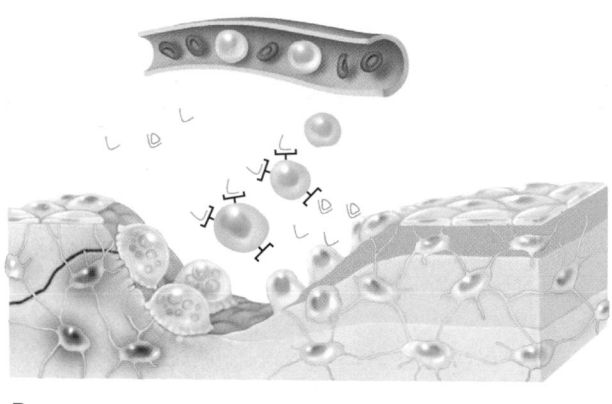

FIGURE 21-8 Bone remodeling. **A.** Osteoclasts resorb matrix, whereas osteoblasts deposit new lamellar bone. Osteoblasts that are trapped in the matrix become osteocytes. Others undergo apoptosis or form new, flattened osteoblast lining cells. Osteoblasts produce the proteins RANKL and OPG. When RANKL binds to RANK, which is a receptor on the surface of osteoclast progenitor cells, this promotes those cells' development, activity, and survival as osteoclasts. This leads to bone resorption. OPG serves as a counterbalance. OPG binds to RANKL, and thereby, RANKL is incapable of binding with RANK to promote osteoclast development. Through this mechanism, bone resorption is limited. **B.** With hypoestrogenism, RANKL production is increased. Excessive levels of RANKL outnumber those of OPG, and osteoclast development and bone resorption is favored. OPG = osteoprotegerin; RANK = receptor activator of nuclear factor kappa-β; RANKL = RANK ligand.

OPG is also secreted by osteoblasts and is a natural inhibitor of RANKL. OPG is able to bind RANKL. When bound to OPG, RANKL is unable then to bind to RANK. In this manner, OPG blocks RANKL-mediated activation of RANK and thereby blocks osteoclast activation and activity. This balances bone remodeling (Kostenuik, 2005).

Many different factors can affect osteoclast activity, but RANKL is required to mediate their effects on bone resorption. Cytokines and certain hormones stimulate the expression of RANKL by osteoblasts and other cells. One regulator of this process is estrogen.

Estrogen Effects on Bone Remodeling

In healthy premenopausal women, estrogen limits the expression of RANKL from osteoblasts and thus limits osteoclast formation and bone resorption. Estrogen also increases OPG production by osteoblasts. The OPG binds to RANKL to further limit RANKL availability to stimulate osteoclasts. The remaining RANKL binds to osteoclast precursors. These fuse, form differentiated osteoclasts, and initiate bone resorption. Resorption is followed by the appearance of osteoblasts that rebuild bone. Ultimately, resorption and formation are balanced in premenopausal women.

In postmenopausal women, decreased estrogen levels lead to increased RANK ligand expression. This overproduction may overwhelm the natural competitive activity of OPG. As a result, excess RANKL is available to bind to RANK on osteoclast precursors. This can lead to an increase in osteoclast number, activity, and life span and may decrease rates of osteoclast apoptosis. Bone resorption follows, but osteoblasts can only partially fill resorption pits. This chronic imbalance of formation and resorption creates ongoing bone loss. Thus, increased RANKL after menopause leads to excessive bone resorption and potentially postmenopausal osteoporosis.

Peak bone mass is influenced by heredity and endocrine factors, and there is only a relatively narrow window of opportunity in the younger years for acquiring bone mass. Almost all bone mass in the hip and the vertebral bodies will be accumulated in young women by late adolescence. Thus, the years immediately following menarche (ages 11 to 14 years) are especially important (Sabatier, 1996; Theintz, 1992). Following this peak, bone resorption is normally coupled to bone formation such that positive bone balance is achieved when skeletal maturity is attained, typically at ages 25 to 35 years.

onto the bone surface. This leads to bone mineral dissolution and degradation of the organic matrix. After detaching from the organic matrix, the osteoclasts can relocate and begin resorption at another site on the bone surface or undergo apoptosis.

Increased osteoclast activity in postmenopausal osteoporosis is mediated by the *receptor activator of nuclear factor kappa-B (RANK) ligand* pathway. The three major components of this pathway are RANK, RANK ligand (RANKL), and osteoprotegerin (OPG) (Table 21-4). First, RANKL is produced by osteoblasts. RANKL binds to RANK found on the surface osteoclasts and osteoclast precursors (Bar-Shavit, 2007). This activation of RANK promotes osteoclast formation, function, and survival. As such, RANKL is the common regulator of osteoclast activity and ultimately, of bone resorption.

TABLE 21-4. Key Components of the RANKL/RANK/ OPG Pathway

RANK ligand (RANKL)
Protein expressed by osteoblasts/bone lining cells
Binds to RANK
Activation of RANK promotes osteoclast formation, function, and survival

RANK
Expressed by osteoclasts and their precursor
Activated by RANKL binding

Osteoprotegerin (OPG)
Protein secreted by osteoblasts/bone lining cells
Natural competitor of RANKL
Blocks RANKL-mediated activation of RANK and thereby blocks osteoclast formation to balance bone remodeling

RANK = receptor activator of nuclear factor kappa-β.

Thereafter, bone mass declines at a slow, steady rate of approximately 0.4 percent each year. During menopause, the rate increases to 2 to 5 percent per year for the first 5 to 10 years and then slows to 1 percent per year. The subsequent risk of fracture from osteoporosis will depend on bone mass at the time of menopause and the rate of bone loss following menopause (Riis, 1996).

Osteopenia and Osteoporosis

Incidence

Osteoporosis is a skeletal disorder that compromises bone strength due to a progressive reduction in bone mass (typically greater in trabecular bone) and can cause an increased risk for fracture. Osteopenia is the precursor to osteoporosis.

The estimated number of individuals with osteoporosis or osteopenia continues to increase. The National Osteoporosis Foundation (NOF) (2002) estimates that more than 10 million Americans currently have osteoporosis and another 33.6 million have osteopenia of the hip. In white women aged 50 years, epidemiologic studies from North America have estimated the remaining lifetime risk of common fragility fractures to be 17.5 percent for hip fracture, 15.6 percent for clinically diagnosed vertebral fracture, and 16.0 percent for distal forearm fracture (Holroyd, 2008).

Osteoporosis Sequelae

Fractures are the most debilitating and costly consequence of osteoporosis. Approximately 1.5 million Americans experience osteoporotic fractures each year. Worldwide it is estimated that there are 9 million osteoporotic fractures per year, leading to 5.8 million person-years of disability or loss of life (Johnell, 2006; Lund, 2008). The spine, hip, and wrists are most commonly fractured (Kanis, 1994). Osteoporotic fractures are associated with significant morbidity and mortality rates, and the risk of dying following a clinical fracture is reportedly twofold higher than for persons without fractures. The overall mortality

rate from hip fracture alone is estimated to be 30 percent. In addition, only 40 percent of those who sustain a hip fracture are capable of returning to their prefracture level of independence. Given the potentially devastating effects of osteoporosis-related fractures, educating patients regarding bone loss prevention, screening to identify bone loss early, and working with patients to develop effective management plans for osteoporosis or osteopenia are critical. Treatments for osteoporosis include calcium therapy coupled with weight-bearing exercise or pharmacologic therapy and are discussed in Chapter 22 (p. 590).

Osteoporosis Pathophysiology

Osteoporosis is a skeletal disease in which bone strength is compromised, resulting in an increased risk for fracture. A major proportion of bone strength is determined by bone mineral density (BMD). This explains why BMD measurements are effective tools for identifying patients at high risk for fractures. BMD refers to the grams of mineral per volume of bone and is assessed relatively easily during dual-energy x-ray absorptiometry (DEXA) measurement. However, bone quality, bone strength, and fracture risk are affected by other qualities of bone. These include rates of remodeling, bone size and geometry, microarchitecture, mineralization, damage accumulation, and matrix quality. These parameters are more difficult to determine accurately (Kiebzak, 2003).

Primary osteoporosis refers to bone loss associated with aging and menopausal estrogen deficiency. As estrogen levels fall after menopause, this hormone's regulatory effect on bone resorption is lost. As a result, bone resorption is accelerated and is usually not balanced by compensatory bone formation. This accelerated bone loss is most rapid in the early postmenopausal years (Gallagher, 2002). If osteoporosis is caused by other diseases or medications, the term *secondary osteoporosis* is used (Stein, 2003).

The amount of bone at any point in time reflects the balance of the osteoblastic (building) and osteoclastic (resorbing) activities, which are influenced by a multitude of stimulating and inhibiting agents (Canalis, 2007). As noted earlier, both aging and a loss of estrogen lead to a significant increase in osteoclastic activity. In addition, a decrease in calcium intake or impaired absorption of calcium from the gut lowers the serum level of ionized calcium. This stimulates parathyroid hormone (PTH) secretion to mobilize calcium from bone by stimulation of osteoclastic activity (Fig. 21-9). Specifically, increased PTH levels prompt the production of vitamin D. In turn, increases in vitamin D levels lead to elevated serum calcium levels by several effects: (1) stimulating osteoclasts to remove calcium from bone, (2) increasing intestinal calcium absorption, and (3) stimulating renal calcium reabsorption (Holick, 2007).

In normal premenopausal women, this series of events leads to increased serum calcium levels, and PTH levels return to normal. In postmenopausal women, however, estrogen deficiency leads to a greater responsiveness of bone to PTH. Thus, for any given level of PTH, there is more calcium removed from bone.

As described in Chapter 22 (p. 595), calcium supplementation is encouraged for postmenopausal women to sustain adequate calcium levels. One effect is to block the effects of PTH

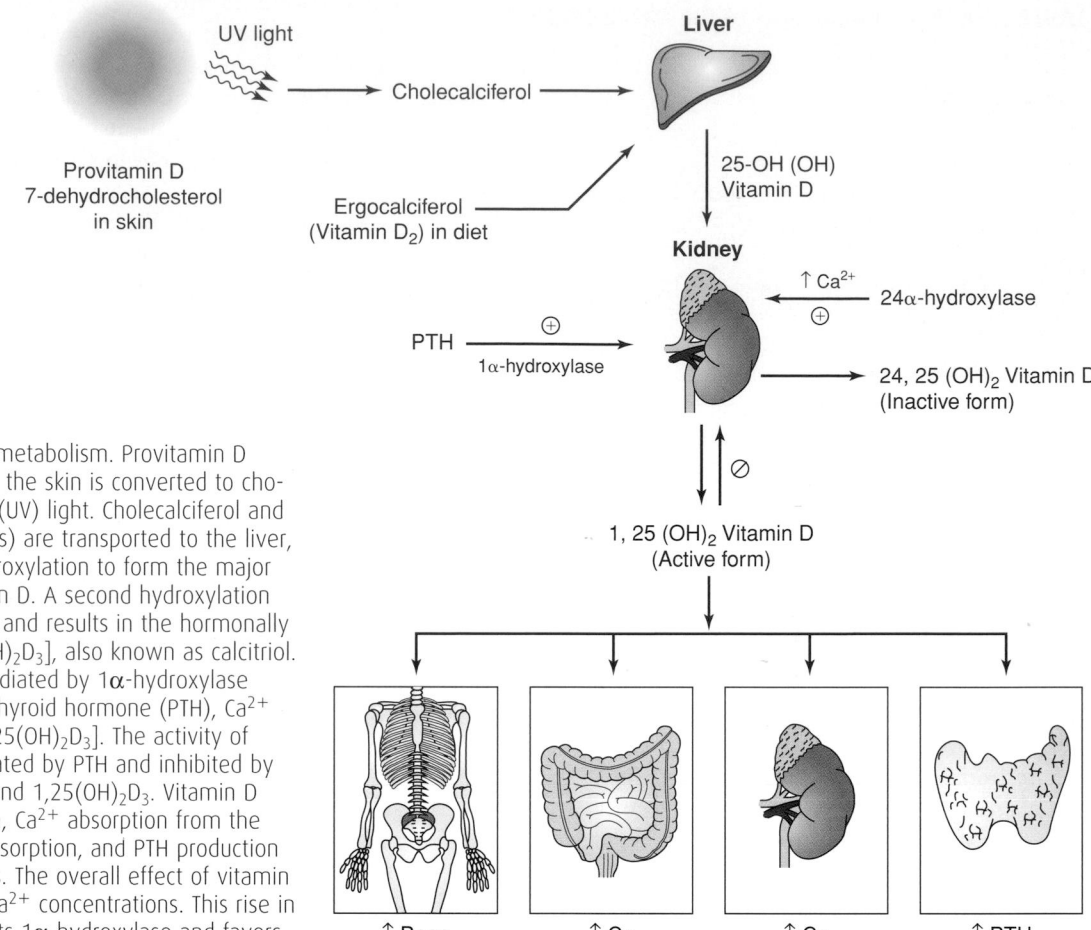

FIGURE 21-9 Vitamin D metabolism. Provitamin D (7-dehydrocholesterol) in the skin is converted to cholecalciferol by ultraviolet (UV) light. Cholecalciferol and ergocalciferol (from plants) are transported to the liver, where they undergo hydroxylation to form the major circulating form of vitamin D. A second hydroxylation step occurs in the kidney and results in the hormonally active vitamin D [1,25(OH)$_2$D$_3$], also known as calcitriol. This activation step is mediated by 1α-hydroxylase and is regulated by parathyroid hormone (PTH), Ca^{2+} levels, and vitamin D [1,25(OH)$_2$D$_3$]. The activity of 1α-hydroxylase is stimulated by PTH and inhibited by sufficient levels of Ca^{2+} and 1,25(OH)$_2$D$_3$. Vitamin D increases bone resorption, Ca^{2+} absorption from the intestine, renal Ca^{2+} reabsorption, and PTH production by the parathyroid glands. The overall effect of vitamin D is to increase plasma Ca^{2+} concentrations. This rise in plasma Ca^{2+} levels inhibits 1α-hydroxylase and favors hydroxylation at C-24. This leads to synthesis of an inactive vitamin D metabolite—24,25(OH)$_2$D$_3$. (*Redrawn from Molina, 2010, with permission.*)

on bone reabsorption. In addition, vitamin D supplementation is also suggested for this group. Although this vitamin activates osteoclasts, its cumulative positive effects on gut absorption and renal calcium reabsorption allow it to serve as one aid in bone loss prevention.

Diagnosis of Osteoporosis

BMD is the standard used for bone mass determination and is assessed with DEXA of the lumbar spine, radius, and hip (Fig. 21-10) (Marshall, 1996). The lumbar spine contains primarily trabecular bone, which comprises 20 percent of skeletal weight. This bone is less dense than cortical bone and has a faster bone remodeling rate. Therefore, early rapid bone loss can be determined by evaluation of this site. Cortical bone is denser and more compact bone and comprises 80 percent of skeletal weight. The greater trochanter and femoral neck contain both cortical and trabecular bone, and these sites are ideal for the prediction of hip fracture risk in older women (Miller, 2002).

Normative bone mineral density values for sex, age, and ethnicity have been determined. For diagnostic purposes, results of BMD testing should be reported as *T-scores*. These measure in standard deviations (SDs) the variance of an individual's BMD

from that expected for a person of the same sex at peak bone mass (25 to 30 years). A T-score of –2.0 in a woman, for example, means that her BMD is two SDs below the average peak bone mass for a young woman. Definitions from the National Osteoporosis Foundation include those found in Table 21-5. A fourth category, "severe osteoporosis," has been suggested to describe patients who have a T-score below –2.5 and who have also suffered a fragility fracture. These are fractures caused by a fall from standing height or lower.

TABLE 21-5. Criteria for Interpretation of Bone Mineral Density

Normal BMD is defined as a T-score between +2.5 and –1.0. As such, the patient's BMD lies between 2.5 standard deviations (SDs) above the young adult mean and 1 SD below the young adult mean.

Osteopenia (low BMD) is associated with a T-score between –1.0 and –2.5, inclusive.

Osteoporosis is defined as a T-score lower than –2.5.

From the National Osteoporosis Foundation, 2010.

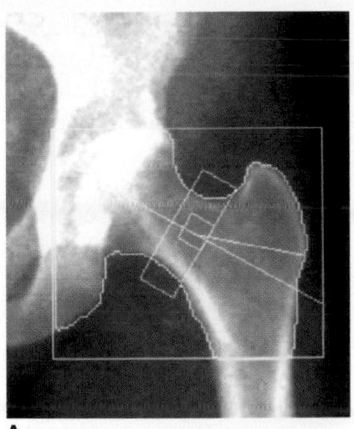

A

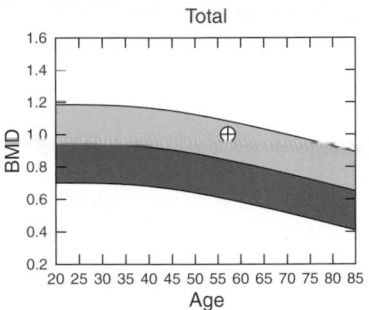

DXA Results Summary:

Region	Area (cm²)	BMC (g)	BMD (g/cm²)	T - Score	Z - Score
Neck	4.59	3.79	0.827	−0.2	1.0
Troch	8.57	6.65	0.775	0.7	1.5
Inter	14.62	17.48	1.196	0.6	1.2
Total	**27.79**	**27.92**	**1.005**	**0.5**	**1.3**
Ward's	1.12	0.71	0.639	−0.8	1.0

Total BMD CV 1.0%, ACF = 1.028, BCF = 0.998, TH = 6.508
WHO Classification: Normal
Fracture Risk: Not Increased

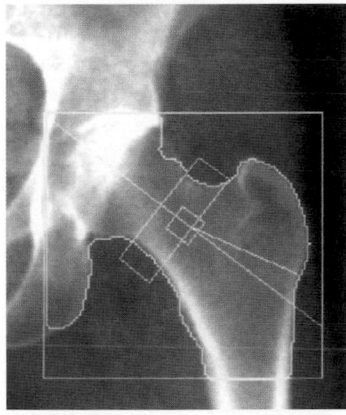

B

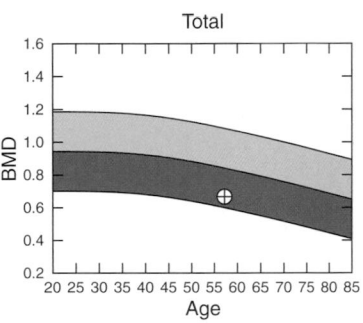

DXA Results Summary:

Region	Area (cm²)	BMC (g)	BMD (g/cm²)	T - Score	Z - Score
Neck	4.97	2.74	0.552	−2.7	−1.4
Troch	11.53	5.62	0.487	−2.1	−1.3
Inter	18.92	14.78	0.781	−2.1	−1.4
Total	**35.43**	**23.14**	**0.653**	**−2.4**	**−1.4**
Ward's	1.16	0.38	0.331	−3.4	−1.5

Total BMD CV 1.0%
WHO Classification: Osteopenia
Fracture Risk: Increased

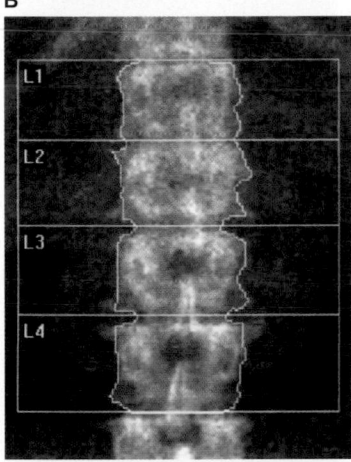

C

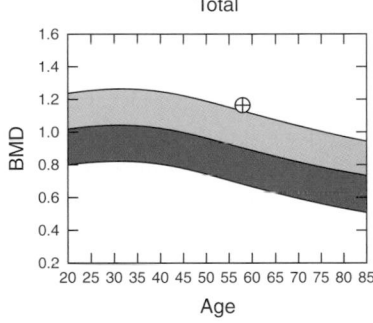

DXA Results Summary:

Region	Area (cm²)	BMC (g)	BMD (g/cm²)	T - Score	Z - Score
L1	12.00	12.73	1.061	1.2	2.3
L2	13.37	14.93	1.116	0.8	2.0
L3	14.03	16.56	1.181	0.9	2.1
L4	15.80	20.23	1.280	1.5	2.8
Total	**55.20**	**64.45**	**1.168**	**1.1**	**2.3**

Total BMD CV 1.0%
WHO Classification: Normal
Fracture Risk: Not Increased

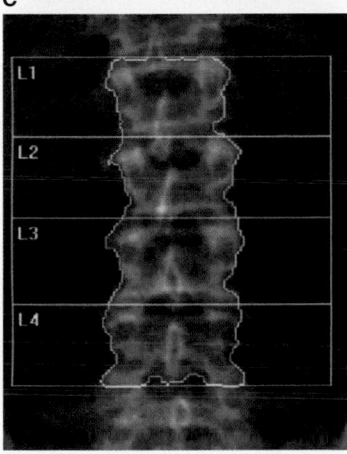

D

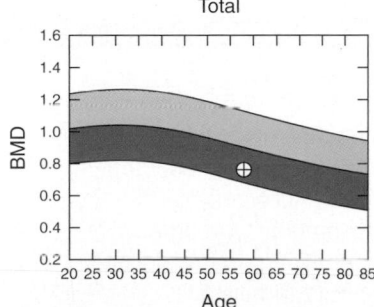

DXA Results Summary:

Region	Area (cm²)	BMC (g)	BMD (g/cm²)	T - Score	Z - Score
L1	11.73	8.03	0.684	−2.2	−1.0
L2	12.60	9.70	0.770	−2.3	−1.0
L3	14.59	11.70	0.802	−2.6	−1.1
L4	14.44	11.01	0.763	−3.2	−1.7
Total	**53.36**	**40.44**	**0.758**	**−2.6**	**−1.2**

Total BMD CV 1.0%, ACF = 1.028, BCF = 0.998, TH = 5.974
WHO Classification: Osteoporosis
Fracture Risk: High

FIGURE 21-10 Dual-energy x-ray absorptiometry (DEXA) scans and scan reports. **A.** DEXA report describing normal hip density. **B.** DEXA report describing osteopenia of the hip. **C.** DEXA report describing normal vertebral body density. **D.** DEXA report describing vertebral body osteoporosis. BMC = bone mineral content; BMD = bone mineral density.

TABLE 21-6. Secondary Causes of Osteoporosis and Recommended Testing

Primary hyper-parathyroidism	Serum levels of: Parathyroid hormone Calcium Phosphorus Alkaline phosphatase
Secondary hyperparathyroidism from chronic renal failure	Renal function tests
Hyperthyroidism	Thyroid function tests
Increased calcium excretion	24-hour urine for Ca^{2+} and creatinine levels
Hypercortisolism Alcohol abuse Metastatic cancer	Careful history Indicated testing
Osteomalacia	Serum levels of: Calcium Phosphorus Alkaline phosphatase 1,25(OH)$_2$ vitamin D

Patients will also be assigned a *Z-score,* which is the standard deviation between the patient's measurement and average bone mass for a patient with the same age and weight. Z-scores lower than –2.0 (2.5 percent of the normal population of the same age) require diagnostic evaluation for secondary osteoporosis, which includes causes other than menopausal bone loss (Faulkner, 1999). Similarly, any patient with osteoporosis should be screened for other conditions that lead to osteoporosis (Table 21-6).

The relation between BMD and fracture risk has been calculated in a large number of studies. A metaanalysis by Marshall and colleagues (1996) showed that BMD is still the most read-ily quantifiable predictor of fracture risk for those who have not yet suffered a fragility fracture. For each standard deviation of BMD below a baseline level (either mean peak bone mass or mean for the reference population of the person's age and sex), the fracture risk approximately doubles.

Fracture Risk Assessment Tool. Accurately measuring bone mass and bone quality and determining best practices for the clinical management of those with low bone mass is difficult. For this reason, the World Health Organization (2004) developed the Fracture Risk Assessment Tool (FRAX) to assess individual 10-year fracture risk. The algorithm, however, is applicable only for patients who have not received pharmacotherapy.

The FRAX tool is accessible online and is available for multiple countries and in different languages at http://www.shef.ac.uk/FRAX/. The online tool incorporates 11 risk factors and the femoral neck raw BMD value in g/cm^2 to calculate the 10-year fracture risk probability. The site also offers downloadable charts for calculating fracture risks using body mass index (BMI) or BMD.

The FRAX algorithm identifies patients who might benefit from pharmacotherapy. It is most useful for recognizing those persons whose BMD falls within the low bone mass range, that is, the osteopenic category.

Prevention

Many factors have been suggested as predictors of risk for osteoporotic fractures (Table 21-7). The most important predictive factors are bone density in combination with age, fracture history, ethnicity, various drug treatments, weight loss, and physical fitness. The presence of a key risk factor should alert a clinician to the need for further assessment and possibly active intervention.

Prophylaxis for osteoporosis with weight-bearing exercise and with vitamin D and calcium intake should begin in adolescence (Recker, 1992). Calcium supplementation in prepubertal and pubertal girls improves bone accrual, an important effect that should have long-lasting beneficial consequences (Bonjour, 2001; Rozen, 2003; Stear, 2003).

TABLE 21-7. Osteoporosis Risk Factors

Major Risk Factors	Minor Risk Factors
Age >65 years	Rheumatoid arthritis
Vertebral compression fracture	Prior history of clinical hyperthyroidism
Fragility fracture after age 40	Chronic anticonvulsant therapy
Family history of osteoporotic fracture	Low dietary calcium intake
Systemic glucocorticoid therapy of >3 months' duration	Smoker
Malabsorption syndrome	Excessive alcohol intake
Primary hyperparathyroidism	Excessive caffeine intake
Propensity to fall	Weight <57 kg
Osteopenia apparent on radiography	>10 percent weight loss at age 25
Hypogonadism	Chronic heparin therapy
Early menopause (before age 45)	

Bone Mineral Density. This characteristic of bone is currently the best quantifiable predictor of osteoporotic fracture. Low BMD and other major risk factors combine to further increase a person's risk of fracture. Therefore, BMD should be measured in a postmenopausal woman older than 50 years with one of the other major risk factors for fracture or in any woman older than 65 (see Table 21-7).

Risk factors for osteoporotic fracture are not independent of one another. They are additive and must be considered in the context of baseline age and sex-related risks of fracture. For example, a 55-year-old woman with low BMD is at significantly less risk than a 75-year-old woman with the same low BMD. Similarly, a woman with low BMD and a prior fragility fracture is at considerably greater risk than another person with the same low BMD and no prior fracture.

Osteoporotic fractures occur most commonly in men and women older than 65 years. Medical interventions have only been demonstrated to be effective in preventing fractures in populations with an average age older than 65 years. However, most currently approved osteoporosis therapies prevent or reverse bone loss if initiated at, or soon after, age 50. Therefore, it seems prudent to begin the identification of people at high risk for osteoporosis in their 50s.

Fragility Fracture. As stated earlier, a prior fragility fracture places a person at increased risk for another fracture. The increased risk is 1.5- to 9.5-fold depending on age at assessment, number of prior fractures, and site of the incident fracture (Melton, 1999). Vertebral fractures have been best studied in this regard. The presence of a vertebral fracture increases the risk of a second vertebral fracture at least fourfold. A study of a placebo group in a major clinical trial showed that 20 percent of those who experienced a vertebral fracture during the period of observation had a second vertebral fracture within 1 year (Lindsay, 2001). Vertebral fractures are also indicators of increased risk of fragility fractures at other sites, such as the hip. Similarly, wrist fractures predict vertebral and hip fractures.

Aging. Age is clearly a major contributor to fracture risk. As summarized in a review by Kanis and associates (2001), the 10-year probability of experiencing a fracture of the forearm, humerus, spine, or hip increases as much as eightfold between ages 45 and 85 years for women.

Race. Osteoporosis is most common in menopausal white women. Although persons of any ethnicity can develop osteoporosis, data from the Third National Health and Nutrition Examination Survey (NHANES III) indicate that the risk is highest among non-Hispanic white and Asian women and lowest among non-Hispanic black women (Looker, 1995).

Genetics. Genetic influence on osteoporosis and BMD is extremely important. It has been estimated that heredity accounts for 50 to 80 percent of BMD variability (Ralston, 2002). These influences have been the subject of major scientific investigations, and a number of genes have been associated with osteoporosis. These discoveries, however, have yet to result in a clinical application. A family history of osteoporotic fracture has been best studied with respect to hip fracture. The Study of Osteoporotic Fractures, for example, identified a maternal history of hip fracture as a key risk factor for hip fracture in a population of elderly women (Cummings, 1995). In addition, a history of hip fracture in a maternal grandmother also carries an increased risk of this fracture.

Fall Precautions. Fractures are frequently associated with falls. Nearly one third of patients over age 65 fall at least once per year. Approximately 1 in 10 falls in this age group results in severe injury such as hip fracture or subdural hematoma (Tinetti, 1988, 2003). To prevent falls in the elderly, the American Geriatric Society and British Geriatric Society (2011) recommend screening questions to include whether a patient: (1) has had two or more falls in the last year, (2) has difficulty with walking or balance, or (3) is presenting for care after an acute fall. An affirmative reply or physical findings of a disturbed gait should prompt a more thorough search and correction of the factors in (Table 21-8).

Systemic Glucocorticoids. Therapy with glucocorticoids lasting more than 2 to 3 months is a major risk factor for bone loss and fracture, particularly among postmenopausal women and men older than 50 years. Most reviews and guidelines consider a daily dose of prednisone that is ≥ 7.5 mg to be the threshold for assessment and clinical intervention to prevent or treat glucocorticoid-induced osteoporosis (Canalis, 1996).

TABLE 21-8. Fall Risk Factors

Physiologic changes
Prior falls
Diminished balance
Reduced muscle mass

Comorbid conditions
Arthritis
Arrhythmia
Alcohol abuse
Gait disorders
Balance disorders
Visual impairment
Cognitive impairment
Orthostatic hypotension

Environmental
Poor lighting
Unsafe footwear
Telephone cords
Cluttered hallways
Loose rugs on floors
Slippery or damaged flooring
No support bars in tub or toilet areas

Medications
Narcotics
Anticonvulsants
Antiarrhythmic agents
Psychiatric medications
Antihypertensive agents

Screening. As a result of these risk factors, programs to confirm osteoporosis and determine disease severity should include BMD measurements in all postmenopausal women who: (1) are aged 65 years or older, (2) have one or more risk factors for osteoporosis, or (3) have sustained fractures. Additionally, screening is recommended for perimenopausal women if they have a specific risk factor such as a prior low-trauma fracture or low body weight, or if they are taking a medication known for increasing the risk of bone loss. If therapy to increase bone mineral density is instituted, density should be monitored.

Cardiovascular Changes

Cardiovascular Disease Risk

Cardiovascular disease (CVD) remains the leading overall cause of death in women. Of all female deaths in 2007, 25 percent were caused by heart disease, and 6.7 percent were linked to stroke (Heron, 2011). An estimated 43 million women, or 35 percent of the total American female population, suffer from CVD (Roger, 2011). Most cardiovascular disease develops from atherosclerotic changes in the major blood vessels. Risk factors are the same for men and women and include nonmodifiable risk factors such as age and family history of cardiovascular disease. Modifiable cardiovascular risk factors include hypertension, dyslipidemia, obesity, diabetes mellitus or glucose intolerance, cigarette smoking, poor diet, and lack of physical activity. As discussed in Chapter 1 (p. 21), the first four of these risks factors are components of the metabolic syndrome, which is in itself a strong predictor of cardiovascular morbidity and mortality (Malik, 2004).

Before menopause, women have a much lower risk for cardiovascular events compared with men their age. Reasons for protection from CVD in premenopausal women are complex, but a significant contribution can be assigned to the greater high-density lipoprotein (HDL) levels in younger women, which is an effect of estrogen. However, after menopause this benefit disappears over time such that a 70-year-old woman begins to have a risk identical to that of a comparably aged male (Matthews, 1989). The risk of CVD increases exponentially for women as they enter the postmenopause and estrogen levels decline (Matthews, 1994; van Beresteijn, 1993). This becomes vitally important for women in menopausal transition, when preventive measures can significantly improve both the quality and the quantity of their lives. Statistics indicate that one in three women older than 65 years has some evidence of CVD. By age 55, 20 percent of all deaths are caused by CVD, and 30 to 40 percent of women eventually die of CVD.

The relationship between menopause and CVD incidence was first examined in the Framingham cohort of 2873 women (Kannel, 1987). There was a trend for a two- to sixfold higher incidence of CVD in postmenopausal women compared with premenopausal women in the same age range. This pattern is similar to that seen with the incidence of osteoporosis, which increases dramatically during menopausal transition. Moreover, the increases in CVD associated with menopausal transition are observed regardless of the age at menopause. These and other data indicate that withdrawal of estrogen may be associated with an increased risk of CVD.

Cardiovascular Disease Prevention

Because most risk factors for CVD are modifiable, significant reduction in cardiovascular morbidity and mortality rates is feasible. Therefore, clinicians should offer strategies to their postmenopausal patients that help to prevent or delay CVD (Table 1-17, p. 22). Since recent data have questioned the widespread prescription of hormonal treatment to avert this common problem, other strategies must be considered. Lifestyle interventions that have been shown to be useful and effective include smoking cessation, physical activity of moderate intensity for 30 minutes per day, maintenance of appropriate weight, and following a heart-healthy diet. More specific effective risk factor interventions include maintaining optimal blood pressure and lipid levels through lifestyle approaches and when necessary, with pharmacotherapy (Mosca, 2011). The cardiovascular benefits of physical activity were studied as a part of the Women's Health Initiative (WHI) study. Manson and colleagues (2002) identified the cardiovascular benefits of physical activity. They determined that walking—as well as vigorous exercise—prevented cardiovascular events in postmenopausal women regardless of age, BMI, or ethnic background. As expected, a sedentary lifestyle correlated directly with an increase in the risk for a coronary event (McKechnie, 2001).

Central adiposity is a risk factor for coronary heart disease in women and is associated with a relatively androgenic hormonal state. Central fat distribution, also termed truncal obesity, in women is positively correlated with increases in total cholesterol, triglyceride, and LDL levels, and negatively correlated with HDL levels (Haarbo, 1989). This atherogenic lipid profile associated with abdominal adiposity is at least partly mediated through interplay with insulin and estrogen. A strong correlation exists between the magnitude of the worsening in cardiovascular risk factors (lipid and lipoprotein changes, blood pressure, and insulin levels) and the amount of weight gained during menopausal transition (Wing, 1991). Davies (2001) and Matthews (2001) and their associates have shown that weight gain at menopause is not an effect of hormonal changes, but rather reflects diet, exercise, and a reduction of metabolic rate associated with aging.

Aspirin Therapy. Aspirin has been shown to be effective in the *secondary* prevention of cardiovascular disease in both men and women (Antithrombotic Trialists' Collaboration, 2002). However, data are limited on the role of low-dose aspirin in *primary* prevention of cardiovascular disease in women. The largest single randomized trial to address this issue indicates that among women 45 and older, there is a nonsignificant reduction in all major cardiovascular events of 9 percent with low-dose aspirin use. There is a significant 17-percent reduction in the risk of stroke. Among women 65 years and older, significant reductions were noted in all categories of cardiovascular events. This included a 30-percent reduction in ischemic stroke and a 34-percent reduction in myocardial infarction (Cook, 2005). In general, aspirin should not be used for primary prevention of heart disease in women under the age of 65 unless individual health benefits are judged to outweigh risks. These risks primarily involve bleeding episodes such as hemorrhagic stroke and gastrointestinal bleeding (Lund, 2008).

Lipids

Physiologic levels of estrogen are known to help maintain favorable lipoprotein profiles in women. Specifically, throughout adulthood, HDL levels are approximately 10 mg/dL higher in women, and this difference continues throughout the postmenopausal years. Moreover, total cholesterol and low-density lipoprotein (LDL) levels are lower in premenopausal women than in men (Jensen, 1990; Matthews, 1989). After menopause and with the subsequent decrease in estrogen, this favorable effect on lipids is lost. High-density lipoprotein levels decrease and total cholesterol levels increase.

After menopause, the risk of coronary heart disease doubles for women and at approximately age 60, the atherogenic lipids reach levels higher than those in men. Brunner (1987) and Jacobs (1990), with their colleagues, have prospectively documented the strong association between total cholesterol and coronary heart disease in women, although coronary heart disease risk appears at higher total cholesterol levels for women than for men. Women with a total cholesterol concentration greater than 265 mg/dL have rates of coronary heart disease three times those of women with low or normal levels. A low HDL-cholesterol level is also a strong predictor of CVD in women. The average HDL cholesterol in women is 55 to 60 mg/dL, and a decrease in HDL cholesterol of 10 mg/dL increases coronary heart disease risk by 40 to 50 percent (Kannel, 1987).

Despite these changes in atherogenic lipids following menopause, total cholesterol and LDL levels can be favorably reduced by dietary modifications, estrogen treatment, and lipid-lowering medications (Chap. 1, p. 23) (Matthews, 1994).

Coagulation

Changes in clotting parameters are known to occur with aging. Fibrinogen, plasminogen activator inhibitor-1, and factor VII levels increase and cause a relatively hypercoagulable state. This is thought to contribute to increases in cardiovascular and cerebrovascular disease in older women.

Weight Gain and Fat Distribution

Weight gain is a common complaint among women in the menopausal transition. With aging, a woman's metabolism slows, reducing her caloric requirements. If eating and exercise habits are not altered, weight is gained (Matthews, 2001). Specifically, Espeland and colleagues (1997) characterized the weight and fat distribution of 875 women in the Postmenopausal Estrogen/Progestin Interventions (PEPI) trial and correlated the impact of lifestyle, clinical, and demographic factors. They found that women aged 45 to 54 years had significantly greater increases in weight and in hip circumference than those aged 55 to 65 years. They reported that overall baseline physical activity and baseline leisure and work activities were strongly related to weight gain in the PEPI cohort. Women who reported more activity gained less weight than less active women.

Weight gain during this period is associated with fat deposition in the abdomen, which increases the likelihood of developing insulin resistance and subsequent diabetes mellitus and heart disease (Dallman, 2004; Wing, 1991). In addition, as reviewed by Baumgartner (1995), data from the Rosetta Study and the New Mexico Aging Process Study show that older adults have higher percentages of body fat than younger adults at any age due to the loss of muscle mass with aging.

Numerous other factors underlie weight gain and include genetic factors, neuropeptides, and adrenergic nervous system activity (Milewicz, 1996). Although many women believe that estrogen therapy causes weight gain, results from clinical trials and epidemiologic studies indicate that the impact of menopausal hormone therapy on body weight and girth, if any, is to decrease slightly the rate of age-related increases (Espeland, 1997; Guthrie, 1999).

Dermatologic Changes

Skin changes that may develop during menopausal transition include hyperpigmentation (age spots), wrinkles, and itching. These are caused in part from skin aging, which results from the synergistic effects of intrinsic aging and photoaging (Guinot, 2005). In addition, hormonal aging of the skin is thought to be responsible for many dermal changes. These include a reduced thickness due to diminished collagen content, a decrease in sebaceous gland secretion, a loss of elasticity, diminished blood supply, and epidermal changes (Wines, 2001). Although the impact of hormone deficiency on skin aging has been widely studied, its distinction from the effects of intrinsic aging, photoaging, and other environmental insults is difficult.

Dental Changes

Dental problems may also develop as estrogen levels wane in late menopausal transition. The buccal epithelium undergoes atrophy due to estrogen deprivation, resulting in decreased saliva and sensation. A bad taste in the mouth, increased incidence of cavities, and tooth loss also may occur (Krall, 1994).

Oral alveolar bone loss is strongly correlated with osteoporosis and can lead to tooth loss. The beneficial effect of estrogen on skeletal bone mass is also manifested on oral bone. Even in women without osteoporosis, there is a correlation between spinal bone density and number of teeth. Tooth loss is also strongly associated with the use of cigarettes and the adverse effect they have on dental health (Krall, 1994).

Breast Changes

The breast undergoes change during menopause mainly because of hormonal withdrawal. In premenopausal women, estrogen and progesterone exert proliferative effects on ductal and glandular structures, respectively. At menopause, withdrawal of estrogen and progesterone leads to a relative reduction in breast proliferation. A significant reduction in the volume and percentage of dense tissue on mammography is noted, and these areas become replaced with adipose tissue.

Central Nervous System Changes
Sleep Dysfunction

Difficulties in sleep onset and sleep maintenance are common in menopausal women. Sleep fragmentation is commonly associated with hot flashes and results in daytime fatigue, mood lability, irritability, and problems with short-term memory (Owens, 1998). Even women with few vasomotor symptoms may experience insomnia and associated menopause-related mood symptoms (Erlik, 1982; Woodward, 1994). At times, short-term use of pharmacologic sleep aids are indicated, and these are listed in Table 1-24 (p. 29).

As women age, they are more likely to experience lighter sleep and are awakened more easily by pain, sound, or bodily urges. Health issues and other chronic conditions experienced by women, or not infrequently by their spouse or bedmate, are likely to further disrupt sleep. Painful orthopedic conditions, chronic lung disease, heartburn, and certain medications that are known to disrupt sleep may dramatically diminish the quality and quantity of restful sleep. Nocturia, urinary frequency, and urgency, all of which are more common in menopausal women, are also important factors.

Sleep disordered breathing (SDB), which includes various degrees of pharyngeal obstruction, is much more common in menopausal women and their mates. In women, SDB is commonly associated with increased body mass and declining estrogen and progesterone levels. Loud snoring may develop due to upper airway obstruction and can range in severity from upper airway resistance to obstructive sleep apnea (Gislason, 1993). In all these examples, treatment of underlying health conditions should be the focus to improve patient sleep.

Cognitive Dysfunction

Memory decreases with advancing age. Although no direct effect of lowered estrogen levels on memory and cognition has been determined, many investigators suspect a relationship to, or an acceleration of, cognitive decline during menopause. Cognitive functioning was assessed in a cohort study of reproductive-aged and postmenopausal women not using hormone replacement therapy. In postmenopausal patients, cognitive performance declined with advancing age. This was not the case for reproductive-aged women. Premenopausal women in their forties were less likely to exhibit cognitive decline compared with postmenopausal patients in the same decade of life. These investigators concluded that there is accelerated deterioration of some forms of cognitive function after menopause (Halbreich, 1995).

Factors accelerating cerebral degenerative changes represent potentially modifiable risks for cognitive decline (Kuller, 2003; Meyer, 1999). Investigators have studied putative risk factors that accelerate subtle cognitive decline and dementia. They have correlated them with repeated measures of cerebral atrophy, computed tomography (CT) densitometry, and cognitive testing among neurologically and cognitively normal, aging volunteers. Risk factors for decreased cerebral perfusion and thinning of gray and white matter densities include transient ischemic attacks (TIAs), hyperlipidemia, hypertension, smoking, excess alcohol consumption, and male gender, which would imply lack of estrogen. The authors suggested interventions to control those risk factors amenable to modification.

■ Psychosocial Changes

Few studies of women's health in the menopausal years have formally assessed well-being and the psychosocial aspects of menopausal transition. Dennerstein and colleagues (1994) studied women during midlife to determine whether menopausal status, social circumstance, health status, interpersonal stress, attitude, and lifestyle behavior correlated with well-being in midlife. These investigators found that menopausal status had little effect on well-being. However, well-being was found to be significantly related to current perceived health status, general psychosomatic symptoms, general respiratory symptoms, history of premenstrual symptoms, and interpersonal stress. Attitudes toward aging and menopause were also significantly associated with well-being scores. Other investigators have found that psychosocial issues are common during this time and do relate them directly to the fluctuation in hormonal levels (Bromberger, 2009; Freeman, 2010; Soares, 2010).

Psychological and cognitive symptoms may develop during menopausal transition and include depression, mood changes, poor concentration, and impaired memory. Although many women perceive these changes as age-related aggravations or attribute them to worsening premenstrual syndrome (PMS), these symptoms may in fact result from changes in reproductive hormones (Bachmann, 1994; Schmidt, 1991).

More importantly, the menopausal transition is a complex sociocultural as well as a hormonal event. Psychosocial factors also may contribute to mood and cognitive symptoms during this phase, since women entering menopausal transition may face additional emotional stress from dealing with adolescents, onset of a major illness, caring for an aging parent, divorce or widowhood, career change, or retirement (LeBoeuf, 1996).

Lock (1991) suggests that part of the stress reported by Western women is clearly culture specific. Western culture emphasizes beauty and youth, and as women grow older, some suffer from a perceived loss of status, function, and control (LeBoeuf, 1996). However, the end of predictable menstruation and the end of fertility may be important to a woman simply because it is a change, no matter how aging and the end of reproductive life are viewed by that woman and by her culture (Frackiewicz, 2000). For some women, the approach of menopause may also be perceived as a significant loss, both to women who have accepted childbearing and rearing as their major life roles and to those who are childless, perhaps not by choice. For these reasons, impending menopause may be perceived as a time of loss, when depression and other psychological disorders may develop (Avis, 2000).

Contemporary findings have dispelled myths that natural menopause itself is associated with depressed mood (Ballinger, 1990; Busch, 1994). That said, in general, there are a high percentage of subjects with recurrent depression at menopause, and a high percentage experiencing their first episode of depression during menopausal transition (Freeman, 2007; Spinelli, 2005).

It has been suggested that the hormonal fluctuations during early menopausal transition are responsible, in part, for this affective instability. Similarly, surgical menopause induces mood changes because of the rapid hormonal loss at this time. Soares (2005) hypothesizes that a major component of the reported emotional distress during menopausal transition may be causally related to high and erratic estradiol levels. For example, Ballinger and colleagues (1990) have shown that increases in stress hormones (and probably symptoms that are stress related) are physiologically linked with high estrogen levels. They also showed that women who had abnormal scores on psychometric tests early after menopause had higher estradiol levels than those with lower scores. In prospective, physiological studies of women reporting severe PMS, Spinelli and associates (2005) have shown that estrogen levels are correlated with the intensity of menopausal symptoms. A randomized, placebo-controlled menopause treatment study evaluated administered standard doses of conjugated equine estrogen (0.625 mg/d), which significantly improved sleep, but also showed an estrogen-related increase of inward-directed hostility (Schiff, 1980).

Libido Changes

Although the relationship between circulating hormones and libido has been extensively investigated, definitive data are lacking. Many studies demonstrate that other factors besides menopause may account for changes in libido (Gracia, 2007). Avis and colleagues (2000) studied sexual function in a subgroup of 200 women in the Massachusetts Women's Health Study II who underwent natural menopause. None took hormone treatment, and all these women had sexual partners. Menopausal status was observed to be significantly related to decreased sexual interest. However, after adjustment for physical and mental health, smoking, and marital satisfaction, menopause status no longer had a significant relationship to libido. Dennerstein and Hayes (2005) prospectively evaluated 438 Australian women during 6 years of their menopausal transition. Menopause was significantly associated with dyspareunia and indirectly with sexual response. Psychological factors of feelings for one's partner, stress, and other social factors also indirectly affected sexual functioning.

Other investigators have demonstrated that sexual problems are more prevalent after menopause. A longitudinal study of women during the menopausal transition until at least 1 year after the final menstrual period demonstrated a significant decrease in the rate of weekly coitus. Patients reported a significant decrease in the quantity of sexual thoughts, sexual satisfactions, and vaginal lubrication after becoming menopausal (McCoy, 1985). In a study of 100 naturally menopausal women, both sexual desire and activity decreased compared with that during the premenopausal period. Women reported loss of libido, dyspareunia, and orgasmic dysfunction, with 86 percent reporting no orgasms after menopause (Tungphaisal, 1991).

Lower Reproductive Tract Changes

Symptoms of urogenital atrophy, including vaginal dryness and dyspareunia, are common in menopausal transition and can pose significant quality-of-life issues, especially among sexually active women. Prevalence estimates range from 10 percent to 50 percent (Levine, 2008). Estrogen receptors have been identified in the vulva, vagina, bladder, urethra, pelvic floor musculature, and endopelvic fascia. These structures thus share a similar hormonal responsiveness and are susceptible to the estrogen deprivation that develops after menopause, in the postpartum period during lactation, or with hypothalamic amenorrhea.

Without estrogen's trophic influence, the vagina loses collagen, adipose tissue, and ability to retain water (Sarrel, 2000). As vaginal walls shrink, rugae flatten, and the vagina becomes flat-surfaced and pale pink. The surface epithelium thins to a few cell layers, markedly reducing the ratio of superficial to basal cells. As a result, the vaginal surface is left friable and prone to bleeding with minimal trauma. The blood vessels in the vaginal walls narrow, and over time, the vagina itself contracts and loses flexibility. In addition, vaginal pH becomes more alkaline, and a pH greater than 4.5 is typically observed with estrogen deficiency (Caillouette, 1997; Roy, 2004). An alkaline pH creates a vaginal environment less hospitable to lactobacilli and more susceptible to infection by urogenital and fecal pathogens.

In addition to vaginal changes, as estrogen production wanes in the later menopausal transition, the vulvar epithelium gradually atrophies and secretions from sebaceous glands diminish. Subcutaneous fat in the labia majora is lost and leads to shrinkage and retraction of clitoral prepuce and the urethra, to fusion of the labia minora, and to introital narrowing and then stenosis (Mehta, 2008). As a result of these changes, the clinical symptoms associated with vulvovaginal atrophy include vaginal dryness, itching, irritation, dyspareunia, and recurrent urinary tract infections (Levine, 2008).

Dyspareunia and Sexual Dysfunction

Complaints of dyspareunia and other forms of sexual dysfunction are common in menopausal patients. Laumann and associates (1999) studied the prevalence of sexual dysfunction in postmenopausal women and found that 25 percent complained of some degree of dyspareunia. They found that painful intercourse correlated with sexual problems, including lack of libido, arousal disorder, and anorgasmia. Dyspareunia in this population is generally attributed to vaginal dryness and mucosal atrophy secondary to loss of ovarian hormones. However, prevalence studies suggest that a decrement in all aspects of female sexual function is associated with midlife (Dennerstein, 2005).

Levine and colleagues (2008) studied 1480 sexually active postmenopausal women and found the prevalence of vulvovaginal atrophy to be 57 percent and female sexual dysfunction to be 55 percent. They found that women with female sexual dysfunction were nearly four times more likely to have vulvovaginal atrophy than women without female sexual dysfunction. The reduction in ovarian estrogen production results in a decline in vaginal lubrication, a greater risk for atrophic vaginitis, and decreased blood flow and vasocongestion with sexual activity. Reduced testosterone levels have been implicated in genital atrophy as well.

Urogenital conditions such as prolapse or incontinence also correlate strongly with sexual dysfunction (Barber, 2002;

Salonia, 2004). Patients with urinary incontinence are likely to have pelvic floor hypotonus dysfunction. This may cause pain with deep penetration due to lack of pelvic stability. Hypertonic or dyssynergic pelvic floor muscles, which are commonly seen in patients with urinary frequency, constipation, and vaginismus, are often associated with superficial pain and friction during intercourse (Handa, 2004). The presence of organ prolapse contributes to dyspareunia as does a history of a gynecologic surgical procedure that may cause dyspareunia by shortening the vagina (Goldberg, 2001).

Other medical conditions such as arthritis, hip or lumbar joint pain, or fibromyalgia may contribute to vaginal or pelvic pain with intercourse. Chronic pelvic pain, which is discussed in detail in Chapter 11 (p. 309), may also be a contributor to sexual dysfunction.

Urogenital

As was stated earlier, there are estrogen and progesterone receptors in most pelvic floor muscles and ligaments. Due to low estrogen production in late menopause or after oophorectomy, genitourinary atrophy may lead to a variety of symptoms that affect quality of life. Urinary symptoms may include dysuria, urgency, and recurrent urinary tract infections (Notelovitz, 1989).

Specifically, thinning of urethral and bladder mucosa may lead to urethritis with dysuria, to urge urinary incontinence, and to urinary frequency. In addition, urethral shortening associated with menopausal atrophic changes may result in genuine stress urinary incontinence. For example, Bhatia and colleagues (1989) showed that estrogen therapy may improve or cure stress urinary incontinence in more than 50 percent of treated women, presumably by exerting a direct effect on urethral mucosal coaptation (Chap. 23, p. 611). Accordingly, a trial of hormone therapy should be considered in select patients prior to surgical correction of incontinence in women with vaginal atrophy.

In 2009, Waetjen and others evaluated women in menopausal transition and found a slight increase in stress and urge urinary incontinence rates. However, other studies have not found an association between incontinence and menopausal status. Sherburn and colleagues (2001) performed a cross-sectional study of women aged 45 to 55 years. They identified a 15-percent prevalence of urinary incontinence. Associated risk factors included gynecologic surgery, higher BMI, urinary tract infections (UTIs), constipation, and multiparity. Subsequently, these investigators studied a subset of 373 premenopausal females during 7 years to determine if menopausal transition itself was associated with an increased incidence of incontinence. In this group of women, the overall incidence of incontinence was 35 percent, with no increase associated with menopause. Incontinence was most closely related to hysterectomy during the course of the study. Importantly, as described in Chapter 23 (p. 607), incontinence incidence does correlate with aging itself.

In addition to incontinence, pelvic organ prolapse rates increase with advancing age. Importantly, vaginal relaxation with cystocele, rectocele, and uterine prolapse are not a direct consequence of estrogen deprivation, as many factors play a role in pelvic floor relaxation (Chap. 24, p. 633).

PATIENT EVALUATION

Clinical goals of the menopausal transition evaluation are to optimize a woman's health and well-being during and after this transition. This is an excellent time for a detailed health evaluation, including a complete medical history, physical examination, and laboratory studies. As described in Chapter 1 (p. 2), risk factors for common health problems such as obesity, osteoporosis, heart disease, diabetes mellitus, and certain cancers should be assessed and then managed. Counseling regarding diet, exercise, alcohol moderation, and smoking cessation are imperative if applicable.

DIAGNOSIS

The diagnosis of menopausal transition can usually be made with documentation of age-appropriate symptoms and careful physical examination (see Table 21-1). However, many symptoms typical of the menopause may also reflect pathologic conditions, and testing to exclude these is indicated in many cases (Table 21-9).

Clearly, a 50-year-old woman with menstrual irregularity, hot flashes, and vaginal dryness should be considered to be in menopausal transition. Other testing such as FSH or estradiol levels can be performed to document ovarian failure. However,

---

TABLE 21-9. Differential Diagnosis of Menopausal Symptoms

Hot flashes, vasomotor symptoms
Hyperthyroidism
Pheochromocytoma
Febrile illness
Anxiety and psychological symptoms

Vaginal dryness, dyspareunia
Bacterial vaginosis
Yeast infection
Pelvic pathology
Poor vaginal lubrication
Marital discord

Primary osteoporosis
Osteomalacia
Primary and secondary hyperparathyroidism
Hyperthyroidism or excess thyroid replacement
Excess corticoid therapy
Increased calcium excretion

Abnormal uterine bleeding
Anovulation
Endometrial cancer
Cervical cancer
Endometrial hyperplasia
Endometrial polyps
Uterine leiomyoma
Urogenital atrophy
Hormone treatment

in the menopausal transition group, FSH and estradiol levels may be normal. Even when much younger women present with similar symptoms, evaluation should also include FSH measurement. If ovarian failure occurs before 40 years, it is usually pathologic. Thus, investigation for chromosomal abnormalities, infections, autoimmune disorders, or iatrogenic causes such as radiation or chemotherapy should be considered (Chap. 16, p. 444).

Physical Examination

A thorough general physical examination should be performed during patient visits to document changes associated with aging and menopausal transition.

Constitutional

Height, weight, and BMI are recorded and can be used to counsel women about physical exercise and weight loss or weight gain. Moreover, assessment of weight distribution and waist circumference may identify those with truncal obesity, who carry greater risks for other comorbidity. Height loss may be associated with osteoporosis and spinal compression fractures. Therefore, yearly height measurement is prudent. Blood pressure monitoring effectively screens for hypertension, which is common in this population.

Cognitive

Cognitive decline is unusual in a woman during menopausal transition, but common complaints of forgetfulness or scattered thinking may be part of normal aging. In patients who are concerned about cognitive decline, brief screening tests can be used (Chap. 1, p. 27).

Psychosocial

Evaluation of psychosocial well-being should be part of transition assessment. Clinicians may inquire directly regarding depression, anxiety, and sexual functioning or may choose to administer a simple questionnaire to screen for specific psychosocial issues (Chap. 13, p. 356).

Dermatologic

Skin changes associated with estrogen deficiency include skin thinning and wrinkling. In addition, various skin lesions are commonly associated with aging and photoaging. Careful inspection for abnormal nevi or excessive sun exposure may prompt referral to a dermatologist for further skin cancer evaluation.

Breast

During menopausal transition, estrogen levels fall and glandular breast tissue is gradually replaced by fatty tissue. Breast tissue and axillae are carefully inspected and palpated. Nipple discharge, skin changes, nipple inversion, and masses should be documented and evaluated as described in Chapter 12 (p. 334).

Pelvic Examination

Examination of the vulva may demonstrate loss of the connective tissue that results in shrinkage of the labia majora. The labia minora may disappear completely, and there is often a narrowing of the introitus. The vulva should be examined for redness, atrophy, or scarring. In those with pain, scar tissue from a past tear or episiotomy or from surgery should be noted. Specific areas of tenderness can often be localized with a methodical evaluation of the vulva. Touch with a cotton swab may locate and reproduce a patient's pain (Fig. 4-1, p. 112).

Vaginal examination will typically reveal a narrow vaginal canal and thin, flat vaginal epithelium. The classic appearance of vaginal atrophy includes loss of rugae and a pale, dry vaginal mucosa. Epithelial tissues are often friable, and submucosal petechial hemorrhages may be seen. Markers of vaginal atrophy include a vaginal pH greater than 5.0 and a change in the vaginal wall's maturation index toward basal cell predominance. Culture of the vagina may reveal pathogenic bacteria not normally found in the vagina.

In addition to a standard gynecologic evaluation—that is, bimanual and speculum examination—external and internal assessment should focus on pelvic muscle and vaginal muscular tone and strength, as well as mobility and integrity of the fascia and connective tissues. The degree of introital flexibility, mucosal dryness, or atrophy is determined. Integrity of the pelvic organs and possible prolapse of the bladder, uterus, or rectum is evaluated by having the patient perform a Valsalva maneuver and observing for bulging of a cystocele, rectocele, or cervical or vaginal prolapse.

Laboratory Testing
Gonadotropin Levels

Biochemical changes may be evident prior to cycle irregularity. For example, in the early follicular phase of the menstrual cycle in many women older than 35 years, FSH levels may rise without a concurrent LH elevation. This finding is associated with a poor prognosis for future fertility. Specifically, a day-3 FSH level greater than 10 mIU/mL is used in some in vitro fertilization (IVF) programs to route patients into donor egg programs (Chap. 19, p. 514). An FSH level greater than 40 mIU/mL has been used to document ovarian failure associated with the menopause.

Estrogen Levels

Estrogen levels may be normal, elevated, or low depending on the stage of menopausal transition. Only at menopause are estrogen levels extremely low or undetectable. Additionally, estrogen levels may be used to assess women's response to hormone treatment. Most clinicians prefer to reach a physiologic serum estradiol range of 50 to 100 pg/mL when selecting and adjusting replacement therapy. Women who receive estradiol pellets as replacement therapy may have elevated serum estradiol values from 300 to 500 pg/mL. These high levels are not uncommon with this replacement method but should be discouraged.

Estrogen Maturation Index

The maturation index is an inexpensive means to evaluate hormonal influences in women. A specimen to measure the maturation index may be collected during a vaginal speculum

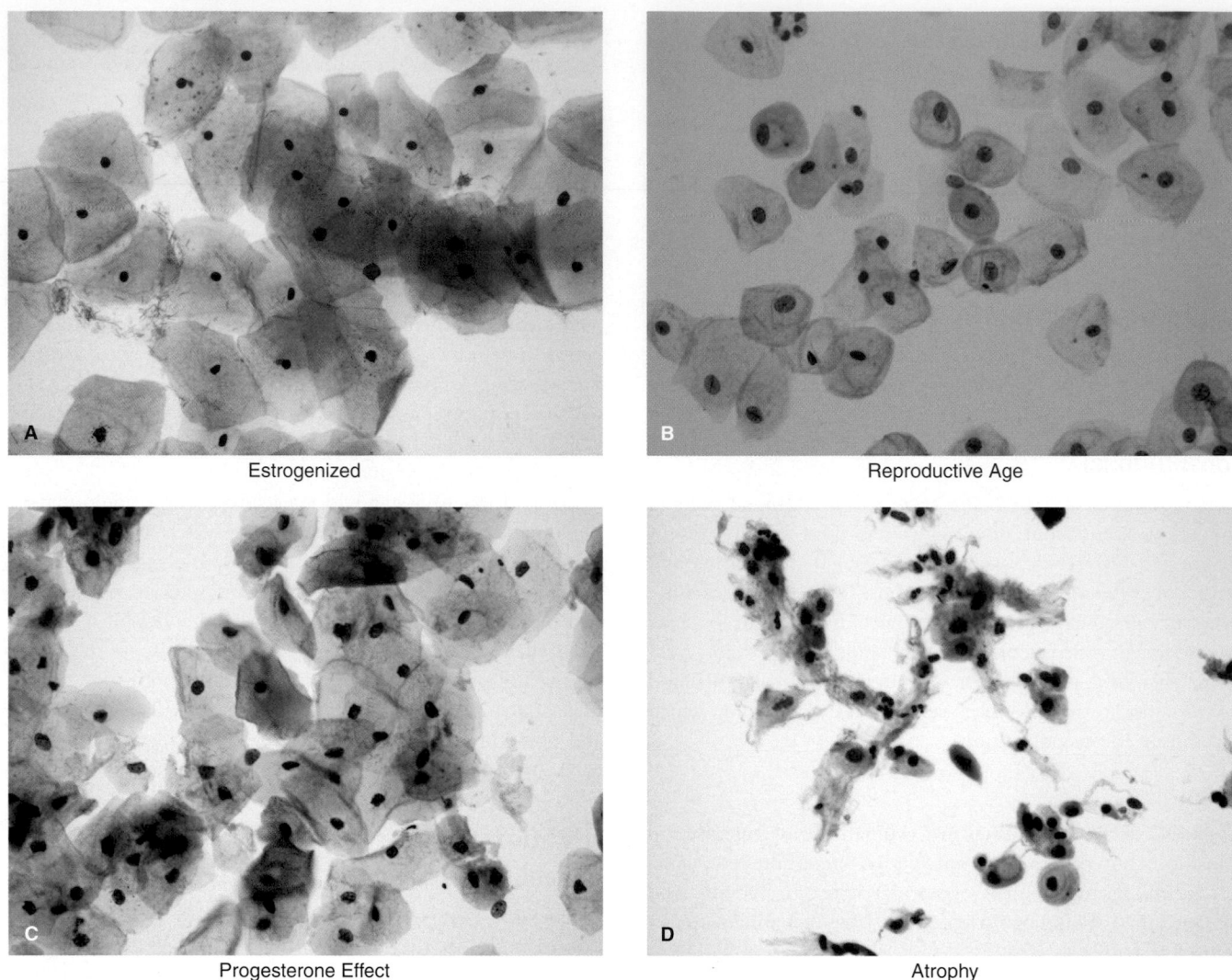

Estrogenized

Reproductive Age

Progesterone Effect

Atrophy

FIGURE 21-11 Photomicrographs of cytologic specimens illustrate key points of the maturation index. This index provides insight into the cytohormonal status of the patient and is based on a count of parabasal, intermediate, and superficial (P:I:S) cells. Generally, a predominance of superficial or superficial and intermediate cells (**A** and **B**) is seen in reproductive-aged women. **C.** A predominance of intermediate cells is seen in the luteal phase, in pregnancy, with amenorrhea, and in newborns, premenarchal girls, and women in early menopausal transition. **D.** A predominance of parabasal cells is seen in menopausal patients with atrophy. *(Photographs contributed by Dr. Raheela Ashfaq.)*

examination at the same time a Pap smear is performed. The index ratio is read from left to right and refers to the percentage of parabasal, intermediate, and superficial squamous cells appearing on a smear. The total sum of all three values equals 100 percent (Fig. 21-11) (Randolph, 2005). For example, a maturation index of 0:40:60 represents 0 percent parabasal cells, 40 percent intermediate cells, and 60 percent superficial cells. This index reflects adequate vaginal estrogenization. A shift to the left indicates an increase in parabasal or intermediate cells, which denotes low estrogen levels. Conversely, a shift to the right reflects an increase in the superficial or intermediate cells, which is associated with higher estrogen levels.

An ideal maturation index vaginal specimen consists of freely exfoliating squamous cells from the upper third of the vaginal wall. Avoiding the cervical area, the vaginal wall secretions are gently scraped with a spatula or saline-moistened swab. Immediately after collection, the specimen is transferred

to a microscope slide. Cells are either suspended in a small amount of saline (as in a wet prep) or smeared to the slide and fixed with 95-percent ethanol spray fixative.

In daily practice, the role of the maturation index in patient assessment has been diminished by the increased use of simpler assays for serum FSH and estradiol. However, the maturation index is still commonly used in research studies to evaluate the efficacy of agents used to treat menopausal symptoms.

Urinary and Serum Markers of Bone Resorption and Formation

Remodeling is a normal, natural process that maintains skeletal strength, enables repair of microfractures, and allows calcium homeostasis. During remodeling, osteoblasts synthesize a number of cytokines, peptides, and growth factors that are released into the circulation. Their concentration thus reflects the rate of bone formation. Bone formation markers found in serum

TABLE 21-10. Analytes Considered Markers of Bone Resorption and Formation

Resorption	Formation
Urinary calcium	Bone-specific alkaline
Tartrate-resistant acid	phosphatase (BALP)
phosphatase	Osteocalcin
Bone sialoprotein	Procollagen I propeptides:
Cross-links	Carboxy terminal (PICP)
Pyridinoline	Amino terminal (PINP)
Deoxypyridinoline	
N-telopeptide (NTX)	
C-telopeptide (CTX)	
C-terminal telopeptide of	
type I collagen	

PICP = procollagen I C-terminal propeptide;
PINP = procollagen I N-terminal propeptide.

include osteocalcin, bone-specific alkaline phosphatase, and two procollagen I propeptides (Table 21-10).

Osteoclasts produce bone degradation products that are also released into the circulation and are eventually cleared via the kidney. These include collagen cross-linking peptides and pyridinolines, which can be measured in the blood or urine and enable estimation of bone resorption rates. Bone resorption markers include urinary hydroxyproline, urinary pyridinoline (PYR), and urinary deoxypyridinoline (DPD), as well as collagen type I cross-linked N telopeptide (NTX) and collagen type I cross-linked C telopeptide (CTX).

Markers of bone formation and resorption are valuable in estimating bone-remodeling rates. These biochemical markers may be used to identify fast bone losers. Numerous cross-sectional studies have shown that bone remodeling rates, as evaluated by markers, increase at menopause and remain elevated. Bone remodeling rates in menopausal women correlate negatively with BMD.

Markers of bone resorption may be useful predictors of fracture risk and bone loss. Elevation of these markers may be associated with an increased fracture risk in elderly women, although data are not uniform. The association of markers of bone resorption with hip fracture risk is independent of BMD, but a low BMD combined with high bone resorption biomarker doubles the risk associated with either of these factors alone. Biomarker measurements are also currently limited by their high variability within individuals. Additional studies with fracture endpoints are needed to confirm the usefulness of these markers in individual patients.

Biomarkers may also be of value in predicting and monitoring response to potent antiresorptive therapy in clinical trials. Normalization of bone formation and resorption marker levels following therapy has been observed in prospective trials. Reduction in biochemical marker levels appears to be correlated with a decrease in vertebral fracture incidence in some studies, but is not necessarily always predictive of response to therapies.

Bone remodeling markers should not yet be used for routine clinical management. Additional studies are needed to confirm their use in individual patients. However, with refinement of assay technology and better understanding of biologic variability, it is likely that they will become a useful adjunct for risk assessment and management.

REFERENCES

American College of Obstetricians and Gynecologists: Depot medroxyprogesterone acetate and bone effects. Committee Opinion No. 415, September 2008

American College of Obstetricians and Gynecologists: The role of transvaginal ultrasonography in the evaluation of postmenopausal bleeding. Committee Opinion No. 440, August 2009

American Geriatrics Society and British Geriatrics Society: Summary of the Updated American Geriatrics Society/British Geriatrics Society clinical practice guideline for prevention of falls in older persons. J Am Geriatr Soc 59(1):148, 2011

Antithrombotic Trialists' Collaboration: Collaborative meta-analysis of randomised trials of antiplatelet therapy for prevention of death, myocardial infarction, and stroke in high risk patients. BMJ 324(7329):71, 2002

Avis NE, Stellato R, Crawford S, et al: Is there an association between menopause status and sexual functioning? Menopause 7:297, 2000

Bachmann G: Physiologic aspects of natural and surgical menopause. J Reprod Med 46(3 Suppl):307, 2001

Bachmann GA: Menopausal vasomotor symptoms: a review of causes, effects and evidence-based treatment options. J Reprod Med 50:155, 2005

Bachmann GA: The changes before "the change." Strategies for the transition to the menopause. Postgrad Med 95:113, 1994

Ballinger CB: Psychiatric aspects of the menopause. Br J Psychiatry 156:773, 1990

Bar-Shavit Z: The osteoclast: a multinucleated, hematopoietic-origin, bone-resorbing osteoimmune cell. J Cell Biochem 102(5):1130, 2007

Barber MD, Visco AG, Wyman JF, et al: Sexual function in women with urinary incontinence and pelvic organ prolapse. Obstet Gynecol 99:281, 2002

Baumgartner RN, Heymsfield SB, Roche AF: Human body composition and the epidemiology of chronic disease. Obes Res 3:73, 1995

Bhatia NN, Bergman A, Karram MM: Effects of estrogen on urethral function in women with urinary incontinence. Am J Obstet Gynecol 160:176, 1989

Bonjour JP, Chevalley T, Ammann P, et al: Gain in bone mineral mass in prepubertal girls 3.5 years after discontinuation of calcium supplementation: a follow-up study. Lancet 358:1208, 2001

Bromberger JT, di Scalea TL: Longitudinal associations between depression and functioning in midlife women. Maturitas 64(3):145, 2009

Brunner D, Weisbort J, Meshulam N, et al: Relation of serum total cholesterol and high-density lipoprotein cholesterol percentage to the incidence of definite coronary events: twenty-year follow-up of the Donolo-Tel Aviv Prospective Coronary Artery Disease Study. Am J Cardiol 59:1271, 1987

Burger HG, Dudley EC, Cui J, et al: A prospective longitudinal study of serum testosterone, dehydroepiandrosterone sulfate, and sex hormone-binding globulin levels through the menopause transition. J Clin Endocrinol Metab 85:2832, 2000

Burger HG, Hale GE, Dennerstein L, et al: Cycle and hormone changes during perimenopause: the key role of ovarian function. Menopause 15(4 Pt 1):603, 2008

Busch CM, Zonderman AB, Costa PT Jr: Menopausal transition and psychological distress in a nationally representative sample: is menopause associated with psychological distress? J Aging Health 6:206, 1994

Caillouette JC, Sharp CF Jr, Zimmerman GJ, et al: Vaginal pH as a marker for bacterial pathogens and menopausal status. Am J Obstet Gynecol 176:1270, 1997

Canalis E: Mechanisms of glucocorticoid action in bone: implications for glucocorticoid-induced osteoporosis. J Clin Endocrinol Metab 81:3441, 1996

Canalis E, Giustina A, Bilezikian JP: Mechanisms of anabolic therapies for osteoporosis. N Engl J Med 357(9):905, 2007

Centers for Disease Control and Prevention: U.S. medical eligibility criteria for contraceptive use, 2010. MMWR 59, 2010

Cook NR, Lee IM, Gaziano JM, et al: Low-dose aspirin in the primary prevention of cancer: the Women's Health Study: a randomized controlled trial. JAMA 294(1):47, 2005

Cummings SR, Nevitt MC, Browner WS, et al: Risk factors for hip fracture in white women. Study of Osteoporotic Fractures Research Group. N Engl J Med 332:767, 1995

Dallman MF, la Fleur SE, Pecoraro NC, et al: Minireview: glucocorticoids—food intake, abdominal obesity, and wealthy nations in 2004. Endocrinology 145:2633, 2004

Davies KM, Heaney RP, Recker RR, et al: Hormones, weight change and menopause. Int J Obes Relat Metab Disord 25:874, 2001

Dennerstein L, Hayes RD: Confronting the challenges: epidemiological study of female sexual dysfunction and the menopause. J Sex Med 2(Suppl 3):118, 2005

Dennerstein L, Smith AM, Morse C, et al: Menopausal symptoms in Australian women. Med J Aust 159:232, 1993

Dennerstein L, Smith AM, Morse C: Psychological well-being, mid-life and the menopause. Maturitas 20:1, 1994

Erlik Y, Meldrum DR, Judd HL: Estrogen levels in postmenopausal women with hot flashes. Obstet Gynecol 59:403, 1982

Espeland MA, Stefanick ML, Kritz-Silverstein D, et al: Effect of postmenopausal hormone therapy on body weight and waist and hip girths. Postmenopausal Estrogen-Progestin Interventions Study Investigators. J Clin Endocrinol Metab 82:1549, 1997

Faulkner KG, von Stetten E, Miller P: Discordance in patient classification using T-scores. J Clin Densitom 2:343, 1999

Finer LB, Henshaw SK: Disparities in rates of unintended pregnancy in the United States, 1994 and 2001. Perspect Sex Reprod Health 38(2):90, 2006

Frackiewicz EJ, Cutler NR: Women's health care during the perimenopause. J Am Pharm Assoc (Wash) 40:800, 2000

Freedman RR: Biochemical, metabolic, and vascular mechanisms in menopausal hot flashes. Fertil Steril 70:332, 1998

Freedman RR: Physiology of hot flashes. Am J Hum Biol 13:453, 2001

Freedman RR, Woodward S, Sabharwal SC: Alpha 2-adrenergic mechanism in menopausal hot flushes. Obstet Gynecol 76:573, 1990

Freeman EW: Associations of depression with the transition to menopause. Menopause 17(4):823, 2010

Freeman EW, Sammel MD, Lin H, et al: Symptoms associated with menopausal transition and reproductive hormones in midlife women. Obstet Gynecol 110(2 Pt 1):230, 2007

Gallagher JC, Rapuri PB, Haynatzki G, et al: Effect of discontinuation of estrogen, calcitriol, and the combination of both on bone density and bone markers. J Clin Endocrinol Metab 87:4914, 2002

Gebbie AE, Hardman SM: Contraception in the perimenopause—old and new. Menopause Int 16(1):33, 2010

Gerber LM, Sievert LL, Warren K, et al: Hot flashes are associated with increased ambulatory systolic blood pressure. Menopause 14(2):308, 2007

Gislason T, Benediktsdottir B, Bjornsson JK, et al: Snoring, hypertension, and the sleep apnea syndrome. An epidemiologic survey of middle-aged women. Chest 103:1147, 1993

Gold EB, Bromberger J, Crawford S, et al: Factors associated with age at natural menopause in a multiethnic sample of midlife women. Am J Epidemiol 153:865, 2001

Gold EB, Colvin A, Avis N, et al: Longitudinal analysis of the association between vasomotor symptoms and race/ethnicity across the menopausal transition: study of women's health across the nation. Am J Public Health 96(7):1226, 2006

Goldberg RP, Tomezsko JE, Winkler HA, et al: Anterior or posterior sacrospinous vaginal vault suspension: long-term anatomic and functional evaluation. Obstet Gynecol 98:199, 2001

Goldstein SR: Modern evaluation of the endometrium. Obstet Gynecol 116(1):168, 2010

Gonzales GF, Carrillo C: Blood serotonin levels in postmenopausal women: effects of age and serum oestradiol levels. Maturitas 17:23, 1993

Gracia CR, Freeman EW, Sammel MD, et al: Hormones and sexuality during transition to menopause. Obstet Gynecol 109(4):831, 2007

Guinot C, Malvy D, Ambroisine L, et al: Effect of hormonal replacement therapy on skin biophysical properties of menopausal women. Skin Res Technol 11:201, 2005

Guthrie JR, Dennerstein L, Dudley EC: Weight gain and the menopause: a 5-year prospective study. Climacteric 2(3):205, 1999

Guthrie JR, Dennerstein L, Taffe JR, et al: Hot flushes during the menopause transition: a longitudinal study in Australian-born women. Menopause 12(4):460, 2005

Haarbo J, Hassager C, Riis BJ, et al: Relation of body fat distribution to serum lipids and lipoproteins in elderly women. Atherosclerosis 80:57, 1989

Halbreich U, Lumley LA, Palter S, et al: Possible acceleration of age effects on cognition following menopause. J Psychiatr Res 29:153, 1995

Hale GE, Zhao X, Hughes CL, et al: Endocrine features of menstrual cycles in middle and late reproductive age and the menopausal transition classified according to the Staging of Reproductive Aging Workshop (STRAW) staging system. J Clin Endocrinol Metab 92(8):3060, 2007

Hale GE, Burger HG: Hormonal changes and biomarkers in late reproductive age, menopausal transition and menopause. Best Pract Res Clin Obstet Gynaecol 23(1):7, 2009

Handa VL, Harvey L, Cundiff GW, et al: Sexual function among women with urinary incontinence and pelvic organ prolapse. Am J Obstet Gynecol 191:751, 2004

Heron MP: Deaths: final data for 2007. Natl Vital Stat Rep 59(8):1, 2011

Holick MF: Vitamin D deficiency. N Engl J Med 357(3):266, 2007

Hollander LE, Freeman EW, Sammel MD, et al: Sleep quality, estradiol levels, and behavioral factors in late reproductive age women. Obstet Gynecol 98:391, 2001

Holroyd C, Cooper C, Dennison E: Epidemiology of osteoporosis. Best Pract Res Clin Endocrinol Metab 22(5):671, 2008

Jacobs DR Jr, Mebane IL, Bangdiwala SI, et al: High density lipoprotein cholesterol as a predictor of cardiovascular disease mortality in men and women: the follow-up study of the Lipid Research Clinics Prevalence Study. Am J Epidemiol 131:32, 1990

Jain A, Santoro N: Endocrine mechanisms and management for abnormal bleeding due to perimenopausal changes. Clin Obstet Gynecol 48:295, 2005

Jensen J, Nilas L, Christiansen C: Influence of menopause on serum lipids and lipoproteins. Maturitas 12(4):321, 1990

Johnell O, Kanis JA: An estimate of the worldwide prevalence and disability associated with osteoporotic fractures. Osteoporos Int 17(12):1726, 2006

Kanis JA: Assessment of fracture risk and its application to screening for postmenopausal osteoporosis: synopsis of a WHO report. WHO Study Group. Osteoporos Int 4:368, 1994

Kanis JA, Johnell O, Oden A, et al: Ten year probabilities of osteoporotic fractures according to BMD and diagnostic thresholds. Osteoporos Int 12:989, 2001

Kannel WB: Metabolic risk factors for coronary heart disease in women: perspective from the Framingham Study. Am Heart J 114:413, 1987

Kiebzak GM, Miller PD: Determinants of bone strength. J Bone Miner Res 18:383, 2003

Klein NA, Illingworth PJ, Groome NP, et al: Decreased inhibin B secretion is associated with the monotropic FSH rise in older, ovulatory women: a study of serum and follicular fluid levels of dimeric inhibin A and B in spontaneous menstrual cycles. J Clin Endocrinol Metab 81:2742, 1996

Kostenuik PJ: Osteoprotegerin and RANKL regulate bone resorption, density, geometry and strength. Curr Opin Pharmacol 5(6):618, 2005

Krall EA, Dawson-Hughes B, Papas A, et al: Tooth loss and skeletal bone density in healthy postmenopausal women. Osteoporos Int 4:104, 1994

Kravitz HM, Ganz PA, Bromberger J, et al: Sleep difficulty in women at midlife: a community survey of sleep and the menopausal transition. Menopause 10:19, 2003

Kronenberg F: Hot flashes: epidemiology and physiology. Ann NY Acad Sci 592:52, 1990

Kuh DL, Wadsworth M, Hardy R: Women's health in midlife: the influence of the menopause, social factors and health in earlier life. Br J Obstet Gynaecol 104:923, 1997

Kuller LH, Lopez OL, Newman A, et al: Risk factors for dementia in the cardiovascular health cognition study. Neuroepidemiology 22:13, 2003

Kwee J, Schats R, McDonnell J, et al: Evaluation of anti-Müllerian hormone as a test for the prediction of ovarian reserve. Fertil Steril 90(3):737, 2008

La Marca A, Sighinolfi G, Radi D, et al: Anti-Mullerian hormone (AMH) as a predictive marker in assisted reproductive technology (ART). Hum Reprod Update 16(2):113, 2010

Labrie F, Belanger A, Cusan L, et al: Marked decline in serum concentrations of adrenal C19 sex steroid precursors and conjugated androgen metabolites during aging. J Clin Endocrinol Metab 82:2396, 1997

Laufer LR, Erlik Y, Meldrum DR, et al: Effect of clonidine on hot flashes in postmenopausal women. Obstet Gynecol 60:583, 1982

Laumann EO, Paik A, Rosen RC: Sexual dysfunction in the United States: prevalence and predictors. JAMA 281:537, 1999

LeBoeuf FJ, Carter SG: Discomforts of the perimenopause. J Obstet Gynecol Neonatal Nurs 25:173, 1996

Levine KB, Williams RE, Hartmann KE: Vulvovaginal atrophy is strongly associated with female sexual dysfunction among sexually active postmenopausal women. Menopause 15(4 Pt 1):661, 2008

Lidor A, Ismajovich B, Confino E, et al: Histopathological findings in 226 women with post-menopausal uterine bleeding. Acta Obstet Gynecol Scand 65:41, 1986

Lindsay R, Silverman SL, Cooper C, et al: Risk of new vertebral fracture in the year following a fracture. JAMA 285:320, 2001

Lock M: Medicine and culture: Contested meanings of the menopause. Lancet 337:1270, 1991

Looker AC, Johnston CC Jr, Wahner HW, et al: Prevalence of low femoral bone density in older U.S. women from NHANES III. J Bone Miner Res 10(5):796, 1995

Lund KJ: Menopause and the menopausal transition. Med Clin North Am 92(5):1253, 2008

Malik S, Wong ND, Franklin SS, et al: Impact of the metabolic syndrome on mortality from coronary heart disease, cardiovascular disease, and all causes in United States adults. Circulation 110(10):1245, 2004

Manson JE, Greenland P, LaCroix AZ, et al: Walking compared with vigorous exercise for the prevention of cardiovascular events in women. N Engl J Med 347:716, 2002

Marshall D, Johnell O, Wedel H: Meta-analysis of how well measures of bone mineral density predict occurrence of osteoporotic fractures. BMJ 312:1254, 1996

Matthews KA, Abrams B, Crawford S, et al: Body mass index in mid-life women: relative influence of menopause, hormone use, and ethnicity. Int J Obes Relat Metab Disord 25:863, 2001

Matthews KA, Meilahn E, Kuller LH, et al: Menopause and risk factors for coronary heart disease. N Engl J Med 321:641, 1989

Matthews KA, Wing RR, Kuller LH, et al: Influence of the perimenopause on cardiovascular risk factors and symptoms of middle-aged healthy women. Arch Intern Med 154:2349, 1994

McCoy NL, Davidson JM: A longitudinal study of the effects of menopause on sexuality. Maturitas 7:203, 1985

McKechnie R, Rubenfire M, Mosca L: Association between self-reported physical activity and vascular reactivity in postmenopausal women. Atherosclerosis 159:483, 2001

McKinlay SM, Brambilla DJ, Posner JG: The normal menopause transition. Maturitas 14:103, 1992

Mehta A, Bachmann G: Vulvovaginal complaints. Clin Obstet Gynecol 51 (3):549, 2008

Melton LJ III, Atkinson EJ, Cooper C, et al: Vertebral fractures predict subsequent fractures. Osteoporos Int 10:214, 1999

Meyer JS, Rauch GM, Crawford K, et al: Risk factors accelerating cerebral degenerative changes, cognitive decline and dementia. Int J Geriatr Psychiatry 14:1050, 1999

Milewicz A, Bidzinska B, Sidorowicz A: Perimenopausal obesity. Gynecol Endocrinol 10:285, 1996

Miller PD, Njeh CF, Jankowski LG, et al: What are the standards by which bone mass measurement at peripheral skeletal sites should be used in the diagnosis of osteoporosis? J Clin Densitom 5(Suppl):S39, 2002

Minino AM, Heron MP, Murphy SL, et al: Deaths: final data for 2004. Natl Vital Stat Rep 55(19):1, 2007

Moen MH, Kahn H, Bjerve KS, et al: Menometrorrhagia in the perimenopause is associated with increased serum estradiol. Maturitas 47:151, 2004

Molina P: Parathyroid gland and Ca^{2+} and PO_4^{3-} regulation. In Endocrine Physiology, 3rd ed. New York, McGraw-Hill, 2010

Molnar WR: Menopausal hot flashes: their cycles and relation to air temperature. Obstet Gynecol 57:52S, 1981

Montan S: Increased risk in the elderly parturient. Curr Opin Obstet Gynecol 19(2):110, 2007

Mosca L, Benjamin EJ, Berra K, et al: Effectiveness-based guidelines for the prevention of cardiovascular disease in women—2011 update: a guideline from the American Heart Association. J Am Coll Cardiol 57(12):1404, 2011

Moschos E, Ashfaq R, McIntire DD, et al: Saline-infusion sonography endometrial sampling compared with endometrial biopsy in diagnosing endometrial pathology. Obstet Gynecol 113(4):881, 2009

National Osteoporosis Foundation: America's bone health: the state of osteoporosis and low bone mass in our nation. 2002. Available at: http://www.osteoporosisnews.org/advocacy/prevalence/index.htm. Accessed January 26, 2011

National Osteoporosis Foundation: Clinician's Guide to Prevention and Treatment of Osteoporosis. Washington, DC, National Osteoporosis Foundation, 2010, p 1

Notelovitz M: Estrogen replacement therapy: indications, contraindications, and agent selection. Am J Obstet Gynecol 161(6 Pt 2):1832, 1989

Ohayon MM. Severe hot flashes are associated with chronic insomnia. Arch Intern Med 166:1262, 2006

Overlie I, Finset A, Holte A: Gendered personality dispositions, hormone values, and hot flushes during and after menopause. J Psychosom Obstet Gynaecol 23(4):219, 2002

Owens JF, Matthews KA: Sleep disturbance in healthy middle-aged women. Maturitas 30:41, 1998

Pinkerton JV, Stovall DW, Kightlinger RS: Advances in the treatment of menopausal symptoms. Womens Health (England) 5(4):361, 2009

Ralston SH: Genetic control of susceptibility to osteoporosis. J Clin Endocrinol Metab 87:2460, 2002

Randolph JF Jr, Sowers M, Bondarenko I, et al: The relationship of longitudinal change in reproductive hormones and vasomotor symptoms during the menopausal transition. J Clin Endocrinol Metab 90:6106, 2005

Rapkin AJ: Vasomotor symptoms in menopause: physiologic condition and central nervous system approaches to treatment. Am J Obstet Gynecol, 196(2):97, 2007

Recker RR, Davies KM, Hinders SM, et al: Bone gain in young adult women. JAMA 268:2403, 1992

Reyes FI, Winter JS, Faiman C: Pituitary-ovarian relationships preceding the menopause. I. A cross-sectional study of serum follicle-stimulating hormone, luteinizing hormone, prolactin, estradiol, and progesterone levels. Am J Obstet Gynecol 129:557, 1977

Richardson SJ, Senikas V, Nelson JF: Follicular depletion during the menopausal transition: evidence for accelerated loss and ultimate exhaustion. J Clin Endocrinol Metab 65:1231, 1987

Riis BJ, Hansen MA, Jensen AM, et al: Low bone mass and fast rate of bone loss at menopause: equal risk factors for future fracture: a 15-year follow-up study. Bone 19:9, 1996

Roger VL, Go AS, Lloyd-Jones DM, et al: Heart disease and stroke statistics—2011 update: a report from the American Heart Association. Circulation 123(4):e18, 2011

Roy S, Caillouette JC, Roy T, et al: Vaginal pH is similar to follicle-stimulating hormone for menopause diagnosis. Am J Obstet Gynecol 190:1272, 2004

Rozen GS, Rennert G, Dodiuk-Gad RP, et al: Calcium supplementation provides an extended window of opportunity for bone mass accretion after menarche. Am J Clin Nutr 78:993, 2003

Sabatier JP, Guaydier-Souquieres G, Laroche D, et al: Bone mineral acquisition during adolescence and early adulthood: a study in 574 healthy females 10-24 years of age. Osteoporos Int 6:141, 1996

Saladin KS: Bone Tissue in Human Anatomy. New York, McGraw-Hill, 2005, p 158

Salonia A, Zanni G, Nappi RE, et al: Sexual dysfunction is common in women with lower urinary tract symptoms and urinary incontinence: results of a cross-sectional study. Eur Urol 45:642, 2004

Santoro N, Brown JR, Adel T, et al: Characterization of reproductive hormonal dynamics in the perimenopause. J Clin Endocrinol Metab 81:1495, 1996

Santoro N, Lasley B, McConnell D, et al: Body size and ethnicity are associated with menstrual cycle alterations in women in the early menopausal transition: the Study of Women's Health across the Nation (SWAN) Daily Hormone Study. J Clin Endocrinol Metab 89(6):2622, 2004

Sarrel PM: Effects of hormone replacement therapy on sexual psychophysiology and behavior in postmenopause. J Womens Health Gend Based Med 9(Suppl 1):S25, 2000

Schiff I, Tulchinsky D, Cramer D, et al: Oral medroxyprogesterone in the treatment of postmenopausal symptoms. JAMA 244:1443, 1980

Schmidt PJ, Rubinow DR: Menopause related affective disorders: a justification for further study. Am J Psychiatry 148:844, 1991

Schoen C, Rosen T: Maternal and perinatal risks for women over 44—a review. Maturitas 64(2):109, 2009

Sherburn M, Guthrie JR, Dudley EC, et al: Is incontinence associated with menopause? Obstet Gynecol 98:628, 2001

Slopien R, Meczekalski B, Warenik-Szymankiewicz A: Relationship between climacteric symptoms and serum serotonin levels in postmenopausal women. Climacteric 6:53, 2003

Soares CN: Menopause and mood disturbance. Psychiatric Times 12:2005

Soares CN, Frey BN: Challenges and opportunities to manage depression during the menopausal transition and beyond. Psychiatr Clin North Am 33(2):295, 2010

Soules MR, Sherman S, Parrott E, et al: Executive summary: stages of reproductive aging workshop (STRAW). Fertil Steril 76:874, 2001

Spinelli MG: Neuroendocrine effects on mood. Rev Endocr Metab Disord 6:109, 2005

Stear SJ, Prentice A, Jones SC, et al: Effect of a calcium and exercise intervention on the bone mineral status of 16- to 18-year-old adolescent girls. Am J Clin Nutr 77:985, 2003

Stearns V, Ullmer L, Lopez JF, et al: Hot flushes. Lancet 360(9348):1851, 2002

Stein E, Shane E: Secondary osteoporosis. Endocrinol Metab Clin North Am 32:115, 2003

Stovall TG, Photopulos GJ, Poston WM, et al: Pipelle endometrial sampling in patients with known endometrial carcinoma. Obstet Gynecol 77:954, 1991

Theintz G, Buchs B, Rizzoli R, et al: Longitudinal monitoring of bone mass accumulation in healthy adolescents: evidence for a marked reduction after 16 years of age at the levels of lumbar spine and femoral neck in female subjects. J Clin Endocrinol Metab 75:1060, 1992

Thurston RC, Sowers MR, Chang Y, et al: Adiposity and reporting of vasomotor symptoms among midlife women: the study of women's health across the nation. Am J Epidemiol 167(1):78, 2008

Tinetti ME: Clinical practice. Preventing falls in elderly persons. N Engl J Med 348(1):42, 2003

Tinetti ME, Speechley M, Ginter SF: Risk factors for falls among elderly persons living in the community. N Engl J Med 319(26):1701, 1988

Treloar AE: Menstrual cyclicity and the pre-menopause. Maturitas 3(3-4):249, 1981

Tungphaisal S, Chandeying V, Sutthijumroon S, et al: Postmenopausal sexuality in Thai women. Asia Oceania J Obstet Gynaecol 17:143, 1991

U.S. Census Bureau: Age and sex composition: 2010. May 2011. Available at: http://www.census.gov/prod/cen2010/briefs/c2010br-03.pdf. Accessed October 14, 2011 van Beresteijn EC, Korevaar JC, Huijbregts PC, et al: Perimenopausal increase in serum cholesterol: a 10-year longitudinal study. Am J Epidemiol 137:383, 1993

Waetjen LE, Ye J, Feng WY, et al: Association between menopausal transition stages and developing urinary incontinence. Obstet Gynecol 114(5):989, 2009

Wallace RB, Sherman BM, Bean JA, et al: Probability of menopause with increasing duration of amenorrhea in middle-aged women. Am J Obstet Gynecol 135:1021, 1979

Wilbur J, Miller AM, Montgomery A, et al: Sociodemographic characteristics, biological factors, and symptom reporting in midlife women. Menopause 5:43, 1998

Wines N, Willsteed E: Menopause and the skin. Australas J Dermatol 42:149, 2001

Wing RR, Matthews KA, Kuller LH, et al: Weight gain at the time of menopause. Arch Intern Med 151:97, 1991

Woodward S, Freedman RR: The thermoregulatory effects of menopausal hot flashes on sleep. Sleep 17:497, 1994

World Health Organization: WHO Scientific Group on the assessment of osteoporosis at primary health care level: summary meeting report. 2004. Available at: http://www.who.int/chp/topics/Osteoporosis.pdf. Accessed January 26, 2011

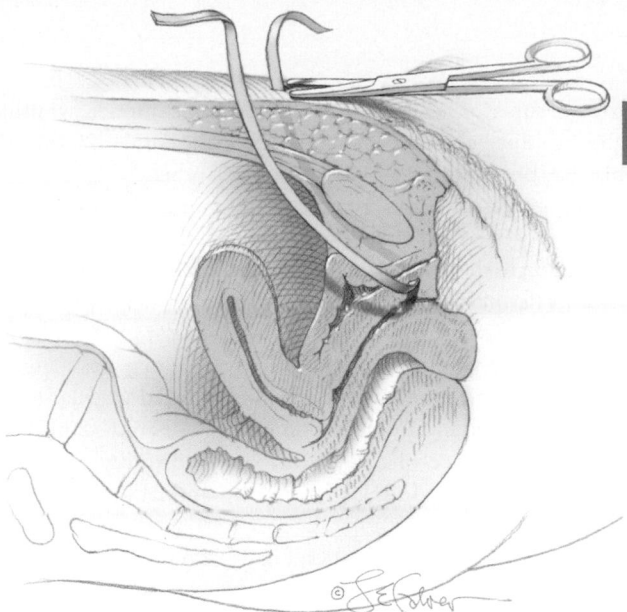

CHAPTER 22

The Mature Woman

The typical "mature woman" is aged 40 years or older and has completed childbearing. During their late 40s, most women enter the menopausal transition. This period of physiologic change is due to ovarian senescence and estrogen decline and is usually completed between ages 51 and 56 (Chap. 21, p. 554). Menopause marks a defining point in this transition. Specifically, menopause is defined by the World Health Organization as the point in time of permanent menstruation cessation due to loss of ovarian function. Clinically, the menopause refers to a point in time that follows 1 year after menstruation cessation.

With ovarian senescence, declining hormone levels have specific effects on many tissues. Some effects lead to physical complaints, such as vasomotor symptoms and vaginal dryness,

whereas others are metabolic and structural changes. These include osteopenia, osteoporosis, skin thinning, fatty replacement of the breast, cardiovascular changes, and genitourinary atrophy. As a result, postmenopausal women have specific issues associated with aging and estrogen loss that may negatively affect their individual health.

For many years menopause was seen as a "deficiency disease" much like hypothyroidism. For this reason, hormone replacement therapy has been used in one form or another for more than 100 years. The history and controversies surrounding this treatment are discussed in detail, as are current recommendations for the treatment of menopausal symptoms.

HORMONE TREATMENT: HISTORY AND CONTROVERSIES

In the recent past, hormone treatment (HT) was widely prescribed, in good faith, to menopausal women for many potential health benefits, based on available observational and epidemiologic studies of the time. The general medical consensus was that HT, in addition to its beneficial role in prevention and treatment of osteoporosis, could protect against cardiovascular disease, stroke, and dementia. However, recent prospective, randomized clinical trials (RCTs) have challenged the validity of earlier observational studies as they were initially reported. Specifically, the type of population studied, the ages and risk-factor status of the women participating, and the hormonal regimens tested are important to this critique. Clinicians should practice evidence-based medicine to ensure the highest quality health care for their patients, and no single study should be relied on solely to guide clinical practice. Understanding that there is a hierarchy of clinical data, the entire literature should be sought to provide the basis on which medicine is practiced (Lobo, 2008). Thus, clinicians should understand the history and controversies surrounding HT as well as the weaknesses and strengths of clinical trials to accurately counsel their patients on the complexities and appropriate use of HT.

Early Estrogen Administration Trends

Estrogen treatment (ET) for menopausal symptom relief gained popularity in the 1960s and 1970s. *Feminine Forever*, the book by author and gynecologist Robert Wilson, was published in 1968. In it, he wrote that "Women who use the drug (estrogen) will be much more pleasant to live with and will not become dull and unattractive" (Bell, 1990). Wilson was a prolific lecturer. His book was widely read and was influential, in part, by creating some of the enthusiasm for ET and its "preservation of youth" and prevention of chronic disease.

By the mid-1970s, more than 30 million prescriptions were written for estrogen each year, and half of all menopausal women were using HT for a median of 5 years. Premarin (conjugated equine estrogen) was the fifth most prescribed drug in the marketplace.

In 1975, a study revealed a connection between endometrial cancer and estrogen replacement. Investigators found a 4.5 times greater risk of this cancer in those using estrogen (Smith, 1975). As a result, the U.S. Food and Drug Administration (FDA) ordered labeling changes to state this higher risk.

Estrogen as a Prevention Tool

In the 1980s, progestins were added to therapy regimens to significantly reduce endometrial cancer risks. During that same time, estrogens were documented by several studies to prevent bone loss (Gambrell, 1983). Additionally, an expanding literature provided a robust affirmation of the effectiveness of menopausal hormone therapy in reducing vasomotor symptoms, preventing and treating vulvovaginal atrophy, and maintaining bone mineral density (Shulman, 2010). A number of observational studies also suggested that estrogens prevented development of coronary heart disease and other conditions such as Alzheimer disease. However, in 1985, conflicting reports from the Framingham Heart Study and the Nurses' Health Study were published.

The Framingham Heart Study, an observational study of 1234 women, showed that those who took hormones had a 50-percent elevated risk of cardiac morbidity and more than a twofold risk for cerebrovascular disease (Wilson, 1985). Critics of the Framingham Study cite the increased incidence of obesity, cigarette smoking, and diabetes in the cohort. In the same edition of the *New England Journal of Medicine,* a much larger observational trial with 121,964 women, The Nurses' Health Study, found significantly lower rates of heart disease in postmenopausal women taking estrogen compared with postmenopausal women not taking estrogen (Stampfer, 1985). Numerous subsequent articles published in medical periodicals reported on the protective effects that combination HT provided menopausal women against cardiovascular disease and osteoporosis.

Current thinking is that that these early nonrandomized, unblinded, observational studies included samples of women who were not necessarily representative of the entire population of postmenopausal women. These hormone users tended to have superior health-care access and to be thinner, wealthier, and healthier overall (Grodstein, 2003; Prentice, 2006). This bias has been termed "the healthy woman bias."

An additional source of confounding and possible selection bias is suggested to be the timing of hormone therapy initiation in relation to the underlying state of the vasculature. Some investigators have hypothesized that estrogen may delay the onset of the earliest stages of atherosclerosis, which are more likely to be present in younger women. However, it may be ineffective or may even trigger events in existing advanced vascular lesions such as those found in older women (Mendelsohn, 2005). The potential existence of a "window of opportunity" to reduce cardiovascular disease is supported by animal and laboratory studies (Grodstein, 2003).

These patient characteristics, biases, and timing in initiation may have led, in part, to favorable outcomes attributed to estrogen in observational trials. When the biases of observational trials are eliminated and the data reanalyzed, the results from earlier observational trials and from existing RCTs are remarkably similar. Importantly, these data should not be extrapolated en bloc to a chronologically distinct younger population experiencing early menopause or to those with oophorectomy prior to the normal age of menopause.

Postmenopausal Estrogen/Progestin Interventions Trial

Because of data available in the late 1980s, estrogens were prescribed, not only for vasomotor symptom relief, but also for prevention of other conditions. In 1995, the Postmenopausal Estrogen/Progestin Interventions (PEPI) Trial results were published and suggested benefit for coronary heart disease risk. In this study, menopausal women with a mean age of 56 years were randomly allocated to one of five treatments: (1) placebo, (2) estrogen alone, (3) estrogen plus cyclic medroxyprogesterone acetate (MPA), (4) estrogen plus cyclic micronized progesterone, or (5) estrogen plus continuous MPA (The Writing Group for the PEPI Trial, 1995). Primary outcomes studied in the 875 women evaluated during 3 years included assessment of systolic blood pressure and measurement of serum lipid, insulin, and fibrinogen levels. The PEPI trial documented that low-density lipoprotein cholesterol levels were decreased similarly in all groups administered estrogen compared with placebo. In addition, high-density lipoprotein levels were increased in the four treatment groups receiving estrogen. Levels were most substantially increased in women solely given estrogen. An intermediate effect was noted in those prescribed conjugated equine estrogen (CEE) and micronized progesterone, whereas the smallest increase followed CEE and MPA administration. Fibrinogen was increased in the placebo group compared with groups given hormones. However, no differences were identified among any treatment groups in systolic blood pressure or glucose-challenged insulin levels. Clinical outcomes were also reported, and complications were few. Of these, all occurred in the HT-treated groups and included one cardiac arrest, two myocardial infarctions, and two cerebrovascular events (American College of Obstetricians and Gynecologists, 2004b).

Heart and Estrogen/Progestin Replacement Study

With results published in 1998, the Heart and Estrogen/Progestin Replacement Study (HERS) described cardiac morbidity in 2763 women with preexisting heart disease (Hulley, 1998). These women received estrogen as secondary prevention for further cardiac disease progression. First-year findings showed an increase in myocardial infarctions (MIs) in women who received CEE with continuous MPA. However, after average treatment duration of 4 years, there was no difference in risks of cardiovascular death or nonfatal MI between treatment groups.

The HERS trial represented the first randomized clinical trial at variance with previous observational data and created significant confusion for both clinicians and their patients. There was still widespread belief that hormones prevented heart disease, but the HERS data caused many clinicians and scientists to begin to seriously question the cardioprotective effects of hormones. In June 2002, the follow-up study HERS II results were published by Grady and colleagues (2002) and also showed that HT was not beneficial in the secondary prevention of heart disease even after 6.8 years. Moreover, a subsequent reanalysis of the Nurse's Health Study focusing on early hazard among women initiating HT during the monitoring period showed a similar time trend, with early harm (Grodstein, 2001).

Women's Health Initiative

After an unsuccessful effort in 1990 to obtain FDA approval for HT as a preventive treatment for coronary heart disease, the need for randomized clinical trials to demonstrate conclusive benefit was widely acknowledged. As a result, before the results from the PEPI trial and HERS trials were available, the National Institutes of Health (NIH) launched the Women's Health Initiative (WHI) in 1993. This was the largest study in women ever performed to evaluate the most common causes of death, disability, and decreased quality of life. Specific endpoints were evaluated: coronary heart disease, venous thrombotic events, breast cancer, colon cancer, and bone fractures. The study had both an observational component and a randomized controlled clinical trial. The clinical trial enrolled postmenopausal women, aged 50 to 79 years, mainly without previous cardiovascular events. The WHI examined the effect of a single combined CEE and MPA drug compared with placebo in 16,608 healthy postmenopausal women who had not had a hysterectomy (Rossouw, 2002). Concurrently, the study also compared CEE with placebo in postmenopausal women without a uterus (the estrogen-only arm).

As part of the original WHI study design, investigators predetermined targets for coronary heart disease (CHD) (anticipated benefit) and breast cancer (anticipated risk) as primary disease endpoints. This design dictated that if the incidence of an endpoint was exceeded within a given period, the study would be terminated. Moreover, combined endpoints were weighted into a "global index," which if exceeded within a given time period, would result in study termination. After a mean 5.2 years of monitoring, the estrogen and progestin arm

of WHI was halted early upon recommendation of its Data and Safety Monitoring board because overall risks exceeded the benefits. In July 2002, results were released to the media. This preceded journal publication of the data and timely education of health-care providers. Chaos ensued while physicians and patients evaluated research facts before recommendations could be made.

In a subsequent detailed analysis of cardiovascular endpoints, the hazard for cardiovascular death or nonfatal MI was 1.24. This translated into 188 actual cases in the hormone group and 147 in the placebo group (Anderson, 2004). However, there were no significant differences in coronary revascularization, hospitalization for angina, confirmed angina, acute coronary syndrome, or congestive heart failure. Table 22-1 includes the calculated net adverse or beneficial health events occurring in 10,000 women taking hormone therapy based on the WHI data.

To explore the issue of timing of hormone therapy initiation and its influence on cardiovascular disease, Rossouw and colleagues (2007) did a secondary analysis of the WHI. They looked specifically at the effect of HT on CHD and stroke across categories of age and years since menopause in the combined trial. They found that women who initiated hormone therapy closer to menopause tended to have reduced CHD risk compared with the increase in CHD risk among women more distant from menopause. For women with less than 10 years since menopause began, the hazard ratio for CHD was 0.76; with 10 to 20 years since menopause, 1.10; and with

TABLE 22-1. Net Adverse Health Events in Women Taking Hormone Therapy[a]

Health Event	E + P	E Alone
Potential risks		
Coronary heart disease event	+7	−5
Stroke	+8	+12
Thromboembolism	+18	+7
Breast cancer	+8	−8
Endometrial cancer	−1	NA
Global index	+19	+2
Death	−1	+3
Dementia	+19	+9
Mild cognitive impairment (MCI)	+1	+18
Dementia or MCI	+27	**+35**
Potential benefits		
Colon cancer	−6	−6
Hip fracture	−5	+1

[a]The calculated number of net adverse health events occurring in 10,000 women taking hormone therapy (either estrogen plus progestin, E + P, or estrogen-only, E alone) compared with placebo for 1 year, based on the Women's Health Initiative trial results.
Bolded numbers reflect statistically significant benefits or risks in the hormone groups compared with the placebo group, $p < 0.05$.
NA = not applicable.
From Lam, 2005, with permission.

20 or more years, 1.28. Specifically, for the age group of 50 to 59 years, the hazard ratio (HR) for CHD was 0.93 or two *fewer* events per 10,000 person years; for the age group 60 to 69 years, 0.98 or 1 *fewer* event per 10,000 person years; and for those 70 to 79 years, 1.26 or 19 *extra* events per 10,000 person years. Rossouw and colleagues concluded that women who initiated hormone therapy closer to menopause tended to have reduced CHD risk compared with the increase in CHD risk among women more distant from menopause. In their analysis, hormone therapy increased the risk of stroke. The hazard ratio was 1.32, and risk did not vary significantly by age or time since menopause.

Whether CEE or CEE plus MPA administration improves the cardiovascular health of women who recently experienced menopause remains to be definitely determined. Presently, there is insufficient evidence to suggest that long-term CEE or CEE plus MPA should be initiated or continued for primary prevention of CHD. Although this was the principal conclusion of the trial, the results led to the restriction of HT use even for healthy women with bothersome vasomotor symptoms at the time of menopause. Concurrent with the WHI, a similarly constructed study, the Women's International Study of Long Duration Oestrogen after Menopause (WISDOM) began enrollment in 1999. This trial was prematurely closed as a result of the publication of the WHI findings. Analyzing data collected from this study, Vickers and colleagues (2007) found that hormone replacement therapy increased cardiovascular and thromboembolic risk when started many years after the menopause.

Concerns regarding the older age of the WHI cohort and the use of continuous combined CEE/MPA in the WHI study have led the Kronos Longevity Research Institute to fund a study in eight major medical centers. The Kronos Early Estrogen Prevention Study (KEEPS) will test the benefit of estradiol (E_2) administered to recently menopausal women ranging in age from 40 to 55 years, whose last menstrual period will have occurred from 6 months to 3 years before entering the study. These women will continuously receive estrogen either orally or transdermally. Micronized progesterone will be added for 10 days each month to mimic the normal menstrual cycle and limit the systemic exposure to progesterone. Alteration in surrogate CHD risk markers, including carotid intimal thickness and the accrual of coronary calcium deposition, will be studied (Miller, 2009). Results will be forthcoming.

CURRENT APPROACH TO HORMONE REPLACEMENT ADMINISTRATION

Summary of Risks and Benefits

As a result of these and other studies, clinicians now know more about the risks and benefits of HT than ever before. In the many reviews and discussions following WHI, most clinicians agree that HT is associated with an increased risk of CHD in older menopausal women, and an increased risk of stroke, venous thromboembolism, and cholecystitis. Breast cancer appears to be a risk factor with long-term use (>5 years). Two studies have shown an increase in ovarian cancer risk with long-

term use (>10 years), but not with short-term use (<5 years) (Danforth, 2007; Lacey, 2006). However, other studies have not confirmed this risk (Noller, 2002).

In contrast, several long-term benefits are noted with HT. These include increased bone mineral density and decreased rates of fracture and colorectal cancer. In addition to its individual benefits, HT's effects on mortality rates have been examined. A metaanalysis done by Salpeter and associates (2004) pooled data from 30 randomized trials from 1966 through April 2003. Calculations from 26,708 participants revealed that the total mortality rate associated with HT was 0.98. Of note, HT reduced mortality rates in women younger than 60 years but not in women older than 60. These investigators suggest that once coronary heart disease is established, HT has no effect in reversing disease progression. Moreover, the incidence of cardiovascular events can potentially increase in older groups due to an increased risk for blood clots. Similarly, Rossouw's group (2007) showed a nonsignificant tendency for the effects of hormone therapy on total mortality rates to be more favorable in younger than older women.

A Cochrane Database review reported on 19 randomized double-blind trials involving 41,904 women through 2007 that compared HT with placebo (Farquhar, 2009). HT included estrogens, with or without progestins, via oral, transdermal, or subcutaneous routes. They found that in relatively healthy women, combined continuous HT significantly increased the risk of venous thromboembolism (VTE) or coronary event (after 1 year's use), stroke (after 3 years), and breast cancer and gallbladder disease. Long-term estrogen-only HT significantly increased the risk of VTE, stroke, and gallbladder disease (after 1 to 2 years, 3 years, and 7 years' use, respectively), but did not significantly increase breast cancer risk. The only statistically significant benefits of HT were a decreased incidence of fractures and (for combined HT) colon cancer, with long-term use. Among women aged older than 65 who were relatively healthy and taking continuous combined HT, there was a statistically significant increase in the incidence of dementia. Among women with cardiovascular disease, long-term use of HT significantly increased the risk of VTE.

In this same database review, Farquhar and her colleagues noted one trial in which a subgroup of 2839 relatively healthy 50- to 59-year-old women taking HT and 1637 taking estrogen only were compared to a similar-sized placebo group. The only significantly increase risk reported was for VTEs in women taking combined continuous HT. However, their absolute risk remained low, at less than 1 in 500. This study was not powered to detect differences between groups of younger women.

Long-term use of HT is associated with an increased risk of breast cancer (Collaborative Group on Hormonal Factors in Breast Cancer, 1997). Observational studies demonstrate a relative risk of approximately 1.3 with long-term HT use, generally defined as greater than 5 years. The WHI trial demonstrated a significant 26-percent increase in the risk of invasive breast cancer in women assigned to combined estrogen and progestin therapy after approximately 5 years of use. No increased risk was seen in short-term or past users (Rossouw, 2002). As stated earlier, the WHI trial of estrogen alone in women with prior hysterectomy demonstrated no increased risk of breast cancer after an average of 7 years of estrogen use. In those from this group surveilled for 10.7 years after the WHI was stopped, a decreased risk of breast cancer was noted (LaCroix, 2011). The proportion of women needing repeat mammograms was significantly increased in both intervention groups in WHI (Stefanick, 2006). However, estrogen-alone therapy was associated with a significantly increased risk of breast cancer after 15 years of current use in the Nurses' Health Study and for current users in the Million Women Observational study of United Kingdom women (Beral, 2003; Chen, 2006).

Summary of Current Use Indications

The past decade has emphasized that HT prescribing is complex and needs to be tailored to the individual symptomatic woman's risk/benefit profile. Thus dose, type, and route of administration need to be carefully evaluated. Based on current literature, HT is indicated today only for treatment of vasomotor symptoms and vaginal atrophy and for osteoporosis prevention or treatment. The current standard of care dictates reevaluation of the need for therapy at 6- to 12-month intervals. Accordingly, bone-specific agents would likely be more appropriate in women requiring long-term osteoporosis prevention or treatment. If estrogen treatment is elected for isolated vaginal symptoms, low-dose local ET is advised and safe for extended treatment. Importantly, HT is not indicated for the routine management of other chronic disease.

Hormone treatment should be prescribed in the lowest effective dose for the shortest period of time (American College of Obstetricians and Gynecologists, 2008). Although providers should note these guidelines, there actually are no arbitrary time limits regarding the duration of HT use in the well-informed symptomatic woman. It can be used for as long as the woman feels the benefits outweigh the risks for her. Clinicians should remind patients that risks do increase with increasing age and duration of use. Annual or semiannual visits to discuss symptoms, side effects, and current scientific literature that verify risks and benefits should be tailored to the individual patient.

For women with a uterus, a progestin should be combined with an estrogen to lower risks of endometrial cancer. Progestins may be prescribed daily with estrogen, and this dosing is termed *continuous therapy*. Amenorrhea typically results from this regimen. Alternatively, estrogen may be administered for 25 days each month and a progestin added for the final 10 days. Drugs are withdrawn for 5 days, and endometrial sloughing and bleeding follows. Another common regimen includes treatment with estrogen continuously with a progestin administered for the first 10 days of each month. These regimens are considered *cyclic therapy*. Of these regimens, cyclic therapy is most commonly used in those during menopausal transition, whereas continuous therapy is usually selected for women following menopause.

If required, progestins are usually prescribed in an oral form, although a progestin-releasing intrauterine device (Mirena) provides another promising option for localized progesterone administration in postmenopausal women (Chap. 5, p. 137)

(Peled, 2007). In addition, combined estrogen and progestin products are available for either oral or transdermal use. Low-dose combination oral contraceptives are effective in the young perimenopausal woman and have the additional benefit of pregnancy prevention.

Estrogen Contraindications

Importantly, estrogen is contraindicated in women who exhibit one or more of the following: known or suspected breast carcinoma, known or suspected estrogen-dependent neoplasia, abnormal genital bleeding of unknown etiology, known or suspected pregnancy, and those with active liver disease (Table 22-2). In addition, data show a twofold increase in the risk of VTE in users of HT. Estrogens, particularly those given orally, stimulate hepatic production of clotting factors. Accordingly, HT is also contraindicated in women with a prior history of VTE.

Ultimately, the decision on whether to initiate HT or to stop it is a personal one and is decided by a patient with guidance from her health-care provider. When stopping HT, it is unclear whether abrupt cessation or a taper is superior. Some recurrence of vasomotor symptoms is to be expected.

SYMPTOMS OF MENOPAUSE

Common early symptoms of menopause are those caused by vasomotor instability and include hot flashes, insomnia, irritability, and mood disorders. In addition to symptoms, vaginal atrophy, stress urinary incontinence, and skin atrophy are among the physical changes. There are long-term health risks attributed to the hormonal changes from menopause in association with natural aging. These include osteoporosis, cardiovascular disease, and in some studies, Alzheimer disease, macular degeneration, and stroke.

Treatment of Vasomotor Symptoms

Vasomotor symptoms, also known as hot flashes or hot flushes, are the most frequent complaint of the menopausal transition (Chap. 21, p. 560). Following menopause, hot flashes are still pervasive and are experienced by 50 to 85 percent of postmenopausal women. Significant distress results for approximately 25 percent of women. Sleep disturbances can lead to lethargy and depressed mood.

The frequency of hot flashes does decrease with time. In the PEPI trial, the percentage of women taking placebo who experienced vasomotor symptoms declined from 56 percent at their entry into the study to 30 percent by their third year in the trial (Greendale, 1998). Only a small percentage of women continue to suffer from hot flashes 10 years after their menopause. Fifteen years after menopause, approximately 3 percent of women report frequent hot flashes, and 12 percent report moderate to severe vasomotor symptoms (Barnabei, 2002; Hays, 2003).

Hormonal Therapy
Estrogen
Therapy Effectiveness. Systemic ET is the most effective treatment for vasomotor symptoms and is the only therapy currently approved by the FDA for this indication (Shifren, 2010).

TABLE 22-2. Warnings and Precautions with Estrogen Administration

Estrogen should not be used in women with any of the following conditions:

Undiagnosed abnormal genital bleeding

Known, suspected, or history of breast cancer

Known or suspected estrogen-dependent neoplasia

Active deep vein thrombosis, pulmonary embolism, or history of these conditions

Active or recent (e.g., within the past year) arterial thromboembolic disease (e.g., stroke or myocardial infarction)

Liver dysfunction or disease

Known hypersensitivity to the ingredients of the estrogen preparation

Known or suspected pregnancy. There is no indication for estrogen in pregnancy. There appears to be little or no
  increased risk of birth defects in children born to women who have used estrogens and progestins from oral
  contraceptives inadvertently during early pregnancy

Estrogen should be used with caution in women with the following conditions:

Dementia

Gallbladder disease

Hypertriglyceridemia

Prior cholestatic jaundice

Hypothyroidism

Fluid retention plus cardiac or renal dysfunction

Severe hypocalcemia

Prior endometriosis

Hepatic hemangiomas

Summarized from U.S. Department of Health and Human Services, 2005.

The value of such treatment has been demonstrated in numerous RCTs (Nelson, 2004). MacLennan and associates (2004) performed a systematic review of 24 RCTs involving 3329 women who had moderate to severe hot flashes. These investigators found that HT reduced the frequency of hot flashes by approximately 18 events per week, that is, approximately 75 percent compared with placebo. The severity of vasomotor symptoms was also reduced significantly. Moreover, in the PEPI trial, all treatment arms were more effective than placebo in reducing vasomotor symptoms. There were no significant differences between specific hormone regimens (Greendale, 1998).

Estrogens Approved for Vasomotor Symptoms. Estrogen can be administered by oral, parenteral, topical, vaginal, or transdermal routes with similar effects (Table 22-3). Within these groups, several different formulation choices are available. Continuous estrogen therapy is recommended, although doses and route of administration can be changed relative to patient preference. In the United States, oral estrogens have been the most popular, although it appears that transdermal administration may be somewhat safer. Specifically, transdermal estrogen patches avoid the liver's first pass effect and offer the convenience of less frequent administration (once or twice weekly). The lowest effective dose and duration of therapy are unknown, but this "mantra" is cited by most major menopause organizations for ensuring safety.

Progestins. These alone are somewhat effective for treatment of hot flashes in women for whom estrogen is contraindicated, such as those with history of venous thromboembolism or breast cancer. However, adverse effects that include vaginal bleeding and weight gain may limit their use.

Beyond mild reduction in hot flashes, progestins used as agents in combined HT offer only one additional benefit—they provide essential protection against estrogen-induced endometrial hyperplasia and cancer in women with a uterus. Clinical trials have shown that progestins provide no meaningful increase in estrogen's benefits to bone. In addition, progestins may attenuate estrogen's beneficial effects on lipids and blood flow.

"Bioidentical" Hormones

FDA-Approved Products. Some women have come to believe that conventional pharmaceutical hormone treatment holds a clear and present danger. The lay press and self-help hormone books are replete with information suggesting that bioidentical hormones offer the relief that women need with fewer attendant risks. By definition, bioidentical HT refers to therapy similar in chemical composition to that made in the human body, and these preparations use 17β-estradiol and/or progesterone. FDA-approved bioidentical products are available in various routes of administration that provide constant, low levels of hormones (see Table 22-2). These products are regulated and monitored by the FDA. They have proven efficacy at relieving menopausal symptoms and have published endometrial safety profiles.

Non-FDA-Approved Compounded Bioidentical Products. These are available by prescription for those who cannot tolerate FDA-approved products. Topical regimens include Tri-est

TABLE 22-3. Selected Estrogen and Progestin Preparations for the Treatment of Menopausal Vasomotor Symptoms

Preparation	Generic Name	Brand Name	Available Strengths
Estrogen			
Oral[a]	CEE	Premarin	0.3, 0.45, 0.625, 0.9, or 1.25 mg
	17β-Estradiol	Estrace[b]	0.5, 1.0, or 2.0 mg
	Estradiol acetate	Femtrace	0.45, 0.9, or 1.8 mg
	10 synthetic estrogens	Enjuvia	0.3, 0.45, 0.625, 0.9, or 1.25 mg
Transdermal patch	17β-Estradiol	Alora[b]	0.025, 0.05, 0.075, or 0.1 mg/d (patch applied twice weekly to abdomen or buttock; 8 patches/box)
	17β-Estradiol	Climara[b]	0.025, 0.0375, 0.05, 0.06 0.075, or 0.1 mg/d (patch applied to abdomen or buttock weekly; 4 patches/box)
	17β-Estradiol	Menostar[b]	14 μg/d (patch applied to abdomen weekly; 4 patches/box)
	17β-Estradiol	Vivelle-dot[b]	0.025, 0.0375, 0.05, or 0.075, 0.1 mg/d (patch applied twice weekly to abdomen; 8 patches/box)
Transdermal gel	17β-Estradiol	Estrogel[b]	1 metered-dose of gel applied daily to arm (64 doses per 93-g can)
	17β-Estradiol	Estrasorb[b]	Gel from 2 packets applied to legs daily (56 packets/carton)
	17β-Estradiol	Divigel[b]	0.25, 0.5, or 1 mg packets Gel from 1 packet applied to thigh daily (30 packets/carton)
	17β-Estradiol	Elestrin[b]	1 metered-dose of gel applied to arm daily (30 doses per 35-g container)
	17β-Estradiol	Evamist[b]	1 to 3 metered-dose sprays to forearm daily (56 doses per pump)
Vaginal	Estradiol acetate	Femring	0.05 or 0.1 mg/d (inserted for 90 days)
Progestin			
Oral	MPA	Provera	2.5, 5.0, or 10.0 mg
	Micronized proge-sterone	Prometrium[b]	200 mg (in peanut oil) (1 daily for 12 days each 28-d cycle)
Vaginal	Progesterone	Prochieve 4%[b]	45 mg
Combination Preparations			
Oral sequential[b]	CEE + MPA	Premphase	0.625 mg CEE (red) plus 0.625 mg CEE/5.0 mg MPA (blue) (28 pills per pack; 14 red & 14 blue)[c]
Oral continuous[a]	CEE+ MPA	Prempro	0.3 mg CEE/1.5 mg MPA, or 0.45 mg CEE/1.5 mg MPA, or 0.625 mg CEE/2.5 mg MPA, or 0.625 mg CEE/5 mg MPA (28 pills per pack)
	17β-Estradiol + drospirenone	Angeliq	1 mg E_2/0.5 mg drospirenone (28 pills per pack)
	17β-Estradiol + NETA	Activella	1 mg E_2/0.5 mg NETA, or 0.5 mg E_2/0.1 mg NETA (28 pills per dial pack)
	Ethinyl estradiol + NETA	femhrt	2.5 μg EE/0.5 mg NETA, or 5 μg EE/1 mg NETA
Transdermal continuous	17β-Estradiol + LNG	Climara Pro	0.045 mg/d E_2 + 0.015 mg/d LNG (patch applied weekly)
	17β-Estradiol + NETA	CombiPatch	0.05 mg/d E_2 + 0.14 mg/d NETA, or 0.05 mg/d E_2/0.25 mg/d NETA (patch applied twice weekly to abdomen)

LNG = levonorgestrel; MPA = medroxyprogesterone acetate; NETA = norethindrone acetate.
[a]One pill daily
[b]Considered a bioidentical preparation.
[c]The first 14 pills contain estrogen and the subsequent pills (15 through 28) contain estrogen with progestin.

(80 percent estriol, 10 percent estrone, 10 percent estradiol) or Bi-est (estriol 80 percent and estradiol 20 percent) in a range of 1.25 to 2.5 mg. These estrogens are compounded with micronized progesterone, 10 to 50 mg daily, in Dermabase, Eucerin, or other similar creams or emollients.

Some compounding pharmacies tout the safety and efficacy of their compounded hormones and advertise treatments individualized to patients based on salivary hormone testing. Unfortunately, salivary testing has tremendous inter- and intra-patient variability and has been found to lack correlation with serum hormone levels (Boothby, 2004). Moreover, these products have not undergone rigorous RCTs regarding safety or efficacy. Thus, patient education is needed regarding potential risks and benefits of these products. Specifically, regarding other types or forms of HT, the FDA has pronounced: "Other doses of CEE and MPA, and other combinations and dosage forms of estrogens and progestins were not studied in the WHI clinical trials, and in the absence of comparable data, these risks should be assumed to be similar." Thus, compounded hormones cannot be assumed to be safer than conventional pharmaceutical estrogen or progestins. Importantly, adequate endometrial protection is needed if compounded estrogens are prescribed (Pinkerton, 2009).

Central Nervous System Agents for Vasomotor Symptoms

No nonhormonal treatments are currently FDA-approved for management of hot flashes, and long-term studies are not available. However, multiple agents and treatments have been used, and data from short-term trials have been published (Table 22-4). These products provide options for women who decline HT or for those in whom estrogen is contraindicated. However, for many, the side effects or ineffectiveness of these agents compared with HT limits their routine use for this indication.

Selective Serotonin-Reuptake Inhibitors, Selective Serotonin, Norepinephrine-Reuptake Inhibitors. Randomized placebo-controlled trials with the antidepressants venlafaxine (Effexor), fluoxetine (Prozac, Sarafem), paroxetine (Paxil), and desvenlafaxine (Pristiq) found modest improve-

ment in hot flashes compared with placebo. Specifically, in a randomized, double-blind, placebo-controlled study, Loprinzi and associates (2000) found that venlafaxine XR decreased hot flash scores by 37 percent with a dosage of 37.5 mg/d, 61 percent with 75 mg/d, and 61 percent with 150 mg/d. Women treated with placebo noted a 27-percent reduction in hot flashes. Later, Loprinzi and colleagues (2002) studied the effects of fluoxetine, 20 mg/d, on hot flashes. They reported that women treated with the selective serotonin-reuptake inhibitor (SSRI) noted only 1.5 fewer vasomotor events compared with those receiving placebo. In a 6-week trial, Stearns and coworkers (2003) evaluated paroxetine CR, 12.5 mg/d and 25 mg/d dosages, compared with placebo. At both dosages, paroxetine led to approximately three fewer hot flashes per day compared with 1.8 fewer hot flashes per day with placebo. Lastly, groups prescribed desvenlafaxine 100 or 150 mg/d noted an approximate 65-percent reduction in hot flashes. However, this equated to only 1 to 2 fewer events per day than with placebo (Archer, 2008, 2009b). Importantly, benefits of SSRIs should be balanced against drug side effects, which can include nausea, diarrhea, headache, insomnia, jitteriness, fatigue, and sexual dysfunction.

Clonidine. The centrally active α_2-adrenergic-receptor agonist clonidine (Catapres and others) has also been shown to be effective in some clinical trials. Nagamani and colleagues (1987) evaluated clonidine 0.1 mg/d transdermally in an 8-week trial. They reported that 12 of 15 women noted a decrease in vasomotor symptoms compared with 5 of 14 receiving placebo. However, hypotension, dry mouth, dizziness, constipation, and sedation have limited its use. For many women, low-dose clonidine is ineffective, and thus adequate therapy may require substantially higher doses that may magnify side effects.

Gabapentin. Gabapentin (Neurontin) is structurally related to the neurotransmitter gamma amino butyric acid (GABA), but its exact mechanism of action is unknown. Currently, gabapentin is FDA-approved to treat partial seizures, neuropathic pain, and postherpetic neuralgia (Brown, 2009). However, it has extensive off-label use for various other neurologic conditions.

Guttuso and associates (2003) evaluated the use of gabapentin, 900 mg orally daily, for treatment of vasomotor symptoms. They found a 45-percent reduction in hot flash frequency compared with a 29-percent reduction with placebo. Adverse effects included dizziness and somnolence. Moreover, Reddy and coworkers (2006) conducted a randomized, double-blinded, placebo-controlled trial in which 60 postmenopausal women received gabapentin, 2400 mg/d; oral conjugated estrogen, 0.625 mg/d; or placebo for 12 weeks. The reductions in the hot flash composite scores for both estrogen (72 percent) and gabapentin (71 percent) were greater than that associated with placebo (54 percent). However, headache, dizziness, and disorientation occurred in almost 25 percent of the women treated with gabapentin. Long-term studies evaluating gabapentin for treatment of hot flashes are not available (Shifren, 2010).

TABLE 22-4. Nonhormonal Agents Used as Therapy for Vasomotor Symptoms

Prescription (Brand Name)	Nonprescription
SSRIs (see Table 13-14, p. 366)	Black cohosh
Fluoxetine (Prozac, Sarafem)	Dong quai
Paroxetine (Paxil)	Red clover isoflavones
Venlafaxine (Effexor)	Soy isoflavones
SNRI: Desvenlafaxine (Pristiq)	Vitamin E
Clonidine (Catapres)	
Gabapentin (Neurontin)	
Mirtazapine (Remeron)	
Trazodone (Desyrel)	

SNRI = selective serotonin and norepinephrine-reuptake inhibitor; SSRI = selective serotonin-reuptake inhibitor.

Alpha-Methyldopa. At doses of 500 to 1000 mg/d, methyldopa, an antihypertensive, has been shown to be twice as effective as placebo for the treatment of vasomotor symptoms. However, in studies evaluating its efficacy, side effects included dizziness, nausea, fatigue, and dry mouth (Fugate, 2004). Because of significant side effects with this drug and modest improvement in vasomotor symptoms, this drug is not recommended for this indication.

Bellergal. Bellergal (Bellergal-S, no longer available in the United States) is a sedative that contains phenobarbital, ergotamine tartrate, and belladonna alkaloids (Loprinzi, 2005). In randomized double-blind studies, this agent showed either modest or no reduction in vasomotor symptoms compared with placebo. Moreover, in these studies, more than 30 percent of participants withdrew due to treatment ineffectiveness or side effects. Moreover, barbiturates are addictive and are not recommended for long-term use. Because of its limited efficacy and significant side effects, this agent is not recommended for this indication.

Sleep Medications. Women who are principally bothered by night sweats and sleep disruption may benefit from a trial of sleep medication. The antihistamine diphenhydramine hydrochloride may serve as an inexpensive, over-the-counter sleep aid. Also, the prescription insomnia treatment eszopiclone (Lunesta) significantly improved sleep and positively affected mood, quality of life, next-day functioning, and menopause-related symptoms in a double-blind, placebo-controlled study of perimenopausal and postmenopausal women (Soares, 2006). A list of available sleep aids is found in Table 1-24 (p. 29).

Complementary and Alternative Medicine (CAM)

In 2005, out-of-pocket expenditures for alternative therapies were estimated at nearly $30 billion, which was more than the out-of-pocket expenditures for all physician services that year (Castelo-Branco, 2005) In 2002, 49 percent of women in the United States and Canada used CAM, and the trend seems to be increasing (Newton, 2002).

Acupuncture. This is one CAM therapy that has been evaluated to control hot flashes in multicenter, randomized controlled trials conducted with perimenopausal and postmenopausal women (Borud, 2009; Kim, 2010). In two trials, treatment groups received 10 or 12 sessions of acupuncture compared with a control group. Significant decreases were found in hot flash frequency and intensity. However, both studies had small study groups and had data from only short-term therapy and follow-up. Despite these limitations, this therapy does show promise.

Adiposity. Competing hypotheses suggest how adiposity may affect menopausal hot flashes. One hypothesis asserts that aromatization of androgens to estrogens in body fat should lead to decreased hot flash frequency. Conversely, thermoregulatory models argue that greater body fat should be associated with increased hot flashes from insulating effects. Germaine to this theory, Thurston and colleagues (2008) found that increased abdominal adiposity, particularly subcutaneous adiposity, was associated with increased odds of hot flashes. Their suggestion is that fat loss and aerobic exercise may improve the severity of hot flashes. However, additional studies are needed.

Phytoestrogens. Phytoestrogens (isoflavones) are plant-derived compounds that bind to estrogen receptors and have both estrogen agonist and antagonist properties. They are found in soy products and red clover. Small studies evaluating their effectiveness for the treatment of vasomotor symptoms have noted no efficacy or mixed results (Krebs, 2004).

Soy Products. The two main soybean isoflavones are genistein and daidzein. Although the mechanisms of action of soy and dietary isoflavones are not fully understood, they appear to involve binding to the estrogen receptor. For this reason, one should not assume these dietary supplements are safe for women with estrogen-dependent cancers.

For treatment of hot flashes, data supporting isoflavone efficacy are mixed. Albertazzi and colleagues (1998) provided a pure dietary soy supplement that contained 40 mg of protein and 76 mg of isoflavones. In women using this supplement, a 45-percent reduction in vasomotor symptoms was noted compared with a 30-percent reduction in women receiving placebo. Cheng and associates (2007) provided 60 mg of isoflavones or placebo for 3 months to symptomatic women. They noted that isoflavone treatment reduced hot flashes by 57 percent. In contrast, in a double-blind clinical trial with breast cancer survivors, Levis and colleagues (2011) found higher rates of vasomotor symptoms in women given soy tablets containing 200 mg of isoflavones per day compared with those administered placebo.

The effects of soy protein found in various food preparations are not bioequivalent. Even soy foods are not necessarily reliable sources of biologically active isoflavones. For example, the alcohol processing often used in the manufacture of tofu and soymilk removes the biologically active forms, the aglyconic isoflavones. Accordingly, soy food producers have recognized public interested in isoflavone supplements, and many indicate in their product labeling the amounts and forms of isoflavones found in the foodstuff.

Flaxseed. Flaxseed or flaxseed oil (*Linum usitatissimum*) is rich in α-linolenic acid, a form of omega-3 fatty acid. Also known as linseed, flaxseed is touted to reduce inflammation, bone turnover, heart disease, cancer, diabetes, and cholesterol levels. For perimenopausal women, it also is purported to protect against breast cancer, hot flashes, and mood disturbances. However, data regarding flaxseed efficacy for treatment of hot flashes are limited. Lewis and coworkers (2006) conducted a double-blinded, randomized controlled trial in which 87 women were assigned to one of three groups, which daily ingested muffins that contained soy, flaxseed, or wheat. This study found no significant difference in vasomotor symptoms among the three groups. In contrast, Lemay and associates (2002) found 40 g of flaxseed as effective as 0.625 mg of CEE for the treatment of mild menopausal symptoms in a randomized cross-over study comparing the two.

Red Clover. *Trifolium pratense* is a member of the legume family. It contains at least four estrogenic isoflavones and is therefore marketed as a source of phytoestrogens. Several studies, however, have failed to demonstrate an effect over placebo in the treatment of menopausal symptoms (American College of Obstetricians and Gynecologists, 2004a; Geller, 2009; Nelson, 2004). For example, a randomized controlled trial of 252 women studied hot flash frequency in women given red clover isoflavone extracts and placebo over 12 weeks. No significant change in hot flash frequency was reported between groups receiving isoflavones and those given placebo (Tice, 2003).

Dong Quai. Also translated as don kwai, dang gui, and tang kuei, this Chinese herbal medicine is derived from the root of *Angelica sinensis* and is the most commonly prescribed Chinese herbal medicine for "female problems." Within traditional Chinese medicine (TCM) practice, dong quai is suggested to regulate and balance the menstrual cycle, strengthen the uterus, and enrich the blood. It is also said to exert estrogenic activity. Most herbal practitioners seem to agree that it is contraindicated during pregnancy and lactation.

In 1997, Hirata and colleagues at Kaiser Permanente conducted a double-blinded controlled clinical trial using a daily dong quai dose of 4.5 g. Women using dong quai and those using placebo *both* reported a 25-percent reduction in hot flashes. Critics of the study have noted that the dose of dong quai was lower than that often used in TCM, and that dong quai is never employed as an isolated intervention. However, its benefit cannot be substantiated based on available evidence.

Dong quai is potentially toxic. It contains numerous coumarin-like derivatives and may cause excessive bleeding or interactions with other anticoagulants. This herbal agent also contains psoralens and is potentially photosensitizing, which increases concerns of sun exposure-related skin cancers.

Black Cohosh. The root of the herb *Cimifuga racemosa* is also thought to have estrogenic properties, although the mechanism of action is unknown. In two randomized placebo-controlled trials, it did not decrease the frequency of vasomotor symptoms compared with placebo (Geller, 2009; Krebs, 2004). Although few adverse effects have been reported, the long-term safety of these products is unknown.

Phytoprogestins. Extracts, tablets, and creams derived from yams are claimed to be progesterone substitutes and are frequently touted as a natural source of dehydroepiandrosterone (DHEA). Sterol structures from the plant do not have inherent biologic activity, but are used as precursors in the biosynthesis of progesterone, DHEA, and other steroids. Specifically, claims are made that the plant sterol *dioscorea* is converted into progesterone in the body and alleviates "estrogen dominance." Yam extracts are also purported to be effective for uterine cramps. However, there is no human biochemical pathway for bioconversion of dioscorea to progesterone or DHEA in vivo.

In contrast, Mexican yam extract *is* estrogenic, containing considerable *diosgenin*, an estrogen-like substance found in plants. Some estrogen effects might be expected from eating these yam species, but only if large quantities of raw yams are consumed. Yams from the grocery store generally are not the varieties known to contain significant amounts of dioscorea or diosgenin.

Based on the lack of bioavailability, the hormones in wild and Mexican yam would not be expected to have efficacy. Wild yam extracts are neither estrogenic nor progestational, and although many yam extract products contain no yam, some are laced with progesterone or medroxyprogesterone. Oral ingestion does not produce serum levels. There are no published reports demonstrating the effectiveness of wild yam cream for postmenopausal symptoms.

Vitamin E. In 125 women with a history of breast cancer, vitamin E produced a 25-percent reduction in hot flashes compared with a 22-percent reduction with placebo. This was a decrease of one hot flash per person per day (Barton, 1998).

Environmental and Lifestyle Changes

Practices that lower core body temperature such as using a fan, dressing in layers, and taking cool showers may temporarily help with night sweats and flashing. Relaxation techniques such as paced respiration can decrease symptoms. Meditation, smoking cessation, and weight loss may also be helpful, as are ingestion of cold foods and beverages.

Therapies based on the relaxation of the mind and the body for the treatment of menopausal symptoms have been shown to reduce hot flash frequency. Irvin and coworkers (1996) randomized symptomatic menopausal women to relaxation, reading, or control groups. The relaxation group had significant reductions in hot flash intensity, tension, anxiety, and depression compared with the control group, which had no significant changes. Freedman and Woodward (1992) evaluated women with frequent hot flashes who were randomized to paced respiration, muscle relaxation, and placebo biofeedback. In the paced respiration group, there was a significant reduction in the hot flash frequency, although muscle relaxation and biofeedback techniques showed no improvement. The proposed mechanism of action is decreased central sympathetic tone.

When deciding among the available interventions for vasomotor symptoms, the safest options should be encouraged first, such as lifestyle changes, and then proceeding to prescription treatments, as needed. Patient preference, symptoms severity, side effects, and the presence of other conditions, such as depression, will influence treatment options.

■ Treatment of Osteoporosis
Treatment Indications

The primary goal of osteoporosis treatment is fracture prevention in women who have low bone mineral density (BMD) or additional risk factors for fracture (Fig. 22-1). Toward this end, therapy aims to stabilize or increase BMD. Treatment includes lifestyle changes and often pharmacologic therapy.

Several organizations offer concordant guidelines for intervening with pharmacologic therapy. Namely, the National

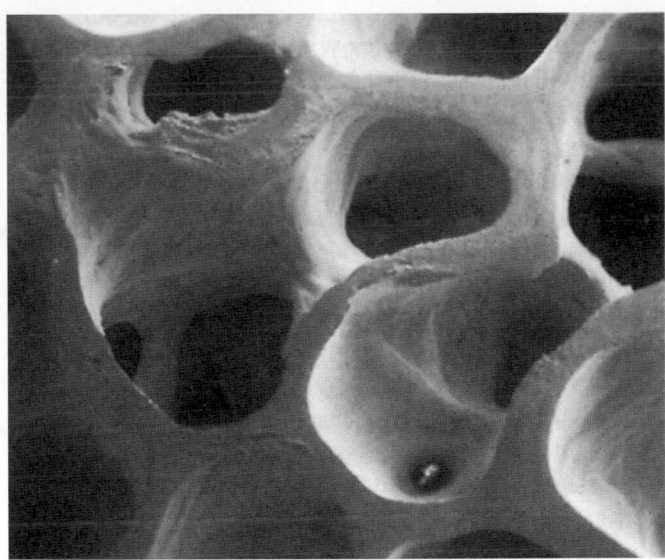 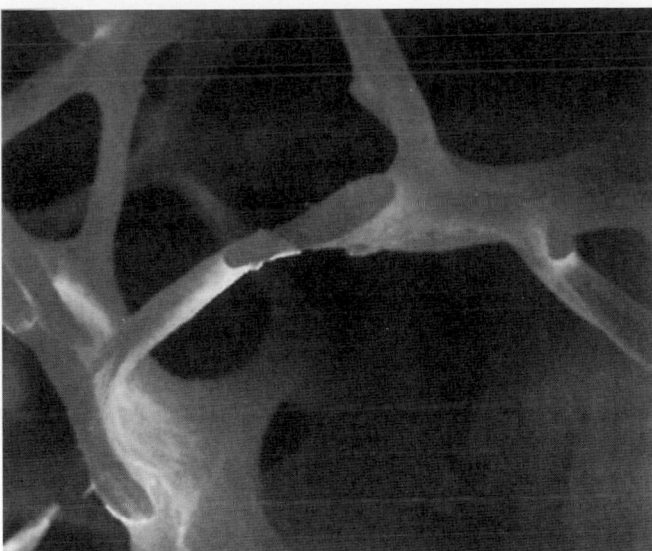

FIGURE 22-1 Electron micrographs of tissue obtained from an iliac crest biopsy. Normal bone architecture is seen in the biopsy from an individual with normal bone mineral density (*left*). Diminished bone architecture is seen in the biopsy from an individual with osteoporosis (*right*). *(From Dempster, 1986, with permission.)*

Osteoporosis Foundation (NOF)(2008), The North American Menopause Society (NAMS) (2010) and American Association of Clinical Endocrinologists (AACE) (Watts, 2010) recommends starting therapy for: (1) all postmenopausal women with total hip or spine T-scores at or below −2.5, (2) those with an osteoporotic vertebral or hip fracture, and (3) all postmenopausal women with total hip or spine T-scores from −2.0 to −2.5 and a 10-year risk of major osteoporotic fracture of at least 20 percent or risk of hip fracture of at least 3 percent. This 10-year risk is derived by the *Fracture Risk Assessment Tool (FRAX)*, which is discussed in greater detail in Chapter 21 (p. 568) and found at: http://www.shef.ac.uk/FRAX/.

Pharmacologic Considerations

Drugs prescribed for fracture prevention attempt to restore and balance bone remodeling by reducing bone resorption or by stimulating bone formation. With therapeutic intervention, BMD improvement varies according to the composition of the bone. For example, therapies that prevent bone resorption will act most quickly on bone that has high trabecular content and rapid turnover, such as the vertebrae. In contrast, the impact of drug therapies on the hip may be delayed because the hip is composed of approximately 50 percent trabecular and 50 percent cortical bone (Fig. 21-7, p. 563).

Therapeutic options include HT for the prevention of osteoporosis. For prevention *and* treatment, bisphosphonates and selective estrogen-receptor modulators (SERMs) are available (Table 22-5). Additionally, calcitonin, one monoclonal antibody, and an injectable recombinant human parathyroid hormone (PTH) have been approved for treatment. Of these, recombinant PTH is the first FDA-approved agent that works by stimulating bone formation rather than slowing bone resorption. Most recently, denosumab (Prolia), a monoclonal antibody against an activator of osteoclast development, has been approved for osteoporosis treatment.

Hormonal Therapy

Estrogen and Progesterone Replacement. As estrogen levels decline, bone-remodeling rates increase and favor bone resorption over bone formation. In observational studies, HT reduces osteoporosis-related fractures by approximately 50 percent if started soon after menopause and continued long term. HT also significantly decreases fracture rates in women with established disease (Tosteson, 2008). Results from more than 50 randomized, placebo-controlled trials show that HT reduces the rate of bone resorption and results in an increase in BMD. The WHI controlled trials confirmed a significant 33-percent reduction in hip fractures in healthy postmenopausal women receiving HT after an average surveillance of 5.6 years. Notably, hip fracture reduction was not limited to women with osteoporosis, as in trials of other pharmacologic agents (The Women's Health Initiative Steering Committee, 2004). Importantly, studies demonstrate that even very-low-dose ET, combined with calcium and vitamin D, produces significant increases in BMD compared with placebo. These dosages include oral E_2 0.25 mg/d, oral conjugated estrogen 0.3 mg/d, or transdermal E_2 0.014 or 0.025 mg/d (Ettinger, 2004; Prestwood, 2003).

Unfortunately, this preventive effect is lost rapidly following discontinuation of HT (Barrett-Connor, 2003). Women participating in the National Osteoporosis Risk Assessment (NORA) trial who had discontinued estrogen therapy within the 5 years preceding the study demonstrated a significantly higher hip fracture risk than did women who had never received estrogen therapy. In addition, current HT users in the NORA trial had a 40-percent reduction in hip fractures, which was lost by past users. Therefore, fracture risk and the potential need for an alternative therapy should be assessed when women discontinue HT.

Selective Estrogen-Receptor Modulators. Estrogen receptors are found in numerous organs (Fig. 15-9, p. 408). Selective

TABLE 22-5. Agents Approved in the United States for the Management of Osteoporosis

Agent	Brand Name	Clinical Indication	
		Prevention	Treatment
Bisphosphonates[a]			
Alendronate	Fosamax	5-mg pill once daily 35-mg pill once weekly	10-mg pill once daily 70-mg pill once weekly 70-mg solution once weekly
Ibandronate	Boniva	2.5-mg pill once daily 150-mg pill once monthly	2.5-mg pill once daily 150-mg pill once monthly
Risedronate	Actonel	5-mg pill once daily 35-mg pill once weekly 150-mg pill once monthly 75-mg pill on two consecutive days as a monthly dose	5-mg pill once daily 35-mg pill once weekly 150-mg pill once monthly 75-mg pill on two consecutive days as a monthly dose
Risedronate (enteric coated)	Atelvia		35-mg pill once weekly
Hormones			
CEE[a]	Premarin	0.3-mg pill daily	
Other estrogens	See Table 22-3		
Monoclonal Antibody			
Denosumab	Prolia		60 mg SC once every 6 months
Recombinant Human PTH			
Teriparatide	Forteo		20 μg SC daily 1 injection pen contains 28 doses
Salmon calcitonin			
Nasal spray	Fortical		1 spray = 200 IU intranasally daily (alternating nostrils daily). 1 bottle contains a 30-day supply.
	Miacalcin		1 spray = 200 IU intranasally daily (alternating nostrils daily). 1 bottle contains a 30-day supply.
Injectable	Miacalcin		100 units SC or IM every other day. 1 vial contains 4 doses.
SERM[a]			
Raloxifene	Evista	60 mg once daily	60 mg once daily

[a]Oral agents.
CEE = conjugated equine estrogen; IM = intramuscular injection; IU = international units; SC = subcutaneous injection;
PTH = parathyroid hormone; SERM = selective estrogen-receptor modulator.

estrogen-receptor modulators are oral nonhormonal compounds that bind to the estrogen receptor but induce different estrogenic responses in these various tissues.

Raloxifene. Of the SERMs, raloxifene (Evista) is the only agent approved for the prevention and treatment of osteoporosis. It activates estrogen receptors in the bone but does not appear to activate those in the breast or uterus. Raloxifene is appropriate for postmenopausal women, but not premenopausal patients. For example, one phase II clinical trial evaluating this SERM found a *decrease* in BMD with its use by a group of premenopausal women at risk for breast cancer (Eng-Wong, 2006).

Raloxifene may be most appropriate for prevention and treatment of vertebral disease. For example, raloxifene prevented vertebral fractures in the Multiple Outcomes of Raloxifene Evaluation (MORE) trial, which enrolled 7705 postmenopausal women with osteoporosis. The beneficial effects of oral raloxifene, 60 mg/d, appeared rapidly, and clinical vertebral fracture risk was reduced by 68 percent following the first year of therapy. In addition, this effect was sustained over time. At 4 years of treatment, dosages of 60 mg daily led to a 36-percent reduction in fractures, and 120 mg each day produced a 43-percent decline (Delmas, 2002; Ettinger, 1999). However, in the MORE trial, Ettinger reported that raloxifene therapy compared with placebo was not associated with significant reductions in *nonvertebral* fracture risks at 3 and 4 years.

In addition to its bone effects, raloxifene may protect against breast cancer, as suggested by observational studies of various clinical trials (Barrett-Connor, 2006). The incidence of breast cancer was evaluated as a secondary endpoint in the MORE trial. Investigators found that raloxifene was associated with a 65-percent relative risk reduction in all breast cancers. Of specific breast cancer subtypes, they noted a 90-percent reduction in estrogen receptor-positive cancers, a 12-percent reduction in estrogen receptor-negative breast cancers, and a 76-percent relative risk reduction in invasive breast cancer.

Raloxifene may not have the same increased cardiovascular risk profile as estrogen. In a MORE post hoc analysis, 4 years of raloxifene therapy had no adverse effect on cardiovascular events in the overall cohort. Advantageously, it did result in a significant 40-percent reduction in the incidence of cardiovascular events among a subgroup of women with increased cardiovascular risk (Barrett-Connor, 2002).

Of side effects, hot flashes are associated with raloxifene therapy, although the incidence is low (Cohen, 2000). Furthermore, raloxifene, 60 mg daily for 4 years, has been associated with an increased risk of thromboembolic events. In one study, the relative risk associated with any dosage of raloxifene was 2.76 for deep-vein thrombosis, 2.76 for pulmonary embolism, and 0.50 for retinal vein thrombosis (Delmas, 2002).

Bazedoxifene. In addition to raloxifene, a new SERM, bazedoxifene (Viviant), is marketed outside the United States under the trade name Conbriza and is undergoing FDA review. Similar to raloxifene, this newer SERM does not stimulate breast or uterine tissue and is effective in osteoporosis treatment. It also shows similar rates of thromboembolic events, vasomotor events, and negative vulvovaginal events (Christiansen, 2010; Silverman, 2008, 2011).

Although effective for treatment of osteoporosis, bazedoxifene is associated with the patient side effects just listed for raloxifene. For this reason, combinations of SERMs plus estrogens are being investigated. Termed *tissue-selective estrogen complexes (TSEC)*, these combinations attempt to achieve a more favorable clinical profile than either group alone. Of these, bazedoxifene plus CEE has shown promise in clinical trials (Archer, 2009a; Lindsay, 2009; Lobo, 2009; Pickar, 2009).

Nonhormonal Antiresorptive Agents

Currently, the main pharmacologic agents for osteoporosis treatment are: (1) those that primarily act by inhibiting resorption, termed *antiresorptives*, and (2) those that act by increasing bone formation, termed *anabolic agents*. Most of the bone-active agents currently available in the United States inhibit bone resorption. These include estrogen, SERMs, bisphosphonates, denosumab, calcitonin, and vitamin D. All have been shown to halt bone loss, and most also increase BMD. Two additional antiresorptive agents undergoing clinical trials currently are odanacatib and saracatinib, both which limit osteoclast activities.

Bisphosphonates. Three bisphosphonates are currently available for the prevention and treatment of osteoporosis. These

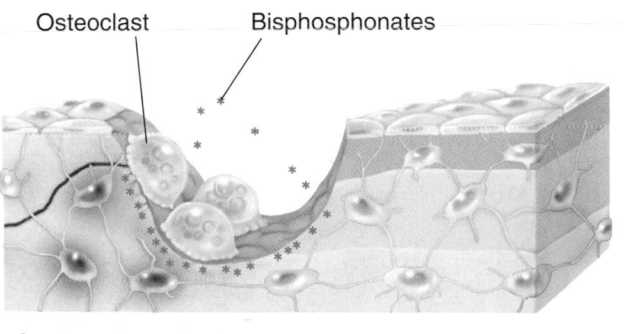

FIGURE 22-2 The molecular structure of bisphosphonates, with two short side chains (R1 and R2) attached to the C core, is similar to that of the naturally occurring pyrophosphates. The R1 side chain determines bone-binding affinity, and the R2 side chain determines antiresorptive potency. Variations in the structure of the side chains determine the strength with which the bisphosphonate binds to bone, the distribution through bone, and the amount of time it remains in the bone after treatment is discontinued.

include alendronate (Fosamax), risedronate (Actonel), and ibandronate (Boniva) (see Table 22-5) (Lambrinoudaki, 2006).

The action of bisphosphonates stems from their structural similarity to pyrophosphate, which is found in bone (Fig. 22-2). Bisphosphonates chemically bind to calcium hydroxyapatite on bone surfaces and then are taken up by osteoclasts (Fig. 22-3). These drugs block the function and survival, but

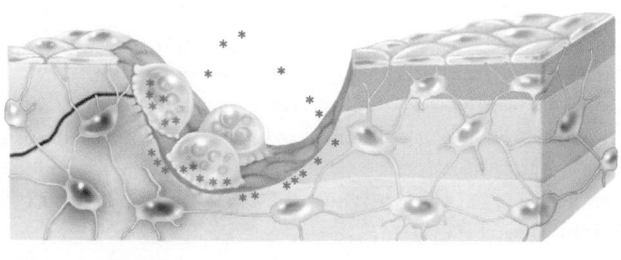

FIGURE 22-3 Bisphosphonates reduce fractures by suppressing bone resorption by osteoclasts. The molecular structure of the bisphosphonates is analogous to that of the naturally occurring pyrophosphates (see Fig. 22-2). **A.** In bone, bisphosphonate concentration is increased eightfold at sites of active bone resorption. **B.** The bisphosphonates enter osteoclasts and reduce resorption through inhibition of farnesyl pyrophosphate synthase. Inhibition of this enzyme leads to disruption of osteoclast attachment to the bone surface. This halts resorption and promotes early osteoclast cell death.

not the formation, of osteoclasts and thereby decrease bone resorption (Russell, 2008).

Bisphosphonates display poor bioavailability and therefore should be taken on an empty stomach with adequate water for proper dissolution and absorption. In general, these agents have a favorable overall safety profile, and adverse event rates arc comparable with placebo (Black, 1996; Harris, 1999). However, bisphosphonates may cause upper gastrointestinal (GI) inflammation, ulceration, and bleeding (Lanza, 2000). Thus, to aid delivery to the stomach and reduce the risk of esophageal irritation, dosing instructions should be reinforced with each patient. First, bisphosphonates should be taken in the morning with a full glass of water. During the 30 minutes following administration, no other food or beverages should be consumed. Finally, women must remain upright (sitting or standing) for at least 30 minutes after ingesting the drug.

In addition to GI effects, bisphosphonate use has been linked with osteonecrosis of the jaw (ONJ), especially following dental extractions (Marx, 2003; Srinivasan, 2007). Fortunately, this complication is rare with oral bisphosphonates (Ruggiero, 2004). More commonly, ONJ is seen with intravenous zoledronate use in those with malignancy-related bone disease (Woo, 2006).

In addition to negative bone effects in the jaw, concern has been raised regarding suppression of bone remodeling at other sites with long-term use of bisphosphonates (Park-Wyllie, 2011). Specifically, rare atypical fractures in the long bones have been reported. Yet, despite these uncommon bone side effects, the FDA (2011) recommends periodic reevaluation of the need for bisphosphonate therapy, especially in those treated for more than 5 years.

Alendronate. This bisphosphonate is approved for the treatment and prevention of osteoporosis. It is available in several forms and dosing regimens (see Table 22-5). Alendronate (Fosamax) has been shown to reduce the risk of vertebral fractures in postmenopausal women with low BMD or osteoporosis, either with or without existing vertebral fractures (Black, 1996). Alendronate also reduces nonvertebral fracture risk in women with osteoporosis. Among women with osteoporosis who participated in the Fracture Intervention Trial (FIT), the risk of nonvertebral fractures was reduced by month 24. In addition, the effects of alendronate are sustained. For example, women who used alendronate for 5 years and then discontinued use for a subsequent 5 years have comparable nonvertebral fracture rates as women using the drug for 10 years (Black, 2006; Bone, 2004).

Ibandronate. This bisphosphonate is approved for the prevention and treatment of postmenopausal osteoporosis. Ibandronate (Boniva) is an effective agent, and data from the Oral Ibandronate Osteoporosis Vertebral Fracture Trial in North America and Europe (BONE) trial showed that daily ibandronate lowered incident vertebral fracture risk by 62 percent (Chesnut, 2004). To improve compliance, this drug was evaluated as a once-monthly therapy. Once-monthly oral ibandronate is at least as effective and as well tolerated as daily treatment (Miller, 2005; Reginster, 2006). Moreover, once-monthly administration may be more convenient and thereby improve compliance rates.

Risedronate. This bisphosphonate is an effective agent in the prevention and treatment of postmenopausal osteoporosis. Several dosing schedules for risedronate (Actonel) are available (see Table 22-5). The strongest data supporting its efficacy stem from the Vertebral Efficacy with Risedronate Therapy (VERT) trials, conducted multinationally and also in North America. In the VERT multinational trial, Reginster and coworkers (2000) showed that risedronate reduced the risk of new vertebral fractures by 61 percent at 1 year and by 49 percent at 3 years of use. Moreover, both VERT trials found significant reductions in vertebral fractures as early as 6 months after initiation of risedronate therapy (Roux, 2004). Two extensions of these trials have provided evidence of sustained efficacy. The continuation of risedronate therapy for 2 additional years (5 years total) in the multinational VERT study was associated with a 59-percent reduction in new vertebral fractures compared with placebo.

Denosumab. Denosumab (Prolia) is a monoclonal antibody against the ligand that binds to RANK (receptor activator of nuclear factor kappa-B) on osteoclast precursors. Fully described and illustrated in Chapter 21 (p. 564), denosumab inhibits the development and activity of osteoclasts. This action thereby decreases bone resorption and increases bone density. In the FREEDOM (Fracture REduction Evaluation of Denosumab in Osteoporosis every 6 Months) trial, 7868 women with osteoporosis were randomly assigned to receive one 60-mg subcutaneous injection of denosumab or placebo every 6 months for 3 years (Cummings, 2009). In this manufacturer-sponsored trial, the relative risk for new radiographically diagnosed vertebral fractures was 68-percent lower in the denosumab group than in the placebo group. Risk for hip fractures was 40-percent lower and for nonvertebral fractures in general was 20-percent lower in the denosumab-treated group. Overall incidence of adverse events, cancer, coronary heart disease, and opportunistic infections was similar between groups. Although cellulitis occurred equally often in both groups, 12 denosumab recipients and one placebo recipient were hospitalized for the infection.

Denosumab seems to be as effective as teriparatide (p. 595) and zolendronic acid and is perhaps more effective than oral bisphosphonates. Uncommon but serious adverse events such as osteonecrosis of the jaw and atypical fractures of the femur associated with long-term bisphosphonate use are unlikely to be linked to short-acting agents such as denosumab. However, because denosumab is an antibody, its potential to affect the immune system requires scrutiny. Long-term adherence to oral bisphosphonate therapy is often poor, making the relative ease of biannual injections with denosumab attractive (Kendler, 2011).

Calcitonin. The polypeptide hormone calcitonin decreases the rate of bone absorption by inhibiting resorptive activity in osteoclasts. Calcitonin is a protein, and as such, oral administration leads to its digestion. For this reason, it is delivered as an injection or nasal spray (Fortical, Miacalcin) (see

Table 22-5). Salmon calcitonin nasal spray has been associated with a reduction in vertebral fracture risk among postmenopausal women with osteoporosis. In the Prevent Recurrence of Osteoporotic Fractures (PROOF) study, calcitonin nasal spray, 200 IU administered daily for up to 5 years, reduced the risk of vertebral fractures by 33 percent compared with placebo. However, vertebral fracture reduction was not seen at lower (100 IU/d) or higher (400 IU/d) dosages (Chesnut, 2000). Moreover, in this study, calcitonin failed to produce significant reductions in nonvertebral fracture.

Some observational data suggest that calcitonin has an analgesic effect independent of its effect on bone (Hauselmann, 2003; Ofluoglu, 2007). This analgesic effect may make this agent particularly useful as an adjunct to other therapies for osteoporosis in women with painful, symptomatic fracture (Blau, 2003). Injectable or intranasal calcitonin is associated with an 8- to 10-percent incidence of nausea or gastric discomfort and a 10-percent incidence of local site reactions. These symptoms tend to decrease in severity with continued use. Nasal symptoms such as rhinitis occur in 3 percent of patients treated with intranasal calcitonin (Cranney, 2002).

Parathyroid Hormone

Recombinant parathyroid hormone (PTH 1–34), known as teriparatide, is given by subcutaneous injection and is approved by the FDA for the treatment of postmenopausal women with established osteoporosis who are at high risk for fracture. Teriparatide (Forteo) increases osteoblast numbers and activity by recruiting new cells and reducing apoptosis of differentiated osteoblasts. At low daily doses of teriparatide, the anabolic effects of PTH predominate. This is in contrast to the catabolic effects generally associated with long-term, higher-dose, and chronic exposure to PTH.

Clinical studies indicate that teriparatide increases bone quality by increasing bone density, turnover, and size (Rubin, 2002). Moreover, improvements in microarchitectural elements are evident in both cancellous and cortical regions. In women with postmenopausal osteoporosis, teriparatide, 20 or 40 μg/day, administered subcutaneously for approximately 21 months, was associated with 65-percent and 69-percent reductions in vertebral fractures, and 35-percent and 40-percent reductions in nonvertebral fractures, respectively (Neer, 2001).

Similar findings were reported in a study of 52 women treated with concomitant teriparatide and HT compared with HT alone (Lindsay, 1997). In this study, at the end of 3 years, increases in spine, total hip, and total body BMD were 13.4 percent, 4.4 percent, and 3.7 percent, respectively, in the combined treatment group. The addition of alendronate to teriparatide, however, does not appear to enhance effects on BMD (Gasser, 2000). The effects of combination use of PTH with other bisphosphonates are not known.

In general, PTH is safe and well tolerated, although additional data from long-term studies are needed. The most frequent treatment-related adverse events in clinical trials of teriparatide were dizziness, leg cramps, nausea, and headache. Toxicity studies with rats have shown an increased risk of osteosarcoma, but as there are significant differences in bone metabolism between rats and humans, it is unlikely that the rat data

are applicable to humans. However, a black box warning has been included on the product labeling in the United States, and use of teriparatide should be avoided by patients at increased risk for skeletal malignancy. Use for more than 2 years is not recommended due to side effect potential (Tashjian, 2002). Although teriparatide is expensive, weekly oral alendronate is available at low cost as a generic, and cost will likely play a central role in determining how these agents are used clinically.

Other anabolic agents have been or are currently being studied for use in the treatment of osteoporosis and include insulin-like growth factor-1; strontium ranelate; calcium-sensing receptor antagonists, which alter PTH release; and modulation of the Wnt signalling pathway, which controls osteoblast differentiation (Rachner, 2011). Full-length PTH (PTH 1–84) is also currently under investigation (Greenspan, 2007).

Nonpharmacologic Therapy

Nonpharmacologic interventions are important cornerstones of osteoporosis prevention. They include dietary modifications, exercise programs, fall prevention strategies, and education.

Calcium. For bone maintenance, adequate daily calcium intake is essential. For women between 31 and 50 years, the recommended dietary reference intake (DRI) is 1000 mg each day, whereas 1200 mg is suggested for those 51 years and older (Institute of Medicine, 2010). Few meet these goals, and calcium deficiency is widespread. For example, more than 90 percent of women fail to take in enough calcium through their diets to meet DRIs put forth by the Food and Nutrition Board of the Institute of Medicine. Although poor calcium intake is observed at all ages, it appears to be most common among older individuals. Specifically, fewer than 1 percent of women 71 years or older actually meet recommended goals.

Calcium supplementation combined with vitamin D administration has been associated with reduced bone loss and decreased risk for fractures in a number of prospective studies (Chapuy, 1992; Dawson-Hughes, 1997; Larsen, 2004). However, supplementation must be continued long term for efficacy to be sustained.

Vitamin D. The DRI of vitamin D is 600 IU daily for a postmenopausal woman who is not at high risk for fractures or falls and 800 IU daily for persons who have a very high risk of osteoporosis or who are older than 70 years (Institute of Medicine, 2010). As with calcium, the prevalence of vitamin D deficiency is high, especially in the elderly. It leads to poor calcium absorption, secondary hyperparathyroidism, increased bone turnover, increased rates of bone loss, and if the deficiency is severe, impaired bone mineralization. In addition, vitamin D deficiency causes muscle weakness and is associated with higher rates of falls. Vitamin D deficiency is defined as a serum level of 25-hydroxyvitamin D below 10 ng/mL, whereas vitamin D "insufficiency" is characterized as a serum level of 25-hydroxyvitamin D of 10 to 30 ng/mL. The metabolite 25-hydroxyvitamin D is considered to be the best clinical measure of vitamin D stores (Rosen, 2011).

Vitamin D supplementation can reverse many of these effects and significantly reduce falls and hip fractures. Although a large study of patients aged 70 years and older failed to demonstrate a decrease in hip fractures using 400 IU/d of vitamin D for 3 years, other studies using approximately 800 IU/d of vitamin D have demonstrated fracture protection (Dawson-Hughes, 1997).

Diet. A relationship between protein intake and BMD has been reported, but a relationship with fractures has not been described. Using data from the Third National Health and Nutrition Examination Survey (NHANES III), Kerstetter and colleagues (2000) demonstrated a significant association between low protein intake and total femur BMD among non-Hispanic white women aged 50 years and older. Moreover, protein supplementation (20 g/d) five times weekly for 6 months following hip fracture was associated with a 50-percent reduction in femoral bone loss at 1 year compared with placebo.

Although no specific recommendations regarding protein intake can be made based on the limited data available, it seems prudent for clinicians to ensure that their patients eat healthy diets that provide the daily DRI of protein. As put forth by the Institute of Medicine, diets should contain at least 46 g/d for women (Dawson-Hughes, 2002). There may be upper limits for desirable protein intake as well. Excess urinary calcium excretion has been observed in association with the large acid loads delivered by very-high-protein diets (Barzel, 1998). Although it is not yet proven, there is concern that these calcium losses may jeopardize bone strength.

Caffeine consumption does not appear to influence bone health in healthy postmenopausal women who maintain an adequate daily intake of calcium and vitamin D. However, one longitudinal study showed that even moderate amounts of caffeine (two to three servings of coffee per day) may lead to bone loss in women with low calcium intake (less than 800 mg/d) (Harris, 1994).

Calcium reabsorption is directly proportional to sodium reabsorption in the renal tubule. Accordingly, increases in dietary sodium have been observed to cause increases in urinary calcium excretion and corresponding increases in biochemical markers of bone turnover. Specifically, a relationship between high sodium intake (more than 1768 mg daily) and lower bone density has been described (Sellmeyer, 2002). This sodium effect appears to be independent of calcium intake and activity levels. As with caffeine, it would be considered practical for all women to moderate sodium intake as a precautionary measure until this relationship is fully understood.

Physical Activity. Small but statistically significant increases in BMD have been observed in postmenopausal women participating in exercise programs, including aerobic exercise and resistance training (heavy weight with few repetitions). A metaanalysis of 18 randomized controlled trials concluded that aerobic, weight-bearing, and resistance exercise were all effective in increasing BMD of the spine. Of these, walking was observed to benefit BMD of both the spine and the hip, and aerobic exercise also increased wrist BMD (Bonaiuti, 2002).

Although an increase in bone density may occur, especially at the sites at which the exercise is directed, it is important to note that the benefits of exercise are likely to be due to factors other than changes in BMD (Carter, 2002). For example,

an association between exercise and reduced falls has been reported. Improvements in balance, stronger muscles, better muscle tone, and stronger, more flexible bone all undoubtedly contribute to fracture reduction.

Fall-Prevention Strategies

Falls are responsible for more than 90 percent of hip fractures (Carter, 2002). Sideways falls appear to be the most detrimental and were independently associated with hip fracture in a study by Greenspan and associates (1998). Therefore, fall prevention is essential for women with osteopenia or osteoporosis (Table 21-8, p. 569). Living conditions should be modified to minimize falls by reducing clutter and implementing nonslip tiles, rugs with nonskid backing, and night lights.

■ Treatment of Sex-Related Issues
Dyspareunia

Estrogen Replacement. Low estradiol levels commonly lead to vaginal atrophy or dryness and subsequent dyspareunia. Data from the Yale Midlife Study showed a close relationship between serum estradiol level and sexual problems. In this study, significantly more women with estradiol levels less than 50 pg/mL reported vaginal dryness, dyspareunia, and pain compared with women whose estradiol levels were greater than 50 pg/mL (Sarrel, 1998). Prospective records of coital behavior and concomitant sex steroid analysis revealed that women with estradiol levels less than 35 pg/mL reported significant reductions in coital activity.

Estrogen replacement effectively reverses atrophic changes. Of these, vaginal atrophy and diminished vaginal mucosal elasticity, vaginal fluid secretion levels, blood flow, and sensorimotor responses are improved by either topical or systemic estrogen (Dennerstein, 2002). Moreover, Cardozo and associates (1998) completed a metaanalysis of randomized, controlled trials from 1969 to 1995. They found that compared with placebo, oral or vaginal estrogens significantly improved vaginal atrophy symptoms, dyspareunia, and vaginal pH. If oral and vaginal estrogens were compared, vaginal products had greater patient acceptance and yielded lower systemic estradiol concentrations, yet significantly improved dyspareunia and pH changes.

Of vaginal topical agents, available forms include creams, continuous-release rings, and tablets (Table 22-6). In comparing types during a 12-week study period, Ayton and colleagues (1996) found that a continuous low-dose estradiol-releasing vaginal ring (Estring) provided relief comparable to CEE vaginal cream used during 12 weeks. In addition, study patients found the vaginal ring significantly more acceptable than the cream. The ring is prescribed as a single unit. Each unit contains 2 mg of estradiol and is worn vaginally for 90 days and then replaced.

Alternatively, a 17β-estradiol tablet (Vagifem) is available for vaginal application. One tablet is inserted daily for an initial 2 weeks of treatment and is followed by twice-weekly application. These tablets and CEE vaginal cream have been found to be equivalent in relieving symptoms of atrophic vaginitis (Rioux, 2000). Advantageously, women using vaginal tablets had less endometrial proliferation or hyperplasia than those

TABLE 22-6. Selected Estrogen Vaginal Preparations for the Treatment of Menopausal Vaginal Symptoms[a]

Preparation	Generic Name	Brand Name	Dose
Vaginal cream	Conjugated estrogens	Premarin	0.625 mg per 1 g cream (0.5 g twice weekly or 0.5 g/d for 3 weeks, with 1 week off therapy. May titrate up to 2 g per application as needed) Available as 42.5 g tube
	17β-Estradiol	Estrace	0.1 mg per 1 g cream (2–4 g/d for 1–2 weeks, then 1–2 g/d for 1–2 weeks, then 1–2 g 1 to 3 times weekly) Available as 42.5-g tube
Vaginal tablet	Estradiol	Vagifem	10 µg or 25 µg tablet (1 tablet/d for 2 weeks, then 1 tablet twice weekly)
Vaginal ring	17β-Estradiol	Estring	0.075 mg/d (inserted every 90 days)

[a]Most products listed in Table 22-3 for the treatment of menopausal hot flashes are also approved for the treatment of vaginal dryness.

using cream. Additionally, tablets were rated significantly more favorable than the cream, and their use was associated with fewer patient withdrawals from the study.

Studies of the vaginal tablets and ring have confirmed endometrial safety at 1 year, but studies of the long-term effects of low dose vaginal ET on the endometrium are lacking. Women using vaginal ET should be told to report any vaginal bleeding, and this bleeding should be evaluated thoroughly. Progestins typically are not prescribed to women using only low-dose vaginal estrogen products (Shifren, 2010).

SERMs. Several studies have investigated the role of SERMs in treating vaginal atrophy. Raloxifene and tamoxifen are used in the chemoprophylaxis of breast cancer and/or the treatment of osteoporosis. However, they have no beneficial or a detrimental effect on vaginal tissue and symptoms of vulvovaginal atrophy (Shelly, 2008).

In contrast, other SERMs appear promising. Ospemifene is in trials. It is effective and well tolerated for the treatment of vaginal dryness and dyspareunia associated with vulvovaginal atrophy but without endometrial proliferation (Bachmann, 2010). Lasofoxifene was also a newer SERM that showed a positive effect on vaginal tissue in the Postmenopausal Evaluation and Risk-Reduction with Lasofoxifene (PEARL) study (Goldstein, 2011). However, the manufacturer has currently withdrawn the drug from the FDA approval process (Schmidt, 2010).

Vaginal Lubricants and Moisturizers. A variety of water-soluble vaginal lubricants are available over the counter for treatment of vaginal dryness with coitus. Most commonly used water-based lubricants include K-Y Jelly, Astroglide, and Slippery Stuff. They can be applied before intercourse to the vaginal introitus.

Alternatively, a polycarbophil-based gel (Replens) offers a more sustained correction of vaginal dryness symptoms. This gel is an acidic hydrophilic insoluble polymer, which can hold water to act as a vaginal moisturizer. The polymer binds to the vaginal epithelium and is sloughed with epithelial layer turnover. In addition, the acidity of the gel helps to lower the vaginal pH to that found in premenopausal women.

Libido

Estrogen Replacement. A randomized, double-blind crossover clinical trial showed significant positive effects of estrogen on mood and sexuality. A 12-month study of 49 women who had undergone oophorectomy reported a significant positive effect of estrogen on both mood and sexuality, apart from vaginal symptomatology. This 12-month trial had four 3-month arms with no hormone washout period: (1) ethinyl estradiol (50 µg), (2) levonorgestrel (250 µg), (3) a combination of these two agents, and (4) placebo. Of these, ethinyl estradiol showed a significant positive effect on mood and sexual desire, enjoyment, and orgasmic frequency. There were no differences between groups in coital rate (Dennerstein, 2002).

Testosterone. Androgen replacement in women with hypoactive sexual desire disorder (HSDD) is a controversial topic. Although studies have documented an association between androgen replacement and improved sexual desire, large, quality trials with long-term follow-up are needed (Pauls, 2005). Shifren and colleagues (2000) demonstrated that women who underwent surgical menopause and who were subsequently treated with systemic estrogen had improved sexual function and psychological well-being if 300 µg of transdermal testosterone was concurrently delivered. However, there was a strong placebo response in this study, and many subjects had evidence of borderline-high androgen levels. Lobo and colleagues (2003) evaluated postmenopausal women to assess effects on HSDD of 0.625 mg oral estrogen with or without 1.25 mg methyltestosterone. At a 16-week reevaluation, therapy with methyltestosterone increased bioavailable testosterone and improved sexual interest and desire in most women.

Symptoms of androgen insufficiency include diminished sense of well-being, persistent fatigue, sexual function changes, and low levels of serum free testosterone. Women with these findings may be offered replacement. Importantly, candidates should be counseled that androgen replacement therapy for treatment of HSDD is off-label and not U.S. FDA-approved. Moreover, most of the available data are based on short-term studies, and long-term safety and efficacy are unknown (Braunstein, 2007). Therapy should be performed under close clinician supervision with monitoring for adverse changes in lipid profiles.

Potential benefits of androgens include increased muscle mass, stimulation of bone formation, diminished hot flash frequency, and improved sense of well being. Increased libido, sexual frequency, and orgasm may also be benefits. Early adverse effects of androgen therapy include acne and hirsutism, with one study reporting a 3-percent increased rate of acne in testosterone-therapy groups (Lobo, 2003). Long-term side effects such as male pattern baldness, voice deepening, and clitoral hypertrophy are infrequent within normal androgen levels. Androgen therapy may adversely affect the lipid profile, and knowledge regarding long-term effects on cardiovascular risk is lacking (Davis, 2000).

Treatment of Depression

Major and minor depression are the two most prevalent forms of acute depressive illness in women with a lifetime prevalence of approximately 18 percent. In the prospective Massachusetts Women's Health Study, during an approximately 2-year observation, women who remained perimenopausal had a higher rate of depression than women who were premenopausal or postmenopausal. This increase was largely explained by the presence of menopausal symptoms. Hot flashes, night sweats, and trouble sleeping were highly related to depression, providing strong support for the "domino" hypothesis that menopausal symptoms are the cause of increased depressed mood at this life stage (Avis, 2001).

Several controlled studies have demonstrated that HT is an effective treatment for depression in perimenopausal women. Most studies involved women with vasomotor symptoms, so it is likely that mood and quality of life improvement was predominantly caused by resolution of bothersome hot flashes, night sweats, and sleep disruption (Soares, 2001; Zweifel, 1997).

Antidepressant medications are highly effective in the treatment of depression (Table 13-14, p. 366). These together with psychotherapy and counseling should be the principal therapeutic intervention for women with depression. Women who present with bothersome vasomotor symptoms and associated disordered mood at the time of the menopausal transition may elect a trial of HT for symptom relief. Although HT should not be considered treatment for depression, improvement of mood symptoms concurrent with resolution of hot flashes and disrupted sleep is likely.

Treatment of Skin Aging

As people age, their skin elasticity decreases and strong collagen fibers weaken. In addition, fatty tissue and collagen beneath the skin shrinks. As a result, the skin lies more loosely, and lines appear where the facial muscles attach to the skin's undersur-

face. Many factors play a role in the rate and degree of this aging. First and foremost is genetics. People with thin, dry, fair skin will realize signs earlier. In addition, overexposure to sunlight and excessive use of tobacco and alcohol accelerate skin aging. Thus, prevention of skin aging includes protection from ultraviolet (UV) light, avoidance of tobacco, and limitation of alcohol intake.

Skin is a hormonally sensitive structure, and both estrogen and androgen receptors have been localized to skin (Hasselquist, 1980; Schmidt, 1990). However, it is difficult to separate hormonal deficiency from chronologic skin aging and age-related environmental insults such a smoking or photo-aging secondary to sun exposure.

The predominant evidence for an estrogen effect on skin has been derived from observational studies using various estrogen preparations with or without cyclic progestin. Thus, it is difficult to clearly separate the effects of estrogen from estrogen and progestin in many of the studies. There have been only two randomized, double-blinded, placebo-controlled trials that have examined the effects of ET or HT on skin. Both trials suggest that ET increases dermis thickness, whereas HT can increase skin collagen fibers (Maheux, 1994; Sauerbronn, 2000). With few randomized studies addressing this topic, the American College of Obstetricians and Gynecologists (2004b) states that "there is insufficient evidence to recommend estrogen treatment to increase skin thickness and collagen content and thereby decrease wrinkling in sun-exposed areas such as the face and forearms."

PREVENTIVE HEALTH CARE

Leading causes of morbidity and mortality for women older than 40 are found in Tables 22-7 and 22-8. Testing and prevention strategies are aimed at reducing the incidence and

TABLE 22-7. Leading Causes of Mortality in Older Women[a]

In those between 40 and 64 years:
Cancer
Heart disease
Cerebrovascular disease
Motor vehicle accident
Chronic obstructive pulmonary disease
Diabetes mellitus

In those older than 65 years:
Heart disease
Cancer
Cerebrovascular disease
Chronic obstructive pulmonary disease
Pneumonia and influenza
Diabetes mellitus
Motor vehicle accident

[a]For each age group, causes are listed by their descending frequency.

TABLE 22-8. Leading Causes of Morbidity for Women Older Than 40 Years[a]

Arthritis
Asthma
Back pain
Cancer
Cardiovascular disease
Chronic obstructive pulmonary disease
Depression
Diabetes mellitus
Headache or migraine
Hypertension
Menopause
Mental disorders
Respiratory infections
Obesity
Osteoporosis
Pneumonia
Sexually transmitted diseases
Skin conditions
Ulcers
Urinary tract infection
Vertigo
Vision impairment

[a]Listed alphabetically.

effects of these causes. In addition to testing, illness prevention requires patient education to enable women to play an active role in maintaining their own health. Through dialogue and counseling, clinicians and their actively participating patients can reap the benefits of preventive care. Although prevention recommendations for many of these causes of morbidity are reviewed in Chapter 1, a select few found commonly in older populations are discussed next.

Prevention of Cardiovascular Disease

Cardiovascular disease is a major health concern for postmenopausal women. It is the leading cause of death for women and accounts for approximately 45 percent of mortalities. Nonmodifiable risk factors include age and family history, whereas modifiable risk factors are smoking, obesity, and a sedentary lifestyle. Medical conditions associated with an increased risk of heart disease include diabetes, hypertension, and hypercholesterolemia. According to the American Heart Association, a high percentage of women between the ages of 45 and 54 have hypertension (30 percent), have hypercholesterolemia (20 percent), and are obese (40 percent) (Perez-Lopez, 2009).

Comprehensive care of midlife women must include a discussion regarding reducing modifiable risk factors and effectively treating associated underlying medical conditions. Currently, there is no role for HT in the prevention of heart disease in women. Assisting women in altering modifiable risk factors and identifying and treating diabetes, hypertension, and

hypercholesterolemia remain the most effective measures to reduce the risk of CHD in postmenopausal women.

Prevention of Alzheimer Senile Dementia

Dementia is defined as a progressive decline in intellectual and cognitive function. Its causes can be categorized into three broad groups: (1) cases in which the brain is the target of a systemic illness; (2) primary structural causes such as tumor; and (3) primary degenerative diseases of the nervous system, such as senile dementia of the Alzheimer type (SDAT). It is estimated that up to 50 percent of women aged 85 years or older may suffer from senile dementia or SDAT.

Early signs of dementia may be subtle. In compensation, women commonly restrict their spheres of activity so that they continue to function well. Consequently, dementia may not become apparent until a woman attempts to function in a broader context. In these instances, she may become lost or show significant confusion.

Prevention or delay of senile dementia includes screening for and early treatment of reversible causes of dementia. One easy screen is the Mini-Cog test in which patients are asked to recall three items. The grading and triage of patients based on test results is described in Chapter 1 (p. 27). For some forms of dementia, identification and treatment of systemic illness such as vitamin B_{12} deficiency, hypothyroidism, opportunistic infections such as cryptococcosis in immunocompromised hosts, and thiamine deficiency may reverse cognitive decline. Central nervous system complications of syphilis are rare. However, in those with acquired immunodeficiency syndrome (AIDS), the frequency of tertiary syphilis has been rising.

The role of estrogen in the prevention of dementia is controversial. Several epidemiologic studies have suggested that HT prevents development of SDAT. Moreover, metaanalyses of observational studies found that HT was associated with a decreased risk of dementia, but it did not improve established disease (Yaffe, 1998; Zandi, 2002). However, data from a large randomized, double-blind, placebo-controlled study found negative findings for a preventive role. Women enrolled in the Women's Health Initiative Memory Study (WHIMS), an ancillary study of the WHI, were noted to have increased rates of dementia compared with those given placebo (Shumaker, 2003, 2004). Although this increased risk was only statistically significant in the group of women >75 years of age, the observation nonetheless is a cause for concern in older postmenopausal women. As with CHD, it is unclear whether the concepts of *critical window* and *timing hypotheses* or the duration of HT has an effect in the prevention of SDAT. Unfortunately, these mixed findings leave unanswered questions regarding HT's efficacy in preventing dementia in postmenopausal women. Currently, HT is not recommended for this indication.

Prevention of Dental Disease Related to Menopause

Dental disease and tooth loss may be an indicator of osteoporosis. Maintenance of good dental hygiene and good bone mineral density will help retard dental disease associated with aging. Evidence of HT's dental benefits comes from the Nurses'

Health Study. The relative risk for tooth loss among current HT users was 0.76 compared with nonusers.

■ Prevention of Urogynecologic Disease

The development of pelvic organ prolapse and urinary incontinence is multifactorial. Thus, the effectiveness of preventive measures such as cesarean delivery, pelvic floor muscle training (Kegel exercises), and estrogen therapy is unclear. Estrogen receptors are found throughout the lower urinary and reproductive tracts. In these areas, hypoestrogenism is associated with collagen changes and diminished vascularity of the urethral subepithelial plexus. However, separating the effects of hypoestrogenism from aging in the genesis of pelvic organ prolapse and urinary incontinence is problematic and discussed in Chapters 23 (p. 607) and 24 (p. 634).

For a woman with obvious lower reproductive tract atrophic changes, a trial of vaginal estrogen treatment for urinary incontinence is reasonable. Vaginal ET reduces irritative urinary symptoms, such as frequency and urgency, and has been demonstrated to reduce the likelihood of recurrent urinary tract infections in postmenopausal women (Eriksen, 1999). However, several other studies evaluating effects of estrogen have noted either de novo development or worsening of incontinence in women using HT (Hendrix, 2005; Jackson, 2006). Accordingly, there is no current indication for the use of HT for the prevention of pelvic organ prolapse or incontinence.

REFERENCES

Albertazzi P, Pansini F, Bonaccorsi G, et al: The effect of dietary soy supplementation on hot flushes. Obstet Gynecol 91(1):6, 1998

American College of Obstetricians and Gynecologists: Hormone therapy and heart disease. Committee Opinion No. 420, November 2008

American College of Obstetricians and Gynecologists Women's Health Care Physicians: Vasomotor symptoms. Obstet Gynecol 104(4 Suppl):106S, 2004a

American College of Obstetricians and Gynecologists Women's Health Care Physicians: Executive summary. Hormone therapy. Obstet Gynecol 104 (4 Suppl):1S, 2004b

Anderson GL, Limacher M, Assaf AR, et al: Effects of conjugated equine estrogen in postmenopausal women with hysterectomy: the Women's Health Initiative randomized controlled trial. JAMA 291(14):1701, 2004

Archer DF, Dupont CM, Constantine GD, et al: Desvenlafaxine for the treatment of vasomotor symptoms associated with menopause: a double-blind, randomized, placebo-controlled trial of efficacy and safety. Am J Obstet Gynecol 200(3):238.e1, 2008

Archer DF, Lewis V, Carr BR, et al: Bazedoxifene/conjugated estrogens (BZA/CE): incidence of uterine bleeding in postmenopausal women. Fertil Steril 92(3):1039, 2009a

Archer DF, Seidman L, Constantine GD, et al: A double-blind, randomly assigned, placebo-controlled study of desvenlafaxine efficacy and safety for the treatment of vasomotor symptoms associated with menopause. Am J Obstet Gynecol 200(2):172.e1, 2009b

Avis NE, Crawford S, Stellato R, et al: Longitudinal study of hormone levels and depression among women transitioning through menopause. Climacteric 4(3):243, 2001

Ayton RA, Darling GM, Murkies AL, et al: A comparative study of safety and efficacy of continuous low dose oestradiol released from a vaginal ring compared with conjugated equine oestrogen vaginal cream in the treatment of postmenopausal urogenital atrophy. Br J Obstet Gynaecol 103(4):351, 1996

Bachmann GA, Komi JO, Ospemifene Study Group: Ospemifene effectively treats vulvovaginal atrophy in postmenopausal women: results from a pivotal phase 3 study. Menopause 17(3):480, 2010

Barnabei VM, Grady D, Stovall DW, et al: Menopausal symptoms in older women and the effects of treatment with hormone therapy. Obstet Gynecol 100(6):1209, 2002

Barrett-Connor E, Grady D, Sashegyi A, et al: Raloxifene and cardiovascular events in osteoporotic postmenopausal women: four-year results from the MORE (Multiple Outcomes of Raloxifene Evaluation) randomized trial. JAMA 287(7):847, 2002

Barrett-Connor E, Mosca L, Collins P, et al: Effects of raloxifene on cardiovascular events and breast cancer in postmenopausal women. N Engl J Med 355(2):125, 2006

Barrett-Connor E, Wehren LE, Siris ES, et al: Recency and duration of postmenopausal hormone therapy: effects on bone mineral density and fracture risk in the National Osteoporosis Risk Assessment (NORA) study. Menopause 10(5):412, 2003

Barton DL, Loprinzi CL, Quella SK, et al: Prospective evaluation of vitamin E for hot flashes in breast cancer survivors. J Clin Oncol 16(2):495, 1998

Barzel US, Massey LK: Excess dietary protein can adversely affect bone. J Nutr 128(6):1051, 1998

Bell SE: Sociological perspectives on the medicalization of menopause. Ann NY Acad Sci 592:173, 1990

Beral V: Breast cancer and hormone-replacement therapy in the Million Women Study. Lancet 362(9382):419, 2003

Black DM, Cummings SR, Karpf DB, et al: Randomised trial of effect of alendronate on risk of fracture in women with existing vertebral fractures. Fracture Intervention Trial Research Group. Lancet 348(9041):1535, 1996

Black DM, Schwartz AV, Ensrud KE, et al: Effects of continuing or stopping alendronate after 5 years of treatment: the Fracture Intervention Trial Long-term Extension (FLEX): a randomized trial. JAMA 296(24):2927, 2006

Blau LA, Hoehns JD: Analgesic efficacy of calcitonin for vertebral fracture pain. Ann Pharmacother 37(4):564, 2003

Bonaiuti D, Shea B, Iovine R, et al: Exercise for preventing and treating osteoporosis in postmenopausal women. Cochrane Database Syst Rev 3:CD000333, 2002

Bone HG, Hosking D, Devogelaer JP, et al: Ten years' experience with alendronate for osteoporosis in postmenopausal women. N Engl J Med 350(12):1189, 2004

Boothby LA, Doering PL, Kipersztok S: Bioidentical hormone therapy: a review. Menopause 11(3):356, 2004

Borud EK, Alraek T, White A, et al: The Acupuncture on Hot Flushes Among Menopausal Women (ACUFLASH) study, a randomized controlled trial. Menopause 16(3):484, 2009

Braunstein GD: Safety of testosterone treatment in postmenopausal women. Fertil Steril 88(1):1, 2007

Brown JN, Wright BR: Use of gabapentin in patients experiencing hot flashes. Pharmacotherapy 29(1):74, 2009

Cardozo L, Bachmann G, McClish D, et al: Meta-analysis of estrogen therapy in the management of urogenital atrophy in postmenopausal women: second report of the Hormones and Urogenital Therapy Committee. Obstet Gynecol 92(4 Pt 2):722, 1998

Carter ND, Khan KM, McKay HA, et al: Community-based exercise program reduces risk factors for falls in 65- to 75-year-old women with osteoporosis: randomized controlled trial. CMAJ 167(9):997, 2002

Castelo-Branco C, Palacios S, Calaf J, et al: Available medical choices for the management of menopause. Maturitas 52 (Suppl 1):S61, 2005

Chapuy MC, Arlot ME, Duboeuf F, et al: Vitamin D_3 and calcium to prevent hip fractures in the elderly women. N Engl J Med 327(23):1637, 1992

Chen WY, Manson JE, Hankinson SE, et al: Unopposed estrogen therapy and the risk of invasive breast cancer. Arch Intern Med 166(9):1027, 2006

Cheng G, Wilczek B, Warner M, et al: Isoflavone treatment for acute menopausal symptoms. Menopause 14(3 Pt 1):468, 2007

Chesnut CH III, Silverman S, Andriano K, et al: A randomized trial of nasal spray salmon calcitonin in postmenopausal women with established osteoporosis: the Prevent Recurrence of Osteoporotic Fractures Study. PROOF Study Group. Am J Med 109(4):267, 2000

Chesnut CH III, Skag A, Christiansen C, et al: Effects of oral ibandronate administered daily or intermittently on fracture risk in postmenopausal osteoporosis. J Bone Miner Res 19:1241, 2004

Christiansen C, Chesnut CH 3rd, Adachi JD, et al: Safety of bazedoxifene in a randomized, double-blind, placebo- and active-controlled Phase 3 study of postmenopausal women with osteoporosis. BMC Musculoskelet Disord 11:130, 2010

Cohen FJ, Lu Y: Characterization of hot flashes reported by healthy postmenopausal women receiving raloxifene or placebo during osteoporosis prevention trials. Maturitas 34(1):65, 2000

Collaborative Group on Hormonal Factors in Breast Cancer: Breast cancer and hormone replacement therapy: collaborative reanalysis of data from 51 epidemiological studies of 52,705 women with breast cancer and 108,411 women without breast cancer. Lancet 350(9084):1047, 1997

Cranney A, Tugwell P, Zytaruk N, et al: Meta-analyses of therapies for postmenopausal osteoporosis. VI. Meta-analysis of calcitonin for the treatment of postmenopausal osteoporosis. Endocr Rev 23(4):540, 2002

Cummings SR, San Martin J, McClung MR, et al: Denosumab for prevention of fractures in postmenopausal women with osteoporosis. N Engl J Med 361(8):756, 2009

Danforth KN, Tworoger SS, Hecht JL, et al: A prospective study of postmenopausal hormone use and ovarian cancer risk. Br J Cancer 96(1):151, 2007

Davis SR: Androgens and female sexuality. J Gend Specif Med 3(1):36, 2000

Dawson-Hughes B, Harris SS: Calcium intake influences the association of protein intake with rates of bone loss in elderly men and women. Am J Clin Nutr 75(4):773, 2002

Dawson-Hughes B, Harris SS, Krall EA, et al: Effect of calcium and vitamin D supplementation on bone density in men and women 65 years of age or older. N Engl J Med 337(10):670, 1997

Delmas PD, Ensrud KE, Adachi JD, et al: Efficacy of raloxifene on vertebral fracture risk reduction in postmenopausal women with osteoporosis: four-year results from a randomized clinical trial. J Clin Endocrinol Metab 87(8):3609, 2002

Dempster DW, Shane E, Horbert W, et al: A simple method for correlative light and scanning electron microscopy of human iliac crest bone biopsies: qualitative observations in normal and osteoporotic subjects. J Bone Miner Res 1(1):15, 1986

Dennerstein L, Randolph J, Taffe J, et al: Hormones, mood, sexuality, and the menopausal transition. Fertil Steril 77(Suppl 4):S42, 2002

Eng-Wong J, Reynolds JC, Venzon D, et al: Effect of raloxifene on bone mineral density in premenopausal women at increased risk of breast cancer. J Clin Endocrinol Metab 91(10):3941, 2006

Eriksen B: A randomized, open, parallel-group study on the preventive effect of an estradiol-releasing vaginal ring (Estring) on recurrent urinary tract infections in postmenopausal women. Am J Obstet Gynecol 180(5):1072, 1999

Ettinger B, Black DM, Mitlak BH, et al: Reduction of vertebral fracture risk in postmenopausal women with osteoporosis treated with raloxifene: results from a 3-year randomized clinical trial. Multiple Outcomes of Raloxifene Evaluation (MORE) Investigators. JAMA 282(7):637, 1999

Ettinger B, Ensrud KE, Wallace R, et al: Effects of ultralow-dose transdermal estradiol on bone mineral density: a randomized clinical trial. Obstet Gynecol 104(3):443, 2004

Farquhar C, Marjoribanks J, Lethaby A, et al: Long term hormone therapy for perimenopausal and postmenopausal women. Cochrane Database Syst Rev 2:CD004143, 2009

Freedman RR, Woodward S: Behavioral treatment of menopausal hot flushes: evaluation by ambulatory monitoring. Am J Obstet Gynecol 167(2):436, 1992

Fugate SE, Church CO: Nonestrogen treatment modalities for vasomotor symptoms associated with menopause. Ann Pharmacother 38(9):1482, 2004

Gambrell RD Jr, Bagnell CA, Greenblatt RB: Role of estrogens and progesterone in the etiology and prevention of endometrial cancer: review. Am J Obstet Gynecol 146(6):696, 1983

Gasser JA, Kneissel M, Thomsen JS, et al: PTH and interactions with bisphosphonates. J Musculoskelet Neuronal Interact 1(1):53, 2000

Geller SE, Shulman LP, van Breemen RB, et al: Safety and efficacy of black cohosh and red clover for the management of vasomotor symptoms: a randomized controlled trial. Menopause 16(6):1156, 2009

Goldstein SR, Neven P, Cummings S, et al: Postmenopausal Evaluation and Risk Reduction With Lasofoxifene (PEARL) trial: 5-year gynecological outcomes. Menopause 18(1):17, 2011

Grady D, Herrington D, Bittner V, et al: Cardiovascular disease outcomes during 6.8 years of hormone therapy: Heart and Estrogen/progestin Replacement Study follow-up (HERS II). JAMA 288(1):49, 2002

Greendale GA, Reboussin BA, Hogan P, et al: Symptom relief and side effects of postmenopausal hormones: results from the Postmenopausal Estrogen/Progestin Interventions Trial. Obstet Gynecol 92(6):982, 1998

Greenspan SL, Bone HG, Ettinger MP, et al: Treatment of Osteoporosis with Parathyroid Hormone Study Group, Effect of recombinant human parathyroid hormone (1-84) on vertebral fracture and bone mineral density in postmenopausal women with osteoporosis: a randomized trial. Ann Int Med 146(5):326, 2007

Greenspan SL, Myers ER, Kiel DP, et al: Fall direction, bone mineral density, and function: risk factors for hip fracture in frail nursing home elderly. Am J Med 104(6):539, 1998

Grodstein F, Clarkson TB, Manson JE: Understanding the divergent data on postmenopausal hormone therapy. N Engl J Med 348(7):645, 2003

Grodstein F, Manson JE, Stampfer MJ: Postmenopausal hormone use and secondary prevention of coronary events in the Nurses' Health Study. A prospective, observational study. Ann Intern Med 135(1):1, 2001

Guttuso T Jr, Kurlan R, McDermott MP, et al: Gabapentin's effects on hot flashes in postmenopausal women: a randomized controlled trial. Obstet Gynecol 101(2):337, 2003

Harris SS, Dawson-Hughes B: Caffeine and bone loss in healthy postmenopausal women. Am J Clin Nutr 60(4):573, 1994

Harris ST, Watts NB, Genant HK, et al: Effects of risedronate treatment on vertebral and nonvertebral fractures in women with postmenopausal osteoporosis: a randomized controlled trial. Vertebral Efficacy With Risedronate Therapy (VERT) Study Group. JAMA 282(14):1344, 1999

Hasselquist MB, Goldberg N, Schroeter A, et al: Isolation and characterization of the estrogen receptor in human skin. J Clin Endocrinol Metab 50(1):76, 1980

Hauselmann HJ, Rizzoli R: A comprehensive review of treatments for postmenopausal osteoporosis. Osteoporos Int 14(1):2, 2003

Hays J, Ockene JK, Brunner RL, et al: Effects of estrogen plus progestin on health-related quality of life. N Engl J Med 348(19):1839, 2003

Hendrix SL, Cochrane BB, Nygaard IE, et al: Effects of estrogen with and without progestin on urinary incontinence. JAMA 293(8):935, 2005

Hirata JD, Swiersz LM, Zell B, et al: Does dong quai have estrogenic effects in postmenopausal women? A double-blind, placebo-controlled trial. Fertil Steril 68(6):981, 1997

Hulley S, Grady D, Bush T, et al: Randomized trial of estrogen plus progestin for secondary prevention of coronary heart disease in postmenopausal women. Heart and Estrogen/progestin Replacement Study (HERS) Research Group. JAMA 280(7):605, 1998

Institute of Medicine: DRIs for Calcium and Vitamin D. 2010. Available at: http://www.iom.edu/Reports/2010/Dietary-Reference-Intakes-for-Calcium-and-Vitamin-D.aspx. Accessed April 20, 2011

Irvin JH, Domar AD, Clark C, et al: The effects of relaxation response training on menopausal symptoms. J Psychosom Obstet Gynaecol 17(4):202, 1996

Jackson SL, Scholes D, Boyko EJ, et al: Predictors of urinary incontinence in a prospective cohort of postmenopausal women. Obstet Gynecol 108(4):855, 2006

Kendler DL, McClung MR, Freemantle N, et al: Adherence, preference, and satisfaction of postmenopausal women taking denosumab or alendronate. Osteoporos Int 22(6):1725, 2011

Kerstetter JE, Looker AC, Insogna KL: Low dietary protein and low bone density. Calcif Tissue Int 66(4):313, 2000

Kim KH, Kang KW, Kim DI, et al: Effects of acupuncture on hot flashes in perimenopausal and postmenopausal women—a multicenter randomized clinical trial. Menopause 17(2):269, 2010

Krebs EE, Ensrud KE, MacDonald R, et al: Phytoestrogens for treatment of menopausal symptoms: a systematic review. Obstet Gynecol 104(4):824, 2004

Lacey JV Jr, Brinton LA, Leitzmann MF, et al: Menopausal hormone therapy and ovarian cancer risk in the National Institutes of Health-AARP Diet and Health Study Cohort. J Natl Cancer Inst 98(19):1397, 2006

LaCroix AZ, Chlebowski RT, Manson JE, et al: Health outcomes after stopping conjugated equine estrogens among postmenopausal women with prior hysterectomy: a randomized controlled trial. JAMA 305(13):1305, 2011

Lam PM, Chung TK, Haines C: Where are we with postmenopausal hormone therapy in 2005? Gynecol Endocrinol 21(5):248, 2005

Lambrinoudaki I, Christodoulakos G, Botsis D: Bisphosphonates. Ann NY Acad Sci 1092(1):397, 2006

Lanza FL, Hunt RH, Thomson AB, et al: Endoscopic comparison of esophageal and gastroduodenal effects of risedronate and alendronate in postmenopausal women. Gastroenterology 119(3):631, 2000

Larsen ER, Mosekilde L, Foldspang A: Vitamin D and calcium supplementation prevents osteoporotic fractures in elderly community dwelling residents: a pragmatic population-based 3-year intervention study. J Bone Miner Res 19(3):370, 2004

Lemay A, Dodin S, Kadri N, et al: Flaxseed dietary supplement versus hormone replacement therapy in hypercholesterolemic menopausal women. Obstet Gynecol 100(3):495, 2002

Levis S, Strickman-Stein N, Ganjei-Azar P, et al: Soy isoflavones in the prevention of menopausal bone loss and menopausal symptoms: a randomized, double-blind trial. Arch Intern Med 171(15):1363, 2011

Lewis JE, Nickell LA, Thompson LU, et al: A randomized controlled trial of the effect of dietary soy and flaxseed muffins on quality of life and hot flashes during menopause. Menopause 13:631, 2006

Lindsay R, Gallagher JC, Kagan R, et al: Efficacy of tissue-selective estrogen complex of bazedoxifene/conjugated estrogens for osteoporosis prevention in at-risk postmenopausal women. Fertil Steril 92(3):1045, 2009

Lindsay R, Nieves J, Formica C, et al: Randomised controlled study of effect of parathyroid hormone on vertebral-bone mass and fracture incidence among postmenopausal women on oestrogen with osteoporosis. Lancet 350(9077):550, 1997

Lobo R: Evidence-based medicine and the management of menopause. Clin Obstet Gynecol 51(3):534, 2008

Lobo RA, Pinkerton JV, Gass ML, et al: Evaluation of bazedoxifene/conjugated estrogens for the treatment of menopausal symptoms and effects on metabolic parameters and overall safety profile. Fertil Steril 92(3):1025, 2009

Lobo RA, Rosen RC, Yang HM, et al: Comparative effects of oral esterified estrogens with and without methyltestosterone on endocrine profiles and dimensions of sexual function in postmenopausal women with hypoactive sexual desire. Fertil Steril 79(6):1341, 2003

Loprinzi CL, Kugler JW, Sloan JA, et al: Venlafaxine in management of hot flashes in survivors of breast cancer: a randomised controlled trial. Lancet 356(9247):2059, 2000

Loprinzi CL, Sloan JA, Perez EA, et al: Phase III evaluation of fluoxetine for treatment of hot flashes. J Clin Oncol 20(6):1578, 2002

Loprinzi CL, Stearns V, Barton D: Centrally active nonhormonal hot flash therapies. Am J Med 118(Suppl 12B):118, 2005

MacLennan AH, Broadbent JL, Lester S, et al: Oral oestrogen and combined oestrogen/progestogen therapy versus placebo for hot flashes. Cochrane Database Syst Rev 4:CD002978, 2004

Maheux R, Naud F, Rioux M, et al: A randomized, double-blind, placebo-controlled study on the effect of conjugated estrogens on skin thickness. Am J Obstet Gynecol 170(2):642, 1994

Marx RE: Pamidronate (Aredia) and zoledronate (Zometa) induced avascular necrosis of the jaws: a growing epidemic. J Oral Maxillofac Surg 61(9):1115, 2003

Mendelsohn ME, Karas RH: Molecular and cellular basis of cardiovascular gender differences. Science 308(5728):1583, 2005

Miller PD, McClung MR, Macovei L, et al: Monthly oral ibandronate therapy in postmenopausal osteoporosis: 1-year results from the MOBILE Study. J Bone Miner Res 20(8):1315, 2005

Miller VM, Black DM, Brinton EA, et al: Using basic science to design a clinical trial: baseline characteristics of women enrolled in the Kronos Early Estrogen Prevention Study (KEEPS). J Cardiovasc Transl Res 2(3):228, 2009

Nagamani M, Kelver ME, Smith ER: Treatment of menopausal hot flashes with transdermal administration of clonidine. Am J Obstet Gynecol 156(3):561, 1987

National Osteoporosis Foundation: Clinician's Guide to Prevention and Treatment of Osteoporosis. Washington, DC: National Osteoporosis Foundation, 2008.

Neer RM, Arnaud CD, Zanchetta JR, et al: Effect of parathyroid hormone (1-34) on fractures and bone mineral density in postmenopausal women with osteoporosis. N Engl J Med 344(19):1434, 2001

Nelson HD: Commonly used types of postmenopausal estrogen for treatment of hot flashes: scientific review. JAMA 291(13):1610, 2004

Newton KM, Buist DS, Keenan NL, et al: Use of alternative therapies for menopause symptoms: results of a population-based survey. Obstet Gynecol 100(1):18, 2002

Noller KL: Estrogen replacement therapy and risk of ovarian cancer. JAMA 288(3):368, 2002

Ofluoglu D, Akyuz G, Unay O, et al: The effect of calcitonin on beta-endorphin levels in postmenopausal osteoporotic patients with back pain. Clin Rheumatol 26(1):44, 2007

Park-Wyllie LY, Mamdani MM, Juurlink DN, et al: Bisphosphonate use and the risk of subtrochanteric or femoral shaft fractures in older women. JAMA 305(8):783, 2011

Pauls RN, Kleeman SD, Karram MM: Female sexual dysfunction: principles of diagnosis and therapy. Obstet Gynecol Surv 60(3):196, 2005

Peled Y, Perri T, Pardo Y, et al: Levonorgestrel-releasing intrauterine system as an adjunct to estrogen for the treatment of menopausal symptoms—a review. Menopause 14(3 Pt 1):550, 2007

Perez-Lopez FR, Chedraui P, Gilbert JJ, et al: Cardiovascular risk in menopausal women and prevalent related co-morbid conditions: facing the post-Women's Health Initiative era. Fertil Steril 92(4):1171, 2009

Pickar JH, Yeh IT, Bachmann G, et al: Endometrial effects of a tissue selective estrogen complex containing bazedoxifene/conjugated estrogens as a menopausal therapy. Fertil Steril 92(3):1018, 2009

Pinkerton JV, Stovall DW, Kightlinger RS: Advances in the treatment of menopausal symptoms. Womens Health (Lond Engl) 5(4):361, 2009

Prentice RL, Langer RD, Stefanick ML, et al: Combined analysis of Women's Health Initiative observational and clinical trial data on postmenopausal hormone treatment and cardiovascular disease. Am J Epidemiol 163(7):589, 2006

Prestwood KM, Kenny AM, Kleppinger A, et al: Ultralow-dose micronized 17beta-estradiol and bone density and bone metabolism in older women: a randomized controlled trial. JAMA 290(8):1042, 2003

Rachner TD, Khosla S, Hofbauer LC: Osteoporosis: now and the future. Lancet 377(9773):1276, 2011

Reddy SY, Warner H, Guttuso T Jr, et al: Gabapentin, estrogen, and placebo for treating hot flashes: a randomized controlled trial. Obstet Gynecol 108(1):41, 2006

Reginster J, Minne HW, Sorensen OH, et al: Randomized trial of the effects of risedronate on vertebral fractures in women with established postmenopausal osteoporosis. Vertebral Efficacy with Risedronate Therapy (VERT) Study Group. Osteoporos Int 11(1):83, 2000

Reginster JY, Adami S, Lakatos P, et al: Efficacy and tolerability of once-monthly oral ibandronate in postmenopausal osteoporosis: 2 year results from the MOBILE study. Ann Rheum Dis 65(5):654, 2006

Rioux JE, Devlin C, Gelfand MM, et al: 17beta-estradiol vaginal tablet versus conjugated equine estrogen vaginal cream to relieve menopausal atrophic vaginitis. Menopause 7(3):156, 2000

Rosen CJ: Clinical practice. Vitamin D insufficiency. N Engl J Med 364(3):248, 2011

Rossouw JE, Anderson GL, Prentice RL, et al: Risks and benefits of estrogen plus progestin in healthy postmenopausal women: principal results from the Women's Health Initiative randomized controlled trial. JAMA 288(3):321, 2002

Rossouw JE, Prentice RL, Manson JE, et al: Postmenopausal hormone therapy and risk of cardiovascular disease by age and years since menopause. JAMA 297(13):1465, 2007

Roux C, Seeman E, Eastell R, et al: Efficacy of risedronate on clinical vertebral fractures within six months. Curr Med Res Opin 20:433, 2004

Ruggiero SL, Mehrotra B, Rosenberg TJ, et al: Osteonecrosis of the jaws associated with the use of bisphosphonates: a review of 63 cases. J Oral Maxillofac Surg 62(5):527, 2004

Russell RG, Watts NB, Ebetino FH, et al: Mechanisms of action of bisphosphonates: similarities and differences and their potential influence on clinical efficacy. Osteoporos Int 19(6):733, 2008

Salpeter SR, Walsh JM, Greyber E, et al: Mortality associated with hormone replacement therapy in younger and older women: a meta-analysis. J Gen Intern Med 19(7):791, 2004

Sarrel P, Dobay B, Wiita B: Estrogen and estrogen-androgen replacement in postmenopausal women dissatisfied with estrogen-only therapy. Sexual behavior and neuroendocrine responses. J Reprod Med 43(10):847, 1998

Sauerbronn AV, Fonseca AM, Bagnoli VR, et al: The effects of systemic hormonal replacement therapy on the skin of postmenopausal women. Int J Gynaecol Obstet 68(1):35, 2000

Schmidt C: Third-generation SERMs may face uphill battle. J Natl Cancer Inst 102(22):1690, 2010

Schmidt JB, Lindmaier A, Spona J: Hormone receptors in pubic skin of premenopausal and postmenopausal females. Gynecol Obstet Invest 30(2):97, 1990

Sellmeyer DE, Schloetter M, Sebastian A: Potassium citrate prevents increased urine calcium excretion and bone resorption induced by a high sodium chloride diet. J Clin Endocrinol Metab 87(5):2008, 2002

Shelly W, Draper MW, Krishnan V, et al: Selective estrogen receptor modulators: an update on recent clinical findings. Obstet Gynecol Surv 63(3):163, 2008

Shifren JL, Braunstein GD, Simon JA, et al: Transdermal testosterone treatment in women with impaired sexual function after oophorectomy. N Engl J Med 343(10):682, 2000

Shifren JL, Schiff I: Role of hormone therapy in the management of menopause. Obstet Gynecol 115(4):839, 2010

Shulman LP: In search of a middle ground: hormone therapy and its role in modern menopause management. Menopause 17(5):898, 2010

Shumaker SA, Legault C, Kuller L, et al: Conjugated equine estrogens and incidence of probable dementia and mild cognitive impairment in postmenopausal women: Women's Health Initiative Memory Study. JAMA 291(24):2947, 2004

Shumaker SA, Legault C, Rapp SR, et al: Estrogen plus progestin and the incidence of dementia and mild cognitive impairment in postmenopausal women: the Women's Health Initiative Memory Study: a randomized controlled trial. JAMA 289(20):2651, 2003

Silverman SL, Christiansen C, Genant HK, et al: Efficacy of bazedoxifene in reducing new vertebral fracture risk in postmenopausal women with osteoporosis: results from a 3-year, randomized, placebo-, and active-controlled clinical trial. J Bone Miner Res 23(12):1923, 2008

Silverman SL, Chines AA, Kendler DL, et al: Sustained efficacy and safety of bazedoxifene in preventing fractures in postmenopausal women with osteoporosis: results of a 5-year, randomized, placebo-controlled study. Osteoporos Int Jul 21, 2011 [Epub ahead of print]

Smith DC, Prentice R, Thompson DJ, et al: Association of exogenous estrogen and endometrial carcinoma. N Engl J Med 293(23):1164, 1975

Soares CN, Almeida OP, Joffe H, et al: Efficacy of estradiol for the treatment of depressive disorders in perimenopausal women: a double-blind, randomized, placebo-controlled trial. Arch Gen Psychiatry 58(6):529, 2001

Soares CN, Joffe H, Rubens R, et al: Eszopiclone in patients with insomnia during perimenopause and early postmenopause: a randomized controlled trial. Obstet Gynecol 108(6):1402, 2006

Srinivasan D, Shetty S, Ashworth D, et al: Orofacial pain—a presenting symptom of bisphosphonate associated osteonecrosis of the jaws. Br Dent J 203(2):91, 2007

Stampfer MJ, Willett WC, Colditz GA, et al: A prospective study of postmenopausal estrogen therapy and coronary heart disease. N Engl J Med 313(17):1044, 1985

Stearns V, Beebe KL, Iyengar M, et al: Paroxetine controlled release in the treatment of menopausal hot flashes: a randomized controlled trial. JAMA 289(21):2827, 2003

Stefanick ML, Anderson GL, Margolis KL, et al: Effects of conjugated equine estrogens on breast cancer and mammography screening in postmenopausal women with hysterectomy. JAMA 295(14):1647, 2006

Tashjian AH Jr, Chabner BA: Commentary on clinical safety of recombinant human parathyroid hormone 1-34 in the treatment of osteoporosis in men and postmenopausal women. J Bone Miner Res 17(7):1151, 2002

The North American Menopause Society: Management of osteoporosis in postmenopausal women: 2010 position statement of The North American Menopause Society. Menopause 17(1):23, 2010

The Women's Health Initiative Steering Committee: Effects of Conjugated Equine Estrogen in Postmenopausal Women with Hysterectomy: The Women's Health Initiative Randomized Controlled Trial. JAMA 291:1701, 2004

The Writing Group for the PEPI Trial. Effects of estrogen or estrogen/progestin regimens on heart disease risk factors in postmenopausal women. The Postmenopausal Estrogen/Progestin Interventions (PEPI) Trial. JAMA 273:199, 1995

Thurston RC, Sowers MR, Sutton-Tyrrell K, et al: Abdominal adiposity and hot flashes among midlife women. Menopause 15(3):429, 2008

Tice JA, Ettinger B, Ensrud K, et al: Phytoestrogen supplements for the treatment of hot flashes: the Isoflavone Clover Extract (ICE) Study: a randomized controlled trial. JAMA 290(2):207, 2003

Tosteson AN, Melton LJ III, Dawson-Hughes B, et al: Cost-effective osteoporosis treatment thresholds: the United States perspective. Osteoporos Int 19(4):437, 2008

U.S. Department of Health and Human Services: Food and Drug Administration Center for Drug Evaluation and Research (CDER): noncontraceptive estrogen drug products for the treatment of vasomotor symptoms and vulvar and vaginal atrophy symptoms—recommended prescribing information for health care providers and patient labeling, 2005. Available at: http://www.fda.gov/downloads/Drugs/DrugSafety/InformationbyDrugClass/UCM135336.pdf. Accessed October 15, 2011

U.S. Food and Drug Administration: FDA drug safety communication: safety update for osteoporosis drugs, bisphosphonates, and atypical fractures. 2010. Available at: <http://www.fda.gov/Drugs/DrugSafety/ucm229009.htm. Accessed December 16, 2011

Vickers MR, MacLennan AH, Lawton B, et al: Main morbidities recorded in the Women's International Study of long Duration Oestrogen after Menopause (WISDOM): a randomised controlled trial of hormone replacement therapy in postmenopausal women. BMJ 335(7613):239, 2007

Watts NB, Bilezikian JP, Camacho PM, et al: American Association of Clinical Endocrinologists Medical Guidelines for Clinical Practice for the diagnosis and treatment of postmenopausal osteoporosis: executive summary of recommendations. Endocr Pract 16(6):1016, 2010

Wilson PW, Garrison RJ, Castelli WP: Postmenopausal estrogen use, cigarette smoking, and cardiovascular morbidity in women over 50. The Framingham Study. N Engl J Med 313(17):1038, 1985

Woo SB, Hellstein JW, Kalmar JR: Narrative review: bisphosphonates and osteonecrosis of the jaws. Ann Intern Med 144(10):753, 2006

Yaffe K, Sawaya G, Lieberburg I, et al: Estrogen therapy in postmenopausal women: effects on cognitive function and dementia. JAMA 279(9):688, 1998

Zandi PP, Carlson MC, Plassman BL, et al: Hormone replacement therapy and incidence of Alzheimer disease in older women: the Cache County Study. JAMA 288(17):2123, 2002

Zweifel JE, O'Brien WH: A meta-analysis of the effect of hormone replacement therapy upon depressed mood. Psychoneuroendocrinology 22(3):189, 1997

SECTION 3

FEMALE PELVIC MEDICINE AND RECONSTRUCTIVE SURGERY

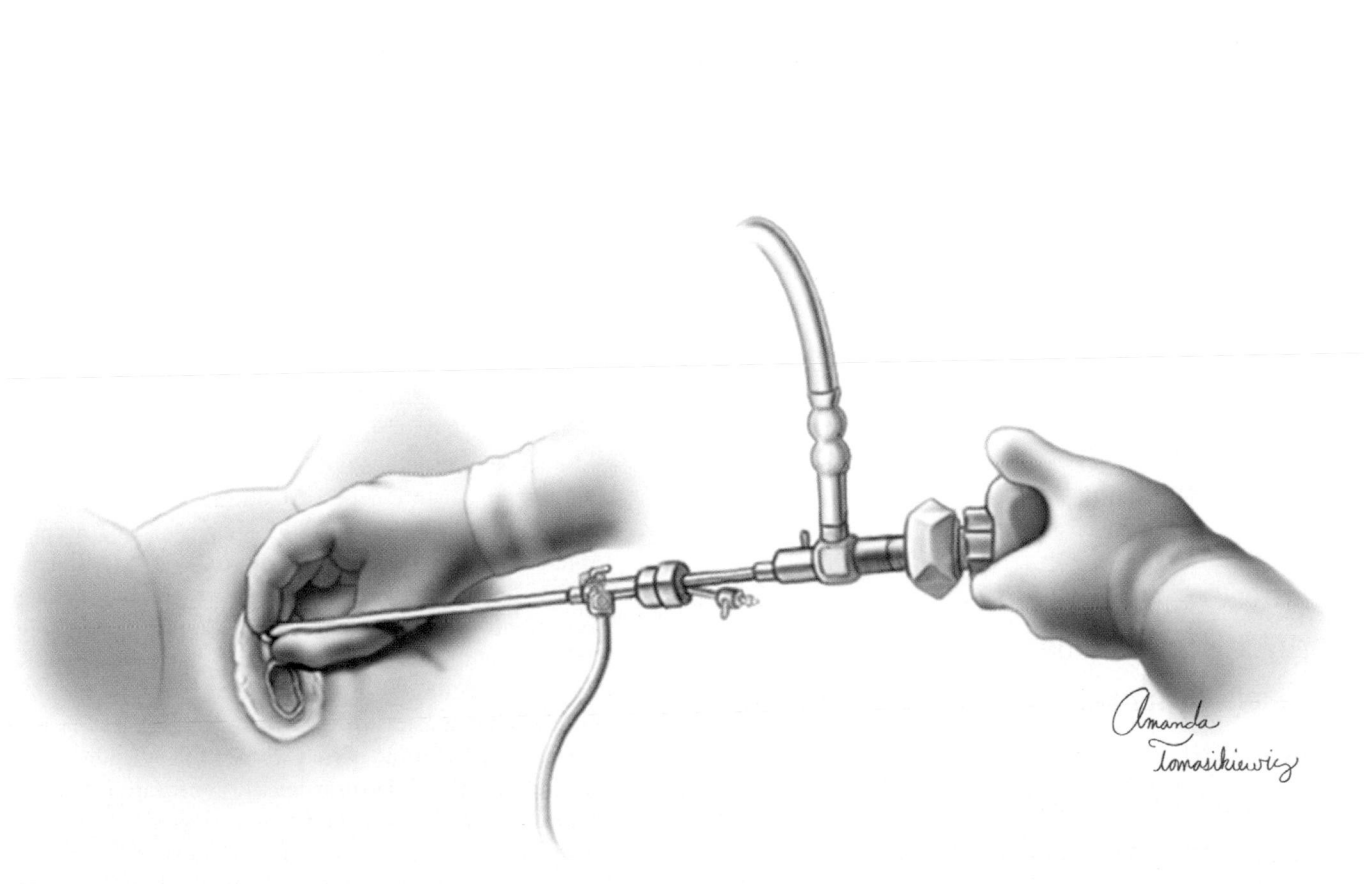

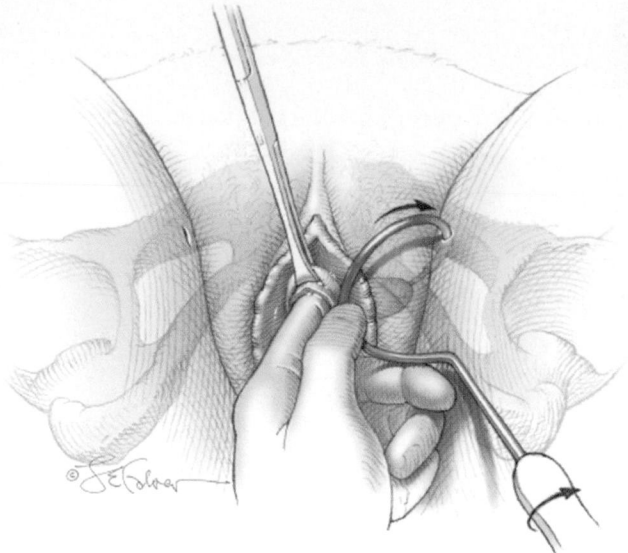

DEFINITIONS

Urinary incontinence is defined as any involuntary leakage of urine. In addition to the urethra, urine may also leak from extraurethral sources, such as fistulas or congenital malformations of the lower urinary tract. Although incontinence is categorized into a number of forms, this chapter will focus on the evaluation and management of stress and urge urinary incontinence. *Stress urinary incontinence* (SUI) is the involuntary leakage of urine with exertion or with sneezing or coughing. *Urge urinary or "urge"—incontinence* is the involuntary leakage accompanied or immediately preceded by a perceived strong imminent need to void. A related condition, overactive bladder, describes urinary urgency *with* or *without* incontinence and usually with increased daytime urinary frequency and nocturia (Abrams, 2009).

According to International Continence Society guidelines, urinary incontinence is a symptom, a sign, and a condition (Abrams, 2002). For example, with SUI, a patient may complain of involuntary urine leakage with exercise or laughing. Concurrent with these symptoms, involuntary leakage from the urethra synchronous with cough or Valsalva may be observed during examination by a provider. And as a condition, SUI is objectively demonstrated during urodynamic testing if involuntary leakage of urine is seen with increased abdominal pressure and absence of detrusor muscle contraction. Under these circumstances, when the symptom or sign of SUI is confirmed with objective testing, the term *urodynamic stress incontinence* (USI), formerly known as *genuine stress incontinence*, is used.

With urge urinary incontinence, women have difficulty postponing urination urges and generally must promptly empty their bladder on cue and without delay. If urge urinary incontinence is objectively demonstrated during urodynamic testing with cystometric evaluation, the condition is termed *detrusor overactivity (DO)*, formerly known as detrusor instability. When both stress and urgency components are present, it is called *mixed urinary incontinence*.

Functional incontinence occurs in situations in which a woman cannot reach a toilet in time because of physical, psychological, or mentation limitations. Often, this group would be continent if these issues were absent.

EPIDEMIOLOGY

In Western societies, epidemiologic studies indicate a prevalence of urinary incontinence of 15 to 55 percent. This wide range is attributed to variations in research methodologies, population characteristics, and definitions of incontinence. As part of the 2005-2006 National Health and Nutrition Examination Survey (NHANES), a cross-sectional group of 1961 nonpregnant, non-institutionalized women in the United States were questioned about pelvic floor disorders. Urinary incontinence that was characterized by participants as moderate to severe leakage was identified in 15.7 percent (Nygaard, 2008). However, current available data are limited by the fact that most women do not seek medical attention for this condition (Hunskaar, 2000). It is estimated that only one in four women will seek medical advice for incontinence due to embarrassment, limited access to health care, or poor screening by health care providers (Hagstad, 1985).

Among ambulatory women with urinary incontinence, the most common condition is SUI, which represents 29 to 75 percent of cases. Urge urinary incontinence accounts for up to 33 percent of incontinence cases, whereas the remainder is attributable to mixed forms (Hunskaar, 2000). In a review of overactive bladder, 15 percent of 64,528 women met criteria for overactive bladder with or without incontinence, and 11 percent had urge urinary incontinence (Hartmann, 2009).

Urinary incontinence can significantly impair a woman's quality of life, leading to disrupted social relationships, psychological distress from embarrassment and frustration, hospitalizations due to skin breakdown and urinary tract infection, and

nursing home admission. An incontinent elderly woman is 2.5 times more likely to be admitted to a nursing home than a continent one (Langa, 2002). Likewise, the monetary ramifications of incontinence are considerable. An estimated $32 billion is spent annually in the United States caring for community-dwelling and institutionalized patients with urinary incontinence (Hu, 2004). Moreover, population projections from the U.S. Census Bureau forecast that the number of American women with urinary incontinence will increase 55 percent from 18.3 million to 28.4 million between 2010 and 2050 (Wu, 2009).

RISKS FOR URINARY INCONTINENCE

Age

The prevalence of incontinence appears to increase gradually during young adult life (Fig. 23-1). A broad peak is noted at middle age and then steadily increases after age 65 (Hannestad, 2000). Similarly, data from the 2005-2006 NHANES demonstrate a steady increase in incontinence prevalence with age: 7 percent in those aged 20 to 40 years, 17 percent for ages 40 to 60, 23 percent for ages 60 to 80, and 32 percent for those older than 80 (Nygaard, 2008).

Incontinence should not be viewed as a normal consequence of aging. However, several physiologic age-related changes in the lower urinary tract may predispose to incontinence, overactive bladder, or other voiding difficulties. First, the prevalence of involuntary detrusor contractions increases with age, and detrusor overactivity is found in 21 percent of healthy,

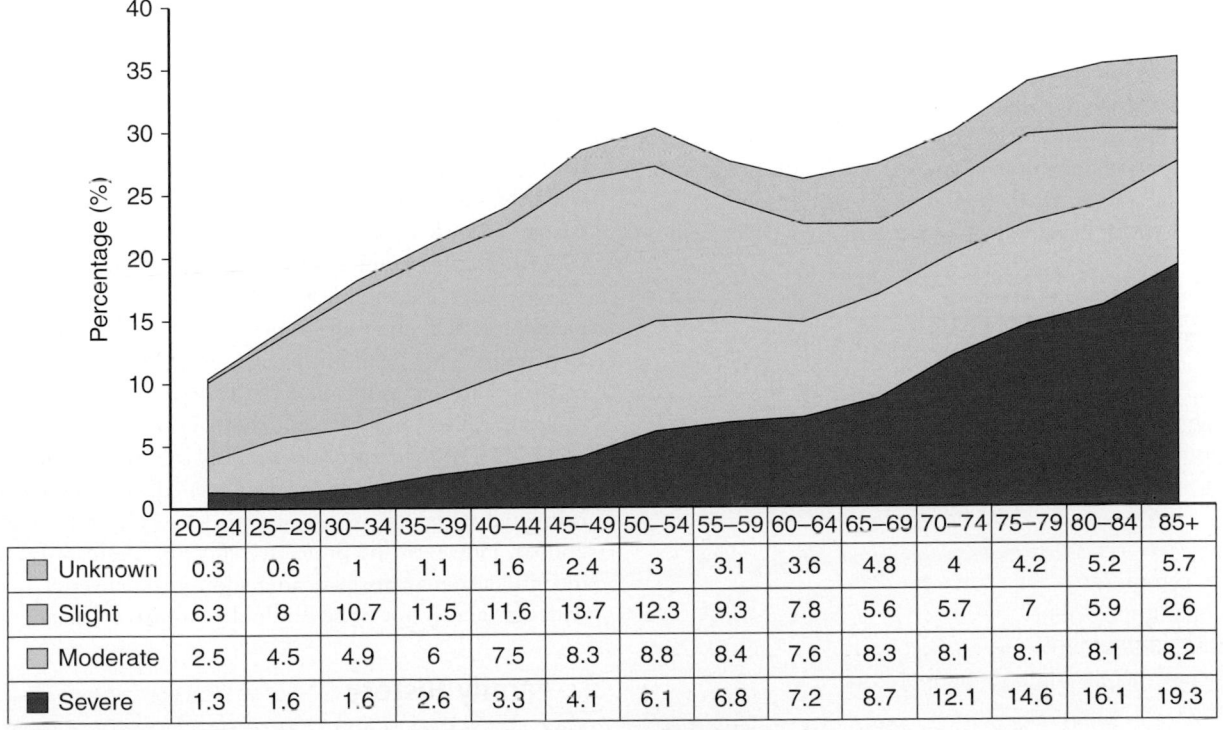

	20–24	25–29	30–34	35–39	40–44	45–49	50–54	55–59	60–64	65–69	70–74	75–79	80–84	85+
☐ Unknown	0.3	0.6	1	1.1	1.6	2.4	3	3.1	3.6	4.8	4	4.2	5.2	5.7
☐ Slight	6.3	8	10.7	11.5	11.6	13.7	12.3	9.3	7.8	5.6	5.7	7	5.9	2.6
☐ Moderate	2.5	4.5	4.9	6	7.5	8.3	8.8	8.4	7.6	8.3	8.1	8.1	8.1	8.2
■ Severe	1.3	1.6	1.6	2.6	3.3	4.1	6.1	6.8	7.2	8.7	12.1	14.6	16.1	19.3

Age (years)

FIGURE 23-1 Prevalence of incontinence by age group (n = 8002). (Adapted from Hannestad, 2000, with permission.)

continent community-dwelling elderly (Resnick, 1995). Total bladder capacity and the ability to postpone voiding decreases, and these declines may lead to urinary frequency. In addition, urinary flow rates are reduced in both older men and women and likely due to an age-associated decrease in detrusor contractility (Resnick, 1984). In women, postmenopausal decreases in estrogen levels result in atrophy of the urethral mucosal seal, loss of compliance, and bladder irritation, which may predispose to both stress and urge urinary incontinence. Finally, there are age-related changes in renal filtration rate and alterations in diurnal levels of antidiuretic hormone and atrial natriuretic factor. These changes shift the diurnal-predominant pattern of fluid excretion toward one with greater urine excretion later in the day (Kirkland, 1983).

Race

Traditionally, white women are believed to have higher rates of stress urinary incontinence than women of other races. In contrast, urge urinary incontinence is believed to be more prevalent among African-American women. Most reports are not population based and thus are not the best estimate of true racial differences. In addition, existing data on racial differences are largely based on small sample sizes (Bump, 1993). However, data from the Nurse's Health Study cohorts, which included more than 76,000 women, did support these racial differences. Investigators found the highest 4-year incidence rates in white participants compared with that in Asian and black women (Townsend, 2010). It is not yet clear whether these differences are biologic, related to health care access, or affected by cultural expectations and symptom tolerance thresholds.

Obesity

Several epidemiologic studies have shown that an increased body mass index (BMI) is a significant and independent risk factor for urinary incontinence of all types (Table 23-1). Moreover, the prevalence of both urge urinary and stress incontinence increases proportionally with BMI (Hannestad, 2003). Theoretically, the increase in intraabdominal pressure that coincides with an increased BMI results in a higher intravesical pressure. This higher pressure overcomes urethral closing pressure and leads to incontinence (Bai, 2002). Accordingly, as a greater portion of our population becomes overweight and obese, we can expect to see an increase in the prevalence of urinary incontinence in the United States (Flegal, 2002). Encouragingly, weight loss for many can be an effective treatment. In overweight or obese women, the prevalence of urinary incontinence significantly declines following weight loss achieved by behavior modification or with bariatric surgery (Burgio, 2007; Deitel, 1988; Subak, 2009).

Menopause

Studies have inconsistently demonstrated an increase in urinary dysfunction after a woman enters her postmenopausal years (Bump, 1998). In those with symptoms, separating hypoestrogenism effects from the effects of aging is difficult.

High-affinity estrogen receptors have been identified in the urethra, pubococcygeal muscle, and bladder trigone but are infrequently found elsewhere in the bladder (Iosif, 1981). Hypoestrogenic-related collagen changes and reductions in urethral vascularity and skeletal muscle volume are factors. They are thought to collectively contribute to impaired urethral function via a decreased resting urethral pressure (Carlile, 1988). Moreover, estrogen deficiency with resulting urogenital atrophy is believed to be responsible in part for urinary sensory symptoms following menopause (Raz, 1993). Despite this current evidence that estrogen plays a role in normal urinary function, it is less clear whether estrogen therapy is useful in the treatment or prevention of incontinence (Cody, 2009; Fantl, 1994, 1996).

Childbirth and Pregnancy

Many studies reveal the prevalence of urinary incontinence to be higher in parous women compared with nulliparas. The effects of childbirth on incontinence may result from direct injury to pelvic muscles and connective tissue attachments. In addition, nerve damage from trauma or stretch injury may result in pelvic muscle dysfunction. Specifically, rates of prolonged pudendal nerve latency after delivery are higher in women with incontinence compared with asymptomatic puerperal women (Snooks, 1986).

One large epidemiologic study identified vaginal delivery parameters that may affect the risk of urinary incontinence later in life. First, fetal birthweight ≥ 4000 g increased the risk of all urinary incontinence types (Rortveit, 2003b). Secondly, cesarean delivery may have a short-term protective effect for preventing urinary incontinence. In this study, the adjusted odds ratio for any incontinence associated with vaginal delivery compared with that with cesarean delivery was 1.7 (Rortveit, 2003a). However, the protective effect of cesarean delivery on incontinence may dissipate after additional deliveries, decreases with age, and is not present in older women (Nygaard, 2006).

Family History

Evidence suggests that the risk of urinary incontinence may be increased in the daughters and sisters of incontinent women. In one large survey, daughters of incontinent women had an increased relative risk of 1.3 and absolute risk of 23 percent

---

TABLE 23-1. Risk Factors for Urinary Incontinence

Age
Pregnancy
Childbirth
Menopause
Hysterectomy
Obesity
Urinary symptoms
Functional impairment
Cognitive impairment
Chronically increased abdominal pressure
   Chronic cough
   Constipation
   Occupational risk
Smoking

of having urinary incontinence. Younger sisters of incontinent women also had a greater likelihood of having any urinary incontinence (Hannestad, 2004).

Smoking and Chronic Lung Disease

In women older than 60 years with chronic obstructive pulmonary disease, a significantly increased risk of urinary incontinence is found (Brown, 1996; Diokno, 1990). Similarly, cigarette smoking is identified as an independent risk factor for urinary incontinence in several studies. Both current and former smokers were noted to have a two- to threefold risk of incontinence compared with nonsmokers (Brown, 1996; Bump, 1992; Diokno, 1990). In another study, investigators also identified an association between current and former smoking and incontinence, but only for those who smoked more than 20 cigarettes daily. Severe incontinence was weakly associated with smoking regardless of cigarette number (Hannestad, 2003). Theoretically, persistently increased intraabdominal pressures are generated from a smoker's chronic cough, and collagen synthesis is diminished by smoking's antiestrogenic effects.

Hysterectomy

Studies have inconsistently shown that hysterectomy is a risk factor for developing urinary incontinence. Those that show an association are retrospective, lack appropriate control groups, and are often based solely on subjective data (Bump, 1998). In contrast, studies that include pre- and postoperative urodynamic testing reveal clinically insignificant changes in bladder function. Moreover, evidence does not support avoidance of clinically indicated hysterectomy or the selection of supracervical hysterectomy as measures to prevent urinary incontinence (Vervest, 1989; Wake, 1980).

PATHOPHYSIOLOGY

Continence

The bladder is a urine storage organ with the capacity to accommodate large increases in volume with minimal or no increases in intravesical pressure. The ability to store urine coupled with convenient and socially acceptable voluntary emptying is *continence*.

Continence requires the complex coordination of multiple components that include: muscle contraction and relaxation, appropriate connective tissue support, and integrated innervation and communication between these structures. Simplistically, during filling, urethral contraction is coordinated with bladder relaxation and urine is stored. During voiding, the urethra relaxes and the bladder contracts. These mechanisms can be challenged by uninhibited detrusor contractions, marked increases in intraabdominal pressure, and changes to the various anatomic components of the continence mechanism.

Bladder Filling
Bladder Anatomy

The bladder wall is multilayered and contains mucosal, submucosal, muscular, and adventitial layers (Fig. 23-2). The bladder

mucosa is comprised of a transitional cell epithelium, supported by a lamina propria. With small bladder volumes, the mucosa is thrown into convoluted folds. However, with bladder filling, it is stretched and thinned. The bladder epithelium, termed *uroepithelium*, is comprised of distinct cell layers. The most superficial is the umbrella cell layer, and its impermeability is thought to provide the primary urine plasma barrier. Covering the uroepithelium is a glycosaminoglycan (GAG) layer. This GAG layer may prohibit bacterial adherence and prevents urothelial damage by acting as a protective barrier. Specifically, theories suggest that this carbohydrate polymer layer may be defective in patients with interstitial cystitis (Chap. 11, p. 320).

The muscular layer, termed the detrusor muscle, is composed of three smooth-muscle layers arranged in a plexiform fashion. This unique arrangement allows for rapid multidimensional expansion during bladder filling and is a key component to the bladder's ability to accommodate large volumes.

Innervation Overview

Normal function of the lower urinary tract requires integration of peripheral and central nervous systems. The peripheral nervous system contains somatic and autonomic divisions (Fig. 23-3). Of these, the somatic component innervates striated muscle, whereas the autonomic division innervates smooth muscle.

The autonomic nervous system controls involuntary motion and is categorized into sympathetic and parasympathetic divisions. The sympathetic system mediates its end-organ effects through epinephrine or norepinephrine acting on α- or β adrenergic receptors (Fig. 23-4). The parasympathetic division acts through acetylcholine binding to muscarinic or nicotinic receptors. In the pelvis, autonomic fibers that supply the pelvic viscera course in the superior and inferior hypogastric plexi (Fig. 23-5).

The somatic nervous system controls voluntary movement, and the portion of this system that is most relevant to lower urinary tract function originates from Onuf somatic nucleus (p. 613). This nucleus is located in the ventral horn gray matter of spinal levels S2–S4 and contains the neurons that innervate the striated urogenital sphincter complex, described next. Nerves involved with that connection include branches of the pudendal and pelvic nerves.

Urogenital Sphincter

As the bladder fills, synchronized contraction of the urogenital sphincter is integral to continence. Composed of striated muscle, this sphincter complex includes: (1) the *sphincter urethrae*, (2) the *urethrovaginal sphincter*, and (3) the *compressor urethrae*. The sphincter urethrae wraps circumferentially around the urethra. In comparison, the urethrovaginal sphincter and the compressor urethrae arch ventrally over the urethra and insert into the fibromuscular tissue of the anterior vaginal wall (Fig. 23-6).

These three muscles function as a single unit and contract to close the urethra. Contraction of these muscles circumferentially constricts the cephalad two thirds of the urethra and laterally compresses the distal one third. The sphincter urethrae is predominantly composed of slow-twitch fibers and remains tonically contracted, contributing substantially to continence at rest. In contrast, the urethrovaginal sphincter and the compressor

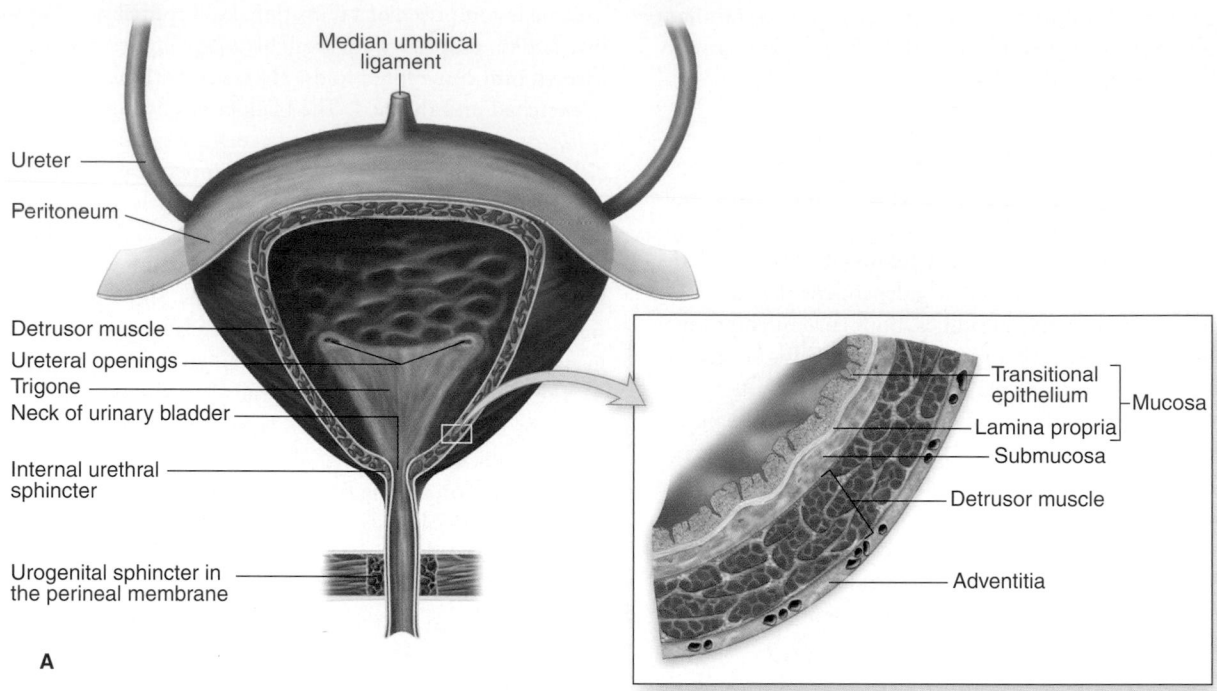

A

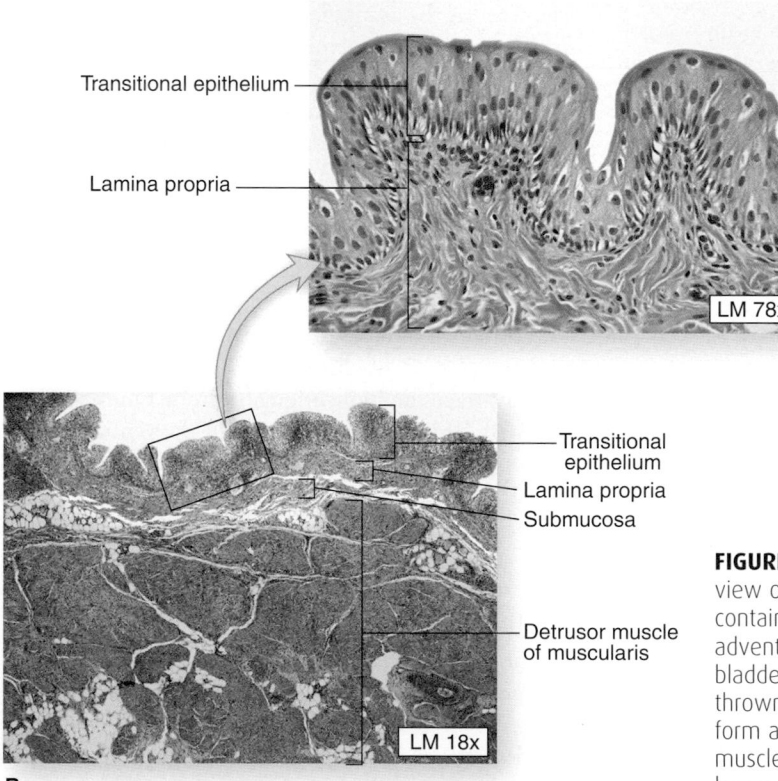

B

FIGURE 23-2 Bladder anatomy. **A.** Anteroposterior view of bladder anatomy. Inset: The bladder wall contains mucosal, submucosal, muscular, and adventitial layers. **B.** Photomicrograph of the bladder wall. The mucosa of an empty bladder is thrown into convoluted folds or rugae. The plexiform arrangement of muscle fibers of the detrusor muscle cause difficulty in defining its three distinct layers. *(From McKinley, 2006, with permission.)*

urethrae are comprised of fast-twitch muscle fibers, which allow brisk contraction and urethra lumen closure when continence is challenged by sudden increases in intraabdominal pressure.

Innervation Important to Storage

The urogenital sphincter receives somatic motor innervation through the pudendal and pelvic nerves (see Figs. 23-5 and 23-7).

Thus, pudendal neuropathy, which may follow obstetric injury, can affect normal sphincter functioning. Additionally, prior pelvic surgery or pelvic radiation therapy may damage nerves, vasculature, and soft tissue. Such injury can lead to ineffective urogenital sphincter action and contribute to incontinence.

Sympathetic fibers are carried through the superior hypogastric nerve plexus and communicate with α- and β-adrenergic

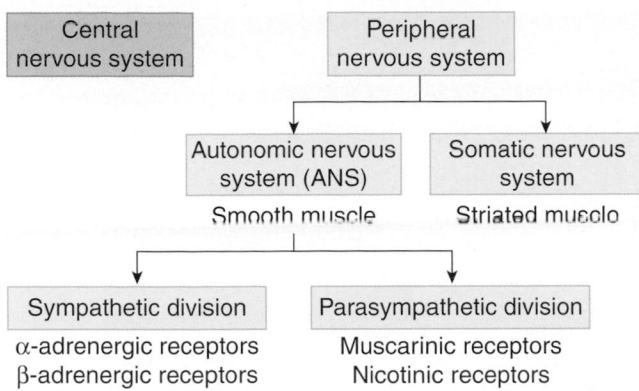

FIGURE 23-3 Divisions of the human nervous system. The peripheral nervous system includes: (1) the somatic nervous system, which mediates voluntary movements through its actions on striated muscle, and (2) the autonomic nervous system, which controls involuntary motion through its actions on smooth muscle. The autonomic nervous system is further divided into the sympathetic division, which acts through epinephrine and norepinephrine binding to adrenergic receptors, and the parasympathetic division, which acts through acetylcholine binding to muscarinic or nicotinic receptors.

receptors within the bladder and urethra. β-Adrenergic receptor stimulation in the bladder dome results in smooth-muscle relaxation and assists with urine storage (Fig. 23-8). In contrast, α-adrenergic receptors predominate in the bladder base and urethra. These receptors are stimulated by norepinephrine, which initiates a cascade of events that preferentially leads to urethral contraction and aids urine storage and continence.

These effects of α-stimulation underlie the treatment of SUI with imipramine, a tricyclic antidepressant with adrenergic agonist properties.

Urethral Coaptation

One key to maintaining continence is adequate urethral mucosal coaptation. The uroepithelium is supported by a connective tissue layer, which is thrown into deep folds, also known as plications. A rich capillary network runs within its subepithelial layer. This vascular network aids in urethral mucosal approximation, also termed *coaptation*, by acting like an "inflatable cushion" (Fig. 23-9). In women who are hypoestrogenic, this submucosal vasculature plexus is less prominent. In part, hormone replacement targets this diminished vascularity and enhances coaptation to improve continence.

Bladder Emptying
Innervation Related to Voiding

When an appropriate time for bladder emptying arises, sympathetic stimulation is reduced and parasympathetic stimulation is triggered. Specifically, neural impulses carried in the pelvic nerves stimulate acetylcholine release and lead to detrusor muscle contraction (Fig. 23-10). Concurrent with detrusor stimulation, acetylcholine also stimulates muscarinic receptors in the urethra and leads to outlet relaxation for voiding.

Within the parasympathetic division, acetylcholine receptors are broadly defined as muscarinic and nicotinic. The bladder is densely supplied with muscarinic receptors, which

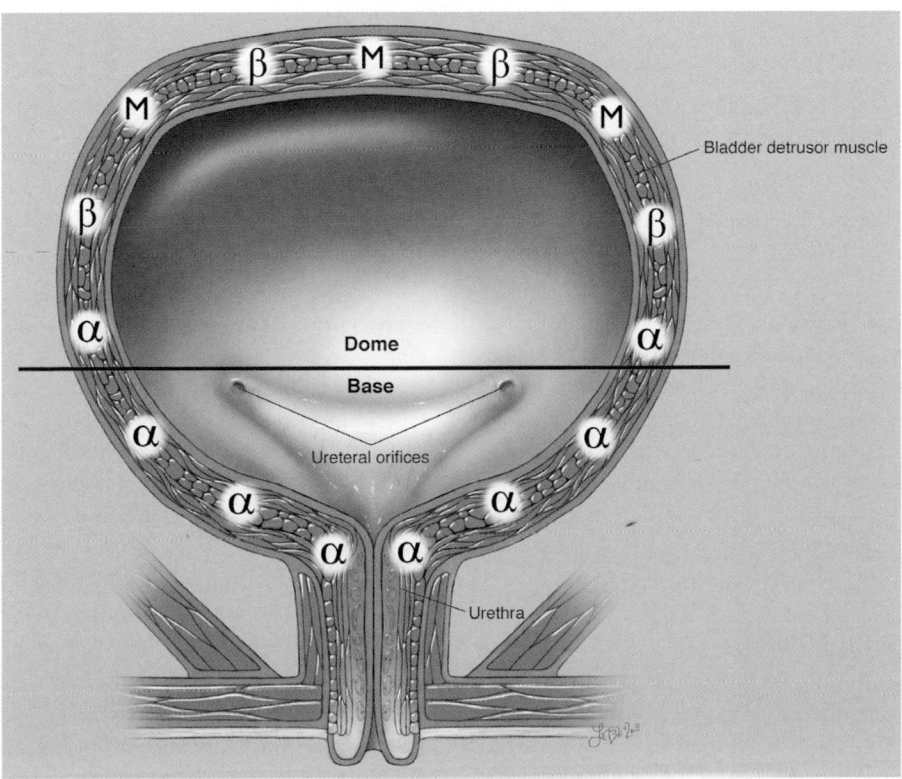

FIGURE 23-4 The bladder dome is rich in parasympathetic muscarinic receptors (M) and sympathetic β-adrenergic receptors (β). The bladder neck contains a greater density of sympathetic α-adrenergic receptors (α).

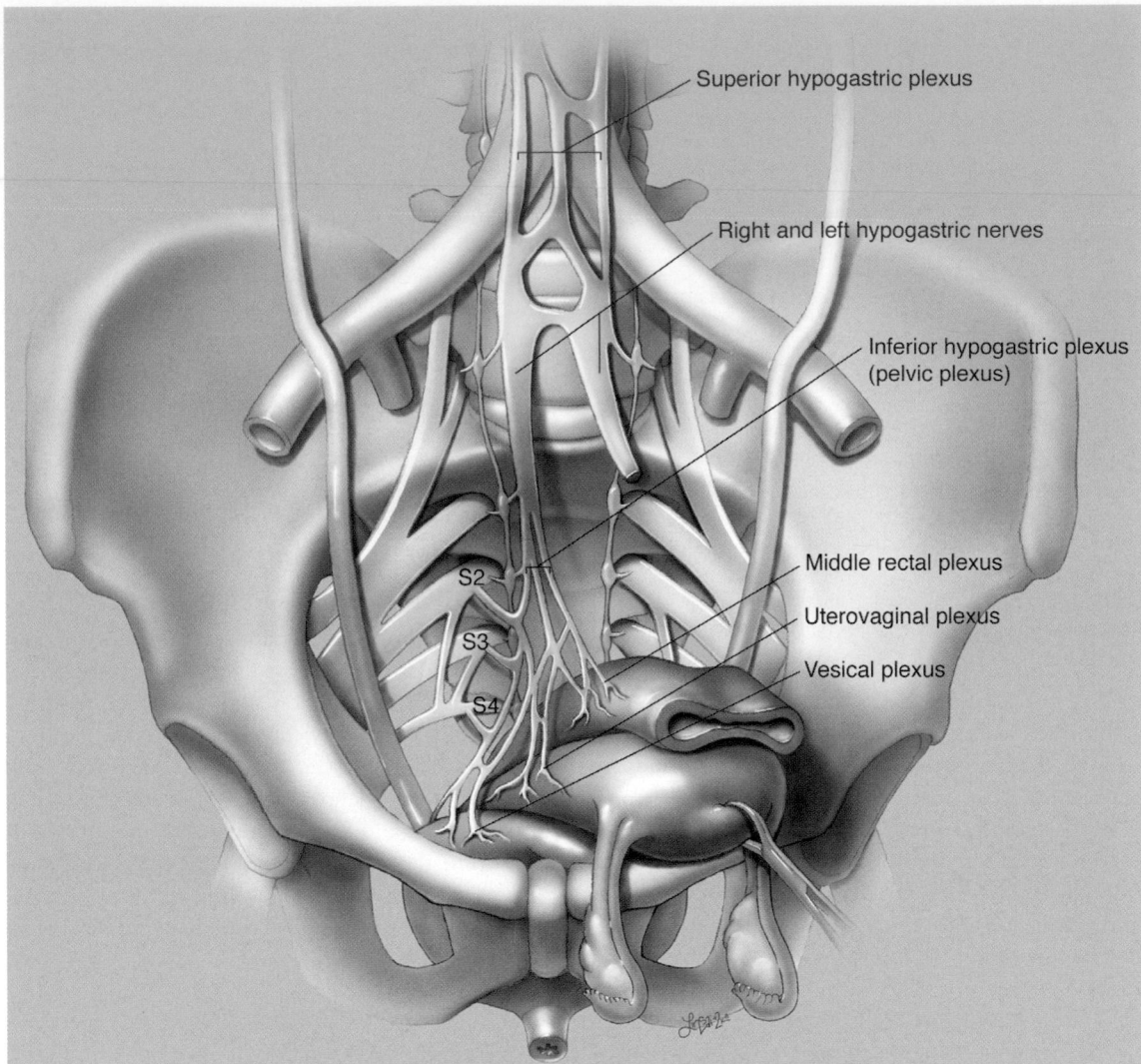

FIGURE 23-5 The inferior hypogastric plexus, also known as the pelvic plexus, is formed by visceral efferents from S2 to S4, which provide the parasympathetic component by way of the pelvic nerves. The superior hypogastric plexus primarily contains sympathetic fibers from the T10 to L2 cord segments and terminates by dividing into right and left hypogastric nerves. The hypogastric nerves and rami from the sacral portion of the sympathetic chain contribute the sympathetic component to the pelvic plexus. The pelvic plexus divides into three portions according to the course and distribution of its fibers: the middle rectal plexus, uterovaginal plexus, and vesical plexus.

when stimulated lead to detrusor contraction. Of the muscarinic receptors, five glycoproteins designated M_1–M_5 have been identified. M_2 and M_3 receptor subtypes have been identified as the ones predominantly responsible for detrusor smooth muscle contraction. Thus, treatment with muscarinic antagonist medication blunts detrusor contraction to improve continence. Specifically, continence drugs that target only the M_3 receptor maximize drug efficacy yet minimize activation of other muscarinic receptors and drug side effects.

Muscular Activity with Voiding

Smooth muscle cells within the detrusor fuse with one another so that low-resistance electrical pathways extend from one muscle cell to the next. Thus, action potentials can spread quickly throughout the detrusor muscle to cause rapid contraction of the entire bladder. In addition, the plexiform arrangement of bladder detrusor fibers allows multidirectional contraction and

is ideally suited for rapid concentric contraction during bladder emptying.

During voiding, all components of the striated urogenital sphincter relax. Importantly, bladder contraction and sphincter relaxation must be coordinated for effective voiding. Occasionally, in a condition known as *detrusor sphincter dyssynergia*, the urethral sphincter fails to relax during contraction of the detrusor, and retention ensues. Women with this condition may be treated with pharmacologic agents such as muscle relaxants. These drugs purportedly relax the urethral sphincter and levator ani muscles to improve coordinated voiding.

■ Continence Theories

Theories on continence abound and vary in their supporting scientific evidence. Most theories can ultimately be distilled down to those that involve the concepts of anatomic stress incontinence and decreased urethral integrity (sphincteric deficiency).

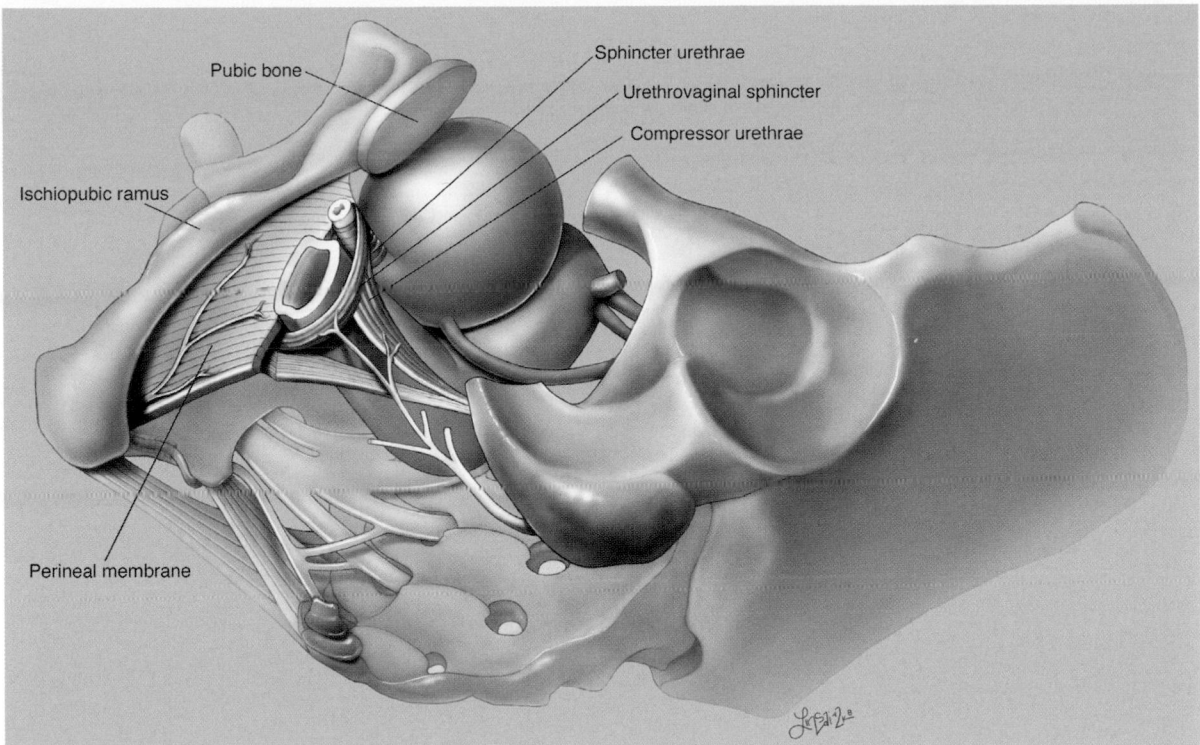

FIGURE 23-6 Striated urogenital sphincter anatomy. The perineal membrane is removed to show the three component muscles of the striated urogenital sphincter. This sphincter receives most of its somatic innervation through the pudendal nerve.

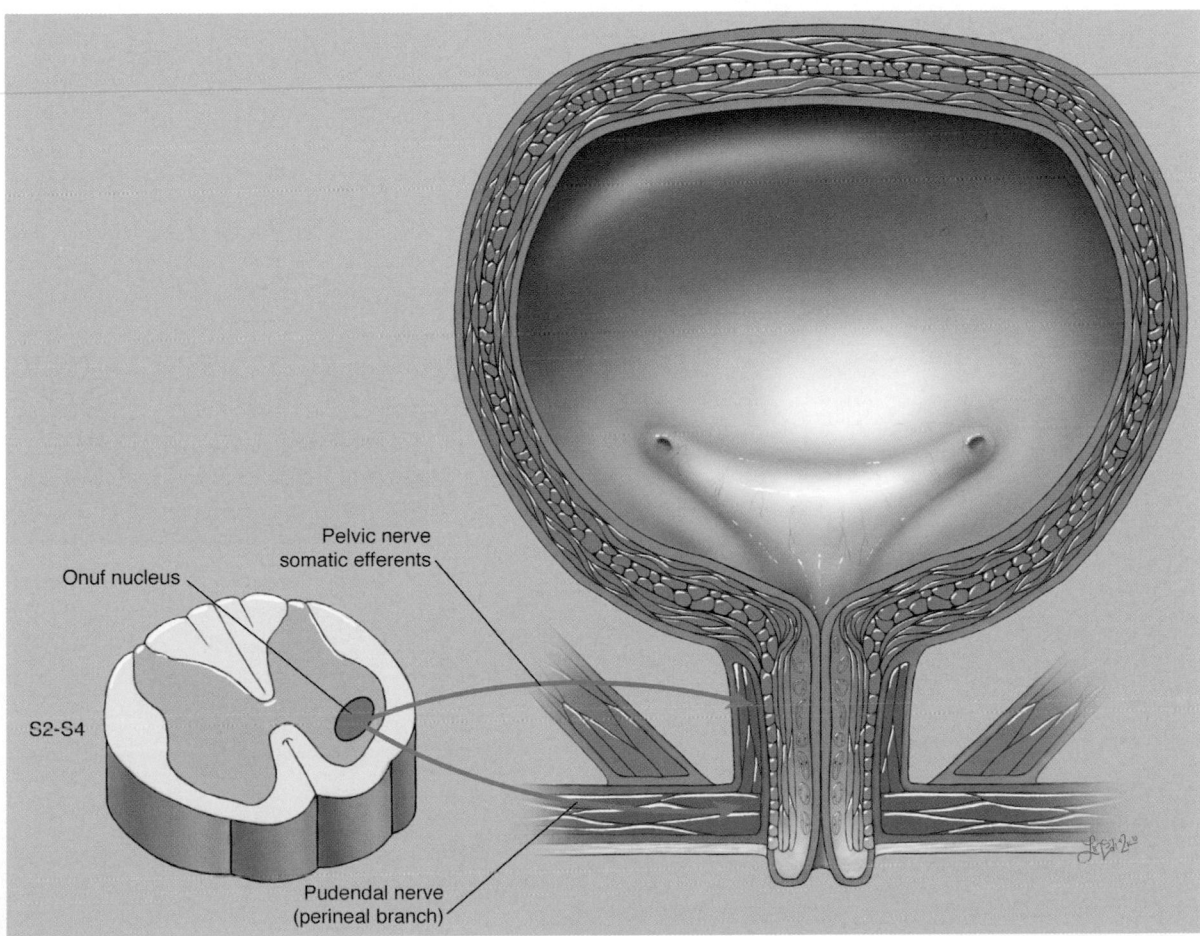

FIGURE 23-7 Onuf nucleus is found in the ventral horn gray matter of S2 through S4. This nucleus contains the neurons whose fibers supply the striated urogenital sphincter. The urethrovaginal sphincter and compressor urethrae are innervated by the perineal branch of the pudendal nerve. The sphincter urethrae is variably innervated by somatic efferents that travel in the pelvic nerves.

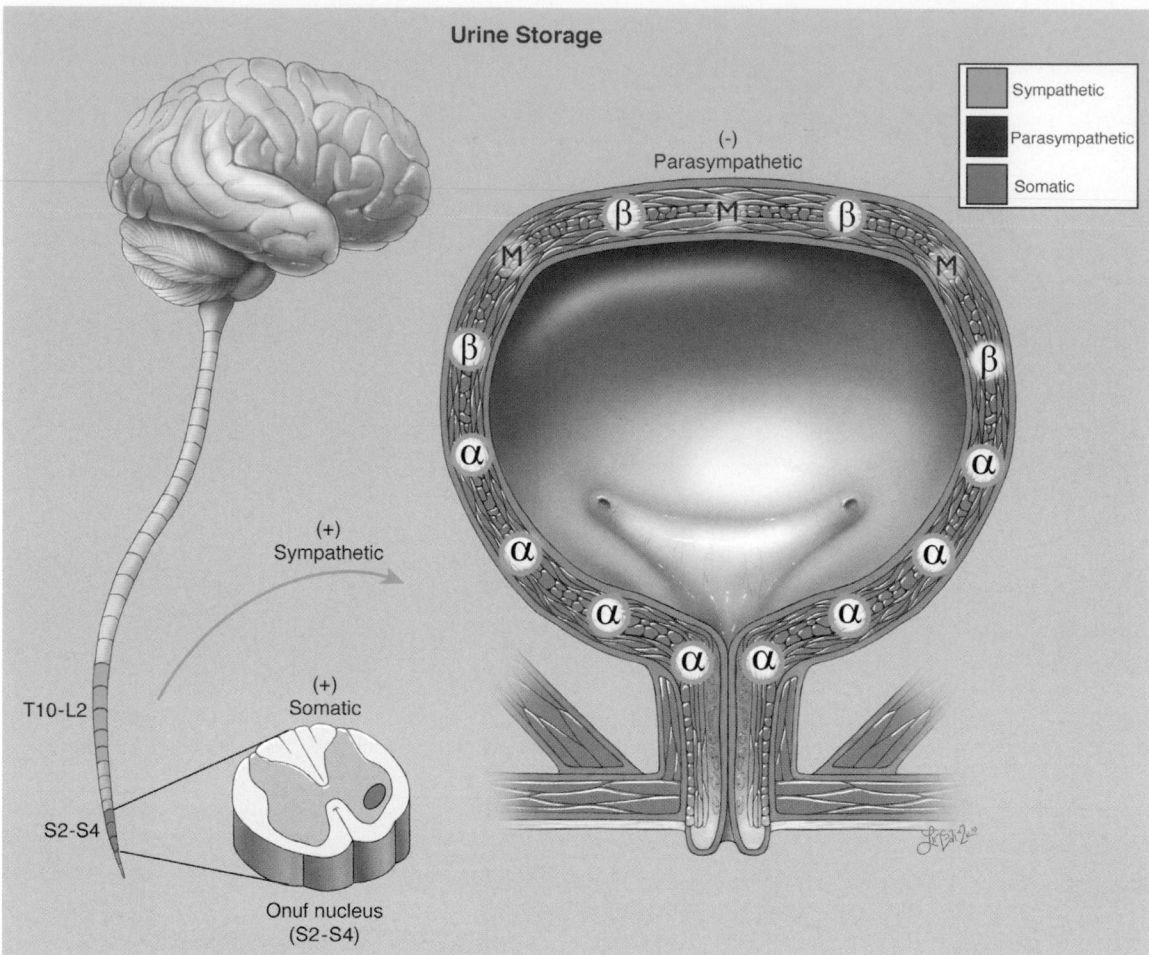

FIGURE 23-8 Physiology of urine storage. Bladder distension from filling leads to: (1) α-adrenergic contraction of the urethral smooth muscle and increased tone at the vesical neck (via the T11-L2 spinal sympathetic reflex); (2) activation of urethral motor neurons in Onuf nucleus with contraction of striated urogenital sphincter muscles (via the pudendal nerve); and (3) inhibited parasympathetic transmission with decreased detrusor pressure. α = alpha adrenergic receptors; β = beta adrenergic; M = muscarinic (cholinergic).

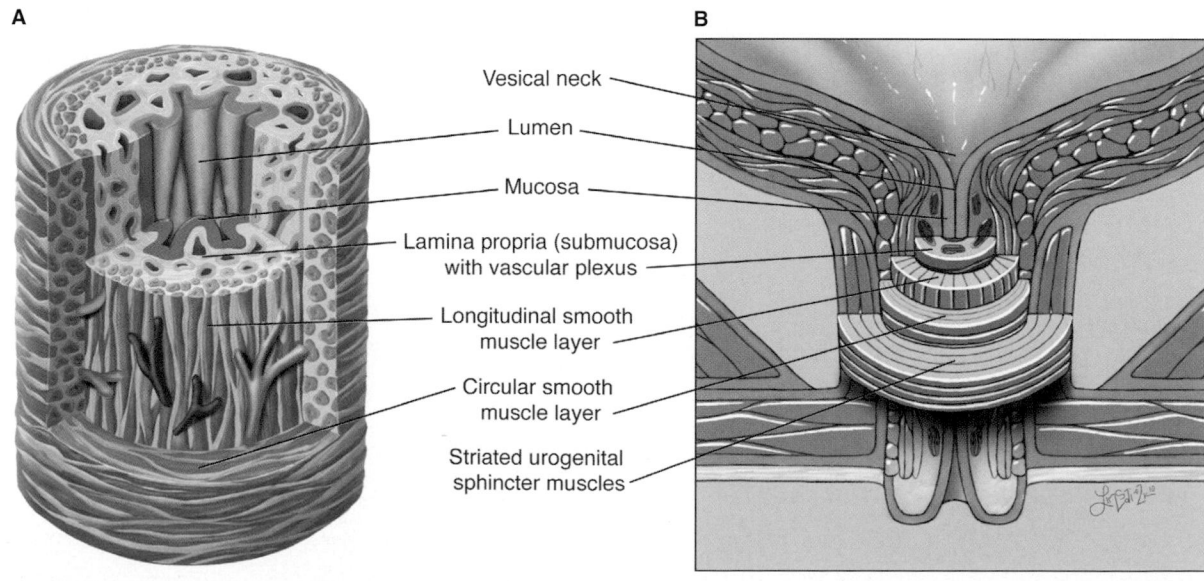

FIGURE 23-9 Drawing of urethral anatomy. **A.** Urethral anatomy in cross section. Urethral coaptation results in part from filling of the rich subepithelial vascular plexus. The urethra contains circular and longitudinal smooth muscle layers. **B.** Vesical neck and urethral anatomy. The striated urogenital sphincter lies external to the urethral smooth muscle layers.

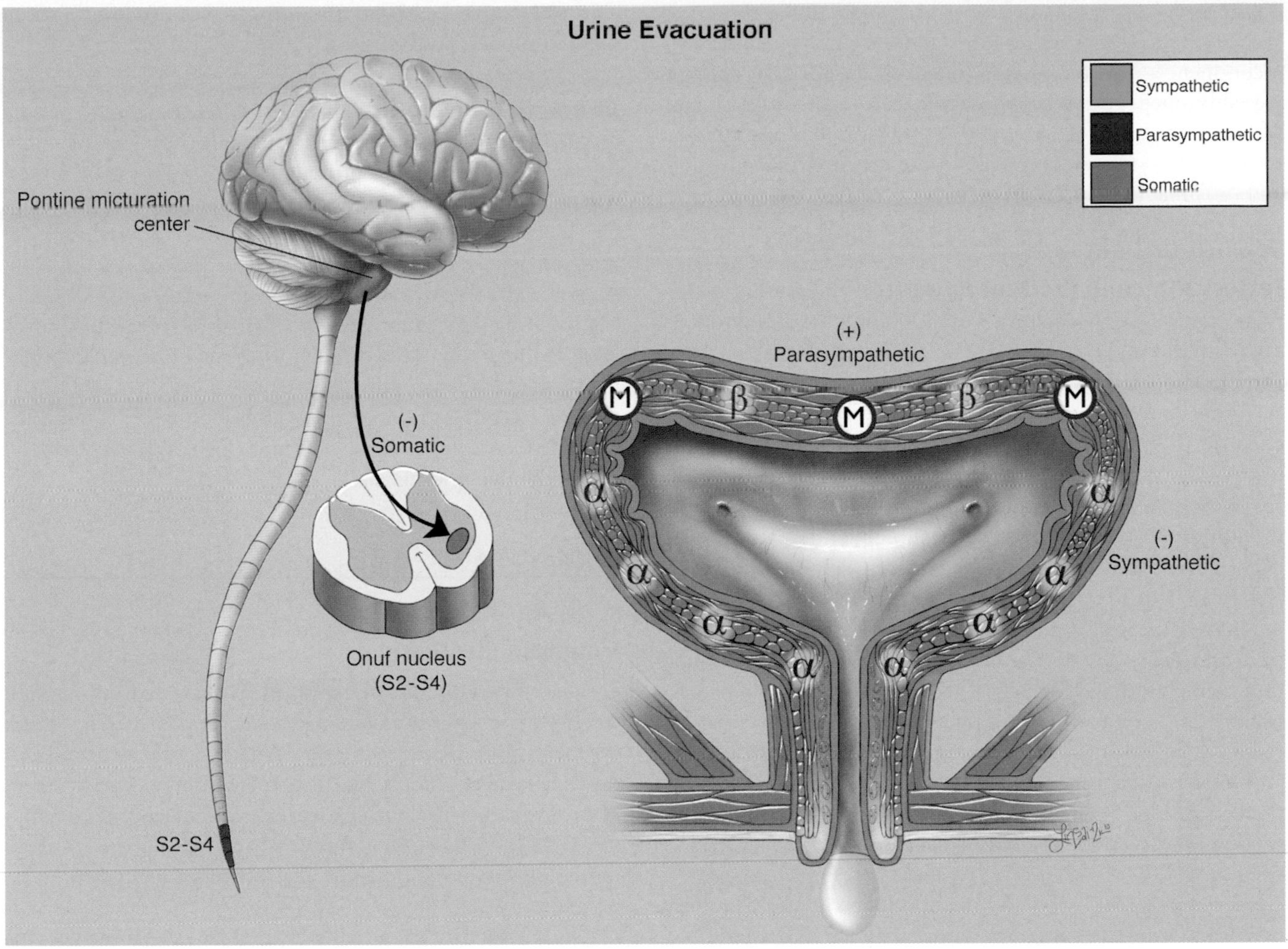

Urine Evacuation

Pontine micturation
center

(−)
Somatic

Onuf nucleus
(S2-S4)

S2-S4

(+)
Parasympathetic

(−)
Sympathetic

| Sympathetic |
| Parasympathetic |
| Somatic |

FIGURE 23-10 Physiology of urine evacuation. Efferent impulses from the pontine micturition center results in inhibition of somatic fibers in Onuf nucleus and voluntary relaxation of the striated urogenital sphincter muscles. These efferent impulses also result in preganglionic sympathetic inhibition with opening of the vesical neck and parasympathetic stimulation, which results in detrusor muscarinic contraction. The net result is relaxation of the striated urogenital sphincter complex causing decreased urethral pressure, followed almost immediately by detrusor contraction and voiding. α = alpha adrenergic receptors; β = beta adrenergic; M = muscarinic (cholinergic).

Anatomic Stress Incontinence

Urethral and bladder neck support is integral to continence. This support stems from: (1) ligaments along the urethra's lateral aspects, termed the pubourethral ligaments; (2) the vagina and its lateral fascial condensation; (3) the arcus tendineus fascia pelvis; and (4) levator ani muscles. A full anatomic description of these ligaments and muscles is found in Chapter 38 (p. 925).

In an ideally supported urogenital tract, increases in intraabdominal pressure are equally transmitted to the bladder, bladder base, and urethra. In women who are continent, increases in downward-directed pressure from cough, laugh, sneeze, and Valsalva maneuver are countered by supportive tissue tone provided by the levator ani muscles and vaginal connective tissue (Fig. 23-11). With loss of support, the ability of the urethra and bladder neck to close against a firm supportive "backboard" is

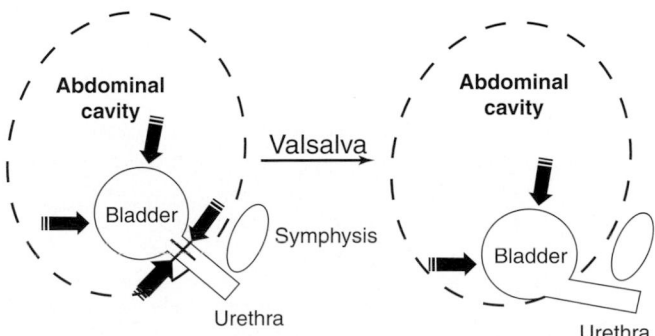

FIGURE 23-11 Drawing describes the pressure transmission theory. In women with normal support (*left image*), increases in intraabdominal pressure are equally distributed to contralateral sides of the bladder and urethra. In those with poor urethral support (*right image*), increases in intraabdominal pressure alter the urethrovesical angle, and continence may be lost.

diminished. This results in reduced urethral closing pressures, an inability to resist increases in bladder pressure, and in turn, incontinence. This mechanistic theory is the basis for surgical reestablishment of this support. Procedures such as Burch and Marshall-Marchetti-Kranz (MMK) colposuspensions attempt to return this anatomic support to the urethrovesical junction and proximal urethra.

Sphincteric Deficiency

Factors Affecting Urethral Integrity. The urethra maintains continence through the combination of urethral mucosal coaptation, the underlying urethral vascular plexus, the combined viscous and elastic properties of the urethral epithelium, and contraction of appropriate surrounding musculature. Defects in any of these components may lead to urine leakage. For example, prior surgery in the retropubic space may cause denervation and scarring of the urethra and its supporting tissue. These effects subsequently prevent urethral closure and lead to incontinence. This urethral state is termed *intrinsic sphincteric defect (ISD)* and colloquially is referred to as a "lead pipe" urethra. With ISD, denervation and/or devascularization of the urethra are common underlying findings. Specific causes are varied and include prior pelvic reconstructive surgeries, prior pelvic radiation therapy, diabetic neuropathy, neuronal degenerative diseases, and hypoestrogenism. In women with atrophic lower genital tracts, vascular changes within the plexus surrounding the urethra lead to poor coaptation and greater risks of incontinence.

As noted earlier, nerve dysfunction following birth trauma may lead to defective urethral sphincter function. In addition, childbirth also commonly injures urethral fascial support. This clinical example highlights the intimate relationship between urethral support and integrity.

Restoration of Urethral Integrity. Treatments to restore urethral integrity include transurethral injection of bulking agents, surgical sling procedures, and pelvic floor muscle strengthening and are described in later sections of this chapter. In brief, bulking agents are placed at the urethrovesical junction to elevate the epithelium and promote coaptation. Alternatively, the partial urethral obstruction created by pubovaginal sling procedures enhances urethral integrity. Lastly, because the urethra exits through urogenital hiatus, conditioning of the levator ani muscles with Kegel exercises can bolster urethral integrity. These muscles can be contracted around the urethra when continence is challenged by sudden increases in intraabdominal pressures.

DIAGNOSIS

■ History
Symptom Clustering

To quantify symptoms, investigators have created various validated patient questionnaires (Kelleher, 1997; Patrick, 1999; Wagner, 1996). Many of these are lengthy and may be impractical for general clinical practice. More simply, assessment of incontinence begins with a patient describing her urinary symptoms. This inventory of complaints may be collected through direct conversation but can be augmented with a patient questionnaire as shown in Table 23-2.

During inquiry, the number of voids and pads used per day, type of pad, frequency of pad changing, and the degree of pad

TABLE 23-2. Review of Systems for Women with Urinary Incontinence

Leak with stress	Y/N	Digital decompression of bowel	Y/N
Leak with urge	Y/N	Digital decompression of bladder	Y/N
Leak with position changes	Y/N	Postvoid dribble	Y/N
Leak with exercise	Y/N	Feeling of incomplete emptying	Y/N
Leak with intercourse/orgasm	Y/N	Recurrent UTI _____/yr	
Unconscious leakage	Y/N	Void with Valsalva	Y/N
Duration of symptoms _____ week(s) _____ month(s) _____ year(s)		Urine stream: strong/normal/weak	
		Childhood enuresis	Y/N
Leaks per _____ day _____ week(s) _____ month(s)		Frequency	Y/N
Pads per day _____ Type of pads _____		Urgency	Y/N
Voids daytime: _____		Dysuria	Y/N
Voids nighttime: _____		Hematuria	Y/N
Constipation Y/N		Back pain	Y/N
Self-medicate with _____		Pelvic pressure/Bulge	Y/N
BMs _____/day _____/week		Dyspareunia	Y/N
Anal incontinence	Y/N	Rectal bleeding	Y/N
Duration _____ month(s) _____ year(s)		Does heavy lifting	Y/N
Flatus _____/week(s) _____/month(s)		Interferes w/lifestyle or quality of life	Y/N
Liquid _____/week(s) _____/month(s)			
Stool _____/week(s) _____/month(s)			

BM = bowel movement; UTI = urinary tract infection.

saturation are important considerations. Although these specifics alone may not establish the exact type of incontinence, it does provide information regarding symptom severity and its effects on patient activities. Obviously, if a woman's symptoms do not diminish her quality of life, then simple observation is reasonable. Conversely, those with disruptive symptoms warrant further evaluation.

Specific to incontinence, information that describes the circumstances in which leakage occurs and specific maneuvers that incite or provoke leakage should be sought. With SUI, provokers may include increases in intraabdominal pressure such as coughing, sneezing, Valsalva maneuver, or thrusting during intercourse (Table 23-3). Alternatively, women with urge urinary incontinence may describe a loss of urine after urge sensations that typically cannot be suppressed. *Overflow incontinence* was a term used in the past to refer to women who had an inability to empty their bladder and had episodes of incontinence associated with urgency. Currently, however, this is considered by most to reflect another presentation of urge urinary incontinence. These women often note a sudden large loss of urine that is preceded by an inability to empty their bladder.

During questioning, symptoms typically cluster into those most frequently seen with SUI or with urge urinary incontinence. Alternatively, a significant overlap of complaints may reflect coexistent SUI and urge urinary incontinence, that is, mixed urinary incontinence. For these reasons, pattern identification is helpful as it may direct diagnostic testing and guide initial empiric therapy.

Bladder Diary

Please record the time and amount of your oral intake, urine output, urine leakage, and pad changes FOR 3 DAYS

Time	Oral Intake	Voided Urine	Urine Leakage or Pad Change

FIGURE 23-12 Example of an abbreviated urinary diary.

Voiding Diary

Typically, patients may not have an entirely accurate recollection of their own voiding habits. Accordingly, to obtain a thorough record, a woman should complete a urinary diary (Fig. 23-12). With this, women are instructed to record for 3 to 7 days the volumes and type of each oral fluid intake, volumes of urine with each void, episodes of urinary leakage, and provokers of incontinence episodes. During each 24-hour period, women should also record times of sleep and awakening. This enables an accurate description of voluntary nocturnal voiding patterns as well as enuresis. Although 5 to 7 days of documentation is desirable, 3 days will suffice in determining the general trend of incontinence. Realistically, most patients are typically not compliant for more than 3 days.

The historical information gained from a voiding/urinary diary is a valuable diagnostic and sometimes therapeutic tool. The first morning void is usually the largest of the day and is a good estimate of bladder capacity. Patients often can identify patterns in intake and voiding and modify behavior. For example, a patient may recognize increased urinary frequency or urge urinary incontinence episodes after caffeine intake. Moreover, this diary information serves as a baseline against which treatment efficacy can be assessed.

Urinary Symptoms

Urinary Frequency. Most women void eight times per day or less. Without a history that reflects increased fluid intake, increased voiding may indicate overactive bladder, urinary tract infection (UTI), calculi, or urethral pathology and should prompt additional evaluation. In addition, urinary frequency is commonly associated with interstitial cystitis (IC). In women with IC, the numbers of voids may commonly exceed 20 per day. In women with urge urinary incontinence or in those with systemic fluid management disorders such as congestive heart failure, nocturia may be noted. In the latter case, treatment of the underlying condition frequently leads to symptom improvement or cure of nighttime frequency.

Urinary Retention. It is important to determine if the patient adequately empties her bladder. Often incomplete emptying can result in incontinence associated with either stress or

TABLE 23-3. Symptom Comparison of Women with Stress or Urge Incontinence

Symptom	Urge Incontinence	Stress Incontinence
Urgency	Yes	No
Frequency with urgency	Yes	No
Urine leakage with increased intraabdominal pressures	No	Yes
Amount of urinary leakage with each incontinence episode	Large	Small
Ability to reach the toilet in time following an urge to void	Often no	Yes
Waking to void at night	Usually	Seldom

urgency. As described earlier, the term *overflow incontinence* is no longer used.

Other Urinary Symptoms. The volume of urine lost with each episode may also provide diagnostic clues. Large volumes are typically lost following a spontaneous detrusor contraction associated with urge urinary incontinence and may often involve loss of the entire bladder volume. In contrast, woman with SUI usually describe smaller volumes lost. Moreover, these women often are able to contract the levator ani muscles to temporarily stop their urine stream.

Postvoid dribbling is classically associated with urethral diverticulum, which may often be mistaken for urinary incontinence (Chap. 26, p. 683). Hematuria, although a common sign of UTI, may also indicate underlying malignancy and can cause irritative voiding symptoms.

The onset of symptoms may also provide information regarding etiology and treatment. For example, onset of symptoms with the menopause may suggest hypoestrogenism as an etiology. These patients may benefit from topical vaginal estrogen. In contrast, symptoms after hysterectomy or childbirth may reflect changes in tissue support or innervation.

Past Medical History

Obstetric trauma may be associated with damage to pelvic floor support, which may lead to SUI. For this reason, information describing a prolonged labor, operative vaginal delivery, macrosomia, postpartum catheterization for urinary retention, and increased parity may be valuable. As alluded to earlier, urinary incontinence may be associated with several medical conditions or their treatments, which could be modified to improve incontinence. To help remember these potential contributors, a useful mnemonic is "DIAPPERS": dementia/delirium, infection, atrophic vaginitis, psychological, pharmacologic, endocrine, restricted mobility, and stool impaction (Swift, 2008).

First, continence requires the cognitive ability to recognize and react appropriately to the sensation of a full bladder, motivation to maintain dryness, sufficient mobility and manual dexterity, and ready access to a toilet. Patients with dementia or significant psychological impairments often do not have the necessary cognitive ability for continence maintenance. Women with severe physical handicaps or restricted mobility may simply not have time to reach the toilet, especially in the setting of urinary urgency/overactive bladder.

Urinary tract infections cause bladder mucosal inflammation. This inflammation is thought to increase sensory afferent activity, which contributes to an overactive bladder. Similarly, estrogen deficiency may lead to atrophic vaginitis and urethritis. These are associated with increased local irritation and greater risks of UTI and overactive bladder.

A detailed medication inventory should be collected. Pertinent drugs may include estrogen, α-adrenergic agonists, and diuretics (Table 23-4).

Diabetes mellitus can lead to osmotic diuresis and polyuria if glucose control is poor. Polydipsia from diabetes insipidus or excessive caffeine or alcohol intake can also lead to polyuria

or urinary frequency. Similarly, other disorders of impaired arginine vasopressin secretion or action may cause polyuria and nocturia (Ouslander, 2004). Conditions such as congestive heart failure, hypothyroidism, venous insufficiency, and the effects of certain medications all contribute to peripheral edema, leading to urinary frequency and nocturia when a patient is supine.

Finally, stool impaction resulting from poor bowel habits and constipation can contribute to overactive bladder symptoms. This is perhaps from local irritation or direct compression against the bladder wall.

Physical Examination
General Inspection and Neurologic Evaluation

Initially, the perineum is inspected for evidence of atrophy, which may be noted throughout the lower genital tract. In addition, suburethral bulging with transurethral expression of fluid during forward-directed compression suggests a urethral diverticulum (Fig. 26-3, p. 683).

A thorough physical examination for a woman with incontinence should also include a detailed neurologic evaluation of the perineum. Because neurologic responses may be altered in an anxious patient who is in a vulnerable setting, signs elicited during examination may not signify true pathology and should be interpreted with caution. Neurologic evaluation begins with an attempt to elicit a *bulbocavernosus reflex*. During this test, one labium majora is stroked with a cotton swab. Normally, both labia equally contract bilaterally. The afferent limb of this reflex is the clitoral branch of the pudendal nerve, whereas its efferent limb is conducted through the inferior hemorrhoidal branch of the pudendal nerve. This reflex is integrated at the S2-S4 spinal cord level (Wester, 2003). Thus, reflex absence may reflect central or peripheral neurologic deficits. Secondly, a normal circumferential anal sphincter contraction, colloquially called an "anal wink," should follow cotton swab brushing of the perianal skin. External urethral sphincter activity requires at least some degree of intact S2-S4 innervation, and this *anocutaneous reflex* is mediated by the same spinal neurologic level. Thus, an absent wink may indicate deficits in this neurologic distribution.

Pelvic Support Assessment

Pelvic Organ Prolapse Evaluation. Poor urethral support commonly accompanies pelvic organ prolapse (POP). For example, women with significant prolapse are often unable to completely empty their bladder due to urethral kinking and obstruction. These women frequently must digitally elevate or reduce their prolapse to allow emptying. Thus, an external evaluation for POP, as described in Chapter 24 (p. 644) is indicated for all women with urinary incontinence. Following this evaluation for vaginal compartment defects, pelvic muscle strength should also be assessed. Women with mild to moderate urinary incontinence often respond well to pelvic floor therapy, and under these circumstances, a trial of this therapy is warranted and often curative (p. 624).

TABLE 23-4. Medications That May Contribute to Incontinence

Medication	Examples	Mechanism	Effect
Alcohol	Beer, wine, liquor	Diuretic effect, sedation, immobility	Polyuria, frequency
α-Adrenergic agonists	Decongestants, diet pills	IUS contraction	Urinary retention
α-Adrenergic blockers	Prazosin, terazosin, doxazosin	IUS relaxation	Urinary leakage
Anticholinergic agents		Inhibit bladder contraction, sedation, fecal impaction	Urinary retention and/or functional incontinence
Antihistamines	Diphenhydramine, scopolamine, dimenhydrinate		
Antipsychotics	Thioridazine, chlorpromazine, haloperidol		
Antiparkinsonians	Trihexyphenidyl, benztropine mesylate		
Miscellaneous	Dicyclomine, disopyramide		
Skeletal muscle relaxants	Orphenadrine, cyclobenzaprine		
Tricyclic antidepressants	Amitriptyline, imipramine, nortriptyline, doxepin		
ACE inhibitors	Enalapril, captopril, lisinopril, losartan	Chronic cough	Urinary leakage
Calcium-channel blockers	Nifedipine, nicardipine, isradipine, felodipine	Relaxes bladder, fluid retention	Urinary retention, nocturnal diuresis
COX-2 inhibitors	Celecoxib	Fluid retention	Nocturnal diuresis
Diuretics	Caffeine, HCTZ, furosemide, bumetanide, acetazolamide, spironolactone	Increases urinary frequency, urgency	Polyuria
Narcotic analgesics	Opiates	Relaxes bladder, fecal impaction, sedation	Urinary retention, and/or functional incontinence
Thiazolidinediones	Rosiglitazone, pioglitazone, troglitazone	Fluid retention	Nocturnal diuresis

ACE = angiotensin-converting enzyme; COX-2 = cyclooxygenase-2; HCTZ = hydrochlorothiazide; IUS — internal urethral sphincter; NSAID = nonsteroidal antiinflammatory drug.

Q-tip Test. If a urethra is poorly supported, it may display hypermobility during increases in intraabdominal pressures. To assess mobility, a clinician places the soft end of a cotton swab into the urethra to the urethrovesical junction. Failure to insert the swab to this depth typically leads to errors in assessment of urethrovesical junction support. Termed the *Q-tip test*, this evaluation may be uncomfortable, and application of intraurethral analgesia may prove helpful. Commonly, 1-percent lidocaine jelly is placed on the cotton swab prior to insertion. Following placement, a Valsalva maneuver is prompted, and the swab-excursion angle at rest and with Valsalva maneuver is measured with a goniometer or standard protractor (Fig. 23-13). An excursion angle from rest and with Valsalva maneuver that

measures >30 degrees above the horizontal plane indicates urethral hypermobility. The utility of this test is controversial given that many asymptomatic women with urethral hypermobility do not have urinary incontinence.

Bimanual and Rectovaginal Examination

In general, these portions of the pelvic examination provide fewer diagnostic clues to underlying incontinence causes. However, bimanual examination may reveal an enlarged pelvic mass or a uterus enlarged by leiomyomas or adenomyosis. These may create incontinence through increased external pressure transmitted to the bladder. In addition, stool impaction is easily identified with rectal examination.

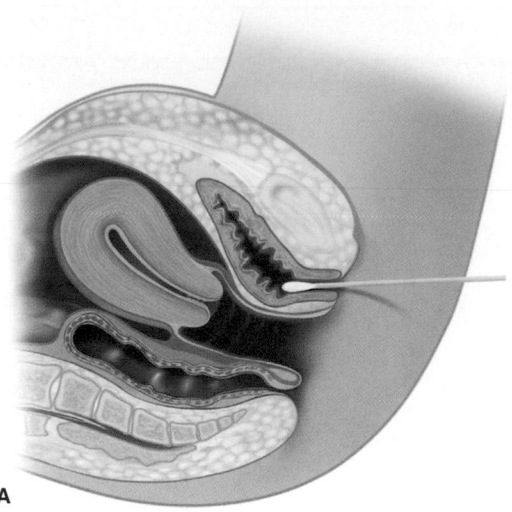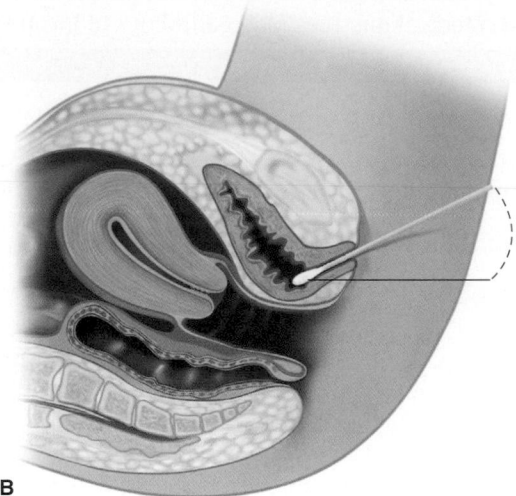

A   **B**

FIGURE 23-13 Drawing depicting Q-tip test in a patient with urethral hypermobility. **A.** Angle of the Q-tip at rest. **B.** Angle of the Q-tip with Valsalva maneuver or other increases in intraabdominal pressure. The urethrovesical junction descends, causing upward deflection of the Q-tip.

Diagnostic Testing

Urinalysis and Culture

In all women with urinary incontinence, infection or urinary tract pathology must be excluded. Urinalysis and urine culture are sent at an initial visit, and infection is treated as described in Table 3-24 (p. 94). Persistent symptoms typically warrant additional evaluation for stress and urge urinary incontinence or for other conditions such as interstitial cystitis.

Postvoid Residual (PVR)

This volume is routinely measured during incontinence evaluation. After a woman voids, the PVR may be measured with a handheld sonographic bladder scanner or by transurethral catheterization. Portable three-dimensional ultrasound devices are used to scan the bladder and provide numerical results (Fig. 23-14). In general, they are quick, easy to use, and more comfortable for the patient. However, if using a handheld scanner, care must be taken in women with an enlarged leiomyomatous uterus as this may falsely record a large PVR. In these instances, or if a scanner is not available, transurethral catheterization may be used to confirm residual bladder volume.

A large postvoid residual may often reflect one of several problems including recurrent infection, urethral obstruction from a pelvic mass, or neurologic deficits. In contrast, a normally small PVR is often found in those with SUI.

Postoperative Postvoid Residual. After antiincontinence surgery, PVR measurement is a helpful indicator of a patient's ability to completely empty her bladder. This evaluation may be completed with a "passive" or an "active" voiding trial.

With a passive trial, a urinary catheter is removed, and the PVR is measured by scanner or by transurethral catheterization after each voluntary void on two occasions. A voided volume of at least 300 mL and PVR less than 100 mL is desirable. However, adequate bladder emptying is assumed if the PVR is less than one third of the voided volume. If the patient does not meet these criteria, or if she is unable to void within 4 to 6 hours

of removing the urinary catheter, then a catheter is replaced, and the test is repeated a day or more later.

During an active bladder trial, the bladder is actively filled with a set volume, and following patient voiding, residual bladder urine volumes are calculated. Initially, the bladder is completely emptied by catheterization. It may be helpful during catheterization for a woman to stand upright to clear the most dependent portions of her bladder. Sterile water is infused under gravity into the

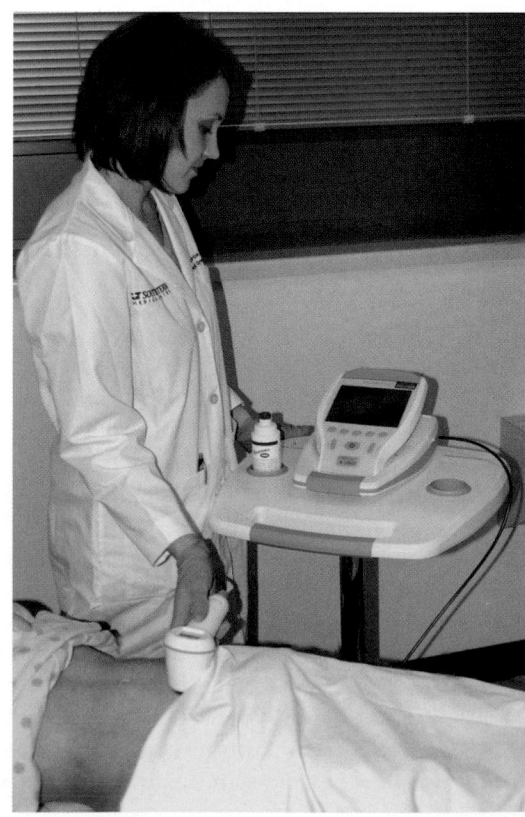

FIGURE 23-14 Handheld bladder scanner aids estimation of bladder volume. *(Photograph courtesy of Dr. Heather Gardow.)*

bladder through the same catheter until approximately 300 mL is used or until a subjective maximum capacity is reached. The patient is then asked to void spontaneously into a urine collection device. The difference between volume infused and volume retrieved is recorded as the PVR. A residual of less than 100 mL or less than one third of the instilled volume—if less than 300 mL is infused—is consistent with adequate bladder emptying.

Urodynamic Studies

Surgical correction of incontinence is invasive and not without risk. However, the "bladder is an unreliable witness," and historical information may not always accurately indicate the true underlying type of incontinence (Blaivas, 1996). Thus, if initial conservative management is unsuccessful or surgical treatment is anticipated, then objective assessment should be pursued. In addition, if symptoms and physical findings are incongruous, then objective urodynamic studies (UDS), using simple or multichannel cystometrics, may also be indicated. For example, in women with mixed urinary incontinence, who have symptoms of both stress and urge urinary incontinence, UDS may reveal that only the urge component is responsible for their incontinence. Most of these women are treated with behavioral, physical, and/or pharmacologic therapy initially. Thus, if identified by UDS, these individuals can avoid unnecessary surgery. Additionally, surgical therapy may be modified if UDS reveals parameters consistent with intrinsic sphincteric defect.

Despite these indications, UDS remains controversial. Leakage noted during testing is not always clinically relevant. In addition, testing may be uninformative if the original offending maneuver or situation that led to incontinence cannot be reproduced during evaluation. Moreover, objective confirmation of the diagnosis is not always necessary, since empiric nonsurgical therapy in women with urge predominant symptoms is reasonable.

Simple Cystometrics. Objective measurements of bladder function are combined in a battery of tests termed cystometrics, which may be *simple* or *multichannel*. Simple cystometrics allows determination of stress incontinence and detrusor overactivity as well as measurement of first sensation, desire to void, and bladder capacity. This procedure is easily performed with room-temperature sterile normal saline, 60-mL catheter-tipped syringe, and urinary catheter, either Foley or Robnell. The urethra is sterilely prepared, the catheter is inserted, and the bladder is drained. A 60-mL syringe with its plunger removed is attached to the catheter and is filled upright with sterile water. Water is added in increments until a woman feels a sensation of bladder filling, urge to void, and bladder maximum capacity. A normal bladder capacity for most women will range from 300 to 700 mL. Changes in the fluid meniscus within the syringe are monitored. In the absence of a cough or Valsalva maneuver that would raise intraabdominal pressure, an abrupt meniscus elevation indicates bladder contraction and suggests a diagnosis of detrusor overactivity. Once bladder capacity is reached, the catheter is removed, and the woman is asked to perform a Valsalva maneuver or cough while standing. Leakage directly linked to these increases in intraabdominal pressure indicates SUI.

Simple cystometrics are easy to perform, require inexpensive equipment, and can typically be completed by most gynecologists. One limitation of simple cystometric testing, however, is its inability to assess for intrinsic sphincteric deficiency (ISD), which may preclude certain surgical options. Multichannel cystometrics can evaluate for ISD and thus may offer advantages.

Multichannel Cystometrics. This objective urodynamic study provides more information on other physiologic bladder parameters that are not afforded by simple cystometrics. Multichannel cystometrics more commonly is performed by urogynecologists or urologists due to the expense and limited availability of the equipment. Testing can be performed with a woman standing or seated upright in a specialized evaluation chair. During testing, two catheters are used. One is placed into the bladder and the other into either the vagina or rectum. The vagina is preferred unless advanced prolapse is evident, as stool in the rectal vault may obstruct catheter sensors and lead to inaccurate readings. Additionally, vaginal placement for most women is more comfortable. From each of these two catheters, distinct pressure readings are obtained or calculated and include: (1) intraabdominal pressure, (2) vesicular pressure, (3) calculated detrusor pressure, (4) bladder volume, and (5) saline infusion flow rate. As shown in Figures 23-15 and 23-16, the different forms of incontinence can be differentiated.

Uroflowmetry. Initially, women are asked to empty their bladder into a commode connected to a flowmeter (uroflowmetry). After a maximal flow rate is recorded, the patient is catheterized to measure a postvoid residual and to ensure an empty bladder prior to further testing. This test provides information on a woman's ability to empty her bladder and can identify women with urinary retention and other types of voiding dysfunction. Presuming that a patient begins with a comfortably full bladder of 200 mL or greater, most patients can empty their bladders over 15 to 20 seconds with flow rates of greater than 20 mL/sec. Maximum flow rates of less than 15 mL/sec, with a voided volume greater than 200 mL, are generally considered abnormally slow. In this setting—especially if accompanied by urinary retention—voiding dysfunction is identified. This may result from obstruction from a kinked urethra in the setting of anterior vaginal wall prolapse or postoperatively after creation of antiincontinence support that is too tight. Voiding dysfunction may also occur in settings of neurologic dysfunction with poor detrusor contractility, as in those with poorly controlled diabetes.

Cystometrography. Following uroflowmetry, cystometrography is performed to determine whether a woman has urodynamic stress incontinence (USI) or detrusor overactivity (DO). Additionally, this test provides information on bladder threshold volumes at which a woman senses bladder capacity. Delayed sensation or sensation of bladder fullness only with large capacities may indicate neuropathy. Conversely, extreme bladder sensitivity may suggest sensory disorders such as interstitial cystitis.

For the cystometrogram, a catheter is inserted transurethrally into the bladder and a second catheter is inserted into the vagina or rectum (see Fig. 23-15). While the patient is seated, the bladder is filled with room-temperature sterile normal saline, and

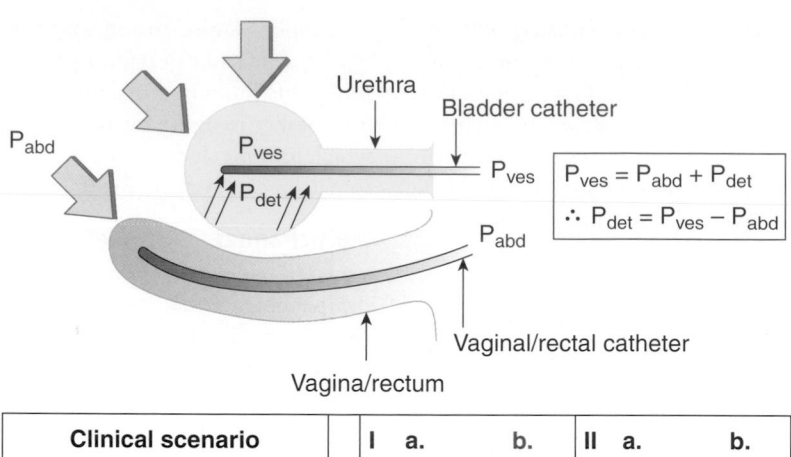

$$P_{ves} = P_{abd} + P_{det}$$
$$\therefore P_{det} = P_{ves} - P_{abd}$$

Clinical scenario	I a.	b.	II a.	b.
P_{abd} (abdominal pressure) [vaginal/rectal catheter]	⌃	⌃	—	⌃
P_{ves} (bladder pressure) [bladder catheter]	⌃	⌃	⌃	⌃
P_{det} (true detrusor pressure) [subtracted/calculated]	—	—	⌃	⌃
Leakage	⊕	⊖	⊕ or ⊖	⊕ or ⊖
Diagnosis	USI	No USI	DO	DO

FIGURE 23-15 Interpretation of multichannel urodynamic evaluation: cystometrogram. A catheter is placed in the bladder to determine the pressure generated within it (P_{ves}). The pressure in the bladder is produced from a combination of the pressure from the abdominal cavity and the pressure generated by the detrusor muscle of the bladder. Bladder pressure (P_{ves}) = pressure in abdominal cavity (P_{abd}) + detrusor pressure (P_{det}). A second catheter is placed in the vagina (or rectum if advanced-stage prolapse is present) to determine the pressure in the abdominal cavity (P_{abd}). As room-temperature saline is instilled into the bladder, the patient is asked to cough every 50 mL and the external urethral meatus is observed for leakage of urine around the catheter. The volume at first desire to void and the bladder capacity is recorded. Additionally, the detrusor pressure (P_{det}) channel is observed for positive deflections to determine if there is detrusor activity during testing. The detrusor pressure (P_{det}) cannot be measured directly by any of the catheters. However, from the first equation, we can calculate the detrusor pressure (P_{det}) by subtracting the abdominal pressure (P_{abd}) from the bladder pressure (P_{ves}):

Detrusor pressure (P_{det}) = bladder pressure (P_{ves}) − pressure in abdominal cavity (P_{abd})

I. Urodynamic Stress Incontinence (USI)

Urodynamic stress incontinence is diagnosed when urethral leakage is seen with increased abdominal pressure, in the *absence* of detrusor pressure.

a. +USI (Column 1): Abdominal pressure is generated with Valsalva maneuver or cough. This pressure is transmitted to the bladder, and a bladder pressure (P_{ves}) is noted. The calculated detrusor pressure is zero. Leakage is observed, and diagnosis of USI is assigned.

b. No USI (Column 2): Abdominal pressure is generated with Valsalva maneuver or cough. This pressure is transmitted to the bladder, and a bladder pressure (P_{ves}) is noted. The calculated detrusor pressure is zero. Leakage is *not* observed. The patient is *not* diagnosed as having USI.

II. Detrusor Overactivity (DO)

Detrusor overactivity is diagnosed when the patient has involuntary detrusor contractions during testing with or without leakage.

a. +DO (Column 3): Although no abdominal pressure is observed, a vesicular pressure is noted. A calculated detrusor pressure is recorded and noted to be present. A diagnosis of DO is made regardless of whether leakage is seen.

b. +DO (Column 4): In this example, an abdominal pressure is observed as well as a vesicular pressure. Using only the P_{abd} and the P_{ves} channels, it is difficult to tell whether or not the detrusor muscle contributed to the pressure generated in the bladder. On subtraction, a calculated detrusor pressure is recorded. Thus, a diagnosis of DO is made, again regardless of whether leakage is seen.

In addition to these channels, occasionally a channel to detect electromyographic activity is used.

P_{abd} = pressure in abdominal cavity; P_{det} = detrusor pressure (calculated); P_{ves} = bladder pressure.

the patient is asked to cough at regular intervals. Additionally, during filling, the volumes at which a first desire to void and maximal bladder capacity is reached are noted. From pressure readings, DO and/or USI may be identified.

After cystometrography, once approximately 200 mL of saline has been instilled, an abdominal *leak point pressure* is measured. The patient is asked to perform a Valsalva maneuver, and the pressure generated by the effort is measured and evidence of urine leakage is sought. If leakage is seen when a pressure of <60 cm H_2O is generated, then criteria have been met for a diagnosis of intrinsic sphincteric deficiency. At our institution, abdominal leak point pressures are measured at a bladder volume

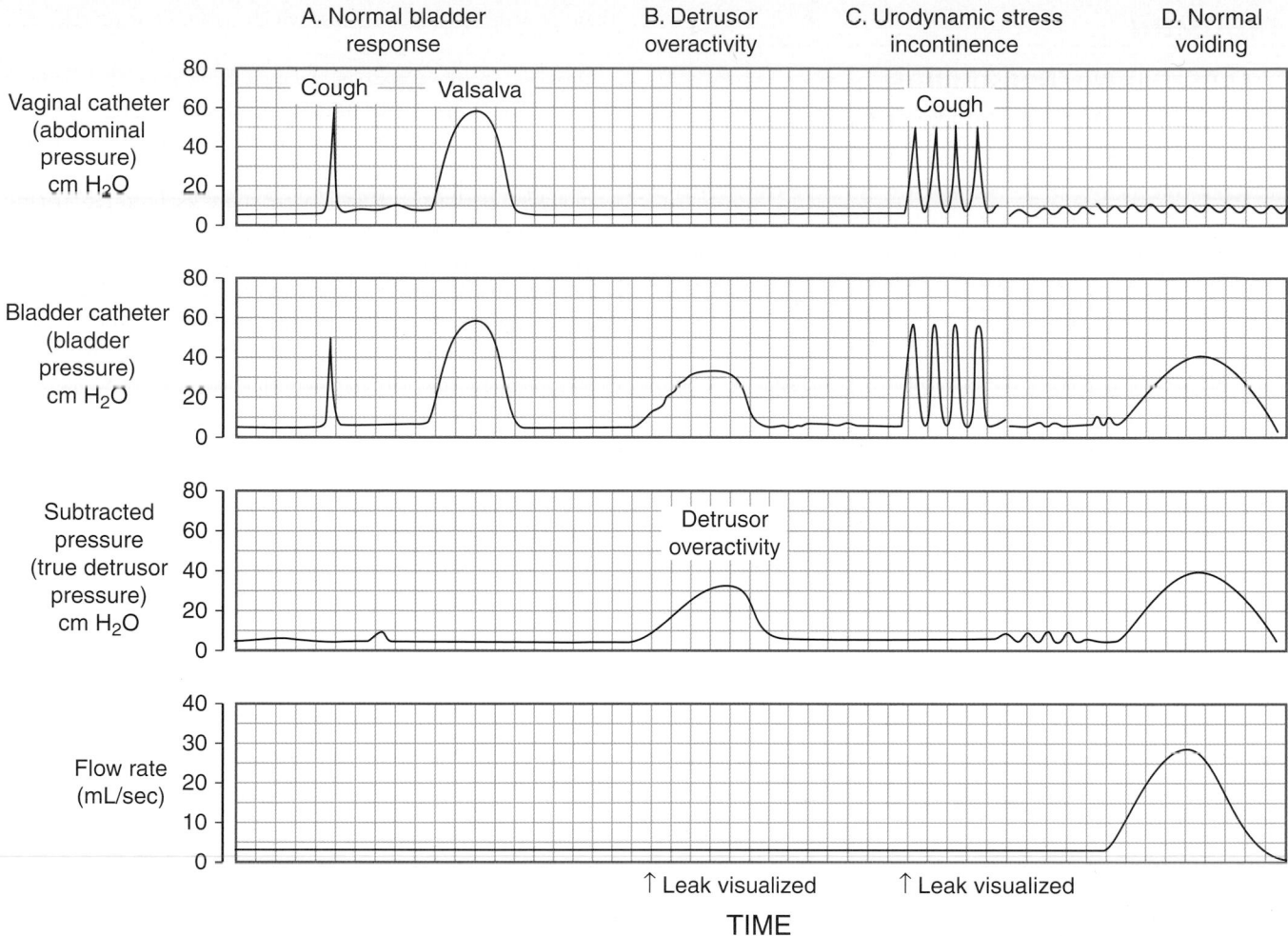

FIGURE 23-16 Urodynamic testing. Cystometrography is reflected by parts A, B, and C. **A.** In a patient with normal function, note that provocation by coughing or Valsalva maneuver does not provoke an abnormal rise in detrusor pressure. **B & C.** In a patient with combined detrusor overactivity and urodynamic stress incontinence. First, spontaneous detrusor activity leads to increased bladder pressure reading in the absence of cough or Valsalva maneuver. Second, a cough alone leads to urine leakage, independent of detrusor muscle activity. **D.** Pressure flowmetry. At maximum capacity and on command, a detrusor contraction is generated, and voiding is initiated.

of 200 mL, using the true zero of intravesical pressure as the baseline. However, the volume at which this test is performed varies among institutions, with some choosing to use bladder capacity and others choosing to use 150 mL as the testing volume.

Pressure Flowmetry. This evaluation usually follows cystometrography and is similar to the uroflowmetry conducted at the beginning of urodynamic testing. A woman is asked to void into a large beaker that rests on a calibrated weighted sensor. Maximum flow rate and postvoid residual are once again recorded. Similar to uroflowmetry, the output from the urodynamics instrumentation provides a graphical representation of the void. However, during voiding, a woman now has a microtip transducer catheter in her bladder, which provides an additional display of detrusor pressure during the void, including at the point of maximum flow rate. This is particularly useful in women who may have incomplete bladder emptying, as the pressure flowmetry may suggest either an obstructive scenario (elevated maximal detrusor pressure with slow flow rate) or poor detrusor contractility (low detrusor pressure and slow flow rate).

Urethral Pressure Profile. The final part of cystometric testing is the urethral pressure profile. At our institution, we usually perform this test in the seated patient with a volume of 200 mL instilled in the bladder. However, again, this volume is often institution dependent. A catheter transducer is positioned within the bladder, and the microtip dual-sensor catheter is pulled through the urethra with the aid of an automated puller arm at a speed of 1 mm/sec. Maximum urethral closure pressure (MUCP) is determined by averaging three pressure profiles. The *functional urethral length* and the *area of continence zone* are also obtained. These values provide important information on the intrinsic properties of the urethra and aid in the diagnosis of ISD. A diagnosis of ISD is made if the MUCP is ≤20 cm H_2O or as described in the last section, if the leak point pressure is <60 cm H_2O (McGuire, 1981). These terms and concepts provide the rationale for procedures aimed at correcting stress incontinence. Importantly, however, the values used to define ISD are not well standardized and have not been consistently found to influence surgical outcomes (Monga, 1997; Weber, 2001).

TREATMENT

Conservative/Nonsurgical

Pelvic Floor Strengthening Exercises

Conservative management is a reasonable initial approach to most patients with urinary incontinence. The rationale behind conservative management is to strengthen the pelvic floor and provide a supportive "backboard" against which the urethra may close. Options include active pelvic floor exercises and passive electrical pelvic floor muscle st.mulation. For both SUI and urge urinary incontinence, these fundamentals prove valuable. With SUI, pelvic floor strengthening attempts to compensate for anatomic defects. For urge urinary incontinence, it improves pelvic floor muscle contraction strength to provide temporary continence during waves of bladder detrusor contraction.

Pelvic Floor Muscle Training. In women who have mild to moderate symptoms, pelvic floor muscle training (PFMT) may improve if not cure urinary incontinence. Also known as *Kegel exercises,* PFMT entails voluntary contraction of the levator ani muscles. As with any muscle building, isometric or isotonic forms of exercise may be selected. Exercise sets should be performed numerous times during the day, with some reporting up to 50 or 60 times each day. However, specific details in performance of these exercises are subject to provider preference and clinical setting.

If isotonic contractions are used for PFMT, a woman is asked to squeeze and hold contracted levator ani muscles. Women, however, often have difficulty isolating these muscles. Frequently, patients will erroneously contract their abdominal wall muscles rather than the levators. To help localize the correct group, an individual may be instructed to identify the muscles that are tightened when snug pants are pulled up and over her hips. Moreover, in an office setting, a provider can determine if the levator ani group is contracted by placing two fingers in the vagina while Kegel exercises are performed.

At our institution, we aim to help patients achieve a sustained pelvic floor contraction of 10 seconds. We begin with the duration of contraction a patient *can* sustain (e.g., 3 seconds), and ask them to hold for this long and then relax for one to two times this duration (e.g., 6 seconds). This squeeze and release is repeated 10 to 15 times. Three sets are performed throughout the day for a total of approximately 45 contractions. Over a series of weeks with frequent follow-up visits, the duration of contraction is steadily increased. Patients, thus, improve the tone of their pelvic floor muscles and are usually able to more forcefully squeeze their muscles in anticipation of sudden increases of intraadominal pressure for SUI.

Alternatively, if isometric contractions are used for PFMT, a woman is asked to rapidly contract and relax the levators. These "quick flicks" of the pelvic floor muscles may prove advantageous if waves of urinary urgency strike. Of note, there is a misconception about the value of stopping urination midstream. Women should be counseled that this practice often worsens voiding dysfunction.

To augment exercise efficacy, weighted vaginal cones or obturators may be placed into the vaginal during Kegel exercises.

These provide resistance against which pelvic floor muscles can work.

Reviewers of the Cochrane database have assessed the effects of PFMT for women with urinary incontinence compared with no treatment, placebo or sham treatments, or other inactive control treatments. Although interventions varied considerably, women who performed PFMT were more likely to report cure or improved incontinence and improved continence-specific quality of life than women who did not use PFMT. The exercising women also objectively demonstrated less leakage during office-based pad testing (Dumoulin, 2010). Prognostic indicators that may predict a poor response to PFMT for the treatment of SUI include severe baseline incontinence, prolapse beyond the hymenal ring, prior failed physiotherapy, a history of prolonged second stage of labor, BMI >30 kg/m^2, high psychological distress, and poor overall physical health (Hendriks, 2010).

Electrical Stimulation. As an alternative to active pelvic floor contraction, a vaginal probe may be used to deliver low-frequency electrical stimulation to the levator ani muscles. Although the mechanism is unclear, electrical stimulation may be used to improve either SUI or urge urinary incontinence (Indrekvam, 2001; Wang, 2004). With urge urinary incontinence, traditionally a low frequency is applied, whereas for SUI, higher frequencies are used. Electrical stimulation may be used alone or more commonly in combination with PFMT.

Biofeedback Therapy. Many behavioral techniques, often considered together as *biofeedback therapy,* measure physiologic signals such as muscle tension and then display them to a patient in real time. In general, visual, auditory, and/or verbal feedback cues are directed to the patient during these therapy sessions. Specifically, during biofeedback for PFMT, a sterile vaginal probe that measures pressure changes within the vagina during levator ani muscle contraction is typically used. Visual readings reflect an estimate of muscle contraction strength. Treatment sessions are individualized, dictated by the underlying dysfunction, and modified based on response to therapy. In many cases, reinforcing sessions at various subsequent intervals may also prove advantageous.

Dietary

Different food groups that may have high acidity or caffeine content may lead to greater urinary frequency and urgency. Dallosso and colleagues (2003) found consumption of carbonated drinks to be associated with development of urge urinary incontinence symptoms. Accordingly, elimination of these dietary irritants may prove beneficial for these women. In addition, certain dietary supplements such as calcium glycerophosphate (Prelief) have been shown to decrease urgency and frequency symptoms (Bologna, 2001). This is a phosphate-based product and is thought to buffer urine acidity.

Scheduled Voiding

Women with urge urinary incontinence may feel voiding urges as frequently as every 10 to 15 minutes. Initial goals extend voidings to half-hour intervals. Tools used to achieve this include Kegel exercises during waves of urgency or mental distraction techniques during these times. Scheduled voiding, although used primarily for urge urinary incontinence, may also be helpful for those with SUI. For these patients, regularly scheduled urination leads to an empty bladder during a greater percentage of the day. Because some women will leak urine only if bladder volumes surpass specific volumes, frequent emptying can significantly decrease incontinence episodes.

Estrogen Replacement

Estrogen has been shown to increase urethral blood flow and increase α-adrenergic receptor sensitivity, thereby increasing urethral coaptation and urethral closure pressure. Hypothetically, estrogen may also increase collagen deposition and increase vascularity of the periurethral capillary plexus. These are purported to improve urethral coaptation. Thus, for incontinent women who are atrophic, administration of exogenous estrogen is reasonable.

Estrogen is commonly administered topically, and many different regimens are appropriate. At our institution, we use conjugated equine estrogen cream (Premarin cream) administered daily for 2 weeks, then twice weekly thereafter. Although no data are available to address the duration of treatment, women may be treated chronically with topical estrogen cream. Alternatively, oral estrogen may be prescribed if other menopausal symptoms for which estrogen would be beneficial coexist (Chap. 22, p. 584).

However, despite these suggested benefits, a consensus regarding estrogen's beneficial effects on the lower urinary tract has not been reached. Specifically, some studies have shown worsening or development of urinary incontinence with systemic estrogen administration (Grady, 2001; Grodstein, 2004; Hendrix, 2005; Jackson, 2006).

■ Treatment of Stress Urinary Incontinence
Medications

Pharmaceutical treatment plays a minor role in the treatment of women with SUI. However, for women with mixed urinary incontinence, a trial of imipramine is reasonable to aid urethral contraction and closure. As discussed earlier, this tricyclic antidepressant has α-adrenergic effects, and the urethra contains a high content of these receptors.

Duloxetine (Cymbalta), a selective serotonin- and norepinephrine-reuptake inhibitor (SSRI), has been evaluated for SUI treatment. In animal studies, serotonergic agonists suppress parasympathetic activity and enhance sympathetic and somatic activity. The sum effect promotes urine storage by relaxing the bladder and increasing outlet resistance. Although considered investigational, in randomized studies, this SSRI has improved symptoms in women with SUI (Dmochowski, 2003a; Millard, 2004; Norton, 2002). Moreover, Ghoniem and coworkers (2005), in a randomized controlled trial, evaluated the benefits of duloxetine, PFMT, and placebo combinations. Pad and quality-of-life data found the combination of duloxetine and PFMT to be more effective than either alone.

Previously, phenylpropanolamine (PPA) was used to treat SUI. However, in 2005, the Food and Drug Administration (FDA) (2009) reclassified PPA as Category II and considered it not generally safe or effective. Specifically, the FDA's decision was prompted by an increased rate of hemorrhagic strokes suffered by women taking this medication.

Pessary and Urethral Inserts

Certain pessaries have been designed to treat incontinence as well as pelvic organ prolapse. Incontinence pessaries are designed to reduce downward excursion or funneling of the urethrovesical junction (Fig. 24-17, p. 648). This provides bladder neck support and thereby helps to reduce incontinence episodes. Dependent on the amount of prolapse present, pessary efficacy for urinary incontinence is variable. Not all women are appropriate candidates for pessaries, nor will all desire long term management of incontinence or prolapse with these devices.

A large prospective trial comparing incontinence pessaries and behavioral therapy for women with SUI demonstrated that 40 and 49 percent of patients were either much or very much improved at 3 months, respectively. The women randomized to behavioral therapy reported greater treatment satisfaction, and a greater percentage reported no bothersome incontinence symptoms (Richter, 2010b).

As an alternative to pessaries, a urethral insert may also be used for SUI control. The only currently commercially available device is the *FemSoft* Insert. As the device is inserted, its sleeve slides into and conforms to the urethra and creates a seal at the bladder neck to prevent accidental urine leakage. During routine bathroom visits, the insert is removed, discarded, and replaced with a fresh insert. Data are limited on the effectiveness of this insert. However, in an observational study of 150 women, Sirls and associates (2002) found significantly reduced rates of incontinence episodes.

Surgical Treatment of Intrinsic Sphincteric Deficiency

Urethral Bulking Agents. Injection of bulking agents has been traditionally indicated for women who have stress incontinence associated with intrinsic sphincteric deficiency. However, the FDA has broadened the criteria for use of bulking agents to include patients with less severe leak point pressures. As a result, those with leak point pressures <100 cm H_2O may also be suitable candidates (McGuire, 2006). Additionally, this office procedure is a useful alternative for women with SUI who have multiple medical problems and are thus poor surgical candidates.

Agents are injected into the urethral submucosa to "bulk up" the mucosa and improve coaptation. Ideally, these injectable bulking agents should be easy to place, effective, durable, safe, and nonimmunogenic. Since few agents satisfy all of these characteristics, newer agents are constantly being developed. The injection location around and along the length of the urethra can vary. Some recommend two locations on either side of the urethra, whereas others advocate injections in three or four quadrants. At our institution, we usually inject at the level of the urethrovesical junction at sites of apparent urethral mucosal defects. However, if a global defect is noted or if a discrete defect is absent, then a two- to four-quadrant approach is used. The specific steps of injection and types of products used are described in Section 43-6 (p. 1198).

TABLE 23-5. Summary of Incontinence Procedures

Procedure	Description	Indication	Comments
Urethral Injection	Bulking agent into urethral submucosa	ISD	Also for SUI in poor surgical candidates; may require a number of repeated injections
Needle suspension	Proximal urethra suspended by anterior abdominal wall	SUI	Low long-term success rates; no longer recommended for SUI
Paravaginal defect repair	Lateral vaginal wall attached to ATFP	Vaginal prolapse	No longer recommended for SUI
Retropubic urethropexy	Pubocervical fascia attached to: Cooper ligament (Burch) or to symphysis pubis (MMK)	SUI	Effective long-term treatment; requires surgeon experience; less reproducible benefits than midurethral sling procedure
Pubovaginal slings	Bladder neck supported by fascial strip attached to anterior abdominal wall	ISD; failed SUI procedure	Effective long-term treatment; may be useful in patients in whom synthetic material is not desirable; requires isolation of graft from anterior abdominal wall or from leg fascia lata
Midurethral slings:	Midurethra supported by mesh placed :		Effective short-term treatment, rapid postoperative recovery; TVT with long-term efficacy data; further study required to determine effectiveness of TOT in patients with ISD
TVT	by retropubic approach or	SUI; ISD	
TOT	by transobturator approach	SUI	

ATFP = arcus tendineus fascia pelvis; ISD = intrinsic sphincteric deficiency; MMK = Marshall-Marchetti-Krantz procedure; SUI = stress urinary incontinence; TOT = transobturator tape; TVT = tension-free vaginal tape.

Surgical Treatment of Anatomic Stress Incontinence

For those who are not adequately improved with or do not desire conservative management, surgery may be an appropriate next step for successful treatment of stress incontinence. As noted earlier, urethral support is integral to continence. Thus, surgical procedures that recreate this support often diminish or cure incontinence. More than 200 procedures have been developed for the surgical correction of SUI, although the complete physiology underlying their success is not entirely clear. In general, these surgical procedures are believed to prevent bladder neck and proximal urethra descent during increases in intraabdominal pressure (Table 23-5).

Transvaginal Needle Procedures and Paravaginal Defect Repair. Surgeries that correct urethral hypermobility are theorized to prevent bladder neck and proximal urethra descent during increases in intraabdominal pressure. In the 1960s through 1980s, needle suspension procedures such as the Raz, Pereyra, and Stamey techniques were popular surgical treatments for SUI but have now largely been replaced by other methods. In brief, these surgeries used specially designed ligature carriers to place sutures through the anterior vaginal wall and/or periurethral tissues and suspend them to various levels of the anterior abdominal wall. These relied on the strength and integrity of the periurethral tissue and abdominal wall strength for successful suspension.

Although initial cure rates were satisfactory, the durability of these procedures decreased with time. Success rates range from 50 to 60 percent, well below rates found with other current

antiincontinence procedures (Moser, 2006). Failure stemmed largely from "pull-through" of sutures at the level of the anterior vaginal wall.

In addition, abdominal paravaginal defect repair (PVDR) is a surgical procedure that corrects lateral support defects of the anterior vaginal wall. The technique involves suture attachment of the lateral vaginal wall to the arcus tendineus fascia pelvis. Currently, PVDR is primarily a prolapse-correcting operation. Although previously used to correct SUI, long-term data have shown this to no longer be a superior method for primary treatment of SUI (Colombo, 1996; Mallipeddi, 2001).

Retropubic Urethropexy. This group of procedures includes the Burch and Marshall-Marchetti-Krantz (MMK) colposuspension procedures, which involve suspension and anchorage of the pubocervical fascia to the musculoskeletal framework of the pelvis (Section 43-2, p. 1189). Long considered the gold standard for surgical treatment of SUI, the Burch technique uses the strength of the iliopectineal ligament (Cooper ligament) to lift the anterior vaginal wall and the periurethral and perivesicular fibromuscular tissue. In contrast, during MMK surgery, the periosteum of the symphysis pubis is used to suspend these tissues.

The retropubic urethropexy is an effective surgical treatment of SUI, with 1-year overall continence rates between 85 and 90 percent and with a 5-year continence rate of approximately 70 percent (Lapitan, 2009). Complications commonly associated with these procedures can include de novo detrusor overactivity, urinary retention, and in the case of the MMK, osteitis pubis. In addition, data suggest that performing a Burch retropubic urethropexy concurrently with abdominal sacrocolpopexy for vaginal vault prolapse may significantly reduce rates of symptomatic postoperative SUI (Chap. 24, p. 655) (Brubaker, 2008a).

Pubovaginal Slings. This surgery is a standard procedure for SUI. It has traditionally been used for SUI stemming from intrinsic sphincteric deficiency. In addition, this procedure may also be indicated for patients with prior failed antiincontinence operations.

With this surgery, a strip of either rectus fascia or fascia lata is placed under the bladder neck and through the retropubic space. The ends are secured at the level of the rectus abdominis fascia (Section 43-5, p. 1196). Previously, cadaveric fascia was used as the suspension material. However, this tissue is eventually degraded and found not to be durable over time (FitzGerald, 1999; Howden, 2006). Currently, autologous fascia is preferred and is obtained from the patient's rectus sheath, although fascia lata from the thigh is an alternative.

Midurethral Slings. These slings surged onto the market in the late 1990s, and their therapeutic mechanism is based on the integral theory hypothesized by Petros and Ulmsten (1993). In brief, control of urethral closure involves the interplay of three structures: the pubourethral ligaments, the suburethral vaginal hammock, and the pubococcygeus muscle. Loss of these support structures is believed to result in urinary incontinence and pelvic floor dysfunction. These slings are believed to reproduce the support provided by these ligamentous support structures.

There are many different variations of these procedures, but all involve midurethral placement of synthetic mesh. Simplistically, they are classified according to the route of placement and can be subdivided into those using a retropubic or a transobturator approach. Of these, popular procedures include: (1) tension-free vaginal tape (TVT), a retropubic method; and (2) transobturator tape (TOT), a transobturator method.

Midurethral slings provide several advantages. First, these techniques are effective, and short-term cure rates approximate 90 percent (Lim, 2006). Of the two, retropubic and transobturator approaches appear to offer comparable short-term continence results (de Tayrac, 2004; Morey, 2006). Laurikainen and coworkers (2007) randomly assigned 267 women to undergo either type and found equal rates of subjective and objective cure.

Despite favorable comparisons, abundant long-term data regarding the efficacy of transobturator approaches are lacking. However, data obtained 17 months postoperatively showed an incontinence improvement rate of 89 percent for those with preoperative SUI (Juma, 2007). In contrast, long-term continence rates are known with the retropubic technique, and these approximate 80 percent (Nilsson, 2004).

In addition to their efficacy, recovery from midurethral sling placement is rapid, and many gynecologists provide this surgery on an outpatient basis. However, as with other antiincontinence surgeries, general risks for midurethral sling procedures include urinary retention, lower urinary tract and vascular injuries, and creation of de novo voiding dysfunction such as urgency and retention.

Retropubic Approach. There are several commercial kits available for this procedure, and one commonly used technique is

the tension-free vaginal tape (TVT). Completed bilaterally, one trocar is placed through a vaginal suburethral incision lateral to the urethra and brought out suprapubically through a skin incision (Section 43-3, p. 1191). Alternatively, needles may be placed through the retropubic space and into the vagina, in a "top-down" approach.

A prospective observational study conducted at three centers in Sweden and Finland confirmed the long-term safety and efficacy of the TVT device, with a 77-percent cure rate at 11.5 years (Nilsson, 2008). Complications vary depending on institution and surgeon expertise and include: urgency, mesh erosion, urinary retention, de novo urge urinary incontinence, and vascular, bowel, and lower urinary tract injury. Of these, bladder perforation is one of the most common, and associated rates range from 3 to 9 percent (Agostini, 2006; Tamussino, 2001; Ward, 2004).

Transobturator Approach. The transobturator (TOT) approach to midurethral sling placement was introduced with the intent to reduce the risks of vascular and lower urinary tract injury that can be associated with traversing the retropubic space. Various kits for this approach are available. Each contains variations in needle and mesh design, but in general, a permanent sling material, usually polypropylene, is placed. Sling material is directed bilaterally through the obturator foramen and underneath the midurethra. The entry point overlies the proximal tendon of the adductor longus muscle.

The two major types of TOT procedures are defined by whether needle placement begins inside the vagina and is directed outward, termed an *in-to-out* approach, or alternatively starts outside and is directed inward, called an *out-to-in* approach (Section 43-4, p. 1194). Initially, this procedure was developed with an out-to-in approach. However, with this direction, bladder and urethral injury were potential complications. In a retrospective study, Abdel-Fattah and colleagues (2006) compared these two approaches. Injury to the bladder or ureter complicated 1 percent of nearly 400 procedures, and all followed the out-to-in technique.

As a result, the in-to-out approach was created and marketed with the assertion of decreased lower urinary tract injury rates. However, with the in-to-out technique, the trocar tip travels closer to the obturator neurovascular bundle (Achtari, 2006; Zahn, 2007). Thus, although each method has its theoretical advantages, the possibility of injury is not entirely eliminated.

The transobturator approach provides an effective day-surgery technique with potentially lower rates of bladder injury. However, some retrospective studies have suggested that it may have limited effectiveness for patients who demonstrate urodynamic criteria for intrinsic sphincteric deficiency (Miller, 2006; O'Connor, 2006). Prospective randomized comparative studies are needed to clarify the efficacy of each transobturator midurethral sling and to confirm the relative safety of each technique. A multicenter randomized study of 597 women compared the retropubic and transobturator techniques for treatment of SUI. No significant differences in objective and subjective success rates at 12 months were found between the retropubic (80.8 and 62.2 percent) and the transobturator (77.7 and 55.8 percent) routes of surgery. The retropubic route had a significantly higher rate of postoperative voiding dysfunction requiring reoperation, whereas the transobturator route resulted in more neurologic symptoms. Overall quality of life and satisfaction with the two procedures were similar (Richter, 2010a).

Minimally Invasive Slings. Modification of the TVT and TOT procedure is seen with the minimally invasive slings, sometimes called "microslings" or "minislings." With this technique, an 8-cm-long strip of polypropylene synthetic mesh is placed across and beneath the midurethra through a small vaginal incision. Mesh is not threaded through the retropubic space and avoids the potential for vascular injury. Currently, the only minimally invasive sling with published data is the TVT-Secur. Initial results have suggested high objective and subjective cure rates (Neuman, 2008). Unfortunately, most of these studies have been case series without comparison or control groups. Additionally, some studies have reported complications such as recurrent UTI (10 percent), de novo urge urinary incontinence (10 percent), and voiding difficulty (8 percent) (Meschia, 2009). Moreover, lower urinary tract injury is not completely averted with this method. As with most technology, data from well-conducted, long-term comparative studies on efficacy and safety should be obtained before complete adoption of any new technique.

Other techniques that have been introduced include microwave ablation of the periurethral tissues. However, current data do not support the efficacy or safety of this method.

■ Treatment of Urge Urinary Incontinence
Anticholinergic Medications

These medications appear to work at the level of the detrusor muscle by competitively inhibiting acetylcholine at muscarinic receptors (M_2 and M_3) (Miller, 2005). These agents thereby blunt detrusor contractions to reduce the number of incontinence episodes and volume lost with each. These medications are significantly better than placebo at improving symptoms of urge urinary incontinence and overactive bladder. However, in a Cochrane database review, Nabi and colleagues (2006) reported that the reduction in baseline urgency incontinence episodes per day reflects only a modest margin of benefit.

Oxybutynin, Tolterodine, and Fesoterodine. These commonly used drugs competitively bind to cholinergic receptors (Table 23-6). As discussed earlier, muscarinic receptors are

TABLE 23-6. Pharmacologic Treatment of Overactive Bladder

Drug Name	Brand Name	Drug Type	Dosage	Available Doses
Oxybutynin (short-acting)	Ditropan	Antimuscarinic	2.5–5 mg PO tid	5-mg tablet, 5 mg/mL syrup
Oxybutynin (long-acting)	Ditropan XL	See above	5–30 mg PO daily	5-, 10-, 15-mg tablet
Oxybutynin (transdermal)	Oxytrol	See above	3.9 mg/d; patch changed twice weekly	36-mg patch, 8 per carton
Oxybutynin (transdermal) 10% gel	Gelnique	See above	Gel applied 1 g daily	1-g packet, 30 per carton 1-g pump dose, 30 doses per bottle
Tolterodine (short-acting)	Detrol	See above	1–2 mg PO bid	1-, 2-mg tablet
Tolterodine (long-acting)	Detrol LA	See above	2–4 mg PO daily	2-, 4-mg capsule
Fesoterodine fumarate	Toviaz	See above	4–8 mg PO daily	4-, 8-mg tablets
Trospium chloride	Sanctura	Antimuscarinic quaternary amine	20 mg PO bid	20-mg tablet
Trospium chloride	Sanctura XR	See above	60 mg PO daily	60-mg tablet
Darifenacin	Enablex	M_3-selective antimuscarinic	7.5–15 mg PO daily	7.5-, 15-mg tablet
Solifenacin	Vesicare	M_3-selective antimuscarinic	5–10 mg PO daily	5-, 10-mg tablets
Imipramine hydrochloride	Tofranil	Tricyclic antidepressant, anticholinergic, α-adrenergic, antihistamine	10–25 mg PO qd-qid	10-, 25-, 50-mg tablets

bid = twice daily; PO = orally; qd = daily; qid = four times daily; tid = three times daily.

TABLE 23-7. Potential Anticholinergic Side Effects

Side Effect	Potential Clinical Consequence
Increased pupil size	Photophobia
Decreased visual accommodation	Blurred vision
Decreased salivation	Gingival and buccal ulceration
Decreased bronchial secretions	Small-airway mucus plugging
Decreased sweating	Hyperthermia
Increased heart rate	Angina, myocardial infarction
Decreased detrusor function	Bladder distension and urinary retention
Decreased gastrointestinal mobility	Constipation

not limited to the bladder. Thus, side effects with these drugs may be significant. Of these, dry mouth, constipation, and blurry vision are the most common (Table 23-7). Patients frequently report that dry mouth is a primary reason for drug discontinuation. Importantly, anticholinergics are contraindicated in those with narrow-angle glaucoma. Because of these effects, the therapeutic goal of bladder M_3 blockade with these antimuscarinic agents is often limited by their anticholinergic side effects. Accordingly, drug selection should be tailored, and efficacy is balanced against tolerability. For example, Diokno and associates (2003) found oxybutynin to be more effective than tolterodine. However, tolterodine was associated with lower side effect rates. Tolterodine and fesoterodine have also been compared in a randomized study of 1135 patients. Fesoterodine was found to perform above tolterodine, although once again, side effects were lowest in the tolterodine group (Chapple, 2008). A population-based study reported that only 56 percent of women felt their overactive bladder medication was effective, and half stopped taking the medication (Diokno, 2006).

Most side effects attributed to oxybutynin stem from its secondary metabolite that follows liver metabolism. Therefore, to minimize oral oxybutynin side effects, a transdermal patch was designed to decrease the "first-pass" effect of this drug. This leads to decreased liver metabolism and fewer systemic cholinergic side effects. Dmochowski and coworkers (2003b) found fewer anticholinergic side effects with transdermal oxybutynin compared with long-acting oral tolterodine.

Transdermal oxybutynin (Oxytrol) is supplied as a 7.6 × 5.7 cm patch that is applied twice weekly to the abdomen, hip, or buttock. Each patch contains 36 mg of oxybutynin and delivers approximately 3.9 mg each day. Application-site pruritus is the most common side effect, and varying the application site may minimize skin reactions (Sand, 2007). A newer trans-

dermal 10-percent oxybutynin gel (Gelnique) is applied daily to skin of the abdomen, upper arms/shoulders, or thigh, and application sites should be rotated. Each sachet contains a 1-g dose of oxybutynin chloride gel, which delivers approximately 4 mg of oxybutynin daily (Staskin, 2009).

Imipramine. This agent is less effective than tolterodine and oxybutynin but displays α-adrenergic and anticholinergic characteristics. Therefore, it is occasionally prescribe for those with mixed urinary incontinence. Importantly, doses of imipramine used to treat incontinence are significantly lower than those used to treat depression or chronic pain. In our experience, this minimizes the theoretical risk of drug-related side effects.

Selective Muscarinic-Receptor Antagonists. Newer anticholinergic medications have been introduced that aim to reduce side effects. The agents are all M_3-receptor selective antagonists and include solifenacin (VESIcare), trospium chloride (Santura), and darifenacin (Enablex). Advantages of increased urgency warning time and decreased muscarinic side effects have been shown in randomized controlled studies (Cardozo, 2004; Chapple, 2005; Haab, 2006; Zinner, 2004). However, although the side-effect profiles of these drugs are attractive, they have not been proved superior to nonselective muscarinic-receptor drugs in randomized controlled trials (Nabi, 2006).

Sacral Neuromodulation

Urine storage and bladder emptying requires a complex coordinated interaction of spinal cord and higher brain centers, peripheral nerves, urethral and pelvic floor muscles, and the detrusor muscle. If any of these levels are altered, normal micturition is lost. To overcome these problems, electrical nerve stimulation, also called neuromodulation, has been used. InterStim is the only implantable neuromodulation system approved by the FDA for treatment of refractory urge urinary incontinence. It is also approved for treatment of anal incontinence. It may be also considered for those with pelvic pain, interstitial cystitis, and defecatory dysfunction, although it is not FDA-approved for these indications. Sacral neuromodulation is not considered primary therapy and is generally offered to women who have typically exhausted pharmacologic and conservative options.

This outpatient surgically implanted device contains a pulse generator and electrical leads that are placed into the sacral foramina to modulate bladder and pelvic floor innervation. Its mode of action is incompletely understood, but may be related to an inhibition of somatic afferents that interrupts abnormal reflex arcs in the sacral spinal cord involved in the filling and evacuation phases of micturition (Leng, 2005).

Implantation is typically a two-stage process. Initially, leads are placed and attached to an externally worn generator (Section 43-12, p. 1212). After placement, frequency and amplitude of electrical impulses can be adjusted and tailored to maximize effectiveness. If a 50-percent or greater improvement in symptoms is noted, then internal implantation of a permanent pulse generator is planned. This procedure is minimally invasive and is typically completed in a day-surgery setting.

Surgical complications are rare but may include pain or infection at the generator insertion site.

Although its use is often reserved for those who have been unsuccessfully treated with behavioral or pharmacologic therapy, this modality has been shown to be effective for treatment of urinary symptoms. Studies have found improvement rates ranging from 60 to 75 percent, and cure rates approximating 45 percent (Janknegt, 2001; Schmidt, 1999; Siegel, 2000). Sustained improvement from baseline incontinence parameters has been shown at long-term follow-up. One 3-year study reported a 57-percent reduction in incontinence episodes per day, and similar findings were found in a separate 5-year study (Kerrebroeck, 2007; Siegel, 2000). A systematic review of 17 case series at follow-up periods of 3 to 5 years similarly reported 39 percent of patients cured and 67 percent with greater than 50-percent improvement in incontinence symptoms (Brazzelli, 2006).

Botulinum Toxin A

Injection of botulinum toxin A into the bladder wall may be used as a treatment for idiopathic detrusor overactivity. Three placebo-controlled studies showed the effectiveness of this treatment (Anger, 2010). All three used cystoscopic injection of 200 units of botulinum toxin A toxin versus placebo, and each demonstrated significant improvement in incontinence. Improvement occurred as early as 4 weeks after injection (Brubaker, 2008b; Flynn, 2009; Khan, 2010; Sahai, 2007). Urinary retention—defined as a >200-mL postvoid residual—is a common side effect and developed in 27 to 43 percent of patients in these randomized trials. Most patients are asymptomatic, but patients receiving botulinum toxin A for overactive bladder or urge urinary incontinence should understand that temporary self-catheterization may be required after injection.

A patient can expect the effects of the toxin to wane over time. In a small study describing the need for repeat injections, 20 patients from a cohort of 34 received a second injection, and 9 patients received up to four injections. These repeat injections appear to be equally effective as the primary injection. Median time between injections is approximately 377 days (Sahai, 2010).

REFERENCES

Abdel-Fattah M, Ramsay I, Pringle S: Lower urinary tract injuries after transobturator tape insertion by different routes: a large retrospective study. BJOG 113:1377, 2006

Abrams P, Artibani W, Cardozo L, et al: Reviewing the ICS 2002 terminology report: the ongoing debate. Neurourol Urodyn 28(4):287, 2009

Abrams P, Cardozo L, Fall M, et al: The standardisation of terminology of lower urinary tract function: report from the Standardisation Sub-committee of the International Continence Society. Am J Obstet Gynecol 187:116, 2002

Achtari C, McKenzie BJ, Hiscock R, et al: Anatomical study of the obturator foramen and dorsal nerve of the clitoris and their relationship to minimally invasive slings. Int Urogynecol J 17(4):330, 2006

Agostini A, Bretelle F, Franchi F, et al: Immediate complications of tension-free vaginal tape (TVT): results of a French survey. Eur J Obstet Gynecol Reprod Biol 124: 237, 2006

Anger JT, Weinberg A, Suttorp MJ, et al: Outcomes of intravesical botulinum toxin for idiopathic overactive bladder symptoms: a systematic review of the literature. J Urol 183:2258, 2010

Bai SW, Kang JY, Rha KH, et al: Relationship of urodynamic parameters and obesity in women with stress urinary incontinence. J Reprod Med 47:559, 2002

Blaivas JG: The bladder is an unreliable witness. Neurourol Urodyn 15:443, 1996

Bologna RA, Gomelsky A, Lukban JC, et al: The efficacy of calcium glycerophosphate in the prevention of food-related flares in interstitial cystitis. Urology 57(6, Suppl 1):119, 2001

Brazzelli M, Murray A, Frasier C: Efficacy and safety of sacral nerve stimulation for urinary urge incontinence. A systematic review. J Urol 175:835, 2006

Brown JS, Seeley DG, Fong J, et al: Urinary incontinence in older women: who is at risk? Study of Osteoporotic Fractures Research Group. Obstet Gynecol 87(5 Pt 1):715, 1996

Brubaker L, Nygaard I, Richter HE, et al: Two-year outcomes after sacrocolpopexy with and without Burch to prevent stress urinary incontinence. Obstet Gynecol 112:49, 2008a

Brubaker L, Richter HE, Visco AG, et al: Refractory idiopathic urge incontinence and botulinum A injection. J Urol 180:217, 2008b

Bump RC: Racial comparisons and contrasts in urinary incontinence and pelvic organ prolapse. Obstet Gynecol 81:421, 1993

Bump RC, McClish DK: Cigarette smoking and urinary incontinence in women. Am J Obstet Gynecol 167:1213, 1992

Bump RC, Norton PA: Epidemiology and natural history of pelvic floor dysfunction. Obstet Gynecol Clin North Am 25:723, 1998

Burgio KL, Richter HE, Clements RH, et al: Changes in urinary and fecal incontinence symptoms with weight loss surgery in morbidly obese women. Obstet Gynecol 110(5):1034, 2007

Cardozo L, Lisec M, Millard R, et al: Randomized, double-blind placebo controlled trial of the once daily antimuscarinic agent solifenacin succinate in patients with overactive bladder. J Urol 172(5, Part 1):1919, 2004

Carlile A, Davies I, Rigby A, et al: Age changes in the human female urethra: a morphometric study. J Urol 139:532, 1988

Chapple CR, Martinez-Garcia R, Selvaggi L, et al: A comparison of the efficacy and tolerability of solifenacin succinate and extended release tolterodine at treating overactive bladder syndrome: results of the STAR Trial. Eur Urol 48:464, 2005

Chapple CR, Van Kerrebroeck PE, Jünemann KP, et al: Comparison of fesoterodine and tolterodine in patients with overactive bladder. BJU Int 102(9):1128, 2008

Cody JD, Richardson K, Moehrer, et al: Oestrogen therapy for urinary incontinence in post-menopausal women. Cochrane Database Syst Rev 4:CD001405, 2009

Colombo M, Milani R, Vitobello D, et al: A randomized comparison of Burch colposuspension and abdominal paravaginal defect repair for female stress urinary incontinence. Am J Obstet Gynecol 175:78, 1996

Dallosso HM, McGrother CW, Matthews RJ, et al: The association of diet and other lifestyle factors with overactive bladder and stress incontinence: a longitudinal study in women. BJU Int 92:69, 2003

de Tayrac R, Deffieux X, Droupy S, et al: A prospective randomized trial comparing tension-free vaginal tape and transobturator suburethral tape for surgical treatment of stress urinary incontinence. Am J Obstet Gynecol 190:602, 2004

Deitel M, Stone E, Kassam HA, et al: Gynecologic-obstetric changes after loss of massive excess weight following bariatric surgery. J Am Coll Nutr 7:147, 1988

Diokno AC, Appell RA, Sand PK, et al: Prospective, randomized, double-blind study of the efficacy and tolerability of the extended-release formulations of oxybutynin and tolterodine for overactive bladder: results of the OPERA trial. Mayo Clin Proc 78:687, 2003

Diokno AC, Brock BM, Herzog AR, et al: Medical correlates of urinary incontinence in the elderly. Urology 36:129, 1990

Diokno AC, Sand PK, Macdiarmid S et al: Perceptions and behaviors of women with bladder control problems. Fam Prac 23 (5):568, 2006

Dmochowski RR, Miklos JR, Norton PA, et al: Duloxetine versus placebo for the treatment of North American women with stress urinary incontinence. J Urol 170(4 Pt 1):1259, 2003a

Dmochowski RR, Sand PK, Zinner NR, et al: Comparative efficacy and safety of transdermal oxybutynin and oral tolterodine versus placebo in previously treated patients with urge and mixed urinary incontinence. Urology 62:237, 2003b

Dumoulin C, Hay-Smith J: Pelvic floor muscle training versus no treatment, or inactive control treatments, for urinary incontinence in women. Cochrane Database Syst Rev 1:CD005654, 2010

Fantl JA, Bump RC, Robinson D, et al: Efficacy of estrogen supplementation in the treatment of urinary incontinence. Obstet Gynecol 88:745, 1996

Fantl JA, Cardozo L, McClish DK: Estrogen therapy in the management of urinary incontinence in postmenopausal women: a meta-analysis. First report of the Hormones and Urogenital Therapy Committee. Obstet Gynecol 83:12, 1994

FitzGerald MP, Mollenhauer J, Bitterman P, et al: Functional failure of fascia lata allografts. Am J Obstet Gynecol 181:1339, 1999

Flegal KM, Carroll MD, Ogden CL, et al: Prevalence and trends in obesity among U.S. adults, 1999–2000. JAMA 288:1723, 2002

Flynn M, Amundsen CL, Perevich M, et al: Short term outcomes of a randomized, double blind placebo controlled trial of botulinum A toxin for the management of idiopathic detrusor overactivity incontinence. J Urol 181(6):2608, 2009

Ghoniem GM, Van Leeuwen JS, Elser DM, et al: A randomized controlled trial of duloxetine alone, pelvic floor muscle training alone, combined treatment and no active treatment in women with stress urinary incontinence. J Urol 173(5):1647, 2005

Grady D, Brown JS, Vittinghoff E, et al: Postmenopausal hormones and incontinence: the heart and estrogen/progestin replacement study. Obstet Gynecol 97:116, 2001

Grodstein F, Lifford K, Resnick, NM, et al: Postmenopausal hormone therapy and risk of developing urinary incontinence. Obstet Gynecol 103:254, 2004

Haab F, Corcos J, Siami P, et al: Long-term treatment with darifenacin for overactive bladder: results of a 2-year, open-label extension study. BJU Int 98:1025, 2006

Hagstad A, Janson PO, Lindstedt G: Gynaecological history, complaints and examinations in a middle-aged population. Maturitas 7:115, 1985

Hannestad YS, Lie RT, Rortveit G, et al: Familial risk of urinary incontinence in women: population based cross sectional study. BMJ 329(7471):889, 2004

Hannestad YS, Rortveit G, Daltveit AK, et al: Are smoking and other lifestyle factors associated with female urinary incontinence? The Norwegian EPINCONT Study. BJOG 110:247, 2003

Hannestad YS, Rortveit G, Sandvik H, et al: A community-based epidemiological survey of female urinary incontinence: the Norwegian EPINCONT study. Epidemiology of Incontinence in the County of Nord-Trondelag. J Clin Epidemiol 53:1150, 2000

Hartmann KE, McPheeters ML, Biller DH, et al: Treatment of overactive bladder in women. Evidence report/technology assessment No. 187, 2009. Rockville, MD, Agency for Healthcare Research and Quality. Available at: http://www.ahrq.gov/downloads/pub/evidence/pdf/bladder/bladder.pdf. Accessed April 29, 2010

Hendriks EJM, Kessels AGH, de Vet HCW, et al: Prognostic indicators of poor short-term outcome of physiotherapy intervention in women with stress urinary incontinence. Neurourol Urodyn 29:336, 2010

Hendrix SL, Cochrane BB, Nygaard IE, et al: Effects of estrogen with and without progestin on urinary incontinence. JAMA 293:935, 2005

Howden NS, Zyczynski HM, Moalli PA, et al: Comparison of autologous rectus fascia and cadaveric fascia in pubovaginal sling continence outcomes. Am J Obstet Gynecol 194:1444, 2006

Hu TW, Wagner TH, Bentkover JD, et al: Costs of urinary incontinence and overactive bladder in the United States: a comparative study. Urology 63(3):461, 2004

Hunskaar S, Arnold EP, Burgio K, et al: Epidemiology and natural history of urinary incontinence. Int Urogynecol J Pelvic Floor Dysfunct 11:301, 2000

Indrekvam S, Sandvik H, Hunskaar S: A Norwegian national cohort of 3198 women treated with home-managed electrical stimulation for urinary incontinence—effectiveness and treatment results. Scand J Urol Nephrol 35:32, 2001

Iosif CS, Batra S, Ek A, et al: Estrogen receptors in the human female lower urinary tract. Am J Obstet Gynecol 141:817, 1981

Jackson SL, Scholes D, Boyko EJ, et al: Predictors of urinary incontinence in a prospective cohort of postmenopausal women. Obstet Gynecol 108:855, 2006

Janknegt RA, Hassouna MM, Siegel SW, et al: Long-term effectiveness of sacral nerve stimulation for refractory urge incontinence. Eur Urol 39:101, 2001

Juma S, Brito CG: Transobturator tape (TOT): two years follow-up. Neurourol Urodyn 26(1):37, 2007

Kelleher CJ, Cardozo LD, Khullar V, et al: A new questionnaire to assess the quality of life of urinary incontinent women. BJOG 1104:1374, 1997

Kerrebroeck PE, Voskuilen A, Heesakkers J, et al: Results of sacral neuromodulation therapy for urinary voiding dysfunction: outcomes of a prospective, worldwide clinical study. J Urol 178:2029, 2007

Khan S, Panicker J, Roosen A, et al: Complete continence after botulinum neurotoxin type A injections for refractory idiopathic detrusor overactivity incontinence: patient-reported outcome at 4 weeks. Eur Urol 57(5):891, 2010

Kirkland JL, Lye M, Levy DW, et al: Patterns of urine flow and excretion in healthy elderly people. Br Med J 287: 1665, 1983

Langa KM, Fultz NH, Saint S, et al: Informal caregiving time and costs for urinary incontinence in older individuals in the United States. J Am Geriatr Soc 50:733, 2002

Lapitan MC, Cody DJ, Grant AM: Open retropubic colposuspension for urinary incontinence in women. Cochrane Database Syst Rev 4:CD002912, 2009

Laurikainen E, Valpas A, Kivela A, et al: Retropubic compared with transobturator tape placement in treatment of urinary incontinence: a randomized controlled trial. Obstet Gynecol 109:4, 2007

Leng WW, Chancellor MB: How sacral nerve stimulation neuromodulation works. Urol Clin North Am 32(1):11, 2005

Lim JL, Cornish A, Carey MP: Clinical and quality-of-life outcomes in women treated by the TVT-O procedure. BJOG 113:1315, 2006

Mallipeddi PK, Steele AC, Kohli N, et al: Anatomic and functional outcome of vaginal paravaginal repair in the correction of anterior vaginal wall prolapse. Int Urogynecol J Pelvic Floor Dysfunct 12:83, 2001

McGuire EJ: Urethral bulking agents. Nat Clin Pract Urol 3(5):234, 2006

McGuire EJ: Urodynamic findings in patients after failure of stress incontinence operations. Prog Clin Biol Res 78: 351, 1981

McKinley M, O'Loughlin VD: Urinary system. In Human Anatomy. New York, McGraw-Hill, 2006, p 843

Meschia M, Barbacini P, Ambrogi V, et al: TVT-secur: a minimally invasive procedure for the treatment of primary stress urinary incontinence. One year data from a multi-centre prospective trial. Int Urogynecol J Pelvic Floor Dysfunct 20:313, 2009

Millard RJ, Moore K, Rencken R, et al: Duloxetine vs placebo in the treatment of stress urinary incontinence: a four-continent randomized clinical trial. BJU Int 93:311, 2004

Miller JJ, Botros SM, Akl MN, et al: Is transobturator tape as effective as tension-free vaginal tape in patients with borderline maximum urethral closure pressure? Am J Obstet Gynecol 195:1799, 2006

Miller JJ, Sand PK: Diagnosis and treatment of overactive bladder. Minerva Ginecol 57:501, 2005

Monga AK, Stanton SL: Urodynamics: prediction, outcome and analysis of mechanism for cure of stress incontinence by periurethral collagen. Br J Obstet Gynaecol 104:158, 1997

Morey AF, Medendorp AR, Noller MW, et al: Transobturator versus transabdominal mid urethral slings: a multi-institutional comparison of obstructive voiding complications. J Urol 175(3 Pt 1):1014, 2006

Moser F, Bjelic-Radisic V, Tamussino K: Needle suspension of the bladder neck for stress urinary incontinence: objective results at 11 to 16 years. Int Urogynecol J 17:611, 2006

Nabi G, Cody JD, Ellis G, et al: Anticholinergic drugs versus placebo for overactive bladder syndrome in adults. Cochrane Database Syst Rev 4:CD0003781, 2006

Neuman M: Perioperative complications and early follow-up with 100 TVT-SECUR procedures. J Minim Invasive Gynecol 15(4):480, 2008

Nilsson CG, Falconer C, Rezapour M: Seven-year follow-up of the tension-free vaginal tape procedure for treatment of urinary incontinence. Obstet Gynecol 104:1259, 2004

Nilsson CG, Palva K, Rezapour M, et al: Eleven years prospective follow-up of the tension-free vaginal tape procedure for treatment of stress urinary incontinence. Int Urogynecol J 19:1043, 2008

Norton PA, Zinner NR, Yalcin I, et al: Duloxetine versus placebo in the treatment of stress urinary incontinence. Am J Obstet Gynecol 187:40, 2002

Nygaard I: Is cesarean delivery protective? Semin Perinatol 30:267, 2006

Nygaard I, Barber MD, Burgio KL, et al: Prevalence of symptomatic pelvic floor disorders in U.S. women. JAMA 300(11):1311, 2008

O'Connor RC, Nanigian DK, Lyon MB, et al: Early outcomes of mid-urethral slings for female stress urinary incontinence stratified by Valsalva leak point pressure. Neurourol Urodyn 25:685, 2006

Ouslander JG: Management of overactive bladder. N Engl J Med 350(8):786, 2004

Patrick DL, Martin ML, Bushnell DM, et al: Quality of life of women with urinary incontinence: further development of the incontinence quality of life instrument (I-QOL). Urology 53:71, 1999

Petros PE, Ulmsten UI: An integral theory of female urinary incontinence. Experimental and clinical considerations. Scand J Urol Nephrol 153(Suppl):1, 1993

Raz R, Stamm WE: A controlled trial of intravaginal estriol in postmenopausal women with recurrent urinary tract infections. N Engl J Med 329:753, 1993

Resnick, NM: Voiding dysfunction in the elderly. In Yalla SV, McGuire EJ, Elbadawi A, et al (eds): Neurourology and Urodynamics: Principles and Practice. New York, Macmillan, 1984, p 303

Resnick NM, Elbadawi A, Yalla SV: Age and the lower urinary tract: what is normal? Neurourol Urodyn 14:577, 1995

Richter HE, Albo ME, Zyczynski HM, et al: Retropubic versus transobturator midurethral slings for stress incontinence. N Engl J Med 362(22):2066, 2010a

Richter HE, Burgio KL, Brubaker L, et al: Continence pessary compared with behavioral therapy or combined therapy for stress incontinence. A randomized controlled trial. Obstet Gynecol 115(3):609, 2010b

Rortveit G, Daltveit AK, Hannestad YS, et al: Urinary incontinence after vaginal delivery or cesarean section. N Engl J Med 348(10):900, 2003a

Rortveit G, Daltveit AK, Hannestad YS, et al: Vaginal delivery parameters and urinary incontinence: the Norwegian EPINCONT study. Am J Obstet Gynecol 189(5):1268, 2003b

Sahai A, Dowson C, Khan MS, et al: Repeated injections of botulinum toxin-A for idiopathic detrusor overactivity. Urology 75(3):552, 2010

Sahai A, Khan MS, Dasgupta P: Efficacy of botulinum toxin-A for treating idiopathic detrusor overactivity: results from a single center, randomized, double-blind, placebo controlled trial. J Urol 177(6):2231, 2007

Sand P, Zinner N, Newman D, et al: Oxybutynin transdermal system improves the quality of life in adults with overactive bladder: a multicentre, community-based, randomized study. BJU Int 99(4):836, 2007

Schmidt RA, Jonas UDO, Oleson KA, et al: Sacral nerve stimulation for treatment of refractory urinary urge incontinence. J Urol 162:352, 1999

Siegel SW, Catanzaro F, Dijkema HE, et al: Long-term results of a multicenter study on sacral nerve stimulation for treatment of urinary urge incontinence, urgency-frequency, and retention. Urology 56(6 Suppl 1):87, 2000

Sirls LT, Foote JE, Kaufman JM, et al: Long-term results of the FemSoft1 Urethral Insert for the management of female stress urinary incontinence. Int Urogynecol J 13:88, 2002

Snooks SJ, Swash M, Henry MM, et al: Risk factors in childbirth causing damage to the pelvic floor innervation. Int J Colorectal Dis 1:20, 1986

Staskin DR, Dmochowski RR, Sand PK, et al: Efficacy and safety of oxybutynin chloride topical gel for overactive bladder: a randomized, double-blind, placebo controlled, multicenter study. J Urol 181(4):1764, 2009

Subak LL, Wing R, West DS, et al: Weight loss to treat urinary incontinence in overweight and obese women. N Engl J Med 360(5):481, 2009

Swift SE, Bent AE: Basic evaluation of the incontinent female patient. In Bent AE, Cundiff GW, Swift SE (eds): Ostergard's Urogynecology and Pelvic Floor Dysfunction, 6th ed. Philadelphia, Lippincott Williams & Wilkins, 2008, p 67

Tamussino KF, Hanzal E, Kolle D, et al: Tension-free vaginal tape operation: results of the Austrian registry. Obstet Gynecol 98(5):732, 2001

Townsend MK, Curhan GC, Resnick, et al: The incidence of urinary incontinence across Asian, black, and white women in the United States. Am J Obstet Gynecol 202:378.e1, 2010

U.S. Food and Drug Administration: Phenylpropanolamine (PPA) Information Page, 2009. Available at: http://www.fda.gov/Drugs/DrugSafety/InformationbyDrugClass/ucm150738.htm. Accessed April 29, 2010

Vervest HA, van Venrooij GE, Barents JW, et al: Non-radical hysterectomy and the function of the lower urinary tract. II: Urodynamic quantification of changes in evacuation function. Acta Obstet Gynecol Scand 68:231, 1989

Wagner TH, Patrick DL, Bavendam TG, et al: Quality of life of persons with urinary incontinence: development of a new measure. Urology 47:67, 1996

Wake CR: The immediate effect of abdominal hysterectomy on intravesical pressure and detrusor activity. Br J Obstet Gynaecol 87:901, 1980

Wang AC, Wang YY, Chen MC: Single-blind, randomized trial of pelvic floor muscle training, biofeedback-assisted pelvic floor muscle training, and electrical stimulation in the management of overactive bladder. Urology 63:61, 2004

Ward KL, Hilton P: A prospective multicenter randomized trial of tension-free vaginal tape and colposuspension for primary urodynamic stress incontinence: two-year follow-up. Am J Obstet Gynecol 190:324, 2004

Weber AM: Leak point pressure measurement and stress urinary incontinence. Curr Womens Health Rep 1:45, 2001

Wester C, Fitzgerald MP, Brubaker L et al: Validation of the clinical bulbocavernosus reflex. Neurourol Urodyn 22:589, 2003

Wu JM, Hundley AF, Fulton RG, et al: Forecasting the prevalence of pelvic floor disorders in U.S. women 2010 to 2050. Obstet Gynecol 114(6):1278, 2009

Zahn CM, Siddique S, Hernandez S, et al: Anatomic comparison of two transobturator tape procedures. Obstet Gynecol 109:701, 2007

Zinner N, Gittelman M, Harris R, et al: Trospium chloride improves overactive bladder symptoms: a multicenter phase III trial. J Urol 171(6 Pt 1):2311, 2004

SECTION 3

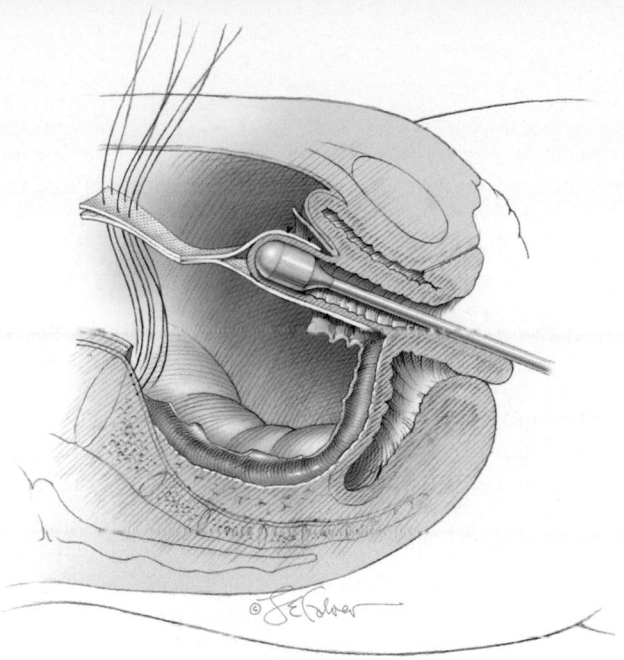

CHAPTER 24

Pelvic Organ Prolapse

Pelvic organ prolapse is a condition of specific signs and symptoms that lead to impairment of normal function and diminished quality of life. *Signs* include descent of one or more of the following: the anterior vaginal wall, posterior vaginal wall, uterus and cervix, the apex of the vagina after hysterectomy, or the perineum (Haylen, 2010). *Symptoms* include vaginal bulging, pelvic pressure, and splinting or digitation. Splinting is manual bolstering of the prolapse to improve symptoms, whereas digitation aids stool evacuation. For pelvic organ prolapse to be considered a disease state in a given individual, symptoms should be attributable to pelvic organ descent such that surgical or nonsurgical reduction relieves the symptoms, restores function, and improves quality of life.

EPIDEMIOLOGY

Pelvic organ prolapse (POP) is a health concern affecting millions of women worldwide. In the United States, it is the third most common indication for hysterectomy. Moreover, a woman has an estimated lifetime risk of 11 percent to undergo surgery for prolapse or incontinence (Olsen, 1997).

Estimation of disease prevalence has been hampered by lack of a consistent definition of pelvic organ prolapse. If the validated Pelvic Organ Prolapse Quantification (POP-Q) examination alone is used to describe pelvic organ support, 30 to 65 percent of women presenting for routine gynecologic care have stage 2 prolapse (Bland, 1999; Swift, 2000, 2005; Trowbridge, 2008). In contrast, studies that define prolapse solely based on patient symptoms show a prevalence ranging from 2.9 to 5.7 percent in the United States (Bradley, 2005; Nygaard, 2008; Rortveit, 2007).

Although data are limited, studies show that the prevalence of pelvic organ prolapse increases steadily with age (Olsen, 1997; Swift, 2005). Given the condition's link to age and the changing demographics in the United States, the prevalence of pelvic organ prolapse will undoubtedly grow.

RISK FACTORS

Table 24-1 summarizes predisposing factors for pelvic organ prolapse. Researchers agree that its etiology is multifactorial and develops gradually over a span of years. The relative importance, however, of each factor is not known.

TABLE 24-1. Risk Factors Associated with Pelvic Organ Prolapse

Pregnancy
Vaginal childbirth
Menopause
   Aging
   Hypoestrogenism
Chronically increased intraabdominal pressure
   Chronic obstructive pulmonary disease (COPD)
   Constipation
   Obesity
Pelvic floor trauma
Genetic factors
   Race
   Connective tissue disorders
Spina bifida

Obstetric-Related Risks

Multiparity

Vaginal childbirth is the most frequently cited risk factor. Although there is some evidence that pregnancy itself predisposes to pelvic organ prolapse, numerous studies have clearly shown that vaginal delivery increases a woman's propensity for developing POP. For example, in the Pelvic Organ Support Study (POSST), increasing parity was associated with advancing prolapse (Swift, 2005). Specifically, the risk of POP increased 1.2 times with each vaginal delivery. In the Reproductive Risks for Incontinence Study at Kaiser (RRISK) study, Rortveit and colleagues (2007) found that the risk of prolapse increased significantly in woman with one vaginal delivery (odds ratio [OR] 2.8), two (OR 4.1), or three or more (OR 5.3) deliveries compared with nulliparas.

Other Obstetric-related Risks

Although vaginal delivery is implicated in a woman's lifetime risk for POP, specific obstetric risk factors remain controversial. These include macrosomia, prolonged second-stage labor, episiotomy, anal sphincter laceration, epidural analgesia, forceps use, and oxytocin stimulation of labor. Each is a proposed risk factor, although not definitively proven. As we await further studies, we can anticipate that although each may have an important effect, it is the cumulative sum of all events occurring as the fetus traverses the birth canal that predisposes to POP.

Currently, two obstetric interventions—elective forceps delivery to shorten second-stage labor and elective episiotomy—are not advocated because of a lack of evidence of benefit and their potential for maternal and fetal harm. First, forceps delivery is directly implicated in pelvic floor injury through its known association with anal sphincter laceration. Secondly, evidence of pelvic floor benefits from shortening the second stage of labor is lacking. For these reasons, elective forceps delivery is not recommended for prevention of pelvic floor disorders. Likewise, at least six randomized controlled tri-

als comparing elective and selective episiotomy have shown no proven benefit, but have shown an association with anal sphincter laceration, postpartum anal incontinence, and postpartum pain (Carroli, 2000).

Elective Cesarean Delivery

Controversy has arisen over the topic of elective cesarean delivery to prevent pelvic floor disorders such as pelvic organ prolapse and urinary incontinence. Theoretically, if all women underwent cesarean delivery, there would be fewer women with pelvic floor disorders. Keeping in mind that most women do *not* develop pelvic floor disorders, elective cesarean delivery would subject many women to a potentially dangerous intervention who would otherwise not develop the problem. Specifically, given the 11-percent lifetime risk of undergoing surgery for incontinence or prolapse, for every one woman who would avoid pelvic floor surgery later in life by undergoing primary elective cesarean delivery, nine women would gain no benefit yet would nevertheless assume the potential risks of the cesarean. Most researchers agree that definitive recommendations will require further clinical studies to define the potential risks and benefits of elective cesarean delivery for primary prevention of pelvic floor dysfunction (American College of Obstetricians and Gynecologists, 2007; Patel, 2006). At this point in time, recommendations regarding elective cesarean delivery to prevent pelvic floor disorders must be individualized.

Age

As described earlier, advancing age is also implicated in the development of POP. In the POSST study, in women aged 20 to 59 years, the incidence of POP roughly doubled with each decade. As with other risks for POP, aging is a complex process. The increased incidence may result from physiologic aging and degenerative processes as well as hypoestrogenism. Clinical and basic investigations clearly demonstrate an important role for reproductive hormones in the maintenance of connective tissues and the extracellular matrix necessary for pelvic organ support. Estrogen and progesterone receptors have been identified in the nuclei of connective tissue and smooth muscle cells of both the levator ani stroma and uterosacral ligaments (Smith, 1990, 1993). Separating the effects of estrogen deprivation from the effects of the aging process is problematic.

Connective Tissue Disease

Women with connective tissue disorders may be more likely to develop POP. Histologic studies have shown that in women with POP, the ratio of collagen I to collagen III and IV is decreased (Moalli, 2004). This relative decrease in well-organized dense collagen is believed to contribute to weakening of vaginal wall tensile strength and an increased susceptibility to vaginal wall prolapse. In a small case series study, one third of women with Marfan syndrome and three fourths of women with Ehlers-Danlos syndrome reported a history of POP (Carley, 2000).

Race

Racial differences in POP prevalence have been demonstrated in several studies (Schaffer, 2005). Black and Asian women show the lowest risk, whereas Hispanic and white women appear to have the highest risk (Hendrix, 2002; Kim, 2005; Whitcomb, 2009). Although differences in collagen content have been demonstrated between races, racial differences in the bony pelvis may also play a role. For instance, black women more commonly have a narrow pubic arch and an android or anthropoid pelvis. These shapes are protective against POP compared with the gynecoid pelvis typical of most white women.

Increased Abdominal Pressure

Chronically elevated intraabdominal pressure is believed to play a role in POP pathogenesis. This condition is present with obesity, chronic constipation, chronic coughing, and repetitive heavy lifting. Higher body mass index (BMI) has been associated with POP. In the Women's Health Initiative (WHI) trial, being overweight (BMI 25–30 kg/m^2) was associated with an increase in POP of 31 to 39 percent, and obesity (BMI >30 kg/m^2) with an increase of 40 to 75 percent (Hendrix, 2002). With regard to lifting, a Danish study demonstrated that nursing assistants who were involved with repetitive heavy lifting were at increased risk to undergo surgical intervention for prolapse, with an odds ratio of 1.6 (Jorgensen, 1994). In addition, cigarette smoking and chronic obstructive pulmonary disease (COPD) have also been implicated in the development of POP (Gilpin, 1989; Olsen, 1997). In a matched case-control study, it was found that chronic pulmonary disease was associated with an increased risk of future pelvic floor repair after hysterectomy (Blandon, 2009). The repetitive increases in intraabdominal pressure resulting from chronic coughing may predispose to POP. Some believe that the inhaled chemical compounds in tobacco may cause tissue changes that lead to POP rather than the chronic cough itself (Wieslander, 2005).

DESCRIPTION AND CLASSIFICATION

Visual Descriptors

Pelvic organ prolapse is descent of the anterior vaginal wall, posterior vaginal wall, uterus (cervix), the apex of the vagina after hysterectomy, or the perineum, alone or in combination. The terms *cystocele, cystourethrocele, uterine prolapse, uterine procidentia, rectocele,* and *enterocele* have traditionally been used to describe the structures behind the vaginal wall thought to be prolapsed (Fig. 24-1). However, these terms are imprecise and misleading, as they focus on what is presumed to be prolapsed rather than what is actually seen.

Although these terms are deeply entrenched in the literature, it is more clinically useful to describe prolapse in terms of what one actually sees: anterior vaginal wall prolapse, apical vaginal wall prolapse, cervical prolapse, posterior vaginal wall prolapse, perineal descent, and rectal prolapse. These descriptors do not presuppose what is behind the vaginal wall, but rather describe the tissues that are objectively noted to be prolapsed.

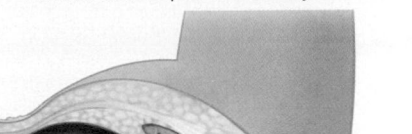

Normal female pelvic anatomy

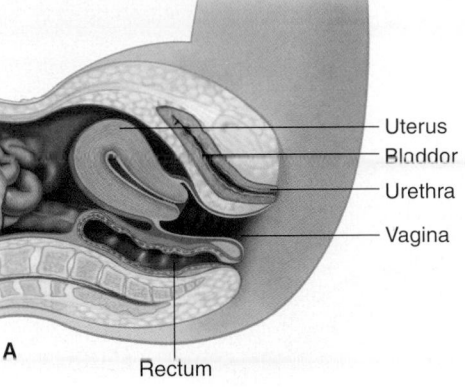

— Uterus
— Bladder
— Urethra
— Vagina
A — Rectum

Anterior vaginal wall prolapse

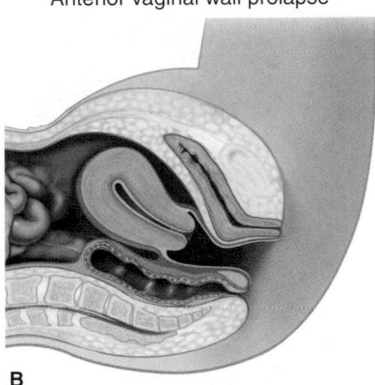

B

Distal posterior wall prolapse

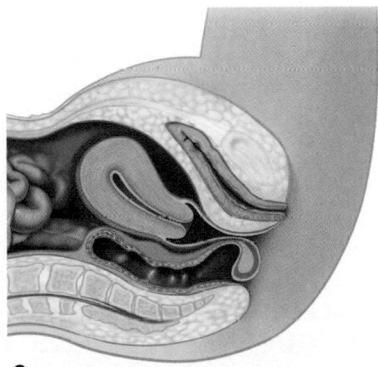

C

Apical posterior wall prolapse

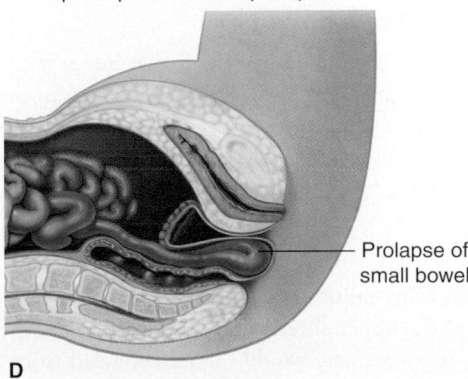

— Prolapse of small bowel
D

FIGURE 24-1 Sagittal view of pelvic anatomy. **A.** Normal pelvic anatomy. **B.** Anterior vaginal wall prolapse or cystocele. **C.** Distal posterior wall prolapse or rectocele. **D.** Apical posterior wall prolapse or enterocele.

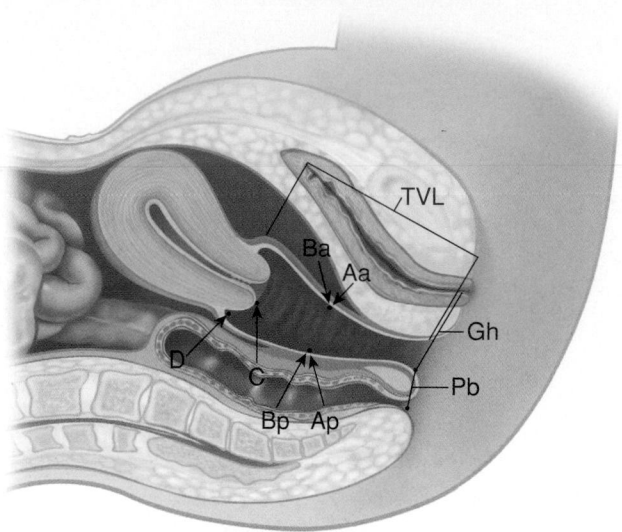

FIGURE 24-2 Drawing displays the anatomic landmarks used during pelvic organ prolapse quantification (POP-Q).

Pelvic Organ Prolapse Quantification (POP-Q)

In 1996, the International Continence Society defined a system of Pelvic Organ Prolapse Quantification (POP-Q) (Bump, 1996). Demonstrating high intra- and interexaminer reliability, the POP-Q system is a major advance in studying prolapse. It allows researchers to report findings in a standardized, easily reproducible fashion. This system contains a series of site-specific measurements of a woman's pelvic organ support. Prolapse in each segment is measured relative to the hymen, which is a anatomic landmark that can be identified consistently. Six points are located with reference to the plane of the hymen: two on the anterior vaginal wall (points Aa and Ba), two in the apical vagina (points C and D), and two on the posterior vaginal wall (points Ap and Bp) (Fig. 24-2). The genital hiatus (Gh), perineal body (Pb), and total vaginal length (TVL) are also measured. All POP-Q points, except TVL, are measured during patient Valsalva and should reflect maximum protrusion.

Anterior Vaginal Wall Points

Point Aa. This term defines a point that lies in the midline of the anterior vaginal wall and is 3 cm proximal to the external urethral meatus. This corresponds to the proximal location of the urethrovesical crease. In relation to the hymen, this point's position ranges, by definition, from −3 (normal support) to +3 cm (maximum prolapse of point Aa).

Point Ba. This point represents the most distal position of any part of the upper anterior vaginal wall, that is, the segment of vagina that normally would extend cephalad from point Aa. It is −3 cm in the absence of prolapse. In a woman with total vaginal eversion posthysterectomy, Ba would have a positive value equal to the position of the cuff from the hymen.

Apical Vaginal Points

Point C. The two apical points, C and D, which are located in the proximal vagina, represent the most proximal locations of a normally positioned lower reproductive tract. Point C defines a point that is at either the most distal edge of the cervix or the leading edge of the vaginal cuff after total hysterectomy.

Point D. This term defines a point that represents the location of the posterior fornix in a woman who still has a cervix. It is omitted in the absence of a cervix. This point represents the level of uterosacral ligament attachment to the proximal posterior cervix and thus differentiates uterosacral-cardinal ligament support failure from cervical elongation. The *total vaginal length* (TVL) is the greatest depth of the vagina in centimeters when point C or D is reduced to its fullest position.

Posterior Vaginal Wall Points

Point Ap. This term defines a point in the midline of the posterior vaginal wall that lies 3 cm proximal to the hymen. Relative to the hymen, this point's range of position is by definition −3 (normal support) to +3 cm (maximum prolapse of point Ap).

Point Bp. This point represents the most distal position of any part of the upper posterior vaginal wall. By definition, this point is at −3 cm in the absence of prolapse. In a woman with total vaginal eversion posthysterectomy, Bp would have a positive value equal to the position of the cuff from the hymen.

Genital Hiatus and Perineal Body. In addition to the hymen, remaining measurements include those of the genital hiatus (Gh) and the perineal body (Pb) (see Fig. 24-2). The genital hiatus is measured from the middle of the external urethral meatus to the midline of the posterior hymenal ring. The perineal body is measured from the posterior margin of the genital hiatus to the midanal opening.

Assessment with POP-Q

With the hymenal plane defined as zero, the anatomic position of these points from the hymen is measured in centimeters. Points above or proximal to the hymen are described with a negative number. Positions below or distal to the hymen are noted using a positive number. The point measurements can be organized using a three-by-three grid as shown in Figure 24-3. Figures 24-4 and 24-5 illustrate the use of POP-Q in evaluating different examples of POP.

The degree of prolapse can also be quantified using a five-stage ordinal system as summarized in Table 24-2 (Bump, 1996). Stages are assigned according to the most severe portion of the prolapse.

Baden-Walker Halfway System

This descriptive tool is also used to classify prolapse during physical examination and is in widespread clinical use. Although not as informative as the POP-Q, it is adequate for clinical use if each compartment (anterior, apical, and posterior) is evaluated (Table 24-3) (Baden, 1972).

anterior wall	anterior wall	cervix or cuff
Aa	**Ba**	**C**
genital hiatus	perineal body	total vaginal length
gh	**pb**	**tvl**
posterior wall	posterior wall	posterior fornix
Ap	**Bp**	**D**

FIGURE 24-3 Grid system used for charting in pelvic organ prolapse quantification (POP-Q).

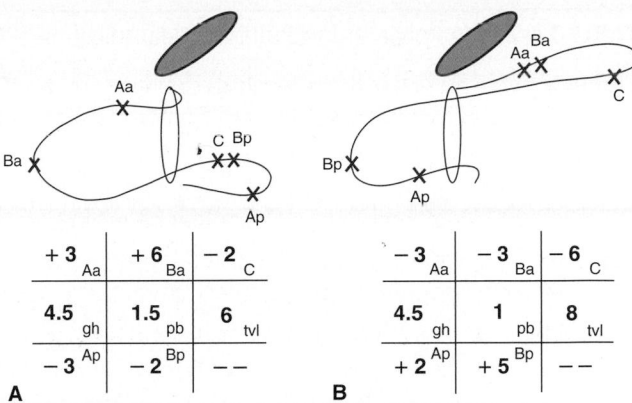

A

+ 3 _Aa_	+ 6 _Ba_	− 2 _C_
4.5 _gh_	1.5 _pb_	6 _tvl_
− 3 _Ap_	− 2 _Bp_	− −

B

− 3 _Aa_	− 3 _Ba_	− 6 _C_
4.5 _gh_	1 _pb_	8 _tvl_
+ 2 _Ap_	+ 5 _Bp_	− −

FIGURE 24-5 Grid and drawing of an anterior support defect **(A)** and posterior support defect **(B)** in patients with prior hysterectomy. *(From Bump, 1996, with permission.)*

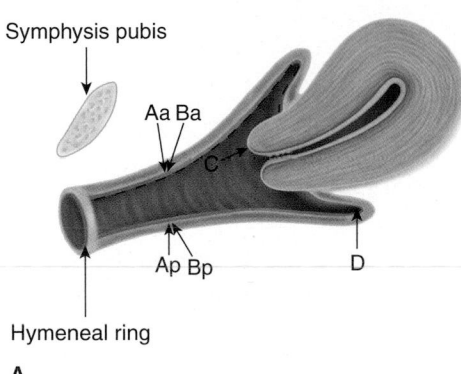

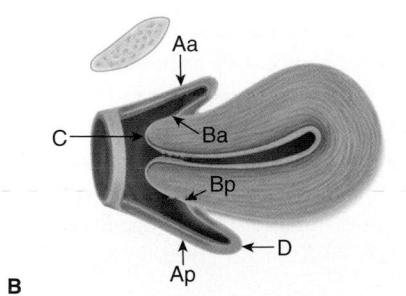

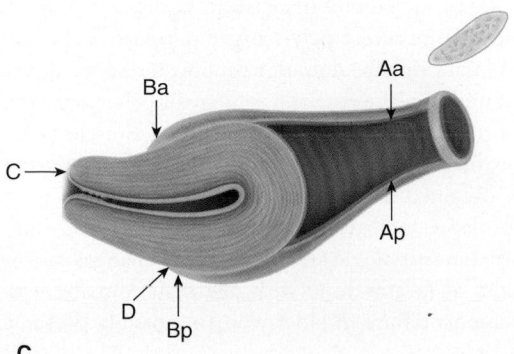

FIGURE 24-4 POP-Q depiction of varying degrees of uterine prolapse **(A–C)**.

PATHOPHYSIOLOGY

Pelvic organ support is maintained by complex interactions among the pelvic floor muscles, pelvic floor connective tissue, and vaginal wall. These work in concert to provide support and also maintain normal physiologic function of the vagina, urethra, bladder, and rectum. Several factors are believed to be involved in pelvic organ support failure. These include genetic predisposition, loss of pelvic floor striated muscle support, vaginal wall weakness, and loss of connective attachments between the vaginal wall and the pelvic floor muscles and pelvic viscera.

Although multiple mechanisms have been hypothesized as contributors to the development of prolapse, none fully explain the origin and natural history of this process. Epidemiologic studies indicate that vaginal birth and aging are two major risk factors for the development of pelvic organ prolapse (Mant, 1997). The loss of support that evolves decades after vaginal delivery may stem from an initial insult compounded by aging and other factors.

Role of Levator Ani Muscle

The levator ani muscle is a pair of striated muscles comprised of three regions. The iliococcygeal portion forms a flat horizontal shelf spanning from one pelvic sidewall to the other (Figs. 38-7 and 38-8, p. 1178). The pubococcygeus muscle arises from the pubic bone on either side; is attached to the walls of the vagina, urethra, anus, and perineal body; and inserts on the coccyx. The pubococcygeus muscle thereby is important in suspending the vaginal wall to the pelvis. The third portion of the levator ani muscle, the puborectalis muscle, forms a sling that originates from the pubic bone. This wraps around and behind the rectum extending to the external anal sphincter. Connective tissue covers the superior and inferior fascia of the levator muscles. In the healthy state, baseline resting contractile activity of the levator ani muscles elevates the pelvic floor and compresses the vagina, urethra, and rectum toward the pubic bone (Fig. 38-10, p. 926). This narrows the genital hiatus and prevents prolapse of the pelvic organs.

TABLE 24-2. The Pelvic Organ Prolapse Quantification (POP-Q) Staging System of Pelvic Organ Support

Stage 0: No prolapse is demonstrated. Points Aa, Ap, Ba, and Bp are all at −3 cm, and either point C or D is between −TVL (total vaginal length) cm and −(TVL−2) cm (i.e., the quantitation value for point C or D is ≤−[TVL−2] cm). Figure 24–2 represents stage 0

Stage I: The criteria for stage 0 are not met, but the most distal portion of the prolapse is >1 cm above the level of the hymen (i.e., its quantitation value is <−1 cm)

Stage II: The most distal portion of the prolapse is ≤1 cm proximal to or distal to the plane of the hymen (i.e., its quantitation value is ≥−1 cm but ≤+1 cm)

Stage III: The most distal portion of the prolapse is >1 cm below the plane of the hymen but protrudes no further than 2 cm less than the total vaginal length in centimeters (i.e., its quantitation value is >+1 cm but <+[TVL−2] cm). Figure 24–5A represents stage III Ba and Figure 24–5B represents stage III Bp prolapse

Stage IV: Essentially, complete eversion of the total length of the lower genital tract is demonstrated. The distal portion of the prolapse protrudes to at least (TVL−2) cm (i.e., its quantitation value is ≥+[TVL−2] cm). In most instances, the leading edge of stage IV prolapse will be the cervix or vaginal cuff scar. Figure 24–4C represents stage IV prolapse

From Bump, 1996, with permission.

When the levator ani muscle has normal tone and the vagina has adequate depth, the upper vagina lies nearly horizontal in the standing female. This creates a "flap-valve" effect in which the upper vagina is compressed against the levator plate during periods of increased intraabdominal pressure. It is theorized that when the levator ani muscle loses tone, the vagina drops from a horizontal to a semivertical position (Fig. 38-11, p. 926). This widens or opens the genital hiatus and predisposes pelvic viscera to prolapse. Without adequate levator ani support, the visceral fascial attachments of the pelvic contents are placed on tension and are thought to stretch and eventually fail.

Changes to the Levator Ani Muscle

It is widely believed that the levator ani muscles sustain either direct muscle or denervation injury during childbirth and that these injuries are involved in the pathogenesis of pelvic organ prolapse. It is hypothesized that during second-stage labor, nerve injury from stretch or compression or both leads to par-

TABLE 24-3. Baden-Walker Halfway System for the Evaluation of Pelvic Organ Prolapse During Physical Examination[a]

Grade	
Grade 0	Normal position for each respective site
Grade 1	Descent halfway to the hymen
Grade 2	Descent to the hymen
Grade 3	Descent halfway past the hymen
Grade 4	Maximum possible descent for each site

[a]Descent of the anterior vaginal wall, posterior vaginal wall, or apical prolapse can be graded with this system. From Baden, 1992, with permission.

tial denervation of the levator ani. Denervated muscle loses tone and the genital hiatus opens, thereby leading to pelvic viscera prolapse (DeLancey, 1993; Harris, 1990; Peschers, 1997; Shafik, 2000).

Experimental evidence for the relationship between denervation-induced injury of the levator ani and pelvic organ prolapse has been difficult to obtain. Investigations using direct assessment of levator ani muscles are not in agreement regarding neuromuscular damage in women with pelvic organ prolapse. Whereas some studies demonstrate histomorphologic abnormalities in the levator ani muscle from women with prolapse and stress incontinence, other studies fail to find histologic evidence of levator ani muscle denervation (Gilpin, 1989; Hanzal, 1993; Heit, 1996; Koelbl, 1989). In addition, levator ani muscle biopsies obtained from parous and nulliparous cadavers failed to find evidence of atrophy or other important muscle changes (Boreham, 2009). This suggests that pregnancy and parturition have little or no effect on levator ani muscle histomorphology.

Additionally, experimental denervation of the levator ani muscle in the squirrel monkey led to significant muscular atrophy but did not affect pelvic organ support. Taken together, experimental evidence does not support a role for denervation-induced injury in the pathophysiology of pelvic organ prolapse.

Importantly, however, loss of skeletal muscle volume and function occurs in virtually all striated muscles during aging. Results obtained from young and older women with pelvic organ prolapse indicate that the levator ani muscle undergoes substantial morphologic and biochemical changes during aging. Thus, loss of levator tone with age may contribute to pelvic organ support failure in older women, possibly those with preexisting defects in connective tissue support. As striated muscles lose tone, ligamentous and connective tissue support of the pelvic organs must sustain more forces conferred by abdominal pressure. As connective tissues bear these loads for long periods, they stretch and may eventually fail, resulting in prolapse.

Role of Connective Tissue

A continuous interdependent system of connective tissues and ligaments surrounds the pelvic organs and attaches them to the levator ani muscle and bony pelvis. The connective tissue of the pelvis is comprised of collagen, elastin, smooth muscle, and microfibers, which are anchored in an extracellular matrix of polysaccharides. The connective tissue that invests the pelvic viscera provides substantial pelvic organ support.

The *arcus tendineus fascia pelvis* is a condensation of the parietal fascia covering the medial aspects of the obturator internus and levator ani muscles (Fig. 38-7, p. 924). It provides the lateral and apical anchor sites for the anterior and posterior vagina. The arcus tendineus fascia pelvis is therefore poised to withstand descent of the anterior vaginal wall, vaginal apex, and proximal urethra. Experts now believe that a major inciting factor for prolapse is loss of connective tissue support at the vaginal apex leading to stretching or tearing of the arcus tendineus fascia pelvis. The result is apical and anterior vaginal wall prolapse.

The *uterosacral ligaments* contribute to apical support by suspending and stabilizing the uterus, cervix, and upper vagina. The ligament is comprised of approximately 20 percent smooth muscle. Several studies have shown a decrease in the fractional area and distribution of smooth muscle in the uterosacral ligaments of women with prolapse (Reisenauer, 2008; Takacs, 2009). These studies suggest that abnormalities in uterosacral ligament support of the pelvic organs contribute to the development of prolapse.

Abnormalities of connective tissue and connective tissue repair may predispose women to prolapse (Norton, 1995; Smith, 1989). As noted, women with connective tissue disorders such as Ehlers-Danlos or Marfan syndrome are more likely to develop POP and urinary incontinence (Carley, 2000; Norton, 1995).

The fascia and connective tissues of the pelvic floor may also lose strength consequent to aging and loss of neuroendocrine signaling in pelvic tissues (Smith, 1989). Estrogen deficiency can affect the biomedical composition, quality, and quantity of collagen. Estrogen influences collagen content by increasing synthesis or decreasing degradation. Exogenous estrogen supplementation has been found to increase the skin collagen content in postmenopausal women who are estrogen deficient (Brincat, 1983). Moreover, estrogen supplementation prior to prolapse surgery and/or postoperatively is considered essential by many pelvic reconstruction surgeons. Although this practice may seem logical and empirically sound, no evidence supports improved surgical outcomes with this use of adjuvant estrogen.

Role of the Vaginal Wall

Abnormalities in the vaginal wall and its attachments to the pelvic floor muscles may be involved in the pathogenesis of pelvic organ prolapse. The vaginal wall is comprised of mucosa (epithelium and lamina propria), a fibroelastic muscularis layer, and an adventitial layer that is composed of loose areolar tissue,

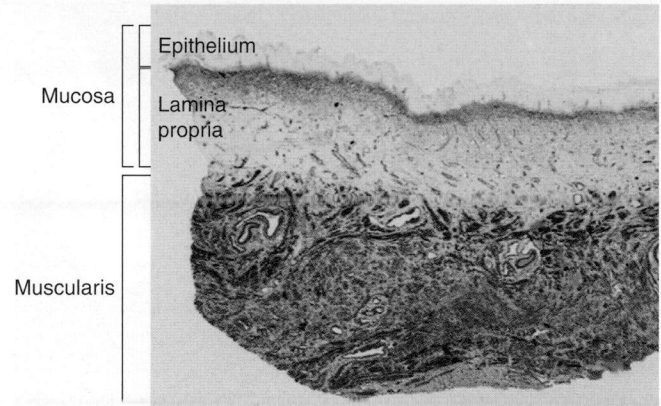

FIGURE 24-6 Photomicrograph shows a cross section of the vaginal wall. Mucosal and muscularis layers are shown here. The adventitia, which is typically seen deep to muscularis, is not shown in this section. The fibromuscular layer is comprised of muscularis and adventitial layers. *(Photograph contributed by Dr. Ann Word.)*

abundant elastic fibers, and neurovascular bundles (Fig. 24-6). The muscularis and adventitial layers together form the *fibromuscular layer*, which was previously referred to as "*endopelvic fascia.*" The fibromuscular layer coalesces laterally and attaches to the arcus tendineus fascia pelvis and superior fascia of the levator ani muscle. In the lower third of the vagina, the vaginal wall is attached directly to the perineal membrane and the perineal body. This suspensory system, together with the uterosacral ligaments, prevents the vagina and uterus from descent when the genital hiatus is open.

Abnormalities in the anatomy, physiology, and cellular biology of vaginal wall smooth muscle may contribute to POP. Specifically, in fibromuscular tissue taken at the vaginal apex from both the anterior and posterior vaginal walls, vaginal prolapse is associated with loss of smooth muscle, myofibroblast activation, abnormal smooth muscle phenotype, and increased protease activity (Boreham, 2001, 2002a,b; Moalli, 2005; Phillips, 2006). Additionally, abnormal synthesis or degradation of vaginal wall collagen and elastin fibers appears to contribute to prolapse.

The Defect Theory of Pelvic Organ Prolapse

This theory states that tears in different sites of the "endopelvic fascia" surrounding the vaginal wall allow herniation of the pelvic organs. The association of POP with vaginal delivery is consistent with this theory. However, the microscopic anatomy of the vaginal wall illustrates that endopelvic fascia does not exist as a specific anatomic tissue, but rather represents the fibromuscular layer of the vaginal wall, that is, vaginal muscularis and adventitia (Boreham, 2001).

Most researchers agree that vaginal delivery predisposes women to POP. However, there is less agreement regarding changes in the pelvic musculature and vaginal wall that result in prolapse. Nichols and Randall (1989) proposed an attenuation of the vaginal wall without loss of fascial attachments. They

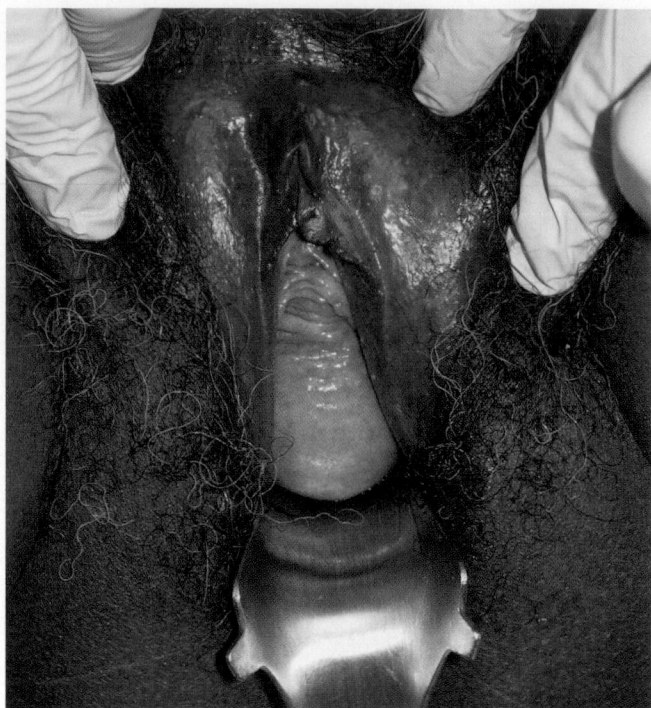

FIGURE 24-7 Photograph shows midline or distension cystocele. Note the characteristic loss of vaginal wall rugae.

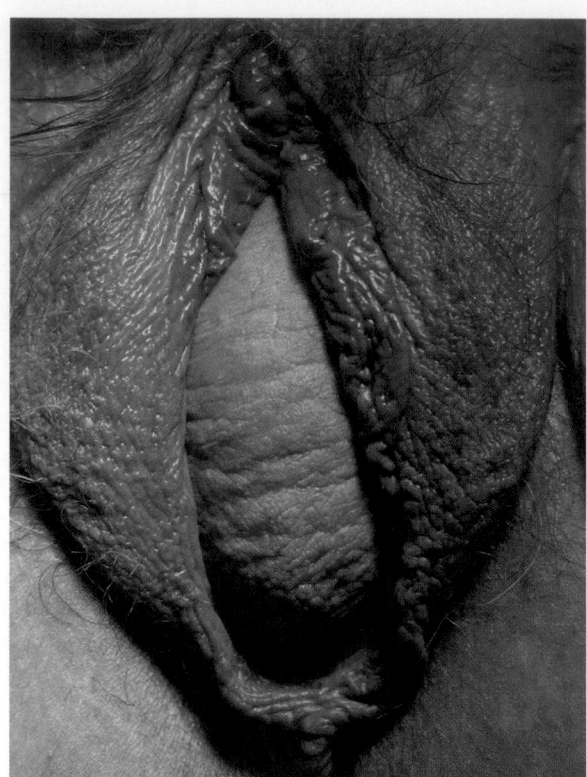

FIGURE 24-8 Photograph shows a lateral cystocele, also termed paravaginal or displacement cystocele. Rugae are present, which indicates that loss of support is lateral rather than central.

term prolapse of this type as *distension* cystocele or rectocele (Fig. 24-7). In contrast, anterior and posterior wall defects due to loss of the connective tissue attachment of the lateral vaginal wall to the pelvic side wall are described as *displacement* (paravaginal) cystocele or rectocele (Fig. 24-8). With distension-type prolapse, the vaginal wall appears smooth and without rugae, due to attenuation. With displacement-type prolapse, vaginal rugae are visible. Both defect types could result from the stretching or tearing of support tissues during second-stage labor.

Many experts now believe the primary "defect" leading to prolapse is often loss of support at the vaginal apex. Although this results in descent of the apical portions of the anterior and posterior vaginal walls, resuspension of the vaginal apex will restore support to both the anterior and posterior walls.

Levels of Vaginal Support

The vagina consists of a fibromuscular, flattened, cylindrical tube with three levels of support, as described by DeLancey (1992). Level I support suspends the upper or proximal vagina. Level II support attaches the midvagina along its length to the arcus tendineus fascia pelvis. Level III support results from fusion of the distal vagina to adjacent structures. Defects in each level of support result in identifiable vaginal wall prolapse: apical, anterior, and posterior.

Level I Support

This level consists of the cardinal and uterosacral ligaments attachment to the cervix and upper vagina (Fig. 38-15, p. 931). The cardinal ligaments fan out laterally and attach to the parietal fascia of the obturator internus and piriformis muscles, the anterior border of the greater sciatic foramen, and the ischial spines. The uterosacral ligaments are posterior fibers that attach to the presacral region at the level of S2 through S4. Together, this dense visceral connective tissue complex maintains vaginal length and horizontal axis. It allows the vagina to be supported by the levator plate and positions the cervix just superior to the level of the ischial spines. Defects in this support complex may lead to apical prolapse. This is frequently associated with small bowel herniation into the vaginal wall, that is, enterocele.

Level II Support

This support consists of the paravaginal attachments that are contiguous with the cardinal/uterosacral complex at the ischial spine. These are the connective tissue attachments of the lateral vagina anteriorly to the arcus tendineus fascia pelvis and posteriorly to the arcus tendineus rectovaginalis. Detachment of this connective tissue from the arcus tendineus fascia pelvis leads to lateral or paravaginal anterior vaginal wall prolapse.

Level III Support

The perineal body, superficial and deep perineal muscles, and fibromuscular connective tissue comprise level III. Collectively, these support the distal one third of the vagina and introitus. The perineal body is essential for distal vaginal support and proper function of the anal canal. Damage to level III support contributes to anterior and posterior vaginal wall prolapse, gaping introitus, and perineal descent.

EVALUATION OF THE PATIENT WITH PELVIC ORGAN PROLAPSE

Symptoms Associated with Pelvic Organ Prolapse

Pelvic organ prolapse involves multiple anatomic and functional systems. Thus, POP is commonly associated with genitourinary, gastrointestinal, and musculoskeletal symptoms (Table 24-4). Prolapse rarely results in severe morbidity or mortality, however, it can greatly diminish quality of life. Therefore, initial evaluation must include a careful assessment of prolapse-related symptoms and their effect on activities of daily living.

Symptoms should be carefully reviewed to determine if they are caused by the prolapse or by other etiologies. "Bulge" symptoms—pelvic pressure, the feeling of sitting on a ball, or heaviness in the vagina—are most likely to correlate with prolapse. Other symptoms, such as back pain, constipation, and abdominal discomfort, may exist in conjunction with prolapse but not result from it. A thorough history and physical examination will often help delineate the relationship between POP and symptoms.

During symptom inventory, several tools may be useful in assessing severity. Two commonly used questionnaires are the Pelvic Floor Distress Inventory (PFDI) and the Pelvic Floor Impact Questionnaire (PFIQ) (Barber, 2005b). The PFDI assesses urinary, colorectal, and prolapse symptoms, whereas the PFIQ assesses the impact of prolapse on quality of life (Tables 24-5 and 24-6).

TABLE 24-4. Symptoms Associated with Pelvic Organ Prolapse

Symptoms	Other Possible Causes
Bulge symptoms	
Sensation of vaginal bulging or protrusion	Rectal prolapse
Seeing or feeling a vaginal or perineal bulge	Vulvar or vaginal cyst/mass
Pelvic or vaginal pressure	Pelvic mass
Heaviness in pelvis or vagina	Hernia (inguinal or femoral)
Urinary symptoms	
Urinary incontinence	Urethral sphincter incompetence
Urinary frequency	Detrusor overactivity
Urinary urgency	Hypoactive detrusor function
Weak or prolonged urinary stream	Bladder outlet obstruction (i.e., postsurgical)
Hesitancy	Excessive fluid intake
Feeling of incomplete emptying	Interstitial cystitis
Manual reduction of prolapse to start or complete voiding	Urinary tract infection
Position change to start or complete voiding	
Bowel symptoms	
Incontinence of flatus or liquid/solid stool	Anal sphincter disruption or neuropathy
Feeling of incomplete emptying	Diarrheal disorder
Hard straining to defecate	Rectal prolapse
Urgency to defecate	Irritable bowel syndrome
Digital evacuation to complete defecation	Rectal inertia
Splinting vagina or perineum to start or complete defecation	Pelvic floor dyssynergia
Feeling of blockage or obstruction during defecation	Hemorrhoids
	Anorectal neoplasm
Sexual symptoms	
Dyspareunia	Vaginal atrophy
Decreased lubrication	Levator ani syndrome
Decreased sensation	Vulvodynia
Decreased arousal or orgasm	Other female sexual disorder
Pain	
Pain in vagina, bladder, or rectum	Interstitial cystitis
Pelvic pain	Levator ani syndrome
Low back pain	Vulvodynia
	Lumbar disc disease
	Musculoskeletal pain
	Other causes of chronic pelvic pain (Table 11-2, p. 309).

Adapted from Barber, 2005a, with permission.

TABLE 24-5. Short Form: Pelvic Floor Impact Questionnaire 7-Item (PFIQ-7)

Please select the best answer to each question below.
Name _____

Has your prolapse affected your:

1. Ability to do household chores (cooking, house cleaning, laundry)?
   _ Not at all   _ Mildly   _ Moderately   _ Severely

2. Physical recreation such as walking, swimming, or other exercises?
   _ Not at all   _ Mildly   _ Moderately   _ Severely

3. Entertainment activities (movies, church)?
   _ Not at all   _ Mildly   _ Moderately   _ Severely

4. Ability to travel by car or bus more than 30 minutes from home?
   _ Not at all   _ Mildly   _ Moderately   _ Severely

5. Participation in social activities outside your home?
   _ Not at all   _ Mildly   _ Moderately   _ Severely

6. Emotional health (nervousness, depression)?
   _ Not at all   _ Mildly   _ Moderately   _ Severely

7. Feeling frustrated?
   _ Not at all   _ Mildly   _ Moderately   _ Severely

From Flynn, 2006, with permission.

TABLE 24-6. Short Form: Pelvic Floor Distress Inventory 22-Item (PFDI-22)[a]

POPDI—6
Do you usually_____, and if so how much are you bothered by:
1. experience pressure in the lower abdomen
2. experience heaviness or dullness in the abdomen or genital area
3. have a bulge or something falling out that you can see or feel in the vaginal area
4. have to push on the vagina or around the rectum to have or complete a bowel movement
5. experience a feeling of incomplete bladder emptying
6. have to push up on a bulge in the vaginal area with your fingers to start or complete urination

CRADI—8
_____, and if so how much are you bothered by it?
1. Do you usually feel you need to strain too hard to have a bowel movement
2. Do you usually feel you have not completely emptied your bowels at the end of bowel movement
3. Do you usually lose stool beyond your control if your stool is well formed
4. Do you usually lose stool beyond your control if your stool is loose or liquid
5. Do you usually lose gas from the rectum beyond your control
6. Do you usually have pain when you pass your stool
7. Do you usually experience a strong sense of urgency and have to rush to the bathroom to have a bowel movement
8. Does part of your bowel ever pass through the rectum and bulge outside during or after a bowel movement

UDI—8
Do you usually have _____, and if so, how much are you bothered by:
1. frequent urination
2. leakage related to feeling of urgency
3. leaking related to activity, coughing, or sneezing
4. leakage when you go from sitting to standing
5. small amounts of urine leakage (i.e., drops)
6. difficulty emptying the bladder
7. pain or discomfort in the lower abdomen or genital area
8. pain in the middle of your abdomen as your bladder fills

[a]For each question, patients fill in the blank with each phrase underneath the question. The same multiple choice responses (not at all, mildly, moderately, and severely) used for the PFIQ-7 are used for the PFDI-22.
From Flynn, 2006, with permission.

Treatment is symptom-directed, and in the absence of symptoms, prolapse generally does not require therapy. However, for those with complaints, treatment may include both nonsurgical and surgical therapy.

Bulge Symptoms

The complaints most strongly associated with prolapse are the sensation or visualization of a vaginal or perineal protrusion, and the sensation of pelvic pressure. Women may comment on feeling a ball in the vagina, sitting on a weight, or noting a bulge rubbing against their clothes. These symptoms worsen with prolapse progression (Ellerkmann, 2001). Specifically, women with prolapse beyond the hymen are more likely to report a vaginal bulge and have more symptoms than those with prolapse above the hymen (Barber, 2005a; Bradley, 2005; Swift, 2000; Tan, 2005; Weber, 2001a). If bulge symptoms are the primary complaint, successful replacement of the prolapse with nonsurgical or surgical therapy will usually provide adequate treatment.

Urinary Symptoms

Patients with POP often have concurrent urinary symptoms. These may include stress urinary incontinence (SUI), urge urinary incontinence, frequency, urgency, urinary retention, recurrent urinary tract infection, or voiding dysfunction. Although these symptoms may be caused or exacerbated by prolapse, it should not be assumed that surgical or nonsurgical correction of prolapse will be curative. For example, irritative bladder symptoms (frequency, urgency, and urge urinary incontinence) do not reliably improve with replacement of prolapse and sometimes worsen after surgical management. Moreover, they may be unrelated to the prolapse and require alternative therapy. In contrast, urinary retention has been found to improve with prolapse treatment if the symptom is due to an obstructed urethra (FitzGerald, 2000).

For these reasons, urodynamic testing is a valuable adjunct in women with urinary symptoms who are undergoing treatment of prolapse (Chap. 23, p. 621). This testing attempts to determine the relationship between urinary symptoms and POP and will help guide therapy. Additionally, consideration may also be given to temporarily placing a pessary prior to surgery to determine if urinary symptoms improve. This may predict whether surgical reduction of prolapse will be beneficial.

Gastrointestinal Symptoms

Constipation is often present in women with pelvic organ prolapse, although it is generally not caused by POP. Thus, surgical repair or treatment with a pessary will not usually cure constipation and may actually worsen it. In one study of defect-directed posterior repair, constipation resolved postoperatively in only 43 percent of patients (Kenton, 1999). Therefore, if a patient's primary symptom is constipation, treatment of prolapse may not be indicated. Constipation should be viewed as a problem distinct from prolapse and evaluated separately (Chap. 25, p. 669).

The need for digital decompression of the posterior vaginal wall, the perineal body, or the distal rectum to evacuate the rectum is the most common defecatory symptom associated with posterior vaginal wall prolapse (Barber, 2003; Burrows, 2004; Ellerkmann, 2001). Surgical approaches to this problem result in variable success, with symptom resolution rates as low as 36 percent (Kenton, 1999).

Anal incontinence of flatus, liquid, or solid stool may also be seen in conjunction with POP. On occasion, prolapse may lead to stool trapping in the distal rectum with subsequent leakage of liquid stool around retained feces. If symptoms are present, a full anorectal evaluation should be performed (Chap. 25, p. 662). Most types of anal incontinence would not be expected to improve with surgical repair of prolapse. However, if evaluation reveals an anal sphincter defect as the cause of anal incontinence, anal sphincteroplasty may be performed concurrently with prolapse repair.

Female Sexual Dysfunction

Female sexual dysfunction is present in women with dyspareunia, low libido, problems with arousal, and inability to achieve orgasm. The etiology is frequently multifactorial and includes psychosocial factors, urogenital atrophy, aging, and male sexual dysfunction (Chap. 13, p. 377). Sexual dysfunction is often also seen in women with POP. However, findings from studies evaluating sexual function in women with prolapse are inconsistent. In one study, a validated sexual function questionnaire was used to compare frequency of intercourse, libido, dyspareunia, orgasmic function, and vaginal dryness in women with and without prolapse (Weber, 1995). No differences were seen between the two groups. In another cross-sectional study of 301 women seeking gynecologic care, pelvic floor symptoms were associated with dyspareunia, reduced arousal, and infrequent orgasm (Handa, 2008). In addition, sexual dysfunction was worse in women with symptomatic prolapse versus those with asymptomatic prolapse.

Accordingly, women with an obstructing bulge as a cause of sexual dysfunction may benefit from therapy to reduce the prolapse. Unfortunately, some prolapse procedures such as posterior repair with levator plication and vaginal placement of mesh may contribute to postoperative dyspareunia. Therefore, care should be taken in planning appropriate surgical procedures for women with concomitant sexual dysfunction.

Pelvic and Back Pain

Many patients with pelvic organ prolapse complain of pelvic and low back pain, but little evidence supports a direct association. A cross-sectional study of 152 consecutive patients with POP did not find an association between pelvic or low back pain and prolapse after controlling for age and prior surgery (Heit, 2002). Swift and colleagues (2003) found that back and pelvic pain were common among 477 women presenting for routine annual gynecologic examination and had no relationship to POP.

Some suggest that low back pain in a patient with prolapse may be caused by altered body mechanics. However, if pain is a primary symptom, other sources should be sought (Chap. 11, p. 309). In the absence of an identifiable etiology, temporary pessary placement is often beneficial to determine whether prolapse reduction will improve pain symptoms. Referral to a physical therapist may also shed light on a connection among prolapse, altered body mechanics, and pain.

Asymptomatic Women

Many women with mild to advanced prolapse lack bothersome symptoms. Because the natural history of prolapse is unknown, it is difficult to predict if prolapse will worsen or if symptoms will develop. In this situation, benefits of treatment should be balanced against risk. Therefore, in the absence of other factors, invasive therapy is typically not selected for asymptomatic women. Pelvic floor muscle rehabilitation may be offered to a patient seeking to prevent prolapse progression. However, no data support the effectiveness of this practice (Adams, 2004; Hagen, 2004).

Comparing Symptoms to Degree and Location of Prolapse

Although POP has been associated with several different types of symptoms, the presence and severity of symptoms does not always correlate well with advancing stages of prolapse. In addition, many common symptoms do not differentiate between compartments. Several studies have shown a poor predictive value among symptoms, the degree of their severity, and the degree of prolapse in a particular vaginal compartment (Ellerkmann, 2001; Jelovsek, 2005; Kahn, 2005; Weber, 1998). Thus, when planning surgical or nonsurgical therapy, realistic expectations should be set with regard to relief of symptoms. A patient should be informed that some symptoms cannot predictably be improved.

■ Physical Examination

Physical examination begins with a full body systems evaluation to identify pathology outside the pelvis. Systemic conditions such as cardiovascular, pulmonary, renal, or endocrinologic disease may affect treatment choices and should be identified early.

Perineal Examination

Initial pelvic examination is performed with a woman in lithotomy position. The vulva and perineum are examined for signs of vulvar or vaginal atrophy, lesions, or other abnormalities. A neurologic examination of sacral reflexes is performed using a cotton swab. First, the *bulbocavernosus reflex* is elicited by tapping or stroking lateral to the clitoris and observing contraction of the bulbocavernosus muscle bilaterally. Secondly, evaluation of anal sphincter innervation is completed by stroking lateral to the anus and observing a reflexive contraction of the anus, known as the *anal wink reflex*. Intact reflexes suggest normal sacral pathways. However, they may be absent in women who are neurologically intact, due to false-negative testing.

Pelvic organ prolapse examination begins by asking a woman to attempt Valsalva maneuver prior to placing a speculum in the vagina (Fig. 24-9). Patients who are unable to adequately complete a Valsalva maneuver are asked to cough. This "hands-off" approach more accurately displays true anatomy. With speculum examination, structures are artificially lifted, supported, or displaced. Importantly, this assessment helps answer three questions: (1) Does the protrusion come beyond the hymen? (2) What is the presenting part of the prolapse (anterior, posterior, or apical)? (3) Does the genital hiatus significantly widen with increased intraabdominal pressure?

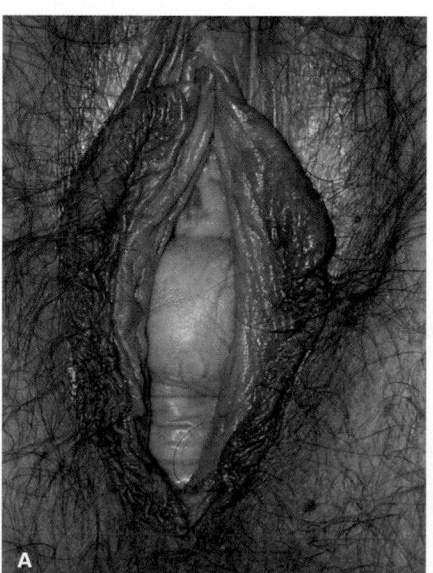 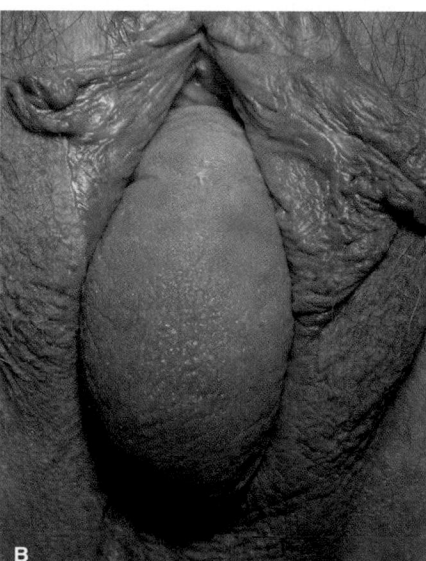 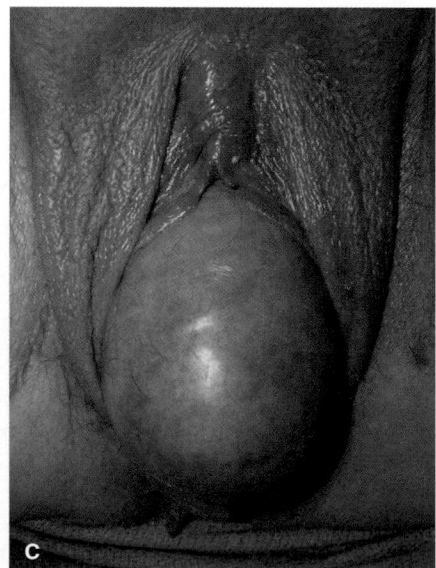

FIGURE 24-9 Photographs of vaginal wall prolapse. **A.** Stage 2. This stage is defined by the most distal edge of the prolapse lying within 1 cm of the hymenal ring. **B.** Stage 3. This stage is defined by the most distal portion of the prolapse being >1 cm below the plane of the hymen, but protruding no farther than 2 cm less than the total vaginal length in centimeters. **C.** Stage 4. This stage is defined as complete or near complete eversion of the vaginal wall.

CHAPTER 24

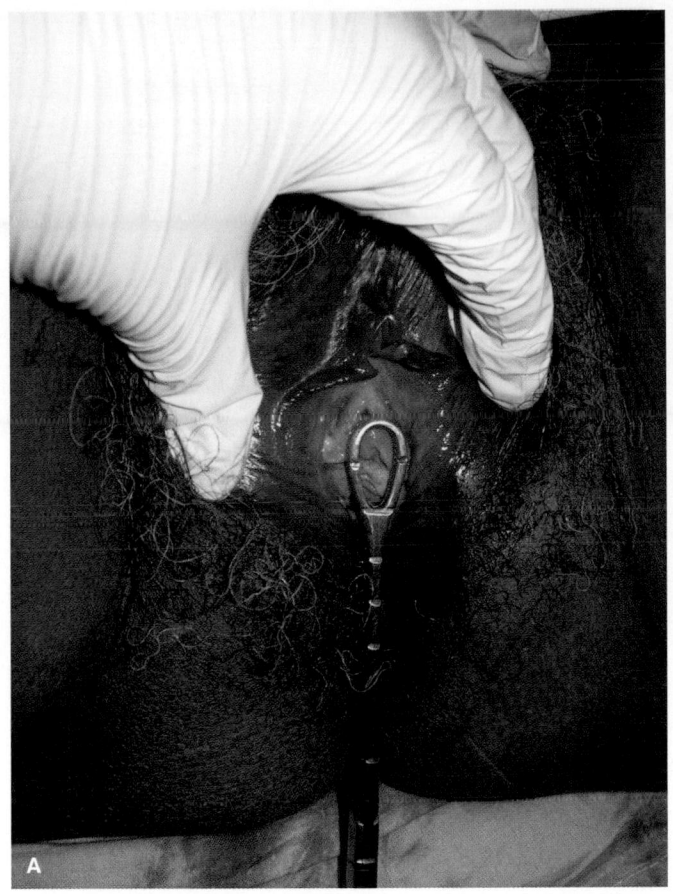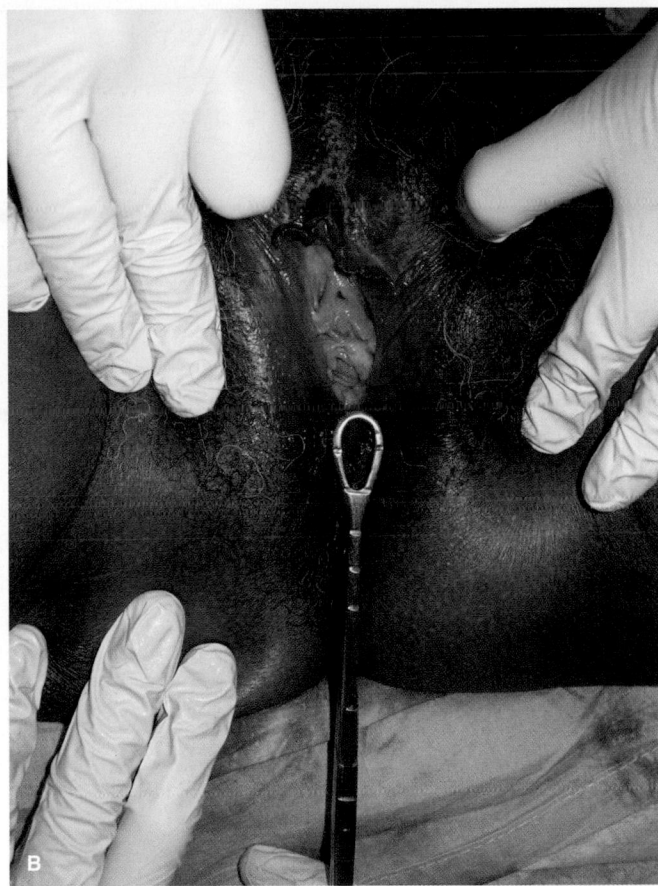

FIGURE 24-10 Photograph displays clinical measurement of the genital hiatus (Gh) and perineal body (Pb). **A.** For POP-Q evaluation, a sponge stick is used that is marked at 1-, 2-, 3-, 4-, 5-, 7.5-, and 10-cm increments. Measurement is obtained with a woman performing maximum Valsalva maneuver. **B.** Measurement of the perineal body.

During examination, a clinician should verify that the full extent of the prolapse is being seen. Specifically, a woman should be asked to describe the extent of prolapse during real-life activities. This degree may be conveyed in terms of inches. Alternatively, a mirror may be placed at the perineum and visual confirmation can be obtained from the patient.

Prolapse is a dynamic condition that responds to the effects of gravity and intraabdominal pressure. It frequently worsens over the course of a day or during physical activity and thus, might not be evident during office examination early in the morning. If the full extent of prolapse cannot be demonstrated, a woman should be examined in a standing position and during Valsalva maneuver.

Vaginal Examination

If the POP-Q examination is performed, the genital hiatus (Gh) and perineal body (Pb) are measured during Valsalva maneuver (Fig. 24-10). The total vaginal length (TVL) is then measured by placing a marked ring forceps, or a ruler, at the vaginal apex and noting the distance to the hymen. A bivalve speculum is then inserted to the vaginal apex. It displaces the anterior and posterior vaginal walls, and points C and D are then measured with Valsalva. The speculum is slowly withdrawn to assess descent of the apex.

A split speculum is then used to displace the posterior vaginal wall and allow for visualization of the anterior wall and measurement of points Aa and Ba (Fig. 24-11). Attempts are

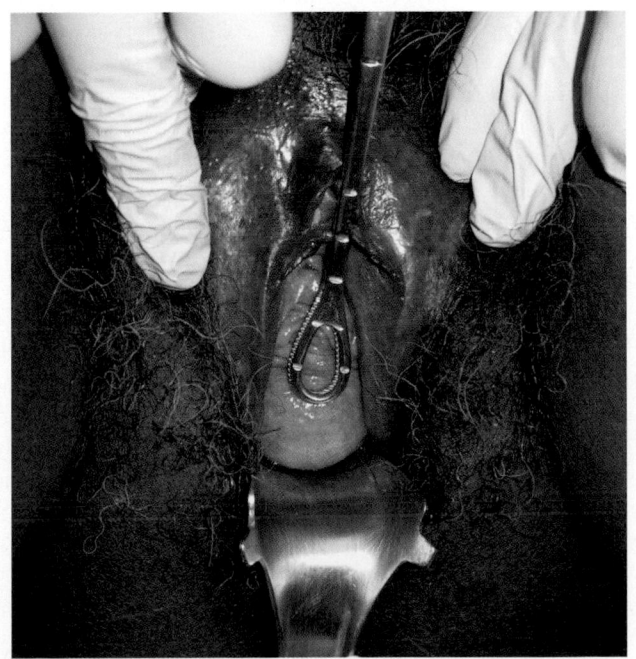

FIGURE 24-11 Photograph shows a split speculum displacing the posterior vaginal wall. This allows for measurement of points Aa and Ba. Aa is always defined as a discrete point lying 3 cm proximal to the urethral meatus and is measured in relation to the hymen. During measurement, downward traction should be avoided, as this causes artificial descent of the anterior vaginal wall.

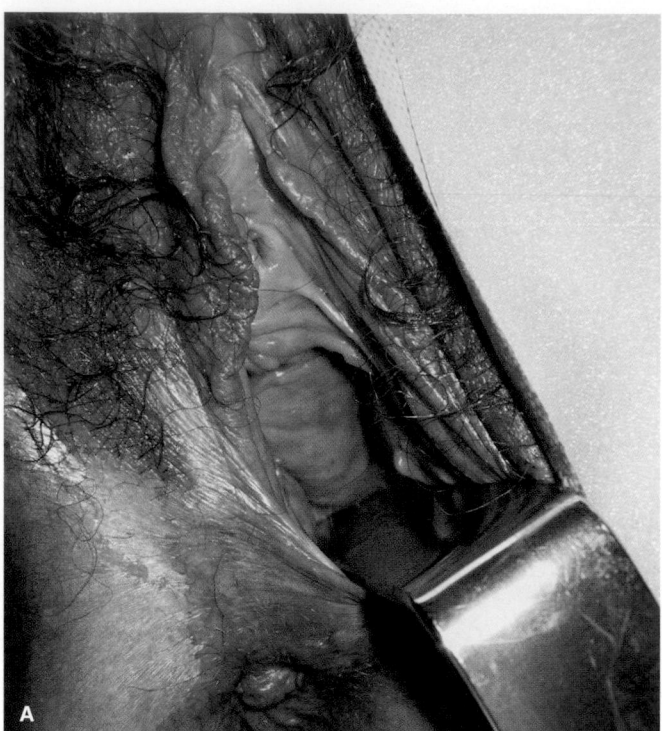
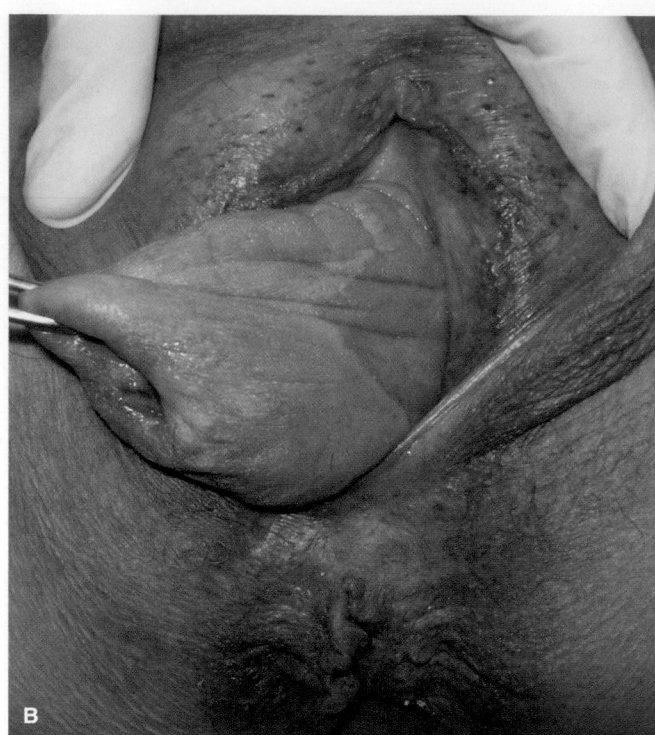

FIGURE 24-12 A. Photograph displays normal lateral support as noted by normal positioning of the vaginal sulci. **B.** Photograph reveals complete loss of lateral support, shown as absent lateral sulci.

made to characterize the nature of the anterior vaginal wall defect. Sagging lateral vaginal sulci with vaginal rugae still present suggest a *paravaginal defect*, that is, a lateral loss of support (Fig. 24-12). A central bulge and loss of vaginal rugae is called a *midline* or *central defect* (see Fig. 24-7). If loss of support appears to arise from detachment of the anterior vaginal wall's apical segment from the apex, it is termed a *transverse* or *anterior apical defect* (Fig. 24-13). Transverse defects are assessed by replacing the anterior apical segment and observing whether the prolapse descends during Valsalva maneuver. The urethra is also evaluated during anterior vaginal wall assessment, and Q-tip testing can be performed to determine urethral hypermobility (Fig. 23-13, p. 620).

The split speculum is then rotated 180 degrees to displace the anterior wall and allow examination of the posterior wall. Points Ap and Bp are measured (Fig. 24-14). If the posterior vaginal wall descends, attempts are made to determine if rectocele or enterocele is present. Enterocele can only definitively be diagnosed by observing small bowel peristalsis behind the vaginal wall (Fig. 24-15). In general, bulges at the apical segment of the posterior vaginal wall should implicate enteroceles, whereas bulges in the distal posterior wall are presumed to be rectoceles. Further distinction may be found during standing rectovaginal examination. A clinician's index finger is placed in the rectum and thumb on the posterior vaginal wall. Small bowel may be palpated between the rectum and vagina, confirming enterocele.

Differentiation of midline, lateral, apical, and distal defects of the anterior and posterior vaginal walls has not been shown to have good inter- or intraexaminer reliability. However, individ-

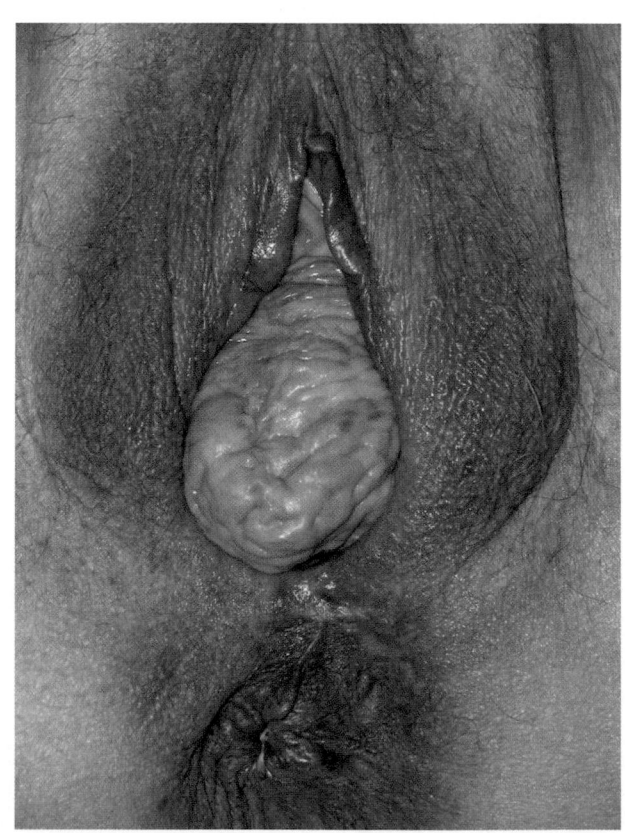

FIGURE 24-13 Photograph displays a transverse vaginal wall defect. Note detachment of the anterior vaginal wall from the apex and the presence of rugae, which suggests that this is not a midline or central defect.

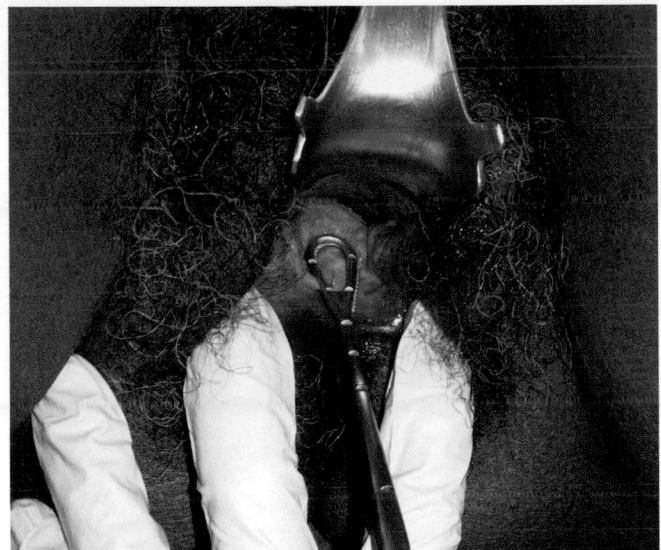

FIGURE 24-14 Photograph showing a split speculum displacing the anterior vaginal wall. This allows for measurement of points Ap and Bp. Ap is always defined as a discrete point lying 3 cm proximal to the hymen.

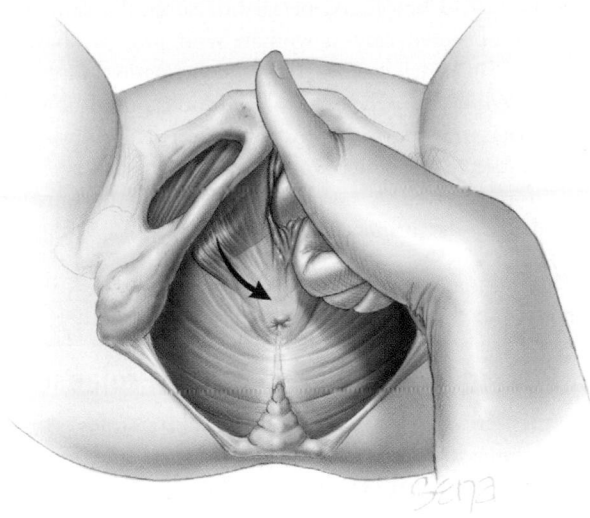

FIGURE 24-16 Drawing depicts pelvic floor muscle assessment. The index finger is placed 2 to 3 cm inside the hymen at 4 and 8 o'clock. Both resting and contraction tone and strength are evaluated. *(Image contributed by Ms. Marie Sena.)*

ual evaluation may help assess prolapse severity and clarify anatomy if surgical correction is planned (Barber, 1999; Whiteside, 2004).

Apical prolapse is believed to be the cause of most anterior and posterior wall descent. Therefore, careful attention is paid

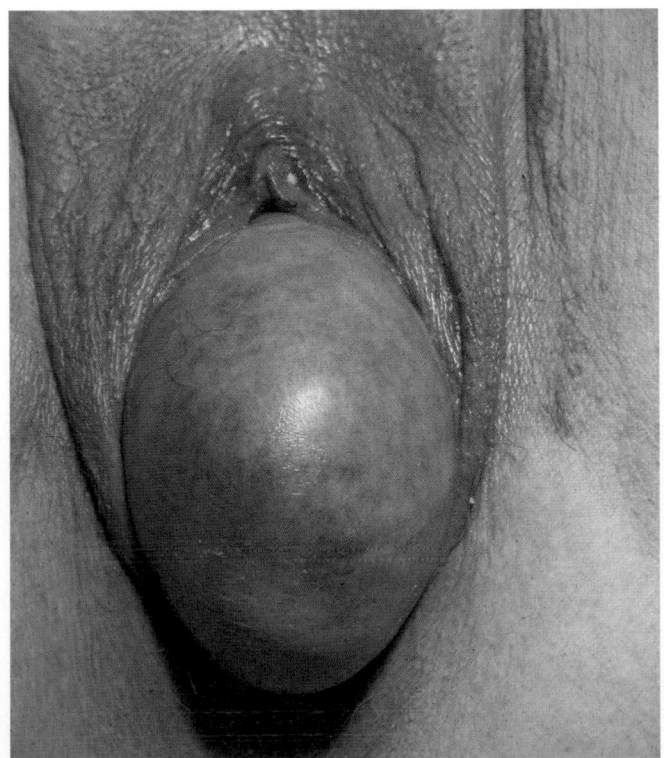

FIGURE 24-15 Photograph of enterocele. During evaluation, small bowel peristalsis may be noted behind the vaginal wall. Enterocele is most commonly noted at the vaginal apex, although anterior and posterior vaginal wall enteroceles may occur.

to the relationship of the apex to these structures. The apex should be replaced to its normal position. If this maneuver restores anterior and posterior support, it can be determined that the primary defect is at the apex.

Bimanual examination is performed to identify other pelvic pathology. In addition, we strongly recommend assessment of pelvic floor musculature (Fig. 11-6, p. 314). This examination is essential if pelvic floor rehabilitation is being considered as treatment. During part of the evaluation, an index finger is placed 1 to 3 cm inside the hymen, at 4 and then 8 o'clock (Fig. 24-16). Muscle resting tone and strength is assessed using the 0 through 5 Oxford grading scale, in which 5 represents normal tone and strength (Laycock, 2002). Muscle symmetry is also evaluated. Asymmetric muscles, with palpable defects or scarring, may be associated with a prior obstetric forceps delivery, episiotomy, or laceration.

APPROACH TO TREATMENT

For women who are asymptomatic or mildly symptomatic, expectant management is appropriate. However, for women with significant prolapse or for those with bothersome symptoms, nonsurgical or surgical therapy may be selected. Treatment choice depends on the type and severity of symptoms, age and medical comorbidities, desire for future sexual function and/or fertility, and risk factors for recurrence. Treatment should strive to provide symptom relief, but therapy benefits should always outweigh risks.

Often a combination of nonsurgical and surgical approaches may be selected. Symptoms should be ranked by severity, and options for each should be discussed. An evidence-based appraisal of each option's success rate should be included. In the simplest case, a patient with prolapse of the vaginal apex beyond the hymen, whose only symptom is bulge or pelvic pressure, could be offered pessary or surgical treatment. In a more complicated case, a woman with prolapse beyond the hymenal ring may note a bulge, constipation, urge urinary incontinence, and pelvic pain. Symptoms would be ranked as to severity and importance of resolution. To address all complaints, therapy might involve pessary or surgery for bulge symptoms, as well as nonsurgical treatment of constipation, urge urinary incontinence, and pelvic pain.

NONSURGICAL TREATMENT

Pessary Use in Pelvic Organ Prolapse

Pessaries are the standard nonsurgical treatment for POP. Throughout history, various vaginal devices and materials for prolapse have been described, including cloth, wood, wax, metal, ivory, bone, sponge, and cork. Today's pessaries are usually made of silicone or inert plastic, and they are safe and simple to manage. Despite a long history of use, literature describing their indications, selection, and management is often anecdotal or contradictory.

Indications for Use

Pelvic organ prolapse is still the most common indication for vaginal pessary. Traditionally, pessaries have been reserved for women either unfit or unwilling to undergo surgery. A survey of the American Urogynecologic Society membership confirmed this sentiment among gynecologists with greater than 20 years in practice (Cundiff, 2000). However, the same survey showed that younger gynecologists, particularly those who described themselves as urogynecologists, used pessaries as a first-line therapy before recommending surgery. Women who have undergone at least one previous attempt at surgical management without relief may often choose a pessary over additional surgery.

Pessaries may also help some women with prolapse and associated incontinence. One multicenter randomized crossover trial compared two pessary types for relief of prolapse symptoms and urinary complaints. This study demonstrated that pessaries provide a modest improvement in urinary obstructive, irritative, and stress symptoms (Schaffer, 2006) (Chap. 23, p. 625).

Pessaries may also be used diagnostically. As previously discussed, symptoms may not correlate with the type or severity of prolapse. Short-term pessary use may be helpful in this process. Even if a patient declines long-term pessary use, she may agree to a short trial to determine if her chief complaint is improved or resolved. A pessary may also be placed diagnostically to identify which women are at risk for urinary incontinence after prolapse-correcting surgery (Chaikin, 2000; Liang, 2004).

Types of Pessaries

Pessaries are divided into two broad categories: support and space-filling pessaries (Fig. 24-17). Support pessaries, such as the ring pessary, use a spring mechanism that rests in the posterior fornix and against the posterior aspect of the symphysis

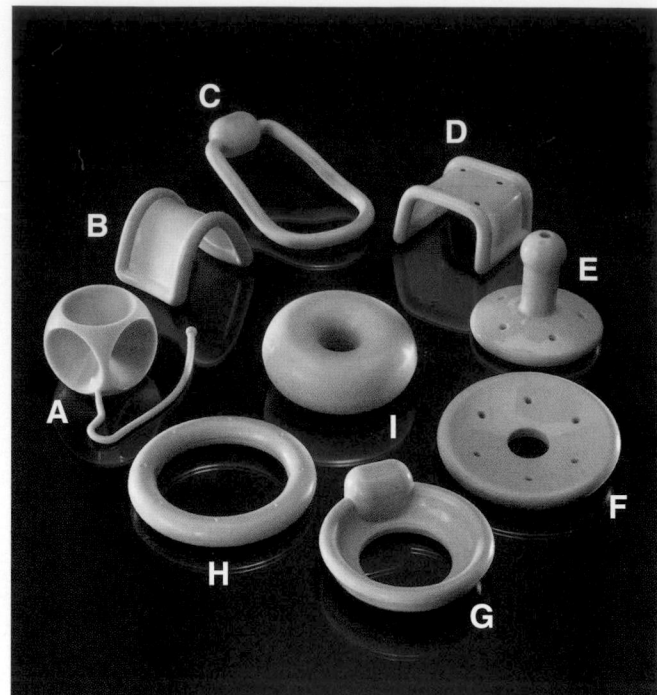

FIGURE 24-17 Photograph displays types of Milex pessaries. **A.** Cube pessary. **B.** Gehrung pessary. **C.** Hodge with knob pessary. **D.** Regula pessary. **E.** Gellhorn pessary. **F.** Shaatz pessary. **G.** Incontinence dish pessary. **H.** Ring pessary. **I.** Donut pessary. *(Reproduced with permission of CooperSurgical, Inc., Trumbull, CT.)*

pubis. Vaginal support results from elevation of the superior vagina by the spring, which is supported by the symphysis pubis. Ring pessaries may be constructed as a simple circular ring or as a ring with support that looks like a large contraceptive diaphragm (Fig. 24-18). These are effective in women with first- and second-degree prolapse. Also, the support ring's diaphragm is especially useful in women with accompanying anterior vaginal wall prolapse. When properly fitted, the device should lie behind the pubic symphysis anteriorly and behind the cervix posteriorly.

In contrast, space-filling pessaries maintain their position by creating suction between the pessary and vaginal walls (cube), by creating a diameter larger than the genital hiatus (donut), or by both mechanisms (Gellhorn). The Gellhorn is often used for moderate to severe prolapse and for complete procidentia. It contains a concave disc that fits against the cervix or vaginal cuff and has a stem that is positioned just cephalad to the introitus. The concave disc supports the vaginal apex by creating suction, and the stem is useful for device removal. Of all pessaries, the two most commonly used and studied devices are the ring and Gellhorn pessaries.

Patient Evaluation and Pessary Placement

A patient must be an active participant in the treatment decision to use a pessary. Its success will depend upon her

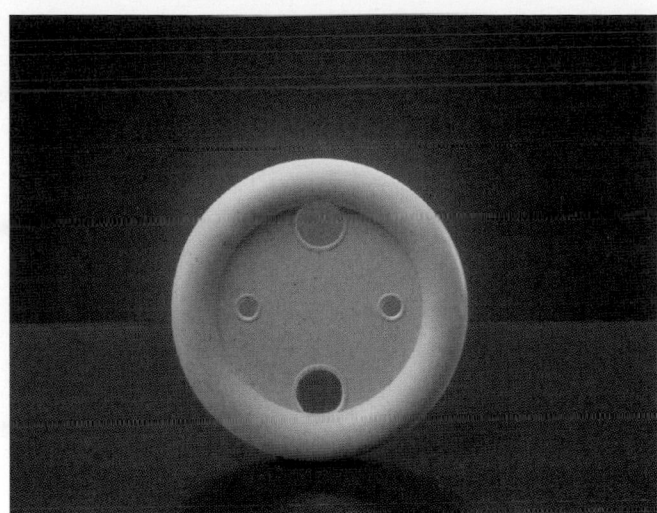

FIGURE 24-18 Milex ring pessary with support. *(Reproduced with permission of CooperSurgical, Inc., Trumbull, CT.)*

ability to care for the pessary—either alone or with the assistance of a caretaker—and her willingness and availability to come for subsequent evaluations. Vaginal atrophy should be treated before or concomitantly with pessary initiation. In women who are suitable candidates for estrogen therapy, vaginal estrogen cream is recommended (Table 22-6, p. 597). In one regimen, 1 g of conjugated equine estrogen cream (Premarin cream) is inserted nightly for 2 weeks, then two times per week thereafter.

The type of device selected may be affected by patient factors such as hormonal status, sexual activity, prior hysterectomy, and stage and site of POP. After a pessary is selected, a woman should be fitted with the largest size that can be comfortably worn. If a pessary is ideally fitted, a patient is not aware of its presence. As a woman ages and gains or loses weight, alternate sizes may be required.

Generally, a patient is fitted with a pessary while in the lithotomy position after she has emptied both her bladder and rectum. A digital examination is performed to assess vaginal length and width, and an initial estimation of pessary size is made. Figure 24-19 shows Gellhorn pessary placement. For ring pessary placement, the device is held in the clinician's dominant hand in a folded position. Lubricant is placed on either the vaginal introitus or the pessary's leading edge. While holding the labia apart, the pessary is inserted by pushing in an inferior, cephalad direction against the posterior vaginal wall. Next, an index finger is directed into the posterior vaginal fornix to ensure that the cervix is resting above the pessary. The clinician's finger should barely slide between the lateral edges of the ring pessary and the vaginal sidewall. The pessary should fit snugly but not tightly against the symphysis pubis and the posterior and lateral vaginal walls. Too much pressure may increase the risk for pain.

Following pessary placement, a woman is prompted to perform a Valsalva maneuver, which might dislodge an improperly fitted pessary. She should be able to stand, walk, cough, and urinate without difficulty or discomfort. Instruction on removal and placement should then follow. For removal of a ring pessary, an index finger is inserted into the vagina to hook the ring's leading edge. Traction is applied along the vaginal axis to bring the ring toward the introitus. Here, it may be grasped by the thumb and index finger and removed.

Ideally, a pessary is removed nightly to weekly, washed in soap and water, and replaced the next morning. Women are sent home from their initial fitting session with instructions describing the management of commonly encountered problems (Table 24-7). After initial placement, a return visit may follow in 1 to 2 weeks. For patients comfortable with their pessary management, return visits may be semiannual. For those unable or unwilling to remove and replace a device themselves, a pessary may be removed and the patient's vagina inspected at the provider's office every 2 or 3 months. Delaying visits longer than this may lead to problematic discharge and odor.

Complications with Pessary Use

Serious complications such as erosion into adjacent organs are rare with proper use and usually result only after years of neglect. At each return visit, the pessary is removed, and the vagina is inspected for erosions, abrasions, ulcerations, or granulation tissue (Fig. 24-20). Vaginal bleeding is usually an early sign and should not be ignored. *Pessary ulcers* or abrasions are treated by changing the pessary type or size to alleviate pressure points or by removing the pessary completely until healing occurs. *Prolapse ulcers* have the same appearance as pessary ulcers, however, the former result from the prolapsed bulge rubbing against patient clothing. These are treated by replacing the prolapse with either a pessary or surgery. Treatment of vaginal atrophy with local estrogen is commonly required. Alternatively, water-based lubricants applied to the pessary may help prevent these complications.

Pelvic pain with pessary use is not normal. This usually indicates that the size is too large and is an indication for substituting a smaller pessary. All pessaries tend to trap vaginal secretions and obstruct normal drainage to some degree. The resultant odor may be managed by encouraging more frequent nighttime device removal, washing, and reinsertion the next day. Alternatively, a woman may use a pH-based deodorant gel (Trimo-San gel) once or twice weekly or may douche with warm water. Trimo-San gel helps restore and maintain normal vaginal acidity that aids in reducing odor-causing bacteria.

■ Pelvic Floor Muscle Exercise

These exercises have been suggested as a therapy that might limit progression and alleviate prolapse symptoms. Also known as Kegel exercises, these muscle-strengthening techniques are described in Chapter 23 (p. 624). There are two hypotheses that describe the benefits of pelvic floor muscle

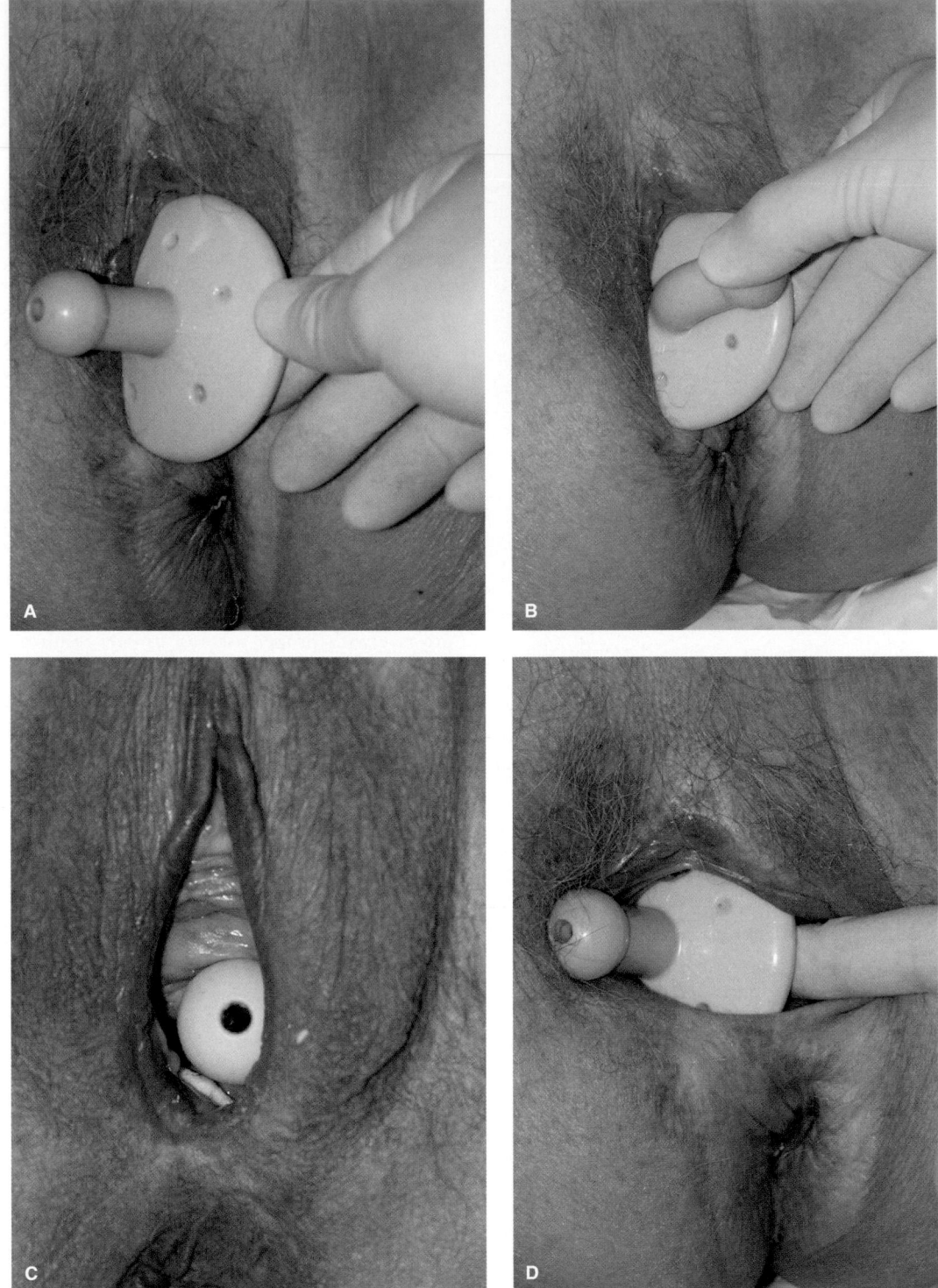

FIGURE 24-19 Photographs display technique for placement and removal of a Gellhorn pessary. Figures **A**, **B**, and **C** show placement. **D**. To remove a Gellhorn pessary, an index finger is placed behind the disc and suction is broken prior to removal.

exercise for prolapse prevention and treatment (Bø, 2004). First, from these exercises, women learn to consciously contract muscles before and during increases in abdominal pressure. This prevents organ descent. Alternatively, regular muscle strength training builds permanent muscle volume and structural support.

Unfortunately, high-quality scientific evidence supporting pelvic exercise for prevention and treatment of prolapse is lacking (Hagen, 2004). However, pelvic floor exercise has minimal risk and low cost. For this reason, it may be offered to asymptomatic or mildly symptomatic women who are interested in prevention of progression and who decline other treatments.

TABLE 24-7. Guidelines for Pessary Care

Pessary type_____
      Size_____

1. After your initial pessary fitting is successful, you will be asked to return for a follow-up appointment in about 2 weeks. The purpose of this visit is to check the pessary and examine the vagina to ensure that it is healthy. Follow-up appointments will follow this schedule:
      1st year: every 3–6 months
      2nd year and beyond: every 6 months
   You may learn to care for the pessary yourself. For those patients who can remove and insert the pessary themselves, we recommend weekly overnight removal and cleansing of the pessary with soap and warm water. These patients should see the doctor at least once per year.
2. The following is a list of problems you may encounter with the pessary and our recommendations for their management.

Problem	Management
A. The pessary falls out.	Keep the pessary and notify your doctor's office. An appointment will be made. It may be possible that a change in the size or the type of pessary is needed.
B. You experience pelvic pain.	Notify your doctor's office. If the pessary has slipped and you can remove it, do so. Otherwise, have your doctor remove the pessary. A change in pessary size or type may be needed.
C. Vaginal discharge and odor.	You can douche with warm water and you may want to try using Trimo-San vaginal gel 1-3 times a week.
D. Vaginal bleeding.	Vaginal bleeding may be a sign that the pessary is irritating the lining of the vagina. Call your doctor's office and arrange an appointment.
E. Leaking from the bladder.	Sometimes, the support provided by the pessary will cause leaking from the bladder. Notify your doctor and discuss this problem.

Trimo-San (Oxyquinolone, Milex Products, Chicago, IL) helps restore and maintain the normal vaginal acidity that helps reduce odor-causing bacteria.
From Farrell, 1997, with permission.

SURGICAL TREATMENT

Obliterative Procedures

The two approaches to prolapse surgery are obliterative and reconstructive. Obliterative approaches include Lefort colpocleisis and complete colpocleisis (Sections 43-24 and 43-25, p. 1246). These procedures involve removing vaginal epithelium, suturing anterior and posterior vaginal walls together, obliterating the vaginal vault, and effectively closing the vagina. Obliterative procedures are only appropriate for elderly or medically compromised patients who have no future desire for coital activity.

Obliterative procedures are technically easier, require less operative time, and offer superior success rates compared with reconstructive procedures. Success rates for colpocleisis range from 91 to 100 percent, although the quality of evidence-based studies supporting these rates is poor (FitzGerald, 2006). Fewer than 10 percent of patients express regret after colpocleisis, often due to loss of coital activity (FitzGerald, 2006; Wheeler, 2005). Therefore, the consent process must include an honest and thoughtful discussion with the patient and her partner regarding future sexual intercourse. Latent stress urinary incontinence can be unmasked with colpocleisis due to downward traction on the urethra. However, the morbidity of a concurrent antiincontinence procedure may outweigh the potential incontinence risk and should be considered before adding surgeries in women who may already be medically compromised.

Reconstructive Procedures

These surgeries attempt to restore normal pelvic anatomy and are more commonly performed for POP than obliterative procedures. Vaginal, abdominal, laparoscopic, and robotic approaches may be used, and selection is individualized. However, in the United States, a vaginal approach is preferred by most for prolapse repair (Boyles, 2003; Brown, 2002; Brubaker, 2005b; Olsen, 1997).

The decision to proceed with a vaginal, abdominal, or minimally invasive approach depends on multiple factors including the patient's unique characteristics and surgeon's expertise. An abdominal approach appears to have advantages in certain instances (Benson, 1996; Maher, 2004a,b). These include women with prior failure of a vaginal approach, those with a

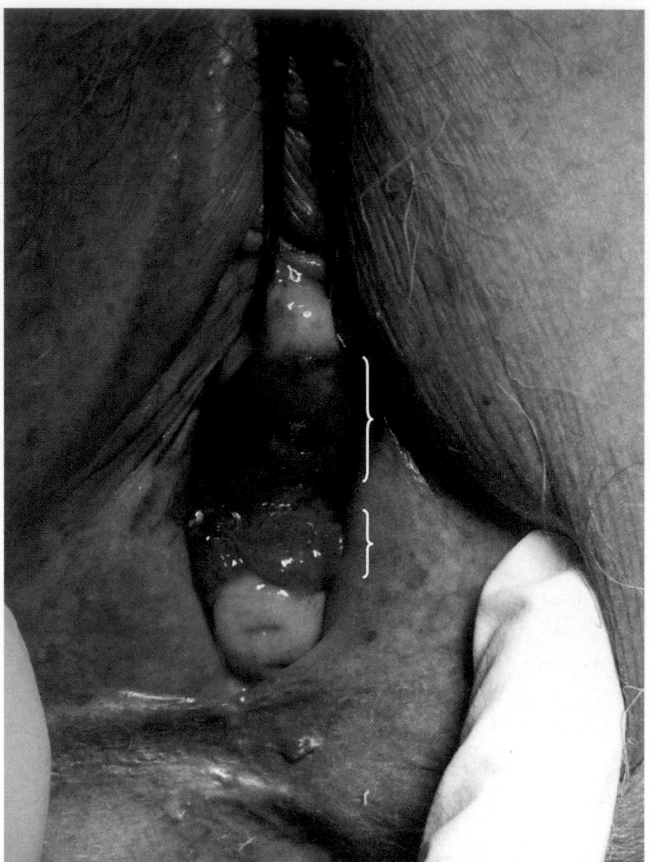

FIGURE 24-20 Photograph shows granulation tissue (*white brackets*) involving the anterior and posterior vaginal wall resulting from pessary trauma.

shortened vagina, or those believed to be at higher risk for recurrence, such as young women with severe prolapse. In contrast, a vaginal approach typically offers shorter operative time and a quicker return to daily activities.

Laparoscopy and Robotic Surgery

Laparoscopic and robotic approaches to prolapse repair are becoming more common. Procedures include sacrocolpopexy, uterosacral ligament vaginal vault suspension, paravaginal repair, and rectocele repair. Outcome studies of laparoscopic pelvic reconstruction, however, are mostly limited to case series (Higgs, 2005). Comparing laparoscopic and open approaches without randomized trials is difficult. However, surgeons with advanced laparoscopic skills who can perform the same operation laparoscopically should have equivalent results. Robotic laparoscopic sacrocolpopexy is currently performed in centers with the da Vinci Surgical System (Section 42-1, p. 1107). However, randomized trials that show equivalence or superiority of the robotic approach currently do not exist.

Surgical Plan

Reconstructive prolapse repair will often involve a combination of procedures in several vaginal compartments. However, the decision regarding which compartments to repair is not always straightforward. In the past, a defect-directed approach to pro-

lapse repair was preferred. With this strategy, all current, latent, or potential compensatory defects are evaluated and repaired. However, current expert opinion suggests that asymptomatic areas of prolapse do not always warrant repair, and in fact, correction can lead to de novo symptoms. For instance, repair of an asymptomatic posterior wall prolapse may lead to dyspareunia. Thus, surgery should be designed to relieve *current* symptoms.

Anterior Compartment

Many procedures for anterior vaginal wall prolapse repair have been described. Historically, anterior colporrhaphy has been the most common operation, yet long-term anatomic success rates are poor. In a randomized trial of three anterior colporrhaphy techniques (traditional midline plication, ultralateral repair, and traditional plication plus lateral reinforcement with synthetic mesh), Weber and associates (2001b) found a low rate of anatomic success. Satisfactory anatomic results were obtained in only 30 percent of the traditional group, 46 percent of the ultralateral group, and 42 percent of the traditional plus mesh group. These differences were not statistically significant. Although still frequently performed, the poor rates of anatomic success with traditional anterior colporrhaphy have prompted reevaluation of repair concepts and development of other procedures.

Despite these limitations, if a central or midline defect is suspected, anterior colporrhaphy may be performed (Section 43-13, p. 1214). Mesh or biomaterial may also be used in conjunction with anterior colporrhaphy or by itself. Mesh is used to reinforce the vaginal wall and is sutured in place laterally. However, the use of mesh and mesh kits for anterior vaginal wall prolapse remains controversial (American College of Obstetricians and Gynecologists, 2007). Although recent studies show improved anatomic success when mesh is used for anterior wall repair, there are significant risks. These include mesh erosion, pain, and dyspareunia and are discussed later on page 654 (Sung, 2008).

In many cases, anterior vaginal wall prolapse results from fibromuscular defects at the anterior apical segment or transverse detachment of the anterior apical segment from the vaginal apex. In these situations, an apical suspension procedure such as an abdominal sacrocolpopexy or uterosacral ligament vaginal vault suspension will resuspend the anterior vaginal wall to the apex and reduce anterior wall prolapse. With these procedures, continuity is also reestablished between the anterior and posterior vaginal fibromuscular layers to prevent enterocele formation.

Alternatively, if a lateral defect is suspected, paravaginal repair can be performed through a vaginal, abdominal, or laparoscopic route (Section 43-14, p. 1217). Paravaginal repair is performed by reattaching the fibromuscular layer of the vaginal wall to the arcus tendineus fascia pelvis.

Vaginal Apex

There is a growing appreciation that support of the vaginal apex provides the cornerstone for a successful prolapse repair. Some experts believe that isolated surgical repair of the anterior and posterior walls is doomed for failure if the apex is not adequately supported (Brubaker, 2005a).

The vaginal apex can be resuspended with a number of procedures including abdominal sacrocolpopexy, sacrospinous ligament fixation, or uterosacral ligament vaginal vault suspension.

Abdominal Sacrocolpopexy. This surgery suspends the vaginal vault to the sacrum using synthetic mesh. Advantages include the procedure's durability over time and conservation of normal vaginal anatomy. For example, compared with other vault suspension procedures, sacrocolpopexy offers greater vaginal apex mobility and avoids vaginal shortening. In addition, sacrocolpopexy provides enduring correction of apical prolapse, and long-term success rates approximate 90 percent. This procedure may be used primarily or as a second surgery for women with recurrences after failure of other prolapse repairs. Sacrocolpopexy may be performed as an abdominal, laparoscopic, or robotic procedure (Section 43-17, p. 1225). When hysterectomy is performed in conjunction with sacrocolpopexy, consideration should be given to performing a supracervical rather than a total abdominal hysterectomy. With the cervix left in situ, the risk of postoperative mesh erosion at the vaginal apex is believed to be diminished. This results from a lack of exposure of the mesh to vaginal bacteria that occurs when the vagina is opened with total abdominal hysterectomy. In addition, the strong connective tissue of the cervix allows for an additional anchoring point for the permanent mesh.

Sacrospinous Ligament Fixation. This is one of the most popular procedures for apical suspension. The vaginal apex is suspended to the sacrospinous ligament unilaterally or bilaterally using a vaginal extraperitoneal approach. After sacrospinous ligament fixation (SSLF), recurrent apical prolapse is uncommon. However, anterior vaginal wall prolapse develops postoperatively in 6 to 28 percent of patients (Benson, 1996; Morley, 1988; Paraiso, 1996). Complications associated with SSLF include buttock pain from nerve involvement with supporting ligatures in 3 percent of patients and vascular injury in 1 percent (Sze, 1997a,b). Although infrequent, significant and life-threatening hemorrhage can follow injury to blood vessels located behind the sacrospinous ligament (Fig. 38-6, p. 923).

Uterosacral Ligament Vaginal Vault Suspension. With this procedure, the vaginal apex is attached to remnants of the uterosacral ligament at the level of the ischial spines or higher (Sections 43-19 and 43-20, p. 1234). Performed vaginally or abdominally, the uterosacral ligament vaginal vault suspension is believed to replace the vaginal apex to a more anatomic position than SSLF, which deflects the vagina posteriorly (Barber, 2000; Maher, 2004b; Shull, 2000).

This procedure has been adopted by many surgeons in the United States in attempts to reduce the rates of anterior vaginal prolapse recurrence following SSLF (Shull, 2000). Although uterosacral ligament vaginal vault suspension has gained wide popularity, studies supporting its use are limited to retrospective case series (Amundsen, 2003; Karram, 2001; Silva, 2006). In these studies and others, anterior vaginal prolapse recurrence rates range from 1 to 7 percent, and overall recurrence rates from 4 to 18 percent.

Hysterectomy at the Time of Prolapse Repair

In the United States, hysterectomy is often performed concurrently with prolapse surgery. Conversely, in many European countries, it is rarely performed during pelvic floor reconstruction. Although arguments exist for both, a comparison has not been performed in randomized prospective trials.

If apical or uterine prolapse is present, hysterectomy will more readily allow the vaginal apex to be resuspended with the previously described apical suspension procedures. If hysterectomy is not performed in the context of apical prolapse, these procedures must be modified or specific uterine suspension procedures performed (not described in this text). Alternatively, if apical or cervical prolapse is not present, hysterectomy need not be incorporated into prolapse repair.

Posterior Compartment

Enterocele Repair. Posterior vaginal wall prolapse may be due to enterocele or rectocele. Enterocele is defined as herniation of the small bowel through the vaginal fibromuscular layer, usually at the vaginal apex. Discontinuity of the anterior and posterior vaginal wall fibromuscular layers allows for this herniation. Accordingly, enterocele repairs have as their goal reattachment of these fibromuscular layers. If posterior wall prolapse is due to enterocele, repair of this defect should reduce the posterior wall prolapse.

Rectocele Repair. Posterior vaginal wall prolapse due to rectocele is repaired with one of several techniques. Traditional posterior colporrhaphy aims to rebuild the fibromuscular layer between the rectum and vagina by performing a midline fibromuscular plication (Section 43-15, p. 1219). The anatomic cure rate is 76 to 96 percent, and most studies report a greater than 75-percent improvement rate of bulge symptoms (Cundiff, 2004). To narrow the genital hiatus and prevent recurrence, some surgeons plicate the levator ani muscles concurrently with posterior repair. However, this practice may contribute to dyspareunia rates of 12 to 27 percent (Kahn, 1997; Mellegren, 1995; Weber, 2000). Thus, it is best avoided in women who are sexually active.

Site-Specific Posterior Repair. This approach to posterior vaginal wall prolapse was first described by Richardson in 1993. This repair is based on the assumption that specific tears exist in the fibromuscular layer, which can be identified and repaired in a discrete fashion (Section 43-15, p. 1219). Defects may be midline, lateral, distal, or superior (Fig. 24-21). This approach is conceptually analogous to a fascial hernia, in which the fascial tear is identified and repaired. Thus, its theoretical advantage lies in its restoration of normal anatomy rather than plication of tissue in the midline.

Site-specific repair has gained wide acceptance, however, anatomic cure rates range from 56 to 100 percent, similar to that with traditional posterior colporrhaphy (Muir, 2007). Moreover, anatomic and functional long-term outcomes are not known.

Mesh Reinforcement. In an effort to reduce prolapse recurrence, graft augmentation with allograft, xenograft, or synthetic

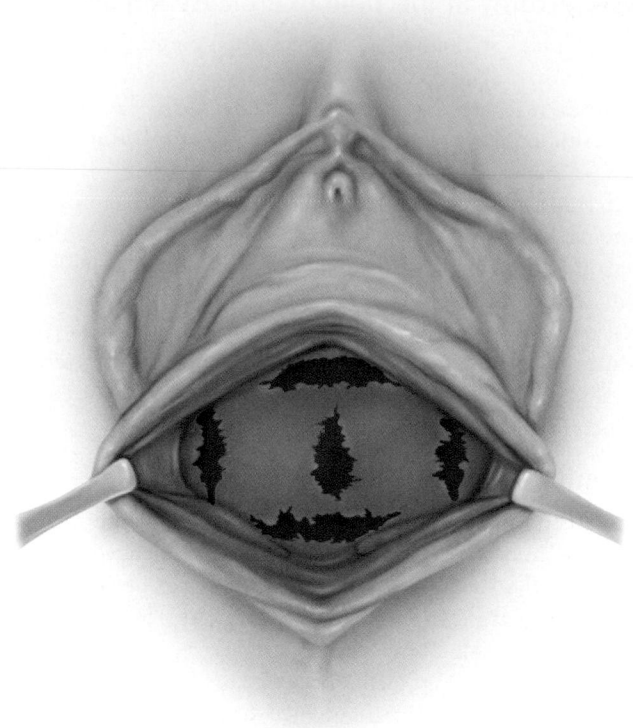

FIGURE 24-21 Drawing depicts posterior vaginal wall defects. These may be midline, lateral, distal, or apical. *(From Richardson, 1993, with permission.)*

mesh has been used in conjunction with posterior colporrhaphy and site-specific repair. Generally, the graft is placed after colporrhaphy or site-specific repair is completed. Moreover, in situations in which the fibromuscular layer cannot be identified to perform a midline plication or site-specific repair, graft augmentation may be the only surgical option.

Mesh is sutured in place laterally with a minimum number of sutures. If technically possible, the graft is attached to the vaginal apex and the uterosacral ligament. Distally, the graft is attached to the perineal body.

The efficacy and safety of graft augmentation in the posterior vaginal wall has not been established. Paraiso and coworkers (2006) randomly assigned 105 women to posterior colporrhaphy, site-specific repair, or site-specific repair plus a graft using porcine small intestine submucosa. After 1 year, those with graft augmentation had a significantly higher anatomic failure rate (46 percent) than those who received site-specific repair alone (22 percent) or posterior colporrhaphy (14 percent). More research is needed to determine the safety, efficacy, and optimal material for posterior wall graft augmentation.

Sacrocolpoperineopexy. This modification of sacrocolpopexy may be selected for correction of posterior vaginal wall descent when an abdominal approach is employed for other prolapse procedures or if treatment of perineal descent is necessary (Cundiff, 1997; Lyons, 1997; Sullivan, 2001; Visco, 2001). With this procedure, the posterior sacrocolpopexy mesh is extended down the posterior vaginal wall to the perineal body. In several case series, anatomic cure rates were greater than 75 percent.

Perineum

The perineum provides distal support to the posterior vaginal wall and anterior rectal wall and anchors these structures to the pelvic floor. A disrupted perineal body will allow descent of the distal vagina and rectum and will contribute to a widened levator hiatus.

Perineorrhaphy is often done in conjunction with posterior colporrhaphy to recreate normal anatomy (Section 43-16, p. 1223). During surgery, the perineum is rebuilt through midline plication of the perineal muscles and connective tissue. Importantly, overly aggressive plication can narrow the introitus, create a posterior vaginal wall ridge, and lead to entry dyspareunia. However, in a woman who is not sexually active, high perineorrhaphy with intentional introital narrowing is believed to decrease the risk of posterior wall prolapse recurrence.

The Use of Mesh and Materials in Reconstructive Pelvic Surgery

Mesh Indications. Approximately 30 percent of women undergoing surgery for prolapse will require a repeat operation for recurrence (Olsen, 1997). As such, there is a continuous effort to improve surgical procedures and outcomes.

Synthetic mesh for sacrocolpopexy and midurethral slings has been widely studied and is safe and effective. Mesh erosion occurs in a small percentage of cases but can be managed with local estrogen therapy and limited vaginal wall mesh excision. Rarely is excision of the entire mesh warranted. In an attempt to limit erosion rates, surgeons have used biologic material grafts, including cadaveric fascia. However, high rates of prolapse recurrence are associated with this material (FitzGerald, 1999, 2004; Gregory, 2005). Therefore, synthetic mesh is recommended for sacrocolpopexy and midurethral slings.

The use of biologic grafts or synthetic mesh for other transvaginal reconstructive pelvic surgery has expanded rapidly in the absence of supporting long-term safety and efficacy data. Some surgeons routinely use graft or mesh augmentation, others never use it, and some use it only for limited indications. Selective use may include: (1) the need to bridge a space, (2) weak or absent connective tissue, (3) connective tissue disease, (4) high risk for recurrence (obesity, chronically increased intraabdominal pressure, and young age), and (5) shortened vagina.

Despite the common use of mesh or grafts, one systematic review on their use in transvaginal prolapse repair found a lack of high-quality scientific data to support this practice (Sung, 2008). Since this review, several randomized prospective study found that mesh use compared with no mesh for anterior colporrhaphy yielded higher short-term rates of successful prolapse treatment. However, more surgical complications and postoperative adverse events were associated with mesh use in these studies (Altman, 2011). In 2011, the U.S. Food and Drug administration (FDA) reported the potentially serious complications associated with surgical mesh for transvaginal repair of POP. Noted complications included mesh erosion, scarring, pain, and dyspareunia. Additionally, synthetic mesh may become ingrown and difficult to remove. Complications may therefore be irreversible. Thus, the FDA urges clinicians to weigh the risks versus theoretical benefit of this practice

TABLE 24-8. Types of Surgical Mesh

Type I:	Macroporous. Pore size >75 μm (size required for infiltration by macrophages, fibroblasts, blood vessels during angiogenesis, and collagen fibers) *GyneMesh, Atrium, Marlex, Prolene*
Type II:	Microporous. Pore size <10 μm in at least one dimension *Gore Tex*
Type III:	Macroporous patch with multifilaments or a microporous component *Teflon, Mersilene, Surgipro, Mycro Mesh*
Type IV:	Submicronic. Pore size <1 μm. Often used in association with type I mesh for intraperitoneal adhesion prevention *Silastic, Cellgard, Preclude*

Compiled from Amid, 1997.

in their patients. The American College of Obstetricians and Gynecologists (2007) echoes these concerns.

Mesh Material. Surgeons using mesh or grafts should be familiar with the different types and their characteristics. Biologic grafts may be autologous, allograft, or xenograft. *Autologous* grafts are harvested from another part of the patient's body such as rectus abdominis fascia or thigh fascia lata. Morbidity is low, but may include increased operative time, pain, hematoma, or weakened fascia at the harvest site. *Allografts* come from a human source other than the patient and include cadaveric fascia or cadaveric dermis. *Xenografts* are biologic tissue obtained from a source or species foreign to the patient such as porcine

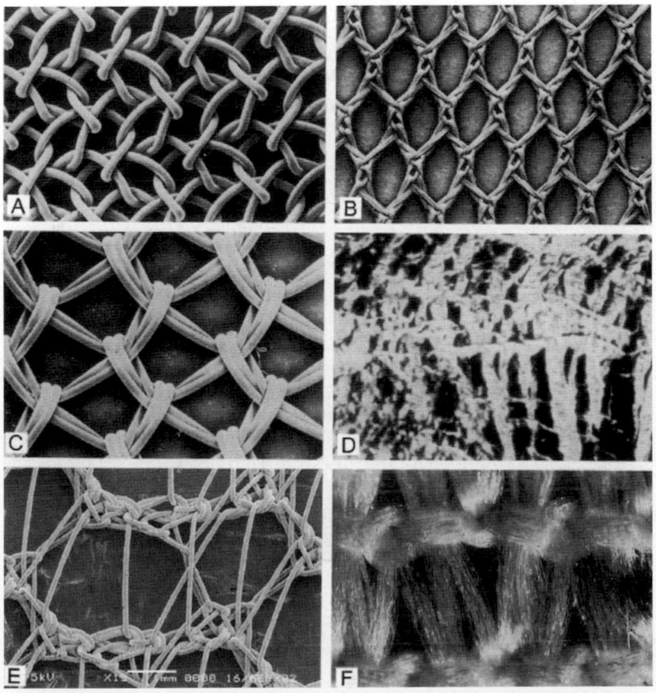

dermis, porcine small intestinal submucosa, or bovine pericardium. Biologic materials have varying biomechanical properties and as noted earlier, are associated with high rates of prolapse recurrence. Thus, recommendations on the appropriate clinical situations for biologic material are limited.

Synthetic mesh is classified as types I through IV, based on pore size (Table 24-8 and Fig. 24-22) (Amid, 1997). Pore size is the most important property of synthetic mesh. Bacteria generally measure less than 1 μm, whereas granulocytes and macrophages are typically larger than 10 μm. Thus, a mesh with pore size <10 μm may allow bacterial but not macrophage infiltration and thereby predispose to infection. Accordingly, type I mesh has the lowest rate of infection compared with types II and III. Pore size is also the basis of tissue ingrowth, angiogenesis, flexibility, and strength. Pore sizes of 50 to 200 μm allow for superior tissue ingrowth and collagen infiltration. This again favors type I. Meshes are either monofilament or multifilament. Multifilament mesh has small intrafiber pores that can harbor bacteria, therefore, monofilament mesh is recommended. From these findings, consensus suggests that if synthetic mesh is used, type I monofilament is the best choice for reconstructive pelvic surgery.

Mesh or graft augmentation will undoubtedly persist due to the current poor cure rates with traditional transvaginal repairs. However, evidence to guide the surgeon and provide a patient with accurate safety and efficacy information is scant. Moreover, industry-driven, premature adoption of untested materials and procedures has historically led to unacceptable complications. For these reasons, randomized, prospective trials comparing traditional repairs with graft or mesh augmentation are needed.

Concomitant Prolapse and Incontinence Surgery

Prior to prolapse surgery, women should be evaluated for stress urinary incontinence (SUI) (Chap. 23, p. 616). Those with bothersome SUI symptoms should be considered for concurrent antiincontinence surgery. However, in women without SUI symptoms, latent stress incontinence may be unmasked or SUI may develop de novo following prolapse repair. Therefore, preoperative urodynamic testing with the prolapse replaced is recommended. If stress incontinence is demonstrated, these

FIGURE 24-22 Photograph depicts different types of surgical mesh. **A.** Marlex. **B.** Mersilene. **C.** Prolene. **D.** Gore-Tex. **E.** Gynemesh-PS. **F.** IVS (intravaginal slingplasty) mesh. (*From Iglesia, 1997, with permission.*)

patients also should be considered for a concurrent anti-incontinence operation. This has been a difficult decision for patients and surgeons because a procedure with known risks is being performed for a problem that does not currently exist and may never develop.

However, the CARE (Colpopexy and Urinary Reduction Efforts) trial has helped clarify this problem (Brubaker, 2006). Women undergoing abdominal sacrocolpopexy for prolapse (anterior vaginal wall stage 2 or greater) who did not exhibit symptoms of stress incontinence were randomized to undergo concurrent Burch colposuspension or not. Preoperative urodynamic testing was performed, but surgeons were blinded to the results. Three months after surgery, 24 percent of women in the Burch group and 44 percent of women in the control group met one or more criteria for stress incontinence. The incontinence was bothersome in 6 percent of the Burch group and 24 percent of the control group.

These data can be interpreted in several ways. It can be argued that all women undergoing sacrocolpopexy for stage 2 or greater anterior vaginal wall prolapse should undergo Burch colposuspension, as 44 percent will develop stress incontinence symptoms. However, the opposing argument is that only 24 percent will develop bothersome incontinence symptoms, thus three quarters of women would be subjected to an unnecessary operation.

Importantly, this study provides Level 1 evidence for a surgeon to share during patient counseling. The authors of this study caution that these data cannot be extrapolated to other prolapse and incontinence surgeries. However, in lieu of other Level 1 evidence, surgeons can still use this information in surgical planning and presurgical patient discussions.

Defining Surgical Success

In preparing for prolapse surgery, the patient should have an understanding of the expected results, and the surgeon should have an understanding of the patient's expectations. Treatment success varies widely based on the definition of success. Thus, the surgeon and the patient must agree on the desired results. Generally, patients seek relief of symptoms, whereas surgeons may view surgical success as restoration of anatomy. In the CARE trial, absence of vaginal bulge symptoms had the strongest relationship to a patient's assessment of overall improvement and surgical success, whereas anatomic success alone did not (Barber, 2009). It is therefore recommended that surgical success be defined as absence of bulge symptoms in addition to anatomic criteria.

REFERENCES

Adams E, Thomson A, Maher C: Mechanical devices for pelvic organ prolapse in women. Cochrane Database Syst Rev 2:CD004010, 2004

Altman D, Väyrynen T, Engh ME, et al: Anterior colporrhaphy versus transvaginal mesh for pelvic-organ prolapse. N Engl J Med 364(19):1826, 2011

American College of Obstetricians and Gynecologists: Cesarean delivery on maternal request. Committee Opinion No. 394, December 2007

American College of Obstetricians and Gynecologists: Pelvic organ prolapse. Practice Bulletin No. 85, September, 2007

Amid PK: Classification of biomaterials and their related complications in abdominal wall hernia surgery. Hernia 1:15, 1997

Amundsen CL, Flynn BJ, Webster GD: Anatomical correction of vaginal vault prolapse by uterosacral ligament fixation in women who also require a pubovaginal sling. J Urol 169:1770, 2003

Baden WF, Walker T: Fundamentals, symptoms and classification. In Surgical Repair of Vaginal Defect. Philadelphia, JB Lippincott, 1992, p 14

Baden WF, Walker TA: Genesis of the vaginal profile: a correlated classification of vaginal relaxation. Clin Obstet Gynecol 15:1048, 1972

Barber MD: Symptoms and outcome measures of pelvic organ prolapse. Clin Obstet Gynecol 48:648, 2005a

Barber MD, Brubaker L, Nygaard I, et al: Defining success after surgery for pelvic organ prolapse. Obstet Gynecol 114:600, 2009

Barber MD, Cundiff GW, Weidner AC, et al: Accuracy of clinical assessment of paravaginal defects in women with anterior wall prolapse. Am J Obstet Gynecol 181:87, 1999

Barber MD, Visco AG, Weidner AC, et al: Bilateral uterosacral ligament vaginal vault suspension with site-specific endopelvic fascia defect repair for treatment of pelvic organ prolapse. Am J Obstet Gynecol 183:1402, 2000

Barber MD, Walters MD, Bump RC: Association of the magnitude of pelvic organ prolapse and presence and severity of symptoms. J Pelvic Med Surg 9:208, 2003

Barber MD, Walters MD, Bump RC: Short forms of two condition-specific quality-of-life questionnaires for women with pelvic floor disorders (PFDI-20 and PFIQ-7). Am J Obstet Gynecol 193:103, 2005b

Benson JT, Lucente V, McClellan E: Vaginal versus abdominal reconstructive surgery for the treatment of pelvic support defects: a prospective randomized study with long-term outcome evaluation. Am J Obstet Gynecol 175:1418, 1996

Bland DR, Earle BB, Vitolins MZ, et al: Use of the Pelvic Organ Prolapse staging system of the International Continence Society, American Urogynecologic Society, and the Society of Gynecologic Surgeons in perimenopausal women. Am J Obstet Gynecol 181:1324, 1999

Blandon RE, Bharucha AE, Melton LJ 3rd, et al: Risk factors for pelvic floor repair after hysterectomy. Obstet Gynecol 113(3):601, 2009

Bø K: Pelvic floor muscle training is effective in treatment of stress urinary incontinence, but how does it work? Int Urogynecol J 15:76, 2004

Boreham M, Marinis S, Keller P, et al: Gene expression profiling of the pubococcygeus in premenopausal women with pelvic organ prolapse. J Pelv Med Surg 4:253, 2009

Boreham MK, Miller RT, Schaffer JI, et al: Smooth muscle myosin heavy chain and caldesmon expression in the anterior vaginal wall of women with and without pelvic organ prolapse. Am J Obstet Gynecol 185:944, 2001

Boreham MK, Wai CY, Miller RT, et al: Morphometric analysis of smooth muscle in the anterior vaginal wall of women with pelvic organ prolapse. Am J Obstet Gynecol 187:56, 2002a

Boreham MK, Wai CY, Miller RT, et al: Morphometric properties of the posterior vaginal wall in women with pelvic organ prolapse. Am J Obstet Gynecol 187:1501, 2002b

Boyles SH, Weber AM, Meyn L: Procedures for pelvic organ prolapse in the United States, 1979–1997. Am J Obstet Gynecol 188:108, 2003

Bradley CS, Nygaard IE: Vaginal wall descensus and pelvic floor symptoms in older women. Obstet Gynecol 106:759, 2005

Brincat M, Moniz CF, Studd JWW, et al: Sex hormone and skin collagen content in postmenopausal women. BMJ 287:1337, 1983

Brown JS, Waetjien LE, Subak LL, et al: Pelvic organ prolapse surgery in the United States, 1997. Am J Obstet Gynecol 186:712, 2002

Brubaker L: Burch colposuspension at the time of sacrocolpopexy in stress continent women reduces bothersome stress urinary symptoms: the CARE randomized trial. J Pelvic Surg 11(Suppl 1):S5, 2005a

Brubaker L, Bump R, Fynes M, et al: Surgery for pelvic organ prolapse. In Abrams P, Cardozo L, Khoury W, et al (eds): 3rd International Consultation on Incontinence. Paris: Health Publication, 2005b, p 1371

Brubaker L, Cundiff GW, Fine P, et al: Pelvic Floor Disorders Network. Abdominal sacrocolpopexy with Burch colposuspension to reduce urinary stress incontinence. N Engl J Med 354:1557, 2006

Bump RC, Mattiasson A, Bø K, et al: The standardization of terminology of female pelvic organ prolapse and pelvic floor dysfunction. Am J Obstet Gynecol 175:10, 1996

Burrows LJ, Meyn LA, Walters MD, et al: Pelvic symptoms in women with pelvic organ prolapse. Obstet Gynecol 104:982, 2004

Carley ME, Schaffer J: Urinary incontinence and pelvic organ prolapse in women with Marfan or Ehlers Danlos syndrome. Am J Obstet Gynecol 182:1021, 2000

Carroli G, Belizan J: Episiotomy for vaginal birth. Cochrane Database Syst Rev 2:CD000081, 2000

Chaikin DC, Groutz A, Blaivas JG: Predicting the need for anti-incontinence surgery in continent women undergoing repair of severe urogenital prolapse. J Urol 163:531, 2000

Cundiff GW, Fenner D: Evaluation and treatment of women with rectocele: focus on associated defecatory and sexual dysfunction. Obstet Gynecol 104:1403, 2004

Cundiff GW, Harris RL, Coates K, et al: Abdominal sacral colpoperineopexy: a new approach for correction of posterior compartment defects and perineal descent associated with vaginal vault prolapse. Am J Obstet Gynecol 177:1345, 1997

Cundiff GW, Weidner AC, Visco AG, et al: A survey of pessary use by the membership of the American Urogynecologic Society. Obstet Gynecol 95:931, 2000

DeLancey JO: Anatomy and biomechanics of genital prolapse. Clin Obstet Gynecol 36:897, 1993

DeLancey JOL: Anatomic aspects of vaginal eversion after hysterectomy. Am J Obstet Gynecol 166:1717, 1992

Ellerkmann RM, Cundiff GW, Melick CF, et al: Correlation of symptoms with location and severity of pelvic organ prolapse. Am J Obstet Gynecol 185:1332, 2001

Farrell SA: Practical advice for ring pessary fitting and management. J SOGC 19:625, 1997

FitzGerald MP, Edwards SR, Fenner D: Medium-term follow-up on use of freeze-dried, irradiated donor fascia for sacrocolpopexy and sling procedures. Int Urogynecol J Pelvic Floor Dysfunct 15(4):238, 2004

FitzGerald MP, Kulkarni N, Fenner D: Postoperative resolution of urinary retention in patients with advanced pelvic organ prolapse. Am J Obstet Gynecol 183:1361, 2000

FitzGerald MP, Mollenhauer J, Bitterman P, et al: Functional failure of fascia lata allografts. Am J Obstet Gynecol 181:1339, 1999

FitzGerald MP, Richter HE, Sohail S, et al: Colpocleisis: a review. Int Urogynecol J 17:261, 2006

Flynn MK, Amundsen CL: Diagnosis of pelvic organ prolapse. In Chapple CR, Zimmern PE, Brubaker L, et al (eds): Multidisciplinary Management of Female Pelvic Floor Disorders. Philadelphia, Elsevier, 2006, p 118

Gilpin SA, Gosling JA, Smith AR, et al: The pathogenesis of genitourinary prolapse and stress incontinence of urine. A histological and histochemical study. Br J Obstet Gynaecol 96:15, 1989

Gregory WT, Otto LN, Bergstrom JO, et al: Surgical outcome of abdominal sacrocolpopexy with synthetic mesh versus abdominal sacrocolpopexy with cadaveric fascia lata. Int Urogynecol J Pelvic Floor Dysfunct 16:369, 2005

Hagen S, Stark D, Maher C, et al: Conservative management of pelvic organ prolapse in women. Cochrane Database Syst Rev (2):CD003882, 2004

Handa VL, Cundiff G, Chang HH, et al: Female sexual function and pelvic floor disorders. Obstet Gynecol 111(5):1045, 2008

Hanzal E, Berger E, Koelbl H: Levator ani muscle morphology and recurrent genuine stress incontinence. Obstet Gynecol 81:426, 1993

Harris T, Bent A: Genital prolapse with and without urinary incontinence. J Reprod Med 35:792, 1990

Haylen BT, de Ridder D, Freeman RM, et al: An International Urogynecologic Association (IUGA)/International Continence Society (ICS) joint report on the terminology for female pelvic floor dysfunction. Int Urogynecol J Pelvic Floor Dysfunct 21:5, 2010

Heit M, Benson JT, Russell B, et al: Levator ani muscle in women with genitourinary prolapse: indirect assessment by muscle histopathology. Neurourol Urodyn 15:17, 1996

Heit M, Culligan P, Rosenquist C, et al: Is pelvic organ prolapse a cause of pelvic or low back pain? Obstet Gynecol 99:23, 2002

Hendrix SL, Clark A, Nygaard I, et al: Pelvic organ prolapse in the Women's Health Initiative: gravity and gravidity. Am J Obstet Gynecol 186:1160, 2002

Higgs PF, Chua HL, Smith AR: Long-term review of laparoscopic sacrocolpopexy. BJOG 112:1134, 2005

Iglesia CB, Fenner DE, Brubaker L: The use of mesh in gynecologic surgery. Int Urogynecol J Pelvic Floor Dysfunct 8(2):105, 1997

Jelovsek JE, Barber MD, Paraiso MFR, et al: Functional bowel and anorectal disorders in patients with pelvic organ prolapse and incontinence. Am J Obstet Gynecol 193:2105, 2005

Jorgensen S, Hein HO, Gyntelberg F: Heavy lifting at work and risk of genital prolapse and herniated lumbar disc in assistant nurses. Occup Med (Lond) 44:47, 1994

Kahn MA, Breitkopf CR, Valley MT, et al: Pelvic Organ Support Study (POSST) and bowel symptoms: straining at stool is associated with perineal and anterior vaginal descent in a general gynecologic population. Am J Obstet Gynecol 192:1516, 2005

Kahn MA, Stanton SL: Posterior colporrhaphy: its effects on bowel and sexual function. Br J Obstet Gynaecol 104:82, 1997

Karram M, Goldwasser S, Kleeman S, et al: High uterosacral vaginal vault suspension with fascial reconstruction for vaginal repair of enterocele and vaginal vault prolapse. Am J Obstet Gynecol 185:1339, 2001

Kenton K, Shott S, Brubaker L: Outcomes after rectovaginal fascia reattachment for rectocele repair. Am J Obstet Gynecol 181:1360, 1999

Kim S, Harvey MA, Johnston S: A review of the epidemiology and pathophysiology of pelvic floor dysfunction: do racial differences matter? J Obstet Gynaecol Cancer 27:251, 2005

Koelbl H, Strasegger H, Riss PA, et al: Morphologic and functional aspects of pelvic floor muscles in patients with pelvic relaxation and genuine stress incontinence. Obstet Gynecol 74:789, 1989

Laycock J: Patient assessment. In Laycock J, Haslam J (eds): Therapeutic Management of Incontinence and Pelvic Pain. Pelvic Organ Disorders. London, Springer-Verlag London, 2002, p 52

Liang CC, Chang YL, Chang SD, et al: Pessary test to predict postoperative urinary incontinence in women undergoing hysterectomy for prolapse. Obstet Gynecol 104:795, 2004

Lyons TL, Winer WK: Laparoscopic rectocele repair using polyglactin mesh. J Am Assoc Gynecol Laparosc 4:381, 1997

Maher C, Baessler K, Glazener CMA, et al: Surgical management of pelvic organ prolapse in women. Cochrane Database Syst Rev 4:CD004014, 2004a

Maher CF, Qatawneh AM, Dwyer PL, et al: Abdominal sacral colpopexy or vaginal sacrospinous colpopexy for vaginal vault prolapse: a prospective randomized study. Am J Obstet Gynecol 190:20, 2004b

Mant J, Painter R, Vessey M: Epidemiology of genital prolapse: observations from the Oxford Family Planning Association Study. Br J Obstet Gynaecol 104:579, 1997

Mellegren A, Anzen B, Nilsson BY, et al: Results of rectocele repair: a prospective study. Dis Colon Rectum 38:7, 1995

Moalli PA, Shand SH, Zyczynski HM, et al: Remodeling of vaginal connective tissue in patients with prolapse. Obstet Gynecol 106:953, 2005

Moalli PA, Talarico LC, Sung VW, et al: Impact of menopause on collagen subtypes in the arcus tendineous fasciae pelvis. Am J Obstet Gynecol 190(3):620, 2004

Morley GW, DeLancey JO: Sacrospinous ligament fixation for eversion of the vagina. Am J Obstet Gynecol 158:872, 1988

Muir TW: Surgical treatment of rectocele and perineal defects. In Walters MD, Karram MM (eds): Urogynecology and Reconstructive Pelvic Surgery, 3rd ed. Philadelphia, Mosby-Elsevier, 2007, p 254

Nichols DH, Randall CL: Types of genital prolapse. In Nichols DH, Randall CL (eds): Vaginal Surgery, 3rd ed. Baltimore, Williams & Wilkins, 1989, p 64

Norton PA, Baker JE, Sharp HC, et al: Genitourinary prolapse and joint hypermobility in women. Obstet Gynecol 85:225, 1995

Nygaard I, Barber MD, Burgio KL, et al: Prevalence of symptomatic pelvic floor disorders in U.S. women. JAMA 300(11):131, 2008

Olsen AL, Smith VJ, Bergstrom JO, et al: Epidemiology of surgically managed pelvic organ prolapse and urinary incontinence. Obstet Gynecol 89:501, 1997

Paraiso MFR, Ballard LA, Walters MD, et al: Pelvic support defects and visceral and sexual function in women treated with sacrospinous ligament suspension and pelvic reconstruction. Am J Obstet Gynecol 175:1423, 1996

Paraiso MFR, Barber MD, Muir TW, et al: Rectocele repair: a randomized trial of three surgical techniques including graft augmentation. Am J Obstet Gynecol 195:1762, 2006

Patel DA, Xu X, Thomason AD, et al: Childbirth and pelvic floor dysfunction: an epidemiologic approach to the assessment of prevention opportunities at delivery. Am J Obstet Gynecol 195:23, 2006

Peschers UM, Schaer GN, DeLancey JO, et al: Levator ani function before and after childbirth. Br J Obstet Gynaecol 104:1004, 1997

Phillips CH, Anthony F, Benyon C, et al: Collagen metabolism in the uterosacral ligaments and vaginal skin of women with uterine prolapse. BJOG 113:39, 2006

Reisenauer C, Shiozawa T, Oppitz M, et al: The role of smooth muscle in the pathogenesis of pelvic organ prolapse—an immunohistochemical and morphometric analysis of the cervical third of the uterosacral ligament. Int Urogynecol J Pelvic Floor Dysfunct 19:383, 2008

Richardson AC: The rectovaginal septum revisited. Its relationship to rectocele and its importance to rectocele repair. Clin Obstet Gynecol 36:976, 1993

Rortveit G, Brown JS, Thom DH, et al: Symptomatic pelvic organ prolapse: prevalence and risk factors in a population-based, racially diverse cohort. Obstet Gynecol 109(6):1396, 2007

Schaffer JI, Cundiff GW, Amundsen CL, et al: Do pessaries improve lower urinary tract symptoms? J Pelvic Med Surg 12:72, 2006

Schaffer JI, Wai CY, Boreham MK: Etiology of pelvic organ prolapse. Clin Obstet Gynecol 48:639, 2005

Shafik A, El-Sibai O: Levator ani muscle activity in pregnancy and the postpartum period: a myolectric study. Clin Exp Obstet Gynecol 27:129, 2000

Shull BL, Bachofen C, Coates KW, et al: A transvaginal approach to repair of apical and other associated sites of pelvic organ prolapse with uterosacral ligaments. Am J Obstet Gynecol 183:1365, 2000

Silva WA, Paulks RN, Segal JL, et al: Uterosacral ligament vault suspension: five-year outcomes. Obstet Gynecol 108:255, 2006

Smith ARB, Hosker GL, Warrell DW: The role of partial denervation of the pelvic floor in the aetiology of genitourinary prolapse and stress incontinence of urine. A neurophysiological study. Br J Obstet Gynecol 96:24, 1989

Smith P, Heimer G, Norgren A, et al: Localization of steroid hormone receptors in the pelvic muscles. Eur J Obstet Gynecol Reprod Biol 50: 83, 1993

Smith P, Heimer G, Norgren A, et al: Steroid hormone receptors in pelvis muscles and ligaments in women. Gynecol Obstet Invest 30: 27, 1990

Sullivan ES, Longaker CJ, Lee PY: Total pelvic mesh repair: a ten-year experience. Dis Colon Rectum 44:857, 2001

Sung VW, Rogers RG, Schaffer JI, et al: Graft use in transvaginal pelvic organ prolapse repair: a systematic review. Obstet Gynecol 112:1131, 2008

Swift S, Woodman P, O'Boyle A, et al: Pelvic Organ Support Study (POSST): the distribution, clinical definition, and epidemiologic condition of pelvic organ support defects. Am J Obstet Gynecol 192:795, 2005

Swift SE: The distribution of pelvic organ support in a population of female subjects seen for routine gynecologic health care. AM J Obstet Gynecol 183:277, 2000

Swift SE, Tate SB, Nicholas J: Correlation of symptoms with degree of pelvic organ support in a general population of women: what is pelvic organ prolapse? Am J Obstet Gynecol 189:372, 2003

Sze HM, Karram MM: Transvaginal repair of vault prolapse: a review. Obstet Gynecol 89:466, 1997a

Sze EH, Miklos JR, Partoll L, et al: Sacrospinous ligament fixation with transvaginal needle suspension for advanced pelvic organ prolapse and stress incontinence. Obstet Gynecol. 89:94, 1997b

Takacs P, Nassiri M, Gualtieri M, et al: Uterosacral ligament smooth muscle cell apoptosis is increased in women with uterine prolapse. Reprod Sci 16: 447, 2009

Tan JS, Lukaz ES, Menefee SA, et al: Predictive value of prolapse symptoms: a large database study. Int Urogynecol J Pelvic Floor Dysfunct 16:203, 2005

Trowbridge ER, Fultz NH, Patel DA, et al: Distribution of pelvis organ support in a population-based sample of middle-aged community-dwelling African American and white women in southeastern Michigan. Am J Obstet Gynecol 198:548, 2008

U.S. Food and Drug Administration: FDA safety communication: UPDATE on serious complications associated with transvaginal placement of surgical mesh for pelvic organ prolapse. Available at: http://www.fda.gov/MedicalDevices/Safety/AlertsandNotices/ucm262435.htm. Accessed October 14, 2011

Visco AG, Weidner AC, Barber MD, et al: Vaginal mesh erosion after abdominal sacral colpopexy. Am J Obstet Gynecol 184:297, 2001

Weber AM, Abrams P, Brubaker L, et al: The standardization of terminology for researchers in female pelvic floor disorders. Int Urogynecol J Pelvic Floor Dysfunct 12:178, 2001a

Weber AM, Walters MD, Ballard LA, et al: Posterior vaginal wall prolapse and bowel function. Obstet Gynecol 179:1446, 1998

Weber AM, Walters MD, Piedmonte MR, et al: Anterior colporrhaphy: a randomized trial of three surgical techniques. Am J Obstet Gynecol 185:1299, 2001b

Weber AM, Walters MD, Piedmonte MR: Sexual function and vaginal anatomy in women before and after surgery for pelvic organ prolapse and urinary incontinence. Am J Obstet Gynecol 182:1610, 2000

Weber AM, Walters MD, Schover LR: Sexual function in women with uterovaginal prolapse and urinary incontinence. Obstet Gynecol 85:483, 1995

Wheeler TL 2nd, Richter HE, Burgio KL, et al: Regret, satisfaction, and symptoms improvement: analysis of the impact of partial colpocleisis for the management of severe pelvic organ prolapse. Am J Obstet Gynecol 193:2067, 2005

Whitcomb EL, Rortveit G, Brown JS, et al: Racial differences in pelvic organ prolapse. Obstet Gynecol 114(6):1271, 2009

Whiteside JL, Weber AM, Meyn LA, et al: Risk factors for prolapse recurrence after vaginal repair. Am J Obstet Gynecol 191:1533, 2004

Wieslander CK, Word RA, Schaffer JI, et al: Smoking is a risk factor for pelvic organ prolapse. J Pelvic Medicine & Surgery 26th Annual Scientific Meeting of the American Urogynecologic Society (AUGS), Atlanta, GA, p S16, 2005

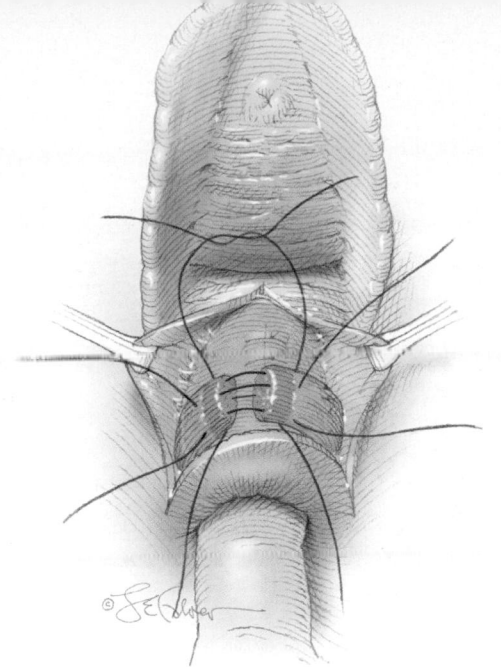

CHAPTER 25

Anal Incontinence and Functional Anorectal Disorders

ANAL INCONTINENCE

Anal incontinence (AI) is an involuntary loss of flatus, liquid, or solid stool that causes a social or hygienic problem (Abrams, 2005). This condition may lead to poor self-image and social isolation, thus significantly impairing quality of life (Johanson, 1996; Perry, 2002). Additionally, AI creates a substantial financial burden on patients and the health care system (Whitehead, 2001).

The definition of AI includes incontinence of flatus, whereas that of *fecal incontinence* (FI) does not. Not included in either definition is *anal mucoid seepage*. This type of fecal leakage tends to develop in those with a fully functional anal sphincter and intact cognition. It most often is associated with organic colonic disease or dietary sensitivity (Abrams, 2005).

Epidemiology

Anal incontinence is common and affects all age groups. In contrast to previous beliefs, it affects men and women similarly (Heymen, 2009; Madoff, 2004; Nelson, 2004). The prevalence of AI increases with age and has been reported to reach 46 percent in older, institutionalized women (Nelson, 1998). In a systematic review of the literature, Macmillan and coworkers (2004) reported that the estimated prevalence of AI among community-dwelling adults ranges between 2 and 24 percent if flatal incontinence is included and between 0.4 and 18 percent if flatal incontinence is not. These wide variations are attributed to differences in definitions and in the surveyed cohort's age and to lack of validated questionnaires. In a multicenter trial that included seven geographically distinct sites in the United States, Boreham and associates (2005) reported the prevalence, risk factors, and quality of life effects of AI in women aged 18 to 65 years presenting for benign gynecologic care. The overall prevalence of AI in this cohort was 28 percent. In a recent study conducted by the Pelvic Floor Disorders Network, a validated FI severity scale was added to the National Health and Nutrition Examination Survey (NHANES) in 2005-2006 (Rockwood, 1999; Whitehead, 2009). The estimated prevalence of FI in the nationally representative sample of noninstitutionalized U.S. adults was 8.3 percent (18 million) and consisted of liquid stool incontinence in 6.2 percent, mucus in 3.1 percent, and solid stool in 1.6 percent. This survey confirmed the strong association between FI and age. The prevalence of FI increased from

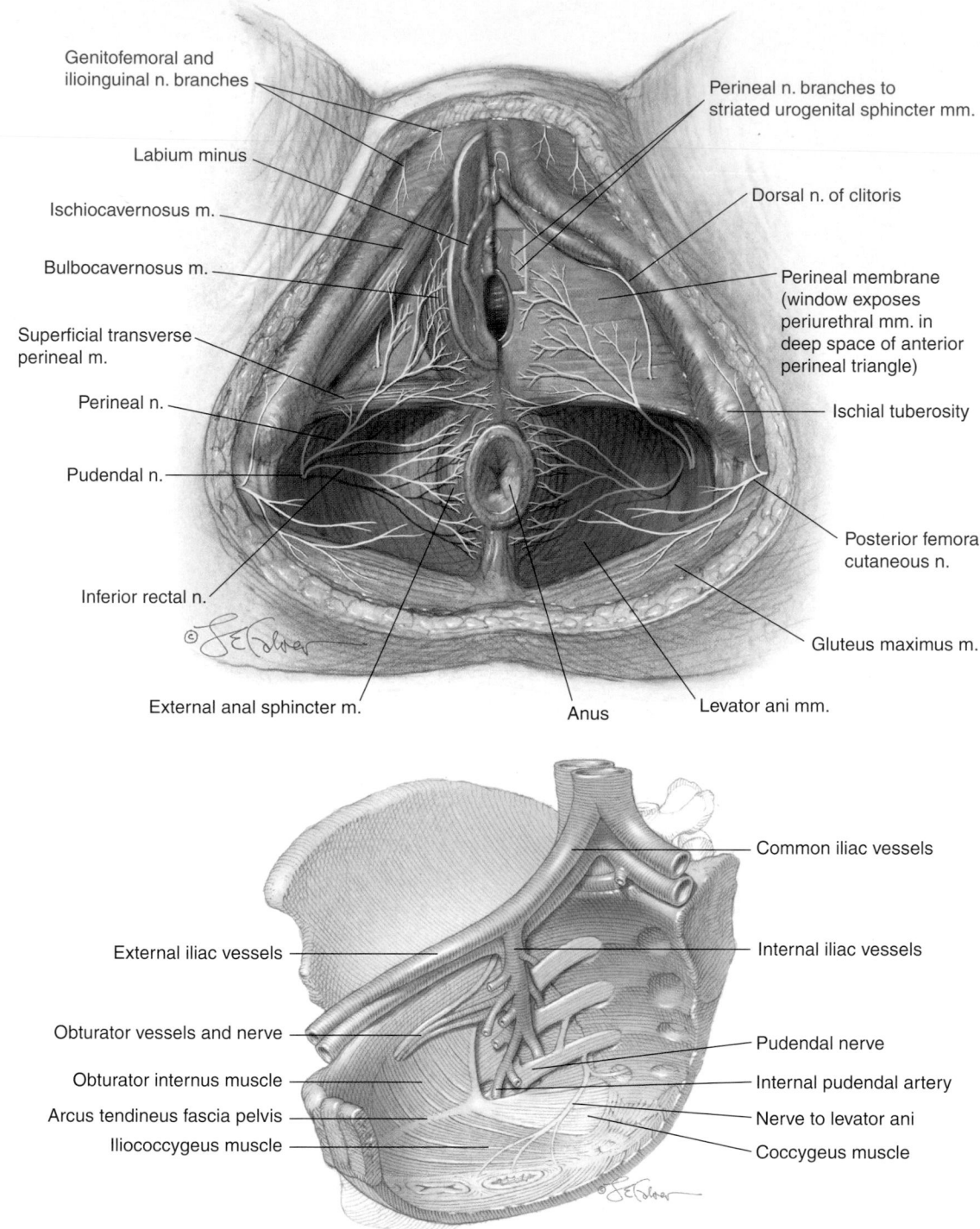

Genitofemoral and ilioinguinal n. branches

Labium minus

Ischiocavernosus m.

Bulbocavernosus m.

Superficial transverse perineal m.

Perineal n.

Pudendal n.

Inferior rectal n.

External anal sphincter m.

Perineal n. branches to striated urogenital sphincter mm.

Dorsal n. of clitoris

Perineal membrane (window exposes periurethral mm. in deep space of anterior perineal triangle)

Ischial tuberosity

Posterior femoral cutaneous n.

Gluteus maximus m.

Anus

Levator ani mm.

External iliac vessels

Obturator vessels and nerve

Obturator internus muscle

Arcus tendineus fascia pelvis

Iliococcygeus muscle

Common iliac vessels

Internal iliac vessels

Pudendal nerve

Internal pudendal artery

Nerve to levator ani

Coccygeus muscle

FIGURE 25-1 Innervation of the anal sphincter complex. **A.** The external anal sphincter is innervated by the pudendal nerve. **B.** Innervation of the female pelvic floor muscles from direct branches of S3–S5.

2.6 percent in those aged 20 to 30 years up to 15.3 percent in subjects aged 70 years or older.

Pathophysiology of Defecation and Anal Continence

Normal defecation and anal continence are complex processes that require a competent anal sphincter complex, normal ano-

rectal sensation, adequate rectal capacity and compliance, and conscious control.

Anal Sphincter Complex

This neuromuscular complex consists of the internal and external anal sphincter muscles and the puborectalis muscle (Figs. 38-9 and 38-21, p. 925). Of these, the internal anal sphincter (IAS) is the thickened distal 3- to 4-cm longitudinal extension of the colon's circular smooth muscle layer. It is innervated by the autonomic nervous system and provides 70 to 85 percent of the anal canal's resting pressure (Frenckner, 1975). As a result, the IAS contributes substantially to the maintenance of fecal continence at rest.

The external anal sphincter (EAS) consists of striated muscle and is primarily innervated by somatic motor fibers that course in the inferior rectal branch of the pudendal nerve (Fig. 25-1A). The EAS provides the anal canal's *squeeze pressure* and is mainly responsible for maintaining fecal continence when continence is threatened. At times, squeeze pressure may be voluntary or may be induced by increased intraabdominal pressure. In addition, although resting sphincter tone is generally attributed to the IAS, the EAS maintains a constant state of resting contraction and may be responsible for approximately 25 percent of anal resting pressure. During defecation, however, the EAS relaxes to allow stool passage.

The puborectalis muscle is part of the levator ani muscle complex and is innervated from its pelvic surface by direct efferents from the third, fourth, and fifth sacral nerve roots (see Fig. 25-1B) (Barber, 2002). Its constant tone contributes to the anorectal angle, which aids in preventing rectal contents from entering the anus (Fig. 38-10, p. 926). Similar to the EAS, this muscle can be contracted voluntarily or in response to sudden increases in abdominal pressure.

The role of the puborectalis in maintaining stool continence remains controversial. However, it is best appreciated in women who remain continent of solid stool despite absence of the anterior portion of the external and internal sphincters, as can be seen in those with chronic fourth-degree lacerations (Fig. 25-2). With normal functioning of this muscle, evacuation is generally associated with a greater (or less obtuse) anorectal angle, and thus better longitudinal alignment of the rectoanal lumen, as the puborectalis relaxes. Conversely, paradoxical contraction of the puborectalis muscle during defecation may lead to impaired evacuation. Moreover, atrophy of this muscle has been associated with FI (Bharucha, 2004).

Anorectal Sensation

Innervation to the rectum and anal canal is derived from the superior, middle, and inferior rectal autonomic nerve plexuses that contain sympathetic and parasympathetic components and by intrinsic nerves present in the rectoanal wall (Fig. 38-13, p. 929). In addition, the inferior rectal branch of the pudendal nerve conveys sensory input from the lower anal canal and the skin around the anus. Sensory receptors within the anal canal and pelvic floor muscles can detect the presence of stool in the rectum as well as the degree of distension. Through these neural pathways, information regarding rectal distension and rectal contents can be transmitted and processed and the action of the sphincteric musculature coordinated.

The *rectoanal inhibitory reflex (RAIR)* refers to the transient relaxation of the IAS and contraction of EAS induced by rectal distension when stool first arrives in the rectum. This reflex is mediated by the intrinsic nerves in the anorectal wall and allows the sensory-rich upper anal canal to come in contact with or "sample" the rectal contents (Whitehead, 1987). Specifically, *sampling* refers to the process whereby the IAS relaxes, often

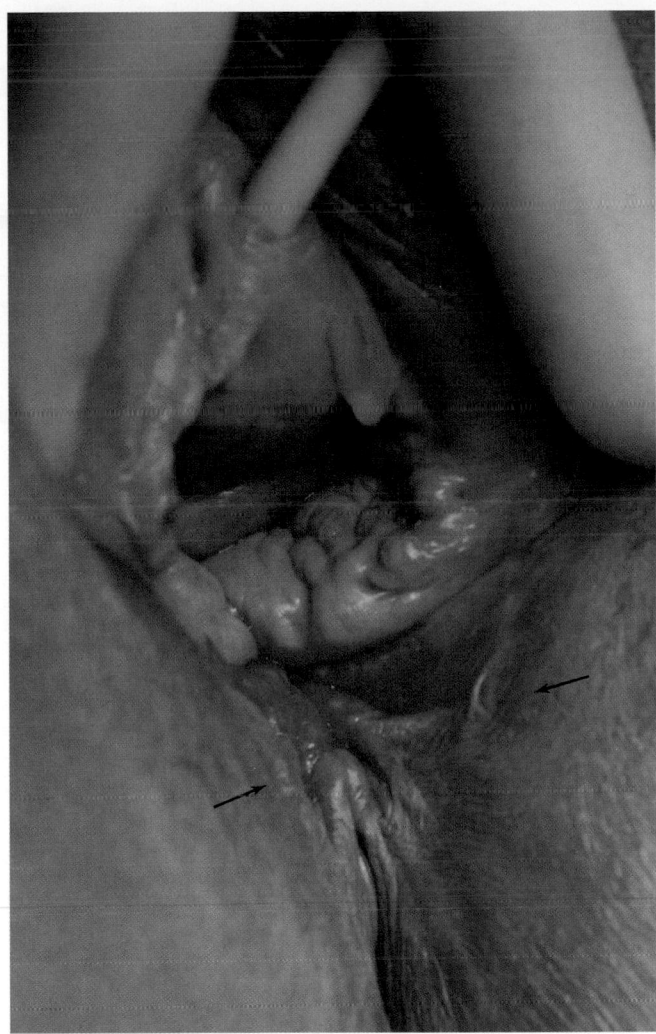

FIGURE 25-2 Chronic fourth-degree laceration with complete absence of the perineal body and absence of the anterior portion of external anal sphincter (cloacal deformity). Skin dimples at 3 and 9 o'clock (*arrows*) indicate sites of retracted ends of the external anal sphincter.

independently of rectal distension, allowing the anal epithelium to ascertain whether rectal contents are gas, liquid, or solid stools (Miller, 1988).

Following integration of this neural information, defecation can ensue in the appropriate social setting. Alternatively, if required, defecation can generally be postponed, as the rectum can accommodate its contents and the EAS or puborectalis muscle or both can be voluntarily contracted. However, if rectal sensation is impaired, contents may enter the anal canal and may leak before the EAS can contract (Buser, 1986).

Evaluation of the RAIR may clarify the underlying etiology of AI. This reflex is absent in those with congenital aganglionosis (Hirschsprung disease) but preserved in patients with cauda equina lesions or after spinal cord transection (Bharucha, 2006).

Rectal Accommodation and Compliance

Following anal sampling, the rectum can relax to admit the increased rectal volume in a process known as accommodation.

The rectum is a highly compliant reservoir that aids storage of stool. As rectal volume increases, an urge to defecate is perceived. If this urge is voluntarily suppressed, the rectum relaxes to continue stool accommodation. A loss of compliance may decrease the ability of the rectal wall to stretch or accommodate, and as a result, rectal pressure may remain high. This may place increased demands on the other components of the continence mechanism such as the anal sphincter complex.

Rectal compliance can be calculated by measuring the sensitivity to and maximal volume tolerated from a fluid-filled balloon during anorectal manometry (p. 665). Rectal compliance may be decreased in those with ulcerative and radiation proctitis. In contrast, increased compliance may be noted in certain patients with constipation, potentially signaling a megarectum.

Incontinence Risks

Causes of AI and defecatory disorders are diverse and are likely multifactorial. These conditions develop if structural and/or functional components of continence or defecatory mechanisms are altered (Table 25-1).

Obstetric

In younger, reproductive-aged women, the most common association with AI is vaginal delivery and damage to the anal sphincter muscles (Snooks, 1985; Sultan, 1993; Zetterstrom, 1999). This damage may be mechanical or neuropathic and can result in early fecal and flatal incontinence.

The rates of sphincter tear during vaginal births in the United States range from 6 to 18 percent (Fenner, 2003; Handa, 2001). A multicenter trial conducted by the Pelvic Floor Disorders Network prospectively evaluated bowel continence status in primiparous women delivered at term in the United States. At both 6 weeks and 6 months postpartum, women who sustained anal sphincter tears during vaginal delivery had twice the risk of FI and reported more severe FI compared with women who delivered vaginally without evidence of sphincter disruption (Borello-France, 2006). In contrast, a retrospective study of 151 women with diverse obstetric histories who delivered 30 years previously reported that women with a prior sphincter disruption were more likely to have "bothersome" flatal incontinence, but were not at increased risk for FI compared with women who had an isolated episiotomy or those who underwent cesarean delivery (Nygaard, 1997). Thus, other mechanisms associated with pregnancy and with aging may contribute to AI regardless of delivery mode or anal sphincter disruption.

Other Factors

Inflammatory bowel conditions and radiation therapy involving the rectum can result in poor compliance and loss of accommodation. Of these patients, those with inflammatory bowel disease and chronic diarrhea are more frequently affected. Liquid stool is more difficult to control than solid, and thus FI may develop in these women even if all components of the continence mechanism are grossly intact. Alternatively, chronic constipation with straining to defecate may result in damage to the muscular and/or neural components of the

TABLE 25-1. Risk Factors for Fecal Incontinence

Obstetric
Increasing parity
Anal sphincter damage

Other Medical Conditions
Increasing age
Increasing body mass index
Postmenopausal status
Diabetes
Chronic hypertension
Chronic obstructive pulmonary disease
Stroke
Scleroderma
Prior pelvic radiation therapy
Medications

Urogynecologic
Urinary incontinence
Pelvic organ prolapse

Gastrointestinal
Constipation
Diarrhea
Fecal urgency
Food intolerance
Irritable bowel syndrome
Prior anal abscess or fistula
Prior anal surgery

Neuropsychiatric
Spinal cord injury
Parkinson disease
Prior spinal surgery
Multiple sclerosis
Myopathies
Cognitive dysfunction
Psychosis

sphincter mechanism. Similarly, other neuromuscular injury to the puborectalis and/or anal sphincter muscles, such as that associated with pelvic organ prolapse, may lead to AI.

Nervous system dysfunction in those with spinal cord injury, back surgery, multiple sclerosis, diabetes, or cerebrovascular accident may lead to poor accommodation, loss of sensation, impaired reflexes, and myopathy. Finally, loss of rectal sensation can be seen with normal aging.

In the NHANES survey, FI was not significantly associated with race or ethnicity, level of education, income, or marital status after adjusting for age (Whitehead, 2009). Independent risk factors in women included advancing age, loose or watery stools, multiple chronic illness, and urinary incontinence.

Diagnosis

Precise identification of the underlying cause and accurate assessment of symptom severity are essential prior to selecting

TABLE 25-2. Fecal Incontinence Severity Index

	Two or More Times Daily	Once Daily	Two or More Times Weekly	Once Weekly	One to Three Times Monthly	Never
Gas	☐	☐	☐	☐	☐	☐
Mucus	☐	☐	☐	☐	☐	☐
Liquid stool	☐	☐	☐	☐	☐	☐
Solid stool	☐	☐	☐	☐	☐	☐

From Rockwood, 1999, with permission.

an appropriate treatment plan. A complete history and physical examination should always be the first step in evaluating patients with AI and often identifies correctable problems. Following examination, anal endosonography can be obtained to identify anal sphincter anatomic defects that may be amenable to surgery. Other selected tests, which are described later, may be added as clinically indicated. However, because current surgical outcomes are less than optimal, most patients, even those with anatomic defects, are initially treated conservatively.

History

A thorough history should include incontinence duration and frequency, stool consistency, timing of incontinent episodes, use of sanitary protection, and social impact of incontinence. Additionally, questioning should address risk factors noted in

Table 25-1. Importantly, urge-related AI should be differentiated from incontinence without awareness, as these may be associated with different underlying pathologies. For example, urgency without incontinence may reflect inability of the rectal reservoir to store stool rather than a sphincteric disorder.

Patient Diaries and Validated Questionnaires. These tools have been developed in an effort to reduce patient recall bias and to help standardize AI scores. Several incontinence-scoring systems have been developed that provide objective measure of a patient's degree of incontinence. Four commonly used symptom severity scores are the Pescatori Incontinence Score; Wexner (Cleveland Clinic) Score; St. Marks (Vaizey) Score; and the Fecal Incontinence Severity Index (FISI) (Tables 25-2 and 25-3) (Jorge, 1993; Pescatori, 1992; Rockwood, 1999;

TABLE 25-3. St. Marks (Vaizey) Incontinence Score

	Never[a]	Rarely[b]	Sometimes[c]	Weekly[d]	Daily[e]
Incontinence for solid stool	0	1	2	3	4
Incontinence for liquid stool	0	1	2	3	4
Incontinence for gas	0	1	2	3	4
Alteration in lifestyle	0	1	2	3	4
				No	Yes
Need to wear a pad or plug				0	2
Taking constipating medicines				0	2
Lack of ability to defer defecation for 15 minutes				0	4

[a]Never = no episodes in the past 4 weeks.
[b]Rarely = 1 episode in the past 4 weeks.
[c]Sometimes = >1 episode in the past 4 weeks but <1 a week.
[d]Weekly = 1 or more episodes a week but <1 a day.
[e]Daily = 1 or more episodes a day.
Add one score from each row: minimum score = 0 = perfect continence
maximum score = 24 = totally incontinent
From Vaizey, 1999, with permission.

TABLE 25-4. Fecal Incontinence Quality of Life Scale Composition

Scale 1: Lifestyle
I cannot do many of the things I want to do
I am afraid to go out
It is important to plan my schedule (daily activities) around my bowel pattern
I cut down on how much I eat before I go out
It is difficult for me to get out and do things like going to a movie or to church
I avoid traveling by plane or train
I avoid traveling
I avoid visiting friends
I avoid going out to eat
I avoid staying overnight away from home

Scale 2: Coping/Behavior
I have sex less often than I would like to
The possibility of bowel accidents is always on my mind
I feel I have no control over my bowels
Whenever I go someplace new, I specifically locate where the bathrooms are
I worry about not being able to get to the toilet in time
I worry about bowel accidents
I try to prevent bowel accidents by staying very near a bathroom
I can't hold my bowel movement long enough to get to the bathroom
Whenever I am away from home, I try to stay near a restroom as much as possible

Scale 3: Depression/Self-perception
In general, how would you say your health is
I am afraid to have sex
I feel different from other people
I enjoy life less
I feel like I am not a healthy person
I feel depressed
During the past month, have you felt so sad, discouraged, hopeless, or had so many problems that you wondered if anything was worthwhile

Scale 4: Embarrassment
I leak stool without even knowing it
I worry about others smelling stool on me
I feel ashamed

Adapted from Rockwood, 2000, with permission.

Vaizey, 1999). Of these, the Vaizey Score and the FISI include symptom weighting. The inclusion of patient-assigned severity scores increases the utility of the FISI compared to other scales. The ability of the Vaizey Score to incorporate a component of fecal urgency makes this scale desirable in certain clinical trials.

In addition to symptom severity, AI should also be characterized by its impact on the patient's quality of life. The validated fecal incontinence quality of life (FI-QOL) questionnaire is a 29-item tool designed to estimate the impact of fecal incontinence on lifestyle, coping behavior, depression/self-perception, and embarrassment (Table 25-4) (Rockwood, 2000). Other quality-of-life scales available, but less widely used, include the Modified Manchester Health Questionnaire and the Gastrointestinal Quality of Life Index (Kwon, 2005; Sailer, 1998). These validated questionnaires may be used diagnostically and also following treatment to determine response.

Bristol Stool Scale. The validated Bristol Stool Scale is commonly used to determine a patient's usual stool consistency (Lewis, 1997). This scale consists of seven descriptions of stool characteristics and includes pictures of each stool type (Fig. 25-3) (Degen, 1996; Heaton, 1994). Such stool consistency categorization has been shown to correlate with objective measures of whole-gut transit time (Heaton, 1994).

Physical Examination

Examination should begin with careful inspection of the anus and perineum looking for stool soiling, scars, perineal body length, hemorrhoids, anal warts, rectal prolapse, dovetail sign, or other anatomic abnormalities (Fig. 25-4). The perianal skin is gently stroked with a cotton-tipped swab, and the cutaneous anal reflex, also colloquially termed *anal wink*, should normally be present. This finding provides gross assessment of pudendal nerve integrity (Chap. 23, p. 618).

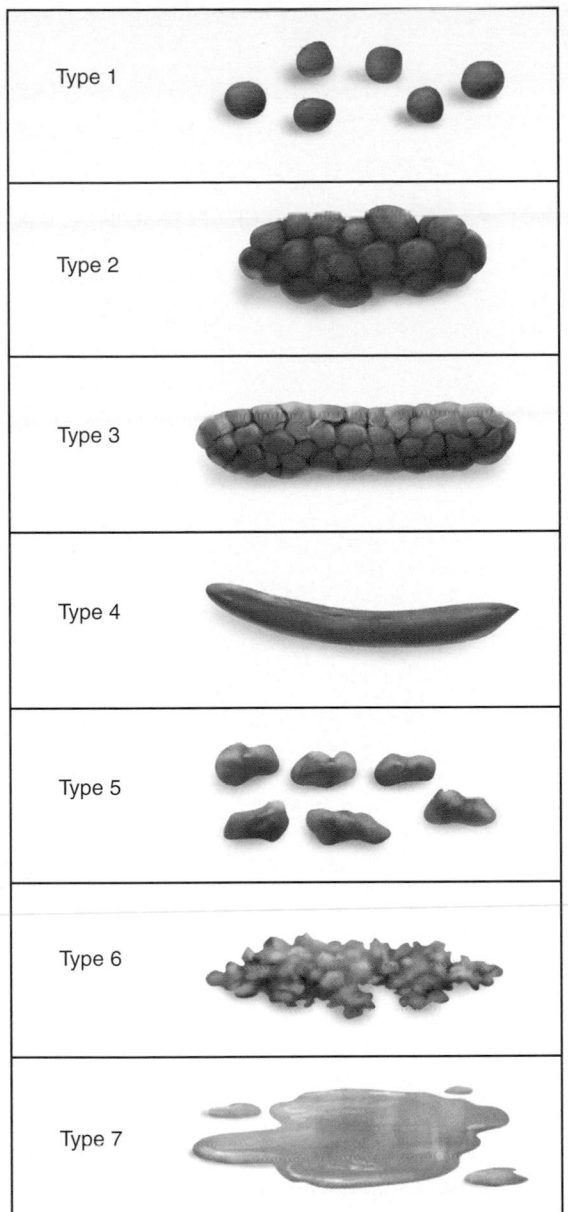

FIGURE 25-3 Bristol Stool Scale. Stools are categorized by their shape and texture. *(Redrawn from Lewis, 1997.)*

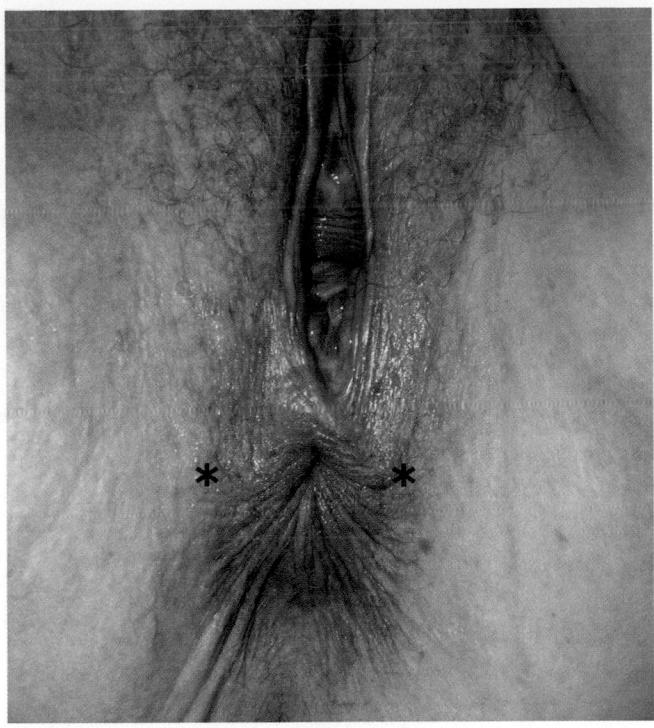

FIGURE 25-4 Photograph showing the "dovetail" sign, which is created by disruption of the anterior portion of external anal sphincter (EAS). Radial skin spikes are typically formed by attachment of skin to the EAS but are commonly absent from 10 to 2 o'clock (*asterisks*) in those with this disruption.

With digital rectal examination, one can assess IAS resting tone, sample for gross or occult blood, and palpate masses or fecal impaction. In addition, squeeze pressure can subjectively be assessed during voluntary patient contraction of the EAS around a gloved finger inserted into the rectum. Lastly, patients performing a Valsalva maneuver can allow inspection for excessive perineal body descent, vaginal wall prolapse, and rectal prolapse (Fig. 25-5).

Diagnostic Testing

Enema. A tap water enema is a simple test that may be used to determine if a patient is truly incontinent. Liquid stool is more difficult to control than solid stool, and thus patients who can hold enema contents for several minutes are not likely to have significant FI. In these instances, other etiologies for their symptoms should be sought.

Anorectal Manometry. During this test, a small flexible tube containing an inflatable balloon tip and pressure transducer is inserted into the rectum. Resting and squeeze pressures of the anal canal are then measured at incremental points as the balloon is slowly withdrawn from the rectum (Fig. 25-6). As an additional test, pressures may also be measured as a patient simulates defecation and expels the catheter balloon tip. In sum, anorectal manometry allows assessment of: (1) anal sphincter function, (2) reflexes, (3) rectal compliance, and (4) rectal sensation (Table 25-5).

During evaluation of the sphincters, manometry objectively measures IAS resting pressure and EAS squeeze pressure. Decreased pressure readings may indicate structural disruption, myopathy, or neuropathy.

Sphincter reflexes are also assessed during pressure measurements. During balloon insufflation, relaxation of the IAS should accompany rectal distension via the recto-anal inhibitory reflex (RAIR) (p. 661).

Rectal compliance and sensation may be determined by sequentially inflating a rectal balloon to various volumes. Decreased rectal compliance may be noted by an inability to inflate a balloon to typical volumes without patient discomfort. This may indicate a rectal reservoir that is unable to appropriately store stool. In contrast, decreased perception of balloon insufflation may indicate neuropathy.

One of the main limitations with manometry is that normal values may be seen in incontinent patients and vice versa. Despite this disadvantage, anal manometry serves an important role in AI evaluation.

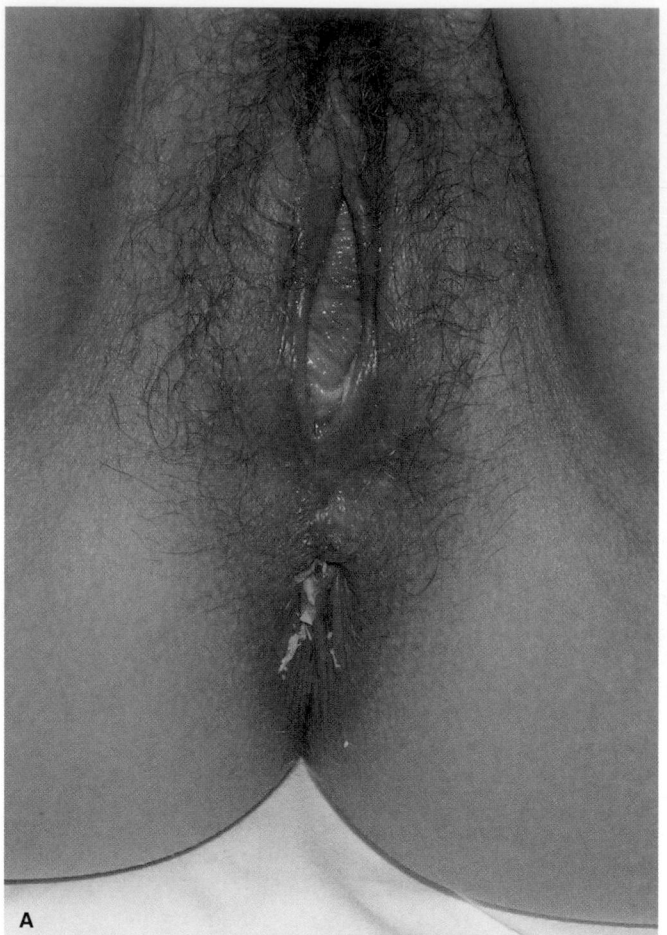
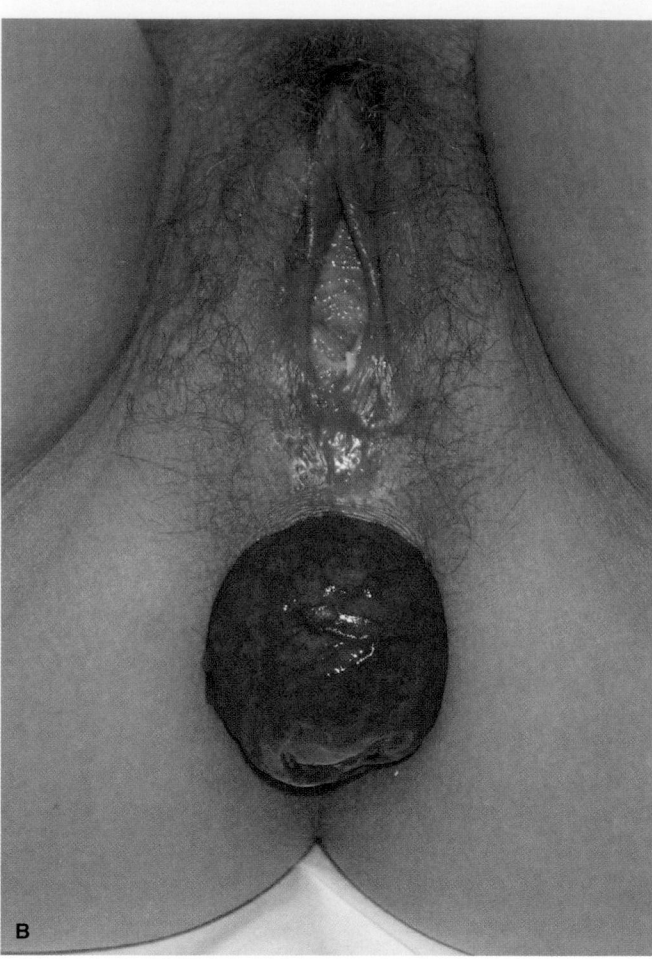

FIGURE 25-5 Patient at rest **(A)** and with Valsalva **(B)**, showing full-thickness rectal prolapse protruding through the anal opening.

Endoanal Ultrasonography (EAUS). Also known as *transanal sonography*, this technique was introduced in 1989 and is now the primary diagnostic imaging technique to evaluate the integrity, thickness, and length of the IAS and EAS (Fig. 25-7). The technique uses a rotating endoprobe with a ≥10-MHz transducer, which provides a 360-degree evaluation of the anal canal. Sonography gel is placed on the probe tip, which is sheathed with a condom prior to insertion into the anus. This tool allows diagnosis of anterior anal sphincter defects in women with a known history of clinically diagnosed anal sphincter disruption and also in those with unrecognized or misdiagnosed defects at the time of delivery. Prior to the common use of endoanal sonography, women with these "occult"—that is, solely sonographically diagnosed—anal sphincter defects were

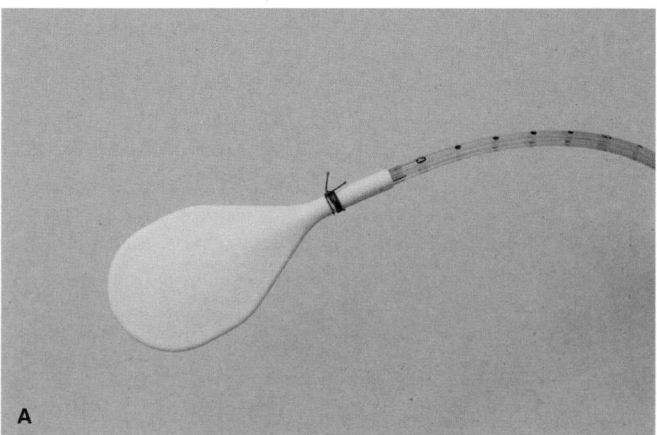
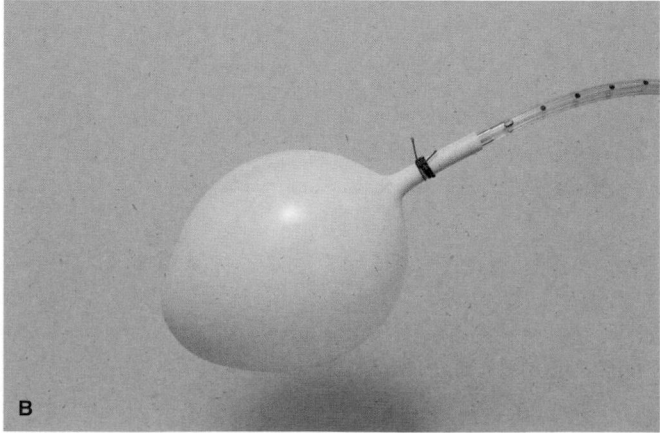

FIGURE 25-6 Manometry tube and balloon, empty **(A)** and after filling **(B)**.

TABLE 25-5. Functional Testing for Patients with Fecal Incontinence[a]

| Factors of Relevance in FI | Manometry | | | | Defecography | EAUS | EMG |
	Anal Resting Pressure	Anal Squeeze Pressure	Rectal Perception	Rectal Compliance			
Anal sphincters							
Internal	+					+	
External		+				+	+
Puborectalis					+		+
Rectum							
Perception			+				
Compliance				+			
Reservoir function			+	+	+		
Megarectum			+		+		
Pelvic floor							
Perineal descent					+		
Anorectal angle					+		
Neural							
Pudendal nerve	+						+

[a]Plus sign indicates an appropriate test for a particular component of continence.
EAUS = Endoanal ultrasonography; EMG = electromyography; FI = fecal incontinence.
From Hinninghofen, 2003, with permission.

labeled as having "idiopathic" FI and were not considered good candidates for surgical correction.

In addition to the anal sphincters, this modality can image the puborectalis muscle and perineal body. Oberwalder and colleagues (2004) showed that in a group of incontinent women, perineal body thickness ≤10 mm was associated with anal sphincter defects in 97 percent of cases, whereas perineal body thicknesses of 10 to 12 mm were associated with sphincter defect in one third of patients with FI. Perineal body thickness >12 mm was infrequently associated with these defects.

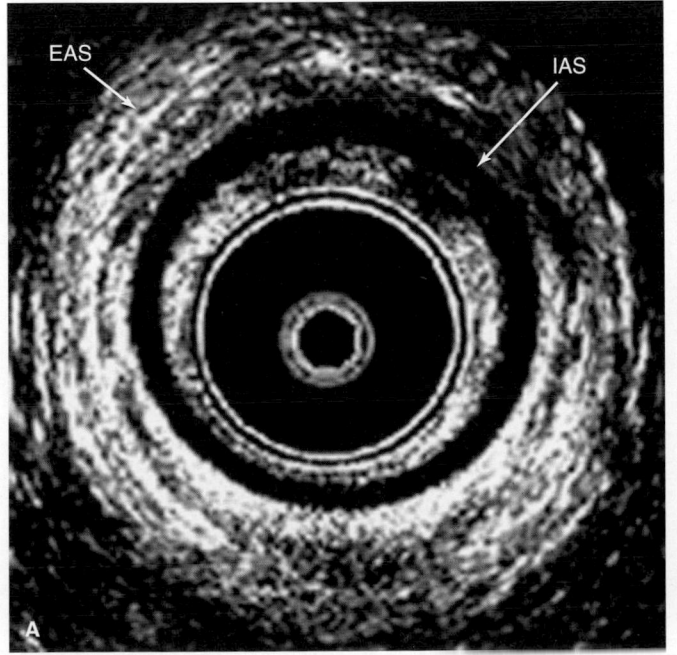
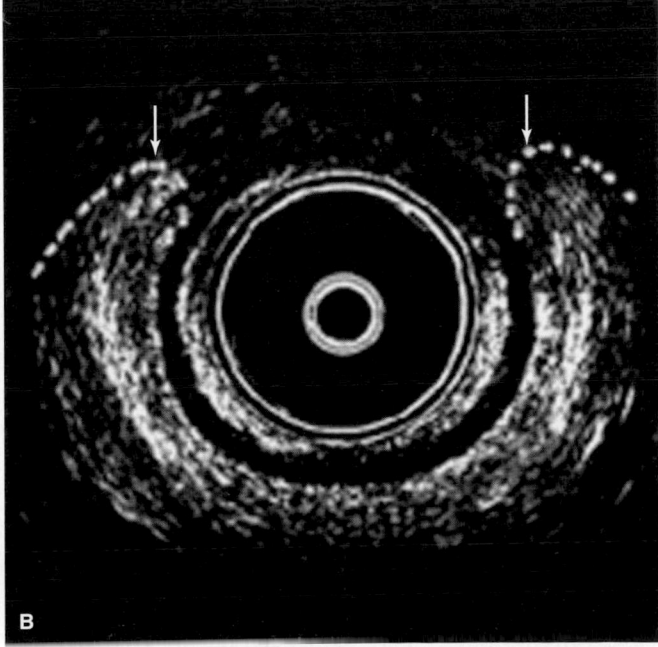

FIGURE 25-7 Anal endosonography. **A.** A woman with normal anal sphincters. **B.** Anterior defects of the external and internal anal sphincter muscles. EAS = external anal sphincter; IAS = internal anal sphincter. Dashed lines and arrows in B illustrate the ends of the torn EAS.

Magnetic Resonance Imaging. Endoanal magnetic resonance (MR) imaging is typically done with an anal endocoil placed within the anus. This modality is more expensive than anal endosonography, and its value for anal sphincter evaluation is controversial. Although sonography has been shown to be more sensitive in detecting IAS abnormalities, MR imaging is more sensitive in visualizing EAS morphology, including atrophy (Beets-Tan, 2001; Rociu, 1999). This may have value preoperatively, as patients with EAS atrophy may have poorer results following anal sphincteroplasty compared with those without atrophy (Briel, 1999). However, the role of endocoil MR imaging in the clinical assessment of AI is yet to be determined. As an alternative to endocoil MR imaging, use of external phased-array MR imaging with an *external* coil has been evaluated for sphincter imaging (Beets-Tan, 2001). Its main advantages are less distortion of the anatomy and greater patient comfort because no intraluminal coil is required. External phased-array MR imaging has been shown to be comparable to endoanal MR imaging in depicting external anal sphincter atrophy and thereby, in selecting patients for anal sphincter repair (Terra, 2006). However, results among interpreters varied considerably depending on experience level. Thus, the authors concluded that both techniques can be recommended in the diagnostic evaluation of FI only if sufficient experience is available.

Another MR imaging modality, termed *dynamic MR imaging,* allows dynamic examination of rectal emptying and evaluation of pelvic floor muscles, including the puborectalis muscle, during rest, squeeze, and defecation (Gearhart, 2004; Kaufman, 2001). It simultaneously permits pelvic organ prolapse assessment. This current research tool, however, is technically difficult. Moreover, other than avoiding the ionizing radiation associated with evacuation proctography, this technique offers no advantage for studying rectal function in the clinical setting. In addition, evidence from a National Institutes of Health (NIH) funded trial within the Pelvic Floor Disorders Network showed that despite standardized central training, the variability of pelvic MR imaging measurements among readers is high (Lockhart, 2008). The authors concluded that this variability adversely affects the utility of many MR imaging measurements for multicenter pelvic floor disorder research.

Evacuation Proctography. During this radiographic test, also known as *defecography,* the rectum is opacified with a thick barium paste, and the small bowel fills with a barium suspension given orally. Radiographic or fluoroscopic imaging is then obtained while a patient is resting, contracting their sphincter, coughing, and straining to expel the barium.

This test of dynamic rectal emptying and anorectal anatomy is not widely used to assess evacuation disorders unless obstructive causes for AI are suspected. Accordingly, it may be obtained if intussusception, internal rectal prolapse, enterocele, or failed relaxation of the puborectalis muscle during defecation is a concern.

Electromyography. This test graphically records electrical activity of muscles at rest and during contraction. During electromyography (EMG), needle electrodes are inserted through the skin into a muscle, and electrical activity detected by these electrodes is displayed graphically. In evaluation of AI, EMG may be used to assess the neuromuscular integrity of the EAS and puborectalis muscle. Specifically, by measuring action potentials from muscle motor units, EMG can help clarify which portions of these muscles are contracting and relaxing appropriately. Additionally, following injury, muscle may be partially or completely denervated, and compensatory reinnervation may then follow. Patterns characteristic of such denervation and reinnervation may be identified with EMG.

For EMG testing, concentric-needle, single-fiber, or surface EMG can be used. Needle EMG is primarily used in research, whereas surface EMG is most commonly used in clinical settings. Unlike needle electrodes, surface patch electrodes are placed on the darker-skinned area of the anus, cause little discomfort to the patient, and carry no risk of infection. Needle EMG provides useful information regarding sphincter innervation and surface EMG can be used during biofeedback to give visual or auditory signals to patients.

Pudendal Nerve Terminal Motor Latency Test. This stimulation test of the pudendal nerve measures the time delay between electrical nerve stimulation and EAS motor response. This delay, also termed *latency,* if prolonged, may indicate pudendal nerve pathology, which may be a cause of AI.

During pudendal nerve terminal motor latency (PNTML) testing, a stimulating electrode positioned on an examiner's gloved fingertip is connected to a pulsed-stimulus generator (Fig. 25-8). The pudendal nerves are transanally stimulated through the lateral walls of the rectum at the level of the ischial spines by this electrode. The action potential response of the EAS is received by recording electrodes at the base of the examining finger and registered on an oscilloscope.

Although PNTML prolongation has been considered a marker of idiopathic fecal incontinence, this test provides little information regarding the etiology of fecal incontinence. Accordingly, it has been replaced by more specific and sensitive tests for sphincter muscle innervation such as EMG (Barnett,

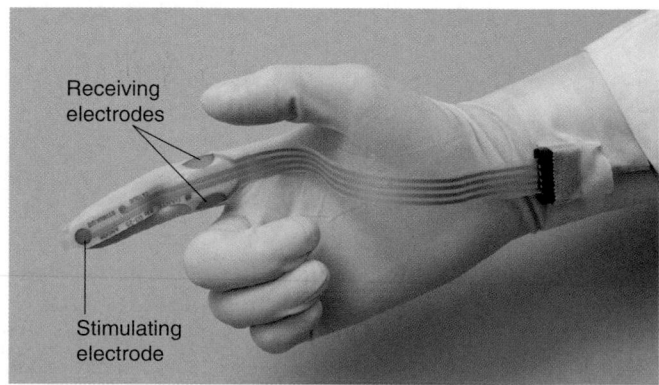

FIGURE 25-8 Pudendal nerve terminal motor latency (PNTML) electrode connected to examiner's gloved finger. The pudendal nerve is stimulated transanally by an electrode at the examiner's fingertip. Response by the external anal sphincter is received by electrodes at the finger's base.

1999). However, in patients with a sphincter defect who are candidates for repair, general sphincter neurologic status can be assessed by this test, and the results used in preoperative counseling. For example, patients with pudendal neuropathy may have poorer outcomes after anatomic sphincter reapproximation compared with those without nerve dysfunction (Gilliland, 1998).

Colonoscopy and Barium Enema. Based on the history and physical examination, these tests may be indicated to exclude inflammatory bowel conditions or malignancy.

Treatment

The goal of treatment is to restore or improve fecal continence and improve patient quality of life. Treatment is highly individualized and dependent on the etiology and severity of AI, available treatment options, and patient health.

Nonsurgical Treatment

Most patients with AI, excluding those with an obvious anal sphincter defect and significant FI, may benefit from conservative management. This may include diet modification, constipating agents, bulking agents, timed enemas or suppositories, and biofeedback.

Medical Management. A Cochrane review of randomized or quasirandomized controlled trials analyzed the use of pharmacologic agents for the treatment of FI in adults. Of these trials, most focused on diarrheal treatment, rather than FI, and thus limited data are available to guide clinicians in drug therapy selection (Cheetham, 2003). However, for patients with minor incontinence, the use of bulking agents can change stool consistency and create feces that are firmer and easier to control (Table 25-6). Common side effects such as abdominal distension and bloating can be improved by starting with smaller doses or switching to a different agent.

Agents that slow fecal intestinal transit time such as loperamide hydrochloride (Imodium) can reduce stool volume in patients with diarrhea and FI by increasing the time available for the colon to reabsorb fluid from stool. This agent has

also shown to increase anal resting tone and therefore, may even be beneficial for patients with FI and no diarrhea (Read, 1982). Side effects are uncommon and include dry mouth. In one double-blind, cross-over study, Lauti and colleagues (2008) prescribed loperamide to 63 patients with the primary complaint of liquid and solid FI. Patients were randomized first to loperamide with fiber supplements and a neutral diet or to loperamide with placebo fiber supplements and a balanced low-residue diet. They then crossed to the alternate treatment after 6 weeks. Both groups improved from their baseline status during the 12-week study, but there were no significant differences in scores when crossing from one diet and fiber regimen to the other.

Diphenoxylate hydrochloride (Lomotil) is used in the same capacity as loperamide hydrochloride, and dosing is similar. Although this is a Schedule V substance, potential for physical dependence is minimal. Finally, amitriptyline is a tricyclic antidepressant that has been used to treat idiopathic FI. Although the mechanism of action is poorly understood, some of its beneficial effects may be related to its anticholinergic properties.

Bowel Management. Daily, timed, tap-water enemas or glycerin or bisacodyl suppositories (Dulcolax) may be used to empty the rectum after eating. These provide acceptable and helpful options for some patients with constipative symptoms associated with AI. These may include women with normal stool consistency but difficulty evacuating due to anatomic reasons such as rectocele with stool trapping or those with denervation and impaired rectal sensation. All these may lead to accumulation of a large mass of solid stool in the rectum and leaking of loose stool around it. Bulking agents can be used concurrently with these evacuation methods to diminish stooling between desired defecations. These agents may also be used in those with frequent bowel movements, loose stools, or diarrheal symptoms associated with AI.

Biofeedback and Pelvic Floor Therapy. Many behavioral techniques, often considered together as biofeedback, measure

TABLE 25-6. Medical Management of Fecal Incontinence

Treatment	Brand Name	Oral Dosage
Bulking agents		
Psyllium	Metamucil	1 tbsp. mixed into 8 oz. of water 1–3 times daily
Psyllium	Konsyl	1 tsp. mixed into 8 oz. of water 1–3 times daily
Methylcellulose	Citrucel	1 tbsp. mixed into 8 oz. of water 1–3 times daily
Loperamide hydrochloride	Imodium	2–4 mg, 1–4 times daily to a maximum daily dose of 16 mg
Diphenoxylate hydrochloride	Lomotil	5 mg, 1–4 times daily to a maximum daily dose of 20 mg
Amitriptyline	Generic	10–25 mg at bedtime; increase by 10–25 mg weekly up to 75–150 mg at bedtime or a therapeutic drug level

physiologic signals such as muscle tension and then display them to a patient in real time. In general, visual, auditory, and/or verbal feedback cues are directed to the patient during these therapy sessions. Thus, candidates typically include those whose cognitive function is intact, who can follow commands, and who are motivated.

Biofeedback is usually selected to increase neuromuscular conditioning. Specifically, for FI, goals of therapy are to improve anal sphincter strength, sensory awareness of stool presence, and coordination between the rectum and the anal sphincter (Rao, 1998). Treatment protocols are individualized and dictated by the underlying dysfunction. Accordingly, the number and frequency of sessions required for improvement varies, but commonly three to six 1-hour, weekly or biweekly appointments are needed. In many cases, reinforcing sessions at various subsequent intervals are also recommended.

Biofeedback has been noted to be an effective treatment for FI, and symptomatic improvement has been reported in up to 80 percent of treated patients (Engel, 1974; Jensen, 1997; Norton, 2001). However, in a Cochrane review of controlled studies of biofeedback or pelvic floor exercises for FI, Norton and colleagues (2001) found insufficient evidence to draw conclusions regarding the benefit of biofeedback for FI. More recently, however, a randomized controlled trial by Heymen and coworkers (2009) provided definitive support for biofeedback's efficacy in treating FI. Investigators initially provided education on pelvic floor muscle anatomy and physiology, a review of anorectal manometry results, and instruction regarding fiber supplements and/or antidiarrheal medication use to participants. Patients who were adequately treated by these strategies (21 percent) were excluded from further study participation. The remaining 108 patients, who remained incontinent and dissatisfied, then progressed to the treatment, either biofeedback or pelvic floor exercises, to which they had been previously randomized. Biofeedback training more effectively reduced fecal incontinence severity and number of days with fecal incontinence. Moreover, 3 months after training, 76 percent of patients treated with biofeedback reported adequate relief of fecal incontinence symptoms compared with only 41 percent of patients treated with pelvic floor exercises. Twelve months later, biofeedback patients continued to show significantly greater reduction in FISI scores, and more patients continued to report adequate relief of fecal incontinence symptoms. The results of this and other trials suggest that biofeedback may not be necessary for patients with milder FI symptoms, as education, medical management, and pelvic floor exercises provide adequate symptom control for many patients. However, for those with more severe FI symptoms, instrument-assisted biofeedback is a highly effective treatment.

Pelvic Floor Muscle Strengthening Exercises. Also known as *Kegel exercises*, this technique alone has been shown to be less effective than instrument-assisted biofeedback in treating patients with chronic and more severe FI symptoms (Heymen, 2009). However, the exercises are safe and inexpensive and may benefit patients with mild symptoms, especially if performed in conjunction with other interventions, such as patient education, diet modification, and medical management.

Performance of these exercises is fully described in Chapter 23 (p. 624).

Surgical Treatment

Given the potential for postoperative morbidity and the less than optimal results presently reported with available surgical procedures, surgery should be reserved for those patients with major structural abnormalities of the anal sphincter(s), those with severe symptoms, and those who fail to respond to conservative management.

Anal Sphincteroplasty. Repair of the EAS and/or IAS is most commonly performed in patients with acquired AI and an anterior sphincter defect following an obstetric or iatrogenic injury. Two methods may be used for sphincter repair and include an end-to-end technique and an overlapping method (Section 43-26, p. 1252). The end-to-end technique is most commonly used by obstetricians to reapproximate torn ends of an anal sphincter at delivery. However, in patients remote from delivery with a sphincter defect and FI, the overlapping technique is preferred by most colorectal surgeons and urogynecologists.

With the overlapping method performed remote from delivery, short-term continence improvements of up to 85 percent were previously reported (Fleshman, 1991; Sitzler, 1996). However, recent reports show significant deterioration of continence during long-term postoperative surveillance (Baxter, 2003; Bravo, 2004; Halverson, 2002; Malouf, 2000). The reason for this deterioration following initial improvement remains unknown. Hypotheses include aging, scarring, and progressive pudendal neuropathy related either to initial injury or to repair. Patients who fail to improve after anal sphincteroplasty and who are found to have a persistent sphincter defect may be candidates for a second sphincteroplasty. However, those with an intact sphincter following repair and persistent symptoms are only considered candidates for conservative management or one of the salvage or minimally invasive surgical procedures described later.

Currently, there is no conclusive evidence that the overlapping method, if used at delivery, leads to results superior to those obtained with the traditional end-to-end method of anal sphincter repair (Fitzpatrick, 2000; Garcia, 2005). Moreover, overlapping repair requires increased technical skills and carries the potential for increased blood loss, operating time, and pudendal neuropathy. For these reasons, the end-to-end technique is likely to remain the standard method for sphincter reapproximation at delivery until further data from randomized controlled trials are available. Importantly, given the strong association between anal sphincter lacerations and development of AI, emphasis should continue to be given to primary prevention of these lacerations.

Postanal Pelvic Floor Repair. This repair is only advocated for patients who have significant FI with no evidence of sphincter defects or neuropathy and who fail to improve with conservative management. The procedure is designed to reestablish the anorectal angle and to lengthen and tighten the anal canal. Through an intersphincteric approach, sutures are

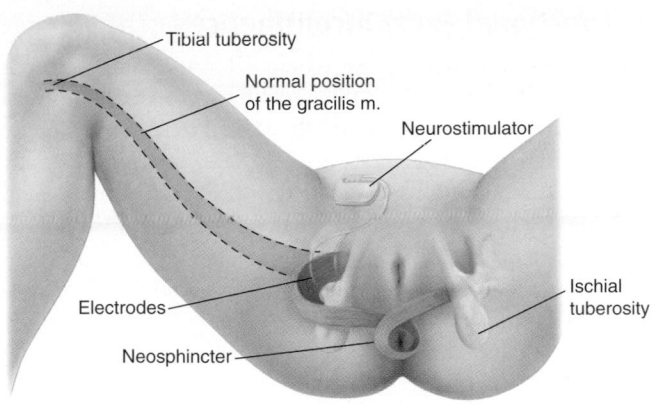

FIGURE 25-9 Dynamic graciloplasty. The gracilis muscle is detached from its insertion to the tibia, is wrapped around the anus, and is attached to contralateral ischial tuberosity. Muscle action is control by the neurostimulation unit.

placed between the ends of the iliococcygeus, pubococcygeus, puborectalis, and external anal sphincter muscles. Although Parks originally reported incontinence improvement in up to 80 percent of patients, similar results have not been replicated (Browning, 1983; Parks, 1975).

Gracilis Muscle Transposition. This procedure is advocated for patients who have failed sphincter repair or those with a sphincter defect too large to allow muscle reapproximation (Baeten, 1991). *Dynamic graciloplasty* involves separating the gracilis tendon from its point of insertion at the knee, wrapping the muscle around the anus, and attaching the tendon to the contralateral ischial tuberosity (Fig. 25-9). The muscle is then stimulated with an electrical pulse generator that is implanted in the abdominal wall.

This procedure has a significant learning curve and is performed in only a few medical centers that have adequate patient volume and surgical experience. Complication rates of greater than 50 percent have been reported and overall success rates range below 35 percent (Chapman, 2002; Matzel, 2001; Thornton, 2004; Wexner, 2002). However, it is an acceptable option for many patients whose only alternative is a permanent stoma. This procedure is not currently performed in the United States, as the generator used to stimulate the gracilis muscle has not been approved by the U.S. Food and Drug Administration (FDA) (Cera, 2005).

Artificial Anal Sphincters. The Acticon Neosphincter is an FDA-approved, fluid-inflated cuff that mimics anal sphincter function. The device is implanted around the anus; its reservoir balloon is placed within the abdominal wall or iliac fossa; and its control pump is placed in the labia (Fig. 25-10). When fully inflated, the cuff occludes the anal canal. When defecation is desired, the control pump in the labia is squeezed to move fluid from the anal cuff into the reservoir balloon. The cuff, when fluid-empty, relaxes pressure around the anus and permits defecation. After several minutes, the fluid within the reservoir returns to the anal cuff to restore circumferential pressure and continence. This procedure was first reported by Christiansen and Lorentzen (1987) and is still considered experimental by

many. It is indicated for patients with severe incontinence who have failed other treatment methods. This procedure carries high rates of complications and subsequent implant removal. Similar to the muscle transposition procedures, it has a considerable learning curve (Devesa, 2002; Parker, 2003).

Diversion (Colostomy or Ileostomy). Diversion is reserved for patients with incapacitating FI who have failed other treatments (Sections 44-19 and 44-21, p. 1319). For these selected patients, such procedures can significantly improve their quality of life.

Minimally Invasive Procedures for Fecal Incontinence

Secca Procedure. This outpatient procedure is currently used in the United States to treat FI in patients with no evidence of sphincter defects or pudendal neuropathy. It involves delivery of temperature-controlled radiofrequency energy to the anal sphincter muscles by means of a specifically designed anoscope. Resulting tissue heating is believed to cause heat-induced collagen contraction followed by focal wound healing, remodeling, and tightening. However, studies to date with this procedure have involved only small cohorts. In a multicenter study, Efron and colleagues (2003) showed a median 70-percent resolution of symptoms in 50 patients. Results also appear to be sustained over time. Specifically, Takahashi-Monroy and associates (2008) noted a >50-percent improvement of fecal incontinence scores 5 years after treatment in 16 of 19 patients.

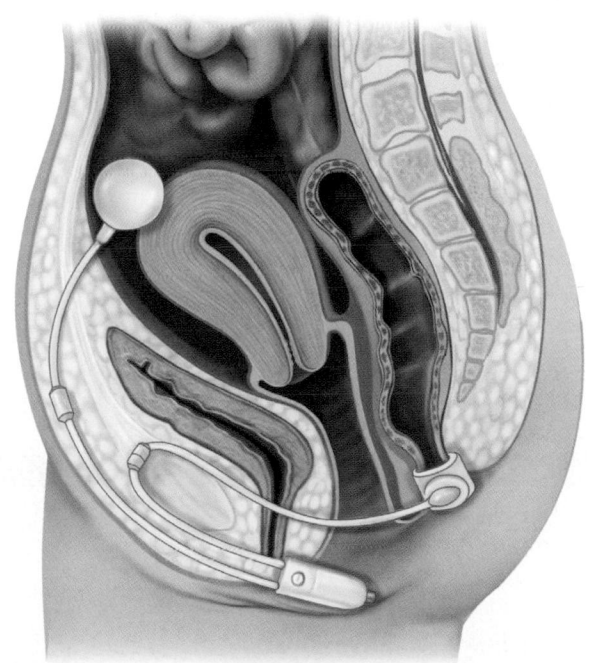

FIGURE 25-10 Artificial anal sphincter. The inflated cuff occludes the anal canal. When defecation is desired, the control pump in the labia is squeezed to remove fluid from the anal cuff into the reservoir balloon. Once emptied, the cuff relieves pressure around the anus and permits defecation. After several minutes, the fluid within the reservoir returns to the anal cuff to restore circumferential pressure and continence.

Sacral Nerve Stimulation (SNS). Sacral neuromodulation is presently used in the United States to treat selected cases of urge urinary incontinence, urgency-frequency syndrome, and idiopathic nonobstructive urinary retention (Section 43-12, p. 1212). In 2011, the U.S. FDA approved SNS for treatment of fecal incontinence. In one multicenter prospective trial, investigators placed the long-term SNS device (InterStim Therapy) only in patients that showed 50 percent or greater improvement during test stimulation. Of these individuals, 83 percent and 85 percent achieved therapeutic success at 12-month and 24-month follow-up, respectively (Wexner, 2010). Therapeutic success was defined as 50-percent or greater reduction of incontinent episodes per week at 12 months compared with baseline.

Percutaneous Tibial Nerve and Pudendal Nerve Stimulation. The *posterior tibial nerve* contains fibers from the sacral nerves. Stimulation of its peripheral fibers that reach the ankle transmits impulses to the sacral nerves and reflexively neuromodulates the rectum and anal sphincters (Shafik, 2003). The *pudendal nerve* innervates the pelvic floor muscles and the external urethral and anal sphincters. With either modality, stimulation of that particular nerve attempts to improve multiple impaired pelvic functions, including FI (Spinelli, 2005). However, limited data exist regarding the clinical indications, safety, and efficacy of each of these modalities for FI.

FUNCTIONAL ANORECTAL DISORDERS

In the current classification of functional gastrointestinal disorders, three functional anorectal disorders are recognized: (1) functional FI, (2) functional anorectal pain, and (3) functional defecation disorders (Table 25-7) (Drossman, 2006). Criteria for these and other functional GI disorders have been defined by the Rome III Foundation expert consensus organization and are primarily diagnosed based on patients' reported symptoms. As with other functional disorders, organic disease should be excluded prior to assignment of these diagnoses.

TABLE 25-7. Rome III Criteria of Functional Gastrointestinal Disorders

Functional Anorectal Disorders

Functional fecal incontinence
Functional anorectal pain
  Chronic proctalgia
    Levator ani syndrome
    Unspecified functional anorectal pain
  Proctalgia fugax
Functional defecation disorders
  Dyssynergic defecation
  Inadequate defecatory propulsion

Abbreviated from Drossman, 2006, with permission.

Functional Fecal Incontinence

Functional FI is defined by Rome III criteria as recurrent uncontrolled passage of fecal material for more than 3 months in an individual with anatomically normal defecatory muscles that function abnormally. As a result, fecal retention or diarrhea is common, and psychologic disorders may be associated. The etiology is varied, and causes may include disturbed intestinal motility, poor rectal compliance, impaired rectal sensation, and weakened pelvic floor muscles (Whitehead, 2001). Once diagnosed, functional FI is primarily treated with medical management or biofeedback, as described earlier.

Functional Anorectal Pain

Categories within this group are differentiated from one another by the duration of pain and by the presence or lack of associated puborectalis muscle tenderness. *Levator ani syndrome,* also known as *levator ani spasm,* usually presents as a pressure sensation or ache in the upper rectum (Chap. 11, p. 326). Rome III criteria require that symptoms be present for more than 3 months; that episodes should last at least 20 minutes; and that symptoms be associated with puborectalis muscle tenderness when palpated. In contrast, *proctalgia fugax* presents as sudden, severe anal or lower rectal pain that lasts for a few seconds to a few minutes. Pain may disrupt normal activities, but episodes rarely occur more than five times a year.

Treatments for levator ani syndrome are varied and may include, among others, trigger-point release maneuvers, biofeedback, local heat, and pharmacologic agents such as non-steroidal antiinflammatory drugs, other analgesics, muscle relaxants, and tranquilizers. In contrast, proctalgia fugax is typically managed with reassurance.

Functional Defecation Disorders

This group of disorders includes dyssynergic defecation and inadequate defecatory propulsion disorders. *Dyssynergic defecation* is also called pelvic floor dyssynergia, anismus, outlet obstruction constipation, or spastic pelvic floor syndrome. It is characterized by failed relaxation of the puborectalis muscle and EAS, which is needed for normal defecation. This condition is common and is thought to account for 25 to 50 percent of chronic constipation cases (Wald, 1990). Symptoms include chronic straining and impaired or incomplete evacuation. Diagnosis requires confirmation by EMG, manometry, or radiologic testing of persistent contraction of these muscles during attempted defecation. Other causes of constipation should also be excluded.

The treatment of constipation is challenging and often ineffective. Schiller and colleagues (1984) showed that only 53 percent of patients were satisfied with traditional medical therapies. Biofeedback interventions for dyssynergic defecation teach patients to relax their pelvic floor and anal sphincter muscles while simultaneously increasing intraabdominal/intrarectal pressures (Valsalva maneuver). The efficacy of biofeedback compared with laxatives in treating dyssynergic defecation was demonstrated in a controlled trial by Chiarioni and coworkers (2006). The benefits of biofeedback in this trial were sustained at 1-year follow-up. In a prospective randomized trial by Rao and associates (2007), biofeedback efficacy (manometric-assisted anal relaxation, muscle coordination, and simulated defecation training) was compared with sham feedback therapy and with standard therapy (diet, exercise, laxatives) in 77 subjects (69 women) with chronic constipation and dyssynergic defecation. Subjects in the biofeedback group had a greater number of complete spontaneous bowel movements and greater satisfaction with bowel function and were more likely to discontinue the use of digital maneuvers than subjects receiving standard treatment or sham feedback treatment. Specifically, dyssynergia patterns were corrected in 79 percent of subjects receiving biofeedback, in 4 percent receiving sham, and in 8.3 percent with standard treatment. Another manometric index, the time taken to expel an artificial stool, also significantly improved in the biofeedback group alone. In addition, colonic transit time significantly improved in subjects who received biofeedback and standard therapy but not in subjects who received sham feedback, suggesting that colonic transit slowing is due to dyssynergia. These findings emphasize the importance of performing neuromuscular conditioning and modifying the underlying physiologic behavior to correct dyssynergia and improve bowel function. Based on current data, biofeedback therapy is the preferred treatment for patients with dyssynergic defecation and chronic constipation, especially for those who have failed diet, exercise, and/or laxative therapy.

Sacral nerve stimulation is a promising therapeutic option for patients with intractable constipation. Although not yet approved in the United States for this indication, a recent prospective study at five European sites showed that SNS is effective in treating idiopathic slow- and normal-transit constipation that is refractory to conservative treatment (Kamm, 2010). In this trial, patients who failed conservative treatment underwent a 21-day test stimulation. Patients with >50-percent improvement in symptoms underwent permanent neurostimulator implantation. Primary endpoints were increased defecation frequency, decreased straining, and decreased sensation of incomplete evacuation. Of 62 patients (55 women) who underwent test stimulation, 45 (73 percent) proceeded to chronic stimulation. Treatment success was achieved in 39 (87 percent) of these patients.

RECTOVAGINAL FISTULA

Definition and Classification

Rectovaginal fistulas (RVFs) are congenital or acquired epithelial lined tracts between the vagina and rectum. They are classified according to their location, size, and etiology. All of these features aid in selecting the appropriate management and in predicting surgical repair outcome. The underlying cause of a fistula is believed to be the most important predictor of a successful outcome as it takes into account tissue and overall patient health.

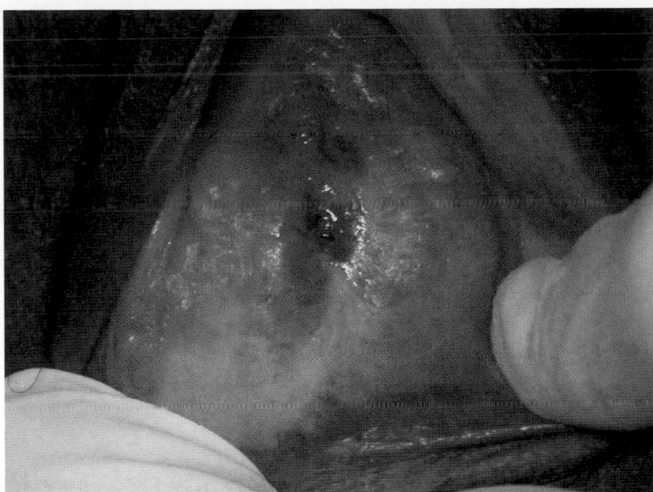

FIGURE 25-11 Rectovaginal fistula in the distal wall of the posterior vagina in a woman who sustained a fourth-degree perineal laceration.

Most RVFs are related to obstetric events and occur in the distal third of the vagina just above the hymen (Fig. 25-11 and Table 25-8) (Greenwald, 1978; Lowry, 1988; Tsang, 1998). Defect diameters can range from less than 1 mm to several centimeters, and most communicate with the rectum at or above the pectinate (dentate) line (Fig. 38-21, p. 937). In contrast, fistulas with an opening below the dentate line are also appropriately called *anovaginal fistulas*. Surgical management of these "low" RVFs depends on the condition of the EAS but is usually achieved by a perineal (transvaginal or transanal) approach. Midlevel RVFs are found in the middle third of the vagina, whereas high rectovaginal fistulas have their vaginal communication close to the cervix or the vaginal cuff. In cases with high RVFs, fistulas may open into the sigmoid colon. These fistulas may not be readily seen on examination. They often require contrast or endoscopic studies for diagnosis and an abdominal approach for repair.

Diagnosis

Patient History

Patients with RVF usually complain of flatus or stool leakage per vagina. They may also present with recurrent bladder or vaginal infection, rectal or vaginal bleeding, and pain. Presenting symptoms are often suggestive of the underlying etiology. For example, patients with obstetric injury and large defects of the anterior portion of the anal sphincters may present with gross fecal incontinence. In contrast, those with an infectious or inflammatory process may complain of diarrhea, abdominal cramping, and fevers.

Physical Examination

Most low RVFs can be visualized during inspection of the perineum and distal portion of the posterior vaginal wall. Rectovaginal examination allows assessment of the thickness of the perineal body and anovaginal wall and may allow

TABLE 25-8. Rectovaginal Fistula Risk Factors

Obstetric complications
Third- or fourth-degree laceration repair dehiscence
Unrecognized vaginal laceration during operative
  vaginal or precipitous delivery

Inflammatory bowel disease
Most commonly Crohn disease
Ulcerative colitis less common, as it is not a
  transmural disease

Infection
Most commonly cryptoglandular abscess located
  in the anterior aspect of the anal canal
Lymphogranuloma venereum
Tuberculosis
Bartholin gland duct abscess
Human immunodeficiency virus infection
Diverticular disease

Previous surgery in the anorectal area
Hemorrhoidectomy
Low anterior resection
Excision of rectal tumors
Hysterectomy
Posterior vaginal wall repairs

Pelvic radiation therapy

Neoplasm
Invasive cervical or vaginal cancer
Anal or rectal cancer

Trauma
Intraoperative
Coital

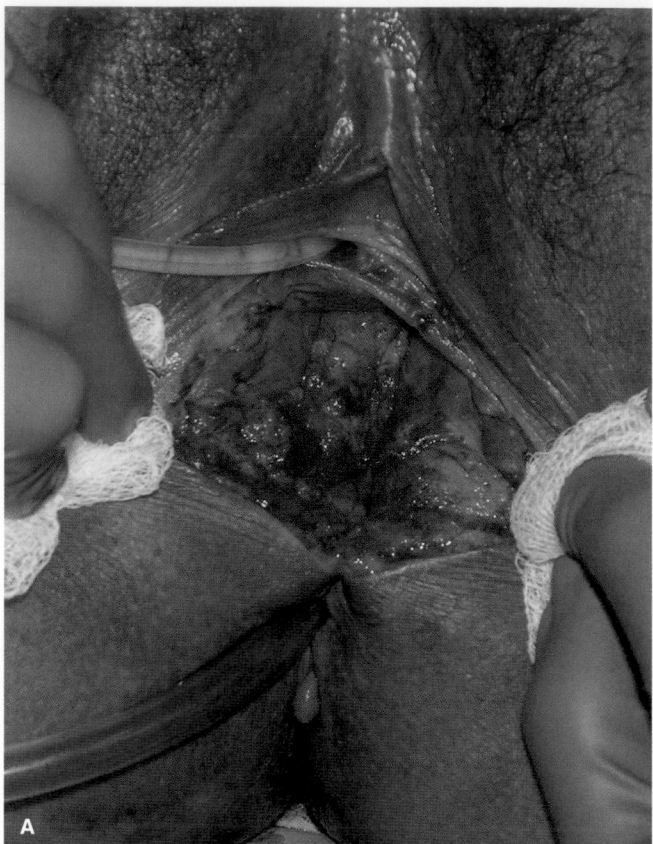

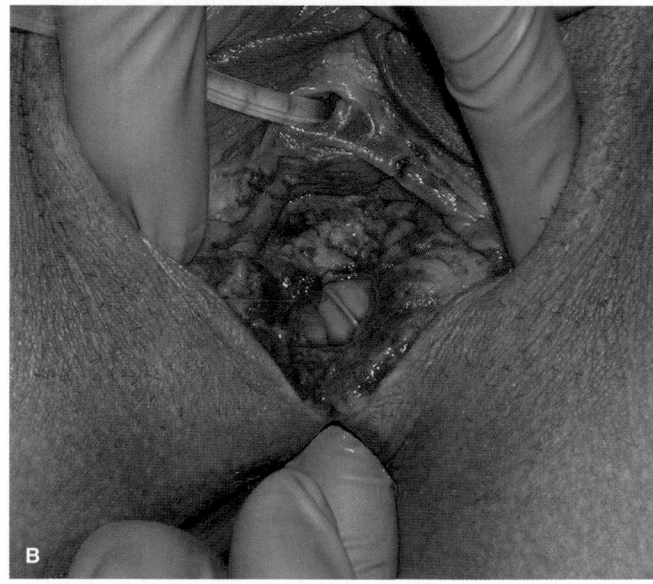

FIGURE 25-12 A. Large rectovaginal fistula in a woman who underwent midline episiotomy. **B.** Note that the fistula is above an intact external anal sphincter.

palpation and visualization of the actual defect. Some RVFs that are not readily seen on initial examination can be identified by noting air bubbles at the fistula's vaginal opening after filling the vagina with water. Alternatively, methylene blue can be instilled in the rectum after a tampon is placed in the vagina. The fistula and a gross assessment of its location can be identified by inspecting the level of blue staining on the tampon following its removal.

Diagnostic Testing

If the fistula site is not determined by the preceding maneuvers, a contrast study is indicated. These include barium enema and computed tomography (CT) scanning. Alternatively, vaginoscopy may be performed. The vagina is filled with sterile water or saline, the labia are closed, and a small endoscope is inserted vaginally to inspect the walls.

Unless RVFs are obviously due to a prior obstetric event, a biopsy of the fistulous tract is indicated to investigate possible malignancy or inflammatory conditions. In addition, proctoscopy or colonoscopy is warranted if inflammatory bowel disease, malignancy, or gastrointestinal infection is suspected.

■ Treatment

Treatment of RVF depends on the underlying etiology and the defect's size and location. Some women with small RVFs following obstetric trauma may be followed conservatively in anticipation of spontaneous healing of the fistulous tract (Goldaber, 1993; Rahman, 2003). If surgical repair is required, it should be delayed until surrounding tissues are free of edema, induration, and infection (Wiskind, 1992).

Larger obstetric-related defects and other low fistulas are most often corrected surgically. Surgical techniques include: (1) a transvaginal or transanal approach through episioproctotomy (conversion of the defect into a complete perineal tear, that is, a fourth-degree laceration), (2) a fistulotomy with a tension-free layered closure without episioproctotomy, or (3) a fistulotomy with transvaginal purse-string method of repair without episioproctotomy (Fig. 25-12). Additionally, endorectal flap advancement is used by colorectal surgeons primarily for the treatment of complex perianal fistulas such as those with tract diameters >2.5 cm or related to trauma or infection (MacRae, 1995). With flap advancement, the fistulous tract is excised, a broad-based flap of rectal wall is employed to obliterate the fistula's origin, and sphincter muscle division is avoided. Of these methods, better outcomes have been shown following RVF repair using anal sphincteroplasties compared with endorectal advancement flap (Tsang, 1998). In patients with low RVFs, preoperative endoanal ultrasonography of the EAS is important. For example, an episioproctotomy should be avoided if the sphincter is intact (Hull, 2007).

Midlevel vaginal fistulas are also often due to obstetric trauma and are repaired transvaginally or transanally by a tension-free layered closure or an endorectal advancement flap. High fistulas are most commonly repaired by a transabdominal approach using bowel resection of the involved segment followed by primary bowel reanastomosis.

Success rates vary depending on the underlying cause and method of repair. Successful repairs following obstetric injury vary from 78 percent to 100 percent (Khanduja, 1999; Tsang, 1998). Success rates of 40 to 50 percent have been reported with the rectal advancement flaps and of 74 percent with episioproctotomy (Mizrahi, 2002; Sonoda, 2002). Fistulas due to other etiologies such as radiation, cancer, or active inflammatory bowel disease are more difficult to treat successfully. In general, success rates are highest with the first surgical attempt at repair (Lowry, 1988).

REFERENCES

Abrams P, Cardozo L, Khoury S, et al: Incontinence. Third International Consultation on Incontinence, Monaco, 2004. Public Health Publications, 2005, p 286

Baeten CG, Konsten J, Spaans F, et al: Dynamic graciloplasty for treatment of faecal incontinence. Lancet 338(8776):1163, 1991

Barber MD, Bremer RE, Thor KB, et al: Innervation of the female levator ani muscles. Am J Obstet Gynecol 187(1):64, 2002

Barnett JL, Hasler WL, Camilleri M: American Gastroenterological Association medical position statement on anorectal testing techniques. American Gastroenterological Association. Gastroenterology 116(3):732, 1999

Baxter NN, Rothenberger DA, Lowry AC: Measuring fecal incontinence. Dis Colon Rectum 46(12):1591, 2003

Beets-Tan RG, Morren GL, Beets GL, et al: Measurement of anal sphincter muscles: endoanal US, endoanal MR imaging, or phased-array MR imaging? A study with healthy volunteers. Radiology 220(1):81, 2001

Bharucha AE: Outcome measures for fecal incontinence: anorectal structure and function. Gastroenterology 126(1 Suppl 1):S90, 2004

Bharucha AE: Pelvic floor: anatomy and function. Neurogastroenterol Motil 18(7):507, 2006

Borcham MK, Richter HE, Kenton KS, et al: Anal incontinence in women presenting for gynecologic care: prevalence, risk factors, and impact upon quality of life. Am J Obstet Gynecol 192(5):1637, 2005

Borello-France D, Burgio KL, Richter HE, et al: Fecal and urinary incontinence in primiparous women. Obstet Gynecol 108(4):863, 2006

Bravo GA, Madoff RD, Lowry AC, et al: Long-term results of anterior sphincteroplasty. Dis Colon Rectum 47(5):727, 2004

Briel JW, Stoker J, Rociu E, et al: External anal sphincter atrophy on endoanal magnetic resonance imaging adversely affects continence after sphincteroplasty. Br J Surg 86(10):1322, 1999

Browning GGP, Parks AG: Post-anal repair for neuropathic fecal incontinence—correlation of clinical-result and anal-canal pressures. Br J Surg 70(2):101, 1983

Buser WD, Miner PB: Delayed rectal sensation with fecal incontinence. Gastroenterology 91:1186, 1986

Cera SM, Wexner SD: Muscle transposition: does it still have a role? Clin Colon Rectal Surg 18(1):46, 2005

Chapman AE, Geerdes B, Hewett P, et al: Systematic review of dynamic grac[]loplasty in the treatment of faecal incontinence. Br J Surg 89(2):138, 2002

Cheetham M, Brazzelli M, Norton C, et al: Drug treatment for faecal incontinence in adults. Cochrane Database Syst Rev 3:CD002116, 2003

Chiarioni G, Whitehead WE, Pezza V, et al: Biofeedback is superior to laxatives for normal transit constipation due to pelvic floor dyssynergia. Gastroenterology 130(3):657, 2006

Christiansen J, Lorentzen M: Implantation of artificial sphincter for anal incontinence. Lancet 2(8553):244, 1987

Degen LP, Phillips SF: How well does stool form reflect colonic transit? Gut 39(1):109, 1996

Devesa JM, Rey A, Hervas PL, et al: Artificial anal sphincter: complications and functional results of a large personal series. Dis Colon Rectum 45(9):1154, 2002

Drossman DA: The functional gastrointestinal disorders and the Rome III process. Gastroenterology 130(5):1377, 2006

Efron JE, Corman ML, Fleshman J, et al: Safety and effectiveness of temperature-controlled radio-frequency energy delivery to the anal canal (Secca procedure) for the treatment of fecal incontinence. Dis Colon Rectum 46(12):1606, 2003

Engel BT, Nikoomanesh P, Schuster MM: Operant conditioning of rectosphincteric responses in the treatment of fecal incontinence. N Engl J Med 290:646, 1974

Fenner DE, Genberg B, Brahma P, et al: Fecal and urinary incontinence after vaginal delivery with anal sphincter disruption in an obstetrics unit in the United States. Am J Obstet Gynecol 189(6):1543, 2003

Fitzpatrick M, Behan M, O'Connell PR, et al: A randomized clinical trial comparing primary overlap with approximation repair of third-degree obstetric tears. Am J Obstet Gynecol 183(5):1220, 2000

Fleshman JW, Peters WR, Shemesh EI, et al: Anal sphincter reconstruction: anterior overlapping muscle repair. Dis Colon Rectum 34(9):739, 1991

Frenckner B, Euler CV: Influence of pudendal block on the function of the anal sphincters. Gut 16(6):482, 1975

Ganio E, Luc AR, Clerico G, et al: Sacral nerve stimulation for treatment of fecal incontinence: a novel approach for intractable fecal incontinence. Dis Colon Rectum 44(5):619, 2001

Garcia V, Rogers RG, Kim SS, et al: Primary repair of obstetric anal sphincter laceration: a randomized trial of two surgical techniques. Am J Obstet Gynecol 192(5):1697, 2005

Gearhart SL, Pannu HK, Cundiff GW, et al: Perineal descent and levator ani hernia: a dynamic magnetic resonance imaging study. Dis Colon Rectum 47:1298, 2004

Gilliland R, Altomare DF, Moreira H Jr, et al: Pudendal neuropathy is predictive of failure following anterior overlapping sphincteroplasty. Dis Colon Rectum 41(12):1516, 1998

Goldaber KG, Wendel PJ, McIntire DD, et al: Postpartum perineal morbidity after fourth-degree perineal repair. Am J Obstet Gynecol 168(2):489, 1993

Greenwald JC, Hoexter B: Repair of rectovaginal fistulas. Surg Gynecol Obstet 146(3):443, 1978

Halverson AL, Hull TL: Long-term outcome of overlapping anal sphincter repair. Dis Colon Rectum 45(3):345, 2002

Handa VL, Danielsen BH, Gilbert WM: Obstetric anal sphincter lacerations. Obstet Gynecol 98(2):225, 2001

Heaton KW, O'Donnell LJ: An office guide to whole-gut transit time. Patients' recollection of their stool form. J Clin Gastroenterol 19(1):28, 1994

Heymen S, Scarlett Y, Jones K, et al: Randomized controlled trial shows biofeedback to be superior to pelvic floor exercises for fecal incontinence. Dis Colon Rectum 52(10):1730, 2009

Hinninghofen H, Enck P: Fecal incontinence: evaluation and treatment. Gastroenterol Clin North Am 32:685, 2003

Hull TL, Bartus C, Bast J, et al: Success of episioproctotomy for cloaca and rectovaginal fistula. Dis Colon Rectum 50(1):97, 2007

Jensen LL, Lowry AC: Biofeedback improves functional outcome after sphincteroplasty. Dis Colon Rectum 40(2):197, 1997

Johanson JF, Lafferty J: Epidemiology of fecal incontinence: the silent affliction. Am J Gastroenterol 91(1):33, 1996

Jorge JMN, Wexner SD: Etiology and management of fecal incontinence. Dis Colon Rectum 36:77, 1993

Kamm MA, Dudding TC, Melenhorst J, et al: Sacral nerve stimulation for intractable constipation. Gut 59(3):333, 2010

Kaufman HS, Buller JL, Thompson JR, et al. Dynamic pelvic magnetic resonance imaging and cystocolpoproctography alter surgical management of pelvic floor disorders. Dis Colon Rectum 44:1575, 2001

Khanduja KS, Padmanabhan A, Kerner BA, et al: Reconstruction of rectovaginal fistula with sphincter disruption by combining rectal mucosal advancement flap and anal sphincteroplasty. Dis Colon Rectum 42(11):1432, 1999

Kwon S, Visco AG, Fitzgerald MP, et al: Validity and reliability of the modified Manchester health questionnaire in assessing patients with fecal incontinence. Dis Colon Rectum. 48(2):323, 2005

Lauti M, Scott D, Thompson-Fawcett MW: Fibre supplementation in addition to loperamide for faecal incontinence in adults: a randomized trial. Colorectal Dis 10(6):553, 2008

Lewis SJ, Heaton KW: Stool form scale as a useful guide to intestinal transit time. Scand J Gastroenterol 32(9):920, 1997

Lockhart ME, Fielding JR, Richter HE: Reproducibility of dynamic MR imaging pelvic measurements: a multi-institutional study. Radiology 249(2):534, 2008

Lowry AC, Thorson AG, Rothenberger DA, et al: Repair of simple rectovaginal fistulas. Influence of previous repairs. Dis Colon Rectum 31(9):676, 1988

Macmillan AK, Merrie AE, Marshall RJ, et al: The prevalence of fecal incontinence in community-dwelling adults: a systematic review of the literature. Dis Colon Rectum 47(8):1341, 2004

MacRae HM, McLeod RS, Cohen Z: et al: Treatment of rectovaginal fistulas that has failed previous repair attempts. Dis Colon Rectum 38(9):921, 1995

Madoff RD, Parker SC, Varma MG, et al: Faecal incontinence in adults. Lancet 364(9434):621, 2004

Malouf AJ, Norton CS, Engel AF, et al: Long-term results of overlapping anterior anal-sphincter repair for obstetric trauma. Lancet 355(9200):260, 2000

Matzel KE, Madoff RD, LaFontaine LJ, et al: Complications of dynamic graciloplasty: incidence, management, and impact on outcome. Dis Colon Rectum 44(10):1427, 2001

Matzel KE, Stadelmaier U, Hohenberger W: Innovations in fecal incontinence: sacral nerve stimulation. Dis Colon Rectum 47(10):1720, 2004

Matzel KE, Stadelmaier U, Hohenfellner M, et al: Electrical stimulation of sacral spinal nerves for treatment of faecal incontinence. Lancet 346(8983):1124, 1995

Miller R, Lewis GT, Bartolo DC, et al: Sensory discrimination and dynamic activity in the anorectum: evidence using a new ambulatory technique. Br J Surg 75(10):1003, 1988

Mizrahi N, Wexner SD, Zmora O, et al: Endorectal advancement flap: are there predictors of failure? Dis Colon Rectum 45(12):1616, 2002

Mowatt G, Glazener C, Jarrett M: Sacral nerve stimulation for faecal incontinence and constipation in adults. Cochrane Database Syst Rev 3:CD004464, 2007

Nelson R, Furner S, Jesudason V: Fecal incontinence in Wisconsin nursing homes: prevalence and associations. Dis Colon Rectum 41(10):1226, 1998

Nelson RL: Epidemiology of fecal incontinence. Gastroenterology 126(1 Suppl 1):S3, 2004

Norton C, Kamm MA: Anal sphincter biofeedback and pelvic floor exercises for faecal incontinence in adults—a systematic review. Aliment Pharmacol Ther 15(8):1147, 2001

Nygaard IE, Rao SS, Dawson JD: Anal incontinence after anal sphincter disruption: a 30-year retrospective cohort study. Obstet Gynecol 89(6):896, 1997

Oberwalder M, Thaler K, Baig MK, et al: Anal ultrasound and endosonographic measurement of perineal body thickness: a new evaluation for fecal incontinence in females. Surg Endosc 18(4):650, 2004

Parker SC, Spencer MP, Madoff RD, et al: Artificial bowel sphincter: long-term experience at a single institution. Dis Colon Rectum 46(6):722, 2003

Parks AG: Anorectal Incontinence. Proc R Soc Med 68(11):681, 1975

Perry S, Shaw C, McGrother C, et al: Prevalence of faecal incontinence in adults aged 40 years or more living in the community. Gut 50(4):480, 2002

Pescatori M, Anastasio G, Bottini C, et al: New grading and scoring for anal incontinence. Evaluation of 335 patients. Dis Colon Rectum 35(5):482, 1992

Rahman MS, Al-Suleiman SA, El-Yahia AR, et al: Surgical treatment of rectovaginal fistula of obstetric origin: a review of 15 years' experience in a teaching hospital. J Obstet Gynaecol 23(6):607, 2003

Rao SS: The technical aspects of biofeedback therapy for defecation disorders. Gastroenterologist 6(2):96, 1998

Rao SS, Seaton K, Miller M, et al: Randomized controlled trial of biofeedback, sham feedback, and standard therapy for dyssynergic defecation. Clin Gastroenterol Hepatol 5(3):331, 2007

Read M, Read NW, Barber DC, et al: Effects of loperamide on anal sphincter function in patients complaining of chronic diarrhea with fecal incontinence and urgency. Dig Dis Sci 27(9):807, 1982

Rociu E, Stoker J, Eijkemans MJ, et al: Fecal incontinence: endoanal US versus endoanal MR imaging. Radiology 212(2):453, 1999

Rockwood TH, Church JM, Fleshman JW, et al: Fecal incontinence quality of life scale: quality of life instrument for patients with fecal incontinence. Dis Colon Rectum 43(1):9, 2000

Rockwood TH, Church JM, Fleshman JW, et al: Patient and surgeon ranking of the severity of symptoms associated with fecal incontinence: the fecal incontinence severity index. Dis Colon Rectum 42(12):1525, 1999

Sailer M, Bussen D, Debus ES, et al: Quality of life in patients with benign anorectal disorders. Br J Surg 85(12):1716, 1998

Schiller LR, Santa Ana CA, Morawski SG, et al: Mechanism of the antidiarrheal effect of loperamide. Gastroenterology 86(6):1475, 1984

Shafik A, Ahmed I, El-Sibai O, et al: Percutaneous peripheral neuromodulation in the treatment of fecal incontinence. Eur Surg Res 35(2):103, 2003

Sitzler PJ, Thomson JP: Overlap repair of damaged anal sphincter. A single surgeon's series. Dis Colon Rectum 39(12):1356, 1996

Snooks SJ, Henry MM, Swash M: Faecal incontinence due to external anal sphincter division in childbirth is associated with damage to the innervation of the pelvic floor musculature: a double pathology. Br J Obstet Gynaecol 92(8):824, 1985

Sonoda T, Hull T, Piedmonte MR, et al: Outcomes of primary repair of anorectal and rectovaginal fistulas using the endorectal advancement flap. Dis Colon Rectum 45(12):1622, 2002

Spinelli M, Malaguti S, Giardiello G, et al: A new minimally invasive procedure for pudendal nerve stimulation to treat neurogenic bladder: description of the method and preliminary data. Neurourol Urodyn 24(4):305, 2005

Sultan AH, Kamm MA, Hudson CN, et al: Anal-sphincter disruption during vaginal delivery. N Engl J Med 329(26):1905, 1993

Takahashi-Monroy T, Morales M, Garcia-Osogobio S, et al: SECCA procedure for the treatment of fecal incontinence: results of five-year follow-up. Dis Colon Rectum 51(3):355, 2008

Terra MP, Beets-Tan RG, van der Hulst VP, et al: MRI in evaluating atrophy of the external anal sphincter in patients with fecal incontinence. AJR Am J Roentgenol 187(4):991, 2006

Thornton MJ, Kennedy ML, Lubowski DZ, et al: Long-term follow-up of dynamic graciloplasty for faecal incontinence. Colorectal Dis 6(6):470, 2004

Tsang CB, Madoff RD, Wong WD, et al: Anal sphincter integrity and function influences outcome in rectovaginal fistula repair. Dis Colon Rectum 41(9):1141, 1998

U.S. Food and Drug Administration: Medtronic® InterStim® Therapy System - P080025. May 25, 2011. Available at: http://www.fda.gov/MedicalDevices/ProductsandMedicalProcedures/DeviceApprovalsandClearances/RecentlyApprovedDevices/ucm249208.htm. Accessed October 25, 2011

Vaizey CJ, Carapeti E, Cahill JA, et al: Prospective comparison of faecal incontinence grading systems. Gut 44(1):77, 1999

Wald A: Surgical treatment for refractory constipation—more hard data about hard stools? Am J Gastroenterol 85(6):759, 1990

Wexner SD, Baeten C, Bailey R, et al: Long-term efficacy of dynamic graciloplasty for fecal incontinence. Dis Colon Rectum 45(6):809, 2002

Wexner SD, Coller JA, Devroede G, et al: Sacral nerve stimulation for fecal incontinence: results of a 120-patient prospective multicenter study. Ann Surg 251(3):441, 2010

Whitehead WE, Borrud L, Goode PS, et al: Fecal incontinence in U.S. adults: epidemiology and risk factors. Gastroenterology 137(2):512.e1, 2009

Whitehead WE, Schuster MM: Anorectal physiology and pathophysiology. Am J Gastroenterol 82(6):487, 1987

Whitehead WE, Wald A, Norton NJ: Treatment options for fecal incontinence. Dis Colon Rectum 44(1):131, 2001

Wiskind AK, Thompson JD: Transverse transperineal repair of rectovaginal fistulas in the lower vagina. Am J Obstet Gynecol 167(3):694, 1992

Zetterstrom JP, Lopez A, Anzen B, et al: Anal incontinence after vaginal delivery: a prospective study in primiparous women. Br J Obstet Gynaecol 106(4):324, 1999

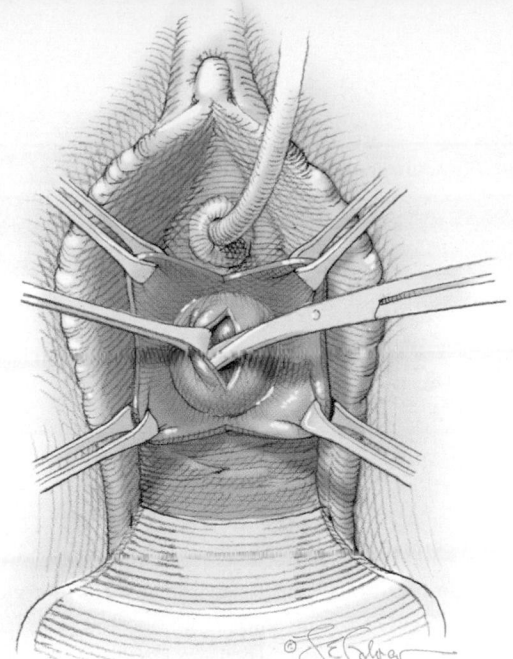

Genitourinary Fistula and Urethral Diverticulum

GENITOURINARY FISTULA

A genitourinary fistula is defined as an abnormal communication between the urinary (ureters, bladder, urethra) and the genital (uterus, cervix, vagina) systems. The true incidence of genitourinary fistula is unknown. However, the generally accepted incidence is derived from surgeries to correct these fistulas and approximates 1 percent or less of all genitourinary operations (Harris, 1995). This is most likely an underestima-

tion because many are unreported or unrecognized. The most common type of genitourinary fistula is the vesicovaginal fistula and is discussed later (Goodwin, 1980).

PATHOPHYSIOLOGY

Knowledge of the principles and phases of wound healing is important in understanding the pathogenesis of genitourinary fistula. After injury, tissue damage and necrosis stimulate inflammation, and the process of cell regeneration begins (Kumar, 2005). Initially, at the injury site, new blood vessels form in a process termed *angiogenesis*. Three to 5 days after injury, fibroblasts proliferate and subsequently synthesize and deposit extracellular matrix, in particular collagen. This *fibrosis phase* determines the final strength of the healed wound. Collagen deposition peaks approximately 7 days after injury and continues for a number of weeks. Subsequent maturation and organization of the scar, termed *remodeling*, augments wound strength. These phases are interdependent and are intrinsically involved in wound healing. Any disruption of this sequence eventually may result in fistula formation. Most fistulas tend to present 1 to 3 weeks after tissue injury, a time during which tissues are most vulnerable to alterations in the healing environment, such as hypoxia, ischemia, malnutrition, radiation, and chemotherapy. Edges of the wound eventual epithelialize, and a chronic fistulous tract is thus formed.

CLASSIFICATION

Although many classification systems exist for genitourinary fistula, there is no single, accepted standardized scheme. Fistulas can develop at any point between the genital and urinary systems. Thus, one method of classification is based on anatomic communication (Table 26-1).

Vesicovaginal fistulas can also be characterized by their size and location in the vagina. They are termed *high vaginal,* when

TABLE 26-1. Classification of Genitourinary Fistula Based on Anatomic Communication

	Urinary Tract		
	Ureter	Bladder	Urethra
Vagina	Ureterovaginal	Vesicovaginal	Urethrovaginal
	Vesicoureterovaginal		
Cervix	Ureterocervical	Vesicocervical	Urethrocervical
Uterus	Ureterouterine	Vesicouterine	Not reported

found proximally in the vagina; *low vaginal,* when noted distally; or *midvaginal,* when identified centrally. For instance, posthysterectomy vesicovaginal fistulas are often proximal, or "high" in the vagina, and located at the level of the vaginal cuff.

Alternatively, some have classified vesicovaginal fistula based on the complexity and extent of involvement (Table 26-2) (Elkins, 1999). In this scheme, complicated vesicovaginal fistulas are those that involve pelvic malignancy, prior radiation therapy, shortened vaginal length, or bladder trigone; those that are distant from the vaginal cuff; or those that are greater than 3 cm in diameter.

In one obstetric classification system, high-risk vesicovaginal fistulas are described by their size (greater than 4 to 5 cm in diameter; involvement of urethra, ureter(s), or rectum; juxtacervical location with an inability to visualize the superior edge; and reformation following a failed repair (Elkins, 1999).

In addition, a surgical classification has been introduced as a method to objectively evaluate the repair of obstetric urinary fistulas (Waaldijk, 1995). In this system, type I fistulas are those that do not involve the urethral closure mechanism, type II fistulas do, and type III fistulas involve the ureter and include other exceptional fistulas. Type II fistulas are divided into: (1) without or (2) with total or subtotal urethra involvement. Type IIB fistulas are further subdivided as (a) without or (b) with a circumferential defect.

A more comprehensive and standardized classification system has been proposed that integrates the fistula location in reference to a fixed point of anatomy, the size of the fistula, and

TABLE 26-2. Classification of Vesicovaginal Fistulas

Classification	Description
Simple	Fistula measures <2 to 3 cm and is located near the cuff (supratrigonal) Patient with no prior radiation or malignancy Vaginal length is normal
Complicated	Patient with prior radiation therapy Pelvic malignancy is present Vaginal length is shortened Fistula measures >3 cm Fistula is distant from cuff or has trigonal involvement

the integrity of the surrounding tissues (Goh, 2004). This system's goal is to aid objective comparisons of surgical outcomes and fistula complications. In this scheme, genitourinary fistulas are initially divided into four types based on their distance from the external urethral meatus. They are further subdivided by fistula size, the extent of scarring that surrounds the defect, and whether the vagina is reduced in length from scarring or from fistula involvement (Table 26-3). Of these systems, the generalist gynecologist most commonly describes fistulas according to their anatomic communication and to their position in the vagina as high, mid, or low.

ETIOLOGY
Congenital

Congenital genitourinary fistulas are rare, with only 10 cases reported in the literature (Asanuma, 2000). It is thought to result either from the abnormal fusion of the ureteric bud and the caudal end of the müllerian duct with the urogenital sinus, or from incorporation of an aborted ureteric bud into a future mesonephric (Wolffian) duct remnant (Fig. 18-2, p. 483). These fistulas are usually associated with other renal or urogenital abnormalities (Dolan, 2004).

Acquired

Most vesicovaginal fistulas do not arise from developmental abnormalities but result from either obstetric trauma or pelvic surgery.

Obstetric Trauma. In developing countries, 90 percent of genitourinary fistulas arise from obstetric trauma, specifically from prolonged or obstructed labor (Arrowsmith, 1996). Their development in this setting often reflects social customs and practices, lifestyle, or accepted obstetric management inherent to a particular society or geographic region. For example, both childbearing at a young age, before the pelvis has completely developed or fully grown, and female circumcision, more recently termed *female genital mutilation* or *cutting,* may lead to a narrow vaginal introitus and can obstruct labor. Obstructed labor or malpresentation of the presenting fetal part may cause pressure or ischemic necrosis of the anterior vaginal wall and bladder, subsequently resulting in fistula formation. Alternatively, vaginal trauma may result from damage by instruments used to deliver stillborn infants or perform abortion. Malnutrition and limited health care in many of these countries further complicates wound healing.

TABLE 26-3. Classification of Genitourinary Fistula

This new classification divides genitourinary fistulas into four main types, depending on the distance of the fistula's distal edge from the external urinary meatus. These four types are further subclassified by the size of the fistula, extent of associated scarring, vaginal length, or special considerations.

Type 1: Distal edge of fistula >3.5 cm from external urinary meatus
Type 2: Distal edge of fistula >2.5–3.5 cm from external urinary meatus
Type 3: Distal edge of fistula 1.5–2.5 cm from external urinary meatus
Type 4: Distal edge of fistula <1.5 cm from external urinary meatus

(a) Size <1.5 cm, in the largest diameter
(b) Size 1.5–3 cm, in the largest diameter
(c) Size >3 cm, in the largest diameter

   i. None or only mild fibrosis (around fistula and/or vagina) and/or vaginal length >6 cm, normal capacity
   ii. Moderate or severe fibrosis (around fistula and/or vagina) and/or reduced vaginal length and/or capacity
   iii. Special consideration, e.g., postradiation, ureteric involvement, circumferential fistula, or previous repair.

From Goh, 2004, with permission.

In contrast, in most developed countries, fistulas uncommonly follow obstetric procedures or deliveries. On rare occasion, cesarean deliveries, usually those accompanied by obstetric complications, have led to complex urinary fistula (Billmeyer, 2001).

Pelvic Surgery. In developed countries, iatrogenic injury during pelvic surgery is responsible for 90 percent of vesicovaginal fistulas, and the accepted incidence of fistula formation after pelvic surgery is 0.1 to 2 percent (Harris, 1995; Lee, 1988; Mattingly, 1978; Tancer, 1992). Eighty to 90 percent of genitourinary fistulas are related to surgery by obstetrician-gynecologists, whereas the remainder result from procedures performed by urologists and by colorectal, vascular, and general surgeons. In industrialized countries, hysterectomy is the most common surgical cause of vesicovaginal fistula, accounting for approximately 75 percent of fistula cases (Symmonds, 1984). When all types of hysterectomy are included, vesicovaginal fistula is estimated to complicate 0.8 per 1000 procedures (Harkki-Siren, 1998). In their review of more than 62,000 hysterectomy cases, laparoscopic hysterectomies were associated with the greatest incidence (2 per 1000), followed by abdominal (1 per 1000), vaginal (0.2 per 1000), and supracervical (0 per 1000) hysterectomies.

Because most genitourinary fistulas have an operative etiology, prevention and intraoperative recognition of lower urinary tract injury is imperative. For this, the use of intraoperative cystoscopy has been shown to improve the detection rate of lower urinary tract injuries. Gilmour (1999) found, in hysterectomies performed without cystoscopy, that ureteric and bladder injuries have crude occurrence rates of 1.6 and 2.6 per 1000 procedures, respectively. With intraoperative cystoscopy, the detection rate of these injuries increased to 6.2 per 1000 cases for ureteral injury and to 10.4 per 1000 cases for bladder injury. A cost analysis by Visco and coworkers (2001) addressed the cost-benefit aspects of performing routine intraoperative cystoscopy after hysterectomy. These investigators suggested that routine cystoscopy is cost effective if the base-line institutional rate of ureteral injury exceeds 1.5 percent for abdominal hysterectomy and 2 percent for vaginal or laparoscopically assisted vaginal hysterectomy. Although routine cystourethroscopy during hysterectomy is not mandatory, studies have underscored its value. Vakili and colleagues (2005) performed cystoscopy in patients undergoing abdominal, vaginal, or laparoscopic hysterectomy for benign disease. Of the 471 patients enrolled, 23 (5 percent) had a lower urinary tract injury. Two had both ureteral and bladder injuries, six had ureteral injuries only, and 15 had bladder injuries only. Of the 23 injuries, only 30 percent (one ureteral and six bladder injuries) were detected prior to cystoscopic survey. Thus, the implementation of routine cystoscopy may be a useful adjunct in the detection of lower urinary tract injury during hysterectomy. This in turn may ultimately result in a lower incidence of genitourinary fistula.

Other Causes. Although surgical and obstetric causes account for most urinary fistulas, other causes have been reported and include radiation therapy, malignancy, trauma, foreign bodies, infections, pelvic inflammation, and inflammatory bowel disease.

Radiation. Radiation therapy induces an endarteritis, which can lead to tissue necrosis and subsequent potential fistula formation. This modality is a frequent cause, and some series have reported that up to 6 percent of genitourinary fistulas can result from radiation (Lee, 1988). Although most damage following radiation treatment develops within weeks or months, fistulas associated with radiation therapy have been reported to present up to 20 years after the original insult (Graham, 1967; Zoubek, 1989).

Malignancy. Tissue necrosis and deterioration of tissue is commonly associated with malignancy and may lead to urinary fistula formation. Emmert and Kohler (1996) found a 1.8-percent incidence of rectovaginal and vesicovaginal fistula in their analysis of nearly 2100 women with cervical cancer.

For this reason, tissue biopsy should routinely be performed in a woman with a fistula and history of malignancy.

Trauma and Foreign Body. Trauma sustained during sexual activity or sexual assault can result in genitourinary fistula formation and has been estimated to precede 4 percent of these defects (Kallol, 2002; Lee, 1988). Foreign bodies such as a neglected pessary, an aerosol cap, and vesical calculi are also documented causes (Binstock, 1990; Dalela, 2003; Grody, 1999). Foreign bodies introduced during surgery such as collagen injected transurethrally and synthetic materials used in urethral sling procedures can also be inciting agents (Kobashi, 1999; Pruthi, 2000). For example, during sling surgeries, placement of the synthetic mesh under excess tension may contribute to increased tissue stress and necrosis. Additionally, initial material selection and patient evaluation for risk factors of poor wound healing play important roles in fistula prevention (Giles, 2005). Materials that minimize the inflammatory foreign body reaction are preferred and will maximize biocompatibility. Ideally, the material should also be nontoxic, nonantigenic, and porous enough to admit immune and phagocytic cells and promote native tissue ingrowth (Birch, 2002). Mesh selection is further discussed in Chapter 24 (p. 654).

Miscellaneous. Other rare causes of fistula formation include infections such as lymphogranuloma venereum, urinary tuberculosis, pelvic inflammation, and syphilis; inflammatory bowel disease; and autoimmune disease (Ba-Thike, 1992; Monteiro, 1995). Additionally, conditions that interfere with healing, such as poorly controlled diabetes mellitus, smoking, local infection, peripheral vascular disease, and chronic corticosteroid use, are potential risk factors.

CLINICAL PRESENTATION

Vesicovaginal fistula classically presents with unexplained continuous urinary leakage from the vagina after a recent operation. Depending on the size and location of the fistula, the amount of urine will vary. Occasionally small-volume, intermittent leakage is mistaken for postoperative stress incontinence. For this reason, patients with new-onset urinary leakage, particularly in the setting of recent pelvic surgery, should be examined thoroughly to exclude fistula formation. Other less specific symptoms of genitourinary fistula include fever, pain, ileus, and bladder irritability.

Vesicovaginal fistula may present days to weeks after the initial inciting surgery, and those following hysterectomy typically present at 1 to 3 weeks. Some fistulas, however, have longer latency and can cause symptoms a number of years later.

DIAGNOSIS

A thorough history and physical examination identifies most cases of vesicovaginal fistula. Accordingly, information regarding obstetric deliveries, prior surgeries, previous management of fistula, and treatment of malignancy, especially involving pelvic surgery and radiation therapy, should be documented.

The physical examination is equally important, and visual inspection during physical examination often will identify the defect. A meticulous assessment for other fistulous tracts should be performed, and their location and size noted. Vaginoscopy has been described by some to aid in fistula identification. With this procedure, a laparoscope is inserted into a vagina in which the walls are held apart by a translucent plastic speculum (Andreoni, 2003).

During evaluation, it is essential to differentiate between urinary leakage that occurs "extraurethrally," as with fistulas, and "transurethral" leakage, that is, through the urethra, as with stress urinary incontinence. Occasionally, the source of fluid present in the vagina is unclear, and a small amount of urine can easily be mistaken for vaginal discharge. Measurement of the vaginal fluid's creatinine content may sometimes be used to confirm its origin. Although levels of creatinine in urine can vary, with mean levels reaching 113.5 mg/dL, a value greater than 17 mg/dL is consistent with urine (Barr, 2005).

Although the ideal method of confirming genitourinary fistula is by direct visualization, there are instances in which physical examination and inspection are unrevealing. In these circumstances, bladder instillation of visually distinct solutions such as sterile milk or dilute methylene blue or indigo carmine can often indicate the presence of a fistula and aid in localizing the fistula site.

When the presence of a urinary fistula is uncertain, or the location in the vagina cannot be identified, a *three-swab test*, which is more commonly known as the *"tampon test,"* is recommended (Moir, 1973). When initially introduced, this test was commonly performed with a tampon. However, we recommend using two to four pieces of gauze sequentially packed into the vaginal canal. A diluted solution of methylene blue or indigo carmine is instilled into the bladder in a retrograde fashion using a urinary catheter. After 15 to 30 minutes of routine activity, the gauze is removed serially from the vagina, and each is inspected for dye. The specific gauze colored with dye suggests fistula location—a proximal or high location in the vagina for the innermost gauze and a low or distal fistula for the outermost. If the distally placed sponge is stained with dye, however, confirmation that it was not contaminated by urine leaking out through the urethra, as in the case of stress urinary incontinence, is essential.

Cystourethroscopy is another valuable diagnostic tool (Fig. 26-1). It allows localization of the fistula, determination of its proximity to the ureteral orifices, evaluation for multiple fistula sites, and assessment of surrounding bladder mucosa viability. In addition, Andreoni and associates (2003) described the use of cystourethroscopy and vaginoscopy concurrently to identify vesicovaginal fistula.

Concomitant ureteral involvement is estimated to complicate 10 to 15 percent of vesicovaginal fistulas and should be excluded in the diagnostic evaluation (Goodwin, 1980). Accordingly, intravenous urography may be used to assess integrity of the upper collecting system and ureteral involvement in a fistula. Retrograde pyelography generally has been reported to have the same diagnostic value as intravenous urography. However, some authors have attested to retrograde pyelography's higher diagnostic accuracy in detecting ureterovaginal fistulas (Dmochowski, 2002).

Alternatively, with some planning ahead, phenazopyridine hydrochloride (Pyridium) can be used in conjunction with the three-swab test to determine if there is ureteral involvement. This

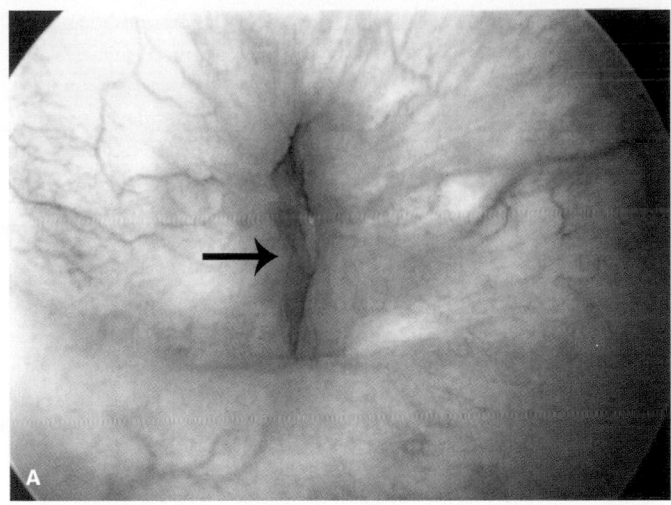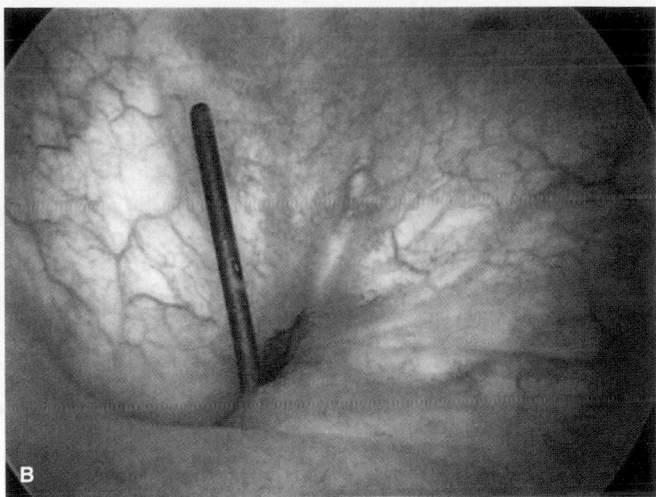

FIGURE 26-1 A. Cystoscopic view of vesicovaginal fistula (*arrow*). **B.** Probe placed through fistulous tract to aid cystoscopic visualization.

agent is administered orally, is excreted renally, acts as a topical bladder analgesic, and as a side effect, stains the urine orange. Women with suspected ureteral involvement are instructed to take a 200-mg dose a few hours before their clinic appointment. Gauze is packed serially into the vagina as described previously. If the most proximal (innermost) sponge is colored with orange dye, ureteral involvement is suspected. If both orange and blue dyes are seen, then there should be a high suspicion for involvement of both the bladder and ureter(s).

Voiding cystourethrography (VCUG) can also demonstrate leakage into the vagina and helps confirm the presence, location, and number of fistulous tracts (Fig. 26-2). Another radiographic tool that has been used to identify genitourinary fistula is sonography with color Doppler flow (Volkmer, 2000). The efficacy of this technique has not been substantiated, and some have documented low sensitivity rates for fistula detection (Adetiloye, 2000).

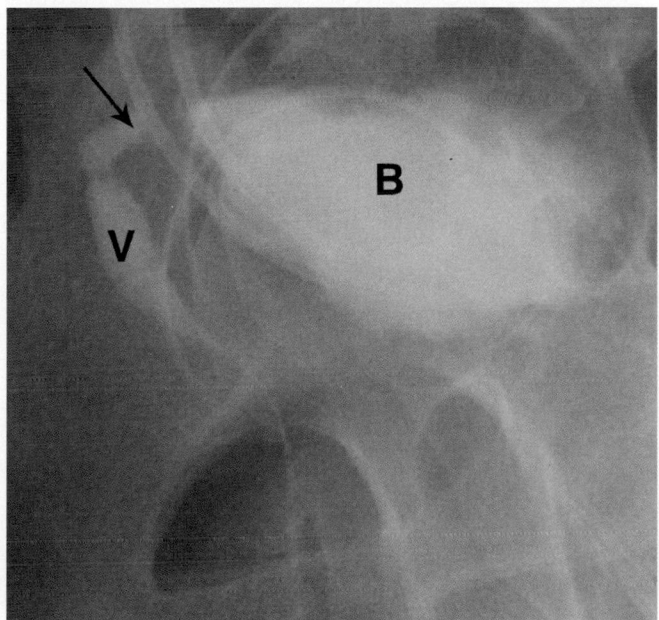

FIGURE 26-2 Voiding cystourethrogram of a vesicovaginal fistula. Arrow = fistula; B = bladder; V = vagina.

At our institution, we perform cystourethroscopy and intravenous pyelography (IVP)/VCUG as the initial diagnostic evaluation.

TREATMENT
Conservative Treatment

Occasionally, genitourinary fistulas may spontaneously close during continuous bladder drainage using an indwelling urinary catheter. Waaldjik (1994) found that 21 of 170 patients (12 percent) treated by catheterization alone had fistulas that healed spontaneously. Romics and colleagues (2002) found that in 10 percent of cases, urinary fistulas closed spontaneously after 2 to 8 weeks of transurethral catheterization, especially if the fistula was small (2 to 3 mm diameter). Another series reported that fistulas up to 2 cm in diameter spontaneously healed in 50 to 60 percent of patients treated with an indwelling catheter (Waaldijk, 1989).

Despite these series, data that correlate fistula size and success of conservative management are limited. Many of the studies reporting successful spontaneous closure with catheter drainage have been limited to fistulas that were 1 cm in size or smaller (Alonso Gorrea, 1985; Chittacharoen, 1993; Lentz, 2005; Ou, 2004). Many studies are vague regarding how fistula size is measured, and there is the potential for considerable bias in the selection criteria and size of fistulas included in each series. However, in general, the larger the fistula, the less likely it is to heal without surgery.

Evidence regarding the duration of catheter drainage has also varied. Regardless, many agree that if the fistula has not closed within 4 weeks, it is unlikely to do so. This may be secondary to epithelialization of the fistulous tract (Davits, 1991; Tancer, 1992). Moreover, continued urinary drainage may lead to further inflammation and irritation of the bladder (Zimmern, 1991). Importantly, if attempting conservative treatment of vesicovaginal fistulas with catheter insertion and chronic drainage, urinary drainage ideally begins shortly after the inciting event.

Although fibrin sealant has been described for the treatment of vesicovaginal fistula, its use has been as a surgical adjunct rather than primary surgical treatment (Evans, 2003). First, data regarding fibrin sealant effectiveness are sparse, and well-designed trials are lacking. Second, compared with surgical treatment, fibrin sealant monotherapy has not been shown to be durable, and recurrences are common (Kanaoka, 2001).

In sum, a trial of conservative therapy is usually warranted and reasonable, especially if instituted shortly after the inciting event and if the fistula is small. However, a balance between a conservative approach and the patient's desire for an expedited repair should be considered. Thus, the timing of intervention should achieve a compromise between reasonable conservative efforts and addressing the patient's immediate distress and quality of life. Indeed, most urinary fistulas ultimately require surgical intervention.

Surgical Treatment

General Principles. Although the first successful repair of a vesicovaginal fistula was reported hundreds of years ago, the principles of repair have withstood the test of time. These fundamentals include appropriate preoperative preparation; timely repair; multilayer, tension-free closure; adequate surrounding tissue viability; and postoperative bladder drainage.

Cure Rates. Surgical repair of genitourinary fistula is associated with high cure rates (67 to 100 percent) (Dmochowski, 2002). Factors that affect this success rate include viability of the surrounding tissue, duration of the fistulous tract, prior irradiation, surgical technique, and surgeon experience. The first attempt at surgical repair is usually associated with the best chance of successful healing (Weed, 1978). Surgical repair of obstetric fistulas also has high success rates. Of these, 81 percent are corrected with the first attempt, and 65 percent with the second (Elkins, 1994; Hilton, 1998).

Timing of Repair. Traditional teaching recommends delayed repair of fistulas at 3 to 6 months after the injury. However, this dictum is probably no longer applicable. Most agree that unless there is severe infection or acute signs of inflammation, waiting is not necessary and potentially subjects the patient to further anxiety (Wein, 1980). Early surgical intervention of uncomplicated fistulas does not affect closure rates, yet appears to reduce social and psychologic patient distress (Blaivas, 1995). Fistulas identified within the first 24 to 48 hours postoperatively can be safely repaired immediately with success rates of 90 to 100 percent (Blandy, 1991; Persky, 1979; Wang, 1990). Otherwise, intervention should be individualized, balancing patient quality of life with viability of surrounding tissue.

Route of Surgical Repair. Although there are many different types of surgical repair for vesicovaginal fistula, data that support an optimal route are limited and the lack of consensus may reflect the disparity in surgeon expertise and experience. Among important surgical considerations, ability to gain access to the fistula is essential and commonly dictates surgery selection. Fortunately, success rates are high whether the route of repair is transvaginal or transabdominal.

Vaginal. The transvaginal approach to genitourinary fistula repair is straightforward and direct. Compared with abdominal approaches, it is associated with shorter operative times, decreased blood loss, less morbidity, and shorter hospital stays (Wang, 1990). The transvaginal route also allows the use of ancillary equipment, such as ureteral stents. This is particularly useful if the fistula is located near the ureteral orifices.

Latzko Technique. This transvaginal approach to vesicovaginal fistula repair has been likened to a partial colpocleisis and is illustrated in Section 43-10 (p. 1206). This analogy stems from the fact that typically during this procedure, the most proximal portions of the anterior and posterior vaginal walls are surgically apposed to close the defect, without removing the fistulous tract. This partially obliterates the upper vagina. Because vaginal depth is potentially compromised, this technique may not be appropriate if vaginal depth has already been compromised or if there is preexisting sexual dysfunction. If use of this technique is anticipated, patient counseling should specifically address these issues and potential sequelae.

Classical Technique. In contrast to the Latzko method, the classical technique involves excision of the fistulous tract. After excision of the fistula, the vaginal epithelium is undermined and widely mobilized. The bladder mucosa is closed, followed by subsequent closure of two layers of fibromuscular tissue. A watertight repair is confirmed, and the vaginal epithelium is reapproximated. There is a school of thought that believes excising the fistulous tract may inherently weaken the repair or may extend the fistula size. Thus, some opt to keep the fistulous tract in situ during repair.

Abdominal (Transperitoneal). With this approach, the fistula is accessed through an intentional cystotomy on the preperitoneal side of the bladder as shown in Section 43-10 (p. 1206). Similar to the transvaginal approach, the bladder and vaginal epithelium at the fistula site are undermined for approximately 1.5 cm in all directions. After adequate mobilization, the fistula site is closed in layers. This approach is used for situations in which: (1) the fistula is located proximally in a narrow vagina, (2) it is in close proximity to the ureteral orifices, (3) a concomitant ureteric fistula is present, (4) previous repairs of the fistula have been unsuccessful and the fistula is recurrent, (5) the vaginal walls are rigid with little mobility, (6) the fistula is large or complex in configuration, or (7) there is a need for an abdominal interpositional graft.

Laparoscopic. Evidence-based support for laparoscopic genitourinary fistula repair has been limited to case reports and expert opinion (Miklos, 1999; Nezhat, 1994; Ou, 2004). The technique was first described by Nezhat and colleagues (1994) and requires advanced laparoscopic surgical skills. As a result, success with this approach appears to be highly dependent on surgeon expertise and experience.

Interpositional Flaps. Viability of the surrounding tissue is an important consideration in the repair of genitourinary fistula. When intervening tissues for fistula closure are weak and poorly vascularized, various tissue flaps may be placed vaginally or abdominally between the bladder and the vagina to lend support and blood supply (Eisen, 1974; Martius, 1928). Section 43-11 (p. 1210) illustrates the Martius bulbocavernosus fat pad flap, whereas Section 44-16 (p. 1314) illustrates the omental J-flap. Although interpositional flaps are useful in situations where the tissue viability is in question, their utility in uncomplicated cases of vesicovaginal fistula is unclear.

Urethrovaginal and Other Genitourinary Fistulas.
Although vesicovaginal fistulas are the most common type of genitourinary fistula, other fistulas can exist and may be described based on their communication between anatomic structures. Urethrovaginal fistulas commonly result from surgery involving the anterior vaginal wall, in particular anterior colporrhaphy and urethral diverticulectomy (Blaivas, 1989; Ganabathi, 1994a). In developing countries, as with vesicovaginal fistula, obstetric trauma remains the most common cause of urethrovaginal fistulas. In these cases, prolonged labor with ensuing tissue necrosis results in fistula development. Frequently, patients present with continuous urinary drainage into the vagina or with stress urinary incontinence. The principles of repair are similar—layered closure, tension-free repair, and postoperative bladder drainage. Other types of genitourinary fistula can also develop (see Table 26-1).

URETHRAL DIVERTICULUM

As shown on the next page, paraurethral glands are found along the anterior vaginal wall and communicate directly with the urethra. A urethral diverticulum is a cystic enlargement of one of these glands (Fig. 26-3). This isolated outpouching is commonly asymptomatic and is frequently diagnosed incidentally on routine examination. However, many present with symptoms and often require surgical excision.

INCIDENCE

Urethral diverticulum is reported to develop in 1 to 5 percent of the general female population. With greater awareness and radiologic advances, rates of diagnosis are increasing (Dmochowski, 2002). However, this incidence may be an underestimation of the true incidence because diverticula are frequently asymptomatic and thus underreported. In women with lower urinary tract symptoms, the incidence dramatically increases and may reach 40 percent (Stewart, 1981).

Urethral diverticulum may be found in any age group but is diagnosed most often in the third to sixth decades of life and more commonly in females than in males (Aldridge, 1978). Although some authors have reported a 6:1 predominance of urethral diverticula in African-Americans compared with whites, others have found no racial predisposition for the condition (Davis, 1970; Leach, 1987).

ETIOLOGY/PATHOPHYSIOLOGY
Congenital Diverticulum

The etiology of urethral diverticula is unclear. Although most are thought to be acquired, diverticula of congenital origin

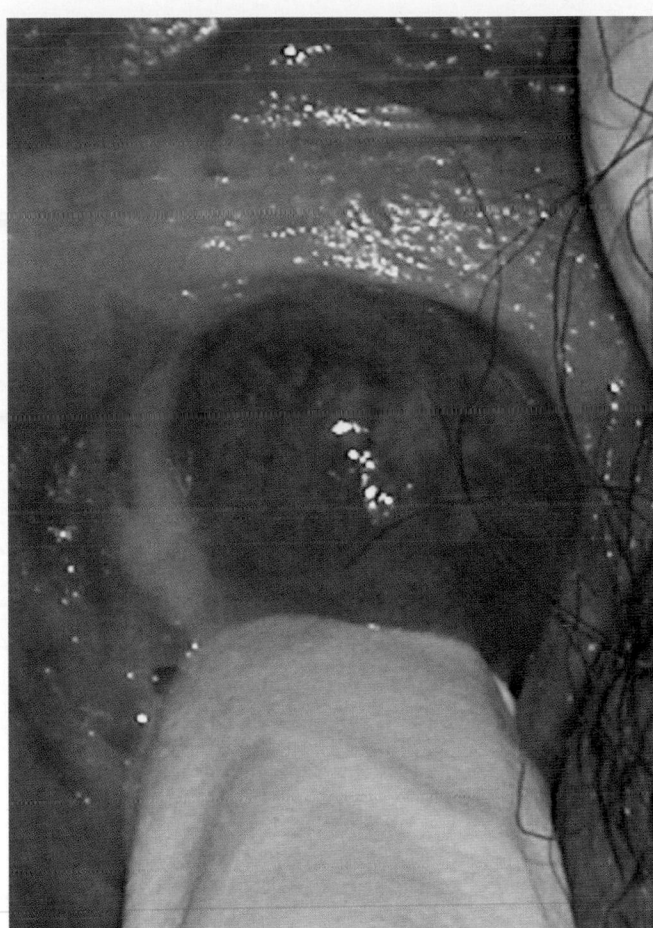

FIGURE 26-3 Transurethral expression of discharge with compression of a urethral diverticulum seen in the anterior vaginal wall.

have been reported (Bhatnagar, 1999; Nel, 1955). Congenital causes of urethral diverticula include persistence of embryologic remnants, defective closure of the ventral portion of the urethra, and congenital dilatation of paraurethral glands (Ratner, 1949).

An appreciation of the embryology and anatomy of the female genital tract and surrounding structures contributes, in part, to our understanding of congenital urethral diverticulum. During development of the vagina, the caudal aspect of the paired müllerian tubes fuses with an evagination of the urogenital sinus. The müllerian tubes form the upper vagina, whereas the urogenital sinus gives rise to the distal vagina and vestibule (Fig. 18-5, p. 486). In the vagina, müllerian mucinous columnar epithelium is replaced by squamous epithelium of the urogenital sinus. Similarly, the epithelium of the female urethra is also derived from the urogenital sinus. When the process of epithelial replacement is arrested, small foci of müllerian epithelium may persist and may form cysts or diverticula.

Acquired Diverticulum

More commonly, diverticula are acquired and may result from infection, birth trauma, and traumatic instrumentation. The most widely held theory regarding urethral diverticular development dates back to Routh (1890) and involves the paraurethral glands and their ducts. The paraurethral glands surround

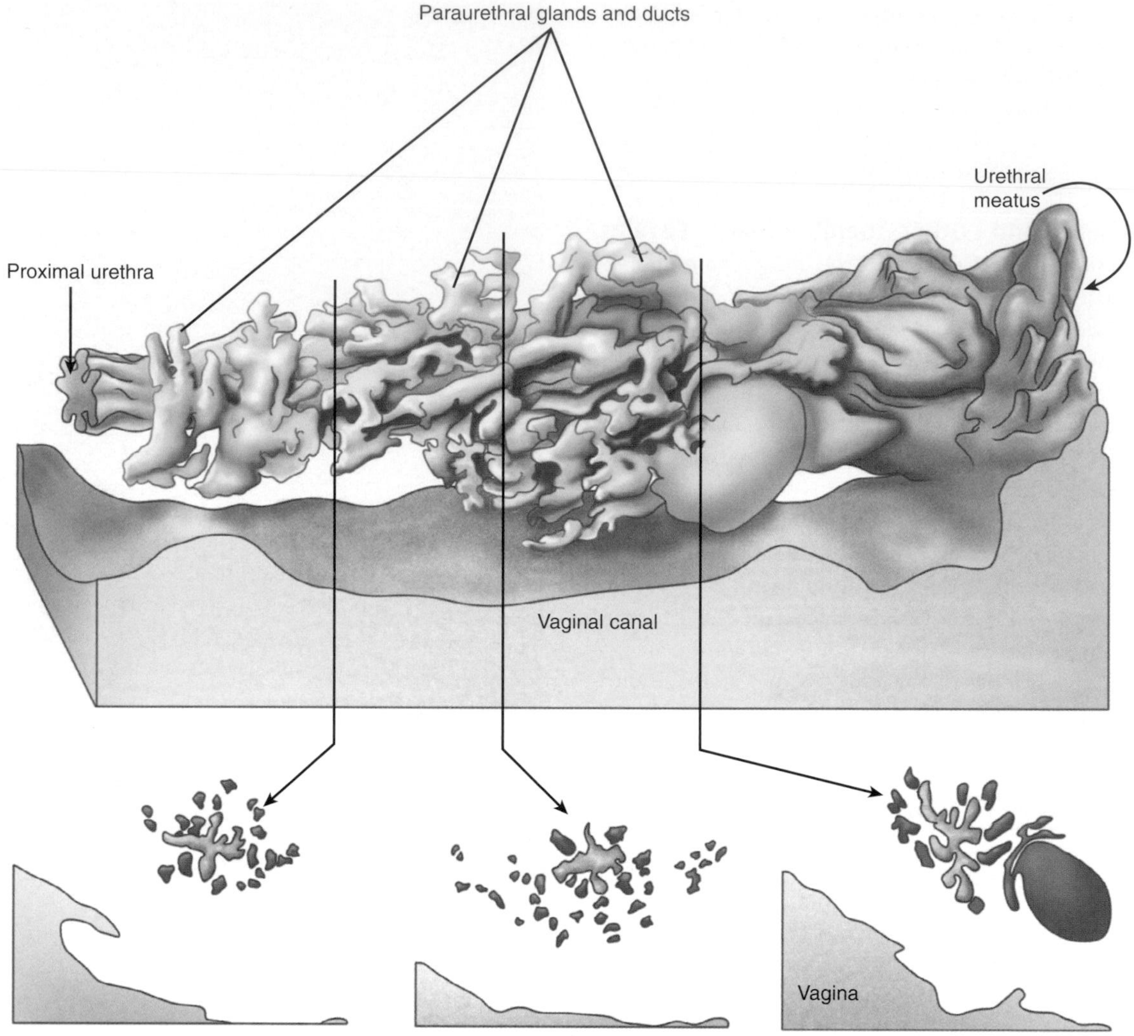

Paraurethral glands and ducts

Urethral meatus

Proximal urethra

Vaginal canal

Vagina

FIGURE 26-4 Complex configuration of paraurethral glands. Three cross sections are taken at different sites along the length of the urethra and show the varying density of paraurethral glands. *(Redrawn from Huffman, 1948, with permission.)*

and cluster most densely along the urethra's inferolateral border (Fig. 26-4). Of these glands, the Skene glands are the most distal and typically the largest. The paraurethral glands connect to the urethral canal via a network of branching ducts. The arborizing pattern in portions of this network helps to explain the complexity of some urethral diverticula (Vakili, 2003).

Routh theorized that infection and inflammation obstructs individual ducts, leading to cystic dilation. If spontaneous resolution does not occur or if intervention is not instituted promptly, abscess formation may ensue. Subsequent abscess progression and continued inflammation can lead to submural rupture of the gland into the urethral lumen, creating a communication between the two (Fig. 26-5). As the infection clears, the dilated diverticular sac and communicating ostium into the urethra persist. Of infectious agents, *Neisseria gonorrhoeae* and *Chlamydia trachomatis* are organisms commonly associated with urethritis and severe inflammation of the paraurethral glands.

In addition to infection, damage to urethral tissue may lead to tissue swelling and paraurethral duct obstruction. Accordingly, urethral trauma sustained during childbirth and during urethral instrumentation has been suggested as an etiology (McNally,

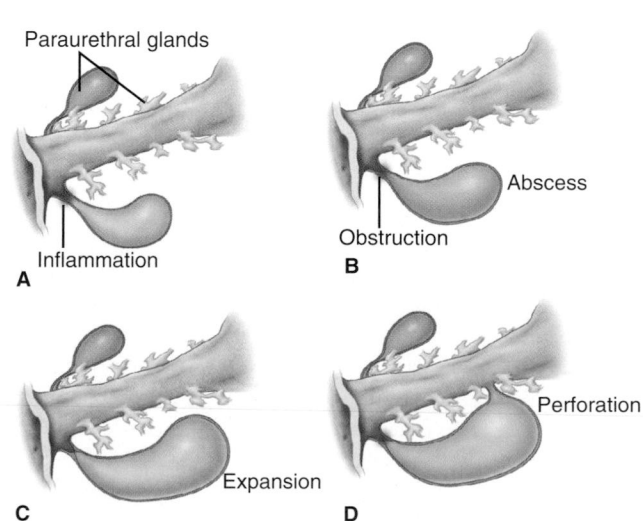

Paraurethral glands

Inflammation

A

Abscess

Obstruction

B

Expansion

C

Perforation

D

FIGURE 26-5 Mechanism of urethral diverticulum development. Inflammation at a paraurethral gland opening (**A**) leads to obstruction and potential abscess formation (**B**). **C.** Abscess expansion can lead to submural rupture into the urethral lumen (**D**). *(Redrawn from Elkins, 1999, with permission.)*

1935). Moreover, different social customs and obstetric practices in the developing world can potentially contribute to urethra trauma and diverticulum development. Obstetric trauma may result from childbirth at an early age, prolonged labor, and vaginal trauma during delivery. However, Pathak and House (1970) found that 40 percent of urethral diverticula in their series developed in nulliparous women, suggesting that causes in addition to childbirth are associated. For example, female genital mutilation or repeated urethral dilatations may traumatize the urethra.

Calculi

The development of stones within the diverticulum may complicate these lesions, and the reported frequency approximates 10 percent (Perlmutter, 1993). Stones may be singular or multiple and are usually composed of calcium oxalate or calcium phosphate. Stagnation of urine and precipitation of salts within the diverticular sac lead to crystal and subsequent stone formation.

Cancer

Malignant transformation within a urethral diverticulum is rare and accounts for only 5 percent of urethral cancer. Although most of these tumors are adenocarcinomas, transitional cell and squamous cell carcinomas have also been identified (Clayton, 1992). These tumors typically are found in women who are in their sixth or seventh decade of life. Although hematuria and irritative voiding complaints are common, palpation of an indurated or fixed mass around the urethra coupled with urinary obstructive symptoms should prompt further diagnostic evaluation and tissue biopsy (Ghoniem, 2004). Because fewer than 100 cases of urethral cancer associated with urethral diverticula have been reported, development of definitive treatment strategies has been limited. Currently, these cancers are treated by anterior exenteration or by diverticulectomy, alone or with adjuvant radiation therapy (Shalev, 2002).

CLASSIFICATION

Early classification systems organized urethral diverticula according to their radiographic complexity and described them as: (1) simple saccular, (2) multiple, or (3) compound or complex with branching sinuses (Lang, 1959). Alternatively, to help standardize surgical treatment, Ginsburg and Genadry (1983) created a preoperative classification system based on urethral location. This system organized diverticula depending on their urethral location and described lesions as type I (proximal third), type 2 (middle third), and type 3 (distal third).

In an attempt to fully incorporate all characteristics necessary to adequately assign treatment, Leach and coworkers (1993) constructed the L/N/S/C3 classification system. In this system, the characteristics of a diverticulum are described according to its location (L), number (N), size (S), and communication, configuration, and continence status of the patient (C3). Determining the location, configuration, and complexity of these lesions is important for surgical planning and aids in the selection of appropriate technique and approach. Location is described in relation to the urethra and is defined as distal,

mid-, or proximal urethral and as with or without extension beneath the bladder neck. In their series of 61 patients, these investigators found that most diverticula were in the midurethra (62 percent). Logically, this distribution reflects the predominance of paraurethral glands along the middle third of the urethra (see Fig. 26-4).

In addition to location, the number of diverticula is an important determination preoperatively. Inadequate excision and symptom persistence may ensue with failure to identify and completely excise multiple diverticula. Diverticulum size similarly may influence treatment options. For example, some authors recommend concomitant interpositional tissue flaps for large diverticula (Dmochowski, 2002). Moreover, urinary incontinence may develop de novo or persist if the diverticulum is extremely large and involves sphincter continence mechanisms.

The configuration of the diverticula may be described as solitary or multiloculated and as simple, saddle-shaped, or circumferential (Fig. 26-6). Preoperative knowledge regarding configuration can assist in complete surgical excision and aids with anticipating the need for an interpositional flap in those cases requiring extensive urethral resection (Rovner, 2003).

Obviously, successful repair of the urethral wall defect depends in great part on identifying the opening of the diverticulum into the urethral canal. Preoperative determination of the communication site is thus important with ostia being classified as proximal, mid-, or distal urethral. Leach and his associates (1993) found midurethral communication sites to be the most common (60 percent), followed by proximal (25 percent), and distal (15 percent).

Finally, in this classification system, the continence status and urethral hypermobility of the patient are documented. Almost half of the patients in their series had stress urinary incontinence, and these authors suggest that the presence of urethral hypermobility is an indication for concomitant antiincontinence surgery. Although several studies have documented the safety of

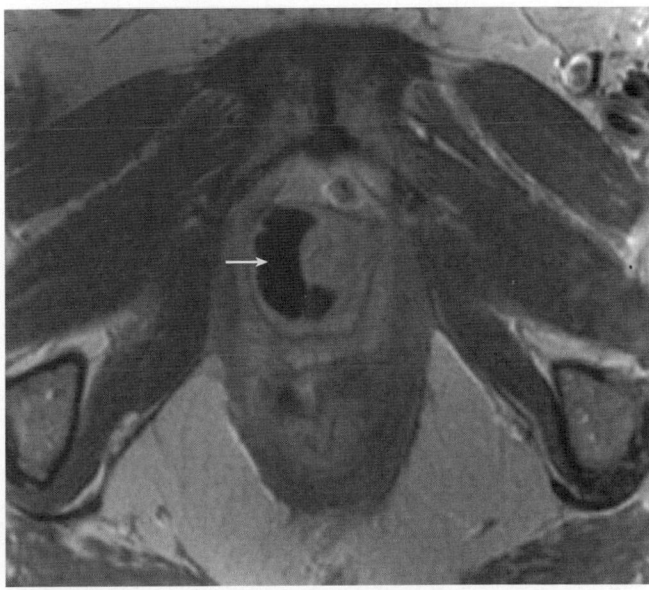

FIGURE 26-6 Magnetic resonance image of a circumferential urethral diverticulum. Arrow shows diverticulum extending around the urethra.

performing concurrent bladder-neck suspension, this approach is still considered by some as controversial due to concerns of urethral erosion (Bass, 1991; Faerber, 1998; Ganabathi, 1994b). However, others have not demonstrated increased erosion with concomitant performance of an antiincontinence procedure (Leng, 1998; Swierzewski, 1993).

Although there is no universal consensus on this issue, it is not unreasonable to treat the diverticulum first and then consider antiincontinence surgery if urinary incontinence persists. Pursuing treatment in this staged fashion is a particularly realistic option because of the current armamentarium of effective minimally invasive surgical procedures for the treatment of urinary incontinence, such as midurethral slings. Regardless of the decision of whether or not to proceed with concomitant antiincontinence surgery, these data and postoperative expectations should be discussed in detail with the patient during preoperative counseling.

SIGNS AND SYMPTOMS

Urethral diverticula are frequently asymptomatic and discovered incidentally on gynecologic or urologic examination for other complaints. However, when symptomatic, their presentations may vary and reflect their characteristics, especially size, location, and extension. Although postvoid dribbling, dysuria, and egress of discharge through the urethra with compression of a suburethral mass are pathognomonic, few women present so classically. For most patients, symptoms are nonspecific and include pain, dyspareunia, and a number of urinary symptoms. In a retrospective review, Romanzi and colleagues (2000) found that pain was one of the most common symptoms reported (48 percent). Pain is thought to result from occlusion of the diverticular neck and cystic dilatation behind the obstruction. In addition, dyspareunia may develop if the diverticulum is sufficiently large, inflamed, or infected. Accordingly, women may note either entry or deep dyspareunia, depending on whether the diverticulum is distal or proximal.

Large diverticula can often be mistaken for early-stage pelvic organ prolapse, especially when the presenting complaint is vaginal fullness, bulge, or pressure. In these cases, the palpable vaginal mass caused by a diverticulum may be mistaken for a cystocele or rectocele. Careful systematic palpation of the vaginal wall will distinguish prolapse from a discrete vaginal wall cyst or diverticulum in most cases.

A variety of lower urinary tract symptoms are commonly associated with urethral diverticulum. Specifically, urinary incontinence is noted by 35 to 60 percent of affected women (Ganabathi, 1994b; Romanzi, 2000). In addition, during micturition, urine may enter the diverticular sac, only to later spill from the sac and present as postvoid dribble or as urinary incontinence. In contrast to urine loss, urinary retention has also been reported to complicate diverticula (Nitti, 1999). Because symptoms of retention frequently accompany cancers growing within a diverticulum or around the urethra, women with urinary retention and an associated periurethral or urethral induration require biopsy to exclude malignancy (von Pechmann, 2003).

Urinary tract infection commonly complicates urethral diverticulum. In their treatment of 18 women with diverticula, Fortunato and associates (2001) noted acute cystitis in 8, dysuria in 7, and recurrent cystitis in 11.

DIAGNOSIS

For many women, urethral diverticula may be diagnosed using simply a detailed history, physical examination, and high index of suspicion. Patient history should focus on the common characteristics and symptoms of diverticula noted earlier. In addition, a history of prior vaginal trauma, infections, or surgery should be sought. However, despite available clinical and radiologic tools, the diagnosis for many women is delayed as women may be treated for stress or urgency incontinence, chronic cystitis, trigonitis, urethral syndrome, vulvovestibulitis, cystocele, and idiopathic chronic pelvic pain prior to identification of a diverticulum (Romanzi, 2000). Moreover, the diverticulum itself may mimic a Gartner duct cyst, vaginal inclusion cyst, ectopic ureterocele, or endometrioma (Chowdhry, 2004).

Physical Examination

With examination, the most common finding is an anterior vaginal mass underlying the urethra and is detected in 50 to 90 percent of symptomatic patients (Ganabathi, 1994b; Gerrard, 2003; Romanzi, 2000). Although urethral expression of purulent material with compression of the mass is common, failure to demonstrate transurethral expression of discharge does not exclude the diagnosis. Stenosis of the diverticular duct may obstruct sac emptying in these cases. Meticulous examination and palpation should be performed along the entire course of the urethra. Once diverticula are identified, their size, borders, consistency, configuration, and number should be determined.

However, if physical examination alone precludes complete delineation of these characteristics, further testing may be required. The diagnosis of urethral diverticulum has increased in the past few decades due to improved diagnostic modalities. Of available tests, each has significant advantages and disadvantages. For this reason, investigators may disagree as to which should be chosen primarily in evaluation of a urethral diverticulum. Accordingly, clinicians should be familiar with each modality's strengths and select whichever best fits the clinical setting.

Cystourethroscopy

Of the diagnostic procedures used to detect urethral diverticula, cystourethroscopy is the only tool that allows direct inspection of the urethra and bladder. During cystourethroscopy, fingers pressed upward against the proximal anterior vaginal wall occlude the bladder neck and allow the distending medium to create positive pressure and open diverticular ostia (Fig. 26-7). Use of a zero-degree cystoscope lens allows complete assessment of the urethra. This aids direct visualization and localization of diverticular ostia and identification of purulent discharge issuing from them.

A primary advantage to cystourethroscopy includes its accuracy in diverticula detection (Summitt, 1992). In addition, many women with diverticula present with nonspecific lower urinary tract symptoms, and endoscopic evaluation of the urethra and bladder allows exclusion of other etiologies for these

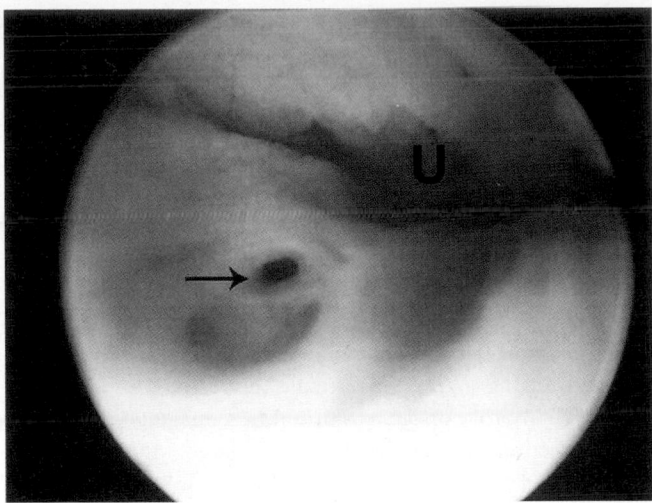

FIGURE 26-7 Diverticular opening visualized on cystourethroscopic examination (*arrow*). U = urethra.

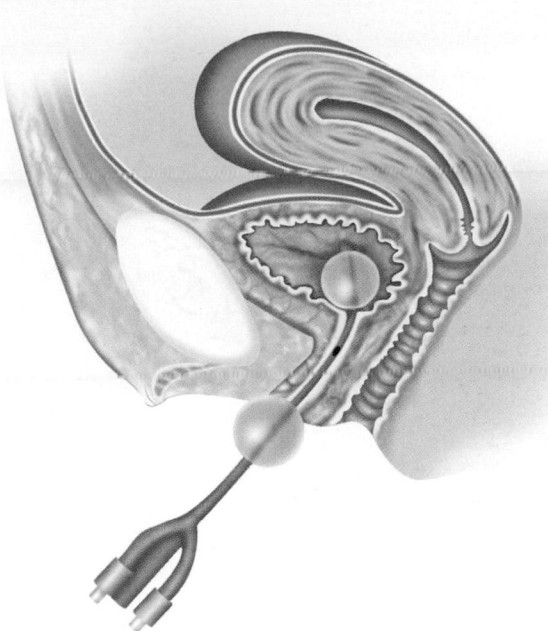

FIGURE 26-8 Trattner double-balloon catheter used to diagnose urethral diverticula. The portion of catheter between the two balloons contains an opening (*black oval*) through which contrast dye can flow to fill the urethra and any diverticula. *(Redrawn from Greenberg, 1981, with permission.)*

symptoms such as urethritis, cystitis, stones, or stenosis. Despite these advantages and its common use by urogynecologists, cystourethroscopy is used less frequently by gynecologic generalists. Obstacles include the need for a general knowledge of bladder and urethral mucosal anatomy, cystoscopic expertise, cost of instrumentation, and challenges in obtaining credentialing. Even for clinicians who are experienced with cystourethroscopy, this tool may still fail to display all diverticula. For example, a poor seal between the cystoscope and distal urethral mucosa may lead to inadequate distension and failure to identify distally located diverticula. Moreover, diverticula whose ostia are stenotic, and thus do not communicate with the urethral lumen, may be missed. Although cystourethroscopy is minimally invasive, patient pain and risk of postprocedural infection are also legitimate concerns. Lastly, important information regarding size, consistency, and circumferential extent of the diverticulum may not be obtained with this tool.

Voiding Cystourethrogram

Voiding cystourethrography (VCUG) is used by many as an initial tool in the evaluation of urethral diverticulum. Radiographic contrast instilled into the bladder will fill the diverticular sac during voiding, and postvoid radiographs demonstrate the presence of the diverticulum.

This test is painless and simple to perform, and its overall reported accuracy approximates 85 percent. However, some prefer positive-pressure urethrography as a primary diagnostic tool, since VCUG requires the diverticular communication to be patent during testing (Blander, 2001; O'Shaughnessy, 2006). Additionally, VCUG involves exposing the patient to ionizing radiation, albeit minimal.

Positive Pressure Urethrography

Following introduction by Davis and Cian (1956), positive pressure urethrography (PPUG) dramatically improved the detection of urethral diverticula. During PPUG, a double balloon, triple-lumen catheter (Trattner catheter) is inserted through the urethra, and its tip enters the bladder (Fig. 26-8).

Inflating the proximal balloon allows it to be pulled snug against and occlude the urethra at the urethrovesical junction. The distal balloon obstructs the distal urethra. A single catheter port between the two balloons allows instillation of radiopaque contrast dye into the urethra. This positive pressure then distends the urethra and expands any diverticula.

Urethrography is an effective modality for accurately identifying diverticula, and its sensitivity surpasses that of VCUG (Jacoby, 1999; Wang, 2000). Golomb and colleagues (2003) in their small series found 100-percent sensitivity with PPUG compared with 66 percent for VCUG. In every case in their study, PPUG defined the location, size, configuration, and communication of the diverticulum to the urethra. However, PPUG can be time consuming, technically difficult, and associated with patient discomfort and risk of postprocedural infection. Moreover, similar to VCUG, diverticula may be missed if thick pus or debris prevents adequate filling with contrast medium or if the ostium is obstructed and prevents communication with the urethral lumen. Accordingly, although PPUG for many has been a primary tool for diagnosing urethral diverticula, it has gradually been replaced by other radiologic modalities due to the lack of necessary equipment and expertise and because of its associated discomfort and invasiveness.

Sonography

This is a relatively new modality used to evaluate urethral diverticula and has been shown to be effective (Gerrard, 2003). Suggested technical advantages of sonography in this setting include visualization of diverticula that did not fill during radiographic contrast studies and characterization of diverticular wall thickness, size, and internal architecture (Fig. 26-9) (Yang,

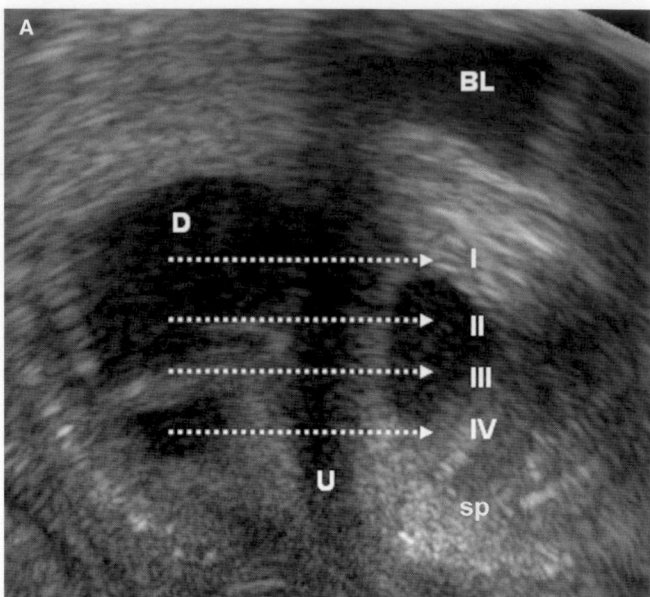

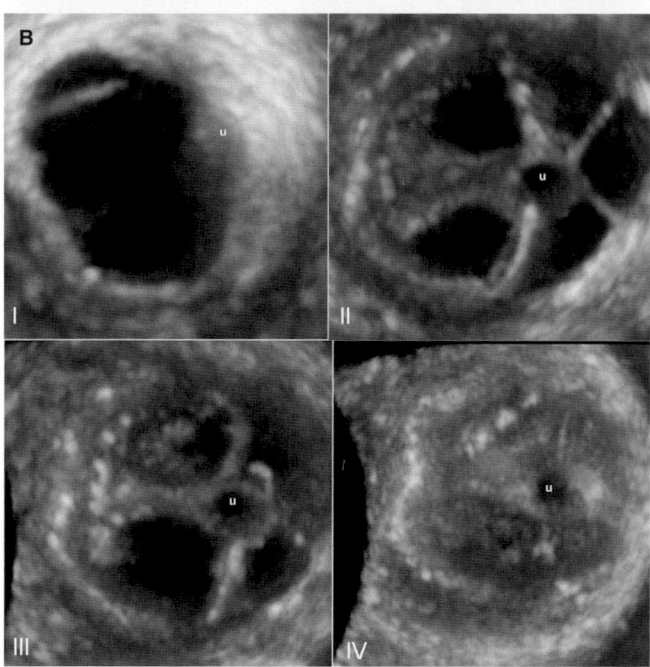

FIGURE 26-9 Transvaginal sonographic view of urethral diverticula. **A.** A sagittal view displaying the urethra and diverticulum. Dotted lines labeled with Roman numerals reflect the urethral level at which the remaining four axial views (**B**) were obtained. D = diverticulum; sp = symphysis pubis; U = urethra. *(From Yang, 2005, with permission.)*

2005). In addition, Siegel and coworkers (1998) noted that sonography provided information on other lesions such periurethral leiomyomas, diffuse urethritis, and periurethral scarring. Transabdominal, -vaginal, -rectal, -perineal, and -urethral sonography have all been reported (Keefe, 1991; Vargas-Serrano, 1997). Although the advantages of sonography include patient comfort, avoidance of ionizing radiation and contrast exposure, relative low cost, and reduced invasiveness, its role in the diagnosis of urethral diverticula has not been clearly established. It remains an academic or adjunctive technique currently.

Magnetic Resonance Imaging

Within the past decade, the use of magnetic resonance (MR) imaging has become more common in the diagnosis of periurethral pathology and is particularly useful in establishing the location, extent, and internal characteristics of periurethral masses (Kim, 1993; Nurenberg, 1997). For this reason, MR imaging is often recommended when diverticular architecture is complex and its entire extent has not been delineated by other modalities (Daneshgari, 1999; Rovner, 2003; Vakili, 2003). In comparison with other imaging tools, MR imaging has been shown to be comparable or have superior sensitivity for detecting urethral diverticula (Lorenzo, 2003; Neitlich, 1998). To improve image resolution, MR imaging may be used in conjunction with an imaging coil placed into the rectum or vagina. The coil, which is housed inside a probe, improves the image quality of structures surrounding the rectum or vagina (Blander, 2001). Alternatively, an external plate or coil for enhancement of image resolution can be used to minimize patient discomfort. However, the two techniques have not been compared with each other. In spite of the advantages of MR imaging, procedure costs should be considered within the clinical context. For a solitary diverticulum with clearly demarcated boundaries and no evidence of extension, costly and extensive imaging is probably not necessary.

Because there is still no consensus on which modality should be used primarily, it is reasonable to begin with cystourethroscopic evaluation followed by VCUG. If the initial evaluation is unrevealing but the diagnostic suspicion remains high or if the lesion appears more complex, then MR imaging combined with an endorectal coil or external plate may improve the resolution of images and add to the information gained.

▪ TREATMENT
Acute Treatment

A urethral diverticulum may present acutely with symptoms of pain, urinary symptoms, or focal tenderness during examination. Conservative management is recommended as initial treatment and includes sitz baths and administration of a broad-spectrum antibiotic such as a cephalosporin or fluoroquinolone.

Observation

Many women with minimal or no symptoms may decline surgery due to its associated risks of urethrovaginal fistula and sphincter defect incontinence. Long-term data on these women regarding rates of subsequent symptom development, diverticulum enlargement, and eventual need for surgical excision, however, are lacking.

Surgical

For many women, especially those with persistent symptoms, surgical correction is often indicated, and procedures include transvaginal partial ablation, marsupialization, and diverticulectomy.

Of these procedures, diverticulectomy is the most commonly used and can be selected to treat diverticula at any site along the urethra (Section 43-9, p. 1203). Excision of the entire diverticulum provides long-term correction of the urethral defect, normal urine stream, and high rates of postoperative continence. Disadvantages, however, include the risk of post-surgical urethral stenosis, urethrovaginal fistula, and potential injury of the urinary sphincter continence mechanism with subsequent development of urinary incontinence.

Alternatively, marsupialization of the diverticulum, also known as the Spence procedure, may be chosen to correct distal diverticula (Spence, 1970). The procedure is a meatotomy that when healed forms a new urethral meatus. Although simple to perform, this procedure alters the configuration of the meatus, and women often note a spray pattern with urination.

For proximal diverticula, partial ablation of the diverticular sac may be preferred to avoid the risk of bladder entry or bladder neck injury, which is associated with sacs in this location. Tancer and associates (1983) described this procedure, during which excess diverticular wall is excised, the diverticular neck is not removed, but remaining diverticular wall tissue is reapproximated to close the defect.

In addition to these approaches, case reports have described other procedures such as urethroscopic transurethral electrosurgical fulguration of the diverticular sac and transurethral incision to widen the diverticular ostia (Miskowiak, 1989; Saito, 2000; Vergunst, 1996). Data regarding long-term efficacy and complication rates with these techniques, however, are lacking.

REFERENCES

Adetiloye VA, Dare FO: Obstetric fistula: evaluation with ultrasonography. J Ultrasound Med 19:243, 2000

Aldridge CW Jr, Beaton JH, Nanzig RP: A review of office urethroscopy and cystometry. Am J Obstet Gynecol 131:432, 1978

Alonso Gorrea M, Fernandez Zuazu J, Mompo Sanchis JA, et al: Spontaneous healing of uretero-vesico-vaginal fistulas. Eur Urol 11: 341, 1985

Andreoni C, Bruschini H, Truzzi JC, et al: Combined vaginoscopy-cystoscopy: a novel simultaneous approach improving vesicovaginal fistula evaluation. J Urol 170:2330, 2003

Arrowsmith S, Hamlin EC, Wall LL: Obstructed labor injury complex: obstetric fistula formation and the multifaceted morbidity of maternal birth trauma in the developing world. Obstet Gynecol Surv 51:568, 1996

Asanuma H, Nakai H, Shishido S, et al: Congenital vesicovaginal fistula. Int J Urol 7:195, 2000

Barr DB, Wilder LC, Caudill SP, et al: Urinary creatinine concentrations in the U.S. population: implications for urinary biologic monitoring measurements. Environ Health Perspect 113:192, 2005

Bass JS, Leach GE: Surgical treatment of concomitant urethral diverticulum and stress incontinence. Urol Clin North Am 18:365, 1991

Ba-Thike K, Than A, Nan O: Tuberculous vesico-vaginal fistula. Int J Gynaecol Obstet 37:127, 1992

Bhatnagar V, Lal R, Mitra DK: Primary reconstruction of a congenital anterior urethral diverticulum. Pediatr Surg Int 15:294, 1999

Billmeyer BR, Nygaard IE, Kreder KJ: Ureterouterine and vesicoureterovaginal fistulas as a complication of cesarean section. J Urol 165:1212, 2001

Binstock MA, Semrad N, Dubow L, et al: Combined vesicovaginal-ureterovaginal fistulas associated with a vaginal foreign body. Obstet Gynecol 76:918, 1990

Birch C, Fynes MM: The role of synthetic and biological prostheses in reconstructive pelvic floor surgery. Curr Opin Obstet Gynecol 14:527, 2002

Blaivas JG: Vaginal flap urethral reconstruction: an alternative to the bladder flap neourethra. J Urol 141:542, 1989

Blaivas JG, Heritz DM, Romanzi LJ: Early versus late repair of vesicovaginal fistulas: vaginal and abdominal approaches. J Urol 153:1110, 1995

Blander DS, Rovner ES, Schnall MD, et al: Endoluminal magnetic resonance imaging in the evaluation of urethral diverticula in women. Urology 57:660, 2001

Blandy JP, Badenoch DF, Fowler CG, et al: Early repair of iatrogenic injury to the ureter or bladder after gynecological surgery. J Urol 146:761, 1991

Chittacharoen A, Theppisai U: Urological injury during gynecologic surgical procedures. J Med Assoc Thai 76(Suppl 1):87, 1993

Chowdhry AA, Miller FH, Hammer RA: Endometriosis presenting as a urethral diverticulum: a case report. J Reprod Med 49:321, 2004

Clayton M, Siami P, Guinan P: Urethral diverticular carcinoma. Cancer 70:665, 1992

Dalela D, Goel A, Shakhwar SN, et al: Vesical calculi with unrepaired vesicovaginal fistula: a clinical appraisal of an uncommon association. J Urol 170:2206, 2003

Daneshgari F, Zimmern PE, Jacomides L: Magnetic resonance imaging detection of symptomatic noncommunicating intraurethral wall diverticula in women. J Urol 161:1259, 1999

Davis BL, Robinson DG: Diverticula of the female urethra: assay of 120 cases. J Urol 104:850, 1970

Davis HJ, Cian LG: Positive pressure urethrography: a new diagnostic method. J Urol 75:753, 1956

Davits RJ, Miranda SI: Conservative treatment of vesicovaginal fistulas by bladder drainage alone. Br J Urol 68:155, 1991

Dmochowski R: Surgery for vesicovaginal fistula, urethrovaginal fistula, and urethral diverticulum. In Walsh PC, Retik AB, Vaughan ED, Wein AJ (eds): Campbell's Urology. Philadelphia, WB Saunders, 2002, p 1196

Dolan LM, Easwaran SP, Hilton P: Congenital vesicovaginal fistula in association with hypoplastic kidney and uterus didelphys. Urology 63:175, 2004

Eisen M, Jurkovic K, Altwein JE, et al: Management of vesicovaginal fistulas with peritoneal flap interposition. J Urol 112:195, 1974

Elkins TE: Surgery for the obstetric vesicovaginal fistula: a review of 100 operations in 82 patients. Am J Obstet Gynecol 170:1108, 1994

Elkins TE, Thompson JR: Lower urinary tract fistulas. In Walters MD, Karram MM (eds): Urogynecology and Reconstructive Pelvic Surgery. St. Louis, MO, Mosby, 1999, p 355

Emmert C, Kohler U: Management of genital fistulas in patients with cervical cancer. Arch Gynecol Obstet 259:19, 1996

Evans LA, Ferguson KH, Foley JP, et al: Fibrin sealant for the management of genitourinary injuries, fistulas and surgical complications. J Urol 169:1360, 2003

Faerber GJ: Urethral diverticulectomy and pubovaginal sling for simultaneous treatment of urethral diverticulum and intrinsic sphincter deficiency. Tech Urol 4:192, 1998

Fortunato P, Schettini M, Gallucci M: Diagnosis and therapy of the female urethral diverticula. Int Urogynecol J Pelvic Floor Dysfunct 12:51, 2001

Ganabathi K, Dmochowski R, Zimmern PE, et al: Prevention and management of urovaginal fistula. Urol Panamer 6:91, 1994a

Ganabathi K, Leach GE, Zimmern PE, et al: Experience with the management of urethral diverticulum in 63 women. J Urol 152:1445, 1994b

Gerrard ER Jr, Lloyd LK, Kubricht WS, et al: Transvaginal ultrasound for the diagnosis of urethral diverticulum. J Urol 169:1395, 2003

Ghoniem G, Khater U, Hairston J, et al: Urinary retention caused by adenocarcinoma arising in recurrent urethral diverticulum. Int Urogynecol J Pelvic Floor Dysfunct 15:363, 2004

Giles DL, Davila GW: Suprapubic-vaginocutaneous fistula 18 years after a bladder-neck suspension. Obstet Gynecol 105:1193, 2005

Gilmour DT, Dwyer PL, Carey MP: Lower urinary tract injury during gynecologic surgery and its detection by intraoperative cystoscopy. Obstet Gynecol 94:883, 1999

Ginsburg D, Genadry R: Suburethral diverticulum: classification and therapeutic considerations. Obstet Gynecol 61:685, 1983

Goh JT: A new classification for female genital tract fistula. Aust N Z J Obstet Gynaecol 44:502, 2004

Golomb J, Leibovitch I, Mor Y, et al: Comparison of voiding cystourethrography and double-balloon urethrography in the diagnosis of complex female urethral diverticula. Eur Radiol 13:536, 2003

Goodwin WE, Scardino PT: Vesicovaginal and ureterovaginal fistulas: a summary of 25 years of experience. J Urol 123:370, 1980

Graham JB: Painful syndrome of postradiation urinary-vaginal fistula. Surg Gynecol Obstet 124:1260, 1967

Greenberg M, Stone D, Cochran ST, et al: Female urethral diverticula: double-balloon catheter study. AJR Am J Roentgenol 136:259, 1981

Grody MH, Nyirjesy P, Chatwani A: Intravesical foreign body and vesicovaginal fistula: a rare complication of a neglected pessary. Int Urogynecol J 10:407, 1999

Harkki-Siren P, Sjoberg J, Tiitinen A: Urinary tract injuries after hysterectomy. Obstet Gynecol 92:113, 1998

Harris WJ: Early complications of abdominal and vaginal hysterectomy. Obstet Gynecol Surv 50:795, 1995

Hilton P, Ward A: Epidemiological and surgical aspects of urogenital fistulae: a review of 25 years' experience in southeast Nigeria. Int Urogynecol J Pelvic Floor Dysfunct 9:189, 1998

Huffman JW: The detailed anatomy of the paraurethral ducts in the adult human female. Am J Obstet Gynecol 55:86, 1948

Jacoby K, Rowbotham RK: Double balloon positive pressure urethrography is a more sensitive test than voiding cystourethrography for diagnosing urethral diverticulum in women. J Urol 162:2066, 1999

Kallol RK, Vaijyanath AM, Sinha A, et al: Sexual trauma—an unusual case of a vesicovaginal fistula. Eur J Obstet Gynecol 101:89, 2002

Kanaoka Y, Hirai K, Ishiko O, et al: Vesicovaginal fistula treated with fibrin glue. Int J Gynaecol Obstet 73:147, 2001

Keefe B, Warshauer DM, Tucker MS, et al: Diverticula of the female urethra: diagnosis by endovaginal and transperineal sonography. AJR Am J Roentgenol 156:1195, 1991

Kim B, Hricak H, Tanagho EA: Diagnosis of urethral diverticula in women: value of MR imaging. AJR Am J Roentgenol 161:809, 1993

Kobashi KC, Dmochowski R, Mee SL, et al: Erosion of woven polyester pubovaginal sling. J Urol 162:2070, 1999

Kumar V, Abbas AK, Fausto N: Tissue renewal and repair: regeneration, healing, and fibrosis. In Kumar V, Abbas AK, Fausto N (eds): Pathologic Basis of Disease. St. Louis, MO, WB Saunders, 2005, p 87

Lang EK, Davis HJ: Positive pressure urethrography: a roentgenographic diagnostic method for urethral diverticula in the female. Radiology 72:401, 1959

Leach GE, Bavendam TG: Female urethral diverticula. Urology 30:407, 1987

Leach GE, Sirls LT, Ganabathi K, et al: L N S C3: a proposed classification system for female urethral diverticula. Neurourol Urodyn 12:523, 1993

Lee RA, Symmonds RE, Williams TJ: Current status of genitourinary fistula. Obstet Gynecol 72:313, 1988

Leng WW, McGuire EJ: Management of female urethral diverticula: a new classification. J Urol 160:1297, 1998

Lentz SS: Transvaginal repair of the posthysterectomy vesicovaginal fistula using a peritoneal flap: the gold standard. J Reprod Med 50: 41, 2005

Lorenzo AJ, Zimmern P, Lemack GE, et al: Endorectal coil magnetic resonance imaging for diagnosis of urethral and periurethral pathologic findings in women. Urology 61:1129, 2003

Martius H: Die operative Wiederherstellung der vollkommen fehlenden Harnröhre und des Schließmuskels derselben. Zentralbl Gynäk 52:480, 1928

Mattingly RF, Borkowf HI: Acute operative injury to the lower urinary tract. Clin Obstet Gynaecol 5:123, 1978

McNally A: A diverticulum of the female urethra. Am J Surg 28:177, 1935

Miklos JR, Sobolewski C, Lucente V: Laparoscopic management of recurrent vesicovaginal fistula. Int Urogynecol J Pelvic Floor Dysfunct 10:116, 1999

Miskowiak J, Honnens dL: Transurethral incision of urethral diverticulum in the female. Scand J Urol Nephrol 23:235, 1989

Moir JC: Vesico-vaginal fistulae as seen in Britain. J Obstet Gynaecol Br Commonw 80:598, 1973

Monteiro H, Nogueira R, de Carvalho H: Behçet's syndrome and vesicovaginal fistula: an unusual complication. J Urol 153:407, 1995

Neitlich JD, Foster HE Jr, Glickman MG, et al: Detection of urethral diverticula in women: comparison of a high resolution fast spin echo technique with double balloon urethrography. J Urol 159:408, 1998

Nel JB: Diverticulum of the female urethra. J Obstet Gynaecol Br Emp 62:90, 1955

Nezhat CH, Nezhat F, Nezhat C, et al: Laparoscopic repair of a vesicovaginal fistula: a case report. Obstet Gynecol 83:899, 1994

Nitti VW, Tu LM, Gitlin J: Diagnosing bladder outlet obstruction in women. J Urol 161:1535, 1999

Nurenberg P, Zimmern PE: Role of MR imaging with transrectal coil in the evaluation of complex urethral abnormalities. AJR Am J Roentgenol 169:1335, 1997

O'Shaughnessy M: Urethral diverticulum. EMedicine 2006. Available at http://www.emedicine.com/med/topic3331.htm. Accessed February 26, 2006

Ou CS, Huang UC, Tsuang M, et al: Laparoscopic repair of vesicovaginal fistula. J Laparoendosc Adv Surg Tech A 14:17, 2004

Pathak UN, House MJ: Diverticulum of the female urethra. Obstet Gynecol 36:789, 1970

Perlmutter S, Huang AB, Hon M, et al: Sonographic demonstration of calculi within a urethral diverticulum. Urology 42:735, 1993

Persky L, Herman G, Guerrier K: Nondelay in vesicovaginal fistula repair. Urology 13:273, 1979

Pruthi RS, Petrus CD, Bundrick WS Jr: New onset vesicovaginal fistula after transurethral collagen injection in women who underwent cystectomy and orthotopic neobladder creation: presentation and definitive treatment. J Urol 164:1638, 2000

Ratner M, Siminovitch M, Ritz I: Diverticulum of the female urethra with multiple calculi. Can Med Assoc J 60:510, 1949

Romanzi LJ, Groutz A, Blaivas JG: Urethral diverticulum in women: diverse presentations resulting in diagnostic delay and mismanagement. J Urol 164:428, 2000

Romics I, Kelemen Z, Fazakas Z: The diagnosis and management of vesicovaginal fistulae. BJU Int 89:764, 2002

Routh A: Urethral diverticulum. BMJ 1:361, 1890

Rovner ES, Wein AJ: Diagnosis and reconstruction of the dorsal or circumferential urethral diverticulum. J Urol 170:82, 2003

Saito S: Usefulness of diagnosis by the urethroscopy under anesthesia and effect of transurethral electrocoagulation in symptomatic female urethral diverticula. J Endourol 14:455, 2000

Shalev M, Mistry S, Kernen K, et al: Squamous cell carcinoma in a female urethral diverticulum. Urology 59:773, 2002

Siegel CL, Middleton WD, Teefey SA, et al: Sonography of the female urethra. AJR Am J Roentgenol 170:1269, 1998

Spence HM, Duckett JW Jr: Diverticulum of the female urethra: clinical aspects and presentation of a simple operative technique for cure. J Urol 104:432, 1970

Stewart M, Bretland PM, Stidolph NE: Urethral diverticula in the adult female. Br J Urol 53:353, 1981

Summitt RL Jr, Stovall TG: Urethral diverticula: evaluation by urethral pressure profilometry, cystourethroscopy, and the voiding cystourethrogram. Obstet Gynecol 80:695, 1992

Swierzewski SJ 3rd, McGuire EJ: Pubovaginal sling for treatment of female stress urinary incontinence complicated by urethral diverticulum. J Urol 149: 1012, 1993

Symmonds RE: Incontinence: vesical and urethral fistulas. Clin Obstet Gynecol 27:499, 1984

Tancer ML, Mooppan MM, Pierre-Louis C, et al: Suburethral diverticulum treatment by partial ablation. Obstet Gynecol 62:511, 1983

Tancer ML: Observations on prevention and management of vesicovaginal fistula after total hysterectomy. Surg Gynecol Obstet 175:501, 1992

Vakili B, Chesson RR, Kyle BL, et al: The incidence of urinary tract injury during hysterectomy: a prospective analysis based on universal cystoscopy. Am J Obstet Gynecol 192:1599, 2005

Vakili B, Wai C, Nihira M: Anterior urethral diverticulum in the female: diagnosis and surgical approach. Obstet Gynecol 102:1179, 2003

Vargas-Serrano B, Cortina-Moreno B, Rodriguez-Romero R, et al: Transrectal ultrasonography in the diagnosis of urethral diverticula in women. J Clin Ultrasound 25:21, 1997

Vergunst H, Blom JH, De Spiegeleer AH, et al: Management of female urethral diverticula by transurethral incision. Br J Urol 77:745, 1996

Visco AG, Taber KH, Weidner AC, et al: Cost-effectiveness of universal cystoscopy to identify ureteral injury at hysterectomy. Obstet Gynecol 97:685, 2001

Volkmer BG, Kuefer R, Nesslauer T, et al: Colour Doppler ultrasound in vesicovaginal fistulas. Ultrasound Med Biol 26:771, 2000

von Pechmann WS, Mastropietro MA, Roth TJ, et al: Urethral adenocarcinoma associated with urethral diverticulum in a patient with progressive voiding dysfunction. Am J Obstet Gynecol 188:1111, 2003

Waaldijk K: Surgical classification of obstetric fistulas. Int J Gynaecol Obstet 49:161, 1995

Waaldijk K: The immediate surgical management of fresh obstetric fistulas with catheter and/or early closure. Int J Gynaecol Obstet 45:11, 1994

Waaldijk K: The (surgical) management of bladder fistula in 775 women in northern Nigeria. Doctoral thesis, University of Utrecht, Utrecht, The Netherlands, 1989, p 85

Wang AC, Wang CR: Radiologic diagnosis and surgical treatment of urethral diverticulum in women. A reappraisal of voiding cystourethrography and positive pressure urethrography. J Reprod Med 45:377, 2000

Wang Y, Hadley HR: Nondelayed transvaginal repair of high lying vesicovaginal fistula. J Urol 144:34, 1990

Weed JC: Surgical management of urethrovaginal and vesicovaginal fistulas. Am J Obstet Gynecol 131:429, 1978

Wein AJ, Malloy TR, Carpiniello VL, et al: Repair of vesicovaginal fistula by a suprapubic transvesical approach. Surg Gynecol Obstet 150:57, 1980

Yang JM, Huang WC, Yang SH: Transvaginal sonography in the diagnosis, management and follow-up of complex paraurethral abnormalities. Ultrasound Obstet Gynecol 25:302, 2005

Zimmern PE, Leach GE: Vesicovaginal fistula repair. Prob Urol 5:171, 1991

Zoubek J, McGuire EJ, Noll F, et al: The late occurrence of urinary tract damage in patients successfully treated by radiotherapy for cervical carcinoma. J Urol 141:1347, 1989

GYNECOLOGIC ONCOLOGY

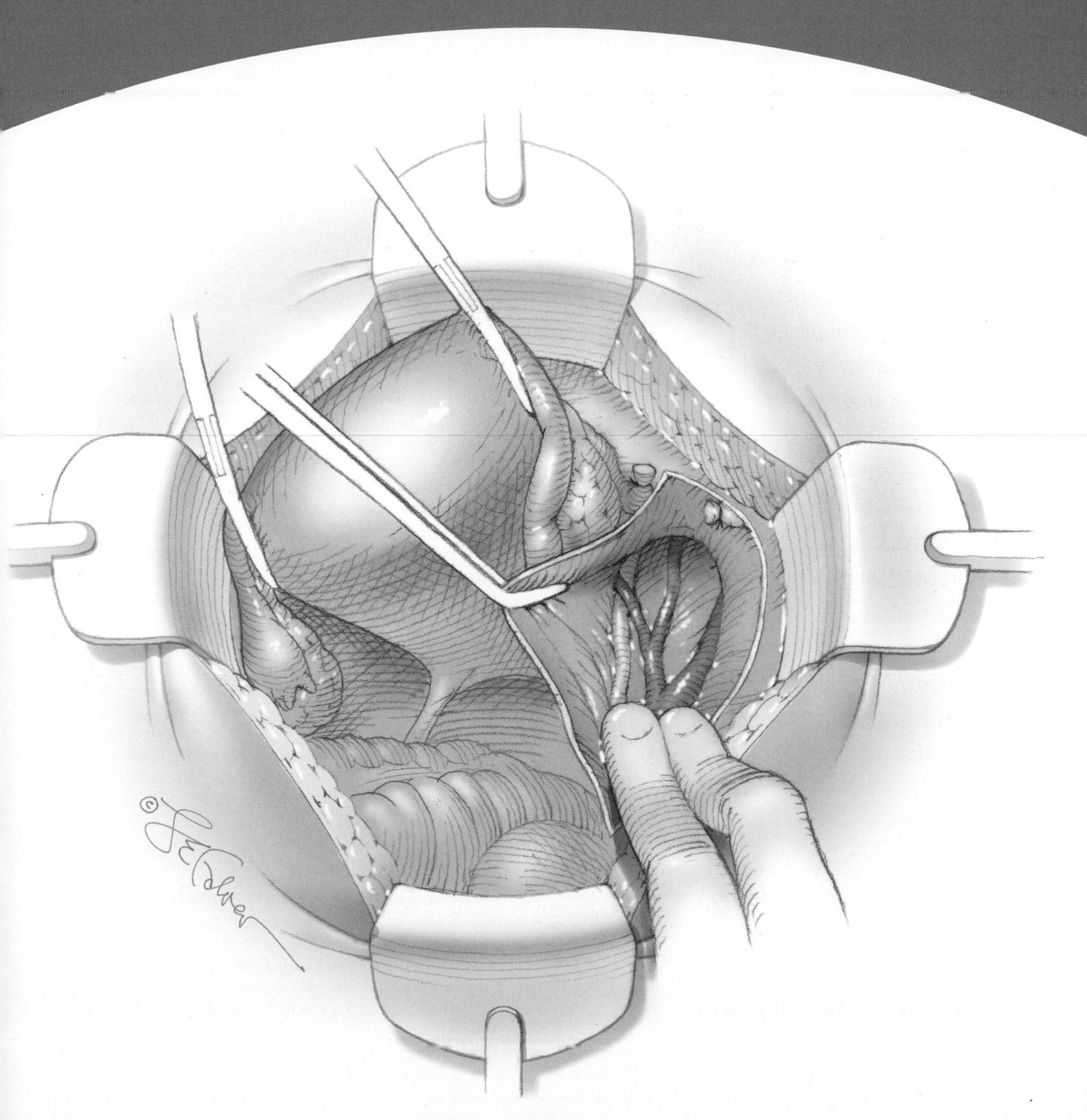

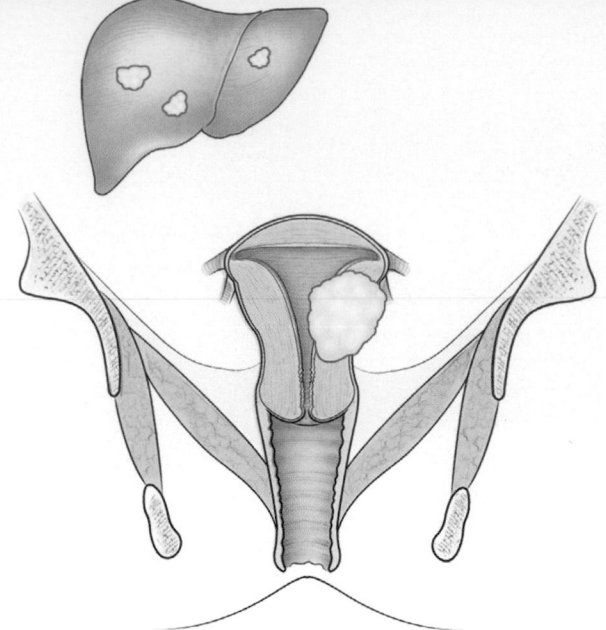

Principles of Chemotherapy

For the past 50 years, the incorporation of chemotherapy into the treatment of gynecologic cancers has perpetually evolved. New advances develop frequently and pose a continual challenge to staying abreast of the field. Thus, a foundation in this important third component of cancer treatment is essential.

BIOLOGY OF CANCER GROWTH

In principle, chemotherapeutic drugs are able to treat cancer and spare normal cells by exploiting inherent differences in their individual growth patterns. Each tumor type has its own

characteristics, which explain why the same chemotherapy regimen is not equally effective for the whole spectrum of gynecologic cancers. Selecting appropriate drugs and limiting toxicity demands an understanding of cellular kinetics and biochemistry.

The Cell Cycle

All dividing cells follow the same basic sequence for replication. The *cell generation time* is the time required to complete the five phases of the cell cycle (Fig. 27-1). The G_1 phase (G = gap) involves various cellular activities, such as protein synthesis, RNA synthesis, and DNA repair. When prolonged, the cell is considered to be in the G_0 phase, that is, the resting phase. G_1 cells may either terminally differentiate into the G_0 phase or reenter the cell cycle after a period of quiescence. During the S phase, new DNA is synthesized. The G_2 (premitotic) phase is characterized by cells having twice the DNA content as they prepare for division. Finally, actual mitosis and chromosomal division takes place during the M phase.

Tumors do *not* typically have faster generation times, but instead have many more cells in the active phases of replication and have dysfunctional apoptosis, hence proliferation. In contrast, normal tissues have a much larger number of cells in the G_0 phase. As a result, cancer cells proceeding through the cell cycle may be more sensitive to chemotherapeutic agents, whereas normal cells in G_0 are protected. This growth pattern disparity underlies the effectiveness of chemotherapeutic agents.

Cancer Cell Growth

Tumors are characterized by a *gompertzian growth* pattern (Fig. 27-2). Fundamentally, a tumor mass requires progressively longer times to double in size as it enlarges. When a cancer is microscopic and nonpalpable, growth is exponential. However, as a tumor enlarges, the number of its cells undergoing replication decreases due to limitations in blood supply and increasing interstitial pressure.

When tumors are in the exponential phase of gompertzian growth, they should be more sensitive to chemotherapy because a larger percentage of cells are in the active phase of the cell

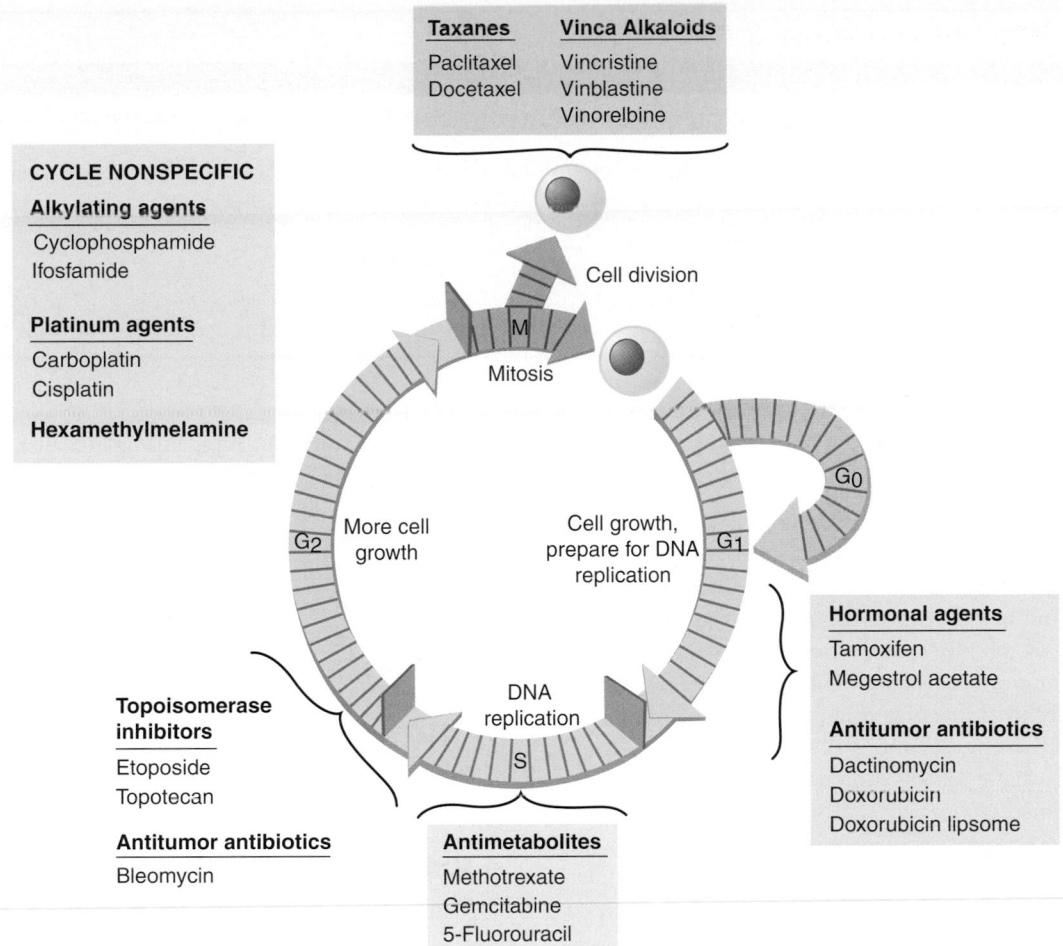

FIGURE 27-1 Diagram of the cell cycle. Agents are organized according to the cell cycle stage in which they are most effective for tumor control.

cycle. For this reason, metastases should be more sensitive to chemotherapy than the primary tumor. To capitalize on this potential benefit, advanced ovarian cancer is usually first treated with surgery to remove the primary tumor, debulk large masses, and leave only microscopic residual disease for the adjuvant chemotherapy to act upon. In addition, when a tumor mass shrinks in response to treatment, the presumption is that a greater number of cells will enter the active phase of the cell cycle to accelerate growth. This larger percentage of replicating cells should also increase the sensitivity of a tumor to chemothrapy.

Doubling Time

The time needed for a tumor to double in size is commonly referred to as its *doubling time*. Whereas the cell cycle generally refers to the activity of individual tumor cells, doubling time refers to the growth of an entire heterogenous tumor mass. In humans, the doubling times of specific tumors vary greatly.

The speed with which tumors grow and double in size is largely regulated by the number of cells that are actively dividing—known as the *growth fraction*. Typically, only a small percentage of the tumor will have cells that are rapidly proliferating. The remaining cells are in the G_0 resting phase. In general, tumors that are cured by chemotherapy are those with a high growth fraction, such as gestational trophoblastic neoplasia. When tumor volume is reduced by surgery or chemotherapy, the remaining tumor cells are theoretically propelled from the G_0 phase into the more vulnerable phases of the cell cycle, rendering them susceptible to chemotherapy.

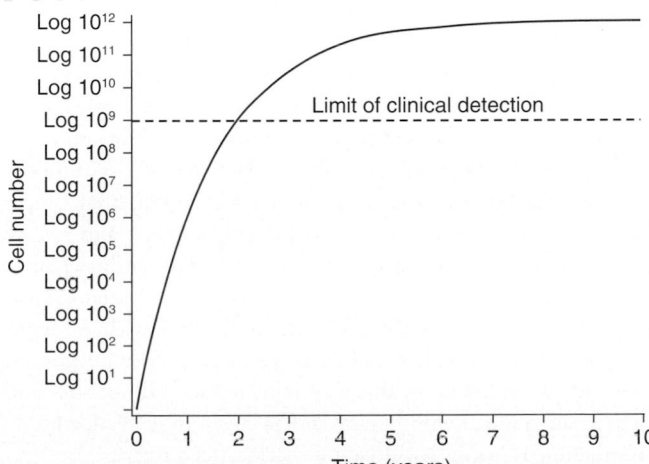

FIGURE 27-2 The gompertzian growth curve. During early stages of tumor expansion, growth is exponential, but with enlargement, tumor growth slows. Consequently, most tumors have completed their exponential growth phase at the time of clinical detection.

TABLE 27-1. Different Clinical Settings for Delivering Chemotherapy

Categories	Gynecologic Oncology Examples
Induction	Metastatic gestational trophoblastic neoplasia
Adjuvant	Platinum-based chemotherapy for advanced ovarian cancer after surgical debulking
Neoadjuvant	Primary platinum-based chemotherapy for advanced ovarian cancer that is initially unresectable
Consolidation	Paclitaxel or bevacizumab for advanced ovarian cancer in remission
Salvage	Recurrent or persistent gynecologic cancer not amenable to curative surgery or radiation

Cell Kinetics

Chemotherapeutic agents typically work by first-order kinetics to kill a constant *fraction* of cells rather than a constant number. For example, one dose of a cytotoxic drug may result in a few logs (10^2 to 10^4) of cell kill. This, however, is not curative since tumor burden may be 10^{12} cells or more. Thus, the magnitude of cell kill necessary to eradicate a tumor typically requires intermittent courses of chemotherapy. In general, a cancer's curability is inversely proportional to the number of viable tumor cells at the beginning of chemotherapy.

Some drugs achieve cell kill at several phases of the cell cycle. These *cell cycle-nonspecific* agents act in all phases of replication from G_0 to the M phase. *Cell cycle-specific* agents act only on cells that are in a specific phase. By combining drugs that act in different phases of the cell cycle, the overall cell kill should be enhanced.

CLINICAL USE OF CHEMOTHERAPY

Clinical Setting

Chemotherapy may be used in at least five different ways (Table 27-1). The term *induction chemotherapy* is defined as primary treatment for patients with an advanced malignancy when no feasible alternative treatment exists. *Adjuvant chemotherapy* is given to destroy remaining microscopic cells that may be present after the primary tumor is removed by surgery. *Neoadjuvant chemotherapy* refers to drug treatment directed at an advanced cancer to decrease preoperatively the extent or morbidity of a subsequent surgical resection. *Consolidation* (or *maintenance*) therapy is given after cancer has disappeared following the initial therapy to prolong the duration of clinical remission or to prevent ultimate relapse. Therapy applied to recurrent disease or to a tumor that is refractory to initial treatment is termed *salvage* (or *palliative*) *chemotherapy*. In these incurable patients, the intent is to achieve tumor shrinkage or stability while maintaining quality of life.

Combination Therapy

With rare exceptions, single drugs administered at clinically tolerable doses do not cure cancer. However, using two or more drugs simultaneously may greatly exacerbate toxicity. Thus, in principle, the goal of combination chemotherapy is to provide maximum cell kill with minimal or tolerable adverse patient side effects. Drugs are selected based on their proven efficacy as single agents, different mechanisms of action, and toxicities that overlap minimally or not at all.

Combination chemotherapy is more effective in attacking heterogeneous populations of cells. Moreover, the use of multiple drugs with different mechanisms of action tends to minimize the emergence of drug resistance. Typically, drugs used in combination should have clinical data indicating that their effects will be synergistic or at least additive. Drugs in combination should be used at their optimal doses and schedules. Dose reductions initiated solely to allow the addition of other agents are counterproductive because most drugs must be used near their maximum tolerated dose to ensure efficacy.

Multimodality Treatment

Frequently, chemotherapy is combined with radiation therapy or sequenced with surgery. For example, the standard of care for locally advanced cervical cancer was transformed by adding weekly cisplatin to standard radiotherapy (Fig. 28-12, p. 724). As a result, patients are more likely to have local control due to enhanced radiosensitivity of the tumor. In addition, concurrent chemoradiation with or without adjuvant chemotherapy is designed to treat micrometastases outside the radiation field.

However, treatment-related toxicity is also increased. Patients previously treated with radiation therapy may have bone marrow, skin, or other body systems that are more susceptible to chemotherapy toxicity. As a result, dose reductions or delays are commonplace. Furthermore, chemotherapy is generally less effective in tumors that lie within a previously irradiated field due to increased fibrosis and capillary destruction.

Combining chemotherapy with surgery has many different applications. For example, a woman with endometrial cancer may have nodal metastases detected during surgery, and receive pelvic radiation preceded or followed by combination chemotherapy. Alternatively, a woman with recurrent ovarian cancer may be treated by combination chemotherapy with or without preceding secondary cytoreductive surgery. The purpose of sequencing treatment in this way is to reduce tumor bulk and thereby augment chemotherapy effectiveness. In general, adjunctive therapy is begun within a few weeks after surgery.

Goals of Treatment

In general, chemotherapy is used with either curative or palliative intent. When implementing chemotherapy with curative intent, the number of courses is typically predefined. For instance, after tumor debulking, an advanced ovarian cancer patient will usually achieve remission with six cycles of platinum-based combination chemotherapy. Emphasis is placed on maintaining curative dosages and adhering closely to the treatment schedule. This may lead to significant toxicity and require growth factor support. However, for the possibility of achieving cure, these side effects are typically deemed acceptable.

Chemotherapy is often not used with curative intent, and the treating clinician must balance several factors to provide effective, compassionate palliation. Thus, in this setting, greater importance is attached to avoiding excessive toxicity. In many ways, the use of chemotherapy for palliation exemplifies the "art" of medicine. Instead of a defined number of treatment courses, a clinician must frequently revisit the treatment effectiveness and alter the dosage and timing of chemotherapy administration accordingly.

Directing Care of the Patient

To effectively counsel a gynecologic cancer patient and then guide her chemotherapeutic treatment course requires a comprehensive understanding of the diagnosis, alternatives, and goals of care. Coexisting conditions or tumor-related complications (e.g., deep-vein thrombosis) may need to be addressed. As the intended therapy is finalized, extensive information regarding side effects should be provided to allay concerns and reduce anxiety. A consent form is usually reviewed and signed by the patient, in addition to clarification of all potential logistical challenges (e.g., intravenous access).

Prior to drug infusion, a complete medical history and comprehensive physical examination are mandatory. Blood work, including a complete blood count, comprehensive metabolic panel, and tumor markers (e.g., CA125) as indicated, should be drawn and reviewed before orders to begin infusion are signed. Drug administration must take place in a setting where staff are immediately available to intervene should the need arise. Afterward, the patient should have contact numbers provided in case of questions, problems, or other concerns that can often occur prior to the next visit.

Typically, regular office visits shortly before or on the day of treatment allow assessment of toxicity and general health. Patient examination and review of blood work, in the context of the tumor response and overall treatment goal, will help determine whether drugs should be changed or their dosages revised. Over time, the treatment strategy should be continually reassessed as circumstances change.

PHARMACOLOGIC PRINCIPLES

Various characteristics determine the appropriate use of chemotherapeutic agents. Overall, treatment effectiveness depends on drug concentration and duration of exposure to critical tumor sites.

Drug Dosing

Chemotherapeutic agents typically have a narrow therapeutic range or "window." Thus, doses must be calculated accurately to achieve an optimal effect above a critical threshold while avoiding undue toxicity.

Most commonly, chemotherapy doses are calculated based on the patient's body surface area (BSA) and are expressed in milligrams per meter squared (mg/m^2). BSA is a better indicator of metabolic mass than body weight because it is less affected by abnormal adipose mass. This calculation ensures that each patient receives proportionally similar amounts of drug. Although height is a fixed variable, patient weights are obtained prior to every therapy course, since significant fluctuations may occur. Rarely, tissue edema or ascites must be factored, since doses should be based on actual weight without these coexisting conditions. The BSA is most often calculated by using a nomogram (standard reference graph table) (Fig. 27-3). Consistent derivation of the BSA at each visit is important, and

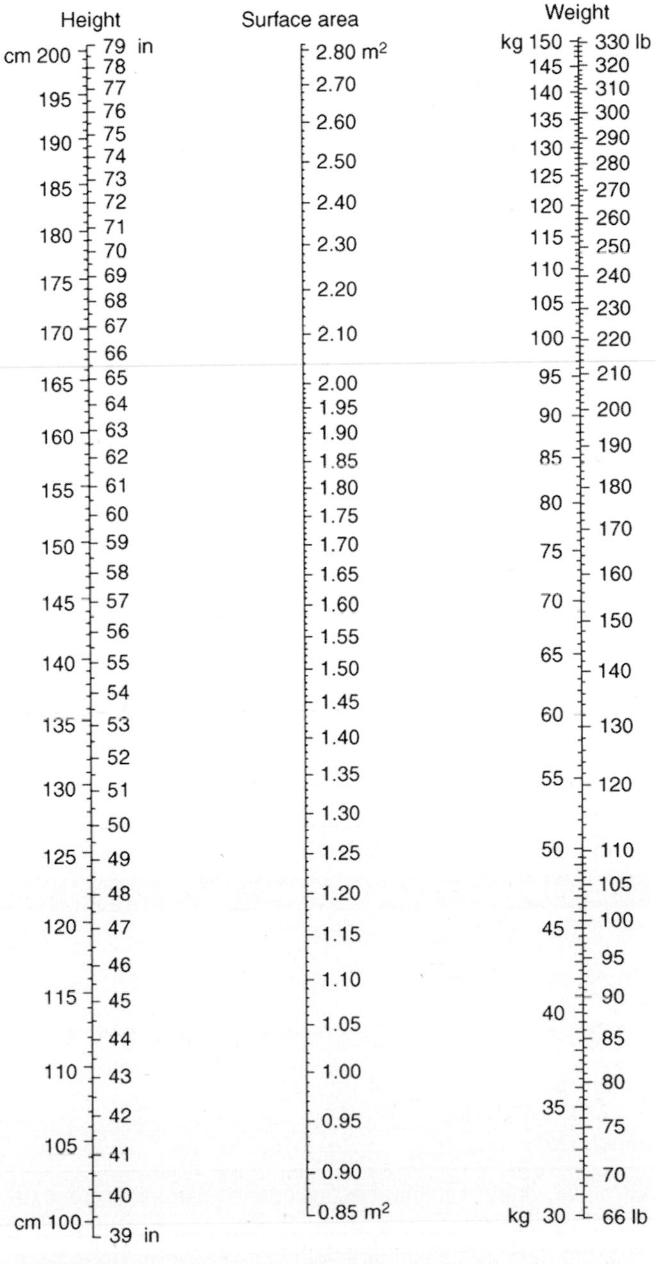

FIGURE 27-3 Nomogram for calculating the body surface area (BSA) of adults. *(From DiSaia, 2002, with permission.)*

various calculators are routinely available via software or online (http://www.globalrph.com/bsa2.htm). "Normal" adult BSA is approximately 1.73 mg/m².

Alternatively, the dosing of some drugs is more specific. For example, bevacizumab is a monoclonal antibody metabolized and eliminated via the reticuloendothelial system. It is dosed only by patient weight (mg/kg). For renally excreted drugs, such as carboplatin, dosing may be based on an estimate of the glomerular filtration rate (Calvert formula).

Dose Intensity

The amount of drug administered over time is known as the *dose intensity* (or *density*). Its primary importance is in highly responsive tumors in which cure can be achieved with chemotherapy. However, in other less sensitive tumors, it may not be possible to increase the dose to a level sufficient to produce demonstrable benefit without producing dose-limiting toxicity. For example, trials using higher-dose chemotherapy with adjunctive peripheral blood stem cell support have not improved outcomes in women with ovarian cancer. However, reducing dose intensity to decrease toxicity can produce inferior therapeutic results.

Route of Administration

Chemotherapy may be administered systemically or regionally. Systemic therapy aims to attain maximal therapeutic cytotoxic effect without extreme toxicity to normal tissues. Oral, intravenous (IV), subcutaneous (SC), or intramuscular (IM) routes comprise systemic treatment options. Regional chemotherapy is aimed at delivering drugs directly into the cavity in which the tumor is located. Clearance for many agents from a body cavity is slower than from systemic circulation. As a result, cancer cells are exposed longer to higher concentrations of active agents. This technique has been most extensively studied in ovarian cancer, in which tumors are usually confined to the intraperitoneal (IP) space. Clinical studies have uniformly demonstrated a pharmacologic advantage favoring administration into the IP compartment. However, penetration into peritoneal tumor nodules by passive diffusion is often limited by the presence of intraabdominal adhesions, poor fluid circulation, fibrotic tumor encapsulation, and coexisting ascites. Because of these limitations in drug penetration, IP chemotherapy is typically administered to women with minimal residual disease.

During intravenous administration, several drugs known as vesicants require special care (Table 27-2). Extravasation of these into the subcutaneous tissue can result in severe pain and necrosis. These drugs require slow infusion either through a rapidly flowing peripheral IV, or preferably via a central venous catheter. If extravasation is suspected, the infusion should be immediately stopped, the affected arm elevated, and ice packs applied. In severe cases, a plastic surgeon should be consulted.

Excretion

Drug inactivation, elimination, or excretion dramatically influences activity and toxicity. For the most part, this takes place primarily via the liver or kidneys. As a result, drug activity may be diminished and toxicity exacerbated when normal hepatic or renal function is impaired.

In addition, drug toxicity is often more pronounced in the elderly or malnourished. For example, a low serum creatinine level in cachectic women may not accurately reflect underlying renal function. If a carboplatin dose is calculated using this falsely low value, the amount may be excessive and result in considerable morbidity. Instead, a preset creatinine level may need to be selected (0.8 or 1.0 mg/dL) to aid safer dosing in some patients.

Drug Interactions

Most women who receive chemotherapy are often prescribed medication for other noncancerous conditions, such as hypertension. Moreover, women also typically receive analgesics, antiemetics, and antibiotics during chemotherapy. Most drug interactions are of little consequence, but some may lead to substantially altered drug toxicity. Often drugs that are metabolized in the liver are at risk for such interactions. For example, using methotrexate in a woman taking warfarin (Coumadin) will usually enhance the anticoagulant effect and thus will require a Coumadin dose reduction.

TABLE 27-2. Chemotherapeutic Agents and Their Association with Extravasation Injury

Vesicants	Exfoliants	Irritants	Inflammants	Neutral
Dactinomycin	Cisplatin	Carboplatin	Methotrexate	Bleomycin
Doxorubicin	Docetaxel	Etoposide		Cyclophosphamide
Paclitaxel	Liposomal doxorubicin			Gemcitabine
Vinblastine	Topotecan			Ifosfamide
Vinorelbine				

Exfoliant, agent capable of causing skin exfoliation on extravasation; *inflammant*, agent capable of causing skin inflammation on extravasation; *irritant*, agent capable of causing skin irritation on extravasation; *vesicant*, agent capable of causing skin ulceration and tissue necrosis on extravasation.
Adapted from Mileshkin, 2004, with permission.

TABLE 27-3. Management of Hypersensitivity Reactions

1. Stop the chemotherapy infusion
2. Assess the patient's airway, breathing, and circulation
3. Administer intravenous normal saline if hypotensive
4. Administer oxygen if dyspneic or hypoxic
5. Administer intravenous antihistamine (e.g., 50 mg intravenous diphenhydramine or 25–50 mg intravenous promethazine)
6. Administer 5 mg of nebulized salbutamol if the patient has bronchospasm
7. Administer intravenous corticosteroids (e.g., 100 mg of hydrocortisone); this may have no effect on the initial reaction, but may prevent rebound or prolonged allergic manifestations
8. If the patient does not promptly improve or has symptoms of persistent or severe hypotension or persistent bronchospasm or laryngeal edema, administer adrenaline or epinephrine (0.1–0.25 mg intravenous); further acute resuscitation measures may be required
9. Reassure the patient that the problem is a recognized and treatable one

Modified from Mileshkin, 2004, with permission.

Allergic Reaction

Despite patient history review and administration of prophylactic medications, an anaphylactic, allergic, or hypersensitivity reaction during or after administration of chemotherapy may occur. Accordingly, a treatment facility must have trained nursing staff and resources to manage these sudden, but common, issues.

Prior to drug administration, a woman is instructed to report symptoms that may precede an anaphylactic reaction such as flushing, pruritus, dyspnea, tachycardia, hoarseness, or lightheadedness. Emergency equipment, such as supplemental oxygen, ventilatory face mask and bag, or intubation equipment must be immediately available. For a localized hypersensitivity response, administration of intravenous diphenhydramine (Benadryl) and/or corticosteroids may be sufficient. However, for a generalized hypersensitivity or anaphylactic response, chemotherapy should be stopped immediately, the emergency team notified, and emergency drugs administered, such as epinephrine (0.1–0.5 mg of a 1:10,000 solution) (Table 27-3).

Drug Resistance

In principle, larger tumor masses have a greater proportion of cells that have already developed resistance. Resistance may be intrinsic or acquired, and it may develop to one drug or to multiple agents. Intrinsic drug resistance is seen if tumors are first exposed to an agent and fail to respond.

In contrast, with acquired drug resistance, tumors no longer respond to drugs to which they were initially sensitive. Sometimes, this develops with a specific drug. For instance, patients with low-risk gestational trophoblastic neoplasia may become resistant to methotrexate yet remain exquisitely sensitive to dactinomycin. More often, however, acquired resistance is "pleiotropic," meaning that a cancer is resistant to multiple chemotherapy agents. This is often mediated by the P-glycoprotein or multidrug resistance pump. Advanced ovarian cancer is a good example. Most patients will initially achieve remission with platinum-based chemotherapy, but 80 percent will ultimately relapse and die from tumors that have become resistant to all cytotoxic therapy.

Evaluating Response to Chemotherapy

The effective use of chemotherapy is a dynamic process whereby a treating clinician is constantly weighing toxicity to the patient against tumor response. In counseling women to continue treatment or switch to a different regimen, a clinician must have objective criteria for response (Table 27-4). The most important indicator is the *complete response rate*. For ovarian cancer, this would include normal CA125 levels (usually <35 U/mL), physical examination findings, and imaging test results (such as computed tomography scans). Ultimately, women who have any possibility of cure are those who first achieve a complete response. However, if chemotherapy results in a partial response,

TABLE 27-4. Clinical Endpoints in Evaluating Response to Chemotherapy

Endpoint	Definition
Complete response (CR)	Disappearance of all measurable "target" lesions
Partial response (PR)	A decrease of ≥30% in the sum of diameters of all target lesions
Progressive disease (PD)	An increase of ≥20% in the sum of diameters of target lesions or the identification of one or more new lesions
Stable disease (SD)	Neither sufficient shrinkage to qualify for PR, nor sufficient increase to qualify for PD

Summarized from Eisenhauer (2009).

TABLE 27-5. Chemotherapy Antimetabolites Used for Gynecologic Cancer

Generic Name	Brand Name	Indications	Routes	Common Dosages	Common Toxicity
Methotrexate (MTX)	Trexall, Rheumatrex	GTN	PO, IM, IV, intrathecal	IM: 30–50 mg/m²/week, or 1 mg/kg on days 1, 3, 5, 7 of 8-day cycle IV: 100 mg/m² during 30 min, then 200 mg/m² during 12 hour	BMD, mucositis, renal toxicity, CNS dysfunction
Gemcitabine	Gemzar	Recurrent ovarian CA, uterine sarcoma	IV	600–1250 mg/m²/week over 30 min × 2–3 weeks	BMD, N/V/D, malaise and fever
5-Fluorouracil	Adrucil	Cervical CA, Vulvar CA	IV	800–1000 mg/m²/day during 96 hour	Mucositis, PPE
	Efudex	VAIN	Vaginal cream	3 mL QOD × 1 week, then weekly up to 10 weeks	Vulvovaginal irritation

BMD = bone marrow depression; CA = cancer; CNS = central nervous system; GTN = gestational trophoblastic neoplasia; IM = intramuscular; IV = intravenous; N/V/D = nausea, vomiting, and diarrhea; PPE = palmar-plantar erythrodysesthesia; PO = orally; QOD = every other day; VAIN = vaginal intraepithelial neoplasia.

many women still view this as advantageous compared with supportive care, even if a survival benefit is unproven.

CHEMOTHERAPEUTIC DRUGS

In gynecologic oncology, diverse compounds that have demonstrated activity include antimetabolites, alkylating agents, antitumor antibiotics, plant alkaloids, taxanes, hormonal agents, and biologic therapies (see Fig. 27-1). These drugs may be used as single agents or in combination regimens.

Antimetabolites

The antimetabolites are structural and chemical analogs of naturally occurring components of the metabolic pathways that lead to the synthesis of purines, pyrimidines, and nucleic acids. In most cases, they are S phase-specific agents that are most effective in rapidly growing tumors associated with short doubling times and large growth fractions (Table 27-5).

Methotrexate

Mechanism of Action. This antimetabolite, historically known as amethopterin, is U.S. Food and Drug Administration (FDA)-approved to be used by itself for treatment of women with gestational trophoblastic neoplasia (GTN). It is also commonly used for the medical management of ectopic pregnancy. Methotrexate (MTX) tightly binds to dihydrofolate reductase, blocking the reduction of dihydrofolate to tetrahydrofolate (the active form of folic acid) (Fig. 27-4). As a result, thymidylate synthetase and various steps in de novo purine synthesis are halted. This leads to arrest of DNA, RNA, and protein synthesis.

Prescribing Information and Toxicity. Methotrexate may be administered orally, IM, IV, or intrathecally. Most commonly, single-agent treatment of GTN involves MTX given IM at

dosages of 30 to 50 mg/m² once each week or an 8-day regimen of 1 mg/kg on treatment days 1, 3, 5, and 7. Combination therapy for high-risk disease includes 100 mg/m² MTX given IV over 30 minutes, followed by a 200 mg/m² IV dose over 12 hours.

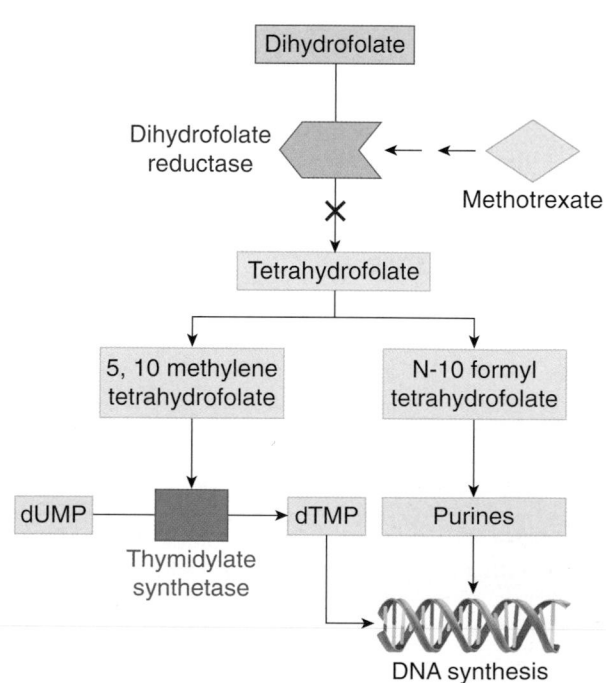

FIGURE 27-4 Methotrexate's primary target is the enzyme dihydrofolate reductase (DHFR). Inhibition of DHFR leads to partial depletion of 5,10 methylene tetrahydrofolic acid and N-10 formyl tetrahydrofolic acid, which are cofactors required for the respective synthesis of thymidylate and purines. As a result, methotrexate leads to arrested DNA, RNA, and protein synthesis. dTMP = deoxythymidine monophosphate; dUMP = deoxyuridine monophosphate.

This agent causes few side effects at typical doses. However, at high doses, although used infrequently, MTX can lead to fatal bone marrow toxicity. This toxicity can be prevented by early administration of leucovorin, and this therapy is termed *leucovorin rescue*. Leucovorin is folinic acid; has activity that is equivalent to folic acid; and thus is readily converted to tetrahydrofolate. Leucovorin, however, does not require dihydrofolate reductase for its conversion. Therefore, its function is unaffected by inhibition of this enzyme by drugs such as methotrexate. Leucovorin, therefore, allows for some purine and pyrimidine synthesis.

Leucovorin rescue is often incorporated into higher-dose regimens. For example, the 8-day alternating MTX schedule usually includes 7.5 mg of leucovorin orally on treatment days 2, 4, 6, and 8. Patients should be counseled to avoid folate-containing supplements unless specifically directed. In addition to myelosuppression, renal toxicity and acute cerebral dysfunction are typically only seen at high MTX doses. Methotrexate is predominantly excreted through the kidneys, and thus women with renal insufficiency should have doses reduced. Serum MTX levels are carefully monitored in these patients, as these women may require prolonged leucovorin rescue.

Gemcitabine

Mechanism of Action. This antimetabolite is FDA approved to be used with other agents for treatment of recurrent ovarian cancer, but is also commonly used for uterine sarcoma. Gemcitabine (Gemzar) is a synthetic nucleoside analog that undergoes multiple phosphorylations to form the active metabolite. The resulting triphosphate is subsequently incorporated into DNA as a fraudulent base pair. Following the insertion of gemcitabine, one additional deoxynucleotide is added to the end of the DNA chain before replication is terminated, and thereby, DNA synthesis is halted.

Prescribing Information and Toxicity. The usual administration of gemcitabine is by 30-minute infusion. Longer durations, such as those greater than 60 min, are associated with increased toxicity due to intracellular accumulation of the triphosphate. Depending on whether it is used as a single agent or in combination, gemcitabine is typically given at doses between 600 and 1250 mg/m^2 once weekly for 2 to 3 weeks, followed by a week off therapy.

Myelosuppression, especially neutropenia, is the main dose-limiting side effect. Gastrointestinal (GI) toxicity, such as nausea, vomiting, diarrhea, or mucositis, is also common. Approximately 20 percent of patients will develop a flu-like syndrome, including fever, malaise, headache, and chills. Pulmonary toxicity is relatively uncommon, but reported.

5-Fluorouracil

Mechanism of Action. This "false" pyrimidine antimetabolite is not FDA approved for gynecologic cancer, but is occasionally paired with cisplatin during chemoradiation of cervical cancer or used in topical form (Efudex) for the treatment of vaginal intraepithelial neoplasia (VAIN). 5-Fluorouracil (5-FU) acts principally as a thymidine synthetase inhibitor to block DNA replication.

Prescribing Information and Toxicity. 5-FU may be administered IV (Adrucil) or topically. The usual dosage is a 96-hour continuous IV infusion of 800 to 1000 mg/m^2/d. Regimens for topical use are discussed in Chapter 29 (p. 756).

Mucositis and/or diarrhea may be severe and dose-limiting for infusion schedules. Hand-foot syndrome (palmar-plantar erythrodysesthesia) is less common, but can also be dose-limiting (p. 702). Myelosuppression, mainly neutropenia and thrombocytopenia, are less frequently observed. Nausea and vomiting are usually mild.

Topical 5-FU used intravaginally may result in dramatic pain, itching, burning, and mucosal inflammation that often causes patients to abort further applications.

Alkylating Agents

The alkylating agents are characterized by positively charged alkyl groups that bind to negatively charged DNA to form adducts (Table 27-6). Binding leads to DNA breaks or cross-links and a halt to DNA synthesis. In general, these drugs are cell cycle-nonspecific agents that work at any phase of active replication.

Cyclophosphamide

Mechanism of Action. This alkylating agent is FDA approved by itself or in combination for epithelial ovarian cancer treatment. Cyclophosphamide (Cytoxan) is the "C" of

TABLE 27-6. Chemotherapy Alkylating Agents Used for Gynecologic Cancer

Generic Name	Brand Name	Indication	Routes	Dosages	Toxicity
Cyclophosphamide	Cytoxan	GTN, recurrent ovarian CA	PO, IV	IV: 500–750 mg/m^2 over 30 min, every 3 weeks PO: 50 mg/day	BMD, cystitis, N/V, alopecia
Ifosfamide	Ifex	Recurrent ovarian CA, cervical CA, uterine sarcoma	IV	1.2–1.6 g/m^2/day, days 1–3 of 3-week cycle	BMD, cystitis, N/V, alopecia, CNS and renal toxicity

BMD = bone marrow depression; CA = cancer; CNS = central nervous system; GTN = gestational trophoblastic neoplasia; IV = intravenous; N/V = nausea and vomiting; PO = orally.

the EMA-CO (etoposide, methotrexate, actinomycin D, cyclophosphamide, oncovin) regimen prescribed for GTN and is also used as salvage therapy for recurrent epithelial ovarian cancer (Bower, 1997; Cantu, 2002). It is a derivative of nitrogen mustard and is activated through a multistep process by microsomal enzymes in the liver. It promotes DNA cross-linking and DNA synthesis inhibition.

Prescribing Information and Toxicity. Cyclophosphamide may be administered IV or orally. It is typically given IV at doses of 500 to 750 mg/m² over 30 minutes every 3 weeks. Orally, a metronomic (repetitive low-dose) regimen of 50 mg daily is commonly used to minimize toxicity and target the tumor endothelium or stroma in combination with a biologic agent, such as bevacizumab (Chura, 2007).

Following IV administration, myelosuppression, mainly neutropenia, is the usual dose-limiting side effect. This agent is exclusively excreted by the kidneys. One of its metabolites, acrolein, can alkylate and inflame the bladder mucosa. As a result, hemorrhagic cystitis is a classic complication that may follow from 24 hours to several weeks after administration. To prevent this effect, adequate hydration is imperative to aid acrolein excretion. In addition, GI toxicity, such as nausea, vomiting, or anorexia, is common. Alopecia is typically severe. Moreover, secondary malignancies are increased, particularly acute myelogenous leukemia and bladder cancer.

Ifosfamide

Mechanism of Action. This alkylating agent is not FDA approved for gynecologic cancers, but is typically administered for salvage treatment of recurrent epithelial ovarian cancer, cervical cancer, and uterine sarcoma. Ifosfamide (Ifex) is a structural analog of cyclophosphamide, differing only slightly. However, its metabolic activation occurs more slowly and leads to a greater production of chloracetaldehyde, a possible neurotoxin.

Prescribing Information and Toxicity. Ifosfamide is administered IV, usually as a short infusion. Common doses of 1.2 to 1.6 gm/m² are given on days 1–3 of a 3-week cycle. As with cyclophosphamide, adequate hydration is recommended to reduce the incidence of drug-induced hemorrhagic cystitis. In addition, concurrent mesna (Mesnex) is used to prevent severe hematuria. A metabolite of mesna chemically binds with acrolein and detoxifies it in the bladder (Fig. 27-5).

Overall, side effects are similar to those of cyclophosphamide. However, neurotoxicity, manifested as lethargy, confusion, seizure, ataxia, hallucinations, and occasionally coma, is more likely. These symptoms are caused by the chloracetaldehyde metabolite and are reversible with removal of the drug and supportive care. The incidence of neurotoxicity is higher in the rare patient receiving high-dose therapy and also in those with impaired renal function, where a dose reduction is necessary.

▪ Antitumor Antibiotics

The antitumor antibiotics are generally derived from microorganisms. Most antitumor antibiotics exert their cytotoxic

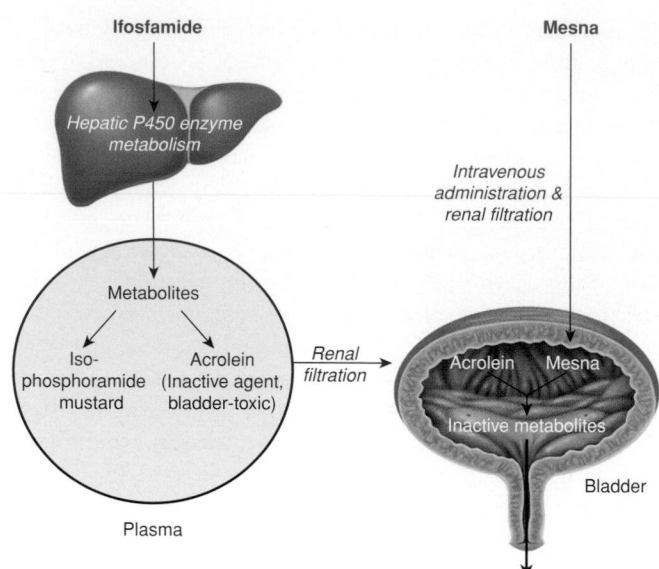

FIGURE 27-5 Ifosfamide is a prodrug, which is ultimately metabolized into active and inactive metabolites. Isophosphoramide mustard is the main active alkylating metabolite. The inactive metabolite, acrolein, is concentrated in the bladder and is bladder toxic. The drug mesna and acrolein join in the bladder to create an inactive compound, which is then excreted by the bladder. This conversion of acrolein to an inactive compound minimizes the bladder toxicity of ifosfamide.

effects by DNA intercalation during multiple phases of the cell cycle. As a group they are considered cell-cycle specific.

Dactinomycin

Mechanism of Action. This agent is FDA approved to treat GTN as a single agent or as part of combination chemotherapy (Table 27-7). Dactinomycin (Cosmegen), also known as actinomycin D, is the "A" of the EMA-CO chemotherapy combination. Dactinomycin is a product of the Streptomyces species and becomes anchored into purine-pyrimidine DNA base pairs, resulting in DNA synthesis inhibition. It also produces toxic oxygen-free radicals that cause DNA breaks. Dactinomycin is mainly excreted through the biliary system.

Prescribing Information and Toxicity. The usual "pulse" dosage of dactinomycin is 1.25 mg IV push every other week or 0.5 mg on days 1–5 every 2 to 3 weeks. Myelosuppression is the main dose-limiting side effect, and it may be severe. Moreover, GI toxicity, including nausea, vomiting, mucositis, and diarrhea, is often significant. Alopecia is common. As with others in the antibiotic group, dactinomycin is a potent vesicant, that is, an agent that can cause skin ulceration and tissue necrosis if extravasated during IV infusion (p. 696).

Bleomycin

Mechanism of Action. This antitumor antibiotic is FDA approved for malignant pleural effusion treatment or for palliative therapy of recurrent squamous cervical cancer, squamous vulvar cancer, and testicular cancer. An off-label use includes

TABLE 27-7. Chemotherapeutic Antibiotics Used for Gynecologic Cancer

Generic Name	Brand Name	Indication	Route	Dosage	Toxicity
Actinomycin D (dactinomycin)	Cosmegen	GTN	IV	1.25 mg IV push every other week or 0.5 mg on days 1–5, every 2–3 weeks	BMD, N/V/D, alopecia, vesicant
Bleomycin	Blenoxane	Germ cell or SCST ovarian CA, GTN	IV, IM, SC, intrapleural	IV: 20 U/m^2 (maximum dose of 30 U), every 3 weeks	Pulmonary toxicity, fever, skin reaction
Doxorubicin	Adriamycin	Endometrial CA, recurrent epithelial ovarian CA	IV	45–60 mg/m^2 every 3 weeks	BMD, cardiac toxicity, alopecia, vesicant
Liposomal doxorubicin	Doxil	Recurrent epithelial ovarian CA	IV	40–50 mg/m^2 over 30 min, every 4 weeks	PPE, stomatitis, infusion reaction

BMD = bone marrow depression; CA = cancer; GTN = gestational trophoblastic neoplasia; IM = intramuscular; IV = intravenous; N/V/D = nausea, vomiting, and diarrhea; PPE = palmar-plantar erythrodysesthesia; SC = subcutaneous; SCST = sex cord-stromal tumor.

bleomycin as the "B" in BEP (bleomycin, etoposide, cisplatin) regimens, which are used as adjuvant treatment of malignant ovarian germ cell or sex cord-stromal tumors (Homesley, 1999; Williams, 1991). Additionally, it is used in salvage treatment of GTN (DuBeshter, 1989).

Bleomycin (Blenoxane), when complexed with iron, creates activated oxygen-free radicals, which cause DNA-strand breaks and cell death. It is maximally effective during the G$_2$ phase.

Prescribing Information and Toxicity. The usual dosage of bleomycin is 20 units/m^2 IV (maximum dose of 30 units), given every 3 weeks. Bleomycin can also be administered IM, SC, or intrapleurally. The dose is quantified by international units of "cytotoxic activity."

Pulmonary toxicity is the main dose-limiting side effect, developing in 10 percent of patients and causing death in 1 percent. Accordingly, for women prescribed bleomycin, chest radiographs and pulmonary function tests (PFTs) should be performed at baseline and obtained regularly before every one or two treatment cycles. The most important PFT measurement is the diffusing capacity of the lung for carbon monoxide (DLCO). The DLCO measures the ability to transfer oxygen from the lungs to the blood stream. If the DLCO decreases by 15 to 30 percent, it indicates the development of restrictive lung disease. In patients receiving bleomycin, therapy may then be stopped before the onset of symptomatic pulmonary fibrosis. Fibrosis often presents clinically as pneumonitis with cough, dyspnea, dry inspiratory crackles, and infiltrates on chest radiograph. This complication is more common in patients older than 70 years and with cumulative doses of greater than 400 units.

Bleomycin is not a myelosuppressive drug. However, skin reactions are common and include hyperpigmentation or erythema.

Doxorubicin

Mechanism of Action. This antitumor antibiotic is FDA approved to treat epithelial ovarian cancer. Doxorubicin (Adriamycin) is also used as the "A" in the combination chemotherapy regimen TAP (taxol, adriamycin, cisplatin), used for endometrial cancer. This agent intercalates into DNA to inhibit DNA synthesis, inhibits topoisomerase II (p. 704), and forms cytotoxic oxygen-free radicals. The drug is metabolized extensively in the liver and eliminated through biliary excretion.

Prescribing Information and Toxicity. The usual dose of doxorubicin is 45 to 60 mg/m^2 IV as part of combination chemotherapy, repeated every 3 weeks. Myelosuppression, particularly neutropenia, is the main dose-limiting side effect. However, cardiotoxicity is a classic complication. Patients should be monitored with a multiple gated acquisition (MUGA) radionuclide scan at baseline and periodically (every other treatment) during therapy. The risk of cardiotoxicity is higher in women older than 70 years and those with cumulative doses exceeding 550 mg/m^2. Ultimately, women may develop an irreversible dilated cardiomyopathy associated with congestive heart failure. Gastrointestinal toxicities are generally mild, but alopecia is universal.

Doxorubicin Hydrochloride Liposome

Mechanism of Action. This antitumor antibiotic is FDA approved for the salvage treatment of recurrent epithelial ovarian cancer (Gordon, 2004a). The liposomal encapsulation of doxorubicin (Doxil) dramatically alters the pharmacokinetic and toxicity profiles of the drug. Researchers developed liposomal doxorubicin to reduce cardiotoxicity and to selectively target tumor tissues.

Prescribing Information and Toxicity. Liposomal doxorubicin may be administered as an IV infusion over 30 to 60 minutes and is dosed at 40 to 50 mg/m² every 4 weeks. Unlike doxorubicin, administration of the encapsulated liposome is associated with minimal nausea, vomiting, alopecia, and cardiotoxicity. Infusion-related reactions develop in less than 10 percent of patients and are most common during the first course of treatment. However, an increased rate of stomatitis and palmar-plantar erythrodysesthesia (PPE) is noted.

PPE is characterized by a cutaneous reaction of varying intensity. Patients may initially complain of tingling sensations on their soles and palms that generally progresses to swelling and tenderness to touch. Erythematous plaques typically develop that can become extremely painful and often lead to desquamation and cracking of the skin. Symptoms result from the prolonged blood levels of this time-released cytotoxic agent and may last several weeks.

Plant-Derived Agents

A common theme in the cytotoxic activity of these agents is disturbance of normal assembly, disassembly, and stabilization of intracellular microtubules to halt cell division during mitosis (Fig. 27-6). The group includes the taxanes, vinca alkaloids, and topoisomerase inhibitors.

Taxanes

Paclitaxel and docetaxel are both cell cycle-specific agents that have maximal activity during the M phase (Table 27-8). They act to "poison" the mitotic spindle by preventing depolymerization of the microtubules and inhibiting cellular replication. Paclitaxel is derived from the needles and bark of the rare Pacific yew tree, *Taxus brevifolia*. Docetaxel is a semisynthetic analog of paclitaxel, derived from the readily available European yew tree.

Paclitaxel. The best-selling cancer drug ever manufactured, paclitaxel (Taxol) is FDA approved for the treatment of primary or recurrent epithelial ovarian cancer. It is also extensively used for endometrial cancers, cervical cancers, and GTN.

Prescribing Information and Toxicity. Paclitaxel is typically administered IV as a 3-hour infusion, but may also be given as an intraperitoneal (IP) dose. The usual IV dosage is 135 to 175 mg/m² every 3 weeks. Weekly paclitaxel is also effective in a regimen of 80 mg/m² IV for 3 consecutive weeks on a 21-day schedule ("dose-dense" regimen) for primary disease or on a 28-day schedule for recurrent disease (Katsumata, 2009; Markman, 2006). For initial therapy of optimally debulked ovarian cancer following a day 1 IV dose, paclitaxel is usually given IP on day 8 at a dose of 60 mg/m² (Armstrong, 2006).

Myelosuppression is the usual dose-limiting side effect. In addition, a hypersensitivity reaction occurs in approximately one third of patients due to its formulation in Cremophor-EL, an emulsifying agent. Typically, the reaction develops within minutes of starting an initial infusion. Fortunately, the

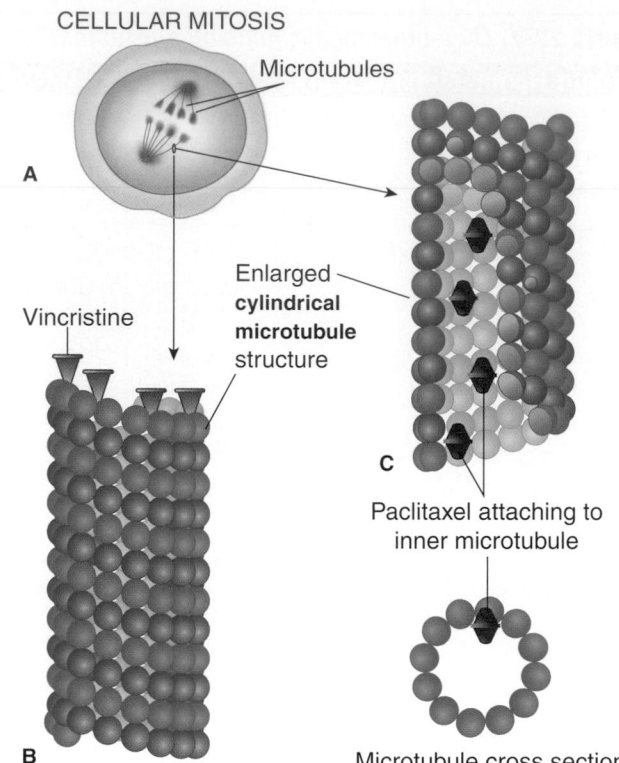

CELLULAR MITOSIS

FIGURE 27-6 Diagram of taxane's and vinca alkaloid's mechanism of action. Parts B and C show magnified microtubule structure. **A.** During cellular mitosis, microtubules are essential for chromosome alignment and separation. **B.** Vincristine, one of the vinca alkaloids, attaches consistently to one end of the microtubule to inhibit microtubule assembly. **C.** Paclitaxel, one of the taxanes, binds to the inner ring of the microtubule and prohibits microtubule disassembly. In both B and C, microtubule function is impaired.

incidence can be decreased 10-fold by premedication with corticosteroids, usually dexamethasone, 20 mg orally 12 and 6 hours before administration. Neurotoxicity is the principal nonhematologic dose-limiting side effect. Common symptoms include numbness, tingling, and/or burning pain in a stocking-glove distribution. Peripheral neuropathy progresses with increased paclitaxel exposure and may become debilitating. Alopecia is almost universal and results in loss of total body hair.

Docetaxel. This taxane is not FDA approved for gynecologic cancers, but is often used to treat recurrent epithelial ovarian cancer and uterine sarcoma (Bay, 2006; Strauss, 2007). In addition, patients with worsening peripheral neuropathy with paclitaxel are often switched to docetaxel. Clinical efficacy is similar, but docetaxel is associated with less neurotoxicity.

Prescribing Information and Toxicity. The usual dosage of docetaxel (Taxotere) is 75 to 100 mg/m² IV, repeated every 3 weeks. For recurrent ovarian cancer, weekly docetaxel is also effective at a dosage of 35 mg/m² IV for 3 consecutive weeks on a 28-day schedule (Tinker, 2007).

TABLE 27-8. Chemotherapeutic Plant Alkaloids Used for Gynecologic Cancer

Generic Name	Brand Name	Indications	Routes	Dosages	Toxicity
Paclitaxel	Taxol	Recurrent epithelial ovarian CA, endometrial CA, cervical CA, GTN	IV, IP	IV: 135–175 mg/m² every 3 weeks, or 80 mg/m²/week for 3 weeks IP: 60 mg/m² on day 8 following a day-1 IV dose	HSR, peripheral neurotoxicity, BMD, alopecia, bradycardia and arrhythmia
Docetaxel	Taxotere	Recurrent epithelial ovarian CA, uterine sarcoma	IV	75–100 mg/m² every 3 weeks, or 35 mg/m²/week for 3 weeks	BMD, peripheral edema, HSR, alopecia
Vincristine	Oncovin	GTN	IV	0.8–1.0 mg/m² every other week	Neurotoxicity, abdominal pain, alopecia
Vinblastine	Velban	GTN	IV	9 mg/m² every 3 weeks	BMD, N/V/D, mucositis, HTN, neurotoxicity, alopecia
Vinorelbine	Navelbine	Recurrent epithelial ovarian CA, cervical CA	IV	30 mg/m² every week	BMD, N/V/D, stomatitis, peripheral neurotoxicity
Etoposide	VP-16	Germ cell or SCST ovarian CA; recurrent epithelial ovarian CA; endometrial CA	IV, PO	IV: 100 mg/m² days 1 & 2, every 2 weeks, or 75–100 mg/m², days 1–5, every 3 weeks PO: 50 mg/m²/day for 3 weeks	BMD, alopecia, secondary cancers
Topotecan	Hycamtin	Recurrent epithelial ovarian CA, cervical CA	IV	1.5 mg/m²/day, days 1–5, every 3 weeks, or 4 mg/m²/week for 3 weeks, or 0.75 mg/m²/day, days 1–3, every 3 weeks	BMD, N/V, alopecia, fever, malaise

BMD = bone marrow depression; CA = cancer; GTN = gestational trophoblastic neoplasia; HSR = hypersensitivity reaction; HTN = hypertension; IV = intravenous; N/V/D = nausea, vomiting, and diarrhea; PO = orally; SCST = sex cord-stromal tumor.

Unlike paclitaxel, myelosuppression is the main dose-limiting side effect. Fluid retention syndrome occurs in approximately half of patients and manifests as weight gain, peripheral edema, pleural effusion, and ascites. Corticosteroid prophylaxis prevents most of this toxicity, as well as dermatologic side effects and hypersensitivity reactions.

Vinca Alkaloids

Vincristine, vinblastine, and vinorelbine are cell cycle-specific drugs derived from the periwinkle plant with maximal activity in the M phase. These compounds inhibit normal microtubular polymerization by binding to the tubulin subunit at a site distinct from the taxane-binding site (see Fig. 27-6). These drugs are among the least commonly used agents in gynecologic oncology.

Vincristine. This vinca alkaloid is not FDA approved for gynecologic cancers, but represents the "O" of EMA-CO com-

bination chemotherapy for GTN treatment. The usual dosage of vincristine (Oncovin) is 0.8 to 1.0 mg/m² given IV every other week. To prevent or delay the development of neurotoxicity, the total individual dose should be capped at 2 mg.

Neurotoxicity is the most common dose-limiting toxicity and may include peripheral neuropathy, autonomic nervous system dysfunction, cranial nerve palsies, ataxia, or seizures. Moreover, concurrent administration with other neurotoxic agents such as cisplatin and paclitaxel may increase severity. Gastrointestinal toxicity is also common, including constipation, abdominal pain, and paralytic ileus. However, myelosuppression is typically mild.

Vinblastine. This vinca alkaloid is FDA approved for the salvage treatment of GTN. The usual dosage of vinblastine (Velban) varies, but one approach administers 9 mg/m² IV every 3 weeks. Myelosuppression is the main dose-limiting side effect. Gastrointestinal toxicity may be severe and include mucositis, stomatitis, nausea, vomiting, anorexia, and diarrhea or constipation. In addition, hypertension may result from autonomic dysfunction. Neurotoxicity develops much less frequently, but is similar to that seen with vincristine.

Vinorelbine. This vinca alkaloid is not FDA approved for gynecologic cancer, but is a semisynthetic derivation of vinblastine used in salvage treatment for recurrent epithelial ovarian cancer and for treatment of cervical cancer. The usual dosage of vinorelbine (Navelbine) is 30 mg/m^2 given IV as a single agent or in combination on a weekly basis, with a week off in a 21- or 28-day schedule.

Myelosuppression is the main dose-limiting side effect. Moreover, GI toxicity is common and may include those similar to vinblastine. Neurotoxicity is usually mild, particularly compared with other vinca alkaloids.

Topoisomerase Inhibitors

Topoisomerase (TOPO) enzymes unwind and rewind DNA to aid DNA replication. Topoisomerase inhibitors interfere with this function and halt DNA synthesis. This group of agents may be further divided into categories based on the specific topoisomerase enzyme they inhibit. The camptothecins inhibit TOPO I and include topotecan. The podophyllotoxins inhibit TOPO II and include etoposide.

Topotecan

Mechanism of Action. This TOPO I inhibiting agent is a semisynthetic analog of the alkaloid extract, camptothecin. It binds to and stabilizes a transient TOPO I-DNA complex, resulting in double-strand breakage and lethal DNA damage. Topotecan (Hycamtin) is FDA approved as salvage therapy of recurrent epithelial ovarian cancer and recurrent cervical cancer (Long, 2005c).

Prescribing Information and Toxicity. Topotecan is usually administered IV, by either of two different schedules. Standard dosage for recurrent ovarian cancer is 1.5 mg/m^2 for days 1–5, given every 3 weeks (Gordon, 2004). However, this schedule is associated with a greater than 80-percent incidence of severe neutropenia. A less toxic regimen is 4 mg/m^2 weekly for 3 weeks during a 28-day schedule (Spannuth, 2007). The usual dosage when combined with cisplatin for recurrent cervical cancer is 0.75 mg/m^2 on days 1–3, given every 3 weeks (Long, 2005b).

Myelosuppression, most commonly neutropenia, is the main dose-limiting side effect. GI toxicity is also common and includes nausea, vomiting, diarrhea, and abdominal pain. Systemic symptoms, such as headache, fever, malaise, arthralgias, and myalgias, are typical. Alopecia is often as complete as that seen with paclitaxel therapy.

Etoposide

Mechanism of Action. Etoposide is a cell-cycle specific agent with maximal activity in the late S and G$_2$ phase. This drug "poisons" the TOPO II enzyme by stabilizing an oth-

erwise transient form of the TOPO II-DNA complex. As a result, DNA cannot unwind and double-strand DNA breaks form.

This agent is FDA approved for testicular cancers, but not gynecologic cancers per se. However, it is often used IV as part of combination chemotherapy. Etoposide (VP-16) represents the "E" of the EMA-CO regimen, which is used for GTN. In addition, it is a component of the BEP regimen, used for ovarian germ cell or sex cord-stromal tumors. Oral etoposide may be efficacious as a single agent for salvage treatment of recurrent epithelial ovarian cancer or endometrial cancer.

Prescribing Information and Toxicity. The usual dosage of etoposide varies. In the EMA-CO regimen, 100 mg/m^2 is administered IV on days 1 and 2, every 2 weeks. In the BEP regimen, it is usually prescribed in dosages of 75 to 100 mg/m^2 IV on days 1–5, given every 3 weeks. The oral dosage is 50 mg/m^2/day for 3 weeks, followed by a week off during a 28-day schedule.

Up to 95 percent of etoposide is protein-bound, mainly to albumin. Thus, decreased albumin levels result in a higher fraction of free drug and potentially a higher incidence of toxicity.

Myelosuppression, most commonly neutropenia, is the main dose-limiting side effect. Gastrointestinal symptoms of nausea, vomiting, and anorexia are usually minor, except with oral administration. Most patients will develop alopecia. With etoposide, particularly if the total dose exceeds 2000 mg/m^2, there is a small but significant risk of secondary malignancies (approximately 1 in 1000). Of these, acute myelogenous leukemia is the most common.

Miscellaneous

Several antineoplastic compounds do not clearly fit into any of the preceding categories. In general, these cell-cycle nonspecific drugs have similarities to alkylating agents.

Carboplatin

Mechanism of Action. Carboplatin (Paraplatin) produces DNA adducts that inhibit DNA synthesis. This agent is one of the most widely used, particularly in adjuvant or salvage treatment of epithelial ovarian cancer, and is FDA approved for this indication. It is also commonly used off-label for endometrial cancer.

Prescribing Information and Toxicity. The usual IV dose of carboplatin is calculated to a target "area under the curve" (AUC) of 6, based on the glomerular filtration rate (GFR). For dose calculation, the Calvert equation is the most frequently used (Carboplatin total dose [mg] = AUC × [GFR + 25]). In clinical practice, the estimated creatinine clearance (CrCl) is usually substituted for the GFR and may be calculated by the Cockcroft-Gault equation (CrCl = [140 − age] × weight [kg]/0.72 × serum creatinine level [mg/100 mL]). The infusion takes 30 to 60 minutes, and dosing is repeated every 3 to 4 weeks.

Myelosuppression, most commonly thrombocytopenia, is the main dose-limiting side effect. Gastrointestinal toxicity and peripheral neuropathy are notably less than those with

TABLE 27-9. Dose and Schedule of Antiemetics to Prevent Emesis Induced by Antineoplastic Therapy of High Emetic Risk

Antiemetics	Brand Name	Single Dose Administered before Chemotherapy	Single Dose Administered Daily
5-HT₃ serotonin-receptor antagonists			
Granisetron	Kytril	Oral: 2 mg IV: 1 mg or 0.01 mg/kg	
Ondansetron	Zofran	Oral: 24 mg IV: 8 mg or 0.15 mg/kg	
Palonosetron	Aloxi	IV: 0.25 mg	
Dexamethasone	Decadron	Oral: 12 mg	Oral: 8 mg, days 2–4
Aprepitant	Emend	Oral: 125 mg	Oral: 80 mg, days 2 and 3

$5-HT_3$ = 5-Hydroxytryptamine-3; IV = intravenous.
Adapted from Hesketh, 2008; Kris, 2006.

cisplatin. Hypersensitivity reactions will eventually develop in up to 25 percent of women receiving more than six cycles.

Cisplatin

Mechanism of Action. Similar to carboplatin, this agent produces DNA adducts that inhibit DNA synthesis (Fig. 28-12, p. 724). Cisplatin is one of the oldest and most widely used agents and is FDA approved for ovarian, cervical, and germ cell cancer. It may be given concomitantly with radiation as a radiosensitizing agent for primary treatment of cervical cancer or either as a single agent or in combination for recurrent cervical cancer. Alternatively, cisplatin is part of combination chemotherapy as the "P" of BEP, given for ovarian germ cell or sex cord-stromal tumors. It is also a member of combination chemotherapy as the "P" of TAP for advanced or recurrent endometrial cancer. However, for use in epithelial ovarian cancer, cisplatin has largely been replaced by carboplatin, except for IP therapy, due to possibly superior tissue penetration.

Prescribing Information and Toxicity. The usual dosage of cisplatin varies, depending on the indication. In cervical cancer, it is given in dosages of 40 mg/m² IV weekly during radiation therapy, or 50 mg/m² IV every 3 weeks for patients with recurrent disease (Long, 2005a). The 50 mg/m² dose is also used in the TAP regimen every 3 weeks (Fleming, 2004). As part of the BEP protocol, cisplatin is administered 20 mg/m² IV on days 1-5 every 3 weeks. Alternatively, for ovarian cancer IP chemotherapy, it is given on day 2 of a 21-day cycle at a dose of 75 to 100 mg/m² (Armstrong, 2006).

Cisplatin has several significant adverse effects associated with administration. Of these, nephrotoxicity is the main dose-limiting side effect. Accordingly, patients must be aggressively hydrated before, during, and after drug administration. Mannitol (10 g) or furosemide (20 to 40 mg) may be necessary to maintain a urine output of at least 100 to 150 mL/hour. With cisplatin administration, electrolyte abnormalities, such as hypomagnesemia and hypokalemia, are

common. In addition, severe, prolonged nausea and vomiting can be dramatic without adequate premedication (Table 27-9). Patients often describe a metallic taste and loss of appetite following treatment. Neurotoxicity, usually in the form of peripheral neuropathy, can also be dose limiting and irreversible. Ototoxicity typically manifests as high-frequency hearing loss and tinnitus. Similar to carboplatin, hypersensitivity reactions may develop with prolonged use. Overall, cisplatin is significantly more toxic than carboplatin, except for reduced hematologic toxicity.

Hexamethylmelamine

This agent forms DNA cross-links, but its exact chemotherapeutic mechanism of action is unknown. Hexamethylmelamine, also known as altretamine (Hexalen), is FDA approved for consolidation therapy of advanced epithelial ovarian cancer and for salvage treatment of recurrent epithelial ovarian cancer (Alberts, 2004; Rustin, 1997).

The usual dose of hexamethylmelamine is 260 mg/m² daily, given as four divided oral doses for 14 to 21 consecutive days in a 28-day cycle. Gastrointestinal side effects, such as nausea and vomiting, are the usual dose-limiting toxicities. Myelosuppression is also common. In addition, approximately one quarter of patients will develop neurotoxicity, manifested as lethargy, agitation, or peripheral neuropathy.

■ Hormonal Agents

Due to their minimal toxicity and reasonable activity, hormonal agents are commonly used for palliative treatment of endometrial and ovarian cancers despite lacking formal FDA approval for these indications.

Tamoxifen

Mechanism of Action. This nonsteroidal prodrug is metabolized into a high-affinity antagonist of the estrogen receptor in breast tissue. It competes with estrogen for receptor binding, but does not activate the receptor, and thereby blocks breast cancer cell growth. The complex is then transported into the tumor cell nucleus, where it binds to DNA and halts cellular growth and proliferation in the G_0 or G_1 phase. Antiangiogenic effects have also been suggested. In addition to breast cancer, tamoxifen (Nolvadex) is occasionally used to treat endometrial and ovarian cancer (Fiorica, 2004; Markman, 2004).

Prescribing Information and Toxicity. Tamoxifen is an orally administered drug, usually prescribed in doses of 20 to 40 mg for continuous daily use.

Toxicity associated with tamoxifen is minimal, mainly consisting of menopausal symptoms such as hot flashes, nausea, and vaginal dryness or discharge. Moreover, some degree of fluid retention and peripheral edema develops in one third of patients.

In women with a uterus, tamoxifen acts as a partial estrogen receptor agonist in the endometrium, and sustained use increases the risk of developing cancer by up to threefold. In addition, the risk of thromboembolic events is increased, especially during and immediately after major surgery or periods of immobility. Reduced cognition and libido may also be noted during therapy.

In contrast, tamoxifen prevents osteoporosis due to its partial agonist properties and has beneficial effects on the serum lipid profile.

Megestrol Acetate

Mechanism of Action. This agent is a synthetic derivative of progesterone that has activity on tumors through its antiestrogenic effects. As such, megestrol acetate (Megace) is most often used to treat endometrial hyperplasia, nonoperable endometrial cancer, and recurrent endometrial cancer, especially in those patients with grade 1 disease (Chap. 33, p. 822).

Prescribing Information and Toxicity. The usual dosage is 40 mg orally four times daily or 80 mg twice daily. Megestrol acetate has minimal toxicity, but commonly patients gain weight from a combination of fluid retention and increased appetite. Thromboembolic events are rarely observed. Patients with diabetes mellitus should be carefully monitored due to the possibility of exacerbating hyperglycemia.

BIOLOGICAL AND TARGETED THERAPY

New knowledge of the differing molecular pathways within normal and malignant cells has led to the development of targeted agents designed to exploit these differences. Targeted therapies

offer the potential for improved long-term disease control with less toxicity. Many of these novel agents are currently being evaluated in clinical trials. Thus, an overview of noncytotoxic drug development is critical for understanding the future medical treatment of gynecologic cancer. Ultimately, the long-term goal is to improve patient outcome, especially in those with tumors that are resistant to standard therapy.

Antiangiogenesis Agents

Angiogenesis is a normal physiologic process involving the formation of new blood vessels and remodeling of vasculature to provide oxygen and nutrients to tissues. This process is usually transient and tightly regulated by a variety of pro- and antiangiogenic factors. However, the homeostatic balance is dysregulated in malignancy. Sustained angiogenesis leads to tumor growth and metastasis. Angiogenesis also provides access to the systemic lymphatic and circulatory systems. Thus, targeted inhibition of angiogenesis is an appealing therapeutic approach.

The binding of vascular endothelial growth factor (VEGF) to the VEGF receptor is a vital first step in stimulating normal angiogenesis. Many malignancies, such as ovarian cancer, are characterized by increased levels of VEGF or other proangiogenic factors. Several novel agents are designed to interfere with this process to halt tumor growth. However, none of these drugs are currently FDA approved for use in gynecologic cancers.

Bevacizumab

This agent is a monoclonal antibody that binds to VEGF to prevent VEGF interaction with its receptor (Fig. 27-7A). Currently, bevacizumab (Avastin) is indicated primarily for treatment of epithelial ovarian cancer (Burger, 2007; Cannistra, 2007; Wright, 2006). Its usual dosage is 15 mg/kg given IV every 3 weeks with or without cytotoxic chemotherapy. In most cases, toxicity with bevacizumab is minimal. However, GI perforation occurs in up to 10 percent of patients. Elevated blood

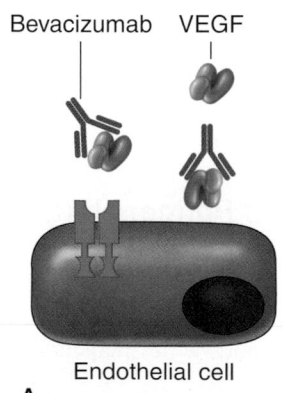

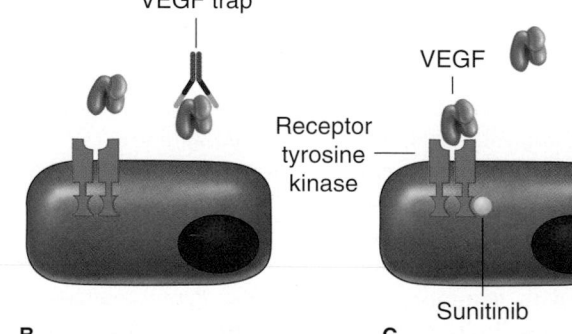

FIGURE 27-7 Mechanisms of action for three antiangiogenesis agents. **A.** Bevacizumab is a monoclonal antibody that binds vascular endothelial growth factor (VEGF). Binding prevents VEGF from combining with its endothelial-bound receptor, which is a receptor tyrosine kinase. **B.** VEGF Trap similarly binds VEGF and prevents receptor binding. **C.** Sunitinib binds with the intracellular ATP-binding sites of receptor tyrosine kinase to inhibit receptor action even though VEGF may be bound. In all three cases, angiogenesis is inhibited, and tumor growth is halted.

pressure is common and may lead to hypertensive crisis. Other possible toxicities include incomplete wound healing, weakness, pain, nosebleed, and proteinuria.

VEGF Trap

VEGF-A is the main isoform of VEGF. It can be bound by bevacizumab, as just described, or by a recombinant "fusion protein" named VEGF Trap (Aflibercept). VEGF Trap is constructed by fusing two specific portions of the VEGF receptor and the "Fc" constant region of the IgG molecule. The receptor portions provide high-affinity binding of VEGF (Fig. 27-7B).

Sunitinib

Receptor tyrosine kinases (RTKs) are proteins that span the plasma membrane of cells and act as receptors (Fig. 27-7C). If two side-by-side receptors bind a ligand, then an active dimer is formed. Ligands for RTKs include cytokines, hormones, and growth factors. The activated dimer then phosphorylates tyrosine residues. Phosphorylation first of the tyrosine kinase itself, and then of other proteins, activates them. Receptor tyrosine kinases are regulators of normal cellular processes, however, these also have a critical role in cancer development and progression.

Sunitinib (Sutent) is an oral agent that inhibits several receptor tyrosine kinases including those that bind proangiogenic growth factors, such as VEGF and platelet-derived growth factor.

Mammalian Target of Rapamycin Inhibitors

The *mammalian target of rapamycin (mTOR)* is a protein kinase that regulates membrane trafficking, transcription, translation, and maintenance of the cell cytoskeleton. mTOR has downstream effects that include increased VEGF production. Thus, efforts to inhibit mTOR signaling also can lead to inhibition of angiogenesis. Rapamycin inhibits mTOR, and analogs of this drug, such as temsirolimus (CCI-779) and everolimus (RAD001), are currently being studied for their efficacy in treating gynecologic cancers.

Poly (ADP) Ribose Polymerase Inhibitors

Another promising group of targeted therapies, poly (ADP) ribose polymerase (PARP) inhibitors, exploit the differences between normal and malignant cells in repairing DNA damage. During the cell cycle, DNA is routinely damaged thousands of times. The BRCA protein repairs double-strand breaks, and PARP repairs single-strand breaks. In the functioning cell, if BRCA does not repair the break, PARP will.

Five to 10 percent of ovarian cancer patients have a germline BRCA1 or BRCA2 mutation, predisposing them to loss of that repair function. Other patients without mutations develop defects in the BRCA pathway that also result in defective repair. Tumor cells in both types of patients are almost entirely dependent on PARP repair. If PARP repair is prevented, cancer cells cannot be repaired and they die. In contrast, normal cells are unaffected. Several PARP inhibitors are currently in development to take advantage of this unique tumor cell sensitivity while sparing healthy surrounding tissues.

Olaparib (AZD2281)

This PARP inhibitor has been tested in a study population enriched in BRCA1- and BRCA2-mutation carriers. Antitumor activity was observed only in those patients with mutations, all of whom had ovarian, breast, or prostate cancer. Encouragingly, few of the adverse effects of conventional chemotherapy were seen (Fong, 2009). Further studies are evaluating olaparib effects in cancer patients without germline mutations, but whose cancers exhibit similar DNA repair defects. Iniparib and veliparib are other PARP inhibitors designed to similarly capitalize on this strategy.

Vaccines

Biologic modifiers, such as therapeutic cancer vaccines, are designed to induce cellular components of the immune system to recognize and attack tumors. Malignant cells that express specific surface antigens can thereby be targeted and destroyed. For example, in cervical cancer, viral peptides derived from human papillomavirus (HPV) E6 and E7 oncoproteins have been clinically targeted (Borysiewicz, 1996). Additionally, ovarian cancer patients have been studied with a vaccine directed against CA125 (Reinartz, 2004).

For the most part, such strategies have not been clinically effective. Only a limited number of shared tumor-associated antigens have been identified, epitopes for cellular immunity have not been adequately defined, and few tumor antigens are unique. Tumors commonly lose their distinctive antigen expression and may undergo mutation. In general, vaccine trials are performed with patients with advanced disease. However, in these situations, clinical response is difficult to evaluate and statistically uninformative. Moreover, inherent systemic immunosuppression in women with advanced disease may prevent an adequate immune response.

In contrast, prophylactic vaccines, such as the HPV vaccine, have shown great promise for preventing cervical cancer (Massad, 2009; Romanowski, 2009). These work by eliciting humoral immune responses to induce the production of antibodies capable of neutralizing a virus before infection (Chap. 29, p. 737).

SIDE EFFECTS

Chemotherapy regimens, especially those including cytotoxic drugs, are universally toxic and display a narrow margin of safety. Several agents are associated with classic toxicities that can often be anticipated, and thereby avoided. Because of their limited therapeutic ranges, most agents require dose adjustments in accordance with the individual patient tolerances. Initial chemotherapy dosing is calculated from BSA, weight, renal function, and hepatic function, using specified guidelines from clinical trials. However, numerous other factors influence toxicity and include the patient's baseline nutrition, overall health, extent of disease, and prior therapy. The Cancer

Therapy Evaluation Program (CTEP) of the National Cancer Institute (NCI), in collaboration with the Food and Drug Administration (FDA), national cooperative groups, and the pharmaceutical industry, has developed a detailed and comprehensive set of guidelines for the description and grading of toxicity. Termed the Common Terminology Criteria for Adverse Events (CTCAE), the most recent revision is version 4 and is available at: http://evs.nci.nih.gov/ftp1/CTCAE/About.html.

In general, treatment modifications depend on the degree (grade) and duration of toxicity experienced during the preceding therapy course. Doses should be reduced if a woman experiences a severe reaction, but then may be subsequently increased if tolerance improves. However, treatment should not resume until toxicity has resolved to baseline or "grade 1" levels and may be delayed on a week-to-week basis to permit recovery. Dose modification and supportive care should be implemented to prevent delays of greater than 2 weeks, which would otherwise compromise therapeutic efficacy. Serious myelosuppression can be partially corrected with the use of hematopoietic growth factors (p. 709). Many of the common toxicities can be prevented with proper use of premedications or alleviated with supportive measures.

Bone Marrow Toxicity

Myelosuppression, especially neutropenia, is the most common dose-limiting side effect of cytotoxic drugs. The absolute neutrophil count (ANC) is the critical measure when determining patient infection risk and may reflect mild ($1000–1500/mm^3$), moderate ($500–1000/mm^3$), or severe ($<500/mm^3$) neutropenia. Frequently, patients receiving therapy will have a nadir (lowest measurement) in the neutropenic range that will recover before the next scheduled course of treatment. However, if they are admitted to the hospital for fever or other condition, neutropenic precautions should be observed. Although guidelines may vary, precautions include assiduous provider hand washing; provider outer gowns, gloves, and masks; and patient isolation from potentially infectious carriers.

Moderate degrees of anemia are common in cancer patients receiving chemotherapy and may contribute to chronic fatigue. Frequent transfusions are not practical or recommended, and many patients will adapt to chronic anemia with minimal symptoms. In some patients, synthetic erythropoietin may be indicated (p. 709).

Thrombocytopenia is less common, but may predispose the patient to serious bleeding if the platelet count is $<10,000/mm^3$. No predetermined platelet value should prompt routine transfusion, but ongoing bleeding in affected patients is a warranted indication.

Gastrointestinal Toxicity

Most anticancer agents are associated with some degree of nausea, vomiting, and anorexia. Typically, the emetogenic potential of a particular drug or regimen will dictate the antiemetic regimen used (Tables 27-10 and 27-11). Mild nausea and vomiting can often be managed effectively by prochlorperazine (Compazine) with or without dexamethasone (Table 39-10, p. 963). For drugs with more severe emetogenic effects such as cisplatin, the 5-hydroxytryptamine antagonists ondansetron,

TABLE 27-10. Emetic Risk of Intravenously Administered Antineoplastic Agents Used in Gynecologic Oncology

Emetic Risk	Incidence of Emesis (without antiemetics)	Agent
High	>90%	Cisplatin Cyclophosphamide ≥ 1500 mg/m^2 Dactinomycin
Moderate	30–90%	Carboplatin Ifosfamide Cyclophosphamide <1500 mg/m^2 Doxorubicin
Low	10–30%	Paclitaxel Docetaxel Topotecan Etoposide Methotrexate Gemcitabine
Minimal	<10%	Bevacizumab Bleomycin Vinblastine Vincristine Vinorelbine

Abbreviated from Hesketh, 2008; Kris, 2006; Roila, 2006.

granisetron, or palonosetron can be given IV before chemotherapy. Ondansetron (Zofran) and granisetron (Kytril) may also be provided orally to manage delayed and/or chronic nausea after chemotherapy. However, these drugs may induce significant constipation as a side effect. Chemotherapy-related diarrhea, oral mucositis, esophagitis, and gastroenteritis are treated with supportive care.

Dermatologic Toxicity

Most drugs can cause a spectrum of toxicity to the skin or subcutaneous tissues, including hyperpigmentation, photosensitivity, nail abnormalities, rashes, urticaria, or erythema. Many of these are drug specific and self-limited, but occasionally, they may be dose limiting. As discussed earlier, palmar-plantar erythrodysesthesia is a known toxicity of liposomal doxorubicin (p. 702). In addition, changes in skin pigmentation are seen with bleomycin, whereas nail discoloration and onycholysis have been associated with docetaxel therapy. Premedication with diphenhydramine hydrochloride, 50 mg IV or orally, will prevent or alleviate mild urticarial reactions.

Neurotoxicity

Peripheral neuropathy occurs commonly with cisplatin, paclitaxel, the vinca alkaloids, and hexamethylmelamine.

TABLE 27-11. Drug Regimens for the Prevention of Chemotherapy-Induced Emesis by Emetic Risk Category

Emetic Risk Category (Incidence of Emesis without Antiemetics)	Antiemetic Regimens and Schedules
High (>90%)	5-HT$_3$ serotonin receptor antagonist: day 1 Dexamethasone: days 1–3 Granisetron: days 1–3
Moderate (30% to 90%)	5-HT$_3$ serotonin receptor antagonist: day 1 Dexamethasone: days 1–3
Low (10% to 30%)	5-HT$_3$ serotonin receptor antagonist: day 1 Dexamethasone: days 1–3
Minimal (<10%)	Prescribe as needed

5-HT$_3$ = 5-Hydroxytryptamine-3.
Adapted from Hesketh, 2008; Kris, 2006.

Cisplatin-induced neurotoxicity usually resolves slowly, due to axonal demyelination and loss. This toxicity is related to cumulative dose and intensity. To counter this toxicity, amifostine (Ethyol) may be administered, but substitution of carboplatin will avoid much of the toxicity. Gabapentin (Neurontin) is the usual treatment for neuropathic pain, starting at a dosage of 300 mg daily. Other options to treat symptomatic peripheral neuropathy that have shown some efficacy include oral glutamine (up to 15 g twice daily) or oral vitamin B$_6$ (up to 50 mg three times daily).

With chemotherapeutic agents in general, drug dosing may need to be adjusted if peripheral neuropathy becomes problematic—for example, if a patient can no longer hold a cup of coffee. More dramatic instances of acute cerebellar syndromes, cranial nerve palsies or paralysis, and occasionally acute and chronic encephalopathies should be managed with supportive care, and usually discontinuation of the offending agent.

Alopecia

One of the most emotionally distressing side effects of many chemotherapeutic agents is scalp alopecia. Fortunately, this is usually reversible. With some drugs such as paclitaxel, women will also experience loss of eyelashes, eyebrows, and other body hair. In general, techniques to minimize alopecia are unsuccessful. Instead, women should be counseled regarding cosmetic options such as false eyelashes and wigs.

GROWTH FACTORS

In several clinical situations, incorporation of hematopoietic drug factors to the administration of chemotherapy is helpful. Epoetin alfa and darbepoetin alfa are synthetic erythropoietins that stimulate red blood cell (RBC) production. Given by subcutaneous injection, these agents are recommended for patients with chemotherapy-associated anemia who have a hemoglobin concentration that is approaching, or has fallen below, 10 g/dL. For this indication, these agents increase hemoglobin levels and decrease transfusions. However, when used at higher hemoglobin levels (between 10 and 12 g/dL), they may actually be associated with tumor progression and shorten survival (Rizzo, 2008).

Filgrastim and pegfilgrastim increase granulocyte production. These growth factors are mainly used to prevent episodes of febrile neutropenia (ANC <1500), particularly in patients with a greater than 20-percent risk for such an event. Regimens such as docetaxel at 75 to 100 mg/m^2 every 3 weeks for recurrent ovarian cancer have a high risk of developing a life-threatening infection (Aapro, 2006; Crawford, 2009). In addition to preventing neutropenic fever, growth factors may also be indicated to permit a patient to maintain her treatment schedule, such as the alternating weeks of EMA-CO therapy.

Epoetin Alfa

This hematopoietic drug is a recombinant glycoprotein that has the same biologic effects as endogenous erythropoietin. Epoetin alfa (Procrit, Eprex, and Epogen) is usually prescribed as 40,000 units SC, given weekly (Case, 2006). Beyond local pain at the injection site, this agent has minimal side effects. Possible toxicity may include diarrhea, nausea, or hypertension (Bohlius, 2006; Khuri, 2007).

Darbepoetin Alfa

This hematopoietic drug is closely related to epoetin alfa and has the same biologic effects as endogenous erythropoietin. Indicated for the treatment of chemotherapy-induced anemia, the usual SC dose of darbepoetin alfa (Aranesp) is 200 µg every other week or 500 µg given every 3 weeks. Darbepoetin alfa has minimal side effects beyond local pain at the injection site.

Filgrastim

This protein is a human granulocyte colony-stimulating factor (G-CSF), produced by recombinant DNA technology. As such, filgrastim (Neupogen) is a cytokine that binds to hematopoietic cells and activates the proliferation, differentiation, and activation of granulocyte progenitor cells. This agent is indicated as an adjunct to chemotherapy. In addition to preventing neutropenic fever, it allows women to continue their chemotherapy schedule without dose delays from myelosuppression and/or speeds resolution of neutropenic fever episodes.

The usual SC dose of filgrastim is 5 μg/kg/d, but typically patients are given either 300 μg or 480 μg, which is the content of manufactured vials. It must be administered at least 24 hours after the completion of chemotherapy. Therapy should be terminated when the white blood count exceeds 10,000/mm^3 or when the absolute neutrophil count exceeds 1000/mm^3 for 3 consecutive days. Toxicity with filgrastim is limited, and transient bone pain is usually mild to moderate.

Pegfilgrastim

This agent acts similar to filgrastim to stimulate production of granulocyte progenitor cells within the bone marrow. The "peg" in pegfilgrastim (Neulasta) refers to a polyethylene glycol unit that prolongs the time it remains in the body. Pegfilgrastim is given as a single 6-mg SC injection once per chemotherapy cycle. This is usually far more convenient than daily filgrastim doses. It should not be administered during the 14 days before and 24 hours after administration of cytotoxic chemotherapy. Transient bone pain is usually mild to moderate, but often more pronounced than with filgrastim.

CHEMOSENSITIVITY AND RESISTANCE ASSAYS

Routinely, the selection of specific chemotherapeutic agents is based on clinical literature describing outcomes for a specific gynecologic cancer. In contrast to this empiric therapy approach, chemotherapy sensitivity and resistance assays are theoretically appealing due to the possibility of tailoring treatment. Using this strategy, viable tumor tissue is collected from the patient during surgery or other intervention (e.g., paracentesis). The sample is shipped to a laboratory (Oncotech or Precision Therapeutics). Here, in vitro analysis determines whether tumor growth is inhibited by a drug or panel of drugs.

The potential of selecting effective cancer treatments while sparing unnecessary ones is intriguing, and patients may even request testing. However, no current assay has demonstrated sufficient efficacy to support its use. Thus, these assays should not be recommended for individual patients outside of a clinical trial (Schrag, 2004).

CANCER DRUG DEVELOPMENT

The only proven way to improve the success of cancer treatment involves testing new agents, higher doses, novel combinations of drugs, or unique ways of administering treatment. Over the past few decades, clinical trial designs have become increasingly sophisticated. Since gynecologic cancers are relatively uncommon, most landmark Phase III studies are conducted within large collaborative groups such as the Gynecologic Oncology Group (GOG). Occasionally, there are astonishing successes.

For example, metastatic gestational choriocarcinoma has gone from a uniformly fatal diagnosis to one being routinely cured with combination chemotherapy. More commonly, gradual improvements in extending patient survival length take years to realize.

The identification of a new and active anticancer drug is a long, complicated, expensive process. Promising drugs are first identified by demonstrating success in cancer cell lines or in animals inoculated with tumor. Next, drugs are subjected to detailed preclinical toxicology tests in animals. After preclinical steps are completed, novel agents proceed through four phases of clinical testing.

Phase I trials use a dose-escalating design to determine the dose-limiting toxicity, maximum tolerated dose (MTD), and pharmacokinetic parameters of the drug. Groups of three to six patients with a variety of tumor types are enrolled and receive escalating dose levels. The MTD is determined as the dose below which two patients experience dose-limiting toxicity (DLT). In a Phase I trial, detecting a tumor response is not critical, since enrolled patients have typically completed extensive prior therapy. However, observed responses would encourage further disease-specific Phase II trials.

After the recommended dose and treatment schedule have been defined in a Phase I trial, the regimen can proceed to Phase II. The primary goal of this trial type is to define the actual response rate in patients with a specific cancer type. Usually a measure of disease (MOD) is required to allow accurate determination of a complete response, partial response, stable disease, or progression. Typically, patients enrolled in Phase II trials have received only one prior chemotherapy regimen. This allows for a reasonable chance of response compared with subjects in Phase I studies. Secondary endpoints of Phase II trials include determination of the "progression-free interval," cumulative incidence of dose-limiting toxicity over multiple cycles, and overall survival.

When a promising regimen is identified in Phase II, it may then progress to Phase III. These randomized trials are designed to directly compare the drug with existing standard regimens in a particular stage and type of cancer. Phase III trials generally require a minimum of 150 patients per "arm" to provide adequate statistical precision.

Phase IV clinical trials evaluate drugs that are already FDA approved. The goal of Phase IV trials is to study long-term drug safety and efficacy.

The emergence of biologic and targeted therapies has necessitated a reanalysis of this traditional paradigm of cancer drug development. For example, antiangiogenic agents and PARP inhibitors do not have dose-dependent toxicities to establish a MTD. Additionally, instead of measuring tumor shrinkage as an indicator of response for these cytostatic agents, new endpoints will need to be developed and validated (6-month progression-free survival). Novel clinical trial designs will be a vital part of drug development in the future.

In general, patients should be strongly encouraged to participate in appropriate Phase I, II, and III clinical trials. By doing so, their options for treatment are expanded. In addition, the results of such studies are the primary method to improve the outcomes of women diagnosed with gynecologic cancer in the future.

REFERENCES

Aapro MS, Cameron DA, Pettengell R, et al: EORTC guidelines for the use of granulocyte-colony stimulating factor to reduce the incidence of chemotherapy-induced febrile neutropenia in adult patients with lymphomas and solid tumours. Eur J Cancer 42(15):2433, 2006

Alberts DS, Jiang C, Liu PY, et al: Long-term follow-up of a phase II trial of oral altretamine for consolidation of clinical complete remission in women with stage III epithelial ovarian cancer in the Southwest Oncology Group. Int J Gynecol Cancer 14(2):224, 2004

Armstrong DK, Bundy B, Wenzel L, et al: Intraperitoneal cisplatin and paclitaxel in ovarian cancer. N Engl J Med 354(1):34, 2006

Bay JO, Ray-Coquard I, Fayette J, et al: Docetaxel and gemcitabine combination in 133 advanced soft-tissue sarcomas: a retrospective analysis. Int J Cancer 119(3):706, 2006

Bohlius J, Wilson J, Seidenfeld J, et al: Recombinant human erythropoietins and cancer patients: updated meta-analysis of 57 studies including 9353 patients. J Natl Cancer Inst 98(10):708, 2006

Borysiewicz LK, Fiander A, Nimako M, et al: A recombinant vaccinia virus encoding human papillomavirus types 16 and 18, E6 and E7 proteins as immunotherapy for cervical cancer. Lancet 347(9014):1523, 1996

Bower M, Newlands ES, Holden L, et al: EMA/CO for high-risk gestational trophoblastic tumors: results from a cohort of 272 patients. J Clin Oncol 15(7):2636, 1997

Burger RA, Sill MW, Monk BJ, et al: Phase III trial of bevacizumab in persistent or recurrent epithelial ovarian cancer or primary peritoneal cancer: a gynecologic oncology group study. J Clin Oncol 25(33):5165, 2007

Cannistra SA, Matulonis UA, Penson RT, et al: Phase III study of bevacizumab in patients with platinum-resistant ovarian cancer or peritoneal serous cancer. J Clin Oncol 25(33):5180, 2007

Cantu MG, Buda A, Parma G, et al: Randomized controlled trial of single-agent paclitaxel versus cyclophosphamide, doxorubicin, and cisplatin in patients with recurrent ovarian cancer who responded to first-line platinum-based regimens. J Clin Oncol 20(5):1232, 2002

Case AS, Rocconi RP, Kilgore LC, et al: Effectiveness of darbepoetin alfa versus epoetin alfa for the treatment of chemotherapy induced anemia in patients with gynecologic malignancies. Gynecol Oncol 101(3):499, 2006

Chura JC, Van Iseghem K, Downs LS Jr, et al: Bevacizumab plus cyclophosphamide in heavily pretreated patients with recurrent ovarian cancer. Gynecol Oncol 107(2):326, 2007

Crawford J, Allen J, Armitage J, et al: Myeloid growth factors. v.1.2010. National Comprehensive Cancer Network, 2009. Available at: http://www.nccn.org/professionals/physician_gls/PDF/myeloid_growth.pdf. Accessed April 1, 2010

DiSaia PJ, Creasman WT: Basic principles of chemotherapy. In Clinical Gynecologic Oncology. St. Louis, MO, Mosby, 2002, p 517

DuBeshter B, Berkowitz RS, Goldstein DP, et al: Vinblastine, cisplatin and bleomycin as salvage therapy for refractory high-risk metastatic gestational trophoblastic disease. J Reprod Med 34(3):189, 1989

Eisenhauer EA, Therasse P, Bogaerts J, et al: New response evaluation criteria in solid tumours: revised RECIST guideline (version 1.1). Eur J Cancer 45:228, 2009

Fiorica JV, Brunetto VL, Hanjani P, et al: Phase II trial of alternating courses of megestrol acetate and tamoxifen in advanced endometrial carcinoma: a Gynecologic Oncology Group study. Gynecol Oncol 92(1):10, 2004

Fleming GF, Brunetto VL, Cella D, et al: Phase III trial of doxorubicin plus cisplatin with or without paclitaxel plus filgrastim in advanced endometrial carcinoma: a Gynecologic Oncology Group Study. J Clin Oncol 22(11):2159, 2004

Fong PC, Boss DS, Yap TA, et al: Inhibition of poly (ADP-ribose) polymerase in tumors from BRCA mutation carriers. N Engl J Med 361(2):123, 2009

Gordon AN, Tonda M, Sun S, et al: Long-term survival advantage for women treated with pegylated liposomal doxorubicin compared with topotecan in a phase 3 randomized study of recurrent and refractory epithelial ovarian cancer. Gynecol Oncol 95(1):1, 2004

Hesketh PJ: Chemotherapy-induced nausea and vomiting. N Engl J Med 358(23):2482, 2008

Homesley HD, Bundy BN, Hurteau JA, et al: Bleomycin, etoposide, and cisplatin combination therapy of ovarian granulosa cell tumors and other stromal malignancies: a Gynecologic Oncology Group study. Gynecol Oncol 72(2):131, 1999

Katsumata N, Yasuda M, Takahashi F, et al: Dose-dense paclitaxel once a week in combination with carboplatin every 3 weeks for advanced ovarian cancer: a phase 3, open-label, randomised controlled trial. Lancet 374(9698):1331, 2009

Khuri FR: Weighing the hazards of erythropoiesis stimulation in patients with cancer. N Engl J Med 356(24):2445, 2007

Kris MG, Hesketh PJ, Somerfield MR, et al: American Society of Clinical Oncology guideline for antiemetics in oncology: update 2006. J Clin Oncol 24(18):1, 2006

Long HJ III, Bundy BN, Grendys EC, Jr., et al: Randomized phase III trial of cisplatin with or without topotecan in carcinoma of the uterine cervix: a Gynecologic Oncology Group Study. J Clin Oncol 23(21):4626, 2005a

Long HJ III, Bundy BN, Grendys EC, Jr., et al: Randomized phase III trial of cisplatin with or without topotecan in carcinoma of the uterine cervix: a Gynecologic Oncology Group Study. J Clin Oncol 23(21):4626, 2005b

Long HJ III, Bundy BN, Grendys EC, Jr., et al: Randomized phase III trial of cisplatin with or without topotecan in carcinoma of the uterine cervix: a Gynecologic Oncology Group Study. J Clin Oncol 23(21):4626, 2005c

Markman M, Blessing J, Rubin SC, et al: Phase II trial of weekly paclitaxel (80 mg/m^2) in platinum and paclitaxel-resistant ovarian and primary peritoneal cancers: a Gynecologic Oncology Group study. Gynecol Oncol 101(3):436, 2006

Markman M, Webster K, Zanotti K, et al: Use of tamoxifen in asymptomatic patients with recurrent small-volume ovarian cancer. Gynecol Oncol 93(2):390, 2004

Massad LS, Einstein M, Myers E, et al: The impact of human papillomavirus vaccination on cervical cancer prevention efforts. Gynecol Oncol 114(2):360, 2009

Mileshkin L, Antill Y, Rischin D: Management of complications of chemotherapy. In Gershenson DM, McGuire WP, Gore M, et al (eds): Gynecologic Cancer Controversies in Management. Philadelphia, Elsevier, 2004, p 618

Reinartz S, Kohler S, Schlebusch H, et al: Vaccination of patients with advanced ovarian carcinoma with the anti-idiotype ACA125: immunological response and survival (phase Ib/II). Clin Cancer Res 10(5):1580, 2004

Rizzo JD, Somerfield MR, Hagerty KL, et al: Use of epoetin and darbepoetin in patients with cancer: 2007 American Society of Clinical Oncology/American Society of Hematology clinical practice guideline update. J Clin Oncol 26(1):132, 2008

Roila F, Hesketh PJ, Herrstedt J, et al: Prevention of chemotherapy- and radiotherapy-induced emesis: results of the 2004 Perugia International Antiemetic Consensus Conference. Ann Oncol 17:20, 2006

Romanowski B, de Borba PC, Naud PS, et al: Sustained efficacy and immunogenicity of the human papillomavirus (HPV)-16/18 AS04-adjuvanted vaccine: analysis of a randomised placebo-controlled trial up to 6.4 years. Lancet 374(9706):1975, 2009

Rustin GJ, Nelstrop AE, Crawford M, et al: Phase II trial of oral altretamine for relapsed ovarian carcinoma: evaluation of defining response by serum CA125. J Clin Oncol 15(1):172, 1997

Schrag D, Garewal HS, Burstein HJ, et al: American Society of Clinical Oncology Technology Assessment: chemotherapy sensitivity and resistance assays. J Clin Oncol 22(17):3631, 2004

Spannuth WA, Leath CA, III, Huh WK, et al: A Phase II trial of weekly topotecan for patients with secondary platinum-resistant recurrent epithelial ovarian carcinoma following the failure of second-line therapy. Gynecol Oncol 104(3):591, 2007

Strauss HG, Henze A, Teichmann A, et al: Phase II trial of docetaxel and carboplatin in recurrent platinum-sensitive ovarian, peritoneal and tubal cancer. Gynecol Oncol 104(3):612, 2007

Tinker AV, Gebski V, Fitzharris B, et al: Phase II trial of weekly docetaxel for patients with relapsed ovarian cancer who have previously received paclitaxel—ANZGOG 02-01. Gynecol Oncol 104(3):647, 2007

Williams SD, Blessing JA, Hatch KD, et al: Chemotherapy of advanced dysgerminoma: trials of the Gynecologic Oncology Group. J Clin Oncol 9(11):1950, 1991

Wright JD, Hagemann A, Rader JS, et al: Bevacizumab combination therapy in recurrent, platinum-refractory, epithelial ovarian carcinoma: a retrospective analysis. Cancer 107(1):83, 2006

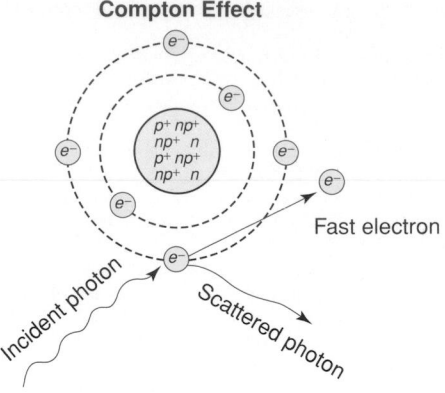

Compton Effect

Fast electron

Incident photon

Scattered photon

Principles of Radiation Therapy

For more than a century, the important biologic effects of ionizing radiation have been noted by scientists and have been applied clinically. Significant advances in technologic innovation coupled with radiobiologic research have firmly established *radiation therapy* as an important modality in cancer treatment. It may be used alone or in conjunction with other therapies in the management of a variety of conditions, both malignant and benign.

Radiation therapy can be delivered: (1) by external beam therapy; (2) by internal cavity placement of radionuclide sources, termed *brachytherapy*; or (3) by instillation of radionuclide solutions. These forms play significant roles in the treatment of various gynecologic malignancies (Table 28-1). For example, external beam therapy and brachytherapy are used in the primary management of inoperable cancers of the cervix, vagina, and vulva. Additionally, radiation therapy may be recommended as adjuvant treatment postoperatively if the probability of regional recurrence is high. For uterine malignancies, external beam therapy or brachytherapy may be recommended for adjuvant posthysterectomy treatment or can occasionally be used as a primary modality for inoperable tumors. For epithelial ovarian cancer, the indications for radiation therapy are few. Similarly, the role currently is limited for external beam therapy in the management of ovarian germ cell tumors and gestational trophoblastic neoplasia (Soper, 2003). Radiation therapy is used frequently in the relief of symptoms caused by metastasis of any gynecologic cancer. Accordingly, pain, bleeding, bronchial obstruction, and neurologic sequelae may often be effectively palliated.

RADIATION PHYSICS

Electromagnetic Radiation

Photons and *gamma rays* are the two types of electromagnetic radiation used in radiation therapy. Both can be considered as *electromagnetic waves* or as discrete *particles* (quanta) of energy. This duality is described in the wave-particle theory of quantum physics, which explains that energy can be transferred either by waves or particles.

Photons also known as *x-rays* are produced when a stream of electrons collides with a high atomic-number target, such as a tungsten target located in the head of a linear accelerator (Fig. 28-1). These photons are used in external beam therapy.

In contrast, gamma rays originate from unstable atomic nuclei and are emitted during decay of radioactive materials,

TABLE 28-1. Role of Radiation Therapy in the Management of Gynecologic Cancers

Intent	Site
Curative	Cervix, vulva, vagina
Adjunctive to surgery	Cervix, vulva, vagina, uterus
Palliative	Metastasis causing symptoms: bleeding, pain, obstruction

also termed radionuclides, which are widely used in brachytherapy (Fig. 28-2).

Particle Radiation

Whereas electromagnetic waves are defined by their wavelengths, particles are defined by their masses. For clinical use, particles include electrons, neutrons, protons, helium ions, heavy charged ions, and pi mesons. Except for electrons, which are available in

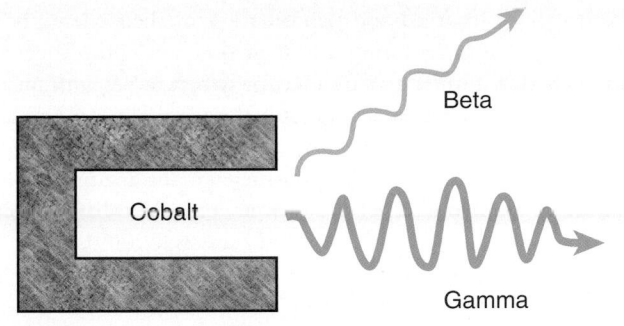

FIGURE 28-2 Gamma rays are emitted during the nuclear decay of cobalt-60. Beta rays are also emitted but are not used clinically.

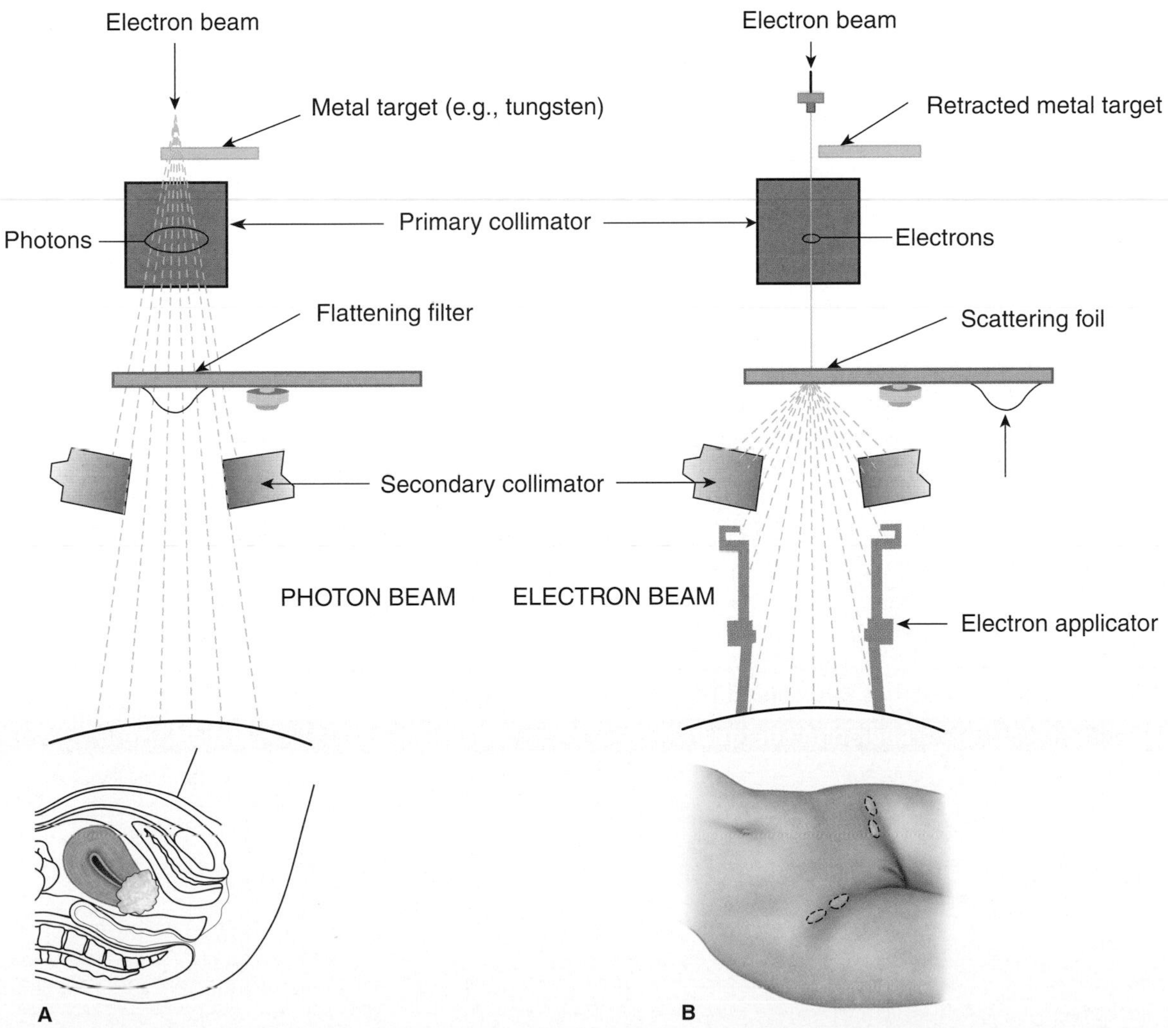

all modern radiation oncology centers, only a few institutions have the capability to use the other particles for clinical therapy.

Particles are produced by linear accelerators or other high-energy generators designed for physics research. Particle radiation is usually delivered by external beam, and each particle type has specific biologic and physical properties. *Electrons*

FIGURE 28-1 Block diagram of a linear accelerator used to create external beam radiation. Either photon beams or electron beams may be produced. **A.** Photon beam therapy is suited for deep tumors such as the cervical cancer shown here. Beam energy is measured in million volts (MV). **B.** Electron beam therapy is indicated for superficial lesions such as inguinal lymph nodes. Beam energy is measured in million electron volts (MeV).

are negatively charged and deposit most of their energy near the surface, thus delivering a limited dose at depth. They are uniquely suited to treat skin cancer or lymph nodes with metastatic disease, such as affected inguinal nodes. Clinical research with neutrons, protons, helium ions, alpha particles, carbon ions, and pi mesons has been pursued for the treatment of a variety of tumors. Except for electrons, particle radiation therapy remains an investigational tool (Terasawa, 2009).

Radionuclides

Radionuclides, also called radioisotopes, undergo nuclear decay and can emit: (1) positively charged alpha particles, (2) negatively charged beta particles (electrons), and (3) gamma rays. Radionuclides commonly used in gynecologic oncology are commercially available as sealed sources such as cobalt, cesium, iridium, gold, and iodine or as unsealed solutions of strontium, iodine, or phosphorus (Table 28-2). Cesium and iridium are commonly used in gynecologic brachytherapy.

Radiation Equipment

Linear Accelerator (Linac).
One of the main types of radiation-producing units is the linear accelerator, also called a *linac*. It is widely used throughout the world to deliver external beam radiation.

A linac can produce both photon and electron beams (see Fig. 28-1). In the *photon-therapy mode*, indicated for deep-seated tumors, the accelerated electron beam is guided to hit a metal target to produce photons with heterogeneous energies. The photon beam intensity must be uniform for clinical use. To that goal, a beam-flattening filter is employed. In the *electron-therapy mode*, indicated for superficial lesions, the electron beam strikes a lead scattering foil instead of the metal target. Applicators or cones then shape the electron beam. In both cases, energy from the linac is directed to the desired target tissues.

The unit used to describe the energy of a photon beam is MV (million volts). The unit for electron beam energy is expressed in MeV (million electron volts). Customarily, a linac is designated by a number corresponding to the highest energy of the electron beam available. For example, the maximum energy of the electron beam produced by a linac 18 is 18 MeV.

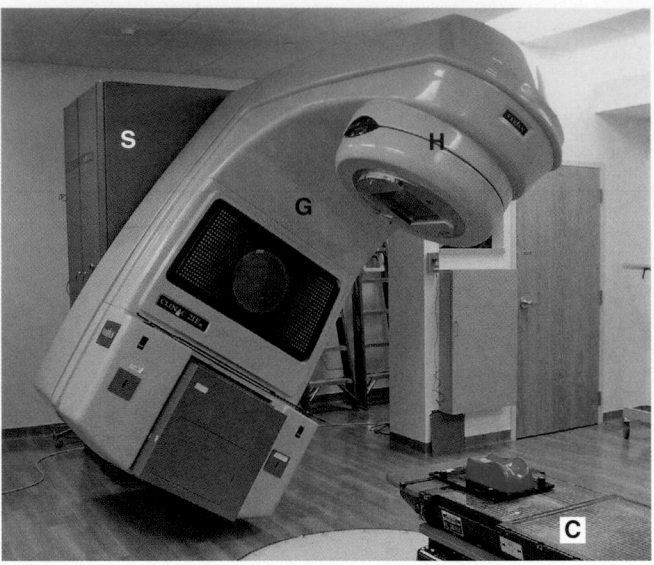

FIGURE 28-3 Photograph of a linear accelerator currently in use at the University of Texas Southwestern Medical Center. The patient lies on the treatment couch (C). The gantry (G), couch, and head (H) can all rotate and allow radiation beams to reach target tissues through different angles. S = stand.

Figure 28-3 displays a linac with four components: stand, gantry, treatment head, and couch. Of these, the gantry, treatment head, and treatment couch can all rotate 360 degrees. Thus, linac mobility allows the use of multiple fields and angles to achieve an optimal dose delivery to a tumor.

Cobalt Machine. Although linacs are widely installed worldwide for cancer treatment, cobalt machines are still used for external beam therapy in a very few centers in the United States and in some developing countries. Cobalt-60 is an artificially created isotope that undergoes nuclear decay, emitting 1.17-MV and 1.33-MV gamma rays, which deposit the maximum energy less than 1 cm below the skin surface. As a result, the skin-sparing effect of a Co-60 beam is less than that of photon beams produced by the linacs. In addition, the half-life of Co-60 is short (5.2 years), and the source requires frequent replacement, every 4 to 5 years.

TABLE 28-2. Physical Properties and Clinical Use of Selected Radionuclides

Element	Radiation Energy in MeV	Half-Life	Clinical Use
Cesium-137	0.6	30 years	Brachytherapy
Iridium-192	0.4	74 days	Brachytherapy
Cobalt-60	1.2	5 years	Brachytherapy
Iodine-125	0.028	60 days	Brachytherapy
Phosphorus-32	1.7	14 days	Intraperitoneal instillation
Gold-196	0.4	2.7 days	Intraperitoneal instillation
Strontium-89	1.4	51 days	Diffuse bone metastasis

MeV = million electron volts.

Electromagnetic Radiation Energy Deposition

When electromagnetic radiation is used in daily clinical practice, it contacts target tissues, and energy is transferred to those tissues. This transfer creates ions by dislodging electrons from atoms within these tissues. During this ionizing process, energy is passed to *fast electrons*. These electrons then collide with surrounding molecules to initiate the biologic process of radiation damage.

There are three mechanisms involved in energy transfer: (1) photoelectric effect, (2) Compton effect, and (3) pair production (Fig. 28-4). Depending on the energy level of the impacting radiation, one of these mechanisms will predominate.

If the impacting energy is low (less than 100 kV), the *photoelectric effect* is dominant. The effect causes ejection of an orbiting electron from its shell. After ejection, the vacancy is filled by an electron from an outer orbiting shell. The ejected fast-electron kinetic energy is then deposited into tissues to cause radiation damage.

The *Compton effect* dominates in the mid- to high-energy range (1 MV to 20 MV) and is the most important of the three in clinical radiation therapy. With this effect, the impacting photon energy is much larger than the binding electron energy. As a result, part of the photon energy is transferred to an electron that is then ejected from the orbiting shell. The newly formed fast electron initiates the chain of events leading to biologic damage.

Pair production occurs when a photon beam with very high energy (beyond 20 MV) impacts the electromagnetic field of the nucleus. The result is formation of a *pair* comprised of a negatively charged electron and a positively charged positron. If the positron slows and interacts with a negatively charged electron, there is mutual annihilation. As a result, two photons going in opposite directions are produced. These photons interact with tissues to transfer energy and cause biologic damage.

Linear Energy Transfer and Relative Biologic Effectiveness

When radiation interacts with tissues, ionizing events occur along the path of energy transfer. The rate of energy deposition along this path is called *linear energy transfer* or LET, which is expressed

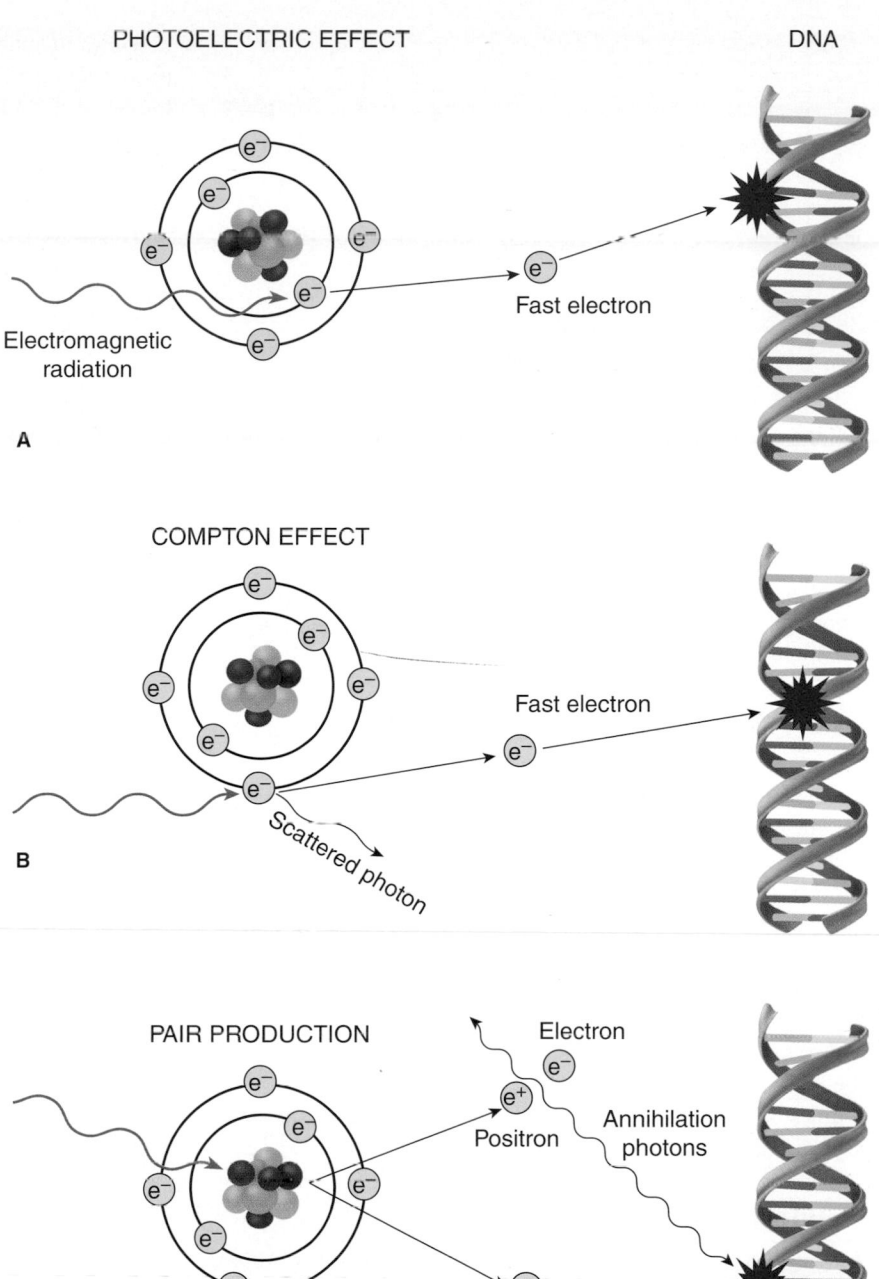

FIGURE 28-4 When electromagnetic radiation impacts target tissues, energy is transferred to those tissues. The three mechanisms involved in this energy transfer are the photoelectric effect, Compton effect, and pair production. Both photoelectric effect **(A)** and Compton effect **(B)** result in creation of fast electrons, which then initiate the biologic process of radiation damage. **A.** With photoelectric effect, radiation interacts with an inner orbital electron. **B.** With Compton effect, interaction occurs with an outer orbital electron. **C.** During pair production, radiation impacts the atom's nuclear forces to produce a positron-electron pair. When a positron later combines with a free electron in these tissues, two photons are created, which can then lead to radiation damage.

as kiloelectronvolts (keV) per micron. Photons, gamma rays, x-rays, electrons, protons, and helium ions are classified as low-LET radiation since the ionizing events tend to be sparse. In contrast, high-LET radiation, such as heavy particles (fast neutrons,

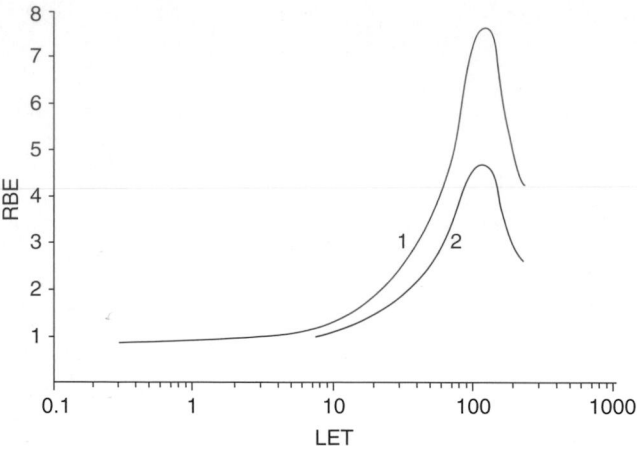

FIGURE 28-5 Graph that displays linear energy transfer as a function of relative biologic effectiveness (RBE). RBE reaches its maximum at approximately 100 keV/micron and varies depending on biologic endpoints. Curve 1 depicts a cell survival rate of 80 percent, whereas the endpoint for curve 2 is a cell survival rate of 10 percent.

heavy charged ions, and pi mesons), creates dense clusters of ionization and as a result, is more biologically damaging.

Due to the ionization-inducing differences, biologists use a parameter called relative biologic effectiveness (RBE) to compare the different radiation types. RBE is the ratio of the *reference* radiation dose (typically x-rays or Co-60) to the *test* radiation dose (e.g., neutrons). Each of the two doses used in the ratio is required to achieve a defined biologic endpoint, say, a given cell surviving fraction. Should one choose a different endpoint, then the RBE value would not be the same (Fig. 28-5). Using x-rays as the reference radiation and cell-killing effects as the biologic endpoint, the RBE of neutrons is 3 to 5. Thus, the x-ray dose needed is 3 to 5 times higher than the neutron dose required to cause the same level of cell death.

Depth-Dose Curve

A depth-dose curve specifically illustrates the dose distribution of a given radiation beam as it penetrates the tissues. Radiation oncologists rely on the characteristics of those curves when choosing the radiation beam with an appropriate energy to reach a tumor.

With electron beam therapy, the maximum dose lies close to the surface, and the dose distribution has a steep taper. For this reason, electron beam therapy is indicated for targets that are close to the skin surface, such as skin cancer or cancer that has metastasized to the inguinal lymph nodes.

With high-energy photons, the maximum dose is deposited well below the surface. Beyond this point, the dose gradually tapers as energy is absorbed by the deep surrounding tissues. This explains the so-called *skin-sparing effect* of high-energy photons. A patient with a pelvic malignancy is usually treated with at least 6-MV photon beams.

Dosimetry

This is the discipline of calculating the radiation dose absorbed by the patient. Dosimetric calculations are based on the depth-dose measurements of the radiation beams used to treat an actual patient. Computers and accurate measurements have dramatically improved the ability to present absorbed dose in two, three, and even four dimensions, with the fourth dimension being time. The dose distribution is usually displayed as a colorful map overlaid on the radiologic images of the patient (p. 721). It is important to note, however, that these calculations merely *predict* the absorbed dose in a given situation. Seldom is it practical to actually measure the dose in vivo since this requires the insertion of probes inside the patient.

Radiation Unit

The biologic effect of radiation correlates well with the amount of energy absorbed by the tissues. Therefore, quantification of the absorbed radiation dose is essential. In older terminology, the rad (radiation absorbed dose) was the unit of absorbed dose. Currently, the standard international unit for absorbed dose is the gray (Gy). One Gy equals 100 rad or 1 joule/kg. Clinically, the radiation doses for curative and palliative treatment are 70 to 85 Gy and 30 to 40 Gy, respectively.

RADIATION BIOLOGY

DNA Molecule as Target of Radiation Therapy's Biologic Effect

Evidence indicates that the DNA molecule is the target for the biologic effect of radiation on mammalian cells. DNA injuries involve its strands, bases, and cross-links, but the hallmark damage is breaking of DNA molecule strands. Single and double strand breaks may occur. Single strand breaks develop when only one strand is damaged, and these are easily repaired. Currently, radiation biologists agree that the most important lesion is the double strand break. Double strand breaks lead to DNA fragmentation when two or more breaks are formed in opposite locations of the DNA ladder. As cells attempt to repair the strand breaks, the DNA pieces may rejoin incorrectly, leading to gene translocation, mutation, or amplification. Increasing numbers of double strand breaks positively correlate with cell death.

Direct versus Indirect Actions of Ionizing Radiation

Whenever radiation, be it particulate or electromagnetic, penetrates a medium, such as tissues in a patient, it can interact *directly* with the atoms in the DNA molecule, creating ions that then initiate the biologic damage process. This *direct* effect is predominant with high-LET particles such as protons, fast neutrons, and heavy ions (Fig. 28-6).

Alternatively, approximately 70 percent of the ionizing effects of low-LET electromagnetic radiation, such as photons used in routine clinical settings, are *indirect*. Namely, energy is transferred from the electromagnetic radiation to the patient's tissues through chemical intermediates.

Tissues are mostly formed of water. The interaction between electromagnetic radiation and water molecules produces

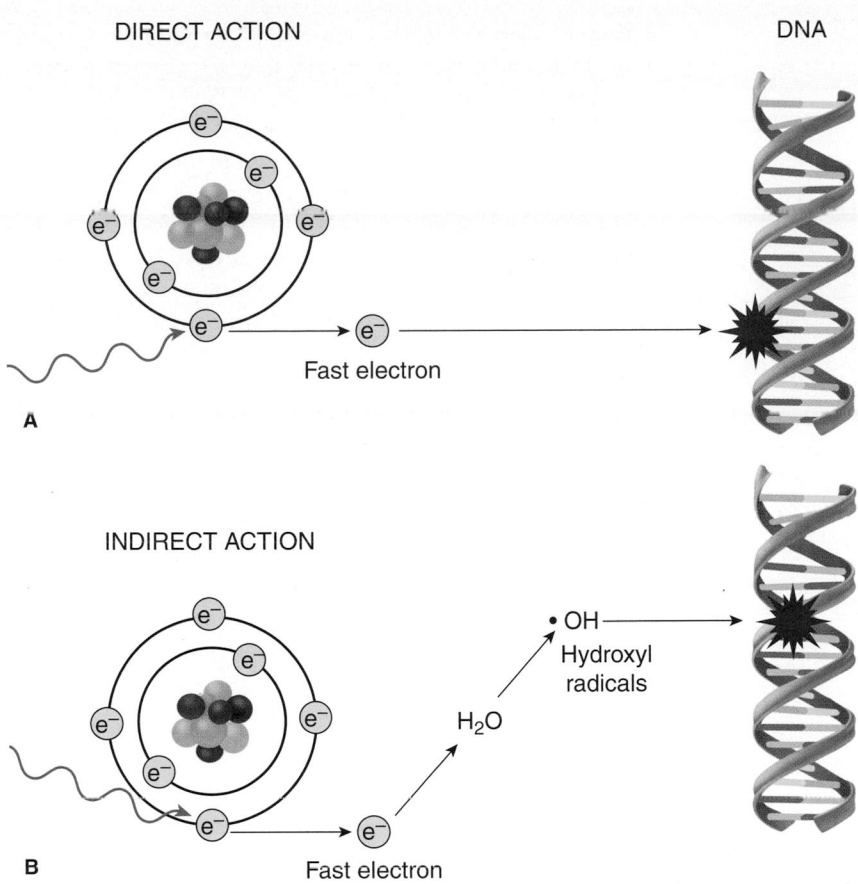

DIRECT ACTION

Fast electron

A

INDIRECT ACTION

• OH
Hydroxyl
radicals

H_2O

Fast electron

B

DNA

FIGURE 28-6 Direct and indirect actions of radiation. **A.** Fast electrons may directly impact DNA to create damage. **B.** Alternatively, a fast electron may interact with water to create a hydroxyl radical, which subsequently interacts with DNA to cause damage.

the H_2O^+ ion, which then reacts with water to form a free radical, the hydroxyl radical ($\bullet OH$). Because of a free radical's unpaired electron, it is highly reactive and easily transfers energy to tissues. It is this interaction between hydroxyl radicals and DNA molecules that leads to biologic damage. However, for the damage within the DNA to be permanent or "fixed," free radicals must interact with oxygen. Without the presence of oxygen, this damage will not be permanent since it can be repaired. This is the basis for the "oxygen fixation" hypothesis. Ninety-five percent of the energy deposited by electromagnetic radiation in tissues occurs within 4 nm of the ionization track, that is, about 2 DNA molecule diameters.

The Importance of Oxygen

The presence of oxygen is critical to the response of mammalian cells to low-LET radiation. The *oxygen enhancing ratio* (OER) is the ratio of doses needed to achieve the same cell survival fraction in hypoxic and oxic environments. The OER depends on the type of radiation. For low-LET radiation, the oxygen enhancing ratio is 2 for doses below 2 Gy and is 2.5 to 3 for higher doses (Fig. 28-7). In contrast, for high-LET heavy particles such as neutrons, the OER is approximately 1.5. This

implies that tumor hypoxia becomes less relevant with high-LET radiation.

Cell Death

After radiation exposure, cell damage triggers competing death and survival signals. How cells deal with that stress will determine their ultimate fate. A cell is considered biologically dead when it has lost its reproductive capacity. The two main cell death pathways are *apoptosis* and *delayed mitotic death*. The latter is more common after radiation exposure and is characteristic of many p53 mutated cancers (Erenpreisa, 2001).

Apoptosis

Apoptosis is also known as programmed cell death or interphase death. It occurs naturally in normal organisms to limit cell proliferation and maintain homeostasis. Dysregulation of the normal apoptotic process is believed to play a role in carcinogenesis and other pathologic conditions.

After an intracellular stress, such as radiation-induced irreparable double strand breaks, a series of events develop rapidly within a few hours. Cell membrane blebbing, apoptotic body formation in the cytoplasm, chromatin condensation, nuclear fragmentation, and DNA laddering can be seen (Okada, 2004). An apoptotic tendency is highly cell dependent and is present in lymphocytes, spermatogonia, salivary glands, and some tumors that are responsive to radiation. Such tissues are believed to have a "proapoptotic phenotype."

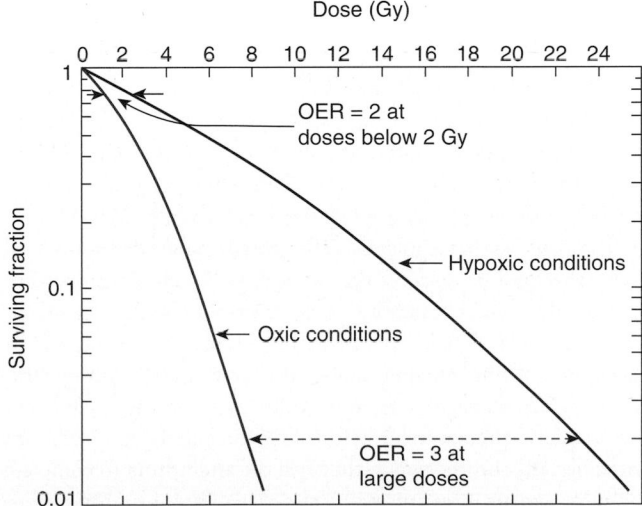

Dose (Gy)

OER = 2 at doses below 2 Gy

Hypoxic conditions

Oxic conditions

OER = 3 at large doses

FIGURE 28-7 Cells in an oxic environment are more sensitive to radiation than are those in hypoxic conditions. To achieve the same drop in the cell survival fraction, lower radiation doses are required in oxic conditions (*red curve*) compared with doses needed in hypoxic conditions (*blue curve*). (*Modified from Hall, 2003, with permission.*)

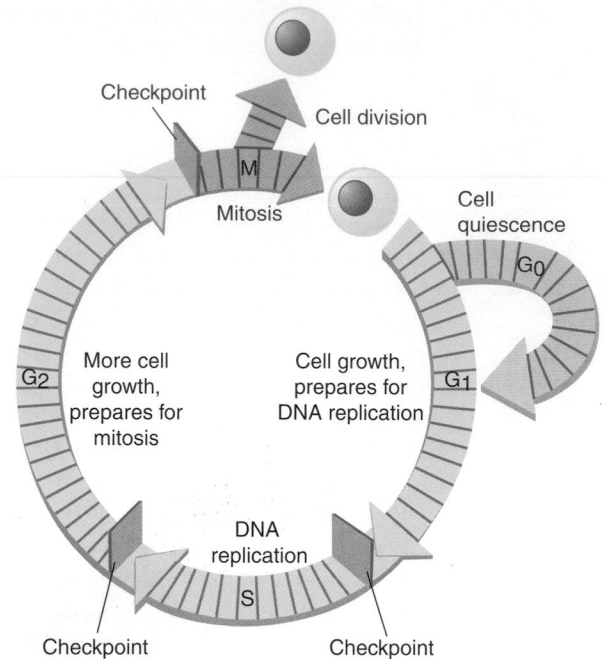

FIGURE 28-8 Mammalian cell cycle. The cycle contains five phases: G_0, G_1, S, G_2, and M. Quiescent cells in G_0 phase, responding to growth signals, can reenter the cell cycle. The critical cellular decision of whether to initiate a cycle or move to G_0 is made during the early part of G_1.

During each cell cycle phase, checkpoints ensure the integrity and fidelity of the steps required for cell division. If a cell sustains DNA damage, the checkpoint will not allow it to proceed to S or M phases until the damage is repaired. In case of irreparable DNA damage, cells undergo apoptosis. Defective checkpoints in many types of cancer cells allow them to proceed unchecked through the cycle and to proliferate.

Conversely, cells with "antiapoptotic phenotype" are resistant to radiation. Thus, factors that direct death pathways determine a cell's intrinsic radiation sensitivity.

Delayed Mitotic Death

A cell cycle has four phases, G_1, S, G_2, and M (Fig. 28-8). Alternatively, cells can be in the G_0 phase, where they remain in a quiescent, nonproliferative state. Cells in mitosis (M) and G_2 are most sensitive to radiation. Conversely, cells in G_1 and S (DNA synthesis) phases are less sensitive (Pawlik, 2004).

The cell cycle regulates cell growth and division. Cell cycle checkpoints ensure the integrity of cell division, and one of their main functions is to assess DNA damage. Cells with damaged DNA are frequently blocked at the G_2/M checkpoint from moving along the cell cycle. During this arrest, DNA damage is repaired. However, if these cells enter the M phase prematurely, before DNA repair is complete and with aberrant chromosomes, they will die attempting to complete the next two to three mitotic cycles. Therefore, a mitotic death is delayed in contrast with the more immediate apoptotic death.

Cancer cells can inactivate their own checkpoints and maintain growth and proliferation. For example, cells such as those in ataxia telangiectasia have defective G_1/S and G_2/M checkpoints, allowing cells with damaged DNA to move along the cell cycle. As a result, they are exquisitely sensitive to radiation. In radioresistant cancer cells that are exposed to radiation, apoptosis is not activated at the G_1/S checkpoint. At the G_2/M checkpoint, the fate of those damaged cells is either survival by DNA damage repair or delayed mitotic death. Specifically, this capacity to repair damage is operational in tumors with p53 mutations (Erenpreisa, 2001). In a study involving a small group of patients with cervical cancer treated with radiation, the patients with a dysfunctional G_2/M checkpoint were at a higher risk for progressive disease compared with those with a functional one (Cerciello, 2005).

Cell Repair

The extent of DNA damage and repair, and thus the radiation response depends, in part, on the cell cycle phase (Pawlik, 2004). After radiation exposure, cells that survive will repair their damage. Two types of repair have been described: sublethal damage repair (SLDR) and potentially lethal damage repair (PLDR). Both have been observed in normal and tumor tissues, and currently, the molecular mechanisms of both are unknown.

Sublethal Damage Repair

When a radiation dose is split into two or more fractions and a few hours separate the fractions, cells have time to *repair* their damage, and their survival rate increases. This type of repair is typically completed within 6 hours after radiation exposure.

During SLDR, a number of characteristic processes have been noted. Following the initial repair of sublethal damage, *reassortment* begins. In a tumor, proliferating cells are located at different phases of the cell cycle. When exposed to radiation, those cells that are in the G_2/M phase are most sensitive and are killed. During reassortment, surviving cell populations restart their progression through the mitotic cycle. In this manner, all cells within a tumor resort or redistribute themselves into different phases of the cycle. Following reassortment, mitosis begins again. The last process seen in SLDR is *repopulation*, which is the tissue's response to replenish the cell pool (Trott, 1999).

Potentially Lethal Damage Repair

After radiation exposure, certain environment conditions can allow extra time for DNA damage repair. Thus, radiation exposure that might otherwise cause cell death is attenuated and becomes "potentially lethal damage." In these environments, cells are able to repair radiation damage and survive. Conditions such as decreased nutrients or lower temperatures, which are suboptimal for growth, allow such increases in time for repair. In these settings, the inability of cells to repair the radiation-induced damages correlates positively with their ultimate radiation sensitivities (Kelland, 1988).

Five R's of Radiation Biology

In addition to cellular repair, reassortment, and repopulation, the fourth "R" of radiation biology theory is *reoxygenation*. A tumor cell population is composed of oxygenated and hypoxic components. Cells that are located within 100 microns of blood capillaries are oxygenated and beyond 100 microns, cells are hypoxic. After a radiation dose, the oxygenated cells are killed by chemical intermediates described earlier (p. 717). Following cell death, the tumor shrinks and allows hypoxic cells to be positioned within the oxygen diffusion range of blood capillaries. Thus, these previously hypoxic cells now become oxygenated and die when another dose of radiation is delivered. The DNA damage repair and consequently the cellular radiation response are influenced by hypoxia (Bristow, 2008).

There is an intricate relationship between the cell cycle, cell repair mechanism, and radiosensitivity. Because these processes are regulated by molecular signaling, some investigators have proposed adding a fifth "R," molecular *regulation*, to the classic four R's of radiation biology (Woodward, 2008).

Cell Survival Curve

The cell survival curve is a graphic representation of the fraction of cells surviving a given dose of radiation. For low-LET radiation, the linear-quadratic curve has been adopted to explain this relationship. The curve is composed of two parts (Fig. 28-9). The initial linear portion of the curve depicts that the probability of cell death is proportional to the radiation dose. This higher survival rate at low radiation doses is due to repair of sublethal DNA damage, described earlier. In the higher dose region, the slope deepens due to multiple DNA damaging events. Here, the curved quadratic portion indicates that the probability of cell death is proportional to the *square* of the dose. The components of the cell survival curve therefore

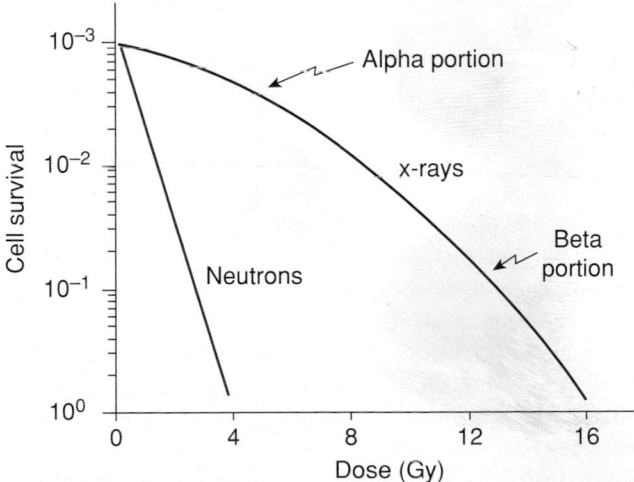

FIGURE 28-9 Linear quadratic mammalian cell survival curve. The cell survival is plotted on a logarithmic scale. The dose (in Gy) is on a linear scale. The typical cell survival curves with low-LET (*blue curve*) and with high-LET radiation (*red line*) are shown. With low-LET x-ray doses, the alpha (linear) portion of the curve is flat and depicts that cell survival is proportional to the dose. However, as the dose increases, the beta (quadratic) portion is bent, which implies that cell survival is proportional to the dose squared. In contrast, with high-LET radiation, such as neutrons, the survival curve is straight.

are expressed as $alphaD$ and $betaD^2$. The dose is denoted by "D," but alpha and beta are constants. At the dose, $D = alpha/beta$, there is an equal contribution to cell death from the linear and quadratic parts.

In contrast, when high-LET radiation such as neutron therapy is used, the shape of the curve is straight.

Clinical Implication of the Alpha/Beta Ratio

Not all normal tissues respond similarly to radiation. Those that manifest reactions to radiation within a few days to weeks after treatment initiation are categorized as *early responding*. Examples are tissues with high proliferation rates such as bone marrow, reproductive organs, and gastrointestinal tract mucosa. Their alpha/beta ratio values are high and are reflected by the steep early slope on the cell survival curve. By administering multiple small radiation dose fractions, the alpha component of the curve is amplified, denoting a repair of sublethal damage. Thus, with treatment protraction, early acute reactions can be decreased. For example, in patients who have radiation delivered to the abdomen, in which the mucosal tissues are early responding, treatment protraction is preferred.

In contrast, *late-responding* tissues only show clinical reactions weeks to months after completion of a radiation therapy course. These tissues are slow to respond by proliferative reaction, and it is postulated that late-responding tissues are composed of cells in G_0, the quiescent stage. Examples are the lung, kidney, spinal cord, and brain. Late-responding tissues have a low alpha/beta ratio. A low ratio value means that the cell survival fraction is markedly decreased when the dose per fraction is high. Also, more time is needed to repair sublethal damage in late-responding than in early-responding tissues. Therefore, the use of high-dose per fraction radiation therapy can easily lead to severe late complications. For example, there is a high incidence of myelitis if the spinal cord receives a high radiation dose in a short period of time, that is, a large dose per fraction.

RADIATION ONCOLOGY PRACTICE

Patient Evaluation

Typically, patients referred for radiation oncology consultation already have an established cancer diagnosis. Initially, they are examined by the radiation oncologist, and their imaging studies reviewed. Further cancer evaluation may be needed and ordered accordingly. If radiation therapy is deemed appropriate, patients are seen at least once a week by the radiation oncologist throughout the radiation course. Once the treatment is completed, usually the patient is followed by both the referring physician and the radiation oncologist.

Background of Fractionated Radiation Therapy
Standard Fractionation

In the early 20th century, controversy grew concerning two different approaches for radiation delivery in the treatment of human cancers. One school recommended the delivery of a massive radiation dose within a short time interval. The assumption was that a rapidly growing tumor would retain the capacity to recover quickly from radiation damage if a tumoricidal dose was not given in the first treatment (Thames, 1992). Alternatively, smaller doses given over many days to weeks were advocated by others as a method to minimize radiation side effects.

The controversy was resolved when Coutard (1932) along with the work of others found success with *fractionated radiation therapy*. As a result, in the United States since the 1950s, the practice of giving 1.8 to 2 Gy each day, 5 days a week, has been considered standard or conventional.

Altered Fractionation

Regimens involving more than once-a-day treatment are reserved for selected cases. In such instances, increased local tumor control and decreased long-term complications may be achieved by manipulating both fraction size and overall treatment time. This manipulation leads to a variety of altered fractionations. Two major strategies have been employed: hyperfractionation and accelerated treatment.

With *hyperfractionation*, the reduction of late damage to normal tissues is sought, and accordingly, a smaller dose per fraction is given. Two or more fractions are administered each day.

There is tumor cell repopulation during a conventional 6- to 7-week course that may lead to treatment failure. To counter this problem, an *accelerated treatment* schedule may be used. This entails shortening the treatment duration with or without a decrease in total dose. The usual weekend break is shortened or even eliminated. With accelerated treatment, however, severe acute reactions are frequently encountered. Thus, often a mandatory rest period in the middle of the treatment course is required (Wang, 1988).

Altered fractionation has been studied in cervical cancer. The tumor control, late toxicity, and survival results were similar to historical rates achieved by standard fractionation (Grigsby, 2002; Komaki, 1994). However, it was poorly tolerated, especially when large-field radiation therapy and chemotherapy or both were added (Grigsby, 1998; Marcial, 1995).

Radiation Therapy
External Beam Radiation Therapy

External beam radiation therapy is indicated when an area to be irradiated is large. For example, the fields needed to treat a locally advanced cervical cancer may cover the whole pelvis and occasionally, the retroperitoneal draining nodes.

Conformal radiation therapy describes the radiation treatment technique that maximizes tumor damage while minimizing injury to the surrounding normal tissues. To this goal, the radiation oncologist must know the precise extent of the cancer to be irradiated and its relationship to surrounding normal tissues.

This process begins with a review of the patient's cancer imaging. During the past few decades, technologic innovation in medical imaging equipment and computers has aided tremendously in radiation therapy planning and delivery. Modern imaging tools include computerized tomography (CT), magnetic resonance (MR) imaging, and functional imaging techniques such as nuclear MR imaging/spectroscopy, positron emission tomography (PET), and single-

photon emission computed tomography (SPECT). These have aided the radiation oncologist in defining 3-dimensional tumor and healthy tissue volumes (Chapman, 2001; Kwee, 2004, Zakian, 2001).

Next, a simulation is performed in a simulation suite to delineate the anticipated therapy fields prior to an actual treatment session. During this process, patient positioning, immobilization techniques, and treatment fields are defined. Whenever feasible, radiation blocks are also planned to shield normal tissues. Both x-ray machines and CT scanners can be used for simulation. For most patients, a simulation using a CT scanner, located in the simulation suite, is preferred.

The patient is placed in a treatment position, and a CT scan of the area of interest is performed. Later, on each of the computer-based CT scan slices, the radiation oncologist carefully delineates the anatomic areas that are to receive a tumoricidal dose as well as those normal tissues that will be exposed to a lesser radiation dose. During this process, potential risks for early and late radiation complications are considered.

Once this step is completed, a radiation dosimetrist employs treatment-planning software to develop an optimal plan. This is often a reiterative process where the physician and the dosimetrist will arrive at an acceptable option, which means an optimal arrangement of the radiation beams in the case of external beam radiation therapy, or radioactive sources in the case of brachytherapy. This step is called dose optimization.

One tool that is particularly helpful in the radiation planning and optimization process is the dose volume histogram (DVH). This is a graphic summary of the entire dose distribution to the cancer and normal structures. Thus, the DVH gives the radiation oncologist information regarding: (1) whether the cancer will be adequately treated with a tumoricidal dose and (2) whether surrounding normal structures are expected to receive an acceptably low dose to minimize treatment complications.

In addition to the DVH, 3-dimensional conformal radiation therapy (3D-CRT) is often used. With 3D-CRT, dose distributions are displayed as computer-generated radiation dose map images that are overlaid on the CT images (Fig. 28-10). This provides a visual dose-anatomy relationship. These dose distributions are produced for the radiation oncologist to review, adjust, and finally approve. The final chosen plan is reviewed by a radiation physicist, who ensures that the physical and technical details can be implemented.

In an effort to further improve the conformality of the dose distribution, especially around concave targets, a more advanced 3D-CRT planning system, called *intensity-modulated radiation therapy (IMRT)*, is used. As a result of this improved conformality, IMRT has the potential to decrease bowel and bladder toxicity during pelvic radiation therapy (Heron, 2003).

To achieve this goal, the radiation oncologist first defines the doses to be delivered to the tumor and normal tissues as well as the dose constraints or limits to those regions. The intensity of the radiation beams to be used is modulated or changed with the help of dedicated computer software. This reiterative process is called *inverse planning*.

On the other hand, in the traditional approach of *forward planning*, the physician designs the actual radiation fields, based

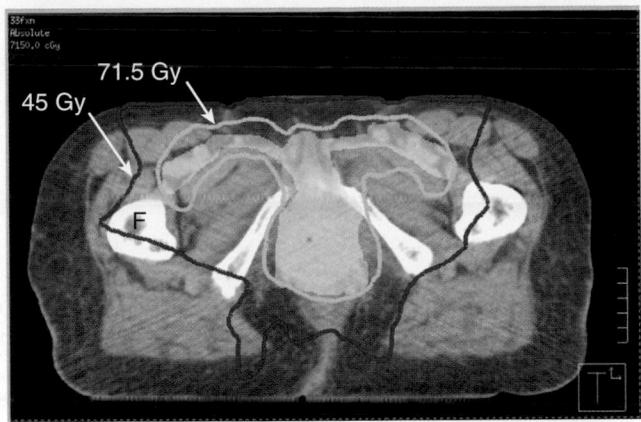

A

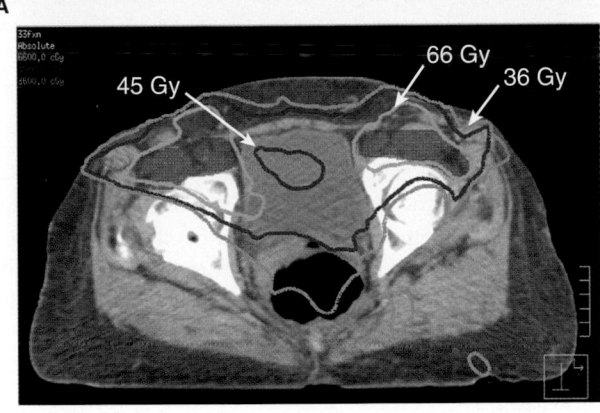

B

FIGURE 28-10 Intensity-modulated radiation therapy (IMRT) dose distribution in a patient with stage T4 N2 M0 cancer of the vulva. This technique allows for the delivery of tumoricidal doses to the vulva and inguinal nodes while minimizing that to normal tissues. **A.** The yellow area displays the actual vulvar cancer and inguinal lymph nodes. Doses to the vulva and femoral heads (F) are shown (*arrows*). The doses to the vulva and femoral heads are 71.5 Gy and 45 Gy, respectively. **B.** Pink shading displays the inguinal nodes. Doses to the inguinal nodes, bladder, and rectum are shown (*arrows*). The doses to the inguinal nodes, bladder, and rectum were 66 Gy, 45 Gy, and 36 Gy, respectively.

on imaging data, and chooses the radiation beams. A computer then calculates and displays the resultant dose distribution. The physician can then either accept it or design another plan. Obviously, this approach is appropriate only for straightforward cases. For example, in forward planning for the more common pelvic malignancies, the radiation oncologist may choose a standard pelvic four-field technique and 10-MV photon beams.

For quality assurance, weekly or sometimes even daily imaging of the treated regions is performed to verify that treatment configurations are correct. These portal images are taken with the actual treatment beam and compared with the original simulation films. If deviations are noticed, adjustments are made. The radiation oncologist also evaluates the patient at least weekly for untoward treatment side effects. If severe acute complications develop, treatment plans may be revised or a break in treatment may be warranted.

Stereotactic Body Radiation Therapy. Over the past decade, a novel external beam radiation therapy technique,

stereotactic body radiation therapy (SBRT), has become commonly used in sites such as the lung, liver, and spine. It uses a hypofractionated regimen of five or fewer fractions (10 to 20 Gy per fraction). With such high doses per treatment, there are significant concerns about potential damage to normal tissues. However, with technology advancements, such as image-guided radiation therapy (IGRT), precise, safe SBRT has become possible. During SBRT, a linac-based IGRT system relies on daily targeted regional imaging guidance. This is performed while the patient is in the treatment room. If the tumor or patient positions have changed since the last treatment, adjustments are made prior to subsequent radiation delivery. This "real time" approach can overcome technical factors such as patient or organ motion and changes in tumor size and shape during a treatment course. As a result, radiation delivery precision is enhanced.

Brachytherapy

Brachytherapy means treatment at a short distance. During this therapy, sealed or unsealed radioisotopes are inserted or instilled into the cancer or its immediate vicinity. Radiation doses decline sharply with increasing distances from the radioactive source. Thus, brachytherapy works best if the cancer volume is small, less than 3 to 4 cm in greatest dimensions. For this reason, brachytherapy is typically practiced after external beam radiation therapy has decreased a large tumor.

Intracavitary, Interstitial, and Intraperitoneal Brachytherapy. During *intracavitary brachytherapy*, applicators that hold sealed radioactive sources such as cesium are inserted into a body cavity such as the uterus. Alternatively, *interstitial brachytherapy* requires the placement of catheters or needles directly into the cancer and surrounding tissues. The typical source used is iridium. With *intraperitoneal brachytherapy*, unsealed sources, such as phosphorus and gold, are available as solutions for instillation into the peritoneal cavity.

Temporary and Permanent Brachytherapy. In *temporary brachytherapy*, the radioisotopes are removed from the patient after a period of time, ranging from minutes to days. All intracavitary and some interstitial implants are temporary. In *permanent brachytherapy*, the radioisotopes are left permanently to decay within the tissues. The time for the delivery of the absorbed dose varies depending on the isotopes used and ranges from 1 week with gold to 6 months with iodine.

Equipment. For routine gynecologic intracavitary implantation, standard equipment includes an applicator, called a *tandem*, which fits into the uterine cavity, and a pair of vaginal applicators, which are known as *ovoids* or alternatively, *colpostats* (Fig. 28-11). Tandems have different curvatures to adapt to varied uterine shapes. Similarly, plastic caps can be fitted onto the ovoids to adapt to varied vaginal anatomy. The tandem and ovoid device (T&O) is inserted under general anesthesia or conscious sedation. Following placement, radioactive sources can then be loaded into both the tandem and ovoids either manually or via remote control. In gynecologic oncology, brachytherapy with T&O is indicated for cervical and endometrial cancer.

Another intracavitary method uses Heyman capsules, which are long plastic holders with a capsule-shaped tip. Used in some

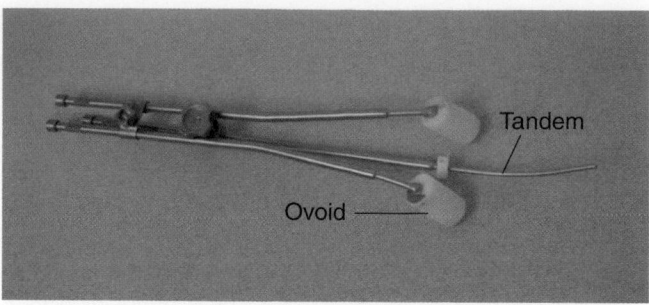

FIGURE 28-11 Photograph of typical tandem and ovoids used for cervical cancer brachytherapy. The long slender portion of the device (tandem) is inserted into the endometrial cavity, and white cylinders (ovoids) are positioned in the proximal vagina. Radioactive sources can be loaded into both the tandem and ovoid reservoirs.

cases of inoperable endometrial cancer, several capsules are packed into the uterine cavity. Miniaturized Ir-192 seeds attached to thin steel rods are then afterloaded through each holder.

For temporary interstitial implantation, flexible plastic catheters or metal needles are surgically placed into the target tissues. These are then afterloaded with Ir-192 seeds. To achieve an optimal dose distribution, the catheters or needles should stay firmly in place. For this reason, a perineal template is often used. Although used less frequently than T&O, templates are suitable in the management of patients with advanced cancer, suboptimal anatomy for T&O application, and selected recurrent cancer.

Manual versus Remote Afterloading. During brachytherapy, once the holding devices for the radioactive sources are optimally positioned, the sources are inserted. Previously, these sources were carried in a shielded cart to the patient's room, loaded into the patient, and then removed and replaced in a storage room following treatment. This *manual afterloading* method increased hospital staff radiation exposure. For this reason, a *remote afterloading* approach was developed and is commonly practiced today. This remote control system delivers a single miniaturized iridium or cobalt source from a shielded safe. A connecting cable, housed in a catheter, precisely positions the miniaturized source within an applicator previously inserted into the patient. When radiation is actually delivered, personnel are outside the patient's treatment room. Following treatment, the cable, with its attached source, is automatically retracted into the shielded safe.

Low Dose-Rate versus High Dose-Rate Brachytherapy. Traditionally, low dose-rate (LDR) brachytherapy is delivered over the course of many days and requires patient hospitalization. Over the last few decades, however, high dose-rate (HDR) brachytherapy has become more popular. With this technique, treatment is shortened to minutes. Low dose is defined as dose rates from 0.4 Gy to 2 Gy/hr, and high dose rate are those higher than 12 Gy/hr. For example, in an intracavitary implant for cervical cancer with an LDR technique, a dose of 30 to 40 Gy is given over several days continuously. In contrast, in an HDR technique, an equivalent dose can be delivered in 3 to 5 weekly fractions. The dose per fraction is 6 to 8 Gy and can be given in 10 to 20 minutes.

The radiobiology differences between LDR and HDR brachytherapy are based on the dose-rate effect. As the dose rate increases, there is increased tumor control and increased damage to the late-responding normal tissues. Therefore, to avoid late complications, the number of fractions is increased from one to two in LDR to three to six in HDR brachytherapy. Increasing the number of fractions allows more time for sublethal damage repair. Furthermore, the total tumor dose delivered in HDR brachytherapy of the cervix is lower than the dose used in LDR (Nag, 2000). This dose is divided into brief fractions that avoid lengthy inpatient hospitalization and minimize patient immobility and thromboembolic events. Advantageously, with either HDR or LDR brachytherapy, long-term analysis has shown similar local tumor control and rates of late complications in patients treated for cervical cancer (Arai, 1991; Hareyama, 2002; Wong, 2003).

Tumor Control Probability

With most epithelial cancers, the probability of radiation therapy to control a cancerous mass depends on: (1) the tumor size and its intrinsic radiosensitivity and (2) the radiation dose and delivery schedule. For example, within a given stage, large tumors are more difficult to control with radiation than smaller ones (Bentzen, 1996; Dubben, 1998).

Intrinsic Radiosensitivity

It is recognized that a tumor's radiosensitivity in general is determined by its pathologic type (Table 28-3). However, even cancers within a similar histology may have variable responses to radiation. Heterogeneity within a given tumor may explain this varied response. Another factor in tumor radiosensitivity is the cancer cell's ability to repair radiation damage. For example, a lower rate of DNA double strand break repair was found to correlate with a higher radiosensitivity of tumors (Schwartz, 1988, 1996; Weichselbaum, 1992). Recent basic translational research indicates that the factors determining tumor radiosensitivity are multiple, probably related, and not all well understood. Current areas of investigation are focusing on pathways of DNA damage repair, hypoxia, microenvironment, and immune response (Glazer, 2011).

Treatment Time

When protracted time intervals are required to complete a fractionated radiation therapy course, tumor control probability decreases, especially in rapidly proliferating epithelial cancers.

TABLE 28-3. Radiosensitivity of Some Selected Cancers

Sensitivity	Cancer Type
Highly sensitive	Lymphoma, dysgerminoma, small cell cancer, embryonal cancer
Moderately sensitive	Squamous cell carcinoma, adenocarcinoma
Poorly sensitive	Osteosarcoma, glioma, melanoma

Therefore, treatment breaks or delays for any reason should be minimized. In a retrospective review of 209 patients with stage I to III cervical cancer treated with radiation therapy, the 5-year pelvic control and overall survival rates were better for those who completed the treatment in less than 55 days (87 percent and 65 percent, respectively) than for those who did so in more than 55 days (72 percent and 54 percent, respectively) (Petereit, 1995).

Tumor Hypoxia

Tumor hypoxia is a major factor leading to poor local tumor control and poor survival in patients with cervical cancer (Brizel, 1999; Nordsmark, 1996). The close relationship between tumor hypoxia, anemia, and angiogenesis was demonstrated in a study involving 87 patients with stage II, III, and IV cervical cancer treated with radiation only. Of these, the patients with a hemoglobin level of less than 11 g/dL, a median tumor oxygen tension pO_2 less than 15 mm Hg, and an increased abnormal tumor microvascular density had decreased 3-year survival rates (Dunst, 2003). For this reason, many strategies have been devised to overcome tumor hypoxia.

Hyperbaric Oxygen. Hyperbaric oxygen used in conjunction with radiation therapy in stage II and III cervical cancer has not been shown to be effective in clinical studies (Dische, 1999). In addition, there is concern that hyperbaric oxygen may actually accelerate tumor growth (Bradfield, 1996).

A more convenient method of increasing the delivery of oxygen to tissues involves manipulating blood vessel hemodynamics with either carbogen or nicotinamide. *Carbogen* (95 percent oxygen and 5 percent carbon dioxide) is an oxygen preparation with increased intratumoral diffusion capabilities. Inhaled during concurrent external beam radiation therapy, carbogen has been shown to increase the tumor oxygen pressure and is well tolerated (Aquino-Parsons, 1999). Alternatively, *nicotinamide* is the amide derivative of vitamin B_3 (niacin) and has been shown to prevent intermittent vascular vasospasm. In combination, inhaled carbogen and oral nicotinamide are thought to increase oxygen delivery to hypoxic regions.

Bioreductive Agents. These drugs serve as adjuncts to radiation therapy and initiate a series of hypoxia-activated biochemical events. These steps lead to cytotoxic agents that selectively kill hypoxic cells. In recent decades, mitomycin C and tirapazamine (TPZ) have been reported to be clinically effective (Craighead, 2000; Nguyen, 1991; Rischin, 2001). Despite earlier promising findings, results of a phase III trial of TPZ, cisplatin, and radiation therapy compared with cisplatin and radiation failed to show improvement of survival rates in patients with head and neck cancers (Rischin, 2005, 2010). The Gynecologic Oncology Group (GOG) has completed data collection from a phase III trial that randomly assigns patients with cervical cancer to receive either cisplatin plus external beam radiation or cisplatin, TPZ, and radiation therapy, although publications are not yet available (National Institutes of Health, 2010).

Blood Transfusion. In clinical practice, a hemoglobin level of at least 12 g/dL is desirable in patients receiving radiation therapy. To this goal, transfusion ameliorates tumor hypoxia and increases radiation response. For example, in a review of a group of 204 women with cervical cancer who were treated with radiation, 26 percent had a hemoglobin level <11 g/dL either before or during the radiation course and received packed red blood cell transfusion. Of the women who received transfusions, only 18 percent were able to maintain a hemoglobin level >11 g/dL throughout the treatment. This subset of women had a similar 5-year disease-free survival rate of 71 percent compared with a group of women who never required transfusion. The disease-free survival rate was only 26 percent for those with persistent anemia. However, not all patients showed marked benefit from transfusion, especially those with nodal metastasis, late stage, and large tumor size (Kapp, 2002). As a caution, blood transfusion may cause immunosuppression and thus may worsen cancer outcome. Many mechanisms have been postulated, including an inflammatory response (Varlotto, 2005).

Recombinant Human Erythropoietin. In addition to transfusion, recombinant human erythropoietin has been used to correct anemia. Clinically, however, this therapy has not proved beneficial. In a Southwest Oncology Group phase II multi-institutional trial, erythropoietin and iron supplements produced an inadequate increase in hemoglobin levels, and there was additional concern that erythropoietin increased the risk of deep-vein thrombosis (Lavey, 2004; Wun, 2003).

Darbepoetin alpha is another erythropoiesis-stimulating protein. It has a longer terminal half-life than recombinant human erythropoietin and allows for less frequent dosing. Darbepoetin alpha was found to be associated with poorer tumor control in a Danish phase III trial of patients with head and neck cancer treated with radiation. The trial was stopped in 2006 when the interim analysis showed poor tumor control (Overgaard, 2009). Similar results with epoetin beta have been published (Henke, 2003). Moreover, in a survey of cancer patients treated from 1991 to 2002 who received epoetin or darbepoetin, the blood transfusion rate remained constant at 22 percent. However, venous thromboembolism developed in 14 percent of those patients who used erythropoietin-stimulating agents compared with 9.8 percent of those who did not (Hershman, 2009).

■ Combination of Ionizing Radiation and Chemotherapy

Ionizing radiation as a single modality rarely controls locally advanced cancers, such as gynecologic cancer. Factors such as tumor hypoxia, distant metastasis, and inability of pelvic tissues to tolerate high radiation doses are purported causes. Accordingly, for many decades, radiation has been combined with chemotherapy or surgery to increase local disease control and decrease distant metastasis. Radiation therapy and chemotherapy can be administered in a concurrent or alternating fashion. However, with such combination therapy, efforts to maximize tumoricidal effects while minimizing overlapping toxicities should be a priority (Steel, 1979). In many controlled studies involving cervical and other cancers, concurrent radiation and chemotherapy have improved local tumor control with acceptable rates of severe complications. In the management of gynecologic cancers, platinum compounds are most commonly used with radiation therapy.

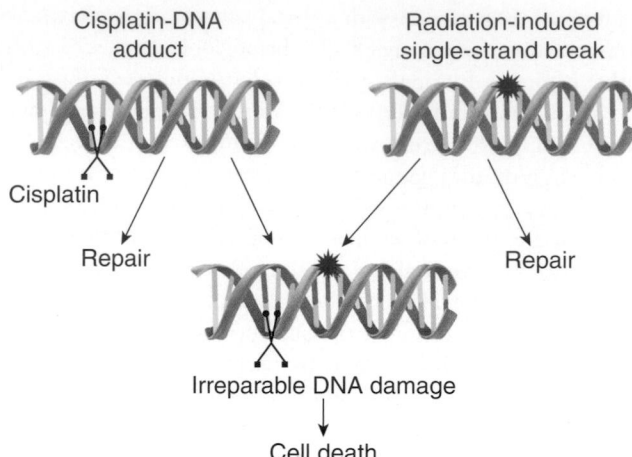

FIGURE 28-12 DNA damage by radiation therapy (*upper right*) and by cisplatin (*upper left*). Cisplatin can bind covalently to DNA bases. Radiation therapy may create single strand breaks. If occurring alone, each damaging event is likely to be repaired. However, if both occur in close proximity, irreparable damage can lead to cell death.

Platinum Compounds

Both radiation and cisplatin have DNA as targets to cause single and double strand breaks and base damage (Fig. 28-12). Although most lesions are repaired, if a cisplatin-induced DNA adduct is in close proximity with a radiation-induced single strand break, then the damage is irreparable and leads to cell death (Amorino, 1999; Begg, 1990). In addition, irradiated cell membranes may be more permeable to carboplatin, allowing an increased cellular uptake of the drug (Yang, 1995). Since the late 1990s, the standard treatment for newly diagnosed locally advanced cancer of the cervix has been radiation therapy and cisplatin (Keys, 1999; Morris, 1999; Rose, 1999).

Nucleoside Analogs

Agents such as fludarabine and gemcitabine inhibit DNA synthesis and metabolism. Cells at the G_1/S junction of the cycle are involved in DNA synthesis and therefore are blocked from progressing. The remaining cell population, however, is synchronized at the G_2/M junction and is sensitive to radiation. Gregoire and associates (1994, 1999) found that radiation was most effective when radiation was delivered 24 to 72 hours after nucleoside analog chemotherapy administration. In a phase III study involving patients with stage IIB to IVA cervical cancer, the progression-free survival rate at 3 years was 74 percent in patients randomized to receive gemcitabine plus cisplatin and radiation followed by adjuvant gemcitabine compared with 65 percent in those treated with concurrent cisplatin and radiation alone. Overall survival rates and time to disease progression were also improved. However, severe toxicity, including two treatment-related deaths, was observed in 86 percent of women in the study arm compared with 46 percent of those treated without gemcitabine (Dueñas-Gonzalez, 2009). As a result, there is serious concern whether this regimen can be accepted as a new paradigm in the treatment of cervical cancer without modifications (Rose, 2011).

Taxanes

The taxanes such as paclitaxel and docetaxel dysregulate microtubule function and block cells at the G_2/M junction, where cells are most sensitive to radiation (Mason, 1999). Taxanes have been administered with platinum agents and radiation therapy in small nonrandomized trials involving patients with locally advanced cervical cancer (Lee, 2007).

Combination of Radiation Therapy and Biologic Therapy

Among the various classes of biologic agents, cetuximab (Erbitux) is a epithelial growth factor receptor (EGFR)-inhibiting monoclonal antibody that interferes with DNA strand break repair. In a phase III trial, cetuximab and radiation therapy improved survival rates in patients with locally advanced head and neck cancers (Bonner, 2010).

The GOG is conducting a phase I study of cetuximab plus cisplatin and radiation therapy in patients with stages IB–IVA cervical cancer. The preliminary results indicated that this combination was feasible only in those patients who received radiation therapy to the pelvis (Moore, 2011). Other agents such as gefitinib and erlotinib, which are EGFR tyrosine kinase inhibitors; bevacizumab, which is a vascular endothelial growth factor (VEGF)-inhibiting monoclonal antibody; and sorafenib, which is a VEGF receptor tyrosine kinase inhibitor are also being investigated (del Campo, 2008; González-Cortijo, 2008).

Combination of Radiation Therapy and Surgery

Radiation therapy can be given before, after, or at the time of surgery. With this combination, surgical resection and its associated morbidity can often be minimized. For example, the combination of radiation and surgery in locally advanced vulvovaginal cancer can allow surgeons to avoid extensive surgery, such as pelvic exenteration (Boronow, 1982). Typically, whenever radiation is indicated with surgery, some form of chemotherapy is also added in an adjuvant fashion.

Preoperative Radiation Therapy

Primary cancers tend to locally infiltrate surrounding normal tissues with microscopic extension. For this reason, radiation can be delivered prior to surgery to decrease the potential of locoregional and distant tumor dissemination and lower the likelihood of having positive surgical margins. To sterilize those areas of subclinical infiltration, doses of 40 to 50 Gy given during 4 to 5 weeks are required. Although preoperative radiation therapy is not expected to render the main tumor mass cancer-free at the time of surgery, it is common to find no evidence of cancer in the surgical specimen. In patients who presented with unresectable cancers, preoperative radiation therapy can transform them into suitable candidates for a surgical attempt (Montana, 2000).

Despite these advantages, administering preoperative radiation therapy may unnecessarily expose patients to radiation because the true pathologic tumor staging is unknown. Moreover, if the nodal status is normal at the time of surgery, the clinician is faced with the question of whether there initially were lymph nodes containing tumor that were sterilized by the preoperative regimen. This is important as patients with initially positive lymph nodes tend to develop distant metastasis and typically would require further treatment. Another problem encountered is the management of those patients with pathologically proven residual cancer within the irradiated areas. The pathologist may not able to adequately ascertain the viability of those residual cells, especially when surgery is performed soon after radiation. Therefore, surgery is usually delayed 4 to 6 weeks after radiation completion. By then, the acute radiation reactions have subsided, and pathologic interpretation of the resected specimen is easier.

Postoperative Radiation Therapy

Often following surgery, a high probability for local recurrence may be predicted by factors such as positive margins, lymph node metastases, lymphovascular invasion, and high-grade cancer. In these cases, postoperative radiation therapy may be advantageous and is ideally delivered 3 to 6 weeks following surgery. This delay allows initial wound healing (Sedlis, 1999). Because the pathologic stage is known, management can be individualized and unnecessary radiation therapy avoided (Rushdan, 2004). The radiation fields should encompass the operative bed due to the possibility of tumor contamination at the time of surgery.

Intraoperative Radiation Therapy

Infrequently, radiation therapy can be delivered during surgery either by interstitial brachytherapy or by an electron beam produced by a dedicated linear accelerator installed in the operating room. This technique is indicated in selected patients with recurrent gynecologic cancers. A single dose of 10 to 20 Gy is typically delivered to the area at risk for recurrence or suspected of harboring residual cancer (Gemignani, 2001; Yap, 2005).

■ Normal Tissue Response to Radiation Therapy

In general, radiation therapy is less well tolerated if: (1) the volume of irradiated tissues is large, (2) the radiation dose is high, (3) the dose per fraction is large, and (4) the patient's age is advanced. Furthermore, the radiation damage to normal tissues can be exacerbated by factors such as previous surgery, concurrent chemotherapy, infection, diabetes mellitus, hypertension, and inflammatory conditions, for example, Crohn disease and ulcerative colitis.

In general, if tissues with a rapid proliferation rate such as epithelium of the small intestine or oral cavity are irradiated, the onset of acute clinical signs and symptoms occurs within a few days to weeks. This contrasts with tissues such as muscular, renal, and neural tissues, which have low proliferation rates and may not display signs of radiation damage for months to years after treatment. To avoid serious complications in practice, radiation oncologists must rely on their own clinical experiences and use published tolerance doses for normal tissues as a guide. For example, to avoid severe rectum and bladder complications in the management of patients with cervical cancer, doses of no more than 65 Gy and 70 Gy are recommended to the rectum and bladder, respectively (Milano, 2007).

Epithelium and Parenchyma

Atrophy is the most consistent sequela of radiation therapy. It affects all lining epithelia—including skin and the epithelia of the gastrointestinal, respiratory and genitourinary tracts, and the endocrine glands. Additionally, necrosis and ulceration may develop.

Within the epithelium, other histologic changes may be found, and atypical and dysplastic transformations are the most frequent. In addition to epithelial changes, within the submucosa and deep soft tissues, fibrosis frequently follows radiation therapy. This clinically leads to tissue contracture and stenosis (Fajardo, 2005).

Of vascular structures, the capillary is the most sensitive to radiation, and ischemia results from endothelial damage, capillary wall rupture, loss of capillary segments, and reduction of microvascular networks. In large arteries, atheroma-like calcifications develop (Friedlander, 2003; Zidar, 1997).

Skin

Four general types of skin reactions may follow radiation therapy. In order of severity, they include erythema, dry desquamation, moist desquamation, and skin necrosis. For many women during a 6- to 7-week radiation therapy course, the first three of these reactions are common. Within 1 week following radiation exposure, the skin develops mild erythema. By the third week, the redness becomes more pronounced and dry desquamation begins. After 5 to 6 weeks, moist desquamation follows. This involves epidermal sloughing, followed by serum and blood oozing through denuded skin. This reaction is mostly pronounced in concealed areas of the body, such as the inguinal, axillary, and inframammary creases.

Preventatively, throughout and after a radiation course, the skin should be kept clean and aerated. For dry desquamative findings, ointments or aloe vera-containing creams promote dermal hydration with an emollient effect. During the moist desquamation phase, hydrogen peroxide and water can be used for wound cleaning. Additional skin treatment may include moisturizers (e.g., Biafine), whirlpool sessions, sitz baths, and silver sulfadiazine-containing, nonadhering dressings (e.g., Vigilon) for weeping areas. Importantly, individuals should avoid applying heating pads, soaps, or alcohol-based lotions to irradiated skin.

Regeneration of the epithelium starts soon after radiation treatment and is usually complete in 4 to 6 weeks. Months after radiation therapy, areas of skin hyper- and hypopigmentation can be seen. The skin remains atrophied, thin, and dry.

Vagina

Radiation therapy directed to the pelvis commonly leads to acute vaginal mucositis. Although mucosal ulceration is rare, discharge is present in most cases. For these women, a dilute hydrogen peroxide and water solution used at the vulva provides symptomatic relief. In contrast to acute changes, delayed reactions to radiation may include vaginal shortening, atrophic vaginitis, and formation of vaginal synechiae or telangiectasia. Preventatively, these complications may be avoided if vaginal intercourse is resumed following treatment or if women are instructed regarding the use of dilators. Lastly, rectovaginal or vesicovaginal fistulas can develop after radiation therapy, especially in advanced stage cancers.

For those women who remain sexually active following radiation therapy, water-based *lubricants* (e.g., Astroglide or K-Y

Jelly) may be of benefit during intercourse. Disadvantageously, lubricants have no sustained effects. Thus, for those with chronic vaginal dryness, *vaginal moisturizers* may prove superior. Vaginal moisturizers form a lubricated coating on the vaginal epithelium and retain moisture for 48 to 72 hours. Moisturizers (e.g., Replens and K-Y Silk-E) can be used daily or several times weekly to maintain moist vaginal tissues. Alternatively, for suitable candidates, topical estrogen cream may be applied to improve atrophic symptoms (Chap. 22, p. 597).

These products may improve vaginal changes following radiation treatment. However, persistent adverse vaginal changes and sexual dysfunction during the 2 years after radiation therapy for cervical cancer have been documented in a longitudinal study of 118 women. Sixty-three percent of those who engaged in sexual activities before radiation therapy continued to do so following treatment, although with less frequency (Jensen, 2003).

Ovary and Pregnancy Outcomes

The effects of radiation on ovarian function depend on the radiation dose and the patient's age. For example, a dose of 4 Gy may sterilize 30 percent of young women, but 100 percent of those older than 40 years. In addition, fractionated radiation therapy appears to be more damaging. Ash (1980) noted that after 10 Gy given in one fraction, 27 percent of the women recovered ovarian function, compared with only 10 percent of those receiving 12 Gy over 6 days. In patients with gynecologic cancers who receive pelvic radiation therapy, symptoms of ovarian failure mirror those of natural menopause, and symptom treatment is similar (Chap. 22, p. 585).

To minimize radiation exposure to the ovaries of premenopausal women, these organs may be surgically repositioned, termed *transposition,* out of the radiation fields. Despite this maneuver, several investigators have reported high rates of ovarian failure when the ovarian dose was more than 3 to 5 Gy. In addition, a birth incidence of only 19 percent was reported among the patients who could conceive (Chambers, 1991; Haie-Meder, 1993).

Among female childhood-cancer survivors who received abdominal irradiation, higher spontaneous abortion rates and lower first-born birth weights were observed compared with cancer survivors who were not irradiated (Hawkins, 1989).

Bladder

Most patients receiving radiation therapy to the pelvis note some symptoms of acute cystitis within 2 to 3 weeks of beginning treatment. Although urinary frequency, spasm, and pain develop commonly, hematuria is rare. Typically, flavoxate hydrochloride (Urispas), oxybutynin (Ditropan), phenazopyridine hydrochloride (Pyridium), or fluid ad lib promptly relieves symptoms. Antibiotics may be used to treat infection when indicated. Major chronic complications following radiation therapy are infrequent and include bladder contracture and hematuria. For severe hematuria, bladder saline irrigation, transurethral cystoscopic fulguration, and temporary urinary diversion are proven techniques. Hyperbaric oxygen therapy has also been described. Fistulas involving the bladder may be a long-term sequela of radiation therapy.

Small Bowel

The small bowel is particularly vulnerable to acute early damage from radiation therapy. After a single dose of 5 to 10 Gy, crypt cells are destroyed, and villi become denuded. An acute malabsorption syndrome ensues and causes nausea, diarrhea, vomiting, and crampy pain. In addition to general instructions of adequate fluid intake and a low-lactose, low-fat, and low-fiber diet, the administration of antinausea and antidiarrhea medications may be warranted (Table 25-6, p. 669, and Table 39-10, p. 963). Additionally, bowel antispasmodics with sedatives (e.g., Donnatal) are particularly helpful.

Patients should be warned about the late, chronic nature of radiation-induced enteritis. Intermittent diarrhea, crampy abdominal pain, and nausea and vomiting, which in combination may mimic a low-grade bowel obstruction, are frequent. Those patients with comorbidities, such as obesity, small-vessel diseases resulting from diabetes or hypertension, previous abdominal surgeries, and inflammatory conditions of the pelvis or bowel, are at increased risk.

Preventatively, several types of devices have been surgically inserted to displace the small bowel from the pelvis. These have included saline-filled tissue expanders, omental slings, and absorbable mesh (Hoffman, 1998; Martin, 2005; Soper, 1988). Furthermore, defining the areas at risk with surgical clips and careful radiation therapy planning, including the use of IMRT may minimize bowel toxicity (Portelance, 2001). More recent advances include the intravenous use of radiation protectors such as amifostine (Athanassiou, 2003). Amifostine is thought to attenuate radiation cell injury through its ability to reduce levels of radiation-induced free radicals. In 2007, guidelines for the prevention and treatment of mucositis were updated. Specifically, for prevention of radiation-induced gastrointestinal mucositis, sulfasalazine orally and amifostine intravenously are suggested. Sucralfate enemas are advised for the treatment of proctitis (Keefe, 2007).

Rectosigmoid

Commonly, within a few weeks after radiation therapy initiation, patients may develop diarrhea, tenesmus, and mucoid discharge, which can be bloody. In these cases, antidiarrheal medications, low-residue diet, steroid-retention or sucralfate enemas, and hydration are management mainstays. Alternatively, rectal bleeding may be seen months to years after radiation therapy. Hemorrhage may at times be severe and require blood transfusion. Moreover, invasive procedures may be needed to control bleeding neovasculature. These include the topical application of 4-percent formalin, cryotherapy, and vessel coagulation with laser (Kantsevoy, 2003; Konishi, 2005; Smith, 2001; Ventrucci, 2001). During the evaluation of late-onset rectal bleeding, barium enema is often indicated. The study usually reveals narrowing of the rectosigmoid lumen and wall thickening. In case of severe obstruction, resection of the involved colonic segment is necessary. In addition, rectovaginal fistulas may result from radiation therapy.

Kidney

Manifestations of acute radiation nephropathy typically appear 6 to 12 months after radiation exposure. The patients develop hypertension, edema, anemia, microscopic hematuria,

TABLE 28-4. Susceptibility of Selected Tissues to Radiation-Induced Cancer

Susceptibility	Tissues
High	Bone marrow, female breast, thyroid
Moderate	Bladder, colon, stomach, liver, ovary
Low	Bone, connective tissue, muscle, cervix, uterus, rectum

proteinuria, and decreased creatinine clearance (Luxton, 1961). Although deteriorating renal function is occasionally reversible, it usually worsens and leads to chronic nephropathy. Patients receiving concurrent radiation and chemotherapy require special consideration, because of the nephrotoxicity associated with many chemotherapeutics.

Radiation-Induced Carcinogenesis

Development of a secondary radiation-induced cancer depends on the patient age at exposure, radiation dose, and susceptibility of specific tissue types to radiation-induced carcinogenesis (Table 28-4). The accepted criteria for the diagnosis of radiation-induced cancer require that the cancer be located within the previously irradiated regions and that its pathology differ from that of the original malignancy. Additionally, there should be a latent period of at least a few years.

In general, those receiving higher radiation doses and those exposed at an earlier age have increased risks for second malignancies. The latency of secondary tumor development also varies depending on the type of second malignancy. For example, the latent period between radiation exposure and the clinical appearance of leukemia is less than 10 years, whereas solid tumors may not develop for decades. Of note, for most radiation-induced malignancies, the clinical appearance of these cancers does not occur until the age when nonirradiated patients would spontaneously develop that particular cancer type. Moreover, radiation-induced and spontaneously developing cancer cells have identical pathologic characteristics. The most common example is development of uterine sarcoma years after pelvic radiation for treatment of cervical cancer (Mark, 1996). However, at the molecular level, a retrospective review unveiled a difference in the mutation patterns of the tumor suppressor gene p53 between spontaneous and radiation-induced sarcomas. More base substitutions were noted in the former, whereas deletions were more frequently observed in the latter (Gonin-Laurent, 2006).

REFERENCES

Amorino GP, Freeman ML, Carbone DP, et al: Radiopotentiation by the oral platinum agent, JM216: role of repair inhibition. Int J Radiat Oncol Biol Phys 44(2):399, 1999

Aquino-Parsons C, Lim P, Green A, et al: Carbogen inhalation in cervical cancer: assessment of oxygenation change. Gynecol Oncol 74(2):259, 1999

Arai T, Nakano T, Fukuhisa K, et al: Second cancer after radiation therapy for cancer of the uterine cervix. Cancer 67(2):398, 1991

Ash P: The influence of radiation on fertility in man. Br J Radiol 53:271, 1980

Athanassiou H, Antonadou D, Coliarakis N, et al: Protective effect of amifostine during fractionated radiotherapy in patients with pelvic carcinomas: results of a randomized trial. Int J Radiat Oncol Biol Phys 56(4):1154, 2003

Begg AC: Cisplatin and radiation: interaction probabilities and therapeutic possibilities. Int J Radiat Oncol Biol Phys 19(5):1183, 1990

Bentzen, SM: Tumor volume and local control probability: clinical data and radiobiological interpretations. Int J Radiat Oncol Biol Phys 36(1):247, 1996

Bonner JA, Harari PM, Giralt J, et al: Radiotherapy plus cetuximab for locoregionally advanced head and neck cancer. 5-year survival data from a phase 3 randomised trial, and relation between cetuximab-induced rash and survival. Lancet Oncol 11:21, 2010

Boronow RC: Combined therapy as an alternative to exenteration for locally advanced vulvo-vaginal cancer: rationale and results. Cancer 49(6):1085, 1982

Bradfield JJ, Kinsella JB, Mader JT, et al: Rapid progression of head and neck squamous carcinoma after hyperbaric oxygenation. Otolaryngol Head Neck Surg 114(6):793, 1996

Bristow RG, Hill RP: Hypoxia and metabolism: Hypoxia, DNA repair and genetic instability. Nat Rev Cancer 8(3):180, 2008

Brizel DM, Dodge RK, Clough RW, et al: Oxygenation of head and neck cancer: changes during radiotherapy and impact on treatment outcome. Radiother Oncol 53(2):113, 1999

Chambers SK, Chambers JT, Kier R, et al: Sequelae of lateral ovarian transposition in irradiated cervical cancer patients. Int J Radiat Oncol Biol Phys 20(6):1305, 1991

Chapman JD, Schneider RF, Urbain JL, et al: Single-photon emission computed tomography and positron-emission tomography assays for tissue oxygenation. Semin Radiat Oncol 11(1):47, 2001

Cerciello F, Hofstetter B, Fatah SA, et al: G2/M cell cycle checkpoint is functional in cervical cancer patients after initiation of external beam radiotherapy. Int J Radiat Oncol Biol Phys 62(5):1390, 2005

Coutard H: Roentgen therapy of epitheliomas of the tonsillar region, hypopharynx and larynx from 1920 to 1926. Am J Roentgenol 28:313, 1932

Craighead PS, Pearcey R, Stuart G: A phase I/II evaluation of tirapazamine administered intravenously concurrent with cisplatin and radiotherapy in women with locally advanced cervical cancer. Int J Radiat Oncol Biol Phys 48(3):791, 2000

del Campo JM, Prat A, Gil-Moreno A, et al: Update on novel therapeutic agents for cervical cancer. 110:S72, 2008

Dische S, Saunders MI, Sealy R, et al: Carcinoma of the cervix and the use of hyperbaric oxygen with radiotherapy: a report of a randomised controlled trial. Radiother Oncol 53(2):93, 1999

Dubben HH: Tumor volume: a basic and specific response predictor in radiotherapy. Radiother Oncol 47(2):167, 1998

Dueñas-González A, Zarba JJ, Alcedo JC, et al: A phase III study comparing concurrent gemcitabine (Gem) plus cisplatin (Cis) and radiation followed by adjuvant Gem plus Cis versus concurrent Cis and radiation in patients with stage IIB to IVA carcinoma of the cervix. Abstract No CRA5507. Presented at the ASCO Annual Meeting. 2009

Dunst J, Kuhnt T, Strauss HG, et al: Anemia in cervical cancers: impact on survival, patterns of relapse, and association with hypoxia and angiogenesis. Int J Radiat Oncol Biol Phys 56(3):778, 2003

Erenpreisa J, Cragg MS: Mitotic death: a mechanism of survival? A review. Cancer Cell Int 1:1, 2001

Fajardo LF: The pathology of ionizing radiation as defined by morphologic patterns. Acta Oncol 44(1):13, 2005

Friedlander AH, Freymiller EG: Detection of radiation-accelerated atherosclerosis of the carotid artery by panoramic radiography. A new opportunity for dentists. J Am Dent Assoc 134(10):1361, 2003

Gemignani ML, Alektiar KM, Leitai M, et al: Radical surgical resection and high-dose intraoperative radiation therapy (HDR-IORT) in patients with recurrent gynecologic cancers. Int J Radiat Oncol Biol Phys 50(3):687, 2001

Glazer PM, Grandis J, Powell SN, et al: Radiation resistance in cancer therapy: meeting summary and research opportunities: report of an NCI workshop held September 1–3, 2010. Radiat Res 176:e0016, 2011

Gonin-Laurent N, Gibaud A, Huygue M, et al: Specific TP53 mutation pattern in radiation-induced sarcomas. Carcinogenesis 27(6):1266, 2006

Gonzáles-Cortijo L, Carballo N, Gonzáles-Martin A, et al: Novel chemotherapy approaches in chemoradiation protocol. Gynecol Oncol 110:S45, 2008

Gregoire V, Hittelman WN, Rosier JF, et al: Chemo-radiotherapy: radiosensitizing nucleoside analogues (review). Oncol Rep 6(5):949, 1999

Gregoire V, Van NT, Stephens LC, et al: The role of fludarabine-induced apoptosis and cell cycle synchronization in enhanced murine tumor radiation response in vivo. Cancer Res 54(23):6201, 1994

Grigsby PW, Lu JD, Mutch DG, et al: Twice-daily fractionation of external irradiation with brachytherapy and chemotherapy in carcinoma of the cervix with positive para-aortic lymph nodes: Phase II study of the Radiation Therapy Oncology Group 92-10. Int J Radiat Oncol Biol Phys 41(4):817, 1998

Grigsby: Long-term follow-up of RTOG 88-05: twice-daily external irradiation with brachytherapy for carcinoma of the cervix. Int J Radiat Oncol Biol Phys 54:51, 2002

Haie-Meder C, Mlika-Cabanne N, Michel G, et al: Radiotherapy after ovarian transposition: ovarian function and fertility preservation. Int J Radiat Oncol Biol Phys 25(3):419, 1993

Hall EJ, Cox JD: Physical and biological basis of radiation therapy. In Cox JD, Ang KK (eds): Radiation Oncology, Rationale, Technique, Results, 8th ed. St. Louis, MO, Mosby, 2003, p 5

Hareyama M, Sakata K, Oouchi A, et al: High-dose-rate versus low-dose-rate intracavitary therapy for carcinoma of the uterine cervix: a randomized trial. Cancer 94(1):117, 2002

Hawkins MM, Smith RA: Pregnancy outcomes in childhood cancer survivors: probable effects of abdominal irradiation. Int J Cancer 43(3):399, 1989

Henke M, Laszig R, Rübe C, et al: Erythropoietin to treat head and neck cancer patients with anaemia undergoing radiotherapy: randomized, double-blind, placebo-controlled trial. Lancet 362:1255, 2003

Heron DE, Gerszten K, Selvaraj RN, et al: Conventional 3D conformal versus intensity-modulated radiotherapy for the adjuvant treatment of gynecologic malignancies: a comparative dosimetric study of dose-volume histograms. Gynecol Oncol 91 (1):39, 2003

Hershman DL, Buono DL, Malin J, et al: Patterns of use and risks associated with erythropoietin-stimulating agents among Medicare patients with cancer. J Natl Cancer Inst 101:1633, 2009

Hoffman JP, Sigurdson ER, Eisenberg BL: Use of saline-filled tissue expanders to protect the small bowel from radiation. Oncology (Williston Park) 12(1):51, 1998

Jensen PT, Groenvold M, Klee MC, et al: Longitudinal study of sexual function and vaginal changes after radiotherapy for cervical cancer. Int J Radiat Oncol Biol Phys 56(4):937, 2003

Kantsevoy SV, Cruz-Correa MR, Vaughn CA, et al: Endoscopic cryotherapy for the treatment of bleeding mucosal vascular lesions of the GI tract: a pilot study. Gastrointest Endosc 57(3):403, 2003

Kapp KS, Poschauko J, Geyer E, et al: Evaluation of the effect of routine packed red blood cell transfusion in anemic cervix cancer patients treated with radical radiotherapy. Int J Radiat Oncol Biol Phys 54(1):58, 2002

Keefe DM, Schubert MM, Elting, et al: Updated clinical practice guidelines for the prevention and treatment of mucositis. Cancer 109:820, 2007

Kelland LR, Edwards SM, Steel GG: Induction and rejoining of DNA double-strand breaks in human cervix carcinoma cell lines of differing radiosensitivity. Radiat Res 116(3):526, 1988

Keys HM, Bundy BM, Stehman FB, et al: A comparison of weekly cisplatin during radiation therapy versus irradiation alone each followed by adjuvant hysterectomy in bulky stage IB cervical carcinoma: a randomized trial of the Gynecologic Oncology Group. N Engl J Med 340:1154, 1999

Komaki: Twice-daily fractionation of external irradiation with brachytherapy in bulky carcinoma of the cervix. Phase I/II study of the Radiation Therapy Oncology Group 88-05. Cancer 73, 2619, 1994

Konishi T, Watanabe T, Kitayama J, et al: Endoscopic and histopathologic findings after formalin application for hemorrhage caused by chronic radiation-induced proctitis. Gastrointest Endosc 61(1):161, 2005

Kwee SA, Coel MN, Lim J, et al: Combined use of F-18 fluorocholine positron emission tomography and magnetic resonance spectroscopy for brain tumor evaluation. J Neuroimaging 14(3):285, 2004

Lavey RS, Liu PY, Greer BE, et al: Recombinant human erythropoietin as an adjunct to radiation therapy and cisplatin for stage IIB-IVA carcinoma of the cervix: a Southwest Oncology Group study. Gynecol Oncol 95(1):145, 2004

Lee MY, Wu HG, Kim K, et al: Concurrent radiotherapy with paclitaxel/carboplatin chemotherapy as a definitive treatment for squamous cell carcinoma of the uterine cervix. Gynecol Oncol 104(1):95, 2007

Luxton RW, Kunkler PB: Radiation nephritis. Acta Radiol Ther Phys Biol 66:169, 1964

Marcial VA, Komaki R: Altered fractionation and extended-field irradiation of carcinoma of the cervix. Cancer 76(10 Suppl):2152, 1995

Mark RJ, Poen J, Tran LM et al: Postirradiation sarcoma of the gynecologic tract. A report of 13 cases and a discussion of the risk of radiation-induced gynecologic malignancies. Am J Clin Oncol 19(1):59, 1996

Martin J, Fitzpatrick K, Horan G, et al: Treatment with a belly-board device significantly reduces the volume of small bowel irradiated and results in low acute toxicity in adjuvant radiotherapy for gynecologic cancer: results of a prospective study. Radiother Oncol 74(3):267, 2005

Mason KA, Kishi K, Hunter N, et al: Effect of docetaxel on the therapeutic ratio of fractionated radiotherapy in vivo. Clin Cancer Res 5:4191, 1999

Milano MT, Constine LS, Okunieff P: Normal tissue tolerance dose metrics for radiation therapy of major organs. Semin Radiat Oncol 17:131, 2007

Montana GS, Thomas GM, Moore DH, et al: Preoperative chemo-radiation for carcinoma of the vulva with N2/N3 nodes: a gynecologic oncology group study. Int J Radiat Oncol Biol Phys 48(4):1007, 2000

Moore KN, Sill D, Miller DS, et al: A phase I trial of concurrent cetuximab (CET), cisplatin (CDDP), and radiation therapy (RT) women with locally advanced cervical cancer (CXCA): a GOG study. J Clin Oncol 29(abstract 5032), 2011

Morris M, Eifel PJ, Watkins EB, et al: Pelvic radiation with concurrent chemotherapy versus pelvic and para-aortic radiation for high risk cervical cancer: a randomized Radiation Therapy Oncology Group clinical trial. N Engl J Med 340:1137, 1999

Nag S, Erickson B, Thomadsen, et al: The American Brachytherapy Society recommendations for high-dose-rate brachytherapy for carcinoma of the cervix. Int J Radiat Oncol Biol Phys 48(1):201, 2000

National Institutes of Health: Cisplatin and Radiation Therapy With or Without Tirapazamine in Treating Patients With Cervical Cancer. 2010. Available at: http://clinicaltrials.gov/ct2/show/record/NCT00262821. Accessed October 20, 2011

Nguyen PD, John B, Munoz AK, et al: Mitomycin-C/5-FU and radiation therapy for locally advanced uterine cervical cancer. Gynecol Oncol 43(3):220, 1991

Nordsmark M, Overgaard M, Overgaard J: Pretreatment oxygenation predicts radiation response in advanced squamous cell carcinoma of the head and neck. Radiother Oncol 41(1):31, 1996

Okada H, Mak TW: Pathways of apoptotic and non-apoptotic death in tumour cells. Nat Rev Cancer 4(8):592, 2004

Overgaard J, Hoff CM, Hansen HS, et al: Randomized study of darbepoetin alfa as modifier of radiotherapy in patients with primary squamous cell carcinoma of the head and neck (HNSCC): final outcome of the DAHANCA 10 trial. J Clin Oncol 27(No 15S):6007, 2009

Pawlik TM, Keyomarsi K: Role of cell cycle in mediating sensitivity to radiotherapy. Int J Radiat Oncol Bio Phys 59(4):928, 2004

Petereit DG, Sarkaria JN, Chappell R, et al: The adverse effect of treatment prolongation in cervical carcinoma. Int J Radiat Oncol Biol Phys 32(5):1301, 1995

Portelance L, Chao KS, Grigsby PW, et al: Intensity-modulated radiation therapy (IMRT) reduces small bowel, rectum, and bladder doses in patients with cervical cancer receiving pelvic and para-aortic irradiation. Int J Radiat Oncol Biol Phys 51(1):261, 2001

Rischin D, Peters L, Fisher R, et al: Tirapazamine, cisplatin, and radiation versus fluorouracil, cisplatin, and radiation in patients with locally advanced head and neck cancer: A randomized phase II trial of the Trans-Tasman Radiation Oncology Group (TROG 98.02). J Clin Oncol 23:79, 2005

Rischin D, Peters L, Hicks R, et al: Phase I trial of concurrent tirapazamine, cisplatin, and radiotherapy in patients with advanced head and neck cancer. J Clin Oncol 19(2):535, 2001

Rischin D, Peters LJ, O'Sullivan B, et al: Tirapazamine, cisplatin, and radiation versus cisplatin and radiation for advanced squamous cell carcinoma of the head and neck (TROG 02.02, HeadSTART): a phase III trial of the Trans-Tasman Radiation Oncology Group. J Clin Oncol 8(18):2989, 2010

Rose PG: Combination therapy: new treatment paradigm for locally advanced cervical cancer? Nat Rev Clin Oncol 8(7): 388, 2011

Rose PG, Bundy BN, Watkins EB, et al: Concurrent cisplatin-based chemoradiation improves progression free and overall survival in advanced cervical cancer: results of a randomized Gynecologic Oncology Group study. N Engl J Med 340:1144, 1999

Rushdan MN, Tay EH, Khoo-Tan HS, et al: Tailoring the field and indication of adjuvant pelvic radiation for patients with FIGO stage Ib lymph nodes-negative cervical carcinoma following radical surgery based on the GOG score—a pilot study. Ann Acad Med Singapore 33(4):467, 2004

Schwartz JL, Mustafi R, Beckett MA, et al: DNA double-strand break rejoining rates, inherent radiation sensitivity and human tumor response to radiotherapy. Br J Cancer 74(1):37, 1996

Schwartz JL, Rotmensch J, Giovanazzi S, et al: Faster repair of DNA double-strand breaks in radioresistant human tumor cells. Int J Radiat Oncol Biol Phys 15(4):907, 1988

Sedlis A, Bundy BN, Rotman MZ, et al: A randomized trial of pelvic radiation therapy versus no further therapy in selected patients with stage IB carcinoma of the cervix after radical hysterectomy and pelvic lymphadenectomy: a Gynecologic Oncology Group Study. Gynecol Oncol 73(2)177, 1999

Smith S, Wallner K, Dominitz JA, et al: Argon plasma coagulation for rectal bleeding after prostate brachytherapy. Int J Radiat Oncol Biol Phys 51(3):636, 2001

Soper JT: Role of surgery and radiation therapy in the management of gestational trophoblastic disease. Best Pract Res Clin Obstet Gynaecol 17(6):943, 2003

Soper JT, Clarke-Pearson DL, Creasman WT: Absorbable synthetic mesh (910-polyglactin) intestinal sling to reduce radiation-induced small bowel injury in patients with pelvic malignancies. Gynecol Oncol 29(3):283, 1988

Steel GG, Peckham MJ: Exploitable mechanisms in combined radiotherapy-chemotherapy: the concept of additivity. Int J Radiat Oncol Biol Phys 5(1):85, 1979

Terasawa T, Dvorak T, Ip Stanley, et al: Systematic review: charged-particle radiation therapy for cancer. Ann Inter Med 151:556, 2009

Thames H: On the origin of dose fractionation regimens in radiotherapy. Semin Radiat Oncol 2(1):3, 1992

Trott KR: The mechanisms of acceleration of repopulation in squamous epithelia during daily irradiation. Acta Oncol 38(2):153, 1999

Varlotto J, Stevenson MA: Anemia, tumor hypoxemia, and the cancer patient. Int J Radiat Oncol Biol Phys 63(1):25, 2005

Ventrucci M, Di Simone MP, Giulietti P, et al: Efficacy and safety of Nd:YAG laser for the treatment of bleeding from radiation proctocolitis. Dig Liver Dis 33(3):230, 2001

Wang CC: Local control of oropharyngeal carcinoma after two accelerated hyperfractionation radiation therapy schemes. Int J Radiat Oncol Biol Phys 14(6):1143, 1988

Weichselbaum RR, Beckett MA, Hallahan DE, et al: Molecular targets to overcome radioresistance. Semin Oncol 19(4 Suppl 11):14, 1992

Wong FC, Tung SY, Leung TW, et al: Treatment results of high-dose-rate remote afterloading brachytherapy for cervical cancer and retrospective comparison of two regimens. Int J Radiat Oncol Biol Phys 55(5):1254, 2003

Woodward WA, Cox JD: Molecular basis of radiation therapy. In Mendelsohn J, Howley PM, Israel MA, et al (eds): The Molecular Basis of Cancer, 3rd ed. Philadelphia, Saunders Elsevier, 2008, p 593

Wun T, Law L, Harvey D, et al: Increased incidence of symptomatic venous thrombosis in patients with cervical carcinoma treated with concurrent chemotherapy, radiation, and erythropoietin. Cancer 98(7):1514, 2003

Yang LX, Douple E, Wang HJ: Irradiation-enhanced binding of carboplatin to DNA. Int J Radiat Biol 68(6):609, 1995

Yap OW, Kapp DS, Teng NN, et al: Intraoperative radiation therapy in recurrent ovarian cancer. Int J Radiat Oncol Biol Phys 63(4):1114, 2005

Zakian KL, Koutcher JA, Ballon D, et al: Developments in nuclear magnetic resonance imaging and spectroscopy: application to radiation oncology. Semin Radiat Oncol 11(1):3, 2001

Zidar N, Ferlunga D, Hvala A, et al: Contribution to the pathogenesis of radiation-induced injury to large arteries. J Laryngol Otol 111(10):988, 1997

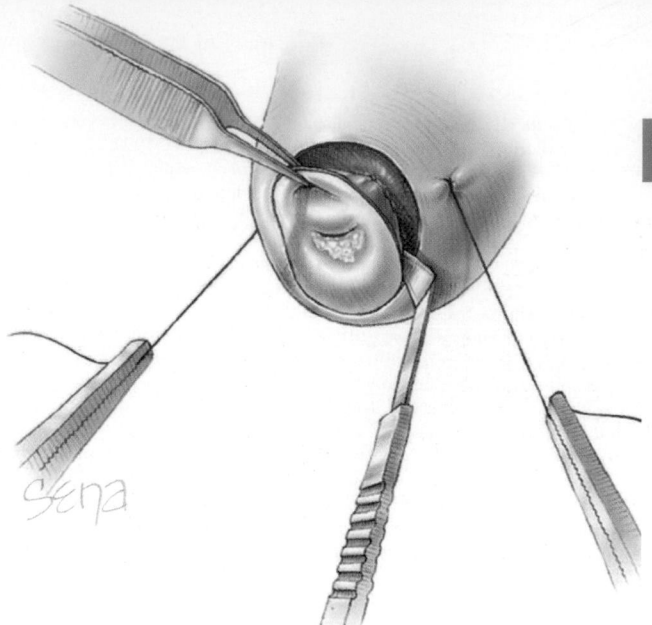

Since the introduction of the Papanicolaou (Pap) test in the 1950s, cytology screening has been associated with a significant reduction in both the incidence of and mortality rate from invasive cervical cancer (Saslow, 2002). Annually, approximately 7 percent of U.S. women who undergo screening will have abnormal cervical cytologic results requiring a clinical response (Jones, 2000). Accordingly, office gynecology frequently involves the diagnosis and management of preinvasive lower genital tract disease.

DISEASE SPECTRUM OF LOWER GENITAL TRACT NEOPLASIA

The term *intraepithelial neoplasia* refers to squamous epithelial lesions of the lower genital tract that are considered to be precursors of invasive cancer. Lesions are diagnosed by biopsy and histologic evaluation. Cervical, vaginal, vulvar, perianal, and anal intraepithelial neoplasia (CIN, VaIN, VIN, PAIN, and AIN, respectively) demonstrate a disease spectrum ranging from mildly dysplastic cytoplasmic and nuclear changes to those of severe dysplasia. There is no invasion through the basement membrane, which would then characterize an invasive cancer.

The severity of an intraepithelial lesion is graded by the proportion of epithelium affected from the basement membrane upward toward the surface. In the case of CIN, abnormal cells confined to the lower third of the squamous epithelium are referred to as *mild dysplasia* or *CIN 1,* extending into the middle third as *moderate dysplasia* or *CIN 2,* into the upper third as *severe dysplasia* or *CIN 3,* and full-thickness involvement as *carcinoma in situ (CIS)* (Fig. 29-1). Squamous lesions of the vagina, vulva, perianal, and anal epithelia are graded similarly with the caveat that VIN 1 is no longer recognized (p. 757). The natural history of these extracervical lesions is less well understood than for CIN.

In contrast, because it is only one cell-layer thick, the cervical columnar epithelium does not demonstrate an analogous neoplastic disease spectrum. Histologic abnormalities are therefore limited to either *adenocarcinoma in situ (AIS)* or *adenocarcinoma.*

New cervical cytology terminology was introduced in 1989 (p. 744) (Kurman, 1994; National Cancer Institute Workshop, 1989). Since then, the term *squamous intraepithelial lesion (SIL)* has been used interchangeably with *intraepithelial neoplasia* and is often used to report histologic diagnoses as well. Because histologic changes of human papillomavirus (HPV) infection and CIN 1 are similar and cannot be distinguished reliably, they may be referred to more generally as *low-grade*

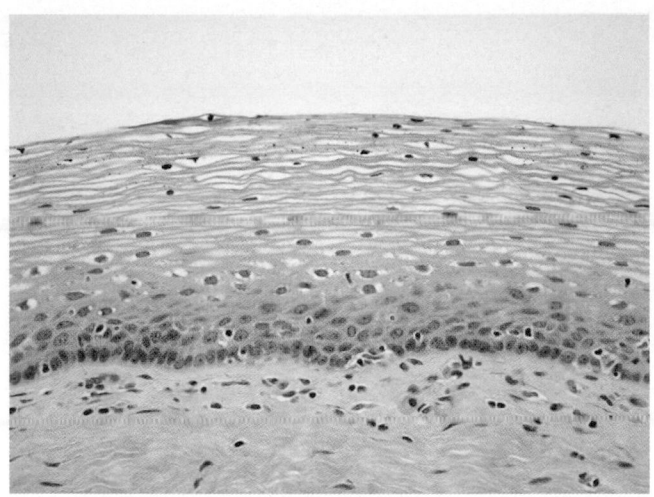

A   Normal squamous epithelium

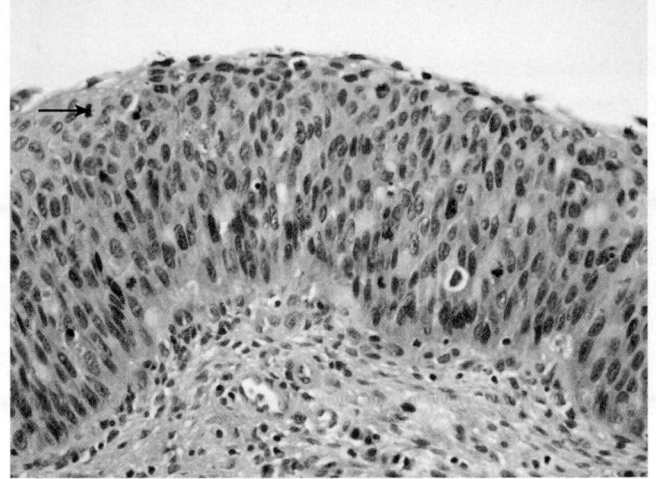

C   CIN 3/Squamous cell carcinoma in situ

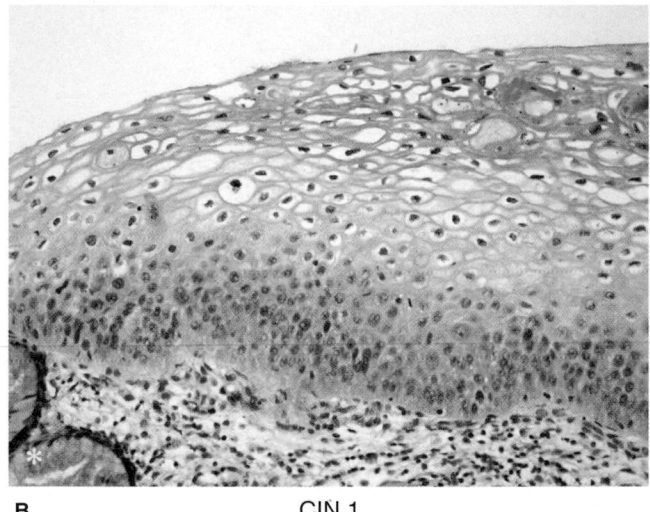

B   CIN 1

FIGURE 29-1 A. Normal ectocervical mucosa. The ectocervical epithelium is a nonkeratinizing, stratified squamous epithelium that matures in response to estrogen stimulation. Mitoses are normally confined to the deeper layers, that is, the basal and parabasal epithelial layers. **B.** Cervical biopsy taken from the transformation zone with mild squamous dysplasia (CIN I). The transformation zone is indicated by the presence of both squamous epithelium and endocervical glands (*yellow asterisk*). CIN 1 is characterized by a disordered proliferation of squamous cells and increased mitotic activity confined to the basal one third of the epithelium, with koilocytotic atypia involving the more superficial epithelium. Koilocytosis is typified by nuclear enlargement, coarse chromatin, nuclear "wrinkling," and perinuclear halos. **C.** Severe squamous dysplasia (CIN 3/squamous cell carcinoma in situ) is characterized by disordered proliferation of atypical squamous cells and increased mitotic activity involving the full thickness of the epithelium. Note the mitotic figure located close to epithelial surface (*arrow*). Abnormal mitoses are sometimes present. (*Photographs contributed by Dr. Kelley Carrick.*)

squamous intraepithelial lesions (LSILs). In contrast, CIN 2 and CIN 3/CIS may be designated as *high-grade SIL (HSIL)*. LSILs lack reproducibility as cytologic or histologic diagnoses, are associated with a wide range of papilloma viral types, and generally portend a benign clinical course. HSILs are more reproducible diagnostically, are caused by a narrower range of carcinogenic viral types, and are more likely to be cancer precursors (Lungu, 1992). Therefore, clinical interventions generally target HSIL lesions.

Regardless of the terminology used, cervical *cytology* is the screening tool that prompts further evaluation and should not be confused with a histologic diagnosis. Cytologic results merely direct the next step in patient evaluation. *Histology*, generally obtained from a colposcopically directed biopsy, is used to diagnose the presence and severity of lower genital tract neoplasia. These histologic results direct appropriate treatment steps.

ANATOMIC CONSIDERATIONS

External Genitalia

Precancerous lesions of the female lower genital tract are often multifocal, can involve any of its structures, and may appear

similar to benign processes. For example, *micropapillomatosis labialis* is a benign variant of normal anatomy characterized by minute epithelial projections on the inner epithelial surface of the labia minora (Fig. 29-2). Each papillary projection arises from its own individual base. These can be easily mistaken for HPV-related lesions. In contrast, HPV lesions tend to be multifocal, asymmetric, and have multiple papillations arising from a single base (Ferris, 2004). Micropapillomatosis often shows spontaneous regression, and treatment is not indicated (Bergeron, 1990).

Vagina

The vagina is lined by nonkeratinized squamous epithelium, and glands are absent. However, areas of columnar epithelium can occasionally be found within the vaginal squamous mucosa, a condition termed *adenosis*. It is most commonly attributable to in utero exposure to exogenous estrogen, particularly diethylstilbestrol (DES) (Trimble, 2001). These areas appear as red patches surrounded by squamous epithelium and can be mistaken for ulcers or other lesions. In addition to inspection, careful palpation of the vagina is warranted, as clear cell adenocarcinoma, also associated with DES, may be palpable before it is visible.

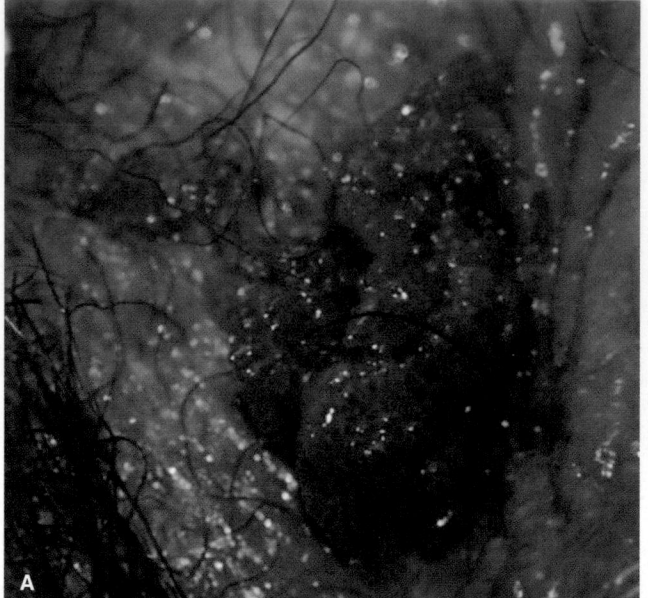

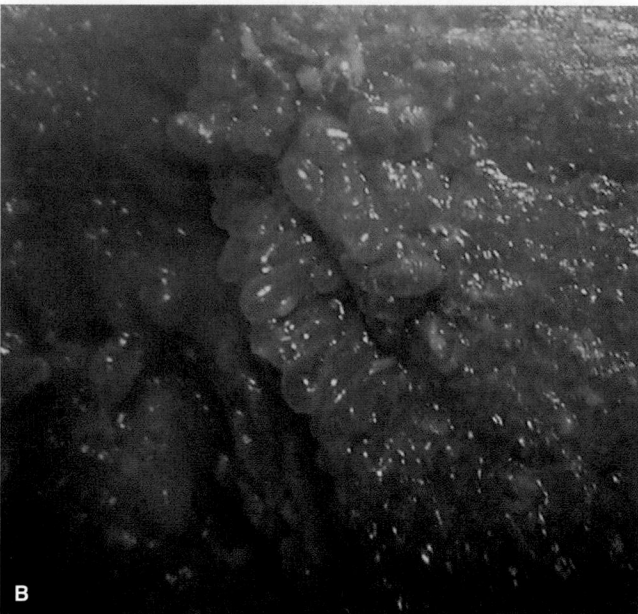

FIGURE 29-2 Benign lower genital tract lesions. **A.** Condylomata tend to be multifocal, asymmetric, and have multiple papillations arising from a single base. **B.** Micropapillomatosis labialis is a normal variant of vulvar anatomy encountered along the inner aspects of the labia minora and lower vagina. In contrast to condylomata, projections are uniform in size and shape and arise singly from their base attachments.

Cervix

Squamocolumnar Junction

During embryogenesis, upward migration of stratified squamous epithelium from the urogenital sinus and vaginal plate is thought to replace müllerian epithelium (Ulfelder, 1976). This process usually terminates near the external cervical os, forming the original (congenital) squamocolumnar junction (SCJ). Here, the pink, smooth squamous epithelium is juxtaposed to the red, velvety columnar epithelium. In a minority of women, this migration may be incomplete and lead to a location of the

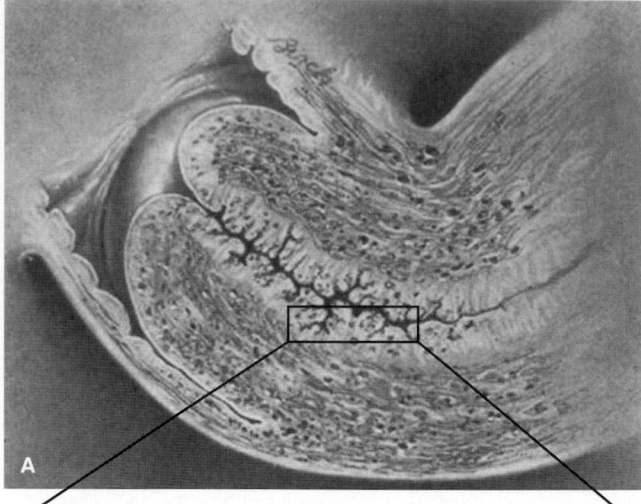

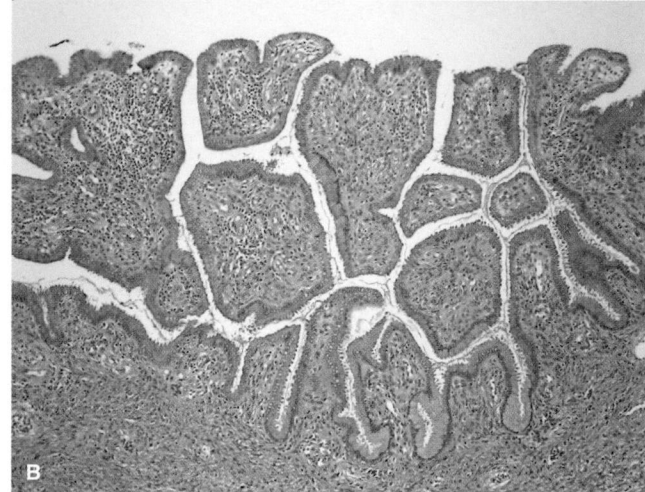

FIGURE 29-3 Endocervical anatomy. **A.** Sagittal view of the cervix. In this drawing, the boxed portion of the endocervical canal reflects the orientation of the photomicrograph. (Modified from Eastman, 1961, with permission.) **B.** The endocervix is lined by a simple columnar, mucin-secreting epithelium. Crypts and small exophytic projections appear pseudopapillary when viewed in cross section. A mild lymphocytic infiltrate, as seen in this case, is usually present and may become marked in the presence of infection or chronic irritation. *(Photograph contributed by Dr. Kelley Carrick.)*

SCJ in the upper vagina. This is seen as a normal variant and also with in utero DES exposure (Kaufman, 2005).

The columnar epithelium is commonly referred to as "glandular" (Solomon, 2002). This is because deep infoldings of the columnar epithelium give a histologic appearance similar to that of glandular tissue (Fig. 29-3). However, the term glandular is technically incorrect, as true glands, consisting of acini and ducts, are not present on the cervix (Ulfelder, 1976).

The location of the SCJ varies with age and hormonal status (Fig. 29-4). Under the influence of estrogen, it everts outward onto the ectocervix during adolescence, pregnancy, and with the use of combination hormone contraceptives. It regresses into the endocervical canal with menopause and other low estrogen states, such as prolonged lactation and the use of progestin-only contraceptives, as well as from the ongoing natural process of squamous metaplasia (Anderson, 1991).

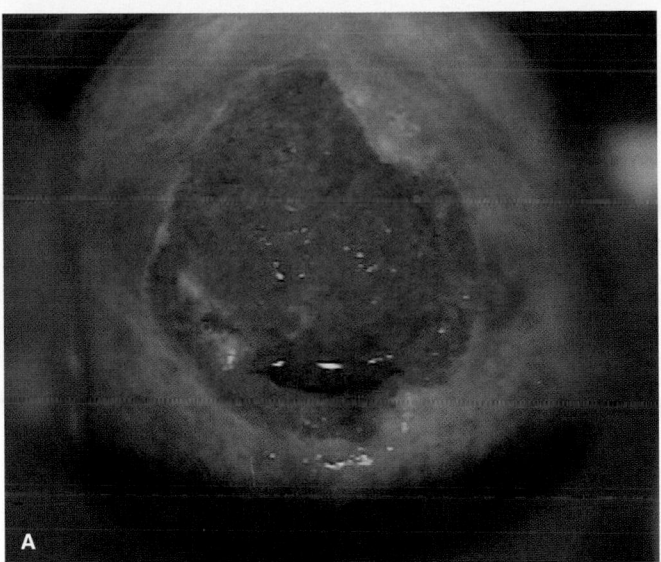 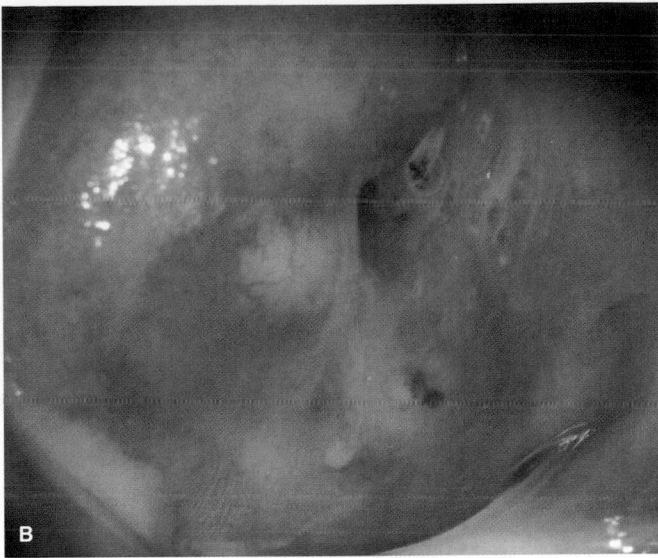

FIGURE 29-4 The location of the squamocolumnar junction (SCJ) is variable. **A.** The SCJ is located on the ectocervix and is fully visualized. **B.** The SCJ is located within the endocervical canal and is not visible.

Squamous Metaplasia

At puberty, the rise in estrogen levels leads to increased glycogen stores in the nonkeratinized squamous epithelium of the lower genital tract. Glycogen provides a carbohydrate source for lactobacilli and leads to domination of the vaginal flora by lactobacilli. These bacteria produce lactic acid, which lowers the vaginal pH to less than 4.5. This lower vaginal pH is the suspected stimulus for *squamous metaplasia*, which is the ongoing replacement of columnar epithelium by squamous epithelium on the cervix. Relatively undifferentiated reserve cells underlying the cervical epithelia are the apparent precursors of the new metaplastic cells, which differentiate further into squamous epithelium. This normal process creates a progressively widening band of metaplastic epithelium termed the *transformation zone* (TZ), lying between the original SCJ and the present columnar epithelium (Fig. 29-5).

Transformation Zone and Cervical Neoplasia

Nearly all cervical neoplasia, both squamous and columnar, develops within the TZ, usually adjacent to the new or current SCJ (Anderson, 1991). Cervical reserve and immature metaplastic cells appear particularly vulnerable to the oncogenic effects of HPV and cocarcinogens (Stanley, 2010). Squamous metaplasia is most active during adolescence and pregnancy. This may explain why early age at sexual activity onset and at first pregnancy are known risk factors for cervical cancer.

HUMAN PAPILLOMAVIRUS

The causative role of this virus in the genesis of essentially all cervical neoplasia and a variable but significant portion of vulvar, vaginal, and anal neoplasia is firmly established.

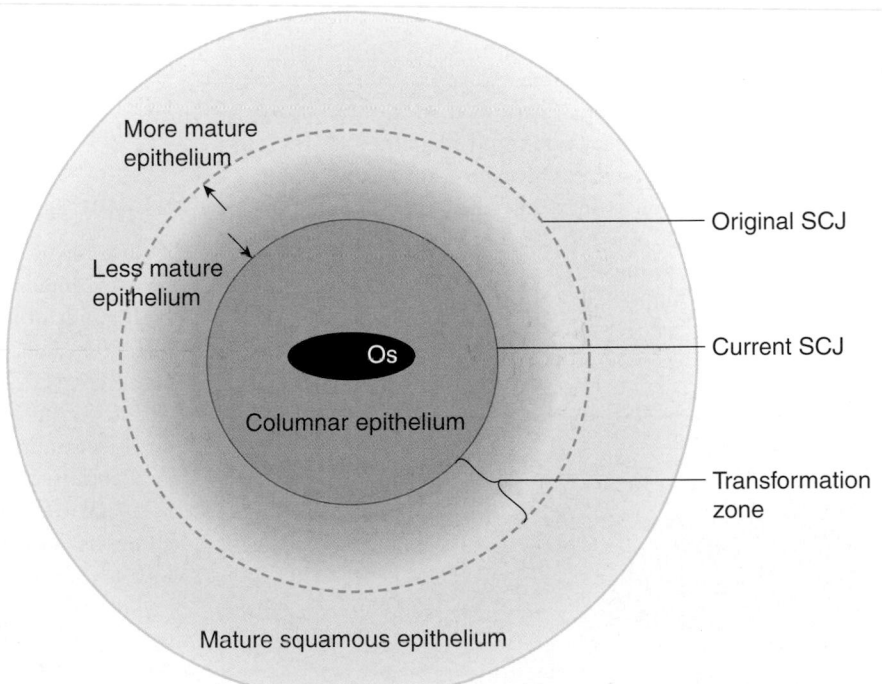

FIGURE 29-5 Schematic describing relevant cervical landmarks. The original squamocolumnar junction (SCJ) marks the terminal site of the upward migration of squamous epithelium from the urogenital sinus during embryonic development. The location of the SCJ moves with age and hormonal status. With higher estrogen states, the SCJ everts outward. With low-estrogen states and with squamous metaplasia, the SCJ is moved closer to the cervical os. The transformation zone consists of the band of squamous metaplasia lying between the original SCJ and new (current) SCJ. As the metaplastic epithelium matures, it moves outward relative to the newer, less mature areas of metaplasia and can become indistinguishable from the original squamous epithelium.

HPV has also become recognized as an important causative agent for a variety of extragenital cancers, including certain head and neck cancers. This virus is responsible for approximately 5 percent of all cancers (D'Souza, 2007; Steben, 2007).

Basic Virology of HPV

Human papillomavirus is a simple, double-stranded DNA virus with a protein capsid. HPV infects human squamous or metaplastic epithelial cells primarily. HPV types and subtypes are distinguished by degree of genetic homology (Coggin, 1979; de Villiers, 2004). Approximately 130 genetically distinct HPV types have been identified. Of these types, 30 to 40 primarily infect the lower anogenital tract.

HPV Life Cycle

The circular, double-stranded HPV genome consists of only nine identified open reading frames (Southern, 1998; Stanley, 2010). In addition to a regulatory region, the six "early" (E) genes govern functions early in the viral life cycle, including DNA maintenance, replication, and transcription. Early genes are expressed in the lower epithelial layers (Fig. 29-6). The two "late" genes encode the major (L1) and minor (L2) capsid proteins and are expressed in the more superficial layers. These proteins are needed late in the viral life cycle to complete assembly into new, infectious viral particles (Beutner, 1997). HPV gene expression occurs in synchrony with and is dependent upon squamous epithelial differentiation. Therefore, completion of the viral life cycle takes place only within an intact, fully differentiating squamous epithelium (Doorbar, 2005). The completely assembled viral particles are shed within the superficial squames. HPV is a nonlytic virus, and therefore infectiousness depends upon the normal desquamation of infected epithelial cells. A new infection is initiated when the L1 and L2 capsid proteins bind to the epithelial basement membrane and/or basal cells, permitting entry of HPV viral particles into new host cells (Sapp, 2009).

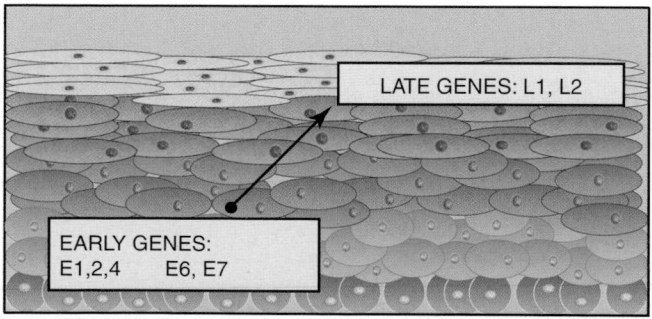

FIGURE 29-6 The human papillomavirus life cycle is completed in synchrony with squamous epithelium differentiation. Early genes, including the *E6* and *E7* oncogenes, are expressed most strongly within the basal and parabasal layers. The late genes encoding capsid proteins are expressed later in the superficial layers. Intact virus is shed during normal desquamation of superficial squames. Late genes are not strongly expressed in high-grade neoplastic lesions.

HPV Types

Clinically, HPV types are classified as high-risk (HR) or low-risk (LR) based on their oncogenicity and strength of association with cervical cancer. Low-risk HPV types 6 and 11 cause nearly all genital warts and a minority of subclinical HPV infections. Low-risk HPV infections are rarely, if ever, oncogenic.

In contrast, persistent HR HPV infection is a requirement for the development of cervical cancer. HR HPV types, including 16, 18, 31, 33, 35, 45, and 58 as well as other less common types, account for approximately 95 percent of cervical cancer cases worldwide (Bosch, 2002; Lorincz, 1992; Muñoz, 2003). HPV 16 is the most carcinogenic of these, likely due to its increased tendency toward persistence compared with other HPV types (Schiffman, 2005). It accounts for the largest percentage of CIN 3 lesions (45 percent) and cervical cancers (55 percent) worldwide and for HPV-related cancers located elsewhere in the anogenital tract and in the oropharynx (Schiffman, 2010; Smith, 2007). The prevalence of HPV 18 is much lower than that of HPV 16 in the general population. However, it is found in 13 percent of squamous cell carcinomas, and in an even higher proportion of cervical adenocarcinomas and adenosquamous carcinomas (37 percent) (Smith, 2007). Together, HPVs 16 and 18 account for approximately 70 percent of cervical cancers.

The HPV types most often found in cervical cancer (HPV types 16, 18, 45, and 31) are also among the most prevalent in the general population. HPV 16 is frequently the most common HPV found among low-grade lesions and in women without neoplasia (Herrero, 2000). Infection with HR HPV does not result in neoplasia in most infected women. This indicates that additional host and environmental factors determine whether or not HR HPV will cause neoplasia.

HPV Transmission

Transmission of genital HPV results from direct, usually sexual, contact with the genital skin, mucous membranes, or body fluids of a partner with either warts or subclinical HPV infection (Abu, 2005; American College of Obstetricians and Gynecologists, 2005).

Little is known regarding the infectivity of subclinical HPV, but it is assumed to be high, especially in the presence of high viral counts. It is generally accepted that HPV gains access to the basal cell layer and basement membrane through microabrasions of the genital epithelium during sexual contact. Once infected, these basal cells become a viral reservoir.

Genital HPV infection is multifocal, involving more than one lower reproductive tract site in most cases (Bauer, 1991; Spitzer, 1989). Therefore, neoplasia at one genital site increases the risk of neoplasia elsewhere within the lower genital tract, although the cervix appears most vulnerable. Also, simultaneous or sequential infection with multiple HPV types is common (Schiffman, 2010).

Modes of HPV Transmission

Most genital HPV infections result from sexual intercourse. High-risk HPV cervical infection is generally limited to women who have experienced penetrative sexual contact. Sexually naïve women occasionally test positive for nononcogenic types at the vulva or vagina, perhaps due to vaginal tampon use or digital penetration (Ley, 1991; Rylander, 1994; Winer, 2003). It has been reported recently that women prior to coitarche can become infected with high-risk types as well, but this is uncommon (Doerfler, 2009). Fomite transmission, known to occur with nongenital warts, is unproven but likely explains some of these cases (Ferenczy, 1989). The role of nonsexual transmission of HPV remains unclear and requires further study.

Oral-to-genital and hand-to-genital HPV transmissions are possible, but appear to be far less common than with genital-to-genital transmission, particularly penile-vaginal penetrative contact (Winer, 2003). Women who have sex with women frequently report past sexual experiences with men. This subgroup of women has rates of HR HPV positivity, abnormal cervical cytology, and high-grade cervical neoplasia similar to those of heterosexual women, but undergoes cervical cancer screening less often (Marrazzo, 2000). Those who have never had sex with men appear to be at similar risk, implying that digital, oral, and object contact places them at risk of HPV infection. Therefore, all women who are sexually active should undergo cervical cancer screening according to current recommendations regardless of sexual orientation.

Congenital HPV Infection

Despite the high prevalence of genital HPV infection, vertical transmission (mother to fetus or newborn) beyond transient skin colonization is rare. Conjunctival, laryngeal, vulvar, or perianal warts present at birth or that develop within 1 to 3 years of birth are most likely due to perinatal exposure to maternal HPV (Cohen, 1990). Infection is not related to the presence of maternal genital warts or route of delivery (Silverberg, 2003; Syrjanen, 2005). Accordingly, cesarean delivery is generally not recommended for maternal HPV infection. Exceptions may include cases of large genital warts that would likely obstruct delivery or avulse and bleed with cervical dilation or vaginal delivery.

Genital warts that develop in children after infancy are always reason to consider the possibility of sexual abuse. However, infection by nonsexual contact, autoinoculation, or fomite transfer appears possible. This is supported by reports of nongenital HPV types in a significant minority of pediatric and adolescent genital wart cases (Cohen, 1990; Doerfler, 2009; Obalek, 1990; Siegfried, 1997).

■ Outcomes of HPV Infection

Genital HPV infection causes a variety of outcomes (Fig. 29-7). Infection may be latent or expressed. Moreover, expression may be productive, leading to formation of new virus, or may be neoplastic, causing preinvasive disease or malignancy. Most productive and neoplastic infections are subclinical, rather than clinically apparent, as with genital warts or obvious malignancy. Finally, HPV infection can be

transient or can be persistent with or without the development of neoplasia (dysplasia or malignancy). Neoplasia is the least common result of genital HPV infection.

Latent HPV Infection

Latent infection refers to that in which cells are infected, but HPV remains quiescent. The viral genome remains episomal, that is, intact and not integrated into the host cell genome. There are no detectable tissue effects, as the virus is not reproducing. Little is known regarding the incidence, natural history, or significance of latent HPV infection, as the virus is present below detectable levels. It is still unknown if apparent clearance of the HPV clinically or by use of current testing methods constitutes true eradication of HPV from infected tissues or whether it reflects a return to latency.

Productive HPV Infection

These infections are characterized by completion of the viral life cycle and increasing the population of infectious viral particles. As described earlier, viral production is completed in synchrony with terminal squamous differentiation, which concludes with programmed squamous cell death and desquamation from the epithelial surface. Thus, these infections have little or no malignant potential. As in latent infection, the circular HPV genome remains episomal, and its oncogenes are expressed at only very low levels (Durst, 1985; Stoler, 1996). Plentiful production of infectious viral particles occurs during a time frame of 2 to 3 weeks (Stanley, 2010).

In both the female and male genital tracts, productive HPV infections produce either visible genital warts, called condyloma acuminata, or much more commonly, cause subclinical infections. Subclinical infections may be indirectly identified by cytology as low-grade squamous intraepithelial lesions

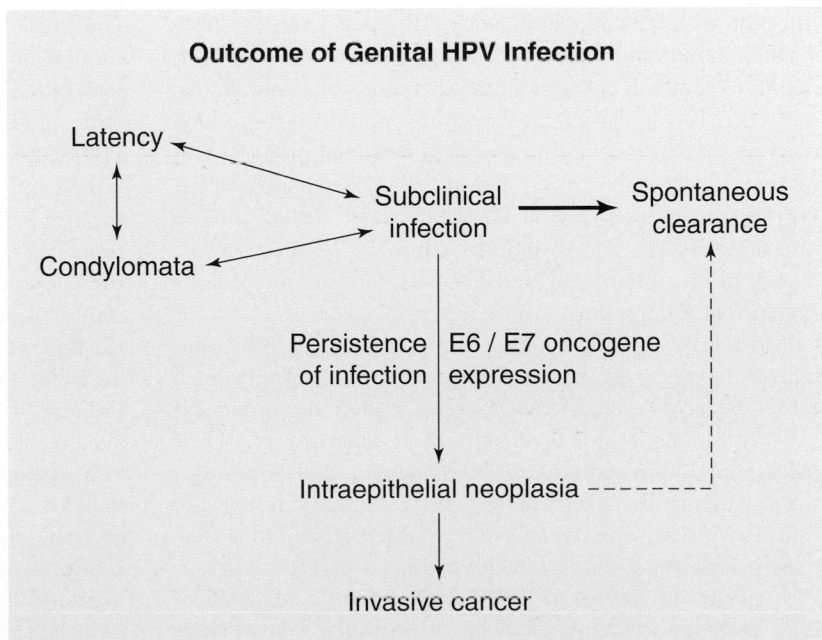

FIGURE 29-7 The natural history of genital HPV infection is variable between individuals and over time. Most infections are subclinical. Spontaneous resolution is the most common outcome. Neoplasia is the least common manifestation of HPV infection, developing as the result of persistent infection.

(LSILs), by colposcopic abnormalities, and by histology as flat condyloma or CIN 1. However, such diagnoses are indirect and do not always accurately reflect the presence or absence of HPV.

Neoplastic HPV Infection

In CIN 3 and cancerous lesions, the circular HPV genome breaks open and integrates linearly at random locations into a host chromosome (Fig. 30-1, p. 771). Unrestrained transcription of the E6 and E7 oncogenes follows (Durst, 1985; Stoler, 1996). The products, the E6 and E7 oncoproteins, interfere with the function of and accelerate degradation of p53 and pRB, which are key host tumor suppressor proteins (Fig. 30-2, p. 772). This leaves the infected cell vulnerable to malignant transformation by loss of cell-cycle control, cellular proliferation, and accumulation of DNA mutations over time (Doorbar, 2005).

In preinvasive lesions, normal epithelial differentiation is curtailed. The degree of abnormal epithelial maturation is used to grade lesion histology as mild, moderate, or severe dysplasia or CIN (see Fig. 29-1). The average age at diagnosis of low-grade cervical disease is younger than that of high-grade lesions and invasive cancers. Thus, it has long been assumed that a disease continuum exists with progression from mild to higher-grade lesions over time. An alternative theory proposes that low-grade lesions are generally transient and not oncogenic, whereas high-grade lesions and cancers are monoclonal, arising de novo without prerequisite low-grade disease (Baseman, 2005; Kiviat, 1996). This may explain why some cancers are diagnosed soon after negative cytologic screening.

Natural History of HPV Infection

Infection with HPV, predominantly HR types, is very common soon after initiation of sexual activity (Brown, 2005; Winer, 2003). Collins and colleagues (2002) conducted a longitudinal study of 242 women recruited within 6 months of beginning their first sexual relationship and who remained monogamous to that one sexual partner. During 3 years of surveillance, 46 percent acquired cervical HPV infection. Median time to infection was less than 3 months. Thus, HPV infection is a marker of the initiation of sexual activity and is not necessarily evidence of promiscuity.

Most HPV lesions, whether clinical or subclinical, spontaneously regress, especially in adolescents and young women (Ho, 1998; Moscicki, 1998). Several studies show that LR HPV infections resolve faster than those involving HR HPV (Moscicki, 2004; Schlecht, 2003; Woodman, 2001). Younger women frequently change HPV types, reflecting transience of infection and sequential reinfection by new partners rather than persistence (Ho, 1998; Rosenfeld, 1992).

Estimates of short-term risk of progression from incident HPV infection to high-grade neoplasia in young women range from 3 to 31 percent (Moscicki, 2004; Wright, 2005). The risk of progression to high-grade neoplasia increases with age, as HPV infection in older women is more likely to be a persistent infection (Hildesheim, 1999).

HPV Prevalence

Genital HPV is the most common sexually transmitted infection. The Centers for Disease Control and Prevention (2002) estimate that the risk of a woman acquiring genital HPV by age 50 is greater than 80 percent. Most incident HPV infections develop in women younger than 25 years. The point prevalence in U.S. females aged 14 to 59 years by single genital HPV testing is 27 percent. It is highest in the 20- to 24-year-old age group (45 percent) and becomes less prevalent with increasing age (Dunne, 2007). By comparison, the prevalence of genital warts is approximately 1 percent, and cytologic abnormalities less than 10 percent. These findings indicate that inapparent (subclinical) infection is far more common than clinically apparent infection (Koutsky, 1997).

Risk Factors for HPV Infection

The most important risk factors for the acquisition of genital HPV infection are the number of lifetime and recent sexual partners and early age at first sexual intercourse (Burk, 1996; Fairley, 1994; Franco, 1995; Melkert, 1993).

Diagnosis of HPV Infection

Infection with HPV is suspected by the appearance of clinical lesions and the results of cytology, histology, and colposcopy, all of which are subjective and often inaccurate. In addition, serology is unreliable and unable to distinguish past from current infection (Carter, 2000; Dillner, 1999). Therefore, a sure diagnosis can be made only by the direct detection of HPV DNA. This can be done histologically by in situ hybridization, by nucleic acid amplification testing, by polymerase chain reaction (PCR), or by other techniques (Molijn, 2005). Currently, two products are approved by the U.S. Food and Drug Administration (FDA) for clinical use. The Digene HC2 High-Risk HPV DNA Test uses a mixture of RNA probes for the detection of 13 oncogenic HPV types. The newer Cervista HPV HR test uses DNA amplification to detect the same 13 HPVs as Digene HC2, plus one additional high-risk HPV type (HPV 66). Both tests detect HR HPV infection caused by any one or more of the HPV types included in the test panel, but do not specifically identify which among those HR HPV types is present. However, a different test, the Cervista HPV 16/18 test, can be used subsequent to a positive Cervista HPV HR test result to specifically identify the presence of HPVs 16 and 18. For all these tests, cells can be collected into a liquid-based cytology medium, namely, PreservCyt Solution (ThinPrep Pap Test). Digene HC2 also allows collection into a specific collection tube.

If typical genital warts are found in a young woman or if high-grade cervical neoplasia or invasive cancer is identified by cytology or histology, then HPV infection is assumed, and confirmation by HPV testing is not necessary. Routine testing for HPV is not currently indicated outside of the following settings: cervical cancer screening in women aged 30 years or older, triage or surveillance of certain abnormal cytology results, and posttreatment surveillance. HPV testing is not indicated for primary screening in women younger than 30 years or for any indication in women under age 21 because of the high prevalence rates and viral clearance rates in these groups. HPV testing is also not FDA approved for use in women after total hysterectomy. There is no longer any clinical indication for low-risk HPV testing; doing so can lead to inappropriate expense, further evaluation, and unnecessary treatment.

■ Treatment of HPV Infection

The indications to treat HPV-related lower genital tract disease are symptomatic warts that cause physical or psychologic discomfort, high-grade neoplasia, or invasive cancer. HPV infection diagnosed by clinical impression, cytology, histology, or HPV DNA testing should not prompt treatment.

Various treatment modalities are available for warts and are chosen according to wart size, location, and number. Mechanical removal or destruction, topical immunomodulators, and chemical or thermal coagulation can be used (Table 3-21, p. 89). There is no effective treatment for subclinical HPV infection. Needless physical damage can be done to the lower genital tract during unrealistic attempts to eradicate HPV infections, which are usually self-limited.

Examination of a male partner does not benefit a female partner either by influencing reinfection or by altering the clinical course or treatment outcome for genital warts or lower genital tract neoplasia (Centers for Disease Control and Prevention, 2002).

■ Prevention of HPV Infection

Behavioral Interventions

Sexual abstinence, delaying coitarche, and limiting the number of sexual partners are logical strategies to avoid or limit genital HPV infection and its adverse effects. However, evidence from trials of counseling and sexual practice modification is lacking.

Condoms. Use of condoms is recommended for prevention of sexually transmitted infections (STIs) in general, but their efficacy specifically in preventing HPV transmission is less certain. Male condoms are more effective at preventing STIs transmitted through body fluids and across mucosal surfaces, and less effective for STIs spread skin-to-skin, as is the case with HPV. Moreover, condoms do not cover all anogenital skin that is potentially infected (Centers for Disease Control and Prevention, 2010b). However, Winer and associates (2003) conducted the first prospective study of male condom use and HPV risk in young women and showed reductions in HPV infection rates even if condoms were not consistently used.

HPV Vaccines

Recent and ongoing development of vaccines offers the greatest promise for prevention of HPV infection and perhaps for limiting or reversing its sequelae in those already infected.

Immunology of HPV Infection. The immunology of HPV infection is only partially understood. It appears that local and humoral immunity protect against initial infection. Cell-mediated immunity likely plays the larger role in HPV infection persistence, as well as progression or regression of benign and neoplastic lesions. HPV evades immune control by a variety of mechanisms. These include limitation of the infection to the epithelium and therefore absence of a viremic phase; low-level expression of early genes; the nonlytic, noninflammatory nature of the infection; and delayed production of the highly immunogenic capsid proteins within the superficial squames (Kanodia, 2007).

Prophylactic HPV Vaccines. Prophylactic vaccines elicit the production of humoral antibodies that neutralize HPV before it can infect host cells (Christensen, 2001). They do not prevent transient HPV positivity or resolve preexistent infection. However, they do prevent the establishment of new and persistent infection and subsequent development of neoplasia.

Currently, two vaccines are FDA approved for prevention of incident HPV infections and cervical neoplasia. They use recombinant technologies for the synthetic production of the L1 capsid proteins of each HPV type included in the vaccine. The resultant virus-like particles are highly immunogenic, but they are not infectious as they lack viral DNA (Stanley, 2006b). The immune response to both vaccines is much stronger and consistent than that seen in response to naturally occurring infections (Stanley, 2006a; Villa, 2006).

Gardasil is a quadrivalent vaccine against HPV types 6, 11, 16, and 18. Cervarix is a bivalent vaccine against HPVs 16 and 18. Each contains a different adjuvant that boosts the immune response of the recipient to the vaccine antigens. Administered in three intramuscular doses during a 6-month period, both vaccines are extremely safe and well tolerated (Table 1-1, p. 8) (Harper, 2006; Mao, 2006). Vaccination strategies should emphasize administration prior to initiation of sexual activity, when the potential benefit is greatest. However, a history of previous sexual intercourse or HPV-related disease is not a contraindication to vaccine administration. This is because previous exposure and the magnitude of natural immune response to the HPV types targeted by the vaccines cannot be determined for any individual. Accordingly, testing for HPV is not recommended prior to vaccination (American College of Obstetricians and Gynecologists, 2010b). The Advisory Committee on Immunization Practices currently recommends that either HPV vaccine be administered routinely to girls aged 11 to 12 years (as early as age 9 years). Vaccination is also recommended for 13- to 26-year-old individuals, ideally before potential exposure through sexual contact (Centers for Disease Control and Prevention, 2010a). Vaccination can be given to lactating women but should not be given during pregnancy (Category B) (American College of Obstetricians and Gynecologists, 2010b). Immunocompromised women are candidates to receive the vaccine but theoretically may not develop antibody titers as high as those of immunocompetent women. Women should be advised that these vaccines are expected to prevent approximately 70 percent of cervical cancers, but they will not protect against the approximately 30 percent caused by oncogenic HPV types not covered in the vaccine. HPV vaccination, therefore, does not negate the need for cervical cancer screening.

Both vaccines show nearly 100-percent efficacy in prevention of incident infection and high-grade cervical neoplasia from HPV types 16 and 18 (Future II Study Group, 2007; Paavonen, 2009). Debate over the superiority of either vaccine center around: (1) the range of HPV infections and clinical lesions prevented, (2) cross-protection against HPV types not covered by the vaccine, and (3) the strength and duration of the provoked immune response (Bornstein, 2009).

First, Gardasil protects additionally against HPVs 6 and 11, which cause nearly all genital warts as well as a significant portion of low-grade cytologic abnormalities requiring evaluation. Gardasil is approved for the prevention of genital warts in both males and females. It is also FDA approved for the prevention of vaginal, vulvar, and anal neoplasia (Centers for Disease Control and Prevention, 2010a). Cervarix does not prevent genital warts and is not yet approved for the prevention of extracervical lower genital tract disease.

Regarding the second debate point, Cervarix has demonstrated cross-protection against HPVs 45, 31, and 52, whereas Gardasil shows cross-reactivity for only HPV 31 (Brown, 2009; Jenkins, 2008). HPV 45 is a significant cause of cervical adenocarcinomas. These tumors are more difficult to detect and prevent than squamous lesions and are increasing in incidence (Huh, 2007). This cross-coverage for HPV types not specifically targeted by either vaccine could potentially protect against an additional 10 to 20 percent of cervical cancers.

If immunogenicity is compared, both vaccines are highly immunogenic and have shown maintenance of protection for at least 5 years after vaccination. Cervarix claims that its adjuvant induces higher and more sustained antibody levels than that of Gardasil. However, antibody levels do not necessarily correlate with duration of clinical protection, and both vaccines have shown excellent immune memory (Bornstein, 2009).

The efficacy of the two vaccines has not been compared in any published clinical trials to date. Although it is clear that both can greatly decrease the burden of HPV-related disease, neither has been proven to decrease the incidence of or mortality rates from cervical cancer compared with routine cytologic screening.

Therapeutic Vaccines. The development of effective therapeutic vaccines for the mitigation or eradication of established HPV-related disease, including genital warts, preinvasive lesions, and invasive cancer, presents far greater challenges. The cell-mediated immunology of HPV is more complex and less understood than its humoral immunity. Persistent HPV infection in any form is an indication that the host-HPV interaction has evaded an individual's immune responsiveness. Research and clinical trials were last reviewed by Padilla-Paz (2005) and to date have shown very limited success of therapeutic vaccines.

CERVICAL INTRAEPITHELIAL NEOPLASIA

Incidence

The true incidence of CIN can only be estimated. Of the approximate 7 percent of Pap tests with epithelial abnormalities found annually during screening in the United States, perhaps half represent any degree of histologic CIN (Jones, 2000). The incidence of CIN will vary by population studied, as it is strongly related to younger age of sexual activity, socioeconomic factors, and a variety of other risk-related behaviors. Moreover, the clinical methods used to diagnose CIN, mainly screening cytology and colposcopy, both lack sensitivity.

Natural History

Preinvasive lesions can spontaneously regress to normal, remain stable for long periods, or progress to a higher degree of dysplasia. Although few CIN lesions have the potential to progress to frankly invasive cancer, neoplastic potential increases with CIN grade. Hall and Walton (1968) observed progression to CIS in 6 percent of histologic "slight" dysplasias, 13 percent of moderate dysplasias, and 29 percent of "marked" dysplasias. Slight dysplasia regressed or disappeared in 62 percent but did so in only 19 percent of those with marked disease. The best available estimates of CIN progression, persistence, and regression are provided in a review by Ostor (1993) and shown in Table 29-1. Recently, Castle and associates (2009b) calculated that approximately 40 percent of CIN 2 regresses spontaneously within 2 years.

Risk Factors

Identifiable risk factors for cervical intraepithelial neoplasia are similar to those of invasive lesions and prove useful in the development of cervical cancer screening and prevention programs (Table 29-2). The risk of cervical neoplasia is most strongly related to persistent genital HR HPV infection and older age (Ho, 1995; Kjaer, 2002; Remmink, 1995; Schiffman, 2005). Other, less robust demographic, behavioral, and medical risk factors for cervical neoplasia have been proposed.

Age

In the United States, the median age of cervical cancer diagnosis is 48 years, approximately a decade later than CIN (National Cancer Institute, 2011). HPV infection in an older woman is more likely to be persistent than transient. Older age also allows

TABLE 29-1. Natural History of Cervical Intraepithelial Neoplasia Lesions

	Regression (%)	Persistence (%)	Progression to CIS (%)	Progression to Invasion (%)
CIN 1	57	32	11	1
CIN 2	43	35	22	5
CIN 3	32	<56	—	>12

CIN = cervical intraepithelial neoplasia; CIS = carcinoma in situ.
From Ostor, 1993, with permission.

TABLE 29-2. Risk Factors for Cervical Neoplasia

Demographic risk factors
Ethnicity (Latin American countries, U.S. minorities)
Low socioeconomic status
Increasing age

Behavioral risk factors
Early coitarche
Multiple sexual partners
Male partner who has had multiple sexual partners
Tobacco smoking
Dietary deficiencies

Medical risk factors
Cervical high-risk human papillomavirus infection
Exogenous hormones (combination oral contraceptives)
Parity
Immunosuppression
Inadequate screening

accumulation of mutations that can lead to cellular malignant transformation. Additionally, decreased needs for prenatal care and contraception cause older women to access cervical cancer prevention programs less often.

Behavior Risk Factors

The most consistently recognized behavioral risk factors for cervical neoplasia are noted in Table 29-2 (Brinton, 1992; Suris, 1999). Such behaviors increase the risk of acquiring oncogenic HPV infection. For many years, epidemiologic evidence has linked sexual behaviors such as early onset of sexual activity, multiple sexual partners, and male partner promiscuity with cervical neoplasia (Buckley, 1981; de Vet, 1994; Kjaer, 1991).

Tobacco Smoking. Cervical cancer is now established as a smoking-related cancer. This is specifically true for squamous cancers, and the relationship to adeno- and adenosquamous cervical cancer is less certain (International Agency for Research on Cancer, 2004). Tobacco use also increases the risks of preinvasive cervical disease, and this relationship persists even after adjustments for HPV positivity and lower socioeconomic status are made (Bosch, 2002; Castle, 2004; Plummer, 2003). Current smoking, higher pack-years of use, and smoking at the time of menarche are all associated with cervical neoplasia (Becker, 1994). The biologic plausibility of a link between tobacco and cervical neoplasia is supported by several points: (1) cervical mucus of smokers contains carcinogens and is mutagenic; (2) genetic alterations in the cervical tissue of smokers are similar to those seen in smoking-related neoplasias at other sites; (3) risk is dose-dependent, increasing with both duration and amount of tobacco use; and (4) risk decreases with cessation of smoking (U.S. Department of Health and Human Services, 2004).

Dietary Deficiencies. Although data are inconclusive, dietary deficiencies of certain vitamins such as A, C, E, beta carotene,

and folic acid may alter cellular resistance to HPV infection and thus may promote viral infection persistence and cervical neoplasia (Paavonen, 1990). However, in the United States, lack of association between dietary deficiencies and cervical disease may reflect the relatively sufficient nutritional status of even lower-income women (Amburgey, 1993).

Medical Risk Factors

Exogenous Hormones. Studies linking cervical neoplasia and exogenous hormones are conflicting and fraught with confounders such as increased sexual activity and Pap screening in users. Moreover, epithelial cell cancers are generally not influenced by hormonal factors. The largest analysis of epidemiological studies to date, the International Collaboration of Epidemiological studies of Cervical Cancer (2007), concludes that there is an increased risk of cervical cancer in current users of combination oral contraceptives (COCs) that is related to duration of use. Moreover, the relative risk nearly doubles at 5 years of COC use. The increased risk declines after COC use ceases, and risk returns to that of nonusers 10 years after use stops. The International Agency for Research on Cancer (2007) therefore classifies COCs as carcinogenic to humans. Possible mechanisms by which COCs might influence cervical cancer risk include increased persistence of infection and HPV oncogene expression (de Villiers, 2003). However, analysis of young women enrolled in the Atypical Squamous Cells of Undetermined Significance-Low Grade Intraepithelial Lesion Triage Study (ALTS) found that noninjectable hormonal contraceptives, pregnancy, and parity had little effect on the acquisition of high-risk HPV infection or development of CIN 3 (Castle, 2005). Harris and associates (2009) found no increased risk of high-grade neoplasia in either depot-medroxyprogesterone or COC users. Finally, there was no increased risk observed among postmenopausal estrogen-progestin users in the Women's Health Initiative Study (Yasmeen, 2006).

Parity. Increasing parity has been correlated with cervical cancer risk, but it is unclear if this is related to earlier sexual activity, a progestin exposure effect, or other factors. Immune suppression during pregnancy, hormonal influences on cervical epithelium, and physical trauma related to vaginal deliveries have been suggested as etiologic factors associated with the development of cervical neoplasia (Brinton, 1989; Muñoz, 2002).

Immunosuppression. Studies consistently suggest that human immunodeficiency virus (HIV)-positive women have higher rates of CIN compared with HIV-negative women (Ellerbrock, 2000; Wright, 1994). In women infected with HIV, up to 60 percent of Pap tests exhibit cytologic abnormalities, and as many as 40 percent have colposcopic evidence of dysplasia (p. 762). As reviewed by Gomez-Lobo (2009), transplant recipients have an increased risk of developing a malignancy after transplantation, including neoplasms of the lower genital tract and anal canal. Women on immunosuppressive medications for other disorders have higher rates of lower genital tract neoplasia. Immunosuppressed women in general show increased severity, multifocal lesion pattern, treatment failure, persistence, and recurrence of lower genital tract disease compared with those who are immunocompetent.

Inadequate Screening

Cervical cancer prevention requires identification and eradication of precursor or early invasive lesions through cytologic screening. It is estimated that half of women diagnosed with cervical cancer have never been screened and an additional 10 percent have not had a Pap test during the prior 5 years (National Institutes of Health, 1996). Lack of screening is a major contributor to higher rates of cervical cancer in socioeconomically disadvantaged women. Minority ethnicity, recent immigration from underdeveloped countries, rural residency within the United States, and older age all increase cervical cancer risk (Benard, 2007).

Differential Diagnosis and Evaluation of Cervical Lesions

In general, preinvasive lesions of the lower genital tract are not visible to unaided inspection. The exception to this is VIN 3, which is often visible or palpable or both. Only cervical lesions at either end of the neoplastic disease spectrum are grossly visible: condylomata and invasive cancers. Accordingly, all grossly visible cervical lesions, particularly ulcers, erosions, or leukoplakias, are justification for colposcopic examination and require biopsy.

Cervical Cytology

Cervical cytologic screening is one of modern medicine's greatest success stories. The Pap test detects most cervical neoplasia during the typically prolonged premalignant or early occult malignant phases, when treatment outcomes are optimal.

Efficacy of Cervical Cancer Screening

The Pap test has never been evaluated in a randomized, controlled or masked trial (Koss, 1989). However, countries with organized screening programs have consistently realized a dramatic decline, generally 60 to 70 percent, in both cervical cancer incidence and mortality rates (Noller, 2005; World Health Organization, 2010). The Pap test's specificity is consistently high, approximating 98 percent. However, estimates of its sensitivity are lower and more variable. Imperfect sensitivity is countered by recommendations for repetitive screening throughout a woman's life. Although the incidence of cervical squamous carcinomas continues to decline, both the relative and absolute incidences of adenocarcinomas have increased, particularly in women younger than age 50 (Herzog, 2007). Adenocarcinomas and adenosquamous carcinomas now account for more than 20 percent of cervical cancers. This increase is believed to be due in large part to the Pap test being less sensitive for the detection of adenocarcinomas than for squamous lesions.

Women should be aware of the imperfect sensitivity of the Pap test and the need for periodic screening. Likewise, providers should use the Pap test appropriately as a screening test in asymptomatic women. Physical findings or symptoms suspicious for cervical cancer should be evaluated immediately with diagnostic studies such as colposcopy and biopsy.

Although up to 60 percent of cervical cancer cases in screened populations are associated with inadequate screening, 30 to 40 percent develop in adequately screened women due to false-negative test results or inadequate management of abnormal results (Carmichael, 1984). False-negative Pap test results may be caused by sampling error, in which abnormal cells are not present in the Pap test; by screening error, in which the cells are present but missed by the screener; or by interpretation error, in which abnormal cells are misclassified as benign (Wilkinson, 1990). Mandated quality assurance measures and computerized slide-screening technologies address the latter two factors. Clinicians must maximize the benefit of screening by obtaining an optimal cytologic specimen and by adhering to evidence-based guidelines for the management of abnormal test results.

Performing a Pap Test

Patient Preparation. Ideally, Pap tests should be scheduled to avoid menstruation. Patients should abstain from vaginal intercourse, douching, and use of vaginal tampons and medicinal or contraceptive creams for a minimum of 24 to 48 hours before a test. Treatment of cervicitis or vaginitis prior to Pap testing is optimal. However, Pap testing should never be deferred due to unexplained discharge or unscheduled bleeding, as these may be caused by cervical or other genital tract cancers.

As shown in Figure 21-11 (p. 576), the appearance of cervical squamous cells varies throughout the menstrual cycle and with hormone status changes. Thus, provision of clinical information on requisition forms is essential to accurate interpretation of a Pap test. This includes date of last menstrual period or current pregnancy, exogenous hormone use, menopausal status, complaints of abnormal bleeding, and any history of abnormal Pap tests, dysplasia, or cancer. Additionally, intrauterine devices (IUDs) can cause reactive cellular changes, and their presence should be noted. Important risk factors such as immune compromise, recent immigration from an underdeveloped country, or prior lack of adequate screening may be helpful.

Adequate visualization of the cervix is essential for detection of gross lesions and identification of the SCJ. Speculum placement should be as comfortable as possible. A thin coating of water-based lubricant can be used on the outside of the speculum blades without compromising Pap quality or interpretation (Griffith, 2005; Harmanli, 2010). Touching the cervix prior to performing a Pap should be avoided, as dysplastic epithelium may be inadvertently removed with minimal trauma. Discharge covering the cervix may be carefully removed with a large swab, with care not to contact the cervix. Vigorous blotting or rubbing may cause scant cellularity or a false-negative Pap test result. When indicated, additional cervical sampling to detect infection should follow Pap test collection.

Location. Sampling of the transformation zone is paramount to the sensitivity of the Pap test. Technique should be adapted and sampling devices chosen according to the location of the SCJ, which varies widely with age, obstetric trauma, and hormonal status. Women known or suspected of in utero DES exposure may also benefit from a separate Pap test of the upper vagina, as these women are at additional risk for vaginal cancers (Chap. 32, p. 813) (Kaufman, 2005).

Sampling Devices. Three types of devices are commonly used to sample the cervix and include the spatula, the broom, and

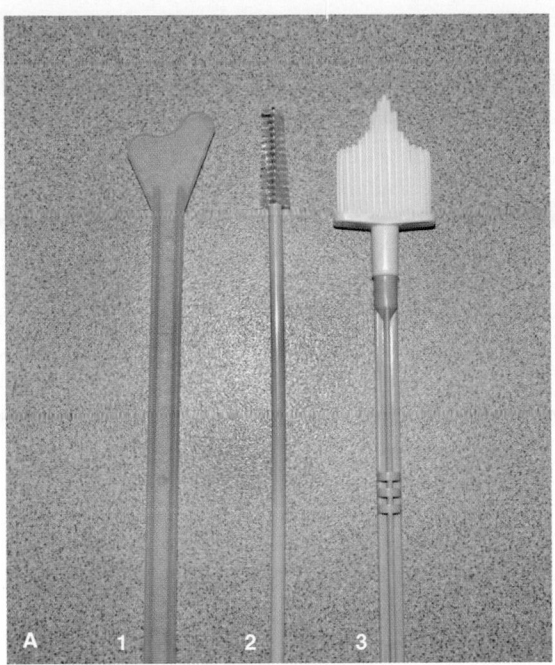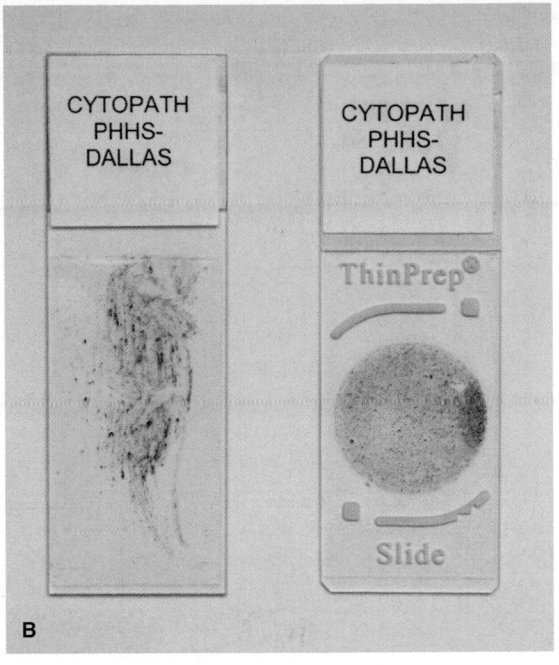

FIGURE 29-8 A. Cervical cytology collection devices. **1.** Plastic spatula. **2.** Endocervical brush. **3.** Plastic broom. **B.** PAP smear preparations. Conventional cervical cytology is prepared by smearing collected cells directly onto a glass slide with the collection device followed by immediate fixation (*left slide*). Thin-layer liquid-based cytology involves transfer of collected cells from the collection device into a liquid transport medium with subsequent processing and transfer onto a glass slide. Cells are distributed over a smaller area, and debris, mucus, blood, and cell overlap are largely eliminated (*right slide*). *(Photograph contributed by Dr. Raheela Ashfaq.)*

the endocervical brush (also known as a cytobrush) (Fig. 29-8) (Saslow, 2002; Spitzer, 1999). A spatula predominantly samples the ectocervix. An endocervical brush samples the endocervical canal and is used in combination with a spatula. A broom samples both endo- and ectocervical epithelia simultaneously, but can be supplemented by an endocervical brush.

A spatula is oriented to best fit the cervical contour, straddle the squamocolumnar junction, and sample the distal endocervical canal. A clinician firmly scrapes the cervical surface, completing at least one full rotation. A plastic spatula is preferred to wood because cells are more easily released from the plastic surface.

The endocervical brush, with its conical shape and plastic bristles, has largely replaced the moistened cotton swab to sample the endocervical canal because of its superior ability to collect and release cells. After the spatula sample is obtained, the endocervical brush is inserted into the endocervical canal only until the outermost bristles remain visible just within the external os. This prevents inadvertent sampling of lower uterine segment cells, which can be mistaken for atypical cervical cells. To avoid obscuring blood, the brush is rotated only one-quarter to one-half turn and is used after the ectocervix has been sampled. If the cervical canal is very wide, the brush is moved so as to contact all surfaces of the endocervical canal.

Broom devices have longer central bristles that are inserted into the endocervical canal. These longer bristles are flanked by shorter bristles that splay out over the ectocervix during rotation. The recommended number of broom rotations varies by device manufacturer but is usually five rotations in the same direction (reversing direction causes loss of cellular material). Broom devices are favored for liquid-based Pap testing.

Conventional Slide Collection. This method requires special care to avoid air drying of cells, which is a leading cause of poor slide quality. The spatula sample should be held while the endocervical brush sampling immediately follows. The spatula sample is then quickly spread as evenly as possible over one half to two thirds of a glass slide (see Fig. 29-8). The endocervical brush is firmly rolled over the remaining area of the slide, after which fixation is quickly carried out by spraying with or immersing in fixative.

Liquid-Based Test Collection. Currently, two liquid-based Pap tests are FDA approved. Sampling and cell transfer to a liquid medium should be performed according to manufacturer specifications. BD SurePath allows for the use of all three device types, but with modified tips that can be broken off and sent to the laboratory in the liquid medium. ThinPrep requires immediate and vigorous agitation of the chosen collection device in the liquid medium, after which the device is discarded.

Comparison of Conventional and Liquid-Based Cytology

FDA approval of the first liquid-based cytology tests (LBCs), ThinPrep in 1996 followed by BD SurePath in 1999, represented the first significant change in Pap testing since its clinical debut in the early 1940s. Scores of published studies lauded the increased sensitivity and readability of liquid-based Pap cytologies compared with conventional glass slide Pap tests. Indeed, both LBCs were FDA approved to claim a greater than 60-percent increased detection of cervical disease compared with conventional Pap testing and lower unsatisfactory rates. As a result, 80 to 90 percent of Pap tests currently performed in the

United States use liquid-based technology. This is largely driven by the volume of supportive studies, difficulty in finding labs that will still read conventional Pap slide tests, and potential medicolegal jeopardy should a case of cervical cancer be diagnosed after a negative conventional Pap test result.

The potential superiority of LBCs seems plausible on two fronts: (1) improved cell collection and preparation quality and (2) random distribution of abnormal cells on the test slide. Goodman and Hutchinson (1996) demonstrated that after a conventional Pap is prepared, most cellular material remains on the collection device and is discarded. Although examination of the excess material ordinarily discarded with the device did not result in additional diagnoses of HSIL or cancer, the loss of most cervical material collected has raised concern. Additionally, conventional Pap quality is very much provider dependent, causing wide variation in smear thickness, cellularity, and compromise by air-drying artifact due to delay in fixation. Patient factors such as presence of inflammatory exudates, atrophy, or bleeding create variability in slide quality as well.

In comparison, automated processing of LBCs produces an even monolayer of cells that covers less area of the slide. The number of cells present is generally less than a conventional Pap. However, obscuring blood, mucus, debris, and cell overlap are largely eliminated. Theoretically, abnormal cells, which might be few in number, clustered, or obscured on a conventional Pap slide, will be randomly and evenly distributed over the LBC slide and thus be more visible for detection. In addition, most of the collected cellular material is available for laboratory processing rather than being discarded.

Despite the theoretical advantages LBC offers, its superior performance over conventional Pap testing has not been demonstrated conclusively. Also of concern are the greatly increased costs of the LBC testing and its decreased specificity (Davey, 2006; Sawaya, 1999). Ronco and coworkers (2006) published the first, largest, and best-designed randomized controlled trial to date comparing conventional Pap testing and LBCs in a screening population. LBC sensitivity was not superior to that of conventional Pap testing and showed a significantly lower positive predictive value. A recent review of all studies published with metaanalysis by Arbyn and associates (2008) found fewer than 10 studies with high-quality study designs and verification of cytologic abnormalities with colposcopy and histology. They conclude that LBC is not more sensitive than conventional cytology. LBCs consistently show a lower rate of unsatisfactory tests, although these represent less than 2 percent of Pap tests in most U.S. labs (Arbyn, 2008; Siebers, 2008). Sawaya (2008) summarizes the disadvantages of LBCs including decreased specificity, particularly in younger women, which is not balanced by increased sensitivity.

At present, the American College of Obstetricians and Gynecologists (2009) deems both cytologic methods as acceptable. It is doubtful that Pap testing will revert back to a predominance of conventional smears despite growing evidence refuting the superiority of LBC and its greater cost. Laboratories generally prefer to read LBCs. Also, LBC permits computerized screening of slides and concomitant testing for infections, including HPV, which can be conveniently performed on residual material. Resource-limited health care systems can be reassured that conventional Pap tests are a cost-effective approach to cervical cancer screening without compromise of disease detection.

Screening Guidelines

Current cervical cancer screening guidelines are more evidence-based and comprehensive than in the past. The three agencies offering guidelines are the American College of Obstetricians and Gynecologists (ACOG) (2009), the American Cancer Society (ACS) (Saslow, 2002), and the U.S. Preventive Services Task Force (USPSTF) (2003). The more recent ACOG guidelines include significant changes in initiation and intervals of screening. The other two agencies are expected to update their screening guidelines in 2012. This section will primarily discuss the updated ACOG guidelines. Adherence to current guidelines should not preclude or delay other indicated gynecologic care. Thus, access to contraception and other medical care should never be contingent upon compliance with cervical cancer screening recommendations or evaluation of cytologic abnormalities.

Initiation of Screening. HPV-related disease acts differently in younger than in older populations, and newer Pap test guidelines reflect these differences. First, adolescents have higher rates of Pap abnormalities than adult women and very high rates of histologic CIN (Case, 2006). However, many Pap abnormalities represent transient HPV infection, and spontaneous regression of even high-grade lesions is common in young women (Moscicki, 2005). Most high-grade lesions are CIN 2 rather than CIN 3 in young women, and cervical cancer has generally not been found in large studies of adolescents (Moscicki, 2008). Additionally, treatment of high-grade CIN in adolescents with excisional procedures is often followed by persistence of Pap abnormalities and thus does not achieve therapeutic goals (Case, 2006; Moore, 2007). Finally, as reviewed by ACOG (2009), cervical cancer does occur in adolescents, but it is rare and not as preventable with screening as in older women.

In response to this improved understanding of cervical disease in adolescents, it is now recommended that screening begin at age 21 years regardless of sexual history (American College of Obstetricians and Gynecologists, 2009). Exceptions to this are conditions of immune compromise, including HIV infection, use of immunosuppressive medications, and organ transplantation. In such cases, screening should begin at sexual activity onset, even if before age 21, and should consist of two Pap tests at 6-month intervals during the first year, then annually (American College of Obstetricians and Gynecologists, 2010a; Centers for Disease Control and Prevention, 2009a,b). Pregnancy or diagnosis of an STI other than HIV does not alter the recommendation to defer initiation of Pap testing until age 21 (American College of Obstetricians and Gynecologists, 2010a).

Screening Interval. Between ages 21 and 29, ACOG (2009) recommends Pap testing at 2-year intervals using either conventional or liquid-based methods. At age 30, women at average risk for cervical cancer can be screened at 3-year intervals if three previous, consecutive, Pap tests have been documented as negative. The cancer risk is very low within this time frame. Women eligible for extended screening intervals should be educated that the Pap test is only one component of preventive health care and does not preclude the need for other health care evaluations. Women at higher than average risk, including those with in utero diethylstilbestrol exposure or immunocompromise, may warrant more frequent screening. Specifically, women with HIV infection should receive annual screening for life (Centers for Disease Control and Prevention, 2009b). Women with prior treatment for CIN 2, CIN 3, or cervical cancer should receive annual screening for at least 20 years as they remain at increased long-term risk of cervical cancer (American College of Obstetricians and Gynecologists, 2009; Strander, 2007).

Discontinuation of Screening.
Screening may be stopped at age 65 or 70 in women with average risk for cervical cancer after three consecutive, negative Pap results during the prior 10 years (American College of Obstetricians and Gynecologists, 2009; Saslow, 2002). The USPSTF (2003) recommends that screening stop at age 65. ACOG (2009) alone recommends that older women who are sexually active and have multiple partners continue routine screening because it is unclear if the postmenopausal cervix remains at increased risk of neoplasia when exposed to new HPV infection.

Hysterectomy.
Vaginal cancers are rare, accounting for less than 2 percent of cancers in women. All three agencies recommend against Pap screening in women who have undergone total hysterectomy for benign disease if there is no past history of high-grade CIN or cervical cancer. The absence of a cervix should be confirmed by examination or pathology report. Women who have undergone supracervical hysterectomy still have a cervix and should continue routine screening. Recommendations for vaginal cytology after hysterectomy in women with histories of high-grade cervical neoplasia or cancer are less clear. Current American Cancer Society (Saslow, 2002) and ACOG (2009) guidelines recommend screening beyond the initial posttreatment surveillance of three Pap tests in 2 years, although the duration and frequency of this continued screening are not specified. In the absence of clear, evidence-based guidelines, it seems prudent that cytologic screening of the vaginal cuff in women with histories of high-grade cervical neoplasia or cancer continue at 1- to 3-year intervals and for a duration decided by provider discretion. HPV testing is not FDA-approved for vaginal testing but is frequently requested in conjunction with vaginal cytology. Clinical data are of limited utility in this setting, and evidence-based recommendations are lacking (Chappell, 2010).

HPV Testing for Primary Cervical Cancer Screening

Cytology and HPV Cotesting.
In 2003, the FDA approved the use of the Hybrid Capture 2 test for HR HPV in combination with cytology for primary cervical cancer screening in women aged 30 years and older. This strategy is not approved for women younger than 30 years due to the high prevalence of HR HPV infection, which makes this strategy ineffective. A cervical sample for HPV can be sent in a collection device separate from the cytology specimen. This allows simultaneous processing of the two components. Alternatively, HPV

testing can be performed from the LBC specimen remaining after the cytology slide is prepared. Testing is performed only for high-risk HPV types. There is no clinical role for low-risk HPV testing. This combination of HR HPV DNA testing with cytology increases the sensitivity of a single Pap test for high-grade neoplasia from 50 to 85 percent, to nearly 100 percent (American College of Obstetricians and Gynecologists, 2005). The lack of sensitivity for cervical adenocarcinoma seen with traditional cytologic testing also supports HPV testing use for primary screening (Castellsagué, 2006).

Due to a near-perfect negative predictive value for high-grade neoplasia, slow progression of new HPV infection to neoplasia, and increased cost, testing is performed at 3-year intervals if both test results are negative. Clinical guidelines have been developed for management of an abnormal HPV DNA test plus cytology result (Wright, 2007b). If cytology is abnormal, current cytology management guidelines are followed (p. 744). Cytology-negative and HPV-positive test results will occur in less than 10 percent of screened patients (Castle, 2009a; Datta, 2008). In such cases, both cytology and HPV DNA testing are repeated 12 months later, as the risk of high-grade neoplasia is less than that of an ASC-US Pap and most HPV infections will resolve during this time (Wright, 2007b). Colposcopy is recommended for persistently positive HPV DNA test results. An abnormal repeat cytology result is managed according to current guidelines regardless of concurrent HPV status.

An alternative strategy is now available for management of a negative cytology but positive HR HPV test result. A reflex test specifically for HPVs 16 and 18 can be performed. If positive, then immediate colposcopy is recommended (American Society for Colposcopy and Cervical Pathology, 2009). This protocol targets those at highest risk for significant disease. Khan and coworkers (2005) followed women with initially negative cytology results for 10 years and showed that the risk of developing CIN 3 or cancer was 17 percent for those positive for HPV 16 at enrollment and 14 percent for those with HPV 18, but only 3 percent for those infected with other HR HPVs. Such evidence provides a sound basis for this strategy.

HPV Testing Alone for Primary Screening.
A growing body of evidence supports the use of HR HPV testing without cytology for primary cervical cancer screening (Cuzick, 2006). HPV testing alone is approximately twice as sensitive (>90 percent) as a single Pap test and leads to earlier detection of high-grade neoplasias. However, there is a significant loss of specificity, particularly in younger women (Mayrand, 2007; Ronco, 2006, 2010). Strategies for surveillance of a positive HPV test result, such as reflex cytology for those who test positive, with or without genotyping for HPVs 16 and 18, are currently being investigated (Wright, 2007a).

Cervical Cancer Screening in Perspective.
The introduction of liquid-based cervical cytology and HPV DNA testing for both primary screening and reflex testing have added complexity and expense to cervical cancer screening to achieve supposed improved sensitivity. Despite widespread use and FDA-approved claims, liquid-based cytology does

not add sensitivity to Pap screening. Reflex HPV testing in response to ASC-US results is similar in sensitivity to repeat cytology (ASCUS-LSIL Triage Study Group, 2003b). HPV cotesting for primary screening appears to be more sensitive than a single Pap test alone and may lead to earlier diagnosis of high-grade neoplasia. However, this has not yet been proven to decrease either the incidence or mortality rate from cervical cancer compared with cytology alone. Of clinical importance, the optimal clinical response to the combination of a negative Pap test result and a positive HPV test result remains uncertain, and current recommendations were not developed by consensus. As screening technologies evolve, it is paramount that clinicians critically assess the complexity and cost posed by these options compared with actual lives saved. Fears of litigation if cervical cancer arises after conventional cytology screening should not drive use of liquid-based cytology. The USPSTF continues to recommend Pap screening every 3 years. It finds no advantage to annual screening intervals and likewise finds insufficient evidence to support liquid-based testing or HPV testing for either primary screening or triage (U.S. Preventive Services Task Force, 2003). Most importantly, these new technologies are less specific than cytology alone, causing potential harm in the form of increased evaluations and procedures with unproven efficacy in preventing additional cervical cancers, which are already rare in screened U.S. women. As reviewed by Sawaya (2010), clinicians and patients alike need to be vigilant and analytical in their approach to cervical cancer screening.

The 2001 Bethesda System

In 1988, standardization of cervical cytology reporting took place with the development of the Bethesda System nomenclature (National Cancer Institute Workshop, 1989). Subsequent revisions led to the 2001 Bethesda System in current use for reporting cervical cytology results. Its components are seen in Table 29-3 (Solomon, 2002). Clinically, the key elements reported are specimen adequacy and epithelial cell abnormalities (Table 29-4).

Specimen Adequacy. Specimen adequacy is reported as satisfactory or unsatisfactory for evaluation and is based primarily on criteria for slide cellularity and the presence of obscuring blood or inflammation. The presence or absence of transformation zone (TZ) components (endocervical or squamous metaplastic cells or both) is also reported. Their presence is not required for test adequacy but provides evidence that the area at risk for neoplasia has been sampled. Their presence is associated with increased detection of cytologic abnormalities, but their absence has not been associated with failure to diagnose CIN. Pap tests lacking TZ components or that are unsatisfactory due to obscuring blood or inflammation should be repeated in 1 year, or earlier if clinically indicated by individual risk factors and adequacy of past screening (American College of Obstetricians and Gynecologists, 2009; Saslow, 2002). In rare cases, obscuring blood and inflammation on cervical cytology indicate the presence of invasive cancer. Therefore, presence of an unexplained vaginal discharge, abnormal bleeding, or abnormal physical findings should

TABLE 29-3. The 2001 Bethesda System Cytology Report Components
Specimen type
Conventional Pap test
Thin-layer liquid-based cytology
Specimen adequacy
Satisfactory for evaluation
Unsatisfactory for evaluation
General categorization (optional)
Negative for intraepithelial lesion or malignancy
Epithelial cell abnormality (see Table 29-4)
Other findings that may indicate increased risk
Interpretation of results
Negative for intraepithelial lesion or malignancy
Organisms:
Trichomonas vaginalis
Fungal organisms consistent with *Candida* species
Shift in flora suggestive of bacterial vaginosis
Cellular change consistent with herpes simplex virus
Bacteria consistent with *Actinomyces* species
Other non-neoplastic findings (optional)
Reactive cellular changes (inflammation, repair, radiation)
Glandular cells posthysterectomy
Atrophy
Epithelial cell abnormalities
Squamous cell
Glandular cell
Other:
Endometrial cells in a woman ≥40 years of age
Automated review and ancillary testing as appropriate
Educational notes and recommendations (optional)

From Solomon, 2002, with permission.

prompt immediate evaluation rather than later repeat Pap testing.

Epithelial Cell Abnormalities: Significance and Management. A cytology report is a medical consultation that interprets a screening test and does not provide a diagnosis. A final diagnosis is determined clinically, often with results from histologic evaluation. Pap tests are interpreted as either negative for intraepithelial lesion or malignancy, or consistent with one or more epithelial cell abnormalities. Examples of normal and abnormal cytologic findings are shown in Figure 29-9. Evidence-based management guidelines have been developed to address epithelial cell abnormalities and are summarized in Table 29-5 (American College of Obstetricians and Gynecologists, 2009; Wright, 2007b). These draw heavily from the results of the ALTS study, which compared HPV testing, immediate colposcopy, and repeat cytology in a large, multicentered, randomized trial (ASCUS-LSIL Triage Study Group, 2003a,b). Alternative management strategies may be

TABLE 29-4. The 2001 Bethesda System: Epithelial Cell Abnormalities

Squamous cell
Atypical squamous cells (ASC)
  of undetermined significance (ASC-US)
  cannot exclude HSIL (ASC-H)
Low-grade squamous intraepithelial lesion (LSIL)
High-grade squamous intraepithelial lesion (HSIL)
Squamous cell carcinoma

Glandular cell
Atypical glandular cells (AGC)
  Endocervical, endometrial, or not otherwise specified
Atypical glandular cells, favor neoplastic
  Endocervical or not otherwise specified
Endocervical adenocarcinoma in situ (AIS)
Adenocarcinoma

From Solomon, 2002, with permission.

appropriate based on individual patient characteristics, available resources, and other clinical factors. General guidelines pertain to adult women 21 years and older. The management of those younger than 21 years and pregnant women are discussed separately (p. 746).

Atypical Squamous Cells Of Undetermined Significance.
The most common cytologic abnormality is atypical squamous cells of undetermined significance (ASC-US). This term indicates cells that are suggestive of, but which do not fulfill the criteria for, SIL. Although an ASC-US result often precedes the diagnosis of CIN 2 or 3, this risk approximates only 5 to

10 percent, and cancer is found in only 1 to 2 per thousand (Solomon, 2002). Therefore, the evaluation of ASC-US is not overly aggressive. Three options for evaluation of ASC-US are reflex HPV DNA testing, colposcopy, or repeat cytologies at 6 and 12 months, with referral to colposcopy if either repeat cytology is abnormal (Wright, 2007b). If LBC is used, reflex HPV DNA testing from the same specimen is preferred. If high-risk HPV DNA types are found, colposcopy is indicated, as the risk of CIN 2 or higher-grade lesions with HPV-positive ASC-US findings equals that of LSIL cytology. If high-risk HPV DNA is absent, a repeat Pap test in 12 months is recommended. Alternatively, immediate colposcopy may be considered in certain patients, such as those for whom compliance with further testing will be problematic.

Atypical Squamous Cells, Cannot Exclude HSIL. Five to 10 percent of ASC is designated as atypical squamous cells, cannot exclude high grade SIL (ASC-H). This finding should not to be confused with ASC-US. ASC-H describes cellular changes that do not fulfill criteria for HSIL cytology, but a high-grade lesion cannot be excluded. Histologic HSIL is found in upward of 25 percent of these cases. This is higher than that seen with ASC-US, and therefore colposcopy is indicated for evaluation (Wright, 2007b).

Low-Grade Squamous Intraepithelial Lesion. Low-grade SIL encompasses the cytologic features of HPV infection and CIN 1 but carries a 15- to 30-percent risk of CIN 2 or 3, similar to the ASC-US, HPV-positive category. Therefore, colposcopy is indicated for most LSIL Pap test results. HPV testing is not useful in reproductive-aged women, as approximately 80 percent will test positive for HPV DNA (ASCUS LSIL Triage Study Group, 2000). In postmenopausal women, due to a lower positive-predictive value of LSIL cytology for CIN 2 or 3 and a lower rate of HPV positivity, alternative

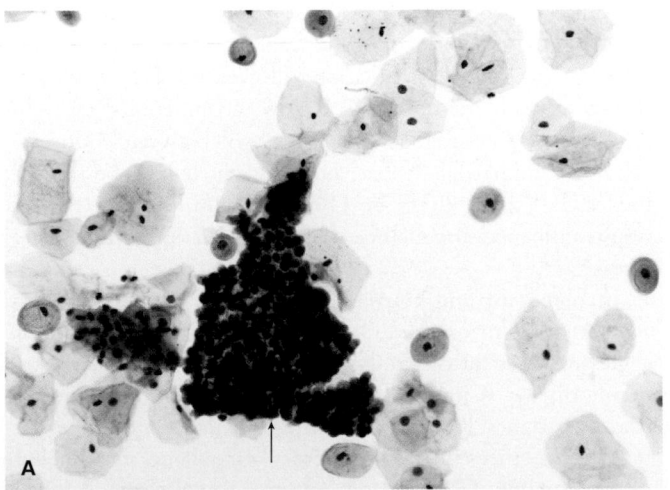
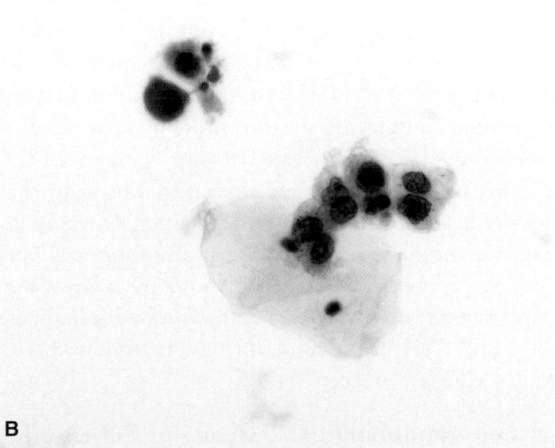

FIGURE 29-9 A. Normal Pap test. A fragment of benign endocervical epithelium with the characteristic "honeycomb" appearance conferred by the presence of cytoplasmic mucin is seen (*arrow*). Benign parabasal, intermediate, and superficial squamous cells are present in the background. **B.** Pap test reflecting high-grade squamous intraepithelial lesion. The dysplastic squamous cells have nuclear membrane irregularities and coarse chromatin. The nuclear to cytoplasmic size ratio would classify this as a moderate squamous dysplasia (CIN 2). (*Photographs contributed by Ann Marie West, MBA, CT [ASCP].*)

TABLE 29-5. Cervical Cytology: Initial Management of Epithelial Cell Abnormalities

Epithelial Cell Abnormality	General Recommendation	Special Circumstances
ASC-US	Repeat cytology at 6 and 12 months Reflex HPV DNA testing Colposcopy	Refer to colposcopy for recurrent abnormal cytology, or positive reflex HPV test; adolescents[a] managed with repeat annual cytology
LSIL	Colposcopy for non-adolescent women	Adolescents[a] managed with repeat annual cytology; HPV DNA test at 12 months or repeat cytology at 6 and 12 months are also acceptable for postmenopausal women
ASC-H, HSIL, squamous cell carcinoma	Colposcopy	
AGC, AIS, adenocarcinoma	Colposcopy, endocervical curettage[b]; HPV DNA testing for AGC	Endometrial sampling[b] indicated if age >35 years, abnormal bleeding, chronic anovulation, or atypical endometrial cells specified

[a]Adolescents = <21 years.
[b]Endocervical curettage and endometrial sampling are contraindicated in pregnancy.
AGC = atypical glandular cells; AIS = adenocarcinoma in situ; ASC-H = atypical squamous cells, cannot exclude high-grade squamous intraepithelial lesion; ASC-US = atypical squamous cells of undetermined significance; HPV = human papillomavirus; HSIL = high-grade squamous intraepithelial lesion; LSIL = low-grade squamous intraepithelial lesion.
Adapted from Wright, 2007b.

management of LSIL includes reflex HR HPV testing or repeat cytology at 6 and 12 months. As with ASC-US, HPV positivity and abnormal repeat cytology are indications for colposcopy (Wright, 2007b).

High-Grade Squamous Intraepithelial Lesion. High-grade SIL, all glandular epithelial cell abnormalities, and suspicion of carcinoma should all be evaluated by prompt colposcopic evaluation. HPV DNA testing is not useful in the management of HSIL cytology. High-grade SIL cytology encompasses features of CIN 2 and CIN 3 and carries a high risk of underlying histologic CIN 2 or CIN 3 (at least 70 percent) or invasive cancer (1 to 2 percent) (Kinney, 1998). Alternative management of HSIL cytology in women 21 years and older includes immediate diagnostic loop electrosurgical excision procedure (LEEP) (referred to as "see and LEEP" approach). This strategy is reasonable because colposcopy may miss a high-grade lesion, and most HSIL cytologies eventually result in excision for diagnosis or treatment. This option should be used judiciously, preferably when colposcopy is consistent with the presence of HSIL, and generally in older patients as some CIN 2 and CIN 2/3 lesions can now be followed with observation in young women.

Glandular Cell Abnormalities. This category carries with it a high risk of neoplasia (Zhao, 2009). As reviewed by Schnatz and associates (2006), compared with glandular disease, squamous neoplasia is more commonly diagnosed upon evaluation of atypical glandular cell (AGC) cytology. There is also an increased risk of endometrial and other reproductive tract can-

cers. Therefore, evaluation of a glandular abnormality includes colposcopy and endocervical curettage. It also includes endometrial sampling in nonpregnant patients older than 35 years or in those younger if there is a history of abnormal bleeding, if risk factors for endometrial disease are noted, or if the cytology report specifies that the atypical glandular cells are of endometrial origin. Approximately half of the pathology diagnosed subsequent to an AGC Pap is endometrial.

Reflex HPV testing is not recommended for the *triage* of glandular cytologic abnormalities. Indeed, a negative reflex HPV test result could dissuade appropriate referral of AGC cytology for further evaluation. However, HPV testing at the *initial evaluation* of AGC is now recommended (Wright, 2007b). HPV testing discriminates well between endocervical and endometrial disease, both of which may be difficult to detect (Castle, 2010; de Oliveira, 2006). Also, HPV test results influence surveillance if initial evaluation fails to reveal disease.

If colposcopy and biopsies are without evidence of neoplasia, management of glandular abnormalities is generally more aggressive than for other abnormalities due to a higher risk of occult disease. Current consensus guidelines should be followed (Wright, 2007b). Depending on the glandular abnormality and other clinical risk factors, surveillance may include postcolposcopic HPV testing, repeat cytologies, or diagnostic excision.

Adolescents. Deferral of initiation of cervical cancer screening until age 21 for those at average risk will largely eliminate evaluation of abnormalities in this age group in the near future. In the interim, ASC-US and LSIL cytologies in adolescents are evaluated differently due to a higher rate of HPV positivity, the rarity of cervical cancer, and the high rates of spontaneous regression of cervical neoplasia in this group (Boardman, 2005; Moscicki, 2005; Wright, 2006). Reflex HPV testing is unacceptable for this age group, and results should be disregarded. Instead, repeat cytology should subsequently be obtained twice at 12-month intervals and colposcopy performed only with a high-grade cytology result or if any cytologic abnormality persists at 2 years (Wright, 2007b). If two negative Pap tests have been obtained since the ASC-US or LSIL result, no further evaluation is needed, and screening is resumed at age 21. Other Pap abnormalities (ASC-H, HSIL, glandular abnormalities) should be managed as per guidelines for the general population.

Pregnancy. Pregnant patients 21 years and older should be screened and their abnormal cytologies managed according to guidelines for the general population. However, deferred evaluation of ASC-US and LSIL cytologies until at least 6 weeks postpartum is acceptable (Wright, 2007b). When indicated, the goal of colposcopy is to exclude invasive cancer, and endocervical curettage is not performed during pregnancy. Preinvasive neoplasia is not treated. It is reevaluated postpartum and managed accordingly as the lesion grade may change. Although infrequently performed, indications for cervical conization during pregnancy are discussed in Chapter 30 (p. 789).

Nonneoplastic Findings. Certain nonneoplastic findings may be reported, and these include findings consistent with, but not conclusively diagnostic of, certain organisms. These findings include *Trichomonas vaginalis*, *Candida* species, *Actinomyces* species, herpes simplex virus, or shift in flora consistent with bacterial vaginosis. Sensitivity is generally limited, and accuracy of diagnosis varies (Fitzhugh, 2008). Therefore, confirmatory tests or clinical correlation should dictate any actions related to these findings. Other nonneoplastic findings are reactive changes associated with inflammation or repair, radiation changes, benign glandular cells posthysterectomy, and atrophy. None of these warrant a specific clinical response.

Because menstrual history is often unknown to the cytologist, endometrial cells that appear benign are reported on Pap reports for all women 40 years and older. As reviewed by Browne and associates (2005), the need for evaluation in normally menstruating women has been controversial and therefore individualized according to clinical history and risk factors. The 2006 Consensus Guidelines state that no evaluation is needed in an asymptomatic, premenopausal woman (Wright, 2007b). However, premenopausal women with abnormal bleeding or the presence of other risk factors for endometrial disease should undergo further evaluation of the endometrium as should all postmenopausal women (Chap. 8, p. 223).

Colposcopy

This is an outpatient procedure that examines the lower anogenital tract with a binocular microscope. Its primary goal is the identification of invasive or preinvasive neoplastic lesions for colposcopically directed biopsy and subsequent management. It remains the clinical gold standard for the evaluation of patients with abnormal cervical cytology and in the past, was assumed to have near-perfect sensitivity. However, its sensitivity, interobserver agreement, and reproducibility have recently come into question (American College of Obstetricians and Gynecologists, 2008; Cox, 2008; Ferris, 2005; Jeronimo, 2007). A more realistic estimate of colposcopy's sensitivity for the detection of high-grade cervical neoplasia after referral for abnormal cytology is 70 percent (Cantor, 2008). This highlights the need for continued cytologic or colposcopic surveillance if colposcopy fails to reveal CIN 2 or higher-grade lesions.

Colposcopy requires specialized knowledge of lower genital tract physiology and disease as well as a clinical skill set encompassing lesion identification, lesion grading, and biopsy techniques. A thorough review of colposcopy and its current procedural components and potential improvements is provided by Chase and associates (2009). As cervical cancer screening technologies become more sensitive, women are referred for colposcopy with earlier, smaller lesions, some beneath the limits of colposcopic visualization. New technologies to improve the positive predictive value and specificity of cervical cytology and histology are needed. Several potential biomarkers, such as staining for $p16^{INK4A}$, a tumor suppressor protein, are under investigation (del Pino, 2009). The development of objective, sensitive, and accurate technologies as adjuncts to colposcopy are also needed. Most promising to date is multimodal hyperspectroscopy, which uses tissue fluorescence to identify high-grade neoplasia (DeSantis, 2007).

Colposcope

There are many styles of colposcopes, but they all operate similarly. The colposcope consists of a stereoscopic lens or digital imaging system that has magnification settings ranging from 3- to 40-fold and that is attached to a moveable stand. A high-intensity light provides illumination. Use of a green (red-free) light filter adds contrast to aid examination of vascular patterns (Fig. 29-10).

Preparation

Prior to colposcopic examination, a woman's medical record, including gynecologic and dysplasia histories, should be reviewed and indications for colposcopy confirmed (Table 29-6). Urine pregnancy testing should be performed if clinically indicated. Colposcopic examination is optimally timed to avoid menses but should not be delayed if a gross lesion suspicious for invasive cancer is present, if a patient is unreliable or cannot easily reschedule the examination, or if the current bleeding is unscheduled or abnormal.

A Pap test at the time of colposcopy is of questionable value, may obscure colposcopic findings, and should be performed only on an individualized basis. In cases of severe cervicitis, a saline wet prep, cervical testing for infection, and treatment of an identified pathogen may be indicated before performing biopsies or endocervical curettage.

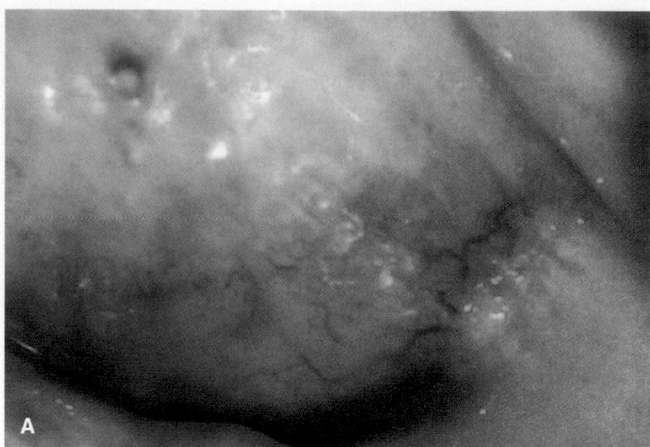

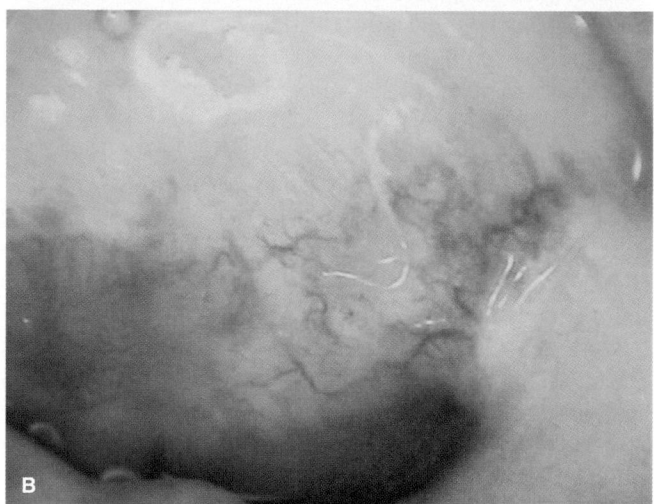

FIGURE 29-10 Evaluation of surface vessels. **A.** Benign surface vessels viewed through a colposcope using usual white light source. **B.** Use of a blue–green (red-free) light filter provides higher contrast and definition of vascular patterns.

Solutions

Normal Saline. Used at the beginning of the colposcopic examination, saline helps remove cervical mucus and allows initial assessment of vascular patterns and surface contours. Abnormal vessels, especially when viewed with green-filtered light, may be more prominent than after acetic acid application.

Acetic Acid. Acetic acid 3- to 5-percent is a mucolytic agent that is thought to exert its effect by reversibly clumping nuclear chromatin. This causes lesions to assume various shades of white depending on the degree of abnormal nuclear density. Applying acetic acid to abnormal epithelium results in the *acetowhite* change characteristic of neoplastic lesions as well as some nonneoplastic conditions. White vinegar sold for cooking is 5-percent acetic acid and is an inexpensive source of acetic acid for colposcopy.

Lugol Solution. Lugol iodine solution stains mature squamous epithelial cells a dark brown color in estrogenized women as a result of high cellular glycogen content. Due to poor cellular differentiation, dysplastic cells have lower glycogen content, fail

TABLE 29-6. Clinical Considerations Directing Colposcopy

Clinical objectives
Provide a magnified view of the lower genital tract
Identify squamocolumnar junction of the cervix
Detect lesions suspicious for neoplasia
Direct biopsy of lesions
Monitor patients with a current or past history of
    lower genital tract neoplasia

Clinical indications
Grossly visible genital tract lesions
Abnormal cervical cytology
History of in utero diethylstilbestrol exposure
Unexplained genital tract bleeding

Contraindications
None

Relative contraindications
Upper or lower reproductive tract infection
Uncontrolled severe hypertension
Uncooperative or overly anxious patient

to fully stain, and appear various shades of yellow (Fig. 29-11). Lugol solution should not be used in patients allergic to iodine, radiographic contrast, or shellfish. This solution is particularly useful when abnormal tissue cannot be found using acetic acid alone. It is also used to define the limits of the active transformation zone, as immature squamous metaplasia does not stain as strongly as mature (fully differentiated) squamous epithelium.

Colposcopic Grading of Lesions

Colposcopically, normal squamous epithelium of the cervix appears as a featureless, smooth, pale-pink surface. Blood vessels lie below this layer and therefore are not visible or are seen only as a fine capillary network. The mucin-secreting columnar epithelium appears red due to its thinness and the close proximity of blood vessels to the surface. It has a polypoid appearance due to infoldings that form peaks and clefts (see Fig. 29-3).

Colposcopists are trained to discriminate between normal and abnormal tissue for biopsy purposes and to choose the site most likely to harbor the highest grade of neoplasia. Several colposcopic grading systems that quantify various lesion characteristics have been developed to improve accuracy (Coppleson, 1993; Reid, 1985). Best known, the Reid Colposcopic Index is based on four colposcopic lesion features: margin, color, vascular patterns, and Lugol solution staining. Each category is scored from 0 to 2, and the summation provides a numeric index that correlates with histology (Table 29-7).

The International Federation for Cervical Pathology and Colposcopy (2011) has approved a nomenclature that standardizes descriptors of colposcopic findings and incorporates them into a graded system. Lesions with low-grade characteristics corresponding to zero scores by Reid Index are labeled grade 1 (minor) lesions; higher-grade characteristics are grade 2 (major) findings.

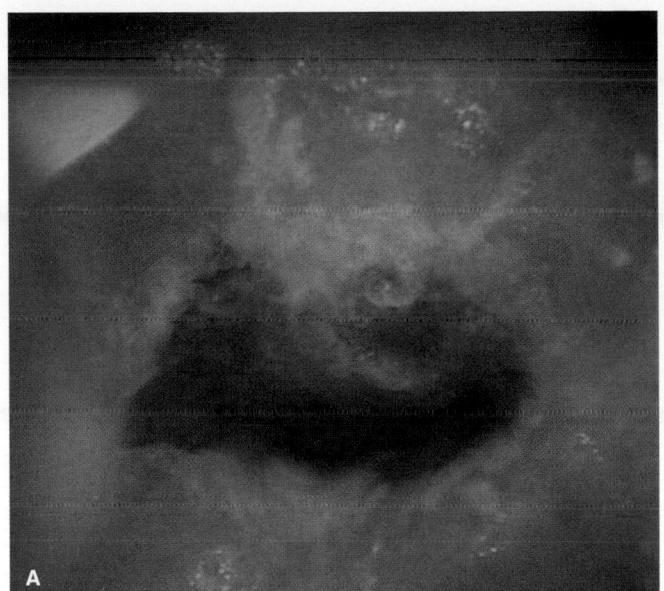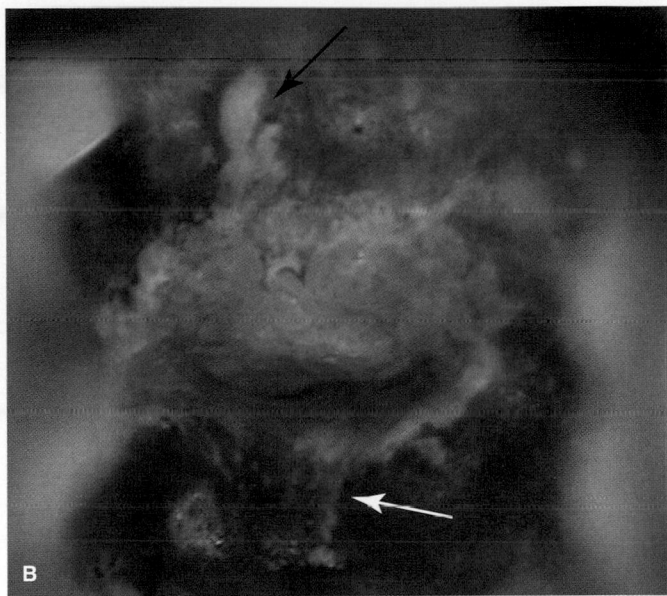

FIGURE 29-11 Solutions used for colposcopy. **A.** Cervix after application of acetic acid. Several areas of acetowhite change adjacent to the squamocolumnar junction are apparent. **B.** Same cervix after application of Lugol iodine solution. Nonstaining of the lesions at the 10 to 11 o'clock positions is seen (*black arrow*), while there is partial iodine uptake of acetowhite areas along the posterior SCJ (*white arrow*).

Lesion Margins and Color. Following application of acetic acid to mucosal epithelium, the color or degree of whiteness obtained, rapidity and duration of acetowhitening, and sharpness of lesion borders are observed. High-grade lesions demonstrate a more persistent, duller shade of white, whereas low-grade lesions are translucent or bright white and fade quickly. Low-grade lesions characteristically have feathery margins, whereas high-grade lesions have straighter, sharper outlines (Figs. 29-12 and 29-13). A lesion with an internal border, that is, a lesion within a lesion, is typically high-grade.

Lesion Vascular Patterns. The vascular patterns associated with abnormal epithelium include punctation, mosaicism, and atypical vessels. Punctate and mosaic patterns are graded on the basis of vessel caliber, intercapillary distance, and the uniformity of each of these. Fine punctation and mosaicism, which are created by narrow vessels and short, uniform intercapillary distances, typify low-grade lesions. A coarse pattern results from wider and more variable vessel diameters and spacing and indicates higher-grade abnormalities. Atypical vessels are irregular in caliber, shape, course, and arrangement (Fig. 29-14). These should raise suspicion of cancer.

TABLE 29-7. Reid Colposcopic Index

Colposcopic Sign	Zero Points	1 Point	2 Points
Margin	Condylomatous Micropapillary Feathery Satellite lesions	Smooth Straight	Rolled Peeling Internal border
Color: acetowhitening	Shiny Snowy Translucent Transient	Duller white	Dull white Gray
Vessels	Fine patterns Uniform caliber and patterns	Absent	Coarse patterns Dilated with variable caliber and intercapillary distances
Iodine staining	Positive	Partial	Negative

Adapted from Reid, 1985, with permission.

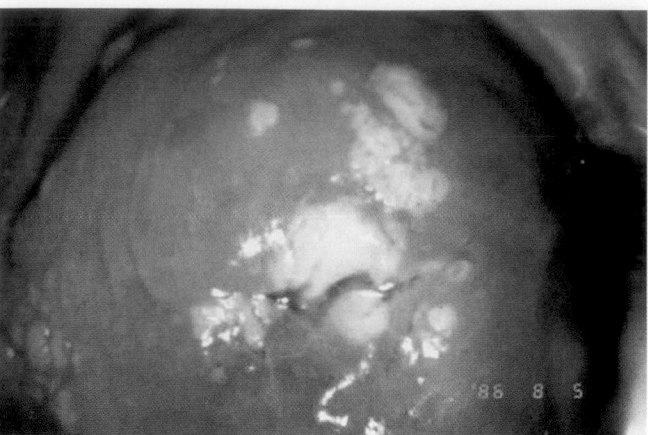

FIGURE 29-12 Low-grade squamous intraepithelial lesions. Seen after 5-percent acetic acid application, HPV/CIN 1 lesions are often multifocal and bright white with irregular borders.

Biopsy

Ectocervical Biopsy. Under direct colposcopic visualization, suspicious lesions on the ectocervix are biopsied using a sharp instrument such as a Tischler biopsy forceps (Fig. 29-15). Generally, cervical biopsy does not require an anesthetic. Thickened Monsel solution (ferric subsulfate) or a silver nitrate applicator, applied with pressure to the biopsy site, provides hemostasis if needed. Extreme cases of bleeding are rare and can be controlled with direct pressure or vaginal packing. For patients requiring chronic anticoagulation, colposcopic biopsies can be taken without a break in their anticoagulant regimen. Ideally, biopsies are taken by an experienced colposcopist in a setting where possible excessive bleeding can be anticipated and addressed safely.

Traditionally, biopsies have been limited to the most severe-appearing lesions. However, there is growing evi-

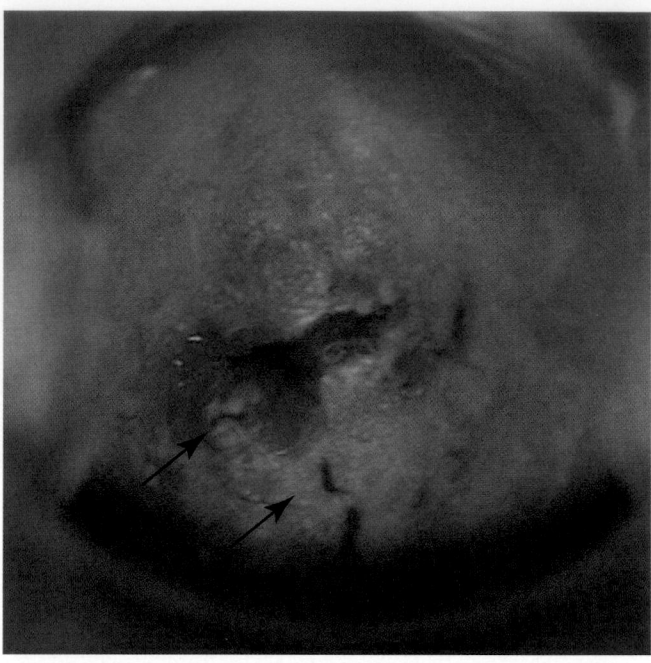

FIGURE 29-14 Mosaic vascular pattern with atypical vessels (*arrows*).

dence that disease detection is strongly correlated with the total number of biopsies taken (Zuchna, 2010). Two studies have shown that colposcopically directed biopsy detects only 60 to 70 percent of high-grade disease present. Disease detection increases with the addition of random biopsies of normal-appearing epithelium and with the total number of biopsies taken (Gage, 2006; Pretorius, 2004). The American College of Obstetricians and Gynecologists (2008) concludes that biopsy of all visualized lesions is indicated regardless of colposcopic impression.

Satisfactory Colposcopy. Within a neoplastic lesion, more severe disease tends to be at the proximal (cephalad) limit of the

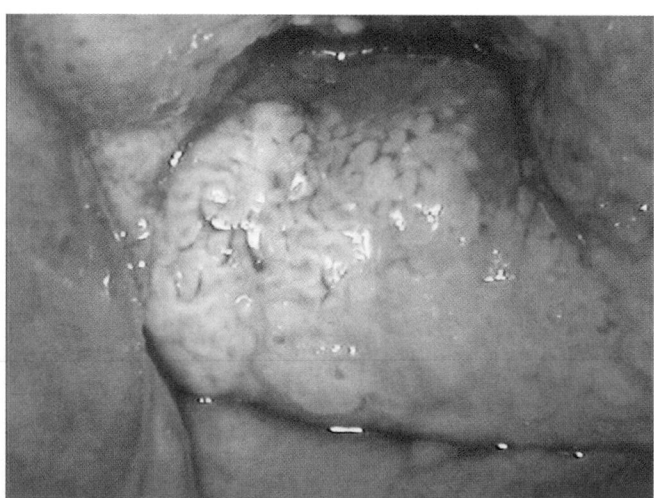

FIGURE 29-13 High-grade squamous intraepithelial lesion. CIN 3 lesion after 5-percent acetic acid application demonstrating large size, well-defined borders, off-white dull coloration, and coarse vascular pattern.

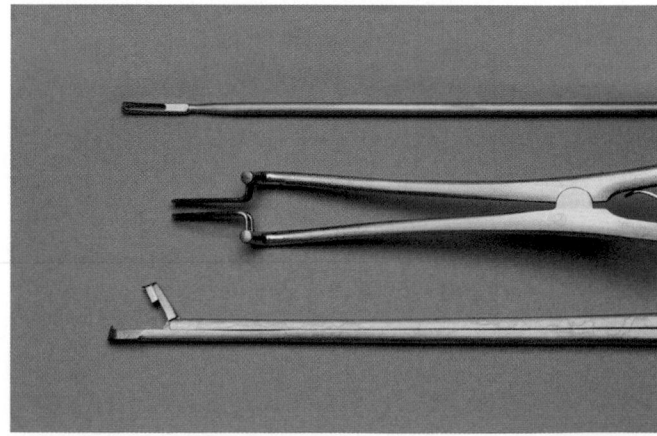

FIGURE 29-15 Tools used for cervical evaluation and biopsy. From top to bottom: endocervical curette, endocervical speculum, and cervical biopsy forceps.

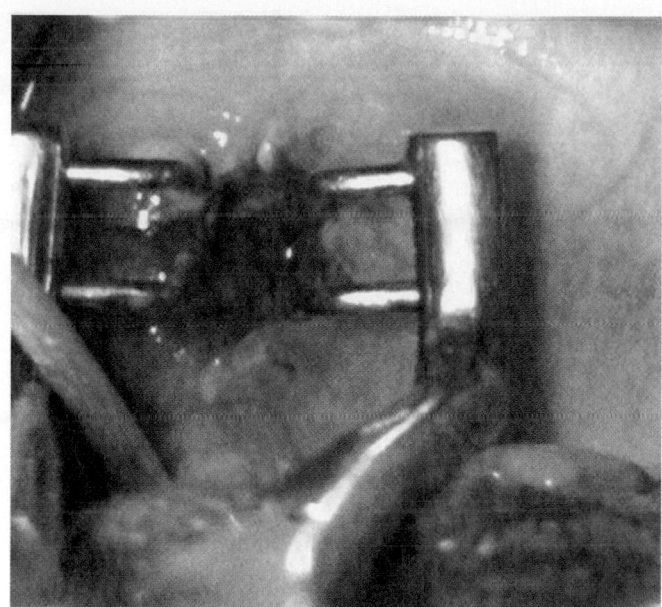

FIGURE 29-16 Use of an endocervical speculum to visualize the endocervical canal during colposcopy.

transformation zone. Thus, adequate visualization of the entire cervical SCJ and upper limits of all lesions defines whether a colposcopic examination is deemed *satisfactory* or *unsatisfactory*. This determination can affect management. Therefore, with initially unsatisfactory colposcopy, an endocervical speculum may be used to attempt full visualization of the current SCJ and lesions that extend cephalad into the endocervical canal (Fig. 29-16).

Endocervical Sampling. For nonpregnant patients, endocervical sampling by curettage (ECC) is used to evaluate tissue within the endocervical canal not visualized by colposcopy. A normal ECC provides an added degree of assurance that a neoplastic endocervical lesion is not present and adds to colposcopic sensitivity (Grainger, 1987; Pretorius, 2004). Despite its common use, there are no randomized trials supporting the performance of ECC routinely during colposcopy, and its routine use has been questioned (Abu, 2005).

Endocervical curettage is currently recommended at the time of colposcopy in the following situations:

- Colposcopy is unsatisfactory, or if colposcopy is satisfactory, but no lesion is identified. ECC is acceptable in other cases at provider discretion (American College of Obstetricians and Gynecologists, 2008; Wright, 2007b).
- Initial evaluation of glandular cell abnormalities (Granai, 1985; Wright, 2007b).
- Ablative treatment is planned (Husseinzadeh, 1989).
- Surveillance after excisional therapy if specimen margins are positive for HSIL (Wright, 2007c).
- Surveillance after conization for adenocarcinoma in situ has been performed. During surveillance of these women, Schorge and associates (2003) found that negative ECC results may postpone repeat conization or definitive hysterectomy in women wanting to preserve fertility.

Endocervical curettage is performed by introducing an endocervical curette 1 to 2 cm into the cervical canal (see Fig. 29-15). The entire length and circumference of the canal is firmly curetted, carefully avoiding sampling of the ectocervix or the lower uterine segment. Endocervical scrapings admix with cervical mucus, which may then be removed using ring forceps or a cytobrush and included with the curettage specimen. Alternatively, vigorous brushing with a cytobrush may be used to obtain an endocervical tissue specimen. Endocervical sampling is often the most painful part of a colposcopic evaluation, and cramping is common.

Management of Cervical Intraepithelial Neoplasia

Management of histologic CIN falls into two general categories: observation and treatment. The objective of all treatment is obliteration of the entire cervical transformation zone, including abnormal tissue. This may be achieved by excision of tissue or by ablation, that is, tissue destruction with cryosurgery or laser. Excisional options include loop electrosurgical excision procedure, laser conization, and cold-knife conization. All treatment modalities, particularly excisional procedures, are suspected of increasing the risk of adverse future reproductive outcomes, such as cervical stenosis, preterm delivery, and premature rupture of membranes (Wright, 2007c). Therefore, treatment should be focused primarily on the eradication of high-grade lesions.

Evidence-based guidelines for the management of women with biopsy-confirmed CIN have been developed and subsequently updated in 2006 through the organizational efforts of the American Society for Colposcopy and Cervical Pathology (Wright, 2007c). In general, histologic CIN 1 can be observed indefinitely, especially in adolescents. Treatment is acceptable if it persists for at least 2 years. Observation is also an option for CIN 2 or CIN 2/3 lesions (distinction between CIN 2 and CIN 3 not made) in adolescents and young women (American College of Obstetricians and Gynecologists, 2010a; Wright, 2007c). CIN 2 in adult women and CIN 3 at any age are treated by excision or ablation. Treatment is deferred during pregnancy. The "see and treat" approach in which loop excision is performed at initial colposcopy is an acceptable option for high-risk, adult patients who present with high-grade cytology and corresponding colposcopic abnormalities. A prospective study using this approach found that 84 percent of patients had CIN 2 or 3 within the excisional biopsy specimen (Numnum, 2005).

Adenocarcinoma in situ of the cervix, although uncommon, is increasing in incidence and typically diagnosed at a younger age (Krivak, 2001). Exclusion of invasive cancer and removal of all affected tissue are the primary goals. Cold-knife conization is recommended to optimize specimen orientation, interpretation of histology, and preservation of margins. The risk of residual AIS is reported to be as high as 80 percent in patients with positive margins, and therefore, repeat conization is advisable (Krivak, 2001). Even with negative conization specimen margins and endocervical curettage, there is risk of residual disease. Therefore, hysterectomy is recommended after childbearing is completed (Krivak, 2001; Poynor, 1995).

Management of Negative Evaluation Subsequent to Abnormal Cytology

When colposcopic and histologic evaluations fail to reveal the presence of high-grade neoplasia, further surveillance is recommended based upon the original abnormal cytology result as listed in Table 29-8.

Treatment of Cervical Intraepithelial Neoplasia

Current treatment of CIN is limited to local ablative or excisional procedures. Whereas ablative procedures destroy cervical tissue, excisional methods provide histologic specimens that allow the evaluation of excised margins and further assurance that invasive cancer is not present. Medical treatment using topical agents is currently investigational and not recognized as standard clinical practice. Selection of treatment modality depends on multiple factors including patient age, parity, desire for future fertility, size and severity of a lesion(s), contour of the cervix, prior treatment for CIN, and coexisting medical conditions such as immune compromise. Most randomized clinical trials evaluating differences in treatment success are underpowered, and no clear evidence shows any treatment technique to be superior (Martin-Hirsch, 2010; Mitchell, 1998). Most reports suggest that surgical treatments

have an approximate 90-percent success rate. An understanding of cervical anatomy, transformation zone topography and histology, and the distribution and pathologic features of CIN is essential for the individualized selection and efficacy of a given treatment modality.

Ablative Treatment Modalities

Ablation of the transformation zone is effective for noninvasive ectocervical disease. Before using ablative treatment modalities, evidence of glandular disease or invasive cancer by cytologic or histologic evaluation or by colposcopic impression should be excluded. Cytologic results, histologic findings, and colposcopic impression should be concordant. Before ablation, colposcopic examination should be satisfactory, and negative endocervical curettage provides added assurance that there is no occult disease in the endocervical canal. The most commonly used ablative treatment modalities are cryosurgery, electrofulguration, and carbon dioxide (CO_2) laser. Prior to the introduction of loop excision in 1989, when cold knife conization was the only excisional option, these ablative techniques were more commonly used (Prendiville, 1989). The relative decreased morbidity and ease of performing loop excision compared with cold knife conization as well as the trends toward observation of CIN 1 and some CIN 2 and CIN 2/3 lesions has led to decreased use of ablative procedures in clinical practice.

Cryosurgery. Cryosurgery delivers a refrigerant gas, usually nitrous oxide, through flexible tubing to a metal probe that

TABLE 29-8. Surveillance of Abnormal Cervical Cytology in the Absence of Histologic High-Grade Neoplasia

Cytology	Colposcopy/Histology	Recommended Surveillance
ASC-US, HPV status unknown	No CIN found	Repeat cytology at 12 months
ASC-US, HPV+; ASC-H; or LSIL	No CIN found	Cytology at 6 and 12 months or HR HPV testing at 12 months
HSIL	No CIN 2/CIN 3 found	Satisfactory colposcopy: review cytology and histology results and colposcopic findings or repeat colposcopy and cytology at 6-month intervals for 1 year or diagnostic excision; Unsatisfactory colposcopy: diagnostic excision
AGC	No CIN or glandular neoplasia	Repeat cytology at 6-month intervals for four times if HPV status unknown; if HPV negative, repeat cytology and HR HPV testing at 12 months; if HPV positive, repeat cytology and HR HPV testing at 6 months
AGC, favor neoplasia	No invasive carcinoma	Diagnostic excisional procedure
AIS	No invasive carcinoma	Diagnostic excisional procedure

AGC = atypical glandular cells; AIS = endocervical adenocarcinoma; ASC-H = atypical squamous cells, cannot exclude high-grade squamous intraepithelial lesion; ASC-US = atypical squamous cells of undetermined significance; CIN = cervical intraepithelial neoplasia; HPV+ = reflex HPV DNA test positive result; HR HPV = high-risk human papillomavirus; HSIL = high-grade squamous intraepithelial lesion; LSIL = low-grade squamous intraepithelial lesion.
Adapted from Wright, 2007c.

TABLE 29-9. Cryosurgery: Clinical Characteristics

Advantages

Favorable safety profile
Outpatient procedure
No anesthetic requirements
Ease of procedure
Low-cost equipment with minimal maintenance
Bleeding complications rare
No proven adverse reproductive effects
Acceptable primary cure rate

Disadvantages

No tissue specimen for histopathologic evaluation
Cannot treat lesions with unfavorable sizes or shapes
Uterine cramping
Potential for vasovagal reaction
Profuse vaginal discharge postprocedure
Cephalad migration of squamocolumnar junction

From Martin-Hirsch, 2010.

freezes tissue on contact (Section 41-26, p. 1078). Cryonecrosis is achieved by crystallizing intracellular water. This treatment is most successful for ectocervical lesions associated with a satisfactory colposcopic examination and with biopsy-proven squamous dysplasia limited to two quadrants of the cervix. Cryosurgery is generally not favored for the treatment of CIN 3 due to higher rates of disease persistence following treatment and lack of a histologic specimen to exclude occult invasive cancer (Table 29-9) (Martin-Hirsch, 2010). Moreover, cryosurgery and other ablative techniques are not favored for HIV-positive women with CIN due to high failure rates (Spitzer, 1999).

Carbon Dioxide Laser Ablation. Treatment with *l*ight *a*mplification by *s*timulated *e*mission of *r*adiation, or *laser,* is delivered using colposcopic guidance with a micromanipulator. This modality is used to vaporize tissue to a depth of 5 to 7 mm to ensure obliteration of all dysplastic tissue (Section 41-26, p. 1081). Laser ablation is appropriate for biopsy-proven squamous intraepithelial lesions associated with a satisfactory colposcopic examination. The laser is well suited for large, irregularly shaped preinvasive lesions of all grades as well as condylomatous and dysplastic lesions at other lower genital tract sites.

Excisional Treatment Modalities

Lesions suspicious for invasive cancer and AIS of the cervix must undergo a diagnostic excisional procedure. In addition, excision is indicated for patients with unsatisfactory colposcopy with histologic CIN who need treatment, or those with unexplained high-grade or recurrent AGC cytology. It is also warranted in cases of cytologic and histologic discordance, if histologic results are significantly less severe. Excision is pru-

dent for any posttreatment recurrence of high-grade CIN to allow complete histologic evaluation of the specimen. Women with recurrent CIN have a higher risk for occult invasive cancer (Paraskevaidis, 1991).

Excisional treatment modalities include LEEP, cold-knife conization, and laser conization. Excisional procedures, and to a lesser extent ablative procedures, are associated with operative and long-term risks including cervical stenosis and adverse pregnancy outcomes. For decades, cold-knife conization has been associated with cervical incompetence and preterm birth. Furthermore, Himes (2007) suggests that women with a shorter conization-to-pregnancy interval, that is, less than 2 to 3 months, are at particularly increased risk for preterm birth. However, the relationship between preterm birth and LEEP continues to be debated. Although some studies show increased risk, others do not (Jakobsson, 2009; Kyrgiou, 2006; Sadler, 2004; Samson, 2005; Werner, 2010). An important study confounder is the increased risk of preterm birth in women with cervical neoplasia compared with the general population even if they have not undergone an excisional procedure (Bruinsma, 2007; Shanbhag, 2009). This implies that CIN and preterm birth have overlapping risk factors. The contribution of treatment to this risk is therefore difficult to ascertain.

Loop Electrosurgical Excision Procedure. This technique uses a thin wire on an insulated handle through which an electrical current is passed. This creates an instrument that simultaneously cuts and coagulates tissue and that can be used during direct colposcopic visualization (Section 41-26, p. 1080). Because LEEP can be performed using local anesthesia, it has become the primary outpatient treatment modality for high-grade cervical lesions, including those that extend into the endocervical canal (Table 29-10). LEEP provides a tissue specimen with margins that can be histologically assessed. Additionally, the size and shape of tissue excision can be customized by varying loop sizes and the order in which loops are used (Figure 41-26.4, p. 1081). This helps conserve cervical stroma volume.

TABLE 29-10. Loop Electrosurgical Excision Procedure: Clinical Characteristics

Advantages

Favorable safety profile
Ease of procedure
Outpatient procedure using local anesthesia
Low-cost equipment
Tissue specimen for histopathologic evaluation

Disadvantages

Thermal damage may obscure specimen margin status
Special training required
Risk of postprocedure bleeding
Theoretical risk of vapor plume inhalation
Possible increased risk of adverse reproductive outcomes

TABLE 29-11. Cold-Knife Conization Clinical Characteristics

Advantages
Anesthetized patient
Tissue specimen for histopathologic evaluation without margin compromise
Enhanced patient support if hemorrhage is encountered
Variety of instruments to individualize conization

Disadvantages
Potential for hemorrhage
Lengthier procedure
Postoperative discomfort
General or regional anesthesia required
Operating room setting
High cost
Larger volume of cervical stroma removed
Increased risk of adverse reproductive outcomes

Cold-Knife Conization. This surgical procedure uses a scalpel to remove the cervical transformation zone including the cervical lesion (Section 41-27, p. 1083). It is performed in an operating room and requires general or regional anesthesia (Table 29-11). Cold-knife conization is often preferred over LEEP for cases with high-grade CIN extending deep into the endocervical canal, for endocervical glandular disease, and for posttreatment CIN recurrences. Patient selection favors those with risks for invasive cancer, which include cervical cytology suspicious for invasive cancer, patients older than 35 years with CIN 3 or CIS, large high-grade lesions, and biopsies showing AIS.

Carbon Dioxide Laser Conization. This method has the disadvantages of expense and some thermal compromise of margins. However, it offers advantages of precise cone size and shape tailoring and less blood loss. Requiring special training, this procedure can be performed under local or general anesthesia (Section 41-27, p. 1084).

Posttreatment Surveillance

Additional patient surveillance is required posttreatment (Wright, 2007b). Patients who have excised margins negative for CIN or who have undergone an ablative procedure may be followed with cytologic testing alone or with colposcopy every 6 months until two negative evaluations are obtained before returning to routine screening. Alternatively, HPV DNA testing may be done between 6 and 12 months posttreatment, and colposcopy performed for persistent HPV infection as this is a sensitive marker of disease persistence. Cytology screening should continue for at least 20 years thereafter due to a persistently increased risk of cervical neoplasia after a diagnosis of high-grade CIN (American College of Obstetricians and Gynecologists, 2009). If excision margins or endocervical curettage performed intraoperatively immediately after an exci-

sion are positive for CIN 2 or CIN 3, then surveillance with repeat cytology and endocervical sampling 4 to 6 months later is preferred. In this instance, repeat excision is also acceptable. Moreover, repeat diagnostic excision is indicated for special circumstances such as AIS or microinvasive carcinoma at the excision margins.

Hysterectomy

Hysterectomy is unacceptable as primary therapy for CIN 1, 2, or 3 (Wright, 2007c). However, it may be considered when treating recurrent high-grade cervical disease if childbearing has been completed or when a repeat cervical excision is strongly indicated but technically not feasible. Although hysterectomy provides the lowest recurrence rate for CIN, invasive cancer must always be excluded beforehand. The choice of either a vaginal or abdominal approach is directed by other clinical factors. Hysterectomy is the preferred treatment of AIS when future fertility is not desired.

Even with negative cervical margins, hysterectomy performed for CIN is not completely protective. Patients, particularly those who are immunosuppressed, are at risk for recurrent disease and require postoperative interval cytologic screening of the vaginal cuff as described on page 743 (Saslow, 2002).

VAGINAL PREINVASIVE LESIONS

Incidence

Vaginal cancer is rare and comprises approximately 1 percent of all gynecologic cancers. Of vaginal cancers, data from the Surveillance, Epidemiology and End Results (SEER) database showed that nearly 50 percent of cases are diagnosed in women aged 70 years and older (Kosary, 2007). Approximately 90 percent of vaginal cancers are squamous. These appear to develop slowly from precancerous epithelial changes, called vaginal intraepithelial neoplasia (VaIN), in a fashion similar to CIN.

Pathophysiology

Vaginal intraepithelial neoplasia has histopathology similar to CIN and VIN. It is rarely found as a primary lesion and most often develops as an extension of CIN, mainly in the upper third of the vagina (Diakomanolis, 2002; Hoffman, 1992a). Unlike the cervix, the vagina lacks an active transformation zone susceptible to HPV-induced neoplasia. However, HPV entry may result from vaginal mucosal abrasions and reparative metaplastic squamous cell activity (Woodruff, 1981). In a recent systematic review of 315 cases of vaginal neoplasia, investigators found HPV DNA in up to 98 percent of VaIN lesions and in three quarters of vaginal cancers. HPV 16 was the most common HPV type (Smith, 2009).

Risk Factors

The natural history of VaIN is less understood than that of CIN, although risk factors for VaIN are similar to those for

CIN, suggesting a similar etiology (see Table 29-2). Thus, HPV prophylactic vaccination against HPV types 16 and 18 has the potential to prevent approximately one half of vaginal cancers (Smith, 2009). As noted, vaginal cancer is primarily found in postmenopausal women (Hoffman, 1992a). However, with recent increases in HPV infection of the lower genital tract in a younger population, VaIN is now also diagnosed in younger women. Cervical and vulvar neoplasia increase the risk for VaIN and vaginal squamous cancer. Moreover, a recent retrospective study suggests that hysterectomy is not definitive therapy for high-grade neoplasia, as researchers have found a subsequent high-grade VaIN recurrence rate greater than 7 percent (Schockaert, 2008).

Diagnosis

Generally, VaIN is asymptomatic. If present, symptoms may include vaginal spotting, discharge, and odor. Abnormal cytology most often is the first indication of VaIN, particularly if the patient lacks a cervix. Integral to management, subsequent examination of the vagina with a colposcope, termed *vaginoscopy*, frequently locates a vaginal lesion for biopsy. Prior to visual evaluation, careful palpation of the vagina is advisable, particularly if the patient has undergone hysterectomy for high-grade cervical neoplasia. In such cases, invasive cancer may present as a nodular lesion buried within the vaginal cuff before it becomes visible.

Vaginoscopy

Because of a large surface area and rugation, examination of the entire vagina using a colposcope can be cumbersome and requires patience. A clear plastic speculum may aid visualization of all quadrants of the vagina. During examination, particular attention should be given to tissue in the upper third of the vaginal vault due to the common relationship of VaIN as an extension of CIN. In women who have undergone hysterectomy for high-grade CIN, the vaginal cuff should be carefully evaluated in response to abnormal vaginal cytology. By applying 3- to 5-percent acetic acid to the vaginal mucosa, acetowhite changes consistent with HPV infection or neoplasia are identified (Fig. 29-17). Vascular patterns are less common in VaIN lesions than with CIN, but coarse punctation and even atypical vessels may be seen in high-grade lesions. High-grade VaIN tends to demonstrate flat, dense acetowhitening with sharply demarcated borders. Half-strength Lugol solution applied to the vagina further delineates abnormal areas. Similar to cervical dysplasia, these nonstaining areas most likely contain abnormal epithelium. Iodine staining can be an important aid in the selection of biopsy site. Biopsies should focus on the areas of least staining and straightest lesion margins. Biopsy may be obtained by means of a cervical biopsy forceps, and an Emmett hook can be used to elevate and stabilize vaginal tissue if needed. Local anesthesia is usually not necessary for biopsies of the upper third of the vagina, but may be needed for more distal biopsies. In premenopausal women, the vaginal mucosa is several millimeters thick, and biopsy using a Tischler biopsy forceps is appropriate. The vagi-

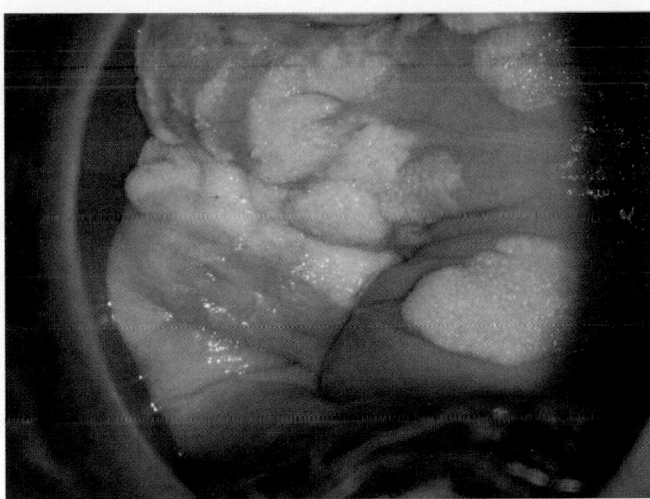

FIGURE 29-17 Vaginoscopy showing multifocal acetowhite HPV lesions after application of 5-percent acetic acid.

nal tissue is grasped and lifted to limit the biopsy depth. Menopausal women may have significant thinning of the vaginal mucosa, and biopsy should be done with greater care or with a smaller biopsy forceps to avoid perforation through the vaginal wall. Hemostasis is achieved using silver nitrate applicators or Monsel paste. Vaginal lesion size, location, and specific biopsy sites are carefully documented for future management and surveillance.

Treatment

Like high-grade CIN, high-grade VaIN is believed to be a precancerous lesion and generally requires eradication (Punnonen, 1989; Rome, 2000). Because vaginal neoplasia is uncommon, most management strategies are derived from small, nonrandomized, retrospective, and statistically underpowered investigations. Management of VaIN depends on the grade of neoplasia and may include observation, excision, ablation, topical antineoplastics, or rarely, radiation therapy. Each treatment method has advantages and disadvantages, and none has proven superior efficacy. Management strategies are determined after physical, colposcopic, and histologic examination of lesions and comprehensive patient counseling.

Low-Grade Vaginal Intraepithelial Neoplasia 1

In a long-term study following 132 patients with VaIN, Rome and associates (2000) found that an observational approach after biopsy resulted in regression of VaIN 1 in seven of eight patients (88 percent). Furthermore, no VaIN 1 lesion progressed to high-grade VaIN or invasive cancer. This lesion most often represents atrophy or a transient HPV infection, and surveillance is reasonable in most cases. Although no evidence-based guidelines are available, surveillance similar to that for CIN with repeat cytology with or without vaginoscopy every 6 to 12 months seems reasonable until abnormalities resolve.

High-Grade Vaginal Intraepithelial Neoplasia 2 to 3

The treatment choice for patients with high-grade VaIN is influenced by several factors. These include the location and number of lesions, the patient's sexual activity status, vaginal length, prior radiation therapy, previous treatment modalities in patients with recurrent VaIN, and clinician experience. Potential adverse effects of treatment on subsequent quality of life such as pain, difficulties with sexual intercourse, and scarring should always be considered when choosing a therapeutic modality.

Excision. Wide local excision of a high-grade unifocal lesion or partial vaginectomy for multifocal lesions may be used. Hoffman (1992a) found that 9 of 32 patients (28 percent) with prior hysterectomy and VaIN 3 had occult invasive cancer in the vaginal cuff. Therefore, surgical excision should be considered for high-grade lesions involving the vaginal cuff region, particularly if any thickening or nodularity of the cuff suggests occult invasive disease.

Excisional procedures have the advantage of providing a surgical specimen for which resected margins can be examined and in which invasive vaginal cancer can be excluded. Moreover, partial vaginectomy has the highest cure rate and fewest recurrences for high-grade disease (Dodge, 2001). Wide local excision carries less morbidity than vaginectomy, but both procedures may be complicated by bladder or rectal injury and hemorrhage. In addition, subsequent vaginal scarring and stenosis may compromise vaginal intercourse or cause dyspareunia.

As an alternative excisional modality, CO_2 laser causes significant thermal damage to the tissue specimen and is not recommended. Likewise, LEEP has poor depth control and carries a substantial risk of thermal damage to underlying pelvic structures, including the bladder and bowel.

Carbon Dioxide Laser Ablation. Laser ablation is well suited for eradication of multifocal lesions and causes less scarring and blood loss than excisional modalities. Rarely, excessive bleeding and thermal damage to the bladder and bowel can occur. A broader explanation of laser ablation techniques is found in Section 41-26 (p. 1081).

Medical Ablation. Before medical treatment, as with any ablative procedure, the possibility of invasive cancer must be excluded. Following this, persistent VaIN 1 or 2 and selected VaIN 3 lesions may be medically treated using 5-percent fluorouracil (5-FU) cream "off-label" as it is not FDA approved for this indication (Efudex) (Krebs, 1989). Its efficacy has not been proven in large, randomized trials, and studies with small numbers of patients have demonstrated mixed results. Treatment regimens vary widely. One dosing schedule calls for a 3-mL dose of cream placed in the vaginal vault by plastic vaginal applicator every other day for 3 days during the first week of treatment and then once weekly thereafter for up to 10 weeks. This cream is often associated with a robust inflammatory reaction that can include vaginal burning and vulvar irritation. To minimize leakage onto the vulva, 5-FU cream is best applied intravaginally at bedtime, when a recumbent position will be maintained for hours. Additionally, an occlusive, water-resistant ointment can be placed on the vulva to protect it from 5-FU's effects. Protective gloves should be worn when handling 5-FU cream. Patients selected for this treatment require thorough counseling, effective contraception as needed, consent for off-label medication use, and close monitoring for excessive inflammation and ulceration, which can lead to vaginal or vulvar scarring and loss of function.

Radiation Therapy. There is a very limited role for radiation treatment of high-grade VaIN. It carries a significant risk of serious morbidity and should be reserved for select cases. In a review of 136 cases of vaginal carcinoma in situ, radiation therapy was used in 27 patients, and a 100-percent cure rate was noted. However, 63 percent developed significant complications including vaginal stenosis, adhesions, ulceration, necrosis, and fistula formation (Benedet, 1984). Furthermore, radiation treatment compromises subsequent cytologic, colposcopic, and histologic interpretation. Disease recurrence often necessitates radical surgery.

Prognosis

In a study of 132 patients treated for high-grade VaIN, excision and CO_2 laser ablation had similar cure rates of 69 percent. Topical 5-fluorouracil cream was curative in 46 percent of cases (Rome, 2000). Patients with any grade of vaginal neoplasia require long-term monitoring as the persistence and recurrence rate for high-grade disease is significant. Currently, there are no evidence-based guidelines available for post-treatment surveillance of VaIN. Monitoring should include collection of vaginal cytology and performance of vaginoscopy approximately 2 months after treatment is completed. Continued surveillance with periodic cytology with or without vaginoscopy at 6- to 12-month intervals for several years thereafter seems prudent. Long-term annual cytologic screening is needed thereafter.

VULVAR PREINVASIVE LESIONS

Incidence

Vulvar cancer is rare. Specifically, the U.S. incidence in 2006 comprised less than 3 to 5 percent of all gynecologic cancers and less than 0.5 percent of all cancers in women. Ninety percent of vulvar cancer is squamous and in some cases, develops slowly through precancerous epithelial changes called vulvar intraepithelial neoplasia (VIN) (Fig. 29-18). However, VIN is not necessarily analogous to CIN, as the vulva lacks a transformation zone, is keratinized, and VIN does not progress to high-grade disease and cancer as often.

A study identifying trends in the incidence of vulvar carcinoma in situ found a 411-percent increase from 1973 to 2000. This trend is particularly pronounced in younger women and is thought to be linked to the increased incidence of sexually

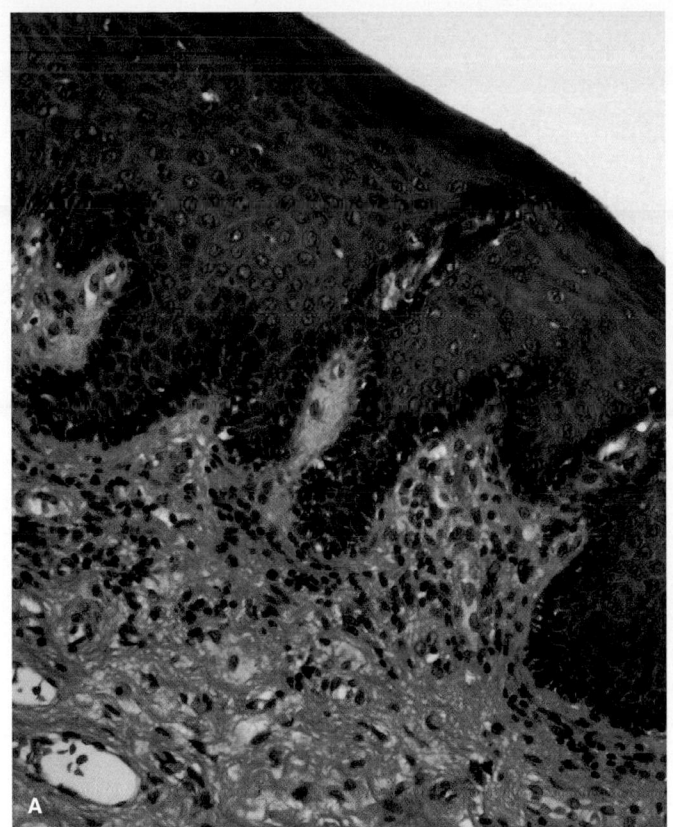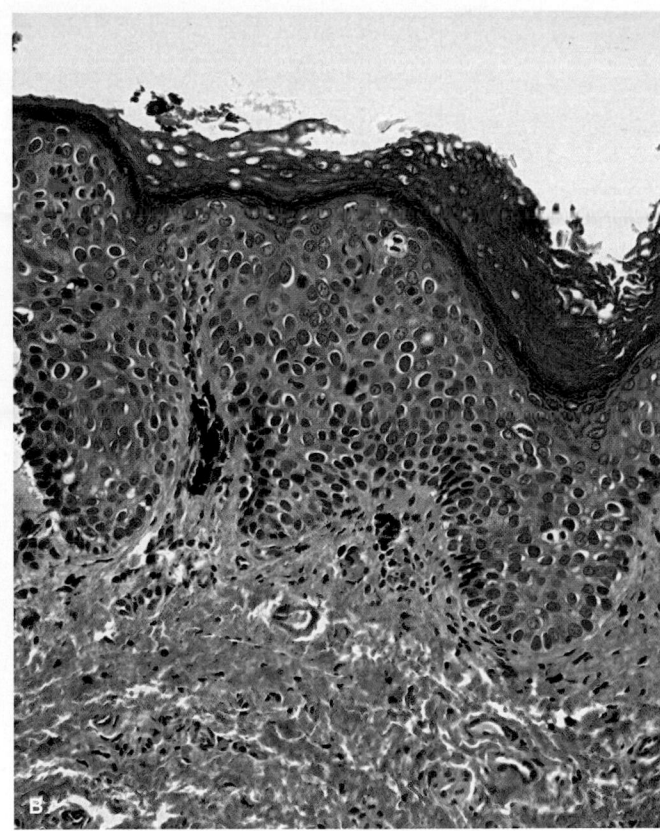

FIGURE 29-18 A. Normal vulvar histology. **B.** VIN 3 histology. *(Photographs contributed by Dr. Raheela Ashfaq.)*

transmitted infections such as that caused by HPV (Howe, 2001). Jones and colleagues (2005) reported that the mean age of women with VIN has decreased from 50 to 39 years since 1980.

Pathophysiology

Although HPV DNA has been found in up to 80 percent of VIN lesions, HPV is less commonly associated with vulvar cancer. Most studies show approximately 40-percent HPV DNA positivity in vulvar cancer specimens worldwide (Madeleine, 1997; Monk, 1995; Smith, 2009). The progression of vulvar carcinoma in situ to invasive cancer has been strongly suggested, although not confirmed conclusively. Therefore, VIN 3 lesions are generally treated (van Seters, 2005).

Original Terminology

Terminology for squamous vulvar intraepithelial neoplasia was introduced by the International Society for the Study of Vulvar Disease (ISSVD) in 1986. Under this classification, VIN grades 1, 2, and 3 were defined by abnormal cellular changes found to varying thicknesses within the squamous epithelium, similar to CIN (Wilkinson, 1986).

Current Terminology

In 2004, classification of VIN was simplified by the ISSVD. The older designation of VIN 1 has been eliminated, whereas VIN 2 and 3 categories have been combined. This redefinition reflects issues of whether lesions are likely to be premalignant or not and therefore, whether lesions require therapy or not. The VIN 1 category has been eliminated because evidence is lacking that such lesions are cancer precursors. These lesions more likely represent benign reactive changes or HPV effect. In support of this view, a recent analysis of type-specific HPV prevalence in VIN 1 lesions demonstrated that the most common type isolated was HPV 6, which is nononcogenic (Smith, 2009). The term *VIN* is now applied only to histologically high-grade squamous cell lesions and combines the previous categories of VIN 2 and 3 (Table 29-12).

Vulvar intraepithelial neoplasia is subcategorized into VIN, *usual type*; VIN, *differentiated type*; and VIN, *unclassified type*. Of these, VIN, *usual type* encompasses the former VIN 2 and 3 categories as well as older histologic terms including carcinoma in situ. VIN, *usual type* lesions can be grouped histologically as warty (condylomatous), basaloid, or mixed and are associated with oncogenic HPV infection. HPV 16 was the most prevalent type found in an analysis of VIN 2/3 and vulvar cancer (Smith, 2009). In general, HPV DNA-positive high-grade VIN lesions morphologically resemble high-grade CIN and tend to be multicentric and multifocal (Haefner, 1995).

The lower genital tract responds to HPV infection as a "field effect," and thus, risk factors for cervical carcinoma may have similar influence on the squamous epithelia of the vulva and vagina. Accordingly, VIN, *usual type* is strongly associated with

TABLE 29-12. Vulvar Intraepithelial Neoplasia: Terminology and Characteristics

VIN Type	Clinical Presentation and Risk Factors

VIN, usual type
  Warty
  Basaloid
  Mixed
	Formerly VIN 2, VIN 3, vulvar CIS
	Younger women
	Multicentric disease
	Oncogenic HPV infection
	Smoking, other STIs, immunosuppression

VIN, differentiated type	2–10% of former VIN 3 lesions Older, postmenopausal women Oncogenic HPV infection uncommon
VIN, unclassified type	Rare pagetoid lesions

CIS = carcinoma in situ; HPV = human papillomavirus; STIs = sexually transmitted infections; VIN = vulvar intraepithelial neoplasia.

TABLE 29-13. Symptoms of Vulvar Intraepithelial Neoplasia

Pruritus, pain, burning
Bleeding
Discharge
Urination discomfort
Persistent ulcer
Abnormal skin color or texture
Existing nevus change in symmetry or color
Lump or wart-like growth

sexually transmissible infections and tobacco smoking, particularly in younger women (Hoffman, 1992b; Jones, 1994, 2005). It is also seen as part of multifocal lower genital tract neoplasia in immune compromised women.

In contrast, VIN, *differentiated type* is less common and accounts for only 2 to 10 percent of all VIN 3 cases (Hart, 2001). Such lesions tend to be unifocal and are typically found in older, nonsmoking, postmenopausal women in their sixth and seventh decade. Infection with oncogenic HPV is uncommon and probably does not play a role in the genesis of these lesions. However, VIN, *differentiated type* is more likely to progress to squamous cell carcinoma than VIN, *usual type.* A recent study noted a five times higher progression of VIN, *differentiated type* to vulvar squamous cell carcinoma compared with VIN, *usual type* (van de Nieuwenhof, 2009). Rare pagetoid types of VIN 2 and 3 cannot be classified in any of the foregoing categories and are termed VIN, *unclassified type* (Sideri, 2005).

Diagnosis

VIN may be asymptomatic and discovered with routine gynecologic examinations or during evaluation of abnormal cervical or vaginal cytology. When present, potentially distressing signs and symptoms may affect a patient's sexuality and quality of life (Table 29-13). Whereas high-grade lesions of the cervix and vagina are generally invisible without acetic acid application and use of a colposcope, clinically significant VIN lesions are usually visible without the use of special techniques. To avoid diagnostic delay, most focal vulvar lesions should be biopsied. This is particularly true of pigmented lesions, genital warts in postmenopausal or immune compromised women, or warts that persist despite topical thera-

pies (American College of Obstetricians and Gynecologists, American Society for Colposcopy and Cervical Pathology, 2011).

Vulvoscopy

A histologic confirmation of diagnosis is necessary before high-grade VIN is managed. Selection of the best location to biopsy is aided by magnification of the vulva and perianus, usually with a colposcope. This examination is termed vulvoscopy. Alternatively, any good light source and a handheld magnifying lens can be used.

Vulvar epithelial changes are enhanced by applying a 3- to 5-percent acetic-acid-soaked gauze pad to the vulva for 5 minutes prior to vulvoscopic examination. This is usually well tolerated but may cause excessive pain or burning in the presence of vulvar irritation, ulceration, or fissures. Acetic acid wash accentuates the surface topography of lesions and may call attention to acetowhite lesions not easily seen with gross inspection. Pigmented VIN lesions tend to turn a dusky gray due to hyperkeratosis. Vascular patterns are generally not seen, but high-grade VIN may rarely demonstrate coarse punctation. As an alternative, 1-percent toluidine blue, a nuclear stain, may be helpful in defining the best site for biopsy or the margins of surgery (Joura, 1998). Its use is technically more challenging and results are fraught with both false positives and negatives.

VIN, *usual type* varies in clinical appearance. Some lesions are raised, hyperkeratotic, and darkly pigmented, whereas others are flat and white (Figs. 29-19 and 29-20). Often, lesions appear bulky, resemble condylomata, and are multifocal with extensive involvement of the perineum and adjacent skin (Fig. 29-21). VIN, *differentiated type* is generally unifocal and may be associated with lichen sclerosis or vulvar squamous cell hyperplasia. A lesion may appear as an ulcer, warty papule, or hyperkeratotic plaque. Any lesion suspicious for invasive carcinoma should be biopsied, particularly lesions that are elevated, roughened, nodular, or ulcerated.

The most abnormal-appearing areas are biopsied, although necrotic areas often yield nondiagnostic findings and should be avoided if possible. Biopsies measuring up to 6 mm diameter can be obtained using a Keyes punch biopsy after provision of a local subcutaneous anesthetic injection with 1- to 2-percent lidocaine with or without epinephrine (Fig. 4-2,

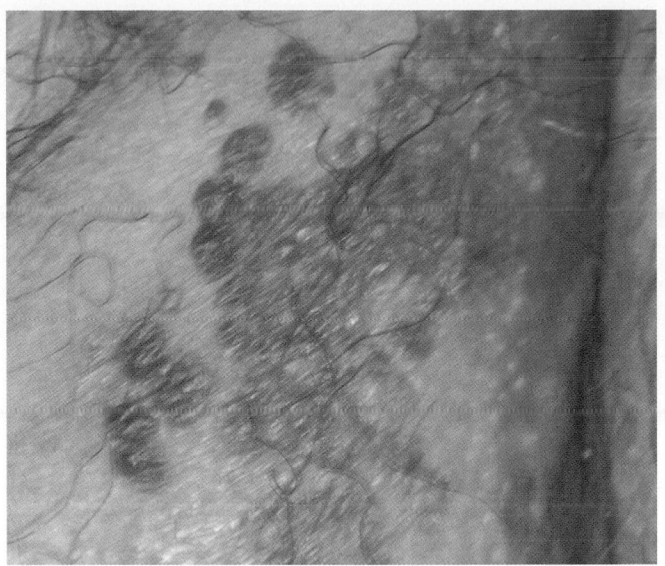

FIGURE 29-19 Pigmented, multifocal, high-grade VIN.

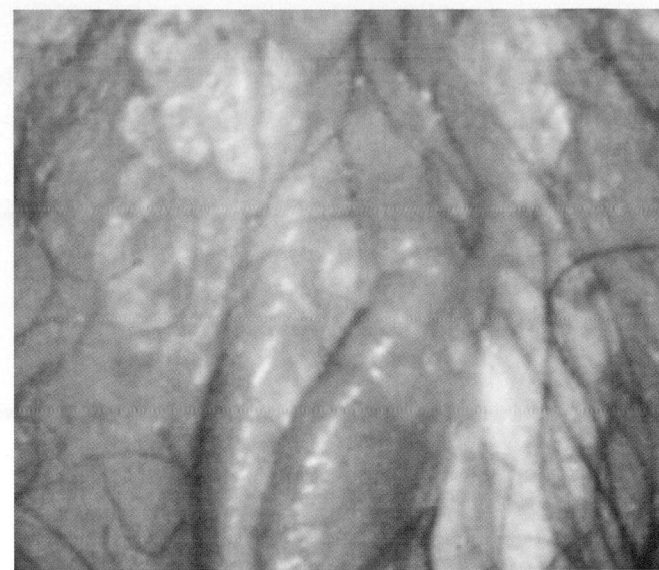

FIGURE 29-20 Multifocal leukoplakia typical of high-grade VIN.

p. 112). Topical anesthetics can be applied several minutes prior to injection of local anesthesia to decrease discomfort. If lesions are close to the clitoral hood, general anesthesia is often warranted due to increased pain with injection of local anesthesia and increased vascularity. Careful documentation and mapping of vulvar biopsy sites aids future management plans.

Management
Vulvar Intraepithelial Neoplasia 1

As previously stated, the progression of VIN 1 to VIN 3 has not been observed, and the modified 2004 ISSVD terminology has eliminated the VIN 1 category entirely. Previously reported

VIN 1 should not be treated but may be reassessed annually in patients at risk for high-grade VIN. Reassessment may include gross inspection or vulvoscopy and biopsy as clinically indicated if high-grade neoplasia is suspected.

Vulvar Intraepithelial Neoplasia 2 and 3

All high-grade VIN should be treated (American College of Obstetricians and Gynecologists, American Society for Colposcopy and Cervical Pathology, 2011). Standard treatment of high-grade lesions of the vulva consists of local destruction or excision. Medical management is currently investigational. Treatment of VIN 2 or 3 is individualized with the goal of preserving normal anatomy and genital function and is based on lesion location and size. VIN involving the hair-bearing areas

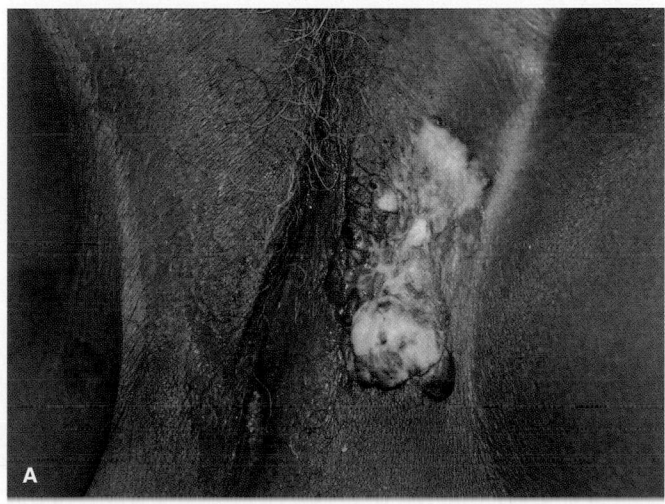

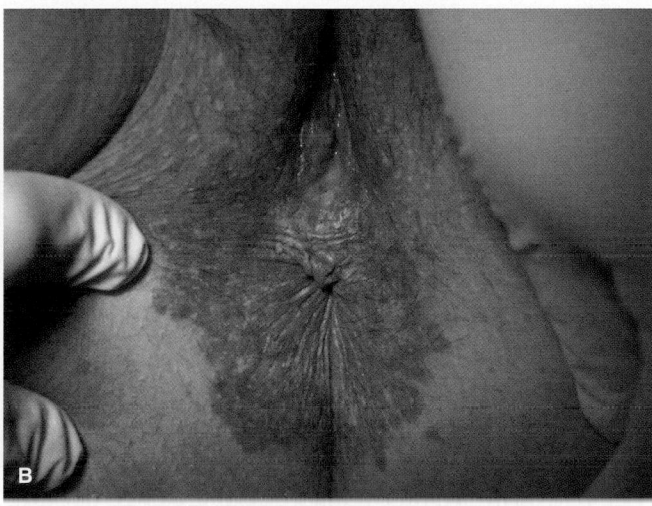

FIGURE 29-21 A. Bulky lesion of VIN 3/carcinoma in situ. **B.** VIN 3 with extensive perineal and perianal involvement.

of the vulva (external to Hart line) may extend deeper into pilosebaceous units, whereas mucosal lesions tend to be more superficial (Wright, 1992). Many patients are best treated by combined excisional and ablative procedures.

Regardless of the modality selected, treatment side effects are common and can include vulvar discomfort, poor wound healing, infection, and scarring that may result in chronic pain or dyspareunia. Thus, treatment objectives should include: (1) improving patient symptoms, (2) preserving the appearance and function of the vulva, and (3) excluding and preventing invasive disease.

Excision. Extensive vulvar surgery for VIN is not always necessary if patients are closely monitored for disease progression or recurrence. VIN 3 or vulvar carcinoma in situ or large VIN lesions in which invasive carcinoma cannot be excluded are best managed by wide local excision (WLE) with a surgical margin of at least 5 mm of normal tissue (Section 41-28, p. 1086). Because disease recurrence is related to surgical margin status, frozen section histology of the specimen margins is advantageous (Friedrich, 1980; Jones, 2005). Hopkins (2001) reported disease recurrence rates of 20 percent for cases with negative surgical margins but 40 percent for those with positive margins.

Wide local excision can be disfiguring and may require plastic surgical techniques or skin grafting to minimize anatomic distortion, pain, and loss of function. All vulvar surgeries require thorough preoperative counseling regarding expected anatomic results and sexual function and should be performed by adequately trained and experienced clinicians.

Ablation. Although it provides good cosmetic results, lesion ablation with CO_2 laser does not allow evaluation of the surgical specimen (Section 41-28, 1088). Therefore, the presence of invasive carcinoma must be excluded beforehand. Laser is generally less disfiguring than WLE, but can result in prolonged, painful healing and wound discharge. Preoperative counseling regarding anticipated postoperative results mirrors that for WLE. VIN recurrence has been reported more commonly following laser vaporization than after WLE (David, 1996; Herod, 1996). However, Hoffman (1992b) reported that 15 of 18 patients (83 percent) with VIN 3 remained free of recurrent disease after CO_2 laser ablation.

Cavitational ultrasonic surgical aspiration (CUSA) may be used in the treatment of high-grade VIN confined solely to non-hair-bearing vulvar skin. With this tool, ultrasound is used to cause cavitation and disruption of affected tissue, which is then aspirated and collected (Section 41-28, p. 1087). This technique offers the advantages of laser, less scarring and pain than WLE, while additionally providing a pathologic specimen (von Gruenigen, 2007). However, the tissue specimen is severely fragmented and lacks the diagnostic accuracy of surgically excised tissue. Miller and colleagues (2002) evaluated this procedure in 37 patients with VIN 2 or 3. They found an overall recurrence of 35 percent within a mean surveillance of 33 months.

VIN involves the pilosebaceous units in up to two thirds of cases, but rarely exceeds 2.5 mm in depth from the epidermal surface (Shatz, 1989). This is important for disease management, particularly if ablative procedures are considered.

Topical Therapy. Topical treatments are currently under investigation and have not yet become recommended clinical therapy. These agents include imiquimod 5-percent cream (Aldara), cidofovir emulsion (Vistide), and 5-percent fluorouracil cream (van Seters, 2008). Cidofovir is not currently FDA approved for use in HPV-related disease, and topical preparations must be compounded. 5-FU is potentially caustic and teratogenic and is not a first-line choice for VIN treatment (National Cancer Institute, 2010). Topical imiquimod (off-label) has garnered the most interest recently. It has lower toxicity, and numerous case reports and two randomized controlled trials have reported favorable regression rates of high-grade VIN (Mahto, 2010). A phase II study on the use of imiquimod in treating VIN 2/3 found a response rate of 77 percent and 20 percent recurrence rate compared with a recurrence rate of 53 percent in a surgically treated cohort (Le, 2007).

Other Therapy. Photodynamic therapy (PDT) using topical 5-aminolevulinic acid (5-ALA) has been used as tissue-conserving treatment for VIN or vulvar carcinoma in situ. Although PDT preserves tissue without scarring or disfigurement, it has low response and high recurrence rates (Hillemanns, 2006; Kurwa, 2000).

Prognosis and Prevention

Case reports describing the invasive potential of untreated, high-grade VIN are accumulating (Jones, 2005). Jones and associates (1994) reviewed the outcome of 113 patients with VIN 3 and their risk for future development of invasive vulvar carcinoma. They found that 87 percent of untreated patients progressed to vulvar cancer, whereas only 3.8 percent of treated patients progressed to invasive carcinoma. It is currently not possible to predict high-grade VIN lesion behavior. Regardless of the treatment modality chosen, recurrence is common (up to 50 percent), particularly in patients with multifocal disease or immune compromise. Indefinite surveillance for multifocal lower genital tract disease is recommended. Moreover, high-grade VIN is considered by some to be an indication for colposcopic evaluation of the cervix and vagina regardless of normal cervical cytology. Posttreatment surveillance consists of careful vulvar reevaluation at 6 and 12 months, with annual vulvar inspection thereafter (American College of Obstetricians and Gynecologists, American Society for Colposcopy and Cervical Pathology, 2011).

For prevention, prophylactic HPV vaccination against types 16 and 18 would has the potential to prevent approximately one third of vulvar cancers (Smith, 2009). Smoking cessation and optimization of compromised immune status are also important strategies.

ANAL INTRAEPITHELIAL NEOPLASIA (AIN)

Incidence

For U.S. women in 2009, 3190 anal cancers and 450 deaths from this cancer were reported (Jemal, 2009). Accordingly, the lifetime risk is low and approximates 1 in 610. Moreover, since

2000, the incidence of anal cancer has decreased slightly in women younger than 50 years (Altekruse, 2009).

Pathophysiology

Anal cancer is strongly associated with anal intraepithelial neoplasia (AIN) (Palefsky, 1994). Of AIN cases, Hampl and coworkers (2006) documented that 89 percent contained HPV DNA. In addition, Santoso and associates (2010) reported a 12-percent prevalence of biopsy-proven AIN in a group of women with HPV-related disease. As with cervical squamous cell cancers, oncogenic HPV types 16 and 18 are thought to be the principal etiologic agents responsible for the development of anal squamous cell cancers and their precursors (Zbar, 2002). Little is known of the natural history of anal HPV infection and its progressive potential in women, but it is suspected to behave similarly to cervicovaginal lesions. Cervical and anal lesions generally are manifested at or near their respective squamocolumnar epithelial junctions, which in the anus is called the *transition zone* (Goldstone, 2001). Anal disease is classified by the same cytologic and histologic nomenclature used to describe cervical disease. Thus, AIN 1, 2, and 3 correspond to mild, moderate, and severe dysplasia, respectively (Fig. 29-22). Although natural history studies for anal HPV disease are lacking, some suggest that eradication of high-grade anal lesions may decrease the incidence of invasive anal cancer (Santoso, 2010). However, in contrast to cervical neoplasia, the protective effect of treating precursor lesions of the anal canal remains unproven (Williams, 1994). The FDA (2010) has approved the vaccine Gardasil for the prevention of anal cancer and precancerous lesions associated with HPV types 6, 11, 16, and 18.

Risk Factors

Risk factors for AIN include anal HPV infection, receptive anal intercourse, tobacco smoking, and history of other sexually transmitted infections, including HIV. Anal cancer and its

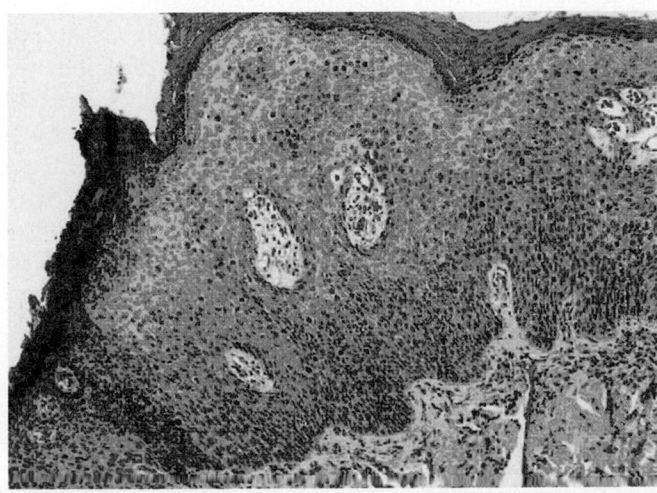

FIGURE 29-22 AIN 3 histology. *(Photograph contributed by Dr. Raheela Ashfaq.)*

likely precursor, AIN 3, are increasing at higher rates in HIV-positive compared with HIV-negative patients (Frisch, 2000; Tandon, 2010).

Diagnosis
Screening Recommendations

As with cervical cancer, prevention by screening persons at risk may be the best approach to decreasing the incidence of anal cancer. Unlike cervical cancer prevention, screening and treatment protocols for AIN are not codified. Approaches may include testing at an undetermined frequency with any of a combination of anal cytology, HPV testing, and anoscopy. Testing would be followed by treatment of high-grade anal lesions (Berry, 2004; Friedlander, 2004; Palefsky, 1997). Some investigators suggest that annual cervical and anal cytology should be offered to all HIV-positive patients, but only if the infrastructure necessary for the evaluation and management of abnormal cytology results and precancerous lesions is available (Palefsky, 2005; Panther, 2005). For the generalist who lacks adequate clinical support for the management of abnormal anal cytology, patients may be referred to tertiary care centers or colorectal surgeons for further evaluation and treatment. Currently, neither the American College of Obstetricians and Gynecologists nor the U.S. Preventive Services Task Force provides screening recommendations for AIN.

Anal Cytology

Some studies suggest that anal cytology lacks efficacy as a screening tool for AIN and anal cancer (Nahas, 2009; Santoso, 2010). If used, anal cytology may be more sensitive using liquid-based preparations than conventional glass slides (Friedlander, 2004; Sherman, 1995). Sampling is obtained by inserting a Dacron swab or endocervical brush moistened with water or a small amount of water-based lubricant approximately 5 cm into the anal canal, which should be above the anal transition zone. The device is then withdrawn with a twirling motion while applying pressure to the anal canal walls. The swab is then either swirled in the cytology solution to release exfoliated cells or smeared on a glass slide and fixed with isopropyl alcohol as with cervical cytology. Nothing per rectum is recommended 24 hours prior to an anal cytology test. Anal cytology is reported using terminology analogous to the Bethesda 2001 nomenclature for cervical cytology.

High-resolution Anoscopy

This technique uses anoscopy, illumination and magnification with a colposcope, and acetic acid application to evaluate the anal canal in a manner similar to colposcopy (Fig. 29-23) (Jay, 1997). It is more challenging to perform than colposcopy for both the patient and the provider, and specific training is recommended. Anal neoplasia demonstrates colposcopic features similar to those of CIN. Therefore, lesion grading and terminology are the same as for cervical lesions. Biopsies are directed at the most abnormal areas. Considered

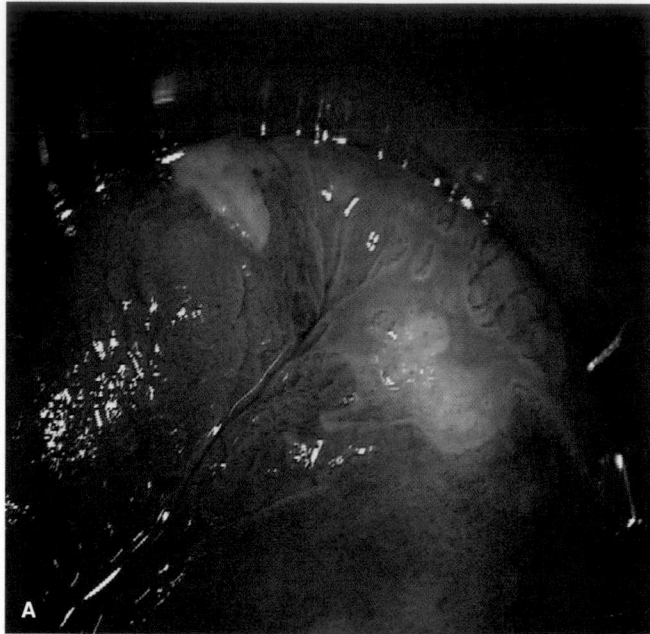

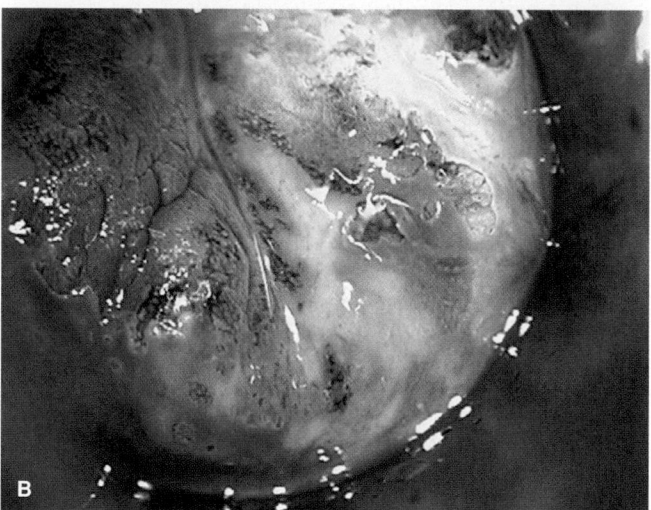

FIGURE 29-23 A. AIN 1 translucent acetowhite lesion. **B.** AIN 3 dense acetowhite lesion. *(Photographs contributed by Naomi Jay, RN NP PhD.)*

by some to be the gold standard for diagnosing AIN, the role of high-resolution anoscopy for primary screening or for the evaluation of abnormal anal cytology is not yet clearly defined. It is presently available in a limited number of health care locales.

Management

The natural history of AIN is not yet established. And, the benefits of screening for, identification of, and eradication of anal cancer precursor lesions are currently under investigation, and clinical guidelines are not currently available. Therefore, clinicians should use their judgment and involve patients in decisions regarding screening for and managing AIN. Abnormal anal cytology is best evaluated with high-resolution anoscopy.

High-grade AIN lesions should be referred to appropriate specialists for possible excision or ablative procedures.

Treatment

Treatment is restricted to locally ablative or excisional procedures that eliminate individual high-grade intraepithelial lesions. Unlike the cervix, the entire anal squamocolumnar junction cannot be destroyed or removed due to potential morbidity. Treatment of biopsy-proven high-grade AIN lesions can be accomplished by a variety of ablative procedures including the CO_2 laser, electrosurgical coagulation performed under general anesthesia, or infrared coagulation as an office procedure (Chang, 2002; Goldstone, 2005). Cryoablation and topically applied 85-percent trichloroacetic acid are alternative treatment methods.

THE HIV-INFECTED PATIENT

Pathophysiology

HIV-infected women are known to have a high burden of HPV-associated anogenital disease. Multiple studies show that HIV-positive women have a higher prevalence and longer persistence of cervical HPV infection (De Vuyst, 2008). The risks of all HPV-associated cancers of the vulva, vagina, and anus have been shown to increase from 5 years prior to 5 years following HIV seroconversion (Chaturvedi, 2009). In addition, these women have a higher probability of simultaneously carrying multiple oncogenic HPV types than those without HIV infection.

Additionally, studies consistently suggest that HIV-positive women have much higher rates of both CIN and VIN compared with rates in HIV-uninfected women (Ellerbrock, 2000; Spitzer, 1999; Wright, 1994). In women infected with HIV, up to 60 percent of Pap tests exhibit cytologic abnormalities and as many as 40 percent have colposcopic evidence of dysplasia. Moreover, a recent study found that HIV-positive women with abnormal cervical cytology and/or cervical HPV results are at increased risk for anal HPV infection and anal neoplasia (Tandon, 2010).

HIV infection influences lower genital tract disease prognosis. For example, during the acquired immunodeficiency disease (AIDS) epidemic, Maiman and associates (1990) noted in a study cohort that all HIV-positive women with cervical cancer died from their cervical cancer compared with only 37 percent of HIV-negative women. Because of the increased risk of cervical cancer and poorer prognosis, cervical cancer was designated as an AIDS-defining condition by the Centers for Disease Control and Prevention (Ahdieh, 2001; Brown, 1994; Centers for Disease Control and Prevention, 2002; Palefsky, 1999).

Management
Screening

Because of a significantly higher risk of developing squamous intraepithelial lesions throughout the lower genital tract, cervical cytologic screening should be obtained every 6 months for the first year after an HIV infection diagnosis. With normal cytologies, annual screening for life is recommended (Kaplan,

2009). In addition, women with HIV may benefit from routine anal Pap screens (Palefsky, 2001). However, evidence-based screening recommendations for AIN have not yet been developed but are expected to evolve as the results of current clinical research become available.

Abnormal Cytology

The 2006 Consensus Guidelines recommend that Pap test abnormalities, including ASC-US, in HIV-positive women be managed in the same manner as for the general population (Wright, 2007b). However, the Centers for Disease Control and Prevention has questioned the utility of HPV testing for the triage of ASC-US in HIV-positive women and therefore recommends referral of all women with ASC-US results for colposcopy (Kaplan, 2009). Because HIV-positive women with cervical intraepithelial neoplasia are often found to have extensive, multifocal dysplastic epithelial disease, any colposcopic examination should include inspection of the entire lower genital tract (Hillemanns, 1996; Tandon, 2010).

Treatment
Treatment Selection

HIV-positive women are at high risk of disease recurrence and progression after treatment of CIN or VIN, and poorer outcomes appear to correlate with degree of immune suppression. Cryotherapy has a particularly high failure rate among treatment methods (Korn, 1996; Spitzer, 1999). Additionally, ablative modalities have an increased risk of obscuring occult invasive cancer in high-grade lesions. Excisional procedures including loop excision, and cold-knife conization provide histologic confirmation and margins for evaluation. Although excisional therapy is effective for eradicating CIN in immune competent patients, the same treatment seems to be effective only in preventing progression to cancer in HIV-infected women (Heard, 2005). Moreover, persistence and recurrence rates for excised lower genital tract disease are higher in women with HIV compared with those without HIV infection.

Highly Active Anti-Retroviral Therapy (HAART)

The therapeutic impact of HAART on HPV infection is poorly understood and conflicting results have been reported (Heard, 2004). To date, HAART has not been shown consistently to improve the natural history of HPV-related diseases. In fact, anal cancer rates in HIV-infected individuals have continued to increase over the past decade (De Vuyst, 2008; Tandon, 2010). Indeed, if HAART leads to increased longevity yet does not alter the incidence or progression of HPV-related disease, individuals on HAART may gain sufficient longevity to develop HPV-related epithelial cancers (de Sanjose, 2002).

REFERENCES

Abu J, Davies Q: Endocervical curettage at the time of colposcopic assessment of the uterine cervix. Obstet Gynecol Surv 60(5):315, 2005

Ahdieh L, Klein RS, Burk R, et al: Prevalence, incidence, and type-specific persistence of human papillomavirus in human immunodeficiency virus (HIV)-positive and HIV-negative women. J Infect Dis 184(6):682, 2001

Altekruse SF, Kosary CL, Krapcho M, et al (eds): SEER Cancer Statistics Review, 1975-2007, National Cancer Institute. 2009. Available at: http://seer.cancer.gov/csr/1975_2007/. Accessed December 27, 2010

Amburgey CF, VanEenwyk J, Davis FG, et al: Undernutrition as a risk factor for cervical intraepithelial neoplasia: a case-control analysis. Nutr Cancer 20(1):51, 1993

American College of Obstetricians and Gynecologists: Cervical cancer in adolescents: screening, evaluation, and management. Committee Opinion No. 463, August 2010a

American College of Obstetricians and Gynecologists: Cervical cytology screening. Practice Bulletin No. 109, December 2009

American College of Obstetricians and Gynecologists: Human papillomavirus. Practice Bulletin No. 61, December 2005

American College of Obstetricians and Gynecologists: Human papillomavirus vaccination. Committee Opinion No. 467, September 2010b

American College of Obstetricians and Gynecologists: Management of abnormal cervical cytology and histology. Practice Bulletin No. 99, December 2008

American College of Obstetricians and Gynecologists, American Society for Colposcopy and Cervical Pathology: Management of vulvar intraepithelial neoplasia. Committee Opinion No. 509, November 2011

American Society for Colposcopy and Cervical Pathology: HPV genotyping 2009 clinical update. 2009. Available at: http://www.asccp.org/pdfs/consensus/clinical_update_20090408.pdf Accessed October 8, 2010

Anderson MC: The cervix, excluding cancer. In Anderson MC (ed): Systematic Pathology—Female Reproductive System. New York, Churchill Livingstone, 1991, p 47

Arbyn M, Bergeron C, Klinkhamer P, et al: Liquid compared with conventional cervical cytology. Obstet Gynecol 111:167, 2008

ASCUS-LSIL Triage Study (ALTS) Group: A randomized trial on the management of low-grade squamous intraepithelial lesion cytology interpretations. Am J Obstet Gynecol 188:1393, 2003a

ASCUS-LSIL Triage Study (ALTS) Group: Human papillomavirus testing for triage of women with cytologic evidence of low-grade squamous intraepithelial lesions: baseline data from a randomized trial. J Natl Cancer Inst 92(5):397, 2000

ASCUS-LSIL Triage Study (ALTS) Group: Results of a randomized trial on the management of cytology interpretations of atypical squamous cells of undetermined significance. Am J Obstet Gynecol 188:1383, 2003b

Baseman JG, Koutsky LA: The epidemiology of human papillomavirus infections. J Clin Virol 32(Suppl 1):S16, 2005

Bauer HM, Ting Y, Greer CE, et al: Genital human papillomavirus infection in female university students as determined by a PCR-based method. JAMA 265(4):472, 1991

Becker TM, Wheeler CM, McGough NS, et al: Cigarette smoking and other risk factors for cervical dysplasia in southwestern Hispanic and non-Hispanic white women. Cancer Epidemiol Biomarkers Prev 3(2):113, 1994

Benard VB, Coughlin SS, Thompson T, et al: Cervical cancer incidence in the United States by area of residence, 1998-2001. Obstet Gynecol 110:681, 2007

Benedet JL, Sanders BH: Carcinoma in situ of the vagina. Am J Obstet Gynecol 148(5):695, 1984

Bergeron C, Ferenczy A, Richart RM, et al: Micropapillomatosis labialis appears unrelated to human papillomavirus. Obstet Gynecol 76(2):281, 1990

Berry JM, Palefsky JM, Welton ML: Anal cancer and its precursors in HIV-positive patients: perspectives and management. Surg Oncol Clin North Am 13(2):355, 2004

Beutner KR, Tyring S: Human papillomavirus and human disease. Am J Med 102(5A):9, 1997

Boardman LA, Stanko C, Weitzen S, et al: Atypical squamous cells of undetermined significance: human papillomavirus testing in adolescents. Obstet Gynecol 105(4):741, 2005

Bornstein J: The HPV vaccines—which to prefer? Obstet Gynecol Surv 64(5):345, 2009

Bornstein J, Bentley J, Bosze P, et al: 2011 IFCPC colposcopic nomenclature. July 5, 2011. Available at: http://www.ifcpc.org/documents/nomenclature7-11.pdf. Accessed October 25, 2011

Bosch FX, Lorincz A, Muñoz N, et al: The causal relation between human papillomavirus and cervical cancer. J Clin Pathol 55(4):244, 2002

Brinton LA: Epidemiology of cervical cancer—overview. IARC Sci Publ (119):3, 1992

Brinton LA, Reeves WC, Brenes MM, et al: Parity as a risk factor for cervical cancer. Am J Epidemiol 130:486, 1989

Brown DR, Bryan JT, Cramer H, et al: Detection of multiple human papillomavirus types in condylomata acuminata from immunosuppressed patients. J Infect Dis 170(4):759, 1994

Brown DR, Kjaer SK, Sigurddson K, et al: The impact of quadrivalent human papillomavirus (HPV; types 6, 11, 16, and 18) L1 virus-like particle vaccine on infection and disease due to oncogenic nonvaccine HPV types in generally HPV-naïve women aged 16-26 years. J Infect Dis 199:926, 2009

Brown DR, Shew ML, Qadadri B, et al: A longitudinal study of genital human papillomavirus infection in a cohort of closely followed adolescent women. J Infect Dis 191(2):182, 2005

Browne TJ, Genest DR, Cibas ES: The clinical significance of benign-appearing endometrial cells on a Papanicolaou test in women 40 years or older. Am J Clin Pathol 124(6):834, 2005

Bruinsma F, Lumley J, Tan J, et al: Precancerous changes in the cervix and risk of subsequent preterm birth. BJOG 114:70, 2007

Buckley JD, Harris RW, Doll R, et al: Case-control study of the husbands of women with dysplasia or carcinoma of the cervix uteri. Lancet 2(8254):1010, 1981

Burk RD, Ho GY, Beardsley L, et al: Sexual behavior and partner characteristics are the predominant risk factors for genital human papillomavirus infection in young women. J Infect Dis 174(4):679, 1996

Cantor SB, Cárdenas-Turanzas, M, Cox DD, et al: Accuracy of colposcopy in the diagnostic setting compared with the screening setting. Obstet Gynecol 111:7, 2008

Carmichael JA, Jeffrey JF, Steele HD, et al: The cytologic history of 245 patients developing invasive cervical carcinoma. Am J Obstet Gynecol 148:685, 1984

Carter JJ, Koutsky LA, Hughes JP, et al: Comparison of human papillomavirus types 16, 18, and 6 capsid antibody responses following incident infection. J Infect Dis 181(6):1911, 2000

Case AS, Rocconi RP, Straughn JM Jr, Wang W, et al: Cervical intraepithelial neoplasia in adolescent women. Obstet Gynecol 108:1369, 2006

Castellsagué X, Diaz M, de Sanjosé S, et al: Worldwide human papillomavirus etiology of cervical adenocarcinoma and its cofactors: implications for screening and prevention. J Natl Cancer Inst 98:303, 2006

Castle PE: Beyond human papillomavirus: the cervix, exogenous secondary factors, and the development of cervical precancer and cancer. J Low Genit Tract Dis 8(3):224, 2004

Castle PE, Fetterman B, Poitras N, et al: Five-year experience of human papillomavirus DNA and Papanicolaou test cotesting. Obstet Gynecol 113:595, 2009a

Castle PE, Fetterman B, Poitras N, et al: Relationship of atypical glandular cell cytology, age, and human papillomavirus detection to cervical and endometrial cancer risks. Obstet Gynecol 115:243, 2010

Castle PE, Schiffman M, Wheeler CM, et al: Evidence for frequent regression of cervical intraepithelial neoplasia-grade 2. Obstet Gynecol 113:18, 2009b

Castle PE, Walker JL, Schiffman M, et al: Hormonal contraceptive use, pregnancy and parity, and the risk of cervical intraepithelial neoplasia 3 among oncogenic HPV DNA-positive women with equivocal or mildly abnormal cytology. Int J Cancer 117(6):1007, 2005

Centers for Disease Control and Prevention: FDA licensure of bivalent human papillomavirus vaccine (HPV2, Cervarix) for use in females and updated HPV vaccination recommendations from the Advisory Committee on Immunization Practices (ACIP). MMWR 59(20):626, 2010a

Centers for Disease Control and Prevention: Guidelines for the prevention and treatment of opportunistic infections among HIV-exposed and HIV-infected children. MMWR 58(11):1, 2009a

Centers for Disease Control and Prevention: Guidelines for the prevention and treatment of opportunistic infections in HIV-infected adults and adolescents. MMWR 58(4):1, 2009b

Centers for Disease Control and Prevention: Sexually transmitted diseases treatment guidelines 2002. MMWR 51(6):1, 2002

Centers for Disease Control and Prevention: Sexually transmitted diseases treatment guidelines, 2010. MMWR 59(12):1, 2010b

Chang GJ, Berry JM, Jay N, et al: Surgical treatment of high-grade anal squamous intraepithelial lesions: a prospective study. Dis Colon Rectum 45(4):453, 2002

Chappell CA, West AM, Kabbani W, et al: Off-label high-risk HPV DNA testing of vaginal ASC-US and LSIL cytologic abnormalities at Parkland Hospital. J Low Genit Tract Dis 14(4):352, 2010

Chase DM, Kalouyan M, DiSaia J: Colposcopy to evaluate abnormal cervical cytology in 2008. Am J Obstet Gynecol 200(5):472, 2009

Chaturvedi AK, Madeleine MM, Biggar RJ: et al: Risk of human papillomavirus-associated cancers among persons with AIDS. J Natl Cancer Inst 101(16):1120, 2009

Christensen ND, Cladel NM, Reed CA, et al: Hybrid papillomavirus L1 molecules assemble into virus-like particles that reconstitute conformational epitopes and induce neutralizing antibodies to distinct HPV types. Virology 291(2):324, 2001

Coggin JR, zur Hausen H: Workshop on papillomavirus and cancer. Cancer Res 39:545, 1979

Cohen BA, Honig P, Androphy E: Anogenital warts in children. Clinical and virologic evaluation for sexual abuse. Arch Dermatol 126(12):1575, 1990

Collins S, Mazloomzadeh S, Winter H, et al: High incidence of cervical human papillomavirus infection in women during their first sexual relationship. BJOG 109(1):96, 2002

Coppleson M, Dalrymple JC, Atkinson KH: Colposcopic differentiation of abnormalities arising in the transformation zone. Obstet Gynecol Clin North Am 20(1):83, 1993

Cox JT: More questions about the accuracy of colposcopy. What does this mean for cervical cancer prevention? Obstet Gynecol 111(6):1266, 2008

Cuzick J, Clavel C, Petry KU, et al: Overview of the European and North American studies on HPV testing in primary cervical cancer screening. Int J Cancer 119:1095, 2006

Datta SD, Koutsky LA, Ratelle S, et al: Human papillomavirus infection and cervical cytology in women screened for cervical cancer in the United States, 2003-2005. Ann intern Med 148:493, 2008

Davey E, Barratt A, Irwig L, et al: Effect of study design and quality on unsatisfactory rates, cytology classifications, and accuracy in liquid-based versus conventional cervical cytology: a systematic review. Lancet 367(9505):122, 2006

David YB: Vulvar intraepithelial neoplasia treatment outcome. Int J Gynecol Cancer 6145, 1996

de Oliveira ERZM, Derchain SFM, Sarian LOZ, et al: Prediction of high-grade cervical disease with human papillomavirus detection in women with glandular and squamous cytologic abnormalities. Int J Gynecol Cancer 16:1055, 2006

de Sanjose S, Palefsky J: Cervical and anal HPV infections in HIV positive women and men. Virus Res 89(2):201, 2002

de Vet HC, Sturmans F: Risk factors for cervical dysplasia: implications for prevention. Public Health 108(4):241, 1994

de Villiers EM: Relationship between steroid hormone contraceptives and HPV, cervical intraepithelial neoplasia and cervical carcinoma. Int J Cancer 103(6):705, 2003

de Villiers EM, Fauquet C, Broker TR, et al: Classification of papillomaviruses. Virology 324(1):17, 2004

De Vuyst H, Lillo F, Broutet N, et al: HIV, human papillomavirus, and cervical neoplasia and cancer in the era of highly active antiretroviral therapy. Eur J Cancer Prev 17:545, 2008

del Pino M, Garcia S, Fusté V, et al: Value of p16INK4a as a marker of progression/regression in cervical intraepithelial neoplasia grade 1. Am J Obstet Gynecol 201:488.e1, 2009

DeSantis T, Chakhtoura N, Twiggs L, et al: Spectroscopic imaging as a triage test for cervical disease: a prospective multicenter clinical trial. J Low Genit Tract Dis 11(1):18, 2007

Diakomanolis E, Stefanidis K, Rodolakis A, et al: Vaginal intraepithelial neoplasia: report of 102 cases. Eur J Gynaecol Oncol 23(5):457, 2002

Dillner J: The serological response to papillomaviruses. Semin Cancer Biol 9(6):423, 1999

Dodge JA, Eltabbakh GH, Mount SL, et al: Clinical features and risk of recurrence among patients with vaginal intraepithelial neoplasia. Gynecol Oncol 83(2):363, 2001

Doerfler D, Bernhaus A, Kottmel A, et al: Human papilloma virus infection prior to coitarche. Am J Obstet Gynecol 200:487.e1, 2009

Doorbar J: The papillomavirus life cycle. J Clin Virol 32(Suppl 1):S7, 2005

D'Souza G, Kreimer AR, Viscidi R, et al: Case-control study of human papillomavirus and oropharyngeal cancer. N Engl J Med 356:1944, 2007

Dunne EF, Unger ER, Sternberg M, et al: Prevalence of HPV infection among females in the United States. JAMA 297:813, 2007

Durst M, Kleinheinz A, Hotz M, et al: The physical state of human papillomavirus type 16 DNA in benign and malignant genital tumours. J Gen Virol 66(Pt 7):1515, 1985

Eastman NJ, Hellman LM: Maternal physiology in pregnancy. In Williams Obstetrics, 12th ed. New York, Appleton-Century-Crofts, 1961, p 230

Ellerbrock TV, Chiasson MA, Bush TJ, et al: Incidence of cervical squamous intraepithelial lesions in HIV-infected women. JAMA 283(8):1031, 2000

Fairley CK, Chen S, Ugoni A, et al: Human papillomavirus infection and its relationship to recent and distant sexual partners. Obstet Gynecol 84(5):755, 1994

Ferenczy A, Bergeron C, Richart RM: Human papillomavirus DNA in fomites on objects used for the management of patients with genital human papillomavirus infections. Obstet Gynecol 74(6):950, 1989

Ferris DG, Cox JT, O'Connor DM: The biology and significance of human papillomavirus infection. In Haefner HK, Krumholz BA, Massad LS (eds): Modern Colposcopy. Dubuque, IA, Kendall/Hunt, 2004, p 454

Ferris DG, Litaker M: Interobserver agreement for colposcopy quality control using digitized colposcopic images during the ALTS trial. J Low Genit Tract Dis 9(1):29, 2005

Fitzhugh VA, Heller DS: Significance of a diagnosis of microorganisms on Pap smear. J Low Genit Tract Dis 12(1):40, 2008

Food and Drug Administration: Gardasil approved to prevent anal cancer. FDA News Release, Dec. 22, 2010. Available at: http://www.fda.gov/NewsEvents/Newsroom/PressAnnouncements/ucm237941.htm. Accessed January 5, 2011

Franco EL, Villa LL, Ruiz A, et al: Transmission of cervical human papillomavirus infection by sexual activity: differences between low and high oncogenic risk types. J Infect Dis 172(3):756, 1995

Friedlander MA, Stier E, Lin O: Anorectal cytology as a screening tool for anal squamous lesions: cytologic, anoscopic, and histologic correlation. Cancer 102(1):19, 2004

Friedrich EG Jr, Wilkinson EJ, Fu YS: Carcinoma in situ of the vulva: a continuing challenge. Am J Obstet Gynecol 136(7):830, 1980

Frisch M, Biggar RJ, Goedert JJ: Human papillomavirus-associated cancers in patients with human immunodeficiency virus infection and acquired immunodeficiency syndrome. J Natl Cancer Inst 92(18):1500, 2000

Future II Study Group. Quadrivalent vaccine against human papillomavirus to prevent high-grade cervical lesions. N Engl J Med 356(19):1915, 2007

Gage JC, Anson VW, Abbey K, et al: Number of cervical biopsies and sensitivity of colposcopy. Obstet Gynecol 108(2):264, 2006

Goldstone SE, Kawalek AZ, Huyett JW: Infrared coagulator: a useful tool for treating anal squamous intraepithelial lesions. Dis Colon Rectum 48(5):1042, 2005

Goldstone SE, Winkler B, Ufford LJ, et al: High prevalence of anal squamous intraepithelial lesions and squamous-cell carcinoma in men who have sex with men as seen in a surgical practice. Dis Colon Rectum 44(5):690, 2001

Gomez-Lobo V: Gynecologic care of the transplant recipient. Postgrad Obstet Gynecol 29(10):1, 2009

Goodman A, Hutchinson ML: Cell surplus on sampling devices after routine cervical cytologic smears. A study of residual cell populations. J Reprod Med 41(4):239, 1996

Grainger DA, Roberts DK, Wells MM, et al: The value of endocervical curettage in the management of the patient with abnormal cervical cytologic findings. Am J Obstet Gynecol 156(3):625, 1987

Granai CO, Jelen I, Louis F, et al: The value of endocervical curettage as part of the standard colposcopic evaluation. J Reprod Med 30(5):373, 1985

Griffith WF, Stuart GS, Gluck KL, et al: Vaginal speculum lubrication and its effects on cervical cytology and microbiology. Contraception 72:60, 2005

Haefner HK, Tate JE, McLachlin CM, et al: Vulvar intraepithelial neoplasia: age, morphological phenotype, papillomavirus DNA, and coexisting invasive carcinoma. Hum Pathol 26(2):147, 1995

Hall JE, Walton L: Dysplasia of the cervix: a prospective study of 206 cases. Am J Obstet Gynecol 100(5):662, 1968

Hampl M, Sarajuuri H, Wentzensen N, et al: Effect of human papillomavirus vaccines on vulvar, vaginal, and anal intraepithelial lesions and vulvar cancer. Obstet Gynecol 108:1361, 2006

Harmanli O, Jones KA: Using lubrication for speculum insertion. Obstet Gynecol 116(No. 2, Part 1):415, 2010

Harper DM, Franco EL, Wheeler CM, et al: Sustained efficacy up to 4.5 years of a bivalent L1 virus-like particle vaccine against human papillomavirus types 16 and 18: follow-up from a randomised control trial. Lancet 367(9518):1247, 2006

Harris TG, Miller L, Kulasingam SL, et al: Depot-medroxyprogesterone acetate and combined oral contraceptive use and cervical neoplasia among women with oncogenic human papillomavirus infection. Am J Obstet Gynecol 200:489.e1, 2009

Hart WR: Vulvar intraepithelial neoplasia: historical aspects and current status. Int J Gynecol Pathol 20(1):16, 2001

Heard I, Palefsky JM, Kazatchkine MD: The impact of HIV antiviral therapy on human papillomavirus (HPV) infections and HPV-related diseases. Antivir Ther 9(1):13, 2004

Heard I, Potard V, Foulot H, et al: High rate of recurrence of cervical intraepithelial neoplasia after surgery in HIV-positive women. J Acquir Immune Defic Syndr 39(4):412, 2005

Herod JJ, Shafi MI, Rollason TP, et al: Vulvar intraepithelial neoplasia: long term follow up of treated and untreated women. Br J Obstet Gynaecol 103(5):446, 1996

Herrero R, Hildesheim A, Bratti C, et al: Population-based study of human papillomavirus infection and cervical neoplasia in rural Costa Rica. J Natl Cancer Inst 92(6):464, 2000

Herzog TJ, Monk BJ: Reducing the burden of glandular carcinomas of the uterine cervix. Am J Obstet Gynecol 197(6):566, 2007

Hildesheim A, Hadjimichael O, Schwartz PE, et al: Risk factors for rapid-onset cervical cancer. Am J Obstet Gynecol 180(3 Pt 1):571, 1999

Hillemanns P, Ellerbrock TV, McPhillips S, et al: Prevalence of anal human papillomavirus infection and anal cytologic abnormalities in HIV-seropositive women. AIDS 10(14):1641, 1996

Hillemanns P, Wang X, Staehle S, et al: Evaluation of different treatment modalities for vulvar intraepithelial neoplasia (VIN): CO(2) laser vaporization, photodynamic therapy, excision and vulvectomy. Gynecol Oncol 100(2):271, 2006

Himes KP, Simhan HN: Time from cervical conization to pregnancy and preterm birth. Obstet Gynecol 109(2 Pt 1):314, 2007

Ho GY, Bierman R, Beardsley L, et al: Natural history of cervicovaginal papillomavirus infection in young women. N Engl J Med 338(7):423, 1998

Ho GY, Burk RD, Klein S, et al: Persistent genital human papillomavirus infection as a risk factor for persistent cervical dysplasia. J Natl Cancer Inst 87(18):1365, 1995

Hoffman MS, DeCesare SL, Roberts WS, et al: Upper vaginectomy for in situ and occult, superficially invasive carcinoma of the vagina. Am J Obstet Gynecol 166(1 Pt 1):30, 1992a

Hoffman MS, Pinelli DM, Finan M, et al: Laser vaporization for vulvar intraepithelial neoplasia III. J Reprod Med 37(2):135, 1992b

Hopkins MP, Morley GW, Nemunaitis-Keller J: Carcinoma of the vulva. Obstet Gynecol Clin North Am 28(4):791, 2001

Howe HL, Wingo PA, Thun MJ, et al: Annual report to the nation on the status of cancer (1973 through 1998), featuring cancers with recent increasing trends. J Natl Cancer Inst 93(11):824, 2001

Huh WK, Kendrick JE, Alvarez RD: New advances in vaccine technology and improved cervical cancer prevention. Obstet Gynecol 109:1187, 2007

Husseinzadeh N, Carter V, Wesseler T: Significance of positive endocervical curettage in predicting endocervical canal involvement in patients with cervical intraepithelial neoplasia. Gynecol Oncol 35(3):358, 1989

International Agency for Research on Cancer: Combined estrogen-progestogen contraceptives and combined estrogen-progestogen menopausal therapy. IARC Monographs on the Evaluation of Carcinogenic risks to Humans. Vol 91, 2007. Available at: http://monographs.iarc.fr/ENG/Monographs/vol91/mono91.pdf. Accessed December 27, 2010

International Agency for Research on Cancer: Tobacco smoke and involuntary smoking. IARC Monographs on the Evaluation of Carcinogenic Risks to Humans. Vol 83. 2004. Available at: http://monographs.iarc.fr/ENG/Monographs/vol83/mono83.pdf. Accessed December 27, 2010

International Collaboration of Epidemiological Studies of Cervical Cancer: Cervical cancer and hormonal contraceptives: collaborative reanalysis of individual data for 16573 women with cervical cancer and 35509 women without cervical cancer from 24 epidemiological studies. Lancet 370:1609, 2007

Jakobsson M, Gissler M, Paavonen J, et al: Loop electrosurgical excision procedure and the risk for preterm birth. Obstet Gynecol 114:504, 2009

Jay N, Berry JM, Hogeboom CJ, et al: Colposcopic appearance of anal squamous intraepithelial lesions: relationship to histopathology. Dis Colon Rectum 40(8):919, 1997

Jemal A, Siegel R, Ward E, et al: Cancer statistics, 2009. CA Cancer J Clin 59:225, 2009

Jenkins D: A review of cross-protection against oncogenic HPV by an HPV-16/18 ASO4-adjuvanted cervical cancer vaccine: importance of virological and clinical endpoints and implications for mass vaccination in cervical cancer prevention. Gynecol Oncol 110:518, 2008

Jeronimo J, Massad LS, Castle PE, et al: Interobserver agreement in the evaluation of digitized cervical images. Obstet Gynecol 110:833, 2007

Jones BA, Davey DD: Quality management in gynecologic cytology using interlaboratory comparison. Arch Pathol Lab Med 124(5):672, 2000

Jones RW, Rowan DM: Vulvar intraepithelial neoplasia III: a clinical study of the outcome in 113 cases with relation to the later development of invasive vulvar carcinoma. Obstet Gynecol 84(5):741, 1994

Jones RW, Rowan DM, Stewart AW: Vulvar intraepithelial neoplasia: aspects of the natural history and outcome in 405 women. Obstet Gynecol 106(6):1319, 2005

Joura EA, Zeisler H, Losch A, et al: Differentiating vulvar intraepithelial neoplasia from nonneoplastic epithelial disorders. The toluidine blue test. J Reprod Med 43(8):671, 1998

Kanodia S, Fahey LM, Kast WM: Mechanisms used by human papillomaviruses to escape the host immune response. Curr Cancer Drug Targets 7:79, 2007

Kaplan JE, Benson C, Holmes KH, et al: Guidelines for prevention and treatment of opportunistic infections in HIV-infected adults and adolescents: recommendations from CDC, the National Institutes of Health, and the HIV Medicine Association of the Infectious Diseases Society of America. Centers for Disease Control and Prevention (CDC); National Institutes of Health; and the HIV Medicine Association of the Infectious Diseases Society of America. MMWR Recomm Rep 58(4):1, 2009

Kaufman RH: Anatomy of the vulva and vagina. In Kaufman RH, Faro S, Brown D (eds): Benign Diseases of the Vulva and Vagina, 5th ed. Philadelphia, Elsevier, 2005, pp 1, 232

Khan MJ, Castle PE, Lorincz AT, et al: The elevated 10-year risk of cervical precancer and cancer in women with human papillomavirus (HPV) type 16 or 18 and the possible utility of type-specific HPV testing in clinical practice. J Natl Cancer Inst 97:1072, 2005

Kinney WK, Manos MM, Hurley LB, et al: Where's the high-grade cervical neoplasia? The importance of minimally abnormal Papanicolaou diagnoses. Obstet Gynecol 91(6):973, 1998

Kiviat N: Natural history of cervical neoplasia: overview and update. Am J Obstet Gynecol 175(4 Pt 2):1099, 1996

Kjaer SK, de Villiers EM, Dahl C, et al: Case-control study of risk factors for cervical neoplasia in Denmark. I: Role of the "male factor" in women with one lifetime sexual partner. Int J Cancer 48(1):39, 1991

Kjaer SK, van den Brule AJ, Paull G, et al: Type specific persistence of high risk human papillomavirus (HPV) as indicator of high grade cervical squamous intraepithelial lesions in young women: population based prospective follow up study. BMJ 325(7364):572, 2002

Korn AP, Abercrombie PD, Foster A: Vulvar intraepithelial neoplasia in women infected with human immunodeficiency virus-1. Gynecol Oncol 61:384, 1996

Kosary C: Cancer of the vagina. In Ries LAG, Young JL, Keel GE, et al (eds): SEER Survival Monograph: Cancer Survival among Adults: U.S. SEER Program, 1988-2001, Patient and Tumor Characteristics. National Cancer Institute, SEER Program, NIH Pub. No. 07-6215, Bethesda, MD, 2007. Available at: seer.cancer.gov/publications/survival/surv_vagina.pdf. Accessed November 25, 2010

Koss LG: The Papanicolaou test for cervical cancer detection. A triumph and a tragedy. JAMA 261(5):737, 1989

Koutsky L: Epidemiology of genital human papillomavirus infection. Am J Med 102(5A):3, 1997

Krebs HB: Treatment of vaginal intraepithelial neoplasia with laser and topical 5-fluorouracil. Obstet Gynecol 73(4):657, 1989

Krivak TC, Rose GS, McBroom JW, et al: Cervical adenocarcinoma in situ: a systematic review of therapeutic options and predictors of persistent or recurrent disease. Obstet Gynecol Surv 56(9):567, 2001

Kurman RJ, Solomon D: The Bethesda System for Reporting Cervical/Vaginal Cytologic Diagnoses: Definitions, Criteria, and Explanatory Notes for Terminology and Specimen Adequacy. New York, Springer, 1994

Kurwa HA, Barlow RJ, Neill S: Single-episode photodynamic therapy and vulval intraepithelial neoplasia type III resistant to conventional therapy. Br J Dermatol 143(5):1040, 2000

Kyrgiou M, Koliopoulos G, Martin-Hirsch P, et al: Obstetric outcomes after conservative treatment for intraepithelial or early invasive cervical lesions: systematic review and meta-analysis. Lancet 367:489, 2006

Le T, Menard C, Hicks-Boucher W, et al: Final results of a phase 2 study using continuous 5% imiquimod cream application in the primary treatment of high-grade vulva intraepithelial neoplasia. Gynecol Oncol 106(3):579, 2007

Ley C, Bauer HM, Reingold A, et al: Determinants of genital human papillomavirus infection in young women. J Natl Cancer Inst 83:997, 1991

Lorincz AT, Reid R, Jenson AB, et al: Human papillomavirus infection of the cervix: relative risk associations of 15 common anogenital types. Obstet Gynecol 79(3):328, 1992

Lungu O, Sun XW, Felix J, et al: Relationship of human papillomavirus type to grade of cervical intraepithelial neoplasia. JAMA 267:2493, 1992

Madeleine MM, Daling JR, Carter JJ, et al: Cofactors with human papillomavirus in a population-based study of vulvar cancer. J Natl Cancer Inst 89(20):1516, 1997

Mahto M, Nathan M, O'Maony C: More than a decade on: review of the use of imiquimod in lower anogenital intraepithelial neoplasia. Int J STD AIDS 21:8, 2010

Maiman M, Fruchter RG, Serur E, et al: Human immunodeficiency virus infection and cervical neoplasia. Gynecol Oncol 38:377, 1990

Mao C, Koutsky LA, Ault KA, et al: Efficacy of human papillomavirus-16 vaccine to prevent cervical intraepithelial neoplasia: a randomized controlled trial. Obstet Gynecol 107(1):18, 2006

Marrazzo JM, Stine K, Koutsky LA: Genital human papillomavirus infection in women who have sex with women: a review. Am J Obstet Gynecol 183(3):770, 2000

Martin-Hirsch PL, Paraskevaidis E, Kitchener H: Surgery for cervical intraepithelial neoplasia. Cochrane Database Syst Rev 6:CD001318, 2010

Mayrand MH, Duarte-Franco E, Rodrigues I, et al: Human papillomavirus DNS versus Papanicolaou screening tests for cervical cancer. N Engl J Med 357(16):1579, 2007

Melkert PW, Hopman E, van den Brule AJ, et al: Prevalence of HPV in cytomorphologically normal cervical smears, as determined by the polymerase chain reaction, is age-dependent. Int J Cancer 53(6):919, 1993

Miller BE: Vulvar intraepithelial neoplasia treated with cavitational ultrasonic surgical aspiration. Gynecol Oncol 85(1):114, 2002

Mitchell MF, Tortolero-Luna G, Cook E, et al: A randomized clinical trial of cryotherapy, laser vaporization, and loop electrosurgical excision for treatment of squamous intraepithelial lesions of the cervix. Obstet Gynecol 92(5):737, 1998

Molijn A, Kleter B, Quint W, et al: Molecular diagnosis of human papillomavirus (HPV) infections. J Clin Virol 32(Suppl 1):S43, 2005

Monk BJ: Prognostic significance of human papillomavirus DNA in vulvar carcinoma. Obstet Gynecol 85(5):709, 1995

Moore K, Cofer A, Elliot L, et al: Adolescent cervical dysplasia: histologic evaluation, treatment, and outcomes. Am J Obstet Gynecol 197:141.e1, 2007

Moscicki AB: Impact of HPV infection in adolescent populations. J Adolesc Health 37:S3, 2005

Moscicki AB, Ma Y, Wibblesman C, et al: Risks for cervical intraepithelial neoplasia 3 among adolescents and young women with abnormal cytology. Obstet Gynecol 112:1335, 2008

Moscicki AB, Shiboski S, Broering J, et al: The natural history of human papillomavirus infection as measured by repeated DNA testing in adolescent and young women. J Pediatr 132(2):277, 1998

Moscicki AB, Shiboski S, Hills NK, et al: Regression of low-grade squamous intra-epithelial lesions in young women. Lancet 364(9446):1678, 2004

Muñoz N, Bosch FX, de Sanjose S, et al: Epidemiologic classification of human papillomavirus types associated with cervical cancer. N Engl J Med 348(6):518, 2003

Muñoz N, Franceschi S, Bosetti C, et al: Role of parity and human papillomavirus in cervical cancer: the IARC multicentric case-control study. Lancet 359:1093, 2002

Nahas CSR, da Silva Filho EV, Segurado AAC, et al: Screening anal dysplasia in HIV-infected patients: is there an agreement between anal Pap smear and high-resolution anoscopy-guided biopsy? Dis Colon Rectum 52:1854, 2009

National Cancer Institute: PDQ® Vulvar cancer treatment. Bethesda, MD: National Cancer Institute. 2010. Available at http://cancer.gov/cancertopics/pdg/treatment/vulvar/HealthProfessional. Accessed December 19, 2010

National Cancer Institute: Surveillance Epidemiology and End Results: SEER Stat Fact Sheets: cervix uteri. 2011. Available at: http://seer.cancer.gov/statfacts/html/cervix.html. Accessed October 25, 2011

National Cancer Institute Workshop: The 1988 Bethesda system for reporting cervical/vaginal cytological diagnoses. JAMA 262(7):931, 1989

National Institutes of Health: Cervical cancer. NIH Consensus Statement 14(1):1, 1996. Available at: http://consensus.nih.gov/1996/1996CervicalCancer102PDF.pdf. Accessed December 27, 2010

Noller KL: Cervical cytology screening and evaluation. Obstet Gynecol 106(2):391, 2005

Numnum TM, Kirby TO, Leath CA III, et al: A prospective evaluation of "see and treat" in women with HSIL Pap smear results: is this an appropriate strategy? J Low Genit Tract Dis 9(1):2, 2005

Obalek S, Jablonska S, Favre M, et al: Condylomata acuminata in children: frequent association with human papillomaviruses responsible for cutaneous warts. J Am Acad Dermatol 23(2 Pt 1):205, 1990

Ostor AG: Natural history of cervical intraepithelial neoplasia: a critical review. Int J Gynecol Pathol 12(2):186, 1993

Paavonen J, Koutsky LA, Kiviat N: Cervical neoplasia and other STD related genital and anal neoplasias. In Holmes KK, Mardh PA, Sparling PG, et al (eds): Sexually Transmitted Diseases, 2nd ed. New York, McGraw-Hill, 1990, p 561

Paavonen J, Naud P, Salmerón J, et al: Efficacy of human papillomavirus (HPV)-16/18 AS04-adjuvanted vaccine against cervical infection and precancer caused by oncogenic HPV types (PATRICIA): final analysis of a double-blind, randomized study in young women. Lancet 374:301, 2009

Padilla-Paz LA: Human papillomavirus vaccine: history, immunology, current status, and future prospects. Clin Obstet Gynecol 48:226, 2005

Palefsky JM: Anal human papillomavirus infection and anal cancer in HIV-positive individuals: an emerging problem. AIDS 8:283, 1994

Palefsky JM, Holly EA, Efirdc JT, et al: Anal intraepithelial neoplasia in the highly active antiretroviral therapy era among HIV-positive men who have sex with men. AIDS 19(13):1407, 2005

Palefsky JM, Holly EA, Hogeboom CJ, et al: Anal cytology as a screening tool for anal squamous intraepithelial lesions. J Acquir Immune Defic Syndr Hum Retrovirol 14(5):415, 1997

Palefsky JM, Holly EA, Ralston ML, et al: Prevalence and risk factors for anal human papillomavirus infection in human immunodeficiency virus (HIV)-positive and high-risk HIV-negative women. J Infect Dis 183(3):383, 2001

Palefsky JM, Minkoff H, Kalish LA, et al: Cervicovaginal human papillomavirus infection in human immunodeficiency virus-1 (HIV)-positive and high-risk HIV-negative women. J Natl Cancer Inst 91(3):226, 1999

Panther LA, Schlecht HP, Dezube BJ: Spectrum of human papillomavirus-related dysplasia and carcinoma of the anus in HIV-infected patients. AIDS Read 15(2):79, 2005

Paraskevaidis E, Jandial L, Mann E, et al: Pattern of treatment failure following laser for cervical intraepithelial neoplasia: implications for follow-up protocol. Obstet Gynecol 78:80, 1991

Plummer M, Herrero R, Franceschi S, et al: Smoking and cervical cancer: pooled analysis of the IARC multi-centric case-control study. Cancer Causes Control 14(9):805, 2003

Poynor EA, Barakat RR, Hoskins WJ: Management and follow-up of patients with adenocarcinoma in situ of the uterine cervix. Gynecol Oncol 57(2):158, 1995

Prendiville W, Cullimore J, Norman S: Large loop excision of the transformation zone (LLETZ). A new method of management for women with cervical intraepithelial neoplasia. Br J Obstet Gynaecol 96:1054, 1989

Pretorius RG, Zhang WH, Belinson JL, et al: Colposcopically directed biopsy, random cervical biopsy, and endocervical curettage in the diagnosis of cervical intraepithelial neoplasia II or worse. Am J Obstet Gynecol 191:430, 2004

Punnonen R, Kallioniemi OP, Mattila J, et al: Primary invasive and in situ vaginal carcinoma. Flow cytometric analysis of DNA aneuploidy and cell proliferation from archival paraffin-embedded tissue. Eur J Obstet Gynecol Reprod Biol 32(3):247, 1989

Reid R, Scalzi P: Genital warts and cervical cancer. VII. An improved colposcopic index for differentiating benign papillomaviral infections from high-grade cervical intraepithelial neoplasia. Am J Obstet Gynecol 153(6):611, 1985

Remmink AJ, Walboomers JM, Helmerhorst TJ, et al: The presence of persistent high-risk HPV genotypes in dysplastic cervical lesions is associated with progressive disease: natural history up to 36 months. Int J Cancer 61(3):306, 1995

Rome RM, England PG: Management of vaginal intraepithelial neoplasia: a series of 132 cases with long-term follow-up. Int J Gynecol Cancer 10:382, 2000

Ronco G, Segnan N, Giorgi-Rossi P, et al: Human papillomavirus testing and liquid-based cytology: results at recruitment from the New Technologies for Cervical Cancer randomized controlled trial. J Natl Cancer Inst 98(11):765, 2006

Ronco G, Giorgi-Rossi P, Carozzi F, et al: Efficacy of human papillomavirus testing for the detection of invasive cervical cancers and cervical intraepithelial neoplasia: a randomized controlled trial. Lancet Oncol 11:249, 2010

Rosenfeld WD, Rose E, Vermund SH, et al: Follow-up evaluation of cervicovaginal human papillomavirus infection in adolescents. J Pediatr 121(2):307, 1992

Rylander E, Ruusuvaara L, Almstromer MW, et al: The absence of vaginal human papillomavirus 16 DNA in women who have not experienced sexual intercourse. Obstet Gynecol 83(5 Pt 1):735, 1994

Sadler L, Saftlas A, Wang W, et al: Treatment for cervical intraepithelial neoplasia and risk of preterm delivery. JAMA 291:2100, 2004

Samson SL, Bentley JR, Fahey TJ, et al: The effect of loop electrosurgical excision procedure on future pregnancy outcome. Obstet Gynecol 105:325, 2005

Santoso J, Long M, Crigger M, et al: Anal intraepithelial neoplasia in women with genital intraepithelial neoplasia. Obstet Gynecol 116(3):578, 2010

Sapp M, Bienkowska-Haba M: Viral entry mechanisms: human papillomavirus and a long journey from extracellular matrix to the nucleus. FEBS J 276:7206, 2009

Saslow D, Runowicz CD, Solomon D, et al: American Cancer Society guideline for the early detection of cervical neoplasia and cancer. CA Cancer J Clin 52(6):342, 2002

Sawaya GF: Evidence-based medicine versus liquid-based cytology. Obstet Gynecol 111(1):2, 2008

Sawaya GF: Rightsizing cervical cancer screening. Arch Intern Med 170(11):986, 2010

Sawaya GF, Grimes DA: New technologies in cervical cytology screening: a word of caution. Obstet Gynecol 94(2):307, 1999

Schiffman M, Herrero R, DeSalle R, et al: The carcinogenicity of human papillomavirus types reflects viral evolution. Virology 337(1):76, 2005

Schiffman M, Wentzensen N: From human papillomavirus to cervical cancer. Obstet Gynecol 116(1):177, 2010

Schlecht NF, Platt RW, Duarte-Franco E, et al: Human papillomavirus infection and time to progression and regression of cervical intraepithelial neoplasia. J Natl Cancer Inst 95(17):1336, 2003

Schnatz PF, Guile M, O'Sullivan DM, et al: Clinical significance of atypical glandular cells on cervical cytology. Obstet Gynecol 107:701, 2006

Schockaert S, Poppe W, Arbyn M, et al: Incidence of vaginal intraepithelial neoplasia after hysterectomy for cervical intraepithelial neoplasia: a retrospective study. Am J Obstet Gynecol 199:113.e1, 2008

Schorge JO, Lea JS, Ashfaq R: Postconization surveillance of cervical adenocarcinoma in situ: a prospective trial. J Reprod Med 48(10):751, 2003

Shanbhag S, Clark H, Timmaraju V, et al: Pregnancy outcome after treatment for cervical intraepithelial neoplasia. Obstet Gynecol 114:727, 2009

Shatz P, Bergeron C, Wilkinson EJ, et al: Vulvar intraepithelial neoplasia and skin appendage involvement. Obstet Gynecol 74(5):769, 1989

Sherman ME, Friedman HB, Busseniers AE, et al: Cytologic diagnosis of anal intraepithelial neoplasia using smears and Cytyc Thin-Preps. Mod Pathol 8(3):270, 1995

Sideri M, Jones RW, Wilkinson EJ, et al: Squamous vulvar intraepithelial neoplasia: 2004 modified terminology, ISSVD Vulvar Oncology Subcommittee. J Reprod Med 50(11):807, 2005

Siebers AG, Klinkhamer PJJM, Arbyn M, et al: Cytologic detection of cervical abnormalities using liquid-based compared with conventional cytology. Obstet Gynecol 112:1327, 2008

Siegfried EC, Frasier LD: Anogenital warts in children. Adv Dermatol 12:141, 1997

Silverberg MJ, Thorsen P, Lindeberg H, et al: Condyloma in pregnancy is strongly predictive of juvenile-onset recurrent respiratory papillomatosis. Obstet Gynecol 101(4):645, 2003

Smith JS, Backes DM, Hoots BF, et al: Human papillomavirus type-distribution in vulvar and vaginal cancers and their associated precursors. Obstet Gynecol 113(4):917, 2009

Smith JS, Lindsay L, Hoots B, et al: Human papillomavirus type distribution in invasive cervical cancer and high-grade cervical lesions: a meta-analysis update. Int J Cancer 121:621, 2007

Solomon D, Davey D, Kurman R, et al: The 2001 Bethesda System: terminology for reporting results of cervical cytology. JAMA 287(16):2114, 2002

Southern SA, Herrington CS: Molecular events in uterine cervical cancer. Sex Transm Infect 74(2):101, 1998

Spitzer M: Lower genital tract intraepithelial neoplasia in HIV-infected women: guidelines for evaluation and management. Obstet Gynecol Surv 54(2):131, 1999

Spitzer M, Krumholz BA, Seltzer VL: The multicentric nature of disease related to human papillomavirus infection of the female lower genital tract. Obstet Gynecol 73(3 Pt 1):303, 1989

Stanley M: Immune responses to human papillomavirus. Vaccine 24S1:S1/16, 2006a

Stanley M: Pathology and epidemiology of HPV infection in females. Gynecol Oncol 117:S5, 2010

Stanley M, Lowy DR, Frazer I: Chapter 12: Prophylactic HPV vaccines: underlying mechanisms. Vaccine 24S3:S3/106, 2006b

Steben M, Duarte-Franco E: Human papillomavirus infection: epidemiology and pathophysiology. Gynecol Oncol 107:S2, 2007

Stoler MH: A brief synopsis of the role of human papillomaviruses in cervical carcinogenesis. Am J Obstet Gynecol 175(4 Pt 2):1091, 1996

Strander B, Andersson-Ellström A, Milson L, et al: Risk of invasive cancer after treatment for cervical intraepithelial neoplasia grade 3: population based cohort study. BMJ 335:1077, 2007

Suris JC: Epidemiology of preinvasive lesions. Eur J Gynaecol Oncol 20(4):302, 1999

Syrjanen S: HPV infections in children. HPV Today 68, 2005

Tandon R, Baranoski AS, Huang F, et al: Abnormal anal cytology in HIV-infected women. Am J Obstet Gynecol 203:21.e1, 2010

Trimble EL: A guest editorial: update on diethylstilbestrol. Obstet Gynecol Surv 56(4):187, 2001

U.S. Department of Health and Human Services: The Health Consequences of smoking: a Report of the Surgeon General. Atlanta, GA, U.S. Department of Health and Human Services, Center for Disease Control and Prevention, National Center for Chronic Disease Prevention and Health Promotion, Office on Smoking and Health, 2004, p 167

U.S. Preventive Services Task Force: Screening for cervical cancer: recommendations and rationale. 2003. Available at: http://www.uspreventiveservicestaskforce.org/uspstf/uspscerv.htm. Accessed December 27, 2010

Ulfelder H, Robboy SJ: The embryologic development of the human vagina. Am J Obstet Gynecol 126(7):769, 1976

van de Nieuwenhof HP, Massuger LF, van der Avoort I, et al: Vulvar squamous cell carcinoma development after diagnosis of VIN increases with age. Eur J Cancer 45(5):851, 2009

van Seters M, van Beurden M, de Craen AJ: Is the assumed natural history of vulvar intraepithelial neoplasia III based on enough evidence? A systematic review of 3322 published patients. Gynecol Oncol 97(2):645, 2005

van Seters M, van Beurden M, ten Kate FJ, et al: Treatment of vulvar intraepithelial neoplasia with topical imiquimod. N Engl J Med 358:1465, 2008

Villa LL, Ault KA, Giuliano AR, et al: Immunologic responses following administration of a vaccine targeting human papillomavirus Types 6, 11, 16, and 18. Vaccine 24:5571, 2006

von Gruenigen VE, Gibbons HE, Gibbins K, et al: Surgical treatments for vulvar and vaginal dysplasia. Obstet Gynecol 109:942, 2007

Werner CL, Lo JY, Heffernan, et al: Loop electrosurgical excision procedure and risk of preterm birth. Obstet Gynecol 115:605, 2010

Wilkinson EJ: Pap smears and screening for cervical neoplasia. Clin Obstet Gynecol 33(4):817, 1990

Wilkinson EJ, Kneale B, Lynch PJ: Report of the ISSVD Terminology Committee. J Reprod Med 31:973, 1986

Williams AB, Darragh TM, Vranizan K, et al: Anal and cervical human papillomavirus infection and risk of anal and cervical epithelial abnormalities in human immunodeficiency virus-infected women. Obstet Gynecol 83(2):205, 1994

Winer RL, Lee SK, Hughes JP, et al: Genital human papillomavirus infection: incidence and risk factors in a cohort of female university students. Am J Epidemiol 157(3):218, 2003

Woodman CB, Collins S, Winter H, et al: Natural history of cervical human papillomavirus infection in young women: a longitudinal cohort study. Lancet 357(9271):1831, 2001

Woodruff JD: Carcinoma in situ of the vagina. Clin Obstet Gynecol 24(2):485, 1981

World Health Organization: Screening and early detection of cancer. Cervical cancer screening. Cytology screening. 2010. Available at: http://www.who.int/cancer/detection/cytologyscreen/en/index.html. Accessed December 27, 2010

Wright JD, Davila RM, Pinto KR, et al: Cervical dysplasia in adolescents. Obstet Gynecol 106(1):115, 2005

Wright JD, Rader JS, Davila R, et al: Human papillomavirus triage for young women with atypical squamous cells of undetermined significance. Obstet Gynecol 107(4):822, 2006

Wright TC Jr: Cervical cancer screening in the 21st century: is it time to retire the Pap smear? Clin Obstet Gynecol 50(2):313, 2007a

Wright TC Jr, Ellerbrock TV, Chiasson MA, et al: Cervical intraepithelial neoplasia in women infected with human immunodeficiency virus: prevalence, risk factors, and validity of Papanicolaou smears. New York Cervical Disease Study. Obstet Gynecol 84(4):591, 1994

Wright TC Jr, Massad S, Dunton CJ, et al: 2006 consensus guidelines for the management of women with abnormal cervical cancer screening tests. Am J Obstet Gynecol 197(4):346, 2007b

Wright TC Jr, Massad S, Dunton CJ, et al: 2006 consensus guidelines for the management of women with cervical intraepithelial neoplasia or adenocarcinoma in situ. Am J Obstet Gynecol 197(4):340, 2007c

Wright VC Chapman W: Intraepithelial neoplasia of the lower female genital tract: etiology, investigation, and management. Semin Surg Oncol 8:180, 1992

Yasmeen S, Romano PS, Pettinger M, et al: Incidence of cervical cytological abnormalities with aging in the Women's Health Initiative. Obstet Gynecol 108:410, 2006

Zbar AP, Fenger C, Efron J, et al: The pathology and molecular biology of anal intraepithelial neoplasia: comparisons with cervical and vulvar intraepithelial carcinoma. Int J Colorectal Dis 17(4):203, 2002

Zhao C, Florea A, Onisko A, et al: Histologic follow-up results in 662 patients with Pap test findings of atypical glandular cells: results from a large academic women's hospital laboratory employing sensitive screening methods. Gynecol Oncol 114:383, 2009

Zuchna C, Hager M, Tringler B, et al: Diagnostic accuracy of guided cervical biopsies: a prospective multicenter study comparing the histopathology of simultaneous biopsy and cone specimen. Am J Obstet Gynecol 203:321.e1, 2010

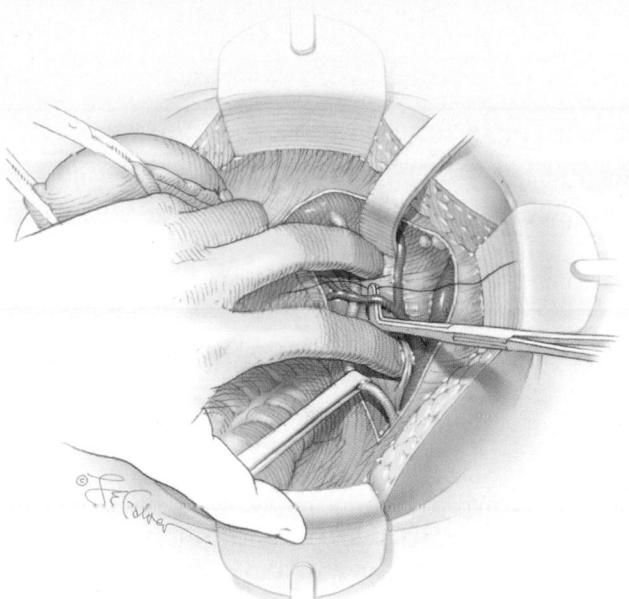

CHAPTER 30

Cervical Cancer

Cervical cancer is the most common gynecologic cancer in women. Most of these cancers stem from infection with the human papillomavirus, although other host factors affect neoplastic progression following initial infection. Compared with other gynecologic malignancies, cervical cancer develops in a younger population of women. Thus, screening for this neoplasia with Pap smear sampling typically begins in young adulthood.

Most early cancers are asymptomatic. Symptoms of advancing cervical cancer may include bleeding, watery discharge, and signs associated with venous, lymphatic, neural, or ureteral compression. Diagnosis of cervical cancer usually follows histologic evaluation of biopsies taken during colposcopic examination or biopsies from a grossly abnormal cervix.

This cancer is staged clinically. Treatment varies and is typically dictated by this staging. In general, early-stage disease is effectively eradicated surgically by either conization or radical hysterectomy. However, for those with advanced disease, chemoradiation is primarily selected. As expected, disease prognosis differs with tumor stage, and stage is the most important indicator of long-term survival. Women with stage I disease typically have high survival and low recurrence rates, whereas those with advanced disease have a poorer long-term prognosis.

Prevention lies mainly in identifying and treating women with high-grade dysplasia. For this reason, regular Pap smear screening is recommended by the American College of Obstetricians and Gynecologists (2009) and by the U.S. Preventive Services Task Force (2003) (Chap. 29, p. 742). It is hoped that the human papillomavirus (HPV) vaccines will prove effective in reducing the incidence of cervical cancer in the future.

INCIDENCE

Cervical cancer is common worldwide and ranks third among all malignancies for women (Ferlay, 2010). In 2008, an estimated 529,000 new cases were identified globally, and 275,000 deaths were recorded. In general, higher incidences are found in developing countries, and these countries contribute 85 percent of reported cases annually. Economically advantaged countries have significantly lower cervical cancer rates and add only 3.6 percent of new cancers. This incidence disparity highlights successes achieved by cervical cancer screening programs in which Pap smears are regularly obtained.

TABLE 30-1. Cervical Cancer Age-Standardized Incidence and Death Rates (per 100,000 women per year)

	All Races	White	Black	Asian American and Pacific Islander	American Indian and Alaskan Native	Hispanic Latino
Incidence	8.1	8.0	10.0	7.3	7.8	11.1
Death	2.4	2.2	4.3	2.1	3.4	3.1

Based on cases diagnosed during 2004 through 2008 from 17 geographic areas in the Surveillance, Epidemiology and End Results (SEER) Program.
From the National Cancer Institute, 2011.

Within the United States, cervical cancer is the third most common gynecologic cancer and the 11th most common solid malignant neoplasm among women. In the United States, women have a 1 in 147 lifetime risk of developing this cancer. In 2011, the American Cancer Society estimated that there will be 12,710 new cases and 4290 deaths from this malignancy (Siegel, 2011). Of U.S. women, African-Americans and women in lower socioeconomic groups have the highest age-standardized death rates from this cancer, and Hispanic and Latino women have the highest incidence rates (Table 30-1). This trend is thought to result mainly from financial and cultural characteristics affecting access to screening and treatment. The age at which cervical cancer develops is in general earlier than that for other gynecologic malignancies, and the median age at diagnosis is 48 years (National Cancer Institute, 2011). In women aged 20 to 39 years, cervical cancer is the second leading cause of cancer deaths (Jemal, 2010).

RISKS

In addition to demographic risks, behavioral risks have been linked with cervical malignancy. Most cervical cancers originate from cells infected with HPV, which is sexually transmitted. As with cervical intraepithelial neoplasia, early coitarche, multiple sexual partners, and increased parity are associated with a substantially greater incidence of cervical cancer (Table 29-2, p. 739). Smokers are also at greater risk, although the mechanism underlying this risk is not known. The greatest risk for cervical cancer is the lack of regular Pap smear screening. Most communities that have adopted such screening have documented decreased incidences of this cancer (Jemal, 2006).

Human Papillomavirus Infection

This virus is the primary etiologic infectious agent associated with cervical cancer (Ley, 1991; Schiffman, 1993). Women who test positive for high-risk HPV subtypes have a relative risk of 189 of developing squamous cell carcinoma and a relative risk of 110 of developing adenocarcinoma of the cervix compared with women who test negative for HPV (International Collaboration of Epidemiological Studies of Cervical Cancer, 2006). Although other sexually transmitted factors, including herpes simplex virus 2, may play a concurrent causative role, 99.7 percent of cervical cancers are associated with an oncogenic HPV subtype (Walboomers, 1999). In a metaanalysis of 243 studies involving more than 30,000 women worldwide,

90 percent of invasive cervical cancers were associated with one of 12 high-risk HPV subtypes (Li, 2010). Specifically in this study, 57 percent of invasive cervical cancer cases were attributable to HPV serotype 16. Serotype 18 was associated with 16 percent of invasive disease. Each of these serotypes can lead to either squamous cell carcinoma or adenocarcinoma of the cervix. However, HPV 16 is more commonly associated with squamous cell carcinoma of the cervix, whereas HPV 18 is a risk factor for adenocarcinoma of the cervix (Bulk, 2006).

Recent trials show that vaccination against HPV 16 and HPV 18 reduces incident and persistent infections with 95-percent and 100-percent efficacy, respectively (The GlaxoSmithKline HPV-007 Study Group, 2009). However, the effective duration of these vaccines is not yet known. Moreover, their ultimate goal of lowering of cervical cancer rates is yet to be realized. A detailed discussion of HPV and vaccination is found in Chapter 29 (p. 733).

Lower Socioeconomic Predictors

Lower educational attainment, older age, obesity, smoking, and neighborhood poverty are independently related to lower rates of cervical cancer screening. Specifically, those living in impoverished neighborhoods have limited access to screening and may benefit from outreach programs that increase Pap smear screening availability (Datta, 2006).

Cigarette Smoking

Both active and passive cigarette smoking increases the risk of cervical cancer. Among HPV-infected women, current and former smokers have a two- to threefold increased incidence of high-grade squamous intraepithelial lesion (HSIL) or invasive cancer. Passive smoking is also associated with increased risk, but to a lesser extent (Trimble, 2005). Of cervical cancer types, current smoking has been associated with a significantly increased rate of squamous cell carcinoma, but not of adenocarcinoma. Interestingly, squamous cell and adenocarcinomas of the cervix share most risk factors with this exception of smoking (International Collaboration of Epidemiological Studies of Cervical Cancer, 2006). Although the mechanism underlying the association between smoking and cervical cancer is unclear, smoking may alter HPV infection in those who smoke. For example, "ever smoking" has been associated with reduced clearance of high-risk HPV (Koshiol, 2006; Plummer, 2003).

Reproductive Behavior

Parity and combination oral contraceptive (COC) pill use has a significant association with cervical cancer. Pooled data from case-control studies indicate that high parity increases the risk of developing cervical cancer. Specifically, women with seven prior full-term pregnancies have an approximately fourfold risk, and those with one or two have a twofold risk compared with nulliparas (Muñoz, 2002).

In addition, long-term COC pill use may be a cofactor. There is a significant positive correlation between a low serum estradiol:progesterone ratio and shorter overall cervical cancer survival in premenopausal women (Hellberg, 2005). In vitro studies suggest that hormones might have a permissive effect for the growth of cervical cancer by promoting cell proliferation and thus allowing cells to be vulnerable to mutations. In addition, estrogen acts as an antiapoptotic agent, permitting proliferation of cells infected with oncogenic HPV. In women who are positive for cervical HPV DNA and who use COCs, risks of cervical carcinoma increase by up to fourfold compared with women who are HPV-positive and never users of COCs (Moreno, 2002). Additionally, current COC users and women who are within 9 years of use have a significantly higher risk of developing both squamous cell and adenocarcinoma of the cervix (International Collaboration of Epidemiological Studies of Cervical Cancer, 2006). Encouragingly, the relative risk in COC users appears to decline after cessation. An analysis of data from 24 epidemiologic studies showed that by 10 or more years following COC cessation, cervical cancer risk returned to that of never users (International Collaboration of Epidemiological Studies of Cervical Cancer, 2007).

Sexual Activity

An increased number of sexual partners and early age of first intercourse have been shown to increase cervical cancer risks. Having more than six lifetime sexual partners imposes a significant increase in the relative risk of cervical cancer. Similarly, an early age of first intercourse before age 20 confers an increased risk of developing cervical cancer, whereas intercourse after age 21 only shows a trend toward an increased risk. Moreover, abstinence from sexual activity and barrier protection during sexual intercourse decrease cervical cancer incidence (International Collaboration of Epidemiological Studies of Cervical Cancer, 2006).

PATHOPHYSIOLOGY

Tumorigenesis

Squamous cell carcinoma of the cervix typically arises at the squamocolumnar junction from a preexisting dysplastic lesion, which in most cases follows infection with HPV (Bosch, 2002). Although most women readily clear HPV, those with persistent infection may develop preinvasive dysplastic cervical disease. In general, progression from dysplasia to invasive cancer requires several years, but wide variation exists. The molecular alterations involved with cervical carcinogenesis are complex and not fully understood. Uncovering these additional common molecular events has been difficult, and studies demonstrate vast heterogeneity. Accordingly, carcinogenesis is suspected to result from the interactive effects between environmental insults, host immunity, and somatic-cell genomic variations (Helt, 2002; Jones, 1997, 2006; Wentzensen, 2004).

HPV plays a major role in the development of cervical cancers. Increasing evidence also suggests that HPV oncoproteins may be a critical component of continued cancer cell proliferation (Mantovani, 1999; Munger, 2001). Unlike low-risk serotypes, oncogenic HPV serotypes can integrate into the human genome (Fig. 30-1). As a result, with infection, oncogenic HPV's early replication proteins E1 and E2 enable the virus to replicate within cervical cells. These proteins are expressed at high levels early in HPV infection. They can lead to cytologic

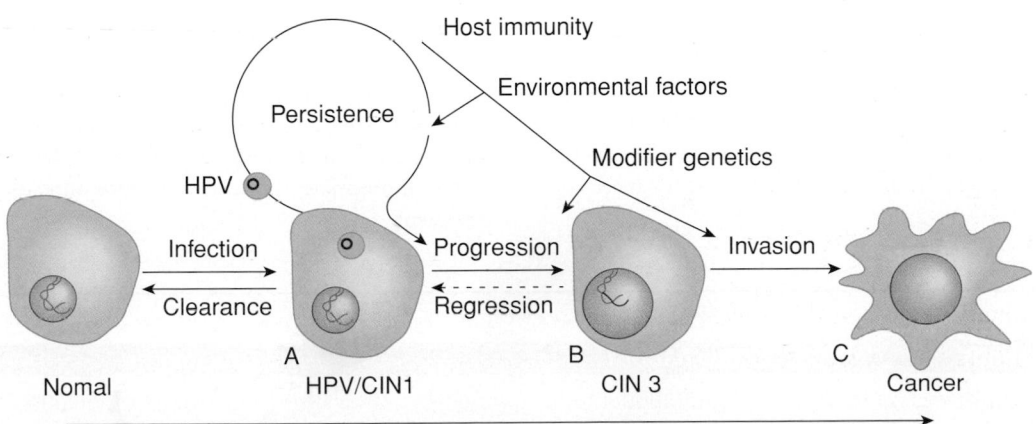

FIGURE 30-1 Diagram illustrating genesis of cervical cancers. There are two critical endpoints on the spectrum of cervical dysplasia. **A.** This initial point represents the cell at risk due to active HPV infection. The HPV genome exists as a plasmid, separate from the host DNA. **B.** The clinically relevant preinvasive lesion, cervical intraepithelial neoplasia 3 (CIN 3) or carcinoma in situ (CIS), represents an intermediate stage in cervical cancer development. The HPV genome (*red DNA strand*) has become integrated into the host DNA, resulting in increased proliferative ability. **C.** Interactive effects between environmental insults, host immunity, and somatic cell genomic variations lead to invasive cervical cancer.

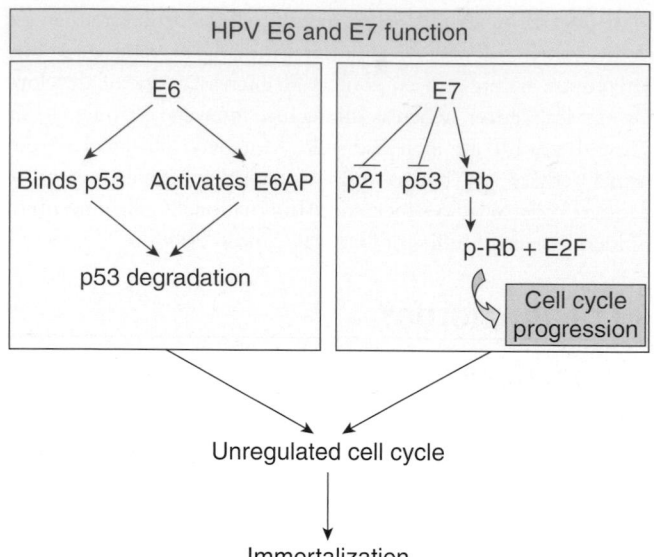

FIGURE 30-2 Diagram of E6 and E7 oncoproteins and p53, p21, and retinoblastoma (Rb) tumor suppressor proteins. On the left, viral oncoprotein E6 directly binds p53 and also activates E6AP to degrade p53 tumor suppressor protein. On the right, E7 onco- protein phosphorylates retinoblastoma tumor suppressor protein, resulting in release of E2F transcription factors, which are involved in cell cycle progression. E7 has also been shown to downregu- late p21 tumor suppressor protein production and to subvert p53 function. The cumulative effect of oncoproteins E6 and E7 even- tually results in cell cycle alteration, promoting uncontrolled cell proliferation.

changes detected as low-grade squamous intraepithelial (LSIL) cytologic findings on Pap smears.

Amplification of viral replication and subsequent transfor- mation of normal cells into tumor cells may follow (Mantovani, 1999). Specifically, viral gene products E6 and E7 oncoproteins are implicated in this transformation (Fig. 30-2). E7 protein binds to the retinoblastoma (Rb) tumor suppressor protein, whereas E6 binds to the p53 tumor suppressor protein. In both instances, binding leads to degradation of these suppressor proteins. The E6 effect of p53 degradation is well studied and linked with the proliferation and immortalization of cervical cells (Jones, 1997, 2006; Mantovani, 1999; Munger, 2001). Other mechanisms of genetic alterations and molecular changes that occur in precancerous and cancerous cervical cancer cells are outlined in Table 30-2.

Tumor Spread

Following tumorigenesis, the pattern of local growth may be exophytic if a cancer arises from the ectocervix, or may be endo- phytic if it arises from the endocervical canal (Fig. 30-3). Lesions lower in the canal and on the ectocervix are more likely to be clinically visible during physical examination. Alternatively, growth may be infiltrative, and in these cases, ulcerated lesions are common if necrosis accompanies this growth.

Lymphatic Spread

Lymph Node Groups. The cervix has a rich network of lymphatics, which follow the course of the uterine artery (Fig. 30-4). These channels drain principally into the paracer- vical and parametrial lymph nodes. Accordingly, these lymph nodes are clinically important and are removed as part of para- metrial resection during radical hysterectomy. The lymphatics that drain the cervix are called the paracervical lymph nodes and are located at the point where the ureter crosses over the uterine artery. The lower uterine segment and fundus drain into the parametrial nodes.

From the parametrial and paracervical nodes, lymph sub- sequently flows into the obturator lymph nodes and into the internal, external, common iliac lymph nodes, and ultimately into the paraaortic lymph nodes. In contrast, lymphatic chan- nels from the posterior cervix course through the rectal pillars and the uterosacral ligaments to the rectal lymph nodes. These nodes are encountered during radical hysterectomy and are removed with the uterosacral ligaments.

The pattern of tumor spread typically follows cervical lymphatic drainage. Thus, lymphatics involving the cardinal ligaments and anterior and posterior parametria are commonly involved. As primary lesions enlarge and lymphatic involvement progresses, local invasion increases and will eventually become extensive.

Lymphovascular Space Involvement. As tumor invades deeper into the stroma, it enters blood capillaries and lymphatic channels (Fig. 30-5). Termed *lymphovascular space involvement* (LVSI), this type of invasive growth is not included in the clini- cal staging of cervical cancer. However, its presence is regarded as a poor prognostic indicator, especially in early-stage cervi- cal cancers. Thus, the presence of LVSI often requires tailoring of the appropriate surgical procedure and adjuvant radiation treatment.

TABLE 30-2. Genetic Alterations in Cervical Cancer

Genetic Alterations	Mechanism	Function
Overexpression of HPV E6 and E7 oncoproteins	Integration into host genome	Cell cycle deregulation; inhibition of apoptosis
Chromosomal aberrations	Regional gains and losses and global aneuploidy	Loss or gain of gene function
Epigenetic modification	Aberrant methylation	Loss of gene function

HPV = Human papillomavirus.

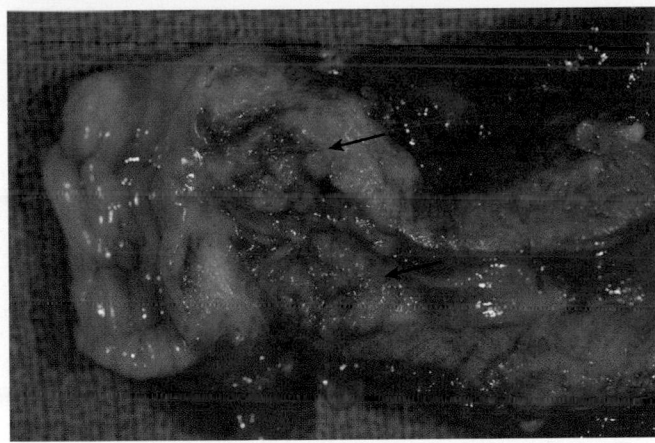

FIGURE 30-3 Radical hysterectomy specimen with exophytic growth of cervical adenocarcinoma (*arrows*) into the endocervical canal. (*Photograph contributed by Dr. John Schorge.*)

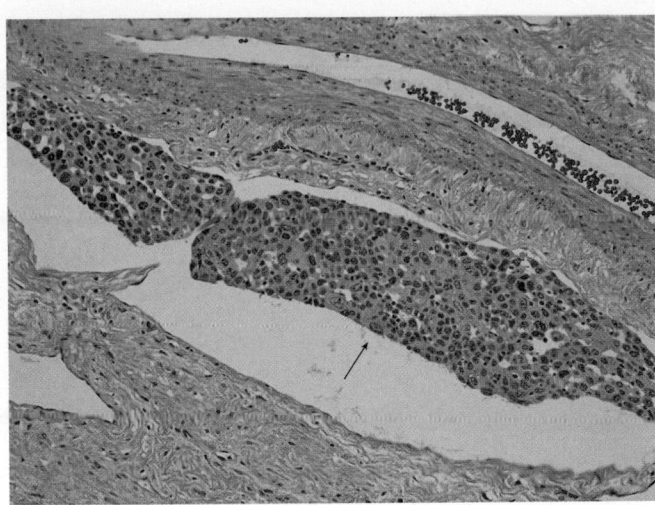

FIGURE 30-5 Photomicrograph of lymphovascular space involvement. A large lymphatic channel plugged with squamous cell carcinoma (*arrow*). (*Photograph contributed by Dr. Raheela Ashfaq.*)

Local and Distant Tumor Extension

With extension through the parametria to the pelvic sidewall, ureteral blockage frequently develops, resulting in hydronephrosis (Fig. 30-6). Additionally, the bladder may be invaded by direct tumor extension through the vesicouterine ligaments (bladder pillars) (Fig. 38-18, p. 934). The rectum is invaded less often because it is anatomically separated from cervix by the posterior cul-de-sac. Distant metastasis results from hematogenous dissemination, and the lungs, ovaries, liver, and bone are the most frequently affected organs.

HISTOLOGIC TYPES

Squamous Cell Carcinoma

The two most common histologic subtypes of cervical cancer are squamous cell and adenocarcinoma (Table 30-3). Of these, squamous cell tumors predominate, comprise 75 percent of all cervical cancers, and arise from the ectocervix. Over the past 30 years, there has been a decrease in the incidence of squamous cell cancers and an increase in the incidence of cervical adenocarcinomas. These changes may be attributed to an improved method of screening for early squamous lesions of the cervix and an increase in the prevalence of HPV (Vizcaino, 2000). Squamous cell carcinomas can be subdivided into keratinizing and nonkeratinizing carcinomas. Keratinizing carcinomas have keratin pearls and nests of neoplastic squamous epithelium (Fig. 30-7). Nonkeratinizing carcinomas have rounded nests of

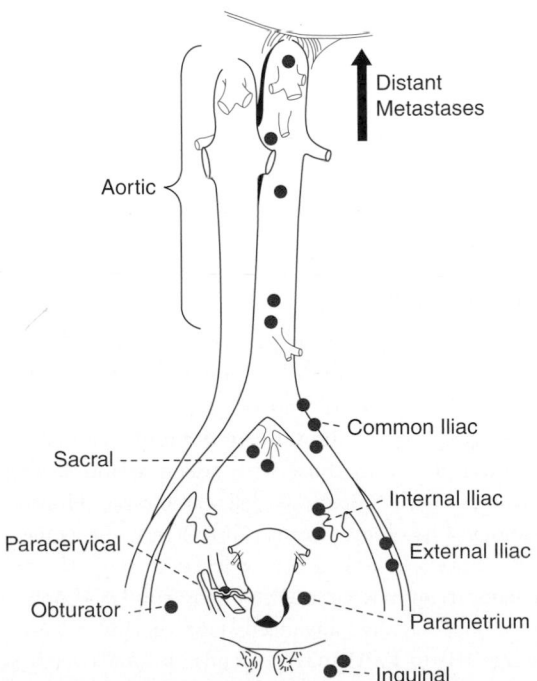

FIGURE 30-4 Drawing of lymphatic drainage of the cervix. The parametrial lymph nodes are removed as part of radical hysterectomy. Lymph node dissection for cervical cancer includes removal of pelvic lymph nodes (from the external iliac artery and vein, the internal iliac artery, and the common iliac artery) with or without paraaortic lymph node dissection to the level of the inferior mesenteric artery. (*From Henriksen, 1949, with permission.*)

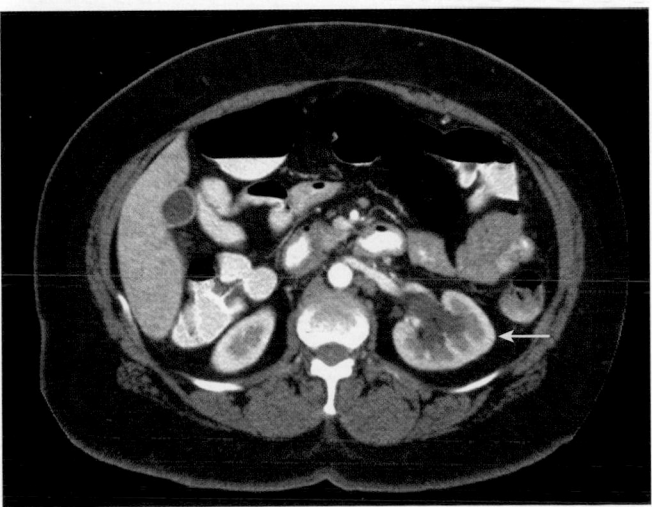

FIGURE 30-6 Computed tomography (CT) scan reveals hydronephrosis (*arrow*) caused by tumor compression of the left ureter. (*Image contributed by Dr. John Schorge.*)

TABLE 30-3. Histologic Subtypes of Cervical Cancer

Squamous	Adenocarcinoma	Mixed Cervical Carcinomas	Neuroendocrine Cervical Tumors	Others
Keratinizing	Mucinous	Adenosquamous	Large cell neuroendocrine	Sarcomas
Nonkeratinizing	Endocervical	Glassy cell	Small cell neuroendocrine	Lymphomas
Papillary	Intestinal			Melanomas
	Minimal deviation			
	Villoglandular			
	Endometrioid			
	Serous			
	Clear cell			
	Mesonephric			

Squamous cell carcinomas represent 75% of all cervical cancer, and adenocarcinomas account for 20–25% of cervical cancers. The other cell types are rare.

neoplastic squamous cells with individual cell keratinization, but lack keratin pearls. Papillary squamous cell carcinoma is a rare variant and resembles transitional cell carcinoma of the bladder.

Adenocarcinomas

Adenocarcinomas are a group of cervical cancers comprised of the subtypes listed in Table 30-3. In contrast to squamous cell cervical carcinoma, adenocarcinomas comprise 20 to 25 percent of cervical cancers and arise from the endocervical mucus-producing columnar cells. Because of this origin within the endocervix, adenocarcinomas are often occult and may be advanced before becoming clinically evident. They often give the cervix a palpable barrel shape during pelvic examination.

Adenocarcinomas exhibit a variety of histologic patterns composed of diverse cell types. Of these, *mucinous adenocarcinomas* are the most common and can be subdivided into endocervical, intestinal, minimal deviation, or villoglandular types

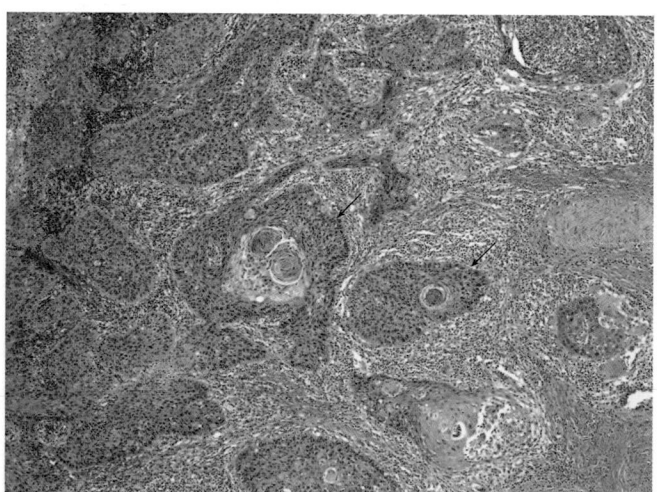

FIGURE 30-7 Photomicrograph of squamous cell cervical cancer. Nests of malignant cells (*arrows*), with brightly eosinophilic keratin pearls centrally, invade the stroma and are accompanied by a brisk lymphocytic response. (*Photograph contributed by Dr. Raheela Ashfaq.*)

(Fig. 30-8). The mucinous endocervical type retains resemblance to normal endocervical tissue, whereas the intestinal type resembles intestinal cells and may include goblet cells. *Minimal deviation adenocarcinoma,* also known as adenoma malignum, is characterized by cytologically bland glands that are abnormal in size and shape. These tumors contain an increased number of glands positioned at a deeper level than normal endocervical glands. *Villoglandular adenocarcinomas* are comprised of surface papillae. The superficial portion often resembles a villous adenoma, while the deeper part is made up of branching glands and an absence of desmoplasia.

Endometrioid adenocarcinomas are the second most frequently identified and display glands resembling those of the endometrium. *Serous carcinoma* is identical to serous carcinomas of the ovaries or uterus and is rare. Clear cell adenocarcinoma accounts for less than 5 percent of cervical adenocarcinomas and is named for its clear cytoplasm (Jaworski, 2009). Rarely, adenocarcinomas arise in mesonephric remnants in the cervix, termed *mesonephric adenocarcinomas.* They often arise laterally and are aggressive.

Prognosis Comparison

Evidence describing the prognosis of squamous cell carcinoma compared with that of adenocarcinoma is contradictory. A randomized study of stage IB and IIA cervical cancer by Landoni and colleagues (1997) showed a statistically significant lower overall survival rate in those with adenocarcinoma compared with women with squamous cell carcinoma. However, the Gynecologic Oncology Group (GOG) in a subsequent study found that overall survival in women with stage IB squamous and adenocarcinomas of the cervix is similar (Look, 1996). Evidence suggests that advanced-stage cervical adenocarcinomas (stage IIB to IVA) may portend a poorer overall survival risk compared with similarly staged squamous cell carcinomas (Eifel, 1990; Lea, 2002). The 2006 International Federation of Obstetricians and Gynecologists (FIGO) annual report, which reported on more than 11,000 squamous carcinomas and 1613 adenocarcinomas, demonstrated that women with adenocarcinomas have worse overall survival rates at every stage compared with those with squamous cell carcinoma (Quinn, 2006).

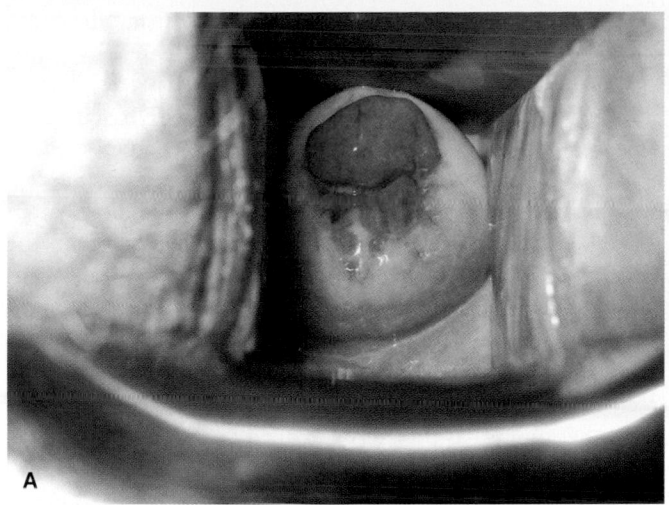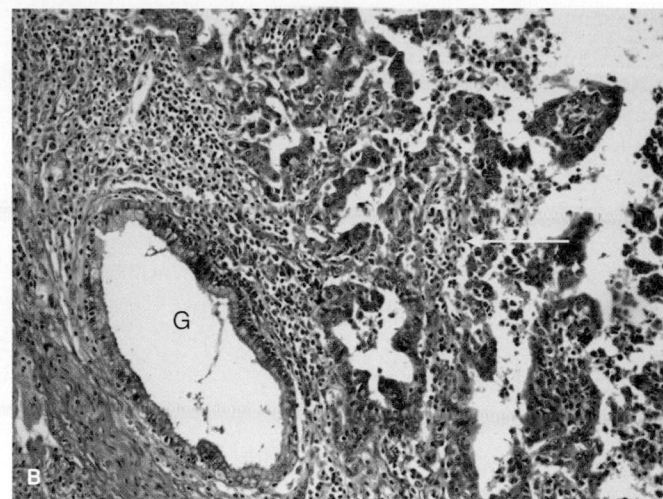

FIGURE 30-8 Cervical adenocarcinoma. **A.** Photograph of invasive cervical cancer originating from the endocervix. *(Photograph contributed by Dr. David Miller.)* **B.** Photomicrograph of adenocarcinoma of the cervix. Note the surface growth of adenocarcinoma *(arrow)* in relation to a normal endocervical gland *(G)*. *(Photograph contributed by Dr. Raheela Ashfaq.)*

In conclusion, the evidence suggests that adenocarcinoma of the cervix is a high-risk cell type.

Mixed Cervical Carcinomas

These cervical malignancies are rare. *Adenosquamous carcinomas* do not differ grossly from adenocarcinomas of the cervix. The squamous component is poorly differentiated and shows little keratinization. *Glassy cell carcinoma* describes a form of poorly differentiated adenosquamous carcinoma in which cells display cytoplasm with a ground-glass appearance and a prominent nucleus with rounded nucleoli.

Neuroendocrine Tumors of the Cervix

These rare malignancies include large cell and small cell tumors of the cervix. Neuroendocrine tumors are highly aggressive, and even early-stage cancers have a relatively low disease-free survival rate despite treatment with radical hysterectomy and adjuvant chemotherapy (Albores-Saavedra, 1997; Viswanathan, 2004). Large cell neuroendocrine tumors form trabecular or solid sheets, and the cells are three to five times the size of erythrocytes. In contrast, small cell neuroendocrine carcinoma contains a uniform population of small cells with a high nuclear:cytoplasm ratio and resemble small cell carcinoma of the lung. Often, neuroendocrine markers, including chromogranin, synaptophysin, and CD56, are used to confirm the diagnosis. Uncommonly, endocrine and paraendocrine tumors are associated with these neuroendocrine tumors.

Other Malignant Tumors

Rarely, the cervix may be the site of sarcomas, malignant lymphomas, and melanomas. Most of these tumors present as a bleeding cervical mass. Initially, differentiation of cervical sarcomas from primary uterine sarcoma requires careful pathologic examination and localization of the tumor's primary bulk. Cervical leiomyosarcomas and cervical stromal sarcomas have

a poor prognosis, similar to uterine sarcomas. Because these tumors are rare, statements regarding treatment of cervical sarcomas are limited. Most cases are managed with multimodality treatment. Melanomas often present as ulcerated blue or black nodules. These tumors have a poor prognosis.

DIAGNOSIS

Symptoms

Some women diagnosed with cervical cancer are asymptomatic. For those with symptoms, early-stage cervical cancer may create a watery, blood-tinged vaginal discharge. Intermittent vaginal bleeding that follows coitus or douching may also be noted. As a malignancy enlarges, bleeding typically intensifies, and occasionally, a woman may present to an emergency room with uncontrolled hemorrhage from a tumor bed. If a woman presents with heavy bleeding from cervical cancer, this bleeding can often be controlled with a combination of Monsel solution and vaginal packing. Topical acetone can also be used to obtain hemostasis, especially in cases refractory to Monsel (Patsner, 1993). A Foley catheter is inserted to drain the bladder when vaginal packing is in place. This allows the bladder to be drained, as the pack may interfere with normal voiding, and it also allows for accurate monitoring of urine output. If bleeding continues, emergent radiation can be delivered. Alternatively, hypogastric artery embolization or ligation can be performed in cases of refractory hemorrhage. However, caution should be used, since oxygenation to the tumor will be decreased if these blood supplies are occluded. A noted in Chapter 28 (p. 723), radiation therapy is more effective in an oxic environment. One study showed a trend toward worsening disease-specific survival rates in patients undergoing embolization prior to definitive chemoradiation (Kapp, 2005). In those with significant bleeding, hemodynamic support of the patient should follow that described in Chapter 40 (p. 1006).

With parametrial invasion and extension to the pelvic sidewall, a tumor may compress adjacent organs to produce symptoms.

For example, lower extremity edema and low back pain, often radiating down the posterior leg, may reflect compression of the sciatic nerve root, lymphatics, veins, or ureter by an expanding tumor. With ureteral obstruction, hydronephrosis and uremia can follow and may occasionally be initial presenting symptoms. In these cases, ureteral stenting or percutaneous nephrostomy tube insertion are usually required. Kidney function is ideally preserved for chemotherapy. Additionally, with tumor invasion into the bladder or rectum, women may note hematuria and/or symptoms of vesicovaginal or rectovaginal fistula.

Physical Examination

Most women with cervical cancer have normal general physical examination findings. However, with advancing disease, enlarged supraclavicular or inguinal lymphadenopathy, lower extremity edema, ascites, or decreased breath sounds with lung auscultation may indicate metastases.

In those with suspected cervical cancer, a thorough external genital and vaginal examination should be performed, looking for concomitant lesions. Human papillomavirus is a common risk factor for cervical, vaginal, vulvar, and anal cancers. With speculum examination, the cervix may appear grossly normal if cancer is microinvasive. Visible disease displays varied appearances. Lesions may appear as exophytic or endophytic growth; as a polypoid mass, papillary tissue, or barrel-shaped cervix; as a cervical ulceration or granular mass; or as necrotic tissue. A watery, purulent, or bloody discharge may also be present. For this reason, cervical cancer may mirror the appearance of different diseases. These include cervical leiomyoma, cervical polyp, prolapsing uterine leiomyoma or sarcoma, vaginitis, cervical eversion, cervicitis, threatened abortion, placenta previa, cervical pregnancy, condyloma acuminata, herpetic ulcer, and chancre.

During bimanual examination, a clinician may palpate an enlarged uterus resulting from tumor invasion and growth. Alternatively, hematometra or pyometra may expand the endometrial cavity following obstruction of fluid egress by a primary cervical cancer. In this case, the uterus may feel enlarged and boggy. Advanced cervical cancer cases may have vaginal involvement, and the extent of disease can be appreciated on rectovaginal examination. In such cases, palpation of the rectovaginal septum between the index and middle finger of an examiner's hand reveals a thick, hard, irregular septum. The proximal posterior vaginal wall is most commonly invaded. In addition, during digital rectal examination, parametrial, uterosacral, and pelvic sidewall involvement may be palpated. Either one or both parametria may be invaded, and involved tissues feel thick, irregular, firm, and less mobile. A fixed mass indicates that tumor has probably extended to the pelvic sidewalls. However, a central lesion can become as large as 8 to 10 cm in diameter before reaching the sidewall.

Papanicolaou Smear

Histologic evaluation of cervical biopsy is the primary tool used to diagnose cervical cancer. Although Papanicolaou (Pap) smears are performed extensively to screen for this cancer, this test does not always detect cervical cancer. Specifically, Pap smear testing has only a 55- to 80-percent sensitivity for detecting high-grade lesions on any given single test (Benoit, 1984; Soost, 1991). Thus, the preventive power of Pap smear testing lies in regular serial screening (Fig. 30-9). Moreover, in women who have stage I cervical cancer, only 30 to 50 percent of single cytologic smears obtained are read as positive for cancer (Benoit, 1984). Hence, the use of Pap smear alone for evaluation of suspicious lesions is discouraged. Importantly, concerning lesions should be directly biopsied with Tischler biopsy forceps or a Kevorkian curette (Fig. 29-15, p. 750). When possible, biopsies should be taken from the periphery of the tumor and should include underlying stroma, so that invasion, if present, can be diagnosed.

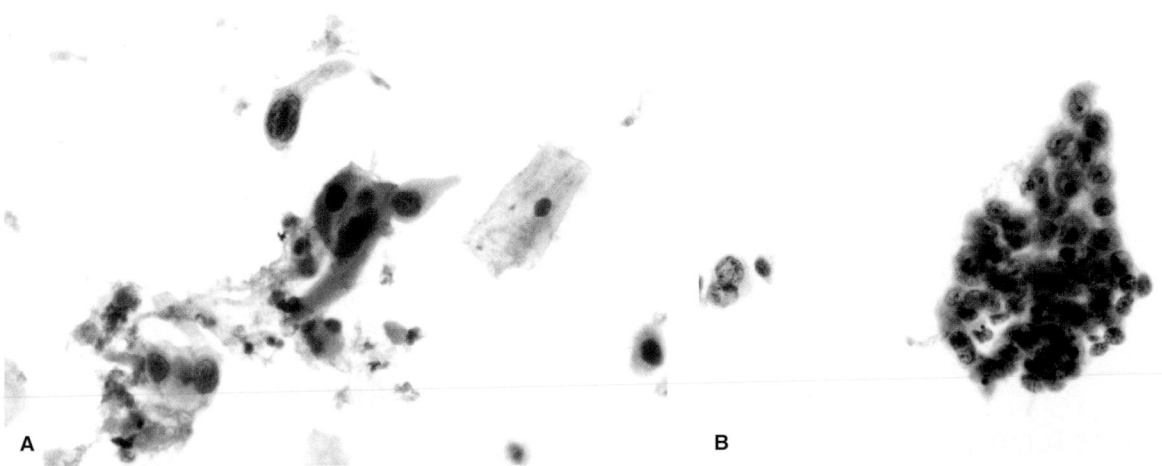

FIGURE 30-9 A. Pap smear, squamous cell carcinoma. Some squamous cell carcinomas like this one show spindled tumor cells and/or cytoplasmic keratinization, as evidenced by dense orangeophilic cytoplasm. **B.** Pap smear, endocervical adenocarcinoma. This example of adenocarcinoma shows malignant cytologic features including nuclear pleomorphism, nuclear membrane abnormalities, and nucleolar prominence. Cytoplasm tends to be more delicate than in squamous carcinoma and may contain mucin. In practice, distinguishing glandular lesions from squamous lesions on Pap smear may be challenging. *(Photographs contributed by Ann Marie West, MBA, CT [ASCP].)*

Colposcopy and Cervical Biopsy

If abnormal Pap smear findings are noted, colposcopy is often performed as described in Chapter 29 (p. 747). During this evaluation, the entire transformation zone is identified, and adequate cervical and endocervical biopsies are obtained. An endocervical speculum can be used to visualize the transformation zone if it has receded into the endocervical canal.

A cold knife cone should be performed in patients with an unsatisfactory colposcopy and high-grade disease. Cervical punch biopsies or conization specimens are the most accurate for allowing assessment of cervical cancer invasion. Both sample types typically contain underlying stroma and enable differentiation between invasive and in situ carcinomas. Of these, conization specimens provide a pathologist with a larger tissue sample and are most helpful in diagnosing in situ cancers and microinvasive cervical cancers.

STAGING

Clinical Staging

Cervical cancers are staged clinically. Allowable components of staging include cold knife conization, pelvic examination under anesthesia, cystoscopy, proctoscopy, intravenous pyelogram (can use this portion of the computed-tomography [CT] scan), and chest radiograph. Table 30-4 lists these and also contains radiologic and laboratory tools that are not included in formal staging but may contribute additional information. Bullous edema is not sufficient for the diagnosis of bladder involvement; bladder involvement must be biopsy proven. Lymph node involvement does not change the stage. The staging system widely used for cervical cancer is that developed by FIGO in collaboration with the World Health Organization (WHO) and the International Union Against Cancer (UICC). This staging was updated in 2009 and is represented in Table 30-5 and Figure 30-10. In this chapter, *early-stage disease* refers to FIGO stages I through IIA. The term *advanced stage disease* describes stages IIB and higher.

RADIOLOGIC IMAGING

As discussed, cervical cancer is staged clinically, and accurate evaluation is critical to appropriate treatment planning. For example, early-stage tumors may be treated surgically, whereas more advanced tumors require radiation and/or chemotherapy. Although imaging does not affect assignment of stage (except lung metastases seen on chest radiograph and hydronephrosis seen on CT scan), results of imaging can be used to tailor treatment for an individual. In addition, lymph node metastases, although not included in the FIGO system, worsen patient prognosis and may be identified with imaging. Thus, radiologic tools such as CT scanning, magnetic resonance (MR) imaging, or positron emission tomography (PET) scanning are commonly used as adjuncts in the initial evaluation of cervical cancer. However, no uniform approach to the use of these tools has been developed.

Magnetic Resonance Imaging

For defining anatomy, this high-resolution imaging tool offers superior contrast resolution at soft-tissue interfaces. Thus, MR imaging is effective for measuring tumor size, even endocervical lesions, and for delineating cervical tumor boundaries. In addition, it aids identification of surrounding bladder, rectal, or parametrial invasion. Unfortunately, MR imaging is less accurate

---

TABLE 30-4. Testing Used During Cervical Cancer Evaluation

Testing	To Identify:
Laboratory	
CBC	Anemia prior to surgery, chemotherapy, or radiotherapy
Urinalysis	Hematuria
Chemistry profile	Electrolyte abnormalities
Liver function	Liver metastasis
Creatinine and BUN levels	Renal impairment or obstruction
Radiologic	
Chest radiograph	Lung metastasis
Intravenous pyelogram	Hydronephrosis
CT scan (abdomen and pelvis)	Lymph node metastasis, metastasis to other distant organs, and hydronephrosis
MR imaging	Local extracervical invasion, lymph node metastasis
PET scan	Lymph node metastasis, distant metastasis
Procedural	
Cystoscopy	Tumor invasion into the bladder
Proctoscopy	Tumor invasion into the rectum
Examination under anesthesia	Extent of pelvic tumor spread, clinical staging

BUN = blood urea nitrogen; CBC = complete blood count; CT = computed tomography; MR = magnetic resonance; PET = positron emission tomography.

TABLE 30-5. FIGO Staging of Cervical Cancer

Stage	Characteristics
I	**Carcinoma is strictly confined to cervix (extension to corpus should be disregarded)**
IA	Invasive carcinoma that can be diagnosed only by microscopy, with deepest invasion ≤5 mm and largest extension ≤7 mm
IA1	Measured invasion of stroma no greater than 3 mm in depth and no wider than 7 mm
IA2	Measured invasion of stroma greater than 3 mm and no greater than 5 mm in depth and no wider than 7 mm
IB	Clinical lesions confined to the cervix or preclinical lesions greater than IA
IB1	Clinical lesions no greater than 4 cm in size
IB2	Clinical lesions greater than 4 cm in size
II	**Carcinoma extends beyond cervix but has not extended to pelvic wall; it involves vagina, but not as far as the lower third**
IIA	No obvious parametrial invasion
IIA1	Clinical lesions no greater than 4 cm in size
IIA2	Clinical lesions greater than 4 cm in size
IIB	Obvious parametrial involvement
III	**Carcinoma has extended to the pelvic wall; on rectal examination there is no cancer-free space between tumor and pelvic wall; tumor involves lower third of vagina; all cases with hydronephrosis or nonfunctioning kidney should be included, unless they are known to be due to another cause**
IIIA	No extension to pelvic wall, but involvement of lower third of vagina
IIIB	Extension to pelvic wall and/or hydronephrosis or nonfunctioning kidney due to tumor
IV	**Carcinoma has extended beyond true pelvis or has clinically involved mucosa of bladder or rectum**
IVA	Spread of growth to adjacent pelvic organs
IVB	Spread to distant organs

FIGO = International Federation of Obstetricians and Gynecologists.

for diagnosing microscopic or deep cervical stromal invasion or identifying minimal parametrial extension (Mitchell, 2006). In addition, false-negative findings occur with small volumes of disease and with tissue foci in which cancer cannot be differentiated from other tissues such as scar or necrosis. In these cases, the ability of PET scanning to identify metabolic rather than anatomic changes can be a complementary tool.

As a tool in the staging of primary cervical cancer, MR imaging is superior to CT for determining cervical carcinoma size, local tumor extension, and lymph node involvement (Bipat, 2003; Mitchell, 2006; Subak, 1995). Overall, however, both MR imaging and CT perform similarly in evaluating cervical cancer (Hricak, 2005). MR imaging is most commonly performed in patients being considered for fertility-sparing radical trachelectomy (Abu-Rustum, 2008; Olawaiye, 2009).

Computed Tomography

This modality is the most widely used imaging tool for the assessment of nodal involvement and distant metastatic disease. It offers high-resolution depiction of anatomy, especially when used with contrast. CT scanning is not a component of FIGO staging. However, it is obtained in many women with cervical

cancer to evaluate tumor size and bulky extension beyond the cervix. CT can also aid detection of enlarged lymph nodes, ureteral obstruction, or distant metastasis (Follen, 2003).

However, CT has limitations similar to those of MR imaging. CT is not accurate for assessing subtle parametrial invasion or deep cervical stromal invasion. This is because of its poor soft-tissue contrast resolution and thus its difficulty in enhancing local tumor invasion from normal parametrium. CT is also limited by its inability to detect small-volume metastatic involvement in normal-size lymph nodes. Moreover, internal node architecture is often poorly defined by CT. This makes distinction between reactive node hyperplasia and true metastatic disease difficult.

Positron Emission Tomography

As described in Chapter 2 (p. 52), PET is a nuclear medicine imaging technique that creates an image of functional processes within the body. With FDG-PET, a radiolabeled analog of glucose, fluorodeoxyglucose (FDG), is injected intravenously and is taken up by metabolically active cells such as tumor cells. PET provides a poor depiction of detailed anatomy, thus scans are frequently read side-by-side CT scans. The combination allows

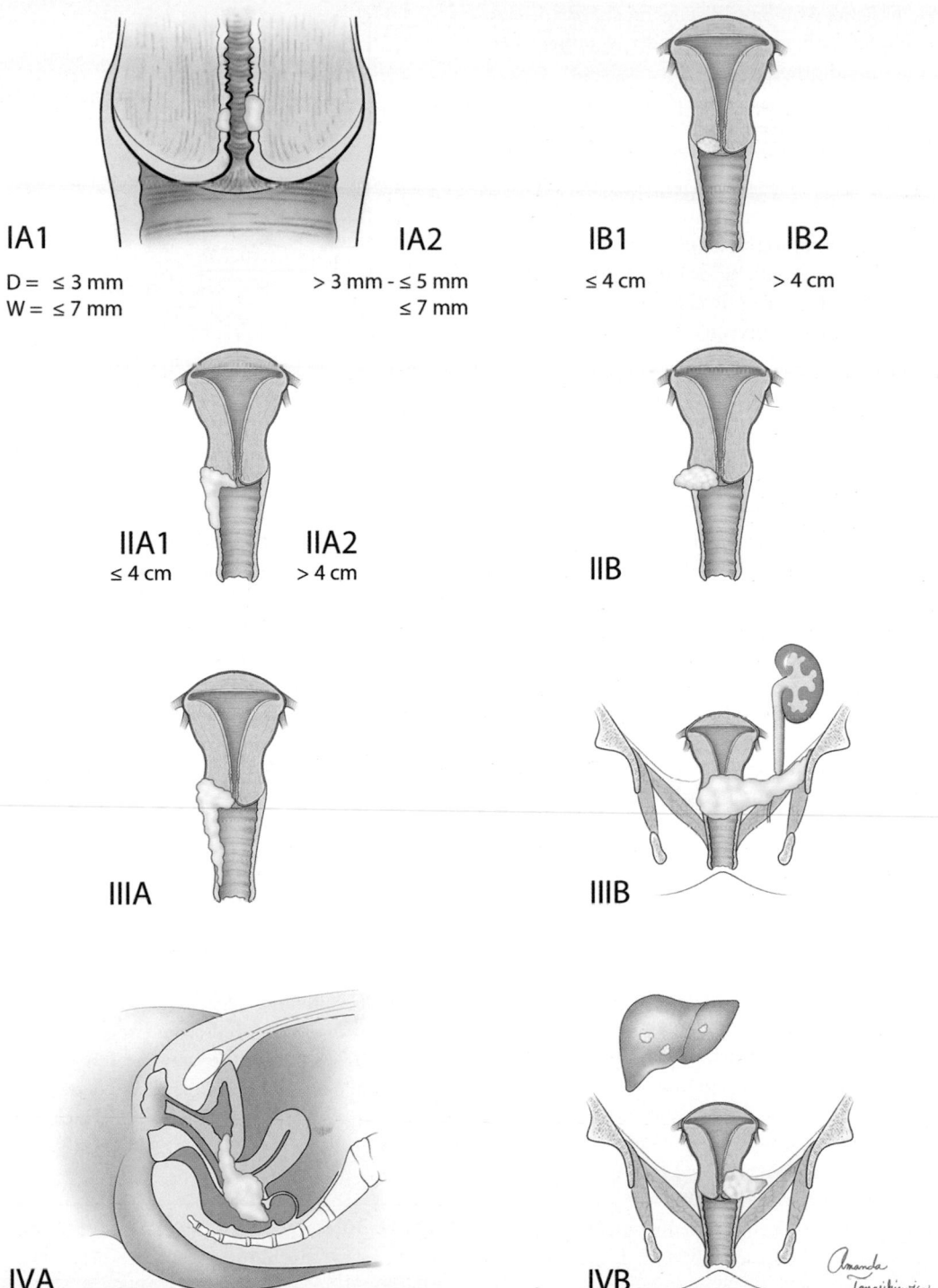

FIGURE 30-10 Drawing illustrates the FIGO stages of cervical cancer.

correlation of metabolic and anatomic data. As a result, current PET scanners are now commonly integrated with CT scanners, and the two scans can be performed during the same session.

FDG-PET is superior to CT or MR imaging for lymph node metastasis identification and is useful in primary lymph node evaluation of locally advanced disease (Belhocine, 2002; Havrilesky, 2005). In one study, Grigsby and colleagues (2001) showed that the survival rate after pelvic radiation therapy for patients with FDG paraaortic nodal uptake (PET+) and with normal paraaortic anatomy identified by

CT scanning was identical to that of patients with PET+ and abnormal paraaortic nodes by CT scanning. However, PET is insensitive for lymphatic metastasis <5 mm. Moreover, its role in early-stage smaller, resectable tumors is limited (Sironi, 2006). Specifically, for stage IA through IIA tumors, Wright and associates (2005) found a sensitivity of 53 percent and specificity of 90 percent for detecting pelvic lymph node metastases and a sensitivity of 25 percent and specificity of 98 percent for paraaortic lymph node metastases. PET scans can be useful in planning treatment fields for radiation and also in identifying those patients who have distant metastatic disease and are candidates for palliative chemotherapy rather than curative-intent chemoradiotherapy.

LYMPH NODE DISSECTION

As previously noted, cervical cancer is staged clinically and not surgically. However, surgical evaluation of retroperitoneal lymph nodes offers accurate detection of pelvic and paraaortic metastasis. In addition, debulking of tumor-laden nodes is also achieved. As a result, lymph node dissection may enhance management of and improve survival rates in patients with advanced-stage cervical cancer.

During this dissection, most experts recommend lymph node dissection in the common iliac and paraaortic region and resection of macroscopic lymph nodes (Querleu, 2000). Traditional laparotomic as well as laparoscopic approaches, either extraperitoneal or intraperitoneal, to these procedures have been studied. Although diagnostically equivalent, laparoscopic approaches offer the postoperative advantages of minimally invasive surgery. In addition, laparoscopic node dissection has been associated with significantly less radiation morbidity than that with radiation following laparotomy (Vasilev, 1995).

One advantage to surgical staging is its improved sensitivity to detect pelvic and paraaortic nodal metastasis more accurately than radiologic techniques (Goff, 1999). Surgical staging enables the detection of microscopic metastasis and confirms macroscopic nodal metastasis. Moreover, for those with locally advanced cervical cancer, surgical staging can be performed with acceptable morbidity, and findings may modify a patient's primary treatment strategy based on the level of nodal metastasis. Retrospective studies have suggested a statistically significant survival benefit to extended chemotherapy and/or extended field radiation therapy if positive pelvic/paraaortic nodes are identified (Hacker, 1995; Holcomb, 1999; Leblanc, 2007). As a result, radiation fields during radiotherapy may be modified, ensuring that patients with negative paraaortic lymph nodes are not overtreated with extended-field radiation and that patients with positive paraaortic lymph nodes are not undertreated.

In addition to its diagnostic power, surgical staging also permits debulking of grossly positive nodes. Several retrospective studies have shown that disease-free survival rates for patients whose macroscopic nodal disease has been resected is similar to that of women with microscopic nodal disease (Cosin, 1998; Downey, 1989; Hacker, 1995). There is virtually no long-term survival for patients with unresectable bulky paraaortic lymph nodes.

Despite these suggested benefits, some experts argue that the benefits of surgical staging, if any, are minimal. These studies estimate only a 4- to 6-percent survival benefit after aggressive surgical debulking of retroperitoneal lymph nodes (Kupets, 2002; Petereit, 1998).

PROGNOSIS

Prognostic Factors

The significance of tumor burden for survival has been well demonstrated, whether measured by FIGO stage, centimeter

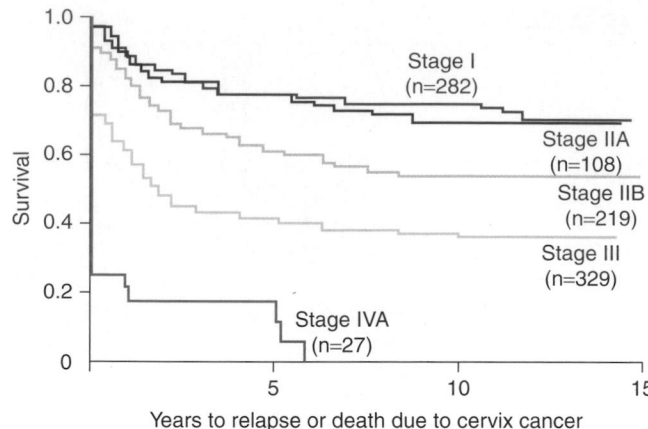

FIGURE 30-11 Graph illustrates decreased 5-year survival with advancing FIGO stage. *(From Fyles, 1995, with permission.)*

size, or surgical staging (Stehman, 1991). Of these definers, FIGO stage is the most significant prognostic factor (Fig. 30-11 and Table 30-6). However, within each stage distribution, lymph node involvement also becomes an important factor in determining prognosis. For example, in early-stage cervical cancer (stages I through IIA), nodal metastases are an independent predictor of survival (Delgado, 1990; Tinga, 1990). One GOG study demonstrated a 3-year survival rate for 86 percent of women with early-stage cervical cancer and negative pelvic lymph nodes. This was compared with a 3-year survival rate of 74 percent in patients who had one or more positive lymph nodes (Delgado, 1990).

In addition, the number of nodal metastases is also predictive. Retrospective studies have demonstrated significantly higher 5-year survival rates in those with one positive lymph node compared with rates in women with multiple involved nodes (Tinga, 1990). Similarly, the negative prognostic impact of lymph node involvement in advanced-stage (stage IIB through IV) cervical cancer has been demonstrated by several authors. In general, microscopic nodal involvement has a better prognosis than macroscopic nodal disease (Cosin, 1998; Hacker, 1995).

TABLE 30-6. Cervical Cancer Survival Rates According to Stage

Stage	5-Year Survival
IA	100%
IB	88%
IIA	68%
IIB	44%
III	18–39%
IVA	18–34%

Compiled from Grigsby, 1991, Komaki, 1995, and Webb, 1980.

TREATMENT

Early-Stage Primary Disease

Stage IA

The term *microinvasive cervical cancer* identifies this subgroup of small tumors. By definition, these tumors are not visible to the naked eye. Specifically, as seen in Table 30-6, criteria for stage IA tumors limit invasion depth to no greater than 5 mm and lateral spread to no wider than 7 mm (Fig. 30-12). Microinvasive cervical cancer carries a minor risk of lymph node involvement and excellent prognosis following treatment. A retrospective study compared tumors with horizontal spread less than or equal to 7 mm and those with greater than 7 mm spread. Higher rates of pelvic lymph node metastasis and recurrence rates were noted as tumor spread further than 7 mm (Takeshima, 1999).

Stage IA tumors are further divided into IA1 and IA2. These cancers are subdivided to reflect increasing depth and width of invasion and increasing risks for lymph node involvement.

Stage IA1. These tumors invade no deeper than 3 mm, spread no wider than 7 mm, and are associated with the lowest risk for lymph node involvement. Squamous cervical cancers with stromal invasion less than 1 mm have a 1-percent risk of nodal metastasis, and those with 1 to 3 mm of stromal invasion carry a 1.5-percent risk. Of 4098 women studied with this tumor stage, less than 1 percent died of disease (Ostor, 1995). Such evidence supports conservative management of stage IA1 squamous cell cancer if lymphovascular space invasion (LVSI) is absent. These lesions may be effectively treated with cervical conization alone (Table 30-7) (Keighley, 1968; Kolstad, 1989; Morris, 1993; Ostor, 1994). However, a total extrafascial hysterectomy (type I hysterectomy) is preferred via an abdominal, vaginal, laparoscopic, or robotic approach for women who have completed childbearing. Hysterectomy types are described in Table 30-8.

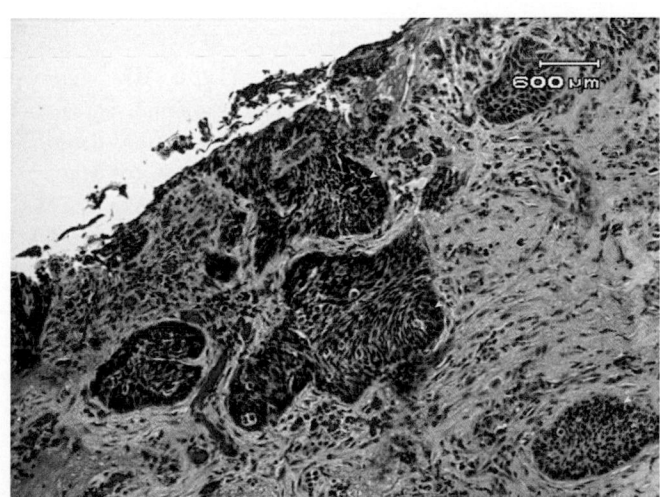

FIGURE 30-12 Photomicrograph of microinvasive squamous cell cervical cancer (*arrows*). Microinvasive squamous cell carcinomas are not grossly visible and are identified microscopically. These foci are not to exceed 5 mm in depth or 7 mm in lateral spread. (*Photograph contributed by Dr. Raheela Ashfaq.*)

The presence of LVSI in stage IA1 microinvasive cancers increases the risk of lymph node metastasis and cancer recurrence to approximately 5 percent. Accordingly, at our institution, these cases are traditionally managed with modified radical hysterectomy (type II hysterectomy) and pelvic lymphadenectomy. Radical trachelectomy with pelvic lymph node dissection can be considered in those patients desiring fertility preservation (Olawaiye, 2009).

Adenocarcinomas are typically diagnosed at a more advanced stage than squamous cell cervical cancers. Thus, microinvasive adenocarcinomas present a unique management dilemma, due to sparse data regarding this tumor stage. However, based on evaluation of Surveillance Epidemiology and End Result (SEER) data provided by the National Cancer Institute, the incidence of lymph node involvement is similar to that of squamous cancers (Smith, 2002). Of microinvasive cervical adenocarcinomas, 36 cases managed with uterine preservation and conization have been reported in the literature (Bisseling, 2007; Ceballos, 2006; McHale, 2001; Schorge, 2000; Yahata, 2010). Of these cases, following conization, no recurrences were identified during surveillance.

Stage IA2. Cervical lesions with 3 to 5 mm of stromal invasion have a 7-percent risk of lymph node metastasis and a greater than 4-percent risk of disease recurrence. In this group of women, the safety of conservative therapy is yet to be proven. Thus, for this degree of invasion, radical hysterectomy (type III hysterectomy) and pelvic lymphadenectomy is typical.

A few authors have reported management of stage IA2 squamous cervical lesions with radical trachelectomy and lymphadenectomy for fertility preservation. Although this technique is promising, it carries a learning curve, and further studies to validate its efficacy are needed. Several studies have also recommended that a nonabsorbable cerclage be placed concurrently with such radical trachelectomy to improve cervical competence during pregnancy. These procedures have high cure rates, and successful pregnancies have been reported. If women are carefully selected for age <45 years, smaller tumor size (<2 cm), and negative nodal involvement, then reported recurrence rates are similar to those of radical hysterectomy (Burnett, 2003; Covens, 1999a,b; Gien, 2010; Olawaiye, 2009). Some experts will offer radical trachelectomy to patients with tumors up to 4 cm (stage IB1), but approximately one third of patients with this tumor stage will need radical hysterectomy or adjuvant chemoradiation due to intermediate- or high-risk features (Abu-Rustum, 2008; Gien, 2010). Preoperative MR imaging to evaluate the parametria and/or CT scan to evaluate extracervical disease is recommended in these cases. If tumor has extended proximally past the internal cervical os, then trachelectomy is contraindicated.

Alternatively, patients with microinvasive carcinoma (stages IA1 and IA2) can be treated with intracavitary brachytherapy alone with excellent results (Grigsby, 1991; Hamberger, 1978). Potential candidates for vaginal brachytherapy include women who are elderly or who are not surgical candidates due to concurrent medical disease.

Hysterectomy

Women with FIGO stage IA2 through IIA cervical cancer may be selected for radical hysterectomy with pelvic lymph node

TABLE 30-7. General Treatment for Primary Invasive Cervical Carcinoma[a]

Cancer Stage	Treatment
IA1[c]	Simple hysterectomy preferred if childbearing completed **or** Cervical conization
IA1[c] (with LVSI)	Modified radical hysterectomy and pelvic lymphadenectomy **or** Radical trachelectomy and pelvic lymphadenectomy for selected patients desiring fertility
IA2[b,c]	Radical hysterectomy and pelvic lymphadenectomy **or** Radical trachelectomy and pelvic lymphadenectomy for selected patients desiring fertility
IB1[b] Some IB2 IIA1	Radical hysterectomy and pelvic lymphadenectomy or radical trachelectomy and pelvic lymphadenectomy for selected patients desiring fertility **or** Chemoradiation
Bulky IB2 IIA2	Chemoradiation
IIB to IVA	Chemoradiation **or** Rarely pelvic exenteration[d]
IVB	Palliative chemotherapy **and/or** Palliative radiotherapy **OR** Best supportive care (hospice)

[a]For individual patients, recommendations for treatment can vary depending on the clinical circumstances.
[b]Some institutions perform modified (type II) radical hysterectomy and pelvic lymphadenectomy for stage IA2 lesions and smaller stage IB tumors.
[c]Intracavitary brachytherapy may be selected for nonsurgical candidates.
[d]A patient with stage IVA lesion with a fistula may be a candidate for a pelvic exenteration.
LVSI = lymphovascular space involvement.

dissection and with or without paraaortic lymph node dissection. Surgery is appropriate for those who are physically able to tolerate an aggressive surgical procedure, those who wish to avoid the long-term effects of radiation therapy, and/or those who have contraindications to pelvic radiotherapy. Typical candidates include young patients who desire ovarian preservation and retention of a functional, nonirradiated vagina.

Historically, there are five types of hysterectomy, as described by Piver and colleagues (1974). However, hysterectomy techniques used clinically today vary depending on the degree of surrounding support that is resected and are categorized as type I, II, or III (see Table 30-8).

Simple Hysterectomy (Type I). Type I hysterectomy, also known as an *extrafascial hysterectomy* or *simple hysterectomy*, removes the uterus and cervix but does not require excision of the parametrium or paracolpium. It is appropriately selected for benign gynecologic pathology, preinvasive cervical disease, and stage IA1 cervical cancer.

Modified Radical Hysterectomy (Type II). Modified radical hysterectomy removes the cervix, proximal vagina, and parametrial and paracervical tissue. This procedure is described in full in Section 44-2 (p. 1265). This hysterectomy is well suited for tumors in patients with stage IA1 cervical cancer and with positive margins following conization in whom there is insufficient cervix to repeat conization. This hysterectomy is also appropriate for patients with stage IA1 cervical cancer with LVSI. Some institutions perform type II hysterectomies in women with stage IA2 tumors and smaller stage IB tumors with good outcomes (Landoni, 2001).

Radical Hysterectomy (Type III). This hysterectomy requires greater resection of the parametria. The paravesical and pararectal spaces are opened. The uterine arteries are ligated at their origin from the internal iliac arteries, and all tissue medial to the origin of the uterine arteries is resected (Fig. 30-13) (Section 44-1, p. 1259). The parametrial excision extends to the pelvic sidewall. The ureters are completely dissected from their beds, and the

TABLE 30-8. Tissues Resected during Simple and Extended Hysterectomy

Hysterectomy Type			Involved Tissues[a]				
Procedure	Type[b]	Corpus[c]	Parametria & Paracolpos	Uterine Vessel Ligation	Uterosacral Ligament Transection	Vagina	Proximal Ureter & Bladder
Simple hysterectomy	I	Remove	Preserve	At uterine isthmus	At uterine insertion	Preserve	Preserve
Modified radical hysterectomy	II	Remove	Remove between uterus & ureter	At level of ureter	Midway between uterus & rectum	Remove 1–2 cm	Preserve
Radical abdominal hysterectomy	III	Remove	Remove from origin of uterine vessels (lateral to ureter)	At origin from internal iliac vessels	Entirely excised[d]	Remove ≥2 cm	Preserve
Type	IV[e]	Remove	Remove from origin of uterine vessels (lateral to ureter)	At origin from internal iliac vessels; ligate superior vesical artery	Entirely excised	Remove 3/4[ths]	Preserve
Type	V[e]	Remove	Remove from origin of uterine vessels (lateral to ureter)	At origin from internal iliac vessels; ligate superior vesical artery	Entirely excised	Remove 3/4[ths]	Remove, requires utereroileoneo-cystotomy
Radical vaginal hysterectomy		Remove	Remove between uterus & ureter	At level of ureter	Partially removed	Remove ≥2 cm	Preserve
Radical vaginal trachelectomy		Preserve	Partially removed	Ligate descending cervico-vaginal branch	Midway between uterus & rectum	Remove 1–2 cm	Preserve
Radical abdominal trachelectomy		Preserve	Remove from origin of uterine vessels (lateral to ureter)	At origin from internal iliac vessels	Near rectum	Remove ≥2 cm	Preserve

[a]Pelvic lymph node dissection accompanies all except simple hysterectomy.
[b]Rutledge classification of extended hysterectomy (Types I-V) (Piver, 1974).
[c]In all procedures listed, the uterine cervix is removed.
[d]Although Piver (1974) described resection of the entire uterosacral ligament, this is not done in practice today due to the high incidence of urinary retention. Instead, the uterosacral ligaments are divided near the rectum.
[e]Although described by Piver (1974), these procedures are currently not used clinically.
Fallopian tubes and ovaries are usually preserved in premenopausal patients but removed in postmenopausal patients.

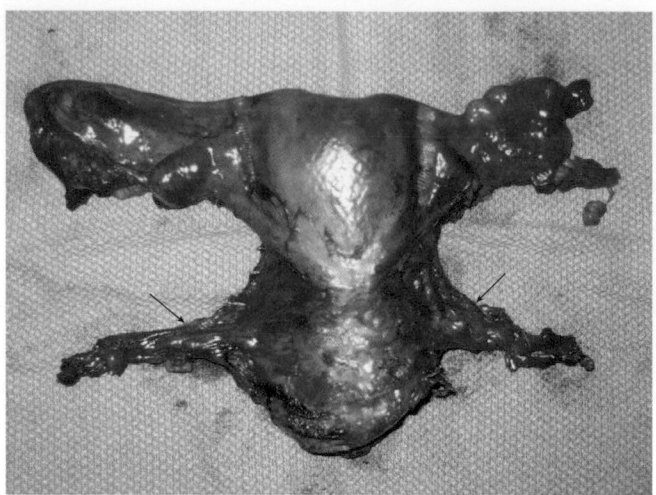

FIGURE 30-13 Gross surgical specimen following radical hysterectomy. The specimen includes the uterus, adnexa, and parametria *(arrows)*. *(Photograph contributed by Dr. John Schorge.)*

bladder and rectum are mobilized to permit this more extensive removal of tissue. The rectovaginal septum is opened to dissect the rectum away from the vagina, and the uterosacral ligaments are divided near the rectum. Although Piver (1974) described resection of the entire uterosacral ligament, this is not done in practice today due to the high incidence of urinary retention. In addition, at least 2 cm of proximal vagina is resected. This procedure is performed for stage IA2, stage IB1, occasionally stage IB2 lesions, for stage IIA1 lesions, and for patients with relative contraindications to radiation such as diabetes, pelvic inflammatory disease, hypertension, collagen disease, inflammatory bowel disease, or adnexal masses.

The approach for types I, II, and III hysterectomies can be abdominal, laparoscopic, robot-assisted, or vaginal, depending on patient characteristics and surgeon preference and experience. Techniques for the laparoscopic radical hysterectomy were described in the early 1990s (Canis, 1990; Nezhat, 1992). Advantages to a minimally invasive approach include less blood loss and shorter hospital stay. Intra- and postoperative complications are similar regardless of approach (Ramirez, 2008). Long-term follow-up of patients undergoing laparoscopic radical hysterectomy demonstrates excellent overall survival rates (Lee, 2010).

Radical Trachelectomy. This is a surgical option to preserve fertility in selected young women with cervical cancer, and the cancer stages appropriate for radical trachelectomy mirror those for radical hysterectomy. Compared with radical hysterectomy, radical trachelectomy is less commonly performed. As of 2008, 990 cases had been recorded in the literature (Shepherd, 2008).

Radical trachelectomy is more commonly completed vaginally, as described by Dargent (2000), but an abdominal approach is also used (Abu-Rustum, 2006). The abdominal approach allows for a larger resection of the parametria and is appropriate for patients with larger tumors (>2 cm). The paravesical and pararectal spaces are opened. Similar to a radical hysterectomy, the uterine vessels are ligated at their origins. The parametria medial to the uterine vessels is resected. A complete ureterolysis is

performed. Again, the rectovaginal septum is opened, and the uterosacral ligaments are divided. The upper vagina is resected. Next, the uterus is incised at or just below the level of the internal os, with the goal to preserve 5 mm of endocervix. At the remaining endocervical margin, a thin tissue sample is sharply excised, termed a *shave margin*, and sent for frozen section. If cancer is absent in this specimen, a cerclage using permanent suture is placed, and the knot is tied posteriorly. The uterus is reconstructed to the vagina using absorbable sutures.

Following radical trachelectomy, women continue to menstruate, and conception can occur naturally. However, cervical stenosis may develop, and thus, intrauterine insemination or in vitro fertilization may be needed. Pregnancies are often complicated by second-trimester loss and higher rates of preterm birth (Plante, 2005; Shepherd, 2008). Cesarean delivery with a classical incision is recommended.

Stage IB to IIA

Stage IB lesions are defined as those extending past the limits of microinvasion yet still confined to the cervix. This stage is subcategorized either as IB1 if tumors measure ≤4 cm or as IB2 if they measure >4 cm (Fig. 30-14).

Stage II cancers extend outside the cervix. They may invade the upper vagina and the parametria but do not reach the pelvic sidewalls. Stage IIA tumors have no parametrial involvement, but do extend vaginally and may extend as far as the proximal two thirds of the vagina. Stage IIA is further subdivided into stage IIA1 for tumor size ≤4 cm and IIA2 for tumor size >4 cm. Stage IIB cancer may invade the vagina to a similar extent as well as invade the parametria.

Treatment of Stage IB to IIA Tumors. These cancers can be managed with either surgery or chemoradiation (Fig. 30-15). In a prospective study of primary therapy, 393 women were randomly assigned to undergo radical hysterectomy and pelvic lymphadenectomy or receive primary radiation therapy. Five-year overall survival and disease-free survival rates were statistically equivalent (83 percent and 74 percent, respectively). Patients who underwent radical surgery followed by radiation had the worst morbidity (Landoni, 1997).

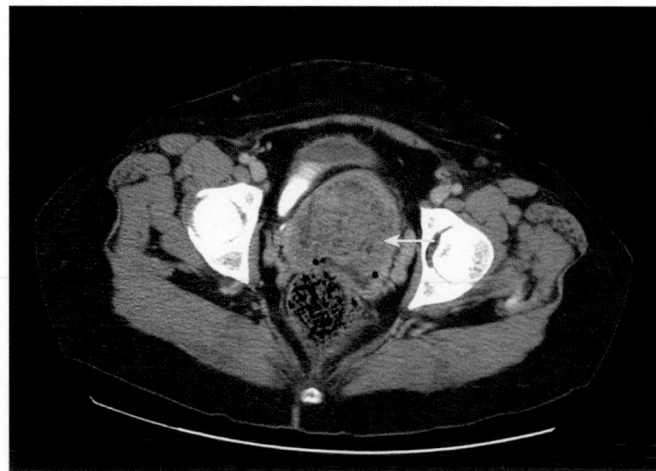

FIGURE 30-14 Computed tomography (CT) scan of stage IB2 cervical cancer. *(Image contributed by Dr. John Schorge.)*

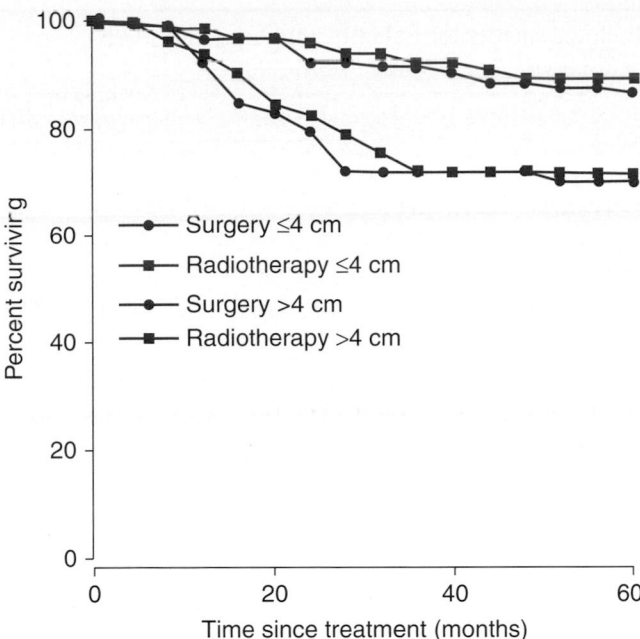

FIGURE 30-15 Graph shows equivalent overall survival rates whether stage IB through IIA tumors are treated surgically or with radiation therapy. *(From Landoni, 1997, with permission.)*

Because chemoradiation and surgery are both viable options, the optimum treatment for each woman ideally should assess clinical factors such as menopausal status, age, concurrent medical illness, tumor histology, and cervical diameter. For stage IB1 and IIA1 cervical cancers, it is left to the physician's discretion and patient preference as to which treatment modality is preferred. Our general approach to patients with bulky stage IB2 and stage II cervical cancers is to manage them primarily with chemoradiation, in a similar fashion to advanced-stage cervical cancers.

In general, radical hysterectomy for stage IB through IIA tumors is usually selected for premenopausal women who wish to preserve ovarian function and for women who have concerns about altered sexual functioning following radiotherapy. Age and weight are not contraindications to surgery. However, in general, older women may have longer hospital stays, and heavier women can have longer operative time, greater blood loss, and higher rates of wound complications. Surgery is contraindicated in patients with severe cardiac or pulmonary disease.

In those electing surgery, oophorectomy may be deferred in younger women. One GOG study evaluated tumor spread to the ovary in those with IB tumors electing radical hysterectomy without adnexectomy. Ovarian metastases were identified in only 0.5 percent of 770 women with stage IB squamous cell cancers and in 2 percent of those with adenocarcinomas (Sutton, 1992). For those electing ovarian preservation, ovarian transposition, accomplished by oophoropexy of the ovary into the upper abdomen, can be performed at the time of radical hysterectomy. This repositioning helps to preserve ovarian function, in case postoperative pelvic radiation is indicated, and is described in Section 44-1 (p. 1263). In addition, consideration can be given to performing an omental J-flap to reduce complications from radiotherapy following radical hysterectomy. After surgery, the small bowel can become fixed due to adhesions, exposing it to

a toxic amount of radiation. The omental J-flap can reduce the risk of adhesions of the small bowel to the vagina. As described in Section 44-16 (p. 1313), once the major portion of the omentum is resected from the stomach, the flap is affixed into the pelvis.

Surgical and Radiotherapy Complications. Complications for early-stage cervical cancer surgery include ureteral stricture, ureterovaginal fistula, bladder dysfunction, constipation, wound breakdown, lymphocyst, and lymphedema. The risk of venous thromboembolism warrants chemoprophylaxis and/or sequential compression devices depending on additional risk factors as outlined in Tables 39-8 and 39-9 (p. 960). If radiotherapy is added as an adjuvant to surgery, the risk of many of these complications is increased.

On the other hand, radiation therapy also may be associated with long-term complications. Altered sexual function secondary to a shortened vagina, dyspareunia, psychological factors, and vaginal stenosis is often encountered. Late urinary and bowel complications such as fistula formation, enteritis, proctitis, and bowel obstruction may also develop following radiotherapy.

Positive Pelvic Lymph Nodes. Approximately 15 percent of patients with stage I through IIA cervical cancers will have positive pelvic nodes. Risk factors for lymph node involvement include those listed in Table 30-9. Of those with involved nodes, 50 percent will have grossly positive pelvic nodes intraoperatively. In most cases involving grossly positive nodes, radical hysterectomy is abandoned. After recovering from surgery, whole-pelvic radiation and brachytherapy with concomitant chemotherapy is administered. The 50 percent of patients with involved nodes not grossly identified intraoperatively are considered to be at high risk of recurrence following their radical hysterectomy. As described subsequently, these women require postoperative adjuvant chemoradiation therapy.

Recurrence Risk
Intermediate Risk of Recurrence. For women who have completed radical surgery for early-stage cervical cancer, the GOG has defined risk factors to help identify women at risk for tumor recurrence. *Intermediate risk* describes those who on average would have a 30-percent risk of cancer recurrence within 3 years. Factors included in this model are depth of tumor invasion, tumor diameter, and LVSI.

To determine appropriate treatment of these at-risk women, patients with these intermediate-risk factors have been studied. In one study, women were randomly assigned to receive pelvic radiation therapy following radical hysterectomy or to undergo radical hysterectomy and observation. A nearly 50-percent reduced risk of recurrence was found in those who received postoperative adjuvant radiation therapy (Sedlis, 1999). However, this adjuvant radiation does not prolong overall survival. Importantly, it should be noted that these patients did not receive chemoradiation. In our practice, these intermediate-risk patients are counseled regarding their risk of recurrence and offered the option of adjuvant chemoradiation therapy.

High Risk of Recurrence. A high-risk category of patients who undergo radical surgery for early-stage cervical cancer has also been described. *High risk* is defined as a 50- to 70-percent

TABLE 30-9. Frequency of Positive Pelvic Lymph Nodes by Pathologic Factors for Patients with Squamous Cell Carcinoma, No Gross Disease Beyond the Uterus and Cervix, and Negative Aortic Nodes

Factor	Frequency with Positive Pelvic Lymph Nodes (%)		p
Histologic grade			
1	9/93	(9.7)	
2	52/373	(13.9)	0.01
3	39/179	(21.8)	
Keratinizing/cell type size classification			
Large cell nonkeratinizing	58/401	(14.5)	
Large cell keratinizing	39/227	(17.2)	0.6
Small cell/other	3/17	(17.6)	
Depth of invasion			
≤5 mm	6/177	(3.4)	
6–10 mm	36/238	(15.1)	
11–15 mm	30/135	(22.2)	0.0001
16–20 mm	19/49	(38.8)	
21+ mm	7/31	(22.6)	
Inner third	9/199	(4.5)	
Middle third	28/210	(13.3)	0.0001
Outer third	60/227	(26.4)	
Uterine extension			
Negative	83/567	(14.6)	
Positive	16/74	(21.6)	0.2
Surgical margins			
Negative	95/623	(15.2)	
Positive	5/20	(25.0)	0.4
Parametrial extension			
Negative	81/599	(13.5)	
Positive	19/44	(43.2)	0.0001
Capillary/lymphatic spaces			
Negative	30/366	(8.2)	
Positive	70/276	(25.4)	0.0001

From Delgado, 1990, with permission.

risk of recurrence within 5 years. These women have positive lymph nodes, positive surgical margins, or microscopically positive parametria (Peters, 2000).

This group is routinely offered adjuvant radiation therapy. Moreover, the GOG demonstrated that the addition of concurrent chemotherapy consisting of cisplatin and 5-fluorouracil (5-FU) would be beneficial for significantly prolonging disease-free and overall survival rates in this group of women with high-risk early-stage cancer (Peters, 2000).

Adjuvant Hysterectomy Following Primary Radiation.
The benefits of treating bulky stage I (IB2) cervical cancers with adjuvant hysterectomy following radiation therapy has been evaluated. Adjuvant hysterectomy reduces locoregional relapse but does not contribute to an overall improvement in survival. However, initial lesion size may affect efficacy. In

one study, those with tumors measuring less than 7 cm who underwent postradiation hysterectomy survived longer compared with women with equivalent tumors in the radiation-only regimen group. In contrast, those with lesions 7 cm or larger who underwent postradiation hysterectomy fared worse than their counterparts receiving only radiotherapy (Keys, 2003).

Early-Stage Cervical Adenocarcinoma
These cancers may be more radioresistant than squamous cell cervical carcinomas. Although some prefer radical hysterectomy to radiotherapy, studies suggest equivalent survival rates with both (Eifel, 1990, 1991, 1995; Hopkins, 1988; Nakano, 1995). However, larger lesions may not regress if managed by radiation alone (Leveque, 1998; Silver, 1998). The centers of bulky tumors may be less radiosensitive due to relative cellular

hypoxia. This effect underscores the advantages of radical hysterectomy for women with stage I cervical adenocarcinoma.

■ Advanced-Stage Primary Disease
Stages IIB through IVA

Advanced-stage cervical cancers extend past the confines of the cervix and often involve adjacent organs and retroperitoneal lymph nodes. As such, treatment for these tumors must be individualized to maximize patient outcome. Most advanced-stage tumors have poor prognosis, and 5-year survival rates are less than 50 percent. Advanced-stage tumors represent a large proportion of invasive cervical cancers treated, depending on the geographic area studied. If untreated, these tumors progress rapidly.

Radiation Therapy. This modality forms the cornerstone of advanced-stage cervical cancer management. Both external beam pelvic radiation and brachytherapy are typically delivered (Chap. 28, p. 720). Of these, external beam radiation usually precedes intracavitary radiation, which is one form of brachytherapy. External beam radiation is commonly administered in 25 fractions during 5 weeks (40-50 Gy). During evaluation, if paraaortic nodal metastases are found, then extended field radiation can be added to treat these affected lymph nodes. During brachytherapy, to limit bladder and rectal doses, bowel and bladder are packed away from the intracavitary source during tandem insertion, using vaginal packing. Treatment is often prescribed to point A—a point 2 cm lateral and 2 cm superior to the external cervical os, and point B—a point 3 cm lateral to point A. Side effects during and following radiation therapy are common, and discussion of these and potential management is found in Chapter 28 (p. 725).

Chemoradiation. Current evidence indicates that chemotherapy given concurrently with radiation therapy significantly improves overall and disease-free survival rates of women with cervical cancer. Chemoradiation is also associated with superior survival rates compared with pelvic and extended field paraaortic region irradiation alone (Morris, 1999). After the publication of five trials demonstrating improved survival, the National Cancer Institute issued a clinical alert in 1999 recommending that cisplatin-based chemotherapy be considered in women undergoing radiation for cervical cancer (Keys, 1999; Morris, 1999; Peters, 2000; Rose, 1999; Whitney, 1999).

Of chemotherapy agents, cisplatin-containing regimens have been associated with the best survival rates (Rose, 1999; Whitney, 1999). The characteristics of this agent are describe in Chapter 27 (p. 705), and Figure 28-12 (p. 724) describes its tumoricidal action. Nonplatinum regimens also have activity but have not been directly compared with cisplatin-containing regimens (Vale, 2008). At our institution, cisplatin is given weekly for 5 weeks. It is administered concurrently with external beam radiation as well as with brachytherapy.

Pelvic Exenteration for Primary Disease. This ultraradical surgery encompasses removal of the bladder, rectum, uterus, fallopian tubes and ovaries (if present), vagina, and surrounding tissues (Section 44-5, p. 1276). Primary exenteration may be considered for women with stage IVA cancer, that is, with direct tumor invasion into bladder and/or bowel but without distant spread. However, it is rarely performed for this indication. Yet for women with stage IVA cervical cancer and extension solely into the bladder, the survival rate can reach 30 percent (Million, 1972; Upadhyay, 1988).

Stage IVB

Patients with stage IVB disease have a poor prognosis and are treated with a goal of palliation. Pelvic radiation is administered to control vaginal bleeding and pain. Systemic chemotherapy is offered to palliate symptoms and prolong overall survival. The chemotherapy regimens used in this group of women are similar to those used in the setting of recurrent cancer.

■ Surveillance
Following Radiotherapy

Women who receive radiotherapy should be closely monitored to assess their response. Tumors may be expected to regress for up to 3 months after therapy. Pelvic examination and/or radiologic scanning should document progressive shrinkage of the cervical mass. The rectovaginal examination should be used to detect nodularity in the ligaments and parametria. If disease progresses locally after this interval, surgery should be considered. Pelvic exenteration may be indicated for this clinical setting.

At each visit, in addition to pelvic examination, a thorough manual nodal survey should include neck, supraclavicular, infraclavicular, axillary, and inguinal lymph nodes. A chest radiograph can be obtained yearly. A cervical or vaginal cuff Pap smear should also be collected every 3 months for 2 years and then every 6 months for 3 years. Findings of low-grade or high-grade squamous intraepithelial lesion should prompt colposcopic evaluation. If high-grade lesion or cancer is noted on cervical biopsy, then CT scanning to assess disease recurrence is indicated.

After completion of radiation, patients should be recommended to use a vaginal dilator or have vaginal intercourse three times per week. This helps the vagina stay patent, aids pelvic examination and Pap smears in the future, and ensures that the patient can remain sexually active if desired. Otherwise, radiation may result in vaginal fibrosis, leading to a shortened, nonfunctional vagina. The use of a water-based lubricant is also recommended.

Following Surgery

After a radical hysterectomy, 80 percent of recurrences are detected within the subsequent 2 years. During patient surveillance, identification of an abnormal pelvic mass or abnormal pelvic examination finding, for example, cervical or vaginal lesion or rectovaginal nodularity; pain radiating down the posterior thigh; or new-onset lower extremity edema, should prompt CT scanning of the abdomen and pelvis. Pelvic recurrences after radical hysterectomy, if diagnosed early, can be treated with radiation therapy. The same schedule of visits and Pap smears as just outlined for surveillance following radiotherapy is then recommended.

Hormone Replacement following Radiotherapy or Surgery

Cervical cancer is not a contraindication for hormone replacement therapy. Hormone therapy may be used for women with a history of cervical cancer to treat menopausal symptoms, taking into account the risks and benefits. Moreover, hormone therapy may be strongly considered in any premenopausal patient undergoing radiation therapy for cervical cancer until the average age of menopause. Either systemic or vaginal forms may be used. Estrogen alone is used if the uterus has been surgically removed, whereas combination hormonal therapy is given if the uterus remains.

■ Secondary Disease

This is defined as either persistent or recurrent cancer. Cervical cancer that has not completely regressed within 3 months of radiotherapy is considered persistent. Disease recurrence is defined as a new lesion after completion of primary therapy.

Treatment of persistent or recurrent disease depends on its location and extent. The intent in these cases is usually palliative. However, in certain instances, a woman may qualify for pelvic radiation if she previously had not received this treatment. Alternatively, a woman may be a candidate for a curative-intent surgical procedure. All chemotherapy-based treatments of metastatic disease are administered with a goal of palliation. In these cases, the primary focus is to maximize existing patient quality of life.

Pelvic Exenteration for Secondary Disease

When curative-intent surgery is contemplated, local disease should be biopsy proven. Clinically, a patient may be considered for pelvic exenteration if the triad of lower extremity edema, back pain, and hydronephrosis is absent. If present, these suggest disease extension to the pelvic sidewalls, which would contraindicate surgery. In addition, regional and distant metastasis should be excluded by both physical examination and radiologic imaging, which typically is a PET/CT scan.

Pelvic exenteration begins with exploratory laparotomy, biopsies of suspicious lesions, and paraaortic lymph node evaluation. Exenteration is completed only if there is no disease in frozen section specimens sampled during surgical evaluation at the beginning of the procedure. A complete surgical description of this procedure is found in Section 44-5 (p. 1276).

Alternatively, in highly selected patients, radical hysterectomy may be considered an alternative to pelvic exenteration (Coleman, 1994). In these circumstances, women should have small cervical recurrences measuring less than 2 cm and have disease-free pelvic lymph nodes both prior to and during surgery. With either surgical procedure, intraoperative and postoperative complications can be significant. Reported 5-year survival rates approximate 50 percent. Most recurrences occur in the first 2 years postoperatively (Berek, 2005; Goldberg, 2006).

Radiotherapy for Secondary Disease

Patients with central or limited peripheral recurrences who are radiotherapy naive are candidates for curative-intent chemoradiation treatment. In these groups, survival rates of 30 to 70 percent have been reported (Ijaz, 1998; Ito, 1997; Lanciano, 1996; Potter, 1990).

Chemotherapy for Secondary Disease

Antineoplastic drugs are used to palliate both disease and symptoms of advanced, persistent, or recurrent cervical cancer (Table 30-10). Cisplatin is considered the single most active cytotoxic agent in this setting (Thigpen, 1995). Overall, response duration to cisplatin is 4 to 6 months, and survival in such women only approximates 7 months (Vermorken, 1993). A four-arm prospective randomized study demonstrated that the combinations of cisplatin with topotecan, vinorelbine, or gemcitabine are not superior to the combination of cisplatin and paclitaxel. Patients treated with the cisplatin and paclitaxel combination had the longest median overall survival (12.9 months) compared with the other three arms (10 to 10.3 months) (Monk, 2009). Ongoing GOG studies aim to determine the best combination cytotoxic chemotherapy for women with recurrent or persistent cervical cancer.

TABLE 30-10. Chemotherapy Regimens and Response Rates of Cervical Cancer

Study	Chemotherapy Agents	Response Rates (%)	Progression-Free Survival (months)	Overall Survival (months)
Moore, 2004	Cisplatin vs.	19	2.8	8.8
	cisplatin and paclitaxel	36	4.8	9.7
Long, 2005	Cisplatin vs.	13	2.9	6.5
	cisplatin and topotecan	27	4.6	9.4
Morris, 2004	Cisplatin and vinorelbine	30	5.5	—
Brewer, 2006	Cisplatin and gemcitabine	22	2.1	—
Monk, 2009	Cisplatin and paclitaxel vs.	29	5.8	12.9
	cisplatin and vinorelbine vs.	26	4	
	cisplatin and gemcitabine vs.	22	4.7	10–10.3
	cisplatin and topotecan	23	4.6	

Palliative Care

Palliative chemotherapy is administered only if this treatment does not cause significant decline in patient quality of life. Any decision for treatment of cervical cancer in a palliative care setting should be assessed against the benefits of supportive care. Women with persistent nausea and vomiting from tumor-associated ileus may benefit from a gastrostomy tube. Bowel obstruction can be managed surgically, provided a patient is an appropriate surgical candidate. Percutaneous nephrostomy tubes may be placed for urinary fistulas or urinary tract obstruction.

Pain management forms the basis of palliation, and an extensive list of pain medications is found in Table 39-12 (p. 965). Cervical cancer patients can experience significant pain, and this should be assessed at each visit. Many patients will require narcotics. If a patient has been using opioids and is hospitalized for inadequate pain control, consideration should be given to using patient-controlled analgesia. The total dose that controls the pain in a 24-hour period should be determined. This dose can then be converted an equivalent dose of long-acting opioids. To allow for incomplete cross-tolerance between narcotics, the dose should be decreased by 25 to 50 percent. A short-acting opioid is then administered for breakthrough pain and is typically prescribed at a dose that is 10 to 20 percent of the total daily dose and given at appropriate intervals. Narcotics can constipate, and patients using these should be given a bowel regimen. This can be individualized. In particular, a combination of stool softeners (docusate sodium) plus laxative (senna) plus polyethylene glycol is often effective.

We recommend discussion of medical directives if a patient has adequate mental capability. Often, such discussion is conducted over time, giving a woman an opportunity to understand the nature and progression of her disease. Home hospice is an invaluable part of terminal care for most of these women, who require intensive pain management and considerable assistance with daily living activities.

Management During Pregnancy

There is no difference in survival between pregnant and non-pregnant women with cervical cancer when matched by age, stage, and year of diagnosis. As with nonpregnant women, clinical stage at diagnosis is the single most important prognostic factor for cervical cancer during pregnancy. Overall survival is slightly better for cervical cancer in pregnancy, because an increased proportion of patients have stage I disease.

Diagnosis

Pap smear screening guidelines for pregnancy follow those for nonpregnant women (Chap. 29, p. 742). Additionally, clinically suspicious lesions should be directly biopsied. If Pap test results reveal HSIL or suspected malignancy, then colposcopy is performed and biopsies are obtained. However, endocervical curettage is excluded. If Pap testing indicates malignant cells and colposcopic-directed biopsy fails to confirm malignancy, then diagnostic conization may be necessary. Cold-knife conization is recommended only during the second trimester and only in patients with inadequate colposcopic findings and strong cyto-

logic evidence of invasive cancer. Conization is deferred in the first trimester, as this surgery is associated with abortion rates of 25 percent in this part of pregnancy. In pregnant patients, the loop electrosurgical excision procedure (LEEP) does not appear to offer an advantage compared with cold-knife conization. Moreover, one study found a surgical complication rate of 25 percent with LEEP, and 47 percent of the women had persistent or recurrent disease (Robinson, 1997).

Stages I and II Cancer in Pregnancy

Women with microinvasive squamous cell cervical carcinoma found during conization and measuring 3 mm or less and containing no LVSI may deliver vaginally and be reevaluated 6 weeks postpartum. Moreover, for those with stage IA or IB disease, studies find no increased maternal risk if treatment is intentionally delayed to optimize fetal maturity regardless of the trimester in which the cancer was diagnosed. Given the outcomes, a planned treatment delay is generally acceptable for women who are 20 or more weeks' gestational age at diagnosis with stage I disease and who desire to continue their pregnancy. However, a patient may be able to delay from earlier gestational ages if she wishes. For patients with stage IA2 through IIA1, a cesarean section via a classical uterine incision may be performed at term, followed immediately by a radical hysterectomy with lymph node dissection.

Advanced Cervical Cancer in Pregnancy

Women with advanced cervical cancer diagnosed prior to fetal viability are offered primary chemoradiation. Spontaneous abortion of the fetus tends to follow whole-pelvis radiation therapy. If cancer is diagnosed after fetal viability is reached and a delay until fetal pulmonary maturity is elected, then a classical cesarean delivery is performed. A classical cesarean incision minimizes the risk of cutting through tumor in the lower uterine segment, which can cause serious blood loss and result in tumor spread. Chemoradiation is administered after uterine involution. For patients with advanced disease and treatment delay, pregnancy may impair prognosis. Women who elect to delay treatment, to provide quantifiable benefit to their fetuses, will have to accept an undefined risk of disease progression.

REFERENCES

Abu-Rustum NR, Neubauer N, Sonoda Y, et al: Surgical and pathologic outcomes of fertility-sparing radical abdominal trachelectomy for FIGO stage IB1 cervical cancer. Gynecol Oncol 111:261, 2008

Abu-Rustum NR, Sonoda Y, Black D, et al: Fertility-sparing radical abdominal trachelectomy for cervical carcinoma: technique and review of the literature. Gynecol Oncol 103:807, 2006

Albores-Saavedra J, Gersell D, Gilks CB, et al: Terminology of endocrine tumors of the uterine cervix: results of a workshop sponsored by the College of American Pathologists and the National Cancer Institute. Arch Pathol Lab Med 121:34, 1997

American College of Obstetricians and Gynecologists: Cervical cytology screening. Practice Bulletin No. 109. December, 2009

Belhocine T, Thille A, Fridman V, et al: Contribution of whole-body 18FDG PET imaging in the management of cervical cancer. Gynecol Oncol 87:90, 2002

Benoit AG, Krepart GV, Lotocki RJ: Results of prior cytologic screening in patients with a diagnosis of stage I carcinoma of the cervix. Am J Obstet Gynecol 148:690, 1984

Berek JS, Howe C, Lagasse LD, et al: Pelvic exenteration for recurrent gynecologic malignancy: survival and morbidity analysis of the 45-year experience at UCLA. Gynecol Oncol 99:153, 2005

Bipat S, Glas AS, van der Velden J, et al: Computed tomography and magnetic resonance imaging in staging of uterine cervical carcinoma: a systemic review. Gynecol Oncol 91:59, 2003

Bisseling KCHM, Bekkers RLM, Rome RM, et al: Treatment of microinvasive adenocarcinoma of the uterine cervix: a retrospective study and review of the literature. Gynecol Oncol 107:424, 2007

Bosch FX, Munoz N: The viral etiology of cervical cancer. Virus Res 89:183, 2002

Brewer CA, Blessing JA, Nagourney RA, et al: Cisplatin plus gemcitabine in previously treated squamous cell carcinoma of the cervix: a phase II study of the Gynecologic Oncology Group. Gynecol Oncol 100(2):385, 2006

Bulk S, Berkhof J, Bulkmans NWJ, et al: Preferential risk of HPV16 for squamous cell carcinoma and of HPV18 for adenocarcinoma of the cervix compared to women with normal cytology in the Netherlands. Br J Cancer 94:171, 2006

Burnett AF, Roman LD, O'Meara AT, et al: Radical vaginal trachelectomy and pelvic lymphadenectomy for preservation of fertility in early cervical carcinoma. Gynecol Oncol 88:419, 2003

Canis M, Mage G, Wattiez A, et al: Does endoscopic surgery have a role in radical surgery of cancer of the cervix uteri? J Gynecol Obstet Biol Reprod 19:921, 1990

Ceballos KM, Shaw D, Daya D: Microinvasive cervical adenocarcinoma (FIGO stage IA tumors), results of surgical staging and outcome analysis. Am J Surg Pathol 30:370, 2006

Coleman RL, Keeney ED, Freedman RS, et al: Radical hysterectomy for recurrent carcinoma of the uterine cervix after radiotherapy. Gynecol Oncol 55:29, 1994

Cosin JA, Fowler JM, Chen MD, et al: Pretreatment surgical staging of patients with cervical carcinoma: the case for lymph node debulking. Cancer 82:2241, 1998

Covens A, Kirby J, Shaw P, et al: Prognostic factors for relapse and pelvic lymph node metastases in early stage I adenocarcinoma of the cervix. Gynecol Oncol 74:423, 1999a

Covens A, Shaw P, Murphy J, et al: Is radical trachelectomy a safe alternative to radical hysterectomy for patients with stage IA-B carcinoma of the cervix? Cancer 86:2273, 1999b

Dargent D, Martin X, Saccetoni A, et al: Laparoscopic vaginal radical trachelectomy. Cancer 88:1877, 2000

Datta GD, Colditz GA, Kawachi I, et al: Individual-, neighborhood-, and state-level socioeconomic predictors of cervical carcinoma screening among U.S. black women: a multilevel analysis. Cancer 106:664, 2006

Delgado G, Bundy B, Zaino R, et al: Prospective surgical-pathological study of disease-free interval in patients with stage IB squamous cell carcinoma of the cervix: a Gynecologic Oncology Group study. Gynecol Oncol 38:352, 1990

Downey GO, Potish RA, Adock LL, et al: Pretreatment surgical staging in cervical carcinoma: therapeutic efficacy of pelvic lymph node resection. Am J Obstet Gynecol 160:1055, 1989

Eifel PJ, Burke TW, Delclos L, et al: Early stage I adenocarcinoma of the uterine cervix: treatment results in patients with tumors less than or equal to 4 cm in diameter. Gynecol Oncol 41:199, 1991

Eifel PJ, Burke TW, Morris M, et al: Adenocarcinoma as an independent risk factor for disease recurrence in patients with stage IB cervical carcinoma. Gynecol Oncol 59:38, 1995

Eifel PJ, Morris M, Oswald MJ, et al: Adenocarcinoma of the uterine cervix. Prognosis and patterns of failure in 367 cases. Cancer 65:2507, 1990

Ferlay J, Shin HR, Bray F, et al: Estimates of worldwide burden of cancer in 2008: GLOBOCAN 2008. Int J Cancer 127(12):2893, 2010

Follen M, Levenback CF, Iyer RB, et al: Imaging in cervical cancer. Cancer 98(9S):2028, 2003

Fyles AW, Pintilie M, Kirkbride P, et al: Prognostic factors in patients with cervix cancer treated by radiation therapy: results of a multiple regression analysis. Radiother Oncol 35:107, 1995

Gien LT, Covens A: Fertility-sparing options for early stage cervical cancer. Gynecol Oncol 117:350, 2010

Goff BA, Muntz HG, Paley PJ, et al: Impact of surgical staging in women with locally advanced cervical cancer. Gynecol Oncol 74:436, 1999

Goldberg GL, Sukumvanich P, Einstein MH, et al: Total pelvic exenteration: the Albert Einstein College of Medicine/Montefiore Medical Center Experience (1987 to 2003). Gynecol Oncol 101:261, 2006

Grigsby PW, Perez CA: Radiotherapy alone for medically inoperable carcinoma of the cervix: stage IA and carcinoma in situ. Int J Radiat Oncol Biol Phys 21:375, 1991

Grigsby PW, Siegel BA, Dehdashti F: Lymph node staging by positron emission tomography in patients with carcinoma of the cervix. J Clin Oncol 19:3745, 2001

Hacker NF, Wain GV, Nicklin JL: Resection of bulky positive lymph nodes in patients with cervical carcinoma. Int J Gynecol Cancer 5:250, 1995

Hamberger AD, Fletcher GH, Wharton JT: Results of treatment of early stage I carcinoma of the uterine cervix with intracavitary radium alone. Cancer 41:980, 1978

Havrilesky LJ, Kulasingam SL, Matchar DB, et al: FDG-PET for management of cervical and ovarian cancer. Gynecol Oncol 97:183, 2005

Hellberg D, Stendahl U: The biological role of smoking, oral contraceptive use and endogenous sexual steroid hormones in invasive squamous epithelial cervical cancer. Anticancer Res 25:3041, 2005

Helt AM, Funk JO, Galloway DA: Inactivation of both the retinoblastoma tumor suppressor and p21 by the human papillomavirus type 16 E7 oncoprotein is necessary to inhibit cell cycle arrest in human epithelial cells. J Virol 76:10559, 2002

Henriksen E: The lymphatic spread of carcinoma of the cervix and of the body of the uterus; a study of 420 necropsies. Am J Obstet Gynecol 58(5):924, 1949

Holcomb K, Abulafia O, Matthews RP, et al: The impact of pretreatment staging laparotomy on survival in locally advanced cervical carcinoma. Eur J Gynaecol Oncol 20:90, 1999

Hopkins MP, Schmidt RW, Roberts JA, et al: The prognosis and treatment of stage I adenocarcinoma of the cervix. Obstet Gynecol 72:915, 1988

Hricak H, Gatsonis C, Chi DS, et al: Role of imaging in pretreatment evaluation of early invasive cervical cancer: results of the intergroup study American College of Radiology Imaging Network 6651—Gynecologic Oncology Group 183. J Clin Oncol 23:9329, 2005

Ijaz T, Eifel PJ, Burke T, et al: Radiation therapy of pelvic recurrence after radical hysterectomy for cervical carcinoma. Gynecol Oncol 70:241, 1998

International Collaboration of Epidemiological Studies of Cervical Cancer: Comparison of risk factors for invasive squamous cell carcinoma and adenocarcinoma of the cervix: collaborative reanalysis of individual data on 8,097 women with squamous cell carcinoma and 1,374 women with adenocarcinoma from 12 epidemiological studies. Int J Cancer 120:885, 2006

International Collaboration of Epidemiological Studies of Cervical Cancer, Appleby P, Beral V, et al: Cervical cancer and hormonal contraceptives: collaborative reanalysis of individual data for 16,573 women with cervical cancer and 35,509 women without cervical cancer from 24 epidemiological studies. Lancet 370(9599):1609, 2007

Ito H, Shigematsu N, Kawada T, et al: Radiotherapy for centrally recurrent cervical cancer of the vaginal stump following hysterectomy. Gynecol Oncol 67:154, 1997

Jaworski RC, Roberts JM, Robboy SJ, et al: Cervical glandular neoplasia. In Robboy SJ, Mutter GL, Prat J, et al (eds): Robboy's Pathology of the Female Reproductive Tract, 2nd ed. Churchill Livingstone Elsevier, 2009, p 273

Jemal A, Siegel R, Ward E, et al: Cancer statistics, 2006. CA Cancer J Clin 56:106, 2006

Jemal A, Siegel R, Ward E, et al: Cancer statistics, 2010. CA Cancer J Clin 60:277, 2010

Jones DL, Munger K: Analysis of the p53-mediated G1 growth arrest pathway in cells expressing the human papillomavirus type 16 E7 oncoprotein. J Virol 71:2905, 1997

Jones EE, Wells SI: Cervical cancer and human papillomaviruses: inactivation of retinoblastoma and other tumor suppressor pathways. Curr Mol Med 6:795, 2006

Kapp KS, Poschauko J, Tauss J, et al: Analysis of the prognostic impact of tumor embolization before definitive radiotherapy for cervical carcinoma. Int J Radiation Oncology Biol Phys 62:1399, 2005

Keighley E: Carcinoma of the cervix among prostitutes in a women's prison. Br J Vener Dis 44:254, 1968

Keys HM, Bundy BN, Stehman FB, et al: Cisplatin, radiation and adjuvant hysterectomy compared with radiation and adjuvant hysterectomy for bulky stage IB cervical carcinoma. N Engl J Med 340:1154, 1999

Keys HM, Bundy BN, Stehman FB, et al: Radiation therapy with and without extrafascial hysterectomy for bulky stage IB cervical carcinoma: a randomized trial of the Gynecologic Oncology Group. Gynecol Oncol 89:343, 2003

Kolstad P: Follow-up study of 232 patients with stage Ia1 and 411 patients with stage Ia2 squamous cell carcinoma of the cervix (microinvasive carcinoma). Gynecol Oncol 33:265, 1989

Komaki R, Brickner TJ, Hanlon AL, et al: Long-term results of treatment of cervical carcinoma in the United States in 1973, 1978, and 1983: Patterns of Care Study (PCS). Int J Radiat Oncol Biol Phys 31:973, 1995

Koshiol J, Schroeder J, Jamieson DJ, et al: Smoking and time to clearance of human papillomavirus infection in HIV-seropositive and HIV-seronegative women. Am J Epidemiol 164:176, 2006

Kupets R, Thomas GM, Covens A: Is there a role for pelvic lymph node debulking in advanced cervical cancer? Gynecol Oncol 87:163, 2002

Lanciano R: Radiotherapy for the treatment of locally recurrent cervical cancer. J Natl Cancer Inst Monogr 21:113, 1996

Landoni F, Maneo A, Colombo A, et al: Randomised study of radical surgery versus radiotherapy for stage Ib-IIa cervical cancer. Lancet 350:535, 1997

Landoni F, Maneo A, Cormio G, et al: Class II versus class III radical hysterectomy in stage IB-IIA cervical cancer: a prospective randomized study. Gynecol Oncol 80:3, 2001

Lea JS, Sheets EE, Wenham RM, et al: Stage IIB-IVB cervical adenocarcinoma: prognostic factors and survival. Gynecol Oncol 84:115, 2002

Leblanc E, Narducci F, Frumovitz M, et al: Therapeutic value of pretherapeutic laparoscopic staging of locally advanced cervical carcinoma. Gynecol Oncol 105:304, 2007

Lee CL, Wu KY, Juang KG, et al: Long-term survival outcomes of laparoscopically assisted radical hysterectomy in treating early-stage cervical cancer. Am J Obstet Gynecol 203:165.e1, 2010

Leveque J, Laurent JF, Burtin F, et al: Prognostic factors of the uterine cervix adenocarcinoma. Eur J Obstet Gynecol Reprod Biol 80:209, 1998

Ley C, Bauer HM, Reingold A, et al: Determinants of genital human papillomavirus infection in young women. J Natl Cancer Inst 83:997, 1991

Li N, Franceschi S, Howell-Jones R, et al: Human papillomavirus type distribution in 30,848 invasive cervical cancers worldwide: variation by geographical region, histological type and year of publication. Int J Cancer, 2010

Long HJ 3rd, Bundy BN, Grendys EC Jr, et al: Randomized phase III trial of cisplatin with or without topotecan in carcinoma of the uterine cervix: a Gynecologic Oncology Group study. J Clin Oncol 23(21):4626, 2005

Look KY, Brunetto VL, Clarke-Pearson DL, et al: An analysis of cell type in patients with surgically staged stage IB carcinoma of the cervix: a Gynecologic Oncology Group study. Gynecol Oncol 63:304, 1996

Mantovani F, Banks L: Inhibition of E6 induced degradation of p53 is not sufficient for stabilization of p53 protein in cervical tumour derived cell lines. Oncogene 18:3309, 1999

McHale MT, Le TD, Burger RA, et al: Fertility sparing treatment for in situ and early invasive adenocarcinoma of the cervix. Obstet Gynecol 98:726, 2001

Million RR, Rutledge F, Fletcher GH: Stage IV carcinoma of the cervix with bladder invasion. Am J Obstet Gynecol 113:239, 1972

Mitchell DG, Snyder B, Coakley F, et al: Early invasive cervical cancer: tumor delineation by magnetic resonance imaging, computed tomography, and clinical examination, verified by pathologic results, in the ACRIN 6651/GOG 183 intergroup study. J Clin Oncol 24:5687, 2006

Monk BJ, Sill MW, McMeekin DS, et al: Phase III trial of four cisplatin-containing doublet combinations in stage IVB, recurrent, or persistent cervical carcinoma: a Gynecologic Oncology Group study. J Clin Oncol 27:1, 2009

Moore DH, Blessing JA, McQuellon RP, et al: Phase III study of cisplatin with or without paclitaxel in stage IVB, recurrent, or persistent squamous cell carcinoma of the cervix: a Gynecologic Oncology Group study. J Clin Oncol 22(15):3113, 2004

Moreno V, Bosch FX, Muñoz N, et al: Effect of oral contraceptives on risk of cervical cancer in women with human papillomavirus infection: the IARC multicentric case-control study. Lancet 359:1085, 2002

Morris M, Blessing JA, Monk BJ, et al: Phase II study of cisplatin and vinorelbine in squamous cell carcinoma of the cervix: a Gynecologic Oncology Group study. J Clin Oncol 22(16):3340, 2004

Morris M, Eifel PJ, Lu J, et al: Pelvic radiation with concurrent chemotherapy compared with pelvic and para-aortic radiation for high-risk cervical cancer. N Engl J Med 340:1137, 1999

Morris M, Mitchell MF, Silva EG, et al: Cervical conization as definitive therapy for early invasive squamous carcinoma of the cervix. Gynecol Oncol 51:193, 1993

Munger K, Basile JR, Duensing S, et al: Biological activities and molecular targets of the human papillomavirus E7 oncoprotein. Oncogene 20:7888, 2001

Muñoz N, Franceschi S, Bosetti C, et al: Role of parity and human papillomavirus in cervical cancer: the IARC multicentric case-control study. Lancet 359:1093, 2002.

Nakano T, Arai T, Morita S, et al: Radiation therapy alone for adenocarcinoma of the uterine cervix. Int J Radiat Oncol Biol Phys 32:1331, 1995

National Cancer Institute: Surveillance Epidemiology and End Results: SEER Stat Fact Sheets: cervix uteri 2011. Available at: http://seer.cancer.gov/statfacts/html/cervix.html. Accessed October 28, 2011

Nezhat CR, Burrell MO, Nezhat FR, et al: Laparoscopic radical hysterectomy with paraaortic and pelvic node dissection. Am J Obstet Gynecol 166:864, 1992

Olawaiye A, Del Carmen M, Tambouret R, et al: Abdominal radical trachelectomy: success and pitfalls in a general gynecologic oncology practice. Gynecol Oncol 112:506, 2009

Ostor AG: Pandora's box or Ariadne's thread? Definition and prognostic significance of microinvasion in the uterine cervix. Squamous lesions. Pathol Annu 30(Pt 2):103, 1995

Ostor AG, Rome RM: Micro-invasive squamous cell carcinoma of the cervix: a clinico-pathologic study of 200 cases with long-term follow-up. Int J Gynecol Cancer 4:257, 1994

Patsner B: Topical acetone for control of life-threatening vaginal hemorrhage from recurrent gynecologic cancer. Eur J Gynaecol Oncol 14:33, 1993

Pecorelli S: Revised FIGO staging for carcinoma of the vulva, cervix, and endometrium. Int J Gynaecol Obstet 105(2):103, 2009

Petereit DG, Hartenbach EM, Thomas GM: Para-aortic lymph node evaluation in cervical cancer: the impact of staging upon treatment decisions and outcome. Int J Gynecol Cancer 8:353, 1998

Peters WA III, Liu PY, Barrett RJ, et al: Concurrent chemotherapy and pelvic radiation therapy compared with pelvic radiation therapy alone as adjuvant therapy after radical surgery in high-risk early-stage cancer of the cervix. J Clin Oncol 18:1606, 2000

Piver MS, Rutledge F, Smith JP: Five classes of extended hysterectomy for women with cervical cancer. Obstet Gynecol 44(2):265, 1974

Plante M, Renaud MC, Hoskins IA, et al: Vaginal radical trachelectomy: a valuable fertility-preserving option in the management of early-stage cervical cancer. A series of 50 pregnancies and review of the literature. Gynecol Oncol 98(1):3, 2005

Plummer M, Herrero R, Franceschi S, et al: Smoking and cervical cancer: pooled analysis of the IARC multi-centric case-control study. Cancer Causes Control 14:805, 2003

Potter ME, Alvarez RD, Gay FL, et al: Optimal therapy for pelvic recurrence after radical hysterectomy for early-stage cervical cancer. Gynecol Oncol 37:74, 1990

Querleu D, Dargent D, Ansquer Y, et al: Extraperitoneal endosurgical aortic and common iliac dissection in the staging of bulky or advanced cervical carcinomas. Cancer 88:1883, 2000

Quinn MA, Benedet JL, Odicino F, et al: Carcinoma of the cervix uteri. Int J Gynecol Obstet 95(suppl 1):S43, 2006

Ramirez PT, Soliman PT, Schmeler KM, et al: Laparoscopic and robotic techniques for radical hysterectomy in patients with early-stage cervical cancer. Gynecol Oncol 110:S21, 2008

Robinson WR, Webb S, Tirpack J, et al: Management of cervical intraepithelial neoplasia during pregnancy with LOOP excision. Gynecol Oncol 64:153, 1997

Rose PG, Adler LP, Rodriguez M, et al: Positron emission tomography for evaluating para-aortic nodal metastasis in locally advanced cervical cancer before surgical staging: a surgicopathologic study. J Clin Oncol 17:41, 1999

Schiffman MH, Bauer HM, Hoover RN, et al: Epidemiologic evidence showing that human papillomavirus infection causes most cervical intraepithelial neoplasia. J Natl Cancer Inst 85:958, 1993

Schorge JO, Lee KR, Sheets EE: Prospective management of stage IA(1) cervical adenocarcinoma by conization alone to preserve fertility: a preliminary report. Gynecol Oncol 78:217, 2000

Sedlis A, Bundy BN, Rotman MZ, et al: A randomized trial of pelvic radiation therapy versus no further therapy in selected patients with stage IB carcinoma of the cervix after radical hysterectomy and pelvic lymphadenectomy: a Gynecologic Oncology Group Study. Gynecol Oncol 73:177, 1999

Shepherd JH, Milliken DA: Conservative surgery for carcinoma of the cervix. Clin Oncol 20(6):395, 2008

Siegel R, Ward E, Brawley O, et al: Cancer statistics, 2011: the impact of eliminating socioeconomic and racial disparities on premature cancer deaths. CA Cancer J Clin 61(4):212, 2011

Silver DF, Hempling RE, Piver MS, et al: Stage I adenocarcinoma of the cervix: does lesion size affect treatment options and prognosis?. Am J Clin Oncol 21:431, 1998

Sironi S, Buda A, Picchio M, et al: Lymph node metastasis in patients with clinical early-stage cervical cancer: detection with integrated FDG PET/CT. Radiology 238:272, 2006

Smith HO, Qualls CR, Romero AA, et al: Is there a difference in survival for IA1 and IA2 adenocarcinoma of the uterine cervix? Gynecol Oncol 85:229, 2002

Soost HJ, Lange HJ, Lehmacher W, et al: The validation of cervical cytology. Sensitivity, specificity and predictive values. Acta Cytol 35:8, 1991

Stehman FB, Bundy BN, DiSaia PJ, et al: Carcinoma of the cervix treated with radiation therapy. I. A multivariate analysis of prognostic variables in the Gynecologic Oncology Group. Cancer 67:2776, 1991

Subak LL, Hricak H, Powell CB, et al: Cervical carcinoma: computed tomography and magnetic resonance imaging for preoperative staging. Obstet Gynecol 86:43, 1995

Sutton GP, Bundy BN, Delgado G, et al: Ovarian metastases in stage IB carcinoma of the cervix: a Gynecologic Oncology Group study. Am J Obstet Gynecol 166(1 Pt 1):50, 1992

Takeshima N, Yanoh K, Tabata T, et al: Assessment of the revised International Federation of Gynecology and Obstetrics staging for early invasive squamous cervical cancer. Gynecol Oncol 74:165, 1999

The GlaxoSmithKline HPV-007 Study Group, Romanowski B, Colares de Borba P, et al: Sustained efficacy and immunogenicity of the human papillomavirus (HPV)-16/18 ASO4-adjuvanted vaccine: analysis of a randomized placebo-controlled trial up to 6.4 years. Lancet 374:1975, 2009

Thigpen JT, Vance R, Puneky L, et al: Chemotherapy as a palliative treatment in carcinoma of the uterine cervix. Semin Oncol 22(2 Suppl 3):16, 1995

Tinga DJ, Timmer PR, Bouma J, et al: Prognostic significance of single versus multiple lymph node metastases in cervical carcinoma stage IB. Gynecol Oncol 39:175, 1990

Trimble CL, Genkinger JM, Burke AE, et al: Active and passive cigarette smoking and the risk of cervical neoplasia. Obstet Gynecol 105:174, 2005

Upadhyay SK, Symonds RP, Haelterman M, et al: The treatment of stage IV carcinoma of cervix by radical dose radiotherapy. Radiother Oncol 11:15, 1988

U.S. Preventive Services Task Force: Screening for cervical cancer: summary of recommendations, 2003. Available at: http://www.uspreventiveservicestaskforce.org/uspstf/uspscerv.htm. Accessed October 8, 2010

Vale C, Chemoradiotherapy for Cervical Cancer Meta-Analysis Collaboration: Reducing uncertainties about the effects of chemoradiotherapy for cervical cancer: a systematic review and meta-analysis of individual patient data from 18 randomized trials. J Clin Oncol 26:5802, 2008

Vasilev SA, McGonigle KF: Extraperitoneal laparoscopic paraaortic lymph node dissection: development of a technique. J Laparoendosc Surg 5:85, 1995

Vermorken JB: The role of chemotherapy in squamous cell carcinoma of the uterine cervix: a review. Int J Gynecol Cancer 3:129, 1993

Vizcaino AP, Moreno V, Bosch FX, et al: International trends in incidence of cervical cancer: II. Squamous-cell carcinoma. Int J Cancer 86:429, 2000

Viswanathan AN, Deavers MT, Jhingran A, et al: Small cell neuroendocrine carcinoma of the cervix: outcome and patterns of recurrence. Gynecol Oncol 93:27, 2004

Walboomers JN, Jacons MV, Manos M, et al: Human papillomavirus is a necessary cause of invasive cervical cancer worldwide. J Pathol 189:12, 1999.

Webb MJ, Symmonds RE: Site of recurrence of cervical cancer after radical hysterectomy. Am J Obstet Gynecol 138(7 Pt 1):813, 1980

Wentzensen N, Vinokurova S, von Knebel DM: Systematic review of genomic integration sites of human papillomavirus genomes in epithelial dysplasia and invasive cancer of the female lower genital tract. Cancer Res 64:3878, 2004

Whitney CW, Sause W, Bundy BN, et al: Randomized comparison of fluorouracil plus cisplatin versus hydroxyurea as an adjunct to radiation therapy in stage IIB-IVA carcinoma of the cervix with negative para-aortic lymph nodes: a Gynecologic Oncology Group and Southwest Oncology Group study. J Clin Oncol 17:1339, 1999

Wright JD, Dehdashti F, Herzog TJ, et al: Preoperative lymph node staging of early-stage cervical carcinoma by [18F]-fluoro-2-deoxy-D-glucose-positron emission tomography. Cancer 104:2484, 2005

Yahata T, Nishino K, Kashmima K, et al: Conservative treatment of stage IA1 adenocarcinoma of the uterine cervix with a long-term follow-up. Int J Gynecol Cancer 20:1063, 2010

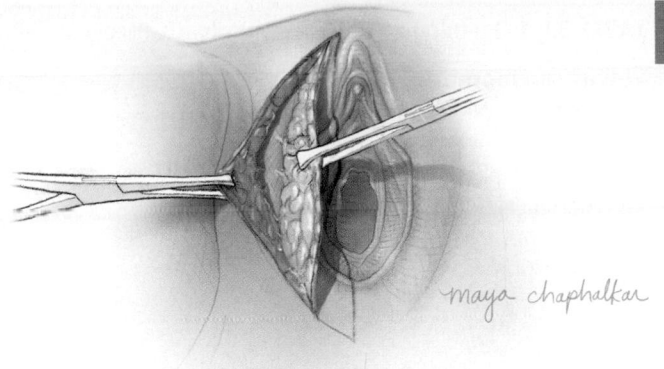

maya chaphalkar

CHAPTER 31

Invasive Cancer of the Vulva

Vulvar cancers are uncommon and comprise approximately 5 percent of all gynecologic malignancies. Most vulvar cancers are diagnosed at an early stage (I and II). Advanced disease is found mainly in older women, perhaps due to clinical and behavioral barriers that lead to diagnostic delays. Thus, early detection of any abnormal vulvar lesion by biopsy is imperative to diagnosing this cancer in its early stages and improving subsequent morbidity and mortality rates.

Approximately 90 percent of vulvar tumors are squamous cell carcinomas (Fig. 31-1). Accordingly, virtually all knowledge regarding prognostic factors, spread patterns, and survival information is derived from women with this histologic type. Although rare, uncommon histologic subtypes such as melanomas, basal cell

carcinomas, Bartholin gland adenocarcinomas, soft tissue sarcomas, and metastatic lesions may also be encountered (Table 31-1).

In the United States, vulvar cancers carry a relatively good prognosis with a 5-year relative survival rate of 78 percent (Stroup, 2008). Traditional therapy includes radical excision of the vulva and inguinal lymphadenectomy. For advanced stages, adjuvant chemoradiation may be used preoperatively or postoperatively to aid tumor control.

Treatment of vulvar cancer frequently results in dramatic anatomic deformity that leads to significant negative effects on patient sexuality. However, during the past decade, management of vulvar cancer has trended toward more conservative surgery and improved psychosexual outcomes.

INCIDENCE

Vulvar cancer is primarily a disease of elderly women but has been observed in premenopausal women as well. In the United States, the age-adjusted incidence of invasive vulvar tumors has trended upward during the past three decades. This increase persists among all age groups and all geographic areas (Bodelon, 2009). Specifically, the age-adjusted incidence of vulvar carcinoma in situ (CIS) has increased by 3.5 percent per year, whereas that of invasive cancers has risen by 1 percent each year. As a result, during the past decade, the incidence of vulvar CIS has been reported at 5 per 100,000 women, and invasive cancer at 2.5 per 100,000. In 2011, there were an estimated 4340 new cases of vulvar cancer and 940 vulvar cancer-related deaths (Siegel, 2011).

RELATED ANATOMY

Vulva

The *external vulva* includes the mons pubis, labia majora and minora, clitoris, vestibule, vestibular bulbs, greater vestibular or Bartholin glands, lesser vestibular glands, Skene or paraurethral

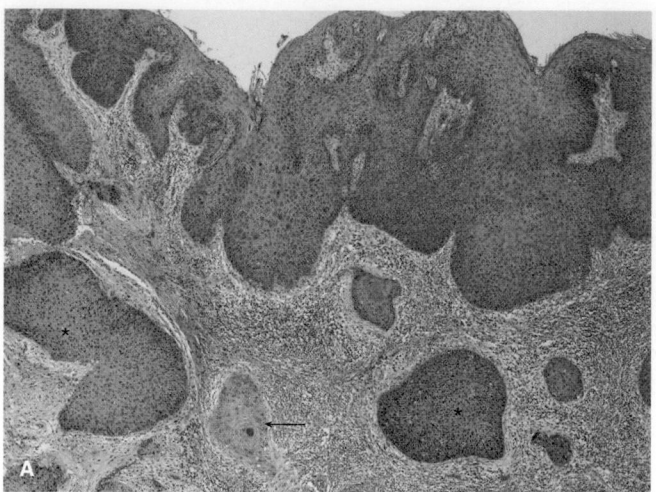

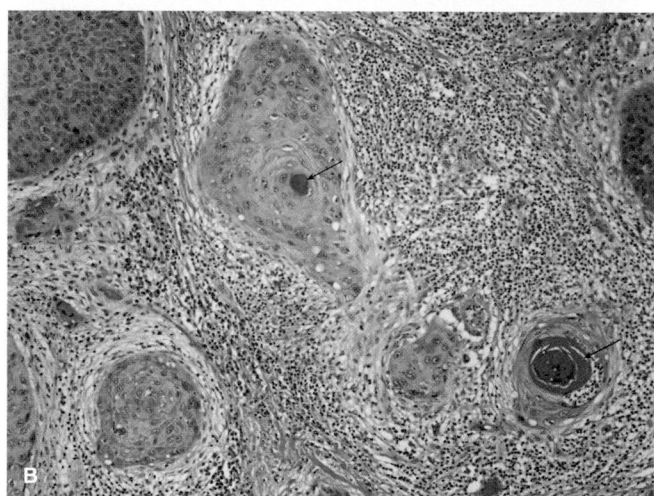

FIGURE 31-1 Vulvar squamous cell carcinoma. **A.** Low-power view. The surface epithelium shows high-grade squamous dysplasia. Nests of invasive squamous cell carcinoma (*arrow*) are present. A brisk chronic inflammatory infiltrate is present as is often the case with invasive squamous cell carcinoma. Portions of the surface epithelium extend deep and are cut tangentially (*asterisks*), giving the false impression of invasive tumor at these sites. **B.** Tumor shows classic diagnostic features of invasive squamous cell carcinoma that include a squamoid appearance, intercellular bridges, and brightly eosinophilic keratin pearls (*arrows*). Nests of invasive tumor are surrounded by chronic inflammation. (*Photographs contributed by Dr. Kelley Carrick.*)

TABLE 31-1. Histologic Subtypes of Vulvar Cancer
Vulvar carcinomas
Squamous cell carcinoma
Adenocarcinoma
Carcinoma of Bartholin gland
Adenocarcinoma
Squamous carcinoma
Transitional cell carcinoma
Vulvar Paget disease
Merkel cell tumors
Verrucous carcinoma
Basal cell carcinoma
Vulvar malignant melanoma
Vulvar sarcoma
Leiomyosarcoma
Malignant fibrous histiocytoma
Epithelial sarcoma
Malignant rhabdoid tumor
Metastatic cancers to vulva
Malignant schwannoma
Yolk sac tumors

During radical vulvectomy, dissection is carried to the depth of the perineal membrane. As a result, contents of the superficial urogenital triangle that lie beneath the mass are removed during tumor excision.

Vulvar Lymphatics

Typically, the lymphatics of the vulva and distal third of the vagina drain into the superficial inguinal node group (Fig. 38-29, p. 945). From here, they travel through the deep inguinal (femoral) lymphatics and the node of Cloquet to the pelvic nodal groups. Cloquet node is the superiormost deep femoral lymph node. Importantly, direct lymphatic drainage to the deep femoral nodes can also occur from the clitoris and the upper part of the labia (Way, 1948). Vulvar lymphatics decussate in the mons pubis and the posterior fourchette. Previous lymphatic mapping of the vulva has demonstrated that lymphatics do not cross the labiocrural folds (Morley, 1976). As a result, metastases to contralateral nodes are rare in the absence of ipsilateral groin metastasis. Also rarely, lymphatic tumor spread within dermal lymphatics occurs before reaching the superficial inguinal nodes and is termed in-transit metastasis.

The superficial inguinal nodes are located within the femoral triangle formed by the inguinal ligament, the medial border of the sartorius muscle, and the lateral border of the adductor longus muscle (Fig. 38-29, p. 945). The deep femoral nodes are found on the medial aspect of the femoral vein, beneath the borders of the fossa ovalis. An *inguinofemoral lymphadenectomy* typically refers to the removal of both the superficial inguinal and deep femoral lymph nodes (Levenback, 1996).

glands, and urethral and vaginal orifices. The lateral margins of the vulva are the labiocrural folds (Fig. 38-25, p. 941). Vulvar cancer may involve any of these external structures.

The *internal vulva* can be divided into superficial and deep urogenital triangle compartments. The superficial space of the urogenital triangle is an enclosed compartment that lies between Colles fascia (superficial perineal fascia) and the perineal membrane (deep perineal fascia). Within this space lie the ischiocavernosus muscles laterally, the bulbocavernosus muscles medially, and the transverse perineal muscle inferiorly. Deep to each bulbocavernosus muscle is a vestibular bulb, and crura of the clitoris lie deep to the ischiocavernosus muscles as illustrated in Figure 38-26 (p. 942).

Vulvar Blood Supply

Blood supply to the vulva is provided primarily by the internal pudendal artery, which is a branch of the internal iliac artery and accompanies the pudendal nerve (Fig. 38-28, p. 944). The internal pudendal vein receives tributaries that correspond to the branches of the internal pudendal artery. Knowledge of vascular anatomy allows for a more hemostatic procedure and enhanced visibility.

The deep external pudendal artery and the superficial external pudendal artery are branches of the femoral artery and drain into the great saphenous vein. Both arteries supply the labia majora and their deep structures and have anastomotic connections with branches of the internal pudendal vessels in areas where their tributaries mutually contribute blood supply. These arteries' corresponding veins are in proximity during superficial inguinofemoral lymphadenectomy. Specifically, the superficial lymph nodes that are removed lie within the fatty tissue along the saphenous, superficial external pudendal, superficial circumflex iliac, and superficial epigastric veins (Fig. 38-29, p. 945).

HISTOLOGIC SUBTYPES OF VULVAR CANCER

The majority of vulvar malignancies arise within the squamous epithelium that covers most of the vulva. Although the vulva does not have an identifiable transformation zone, squamous neoplasias arise most frequently on the vestibule at the border between the vulvar keratinized stratified squamous epithelium, which lies laterally, and the nonkeratinized squamous mucosa, which lies medially. This demarcation line is termed *Hart line*.

Table 31-1 describes other histologic subtypes of vulva cancers. Malignant melanoma of the vulva is the second most common vulvar cancer and usually arises from the epidermal layer of the external vulva.

EPIDEMIOLOGY AND RISK FACTORS

Risk factors for vulvar cancer can be divided into two distinct profiles, which are age dependent. Vulvar cancers that develop in younger women (<55 years) tend to have the same risk profile as other anogenital cancers. Accordingly, women with low socioeconomic status, high-risk sexual behaviors, human papillomavirus (HPV) infection, and cigarette use are disproportionately affected (Madeleine, 1997). These cancers are usually described histologically as being basaloid or warty and are associated with HPV in 50 percent of cases.

In contrast, older women (55 to 85 years) with late-onset vulvar cancers typically do not have a history of prior sexually transmitted infections and tend not to be smokers. These cancers are largely keratinizing, and HPV DNA is found in only 15 percent (Canavan, 2002; Madeleine, 1997).

Infection
Human Papillomavirus Infection

High-risk human papillomavirus has been associated with vulvar cancer. Serotype 16 predominates, although HPV serotypes 18, 31, 33, and 45 have also been reported (Hildesheim,

1997). Although implicated in some cases of vulvar cancer, HPV infection has stronger correlations with preinvasive vulvar lesions than with frankly invasive cancers (Hildesheim, 1997). Specifically, HPV DNA is identified in only 20 to 50 percent of invasive lesions, but is seen in 70 to 80 percent of vulvar intraepithelial neoplasia (VIN) lesions. Additional discussions of HPV and VIN are found in Chapter 29 (p. 756).

The presence of HPV becomes a stronger risk for vulvar cancer when combined with other cofactors such as smoking and herpes simplex virus (HSV) infection (Madeleine, 1997). Women who have smoked and have a history of genital warts have a 35-fold increased risk for developing vulvar cancer compared with women without these factors (Brinton, 1990; Kirschner, 1995).

Herpes Simplex Virus

Herpes simplex virus has been shown to have a strong association with vulvar cancer in several studies. However, the association is more prominent when combined with other cofactors such as smoking (Madeleine, 1997). Thus, the association of HSV alone being a causative factor for vulvar cancer should not be considered conclusive.

Immunosuppression

Chronic immunosuppression has been indirectly associated with vulvar cancer. Specifically, vulvar cancer rates have been shown to be increased in women with human immunodeficiency virus (HIV) (Elit, 2005; Frisch, 2000). A possible explanation is the association of HIV and high-risk HPV subtypes. However, vulvar cancers are not considered an acquired immunodeficiency syndrome (AIDS)-defining malignancy.

Lichen Sclerosus

This chronic vulvar inflammatory disease has been particularly linked to the development of vulvar cancer. Although not validated as a causative or precursor lesion, current evidence suggests a correlative relationship between the two. Keratinocytes affected by lichen sclerosus show a proliferative phenotype and can exhibit markers of neoplastic progression. This suggests that lichen sclerosus may be a precursor lesion in some cases of invasive squamous vulvar cancer (Rolfe, 2001). Vulvar cancers that coexist with lichen sclerosus have been shown to develop in older women, predominate in near the clitoris, and lack association with VIN 3.

Vulvar Intraepithelial Neoplasia

The natural history of VIN 3 is unclear. On one hand, the progression of VIN 3 to invasive cancer has been strongly suggested. Although most VIN 3 lesions do not progress, several reports have demonstrated that in a small percentage of women older than 30 years, untreated lesions can progress to invasive cancer within a mean of 4 years (Jones, 2005; van Seters, 2005).

However, some cases of progression may reflect misdiagnosis. For example, one metaanalysis of 3322 women who were treated for VIN 3 revealed that occult carcinomas were diagnosed in the final pathology specimen in 3.2 percent of patients, and 3.3 percent of carcinomas were diagnosed during postoperative

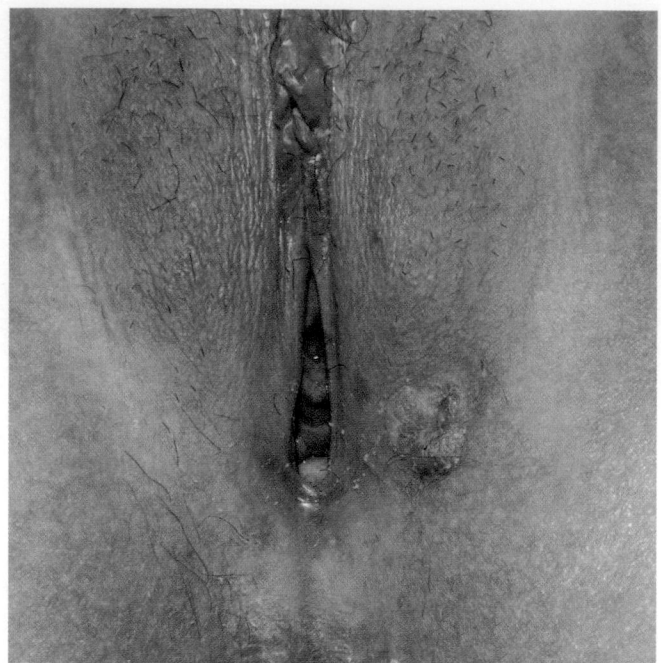

FIGURE 31-2 Early-stage squamous cell cancer of the vulva.

surveillance (van Seters, 2005). Although progression from VIN 3 to invasive cancer cannot be conclusively validated, we recommend that patients with moderate and severe vulvar dysplasia receive early definitive treatment (Chap. 29, p. 759).

SYMPTOMS

Women with VIN and vulvar cancer commonly present with pruritus and a visible lesion (Fig. 31-2). However, pain, bleeding, and ulceration may also be initial complaints. Most patients experience symptoms for weeks or months before diagnosis. Many may be embarrassed or not recognize their symptoms' significance. Thus, minor symptoms may be initially ignored by women, contributing to a diagnostic delay. Additionally, clinicians may also contribute to delays by providing medical treatment for up to 12 months before obtaining a biopsy or considering referral (Canavan, 2002).

A well-defined mass is not always present, especially in younger women with multifocal disease. Moreover, selecting the appropriate site for tissue sampling may be challenging in such cases and may require multiple biopsies. Colposcopic examination of the vulva, termed *vulvoscopy,* can direct biopsy site selection. Other clinical entities may present similarly and include preinvasive neoplasia, infection, chronic inflammatory disease, and granulomatous disease. Thus, the goal of evaluation should be to obtain an accurate and definitive pathologic diagnosis.

DIAGNOSIS

Lesion Evaluation

At the initiation of vulvoscopy, the vulva is soaked with 3-percent acetic acid for 5 minutes to allow adequate penetration into the keratin layer. This aids identification of acetowhite areas and

abnormal vascular patterns, which are characteristics of vulvar neoplasia (Chap. 29, p. 758). The entire vulva and perianal skin should be systematically examined. Lesions may be raised, ulcerated, pigmented, or warty, and biopsies of the most suspicious-appearing areas are obtained as described in Chapter 4 (p. 112). Specimens removed with a Keyes punch should include the surface epithelial lesion and the underlying stroma to evaluate for presence and depth of lesion invasion. Colposcopic examination of the cervix and vagina and careful evaluation of the perianal area are recommended to diagnose any synchronous lesions or associated neoplasm of the lower genital tract.

Cancer Patient Evaluation

Following histologic diagnosis, a patient with vulvar cancer is assessed for the clinical extent of disease and for coexisting medical illnesses. Thus, detailed physical examination includes measurement of the primary tumor and evaluation of extension into other areas of the genitourinary system, the anal canal, the bony pelvis, and the inguinal lymph nodes. At our institution, if a thorough physical examination is not possible because of patient discomfort or disease extent, an examination under anesthesia is performed together with cystourethroscopy or proctosigmoidoscopy or both if suspicion of tumor invasion into the urethra, bladder, or anal canal is high (Fig. 31-3).

Women with small tumors and clinically negative groin nodes require few additional diagnostic studies other than those needed for surgical preparation (Chap. 39, p. 958). Additional radiologic studies such as computed tomography (CT) scanning, magnetic resonance (MR) imaging, or positron emission tomography (PET) are recommended in women with larger tumors to assess for local invasion, lymph node involvement, and distant metastatic disease. For some patients with advanced tumors, fine-needle aspiration biopsy from sites of suspected metastases in the groins and/or direct biopsy of a vulvar mass can provide a pathologic diagnosis to guide appropriate treatment.

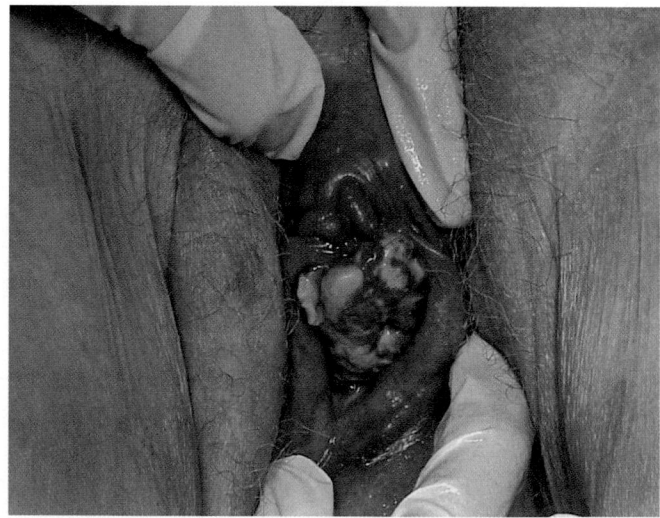

FIGURE 31-3 Photograph of invasive vulvar cancer. The lesion seen involves the labia minora bilaterally, urethral orifice, and anterior lower vagina, and abuts the clitoris. *(Photograph contributed by Dr. David Miller.)*

TABLE 31-2. FIGO Staging of Invasive Cancer of the Vulva

Stage	Characteristics
I	**Tumor confined to the vulva**
IA	Lesions ≤2 cm in size, confined to the vulva or perineum and with stromal invasion ≤1.0 mm[a], no nodal metastasis
IB	Lesions >2 cm in size or with stromal invasion >1.0 mm[a], confined to the vulva or perineum, with negative nodes
II	**Tumor of any size with extension to adjacent perineal structures (1/3 lower urethra, 1/3 lower vagina, anus) with negative nodes**
III	**Tumor of any size with or without extension to adjacent perineal structures (1/3 lower urethra, 1/3 lower vagina, anus) with positive inguinofemoral lymph nodes**
IIIA	(i) With 1 lymph node metastasis (≥5 mm), or (ii) 1–2 lymph node metastasis(es) (<5 mm)
IIIB	(i) With 2 or more lymph node metastases (≥5 mm), or (ii) 3 or more lymph node metastases (<5 mm)
IIIC	With positive nodes with extracapsular spread
IV	**Tumor invades other regional (2/3 upper urethra, 2/3 upper vagina), or distant structures**
IVA	Tumor invades any of the following: (i) upper urethral and/or vaginal mucosa, bladder mucosa, rectal mucosa, or fixed to pelvic bone, or (ii) fixed or ulcerated inguinofemoral lymph nodes
IVB	Any distant metastasis including pelvic lymph nodes

[a]The depth of invasion is defined as the measurement of the tumor from the epithelial–stromal junction of the adjacent most superficial dermal papilla to the deepest point of invasion (Fig. 31-5).
FIGO = International Federation of Gynecology and Obstetrics.

Staging Systems

The International Federation of Gynecology and Obstetrics (FIGO) advocate surgically staging of the patient with vulvar cancer and in 1988, adopted a staging system that is based on a tumor, nodal, metastatic (TNM) classification. Thus, staging involves: (1) primary tumor resection to obtain tumor dimensions and (2) dissection of superficial and deep inguinal lymph nodes to evaluate tumor spread. In patients with larger tumors or with clinically obvious metastatic disease involving the inguinal lymph nodes, a chest radiograph in combination with CT scanning, PET scanning, or MR imaging of the abdomen and pelvis are also obtained preoperatively to determine the presence or absence of metastatic disease. Importantly, despite the frequent use of imaging tests to guide treatment planning, these are not a formal part of vulvar cancer staging.

The FIGO staging for vulvar cancer was revised in 2009 (Pecorelli, 2009). The updated system better predicts prognosis and accounts for the differences in survival observed, based on the number and morphology of positive inguinal lymph nodes (van der Steen, 2010). Table 31-2 and Figure 31-4 describe 2009 FIGO staging criteria.

PROGNOSIS AND PROGNOSTIC FACTORS

The overall survival rates of women with squamous cell carcinoma of the vulva are relatively good. Five-year survival rates of 75 to 90 percent are routinely reported for stage I and II disease. As anticipated, 5-year survival rates for higher stages are poorer, and rates of 50 percent for stage III and 15 percent for stage IV have been noted. Numerous studies indicate important prognostic factors for women with vulvar cancer including tumor FIGO stage, lesion size, depth of invasion, lymph node involvement and morphology, lymphatic vascular space involvement (LVSI), and resection-margin status (Tables 31-3 and 31-4).

Lymph Node Metastasis

Of the prognostic factors, lymph node metastasis is the single most important in vulvar cancer, and inguinal node metastasis reduces long-term survival by 50 percent (Farias-Eisner, 1994;

TABLE 31-3. Depth of Invasion as Prognostic Predictor

Depth of Invasion (mm)	Positive Nodes (%)
1	3
2	9
3	19
4	31
5	33
≥ 5	48

Abbreviated from Homesley, 1993, with permission.

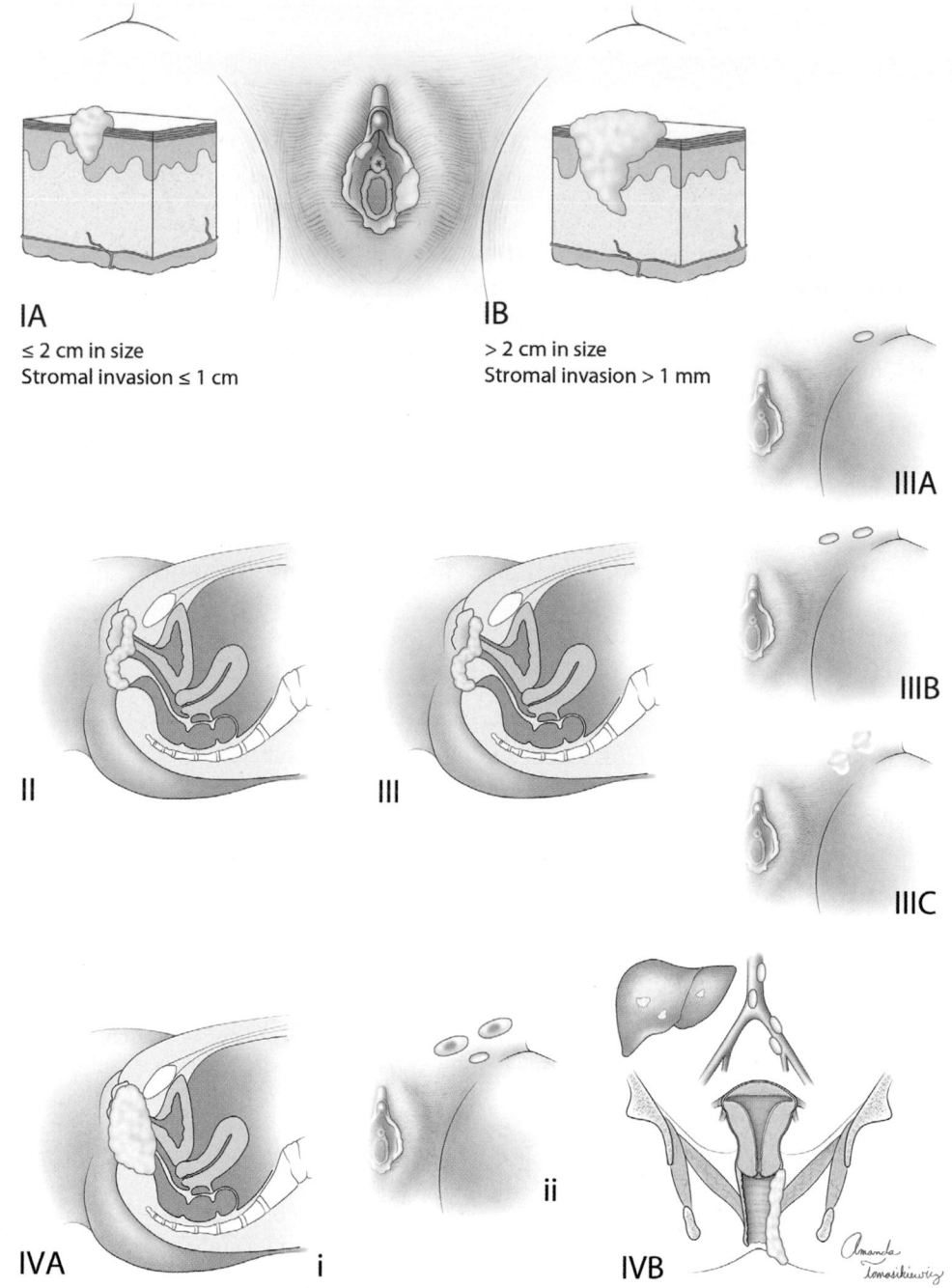

IA
≤ 2 cm in size
Stromal invasion ≤ 1 cm

IB
> 2 cm in size
Stromal invasion > 1 mm

II

III

IIIA

IIIB

IIIC

IVA

i

IVB

ii

FIGURE 31-4 FIGO (International Federation of Gynecology and Obstetrics) staging of invasive vulvar cancer.

TABLE 31-4. Tumor Size as Prognostic Predictor

Tumor Diameter (cm)	5-Year Survival (%)
0–1	90
1–2	89
2–3	83
3–4	63
>4	44

Abbreviated from Stehman, 2006, with permission.

Figge, 1985). Nodal status is determined by surgical resection and pathologic evaluation.

Independent predictors that increase the risk for nodal metastasis include larger tumor size, presence of LVSI, older patient age, and greater tumor depth of invasion (Homesley, 1993; Stehman, 2006). Depth of invasion is measured from the basement membrane to the deepest point of invasion as specified by the International Society of Gynecological Pathologists, the World Health Organization, and FIGO (Fig. 31-5) (Creasman, 1995; Kalnicki, 1987; Scully, 1994). Tumors with a depth of invasion less than 1 mm carry little or no risk of inguinal lymph node metastasis, and increasing rates of metastasis are associated with increasing invasion.

Among patients who have inguinal lymph node metastasis, there are factors that further delineate a poorer prognosis. These include a high number of lymph nodes involved, large size of metastasis, extracapsular invasion, and fixed or ulcerated nodes (Homesley, 1991; Origoni, 1992).

Surgical Margins

The risk of local recurrence is related to surgical margin adequacy. Traditionally a 1- to 2-cm tumor-free surgical margin has been desired. Two large retrospective, institutional series demonstrated that a tumor-free surgical margin ≥8 mm resulted in a high rate of local control. In contrast, margins <8 mm were associated with a 23- to 48-percent chance of recurrence (Chan, 2007; Heaps, 1990). Hence, when lesions are close to the clitoris, anus, urethra, or vagina, a 1-cm surgical tumor-free margin may be used to preserve important anatomy yet still provide an optimal resection.

Lymphatic Vascular Space Invasion

Histologic identification of tumor cells within lymphatic vessels, termed lymphatic vascular space invasion (LVSI), is also a predictor of early disease recurrence (Preti, 2005). LVSI is

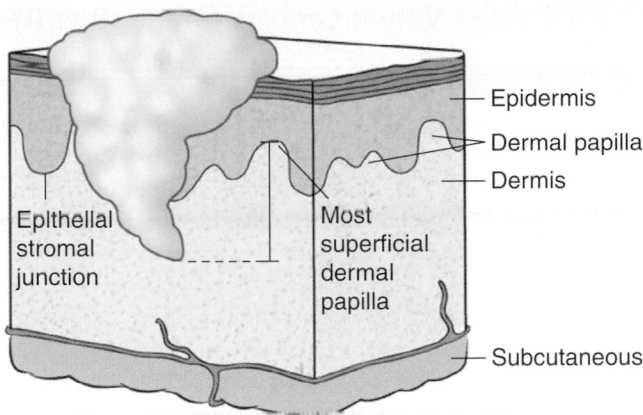

FIGURE 31-5 Histologic measurement of invasive vulvar cancer. Depth of invasion is measured from the junction between the epithelium and stroma of the most superficial dermal papilla to the greatest depth of tumor invasion.

associated with a higher frequency of lymph node metastasis and a lower overall 5-year survival rate (Hoskins, 2000).

TREATMENT

Surgical Procedures

Procedures for the treatment of invasive vulvar neoplasia include wide local excision (WLE), radical partial vulvectomy, and radical complete vulvectomy. Wide local excisions can be used for microinvasive tumors of the vulva. With *wide local excision*, also termed *simple partial vulvectomy*, 1- to 2-cm surgical margins are obtained around the lesion. Deep surgical margins of 1 cm are also preferred. This deep margin usually corresponds to the superficial perineal fascia, that is, Colles fascia (Fig. 38-25, p. 941). Extended WLE, termed *skinning vulvectomy* (Section

44-26, p. 1335), refers to removal of only the skin and superficial subcutaneous tissue. Currently, this disfiguring procedure is rarely performed except in unique circumstances of confluent VIN 3. However, if foci of microinvasive disease are identified on final pathology, it may be considered definitive treatment.

With *radical partial vulvectomy* (Section 44-27, p. 1337), tumor-containing portions of the vulva are completely removed, wherever they are located. Skin margins are 1 to 2 cm, and excision extends deep to the perineal membrane (Figure 31-6). Lastly, with *radical complete vulvectomy* (Section 44-28, p. 1340), again 1- to 2-cm margins are obtained around large vulvar tumors and dissection is completed down to the perineal membrane. Occasionally, flap reconstruction of a surgical defect is needed. Skin grafts, advancement flaps, or rotational flaps are options for closing vulvar defects as described in Section 44-30 (p. 1346). Of the three procedures shown in Figure 31-7, the en bloc incision, colloquially termed the *butterfly* or *longhorn* incision, has largely been abandoned. It has survival rates equivalent to radical complete vulvectomy but carries significantly greater morbidity.

Lymphadenectomy accompanies radical partial or radical complete vulvectomy procedures. Although lymphatic drainage rarely bypasses the superficial inguinal nodes, the dissection usually includes excision of both the superficial inguinal and deep femoral lymph nodes to maximize detection of metastatic disease (Gordinier, 2003).

Microinvasive Tumors (Stage IA)

FIGO surgical staging for vulvar cancer contains a subclassification of stage I tumors. Stage IA lesions are 2 cm or smaller, are confined to the vulva or perineum, and displayed stromal invasion no greater than 1 mm. These lesions, termed *microinvasive cancers*, reflect a subpopulation in which the risk of inguinal metastasis is negligible (Binder, 1990; Donaldson, 1981; Hacker, 1984).

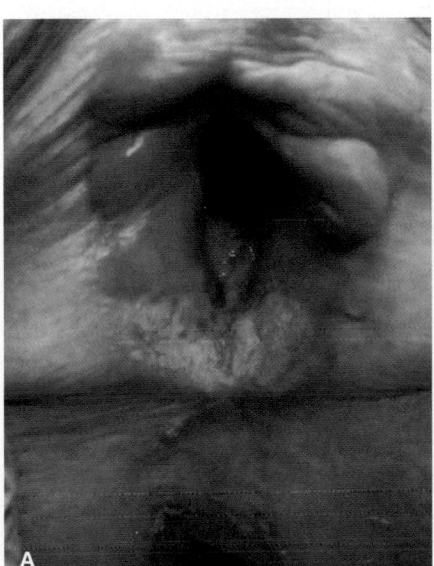
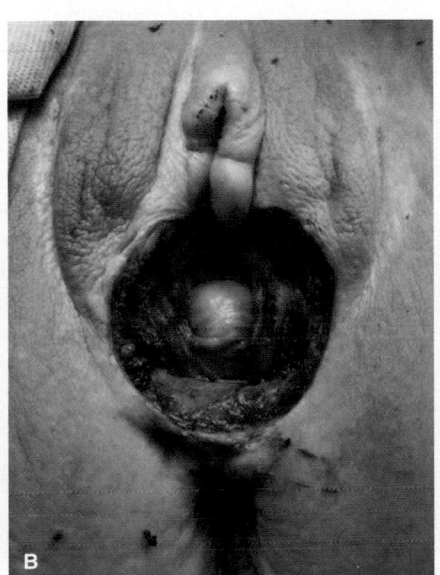
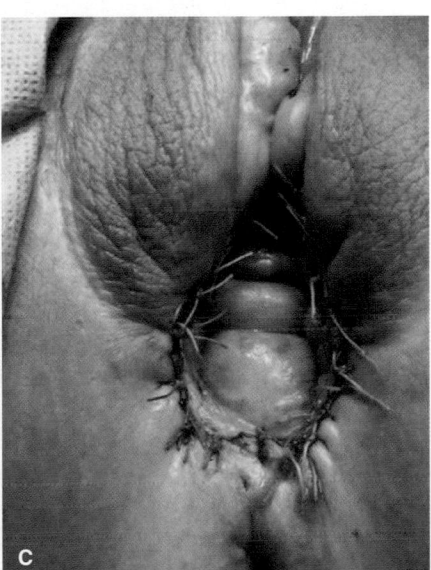

FIGURE 31-6 A. Vulvar cancer following radiation therapy and in preparation for surgical excision. **B.** Radical partial vulvectomy. **C.** Final surgical closure. *(Photographs contributed by Dr. David Miller.)*

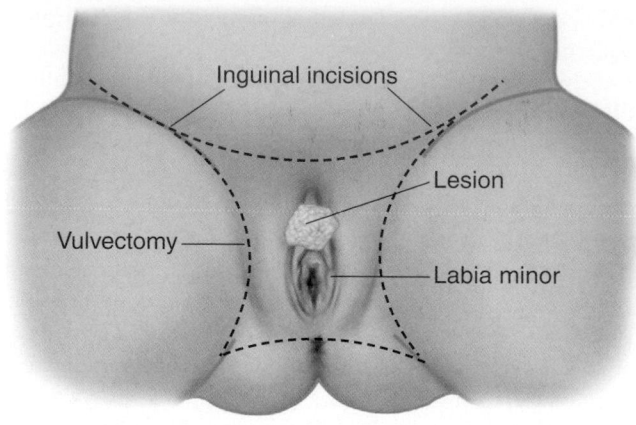

A

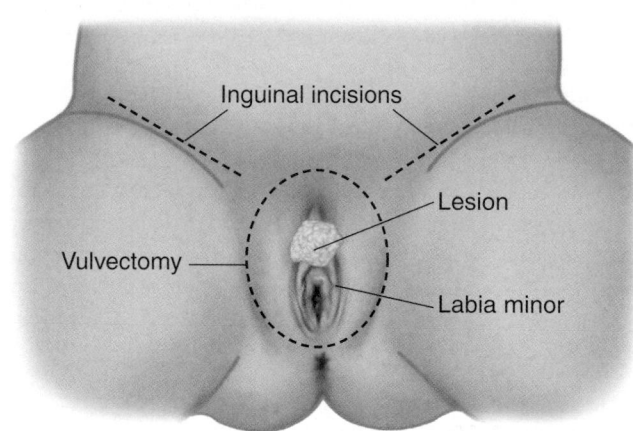

B

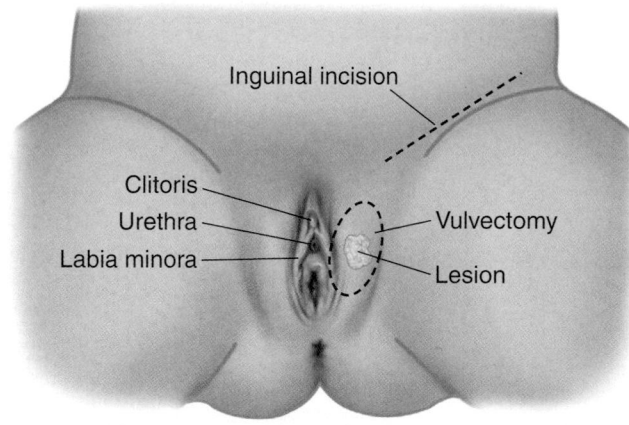

C

FIGURE 31-7 Types of vulvectomy used in the treatment of vulvar cancer. **A.** En bloc radical vulvectomy with bilateral inguinofemoral lymphadenectomy. **B.** Radical complete vulvectomy with bilateral inguinofemoral lymphadenectomy. **C.** Radical partial vulvectomy with ipsilateral inguinofemoral lymphadenectomy.

Women with microinvasive stage IA tumors tend to be younger and have multifocal disease associated with HPV. As curative resection, these patients can undergo wide local excision. Lymphadenectomy is not indicated for these patients with very low risk for lymph node metastasis.

■ Early Stage Vulvar Cancers (Stage IB to II)

Most patients with early-stage vulvar cancer require radical resection of the primary tumor and inguinofemoral nodal assessment. Surgical treatment has favored a more conservative approach that offers similar cure rates and reduced surgical morbidity (Tantipalakorn, 2009). Lesions measuring ≤2 cm in diameter but that invade >1 mm are stage IB. These can be managed with radical partial vulvectomy. By obtaining adequate margins and maintaining a similar depth of dissection, radical local excisions result in similar recurrence rates as radical complete vulvectomy.

Traditionally, an inguinofemoral lymphadenectomy is performed and is either ipsilateral or bilateral depending on the location of the vulvar lesion. Most ipsilateral vulvar lesions, defined as lesions located 1 to 2 cm lateral to the midline, can be managed with an ipsilateral inguinofemoral lymphadenectomy (Gonzalez Bosquet, 2007). Midline lesions (within 1 to 2 cm of the midline) warrant bilateral inguinofemoral lymphadenectomy.

Lesions >2 cm (stage IB) or with extension to lower perineal structures (stage II) are most often managed with a larger radical partial excision, that is, anterior hemivulvectomy with distal urethrectomy and bilateral inguinofemoral lymphadenectomy. Occasionally, a radical complete vulvectomy is required, depending on the location of the tumor. Reported experience with conservative surgery suggests identical local recurrence rates as long as 1- to 2-cm surgical margins are obtained (Burke, 1995; Farias–Eisner, 1994; Tantipalakorn, 2009).

Inguinofemoral Lymphadenectomy

The superficial inguinal lymph nodes are accessed by dissecting below the inguinal ligament along the fascia lata to reach the fossa ovalis (Section 44-29, p. 1343). During dissection, the saphenous vein can be spared in some cases in an attempt to minimize the risk for postoperative lymphedema and other morbidity (Dardarian, 2006).

Deep femoral nodes are excised from their location medial to the femoral vein. In reaching these nodes, a modified approach to inguinofemoral lymphadenectomy preserves the fascia lata by removing the deep femoral nodes through the fossa ovalis. This modified approach is associated with recurrence rates comparable to those obtained following classic inguinofemoral node dissection (Bell, 2000; Hacker, 1983). Advantageously, complications described in Table 31-5 of wound breakdown, infection, and lymphedema are significantly decreased.

On occasion, a classic inguinofemoral node dissection is required to reach the deep femoral lymph nodes. In such cases, the fascia lata (cribriform fascia) is excised, lymph nodes are removed, and the sartorius muscle may then be transposed over the femoral vessels. This transposition may reduce the risk of postoperative erosion into the skeletonized femoral vessels in the event of dehiscence of the overlying skin incision, but does not reduce overall postoperative wound morbidity (Judson, 2004; Rouzier, 2003).

Sentinel-Node Biopsy

One of the most important innovations in the treatment of vulvar cancer is the emerging recognition that selective dissection of a solitary node or nodes, termed *sentinel-node biopsy*, can dramatically reduce surgical morbidity and yet accurately assess nodal involvement. The basic principle of this procedure

TABLE 31-5. Postoperative Complications of Inguinofemoral Lymphadenectomy

Complication	No. of Events	Percent of Groins
Lymphedema	13	14.0
Lymphocele	11	11.8
Groin infection	7	7.5
Groin necrosis	2	2.2
Groin separation	7	7.5

From Bell, 2000, with permission.

is that the first lymph node to receive lymphatic drainage from the tumor site, termed the *sentinel lymph node*, should be the first site of malignant lymphatic spread. Therefore, a sentinel lymph node devoid of disease implies absence of lymph node metastases in the entire draining basin. Currently, both lymphoscintigraphy and isosulfan blue dye techniques are recommended when performing sentinel-node biopsy of vulvar cancer (Levenback, 2008).

Intraoperative lymphatic mapping is accomplished by injecting radionuclide intradermally at the border of the primary tumor that is closest to the groin. For midline tumors, both sides of the tumor are injected. A handheld gamma counter aids attempts to identify the sentinel node subcutaneously, and the skin is marked. Next, isosulfan blue dye is injected at the same primary tumor location (Fig. 31-8), followed by groin skin incision approximately 5 minutes later. The tracer and dye are taken up by the specific node that drains the tumor site. The handheld gamma counter may assist in localizing the sentinel node, and/or it can be visually identified by its blue color and separated from the other nodes within the regional group.

Several studies have confirmed the accuracy of sentinel-node biopsy to predict vulvar cancer metastasis in the inguinal lymph nodes. The GROningen International Study on Sentinel nodes in Vulvar cancer (GROINSS-V) multicenter observational study on sentinel-node detection used radioactive tracer and blue dye in patients with squamous cell cancer of the vulva measuring <4 cm. In 259 patients with unifocal vulvar disease and a negative sentinel-node biopsy, six groin recurrences were diagnosed (2.3 percent), and the 3-year survival rate was 97 percent. In addition to evaluation of biopsy's predictive value, this study concluded that the risk of metastasis to additional inguinal lymph nodes increased with the size of the sentinel-node metastasis. The prognosis of patients with a sentinel-node metastasis measuring >2 mm was significantly worse than those with metastasis <2 mm (Oonk, 2010; Van der Zee, 2008).

The Gynecologic Oncology Group (GOG) has also conducted a multicenter trial to evaluate the benefit of sentinel-node biopsy for vulvar cancer (protocol #173). Preliminary data of 459 evaluable patients with lesions at least 2 cm in size and >1 mm invasive depth showed a sensitivity of >90 percent, negative predictive value of >95 percent, and a false negative rate of 4.3 percent. Moreover, the combination of lymphoscintigraphy and blue dye were superior to blue dye alone (Levenback, 2009a). Because of the promising data from the foregoing trials, sentinel-node biopsy for vulva cancer is a reasonable alternative to inguinofemoral lymphadenectomy when performed by a skilled multidisciplinary team in well-selected patients (Levenback, 2009b).

Stage III Vulvar Cancer

By definition, stage III vulvar cancers include node-positive tumors. Patients with resectable primary vulvar cancer that is metastatic to the inguinal lymph nodes benefit from postoperative pelvic and groin irradiation. Typically, radiation begins 3 to 4 weeks after surgery to allow for adequate wound healing. In a prospective randomized GOG trial of 114 patients, this strategy proved superior to extended pelvic node resection, especially in cases with clinically suspicious or fixed ulcerated inguinal nodes and two or more cancer-positive groin nodes (Homesley, 1986; Kunos, 2009).

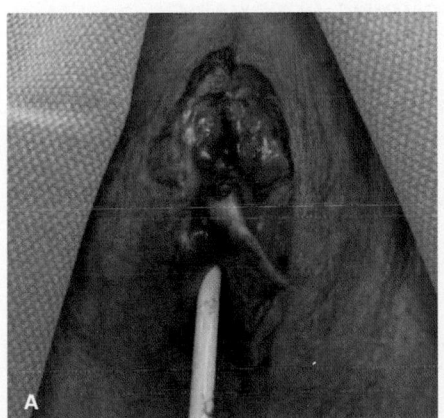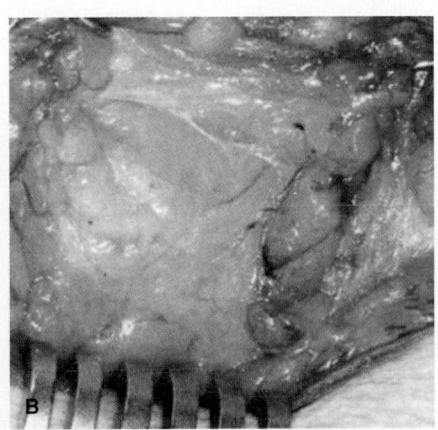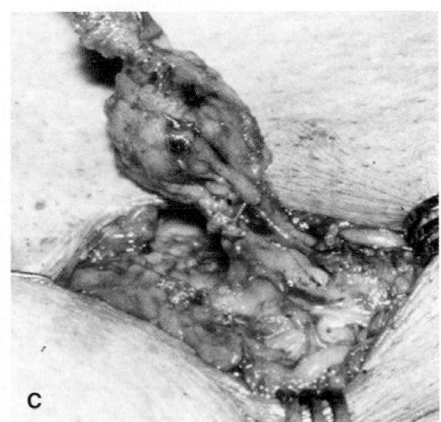

FIGURE 31-8 Sentinel lymph node evaluation. **A.** Blue dye and radiotracer are injected at the tumor periphery. (*Photograph contributed by Dr. John Schorge.*) **B.** Blue dye is taken up by the specific node that drains the tumor site. **C.** This sentinel node can be visually identified, separated from the other nodes within the regional group, and removed for evaluation.

The addition of platinum-based chemotherapy concurrent with radiation therapy has been heavily influenced by advances in the treatment of cervical cancer and squamous cell carcinoma of the anal canal. Moreover, extrapolation of apparent efficacy in phase II trials of more locally advanced vulvar cancer suggests a role in postoperative patients with lymph node metastases. However, the rarity of vulvar cancer precludes completion of a more definitive trial in this setting.

Stage IVA Vulvar Cancer

These locally advanced vulvar cancers involve the upper urethra, bladder or rectal mucosa, or pelvic bone and may or may not have associated positive inguinal lymph nodes or fixed ulcerated lymph nodes. Occasionally, patients with stage IVA vulvar cancers can be treated with radical primary surgery. Much more often, the size and location of the tumor would necessitate some form of exenterative surgical procedure to remove the entire lesion with adequate margins. Such unresectable, locally advanced vulvar cancers can be effectively treated with chemoradiation to drastically minimize the surgical resection required. Two phase II studies conducted by the GOG have demonstrated the feasibility of this approach.

In the first trial (protocol #101), 73 patients with clinically unresectable stage III-IV squamous vulvar cancer were treated with a split course of cisplatin/5-fluoruouracil and received a planned radiation dose of 4760 cGy (Moore, 1998). The second study (protocol #205) evaluated 58 comparable patients treated with weekly cisplatin and a total radiation dose of 5760 cGy (Moore, 2011). This latter trial yielded a higher response rate (64 versus 48 percent) compared with the initial study. However, it is unclear whether the chemotherapy regimen or increased radiation dose was most responsible for the observed benefit.

In our practice, we offer preoperative cisplatin-based chemoradiation if patients have: (1) extensive primary lesions that would require pelvic exenteration, or (2) inoperable primary tumors. In cases in which a patient does not have fixed groin nodes, pretreatment inguinofemoral lymphadenectomy may help determine the need for groin irradiation. If residual disease remains following chemoradiation, then local resection is indicated. For those patients with no gross disease and an apparent complete response to chemoradiation, the need for surgery is unclear.

Stage IVB Vulvar Cancer

Treatment of patients with distant metastases should be individualized. A multimodality approach is used to achieve palliation.

SURVEILLANCE

After completing primary treatment, all patients receive thorough physical examination, including inguinal lymph node palpation and pelvic examination every 3 months for the first 2 to 3 years. Surveillance examinations are then scheduled every 6 months to complete a total of 5 years. Thereafter,

disease-free patients may be seen annually. Vulvoscopy and biopsies are performed if areas of concern are noted during history or physical examination. Radiologic imaging and biopsies to diagnose possible tumor recurrence are performed as indicated.

RECURRENT DISEASE

In a patient who presents with a suspected recurrence, a careful evaluation should be completed to define the extent of disease.

Vulvar Recurrences

For the most common local vulvar recurrences, surgical reexcision is usually the best option. Radical partial vulvectomy is appropriate for smaller lesions. For large central recurrences involving the urethra, vagina, or rectum that lie in a previously radiated field, a total pelvic exenteration with myocutaneous flap may be required. To maintain sexual function, vaginal reconstruction can be completed as described in Section 44-10 (p. 1292) at the time of surgery or after a short postoperative interval.

For patients who are not surgical candidates, external beam radiation combined with interstitial brachytherapy can be used. However, with previous radiation therapy, this is not always a possibility, and supportive care may be most appropriate.

Distant Recurrences

Inguinal lymph node recurrences carry a dismal prognosis and are virtually always associated with fatal disease. Few of these patients are alive at the end of the first year following this diagnosis.

Palliative chemotherapy can be offered to patients with pelvic or distant metastases. However, there are few data to indicate that chemotherapy provides an effective palliative intervention. Only doxorubicin and bleomycin appear to have reproducible activity as single agents. Combination platinum-based chemotherapy has also been shown to have very modest activity in recurrent vulvar cancers (Cunningham, 1997; Moore, 1998).

MANAGEMENT DURING PREGNANCY

Squamous cell cancer of the vulva diagnosed and surgically treated during pregnancy is rare, and an incidence of 1 per 20,000 deliveries has been reported (DiSaia, 1997). Nevertheless, all suspicious lesions should be examined and biopsied, even during pregnancy, to prevent a delayed diagnosis.

Radical complete or partial vulvectomy and inguinofemoral lymphadenectomy can be performed when indicated after the first trimester. During the third trimester, markedly increased genital vasculature may increase surgical morbidity. In general, when diagnosis is made during the late third trimester, lesions may be removed by wide local excision, and definitive surgery postponed until after delivery. In cases in which diagnosis is not made until delivery, definitive surgery should be started as soon as deemed appropriate by the treating physician, which in most reported cases has been 2 to 3 weeks.

The mode of delivery following surgery is left to the discretion of the obstetrician and heavily influenced by the state of the postsurgical vulva. In instances of vaginal stenosis, significant fibrosis, or tumor involvement, a cesarean delivery is recommended.

MELANOMA

Melanoma of the vulva is the second most common malignancy arising within the vulva and accounts for 8 to 10 percent of all vulvar malignancies. Vulvar melanoma is a disease of the elderly, and its incidence peaks in the fifth to eighth decades of life (Piura, 1992; Podratz, 1983). It develops more commonly among whites than among Asians, African-Americans, or other more heavily pigmented races (Evans, 1994; Franklin, 1991; Piura, 1992).

Malignant vulvar melanoma will most commonly arise from the labia minora, labia majora, or clitoris (Figs. 31-9 and 31-10) (Moore, 1998; Piura, 1992; Woolcott, 1988). Similarly, various benign pigmented lesions including lentigo simplex, vulvar melanosis, acanthosis nigricans, seborrheic keratosis, and junctional, compound, intradermal, or dysplastic nevi may also be found in these areas (Chap. 4, p. 120). In addition, pigmented vulvar neoplasia may include VIN, squamous cell carcinoma, and Paget disease. Thus, tissue sampling is mandatory, and immunohistochemical studies or electron microscopy may help to clarify the diagnosis. Three histologic subtypes of vulvar melanoma have been described: superficial spreading melanoma (SS), nodular melanoma (NM), and acral lentiginous melanoma (AL).

Vulvar melanomas have been staged by several microstaging systems including the Chung, the Clark, and the Breslow systems (Table 31-6). The Clark system of staging cutaneous melanomas is based on depth of invasion. Agreeing that depth of invasion was important, Breslow published an alternative list

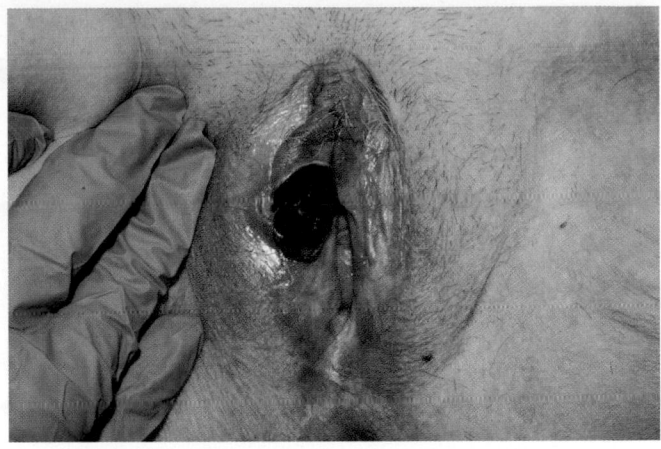

FIGURE 31-9 Photograph of vulvar melanoma. *(Photograph contributed by Dr. Debra Richardson.)*

of prognostic indicators, but added tumor size and used tumor thickness as the most significant measure of size. All three systems have been found to correlate with prognosis in patients with cutaneous melanoma.

There are no prospective data from randomized clinical trials evaluating the extent of negative margins in patients with vulvar melanoma, and surgical techniques do not seem to alter the prognosis (Verschraegen, 2001). We recommend patients undergo a radical partial vulvectomy with a 1- to 2-cm margin (Irvin, 2001).

The presence and number of nodal metastases is a major predictor of prognosis. The incidence of occult inguinal lymph node metastases is less than 5 percent for thin melanomas measuring <1 mm and greater than 70 percent for lesions >4 mm (Hoskins, 2000). The decision to perform inguinofemoral lymphadenectomy or sentinel-node biopsy should balance the potential morbidity of the procedure against the limited range

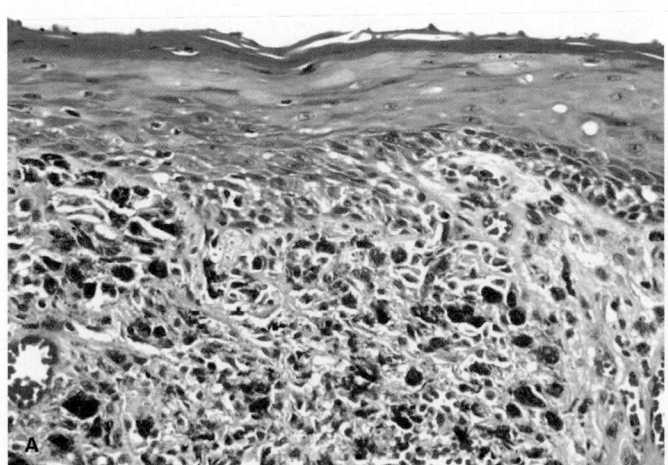
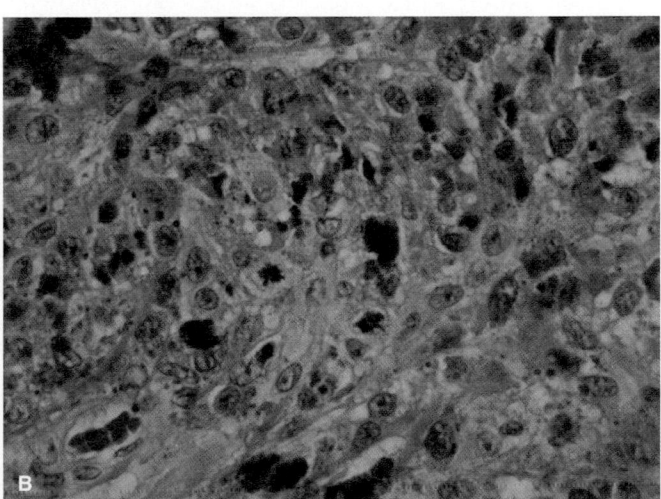

FIGURE 31-10 Photomicrographs of vulvar melanoma. **A.** Medium-power view. Atypical, hyperchromatic melanoma cells are identified within the basal portion of the surface epithelium. Melanoma cells containing intracytoplasmic melanin pigment invade subepithelial stroma in a broad swathe. **B.** High-power view. The malignant melanoma cells in this case have occasionally prominent nucleoli, abundant intracytoplasmic melanin pigment, and frequent mitoses including abnormal mitoses. *(Photographs contributed by Dr. Kelley Carrick.)*

TABLE 31-6. Microstaging of Vulvar Melanomas

	Clark Levels	Chung et al	Breslow
I	Intraepithelial	Intraepithelial	<0.76 mm
II	Into papillary dermis	≤1 mm from granular layer	0.76–1.50 mm
III	Filling dermal papillae	1.1–2 mm from granular layer	1.51–2.25 mm
IV	Into reticular dermis	>2 mm from granular layer	2.26–3.0 mm
V	Into subcutaneous fat	Into subcutaneous fat	>3 mm

From Hacker, 2005, with permission.

of adjuvant therapy for metastatic disease. Our current practice is to perform the appropriate inguinofemoral lymphadenectomy, based on lesion thickness, along with a radical partial vulvectomy.

In certain patients with cutaneous melanoma involving other body surfaces, trials have suggested that adjuvant therapy may be of benefit in preventing recurrence. Specifically, high-dose adjuvant alpha interferon has been shown to increase both progression-free and overall survival rates in patients with cutaneous melanoma (Lens, 2002). However, given the small number of patients with vulvar melanoma, no trials have yet evaluated the benefit of this adjuvant therapy in these women. Moreover, tolerability of the interferon regimen has remained a barrier to patient acceptance.

In general, vulvar melanomas carry a poor prognosis and show a tendency to recur locally and develop distant metastases through hematogenous dissemination. Deaths from vulvar melanoma more commonly result from the effects of widespread metastatic disease, most commonly involving the lungs, liver, or brain. In a Surveillance Epidemiology and End Results (SEER) database study of 644 patients, the 5-year disease-specific survival rates for those with localized, regional, and distant disease were 75, 39, and 22 percent, respectively (Sugiyama, 2007).

BASAL CELL CARCINOMA

Basal cell carcinoma (BCC) of the vulva accounts for less than 2 percent of all vulvar cancers and is most commonly found in elderly women (DiSaia, 1997). The lesions typically arise on the labia majora. On the vulva, BCC is characterized by poor pigmentation, pruritus, and a clinical appearance often mimicking other dermatopathologies such as eczema, psoriasis, or intertrigo. As a result, correct diagnosis is often delayed and typically follows treatment for other presumed inflammatory or infectious dermatoses.

Although ultraviolet radiation is thought to be the primary risk factor for BCC on sun-exposed areas, its development on areas protected from sunlight raises the possibility of other, yet undefined, etiologic agents. The literature suggests that local trauma and advancing age may contribute to the development of BCC in these sites (LeSueur, 2003; Wermuth, 1970).

Basal cell carcinoma should be removed by wide local excision using a minimum surgical margin of 1 cm. Deep margins of 1 cm should also be obtained. Lymphatic or distant spread is rare. However, local recurrences may occur, particularly in tumors removed with suboptimal resection margins.

VULVAR SARCOMA

Sarcoma of the vulva is rare, and leiomyosarcoma, malignant fibrous histiocytoma, epithelioid sarcoma, and malignant rhabdoid tumor are some of the more frequently encountered histologic types. Tumors typically develop as isolated masses in labia majora, clitoris, or Bartholin gland (Fig. 31-11). Unlike squamous cell carcinoma of the vulva, the age of affected women is significantly broader and varies between histologic types. There are no large series reporting the management of vulvar sarcoma. Recommended treatment for most types is primary surgery followed by adjuvant radiation or chemotherapy or both.

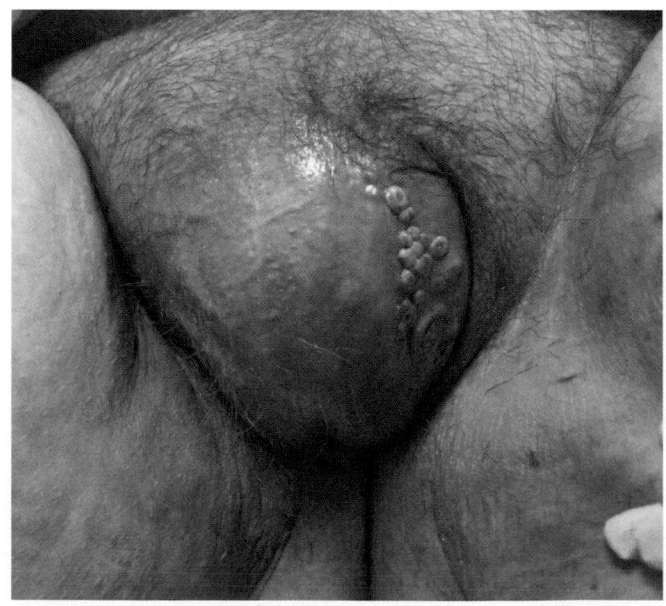

FIGURE 31-11 Vulvar epithelioid sarcoma.

BARTHOLIN GLAND CARCINOMA

Primary malignant tumors arising from the Bartholin gland can be adenocarcinomas, squamous cell carcinomas, or transitional cell carcinomas. The incidence of Bartholin gland carcinomas peaks in women in their mid-60s. Soft, distensible tissue normally surrounds these glands, and tumors may reach considerable size before patients develop symptoms. Dyspareunia is a common first complaint. Bartholin gland enlargement in a woman older than 40 years and recurrent cysts or abscesses warrant a biopsy or excision (Section 41-20, p. 1066). Similarly, all solid masses require fine-needle aspiration or biopsy to establish definitive diagnosis.

Bartholin gland carcinomas tend to spread into the ischiorectal fossa and have a propensity for lymphatic spread into the inguinal and pelvic lymph nodes. Therapy includes a radical partial vulvectomy with inguinofemoral lymphadenectomy. Decisions to perform ipsilateral or bilateral groin dissection follow the same criteria as for squamous cell tumors. Postoperative chemoradiation has been shown to reduce the likelihood of local recurrence for all stages. If the initial lesion impinges on the rectum or anal sphincter, preoperative chemoradiation can be used to avoid extensive surgery.

VULVAR PAGET DISEASE

Extramammary Paget disease is a heterogeneous group of intraepithelial neoplasias and when present on the vulva, appears as an eczematoid, red, weeping area (Fig. 31-12). These are often localized to the labia majora, perineal body, or clitoral area. This disease typically develops in older white women and accounts for approximately 2 percent of all vulvar tumors. Vulvar Paget disease is accompanied by invasive adenocarcinoma in 10 to 20 percent of cases (Hoskins, 2000). In addition, 20 to 30 percent of patients will have or will later develop an adenocarcinoma at another nonvulvar location.

A histologic classification proposed by Williamson and Brown includes: (1) primary vulvar cutaneous Paget disease, (2) Paget disease as an extension of transitional cell carcinoma of the bladder or urethra, and (3) Paget disease as an extension of an associated adjacent primary cancer such as vulvar, anal, or rectal cancers. The histologic differentiation of these Paget disease types is important because the specific diagnosis significantly influences treatment selection.

Primary cutaneous vulvar Paget disease displays slow growth. Diseased areas should be resected with a wide local excision. Positive margins occur frequently, and disease recurrence is common regardless of the surgical margin status (Black, 2007). If invasive disease is suspected, radical partial vulvectomy is warranted by extending the deep margins to the perineal membrane. Recurrent Paget disease is common, and long-term surveillance is prudent since repeat surgical excision is often necessary. Moreover, screening and surveillance for tumors at nongynecologic sites should be considered, including evaluation of the breasts and the gastrointestinal and genitourinary tracts. A detailed discussion of Paget disease of the breast is presented in Chapter 12 (p. 345).

CANCER METASTATIC TO THE VULVA

Metastatic tumors comprise approximately 8 percent of all vulvar cancers. Tumors may extend from primary cancers of the bladder, urethra, vagina, or rectum. Less proximate cancers include those from the breast, kidney, lung, stomach, and gestational choriocarcinoma (Fig. 31-13) (Wilkinson, 2011).

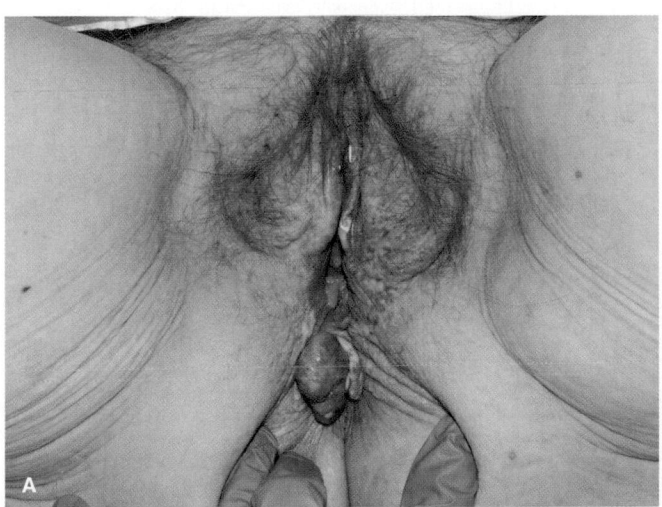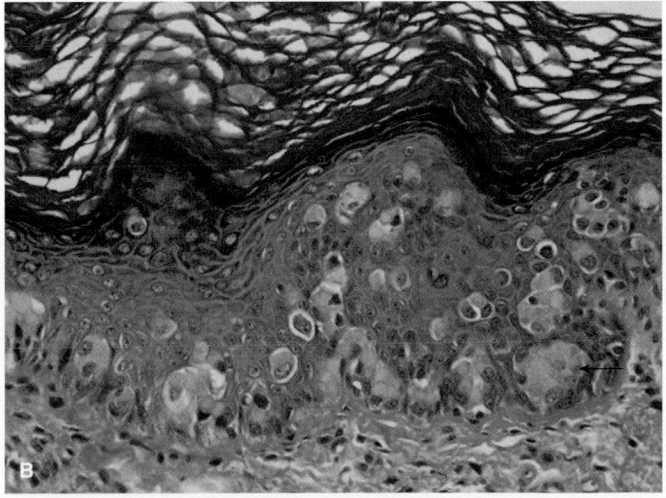

FIGURE 31-12 Vulvar Paget disease. **A.** Vulvar Paget disease involving the labia bilaterally, perineum, perianus, and solid right perianal mass. *(Photograph contributed by Dr. Claudia Werner.)* **B.** Photomicrograph of primary cutaneous vulvar Paget disease. This is characterized microscopically by the presence of relatively large atypical cells with prominent nucleoli and abundant delicate cytoplasm *(arrow)*. These cells are disposed singly or in clusters at various levels within the epithelium. The neoplastic cells are most often confined to the epithelium and would in these instances be classified as an adenocarcinoma in situ. *(Photograph contributed by Dr. Kelley Carrick.)*

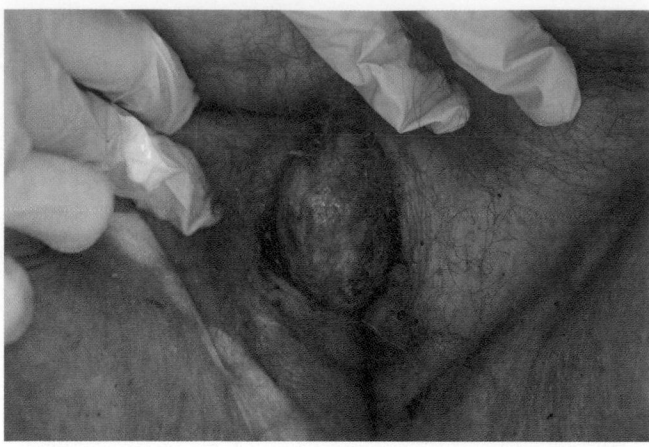

FIGURE 31-13 Solid vulvar tumor. Biopsy revealed endometrial cancer metastatic to the clitoris. *(Photograph contributed by Dr. William Griffith.)*

REFERENCES

Bell JG, Lea JS, Reid GC: Complete groin lymphadenectomy with preservation of the fascia lata in the treatment of vulvar carcinoma. Gynecol Oncol 77:314, 2000

Binder SW, Huang I, Fu YS, et al: Risk factors for the development of lymph node metastasis in vulvar squamous cell carcinoma. Gynecol Oncol 37:9, 1990

Black D, Tornos C, Soslow RA, et al: The outcomes of patients with positive margins after excision for intraepithelial Paget's disease of the vulva. Gynecol Oncol 104:547, 2007

Bodelon C, Madeleine MM, Voigt LF, et al: Is the incidence of invasive vulvar cancer increasing in the United States? Cancer Causes Control 20:1779, 2009

Brinton LA, Nasca PC, Mallin K, et al: Case-control study of cancer of the vulva. Obstet Gynecol 75:859, 1990

Burke TW, Levenback C, Coleman RL, et al: Surgical therapy of T1 and T2 vulvar carcinoma: further experience with radical wide excision and selective inguinal lymphadenectomy. Gynecol Oncol 57:215, 1995

Canavan TP, Cohen D: Vulvar cancer. Am Fam Physician 66(7):1269, 2002

Chan JK, Sugiyama V, Pham H, et al: Margin distance and other clinico-pathologic prognostic factors in vulvar carcinoma: a multivariate analysis. Gynecol Oncol 104:636, 2007

Creasman WT: New gynecologic cancer staging. Gynecol Oncol 58:157, 1995

Cunningham MJ, Goyer RP, Gibbons SK, et al: Primary radiation, cisplatin, and 5-fluorouracil for advanced squamous carcinoma of the vulva. Gynecol Oncol 66:258, 1997

Dardarian TS, Gray JT, Morgan MA, et al: Saphenous vein sparing during inguinal lymphadenectomy to reduce morbidity in patients with vulvar carcinoma. Gynecol Oncol 101(1):140, 2006

DiSaia PJ, Creasman WT (eds): Invasive cancer of the vulva. In Clinical Gynecologic Oncology, 5th ed. St. Louis, MO, Mosby–Year Book, 1997, pp 202, 229

Donaldson ES, Powell DE, Hanson MB, et al: Prognostic parameters in invasive vulvar cancer. Gynecol Oncol 11:184, 1981

Elit L, Voruganti S, Simunovic M: Invasive vulvar cancer in a woman with human immunodeficiency virus: case report and review of the literature. Gynecol Oncol 98:151, 2005

Evans RA: Review and current perspectives of cutaneous malignant melanoma. J Am Coll Surg 179:764, 1994

Farias-Eisner R, Cirisano FD, Grouse D, et al: Conservative and individualized surgery for early squamous carcinoma of the vulva: the treatment of choice for stage I and II (T$_{1-2}$N$_{0-1}$M$_0$) disease. Gynecol Oncol 53:55, 1994

Figge DC, Tamimi HK, Greer BE: Lymphatic spread in carcinoma of the vulva. Am J Obstet Gynecol 152:387, 1985

Franklin EW III, Weiser EB: Surgery for vulvar cancer. Surg Clin North Am 71:911, 1991

Frisch M, Biggar RJ, Goedert JJ: Human papillomavirus-associated cancers in patients with human immunodeficiency virus infection and acquired immunodeficiency syndrome. J Natl Cancer Inst 92:1500, 2000

Gonzalez Bosquet J, Magrina JF, Magtibay PM, et al: Patterns of inguinal groin metastases in squamous cell carcinoma of the vulva. Gynecol Oncol 105:742, 2007

Gordinier ME, Malpica A, Burke TW, et al: Groin recurrence in patients with vulvar cancer with negative nodes on superficial inguinal lymphadenectomy. Gynecol Oncol 90:625, 2003

Hacker NF: Vulvar cancer. In Berek JS, Hacker NF (eds): Practical Gynecologic Oncology. Philadelphia, Lippincott Williams & Wilkins, 2005, p 471

Hacker NF, Berek JS, Lagasse LD, et al: Individualization of treatment for stage I squamous cell vulvar carcinoma. Obstet Gynecol 63:155, 1984

Hacker NF, Berek JS, Lagasse LD, et al: Management of regional lymph nodes and their prognostic influence in vulvar cancer. Obstet Gynecol 61:408, 1983

Heaps JM, Fu YS, Montz FJ, et al: Surgical-pathologic variables predictive of local recurrence in squamous cell carcinoma of the vulva. Gynecol Oncol 38(3):309, 1990

Hildesheim A, Han CL, Brinton LA, et al: Human papillomavirus type 16 and risk of preinvasive and invasive vulvar cancer: results from a seroepidemiological case-control study. Obstet Gynecol 90:748, 1997

Homesley HD, Bundy BN, Sedlis A, et al: Assessment of current International Federation of Gynecology and Obstetrics staging of vulvar carcinoma relative to prognostic factors for survival (a Gynecologic Oncology Group study). Am J Obstet Gynecol 164(4):997, 1991

Homesley HD, Bundy BN, Sedlis A, et al: Prognostic factors for groin node metastasis in squamous cell carcinoma of the vulva. A Gynecologic Oncology Group study. Gynecol Oncol 49:279, 1993

Homesley HD, Bundy BN, Sedlis A, et al: Radiation therapy versus pelvic node resection for carcinoma of the vulva with positive groin nodes. Obstet Gynecol 68:733, 1986

Hoskins WJ, Perez CA, Young RC (eds): Vulva. In Principles and Practice of Gynecologic Oncology, 3rd ed. Philadelphia, Lippincott Williams & Wilkins, 2000, p 665

Irvin WP Jr, Legallo RL, Stoler MH, et al: Vulvar melanoma: a retrospective analysis and literature review. Gynecol Oncol 83:457, 2001

Jones RW, Rowan DM, Stewart AW: Vulvar intraepithelial neoplasia: aspects of the natural history and outcome in 405 women. Obstet Gynecol 106:1319, 2005

Judson PL, Jonson AL, Paley PJ, et al: A prospective, randomized study analyzing Sartorius transposition following inguinal-femoral lymphadenectomy. Gynecol Oncol 95:226, 2004

Kalnicki S, Zide A, Maleki N, et al: Transmission block to simplify combined pelvic and inguinal radiation therapy. Radiology 164:578, 1987

Kirschner CV, Yordan EL, De Geest K, et al: Smoking, obesity, and survival in squamous cell carcinoma of the vulva. Gynecol Oncol 56:79, 1995

Kunos C, Simpkins F, Gibbons H, et al: Radiation therapy compared with pelvic node resection for node-positive vulvar cancer: a randomized controlled trial. Obstet Gynecol 114:537, 2009

Lens MB, Dawes M: Interferon alfa therapy for malignant melanoma: a systematic review of randomized controlled trials. J Clin Oncol 20(7):1818, 2002

LeSueur BW, DiCaudo DJ, Connolly SM: Axillary basal cell carcinoma. Dermatol Surg 29:1105, 2003

Levenback C: Update on sentinel lymph node biopsy in gynecologic cancers. Gynecol Oncol 111(2 Suppl):S42, 2008

Levenback C, Morris M, Burke TW, et al: Groin dissection practices among gynecologic oncologists treating early vulvar cancer. Gynecol Oncol 62(1):73, 1996

Levenback CF, Tian C, Coleman RL, et al: Sentinel node (SN) biopsy in patients with vulvar cancer: a Gynecologic Oncology Group (GOG) study. Abstract No. 5505. Presented at the Annual Meeting of the American Society of Clinical Oncology. June 2009a

Levenback CF, van der Zee AGJ, Lukas R, et al: Sentinel lymph node biopsy in patients with gynecologic cancers. Expert panel statement from the International Sentinel Node Society Meeting, February 21, 2008. Gynecol Oncol 114:151, 2009b

Madeleine MM, Daling JR, Carter JJ, et al: Cofactors with human papillomavirus in a population-based study of vulvar cancer. J Natl Cancer Inst 89:1516, 1997

Moore D, Ali S, Barnes M, et al: A phase II trial of radiation therapy and weekly cisplatin chemotherapy for the treatment of locally advanced squamous cell carcinoma of the vulva: a Gynecologic Oncology Group study. Abstract No. 1. Presented at the 42nd Annual Meeting of the Society of Gynecologic Oncologists. March 6, 2011

Moore DH, Thomas GM, Montana GS, et al: Preoperative chemoradiation for advanced vulvar cancer: a phase II study of the Gynecologic Oncology Group. Int J Radiat Oncol Biol Phys 42:79, 1998

Morley GW: Infiltrative carcinoma of the vulva: results of surgical treatment. Am J Obstet Gynecol 124:874, 1976

Oonk MH, van Hemel BM, Hollema H, et al: Size of sentinel-node metastasis and chances of non-sentinel-node involvement and survival in early stage vulvar cancer: results from GROINSS-V, a multicentre observational study. Lancet Oncol 11:646, 2010

Origoni M, Sideri M, Garsia S, et al: Prognostic value of pathological patterns of lymph node positivity in squamous cell carcinoma of the vulva stage III and IVA FIGO. Gynecol Oncol 45:313, 1992

Pecorelli S: Revised FIGO staging for carcinoma of the vulva, cervix, and endometrium. Int J Gynaecol Obstet 105(2):103, 2009

Piura B, Egan M, Lopes A, et al: Malignant melanoma of the vulva: a clinicopathologic study of 18 cases. J Surg Oncol 50:234, 1992

Podratz KC, Gaffey TA, Symmonds RE, et al: Melanoma of the vulva: an update. Gynecol Oncol 16:153, 1983

Preti M, Rouzier R, Mariani L, et al: Superficially invasive carcinoma of the vulva: diagnosis and treatment. Clin Obstet Gynecol 48:862, 2005

Rolfe KJ, Crow JC, Benjamin E, et al: Cyclin D1 and retinoblastoma protein in vulvar cancer and adjacent lesions. Int J Gynecol Cancer 11:381, 2001

Rouzier R, Haddad B, Dubernard G, et al: Inguinofemoral dissection for carcinoma of the vulva: effect of modifications of extent and technique on morbidity and survival. J Am Coll Surg 196:442, 2003

Scully RE, Bonfiglio TA, Kurman RJ, et al: Histological typing of female genital tract tumors. In World Health Organization International Histological Classification of Tumors. New York, Springer, 1994

Siegel R, Ward E, Brawley O, et al: Cancer statistics, 2011: the impact of eliminating socioeconomic and racial disparities on premature cancer deaths. CA Cancer J Clin 61(4):212, 2011

Stehman FB, Look KY: Carcinoma of the vulva. Obstet Gynecol 107(3):719, 2006

Stroup AM, Harlan LC, Trimble EL: Demographic, clinical, and treatment trends among women diagnosed with vulvar cancer in the United States. Gynecol Oncol 108(3):577, 2008

Sugiyama VE, Chan JK, Shin JY, et al: Vulvar melanoma: a multivariable analysis of 644 patients. Obstet Gynecol 110:296, 2007

Tantipalakorn C, Robertson G, Marsden DE, et al: Outcome and patterns of recurrence for International Federation of Gynecology and Obstetrics (FIGO) stages I and II squamous cell vulvar cancer. Obstet Gynecol 113(4):895, 2009

Van der Steen S, de Nieuwenhof HP, Massuger L, et al: New FIGO staging system of vulvar cancer indeed provides a better reflection of prognosis. Gynecol Oncol 119(3):520, 2010

Van der Zee AG, Oonk MH, De Hullu JA, et al: Sentinel node dissection is safe in the treatment of early-stage vulvar cancer. J Clin Oncol 26:884, 2008

van Seters M, van Beurden M, de Craen AJ: Is the assumed natural history of vulvar intraepithelial neoplasia III based on enough evidence? A systematic review of 3322 published patients. Gynecol Oncol 97:645, 2005

Verschraegen CF, Benjapibal M, Supakarapongkul W, et al: Vulvar melanoma at the M. D. Anderson Cancer Center: 25 years later. Int J Gynecol Cancer 11:359, 2001

Way S: The anatomy of the lymphatic drainage of the vulva and its influence on the radical operation for carcinoma. Ann R Coll Surg Engl 3(4):187, 1948

Wermuth BM, Fajardo LF: Metastatic basal cell carcinoma: a review. Arch Pathol 90:458, 1970

Wilkinson EJ: Premalignant and malignant tumors of the vulva. In Kurman RJ, Ellenson LH, Ronnett BM (eds): Blaustein's Pathology of the Female Genital Tract. New York, Springer, 2011, p 95

Woolcott RJ, Henry RJ, Houghton CR: Malignant melanoma of the vulva: Australian experience. J Reprod Med 33:699, 1988

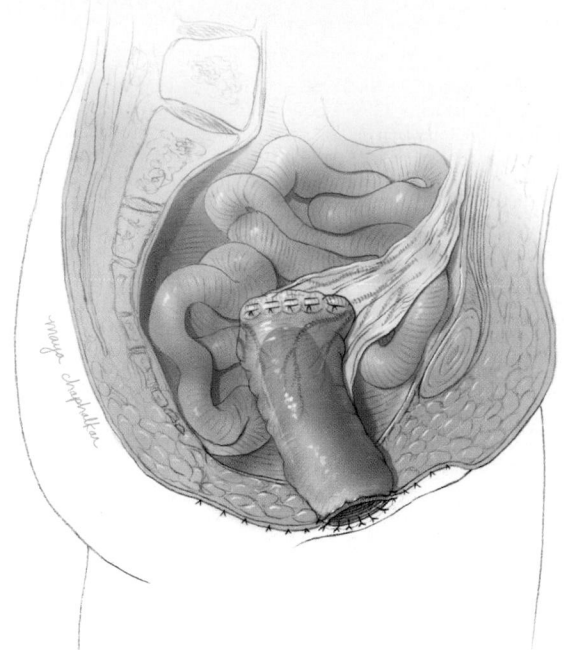

CHAPTER 32

Vaginal Cancer

Primary vaginal carcinoma is rare and comprises only 1 to 2 percent of all gynecologic malignancies (National Cancer Institute, 2011). This low incidence reflects the infrequency with which primary carcinoma arises in the vagina as well as the strict criteria for its diagnosis. According to International Federation of Gynecology and Obstetrics (FIGO) staging criteria, a lesion in the vagina that involves adjacent organs such as the cervix or vulva is, by convention, deemed primary cervical or vulvar, respectively (Pecorelli, 1999). Cancer found in the vagina is more likely to be metastatic disease than primary disease. Of

these, cancers from the cervix, endometrium, and colon/rectum are the most frequent. The most common histologic type of primary vaginal cancer is squamous cell carcinoma, followed by adenocarcinoma (Platz, 1995).

ANATOMY

Vaginal Epithelium

Embryologically, both the müllerian ducts and the urogenital sinus contribute to form the vagina (Fig. 18-5, p. 486). Early in fetal development, the caudal ends of the müllerian ducts fuse to form the uterovaginal canal, which is lined by columnar epithelium. Subsequently, squamous cells from the urogenital sinus migrate along the uterovaginal canal and replace this original columnar epithelium. These squamous cells stratify, and the vagina begins to mature and thicken. Underlying this epithelium, muscularis and adventitial layers are found.

Vascular and Lymphatic Supply

Local extension and lymphatic invasion are common patterns of vaginal cancer spread. The lymphatic channels that drain the vagina form extensive, complex, and variable anastomoses. As a result, any node in the pelvis, groin, or anorectal area may drain any part of the vagina. Of these, the external, internal, and common iliac lymph nodes are the primary sites of vaginal lymphatic drainage. Alternatively, the posterior vagina may drain to the inferior gluteal, presacral, or perirectal lymph nodes, and the distal third of the vagina may drain to the superficial and deep inguinal lymph nodes (Frank, 2005).

Hematogenous spread of vaginal cancer is less frequent, and venous drainage consists of the uterine, pudendal, and rectal veins, which drain into the internal iliac vein. Arterial blood supply to the vagina comes primarily from branches of the internal iliac artery, which include the uterine, vaginal, middle rectal, and internal pudendal arteries (Fig. 38-12, p. 927).

INCIDENCE

In 2011, it is estimated that 2570 new cases of vaginal cancer will be diagnosed in the United States, and there will be 780 deaths (Siegel, 2011). The overall incidence is 0.45 cases per 100,000 women, but notably lower in whites (0.42) compared with black and Hispanic women (0.73 and 0.56, respectively) (Watson, 2009).

Rates of vaginal cancer increase with age and peak among women ≥80 years. The median age at diagnosis is 58 (Watson, 2009). Of the histologic forms of vaginal cancer, squamous cell carcinoma accounts for 70 to 80 percent of all primary cases (Beller, 2003; Platz, 1995).

SQUAMOUS CELL CARCINOMA

Risks

Squamous cell cancer of the vagina arises within its stratified nonkeratinized epithelium (Fig. 32-1). As with other cancers of the lower reproductive tract, the human papillomavirus (HPV) has been closely linked with squamous cell vaginal cancer. For example, Daling and colleagues (2002) analyzed results from a case-control study of 156 women with squamous cell carcinoma in situ or invasive vaginal carcinoma. Human papillomavirus DNA was detected in 82 percent of the in situ lesions and 64 percent of the invasive tumors. Specifically, antibodies to HPV serotypes 16 and 18 were identified in more than 50 percent of all patients. Because of this association with HPV infection, vaginal in situ and invasive squamous cell carcinoma share risk factors similar to cervical cancer. Some of these include five or more lifetime sexual partners, early age at first intercourse, and current cigarette smoking. Women with a history of vulvar or cervical cancer are also at increased risk. This last association may stem from the field effect of HPV affecting multiple lower genital tract epithelia or may result from direct tumor spread.

Vaginal intraepithelial neoplasia (VAIN) is a precursor to invasive vaginal cancer, and approximately 2 percent of patients with VAIN will progress to invasive cancer (Dodge, 2001). The quadrivalent HPV vaccine is effective in preventing VAIN 2 and 3 associated with HPV 16 or 18 (Joura, 2007). It is possible that use of HPV vaccines will decrease invasive vaginal cancer rates in the future.

Diagnosis

Vaginal bleeding is the most common complaint associated with vaginal cancer, although pelvic pain and vaginal discharge also may be noted. Less frequently, lesions involving the anterior vaginal wall may lead to dysuria, hematuria, retention, or urgency. Alternatively, constipation may result from

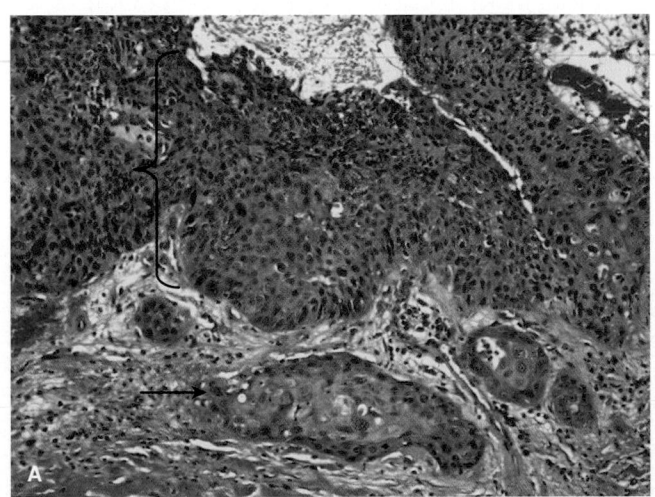

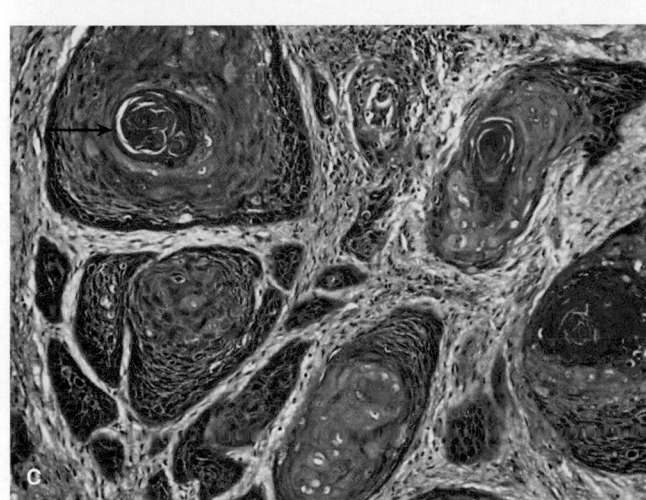

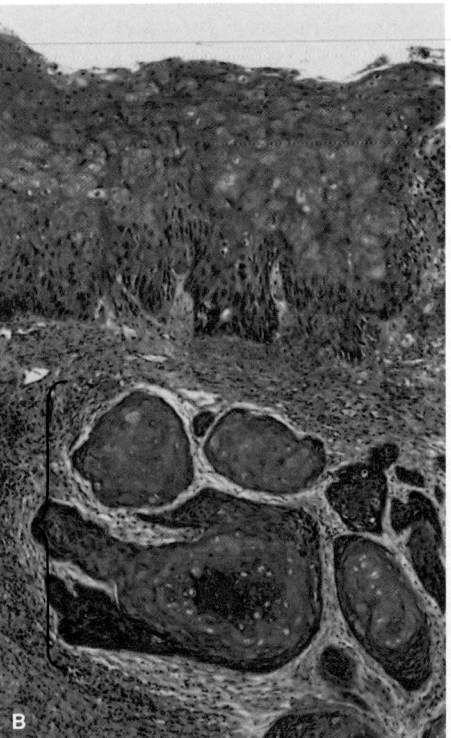

FIGURE 32-1 Sections showing invasive squamous cell carcinoma of the vagina. **A.** Superficially invasive squamous cell carcinoma of the vagina (*arrow*) with overlying squamous cell carcinoma in situ (*bracket*) (×10). **B.** Invasive, well-differentiated squamous cell carcinoma of the vagina (*bracket*) (×4). **C.** Invasive, well-differentiated squamous cell carcinoma of the vagina (×10). Invasive tumor is composed of irregular nests of malignant squamous cells with keratin pearls (*arrow*) and intercellular bridges. (*Photographs contributed by Dr. Kelley Carrick.*)

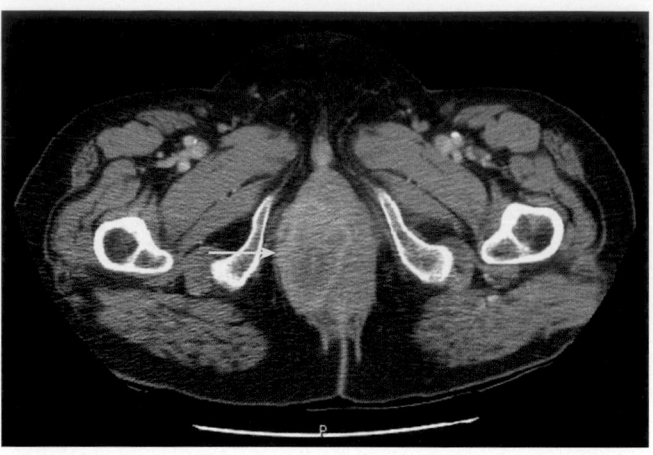

FIGURE 32-2 Computed tomography (CT) scan reveals size and extent of vaginal mass (*arrow*).

TABLE 32-1. Vaginal Cancer Evaluation

Vaginal biopsy
Physical examination
Endocervical curettage[b]
Endometrial biopsy[b]
Cystourethroscopy
Proctosigmoidoscopy
Chest radiograph
Abdominal/pelvic CT scan or MR imaging[a]

[a]Useful for treatment planning but not used to assign FIGO stage.
[b]Performed to excude primary endometrial or cervical cancer that is metastatic to the vagina.
CT = computed tomography; MR = magnetic resonance.

those of the posterior wall. Most vaginal cancers develop in the upper third of the vagina. Moreover, of those with cancers, women who have had a prior hysterectomy are significantly more likely to have lesions in the upper vagina (70 percent) than those without prior hysterectomy (36 percent) (Chyle, 1996).

During pelvic evaluation in all women, the vagina should be inspected as the speculum is being inserted or removed. If a gross lesion is found, vaginal cancer usually can be diagnosed by punch biopsy in the office. Biopsy may be obtained with a Tischler biopsy forceps (Fig. 29-15, p. 750). An Emmett hook, one type of skin hook, may be useful to elevate and stabilize vaginal tissue during biopsy. If a gross lesion is not detectable, vaginoscopy may aid directed biopsy, as described in Chapter 29 (p. 755). Bimanual examination can assist in determining the tumor size, and rectovaginal examination is especially important for posterior wall lesions.

Once cancer is diagnosed, no specific laboratory testing other than that used generally for preoperative preparation such as complete blood count and serum chemistry panel is required. Computed tomographic (CT) scanning can delineate the size and extent of many tumors (Fig. 32-2). However, if the extent of cancer expansion is unclear, magnetic resonance (MR) imaging is the most useful radiologic tool available to

visualize the vagina. Fluorodeoxyglucose-positron emission tomography (FDG-PET) can also be selected to evaluate lymph node involvement and distant metastases. In one study, FDG-PET was more sensitive than CT for detection of abnormal lymph nodes (Lamoreaux, 2005).

As in cervical cancer, an examination under anesthesia may be helpful to clinically stage the patient and further guide treatment. Proctosigmoidoscopy to a depth of at least 15 cm can detect local bowel invasion, whereas cystourethroscopy should be performed in the presence of anterior tumors to exclude bladder or urethral involvement.

Staging and Classification

Staging of vaginal cancer is similar to that for cervical cancer and is completed clinically by physical examination and with the assistance of cystourethroscopy, proctosigmoidoscopy, and chest radiography (Table 32-1, Table 32-2, and Fig. 32-3). CT scanning, MR imaging, and FDG-PET may also be useful in treatment planning but are not used to determine disease stage.

Prognosis

The prognosis of squamous cell carcinoma of the vagina has improved since the 1950s. At that time, Palmer published a

TABLE 32-2. FIGO Staging of Carcinoma of the Vulva

Stage	Characteristics
I	The carcinoma is limited to the vaginal wall
II	The carcinoma has involved the subvaginal tissue but has not extended to the pelvic wall
III	The carcinoma has extended to the pelvic wall
IV	The carcinoma has extended beyond the true pelvis or has involved the mucosa of the bladder or rectum; bullous edema as such does not permit a case to be allotted to stage IV
IVA	Tumor invades bladder and/or rectal mucosa and/or direct extension beyond the true pelvis
IVB	Spread to distant organs

FIGO = International Federation of Gynecology and Obstetrics.

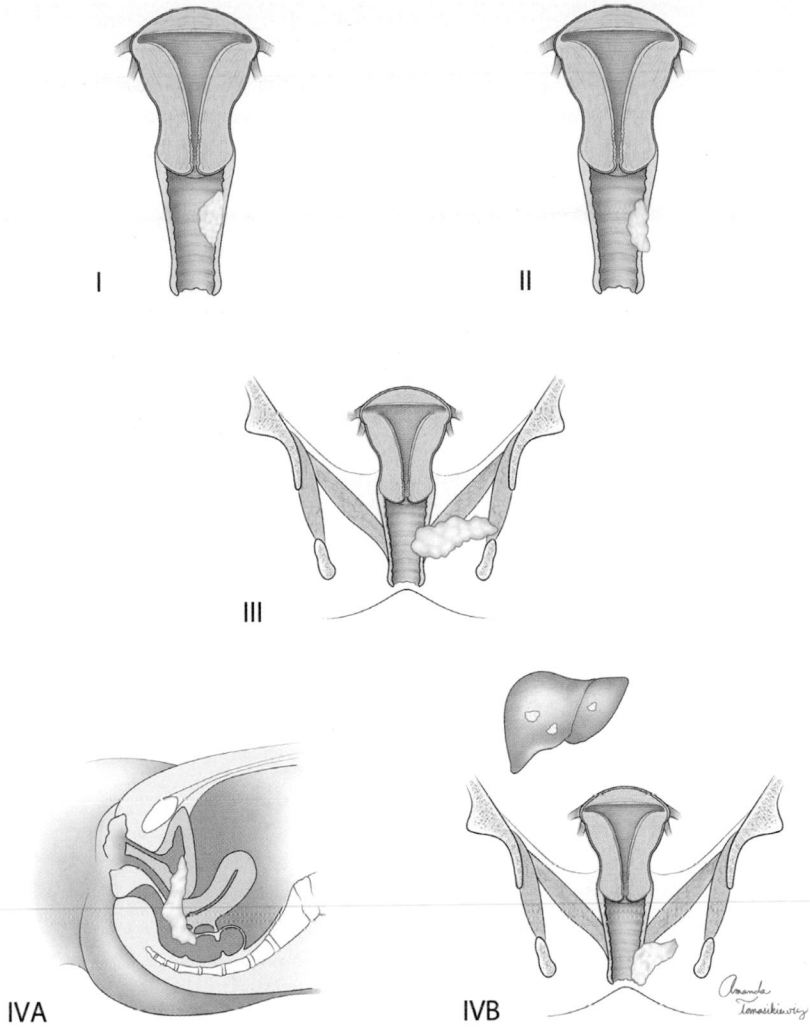

FIGURE 32-3 FIGO (International Federation of Gynecology and Obstetrics) staging of vaginal cancer.

Stage I

Both surgery and radiotherapy are options for stage I disease. However, surgery is preferred for most if negative surgical margins can be achieved. Surgery includes radical vaginectomy and pelvic lymphadenectomy for most tumors located in the upper third of the vaginal vault. A review of the National Cancer Data Base showed that women with stage I disease treated with surgery alone had a significantly improved 5-year survival rate compared with those treated with radiation (90 percent versus 63 percent) (Creasman, 1998). However, other reports have found no significant difference in disease-free survival rates in women with stage I disease treated with surgery compared with radiation alone (Stock, 1995). Radiotherapy may be delivered by external beam, with or without brachytherapy, as described in Chapter 28 (p. 720). Further, brachytherapy alone has been used successfully to treat selected small stage I lesions (Nori, 1983; Perez, 1999; Prempree, 1985; Reddy, 1991).

Stage II

Depending on circumstances and at the discretion of the treating clinician, stage II patients may be treated with primary surgery or radiation. Stock and colleagues (1995) found a significant survival advantage at 5 years in those with stage II disease treated with surgery compared with those treated with radiation (62 percent versus 53 percent). Review of the National Cancer Data Base showed that the 5-year survival rate for women with stage II disease treated with surgery alone was 70 percent; with radiotherapy alone 57 percent; and with a combination of surgery and radiotherapy 58 percent (Creasman, 1998). However, other researchers have found no survival advantage of surgery compared with radiotherapy in stage II disease (Davis, 1991; Rubin, 1985).

If primary radiation is to be administered, it is given most often as a combination of external beam radiation and brachytherapy. External beam radiation generally is given first, and depending on tumor response, brachytherapy is tailored to remaining disease. Radiation is generally recommended if negative margins cannot be achieved with surgery due to the anatomic location or size of the tumor or if a woman has medical comorbidities and is deemed not to be a surgical candidate. Although not proven to be advantageous as a vaginal cancer adjuvant, concurrent chemotherapy with cisplatin can be considered because of its proven efficacy in cervical cancer treatment. The characteristics of this agent are describe in Chapter 27 (p. 705), and Figure 28-12 (p. 724) describes its tumoricidal action.

review of 992 cases, which showed a dismal 5-year survival rate of only 18 percent. Advances in radiation technology and earlier diagnosis are largely responsible for the improved 5-year survival rate, which now ranges from 45 to 68 percent for all stages (Gia, 2011; Hellman, 2006).

The prognosis of squamous cell carcinoma of the vagina depends primarily on FIGO stage (Frank, 2005; Peters, 1985b). Other factors that have been reported to be associated with poor prognosis include larger tumor size, adenocarcinoma cell type, and older age (Chyle, 1996; Hellman, 2006; Tjalma, 2001; Tran, 2007). The 5-year disease-specific survival rate is 85 to 92 percent for women with stage I disease, 68 to 78 percent for those with stage II, and 13 to 58 percent for those with stage III or IV (Fig. 32-4) (Frank, 2005; Tran, 2007).

■ Treatment

Because of vaginal cancer's rarity, data to provide a basis for treatment decisions are limited. Therefore, therapy is individualized and based on factors such as tumor type, stage, location, and size.

Stage III and IVA

For advanced disease, external beam radiation alone or combined with brachytherapy is usually administered (Frank, 2005). Concurrent chemotherapy with cisplatin as a radiation adjunct is generally also recommended.

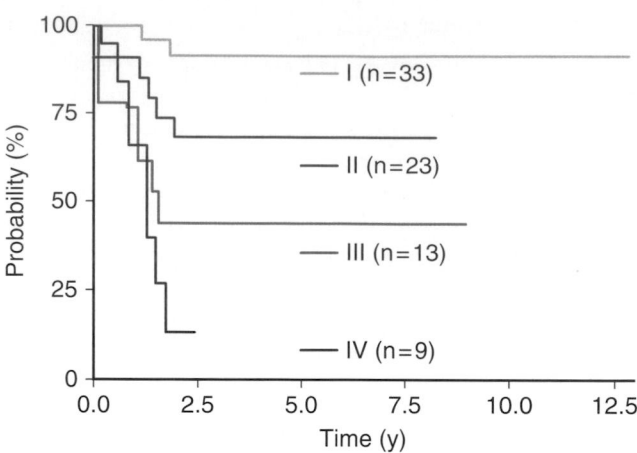

FIGURE 32-4 Disease-specific survival stratified by International Federation of Gynecology and Obstetrics (FIGO) stage. *(From Tran, 2007, with permission.)*

Stage IVB

Metastatic vaginal cancer is not curable, and treatment may include systemic chemotherapy or supportive hospice care. The most common sites of distant spread include liver, lungs, and bones. The choice of chemotherapeutic agents is again commonly extrapolated from cervical cancer data, given the rarity of vaginal cancer.

Chemoradiation

The numbers of women with vaginal cancer have been too small to make a prospective, randomized trial feasible. However, it is generally considered that the addition of chemotherapy to radiation treatment would be beneficial in those with locally advanced vaginal cancer. In a small series, it was found that the addition of concurrent chemotherapy provided a 10 to 33 percent decrease in the total amount of radiation delivered (Dalrymple, 2004). Although the authors were not intending to show an improved survival with chemoradiation, they found that local control of tumor growth and survival rates were comparable with those who had received higher doses of radiation alone. Decreases in the total dose of radiation may lead to lower rates of vaginal stenosis and fistula formation.

In a recent Surveillance Epidemiology and End Result (SEER) database analysis of 326 patients treated with external beam radiation and/or brachytherapy between 1991 and 2005, a notable increase in the usage of sensitizing chemotherapy was observed since the 1999 National Cancer Institute announcement confirmed the efficacy of chemoradiation in cervical cancer. Interestingly, the authors did not observe any survival advantage among those vaginal cancer patients who received chemoradiation compared with radiation alone (Gia, 2011).

Chemotherapy

In general, chemotherapy alone is ineffective in the treatment of vaginal cancer, although data are limited. The Gynecologic Oncology Group (GOG) performed a phase II trial evaluating 50 mg/m^2 cisplatin every 3 weeks for advanced or recurrent cancer of the vagina in 26 patients. Only one woman with squamous cell carcinoma achieved a complete response. Five of 16 patients

with squamous cell carcinoma had stable disease, and 10 had progression of disease. Based on this trial, single-agent cisplatin is considered to have insignificant activity at that dose and schedule (Thigpen, 1986). To date, this has been the only prospective GOG trial evaluating chemotherapy alone for vaginal cancer.

Radiation Therapy

This therapy to the primary tumor usually involves pelvic external beam radiation with or without brachytherapy, and often concurrent platinum-based sensitizing chemotherapy depending on the stage and other factors described earlier. Additionally, groin radiation is effective in patients with palpable nodal metastases. Moreover, elective irradiation may be delivered to clinically negative inguinal lymph nodes if the distal third of the vagina is involved. In a retrospective review, Perez and colleagues (1999) found that of 100 women who did not receive groin radiation, if disease was confined to the upper two thirds of the vagina, then none developed groin metastases. However, 10 percent of patients with lower-third primary tumors and 5 percent with tumors involving the entire length of the vagina developed inguinal node metastases.

Surveillance

Treatment failures usually occur within 2 years of primary therapy completion. Thus, patients usually are examined every 3 months for the first 2 years and then every 6 months until 5 years of surveillance is completed (Pingley, 2000; Rubin, 1985). After 5 years following treatment, women can be seen annually. A Pap smear and pelvic examination with careful attention to the inguinal and scalene nodes are performed. Surveillance imaging with CT scanning or MR imaging is at the clinician's discretion.

Recurrent Disease

Disease recurrence should be confirmed by biopsy if further treatment is planned. Therapeutic options in women with central pelvic recurrence who have had prior pelvic radiation are limited. Pelvic exenteration can be considered if a patient is psychologically and medically fit to undergo a radical surgery with high morbidity. However, it should be attempted only in those whose disease is limited to the central pelvis. Therefore, clinicians should be alert to the triad of sciatic pain, leg edema, and hydronephrosis, which is suggestive of pelvic sidewall disease. These women are not surgical candidates but can be managed with chemoradiation or with chemotherapy alone for women previously irradiated.

Survival after relapse is poor. In a review of 301 patients, 5-year survival was 20 percent for local recurrence and 4 percent for metastatic disease recurrence (Chyle, 1996).

Squamous Cell Vaginal Cancer in Pregnancy

This clinical situation is rare, and only 13 cases have been reported in the literature (Fujita, 2005). Women may be treated with surgical resection, radiation, chemoradiation, or a combination of these, and survival rates mirror those of nonpregnant women. Typically, treatment and timing of delivery must be tailored to the individual patient because there is limited evidence to support a general recommendation. To promptly begin treatment, women may elect to terminate their pregnancies or effect delivery at the time of cancer diagnosis. However, this does not appear to improve survival rates. Alternatively, a woman may choose to continue her pregnancy, and most who do, ultimately undergo cesarean delivery.

Verrucous Carcinoma

This carcinoma of the vagina is a rare variant of squamous cell carcinoma. Grossly, verrucous carcinoma is a warty, fungating mass that grows slowly and pushes into rather than invades contiguous structures (Isaacs, 1976). The diagnosis may be difficult to determine and may not be possible with a superficial biopsy. For this reason, multiple, large biopsies are recommended to avoid misdiagnosis and inadequate treatment.

Treatment requires surgical resection with either wide local excision for smaller lesions or radical surgery for larger tumors (Crowther, 1988). Verrucous carcinomas are resistant to radiotherapy and actually may transform to conventional squamous cell carcinoma after radiation (Zaino, 2011). Therefore, radiation treatment is contraindicated for these tumors.

Verrucous carcinoma has a tendency for local recurrence but rarely metastasizes to lymph nodes. This cancer may coexist with squamous cell carcinoma. When it does, it should be managed as a squamous cell carcinoma.

VAGINAL ADENOSIS- AND DES-RELATED TUMORS

Vaginal adenosis is a condition common in females exposed to diethylstilbestrol (DES) (Chap. 18, p. 502). *Adenosis* found in the vagina is defined by the presence of subepithelial glandular structures lined by mucinous columnar cells that resemble endocervical cells (Sandberg, 1965). These represent residual glands of müllerian origin. Clinically, adenosis appears as red granular spots or patches and does not stain following Lugol solution application.

Adenocarcinoma

Primary adenocarcinoma of the vagina is rare, comprising only 13 percent of all vaginal cancers (Platz, 1995). When the vagina is the primary site, it is believed to arise from adenosis. More commonly, vaginal adenocarcinoma is metastatic disease, typically from a lesion higher in the genital tract. Metastatic disease frequently arises from the endometrium, although it also may originate in the cervix or ovary (Saitoh, 2005). In addition, adenocarcinoma metastases from the breast, pancreas, kidney, and colon also have been identified in the vagina.

Treatment is similar to that for squamous cell carcinoma. Thus, surgery, radiation, or a combination of both can be used. Primary adenocarcinoma of the vagina is a more aggressive tumor than squamous cell carcinoma. In one series of 30 patients, it was associated with greater than twice the local and metastatic relapse rates of squamous cell carcinoma (Chyle, 1996).

Clear Cell Adenocarcinoma

In 1971, clear cell adenocarcinoma of the vagina was linked initially to in utero exposure to DES. DES was used off label to prevent miscarriage in the United States starting around 1940 and was approved for this use by the U.S. Food and Drug Administration (FDA) in 1947. In 1971, the FDA withdrew this indication, and pregnancy was a contraindication to DES usage (Food and Drug Administration, 1975).

It is estimated that 1 to 4 million women used DES and that approximately 0.01 percent of females exposed in utero developed clear cell adenocarcinoma of the vagina (Melnick, 1987). Most DES-exposed patients with vaginal cancer were born between 1951 and 1953, when the drug was prescribed most frequently. The median age at diagnosis of vaginal clear cell carcinoma in the United States is 19 years.

However, in the Netherlands, a bimodal distribution of vaginal clear cell carcinoma has been observed—the first peak occurring with a mean age of 26 years and the second at 71 years. The younger group all had been exposed in utero to DES, whereas the older group, born before 1947, had not been exposed (Hanselaar, 1997). It remains to be seen if the incidence of vaginal clear cell carcinoma will rise as the DES-exposed population ages.

Treatment is similar to that for squamous cell carcinoma of the vagina. The 5-year survival rate for 219 patients with stage I disease was 92 percent and was equivalent regardless of mode of therapy (Senekjian, 1987). The reported 5-year survival for 76 patients with stage II disease was 83 percent (Senekjian, 1988).

EMBRYONAL RHABDOMYOSARCOMA (SARCOMA BOTRYOIDES)

Embryonal rhabdomyosarcoma is the most common malignancy of the vagina in infants and children. Most are of the subtype sarcoma botryoides. This rare tumor develops almost exclusively in girls aged younger than 5 years, although vaginal and cervical sarcoma botryoides have been reported in females aged 15 to 20 years (Copeland, 1985a).

In infants and children, sarcoma botryoides usually is found in the vagina; in reproductive-aged women, within the cervix; and after menopause, within the uterus. Its name, derived from the Greek word *botrys,* which means "bunch of grapes," describes its appearance (Fig. 32-5). The gross specimen can exhibit multiple polyp-like structures or can be a solitary growth with a nodular, cystic, or pedunculated appearance (Hilgers, 1970). Although this distinctive appearance may guide diagnosis, the classic histologic finding of this tumor is the rhabdomyoblast (Fig. 32-6). Bleeding or a vaginal mass are typical complaints.

Embryonal rhabdomyosarcomas have a poor prognosis, but the subtype sarcoma botryoides is the easiest to treat and has the best chance of cure. It may be that its superficial location allows earlier detection (Copeland, 1985a).

As the result of work by the Intergroup Rhabdomyosarcoma Study (IRS) group, treatment of sarcoma botryoides has undergone dramatic revision. Before 1972, vaginal sarcoma botryoides was treated with pelvic exenteration (Hilgers, 1975). Since that time, four sequential prospective clinical trials to optimize the treatment and survival of childhood rhabdomyosarcoma have

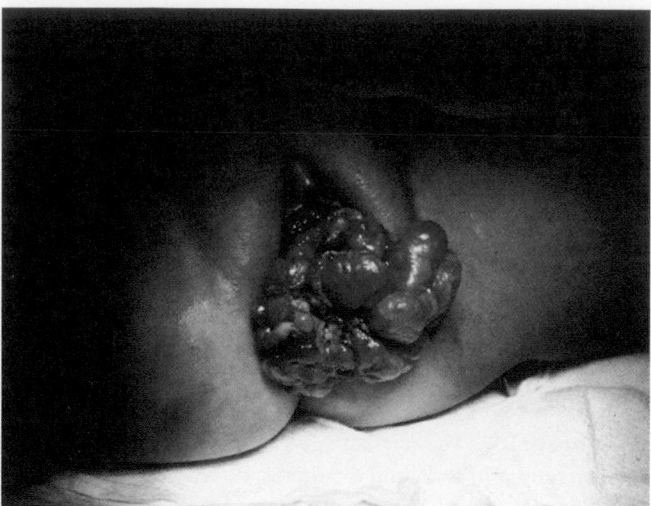

FIGURE 32-5 Sarcoma botryoides protruding through the vaginal introitus. *(From North American Society for Pediatric and Adolescent Gynecology, 2001, with permission.)*

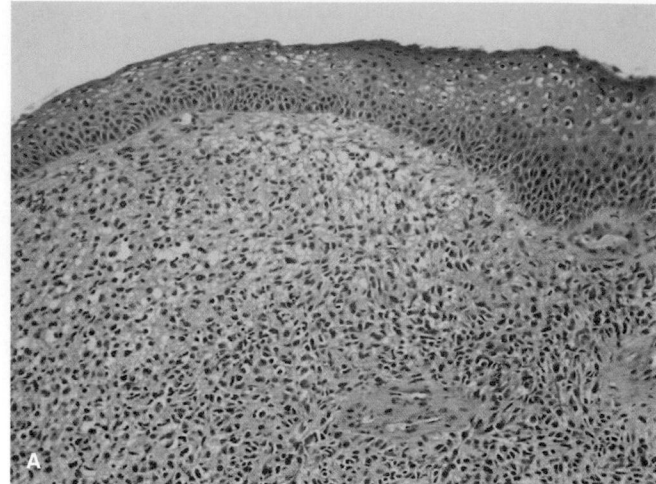

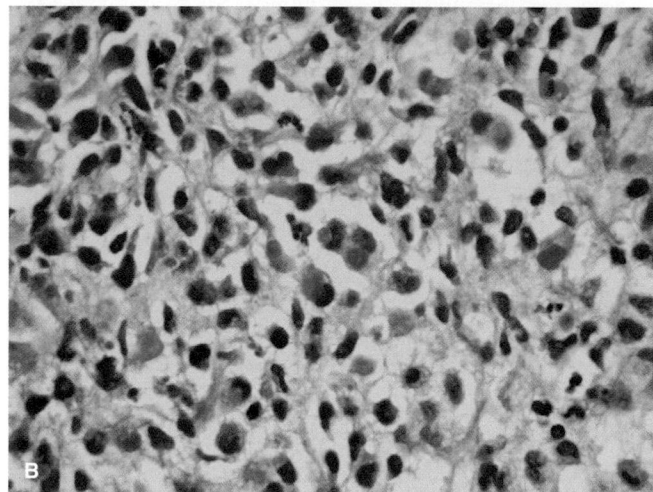

FIGURE 32-6 A. Embryonal rhabdomyosarcoma, botryoid type (×10). Malignant embryonal rhabdomyoblasts lie within a fibromyxoid stroma beneath the vaginal epithelium and cluster around blood vessels. **B.** Seen at higher power, undifferentiated round and spindled cells, some with brightly eosinophilic granular cytoplasm, are suggestive of rhabdomyoblastic differentiation. *(Photographs contributed by Dr. Kelley Carrick.)*

been completed. Within this series of four trials, each phase gradually shifted disease management away from radical surgery and toward primary chemotherapy followed by conservative surgery to excise residual tumor (Andrassy, 1995, 1999; Hays, 1981, 1985). In the last trial (IRS-IV), patients underwent primary chemotherapy. All but one patient, who died of chemotherapy-related toxicity, are alive without evidence of disease (Andrassy, 1999). The authors concluded that primary chemotherapy without surgery is adequate for most patients.

YOLK SAC TUMOR (ENDODERMAL SINUS TUMOR)

This type of adenocarcinoma is a germ cell tumor (Chap. 36, p. 883). Although most often developing in the gonads, yolk sac tumors rarely may arise in the vagina and usually in children aged 2 years or younger (Young, 1984). The clinical presentation is similar to that of sarcoma botryoides, and the most common symptom is bloody vaginal discharge. Grossly, the tumor differs from sarcoma botryoides, and a yolk sac tumor appears polypoid or sessile and often ulcerated (Young, 1984). On microscopic examination, these tumors most commonly have a reticular pattern. A classic finding, although not always present, is the Schiller-Duval body. This is a papilla with a single central vessel (Fig. 36-6, p. 883).

Serum alpha-fetoprotein (AFP) is a useful tumor marker, and levels are measured preoperatively if a yolk sac tumor is suspected. It can be used to monitor response to treatment and to detect disease recurrence before it becomes clinically evident (Copeland, 1985b).

Earlier studies demonstrated success with the chemotherapy regimen vincristine, adriamycin, and cyclophosphamide (VAC) for the treatment of yolk sac tumors (Copeland, 1985b; Young, 1984). More recently, the combination of bleomycin, etoposide, and cisplatin (BEP) has been used with excellent results (Arora, 2002; Handel, 2002; Terenziani, 2007). Neoadjuvant chemotherapy has been used to shrink the tumor and minimize

or obviate surgical resection. Yolk sac tumors are also responsive to radiation. However, radiotherapy should be used with caution in this age group given the severe side effects, such as loss of reproductive and sexual function, femoral head necrosis, and abnormal pelvic bone growth (Aartsen, 1993; Arora, 2002).

LEIOMYOSARCOMA

Leiomyosarcoma is the most common type of vaginal sarcoma in adults. However, it is estimated to comprise no more than 1 percent of vaginal malignancies, and only 138 cases have been described in the literature to date (Ahram, 2006). The age of affected individuals is broad, but most are older than 40 years (Zaino, 2011).

Because of the small number of these tumors, their epidemiology has not been widely studied, and few risk factors have been identified. However, patients previously treated with pelvic radiotherapy for cervical cancer appear to be at risk.

Affected women most often complain of an asymptomatic vaginal mass. However, vaginal, rectal, or bladder pain; bleeding or discharge from the vagina or rectum; dyspareunia; or difficult micturition also may be noted. Any wall of the vagina may be affected, but most tumors develop posteriorly (Ahram, 2006). Microscopically, tumors resemble uterine leiomyosarcoma (Fig. 34-2, p. 842). Tumors spread by local invasion and hematogenous dissemination.

Surgical resection with negative margins is the preferred primary treatment. The benefit of adjuvant radiation is unclear due to a lack of controlled trials. However, some clinicians recommend adjuvant radiation for those with high-grade tumor or local recurrence (Curtin, 1995).

CARCINOSARCOMA (MALIGNANT MIXED MÜLLERIAN TUMOR)

Carcinosarcoma contains both malignant epithelial (carcinomatous) and malignant stromal (sarcomatous) elements. Although most commonly developing in the uterus, it can arise from other sites such as the ovaries or peritoneum. Rarely found in the vagina, these highly aggressive tumors have been described in only eight cases in the literature (Neesham, 1998; Shibata, 2003). Of these eight women, four had received prior pelvic radiation.

Given the rarity of this tumor and the lack of controlled trials, optimal treatment is unknown. Most patients have been treated with surgical resection alone, whereas others have received primary radiotherapy or combined surgery and adjuvant radiation. The 5-year survival rate is reported to be only 17 percent (Peters, 1985a).

MELANOMA

Primary malignant melanoma in the vagina is rare, accounting for less than 3 percent of all vaginal cancers. In women, 1.6 percent of melanomas are genital. The most common site is the vulva (70 percent), followed by the vagina (21 percent) and the cervix (9 percent) (Miner, 2004). Using data from the SEER database, Weinstock (1994) estimated that the incidence of vaginal melanoma is 0.26 per 10,000 women per year. Both U.S. and Swedish studies have shown the mean age at diagnosis to be 66 years (Ragnarsson-Olding, 1993; Reid, 1989).

The most common presenting symptoms include vaginal bleeding, vaginal mass, and vaginal discharge (Gupta, 2002; Reid, 1989). Most are located in the distal vagina (Frumovitz, 2010). Vaginal melanoma is often detected late, and this may be largely responsible for poor treatment outcomes.

Cutaneous melanomas at other body sites are staged by a variety of microstaging systems, including the Chung, the Clark, and the Breslow systems, which use staging criteria such as depth of invasion, tumor size, and tumor thickness (Chap. 31, p. 803). However, Clark levels are not applicable to vaginal melanoma because the typical microscopic skin landmarks used are not present. Therefore, staging is based on tumor thickness, as described by Breslow or Chung.

With a reported 5-year survival rate ranging from 10 to 20 percent, the prognosis is among the worst of vaginal malignancies (Beller, 2003; Ragnarsson-Olding, 1993; Signorelli, 2005; Weinstock, 1994). Although survival rates are significantly better for those with vaginal lesions measuring less than 3 cm, FIGO staging of vaginal melanomas does not accurately predict survival (Reid, 1989).

An effective treatment for vaginal melanoma has not yet been identified. Both wide local excision and radical surgery have been used, as well as radiotherapy and chemotherapy. One study demonstrated a survival benefit to surgical management (Frumovitz, 2010). Melanomas generally are thought to be radioresistant. However, in one series, radiation therapy was found to provide local tumor control in women who had surgically unresectable disease (Miner, 2004).

REFERENCES

Aartsen EJ, Delemarre JF, Gerretsen G: Endodermal sinus tumor of the vagina: radiation therapy and progeny. Obstet Gynecol 81:893, 1993

Ahram J, Lemus R, Schiavello HJ: Leiomyosarcoma of the vagina: case report and literature review. Int J Gynecol Cancer 16:884, 2006

Andrassy RJ, Hays DM, Raney RB, et al: Conservative surgical management of vaginal and vulvar pediatric rhabdomyosarcoma: a report from the Intergroup Rhabdomyosarcoma Study III. J Pediatr Surg 30:1034, 1995

Andrassy RJ, Wiener ES, Raney RB, et al: Progress in the surgical management of vaginal rhabdomyosarcoma: a 25-year review from the Intergroup Rhabdomyosarcoma Study Group. J Pediatr Surg 34:731, 1999

Arora M, Shrivastav RK, Jaiprakash MP: A rare germ-cell tumor site: vaginal endodermal sinus tumor. Pediatr Surg Int 18:521, 2002

Beller U, Maisonneuve P, Benedet JL, et al: Carcinoma of the vagina. Int J Gynaecol Obstet 83 Suppl 1:27, 2003

Chyle V, Zagars GK, Wheeler JA, et al: Definitive radiotherapy for carcinoma of the vagina: outcome and prognostic factors. Int J Radiat Oncol Biol Phys 35:891, 1996

Copeland LJ, Gershenson DM, Saul PB, et al: Sarcoma botryoides of the female genital tract. Obstet Gynecol 66:262, 1985a

Copeland LJ, Sneige N, Ordonez NG, et al: Endodermal sinus tumor of the vagina and cervix. Cancer 55:2558, 1985b

Creasman WT, Phillips JL, Menck HR: The National Cancer Data Base report on cancer of the vagina. Cancer 83:1033, 1998

Crowther ME, Lowe DG, Shepherd JH: Verrucous carcinoma of the female genital tract: a review. Obstet Gynecol Surv 43:263, 1988

Curtin JP, Saigo P, Slucher B, et al: Soft-tissue sarcoma of the vagina and vulva: a clinicopathologic study. Obstet Gynecol 86:269, 1995

Daling JR, Madeleine MM, Schwartz SM, et al: A population-based study of squamous cell vaginal cancer: HPV and cofactors. Gynecol Oncol 84:263, 2002

Dalrymple JL, Russell AH, Lee SW, et al: Chemoradiation for primary invasive squamous carcinoma of the vagina. Int J Gynecol Cancer 14:110, 2004

Davis KP, Stanhope CR, Garton GR, et al: Invasive vaginal carcinoma: analysis of early-stage disease. Gynecol Oncol 42:131, 1991

Dodge JA, Eltabbakh GH, Mount SL, et al: Clinical features and risk of recurrence among patients with vaginal intraepithelial neoplasia. Gynecol Oncol 83:363, 2001

FIGO Committee on Gynecologic Oncology: Current FIGO staging for cancer of the vagina, fallopian tube, ovary, and gestational trophoblastic neoplasia. Int J Gynaecol Obstet 105(1):3, 2009

Food and Drug Administration: Certain estrogens for oral use. Notice of withdrawal of approval of new drug applications. Fed Regist 40: 5384, 1975

Frank SJ, Jhingran A, Levenback C, et al: Definitive radiation therapy for squamous cell carcinoma of the vagina. Int J Radiat Oncol Biol Phys 62:138, 2005

Frumovitz M, Etcheparreborda M, Sun CC, et al: Primary malignant melanoma of the vagina. Obstet Gynecol 116:1358, 2010

Fujita K, Aoki Y, Tanaka K: Stage I squamous cell carcinoma of vagina complicating pregnancy: successful conservative treatment. Gynecol Oncol 98:513, 2005

Gia AJ, Gonzalez VJ, Tward JD, et al: Primary vaginal cancer and chemoradiotherapy: a patterns-of-care analysis. Int J Gynecol Cancer 21:378, 2011

Gupta D, Malpica A, Deavers MT, et al: Vaginal melanoma: a clinicopathologic and immunohistochemical study of 26 cases. Am J Surg Pathol 26:1450, 2002

Handel LN, Scott SM, Giller RH, et al: New perspectives on therapy for vaginal endodermal sinus tumors. J Urol 168:687, 2002

Hanselaar A, van Loosbroek M, Schuurbiers O, et al: Clear cell adenocarcinoma of the vagina and cervix: an update of the central Netherlands registry showing twin age incidence peaks. Cancer 79:2229, 1997

Hays DM, Raney RB Jr, Lawrence W Jr, et al: Rhabdomyosarcoma of the female urogenital tract. J Pediatr Surg 16:828, 1981

Hays DM, Shimada H, Raney RB Jr, et al: Sarcomas of the vagina and uterus: the Intergroup Rhabdomyosarcoma Study. J Pediatr Surg 20:718, 1985

Hellman K, Lundell M, Silfversward C, et al: Clinical and histopathologic factors related to prognosis in primary squamous cell carcinoma of the vagina. Int J Gynecol Cancer 16:1201, 2006

Hilgers RD: Pelvic exenteration for vaginal embryonal rhabdomyosarcoma: a review. Obstet Gynecol 45:175, 1975

Hilgers RD, Malkasian GD Jr, Soule EH: Embryonal rhabdomyosarcoma (botryoid type) of the vagina: a clinicopathologic review. Am J Obstet Gynecol 107:484, 1970

Isaacs JH: Verrucous carcinoma of the female genital tract. Gynecol Oncol 4(3):259, 1976

Joura EA, Leodolter S, Hernandez-Avila M, et al: Efficacy of a quadrivalent prophylactic human papillomavirus (types 6, 11, 16, and 18) L1 virus-like-particle vaccine against high-grade vulval and vaginal lesions: a combined analysis of three randomized clinical trials. Lancet 369(9574):1693, 2007

Lamoreaux WT, Grisby PW, Dehdashti F, et al: FDG-PET evaluation of vaginal carcinoma. Int J Radiation Oncology Biol Phys 62:733, 2005

Melnick S, Cole P, Anderson D, et al: Rates and risks of diethylstilbestrol-related clear-cell adenocarcinoma of the vagina and cervix: an update. N Engl J Med 316:514, 1987

Miner TJ, Delgado R, Zeisler J, et al: Primary vaginal melanoma: a critical analysis of therapy. Ann Surg Oncol 11:34, 2004

National Cancer Institute: General information about vaginal cancer. 2011. Available at: http://www.cancer.gov/cancertopics/pdq/treatment/vaginal/HealthProfessional. Accessed October 25, 2011

Neesham D, Kerdemelidis P, Scurry J: Primary malignant mixed mullerian tumor of the vagina. Gynecol Oncol 70:303, 1998

Nori D, Hilaris BS, Stanimir G, et al: Radiation therapy of primary vaginal carcinoma. Int J Radiat Oncol Biol Phys 9:1471, 1983

North American Society for Pediatric and Adolescent Gynecology: The PediGYN teaching slide set. Philadelphia, 2001, slide 124

Pecorelli S, Benedet JL, Creasman WT, et al: FIGO staging of gynecologic cancer. 1994–1997 FIGO Committee on Gynecologic Oncology. International Federation of Gynecology and Obstetrics. Int J Gynaecol Obstet 65:243, 1999

Perez CA, Grigsby PW, Garipagaoglu M, et al: Factors affecting long-term outcome of irradiation in carcinoma of the vagina. Int J Radiat Oncol Biol Phys 44:37, 1999

Peters WA III, Kumar NB, Andersen WA, et al: Primary sarcoma of the adult vagina: a clinicopathologic study. Obstet Gynecol 65:699, 1985a

Peters WA III, Kumar NB, Morley GW: Carcinoma of the vagina: factors influencing treatment outcome. Cancer 55:892, 1985b

Pingley S, Shrivastava SK, Sarin R, et al: Primary carcinoma of the vagina: Tata Memorial Hospital experience. Int J Radiat Oncol Biol Phys 46:101, 2000

Platz CE, Benda JA: Female genital tract cancer. Cancer 75:270, 1995

Prempree T, Amornmarn R: Radiation treatment of primary carcinoma of the vagina: patterns of failures after definitive therapy. Acta Radiol Oncol 24:51, 1985

Ragnarsson-Olding B, Johansson H, Rutqvist LE, et al: Malignant melanoma of the vulva and vagina: trends in incidence, age distribution, and long-term survival among 245 consecutive cases in Sweden 1960–1984. Cancer 71:1893, 1993

Reddy S, Saxena VS, Reddy S, et al: Results of radiotherapeutic management of primary carcinoma of the vagina. Int J Radiat Oncol Biol Phys 21:1041, 1991

Reid GC, Schmidt RW, Roberts JA, et al: Primary melanoma of the vagina: a clinicopathologic analysis. Obstet Gynecol 74:190, 1989

Rubin SC, Young J, Mikuta JJ: Squamous carcinoma of the vagina: treatment, complications, and long-term follow-up. Gynecol Oncol 20:346, 1985

Saitoh M, Hayasaka T, Ohmichi M, et al: Primary mucinous adenocarcinoma of the vagina: possibility of differentiating from metastatic adenocarcinomas. Pathol Int 55:372, 2005

Sandberg EC, Danielson Rw, Cauwet RW, et al: Adenosis vaginae. Am J Obstet Gynecol 93:209, 1965

Senekjian EK, Frey KW, Anderson D, et al: Local therapy in stage I clear cell adenocarcinoma of the vagina. Cancer 60:1319, 1987

Senekjian EK, Frey KW, Stone C, et al: An evaluation of stage II vaginal clear cell adenocarcinoma according to substages. Gynecol Oncol 31:56, 1988

Shibata R, Umezawa A, Takehara K, et al: Primary carcinosarcoma of the vagina. Pathol Int 53:106, 2003

Siegel R, Ward E, Brawley O, et al: Cancer statistics, 2011: the impact of eliminating socioeconomic and racial disparities on premature cancer deaths. CA Cancer J Clin 61(4):212, 2011

Signorelli M, Lissoni AA, Garbi A, et al: Primary malignant vaginal melanoma treated with adriamycin and ifosfamide: a case report and literature review. Gynecol Oncol 97:700, 2005

Stock RG, Chen AS, Seski J: A 30-year experience in the management of primary carcinoma of the vagina: analysis of prognostic factors and treatment modalities. Gynecol Oncol 56:45, 1995

Terenziani M, Spreafico F, Collini P, et al: Endodermal sinus tumor of the vagina. Pediatr Blood Cancer 48(5):577, 2007

Thigpen JT, Blessing JA, Homesley HD, et al: Phase II trial of cisplatin in advanced or recurrent cancer of the vagina: a Gynecologic Oncology Group Study. Gynecol Oncol 23:101, 1986

Tjalma WA, Monaghan JM, de Barros Lopes A, et al: The role of surgery in invasive squamous carcinoma of the vagina. Gynecol Oncol 81:360, 2001

Tran PT, Su Z, Lee P, et al: Prognostic factors for outcomes and complications for primary squamous cell carcinoma of the vagina treated with radiation. Gynecol Oncol 105:641, 2007

Watson M, Saraiya M, Wu X: Update of HPV-associated female genital cancers in the United States, 1999-2004. J Womens Health 18:1731, 2009

Weinstock MA: Malignant melanoma of the vulva and vagina in the United States: patterns of incidence and population-based estimates of survival. Am J Obstet Gynecol 171:1225, 1994

Young RH, Scully RE: Endodermal sinus tumor of the vagina: a report of nine cases and review of the literature. Gynecol Oncol 18:380, 1984

Zaino RJ, Nucci M, Kurman RJ: Diseases of the vagina. In Kurman RJ, Ellenson LH, Ronnett BM (eds): Blaustein's Pathology of the Female Genital Tract, New York, Springer, 2011, p 137

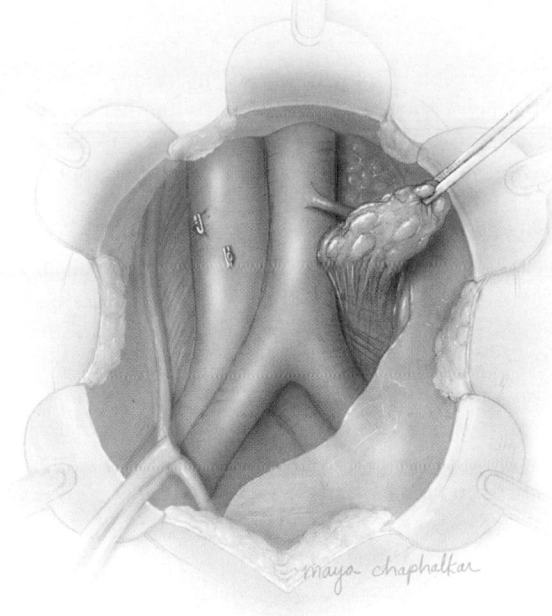

CHAPTER 33

Endometrial Cancer

In the United States, endometrial cancer is the most common gynecologic malignancy. Worldwide each year, 287,100 women are diagnosed with this disease (Jemal, 2011). Risk factors include obesity and advancing age. Moreover, as both of these become more prevalent, the incidence of endometrial cancer will likely similarly increase. Fortunately, patients typically seek medical attention early due to vaginal bleeding, and endometrial biopsy leads quickly to diagnosis. The primary treatment is hysterectomy with bilateral salpingo-oophorectomy (BSO) and staging lymphadenectomy for most women.

Three quarters will have stage I disease that is curable by surgery alone. Patients with more advanced disease typically require postoperative combination chemotherapy, radiotherapy, or both.

EPIDEMIOLOGY AND RISK FACTORS

During their lifetime, one in 38 American women (3 percent) will develop endometrial cancer. In the United States, 46,470 new cases are estimated to develop in 2011, but only 8120 deaths are expected. Most patients are diagnosed early and are subsequently cured. As a result, endometrial cancer is the fourth leading cause of cancer, but only the eighth leading cause of cancer deaths among women (Siegel, 2011). The average age at diagnosis is in the early 60s (Creasman, 1998; Farley, 2000; Madison, 2004).

Numerous risk factors for developing endometrial cancer have been described (Table 33-1). In general, most risk factors are associated with direct or indirect creation of an excessive estrogen environment.

Of these, *obesity* is the most common cause of endogenous overproduction of estrogen. Excessive adipose tissue increases peripheral aromatization of androstenedione to estrone. In premenopausal women, elevated estrone levels trigger abnormal feedback in the hypothalamic-pituitary-ovarian axis. The clinical result is oligo- or anovulation. In the absence of ovulation, the endometrium is exposed to virtually continuous estrogen stimulation without subsequent progestational effect and without menstrual withdrawal bleeding.

Unopposed estrogen therapy is the next most important potential inciting factor. Fortunately, the malignant potential of continuous or sequentially administered estrogen was recognized more than three decades ago (Smith, 1975). Currently, it is rare to encounter a woman with a uterus who has taken unopposed estrogen for years. Instead, combined estrogen plus progestin hormonal therapy is routinely prescribed for

TABLE 33-1. Risk Factors for Endometrial Cancer

Factors Influencing Risk	Estimated Relative Risk[a]
Obesity	2–5
Polycystic ovarian syndrome	>5
Long-term use of high-dose menopausal estrogens	10–20
Early age of menarche	1.5–2
Late age of natural menopause	2–3
History of infertility	2–3
Nulliparity	3
Menstrual irregularities	1.5
Residency in North America or northern Europe	3–18
Higher level of education or income	1.5–2
White race	2
Older age	2–3
High cumulative doses of tamoxifen	3–7
History of diabetes, hypertension, or gallbladder disease	1.3–3
Long-term use of high-dose COCs	0.3–0.5
Cigarette smoking	0.5

[a]Relative risks depend on the study and referent group employed.
COCs = combination oral contraceptives.
From Brinton, 2004, with permission.

postmenopausal women with a uterus to reduce their risk of endometrial cancer (Strom, 2006). There remain questions about how effective this combination strategy is at preventing endometrial cancer, but certainly, it is superior to unopposed estrogen (Allen, 2010; Karageorgi, 2010; Lacey, 2005).

Menstrual and reproductive factors are commonly associated with endometrial cancer whenever anovulation is present or the duration of uninterrupted menstrual cycles is prolonged. For example, early age at menarche or late age of menopause are both associated with increased risk (Wernli, 2006). Classically, women with polycystic ovarian syndrome are anovulatory and thus have an increased risk of developing endometrial cancer (Fearnley, 2010; Pillay, 2006).

Environment is another factor that has been associated with endometrial cancer in several ways. Women in Western and developed societies have a much higher incidence (Parkin, 2005). Obvious confounding variables within these populations, such as obesity and low parity, account for much of this effect.

However, a possible etiologic role for nutrition—especially a diet with a high content of animal fat—is another explanation (Goodman, 1997). Immigrant populations tend to assume the risks of native populations within one or two generations, highlighting the importance of environmental factors (Liao, 2003).

Older age is an associated risk factor for developing endometrial cancer with a peak incidence among women in their 70s. Overall, approximately 80 percent of diagnoses occur in postmenopausal women older than 55 years (Schottenfeld, 1995). Fewer than 5 percent of endometrial cancers develop in patients younger than 40 years.

Family history is another risk factor for endometrial cancer. Endometrial cancer is the most common extracolonic manifestation in hereditary nonpolyposis colorectal cancer (HNPCC), also known as Lynch syndrome (Hemminki, 2005). This autosomal-dominant syndrome results primarily from mutations in the mismatch repair genes *MLH1* and *MSH2* (Bansal, 2009). Mutation in one of these genes prevents repair of base mismatches, which are commonly produced during DNA replication. Inactivity of this DNA mismatch repair system leads to mutations that can promote carcinogenesis. Mutation carriers have a risk of developing endometrial cancer that ranges from 40 to 60 percent. Among affected women, the endometrial cancer risk actually exceeds that for colorectal cancer (Aarnio, 1999; Delin, 2004; Dunlop, 1997). However, fewer than 5 percent of endometrial cancers are attributable to HNPCC (Hampel, 2006). In general, most familial cases develop in premenopausal women (Gruber, 1996).

BRCA1 and BRCA2 mutation carriers also have a slightly elevated risk, but only because of frequent tamoxifen treatment of previous breast cancers (Beiner, 2007; Thai, 1998). In general, these mutations mainly predispose women to breast and ovarian cancer—not endometrial.

Tamoxifen causes a two- to threefold higher risk of developing endometrial cancer by having a modest "unopposed" estrogenic effect on the endometrium (Chap. 27, p. 705). The level of risk also increases linearly with the duration of therapy and the cumulative dose (van Leeuwen, 1994). Most data suggest that endometrial cancers that develop in patients receiving tamoxifen exhibit the same stage, grade, and prognosis distribution as those in nonusers (Fisher, 1994). The increased risk of endometrial cancer occurs almost exclusively in postmenopausal women (Fisher, 1998). Unless a patient is identified to be at otherwise high risk for endometrial cancer, routine endometrial surveillance has not been effective in increasing early detection of endometrial cancer in women using tamoxifen (American College of Obstetricians and Gynecologists, 2006).

Coexisting medical conditions such as diabetes mellitus, hypertension, and gallbladder disease are more commonly associated with endometrial cancer (Morimoto, 2006; Soliman, 2005). In general, these are frequent sequelae of obesity and an environment of chronic excess estrogen.

Combination oral contraceptive (COC) use for a period of at least 1 year confers as much as a 30- to 50-percent reduced risk of endometrial cancer, and risk reduction extends for 10 to 20 years (Dossus, 2010; Stanford, 1993). In essence, the progestin component has a chemopreventive biologic effect on the endometrium. The potency of the progestin in most oral contraceptives is adequate, but higher progestin potency may be more protective among obese women (Maxwell, 2006). Progesterone intrauterine devices (IUDs) also confer long-term protection against endometrial cancer (Tao, 2006).

Smokers have a lower risk of developing endometrial cancer. The biologic mechanism is multifactorial, but in part involves reduced levels of circulating estrogens through weight reduction, an earlier age at menopause, and altered hormonal metabolism. Both current and past smoking has a long-lasting influence (Viswanathan, 2005).

ENDOMETRIAL HYPERPLASIA

Most endometrial cancers arise following progression of histologically distinguishable hyperplastic lesions. In fact, endometrial hyperplasia is the only known direct precursor of invasive disease. Endometrial hyperplasia is defined as endometrial thickening with a proliferation of irregularly sized and shaped glands and an increased gland-to-stroma ratio (Ellenson, 2011a) (Fig. 33-1). In the absence of such thickening, lesions are best designated as *disorderly proliferative endometrium* or *focal glandular crowding*. Endometrial hyperplasia represents a continuum of histopathologic findings that are difficult to differentiate by standard characteristics. These lesions range from anovulatory endometrium to monoclonal precancers.

Classification
World Health Organization

The classification system used by the World Health Organization (WHO) and International Society of Gynecological Pathologists designates four different types with varying

TABLE 33-2. World Health Organization Classification of Endometrial Hyperplasia

Types	Progressing to Cancer (%)
Simple hyperplasia	1
Complex hyperplasia	3
Simple atypical hyperplasia	8
Complex atypical hyperplasia	29

From Kurman, 1985, with permission.

malignant potential (Table 33-2) (Kurman, 1985; Silverberg, 2003). Hyperplasias are classified as *simple* or *complex*, based on the absence or presence of architectural abnormalities such as glandular complexity and crowding (Fig. 33-2). Most importantly, hyperplasias are further designated as *atypical* if they demonstrate cytologic, that is, nuclear, atypia. Only atypical endometrial hyperplasias are clearly associated with the subsequent development of adenocarcinoma. Simple atypical hyperplasia is a relatively uncommon diagnosis. In general, most have a complex architecture.

Although endometrial hyperplasias are formally classified in these four different groups, they tend to be morphologically heterogeneous, both within and between individual patients. This histologic diversity explains why only a small number of conserved features are useful as diagnostic criteria. As a result, reproducible scoring of cytologic atypia is often challenging, particularly with a small amount of tissue from a biopsy sample.

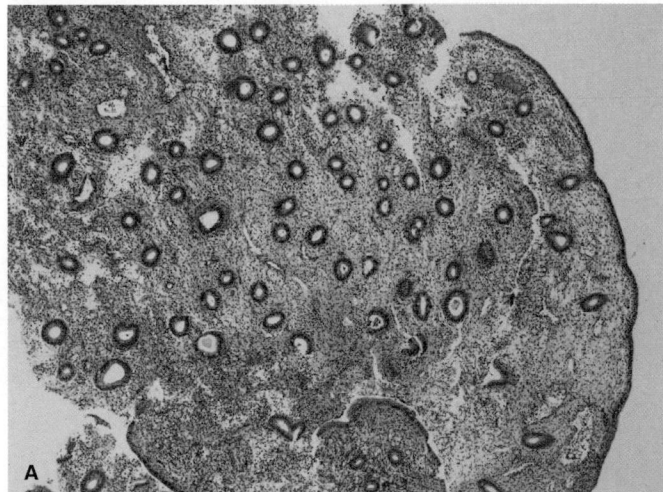
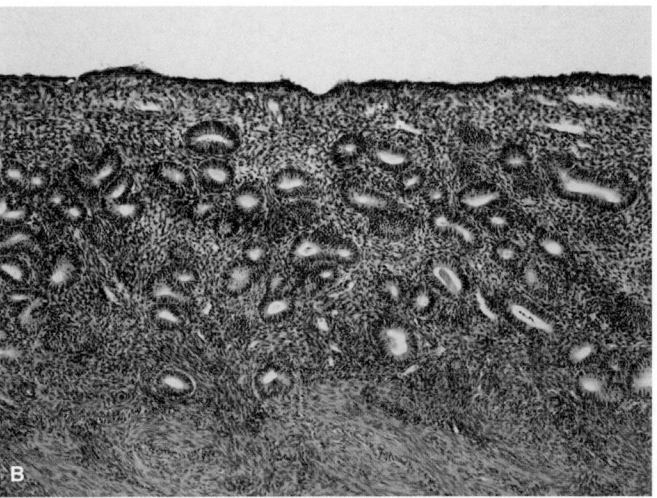

FIGURE 33-1 Photomicrographs display normal proliferative endometrium contrasted with hyperplastic endometrium. **A.** This low-power view of normal proliferative endometrium shows endometrial glands (cut in cross section) with predominantly round regular contours, regular spacing, and a gland-to-stroma ratio of less than 1:1. **B.** Endometrial hyperplasia is characterized by a proliferation of endometrial glands such that the glands are more crowded than usual, resulting in a gland-to-stroma ratio greater than 1:1. The terms *simple* and *complex* refer to the degree of gland crowding and architectural abnormality. The term *atypia* refers to the presence of nuclear atypia within the endometrial glands. In this example, endometrial glands are modestly, irregularly crowded but do not display nuclear atypia. *(Photographs contributed by Dr. Kelley Carrick.)*

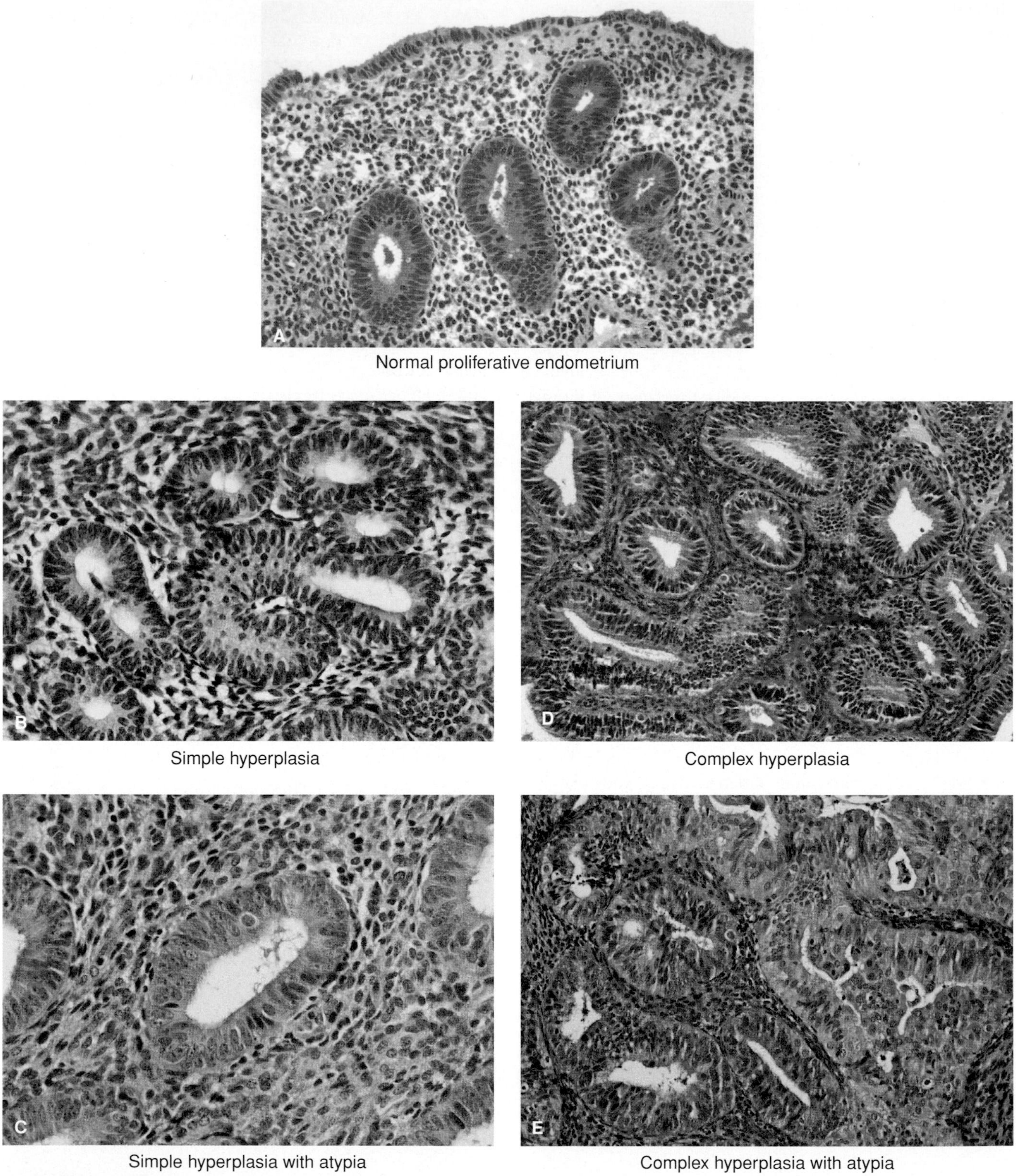

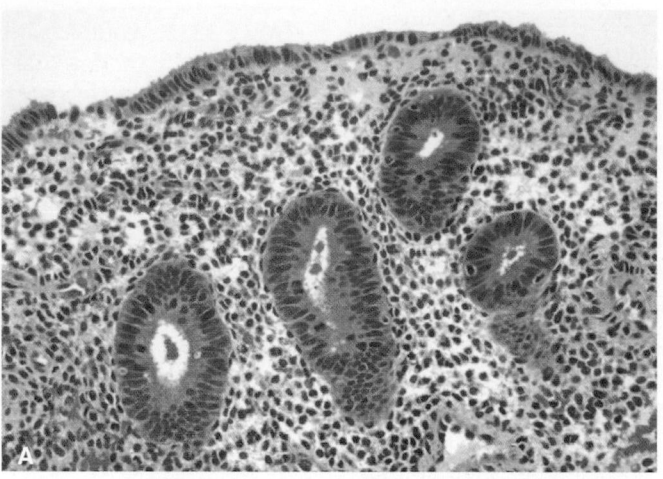

Normal proliferative endometrium

Simple hyperplasia

Complex hyperplasia

Simple hyperplasia with atypia

Complex hyperplasia with atypia

FIGURE 33-2 Photomicrographs display normal proliferative endometrium contrasted with different types of hyperplastic endometrium. **A.** This high-power view of normal proliferative endometrium shows regularly spaced glands composed of stratified columnar epithelium with bland, slightly elongate nuclei and mitotic activity. **B.** In simple hyperplasia, glands are modestly crowded and typically display normal tubular shape or mild gland-shape abnormalities. Nuclei are bland. **C.** In this case, glands are only mildly crowded, but occasional glands, such as the one pictured in this high-power view, have nuclear atypia characterized by nuclear rounding and visible nucleoli. Cytologic atypia accompanies complex hyperplasia more often than it does simple hyperplasia. **D.** In complex hyperplasia, glands are more markedly crowded and sometimes show architectural abnormalities such as papillary infoldings. In this case, gland profiles are fairly regular but the glands are markedly crowded. **E.** Glands are markedly crowded and some show papillary infoldings. Nuclei show variable nuclear atypia. Some of the atypical glands have an eosinophilic cytoplasmic change. *(Photographs contributed by Dr. Kelley Carrick.)*

Endometrial Intraepithelial Neoplasia

The term *endometrial intraepithelial neoplasia* (EIN) has been introduced to more accurately distinguish the two very different clinical categories of hyperplasia: (1) normal polyclonal endometria diffusely responding to an abnormal hormonal environment and (2) intrinsically proliferative monoclonal lesions that arise focally and confer an elevated risk of adenocarcinoma (Mutter, 2000). This nomenclature emphasizes the malignant potential of endometrial precancers, in keeping with similar precedents in the cervix, vagina, and vulva.

Using this system, anovulatory or prolonged estrogen-exposed endometria without atypia are generally designated as *endometrial hyperplasias*. In contrast, *endometrial intraepithelial neoplasia* is used to describe all endometria delineated as premalignant by a combination of three morphometric features that reflect glandular volume, architectural complexity, and cytologic abnormality. The EIN classification system is a more accurate and reproducible way of predicting progression to cancer, but has not been universally implemented (Baak, 2005; Hecht, 2005).

Clinical Features

The risk factors for developing endometrial hyperplasia generally mirror those for invasive carcinoma (Anastasiadis, 2000; Ricci, 2002). Two thirds of women present with postmenopausal bleeding (Horn, 2004). However, almost any type of abnormal uterine bleeding should prompt diagnostic evaluation (Chap. 8, p. 223).

In those with abnormal bleeding, transvaginal sonography of endometrial thickness is a feasible method for predicting endometrial hyperplasia (Goldstein, 1990; Granberg, 1991; Jacobs, 2011). In postmenopausal women, endometrial stripe thickness measurements less than 5 mm have been associated in sonographic-pathologic studies with bleeding that can be attributed to endometrial atrophy (American College of Obstetricians and Gynecologists, 2009). Those with a thicker endometrium warrant biopsy. Sonography may also identify abnormal echostructural changes in the endometrium. Cystic endometrial changes suggest polyps, homogeneously thickened endometrium may indicate hyperplasia, and a heterogeneous structural pattern is suspicious for malignancy (Figs. 33-3 and 33-4). However, these sonographic findings show much overlap and cannot be used alone.

For premenopausal women, transvaginal sonography is often performed to exclude structural sources of abnormal bleeding. Similarly, researchers have attempted to create endometrial thickness guidelines. However, endometrial thicknesses can vary considerably among premenopausal women, and suggested evidence-based abnormal thresholds range from ≥4 mm to >16 mm (Breitkopf, 2004; Goldstein, 1997; Shi, 2008). Thus, consensus for endometrial thickness guidelines has not been established for this group. At our institution, no additional evaluation is recommended for a normal-appearing endometrium measuring ≤10 mm in a premenopausal female experiencing abnormal uterine bleeding if she has no other risk factors to prompt further testing.

As an alternative to sonography, Pipelle office biopsy or outpatient dilatation and curettage (D&C) may be initially

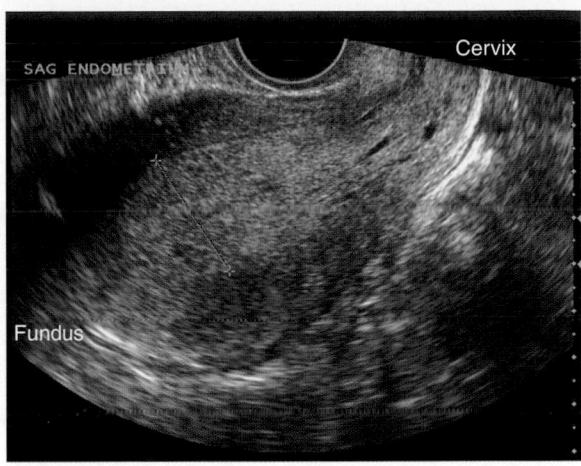

FIGURE 33-3 Transvaginal sonographic image of a uterus. In this sagittal view, the markedly thickened endometrium, which is measured by the calipers, suggests endometrial hyperplasia. *(Image contributed by Dr. Elysia Moschos.)*

selected for evaluation of abnormal bleeding (Merisio, 2005). Grossly, hyperplastic endometrium is not distinctive, and thus, direct visual identification using hysteroscopy is inaccurate (Garuti, 2006).

Occasionally, an adnexal mass may be palpable on examination. Although this most likely is a benign ovarian cyst, any solid features noted during transvaginal sonography should raise the possibility of a coexisting ovarian granulosa cell tumor. These tumors produce an excessive estrogenic environment that results in up to a 30-percent risk of endometrial hyperplasia or less commonly, carcinoma (Chap. 36, p. 889) (Ayhan, 1994).

Treatment

Management of women with endometrial hyperplasia mainly depends on a patient's age, presence or absence of cytologic atypia, and risks for surgery. However, nonsurgical therapy is inherently risky due to the inconsistency of diagnosis and uncertainty in predicting the stability or progression of individual lesions. Specifically, a number of studies have documented

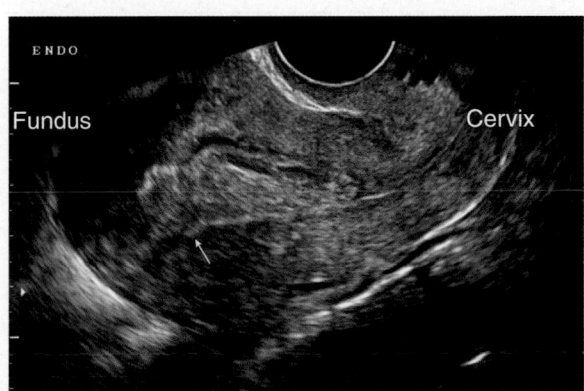

FIGURE 33-4 Transvaginal sonographic image of a uterus. In this sagittal view, a markedly thickened endometrium and evidence of myometrial invasion at the fundus (*arrow*) suggest endometrial cancer. *(Image contributed by Dr. Elysia Moschos.)*

low reproducibility for WHO classifications of endometrial hyperplasia (Allison, 2008; Sherman, 2008; Zaino, 2006). In addition, there is no way to anticipate which types will involute with progestin therapy. However, as long as an endometrial sample is representative and a provider has no reason to suspect a coexisting invasive carcinoma, the decision to treat endometrial hyperplasia through hormonal or surgical means relies on clinical judgment.

Nonatypical Endometrial Hyperplasia

Premenopausal Women. Premenopausal women with nonatypical endometrial hyperplasia typically require a 3- to 6-month course of low-dose progestin therapy. Cyclic medroxyprogesterone acetate (MPA) (Provera) given orally for 12 to 14 days each month at a dose of 10 to 20 mg daily is commonly used. Another frequently used option is to initiate a combination oral contraceptive pill in those without contraindications. Progesterone-containing IUDs have been shown to be effective in small case series (Gallos, 2010; Scarselli, 2011; Wildemeersch, 2007). Although lesions may spontaneous regress without therapy, progestins are generally used to address the underlying etiology, that is, chronic anovulation and excess estrogen (Terakawa, 1997). If there is no residual hyperplastic endometrium found during surveillance biopsy, then patients should be continued on progestins and observed until menopause. Additional endometrial biopsy is required for new bleeding.

In general, biopsies should be avoided when a patient is taking progestins, as this hormone confounds the pathologic diagnosis through modification of endometrial morphology. Endometrial shedding during a withdrawal bleed is also an integral component of the medical ablation process that should be completed before assessing persistence. Waiting 2 to 6 weeks after hormonal withdrawal and abstaining from restarting progestins before biopsy solves these problems. In those with a levonorgestrel-releasing IUD, endometrial biopsy can be performed without device removal.

Postmenopausal Women. Postmenopausal women with nonatypical endometrial hyperplasia may also be treated with low-dose cyclic MPA or a continuous 2.5-mg daily regimen. However, it is particularly important in older women to be confident that an adequate sample has been obtained to exclude cytologic atypia. A D&C may be indicated in some circumstances. For instance, occasionally tissue volume with Pipelle sampling is scant, or bleeding symptoms are more prominent than expected.

In practice, postmenopausal patients with simple hyperplasia are often followed without therapy. Complex hyperplasia without atypia is usually treated chronically with progestins. Office endometrial biopsy is performed annually.

Response of Nonatypical Endometrial Hyperplasia to Progestins. The overall clinical and pathologic regression rates of progestin therapy exceed 90 percent for nonatypical endometrial hyperplasia (Rattanachaiyanont, 2005). Patients with persistent disease on repeated biopsy should be switched to a higher dose regimen such as MPA, 40 to 100 mg daily, or megestrol acetate (Megace), 160 mg daily. Again, a clinician must confirm that hormonal ablation has occurred by resampling the endometrium after a suitable therapeutic interval. Hysterectomy should also be reconsidered for lesions that are refractory to medical management.

Minimally invasive surgical approaches such as total laparoscopic hysterectomy are appropriate options. However, in cases in which there is any suspicion for atypical hyperplasia, removal of the uterus in toto and without morcellation is preferred. Because the lesion may extend into the lower uterine segment or upper endocervix, supracervical hysterectomy is not appropriate for women undergoing hysterectomy for treatment of endometrial hyperplasia.

Atypical Endometrial Hyperplasia

Hysterectomy is the best treatment for women at any age with atypical endometrial hyperplasia because the risk of concurrent subclinical invasive malignancy is high (Horn, 2004; Trimble, 2006). Premenopausal women who strongly wish to preserve fertility are the main exception. High-dose progestin therapy may be most appropriate for highly motivated patients (Randall, 1997). Poor surgical candidates may also warrant an attempt at hormonal ablation with progestins. Resolution of the hyperplasia must be confirmed by serial endometrial biopsies every 3 months until response is documented. Otherwise, hysterectomy should be recommended (American College of Obstetricians and Gynecologists, 2005). Following hyperplasia resolution, surveillance and progestins should continue long-term due to the potential for eventual progression to carcinoma (Rubatt, 2005).

The Gynecologic Oncology Group (GOG) performed a prospective cohort study of 289 patients who had a diagnosis of atypical endometrial hyperplasia in the community. Participants underwent hysterectomy within 3 months of their biopsy, and 43 percent were found to have a concurrent endometrial carcinoma (Trimble, 2006). Suh-Burgmann and associates (2009) found a similarly high number of 48 percent. Results demonstrate the difficulty of trying to make an accurate diagnosis before hysterectomy and the potential risks of conservative hormonal treatment.

Generalists in obstetrics and gynecology who perform hysterectomy for atypical endometrial hyperplasia should be especially wary of the possibility of invasive malignancy and the need for surgical staging. At a minimum, peritoneal washings should be obtained prior to performing a hysterectomy. In addition, the uterus should be opened and examined in the operating room, and frozen section can be performed. Any suspicion for myometrial invasion is an appropriate indication for intraoperative consultation with a gynecologic oncologist.

ENDOMETRIAL CANCER

Pathogenesis

Endometrial cancer is a biologically and histologically diverse group of neoplasms characterized by a dualistic model of pathogenesis. Type I endometrioid adenocarcinomas comprise 75 percent of all cases. They are estrogen-dependent, low grade, and derived from atypical endometrial hyperplasia. In contrast, type II cancers usually have serous or clear cell histology, no precursor lesion, and a more aggressive clinical course (Table 33-3).

TABLE 33-3. Type I and II Endometrial Carcinoma: Distinguishing Features

Feature	Type I	Type II
Unopposed estrogen	Present	Absent
Menopausal status	Pre- and perimenopausal	Postmenopausal
Hyperplasia	Present	Absent
Race	White	Black
Grade	Low	High
Myometrial invasion	Minimal	Deep
Specific subtypes	Endometrioid	Serous, clear cell
Behavior	Stable	Aggressive

From Kurman, 1994, with permission.

The morphologic and clinical differences are paralleled by genetic distinctions, in that type I and II tumors carry mutations of independent sets of genes (Bansal, 2009; Hecht, 2006).

The two pathways of endometrial cancer pathogenesis obviously have significant overlap and result in a spectrum of histologic features. However, this dualistic view has therapeutic ramifications for novel treatment strategies that target high-risk disease (Cerezo, 2006).

Prevention
Screening

There is currently no role for routine screening of endometrial cancer for women at average risk or increased risk. Instead, at the onset of menopause, women should be informed about the risks and symptoms of endometrial cancer and strongly encouraged to report any unexpected bleeding or spotting to their health care provider (American College of Obstetricians and Gynecologists, 2006; Smith, 2011).

However, annual screening by endometrial sampling should begin at age 35 years in women at high risk for endometrial cancer due to HNPCC (Burke, 1997; Smith, 2011). Criteria for screening potential mutation carriers of this syndrome include colorectal or other Lynch syndrome-associated cancers in three first-degree relatives, occurring in at least two successive generations, and in one individual under the age of 50 years. Lynch syndrome cancers include colon, endometrium, small bowel, renal pelvis and ureter, and ovary, among others (Vasen, 1999). Referral for genetic counseling can further clarify the risk to predict which patients may benefit from specific germline testing (Balmana, 2006; Chen, 2006). Endometrial cancer is the most common "sentinel cancer," thus, obstetrician-gynecologists play a pivotal role in the identification of women with HNPCC (Lu, 2005).

Prophylactic Surgery

Since women with HNPCC have such a high lifetime risk of developing endometrial cancer (40 to 60 percent), prophylactic hysterectomy is another option. In a cohort of 315 HNPCC-

mutation carriers, Schmeler (2006) confirmed the benefit of this approach by reporting a 100-percent risk reduction. In general, BSO should also be performed due to the 10- to 12-percent lifetime risk of ovarian cancer.

Diagnosis
Signs and Symptoms

Early diagnosis of endometrial cancer is almost entirely dependent on the prompt recognition and evaluation of irregular vaginal bleeding. In premenopausal women, a clinician must maintain a high index of suspicion for a history of prolonged, heavy menstruation or intermenstrual spotting, because many other benign disorders give rise to similar symptoms (Table 8-2, p. 225). Postmenopausal bleeding is particularly worrisome, leading to a 5- to 10-percent likelihood of diagnosing endometrial carcinoma (Gredmark, 1995; Iatrakis, 1997). Abnormal vaginal discharge may be another symptom in older women.

Unfortunately, some patients do not seek medical attention despite months or years of heavy, irregular bleeding. In more advanced disease, pelvic pressure and pain may reflect uterine enlargement or extrauterine tumor spread. Patients with serous or clear cell tumors often present with signs and symptoms suggestive of advanced epithelial ovarian cancer (Chap. 35, p. 860).

Papanicolaou Test

Historically, the Pap smear has not been a sensitive tool to diagnose endometrial cancer, and 50 percent of women with endometrial cancer will have normal findings (Gu, 2001). Liquid-based cytology appears to increase the detection of glandular abnormalities, but not enough to cause a shift in clinical practice (Guidos, 2000; Schorge, 2002).

Benign endometrial cells are occasionally recorded on a routine Pap smear report in women 40 years and older. In premenopausal women, this is often a finding of limited importance, especially if a smear is obtained following menses. However, postmenopausal women with such findings have nearly a

3- to 5-percent risk of endometrial cancer (Simsir, 2005). In those using hormone replacement therapy, the prevalence of benign endometrial cells on smears is increased, and the risk of malignancy is less (1 to 2 percent) (Mount, 2002). Although endometrial biopsy should be considered in asymptomatic postmenopausal women if this finding is reported, most patients ultimately diagnosed with hyperplasia or cancers have concomitant abnormal bleeding (Ashfaq, 2001).

In contrast, atypical glandular cells found during Pap smear screening carry higher risks for underlying cervical or endometrial neoplasia. Accordingly, evaluation of a glandular abnormality includes colposcopy and endocervical curettage. It may also include endometrial sampling in nonpregnant patients older than 35 years or in those younger if there is a history of abnormal bleeding, if risk factors for endometrial disease are noted, or if the cytology specifies that the atypical glandular cells are of endometrial origin.

Endometrial Sampling

Office Pipelle biopsy is preferred for the initial evaluation of women with bleeding suspicious for malignancy (Feldman, 1993). However, if sampling techniques fail to provide sufficient diagnostic information or if abnormal bleeding persists, D&C may be required to clarify the diagnosis (Gordon, 1999).

Outpatient hysteroscopy is more sensitive for focal endometrial lesions and thus has proved less helpful in diagnosing hyperplasia (Ben Yehuda, 1998). Moreover, in those cases in which hysteroscopy is used to evaluate abnormal bleeding and in which cancer is ultimately diagnosed, an increased incidence of positive peritoneal cytology has been noted during subsequent staging surgery (Obermair, 2000; Polyzos, 2010; Zerbe, 2000). Although there may be a risk of peritoneal contamination by cancer cells with hysteroscopy, patient prognosis overall does not appear to be worsened (Cicinelli, 2010; Revel, 2004).

Laboratory Testing

The only clinically useful tumor marker in the management of endometrial cancer is measurement of a serum CA125 level.

Preoperatively, an elevated level indicates the possibility of more advanced disease (Powell, 2005). In practice, it is most useful in patients with advanced disease or serous subtypes to assist in monitoring response to therapy or during posttreatment surveillance. However, even in this setting, its utility in the absence of other clinical findings is limited (Price, 1998).

Imaging Studies

In general, for women with a well-differentiated type I endometrioid tumor, chest radiography is the only required preoperative imaging study. All other preoperative testing is directed toward surgical preparation in general (Chap. 39, p. 958).

Computed tomography (CT) or magnetic resonance (MR) imaging is usually not necessary (American College of Obstetricians and Gynecologists, 2005). However, MR imaging can occasionally help distinguish an endometrial cancer with cervical extension from a primary endocervical adenocarcinoma (Nagar, 2006). Moreover, women with serous features or other high-risk histology on preoperative biopsy and those with physical examination findings suggesting advanced disease are most appropriate for abdominopelvic CT scanning (Fig. 33-5). In these cases, advance knowledge of intraabdominal disease may be helpful in guiding treatment.

■ Role of the Generalist

Although most endometrial cancers are cured by hysterectomy and BSO, primary management by gynecologic oncologists results in an efficient use of health care resources, minimizes potential morbidity, more likely leads to staging, and improves the survival of patients with high-risk disease (Chan, 2011; Roland, 2004). Therefore, preoperative consultation is generally advisable for any patient with endometrial cancer who is being prepared for surgery by a generalist in obstetrics and gynecology. Young or perimenopausal women with grade 1 endometrioid adenocarcinoma in a background of atypical endometrial hyperplasia are possible exceptions. However,

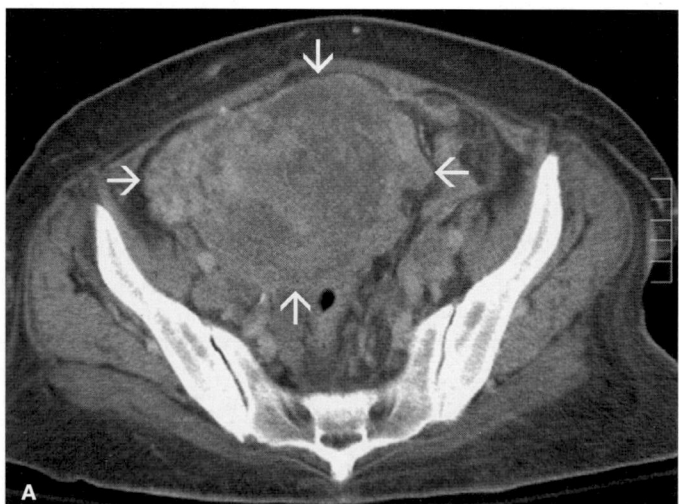
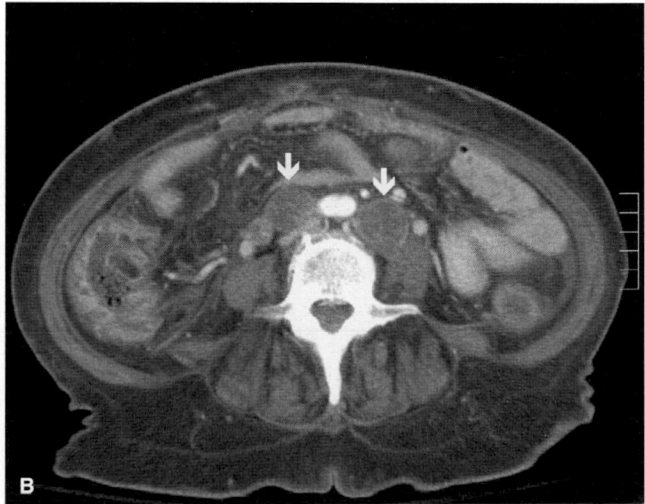

FIGURE 33-5 Computed-tomographic (CT) images in the axial plane of a 61-year-old woman with endometrial cancer. **A.** Massively enlarged and inhomogeneous uterus (*arrows*) in the upper pelvis. **B.** At the level of the aortic bifurcation, enlarged lymph nodes are seen bilaterally (*arrows*) consistent with lymph node involvement. *(Images contributed by Dr. Diane Twickler.)*

the old axiom of a nodal dissection not being required for a grade 1 tumor no longer applies because many patients will have more advanced disease than predicted by preoperative prognostic factors. In addition, intraoperative evaluation of depth of invasion is less accurate than previously thought (Frumovitz, 2004a; Leitao, 2008).

Postoperatively, a gynecologic oncologist should be consulted whenever there is evidence for cervical extension, extrauterine disease, or positive peritoneal washings. In many cases, early-stage patients treated by surgery alone will return to their primary obstetrician-gynecologist for surveillance. Consultation is again recommended if recurrent disease is diagnosed or suspected.

When an endometrial cancer is unexpectedly diagnosed after hysterectomy performed by a generalist for other indications, consultation is also recommended. Possible therapeutic options include no further therapy and surveillance only, reoperation to complete surgical staging, or radiotherapy to prevent local recurrence. In general, the survival advantages of staging must be weighed against the complications from another surgical procedure (American College of Obstetricians and Gynecologists, 2005). Fortunately, the advent of laparoscopic and robotic restaging has resulted in the potential for less morbidity in selected cases (Spirtos, 2005).

Pathology

There is a broad spectrum of aggressiveness within the histopathologic types of endometrial cancer (Table 33-4). Most patients have endometrioid adenocarcinomas that behave indolently. However, some will have an unfavorable histology that portends a much more aggressive tumor. In addition, the degree of tumor differentiation is an important predictor of disease spread. Tumors that arise following pelvic radiation differ from sporadic endometrial cancers by having a preponderance of high-stage, high-grade, and high-risk histologic subtypes (Pothuri, 2003). Effectively managing women with endometrial cancer requires an understanding of these interrelated clinical features.

TABLE 33-4. World Health Organization Histologic Classification of Endometrial Carcinoma

Endometrioid adenocarcinoma
  Variant with squamous differentiation
  Villoglandular variant
  Secretory variant
  Ciliated cell variant
Mucinous carcinoma
Serous carcinoma
Clear cell carcinoma
Mixed cell carcinoma
Squamous cell carcinoma
Small cell carcinoma
Undifferentiated carcinoma
Others

From Silverberg, 2003.

TABLE 33-5. Histopathologic Criteria for Assessing Grade

Grade	Definition
1	≤5% of a nonsquamous or nonmorular solid growth pattern
2	6–50% of a nonsquamous or nonmorular solid growth pattern
3	>50% of a nonsquamous or nonmorular solid growth pattern

From Pecorelli, 1999.

Histologic Grade

The most widely used grading system for endometrial carcinoma is the three-tiered International Federation of Gynecology and Obstetrics (FIGO) system (Table 33-5). Grade 1 lesions typically are indolent with little propensity to spread outside the uterus or recur. Grade 2 tumors have an intermediate prognosis. Grade 3 cancers are associated with an increased potential for myometrial invasion and nodal metastasis.

Histologic grading should primarily be determined microscopically by the tumor's architectural growth pattern (Zaino, 1994). However, there are a few exceptions, and the optimal method for determining grade is somewhat controversial. Nuclear atypia that is inappropriately advanced relative to the architectural grade raises a grade 1 or 2 tumor by one level. For example, a grade 2 lesion based on architectural features may be increased to a grade 3 lesion if significant nuclear atypia is present. This modification was shown to have prognostic utility in a GOG study of 715 endometrioid adenocarcinomas (protocol #33) (Zaino, 1995). Based on the FIGO system, nuclear grading is also used for all serous and clear cell adenocarcinomas (Pecorelli, 1999).

In an effort to improve the reproducibility and prognostic importance of the FIGO system, a binary architectural grading system has been proposed (Lax, 2000; Scholten, 2004). The simplicity of dividing tumors into low-grade lesions and high-grade lesions based on the proportion of solid growth (≤50 percent or >50 percent, respectively) is attractive and appears to have value. This approach, however, has not been widely implemented in clinical practice.

Histologic Type

Endometrioid Adenocarcinoma. The most common histologic type of endometrial cancer is endometrioid adenocarcinoma, accounting for more than 75 percent of cases. This tumor characteristically contains glands that resemble those of the normal endometrium (Fig. 33-6). The concomitant presence of hyperplastic endometrium correlates with a low-grade tumor and a lack of myometrial invasion. However, when the glandular component decreases and is replaced by solid nests and sheets of cells, the tumor is classified as a higher grade (Silverberg, 2003). In addition, an atrophic endometrium is more frequently associated with high-grade lesions that are commonly metastatic (Kurman, 1994).

In addition to the characteristic appearance described, endometrioid adenocarcinomas may display variant forms. These

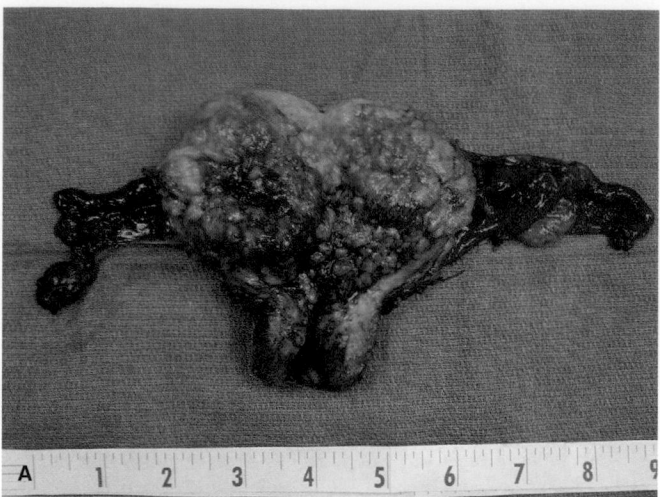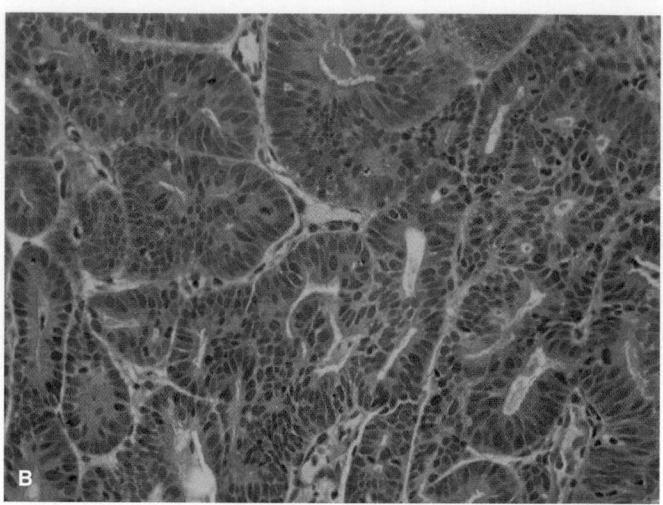

FIGURE 33-6 Endometrioid adenocarcinoma. **A.** Photograph of a uterine specimen with endometrioid adenocarcinoma. Tumor is seen filling the endometrial cavity and invading myometrial walls. **B.** Photomicrograph of endometrioid adenocarcinoma. These tumors are composed of neoplastic glands resembling those of the normal endometrium. Cells are typically tall columnar with mild to moderate nuclear atypia. They form glands that are abnormally crowded or "back-to-back." Gland cribriforming, confluence, and villous structures are also common. It is these architectural forms, with the associated disappearance of intervening stroma, that distinguish well-differentiated endometrioid adenocarcinoma from complex hyperplasia. Better-differentiated endometrioid adenocarcinomas like this example are composed exclusively of glandular structures. In less well-differentiated tumors, cells form solid sheets that may comprise various proportions of the tumor. *(Photograph contributed by Dr. Kelley Carrick.)*

include endometrioid adenocarcinoma with squamous differentiation and villoglandular, secretory, and ciliated cell variants (see Table 33-4 and Fig. 33-7). In general, the biologic behavior of these variant tumors reflects that of classic endometrial adenocarcinoma.

Serous Carcinoma. Accounting for 5 to 10 percent of endometrial cancers, serous carcinoma typifies the highly aggressive type II tumors that arise from the atrophic endometrium

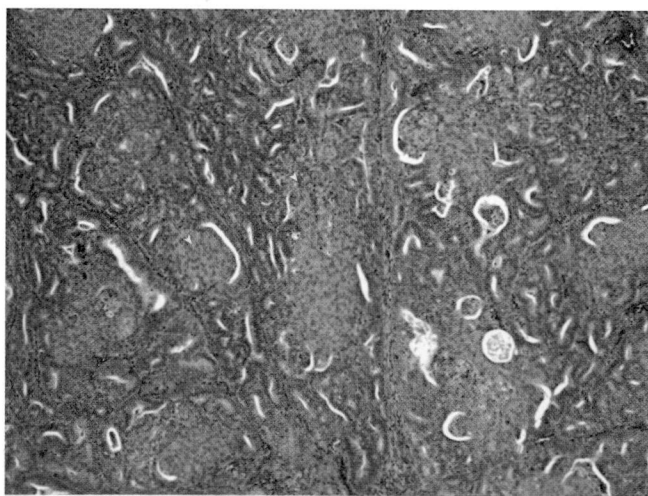

FIGURE 33-7 Endometrioid adenocarcinoma with squamous differentiation. A common feature of endometrioid adenocarcinomas is the presence of foci of squamous differentiation, which may be focal or relatively prominent. The squamous elements may have obvious squamous features such as keratinization or intercellular bridges or may be represented by less well-differentiated squamous morules (*arrows*), as in this example. The squamous elements do not alter the grading of the tumor and are not clinically significant. *(Photograph contributed by Dr. Raheela Ashfaq.)*

of older women (Jordan, 2001). There is typically a complex pattern of papillary growth with cells demonstrating marked nuclear atypia (Fig. 33-8). Commonly referred to as uterine papillary serous carcinoma (UPSC), its histologic appearance resembles epithelial ovarian cancer, and psammoma bodies are seen in 30 percent of cases (Silverberg, 2003).

Grossly, the tumor is exophytic with a papillary appearance emerging from a small, atrophic uterus (see Fig. 33–8). These tumors may occasionally be confined within a polyp and have no evidence for spread (Carcangiu, 1992). However, UPSC has a known propensity for myometrial and lymphatic invasion. Intraperitoneal spread, such as omental caking, which is unusual for typical endometrioid adenocarcinoma, is also common even when myometrial invasion is minimal or absent (Fig. 33-9) (Sherman, 1992). As a result, it may be impossible to distinguish UPSC from epithelial ovarian cancer during surgery. Similar to ovarian carcinoma, these tumors usually secrete CA125. Thus, serial serum measurements are a useful marker to monitor the disease postoperatively. Uterine papillary serous carcinoma is an aggressive cell type, and women with mixed endometrial cancers containing as little as 25 percent of UPSC have the same survival as those with pure uterine serous carcinoma (Ellenson, 2011b).

Clear Cell Carcinoma. Fewer than 5 percent of endometrial cancers are clear cell variants, but this is the other major type II tumor (Abeler, 1991). The microscopic appearance may be predominantly solid, cystic, tubular, or papillary. Most frequently, it consists of a mixture of two or more of these patterns (Fig. 33-10) (Silverberg, 2003).

Endometrial clear cell adenocarcinomas are similar to those arising in the ovary, vagina, and cervix. Grossly, there are no characteristic features, but like UPSC, they tend to be high-grade, deeply invasive tumors. Patients are often diagnosed with advanced disease and have a poor prognosis (Hamilton, 2006).

Mucinous Carcinoma. One to 2 percent of endometrial cancers have a mucinous appearance that comprises more than half of the tumor. However, many endometrioid adenocarcinomas will have this as a focal component (Ross, 1983). Typically, mucinous tumors have a glandular pattern with uniform columnar cells and minimal stratification (Fig. 33-11). Almost all are stage I grade 1 lesions with a good prognosis (Melhem, 1987). Since endocervical epithelium merges with the lower uterine segment, the main diagnostic dilemma is differentiating this tumor from a primary cervical adenocarcinoma. Immunostaining may be helpful, but MR imaging may be required to further clarify the most likely site of origin. For defining anatomy, MR imaging tool offers superior contrast resolution at soft-tissue interfaces.

Mixed Carcinoma. An endometrial cancer may demonstrate combinations of two or more pure types. To be classified as a mixed carcinoma, a component must comprise at least 10 percent of the tumor. Except for serous and clear cell histology, the combination of other types usually has no clinical significance. As a result, mixed carcinoma usually refers to an admixture of a type I (endometrioid adenocarcinoma and its variants) and a type II carcinoma (Silverberg, 2003).

Undifferentiated Carcinoma. In 1 to 2 percent of endometrial cancers, there is no evidence of glandular, sarcomatous, or squamous differentiation. These undifferentiated tumors are characterized by proliferation of medium-sized, monotonous epithelial cells growing in solid sheets with no specific pattern (Silva, 2007). Overall, the prognosis is worse than in patients with poorly differentiated endometrioid adenocarcinomas (Altrabulsi, 2005).

Rare Histologic Types. Fewer than 100 cases of *squamous cell carcinoma* of the endometrium have been reported. Diagnosis requires exclusion of an adenocarcinoma component and no connection with the squamous epithelium of the cervix (Varras, 2002). Typically, the prognosis is poor (Goodman, 1996). *Transitional cell carcinoma* of the endometrium is also rare, and metastatic disease from the bladder or ovary must be excluded during diagnosis (Ahluwalia, 2006).

Patterns of Spread

Endometrial cancers have several different potential ways to spread beyond the uterus (Morrow, 1991). Type I endometrioid tumors and their variants most commonly spread, in order of frequency, by: (1) direct extension, (2) lymphatic metastasis, (3) hematogenous dissemination, and (4) intraperitoneal exfoliation. Type II serous and clear cell carcinomas have a particular propensity for extrauterine disease, in a pattern that closely resembles epithelial ovarian cancer. In general, the various patterns of spread are interrelated and often develop simultaneously.

Invasion of the endometrial stroma and exophytic expansion within the uterine cavity follows initial growth of an early cancer. Over time, the tumor invades the myometrium and may

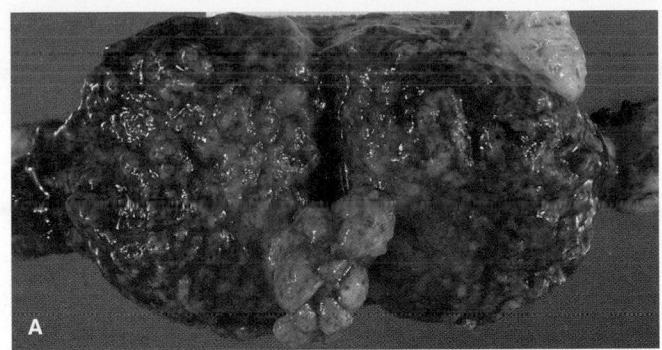
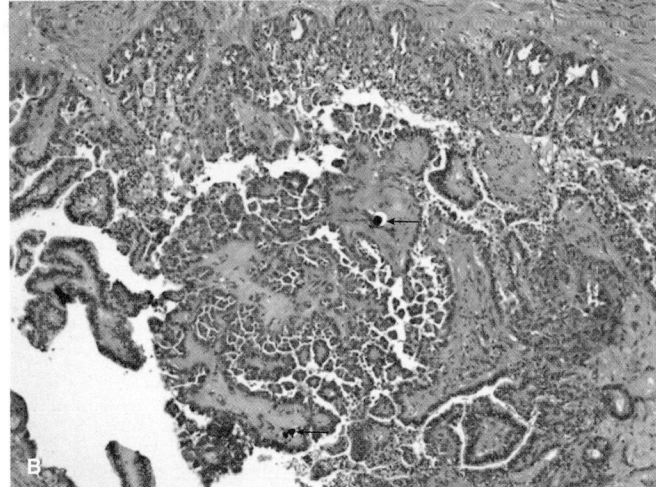
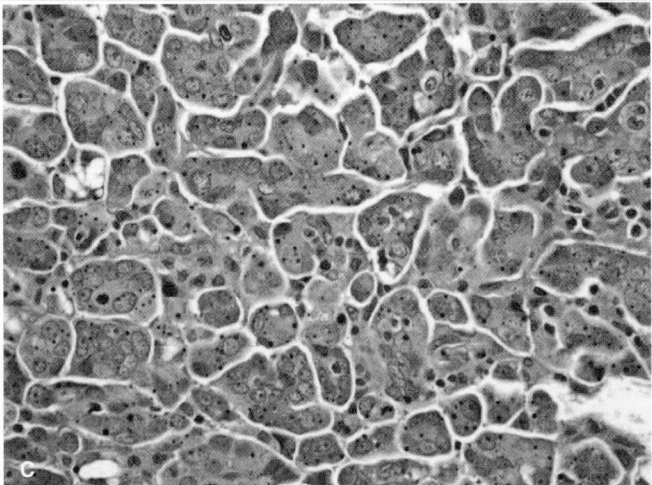

FIGURE 33-8 Uterine papillary serous carcinoma. **A.** Photograph of a uterine specimen. *(Photograph contributed by Dr. Raheela Ashfaq.)* **B.** Photomicrographs of uterine papillary serous carcinoma. This cancer is a high-grade adenocarcinoma with a morphologic appearance similar to its more common counterpart in the ovary or fallopian tube. The tumor is typically characterized by a papillary architecture. Psammoma bodies, which are concentrically laminated calcifications *(arrows)*, may be present. **C.** Cells are typically rounded as opposed to columnar. They have high-grade nuclear features including relatively large, pleomorphic nuclei; prominent nucleoli; and frequent, abnormal mitoses. Multinucleate tumor cells are also common. *(Photomicrographs contributed by Dr. Kelley Carrick.)*

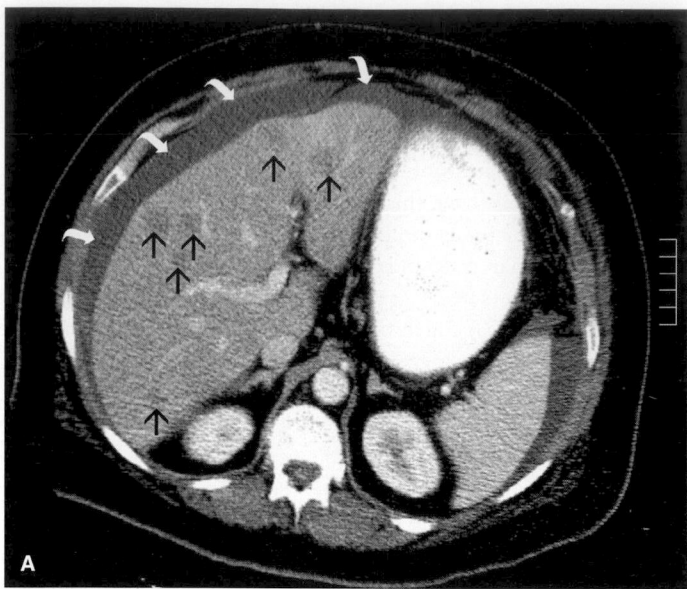
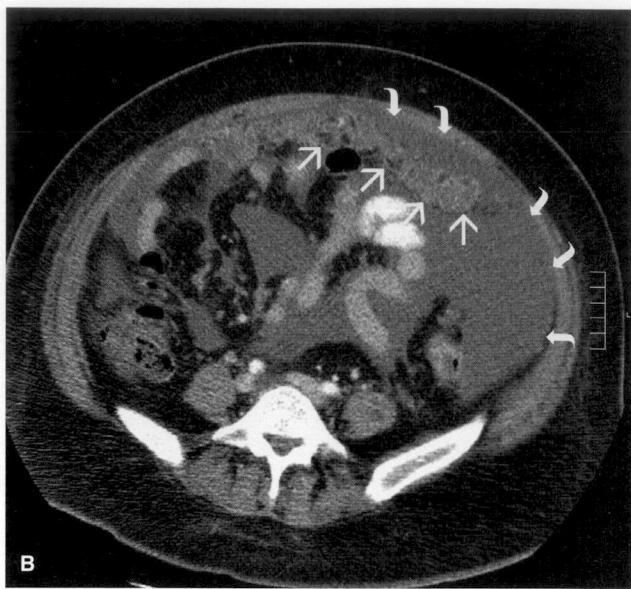

FIGURE 33-9 Computed-tomographic (CT) images of liver metastases, ascites, and omental caking in a 51-year-old woman with endometrial cancer. **A.** Black arrows demarcate multiple low-density areas in the liver that are consistent with a metastatic process and ascites *(curved, white arrows)* surrounding the liver. **B.** A more caudal image reveals omental caking *(white arrows)*, surrounded by massive ascites *(curved, white arrows)*. *(Images contributed by Dr. Diane Twickler.)*

ultimately perforate the serosa (Table 33-6). Tumors situated in the lower uterine segment tend to involve the cervix early, whereas those in the upper corpus tend to extend to the fallopian tubes or serosa. Advanced regional growth may lead to direct invasion into adjacent pelvic structures, including the bladder, large bowel, vagina, and broad ligament.

Lymphatic channel invasion and metastasis to the pelvic and paraaortic nodal chains can follow tumor penetration of the myometrium (Table 33-7). The lymphatic network draining the uterus is complex, and patients can have metastases to any single nodal group as well as combinations of groups (Burke, 1996). This haphazard pattern is in contrast to cervical cancer, in which lymphatic spread usually follows a stepwise progression from pelvic to paraaortic to scalene nodal groups.

Hematogenesis dissemination most commonly results in metastases to the lung and less commonly, to the liver, brain, bone, and other sites. Deep myometrial invasion is the strongest predictor of this pattern of spread (Mariani, 2001a).

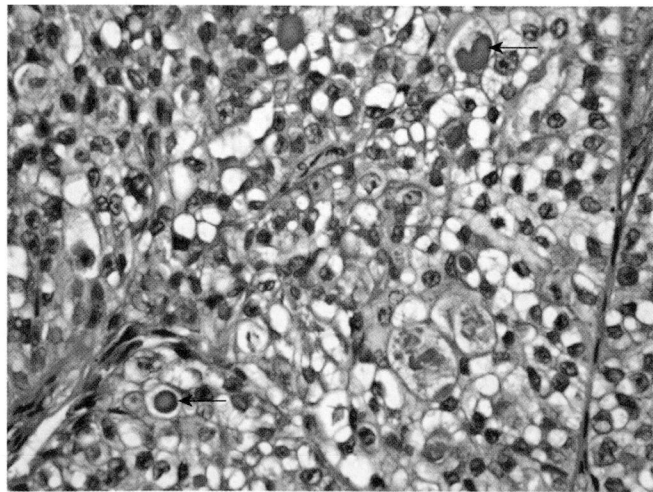

FIGURE 33-10 Clear cell adenocarcinoma–solid type. This tumor is composed of cells with clear to eosinophilic granular cytoplasm. Cells are arranged in papillae, sheets, tubulocystic structures, or some combination of these. Eosinophilic hyaline globules *(arrows)* are a common feature. Here, cells have the clear cytoplasm and distinct cell membranes characteristic of this tumor. Nuclei are moderately pleomorphic, with nucleolar prominence. *(Photograph contributed by Dr. Kelley Carrick.)*

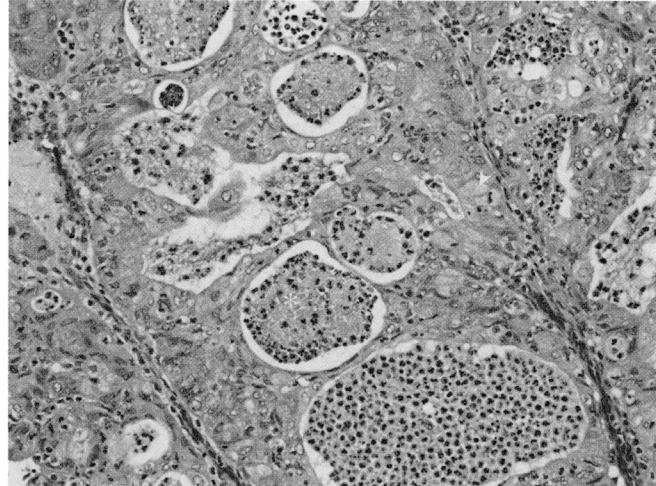

FIGURE 33-11 Photomicrograph of mucinous carcinoma. Mucinous adenocarcinoma of the endometrium is a relatively rare type of endometrial adenocarcinoma in which most of the tumor cells contain intracytoplasmic mucin. In this example, tumor cells form sheets and cribriform structures, and many contain delicate bluish intracytoplasmic mucin *(arrow)*. Cribriform spaces in the tumor contain bluish mucin *(asterisk)* and numerous neutrophils. *(Photograph contributed by Dr. Kelley Carrick.)*

TABLE 33-6. Correlation of Histologic Grade and Depth of Myometrial Invasion in Stage I Patients (*n* = 5095)

Myometrial Invasion	Grade		
	1	2	3
None	29%	11%	15%
≤50%	51%	59%	46%
>50%	20%	30%	39%

Modified from Creasman, 2006, with permission.

Retrograde transtubal transport of exfoliated endometrial cancer cells is one mechanism by which malignant cells reach the peritoneal cavity. Serosal perforation of the tumor is another possible pathway. Most types of endometrial cancer cells found in the peritoneal cavity disappear within a short time and have low malignant potential (Hirai, 2001). Alternatively, in the presence of other high-risk features, such as adnexal metastases or serous histology, widespread intraabdominal disease may result.

Port-site metastasis is a rare but potential method of cancer spread. Martínez and coworkers (2010) evaluated nearly 300 laparoscopic staging procedures for endometrial cancer. Port-site metastases complicated 0.33 percent of cases.

Treatment

Surgical Staging

Patients with endometrial cancer should undergo hysterectomy, BSO, and surgical staging using the revised FIGO system (Table 33-8 and Fig. 33-12) (Mutch, 2009). Almost three quarters of patients are stage I at diagnosis (Table 33-9). Only a few circumstances contraindicate primary surgery and include a desire to preserve fertility, massive obesity, high operative risk, and clinically unresectable disease. In general, an extrafascial hysterectomy, also known as type I or simple hysterectomy, is sufficient. However, radical hysterectomy (type III hysterectomy) may be preferable for patients with clinically obvious cervical extension of endometrial cancer (Cornelison, 1999; Mariani, 2001b). Differences in these hysterectomy types are outlined in Table 30-8 (p. 783). Vaginal hysterectomy with or without BSO is another option for those women who can-

not undergo systematic surgical staging due to comorbidities (American College of Obstetricians and Gynecologists, 2005).

For optimal patient management, the histopathologic description of the preoperative biopsy findings is carefully reviewed. For example, papillary serous features should suggest the possibility of intraperitoneal disease in the upper abdomen that may make a vertical incision most appropriate (American College of Obstetricians and Gynecologists, 2005). Traditionally, laparotomy has been the standard approach, but laparoscopic and robotic approaches to surgical staging have become increasingly used for endometrial cancer that appears clinically confined to the uterus.

Staging Laparotomy. Surgery begins with an adequate abdominal incision, most commonly vertical, but targeted to specific patient circumstances. Upon entering the peritoneal cavity, washings are obtained by pouring 50 to 100 mL of sterile saline into the abdomen, manually circulating the fluid, and collecting it for cytologic assessment. Retrieval of ascitic fluid is a perfectly acceptable alternative, but ascites is infrequently encountered. Next, a thorough intraabdominal and pelvic exploration is performed, and suspicious lesions are biopsied or excised.

These preliminary procedures are followed by hysterectomy and BSO. The uterus is opened away from the operating table, and the depth of myometrial penetration may be determined by intraoperative gross examination or microscopic frozen section (Sanjuan, 2006; Vorgias, 2002). Historically, the combination of preoperative biopsy grade and intraoperative assessment of the depth of myometrial invasion were the two factors that a surgeon used to determine whether to proceed with pelvic and paraaortic lymph node dissection. However, more recent studies have challenged this paradigm.

This approach is inconsistent and frequently inadequate. It is difficult to predict with certainty the final histologic grade based on the preoperative biopsy or intraoperative frozen section (Eltabbakh, 2005; Leitao, 2008; Papadia, 2009). In addition, the depth of myometrial invasion determined in the operative room is often inaccurate (Frumovitz, 2004a,b). As a result, complete surgical staging with pelvic and paraaortic lymphadenectomy is recommended by the American College of Obstetricians and Gynecologists (2005) for *all* patients with endometrial cancer. However, nodal staging for all cases of endometrial cancer is controversial (Miller, 2006). Two recent trials did not show improvement in disease-free or overall

TABLE 33-7. Correlation of Histologic Grade and Depth of Myometrial Invasion with Risk of Nodal Metastases

Myometrial Invasion	Pelvic Lymph Nodes			Paraaortic Lymph Nodes		
	G1	G2	G3	G1	G2	G3
None	1%	7%	16%	<1%	2%	5%
≤50%	2%	6%	10%	<1%	2%	4%
>50%	11%	21%	37%	2%	6%	13%

Modified from Creasman, 2006, with permission.

TABLE 33-8. FIGO Staging of Carcinoma of the Endometrium

Stage[a]	Characteristics
I	**Tumor confined to the corpus uteri**
IA	No or less than half myometrial invasion
IB	Invasion equal to or more than half of the myometrium
II	**Tumor invades cervical stroma, but does not extend beyond the uterus[b]**
III	**Local and/or regional spread of the tumor**
IIIA	Tumor invades the serosa of the corpus uteri and/or adnexae[c]
IIIB	Vaginal and/or parametrial involvement[c]
IIIC	Metastases to pelvic and/or paraaortic lymph nodes[c]
IIIC1	Positive pelvic nodes
IIIC2	Positive paraaortic lymph nodes with or without positive pelvic lymph nodes
IV	**Tumor invades bladder and/or bowel mucosa, and/or distant metastases**
IVA	Tumor invasion of bladder and/or bowel mucosa
IVB	Distant metastases, including intraabdominal metastases and/or inguinal lymph nodes

[a]Either G1, G2, or G3.
[b]Endocervical glandular involvement only should be considered as stage I and no longer as stage II.
[c]Positive cytology has to be reported separately without changing the stage.
FIGO = International Federation of Gynecology and Obstetrics.

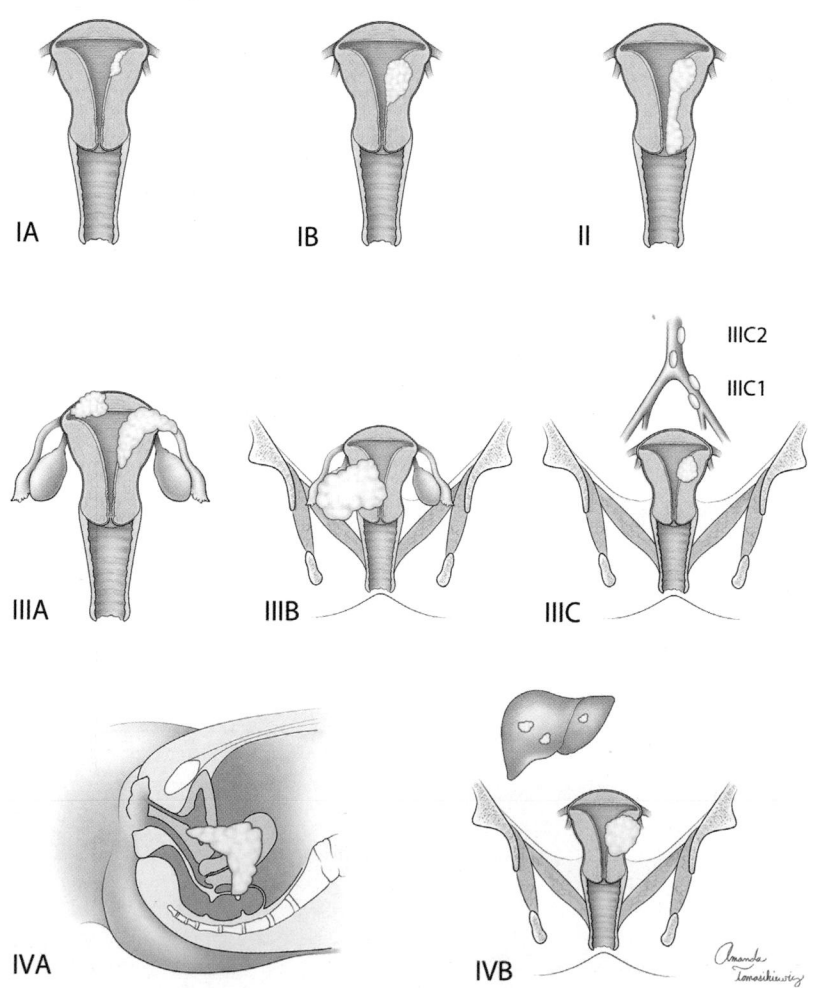

FIGURE 33-12 FIGO (International Federation of Gynecology and Obstetrics) staging of endometrial cancer.

survival rates after lymphadenectomy in early-stage disease (Benedetti Panici, 2008; Kitchener, 2009). Regardless, the concern exists that omitting lymphadenectomy may lead to inappropriate postoperative treatment. At minimum, any suspicious pelvic or paraaortic lymph nodes should be removed. Sentinel lymph node evaluation, as done in vulvar and breast cancers, is being investigated and may become a useful technique in endometrial cancer (Chap. 31, p. 800) (Abu-Rustum, 2009).

Higher nodal counts correlate with improved survival, most likely because of improved staging (Lutman, 2006). In addition, evidence suggests the possibility of a therapeutic benefit from multiple-site lymphadenectomy (Kilgore, 1995). Removal of grossly involved lymph nodes leads to a survival advantage (Havrilesky, 2005). Moreover, microscopic nodal disease may be unknowingly resected and prevent future relapse.

Those patients with serous or clear cell features on preoperative biopsy should have extended surgical staging with an infracolic omentectomy and bilateral peritoneal biopsies of the pelvis, pericolic gutter, and diaphragm (Bristow, 2001a). As in ovarian cancer, a surgeon should also be prepared to resect any metastases (Bristow, 2000).

Laparoscopic Staging. An alternative method of surgical staging combines a laparoscopic approach to both hysterectomy and lymphadenectomy. In general, this approach is best

TABLE 33-9. Distribution of Endometrial Cancer by FIGO Stage (n = 5281 patients)

FIGO Stage	%
I	73
II	11
III	13
IV	3

FIGO = International Federation of Gynecology and Obstetrics.
From Creasman, 2006, with permission.

suited to a select group of women with clinical stage I disease. Previous GOG and other reports described the feasibility of laparoscopic staging of gynecologic cancers (Childers, 1994; Spirtos, 2005). Those studies led to GOG LAP2, the first multicenter randomized trial of laparoscopy for gynecologic cancer. This study addressed the important question of the equivalency of conventional surgery with total abdominal hysterectomy, BSO, and pelvic and paraaortic lymph node dissection versus laparoscopic pelvic and paraaortic lymph node dissection, BSO, and vaginal hysterectomy or total laparoscopic hysterectomy for clinical stage I and IIA endometrial carcinoma. Laparoscopy was completed without conversion in 74 percent of patients randomized to this approach. Advantageously, compared with those undergoing laparotomy, laparoscopy patients had similar rates of intraoperative injuries (9 vs 8 percent), fewer moderate to severe complications (14 vs 21 percent), shorter hospital stays (median 3 vs 4 days), and better quality of life at 6 weeks postoperatively. However, laparoscopic staging was linked with longer operative times (Kornblith, 2009; Walker, 2009). Long-term treatment success is not compromised with laparoscopic staging, and overall survival and recurrence rates in early reports are similar to those for a traditional abdominal approach (Ghezzi, 2010; Magrina, 1999; Zullo, 2009).

Robot-assisted laparoscopic staging of endometrial cancer has been embraced by many gynecologic oncologists to overcome the technical challenges of minimally invasive surgery in an obese patient population. It appears to be feasible and safe (Hoekstra, 2009). Compared with a laparoscopic approach for endometrial cancer staging, both major complication rates and mean number of lymph nodes removed are comparable. However, the robotic approach results in lower blood loss (Cardenas-Goicoechea, 2010; Seamon, 2009).

As described in Section 44-3 (p. 1267), not all women are candidates for minimally invasive surgery. First, extensive adhesive disease may significantly lengthen operative times and obstruct necessary visualization. Additionally, in those with a large bulky uterus, uterine manipulation and visualization may be inadequate. Moreover, morcellation should be avoided in cancer cases. Lastly, as described in Chapter 42 (p. 1095), those with significant cardiopulmonary disease may not tolerate the hypercarbia created by pneumoperitoneum or steep Trendelenburg positioning.

Surveillance

Most surgically treated patients can simply be followed by pelvic examination every 3 to 4 months for the first 2 years and twice yearly for an additional 3 years before returning to annual visits (American College of Obstetricians and Gynecologists, 2005; National Comprehensive Cancer Network, 2010). Pap tests are not a mandatory part of surveillance since they identify an asymptomatic vaginal recurrence in less than 1 percent of patients and are not cost effective (Bristow, 2006a; Cooper, 2006).

Women who have more advanced disease that requires postoperative radiation or chemotherapy or both warrant more aggressive monitoring. Serum CA125 measurements may be valuable, particularly for UPSC. Intermittent imaging using CT scanning or MR imaging may also be indicated. In general, the pattern of recurrent disease depends on the original sites of metastasis and the treatment received.

Chemotherapy

Only three cytotoxic drugs with definite activity have been identified to date: doxorubicin, cisplatin, and paclitaxel (Barrena Medel, 2009). Other agents, 5-fluorouracil, vincristine, ifosfamide, and ixabepilone, have possible activity based on collected data (Miller, 2009a). Paclitaxel (Taxol), doxorubicin (Adriamycin), and cisplatin (TAP) chemotherapy is the adjuvant treatment of choice for advanced endometrial cancer following surgery. In a randomized phase III GOG trial of 273 women (protocol #177), administration of seven courses of TAP was superior to doxorubicin and cisplatin (AP), but toxicity was increased—particularly peripheral neuropathy (Fleming, 2004). A less toxic alternative to TAP chemotherapy is the combination of paclitaxel and carboplatin. Routinely used for the treatment of ovarian cancer, this regimen has also demonstrated efficacy in advanced-stage endometrial cancer and is the community standard (Hoskins, 2001; Sovak, 2006, 2007). A GOG trial comparing TAP to carboplatin and paclitaxel, protocol #209, has recently completed accrual and is awaiting analysis (King, 2009).

In practice, cytotoxic chemotherapy is frequently combined, sequenced, or sandwiched with radiotherapy in patients with advanced endometrial cancer following surgery. To reduce toxicity, directed pelvic or paraaortic radiation is usually employed rather than whole abdominal irradiation (Homesley, 2009; Miller, 2009b).

Radiation

Primary Therapy. Primary radiation therapy is usually considered only in rare instances in which a patient is an exceptionally poor surgical candidate. Intracavitary brachytherapy such as Heyman capsules with or without external beam pelvic radiation is the typical method (Chap. 28, p. 721). In general, the survival rate is 10 to 15 percent lower than that with surgical treatment (Chao, 1996; Fishman, 1996). These poor results suggest that a careful preoperative evaluation and appropriate consultation be undertaken before denying any woman the benefits of hysterectomy (American College of Obstetricians and Gynecologists, 2005).

Adjuvant Therapy. As with many other malignancies, patients with grossly resected endometrial cancer who are thought to be at risk for recurrence because of uterine factors or extrauterine metastasis are offered adjuvant therapy. Traditionally, patients in these circumstances have been offered radiation therapy, particularly if the volume of tissue at risk could be safely contained within a radiation treatment field. If not, hormonal or chemotherapy might have been offered. Recent trials have suggested that these approaches could be improved with the addition of or substitution with chemotherapy (Miller, 2009b).

The use of postoperative radiation in women with stage I disease is highly controversial due to the low relapse rate and the scarcity of data from randomized trials. Most patients with lower-risk surgical stage I disease may be counseled that postoperative radiation therapy can reduce the risk of recurrence in the vagina and pelvis. However, the cost and toxicity should be balanced with the evidence that does not support improved survival or reduced distant metastasis rates. The use of radiation in early-stage disease has been evaluated in three major trials, all of which demonstrated that adjuvant radiation improved local disease control and recurrence-free survival rates but did not decrease the rate of distant metastases or improve overall survival rates at 5 years (Aalders, 1980; Creutzberg, 2001, 2004; Keys, 2004). The Gynecologic Oncology Group (GOG) trial found that the reduction in recurrence risk was particularly evident in a high-intermediate risk subgroup of women with three risk factors (grade 2 or 3 tumors, lymphovascular invasion, and invasion of the outer third of the myometrium); in those ≥50 years with two of these risk factors; and in those ≥70 years with one risk factor (Keys, 2004). These risk factors have found their way into both clinical management and the design of more contemporary endometrial cancer trials.

The efficacy of postoperative radiotherapy is even harder to decipher among women with surgical stage II endometrial adenocarcinoma. Most data consist of retrospective, single-institution experiences, and there is evidence to support external beam pelvic radiation, vaginal brachytherapy, both, or no further treatment (Ayhan, 2004; Calvin, 1999; Cannon, 2009; Rittenberg, 2005). Currently, there is no standard approach, and most patients are treated individually based on analysis of coexisting risk factors (Feltmate, 1999).

In most women with stage III endometrial cancer, chemotherapy and/or tumor-directed postoperative external beam radiation is indicated (Barrena-Medel, 2009; Homesley, 2009). Most commonly, radiation therapy is specifically directed at pelvic disease, but may be extended to the paraaortic area if metastases are detected.

Few patients with stage IV disease are candidates for radiotherapy with curative intent. Infrequently, a locally confined stage IVA tumor may be an exception. With stage IV disease, intraperitoneal metastases most often lie outside a tolerated radiation field. Therefore, whole abdominal irradiation is not generally preferable to chemotherapy (Randall, 2006). As a result, the role of radiotherapy is generally palliative in these women (Goff, 1994).

Hormonal Therapy

Primary Treatment. One of the unique characteristics of endometrial cancer is its hormonal responsiveness. Rarely, progestin treatment is used for primary treatment of women with excessively high operative risk. This may be the only feasible palliative option in a few exceptional circumstances. In other uncommon situations of clinical stage I disease and grade 1 adenocarcinoma in a poor surgical candidate, an intrauterine progestational device may be useful. In general, this strategy should be used with great caution (Dhar, 2005; Montz, 2002).

Adjuvant Hormonal Therapy. Single-agent progestins have shown activity in women with advanced disease (Lentz, 1996; Thigpen, 1999). Tamoxifen modulates the expression of the progesterone receptor and is postulated to thereby improve progestin therapy efficacy. Clinically, high response rates have been noted with tamoxifen used adjunctively with progestin therapy (Fiorica, 2004; Whitney, 2004). In general, toxicity is very low, but this combination is most commonly used for recurrent disease.

Estrogen Replacement Therapy. Due to the presumed role of excess estrogen in the development of endometrial cancer, there has historically been great concern that use of estrogen in women with known endometrial cancer could feasibly increase the risk of recurrence or death. However, such an effect has not been observed (Suriano, 2001). The GOG attempted to determine the effect of estrogen replacement therapy by randomly assigning 1236 women who had undergone surgery for stage I and II endometrial cancer to receive either estrogen or placebo. Although the study did not meet its enrollment goals, the low recurrence rate (2 percent) was promising (Barakat, 2006). Because of the potential risks and lack of proven safety, women should be carefully counseled before beginning a regimen of postoperative estrogen for menopausal symptoms.

Management of Uterine Papillary Serous Carcinoma

This most aggressive type of endometrial carcinoma is rare, and thus, randomized trials are difficult to perform. As a result, most data are single-institution, retrospective analyses. Treatment is usually individualized but is often different from typical endometrioid adenocarcinoma.

If a preoperative biopsy demonstrates serous features, comprehensive surgical staging for UPSC is recommended. This includes total abdominal hysterectomy, BSO, peritoneal washings, pelvic/paraaortic lymph node dissection, infracolic omentectomy, and peritoneal biopsies (Chan, 2003). Even noninvasive disease is often widely metastatic (Gehrig, 2001). Fortunately, patients tend to have a good prognosis if surgical staging confirms that disease is confined to the uterus (stage I/II) (Grice, 1998).

Occasionally, no residual UPSC is evident on the hysterectomy specimen, or the tumor minimally involves the tip of a polyp. These women with surgical stage IA can safely be observed. However, all other patients with stage I disease should be considered for adjuvant treatment. One effective strategy is to treat women with stage I disease postoperatively using paclitaxel and carboplatin for three to six cycles along with concomitant vaginal brachytherapy (Dietrich, 2005; Kelly, 2005). However, some data suggest an intrinsic radioresistance for UPSC tumors (Martin, 2005). In addition, based on the largest reported retrospective review of surgical stage I patients, Huh and coworkers (2003) questioned the benefit of any radiation therapy.

Women with stage II UPSC are more likely to benefit from pelvic radiotherapy with or without chemotherapy following surgery. Those having stage III disease are especially prone to have recurrent disease at distant sites. Accordingly, paclitaxel and carboplatin should be considered in addition to tumor-directed radiotherapy after surgery (Bristow, 2001a; Slomovitz, 2003).

In practice, many patients will have stage IVB disease. Aggressive surgical cytoreduction is perhaps most important, because one of the strongest predictors of overall survival is the amount of residual disease. Postoperatively, at least six cycles of paclitaxel and carboplatin chemotherapy are indicated (Barrena-Medel, 2009; Bristow, 2001b; Moller, 2004). Alternatively, enrollment in a clinical trial is another option for eligible patients.

Fertility-Sparing Management

Hormonal therapy without hysterectomy is an option in carefully selected young women with endometrial cancer who desperately wish to preserve their fertility. Careful selection can be aided by a reproductive endocrinology consultation that can clarify for the patient what her likelihood of conception is. Importantly, many of the biologic processes that lead to the endometrial cancer also contribute to decreased fertility. In general, this strategy should only apply to those with grade 1 [type I tumors] adenocarcinomas and no imaging evidence of myometrial invasion. Rarely, women with grade 2 lesions may be considered candidates, although it may advisable to further assess their disease laparoscopically (Morice, 2005). The aim of hormonal treatment is to reverse the lesion. However, any type of medical management obviously involves inherent risk that a patient must be willing to accept (Yang, 2005).

Progestins are the most commonly used agents. Megestrol acetate, 160 mg given orally daily, has demonstrated efficacy. Alternatively, MPA may be delivered by oral or intramuscular administration at varying doses (Gotlieb, 2003). Combinations of progestin therapy with tamoxifen and gonadotropin-releasing hormone agonists are less frequently used (Wang, 2002). Regardless of the hormonal agent, recurrence rates are high during long-term observation (Gorlieb, 2003; Niwa, 2005).

Women receiving fertility-sparing conservative management must be carefully monitored by repeated endometrial biopsy or D&C every 3 months to assess treatment efficacy. If there is evidence for persistence, then the regimen may need to be changed or the dose increased. Hysterectomy and operative staging should be recommended if a lesion does not regress with hormonal therapy or if disease progression is suspected.

Delivery of a healthy infant is a feasible expectation for those patients who respond to treatment and have normal histologic findings in surveillance endometrial samplings. However, assisted reproductive technologies may be required to achieve pregnancy in some cases. Postpartum, patients should again be regularly monitored for recurrent endometrial adenocarcinoma (Ferrandina, 2005). In general, women should undergo hysterectomy at completion of childbearing or whenever the preservation of fertility is no longer desired.

Prognostic Factors

Many clinical and pathologic factors influence the likelihood of endometrial cancer recurrence and survival (Table 33-10) (Lurain, 1991; Schink, 1991). Of these, FIGO surgical stage is the most important overriding variable because it incorporates many of the most important risk factors (Table 33-11).

TABLE 33-10. Poor Prognostic Variables in Endometrial Cancer

Advanced surgical stage
Older age
Histologic type: UPSC or clear cell adenocarcinoma
Advanced tumor grade
Presence of myometrial invasion
Presence of lymphovascular space invasion
Peritoneal cytology positive for cancer cells
Increased tumor size
High tumor expression levels of ER and PR

ER = estrogen receptor; PR = progesterone receptor; UPSC = uterine papillary serous carcinoma.

TABLE 33-11. Endometrial Cancer 5-Year Survival Rates for Each Surgical Stage (n = 5562 Patients)

FIGO Stage	Survival (%)
IA	91
IB	88
IC	81
IIA	77
IIB	67
IIIA	60
IIIB	41
IIIC	32
IVA	20
IVB	5

FIGO = International Federation of Gynecology and Obstetrics.
From Creasman, 2006, with permission.

Metastatic disease to the adnexa, pelvic/paraaortic lymph nodes, and peritoneal surfaces is reflected by the FIGO stage.

Relapse

Patients with recurrent endometrial cancer generally require individualized treatment. In general, the site of relapse is the most important predictor of survival. Depending on the circumstances, surgery, radiation, chemotherapy, or a combination of modalities may be the best strategy. The most curable scenario is an isolated relapse at the vaginal apex in a previously unirradiated patient. These women are usually effectively treated by external beam pelvic radiotherapy. In patients who were previously irradiated, exenteration is often the only curative option (Section 44-5, p. 1276) (Barakat, 1999; Morris, 1996). Nodal recurrences or isolated pelvic disease is more likely to result in progressive disease, regardless of treatment modality. However, either is often an appropriate indication for external beam radiotherapy. Salvage cytoreductive surgery may also be beneficial in selected patients (Awtrey, 2006; Bristow, 2006b).

Widely disseminated endometrial cancer or a relapse not amenable to radiation or surgery is an indication for systemic chemotherapy (Barrena-Medel, 2009). Such patients should be enrolled in an experimental trial, if possible, due to the limited duration of response and the urgent need for more effective therapy. Currently, TAP is thought to be the most active cytotoxic regimen (Fleming, 2004). Paclitaxel and carboplatin is another useful combination widely used in the community that is being compared with TAP in GOG protocol #209 (King, 2009; Sovak, 2007). Progestin therapy with or without tamoxifen is a less toxic option that is particularly useful in selected cases (Fiorica, 2004; Whitney, 2004).

In general, effective palliation of women with incurable, recurrent endometrial cancer requires an ongoing dialogue to achieve the optimal balance between symptomatic relief and treatment toxicity.

REFERENCES

Aalders J, Abeler V, Kolstad P, et al: Postoperative external irradiation and prognostic parameters in stage I endometrial carcinoma: clinical and histopathologic study of 540 patients. Obstet Gynecol 56(4):419, 1980

Aarnio M, Sankila R, Pukkala E, et al: Cancer risk in mutation carriers of DNA-mismatch-repair genes. Int J Cancer 81(2):214, 1999

Abeler VM, Kjorstad KE: Clear cell carcinoma of the endometrium: a histopathological and clinical study of 97 cases. Gynecol Oncol 40(3):207, 1991

Abu-Rustum NR, Khoury-Collado F, Pandit-Taskar N, et al: Sentinel lymph node mapping for grade 1 endometrial cancer: is it the answer to the surgical staging dilemma? Gynecol Oncol 113(2):163, 2009

Ahluwalia M, Light AM, Surampudi K, et al: Transitional cell carcinoma of the endometrium: a case report and review of the literature. Int J Gynecol Pathol 25(4):378, 2006

Allen NE, Tsilidis KK, Key TJ, et al: Menopausal hormone therapy and risk of endometrial carcinoma among postmenopausal women in the European Prospective Investigation into Cancer and Nutrition. Am J Epidemiol 172(12):1394, 2010

Allison KH, Reed SD, Voigt LF, et al: Diagnosing endometrial hyperplasia: why is it so difficult to agree? Am J Surg Pathol 32(5):691, 2008

Altrabulsi B, Malpica A, Deavers MT, et al: Undifferentiated carcinoma of the endometrium. Am J Surg Pathol 29(10):1316, 2005

Amant F, Moerman P, Neven P, et al: Endometrial cancer. Lancet 366(9484):491, 2005

American College of Obstetricians and Gynecologists: Management of endometrial cancer. Practice Bulletin No. 65, August 2005

American College of Obstetricians and Gynecologists: Tamoxifen and uterine cancer. Committee opinion No. 336, June 2006

American College of Obstetricians and Gynecologists: The role of transvaginal ultrasonography in the evaluation of postmenopausal bleeding. Committee Opinion No. 440, August 2009

Anastasiadis PG, Skaphida PG, Koutlaki NG, et al: Descriptive epidemiology of endometrial hyperplasia in patients with abnormal uterine bleeding. Eur J Gynaecol Oncol 21(2):131, 2000

Ashfaq R, Sharma S, Dulley T, et al: Clinical relevance of benign endometrial cells in postmenopausal women. Diagn Cytopathol 25(4):235, 2001

Awtrey CS, Cadungog MG, Leitao MM, et al: Surgical resection of recurrent endometrial carcinoma. Gynecol Oncol 102(3):480, 2006

Ayhan A, Taskiran C, Celik C, et al: The long-term survival of women with surgical stage II endometrioid type endometrial cancer. Gynecol Oncol 93(1):9, 2004

Ayhan A, Tuncer ZS, Tuncer R, et al: Granulosa cell tumor of the ovary. A clinicopathological evaluation of 60 cases. Eur J Gynaecol Oncol 15(4):320, 1994

Baak JP, Mutter GL, Robboy S, et al: The molecular genetics and morphometry-based endometrial intraepithelial neoplasia classification system predicts disease progression in endometrial hyperplasia more accurately than the 1994 World Health Organization classification system. Cancer 103(11):2304, 2005

Balmana J, Stockwell DH, Steyerberg EW, et al: Prediction of MLH1 and MSH2 mutations in Lynch syndrome. JAMA 296(12):1469, 2006

Bansal N, Yendluri V, Wenham RM: The molecular biology of endometrial cancers and the implications for pathogenesis, classification, and targeted therapies. Cancer Control 16(1):8, 2009

Barakat RR, Bundy BN, Spirtos NM, et al: Randomized double-blind trial of estrogen replacement therapy versus placebo in stage I or II endometrial cancer: a Gynecologic Oncology Group Study. J Clin Oncol 24(4):587, 2006

Barakat RR, Goldman NA, Patel DA, et al: Pelvic exenteration for recurrent endometrial cancer. Gynecol Oncol 75(1):99, 1999

Barrena Medel NI, Bansal S, Miller DS, et al: Pharmacotherapy of endometrial cancer. Expert Opin Pharmacother 10(12):1939, 2009

Beiner ME, Finch A, Rosen B, et al: The risk of endometrial cancer in women with BRCA1 and BRCA2 mutations. A prospective study. Gynecol Oncol 104(1):7, 2007

Ben Yehuda OM, Kim YB, Leuchter RS: Does hysteroscopy improve upon the sensitivity of dilatation and curettage in the diagnosis of endometrial hyperplasia or carcinoma? Gynecol Oncol 68:4, 1998

Benedetti Panici P, Basile S, Maneschi F, et al: Systematic pelvic lymphadenectomy vs. no lymphadenectomy in early stage endometrial carcinoma: randomized clinical trial. J Natl Cancer Inst 100:1707, 2008

Breitkopf DM, Frederickson RA, Snyder RR: Detection of benign endometrial masses by endometrial stripe measurement in premenopausal women. Obstet Gynecol 104(1):2004

Brinton LA, Lacey JV Jr, Devesa SS, et al: Epidemiology of uterine corpus cancer. In Gershenson DM, McGuire WP, Gore M, et al (eds): Gynecologic Cancer: Controversies in Management. New York, Churchill Livingstone, 2004, p 190

Bristow RE, Asrari F, Trimble EL, et al: Extended surgical staging for uterine papillary serous carcinoma: survival outcome of locoregional (stage I-III) disease. Gynecol Oncol 81(2):279, 2001a

Bristow RE, Duska LR, Montz FJ: The role of cytoreductive surgery in the management of stage IV uterine papillary serous carcinoma. Gynecol Oncol 81(1):92, 2001b

Bristow RE, Purinton SC, Santillan A, et al: Cost-effectiveness of routine vaginal cytology for endometrial cancer surveillance. Gynecol Oncol 103(2):709, 2006a

Bristow RE, Santillan A, Zahurak ML, et al: Salvage cytoreductive surgery for recurrent endometrial cancer. Gynecol Oncol 103(1):281, 2006b

Bristow RE, Zerbe MJ, Rosenshein NB, et al: Stage IVB endometrial carcinoma: the role of cytoreductive surgery and determinants of survival. Gynecol Oncol 78(2):85, 2000

Burke TW, Levenback C, Tornos C, et al: Intraabdominal lymphatic mapping to direct selective pelvic and paraaortic lymphadenectomy in women with high-risk endometrial cancer: results of a pilot study. Gynecol Oncol 62(2):169, 1996

Burke W, Petersen G, Lynch P, et al: Recommendations for follow-up care of individuals with an inherited predisposition to cancer. I. Hereditary nonpolyposis colon cancer. Cancer Genetics Studies Consortium. JAMA 277(11):915, 1997

Calvin DP, Connell PP, Rotmensch J, et al: Surgery and postoperative radiation therapy in stage II endometrial carcinoma. Am J Clin Oncol 22(4):338, 1999

Cannon GM, Geye H, Terakedis BE, et al: Outcomes following surgery and adjuvant radiation in stage II endometrial adenocarcinoma. Gynecol Oncol 113(2):176, 2009

Carcangiu ML, Chambers JT: Uterine papillary serous carcinoma: a study on 108 cases with emphasis on the prognostic significance of associated endometrioid carcinoma, absence of invasion, and concomitant ovarian carcinoma. Gynecol Oncol 47(3):298, 1992

Cardenas-Goicoechea J, Adams S, Bhat SB, et al: Surgical outcomes of robotic-assisted surgical staging for endometrial cancer are equivalent to traditional laparoscopic staging at a minimally invasive surgical center. Gynecol Oncol 117(2):224, 2010

Cerezo L, Cardenes H, Michael H: Molecular alterations in the pathogenesis of endometrial adenocarcinoma. Therapeutic implications. Clin Transl Oncol 8(4):231, 2006

Chan JK, Loizzi V, Youssef M, et al: Significance of comprehensive surgical staging in noninvasive papillary serous carcinoma of the endometrium. Gynecol Oncol 90(1):181, 2003

Chan JK, Sherman AE, Kapp DS, et al: Influence of gynecologic oncologists on the survival of patients with endometrial cancer. J Clin Oncol 29(7):832, 2011

Chao CK, Grigsby PW, Perez CA, et al: Medically inoperable stage I endometrial carcinoma: a few dilemmas in radiotherapeutic management. Int J Radiat Oncol Biol Phys 34(1):27, 1996

Chen S, Wang W, Lee S, et al: Prediction of germline mutations and cancer risk in the Lynch syndrome. JAMA 296(12):1479, 2006

Childers JM, Spirtos NM, Brainard P, et al: Laparoscopic staging of the patient with incompletely staged early adenocarcinoma of the endometrium. Obstet Gynecol 83(4):597, 1994

Cicinelli E, Tinelli R, Colafiglio G, et al: Risk of long-term pelvic recurrences after fluid minihysteroscopy in women with endometrial carcinoma: a controlled randomized study. Menopause 17(3):511, 2010

Cooper AL, Dornfeld-Finke JM, Banks HW, et al: Is cytologic screening an effective surveillance method for detection of vaginal recurrence of uterine cancer? Obstet Gynecol 107(1):71, 2006

Cornelison TL, Trimble EL, Kosary CL: SEER data, corpus uteri cancer: treatment trends versus survival for FIGO stage II, 1988-1994. Gynecol Oncol 74(3):350, 1999

Creasman W, Odicino F, Maisonneuve P, et al: FIGO 26th Annual Report on the Results of Treatment in Gynecological Cancer. 2006, p 5105

Creasman W, Odicino F, Maisonneuve P, et al: FIGO Annual Report on the Results of Treatment in Gynaecological Cancer. 1998, p 335

Creutzberg CL, van Putten WL, Koper PC, et al: The morbidity of treatment for patients with stage I endometrial cancer: results from a randomized trial. Int J Radiat Oncol Biol Phys 51(5):1246, 2001

Creutzberg CL, van Putten WL, Warlam-Rodenhuis CC, et al: Outcome of high-risk stage IC, grade 3, compared with stage I endometrial carcinoma patients: the Postoperative Radiation Therapy in Endometrial Carcinoma Trial. J Clin Oncol 22(7):1234, 2004

Delin JB, Miller DS, Coleman RL: Other primary malignancies in patients with uterine corpus malignancy. Am J Obstet Gynecol 190:1429, 2004

Dhar KK, NeedhiRajan T, Koslowski M, et al: Is levonorgestrel intrauterine system effective for treatment of early endometrial cancer? Report of four cases and review of the literature. Gynecol Oncol 97(3):924, 2005

Dietrich CS III, Modesitt SC, DePriest PD, et al: The efficacy of adjuvant platinum-based chemotherapy in stage I uterine papillary serous carcinoma (UPSC). Gynecol Oncol 99(3):557, 2005

Dossus L, Allen N, Kaaks R, et al: Reproductive risk factors and endometrial cancer: the European Prospective Investigation into Cancer and Nutrition. Int J Cancer 127(2):442, 2010

Dunlop MG, Farrington SM, Carothers AD, et al: Cancer risk associated with germline DNA mismatch repair gene mutations. Hum Mol Genet 6(1):105, 1997

Ellenson LH, Ronnett BM, Kurman RJ: Precursor lesions of endometrial carcinoma. In Kurman RJ, Ellenson LH, Ronnett BM (eds): Blaustein's Pathology of the Female Genital Tract. New York, Springer, 2011a, p 360

Ellenson LH, Ronnett BM, Soslow RA: Endometrial cancer. In Kurman RJ, Ellenson LH, Ronnett BM (eds): Blaustein's Pathology of the Female Genital Tract. New York, Springer, 2011b, p 422

Eltabbakh GH, Shamonki J, Mount SL: Surgical stage, final grade, and survival of women with endometrial carcinoma whose preoperative endometrial biopsy shows well-differentiated tumors. Gynecol Oncol 99(2):309, 2005

Farley JH, Nycum LR, Birrer MJ, et al: Age-specific survival of women with endometrioid adenocarcinoma of the uterus. Gynecol Oncol 79(1):86, 2000

Fearnley EJ, Marquart L, Spurdle AB, et al: Polycystic ovary syndrome increases the risk of endometrial cancer in women aged less than 50 years: an Australian case-control study. Cancer Causes Control 12:2303, 2010

Feldman S, Berkowitz RS, Tosteson AN: Cost-effectiveness of strategies to evaluate postmenopausal bleeding. Obstet Gynecol 81(6):968, 1993

Feltmate CM, Duska LR, Chang Y, et al: Predictors of recurrence in surgical stage II endometrial adenocarcinoma. Gynecol Oncol 73(3):407, 1999

Ferrandina G, Zannoni GF, Gallotta V, et al: Progression of conservatively treated endometrial carcinoma after full term pregnancy: a case report. Gynecol Oncol 99(1):215, 2005

FIGO Committee on Gynecologic Oncology: Revised FIGO staging for carcinoma of the vulva, cervix, and endometrium. Int J Gynaecol Obstet 105(2):103, 2009

Fiorica JV, Brunetto VL, Hanjani P, et al: Phase II trial of alternating courses of megestrol acetate and tamoxifen in advanced endometrial carcinoma: a Gynecologic Oncology Group study. Gynecol Oncol 92(1):10, 2004

Fisher B, Costantino JP, Redmond CK, et al: Endometrial cancer in tamoxifen-treated breast cancer patients: findings from the National Surgical Adjuvant Breast and Bowel Project (NSABP) B-14. J Natl Cancer Inst 86(7):527, 1994

Fisher B, Costantino JP, Wickerham DL, et al: Tamoxifen for prevention of breast cancer: report of the National Surgical Adjuvant Breast and Bowel Project P-1 Study. J Natl Cancer Inst 90(18):1371, 1998

Fishman DA, Roberts KB, Chambers JT, et al: Radiation therapy as exclusive treatment for medically inoperable patients with stage I and II endometrioid carcinoma with endometrium. Gynecol Oncol 61(2):189, 1996

Fleming GF, Brunetto VL, Cella D, et al: Phase III trial of doxorubicin plus cisplatin with or without paclitaxel plus filgrastim in advanced endometrial carcinoma: a Gynecologic Oncology Group Study. J Clin Oncol 22(11):2159, 2004

Frumovitz M, Singh DK, Meyer L, et al: Predictors of final histology in patients with endometrial cancer. Gynecol Oncol 95(3):463, 2004a

Frumovitz M, Slomovitz BM, Singh DK, et al: Frozen section analyses as predictors of lymphatic spread in patients with early-stage uterine cancer. J Am Coll Surg 199(3):388, 2004b

Gallos ID, Shehmar M, Thangaratinam S, et al: Oral progestogens vs levonorgestrel-releasing intrauterine system for endometrial hyperplasia: a systematic review and metaanalysis. Am J Obstet Gynecol 203(6):547.e1, 2010

Garuti G, Mirra M, Luerti M: Hysteroscopic view in atypical endometrial hyperplasias: a correlation with pathologic findings on hysterectomy specimens. J Minim Invasive Gynecol 13(4):325, 2006

Gehrig PA, Groben PA, Fowler WC Jr, et al: Noninvasive papillary serous carcinoma of the endometrium. Obstet Gynecol 97(1):153, 2001

Ghezzi F, Cromi A, Uccella S, et al: Laparoscopic versus open surgery for endometrial cancer: a minimum 3-year follow-up study. Ann Surg Oncol 17(1):271, 2010

Goff BA, Goodman A, Muntz HG, et al: Surgical stage IV endometrial carcinoma: a study of 47 cases. Gynecol Oncol 52(2):237, 1994

Goldstein SR, Nachtigall M, Snyder JR, et al: Endometrial assessment by vaginal ultrasonography before endometrial sampling in patients with postmenopausal bleeding. Am J Obstet Gynecol 163:119, 1990

Goldstein SR, Zeltser I, Horan CK, et al: Ultrasonography-based triage for perimenopausal patients with abnormal uterine bleeding. Am J Obstet Gynecol 177(1):102, 1997

Goodman A, Zukerberg LR, Rice LW, et al: Squamous cell carcinoma of the endometrium: a report of eight cases and a review of the literature. Gynecol Oncol 61(1):54, 1996

Goodman MT, Hankin JH, Wilkens LR, et al: Diet, body size, physical activity, and the risk of endometrial cancer. Cancer Res 57(22):5077, 1997

Gordon SJ, Westgate J: The incidence and management of failed Pipelle sampling in a general outpatient clinic. Aust N Z J Obstet Gynaecol 39(1):115, 1999

Gotlieb WH, Beiner ME, Shalmon B, et al: Outcome of fertility-sparing treatment with progestins in young patients with endometrial cancer. Obstet Gynecol 102(4):718, 2003

Granberg S, Wikland M, Karlsson B, et al: Endometrial thickness as measured by endovaginal ultrasonography for identifying endometrial abnormality. Am J Obstet Gynecol 164:47, 1991

Gredmark T, Kvint S, Havel G, et al: Histopathological findings in women with postmenopausal bleeding. Br J Obstet Gynaecol 102(2):133, 1995

Grice J, Ek M, Greer B, et al: Uterine papillary serous carcinoma: evaluation of long-term survival in surgically staged patients. Gynecol Oncol 69(1):69, 1998

Gruber SB, Thompson WD: A population-based study of endometrial cancer and familial risk in younger women. Cancer and Steroid Hormone Study Group. Cancer Epidemiol Biomarkers Prev 5(6):411, 1996

Gu M, Shi W, Barakat RR, et al: Pap smears in women with endometrial carcinoma. Acta Cytol 45(4):555, 2001

Guidos BJ, Selvaggi SM: Detection of endometrial adenocarcinoma with the ThinPrep Pap test. Diagn Cytopathol 23(4):260, 2000

Hamilton CA, Cheung MK, Osann K, et al: Uterine papillary serous and clear cell carcinomas predict for poorer survival compared to grade 3 endometrioid corpus cancers. Br J Cancer 94(5):642, 2006

Hampel H, Frankel W, Panescu J, et al: Screening for Lynch syndrome (hereditary nonpolyposis colorectal cancer) among endometrial cancer patients. Cancer Res 66(15):7810, 2006

Havrilesky LJ, Cragun JM, Calingaert B, et al: Resection of lymph node metastases influences survival in stage IIIC endometrial cancer. Gynecol Oncol 99(3):689, 2005

Hecht JL, Ince TA, Baak JP, et al: Prediction of endometrial carcinoma by subjective endometrial intraepithelial neoplasia diagnosis. Mod Pathol 18(3):324, 2005

Hecht JL, Mutter GL: Molecular and pathologic aspects of endometrial carcinogenesis. J Clin Oncol 24(29):4783, 2006

Hemminki K, Bermejo JL, Granstrom C: Endometrial cancer: population attributable risks from reproductive, familial and socioeconomic factors. Eur J Cancer 41(14):2155, 2005

Hirai Y, Takeshima N, Kato T, et al: Malignant potential of positive peritoneal cytology in endometrial cancer. Obstet Gynecol 97(5 Pt 1):725, 2001

Hoekstra AV, Jairam-Thodla A, Rademaker A, et al: The impact of robotics on practice management of endometrial cancer: transitioning from traditional surgery. Int J Med Robot 5(4):392, 2009

Homesley HD, Filiaci V, Gibbons SK et al: A randomized phase III trial in advanced endometrial carcinoma of surgery and volume directed radiation followed by cisplatin and doxorubicin with or without paclitaxel: a Gynecologic Oncology Group study. Gynecol Oncol 112:543, 2009

Horn LC, Schnurrbusch U, Bilek K, et al: Risk of progression in complex and atypical endometrial hyperplasia: clinicopathologic analysis in cases with and without progestogen treatment. Int J Gynecol Cancer 14(2):348, 2004

Hoskins PJ, Swenerton KD, Pike JA, et al: Paclitaxel and carboplatin, alone or with irradiation, in advanced or recurrent endometrial cancer: a phase II study. J Clin Oncol 19(20):4048, 2001

Huh WK, Powell M, Leath CA III, et al: Uterine papillary serous carcinoma: comparisons of outcomes in surgical stage I patients with and without adjuvant therapy. Gynecol Oncol 91(3):470, 2003

Iatrakis G, Diakakis I, Kourounis G, et al: Postmenopausal uterine bleeding. Clin Exp Obstet Gynecol 24(3):157, 1997

Jacobs I, Gentry-Maharaj A, Burnell M, et al: Sensitivity of transvaginal ultrasound screening for endometrial cancer in postmenopausal women: a case-control study within the UKCTOCS cohort. Lancet Oncol 12(1):38, 2011

Jemal A, Bray F, Center MM, et al: Global cancer statistics. CA Cancer J Clin 61(2):69, 2011

Jordan LB, Abdul-Kader M, Al Nafussi A: Uterine serous papillary carcinoma: histopathologic changes within the female genital tract. Int J Gynecol Cancer 11(4):283, 2001

Karageorgi S, Hankinson SE, Kraft P, et al: Reproductive factors and postmenopausal hormone use in relation to endometrial cancer risk in the Nurses' Health Study cohort 1976-2004. Int J Cancer 126(1):208, 2010

Kelly MG, O'Malley DM, Hui P, et al: Improved survival in surgical stage I patients with uterine papillary serous carcinoma (UPSC) treated with adjuvant platinum-based chemotherapy. Gynecol Oncol 98(3):353, 2005

Keys HM, Roberts JA, Brunetto VL, et al: A phase III trial of surgery with or without adjunctive external pelvic radiation therapy in intermediate risk endometrial adenocarcinoma: a Gynecologic Oncology Group study. Gynecol Oncol 92(3):744, 2004

Kilgore LC, Partridge EE, Alvarez RD, et al: Adenocarcinoma of the endometrium: survival comparisons of patients with and without pelvic node sampling. Gynecol Oncol 56(1):29, 1995

King LP, Miller DS: Recent progress: gynecologic oncology group trials in uterine corpus tumors. Rev Recent Clin Trials 4(2):70, 2009

Kitchener H, Swart AM, Qian Q, et al: Efficacy of systematic pelvic lymphadenectomy in endometrial cancer (MRC ASTEC trial): a randomized study. Lancet 373:125, 2009

Kornblith AB, Huang HQ, Walker JL, et al: Quality of life of patients with endometrial cancer undergoing laparoscopic International Federation of Gynecology and Obstetrics staging compared with laparotomy: a Gynecologic Oncology Group study. J Clin Oncol 27(32):5337, 2009

Kurman RJ, Kaminski PF, Norris HJ: The behavior of endometrial hyperplasia. A long-term study of "untreated" hyperplasia in 170 patients. Cancer 56(2):403, 1985

Kurman RJ, Norris HJ: Endometrial hyperplasia and related cellular changes. In Kurman RJ (ed): Blaustein's Pathology of the Female Genital Tract. New York, Springer, 1994, p 411

Lacey J Jr, Brinton LA, Lubin JH, et al: Endometrial carcinoma risks among menopausal estrogen plus progestin and unopposed estrogen users in a cohort of postmenopausal women. Cancer Epidemiol Biomarkers Prev 14(7):1724, 2005

Lax SF, Kurman RJ, Pizer ES, et al: A binary architectural grading system for uterine endometrial endometrioid carcinoma has superior reproducibility compared with FIGO grading and identifies subsets of advance-stage tumors with favorable and unfavorable prognosis. Am J Surg Pathol 24(9):1201, 2000

Leitao MM, Kehoe S, Barakat RR, et al: Accuracy of preoperative endometrial sampling diagnosis of FIGO grade 1 endometrial adenocarcinoma. Gynecol Oncol 111:244, 2008

Lentz SS, Brady MF, Major FJ, et al: High-dose megestrol acetate in advanced or recurrent endometrial carcinoma: a Gynecologic Oncology Group Study. J Clin Oncol 14(2):357, 1996

Liao CK, Rosenblatt KA, Schwartz SM, et al: Endometrial cancer in Asian migrants to the United States and their descendants. Cancer Causes Control 14(4):357, 2003

Lu KH, Dinh M, Kohlmann W, et al: Gynecologic cancer as a "sentinel cancer" for women with hereditary nonpolyposis colorectal cancer syndrome. Obstet Gynecol 105(3):569, 2005

Lurain JR, Rice BL, Rademaker AW, et al: Prognostic factors associated with disease recurrence in clinical stage I adenocarcinoma of the endometrium. Obstet Gynecol 78:63, 1991

Lutman CV, Havrilesky LJ, Cragun JM, et al: Pelvic lymph node count is an important prognostic variable for FIGO stage I and II endometrial carcinoma with high-risk histology. Gynecol Oncol 102(1):92, 2006

Madison T, Schottenfeld D, James SA, et al: Endometrial cancer: socioeconomic status and racial/ethnic differences in stage at diagnosis, treatment, and survival. Am J Public Health 94(12):2104, 2004

Magrina JF, Mutone NF, Weaver AL, et al: Laparoscopic lymphadenectomy and vaginal or laparoscopic hysterectomy with bilateral salpingo-oophorectomy for endometrial cancer: morbidity and survival. Am J Obstet Gynecol 181(2):376, 1999

Mariani A, Webb MJ, Keeney GL, et al: Hematogenous dissemination in corpus cancer. Gynecol Oncol 80(2):233, 2001a

Mariani A, Webb MJ, Keeney GL, et al: Role of wide/radical hysterectomy and pelvic lymph node dissection in endometrial cancer with cervical involvement. Gynecol Oncol 83(1):72, 2001b

Martin JD, Gilks B, Lim P: Papillary serous carcinoma—a less radio-sensitive subtype of endometrial cancer. Gynecol Oncol 98(2):299, 2005

Martínez A, Querleu D, Leblanc E, et al: Low incidence of port-site metastases after laparoscopic staging of uterine cancer. Gynecol Oncol 118(2):145, 2010

Maxwell GL, Schildkraut JM, Calingaert B, et al: Progestin and estrogen potency of combination oral contraceptives and endometrial cancer risk. Gynecol Oncol 103(2):535, 2006

Melhem MF, Tobon H: Mucinous adenocarcinoma of the endometrium: a clinico-pathological review of 18 cases. Int J Gynecol Pathol 6(4):347, 1987

Merisio C, Berretta R, De Ioris A, et al: Endometrial cancer in patients with preoperative diagnosis of atypical endometrial hyperplasia. Eur J Obstet Gynecol Reprod Biol 122(1):107, 2005

Miller, DS: Advanced endometrial cancer: is lymphadenectomy necessary or sufficient? Gynecol Oncol 101(2):191, 2006

Miller DS, Blessing JA, Drake RD, et al: A phase II evaluation of pemetrexed (Alimta, LY31514, IND #40061) in the treatment of recurrent or persistent endometrial carcinoma: a phase II study of the Gynecologic Oncology Group. Gynecol Oncol 115:443, 2009a

Miller DS, Fleming G, Randall ME: Chemo- and radiotherapy in adjuvant management of optimally debulked endometrial cancer. J Natl Compr Cancer Netw 7(5):535, 2009b

Moller KA, Gehrig PA, Van Le L, et al: The role of optimal debulking in advanced stage serous carcinoma of the uterus. Gynecol Oncol 94(1):170, 2004

Montz FJ, Bristow RE, Bovicelli A, et al: Intrauterine progesterone treatment of early endometrial cancer. Am J Obstet Gynecol 186(4):651, 2002

Morice P, Fourchotte V, Sideris L, et al: A need for laparoscopic evaluation of patients with endometrial carcinoma selected for conservative treatment. Gynecol Oncol 96(1):245, 2005

Morimoto LM, Newcomb PA, Hampton JM, et al: Cholecystectomy and endometrial cancer: a marker of long-term elevated estrogen exposure? Int J Gynecol Cancer 16(3):1348, 2006

Morris M, Alvarez RD, Kinney WK, et al: Treatment of recurrent adenocarcinoma of the endometrium with pelvic exenteration. Gynecol Oncol 60(2):288, 1996

Morrow CP, Bundy BN, Kurman RJ, et al: Relationship between surgical-pathological risk factors and outcome in clinical stage I and II carcinoma of the endometrium: a Gynecologic Oncology Group study. Gynecol Oncol 40(1):55, 1991

Mount SL, Wegner EK, Eltabbakh GH, et al: Significant increase of benign endometrial cells on Papanicolaou smears in women using hormone replacement therapy. Obstet Gynecol 100(3):445, 2002

Mutch DG: The new FIGO staging system for cancers of the vulva, cervix, endometrium and sarcomas. Gynecol Oncol 115(3):325, 2009

Mutter GL: Endometrial intraepithelial neoplasia (EIN): will it bring order to chaos? The Endometrial Collaborative Group. Gynecol Oncol 76(3):287, 2000

Nagar H, Dobbs S, McClelland HR, et al: The diagnostic accuracy of magnetic resonance imaging in detecting cervical involvement in endometrial cancer. Gynecol Oncol 103(2):431, 2006

National Comprehensive Cancer Network: Uterine neoplasms, version 1.2011. In NCCN Clinical Practice Guidelines in Oncology. National Comprehensive Cancer Network, 2010, p. MS-9

Niwa K, Tagami K, Lian Z, et al: Outcome of fertility-preserving treatment in young women with endometrial carcinomas. BJOG 112(3):317, 2005

Obermair A, Geramou M, Gucer F, et al: Does hysteroscopy facilitate tumor cell dissemination? Incidence of peritoneal cytology from patients with early stage endometrial carcinoma following dilatation and curettage (D & C) versus hysteroscopy and D & C. Cancer 88(1):139, 2000

Papadia A, Azioni G, Brusaca B, et al: Frozen section underestimates the need for surgical staging in endometrial cancer patients. Int J Gynecol Cancer 19(9):1570, 2009

Parkin DM, Bray F, Ferlay J, et al: Global cancer statistics, 2002. CA Cancer J Clin 55(2):74, 2005

Pecorelli S, Benedet JL, Creasman WT, et al: FIGO staging of gynecologic cancer. 1994-1997 FIGO Committee on Gynecologic Oncology. International Federation of Gynecology and Obstetrics. Int J Gynaecol Obstet 64(1):5, 1999

Pillay OC, Te Fong LF, Crow JC, et al: The association between polycystic ovaries and endometrial cancer. Hum Reprod 21(4):924, 2006

Polyzos NP, Mauri D, Tsioras S, et al: Intraperitoneal dissemination of endometrial cancer cells after hysteroscopy: a systematic review and meta-analysis. Int J Gynecol Cancer 20(2):261, 2010

Pothuri B, Ramondetta L, Martino M, et al: Development of endometrial cancer after radiation treatment for cervical carcinoma. Obstet Gynecol 101(5 Pt 1):941, 2003

Powell JL, Hill KA, Shiro BC, et al: Preoperative serum CA-125 levels in treating endometrial cancer. J Reprod Med 50(8):585, 2005

Price FV, Chambers SK, Carcangiu ML, et al: CA 125 may not reflect disease status in patients with uterine serous cancer. Cancer 82(9):1720, 1998

Randall ME, Filiaci VL, Muss H, et al: Randomized phase III trial of whole-abdominal irradiation versus doxorubicin and cisplatin chemotherapy in advanced endometrial carcinoma: a Gynecologic Oncology Group Study. J Clin Oncol 24(1):36, 2006

Randall TC, Kurman RJ: Progestin treatment of atypical hyperplasia and well-differentiated carcinoma of the endometrium in women under age 40. Obstet Gynecol 90(3):434, 1997

Rattanachaiyanont M, Angsuwathana S, Techatrisak K, et al: Clinical and pathological responses of progestin therapy for non-atypical endometrial hyperplasia: a prospective study. J Obstet Gynaecol Res 31(2):98, 2005

Revel A, Tsafrir A, Anteby SO, et al: Does hysteroscopy produce intraperitoneal spread of endometrial cancer cells? Obstet Gynecol Surv 59:280, 2004

Ricci E, Moroni S, Parazzini F, et al: Risk factors for endometrial hyperplasia: results from a case-control study. Int J Gynecol Cancer 12(3):257, 2002

Rittenberg PV, Lotocki RJ, Heywood MS, et al: Stage II endometrial carcinoma: limiting post-operative radiotherapy to the vaginal vault in node-negative tumors. Gynecol Oncol 98(3):434, 2005

Roland PY, Kelly FJ, Kulwicki CY, et al: The benefits of a gynecologic oncologist: a pattern of care study for endometrial cancer treatment. Gynecol Oncol 93(1):125, 2004

Ross JC, Eifel PJ, Cox RS, et al: Primary mucinous adenocarcinoma of the endometrium. A clinicopathologic and histochemical study. Am J Surg Pathol 7(8):715, 1983

Rubatt JM, Slomovitz BM, Burke TW, et al: Development of metastatic endometrial endometrioid adenocarcinoma while on progestin therapy for endometrial hyperplasia. Gynecol Oncol 99(2):472, 2005

Sanjuan A, Cobo T, Pahisa J, et al: Preoperative and intraoperative assessment of myometrial invasion and histologic grade in endometrial cancer: role of magnetic resonance imaging and frozen section. Int J Gynecol Cancer 16(1):385, 2006

Scarselli G, Bargelli G, Taddei GL, et al: Levonorgestrel-releasing intrauterine system (LNG-IUS) as an effective treatment option for endometrial hyperplasia: a 15-year follow-up study. Fertil Steril 95(1):420, 2011

Schink JC, Rademaker AW, Miller DS, et al: Tumor size in endometrial cancer. Cancer 67(11):2791, 1991

Schmeler KM, Lynch HT, Chen LM, et al: Prophylactic surgery to reduce the risk of gynecologic cancers in the Lynch syndrome. N Engl J Med 354(3):261, 2006

Scholten AN, Smit VT, Beerman H, et al: Prognostic significance and interobserver variability of histologic grading systems for endometrial carcinoma. Cancer 100(4):764, 2004

Schorge JO, Hossein SM, Hynan L, et al: ThinPrep detection of cervical and endometrial adenocarcinoma: a retrospective cohort study. Cancer 96(6):338, 2002

Schottenfeld D: Epidemiology of endometrial neoplasia. J Cell Biochem Suppl 23:151, 1995

Seamon LG, Cohn DE, Henretta MS, et al: Minimally invasive comprehensive surgical staging for endometrial cancer: robotics or laparoscopy? Gynecol Oncol 113(1):36, 2009

Sherman ME, Bitterman P, Rosenshein NB, et al: Uterine serous carcinoma. A morphologically diverse neoplasm with unifying clinicopathologic features. Am J Surg Pathol 16(6):600, 1992

Sherman ME, Ronnett BM, Ioffe OB, et al: Reproducibility of biopsy diagnoses of endometrial hyperplasia: evidence supporting a simplified classification. Int J Gynecol Pathol 27(3):318, 2008

Shi AA, Lee SI: Radiological reasoning: algorithmic workup of abnormal vaginal bleeding with endovaginal sonography and sonohysterography. AJR Am J Roentgenol 191(6 Suppl):S68, 2008

Siegel R, Ward E, Brawley O, et al: Cancer statistics, 2011: the impact of eliminating socioeconomic and racial disparities on premature cancer deaths. CA Cancer J Clin 61(4):212, 2011

Silva EG, Deavers MT, Malpica A: Undifferentiated carcinoma of the endometrium: a review. Pathology 39(1):134, 2007

Silverberg SG, Kurman RJ, Nogales F, et al: Tumors of the uterine corpus [Epithelial tumors and related lesions]. In Tavassoli FA, Devilee P (eds): World Health Organization Classification of Tumours. Lyon, France, IARC Press, 2003, p 221

Simsir A, Carter W, Elgert P, et al: Reporting endometrial cells in women 40 years and older: assessing the clinical usefulness of Bethesda 2001. Am J Clin Pathol 123(4):571, 2005

Slomovitz BM, Burke TW, Eifel PJ, et al: Uterine papillary serous carcinoma (UPSC): a single institution review of 129 cases. Gynecol Oncol 91(3):463, 2003

Smith DC, Prentice R, Thompson DJ, et al: Association of exogenous estrogen and endometrial carcinoma. N Engl J Med 293 (23):1164, 1975

Smith RA, Cokkinides V, Brooks D, et al: Cancer screening in the United States, 2011: a review of current American Cancer Society guidelines and issues in cancer screening. CA Cancer J Clin 61(1):8, 2011

Soliman PT, Oh JC, Schmeler KM, et al: Risk factors for young premenopausal women with endometrial cancer. Obstet Gynecol 105(3):575, 2005

Sovak MA, Dupont J, Hensley ML, et al: Paclitaxel and carboplatin in the treatment of advanced or recurrent endometrial cancer: a large retrospective study. Int J Gynecol Cancer 17(1):197, 2007

Sovak MA, Hensley ML, Dupont J, et al: Paclitaxel and carboplatin in the adjuvant treatment of patients with high-risk stage III and IV endometrial cancer: a retrospective study. Gynecol Oncol 103(2):451, 2006

Spirtos NM, Eisekop SM, Boike G, et al: Laparoscopic staging in patients with incompletely staged cancers of the uterus, ovary, fallopian tube, and primary peritoneum: a Gynecologic Oncology Group (GOG) study. Am J Obstet Gynecol 193(5):1645, 2005

Stanford JL, Brinton LA, Berman ML, et al: Oral contraceptives and endometrial cancer: do other risk factors modify the association? Int J Cancer 54(2):243, 1993

Strom BL, Schinnar R, Weber AL, et al: Case-control study of postmenopausal hormone replacement therapy and endometrial cancer. Am J Epidemiol 164(8):775, 2006

Suh-Burgmann E, Hung YY, Armstrong MA: Complex atypical endometrial hyperplasia: the risk of unrecognized adenocarcinoma and value of preoperative dilation and curettage. Obstet Gynecol 114(3):523, 2009

Suriano KA, McHale M, McLaren CE, et al: Estrogen replacement therapy in endometrial cancer patients: a matched control study. Obstet Gynecol 97(4):555, 2001

Tao MH, Xu WH, Zheng W, et al: Oral contraceptive and IUD use and endometrial cancer: a population-based case-control study in Shanghai, China. Int J Cancer 119(9):2142, 2006

Terakawa N, Kigawa J, Taketani Y, et al: The behavior of endometrial hyperplasia: a prospective study. Endometrial Hyperplasia Study Group. J Obstet Gynaecol Res 23(3):223, 1997

Thai TH, Du F, Tsan JT, et al: Mutations in the BRCA1-associated ring domain (BARD1) gene in primary breast, ovarian and uterine cancers. Hum Mole Genet 7(2):195, 1998

Thigpen JT, Brady MF, Alvarez RD, et al: Oral medroxyprogesterone acetate in the treatment of advanced or recurrent endometrial carcinoma: a dose-response study by the Gynecologic Oncology Group. J Clin Oncol 17(6):1736, 1999

Trimble CL, Kauderer J, Zaino R, et al: Concurrent endometrial carcinoma in women with a biopsy diagnosis of atypical endometrial hyperplasia: a Gynecologic Oncology Group study. Cancer 106(4):812, 2006

van Leeuwen FE, Benraadt J, Coebergh JW, et al: Risk of endometrial cancer after tamoxifen treatment of breast cancer. Lancet 343(8895):448, 1994

Varras M, Kioses E: Five-year survival of a patient with primary endometrial squamous cell carcinoma: a case report and review of the literature. Eur J Gynaecol Oncol 23(4):327, 2002

Vasen HF, Watson P, Mecklin JP, et al: New clinical criteria for hereditary nonpolyposis colorectal cancer (HNPCC, Lynch syndrome) proposed by the International Collaborative Group on HNPCC. Gastroenterology 116(6):1453, 1999

Viswanathan AN, Feskanich D, De Vivo I, et al: Smoking and the risk of endometrial cancer: results from the Nurses' Health Study. Int J Cancer 114(6):996, 2005

Vorgias G, Hintipas E, Katsoulis M, et al: Intraoperative gross examination of myometrial invasion and cervical infiltration in patients with endometrial cancer: decision-making accuracy. Gynecol Oncol 85(3):483, 2002

Walker JL, Piedmonte MR, Spirtos, NM, et al: Laparoscopy compared with laparotomy for comprehensive surgical staging of uterine cancer: Gynecologic Oncology Group Study (LAP2). J Clin Oncol 27(32): 5331, 2009

Wang CB, Wang CJ, Huang HJ, et al: Fertility-preserving treatment in young patients with endometrial adenocarcinoma. Cancer 94(8):2192, 2002

Wernli KJ, Ray RM, Gao DL, et al: Menstrual and reproductive factors in relation to risk of endometrial cancer in Chinese women. Cancer Causes Control 17(7):949, 2006

Whitney CW, Brunetto VL, Zaino RJ, et al: Phase II study of medroxyprogesterone acetate plus tamoxifen in advanced endometrial carcinoma: a Gynecologic Oncology Group study. Gynecol Oncol 92(1):4, 2004

Wildemeersch D, Janssens D, Pylyser K, et al: Management of patients with non-atypical and atypical endometrial hyperplasia with a levonorgestrel-releasing intrauterine system: long-term follow-up. Maturitas 57(2):210, 2007

Yang YC, Wu CC, Chen CP, et al: Reevaluating the safety of fertility-sparing hormonal therapy for early endometrial cancer. Gynecol Oncol 99(2):287, 2005

Zaino RJ, Kauderer J, Trimble CL, et al: Reproducibility of the diagnosis of atypical endometrial hyperplasia: a Gynecologic Oncology Group study. Cancer 106(4):804, 2006

Zaino RJ, Kurman RJ, Diana KL, et al: The utility of the revised International Federation of Gynecology and Obstetrics histologic grading of endometrial adenocarcinoma using a defined nuclear grading system. A Gynecologic Oncology Group study. Cancer 75(1):81, 1995

Zaino RJ, Silverberg SG, Norris HJ, et al: The prognostic value of nuclear versus architectural grading in endometrial adenocarcinoma: a Gynecologic Oncology Group study. Int J Gynecol Pathol 13(1):29, 1994

Zerbe MJ, Zhang J, Bristow RE, et al: Retrograde seeding of malignant cells during hysteroscopy in presumed early endometrial cancer. Gynecol Oncol 79(1):55, 2000

Zullo F, Palomba S, Falbo A, et al: Laparoscopic surgery vs laparotomy for early stage endometrial cancer: long-term data of a randomized controlled trial. Am J Obstet Gynecol 200(3):296.e1, 2009

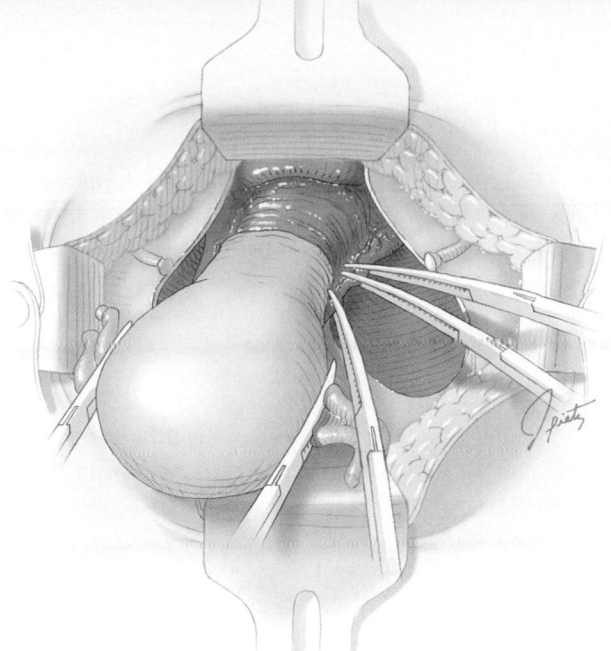

Uterine Sarcoma

Malignant tumors of the uterine corpus are broadly divided into three main types: carcinomas (Chap. 33, p. 822), sarcomas, and carcinosarcomas. Although the latter two categories are rarely encountered, they tend to behave more aggressively and contribute to a disproportionately higher number of uterine cancer deaths. Pure sarcomas are mainly characterized by differentiation toward smooth muscle (leiomyosarcoma) or stromal tissue within the endometrium (endometrial stromal tumors). Carcinosarcomas are mixed tumors demonstrating both epithelial and stromal components and have also been known as malignant mixed müllerian tumor (MMMT). In general, uterine sarcomas and carcinosarcomas grow quickly, lymphatic or hematogenous spread occurs early, and the overall prognosis is poor. However, there are several notable exceptions among these tumors.

EPIDEMIOLOGY AND RISK FACTORS

Sarcomas account for approximately 3 to 8 percent of all malignancies of the uterine corpus (Brooks, 2004; Major, 1993). Historically, uterine sarcomas included carcinosarcomas, comprising 40 percent of cases; leiomyosarcomas, 40 percent; endometrial stromal sarcomas, 10 to 15 percent; and undifferentiated sarcomas, 5 to 10 percent. Recently, carcinosarcomas have been reclassified as a metaplastic form of endometrial carcinoma. Despite this, carcinosarcomas are still commonly included in most retrospective studies of uterine sarcomas as well as in the 2003 World Health Organization (WHO) classification (Greer, 2011; McCluggage, 2002; Tavassoli, 2003). After excluding carcinosarcomas, leiomyosarcomas have become the most common subtype of true uterine sarcomas (D'Angelo, 2010).

Because of their relative infrequency, the epidemiology of uterine sarcomas and carcinosarcomas has not been extensively studied. As a result, relatively few risk factors have been identified, but they include chronic excess estrogen exposure, tamoxifen use, African American race, and prior pelvic radiation. In contrast, combination oral contraceptive pill use and smoking appear to lower risks for some of these tumors.

PATHOGENESIS

Leiomyosarcomas have a monoclonal origin, and although commonly believed to arise from benign leiomyomas, for the most part, they do not. Instead, they appear to develop de novo as solitary lesions (Zhang, 2006). They are, however, often found in proximity to leiomyomas. Supporting this theory, leiomyosarcomas have molecular pathways that have been shown to be distinct from those of leiomyomas or normal myometrium (Quade, 2004; Skubitz, 2003).

Endometrial stromal tumors have heterogeneous chromosomal aberrations (Halbwedl, 2005). However, the pattern of rearrangements is clearly nonrandom, with chromosomal arms 6p and 7p frequently involved (Micci, 2006). A loss of tumor suppressor gene function(s) is suspected. However, too few cases have been studied to generate a working hypothesis (Moinfar, 2004).

Uterine carcinosarcomas are monoclonal, biphasic neoplasms composed of distinctive and separate, but admixed, malignant epithelial and malignant stromal elements (D'Angelo, 2010; Wada, 1997). The sarcomatous component is derived from the carcinomatous element, which is the driving force (McCluggage, 2002). Several identifiable risk factors parallel those observed in endometrial carcinoma, thus it would seem plausible that these tumors have a similar pathogenesis. However, their morphologic diversity suggests a variety of potential pathways. Both the carcinoma and sarcoma components are thought to arise from a common epithelial progenitor cell. Acquisition of any number of genetic mutations, including defects in the p53 and DNA mismatch repair genes, may be sufficient to trigger tumorigenesis (Liu, 1994). These early molecular defects will be shared by both components as the tumor undergoes divergent carcinomatous and sarcomatous differentiation. Thereafter, acquired molecular defects will be discordant between the two components (Taylor, 2006). This genetic progression and subsequent diversion parallels the varying phenotypes observed in these tumors (Fujii, 2000).

DIAGNOSIS

Signs and Symptoms

As in endometrial cancer, abnormal vaginal bleeding is the most frequent presenting symptom for uterine sarcomas and carcinosarcomas (Gonzalez-Bosquet, 1997). Pelvic or abdominal pain is also common. Specifically, up to one third of women will describe significant discomfort that may result from passage of clots, rapid uterine enlargement, or prolapse of a sarcomatous polyp through an effaced cervix (De Fusco, 1989). In addition, a profuse, foul-smelling discharge may be obvious, and gastrointestinal and genitourinary complaints are also common. Importantly, degenerating leiomyomas with necrosis can mimic all of these signs and symptoms.

With rapid growth, a uterus may extend out of the pelvis into the mid- or upper abdomen (Fig. 34-1). Fortunately, the incidence of malignancy in such cases is still extremely low (<0.5 percent), and in most instances, benign enlarging leiomyomas are found (Leibsohn, 1990; Parker, 1994). Although uterine leiomyosarcomas do tend to grow quickly, no criteria define what constitutes significant growth. Despite these often-dramatic presentations, many women with uterine sarcoma and carcinosarcoma will have few symptoms other than abnormal vaginal bleeding and a seemingly normal uterus on physical examination.

Endometrial Sampling

The sensitivity of an office endometrial biopsy or dilatation and curettage (D&C) to detect sarcomatous elements is lower than that for endometrial carcinomas. Specifically, with leiomyosarcoma, symptomatic women receive a correct preoperative diagnosis in only 25 to 50 percent of cases. This inability to accurately sample the tumor is probably related to the origin of these neoplasms in the myometrium, rather than the endometrium. Similarly, endometrial stromal nodules and endometrial stromal sarcomas may be undetectable by Pipelle biopsy, especially if the neoplasm is entirely intramural (Yang, 2002). For those with carcinosarcoma, sampling will more often lead to a correct diagnosis, although in many cases only the carcinomatous features are evident. The reverse is also true, and occasionally a uterine carcinosarcoma is suspected based on endometrial biopsy findings, but no sarcomatous features are found within the hysterectomy specimen.

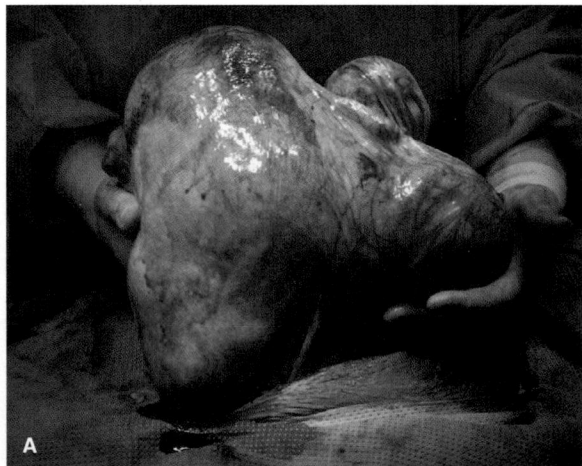 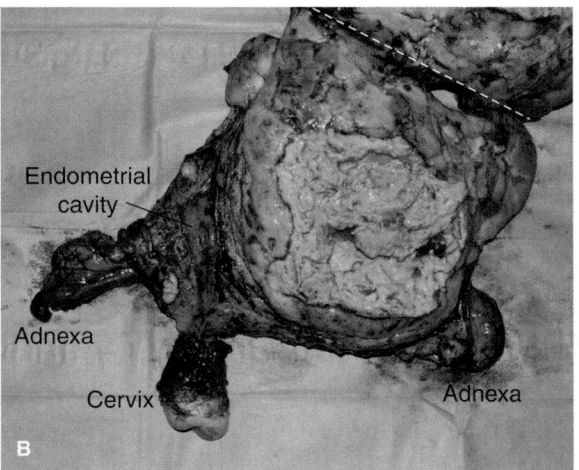

FIGURE 34-1 Leiomyosarcoma. **A.** Intraoperative photograph of a uterine corpus. **B.** Photograph of the surgical specimen after it has been bivalved and remains joined at the fundus. The other half of the specimen lies above the white dashed and out of the field of view. The large tumor lies to the right of the endometrial cavity. It has central necrosis seen as yellow amorphous debris with the tumor borders. *(Photographs contributed by Dr. Martha Rac.)*

Laboratory Testing

Elevated preoperative serum CA125 levels may indicate extrauterine disease and deep myometrial invasion in patients with carcinosarcoma. After surgery, CA125 measurement may be a somewhat useful marker to monitor disease response (Huang, 2007).

Imaging Studies

Unlike most women with endometrial carcinoma, who only require a preoperative chest radiograph, additional imaging studies are often helpful if sarcoma is diagnosed before hysterectomy. In most cases, a computed tomography (CT) scan of the abdomen and pelvis should be routinely performed. This serves at least two purposes. First, sarcomas often violate normal soft tissue planes in the pelvis, and therefore, unresectable tumors may be identified preoperatively. Secondly, extrauterine metastases may be visualized. In either case, treatment may be altered based on radiographic findings.

If a diagnosis is still in question, magnetic resonance (MR) imaging is often useful for distinguishing uterine sarcoma from a benign "mimic." For example, MR imaging can assist in determining whether a pedunculated mass is a submucosal leiomyoma or a prolapsing endometrial stromal tumor (Kido, 2003). As a diagnostic tool for sarcoma, sonography is far less helpful. Positron emission tomography (PET) scanning is most effectively used for disease monitoring after completion of treatment.

Role of the Generalist

Preoperative consultation with a gynecologic oncologist is recommended for any patient with a biopsy suggesting uterine sarcoma or carcinosarcoma. The potential for intraabdominal metastases and disruption of tissue planes within the pelvis increases the technical difficulty and surgical risks. Moreover, if a patient undergoes inadvertent myomectomy or hysterectomy with morcellation, it may worsen her prognosis (Perri, 2009). Just as importantly, the approach to staging is subtly dissimilar to that of endometrial carcinomas. For example, due to the low rate of metastasis, it may be appropriate to only sample nodes suspicious for leiomyosarcomas, instead of performing a complete pelvic and paraaortic lymphadenectomy (Leitao, 2003; Major, 1993). In addition, it may be prudent to preserve the ovaries in a young woman with an endometrial stromal sarcoma or leiomyosarcoma because the risk of adnexal metastasis with these is minimal (Kapp, 2008; Li, 2005). In general, a treatment plan is best organized preoperatively, if possible.

Many uterine sarcomas and carcinosarcomas are not diagnosed until surgery or several days later when a pathology report is available. As a result, unstaged cases are common, and a gynecologic oncologist should be consulted at the earliest feasible time. If the diagnosis is made postoperatively, the criteria to recommend surveillance only, reoperation, or radiotherapy vary widely, depending on the sarcoma type and other clinical circumstances. In general, these options are less straightforward than in typical endometrial carcinomas, largely due to the rarity of these tumors and the comparatively limited data supporting one strategy over another.

PATHOLOGY

Uterine mesenchymal tumors are classified broadly into pure and mixed tumors (Table 34-1). Pure sarcomas are virtually all homologous, differentiating into mesenchymal tissue that is normally present within the uterus, such as smooth muscle (leiomyosarcoma) or stromal tissue within the endometrium (endometrial stromal tumors). Pure heterologous sarcomas, such as chondrosarcoma, are exceedingly rare.

Mixed sarcomas contain a malignant mesenchymal component admixed with an epithelial element. If the epithelial element is also malignant, the tumor is termed *carcinosarcoma*. If the epithelial element is benign, the term *adenosarcoma* is used.

TABLE 34-1. World Health Organization Histological Classification of Mesenchymal Tumors of the Uterus

Mesenchymal tumors
Endometrial stromal and related tumors
  Endometrial stromal sarcoma, low grade
  Endometrial stromal nodule
  Undifferentiated endometrial sarcoma
Smooth muscle tumors
  Leiomyosarcoma
    Epithelial variant
    Myxoid variant
Smooth muscle tumor of uncertain malignant potential
Leiomyoma, not otherwise specified
  Histologic variants
    Mitotically active variant
    Cellular variant
    Hemorrhagic cellular variant
    Epithelioid variant
    Myxoid
    Atypical variant
    Lipoleiomyoma variant
  Growth pattern variants
    Diffuse leiomyomatosis
    Dissecting leiomyoma
    Intravenous leiomyomatosis
    Metastasizing leiomyoma
Miscellaneous mesenchymal tumors
  Mixed endometrial stromal and smooth muscle tumor
  Perivascular epithelioid cell tumor
  Adenomatoid tumor
  Other malignant mesenchymal tumors
  Other benign mesenchymal tumors

Mixed epithelial and mesenchymal tumors
Carcinosarcoma (malignant müllerian mixed tumor, metaplastic carcinoma)
Adenosarcoma
Carcinofibroma
Adenofibroma
Adenomyoma
  Atypical polypoid variant

Carcinosarcomas can be either homologous or heterologous, reflecting the potentiality of the uterine primordium.

Leiomyosarcoma

Leiomyosarcomas account for 1 to 2 percent of all uterine malignancies. In a Surveillance, Epidemiology and End Results (SEER) database study of 1396 patients, the median age at presentation was 52 years. Most tumors (68 percent) were stage I at the time of diagnosis, whereas stage II (3 percent), stage III (7 percent), and stage IV cancer (22 percent) comprised the remainder (Kapp, 2008).

The histopathologic criteria for diagnosing leiomyosarcoma are somewhat controversial, but include the frequency of mitotic figures, extent of nuclear atypia, and presence of any coagulative tumor cell necrosis (Fig. 34-2). Each row of Table 34-2,

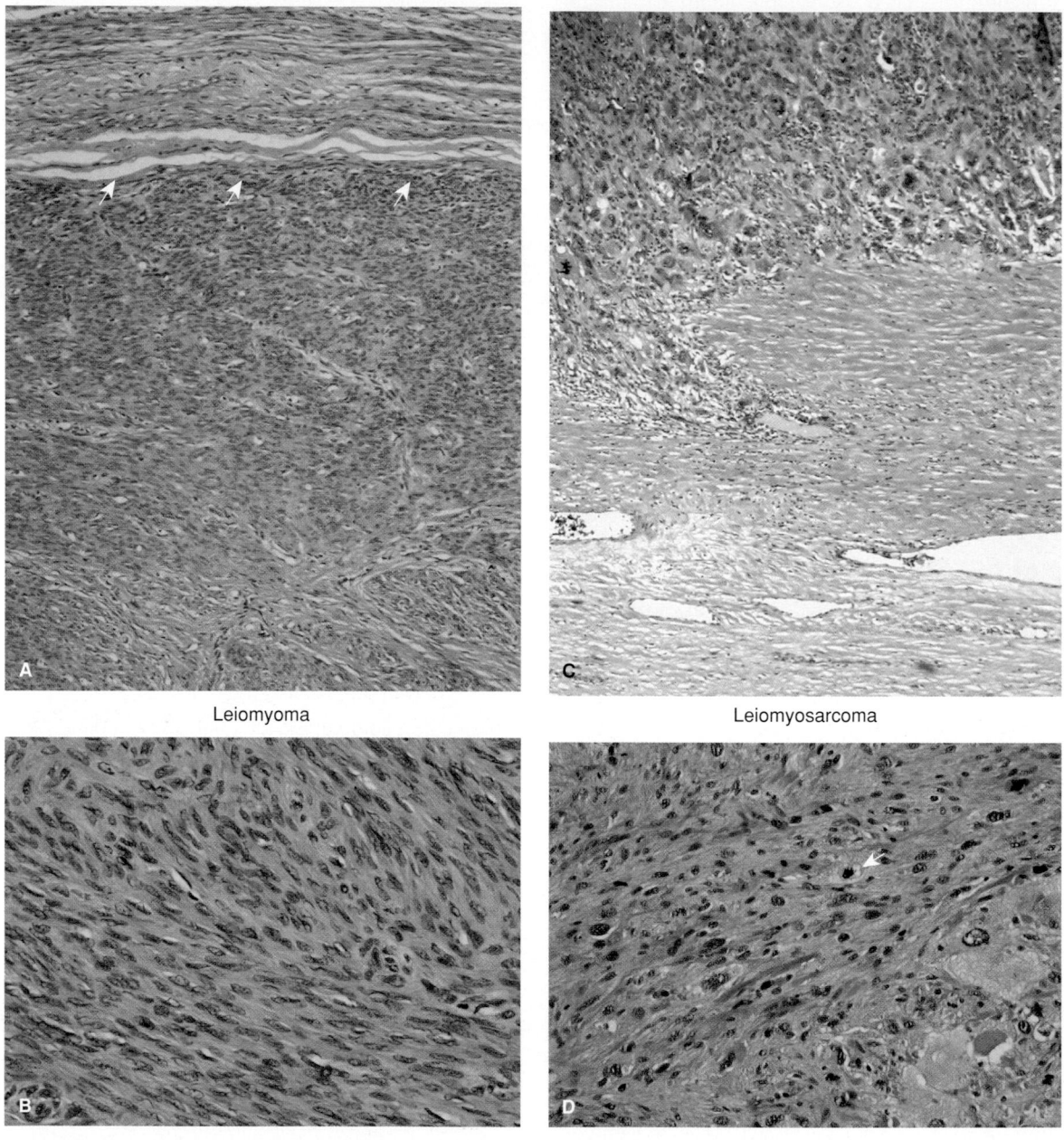

Leiomyoma   Leiomyosarcoma

FIGURE 34-2 Photomicrographs of leiomyoma **(A, B)** and leiomyosarcoma **(C, D)**. **A.** Low-power view of uterine leiomyoma. Leiomyomas tend to be well-circumscribed masses. This relatively cellular leiomyoma shows a well-demarcated interface (*arrows*) with the adjacent, less cellular myometrium. **B.** High-power view of leiomyoma. Although leiomyomas may have variable histologic features, most leiomyomas are composed of bland spindled cells with blunt-ended nuclei and limited mitotic activity. **C.** Leiomyosarcoma. Leiomyosarcoma is a malignant smooth muscle neoplasm that may differ markedly in its microscopic appearance from case to case. Generally, uterine leiomyosarcoma shows some combination of "malignant" histologic features, which include coagulative tumor necrosis (in contrast to the hyaline-type necrosis often found in benign leiomyomas), increased mitotic activity, and/or nuclear atypia. This example has marked nuclear atypia and pleomorphism and an infiltrative growth pattern at its periphery. This differs from the usually smooth, pushing border of typical leiomyomas. **D.** This particular example has moderate to marked nuclear atypia and a mitosis (*arrow*). *(Photographs contributed by Drs. Kelley Carrick and Raheela Ashfaq.)*

TABLE 34-2. Diagnostic Criteria for Uterine Leiomyosarcoma

Coagulative Tumor Cell Necrosis	Mitotic Index[a]	Degree of Atypia
Present	≥10 MF/10 HPF	None
Present	Any	Diffuse, significant
Absent	≥10 MF/10 HPF	Diffuse, significant

[a]MF/10 HPF = the total number of mitotic figures counted when 10 high-powered field are examined.
From Hendrickson, 2003.

illustrates combinations of histologic findings that may be found in leiomyosarcomas. In most cases, the mitotic index exceeds 15 mitotic figures total when 10 high-power fields are examined, moderate to severe cytologic atypia is seen, and tumor cell necrosis is prominent (Hendrickson, 2003; Zaloudek, 2011). Occasionally, a leiomyosarcoma will be reported as low-, intermediate- or high-grade, but the overall utility of grading is controversial, and no universally accepted grading system exists.

Smooth Muscle Tumor of Uncertain Malignant Potential (STUMP)

Tumors that show some worrisome histologic features, such as necrosis or nuclear atypia, but cannot be diagnosed reliably as benign or malignant based on generally applied criteria fall into this category. The diagnosis should be used sparingly and is reserved for smooth muscle neoplasms whose appearance is ambiguous (Hendrickson, 2003).

Endometrial Stromal Tumors

Significantly less common than leiomyosarcomas, endometrial stromal tumors comprise fewer than 10 percent of all uterine sarcomas. In a SEER database study of 831 patients, the median age at diagnosis was 52 years (Chan, 2008). Although constituting a wide morphologic spectrum, endometrial stromal tumors are composed exclusively of cells that resemble the endometrial stroma and include both benign stromal nodules and malignant stromal tumors (see Table 34-1).

Historically, there has been controversy regarding subdivision of these tumors. The division of endometrial stromal sarcomas into low-grade and high-grade categories has fallen out of favor. In its place, the designation *endometrial stromal sarcoma* is now best restricted to neoplasms that were formerly referred to as low-grade. Alternatively, the term *high-grade undifferentiated sarcoma* is believed to more accurately reflect those tumors without recognizable evidence of a definite endometrial stromal phenotype. These lesions are almost invariably high grade and often resemble the mesenchymal component of a uterine carcinosarcoma (Oliva, 2000). In this revised classification, the distinctions are not determined by mitotic count, but by features such as nuclear pleomorphism and necrosis (Evans, 1982; Hendrickson, 2003).

Endometrial Stromal Nodule

Representing less than a quarter of endometrial stromal tumors, these rare nodules are benign, characterized by a well-delineated

margin, and composed of neoplastic cells that resemble proliferative-phase endometrial stromal cells. Grossly, the tumor is a solitary, round or oval, fleshy nodule measuring a few centimeters. Histologically, they are distinguished from endometrial stromal sarcomas by a lack of myometrial infiltration (Dionigi, 2002). These nodules are benign, and myomectomy is an appropriate option. However, because differentiation between endometrial stromal sarcoma and this benign lesion cannot be determined clinically, it is important to remove the entire nodule. Thus, for large lesions, hysterectomy may be required (Hendrickson, 2003).

Endometrial Stromal Sarcoma

The precise frequency of these tumors is difficult to estimate because they are excluded from some reports and included in others, and the terminology used has been inconsistent. In general, endometrial stromal sarcomas (formerly called low-grade) are thought to be the most frequently encountered stromal tumor variant and are twice as common as high-grade undifferentiated sarcomas.

Typically, they extensively invade the myometrium and extend to the serosa in approximately half of cases (Fig. 34-3). Less often, they present as a solitary well-delineated, predominantly intramural mass that is difficult to grossly distinguish from an endometrial stromal nodule. Microscopically, endometrial stromal sarcomas resemble the stromal cells of proliferative phase endometrium (Fig. 34-4).

Metastases are rarely detected prior to the diagnosis of the primary lesion. However, permeation of the lymphatic and vascular channels is characteristic. In up to one third of cases, extrauterine extension is present, often appearing as "worm-like" plugs of tumor within the vessels of the broad ligament and adnexa. At operation, this may resemble intravenous leiomyomatosis or a broad ligament leiomyoma, but frozen section analysis can usually make the distinction (Chap. 9, p. 250).

High-Grade Undifferentiated Sarcoma

Compared with endometrial stromal sarcomas, these tumors tend to be larger and more polypoid, often filling the uterine cavity. Instead of an infiltrating pattern, high-grade undifferentiated sarcomas displace the myometrium more destructively, leading to prominent hemorrhage and necrosis.

Microscopically, the cells are larger and more pleomorphic. The presence of marked cellular atypia is characteristic (Fig. 34-5). Typically, there are more than 10 mitoses per 10 high power fields, but frequently there are more than 20 in the most active areas. These tumors lack specific differentiation and bear

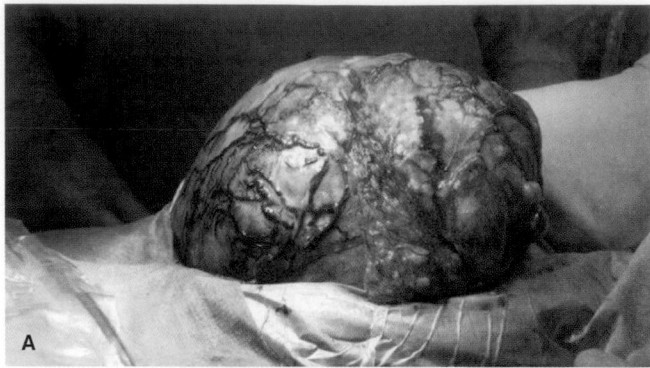

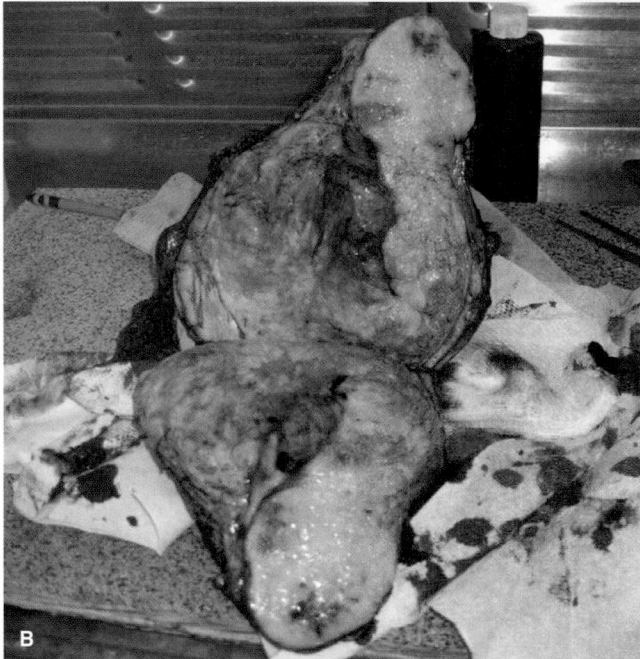

FIGURE 34-3 Endometrial stromal sarcoma. **A.** Intraoperative photograph of the uterine corpus. **B.** Photograph of the surgical specimen after it has been bivalved and remains joined at the fundus. The large tumor extends to involve the cervix.

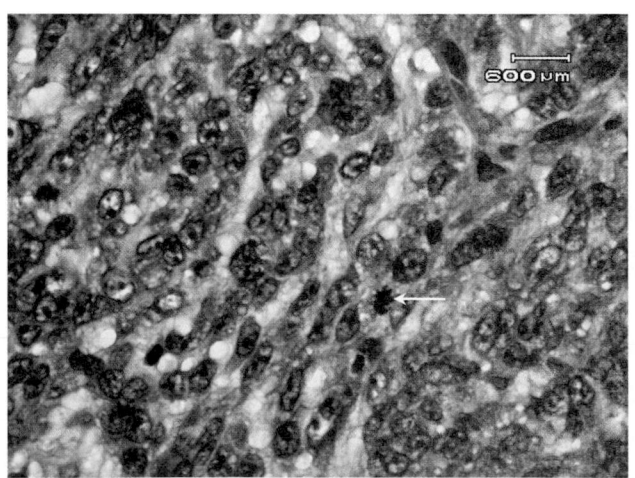

FIGURE 34-5 Undifferentiated uterine sarcoma. This is a high-grade mesenchymal neoplasm that lacks specific differentiation. These tumors usually show marked nuclear atypia and frequent mitotic activity (*arrow*). (*Photograph contributed by Dr. Raheela Ashfaq.*)

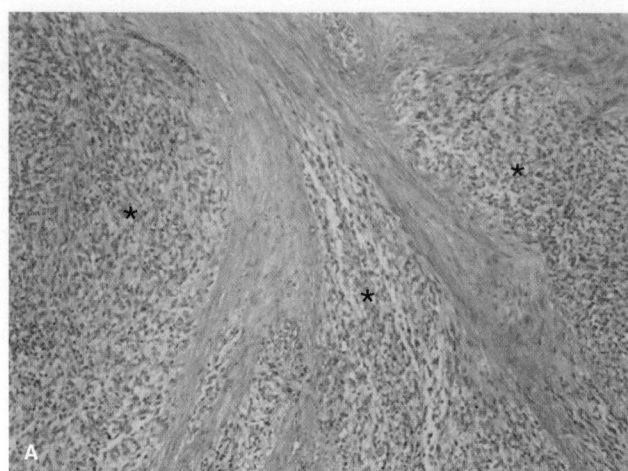

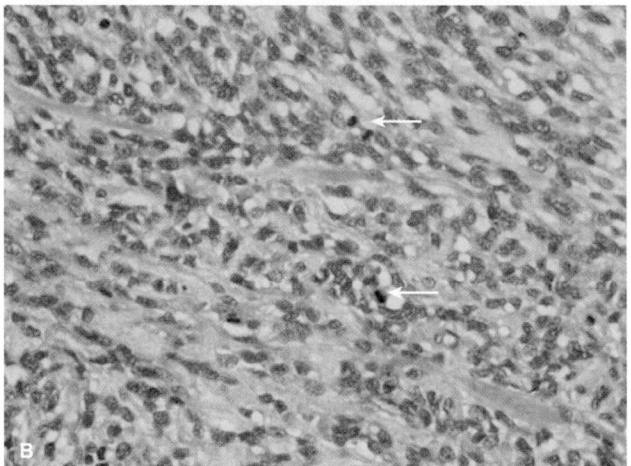

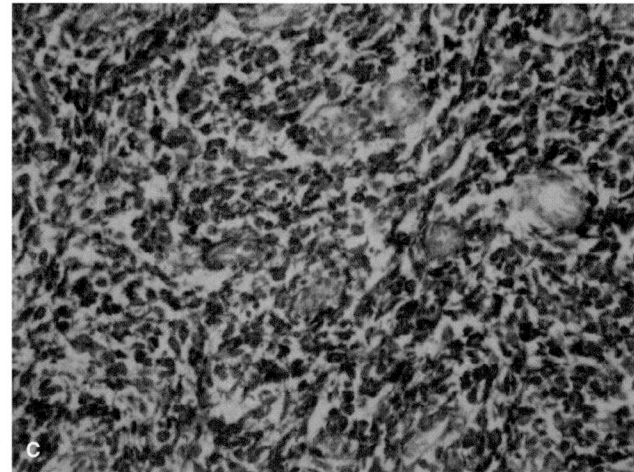

FIGURE 34-4 Endometrial stromal sarcoma (ESS), same patient as in Figure 34-3. **A.** ESS is a malignant neoplasm composed of cells morphologically similar to proliferative-phase endometrial stromal cells. In this low-power view of an ESS that involved the corpus and cervix, irregular tongues of tumor (*asterisks*) are seen dissecting into the cervical stroma. **B.** The tumor cells are spindled and relatively bland, similar to normal endometrial proliferative-phase stroma. Two mitoses (*arrows*) are identified in this single medium-power field. **C.** Immunohistochemical stain, CD10. Endometrial stroma marks positively with CD10, as does ESS. A battery of immunostains, including CD10, may be used to help distinguish ESS from other spindle cell neoplasms. (*Photographs contributed by Dr. Kelley Carrick.*)

no histologic resemblance to endometrial stroma (Hendrickson, 2003; Zaloudek, 2011).

Carcinosarcoma

Accumulating clinical and pathologic evidence suggests that carcinosarcomas actually represent endometrial carcinomas that have undergone clonal evolution, resulting in the acquisition of sarcomatous features. In principle, these tumors are metaplastic carcinomas. Clinically, their pattern of spread more closely mirrors that of aggressive endometrial carcinomas than that of sarcomas. In addition, metastases usually show carcinomatous elements, with or without sarcomatous differentiation.

However, by convention, carcinosarcomas are usually grouped with uterine sarcomas, accounting for 2 to 3 percent of all uterine malignancies. Patients are often elderly, having an average age of 65 years. Fewer than 5 percent are diagnosed in women younger than 50 years. Most cancers (40 percent) are stage I at the time of diagnosis; stage II (10 percent), stage III (25 percent), and stage IV disease (25 percent) comprise the remainder (Sartori, 1997; Vaidya, 2006).

Grossly, the tumor is sessile or polypoid, bulky, necrotic, and often hemorrhagic (Fig. 34-6). It often fills the endometrial cavity and deeply invades the myometrium. On occasion, a large tumor protrudes through the external cervical os and fills the vaginal vault.

Microscopically, carcinosarcomas have an admixture of epithelial and mesenchymal differentiation. The malignant epithelial element is typically an adenocarcinoma of endometrioid type, but serous, clear cell, mucinous, squamous cell, and undifferentiated carcinoma are also common (Fig. 34-7) (Chap. 33, p. 825). Mesenchymal components can be homologous, usually resembling endometrial stromal sarcomas or fibrosarco-

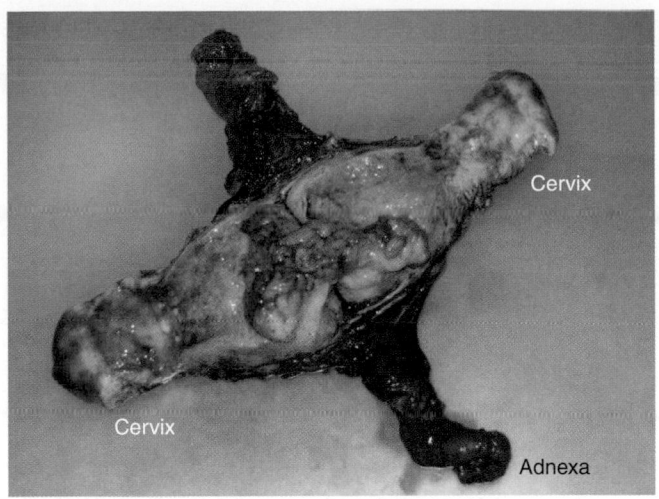

FIGURE 34-6 Carcinosarcoma. Photograph of the surgical specimen after it has been bivalved and remains joined at the fundus.

mas. Alternatively, heterologous mesenchymal differentiation can be found in association with areas of endometrial stromal or undifferentiated sarcomas. Most commonly, rhabdomyosarcoma or chondrosarcoma comprise these cases of heterologous mesenchymal differentiation (Fig. 34-8). Although interesting, there is no clinical importance to designating a uterine carcinosarcoma as homologous or heterologous (McCluggage, 2003).

Adenosarcoma

This rare, biphasic neoplasm is characterized by a benign epithelial component and a sarcomatous mesenchymal component. Tumors may develop in women of all ages. Grossly,

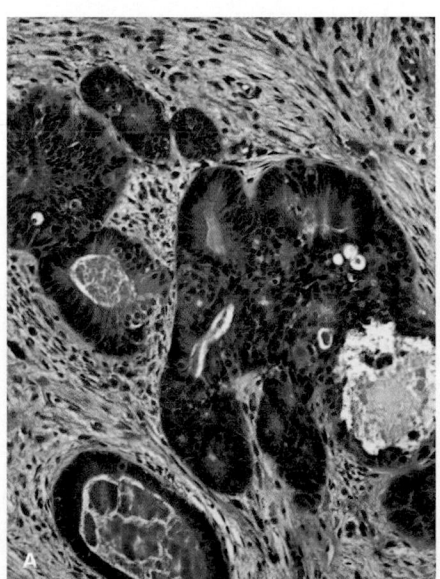 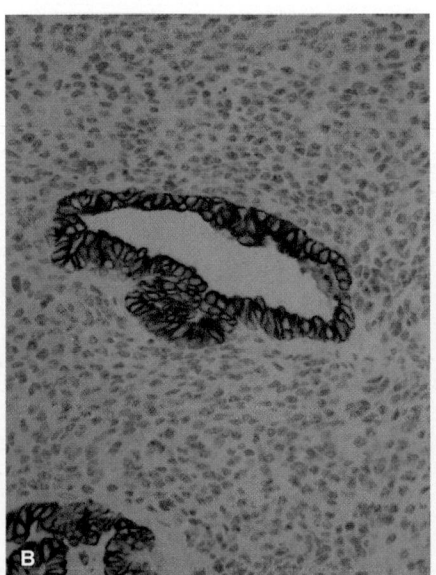 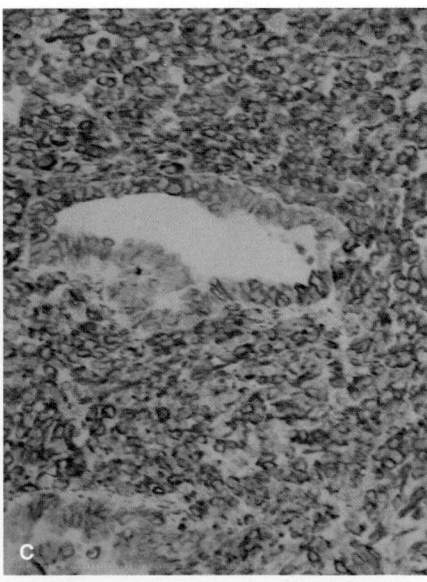

FIGURE 34-7 Carcinosarcoma, also known as malignant mixed müllerian tumor (MMMT). **A.** Carcinosarcoma is a biphasic malignant neoplasm composed of both carcinomatous and sarcomatous elements. In this example, malignant endometrioid-type glands are present within an atypical spindled stroma. **B.** Immunohistochemical stain for cytokeratin. Keratin marks the epithelial component but not the stromal component. **C.** Conversely, an immunohistochemical stain for vimentin (a mesenchymal marker) stains the sarcomatous component. *(Photographs contributed by Dr. Raheela Ashfaq.)*

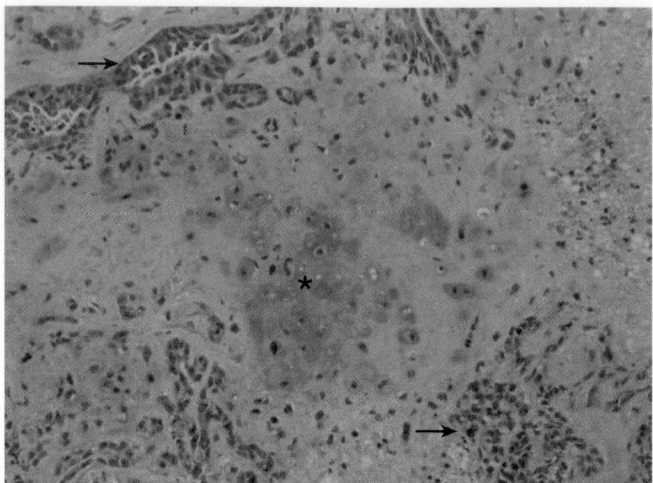

FIGURE 34-8 Carcinosarcoma with heterologous elements. In this medium-power view of a carcinosarcoma with cartilaginous differentiation, malignant glands are present at the periphery (*arrows*) of a focus of malignant cartilage (*asterisk*), with its characteristic lacunae embedded within a bluish chondroid matrix. (*Photograph contributed by Dr. Kelley Carrick.*)

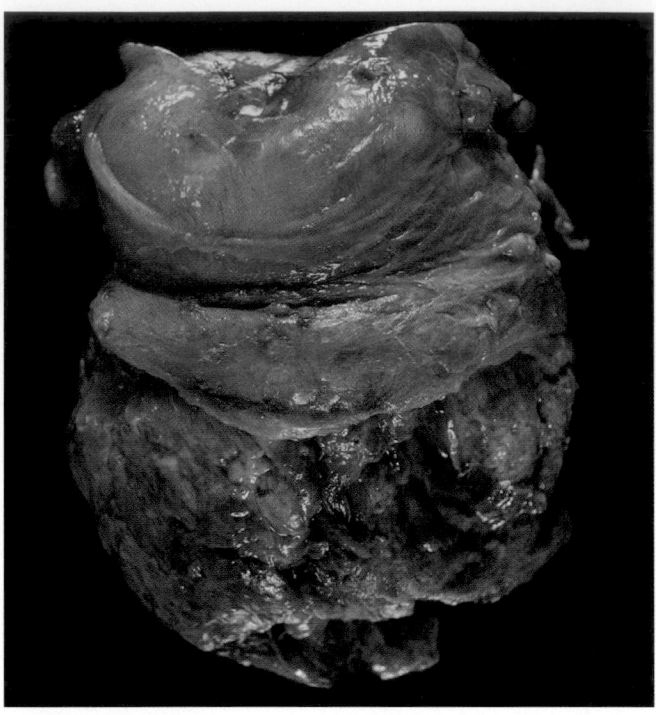

FIGURE 34-10 Gross uterine surgical specimen containing a large adenosarcoma.

adenosarcomas grow as exophytic polypoid masses that extend into the uterine cavity. Rarely, they may arise in the myometrium, presumably from adenomyosis. Microscopically, isolated glands are dispersed throughout the mesenchymal component and are often dilated or compressed into thin slits. Typically, the mesenchymal component resembles an endometrial stromal sarcoma or fibrosarcoma and contains varying amounts of fibrous tissue and smooth muscle (Fig. 34-9). In general, these are considered low-grade tumors with mild atypia and relatively few mitotic figures. However, 10 percent have a more malignant behavior due to one-sided proliferation of the sarcomatous, often high-grade, component. These adenosarcomas are designated as having "sarcomatous overgrowth," and patients

have a poor prognosis, similar to that of carcinosarcomas (Fig. 34-10) (Krivak, 2001; McCluggage, 2003).

PATTERNS OF SPREAD

Uterine sarcomas generally fall into two categories of malignant behavior. Leiomyosarcomas, high-grade undifferentiated sarcomas, and carcinosarcomas are consistently characterized by an aggressive growth pattern, early lymphatic or hematogenous dissemination, and rapid disease progression despite treatment.

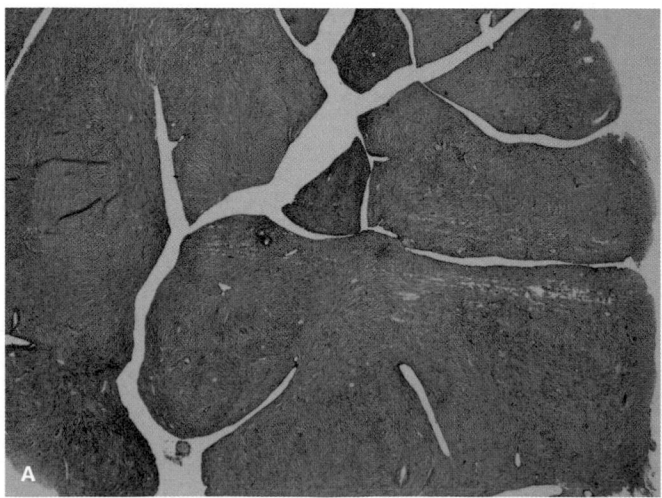
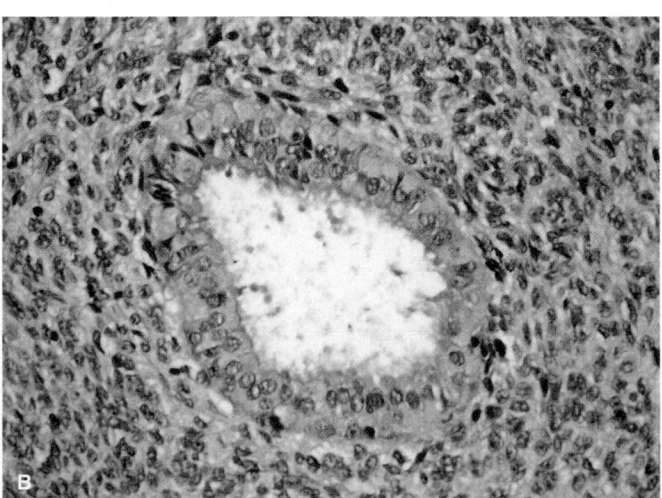

FIGURE 34-9 Photomicrographs of adenosarcoma. **A.** A broad-based villous architecture is typically seen at low magnification. **B.** A normal endometrial gland is surrounded by a cellular stroma consisting of a low-grade sarcoma—in this case, an endometrial stromal sarcoma. (*Photographs contributed by Dr. Raheela Ashfaq.*)

In contrast, endometrial stromal sarcomas and adenosarcomas have an indolent growth pattern with long disease-free intervals. All of these tumors grow, to some degree, by direct extension.

Leiomyosarcomas have a propensity for hematogenous dissemination. For example, lung metastases are particularly common, and more than half of patients will have distant spread if diagnosed with recurrent disease. To a lesser extent, leiomyosarcomas metastasize via lymphatic channels (Leitao, 2003). In a clinicopathologic Gynecologic Oncology Group (GOG) study, fewer than 5 percent of clinical stage I and II patients had nodal involvement (Major, 1993).

The opposite is true for carcinosarcomas, in which one third of patients with clinically stage I tumors will have nodal metastases (Park, 2010). Thus, comprehensive pelvic and paraaortic

lymphadenectomy is particularly important (Temkin, 2007). Extraabdominal spread is less common, and most recurrences are found in the pelvis or abdomen.

STAGING

There is now a specific staging system for uterine sarcomas. Formerly, most clinicians used the FIGO surgical staging system for endometrial cancer to stage uterine sarcomas. However, beginning in 2009, only carcinosarcomas share the same staging criteria as carcinomas of the endometrium (Table 33-8, p. 830). Endometrial stromal sarcomas and adenosarcomas share new criteria, whereas leiomyosarcomas have a different system for stage I (Table 34-3 and Fig. 34-11).

TABLE 34-3. FIGO Staging for Uterine Sarcomas (Leiomyosarcomas, Endometrial Stromal Sarcomas, Adenosarcomas, and Carcinosarcomas)

Stage	Characteristics
Leiomyosarcomas	
I	**Tumor limited to uterus**
IA	<5 cm
IB	>5 cm
II	**Tumor extends to the pelvis**
IIA	Adnexal involvement
IIB	Tumor extends to extrauterine pelvic tissue
III	**Tumor invades abdominal tissues (not just protruding into the abdomen)**
IIIA	One site
IIIB	>One site
IIIC	Metastasis to pelvic and/or paraaortic lymph nodes
IV	
IVA	Tumor invades bladder and/or rectum
IVB	Distant metastasis
Adenosarcomas and endometrial stromal sarcomas[a]	
I	**Tumor limited to uterus**
IA	Tumor limited to endometrium/endocervix with no myometrial invasion
IB	Less than or equal to half myometrial invasion
IC	More than half myometrial invasion
II	**Tumor extends to the pelvis**
IIA	Adnexal involvement
IIB	Tumor extends to extrauterine pelvic tissue
III	**Tumor invades abdominal tissues (not just protruding into the abdomen)**
IIIA	One site
IIIB	> One site
IIIC	Metastasis to pelvic and/or paraaortic lymph nodes
IV	
IVA	Tumor invades bladder and/or rectum
IVB	Distant metastasis
Carcinosarcomas	
Carcinosarcomas should be staged as carcinomas of the endometrium (see Table 33-8, p. 830)	

[a]Note: Simultaneous tumors of the uterine corpus and ovary/pelvis in association with ovarian/pelvic endometriosis should be classified as independent primary tumors.
FIGO = International Federation of Gynecology and Obstetrics.

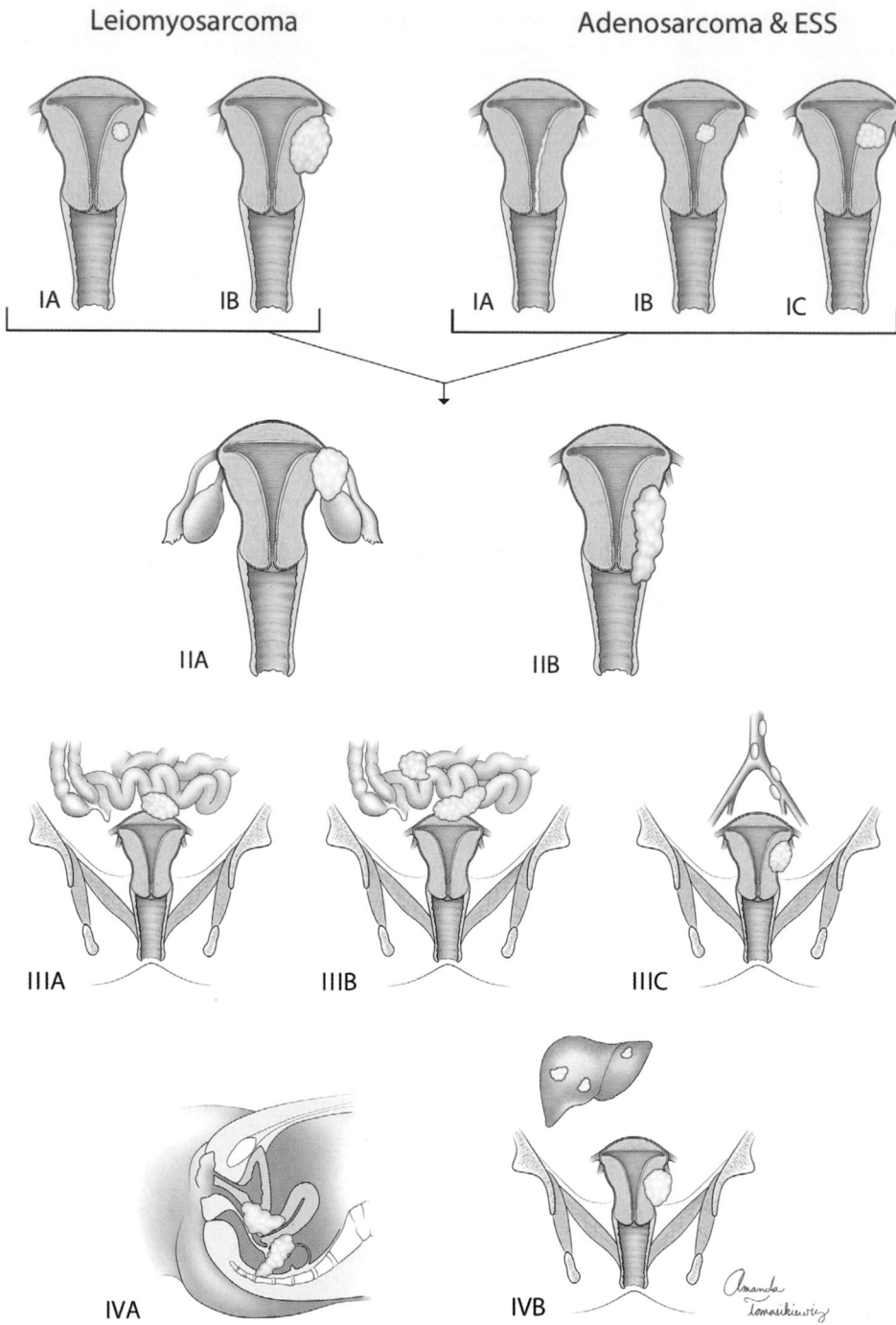

FIGURE 34-11 FIGO staging of leiomyosarcoma and that for adenosarcoma and endometrial stromal sarcoma (ESS).

The staging laparotomy described for endometrial cancer can be revised in several ways to incorporate the unique spread patterns of uterine sarcomas (Chap. 33, p. 829). For instance, peritoneal washings may be easily obtained upon opening the abdomen, but are not part of the staging system and have limited value regardless of the result (Kanbour, 1989). Exploration is particularly important to assess the abdomen for unresectable or widely metastatic disease that might indicate a need to abort the procedure. As in endometrial carcinomas, there is some evidence of benefit with aggressive cytoreductive surgery (Dinh, 2004; Leath, 2007; Thomas, 2009).

With uterine leiomyosarcoma, all patients should undergo a hysterectomy, if feasible. A modified radical or radical procedure may be occasionally required if there is parametrial infiltration. In the absence of other gross disease, fewer than 5 percent will have ovarian or nodal metastases. Ovarian preservation is therefore an option for premenopausal women. In addition, lymph node dissection should be reserved for patients with clinically suspicious nodes (Kapp, 2008; Leitao, 2003; Major, 1993). For STUMP, hysterectomy alone is sufficient.

Endometrial stromal tumors and adenosarcomas are also best treated by hysterectomy. Again, a more radical procedure may be required to encompass local disease. Preservation of the ovaries is generally accepted for endometrial stromal sarcomas or adenosarcomas in the absence of extrauterine disease (Chan, 2008; Li, 2005; Shah, 2008). However, bilateral salpingo-oophorectomy (BSO) is indicated for high-grade undifferentiated sarcomas (Leibsohn, 1990). Unlike leiomyosarcoma, lymph node dissection is typically more informative. Although nodal metastases are most often identified in patients with obvious extrauterine disease, they do occur in 5 to 10 percent of patients with no evidence for intraabdominal spread (Dos Santos, 2011; Goff, 1993; Signorelli, 2010).

For uterine carcinosarcoma, hysterectomy and BSO are mandatory. Lymph node metastases will be found in up to one third of patients with clinical stage I disease, and thus, comprehensive lymphadenectomy should be performed as for poorly differentiated endometrial cancers (Major, 1993; Nemani,

TREATMENT OF EARLY-STAGE DISEASE (STAGE I AND II)

Surgery

The highest chance of cure is achieved by complete surgical resection of a sarcoma that is confined to the uterus. In general, a laparotomy is performed due to the typical features of sarcomas, which include uterine enlargement, parametrial extension, and tumor metastasis. Laparoscopic or vaginal approaches have not yet been shown to yield equivalent outcomes.

2008; Park, 2010; Temkin, 2007). Typically, disease spread is histologically consistent with the carcinomatous element of this mixed tumor. Because this component may be serous or clear cell, extended surgical staging with infracolic omentectomy and random peritoneal biopsies is also advisable (Greer, 2011).

Surveillance

In women with early-stage uterine sarcoma, adjuvant treatment is routinely employed, but has not been demonstrated to improve survival (Greer, 2011; Reed, 2008). However, because the recurrence rate for the clinically aggressive types is excessive, enrollment in an experimental clinical trial should be carefully considered, if available. In practice, many patients receive postoperative radiation with or without chemotherapy.

After surgery, menopausal symptoms such as hot flashes may be treated as appropriate for uterine leiomyosarcomas, high-grade undifferentiated sarcomas, and adenosarcomas. However, although it is considered safe to preserve the ovaries in a premenopausal woman with endometrial stromal sarcoma, the use of estrogen replacement therapy has been associated with disease progression and should be avoided (Chu, 2003; Pink, 2006). Similar caution is warranted for patients with uterine carcinosarcoma.

Surgically treated patients with uterine sarcoma should have a physical examination every 3 months for the first 2 years and then at 6- to 12-month intervals thereafter. Most recurrences will be distant, and thus Pap tests are largely irrelevant. In addition, serum CA125 levels are not routinely recommended, unless initially elevated prior to surgery. Depending on the type of sarcoma, a chest radiograph or CT imaging should be performed every 6 to 12 months for 2 years, then annually. When clinically indicated, intermittent CT or MR imaging may also be helpful (Greer, 2011).

Adjuvant Radiation

Approximately half of patients with stage I disease who are observed without adjuvant therapy will relapse (Leath, 2009). Due to the rarity of these tumors and limited data to support a consistent approach, the use of postoperative therapy is usually individualized.

The role of postoperative radiotherapy for nonmetastatic disease is controversial. Prior retrospective studies of adjuvant external beam pelvic radiotherapy suggested a reduction in pelvic recurrence for carcinosarcoma, leiomyosarcoma, and endometrial stromal sarcoma (Callister, 2004; Hornback, 1986; Mahdavi, 2009; Malouf, 2010). However, results from a prospective trial that randomly assigned 224 women over 13 years with all subtypes of surgical stage I or II uterine sarcomas to receive either pelvic radiation or no further treatment have been reported. Although a reduction in pelvic relapse for those with carcinosarcomas was noted, there was no benefit for those with leiomyosarcomas and no significant increase in survival rates for either group. Unfortunately, the number of patients with endometrial stromal sarcoma was too small to permit analysis (Reed, 2008).

Pelvic radiation does not prevent distant recurrences and has yet to be shown to improve survival (Nemani, 2008). In many circumstances, vaginal brachytherapy may be an alter-native, especially if paired with systemic chemotherapy (Greer, 2011). However, whole abdominal radiotherapy (WAR) has been proposed as a more definitive option. In one randomized phase III study of 232 patients with stage I-IV carcinosarcoma, WAR was compared with ifosfamide and cisplatin chemotherapy. Although no survival advantage was demonstrated, the observed differences favored the use of combination chemotherapy in future trials (Wolfson, 2007).

Adjuvant Chemotherapy

There is no proven survival benefit for using adjuvant chemotherapy in patients with stage I uterine sarcoma (Omura, 1985). However, because most patients will recur distantly, systemic treatment is frequently used. For completely resected stage I and II leiomyosarcomas, high-grade undifferentiated sarcomas, and carcinosarcomas, chemotherapy regimens used for more advanced disease should be considered. Observation is recommended for stages I and II endometrial stromal sarcoma and adenosarcoma (Greer, 2011).

Fertility-Sparing Management

Rarely, young patients may desire to put off definitive hysterectomy after a fertility-sparing "myomectomy" demonstrates sarcomatous features on final pathology (Lissoni, 1998; Yan, 2010). Although expectant management following tumor resection can result in successful pregnancies in select patients, it is risky not to perform a hysterectomy, and eventually all such women should undergo hysterectomy (Lissoni, 1998). Most patients, even those with negative margins, should be counseled regarding definitive surgery and ovarian preservation during surgery for clinical stage I uterine leiomyosarcomas or endometrial stromal sarcomas. Egg retrieval and assisted reproductive technologies would still be possible. For more advanced disease, fertility-sparing management is not a reasonable option.

TREATMENT OF ADVANCED (STAGE III AND IV)/RECURRENT DISEASE

Patients with advanced or recurrent uterine sarcoma generally have a dismal prognosis. In some circumstances, secondary cytoreductive surgery may be feasible (Giuntoli, 2007). Palliative radiation may also have a role, depending on the site and distribution of the tumor. In general, uterine sarcomas have a propensity for relapse at distant sites, and chemotherapy is required. Since current treatment options have only modest efficacy, patients should be encouraged to enroll in experimental clinical trials.

Leiomyosarcoma

Doxorubicin is considered the most active single agent (Miller, 2000; Omura, 1983). However, treatment with the combination of gemcitabine and docetaxel currently has the highest proven response rate (36 percent) (Hensley, 2008).

For late recurrences of leiomyosarcoma, surgery must be individualized. Five-year survival rates of 30 to 50 percent have been reported following pulmonary resection for lung metastases.

Local and regional recurrences may also be amenable to surgical resection (Giuntoli, 2007).

Endometrial Stromal Tumors

Surgical resection may be feasible for some patients with recurrent endometrial stromal sarcoma, but hormonal therapy is known to be particularly useful. In general, these tumors are estrogen- and progesterone-receptor (ER/PR) positive (Sutton, 1986). Progestins such as megestrol acetate and medroxyprogesterone acetate are most commonly used either postoperatively for advanced-stage disease or for relapses (Reich, 2006). Using this strategy, complete responses are often possible. Aromatase inhibitors and gonadotropin-releasing hormone (GnRH) agonist have also demonstrated activity (Burke, 2004; Leunen, 2004).

High-grade undifferentiated sarcomas do not exhibit the same level of sensitivity to hormonal agents, primarily because they are usually ER/PR negative. Advanced disease or recurrences of these rare tumors are also typically not amenable to surgical resection, although palliative radiation may have some utility. Systemic chemotherapy is usually the only option, and ifosfamide is the only cytotoxic drug with proven activity (Sutton, 1996).

Carcinosarcoma

Ifosfamide is the most active single agent for carcinosarcoma. The combination of ifosfamide and paclitaxel is the current treatment of choice for advanced or recurrent uterine carcinosarcoma (Galaal, 2011). In a recent phase III GOG trial randomizing 179 patients, this regimen demonstrated a superior response rate (45 versus 29 percent) and survival advantage compared with ifosfamide alone (protocol #161) (Homesley, 2007). The combination of carboplatin and paclitaxel is also active and is being compared with ifosfamide and paclitaxel in an ongoing GOG trial (protocol #261) (King, 2009; Powell, 2010).

SURVIVAL AND PROGNOSTIC FACTORS

In general, women with uterine sarcoma have a poor prognosis (Table 34-4). In a study of 141 women followed for a median of 3 years, 74 percent died of disease progression.

TABLE 34-4. Overall Survival of Uterine Sarcomas (All Stages)

Type	5-Year Survival
Carcinosarcoma	35%
Leiomyosarcoma	25%
Endometrial stromal tumors	
Endometrial stromal sarcoma	60%
High-grade undifferentiated sarcoma	25%

Compiled from Acharya, 2005.

FIGO stage is the most important independent variable associated with survival (Livi, 2003). Other poor prognostic factors across all subtypes include older age, African-American race, and lack of primary surgery (Chan, 2008; Kapp, 2008; Nemani, 2008).

Tumor histology is the other main predictor of clinical outcome. Leiomyosarcomas have the worst prognosis and are followed by carcinosarcoma and endometrial stromal tumors (Livi, 2003). Endometrial stromal sarcomas and uterine adenosarcomas without sarcomatous overgrowth are the two notable exceptions. Patients with these tumors tend to have a good prognosis with an indolent growth pattern (Pautier, 2000; Verschraegen, 1998).

REFERENCES

Acharya S, Hensley ML, Montag AC, et al: Rare uterine cancers. Lancet Oncol 6(12):961, 2005

Brooks SE, Zhan M, Cote T, et al: Surveillance, epidemiology, and end results analysis of 2677 cases of uterine sarcoma 1989-1999. Gynecol Oncol 93(1):204, 2004

Burke C, Hickey K: Treatment of endometrial stromal sarcoma with a gonadotropin-releasing hormone analogue. Obstet Gynecol 104(5 Pt 2):1182, 2004

Callister M, Ramondetta LM, Jhingran A, et al: Malignant mixed Mullerian tumors of the uterus: analysis of patterns of failure, prognostic factors, and treatment outcome. Int J Radiat Oncol Biol Phys 58(3):786, 2004

Chan JK, Kawar NM, Shin JY, et al: Endometrial stromal sarcoma: a population-based analysis. Br J Cancer 99:1210, 2008

Chu MC, Mor G, Lim C, et al: Low-grade endometrial stromal sarcoma: hormonal aspects. Gynecol Oncol 90(1):170, 2003

D'Angelo E, Prat J: Uterine sarcomas: a review. Gynecol Oncol 116:131, 2010

De Fusco PA, Gaffey TA, Malkasian GD Jr, et al: Endometrial stromal sarcoma: review of Mayo Clinic experience, 1945-1980. Gynecol Oncol 35(1):8, 1989

Dinh TA, Oliva EA, Fuller AF Jr, et al: The treatment of uterine leiomyosarcoma. Results from a 10-year experience (1990-1999) at the Massachusetts General Hospital. Gynecol Oncol 92:648, 2004

Dionigi A, Oliva E, Clement PB, et al: Endometrial stromal nodules and endometrial stromal tumors with limited infiltration: a clinicopathologic study of 50 cases. Am J Surg Pathol 26(5):567, 2002

Dos Santos LA, Garg K, Diaz JP, et al: Incidence of lymph node and adnexal metastasis in endometrial stromal sarcoma. Gynecol Oncol 121(2):319, 2011

Evans HL: Endometrial stromal sarcoma and poorly differentiated endometrial sarcoma. Cancer 50(10):2170, 1982

Fujii H, Yoshida M, Gong ZX, et al: Frequent genetic heterogeneity in the clonal evolution of gynecological carcinosarcoma and its influence on phenotypic diversity. Cancer Res 60(1):114, 2000

Galaal K, Godfrey K, Naik R, et al: Adjuvant radiotherapy and/or chemotherapy after surgery for uterine carcinosarcoma. Cochrane Database Syst Rev 1:CD006812, 2011

Giuntoli RL 2nd, Garrett-Mayer E, Bristow RE, et al: Secondary cytoreduction in the management of recurrent uterine leiomyosarcoma. Gynecol Oncol 106(1):82, 2007

Goff BA, Rice LW, Fleischhacker D, et al: Uterine leiomyosarcoma and endometrial stromal sarcoma: lymph node metastases and sites of recurrence. Gynecol Oncol 50(1):105, 1993

Gonzalez-Bosquet E, Martinez-Palones JM, Gonzalez-Bosquet J, et al: Uterine sarcoma: a clinicopathological study of 93 cases. Eur J Gynaecol Oncol 18(3):192, 1997

Greer BE, Koh WJ, Abu-Rustum NR, et al: Uterine Neoplasms. NCCN Clinical Practice Guidelines in Oncology. Version I. 2011. Available at: www.nccn.org. Accessed April 14, 2011

Gynecologic Oncology Group: Histologic classification of malignant neoplasm of uterine corpus. Available at: https://gogmember.gog.org/committees/pathology/TOC_Path_Manual.html. Accessed April 14, 2011

Halbwedl I, Ullmann R, Kremser ML, et al: Chromosomal alterations in low-grade endometrial stromal sarcoma and undifferentiated endometrial sarcoma as detected by comparative genomic hybridization. Gynecol Oncol 97(2):582, 2005

Hendrickson MR, Tavassoli FA, Kempson RL, et al: Tumors of the Uterine Corpus [Mesenchymal tumors and related lesions]. In Tavassoli FA, Devilee P (eds): World Health Organization Classification of Tumours. Lyon, France, IARC Press, 2003, p 233

Hensley ML, Blessing JA, Mannel R, et al: Fixed-dose rate gemcitabine plus docetaxel as first-line therapy for metastatic uterine leiomyosarcoma: a Gynecologic Oncology Group phase II trial. Gynecol Oncol 109:329, 2008

Homesley HD, Filiaci V, Markman M, et al: Phase III trial of ifosfamide with or without paclitaxel in advanced uterine carcinosarcoma: a Gynecologic Oncology Group Study. J Clin Oncol 25:526, 2007

Hornback NB, Omura G, Major FJ: Observations on the use of adjuvant radiation therapy in patients with stage I and II uterine sarcoma. Int J Radiat Oncol Biol Phys 12(12):2127, 1986

Huang GS, Chiu LG, Gebb JS, et al: Serum CA125 predicts extrauterine disease and survival in uterine carcinosarcoma. Gynecol Oncol 107:513, 2007

Kanbour AI, Buchsbaum HJ, Hall A, et al: Peritoneal cytology in malignant mixed mullerian tumors of the uterus. Gynecol Oncol 33(1):91, 1989

Kapp DS, Shin JY, Chan JK: Prognostic factors and survival in 1396 patients with uterine leiomyosarcomas: emphasis on impact of lymphadenectomy and oophorectomy. Cancer 112(4):820, 2008

Kido A, Togashi K, Koyama T, et al: Diffusely enlarged uterus: evaluation with MR imaging. Radiographics 23(6):1423, 2003

King LP, Miller DS: Recent progress: gynecologic oncology group trials in uterine corpus tumors. Rev Recent Clin Trials 4(2):70, 2009

Krivak TC, Seidman JD, McBroom JW, et al: Uterine adenosarcoma with sarcomatous overgrowth versus uterine carcinosarcoma: comparison of treatment and survival. Gynecol Oncol 83(1):89, 2001

Leath CA 3rd, Huh WK, Hyde J Jr, et al: A multi-institutional review of outcomes of endometrial stromal sarcoma. Gynecol Oncol 105:630, 2007

Leath CA 3rd, Numnum TM, Kendrick JE 4th, et al: Patterns of failure for conservatively managed surgical stage I uterine carcinosarcoma: implications for adjuvant therapy. Int J Gynecol Cancer 19:888, 2009

Leibsohn S, d'Ablaing G, Mishell DR Jr, et al: Leiomyosarcoma in a series of hysterectomies performed for presumed uterine leiomyomas. Am J Obstet Gynecol 162(4):968, 1990

Leitao MM, Sonoda Y, Brennan MF, et al: Incidence of lymph node and ovarian metastases in leiomyosarcoma of the uterus. Gynecol Oncol 91(1):209, 2003

Leunen M, Breugelmans M, De Sutter P, et al: Low-grade endometrial stromal sarcoma treated with the aromatase inhibitor letrozole. Gynecol Oncol 95(3):769, 2004

Li AJ, Giuntoli RL, Drake R, et al: Ovarian preservation in stage I low-grade endometrial stromal sarcomas. Obstet Gynecol 106(6):1304, 2005

Lissoni A, Cormio G, Bonazzi C, et al: Fertility-sparing surgery in uterine leiomyosarcoma. Gynecol Oncol 70(3):348, 1998

Liu FS, Kohler MF, Marks JR, et al: Mutation and overexpression of the p53 tumor suppressor gene frequently occurs in uterine and ovarian sarcomas. Obstet Gynecol 83(1):118, 1994

Livi L, Paiar F, Shah N, et al: Uterine sarcoma: twenty-seven years of experience. Int J Radiat Oncol Biol Phys 57(5):1366, 2003

Mahdavi A, Monk BJ, Ragazzo J, et al: Pelvic radiation improves local control after hysterectomy for uterine leiomyosarcoma: a 20-year experience. Int J Gynecol Cancer 19:1080, 2009

Major FJ, Blessing JA, Silverberg SG, et al: Prognostic factors in early-stage uterine sarcoma. A Gynecologic Oncology Group study. Cancer 71 (4 Suppl):1702, 1993

Malouf GG, Duclos J, Rey A, et al: Impact of adjuvant treatment modalities on the management of patients with stage I-II endometrial stromal sarcoma. Ann Oncol 21:2102, 2010

McCluggage WG: Uterine carcinosarcomas (malignant mixed Mullerian tumors) are metaplastic carcinomas. Int J Gynecol Cancer 12:687, 2002

McCluggage WG, Haller U, Kurman RJ, et al: Tumors of the Uterine Corpus [Mixed epithelial and mesenchymal tumors]. In Tavassoli FA, Devilee P (eds): World Health Organization Classification of Tumours. Lyon, France, IARC Press, 2003, p 245

Micci F, Panagopoulos I, Bjerkehagen B, et al: Consistent rearrangement of chromosomal band 6p21 with generation of fusion genes JAZF1/PHF1 and EPC1/PHF1 in endometrial stromal sarcoma. Cancer Res 66(1):107, 2006

Miller DS, Blessing JA, Kilgore LC, et al: Phase II trial of topotecan in patients with advanced, persistent, or recurrent uterine leiomyosarcomas: a Gynecologic Oncology Group Study. Am J Clin Oncol 23(4):355-7, 2000

Moinfar F, Kremser ML, Man YG, et al: Allelic imbalances in endometrial stromal neoplasms: frequent genetic alterations in the nontumorous normal-appearing endometrial and myometrial tissues. Gynecol Oncol 95(3):662, 2004

Nemani D, Mitra N, Guo M, et al: Assessing the effects of lymphadenectomy and radiation therapy in patients with uterine carcinosarcoma: a SEER analysis. Gynecol Oncol 111:82, 2008

Oliva E, Clement PB, Young RH: Endometrial stromal tumors: an update on a group of tumors with a protean phenotype. Adv Anat Pathol 7(5):257, 2000

Omura GA, Blessing JA, Major F, et al: A randomized clinical trial of adjuvant adriamycin in uterine sarcomas: a Gynecologic Oncology Group Study. J Clin Oncol 3(9):1240, 1985

Omura GA, Major FJ, Blessing JA, et al: A randomized study of adriamycin with and without dimethyl triazenoimidazole carboxamide in advanced uterine sarcomas. Cancer 52(4):626, 1983

Park JY, Kim DY, Kim JH, et al: The role of pelvic and/or para-aortic lymphadenectomy in surgical management of apparently early carcinosarcoma of uterus. Ann Surg Oncol 17:861, 2010

Parker WH, Fu YS, Berek JS: Uterine sarcoma in patients operated on for presumed leiomyoma and rapidly growing leiomyoma. Obstet Gynecol 83(3):414, 1994

Pautier P, Genestie C, Rey A, et al: Analysis of clinicopathologic prognostic factors for 157 uterine sarcomas and evaluation of a grading score validated for soft tissue sarcoma. Cancer 88(4):1425, 2000

Perri T, Korach J, Sadetzki S, et al: Uterine leiomyosarcoma: does the primary surgical procedure matter? Int J Gynecol Cancer 19:257, 2009

Pink D, Lindner T, Mrozek A, et al: Harm or benefit of hormonal treatment in metastatic low-grade endometrial stromal sarcoma: single center experience with 10 cases and review of the literature. Gynecol Oncol 101(3):464, 2006

Powell MA, Filiaci VL, Rose PG, et al: Phase II evaluation of paclitaxel and carboplatin in the treatment of carcinosarcoma of the uterus: a Gynecologic Oncology Group study. J Clin Oncol 28(16):2727, 2010

Quade BJ, Wang TY, Sornberger K, et al: Molecular pathogenesis of uterine smooth muscle tumors from transcriptional profiling. Genes Chromosomes Cancer 40(2):97, 2004

Reed NS, Mangioni C, Malmstrom H, et al: Phase III randomised study to evaluate the role of adjuvant pelvic radiotherapy in the treatment of uterine sarcomas stages I and II: a European Organisation for Research and Treatment of Cancer Gynaecological Cancer Group Study (protocol 55874). Eur J Cancer 44:808, 2008

Reich O, Regauer S: Survey of adjuvant hormone therapy in patients after endometrial stromal sarcoma. Eur J Gynaecol Oncol 27(2):150, 2006

Sartori E, Bazzurini L, Gadducci A, et al: Carcinosarcoma of the uterus: a clinicopathological multicenter CTF study. Gynecol Oncol 67:70, 1997

Shah JP, Bryant CS, Kumar S, et al: Lymphadenectomy and ovarian preservation in low-grade endometrial stromal sarcoma. Obstet Gynecol 112:1102, 2008

Signorelli M, Fruscio R, Dell-Anna T, et al: Lymphadenectomy in uterine low-grade endometrial stromal sarcoma: an analysis of 19 cases and a literature review. Int J Gynecol Cancer 20:1363, 2010

Skubitz KM, Skubitz APN: Differential gene expression in leiomyosarcoma. Cancer 98 (5):1029, 2003

Sutton G, Blessing JA, Park R, et al: Ifosfamide treatment of recurrent or metastatic endometrial stromal sarcomas previously unexposed to chemotherapy: a study of the Gynecologic Oncology Group. Obstet Gynecol 87 (5 Pt 1):747, 1996

Sutton GP, Stehman FB, Michael H, et al: Estrogen and progesterone receptors in uterine sarcomas. Obstet Gynecol 68(5):709, 1986

Tavassoli FA, Devilee P (eds): World Health Organization Classification of Tumours, Pathology and Genetics of Tumours of the Breast and Female Genital Organs. Lyon, France, IARC Press, 2003

Taylor NP, Zighelboim I, Huettner PC, et al: DNA mismatch repair and TP53 defects are early events in uterine carcinosarcoma tumorigenesis. Mod Pathol 19(10):1333, 2006

Temkin SM, Hellmann M, Lee YC, et al: Early-stage carcinosarcoma of the uterus: the significance of lymph node count. Int J Gynecol Cancer 17:215, 2007

Thomas MB, Keeney GL, Podratz KC, et al: Endometrial stromal sarcoma: treatment and patterns of recurrence. Int J Gynecol Cancer 19:253, 2009

Vaidya AP, Horowitz NS, Oliva E, et al: Uterine malignant mixed mullerian tumors should not be included in studies of endometrial carcinoma. Gynecol Oncol 103:684, 2006

Verschraegen CF, Vasuratna A, Edwards C, et al: Clinicopathologic analysis of mullerian adenosarcoma: the M.D. Anderson Cancer Center experience. Oncol Rep 5(4):939, 1998

SECTION 4

Wada H, Enomoto T, Fujita M, et al: Molecular evidence that most but not all carcinosarcomas of the uterus are combination tumors. Cancer Res 57(23):5379, 1997

Wolfson AH, Brady MF, Rocereto T, et al: A Gynecologic Oncology Group randomized phase III trial of whole abdominal irradiation (WAI) vs. cisplatin-ifosfamide and mesna (CIM) as post-surgical therapy in stage I-IV carcinosarcoma (CS) of the uterus. Gynecol Oncol 107:177, 2007

Yan L, Tian Y, Zhao X: Successful pregnancy after fertility-preserving surgery for endometrial stromal sarcoma. Fertil Steril 93:269.e1, 2010

Yang GC, Wan LS, Del Priore G: Factors influencing the detection of uterine cancer by suction curettage and endometrial brushing. J Reprod Med 47(12):1005, 2002

Zaloudek C, Hendrickson MR, Soslow RA: Mesenchymal tumors of the uterus. In Kurman RJ, Ellenson LH, Ronnett BM (eds): Blaustein's Pathology of the Female Genital Tract, 6th ed. New York, Springer, 2011, p 453

Zhang P, Zhang C, Hao J, et al: Use of X-chromosome inactivation pattern to determine the clonal origins of uterine leiomyoma and leiomyosarcoma. Hum Pathol 37(10):1350, 2006

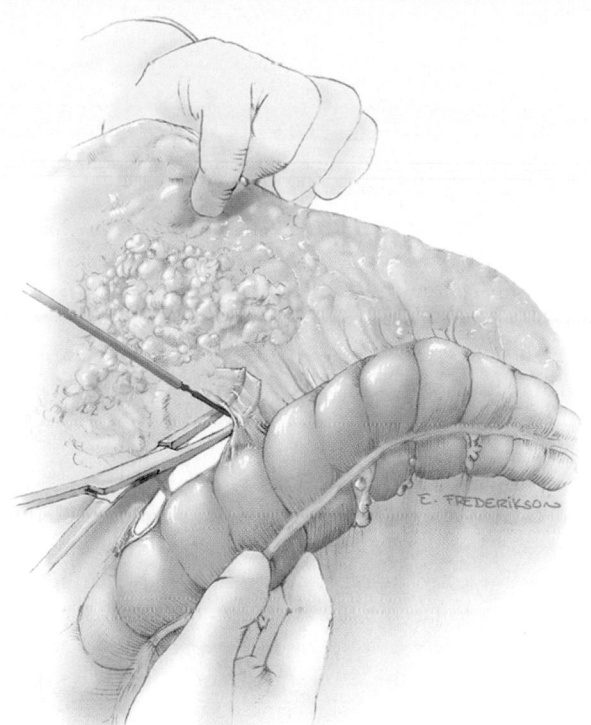

CHAPTER 35

Epithelial Ovarian Cancer

In the United States, ovarian cancer accounts for more deaths than all other gynecologic malignancies combined. Worldwide each year, more than 225,000 women are diagnosed, and 140,000 women die from this disease (Jemal, 2011). Of these, epithelial ovarian carcinomas comprise 90 to 95 percent of all cases, including the more indolent low-malignant-potential

(borderline) tumors (Quirk, 2005). The remainder includes germ cell and sex cord-stromal tumors, which are described in Chapter 36 (p. 879). Due to the similarities of primary peritoneal carcinomas and fallopian tube cancers, they are included within this section for simplicity.

Approximately one quarter of patients will have stage I disease and an excellent long-term survival. However, there are no effective screening tests for ovarian cancer and few notable early symptoms. As a result, two thirds of patients have advanced disease when they are diagnosed. Aggressive debulking surgery, followed by platinum-based chemotherapy, usually results in clinical remission. However, up to 80 percent of these women will develop a relapse that eventually leads to disease progression and death.

EPIDEMIOLOGY AND RISK FACTORS

One in 78 American women (1.3 percent) will develop ovarian cancer during their lifetime. Because the incidence has been slowly declining since the early 1990s, ovarian cancer has dropped to the ninth leading cause of cancer in women. In 2011, 21,990 new cases are estimated to develop in the United States. However, few patients are diagnosed early and subsequently cured. As a result, 15,460 deaths are expected, and ovarian cancer remains the fifth leading cause of cancer-related death (Siegel, 2011). Overall, the average age at diagnosis is in the early 60s.

Numerous reproductive, environmental, and genetic risk factors have been associated with the development of ovarian cancer (Table 35-1). The most important is a *family history* of breast or ovarian cancer, and 5 to 10 percent of patients have an inherited genetic predisposition. For the other 90 to 95 percent with no identifiable genetic link for their ovarian cancer, most risk factors are related to a pattern of uninterrupted ovulatory cycles during the reproductive years (Pelucchi, 2007). Repeated stimulation of the ovarian surface

TABLE 35-1. Risk Factors for Developing Epithelial Ovarian Cancer

Nulliparity
Early menarche
Late menopause
White race
Increasing age
Residence in North America and Northern Europe
Family history
Personal history of breast cancer
Ethnic background (European Jewish, Icelandic, Hungarian)

Abbreviated from Schorge, 2010a, with permission.

epithelium is hypothesized to lead to malignant transformation (Schildkraut, 1997).

Nulliparity is associated with long periods of repetitive ovulation, and patients without children have double the risk of developing ovarian cancer (Purdie, 2003). Among nulliparous women, those with a history of infertility have an even higher risk. Although the reasons are unclear, it is more likely to be an inherent ovarian predisposition rather than an iatrogenic effect of ovulation-inducing drugs. For example, women treated for infertility who successfully achieve a live birth do not have an increased risk of ovarian cancer (Rossing, 2004). In general, risks decrease with each live birth, eventually plateauing in women delivering five times (Hinkula, 2006). One interesting theory to explain this protective effect is that pregnancy may induce shedding of premalignant ovarian cells (Rostgaard, 2003).

Early menarche and *late menopause* have also been associated with an increased risk of ovarian cancer. In contrast, breastfeeding has a protective effect, perhaps by prolonging amenorrhea (Yen, 2003). Presumably by also preventing ovulation, long-term combination oral contraceptive use reduces the risk of ovarian cancer by 50 percent. The duration of protection lasts up to 25 years after the last use (Riman, 2002). In contrast, estrogen replacement therapy after the menopause has an elevated associated risk (Lacey, 2006).

White women have the highest incidence of ovarian cancer among all racial and ethnic groups (Quirk, 2005). Compared with that of black and Hispanic women, the risk is elevated by 30 to 40 percent (Goodman, 2003). Although exact reasons are unknown, racial discrepancies in parity and rates of gynecologic surgery may account for some of the differences.

Tubal ligation and *hysterectomy* have each been associated with a substantial reduction in risk of developing ovarian cancer (Hankinson, 1993). It has been postulated that any type of gynecologic procedure that precludes irritants from reaching the ovaries via ascension from the lower genital tract might plausibly exert a similar protective effect. For example, women who regularly use perineal talc may have an elevated risk (Gertig, 2000; Rosenblatt, 2011).

The overall incidence of ovarian cancer rises with *increasing age* up to the mid-70s, before declining slightly among women beyond 80 years (Goodman, 2003). In general, aging allows an extended period to accumulate random genetic alterations within the ovarian surface epithelium.

Women *residing in North America, Northern Europe, or any industrialized Western country*, for example, Israel, have a higher risk of ovarian cancer. Globally, the incidence varies greatly, but developing countries and Japan have the lowest rates (Jemal, 2011). Regional dietary habits may be partly responsible (Kiani, 2006). For example, consumption of foods low in fat but high in fiber, carotene, and vitamins appears protective (Zhang, 2004).

A *family history* of ovarian cancer in a first-degree relative, that is, a mother, daughter, or sister, triples a woman's lifetime risk of developing ovarian cancer. The risks further escalate with two or more afflicted first-degree relatives. Identification of high-risk patients with family members having ovarian, breast, or colon cancer is currently the best prevention strategy (National Cancer Institute, 2011a). If a family history is mainly comprised of colon cancer, clinicians should be aware of the possibility of *hereditary nonpolyposis colorectal cancer* (HNPCC), also known as Lynch syndrome. Patients with this syndrome have a high lifetime risk of colon cancer (85 percent) and ovarian cancer (10 to 12 percent). Because the predominant gynecologic malignancy is endometrial cancer (40 to 60 percent lifetime risk), HNPCC is described in more detail in Chapter 33 (p. 823).

Hereditary Breast and Ovarian Cancer
Genetic Screening

More than 90 percent of inherited ovarian cancers result from germline mutations in the *BRCA1* or *BRCA2* genes. Thus, any patient with a personal risk of greater than 20 to 25 percent *should* undergo genetic risk assessment (Table 35-2). Moreover, it is reasonable to *offer* genetic risk assessment to any individual with greater than a 5 to 10 percent chance of having an inherited predisposition (Table 35-3) (American College of Obstetricians and Gynecologists, 2009; Lancaster, 2007).

Typically, a patient is referred to a certified genetic counselor where a comprehensive pedigree is constructed first. Then, risk assessment is performed using one of several validated population models. These include the BRCAPRO and Tyrer-Cuzick programs, which are available, respectively, at: http://www4.utsouthwestern.edu/breasthealth/cagene/default.asp, and by contacting the International Breast Cancer Intervention Study (IBIS) at ibis@cancer.org.uk. These models evaluate an individual's risk for carrying a germline deleterious mutation of the *BRCA1* and *BRCA2* genes. These models and their associated software allow accurate quantification of this risk, and the results determine whether a patient should undergo genetic testing (Euhus, 2002; James, 2006; Parmigiani, 2007).

BRCA1 and *BRCA2* Genes

These are two tumor-suppressor genes, whose protein products are BRCA1 and BRCA2. These two proteins interact with recombination/DNA repair proteins to preserve intact chromosomal structure. Mutations of *BRCA1* and *BRCA2*

TABLE 35-2. Patients with Greater Than 20–25% Chance of Having an Inherited Predisposition to Breast and Ovarian Cancer and For Whom Genetic Risk Assessment Is Recommended

Women with a personal history of both breast and ovarian[a] cancer
Women with ovarian cancer[a] and a close relative[b] with breast cancer at ≤50 years or ovarian cancer at any age
Women with ovarian cancer[a] at any age who are of Ashkenazi Jewish ancestry
Women with breast cancer at ≤50 years and a close relative[b] with ovarian[a] or male breast cancer at any age
Women of Ashkenazi Jewish ancestry and breast cancer at ≤40 years
Women with a first- or second-degree relative with a known *BRCA1* or *BRCA2* gene mutation

[a]Peritoneal and fallopian tube cancer should be considered as part of the spectrum of the Hereditary Breast/Ovarian Cancer syndrome.
[b]*Close relative* is defined as a first-, second-, or third-degree relative (i.e., mother, sister, daughter, aunt, niece, grandmother, granddaughter, first cousin, great grandmother, great aunt).
From Lancaster, 2007, with permission.

genes lead to BRCA1 and BRCA2 protein dysfunction, which results in genetic instability and subjects cells to a higher risk of malignant transformation (Fig. 35-1) (Deng, 2006; Scully, 2000). The *BRCA1* gene is located on chromosome 17q21. Patients with a proven mutation have a dramatically elevated risk of developing ovarian cancer (39 to 46 percent). *BRCA2* is located on chromosome 13q12 and in general, is less likely to lead to ovarian cancer (12 to 20 percent). The estimated lifetime risk of breast cancer with a *BRCA1* or *BRCA2* mutation is 65 to 74 percent (American College of Obstetricians and Gynecologists, 2009; Chen, 2006; Risch, 2006). Both genes are inherited in an autosomal dominant fashion, but with variable penetrance. In essence, a carrier has a 50:50 chance of passing the gene to a son or daughter, but it is uncertain whether anyone with the gene mutation will actually develop breast or ovarian cancer. As a result, manifestations of *BRCA1* or *BRCA2* mutations can appear to skip generations.

Genetic Testing

The main purpose of genetic testing is to identify women with deleterious *BRCA1* and *BRCA2* mutations, to intervene with prophylactic surgery, and to thereby prevent ovarian cancer. Three distinct results are possible with this testing. A "positive" test suggests the presence of a deleterious mutation. The most common are the three "Jewish founder" mutations: 185delAG or 5382insC in *BRCA1* and 6174delT in *BRCA2*. Each of these "frameshift" mutations significantly alters the downstream amino acid sequence, resulting in alteration of the BRCA1 or BRCA2 tumor suppressor protein. As suggested, these three specific mutations are thought to have originated from within the Ashkenazi population thousands of years ago. Although Jewish founder mutations are most common, any frameshift mutation within the BRCA genes may result in a deleterious predisposition to developing breast and ovarian cancer.

Second, "variants of uncertain clinical significance" may actually be pathogenic (true mutations) or just polymorphisms (normal variants found in at least 1 percent of alleles in the general population). These unclassified variants are common, representing approximately one third of BRCA1 test results and half of those for BRCA2. Most are missense mutations, which result in a single amino acid change in the protein, without a frameshift. Due to their uncertain clinical relevance, it is

TABLE 35-3. Patients with Greater Than 5–10% Chance of Having an Inherited Predisposition to Breast and Ovarian Cancer and For Whom Genetic Risk Assessment May Be Helpful[a]

Women with breast cancer at ≤40 years
Women with bilateral breast cancer (particularly if the first cancer was at ≤50 years)
Women with breast cancer at ≤50 years and a close relative[b] with breast cancer at ≤50 years
Women of Ashkenazi Jewish ancestry with breast cancer at ≤50 years
Women with breast or ovarian cancer at any age and two or more close relatives[b] with breast cancer at any age
    (particularly if at least one breast cancer was at ≤50 years)
Unaffected women with a first- or second-degree relative that meets one of the above criteria

[a]In families with a paucity of female relatives in either lineage, it may also be reasonable to consider genetic risk assessment even in the setting of either an isolated case of breast cancer at ≥50 years or an isolated case of ovarian, fallopian tube, or peritoneal cancer at any age.
[b]*Close relative* is defined as a first-, second-, or third-degree relative (i.e., mother, sister, daughter, aunt, niece, grandmother, granddaughter, first cousin, great grandmother, great aunt).
From Lancaster, 2007, with permission.

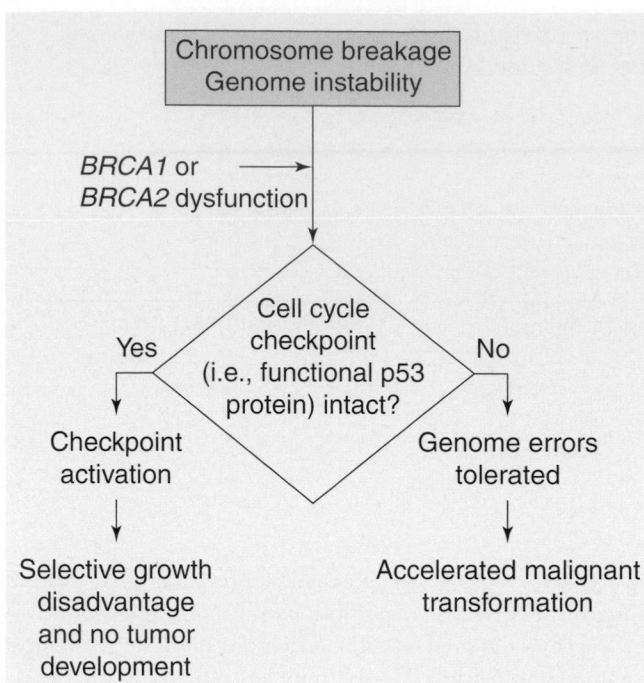

FIGURE 35-1 Diagram describing the role of the *BRCA* mutation in tumor development. Cells with damaged DNA are frequently blocked at checkpoints along the cell cycle and thereby prohibited from moving to the mitotic phase. If these checkpoints are non-functional, then these genomic errors may be tolerated and lead to malignant transformation. *(Modified from Scully, 2000, with permission.)*

reasonable to ignore them and base patient counseling on family history (Gomez-Garcia, 2005).

The third potential and most reassuring genetic test result is "negative." However, due to the large size of the *BRCA1* and *BRCA2* genes, there is a false-negative rate of approximately 10 percent.

PREVENTION

Ovarian Cancer Screening

In addition to genetic testing, other screening strategies for ovarian cancer have been evaluated. However, despite enormous effort, there is no proof that routine screening with serum markers, sonography, or pelvic examinations decreases mortality rates (American College of Obstetricians and Gynecologists, 2009; Morgan, 2011; Schorge, 2010a). Hundreds of possible markers have been identified, yet no test currently available approaches sufficient levels of accuracy (American College of Obstetricians and Gynecologists, 2011).

High-Risk Women

For the most part, screening strategies are directed at *BRCA1* or *BRCA2* carriers, in addition to women with a strong family history of breast and ovarian cancer. Most commonly, cancer antigen 125 (CA125) level measurements and/or transvaginal sonography have been tested, albeit with marginal success.

Thus, in *BRCA1* or *BRCA2* mutation carriers who do not wish to undergo prophylactic surgery, a screening strategy that combines thorough pelvic examination, transvaginal sonographic evaluation, and CA125 blood testing may be offered (American College of Obstetricians and Gynecologists, 2009).

CA125 is a glycoprotein that is not produced by normal ovarian epithelium, but may be produced by both benign and malignant ovarian tumors. CA125 is synthesized within affected ovarian epithelial cells and often secreted into cysts. In benign tumors, excess antigen is released into and may accumulate within cyst fluid. Hypothetically, abnormal tissue architecture associated with malignant tumors allows antigen release into the vascular circulation (Verheijen, 1999).

By itself, CA125 is not a useful marker for detecting ovarian cancer. However, recently, a more sensitive *R*isk of *O*varian *C*ancer *A*lgorithm (ROCA) has been developed and is based on the slope of serial CA125 measurements drawn at regular intervals (Skates, 2003). If a ROCA score exceeds a 1-percent risk of having ovarian cancer, patients then undergo transvaginal sonography to determine whether additional intervention is warranted. This strategy is currently being studied in a prospective, international trial of 2605 high-risk women who initially chose to undergo either risk-reducing salpingo-oophorectomy or screening alone (Greene, 2008).

General Population

Because no sufficiently accurate early detection tests are currently available, routine screening for women at average risk is not recommended. For example, in the United States' prospective Prostate, Lung, Colorectal and Ovarian (PLCO) Trial of screening versus usual care, 34,261 women without prior oophorectomy were randomly assigned to annual CA125 level measurement and transvaginal sonographic examination. Of those with an abnormal screen, approximately 1 percent had invasive ovarian cancer, demonstrating a relatively low predictive value of both tests (Buys, 2005, 2011; Partridge, 2009).

To evaluate the efficacy, cost, morbidity, compliance, and acceptability of ROCA-based CA125 screening and study-directed sonography, a randomized trial of 202,638 patients was conducted. Asymptomatic, average-risk postmenopausal women aged 50 to 74 years were randomly assigned to no treatment, to annual CA125 screening with transvaginal sonography as a second-line test if indicated by ROCA interpretation, or to annual screening with transvaginal sonography. The ROCA-directed approach demonstrated a 35-percent positive predictive value, more than 10 times higher than annual sonography (3 percent). Although in this study ROCA-directed sonography was shown to be feasible, the results of ongoing screening are awaited to determine whether there is any meaningful effect on mortality rates (Menon, 2009).

New Biomarkers and Proteomics

To identify a more accurate screening test for the early detection of ovarian cancer, a variety of potential biomarkers have been described. Dozens have been evaluated alone and in combination with CA125 (Cramer, 2011; Yurkovetsky, 2010). Although the description of such novel, seemingly promising biomarkers often leads to initial enthusiasm, rigorous validation studies are necessary to establish the clinical utility of any such test.

One notable example, based on a preliminary study published in 2002, suggested that the nascent field of proteomics was a promising new technology for the detection of early-stage ovarian cancer (Petricoin, 2002). By profiling the patterns of thousands of proteins with a high degree of sensitivity and specificity, it was hoped that an accurate test, such as OvaCheck, would reliably distinguish those with early ovarian cancer from unaffected women.

Another more recent entry, the OvaSure blood test, also generated enthusiasm. Based on the simultaneous evaluation of six analytes (leptin, osteopontin, insulin-like growth factor-II, macrophage inhibitory factor, and CA125), it was reported to yield high sensitivity and specificity for the detection of ovarian cancer (Mor, 2005; Visintin, 2008).

Prospective clinical trials must be designed and completed before any of these new diagnostic tests can be offered outside of a trial. Unfortunately, neither proteomics nor any other screening strategy is currently near implementation into routine clinical practice.

Physical Examination

For the near future, the only recommendation for prevention of ovarian cancer in asymptomatic women is an annual pelvic examination. There are no additional techniques that have proved to be effective in routine screening (American College of Obstetricians and Gynecologists, 2011). In general, the pelvic examination can only occasionally detect ovarian cancer, generally when the disease is already in advanced stages.

Chemoprevention

Oral contraceptive use is associated with a 50-percent decreased risk of developing ovarian cancer. However, there is a short-term increased risk of developing breast cancer and cervical cancer that should be considered when counseling patients (International Collaboration of Epidemiological Studies of Cervical Cancer, 2006, 2007; National Cancer Institute, 2011b).

Prophylactic Surgery

The only proven way to directly prevent ovarian cancer is surgical oophorectomy. As another possible site of disease among high-risk patients, the fallopian tubes should also be removed (Levine, 2003). In *BRCA1* or *BRCA2* carriers, prophylactic bilateral salpingo-oophorectomy (BSO) may be performed either upon completion of childbearing or at age 35 (American College of Obstetricians and Gynecologists, 1999). In these patients, the procedure is approximately 90-percent effective in preventing epithelial ovarian cancer (Kauff, 2002; Rebbeck, 2002). In women with HNPCC, the risk reduction approaches 100 percent (Schmeler, 2006).

The term *prophylactic* implies that the ovaries are normal at the time of removal. However, approximately 5 percent of *BRCA* mutation carriers undergoing prophylactic BSO will have an otherwise undetected, often microscopic, cancer at the time of sur-

gery (Lu, 2000). In fact, the distal fallopian tube seems to be the dominant site of origin for occult malignancies detected during risk-reducing surgery (Callahan, 2007). To account for this possibility, cytologic washings, peritoneal biopsies, and an omental sample may be routinely collected during surgery. When submitting the final surgical specimen, the pathology report should clearly state that the BSO was performed for a prophylactic indication. In these cases, the ovaries and tubes undergo more intensive scrutiny and are serially sectioned to identify occult disease. Utilizing a rigorous operative and pathologic protocol such as this can significantly increase the detection rate of occult tubal or ovarian malignancy in *BRCA* mutation carriers (Powell, 2005). Typically, the excision, washings, and biopsies can all be completed by minimally invasive laparoscopic surgery.

Prophylactic BSO in young women will induce premature menopause and its associated effects of vasomotor and urogenital symptoms, decline in sexual interest, and osteoporosis (National Cancer Institute, 2011b). Estrogen replacement therapy is commonly used to alleviate these symptoms, but may be less effective than is often assumed (Chap. 22, p. 585) (Madalinska, 2006). Overall, mainly due to the favorable impact in reducing cancer worries, prophylactic BSO does not adversely affect quality of life (Madalinska, 2005).

In addition to preventing ovarian cancer, prophylactic BSO reduces a woman's risk of developing breast cancer by 50 percent (Rebbeck, 2002). Predictably, the protective effect is strongest among premenopausal women (Kramer, 2005).

Hysterectomy is mandatory when performing prophylactic BSO in women with the HNPCC syndrome because of coexisting endometrial cancer risks. In *BRCA* mutation carriers, it is not required. Theoretically, not removing the uterus leaves some residual adnexal tissue that could potentially give rise to "ovarian" cancer. In practice, this concern is unproven. Relatively few reports have suggested an association between *BRCA* mutations and an increased risk of endometrial cancer. Mainly, these develop in patients taking tamoxifen for breast cancer treatment or breast cancer chemoprevention (Beiner, 2007).

LOW-MALIGNANT-POTENTIAL (LMP) TUMORS

Ten to 15 percent of epithelial ovarian cancers have histologic and biologic features that are intermediate between clearly benign cysts and frankly invasive carcinomas. In general, these low-malignant-potential tumors, also termed *borderline tumors*, are associated with risk factors that are similar to those for epithelial ovarian cancer (Huusom, 2006). Typically, they are not considered part of any of the hereditary breast-ovarian cancer syndromes. Although LMP tumors may develop at any age, on average, patients are in their mid-40s, which is 15 years younger than women with invasive ovarian carcinoma. For a variety of reasons, their diagnosis and optimal management are frequently problematic.

Pathology

Histologically, LMP tumors are distinguished from benign cysts by having at least two of the following features: nuclear

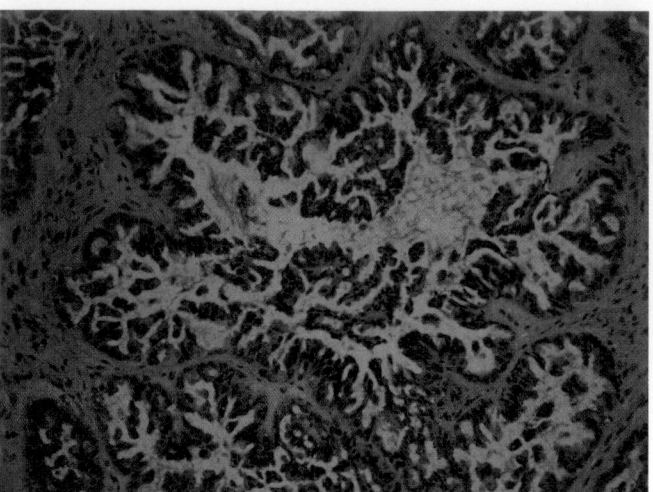

FIGURE 35-2 Serous borderline tumor, also termed serous tumor of low malignant potential. Serous tumors have epithelium resembling tubal-type epithelium. In contrast to benign serous cystadenomas, serous borderline tumors are characterized microscopically by the presence of epithelial proliferation and mild to moderate cytologic atypia. In this low-power view of a serous borderline tumor, cysts are lined by relatively bland serous-type cells with epithelial tufting, reflecting epithelial proliferation. (*Photograph contributed by Dr. Raheela Ashfaq.*)

atypia, stratification of the epithelium, formation of microscopic papillary projections, cellular pleomorphism, or mitotic activity (Figs. 35-2 and 35-3). Unlike invasive carcinomas, LMP tumors are characterized by the *absence* of stromal invasion. However, up to 10 percent of LMP tumors will exhibit areas of microinvasion, defined as foci measuring less than 3 mm in diameter and comprising less than 5 percent of the tumor (Buttin, 2002). Due to

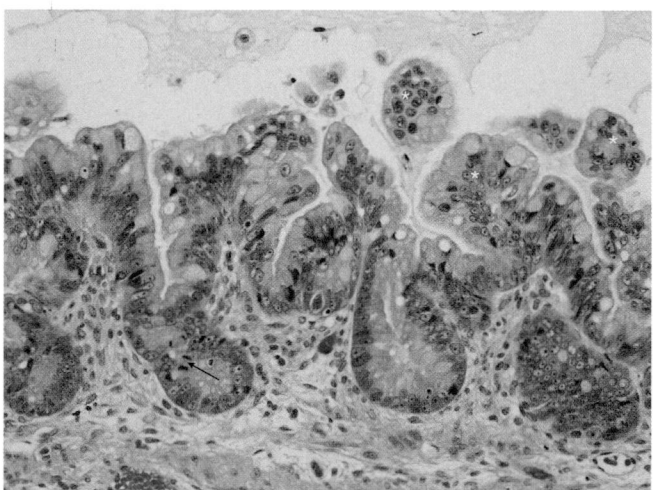

FIGURE 35-3 Mucinous borderline tumor, also termed mucinous tumor of low malignant potential. These tumors are distinguished from benign mucinous cystadenomas by the presence of epithelial proliferation and nuclear atypia. This example has mild to moderate nuclear atypia as evidenced by limited nuclear pleomorphism and visible nucleoli. A mitotic figure is also seen (*arrow in lower left*). Epithelial proliferation is indicated by epithelial tufts (*asterisks*), which are unsupported by fibrovasular cores. (*Photograph contributed by Dr. Kelley Carrick.*)

the subtle nature of many of these findings, it is challenging to diagnose an LMP tumor with certainty based on frozen section.

Clinical Features

Ovarian LMP tumors present in the same manner as other adnexal masses. Patients may have pelvic pain, distension, or increasing abdominal girth. Alternatively, an asymptomatic mass may be palpated during a routine pelvic examination. These tumors are occasionally detected as an incidental finding during routine obstetric sonographic examination or at the time of cesarean delivery.

As with other ovarian tumors, size varies widely from a serous tumor less than 1 cm to a greater than 30 cm mucinous tumor filling the entire abdomen. Preoperatively, there is no pathognomic sonographic appearance, and serum CA125 levels are nonspecific. Depending on the clinical setting, computed tomography (CT) scanning may be indicated to exclude ascites or omental caking, which would suggest typical ovarian cancer. Regardless, any woman with a suspicious adnexal mass should have it removed.

Treatment

Surgery is the cornerstone management for LMP tumors. The operative plan will vary, depending on circumstances, and patients should be carefully counseled beforehand. All women should be prepared for the operating room with the intent to perform complete ovarian cancer surgical staging or debulking, if necessary. In many cases, a laparoscopic approach is appropriate. If laparotomy is planned, then a vertical incision is selected to allow access to the upper abdomen and paraaortic nodes, if needed, for cancer staging.

During surgery, peritoneal washings should be immediately collected upon entrance into the abdomen, followed by exploration. The ovarian mass should be removed intact and submitted to pathology for frozen section. However, it is almost impossible to know with certainty whether a patient has a benign adnexal mass, LMP tumor, or invasive ovarian cancer until final histologic slides have been reviewed (Houck, 2000; Tempfer, 2007). Accordingly, in those with LMP diagnosed intraoperatively, premenopausal women who have not completed childbearing may undergo fertility-sparing surgery with preservation of the uterus and contralateral ovary (Park, 2009; Zanetta, 2001). This is a reasonable approach even if the final diagnosis shows invasive stage I cancer (Schilder, 2002). Alternatively, postmenopausal women should undergo hysterectomy with BSO.

Limited staging biopsies of the peritoneum and omentum should be considered. Additionally, the appendix should also be examined and potentially removed, especially if the tumor has mucinous histology (Timofeev, 2010). In the absence of enlarged nodes or a frozen section suggestive of frankly invasive disease, routine pelvic and paraaortic lymph node dissection may not be necessary (Rao, 2004).

LMP tumors are staged with the same FIGO criteria used for invasive ovarian cancer (p. 869). For the most part, surgical staging has limited value in altering the prognosis of those with LMP tumors unless invasive cancer is ultimately diagnosed

(Wingo, 2006). Although 97 percent of gynecologic oncologists advocate comprehensive surgical staging of LMP tumors, in current practice, it is only performed in 12 percent of patients (Lin, 1999; Menzin, 2000). This disparity stems from the fact that often the diagnosis is not suspected intraoperatively, no frozen section is requested or it is inaccurate, and a clinician is alerted only when the final pathology report has been completed. In this circumstance, consultation with a gynecologic oncologist is recommended, but comprehensive surgical restaging is not necessarily required if the tumor appears confined to a single ovary (Zapardiel, 2010). However, if a cystectomy has been performed, the risk of residual disease should prompt a discussion regarding removal of the entire adnexa with washings and limited staging (Poncelet, 2006).

For patients with stage II-IV disease, usually demonstrated by noninvasive implants (Fig. 35-4) or nodal metastases, the utility of adjuvant chemotherapy is speculative (Shih, 2010; Sutton, 1991). The most worrisome finding is the presence of invasive peritoneal implants. In general, these patients should be treated like those with typical epithelial ovarian carcinoma, including debulking and postoperative chemotherapy.

Prognosis

The prognosis is excellent for patients with ovarian LMP tumors (Table 35-4). Overall, more than 80 percent have stage I disease, and if treated by hysterectomy and BSO, stage I tumors rarely, if ever, recur (Barnhill, 1995). Fertility-sparing surgery is associated with up to a 15-percent risk of relapse, usually in the contralateral ovary, but remains highly curable by reoperation and resection (Park, 2009; Rao, 2005).

Approximately 15 percent of LMP tumors have stage II and III disease, almost invariably of serous histology. Stage IV ovarian LMP tumors account for fewer than 5 percent of diagnoses

TABLE 35-4. Survival of Women with Ovarian Low Malignant Potential Tumors

Stage	5-Year Survival (%)
I	99
II	98
III	96
IV	77

From Trimble, 2002, with permission.

and have the worst prognosis (Trimble, 2002). For advanced-stage tumors, the most reliable prognostic indicator is the presence of invasive peritoneal implants (Seidman, 2000).

Due to their indolent nature, symptomatic recurrence and death may develop as many as 20 years after therapy (Silva, 2006). For most relapses, surgical excision is the most effective therapy. Chemotherapy is typically reserved for patients who develop ascites, have significant changes in the histologic features of the tumor, or demonstrate rapid tumor growth.

EPITHELIAL OVARIAN CANCER

Pathogenesis

There are at least three distinct tumorigenic pathways to account for the heterogeneity of epithelial ovarian cancer. First, relatively few cases seem to arise from an accumulation of genetic alterations leading to malignant transformation of benign cysts to LMP tumors and ultimately progressing to invasive ovarian carcinoma (Makarla, 2005). Typically, these invasive tumors are low-grade and clinically indolent. In these tumors, K-*ras* oncogenic mutations occur early. The *ras* family of oncogenes includes K-*ras*, H-*ras*, and N-*ras*. Their protein products participate in cell cycle regulation and control of cell proliferation. As such, *ras* mutations have been implicated in carcinogenesis by their inhibition of cellular apoptosis and promotion of cellular proliferation (Mammas, 2005). In contrast, invasive cancers arising from LMP tumors have usually acquired mutations in the p53 tumor-suppressor gene.

Second, 5 to 10 percent of epithelial ovarian carcinomas, invariably high-grade serous tumors, result from an inherited predisposition. Women born with a *BRCA* mutation only require one "hit" to the other normal copy (allele) to "knock out" the *BRCA* tumor-suppressor gene product. As a result, *BRCA*-related cancers develop approximately 15 years before sporadic cases. Current data suggests that serous tubal intraepithelial carcinoma is a precursor condition for a significant percentage of serous carcinomas, which were formerly thought to arise spontaneously on

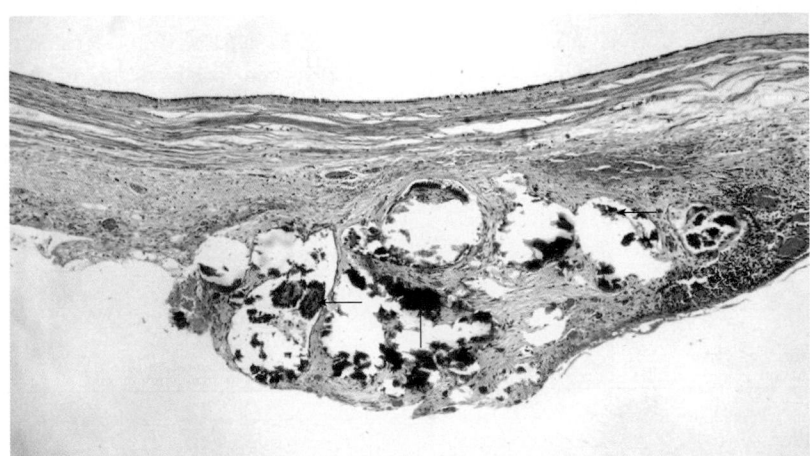

FIGURE 35-4 Noninvasive implant from a patient with an ovarian serous borderline tumor. A noninvasive implant does not have destructive invasion of the underlying tissue. In this noninvasive implant, proliferative serous-type epithelium (*black arrows*) and psammoma bodies (*red arrow*) typical of serous proliferations appear to adhere to the peritoneal tissue, but do not invade it. Psammoma bodies are fragmented in this tissue because calcified material often shatters when sectioned if not decalcified prior to sectioning. (*Photograph contributed by Dr. Raheela Ashfaq.*)

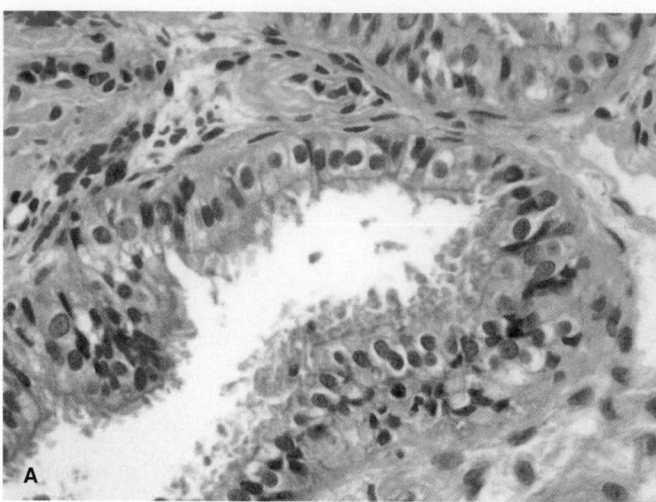
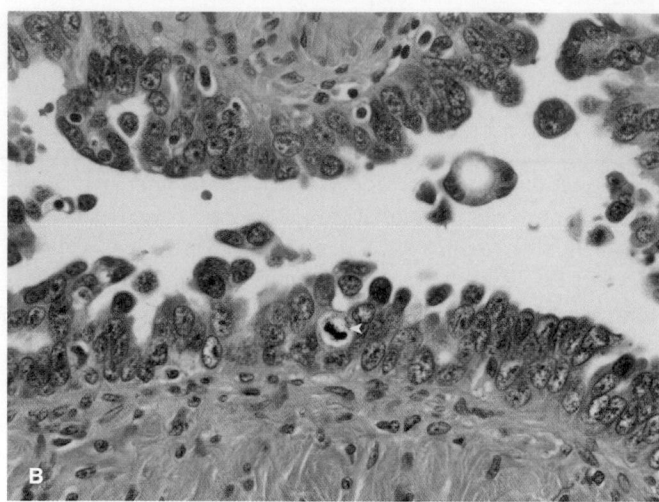

FIGURE 35-5 A. Normal tubal epithelium is composed of three cell types, with bland nuclei and cilia. **B.** Serous tubal intraepithelial carcinoma. The cells lining this fallopian tube are markedly atypical, with nuclear pleomorphism, chromatin coarseness, loss of nuclear polarity, mitotic activity (*arrow*), and epithelial proliferation/tufting. *(Photographs contributed by Dr. Kelley Carrick.)*

the ovarian or peritoneal surface (Fig. 35-5) (Levanon, 2008). Thereafter, *BRCA*-related serous cancers appear to have a unique molecular pathogenesis, requiring p53 inactivation to progress (Buller, 2001; Landen, 2008; Schorge, 2000). *p53* is a tumor suppressor gene. Its protein product prohibits cells from entering subsequent stages of cell division and thereby halts uncontrolled tumor cell replication. Mutations in *p53* are linked with a variety of cancers. In fact, loss of BRCA and p53 protein function has been detected prior to invasion, further supporting its importance as an early triggering event (Werness, 2000).

Third, most carcinomas appear to originate de novo from ovarian surface epithelial cells that are sequestered in cortical inclusion cysts (CICs) within the ovarian stroma. Numerous inciting events and subsequent pathways have been proposed. For example, cyclic repair of the ovarian surface during long periods of repetitive ovulation requires abundant cellular proliferation. In these women, spontaneous *p53* mutations arising during the DNA synthesis that accompanies this proliferation appear to play a primary role in carcinogenesis (Schildkraut, 1997). Certainly, several developmental pathways are possible, stemming from early inactivation of innumerable genes. Ultimately, the replicative stress and DNA damage allows the entrapped surface epithelial cells within CICs to be transformed into any of the histologic variants seen in ovarian carcinoma (Levanon, 2008).

Diagnosis
Signs and Symptoms

Ovarian cancer is typically portrayed as a "silent" killer, without appreciable signs or symptoms until advanced disease is clinically obvious. This is a misconception. Actually, patients are often symptomatic for several months before the diagnosis, even with early-stage disease (Goff, 2000). The difficulty is distinguishing these symptoms from those that normally occur in women.

In general, persistent symptoms that are more severe or frequent than expected and have a recent onset warrant further diagnostic investigation. Women with malignant masses typically experience symptoms of notable severity 20 to 30 times per month. Commonly, increased abdominal size, bloating, urinary urgency, and pelvic pain are reported. Additionally fatigue, indigestion, inability to eat normally, constipation, and back pain may be noted (Goff, 2004). Abnormal vaginal bleeding occurs rarely. Occasionally, patients may present with nausea, vomiting, and a partial bowel obstruction if carcinomatosis is particularly widespread. Unfortunately, many women and clinicians are quick to attribute most symptoms to menopause, aging, dietary changes, stress, depression, or functional bowel problems. As a result, weeks or months often pass before medical advice is sought or diagnostic studies are performed.

Physical Examination

A pelvic or pelvic-abdominal mass is palpable in most patients with ovarian cancer (Fig. 35-6). In general, malignant tumors tend

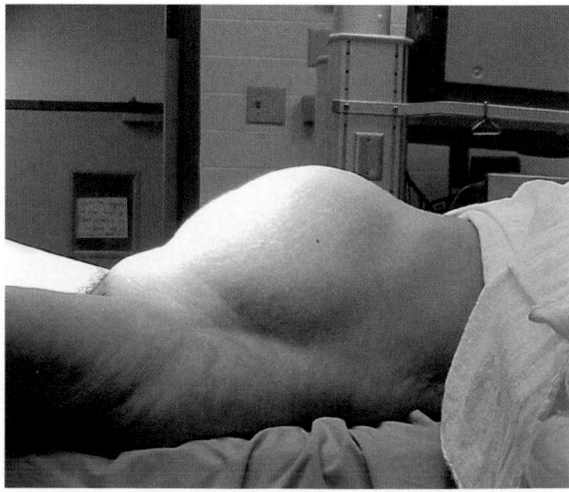

FIGURE 35-6 Photograph of a woman with a distended abdomen from a large ovarian mass.

to be solid, nodular, and fixed, but there are no pathognomonic findings that distinguish these growths from benign tumors. Paradoxically, a huge mass filling the pelvis and abdomen more often represents a benign or borderline tumor. To aid surgical planning, a rectovaginal examination should also be performed. For example, a woman with tumor involving the rectovaginal septum may need to be positioned in dorsal lithotomy to perform a low anterior resection (Section 44-23, p. 1327).

The presence of a fluid wave, or less commonly, flank bulging, suggests the presence of significant ascites. In a woman with a pelvic mass and ascites, the diagnosis is ovarian cancer until proven otherwise. However, ascites without an identifiable pelvic mass suggests the possibility of cirrhosis or other primary malignancies such as gastric or pancreatic cancers. In advanced disease, examination of the upper abdomen usually reveals a central mass signifying omental caking.

Auscultation of the chest is also important, since patients with malignant pleural effusions may not be overtly symptomatic. The remainder of the examination should include palpation of the peripheral nodes in addition to a general physical assessment.

Laboratory Testing

A routine complete blood count and metabolic panel often demonstrates a few characteristic features. For example, 20 to 25 percent of patients will present with thrombocytosis (platelet count $>400 \times 10^9$/L) (Li, 2004). This is believed to result from malignant ovarian cells releasing cytokines that increase rates of platelet production. Hyponatremia, typically ranging between 125 and 130 mEq/L, is another common finding. In these patients, tumor secretion of a vasopressin-like substance can cause a clinical picture suggestive of a syndrome of inappropriate antidiuretic hormone (SIADH).

The serum CA125 test is integral to the management of epithelial ovarian cancer. In 90 percent of patients presenting with malignant nonmucinous tumors, CA125 levels are elevated. However, preoperatively, it should not be used alone in the management of an adnexal mass. Half of stage I ovarian cancers will have a normal CA125 measurement (false-negative). In contrast, an elevated value (false-positive) may be associated with a variety of common benign indications, such as pelvic inflammatory disease, endometriosis, leiomyomas, pregnancy, and even menstruation.

In postmenopausal women with a pelvic mass, a CA125 measurement may be helpful in predicting a higher likelihood of malignancy (Im, 2005). With mucinous tumors, the serum tumor markers cancer antigen 19-9 (CA19-9) and carcinoembryonic antigen (CEA) may be better indicators of disease than CA125. In addition, the OVA1 test appears to improve the predictability of ovarian cancer in women with pelvic masses (American College of Obstetricians and Gynecologists, 2011).

OVA1 is a biomarker blood test that may be used for the preoperative triage of women with an identified ovarian mass for which surgery is planned. The test is indicated for women who are older than 18 years, have an ovarian mass that warrants surgery, and have not yet been referred to an oncologist. If preoperative clinical and radiologic evaluation indicates a high risk for malignancy, then direct referral is indicated, and OVA1 testing is not indicated. However, if clinical assessment points to a low risk of malignancy, then this assay can further assess cancer risk and thus assist in the decision of whether to refer to a gynecologic oncologist (Ueland, 2011; Ware Miller, 2011). Scores $\geq$5.0 in premenopausal and scores $\geq$4.4 in postmenopausal women suggest malignancy. Importantly, this test is not a screening tool and is reserved for those with a known surgical mass to aid preoperative triage (Vermillion Inc, 2011; Zhang, 2010). Randomized studies evaluating this test are limited, and its role in preoperative triage is yet to be clearly defined.

Imaging

Sonography. To differentiate benign tumors and early-stage ovarian cancers, transvaginal sonography is typically the most useful imaging test (Chap. 2, p. 41). In general, malignant tumors are multiloculated, solid or echogenic, and large (>5 cm), and they have thick septae with areas of nodularity (Fig. 35-7A). Other features may include papillary projections or neovascularization–demonstrated by Doppler flow (Figs. 35-7B and 35-7C). Although several presumptive models have been described in an attempt to distinguish benign masses from ovarian cancers preoperatively, none have been universally implemented (Timmerman, 2005; Twickler, 1999).

In patients with advanced disease, sonography is less helpful. The pelvic sonogram may be particularly difficult to interpret if a large mass encompasses the uterus, adnexa, and surrounding structures. Ascites, if present, is easily detected, but in general, abdominal sonography has limited use.

Radiography. Patients with suspected ovarian cancer should have a chest radiograph to detect pulmonary effusions or infrequently, pulmonary metastases. Rarely, a barium enema is clinically helpful in excluding diverticular disease or colon cancer, or in identifying involvement of the rectosigmoid by ovarian cancer.

Computed Tomography Scanning. The main role of CT scanning is in the treatment planning of women with advanced ovarian cancer. Preoperatively, it may detect disease in the liver, retroperitoneum, omentum, or elsewhere in the abdomen and thereby guide surgical cytoreduction (Fig. 35-8). However, CT is not particularly reliable in detecting intraperitoneal disease smaller than 1 to 2 cm in diameter. As a result, almost invariably, tumor sites not detected by CT are identified intraoperatively. Moreover, the accuracy of CT scanning is poor for differentiating a benign ovarian mass from a malignant tumor when disease is limited to the pelvis. In these cases, transvaginal sonography is superior.

In general, other radiologic studies such as magnetic resonance (MR) imaging, bone scans, and positron emission tomography (PET) provide limited additional information preoperatively.

Paracentesis

A woman with a pelvic mass and ascites can be assumed to have ovarian cancer until surgically proven otherwise. Thus, few

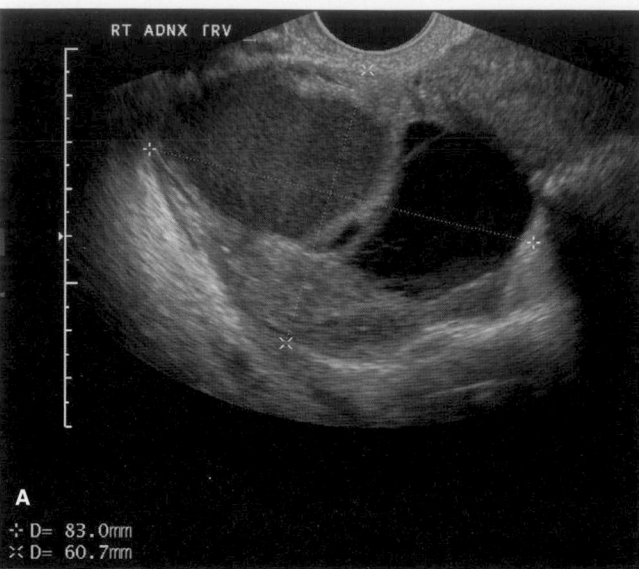

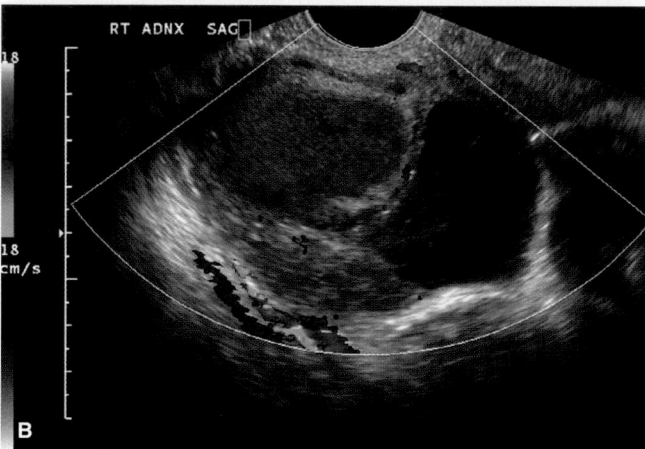

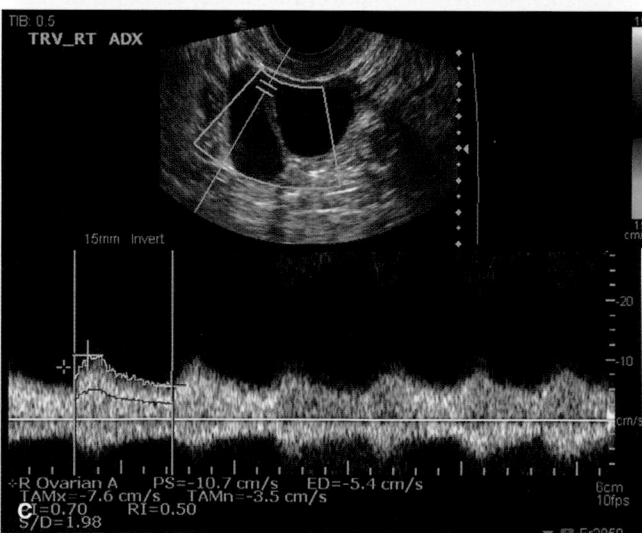

FIGURE 35-7 Sonographic image of an ovarian cyst. **A.** Transvaginal sonogram depicts a complex ovarian mass. Cystic and solid components as well as a thick intracystic septum are seen. These findings increase clinical concern for malignancy. **B.** Color Doppler transvaginal sonogram shows neovascularization within this ovarian tumor. **C.** Transvaginal Doppler study of ovarian mass vessels reveals decreased impedance. *(Images contributed by Dr. Diane Twickler.)*

patients require a diagnostic paracentesis to guide treatment. Moreover, this procedure is typically avoided diagnostically as cytologic results are usually nonspecific and abdominal wall metastases may form at the needle entry site (Kruitwagen, 1996). However, paracentesis may be indicated for those with ascites and the *absence* of a pelvic mass.

Role of the Generalist

There is often tremendous difficulty in distinguishing benign from malignant using the currently available diagnostic modalities. However, the presence of ascites or evidence of abdominal or distant metastases should prompt consideration of referral (American College of Obstetricians and Gynecologists, 2011). Additionally, premenopausal women with elevated CA125 levels (i.e., >200 U/mL) or an OVA1 score ≥5.0 and postmenopausal women with any CA125 elevation or an OVA1 score ≥4.4 are at higher risk.

Ideally, for patients with suspicious adnexal masses, surgery should be performed in a hospital with a pathologist able to reliably interpret an intraoperative frozen section. At minimum, samples for peritoneal cytology should be obtained when the abdomen is entered. The mass should then be removed intact through an incision that permits thorough staging and resection of possible metastatic sites (American College of Obstetricians and Gynecologists, 2011).

If a malignancy is diagnosed, then surgical staging should be performed. However, in a study of more than 10,000 women with ovarian cancer, almost half of those with early-stage disease did not undergo the recommended surgical procedures (Goff, 2006). Surgeons should be prepared to appropriately stage and potentially debulk ovarian cancer or have a gynecologic oncologist immediately available. This type of careful planning has been shown to achieve the best possible surgical result and improve survival rates (Earle, 2006; Engelen, 2006; Mercado, 2010). Moreover, since broader resources are usually available, patients cared for at high-volume hospitals tend to have better outcomes as well (Bristow, 2010).

For women with malignancy only identified postoperatively or intraoperatively and without adequate staging, management will vary according to the clinical circumstances. Women with suspected early-stage disease may be staged laparoscopically. Those with advanced disease may undergo a second laparotomy to obtain optimal tumor debulking. However, if extensive disease is found at the initial surgery, then chemotherapy may be selected first and followed by laparotomy to obtain optimal interval cytoreduction of tumor.

At some point during postoperative surveillance, many patients with early-stage disease, depending on the diagnosis, will return to their referring physician. Monitoring for relapse is often coordinated between the gynecologic oncologist and generalist in obstetrics and gynecology, especially if no chemotherapy is required following surgery.

Pathology

Although epithelial ovarian cancer is often thought of as a single entity, the different histologic types are variable in their behavior

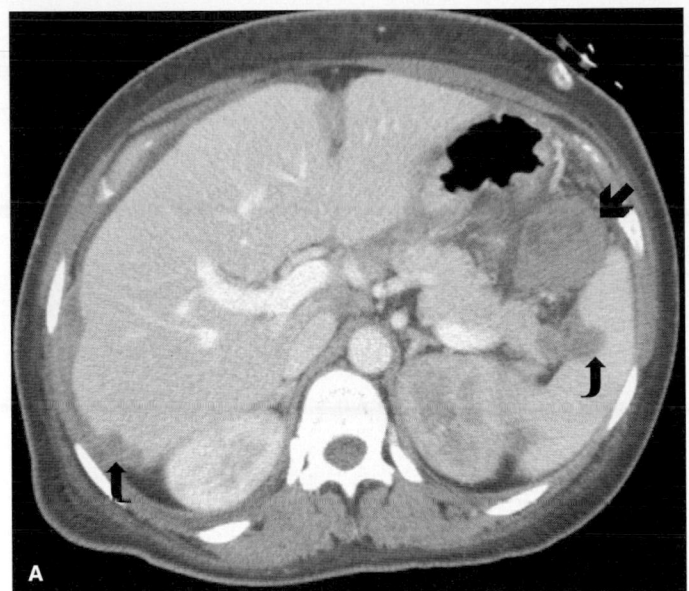 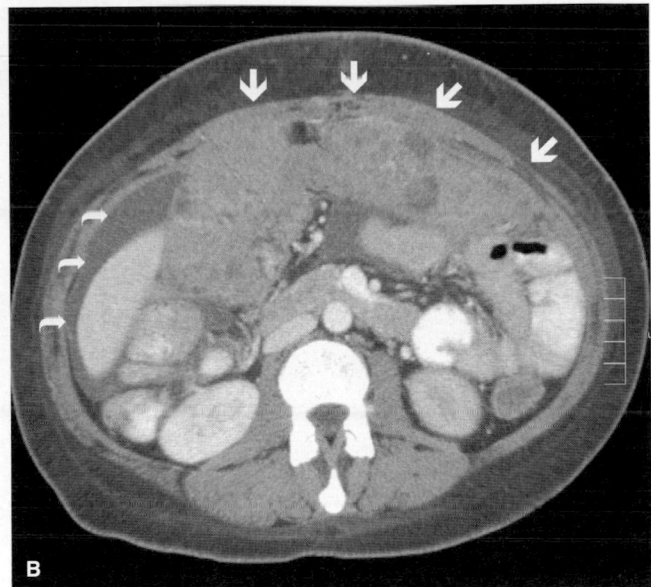

FIGURE 35-8 Computed tomographic scans in a woman with ovarian cancer. **A.** Axial CT scan image at the level of the liver and spleen reveals metastatic lesions in the spleen and liver (*curved arrows*) and a bulky lesion at the splenorenal ligament (*arrow*). **B.** More caudal axial CT image reveals ascites (*curved arrows*) and marked omental caking (*arrows*). (*Images contributed by Dr. Diane Twickler.*)

(Table 35-5). Commonly, two or more cell types are mixed. Within each histologic type, tumors are further categorized as benign, borderline (low malignant potential), or malignant.

Histologic Grade

Mainly in early-stage disease, grade is an important prognostic factor that affects treatment planning (Morgan, 2011). Unfortunately, there is no universally accepted grading system for epithelial ovarian carcinoma. Instead, numerous different systems are currently used to assign grade. Most of these are based on architectural features and/or nuclear pleomorphism, with or without additional histopathologic criteria. In general, tumors are classified as grade

---

TABLE 35-5. World Health Organization Histological Classification of Ovarian Carcinoma

Serous adenocarcinoma
Mucinous tumors
   Adenocarcinoma
   Pseudomyxoma peritonei
Endometrioid tumors
   Adenocarcinoma
   Malignant mixed müllerian tumor (carcinosarcoma)
Clear cell adenocarcinoma
Transitional cell tumors
   Malignant Brenner tumor
   Transitional cell carcinoma
Squamous cell carcinoma
Mixed carcinoma
Undifferentiated carcinoma
Small cell carcinoma

From Tavassoli, 2003.

---

1 (well-differentiated), grade 2 (moderately differentiated), and grade 3 (poorly differentiated) lesions (Pecorelli, 1999).

Histologic Type

Grossly, there are no distinguishing features among the types of epithelial ovarian cancer. In general, each has solid and cystic areas of varying sizes (Fig. 35-9).

Serous Tumors
Adenocarcinoma. More than half of all epithelial ovarian cancers have serous histology. Microscopically, the cells may resemble fallopian tube epithelium in well-differentiated tumors or anaplastic cells with severe nuclear atypia in poorly differentiated tumors (Fig. 35-10). During frozen section, psammoma bodies are essentially pathognomonic of an ovarian-type serous carcinoma. Often, these tumors contain a variety of other cell types as a minor component (less than 10 percent) that may cause diagnostic problems, but do not influence outcome (Lee, 2003).

Endometrioid Tumors
Adenocarcinoma. Fifteen to 20 percent of epithelial ovarian cancers are endometrioid adenocarcinomas, the second most common histologic type (Fig. 35-11). The lower frequency results largely because poorly differentiated endometrioid and serous tumors cannot be easily distinguished and such cases are usually classified as serous. As a result, well-differentiated endometrioid tumors are proportionally more common, which may also explain their overall relatively good prognosis.

In 15 to 20 percent of cases, there is a coexisting endometrial adenocarcinoma. This is usually regarded as a synchronous tumor, but metastasis from one site to the other is difficult to exclude (Soliman, 2004). It has been hypothesized that a müllerian "field effect" accounts for these independently occurring, histologically similar tumors. In addition, many such patients are noted to have pelvic endometriosis.

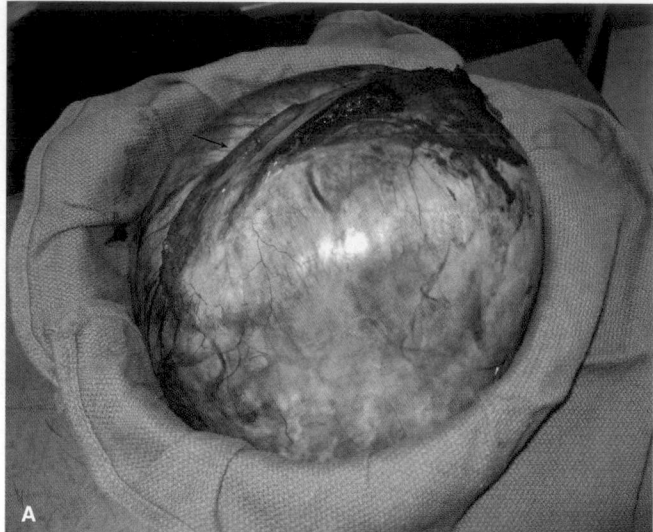

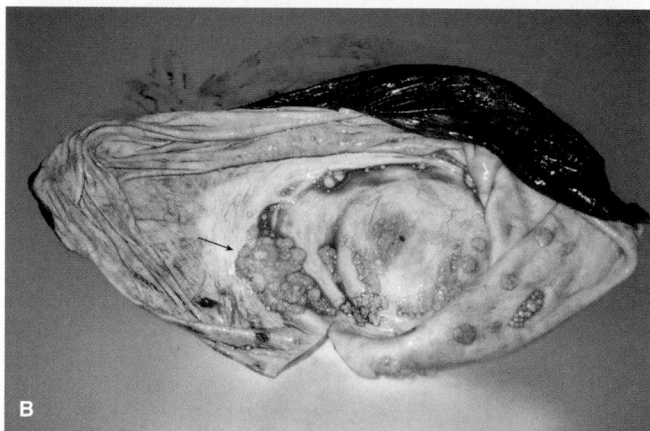

FIGURE 35-9 Gross photographs of an ovarian cystadenofibroma. **A.** Excised cystic ovarian mass. Note the fallopian tube stretched over the ovarian capsule (*arrow*). **B.** Opened tumor reveals the inner cyst wall and scattered papillary tumor growth (*arrow*). (*Photographs contributed by Dr. David Miller.*)

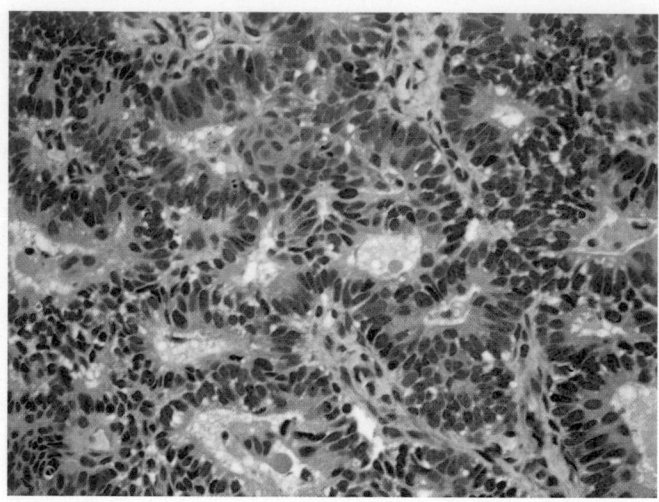

FIGURE 35-11 Endometrioid adenocarcinoma. Ovarian endometrioid adenocarcinomas are morphologically similar to their more common counterparts arising in the endometrium. Better-differentiated tumors like this one have glands resembling proliferative endometrial glands, which grow in a confluent pattern. More poorly differentiated tumors have a variable percentage of solid growth and/or increased nuclear atypia. Like their endometrial counterparts, these tumors may show squamous differentiation. (*Photograph contributed by Dr. Raheela Ashfaq.*)

Malignant Mixed Müllerian Tumor (Carcinosarcoma).

These rare tumors represent less than 1 percent of ovarian cancers, have a poorer prognosis, and are histologically similar to uterine primary tumors (Rauh-Hain, 2011). By definition, they contain malignant epithelial and mesenchymal elements.

Mucinous Tumors

Adenocarcinoma. Five to 10 percent of true epithelial ovarian cancers are mucinous adenocarcinomas. The frequency is usually overestimated because of undetected primary intestinal sites, such as the appendix or colon. Well-differentiated ovarian mucinous

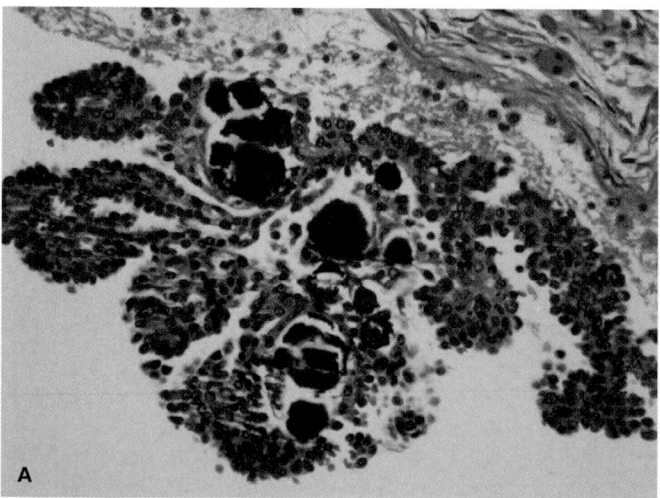

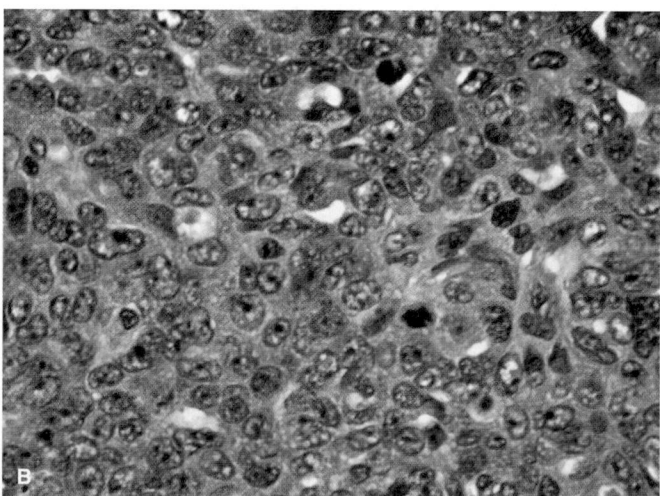

FIGURE 35-10 Serous carcinoma. Serous carcinomas vary in regard to their degree of differentiation, as manifested by their architecture, degree of cytologic atypia and pleomorphism, and mitotic rate. **A.** In this relatively well-differentiated example of serous carcinoma, serous-type cells with moderate nuclear atypia form papillae and project into a cystic space. Numerous psammoma bodies, which are extracellular round laminar dark eosinophilic collections of calcium, are seen here. **B.** In this less well-differentiated example of serous carcinoma, moderately to markedly atypical cells form sheets, as opposed to the glands and papillae formed by better-differentiated tumors. (*Photographs contributed by Dr. Kelley Carrick.*)

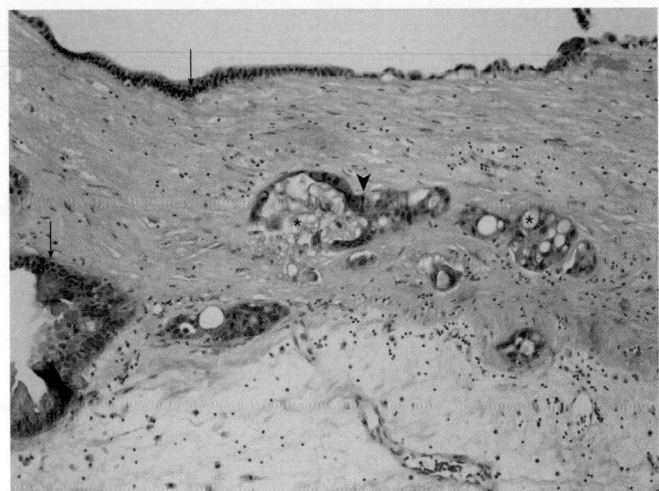

FIGURE 35-12 Ovarian mucinous adenocarcinoma. This mucinous carcinoma arose within a 15-cm mucinous cystadenoma. Benign mucinous-type epithelium lining cystic spaces of the background cystadenoma is seen (*arrows*). A carcinomatous component (*arrowhead*) invades the stroma in a haphazard fashion at the center of the photomicrograph. The malignant cells are arranged in clusters and poorly formed glands and have intracytoplasmic and intraluminal mucin (*asterisks*). (*Photograph contributed by Dr. Kelley Carrick.*)

tumors closely resemble mucin-secreting adenocarcinomas of intestinal or endocervical origin (Fig. 35-12). Histologically, the distinction may be impossible without clinical correlation (Lee, 2003). Advanced-stage mucinous ovarian carcinomas are rare, tend to be resistant to platinum chemotherapy, and have a prognosis significantly worse than serous tumors (Zaino, 2011).

Pseudomyxoma Peritonei. *Pseudomyxoma peritonei* is a clinical term used to describe the rare finding of abundant mucoid or gelatinous material in the pelvis and abdominal cavity, surrounded by thin fibrous capsules. An ovarian mucinous carcinoma with ascites rarely results in this condition, and evidence suggests that ovarian mucinous tumors associated with pseudomyxoma peritonei are almost all metastatic rather than primary. As a result, appendiceal or other intestinal sites of origin should be excluded (Ronnett, 1997). The primary appendiceal tumor may be small relative to the ovarian tumor(s) and may not be appreciated macroscopically. Thus, removal and thorough histologic examination of the appendix is indicated in all cases of pseudomyxoma peritonei.

If the peritoneal epithelial cells are benign or borderline-appearing, the condition is referred to as *disseminated peritoneal adenomucinosis*. Patients with this diagnosis have a benign or protracted, indolent clinical course (Ronnett, 2001). When the peritoneal epithelial cells appear malignant, the clinical course is invariably fatal.

Clear Cell Adenocarcinoma. Comprising 5 to 10 percent of epithelial ovarian cancers, clear cell adenocarcinomas are the most frequently associated with pelvic endometriosis. These tumors appear similar to clear cell carcinomas that develop sporadically in the uterus, vagina, and cervix. Typically tumors are confined to the ovary and generally are cured by surgery alone. However, the 20 percent presenting with advanced disease tend to be platinum resistant and carry a worse prognosis than serous carcinoma (Al-Barrak, 2011).

Microscopically, both clear and "hobnail" cells are characteristic (Fig. 35-13). In clear cells, the visibly clear cytoplasm results from the dissolution of glycogen as the tissue specimen is histologically prepared. Hobnail cells have bulbous nuclei that protrude far into the cystic lumen beyond the apparent cytoplasmic limits of the cell (Lee, 2003).

Transitional Cell Tumors
Malignant Brenner Tumor. These rare ovarian cancers are characterized by the coexistence of a poorly differentiated transitional cell carcinoma and interspersed foci of a benign or borderline Brenner tumor. Microscopically, the transitional cell component resembles carcinomas arising from the urinary tract, often having squamous differentiation. Brenner tumors are characterized by having a dense, unusually abundant, fibrous stroma with embedded nests of transitional epithelium (Fig. 9-21, p. 269).

Transitional Cell Carcinoma. Accounting for fewer than 5 percent of ovarian cancers, these tumors are histologically characterized by the absence of a demonstrable Brenner component. Patients with transitional cell carcinoma have a worse prognosis than those with malignant Brenner tumors, but better than other histologic types of epithelial ovarian cancer (Gershenson, 1993). Microscopically, transitional cell carcinoma resembles a primary bladder carcinoma, but has an immunoreactive pattern consistent with ovarian origin (Lee, 2003).

Squamous Cell Carcinoma. Rarely, ovarian tumors may be classified as primary squamous cell carcinoma. In fact, this is the newest category to be recognized, and typically, the prognosis is poor for most patients with advanced disease (Park, 2010). More commonly, squamous cell carcinomas arise from mature cystic teratomas (dermoid cysts) and are classified as malignant ovarian germ cell tumors (Pins, 1996). In other cases, ovarian endometrioid variants may have extensive squamous differentiation, or alternatively, metastases from a cervical primary are present.

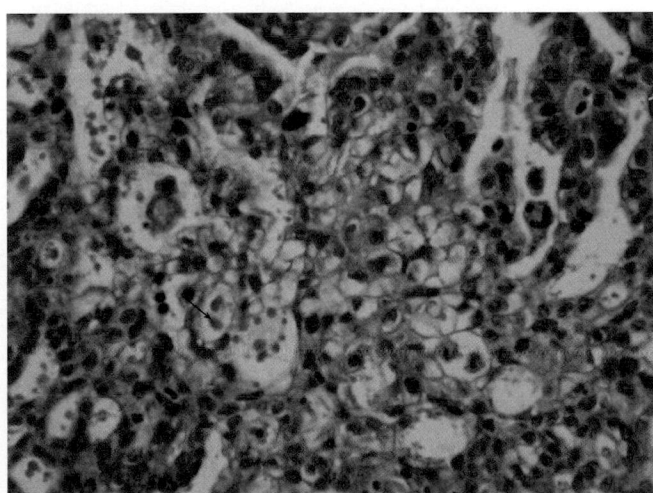

FIGURE 35-13 Ovarian clear cell carcinoma. Clear cell adenocarcinoma is typically composed of cells with clear to eosinophilic cytoplasm that are arranged in cysts, tubules, papillae, and/or sheets. In the ovary, it looks similar to its counterparts in the endometrium and cervix/vagina. This example has the eosinophilic hyaline globules (*arrow*) that are often present in this tumor. (*Photograph contributed by Dr. Kelley Carrick.*)

Mixed Carcinoma. If more than 10 percent of an ovarian cancer exhibits a second cell type, it is classified as a mixed tumor. Common combinations include mixed clear cell/endometrioid or serous/endometrioid adenocarcinomas.

Undifferentiated Carcinoma. Epithelial ovarian tumors rarely are too poorly differentiated to be classified into any of the müllerian types described previously. Microscopically, the cells are arranged in solid groups or sheets with numerous mitotic figures and marked cytologic atypia. Typically, there are foci of müllerian carcinoma, usually serous, within the tumor. Overall, undifferentiated carcinomas of the ovary have a poor prognosis compared with the other histologic types (Silva, 1991).

Small Cell Carcinoma. These tumors are rare, extremely malignant, and consist of two subgroups. Most patients have a *hypercalcemic type*, typically developing in young women during their 20s. Nearly all of these tumors are unilateral, and two thirds are associated with elevated serum calcium levels that resolve postoperatively (Young, 1994). The *pulmonary type* resembles oat-cell carcinoma of the lung and develops in older women. Half of these women have bilateral ovarian disease (Eichhorn, 1992). In general, patients with small cell carcinoma die within 2 years from rapid disease progression.

Primary Peritoneal Carcinoma

Up to 15 percent of "typical" epithelial ovarian cancers are actually primary peritoneal carcinomas that seem to arise de novo from the lining of the pelvis and abdomen. In some cases, especially among *BRCA1* mutation carriers, independent malignant transformation occurs at multiple peritoneal sites simultaneously (Schorge, 1998). However, more recent data suggest that nearly one half of presumed cases actually arise in the tubal fimbria (Carlson, 2008).

Clinically and histologically, these tumors are virtually indistinguishable from epithelial ovarian cancer. However, primary peritoneal carcinoma may develop in a woman years after having a BSO. If ovaries are still present, several criteria are required to make the diagnosis (Table 35-6). By far the most common variant is papillary serous, but any of the other histologic types are possible. In general, the staging, treatment, and prognosis of primary peritoneal carcinoma are the same as that for epithelial ovarian cancer (Mok, 2003). The differential diagnosis mainly includes malignant mesothelioma.

TABLE 35-6. Criteria for Diagnosing Primary Peritoneal Carcinoma When Ovaries Are Present

Both ovaries must be normal in size or enlarged by a benign process

The involvement in the extraovarian sites must be greater than the involvement on the surface of either ovary

The ovarian tumor involvement must be either nonexistent, confined to the ovarian surface epithelium without stromal invasion, or involving the cortical stroma with tumor size less than 5 × 5 mm

---

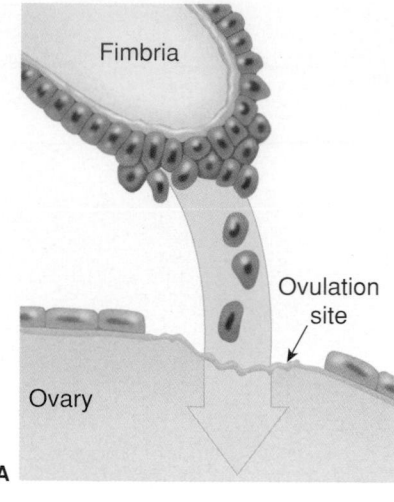

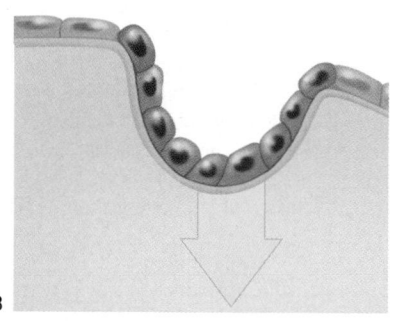

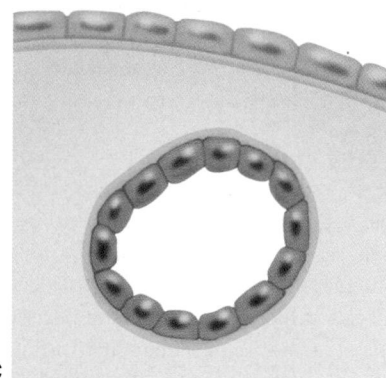

FIGURE 35-14 A. Epithelial cells from the fimbria are released and implant on the denuded surface of the ovary at the site of ovulation. **B & C.** Subsequently, an inclusion cyst is formed.

Fallopian Tube Carcinoma

Historically, this carcinoma was assumed to be rarer than epithelial ovarian cancer. However, the fallopian tube fimbria has recently been identified as an origin for many high-grade pelvic serous carcinomas that were previously assumed to arise from the ovary or peritoneum (Fig. 35-14) (Levanon, 2008).

Clinically, there are many similarities with epithelial ovarian cancer. For the most part, risk factors, histologic types, surgical staging, pattern of spread, treatment, and prognosis are comparable (Table 35-7). To be considered a primary fallopian tube carcinoma, the tumor must be located macroscopically within the tube or its fimbriated end. Additionally, the uterus and ovary must not contain carcinoma, or if they do, it must be clearly different from the fallopian tube lesion (Alvarado-Cabrero, 2003).

TABLE 35-7. FIGO Staging of Carcinoma of the Fallopian Tube

Stage	Characteristics
I	**Growth limited to the fallopian tubes**
IA	Growth is limited to one tube, with extension into the submucosa and/or muscularis, but not penetrating the serosal surface; no ascites
IB	Growth is limited to both tubes, with extension into the submucosa and/or muscularis, but not penetrating the serosal surface; no ascites
IC	Tumor either stage IA or IB, but with tumor extension through or onto the tubal serosa, or with ascites present containing malignant cells, or with positive peritoneal washings
II	**Growth involving one or both fallopian tubes with pelvic extension**
IIA	Extension and/or metastasis to the uterus and/or ovaries
IIB	Extension to other pelvic tissues
IIC	Tumor either stage IIA or IIB and with ascites present containing malignant cells or with positive peritoneal washings
III	**Tumor involves one or both fallopian tubes, with peritoneal implants outside the pelvis and/or positive regional lymph nodes. Superficial liver metastasis equals stage III. Tumor appears limited to the true pelvis, but with histologically-proven malignant extension to the small bowel or omentum**
IIIA	Tumor is grossly limited to the true pelvis, with negative nodes, but with histologically confirmed microscopic seeding of abdominal peritoneal surfaces
IIIB	Tumor involving one or both tubes, with histologically confirmed implants of abdominal peritoneal surfaces, none exceeding 2 cm in diameter. Lymph nodes are negative
IIIC	Abdominal implants >2 cm in diameter and/or positive retroperitoneal or inguinal nodes
IV	**Growth involving one or both Fallopian tubes with distant metastases. If pleural effusion is present, there must be positive cytology to be stage IV. Parenchymal liver metastases equals stage IV**

FIGO = International Federation of Gynecology and Obstetrics.

Secondary Tumors

Malignant tumors that metastasize to the ovary are almost invariably bilateral. The term *Krukenberg tumor* refers to a metastatic mucinous/signet ring cell adenocarcinoma of the ovaries that typically originates from primary tumors of the intestinal tract, characteristically the stomach (Fig. 35-15). Ovarian metastases often represent a late disseminated stage of the disease in which other hematogenous metastases are also found (Prat, 2003).

Patterns of Spread

In general, epithelial ovarian cancers predominantly metastasize by *exfoliation*. Malignant cells are first released into the peritoneal cavity when the tumor penetrates through the ovarian capsule surface. By following the normal circulation of peritoneal fluid, implants may then develop anywhere in the abdomen. A unique characteristic of ovarian cancer is that metastatic tumors do not usually infiltrate visceral organs, but exist as surface implants. As a result, aggressive debulking is possible with reasonable morbidity.

Due to its marked vascularity, the omentum is the most frequent location for disease spread and is often extensively involved with tumor (Fig. 35-16). Nodules are also commonly present on the undersurface of the right hemidiaphragm and small bowel serosa, but all intraperitoneal surfaces are at risk.

Lymphatic dissemination is the other primary mode of spread. Malignant cells may spread via channels that follow the ovarian blood supply along the infundibulopelvic ligament, terminating in paraaortic lymph nodes up to the level of the renal vessels. Other lymphatics pass laterally through the broad ligament and parametrium to the external iliac, obturator, and hypogastric nodal chains. Infrequently, metastases may also follow the round ligament to the inguinal nodes (Lee, 2003).

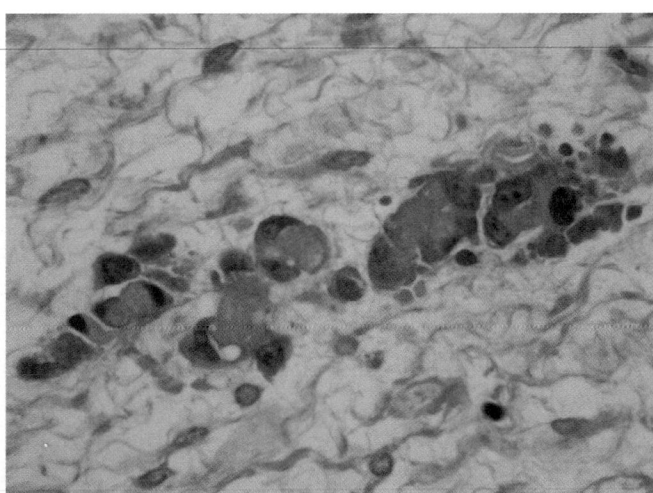

FIGURE 35-15 Krukenberg tumor. This metastatic, poorly differentiated adenocarcinoma is characterized by singly disposed cells with an intracytoplasmic mucin globule that displaces the nucleus to the cell periphery, producing a signet-ring-like cytomorphology. *(Photograph contributed by Dr. Raheela Ashfaq.)*

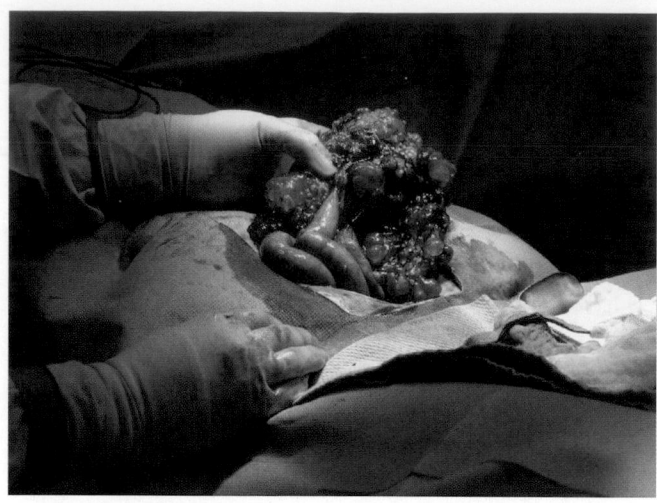

FIGURE 35-16 Omental caking caused by tumor invasion.

Direct extension of a progressively enlarging ovarian cancer may result in confluent tumor involvement of the pelvic peritoneum and adjacent structures, including the uterus, rectosigmoid colon, and fallopian tubes. Usually, this is associated with significant induration of the surrounding tissues.

In advanced disease, several liters of ascites may be present. Generally, this is believed to result from either increased production of carcinomatous fluid or decreased clearance by obstructed lymphatic channels. Similarly, by traversing the diaphragm, a malignant pleural effusion may develop.

Hematogenous spread is atypical. In most cases, metastases to the liver or lung parenchyma, brain, or kidneys are observed in patients with recurrent disease, and not at initial diagnosis.

Staging

Ovarian cancer is surgically staged, and stage is assigned according to findings before tumor removal and debulking (Fig. 35-17). The International Federation of Gynecology and Obstetrics (FIGO) stages reflect the typical patterns of ovarian cancer spread (Table 35-8). Even if a tumor appears clinically confined to the ovary, in many cases it will have detectable metastases. Therefore, accurate surgical staging is crucial to guide treatment. Approximately one third of patients have surgical stage I or II disease (Table 35-9).

Management of Early-Stage Ovarian Cancer
Surgical Staging

If a malignancy appears clinically confined to the ovary, surgical removal and comprehensive staging should be performed. Typically, the abdominal incision must be adequate to identify and resect any disease that may have been missed on physical examination or by imaging. The operation begins by aspirating free ascitic fluid or collecting peritoneal washings. This is followed by inspection and palpation of all peritoneal surfaces. Next, an extrafascial hysterectomy and BSO are performed. In the absence of gross extraovarian disease, the infracolic omentum should be removed or at least biopsied (Section 44-16, p. 1313). Additionally, random peritoneal biopsies or scrapings are obtained, ideally near the diaphragms (Timmers, 2010). The most prognostically important step, a pelvic

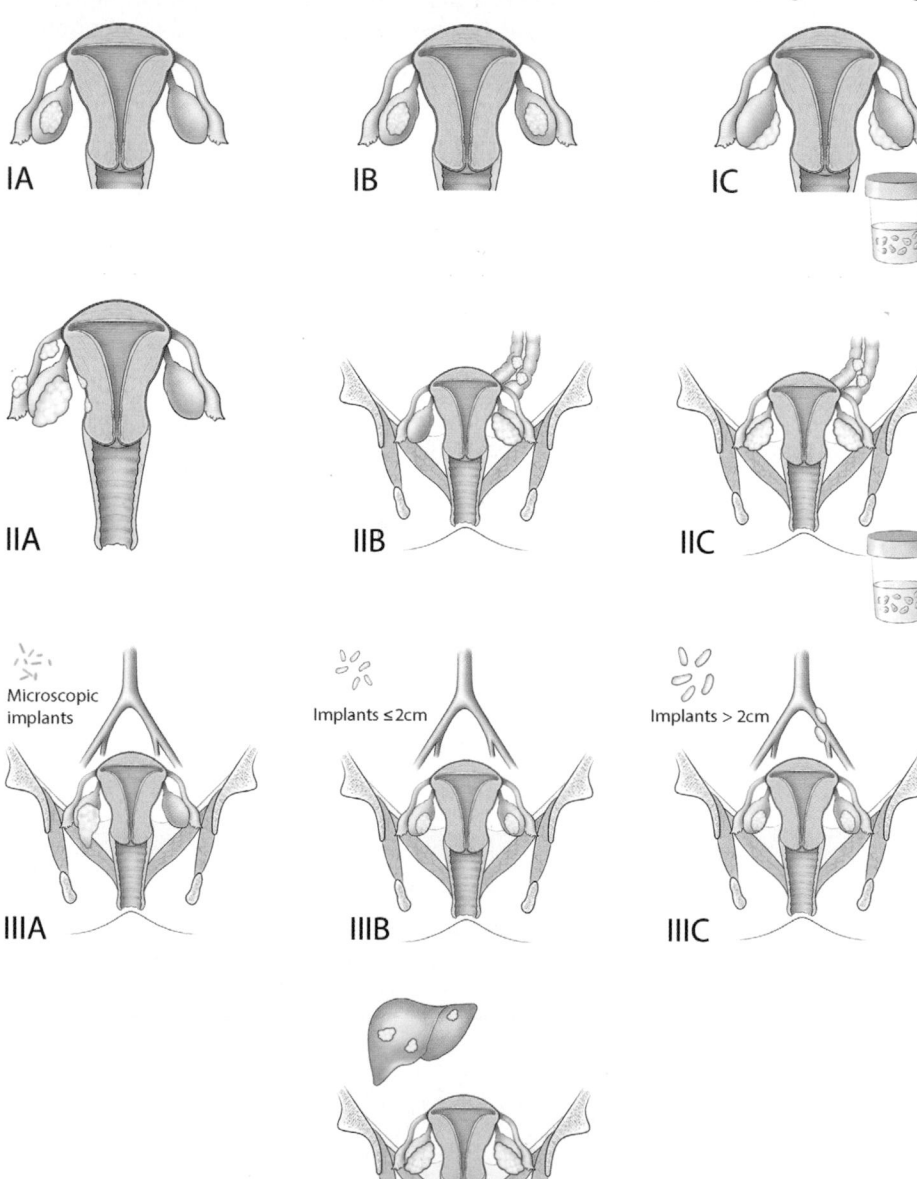

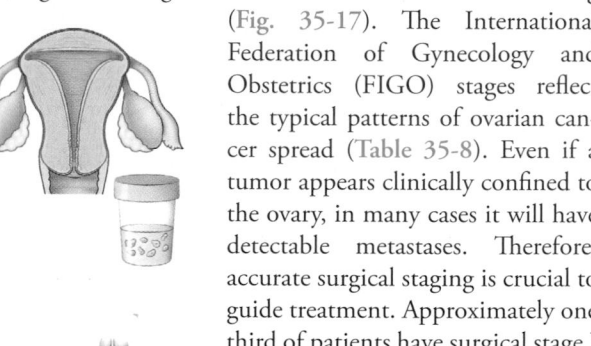

FIGURE 35-17 FIGO staging for ovarian cancer.

TABLE 35-8. FIGO Staging of Carcinoma of the Ovary

Stage	Characteristics
I	**Growth limited to the ovaries**
IA	Growth limited to one ovary; no ascites present containing malignant cells. No tumor on the external surface; capsule intact
IB	Growth limited to both ovaries, no ascites present containing malignant cells. No tumor on the external surface; capsule intact
IC[a]	Tumor either stage IA or IB, but with tumor on surface of one or both ovaries, or with capsule ruptured, or with ascites present containing malignant cells, or with positive peritoneal washings
II	**Growth involving one or both ovaries with pelvic extension**
IIA	Extension and/or metastasis to the uterus and/or tubes
IIB	Extension to other pelvic tissues
IIC[a]	Tumor either stage IIA or IIB, but with tumor on surface of one or both ovaries, or with capsule(s) ruptured, or with ascites present containing malignant cells, or with positive peritoneal washings
III	**Tumor involving one or both ovaries with histologically confirmed peritoneal implants outside the pelvis and/or positive regional lymph nodes. Superficial liver metastasis equal stage III. Tumor is limited to the true pelvis, but with histologically proven malignant extension to the small bowel or omentum**
IIIA	Tumor is grossly limited to the true pelvis, with negative nodes, but with histologically confirmed microscopic seeding of abdominal peritoneal surfaces, or histologically proven extension to small bowel or mesentery
IIIB	Tumor of one or both ovaries with histologically confirmed implants, peritoneal metastases of abdominal peritoneal surfaces, none exceeding 2 cm in diameter; nodes are negative
IIIC	Peritoneal metastasis beyond the pelvis >2 cm in diameter and/or positive regional lymph nodes
IV	**Growth involving one or both ovaries with distant metastases. If pleural effusion is present, there must be positive cytology to allot a case to stage IV. Parenchymal liver metastasis equals stage IV**

[a]To evaluate the impact on prognosis of the different criteria for allotting cases to stage IC or IIC, it would be of value to know if rupture of the capsule was spontaneous, or caused by the surgeon; and if the source of malignant cells detected was peritoneal washings, or ascites.
FIGO = International Federation of Gynecology and Obstetrics.

and infrarenal paraaortic lymphadenectomy, is also completed (Sections 44-11 through 44-14, p. 1296) (Chan, 2007; Cress, 2011; Whitney, 2011).

Laparoscopic staging is particularly valuable as a primary treatment in women who have an apparent stage I ovarian cancer. Alternatively, unstaged patients may have completion of staging by laparoscopy. In general, for laparoscopic staging, all of the required procedures can be safely performed (Chi, 2005). The main putative benefits are a shorter hospital stay and quicker recovery (Tozzi, 2004). However, nodal counts may be inferior, and exploration of the abdomen is unavoidably limited.

One third of patients who appear to have disease confined to the ovary will be "up-staged" by surgical staging and require postoperative chemotherapy. In those with stage IA or IB, grade 1 or 2 epithelial ovarian carcinoma, observation without further treatment following surgery is appropriate (Young, 1990).

Fertility-Sparing Management

Approximately 10 percent of epithelial ovarian cancers develop in women younger than 40 years. In selected cases, fertility-sparing surgery may be an option if disease appears confined to one ovary.

Although many patients will be up-staged as a result of the operative findings, those with surgical stage I disease have an excellent long-term survival with unilateral adnexectomy. In some cases, postoperative chemotherapy may be required, but

TABLE 35-9. Distribution of Epithelial Ovarian Cancer by FIGO Stage (n = 4825 patients)

FIGO Stage	Percent
I	28
II	8
III	50
IV	13

FIGO = International Federation of Gynecology and Obstetrics.
Data from Heintz, 2006.

patients will usually retain their ability to conceive and ultimately carry a pregnancy to term (Schilder, 2002).

Adjuvant Chemotherapy

As noted, patients with stage IA or IB, grades 1 and 2 are adequately treated with surgery alone. However, women with stage IA or IB, grade 3 epithelial ovarian cancer and all stage IC and II tumors should be treated with three to six cycles of carboplatin (Paraplatin) and paclitaxel (Taxol) chemotherapy (Morgan, 2011; Trimbos, 2003). In a phase III Gynecologic Oncology Group (GOG) trial (protocol #157), women with early-stage disease were randomly assigned to either three or six cycles of this combination. Overall, three cycles resulted in a relapse rate comparable to that for six cycles, but was associated with less toxicity (Bell, 2006). However, in a sub-analysis of patients in this study who had serous tumors, treatment with six cycles decreased the risk of relapse (Chan, 2010a).

Despite chemotherapy, more than 20 percent of women with early-stage disease develop recurrences within 5 years, suggesting the need for a better treatment strategy. In response, the GOG conducted a randomized phase III trial of postoperative carboplatin and paclitaxel chemotherapy followed by observation or weekly paclitaxel for 24 weeks (protocol #175). Unfortunately, there was no observed benefit to maintenance paclitaxel for early-stage patients (Mannel, 2011).

Surveillance

After completion of treatment, patients with early-stage ovarian cancer may be followed every 2 to 4 months for the first 2 years, then twice yearly for an additional 3 years, then annually. At each visit, complete physical and pelvic examinations should be performed. In addition, a serum CA125 level may be indicated if it was initially elevated (Morgan, 2011).

However, a multiinstitutional European trial evaluated the utility of CA125 levels in the monitoring of ovarian cancer after completion of primary therapy. The study demonstrated that women with relapsed ovarian cancer did not live longer if chemotherapy was started earlier based on a rising CA125 level, as opposed to delaying treatment until symptoms developed. The group closely monitored with CA125 tests received 5 more months of chemotherapy overall, whereas women who were diagnosed and treated later for clinically evident recurrence had higher quality-of-life measures (Rustin, 2010).

Whether suspected by examination, CA125 level elevation, or new symptoms, recurrent disease may also identified with the aid of imaging tests. Of modalities, CT is initially most helpful to locate recurrent pelvic and metastatic disease.

Management of Advanced Ovarian Cancer

Approximately two thirds of patients will have stage III-IV disease, thus multimodality therapy is particularly important to achieve the most successful outcome (Earle, 2006). Ideally, surgical cytoreduction is initially performed to remove all gross disease, followed by six courses of platinum-based chemotherapy. However, some women will not be appropriate candidates for primary surgery due to their medical condition, and others

will have unresectable tumor. Additionally, a recent randomized trial conducted in Europe concluded that initial treatment with chemotherapy followed by interval debulking surgery might achieve equivalent results (Vergote, 2010). To effectively balance all clinical factors, each patient should be individually assessed before embarking on a treatment strategy.

Primary Cytoreductive Surgery

Residual Disease. Since the initial report by Griffiths (1975) suggested the value of debulking, its value has been largely assumed. Numerous retrospective studies have subsequently supported the apparent survival advantage in women with advanced ovarian cancer if less than 2 cm residual disease can be achieved by cytoreduction. Specifically, 2 cm residual disease describes a surgical result in which none of multiple remaining areas of tumor individually measures greater than 2 cm. Additional incremental improvements in survival have been demonstrated if residual disease is less than 1.5 cm, less than 1 cm, or less than 0.5 cm. Longest survival durations are reported if no residual disease remains at the surgery completion (Chi, 2006). By definition, for patients to be considered "optimally debulked," they must have less than 1 cm residual disease.

There are several reasons why resecting ovarian cancer implants is believed to prolong survival. First, surgery removes large volumes of chemoresistant tumor cell clones. Second, the removal of necrotic masses improves drug delivery to remaining well-vascularized cells. Third, small residual tumor implants should be faster growing and therefore more susceptible to chemotherapy. Fourth, reducing the numbers of cancer cells should require fewer cycles of chemotherapy and reduce the chances of chemoresistance. Finally, removal of bulky disease potentially enhances the immune system.

Whether any of these supposed advantages to debulking are actually clinically relevant is debatable (Covens, 2000). However, because of the presumed benefits, primary surgical cytoreduction is generally performed whenever clinically feasible. Since the goal is the maximal resection of ovarian cancer and all metastatic disease, laparoscopic or robotic surgery has only a limited role (Magrina, 2011; Nezhat, 2010). Typically, a variety of procedures are required to achieve minimal residual disease, as described subsequently.

Surgical Approach to Cytoreductive Surgery. In general, a vertical incision is recommended to provide access to the entire abdomen. Patients with advanced disease do not require peritoneal washings or cytologic assessment of fluid, but often several liters of ascites will need to be evacuated to improve access. Next, the abdomen is carefully explored to quickly determine if optimal debulking is feasible. It is preferable to perform a limited surgical procedure rather than extensive debulking if it is obvious that tumors larger than 2 cm will be left behind. If hysterectomy and BSO is not possible, a biopsy of the ovary and sampling of the endometrium by dilatation and curettage should be performed to confirm an ovarian primary and exclude the possibility of widely metastatic uterine papillary serous carcinoma. However, if disease is resectable, then surgery should begin with the least complicated procedure.

Often, an infracolic omentectomy can be easily performed and extended (i.e., gastrocolic), if necessary, to encompass the disease. A frozen section may then be obtained to confirm the presumptive diagnosis of epithelial ovarian cancer. The pelvis is assessed next. Usually, an extrafascial type I abdominal hysterectomy and BSO is sufficient. However, when the tumor is confluent or invading the rectosigmoid, an en bloc resection, low anterior resection, or modified posterior pelvic exenteration may be required. These and other surgeries mentioned in this section are described and illustrated in Chapter 44 (p. 1259).

Patients with abdominal tumor nodules that are less than 2 cm (apparent stage IIIB) should have bilateral pelvic and paraaortic node biopsies to provide the most accurate surgical staging. In patients with stage IV disease and those with abdominal tumor nodules at least 2 cm (already stage IIIC disease), nodal dissection is not necessarily required (Whitney, 2011). However, if it is not performed, a significant percentage of patients will have unrecognized macroscopic nodal disease (Eisenkop, 2001). Thus, systematic lymphadenectomy in advanced ovarian cancer appears to mainly benefit patients with complete intraperitoneal debulking (du Bois, 2010; Panici, 2005).

Optimal surgical cytoreduction may also require various other radical procedures, including splenectomy, diaphragm stripping/resection, and small or large bowel resection (Aletti, 2006; McCann, 2011). Surgically aggressive centers experienced in such techniques report higher rates of achieving minimal residual disease that correspond to better outcomes (Aletti, 2009; Chi, 2009a; Wimberger, 2007). For diagnostic purposes and since it is a frequent site of disease, an appendectomy is also commonly included (Timofeev, 2010).

Neoadjuvant Chemotherapy and Interval Cytoreductive Surgery

Many patients do not undergo initial optimal surgical debulking (Everett, 2006). In some cases, imaging studies may suggest unresectable disease. Other patients may be too medically compromised, may not have received initial care by a gynecologic oncologist, or may have large-volume "suboptimal" residual disease despite attempted debulking. In such circumstances, three to four courses of chemotherapy are used to shrink the disease before attempting an "interval" cytoreductive surgery.

Neoadjuvant chemotherapy with an interval procedure has been associated with less perioperative morbidity, increased rates of optimal cytoreduction, and similar survival, but had never been directly compared with primary debulking (Hou, 2007; Kang, 2009). However, Vergote and colleagues (2010) recently reported results of a randomized phase III trial of 634 patients with stage IIIC or IV epithelial ovarian cancer, many of whom had bulky upper abdominal disease. In that study, neoadjuvant chemotherapy followed by interval debulking was *not* inferior to primary cytoreductive surgery. Since fewer than half of the primary surgery patients had an optimal debulking procedure, the survival rates were comparable to those in other chemotherapy trials of patients with large-volume residual disease (Ozols, 2003). Of interest, the strongest variable predicting overall survival was complete resection of all macroscopic disease, whether performed as primary treatment or after three cycles of chemotherapy (Vergote, 2010).

Thus, the benefits of interval debulking mainly occur in patients who have very advanced, unresectable disease or who did not initially have a maximal surgical effort by a gynecologic oncologist (Rose, 2004; Tangjitgamol, 2009; van der Burg, 1995).

Adjuvant Chemotherapy

Advanced ovarian cancer is considered to be relatively sensitive to cytotoxic agents. Largely due to recent advances in identifying active drugs, the duration of survival among patients has increased over the past two decades. Despite such improvements, fewer than 20 percent of those requiring chemotherapy will be cured. This is largely due to clinically occult residual chemoresistant tumor cells.

Intravenous Chemotherapy. Platinum-based chemotherapy is the foundation for systemic treatment of most epithelial ovarian cancer types, although alternative regimens are currently being studied for advanced mucinous and clear cell carcinomas because of their known resistance. In two large collaborative group trials (GOG protocol #158 and Arbeitsgemeinschaft Gynäkologische Onkologie [AGO] protocol OVAR-3), the combination of carboplatin and paclitaxel was easier to administer, similarly efficacious, and less toxic (du Bois, 2003; Ozols, 2003). As a result, the most widely used intravenous (IV) regimen in the United States is six courses of carboplatin and paclitaxel. If additional cycles are required to achieve clinical remission, this suggests relative tumor chemoresistance and usually leads to an earlier relapse. In Europe, single-agent carboplatin is often used. This preference is based on two large phase III trials of the International Collaborative Ovarian Neoplasm (ICON) Group, which did not detect a survival advantage for combination chemotherapy (The ICON Collaborators, 1998; The ICON Group, 2002).

Although the combination of carboplatin and paclitaxel is undoubtedly effective, other modifications have been studied. For instance, the addition of a third cytotoxic agent was postulated to further improve outcome. Unfortunately, none of the experimental regimens demonstrated superiority compared with the control group (Bookman, 2009). Addition of the biologic agent bevacizumab (Avastin) during primary chemotherapy, followed by use as maintenance therapy, has recently shown to provide only a modest improvement in progression-free survival (GOG protocol #218 and ICON-7). Finally, administering paclitaxel in a dose-dense weekly schedule may have some advantages at the cost of additional toxicity (Katsumata, 2009). The GOG is currently conducting a definitive phase III trial comparing dose-dense paclitaxel with carboplatin versus every-3-week paclitaxel and carboplatin. In addition, suboptimally debulked patients in both groups receive optional bevacizumab (protocol #262).

Intraperitoneal Chemotherapy. In January 2006, the National Cancer Institute issued a rare Clinical Announcement encouraging the use of intraperitoneal (IP) chemotherapy. This coincided with the publication of results from a phase III GOG

TABLE 35-10. Intraperitoneal Chemotherapy Regimen for Ovarian Cancer

Day 1	Paclitaxel 135 mg/m² IV over 24 hour
Day 2	Cisplatin 100 mg/m² intraperitoneal
Day 8	Paclitaxel 60 mg/m² intraperitoneal

From Armstrong, 2006.

trial (protocol #172) of optimally debulked stage III ovarian cancer patients who were randomly assigned to receive either IV or combination IV/IP paclitaxel and cisplatin chemotherapy (Table 35-10). The median duration of overall survival was 66 months in the IV/IP group compared with 50 months in the IV group (Armstrong, 2006). By comparison, survival in both groups far exceeded patients treated in the Vergote trial (29 to 30 months median survival), described on page 871 (Vergote, 2010). Despite this dramatic improvement in survival, many clinicians still consider IP chemotherapy to be an experimental treatment and do not routinely recommend it (Gore, 2006).

The theoretical advantages of IP chemotherapy are dramatic. In general, epithelial ovarian cancer mainly spreads along peritoneal surfaces. In postoperative patients with minimal residual disease, a much higher dose of chemotherapy can be achieved at the tumor site by administration directly into the abdomen (Alberts, 1996; Markman, 2001).

Obviously, not every woman with advanced ovarian cancer is an appropriate candidate for IP chemotherapy. Stage IV patients and those with large-volume residual disease are least likely to benefit. In addition, toxicity is generally higher with IP therapy, catheter-related problems are common, and the true long-term survival advantage remains controversial (Walker, 2006). Regardless, the current consensus is that IP therapy should certainly be considered for low-volume, optimally debulked disease (Morgan, 2011). However, the choice to receive or not receive IP chemotherapy should ultimately be a decision made by an informed patient (Alberts, 2006).

In light of the National Cancer Institute Clinical Announcement and ensuing debate, newer IP regimens are currently being tested. One current randomized phase III GOG trial (protocol #252) is comparing: (1) dose-dense paclitaxel and IV carboplatin, (2) dose-dense paclitaxel and IP carboplatin, and (3) a modified GOG protocol #172 IP cisplatin regimen. All groups receive concurrent bevacizumab followed by maintenance bevacizumab. It is anticipated that these data will shape future applications of ovarian cancer IP therapy.

Management of Patients in Remission

In most women with advanced ovarian cancer, the combination of surgery and platinum-based chemotherapy will result in clinical remission (normal examination, CA125 levels, and CT scan findings). However, up to 80 percent will eventually relapse and die from disease progression. Lower CA125 levels, that is, single-digit values, are generally associated with fewer relapses and longer survival (Juretzka, 2007). Since most patients achieving remission will have residual, clinically occult

drug-resistant cells, several options are appropriate to consider. Unfortunately, there is no solid proof that any intervention is beneficial.

Surveillance. After completion of treatment, patients may be followed regularly with examinations and CA125 levels, as in early-stage disease. To monitor advanced ovarian cancer patients, imaging tests may be indicated more frequently. In general, clinicians should maintain a more heightened suspicion for relapse.

Second-Look Surgery. The "gold standard" for identifying residual disease is a second-look laparotomy. In general, the main indications are to assess the completeness of response and resect residual tumor.

A true second-look operation consists of several steps. First, ascitic fluid or cytologic washings should be collected unless biopsy-proven disease is discovered. Second, all peritoneal surfaces must be visually examined, including direct inspection of the diaphragm, to aid removal of any suspicious nodules, adhesions, or tumors. Third, in the absence of gross disease, routine biopsies are performed from peritoneal surfaces and residual omentum. Finally, pelvic and paraaortic nodal sampling is required unless it was initially performed and no disease was found (Whitney, 2011). Second-look laparoscopy is an acceptable, less morbid alternative for selected patients (Husain, 2001; Littell, 2006).

For numerous reasons, however, neither type of second-look surgery is routinely performed. Although nonrandomized studies have occasionally reported a clinical advantage to identifying patients with residual disease, two European multicenter randomized trials of second-look laparotomy failed to demonstrate survival benefit (Luesley, 1988; Nicoletto, 1997). In addition, a recent nonrandomized comparison of patients from a prior GOG trial who had undergone second-look surgery was not associated with longer survival (Greer, 2005).

In summary, second-look laparotomy primarily serves as a useful early endpoint in assessing the effectiveness of treatment within an experimental protocol. Otherwise, no prospective clinical trials have demonstrated a survival advantage. Second-look surgery does have prognostic value, since a procedure that reveals no recurrent disease is associated with an improved survival rate. In summary, the additional morbidity and cost must be weighed against the expected benefit for an individual patient (American College of Obstetricians and Gynecologists, 1995).

Maintenance Chemotherapy. There is limited evidence to suggest any advantage for additional treatment in women who achieve clinical remission after six courses of platinum-based chemotherapy. However, due to the known high rate of recurrence, several agents have been tested as maintenance therapy, also termed *consolidation therapy*, in nonrandomized studies.

Monthly paclitaxel for 12 cycles was observed to extend progression-free survival by 7 months when compared with only three courses of treatment. Interestingly, this benefit appeared to be limited mainly to patients with the lowest CA125 levels and presumably, the lowest tumor burdens at study entry (Markman, 2006). In addition, cumulative toxicity, most notably neuropathy, was substantial and resulted in frequent dose reductions. Unfortunately, the trial did not demonstrate prolonged survival of patients receiving prolonged maintenance therapy (Markman, 2003, 2009).

To determine whether lower-dose paclitaxel or CT-2103 (Xyotax) can actually reduce the death rate compared with no maintenance therapy, the GOG is currently conducting a phase III trial of women with advanced ovarian cancer who achieved a clinical remission after standard platinum-based chemotherapy (protocol #212). Bevacizumab is also being studied as maintenance therapy in several ongoing phase III trials.

Radiation Therapy. In the United States, patients in remission after primary therapy are rarely treated with whole abdominal radiotherapy due to unproven benefit and fears of excessive toxicity such as radiation enteritis (Sorbe, 2003). However, the long-term effectiveness of this consolidation strategy is comparable to that achieved in women treated with other modalities. As a result, it may be considered for selected patients with microscopic disease detected at second-look surgery (Morgan, 2011). In general, this practice is much more common in Europe (Petit, 2007).

Prognostic Factors

The overall 5-year survival rate of all stages of epithelial ovarian cancer is 45 percent, far lower than uterine (84 percent) or cervical cancer (73 percent) (National Cancer Institute, 2011c). Survival rates largely depend on whether the disease has metastasized or not (Table 35-11), mirroring the assigned FIGO stage. Additional prognostic factors are shown in Table 35-12. Interestingly, *BRCA* mutation carriers have a better prognosis, chiefly due to increased platinum sensitivity (Cass, 2003; Lacour, 2011). However, even with favorable prognostic factors and despite recent innovations, most patients will ultimately relapse.

Management of Recurrent Ovarian Cancer

Gradual elevation of the CA125 level is usually the first sign of relapse. Tamoxifen is frequently administered when there is only "biochemical" evidence for disease progression, because it has some activity in treating recurrent disease and toxicity is minimal (Hurteau, 2010). Alternatively, patients may be offered participation in a clinical trial, started on cytotoxic chemotherapy, or observed until clinical symptoms arise. Without treatment, the recurrence will usually become clinically obvious within 2 to 6 months. Almost invariably, the tumor will be

TABLE 35-12. Most Important Favorable Prognostic Factors for Ovarian Cancer

Younger age
Good performance status
Cell type other than mucinous and clear cell
Well-differentiated tumor
Smaller disease volume prior to surgical debulking
Absence of ascites
Smaller residual tumor following primary cytoreductive surgery

From National Cancer Institute, 2011c.

located somewhere within the abdomen. Women who progress during primary chemotherapy are classified as having "platinum-refractory" disease. Those who relapse within 6 months have "platinum-resistant" ovarian cancer (National Cancer Institute, 2011c). In general, patients in either category have a dismal prognosis, and palliative nonplatinum chemotherapy is effectively the only option. Participation in an experimental clinical trial should be offered whenever possible. Otherwise, response rates typically range from 5 to 15 percent using conventional cytotoxic drugs such as paclitaxel, pegylated liposomal doxorubicin (Doxil), docetaxel (Taxotere), topotecan (Hycamtin), or gemcitabine (Gemzar).

Women who relapse more than 6 to 12 months after completion of primary therapy are considered "platinum-sensitive." These patients, especially those in prolonged remission beyond 18, 24, or 36 months, have the greatest number of potential options (Morgan, 2011). Of interest, although patients with primary early-stage ovarian cancer have a more favorable overall prognosis, survival after relapse is comparable to those who initially had advanced-stage disease (Chan, 2010b).

Secondary Cytoreductive Surgery

Although patient selection is somewhat arbitrary, the best candidates for secondary cytoreductive surgery have: (1) platinum-sensitive disease, (2) a prolonged disease-free interval, (3) a solitary-site recurrence, and (4) no ascites (Chi, 2006). To achieve a maximal survival benefit, debulking must result in minimal residual disease (Harter, 2006; Schorge, 2010b). However, approximately half of patients will be explored without achieving this goal.

The overall survival benefit of this approach is currently being studied in a phase III GOG trial (protocol #213). This randomizes surgical candidates with platinum-sensitive relapsed disease to secondary debulking or not, followed by carboplatin and paclitaxel with or without additional bevacizumab. Of patients enrolled in this study, only 15 to 20 percent have thus far been considered surgical candidates.

Salvage Chemotherapy

Regardless of whether patients undergo additional surgery, retreatment with a platinum drug is the treatment of choice for patients with recurrent, platinum-sensitive ovarian cancer. Carboplatin combined with either paclitaxel or gemcitabine has

TABLE 35-11. Epithelial Ovarian Cancer 5-Year Survival Rates

Stage	5-Year Survival (%)
Localized (confined to primary site)	92
Regional (spread to regional nodes)	72
Distant (cancer has metastasized)	27
Unknown (unstaged)	22

From National Cancer Institute, 2011c.

demonstrated modest superiority compared with carboplatin alone (Parmar, 2003; Pfisterer, 2006). Moreover, in one randomized phase III trial, the novel combination of carboplatin and pegylated liposomal doxorubicin was superior to carboplatin and paclitaxel (Pujade-Lauraine, 2010). However, giving these drugs sequentially as single agents might be equally successful and less toxic (National Cancer Institute, 2011c). Topotecan or docetaxel are other commonly used agents. Recently, bevacizumab has also demonstrated promising activity (Burger, 2007; Cannistra, 2007).

Regardless of which regimen is selected initially, reevaluation should usually follow two to three cycles of chemotherapy to determine the clinical benefit (Morgan, 2011). Typically, a CA125 response with or without confirmation of tumor shrinkage by CT provides sufficient reassurance to continue therapy. Nonresponders should be changed to a different regimen that may be more efficacious.

Chemotherapy selection is based on overall response rates for all of the epithelial ovarian cancer histologic variants. It would seem plausible that targeting therapy for an individual patient's disease might be more effective than empiric drug selection. In vitro chemosensitivity testing is occasionally used for this purpose. In principle, different agents are tested against the patient's tumor, and the chemotherapeutic drug demonstrating the best response should result in a better outcome. Unfortunately, this approach lacks demonstrable efficacy (Morgan, 2011).

Palliation of End-Stage Ovarian Cancer

During treatment, intermittent episodes of partial small- and large-bowel obstruction are common. However, at some point, patients with recurrent disease will develop worsening symptoms that warrant reevaluation of their overall treatment strategy.

Bowel obstruction that does not resolve with nasogastric suction can be managed in two very different ways. Frequently, a patient may desire an aggressive approach with surgical intervention, initiation of total parenteral nutrition, and continued chemotherapy. A colostomy, ileostomy, or intestinal bypass will often relieve symptoms (Chi, 2009b). Unfortunately, a satisfactory surgical result is sometimes impossible due to multiple sites of partial or complete obstruction. In addition, successful palliation is rarely achieved when the transit time is prolonged due to diffuse peritoneal carcinomatosis or when the anatomy requires a bypass that results in the short bowel syndrome (National Cancer Institute, 2011c). Further, recovery is often complicated by an enterocutaneous fistula, reobstruction, or other morbid event (Pothuri, 2004). For some patients, the best approach to managing a refractory bowel obstruction may be placement of a palliative gastrostomy tube, IV hydration, and hospice care. The final decision regarding how to proceed should be based on a frank discussion. Topics include treatment options, the natural history of progressive ovarian cancer, and the realistic possibility of further disease response by switching to a different therapy.

Another common scenario is a woman with symptomatic, rapidly reaccumulating ascitic fluid. This may be alleviated by repeated paracenteses or placement of an indwelling peritoneal catheter (Pleurx). Similarly, a refractory malignant pleural effu-sion can usually be managed by thoracentesis, pleurodesis, or indwelling pleural catheter placement.

Although these procedures and others may be appropriate in selected patients, the inability to halt disease progression should be acknowledged. In addition, any intervention has the potential to result in an unanticipated, catastrophic complication. Overall, palliative procedures are most compassionately used when incorporated into the overall treatment plan. For example, in a woman with stable disease and normal renal function, tumor-induced ureteral compression and hydronephrosis does not necessarily require stent placement or a nephrostomy tube.

All patients deserve a positive, hopeful, but honest approach to the management of progressive, incurable disease. Often, there are unrealistic expectations regarding the benefit of palliative chemotherapy, but emotionally it may be preferable to the idea of "giving up" (Doyle, 2001). There is no substitute for mutual trust in the doctor–patient relationship when making sound decisions aimed at improving the quality of life of women with end-stage ovarian cancer.

REFERENCES

Al-Barrak J, Santos JL, Tinker A, et al: Exploring palliative treatment outcomes in women with advanced or recurrent ovarian clear cell carcinoma. Gynecol Oncol 122(1):107, 2011

Alberts DS, Liu PY, Hannigan EV, et al: Intraperitoneal cisplatin plus intravenous cyclophosphamide versus intravenous cisplatin plus intravenous cyclophosphamide for stage III ovarian cancer. N Engl J Med 335:1950, 1996

Alberts DS, Markman M, Muggia F, et al: Proceedings of a GOG workshop on intraperitoneal therapy for ovarian cancers. Gynecol Oncol 103(3):738, 2006

Aletti GD, Dowdy SC, Gostout BS, et al: Quality improvement in the surgical approach to advanced ovarian cancer: the Mayo Clinic experience. J Am Coll Surg 208:614, 2009

Aletti GD, Dowdy SC, Podratz KC, et al: Surgical treatment of diaphragm disease correlates with improved survival in optimally debulked advanced stage ovarian cancer. Gynecol Oncol 100:283, 2006

Alvarado-Cabrero I, Cheung A, Caduff R: Tumours of the fallopian tube and uterine ligaments [Tumours of the fallopian tube]. In Tavassoli FA, Devilee P (eds): World Health Organization Classification of Tumours. Geneva, WHO, 2003, p 206

American College of Obstetricians and Gynecologists: Hereditary breast and ovarian cancer syndrome. Practice Bulletin No. 103, April 2009

American College of Obstetricians and Gynecologists: Prophylactic oophorectomy. Practice Bulletin No. 7, September 1999

American College of Obstetricians and Gynecologists: The role of the generalist obstetrician-gynecologist in the early detection of ovarian cancer. Committee Opinion No. 477, March 2011

American College of Obstetricians and Gynecologists: Second-look laparotomy for epithelial ovarian cancer. Committee Opinion No. 165, December 1995

Armstrong DK, Bundy B, Wenzel L, et al: Intraperitoneal cisplatin and paclitaxel in ovarian cancer. N Engl J Med 354:34, 2006

Barnhill DR, Kurman RJ, Brady MF, et al: Preliminary analysis of the behavior of stage I ovarian serous tumors of low malignant potential: a Gynecologic Oncology Group study. J Clin Oncol 13:2752, 1995

Beiner ME, Finch A, Rosen B, et al: The risk of endometrial cancer in women with BRCA1 and BRCA2 mutations: a prospective study. Gynecol Oncol 104(1):7, 2007

Bell J, Brady MF, Young RC, et al: Randomized phase III trial of three versus six cycles of adjuvant carboplatin and paclitaxel in early stage epithelial ovarian carcinoma: a Gynecologic Oncology Group study. Gynecol Oncol 102:432, 2006

Bookman MA, Brady MF, McGuire WP, et al: Evaluation of new platinum-based treatment regimens in advanced-stage ovarian cancer: a phase III trial of the Gynecologic Cancer Intergroup. J Clin Oncol 27:1419, 2009

Bristow RE, Palis BE, Chi DS, et al: The National Cancer Database report on advanced-stage epithelial ovarian cancer: impact of hospital surgical case volume on overall survival and surgical treatment paradigm. Gynecol Oncol 118:262, 2010

Buller RE, Lallas TA, Shahin MS, et al: The *p53* mutational spectrum associated with *BRCA1* mutant ovarian cancer. Clin Cancer Res 7:831, 2001

Burger RA, Sill MW, Monk BJ, et al: Phase II trial of bevacizumab in persistent or recurrent epithelial ovarian cancer or primary peritoneal cancer: a Gynecologic Oncology Group study. J Clin Oncol 25:5165, 2007

Buttin BM, Herzog TJ, Powell MA, et al: Epithelial ovarian tumors of low malignant potential: the role of microinvasion. Obstet Gynecol 99:11, 2002

Buys SS, Partridge E, Black A, et al: Effect of screening on ovarian cancer mortality: the Prostate, Lung, Colorectal and Ovarian (PLCO) Cancer Screening Randomized Controlled Trial. JAMA 305(22):2295, 2011

Buys SS, Partridge E, Greene MH, et al: Ovarian cancer screening in the Prostate, Lung, Colorectal and Ovarian (PLCO) cancer screening trial: findings from the initial screen of a randomized trial. Am J Obstet Gynecol 193:1630, 2005

Callahan MJ, Crum CP, Medeiros F, et al: Primary fallopian tube malignancies in BRCA-positive women undergoing surgery for ovarian cancer risk reduction. J Clin Oncol 25:3985, 2007

Cannistra SA, Matulonis UA, Penson RT, et al: Phase II study of bevacizumab in patients with platinum-resistant ovarian cancer or peritoneal serous cancer. J Clin Oncol 25:5180, 2007

Carlson JW, Miron A, Jarboe EA, et al: Serous tubal intraepithelial carcinoma: its potential role in primary peritoneal serous carcinoma and serous cancer prevention. J Clin Oncol 26:4160, 2008

Cass I, Baldwin RL, Varkey T, et al: Improved survival in women with BRCA-associated ovarian carcinoma. Cancer 97:2187, 2003

Chan JK, Munro EG, Cheung MK, et al: Association of lymphadenectomy and survival in stage I ovarian cancer patients. Obstet Gynecol 109:12, 2007

Chan JK, Tian C, Fleming GF, et al: The potential benefit of 6 vs. 3 cycles of chemotherapy in subsets of women with early-stage high-risk epithelial ovarian cancer: an exploratory analysis of a Gynecologic Oncology Group study. Gynecol Oncol 116:301, 2010a

Chan JK, Tian C, Teoh D, et al: Survival after recurrence in early-stage high-risk epithelial ovarian cancer: a Gynecologic Oncology Group study. Gynecol Oncol 116:307, 2010b

Chen S, Iversen ES, Friebel T, et al: Characterization of *BRCA1* and *BRCA2* mutations in a large United States sample. J Clin Oncol 24:863, 2006

Chi DS, Abu-Rustum NR, Sonoda Y, et al: The safety and efficacy of laparoscopic surgical staging of apparent stage I ovarian and fallopian tube cancers. Am J Obstet Gynecol 192:1614, 2005

Chi DS, Eisenhauer EL, Zivanovic O, et al: Improved progression-free and overall survival in advanced ovarian cancer as a result of a change in surgical paradigm. Gynecol Oncol 114:26, 2009a

Chi DS, McCaughty K, Diaz JP, et al: Guidelines and selection criteria for secondary cytoreductive surgery in patients with recurrent, platinum-sensitive epithelial ovarian carcinoma. Cancer 106:1933, 2006

Chi DS, Phaeton R, Miner TJ, et al: A prospective outcomes analysis of palliative procedures performed for malignant intestinal obstruction due to recurrent ovarian cancer. Oncologist 14:835, 2009b

Covens AL: A critique of surgical cytoreduction in advanced ovarian cancer. Gynecol Oncol 78:269, 2000

Cramer DW, Bast RC Jr, Berg CD, et al: Ovarian cancer biomarker performance in prostate, lung, colorectal, and ovarian cancer screening trial specimens. Cancer Prev Res 4:65, 2011

Cress RD, Bauer K, O'Malley CD, et al: Surgical staging of early stage epithelial ovarian cancer: results from the CDC-NPCR ovarian patterns of care study. Gynecol Oncol 121:94, 2011

Deng CX: *BRCA1*: cell cycle checkpoint, genetic instability, DNA damage response and cancer evolution. Nucleic Acids Res 34:1416, 2006

Doyle C, Crump M, Pintilie M, et al: Does palliative chemotherapy palliate? Evaluation of expectations, outcomes, and costs in women receiving chemotherapy for advanced ovarian cancer. J Clin Oncol 19:1266, 2001

du Bois A, Luck HJ, Meier W, et al: A randomized clinical trial of cisplatin/paclitaxel versus carboplatin/paclitaxel as first-line treatment of ovarian cancer. J Natl Cancer Inst 95:1320, 2003

du Bois A, Reuss A, Harter P, et al: Potential role of lymphadenectomy in advanced ovarian cancer: a combined exploratory analysis of three prospectively randomized phase III multicenter trials. J Clin Oncol 28:1733, 2010

Earle CC, Schrag D, Neville BA, et al: Effect of surgeon specialty on processes of care and outcomes for ovarian cancer patients. J Natl Cancer Inst 98:172, 2006

Eichhorn JH, Young RH, Scully RE: Primary ovarian small cell carcinoma of pulmonary type: a clinicopathologic, immunohistologic, and flow cytometric analysis of 11 cases. Am J Surg Pathol 16:926, 1992

Eisenkop SM, Spirtos NM: The clinical significance of occult macroscopically positive retroperitoneal nodes in patients with epithelial ovarian cancer. Gynecol Oncol 82:143, 2001

Engelen MJ, Kos HE, Willemse PH, et al: Surgery by consultant gynecologic oncologists improves survival in patients with ovarian carcinoma. Cancer 106:589, 2006

Euhus DM, Smith KC, Robinson L, et al: Pretest prediction of *BRCA1* or *BRCA2* mutation by risk counselors and the computer model BRCAPRO. J Natl Cancer Inst 94:844, 2002

Everett EN, French AE, Stone RL, et al: Initial chemotherapy followed by surgical cytoreduction for the treatment of stage III/IV epithelial ovarian cancer. Am J Obstet Gynecol 195:568, 2006

Gershenson DM, Silva EG, Mitchell MF, et al: Transitional cell carcinoma of the ovary: a matched control study of advanced-stage patients treated with cisplatin based chemotherapy. Am J Obstet Gynecol 168:1178, 1993

Gertig DM, Hunter DJ, Cramer DW, et al: Prospective study of talc use and ovarian cancer. J Natl Cancer Inst 92:249, 2000

Goff BA, Mandel L, Muntz HG, et al: Ovarian carcinoma diagnosis. Cancer 89:2068, 2000

Goff BA, Mandel LS, Melancon CH, et al: Frequency of symptoms of ovarian cancer in women presenting to primary care clinics. JAMA 291:2705, 2004

Goff BA, Matthews BJ, Wynn M, et al: Ovarian cancer: patterns of surgical care across the United States. Gynecol Oncol 103:383, 2006

Gomez-Garcia EB, Ambergen T, Blok MJ, et al: Patients with an unclassified genetic variant in the *BRCA1* or *BRCA2* genes show different clinical features from those with a mutation. J Clin Oncol 23:2185, 2005

Goodman MT, Howe HL, Tung KH, et al: Incidence of ovarian cancer by race and ethnicity in the United States, 1992–1997. Cancer 97:2676, 2003

Gore M, du BA, Vergote I: Intraperitoneal chemotherapy in ovarian cancer remains experimental. J Clin Oncol 24:4528, 2006

Greene MH, Piedmonte M, Alberts D, et al: A prospective study of risk-reducing salpingo-oophorectomy and longitudinal CA-125 screening among women at increased genetic risk of ovarian cancer: design and baseline characteristics: a Gynecologic Oncology Group study. Cancer Epidemiol Biomarkers Prev 17:594, 2008

Greer BE, Bundy BN, Ozols RF, et al: Implications of second-look laparotomy in the context of optimally resected stage III ovarian cancer: a non-randomized comparison using an explanatory analysis. A Gynecologic Oncology Group study. Gynecol Oncol 99:71, 2005

Griffiths CT: Surgical resection of tumor bulk in the primary treatment of ovarian carcinoma. Natl Cancer Inst Monogr 42:101, 1975

Hankinson SE, Hunter DJ, Colditz GA, et al: Tubal ligation, hysterectomy, and risk of ovarian cancer: a prospective study. JAMA 270:2813, 1993

Harter P, Bois A, Hahmann M, et al: Surgery in recurrent ovarian cancer: the Arbeitsgemeinschaft Gynaekologische Onkologie (AGO) DESKTOP OVAR Trial. Ann Surg Oncol 13:1702, 2006

Heintz APM, Odicino F, Maisonneuve P, et al: Carcinoma of the ovary. In FIGO annual report on the results of treatment in gynaecological cancer. Int J Obstet Gynecol 95(Suppl 1):S161, 2006

Hinkula M, Pukkala E, Kyyronen P, et al: Incidence of ovarian cancer of grand multiparous women: a population-based study in Finland. Gynecol Oncol 103:207, 2006

Hou JY, Kelly MG, Yu H, et al: Neoadjuvant chemotherapy lessens surgical morbidity in advanced ovarian cancer and leads to improved survival in stage IV disease. Gynecol Oncol 105:211, 2007

Houck K, Nikrui N, Duska L, et al: Borderline tumors of the ovary: correlation of frozen and permanent histopathologic diagnosis. Obstet Gynecol 95:839, 2000

Hurteau JA, Brady MF, Darcy KM, et al: Randomized phase III trial of tamoxifen versus thalidomide in women with biochemical-recurrent-only epithelial ovarian, fallopian tube or primary peritoneal carcinoma after a complete response to first-line platinum/taxane chemotherapy with an evaluation of serum vascular endothelial growth factor (VEGF): a Gynecologic Oncology Group study. Gynecol Oncol 119:444, 2010

Husain A, Chi DS, Prasad M, et al: The role of laparoscopy in second-look evaluations for ovarian cancer. Gynecol Oncol 80:44, 2001

Huusom LD, Frederiksen K, Hogdall EV, et al: Association of reproductive factors, oral contraceptive use and selected lifestyle factors with the risk of ovarian borderline tumors: a Danish case-control study. Cancer Causes Control 17:821, 2006

Im SS, Gordon AN, Buttin BM, et al: Validation of referral guidelines for women with pelvic masses. Obstet Gynecol 105:35, 2005

International Collaboration of Epidemiological Studies of Cervical Cancer: Comparison of risk factors for invasive squamous cell carcinoma and adenocarcinoma of the cervix: collaborative reanalysis of individual data on 8,097 women with squamous cell carcinoma and 1,374 women with adenocarcinoma from 12 epidemiological studies. Int J Cancer 120:885, 2006

International Collaboration of Epidemiological Studies of Cervical Cancer, Appleby P, Beral V, et al: Cervical cancer and hormonal contraceptives: collaborative reanalysis of individual data for 16,573 women with cervical cancer and 35,509 women without cervical cancer from 24 epidemiological studies. Lancet 370(9599):1609, 2007

James PA, Doherty R, Harris M, et al: Optimal selection of individuals for *BRCA* mutation testing: a comparison of available methods. J Clin Oncol 24:707, 2006

Jemal A, Bray F, Center MM, et al: Global cancer statistics. CA Cancer J Clin 61:69, 2011

Juretzka MM, Barakat RR, Chi DS, et al: CA-125 level as a predictor of progression-free survival and overall survival in ovarian cancer patients with surgically defined disease status prior to the initiation of intraperitoneal consolidation therapy. Gynecol Oncol 104(1):176, 2007

Kang S, Nam BH: Does neoadjuvant chemotherapy increase optimal cytoreduction rate in advanced ovarian cancer? Meta-analysis of 21 studies. Ann Surg Oncol 16:2315, 2009

Katsumata N, Yasuda M, Takahashi F, et al: Dose-dense paclitaxel once a week in combination with carboplatin every 3 weeks for advanced ovarian cancer: a phase 3, open-label, randomized controlled trial. Lancet 374:1331, 2009

Kauff ND, Satagopan JM, Robson ME, et al: Risk-reducing salpingo-oophorectomy in women with a *BRCA1* or *BRCA2* mutation. N Engl J Med 346:1609, 2002

Kiani F, Knutsen S, Singh P, et al: Dietary risk factors for ovarian cancer: the Adventist Health Study (United States). Cancer Causes Control 17:137, 2006

Kramer JL, Velazquez IA, Chen BE, et al: Prophylactic oophorectomy reduces breast cancer penetrance during prospective, long-term follow-up of *BRCA1* mutation carriers. J Clin Oncol 23:8629, 2005

Kruitwagen RF, Swinkels BM, Keyser KG, et al: Incidence and effect on survival of abdominal wall metastases at trocar or puncture sites following laparoscopy or paracentesis in women with ovarian cancer. Gynecol Oncol 60:233, 1996

Lacey JV Jr, Brinton LA, Leitzmann MF, et al: Menopausal hormone therapy and ovarian cancer risk in the National Institutes of Health–AARP Diet and Health Study cohort. J Natl Cancer Inst 98:1397, 2006

Lacour RA, Westin SN, Meyer LA, et al: Improved survival in non-Ashkenazi Jewish ovarian cancer patients with BRCA1 and BRCA2 gene mutations. Gynecol Oncol 121:358, 2011

Lancaster MJ, Powell CB, Kauff ND, et al: Society of Gynecologic Oncologists Education Committee statement on risk assessment for inherited gynecologic cancer predispositions. Gynecol Oncol 107:159, 2007

Landen CN Jr, Birrer MJ, Sood AK: Early events in the pathogenesis of epithelial ovarian cancer. J Clin Oncol 26:995, 2008

Lee KR, Tavassoli FA, Prat J, et al: Tumours of the ovary and peritoneum [Surface epithelial-stromal tumours]. In Tavassoli FA, Devilee P (eds): World Health Organization Classification of Tumours. Geneva, WHO, 2003, p 117

Levanon K, Crum C, Drapkin R: New insights into the pathogenesis of serous ovarian cancer and its clinical impact. J Clin Oncol 26:5284, 2008

Levine DA, Argenta PA, Yee CJ, et al: Fallopian tube and primary peritoneal carcinomas associated with *BRCA* mutations. J Clin Oncol 21:4222, 2003

Li AJ, Madden AC, Cass I, et al: The prognostic significance of thrombocytosis in epithelial ovarian carcinoma. Gynecol Oncol 92:211, 2004

Lin PS, Gershenson DM, Bevers MW, et al: The current status of surgical staging of ovarian serous borderline tumors. Cancer 85:905, 1999

Littell RD, Hallonquist H, Matulonis U, et al: Negative laparoscopy is highly predictive of negative second-look laparotomy following chemotherapy for ovarian, tubal, and primary peritoneal carcinoma. Gynecol Oncol 103:570, 2006

Lu KH, Garber JE, Cramer DW, et al: Occult ovarian tumors in women with *BRCA1* or *BRCA2* mutations undergoing prophylactic oophorectomy. J Clin Oncol 18:2728, 2000

Luesley D, Lawton F, Blackledge G, et al: Failure of second-look laparotomy to influence survival in epithelial ovarian cancer. Lancet 2:599, 1988

Madalinska JB, Hollenstein J, Bleiker E, et al: Quality-of-life effects of prophylactic salpingo-oophorectomy versus gynecologic screening among women at increased risk of hereditary ovarian cancer. J Clin Oncol 23:6890, 2005

Madalinska JB, van Beurden M, Bleiker EM, et al: The impact of hormone replacement therapy on menopausal symptoms in younger high-risk women after prophylactic salpingo-oophorectomy. J Clin Oncol 24:3576, 2006

Magrina JF, Zanagnolo V, Noble BN, et al: Robotic approach for ovarian cancer: perioperative and survival results and comparison with laparoscopy and laparotomy. Gynecol Oncol 121:100, 2011

Makarla PB, Saboorian MH, Ashfaq R, et al: Promoter hypermethylation profile of ovarian epithelial neoplasms. Clin Cancer Res 11:5365, 2005

Mammas IN, Zafiropoulos A, Spandidos DA: Involvement of the ras genes in female genital tract cancer. Int J Oncol 26:1241, 2005

Mannel RS, Brady MF, Kohn EC, et al: A randomized phase III trial of IV carboplatin and paclitaxel × 3 courses followed by observation versus weekly maintenance low-dose paclitaxel in patients with early-stage ovarian carcinoma: a Gynecologic Oncology Group study. Gynecol Oncol 122(1):89, 2011

Markman M, Bundy BN, Alberts DS, et al: Phase III trial of standard-dose intravenous cisplatin plus paclitaxel versus moderately high-dose carboplatin followed by intravenous paclitaxel and intraperitoneal cisplatin in small-volume stage III ovarian carcinoma: an intergroup study of the Gynecologic Oncology Group, Southwestern Oncology Group, and Eastern Cooperative Oncology Group. J Clin Oncol 19:1001, 2001

Markman M, Liu PY, Moon J, et al: Impact on survival of 12 versus 3 monthly cycles of paclitaxel (175 mg/m^2) administered to patients with advanced ovarian cancer who attained a complete response to primary platinum-paclitaxel: follow-up of a Southwest Oncology Group and Gynecologic Oncology Group phase III trial. Gynecol Oncol 114(2):195, 2009

Markman M, Liu PY, Rothenberg ML, et al: Pretreatment CA-125 and risk of relapse in advanced ovarian cancer. J Clin Oncol 24:1454, 2006

Markman M, Liu PY, Wilczynski S, et al: Phase III randomized trial of 12 versus 3 months of maintenance paclitaxel in patients with advanced ovarian cancer after complete response to platinum and paclitaxel-based chemotherapy: a Southwest Oncology Group and Gynecologic Oncology Group trial. J Clin Oncol 21:2460, 2003

McCann CK, Growdon WB, Munro EG, et al: Prognostic significance of splenectomy as part of initial cytoreductive surgery in ovarian cancer. Ann Surg Oncol 2011 Mar 22 [Epub ahead of print]

Menon U, Gentry-Maharaj A, Hallett R, et al: Sensitivity and specificity of multimodal and ultrasound screening for ovarian cancer, and stage distribution of detected cancers: results of the prevalence screen of the UK Collaborative Trial of Ovarian Cancer Screening (UKCTOCS). Lancet Oncol 10:327, 2009

Menzin AW, Gal D, Lovecchio JL: Contemporary surgical management of borderline ovarian tumors: a survey of the Society of Gynecologic Oncologists. Gynecol Oncol 78:7, 2000

Mercado C, Zingmond D, Karlan BY, et al: Quality of care in advanced ovarian cancer: the importance of provider specialty. Gynecol Oncol 117:18, 2010

Mok SC, Schorge JO, Welch WR, et al: Tumours of the ovary and peritoneum [Peritoneal tumours]. In Tavassoli FA, Devilee P (eds): World Health Organization Classification of Tumours. Geneva, WHO, 2003, p 197

Mor G, Visintin I, Lai Y, et al: Serum protein markers for early detection of ovarian cancer. Proc Natl Acad Sci USA 102:7677, 2005

Morgan RJ Jr, Alvarez RD, Armstrong DK, et al: NCCN Clinical Practice Guidelines in Oncology. Ovarian cancer, including fallopian tube cancer and primary peritoneal cancer. Version 2. 2011. www.nccn.org. Accessed May 12, 2011

National Cancer Institute: Genetics of breast and ovarian cancer (PDQ). Available at: www.cancer.gov/cancertopics/pdq/genetics/breast-and-ovarian/healthprofessional. Accessed May 12, 2011a

National Cancer Institute: National Cancer Institute issues clinical announcement for preferred method of treatment for advanced ovarian cancer. January 4, 2006. Available at: www.cancer.gov/newscenter/pressreleases/IPchemotherapyrelease. Accessed May 12, 2011

National Cancer Institute: Ovarian cancer prevention (PDQ): Available at: http://www.cancer.gov/cancertopics/pdq/prevention/ovarian/HealthProfessional. Accessed May 12, 2011b

National Cancer Institute: Ovarian epithelial cancer treatment (PDQ). Available at: www.cancer.gov/cancertopics/pdq/treatment/ovarianepithelial/healthprofessional. Accessed May 12, 2011c

Nezhat FR, DeNoble SM, Liu CS, et al: The safety and efficacy of laparoscopic surgical staging and debulking of apparent advanced stage ovarian, fallopian tube, and primary peritoneal cancers. JSLS 14:155, 2010

Nicoletto MO, Tumolo S, Talamini R, et al: Surgical second look in ovarian cancer: a randomized study in patients with laparoscopic complete remission. A Northeastern Oncology Cooperative Group-Ovarian Cancer Cooperative Group study. J Clin Oncol 15:994, 1997

Ozols RF, Bundy BN, Greer BE, et al: Phase III trial of carboplatin and paclitaxel compared with cisplatin and paclitaxel in patients with optimally resected stage III ovarian cancer: a Gynecologic Oncology Group study. J Clin Oncol 21:3194, 2003

Panici PB, Maggioni A, Hacker N, et al: Systematic aortic and pelvic lymphadenectomy versus resection of bulky nodes only in optimally debulked advanced ovarian cancer: a randomized trial. J Natl Cancer Inst 97:560, 2005

Park JY, Kim DY, Kim JH, et al: Surgical management of borderline ovarian tumors: the role of fertility-sparing surgery. Gynecol Oncol 113:75, 2009

Park JY, Song JS, Choi G, et al: Pure primary squamous cell carcinoma of the ovary: a report of two cases and review of the literature. Int J Gynecol Pathol 29:328, 2010

Parmar MK, Ledermann JA, Colombo N, et al: Paclitaxel plus platinum-based chemotherapy versus conventional platinum-based chemotherapy in women with relapsed ovarian cancer: the ICON4/AGO-OVAR-2.2 trial. Lancet 361:2099, 2003

Parmigiani G, Chen S, Iversen Jr ES, et al: Validity of models for predicting BRCA1 and BRCA2 mutations. Ann Intern Med 147:441, 2007

Partridge E, Kreimer AR, Greenlee RT, et al: Results from four rounds of ovarian cancer screening in a randomized trial. Obstet Gynecol 113:775 2009

Pecorelli S, Benedet JL, Creasman WT, et al: FIGO staging of gynecologic cancer, 1994–1997. FIGO Committee on Gynecologic Oncology, International Federation of Gynecology and Obstetrics. Int J Gynaecol Obstet 65:243, 1999

Pelucchi C, Galeone C, Talamini R, et al: Lifetime ovulatory cycles and ovarian cancer risk in 2 Italian case-control studies. Am J Obstet Gynecol 196(1):83.e1, 2007

Petit T, Velten M, d'Hombres A, et al: Long-term survival of 106 stage III ovarian cancer patients with minimal residual disease after second-look laparotomy and consolidation radiotherapy. Gynecol Oncol 104(1):104, 2007

Petricoin EF, Ardekani AM, Hitt BA, et al: Use of proteomic patterns in serum to identify ovarian cancer. Lancet 359:572, 2002

Pfisterer J, Plante M, Vergote I, et al: Gemcitabine plus carboplatin compared with carboplatin in patients with platinum-sensitive recurrent ovarian cancer: an intergroup trial of the AGO OVAR, the NCIC CTG, and the EORTC GCG. J Clin Oncol 24:4699, 2006

Pins MR, Young RH, Daly WJ, et al: Primary squamous cell carcinoma of the ovary. Report of 37 cases. Am J Surg Pathol 20:823, 1996

Poncelet C, Fauvet R, Boccara J, et al: Recurrence after cystectomy for borderline ovarian tumors: results of a French multicenter study. Ann Surg Oncol 13:565, 2006

Pothuri B, Meyer L, Gerardi M, et al: Reoperation for palliation of recurrent malignant bowel obstruction in ovarian carcinoma. Gynecol Oncol 95:193, 2004

Powell CB, Kenley E, Chen LM, et al: Risk-reducing salpingo-oophorectomy in BRCA mutation carriers: role of serial sectioning in the detection of occult malignancy. J Clin Oncol 23:127, 2005

Prat J, Morice P: Tumours of the ovary and peritoneum [Secondary tumours of the ovary]. In Tavassoli FA, Devilee P (eds): World Health Organization Classification of Tumours. Geneva, WHO, 2003, p 193

Pujade-Lauraine E, Wagner U, Aavall-Lundqvist E, et al: Pegylated liposomal doxorubicin and carboplatin compared with paclitaxel and carboplatin for patients with platinum-sensitive ovarian cancer in late relapse. J Clin Oncol 28:3323, 2010

Purdie DM, Bain CJ, Siskind V, et al: Ovulation and risk of epithelial ovarian cancer. Int J Cancer 104:228, 2003

Quirk JT, Natarajan N: Ovarian cancer incidence in the United States, 1992–1999. Gynecol Oncol 97:519, 2005

Rao GG, Skinner E, Gehrig PA, et al: Surgical staging of ovarian low malignant potential tumors. Obstet Gynecol 104:261, 2004

Rao GG, Skinner EN, Gehrig PA, et al: Fertility-sparing surgery for ovarian low malignant potential tumors. Gynecol Oncol 98:263, 2005

Rauh-Hain JA, Growdon WB, Rodriguez N, et al: Carcinosarcoma of the ovary: a case-control study. Gynecol Oncol 121(3):477, 2011

Rebbeck TR, Lynch HT, Neuhausen SL, et al: Prophylactic oophorectomy in carriers of BRCA1 or BRCA2 mutations. N Engl J Med 346:1616, 2002

Riman T, Dickman PW, Nilsson S, et al: Risk factors for invasive epithelial ovarian cancer: results from a Swedish case-control study. Am J Epidemiol 156:363, 2002

Risch HA, McLaughlin JR, Cole DE, et al: Population BRCA1 and BRCA2 mutation frequencies and cancer penetrances: a kin-cohort study in Ontario, Canada. J Natl Cancer Inst 98:1694, 2006

Ronnett BM, Shmookler BM, Sugarbaker PH, et al: Pseudomyxoma peritonei: new concepts in diagnosis, origin, nomenclature, and relationship to mucinous borderline (low malignant potential) tumors of the ovary. Anat Pathol 2197, 1997

Ronnett BM, Yan H, Kurman RJ, et al: Patients with pseudomyxoma peritonei associated with disseminated peritoneal adenomucinosis have a significantly more favorable prognosis than patients with peritoneal mucinous carcinomatosis. Cancer 92:85, 2001

Rose PG, Nerenstone S, Brady MF, et al: Secondary surgical cytoreduction for advanced ovarian carcinoma. N Engl J Med 351:2489, 2004

Rosenblatt KA, Weiss NS, Cushing-Haugen KL, et al: Genital powder exposure and the risk of epithelial ovarian cancer. Cancer Causes Control 22:737, 2011

Rossing MA, Tang MT, Flagg EW, et al: A case-control study of ovarian cancer in relation to infertility and the use of ovulation-inducing drugs. Am J Epidemiol 160:1070, 2004

Rostgaard K, Wohlfahrt J, Andersen PK, et al: Does pregnancy induce the shedding of premalignant ovarian cells? Epidemiology 14:168, 2003

Rustin GJS, van der Burg MEL, Griffin CL, et al: Early versus delayed treatment of relapsed ovarian cancer (MRC OV05/EORTC 55955): a randomized trial. Lancet 376:1155, 2010

Schilder JM, Thompson AM, DePriest PD, et al: Outcome of reproductive age women with stage IA or IC invasive epithelial ovarian cancer treated with fertility-sparing therapy. Gynecol Oncol 87:1, 2002

Schildkraut JM, Bastos E, Berchuck A: Relationship between lifetime ovulatory cycles and overexpression of mutant p53 in epithelial ovarian cancer. J Natl Cancer Inst 89:932, 1997

Schmeler KM, Lynch HT, Chen LM, et al: Prophylactic surgery to reduce the risk of gynecologic cancers in the Lynch syndrome. N Engl J Med 354:261, 2006

Schorge JO, Modesitt SC, Coleman RL, et al: SGO White Paper on ovarian cancer: etiology, screening and surveillance. Gynecol Oncol 119:7, 2010a

Schorge JO, Muto MG, Lee SJ, et al: BRCA1-related papillary serous carcinoma of the peritoneum has a unique molecular pathogenesis. Cancer Res 60:1361, 2000

Schorge JO, Muto MG, Welch WR, et al: Molecular evidence for multifocal papillary serous carcinoma of the peritoneum in patients with germline BRCA1 mutations. J Natl Cancer Inst 90:841, 1998

Schorge JO, Wingo SN, Bhore R, et al: Secondary cytoreductive surgery for platinum-sensitive ovarian cancer. Int J Gynaecol Obstet 108:123, 2010b

Scully R, Livingston DM: In search of the tumour-suppressor functions of BRCA1 and BRCA2. Nature 408:429, 2000

Seidman JD, Kurman RJ: Ovarian serous borderline tumors: a critical review of the literature with emphasis on prognostic indicators. Hum Pathol 31:539, 2000

Shih KK, Zhou QC, Aghajanian C, et al: Patterns of recurrence and role of adjuvant chemotherapy in stage II-IV serous ovarian borderline tumors. Gynecol Oncol 119:270, 2010

Siegel R, Ward E, Brawley O, et al: Cancer statistics, 2011: the impact of eliminating socioeconomic and racial disparities on premature cancer deaths. CA Cancer J Clin 61(4):212, 2011

Silva EG, Gershenson DM, Malpica A, et al: The recurrence and the overall survival rates of ovarian serous borderline neoplasms with noninvasive implants is time dependent. Am J Surg Pathol 30:1367, 2006

Silva EG, Tornos C, Bailey MA, et al: Undifferentiated carcinoma of the ovary. Arch Pathol Lab Med 115:377, 1991

Skates SJ, Menon U, MacDonald N, et al: Calculation of the risk of ovarian cancer from serial CA-125 values for preclinical detection in postmenopausal women. J Clin Oncol 21:206, 2003

Soliman PT, Slomovitz BM, Broaddus RR, et al: Synchronous primary cancers of the endometrium and ovary: a single institution review of 84 cases. Gynecol Oncol 94:456, 2004

Sorbe B: Consolidation treatment of advanced (FIGO stage III) ovarian carcinoma in complete surgical remission after induction chemotherapy: a randomized, controlled, clinical trial comparing whole abdominal radiotherapy, chemotherapy, and no further treatment. Int J Gynecol Cancer 13:278, 2003

Sutton GP, Bundy BN, Omura GA, et al: Stage III ovarian tumors of low malignant potential treated with cisplatin combination therapy: a Gynecologic Oncology Group study. Gynecol Oncol 41:230, 1991

Tangjitgamol S, Manusirivithaya S, Laopaiboon M, et al: Interval debulking surgery for advanced epithelial ovarian cancer. Cochrane Database Syst Rev 2:CD006014, 2009

Tavassoli FA, Devilee P: Tumours of the ovary and peritoneum. In World Health Organization Classification of Tumours: Pathology and Genetics of Tumours of the Breast and Female Genital Organs. Lyon, France, International Agency for Research on Cancer, 2003, p 114

Tempfer CB, Polterauer S, Bentz EK, et al: Accuracy of intraoperative frozen section analysis in borderline tumors of the ovary: a retrospective analysis of 96 cases and review of the literature. Gynecol Oncol 107:248, 2007

The ICON Collaborators: ICON2: Randomised trial of single-agent carboplatin against three-drug combination of CAP (cyclophosphamide, doxorubicin, and cisplatin) in women with ovarian cancer. International Collaborative Ovarian Neoplasm Study. Lancet 352:1571, 1998

The ICON Group: Paclitaxel plus carboplatin versus standard chemotherapy with either single-agent carboplatin or cyclophosphamide, doxorubicin, and cisplatin in women with ovarian cancer: the ICON3 randomised trial. Lancet 360:505, 2002

Timmerman D, Testa AC, Bourne T, et al: Logistic regression model to distinguish between the benign and malignant adnexal mass before surgery: a multicenter study by the International Ovarian Tumor Analysis Group. J Clin Oncol 23:8794, 2005

Timmers PJ, Zwinderman K, Coens C, et al: Lymph node sampling and taking of blind biopsies are important elements of the surgical staging of early ovarian cancer. Int J Gynecol Cancer 20:1142, 2010

Timofeev J, Galgano MT, Stoler MH, et al: Appendiceal pathology at the time of oophorectomy for ovarian neoplasms. Obstet Gynecol 116:1348, 2010

Tozzi R, Kohler C, Ferrara A, et al: Laparoscopic treatment of early ovarian cancer: surgical and survival outcomes. Gynecol Oncol 93:199, 2004

Trimble CL, Kosary C, Trimble EL: Long-term survival and patterns of care in women with ovarian tumors of low malignant potential. Gynecol Oncol 86:34, 2002

Trimbos JB, Parmar M, Vergote I, et al: International Collaborative Ovarian Neoplasm trial 1 and Adjuvant ChemoTherapy in Ovarian Neoplasm trial: Two parallel randomized phase III trials of adjuvant chemotherapy in patients with early-stage ovarian carcinoma. J Natl Cancer Inst 95:105, 2003

Twickler DM, Forte TB, Santos-Ramos R, et al: The ovarian tumor index predicts risk for malignancy. Cancer 86:2280, 1999

Ueland FR, Desmone CP, Seamon LG, et al: Effectiveness of a multivariate index assay in the preoperative assessment of ovarian tumors. Obstet Gynecol 117(6):1289, 2011

van der Burg ME, van Lent M, Buyse M, et al: The effect of debulking surgery after induction chemotherapy on the prognosis in advanced epithelial ovarian cancer. Gynecological Cancer Cooperative Group of the European Organization for Research and Treatment of Cancer. N Engl J Med 332:629, 1995

Vergote I, Trope CG, Amant F, et al: Neoadjuvant chemotherapy or primary surgery in stage IIIC or IV ovarian cancer. N Engl J Med 363:943, 2010

Verheijen RH, Mensdorff-Pouilly S, van Kamp GJ, et al: CA-125: fundamental and clinical aspects. Semin Cancer Biol 9:117, 1999

Vermillion Inc: OVA1™ package insert: executive summary. http://ova-1.com/physicians/package-insert. Accessed May 7, 2011

Visintin I, Feng Z, Longton G, et al: Diagnostic markers for early detection of ovarian cancer. Clin Cancer Res 14:1065, 2008

Walker JL, Armstrong DK, Huang HQ, et al: Intraperitoneal catheter outcomes in a phase III trial of intravenous versus intraperitoneal chemotherapy in optimal stage III ovarian and primary peritoneal cancer: a Gynecologic Oncology Group study. Gynecol Oncol 100:27, 2006

Ware Miller R, Smith A, DeSimone CP, et al: Performance of the American College of Obstetricians and Gynecologists' ovarian tumor referral guidelines with a multivariate index assay. Obstet Gynecol 117(6):1298, 2011

Werness BA, Parvatiyar P, Ramus SJ, et al: Ovarian carcinoma in situ with germline *BRCA1* mutation and loss of heterozygosity at *BRCA1* and *TP53*. J Natl Cancer Inst 92:1088, 2000

Whitney CW: Gynecologic Oncology Group Surgical Procedures Manual. Gynecologic Oncology Group. Available at: https://gogmember.gog.org/manuals/pdf/surgman.pdf. Accessed May 12, 2011

Wimberger P, Lehmann N, Kimmig R, et al: Prognostic factors for complete debulking in advanced ovarian cancer and its impact on survival. An exploratory analysis of a prospectively randomized phase III study of AGO-OVAR. Gynecol Oncol 106:69, 2007

Wingo SN, Knowles LM, Carrick KS, et al: Retrospective cohort study of surgical staging for ovarian low malignant potential tumors. Am J Obstet Gynecol 194:e20, 2006

Yen ML, Yen BL, Bai CH, et al: Risk factors for ovarian cancer in Taiwan: a case-control study in a low-incidence population. Gynecol Oncol 89:318, 2003

Young RC, Walton LA, Ellenberg SS, et al: Adjuvant therapy in stage I and stage II epithelial ovarian cancer: results of two prospective, randomized trials. N Engl J Med 322:1021, 1990

Young RH, Oliva E, Scully RE: Small cell carcinoma of the ovary, hypercalcemic type: a clinicopathological analysis of 150 cases. Am J Surg Pathol 18:1102, 1994

Yurkovetsky Z, Skates S, Lomakin A, et al: Development of a multimarker assay for early detection of ovarian cancer. J Clin Oncol 28:2159, 2010

Zaino RJ, Brady MF, Lele SM, et al: Advanced stage mucinous adenocarcinoma of the ovary is both rare and highly lethal: a Gynecologic Oncology Group study. Cancer 117:554, 2011

Zanetta G, Rota S, Chiari S, et al: Behavior of borderline tumors with particular interest to persistence, recurrence, and progression to invasive carcinoma: a prospective study. J Clin Oncol 19:2658, 2001

Zapardiel I, Rosenberg P, Peiretti M, et al: The role of restaging borderline ovarian tumors: single institution experience and review of the literature. Gynecol Oncol 119:274, 2010

Zhang M, Lee AH, Binns CW: Reproductive and dietary risk factors for epithelial ovarian cancer in China. Gynecol Oncol 92:320, 2004

Zhang Z, Chan DW: The road from discovery to clinical diagnostics: lessons learned from the first FDA-cleared in vitro diagnostic multivariate index assay of proteomic biomarkers. Cancer Epidemiol Biomarkers Prev 19(12):2995, 2010

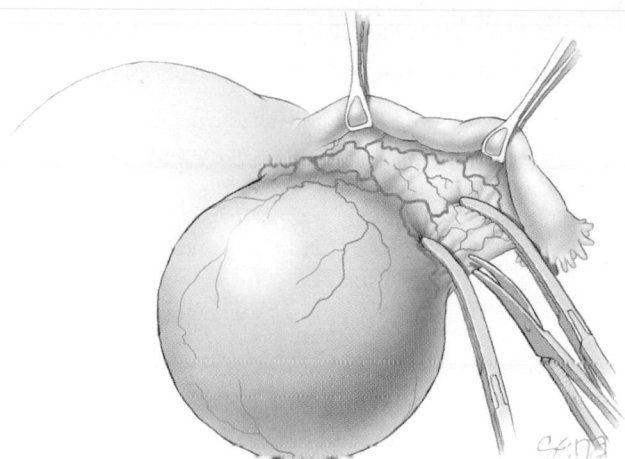

CHAPTER 36

Ovarian Germ Cell and Sex Cord-Stromal Tumors

Three major categories account for virtually all malignant ovarian tumors. Organization of these groups is based on the anatomic structures from which the tumors originate (Fig. 36-1). Epithelial ovarian cancers account for 90 to 95 percent of malignant ovarian tumors (Chap. 35, p. 853). Germ cell and sex cord-stromal ovarian tumors account for the remaining 5 to 10 percent and have unique qualities that require a special management approach (Quirk, 2005).

MALIGNANT OVARIAN GERM CELL TUMORS

Germ cell tumors arise from the ovary's germinal elements and comprise one third of all ovarian neoplasms. The mature cystic teratoma, also called *dermoid cyst,* is by far the most common subtype. This accounts for 95 percent of all germ cell tumors and is clinically benign (Chap. 9, p. 266). In contrast, malignant germ cell tumors comprise fewer than 5 percent of malignant ovarian cancers in Western countries and include *dysgerminoma, yolk sac tumor, immature teratoma,* and other less common types.

Three features typically distinguish malignant germ cell tumors from epithelial ovarian cancers. First, individuals typically present at a younger age, usually in their teens or early 20s. Second, most have stage I disease at diagnosis. Third, prognosis is excellent—even for those with advanced disease—due to exquisite tumor chemosensitivity.

Fertility-sparing surgery is the primary treatment for women seeking future pregnancy, and most will not require postoperative chemotherapy.

Epidemiology

The age-adjusted incidence rate of malignant ovarian germ cell tumors in the United States is much lower (0.4 per 100,000 women) than that of epithelial ovarian carcinomas (15.5), but twice that of sex cord-stromal tumors (0.2) (Quirk, 2005). Smith and associates (2006) analyzed 1262 cases of malignant ovarian germ cell from 1973 to 2002 and observed that incidence rates have declined 10 percent during the past 30 years. Unlike a small proportion of epithelial ovarian carcinomas, malignant germ cell tumors are not generally considered heritable, although rare familial cases are reported (Galani, 2005; Stettner, 1999).

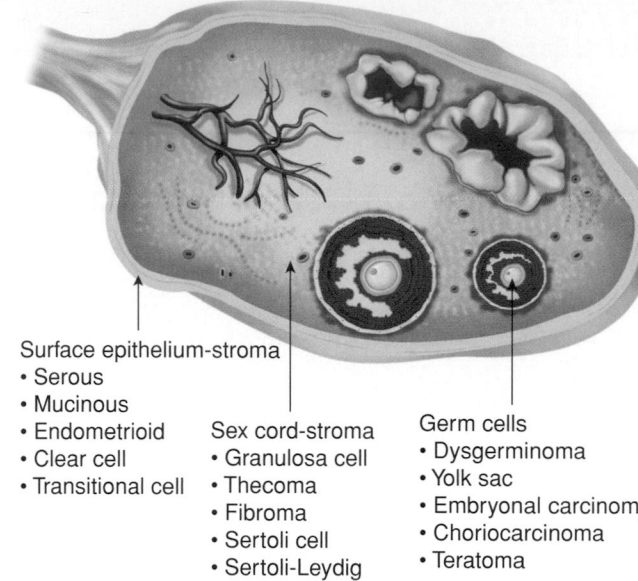

Surface epithelium-stroma
• Serous
• Mucinous
• Endometrioid
• Clear cell
• Transitional cell

Sex cord-stroma
• Granulosa cell
• Thecoma
• Fibroma
• Sertoli cell
• Sertoli-Leydig
• Steroid

Germ cells
• Dysgerminoma
• Yolk sac
• Embryonal carcinoma
• Choriocarcinoma
• Teratoma

FIGURE 36-1 Origins of the three main types of ovarian tumors. *(Redrawn from Chen, 2003, with permission.)*

These tumors are the most common ovarian malignancies diagnosed during childhood and adolescence, although only 1 percent of all ovarian cancers develop in these age groups. At age 20, however, the incidence of epithelial ovarian carcinoma begins to rise and exceeds that of germ cell tumors (Young, 2003).

■ Diagnosis

Signs and Symptoms

The signs and symptoms associated with these tumors are varied, but in general, most arise from tumor growth and the hormones they produce. Subacute abdominal pain is the presenting symptom in 85 percent of patients and reflects rapid growth of a large, unilateral tumor undergoing capsular distension, hemorrhage, or necrosis. Less commonly, cyst rupture, torsion, or intraperitoneal hemorrhage leads to an acute abdomen in 10 percent of cases (Gershenson, 2007a). In more advanced disease, ascites may develop and cause abdominal distension. Because of the hormonal changes that frequently accompany these tumors, menstrual irregularities may also develop. Although most individuals note one or more of these symptoms, one quarter of individuals are asymptomatic, and a pelvic mass is noted unexpectedly during physical or sonographic examination (Curtin, 1994).

History

Individuals typically seek care within 1 month of the onset of abdominal complaints, although some note subtle waxing and waning of symptoms for more than a year. Most young women with these tumors are nulligravidas with normal periods, but as discussed later, individuals with dysgenetic gonads are at significant risk for development of these tumors (Curtin, 1994). Therefore, adolescents who present with pelvic masses and delayed menarche should be evaluated for gonadal dysgenesis (Chap. 16, p. 444).

Differential Diagnosis

Vague pelvic symptoms are common during adolescence due to initiation of ovulation and menstrual cramping. As a result, early symptoms may be missed. Moreover, young girls may be silent about changes to their normal pattern, fearful of their significance. Early symptoms can be misinterpreted as those of pregnancy, and acute pain may be confused with appendicitis.

Finding an adnexal mass is the first diagnostic step. In most cases, sonography can adequately display those qualities that typically characterize benign and malignant ovarian masses (Chap. 2, p. 41). Functional ovarian cysts are vastly more common in young women and once identified as hypoechoic, smooth-walled cysts by sonography, may be observed. In contrast, malignant germ cell tumors are usually larger with solid components. Elevated levels of serum human chorionic gonadotropin (hCG) or alpha-fetoprotein (AFP) tumor markers may narrow the diagnostic possibilities and suggest the potential need for surgical intervention.

Physical Examination

Distinguishing physical findings are typically lacking in individuals with malignant germ cell tumors. A palpable mass on pelvic examination is the most common finding. In children and adolescents, however, completing a comprehensive pelvic or transvaginal sonographic examination can be difficult and can lead to diagnostic delay. Accordingly, premenarchal patients may require examination under anesthesia to adequately assess a suspected adnexal tumor. The remainder of the physical examination should search for signs of ascites, pleural effusion, and organomegaly.

Laboratory Testing

Patients with a suspected malignant germ cell tumor should have serum hCG and AFP tumor markers, complete blood count, and liver function tests drawn before treatment. Alternatively, the appropriate tumor markers may be ordered in the operating room if the diagnosis was not previously suspected (Table 36-1). Preoperative karyotyping of young women with primary amenorrhea and a suspected germ cell tumor can clarify whether both ovaries should be removed, as in the case of women with gonadal dysgenesis (p. 882) (Hoepffner, 2005).

Imaging

Mature cystic teratomas (dermoid cysts) usually display characteristic features when imaged with sonography or computed tomography (CT) (Chap. 9, p. 269). However, the appearance of malignant germ cell tumors differs, and a multilobulated complex ovarian mass is typical (Fig. 36-2). Moreover, prominent blood flow in the fibrovascular septa may be seen using color flow Doppler sonography and suggests the likelihood of malignancy (Kim, 1995). Additional preoperative CT or magnetic resonance (MR) imaging may be indicated based on clinical suspicion. Chest radiography is warranted upon diagnosis to search for tumor metastases in the lungs or mediastinum.

TABLE 36-1. Serum Tumor Markers in Malignant Ovarian Germ Cell Tumors

Histology	AFP	hCG
Dysgerminoma	−	±
Yolk sac tumor	+	−
Immature teratoma	±	−
Choriocarcinoma	−	+
Embryonal carcinoma	+	+
Mixed germ cell tumor	±	±
Polyembryoma	±	±

AFP = alpha-fetoprotein; hCG = human chorionic gonadotropin.

Diagnostic Procedures

A sonographically or CT-guided percutaneous biopsy has no role in the management of patients with an ovarian mass suspicious for malignancy. Surgical resection is required for definitive tissue diagnosis, staging, and treatment. The surgeon should request a frozen section to confirm the diagnosis, but discrepancies between frozen section interpretations and the final paraffin histology are commonplace (Kusamura, 2000). In addition, specific immunostaining is often required to resolve equivocal cases (Cheng, 2004; Ramalingam, 2004; Ulbright, 2005).

Role of the Generalist

Most patients will initially be seen by a generalist gynecologist. Initial symptoms may point to the more common functional ovarian cyst. Persistent symptoms or an enlarging pelvic mass, however, should prompt sonographic evaluation. If a complex ovarian mass with solid features is noted in this young age group, then measurement of serum hCG and AFP levels and

referral to a gynecologic oncologist for primary surgical management should ensue.

If a specialist is unavailable or the diagnosis is not anticipated beforehand, intraoperative decision making is crucial to adequately treat the patient without compromising future fertility. Peritoneal washings are obtained and set aside before proceeding with dissection of any suspicious adnexal mass. These can be discarded later if malignancy is excluded. Initially, the decision to perform cystectomy or oophorectomy depends on the clinical circumstances (Chap. 9, p. 263). In general, the entire adnexa should be removed once a malignant ovarian germ cell tumor is diagnosed. A generalist gynecologist should request intraoperative assistance with staging from a gynecologic oncologist or refer the patient postoperatively if a specialist is not immediately available. At minimum, the abdomen should be explored. Palpation of the omentum and upper abdomen and inspection of the pelvis—especially the contralateral ovary—is easy to perform and document.

Pathology
Classification

The modified World Health Organization (WHO) classification of ovarian germ cell tumors is presented in Table 36-2 (Nogales, 2003). These tumors are composed of several histologically different tumor types derived from primordial germ cells of the embryonic gonad. There are two major categories: primitive malignant germ cell tumors (dysgerminomas) and teratomas—almost all of which are accounted for by mature cystic teratomas (dermoid cysts).

TABLE 36-2. Modified World Health Organization Classification of Ovarian Germ Cell Tumors

Primitive germ cell tumors
Dysgerminoma
Yolk sac tumor (endodermal sinus tumor)
Embryonal carcinoma
Polyembryoma
Nongestational choriocarcinoma

Teratomas
Immature
Mature
  Solid
  Cystic (dermoid cyst)
Monodermal and highly specialized
  Thyroid tumors (struma ovarii: benign or malignant)
  Carcinoids
  Neuroectodermal tumors
  Carcinomas (squamous cell or adeno-)
  Melanocytic group
  Sarcomas
  Sebaceous tumors

Mixed forms (tumors composed of two or more of the above pure types)

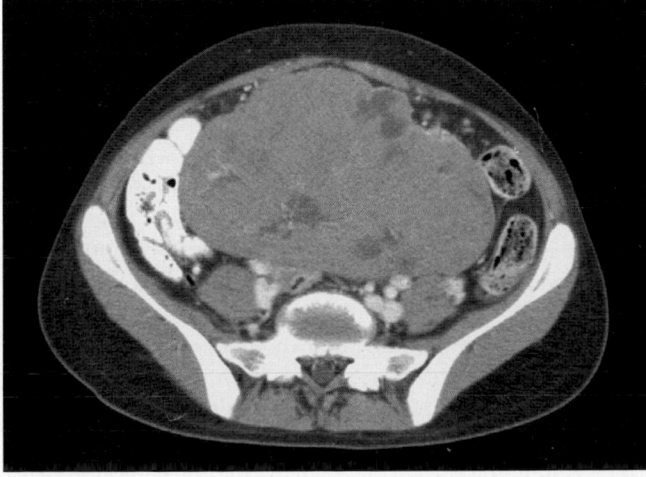

FIGURE 36-2 Computed tomographic (CT) scan of a germ cell tumor.

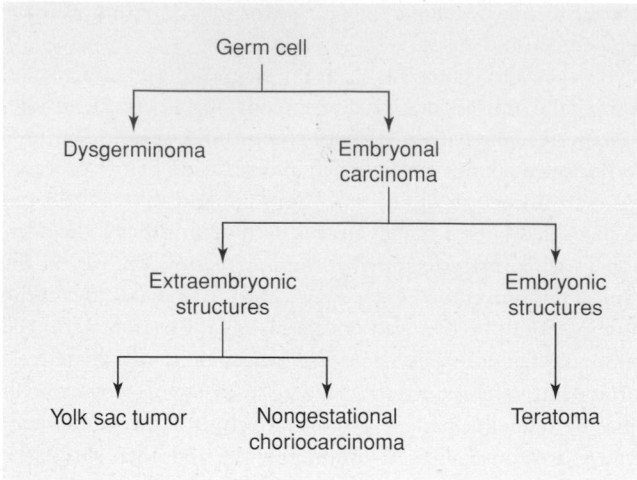

FIGURE 36-3 Differentiation pathway of germ cell tumors.

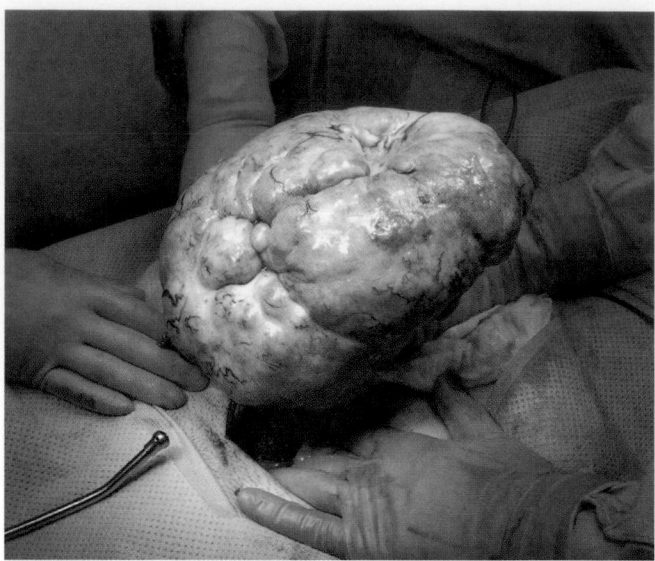

FIGURE 36-4 Intraoperative photograph of a dysgerminoma.

Histogenesis

Primitive germ cells migrate from the wall of the yolk sac to the gonadal ridge (Fig. 18-1, p. 482). As a result, most germ cell tumors arise in the gonad. Rarely, these tumors may develop primarily in extragonadal sites such as the central nervous system, mediastinum, or retroperitoneum (Hsu, 2002).

Ovarian germ cell tumors have a variable pattern of differentiation (Fig. 36-3). Dysgerminomas are primitive neoplasms that do not have the potential for further differentiation. Embryonal carcinomas are composed of multipotential cells that are capable of further differentiation. This lesion is the precursor of several other types of extraembryonic (yolk sac tumor, choriocarcinoma) or embryonic (teratoma) germ cell tumors. The process of differentiation is dynamic, and the resulting neoplasms may be composed of different elements showing various stages of development (Teilum, 1965).

Dysgerminoma

Because their incidence has declined by approximately 30 percent over the past few decades, dysgerminomas currently account for only approximately one third of all malignant ovarian germ cell tumors (Chan, 2008; Smith, 2006). Dysgerminomas are the most common ovarian malignancy detected during pregnancy. This is believed to be an age-related coincidence, however, and not due to some particular characteristic of gestation.

Five percent of dysgerminomas are discovered in phenotypic females with karyotypically abnormal gonads, specifically, with the presence of a normal or abnormal Y-chromosome (Morimura, 1998). Commonly, this group includes those with Turner syndrome mosaicism (45,X/46,XY), and Swyer syndrome (46,XY, pure gonadal dysgenesis) (Chap. 16, p. 444). The dysgenetic gonads of these individuals often contain gonadoblastomas, which are benign germ cell neoplasms. These tumors may regress or alternatively may undergo malignant transformation, most commonly to dysgerminoma. Because approximately 40 percent of gonadoblastomas in these individuals undergo malignant transformation, both ovaries should be removed (Hoepffner, 2005; Pena-Alonso, 2005).

Dysgerminomas are the only germ cell malignancy with a significant rate of bilateral ovarian involvement—15 to 20 percent. Half of patients with bilateral lesions will have grossly obvious disease, whereas cancer in the remainder will only be detected microscopically. Five percent of women have elevated serum hCG levels due to intermingled syncytiotrophoblasts. Similarly, serum lactate dehydrogenase (LDH) and the isoenzymes LDH-1 and LDH-2 may also be useful in monitoring individuals for disease recurrence (Pressley, 1992; Schwartz, 1988).

Dysgerminomas have a variable gross appearance, but in general are solid, pink to tan to cream-colored lobulated masses (Fig. 36-4). Microscopically, there is a monotonous proliferation of large, rounded, polyhedral clear cells that are rich in cytoplasmic glycogen and contain uniform central nuclei with one or a few prominent nucleoli (Fig. 36-5). The tumor cells resemble closely the primordial germ cells of the embryo and are histologically identical to seminoma of the testis.

The standard treatment of dysgerminoma usually involves fertility-sparing surgery with unilateral salpingo-oophorectomy (USO). In some extenuating circumstances, ovarian cystectomy may be considered (Vicus, 2010). Surgical staging is generally extrapolated from epithelial ovarian cancer (Chap. 35, p. 870), but lymphadenectomy is particularly important. Of the malignant germ cell tumors, dysgerminoma has the highest rate of nodal metastases, approximately 25 to 30 percent (Kumar, 2008). Although staging deviations do not adversely affect survival, comprehensive staging allows a safe observation strategy for stage IA tumors (Billmire, 2004; Palenzuela, 2008).

Preservation of the contralateral ovary leads to "recurrent" dysgerminoma in 5 to 10 percent of retained gonads during the next 2 years. This finding in many cases is thought to reflect the high rate of clinically occult disease in the remaining ovary rather than true recurrence. Indeed, at least 75 percent of recurrences develop within the first year of diagnosis (Vicus, 2010). Other common recurrence sites are within the peritoneal cavity or retroperitoneal lymph nodes. Despite this significant incidence of recurrent disease, a conservative surgical approach

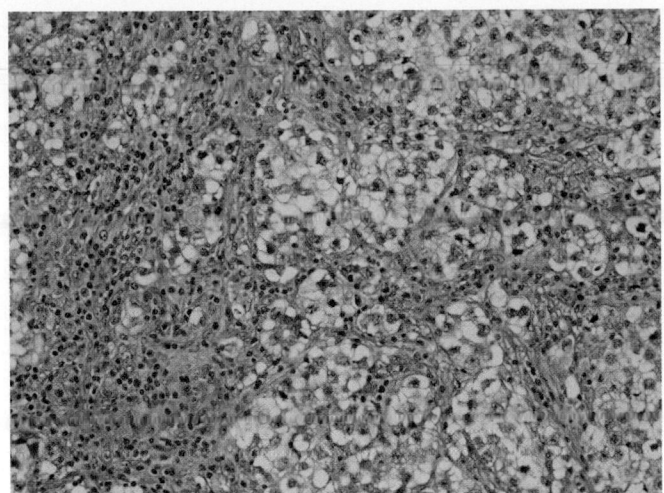

FIGURE 36-5 Photomicrograph of a dysgerminoma. Dysgerminoma is characterized microscopically by a relatively monotonous population of cells resembling primordial germ cells, with a central rounded or square-edged nucleus and abundant clear, glycogen-rich cytoplasm. As in this case, the tumor often contains fibrous septa, seen here as eosinophilic strands, which are infiltrated by chronic inflammatory cells including lymphocytes, macrophages, and occasional plasma cells. *(Photograph contributed by Dr. Kelley Carrick.)*

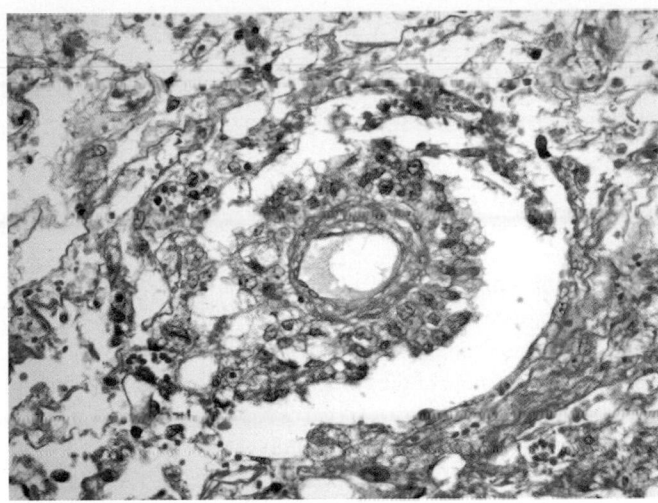

FIGURE 36-6 Schiller-Duval body. This structure consists of a central capillary surrounded by tumor cells, present within a cystic space that may be lined by flat to cuboidal tumor cells. When present, the Schiller-Duval body is pathognomonic for yolk sac tumor, although they are conspicuous in only a minority of cases. In any given case, Schiller-Duval bodies may be few in number, absent, or have atypical morphologic features. *(Photograph contributed by Dr. Kelley Carrick.)*

does not adversely affect long-term survival because of this cancer's sensitivity to chemotherapy.

Dysgerminomas have the best prognosis of all malignant ovarian germ cell tumor variants. Two thirds are stage I at diagnosis, and the 5-year disease-specific survival approximates 99 percent (Table 36-3). Even those with advanced disease have high survival rates following chemotherapy. For example, those with stage II-IV disease have a greater than 98-percent survival rate with platinum-based agents (Chan, 2008).

Yolk Sac Tumors

These tumors account for 10 to 20 percent of all malignant ovarian germ cell tumors. These lesions were previously called endodermal sinus tumors, but the terminology has been revised. One third of individuals are premenarchal at the time of initial presentation. Involvement of both gonads is rare, and the other ovary is usually involved with metastatic disease only when there are other metastases in the peritoneal cavity.

Grossly, these tumors form solid masses that are more yellow and friable than dysgerminomas. They are often focally necrotic

and hemorrhagic, with cystic degeneration and rupture. The microscopic appearance of yolk sac tumors is often diverse. The most common appearance, the reticular pattern, reflects extraembryonic differentiation, with the formation of a network of irregular anastomosing spaces that are lined by primitive epithelial cells. *Schiller-Duval bodies* are pathognomonic when present (Fig. 36-6). These characteristically have a single papilla, which is lined by tumor cells and contains a central vessel. Alpha-fetoprotein is commonly produced. As a result, yolk-sac tumors usually contain cells that stain immunohistochemically for AFP, and serum levels can serve as a reliable tumor marker in posttreatment surveillance.

Yolk sac tumors are the deadliest malignant ovarian germ cell tumor type. As a result, all patients are treated with chemotherapy regardless of stage. Fortunately, more than half present with stage I disease, corresponding to a 5-year disease-specific survival of approximately 93 percent (Chan, 2008). Unfortunately, yolk sac tumors have more of a propensity for rapid growth, peritoneal spread, and distant hematogenous dissemination to the lungs. Accordingly, individuals with stage II-IV disease have a 5-year survival rate ranging from 64 to 91 percent. Of patients

TABLE 36-3. Stage and Survival of Common Malignant Ovarian Germ Cell Tumors

	Dysgerminoma	Yolk Sac Tumor	Immature Teratoma
Stage at diagnosis			
I	66%	61%	72%
II–IV	34%	39%	28%
Five-year survival			
Stage I	99%	93%	98%
Stage II–IV	>98%	64–91%	73–88%

Sources for survival figures are referenced within the text.

with tumor recurrence, most will do so within the first year, and treatment is usually ineffective (Cicin, 2009).

Other Primitive Germ Cell Tumors

The rarest subtypes of nondysgerminomatous tumors are typically mixed with other more common variants and usually are not found in pure form.

Embryonal Carcinoma. Patients diagnosed with embryonal carcinoma are characteristically younger, with a mean age of 14 years, than those having other types of germ cell tumors. Epithelial cells resembling those of the embryonic disc comprise these primitive tumors. The solid disorganized sheets of large anaplastic cells, gland-like spaces, and papillary structures are distinctive and allow easy identification of these tumors (Ulbright, 2005). Although dysgerminomas are the most common germ cell tumor resulting from malignant transformation of gonadoblastomas in individuals with dysgenetic gonads, occasionally embryonal "testicular" tumors may also originate (LaPolla, 1990). Embryonal carcinomas typically produce hCG, and 75 percent also secrete AFP.

Polyembryoma. These tumors characteristically contain many embryolike bodies. Each has a small central "germ disc" positioned between two cavities, one mimicking an amnionic cavity and the other a yolk sac. Syncytiotrophoblast giant cells are frequent, but elements other than the embryoid bodies should constitute less than 10 percent of the tumor for the "polyembryoma" designation to be used. Conceptually, these tumors may be viewed as a bridge between the primitive (dysgerminoma) and differentiated (teratoma) germ cell tumor types. For this reason, polyembryomas are often considered to be the most immature of all teratomas (Ulbright, 2005). Serum AFP or hCG levels or both may be elevated in these individuals due to the yolk sac and syncytial components (Takemori, 1998).

Choriocarcinoma. Primary ovarian choriocarcinoma arising from a germ cell appears similar to gestational choriocarcinoma with ovarian metastases, which is discussed in Chapter 37 (p. 905). The distinction is important because nongestational tumors have a poorer prognosis (Corakci, 2005). The detection of other germ cell components indicates nongestational choriocarcinoma, whereas a concomitant or proximate pregnancy suggests a gestational form (Ulbright, 2005). Clinical manifestations are common and result from high hCG levels produced by these tumors. These elevated levels may induce sexual precocity in prepubertal girls or menometrorrhagia in reproductive-aged women (Oliva, 1993).

Mixed Germ Cell Tumors

Ovarian germ cell tumors have a mixed pattern of cellular differentiation in 25 to 30 percent of cases, although the incidence of these tumors has also declined by approximately 30 percent over the past few decades (Smith, 2006). Dysgerminoma is the most common component and is typically seen with yolk sac tumor or immature teratoma or both. The frequency of bilateral ovarian involvement depends on the presence or absence of a dysgerminoma component and increases when it is present. However, treatment and prognosis are determined by the nondysgerminomatous component (Low, 2000). For this reason, elevated serum

hCG and particularly AFP levels in a woman with a presumed pure dysgerminoma should prompt a search for other germ cell components by more extensive histologic evaluation (Aoki, 2003).

Immature Teratomas

Due to a 60-percent increased incidence over the past few decades, immature teratomas are now the most common variant and account for 40 to 50 percent of all malignant ovarian germ cell tumors (Chan, 2008; Smith, 2006). They are composed of tissues derived from the three germ layers: ectoderm, mesoderm, and endoderm. The presence of immature or embryonal structures, however, distinguishes these tumors from the much more common and benign mature cystic teratoma (dermoid cyst). Bilateral ovarian involvement is rare, but 10 percent have a mature teratoma in the contralateral ovary. Tumor markers are often not elevated unless the immature teratoma is commingled with other germ cell tumor types. Alpha-fetoprotein, cancer antigen 125 (CA125), CA19-9, and carcinoembryonic antigen (CEA) may be helpful in some cases (Li, 2002).

On gross external inspection, these tumors appear as large, rounded or lobulated, soft or firm masses. They frequently perforate the ovarian capsule and invade locally. The most frequent site of dissemination is the peritoneum and much less commonly the retroperitoneal lymph nodes. With local invasion, surrounding adhesions commonly form and are thought to explain the lower rates of torsion with this tumor compared with that of its benign mature counterpart (Cass, 2001). On cut surface, the interior is typically solid with intermittent cystic areas, but occasionally the reverse is seen, with solid nodules present only in the cyst wall (Fig. 36-7). Solid parts may correspond to the immature elements, cartilage, bone, or a combination of these. Cystic areas are filled with serous or mucinous fluid or sebaceous material and hair.

Microscopic examination reveals a disorderly mixture of tissues. Of the immature elements, neuroectodermal tissues almost always predominate and are arranged as primitive tubules and sheets of small, round, malignant cells that may be

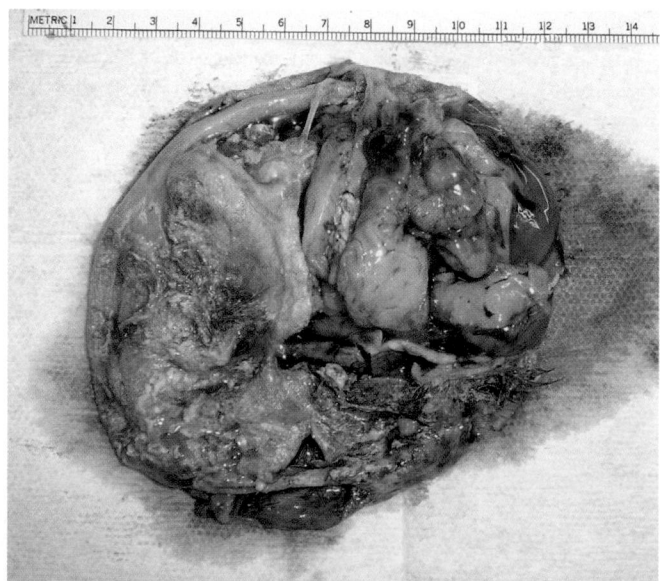

FIGURE 36-7 Photograph of an immature teratoma.

associated with glia formation. The diagnosis is characteristically difficult to confirm at frozen section, and most tumors will be confirmed only on final pathologic review (Pavlakis, 2009). Tumors are graded 1 to 3 primarily by the amount of immature neural tissue they contain. O'Connor and Norris (1994) analyzed 244 immature teratomas and noted significant inconsistencies in grade assignment by different observers. For this reason, they proposed changing the system to two grades: low (previous grades 1 and 2) and high (previous grade 3). This practice, however, has not been universally accepted.

In general, survival is predicted most accurately by the histologic grade of the tumor. For example, almost three quarters of immature teratomas are stage I at diagnosis and have a 5-year survival rate of 98 percent (Chan, 2008). Those with stage IA grade 1 immature teratomas have an excellent prognosis and do not require adjuvant chemotherapy (Bonazzi, 1994; Marina, 1999). Patients with stage II-IV disease have a 5-year survival rate ranging from 73 to 88 percent (Chan, 2008).

Unilateral salpingo-oophorectomy is the standard care for these and other malignant germ cell tumors in reproductive-aged women. Beiner and colleagues (2004), however, treated eight women with early-stage immature teratoma with ovarian cystectomy and adjuvant chemotherapy and noted no recurrences.

Immature teratomas may be associated with mature tissue implants studding the peritoneum that do not increase the stage of the tumor or diminish the prospect of survival. However, these implants of mature teratomatous elements, even though benign, are resistant to chemotherapy and can enlarge during or after chemotherapy. Termed the *growing teratoma syndrome,* these implants require second-look surgery and resection to exclude recurrent malignancy (Zagame, 2006).

Malignant Transformation of Mature Cystic Teratomas (Dermoid Cysts)

These rare tumors are the only germ cell variants that typically develop in postmenopausal women. Malignant areas are usually found as small nodules in the cyst wall or a polypoid mass within the lumen after removal of the entire mature cystic teratoma (Pins, 1996). Squamous cell carcinoma is most common and is found in approximately 1 percent of mature cystic teratomas (Fig. 36-8). Platinum-based chemotherapy with or without pelvic radiation is

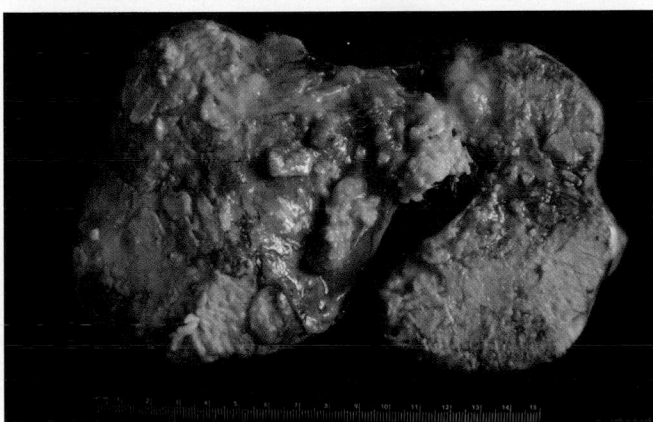

FIGURE 36-8 Photograph of squamous cell carcinoma malignant transformation within a mature cystic teratoma.

most commonly used for adjuvant treatment of early-stage disease (Dos Santos, 2007). However, regardless of treatment received, patients with advanced disease do poorly (Gainford, 2010).

Other types of malignant features may include basal-cell carcinomas, sebaceous tumors, malignant melanomas, adenocarcinomas, sarcomas, and neuroectodermal tumors. Moreover, endocrine-type neoplasms such as struma ovarii (teratoma composed mainly of thyroid tissue) and carcinoid may also be found within mature cystic teratomas. These are malignant in fewer than 5 percent of cases.

Treatment
Surgery

A vertical abdominal incision is traditionally recommended if ovarian malignancy is suspected. However, increasingly, investigators with advanced endoscopic skills have noted laparoscopy to be a safe and effective alternative for women with smaller ovarian masses and apparent stage I disease (Chi, 2005). If present, ascites is evacuated and sent for cytologic evaluation. Otherwise, washings of the pelvis and paracolic gutters are collected for analysis prior to manipulation of the intraperitoneal contents. The washings can be discarded later if the intraoperative evaluation or frozen section interpretation is unequivocally benign. Regardless of the surgical approach, the entire peritoneal cavity should be systematically inspected. The ovaries should be assessed for size, tumor involvement, capsular rupture, external excrescences, and adherence to surrounding structures.

Fertility-sparing USO should be performed in all reproductive-aged women diagnosed with malignant ovarian germ cell tumors, as this conservative approach in general does not adversely affect survival (Chan, 2008; Lee, 2009). Following USO, blind biopsy or wedge resection of a normal-appearing contralateral ovary is not recommended. For those who have completed childbearing, hysterectomy with bilateral salpingo-oophorectomy (BSO) is appropriate. In either case, following removal of the affected ovary, surgical staging by laparotomy or laparoscopy proceeds as previously described for epithelial ovarian cancer (Chap. 35, p. 868) (Gershenson, 2007a). Because of tumor dissemination patterns, lymphadenectomy is most important for dysgerminomas, whereas staging peritoneal and omental biopsies are particularly valuable for yolk sac tumors and immature teratomas (Gershenson, 1983).

Cytoreductive surgery is generally recommended for malignant ovarian germ cell tumors if extensive disease is encountered at initial surgery. Tumor debulking to a level of minimal residual disease improves the likelihood of response to chemotherapy and cure (Bafna, 2001; Nawa, 2001; Suita, 2002). The same general principles for debulking are applied as described for epithelial ovarian cancer (Chap. 35, p. 870). Because of the exquisite chemosensitivity of most malignant germ cell tumors, however, surgeons may choose to be less aggressive in performing radical debulking procedures (Gershenson, 2007a).

Many women will be referred after USO with a tumor that was clinically confined to the excised ovary. For such patients, if initial surgical staging was incomplete, options may include a second surgery for primary staging, regular surveillance, or adjuvant chemotherapy. Unfortunately, there are few data to support a preferred approach. Because of its minimally invasive qualities, laparoscopy is a particularly attractive option for delayed surgical staging following primary excision and has been shown to accurately detect those women who require chemotherapy (Leblanc, 2004). Surgical staging following primary excision, however, is less important for scenarios in which chemotherapy will be administered regardless of surgical findings such as clinical stage I yolk sac tumors and high-grade clinical stage I immature teratomas (Stier, 1996). In such patients, reassurance of no abnormalities by CT imaging is often sufficient prior to proceeding with adjuvant chemotherapy (Gershenson, 2007a).

Surveillance

Patients with malignant ovarian germ cell tumors should be followed by careful clinical, radiologic, and serologic surveillance every 3 months for the first 2 years after therapy completion (Dark, 1997). Ninety percent of recurrences develop within this time frame (Messing, 1992). Second-look surgery at the completion of therapy is not necessary in women with completely resected disease or in those individuals with advanced tumor that does not contain teratoma. However, incompletely resected immature teratoma is the one circumstance among all types of ovarian cancer in which patients clearly benefit from second-look surgery and excision of chemorefractory tumor (Culine, 1996; Rezk, 2005; Williams, 1994b).

Chemotherapy

Stage IA dysgerminomas and stage IA grade 1 immature teratomas do not require additional chemotherapy. More advanced disease and all other histologic types of malignant ovarian germ cell tumors have historically been treated with combination chemotherapy (Suita, 2002; Tewari, 2000). However, there is a strong trend toward exploring the feasibility of surgery followed by close surveillance in a much broader group of patients (Gershenson, 2007a). Because chemotherapy remains effective when used at the time of relapse, some investigators are attempting to identify additional low-risk, early stage subgroups that may be observed postoperatively and thereby avoid treatment-related toxicity (Bonazzi, 1994; Cushing, 1999; Dark, 1997). However, before this strategy can be incorporated into general practice, additional large studies are necessary.

The standard regimen is a 5-day course of bleomycin, etoposide, and cisplatin (BEP) given every 3 weeks (Gershenson, 1990; Williams, 1987). Modified 2- or 3-day BEP combinations have also recently been shown to be safe and effective in pilot studies but are not routinely used in practice (Dimopoulos, 2004; Tay, 2000). For women with accurate staging and completely resected ovarian germ cell tumors, three courses of BEP will prevent recurrence in nearly all (Williams, 1994a). Carboplatin and etoposide, given in three cycles, has shown promise as an alternative for selected patients but warrants further study before it can be considered standard treatment (Williams, 2004). For women with incompletely resected disease, at least four courses of BEP are currently recommended (Williams, 1991).

Radiation

Chemotherapy has replaced radiation as the preferred adjuvant treatment for all types of malignant ovarian germ cell tumors. This transition was prompted primarily by the exquisite sensitivity of these tumors to either modality, but higher likelihood of retained ovarian function using chemotherapy (Mitchell, 1991). Occasional situations may still exist in which radiotherapy should be considered. However, the main role currently is palliation of a germ cell tumor that has demonstrated resistance to chemotherapy.

Relapse

At least four courses of BEP chemotherapy is the preferred treatment for recurrent ovarian germ cell tumors in women initially managed with surgery alone. Patients who achieved a sustained clinical remission of greater than 6 months after completing BEP or another platinum-based chemotherapy regimen may be treated again with BEP. Because their tumors are generally more responsive, these "platinum-sensitive" patients have a much better prognosis. However, women who do not achieve remission with BEP chemotherapy or relapse within a few months (fewer than 6) are considered "platinum-resistant," and treatment options are limited. Chemorefractory cases with dysgerminoma or immature teratoma appear to have a better outcome than other subtypes, and surgical salvage aimed at achieving no residual disease may benefit some patients (Li, 2007). Another option for this group is vincristine, dactinomycin, and cyclophosphamide (VAC) (Gershenson, 1985). Other potentially active drugs include paclitaxel, gemcitabine, and oxaliplatin (Hinton, 2002; Kollmannsberger, 2006).

Second-look procedures with surgical debulking have a limited role because of the inherent chemosensitivity of these recurrent tumors. Chemorefractory immature teratomas are notable exceptions (Munkarah, 1994). Growth or persistence of a tumor after chemotherapy does not necessarily imply progression of malignancy, but these masses should still be resected (Geisler, 1994).

Prognosis

Malignant ovarian germ cell tumors have an excellent overall prognosis (see Table 36-3) (Chan, 2008; Smith, 2006). Moreover, the number of cases with distant and unstaged disease has dramatically declined, suggesting that germ cell tumors are being diagnosed earlier. In addition, the survival rates have significantly improved for all subtypes, especially with the demonstrated efficacy of cisplatin-based combination therapy (Smith, 2006). Histologic cell type, elevation of serum markers, surgical stage, and the amount of residual disease at initial surgery are the major variables affecting prognosis (Murugaesu, 2006; Smith, 2006). Typically, pure dysgerminomas recur within 2 years and are highly treatable (Vicus, 2010). However, for nondysgerminomatous tumors, outcome after relapse is poor, and fewer than 10 percent of patients achieve long-term survival (Murugaesu, 2006).

Most women treated with fertility-sparing surgery, with or without chemotherapy, will resume normal menses and are able to conceive and bear children (Gershenson, 2007b; Zanetta, 2001). In addition, none of the reported studies has noted an increased rate of birth defects or spontaneous abortion in those treated with chemotherapy (Brewer, 1999; Low, 2000; Tangir, 2003; Zanetta, 2001).

Management During Pregnancy

Persistent adnexal masses are detected in 1 to 2 percent of all pregnancies. These neoplasms are usually seen during routine obstetric sonographic examination, but occasionally a dramatically elevated maternal serum alpha-fetoprotein (MSAFP) level is the presenting sign of a malignant germ cell tumor (Horbelt, 1994; Montz, 1989). Mature cystic teratomas (dermoid cysts) comprise one third of tumors resected during pregnancy. In contrast, dysgerminomas account for only 1 to 2 percent of such neoplasms but still are the most common ovarian malignancy during pregnancy. Development of other germ cell tumors is rare (Shimizu, 2003).

Initial surgical management including surgical staging is the same as for the nonpregnant woman (Horbelt, 1994; Zhao, 2006). Fortunately, very few patients have advanced disease necessitating radical dissection for cytoreduction. The decision to administer chemotherapy during pregnancy is controversial. Malignant ovarian germ cell tumors have the propensity to grow rapidly, and delaying treatment until after delivery is potentially hazardous. Treatment with BEP appears to be safe during pregnancy, but some reports have speculated that fetal complications are possible (Elit, 1999; Horbelt, 1994). For this reason, some advocate postponing treatment until the puerperium (Shimizu, 2003). Unfortunately, there are no results from large studies to resolve this dilemma. Although BEP administration may be delayed until the puerperium for completely resected dysgerminomas, patients with nondysgerminomatous tumors (mainly yolk sac tumors and immature teratomas) and incompletely resected disease warrant strong consideration of chemotherapy during pregnancy.

OVARIAN SEX CORD-STROMAL TUMORS

Sex cord-stromal tumors (SCSTs) are a heterogeneous group of rare neoplasms that originate from the ovarian matrix. Cells within this matrix have the potential for hormone production, and nearly 90 percent of hormone-producing ovarian tumors are SCSTs. As a result, individuals with these tumors typically present with signs and symptoms of estrogen or androgen excess.

Surgical resection is the primary treatment, and SCSTs are generally confined to one ovary at the time of diagnosis. Moreover, the majority have an indolent growth pattern and low malignant potential. For these reasons, few patients ever require platinum-based chemotherapy. Although recurrent disease often responds poorly to treatment, patients may live for many years because of characteristically slow tumor progression.

The overall prognosis of ovarian SCSTs is excellent—primarily due to early stage disease at diagnosis and curative surgery. The scarcity of these tumors, however, limits the understanding of their natural history, treatment, and prognosis.

Epidemiology

Sex cord-stromal tumors account for less than 5 percent of ovarian malignancies and are the least common major subtype of ovarian cancer. The age-adjusted incidence rate is much lower (0.20 per 100,000 women) than epithelial ovarian carcinomas (15.48) and half of that for malignant germ cell tumors (0.41). These tumors are more than twice as likely to develop in black women for reasons that are unclear (Quirk, 2005).

In contrast with epithelial ovarian cancers or malignant germ cell tumors, ovarian SCSTs typically affect women of all ages. This range contains a unique bimodal distribution that reflects inherent tumor heterogeneity. For example, juvenile granulosa cell tumors, Sertoli-Leydig cell tumors, and sclerosing stromal tumors are found predominantly in prepubertal girls and women within the first three decades of life (Schneider, 2005). Adult granulosa cell tumors commonly develop in older women, at an average age of approximately 50 years (Boyce, 2009; Fotopoulou, 2010).

There are no proven risk factors for SCSTs. However, in a hypothesis-generating case-control study, Boyce and coworkers (2009) observed that obesity as a hyperestrogenic state was independently associated, whereas parity, smoking, and oral contraceptive use were protective. The etiology of SCSTs is unknown. However, a single, recurrent *FOXL2* gene mutation (402C→G) has recently been shown to be present in virtually all adult-type granulosa cell tumors, but not in a wide variety of other solid tumors. Thus, mutant *FOXL2* appears to be a highly specific event in the pathogenesis of these rare tumors (Schrader, 2009; Shah, 2009).

There is no known inherited predisposition for the development of these tumors, and familial cases are rare (Stevens, 2005). However, ovarian SCSTs do develop in association with several defined hereditary disorders at a frequency that exceeds mere chance. Associated disorders include Ollier disease, which is characterized by multiple benign but disfiguring cartilaginous neoplasms, and Peutz-Jeghers syndrome, characterized by intestinal hamartomatous polyps (Stevens, 2005).

Diagnosis
Signs and Symptoms

Isosexual precocious puberty is the presenting sign in more than 80 percent of prepubertal girls ultimately diagnosed with an ovarian SCST (Kalfa, 2005). Adolescents often report secondary amenorrhea. As a result, these young individuals presenting with endocrinologic symptoms tend to be diagnosed at earlier stages. Abdominal pain and distension are other common complaints in this age group (Schneider, 2003a).

In adult women, menometrorrhagia and postmenopausal bleeding are the most frequent symptoms. In addition, mild hirsutism that rapidly progresses to frank virilization should prompt evaluation to exclude these tumors. The classic presentation is a postmenopausal woman with rapidly evolving stigmata of androgen excess and a complex adnexal mass. Abdominal pain or a mass palpable by the patient herself are other telling signs and symptoms (Chan, 2005).

Physical Examination

The size of SCSTs is widely variable, but most women have a palpable abdominal or pelvic mass on examination regardless of their age. A fluid wave or other physical findings suggestive of advanced disease, however, are rare.

Laboratory Testing

Elevated circulating levels of testosterone or androstenedione or both are strongly suggestive of an ovarian SCST in a woman with signs and symptoms of virilization. Clinical hyperandrogenism is more likely to be idiopathic or related to polycystic ovarian syndrome, but serum testosterone levels >150 g/dL or dehydroepiandrosterone sulfate (DHEAS) levels >8000 g/L

TABLE 36-4. Tumor Markers for Ovarian Sex Cord-Stromal Tumors with Malignant Potential

Granulosa cell tumors (adult and juvenile)	Inhibin A and B, estradiol (not as reliable)
Sertoli–Leydig cell tumors	Inhibin A and B, alpha-fetoprotein (occasionally)
Sex cord tumor with annular tubules	Inhibin A and B
Steroid cell tumors not otherwise specified	Steroid hormones elevated pretreatment

should strongly suggest the possibility of an androgen-secreting tumor (Carmina, 2006). In most instances, tumor marker studies are not usually obtained preoperatively, because the diagnosis of ovarian SCST is often not suspected. When the diagnosis is confirmed, the appropriate tumor markers may be drawn during or following surgery (Table 36-4).

Imaging

The gross appearances of SCSTs range from large multicystic masses to small solid masses—effectively precluding a specific radiologic diagnosis. Granulosa cell tumors often sonographically demonstrate semisolid features but are not reliably discernible from epithelial tumors (Sharony, 2001). In addition, the endometrium may be thickened from increased tumor estrogen production. Although CT or MR imaging has been used to clarify indeterminate sonograms, there is no definitive radiologic study to diagnose these tumors (Fig. 36-9) (Jung, 2005).

Diagnostic Procedures

Patients with an ovarian mass suspicious for malignancy based on clinical and sonographic findings require surgical resection for definitive tissue diagnosis, staging, and treatment. Sonographically or CT-guided percutaneous biopsy has no role. Moreover, diagnostic laparoscopy or laparotomy with visual assessment of the adnexal mass alone is inadequate; excision and pathologic evaluation are necessary. Following removal, ovarian SCSTs can usually be distinguished histologically from germ cell tumors, epithelial ovarian cancers, or other spindle-cell neoplasms by immunostaining for inhibin (Cathro, 2005; Schneider, 2005).

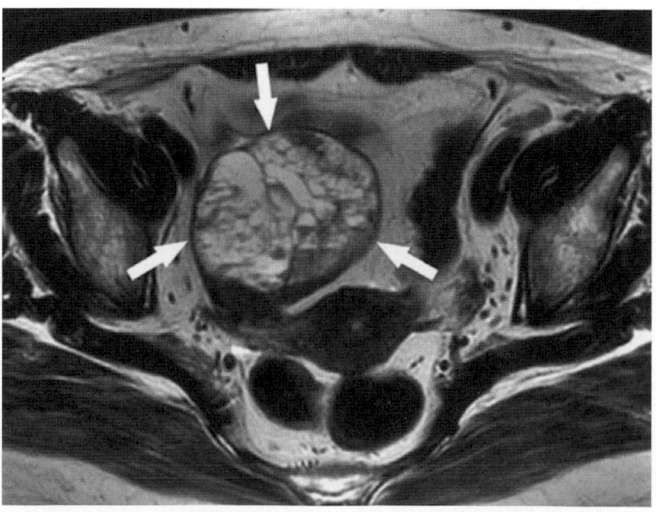

FIGURE 36-9 Computed tomographic (CT) scan of a granulosa cell tumor. *(From Jung, 2005, with permission.)*

Role of the Generalist

Preoperatively, patients with a potentially malignant ovarian SCST should be referred to a gynecologic oncologist for evaluation. Most ovarian SCSTs, however, are diagnosed by generalist gynecologists following resection of a seemingly benign but complex mass in a woman with a CA125 level that is typically normal, if known beforehand. The initial surgery is often performed in a community-based hospital and without adequate staging. In this setting, prior to referral, histologic results should be reviewed and confirmed by an experienced pathologist. Following referral to a gynecologic oncologist, surgical staging via laparotomy or laparoscopy may be indicated.

Pathology
Classification

Ovarian SCSTs arise from sex cord and mesenchymal cells of the embryonic gonad (Chap. 18, p. 485). Granulosa and Sertoli cells develop from the sex cords and thus from the coelomic epithelium. In contrast, theca cells, Leydig cells, and fibroblasts are derived from the mesenchyme (future stroma). This primitive gonadal stroma possesses sexual bipotentiality. Therefore, developing tumors may be composed of a male-directed cell type (Sertoli or Leydig cell) or a female-directed cell type (granulosa or theca cell). Although distinct categories of SCSTs have been defined, mixed tumors are relatively common (Table 36-5). For example, ovarian granulosa cell tumors may have admixed Sertoli components. Similarly, tumors that are predominantly Sertoli or Sertoli-Leydig cells may contain minor granulosa elements. These mixed tumors are believed to arise from a common lineage with variable differentiation and do not represent two concurrent separate entities (McKenna, 2005; Vang, 2004).

Histologic Grading

Ovarian granulosa cell tumors are universally considered to have malignant potential, but most other SCST subtypes do not have definitive criteria for clearly defining benign and malignant. Attempts to grade these tumors using nuclear characteristics or mitotic activity counts have produced inconsistent results (Chen, 2003).

Patterns of Growth and Spread

The natural history of SCSTs in general differs greatly from that of epithelial ovarian carcinomas. For example, most of these tumors have low malignant potential. They are typically unilateral and remain localized, retain hormone-secreting functions, and infrequently relapse. Recurrences tend to be late and usually develop in the abdomen or pelvis (Abu-Rustum, 2006). Bone metastases are rare (Dubuc-Lissoir, 2001).

TABLE 36-5. World Health Organization Classification of Ovarian Sex Cord–Stromal Tumors

Granulosa-stromal cell tumors
Granulosa cell tumor
   Adult type
   Juvenile type
Thecoma-fibroma group
   Thecoma
   Fibroma/fibrosarcoma
   Sclerosing stromal tumor

Sertoli–stromal cell tumors
Sertoli cell tumor
Sertoli–Leydig cell tumor

Sex cord tumor with annular tubules

Steroid cell tumors
Stromal luteoma
Leydig cell tumor
Steroid cell tumor not otherwise specified

Unclassified

Gynandroblastoma

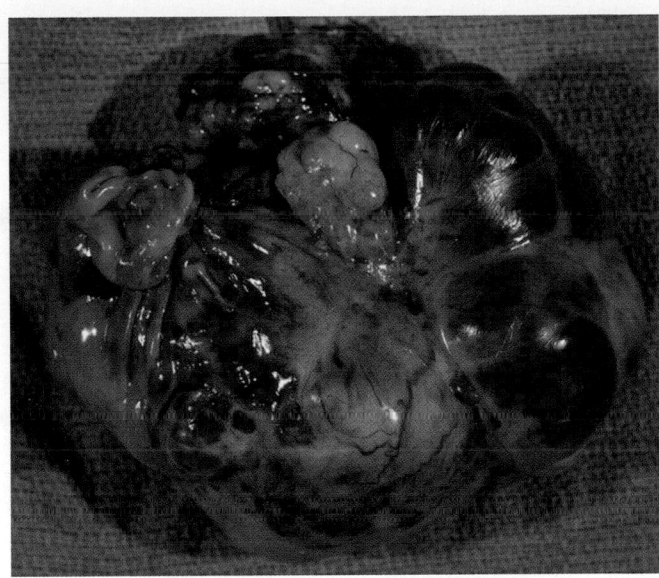

FIGURE 36-10 Adult granulosa cell tumor. *(Photograph contributed by Dr. Raheela Ashfaq.)*

Granulosa Cell Tumors

Seventy percent of ovarian SCSTs are granulosa cell tumors (Colombo, 2007). These tumors are formed by cells believed to arise from those surrounding the germinal cells within ovarian follicles. There are two clinically and histologically distinct types: the adult form, which comprises 95 percent of cases, and the juvenile type, comprising 5 percent.

Adult Granulosa Cell Tumors. Most women with an adult granulosa cell tumor are diagnosed after age 30, with the average age being approximately 50 years. Menometrorrhagia and postmenopausal bleeding are common signs and reflect a prolonged exposure of the endometrium to estrogen. Related to this estrogen excess, coexisting pathology such as endometrial hyperplasia or adenocarcinoma has been found in one quarter of patients with adult granulosa cell tumor. Similarly, breast enlargement and tenderness are common associated complaints, and secondary amenorrhea has been reported (Kurihara, 2004). Alternatively, symptoms may stem from the mass of the ovary rather than from hormones produced. An enlarging and potentially hemorrhagic tumor may cause abdominal pain and distension. Acute pelvic pain may suggest adnexal torsion, or tumor rupture with hemoperitoneum can mimic ectopic pregnancy.

During surgery, if an adult granulosa cell tumor is confirmed, tumor markers may be requested. Of these, inhibin B seems to be more accurate than inhibin A, frequently being elevated months before clinical detection of recurrence (Mom, 2007). The diagnostic value of these markers, however, is often hampered by their physiologically broad normal ranges (Schneider, 2005). Estradiol also has limited use in surveil-

lance, particularly in the younger patient wishing to preserve fertility and having the contralateral ovary left in situ.

Grossly, adult granulosa cell tumors are large, multicystic, and often exceed 10 to 15 cm in diameter (Fig. 36-10). The surface is frequently edematous and unusually adherent to other pelvic organs. For this reason, more extensive dissection is typically required than for epithelial ovarian cancers or malignant germ cell tumors. During excision, inadvertent rupture and intraoperative bleeding from the tumor itself is also common.

The interior of the tumor is highly variable. Solid components may predominate with large areas of hemorrhage and necrosis. Alternatively, it can be cystic, with numerous locules filled with serosanguinous or gelatinous fluid (Colombo, 2007). Microscopic examination shows predominately granulosa cells with pale, grooved, "coffee bean" nuclei. The characteristic microscopic feature is the *Call-Exner body*— a rosette arrangement of cells around an eosinophilic fluid space (Fig. 36-11).

Adult granulosa cell tumors are low-grade malignancies that typically demonstrate indolent growth. Ninety-five percent are unilateral, and 70 to 90 percent are stage I at diagnosis (Table 36-6). The 5-year survival for patients with stage I disease is 90 to 95 percent (Colombo, 2007; Zhang, 2007). However, 15 to 25 percent of stage I tumors will eventually relapse. The median time to recurrence is 5 to 6 years, but may be several decades (Abu-Rustum, 2006; East, 2005). Fortunately, these indolent tumors usually progress slowly thereafter, and the median length of survival after relapse is another 6 years. Advanced tumor stage and residual disease are poor prognostic factors (Al Badawi, 2002; Sehouli, 2004). Patients with stage II-IV tumors have a 5-year survival of 30 to 50 percent (Malmstrom, 1994; Miller, 1997; Piura, 1994). Cellular atypia and mitotic count may help in determining the prognosis but are difficult to reproducibly quantify (Miller, 2001).

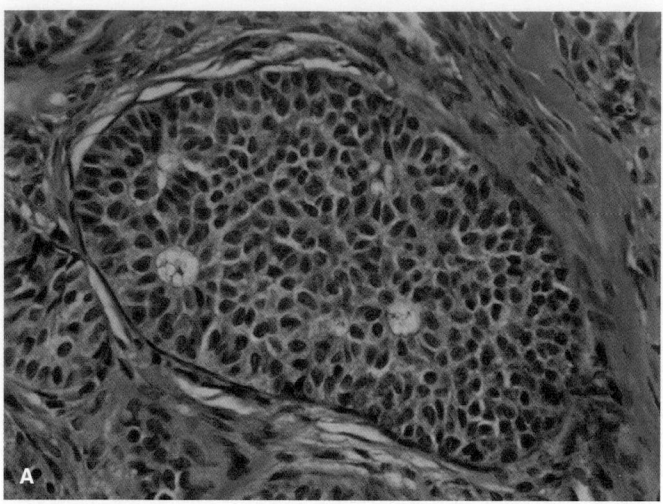
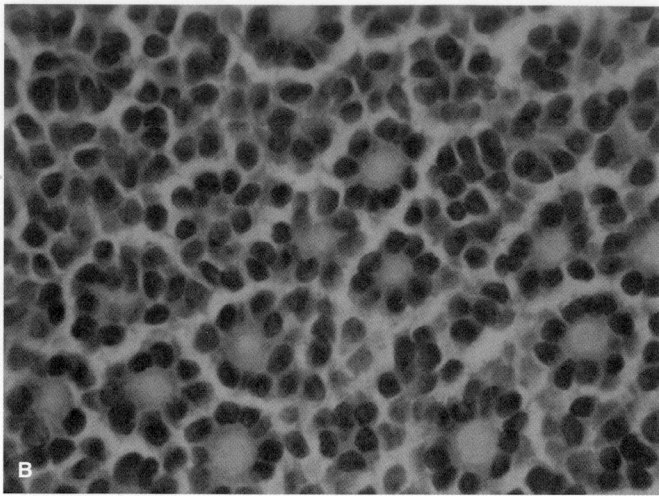

FIGURE 36-11 A. Adult granulosa cell tumor. **B.** Call-Exner bodies are identified by their rosette appearance. *(Photographs contributed by Dr. Raheela Ashfaq.)*

Juvenile Granulosa Cell Tumors. These rare neoplasms develop primarily in children and young adults, and approximately 90 percent are diagnosed before puberty (Colombo, 2007). The mean age at diagnosis is 13 years, but patient ages range from newborn to 67 years (Young, 1984). Juvenile granulosa cell tumors are sometimes associated with Ollier disease or with Maffucci syndrome, which is characterized by endochondromas and hemangiomas (Young, 1984; Yuan, 2004).

In affected females, estrogen, progesterone, and testosterone levels may be elevated and lead to suppression of gonadotropins. As a result, menstrual irregularities or amenorrhea are common. Prepubertal girls typically display isosexual precocious puberty, which is characterized by breast enlargement and development of pubic hair, vaginal secretions, and other secondary sexual characteristics. These tumors infrequently secrete androgens, but in such cases may induce virilization. Despite these endocrinologic signs, a delayed diagnosis of juvenile granulosa cell tumors in pre- and postpubertal girls is common and associated with a higher risk of peritoneal tumor spread (Kalfa, 2005).

In addition to hormonal changes, individuals may display tumor effects. For example, older patients usually seek medical attention for abdominal pain or swelling. Preoperative rupture with resulting hemoperitoneum may create acute abdominal

symptoms in 5 to 10 percent of cases (Colombo, 2007). Ascites is present in 10 percent (Young, 1984).

Juvenile granulosa cell tumors are grossly similar to the adult-type tumor and display variable solid and cystic components. They can attain significant size and have an average diameter of approximately 12 cm. Microscopically, cytologic features that distinguish these tumors from the adult type are their rounded, hyperchromatic nuclei without "coffee-bean" grooves. Call-Exner bodies are rare, but often there is a theca cell component (Young, 1984).

Prognosis is excellent, and the 5-year survival rate is 95 percent. Similar to adult-type tumors, 95 percent of juvenile granulosa cell tumors are unilateral and stage I at diagnosis (Young, 1984). However, the juvenile type is more aggressive in advanced stages, and the time to relapse and death is much shorter. Recurrences typically develop within 3 years and are highly lethal. Later recurrences are unusual (Frausto, 2004).

Thecoma-Fibroma Group

Thecomas. These are relatively common SCSTs and are rarely malignant. Thecomas are unique because they typically develop in postmenopausal women in their mid-60s and develop infrequently before age 30. These solid tumors are among the most hormonally active of the SCSTs and usually produce excess estrogen. As a result, the primary signs and symptoms are abnormal vaginal bleeding or pelvic mass or both. Many women also present with concurrent endometrial hyperplasia or adenocarcinoma (Aboud, 1997). These tumors are composed of lipid-laden stromal cells that are occasionally luteinized. Half of these luteinized thecomas are either hormonally inactive or androgenic with the potential for inducing masculinization.

Thecomas are solid tumors whose cells resemble the theca cells that normally surround the ovarian follicles (Chen, 2003). Because of this texture, these tumors appear sonographically as solid adnexal masses and may mimic extrauterine leiomyomas.

Bilateral ovarian involvement and extraovarian spread are rare. Fortunately, ovarian thecomas are clinically benign, and surgical resection is curative.

TABLE 36-6. Stage and Survival of Common Ovarian Sex Cord–Stromal Tumors

	Adult Granulosa Cell	Sertoli-Leydig Cell
Stage at diagnosis		
I	70–90%	97%
II–IV	10–20%	2–3%
Five-year survival		
Stage I	90–95%	90–95%
Stage II–IV	30–50%	10–20%

Sources for survival figures are referenced within the text.

Fibromas-Fibrosarcomas. Fibromas are relatively common, hormonally inactive SCST variants that usually occur in perimenopausal and menopausal women (Chechia, 2008). These solid, generally benign ovarian neoplasms arise from the spindled stromal cells that form collagen. Most fibromas are found incidentally on pelvic or sonographic examination. They are round, oval, or lobulated solid tumors associated with free fluid or less commonly, with frank ascites and possess minimal to moderate vascularization (Paladini, 2009).

Perhaps 1 percent of women present with *Meigs syndrome,* which is a triad of pleural effusion, ascites, and a solid ovarian mass (Siddiqui, 1995). Pleural effusions are usually right-sided, and these, as well as accompanying ascites, are typically transudative and resolve after tumor resection (Majzlin, 1964). Despite this association of ascites with benign fibromas, when ascites and a pelvic mass coexist, evaluation is based on an assumption of malignancy.

The prognosis following excision of fibromas is that for any benign tumor. However, ten percent will demonstrate increased cellularity and varying degrees of pleomorphism and mitotic activity that indicate a tumor better characterized as having low malignant potential. In 1 percent of cases, malignant transformation to fibrosarcoma is found.

Sclerosing Stromal Tumors. These tumors are rare and account for less than 5 percent of SCSTs. The average patient age is approximately 20 years, and 80 percent develop before age 30. Sclerosing stromal tumors are clinically benign and typically unilateral. Menstrual irregularities and pelvic pain are both common symptoms (Marelli, 1998). Ascites is seldom encountered (unlike fibromas), and sclerosing stromal tumors are hormonally inactive (unlike thecomas). Tumor size ranges from microscopic to 20 cm. Histologically, the presence of pseudolobulation of cellular areas separated by edematous connective tissue, increased vascularity, and prominent areas of sclerosis are distinguishing features.

Sertoli-Stromal Cell Tumors

Sertoli Cell Tumors. Ovarian Sertoli cell tumors are rare and account for less than 5 percent of all SCSTs. The mean patient age at diagnosis is 30 years, but ages range from 2 to 76 years. One quarter of patients present with estrogenic or androgenic manifestations, but most tumors are clinically nonfunctional.

Sertoli cell tumors are typically unilateral, solid, yellow and measure 4 to 12 cm. Derived from the cell type that gives rise to the seminiferous tubules, these tumor cells often organize into histologically characteristic tubules (Young, 2005). Sertoli cell tumors, however, may also mimic many different tumors, and immunostaining in these cases is invaluable to confirm the diagnosis.

More than 80 percent are stage I at diagnosis, and most are clinically benign. Moderate cytologic atypia, brisk mitotic activity, and tumor cell necrosis are indicators of greater malignant potential and are found in 10 percent of individuals with stage I disease and most of those with stage II-IV tumors. The risk of recurrence is higher when these features are identified (Oliva, 2005).

Sertoli-Leydig Cell Tumors. Sertoli-Leydig cell tumors comprise only 5 to 10 percent of ovarian SCSTs (Zhang, 2007).

Their incidence mirrors that of Sertoli cell tumors, and the average age is 25 years. Although Sertoli-Leydig cell tumors have been identified in children and postmenopausal females, more than 90 percent develop during the reproductive years.

These tumors frequently produce sex-steroid hormones, most commonly androgens. As a result, frank virilization develops in one third of women, and another 10 percent have clinical manifestations of androgen excess characterized by hirsutism, temporal balding, deepening of the voice, and clitoral enlargement (Young, 1985). Menstrual disorders are also common. Accordingly, Sertoli-Leydig cell tumors should be suspected preoperatively in a patient with a unilaterally palpable adnexal mass and androgenic manifestations. For these women, an elevated serum testosterone-to-androstenedione ratio further suggests the diagnosis.

Although these hormonal effects frequently develop, one half of patients will have nonspecific abdominal mass symptoms as their only presenting complaint. Associated ascites is infrequent (Outwater, 2000). Thyroid abnormalities also coexist with Sertoli-Leydig cell tumors at a frequency that exceeds mere chance.

These tumors tend to be large at the time of excision with an average diameter of 13.5 cm, but ranges from 1 to 50 cm have been reported. In most cases, Sertoli-Leydig cell tumors appear yellow and lobulated. Tumors can be solid, partially cystic, or completely cystic, and they may or may not have polypoid or vesicular structures in their interior (Fig. 36-12). Microscopically, these morphologically diverse tumors contain cells resembling epithelial and stromal testicular cells in varying proportions. The five subtypes of differentiation (well, intermediate, poor, retiform, heterologous) have considerable overlap. Well-differentiated tumors are all clinically benign (Chen, 2003; Young, 2005).

Overall, 15 to 20 percent of Sertoli-Leydig cell tumors are clinically malignant. Prognosis depends predominantly on the stage and degree of tumor differentiation in these malignant variants. For example, Young and Scully (1985) performed a clinicopathologic analysis of 207 cases and identified stage I disease in 97 percent. The 5-year survival for patients with stage I disease exceeds 90 percent (Zaloudek, 1984). Malignant features were observed in approximately 10 percent of tumors with intermediate differentiation and

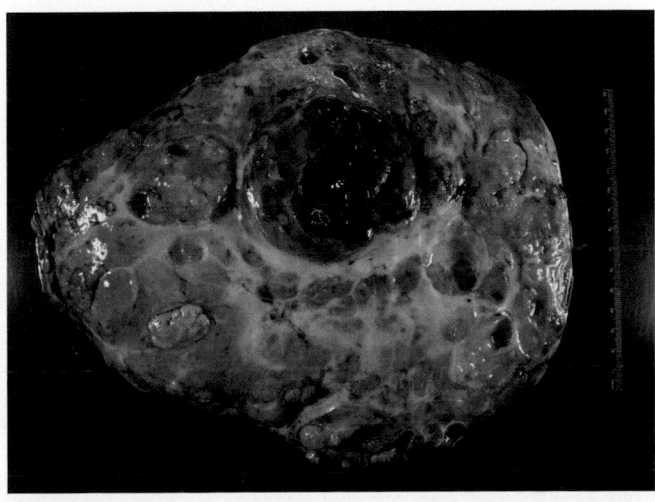

FIGURE 36-12 Sertoli-Leydig tumor.

60 percent of poorly differentiated tumors. Retiform and heterologous elements are seen only in intermediate or poorly differentiated Sertoli-Leydig cell tumors and typically are associated with poorer prognosis. Overall, the 2 to 3 percent of patients with stage II-IV disease have a dismal prognosis (Young, 1985).

Sex Cord Tumors with Annular Tubules

Sex cord tumors with annular tubules account for 5 percent of SCSTs and are characterized by ring-shaped tubules and distinctive cellular elements that are histologically intermediate between Sertoli-cell and granulosa cell tumors. There are two clinically distinct types. One third is clinically benign and develops in patients with Peutz-Jeghers syndrome (PJS). These tumors are typically small, multifocal, calcified, bilateral, and diagnosed incidentally. Fifteen percent of PJS-associated cases will also develop adenoma malignum of the cervix, which is a rare, extremely well-differentiated adenocarcinoma (Chap. 30, p. 774). In contrast, two thirds of tumors are not associated with PJS. These tumors are usually larger, unilateral, and symptomatic and carry a clinical malignancy rate of 15 to 20 percent (Young, 1982).

Steroid-Cell Tumors

Fewer than 5 percent of SCSTs are steroid-cell tumors. The average age at diagnosis is the mid-20s, but patients can present at virtually any age. These tumors are composed entirely or predominantly of cells that resemble steroid hormone-secreting cells and are categorized according to the histologic composition of these cells. *Stromal luteomas* are clinically benign tumors that by definition lie completely within the ovarian stroma. They are usually seen in postmenopausal women. Estrogenic effects are common, but occasional individuals have androgenic manifestations. *Leydig-cell tumors* are also benign and typically are seen in postmenopausal women. They are distinguished microscopically by rectangular, crystal-like cytoplasmic inclusions, termed *crystals of Reinke*. Leydig cells secrete testosterone, and these tumors are usually associated with androgenic effects. *Steroid-cell tumors not otherwise specified (NOS)* are the most common subtype within this group and typically present in younger reproductive-aged women. Some of these cases may represent large stromal luteomas that have grown to reach the ovarian surface or Leydig-cell tumors in which Reinke crystals cannot be identified. These tumors are typically associated with androgenic excess, but estrogenic or cortisol overproduction (i.e., Cushing syndrome) has also been reported. One third of steroid-cell tumors NOS are clinically malignant and have a dismal prognosis (Oliva, 2005).

Unclassified Sex Cord-Stromal Tumors

Unclassified tumors account for 5 percent of SCSTs and have no clearly predominant pattern of testicular (Sertoli cells) or ovarian (granulosa cells) differentiation. These ill-defined tumors are especially common during pregnancy due to alterations in their usual clinical and pathologic features (Young, 2005). They may be estrogenic, androgenic, or nonfunctional. The prognosis is similar to that of granulosa cell tumors and Sertoli-Leydig cell tumors of similar degrees of differentiation.

Gynandroblastomas

These are the rarest type of ovarian SCST. Patients present at a mean age of 30 years and typically have menstrual irregularities or evidence of hormonal excess. The tumors are characterized by intermingled granulosa cells and tubules of Sertoli cells. Theca or Leydig cells or both may also be present in varying degrees. Gynandroblastomas have low malignant potential, and only one death has been reported (Martin-Jimenez, 1994).

■ Treatment

Surgery

The mainstay of treatment for patients with an ovarian SCST is complete surgical resection. Due to their relative insensitivity to adjuvant chemotherapy or radiation, the goals of surgery are not only to establish a definitive tissue diagnosis and determine the extent of disease, but also to remove all grossly visible tumors in those infrequent patients with advanced stage disease. Moreover, in planning surgery, clinicians should consider the patient's age and desire for future fertility. Hysterectomy with BSO is performed for those who have completed childbearing, whereas fertility-sparing USO with preservation of the uterus and remaining ovary may be appropriate in the absence of obvious disease spread to these organs (Zanagnolo, 2004). Endometrial sampling should be performed especially when fertility-sparing surgery is planned in women with granulosa cell tumors or thecomas, since many of these patients will have coexisting hyperplasia or adenocarcinoma that may affect the decision for hysterectomy.

Minimally invasive laparoscopic surgery has a variety of relevant applications. For some, the diagnosis of SCST may not be discovered until the mass is laparoscopically removed and sent for frozen section. Laparoscopic surgical staging can then proceed. When the diagnosis is not made until the final pathology report is confirmed postoperatively, laparoscopic staging may be proposed to determine whether metastatic disease is present while reducing the morbidity of another operation (Kriplani, 2001).

Although staging laparotomy or laparoscopy is essential to determine the extent of disease and the need for adjuvant therapy in most individuals with potentially malignant SCST subtypes, only approximately 20 percent of cases have complete staging (Fig. 36-13) (Abu-Rustum, 2006; Brown, 2009). More recent data suggest that, due to surface and hematogenous routes of spread, the standard ovarian cancer procedure can be modified. Pelvic washings, exploration of the abdomen, peritoneal biopsies and partial omentectomy remain important. However, the utility of routine pelvic and paraaortic lymphadenectomy has been increasingly challenged. In a study of 262 ovarian SCSTs, none of the 58 patients undergoing nodal dissection had positive nodes (Brown, 2009). Additionally, performing a lymphadenectomy has not been shown to improve survival for SCSTs (Chan, 2007).

Surgical removal of hormone-producing SCSTs results in an immediate drop in elevated preoperative sex-steroid hormone levels. Physical manifestations of these elevated levels, however, partially or completely resolve more gradually.

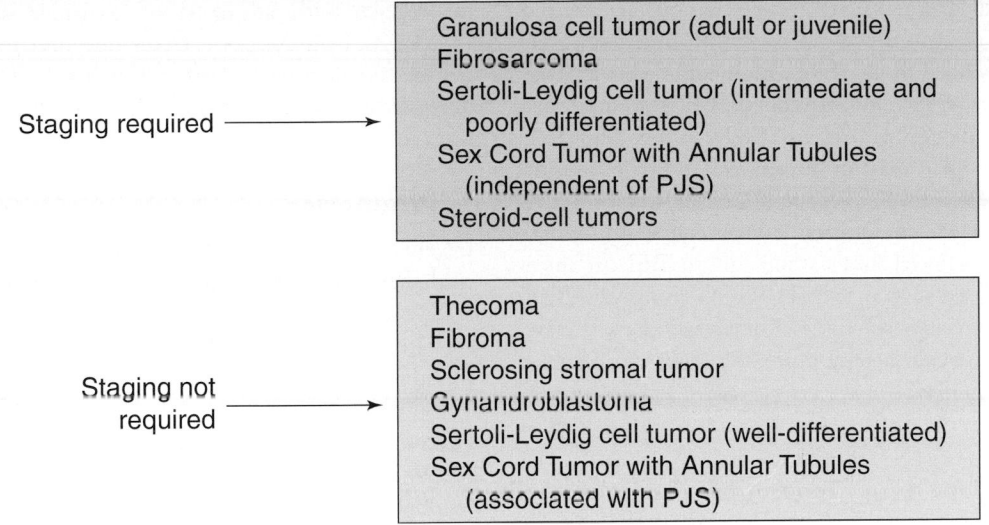

Staging required →
- Granulosa cell tumor (adult or juvenile)
- Fibrosarcoma
- Sertoli-Leydig cell tumor (intermediate and poorly differentiated)
- Sex Cord Tumor with Annular Tubules (independent of PJS)
- Steroid-cell tumors

Staging not required →
- Thecoma
- Fibroma
- Sclerosing stromal tumor
- Gynandroblastoma
- Sertoli-Leydig cell tumor (well-differentiated)
- Sex Cord Tumor with Annular Tubules (associated with PJS)

FIGURE 36-13 Staging of sex cord-stromal tumors. PJS = Peutz-Jeghers syndrome.

Surveillance

In general, women with stage I ovarian SCSTs have an excellent prognosis following surgery alone and can usually be followed at regular intervals without the need for further treatment (Schneider, 2003a). Surveillance includes a general physical and pelvic examination, serum marker testing, and imaging tests as clinically indicated.

Chemotherapy

The decision to administer postoperative therapy depends on a variety of factors (Fig. 36-14). Although typically treated solely with surgery, malignant stage I ovarian SCSTs may require adjuvant chemotherapy when large tumor size, high mitotic index, capsular excrescences, tumor rupture, incomplete staging, or equivocal pathology results are noted. Women with one or more of these suspicious features are thought to be at higher risk of relapse and should be considered for platinum-based chemotherapy (Schneider, 2003b). In addition, stage II-IV disease warrants postoperative treatment. In general, SCSTs display less sensitivity to chemotherapy than other ovarian malignancies, but most women at high risk for disease progression can be treated successfully with adjuvant platinum-based chemotherapy (Schneider, 2005).

The 5-day bleomycin, etoposide, and cisplatin (BEP) regimen is the most widely used first-line chemotherapy combination

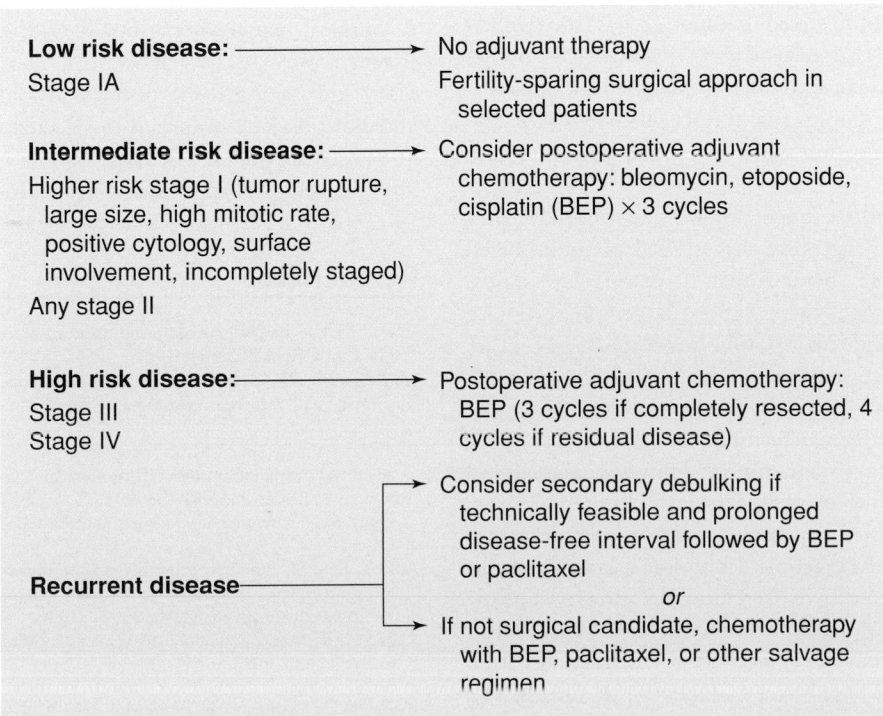

Low risk disease: → No adjuvant therapy
Stage IA   Fertility-sparing surgical approach in selected patients

Intermediate risk disease: → Consider postoperative adjuvant chemotherapy: bleomycin, etoposide, cisplatin (BEP) × 3 cycles
Higher risk stage I (tumor rupture, large size, high mitotic rate, positive cytology, surface involvement, incompletely staged)
Any stage II

High risk disease: → Postoperative adjuvant chemotherapy: BEP (3 cycles if completely resected, 4 cycles if residual disease)
Stage III
Stage IV

Recurrent disease → Consider secondary debulking if technically feasible and prolonged disease-free interval followed by BEP or paclitaxel
or
→ If not surgical candidate, chemotherapy with BEP, paclitaxel, or other salvage regimen

FIGURE 36-14 Postoperative treatment of sex cord-stromal tumors.

(Gershenson, 1996; Homesley, 1999). For completely resected disease, three courses given every 3 weeks are sufficient. Four cycles are recommended for patients with incompletely resected tumor (Homesley, 1999). In addition to BEP, taxanes have demonstrated activity against ovarian SCSTs, and combination paclitaxel and carboplatin chemotherapy has shown promising results (Brown, 2004, 2005). To determine the most effective regimen, a prospective randomized study is currently underway, comparing paclitaxel and carboplatin to BEP in those with newly diagnosed ovarian SCSTs (GOG protocol #264). Unfortunately, the relative scarcity of women who have ovarian SCST and receive chemotherapy limits the ability to conduct large randomized studies.

Radiation

Postoperative radiation therapy currently has a limited role in the management of ovarian SCSTs. There is some evidence indicating a prolonged survival in at least some women with newly diagnosed disease who received whole-abdominal radiotherapy (Wolf, 1999). However, chemotherapy is usually the primary postoperative treatment because it is generally better tolerated, more widely accessible, and easier to administer. Radiation is best reserved for palliation of local symptoms (Dubuc-Lissoir, 2001).

Relapse

The management of recurrent ovarian SCST depends on the clinical circumstances. Secondary surgical debulking should be strongly considered due to the indolent growth pattern, the typically long disease-free interval after initial treatment, and the inherent insensitivity to chemotherapy (Crew, 2005; Powell, 2001). Platinum-based combination chemotherapy is the primary treatment chosen for recurrent disease with or without surgical debulking (Uygun, 2003). Of regimens, BEP is most frequently administered because it has the highest known response rate (Homesley, 1999). Paclitaxel is another promising agent that is currently being evaluated in a phase II Gynecologic Oncology Group trial (GOG protocol #187) and warrants further investigation when combined with platinum (Brown, 2005).

There is no standard treatment for women who have progressive disease despite aggressive surgery and platinum-based chemotherapy. Notably, bevacizumab (Avastin) has shown significant activity in small series, and a larger phase II trial is currently being conducted (GOG protocol #251) (Tao, 2009). Vincristine, actinomycin D, and cyclophosphamide (VAC) regimen has limited activity (Ayhan, 1996; Zanagnolo, 2004). Hormonal therapy may be useful and is minimally toxic in women with chemoresistant tumors. However, the clinical experience with this approach is extremely limited (Hardy, 2005). Medroxyprogesterone acetate and the gonadotropin-releasing hormone (GnRH) agonist leuprolide acetate (Lupron) have each demonstrated activity in halting the growth of recurrent ovarian SCSTs (Fishman, 1996; Homesley, 1999). GnRH antagonists, however, may not be as effective (Ameryckx, 2005).

In addition to traditional drugs, discovery of the *FOXL2* 402C→G mutation occurring exclusively in all adult granulosa cell tumors may lead to the development of targeted therapies for women with advanced or recurrent disease. Although FOXL2 as a transcription factor does not represent a perfect pharmacologic target, further insights into its function and downstream effects may identify targetable molecular alterations in these tumors (Kobel, 2009).

Prognosis

In general, ovarian SCSTs portend a much better prognosis than epithelial ovarian carcinomas chiefly because most women with SCSTs are diagnosed with stage I disease. Stage II-IV tumors are rare, but women with these cancers have a poor prognosis similar to their epithelial counterparts. Unfortunately, improvements in survival have not been observed in ovarian SCSTs over the past few decades (Chan, 2006).

Of the clinical factors affecting prognosis, surgical stage and residual disease are the most important (Lee, 2008; Zanagnolo, 2004). Further, in a Surveillance, Epidemiology and End Results (SEER) database study, Zhang and colleagues (2007) performed a multivariate analysis of 376 women with SCSTs and concluded that age younger than 50 years was also an independent predictor of improved survival.

Management During Pregnancy

Ovarian SCSTs are rarely detected during pregnancy (Okada, 2004). In a California population-based study of more than 4 million obstetric patients, one granulosa cell tumor was diagnosed among 202 women with an ovarian malignancy (Leiserowitz, 2006). Granulosa cell tumors are most common, but only 10 percent are diagnosed during pregnancy (Hasiakos, 2006). One third of pregnant women with SCSTs are incidentally diagnosed at cesarean delivery, one third have abdominal pain or swelling, and the remainder may present with hemoperitoneum, virilization, or vaginal bleeding (Young, 1984).

Surgical management should be the same as for the nonpregnant woman. For most, conservative management with USO and staging is the primary procedure, but hysterectomy and BSO may be indicated in selected circumstances (Young, 1984). Postoperative chemotherapy is typically withheld until after delivery because SCSTs have an indolent growth pattern.

REFERENCES

Aboud E: A review of granulosa cell tumours and thecomas of the ovary. Arch Gynecol Obstet 259:161, 1997

Abu-Rustum NR, Restivo A, Ivy J, et al: Retroperitoneal nodal metastasis in primary and recurrent granulosa cell tumors of the ovary. Gynecol Oncol 103:31, 2006

Al Badawi IA, Brasher PM, Ghatage P, et al: Postoperative chemotherapy in advanced ovarian granulosa cell tumors. Int J Gynecol Cancer 12:119, 2002

Ameryckx L, Fatemi HM, De Sutter P, et al: GnRH antagonist in the adjuvant treatment of a recurrent ovarian granulosa cell tumor: a case report. Gynecol Oncol 99:764, 2005

Aoki Y, Kase H, Fujita K, et al: Dysgerminoma with a slightly elevated alpha-fetoprotein level diagnosed as a mixed germ cell tumor after recurrence. Gynecol Obstet Invest 55:58, 2003

Ayhan A, Tuncer ZS, Hakverdi AU, et al: Sertoli–Leydig cell tumor of the ovary: a clinicopathologic study of 10 cases. Eur J Gynaecol Oncol 17:75, 1996

Bafna UD, Umadevi K, Kumaran C, et al: Germ cell tumors of the ovary: is there a role for aggressive cytoreductive surgery for nondysgerminomatous tumors? Int J Gynecol Cancer 11:300, 2001

Beiner ME, Gotlieb WH, Korach Y, et al: Cystectomy for immature teratoma of the ovary. Gynecol Oncol 93:381, 2004

Billmire D, Vinocur C, Rescorla F, et al: Outcome and staging evaluation in malignant germ cell tumors of the ovary in children and adolescents: an intergroup study. J Pediatr Surg 39:424, 2004

Bonazzi C, Peccatori F, Colombo N, et al: Pure ovarian immature teratoma, a unique and curable disease: 10 years' experience of 32 prospectively treated patients. Obstet Gynecol 84:598, 1994

Boyce EA, Costaggini I, Vitonis A, et al: The epidemiology of ovarian granulosa cell tumors: a case-control study. Gynecol Oncol 115:221, 2009

Brewer M, Gershenson DM, Herzog CE, et al: Outcome and reproductive function after chemotherapy for ovarian dysgerminoma. J Clin Oncol 17:2670, 1999

Brown J, Shvartsman HS, Deavers MT, et al: The activity of taxanes compared with bleomycin, etoposide, and cisplatin in the treatment of sex cord–stromal ovarian tumors. Gynecol Oncol 97:489, 2005

Brown J, Shvartsman HS, Deavers MT, et al: The activity of taxanes in the treatment of sex cord–stromal ovarian tumors. J Clin Oncol 22:3517, 2004

Brown J, Sood AK, Deavers MT, et al: Patterns of metastasis in sex cord-stromal tumors of the ovary: can routine staging lymphadenectomy be omitted? Gynecol Oncol 113:86, 2009

Carmina E, Rosato F, Janni A, et al: Extensive clinical experience: relative prevalence of different androgen excess disorders in 950 women referred because of clinical hyperandrogenism. J Clin Endocrinol Metab 91:2, 2006

Cass DL, Hawkins E, Brandt ML, et al: Surgery for ovarian masses in infants, children, and adolescents: 102 consecutive patients treated in a 15-year period. J Pediatr Surg 36:693, 2001

Cathro HP, Stoler MH: The utility of calretinin, inhibin, and WT1 immunohistochemical staining in the differential diagnosis of ovarian tumors. Hum Pathol 36:195, 2005

Chan JK, Cheung MK, Husain A, et al: Patterns and progress in ovarian cancer over 14 years. Obstet Gynecol 108:521, 2006

Chan JK, Munro EG, Cheung MK, et al: Association of lymphadenectomy and survival in stage I ovarian cancer patients. Obstet Gynecol 109:12, 2007

Chan JK, Tewari KS, Waller S, et al: The influence of conservative surgical practices for malignant ovarian germ cell tumors. J Surg Oncol 98:111, 2008

Chan JK, Zhang M, Kaleb V, et al: Prognostic factors responsible for survival in sex cord stromal tumors of the ovary: a multivariate analysis. Gynecol Oncol 96:204, 2005

Chechia A, Attia L, Temime RB, et al: Incidence, clinical analysis, and management of ovarian fibromas and fibrothecomas. Am J Obstet Gynecol 199:473e1, 2008

Chen VW, Ruiz B, Killeen JL, et al: Pathology and classification of ovarian tumors. Cancer 97:2631, 2003

Cheng L, Thomas A, Roth LM, et al: OCT4: a novel biomarker for dysgerminoma of the ovary. Am J Surg Pathol 28:1341, 2004

Chi DS, Abu-Rustum NR, Sonoda Y, et al: The safety and efficacy of laparoscopic surgical staging of apparent stage I ovarian and fallopian tube cancers. Am J Obstet Gynecol 192:1614, 2005

Cicin I, Saip P, Guney N, et al: Yolk sac tumours of the ovary: evaluation of clinicopathological features and prognostic factors. Eur J Obstet Gynecol Reprod Biol 146:210, 2009

Colombo N, Parma G, Zanagnolo V, et al: Management of ovarian stromal cell tumors. J Clin Oncol 25:2944, 2007

Corakci A, Ozeren S, Ozkan S, et al: Pure nongestational choriocarcinoma of ovary. Arch Gynecol Obstet 271:176, 2005

Crew KD, Cohen MH, Smith DH, et al: Long natural history of recurrent granulosa cell tumor of the ovary 23 years after initial diagnosis: a case report and review of the literature. Gynecol Oncol 96:235, 2005

Culine S, Lhomme C, Michel G, et al: Is there a role for second-look laparotomy in the management of malignant germ cell tumors of the ovary? Experience at Institut Gustave Roussy. J Surg Oncol 62:40, 1996

Curtin JP, Morrow CP, D'Ablaing G, et al: Malignant germ cell tumors of the ovary: 20-year report of LAC-USC Women's Hospital. Int J Gynecol Cancer 4:29, 1994

Cushing B, Giller R, Ablin A, et al: Surgical resection alone is effective treatment for ovarian immature teratoma in children and adolescents: a report of the Pediatric Oncology Group and the Children's Cancer Group. Am J Obstet Gynecol 181:353, 1999

Dark GG, Bower M, Newlands ES, et al: Surveillance policy for stage I ovarian germ cell tumors. J Clin Oncol 15:620, 1997

Dimopoulos MA, Papadimitriou C, Hamilos G, et al: Treatment of ovarian germ cell tumors with a 3-day bleomycin, etoposide, and cisplatin regimen: a prospective multicenter study. Gynecol Oncol 95:695, 2004

Dos Santos L, Mok E, Iasonos A, et al: Squamous cell carcinoma arising in mature cystic teratoma of the ovary: a case series and review of the literature. Gynecol Oncol 105:321, 2007

Dubuc-Lissoir J, Berthiaume MJ, Boubez G, et al: Bone metastasis from a granulosa cell tumor of the ovary. Gynecol Oncol 83:400, 2001

East N, Alobaid A, Goffin F, et al: Granulosa cell tumour: a recurrence 40 years after initial diagnosis. J Obstet Gynaecol Can 27:363, 2005

Elit L, Bocking A, Kenyon C, et al: An endodermal sinus tumor diagnosed in pregnancy: case report and review of the literature. Gynecol Oncol 72:123, 1999

Fishman A, Kudelka AP, Tresukosol D, et al: Leuprolide acetate for treating refractory or persistent ovarian granulosa cell tumor. J Reprod Med 41:393, 1996

Fotopoulou C, Savvatis K, Braicu EI, et al: Adult granulosa cell tumors of the ovary: tumor dissemination pattern at primary and recurrent situation, surgical outcome. Gynecol Oncol 119:285, 2010

Frausto SD, Geisler JP, Fletcher MS, et al: Late recurrence of juvenile granulosa cell tumor of the ovary. Am J Obstet Gynecol 1:366, 2004

Gainford MC, Tinker A, Carter J, et al: Malignant transformation within ovarian dermoid cysts: an audit of treatment received and patient outcomes. An Australia New Zealand gynaecological oncology group (ANZGOG) and gynaecologic cancer intergroup (GCIG) study. Int J Gynecol Cancer 20:75, 2010

Galani E, Alamanis C, Dimopoulos MA: Familial female and male germ cell cancer: a new syndrome? Gynecol Oncol 96:254, 2005

Geisler JP, Goulet R, Foster RS, et al: Growing teratoma syndrome after chemotherapy for germ cell tumors of the ovary. Obstet Gynecol 84:719, 1994

Gershenson DM: Management of ovarian germ cell tumors. J Clin Oncol 25:2938, 2007a

Gershenson DM, Copeland LJ, Kavanagh JJ, et al: Treatment of malignant nondysgerminomatous germ cell tumors of the ovary with vincristine, dactinomycin, and cyclophosphamide. Cancer 56:2756, 1985

Gershenson DM, del Junco G, Herson J, et al: Endodermal sinus tumor of the ovary: the M.D. Anderson experience. Obstet Gynecol 61:194, 1983

Gershenson DM, Miller AM, Champion VL, et al: Reproductive and sexual function after platinum-based chemotherapy in long-term ovarian germ cell tumor survivors: a Gynecologic Oncology Group Study. J Clin Oncol 25:2792, 2007b

Gershenson DM, Morris M, Burke TW, et al: Treatment of poor-prognosis sex cord–stromal tumors of the ovary with the combination of bleomycin, etoposide, and cisplatin. Obstet Gynecol 87:527, 1996

Gershenson DM, Morris M, Cangir A, et al: Treatment of malignant germ cell tumors of the ovary with bleomycin, etoposide, and cisplatin. J Clin Oncol 8:715, 1990

Hardy RD, Bell JG, Nicely CJ, et al: Hormonal treatment of a recurrent granulosa cell tumor of the ovary: case report and review of the literature. Gynecol Oncol 96:865, 2005

Hasiakos D, Papakonstantinou K, Goula K, et al: Juvenile granulosa cell tumor associated with pregnancy: report of a case and review of the literature. Gynecol Oncol 100(2):426, 2006

Hinton S, Catalano P, Einhorn LH, et al: Phase II study of paclitaxel plus gemcitabine in refractory germ cell tumors (E9897): a trial of the Eastern Cooperative Oncology Group. J Clin Oncol 20:1859, 2002

Hoepffner W, Horn LC, Simon E, et al: Gonadoblastomas in 5 patients with 46,XY gonadal dysgenesis. Exp Clin Endocrinol Diabetes 113:231, 2005

Homesley HD, Bundy BN, Hurteau JA, et al: Bleomycin, etoposide, and cisplatin combination therapy of ovarian granulosa cell tumors and other stromal malignancies: a Gynecologic Oncology Group study. Gynecol Oncol 72:131, 1999

Horbelt D, Delmore J, Meisel R, et al: Mixed germ cell malignancy of the ovary concurrent with pregnancy. Obstet Gynecol 84:662, 1994

Hsu YJ, Pai L, Chen YC, et al: Extragonadal germ cell tumors in Taiwan: an analysis of treatment results of 59 patients. Cancer 95:766, 2002

Jung SE, Rha SE, Lee JM, et al: CT and MRI findings of sex cord–stromal tumor of the ovary. AJR Am J Roentgenol 185:207, 2005

Kalfa N, Patte C, Orbach D, et al: A nationwide study of granulosa cell tumors in pre- and postpubertal girls: missed diagnosis of endocrine manifestations worsens prognosis. J Pediatr Endocrinol Metab 18:25, 2005

Kim SH, Kang SB: Ovarian dysgerminoma: color Doppler ultrasonographic findings and comparison with CT and MR imaging findings. J Ultrasound Med 14:843, 1995

Kobel M, Gilks CB, Huntsman DG: Adult-type granulosa cell tumors and FOXL2 mutation. Cancer Res 69:9160, 2009

Kollmannsberger C, Nichols C, Bokemeyer C: Recent advances in management of patients with platinum-refractory testicular germ cell tumors. Cancer 106(6):1217, 2006

Kriplani A, Agarwal N, Roy KK, et al: Laparoscopic management of Sertoli–Leydig cell tumors of the ovary: a report of two cases. J Reprod Med 46:493, 2001

Kumar S, Shah JP, Bryant CS, et al: The prevalence and prognostic impact of lymph node metastasis in malignant germ cell tumors of the ovary. Gynecol Oncol 110:125, 2008

Kurihara S, Hirakawa T, Amada S, et al: Inhibin-producing ovarian granulosa cell tumor as a cause of secondary amenorrhea: case report and review of the literature. J Obstet Gynaecol Res 30:439, 2004

Kusamura S, Teixeira LC, dos Santos MA, et al: Ovarian germ cell cancer: clinicopathologic analysis and outcome of 31 cases. Tumori 86:450, 2000

LaPolla JP, Fiorica JV, Turnquist D, et al: Successful therapy of metastatic embryonal carcinoma coexisting with gonadoblastoma in a patient with 46,XY pure gonadal dysgenesis (Swyer's syndrome). Gynecol Oncol 37:417, 1990

Leblanc E, Querleu D, Narducci F, et al: Laparoscopic restaging of early stage invasive adnexal tumors: a 10-year experience. Gynecol Oncol 94:624, 2004

Lee KH, Lee IH, Kim BG, et al: Clinicopathologic characteristics of malignant germ cell tumors in the ovaries of Korean women: a Korean Gynecologic Oncology Group Study. Int J Gynecol Cancer 19:84, 2009

Lee YK, Park NH, Kim JW, et al: Characteristics of recurrence in adult-type granulosa cell tumor. Int J Gynecol Cancer 18:642, 2008

Leiserowitz GS, Xing G, Cress R, et al: Adnexal masses in pregnancy: how often are they malignant? Gynecol Oncol 101(2):315, 2006

Li H, Hong W, Zhang R, et al: Retrospective analysis of 67 consecutive cases of pure ovarian immature teratoma. Chin Med J (Engl) 115:1496, 2002

Li J, Yang W, Wu X: Prognostic factors and role of salvage surgery in chemorefractory ovarian germ cell malignancies: a study in Chinese patients. Gynecol Oncol 105:769, 2007

Low JJ, Perrin LC, Crandon AJ, et al: Conservative surgery to preserve ovarian function in patients with malignant ovarian germ cell tumors: a review of 74 cases. Cancer 89:391, 2000

Majzlin G, Stevens FL: Meigs' syndrome. Case report and review of literature. J Int Coll Surg 42:625, 1964

Malmstrom H, Hogberg T, Risberg B, et al: Granulosa cell tumors of the ovary: prognostic factors and outcome. Gynecol Oncol 52:50, 1994

Marelli G, Carinelli S, Mariani A, et al: Sclerosing stromal tumor of the ovary: report of eight cases and review of the literature. Eur J Obstet Gynecol Reprod Biol 76:85, 1998

Marina NM, Cushing B, Giller R, et al: Complete surgical excision is effective treatment for children with immature teratomas with or without malignant elements: a Pediatric Oncology Group/Children's Cancer Group Intergroup study. J Clin Oncol 17:2137, 1999

Martin-Jimenez A, Condom-Munro E, Valls-Porcel M, et al: [Gynandroblastoma of the ovary: review of the literature.] French. J Gynecol Obstet Biol Reprod (Paris) 23:391, 1994

McKenna M, Kenny B, Dorman G, et al: Combined adult granulosa cell tumor and mucinous cystadenoma of the ovary: granulosa cell tumor with heterologous mucinous elements. Int J Gynecol Pathol 24:224, 2005

Messing MJ, Gershenson DM, Morris M, et al: Primary treatment failure in patients with malignant ovarian germ cell neoplasms. Int J Gynecol Cancer 2:295, 1992

Miller BE, Barron BA, Dockter ME, et al: Parameters of differentiation and proliferation in adult granulosa cell tumors of the ovary. Cancer Detect Prev 25:48, 2001

Miller BE, Barron BA, Wan JY, et al: Prognostic factors in adult granulosa cell tumor of the ovary. Cancer 79:1951, 1997

Mitchell MF, Gershenson DM, Soeters RP, et al: The long-term effects of radiation therapy on patients with ovarian dysgerminoma. Cancer 67:1084, 1991

Mom CH, Engelen MJ, Willemse PH, et al: Granulosa cell tumors of the ovary: the clinical value of serum inhibin A and B levels in a large single center cohort. Gynecol Oncol 105:365, 2007

Montz FJ, Horenstein J, Platt LD, et al: The diagnosis of immature teratoma by maternal serum alpha-fetoprotein screening. Obstet Gynecol 73:522, 1989

Morimura Y, Nishiyama H, Yanagida K, et al: Dysgerminoma with syncytiotrophoblastic giant cells arising from 46,XX pure gonadal dysgenesis. Obstet Gynecol 92:654, 1998

Munkarah A, Gershenson DM, Levenback C, et al: Salvage surgery for chemorefractory ovarian germ cell tumors. Gynecol Oncol 55:217, 1994

Murugaesu N, Schmid P, Dancey G, et al: Malignant ovarian germ cell tumors: identification of novel prognostic markers and long-term outcome after multimodality treatment. J Clin Oncol 24:4862, 2006

Nawa A, Obata N, Kikkawa F, et al: Prognostic factors of patients with yolk sac tumors of the ovary. Am J Obstet Gynecol 184:1182, 2001

Nogales F, Talerman A, Kubik-Huch R et al: Germ cell tumours. In Tavassoli F, Devilee P (eds): World Health Organization Classification of Tumours. Lyon, France, International Agency for Research on Cancer Press, 2003, p 163

O'Connor DM, Norris HJ: The influence of grade on the outcome of stage I ovarian immature (malignant) teratomas and the reproducibility of grading. Int J Gynecol Pathol 13:283, 1994

Okada I, Nakagawa S, Takemura Y, et al: Ovarian thecoma associated in the first trimester of pregnancy. J Obstet Gynaecol Res 30:368, 2004

Oliva E, Alvarez T, Young RH: Sertoli cell tumors of the ovary: a clinicopathologic and immunohistochemical study of 54 cases. Am J Surg Pathol 29:143, 2005

Oliva E, Andrada E, Pezzica E, et al: Ovarian carcinomas with choriocarcinomatous differentiation. Cancer 72:2441, 1993

Outwater EK, Marchetto B, Wagner BJ: Virilizing tumors of the ovary: imaging features. Ultrasound Obstet Gynecol 15:365, 2000

Paladini D, Testa A, Van Holsbeke C, et al: Imaging in gynecological disease (5): clinical and ultrasound characteristics in fibroma and fibrothecoma of the ovary. Ultrasound Obstet Gynecol 34:188, 2009

Palenzuela G, Martin E, Meunier A, et al: Comprehensive staging allows for excellent outcome in patients with localized malignant germ cell tumor of the ovary. Ann Surg 248:836, 2008

Pavlakis K, Messini I, Vrekoussis T, et al: Intraoperative assessment of epithelial and non-epithelial ovarian tumors: a 7-year review. Eur J Gynaecol Oncol 30:657, 2009

Pena-Alonso R, Nieto K, Alvarez R, et al: Distribution of Y-chromosome-bearing cells in gonadoblastoma and dysgenetic testis in 45,X/46,XY infants. Mod Pathol 18:439, 2005

Pins MR, Young RH, Daly WJ, et al: Primary squamous cell carcinoma of the ovary: report of 37 cases. Am J Surg Pathol 20:823, 1996

Piura B, Nemet D, Yanai-Inbar I, et al: Granulosa cell tumor of the ovary: a study of 18 cases. J Surg Oncol 55:71, 1994

Powell JL, Connor GP, Henderson GS: Management of recurrent juvenile granulosa cell tumor of the ovary. Gynecol Oncol 81:113, 2001

Pressley RH, Muntz HG, Falkenberry S, et al: Serum lactic dehydrogenase as a tumor marker in dysgerminoma. Gynecol Oncol 44:281, 1992

Quirk JT, Natarajan N: Ovarian cancer incidence in the United States, 1992–1999. Gynecol Oncol 97:519, 2005

Ramalingam P, Malpica A, Silva EG, et al: The use of cytokeratin 7 and EMA in differentiating ovarian yolk sac tumors from endometrioid and clear cell carcinomas. Am J Surg Pathol 28:1499, 2004

Rezk Y, Sheinfeld J, Chi DS: Prolonged survival following salvage surgery for chemorefractory ovarian immature teratoma: a case report and review of the literature. Gynecol Oncol 96:883, 2005

Schneider DT, Calaminus G, Harms D, et al: Ovarian sex cord–stromal tumors in children and adolescents. J Reprod Med 50:439, 2005

Schneider DT, Calaminus G, Wessalowski R, et al: Ovarian sex cord–stromal tumors in children and adolescents. J Clin Oncol 21:2357, 2003a

Schneider DT, Janig U, Calaminus G, et al: Ovarian sex cord–stromal tumors: a clinicopathological study of 72 cases from the Kiel Pediatric Tumor Registry. Virchows Arch 443:549, 2003b

Schrader KA, Gorbatcheva B, Senz J, et al: The specificity of the FLXL2 c.402G>G somatic mutation: a survey of solid tumors [Abstract]. PLoS One 4:e7988, 2009

Schwartz PE, Morris JM: Serum lactic dehydrogenase: a tumor marker for dysgerminoma. Obstet Gynecol 72:511, 1988

Sehouli J, Drescher FS, Mustea A, et al: Granulosa cell tumor of the ovary: 10 years follow-up data of 65 patients. Anticancer Res 24:1223, 2004

Shah SP, Kobel M, Senz J, et al: Mutation of FOXL2 in granulosa-cell tumors of the ovary. N Engl J Med 360:2719, 2009

Sharony R, Aviram R, Fishman A, et al: Granulosa cell tumors of the ovary: do they have any unique ultrasonographic and color Doppler flow features? Int J Gynecol Cancer 11:229, 2001

Shimizu Y, Komiyama S, Kobayashi T, et al: Successful management of endodermal sinus tumor of the ovary associated with pregnancy. Gynecol Oncol 88:447, 2003

Siddiqui M, Toub DB: Cellular fibroma of the ovary with Meigs' syndrome and elevated CA-125: a case report. J Reprod Med 40:817, 1995

Smith HO, Berwick M, Verschraegen CF, et al: Incidence and survival rates for female malignant germ cell tumors. Obstet Gynecol 107:1075, 2006

Stettner AR, Hartenbach EM, Schink JC, et al: Familial ovarian germ cell cancer: report and review. Am J Med Genet 84:43, 1999

Stevens TA, Brown J, Zander DS, et al: Adult granulosa cell tumors of the ovary in two first-degree relatives. Gynecol Oncol 98:502, 2005

Stier EA, Barakat RR, Curtin JP, et al: Laparotomy to complete staging of presumed early ovarian cancer. Obstet Gynecol 87:737, 1996

Suita S, Shono K, Tajiri T, et al: Malignant germ cell tumors: clinical characteristics, treatment, and outcome. A report from the study group for Pediatric Solid Malignant Tumors in the Kyushu Area, Japan. J Pediatr Surg 37:1703, 2002

Takemori M, Nishimura R, Yamasaki M, et al: Ovarian mixed germ cell tumor composed of polyembryoma and immature teratoma. Gynecol Oncol 69:260, 1998

Tangir J, Zelterman D, Ma W, et al: Reproductive function after conservative surgery and chemotherapy for malignant germ cell tumors of the ovary. Obstet Gynecol 101:251, 2003

Tao X, Sood AK, Deavers MT, et al: Anti-angiogenesis therapy with bevacizumab for patients with ovarian granulosa cell tumors. Gynecol Oncol 114:431, 2009

Tay SK, Tan LK: Experience of a 2-day BEP regimen in postsurgical adjuvant chemotherapy of ovarian germ cell tumors. Int J Gynecol Cancer 10:13, 2000

Teilum G: Classification of endodermal sinus tumour (mesoblastoma vitellinum) and so-called "embryonal carcinoma" of the ovary. Acta Pathol Microbiol Scand 64:407, 1965

Tewari K, Cappuccini F, DiSaia PJ, et al: Malignant germ cell tumors of the ovary. Obstet Gynecol 95:128, 2000

Ulbright TM: Germ cell tumors of the gonads: a selective review emphasizing problems in differential diagnosis, newly appreciated, and controversial issues. Mod Pathol 18 (Suppl 2):S61, 2005

Uygun K, Aydiner A, Saip P, et al: Clinical parameters and treatment results in recurrent granulosa cell tumor of the ovary. Gynecol Oncol 88:400, 2003

Vang R, Herrmann ME, Tavassoli FA: Comparative immunohistochemical analysis of granulosa and Sertoli components in ovarian sex cord–stromal tumors with mixed differentiation: potential implications for derivation of Sertoli differentiation in ovarian tumors. Int J Gynecol Pathol 23:151, 2004

Vicus D, Beiner ME, Klachook S, et al: Pure dysgerminoma of the ovary 35 years on: a single institutional experience. Gynecol Oncol 117:23, 2010

Williams S, Blessing JA, Liao SY, et al: Adjuvant therapy of ovarian germ cell tumors with cisplatin, etoposide, and bleomycin: a trial of the Gynecologic Oncology Group. J Clin Oncol 12:701, 1994a

Williams SD, Birch R, Einhorn LH, et al: Treatment of disseminated germ cell tumors with cisplatin, bleomycin, and either vinblastine or etoposide. N Engl J Med 316:1435, 1987

Williams SD, Blessing JA, DiSaia PJ, et al: Second-look laparotomy in ovarian germ cell tumors: the Gynecologic Oncology Group experience. Gynecol Oncol 52:287, 1994b

Williams SD, Blessing JA, Hatch KD, et al: Chemotherapy of advanced dysgerminoma: trials of the Gynecologic Oncology Group. J Clin Oncol 9:1950, 1991

Williams SD, Kauderer J, Burnett AF, et al: Adjuvant therapy of completely resected dysgerminoma with carboplatin and etoposide: a trial of the Gynecologic Oncology Group. Gynecol Oncol 95:496, 2004

Wolf JK, Mullen J, Eifel PJ, et al: Radiation treatment of advanced or recurrent granulosa cell tumor of the ovary. Gynecol Oncol 73:35, 1999

Young JL Jr, Cheng W, X, Roffers SD, et al: Ovarian cancer in children and young adults in the United States, 1992-1997. Cancer 97:2694, 2003

Young RH: Sex cord–stromal tumors of the ovary and testis: their similarities and differences with consideration of selected problems. Mod Pathol 18:S81, 2005

Young RH, Dudley AG, Scully RE: Granulosa cell, Sertoli–Leydig cell, and unclassified sex cord–stromal tumors associated with pregnancy: a clinicopathological analysis of thirty-six cases. Gynecol Oncol 18:181, 1984

Young RH, Scully RE: Ovarian Sertoli–Leydig cell tumors: a clinicopathological analysis of 207 cases. Am J Surg Pathol 9:543, 1985

Young RH, Welch WR, Dickersin GR, et al: Ovarian sex cord tumor with annular tubules: review of 74 cases including 27 with Peutz-Jeghers syndrome and four with adenoma malignum of the cervix. Cancer 50:1384, 1982

Yuan JQ, Lin XN, Xu JY, et al: Ovarian juvenile granulosa cell tumor associated with Maffucci's syndrome: case report. Chin Med J 117:1592, 2004

Zagame L, Pautier P, Duvillard P, et al: Growing teratoma syndrome after ovarian germ cell tumors. Obstet Gynecol 108:509, 2006

Zaloudek C, Norris HJ: Sertoli-Leydig tumors of the ovary: a clinicopathologic study of 64 intermediate and poorly differentiated neoplasms. Am J Surg Pathol 8:405, 1984

Zanagnolo V, Pasinetti B, Sartori E: Clinical review of 63 cases of sex cord stromal tumors. Eur J Gynaecol Oncol 25:431, 2004

Zanetta G, Bonazzi C, Cantu M, et al: Survival and reproductive function after treatment of malignant germ cell ovarian tumors. J Clin Oncol 19:1015, 2001

Zhang M, Cheung MK, Shin JY, et al: Prognostic factors responsible for survival in sex cord stromal tumors of the ovary—an analysis of 376 women. Gynecol Oncol 104:396, 2007

Zhao XY, Huang HF, Lian LJ, et al: Ovarian cancer in pregnancy: a clinicopathologic analysis of 22 cases and review of the literature. Int J Gynecol Cancer 16:8, 2006

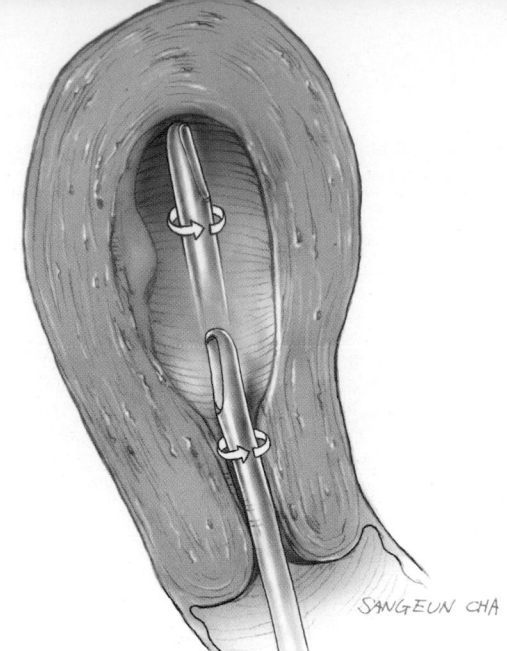

SANGEUN CHA

Gestational Trophoblastic Disease

Gestational trophoblastic disease refers to a spectrum of interrelated but histologically distinct tumors originating from the placenta (Table 37-1). These diseases are characterized by a reliable tumor marker, which is the β-subunit of human chorionic gonadotropin (β-hCG), and have varying tendencies toward local invasion and spread.

Gestational trophoblastic neoplasia (GTN) refers to the subset of gestational trophoblastic disease that develops malignant sequelae. These tumors require formal staging and typically respond favorably to chemotherapy. Most commonly, GTN develops after a molar pregnancy, but may follow any gestation.

The prognosis for most cases of GTN is excellent, and patients are routinely cured even in the presence of widespread metastases. The outlook for preservation of fertility and for successful subsequent pregnancy outcomes is equally bright (Garrett, 2008). Accordingly, although gestational trophoblastic disease is uncommon, because the opportunity for cure is great, clinicians should be familiar with its presentation, diagnosis, and management.

EPIDEMIOLOGY AND RISK FACTORS

Incidence

The incidence of gestational trophoblastic disease has remained fairly constant at approximately 1 to 2 per 1000 deliveries in North America and Europe (Drake, 2006; Loukovaara, 2005; Savage, 2010; Smith, 2003). A similar frequency has been observed in South Africa and Turkey (Moodley, 2003; Ozalp, 2003). Although historically higher incidence rates have been reported in parts of Asia, this may have largely reflected discrepancies between population-based and hospital-based data collection. For example, a South Korean population-based study noted a drop in the incidence from 40 per 1000 deliveries to 2 per 1000 that was coincident with refinement in disease terminology and classification (Kim, 2004). Similarly, hospital-based studies in Japan and Singapore have shown a decreased incidence (Chong, 1999; Matsui, 2003). Improved socioeconomic conditions and dietary changes may be partly responsible as well. Some ethnic groups, however, appear to be at higher risk of developing gestational trophoblastic disease. Hispanics and Native Americans living in the United States reportedly have an increased incidence, as do certain

TABLE 37-1. Modified World Health Organization Classification of Gestational Trophoblastic Disease

Hydatidiform moles
Hydatidiform mole
  Complete
  Partial
Invasive mole

Trophoblastic tumors
Choriocarcinoma
Placental site trophoblastic tumor
Epithelioid trophoblastic tumor

Modified from Ie-Ming, 2011, with permission.

population groups living in Southeast Asia (Drake, 2006; Smith, 2003; Tham, 2003).

Maternal Age

Maternal age at the upper and lower extremes has been found to carry a higher risk of gestational trophoblastic disease (Altman, 2008; Loukovaara, 2005; Tham, 2003). This association is much greater for complete moles, whereas the risk of partial molar pregnancy varies relatively little with age. Moreover, compared with the risk of those with maternal age of 15 years or younger, the degree of risk is much greater for women 45 years (1 percent) or older (17 percent at age 50) (Savage, 2010; Sebire, 2002a). One explanation may relate to ova from older women having higher rates of abnormal fertilization. Similarly, older paternal age has also been associated with increased risk (La Vecchia, 1984; Parazzini, 1986).

Obstetric History

In addition to age, a history of prior unsuccessful pregnancies increases the risk of gestational trophoblastic disease. For example, previous spontaneous abortion at least doubles the risk of molar pregnancy (Parazzini, 1991). More significant, a personal history of gestational trophoblastic disease increases the risk of developing a molar gestation in a subsequent pregnancy by at least 10-fold.

The frequency in a subsequent conception is approximately 1 percent, and most cases mirror the same type of mole as the preceding pregnancy (Garrett, 2008; Sebire, 2003). Furthermore, following two episodes of molar pregnancy, 23 percent of later conceptions result in another molar gestation (Berkowitz, 1998). For this reason, women with a prior history of gestational trophoblastic disease should undergo first-trimester sonographic examination in subsequent pregnancies. Familial molar pregnancies, however, are exceedingly rare (Fallahian, 2003).

Other Factors

In several case-control studies, oral contraceptive pill use has been associated with an increased risk of gestational trophoblastic disease. Specifically, prior oral contraceptive pill use approximately doubles the risk, and a longer duration of use also seems to correlate positively with risk (Palmer, 1999; Parazzini, 2002). Moreover, women who used oral contraceptive pills during the cycle in which they became pregnant appear to have a higher risk in some but not all studies (Costa, 2006; Palmer, 1999). Many of these associations, however, are weak and could be explained by confounding factors other than causality (Parazzini, 2002).

Certain other epidemiologic characteristics also appear to differ markedly between complete and partial moles. For example, vitamin A deficiency and low dietary intake of carotene are associated with an increased risk of only complete moles (Berkowitz, 1985, 1995; Parazzini, 1988). Partial moles have been linked to higher educational levels, smoking, irregular menstrual cycles, and obstetric histories in which only male infants are among the prior live births (Berkowitz, 1995; Parazzini, 1986).

HYDATIDIFORM MOLE (MOLAR PREGNANCY)

Hydatidiform moles are abnormal pregnancies characterized histologically by aberrant changes within the placenta. Classically, the chorionic villi in these placenta show varying degrees of trophoblastic proliferation and edema of the villous stroma (Fig. 37-1). Based on the degree and extent of the tissue changes, hydatidiform moles are categorized as either *complete hydatidiform moles* or *partial hydatidiform moles* (Table 37-2). Cytogenetic

TABLE 37-2. Features of Complete and Partial Hydatidiform Moles

Feature	Complete Mole	Partial Mole
Karyotype	46,XX or 46,XY	69,XXX or 69,XXY
Pathology		
Fetus/embryo	Absent	Present
Villous edema	Diffuse	Focal
Trophoblastic proliferation	Variable, may be marked	Focal and minimal
p57Kip2 immunostaining	Negative	Positive
Clinical presentation		
Typical diagnosis	Molar gestation	Missed abortion
Postmolar malignant sequelae	15%	4–6%

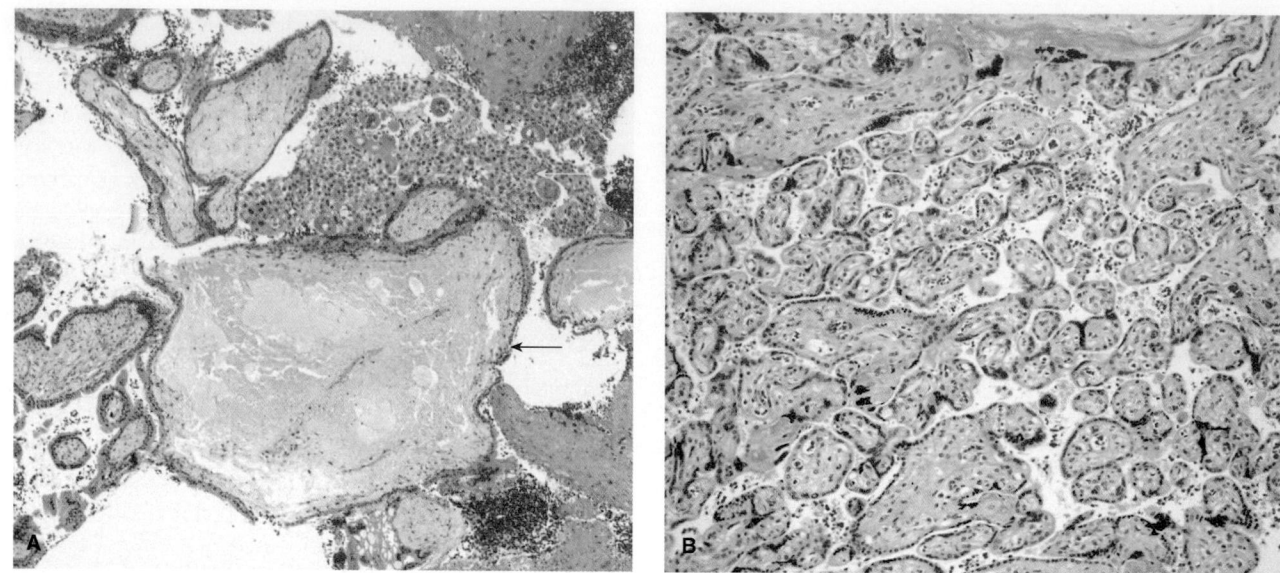

FIGURE 37-1 A. Complete hydatidiform mole. Complete moles are characterized by diffuse placental villous edema, which produces villous enlargement and cistern formation in some villi (*black arrow*). This striking villous edema is the etiology of the vesicle-like villous morphology noted grossly in complete moles (see Fig. 37-3). Complete moles also typically show trophoblastic proliferation (*yellow arrow*), which may be focal or widespread. *(Photograph contributed by Dr. Erika Fong.)* **B.** Normal term placenta showing smaller, nonedematous villi and absence of trophoblastic proliferation. *(Photograph contributed by Dr. Kelley Carrick.)*

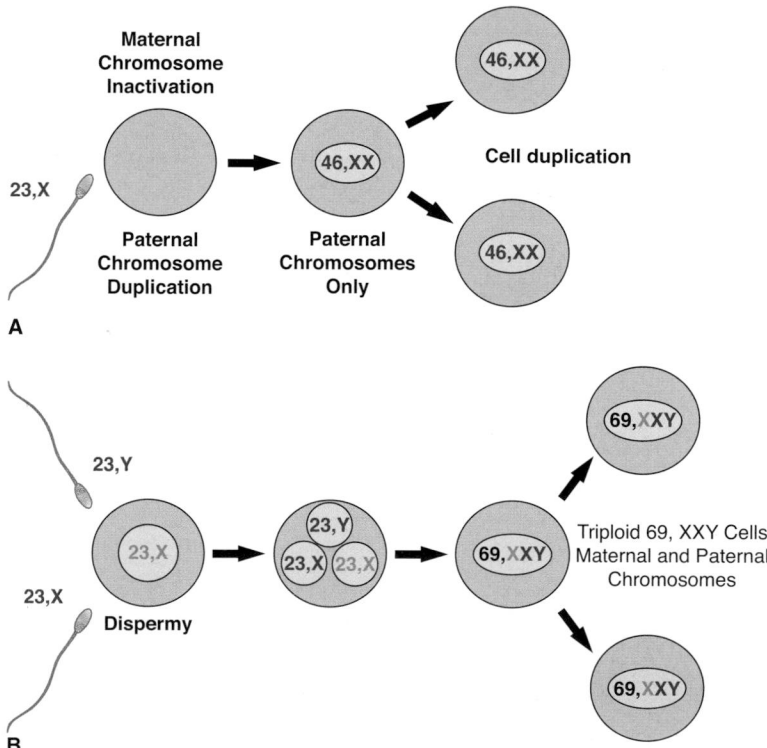

FIGURE 37-2 A. A 46,XX complete mole may be formed if a 23,X-bearing haploid sperm penetrates a 23,X-containing haploid egg whose genes have become "inactive." Paternal chromosomes then duplicate to create a 46,XX diploid chromosomal complement solely of paternal origin. Alternatively, this same type of inactivated egg can be fertilized independently by two sperm, either 23,X- or 23,Y-bearing, to create a 46,XX or 46,XY chromosomal complement, again of paternal origin only. **B.** Partial moles may be formed if two sperm, either 23,X- or 23,Y-bearing, both fertilize a 23,X-containing haploid egg, whose genes have not been inactivated. The resulting fertilized egg is triploid. Alternatively, a similar haploid egg may be fertilized by an unreduced diploid 46,XY sperm.

studies have shown that chromosomal abnormalities play an integral role in the development of hydatidiform moles (Lage, 1992).

Complete Hydatidiform Mole

Karyotyping and Histology

Classically, these molar pregnancies differ from partial moles with regard to their karyotype, their histologic appearance, and their clinical presentation.

Complete moles typically have a complete diploid karyotype, and 85 to 90 percent of cases are 46,XX. The chromosomes, however, in these pregnancies are entirely of paternal origin. In a process termed *androgenesis*, the ovum is fertilized by a haploid sperm, which then duplicates its own chromosomes after meiosis (Fig. 37-2) (Fan, 2002; Kajii, 1977). Most of these moles are 46,XX, but dispermic fertilization of a single ovum can produce a 46,XY karyotype (Lawler, 1987). Although nuclear DNA is entirely paternal, mitochondrial DNA remains maternal in origin (Azuma, 1991).

Microscopically, complete moles display enlarged, edematous villi and abnormal trophoblastic proliferation that diffusely involve the entire placenta (see Fig. 37-1). Macroscopically, these changes transform the chorionic villi into clusters of vesicles with variable dimensions. Indeed, the name *hydatidiform mole* stems from this "bunch of grapes" appearance. In these pregnancies, no fetal tissue or amnion is produced. As a result, this mass of placental tissue completely fills the endometrial cavity (Fig. 37-3).

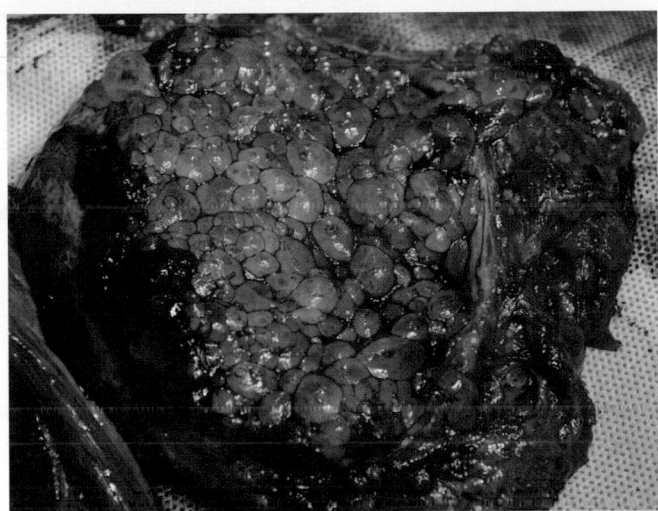

FIGURE 37-3 Photograph of a complete hydatidiform mole specimen. Note the grape-like fluid-filled clusters of chorionic villi. *(Photograph contributed by Dr. Sasha Andrews.)*

Clinical Findings

The clinical presentation of a complete mole has changed considerably over the past few decades. More than half of patients diagnosed in the 1960s and 1970s had anemia and uterine sizes in excess of that predicted for their gestational age. In addition, hyperemesis gravidarum, preeclampsia, and theca-lutein cysts developed in approximately one quarter of women (Montz, 1988; Soto-Wright, 1995). As described in Chapter 9 (p. 266), theca-lutein cysts develop with prolonged exposure to luteinizing hormone (LH) or β-hCG (Fig. 37-4). These cysts may range in size from 3 to 20 cm, and most regress with falling β-hCG titers after molar evacuation. If present, and especially if bilateral, the risk of postmolar GTN is increased.

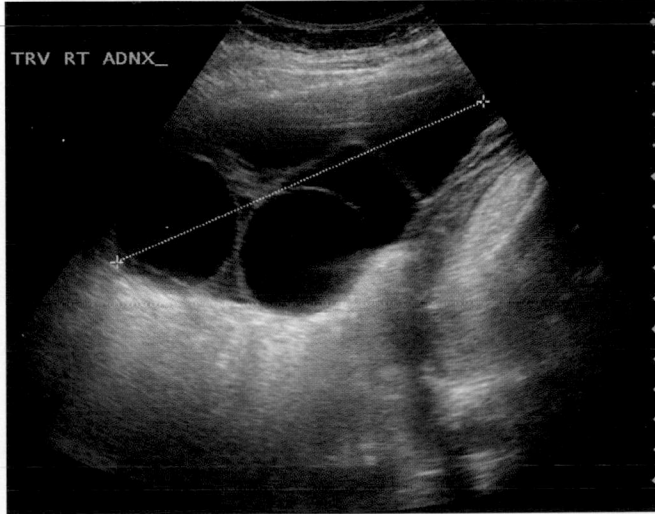

FIGURE 37-4 Transvaginal sonogram of multiple theca lutein cysts within one ovary of a woman with a complete molar pregnancy. Bilateral, multiple simple cysts are characteristic findings. *(Image contributed by Dr. Diane Twickler.)*

Complete moles, however, infrequently present today with these traditional signs and symptoms (Ben-Arie, 2009; Mangili, 2008). As a result of β-hCG testing and sonography, the mean gestational age at evacuation currently approximates 12 weeks, compared with 16 to 17 weeks in the 1960s and 1970s (Drake, 2006; Soto-Wright, 1995). Vaginal bleeding remains the most common symptom, and β-hCG levels are commonly greater than expected. One quarter of women will present with uterine size greater than dates, but the incidence of anemia is less than 10 percent. Moreover, hyperemesis gravidarum, preeclampsia, and symptomatic theca-lutein cysts are rarely observed (Lazarus, 1999; Mosher, 1998; Soto-Wright, 1995). Currently, these sequelae typically develop chiefly in patients without early prenatal care who present with a more advanced gestational age and markedly elevated serum β-hCG levels.

Plasma thyroxine levels are often increased in women with complete moles, but clinical hyperthyroidism is infrequent. In these circumstances, serum free thyroxine levels are elevated as a consequence of the thyrotropin-like effect of β-hCG (Chap. 15, p. 401) (Hershman, 2004).

Partial Hydatidiform Mole

These moles vary from complete hydatidiform moles clinically, genetically, and histologically. The degree and extent of trophoblastic proliferation and villous edema is decreased compared with that of complete moles. Moreover, most partial moles contain fetal tissue and amnion, in addition to placental tissues.

As a result, patients with partial moles typically present with signs and symptoms of an incomplete or missed abortion. Most women will have vaginal bleeding, but because trophoblastic proliferation is slight and only focal, uterine enlargement in excess of gestational age is uncommon. Similarly, preeclampsia, theca-lutein cysts, hyperthyroidism, or other dramatic clinical features are rare (Stefos, 2002). Preevacuation β-hCG levels are typically much lower than those for complete moles and often do not exceed 100,000 mIU per milliliter. For this reason, partial moles are often not identified until after a histologic review of a curettage specimen.

Partial moles have a triploid karyotype (69,XXX, 69,XXY, or less commonly 69,XYY) that is composed of one maternal and two paternal haploid sets of chromosomes (see Fig. 37-2) (Lawler, 1991). Nontriploid partial moles have been reported, but probably do not actually exist (Genest, 2002b). The coexisting fetus present with a partial mole is nonviable and typically has multiple malformations with abnormal growth (Jauniaux, 1999).

Diagnosis
β-hCG Measurement

In reproductive-aged women with vaginal bleeding, diagnoses may include gynecologic causes of bleeding and complications of first-trimester pregnancy. An important characteristic of molar pregnancy is its tendency to produce β-hCG in excess of that expected for the gestational age (Fig. 6-3, p. 176) (Sasaki, 2003). β-hCG is produced by trophoblast, and elevated levels reflect their proliferation. Accordingly, initial urine or serum β-hCG measurement and transvaginal sonography are invaluable in

SECTION 4

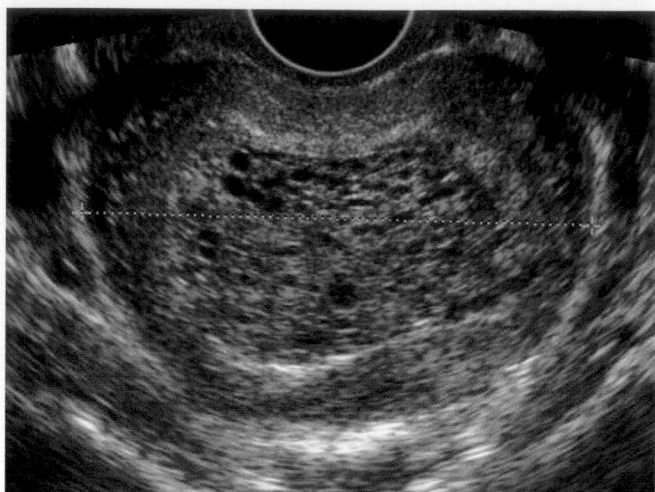

FIGURE 37-5 Transverse sonographic view of a uterus with a complete hydatidiform mole. The classic "snowstorm" appearance is created by the multiple placental vesicles. The mole completely fills this uterine cavity, and calipers are placed on the outer uterine borders.

guiding evaluation. And because of these, first-trimester diagnosis of hydatidiform mole is now common.

Transvaginal Sonography

Although β-hCG levels are helpful, the diagnosis of molar pregnancy is more frequently found sonographically because of the identifiable diffuse swelling and enlargement of the chorionic villi. Most first-trimester complete moles demonstrate a typical sonographic appearance: a complex, echogenic, intrauterine mass containing many small cystic spaces. Fetal tissues and amnionic sac are absent (Fig. 37-5) (Benson, 2000). In contrast, sonographic features of a partial molar pregnancy include a thickened, hydropic placenta with a concomitant fetus (Zhou, 2005).

Despite the utility of these tools, there are diagnostic limitations. For example, Lazarus and colleagues (1999) reported that β-hCG levels in early molar pregnancies may not always be elevated in the first trimester. These same investigators also found that sonography could lead to a false-negative diagnosis if performed at very early gestational ages, before the chorionic villi have attained their characteristic vesicular pattern. For example, only 20 to 30 percent of patients may have sonographic evidence to suspect a partial mole (Johns, 2005; Lindholm, 1999; Sebire, 2001). Consequently, the preoperative diagnosis in early gestations is usually difficult and commonly is not made until after a histologic review of the abortal specimen.

Histopathology

In early pregnancy, it may be histologically difficult to distinguish among complete moles, partial moles, and hydropic abortuses. The histopathologic changes typical of a complete and partial mole are listed in Table 37-2. Hydropic abortuses are pregnancies formed by the traditional union of one haploid egg and one haploid sperm but are pregnancies that have failed. Their placentas may display hydropic degeneration,

which can mimic some villous features of hydatidiform moles. Unfortunately, there is no single criterion that distinguishes these three. But, in general, complete moles characteristically have two prominent features: (1) trophoblastic proliferation and (2) hydropic villi. There are striking differences, however, from these classic findings in gestations younger than 10 weeks. In these early gestations, hydropic villi may not be apparent, and molar stroma may still be vascular (Paradinas, 1997). As a result, complete moles must now often be characterized by more subtle morphologic alterations. Unfortunately, this can result in their misclassification as partial moles or nonmolar hydropic abortuses (Fukunaga, 2005; Mosher, 1998). Partial moles are reliably diagnosed when three or four major diagnostic criteria are demonstrated: (1) two populations of villi, (2) enlarged, irregular, dysmorphic villi (with trophoblast inclusions), (3) enlarged, cavitated villi (≥3-4 mm), and (4) syncytiotrophoblast hyperplasia/atypia (Chew, 2000). Good diagnostic reproducibility can still be achieved in most circumstances using these histologic distinctions of complete and partial mole.

Ploidy Determination

Determination of the type of molar gestation can clearly be enhanced by combining histopathology with determination of ploidy, that is, the number of complete sets of chromosomes. *Flow cytometry* is a technique for counting, examining, and sorting cells that are suspended in a stream of fluid. With this tool, multiple physical or chemical characteristics of single cells can be simultaneously analyzed as they flow through an optical electronic detection apparatus. A second cytometry method, *automated image cytometry*, uses optical images of several hundred cell nuclei to identify subtle morphologic changes within tissues. Both techniques can analyze cellular ploidy and can be used to distinguish complete moles (diploid) from partial moles (triploid) (Fig. 37-6). Automated image cytometry, however, has been shown to be more sensitive than flow cytometry in making this distinction (Crisp, 2003).

Immunostaining

In addition to ploidy analysis, histologic immunostaining techniques can also clarify the diagnosis. p57KIP2 is a nuclear protein whose gene is paternally imprinted and maternally expressed. This means that the gene product is produced only in tissues containing a maternal allele. Because complete moles contain only paternal genes, the p57KIP2 protein is absent in complete moles (Merchant, 2005). In contrast, this nuclear protein is strongly expressed in normal placentas, spontaneous pregnancy losses with hydropic change, and partial hydatidiform moles (Castrillon, 2001). Accordingly, immunostaining for this nuclear protein is a practical and accurate adjunct to ploidy analysis in the pathologic classification of hydatidiform moles (Castrillon, 2001; Genest, 2002a; Jun, 2003). p57KIP2 staining has the additional advantage of differentiating hydropic abortuses from complete moles, a distinction not made by ploidy analysis (Merchant, 2005). As a result, complementary use of ploidy analysis and p57KIP2 status can now help to distinguish among a diploid hydropic spontaneous abortion (p57KIP2-positive), diploid complete mole (p57KIP2-negative),

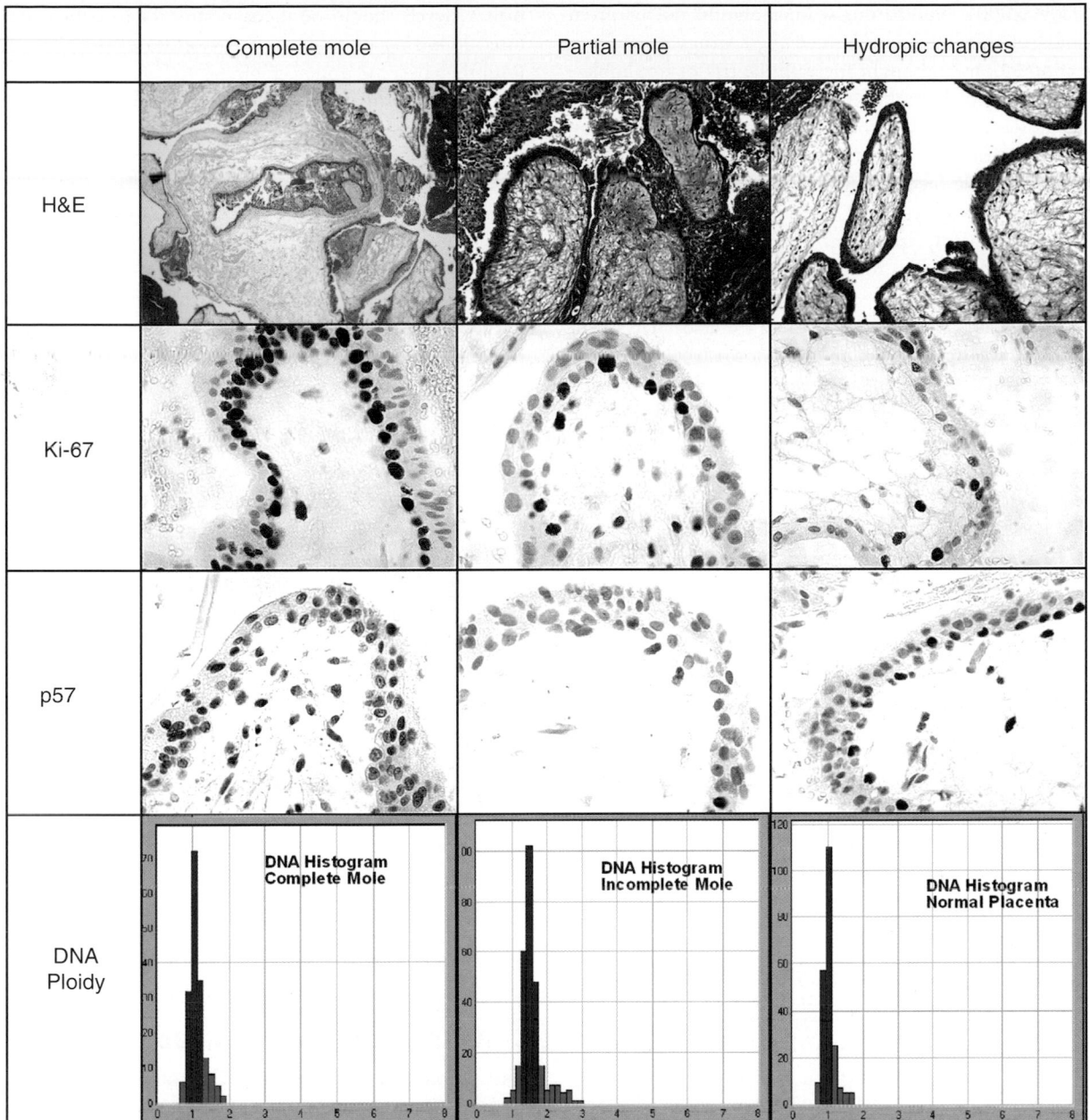

FIGURE 37-6 Composite diagram of differences between normal hydropic abortuses and partial or complete hydatidiform moles. Tissues that are negative for staining are blue, whereas those positive for staining are brown. The extent (percent of cells staining) equates to low, medium, or high expression. Note the progressive increase in Ki-67 and a progressive reduction in p57KIP2 (p57) staining when comparing normal hydropic products of conception with partial and complete moles. First, Ki-67 is a proliferation marker and is most prominently expressed in complete moles. In contrast, p57 is a nuclear protein whose gene is paternally imprinted and maternally expressed, meaning that the gene product is produced only in tissues containing a maternal allele. Because complete moles contain only paternal genes, the p57 protein is absent in complete moles. However, this nuclear protein is strongly expressed in spontaneous pregnancy losses with hydropic change. Finally, the DNA ploidy graphs show normal diploid pattern in hydropic abortuses and in complete moles, whereas the DNA peak is triploid (DNA index 1.5) in partial moles. (*Image contributed by Dr. Raheela Ashfaq.*)

and triploid partial mole (p57KIP2-positive) (see Fig. 37-6) (Crisp, 2003).

In summary, most complete and partial moles are readily identifiable histologically and present little diagnostic difficulty. Those with borderline histology can be resampled in an attempt to confirm the classic features shown in Table 37-2. Ancillary testing with ploidy analysis or p57KIP2 staining is useful for diagnostic, educational, and quality assurance purposes, but

these adjunctive tests should not become the mandatory gold standard for routine clinical practice, because they are neither perfect nor universally available (Genest, 2001).

■ Treatment

Suction curettage is the preferred method of evacuation regardless of uterine size in patients who wish to remain fertile (Soper,

2004; Tidy, 2000). Nulliparous women should not be given prostanoids to ripen the cervix since these drugs can induce uterine contractions and might increase the risk of trophoblastic embolization to the pulmonary vasculature (Seckl, 2010). Hysterectomy is rarely recommended unless the patient wishes surgical sterilization or is approaching menopause (Elias, 2010). Symptomatic theca-lutein ovarian cysts are an unusual finding and tend to regress after molar evacuation. In extreme cases, these may be aspirated, but oophorectomy should not be performed except when torsion leads to extensive ovarian infarction (Mungan, 1996).

Prior to surgery, patients are evaluated for associated medical complications. Fortunately, thyroid storm from untreated hyperthyroidism, respiratory insufficiency from trophoblastic emboli, and other severe coexisting conditions are rare. Because of the tremendous vascularity of these placentas, blood products should be available prior to the evacuation of larger moles, and adequate infusion lines established.

At the beginning of the evacuation, the cervix is dilated to admit a 10- to 12-mm plastic suction curette. As aspiration of molar tissues ensues, intravenous oxytocin is given. At our institution, 20 units of synthetic oxytocin are mixed with 1 L of crystalloid and infused at rates to achieve uterine contraction. In some cases, intraoperative sonography may be indicated to help reduce the risk of uterine perforation and assist in confirming complete evacuation. Finally, a thorough, gentle curettage is performed.

Following curettage, because of the possibility of partial mole and its attendant fetal tissue, Rh immune globulin should be given to nonsensitized Rh D-negative women. Rh immune globulin, however, may be withheld if the diagnosis of complete mole is certain (Fung Kee, 2003).

Postmolar Surveillance

Postmolar Gestational Trophoblastic Neoplasia

Gestational trophoblastic neoplasia develops after evacuation in 15 percent of complete moles (Golfier, 2007; Wolfberg, 2004). Despite the trend of diagnosing these abnormal pregnancies at earlier gestational ages, this incidence has not decreased (Seckl, 2004). Of those women who develop GTN, three quarters have locally invasive molar disease and the remaining one quarter develop metastases.

In contrast, GTN develops in only 4 to 6 percent of partial moles following evacuation (Feltmate, 2006; Lavie, 2005). The lower reported incidence (0.5 to 1.0 percent) of GTN following partial mole in the United Kingdom may reflect more stringent diagnostic criteria (Hancock, 2006; Seckl, 2000). Malignant transformation into metastatic choriocarcinoma does occur after partial mole evacuation, but fortunately this is exceedingly rare (0.1 percent) (Cheung, 2004; Seckl, 2000).

Surveillance Practices

No pathologic or clinical features at presentation accurately predict which patients will ultimately develop GTN. Because of the trophoblastic proliferation that characterizes these neoplasms, serial serum β-hCG levels following evacuation can be used to effectively monitor patients for development of GTN. Therefore, postmolar surveillance with serial quantitative serum β-hCG levels should be the standard. Titers should be monitored following uterine evacuation at least every 1 to 2 weeks until they become undetectable.

After achieving undetectable β-hCG levels, it is generally recommended that monthly levels be drawn during 6 months of surveillance for all patients with molar gestation (Sebire, 2007). However, poor compliance with prolonged monitoring has been reported—especially among indigent women and certain ethnic groups in the United States (Allen, 2003; Massad, 2000). A single blood sample demonstrating an undetectable level of β-hCG following molar evacuation is sufficient to exclude the possibility of progression to GTN in most patients. Thus, some women, especially those with a partial mole, may be safely discharged from routine surveillance once an undetectable value is achieved (Batorfi, 2004; Feltmate, 2003; Lavie, 2005; Wolfberg, 2004). Shortened surveillance could enable women to attempt a subsequent pregnancy sooner. However, GTN may still rarely develop after an hCG level has returned to normal, potentially leading to increased morbidity (Kerkmeijer, 2007; Sebire, 2007).

When pregnancies occur during the monitoring period, the resulting normal β-hCG production can hinder detection of postmolar progression to GTN (Allen, 2003). But other than complicating the monitoring schedule, these pregnancies fortunately are otherwise uneventful (Tuncer, 1999). To prevent difficulties with interpretation, women are encouraged to use effective contraception until achieving a β-hCG titer less than 5 mIU/mL or below the threshold of the individual assay. Oral contraceptive pills decrease the likelihood of pregnancy compared with less effective barrier contraception and do not increase the risk of GTN (Costa, 2006; Gaffield, 2009). Injectable medroxyprogesterone acetate is particularly useful when poor compliance is anticipated (Massad, 2000). In contrast, intrauterine devices are not be inserted until the β-hCG level is undetectable because of the risk of uterine perforation if an invasive mole is present.

Prophylactic Chemotherapy

The purpose of administering chemotherapy at the time of molar evacuation is mainly to prevent GTN development in high-risk patients who are unlikely to be compliant or for whom β-hCG surveillance is not available. In clinical practice, the correct classification of high-risk complete moles, however, is extremely difficult, as there is no universally accepted combination of risk factors that accurately predict GTN development. Typical patients have complete moles and multiple risk factors, such as age greater than 40 years, previous history of molar pregnancy, or an excessively high β-hCG titer prior to evacuation. Regardless of how a high-risk complete mole is defined, few women will be ultimately be assigned to this group, and fatalities have been described using prophylactic chemotherapy (Soper, 2004). Thus, identification of women who could potentially benefit is of marginal clinical importance. For this reason, prophylactic chemotherapy is not routinely offered in the United States and Europe.

However, a single dose of dactinomycin has been shown to reduce the incidence of postmolar GTN in certain populations. For example, in a prospective, double-blinded clinical trial of 60 women who had high-risk complete moles,

Limpongsanurak and associates (2001) randomly assigned Thai women to receive either prophylactic dactinomycin or placebo at the time of evacuation. Treatment reduced the incidence of GTN from 50 percent to 14 percent, but toxicity was significant. As a result, prophylactic chemotherapy is generally only used in those countries with limited resources to reliably monitor patients after evacuation (Uberti, 2009).

Ectopic Molar Pregnancy

The true incidence of ectopic gestational trophoblastic disease approximates 1.5 per 1 million births (Gillespie, 2004). More than 90 percent of suspected cases will reflect an overdiagnosis of florid extravillous trophoblastic proliferation in the fallopian tube (Burton, 2001; Sebire, 2005b). Other sites of ectopic implantation are even less common (Bailey, 2003). As with any ectopic pregnancy, initial management usually involves surgical removal of the conceptus and histopathologic evaluation.

Coexistent Fetus

The estimated incidence of twin pregnancy consisting of hydatidiform mole and a coexisting fetus is 1 per 20,000 to 100,000 pregnancies (Fig. 37-7). Sebire and colleagues (2002b) described the outcome of 77 twin pregnancies, each composed of a complete mole and a healthy co-twin. Of this group, 24 women chose to have an elective termination, and 53 continued their pregnancies. Twenty-three gestations spontaneously aborted at less than 24 weeks, two were terminated due to severe preeclampsia, and 28 pregnancies lasted at least 24 weeks—resulting in 20 live births. The authors demonstrated that coexisting complete moles and healthy co-twin pregnancies have a high risk of spontaneous abortion, but approximately 40 percent result in live births. The risk of progression to GTN was 16 percent in first-trimester terminations and not significantly higher (21 percent) in women who continued their pregnancies. Because the risk of malignancy is unchanged with advancement of gestational age, pregnancy continuation may be allowed, provided that severe maternal complications are controlled and fetal growth is normal. Fetal karyotyping to confirm a normal fetal chromosomal pattern is also recommended (Marcorelles, 2005; Matsui, 2000).

GESTATIONAL TROPHOBLASTIC NEOPLASIA

This term primarily encompasses pathologic entities that are characterized by aggressive invasion of the endometrium and myometrium by trophoblastic cells. Histologic categories include common tumors such as the invasive mole and gestational choriocarcinoma, as well as the rare placental-site trophoblastic tumor and epithelioid trophoblastic tumor. Although these histologic types have been characterized and described, in most cases of GTN no tissue is available for pathologic study. For this reason, most cases of GTN are diagnosed based on elevated β-hCG levels and managed clinically.

Gestational trophoblastic neoplasia typically develops with or follows some form of pregnancy, but occasionally the antecedent gestation cannot be confirmed with certainty. Many of the reported nonmolar cases may actually represent disease due to an unrecognized early molar pregnancy (Sebire, 2005a). Most cases follow a hydatidiform mole. Rarely, GTN develops after a live birth, miscarriage, or termination.

Histologic Classification
Invasive Mole

This is a common manifestation of GTN characterized by whole chorionic villi that accompany excessive trophoblastic overgrowth and invasion. These tissues penetrate deep into the myometrium, sometimes to involve the peritoneum, adjacent parametrium, or vaginal vault. Such moles are locally invasive, but generally lack the pronounced tendency to develop widespread metastases typical of choriocarcinoma. Invasive moles originate almost exclusively from complete or partial molar gestations (Sebire, 2005a).

Gestational Choriocarcinoma

This extremely malignant tumor is comprised of sheets of anaplastic cytotrophoblast cells and syncytiotrophoblast with prominent hemorrhage, necrosis, and vascular invasion (Fig. 37-8). Unlike molar disease, however, formed chorionic villi are characteristically absent. Gestational choriocarcinomas initially

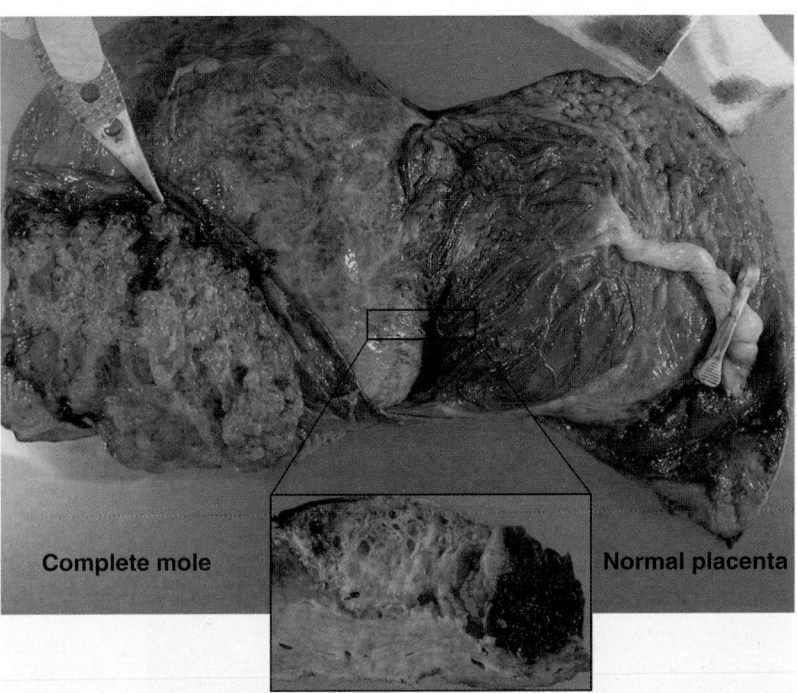

FIGURE 37-7 Photograph of placentas from a twin pregnancy with one normal twin and with a complete mole. The complete mole (*left*) shows the characteristic vesicular structure. The placenta on the *right* appears grossly normal. A transverse section through the border between these two is shown (*inset*). (*Photograph contributed by Drs. April Bleich and Brian Levenson.*)

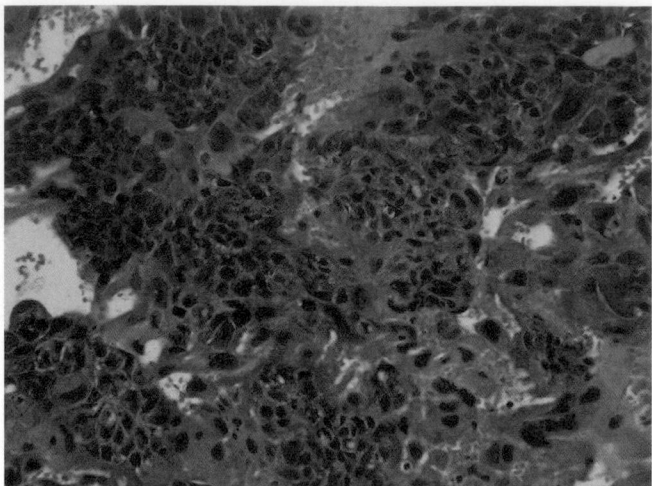

FIGURE 37-8 Photomicrograph of choriocarcinoma. Characteristic histologic features include abnormal cytotrophoblastic proliferation capped by syncytiotrophoblast. These tumors are very vascular; note abundant blood in the background. *(Photograph contributed by Dr. Raheela Ashfaq.)*

invade the endometrium and myometrium, but tend to develop early blood-borne systemic metastases (Fig. 37-9).

Although most cases develop following evacuation of a molar pregnancy, these tumors may also less commonly follow a nonmolar pregnancy. Alternatively, primary "nongestational" choriocarcinoma ovarian germ cell tumors, although rare, have an identical histologic appearance and are in part distinguished by the absence of any preceding pregnancy event (Chap. 36, p. 884) (Lee, 2009).

Gestational choriocarcinoma develops in approximately 1 in 30,000 nonmolar pregnancies. Two thirds of such cases follow term pregnancies, and one third develop after a spontaneous

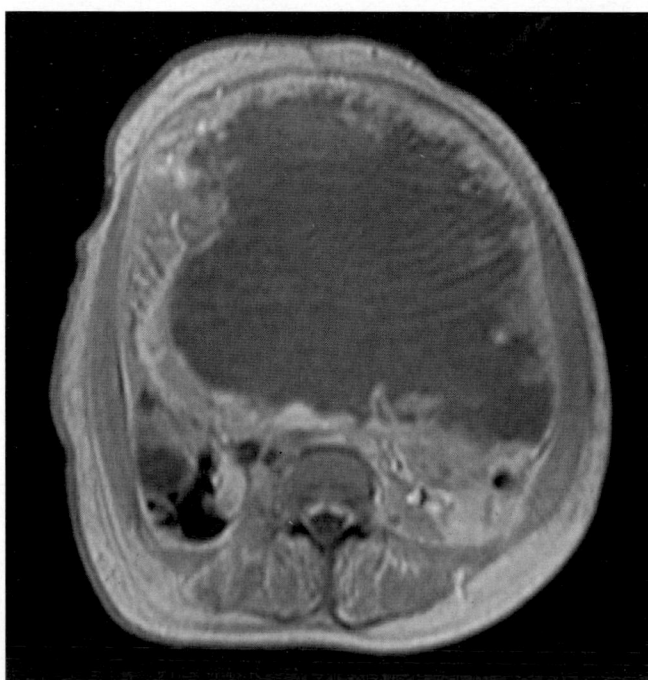

FIGURE 37-9 Computed-tomography (CT) scan of choriocarcinoma invading the uterus.

abortion or pregnancy termination. Tidy and coworkers (1995) reviewed data from 100 patients with nonmolar gestational choriocarcinoma and found that 62 presented after a live birth, 6 after a live birth preceded by a molar pregnancy, and 32 after a nonmolar abortion. Vaginal bleeding was the most common symptom in all groups. For this reason, abnormal bleeding for more than 6 weeks following any pregnancy should be evaluated with β-hCG testing to exclude a new pregnancy or GTN (Soper, 2004).

When choriocarcinoma is diagnosed after a live birth, the antecedent pregnancy is usually found to have proceeded normally to term. For example, Rodabaugh and colleagues (1998) found that in 89 percent of cases, the preceding pregnancy had produced an uncomplicated live birth. Hydrops, however, was a notable complication in the remaining fetuses. Occasionally, unanticipated choriocarcinoma is detected in an otherwise normal-appearing placenta at delivery. More commonly, however, the diagnosis of choriocarcinoma is delayed for months due to subtle signs and symptoms of disease. Most patients ultimately present with metrorrhagia and high β-hCG levels (Lok, 2006). In part because of the typical delay to diagnosis, choriocarcinomas following term pregnancies have a significantly higher mortality rate than GTN following nonmolar abortions (Tidy, 1995). In two separate retrospective studies, each describing 44 patients diagnosed with choriocarcinoma following a term pregnancy, the mortality rate was 14 percent (Lok, 2006; Rodabaugh, 1998).

More than half of patients presenting with brain metastases or placental site trophoblastic tumors have a preceding term gestation (Feltmate, 2001; Newlands, 2002). The frequency of these high-risk features also helps to explain the poorer prognosis for choriocarcinoma following a term pregnancy.

Placental-Site Trophoblastic Tumor

This tumor consists predominantly of intermediate trophoblasts at the placental site and is a rare variant of GTN with unique disease behavior. Placental-site trophoblastic tumors can follow any type of pregnancy, but develop most commonly following a term gestation (Papadopoulos, 2002). Typically, patients have irregular bleeding months or years after the antecedent pregnancy, and the diagnosis is not entertained until endometrial sampling has been performed (Feltmate, 2001). Placental-site trophoblastic tumors tend to infiltrate only within the uterus, disseminate late in their course, and produce low levels of β-hCG. Of interest, an elevated proportion of free β-subunit (>30 percent of total hCG) may be helpful to discriminate from other forms of GTN if the endometrial biopsy is equivocal (Cole, 2008; Harvey, 2008). When this tumor does spread, the pattern mirrors that of gestational choriocarcinoma, with metastases often to the lungs, liver, or vagina (Baergen, 2006).

Hysterectomy is the primary treatment for nonmetastatic placental site trophoblastic tumor due to a relative insensitivity to chemotherapy, although fertility-sparing procedures have been reported in particularly motivated patients (Feltmate, 2001; Machtinger, 2005; Papadopoulos, 2002; Pfeffer, 2007).

Metastatic placental site trophoblastic tumor has a much poorer prognosis than its postmolar GTN counterpart. As a result, aggressive combination chemotherapy is indicated. Regimens of etoposide, methotrexate, and dactinomycin, alternating with etoposide and cisplatin (EMA/EP), are considered the most effective treatment (Newlands, 2000). Radiation, however, may also have a role in some situations. The overall 10-year survival is 70 percent, but patients with metastatic disease or those with more than 4 years after the antecedent pregnancy have a much poorer prognosis (Hassadia, 2005; Schmid, 2009).

Epithelioid Trophoblastic Tumor

This rare trophoblastic tumor is distinct from gestational choriocarcinoma and placental site trophoblastic tumor. The preceding pregnancy event may be remote, or in some cases, a prior gestation cannot be confirmed (Palmer, 2008). Epithelioid trophoblastic tumor develops from neoplastic transformation of chorionic-type intermediate trophoblast. Microscopically, this tumor resembles placental-site trophoblastic tumor, but the cells are smaller and display less nuclear pleomorphism. Grossly, epithelioid trophoblastic tumor grows in a nodular fashion rather than the infiltrative pattern of placental-site trophoblastic tumor (Shih, 1998). Hysterectomy is again the primary method of treatment due to presumed chemoresistance and since the diagnosis is usually confirmed in advance by endometrial biopsy. Approximately one third of patients will present with metastatic disease, but there are too few reported cases to evaluate the efficacy of chemotherapy (Palmer, 2008).

Clinical Classification

Diagnosis

Most GTN cases are clinically diagnosed, using β-hCG evidence of persistent trophoblastic tissue (Table 37-3). Tissue is infrequently available for pathologic diagnosis, unless a diagnosis of placental-site or nongestational tumor is being considered. As a result, most centers in the United States diagnose GTN on the basis of rising β-hCG values or a persistent plateau of β-hCG values for at least 3 weeks. Unfortunately, uniformity is lacking in the definition of a persistent plateau. Additionally, the diagnostic criteria are less stringent in the United States than in Europe, partly because of concern that some patients may be lost to follow-up if stricter criteria are used.

When serologic criteria are met for GTN, a new intrauterine pregnancy should be excluded using β-hCG levels correlated with sonographic findings. This is especially true if there has been a long delay in monitoring of serial β-hCG levels or noncompliance with contraception or both.

Diagnostic Evaluation

Patients with GTN undergo a thorough pretreatment assessment to determine the extent of disease. The initial evaluation may be limited to pelvic examination, chest radiograph, and pelvic sonography or abdominal-pelvic computed tomography (CT) scanning. Although approximately 40 percent of patients will have micrometastases not otherwise visible on chest radiography, chest CT is not needed because these small lesions do not affect outcome (Darby, 2009; Garner, 2004). However, pulmonary lesions identified on chest radiograph should prompt CT of the chest and magnetic resonance (MR) imaging of the brain. Fortunately, central nervous system involvement is rare in the absence of neurologic symptoms or signs (Price, 2010). Position emission tomography (PET) may occasionally be useful in the evaluation of occult choriocarcinoma or relapse from previously treated GTN when conventional imaging is equivocal or fails to identify metastatic disease (Dhillon, 2006; Numnum, 2005).

Staging

Gestational trophoblastic neoplasia is anatomically staged based on a system adopted by the International Federation of Gynecology and Obstetrics (FIGO) (Table 37-4 and Fig. 37-10). Patients at low risk for therapeutic failure are distinguished from those at high risk using the modified prognostic scoring system of the World Health Organization (WHO) (Table 37-5). Those patients with WHO scores of 0 to 6 are considered to have low-risk disease, whereas those with a score of 7 or higher are assigned to the high-risk GTN group. For the most accurate description of these patients, the Roman numeral corresponding to FIGO stage is separated by a colon from the sum of all the actual risk factor scores, for example, stage II:4 or stage IV:9 (FIGO, 2009; Petru, 2009). This addition of risk scoring to anatomic staging has been shown to best reflect disease behavior (Ngan, 2004). Women with high-risk scores are more likely to have tumors that are resistant to single-agent chemotherapy. They are therefore treated initially with combination chemotherapy. Although patients with stage I disease infrequently have a high-risk score, those with stage IV disease invariably have a high-risk score. Women diagnosed with FIGO stage I, II, or III GTN have a survival rate approaching 100 percent (Lurain, 2010).

Nonmetastatic Disease

Invasive moles arising from complete molar gestations comprise most nonmetastatic GTN cases. Approximately 12 percent of complete moles develop locally invasive disease after evacuation,

---

TABLE 37-3. Criteria for the Diagnosis of Gestational Trophoblastic Neoplasia

1. Plateau of β-hCG lasts for four measurements over a period of 3 weeks or longer (days 1, 7, 14, and 21).
2. Rise of β-hCG of 3 weekly consecutive measurements or longer, over a period of 2 weeks or more (days 1, 7, and 14).
3. β-hCG remains elevated for 6 months or more.
4. Histologic diagnosis of choriocarcinoma.

β-hCG = beta human chorionic gonadotropin; FIGO = International Federation of Gynecology and Obstetrics.
From FIGO Oncology Committee, 2002, with permission.

TABLE 37-4. FIGO Staging of Gestational Trophoblastic Neoplasia

Stage	Characteristics
I	Disease confined to the uterus
II	GTN extends outside of the uterus but is limited to the genital structures (adnexa, vagina, broad ligament)
III	GTN extends to the lungs, with or without known genital tract involvement
IV	All other metastatic sites

FIGO = International Federation of Gynecology and Obstetrics; GTN = gestational trophoblastic neoplasia.

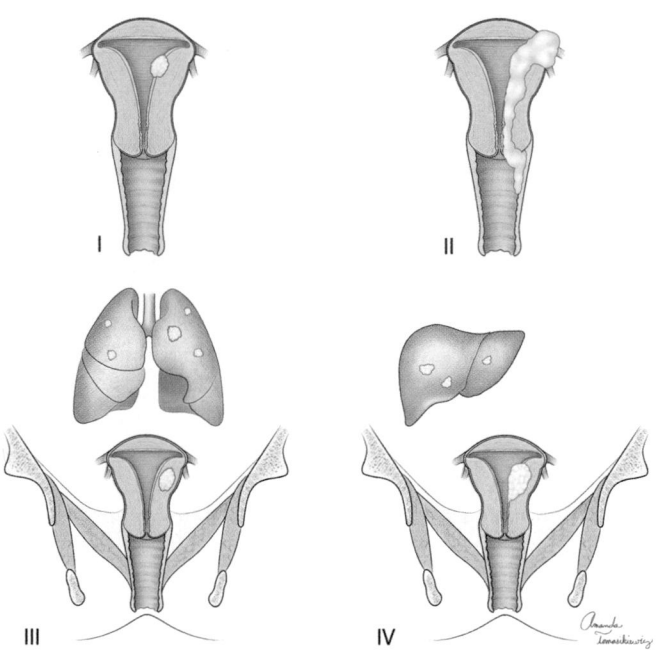

FIGURE 37-10 FIGO staging of gestational trophoblastic neoplasia.

compared with only 4 to 6 percent of partial moles. Placental-site trophoblastic tumors and epithelioid trophoblastic tumors are other rarer causes of nonmetastatic GTN. Locally invasive trophoblastic tumors may perforate through the myometrium and lead to intraperitoneal bleeding (Mackenzie, 1993). Alternatively, vaginal hemorrhage can follow tumor erosion into uterine vessels, or necrotic tumor may involve the uterine wall and serve as a nidus for infection. Fortunately, the prognosis is excellent for all types of nonmetastatic disease despite these possible manifestations.

Metastatic Disease

Choriocarcinomas originating from complete molar gestations comprise most cases of metastatic GTN. Three to 4 percent of complete moles develop metastatic choriocarcinoma after evacuation. The incidence following any other type of molar or nonmolar gestation is exceedingly rare. Choriocarcinomas have a propensity to distant spread and should be suspected in any woman of reproductive age with metastatic disease from an unknown primary (Tidy, 1995). Moreover, because of this tendency, chemotherapy is indicated whenever choriocarcinoma is diagnosed histologically.

TABLE 37-5. Modified WHO Prognostic Scoring System as Adapted by FIGO

Scores	0	1	2	4
Age (yr)	<40	≥40	—	—
Antecedent pregnancy	Mole	Abortion	Term	—
Interval months from index pregnancy	<4	4–6	7–12	>12
Pretreatment serum (β-hCG (mIU/mL)	$<10^3$	$10^3–<10^4$	$10^4–<10^5$	$≥10^5$
Largest tumor size (including uterus)	<3 cm	3–4 cm	≥5 cm	—
Site of metastases		Spleen, kidney	GI	Liver, brain
Number of metastases	—	1–4	5–8	>8
Previous failed chemotherapy drugs	—	—	1	≥2

Low risk = WHO score of 0 to 6; high risk = WHO score of ≥7.
β-hCG = beta human chorionic gonadotropin; FIGO = International Federation of Gynecology and Obstetrics; GI = gastrointestinal; WHO = World Health Organization.

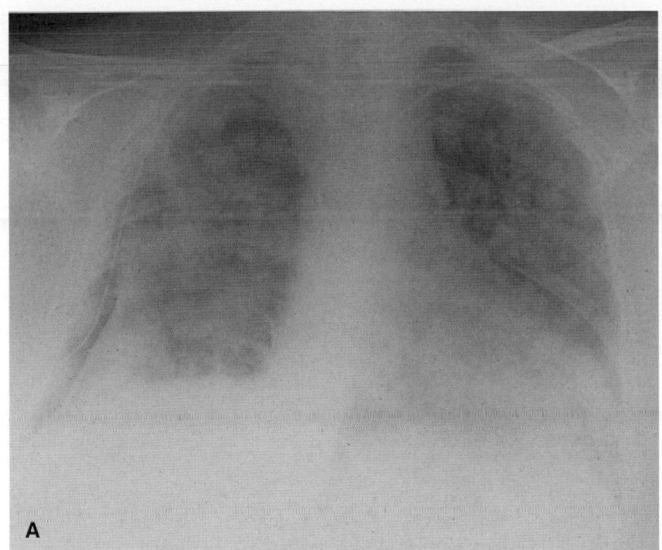

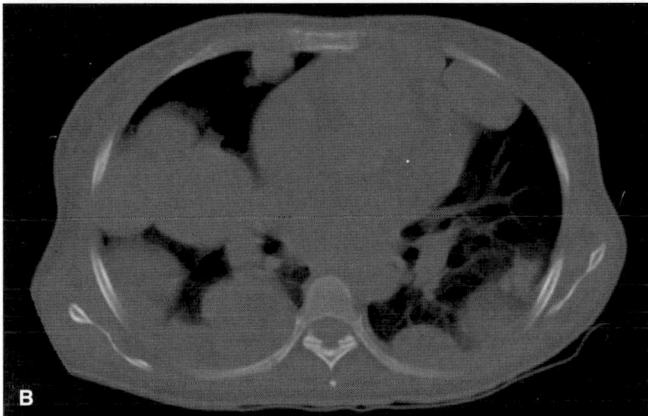

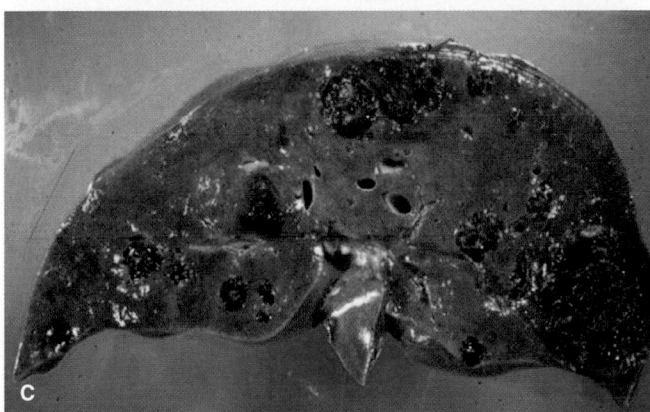

FIGURE 37-11 Common sites of GTN metastasis. **A.** Chest radiography demonstrates widespread metastatic lesions. *(Photograph contributed by Dr. Michael G. Connor.)* **B.** Computed tomography (CT) scan of metastatic disease to the lung. **C.** Autopsy specimen shows multiple hemorrhagic hepatic metastases. *(Photograph contributed by Dr. Michael G. Connor.)*

Although many patients are largely asymptomatic, metastatic GTN is highly vascular and prone to severe hemorrhage either spontaneously or during biopsy. Menorrhagia is a common presenting symptom. The most common sites of spread are the lungs (80 percent), vagina (30 percent), pelvis (20 percent), liver (10 percent) and brain (10 percent) (Fig. 37-11). Patients

with pulmonary metastases typically have asymptomatic lesions identified on routine chest radiograph and infrequently present with cough, dyspnea, hemoptysis, pleuritic chest pain, or signs of pulmonary hypertension (Seckl, 1991). In patients with the early development of respiratory failure that requires intubation, the overall outcome is poor. Hepatic or cerebral involvement is encountered almost exclusively in patients who have had an antecedent nonmolar pregnancy and a protracted delay in tumor diagnosis (Newlands, 2002). These women may present with associated hemorrhagic events. Virtually all patients with hepatic or cerebral metastases have concurrent pulmonary or vaginal involvement or both. Great caution is used in attempting excision of any metastatic disease site due to the risk of profuse hemorrhage. Thus, this practice is almost uniformly avoided except in extenuating circumstances of life-threatening brainstem herniation or chemotherapy-resistant disease.

Treatment

Surgical Management

Most patients diagnosed with postmolar GTN have persistent tumor confined to the endometrial cavity and are treated primarily with chemotherapeutic agents. Repeat dilatation and curettage is generally avoided to prevent morbidity and mortality caused by uterine perforation, hemorrhage, infection, uterine adhesions, and anesthetic complications (Soper, 2004). Accordingly, second evacuations are not typically performed in the United States unless patients have persistent uterine bleeding and substantial amounts of retained molar tissue. Repeat uterine curettage is a more standard part of the management of postmolar GTN in Europe. This practice has been shown to significantly reduce both the number of patients needing any further treatment and the number of courses in those who do require chemotherapy (Pezeshki, 2004; van Trommel, 2005). A second evacuation followed by continued surveillance, however, is a less attractive option, even for poorly compliant patients, than single-agent chemotherapy (Allen, 2003; Massad, 2000).

Hysterectomy may play several roles in the treatment of GTN. First, it may be performed to primarily treat placental-site trophoblastic tumors, epithelioid trophoblastic tumors, or other types of chemotherapy-resistant disease. Fortunately declining in incidence, severe uncontrollable vaginal or intraabdominal bleeding may necessitate hysterectomy as an emergency procedure (Chao, 2002; Clark, 2010). Because of these more extreme indications, most women undergoing hysterectomy have elevated pretreatment risk scores, unusual pathology, and higher mortality rates (Pisal, 2002). Finally, adjuvant hysterectomy decreases the total dose of chemotherapy needed to achieve clinical remission in low-risk GTN. Patients with disease apparently confined to the uterus who do not desire future fertility should be counseled about this option (Suzuka, 2001). However, the risk of GTN persistence after hysterectomy remains approximately 3 to 5 percent, and these patients should be monitored postoperatively (Soper, 2004).

Residual lung metastases may persist in 10 to 20 percent of patients achieving clinical remission of GTN after completion of chemotherapy. These patients do not appear to have an increased risk of relapse compared with those having normal chest radiographs or CT scans. Thus, thoracotomy is not

TABLE 37-6. Intramuscular Methotrexate Regimens for Treatment of Low-Risk GTN

Frequency	Dose	Population Studied	CR Rate (%)	First Author
Weekly	30–50 mg/m²	Nonmetastatic GTN	74–81	Homesley, 1988, 1990
	50 mg/m²	Low-risk GTN	70	Kang, 2010
Days 1, 3, 5, 7	1 mg/kg	Low-risk GTN	67–72	McNeish, 2002
				Khan, 2003
				Kang, 2010
		Low-risk GTN	78	Chalouhi, 2009

CR = clinical remission (calculated for first-line treatment without needing alternative chemotherapy); GTN = gestational trophoblastic neoplasia.

usually necessary unless remission cannot otherwise be achieved (Powles, 2006). In general, the optimal patient to be counseled for thoracotomy will have stage III GTN, a preoperative β-hCG level <1500 mIU/mL, and a solitary lung nodule resistant to chemotherapy (Cao, 2009; Fleming, 2008; Lurain, 2006).

Chemotherapy for Low-Risk GTN

Methotrexate. Approximately 95 percent of patients with hydatidiform mole who develop GTN are at low risk of chemotherapy resistance (score 0-6) (Seckl, 2010). Single-agent methotrexate is the most common treatment, and complete response rates ranging from 67 to 81 percent have been reported for variations of the two most common intramuscular methotrexate regimens (Table 37-6). The remaining 19 to 33 percent of women develop methotrexate resistance and are switched to other agents, described subsequently. With methotrexate, the Gynecologic Oncology Group (GOG) conducted a prospective cohort dose-escalation study (protocol #79) of weekly administration that established a maximum dose of 50 mg/m² with minimal toxicity (Homesley, 1988, 1990). This regimen is continued weekly until β-hCG levels are undetectable, and then two additional weekly doses are given. Alternatively, Charing Cross Hospital and University of Sheffield investigators use an 8-day alternating regimen of methotrexate, 1 mg/kg on treatment days 1, 3, 5, and 7, and oral folinic acid, 7.5 mg taken orally on days 2, 4, 6, and 8. Treatment is repeated every 2 weeks (Khan, 2003; McNeish, 2002).

As discussed more fully in Chapter 27 (p. 698), methotrexate is a folic acid antagonist that inhibits DNA synthesis. Mild stomatitis is the most common side effect, but other serosal symptoms, especially pleurisy, develop in up to one quarter of patients treated with low-dose methotrexate. Pericarditis, peritonitis, and pneumonitis are infrequent (Sharma, 1999). Toxicity develops more frequently with the more intense 8-day regimens compared with weekly administration despite routine folinic acid "rescue," which is provided for normal mucosal and serosal cells (Chap. 27, p. 699) (Gleeson, 1993).

Compared with intramuscular administration, methotrexate intravenous infusion appears somewhat less effective. For example, a 100 mg/m² bolus followed by 200 mg/m² given over 12 hours has a 65-percent complete response rate (Garrett,

2002). Folinic acid rescue is not necessary using this regimen due to the nontoxic levels of methotrexate reached 24 hours after infusion (Allen, 2003; Wong, 2000). Because this regimen is usually successful with a single dose, it reduces the number of required visits and may be most appropriate in poorly compliant patients (Schorge, 2003). Oral methotrexate has few indications in the management of GTN (Farley, 2005).

Dactinomycin. Due to toxicity concerns, dactinomycin is less commonly used for the primary treatment of low-risk disease, but may have superior efficacy as a single agent (Alazzam, 2009; Gilani, 2005; Yarandi, 2008). In a prospective GOG trial (protocol #174) of low-risk GTN, patients were randomly assigned to biweekly "pulse" 1.25-mg dose dactinomycin or to weekly methotrexate, 30 mg/m². Among 215 eligible patients, a complete response was observed in 69 percent given dactinomycin and in 53 percent given methotrexate. However, advocates of methotrexate have speculated that the unexpectedly low efficacy of methotrexate observed in this study may be due to subtherapeutic dosing. Moreover, those randomized to dactinomycin were twice as likely to develop alopecia and were the only patients to develop grade 4 toxicity (Chap. 27, p. 700) (Osborne, 2008). As yet, no trials have directly compared pulse dactinomycin and the widely used 8-day methotrexate regimen. Since survival rates are so high, methotrexate is usually tried first because most clinicians consider it to be the least toxic therapy.

Patients who do not respond to an initial single-agent chemotherapeutic regimen fail to have persistently dropping β-hCG levels. These women should have their score recalculated using the modified WHO prognostic scoring system. Most women will still be considered low-risk and may be switched to a single-agent second-line therapy. Methotrexate-resistant GTN often responds to dactinomycin (Chen, 2004). The GOG recently demonstrated a 74-percent success rate in a phase II trial (protocol #176) of pulse dactinomycin as salvage treatment in 38 patients with methotrexate-resistant GTN (Covens, 2006). Etoposide is less commonly used in this setting, but is also effective (Mangili, 1996). Patients initially treated with pulse dactinomycin who develop resistant GTN may still be successfully treated with the 5-day course of dactinomycin (Kohorn, 2002). Alternatively, single-agent methotrexate or etoposide is effective in these cases (Matsui, 2005).

Chemotherapy for High-Risk GTN. Most high-risk GTN patients present with numerous metastases months or years after the causative pregnancy of any type. Such patients are at high risk of developing drug resistance and are very unlikely to be cured with single-agent chemotherapy (Seckl, 2010). Etoposide, methotrexate, and dactinomycin (actinomycin D) alternating with cyclophosphamide and vincristine (Oncovin) (EMA/CO) chemotherapy is a well-tolerated and highly effective regimen for high-risk GTN. It should be considered the preferred treatment in most circumstances. Bower and associates (1997) at Charing Cross Hospital reported a 78-percent complete remission rate in 272 consecutive women. Similarly, other investigators have observed a 71- to 78-percent complete response rate with the EMA/CO regimen (Escobar, 2003; Lu, 2008). Response rates are comparable whether patients are treated primarily or after failure of single-agent methotrexate and/or dactinomycin.

Patients with high-risk disease have an overall survival of 86 to 92 percent, although approximately one quarter become refractory to or relapse from EMA/CO (Bower, 1997; Escobar, 2003; Lu, 2008; Lurain, 2010). Secondary treatment usually involves platinum-based chemotherapy combined with possible surgical excision of resistant disease. Newlands and colleagues (2000) at Charing Cross Hospital reported an 88-percent survival rate among 34 patients by replacing the cyclophosphamide and vincristine component with etoposide and cisplatin (EMA/EP). Although EMA/EP is an effective option in patients resistant to EMA/CO, paclitaxel and alternating platinum and etoposide (TP/TE) has also demonstrated comparable efficacy and appears less toxic (Kim, 2007; Mao, 2007; Osborne, 2004; Patel, 2010; Wang, 2008). Bleomycin, etoposide, and cisplatin (BEP) is another potentially effective regimen (Lurain, 2005; Patel, 2010).

Brain Metastases. Patients with cerebral metastases may present with seizures, headaches, or hemiparesis (Newlands, 2002). Occasionally, they are moribund on arrival after not recognizing the significance of their symptoms or following an extended delay in diagnosis. In such extenuating circumstances, emergency craniotomy may be indicated to stabilize the patient and is followed by critical care support throughout the active phase of treatment (Yang, 2005). In experienced centers, virtually all GTN-related deaths occur in stage IV patients with WHO risk scores of 12 or more (Lurain, 2010).

Fortunately, the cure rate for those with brain metastases is high if neurologic deterioration does not occur within the first couple of weeks after diagnosis. The sequence of aggressive multimodality therapy is controversial, but may include chemotherapy, surgery, and radiation (Soper, 2004). Newlands and coworkers (2002) at Charing Cross Hospital reported an 80-percent survival rate among 39 patients treated by EMA/CO with an escalated dose of methotrexate and folinic acid. Intrathecal methotrexate was also administered until β-hCG levels were undetectable. Surgical removal of the main active site of disease was performed in 16 patients. Of these, four women died within 8 days of presentation. The presence of both liver and brain metastases was a particularly adverse prognostic combination with only one of five patients surviving (Newlands, 2002). Whole-brain radiation therapy may also be an efficacious adjunct to combination

chemotherapy and surgery, but can induce permanent intellectual impairment (Cagayan, 2006; Schechter, 1998).

Posttreatment Surveillance. Monitoring of patients with low-risk GTN consists of weekly β-hCG measurements until the level is undetectable for 3 consecutive weeks. This is followed by monthly titers until the level is undetectable for 12 months. Patients with high-risk disease are followed for 24 months due to the greater risk of late relapse. Patients are encouraged to use effective contraception, as outlined earlier, during the entire surveillance period.

Psychological Consequences

The diagnosis of gestational trophoblastic disease can have a devastating impact on a woman's life. Increased anxiety, anger, fatigue, and confusion are commonplace. Despite the favorable prognosis, patients and their partners carry pregnancy concerns for a protracted time (Wenzel, 1992, 1994). Sexual dysfunction is another common but underreported complication (Cagayan, 2008). These and other potential sequelae highlight the importance of a multidisciplinary approach to management (Ferreira, 2009).

Subsequent Pregnancy Outcome

Although patients may expect a normal reproductive outcome after achieving remission from gestational trophoblastic disease, some evidence suggests that adverse maternal outcomes and spontaneous abortion occur more frequently among those who conceive within 6 months of chemotherapy completion (Braga, 2009). Women having a pregnancy affected by a histologically confirmed complete or partial mole may be counseled that the risk of a repeat mole in a subsequent pregnancy approximates 1 percent (Garrett, 2008). Most will be of the same type of mole as the preceding pregnancy (Sebire, 2003). Pregnancy after combination EMA/CO chemotherapy for GTN also has a high probability of success and favorable outcome (Lok, 2003). Although chemotherapy for GTN induces menopause on average 3 years earlier, fertility is not thought to be greatly affected (Bower, 1998).

Secondary Tumors

Etoposide-based combination chemotherapy has been associated with an increased risk of leukemia, colon cancer, melanoma, and breast cancer up to 25 years after treatment for GTN. An overall 50-percent excess risk was observed (Rustin, 1996). Etoposide is therefore reserved to treat patients who are likely to be resistant to single-agent chemotherapy and in particular, those with high-risk metastatic disease.

Phantom β-hCG

Occasionally, persistent mild elevations of serum β-hCG are detected that lead physicians to erroneously treat patients with cytotoxic chemotherapy or hysterectomy or both, which in reality no true β-hCG or trophoblastic disease is present (Cole, 1998; Rotmensch, 2000). This "phantom" β-hCG reading results from heterophilic antibodies in the serum that interfere with the β-hCG immunoassay and cause a false-positive result (Soper, 2004).

There are several ways to clarify the diagnosis. First, a urine pregnancy test can be performed. With phantom β-hCG, the heterophilic antibodies are not filtered or renally excreted. Thus, the urine test will show negative results for β-hCG. Importantly, to conclusively exclude trophoblastic disease by this method, the index serum β-hCG level must be significantly higher than the detection threshold of the urine test. Second, performing serial dilutions of the serum sample results in a proportional decrease in the β-hCG level if β-hCG is truly present. However, phantom β-hCG measurements will be unchanged by dilution. In addition, if phantom β-hCG is suspected, some specialized laboratories may be able to block the heterophilic antibodies. Lastly, a different β-hCG assay performed using an alternate method may accurately demonstrate the absence of true β-hCG (Cole, 1998; Olsen, 2001; Rotmensch, 2000).

Quiescent Gestational Trophoblastic Disease

Patients with persistent mild elevations (usually in the range of 50 mIU/mL or less) of true β-hCG may have a dormant premalignant condition if no tumor is identified by physical examination or imaging studies (Khanlian, 2003). In this instance, phantom β-hCG should also be conclusively excluded as a possibility. The low β-hCG titers may persist for months or years before disappearing. Chemotherapy and surgery usually have no effect. Hormonal contraception may be helpful in lowering titers to an undetectable level, but patients should be closely monitored since metastatic GTN may eventually develop (Khanlian, 2003; Kohorn, 2002; Palmieri, 2007).

REFERENCES

Alazzam M, Tidy J, Hancock BW, et al: First line chemotherapy in low risk gestational trophoblastic neoplasia. Cochrane Database Syst Rev 1:CD007102, 2009

Allen JE, King MR, Farrar DF, et al: Postmolar surveillance at a trophoblastic disease center that serves indigent women. Am J Obstet Gynecol 188:1151, 2003

Altman AD, Bentley B, Murray S, et al: Maternal age-related rates of gestational trophoblastic disease. Obstet Gynecol 112:244, 2008

Azuma C, Saji F, Tokugawa Y, et al: Application of gene amplification by polymerase chain reaction to genetic analysis of molar mitochondrial DNA: the detection of anuclear empty ovum as the cause of complete mole. Gynecol Oncol 40:29, 1991

Baergen RN, Rutgers JL, Young RH, et al: Placental site trophoblastic tumor: a study of 55 cases and review of the literature emphasizing factors of prognostic significance. Gynecol Oncol 100:511, 2006

Bailey JL, Hinton EA, Ashfaq R, et al: Primary abdominal gestational choriocarcinoma. Obstet Gynecol 102:988, 2003

Batorfi J, Vegh G, Szepesi J, et al: How long should patients be followed after molar pregnancy? Analysis of serum hCG follow-up data. Eur J Obstet Gynecol Reprod Biol 112:95, 2004

Ben-Arie A, Deutsch H, Volach V, et al: Reduction of postmolar gestational trophoblastic neoplasia by early diagnosis and treatment. J Reprod Med 54(3):151, 2009

Benson CB, Genest DR, Bernstein MR, et al: Sonographic appearance of first trimester complete hydatidiform moles. Ultrasound Obstet Gynecol 16:188, 2000

Berkowitz RS, Bernstein MR, Harlow BL, et al: Case-control study of risk factors for partial molar pregnancy. Am J Obstet Gynecol 173:788, 1995

Berkowitz RS, Cramer DW, Bernstein MR, et al: Risk factors for complete molar pregnancy from a case-control study. Am J Obstet Gynecol 152:1016, 1985

Berkowitz RS, Im SS, Bernstein MR, et al: Gestational trophoblastic disease: subsequent pregnancy outcome, including repeat molar pregnancy. J Reprod Med 43:81, 1998

Bower M, Newlands ES, Holden L, et al: EMA/CO for high-risk gestational trophoblastic tumors: results from a cohort of 272 patients. J Clin Oncol 15:2636, 1997

Bower M, Rustin GJ, Newlands ES, et al: Chemotherapy for gestational trophoblastic tumours hastens menopause by 3 years. Eur J Cancer 34:1204, 1998

Braga A, Maesta I, Michelin OC, et al: Maternal and perinatal outcomes of first pregnancy after chemotherapy for gestational trophoblastic neoplasia in Brazilian women. Gynecol Oncol 112:568, 2009

Burton JL, Lidbury EA, Gillespie AM, et al: Overdiagnosis of hydatidiform mole in early tubal ectopic pregnancy. Histopathology 38:409, 2001

Cagayan MS: Sexual dysfunction as a complication of treatment of gestational trophoblastic neoplasia. J Reprod Med 53:595, 2008

Cagayan MS, Lu-Lasala LR: Management of gestational trophoblastic neoplasia with metastasis to the central nervous system: a 12-year review at the Phillippe General Hospital. J Reprod Med 51:785, 2006

Cao Y, Xiang Y, Feng F, et al: Surgical resection in the management of pulmonary metastatic disease of gestational trophoblastic neoplasia. Int J Gynecol Cancer 19:798, 2009

Castrillon DH, Sun D, Weremowicz S, et al: Discrimination of complete hydatidiform mole from its mimics by immunohistochemistry of the paternally imprinted gene product p57KIP2. Am J Surg Pathol 25:1225, 2001

Chalouhi GE, Golfier F, Soignon P, et al: Methotrexate for 2000 FIGO low-risk gestational trophoblastic neoplasia patients: efficacy and toxicity. Am J Obstet Gynecol 200(6):643.e1-6, 2009

Chao A, Lin CT, Chang TC, et al: Choriocarcinoma with diffuse intra-abdominal abscess and disseminated intravascular coagulation: a case report. J Reprod Med 47:689, 2002

Chen LM, Lengyel ER, Bethan PC: Single-agent pulse dactinomycin has only modest activity for methotrexate-resistant gestational trophoblastic neoplasia. Gynecol Oncol 94:204, 2004

Cheung AN, Khoo US, Lai CY, et al: Metastatic trophoblastic disease after an initial diagnosis of partial hydatidiform mole: genotyping and chromosome in situ hybridization analysis. Cancer 100:1411, 2004

Chew SH, Perlman EJ, Williams R, et al: Morphology and DNA content analysis in the evaluation of first trimester placentas for partial hydatidiform mole (PHM). Hum Pathol 31:914, 2000

Chong CY, Koh CF: Hydatidiform mole in Kandang Kerbau Hospital: a 5-year review. Singapore Med J 40:265, 1999

Clark RM, Nevadunsky NS, Ghosh S, et al: The evolving role of hysterectomy in gestational trophoblastic neoplasia at the New England Trophoblastic Disease Center. J Reprod Med 5:194, 2010

Cole LA: Phantom hCG and phantom choriocarcinoma. Gynecol Oncol 71:325, 1998

Cole LA, Khanlian SA, Muller CY: Blood test for placental site trophoblastic tumor and nontrophoblastic malignancy for evaluating patients with low positive human chorionic gonadotropin results. J Reprod Med 53:457, 2008

Costa HL, Doyle P: Influence of oral contraceptives in the development of post-molar trophoblastic neoplasia—a systematic review. Gynecol Oncol 100:579, 2006

Covens A, Filiaci VL, Burger RA, et al: Phase II trial of pulse dactinomycin as salvage therapy for failed low-risk gestational trophoblastic neoplasia: a Gynecologic Oncology Group study. Cancer 107(6):1280, 2006

Crisp H, Burton JL, Stewart R, et al: Refining the diagnosis of hydatidiform mole: image ploidy analysis and p57KIP2 immunohistochemistry. Histopathology 43:363, 2003

Darby S, Jolley I, Pennington S: Does chest CT matter in the staging of GTN? Gynecol Oncol 112:155, 2009

Dhillon T, Palmieri C, Sebire NJ, et al: Value of whole body 18FDG-PET to identify the active site of gestational trophoblastic neoplasia. J Reprod Med 51:979, 2006

Drake RD, Rao GG, McIntire DD, et al: Gestational trophoblastic disease among Hispanic women: a 21-year hospital-based study. Gynecol Oncol 103(1):81, 2006

Elias KM, Goldstein DP, Berkowitz RS: Complete hydatidiform mole in women older than age 50. J Reprod Med 55:208, 2010

Escobar PF, Lurain JR, Singh DK, et al: Treatment of high-risk gestational trophoblastic neoplasia with etoposide, methotrexate, actinomycin D, cyclophosphamide, and vincristine chemotherapy. Gynecol Oncol 91:552, 2003

Fallahian M: Familial gestational trophoblastic disease. Placenta 24:797, 2003

Fan JB, Surti U, Taillon-Miller P, et al: Paternal origins of complete hydatidiform moles proven by whole genome single-nucleotide polymorphism haplotyping. Genomics 79:58, 2002

Farley JH, Heathcock RB, Branch W, et al: Treatment of metastatic gestational choriocarcinoma with oral methotrexate in a combat environment. Obstet Gynecol 105:1250, 2005

Feltmate CM, Batorfi J, Fulop V, et al: Human chorionic gonadotropin follow-up in patients with molar pregnancy: a time for reevaluation. Obstet Gynecol 101:732, 2003

Feltmate CM, Genest DR, Wise L, et al: Placental site trophoblastic tumor: a 17-year experience at the New England Trophoblastic Disease Center. Gynecol Oncol 82:415, 2001

Feltmate CM, Growdon WB, Wolfberg AJ, et al: Clinical characteristics of persistent gestational trophoblastic neoplasia after partial hydatiform molar pregnancy. J Reprod Med 51:902, 2006

Ferreira EG, Maesta I, Michelin OC, et al: Assessment of quality of life and psychologic aspects in patients with gestational trophoblastic disease. J Reprod Med 54:239, 2009

FIGO Committee on Gynecologic Oncology: Current FIGO staging for cancer of the vagina, fallopian tube, ovary, and gestational trophoblastic neoplasia. Int J Gynaecol Obstet 105:3, 2009

FIGO Oncology Committee: FIGO staging for gestational trophoblastic neoplasia 2000. Int J Gynaecol Obstet 77:285, 2002

Fleming EL, Garrett L, Growdon WB, et al: The changing role of thoracotomy in gestational trophoblastic neoplasia at the New England Trophoblastic Disease Center. J Reprod Med 53:493, 2008

Fukunaga M, Katabuchi H, Nagasaka T, et al: Interobserver and intraobserver variability in the diagnosis of hydatidiform mole. Am J Surg Pathol 29:942, 2005

Fung Kee FK, Eason E, Crane J, et al: Prevention of Rh alloimmunization. J Obstet Gynaecol Can 25:765, 2003

Gaffield ME, Kapp N, Curtis KM: Combined oral contraceptive and intrauterine device use among women with gestational trophoblastic disease. Contraception 80:363, 2009

Garner EI, Garrett A, Goldstein DP, et al: Significance of chest computed tomography findings in the evaluation and treatment of persistent gestational trophoblastic neoplasia. J Reprod Med 49:411, 2004

Garrett LA, Garner EI, Feltmate CM, et al: Subsequent pregnancy outcomes in patients with molar pregnancy and persistent gestational trophoblastic neoplasia. J Reprod Med 53(7):481, 2008

Garrett AP, Garner EO, Goldstein DP, et al: Methotrexate infusion and folinic acid as primary therapy for nonmetastatic and low-risk metastatic gestational trophoblastic tumors: 15 years of experience. J Reprod Med 47:355, 2002

Genest DR: Partial hydatidiform mole: clinicopathological features, differential diagnosis, ploidy and molecular studies, and gold standards for diagnosis. Int J Gynecol Pathol 20:315, 2001

Genest DR, Dorfman DM, Castrillon DH: Ploidy and imprinting in hydatidiform moles: complementary use of flow cytometry and immunohistochemistry of the imprinted gene product p57KIP2 to assist molar classification. J Reprod Med 47:342, 2002a

Genest DR, Ruiz RE, Weremowicz S, et al: Do nontriploid partial hydatidiform moles exist? A histologic and flow cytometric reevaluation of nontriploid specimens. J Reprod Med 47:363, 2002b

Gilani MM, Yarandi F, Eftekhar Z, et al: Comparison of pulse methotrexate and pulse dactinomycin in the treatment of low-risk gestational trophoblastic neoplasia. Aust N Z J Obstet Gynaecol 45:161, 2005

Gillespie AM, Lidbury EA, Tidy JA, et al: The clinical presentation, treatment, and outcome of patients diagnosed with possible ectopic molar gestation. Int J Gynecol Cancer 14:366, 2004

Gleeson NC, Finan MA, Fiorica JV, et al: Nonmetastatic gestational trophoblastic disease: weekly methotrexate compared with 8-day methotrexate-folinic acid. Eur J Gynaecol Oncol 14:461, 1993

Golfier F, Raudrant D, Frappart L, et al: First epidemiological data from the French Trophoblastic Disease Reference Center. Am J Obstet Gynecol 196:172.e1-5, 2007

Hancock BW, Nazir K, Everard JE: Persistent gestational trophoblastic neoplasia after partial hydatidiform mole incidence and outcome. J Reprod Med 51:764, 2006

Harvey RA, Pursglove HD, Schmid P, et al: Human chorionic gonadotropin free beta-subunit measurement as a marker of placental site trophoblastic tumors. J Reprod Med 53:643, 2008

Hassadia A, Gillespie A, Tidy J, et al: Placental site trophoblastic tumour: clinical features and management. Gynecol Oncol 99:603, 2005

Hershman JM: Physiological and pathological aspects of the effect of human chorionic gonadotropin on the thyroid. Best Pract Res Clin Endocrinol Metab 18:249, 2004

Homesley HD, Blessing JA, Rettenmaier M, et al: Weekly intramuscular methotrexate for nonmetastatic gestational trophoblastic disease. Obstet Gynecol 72:413, 1988

Homesley HD, Blessing JA, Schlaerth J, et al: Rapid escalation of weekly intramuscular methotrexate for nonmetastatic gestational trophoblastic disease: a Gynecologic Oncology Group study. Gynecol Oncol 39:305, 1990

Jauniaux E: Partial moles: from postnatal to prenatal diagnosis. Placenta 20:379, 1999

Johns J, Greenwold N, Buckley S, et al: A prospective study of ultrasound screening for molar pregnancies in missed miscarriages. Ultrasound Obstet Gynecol 25:493, 2005

Jun SY, Ro JY, Kim KR: p57kip2 is useful in the classification and differential diagnosis of complete and partial hydatidiform moles. Histopathology 43:17, 2003

Kajii T, Ohama K: Androgenetic origin of hydatidiform mole. Nature 268:633, 1977

Kang WD, Choi HS, Kim SM: Weekly methotrexate (50mg/m²) without dose escalation as a primary regimen for low-risk gestational trophoblastic neoplasia. Gynecol Oncol 117(3):477, 2010

Kerkmeijer LG, Wielsma S, Massuger LF, et al: Recurrent gestational trophoblastic disease after hCG normalization following hydatidiform mole in The Netherlands. Gynecol Oncol 106:142, 2007

Khan F, Everard J, Ahmed S, et al: Low-risk persistent gestational trophoblastic disease treated with low-dose methotrexate: efficacy, acute and long-term effects. Br J Cancer 89:2197, 2003

Khanlian SA, Smith HO, Cole LA: Persistent low levels of human chorionic gonadotropin: a premalignant gestational trophoblastic disease. Am J Obstet Gynecol 188:1254, 2003

Kim SJ, Lee C, Kwon SY, et al: Studying changes in the incidence, diagnosis and management of GTD: the South Korean model. J Reprod Med 49:643, 2004

Kim SJ, Na YJ, Jung SG, et al: Management of high-risk hydatidiform mole and persistent gestational trophoblastic neoplasia: the Korean experience. J Reprod Med 52:819, 2007

Kohorn EI: Persistent low-level "real" human chorionic gonadotropin: a clinical challenge and a therapeutic dilemma. Gynecol Oncol 85:315, 2002

La Vecchia C, Parazzini F, Decarli A, et al: Age of parents and risk of gestational trophoblastic disease. J Natl Cancer Inst 73:639, 1984

Lage JM, Mark SD, Roberts DJ, et al: A flow cytometric study of 137 fresh hydropic placentas: correlation between types of hydatidiform moles and nuclear DNA ploidy. Obstet Gynecol 79:403, 1992

Lavie I, Rao GG, Castrillon DH, et al: Duration of human chorionic gonadotropin surveillance for partial hydatidiform moles. Am J Obstet Gynecol 192:1362, 2005

Lawler SD, Fisher RA: Genetic studies in hydatidiform mole with clinical correlations. Placenta 8:77, 1987

Lawler SD, Fisher RA, Dent J: A prospective genetic study of complete and partial hydatidiform moles. Am J Obstet Gynecol 164:1270, 1991

Lazarus E, Hulka C, Siewert B, et al: Sonographic appearance of early complete molar pregnancies. J Ultrasound Med 18:589, 1999

Lee KH, Lee IH, Kim BG, et al: Clinicopathologic characteristics of malignant germ cell tumors in the ovaries of Korean women: a Korean Gynecologic Oncology Group Study. Int J Gynecol Cancer 19:84, 2009

le-Ming S, Mazur MT, Kurman RJ: Gestational trophoblastic disease and related tumor-like lesions. In Kurman RJ, Ellenson LH, Ronnett BM (eds): Blaustein's Pathology of the Female Genital Tract, 6th ed. New York, Springer, 2011, p 1076

Limpongsanurak S: Prophylactic actinomycin D for high-risk complete hydatidiform mole. J Reprod Med 46:110, 2001

Lindholm H, Flam F: The diagnosis of molar pregnancy by sonography and gross morphology. Acta Obstet Gynecol Scand 78:6, 1999

Lok CA, Ansink AC, Grootfaam D, et al: Treatment and prognosis of post term choriocarcinoma in The Netherlands. Gynecol Oncol 103:698, 2006

Lok CA, van der Houwen C, ten Kate-Booij MJ, et al: Pregnancy after EMA/CO for gestational trophoblastic disease: a report from The Netherlands. Br J Obstet Gynaecol 110:560, 2003

Loukovaara M, Pukkala E, Lehtovirta P, et al: Epidemiology of hydatidiform mole in Finland, 1975 to 2001. Eur J Gynaecol Oncol 26:207, 2005

Lu WG, Ye F, Shen YM, et al: EMA-CO chemotherapy for high-risk gestational trophoblastic neoplasia: a clinical analysis of 54 patients. Int J Gynecol Cancer 18:357, 2008

Lurain JR, Nejad B: Secondary chemotherapy for high-risk gestational trophoblastic neoplasia. Gynecol Oncol 97:618, 2005

Lurain JR, Singh DK, Schink JC: Management of metastatic high-risk gestational trophoblastic neoplasia: FIGO stage II-IV: risk factor score > or = 7. J Reprod Med 55:199, 2010

Lurain JR, Singh DK, Schink JC: Role of surgery in the management of high-risk gestational trophoblastic neoplasia. J Reprod Med 51:773, 2006

Machtinger R, Gotlieb WH, Korach J, et al: Placental site trophoblastic tumor: outcome of five cases including fertility-preserving management. Gynecol Oncol 96:56, 2005

Mackenzie F, Mathers A, Kennedy I: Invasive hydatidiform mole presenting as an acute primary haemoperitoneum. Br J Obstet Gynaecol 100:953, 1993

Mangili G, Garavaglia E, Cavoretto P, et al: Clinical presentation of hydatidiform mole in northern Italy: has it changed in the last 20 years? Am J Obstet Gynecol 2008 198(3):302.e1-4, 2008

Mangili G, Garavaglia E, Frigerio L, et al: Management of low-risk gestational trophoblastic tumors with etoposide (VP16) in patients resistant to methotrexate. Gynecol Oncol 61:218, 1996

Mao Y, Wan X, Lv W, et al: Relapsed or refractory gestational trophoblastic neoplasia treated with etoposide and cisplatin/etoposide, methotrexate, and actinomycin D (EP-EMA) regimen. Int J Gynaecol Obstet 98:44, 2007

Marcorelles P, Audrezet MP, Le Bris MJ, et al: Diagnosis and outcome of complete hydatidiform mole coexisting with a live twin fetus. Eur J Obstet Gynecol Reprod Biol 118:21, 2005

Massad LS, Abu-Rustum NR, Lee SS, et al: Poor compliance with postmolar surveillance and treatment protocols by indigent women. Obstet Gynecol 96:940, 2000

Matsui H, Iitsuka Y, Yamazawa K, et al: Changes in the incidence of molar pregnancies: a population-based study in Chiba Prefecture and Japan between 1974 and 2000. Hum Reprod 18:172, 2003

Matsui H, Sekiya S, Hando T, et al: Hydatidiform mole coexistent with a twin live fetus: a national collaborative study in Japan. Hum Reprod 15:608, 2000

Matsui H, Suzuka K, Yamazawa K, et al: Relapse rate of patients with low-risk gestational trophoblastic tumor initially treated with single-agent chemotherapy. Gynecol Oncol 96:616, 2005

McNeish IA, Strickland S, Holden L, et al: Low-risk persistent gestational trophoblastic disease: outcome after initial treatment with low-dose methotrexate and folinic acid from 1992 to 2000. J Clin Oncol 20:1838, 2002

Merchant SH, Amin MB, Viswanatha DS, et al: p57KIP2 immunohistochemistry in early molar pregnancies: emphasis on its complementary role in the differential diagnosis of hydropic abortuses. Hum Pathol 36:180, 2005

Montz FJ, Schlaerth JB, Morrow CP: The natural history of theca lutein cysts. Obstet Gynecol 72:247, 1988

Moodley M, Tunkyi K, Moodley J: Gestational trophoblastic syndrome: an audit of 112 patients. A South African experience. Int J Gynecol Cancer 13:234, 2003

Mosher R, Goldstein DP, Berkowitz R, et al: Complete hydatidiform mole: comparison of clinicopathologic features, current and past. J Reprod Med 43:21, 1998

Mungan T, Kuscu E, Dabakoglu T, et al: Hydatidiform mole: clinical analysis of 310 patients. Int J Gynaecol Obstet 52:233, 1996

Newlands ES, Holden L, Seckl MJ, et al: Management of brain metastases in patients with high-risk gestational trophoblastic tumors. J Reprod Med 47:465, 2002

Newlands ES, Mulholland PJ, Holden L, et al: Etoposide and cisplatin/etoposide, methotrexate, and actinomycin D (EMA) chemotherapy for patients with high-risk gestational trophoblastic tumors refractory to EMA/cyclophosphamide and vincristine chemotherapy and patients presenting with metastatic placental site trophoblastic tumors. J Clin Oncol 18:854, 2000

Ngan HY: The practicability of FIGO 2000 staging for gestational trophoblastic neoplasia. Int J Gynecol Cancer 14:202, 2004

Numnum TM, Leath CA III, Straughn JM Jr, et al: Occult choriocarcinoma discovered by positron emission tomography/computed tomography imaging following a successful pregnancy. Gynecol Oncol 97:713, 2005

Olsen TG, Hubert PR, Nycum LR: Falsely elevated human chorionic gonadotropin leading to unnecessary therapy. Obstet Gynecol 98:843, 2001

Osborne R, Covens A, Mirchandani D, et al: Successful salvage of relapsed high-risk gestational trophoblastic neoplasia patients using a novel paclitaxel-containing doublet. J Reprod Med 49:655, 2004

Osborne R, Filiaci V, Schink J, et al: A randomized phase III trial comparing weekly parenteral methotrexate and "pulsed" dactinomycin as primary management for low-risk gestational trophoblastic neoplasia: a gynecologic oncology group study. Gynecol Oncol 108:S2, 2008

Ozalp S, Metintas S, Arslantas D, et al: Frequency of hydatidiform mole in the rural part of Eskisehir: the first community-based epidemiological study in Turkey. Eur J Gynaecol Oncol 24:315, 2003

Palmer JR, Driscoll SG, Rosenberg L, et al: Oral contraceptive use and risk of gestational trophoblastic tumors. J Natl Cancer Inst 91:635, 1999

Palmer JE, Macdonald M, Wells M, et al: Epithelioid trophoblastic tumor: a review of the literature. J Reprod Med 53:465, 2008

Palmieri C, Dhillon T, Fisher RA, et al: Management and outcome of healthy women with a persistently elevated beta-hCG. Gynecol Oncol 106:35, 2007

Papadopoulos AJ, Foskett M, Seckl MJ, et al: Twenty-five years' clinical experience with placental site trophoblastic tumors. J Reprod Med 47:460, 2002

Paradinas FJ, Fisher RA, Browne P, et al: Diploid hydatidiform moles with fetal red blood cells in molar villi: 1. Pathology, incidence, and prognosis. J Pathol 181:183, 1997

Parazzini F, Cipriani S, Mangili G, et al: Oral contraceptives and risk of gestational trophoblastic disease. Contraception 65:425, 2002

Parazzini F, La Vecchia C, Mangili G, et al: Dietary factors and risk of trophoblastic disease. Am J Obstet Gynecol 158:93, 1988

Parazzini F, La Vecchia C, Pampallona S: Parental age and risk of complete and partial hydatidiform mole. Br J Obstet Gynaecol 93:582, 1986

Parazzini F, Mangili G, La Vecchia C, et al: Risk factors for gestational trophoblastic disease: a separate analysis of complete and partial hydatidiform moles. Obstet Gynecol 78:1039, 1991

Patel SM, Desai A: Management of drug resistant gestational trophoblastic neoplasia. J Reprod Med 55:296, 2010

Petru E, Luck JH, Stuart G, et al: Gynecologic Cancer Intergroup (GCIG) proposals for changes of the current FIGO staging system. Eur J Obstet Gynecol Reprod Biol 143:69, 2009

Pezeshki M, Hancock BW, Silcocks P, et al: The role of repeat uterine evacuation in the management of persistent gestational trophoblastic disease. Gynecol Oncol 95:423, 2004

Pfeffer PE, Sebire N, Lindsay I, et al: Fertility-sparing partial hysterectomy for placental-site trophoblastic tumour. Lancet Oncol 8:744, 2007

Pisal N, North C, Tidy J, et al: Role of hysterectomy in management of gestational trophoblastic disease. Gynecol Oncol 87:190, 2002

Powles T, Savage P, Short D, et al: Residual lung lesions after completion of chemotherapy for gestational trophoblastic neoplasia: should we operate? Br J Cancer 94:51, 2006

Price JM, Hancock BW, Tidy J, et al: Screening for central nervous system disease in metastatic gestational trophoblastic neoplasia. J Reprod Med 55:301, 2010

Rodabaugh KJ, Bernstein MR, Goldstein DP, et al: Natural history of postterm choriocarcinoma. J Reprod Med 43:75, 1998

Rotmensch S, Cole LA: False diagnosis and needless therapy of presumed malignant disease in women with false-positive human chorionic gonadotropin concentrations. Lancet 355:712, 2000

Rustin GJ, Newlands ES, Lutz JM, et al: Combination but not single-agent methotrexate chemotherapy for gestational trophoblastic tumors increases the incidence of second tumors. J Clin Oncol 14:2769, 1996

Sasaki S: Clinical presentation and management of molar pregnancy. Best Pract Res Clin Obstet Gynaecol 17:885, 2003

Savage P, Williams J, Wong SL, et al: The demographics of molar pregnancies in England and Wales from 2000-2009. J Reprod Med 5:341, 2010

Schechter NR, Mychalczak B, Jones W, et al: Prognosis of patients treated with whole-brain radiation therapy for metastatic gestational trophoblastic disease. Gynecol Oncol 68:183, 1998

Schmid P, Nagai Y, Agarwal R, et al: Prognostic markers and long-term outcome of placental-site trophoblastic tumors: a retrospective observational study. Lancet 374:48, 2009

Schorge JO, Lea JS, Farrar DF, et al: Management of low-risk gestational trophoblastic neoplasia in indigent women. J Reprod Med 48:780, 2003

Sebire NJ, Fisher RA, Foskett M, et al: Risk of recurrent hydatidiform mole and subsequent pregnancy outcome following complete or partial hydatidiform molar pregnancy. Br J Obstet Gynaecol 110:22, 2003

Sebire NJ, Foskett M, Fisher RA, et al: Persistent gestational trophoblastic disease is rarely, if ever, derived from nonmolar first-trimester miscarriage. Med Hypoth 64:689, 2005a

Sebire NJ, Foskett M, Fisher RA, et al: Risk of partial and complete hydatidiform molar pregnancy in relation to maternal age. Br J Obstet Gynaecol 109:99, 2002a

Sebire NJ, Foskett M, Paradinas FJ, et al: Outcome of twin pregnancies with complete hydatidiform mole and healthy cotwin. Lancet 359:2165, 2002b

Sebire NJ, Foskett M, Short D, et al: Shortened duration of human chorionic gonadotrophin surveillance following complete or partial hydatidiform mole: evidence for revised protocol of a UK regional trophoblastic disease unit. BJOG 114:760, 2007

Sebire NJ, Lindsay I, Fisher RA, et al: Overdiagnosis of complete and partial hydatidiform mole in tubal ectopic pregnancies. Int J Gynecol Pathol 24:260, 2005b

Sebire NJ, Rees H, Paradinas F, et al: The diagnostic implications of routine ultrasound examination in histologically confirmed early molar pregnancies. Ultrasound Obstet Gynecol 18:662, 2001

Seckl MJ, Dhillon T, Dancey G, et al: Increased gestational age at evacuation of a complete hydatidiform mole: does it correlate with increased risk of requiring chemotherapy? J Reprod Med 49:527, 2004

Seckl MJ, Fisher RA, Salerno G, et al: Choriocarcinoma and partial hydatidiform moles. Lancet 356:36, 2000

Seckl MJ, Rustin GJS, Newlands ES, et al : Pulmonary embolism, pulmonary hypertension, and choriocarcinoma. Lancet 338:1313, 1991

Seckl MJ, Sebire NJ, Berkowitz RS: Gestational trophoblastic disease. Lancet 376:717, 2010

Sharma S, Jagdev S, Coleman RE, et al: Serosal complications of single-agent low-dose methotrexate used in gestational trophoblastic diseases: first reported case of methotrexate-induced peritonitis. Br J Cancer 81:1037, 1999

Shih IM, Kurman RJ: Epithelioid trophoblastic tumor: a neoplasm distinct from choriocarcinoma and placental site trophoblastic tumor simulating carcinoma. Am J Surg Pathol 22:1393, 1998

Smith HO, Hilgers RD, Bedrick EJ, et al: Ethnic differences at risk for gestational trophoblastic disease in New Mexico: a 25-year population-based study. Am J Obstet Gynecol 188:357, 2003

Soper JT, Mutch DG, Schink JC: Diagnosis and treatment of gestational trophoblastic disease. ACOG Practice Bulletin No. 53. Gynecol Oncol 93:575, 2004

Soto-Wright V, Bernstein M, Goldstein DP, et al: The changing clinical presentation of complete molar pregnancy. Obstet Gynecol 86:775, 1995

Stefos T, Plachouras N, Mari G, et al: A case of partial mole and atypical type I triploidy associated with severe HELLP syndrome at 18 weeks' gestation. Ultrasound Obstet Gynecol 20:403, 2002

Suzuka K, Matsui H, Iitsuka Y, et al: Adjuvant hysterectomy in low-risk gestational trophoblastic disease. Obstet Gynecol 97:431, 2001

Tham BW, Everard JE, Tidy JA, et al: Gestational trophoblastic disease in the Asian population of northern England and North Wales. Br J Obstet Gynaecol 110:555, 2003

Tidy JA, Gillespie AM, Bright N, et al: Gestational trophoblastic disease: a study of mode of evacuation and subsequent need for treatment with chemotherapy. Gynecol Oncol 78:309, 2000

Tidy JA, Rustin GJ, Newlands ES, et al: Presentation and management of choriocarcinoma after nonmolar pregnancy. Br J Obstet Gynaecol 102:715, 1995

Tuncer ZS, Bernstein MR, Goldstein DP, et al: Outcome of pregnancies occurring within 1 year of hydatidiform mole. Obstet Gynecol 94:588, 1999

Uberti EMH, Fajardo MDC, da Cunha AGV, et al: Prevention of postmolar gestational trophoblastic neoplasia using prophylactic single bolus dose of actinomycin D in high-risk hydatidiform mole: a simple, effective, secure and low-cost approach without adverse effects on compliance to general follow-up or subsequent treatment. Gynecol Oncol 114:299, 2009

van Trommel NE, Massuger LF, Verheijen RH, et al: The curative effect of a second curettage in persistent trophoblastic disease: a retrospective cohort survey. Gynecol Oncol 99:6, 2005

Wang J, Short D, Sebire NJ, et al: Salvage chemotherapy of relapsed or high-risk gestational trophoblastic neoplasia (GTN) with paclitaxel/cisplatin alternating with paclitaxel/etoposide (TP/TE). Ann Oncol 19:1578, 2008

Wenzel LB, Berkowitz RS, Robinson S, et al: Psychological, social and sexual effects of gestational trophoblastic disease on patients and their partners. J Reprod Med 39:163, 1994

Wenzel L, Berkowitz R, Robinson S, et al: The psychological, social, and sexual consequences of gestational trophoblastic disease. Gynecol Oncol 46:74, 1992

Wolfberg AJ, Feltmate C, Goldstein DP, et al: Low risk of relapse after achieving undetectable hCG levels in women with complete molar pregnancy. Obstet Gynecol 104:551, 2004

Wong LC, Ngan HY, Cheng DK, et al: Methotrexate infusion in low-risk gestational trophoblastic disease. Am J Obstet Gynecol 183:1579, 2000

Yang JJ, Xiang Y, Yang XY, et al: Emergency craniotomy in patients with intracranial metastatic gestational trophoblastic tumor. Int J Gynaecol Obstet 89:35, 2005

Yarandi F, Eftekhar Z, Shojaei H, et al: Pulse methotrexate versus pulse actinomycin D in the treatment of low-risk gestational trophoblastic neoplasia. Int J Gynaecol Obstet 103:33, 2008

Zhou Q, Lei XY, Xie Q, et al: Sonographic and Doppler imaging in the diagnosis and treatment of gestational trophoblastic disease: a 12-year experience. J Ultrasound Med 24:15, 2005

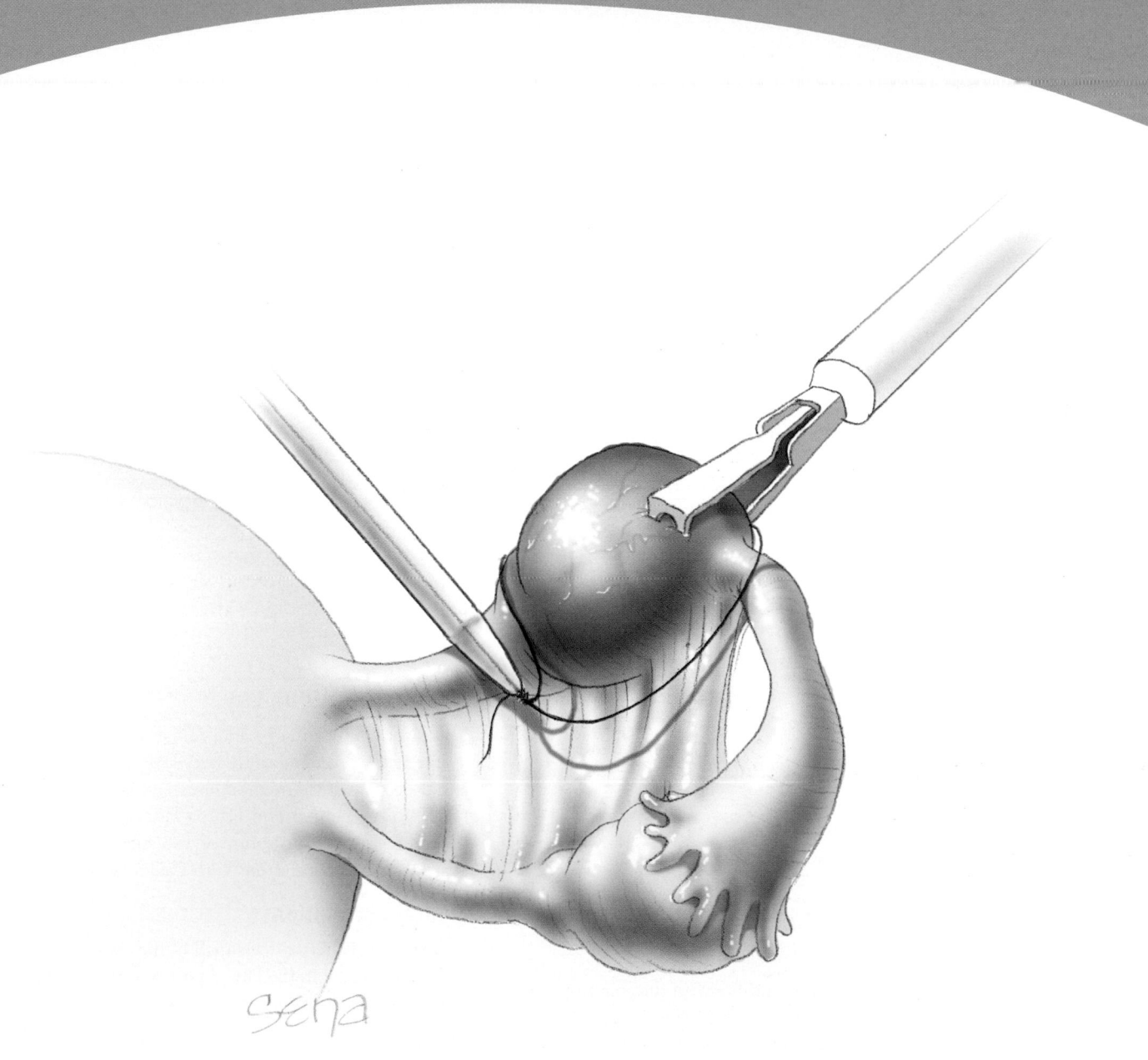

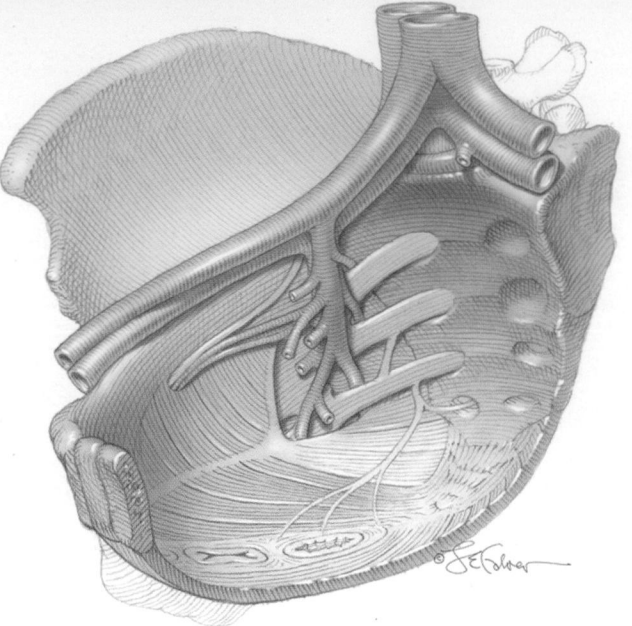

Anatomy

A gynecologic surgeon must be familiar with the anatomy of the female pelvis and lower abdominal wall. Over the past 20 years, the rote knowledge of pelvic anatomy has been complemented by a better understanding of the neuromuscular physiology that governs pelvic function. In this chapter, a broad overview of these relationships is presented.

ANTERIOR ABDOMINAL WALL

The anterior abdominal wall provides core support to the human torso, confines abdominal viscera, and contributes muscular action for functions such as respiration and elimination. In gynecology,

comprehensive knowledge of the layered structure of the anterior abdominal wall is needed to effectively enter the peritoneal cavity for surgery without neurovascular complications.

Skin

The term *Langer lines* describes the orientation of dermal fibers within the skin. In the anterior abdominal wall, they are arranged in a primarily transverse orientation (Fig. 38-1). As a result, vertical skin incisions sustain more lateral tension and thus, in general, develop wider scars compared with transverse skin incisions.

Subcutaneous Layer

This layer of the anterior abdominal wall can be separated into a superficial, predominantly fatty layer known as *Camper fascia* and a deeper, more membranous layer known as *Scarpa fascia* (Fig. 38-2). Camper and Scarpa fasciae are not discrete layers but represent a continuum of the subcutaneous tissue layer. Scarpa fascia is continuous with Colles fascia in the perineum.

Clinical Correlation

Scarpa fascia is better developed in the lower abdomen and can be best identified in the lateral portions of a low transverse incision, just superficial to the rectus fascia. In contrast, this fascia is rarely recognized during midline incisions.

Rectus Sheath

The aponeuroses of the *external oblique, internal oblique,* and *tranversus abdominis muscles* (flank muscles) conjoin, and their layers create the rectus sheath (see Fig. 38-2). In the midline, these aponeurotic layers fuse to create the linea alba. In the lower abdomen, transition from the muscular to the aponeurotic component of the external oblique muscle takes place along a vertical line through the anterior superior iliac spine. Transition from muscle to aponeurosis

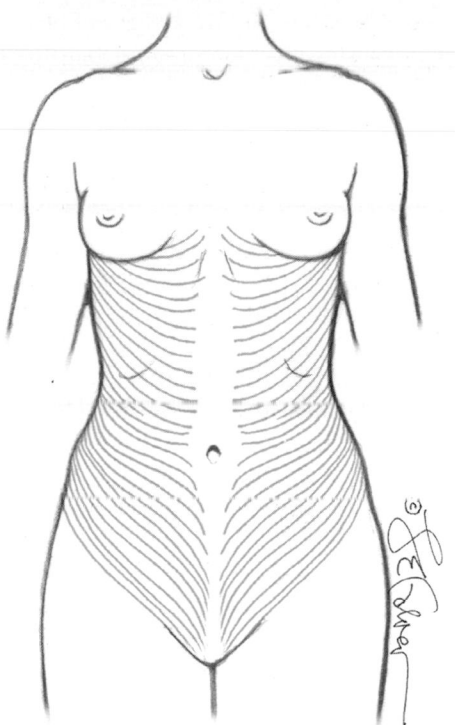

FIGURE 38-1 Langer lines of skin tension.

for the internal oblique and transversus abdominis muscles takes place at a more medial site. For this reason, muscle fibers of the internal oblique muscle are often noted below the aponeurotic layer of the external oblique muscle during low transverse incisions.

The anatomy of the rectus sheath above and below the *arcuate line* has significance to the surgeon (see Fig. 38-2). This horizontal line defines the level at which the rectus sheath passes entirely anterior to the rectus abdominis muscle, and this line typically lies midway between the umbilicus and pubic symphysis. Cephalad to the arcuate line, the rectus sheath lies both anterior and posterior to the rectus abdominis muscle. At this level, the anterior rectus sheath is formed by the aponeurosis of the external oblique muscle and the split aponeurosis of the internal oblique muscle. The posterior rectus sheath is formed by the split aponeurosis of the internal oblique muscle and aponeurosis of the transversus abdominis muscle. Caudad to the arcuate line, all aponeurotic layers pass anterior to the rectus abdominis muscle. Thus, in the lower abdomen, the posterior surface of the rectus abdominis muscle is in direct contact with the transversalis fascia.

Clinical Correlation

In the lower abdomen, the aponeuroses of the internal oblique and transversus abdominis muscles fuse. Therefore, only two layers are identified during low transverse fascial incisions (Sections 41-2, p. 1022). In contrast, during midline vertical incision through the linea alba, only one fascial layer is encountered.

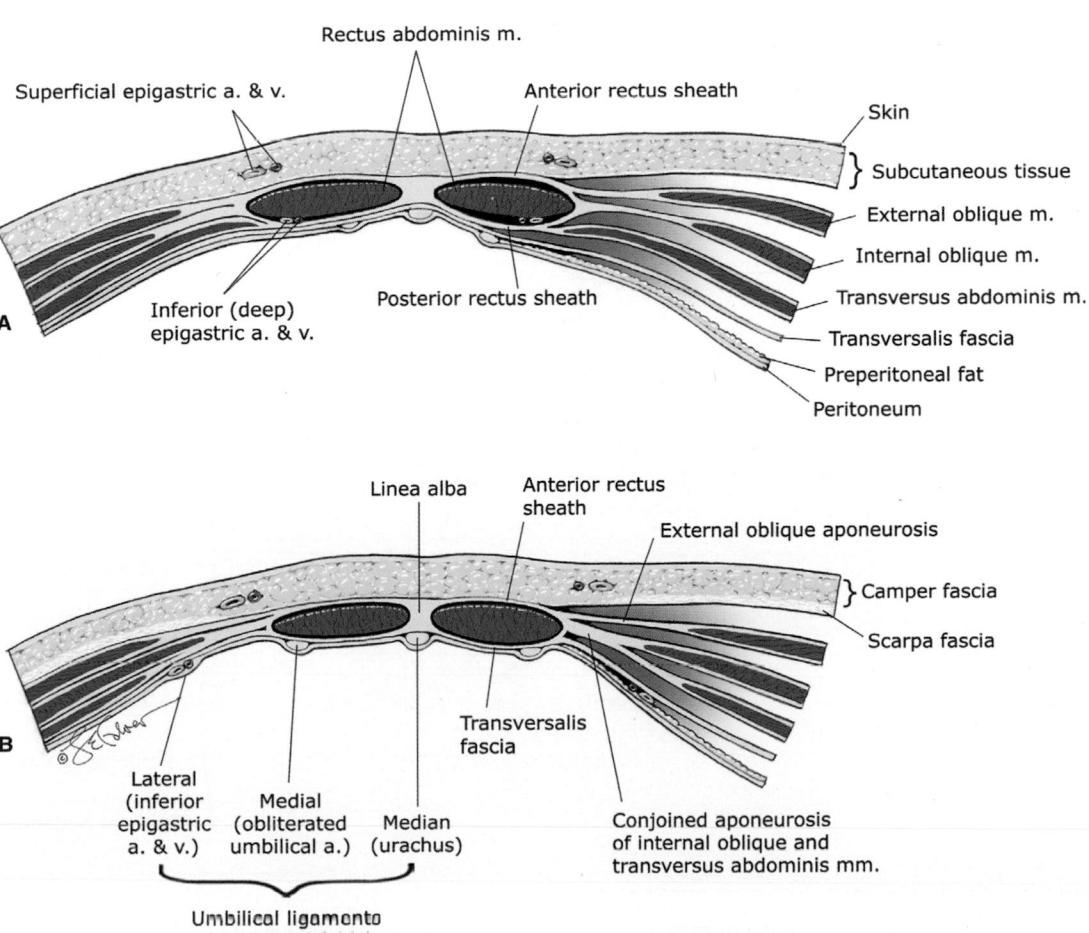

FIGURE 38-2 Transverse sections of the anterior abdominal wall above **(A)** and below **(B)** the arcuate line.

Similar to the fibers of the skin, the flank muscle fibers are oriented primarily transversely. Therefore, suture lines placed in a vertical fascial incision must withstand more tension than those in a transverse incision. As a result, vertical fascial incisions are more prone to dehiscence and hernia formation. In addition to incisional hernias, ventral wall hernias are most common along the linea alba. Another type of anterior abdominal wall hernia, the Spiegelian hernia, is rare and forms at the lateral rectus abdominis border, typically at the level of the arcuate line (Fig. 11-9, p. 324).

Tranversalis Fascia

This thin layer of fibrous tissue lies between the inner surface of the transversus abdominis muscle and preperitoneal fat. Thus, it serves as part of the general fascial layer that lines the abdominal cavity (see Fig. 38-2) (Memon, 1999). Inferiorly, the transversalis fascia blends with the periosteum of the symphysis pubis at a point lateral to the insertion of the rectus abdominis muscle.

Clinical Correlation

This fascia is best recognized as the layer bluntly or sharply dissected off the anterior surface of the bladder during entry into the abdominal cavity. This is the layer of tissue that is last penetrated to gain extraperitoneal entry into the retropubic space (p. 936).

Peritoneum

The peritoneum that lines the inner surface of the abdominal walls is termed *parietal peritoneum*. In the anterior abdominal wall, there are five elevations of parietal peritoneum that are raised by different structures (see Fig. 38-2). All five converge toward the umbilicus and are known as *umbilical ligaments*.

The single *median umbilical ligament* is formed by the *urachus*, an obliterated tube that extends from the apex of the bladder to the umbilicus. In fetal life, the urachus, which is a fibrous remnant of the allantois, extends from the fetal hindgut to the umbilical cord. The paired *medial umbilical ligaments* are formed by the obliterated umbilical arteries that connected the internal iliac arteries to the umbilical cord in fetal life. The paired *lateral umbilical ligaments* contain the patent inferior epigastric vessels. The initial course of these vessels is just medial to the round ligament as the ligament enters the deep inguinal ring (Fig. 38-3).

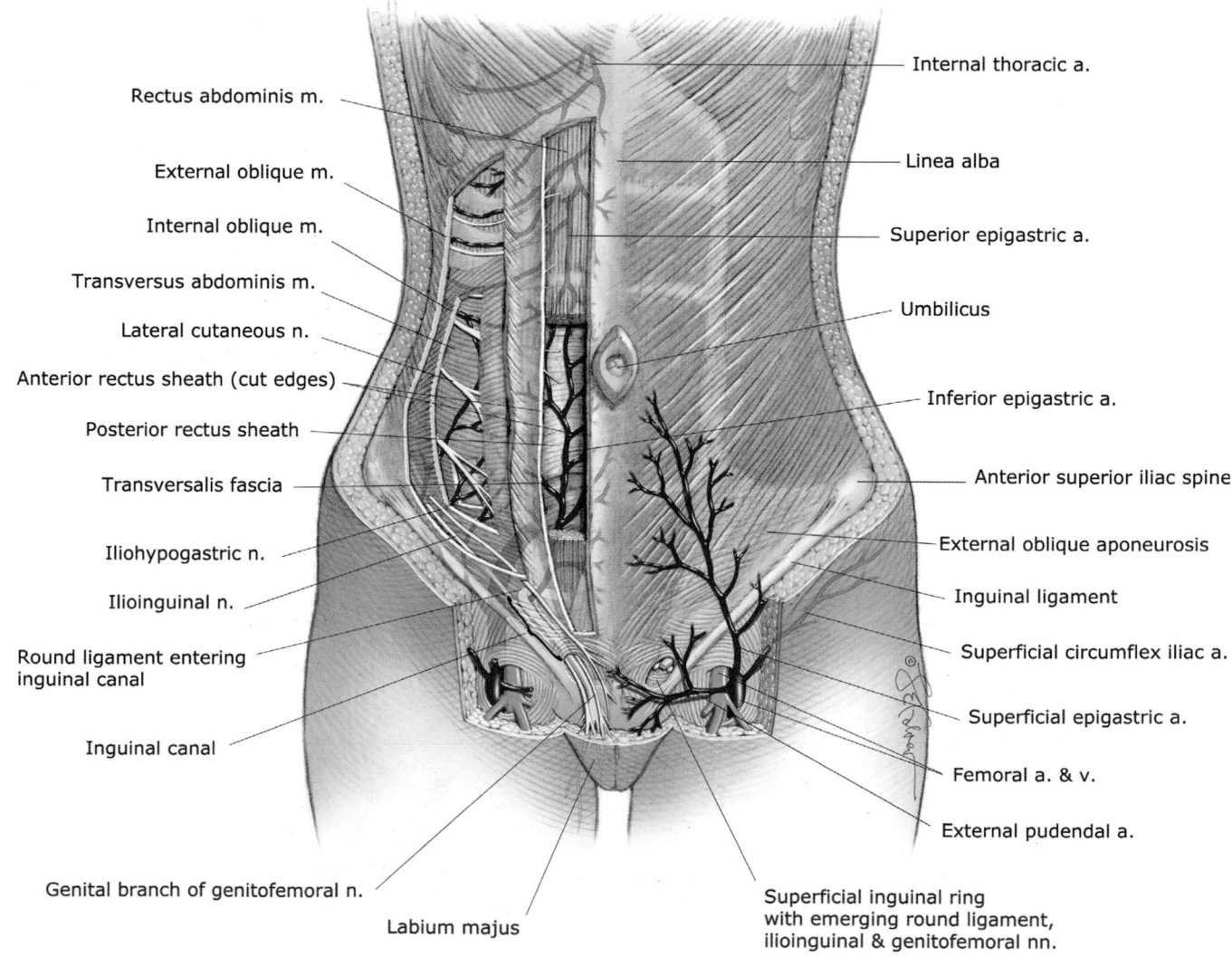

Rectus abdominis m.
External oblique m.
Internal oblique m.
Transversus abdominis m.
Lateral cutaneous n.
Anterior rectus sheath (cut edges)
Posterior rectus sheath
Transversalis fascia
Iliohypogastric n.
Ilioinguinal n.
Round ligament entering inguinal canal
Inguinal canal
Genital branch of genitofemoral n.
Labium majus

Internal thoracic a.
Linea alba
Superior epigastric a.
Umbilicus
Inferior epigastric a.
Anterior superior iliac spine
External oblique aponeurosis
Inguinal ligament
Superficial circumflex iliac a.
Superficial epigastric a.
Femoral a. & v.
External pudendal a.
Superficial inguinal ring with emerging round ligament, ilioinguinal & genitofemoral nn.

FIGURE 38-3 Anterior abdominal wall anatomy.

Clinical Correlation

Transection of a patent urachus can result in extravasation of urine into the abdominal cavity. In addition, the differential diagnosis of a midline anterior abdominal wall cyst should include urachal cyst, urachal sinus, and urachal diverticulum.

The umbilical ligaments serve as valuable laparoscopic landmarks (Fig. 42-1.17, p. 1109). First, the inferior epigastric vessels can be injured during accessory trocar placement (Hurd, 1994; Rahn, 2010). Thus, direct visualization of the lateral umbilical folds can prevent injury to these vessels during laparoscopic port placement. Secondly, the medial umbilical ligaments, if followed proximally, can guide a surgeon to the internal iliac artery and uterine arteries. The medial umbilical ligament also forms the medial border of the paravesical space, which is developed during radical hysterectomy to isolate the parametrium (Fig. 44-3.2, p. 1269).

■ Blood Supply

Laceration of abdominal wall vessels can increase blood loss and the risk of postoperative hematoma formation. Accordingly, familiarity with the origin and course of vessels that supply the anterior abdominal wall structures is essential.

Femoral Branches

The *superficial epigastric, superficial circumflex iliac,* and *external pudendal arteries* arise from the femoral artery just below the inguinal ligament in the region of the femoral triangle (see Fig. 38-3). These vessels supply the skin and subcutaneous layers of the anterior abdominal wall and mons pubis. The superficial epigastric vessels course diagonally toward the umbilicus, similar to the inferior "deep" epigastric vessels.

Clinical Correlation. During low transverse skin incisions, the superficial epigastric vessels can usually be identified halfway between the skin and the rectus fascia, several centimeters from the midline. During laparoscopic procedures in thin patients, these vessels can be identified by transillumination (Chap. 42, p. 1116).

The external pudendal vessels form rich anastomoses with their contralateral equivalents and with other superficial branches. These anastomoses account for the extensive bleeding often encountered with incisions made in the mons pubis area such as for retropubic midurethral sling incisions.

External Iliac Branches

The *inferior "deep" epigastric vessels* and *deep circumflex iliac vessels* are branches of the external iliac vessels (see Fig. 38-3). They supply the muscles and fascia of the anterior abdominal wall. The inferior epigastric vessels initially course lateral to, then posterior to the rectus abdominis muscle, which they supply. They then pass anterior to the posterior rectus sheath and course between the sheath and the rectus muscles (see Figs. 38-2 and 38-3). Near the umbilicus, the inferior epigastric vessels anastomose with the superior epigastric artery and veins, which are branches of the internal thoracic vessels.

Hesselbach triangle is the region in the anterior abdominal wall bounded inferiorly by the inguinal ligament, medially by the lateral border of the rectus muscles, and laterally by the inferior epigastric vessels (Fig. 38-4).

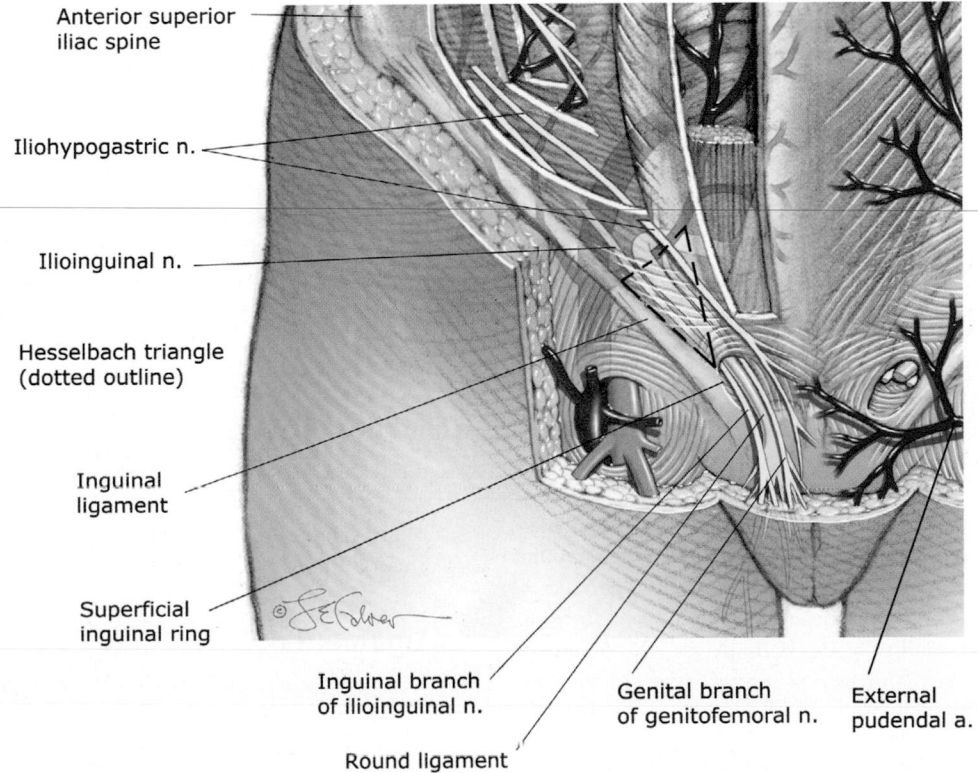

Anterior superior iliac spine

Iliohypogastric n.

Ilioinguinal n.

Hesselbach triangle (dotted outline)

Inguinal ligament

Superficial inguinal ring

Inguinal branch of ilioinguinal n.

Round ligament

Genital branch of genitofemoral n.

External pudendal a.

FIGURE 38-4 Inguinal and upper thigh anatomy.

Clinical Correlation. Low transverse abdominal incisions that extend beyond the lateral margins of the rectus muscles can lead to inferior epigastric vessel laceration with severe hemorrhage or anterior abdominal wall hematoma formation. These vessels should be identified and ligated when performing a Maylard incision (Section 41-4, p. 1025). The deep circumflex iliac vein serves as the caudal border during pelvic lymph node dissection described in Section 44-11 (p. 1296).

Direct hernias protrude through the abdominal wall within Hesselbach triangle. In contrast, indirect hernias protrude through the deep inguinal ring lying lateral to this triangle (Fig. 11-10, p. 325).

Nerve Supply

The anterior abdominal wall is innervated by the abdominal extensions of the intercostal nerves (T7-11), the subcostal nerve (T12), and the iliohypogastric and the ilioinguinal nerves (L1) (see Fig. 38-3). The T10 dermatome approximates the level of the umbilicus.

The iliohypogastric nerve provides sensation to the skin over the suprapubic area. The ilioinguinal nerve supplies the skin of the lower abdominal wall and upper portion of the labia majora and medial portion of the thigh through its inguinal branch (see Fig. 38-4). These two nerves enter the anterior abdominal wall at a site 2 to 3 cm medial to the anterior superior iliac spine and then course between the layers of the rectus sheath (Whiteside, 2003).

Clinical Correlation

The ilioinguinal and iliohypogastric nerves can be entrapped during closure of low transverse incisions, especially if incisions extend beyond the lateral borders of the rectus muscle. They may also be injured by placement of lower abdominal accessory trocars. The risk of iliohypogastric and ilioinguinal nerve injury can be minimized if lateral trocars are placed superior to the anterior superior iliac spines and low transverse fascial incisions are not extended beyond the lateral borders of the rectus muscle (Rahn, 2010).

PELVIC ANATOMY

Bony Pelvis and Pelvic Joints

The bony pelvis is comprised of the *sacrum;* the *coccyx;* and two hip bones, termed the *innominate bones* (Fig. 38-5). The innominate bones consist of the *ilium, ischium,* and *pubis,* which fuse at the *acetabulum,* a cup-shaped structure that articulates with the femoral head. The ilium articulates with the sacrum posteriorly at the sacroiliac joint, and the pubic bones articulate with each other anteriorly at the symphysis pubis. The sacroiliac joint is a synovial joint that connects the articular surfaces of the sacrum and ilium. This joint and its ligaments contribute significantly to the stability of the bony pelvis. The symphysis pubis is a cartilaginous joint, which connects the articular surfaces of the pubic bones by way of a fibrocartilaginous disc. The ischial spines are clinically important bony prominences that project posteromedially from the medial surface of the ischium approximately at the level of the fifth sacral vertebra (S5).

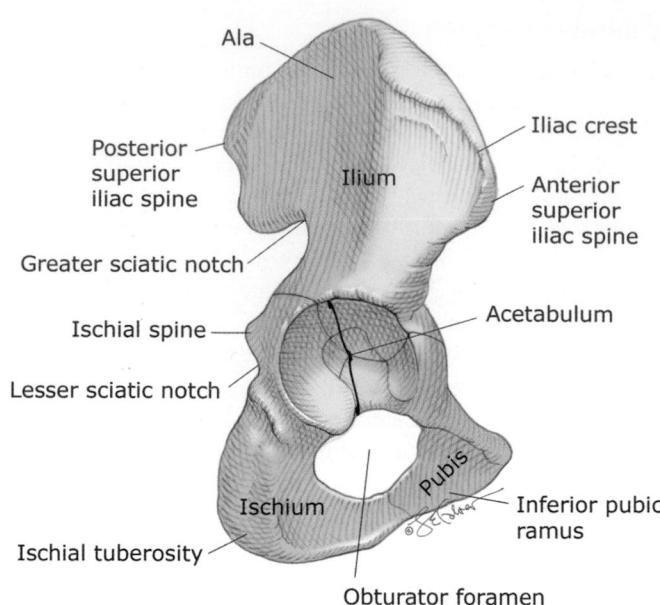

FIGURE 38-5 Right os coxae.

Pelvic Openings

The posterior, lateral, and inferior walls of the pelvis have several openings through which many important structures pass. The large *obturator foramen* between the ischium and pubis is filled almost completely by the obturator membrane. In the superior portion of this membrane, a small aperture known as the *obturator canal* allows passage of the obturator neurovascular bundle into the medial (adductor) compartment of the thigh (Fig. 38-6).

The posterolateral walls of the pelvis are not covered by bone. Instead, two important accessory ligaments, the *sacrospinous* and *sacrotuberous ligaments,* divide the greater and lesser sciatic notches of the ischium into the *greater sciatic foramen* and *lesser sciatic foramen.* The piriformis muscle, internal pudendal and inferior gluteal vessels, sciatic nerve, and other branches of the sacral nerve plexus pass through the greater sciatic foramen in close proximity to the ischial spines.

The internal pudendal vessels, pudendal nerve, and obturator internus tendon pass through the lesser sciatic foramen. Posteriorly, four pairs of pelvic sacral foramina allow passage of the anterior divisions of the first four sacral nerves and lateral sacral arteries and veins.

Clinical Correlation

Anatomic knowledge of the greater sciatic foramen area is critical to avoid neurovascular injury during sacrospinous fixation procedures and when administering pudendal nerve blockade (Roshanravan, 2007).

Ligaments

The term *ligament* is most often used to describe dense connective tissue that connects two bones. However, the ligaments of the pelvis are variable in composition and function. They range from connective tissue structures that support the bony pelvis and pelvic organs to smooth muscle and loose areolar tissue

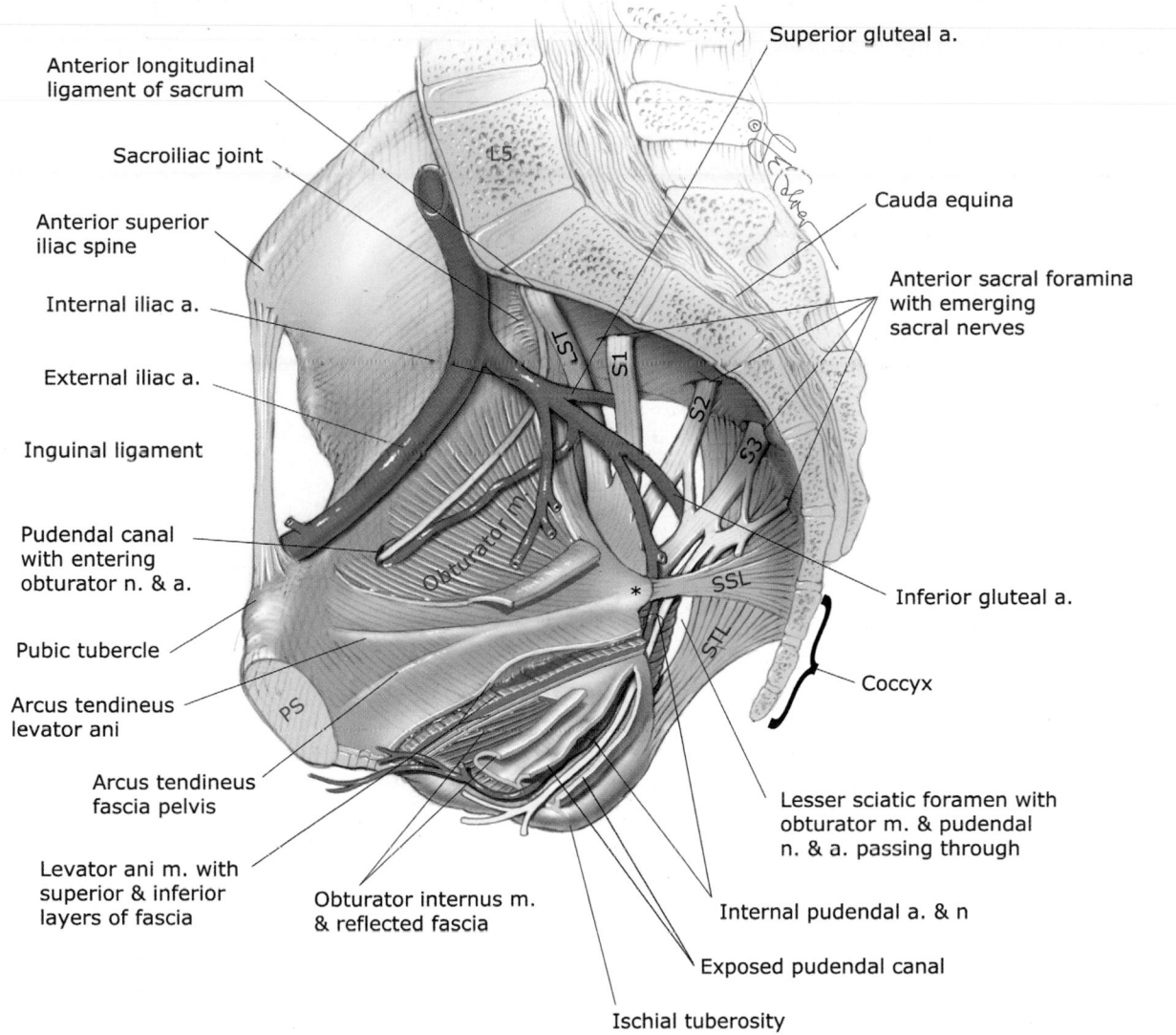

FIGURE 38-6 Bones, ligaments, and openings of the pelvic walls and associated structures. Note the obturator internus muscle extending below the levator ani muscle and then exiting through the lesser sciatic foramen to insert into the lateral femoral trochanter. Ischial spine is marked by an asterisk. L5 = fifth lumbar vertebra; LST = lumbosacral trunk; PS = pubic symphysis; S1–S3 = first through third sacral nerves; SSL = sacrospinous ligament; STL = sacrotuberous ligament.

that add no significant support. The *sacrospinous, sacrotuberous*, and *anterior longitudinal ligaments* of the sacrum consist of dense connective tissue that join bony structures and contribute significantly to bony pelvis stability (see Fig. 38-6).

The round and broad ligaments consist of smooth muscle and loose areolar tissue, respectively. Although they connect the uterus and adnexa to the pelvic walls, they do not contribute to the support of these organs. In contrast, the cardinal and uterosacral ligaments do aid in pelvic organ support and are discussed later (p. 930).

Clinical Correlation

The sacrospinous and anterior longitudinal ligament serve as suture fixation sites in suspensory procedures used to correct pelvic organ prolapse. The iliopectineal ligament, also termed Cooper ligament, is a thickening in the pubic bone periosteum, which is often used to anchor sutures in retropubic bladder neck suspension procedures (Fig. 38-7).

Pelvic Wall Muscles and Fascia
Muscles

The posterior, lateral, and inferior walls of the pelvis are partially covered by striated muscles and their investing layers of fasciae (see Fig. 38-7). The *piriformis muscle* arises from the anterior and lateral surface of the sacrum and partially fills the posterolateral pelvic walls. It exits the pelvis through the greater sciatic foramen, attaches to the greater trochanter of the femur, and functions as an external or lateral hip rotator. The obturator internus muscle partially fills the sidewalls of the pelvis. This muscle arises from the pelvic surfaces of the ilium and ischium and from the obturator membrane. It exits the pelvis through the lesser sciatic foramen, attaches to the greater trochanter of the femur, and also functions as an external hip rotator.

The urogenital hiatus is the U-shaped opening in the pelvic floor muscles through which the urethra, vagina, and rectum pass (Fig. 38-8).

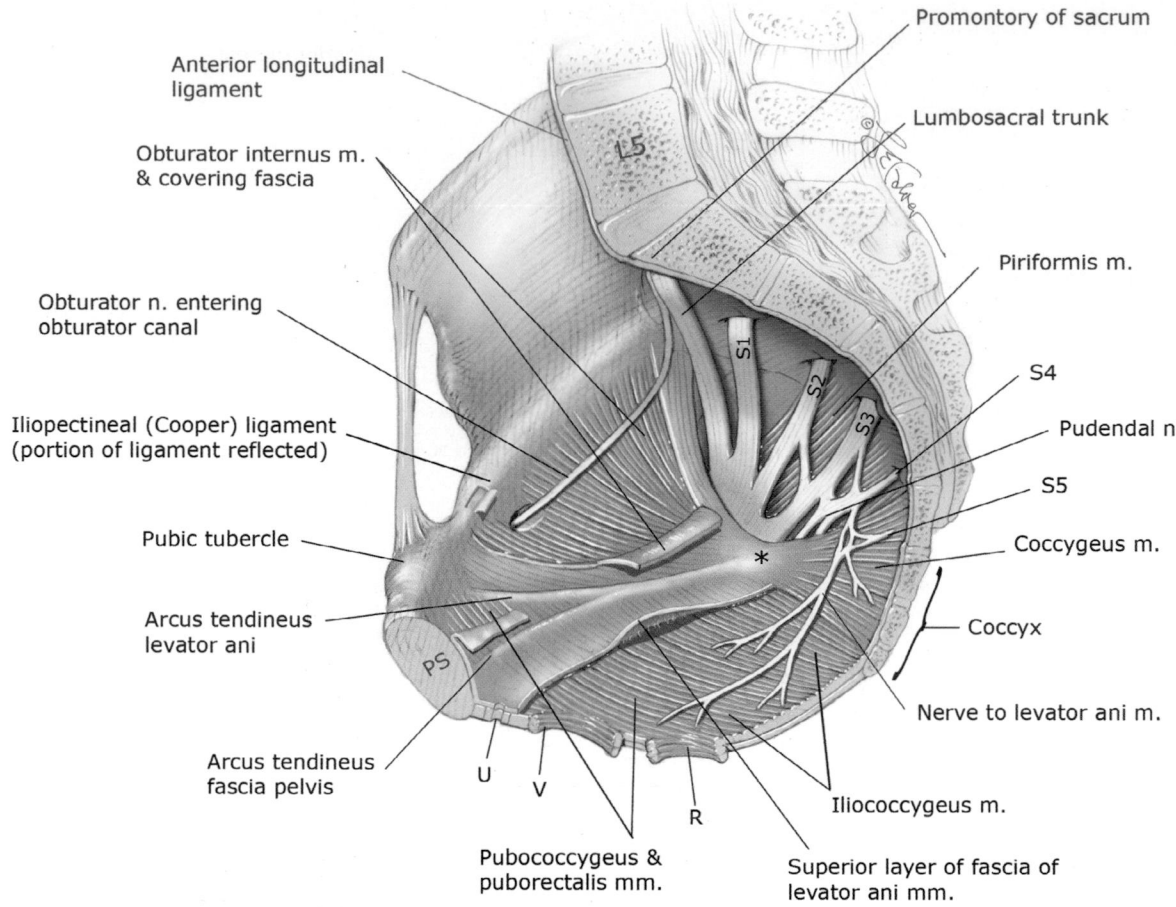

FIGURE 38-7 Muscles and fascia of the pelvic walls and pelvic floor innervation. Ischial spine is marked by an asterisk. L5 = fifth lumbar vertebra; PS = pubic symphysis; R = rectum; S1–S5 = first through fifth sacral nerves; U = urethra; V = vagina.

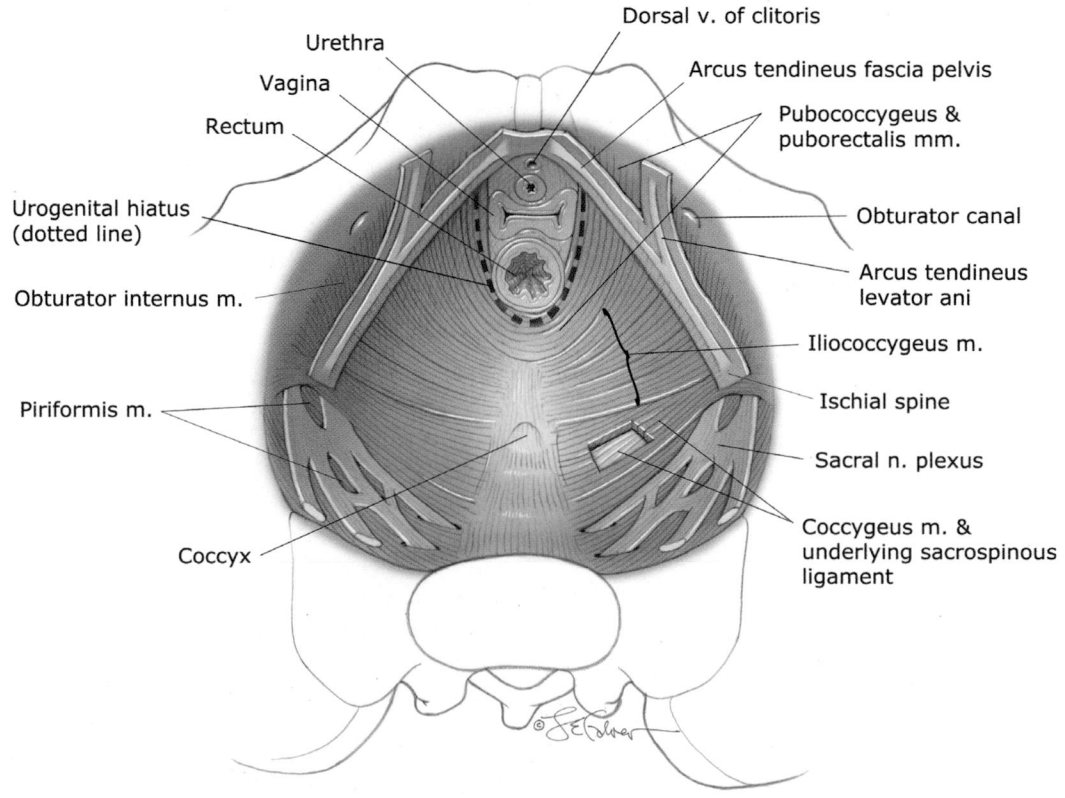

FIGURE 38-8 Superior view of pelvic floor and pelvic wall muscles.

Clinical Correlation. Stretch injury to the piriformis muscle may cause persistent hip pain that can be confused with other hip or pelvic pathology. Weakening and opening of the urogenital hiatus from neuromuscular injury to pelvic floor muscles allows urogenital prolapse as subsequently described.

Fascia

The fascia that invests striated muscles is termed *parietal fascia*. Histologically, this tissue consists of regular arrangements of collagen. Pelvic parietal fascia provides muscle attachment to the bony pelvis and serves as anchoring points for *visceral fascia*, also termed *endopelvic fascia*. The *arcus tendineus levator ani* is a condensation of parietal fascia covering the medial surface of the obturator internus muscle (see Figs. 38-7 and 38-8). This structure serves as the point of origin for parts of the very important levator ani muscle. Also shown Is the *arcus tendineus fascia pelvis*, a condensation of parietal fascia covering the medial aspects of the obturator internus and levator ani muscles. It represents the lateral point of attachment of the anterior vaginal wall.

Pelvic Floor

The muscles that span the pelvic floor are collectively known as the *pelvic diaphragm* (Figs. 38-7, 38-8, and 38-9). This diaphragm consists of the levator ani and coccygeus muscles, along with their superior and inferior investing layers of fasciae. Inferior to the pelvic diaphragm, the perineal membrane and perineal body also contribute to the pelvic floor (p. 942).

Levator Ani Muscles

These are the most important muscles in the pelvic floor and represent a critical component of pelvic organ support (see Figs. 38-7 through 38-9). Physiologically, normal levator ani muscles maintain a constant state of contraction, thus providing a stable floor, which supports the weight of the abdominopelvic contents against intraabdominal forces.

The levator ani muscle is a complex unit, which consists of several muscle components with different origins and insertions and therefore different functions. The *pubococcygeus, puborectalis*, and *iliococcygeus muscles* are the three components of this muscle recognized in the *Terminologia Anatomica* (1998). The pubococcygeus muscle is further divided into the *pubovaginalis, puboperinealis*, and *puboanalis muscles* according to their fiber attachments. Due to the significant attachments of the pubococcygeus muscle to the walls of the pelvic viscera, the term *pubovisceral muscle* is frequently used to describe this muscle (Kerney, 2004; Lawson, 1974).

Pubococcygeus Muscle. The anterior ends of the pubococcygeus (pubovisceral muscle) arise on either side from the inner surface of the pubic bone. The *pubovaginalis* refers to the medial fibers that attach to the lateral walls of the vagina (see Fig. 38-9). Although there are no direct attachments of the levator ani muscles to the urethra in females, those fibers of the muscle that attach to the vagina are responsible for elevating the urethra during a pelvic muscle contraction and hence may contribute to urinary continence (DeLancey, 1990). The *puboperinealis* refers to the fibers that attach to the perineal body and draw this structure toward the pubic symphysis. The *puboanalis* refers to the fibers that attach to the anus at the intersphincteric groove between the internal and external anal sphincters. These fibers elevate the anus and along with the rest of the pubococcygeus and puborectalis fibers, keep the urogenital hiatus narrowed (see Fig. 38-8).

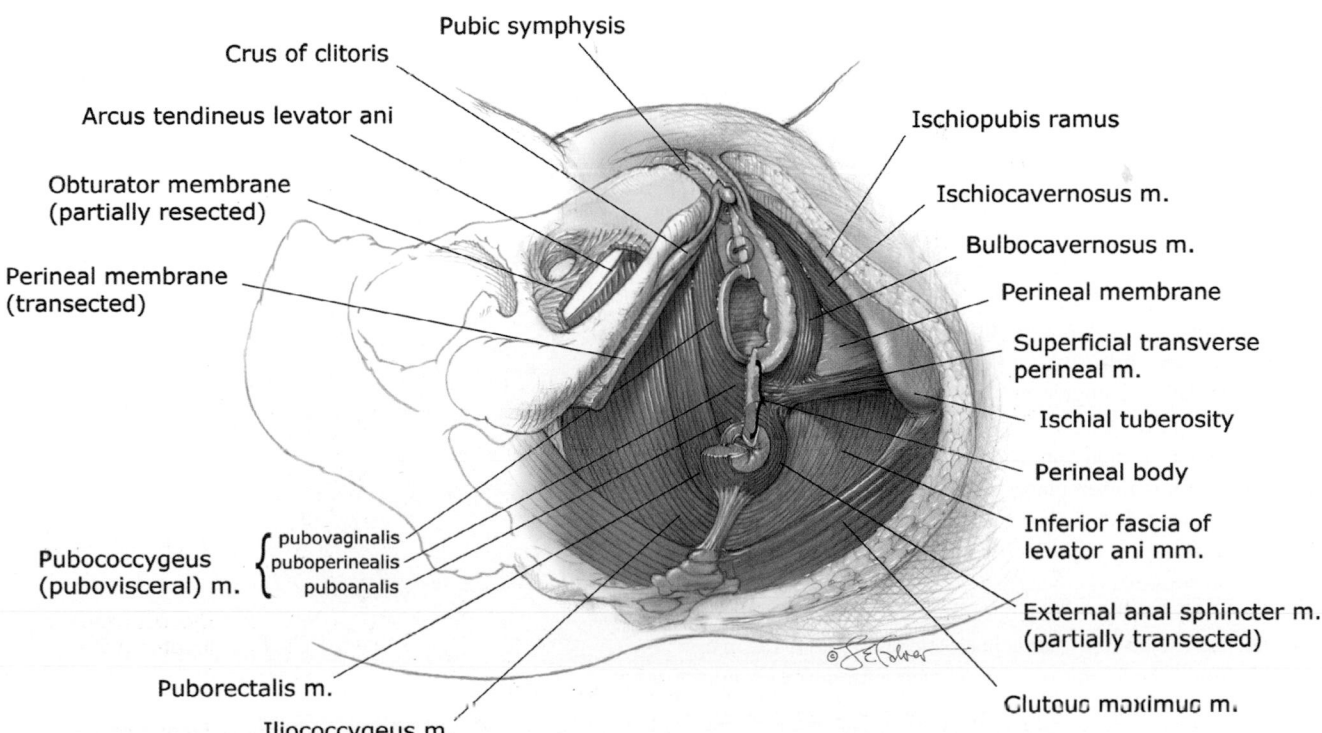

FIGURE 38-9 Inferior view of pelvic floor.

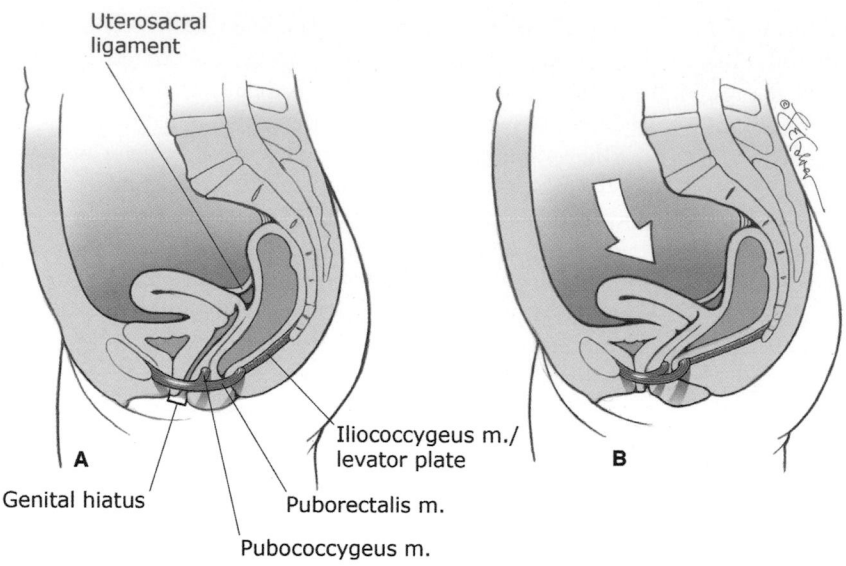

FIGURE 38-10 Pelvic organs and pelvic floor muscle and connective tissue interaction at rest **(A)** and with increasing intraabdominal pressure **(B)**.

Puborectalis Muscle. The puborectalis represents the medial and inferior fibers of the levator ani muscle that arise on either side from the pubic bone and form a U-shaped sling behind the anorectal junction (Figs. 38-8 through 38-10). The action of the puborectalis draws the anorectal junction toward the pubis, contributing to the anorectal angle. This muscle is considered part of the anal sphincter complex and may contribute to maintenance of fecal continence (Chap. 25, p. 660).

Iliococcygeus Muscle. This muscle is the most posterior and thinnest part of the levator ani muscle and has a primarily supportive role. It arises laterally from the arcus tendineus levator ani and the ischial spines (see Figs. 38-7 through 38-10). Muscle fibers from one side join those from the opposite side in the midline region between the anus and the coccyx. This meeting line is termed the *iliococcygeal* or *anococcygeal raphe*. In addition to the iliococcygeus muscle, some fibers of the pubococcygeus muscle pass behind the rectum and attach to the coccyx. These muscle fibers course cephalad or deep to the iliococcygeus muscle and may also contribute to the anococcygeal raphe.

The *levator plate* is the clinical term used to describe the anococcygeal raphe (see Fig. 38-10). This portion of the levator muscles forms a supportive shelf upon which the rectum, upper vagina, and uterus rest.

An important radiographic levator myography study by Berglas and Rubin (1953) led to the long-standing belief that in women with normal support, the levator plate lies almost parallel to the horizontal plane in the standing position. Their study also showed that the levator plate is displaced more vertically during straining in women with prolapse than in women with normal support.

In contrast to the horizontal position of the levator plate previously described, a recent dynamic magnetic resonance (MR) imaging study found the levator plate in women with normal support to have a mean angle of 44 degrees relative to a horizontal reference line during Valsalva (Hsu, 2006). Similar to previous observations, the authors also showed that during Valsalva, women with prolapse have a statistically greater levator plate angle compared with con-

trols. This larger angle showed moderate correlation with larger levator hiatus length and greater displacement of the perineal body in women with prolapse compared with controls.

One theory suggests that levator plate support prevents excessive tension or stretching of the connective tissue pelvic ligaments and fasciae (Paramore, 1908). Accordingly, neuromuscular injury to the levator muscles may lead to eventual sagging or vertical inclination of the levator plate and opening of the urogenital hiatus. Consequently, the vaginal axis becomes more vertical, and the cervix is oriented over the opened hiatus (Fig. 38-11). The mechanical effect of this change is to increase strain on connective tissues that support the pelvic viscera. Increased urogenital hiatus size has been shown to correlate with increased prolapse severity (DeLancey, 1998).

Pelvic Floor Innervation

The pelvic diaphragm muscles are primarily innervated by direct somatic efferents from the second through the fifth sacral nerve roots (S2-5) (see Fig. 38-7) (Barber, 2002; Roshanravan, 2007).

Traditionally, a dual innervation has been described. The pelvic or superior surface of the muscles is supplied by direct efferents from S2-5, collectively known as the nerve to the levator ani muscle. The perineal or inferior surface is supplied by branches of the pudendal nerve. This latter relationship has been recently challenged, with the suggestion that the pudendal nerve does not contribute to levator muscle innervation (Barber, 2002). Pudendal branches do, however, innervate parts of the striated urethral sphincter and external anal sphincter muscles (p. 944).

Separate innervation of the levator ani muscle and of the striated urethral and anal sphincters may explain why some women develop pelvic organ prolapse and others develop urinary or fecal incontinence (Heit, 1996).

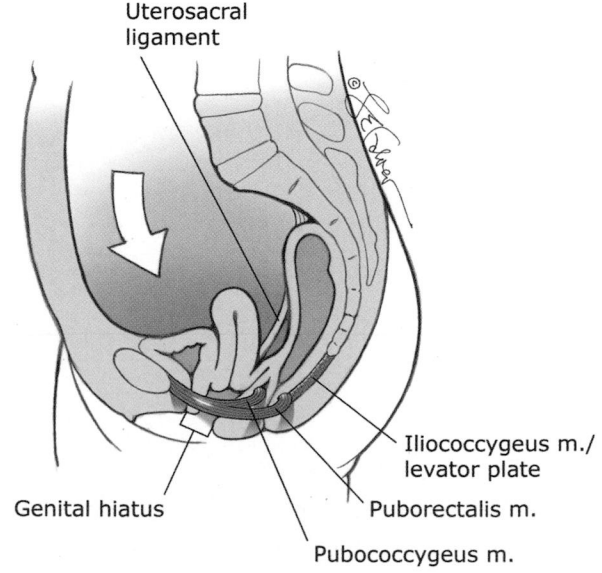

FIGURE 38-11 Pelvic floor muscles and connective tissue interaction in setting of pelvic organ prolapse.

TABLE 38-1. Differences between Visceral and Parietal Fascia of the Pelvic Floor Muscles

	Type of Fascia	
Characteristic	**Visceral or Endopelvic**	**Parietal**
Histologic	Loose arrangements of collagen, elastin, and adipose tissue	Organized collagen arrangements
Function	Allows expansion and contraction of invested structures	Provides muscle attachment to bones
Supportive role	Condensations lend some support to invested organs; encases neurovascular structures	Invests muscles to provide pelvic floor stability and function
Tensile strength	Elastic	Rigid

Pelvic Connective Tissue

Subperitoneal perivascular connective tissue and loose areolar tissue are found throughout the pelvis. This tissue connects the pelvic viscera to the pelvic walls and is termed *visceral* or *endopelvic "fascia."* Recall that visceral fascia differs anatomically and histologically from parietal fascia, which invests most striated muscles (Table 38-1). Visceral fascia is intimately associated with the walls of the viscera and cannot be dissected in the same fashion that parietal fascia—for example, rectus fascia—can be separated from the corresponding skeletal muscle.

Condensations of visceral connective tissue that have assumed special supportive roles have been given different names. Some examples include the cardinal and uterosacral ligaments and the vesicovaginal and rectovaginal fascia. These are described further in later sections.

Pelvic Blood Supply

The pelvic organs are supplied by the visceral branches of the internal iliac (hypogastric) artery and by direct branches from the abdominal aorta (Fig. 38-12). The internal iliac artery gen-

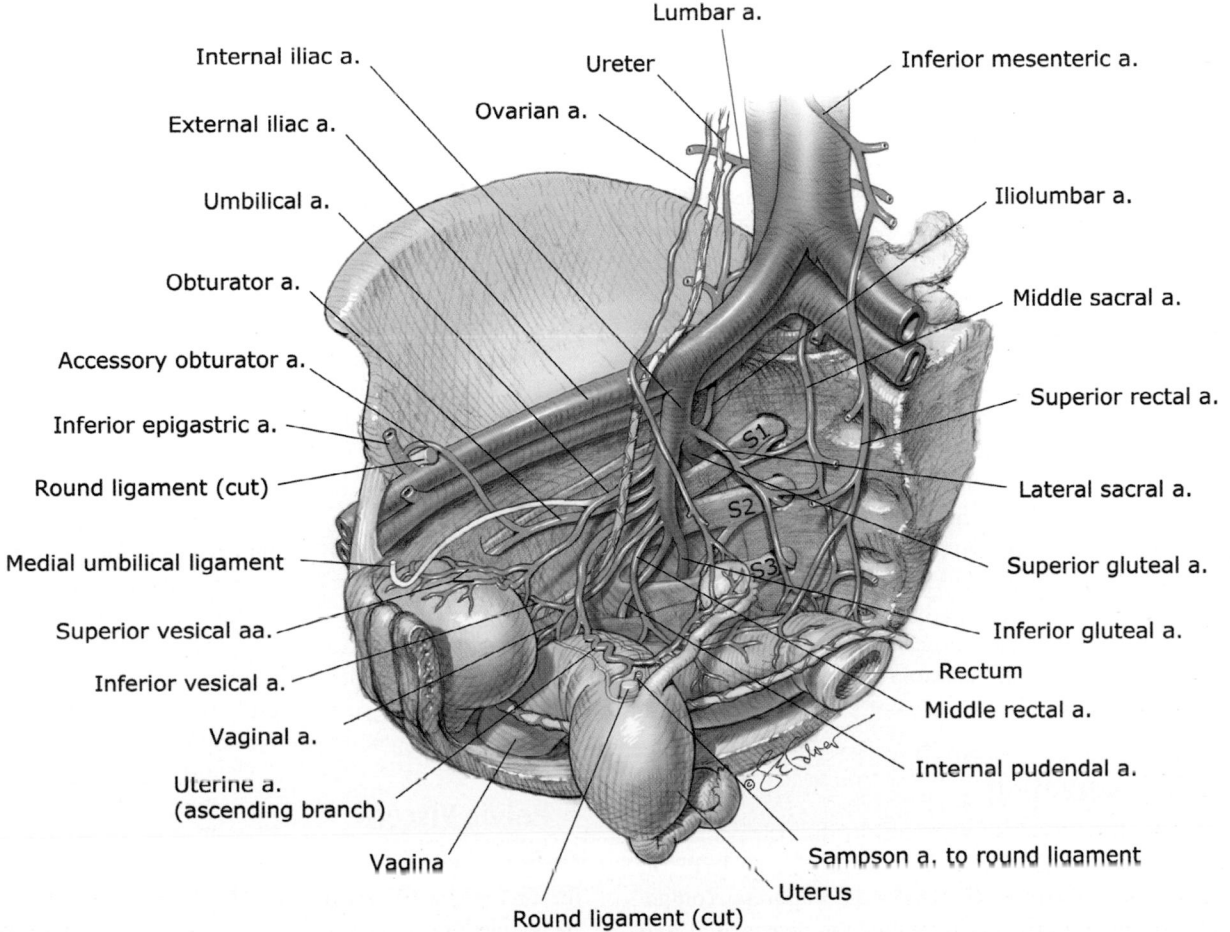

FIGURE 38-12 Pelvic arteries. In this image, the uterus and rectum are reflected to the left.

TABLE 38-2. Pelvic Blood Supply

Internal Iliac Artery[a]			
Anterior Division		**Posterior Division**	
Parietal Branches	**Visceral Branches**	**Parietal Branches**	**Visceral Branches**
Obturator	Superior vesical (from patent segment of umbilical)	Iliolumbar	None
Internal pudendal	Uterine	Lateral sacral	
Inferior gluteal	Vaginal	Superior gluteal	
	Middle rectal		
	Inferior vesical (+/−)		

Direct Branches of Aorta	
Parietal Branches	**Visceral Branches**
Middle sacral	Ovarian
	Superior rectal (terminal branch of inferior mesenteric)

Aortic to Internal Iliac Artery Anastomoses	
Ovarian to uterine	Middle sacral to lateral sacral
Superior rectal to middle rectal	Lumbar to iliolumbar

[a]Note that great variability exists in the origin and distribution of internal iliac branches.

erally divides into an anterior and posterior division in the area of the greater sciatic foramen (see Fig. 38-6). Each division has three parietal branches that supply nonvisceral structures. The *iliolumbar, lateral sacral,* and *superior gluteal arteries* are the three parietal branches of the posterior division. The *internal pudendal, obturator,* and *inferior gluteal arteries* are parietal branches that most commonly arise from the anterior division. The remaining branches of the anterior division supply the pelvic viscera (bladder, uterus, vagina, and rectum). These include the *uterine, vaginal,* and *middle rectal arteries* and the *superior vesical arteries.* These latter vessels commonly arise from the patent part of the umbilical arteries (Table 38-2).

The two most important direct branches of the aorta that contribute to pelvic organ blood supply are the superior rectal and ovarian arteries. The *superior rectal artery,* which is the terminal branch of the inferior mesenteric artery, anastomoses with the middle rectal arteries, thus contributing blood supply to the rectum and vagina. The *ovarian arteries,* which arise directly from the aorta just inferior to the renal vessels, anastomose with the ascending branch of the uterine artery. These anastomoses contribute to the blood supply of the uterus and adnexa.

Other important anastomoses between the aorta and internal iliac arteries include anastomoses between the middle sacral and lateral sacral arteries and anastomoses between the lumbar and iliolumbar arteries.

■ Pelvic Innervation

Nerve supply to the visceral structures in the pelvis (bladder, urethra, vagina, uterus, adnexa, and rectum) arises from the autonomic nervous system. The two most important components of this system in the pelvis include the *superior* and *infe-*

rior hypogastric plexuses. The superior hypogastric plexus, also known as the *presacral nerve,* is an extension of the aortic plexus found below the aortic bifurcation (Fig. 38-13). This plexus primarily contains sympathetic fibers and sensory afferent fibers from the uterus.

The superior hypogastric plexus terminates by dividing into the hypogastric nerves. These nerves join parasympathetic efferents from the second through the fourth sacral nerve roots (pelvic splanchnic nerves, also termed nervi erigentis) to form the *inferior hypogastric plexus,* also known as the *pelvic plexus.*

Fibers of the inferior hypogastric plexus accompany the branches of the internal iliac artery to the pelvic viscera. Accordingly, they are divided into three portions: the vesical, uterovaginal (Frankenhäuser ganglion), and middle rectal plexuses. Extensions of the inferior hypogastric plexus reach the perineum along the vagina and urethra to innervate the clitoris and vestibular bulbs.

Clinical Correlation

The sensory afferent fibers contained within the superior hypogastric plexus are targeted in presacral neurectomy, a surgical procedure performed to treat dysmenorrhea and central pelvic pain refractory to medical management (Chap. 11, p. 316).

Injury to the branches of the inferior hypogastric plexus during cancer debulking or other extensive pelvic surgeries can lead to varying degrees of voiding, sexual, and defecatory dysfunction.

■ Pelvic Viscera
Uterus

The uterus is a fibromuscular hollow organ situated between the bladder and the rectum. The uterus is divided structurally

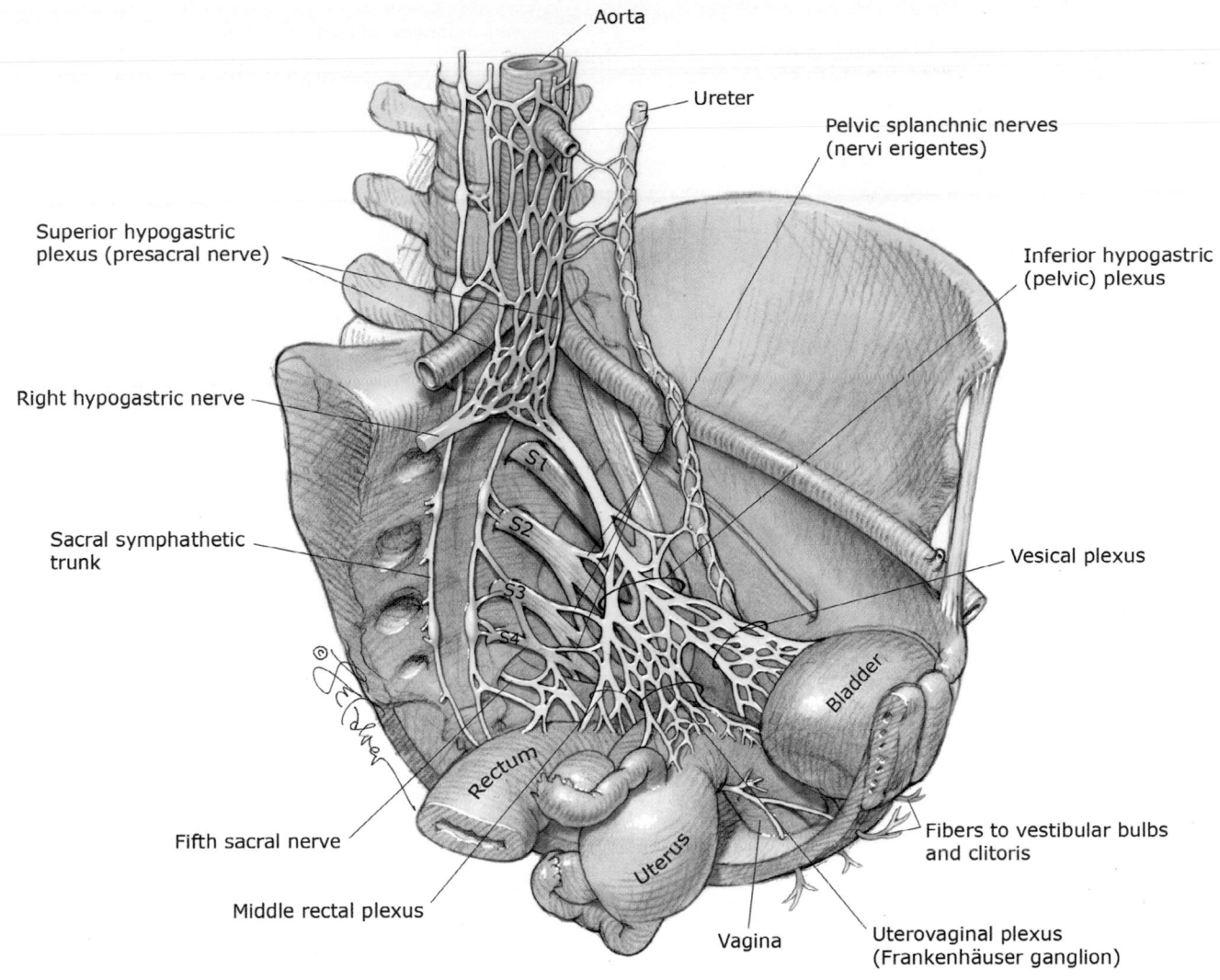

FIGURE 38-13 Pelvic autonomic nerves. Superior and inferior hypogastric plexuses. S1–S4 = first through fourth sacral nerves.

and functionally into two portions: an upper muscular body, the *corpus*, and a lower fibrous *cervix* (Fig. 38-14). The transition between the corpus and the cervix is known as the *uterine isthmus*. This also marks the transition from endocervical canal to endometrial cavity. The portion of the corpus that extends above the level of entry of the fallopian tubes into the endometrial cavity is known as the *fundus*.

The shape, weight, and dimensions of the uterus vary according to parity and estrogen stimulation. Before menarche and after menopause, the corpus and cervix are approximately equal in size, but during the reproductive years, the uterine corpus is significantly larger than the cervix. In the adult, nonpregnant woman, the uterus measures approximately 7 cm in length and 5 cm in width at the fundus.

Endometrium and Serosa. The uterus consists of an inner layer of mucosa called the *endometrium*, which surrounds the endometrial cavity and a thick muscular wall known as the *myometrium*. The endometrium consists of columnar epithelium and specialized stroma. The superficial portion of the endometrium undergoes cyclic changes with the menstrual cycle (Fig. 15-19, p. 423).

The spiral arterioles located in the endometrium undergo hormonally mediated constriction or spasms that cause shedding of the superficial portion of the endometrium with each menstrual cycle. The deeper basalis layer of the endometrium is preserved after the menstrual cycle and is the one responsible for regeneration of a new superficial layer (Fig. 8-3, p. 222).

Peritoneal serosa overlies the outer wall with the exception of two sites. First, the anterior portion of the cervix is covered by the bladder. Second, the lateral portions of the corpus and cervix attach to the broad and cardinal ligaments.

Cervix. The uterine cervix begins caudal to the uterine isthmus and is approximately 3 cm in length. The wall of the cervix consists primarily of fibrous tissue and a smaller amount (approximately 10 percent) of smooth muscle. The smooth muscle is found on the periphery of the cervical wall and serves as the point of attachment for the cardinal and uterosacral ligaments and the fibromuscular walls of the vagina.

The attachments of the vaginal walls to the periphery of the cervix divide it into a vaginal part known as the *portio vaginalis* and a supravaginal part known as the *portio supravaginalis* (see

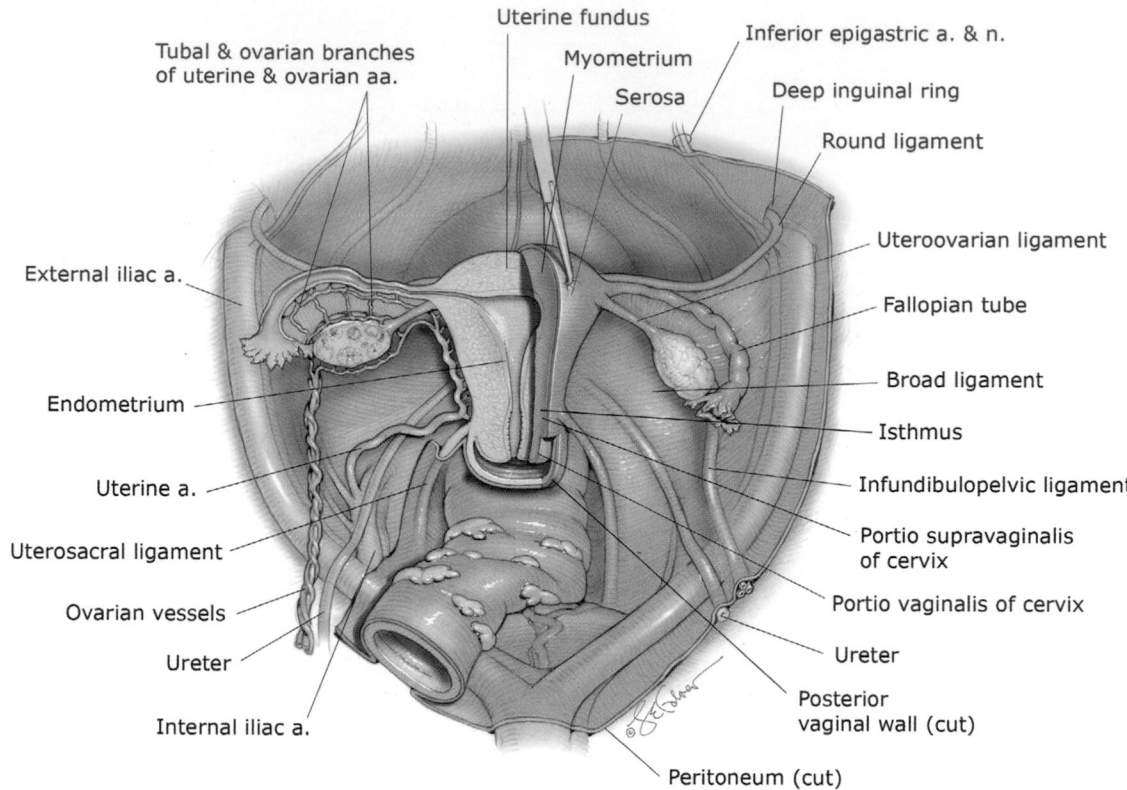

FIGURE 38-14 Uterus, adnexa, and associated anatomy.

Fig. 38-14). The portio vaginalis is covered by nonkeratinizing squamous epithelium.

The endocervical canal is lined by columnar, mucus-secreting epithelium. The lower border of the canal, called the external cervical os, contains a transition from the squamous epithelium of the portio vaginalis to the columnar epithelium of the cervical canal. The exact location of this transition, termed the *squamocolumnar junction,* varies depending on hormonal status (Fig. 29-5, p. 733). At the upper border of the endocervical canal is the internal cervical os, where the narrow cervical canal becomes continuous with the wider endometrial cavity.

Uterine Support. The main support of the uterus and cervix is provided by the interaction between the levator ani muscles and the connective tissue that attaches the walls of the cervix to the pelvic walls. The connective tissue that attaches lateral to the uterus and cervix is called the *parametria* and continues down along the vagina as the *paracolpium.* The parametrium consists of what is clinically known as the *cardinal ligament* and *uterosacral ligament* (Fig. 38-15).

These ligaments are condensations of visceral connective tissue that have assumed special supportive roles. The cardinal ligaments, also termed *transverse cervical ligaments* or *Mackenrodt ligaments,* consist primarily of perivascular connective tissue (Range, 1964). They attach to the posterolateral pelvic walls near the origin of the internal iliac artery and surround the vessels supplying the uterus and vagina.

The uterosacral ligaments insert into a broad area of the pelvic walls and sacrum posteriorly and form the lateral boundaries of the posterior cul-de-sac of Douglas. Although the name

of these ligaments implies attachments to the sacrum posteriorly, one MR imaging study showed their insertion on the pelvic sidewall occurred to the coccygeus muscle/sacrospinous ligament complex in 82 percent of cases reviewed, to the piriformis muscle in 11 percent, and to the sacrum in only 7 percent. These ligaments originate from the posterior inferior surface of the cervix, but may also originate, in part, from the proximal posterior vagina (Umek, 2004). They consist primarily of smooth muscle and contain some of the pelvic autonomic nerves (Campbell, 1950).

Clinical Correlation. The rectum lies medial to the uterosacral ligaments. The ureter and pelvic sidewall vessels run lateral and also in close proximity to these ligaments. Thus, during pelvic reconstructive surgeries that use the uterosacral ligaments as attachment sites for the vaginal apex, these surrounding structures are especially vulnerable for injury (Wieslander, 2007).

Round Ligaments. The round ligaments of the uterus are smooth muscle extensions of the uterine corpus and represent the homolog of the gubernaculum testis. The round ligaments arise from the lateral aspect of the corpus just below and anterior to the origin of the fallopian tubes. They extend laterally to the pelvic sidewall (see Fig. 38-14). They enter the retroperitoneal space and pass lateral to the inferior epigastric vessels before entering the inguinal canal through the internal inguinal ring. After coursing through the inguinal canal, the round ligaments exit through the external inguinal ring to terminate in the subcutaneous tissue of the labia majora (see Fig. 38-4). The round ligaments do not significantly contribute to

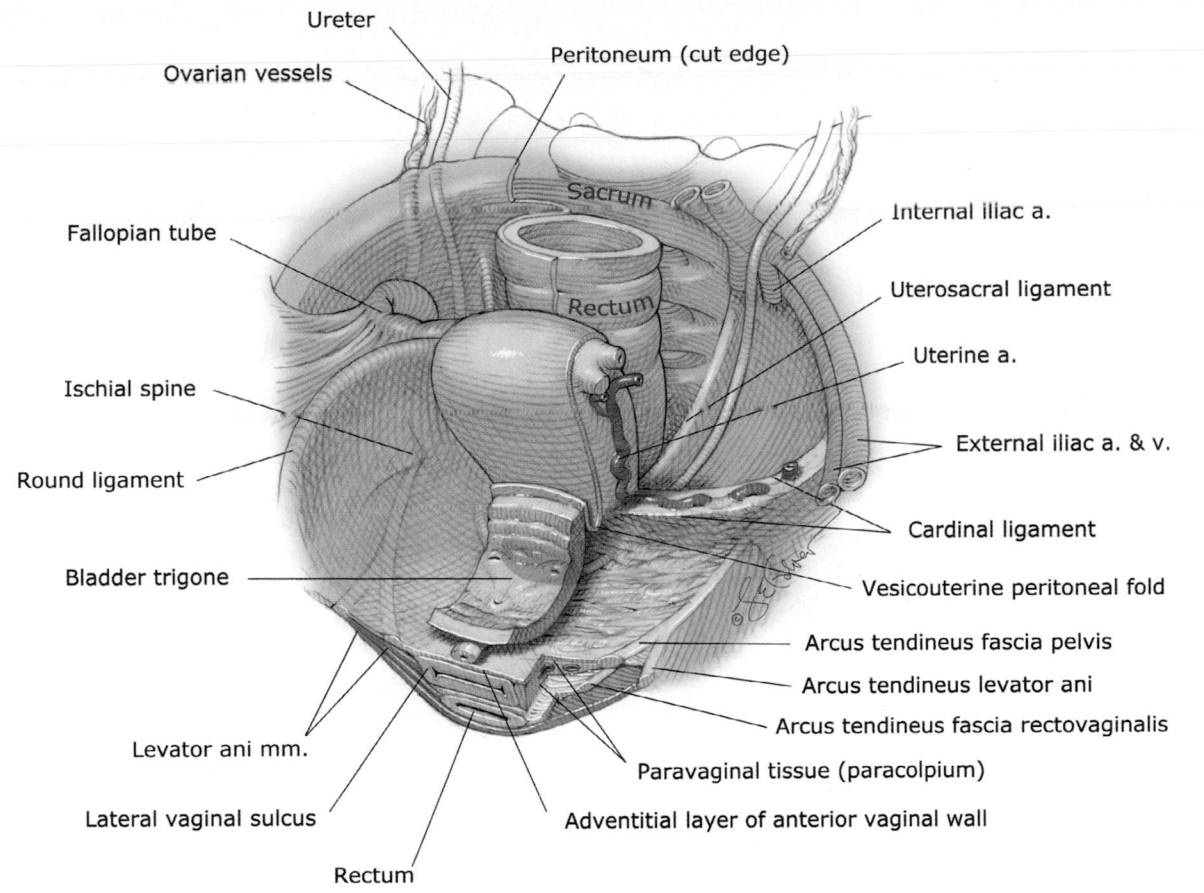

Ureter

Ovarian vessels

Peritoneum (cut edge)

Sacrum

Rectum

Fallopian tube

Internal iliac a.

Uterosacral ligament

Uterine a.

Ischial spine

Round ligament

External iliac a. & v.

Cardinal ligament

Bladder trigone

Vesicouterine peritoneal fold

Arcus tendineus fascia pelvis

Arcus tendineus levator ani

Arcus tendineus fascia rectovaginalis

Levator ani mm.

Paravaginal tissue (paracolpium)

Lateral vaginal sulcus

Adventitial layer of anterior vaginal wall

Rectum

FIGURE 38-15 Pelvic viscera and their connective tissue support. Relationship of the urethra, bladder trigone, and distal ureter to the anterior vaginal wall and to the uterine cervix.

uterine support. They receive their blood supply from a small branch of the uterine or ovarian artery known as Sampson artery (p. 927).

Clinical Correlation. The location of the round ligament anterior to the fallopian tube can assist a surgeon during tubal sterilization through a minilaparotomy incision. This may be especially true if pelvic adhesions limit tubal mobility and thus identification of fimbria prior to tubal ligation.

Division of the round ligament is typically an initial step in abdominal and laparoscopic hysterectomy. Transection opens the broad ligaments and provides access to the pelvic sidewall retroperitoneum. This access allows direct visualization of the ureter and permits "skeletonizing" of the uterine artery for safe ligation and division.

Broad Ligaments. The *broad ligaments* are double layers of peritoneum that extend from the lateral walls of the uterus to the pelvic walls (see Fig. 38-14). Within the upper portion of these two layers, the fallopian tube and the ovarian and round ligaments are found. The fallopian tubes, ovaries, and round ligaments each have their separate mesentery, called the *meso-salpinx, mesovarium,* and *mesoteres,* respectively, which carry nerves and vessels to these structures. At the lateral border of the fallopian tube and the ovary, the broad ligament ends where the infundibulopelvic ligament, described on page 932, blends

with the pelvic wall. The cardinal and uterosacral ligaments lie within the lower portion or "base" of the broad ligaments.

Uterine Blood Supply. The blood supply to the uterine corpus arises from the ascending branch of the uterine artery and from the medial or uterine branch of the ovarian artery (see Figs. 38-14 and 38-15). The uterine artery may originate directly from the internal iliac artery as an independent branch or it may have a common origin with the internal pudendal or with the vaginal artery (see Fig. 38-12).

The uterine artery approaches the uterus in the area of the uterine isthmus. In this area, the uterine artery courses over the ureter and provides a small branch to this structure. Several uterine veins course along the side of the artery and are variably found over or under the ureter. The uterine artery then divides into a larger ascending and a smaller descending branch that course along the side of the uterus and cervix, respectively. These vessels connect on the lateral border of the uterus but form an anastomotic arterial arcade that supplies the uterine walls (Fig. 8-4, p. 222).

The cervix is supplied by the descending or cervical branch of the uterine artery and by ascending branches of the vaginal artery.

Clinical Correlation. The uterus receives dual blood supply from both ovarian and uterine vessels. For this reason, some

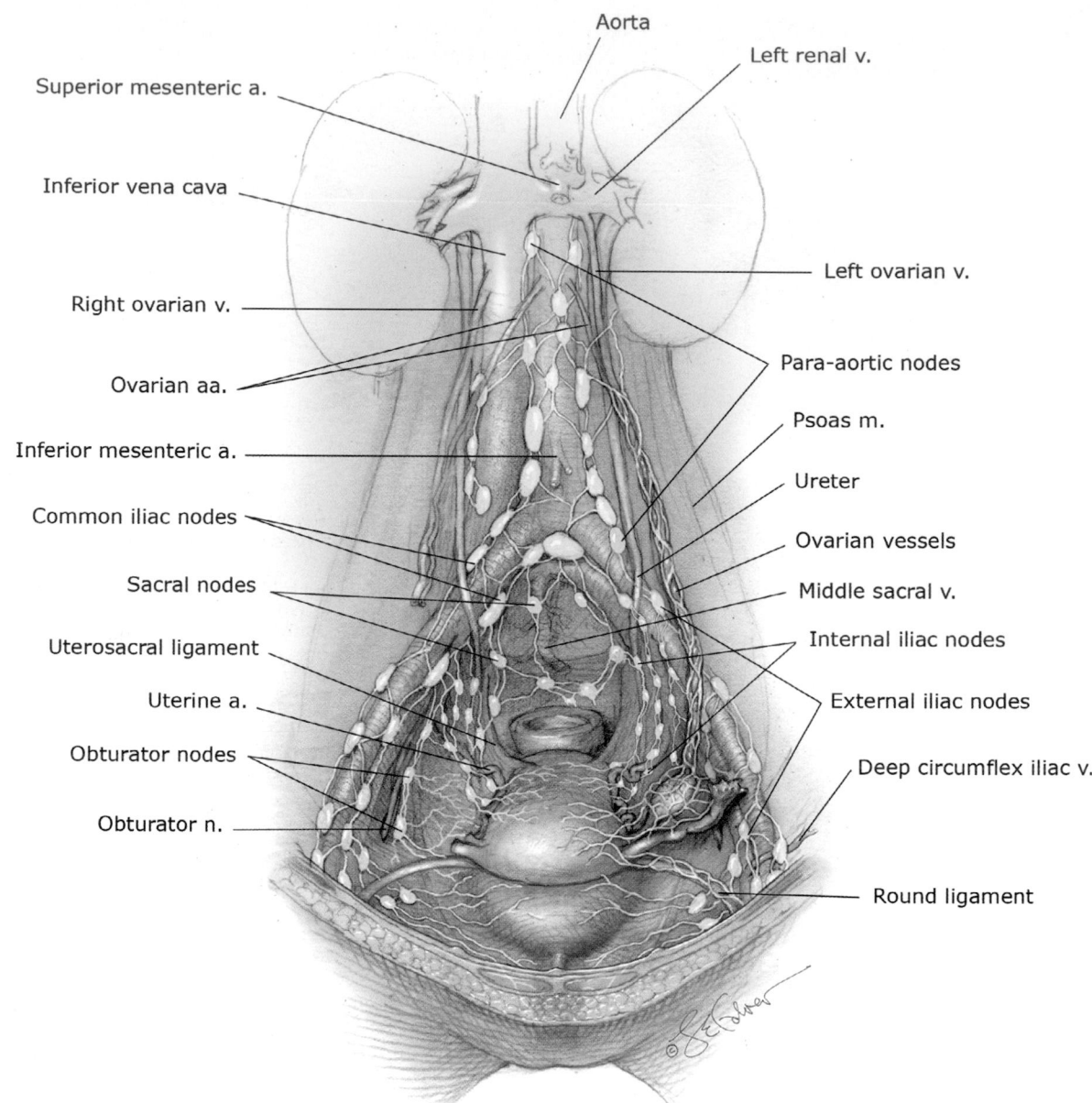

Superior mesenteric a.

Inferior vena cava

Right ovarian v.

Ovarian aa.

Inferior mesenteric a.

Common iliac nodes

Sacral nodes

Uterosacral ligament

Uterine a.

Obturator nodes

Obturator n.

Aorta

Left renal v.

Left ovarian v.

Para-aortic nodes

Psoas m.

Ureter

Ovarian vessels

Middle sacral v.

Internal iliac nodes

External iliac nodes

Deep circumflex iliac v.

Round ligament

FIGURE 38-16 Pelvic lymph nodes and the course of the ureter and ovarian vessels.

surgeons during myomectomy place tourniquets at both the infundibulopelvic ligament and uterine isthmus to decrease blood flow from the ovarian and uterine arteries, respectively.

Uterine Lymphatic Drainage. Lymphatic drainage of the uterus is primarily to the obturator and internal and external iliac nodes (Fig. 38-16). However, some lymphatic channels from the uterine corpus may pass along the round ligaments to the superficial inguinal nodes, and others may extend along the uterosacral ligaments to the lateral sacral nodes.

Uterine Innervation. The uterus is innervated by fibers of the *uterovaginal plexus*, also known as *Frankenhäuser ganglion*. These fibers travel along the uterine arteries and are found in the connective tissue of the cardinal ligaments (see Fig. 38-13).

Ovaries and Fallopian Tubes

Ovaries. The ovaries and fallopian tubes constitute the *uterine adnexa*. The size and hormonal activity of the ovaries are dependent on age, time of the menstrual cycle, and exogenous hormonal suppression. During reproductive years, the ovaries measure 2.5 to 5 cm in length, 1.5 to 3 cm in thickness, and 0.7 to 1.5 cm in width.

The ovaries consist of an *outer cortex* and an *inner medulla*. The ovarian cortex is comprised of a specialized stroma punctuated with follicles, corpora lutea, and corpora albicantia (Fig. 15-20, p. 424). A single layer of mesothelial cells covers this cortex as a surface epithelium. The medullary portion of the ovary primarily consists of fibromuscular tissue and blood vessels. The medial aspect of the ovary is connected to the uterus by the *uteroovarian ligament* (see Fig. 38-14). Laterally, each ovary is attached to the pelvic wall by an *infundibulopelvic ligament,* also termed *suspensory ligament* of the ovary, which contains the ovarian vessels and nerves.

Ovarian Blood Supply, Lymphatics, and Innervation.

The blood supply to the ovaries comes from the *ovarian arteries,* which arise from the anterior surface of the abdominal aorta just below the origin of the renal arteries and from the ovarian branches of the uterine arteries (see Fig. 38-16). The *ovarian veins* follow the same retroperitoneal course as the arteries. The right ovarian vein drains into the inferior vena cava, and the left ovarian vein drains into the left renal vein.

Lymphatic drainage of the ovaries follows the ovarian vessels to the lower abdominal aorta, where they drain into the paraaortic nodes. For their innervation, the ovaries are supplied by extensions of the renal plexus that course along the ovarian vessels in the infundibulopelvic ligament.

Fallopian Tubes.

The fallopian tubes are tubular structures that measure 7 to 12 cm in length (see Fig. 38-14). Each tube has four identifiable portions (Fig. 7-1, p. 199). The *interstitial portion* passes through the body of the uterus at the region known as the *cornua.* The *isthmic portion* begins adjacent to the uterine corpus. It consists of a narrow lumen and a thick muscular wall. The *ampullary portion* is recognized as the lumen of the isthmic portion of the tube widens. In addition to the wider lumen, this segment has a more convoluted mucosa (Fig. 7-4, p. 202). The *fimbriated portion* is the distal continuation of the ampullary segment. The fimbriated end

has many frondlike projections that provide a wide surface area for ovum pickup. The *fimbria ovarica* is the projection that is in contact with the ovary.

The ovarian artery runs along the hilum of the ovary and sends several branches through the mesosalpinx to supply the fallopian tubes (see Fig. 38-14). The venous plexus, lymphatic drainage, and nerve supply of the fallopian tubes follow a similar course to that of the ovaries.

Vagina

The vagina is a hollow viscus whose shape is determined by the structures that surround it and by the attachments of its lateral walls to the pelvic walls as described later. The distal portion of the vagina is constricted by the action of the levator ani muscles (see Fig. 38-10). Above the pelvic floor, the vaginal lumen is much more capacious and distensible. In the standing or anatomic position, the apex of the vagina is directed posteriorly toward the ischial spines, and the upper two thirds of the vaginal tube lie almost parallel to the plane of the levator plate.

Although great variability in length of the vaginal walls is reported, the average length of the anterior vaginal wall is 7 cm and that of the posterior wall is 9 cm. The shorter distance of the anterior vaginal wall results from the anterior position of the uterine cervix in most women. The recesses within the vaginal lumen in front of and behind the cervix are known as the *anterior fornix* and *posterior fornix*, respectively (Fig. 38-17).

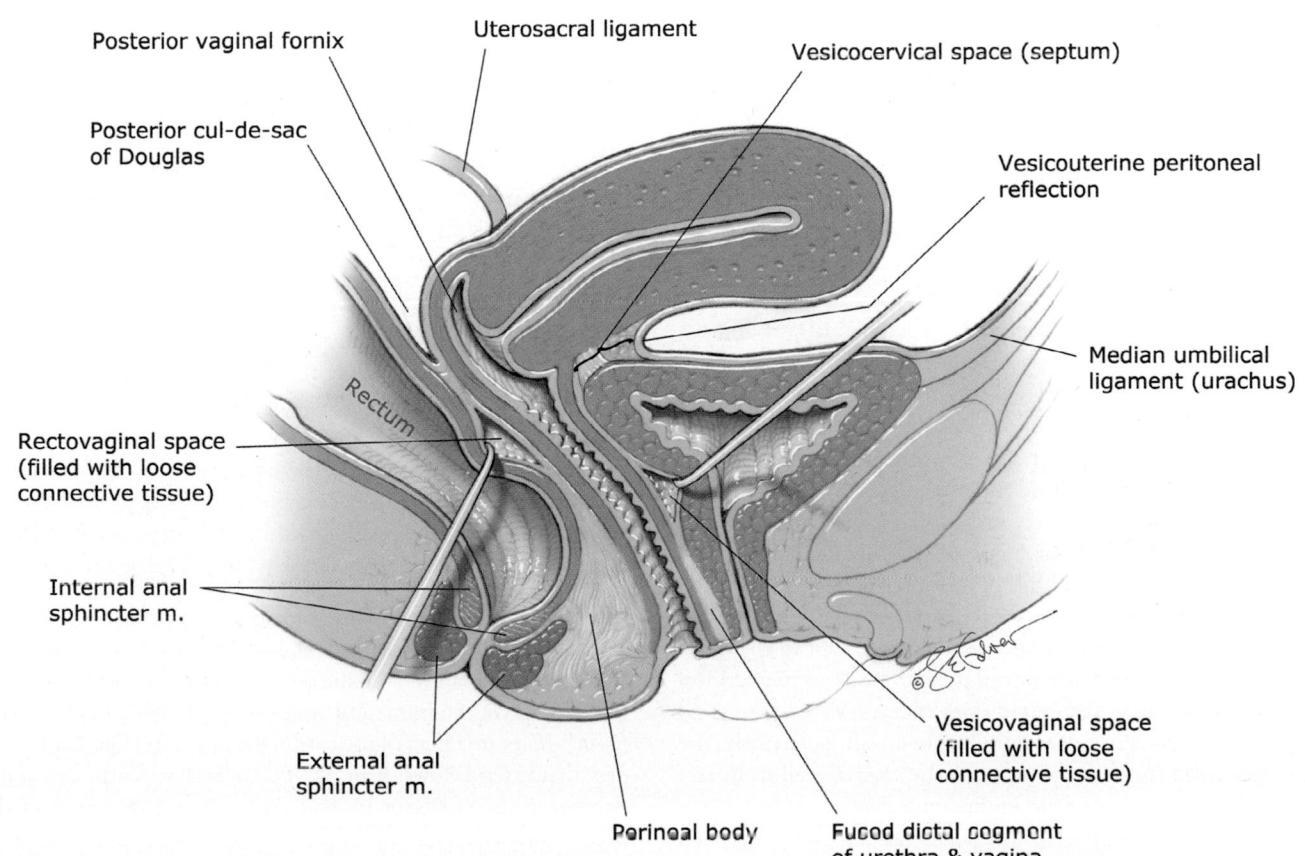

FIGURE 38-17 Surgical cleavage planes and vaginal wall layers.

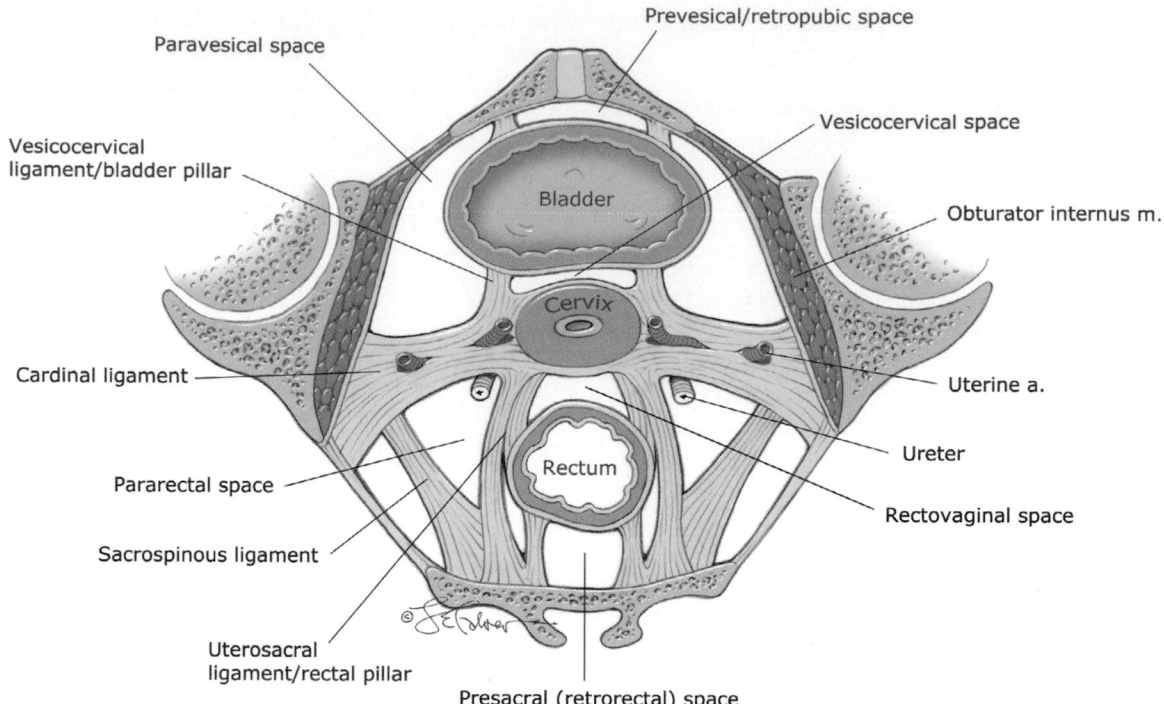

Paravesical space

Prevesical/retropubic space

Vesicocervical ligament/bladder pillar

Vesicocervical space

Bladder

Obturator internus m.

Cervix

Cardinal ligament

Uterine a.

Ureter

Pararectal space

Rectum

Rectovaginal space

Sacrospinous ligament

Uterosacral ligament/rectal pillar

Presacral (retrorectal) space

FIGURE 38-18 Connective tissue and surgical spaces of the pelvis.

The vaginal walls consist of three layers: adjacent to the lumen, a mucosal layer consisting of nonkeratinized squamous epithelium overlying a lamina propria; a muscular layer consisting of smooth muscle, collagen, and elastin; and an adventitial layer consisting of collagen and elastin (Fig. 24-6, p. 639) (Weber, 1995, 1997).

The vagina lies between the bladder and rectum and along with its connections to the pelvic walls, provides support to these structures (see Figs. 38-15 and 38-17). The vagina is separated from the bladder anteriorly and the rectum posteriorly by the vaginal adventitia. The lateral continuation of the adventitial layer constitutes the paravaginal tissue that attaches the walls of the vagina to the pelvic walls. This tissue consists of loose areolar and fatty tissue containing blood vessels, lymphatics, and nerves. The anterior fibromuscular vaginal wall and its paravaginal attachments represent the layer that supports the bladder and urethra and is clinically referred to as pubovesicocervical fascia (see Fig. 38-15).

The lateral attachments of the posterior vaginal walls are to the fascia covering the upper surface of the levator ani muscles. The posterior vaginal wall and its connective tissue attachments to the sidewall support the rectum. This layer is clinically known as the rectovaginal fascia or fascia of Denonvilliers. However, similar to microscopic findings of the anterior vaginal wall, histologic studies have failed to show a separate layer between the posterior wall of the vagina and the rectum except in the distal 3 to 4 cm. Here, the dense fibromuscular tissue of the perineal body separates these structures (DeLancey, 1999). Similar to surgical dissections in the anterior vaginal wall, posteriorly, the plane dissected surgically to separate the vaginal wall from rectum includes portions of the vaginal muscularis.

Because there is no true histologic "fascial" layer between the vagina and the bladder and between the vagina and the rectum, some recommend that terms such as "pubocervical/

pubovesicalfascia" or "rectovaginal fascia" be abandoned. They propose that these be replaced by more accurate descriptive terms such as *vaginal muscularis* or *fibromuscular layer of the anterior and posterior vaginal walls*.

Vesicocervical and Vesicovaginal "Potential" Spaces.
The *vesicocervical space* begins below the vesicouterine peritoneal fold or reflection, which represents the loose attachments of the peritoneum in the region of the anterior cul-de-sac (see Figs. 38-17 and 38-18). The vesicocervical space continues down as the *vesicovaginal space*, which extends to the junction of the proximal and middle thirds of the urethra. Below this point, the urethra and vagina fuse.

Clinical Correlation.
The vesicouterine peritoneal fold can easily be lifted and incised to create a bladder flap during an abdominal hysterectomy or cesarean delivery. During vaginal hysterectomies, the distance between the anterior cul-de-sac peritoneum and the anterior vaginal fornix spans several centimeters, and this relationship is important. Therefore, to successfully enter the peritoneal cavity, proper identification and sharp dissection of the loose connective tissue that lies within the vesicovaginal and vesicocervical spaces is necessary (see Fig. 38-17) (Balgobin, 2011).

Rectovaginal Space.
This is adjacent to the posterior surface of the vagina. It extends from the cul-de-sac of Douglas down to the superior border of the perineal body, which extends 2 to 3 cm above the hymeneal ring (see Figs. 38-17 and 38-18). *Rectal pillars* are fibers of the cardinal-uterosacral ligament complex that extend down from the cervix and attach to the upper portion of the posterior vaginal wall. These fibers connect the vagina to the lateral walls of the rectum and to the sacrum. These pillars also separate the midline rectovaginal space from the pararectal space.

Clinical Correlation. The rectovaginal space contains loose areolar tissue and is easily opened with finger dissection during abdominal surgery (see Fig. 38-18). Perforation of the rectal pillar fibers allows access to the sacrospinous ligaments used in vaginal suspension procedures (Section 43-21, p. 1238).

The posterior cul-de-sac peritoneum extends down the posterior vaginal wall 2 to 3 cm inferior to the posterior vaginal fornix (Kuhn, 1982). Thus, during vaginal hysterectomy, in contrast to anterior peritoneal cavity entry, entering the peritoneal cavity posteriorly is readily done by incising the vaginal wall in the area of the posterior fornix (see Fig. 38-17).

Vaginal Support. The main support of the vagina is provided by the interaction between the levator ani muscles and the connective tissue that attaches the lateral walls of the vagina to the pelvic walls. This tissue consists of the distal extensions of what we clinically know as the cardinal and uterosacral ligaments. Although the visceral connective tissue in the pelvis is continuous and interdependent, DeLancey (1992) has described three levels of vaginal connective tissue support that help explain various clinical manifestations of pelvic support dysfunction.

Upper Vaginal Support. The parametria continues down the vagina as the paracolpium (see Fig. 38-15). This tissue attaches the upper vagina to the pelvic wall, suspending it over the pelvic floor. These attachments are also known as *level I support* or *suspensory axis* and provide connective tissue support to the vaginal apex after hysterectomy. In the standing position, level I support fibers are vertically oriented. Clinical manifestations of level I support defects include posthysterectomy vaginal vault prolapse.

Midvaginal Support. The lateral walls of the midportion of the vagina are attached to the pelvic walls on each side by visceral connective tissue known as endopelvic fascia. These lateral attachments of the vaginal walls blend into the arcus tendineus fascia pelvis and to the medial aspect of the levator ani muscles, and in doing so create the anterior and posterior lateral vaginal sulci (see Fig. 38-15). These grooves run along the vaginal sidewalls and give the vagina an "H" shape when viewed in cross section. The arcus tendineus fascia pelvis is a condensation of fascia covering the medial aspect of the obturator internus and levator ani muscles. It spans from the inner surface of the pubic bones to the ischial spines (see Figs. 38-7 and 38-15).

Attachment of the anterior vaginal wall to the levator ani muscles is responsible for the bladder neck elevation noted with cough or Valsalva maneuver (see Fig. 38-10). Therefore, these attachments may have significance for stress urinary continence. The midvaginal attachments are referred to as *level II support* or the *attachment axis*. Clinical manifestations of level II support defects include anterior and posterior vaginal wall prolapse and stress urinary incontinence.

Distal Vaginal Support. The distal third of the vagina is directly attached to its surrounding structures (see Fig. 38-9). Anteriorly, the vagina is fused with the urethra. Laterally it attaches to the pubovaginalis muscle and perineal membrane, and posteriorly to the perineal body. These vaginal attachments are referred to as *level III support* or *fusion axis*, and they are considered the strongest of the vaginal support components.

Failure of this level of support can result in distal rectoceles or perineal descent. Anal incontinence may also result if the perineal body is absent, as may follow obstetric trauma.

Vaginal Blood Supply, Lymphatics, and Innervation. The main blood supply to the vagina arises from the descending or cervical branch of the uterine artery and from the vaginal artery, a branch of the internal iliac artery (see Fig. 38-12). These vessels form an anastomotic arcade along the lateral sides of the vagina at the level of the vaginal sulci, and they anastomose with the contralateral vessels on the anterior and posterior walls of the vagina. Additionally, the middle rectal artery from the internal iliac artery contributes to supply the posterior vaginal wall. The distal walls of the vagina also receive contributions from the internal pudendal artery (p. 944).

Lymphatic drainage of the upper two thirds of the vagina is similar to that of the uterus as described on page 932. The distal part of the vagina drains with the vulvar lymphatics to the inguinal nodes. A more detailed description of the vulvar lymphatics is presented on page 945.

The vagina receives its nerve supply from the inferior extensions of the uterovaginal plexus, a component of the inferior hypogastric or pelvic plexus (see Fig. 38-13).

Lower Urinary Tract Structures

Bladder. The bladder is a hollow organ that allows storage and evacuation of urine (Fig. 38-19). Anteriorly, the bladder rests against the anterior abdominal wall. Posteriorly, it rests against the vagina and cervix. Inferiorly and laterally, the bladder is in contact with the inner surface of the pubic bones. In these areas, the bladder is devoid of peritoneal covering. The reflection of the bladder onto the abdominal wall is triangular in shape, and the apex of this triangle is continuous with the median umbilical ligament.

The bladder wall consists of coarse bundles of smooth muscle known as the *detrusor muscle*, which extends into the upper part of the urethra. Although separate layers of the detrusor are described, they are not as well defined as the layers of other viscous structures such as the bowel or the ureter (Fig. 23-2, p. 610). The innermost layer of the bladder wall is plexiform, which can be seen from the pattern of trabeculations noted during cystoscopy. The mucosa of the bladder consists of transitional epithelium.

The bladder can be divided into a *dome* and a *base* approximately at the level of the ureteral orifices. The dome is thin walled and distensible. The base has a thicker wall that undergoes less distension during filling (see Fig. 38-15). The bladder base consists of the *vesical trigone* and the *detrusor loops*. These loops are two U-shaped bands of fibers found at the *vesical neck*, where the urethra enters the bladder wall.

The blood supply to the bladder arises from the superior vesical arteries, which are branches of the patent portion of the umbilical artery, and from the inferior vesical artery, which when present, often arises from either the internal pudendal or the vaginal arteries (see Fig. 38-12). The nerve supply to the bladder arises from the vesical plexus, a component of the inferior hypogastric plexus (see Fig. 38-13).

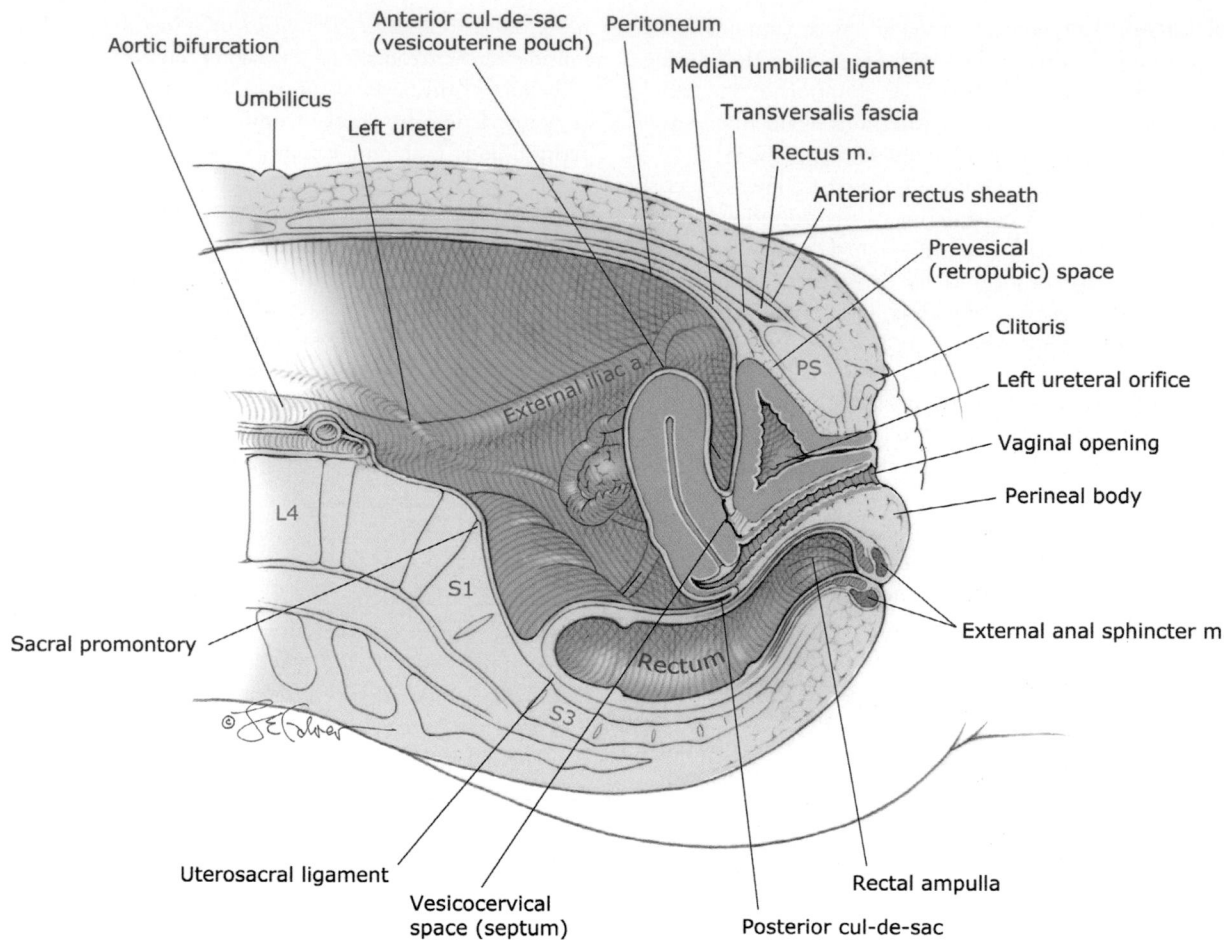

FIGURE 38-19 Midsagittal view of pelvic structures and associated anatomy.

Urethra. The female urethra is a complex organ that is 3 to 4 cm in length. The lumen of the urethra begins at the internal urinary meatus within the bladder, and then courses through the bladder base for less than a centimeter. This region of the bladder where the urethral lumen traverses the bladder base is called the *bladder neck*. The distal two thirds of the urethra are fused with the anterior vaginal wall.

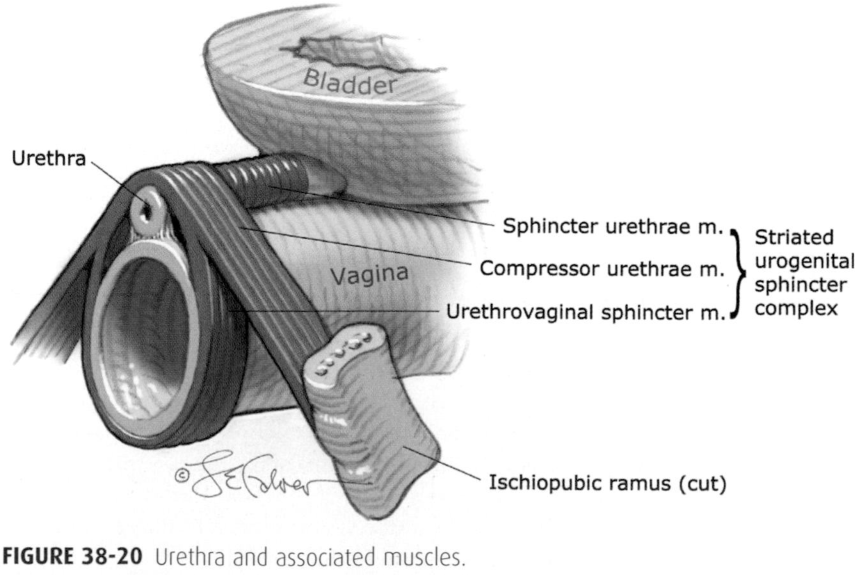

The walls of the urethra begin outside the bladder wall. They consist of two layers of smooth muscle, an inner longitudinal and an outer circular, which is in turn surrounded by a circular layer of skeletal muscle referred to as the *sphincter urethrae* or *rhabdosphincter* (Fig. 38-20). Approximately at the junction of the middle and lower third of the urethra, and just above or deep to the perineal membrane, two strap skeletal muscles known as the *urethrovaginal sphincter* and *compressor urethrae* are found. These muscles were previously known as the *deep transverse perineal muscles* in females and together with the sphincter urethrae constitute the *striated urogenital sphincter complex.* Together, these three muscles function as a unit and have a complex and controversial innervation. Their fibers combine to supply constant tonus and to provide emergency reflex activity mainly in the distal half of the urethra to sustain continence.

Distal to the depth of the perineal membrane, the walls of the urethra consist of fibrous tissue, serving as the nozzle that directs the urine stream. The urethra has a prominent submucosal layer that is lined by hormonally sensitive stratified squamous epithelium (Fig. 23-9, p. 614). Within the

FIGURE 38-20 Urethra and associated muscles.

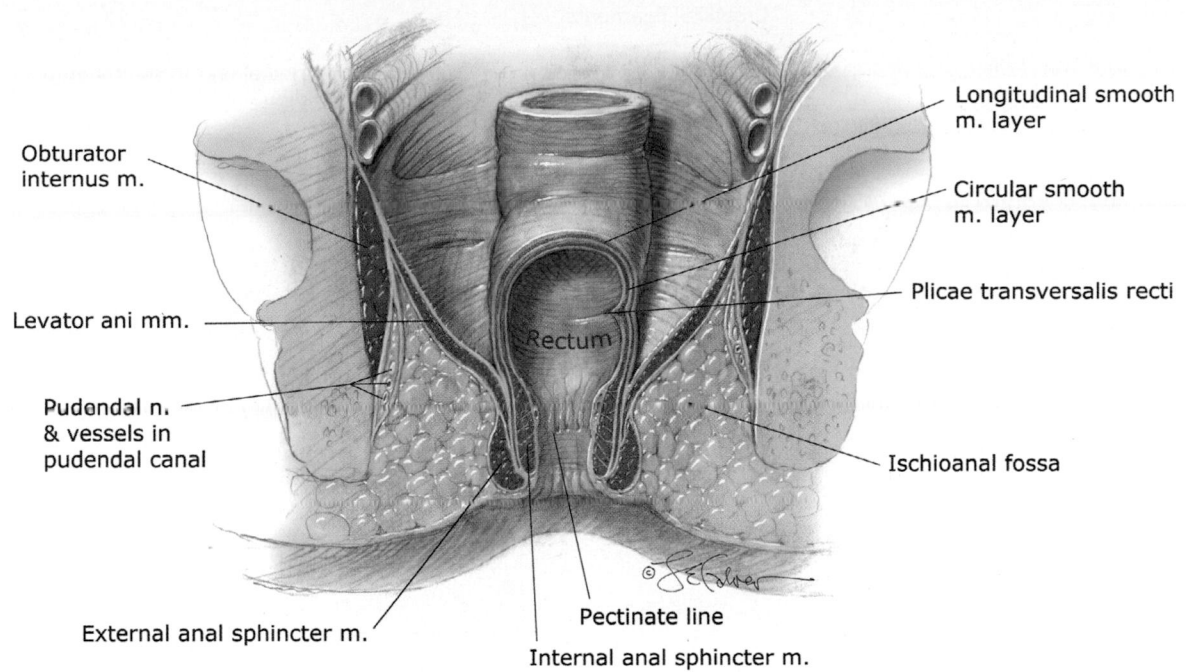

Obturator
internus m.

Levator ani mm.

Pudendal n.
& vessels in
pudendal canal

External anal sphincter m.

Longitudinal smooth
m. layer

Circular smooth
m. layer

Plicae transversalis recti

Ischioanal fossa

Pectinate line

Internal anal sphincter m.

Rectum

FIGURE 38-21 Ischioanal fossa and anal sphincter complex.

submucosal layer on the dorsal (vaginal) surface of the urethra is a group of glands known as the paraurethral glands, which open into the urethral lumen via its dorsal surface (Fig. 26-4, p. 684). Duct openings of the two most prominent glands, termed Skene glands, are seen on the inner surface of the external urethral orifice (p. 941).

The urethra receives its blood supply from branches of the inferior vesical/vaginal and internal pudendal arteries. Although still controversial, the pudendal nerve is believed to innervate the most distal part of the striated urogenital sphincter complex. Somatic efferent branches of the pelvic nerve, a component of the inferior hypogastric or pelvic plexus, variably innervate the sphincter urethrae. An additional discussion of lower urinary tract innervation is found in Chapter 23 (p. 609).

Clinical Correlation. Chronic infection of the paraurethral glands can lead to development of urethral diverticula. Due to the multiple openings of these glands along the length of the urethra, diverticula may develop at various sites along the urethra (Chap. 26, p. 683).

Ureters. A detailed description of the pelvic ureter appears in the pelvic sidewall retroperitoneum discussion on page 938.

Rectum

The rectum is continuous with the sigmoid colon approximately at the level of the third sacral vertebra (see Fig. 38-19). It descends on the anterior surface of the sacrum for approximately 12 cm and ends in the anal canal after passing through the levator hiatus. The anterior and lateral portions of the proximal two thirds of the rectum are covered by peritoneum. The peritoneum is then reflected onto the posterior vaginal wall to form the posterior *cul-de-sac of Douglas*, also termed *rectouterine pouch*. In women, the cul-de-sac is located approximately 5 to

6 cm from the anal orifice and can be palpated manually during rectal or vaginal examination. At its commencement, the rectal wall is similar to that of the sigmoid, but near its termination it becomes dilated to form the rectal ampulla, which begins below the posterior cul-de-sac peritoneum.

The rectum contains several, usually three, transverse folds called the *plicae transversales recti*, also termed valves of Houston (Fig. 38-21). The largest and most constant of these folds is located anteriorly and to the right, approximately 8 cm from the anal orifice. These folds may contribute to fecal continence by supporting fecal matter above the anal canal.

Clinical Correlation. In the empty state, the transverse rectal folds overlap each other, making it difficult at times to manipulate an examining finger or endoscopy tube past this level.

Retroperitoneal Surgical Spaces
Pelvic Sidewall

Knowledge of a number of retroperitoneal spaces is important for the pelvic surgeon. Of these, the retroperitoneal space of the pelvic sidewalls contains the internal iliac vessels and pelvic lymphatics, pelvic ureter, and obturator nerve.

Clinical Correlation. Entering the retroperitoneum at the pelvic sidewalls can be used to identify the ureter (Fig. 38-22). Moreover, it is an essential step for many of the surgeries described in gynecologic oncology and for uterine or internal iliac artery ligation in the setting of hemorrhage.

Vessels. The major pelvic vessels are shown in Figures 38-12, 38-14, and 38-22. The internal iliac and external iliac vessels and their corresponding lymph node groups lie within the pelvic sidewall retroperitoneal space (see Fig. 38-16).

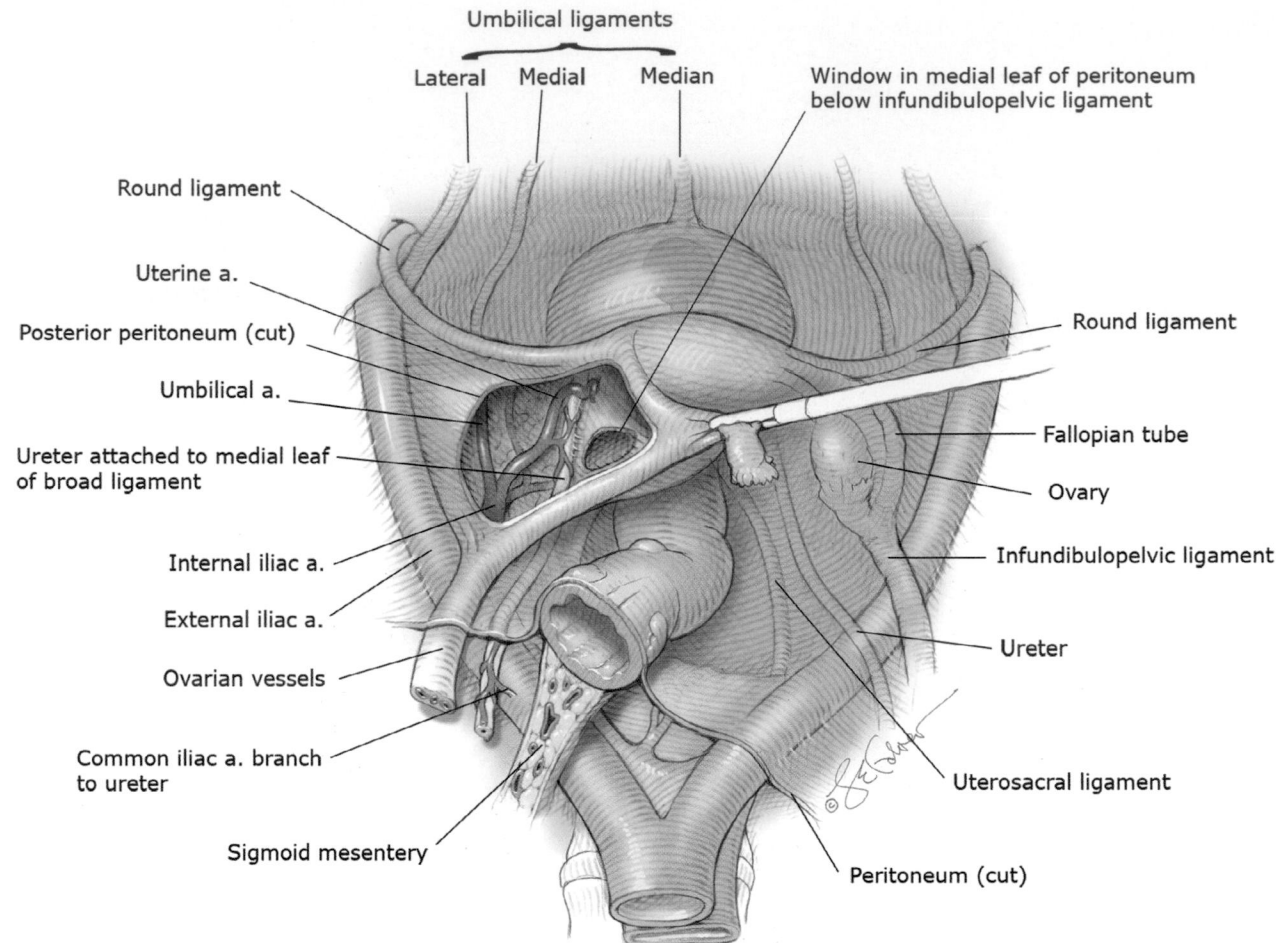

Umbilical ligaments

Lateral   Medial   Median

Window in medial leaf of peritoneum
below infundibulopelvic ligament

Round ligament

Uterine a.

Posterior peritoneum (cut)

Umbilical a.

Ureter attached to medial leaf
of broad ligament

Internal iliac a.

External iliac a.

Ovarian vessels

Common iliac a. branch
to ureter

Sigmoid mesentery

Round ligament

Fallopian tube

Ovary

Infundibulopelvic ligament

Ureter

Uterosacral ligament

Peritoneum (cut)

FIGURE 38-22 Surgical view of left pelvic sidewall retroperitoneal space showing the ureter attached to medial leaf of broad ligament.

Clinical Correlation. If hemorrhage is encountered during pelvic surgery, the internal iliac artery may be ligated to decrease the pulse pressure to pelvic organs. When this vessel is dissected, the ureter should be identified and avoided. The internal iliac artery is ligated distal to the origin of its posterior division branches. This helps to prevent significant devascularization of the gluteal muscles. These posterior division branches generally arise from the posterolateral wall of the internal iliac artery at a site 3 to 4 cm from its origin off the common iliac artery (Bleich, 2007).

Pelvic Ureter. The ureter enters the pelvis by crossing over the bifurcation of the common iliac artery into the internal iliac and external iliac arteries and just medial to the ovarian vessels (see Fig. 38-15). It descends into the pelvis attached to the medial leaf of the pelvic sidewall peritoneum. Along this course, the ureter lies medial to the internal iliac branches and anterolateral to the uterosacral ligaments (see Figs. 38-14, 38-15, and 38-22). The ureter then traverses the cardinal ligament approximately 1 to 2 cm lateral to the cervix. Near the level of the uterine isthmus it courses below the uterine artery ("water under the bridge"). It then travels anteromedially toward the base of the bladder (see Fig. 38-15). In this path, it runs close to the upper third of the anterior vaginal wall (Rahn, 2007). Finally, the ureter enters the bladder and travels obliquely for approximately 1.5 cm before opening at the ureteral orifices.

The pelvic ureter receives blood supply from the vessels it passes: the common iliac, internal iliac, uterine, and superior vesical vessels. Vascular anastomoses on the connective tissue sheath enveloping the ureter form a longitudinal network of vessels.

Clinical Correlation. Because of the pelvic ureter's proximity to many structures encountered during gynecologic surgery, emphasis should be placed on its precise intraoperative identification. Most ureters are injured during gynecologic surgery for benign disease. More than 50 percent of these injuries are not diagnosed intraoperatively (Ibeanu, 2009). The most common sites of injury include: (1) the pelvic brim area during clamping of the infundibulopelvic ligament; (2) the isthmic region during uterine artery ligation, (3) the pelvic sidewall during suturing of the uterosacral ligament, and (4) the vaginal apex during clamping or suturing of the vaginal cuff.

Presacral Space

This retroperitoneal space is located between the rectosigmoid and posterior abdominal wall peritoneum and the sacrum (Figs. 38-18 and 38-23). It begins below the aortic bifurcation and extends inferiorly to the pelvic floor. Laterally, this space is bounded by the internal iliac vessels and branches. Contained within the loose areolar and connective tissue of this space are

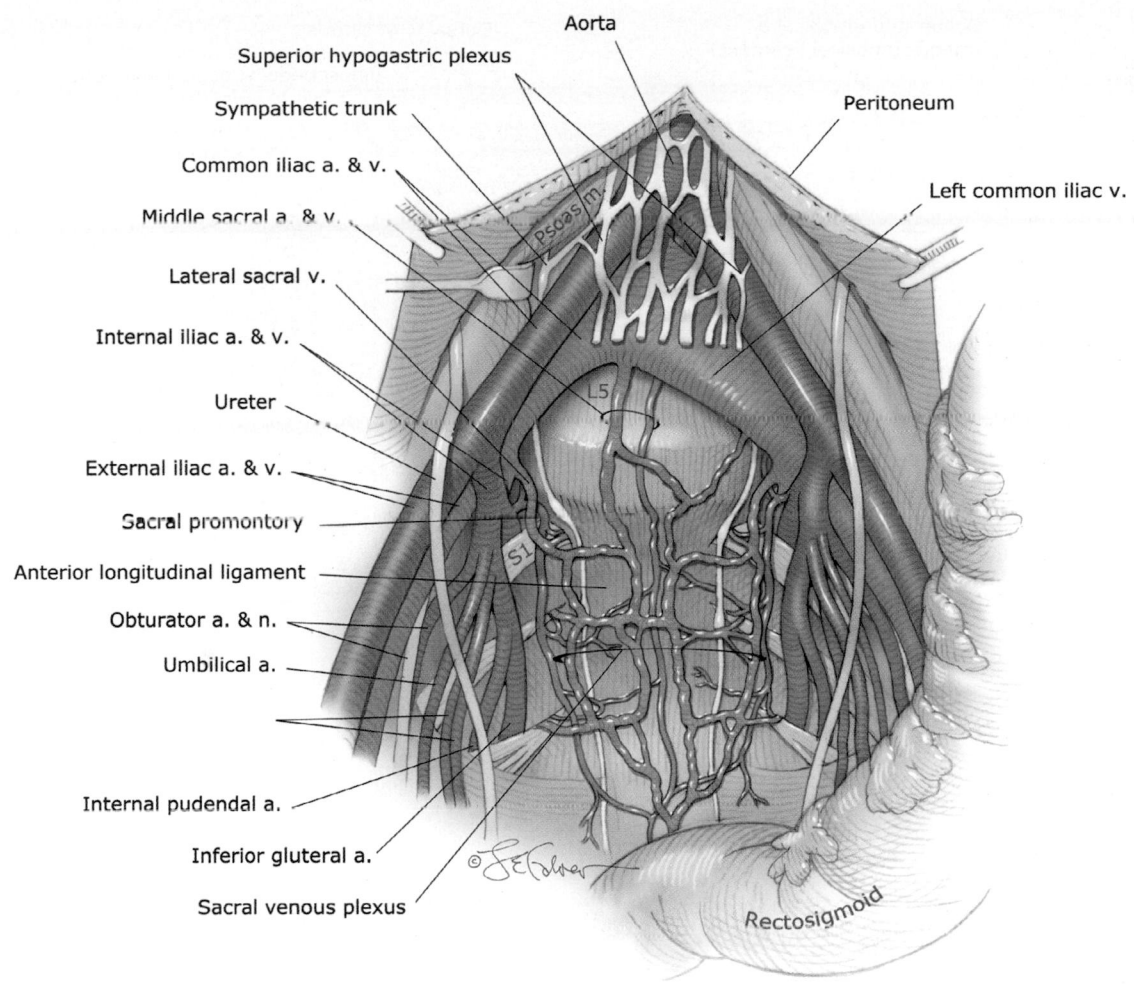

FIGURE 38-23 Presacral space. L5 = fifth lumbar vertebra; S1 = first sacral nerve.

the superior hypogastric plexus, hypogastric nerves, and portions of the inferior hypogastric plexus (see Figs. 38-14 and 38-23). The sacral lymph node group is also found here (see Fig. 38-16).

The vascular anatomy of the presacral space is complex and includes an extensive and intricate venous plexus, termed the *sacral venous plexus*. This plexus is formed primarily by the anastomoses of the middle and lateral sacral veins on the anterior surface of the sacrum. The *middle sacral vein* commonly drains into the left common iliac vein, whereas the each *lateral sacral vein* opens into its respective internal iliac vein. Ultimately, these vessels drain into the caval system. The sacral venous plexus also receives contributions from the *lumbar veins* of the posterior abdominal wall and from the *basivertebral veins* that pass through the pelvic sacral foramina. The *middle sacral artery*, which courses in proximity to the *middle sacral vein*, arises from the posterior and distal part of the abdominal aorta.

In one study of presacral space vascular anatomy, the left common iliac vein was the closest major vessel identified both cephalad and lateral to the midsacral promontory. The average distance of the left common iliac vein to the midsacral promontory in this study was 2.7 cm (range 0.9-5.2 cm) (Wieslander, 2006). The proximity of the left common iliac vein to the sacral promontory makes this vessel especially vulnerable to injury during entrance and dissection in this space.

Clinical Correlation. The presacral space is most commonly entered to perform abdominal sacrocolpopexy (Section 43-17, p. 1225). It may also be entered for presacral neurectomies (Chap. 11, p. 316). Importantly, during these procedures, bleeding from the sacral venous plexus may be difficult to control as the veins may retract into the sacral foramina.

Prevesical Space

This space is also called the retropubic space or *space of Retzius*. It can be entered by perforating the transversalis fascial layer of the anterior abdominal wall (see Fig. 38-19). This space is bounded by the bony pelvis and muscles of the pelvic wall anteriorly and laterally and by the anterior abdominal wall superiorly (Figs. 38-18, 38-19, and 38-24). The bladder and proximal urethra lie posterior to this space. Attachments of the paravaginal connective tissue to the arcus tendineus fascia pelvis constitute the posterolateral limit of the space as well as separate it from the vesicovaginal and vesicocervical spaces.

There are a number of vessels and nerves in this space. The *dorsal vein of the clitoris* passes under the lower border of the pubic symphysis and drains into the *periurethral-perivesical venous plexus*, also termed the *plexus of Santorini* (Pathi, 2009). The *obturator neurovascular bundle* courses along the lateral pelvic walls and enters the obturator canal to reach the medial

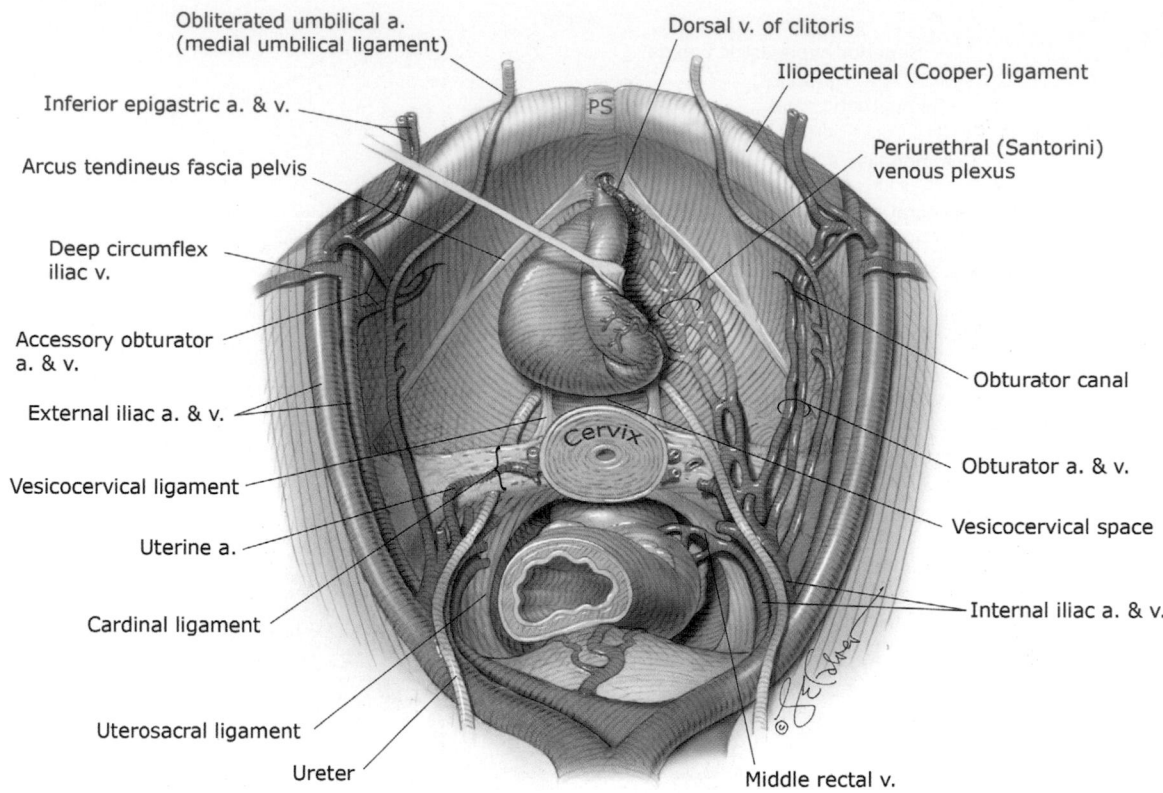

Obliterated umbilical a.
(medial umbilical ligament)

Inferior epigastric a. & v.

Arcus tendineus fascia pelvis

Deep circumflex
iliac v.

Accessory obturator
a. & v.

External iliac a. & v.

Vesicocervical ligament

Uterine a.

Cardinal ligament

Uterosacral ligament

Ureter

Dorsal v. of clitoris

Iliopectineal (Cooper) ligament

Periurethral (Santorini)
venous plexus

Obturator canal

Obturator a. & v.

Vesicocervical space

Internal iliac a. & v.

Middle rectal v.

PS

Cervix

FIGURE 38-24 Retropubic space. PS = pubic symphysis.

compartment of the thigh. The autonomic nerve branches that supply the bladder and urethra course on the lateral borders of these structures. Additionally, in most women, accessory obturator vessels that arise from or open into the inferior epigastric or external iliac vessels are found crossing the superior pubic rami and connecting with the obturator vessels near the obturator canal.

Clinical Correlation. Injury to the obturator neurovascular bundle or accessory obturator vessels is most often associated with pelvic lymph node dissection, paravaginal defect repair procedures, and pelvic fractures. Thus, knowledge of the approximate location of these vessels and of the obturator canal is critical when this space is dissected. The obturator canal is found approximately 5 to 6 cm from the midline of the pubic symphysis, and 1 to 2 cm below the upper margin of the iliopectineal ligament (Drewes, 2005).

Bleeding from the periurethral-perivesical venous plexus is often encountered while placing sutures or passing needles into this space during retropubic bladder neck suspensions and midurethral retropubic procedures, respectively. This venous ooze usually stops when pressure is applied or sutures are tied.

VULVA AND PERINEUM

Vulva

The external female genitalia, collectively known as the *vulva*, lie on the pubic bones and extend posteriorly. Structures included are the mons pubis, labia majora and minora, clitoris, vestibule, vestibular bulbs, greater vestibular glands (Bartholin glands), lesser vestibular glands, Skene and paraurethral glands,

and the urethral and vaginal orifices (Fig. 38-25). The embryologic development and homologs of these structures can be found in Table 18-1 (p. 484).

Mons Pubis and Labia Majora

The *mons pubis*, or *mons veneris*, is the rounded eminence that lies anterior to the pubic symphysis. The labia majora are two prominent folds that extend from the mons pubis toward the perineal body posteriorly. Skin over the mons pubis and labia majora contains hair and has a subcutaneous layer similar to that of the anterior abdominal wall. The subcutaneous layer consists of a superficial fatty layer similar to Camper fascia, and a deeper membranous layer, *Colles fascia* (see Fig. 38-25). Also known as the *superficial perineal fascia*, Colles fascia is similar to and continuous with Scarpa fascia of the anterior abdominal wall.

The round ligament and obliterated *processus vaginalis*, also termed the *canal of Nuck*, exit the inguinal canal and attach to the adipose tissue or skin of the labia majora.

Clinical Correlation. Colles fascia attaches firmly to the ischiopubic rami laterally and the perineal membrane posteriorly. These attachments prevent the spread of fluid, blood, or infection from the superficial perineal space to the thighs or posterior perineal triangle. Anteriorly, Colles fascia has no attachments to the pubic rami and it is therefore continuous with the lower anterior abdominal wall (see Fig. 38-25). This continuity may allow the spread of fluid, blood, and infection between these compartments.

In the labium majus, the differential diagnosis of a mass should include a leiomyoma arising from the round ligament

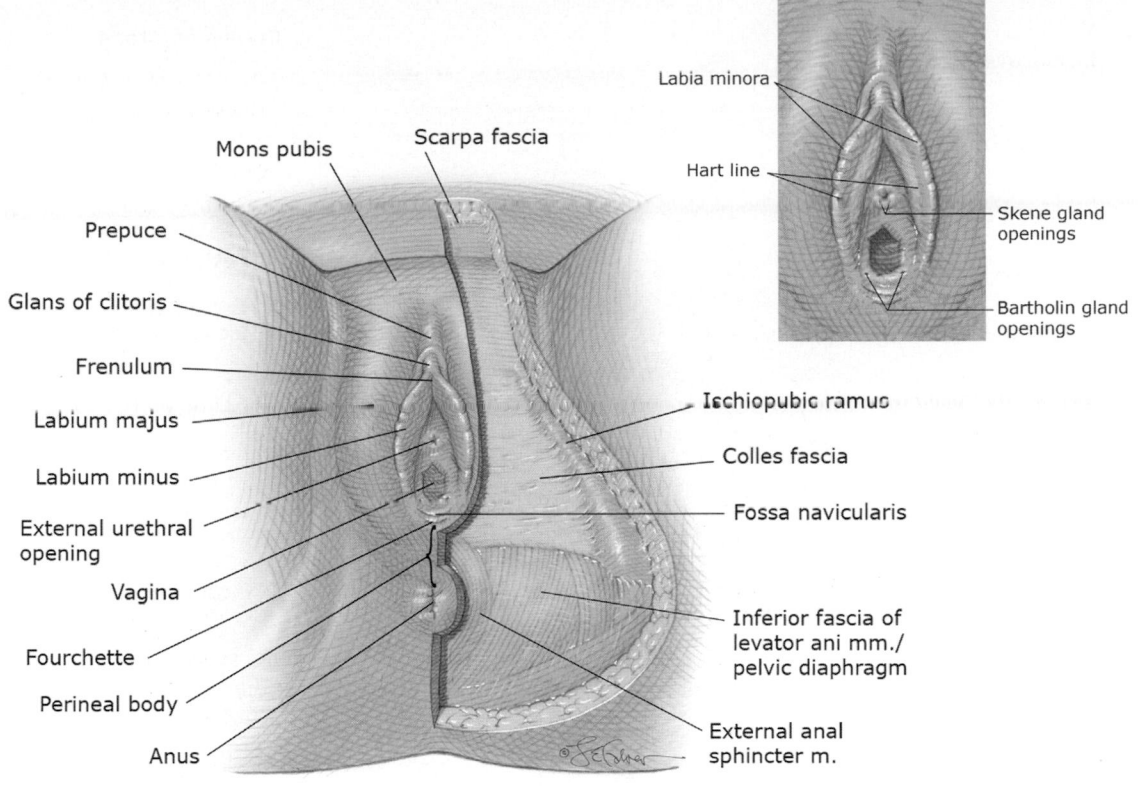

FIGURE 38-25 Vulvar structures and subcutaneous layer of anterior perineal triangle. Note the continuity of Colles and Scarpa fasciae. Inset: Vestibule boundaries and openings onto vestibule.

or a persistent processus vaginalis. An indirect inguinal hernia may also reach the labium majus by passing through the deep inguinal ring and inguinal canal. In contrast to direct inguinal hernias, which usually result from acquired defects of anterior abdominal wall fascia, indirect inguinal hernias are generally congenital.

Labia Minora

These two cutaneous folds lie between the labia majora (see Fig. 38-25). Anteriorly, each labia minora bifurcates to form two folds that surround the glans of the clitoris. The prepuce is the anterior fold that overlies the glans, and the frenulum is the fold that passes below the clitoris. Posteriorly, the labia minora end at the fourchette.

In contrast to the skin that overlies the labia majora, the skin of the labia minora does not contain hair. Also, the subcutaneous tissue is devoid of fat and consists primarily of loose connective tissue. This latter attribute allows mobility of the skin during sex and accounts for the ease of dissection with vulvectomy.

Clinical Correlation. Typically, labia minora are symmetric, but their size and shape can vary widely between women. In some, these winglike structures are pendulous and can be drawn into the vagina during coitus. If associated with dyspareunia in this setting, the labia can be surgically reduced (Section 41-23, p. 1072). Moreover, chronic dermatologic diseases such as lichen sclerosus may lead to significant atrophy or disappearance of the labia minora (Chap. 4, p. 113).

Clitoris

This is the female erectile structure homologous to the penis. It consists of a glans, a body, and two crura. The glans contains many nerve endings and is covered by a thinly keratinized stratified squamous epithelium. The body measures approximately 2 cm and is connected to the pubic ramus by the crura (Fig. 38-26).

Vaginal Vestibule

This is the area between the two labia minora. It is bounded laterally by the line of Hart and medially by the hymenal ring. Hart line represents the demarcation between the skin and the mucous membrane on the inner surface of the labia minora. The vestibule extends from the clitoris anteriorly to the fourchette posteriorly (see Fig. 38-25 inset). It contains the openings of the urethra; vagina; greater vestibular glands, also known as Bartholin glands; and Skene glands, which are the largest pair of paraurethral glands. It also contains the numerous openings of the lesser vestibular glands. A shallow vestibular depression known as the navicular fossa lies between the vaginal orifice and the fourchette.

Clinical Correlation. Localized vulvar dysesthesia—also termed vulvar vestibulitis—is characterized by pain with vaginal penetration, localized point tenderness, and erythema of the vestibular mucosa.

The Hart line is clinically relevant when choosing incision sites for Bartholin gland drainage or marsupialization (Sections 41-18 and 41-19, p. 1063). In attempts to recreate near-normal gland duct anatomy following these procedures,

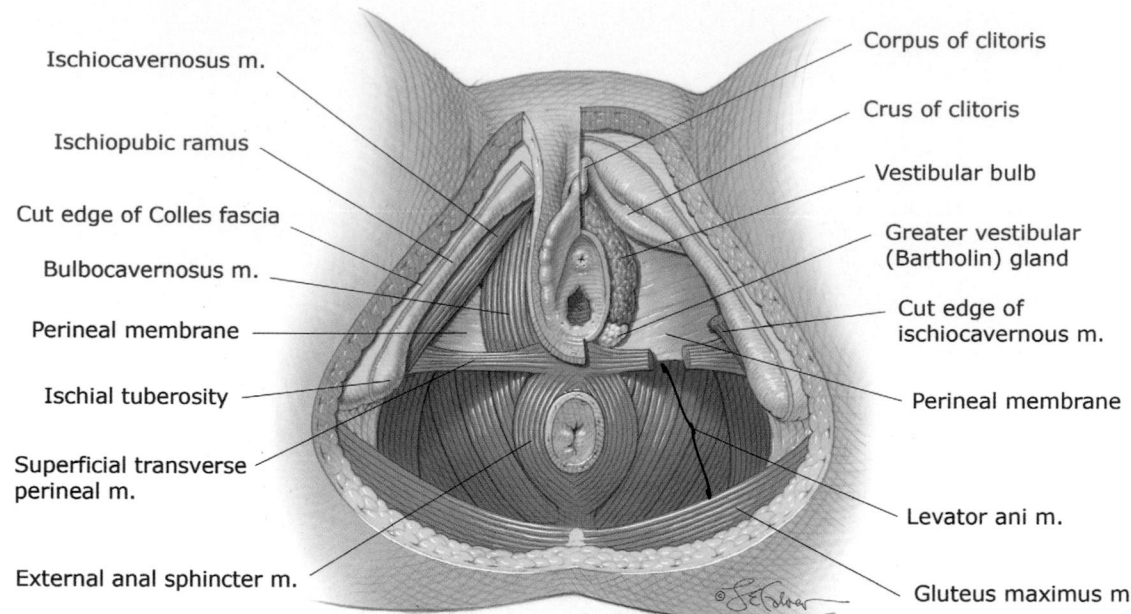

Ischiocavernosus m.

Ischiopubic ramus

Cut edge of Colles fascia

Bulbocavernosus m.

Perineal membrane

Ischial tuberosity

Superficial transverse perineal m.

External anal sphincter m.

Corpus of clitoris

Crus of clitoris

Vestibular bulb

Greater vestibular (Bartholin) gland

Cut edge of ischiocavernous m.

Perineal membrane

Levator ani m.

Gluteus maximus m.

FIGURE 38-26 Anterior (superficial space of anterior triangle) and posterior perineal triangles. On the image's left are the structures noted after removal of Colles fascia. On the image's right are the structures noted after removal of the superficial perineal muscles.

incisions placed external to Hart line should be avoided (Kaufman, 1994).

Vestibular Bulbs

These are homologs to the male penile bulb and corpus spongiosum. They are two elongated, approximately 3-cm long, richly vascular erectile masses that surround the vaginal orifice (see Fig. 38-26). Their posterior ends are in contact with the Bartholin glands. Their anterior ends are joined to one another and to the clitoris. Their deep surfaces are in contact with the perineal membrane, and their superficial surfaces are partially covered by the bulbocavernosus muscles.

Clinical Correlation. The proximity of the Bartholin glands to the vestibular bulbs accounts for the significant bleeding often encountered with Bartholin gland excision (Section 41-20, p. 1066).

Greater Vestibular or Bartholin Glands

These are the homologs of the male bulbourethral or Cowper glands. They are in contact with and often overlapped by the posterior ends of the vestibular bulbs (see Fig. 38-26). Each gland is connected to the vestibule by an approximately 2-cm long duct. The ducts open in the groove between the labia minora and the hymen—the vestibule—at approximately 5 and 7 o'clock positions.

The glands contain columnar cells that secrete clear or whitish mucus with lubricant properties. These glands are stimulated by sexual arousal. Contraction of the bulbocavernosus muscle, which covers the superficial surface of the gland, stimulates gland secretion.

Clinical Correlation. Obstruction of the Bartholin ducts by proteinaceous material or by inflammation from infection can lead to cysts of variable sizes. An infected cyst can lead to an abscess, which typically requires surgical drainage. Symptomatic or recurrent cysts may require marsupialization or gland excision.

Perineum

The *perineum* is the diamond-shaped area between the thighs (see Fig. 38-25). It is bounded deeply by the inferior fascia of the pelvic diaphragm and superficially by the skin between the thighs. The anterior, posterior, and lateral boundaries of the perineum are the same as those of the bony pelvic outlet: the pubic symphysis anteriorly, ischiopubic rami and ischial tuberosities anterolaterally, coccyx posteriorly, and sacrotuberous ligaments posterolaterally. An arbitrary line joining the ischial tuberosities divides the perineum into the anterior or *urogenital triangle,* and a posterior or *anal triangle.*

Anterior (Urogenital) Triangle

Structures that comprise the vulva or external female genitalia lie in the anterior triangle of the perineum. The base or posterior border of this triangle is the *interischial line,* which usually overlies the *superficial transverse perineal muscles* (see Fig. 38-26).

The anterior perineal triangle can be further divided into a *superficial* and a *deep pouch* or *space* by the *perineal membrane.* The superficial perineal pouch lies superficial to the perineal membrane and the deep pouch lies above or deep to the membrane.

Superficial Space. This space of the anterior triangle is an enclosed compartment that lies between Colles fascia and the perineal membrane. It contains the ischiocavernosus, bulbocavernosus, and superficial transverse perineal muscles; Bartholin glands; vestibular bulbs; clitoris; and branches of the pudendal vessels and nerve. The urethra and vagina traverse this space.

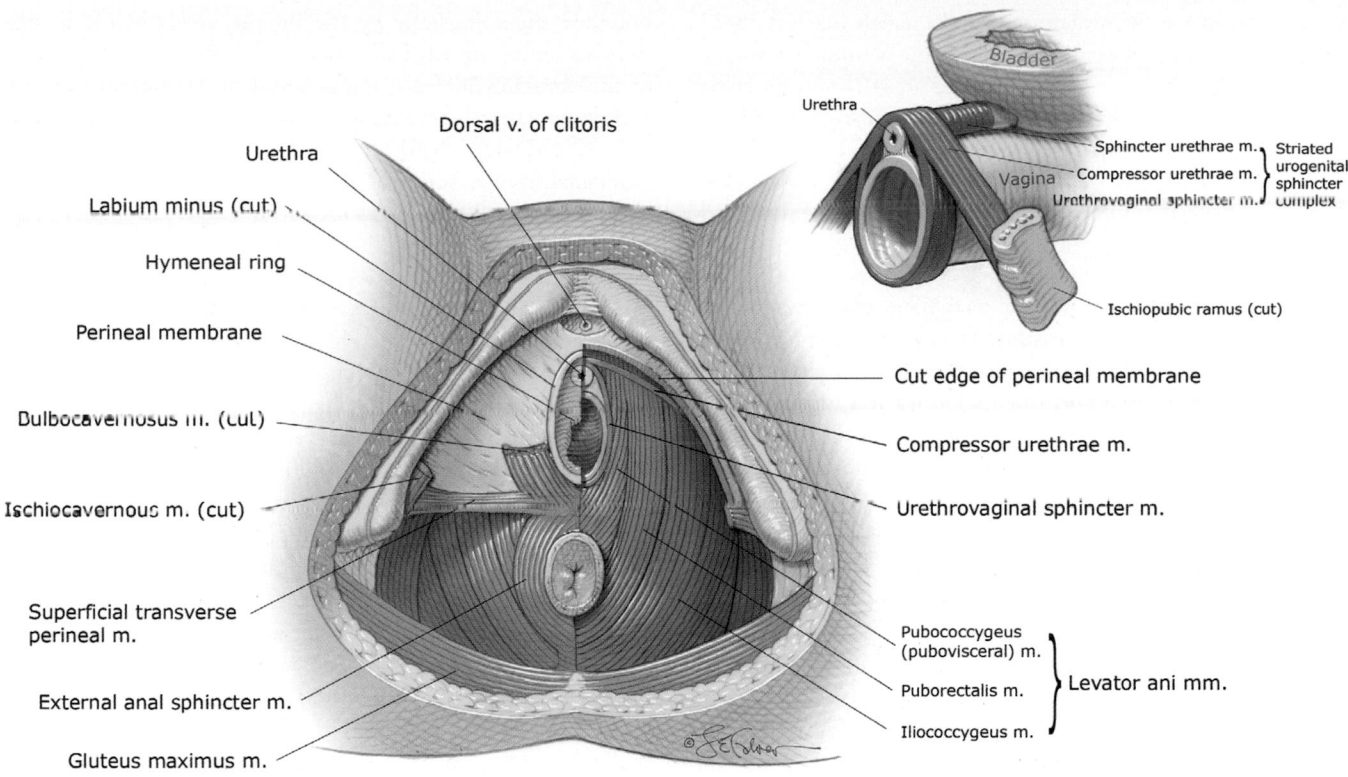

FIGURE 38-27 Deep space of anterior perineal triangle. One the image's right are structures noted after removal of the perineal membrane. Inset: Striated urogenital sphincter muscles. Also shown are all structures that attach to perineal body: bulbocavernosus, superficial transverse perineal, external anal sphincter, and puboperinealis muscles, perineal membrane, and urethrovaginal sphincter.

The *ischiocavernosus muscle* attaches to the medial aspect of the ischial tuberosities posteriorly and the ischiopubic rami laterally. Anteriorly, it attaches to the crus of the clitoris. This muscle may help maintain clitoral erection by compressing the crus of the clitoris, thus retarding venous drainage.

The *bulbocavernosus muscle*, also termed *bulbospongiosus muscle*, covers the superficial portion of the vestibular bulbs and Bartholin glands. These muscles attach to the body of the clitoris anteriorly and the perineal body posteriorly. The muscles act to constrict the vaginal lumen, contributing to the release of secretions from Bartholin glands. They may also contribute to clitoral erection by compressing the deep dorsal vein of the clitoris. The bulbocavernosus muscle, along with the ischiocavernosus muscle, acts to pull the clitoris downward.

The *superficial transverse perineal muscles* are narrow strips that attach to the ischial tuberosity laterally and the perineal body medially. They may be attenuated or even absent, but when present, they contribute to the perineal body.

Deep Perineal Space. This pouch lies deep or superior to the perineal membrane (Fig. 38-27). In contrast to the superficial pouch, which is a closed compartment, the deep space is continuous superiorly with the pelvic cavity. It contains the compressor urethrae and urethrovaginal sphincter muscles, parts of urethra and vagina, branches of the internal pudendal artery, and the dorsal nerve and vein of the clitoris.

Perineal Membrane (Urogenital Diaphragm). Traditionally, a trilaminar, triangular urogenital diaphragm has been described as the main component of the deep perineal space. According to this concept, the urogenital diaphragm consisted of the deep transverse perineal muscles and sphincter urethrae muscles between the perineal membrane (inferior fascia of the urogenital diaphragm) and a superior layer of fascia (superior fascia of the urogenital diaphragm). However, the term *diaphragm* is used to describe a closed compartment. As described earlier, the deep perineal space is an open compartment. It is bounded inferiorly by the perineal membrane and extends up into the pelvis (Oelrich, 1980, 1983). As a result, when describing perineal anatomy, the terms *urogenital diaphragm* or *inferior fascia of the urogenital diaphragm* are misnomers and have been replaced by the anatomically correct term, *perineal membrane.*

The perineal membrane constitutes the deep boundary of the superficial perineal space (see Fig. 38-27). It attaches laterally to the ischiopubic rami, medially to the distal third of the urethra and vagina, and posteriorly to the perineal body. Anteriorly, it attaches to the arcuate ligament of the pubis. In this area, the perineal membrane is particularly thick and is often referred to as the *pubourethral ligament.*

The perineal membrane has recently been shown to consist of two histologically and probably functionally distinct portions that span the opening of the anterior pelvic triangle (Stein, 2008). The dorsal or posterior portion consists of a sheet of dense fibrous tissue that attaches laterally to the ischiopubic rami and medially to the distal third of the vagina and to the perineal body (see Fig. 38-27). The ventral or anterior portion of the perineal membrane is intimately associated with the compressor urethrae and urethrovaginal sphincter muscles, previously called the deep transverse perineal muscles in the female (see Fig. 38-27 inset). In addition, the ventral portion of the perineal membrane is continuous with the insertion of the arcus tendineus fascia pelvis to the pubic bones (see Fig. 38-20). In this same histologic study, the deep or superior surface of the perineal membrane was shown to have direct connections to the levator ani muscles, and the superficial or inferior surface of the membrane was fused with the vestibular bulb and clitoral crus.

Clinical Correlation. The perineal membrane attaches to the lateral walls of the vagina approximately at level of the hymen. It provides support to the distal vagina and urethra by attaching these structures to the bony pelvis. In addition, its attachments to the levator ani muscles suggest that the perineal membrane may play a more active role in support than was previously thought.

Posterior (Anal) Triangle

This triangle contains the ischioanal fossa, anal canal, anal sphincter complex, and branches of the internal pudendal vessels and pudendal nerve (see Figs. 38-21, 38-27, and 38-28). It is bounded deeply by the fascia overlying the inferior surface of the levator ani muscles, and laterally by the fascia overlying the medial surface of the obturator internus muscles. A splitting of the obturator internus fascia in this area is known as the *pudendal* or *Alcock canal* (see Figs. 38-6 and 38-21). This canal allows passage of the internal pudendal vessels and pudendal nerve before these structures split into terminal branches to supply the structures of the vulva and perineum (see Fig. 38-28).

The *ischioanal* or *ischiorectal fossa* fills most of the anal triangle (see Figs. 38-21 and 38-28). It contains adipose tissue and occasional blood vessels. The anal canal and anal sphincter complex lie in the center of this fossa. The ischioanal fossa is

bounded superomedially by the inferior fascia of the levator muscles; anterolaterally by the fascia covering the medial surface of the obturator internus muscles and the ischial tuberosities; and posterolaterally by the lower border of the gluteus maximus muscles and sacrotuberous ligaments. At a superficial level, the ischioanal fossa is bounded anteriorly by the superficial transverse perineal muscles. At a superior or deeper level, there is no fascial boundary between the fossa and the tissues deep to the perineal membrane. Posterior to the anus, the contents of the fossa are continuous across the midline except for the attachments of the external anal sphincter fibers to the coccyx. This continuity of the ischioanal fossa across perineal compartments allows fluid, infection, and malignancy to spread from one side of the anal canal to the other, and also into the anterior perineal compartment deep to the perineal membrane.

The anal sphincter complex consists of two sphincters and the puborectalis muscle. The external anal sphincter consists of striated muscle that surrounds the distal anal canal. It consists of a superficial and a deep portion. The more superficial fibers lie caudal to the internal sphincter and are separated from the anal epithelium only by submucosa. The deep fibers blend with the lowest fibers of the puborectalis muscle. The external sphincter is primarily innervated by the inferior anal branch of the pudendal nerve. The external anal sphincter is responsible for the squeeze pressure of the anal canal.

The internal anal sphincter is the thickening of the circular smooth muscle layer of the anal wall (see Fig. 38-21). It is under the control of the autonomic nervous system and is responsible for approximately 80 percent of the resting pressure of the anal canal.

The puborectalis muscle comprises the medial portion of the levator ani muscle that arises on either side from the inner surface

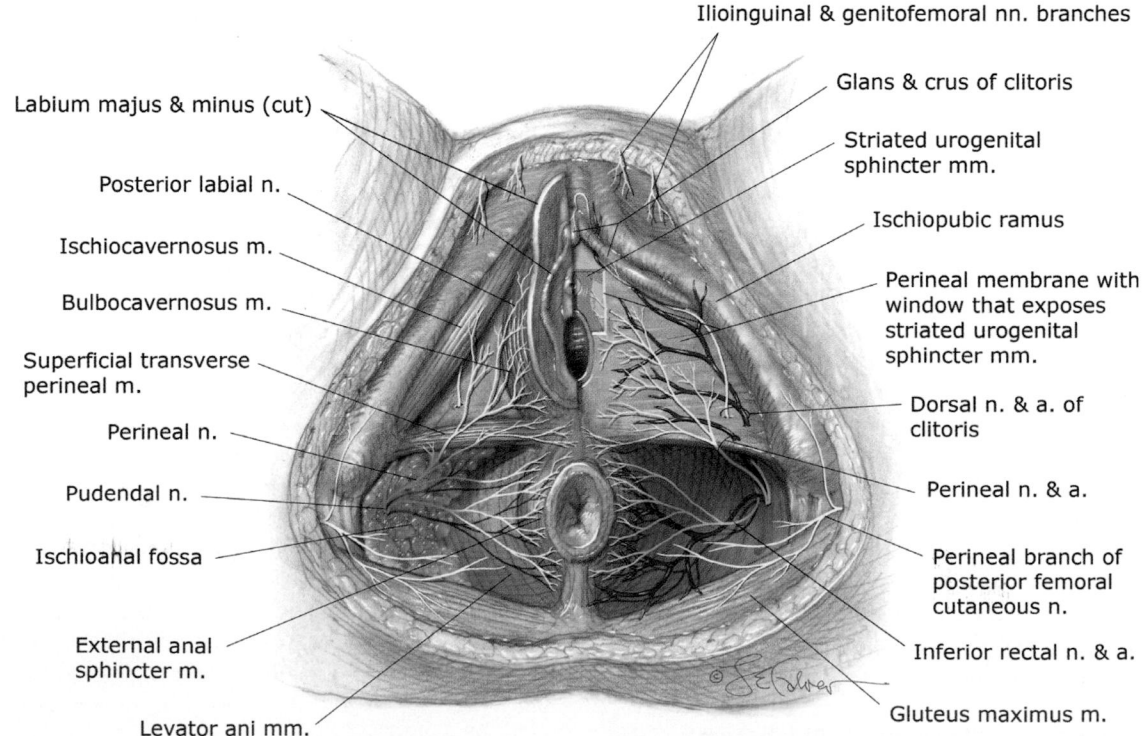

FIGURE 38-28 Pudendal nerve and vessels. Nerve supply to striated urogenital sphincter and external anal sphincter muscles.

of the pubic bones. It passes behind the rectum and forms a sling behind the anorectal junction, contributing to the anorectal angle and possibly to fecal continence (see Figs. 38-9, 38-10, and 38-27).

Perineal Body

This is a mass of fibromuscular tissue found between the distal part of the posterior vaginal wall and the anus. It is formed by the attachment of several structures. Inferiorly or superficially, the structures that attach to and contribute to the perineal body include the bulbocavernosus, superficial transverse perineal, and external anal sphincter muscles (see Fig. 38-26). Structures that attach at a superior or deeper level are the perineal membrane, levator ani muscles and covering fascia, urethrovaginal sphincter muscles, and distal part of the posterior vaginal wall (see Fig. 38-27). The anterior-to-posterior as well as the superior-to-inferior extents of the perineal body measure approximately 2 to 4 cm (see Fig. 38-17).

Clinical Correlation. During episiotomy and other vaginal laceration repairs, and with pelvic reconstructive procedures, particular attention should be paid to reconstruction of the perineal body. Support from the perineal body helps to prevent pelvic organ prolapse and other pelvic floor dysfunction.

Blood Supply, Lymphatics, and Innervation

The vulva and perineum, and contained structures, have an intricate pattern and a number of anatomic variants.

Blood Vessels

The external pudendal artery is a branch of the femoral artery and supplies the skin and subcutaneous tissue of the mons pubis (see Fig. 38-3). The internal pudendal artery is one of the terminal branches of the internal iliac artery (see Fig. 38-6). It has a long course from its origin, and the association of this vessel to other structures has clinical importance. It exits the pelvis through the greater sciatic foramen, passes behind the ischial spines, and reenters the perineum through the lesser sciatic foramen. It then has a variable course, usually 2 to 3 cm, through the pudendal or Alcock canal, and then divides into terminal branches. These are the inferior rectal, perineal, and clitoral arteries (see Fig. 38-28). Branches to the perineum sometimes arise from the pudendal artery before it exits the pelvis. These vessels are called accessory pudendal arteries. Other accessory vessels may also arise directly from the anterior or posterior division of the internal iliac artery.

The veins that drain the structures of the vulva and perineum have courses and names similar to those of the arteries. Venous blood from the vestibular bulbs and other structures, with the exception of the erectile tissue of the clitoris, drains into the internal pudendal veins. The erectile tissue drains into the dorsal vein of the clitoris (see Fig. 38-27). This vein courses backward into the pelvis and terminates in the periurethral–perivesical venous plexus (see Fig. 38-24). The venous plexus that drains the rectum and anal canal empty into the superior, middle, and inferior rectal veins. The superior rectal vein drains into the inferior mesenteric vein, a tributary of the portal vein. The middle rectal vein drains into the internal iliac vein. The inferior rectal vein drains into the internal pudendal and then the internal iliac vein.

Lymphatic Drainage

Structures of the vulva and perineum drain into the inguinal lymph nodes, which are located below the inguinal ligament in the upper anterior and medial thigh (Fig. 38-29). There are

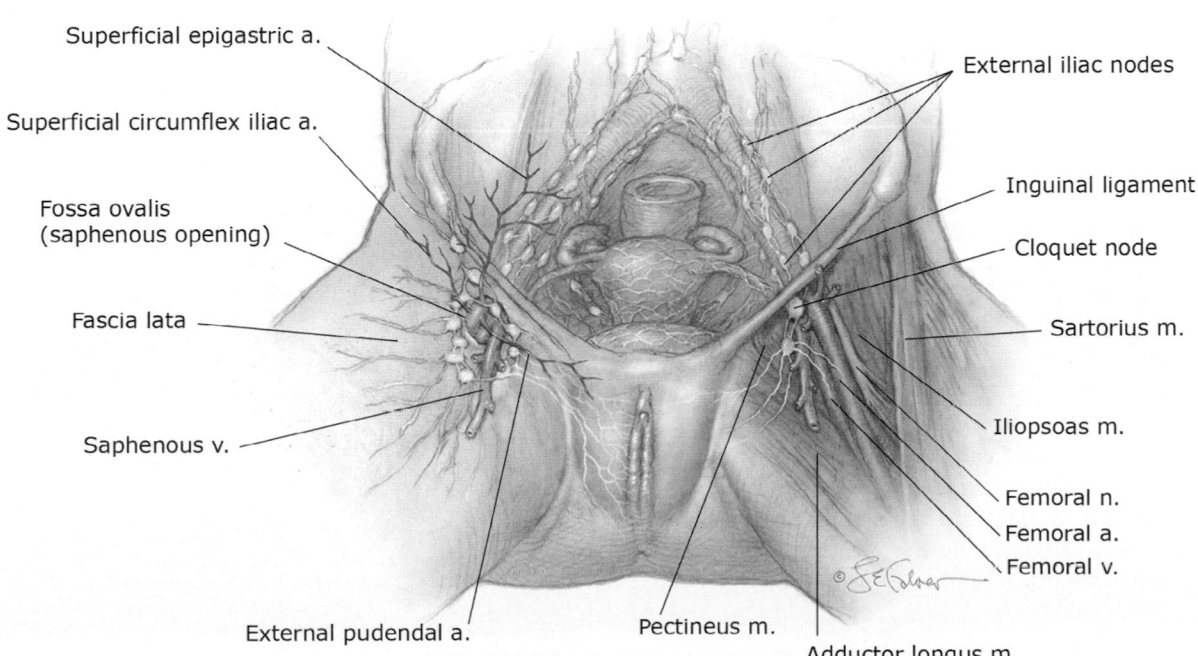

Superficial epigastric a.

Superficial circumflex iliac a.

Fossa ovalis (saphenous opening)

Fascia lata

Saphenous v.

External pudendal a.

Pectineus m.

Adductor longus m.

External iliac nodes

Inguinal ligament

Cloquet node

Sartorius m.

Iliopsoas m.

Femoral n.

Femoral a.

Femoral v.

FIGURE 38-29 Inguinal lymph nodes and contents of femoral triangle. Superficial inguinal nodes are shown on the image's left, and deep inguinal nodes appear on the image's right.

10 to 20 inguinal nodes, which are divided into a superficial and a deep group. Nodes of the superficial inguinal group are more numerous, and they are found in the membranous layer of the subcutaneous tissue of the anterior thigh, just superficial to the fascia lata.

The deep inguinal nodes vary from one to three in number, and are located deep to the fascia lata in the femoral triangle. This triangle is bordered superiorly by the inguinal ligament, laterally by the medial border of the *sartorius muscle* and medially by the medial border of the *adductor longus muscle*. The *iliopsoas* and *pectineus muscles* form its floor. From lateral to medial, the structures found in this triangle are the femoral nerve, artery, vein, and deep inguinal lymphatics. The femoral canal is the space that lies on the medial side of the femoral vein and that contains the deep inguinal nodes. The femoral ring is the abdominal opening of the femoral canal. The *fossa ovalis* or *saphenous opening* is an oval opening in the fascia lata and allows communication between superficial and deep inguinal nodes. Of the deep inguinal nodes, the highest one–*Cloquet node*–is located in the lateral part of the femoral ring. Efferent channels from the deep inguinal nodes pass through the femoral canal and femoral ring to the external iliac nodes. Lymphatics from the skin of the labia, clitoris, and remainder of the perineum drain into the superficial inguinal nodes. The glans and corpora cavernosa of the clitoris may drain directly to the deep inguinal nodes.

Clinical Correlation. Sampling of the superficial, and sometimes also the deep, inguinal nodes is completed as one part of radical vulvectomy (Section 44-29, p. 1343). Familiarity with the surrounding anatomy is essential.

Innervation

Somatic Innervation. Branches of the pudendal nerve–inferior anal, perineal, and dorsal nerve of the clitoris–provide sensory and motor innervation to the perineum (see Fig. 38-28). The pudendal nerve is a branch of the sacral plexus and is formed by the anterior rami of the second through the fourth sacral nerve roots (see Fig. 38-6). It has a course and distribution similar to the internal pudendal artery.

Clinical Correlation. Pudendal nerve blocks can be performed transvaginally or transgluteally by injecting local anesthesia just medial and inferior to the ischial spine. Importantly, inadvertent injection of local anesthetic into the internal pudendal vessels may lead to seizure activity and other complications (Chap. 40, p. 981).

Postsurgical pain in the distribution of the dorsal nerve of the clitoris has been reported following midurethral sling procedures. However, anatomic studies have shown that this nerve courses superficial or caudal to the perineal membrane, and trocar and mesh placement during these procedures remain deep or cephalad to the membrane (Montoya, 2011; Rahn, 2006).

Visceral Innervation. Clitoral erection requires parasympathetic visceral efferents derived from the pelvic plexus nerves or *nervi erigentes*. These arise from the second to the fourth sacral spinal cord segments. They reach the perineum along the urethra and vagina, passing through the urogenital hiatus (see Fig. 38-13). Sympathetic fibers reach the perineum with the pudendal nerve.

REFERENCES

Balgobin S, Carrick KS, Montoya TI, et al: Surgical dimensions and histology of the vesicocervical space. 37th Annual SGS Scientific Meeting, San Antonio, TX, Poster presentation, April 2011

Barber MD, Bremer RE, Thor KB, et al: Innervation of the female levator ani muscles. Am J Obstet Gynecol 187:64, 2002

Berglas B, Rubin IC: The study of the supportive structures of the uterus by levator myography. Surg Gynecol Obstet 97:677, 1953

Bleich AT, Rahn DD, Wieslander CK, et al: Posterior division of the internal iliac artery: anatomic variations and clinical applications. Am J Obstet Gynecol 197(6):658.e1–5, 2007

Campbell RM: The anatomy and histology of the sacrouterine ligaments. Am J Obstet Gynecol 59:1, 1950

DeLancey JOL: Anatomic aspects of vaginal eversion after hysterectomy. Am J Obstet Gynecol 166:1717, 1992

DeLancey JOL: Structural anatomy of the posterior pelvic compartment as it relates to rectocele. Am J Obstet Gynecol 180:815, 1999

DeLancey JOL, Hurd WW: Size of the urogenital hiatus in the levator ani muscles in normal women and women with pelvic organ prolapse. Obstet Gynecol 91:364, 1998

DeLancey JOL, Starr RA: Histology of the connection between the vagina and levator ani muscles: implications for the urinary function. J Reprod Med 35:765, 1990

Drewes PG, Marinis SI, Schaffer JI, et al: Vascular anatomy over the superior pubic rami in female cadavers. Am J Obstet Gynecol 193(6):2165, 2005

Federative Committee on Anatomical Terminology: Terminologia Anatomica. New York, Thieme Stuttgart, 1998

Heit M, Benson T, Russell B, et al: Levator ani muscle in women with genitourinary prolapse: indirect assessment by muscle histopathology. Neurourol Urodyn 15:17, 1996

Hsu Y, Summers A, Hussain HK, et al: Levator plate angle in women with pelvic organ prolapse compared to women with normal support using dynamic MR imaging. Am J Obstet Gynecol 194:1427, 2006

Hurd WW, Bud RO, DeLancey JOL, et al: The location of abdominal wall blood vessels in relationship to abdominal landmarks apparent at laparoscopy. Am J Obstet Gynecol 171 (3):642, 1994

Ibeanu OA, Chesson RR, Echols KT, et al: Urinary tract injury during hysterectomy based on universal cystoscopy. Obstet Gynecol 113:6, 2009

Kaufman RH: Cystic tumors. In Kaufman RH, Faro S (eds): Benign Diseases of the Vulva and Vagina. St Louis, MO, Mosby, 1994, p 238

Kerney R, Sawhney R, DeLancey JOL: Levator ani muscle anatomy evaluated by origin-insertion pairs. Obstet Gynecol 104:168, 2004

Kuhn RJP, Hollyock VE: Observations of the anatomy of the rectovaginal pouch and rectovaginal septum. Obstet Gynecol 59:445, 1982

Lawson JO: Pelvic anatomy: I. Pelvic floor muscles. Ann R Coll Surg Engl 54:244, 1974

Memon MA, Quinn TH, Cahill DR: Transversalis fascia: historical aspects and its place in contemporary inguinal herniorrhaphy. J Laparoendosc Adv Surg Tech A 9:267, 1999

Montoya TI, Calver L, Carrick KS, et al: Anatomic relationships of the pudendal nerve branches: assessment of injury risk with common surgical procedures. Am J Obstet Gynecol Jul 20, 2011 [Epub ahead of print]

Oelrich T: The striated urogenital sphincter muscle in the female. Anat Rec 205:223, 1983

Oelrich TM: The urethral sphincter muscle in the male. Am J Anat 158:229, 1980

Paramore RH: The supports-in-chief of the female pelvic viscera. Br J Obstet Gynaecol 13:391, 1908

Pathi SD, Castellanos ME, Corton MM: Variability of the retropubic space anatomy in female cadavers. Am J Obstet Gynecol. 201(5):524.e1, 2009

Rahn DD, Bleich AT, Wai CY, et al: Anatomic relationships of the distal third of the pelvic ureter, trigone, and urethra in unembalmed female cadavers. Am J Obstet Gynecol 197:668.e1, 2007

Rahn DD, Marinis SI, Schaffer JI, et al: Anatomical path of the tension-free vaginal tape: reassessing current teachings. Am J Obstet Gynecology 195(6):1809, 2006

Rahn DD, Phelan JN, White AB, et al: Clinical correlates of anterior abdominal wall neurovascular anatomy in gynecologic surgery. Am J Obstet Gynecol 202:234.e1, 2010

Range RL, Woodburne RT: The gross and microscopic anatomy of the transverse cervical ligaments. Am J Obstet Gynecol 90:460, 1964

Roshanravan SM, Wieslander CK, Schaffer JI, et al: Neurovascular anatomy of the sacrospinous ligament region in female cadavers: implications in sacrospinous ligament fixation. Am J Obstet Gynecol 197(6):660.e1, 2007

Stein TA, DeLancey JO: Structure of the perineal membrane in females: gross and microscopic anatomy. Obstet Gynecol 111:686, 2008

Umek WH, Morgan DM, Ashton-Miller JA, et al: Quantitative analysis of uterosacral ligament origin and insertion points by magnetic resonance imaging. Obstet Gynecol 103(3):447, 2004

Weber AM, Walters MD: Anterior vaginal prolapse: review of anatomy and techniques of surgical repair. Obstet Gynecol 89:311, 1997

Weber AM, Walter MD: What is vaginal fascia? AUGS Q Rep 13, 1995

Whiteside JL, Barber MD, Walters MD, et al: Anatomy of ilioinguinal and iliohypogastric nerves in relation to trocar placement and low transverse incisions. Am J Obstet Gynecol 189:1574, 2003

Wieslander CK, Rahn DD, McIntire DD, et al: Vascular anatomy of the presacral space in unembalmed female cadavers. Am J Obstet Gynecol 195(6):1736, 2006

Wieslander CK, Roshanravan SM, Wai CY, et al: Uterosacral ligament suspension sutures: anatomic relationships in unembalmed female cadavers. Am J Obstet Gynecol 197:672.e1, 2007

CHAPTER 38

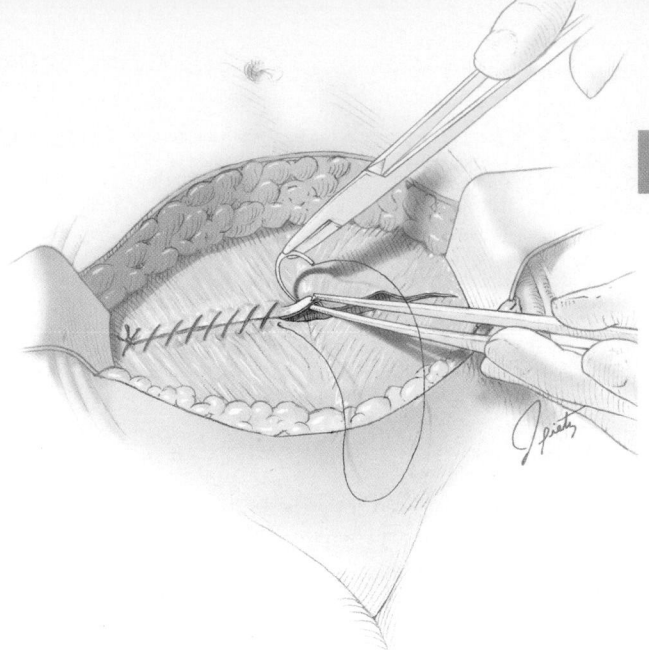

Each year, more than 30 million surgical procedures are performed. During these, nearly 1 million patients suffer a postoperative complication (Mangano, 2004). As surgeons, gynecologists assume responsibility for assessing a patient's clinical status to identify modifiable risk factors and prevent perioperative morbidity. However, clinicians should also be prepared to diagnose and manage such complications, if they arise.

PREOPERATIVE PATIENT EVALUATION

A properly performed preoperative evaluation serves two important functions. It uncovers comorbidities that require further evaluation and optimization to avert perioperative complications (Johnson, 2008). Second, evaluation allows improved use of operating room resources (Correll, 2009; Roizen, 2000).

Medical Consultation

In many cases, a gynecologist can perform a thorough preoperative history and physical examination, averting the need for medical consultation in many cases. However, if a poorly controlled or previously undiagnosed disease is discovered, consultation with an internist can be beneficial. The purpose of a preoperative internal medicine consultation is not to obtain "medical clearance" but rather to provide a risk assessment of a woman's current medical state. With consultation, a summary of the surgical illness is provided, and clear questions are posed to the consultant (Eagle, 2002; Fleisher, 2009; Goldman, 1983). In addition, a complete history and physical examination and medical records that report prior diagnostic testing should be available to the consulting physician. This can prevent unnecessary surgical delays and cost due to redundant testing.

Pulmonary Evaluation

Common postoperative pulmonary morbidities include atelectasis, pneumonia, and exacerbation of chronic lung diseases. Incidences of such complications following surgery are estimated between 20 and 70 percent (Bernstein, 2008; Brooks-Brunn, 1997; Qaseem, 2006).

Risk Factors for Pulmonary Complications

Procedure-Related Factors. Risk factors for pulmonary complications fall into one of two major categories—procedure-related and patient-related. For example, upper abdominal incisions as they approach the diaphragm can alter pulmonary function through three mechanisms, as shown in Figure 39-1. First, intraoperative stimulation of the viscera leads to decreased phrenic motoneuron output, which then lessens diaphragmatic descent. Second, disruption of abdominal wall muscles can hinder effective respiratory efforts. Finally, pain may limit effective voluntary use of respiratory muscles. As a result, poor diaphragmatic function may produce persistent decreases in vital capacity and in functional residual capacity. These predispose patients to atelectasis (Warner, 2000). Surgery duration is another procedure-associated factor. Procedures in which

patients receive general anesthesia for longer than 3 hours are associated with nearly double the risk of developing a postoperative pulmonary complication. Finally, emergency surgery remains a significant independent predictor of postoperative pulmonary complications. Although these procedure-related risk factors are largely unmodifiable, an appreciation of their associated sequelae should prompt increased postoperative vigilance.

Age. Individuals older than 60 years are at increased risk for developing postoperative pulmonary complications. After stratifying patients for comorbidities, those between 60 and 69 years have a twofold increased risk. In those older than 70 years, risk is increased threefold (Qaseem, 2006). Baseline cognition should be documented and postoperative sensorium should be monitored, as changes may be an early indicator of pulmonary function compromise following surgery.

Smoking. A greater than 20-pack-year smoking history confers a high incidence of postoperative pulmonary complications. Fortunately, this risk can be reduced with smoking abstinence before surgery. Specifically, in preparation for elective surgery, smoking cessation for at least 4 to 8 weeks offers risk reduction (Warner, 1984). Short-term benefits may be related to reduced nicotine and carboxyhemoglobin levels, improved mucociliary function, decreased upper airway hypersensitivity, and improved wound healing (Moller, 2002; Nakagawa, 2001). Patients with a history of smoking cessation for 6 or more months have complication risks similar to those who have never smoked.

Patients often see surgery as an opportunity for positive change (Shi, 2010). Education alone may prompt successful behavior modification. For others, agents to assist with smoking cessation can be found in Table 1-23 (p. 28).

Chronic Obstructive Pulmonary Disease (COPD). Inflammatory mediators may account for the intra- and extrapulmonary complications observed in patients with COPD (Agostini, 2010; Maddali, 2008). Although simple optimization of COPD may not reduce the incidence of postoperative pulmonary complications, incentive spirometry with inspiratory muscle training and postoperative physiotherapy have been shown to reduce the frequency of complications (Agostini, 2010).

Obstructive Sleep Apnea (OSA). Obesity is a well-recognized risk factor for peri- and postoperative complications. In particular, unrecognized obstructive sleep apnea (OSA) has been associated with hypoxemia, myocardial infarction, unanticipated admission to an intensive care unit, and even sudden death (Adesanya, 2011; Liao, 2009). A few clinical questionnaires have been validated to assist with the outpatient screening of OSA. Chung and colleagues (2008) developed a brief yes/no questionnaire, known as the STOP-Bang survey, that reliably predicts postoperative respiratory complications. The mnemonic uses yes/no questions for STOP (snoring, tiredness, observed apnea, and elevated blood pressure) and Bang (BMI >35, age >50, neck circumference >40 cm, and male gender). A high-risk patient is defined as one who answers yes to three or more questions.

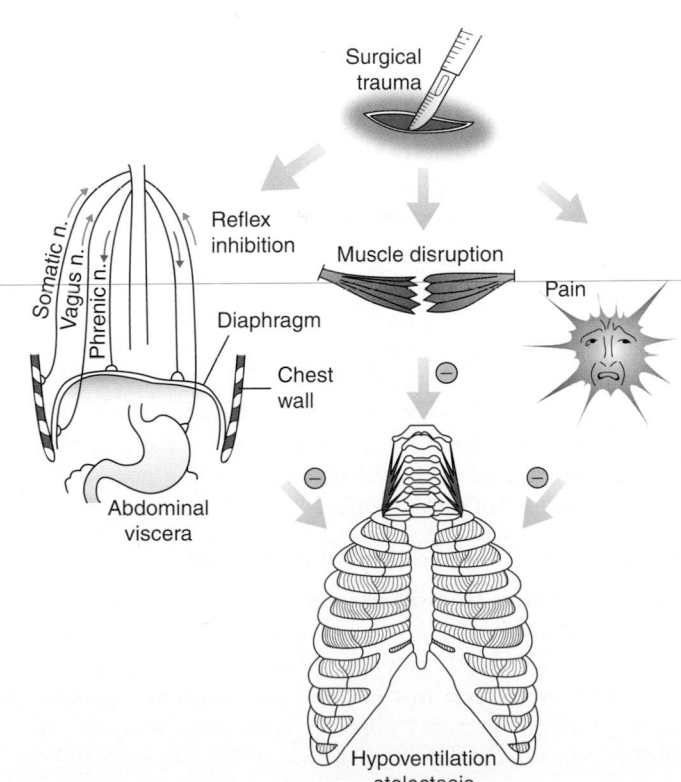

FIGURE 39-1 Surgical factors producing respiratory muscle dysfunction. These factors can reduce lung volumes and produce hypoventilation and atelectasis. *(From Warner, 2000, with permission.)*

Obesity. Decreases in chest wall compliance and in functional residual capacity predispose patients with a body mass index (BMI) ≥30 kg/m^2 to intra- and postoperative atelectasis (Agostini, 2010; Zerah, 1993). Eichenberger and colleagues (2002) observed that pulmonary changes in these patients may persist for more than 24 hours and require aggressive postoperative lung expansion modalities. Moreover, in obese patients undergoing laparoscopy, these pulmonary parameters are further compromised by increased intraabdominal pressures from pneumoperitoneum, as described in Chapter 42 (p. 1095).

Asthma. Well-controlled asthma is not a risk factor for postoperative pulmonary complications. Warner and coworkers (1996) reported that rates of bronchospasm were less than 2 percent in asthmatic patients.

American Society of Anesthesiologist (ASA) Classification. Although this classification was created to help predict perioperative mortality rates, it has also been shown to assess risks for cardiovascular and pulmonary complications (Wolters, 1996). Table 39-1 summarizes the American Society of Anesthesiologist (ASA) classification and associated rates of postoperative pulmonary complications (Qaseem, 2006).

History and Physical Examination

Elements in a pulmonary review of systems that may serve as harbingers of underlying disease include poor exercise tolerance, chronic cough, and otherwise unexplained dyspnea (Smetana, 1999). Physical examination findings of decreased breath sounds, dullness to percussion, rales, wheezes, rhonchi, and a prolonged expiratory phase may carry a nearly sixfold increase in pulmonary complications (Lawrence, 1996; Straus, 2000).

TABLE 39-1. American Society of Anesthesiologists (ASA) Classification

ASA Class	Class Definition	Rates of PPCs by Class (%)
I	Normally healthy patient	1.2
II	With mild systemic disease	5.4
III	With systemic disease that is not incapacitating	11.4
IV	With an incapacitating systemic disease that is a constant threat to life	10.9
V	Moribund patient who is not expected to survive for 24 hours with or without operation	NA

NA = not applicable; PPCs = postoperative pulmonary complications.
Modified from Qaseem, 2006, with permission.

Diagnostic Testing

Pulmonary Function Tests and Chest Radiography. In general, pulmonary function tests (PFTs) offer little information during preoperative pulmonary assessment of patients undergoing nonthoracic procedures. Outside of diagnosing COPD, PFTs are not superior to a through history and physical examination (Johnson, 2008; Lawrence, 1996; Qaseem, 2006). However, if the etiology of symptoms, such as exercise intolerance or dyspnea, remains unclear after clinical examination, then PFTs may provide information that will alter perioperative management.

Chest radiography is not routinely obtained to assist in perioperative management. Compared with a clinical history and physical examination, preoperative chest radiographs rarely provide evidence to modify therapy (Archer, 1993). Although not exhaustive, conditions for which radiography may be reasonable include acute or chronic cardiovascular or pulmonary disease, cancer, ASA status >3, heavy smoking, immunosuppression, history of recent chest radiation therapy, recent emigration from areas with endemic pulmonary disease, and recent symptoms suggestive of cardiopulmonary disease.

Biochemical Markers. The National Veterans Administration Surgical Quality Improvement Program reported that serum albumin levels less than 35 mg/dL were significantly associated with increased perioperative pulmonary morbidity and mortality rates (Arozullah, 2000; Lee, 2009). For each 1 mg/dL decrease in serum albumin concentration, the odds of mortality are increased by 137 percent and morbidity by 89 percent (Vincent, 2004). Serum albumin's association with morbidity and mortality may be due to comorbidity and thus is a marker of malnutrition and disease (Goldwasser, 1997). Although measurement of serum albumin is not routinely recommended for gynecologic procedures, the information may be predictive in the elderly or in those with multiple comorbidities. In addition, serum blood urea nitrogen (BUN) levels greater than 21 mg/dL similarly correlate with increased pulmonary-related morbidity and mortality rates, but not to the same degree as serum albumin levels.

More recently, there has been an interest in finding new markers of asthma and COPD. C-reactive protein (CRP) is an acute-phase reactant, and its levels rise dramatically during inflammation. In the future, CRP may allow clinicians to identify individuals with a low, medium, or high risk of developing COPD (Dahl, 2009). Until this marker is fully validated in a prospective manner, CRP measurement as a preoperative screening test is not recommended.

Prevention of Pulmonary Complications

Lung Expansion Modalities. Techniques aimed at reducing anticipated postoperative decreases in lung volumes can be simple and include deep breathing exercises, incentive spirometry, and early ambulation. In conscious and cooperative patients, deep breathing effectively improves lung compliance and gas distribution (Chumillas, 1998; Ferris, 1960; Thomas, 1994). With these exercises, a woman is asked to take five sequential deep breaths every hour while awake and hold each for 5 seconds. An incentive spirometer can be added to assist by providing direct visual feedback of her efforts. In addition to deep breathing, early ambulation can enhance lung expansion as well as provide some protection from venous thromboembolism. Meyers and associates (1975) demonstrated an increase in functional residual lung capacity of up to 20 percent by simply maintaining an upright posture. Alternatively, formal respiratory physiotherapy may include chest physical therapy in the form of percussion, clapping, or vibration; intermittent positive-pressure breathing (IPPB); and continuous positive-airway pressure (CPAP).

Prophylactic methods, whether simple or more formal, are all effective in preventing postoperative pulmonary morbidity, and no method is superior to another. Thomas and colleagues (1994) performed a metaanalysis to compare incentive spirometry (IS), IPPB, and deep-breathing exercises (DBE). In comparison with no therapy, IS and DBE are superior in preventing postoperative pulmonary complications, and greater than 50-percent reductions were observed. In addition, no significant differences were noted comparing IS to DBE, IS to IPPB, and DBE to IPPB (Thomas, 1994). However, chest physical therapy, IPPB, and CPAP are more expensive and labor intensive (Pasquina, 2006). Accordingly, these methods are typically reserved for patients who are unable to perform simpler effort-dependent therapies.

Nasogastric Decompression. Postoperatively, nasogastric tubes (NGTs) are often placed for gastric decompression. However, nasogastric intubation bypasses normal upper and lower respiratory tract mucosal defenses and exposes patients to risks for nosocomial sinusitis and pneumonia. Routine use of NGT after surgery is associated with increased cases of pneumonia, atelectasis, and aspiration compared with selective use (only in the case of symptomatic abdominal distension or significant postoperative nausea and vomiting) (Cheatham, 1995). Accordingly, the choice to implement this drainage method should be balanced against respiratory risks.

Cardiac Evaluation

Coronary heart disease is the leading cause of death in most industrialized countries and contributes significantly to perioperative mortality rates in patients undergoing cardiac and noncardiac surgery.

Risk Factors for Cardiac Complications

Valvular Heart Disease. Careful chest auscultation will reveal findings suspicious for native valvular lesions. Of the most commonly found defects, aortic stenosis carries the highest independent risk factor for perioperative complications (Kertai, 2004). For other lesions, the degree of heart failure and associated cardiac arrhythmias are the best indicators of risk. If cardiac sounds are suggestive of valvular disease, echocardiography will assist in defining the abnormality.

Guidelines for endocarditis prophylaxis during gastrointestinal (GI) or genitourinary (GU) procedures have changed. The transient enterococcal bacteremia caused by these procedures has not been irrefutably correlated to the development of infective endocarditis. Hence, antibiotic prophylaxis directed at preventing infective endocarditis after GI or GU tract procedures is no longer recommended by the American Heart Association (Wilson, 2007).

Heart Failure. In patients with a history of significant congestive heart failure, a cardiologist may employ strategies aimed at maximizing hemodynamic function, such as preoperative coronary revascularization or perioperative medical therapy (Fleisher, 2009). In addition, judicious use of diuretics will usually avoid intraoperative hypovolemia and related hypotension.

Arrhythmias. These are usually symptoms of underlying cardiopulmonary disease or electrolyte abnormalities. Accordingly, preoperative management should focus on correcting the primary process. However, if pacemakers and implantable cardioverter-defibrillators are required for arrhythmia treatment prior to surgery, they are typically placed for the same indications as in nonoperative circumstances (Gregoratos, 2002).

For those with pacemakers in place, electrosurgery can create electromagnetic interference even during noncardiac surgical and endoscopic procedures. Although encountered less frequently with newer devices, such interference can lead to pacing failure or complete system malfunction (Cheng, 2008). Thus, current guidelines recommend that all systems be evaluated by an appropriately trained physician before and after any invasive procedure (Fleisher, 2009). In addition, as discussed in Chapter 40 (p. 1001), intraoperative efforts by the surgeon should minimize the chance for electromagnetic interference by using bipolar electrosurgery if possible, by using short intermittent bursts of electrosurgical energy at the lowest possible energy levels, by maximizing the distance between the electrosurgical tool and the cardiac device, and by placing the grounding pad in a position to minimize current flow toward the device.

Hypertension. Except in the setting of systolic blood pressures >180 mm Hg and diastolic blood pressures >110 mm Hg, hypertension is not predictive of perioperative cardiac events and should not postpone surgical intervention (Casadei, 2005; Goldman, 1979; Weksler, 2003). If possible, to lower postoperative cardiac complications related to hypertension, blood pressure should be lowered several months prior to an anticipated procedure (Fleisher, 2002). Preoperatively, patients on angiotensin-converting enzyme inhibitors and angiotensin-receptor antagonists should have their morning dose held to reduce the risk of immediate postinduction hypotension (Comfere, 2005). In all patients with hypertension, avoiding hypo- or hypertension intraoperatively with careful postoperative monitoring is recommended. Importantly, intravascular volume expansion, pain, and agitation may exacerbate postoperative hypertension.

Diagnostic Testing and Algorithm

Preoperative guidelines have been developed by several groups to help predict the risk of perioperative cardiac complications. The three most prominent lists used in clinical practice are: (1) those jointly developed by the American College of Cardiology and the American Heart Association (ACC/AHA), (2) guidelines published by the American College of Physicians (ACP), and (3) the Revised Cardiac Risk Index (RCRI) (American College of Physicians, 1997; Fleisher, 2009; Lee,

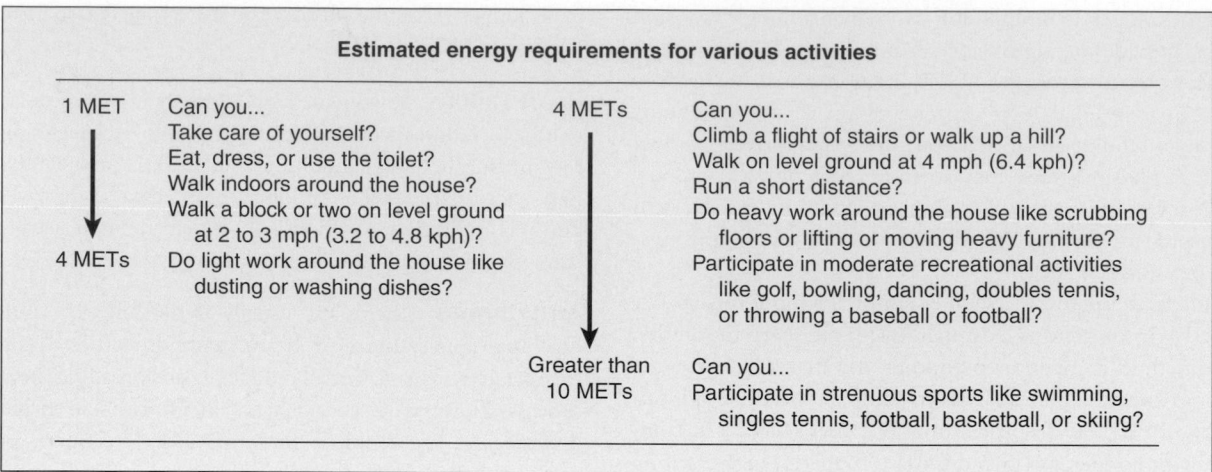

FIGURE 39-2 Questions used to assess functional capacity. METs are used in Figure 39-3. kph = kilometers per hour; MET = metabolic equivalent; mph = miles per hour. *(Modified from Hlatky, 1989, with permission; adapted from Fleisher, 2009, with permission.)*

1999). Each defines major and minor clinical predictors to help guide decision making and specific recommendations.

American College of Cardiology and the American Heart Association Guidelines.

First published in 1996 and last updated in 2009, the ACC/AHA guidelines represent an extensive review of the literature by 12 committee members from various areas of cardiovascular care (Fleisher, 2009). This stepwise strategy centers on assessment of three major considerations—clinical predictors, functional capacity, and surgery-specific risk—to ascertain who is a candidate for cardiac testing (Figs. 39-2 and 39-3). In general, for gynecologic surgery, cardiac complication risks are greatest with major emergency procedures and operations associated with large intravascular fluid shifts. In contrast, lowest risks are found with brief endoscopic procedures.

Revised Cardiac Risk Index (RCRI).

The Revised Cardiac Risk Index is an easy assessment of clinical predictors. It has been tested extensively and offers accurate estimates of cardiac risk (Lee, 1999). The major difference between the RCRI and the ACC/AHA guidelines is the incorporation of exercise capacity in the ACC/AHA tool. Creators of the RCRI suggest that cardiac risk may be overestimated by a patient's noncardiac limitations in exercise function, such as musculoskeletal pain. Thus, these investigators place greater emphasis on cardiac and vascular disease markers.

Prevention Strategies

Perioperative Beta-Blockers.

Lindenauer and associates (2005) retrospectively assessed the impact of perioperative beta-blocker use and its affect on in-hospital mortality rates. In patients with an RCRI of 2 or more, mortality rates were significantly reduced among those undergoing major noncardiac procedures who were given beta-blockers perioperatively. More recently, the Perioperative Ischemic Evaluation (POISE) trial found lower risks for cardiac events (such as ischemia) but an overall higher risk of stroke and noncardiac-related mortality if beta-blockers are used preoperatively (POISE Study Group, 2008). Hence, the use of beta-blockers should be restricted to those patients who are

already taking these or who are identified preoperatively to be candidates for lifelong use (Auerbach, 2008).

Coronary Revascularization.

Diagnostic cardiac catheterization should be considered in high-risk cardiac patients if noninvasive stress testing suggests advanced disease. In such cases, revascularization through coronary artery bypass grafting or percutaneous angioplasty offers comparable benefits perioperatively (Hassan, 2001).

Anemia and Cardiac Risk.

Anemia has been shown to be an independent risk factor for congestive heart failure (Kannel, 1987). A study by Silverberg and associates (2001) found that correction of even mild anemia offered significant improvements in cardiac function. Iron therapy is not a substitution for appropriate cardiac disease treatment, but extrapolated data suggest that maintaining a hemoglobin level above 10 percent is important and reduces perioperative morbidity and mortality rates for those with cardiac disease.

Hepatic Evaluation

The liver plays a central role in drug metabolism; synthesis of proteins, glucose, and coagulation factors; and excretion of endogenous compounds. In patients with suspected hepatic disease, inquiry should include family histories of jaundice or anemia, recent travel history, exposure to alcohol or other hepatotoxins, and medication use (Suman, 2006). Physical findings suggestive of underlying liver disease include jaundice, scleral icterus, spider angiomas, ascites, hepatomegaly, asterixis, and cachexia.

Of liver diseases, acute and chronic hepatitis are commonly encountered. With acute hepatitis, regardless the cause, high associated perioperative mortality rates have been documented by multiple investigators. For this reason, primary management involves supportive care and delay of elective surgical intervention until the acute process has subsided (Patel, 1999). In those with chronic hepatitis, variable levels of hepatic dysfunction are found. Compensated disease carries a low risk of perioperative complications (Sirinek, 1987).

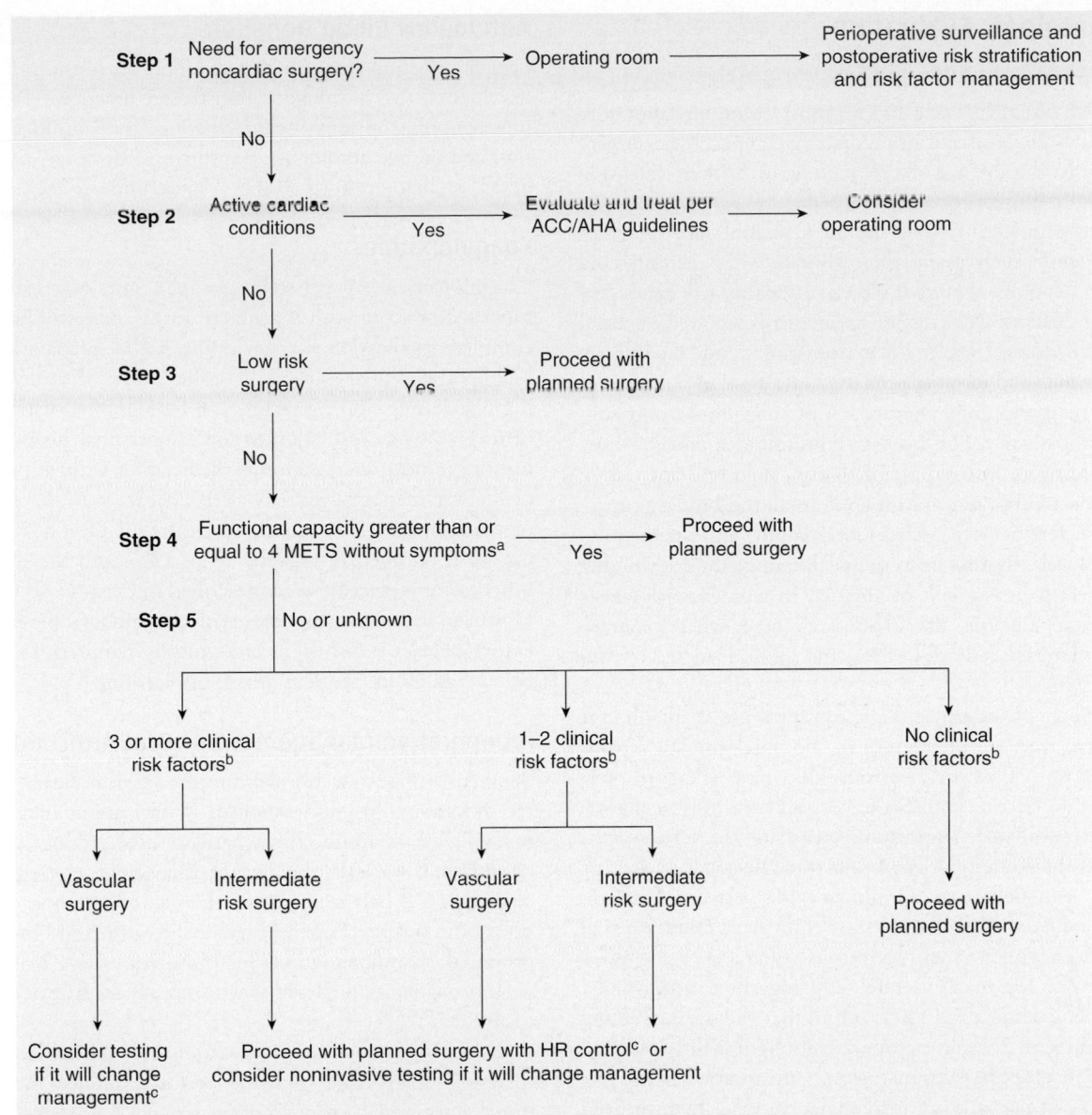

FIGURE 39-3 Cardiac Evaluation and Care Algorithm for Noncardiac Surgery. ACC/AHA = American College of Cardiology/American Heart Association; MET = metabolic equivalent. *(From Fleisher, 2009, with permission.)*
[a]See Figure 39-2 for MET assessment.
[b]Ischemic heart disease, compensated/prior heart failure, diabetes mellitus, renal insufficiency, cerebrovascular disease.
[c]Consider perioperative beta blockade for appropriate individuals (p. 952).

If underlying liver disease is known or suspected, hepatic function should be assessed. In addition to liver function tests, prothrombin time (PT), partial thromboplastin time (PTT), serum albumin level, and a serum chemistry panel are valuable adjuncts.

The Child-Pugh score is a useful tool to predict perioperative survival rates in patients with cirrhosis undergoing abdominal surgery. The risk of mortality based on Child-Pugh class is as follows: class A—10 percent; class B—30 percent; class C—70 percent (Mansour, 1997).

■ Renal Evaluation

The kidney is involved with excretion of metabolic waste, hematologic processes, and fluid and electrolyte balance.

Accordingly, patients with known renal insufficiency should have a serum chemistry panel and complete blood count (CBC) evaluated prior to surgery. Chronic anemia due to renal insufficiency will typically require preoperative administration of erythropoietin or perioperative transfusion depending on the procedure planned and degree of anemia. Dialysis patients require intensive pre- and postoperative surveillance for signs of electrolyte abnormalities and fluid overload. Ideally, these patients' volume status and electrolytes (potassium in particular) can be optimized by performing dialysis the day prior to surgery. Additionally, further renal insult is averted by avoiding nephrotoxic agents. Pharmacokinetic consultation may be warranted to adjust other medication dosages, as serum levels in these patients may be unpredictable postoperatively.

Hematologic Evaluation

Anemia

Preoperative anemia is one of the most common laboratory abnormalities encountered in preoperative gynecologic surgery evaluation. In the absence of a clear etiology, further evaluation is necessary to correct reversible causes.

The preoperative interview should focus on signs of symptomatic anemia such as fatigue, dyspnea with exertion, and palpitations. Inquiry should also seek to identify risk factors for underlying cardiovascular disease as anemia is less well tolerated in these individuals. The physical examination should incorporate thorough pelvic and rectal examination and stool guaiac testing.

For women with mild anemia, a CBC may be the only suggested diagnostic test. For those with profound anemia or those not responding to iron supplementation, then relevant testing may include a CBC, serum iron level, total iron binding capacity (TIBC), ferritin level, reticulocyte count, and vitamin B_{12} and folate levels. Results from these laboratory studies will dictate preoperative treatment of anemia. In women with classic iron deficiency anemia, the TIBC is elevated, whereas hemoglobin, hematocrit, red cell indices, and serum iron and ferritin levels are depressed.

A number of pharmacologic options are available for preoperative iron supplementation. For oral intake, ferrous sulfate (Feosol, Slow Fe), ferrous gluconate (Fergon), ferrous fumarate (Ircon, Fero-Sequels), and iron polysaccharide (Ferrex) are available. Importantly, each of the ferrous salts has a different content of *elemental iron*. In general, therapy to correct iron deficiency should provide between 150 and 200 mg elemental iron daily. Thus, equivalent common oral replacement regimens include ferrous sulfate, 325 mg three times daily or ferrous fumarate, 200 mg three times daily. Okuyama and associates (2005) found that the use of 200 mg of elemental iron 2 weeks preoperatively significantly reduced a need for intraoperative transfusion. Constipation is the primary source of preparation intolerance and can be improved with dietary changes, bulk laxatives, and stool softeners.

In addition to oral forms, there are five U.S. Food and Drug Administration (FDA)-approved intravenous (IV) iron preparations currently available. The newer preparations have a much lower risk of anaphylactic reactions and are considered safe (Shander, 2010). The hemoglobin effects can be seen as quickly as 1 week after the first dose. For most women, iron therapy administered orally is effective to correct anemia. However, these IV forms may be most appropriate for women with poor absorption secondary to gastrointestinal disease, those with chronic renal disease, or those with an intolerance or lack of response to oral iron.

The perioperative decision to transfuse a patient depends in part on a patient's cardiac status. If significant cardiac disease is absent and significant ongoing blood loss is not anticipated, then an otherwise healthy woman can tolerate a postoperative hemoglobin level as low as 6 to 7 g/dL (Simon, 1998). Conversely, transfusions should be considered if hypotension and tachycardia fail to respond to crystalloid or colloid volume expansion (Chap. 40, p. 1007).

Autologous Blood Donation

Fear of infection from allogeneic blood transfusions has led to development of autologous transfusion practices. Two of the most popular options include preoperative autologous donation and salvage autologous transfusions. Both are discussed in detail in Chapter 40 (p. 1002) (Vanderlinde, 2002).

Coagulopathies

Coagulopathies are generally grouped into two categories—inherited or acquired. Of acquired forms, a careful history and complete medication list, including herbal preparations, may highlight potential causes. In either form, disorders involving platelets or clotting factors can be identified with a careful history and physical examination. A personal history of easy bruising, unexpected amounts of bleeding with minor injury, or lifelong menorrhagia may alert a clinician to the possibility of coagulopathy. Screening and treatment of von Willebrand disease is outlined in Chapter 8 (p. 235), and the specifics of other factor replacement are described in Chapter 40 (p. 1010). However, in general, for those with thrombocytopenia, perioperative platelet transfusions are typically required if counts are below 50,000 in a patient at risk of bleeding.

Preoperative Management of Oral Anticoagulation

Women with atrial fibrillation, mechanical heart valve, or recent venous thromboembolism (VTE) are at increased risk for VTE. As a result, these patients are typically prescribed chronic oral warfarin therapy. In this group, a need for anticoagulation is balanced against the risk of bleeding complications from surgery. For these reasons, Kearon and Hirsh (1997) proposed recommendations for the preoperative management of anticoagulants in patients who use these drugs chronically (Table 39-2).

Following temporarily cessation of oral anticoagulation therapy, surgery can safely be performed once the international normalized ratio (INR) reaches 1.5 (Douketis, 2008; Tinker, 1978; White, 1995). If an INR is between 2.0 and 3.0, approximately 5 to 6 days are required for this ratio to reach 1.5. If more rapid reversal of warfarin anticoagulation is needed (within 18 to 24 hours), then 2.5 to 5 mg of vitamin K can be administered by slow intravenous infusion. If emergent reversal (within 12 hours) is required, then vitamin K infusion is augmented with administration of fresh frozen plasma, with prothrombin complex concentrate, or with factor VIIa (Douketis, 2008).

After postoperative reinstitution of anticoagulation, approximately 3 days are required to reach therapeutic levels (Harrison, 1997; White, 1995). Importantly, postoperative heparin should not be restarted until at least 12 hours after major surgery and longer if there is evidence of bleeding. An example of an anticoagulation bridging protocol is given on Table 39-3.

In patients who are on anticoagulants following a VTE, the timing of surgery can often lower the risk of postoperative VTE. After an acute VTE, the recurrence risk without anticoagulation is between 40 and 50 percent. However, the risk of recurrent disease drops significantly after 3 months of

TABLE 39-2. Recommendations for Preoperative and Postoperative Anticoagulation in Patients Who Are Taking Oral Anticoagulants[a]

Indication	Before Surgery	After Surgery
Acute venous thromboembolism		
Month 1	IV heparin[b]	IV heparin[b]
Months 2 and 3	No change[c]	IV heparin
Recurrent venous thromboembolism[d]	No change[c]	SC heparin
Acute arterial embolism		
Month 1	IV heparin	IV heparin[e]
Mechanical heart valve	No change[c]	SC heparin
Nonvalvular atrial fibrillation	No change[c]	SC heparin

[a]IV heparin denotes intravenous heparin at therapeutic doses, and SC heparin denotes subcutaneous unfractionated or low-molecular-weight heparin in doses recommended for prophylaxis against venous thromboembolism in high-risk patients.
[b]A vena caval filter should be considered if acute venous thromboembolism has occurred within 2 weeks or if the risk of bleeding during intravenous heparin therapy is high.
[c]If patients are hospitalized, subcutaneous heparin may be administered, but hospitalization is not recommended solely for this purpose.
[d]The term refers to patients whose last episode of venous thromboembolism occurred more than 3 months before evaluation but who require long-term anticoagulation because of a high risk of recurrence.
[e]Intravenous heparin should be used after surgery only if the risk of bleeding is low.
From Kearon, 1997, with permission.

TABLE 39-3. Anticoagulation Bridging Protocol

7 days prior to surgery	Stop aspirin or other antiplatelets (clopidogrel, ticlopidine, etc.)
5–6 days prior to surgery	Stop warfarin
24 to 48 hours after stopping warfarin	Check INR
3–4 days prior to surgery or when INR is subtherapeutic	Start enoxaparin or UFH at appropriate dose
1 day prior to surgery	Give last preop enoxaparin dose 12–24 (24 hours for 1.5 mg/kg enoxaparin dose) hours prior to surgery (patients with morning surgeries will need to hold their evening dose the night before), or stop UFH at least 6 hours prior to surgery. INR should be checked to determine if vitamin K will need to be given.
Surgery day	INR should be rechecked if it was above surgery goal the day prior. Start warfarin on POD 0.
1 day after surgery	Start enoxaparin or UFH dosing 12–24 hours after surgery, if bleeding risk is low.
5–6 days after surgery	Stop enoxaparin or UFH after INR is >2 for 2 days.

INR = international normalized ratio; UFH = unfractionated heparin; POD = postoperative day.
From Dunn, 2007.

warfarin therapy (Coon, 1973; Kearon, 1997; Levine, 1995). Specifically, a delay in surgery and continued warfarin therapy for an additional 2 to 3 months drops the recurrence risk to 5 to 10 percent and avoids a need for preoperative heparin (Kearon, 1997; Levine, 1995). Thus, in those with recent VTE, a surgical delay, if feasible, may be advantageous and should be considered.

■ Endocrine Evaluation

The pathophysiologic stress of surgery can exacerbate endocrine conditions such as thyroid dysfunction, diabetes mellitus, and adrenal insufficiency.

Hyperthyroidism and Hypothyroidism

Both hyper- and hypothyroidism have anesthetic and metabolic derangements unique to each disease state. Nevertheless, the management goal for both aims to achieve a euthyroid state before surgery.

Hyperthyroidism carries the risk of developing thyroid storm perioperatively. Moreover, airway compromise is a risk in those with a large goiter. Thus, during physical examination, special attention should be given to evaluating for tracheal deviation. In addition to thyroid function tests, an electrocardiogram (EKG) and serum electrolyte levels can help predict signs of preexisting metabolic stress. Patients should be encouraged to maintain their usual medications at prescribed dosages until the day of surgery.

Newly diagnosed hypothyroidism generally does not require preoperative therapy except in cases of severe disease with signs of cardiac depression, electrolyte irregularities, and hypoglycemia.

Diabetes Mellitus

Long-term complications of diabetes mellitus may include vascular, neurologic, cardiac, and renal dysfunction. Thus, a vigilant preoperative risk assessment of these comorbidi-ties in patients with diabetes mellitus is essential. In addition, increased postoperative morbidity rates have been linked with poor preoperative glycemic control. Specifically, glucose levels >200 mg/dL and hemoglobin A_{1C} levels >7 are both associated with significantly increased rates of postoperative wound infection (Dronge, 2006; Trick, 2000).

At minimum, diabetic patients undergoing major surgical procedures would benefit from three diagnostic tests—serum electrolyte levels, urinalysis, and an EKG. These screen for metabolic disturbances, undiagnosed nephropathy, and unrecognized cardiac ischemia in the form of abnormal Q waves, respectively.

In general, stress induced by surgery and anesthesia can lead to elevations in catecholamine levels, relative insulin deficiency, and hyperglycemia (Devereaux, 2005). Although glycemic responses may vary with surgery, overt hyperglycemia should be avoided to minimize postoperative complications related to dehydration, electrolyte abnormalities, diminished wound healing, and even ketoacidosis in type 1 diabetics (Jacober, 1999). However, fluctuations in oral intake and metabolic needs make optimal glycemic control labor intensive. Moreover, clear evidence for glucose targets are lacking. As a result, most providers aim for glucose readings below 200 g/dL (Table 39-4) (Finney, 2003; Garber, 2004; Hoogwerf 2006). Table 39-5 and Figure 39-4 summarize perioperative recommendations set forth by Jacober and coworkers (1999) based on disease severity.

Adrenal Insufficiency

Inadequacy of the hypothalamic-pituitary-adrenal (HPA) axis due to secondary suppression from chronic steroid use can lead to perioperative hypotension. Despite this physiologic understanding, controversy surrounds perioperative corticosteroid supplementation.

Corticosteroid users who undergo minor surgical procedures or who use lower doses are generally assumed not to be at risk for adrenal suppression, and additional corticosteroid therapy is not recommended. Lower doses are considered less than 5 mg of prednisone per day for no more than 2 weeks within the

TABLE 39-4. Sliding-Scale Insulin Order Example[a]

Blood Glucose, mmol/L (mg/dL)[b]	Increment Formula	Calculation	Short-Acting Insulin, units
0–11.0 (0-200)	0	0	0
11.1–14.0 (201–250)	1 × (TDI/30)	1 × (120/30)	4
14.1–17.0 (251–300)	2 × (TDI/30)	2 × (120/30)	4
17.1–20.0 (301–350)	3 × (TDI/30)	3 × (120/30)	12
20.1–23.0 (251–400)	4 × (TDI/30)	1 × (120/30)	16
23.1–26.0 (401–450)	5 × (TDI/30)	5 × (120/30)	20
>26.0 (>450)	Call physician	Call physician	Call physician

[a]Example uses a preoperative total daily insulin dose (TDI) of 120 units.
[b]For convenience, conversions of millimoles per liter to milligrams per deciliter are approximate.
From Jacober, 1999, with permission.

TABLE 39-5. Perioperative Management of Diabetes Mellitus by Disease Type

Disease	Preoperative Management	Postoperative Management
Type 2 DM treated with diet alone	No additional care with PRN subcutaneous regular insulin for AM hyperglycemia	PRN subcutaneous regular insulin
Type 2 DM treated with oral hypoglycemic agents	Discontinue all agents on the day of surgery	Supplemental subcutaneous insulin until return of normal diet, at which time preoperative therapy can be reinstituted
Type 1 or 2 DM treated with insulin	See Figure 39-4	Sliding-scale insulin (Table 39-4)

DM = diabetes mellitus; PRN = as needed.
Adapted from Jacober, 1999.

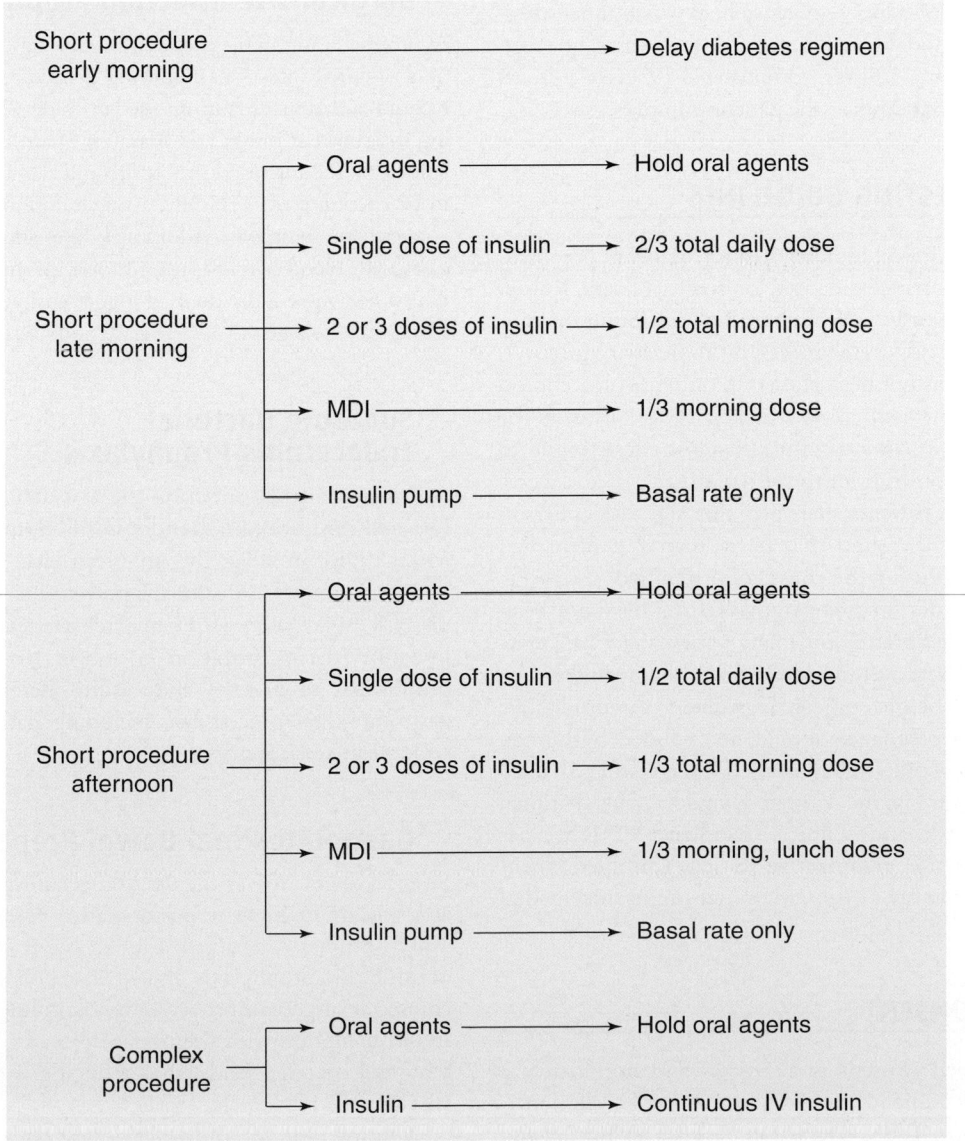

FIGURE 39-4 Perioperative management recommendations for surgical patients with diabetes mellitus. IV = Intravenous; MDI = multiple doses of short-acting insulin. *(From Jacober, 1999, with permission.)*

past year. However, those taking 5 to 20 mg of prednisone per day for more than 3 weeks may be at risk for HPA-axis suppression. In these patients, an adrenocorticotropic hormone (ACTH) stimulation test can verify adrenal suppression and identify those who may benefit from perioperative corticosteroid supplementation.

The value of perioperative supplementation remains an area of chronic debate (Bromberg, 1991; Marik, 2008). For example, patients who took at least 7.5 mg of prednisone daily for several months and who had secondary adrenal insufficiency documented by ACTH testing were randomized to placebo versus high-dose cortisol supplementation. Simply continuing the patient's usual daily dose of corticosteroids perioperatively resulted in no increased rates of hypotension or other perioperative signs of adrenal insufficiency (Glowniak, 1997). Marik and Varon (2008) performed a systematic review of the literature regarding perioperative supplemental doses of corticosteroids and ultimately found no evidence to support additional supratherapeutic doses as long as patients continued to receive their usual daily dose. Close hemodynamic monitoring should be performed to look for volume-refractory hypotension, at which time, stress-dose corticosteroids should be initiated. For these cases, one regimen is hydrocortisone, 100 mg administered IV every 8 hours and titrated to reduced doses as the patient improves.

DIAGNOSTIC TESTING GUIDELINES

In the absence of a clinical indication, a rote panel of preoperative tests does not enhance the safety or quality of care. Roizen (2000) noted that nearly half of abnormalities found on routine preoperative testing were ignored by clinicians. Moreover, diagnostic testing has not been shown to outperform a clinical history and physical examination (Rucker, 1983). Thus, in the absence of changes in clinical status, diagnostic tests found to be normal 4 to 6 months prior to surgery may be used as "preoperative tests." In patients managed this way, Macpherson and coworkers (1990) found that fewer than 2 percent had significant changes during the course of 4 months.

Codified guidelines for preoperative testing have not been crafted in the United States. For many patients, a CBC, electrolyte panel, BUN/creatinine levels, and blood glucose are frequently ordered before surgery. In women of reproductive age with a uterus, pregnancy should be excluded by human chorionic gonadotropin (hCG) assay. Other testing is individualized. However, in the United Kingdom, the National Institute for Health and Clinical Excellence (NICE) has specific indications for preoperative testing. Complete documents are available at: http://www.nice.org.uk/nicemedia/live/10920/29094/29094.pdf.

INFORMED CONSENT

Obtaining informed consent is a process and not merely a medical record document (Kondziolka, 2006; Lavelle-Jones, 1993; Nandi, 2000). This conversation between a clinician and patient should enhance a woman's awareness of her diagnosis and contain a discussion of medical and surgical care alternatives, procedure goals and limitations, and surgical risks. When informed consent cannot be obtained from the patient, an independent surrogate should be identified to represent the patient's best interest and wishes. Written documentation serves as a historical record of a patient's understanding and agreement.

Despite a clinician's recommendations, an informed patient may decline a particular intervention. A woman's decision-making autonomy must be respected, and a clinician should document informed refusal in the medical record. Appropriate documentation should include: (1) a patient's refusal to consent to the recommended intervention, (2) notation that the value of the intervention has been explained to the patient, (3) a patient's reasons for refusal, and (4) a statement describing the health consequences as described to the patient (American College of Obstetricians and Gynecologists, 2009b).

SPECIAL CONSIDERATIONS

Surgical Site Infection Prophylaxis

Appropriate antibiotic prophylaxis can significantly reduce hospital-acquired infections following gynecologic surgery. Selection recommendations are summarized in Table 39-6. Decisions regarding the choice, timing, and duration of antibiotic prophylaxis are guided by the intended procedure and the anticipated organisms to be encountered. Typically, a single dose of antibiotics is given at anesthesia induction. Additional doses should be considered in cases with blood loss >1500 mL or with duration longer than 3 hours. For obese individuals, a higher antibiotic dose is suggested (American College of Obstetricians and Gynecologists, 2009a).

Subacute Bacterial Endocarditis Prophylaxis

Sufficient evidence supports the association between bacteremia and postprocedural endocarditis (Durack, 1995; van der Meer, 1992). In 2007, the American Heart Association revised their recommendations for the prevention of infective endocarditis (Wilson, 2007). After an extensive review of the pertinent literature, the organization no longer recommends antibiotic prophylaxis to prevent endocarditis before genitourinary or gastrointestinal procedures, including patients with infective endocarditis risk factors.

Gastrointestinal Bowel Preparation

Surgical dogma drives the use of mechanical bowel preparation as a means to prevent postoperative complications (Bucher, 2004). Studies conducted prior to the routine administration of antibiotic prophylaxis argued that bowel cleansing prior to colorectal surgery improved bowel handling, prevented anastomosis disruption with the passage of hard feces, and decreased fecal and bacterial loads, thus reducing wound infection rates (Barker, 1971; Nichols, 1971).

Multiple studies, however, question the routine use of mechanical bowel preparations (Duncan, 2009; Platell, 1998).

TABLE 39-6. Antimicrobial Prophylactic Regimens by Procedure[a]

Procedure	Antibiotic	Dose (single dose)
Hysterectomy Urogynecology procedures, including those involving mesh	Cefazolin[b]	1 g or 2 g[c] IV
	Clindamycin[d] ***plus*** Gentamicin ***or*** Quinolone[e] ***or*** Aztreonam	600 mg IV 1.5 mg/kg IV 400 mg IV 1 g IV
	Metronidazole[d] ***plus*** Gentamicin ***or*** Quinolone[e]	500 mg IV 1.5 mg/kg IV 400 mg IV
Laparoscopy: diagnostic, operative, or tubal sterilization	None	
Laparotomy	None	
Hysteroscopy: diagnostic, operative, endometrial ablation, or Essure	None	
Hysterosalpingogram or chromotubation	Doxycycline[f]	100 mg orally, twice daily for 5 days
IUD insertion	None	
Endometrial biopsy	None	
Induced abortion/dilatation and evacuation	Doxycycline Metronidazole	100 mg orally 1 hour before procedure and 200 mg orally after procedure 500 mg orally twice daily for 5 days
Urodynamics	None	

[a]A convenient time to administer antibiotic prophylaxis is just before induction of anesthesia.
[b]Acceptable alternatives include cefotetan, cefoxitin, cefuroxime, or ampicillin-sulbactam.
[c]A 2-g dose is recommended in women with a body mass index >35 or weight >100 kg or 220 lb.
[d]Antimicrobial agents of choice in women with a history of immediate hypersensitivity to penicillin.
[e]Ciprofloxacin or levofloxacin or moxifloxacin.
[f]If patient has a history of pelvic inflammatory disease or procedure demonstrates dilated fallopian tubes.
No prophylaxis is indicated for a study without dilated tubes.
IV = intravenously; IUD = intrauterine device.
From American College of Obstetricians and Gynecologists, 2009a, with permission.

Guenaga and coworkers (2009) performed a metaanalysis of trials to determine the effectiveness of mechanical bowel preparation on morbidity and mortality rates in colorectal surgery. They found no evidence to support the perceived benefit from mechanical bowel preparation. Similar results have been found following gynecologic and urologic procedures (Muzii, 2006; Shafii, 2002). Moreover, another report contradicts the belief that mechanical bowel preparation decreases microbial contamination of the peritoneal cavity and subcutis after elective open colon surgery (Fa-Si-Oen, 2005).

Although its routine use should be limited, mechanical bowel preparation is often preferred for many advanced laparoscopic procedures and for female pelvic reconstructive procedures involving the posterior vaginal wall and anal sphincter. In these cases, evacuation of rectal stool provides additional operating space and undistorted anatomy. Moreover, following sphincteroplasty, preoperative evacuation typically delays stooling and allows initial healing. Other instances in which mechanical bowel preparation may be recommended include those in which the entire colon may be palpated during surgery for evaluation of tumor involvement. Table 39-7 provides a summary of various commercially available agents commonly used for bowel preparation (Valantas, 2004).

TABLE 39-7. Colon Cleansing Preparation Methods

Diet and Cathartics

Diet	Clear liquids for 3 days or a diet designed to leave a minimal colonic fecal residue for 1–3 days
Cathartics	Extract of senna fruit (X-Prep) 240 mL or magnesium citrate 240 mL
Other cathartic	Bisacodyl 20 mg orally and suppositories
Enemas	Sodium phosphate or tap water
Kits	Liqui Prep, LoSo Prep System, Nutra Prep

Gut Lavage Methods

Polyethylene glycol–electrolyte lavage solution (PEG-ELS)

Sodium sulfate and polyethylene glycol (PEG)
    GoLYTELY, CoLyte

Sulfate-free–electrolyte lavage solution (SF-ELS)

PEG without sulfate
    NuLYTELY

Reduced volume with bisacodyl or magnesium citrate
    Half Lytely

Phosphate preps
    Oral sodium phosphate
    Fleet's Phosphosoda
    Phosphate tablets
    Visicol

From Valantas, 2004, with permission.

TABLE 39-8. Risk Factors for Venous Thromboembolism

Surgery
Trauma (major trauma or lower-extremity injury)
Immobility, lower-extremity paresis
Cancer (active or occult)
Cancer therapy (hormonal, chemotherapy, angiogenesis inhibitors, radiotherapy)
Venous compression (tumor, hematoma, arterial abnormality)
Previous venous thromboembolism
Increasing age
Pregnancy and the postpartum period
Estrogen-containing oral contraceptives or hormone replacement therapy
Controlled ovarian hyperstimulation for fertility
Selective estrogen-receptor modulators
Erythropoiesis-stimulating agents
Acute medical illness
Inflammatory bowel disease
Nephrotic syndrome
Myeloproliferative disorders
Paroxysmal nocturnal hemoglobinuria
Obesity
Central venous catheterization
Inherited or acquired thrombophilia

Adapted from Geerts, 2008, with permission.

Along the lines of GI preparation, the widely accepted dogma that patients should remain without oral intake beginning at midnight prior to the procedure has been challenged. The European Society of Anaesthesiology reviewed the literature and updated their guidelines. They now recommend that solid foods should be avoided for 6 hours prior to elective surgery but that adults and children should be encouraged to drink clear fluids (water, pulp-free juice) up to 2 hours before all elective surgical procedures, including cesarean delivery (Smith, 2011). The systematic review also validated the safety of carbohydrate-rich drinks up to 2 hours prior to elective surgery in all patients, including diabetics. The use of preoperative oral carbohydrates was found to shift the body's metabolism from a fasting to a fed state, thus reducing postoperative insulin resistance and resulting hyperglycemia. However, guidelines in the United States have not been similarly modified.

Thromboembolism Prevention

Prophylaxis against venous thromboembolism (VTE) ranks in the top 10 patient safety practices recommended by the Agency for Healthcare Research and Quality (AHRQ) and the National Quality Forum (Kaafarani, 2011). In the United States alone, the annual incidence of deep-vein thrombosis (DVT) and pulmonary thromboembolism is estimated to approach 600,000, with more than 100,000 deaths each year (U.S. Department of Health and Human Services, 2008). National recommendations for prophylaxis against VTE follow a risk-based approach. Geerts and associates (2008) provide a summary of relevant VTE risk factors (Table 39-8).

Thrombophilias

Of these VTE risk factors, thrombophilias are inherited or acquired deficiencies of inhibitory proteins in the coagulation cascade. These can lead to hypercoagulability and recurrent venous thromboembolism.

Guidelines that direct selection of patients for thrombophilia testing are lacking in the United States, although a UK-based guideline group has published recommendations (Baglin, 2010). In general, indiscriminate testing for heritable thrombophilias in unselected patients presenting with a first episode of venous thrombosis is not indicated. Selected candidates for testing, among others, may include those with unprovoked venous thrombosis at an early age (<50 years), those from thrombosis-prone families, those with recurrent VTE, or those with VTE despite adequate anticoagulation.

Antithrombin Deficiency. Thrombin is produced by the enzymatic cleavage of prothrombin (Fig. 39-5). Thrombin

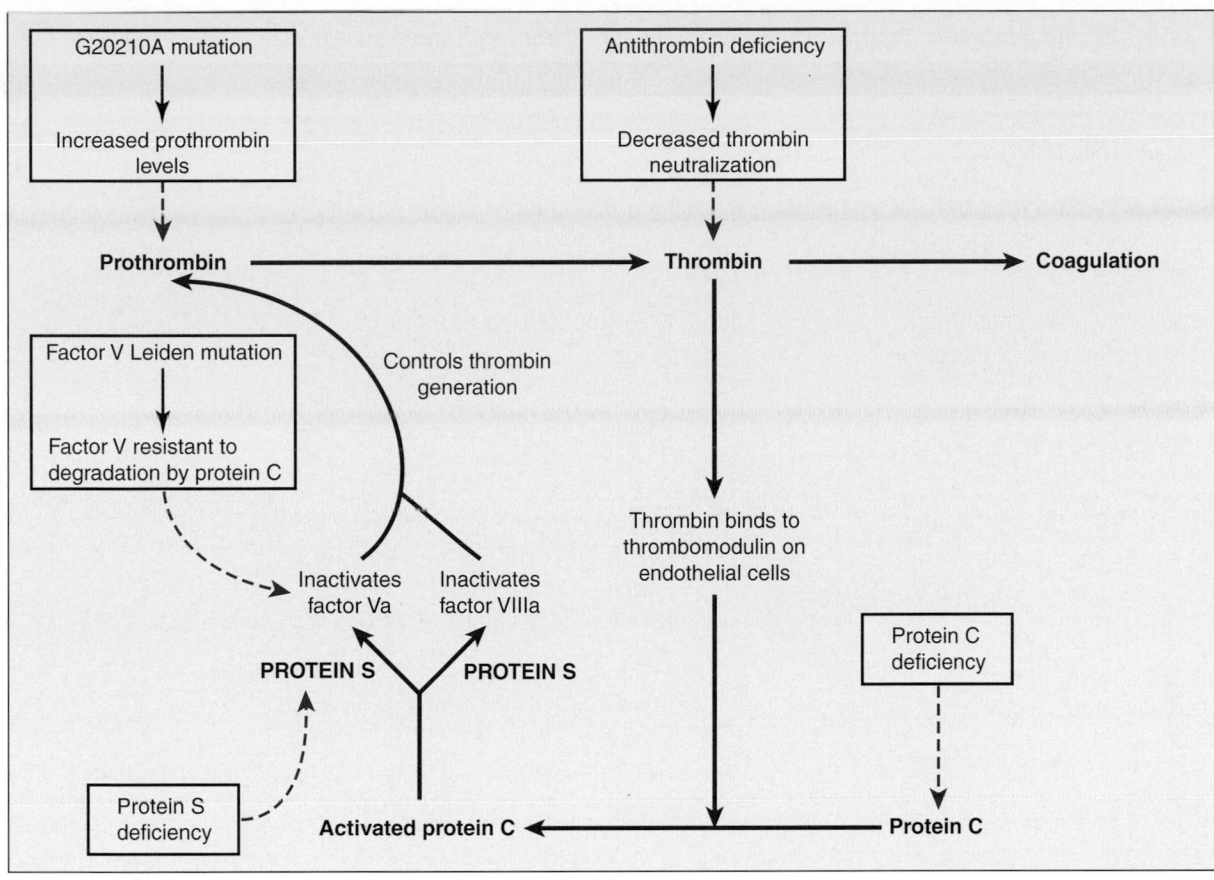

FIGURE 39-5 Points of the coagulation cascade affected by some of the thrombophilias. *(From Cunningham, 2010, with permission).*

converts fibrinogen to an active form that assembles into fibrin for clot formation. Antithrombin, previously known as antithrombin III, is one of the most important inhibitors of thrombin. Antithrombin functions as a natural anticoagulant by binding to and inactivating thrombin as well as the activated coagulation factors IXa, Xa, XIa, and XIIa. If thrombin is not inactivated, then coagulation is favored. Although rare, this deficiency is the most thrombogenic of the heritable coagulopathies.

Protein C or Protein S Deficiency. When thrombin is bound to thrombomodulin on the intact endothelium of small vessels, its procoagulant activities are neutralized. In this bound state, thrombin also activates protein C, a natural anticoagulant. Protein C and its cofactor, protein S, limit coagulation, in part, by inactivating factors Va and VIIIa.

Activated Protein C Resistance (Factor V Leiden Mutation). This is the most prevalent of the known thrombophilias and is caused by a single mutation in the factor V gene. The mutation conveys to FVa a resistance to degradation by activated protein C. The unimpeded abnormal factor V protein retains its procoagulant activity and predisposes to thrombosis.

Prothrombin G20210A Mutation. This is a missense mutation in the prothrombin gene. Mutation leads to excessive accumulation of prothrombin. This may then be converted to thrombin to create a hypercoagulable state.

Hormone Discontinuation

Of risks, hormone use is one factor that can be modified prior to elective surgery. Combined oral contraceptive pills (COCs) induce hypercoagulable changes that are reversed if COCs are stopped at least 6 weeks prior to surgery (Robinson, 1991; Vessey, 1986). To balance the risk of unintended pregnancy in women halting COCs, a suitable alternative is recommended with clear instructions on use. In the decision to halt COCs prior to surgery, the American College of Obstetricians and Gynecologists (2007) notes that the risk of VTE in an individual must be weighed against the risk of unintended pregnancy.

Postmenopausal hormone replacement therapy (HRT) appears also to increase the incidence of postsurgical VTE. Grady and colleagues (2000) estimate a fivefold increase in the risk of developing a venous thrombotic event during the first 90 days after inpatient surgery. Thus, women should be appropriately counseled on this additional postoperative risk, but the value and duration of HRT cessation to negate this increased risk is unclear.

Prophylaxis Options

Various modalities for prophylaxis exist. Early ambulation, although encouraged after surgery, is not regarded as a primary strategy for DVT prophylaxis (Michota, 2006). Graded compression stockings (T.E.D. hose) prevent pooling of blood in the calves. If these are used alone and fitted properly, DVT rates are reduced 50 percent. If they are used in conjunction with

TABLE 39-9. Thromboembolism Prophylaxis Recommendations from the American College of Chest Physicians

Clinical Setting	Recommendation
Patients without VTE risks undergoing minor surgery	Early ambulation
Patients without VTE risks undergoing entirely laparoscopic procedures[a]	Early ambulation
Patients with VTE risks undergoing entirely laparoscopic procedures	LMWH or LDUH or IPC[b] or GCS
Patients without VTE risks undergoing major gynecologic surgery	Prophylaxis continued until hospital discharge LMWH or LDUH or IPC[b]
Patients with VTE risks undergoing major gynecologic surgery	Prophylaxis continued until hospital discharge[c] LMWH or LDUH, 3 times daily, or IPC[b] ***or*** LMWH or LDUH plus IPC[b] or GCS; or fondaparinux alone
Patients undergoing major gynecologic surgery for malignancy	Prophylaxis continued until hospital discharge[c] LMWH or LDUH, 3 times daily, or IPC[b] ***or*** LMWH or LDUH plus IPC[b] or GCS; or fondaparinux alone

GCS = graduated compression stockings; IPC = intermittent pneumatic compression; LDUH = low-dose unfractionated heparin; LMWH = low-molecular-weight heparin; VTE = venous thromboembolism.
[a]With laparoscopic gynecologic surgery, the decision to provide or withhold prophylaxis should factor patient- and procedure-related risks for VTE.
[b]Started before surgery and used continuously while the patient is not ambulatory.
[c]For selected high-risk patients, including those who have undergone major cancer surgery or have previously had VTE, continuing prophylaxis with LMWH for 28 days following hospital discharge is suggested.
Data from Geerts, 2008.

other methods of prophylaxis, additional benefit is achieved (Amaragiri, 2000). Intermittent pneumatic compression (IPC) primarily works by improving venous flow. It appears to be effective in moderate- and high-risk patients, if initiated prior to the induction of anesthesia and continued until patients are fully ambulatory (Clarke-Pearson, 1993; Geerts, 2008). Pharmacologic methods of VTE prophylaxis include low-dose unfractionated heparin, low-molecular-weight heparin, and new classes of medications such as factor Xa inhibitors. Table 39-9 summarizes appropriate treatment strategies based on risk status.

Postoperative Nausea and Vomiting

This is one of the most common complaints following surgery, and its incidence ranges from 30 to 70 percent in high-risk patients (Moller, 2002). Those at risk for postoperative nausea and vomiting (PONV) include females, nonsmokers, those with a history of motion sickness or PONV, those with extended surgeries, and those undergoing laparoscopic or other gynecologic surgery (Apfelbaum , 2003).

A multimodal approach to prevention is recommended (Apfel, 2004). Currently, combinations of 4 to 8 mg of dexamethasone prior to anesthesia induction are followed, toward

the end of surgery, by less than 1 mg of droperidol (Inapsine) and 4 mg of ondansetron (Zofran). This pretreatment significantly reduces symptoms by 25 percent. However, if symptoms develop within 6 hours of surgery, antiemetics from a different pharmacologic class than previously administered should be considered (Habib, 2004). Persistent nausea may benefit from combining agents from different classes (Table 39-10).

POSTOPERATIVE CONSIDERATIONS

Thorough preoperative planning, awareness of common postoperative complications, and vigilance to details will ensure successful convalescence for most patients.

Postoperative Orders

Postoperative orders provide instruction regarding support of each organ system, while normal function is gradually reestablished. Although orders are customized for each woman, goals are common among all surgical patients—resuscitation, pain control, and resumption of daily activities. Table 39-11 offers a template for both inpatient and outpatient postoperative orders.

TABLE 39-10. Commonly Used Medications for Nausea and Vomiting

Class/Medication	Usual Dosage	Route(s)	Adverse Effects
Anticholinergic			
Scopolamine (Transderm Scop)	1 patch every 3 day	Transdermal	Dry mouth, drowsiness, impaired eye accommodation
Antihistamines			
Diphenhydramine (Benadryl)	25–50 mg q4–6h	IM, IV, PO	Sedation, dry mouth, constipation, blurred vision, urinary retention
Hydroxyzine (Atarax, Vistaril)	25–100 mg q6h	IM, PO	
Meclizine (Antivert)	25–50 mg q6h	PO	
Promethazine (Phenergan)	12.5–25 mg q4–6h	IM, IV, PO, PR	
Benzamides			
Metoclopramide (Reglan)	5–15 mg q6h	IM, IV, PO	Sedation or agitation, diarrhea, extrapyramidal effects, hypotension
Trimethobenzamide (Tigan)	250 mg q6–8h	IM, PO, PR	
Benzodiazepines			
Lorazepam (Ativan)[a]	0.5–2.5 mg q8–12h	IM, IV, PO	Sedation, amnesia, respiratory depression, blurred vision, hallucinations
Corticosteroids			
Dexamethasone (Decadron)[a]	4 mg q6h	IM, IV, PO	GI upset, anxiety, insomnia, hyperglycemia
Phenothiazines			
Prochlorperazine (Compazine)	5–10 (25 PR) mg q6h	IM, IV, PO, PR	Sedation, extrapyramidal effects, cholestatic jaundice, hyperprolactinemia
5-HT3 Serotonin Antagonists			
Ondansetron (Zofran)	8 mg q8h	IV, PO	Headache, fever, arrhythmias, ataxia, somnolence or nervousness, elevated hepatic transaminases
Granisetron (Kytril)	2 mg per 24 h	IV, PO	
Dolasetron (Anzemet)	100 mg per 24 h	IV, PO	

[a]Not FDA approved for this indication.
GI = gastrointesinal; HT = hydroxytryptamine; IM = intramuscular; IV = intravenous; PO = orally; PR = per rectum.
From Kraft, 2010, with permission.

Pain Management

Postoperative pain management remains undervalued, and many patients continue to experience intense pain after surgery. A survey by Apfelbaum and colleagues (2003) revealed that more than 85 percent of respondents following surgery have moderate to severe pain. Poor pain control leads to decreased satisfaction with care, prolonged recovery time, increased use of health care resources, and increased health care costs (Joshi, 2005; McIntosh, 2009).

Nonopioid Treatment Options

The two major classes of nonopioid therapies are acetaminophen and nonsteroidal antiinflammatory drugs (NSAIDs). If given preoperatively, NSAIDs reduce postoperative pain, lower the amount of required opiates, and decrease the incidence of PONV by as much as 30 percent (Akarsu, 2004; Chan, 1996;

Mixter, 1998). In general, these drugs are well tolerated and carry a low risk of serious side effects. However, acetaminophen can be toxic to the liver in high doses. For this reason, the U.S. FDA (2011) now limits the amount of acetominophen per tablet or capsule to 325 mg. Moreover, they recommend that dosages greater than 4000 mg/day should be avoided, especially if providing combination therapy with oral opioids and nonopioid drugs.

Opioid Treatment Options

Despite the common side effects that all opiates share—respiratory depression and nausea and vomiting—opiate therapy is the primary choice for managing moderate to severe pain. The three most common opiates prescribed after gynecologic surgeries are morphine, fentanyl, and hydromorphone. Meperidine, although commonly administered in many obstetric units, is

TABLE 39-11. Typical Postoperative Orders (Inpatient and Outpatient)

Postoperative Orders (Inpatient)	Postoperative Orders (Outpatient)
Admit to: recovery room/assigned hospital floor/ attending physician's name	Admit to: recovery room; transfer to DSU when cleared by anesthesia
Diagnosis: s/p what surgical procedure	Diagnosis: s/p what surgical procedure
Condition: stable	Condition: stable
Vital signs: q1h × 4, q2h × 2, then q4h	VS per routine
Activity: bed rest	Allergies: NKDA
Allergies: NKDA	Bed rest until A&A, then activity ad lib
Notify MD for: T > 101°F; BP > 160/110, <90/60; P > 130; RR > 30, <10; UOP < 120 mL/4 h; acute changes	NPO until A&A, then clear liquids
Diet: NPO except ice chips	IV fluids: LR at 125 mL/h until tolerating PO, then discontinue IV
IV fluids: LR at 125/h	Notify MD for: T > 101°F; BP > 160/110, <90/60; P > 130; RR > 30, <10; acute changes
Special:	D/C patient home when A&A, cleared by anesthesia, taking PO, ambulating, & able to void
Strict I/Os	
Turn, cough, deep breath q1h while awake	
IS to BS, q1h while awake	F/U at _____ clinic in _____ weeks
Foley to gravity	
SCD hose to pump	Write any necessary prescriptions

Medications:
1. PCA orders: mix 30 mg morphine sulfate in 30 mL NS; load 4–6 mg, then IV q6min on demand; lockout 20 mg in 4 hours
2. Phenergan 25 mg IV q6h prn N/V
3. ±Toradol 30 mg IM q6h × 24 h (only if Cr is okay)

Labs: H & H in am (or that afternoon if necessary)

A&A = awake and alert; BP = blood pressure; BS = bedside; Cr = creatinine; D/C = discharge; DSU = day surgery unit; F/U = follow-up; H&H = hemoglobin and hematocrit; I/Os = input and output; IM = intramuscular; IS = incentive spirometry; IV = intravenous; LR = lactated Ringer's; NKDA = no known drug allergies; NPO = nil per os; NS = normal saline; N/V = nausea and vomiting; P = pulse; PCA = patient-controlled analgesia; PO = per os; RR = respiratory rate; SCD = sequential compression device; s/p = status post; UOP = urine output; VS = vital signs.

avoided in part because of neurologic side effects associated with its active metabolite, normeperidine. Normeperidine is a cerebral irritant that can cause effects ranging from irritability and agitation to seizure.

Morphine. Morphine, the most common opiate prescribed following gynecologic surgery, is a potent μ-opiate-receptor agonist. Action at this receptor accounts for the analgesia, euphoria, respiratory depression, and decreased gastrointestinal motility seen with morphine. Onset of action is rapid, with the peak effects being seen within 20 minutes of IV administration. Its action typically lasts for 3 to 4 hours. Its active metabolite, morphine-6-glucuronide, is renally excreted and thus is well tolerated in low doses in those with liver disease.

Pruritus is common following administration, although its genesis is poorly understood. Some investigators theorize that central opiate receptors are stimulated, whereas others speculate a histamine release as evidenced by concurrent urticaria, wheals, and flushing (Bergasa, 1991). In these cases, changing to another pain medication is logical. For pruritus treatment, most evidence-based data derives from studies of regional analgesia. Success has been found with ondansetron (Zofran), 4 mg IV (George, 2009). Antihistamines, such as diphenhydramine (Benadryl) 25 mg IV, are another option. Naloxone, an opioid antagonist, can be used but may reverse the analgesia provided by morphine.

Fentanyl. Fentanyl, a potent synthetic opiate, is more lipophilic than morphine and displays a shorter duration of action and half-life. Peak analgesia occurs within minutes of IV administration and lasts for 30 to 60 minutes. Many conscious sedation protocols used during office gynecologic procedures combine fentanyl with a sedative such as midazolam (Versed).

Hydromorphone. Hydromorphone (Dilaudid), another semisynthetic analog of morphine, is less lipophilic than fentanyl. It is available for delivery by multiple routes, including oral, intramuscular, intravenous, rectal, and subcutaneous. Hydromorphone achieves its peak analgesia 15 minutes after IV administration, and its effects last 3 to 4 hours. Although commonly used during epidural analgesia, hydromorphone is a suitable patient-controlled analgesia (PCA) alternative in patients with a morphine allergy. Table 39-12 provides a summary of various pain medications with equivalent dosages listed.

TABLE 39-12. Opioid Equivalency Chart/Dosing Data for Opioids

Drugs	Approximate Opioid Equianalgesic Dose			Usual Starting Dose			
	Parenteral (mg)	Oral (mg)	Duration (h)	Adults > 50 kg Body Wt.		Children and Adults < 50 kg	
				Parenteral	Oral	Parenteral	Oral
Morphine IR (Roxanol)	10	30	3–4	10 mg	30 mg	0.1 mg/kg	0.3 mg/kg
Morphine SR (Oramorph) (MS contin)	—	30	8–12	—	30 mg	—	0.3 mg/kg
Meperidine (Demerol)	75	300	2–3	100 mg	NR	0.75 mg/kg	NR
Hydromorphone (Dilaudid)	1.5	7.5	3–4	1.5 mg	6 mg	0.015 mg/kg	0.06 mg/kg
Codeine	130	200	3–4	60 mg (IM/SC)	60 mg	NR	1 mg/kg
Oxycodone IR (Roxicet)[a] (Percocet)[a]	—	30	3–4	NA	10 mg	NA	0.2 mg/kg
Oxycodone SR (OxyContin)	—	30	8–12	NA	10 mg	NA	0.2 mg/kg
Hydrocodone (Lorcet)[a] (Norco)[a]	NA	30	6–8	NA	10 mg	NA	0.2 mg/kg
Methadone (Dolophine)	10	20	3–4	10 mg	20 mg	0.1 mg/kg	0.2 mg/kg
Fentanyl (Sublimaze) (Duragesic)	0.1	—	1	0.1 mg	—	—	—

[a]Narcotic/nonnarcotic combination product.
IM = intramuscular; IR = immediate release; NA = not available; NR = not recommended; SC = subcutaneous; SR = sustained release.

Hormone Replacement Therapy

Some women will have significant menopausal symptoms after surgical removal of both ovaries. Symptoms can range from severe hot flashes to headaches or sudden mood swings. In these women, consideration should be given to starting estrogen replacement therapy in those without contraindications (Chap. 22, p. 584).

SYSTEM-BASED COMPLICATIONS

Oliguria

Postoperative oliguria is defined as less than 0.5 mL/kg/hr of urine produced. Oliguria can be caused by a prerenal, intrarenal, or postrenal insult, and a systematic approach typically allows efficient differentiation among these.

Prerenal Oliguria

This is a physiologic response to hypovolemia. Coexistent tachycardia and orthostatic hypotension reflect this volume depletion and are commonly seen. Causes of hypovolemia in the postoperative period are varied and include acute hemorrhage, vomiting, severe diarrhea, and inadequate intraoperative volume replacement. In response to hypovolemia, the renin-angiotensin system is activated, and antidiuretic hormone is released to prompt reabsorption of sodium and water by the renal tubules. Prerenal oliguria is the result of this sequence.

Treatment focuses on correcting the patient's volume status. Accordingly, an accurate assessment of the fluid deficit is critical. Adding the estimated blood loss and data from the intraoperative fluid logs kept by the anesthesiologist will help begin the calculations. Insensible loss during open abdominal surgery is approximately 150 mL/hr.

Intrarenal Oliguria

Ischemic injury can lead to necrosis of the renal tubules and decreased filtration. This injury may be more common in a prerenal setting, as the renal tubules are more vulnerable to insult from nephrotoxic agents such as NSAIDs, aminoglycosides, and contrast media. In many cases, differentiating between intrarenal and prerenal oliguria can be achieved by calculating the fractional excretion of sodium (FENa). This is defined as:

(Urine Na$^+$ level/plasma Na$^+$ level) ÷ (Urine creatinine level/plasma creatinine level).

A ratio of <1 suggests a prerenal source, whereas a ratio of >3 indicates an intrarenal insult. Another difference is urine sodium levels. In prerenal oliguria, it is <20 mEq/L, whereas in intrarenal states, it is >80 mEq/L.

Postrenal Oliguria

The most common cause of postrenal oliguria is urinary catheter obstruction. More seriously, ligation or laceration to the ureter or bladder may be sources. Importantly, partial or unilateral obstruction may exist despite adequate urine output. Associated findings may include hematuria, flank or abdominal pain, ileus, or signs of uremia.

For diagnosis, renal sonography is highly sensitive and specific for confirming hydronephrosis. Additional diagnostic tools to identify ureteral obstruction include computed tomography (CT) with IV contrast or retrograde pyelography. Importantly, IV contrast can be nephrotoxic, and thus CT with contrast may a less than ideal choice for those with already elevated creatinine levels. As discussed in Chapter 40 (p. 1011), the obstruction may be relieved with ureteral stenting alone or may require surgical repair.

Postoperative Urinary Retention

Inability to void with a full bladder is a common problem after gynecologic surgery, and incidences range from 7 to 80 percent depending on the definition used and surgical procedure (Stanton, 1979; Tammela, 1986). Overdistension can lead to prolonged difficulty with micturition and even permanent detrusor damage (Mayo, 1973). In addition to patient discomfort, recatheterization to treat retention increases the risk of urinary tract infection and may extend hospitalization.

Keita and colleagues (2005) prospectively evaluated risk factors potentially predictive of early postoperative urinary retention. Three major factors were independently associated with an increased risk—age older than 50 years, intraoperative fluid administration greater than 750 mL, and bladder urine volume greater than 270 mL measured upon entry to the recovery room. Among gynecologic procedures, the risk is higher after laparotomy compared with laparoscopy (Bodker, 2003).

Despite identifiable risks, all women should be advised on the need for immediate evaluation in the event of absent or difficult voiding. Clinical markers that include pain, tachycardia, urge to void without success, and bladder enlargement by palpation or percussion are equivalent diagnostically to evaluation using bedside bladder sonography (Bodker, 2003).

Once retention is identified, catheterization and bladder drainage should follow. Lau and Lam (2004) sought to determine the best catheterization strategy for managing postoperative urinary retention. Compared with overnight bladder decompression with an indwelling catheter, episodic in-and-out catheterization is equally effective. Moreover, infectious morbidity rates between the two approaches do not significantly differ.

Voiding Trials

Normal urination requires appropriate bladder contractility in the absence of significant urethral resistance (Abrams, 1999). Objective criteria that define "normal function" postoperatively vary and may be assessed using either active or passive voiding trials.

Active Voiding Trial. During this test, the bladder is actively filled with a set volume, and following patient voiding, residual bladder urine volumes are calculated. Initially, the bladder is completely emptied by catheterization. It may be helpful during catheterization for a woman to stand upright to clear the most dependent portions of her bladder. Sterile water infused under gravity is then instilled into the bladder through the same catheter until approximately 300 mL is used or until a subjective maximum capacity is reached. A patient is then given up to 30 minutes to void spontaneously into a urine collection device. The difference between volume infused and volume retrieved is recorded as the postvoid residual.

The only published study evaluating the effectiveness of this strategy was reported by Kleeman and associates (2002). They evaluated women following surgery for incontinence and prolapse. In their study, a postvoid residual of less than 50 percent carried a recatheterization rate of 8 percent. If patients could spontaneously void greater than 70 percent of the instilled volume, there were no failures.

Passive Voiding Trial. As an alternative to active saline instillation, voiding and residuals may be assessed following passive, physiologic filling of the bladder. Initially, a Foley catheter is removed, and a woman is encouraged to drink increased amounts of liquid. She is encouraged to void spontaneously at her first urge to urinate or after 4 hours, whichever is first. Urine volumes in a collection device are measured. An in-and-out catheterization or bladder sonogram is then performed to measure the postvoid residual (Fig. 23-14, p. 620).

An easy rule to remember for evaluating either active or passive voiding trials is the "75/75 rule"—spontaneously voiding greater than 75 mL *and* voiding greater than 75 percent of the total volume. This constitutes a successful voiding trial and obviates the need for Foley catheter reinsertion. Alternatively, on the Urogynecology Service at Parkland Memorial Hospital, a postvoid residual of less than 100 mL constitutes a success.

Pulmonary Complications

Broad definitions hinder our ability to accurately assess the incidence of postoperative pulmonary complications, but reported estimates range from 9 to 69 percent (Calligaro, 1993; Hall, 1991). Common pulmonary complications encountered by gynecologists are atelectasis and pneumonia. Five significant risk factors for pulmonary complications following abdominal surgery include age older than 60 years, BMI greater than 27, a history of cancer, smoking within the past 8 weeks, and a surgical incision involving the upper abdomen (Brooks-Brunn, 1997).

Atelectasis

Clinical Features. Atelectasis is a reversible closure or collapse of alveoli that is seen in 90 percent of surgical patients (Lundquist, 1995). Development is associated with decreased lung compliance, gas exchange abnormalities, and increased pulmonary vascular resistance. Thus, characteristic signs include diminished breath sounds, dullness to percussion over affected lung fields, and decreased oxygenation. In addition, linear densities in the lower lung fields typify chest radiographic features

(Hall, 1991). Classically, atelectasis is associated with low-grade fevers. However, Engoren (1995) evaluated 100 consecutive adult postoperative patients with radiographically diagnosed atelectasis and found no association between atelectasis and postoperative fever. Pulse oximetry of >92 percent represents adequate oxygenation, however, a PaO_2 measurement by arterial blood gas will most accurately assess a patient with hypoxic respiratory failure. Despite its common occurrence after abdominal operations, atelectasis is usually temporary (up to 2 days), self-limited, and rarely slows patient recovery or hospital discharge (Platell, 1997). Severe cases of atelectasis can be prevented in many instances using lung expansion therapies described earlier (p. 950).

Importantly, atelectasis may clinically mimic pulmonary embolism or less commonly, pneumonia. All can manifest with respiratory compromise and fever. Thus, risk factors for thromboembolic complications, greater respiratory compromise, fever, and tachycardia may prompt evaluation for pulmonary embolism and pneumonia.

Hospital-Acquired Pneumonia

This is the second most common nosocomial infection in the United States and carries high associated morbidity and mortality rates (Tablan, 2004). Its incidence in surgical patients varies and ranges from 1 to 19 percent depending upon surgical procedure and hospital surveyed (Kozlow, 2003). With these infections, the bacterial pathogens most typically responsible include aerobic gram-negative bacilli, such as *Pseudomonas aeruginosa*, *Escherichia coli*, *Klebsiella pneumoniae*, and *Acinetobacter* species.

Clinically, pneumonia is diagnosed if chest radiography reveals a new or progressive radiographic infiltrate and if two of three clinical features (leukocytosis, fever >38°C, or purulent secretions) are present. Broad-spectrum antibiotic regimens are recommended for hospital-acquired pneumonia treatment. An expanded-spectrum beta-lactam agent, such as piperacillin-tazobactam (Zosyn) or ticarcillin-clavulanate (Timentin), coupled with an aminoglycoside is an approved combination (Table 3-4, p. 68). If aspiration is highly suspected, specific treatment for anaerobes with metronidazole or clindamycin should be considered. An algorithm supported by the American Thoracic Society is shown in Figure 39-6. As discussed earlier, prevention can be accomplished by using oral endotracheal and orogastric tubes in place of nasal tubes; elevating the head of the bed 30 to 45 degrees, particularly during feeding; and removal

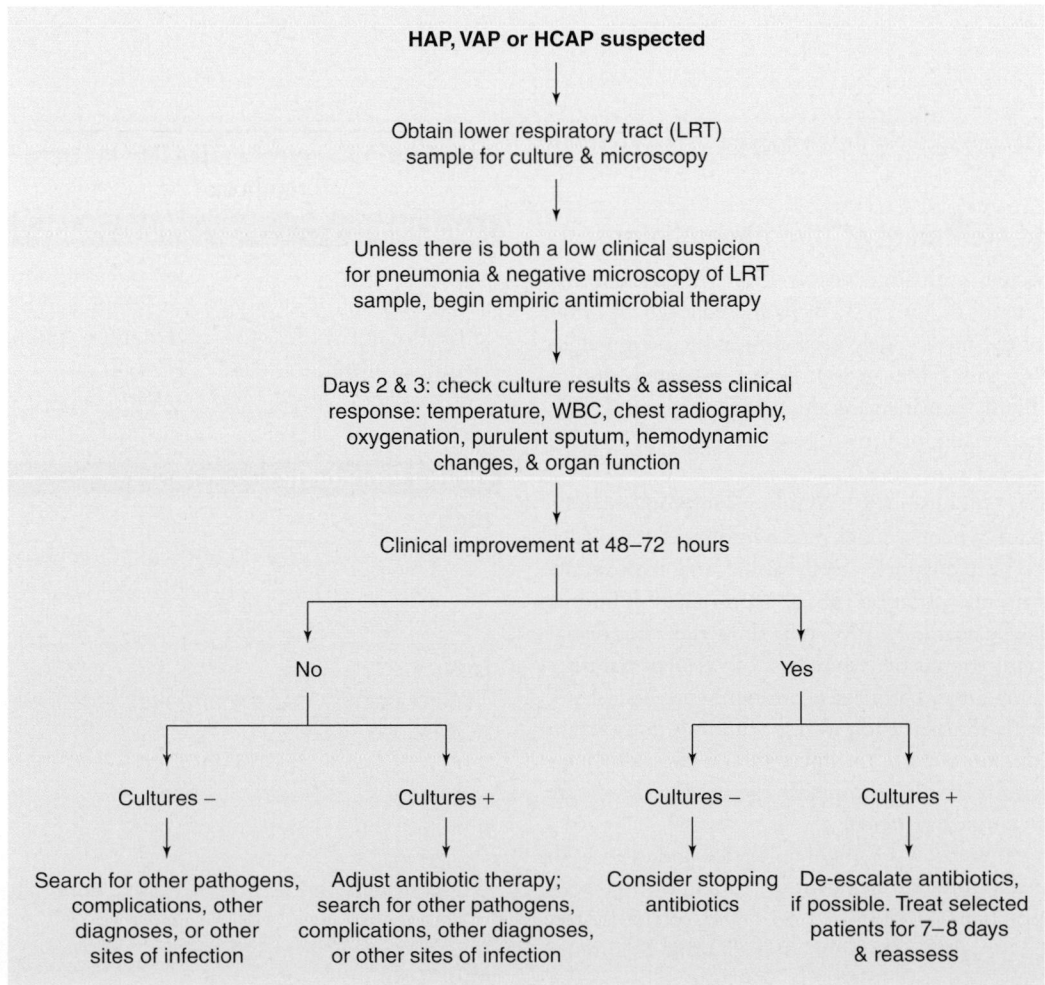

HAP, VAP or HCAP suspected

Obtain lower respiratory tract (LRT)
sample for culture & microscopy

Unless there is both a low clinical suspicion
for pneumonia & negative microscopy of LRT
sample, begin empiric antimicrobial therapy

Days 2 & 3: check culture results & assess clinical
response: temperature, WBC, chest radiography,
oxygenation, purulent sputum, hemodynamic
changes, & organ function

Clinical improvement at 48–72 hours

No / Yes

Cultures − / Cultures + / Cultures − / Cultures +

Search for other pathogens, complications, other diagnoses, or other sites of infection / Adjust antibiotic therapy; search for other pathogens, complications, other diagnoses, or other sites of infection / Consider stopping antibiotics / De-escalate antibiotics, if possible. Treat selected patients for 7–8 days & reassess

FIGURE 39-6 Algorithm describes management strategies for hospital-acquired pneumonia. HAP = Hospital-acquired pneumonia; HCAP = health care-associated pneumonia; VAP = ventilator-associated pneumonia; WBC = white blood cell count. *(From the American Thoracic Society, 2005, with permission.)*

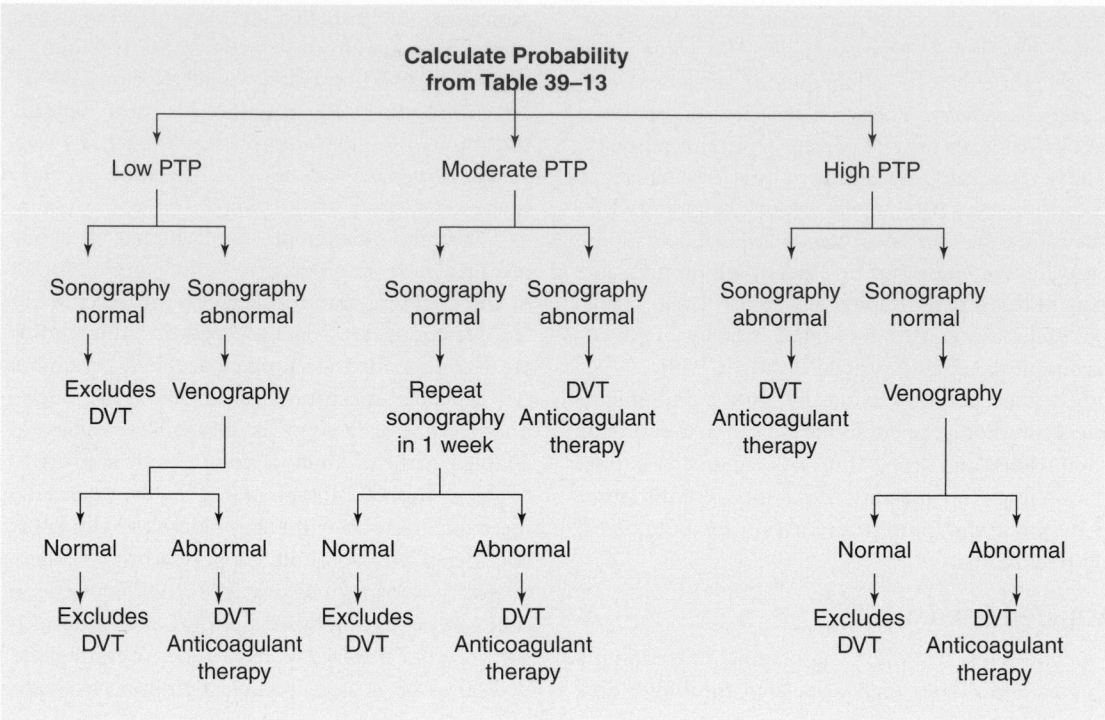

FIGURE 39-7 Algorithm for evaluation of suspected deep-vein thrombosis (DVT). PTP = pretest probability. *(From Wells, 1995, with permission.)*

of subglottic secretions in those unable to clear these (American Thoracic Society, 2005).

Diagnosis and Treatment of Thromboembolism

If VTE is suspected, evaluation begins with clinical examination and risk estimation. For DVT, Wells and colleagues (1995) published one of the most widely used clinical prediction algorithms (Fig. 39-7 and Table 39-13). When indicated, duplex sonography is highly sensitive for detecting proximal DVTs, with a false-negative rate of 0 to 6 percent (Fig. 2-27, p. 49) (Gottlieb, 1999).

For pulmonary embolism (PE), common symptoms include dyspnea, chest pain, syncope, cough, and hemoptysis. Clinically, the patient may be tachypneic, tachycardic, and hypoxemic. With auscultation, rales, friction rub, or accentuated pulmonic valve closure may be heard. An EKG may show right axis deviation, and chest radiographs may show loss of vascular markings in the affected lung areas. Clinicians commonly use helical CT scanning or ventilation/perfusion (V/Q) scanning to ascertain the diagnosis. Measurement of D-dimers are not clinically helpful for the diagnosis of PE postoperatively as these levels are often elevated in surgical patients.

Acute management of VTE involves anticoagulation with intravenous unfractionated heparin or subcutaneous low-molecular-weight heparin (Tables 39-14 and 39-15). After achieving adequate anticoagulation, oral vitamin K antagonists such as warfarin are initiated. Warfarin is generally started at a daily oral dose of 2.5 to 10 mg and adjusted to reach an INR of 2.5 (Kearon, 2008). To avoid paradoxical hypercoagulability, heparin is continued for at least 5 days

TABLE 39-13. Pretest Probability for Deep-Vein Thrombosis	
Major Points	**Minor Points**
Cancer	Recent trauma to
Immobilization	symptomatic leg
Recent major surgery	Unilateral edema
Thigh or calf tenderness	Erythema
Calf swelling	Dilated superficial veins
Family history of DVT	Hospitalized in last 6 months

Clinical Probability

High
>3 major points and no alternative diagnosis
>2 major points and >2 minor points + no alternative diagnosis

Low
1 major point + >2 minor points + has an alternative diagnosis
1 major point + >1 minor point + no alternative diagnosis
0 major points + >3 minor points + has an alternative diagnosis
0 major points + >2 minor points + no alternative diagnosis

Moderate
All other combinations

Modified from Wells, 1995, with permission.

TABLE 39-14. Parkland Hospital Protocol for Continuous Heparin Infusion for Patients with Venous Thromboembolism

Initial Heparin Dose:
__ units IV push (recommended 80 units/kg rounded to nearest 100, maximum 7500 units), then
__ units/hr by infusion (recommended 18 units/kg/hr rounded to nearest 50).

Infusion Rate Adjustments—based on partial thromboplastin time (PTT):

PTT (sec)[a]	Intervention[b]	Baseline Infusion Rate Change[c]
<45	80 units/kg bolus	↑by 4 units/kg/hr
45–54	40 units/kg bolus	↑by 2 units/kg/hr
55–84	None	None
85–100	None	↓by 2 units/kg/hr
>100	Stop infusion 60 minutes	↓by 3 units/kg/hr

[a]PTT goal 55–84.
[b]Rounded to nearest 100.
[c]Rounded to nearest 50.
From Cunningham, 2010, with permission.

after the initiation of warfarin (Fekrazad, 2009). Long term, anticoagulation therapy duration is dictated by clinical circumstance and typically is administered for: (1) 3 to 6 months for a first idiopathic DVT, (2) 6 months for PEs, and (3) indefinite treatment for those with a thrombophilic condition or a second VTE.

Gastrointestinal Considerations
Resumption of Bowel Function

Following intraabdominal surgery, dysfunction of enteric neural activity typically disrupts normal propulsion. Activity first returns in the stomach and is noted typically within 24 hours. The small intestine also exhibits contractile activity within 24 hours after surgery, but normal function may be delayed for 3 to 4 days (Condon, 1986; Dauchel, 1976). Rhythmic colonic motility resumes last, at approximately 4 days following intraabdominal surgery (Huge, 2000). Passage of flatus characteristically marks this return of function, and stool passage typically follows in 1 to 2 days.

Resumption of Diet

Early initiation of postoperative feeding has been found to be most effective. Early feeding has been shown to improve wound healing, stimulate gut motility, decrease intestinal stasis, increase splanchnic blood flow, and stimulate reflexes that elicit secretion of gastrointestinal hormones that can shorten postoperative ileus (Anderson, 2003; Braga, 2002; Correia, 2004; Lewis, 2001). The decision to initiation "early feeding" with liquids or with solid food has been studied prospectively (Jeffery, 1996). In patients who were given solid food as the first postoperative meal, the number of calories and protein consumed on the first postoperative day were higher. In addition, the number of patients requiring diet changes to NPO was not statistically different (7.5 percent in regular diet and 8.1 percent in the clear diet groups). The improved tolerance and better palatability of solids make this a reasonable option.

Ileus

Postoperative ileus (POI) is a transient impairment of gastrointestinal activity that leads to abdominal distension, hypoactive

TABLE 39-15. Characteristics of Some Low-Molecular-Weight Heparins

Name (Brand Name)	Dose	Therapeutic Peak
Enoxaparin (Lovenox)	1 mg/kg q 12 h	0.6–1 IU/mL
	1.5 mg/kg daily	1 1.5 IU/mL
Tinzaparin (Innohep)	175 IU/kg daily	0.85–1 IU/mL
Dalteparin (Fragmin)	100 IU/kg q 12 h	0.4–1.1 IU/mL
	200 IU/kg daily	1–2 IU/mL

bowel sounds, nausea and/or vomiting related to GI gas and fluid accumulation, and delayed passage of flatus and/or stool (Livingston, 1990).

The genesis of POI is multifactorial. First, bowel manipulation during surgery leads to production of factors that contribute to POI. These include: (1) neurogenic factors related to sympathetic overactivity, (2) hormonal factors related to the release of hypothalamic corticotropin-releasing factor, which plays a key role in the stress response, and (3) inflammatory factors (Tache, 2001). Perioperative opioid use also has a significant role in the etiology of POI. Thus, in selecting these agents, clinicians should balance the beneficial analgesia produced by central opioid receptor binding against the GI dysfunction that results from peripheral receptor binding effects (Holzer, 2004).

No single treatment defines the management of POI. Electrolyte repletion and intravenous fluids to reestablish a euvolemic state is traditional therapy. In contrast, routine nasogastric tube (NGT) decompression to promote bowel rest has been challenged by multiple prospective randomized trials. A metaanalysis including nearly 4200 patients found routine NGT decompression unsuccessful and inferior to its selective use in symptomatic patients. Specifically, patients without NGTs had significantly earlier return of normal bowel function and decreased risks of wound infection and ventral hernia (Nelson, 2005). Additionally, tube-related discomfort, nausea, and hospital stays were reduced. For these reasons, postoperative NGTs are recommended only for symptomatic relief of abdominal bloating and recurrent vomiting (Nunley, 2004).

Gum chewing as a preventative modality for POI has been the focus of several studies. Most authors conclude that gum chewing offers no therapeutic value given that there was no significant difference in hospitalization length or in time to first gas or stool passage (Matros, 2006).

Small Bowel Obstruction

Obstruction of the small intestines may be partial or complete and can result from adhesions following intraabdominal surgery, infection, or malignancy. Of these, surgical adhesions are the most common cause (Krebs, 1987; Monk, 1994). Small bowel obstruction (SBO) is estimated to develop following 1 to 2 percent of total abdominal hysterectomies, and nearly 75 percent of obstructions are complete (Al Sunaidi, 2006). The mean interval between a primary intraabdominal procedure and SBO is approximately 5 years (Al Took, 1999).

Although the initial management of a small bowel obstruction is similar to that of postoperative ileus, distinguishing between the two entities is important to prevent serious SBO sequelae. During SBO, the bowel lumen dilates proximal to the obstruction, whereas decompression may develop distally. Bacterial overgrowth in the proximal small bowel may lead to bacterial fermentation and worsening dilation. The bowel wall continues to become edematous and dysfunctional (Wright, 1971). Progressive increases in bowel pressure can compromise perfusion to the intestinal segment and lead to ischemia or rupture (Megibow, 1991).

Clinical signs that may help distinguish small bowel obstruction from POI include tachycardia, oliguria, and fever. Physical examination may reveal abdominal distension, high-pitched bowel sounds, and an empty rectal vault on digital examination. Finally, leukocytosis with a dominance of neutrophils should alert to possible coexistent bowel ischemia.

Computed tomography scanning is the primary imaging tool to identify SBO. Water-soluble contrast can safely help identify the cause and severity of an obstruction. Gastrografin, the most commonly used water-soluble dye, is a mixture of sodium amidotrizoate and meglumine amidotrizoate and may aid resolution of small bowel edema due to its high osmotic pressure. Gastrografin is also theorized to enhance smooth muscle contractility (Assalia, 1994). Although the use of oral Gastrografin does appear to reduce hospital length of stay, it has no therapeutic benefit in adhesion-related small bowel obstruction (Abbas, 2005).

Treatment of small bowel obstruction varies with the degree of obstruction. For those with partial obstruction, feedings are held, intravenous fluids and antiemetics are initiated, and an NGT is placed for significant nausea and vomiting. Continued surveillance should monitor for signs of bowel ischemia, which include fever, tachycardia, increasing abdominal pain, and WBC elevation. Symptoms in most cases of partial SBO should improve within 48 hours. In contrast, for those with complete bowel obstruction, surgery to relieve the obstruction is indicated for most.

Nutrition

The primary goals of postoperative nutrition are to improve immune function, promote wound healing, and minimize metabolic disturbances. Despite the additional stress in the immediate postoperative period, underfeeding is accepted for a brief period (Seidner, 2006). Table 39-16 offers a summary of the basic metabolic needs in the immediate postoperative period. Extended protein calorie restriction in a surgical patient, however, can lead to impaired wound healing, diminished cardiac and pulmonary function, bacterial overgrowth within the GI tract, and other complications that increase hospital stays and

TABLE 39-16. Postoperative Nutritional Requirements

Nutritional Requirements	Recommendations
Basal energy expenditure (BEE) in women	655 + 1.9 × (height in cm) + 9.6 × (weight in kg) − 4.7 × (age in years)
Total calories	100% to 120% BEE
Glucose	50–70% total caloric intake Maintain blood glucose level <200 mg/dL
Protein	1.5 g/kg/d of current weight (BMI < 25) 2.0 g/kg/d of ideal weight (BMI > 25)

BMI = body mass index.
Compiled from Nehra, 2002.

patient morbidity (Elwyn, 1975; Kinney, 1986; Seidner, 2006). If substantial oral caloric intake is delayed for 7 to 10 days, nutritional support is warranted.

Enteral versus Parenteral Nutrition

In the absence of contraindications, enteral nutrition is preferred to a parenteral route, especially when infectious complications are compared (Kudsk, 1992; Moore, 1992). Other advantages of enteral nutrition include fewer metabolic disturbances and lower cost (Nehra, 2002).

Hypovolemic Shock
Diagnosis of Hypovolemic Shock

Circulatory dysfunction causes decreased tissue oxygenation and results in multiorgan failure if not recognized and treated promptly. In gynecology, the most common cause of shock is hemorrhage-related hypovolemia, although cardiogenic, septic, and neurogenic shock should be considered during patient evaluation. Assessment begins with evaluation of the patient's mental status, vital signs, urine output, and hematocrit. Unfortunately, markers such as blood pressure and resting heart rate may be unaffected through early compensation. For example, after an acute blood loss of greater than 25 to 30 percent of total blood volume, hypotension typically lags other markers of multiorgan dysfunction, including oliguria and altered mental status.

In addition to a heightened clinical suspicion of hypovolemia, serum markers may help provide objective evidence of decreased perfusion and oxygenation. Serum lactate levels have been shown to be more sensitive than blood pressure and cardiac output in predicting severe hemorrhage (Broder, 1964; Dunham, 1991). In addition, serum lactate levels can be used to guide the effectiveness of resuscitation. Blood gas analysis can also provide a rapid estimate of the serum base deficit. Hemorrhage severity can be accurately predicted using the following stratification of these base deficits: 2 to –5 (mild hemorrhage), –6 to –14 (moderate hemorrhage), and –15 or less (severe hemorrhage). If patients continue to have dropping base deficits despite aggressive resuscitation, ongoing hemorrhage should be assumed (Davis, 1988). Of note, immediate hematocrit levels do not predict the severity of acute blood loss as accurately as serial trends (Chap. 40, p. 1006).

Treatment of Hypovolemic Shock

Treatment of hypovolemic shock centers on control of ongoing hemorrhage and restoration of intravascular volume. One easy mnemonic used to describe treatment is "ORDER," which represents oxygenate, restore, drug therapy, evaluate, and remedy (American College of Obstetricians and Gynecologists, 1997). Initially, supplemental oxygen is provided to avoid tissue desaturation (Wilson, 2003). Simultaneously, a rapid infusion of isotonic crystalloid solutions through two large-bore intravenous lines can quickly replace volume. In the face of refractory hypotension, supplemental colloids and red blood cell transfusion may be necessary (Chap. 40, p. 1007). In the presence of hypovolemia, vasopressors are generally not recommended except to temporarily assist with an unstable condition while fluid resuscitation is administered.

During treatment, blood pressure, urine output, and a patient's general status provide information regarding resuscitation efforts. Findings will allow augmentation of treatment to prevent or minimize end-organ damage. Finally, if ongoing bleeding is suspected, the benefits of operative intervention may outweigh the risks of continued conservative therapy. Intraoperatively, isolation and control of hemorrhage should be approached systematically as described in Chapter 40 (p. 1003). After a patient is stabilized, close surveillance for electrolyte abnormalities, coagulation imbalance, and ischemic organ injury is essential.

Postoperative Fever Evaluation

One of the most common problems encountered postoperatively is fever. Although fever may reflect an infectious process, most are self-limited (Garibaldi, 1985). However, for those with persistent symptoms, a systematic approach to patient evaluation will help to differentiate inflammatory from infectious etiologies.

Pathophysiology of the Febrile Response

Fever is a response to inflammatory mediators, termed *pyrogens*, which originate either endogenously or exogenously. Circulating pyrogens lead to the production of prostaglandins (primarily PGE_2), which elevates the thermoregulatory set point. The inflammatory cascade produces a number of cytokines (IL-1, IL-6, TNF-α) found in the circulation after a variety of events—surgery, cancer, trauma, and infection (Wortel, 1993). Thus, a differential diagnosis of a postoperative fever should include noninfectious and infectious causes.

Etiology

Postoperative fevers that develop more than 2 days following surgery are more likely to be infectious. The most common causes may be broadly categorized and are reflected in the mnemonic, the "Five Ws," which represent wind, water, walking, wound, and "wonder" drug. First, pneumonia should be considered, and women at greatest risk are those who have been mechanically ventilated for a prolonged period, have an NGT in place, or have preexisting COPD. Additionally, catheterization places women at risk for developing a urinary tract infection. Logically, duration of catheterization correlates positively with the risk for this infection. Venous thromboembolic disease may present with low-grade fever, and patients with VTEs commonly present with other disease-specific symptoms (p. 968) (Stein, 2000). Fever related to surgical site infections usually develops 5 to 7 days after surgery. These infections may involve the pelvis or abdominal wall layers, and their management is discussed later in this chapter and in Chapter 3 (p. 99). Finally, medications commonly used postoperatively—such as heparin, beta-lactam antibiotics, and sulfonamide antibiotics—may cause a rash, eosinophilia, or drug fever.

Clinical Evaluation

Evaluations that rotely include CBC, urinalysis, blood cultures, and chest radiographs have been evaluated in multiple studies and are inefficient and ineffective (Badillo, 2002; de la Torre, 2003; Schey, 2005). Thus, initial assessment of a woman with

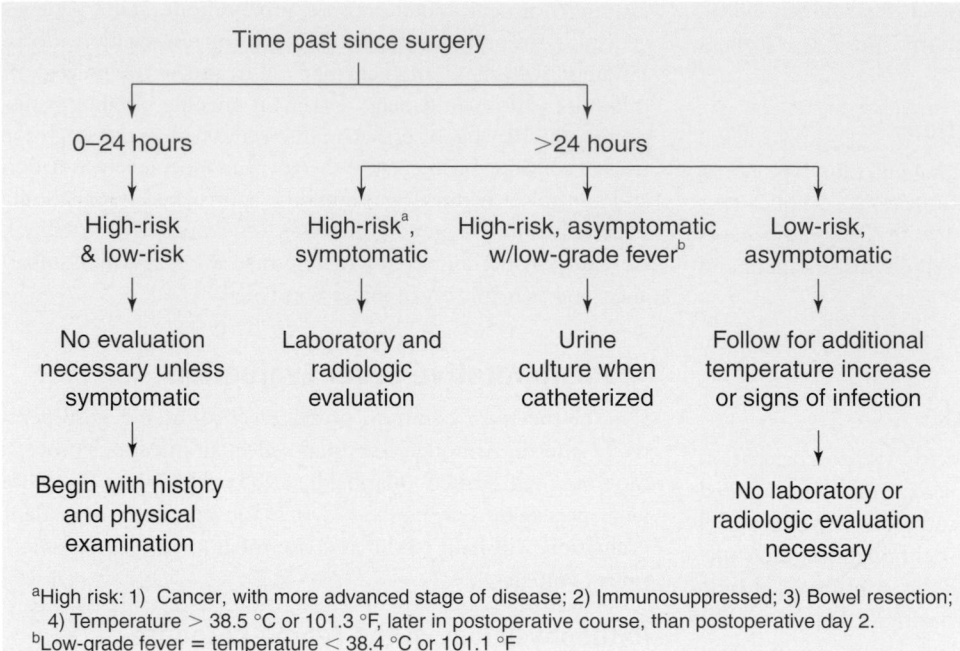

FIGURE 39-8 Algorithm for evaluation of postoperative fever. *(From de la Torre, 2003, with permission.)*

postoperative fever should be individualized and begin with a focused history and physical examination. The simple diagnostic algorithm presented in Figure 39-8 can be used as one high-yield, cost-effective strategy for the management of a woman with postoperative fever.

Postoperative Wound
Acute Wound Healing

Wound healing has been described as a three-phase process—inflammatory reaction, proliferation, and remodeling (Li, 2007). Hemostasis by coagulation initiates the first step in the *inflammatory phase*. The infiltration of leukocytes and release of cytokines helps initiate the *proliferative phase* of wound repair. Two activities happen simultaneously—the growth of granulation tissue to fill the wound along with the formation of epithelium to cover the wound surface. The final stage, *remodeling*, restores the structural integrity and functional aptitude of the new tissue.

Wound Dehiscence

Despite the clinical advances made in the arenas of anesthesia, preoperative antibiotics, suture technology, and postoperative care, the incidence of wound disruptions remains largely unchanged (Cliby, 2002). Dehiscence prolongs hospital stays and requires labor-intensive care. Thus, a surgeon should have knowledge of modifiable risk factors and treatment options for these complications.

Classification and Incidence. The level to which a wound may open varies and may involve the subcutaneous and skin layers. Superficial separation may result solely from a hematoma or seroma, but more commonly is a consequence of a wound

infection. The reported incidence of superficial separations is between 3 and 15 percent (Owen, 1994; Taylor, 1998).

More seriously, separation may also include the abdominal wall fascia. Fascial dehiscence occurs less frequently and is fatal in nearly 25 percent of cases (Carlson, 1997). Infection or sutures held under too much tension are common causes and lead to fascial necrosis. Sutures remain poorly anchored in necrotic fascia (Bartlett, 1985). These layers then separate with only minimal increases in intraabdominal pressure.

Prevention. Important factors for developing a wound dehiscence include general patient health, proper surgical technique, and risks associated with wound infections.

General Patient Health. Riou and coworkers (1992) found that age greater than 65 years, pulmonary disease, malnutrition, obesity, malignancy, and hypertension contribute to a patient's risk of developing subsequent wound disruption.

Proper Surgical Technique. In the operating room, the surgeon has multiple opportunities to modify risks associated with wound disruption. Proper surgical technique advocates hemostasis, gentle tissue handling, removal of devitalized tissue, closure of dead space, use of monofilament suture, indicated placement of closed suction drains, and sustained normothermia (Mangram, 1999). For example, Kurz and colleagues (1996) demonstrated that maintaining normothermia in patients undergoing abdominal surgery significantly reduced postoperative wound infection rates from 19 percent to 6 percent.

Use of electrosurgery instead of scalpel for abdominal entry is common and offers speed, hemostasis, comparable wound healing, and decreased requirements for postoperative analgesia (Chap. 40, p. 999) (Chrysos, 2005). The cutting properties of electrosurgery cause cells to explode by conversion of cell water to steam. This method of heat dissipation leads to minimal lateral thermal tissue damage. Coagulation mode, on the other hand, achieves hemostasis through formation of a superficial eschar and desiccation (the fibrous binding between dehydrated, denatured cells of vessel endothelium). Therefore, tissue dissection should be performed using a cutting mode, whereas hemostasis is best achieved with minimal directed coagulation. In addition, less tissue damage and fewer tracts for bacterial overgrowth result from minimizing the number of surgical strokes during incision.

Dead space closure using a subcutaneous suture in Camper fascia at the time of cesarean delivery has been shown to

TABLE 39-17. Selected Interventions for Prevention of Surgical Site Infection

INTERVENTION
Preoperative
Reduce hemoglobin A1c levels to <7% before operation
Smoking cessation 30 days before operation (see Table 1-23, p. 28 for medication aids)
Administer specialized nutritional supplements or enteral nutrition for severe malnutrition for 7–14 days preoperatively
Adequately treat preoperative infections, such as urinary tract infection or cervicitis
Identification and decolonization of *S aureus* carriers may be a potentially useful intervention
Perioperative
Remove hair only if it will interfere with the operation; hair removal by clipping immediately before the operation or with depilatories; no pre- or perioperative shaving of surgical site
Use an antiseptic surgical scrub or alcohol-based hand antiseptic for preoperative cleansing of the operative team members' hands and forearms
Prepare the skin around the operative site with an appropriate antiseptic agent, including preparations based on alcohol, chlorhexidine,[a] or iodine/iodophors
Administer prophylactic antibiotics for most clean-contaminated and contaminated procedures, and selected clean procedures (see Table 39-6, p. 959).
Administer prophylactic antibiotics within 1 h before incision (2 h for vancomycin and fluoroquinolones)
Use higher dosages of prophylactic antibiotics for morbidly obese patients
Use vancomycin as a prophylactic agent only when there is a significant risk of MRSA infection
Provide adequate ventilation, minimize operating room traffic, and clean instruments and surfaces with approved disinfectants
Avoid flash sterilization
Intraoperative
Carefully handle tissue, eradicate dead space, and adhere to standard principles of asepsis
Avoid use of surgical drains unless absolutely necessary
Leave contaminated or dirty-infected wounds open
Redose prophylactic antibiotics with short half-lives intraoperatively if operation is prolonged (for cefazolin if operation is >3 h) or if there is extensive blood loss
Maintain intraoperative normothermia
Postoperative
Maintain serum glucose levels <200 mg/dL on postoperative days 1 and 2
Monitor wound for the development of SSI

[a]Preferred for laparotomy.
MRSA = methicillin-resistant *Staphylococcus aureus*; *S aureus* = *Staphylococcus aureus*; SSI = surgical site infection.
Modified from Kirby, 2009, with permission.

significantly reduce superficial wound disruptions in those with subcutaneous layers thicker than 2 cm (Naumann, 1995; Ramsey, 2005). However, well-designed prospective studies in gynecologic populations are lacking. Skin closure using subcuticular suturing has lower wound separation rates than staples (Johnson, 2006).

Infection. Infection is a common underlying cause of wound disruption. Risk factors for infection are numerous and are listed in Table 3-29 (p. 99). Of these, many conditions can be improved preoperatively (Table 39-17).

Diagnosis. Superficial wound separations usually present 3 to 5 days after surgery, with wound erythema and new-onset drainage. A delay in evacuating the inflammatory exudates from subcutaneous layer dead space can lead to fascial weakening and an increased risk of fascial dehiscence.

Fascial dehiscence generally presents within the first 10 days postoperatively. Superficial disruption of the subcutaneous layer and extensive leakage of peritoneal fluid or purulent drainage are indicative. Given the high mortality risk associated with fascial dehiscence and bowel evisceration, examination under anesthesia to estimate the extent of separation is often warranted.

Treatment of Superficial Wound Dehiscence. The focus of wound management should be to expedite healing while minimizing costs and complications. If a concomitant wound cellulitis is identified, systemic antibiotics can be used to treat the infection.

Wet to Dry Dressing Changes. The initial focus of wound management is evacuation of all hematomas and/or seromas and treatment of underlying infection. As discussed in Chapter 3 (p. 99), most abdominal wound infections following clean cases originate from *Staphylococcus aureus*. In contrast, those following clean-contaminated cases have a greater chance of being polymicrobial. Thus, suitable antibiotic selection in these cases should cover gram-positive, gram-negative, and anaerobic organisms. Antibiotics found in Table 3-31 (p. 103) are suitable regimens. Importantly, the number of infections caused by methicillin-resistant *S aureus* (MRSA) has increased dramatically, and coverage for this pathogen should be considered.

Irrigation used for wound dressings should remove surface bacteria without disrupting normal healing components. Povidone iodine, iodophor gauze, dilute hydrogen peroxide, and Daiken solution are cytotoxic to white blood cells and are not typically used in wound care (Bennett, 2001; O'Toole, 1996).

Ideally, wound dressings are removed daily and replaced with properly hydrated materials. In very necrotic wounds, allowing gauze to dry and pulling tissue adherent to the gauze with each change is acceptable. More frequent changes should be avoided as they lead to aggressive debridement of vital tissues and slow wound healing. Table 39-18 lists products used in modern wound care.

Negative-Pressure Wound Therapy. This therapy is primarily used for chronic wounds that have been resistant to other forms of wound care and for minimizing scarring of acute wounds. The five mechanisms by which this technology helps wound healing are wound retraction, continuous wound cleaning, stimulation of granulation tissue formation, reduction of interstitial edema, and removal of exudates (Fabian, 2000; Morykwas, 1997; Sullivan, 2009).

The two most commonly used dressings are foam and moistened nonadherent cotton gauze. After the initial application, the dressing is typically changed within 48 hours and then two to three times a week thereafter.

After the dressing is covered with an adhesive film, an evacuation tube runs through the dressing to help draw excessive exudates away from the wound and into a canister attached at the other end (Fig. 39-9). The vacuum pump offers either continuous or intermittent negative pressure (-5 to -125 mm Hg depending on the device recommendations).

Delayed Primary Closure. Approximately 4 days after wound disruption and resolution of any subcutaneous infection, a superficial vertical mattress closure with delayed-absorbable suture may be used to reapproximate tissue edges (Wechter, 2005). Depending on wound depth and patient tolerances, this can be completed in the operating room or at the bedside using a local anesthetic complemented by IV analgesia. Overall, this strategy reduces healing time and significantly decreases the number of postoperative visits.

Treatment of Fascial Dehiscence. Early recognition of abdominal wall separation is critical in reducing the serious

TABLE 39-18. Wound Care Products

Product	Description
Antifungal cream	Topical cream used as treatment for superficial fungal infections of the periwound skin; contains 2% miconazole nitrate.
Calcium alginate	Calcium alginate is a solid that exchanges calcium ions for sodium ions when it contacts any substance containing sodium such as wound fluid. The resulting sodium alginate is a gel that is nonadhesive, nonocclusive, and conformable to wound bed. Indicated for moderately or highly draining wounds.
Enzymatic debrider	Topical solution that breaks down necrotic tissue by directly digesting the components of slough or by dissolving the collagen that holds necrotic tissue to the underlying wound bed.
Film	Thin, transparent polyurethane sheets coated on one side with acrylic, hypoallergenic adhesive. The adhesive will not stick to moist surfaces, and the film is impermeable to fluids and bacteria, but semipermeable to oxygen and water vapor. Indicated in superficial wounds with little or no exudate.
Foam	Polyurethane sheets containing open cells capable of holding fluids and pulling them away from the wound bed. Foams provide absorbency while keeping the wound moist. Indicated in moderately or highly draining wounds.
Gauze	Woven or nonwoven cotton or synthetic blends.
Hydrogel	Formulated in sheets or gels. Glycerin-, saline-, or water-based to hydrate the wound. Indicated in dry or minimally draining wounds.
Silver nitrate	Used to treat overgrown granulation tissue. Apply stick to hypergranulation tissue.

From Sarsam, 2005, with permission.

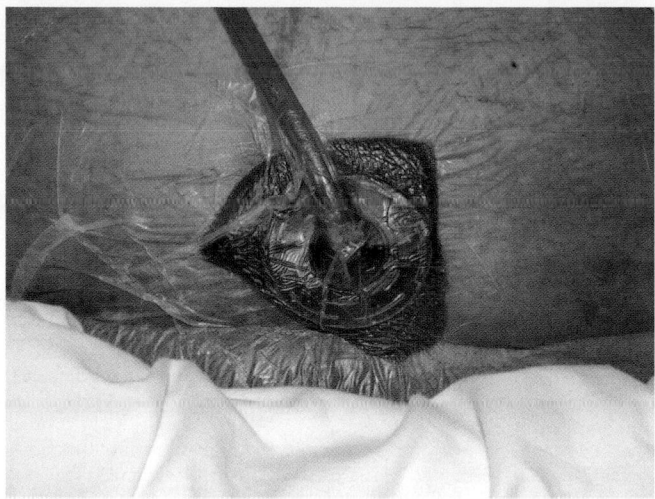

FIGURE 39-9 Photograph of wound vacuum in place. Porous synthetic sponge fills the wound. Negative pressure is created by one end of tubing placed within the sponge and the other attached to a suction-generating device. The sponge and wound are covered by an occlusive adhesive dressing, which helps to maintain the suction seal.

morbidity and mortality rates associated with fascial dehiscence. Faced with this surgical emergency, a gynecologist must first determine if the fascial dehiscence is associated with evisceration of abdominal content. If discharge of abdominal contents is noted, an abdominal binder with sterile towels soaked in saline can be use to replace abdominal contents and temporize the situation. Broad-spectrum antibiotics are generally recommended to minimize ensuing peritonitis.

The final goal of treatment is closure. For critically ill patients with significant edema, temporarily maintaining anterior abdominal wall integrity until a patient is stable enough to tolerate a definitive operative closure is reasonable. Fascial closure under general anesthesia is performed after sufficient debridement of necrotic or infected tissue. An interrupted mass closure using a No. 2 permanent suture is typically recommended. However, if primary closure is under significant tension, a synthetic mesh bridge may be required. If the subcutaneous wound is left open, wet-to-dry dressing changes may be performed until the decision has been made to proceed with a delayed primary closure or allow secondary intention to compete the process (Cliby, 2002).

REFERENCES

Abbas S, Bissett IP, Parry BR: Oral water soluble contrast for the management of adhesive small bowel obstruction. Cochrane Database Syst Rev 1:CD004651, 2005

Abrams P: Bladder outlet obstruction index, bladder contractility index and bladder voiding efficiency: three simple indices to define bladder voiding function. Br J Urol Int 84:14, 1999

Adesanya AO, Lee W, Greilich NB, et al: Perioperative management of obstructive sleep apnea. Chest 138(6):1489, 2010

Agostini P, Cieslik, H, Rathinam S, et al: Postoperative pulmonary complications following thoracic surgery: are there any modifiable risk factors? Thorax 65(9):815, 2010

Akarsu T, Karaman S, Akercan F, et al: Preemptive meloxicam for postoperative pain relief after abdominal hysterectomy. Clin Exp Obstet Gynecol 31:133, 2004

Al Sunaidi M, Tulandi T: Adhesion-related bowel obstruction after hysterectomy for benign conditions. Obstet Gynecol 108:1162, 2006

Al Took S, Platt R, Tulandi T: Adhesion-related small-bowel obstruction after gynecologic operations. Am J Obstet Gynecol 180:313, 1999

Amaragiri SV, Lees TA: Elastic compression stockings for prevention of deep vein thrombosis. Cochrane Database Syst Rev 3:CD001484, 2000

American College of Obstetricians and Gynecologists: Antibiotic prophylaxis for gynecologic procedures. Practice Bulletin No. 104, May 2009a

American College of Obstetricians and Gynecologists: Hemorrhagic shock. Practice Bulletin No. 235, April 1997

American College of Obstetricians and Gynecologists: Informed consent. Committee Opinion No. 439, August 2009b

American College of Obstetricians and Gynecologists: Prevention of deep vein thrombosis and pulmonary embolism. Practice Bulletin No. 84, August 2007

American College of Physicians: Guidelines for assessing and managing the perioperative risk from coronary artery disease associated with major noncardiac surgery. Ann Intern Med 127(4):309, 1997

American Thoracic Society: Guidelines for the management of adults with hospital-acquired, ventilator-associated, and healthcare-associated pneumonia. Am J Respir Crit Care Med 171:388, 2005

Anderson AD, McNaught CE, MacFie J, et al: Randomized clinical trial of multimodal optimization and standard perioperative surgical care. Br J Surg 90:1497, 2003

Apfel CC, Korttila K, Abdalla M, et al: A factorial trial of six interventions for the prevention of postoperative nausea and vomiting. N Engl J Med 350:2441, 2004

Apfelbaum JL, Chen C, Mehta SS, et al: Postoperative pain experience: results from a national survey suggest postoperative pain continues to be undermanaged. Anesth Analg 97:534, 2003

Archer C, Levy AR, McGregor M: Value of routine preoperative chest x-rays: a meta-analysis. Can J Anaesth 40:1022, 1993

Arozullah AM, Daley J, Henderson WG, et al: Multifactorial risk index for predicting postoperative respiratory failure in men after major noncardiac surgery. The National Veterans Administration Surgical Quality Improvement Program. Ann Surg 232:242, 2000

Assalia A, Schein M, Kopelman D, et al: Therapeutic effect of oral Gastrografin in adhesive, partial small-bowel obstruction: a prospective, randomized trial. Surgery 115:433, 1994

Auerbach, AD: Changing the practice of perioperative cardioprotection: perioperative beta-blockers after POISE (Peri-Operative Ischemic Evaluation). Circ Cardiovasc Qual Outcomes 1(1):58, 2008

Badillo AT, Sarani B, Evans SR: Optimizing the use of blood cultures in the febrile postoperative patient. J Am Coll Surg 194:477, 2002

Baglin T, Gray E, Greaves M, et al: Clinical guidelines for testing for heritable thrombophilia. Br J Haematol 149(2):209, 2010

Barker K, Graham NG, Mason MC, et al: The relative significance of preoperative oral antibiotics, mechanical bowel preparation, and preoperative peritoneal contamination in the avoidance of sepsis after radical surgery for ulcerative colitis and Crohn's disease of the large bowel. Br J Surg 58:270, 1971

Bartlett LC: Pressure necrosis is the primary cause of wound dehiscence. Can J Surg 28:27, 1985

Bennett LL, Rosenblum RS, Perlov C, et al: An in vivo comparison of topical agents on wound repair. Plast Reconstr Surg 108:675, 2001

Bergasa NV, Jones EA: Management of the pruritus of cholestasis: potential role of opiate antagonists. Am J Gastroenterol 86:1404, 1991

Bernstein WK, Deshpande S: Preoperative evaluation for thoracic surgery. Semin Cardiothorac Vasc Anesth 12(2):109, 2008

Bodker B, Lose G: Postoperative urinary retention in gynecologic patients. Int Urogynecol J 14:94, 2003

Braga M, Gianotti L, Gentilini O, et al: Feeding the gut early after digestive surgery: results of a nine-year experience. Clin Nutr 21:59, 2002

Broder G, Weil MH: Excess lactate: an index of reversibility of shock in human patients. Science 143:1457, 1964

Bromberg JS, Alfrey EJ, Barker CF, et al: Adrenal suppression and steroid supplementation in renal transplant recipients. Transplantation 51:385, 1991

Brooks-Brunn JA: Predictors of postoperative pulmonary complications following abdominal surgery. Chest 111:564, 1997

Bucher P, Mermillod B, Gervaz P, et al: Mechanical bowel preparation for elective colorectal surgery: a meta-analysis. Arch Surg 139:1359, 2004

Calligaro KD, Azurin DJ, Dougherty MJ, et al: Pulmonary risk factors of elective abdominal aortic surgery. J Vasc Surg 18:914, 1993

Carlson MA: Acute wound failure. Surg Clin North Am 77:607, 1997

Casadei B, Abuzeid H: Is there a strong rationale for deferring elective surgery in patients with poorly controlled hypertension? J Hypertens 23:19, 2005

Chan A, Dore CJ, Ramachandra V: Analgesia for day surgery: evaluation of the effect of diclofenac given before or after surgery with or without bupivacaine infiltration. Anaesthesia 51:592, 1996

Cheatham ML, Chapman WC, Key SP, et al: A meta-analysis of selective versus routine nasogastric decompression after elective laparotomy. Ann Surg 221:469, 1995

Cheng A, Nazarian S, Spragg DD, et al: Effects of surgical and endoscopic electrocautery on modern-day permanent pacemaker and implantable cardioverter-defibrillator systems. Pacing Clin Electrophysiol 31(3):344, 2008

Chrysos E, Athanasakis E, Antonakakis S, et al: A prospective study comparing diathermy and scalpel incisions in tension-free inguinal hernioplasty. Am Surgeon 71:326, 2005

Chumillas S, Ponce JL, Delgado F, et al: Prevention of postoperative pulmonary complications through respiratory rehabilitation: a controlled clinical study. Arch Phys Med Rehabil 79:5, 1998

Chung F, Yegneswaran B, Liao P, et al: STOP questionnaire: a tool to screen patients for obstructive sleep apnea. Anesthesiology 108(5):812, 2008

Clarke-Pearson DL, Synan IS, Dodge R, et al: A randomized trial of low-dose heparin and intermittent pneumatic calf compression for the prevention of deep venous thrombosis after gynecologic oncology surgery. Am J Obstet Gynecol 168:1146, 1993

Cliby WA: Abdominal incision wound breakdown. Clinical Obstet Gynecol 45:507, 2002

Comfere T, Sprung J, Kumar M, et al: Angiotensin system inhibitors in a general surgical population. Anesth Analg 100(3):636, 2005

Condon RE, Frantzides CT, Cowles VE, et al: Resolution of postoperative ileus in humans. Ann Surg 203:574, 1986

Coon WW, Willis PW III: Recurrence of venous thromboembolism. Surgery 73:823, 1973

Correia MI, da Silva RG: The impact of early nutrition on metabolic response and postoperative ileus. Curr Opin Clin Nutr Metab Care 7:577, 2004

Correll DJ, Hepner DL, Chang C, et al: Preoperative electrocardiograms: patient factors predictive of abnormalities. Anesthesiology 110(6):1217, 2009

Cunningham FG, Leveno, KL, Bloom SL, et al (eds): Thromboembolic disorders. In Williams Obstetrics, 23rd ed, New York, McGraw-Hill, 2010, pp 1016, 1021

Dahl M: Genetic and biochemical markers of obstructive lung disease in the general population. Clin Respir J 3(2):121, 2009

Dauchel J, Schang JC, Kachelhoffer J, et al: Gastrointestinal myoelectrical activity during the postoperative period in man. Digestion 14:293, 1976

Davis JW, Shackford SR, Mackersie RC, et al: Base deficit as a guide to volume resuscitation. J Trauma Inj Infect Crit Care 28:1464, 1988

de la Torre SH, Mandel L, Goff BA: Evaluation of postoperative fever: usefulness and cost-effectiveness of routine workup. Am J Obstet Gynecol 188:1642, 2003

Devereaux PJ, Goldman L, Cook DJ, et al: Perioperative cardiac events in patients undergoing noncardiac surgery: a review of the magnitude of the problem, the pathophysiology of the events and methods to estimate and communicate risk. CMAJ 173 (6):627, 2005

Douketis JD, Berger PB, Dunn AS, et al: The perioperative management of antithrombotic therapy. Chest 133(6 Suppl):299S, 2008

Dronge AS, Perkal MF, Kancir S, et al: Long-term glycemic control and postoperative infectious complications. Arch Surg 141:375, 2006

Duncan JE, Quietmeyer CM: Bowel preparation: current status. Clin Colon Rectal Surg 22(1):14, 2009

Dunham CM, Siegel JH, Weireter L, et al: Oxygen debt and metabolic acidemia as quantitative predictors of mortality and the severity of the ischemic insult in hemorrhagic shock. Crit Care Med 19:231, 1991

Dunn AS, Spyropoulos AC, Turpie AGG: Bridging therapy in patients on long-term oral anticoagulants who require surgery: the Prospective Peri-operative Enoxaparin Cohort Trial (PROSPECT). J Thromb Haemost 5(11):2211, 2007

Durack DT: Prevention of infective endocarditis. N Engl J Med 332:38, 1995

Eagle KA, Berger PB, Calkins H, et al: ACC/AHA guideline update for perioperative cardiovascular evaluation for noncardiac surgery: executive summary. A report of the American College of Cardiology/American Heart Association Task Force on Practice Guidelines (Committee to Update the 1996 Guidelines on Perioperative Cardiovascular Evaluation for Noncardiac Surgery). Circulation 105:1257, 2002

Eichenberger A, Proietti S, Wicky S, et al: Morbid obesity and postoperative pulmonary atelectasis: an underestimated problem. Anesth Analg 95:1788, 2002

Elwyn DH, Bryan-Brown CW, Shoemaker WC: Nutritional aspects of body water dislocations in postoperative and depleted patients. Ann Surg 182:76, 1975

Engoren M: Lack of association between atelectasis and fever. Chest 107:81, 1995

Fa-Si-Oen P, Roumen R, Buitenweg J, et al: Mechanical bowel preparation or not? Outcome of a multicenter, randomized trial in elective open colon surgery. Dis Colon Rectum 48:1509, 2005

Fabian TS, Kaufman HJ, Lett ED, et al: The evaluation of subatmospheric pressure and hyperbaric oxygen in ischemic full-thickness wound healing. Am Surg 66:1136, 2000

Fekrazad HM, Lopes RD, Stashenko GJ, et al: Treatment of venous thromboembolism: guidelines translated for the clinician. J Thromb Thrombolysis 28(3):270, 2009

Ferris BG Jr, Pollard DS: Effect of deep and quiet breathing on pulmonary compliance in man. J Clin Invest 39:143, 1960

Finney SJ, Zekveld C, Elia A, et al: Glucose control and mortality in critically ill patients. JAMA 290:2041, 2003

Fleisher LA: Preoperative evaluation of the patient with hypertension. JAMA 287:2043, 2002

Fleisher LA, Beckman JA, Brown KA, et al: 2009 ACCF/AHA focused update on perioperative beta blockade incorporated into the ACC/AHA 2007 guidelines on perioperative cardiovascular evaluation and care for noncardiac surgery: a report of the American College of Cardiology Foundation/American Heart Association Task Force on Practice Guidelines. Circulation 120(21):e169, 2009

Garber AJ, Moghissi ES, Bransome ED Jr, et al: American College of Endocrinology position statement on inpatient diabetes and metabolic control. Endocr Pract 10:77, 2004

Garibaldi RA, Brodine S, Matsumiya S, et al: Evidence for the non-infectious etiology of early postoperative fever. Infect Contr 6:273, 1985

Geerts WH, Bergqvist D, Pineo GF, et al: Prevention of venous thromboembolism: American College of Chest Physicians Evidence-Based Clinical Practice Guidelines (8th ed). Chest 133(6 Suppl):381S, 2008

George RB, Allen TK, Habib AS: Serotonin receptor antagonists for the prevention and treatment of pruritus, nausea, and vomiting in women undergoing cesarean delivery with intrathecal morphine: a systematic review and meta-analysis. Anesth Analg 109(1):174, 2009

Glowniak JV, Loriaux DL: A double-blind study of perioperative steroid requirements in secondary adrenal insufficiency. Surgery 121:123, 1997

Goldman L, Caldera DL: Risks of general anesthesia and elective operation in the hypertensive patient. Anesthesiology 50:285, 1979

Goldman L, Lee T, Rudd P: Ten Commandments for effective consultations. Arch Intern Med 143:1753, 1983

Goldwasser P, Feldman J: Association of serum albumin and mortality risk. J Clin Epidemiol 50:693, 1997

Gottlieb RH, Widjaja J, Tian L, et al: Calf sonography for detecting deep venous thrombosis in symptomatic patients: experience and review of the literature. J Clin Ultrasound 27:415, 1999

Grady D, Wenger NK, Herrington D, et al: Postmenopausal hormone therapy increases risk for venous thromboembolic disease. The Heart and Estrogen/progestin Replacement Study. Ann Intern Med 132:689, 2000

Gregoratos G, Abrams J, Epstein AE, et al: ACC/AHA/NASPE 2002 guideline update for implantation of cardiac pacemakers and antiarrhythmia devices: summary article: a report of the American College of Cardiology/American Heart Association Task Force on Practice Guidelines (ACC/AHA/NASPE Committee to Update the 1998 Pacemaker Guidelines). Circulation 106:2145, 2002

Guenaga KF, Matos D, Castro AA, et al: Mechanical bowel preparation for elective colorectal surgery. Cochrane Database Syst Rev 2:CD001544, 2009

Habib AS, Gan TJ: Evidence-based management of postoperative nausea and vomiting: a review. Can J Anaesth 51:326, 2004

Hall JC, Tarala RA, Hall JL, et al: A multivariate analysis of the risk of pulmonary complications after laparotomy. Chest 99:923, 1991

Harrison L, Johnston M, Massicotte MP, et al: Comparison of 5-mg and 10-mg loading doses in initiation of warfarin therapy. Ann Intern Med 126:133, 1997

Hassan SA, Hlatky MA, Boothroyd DB, et al: Outcomes of noncardiac surgery after coronary bypass surgery or coronary angioplasty in the Bypass Angioplasty Revascularization Investigation (BARI). Am J Med 110:260, 2001

Hlatky MA, Boineau RE, Higginbotham MB, et al: A brief self-administered questionnaire to determine functional capacity (the Duke Activity Status Index). Am J Cardiol 64(10):651, 1989

Holzer P: Opioids and opioid receptors in the enteric nervous system: from a problem in opioid analgesia to a possible new prokinetic therapy in humans. Neurosci Lett 361:192, 2004

Hoogwerf BJ: Perioperative management of diabetes mellitus: how should we act on the limited evidence? Cleve Clin J Med 73(Suppl 1):S95, 2006

Huge A, Kreis ME, Zittel TT, et al: Postoperative colonic motility and tone in patients after colorectal surgery. Dis Colon Rectum 43:932, 2000

Jacober SJ, Sowers JR: An update on perioperative management of diabetes. Arch Intern Med 159:2405, 1999

Jeffery KM, Harkins B, Cresci GA, et al: The clear liquid diet is no longer a necessity in the routine postoperative management of surgical patients. Am Surg 62:167, 1996

Johnson A, Young D, Reilly J: Caesarean section surgical site infection surveillance. J Hosp Infect 64:30, 2006

Johnson BE, Porter J: Preoperative evaluation of the gynecologic patient: considerations for improved outcomes. Obstet Gynecol 111(5):1183, 2008

Joshi GP, Ogunnaike BO: Consequences of inadequate postoperative pain relief and chronic persistent postoperative pain. Anesthesiol Clin North Am 23:21, 2005

Kaafarani HMA, Borzecki AM, Itani KMF, et al: Validity of selected patient safety indicators: opportunities and concerns. J Am Coll Surg 212(6):924, 2011

Kannel WB: Epidemiology and prevention of cardiac failure: Framingham Study insights. Eur Heart J 8:23, 1987

Kearon C, Hirsh J: Management of anticoagulation before and after elective surgery. N Engl J Med 336:1506, 1997

Kearon C, Kahn SR, Agnelli G, et al: Antithrombotic therapy for venous thromboembolic disease: American College of Chest Physicians Evidence-Based Clinical Practice Guidelines (8th Edition). Chest 133(6 Suppl):454S, 2008

Keita H, Diouf E, Tubach F, et al: Predictive factors of early postoperative urinary retention in the postanesthesia care unit. Anesth Analg 101:592, 2005

Kertai MD, Bountioukos M, Boersma E, et al: Aortic stenosis: an underestimated risk factor for perioperative complications in patients undergoing noncardiac surgery. Am J Med 116:8, 2004

Kinney JM, Weissman C: Forms of malnutrition in stressed and unstressed patients. Clin Chest Med 7:19, 1986

Kirby JP, Mazuski JE: Prevention of surgical site infection. Surg Clin North Am 89(2):365, 2009

Kleeman S, Goldwasser S, Vassallo B, et al: Predicting postoperative voiding efficiency after operation for incontinence and prolapse. Am J Obstet Gynecol 187:49, 2002

Kondziolka DS, Pirris SM, Lunsford LD: Improving the informed consent process for surgery. Neurosurgery 58:1184, 2006

Kozlow JH, Berenholtz SM, Garrett E, et al: Epidemiology and impact of aspiration pneumonia in patients undergoing surgery in Maryland, 1999–2000. Crit Care Med 31:1930, 2003

Kraft R: Nausea and Vomiting. In Bope ET, Rakel RE, Kellerman R (eds): Conn's Current Therapy 2010, 1st ed, Philadelphia, Saunders Elsevier, 2010

Krebs HB, Goplerud DR: Mechanical intestinal obstruction in patients with gynecologic disease: a review of 368 patients. Am J Obstet Gynecol 157:577, 1987

Kudsk KA, Croce MA, Fabian TC, et al: Enteral versus parenteral feeding: effects on septic morbidity after blunt and penetrating abdominal trauma. Ann Surg 215:503, 1992

Kurz A, Sessler DI, Lenhardt R: Perioperative normothermia to reduce the incidence of surgical-wound infection and shorten hospitalization. Study of Wound Infection and Temperature Group. N Engl J Med 334:1209, 1996

Lau H, Lam B: Management of postoperative urinary retention: a randomized trial of in-out versus overnight catheterization. Aust N Z J Surg 74:658, 2004

Lavelle-Jones C, Byrne DJ, Rice P, et al: Factors affecting quality of informed consent. Br Med J 306:885, 1993

Lawrence VA, Dhanda R, Hilsenbeck SG, et al: Risk of pulmonary complications after elective abdominal surgery. Chest 110:744, 1996

Lee HP, Chang YY, Jean YH, et al: Importance of serum albumin level in the preoperative tests conducted in elderly patients with hip fracture. Injury 40(7):756, 2009

Lee TH, Marcantonio ER, Mangione CM, et al: Derivation and prospective validation of a simple index for prediction of cardiac risk of major noncardiac surgery. Circulation 100:1043, 1999

Levine MN, Hirsh J, Gent M, et al: Optimal duration of oral anticoagulant therapy: a randomized trial comparing four weeks with three months of warfarin in patients with proximal deep vein thrombosis. Thromb Haemost 74:606, 1995

Lewis SJ, Egger M, Sylvester PA, et al: Early enteral feeding versus "nil by mouth" after gastrointestinal surgery: systematic review and meta-analysis of controlled trials. Br Med J 323:773, 2001

Li J, Chen J, Kirsner R: Pathophysiology of acute wound healing. Clin Dermatol 25(1):9, 2007

Liao P, Yegneswaran B, Vairavanathan S, et al: Postoperative complications in patients with obstructive sleep apnea: a retrospective matched cohort study. Can J Anaesth 56(11):819, 2009

Lindenauer PK, Pekow P, Wang K, et al: Perioperative beta-blocker therapy and mortality after major noncardiac surgery. N Engl J Med 353:349, 2005

Livingston EH, Passaro EP, Jr: Postoperative ileus. Dig Dis Sci 35:121, 1990

Lundquist H, Hedenstierna G, Strandberg A, et al: CT assessment of dependent lung densities in man during general anaesthesia. Acta Radiol 36:626, 1995

Macpherson DS, Snow R, Lofgren RP: Preoperative screening: value of previous tests. Ann Intern Med 113:969, 1990

Maddali MM: Chronic obstructive lung disease: perioperative management. Middle East J Anesthesiol 19(6):1219, 2008

Mangano DT: Perioperative medicine: NHLBI working group deliberations and recommendations. J Cardiothorac Vasc Anesth 18:1, 2004

Mangram AJ, Horan TC, Pearson ML, et al: Guideline for prevention of surgical site infection, 1999. Centers for Disease Control and Prevention (CDC) Hospital Infection Control Practices Advisory Committee. Am J Infect Control 27(2):97, 1999

Mansour A, Watson W, Shayani V, et al: Abdominal operations in patients with cirrhosis: still a major surgical challenge. Surgery 122(4):730, 1997

Marik PE, Varon J: Requirement of perioperative stress doses of corticosteroids: a systematic review of the literature. Arch Surg 143(12):1222, 2008

Matros E, Rocha F, Zinner M, et al: Does gum chewing ameliorate postoperative ileus? Results of a prospective, randomized, placebo-controlled trial. J Am Coll Surg 202:773, 2006

Mayo ME, Lloyd-Davies RW, Shuttleworth KE, et al: The damaged human detrusor: functional and electron microscopic changes in disease. Br J Urol 45:116, 1973

McIntosh CA, Macario A: Managing quality in an anesthesia department. Curr Opin Anaesthesiol 22(2):223, 2009

Megibow AJ, Balthazar EJ, Cho KC, et al: Bowel obstruction: evaluation with CT. Radiology 180:313, 1991

Meyers JR, Lembeck L, O'Kane H, et al: Changes in functional residual capacity of the lung after operation. Arch Surg 110:576, 1975

Michota FA Jr: Preventing venous thromboembolism in surgical patients. Clev Clin J Med 73:S88, 2006

Mixter CG III, Meeker LD, Gavin TJ: Preemptive pain control in patients having laparoscopic hernia repair: a comparison of ketorolac and ibuprofen. Arch Surg 133:432, 1998

Moller AM, Villebro N, Pedersen T, et al: Effect of preoperative smoking intervention on postoperative complications: a randomised clinical trial. Lancet 359:114, 2002

Monk BJ, Berman ML, Montz FJ: Adhesions after extensive gynecologic surgery: clinical significance, etiology, and prevention. Am J Obstet Gynecol 170:1396, 1994

Moore FA, Feliciano DV, Andrassy RJ, et al: Early enteral feeding, compared with parenteral, reduces postoperative septic complications: the results of a meta-analysis. Ann Surg 216:172, 1992

Morykwas MJ, Argenta LC, Shelton-Brown EI, et al: Vacuum-assisted closure: a new method for wound control and treatment: animal studies and basic foundation. Ann Plastic Surg 38:553, 1997

Muzii L, Bellati F, Zullo MA, et al: Mechanical bowel preparation before gynecologic laparoscopy: a randomized, single-blind, controlled trial. Fertil Steril 85:689, 2006

Nakagawa M, Tanaka H, Tsukuma H, et al: Relationship between the duration of the preoperative smoke-free period and the incidence of postoperative pulmonary complications after pulmonary surgery. Chest 120:705, 2001

Nandi PL: Ethical aspects of clinical practice. Arch Surg 135:22, 2000

Naumann RW, Hauth JC, Owen J, et al: Subcutaneous tissue approximation in relation to wound disruption after cesarean delivery in obese women. Obstet Gynecol 85:412, 1995

Nehra V: Fluid electrolyte and nutritional problems in the postoperative period. Clinical Obstet Gynecol 45:537, 2002

Nelson R, Edwards S, Tse B: Prophylactic nasogastric decompression after abdominal surgery. Cochrane Database Syst Rev 1:CD004929, 2005

Nichols RL, Condon RE: Preoperative preparation of the colon. Surg Gynecol Obstet 132:323, 1971

Nunley JC, FitzHarris GP: Postoperative ileus. Curr Surg 61:341, 2004

Okuyama M, Ikeda K, Shibata T, et al: Preoperative iron supplementation and intraoperative transfusion during colorectal cancer surgery. Surg Today 35(1):36, 2005

O'Toole EA, Goel M, Woodley DT: Hydrogen peroxide inhibits human keratinocyte migration. Dermatol Surg 22:525, 1996

Owen J, Andrews WW: Wound complications after cesarean sections. Clin Obstet Gynecol 37:842, 1994

Pasquina P, Tramer MR, Granier JM, et al: Respiratory physiotherapy to prevent pulmonary complications after abdominal surgery: a systematic review. Chest 130:1887, 2006

Patel T: Surgery in the patient with liver disease. Mayo Clin Proc 74:593, 1999

Platell C, Hall J: What is the role of mechanical bowel preparation in patients undergoing colorectal surgery? Dis Colon Rectum 41:875, 1998

Platell C, Hall JC: Atelectasis after abdominal surgery. J Am Coll Surg 185:584, 1997

POISE Study Group: Effects of extended-release metoprolol succinate in patients undergoing non-cardiac surgery (POISE trial): a randomised controlled trial. Lancet 371(9627):1839, 2008

Qaseem A, Snow V, Fitterman N, et al: Risk assessment for and strategies to reduce perioperative pulmonary complications for patients undergoing noncardiothoracic surgery: a guideline from the American College of Physicians. Ann Intern Med 144:575, 2006

Ramsey PS, White AM: Subcutaneous tissue approximation, alone or in combination with drain, in obese women undergoing cesarean delivery. Obstet Gynecol 105:967, 2005

Riou JP, Cohen JR, Johnson H Jr: Factors influencing wound dehiscence. Am J Surg 163:324, 1992

Robinson GE, Burren T, Mackie IJ, et al: Changes in haemostasis after stopping the combined contraceptive pill: implications for major surgery. Br Med J 302:269, 1991

Roizen MF: More preoperative assessment by physicians and less by laboratory tests. N Engl J Med 342:204, 2000

Rucker L, Frye EB, Staten MA: Usefulness of screening chest roentgenograms in preoperative patients. JAMA 250:3209, 1983

Sarsam SE, Elliott JP, Lam GK: Management of wound complications from cesarean delivery. Obstet Gynecol Surv 60:462, 2005

Schey D, Salom EM, Papadia A, et al: Extensive fever workup produces low yield in determining infectious etiology. Am J Obstet Gynecol 192:1729, 2005

Seidner DL: Nutritional issues in the surgical patient. Cleve Clin J Med 73:S77, 2006

Shafii M, Murphy DM, Donovan MG, et al: Is mechanical bowel preparation necessary in patients undergoing cystectomy and urinary diversion? Br J Urol Intl 89:879, 2002

Shander A, Spence RK, Auerbach M: Can intravenous iron therapy meet the unmet needs created by the new restrictions on erythropoietic stimulating agents? Transfusion 50(3):719, 2010

Shi Y, Warner DO: Surgery as a teachable moment for smoking cessation. Anesthesiology 112(1):102, 2010

Silverberg DS, Wexler D, Sheps D, et al: The effect of correction of mild anemia in severe, resistant congestive heart failure using subcutaneous erythropoietin and intravenous iron: a randomized, controlled study. J Am Coll Cardiol 37:1775, 2001

Simon TL, Alverson DC, AuBuchon J, et al: Practice parameter for the use of red blood cell transfusions: developed by the Red Blood Cell Administration Practice Guideline Development Task Force of the College of American Pathologists. Arch Pathol Lab Med 122:130, 1998

Sirinek KR, Burk RR, Brown M, et al: Improving survival in patients with cirrhosis undergoing major abdominal operations. Arch Surg 122:271, 1987

Smetana GW: Preoperative pulmonary evaluation. N Engl J Med 340:937, 1999

Smith I, Kranke P, Murat I, et al: Perioperative fasting in adults and children: guidelines from the European Society of Anaesthesiology. Eur J Anaesthesiol 28(8):556, 2011

Stanton SL, Cardozo LD, Kerr-Wilson R: Treatment of delayed onset of spontaneous voiding after surgery for incontinence. Urology 13:494, 1979

Stein PD, Afzal A, Henry JW, et al: Fever in acute pulmonary embolism. Chest 117:39, 2000

Straus SE, McAlister FA, Sackett DL, et al: The accuracy of patient history, wheezing, and laryngeal measurements in diagnosing obstructive airway disease. CARE-COAD1 Group. Clinical Assessment of the Reliability of the Examination—Chronic Obstructive Airways Disease. JAMA 283:1853, 2000

Sullivan N, Snyder DL, Tipton K, et al: Negative pressure wound therapy device. Technology assessment report. ECRI Institute. 2009. Available at: http://www.ahrq.gov/clinic/ta/negpresswtd/negpresswtd.pdf. Accessed December 30, 2010

Suman A, Carey WD: Assessing the risk of surgery in patients with liver disease. Cleve Clin J Med 73(4):398, 2006

Tablan OC, Anderson LJ, Besser R, et al: Guidelines for preventing health-care—associated pneumonia, 2003: Recommendations of CDC and the Healthcare Infection Control Practices Advisory Committee. MMWR 53:1, 2004

Tache Y, Martinez V, Million M, et al: Stress and the gastrointestinal tract: III. Stress-related alterations of gut motor function: role of brain corticotropin-releasing factor receptors. Am J Physiol Gastrointest Liver Physiol 280:G173, 2001

Tammela T, Kontturi M, Lukkarinen O: Postoperative urinary retention: I. Incidence and predisposing factors. Scand J Urol Nephrol 20:197, 1986

Taylor G, Herrick T, Mah M: Wound infections after hysterectomy: opportunities for practice improvement. Am J Infect Control 26:254, 1998

Thomas JA, McIntosh JM: Are incentive spirometry, intermittent positive pressure breathing, and deep breathing exercises effective in the prevention of postoperative pulmonary complications after upper abdominal surgery? A systematic overview and meta-analysis. Phys Ther 74:3, 1994

Tinker JH, Tarhan S: Discontinuing anticoagulant therapy in surgical patients with cardiac valve prostheses: observations in 180 operations. JAMA 239:738, 1978

Trick WE, Scheckler WE, Tokars JI, et al: Modifiable risk factors associated with deep sternal site infection after coronary artery bypass grafting. J Thorac Cardiovasc Surg 119:108, 2000

U.S. Department of Health and Human Services: Surgeon General's call to action to prevent deep vein thrombosis and pulmonary embolism. 2008. Available at: http://www.surgeongeneral.gov/topics/deepvein/. Accessed December 12, 2010

Valantas MR, Beck DE, Di Palma JA: Mechanical bowel preparation in the older surgical patient. Curr Surg 61:320, 2004

van der Meer JT, Thompson J, Valkenburg HA, et al: Epidemiology of bacterial endocarditis in The Netherlands: I. Patient characteristics. Arch Intern Med 152:1863, 1992

Vanderlinde ES, Heal JM, Blumberg N: Autologous transfusion. Br Med J 324:772, 2002

Vessey M, Mant D, Smith A, et al: Oral contraceptives and venous thromboembolism: findings in a large prospective study. Br Med J (Clin Res Ed) 292:526, 1986

Vincent JL, Navickis RG, Wilkes MM: Morbidity in hospitalized patients receiving human albumin: a meta-analysis of randomized, controlled trials. Crit Care Med 32(10):2029. 2004

Warner DO: Preventing postoperative pulmonary complications: the role of the anesthesiologist. Anesthesiology 92:1467, 2000

Warner DO, Warner MA, Barnes RD, et al: Perioperative respiratory complications in patients with asthma. Anesthesiology 85:460, 1996

Warner MA, Divertie MB, Tinker JH: Preoperative cessation of smoking and pulmonary complications in coronary artery bypass patients. Anesthesiology 60:380, 1984

Wechter ME, Pearlman MD, Hartmann KE: Reclosure of the disrupted laparotomy wound: a systematic review. Obstet Gynecol 106:376, 2005

Weksler N, Klein M, Szendro G, et al: The dilemma of immediate preoperative hypertension: to treat and operate or to postpone surgery? J Clin Anesth 15:179, 2003

Wells PS, Hirsh J, Anderson DR, et al: Accuracy of clinical assessment of deep-vein thrombosis. Lancet 345:1326, 1995

White RH, McKittrick T, Hutchinson R, et al: Temporary discontinuation of warfarin therapy: changes in the international normalized ratio. Ann Intern Med 122:40, 1995

Wilson M, Davis DP, Coimbra R: Diagnosis and monitoring of hemorrhagic shock during the initial resuscitation of multiple trauma patients: a review. J Emerg Med 24:413, 2003

Wilson W, Taubert KA, Gewitz M, et al: Prevention of infective endocarditis: guidelines from the American Heart Association: a guideline from the American Heart Association Rheumatic Fever, Endocarditis, and Kawasaki Disease Committee, Council on Cardiovascular Disease in the Young, and the Council on Clinical Cardiology, Council on Cardiovascular Surgery and Anesthesia, and the Quality of Care and Outcomes Research Interdisciplinary Working Group. Circulation 116(15):1736, 2007

Wolters U, Wolf T, Stutzer H, et al: ASA classification and perioperative variables as predictors of postoperative outcome. Br J Anaesth 77:217, 1996

Wortel CH, van Deventer SJ, Aarden LA, et al: Interleukin-6 mediates host defense responses induced by abdominal surgery. Surgery 114:564, 1993

Wright HK, O'Brien JJ, Tilson MD: Water absorption in experimental closed segment obstruction of the ileum in man. Am J Surg 121:96, 1971

Zerah F, Harf A, Perlemuter L, et al: Effects of obesity on respiratory resistance. Chest 103:1470, 1993

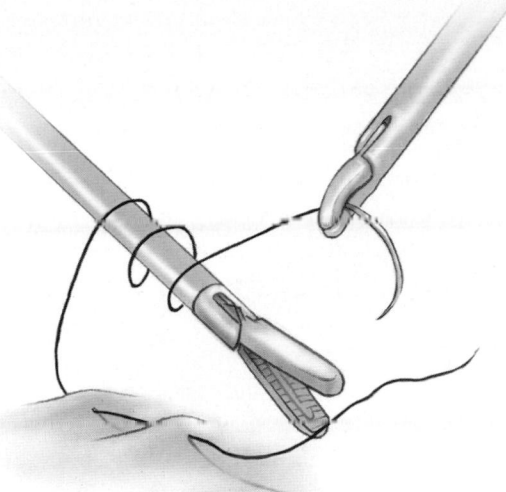

Intraoperative Considerations

Gynecologic surgery is used to treat a broad spectrum of underlying pathology. As a result, the list of surgical procedures used in gynecology is extensive, but in general, techniques maximize tissue healing and patient recovery. Successful outcomes depend upon appropriate patient and procedure selection as well as anticipation and preparation for possible complicating factors. During any procedure, intraoperative complications may be encountered, and surgeons should be familiar with these challenges and their management.

ANESTHESIA SELECTION

Perioperative morbidity and mortality rates may be significantly lowered by thorough preoperative evaluation and management. This process is the responsibility of the surgeon in concert with appropriate consultants and is discussed in detail in Chapter 39 (p. 948).

Many anesthetic options are available for patients undergoing gynecologic procedures. Typically, general anesthesia, regional epidural, or spinal technique is selected. However, paracervical blockade using local anesthetic agents may be used alone or more commonly with conscious sedation for dilation and curettage or hysteroscopy.

The delivery of these anesthetic techniques should be provided by clinicians who are skilled with their placement and are capable of managing their side effects. In general, paracervical blockade and intravenous sedation may be provided by gynecologists. General, epidural, and spinal anesthesia typically are delivered and managed by anesthesiology staff.

The selection of anesthesia for gynecologic surgery is complex. Clinical factors such as the procedure planned, extent of disease, and patient comorbidities weigh heavily in the decision process. Moreover, personal preferences of the patient, anesthesiologist, and surgeon influence choice. Lastly, the providing hospital or clinic may further define options based on their practicing norms and availability of personnel or equipment. For example, an outpatient gynecology clinic may have supporting personnel and equipment sufficient for paracervical blockade or intravenous conscious sedation but may lack sophisticated equipment or expertise required for regional or general anesthesia.

In all cases, both the anesthesia provider and the surgeon should be prepared for potential problems. Difficult patient intubation may complicate general anesthesia, whereas regional anesthetic procedures may lead to higher than anticipated levels of blockade and respiratory muscle dysfunction. Cases using paracervical blockade may be complicated by inadequate levels of anesthesia, or conversely by anesthetic toxicity. Conscious sedation may also fail to provide adequate analgesia, or alternatively, may lead to respiratory depression. Thus, no procedure is free of potential risk, and contingency plans for each should be in place.

Paracervical Block

Usage

Paracervical block is used most commonly during first-trimester pregnancy evacuation but also may be selected for cervical ablative or excisional procedures, transvaginal sonographically guided oocyte retrieval, and in-office hysteroscopy. Studies have also demonstrated improved postoperative pain control in women given preemptive analgesia with paracervical blockade prior to general anesthesia for vaginal hysterectomy (Long, 2009; O'Neal, 2003).

Paracervical blockade is often combined with nonsteroidal antiinflammatory drugs (NSAIDs) or intravenous conscious sedation or both. Conscious sedation may be achieved with several agents, but intravenous midazolam (Versed) combined with fentanyl (Sublimaze) is used frequently (Lichtenberg, 2001).

Anatomy

The cervix, vagina, and uterus are richly supplied by nerves of the uterovaginal plexus (see Fig. 38-13, p. 929). Also known as *Frankenhaüser plexus*, this plexus lies within the connective tissue lateral to the uterosacral ligaments. For this reason, paracervical injections are most effective if placed at a site immediately lateral to the insertion of the uterosacral ligaments into the uterus (Rogers, 1998).

Technique

Injection of divided doses may be given at 4 and 8 o'clock at the cervical base (Figs. 40-1 and 40-2). Alternatively, injections may be placed at 3, 6, 9, and 12 o'clock sites. However, this increased number of sites appears not to improve analgesic effects (Glantz, 2001). Importantly, anatomic structures in proximity to injection sites can lead to potential procedural risks. For example, injecting at the 3 and 9 o'clock sites risks injury to or intravascular injection into the uterine arteries. Injection at the anterolateral fornix near 2 and 10 o'clock poses potential risk to the ureters.

In most cases, total doses of 10 mL of 0.25-percent bupivacaine, 1-percent mepivacaine, or 1- or 2-percent lidocaine may be administered (Cicinelli, 1998; Hong, 2006; Lau, 1999). However, specific calculation of a maximum safe dose for each patient before injection is recommended (Dorian, 2005). The toxic dose of lidocaine approximates 4.5 mg/kg (Table 40-1). For a 50-kg woman, this would equal 225 mg. Thus, if a 1-percent lidocaine solution is used, the calculated allowed amount would be: 225 mg ÷ 10 mg/mL = 22.5 mL. Of note, for any drug solution, 1-percent = 10 mg/mL.

Anesthesia is presumed to result from pharmacologic nerve conduction blockade by the local anesthetic agent (Chanrachakul, 2001). Each drug has a different recovery time based on its individual solubility and tissue binding. Moreover, addition of epinephrine to these solutions leads to local vaso-

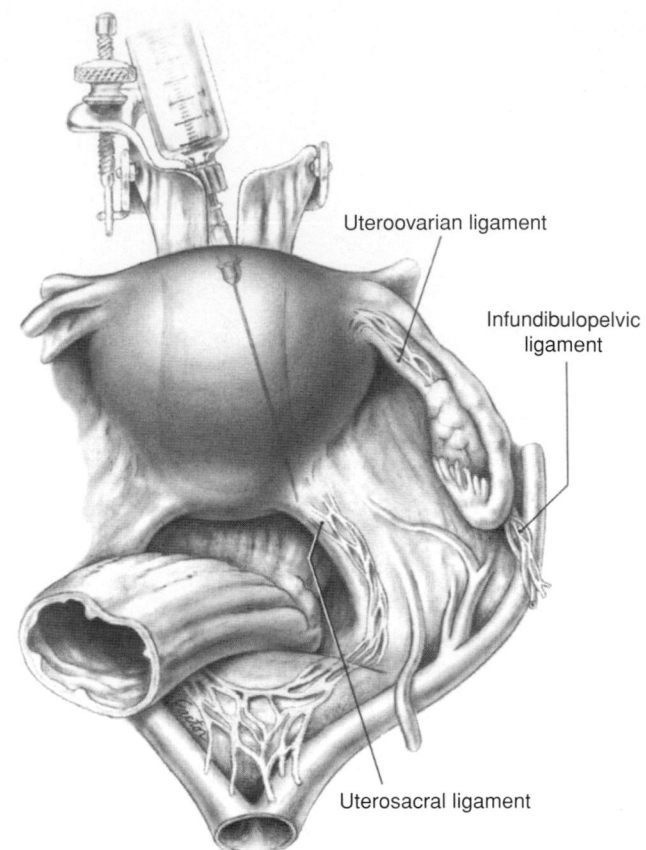

FIGURE 40-1 Abdominal view of paracervical blockade. Local anesthetics are infiltrated near sensory innervation of the cervix, which lies lateral to the uterosacral ligament. *(From Penfield, 1986, with permission.)*

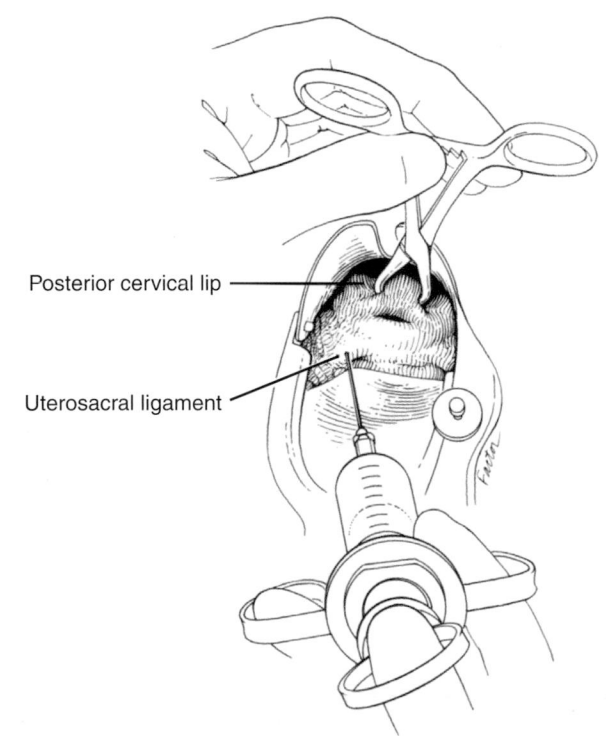

FIGURE 40-2 Vaginal approach to the injection of local anesthetics into the cervical base at 4 and 8 o'clock. *(From Penfield, 1986, with permission.)*

TABLE 40-1. Characteristics of Local Anesthetics

Drug (Brand Name)	Available Concentrations, %	Maximum, mg/kg	Maximum Dose with Epinephrine Combined, mg/kg	Duration, hour
Moderate-Duration				
Lidocaine (Xylocaine)	0.5, 1, 2	4.5	7	0.5–1
Mepivacaine (Carbocaine)	1, 1.5, 2	4	7	0.75–1.5
Prilocaine (Citanest)	0.5, 1	7	8.5	0.5–1.5
Long-Duration				
Bupivacaine (Marcaine)	0.25, 0.5, 0.75	2.5	3	2–4
Etidocaine (Duranest)	0.5, 1	4	5.5	2–3

constriction, which enhances the quality of analgesia, prolongs the duration of action, and decreases toxicity. Return of neural function is spontaneous as the drug is metabolized.

Alternatively, injection itself may have an immediate anesthetic effect by swelling surrounding tissue and exerting mechanical pressure on nerves to disrupt neural transmission. In support of this, similar pain scores were noted in women undergoing elective abortion whether a procedure began immediately after paracervical injection or following a several-minute delay to allow pharmacologic blockade (Phair, 2002; Wiebe, 1995).

Toxicity

Increased doses of local anesthetics may lead to clinically significant conduction blockade within the central nervous system (CNS) and heart. Signs range from drowsiness, tinnitus, perioral tingling, and visual disturbances to confusion, seizure, coma, and ventricular arrhythmia. In monitoring patients, surveillance for the subtle symptoms of CNS toxicity is important because the therapeutic-to-toxic ratios are often narrow with these agents.

When toxicity develops, cardiac effects are potentiated by acidosis, hypercapnia, and hypoxia. Thus, treatment of toxicity typically includes intravenous access, adequate oxygenation, and seizure control. A benzodiazepine such as diazepam (Valium) given intravenously is effective anticonvulsant therapy (Naguib, 1998). For treatment, diazepam, 2 mg/min, is administered until seizures stop or a total dose of 20 mg is delivered.

▪ Intrauterine Instillation

Although not commonly used, injection of local anesthetic through a catheter into the uterine cavity has been reported to lower pain scores in women undergoing in-office hysteroscopy or endometrial biopsy (Cicinelli, 1997; Trolice, 2000). The presumed mechanism is anesthetic blockade of nerve endings within the endometrial mucosa. Studies have used 5-mL doses of 2-percent lidocaine or of 2-percent mepivacaine.

SURGICAL SAFETY

Communication between all members of the team is vital to the success of an operation and avoidance of patient harm. The Joint Commission established the *Universal Protocol for Preventing Wrong Site, Wrong Procedure, and Wrong Person Surgery* (Joint Commission, 2009). This protocol encompasses three components: (1) preprocedure verification of all relevant documents, (2) marking the operative site, and (3) completion of a "time out" prior to procedure initiation. The "time out" requires attention of the entire team to assess that patient, site, and procedure are correctly identified. Important interactions also include introduction of the patient care team members, verification of prophylactic antibiotics, anticipated length of procedures, and communication of anticipated complications such as potential for large blood loss. Additionally, requests for special instrumentation should be addressed preoperatively to prevent the potential patient compromise that accompanies lacking an instrument at the time it is needed.

Breakdowns in communication are common across the pre-, intra-, and postoperative phases of care and are linked to adverse events and patient harm (Greenberg, 2007; Nagpal, 2010). Specifically, the transfer of a patient to a new care team or new location has been identified as a time particularly vulnerable to communication breakdowns.

SURGICAL ASSISTANT

A gynecology resident may sometimes feel that the assistant is an unimportant participant and may take a more passive role. However, the experienced surgeon is well aware of the critical difference that good assistance can provide to the flow of an operation and to patient outcomes.

The role of the assistant is to anticipate the needs of the surgeon and aid the progress of an operation. Therefore, the assistant must be familiar with the steps of the procedure to be performed, the relevant anatomy, and the details of the patient's history and physical examination.

Maintaining exposure by proper retraction and keeping the operative field clear of obstruction are the most important assistant functions. Laparotomy sponge or suction use should be timed to avoid interfering with the surgeon, and the sponge should be used to blot rather than wipe. Immediate pressure should be placed on bleeding surfaces until the situation can be assessed systematically. Clamps should be released slowly to avoid slippage of tissues. Keeping attention fixed on the procedure is imperative. Thus, if music or conversation is distracting, they should be avoided.

PATIENT POSITIONING

Anesthetized patients who undergo prolonged gynecologic procedures are at risk for peripheral neuropathy of their upper or lower extremities. These neuropathies are uncommon, and cited incidences approximate 2 percent of gynecologic cases (Cardosi, 2002). Neurologic deficits typically are mild, transient, and resolve spontaneously. However, infrequently, prolonged or permanent disability may result.

During gynecologic surgery, lower extremity injuries may involve nerves of the lumbosacral plexus (Table 40-2). In most cases, peripheral neuropathy follows improper placement of self-retaining retractors, radical pelvic dissection, or improper patient positioning, especially in the lithotomy position. Mechanisms of injury include surgical nerve transection, rupture following increased stretch, or nerve ischemia. Ischemia may result from compromise of perineural vessels during prolonged or pronounced nerve stretch or compression.

Although any patient may develop postoperative neuropathy, higher rates have been noted in patients who smoke, who have anatomic abnormalities, or who are thin, diabetic, or alcoholic. Use of self-retaining retractors and prolonged surgical duration are additional risks (Warner, 2000).

Symptoms reflect functional loss of the affected nerve. Motor loss typically manifests as muscle weakness, whereas sensory loss may be noted as anesthesia, paresthesia, or pain in the nerve's sensory distribution (Fig. 40-3). Therefore, a detailed neurologic examination allows clinical identification of most peripheral neuropathies. Electrodiagnostic testing is indicated if motor function is diminished, but in cases of sensory loss, this lacks adequate sensitivity (Knockaert, 1996). Generally, electromyography, if used, is most informative after a 2- to 3-week delay to permit denervational changes to fully develop within the affected muscles (Winfree, 2005).

Treatment will vary depending on whether motor or sensory function is affected. If motor function is impaired, neurologic consultation is typically warranted. Physical therapy should begin immediately to minimize contracture and muscle atrophy. Alternatively, for those with only mild sensory losses, observation alone for return of function is reasonable. For those with pain, treatments may include serial trigger point injection with local anesthetics, oral analgesics, biofeedback, or gabapentin.

■ Laparotomy

Nerve injury may occur at the time of laparotomy and more commonly results from poor retractor placement, wide transverse abdominal incisions, and extensive dissections at the pelvic sidewall.

Femoral Nerve Injury

The femoral nerve perforates the psoas muscle early in its course to provide motor function to the iliacus, pectineus, sartorius, and quadriceps muscles. It provides sensory function to the anteromedial thigh and to the medial leg through its cutaneous branch, the saphenous nerve. Before exiting the pelvis, the femoral nerve passes medially beneath the inguinal ligament to enter the femoral triangle lateral to the femoral artery and vein. This nerve can be compressed anywhere along its course but is particularly susceptible within the body of the psoas muscle and at the inguinal ligament. Improper placement of a self-retaining retractor is the most common cause of surgical femoral nerve injury, and rates following abdominal hysterectomy may reach 10 percent (Fig. 40-4) (Goldman, 1985; Kvist-Poulsen, 1982).

TABLE 40-2. The Lumbosacral Nerve Plexus (L1–S4)

Nerve	Origin	Motor Function	Sensory Function
Ilioinguinal	L1	None	Inferior abdominal wall, mons pubis, labia majora
Iliohypogastric	L1	None	Inferior abdominal wall, upper lateral gluteal region
Genitofemoral	L1–2	None	Labia majora, anterior superior thigh
Lateral femoral cutaneous	L2–3	None	Anterolateral thigh
Femoral	L2–4	Hip flexion, adduction; knee extension	Anterior and inferomedial thigh, medial calf
Obturator	L2–4	Thigh adduction, lateral rotation	Superomedial thigh
Pudendal	S2–4	Muscles of perineum; external anal and urethral sphincters	Perineum
Sciatic	L4–S3		
Common peroneal	L4–S2	Knee flexion; foot dorsiflexion, eversion; toe extension	Lateral calf, foot dorsum
Tibial	L4–S3	High extension; knee flexion; foot plantar flexion; inversion	Foot plantar surface, toes

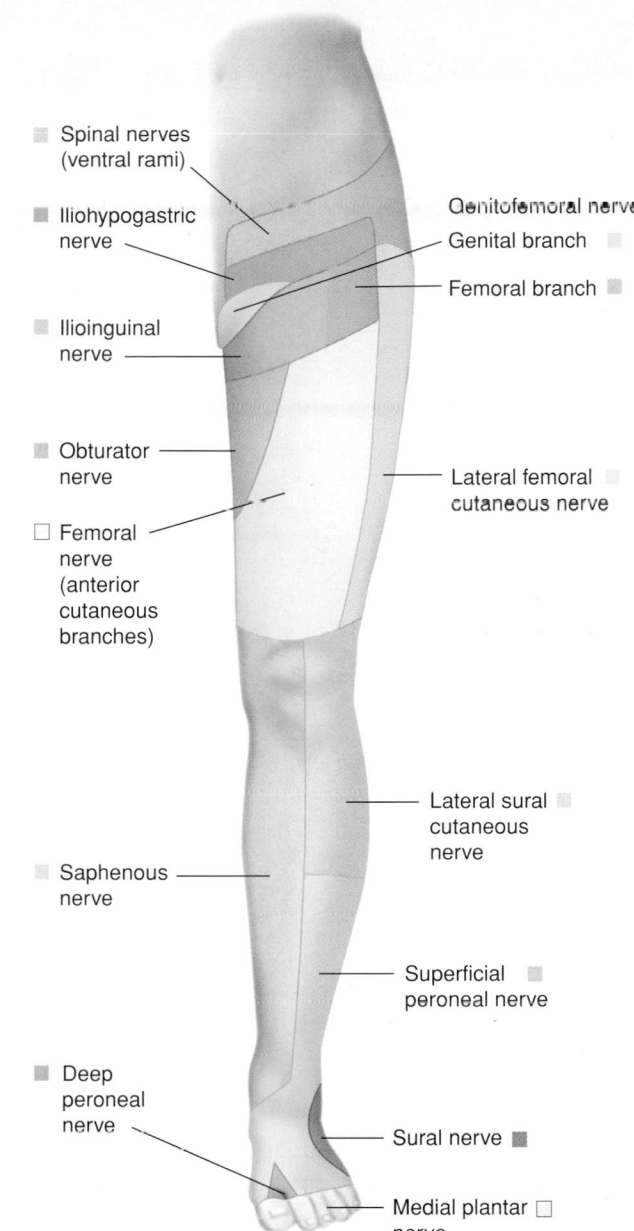

- Spinal nerves (ventral rami)
- Iliohypogastric nerve
- Ilioinguinal nerve
- Obturator nerve
- Femoral nerve (anterior cutaneous branches)
- Saphenous nerve
- Deep peroneal nerve

Genitofemoral nerve:
- Genital branch
- Femoral branch
- Lateral femoral cutaneous nerve
- Lateral sural cutaneous nerve
- Superficial peroneal nerve
- Sural nerve
- Medial plantar nerve

FIGURE 40-3 Peripheral nerves and their corresponding areas of sensory innervation.

Genitofemoral Nerve Injury

The genitofemoral nerve pierces the medial border of the psoas muscle and traverses beneath the peritoneum on this muscle's surface. Above the inguinal ligament, it divides into genital and femoral branches. The femoral branch follows the external iliac artery, continues beneath the inguinal ligament, and exits through the fascia lata to provide sensory function to the femoral triangle. The genital branch enters the inguinal canal to supply sensation to the labia majora and mons pubis. Similar to the femoral nerve, the genitofemoral nerve may suffer injury with compression of the psoas muscle, and sensory symptoms follow the distribution of the nerve (see Fig. 40-3) (Murovic, 2005). In addition, this nerve may be injured during removal of a large pelvic mass adhered to the sidewall or during pelvic lymph node dissection (Irvin, 2004).

Lateral Femoral Cutaneous Nerve Injury

This nerve appears at the lateral border of the psoas major muscle just above the crest of the ilium. It courses obliquely across the anterior surface of the iliacus muscle and dips beneath the inguinal ligament laterally as the nerve exits the pelvis. The lateral femoral cutaneous nerve may be compressed along its portion that traverses along the pelvic wall (Aszmann, 1997). Sensory symptoms extend over the anterolateral hip and thigh. Painful neuropathy specifically involving the lateral femoral cutaneous nerve carries the specific name *meralgia paresthetica*.

Transverse Incisions

Nerve injury during transverse abdominal entry is common. It typically involves the ilioinguinal and iliohypogastric nerves or less frequently, branches of the genitofemoral nerve. The ilioinguinal and iliohypogastric nerves emerge through the internal

Women with femoral neuropathy may display impaired motor function with weakness or inability to flex the hip or extend the knee. The patellar reflex is usually absent. Impaired sensory function is characterized by paresthesia over the anteromedial thigh and medial calf.

In prevention, lateral retractor blades should be selected and positioned such that only the rectus abdominis muscle and not the psoas muscle is retracted (Chen, 1995). The retractor blades should be evaluated at the time of placement to assess that they are not resting on the psoas muscle. For thin patients, folded laparotomy towels may be placed between the retractor rim and skin to elevate blades away from the psoas muscle. Importantly, a small percentage of cases occur when a retractor has not been used.

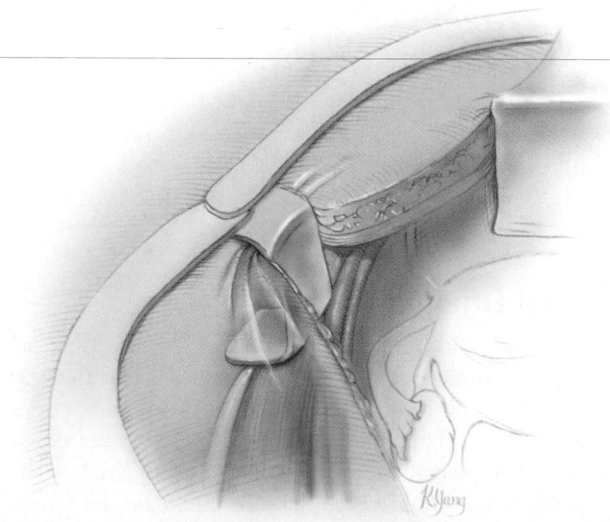

FIGURE 40-4 If poorly positioned, the lateral blade of a self-retaining retractor, pressing against the psoas major muscle, can harm the femoral nerve. Shown here in yellow, the nerve at this level runs lateral to the psoas major muscle.

oblique muscle approximately 2 to 3 cm inferomedial to the anterosuperior iliac spine (Whiteside, 2003). The iliohypogastric nerve extends a lateral branch to innervate the lateral gluteal skin. An anterior branch reaches horizontally toward the midline and runs deep to the external oblique muscle. Near the midline, this nerve perforates the external oblique muscle and becomes cutaneous to innervate the superficial tissues and skin in the region above the symphysis pubis (see Fig. 38-4, p. 921). The ilioinguinal nerve extends medially to enter the inguinal canal and innervates the lower abdomen, labia majora, and upper thigh.

These are sensory nerves, and fortunately, most skin anesthesia or paresthesias that follow their injury resolves with time. Thus, injuries frequently are underreported by both patients and clinicians. To avoid compromising these nerves, surgeons should try to avoid extending the fascial incision beyond the lateral border of the rectus muscles (Rahn, 2010).

In some cases, however, pain may result and may begin immediately following surgery or many years later. It is usually sharp and episodic and radiates to the upper thigh, labia, or upper gluteal region. Later, sensations may become chronic and burning (Ducic, 2006). Ilioinguinal/iliohypogastric nerve involvement is confirmed if an anesthetic injection placed 2 cm inferomedial to the anterosuperior iliac spine and at the depth of the external oblique muscle relieves the pain.

Pelvic Sidewall Dissection

Lymph node dissection, tumor excision, or endometriosis resection performed at the pelvic sidewall may injure the obturator or genitofemoral nerves. Moreover, the obturator nerve also can be injured during surgeries within the space of Retzius (Fig. 38-24, p. 940).

Obturator Nerve Injury

This nerve pierces the medial border of the psoas muscle and extends anteriorly along the lesser wall of the pelvis. The obturator nerve exits through the obturator foramen to supply adductor muscles of the thigh and the obturator externus muscle, which rotates the thigh laterally. Sensory innervation covers the superomedial thigh. Women with obturator neuropathy display weakness of hip adduction and of external rotation. Sensory symptoms extend over the medial thigh (Vasilev, 1994).

Dorsal Lithotomy

This surgical position is used for vaginal, laparoscopic, and hysteroscopic surgeries. It is modified and described as high, standard, or low lithotomy positions (Fig. 40-5). Dorsal lithotomy may be associated with injury to several nerves derived from the lumbosacral plexus, including the femoral, sciatic, and common peroneal nerves. For example, compression and ischemic injury of the femoral nerve beneath the rigid inguinal ligament can follow prolonged sharp flexion, abduction, and external hip rotation in dorsal lithotomy (Fig. 40-6) (Ducic, 2005; Hsieh, 1998). Ideal positioning as shown can minimize these injuries.

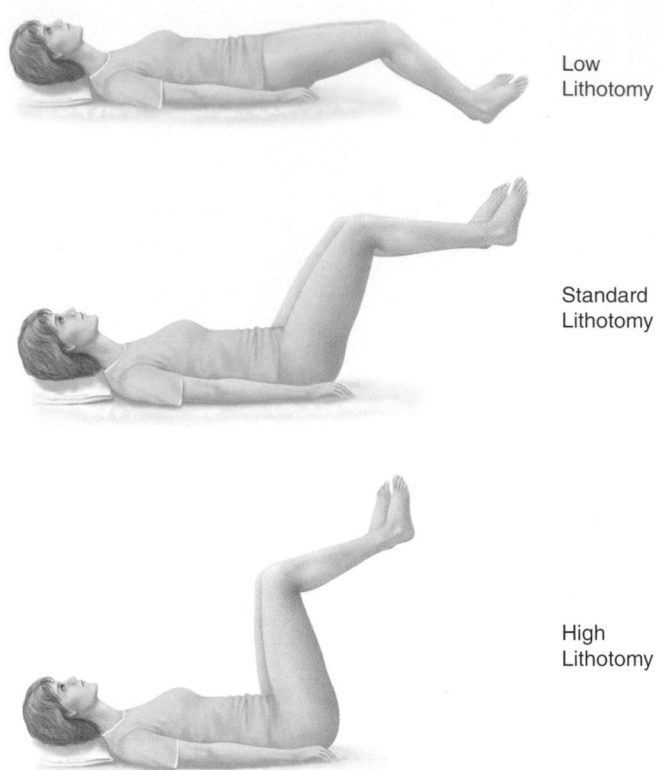

Low Lithotomy

Standard Lithotomy

High Lithotomy

FIGURE 40-5 Lithotomy positions used in gynecologic surgery.

Sciatic Nerve

Derived from the lower sacral plexus, this nerve exits the pelvis through the greater sciatic foramen. It extends down the posterior thigh and branches into the tibial nerve and common peroneal nerve above the popliteal fossa. The sciatic and common peroneal nerves are anatomically fixed at the sciatic notch and head of the fibula, respectively. Thus, stretch injury to the sciatic nerve can develop if a patient's hips are placed in sharp flexion or pronounced external rotation or both. Moreover, even an appropriately positioned patient may be injured if a surgical assistant during vaginal surgery leans against the thigh and creates extreme hip flexion.

The sciatic nerve contains tibial and common peroneal divisions, and injury may reflect impaired function of the entire sciatic nerve or only the common peroneal division. If the entire nerve is injured, impaired hip extension, knee flexion, and foot flexion are seen. In addition, sensory loss of the foot may be noted (McQuarrie, 1972). If only the common peroneal division is injured, then losses reflect those described in the next section.

Common Peroneal Nerve

Now also termed the *common fibular nerve,* the common peroneal nerve is a lateral branch of the sciatic nerve. From its origin above the popliteal fossa, this nerve crosses the lateral head of the fibula before it descends down the lateral calf. At the lateral fibular head, this nerve is at risk for compression against leg stirrups. Therefore, patient positioning that avoids pressure at this point or the addition of cushioned padding is warranted (Philosophe, 2003).

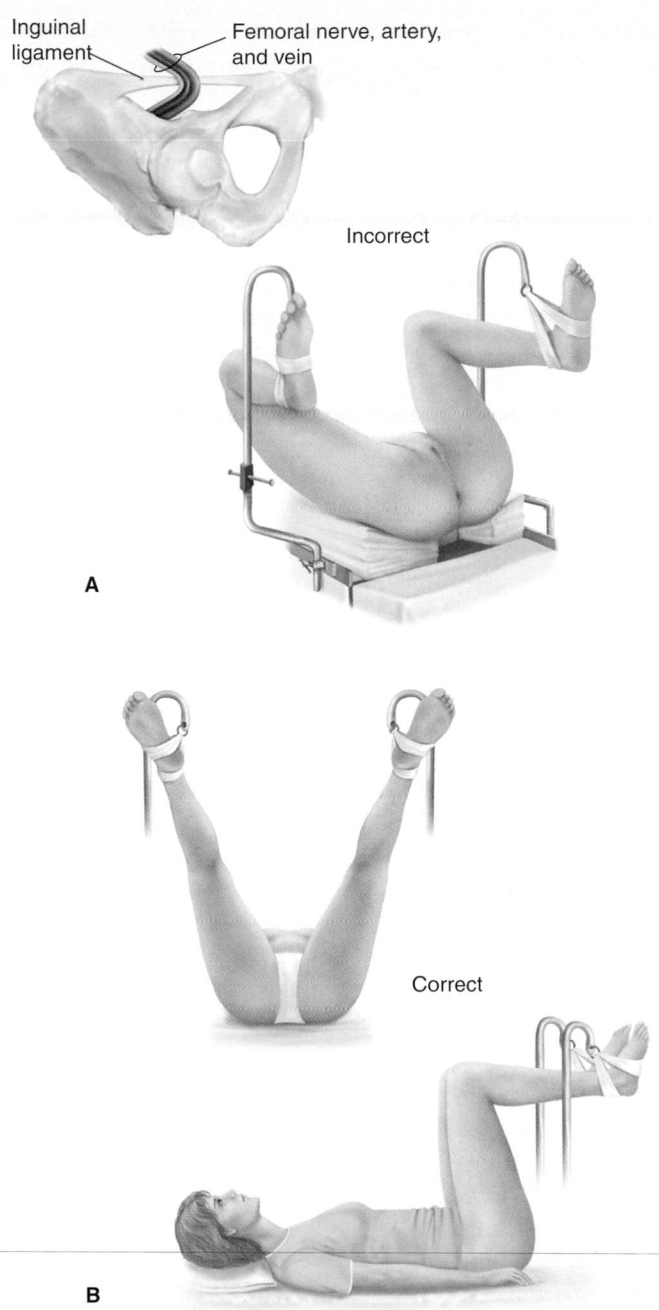

FIGURE 40-6 A. Hyperflexion of the hip can lead to compression of the femoral nerve against the inguinal ligament. *(Redrawn from Anderton, 1988, with permission.)* **B.** Ideal dorsal lithotomy positioning with limited hip flexion, abduction, and external rotation. *(Redrawn from Irvin, 2004, with permission.)*

Injury to the common peroneal nerve may have motor and sensory consequences. An inability to flex or evert the foot or extend the toes may be noted as a "foot drop" with walking. Sensory loss encompasses the foot dorsum and anterolateral leg (Tikoo, 1994).

Brachial Plexus

This plexus derives from the ventral rami of C5-T1. It traverses the neck and axilla to supply the arm and shoulder. Positioning injuries may result from hyperextension of the upper extrem-

ity, for example, when the arm is positioned at an angle to the body that exceeds 90 degrees. Additionally, even in situations in which the arm has been positioned appropriately, injury may result from inadvertently leaning up against the arm to hyperextend it. Moreover, placing the patient in steep Trendelenburg position may push the extremity into hyperextension. Injury may result in motor or sensory losses (Warner, 1998).

Peripheral ulnar neuropathies can also develop by external compression if the arm is placed at the patient's side. Padding the elbow may help to avoid this complication, although factors other than patient malpositioning may be implicated (Warner, 1998).

SURGICAL INCISIONS

In women for whom laparotomy is selected, an ideal abdominal incision allows rapid entry, affords adequate exposure, permits early ambulation, promotes strong wound healing, does not compromise pulmonary function, and maximizes cosmetic results. These criteria should form the foundation in choosing the best incision for each patient. In gynecology, entry into the abdomen typically is achieved using a midline vertical incision or one of three transverse incisions, the Pfannenstiel, Cherney, or Maylard incisions.

Midline Vertical Incision

This incision is used frequently if access to the upper abdomen and generous operating space are required. It can be extended up and above the umbilicus and thus is preferred when the preoperative diagnosis is uncertain. Moreover, simple midline anatomy allows quick entry into the abdomen and low rates of neurovascular injury to the anterior abdominal wall (Greenall, 1980; Lacy, 1994). Moreover, because of decreased midline vascularity, Nygaard and Squatrito (1996) recommend this incision in patients who have coagulopathy, decline transfusion, or are administered systemic anticoagulation.

Its greatest disadvantage stems from increased tension on the incision when abdominal muscles contract. For this reason, compared with transverse incisions, midline vertical incisions are associated with higher rates of fascial dehiscence and incisional hernia formation and poorer cosmetic results (Grantcharov, 2001; Kisielinski, 2004). Additionally, patients who have repeat vertical incisions for gynecologic indications tend to develop more adhesive disease than with transverse incisions (Brill, 1995).

Transverse Incisions

These incisions are used commonly in benign gynecologic surgery and provide several advantages. They follow Langer lines of skin tension and thus offer superior cosmetic results (Fig. 38-1, p. 919). They also carry low rates of incisional hernia formation (Luijendijk, 1997). In addition, their placement in the lower abdomen is associated with decreased postoperative pain and improved pulmonary function compared with midline vertical incisions. Of transverse incisions, Pfannenstiel incision is typically the simplest to perform, and for this reason, it is selected most commonly.

Despite these advantages, transverse incisions have limitations. These incisions limit access to the upper abdomen, and they offer smaller operating space compared with midline incisions. This is especially true of the Pfannenstiel incision and results from narrowing of the surgical field by intact rectus abdominis muscle bellies, which straddle the incision (Section 41-2, p. 1022).

Consequently, Cherney and Maylard incisions were developed to overcome this restriction, and to some degree, they do improve exposure. The Cherney incision releases the rectus abdominis muscle at its inferior tendinous insertion (Section 41-3, p. 1024). This approach affords greater exposure of pelvic organs as well as access to the space of Retzius. Its use therefore is considered when such operating exposure is needed. The Cherney incision may also be used preferentially to the Maylard incision if a Pfannenstiel incision has already been initiated, but then additional exposure is required. This is because with the Maylard incision, rectus abdominis muscles must remain invested by their fascial rectus sheath. However, if a Pfannenstiel incision has been initiated, the fascia will have already been dissected off the underlying rectus abdominis muscles.

The Maylard incision transects the rectus abdominis muscle and provides greater operative exposure and maneuvering space (Section 41-4, p. 1025). However, it is technically more difficult to perform because isolation and ligation of the inferior epigastric arteries are required. The incision is used infrequently because of concerns regarding operative pain, decreased abdominal wall strength, longer operating times, and increased febrile morbidity. Randomized studies, however, have not supported these concerns (Ayers, 1987; Giacalone, 2002). The Maylard incision should be avoided in those patients in whom the superior epigastric vessels have been interrupted, as this leaves the rectus abdominis muscles with inadequate blood supply. Also, patients with significant peripheral vascular disease may rely on the inferior epigastric arteries for collateral blood supply to their lower extremities. Ligation of this artery may lead to claudication (Salom, 2007).

Incision Creation

Entry into the abdomen begins with scalpel incision of the skin, and scars should be excised to improve wound healing and cosmetic results. Although an electrosurgical blade may be used to incise the skin, faster healing and improved appearance in general follow scalpel incision (Hambley, 1988; Singer, 2002a).

For the remaining layers, scalpel or electrosurgical blade may be selected, and investigations have found no differences in short- or long-term wound healing if either is chosen (Franchi, 2001). However, in evaluating surgical bleeding and postoperative pain, Jenkins (2003), in his review, noted an advantage with electrosurgical blade use. Regardless of type of incision or instrument used, adherence to proper technique must be emphasized: obtaining meticulous hemostasis, minimizing devitalized tissue, and avoiding creation of dead space.

WOUND CLOSURE

Following laparotomy, closure of a laparotomy incision must address the peritoneum, fascia, subcutaneous layer, and skin.

Wound closure may be broadly categorized as either primary or secondary. With primary closure, materials are used to approximate tissue layers. In closure by secondary intention, wound layers remain open and heal by a combination of contraction, granulation, and epithelialization. Secondary closure is used infrequently in gynecologic surgery and typically is indicated if tissues planned for closure contain significant infection. The option of delayed primary closure is also available in these situations once infection has resolved.

Optimal closure of a laparotomy incision is the subject of much debate. Most data on the subject stem from general surgery and gynecologic oncology studies on midline abdominal incision closure and from obstetric investigations of cesarean delivery technique. Ideally, closure avoids wound infection, dehiscence, and hernia or sinus tract formation; minimizes patient discomfort; yet preserves cosmesis to the extent possible.

Peritoneum

Neither visceral nor parietal peritoneum may require suturing, as this layer typically regenerates within days following surgery (Lipscomb, 1996). Several studies have shown that nonclosure of the peritoneum compared with closure decreases operating time without increasing adhesion formation, wound complications, or infection (Franchi, 1997; Gupta, 1998; Tulandi, 1988). However, few well-done randomized controlled trials have assessed long-term adhesion formation.

Adhesions may commonly develop between the peritoneum and adjacent organs following surgery. Scarring can be reduced by delicately handling tissues, and achieving hemostasis, and by minimizing tissue ischemia, infection, and foreign-body reaction (American Society for Reproductive Medicine, 2008).

Fascia

In many cases, the first tissue closed is fascia. Many studies have supported the use of a continuous running-stitch closure of abdominal incisions compared with interrupted closure of the fascia (Colombo, 1997; Orr, 1990; Shepherd, 1983). Continuous closure usually is faster and associated with comparable rates of dehiscence, wound infection, and hernia formation. Suture material selection tends to favor delayed-absorbable suture compared with nonabsorbable. Delayed-absorbable sutures appear to afford adequate wound support yet lead to less pain and lower rates of sinus tract formation (Carlson, 1995; Leaper, 1977; Wissing, 1987). However, the use of nonabsorbable suture should be considered in situations in which a hernia is identified or the incision has cut through previously placed mesh. A 0 gauge or No. 1 suture is suitable for closure of most fascial incisions. Sutures are placed approximately 1 cm apart and 1.2 to 1.5 cm from the fascial edge. Little additional security is attained beyond 1.5 cm (Campbell, 1989). Stitches should appose fascial edges and allow tissues to swell postoperatively without cutting through fascia or causing avascular necrosis.

Subcutaneous Adipose Layer

Collections of blood and fluid serve as potential accelerants to bacterial growth. For this reason, to decrease rates of hematoma or seroma, investigators have addressed the use of sub-cutaneous layer suture closure or drains. In those with layers less than 2 cm thick, most studies have found no advantage to either practice. However, wound infection and fat thickness are the greatest risk factors for subcutaneous layer dehiscence (Soper, 1971; Vermillion, 2000). For patients with subcuta-neous layers 2 cm or thicker, closing the subcutaneous layer has been shown to be effective (Gallup, 1996; Guvenal, 2002; Naumann, 1995). The ideal suture and technique for closure of this layer are unknown, but efforts should be made to close the dead space with attention to minimizing the suture burden and inflammatory reaction. A 2-0 gauge plain gut suture is one suitable choice, although some may favor a synthetic suture to avoid the inflammatory effects of biologic suture.

Skin

Skin may be closed effectively with staples, subcuticular sutur-ing, wound tape, or tissue adhesive. Thus, in most instances, this layer is closed according to surgeon preference. Technically, it is important that the incision line not be on tension when approximating skin. This may require subcutaneous adipose or deep dermal suturing to remove tension from the skin closure.

Subcuticular Suturing

The running subcuticular suture is placed by taking horizon-tal bites through the dermis on alternating sides of the wound using absorbable suture (Fig. 40-7). Delayed-absorbable mate-rial such as polyglactin (Vicryl) or poliglecaprone (Monocryl) in a fine gauge, such as 3-0 or 4-0, is suitable suture. Advantages include decreased cost, effective skin approximation, and no required suture removal. Of skin closure techniques, however, this method typically requires the greatest amount of time and technical expertise.

Staples

Automatic stapling devices are used commonly for surgical inci-sions and are favored because of their fast application and secure wound closure. However, they do not allow as meticulous a closure as sutures, and wounds requiring accurate approxima-tion of tissue are not ideal candidates for staple closure (Singer, 1997). Staples may be uncomfortable, may be associated with discomfort during removal, and require the patient to return for staple removal.

Before stapling, the wound edges should be everted, preferably by a second operator. The assistant precedes the operator along the wound and everts the wound edges with forceps. If the edges of a wound invert or if one edge rolls under the opposite side, a poorly formed, deep noticeable scar will result. Additionally, pressing too hard against the skin surface with the stapler should be avoided to prevent placing the staple too deep and causing ischemia within the staple loop. When placed properly, the cross-bar of the staple is elevated a few millimeters above the skin sur-face (Lammers, 2004). Staples are usually removed in 4 to 7 days. Longer periods can be linked with "track mark" scarring.

Topical Skin Adhesives

Octyl-2-cyanoacrylate (Dermabond) is a topical tissue adhesive that is applied as a liquid and polymerizes to a firm pliable film that binds to epithelium and bridges wound edges (Fig. 40-8). It can be used for closure of skin incisions that carry minimal tension such as laparoscopy trocar or transverse laparotomy incisions, or as an adjunct protective layer in larger incisions. Tissue adhesives achieve results similar to those for traditional sutures (Blondeel, 2004; Singer, 2002b).

Following approximation of deeper incision layers, the adhe-sive is applied in three thin layers superficial to apposed skin edges. The adhesive extends at least ½ cm on each side of the apposed wound edges. Attention is required to avoid placement of the liquid between skin edges because the adhesive may retard healing (Quinn, 1997). Although 30 seconds between layers for drying is required, application is fast. Moreover, adhesives cre-ate their own dressing and appear to afford some antibacterial protection (Bhende, 2002). Suture or staple removal is avoided, and the adhesive sloughs in 7 to 10 days. Showering and gentle

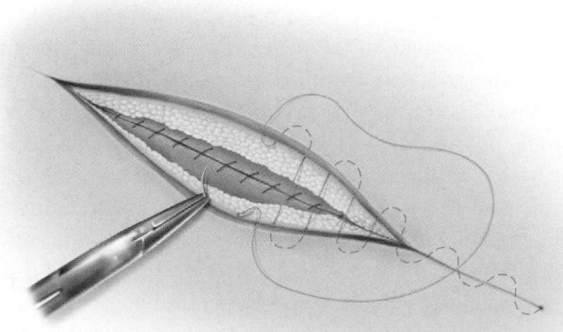

FIGURE 40-7 During subcuticular suturing, stitches are placed with a needle horizontal to the dermis. Suturing is advanced by sequentially piercing just below the dermis on alternating sides. The spot where the first stitch exits the subcutis marks the site along the wound length at which the needle should enter on the opposite side.

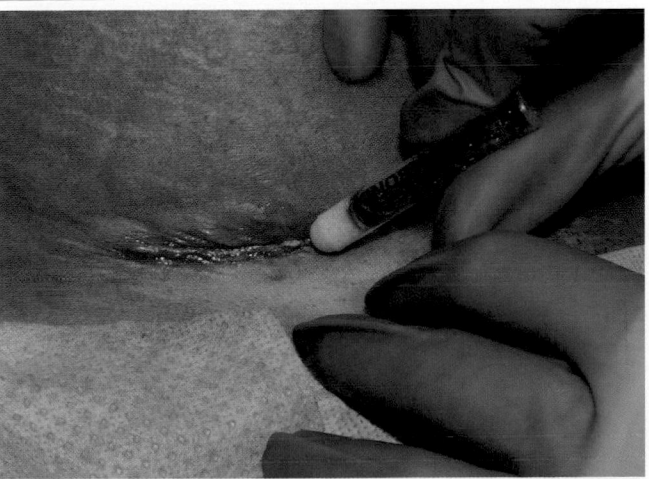

FIGURE 40-8 Application of topical skin adhesive to incision. Adhesive should be spread on top of apposed skin edges. Application should extend out approximately 0.5 cm laterally from the incision. *(Photograph contributed by Dr. Christine Wan.)*

washing of the site are allowed, but swimming is discouraged. Petroleum-based products on the wound can decrease adhesive tensile strength and should be avoided.

Adhesive Wound Tape

The primary indication for tape closure is a superficial straight laceration under little tension. Thus, it is appropriate for closure of laparoscopy trocar sites or laparotomy incisions in which deep layer closure has brought skin edges into close proximity.

Tissue closure is fast, inexpensive, and associated with high patient satisfaction. Tapes typically are removed by the patient several days following surgery. They may also be used after staple removal to provide additional strength, as wounds have only regained approximately 3 percent of their final strength at 1 week.

Prior to application, skin edges should be thoroughly dry for proper adhesion. Adhesive tape strips are applied in a parallel, nonoverlapping fashion after coating the entire application area with adjuvant adhesive such as tincture of benzoin (Katz, 1999). Tape may not be appropriate for a wet or oozing wound, for concave surfaces such as the umbilicus, for areas of significant tissue tension, or for areas of marked tissue laxity. Moreover, tape may loosen prematurely in approximately 3 percent of cases. Importantly, skin blistering may develop if tape is stretched excessively taught across the wound (Lammers, 2004; Rodeheaver, 1983).

INSTRUMENTS

Surgical instruments have been designed to extend the capability of a surgeon's hands and thus are crafted to retract, cut, grasp, and clear the operative field. It is important that operating room lighting be adjusted before the team is scrubbed and that surgeons be positioned at the table to provide the most ergonomic access for the planned procedure. Traditional instrument handling is meant to maximize efficient use of tools, although variations exist to accomplish specific tasks. Tissue types encountered in gynecologic surgery vary, and accordingly, so too do the size, fineness, and strength of the tools used.

■ Scalpel and Blades

Typical surgical blades used in gynecologic surgery are pictured in Figure 40-9 and include No. 10, 11, 15, and 20 blades.

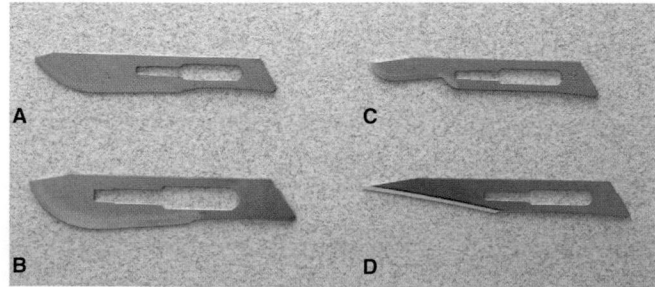

FIGURE 40-9 Photograph of surgical blades commonly used in gynecology. **A.** No. 10. **B.** No. 20. **C.** No. 15. **D.** No. 11. *(Photograph contributed by Dave Gresham.)*

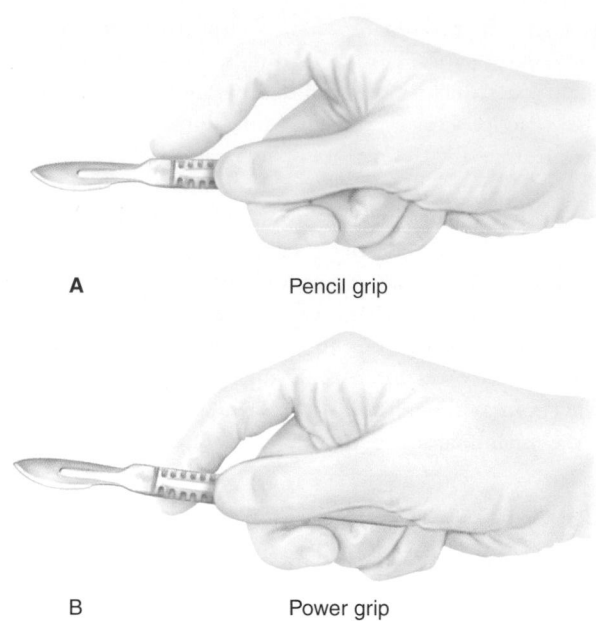

A   Pencil grip

B   Power grip

FIGURE 40-10 A. The scalpel is held as one would a pencil, and movement is directed by the thumb and index finger. **B.** The scalpel is held between the thumb and index finger. Both exert downward pressure, and the end of the blade is forced up against the thenar muscles of the hand. *(From Wind, 1987, with permission.)*

Function follows form, and larger blades are used for coarser tissues or larger incisions, whereas a No. 15 blade is selected for finer incisions. The acute angle and pointed tip of a No. 11 blade can easily incise tough-walled abscesses for drainage, such as those of the Bartholin gland duct.

With correct scalpel grasping, a surgeon can direct blade movement. Fingers may be positioned to straddle the scalpel, termed the "power grip," "violin grip," or "bow grip," which maximizes the use of the knife belly. Alternatively, the scalpel is held like a pencil, termed the "pencil grip" or "precision grip" (Fig. 40-10).

With the No. 10 and No. 20 blades, the scalpel is held at a 20- to 30-degree angle to the skin and drawn firmly along the skin using the arm with minimal wrist and finger movement. This motion aids cutting with the full length of the scalpel belly and avoids burying the tip. In general, a surgeon cuts toward him or herself and from nondominant to dominant sides. The initial incision should penetrate the dermis, maintaining the scalpel perpendicular to the surface to prevent beveling of the skin edge. Firm and symmetrical traction on the lateral aspect of the incision keeps the incision straight and helps avoid multiple tracks and irregular skin edges.

The No. 15 and No. 11 blades, in contrast, are typically held using the pencil grip to make fine, precise incisions. With the No. 15 blade, the scalpel is held approximately 45 degrees to the skin surface. Fine knife dissection is best controlled using the fingers, and the heel of the hand can be stabilized on adjacent tissue. The No. 11 blade scalpel is ideal for stab incisions and is held upright at nearly 90 degrees

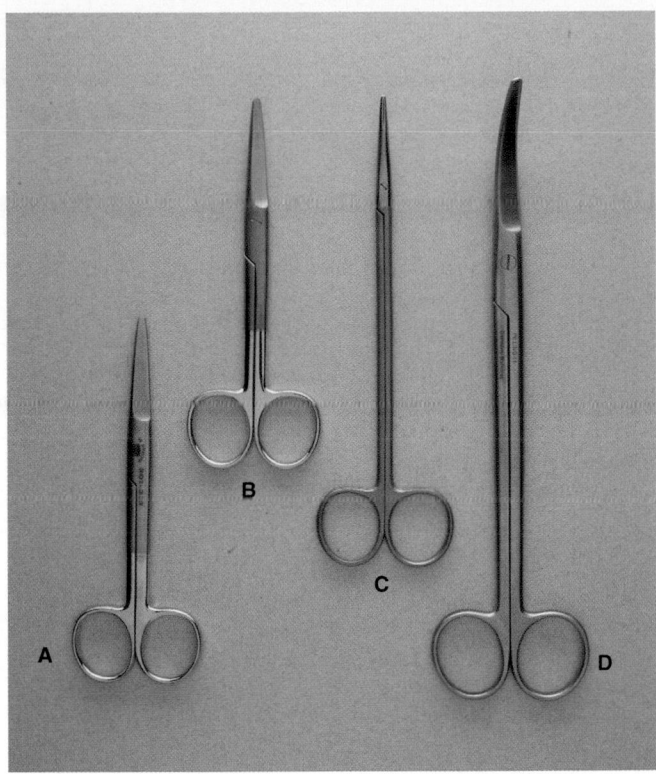

FIGURE 40-11 Scissors. **A.** Straight Mayo. **B.** Curved Mayo. **C.** Metzenbaum. **D.** Jorgenson. *(Photograph contributed by U.S. Surgitech, Inc.)*

to the surface. Creating tension at the skin surface is important to reduce the amount of force required for penetration. Omission of this can result in uncontrolled penetration of underlying structures.

Scissors

Scissors are used commonly to divide tissues, and modification in blade shape and size allows their use in a variety of tissue textures (Fig. 40-11). For correct positioning, the thumb and fourth finger are placed within the instrument's rings, and the index finger is set against the crosspiece of the scissors for greater control. This "tripod" grip allows maximum shear, torque, and closing forces to be applied and provides superior stability and control. In general, surgeons cut away from themselves and from dominant to nondominant sides.

The fine blades of Metzenbaum or iris scissors are used routinely to dissect or define natural tissue planes such as dividing thin adhesions or incising peritoneum or vaginal epithelium. During dissection, traction on opposing poles of the tissue to be dissected typically simplifies the process, and a small nick is often necessary to enter the correct tissue plane. The blades are closed and inserted between planes, following the natural curves of tissues being dissected (Fig. 40-12). The blades are opened and then withdrawn. After turning both wrist and blades 90 degrees, the surgeon reinserts the lower blade, and tissues are divided. When dissecting around a curve, the scissors should follow the natural curve of the structure. Dissection proceeds in the same plane to avoid burrowing into the structure or deviating away and toward unintended adjacent tissues.

Sturdier scissors such as curved Mayo scissors are used on thicker, denser tissues. Similarly, Jorgenson scissors have thick blades and tips that are curved at a 90-degree angle. These are used commonly to separate the vagina and uterus during the final steps of hysterectomy. Suture-cutting scissors have blunt, flat blades and should be reserved for this function. Use of tissue scissors for suture cutting often can dull their blades and should be avoided.

Needle Holders

These may be straight or curved, and commonly, one with straight, blunt jaws is chosen during routine tissue approximation and pedicle ligation (Fig. 40-13). Needles ideally pierce tissues perpendicularly. Thus, in most cases, the needle holder grasps a needle at a right angle and at a site approximately two-thirds from the needle tip.

Alternatively, some needle holders, such as the Heaney needle holder, are curved and aid needle placement in confined or

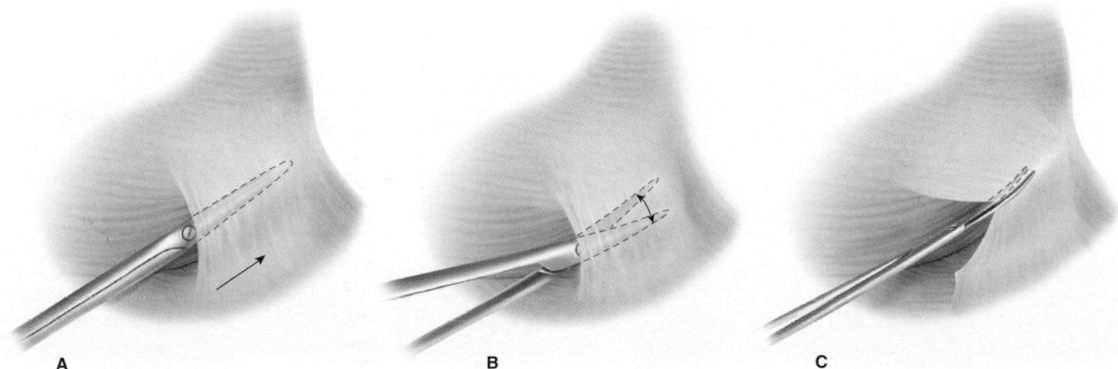

FIGURE 40-12 A. During development of tissue planes, the tips of closed Metzenbaum scissors are placed at the border between two tissues, and forward pressure is applied to advance the tips. **B.** Scissors are spread to expand the tissue plane. **C.** The scissors are retracted and rotated 90 degrees. The lower blade is reinserted into the newly created tissue plane, and tissues are divided.

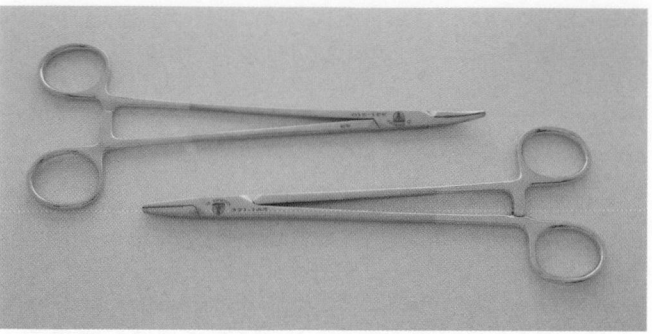

FIGURE 40-13 Needle drivers. Curved needle driver (*above*). Straight needle driver (*below*). (*Photograph contributed by U.S. Surgitech, Inc.*)

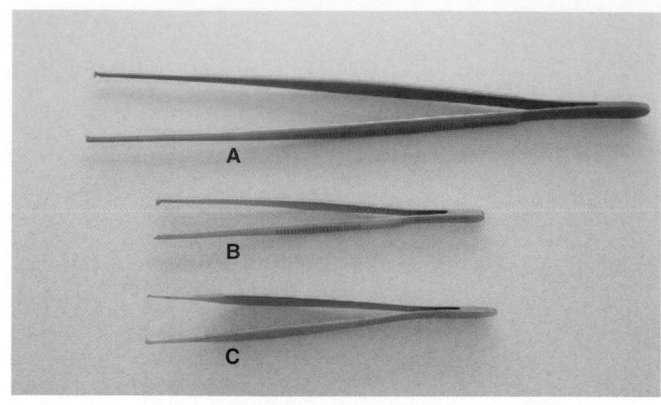

FIGURE 40-15 Toothed thumb forceps. **A** & **B.** Long and short tissue. **C.** Adson. (*Photograph contributed by U.S. Surgitech, Inc.*)

angled areas. If a curved holder is used, the needle is grasped similarly, and the inner curve of the holder faces the needle swage (Fig. 40-14).

Traditionally, the needle holder is held with the thumb and fourth finger in the rings. The greatest advantage of this grip is the precision afforded when manipulating needles. The spring tension of the handles can be relieved from the lock in a controlled fashion, thereby releasing and regrasping the needle more precisely.

Alternatively, with the "palmar grip," the needle holder is held between the ball of the thumb and the remaining fingers, and no fingers enter the instrument rings. This grip allows a simple rotating motion for driving curved needles through an arc. Its greatest advantage is the time saved during continuous suturing, as the needle can be released, regrasped, and redirected efficiently without replacing fingers into the instrument rings. Disadvantageously, this grip has the potential to lack precision during needle release. When unlocking the needle driver, release of the spring lock should be smooth and gradual. This avoids an abrupt release, which may suddenly pop the handles apart with potential for awkwardness, loss of needle control, and tissue injury.

Tissue Forceps

Forceps function to hold tissue during cutting, to retract tissue for exposure, stabilize tissue during suturing, extract needles, grasp vessels for electrosurgical coagulation, pass ligatures around hemostats, and pack sponges. Forceps are held so that one blade functions as an extension of the thumb and the other as an extension of the opposing fingers. Alternate grips may appear awkward and limit the full range of wrist motion, leading to suboptimal instrument use.

Heavy-toothed forceps, such as the Potts-Smith single-toothed forceps, Bonney forceps, and Ferriss-Smith forceps, are used when a firm grasp is more important than gentle tissue handling. These tools are most commonly used to hold fascia for abdominal wound closure (Fig. 40-15).

Light-toothed forceps, such as the single-toothed Adson, concentrate force on a tiny area and give more holding power with less tissue destruction. These are used for more delicate work on moderately dense tissue such as skin. Nontoothed forceps, also known as smooth forceps, exert their grip through serrations on the opposing tips (Fig. 40-16). They are typically used for delicate tissue handling and provide some holding power with minimal injury. DeBakey forceps are another type of smooth forceps originally designed as vascular forceps but can be occasionally used for other delicate tissues. In contrast, the broader, shallow-grooved tips of Russian forceps and Singley forceps may be preferred if a broader or thicker area of tissue is manipulated.

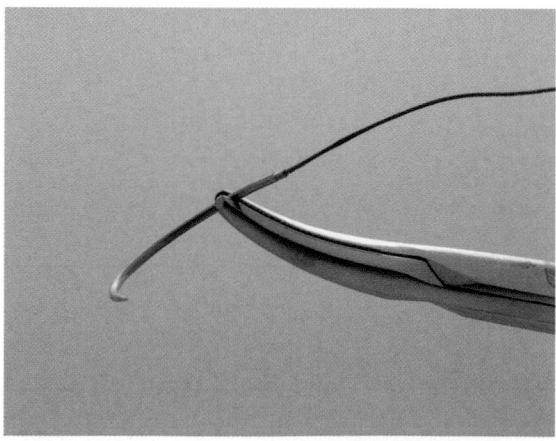

FIGURE 40-14 Correct grasp of a needle using a curved needle holder. The curve of the tips faces the needle swage. (*Photograph contributed by U.S. Surgitech, Inc.*)

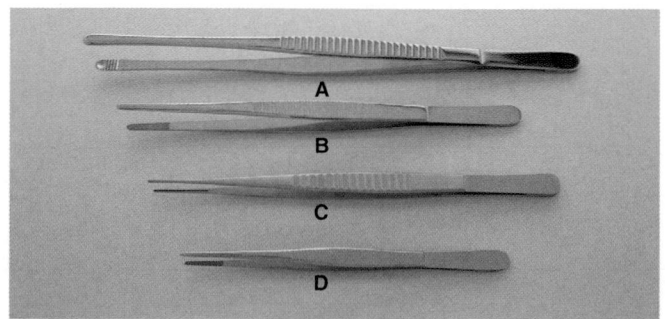

FIGURE 40-16 Smooth tissue forceps. **A.** Russian. **B** & **D.** Long and short dressing. **C.** DeBakey. (*Photograph contributed by U.S. Surgitech, Inc.*)

Retractors

Clear visualization is essential during surgery, and retractors conform to body and organ angles to allow tissues to be pulled back from an operative field. In gynecology, retractors may be grouped broadly as self-retaining or handheld and as abdominal or vaginal.

Retractors Used in Abdominal Surgery

Self-Retaining Retractors. Abdominal surgery often requires active participation of an assistant surgeon around a confined incision. Thus, retractors that by themselves hold abdominal wall muscles apart, termed *self-retaining*, are used commonly during laparotomy. Styles such as the Kirschner and O'Connor-O'Sullivan contain four broad, gently curved blades and retract in four directions. Blades pull the bladder caudally, the anterior abdominal wall muscles laterally, and the packed upper abdominal contents cephalad. The Balfour retractor retracts in three directions, but can be made to retract in four with the addition of an upper arm attachment (Fig. 40-17). Alternatively, ring-shaped retractors such as the Bookwalter and Denis Browne styles offer greater variability in the number and positioning of retractor blades. However, these usually require more time to assemble and place. With most of these styles, deep or shallow blades can be attached to the outer metal frame according to the abdominal cavity depth. As discussed earlier, blades should be shallow enough to avoid compression of the femoral and genitofemoral nerves.

Handheld Retractors. Handheld retractors may be used in addition to or in place of self-retaining styles. These instruments allow retraction in only one direction but can be placed and repositioned quickly (Fig. 40-18). The Richardson retractor has a sturdy, shallow right-angled blade that can hook around an incision for abdominal wall retraction. Alternatively, Deaver retractors have a gentle arching shape and conform easily to the curve of the anterior abdominal wall. Compared with Richardson retractors, they offer increased blade depth and are used commonly to retract bowel, bladder, or anterior abdominal wall muscles. A Harrington retractor, also called a *sweetheart retractor,* has a broader tip that also effectively holds back packed bowel.

In certain instances, such as during suturing of the vaginal cuff, a thin, deep retractor blade, termed a *malleable retractor,* may be required to retract or protect surrounding organs.

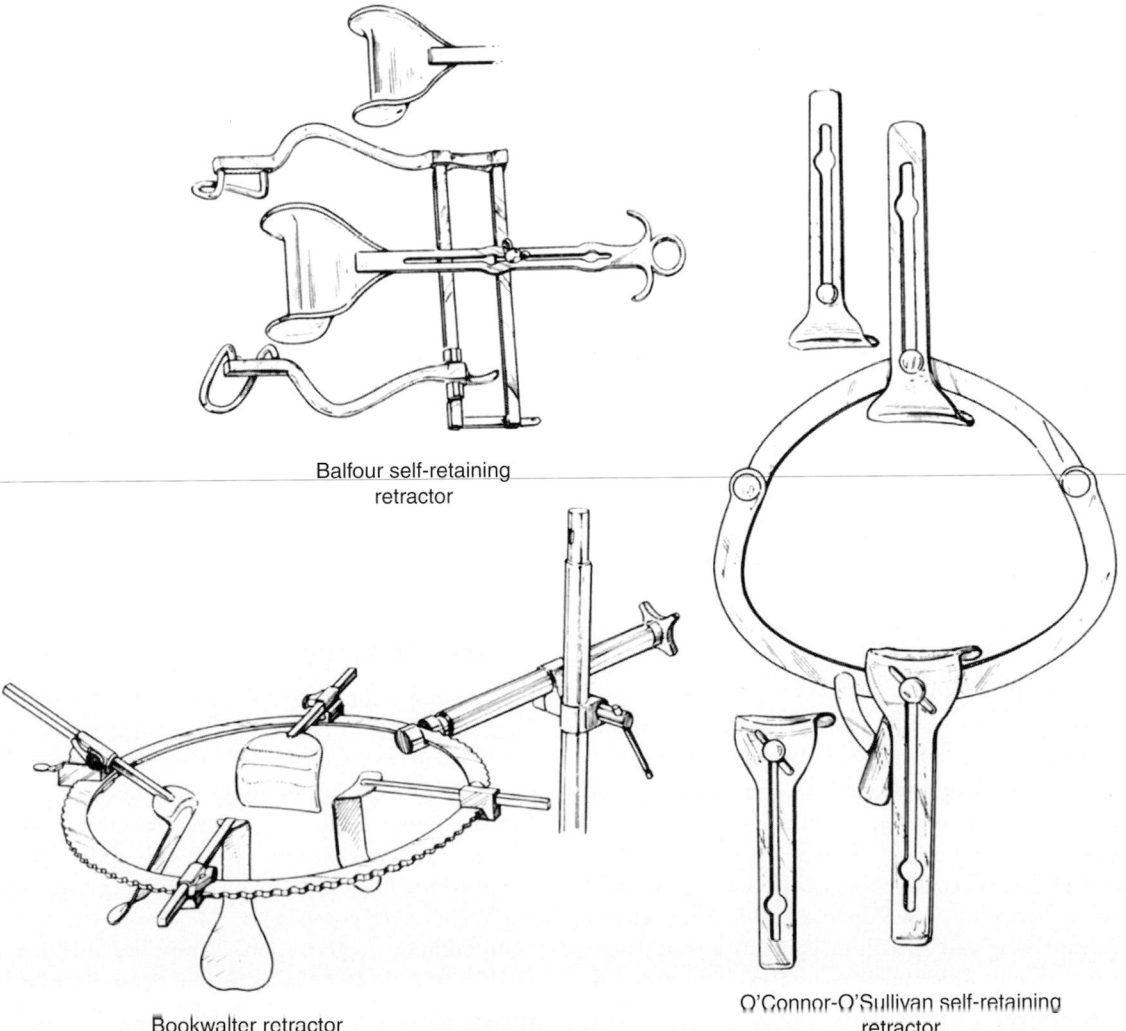

Balfour self-retaining
retractor

Bookwalter retractor

O'Connor-O'Sullivan self-retaining
retractor

FIGURE 40-17 Abdominal self-retaining retractors. *(From Lipscomb, 1997, with permission.)*

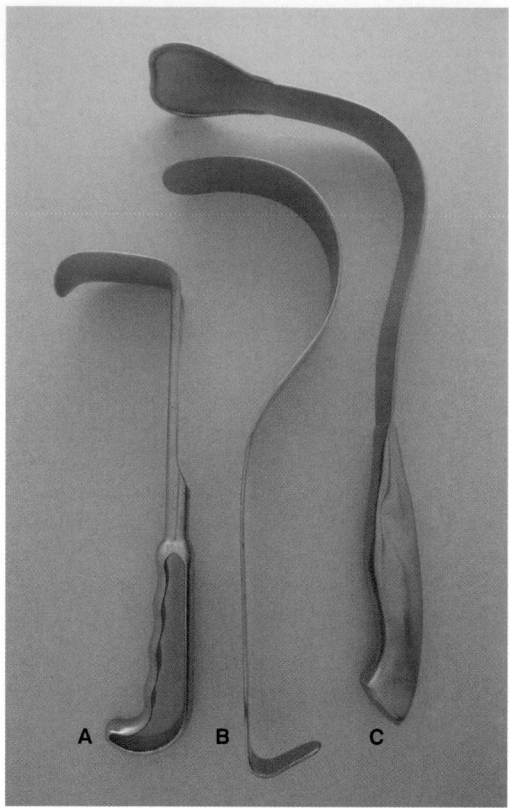

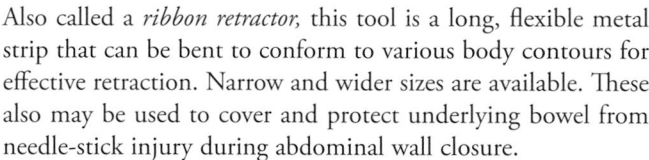

FIGURE 40-18 Long handheld abdominal retractors. **A.** Richardson. **B.** Deaver. **C.** Harrington. *(Photograph contributed by U.S. Surgitech, Inc.)*

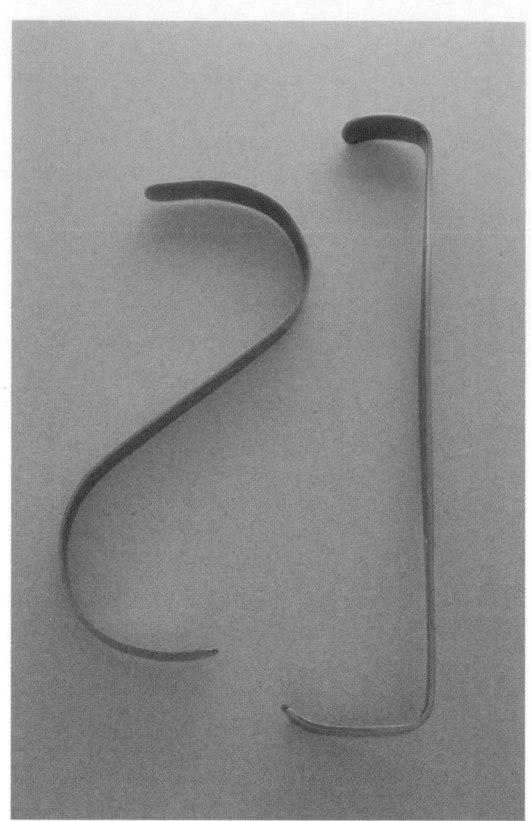

FIGURE 40-19 Short handheld abdominal retractors. S-retractor *(left)*. Army–Navy *(right)*. *(Photograph contributed by U.S. Surgitech, Inc.)*

Also called a *ribbon retractor,* this tool is a long, flexible metal strip that can be bent to conform to various body contours for effective retraction. Narrow and wider sizes are available. These also may be used to cover and protect underlying bowel from needle-stick injury during abdominal wall closure.

For laparoscopy or minilaparotomy incisions, the preceding retractors are too large, and those with smaller blades such as the Army-Navy retractor or S-retractor are selected. S-retractors offer thinner, deeper blades, whereas the sturdier blades of the Army–Navy style allow stronger retraction (Fig. 40-19). Additionally, a metal Weitlaner or synthetic Alexis or Mobius self-retaining retractor may be used for minilaparotomy incisions as well (Fig. 42-9.8, p. 1143).

Retractors Used in Vaginal Surgery

Vaginal surgery requires separation of the vaginal walls, and several self-retaining models have been designed for this purpose. The Gelpi retractor has two narrow teeth that are placed distally against opposing lateral vaginal walls and is most appropriate for perineal procedures (Fig. 40-20). The Rigby retractor, with its longer blades, effectively separates lateral vaginal walls, whereas a Graves speculum holds apart anterior and posterior walls. An Auvard weighted speculum contains a long single blade and ballasted end, which uses gravity to pull the posterior vaginal wall downward (Fig. 40-21).

The degree of retraction offered by vaginal self-retaining retractors, however, at times may be limited. Therefore, hand-

held retractors are often required to augment or replace these instruments. Handheld retractors used in vaginal surgery include the Heaney right-angle retractor, the narrow Deaver retractor, and the Breisky-Navratil retractor (Fig. 40-22).

During vaginal procedures, the cervix often must be manipulated. Lahey thyroid clamps offer a secure grip during vaginal hysterectomy, but their several sharp teeth can cause significant trauma. These are therefore less than ideal in patients in whom the cervix will remain. In these patients, in whom curettage or laparoscopy is performed, a single-toothed tenaculum can afford a firm grip but with less cervical damage (Fig. 40-23).

■ Tissue Clamps

Retraction is a fundamental requirement during most gynecologic surgery. As a result, various shapes, sizes, and strengths of clamps have been created to manipulate the different tissues encountered. For example, the smooth, cupped jaws of a Babcock clamp are ideal for gentle elevation of fallopian tubes, whereas the serrated teeth of the Allis and Allis-Adair clamps can provide a fine, firm grip on covering epithelia or serosa during dissection (Fig. 40-24).

In addition to retraction, clamps are also used to occlude vascular and tissue pedicles during organ excision. Hemostats and Mixter right-angle clamps have small, slender jaws with fine inner transverse ridges to atraumatically grasp delicate tissue, especially vessels (Fig. 40-25).

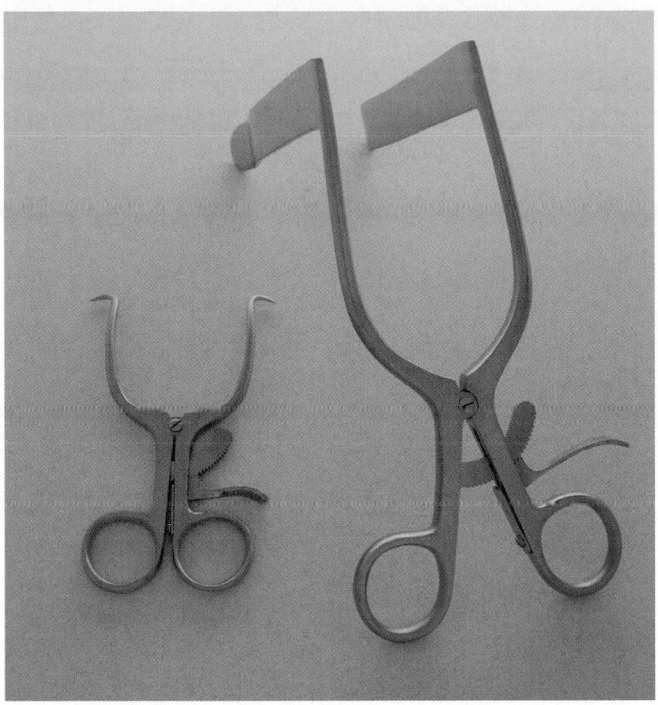

FIGURE 40-20 Vaginal self-retaining retractors. Gelpi retractor (*left*). Rigby retractor (*right*). (*Photograph contributed by U.S. Surgitech, Inc.*)

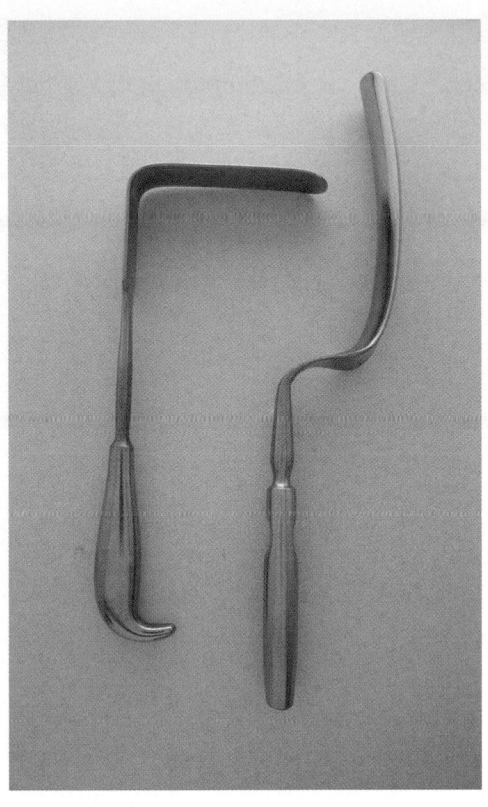

FIGURE 40-22 Vaginal handheld retractors. Heaney right-angle retractor (*left*). Breisky-Navratil retractor (*right*). (*Photograph contributed by U.S. Surgitech, Inc.*)

Heavier clamps are required to grasp and manipulate stiffer tissues such as fascia and include Pean (also termed Kelly) and Kocher (also termed Oschner) clamps (Fig. 40-26). These clamps have finely spaced transverse grooves along their inner jaws to minimize tissue slippage. They may be straight or curved to fit tissue contours and as with Kocher clamps, may contain a set of inter-

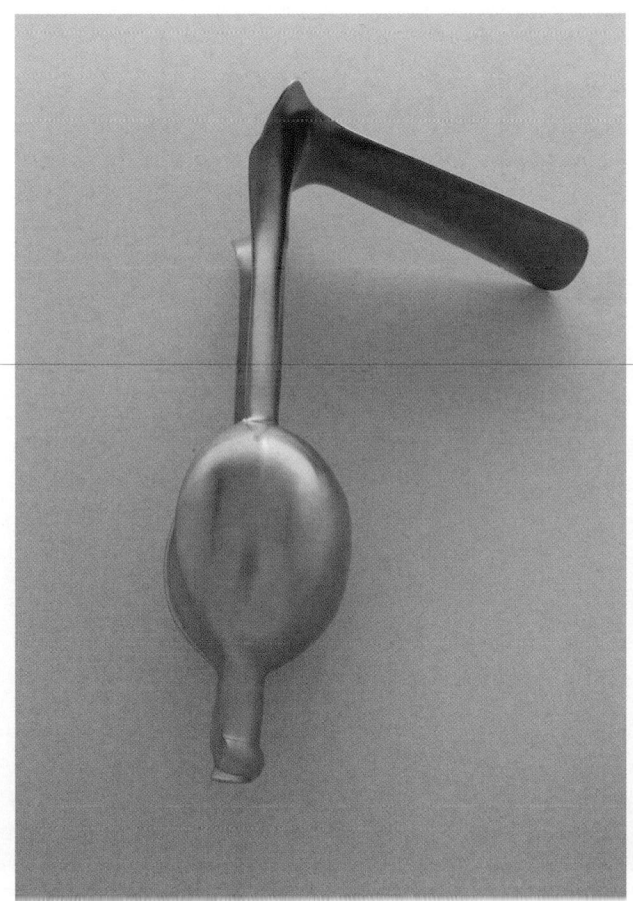

FIGURE 40-21 Auvard weighted vaginal speculum. (*Photograph contributed by U.S. Surgitech, Inc.*)

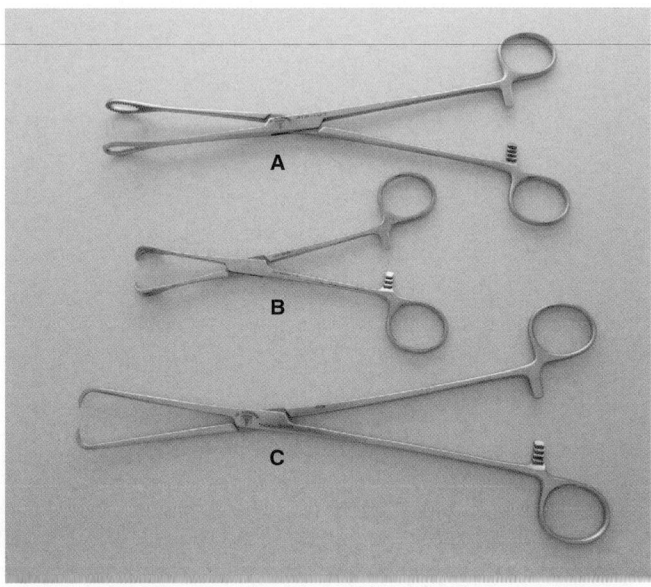

FIGURE 40-23 **A.** Ring forceps. **B.** Lahey-thyroid clamp. **C.** Single-toothed tenaculum. (*Photograph contributed by U.S. Surgitech, Inc.*)

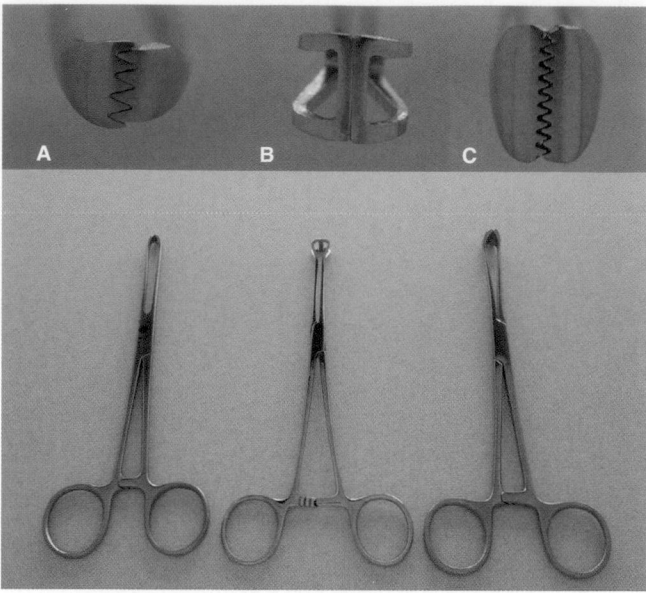

FIGURE 40-24 Tissue clamps. **A.** Allis. **B.** Babcock. **C.** Allis-Adair. *(Photograph contributed by U.S. Surgitech, Inc.)*

locking teeth at the tip for additional grip security. Another choice, the ring forceps, has large circular jaws with fine transverse grooves. These may be used to grasp broad, flat surfaces. Additionally, a folded gauze sponge can be placed between its jaws and used to absorb blood from the operative field or gently retract tissues.

Ligaments that support the uterus and vagina are fibrous and vascular. Thus, a sturdy clamp that resists tissue slippage from its jaws is required during hysterectomy. A number of clamps, including Heaney, Ballantine, Rogers, Zeppelin, and Masterson clamps, are effective (Fig. 40-27). The thick, durable jaws of these clamps carry deep, finely spaced grooves or serra-

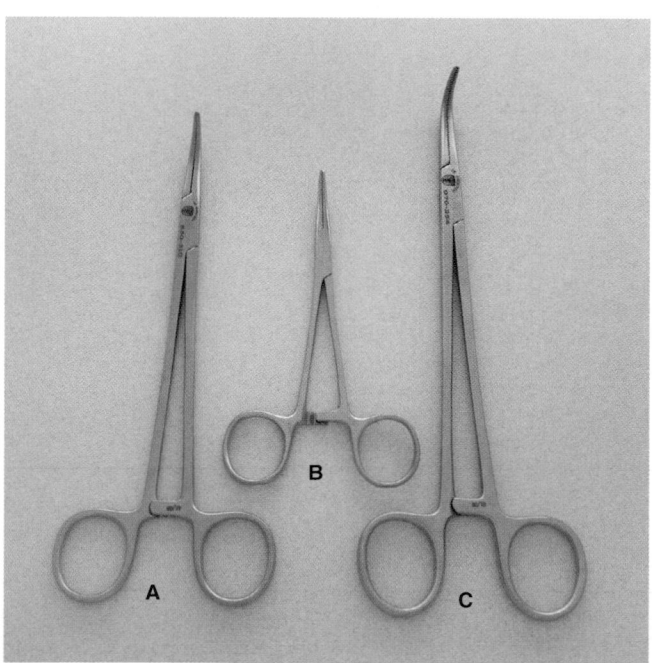

FIGURE 40-25 Vascular clamps. **A.** Tonsil. **B.** Hemostat. **C.** Mixter right-angle clamp. *(Photograph contributed by U.S. Surgitech, Inc.)*

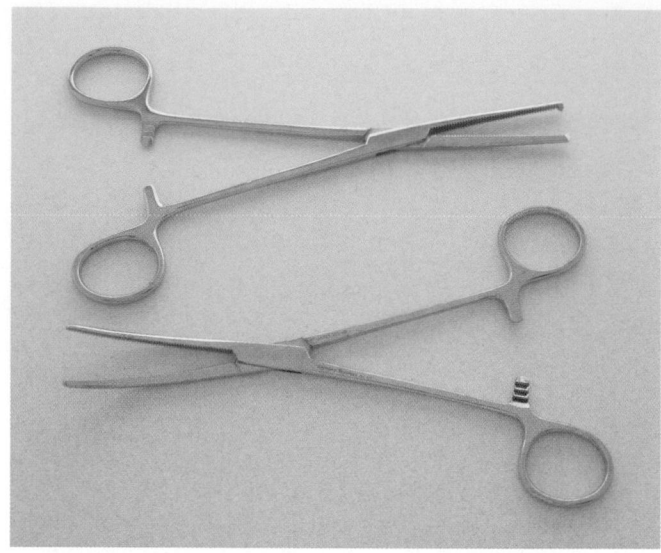

FIGURE 40-26 Curved Kocher clamp (*above*). Pean clamp (*below*). *(Photograph contributed by U.S. Surgitech, Inc.)*

tions arranged either transversely or longitudinally for secure tissue grasping. Additionally, some contain a set of interlocking teeth at the tip or heel or both. Although this modification improves grip, it also may increase tissue trauma. These clamps are also constructed with varying degrees of angling at the tip (Fig. 40-28). More acutely angled clamps are typically selected when available operating space is cramped.

Suction Tips

During gynecologic surgery, bleeding, peritoneal fluids, pus, ovarian cyst contents, and irrigants may obscure the operating field. Accordingly, choice of suction tip typically is dictated by the type and amount of fluid encountered. Adson and Frazier suction tips are fine bore and are useful in shallow or confined areas and when little bleeding is noted (Fig. 40-29).

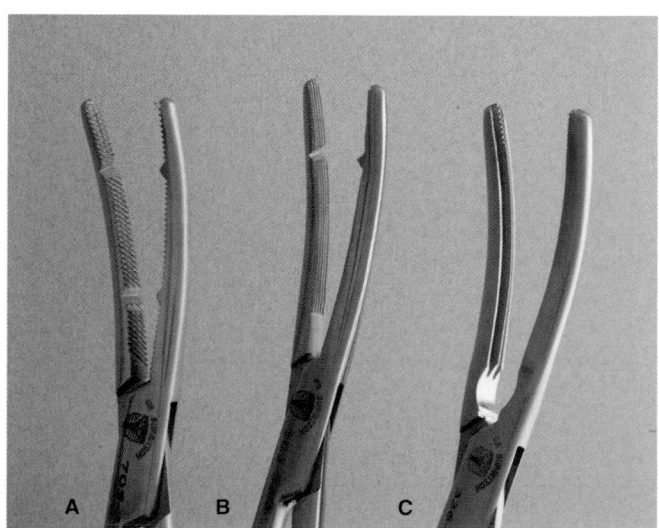

FIGURE 40-27 Heavy tissue clamps. **A.** Heaney. **B.** Heaney-Ballantine. **C.** Zeppelin. *(Photograph contributed by U.S. Surgitech, Inc.)*

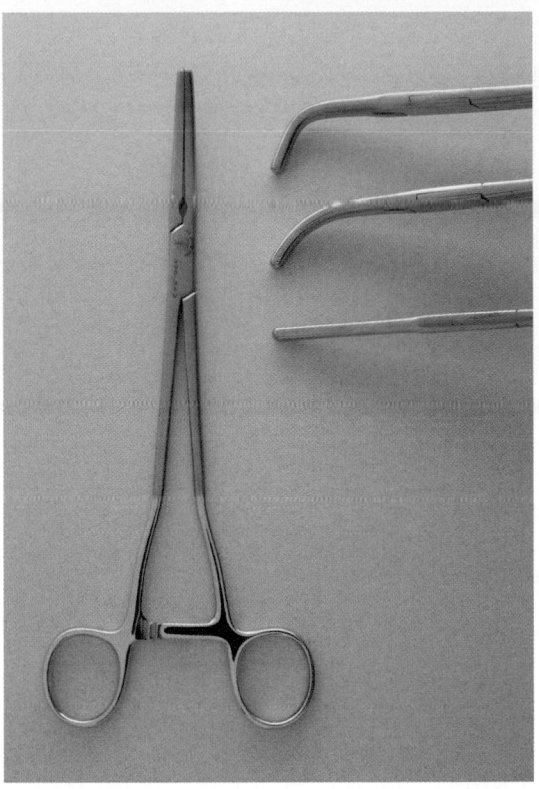

FIGURE 40-28 Heavy tissue clamps, such as the Heaney clamp, are available with increasingly curved tips. Tips with a right angle are helpful for clamping tissue deep in the pelvis when space is limited. *(Photograph contributed by U.S. Surgitech, Inc.)*

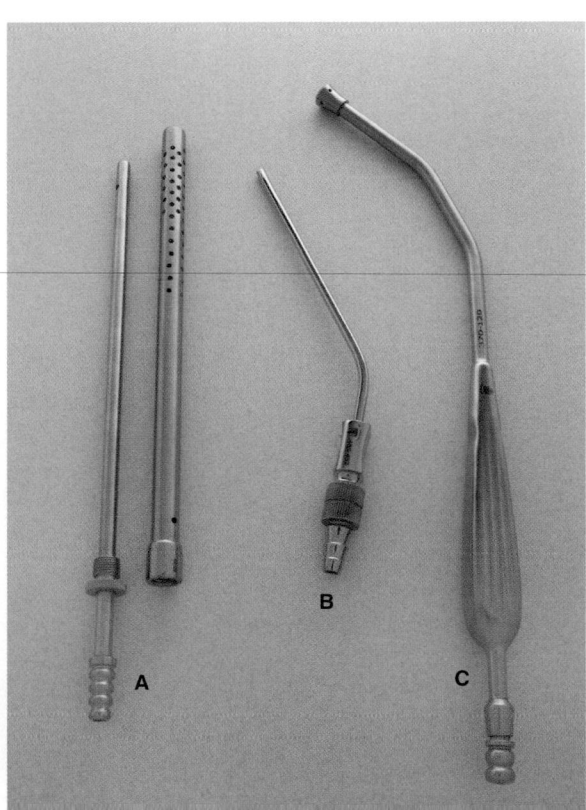

FIGURE 40-29 Suction tips. **A.** Poole. **B.** Frazier. **C.** Yankauer. *(Photograph contributed by U.S. Surgitech, Inc.)*

Alternatively, a Yankauer suction tip offers a midrange-sized tip and is used commonly in general gynecology cases. However, if a larger volume of fluid or blood is expected, then a Poole suction tip may be desired. Its multiple pores allow continued suction even if some are obstructed with clot or tissue. In addition to removing large volumes of fluid quickly, this suction tip's sieved sheath may be removed. The thinner-bore inner suction cannula can then be used for finer suctioning. Larger-bore Karman suction cannulas are used for products of conception evacuation and are discussed in Section 41-16 (p. 1059).

NEEDLES, SUTURES, AND KNOTS

These are foundational tools of tissue approximation, vessel ligation, and wound closure. They are crafted in a variety of strengths, shapes, and sizes to meet surgical needs. Appropriate selection can profoundly affect wound healing and patient recovery. Thus, surgeons should be familiar with their characteristics and most appropriate applications.

Needles

The ideal surgical needle pierces tissue with ease, with minimal tissue damage, and without bending or breaking. Tissues differ in their density and location, and thus needles are designed with variable sizes, shapes, and tips.

Needle Construction

The anatomy of a needle is simple, and each contains a tip, body, and site of suture attachment (Fig. 40-30). For most gynecologic cases, the suture and needle used are attached as a continuous unit, which is described as *swaged*. This contrasts with needles that have eyes for suture threading. Swaged needles may be firmly

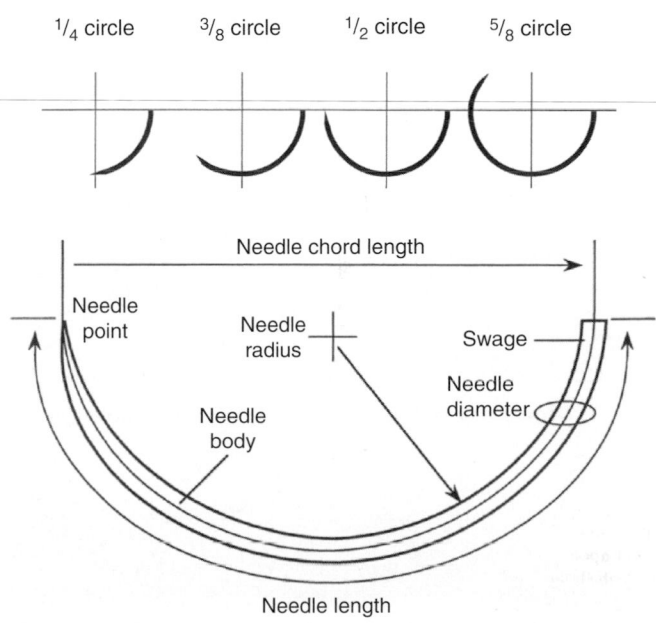

FIGURE 40-30 Various needle configurations and characteristics of a curved surgical needle. *(Modified from Dunn, 2005, with permission.)*

secured to the suture and require cutting at the end of suturing. Alternatively, *controlled-release*, or "pop-off," swaged needles detach from the suture with a brisk tug. Controlled-release needles are used commonly when securing vascular pedicles or placing interrupted sutures. Continuous running suturing typically requires a swaged needle without the controlled-release feature.

In certain urogynecologic procedures, such as abdominal sacrocolpopexy, *double-armed suture* is often chosen. This suture contains identical swaged needles at each of its ends. This design enables surgeons to suture distant tissues with different ends of the suture before approximating them.

Descriptors of needle size and shape are noted in Figure 40-30. Of these, needle radius, circle configuration, and gauge more frequently influence selection. For example, a needle should be large enough to pass completely through the tissue and exit far enough to allow the needle holder to be repositioned on the end of the needle at a safe distance from the tip. Repeated grasping of the needle tip leads to a dulled tip. A dulled tip subsequently leads to difficult tissue penetration and greater tissue trauma.

For thicker tissues, a larger radius and gauge are warranted. For confined surgical spaces, a needle with smaller radius and greater circle configuration typically is required. Thus, for most gynecologic procedures, a three-eighths or one-half circle configuration is used. For some urogynecologic operations, a five-eighths circle configuration is preferred.

Needle Point

The tip should allow passage of the needle through tissue with the smallest degree of tissue damage. Those with tapered points are used for suturing thin tissues, such as peritoneum (Figs. 40-31 and 40-32). Alternatively, cutting needles are preferred for denser tissue such as fascia and ligaments.

Cutting points have sharp edges laterally and a third sharp edge extending either toward or away from the needle's inner curve. A conventional cutting needle features the third cutting edge on the inside curve and provides shallower tissue bites. In contrast, reverse cutting needles have the third cutting edge

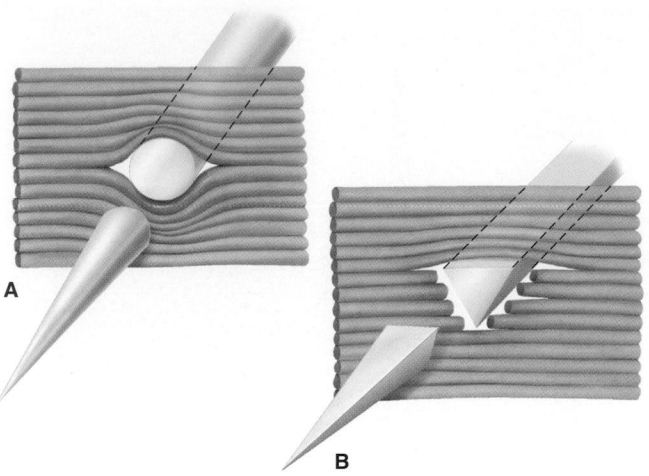

FIGURE 40-32 The bodies of these needles are cut to show the tissue cutting effects of different needles. Taper needles **(A)** pierce through tissue with less trauma than cutting needles **(B)**.

directed away from the inner curve of the needle and are used for particularly tough tissues.

Sutures

Sutures should maximize wound healing and tissue support. Thus, surgeons should be familiar with the qualities of a particular suture for a given clinical setting (Table 40-3 and 40-4). In addition, sutures may be categorized by their biologic or synthetic derivation, their filamentous structure, and their ability to be degraded and reabsorbed.

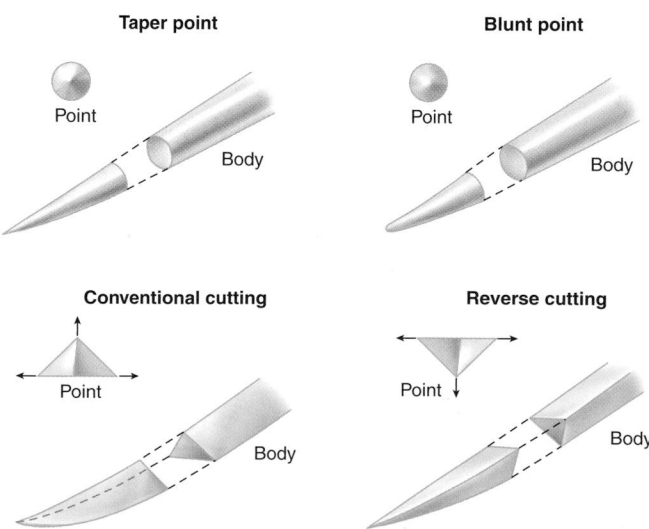

FIGURE 40-31 Configurations of various needle tips and bodies. *(Modified from Dunn, 2005, with permission.)*

TABLE 40-3. Characteristics of Suture Material

I. Physical characteristics
Physical configuration
Capillarity
Fluid absorption ability
Diameter (caliber)
Tensile strength
Knot strength
Elasticity
Plasticity
Memory

II. Handling characteristics
Pliability
Tissue drag
Knot tying
Knot slippage

III. Tissue reaction characteristics
Inflammatory and fibrous cell reaction
Absorption
Potentiation of infection
Allergic reaction

From Bennett, 1988, with permission.

CHAPTER 40

TABLE 40-4. Specific Suture Material Characteristics

Type	Configuration	Tensile Strength	Handling	Knot Security	Reactivity
Nonabsorbable					
Silk	Braided	Good	Good	Good	High
Nylon	Monofilament	High	Fair	Fair	Low
Prolene	Monofilament	Good	Poor	Poor	Low
Mersilene	Braided synthetic	High	Good	Good	Moderate
Ethibond	Braided, coated	High	Fair	Fair	Moderate
Stainless steel wire	Monofilament	High	Poor	Good	Low
Novafil	Monofilament	High	Fair	Poor	Low
Absorbable					
Gut (plain)	Twisted	Poor	Fair	Poor	Low
Chromic (gut)	Twisted	Poor	Fair	Poor	High
Dexon	Braided	Good	Good	Good	Low
Vicryl	Braided	Good	Good	Fair	Low
PDS II	Monofilament	Good	Fair	Poor	Low
Monocryl	Monofilament	Fair	Good	Good	Low

Biologic or Synthetic Sutures

Sutures such as catgut, silk, linen, and cotton are derived from biologic sources. As a group, biologic sutures produce the greatest tissue reaction and have the lowest tensile strength profile. Accordingly, most suture materials currently used in gynecologic surgery are synthetic.

Monofilament or Multifilament Suture

The number of strands that comprise a given suture defines it either as *monofilament* or *multifilament*. Monofilament suture is constructed as a single strand, whereas multifilament suture contains multiple strands that are braided or twisted. Monofilament sutures have lower friction coefficients and therefore pull more easily through tissues. As a result, they create less tissue injury and as a group, tend to incite less tissue reaction. Moreover, braid crevices are absent, and bacteria therefore are less likely to adhere (Bucknall, 1983; Sharp, 1982). However, monofilament sutures are in general less pliant for knot tying and if nicked by instruments, are more prone to breakage.

Absorbable or Nonabsorbable Suture

The rate at which tensile strength is lost differentiates suture types, and suture that has lost most of its tensile strength by 60 days following surgery is considered to be *absorbable* (Bennett, 1988). Absorbable suture is destroyed enzymatically or hydrolyzed, whereas nonabsorbable suture persists and ultimately is encapsulated.

Ideally, absorbable suture material remains throughout wound healing but no longer. Individual tissue characteristics typically dictate whether short- or long-term sutures are required for adequate wound healing. Thus, nonabsorbable suture is indicated when long-term approximation or support is required. Accordingly, nonabsorbable material plays a greater role in pelvic floor reconstruction procedures, whereas absorbable suture is used routinely in general gynecologic surgery.

Reactivity

All sutures, when placed within tissue, will incite inflammation. This response mirrors the total amount of suture placed and the suture's chemical composition (Edlich, 1973). In general, lower inflammatory responses are elicited by monofilament structure compared with multifilament, and by synthetically derived compared with natural fiber (Lin, 2006; Sharp, 1982).

Capillarity and Fluid Absorption

The ease with which fluid wicks from the wet end of a suture to its dry end defines its *capillarity*. A suture's *fluid absorption ability* describes the amount of fluid it absorbs when immersed. Both properties are presumed to have an impact on the access of contaminating bacteria. Increased capillarity and fluid absorption ability greatly increase the number of bacteria similarly absorbed (Blomstedt, 1977). In general, multifilament sutures, even those with coatings, display greater capillarity compared with synthetic monofilament sutures (Geiger, 2005).

Caliber

The diameter of a suture reflects its size and is measured in tenths of a millimeter (Table 40-5). A midpoint diameter size is designated as 0, and as suture diameter increases above this, Arabic numbers are assigned. For example, No. 1 catgut is thicker than 0 catgut.

As suture diameter decreases from this midpoint, 0s are added. By convention, an Arabic number followed by a 0 also may be used to reflect the total number of 0s. For example, 3-0 suture also may be represented as 000. Moreover, 3-0 suture is greater in diameter than 4-0 (0000) suture.

Ideally, the appropriate suture caliber is fine enough to limit tissue damage during placement and minimize subsequent

TABLE 40-5. Suture Designation

U.S.P. Designation	Synthetic Absorbable Diameter (mm)
5	0.7
4	0.6
3	0.6
2	0.5
1	0.4
0	0.35
2-0	0.3
3-0	0.2
4-0	0.15
5-0	0.1
6-0	0.07
7-0	0.05
8-0	0.04
9-0	0.03
10-0	0.02

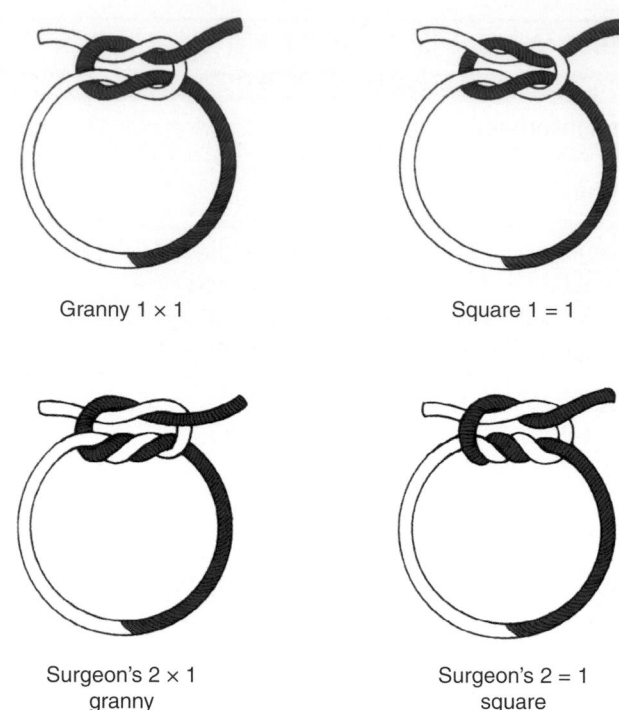

Granny 1 × 1   Square 1 = 1

Surgeon's 2 × 1 granny   Surgeon's 2 = 1 square

FIGURE 40-33 Surgical knots. *(From Cunningham, 2002, with permission.)*

tissue reaction yet provide ample tensile strength to support and approximate involved tissues.

Tensile Strength

Defined as the amount of weight necessary to break a suture divided by its cross-sectional area, *tensile strength* is an important characteristic for suture selection. Ideally, the tensile strength of material chosen should approximate the strength of the tissues being sutured.

Elasticity, Plasticity, Memory

The ability of a material to return to its prior length following stretch defines its *elasticity. Plasticity,* however, describes the tendency of material to retain its new shape once stretched. For tissues in which swelling or movement is expected postoperatively, a suture with increased elasticity is preferred because it will stretch rather than cut into approximated tissues. *Memory* defines the ability of material to return to original form following deformation. Sutures with greater memory tend to untie more easily during knot tying.

Knots

Knot tying is an essential skill for surgeons, and sound technique and knowledge of the various knot types are important aspects of gynecological surgery. A knot is the weakest link in a tied suture loop, and the force necessary to break a knotted suture is less than that to break an individual suture strand (Batra, 1993). Knot failure can lead to serious complications such as bleeding, hernias, and wound dehiscence (Batra, 1993; Trimbos, 1984).

A surgical knot consists of a loop, which maintains tissue apposition, and a knot, which is composed of a number of

throws snugged against each other. One strand is wrapped around the other one time for a single throw, and twice for a double throw (Zimmer, 1991). This latter double weave forms the basis of a surgeon's knot. In characterizing knots, each throw is given a numerical description, with single throws designated as number 1, and double throws as number 2. If successive throws are identical, a multiplication sign is placed between the numbers. If throws mirror one another, then an equal sign is used. Thus, a square knot is described as 1 = 1; granny knot, 1 × 1; and square surgeon's knot, 2 = 1 (Fig. 40-33). Alternative nomenclature schemes exist, but understanding the basic principles of knot construction is more clinically relevant than these descriptive definitions (Dinsmore, 1995).

Flat Knots

Surgical knots can have flat or sliding configurations. Flat configurations include square, granny, and surgeon's knots. To construct a flat square knot, forehanded and backhanded throws are alternated, and the suture strands are pulled with equal tension in opposite directions in the same plane. In addition, the suture strands or the hands may have to cross with each throw to ensure that the knot lies flat.

Sliding Knots

These knots, also termed slip knots, are characterized as identical, nonidentical, and parallel. They are created when unequal tension is applied to the strands, such as during one-hand knot tying. Sliding knots are useful in situations when flat square knotting is difficult or cumbersome, such as in the deep pelvis or vagina (Ivy, 2004b). In general, sliding knots have been shown to have a higher failure rate than do flat knots (Hurt, 2005; Schubert, 2002).

Identical sliding knots are created by holding one strand constantly under tension and repeating identical tying maneuvers with the other hand. Unfortunately, these identical sliding knots carry a high failure rate and are not recommended for general use (Schubert, 2002, Trimbos, 1984, 1986).

Nonidentical sliding knots are formed when a suture strand is held under constant tension, and one hand alternates forehanded and backhanded tying around this strand (Trimbos, 1986). This knot is the most frequent and practical knot used for vaginal surgery. Although these knots can unravel, additional throws can drastically improve their security (Ivy, 2004a; Trimbos, 1984; van Rijssel, 1990).

The loop-to-strand variation of the nonidentical sliding knot is used when the final loop of a continuous suture line is held under traction and alternate throws are made around the loop with the remaining single strand. There are scant data evaluating the properties of this knot type in gynecologic surgery, but it has recently been recognized as having an unacceptably high failure rate when tied with monofilament suture (Hurt, 2005).

Finally, in a *parallel sliding knot*, the suture strand under tension is alternated with each throw, causing alternate throws to slide down the other strand each time. Existing studies have demonstrated that this knot is exceptionally strong and reliable (Ivy, 2004b; Trimbos, 1986).

Surgical Knot Effectiveness

The effectiveness of surgical knots depends mainly on two parameters: initial loop security and knot security. *Loop security* describes the ability to maintain a tight suture loop around the tissue as the initial knot throws are placed (Lo, 2004). Suture loops that are initially loose will fail to secure tissues no matter how tightly the knot is tied and will result in ineffective knots, colloquially termed "air knots" (Burkhart, 1998). Three ways to optimize loop security include maintenance of tension on both strands during tying, use of an initial surgeon's throw, and slip knots (Anderson, 1980). If slip knots are placed initially, they can be converted to square knots or reinforced with a square knot once the pedicle or vessel is secured. Importantly, upward tension on both strands deep within a body cavity should be limited. Excessive force can avulse the pedicle or cause the suture loop to pull completely off (Nichols, 2000).

For *knot security*, the tension with which a given throw is tied is the most important. A knot laid down tightly under great tension is less likely to slip than a knot with more throws tied loosely with the same configuration (Gunderson, 1987).

The number and type of knots required to secure various suture materials vary. Qualities such as elasticity, plasticity, and memory often direct these recommendations. In general, multifilament sutures are easier to handle and display less memory, whereas synthetic monofilament suture materials or multifilament sutures with coatings have increased memory and may hold a knot poorly. For most sutures, four to six throws appear to be adequate, but the exact number depends on the type of suture and whether a flat or sliding knot is formed. Up to a point, additional throws provide more security to knots, but this benefit must be balanced against the corresponding elevated infection risk from increased knot volume (van Rijssel, 1990).

ELECTROSURGERY

Electrosurgery is one of the most commonly used surgical tools and enables surgeons to coagulate vessels and incise tissues rapidly. Familiarity with the basic principles of this modality can increase its effective use and minimize tissue injury.

Semantically, *electrosurgery* differs from *electrocautery,* although the terms are often incorrectly interchanged. With electrocautery, electric current passes through a metal object, such as a wire loop, with internal resistance. Passage of the current through the resistance heats the loop, which then may be used surgically. The flow of current is limited to the metal being heated, and no current enters surgical tissues.

In contrast, electrosurgery directs the flow of current to the tissues themselves and produces localized tissue heating and destruction. As a result, electric current must pass through tissues to produce the desired effect (Amaral, 2005). The electrosurgical circuit contains four main parts: the generator, the active electrode, the patient, and the return electrode.

Monopolar Electrosurgery

Electric current is the flow of electrons through a circuit (Fig. 40-34). *Voltage* is the force that drives those charges around the circuit. *Impedance* is the combination of resistance, inductance, and capacitance that alternating current meets along the way (Morris, 2006). In monopolar electrosurgery, the return electrode in clinical use is the grounding pad. Current therefore flows: (1) from the generator, which is the source of voltage, (2) through the electrosurgical tip to the patient, the source of impedance, and then (3) onto the grounding pad, where it is dispersed. Current leaves the pad to return to the generator, and the circuit is completed (Deatrick, 2010).

In electrosurgery, tissue impedance converts electric current into thermal energy that causes tissue temperatures to rise. It is these thermal increases that create electrosurgery's tissue effects.

The current from a wall outlet that powers electrosurgical generators has a frequency of 60 Hz (in the United States) or 50 Hz (in other parts of the world). Extreme neuromuscular stimulation can result from this lower frequency, as with electrocution. However, at frequencies above 100 Hz, excitable membranes are not depolarized, and thus nerve and muscle responses are bypassed. For safe use during electrosurgery, modern surgical generators increase frequencies to greater than 200 Hz (Valleylab, 2006).

Surgical Effects

Differing tissue effects are created by altering the manner in which current is produced and delivered. First, altering

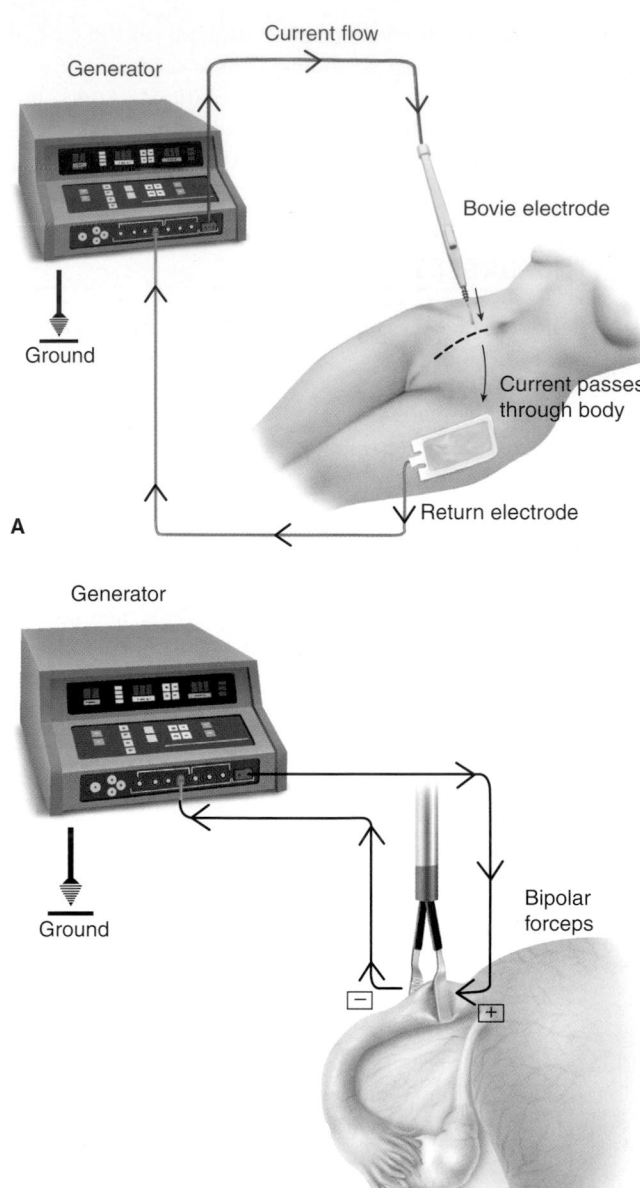

A

B

FIGURE 40-34 Circuits in electrosurgery. **A.** Monopolar electrosurgical circuit. **B.** Bipolar electrosurgical circuit.

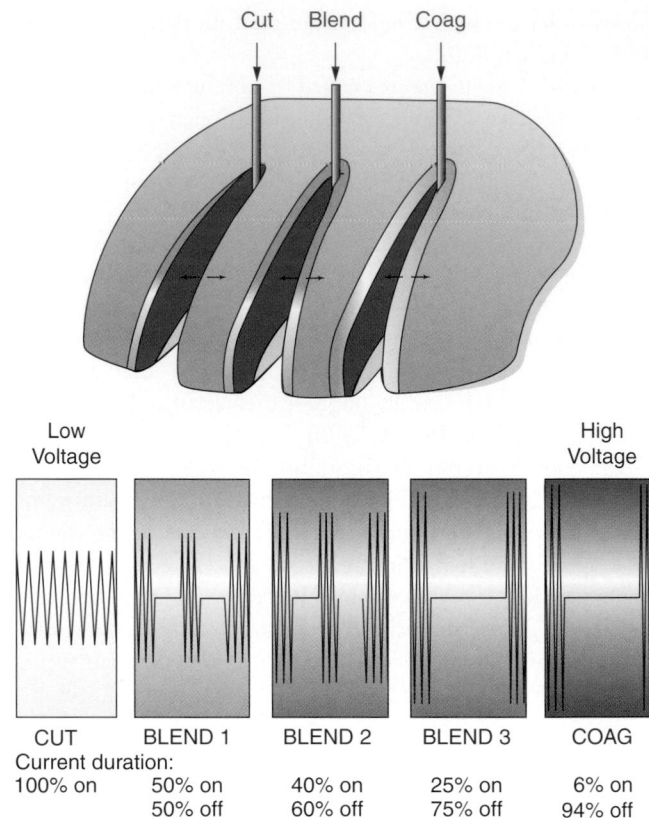

FIGURE 40-35 Tissue effects vary with cutting, blended, and coagulation currents. There is more lateral thermal damage with a pure coagulation current compared with a pure cutting or blended current. The duration of applied energy varies between current types.

the current wave pattern can affect tissue temperatures. For example, the high-frequency continuous sinusoidal waveform produced with cutting current creates higher tissue temperatures than that with coagulation current (Fig. 40-35). Second, the extent to which current is spread over an area, also termed *current density,* alters the rate of heat generation (Fig. 40-36). Thus, if current is concentrated onto a small area, such as a needle-tip electrode, greater tissue temperatures are generated than if delivered over a wider area, such as an electrosurgical blade. In addition to current density, voltage can alter tissue effects. As voltage increases, the degree of thermal tissue damage similarly increases. And finally, the qualities and impedance of the tissues themselves affect energy transfer and heat dissipation. For example, water has low electrical impedance and liberates little heat, whereas skin with its greater

impedance generates significantly higher tissue temperatures (Amaral, 2005).

Cutting Current

With electrosurgical cutting, a continuous sine wave of current is produced. The flow of high-frequency current typically is concentrated through an electrosurgical needle or blade and meets tissue impedance. Sparks are created between the tissue and electrode, intense heat is produced, cellular water vaporizes, and cells in the immediate area burst. Tissues are cut cleanly, and there is minimal coagulum production. As a result, few vessels are sealed, and minimal hemostasis accompanies electrosurgical cutting.

Coagulation Current

In contrast, coagulation current does not produce a constant waveform. Less heat is produced than with cutting current. However, tissue temperature still rises sufficiently to denature protein and disrupt normal cellular architecture. Cells are not vaporized instantly, and cellular debris remains associated with wound edges. This coagulum seals smaller blood vessels and controls local bleeding (Singh, 2006).

Blended Current

Variations in the percentage of time that current is flowing can create electrosurgical effects that contain both cutting and

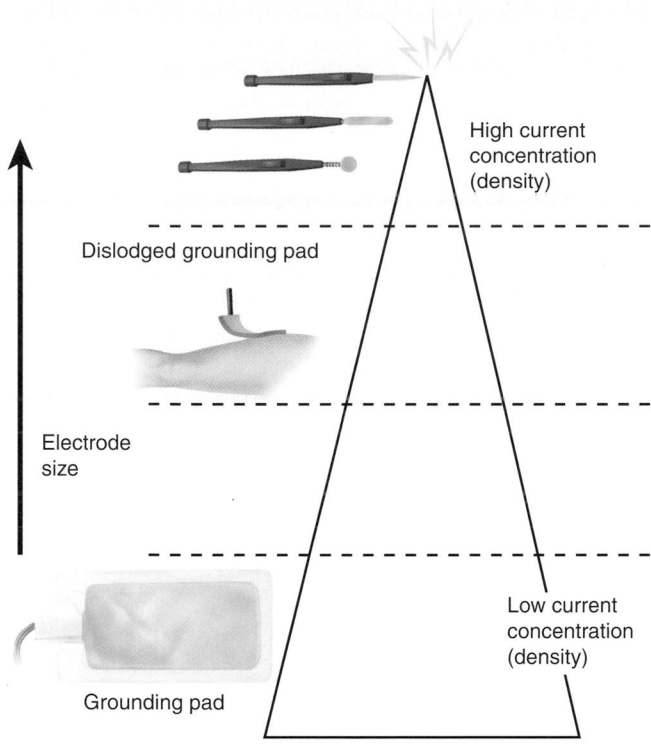

FIGURE 40-36 Current concentration and its effects. Thermal energy and risk for tissue injury rise as current density increases and electrode area decreases.

coagulating features. Such *blended currents* are used commonly in gynecologic surgery. In most cases, selection of specific percentages of cutting and coagulation current is affected by surgeon preference and type of tissues encountered. Thinner vascular tissue may be best suited for a blend with less active current time, whereas denser avascular tissues may require a greater percentage of active current.

Patient Grounding

As discussed earlier, current is concentrated at the electrode tip and enters the patient at a small site. Current follows the path of least resistance and exits the body through a grounding pad that is designed to have a large surface area, high conductivity, and low resistance (see Fig. 40-36). Dissipation across this large surface area allows current to leave the body without generating significant tissue temperatures across the exit site.

However, patient burns may result if current is concentrated through a return electrode. Clinically, this may occur if a grounding pad is partially dislodged. In this setting, the surface area is decreased, and exiting current concentration and tissue temperatures rise at the exit site. In addition, patient jewelry, metal candy cane stirrups, or other surfaces with high conductivity and low resistance may serve as a return electrode. In such cases, patients may be burned by concentrated current exiting through these small contact sites.

Ideally, grounding pads should be firmly adhered to a relatively flat body surface that is near the operative field. Thus, in most gynecology procedures, grounding pads are placed along the lateral upper thigh.

Bipolar Electrosurgery

This form of electrosurgery differs from monopolar electrosurgery in that the tip of a bipolar device contains both an active electrode and a return electrode (see Fig. 40-34B). For this reason, a distant grounding return pad is not required. Coagulation current is concentrated on tissues grasped between the electrodes, and tissue must remain between them. If tissue slips from between the tips, then active and return electrodes contact and create a short circuit. Coagulation will not occur (Michelassi, 1997). Bipolar electrosurgery uses only coagulation current and lacks cutting capability. However, it is useful for vessel coagulation and also is used during laparoscopic sterilization to coagulate fallopian tubes (Section 42-3, p. 1124).

Argon Beam Coagulation

This tool represents a modification of conventional electrosurgical coagulation. With argon beam coagulation (ABC), radiofrequency energy is transferred to tissues through a jet of inert argon gas to create noncontact monopolar electrothermal coagulation. Additionally, the gas jet clears blood and tissue debris during coagulation. Advantages of ABC include the ability to coagulate broad surface areas and larger vessels (Beckley, 2004). In gynecologic surgery, ABC is used most commonly during ovarian staging cases in which extensive debulking may be required.

Coexisting Electrical Devices

Patients with pacemakers, implantable cardioverter-defibrillators, or other electrical implants require special precautions. Stray electrosurgical current may be interpreted as an intracardiac signal by an implanted device and lead to pacing changes. In addition, myocardial electrical burns may result from conduction of current through the pacing electrode rather than through the grounding pad (Pinski, 2002). Accordingly, for patients with these devices, preventative recommendations include pre- and postoperative cardiology consultation, continuous cardiac monitoring, and contingency plans for arrhythmias. During surgery, use of bipolar electrosurgical instruments or Harmonic scalpel is preferred. If monopolar tools are used, then minimal settings are selected, and the active and return electrodes are placed in close proximity (El-Gamal, 2001).

ULTRASONIC ENERGY

Sound waves are mechanical waves that transport energy through a medium. Those above audible range are described as *ultrasound* or *ultrasonic*. In medicine, ultrasound waves that are applied at low levels, such as those used in diagnostic sonography, are harmless. However, if higher power levels are used, then mechanical energy is transferred to the impacted tissues. This energy is of sufficient strength that cutting, coagulation, or tissue cavitation is produced.

Ultrasonic Scalpel

The tip of an ultrasonic scalpel, also known as a *Harmonic scalpel*, vibrates at high frequency. This allows the surgical device to be used effectively for both cutting or coagulating during laparotomy or laparoscopy (Gyr, 2001; Wang, 2000). The vibrating tip transfers mechanical energy to tissues. Mechanical energy breaks hydrogen bonds and generates heat within tissues. High energy levels will allow cutting, whereas lower levels will denature protein and form a sticky coagulum that produces hemostasis. A balance between cutting and coagulation is created by controlling three factors: power levels, tissue tension, and blade sharpness. Higher power level, greater tissue tension, and a sharp blade will lead to cutting. Lower power, decreased tissue tension, and a blunt blade will create slower cutting and greater hemostasis (Sinha, 2003).

Used most commonly in laparoscopic surgery, the ultrasonic scalpel serves as an alternative to suture ligation, electrosurgical coagulation, laser, and stapling or clipping devices (Fig. 42-1.14, p. 1105). However, only a few studies have been published comparing the clinical effectiveness of this method with other methods of hemostasis (Kauko, 1998).

Cavitational Ultrasonic Surgical Aspiration

An ultrasonic surgical aspirator hand piece contains three main components: a high-frequency vibrator, which transfers ultrasonic energy to tissues; irrigation tubing, which directs cooling saline to the tip; and a suction system, which draws tissue up to the tip for contact with the vibrator and which also clears away tissue fragments and irrigant. Ultrasound energy can be used to raise tissue temperatures dramatically and thereby disrupt tissue architecture by a process termed *cavitation*. For cavitation, a rapidly oscillating cavitational ultrasonic surgical aspiration (CUSA) tip produces mechanical waves that create heat and vapor pockets around cells in tissues with high water content such as adipose, muscle, and carcinomas. Collapse of these pockets leads to disruption of cell architecture (Jallo, 2001). Affected tissues are removed subsequently by suction aspiration. However, tissues containing less water and higher contents of collagen and elastic fibers, such as blood vessels, nerves, ureters, and serosa, are more resistant to damage (van Dam, 1996).

In gynecology, CUSA has a limited surgical role. It may be used effectively in the treatment of vulvar intraepithelial neoplasia, bulky condyloma acuminata, and cytoreductive ovarian cancer surgery (Section 41-28, p. 1087) (Aletti, 2006; Deppe, 1988; Robinson, 2000; van Dam, 1996).

MANAGEMENT OF HEMORRHAGE

Ideally, problematic bleeding is avoided during surgery by optimizing preoperative preparations, ensuring adequate operative exposure, and using proper surgical technique. However, if hemorrhage does occur, surgeons should be familiar with its appropriate management.

Optimizing Preoperative Preparations

Although the risk of hemorrhage accompanies most gynecologic procedures, certain factors are associated with higher rates of bleeding and should be assessed prior to surgery. Specifically, obesity, the presence of a large pelvic mass,

adhesions such as those from endometriosis or pelvic inflammatory disease, cancer or prior radiation, and coagulation dysfunction all have been linked with an increased risk of hemorrhage. For those identified to be at risk, intraoperative red cell salvage or preoperative autologous blood donation may be considered.

Red Blood Cell Salvage

Red blood cell (RBC) salvage machines (Autolog; Cell Saver) collect, filter, and centrifuge blood lost during surgery and may be helpful in patients in whom increased intraoperative hemorrhage is anticipated. RBCs are heavier and are separated from plasma and smaller blood components during centrifugation and are then reinfused into the patient. Anticoagulants such as heparin or citrate are added to prevent clotting (Karger, 2005).

Salvage efficiencies approximate 60 percent with good technique. However, vacuum levels, suction tip size, and thoroughness of salvaging efforts can affect this value. For example, turbulence destroys RBCs. Thus, suction tips with greater diameters and lower suction force can minimize hemolysis (Waters, 2005). Additionally, laparotomy sponges can be rinsed in sterile saline to maximize RBC removal. The RBC-containing saline then is suctioned into the salvage device for processing. The filtering systems in these devices have limitations. Accordingly, RBC salvage is not appropriate for contaminated cases or those in which malignancy, topical hemostatic agents, or amnionic fluid may be present (Waters, 2004).

Preoperative Autologous Donation

To avoid potential transfusion reaction or blood-borne infection, a patient may elect to donate her own blood for personal use approximately once a week for 3 to 5 weeks preceding surgery. Patient hemoglobin levels should be greater than 11.0 g/dL before each donation. Moreover, units should not be collected within 72 hours before surgery. This allows intravascular volume to be replenished by the patient and units to be processed by the blood bank (Goodnough, 2005). Disadvantageously, this process has been associated with preoperative anemia secondary to donation, more liberal transfusion, transfusion reaction following clerical error, volume overload, and bacterial contamination of blood products during processing (Henry, 2002; Kanter, 1996, 1999).

Improved blood banking safety has accompanied a decline in preoperative autologous donation (Brecher, 2002). Moreover, for most gynecologic cases, the risk of transfusion is low. For these reasons, autologous donation typically is reserved for selected instances in which the risk of transfusion is significant, such as radical hysterectomy or surgery for patients with coagulopathies. Additionally, patients with rare blood phenotypes in whom acquisition of compatible blood may be difficult may benefit from autologous donation.

Proper Surgical Method

In many instances, proper surgical technique may minimize vascular injury and hemorrhage. Thus, prior to ligation, vessels should have excess connective tissue removed with fine

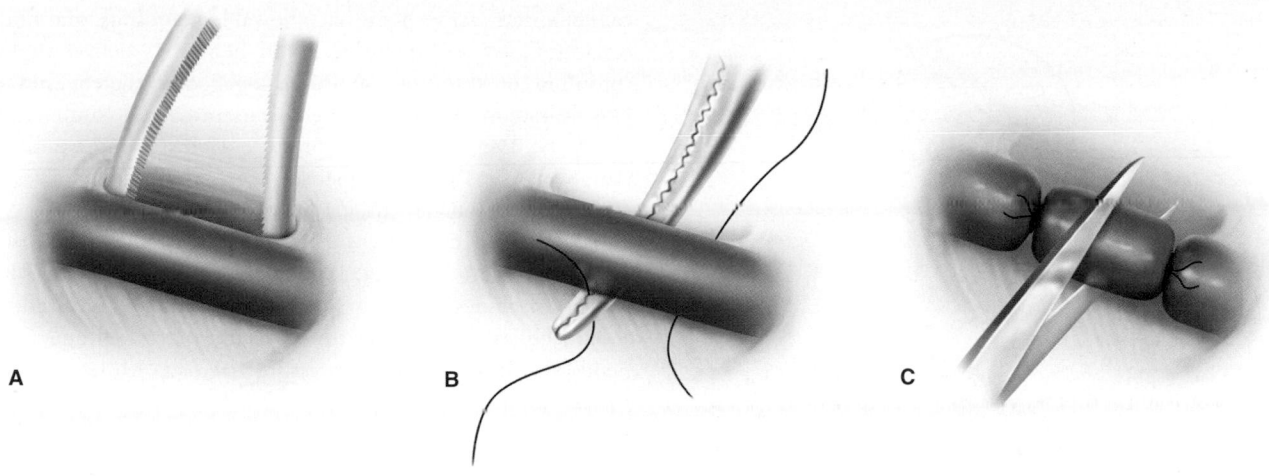

FIGURE 40-37 Steps in vessel isolation, ligation, and transection. **A.** During vessel isolation, a clamp tip can be opened and closed parallel to the side of the vessel to dissect away loose surrounding tissue. **B.** The tip of the clamp is insinuated beneath the vessel, and the jaws are opened. A suture ligature can then be grasped and pulled beneath the vessel. **C.** Two sutures are placed around the vessel, and it is transected between these ligation points.

scissors in a process called *skeletonizing*. Additionally, tissue clamps selected for grasping a vascular pedicle should be large enough to contain the entire pedicle in the distal portion of the clamp. Large pedicles that force excess tissue toward the clamp's heel carry greater risk of tissue slipping from the heel and bleeding. Once secure, sutures placed on vascular pedicles should not be used for traction because the risk of avulsing the suture or vessel increases.

Tying an intact vessel at two places along its length before tissue cutting should be considered in certain situations. This technique may be appropriate if a vessel is on tension or if space for a clamp is limited, such as when the ureter or bowel is in close proximity to the vessel. A window is created below the vessel and ties are passed beneath the vessel before doubly ligating and dividing it (Fig. 40-37).

Steps of Hemorrhage Management

A methodical approach to intraoperative hemorrhage is critical to minimize patient injury. If an isolated vessel is clearly identified, then grasping it with a hemostat, vascular clamp, or fine forceps may allow ligation, electrosurgical coagulation, or vascular clip application.

In contrast, venous bleeding in the pelvis is typically from a venous plexus and rarely stems from a single vessel. A venous plexus often contains thin-walled veins. Thus, indiscriminate clamping, suturing, clipping, and electrosurgical coagulation may cause further laceration and bleeding. However, if other vulnerable structures have been retracted and protected, a few shallow stitches that incorporate the bleeding area may be placed using fine absorbable suture.

If these initial efforts are unsuccessful and significant hemorrhage continues, the bleeding site is compressed with fingertip, sponge stick, or laparotomy sponges. Anesthesia staff should be informed of events to allow for additional monitoring. Nursing staff should also be informed, as significant additional resources, such as specialized instruments, suture, and clips,

may be required. Resuscitative efforts with crystalloid or blood products are individualized depending on the degree of hemorrhage and other patient factors.

Adequate exposure of the site typically is needed to gain control of bleeding. The operative field should be assessed and increased as needed by extending a vertical incision cephalad, converting a Pfannenstiel incision to a Cherney incision, adding retractors, or converting a vaginal or laparoscopic approach to laparotomy. A second suctioning system may be needed, and appropriate clips or suture should be made available before removing pressure. Additional dissection of avascular planes around the bleeding site may improve isolation and ligation of a lacerated vessel. Furthermore, nearby vulnerable structures such as the bladder, ureter, or other vessels should be identified and protected. After these steps, the surgeon may remove the tamponading tool to assess the location, amount, and character of bleeding. The most appropriate technique for control, as described in the next sections, is then selected.

Vessel Ligation

Suture Ligature. Surgical knots have been used since the beginning of surgery to prevent blood loss during operative dissection and resection. Advantages to suture ligation include low cost and effectiveness over a broad range of vessel diameters. However, knot tying in general is time-consuming, difficult in narrow spaces, and less commonly, associated with ligature slippage or breakage.

Small vessels may be ligated by a free-tie suture placed around the heel and tip of a vascular clamp and then secured with knots (Fig. 40-38). Alternatively, surgeons often prefer to secure larger vascular pedicles with two separate sutures. The first ligature is a free tie placed around the toe and heel of a vascular clamp and tied. The second ligature is distal to the first and typically incorporates a bite through the tissue pedicle (see Fig. 40-31B, C). Such *transfixion* of the ligature to the pedicle decreases the risk of it slipping off the pedicle's end. Importantly, this second

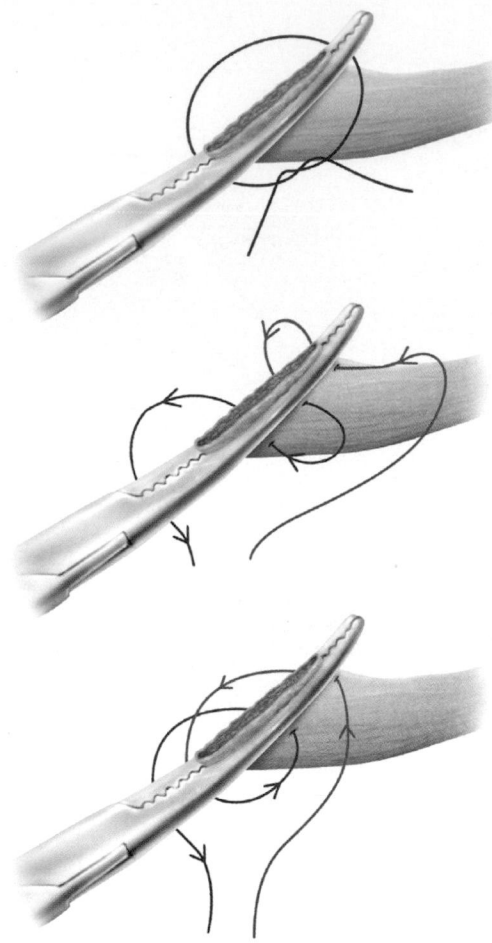

FIGURE 40-38 Different pedicle ligation techniques. The second and third examples are transfixing ligatures.

ligature is placed distal to the first to avert hematoma formation if a vessel is pierced during transfixion.

Clips. Titanium clips seal vessels by direct compression. They are used more commonly during gynecologic oncology cases and offer the advantage of speed. However, clips are expensive, require surgical dissection of the vessel prior to application, and may dislodge from a vessel. Their use in routine gynecology is limited by these factors and surgeon preference.

Electrosurgical Seal. Electrical and ultrasound energy also may be used to seal vessels. Ultrasonic coagulating shears (Autosonix; Harmonic scalpel; SonoSurg) and electrosurgical bipolar vessel sealing clamps (EnSeal; Ligasure) transfer energy that denatures vascular collagen and elastin and seal vessels (Heniford, 2001). Damaging lateral thermal spread for both types is comparable and averages 2.5 mm (Harold, 2003). These tools are useful for laparoscopic surgeries, in which knot tying is time-consuming.

Local Topical Hemostats

These topical products may be placed on bleeding sites where other methods are not possible or have been ineffective. Topical hemostats are most effective in controlling low-pressure bleeding, such as from veins, capillaries, and small arteries. Commercially available materials are categorized as mechani-

cal hemostats, active hemostats, flowable hemostats, and fibrin sealants (Table 40-6). Some liquid hemostats deliver topical thrombin or thrombin and fibrinogen and thereby induce clot formation. Mechanical hemostats provide a combination of effects. They create direct pressure against wound surfaces, entrap platelets, promote platelet aggregation, and serve as a scaffold on which clot can organize.

Although effective, these agents do have disadvantages. They should not be introduced intravascularly or used with RBC salvage machines. Packing agents tightly into bony foramina should be avoided because these agents may swell and cause neurologic dysfunction or pressure necrosis. Moreover, they should not be placed within skin edges because they may retard edge reapproximation. Those composed of gelatin, collagen, or cellulose can serve as an infection nidus and thus, may not be appropriate in grossly infected tissue (Baxter Healthcare, 2005; C.R. Bard, Inc., 2002; Pfizer, 2008). Few data support the use of one agent over another. Selection typically is dictated by surgeon preference and operating room availability of an agent.

Specific Sites of Bleeding

Bleeding can develop during any type of gynecologic surgery. However, there are vascular complications that characteristically may complicate specific procedures, and surgeons may benefit from a familiarity with their management.

Infundibulopelvic Ligament

During or after ligation of this vascular pedicle, a lacerated ovarian vessel within the infundibulopelvic ligament may retract into the retroperitoneum to create a hematoma (Chap. 38, p. 932). In most cases, isolation of the bleeding vessel is required to halt hematoma expansion.

Initially, the pelvic sidewall peritoneum lateral to the ureter and the hematoma is opened, and the incision is extended cephalad to the upper pole of the hematoma. The incision in the peritoneum may be carried up the white line of Toldt, lateral to the ascending or descending colon. The upper pole of the hematoma is identified by the normalization (narrowing) of the vessels above the hematoma. The ovarian vessels are identified, and a closed Mixter right-angle clamp is placed beneath them. A tie on a pass then is threaded beneath and used to ligate these vessels. If large, the hematoma then is evacuated to minimize infection risk (Tomacruz, 2001). In rare cases in which vascular or ureteral anatomy is unclear, an ovarian artery may require ligation as proximal as its aortic origin below the renal arteries (Masterson, 1995).

Presacral Venous Plexus

Sacrocolpopexy requires entry into the retroperitoneum and the presacral space (Fig. 38-23, p. 939). During entry, the presacral venous plexus can be injured during dissection or suturing. Vessels may retract into the vertebral bone, and problematic bleeding may result. Initially, injury to the plexus is managed with constant pressure over several minutes. As pressure is removed, an isolated vessel may be identified and sutured with fine absorbable suture. Extensive suturing, however, is discouraged because this can lead to additional vessel

TABLE 40-6. Topical Hemostatic Agents

Type of Agent	Brand Name	Material
Mechanical Hemostats		
Oxidized, regenerated methylcellulose	Surgicel,	Flat loose woven fabric
	Surgicel Fibrillar,	Flat peelable layers and tufts
	Surgicel Nu-knit,	Flat loose woven fabric
	Surgicel SNoW	Flat nonwoven fabric
Porcine gelatin	Surgifoam	Powder or flat sponge
	Gelfoam	Powder or flat sponge
	Surgiflo	Powder
Bovine collagen	Avitene,	Powder, sheet, or flat sponge
	Instat	Powder
Microporous polysaccharide hemosphere	Arísta	Powder
	Vitasure	Powder
Active Hemostats		
Bovine thrombin	Thrombin-JMI	Liquid spray
Bovine thrombin + gelatin	Thrombi-Gel	Flat sponge
Bovine thrombin + methylcellulose	Thrombi-Pad	Flat sheet
Human thrombin	Evithrom	Liquid
Recombinant thrombin	Recothrom	Liquid
Flowable Hemostats		
Bovine gelatin + human thrombin	FloSeal Matrix	Liquid
Porcine gelatin + Human thrombin	Surgiflo + Evithrom	Liquid
Fibrin Sealants		
Human thrombin, fibrinogen, plasminogen	Tisseel	Spray or drip application
Human thrombin, fibrinogen	Evicel	Spray or drip application
Bovine thrombin, bovine collagen, autologous plasma	Vitagel	Spray or drip application

laceration and bleeding. Alternative methods of control have included the use of bone wax, which is a small ball of beeswax like material that is pressed and flattened against the sacrum to compress vessels; insertion of a sterile thumbtack through the vessel and into the vertebral bone to compress the vessel; and placement of topical hemostatic agents such as Floseal Hemostatic Matrix. In rare refractory cases, patient packing as described later may be required.

Space of Retzius

This space is commonly entered during urogynecologic procedures and contains important vascular structures such as the venous plexus of Santorini, the obturator vessels, and the aberrant obturator vessel (Fig. 38-24, p. 940). Bleeding complications may develop, and approximately 2 percent of tension-free vaginal tape procedures are complicated by bleeding in this space (Kolle, 2005; Kuuva, 2002). In most instances, bleeding is controlled with pressure or suturing.

Major Pelvic Vessels

High-volume vessels within the pelvic sidewall include the internal, external, and common iliac vessels; the inferior vena cava; and the aorta. These may be lacerated during tumor removal, endometriosis excision, or laparoscopic trocar placement.

Initially following large vessel injury, pressure is applied for several minutes. Although gynecologic surgeons may attempt to repair these injuries, excessive delay in obtaining vascular surgery assistance often leads to greater blood loss (Oderich, 2004). Therefore, in many instances, pressure is applied, a vascular surgeon is consulted for repair, blood products are made available, and exposure is maximized. If a large vessel is punctured by a trocar or needle during laparoscopic entry, the instrument should remain in place to act as a plug while preparations for repair are made ready.

As discussed later, internal iliac artery ligation does not lead to ischemia of central pelvic organs due to collateral blood supply (Table 38-2, p. 928). However, injury to the external or common iliac arteries requires repair to maintain blood supply to the lower extremity. Similarly, ligation of the internal iliac vein may not result in severe sequelae, but ligation of the external or common iliac veins may result in lower extremity compromise. Consultation with a vascular surgeon may be indicated depending on the degree of laceration and surgeon skill. Maneuvers that may extend the injury should be avoided until appropriate assistance is available.

If repair is undertaken, familiarity with this vascular anatomy is essential. On the left, the common and external iliac arteries remain lateral to their respective veins. On the right, however, the common iliac artery runs medial to the vein and then courses laterally as it approaches the femoral canal.

These arteries can be repaired by placing vascular clamps 2 to 3 cm proximal and distal to the tear, then closing the defect with a continuous suture line using monofilament synthetic 5-0 suture (Gostout, 2002; Tomacruz, 2001). The proximal clamp should be removed first to allow air and debris to exit the suture line, and then the distal clamp should be removed.

Parametrial and Paravaginal Vessels

During obstetric and gynecologic surgery, vessels supplying the uterus and vagina, especially venous plexuses, can be lacerated. Bleeding may not be easily identified and controlled following application of direct pressure, suturing, or clips. In these extreme situations, ligation of the internal iliac artery, which is a main source of blood supply to the pelvis, may decrease pooling of blood and afford a better opportunity to find a bleeding source. Alternatively, if resources are available, pelvic artery embolization has been shown to be effective in controlling pelvic hemorrhage. Despite these techniques, in rare persistent situations, pelvic packing and termination of surgery may be indicated.

◼ Internal Iliac (Hypogastric) Artery Ligation

The internal iliac artery, also known as the *hypogastric artery,* contains anterior and posterior divisions. Its anterior division supplies blood to central pelvic viscera (Fig. 38-12, p. 927). The female pelvis has extensive collateral circulation, and the internal iliac artery shares arterial anastomoses with branches of the aorta, external iliac artery, and femoral artery. For this reason, ligation of the internal iliac's anterior division can be performed without compromise to pelvic organ viability. Several studies have described normal postligation fertility in these women. One investigation evaluating flow with color Doppler sonography showed recanalization of ligated arteries within an average of 5 months (Demirci, 2005; Khelifi, 2000; Nizard, 2003). Occlusion of the internal iliac artery decreases mean blood flow in branches distal to ligation by 48 percent, which in many cases, slows hemorrhage sufficiently to allow identification of specific bleeding sites (Burchell, 1968).

To perform ligation, the round ligament is divided, and the pelvic sidewall peritoneum lateral to the infundibulopelvic ligament is incised cephalad. Identification of the internal iliac artery is essential because ligation of the common or external iliac arteries will have vascular consequences to the lower extremity.

Once the internal iliac artery is located, a Mixter right-angle clamp is placed under the vessel at a point 2 to 3 cm distal to its origin from the common iliac artery. If the internal iliac is ligated at this site, its posterior division should be spared (Bleich, 2007). Two free ties of No. 1 or 0 absorbable suture are passed beneath the artery and then secured (Fig. 40-39). The artery is ligated but not transected (Gilstrap, 2002). Care is required in passing instruments beneath the artery because the adjacent thin-walled internal iliac vein is easily lacerated. For this reason, it is recommended that clamps be placed with their tips directed medially to avoid vein puncture.

◼ Pelvic Artery Embolization

As described in Chapter 9 (p. 256), embolization similar to that used to treat symptomatic leiomyomas can be used to occlude either the internal iliac artery or the uterine artery. This technique has been described in the management of hemorrhage in both gynecologic and obstetric cases.

◼ Pelvic Packing

In patients with persistent heavy bleeding despite attempts at control, pelvic packing with gauze and termination of the operation may be warranted. Rolls of gauze are packed against the bleeding site to provide constant local pressure. Typically, 24 to 48 hours later, if the patient is stable and bleeding appears to have stopped clinically, packing may be removed. Some surgeons recommend leaving one end of the gauze outside the wound. After administration of general anesthesia, packing is pulled slowly through a small opening left in the incision. Alternatively, entire gauze rolls may be packed into the abdomen and removed during a second laparotomy (Newton, 1988).

FLUID RESUSCITATION AND BLOOD TRANSFUSION

With acute hemorrhage, priorities include control of additional losses and replacement of sufficient intravascular volume for tissue perfusion and oxygenation. In hypoperfused areas, progressive failure of oxidative metabolism with lactate production leads to worsening systemic metabolic acidosis and eventual organ damage (Manning, 2004). To avoid these effects, resuscitation should begin with an assessment of the patient's clinical status, calculation of total blood volume, and estimation of blood loss.

◼ Clinical Assessment

Total blood volume for an adult approximates 70 mL/kg, and thus a 50-kg woman's calculated blood volume is 3500 mL. Of this volume, 15 percent can be lost by most patients with no changes in arterial pressure or heart rate. A 15-percent blood loss can be roughly calculated by multiplication of a patient's weight in kilograms by 10. Thus, for a 50-kg woman, a 15-percent loss approximates 500 mL.

With losses of 15 to 30 percent (500 to 1000 mL for a 50-kg woman), tachycardia and narrowing of the pulse pressure are seen (Table 40-7). Peripheral vasoconstriction leads to pale, cool extremities and poor capillary refill. In unanesthetized patients, there may be mild confusion or lethargy. In most women with normal preoperative hemoglobin levels, this amount of blood loss requires fluid volume replacement, but RBC transfusion typically is not required. Greater losses, however, lead to worsening perfusion, hypotension, and tachycardia. In these cases, blood transfusion in combination with fluid resuscitation typically is indicated (Murphy, 2001).

During surgery, blood collects in suction canisters and laparotomy sponges. Although calculations from these sources provide surgeons with an approximation, blood loss estimates

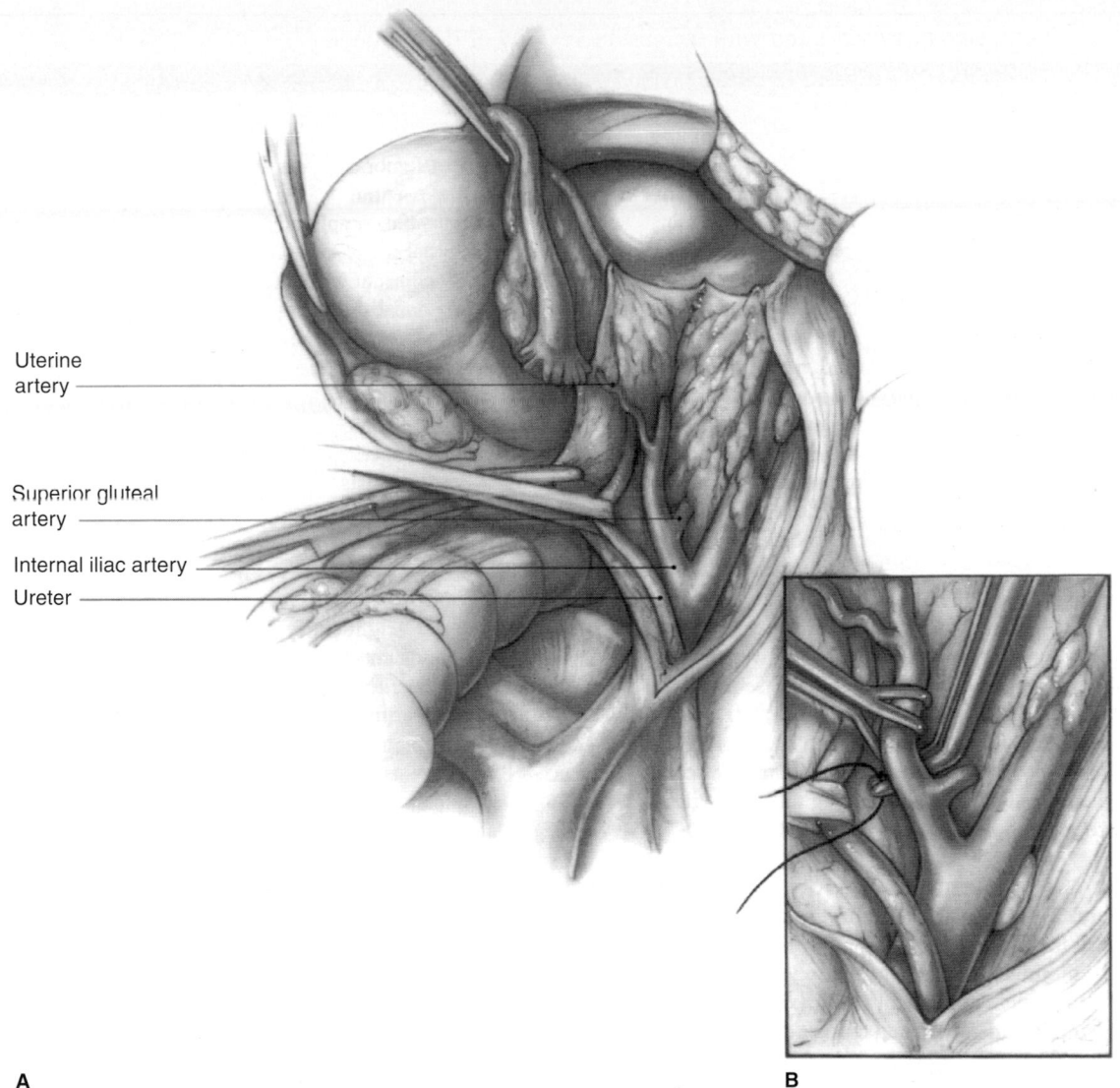

Uterine
artery

Superior gluteal
artery

Internal iliac artery

Ureter

A   **B**

FIGURE 40-39 Internal iliac artery ligation. **A.** After opening the retroperitoneal space, the ureter is identified and retracted medially. **B.** The internal iliac artery is identified and gently elevated with a Babcock clamp. A Mixter right-angle clamp is placed beneath the artery to receive a free tie for ligation. *(From Cunningham, 2010b, with permission.)*

typically are low, and inaccuracy increases as the length and extent of a procedure increase (Bose, 2006; Santoso, 2001). Additionally, a hematocrit may be measured to assess hemorrhage. However, hematocrit values typically lag true losses, and values may reflect only the degree of hemorrhage. For example, following a blood loss of 1000 mL, hematocrit levels typically fall only 3 volumes percent in the first hour but usually show an 8 volume percent drop at 72 hours (Schwartz, 2006).

■ Fluid Resuscitation

If hypovolemia is identified, fluid resuscitation should begin with crystalloid solutions. If hypotension and tachycardia are present, rapid replacement is warranted, and 1 or 2 liters, as indicated, may be infused over several minutes in most patients. Normal saline and lactated Ringer solutions are the two crystalloids used commonly. For moderate hemorrhage, both perform equally well as fluid replacements (Healey, 1998).

Although crystalloids have an immediate effect to expand intravascular volume, a portion will extravasate into extracellular tissues. Thus, in the setting of hemorrhage, crystalloid volume should be administered in a 3:1 ratio of blood lost (Moore, 2004). Clinically, urine output of 0.5 mL/kg/per hour or 30 mL or more per hour, heart rate less than 100 beats per minute, and systolic blood pressure greater than 90 mm Hg may be used as general indicators of volume improvement. If rapid crystalloid infusion fails to correct hypotension or tachycardia, then RBC transfusion usually is warranted.

In addition to crystalloid solutions, colloids also may be used for volume expansion. These fluids have higher molecular weights than crystalloids. As a result, a greater portion remains intravascularly and is not lost to extracellular extravasation. Despite this perceived advantage, studies comparing survival rates if crystalloids or colloids are administered find no superiority with colloids but greater expense (Roberts, 2004).

TABLE 40-7. Clinical Findings Associated with Increasing Severity of Hemorrhage

Hemorrhage Class	Class I	Class II	Class III	Class IV
Blood loss				
Percentage	<15	15–30	30–40	>40
Volume (mL)	750	800–1500	1500–2000	>2000
Blood pressure				
Systolic	Unchanged	Normal	Reduced	Very low
Diastolic	Unchanged	Raised	Reduced	Very low, unrecordable
Pulse (beats/min)	Slight tachycardia	100–120	120 (thready)	>120 (very thready)
Capillary refill	Normal	Slow (>2 s)	Slow (>2 s)	Undetectable
Respiratory rate	Normal	Normal	Tachypnea (>20/min)	Tachypnea (>20/min)
Urinary flow rate (mL/h)	>30	20–30	10–20	0–10
Extremities	Normal color	Pale	Pale	Pale and cold
Complexion	Normal	Pale	Pale	Ashen
Mental state	Alert	Anxious or aggressive	Anxious, aggressive, or drowsy	Drowsy, confused, or unconscious

From Baskett, 1990, with permission.

Red Blood Cell Replacement

Clinical Assessment

The decision to administer RBCs is complex and must balance the risks of transfusion with needs for adequate tissue oxygenation. These needs will vary depending on the clinical setting. An assessment should include hemoglobin level, vital signs, patient age, risks for further blood loss, and underlying medical conditions, especially cardiac disease. Accordingly, no specific hemoglobin threshold dictates when RBCs should be administered. Consensus guidelines suggest that in those without significant cardiac disease, transfusion to a hemoglobin level above 10 g/dL is rarely indicated (Hill, 2002). If hemoglobin levels drop to 6 g/dL, transfusion almost always is required (Madjdpour, 2006). Hemoglobin levels between 6 and 10 g/dL are more problematic, and patient factors and risk for continued hemorrhage should dictate therapy (American Society of Anesthesiologists, 1996). In one randomized study of 838 critically ill patients, one group of euvolemic patients received transfusion when their hemoglobin levels fell below 7 g/dL. These individuals fared better than those transfused at an earlier threshold (hemoglobin below 10 g/dL), excepting those with significant cardiac disease (Hébert, 1999).

Transfusion

Compatibility Testing. When the possible need for transfusion is present, an order for a *type and screen* informs blood bank personnel that blood products may be required and initiates two tests to characterize a patient's RBCs. The first evaluation, termed *typing*, mixes commercially available standardized controls with a patient's blood sample to determine her ABO type and Rh phenotype. The second test, or *screen*, combines a patient's plasma

sample with control RBCs that express clinically significant RBC antigens. If a patient has formed antibodies to any of these specific RBC surface antigens, then agglutination or hemolysis of the sample is seen. However, if blood is needed immediately and a full screen is not possible, then ABO type-specific blood or O-negative blood may be used.

Typing and screening require approximately 45 minutes to complete and are valid for 3 days in patients who do receive transfusion. In those who are not transfused, the validity is considerably longer and typically is determined by individual blood banks.

Alternatively, an order to *type and crossmatch* blood products alerts blood bank personnel to designate specific units of blood solely for one individual's use. Those specific units are tested against the patient's for specific antigen reactions.

Packed Red Blood Cells. Previously, whole-blood transfusion was used commonly to provide RBCs, coagulation factors, and plasma proteins. This largely has been replaced by component therapy. Packed RBCs are the primary product used for most clinical situations, and concentrated RBC suspensions can be prepared by removing most of the supernatant plasma after centrifugation. One unit of packed RBCs contains the same red cell mass as 1 unit of whole blood at approximately half the volume and twice the hematocrit (70 to 80 percent). One unit of packed RBCs raises the hematocrit approximately 3 volume percent in an adult or increases the hemoglobin level of a 70-kg individual by 1 g/dL (Table 40-8) (Gorgas, 2004).

Complications

Transfusion Reactions. Despite numerous tests for compatibility, adverse reactions to blood products can develop

TABLE 40-8. Characteristics of Blood Components

Component	Volume, mL	Content	Clinical Response
PRBCs	180–200	RBCs	Increases Hb 1 g/dL and Hct 3%
Platelets			Increases platelet count
Random-donor unit	50–70	5.5×10^{10}	$5–10 \times 10^9/L$
Single-donor collection	200–400	3.0×10^{11}	$>10 \times 10^9/L$ within 1 h and $>7.5 \times 10^9/L$ within 24 h posttransfusion
FFP	200–250	Coagulation factors, including fibrinogen, proteins C and S, antithrombin	Increases coagulation factors ~2%
Cryoprecipitate	10–15	Fibrinogen, factor VIII, vWF	Increases fibrinogen level 0.1 g/L

FFP = Fresh-frozen plasma; Hct = hematocrit; Hb = hemoglobin; PRBCs = packed red blood cells; RBCs = red blood cells; vWF = von Willebrand factor.

and may include an acute or delayed hemolytic transfusion reaction, febrile nonhemolytic transfusion reaction, or allergic reaction.

Acute Hemolytic Transfusion Reaction. Acute immune-mediated hemolysis usually involves destruction of transfused RBCs by patient antibodies and most commonly results from ABO incompatibility. Symptoms begin within minutes or hours of transfusion and may include chills, fever, urticaria, tachycardia, dyspnea, nausea and vomiting, hypotension, and chest and back pain. In addition, these reactions can lead to acute tubular necrosis or disseminated intravascular coagulopathy, and treatment is directed to these serious complications.

If acute hemolysis is suspected, transfusion should be halted immediately. A sample of the patient's blood should be sent with the remaining donor unit for evaluation in the blood bank. In patients with significant hemolysis, laboratory values will be altered. Specifically, hemoglobin levels and serum haptoglobin levels will be lowered; serum lactate dehydrogenase and indirect bilirubin levels will be increased; and hemoglobinemia and hemoglobinuria may be noted. Serum creatinine and electrolyte levels and coagulation studies additionally are ordered.

To prevent renal toxicity, diuresis is prompted with intravenous crystalloids and administration of furosemide or mannitol. Alkalinization of urine may prevent precipitation of hemoglobin within the renal tubules, and therefore, intravenous bicarbonate also may be given.

In contrast to acute hemolytic transfusion reaction, delayed hemolytic transfusion reactions may develop days or weeks later. Patients often lack acute symptoms, but lowered hemoglobin levels, fever, jaundice, and hemoglobinemia may be noted. Clinical intervention typically is not required in these cases.

Nonhemolytic Transfusion Reactions. Febrile nonhemolytic transfusion reaction is characterized by chills and a greater than 1°C rise in temperature and is the most common transfusion reaction. Blood transfusion typically is stopped to exclude a hemolytic reaction, and treatment is supportive. For patients with a previous history of febrile reaction, premedication with an antipyretic such as acetaminophen prior to transfusion is reasonable.

Urticaria alone may develop during transfusion and typically is not associated with serious sequelae. It is generally attributed to an allergic, antibody-mediated response to donor plasma proteins. The transfusion does not need to be stopped, and treatment with an antihistamine, such as diphenhydramine (Benadryl) 50 mg orally or intramuscularly, usually is sufficient. Rarely, an anaphylactic reaction may complicate transfusion, and treatment follows that for classic anaphylaxis (Table 27-3, p. 697).

Infection. Infectious complications associated with packed RBC transfusion are uncommon and are listed in Table 40-9. The risk for transmission of human immunodeficiency virus and hepatitis B and C virus has diminished over the past decade, and bacterial contamination now stands as a greater infection risk. In addition, emerging infection concerns include transmission of the Creutzfeld-Jakob prion, dengue virus, Babesia protozoal species, and Chikungunya virus (Dodd, 2009; Stramer, 2009).

Transfusion-Related Acute Lung Injury. This infrequent but serious complication of blood component therapy is similar clinically to acute respiratory distress syndrome. Symptoms develop within 6 hours of transfusion and may include extreme respiratory distress, frothy sputum, hypotension, fever, and tachycardia. Noncardiogenic pulmonary edema with diffuse bilateral pulmonary infiltrates on chest radiography is characteristic (Toy, 2005). Treatment of transfusion-related acute lung injury is supportive and focuses on oxygenation and fluid volume status management that avoids overload (Benson, 2009; Swanson, 2006).

Platelets

For patients with moderate hemorrhage, RBC transfusion typically is sufficient, but for patients with severe hemorrhage, platelet transfusion also may be indicated. Donor plasma must

TABLE 40-9. Blood Product Transfusion Risks

Type of Risk/Complication	Incidence
Allergic reactions	1:2000
Transfusion-related acute lung injury	1:4000
ABO-incompatible transfusion	
Mistransfusion	1:14,000–1:18,000
Acute hemolytic reaction	1:6000–1:33,000
Delayed hemolytic reaction	1:2000–11,000
Infections	
Viral	
Hepatitis A	1:1 million
Hepatitis B	1:6000–1:320,000
Hepatitis C	1:1.2 million–<1:13 million
Human cytomegalovirus (CMV)	1:10–1:30
Epstein–Barr virus (EBV)	1:200
Human immunodeficiency virus (HIV)	1:1.4 million–1:11 million
West Nile virus	1:3000–1:5,000
Bacterial	
Yersinia enterocolitica, Serratia marcescens, Pseudomonas aeruginosa, Enterobacter	1:200,000–1:4.8 million
Parasites	
Malaria	1:4 million
Prions	
Creutzfeldt–Jakob disease	Unknown
Immunomodulation/suppression	Unknown

From Strumper-Groves, 2006, with permission.

be compatible with recipient erythrocytes because a few RBCs are invariably transfused along with the platelets. Platelets may be acquired from a single individual during plateletpheresis and are termed *single-donor platelets*. Alternatively, platelets may be derived from random units of whole blood and are referred to as *random-donor platelets*.

Fewer platelets are harvested from a unit of whole blood compared with the amount removed during donor plateletpheresis. Specifically, a single-donor platelet dose contains at least 3×10^{11} platelets in 250 to 300 mL of plasma, and this approximates the dose from six random-donor platelet concentrates.

Each random-donor platelet concentrate contain 5.5×10^{10} platelets suspended in approximately 50 mL of plasma. Each concentrate transfused should raise the platelet count by 5 to 10×10^9/L, and the usual therapeutic dose is one platelet concentrate per 10 kg of body weight. Five to six concentrates provide a typical adult dose.

Surgical patients with bleeding usually require platelet transfusion if the platelet count is less than 50×10^9/L and rarely require therapy if it is greater than 100×10^9/L. With counts between 50 and 100×10^9/L, the decision to provide platelet transfusion is based on a patient's risk for additional significant bleeding (American Society of Anesthesiologists, 1996). In patients requiring a large transfusion, a standard 6-unit pack of platelets may be indicated for every 7.5 units of RBCs transfused (Ketchum, 2006).

Fresh-Frozen Plasma

This component is prepared from whole blood or by plasmapheresis and is stored frozen. Approximately 30 minutes are required for the frozen plasma to thaw. One unit contains all coagulation factors, including fibrinogen, in 250 mL of volume.

Fresh-frozen plasma is used commonly as first-line hemostatic therapy in massive hemorrhage because it replaces multiple coagulation factors. It should be considered in a bleeding woman with a fibrinogen level below 100 mg/dL (normal 150 to 400 mg/dL) or with abnormal prothrombin and partial thromboplastin times (Cunningham, 2005).

Cryoprecipitate

This component is prepared from fresh-frozen plasma and contains fibrinogen, factor VIII, von Willebrand factor, factor XIII, and fibronectin. Cryoprecipitate was developed and used originally for treatment of hemophilia A and von Willebrand disease. However, specific factor concentrates are now available for these disorders, and thus, the clinical indications for cryoprecipitate are limited.

Fresh-frozen plasma provides all coagulation factors and is favored in severe hemorrhage over cryoprecipitate. However, cryoprecipitate is an excellent source of fibrinogen and may be indicated if fibrinogen levels persist below 100 mg/dL despite administration of fresh-frozen plasma, such as in disseminated intravascular coagulopathy.

ADJACENT ORGAN SURGICAL INJURY

Adequate operating exposure, comprehensive knowledge of anatomy, meticulous technique, and experience are important to prevent injury to surrounding organs during gynecologic surgery. However, these complications may arise especially in cases in which anatomy is distorted or the operating field is obscured by adhesions, blood, or tumor spread.

Injuries can often be prevented by initiating surgical dissection in areas free of distortion and by restoring normal anatomy. Dense adhesions should be divided sharply rather than bluntly to avoid tearing into organs and vessels. Once an injury has occurred, identification and repair at the initial surgery generally results in superior outcomes compared with delayed repair. Repairs should be tension free and should maintain adequate vascular support to the injured structure.

■ Bladder and Urethra
Bladder Injury

This complication may include laceration or perforation by sutures. It most commonly occurs during hysterectomy and urogynecologic procedures. Specifically, bladder injury complicates 1 to 2 percent of hysterectomies and is more commonly associated with a vaginal approach (Carley, 2002; Harris, 1997). Risk factors include prior pelvic reconstructive surgeries and prior cesarean delivery with scarring between the bladder and anterior uterus (Neumann, 2004; Rooney, 2005).

During vaginal hysterectomy, the bladder is at risk during dissection to enter the anterior cul de sac, during extraction of the uterus, or during excessive retractor tension. The location of bladder injury during vaginal hysterectomy is mainly the posterior bladder base (Mathevet, 2001). The bladder may also be injured during dissection of the vaginal epithelium when performing anterior colporrhaphy or during bladder neck suspension procedures.

With laparotomy, bladder injury may occur during initial abdominal entry when incising the anterior parietal peritoneum or during dissection within the space of Retzius. With hysterectomy, injury may occur during: (1) dissection of the bladder off the lower uterine segment, cervix, and vagina, (2) entry into the vagina, or (3) suturing of the vaginal cuff. These injuries primarily involve the dome.

With laparoscopic procedures, the incidence of bladder injury ranges from 0.02 to 8.3 percent (Francis, 2002). These are often at the dome and may result from trocar injuries or from dissection of the bladder off the cervix during laparoscopic hysterectomy.

Bladder injury prevention starts with maintaining a drained bladder throughout the procedure (Popert, 2004). A Foley catheter is typically placed for procedures anticipated to last longer than 30 minutes; otherwise in-and-out catheterization should suffice.

Diagnosis. Bladder injury is commonly identified intraoperatively by a gush of clear fluid into the field or by visualization of the Foley bulb. Alternatively, hematuria may be noted in the Foley bag. If the diagnosis is unclear, sterile infant formula may be instilled into the bladder to identify a leak. During instillation, a 60-mL syringe is filled with milk, and the syringe is attached to the distal end of the indwelling Foley catheter. Retrograde injection of milk from the syringe, through the catheter, and into the bladder will fill an intact bladder. However, spill into the operative field quickly identifies a laceration and aids in its localization. Alternatively, indigo carmine or methylene blue may be added to water for bladder instillation to identify leaks, however, these dyes tend to stain the surrounding tissues blue as well. Additionally, cystoscopy may be indicated to further define bladder injury, exclude concurrent ureteral injury, or identify sutures placed through the bladder mucosa. Once ureteral integrity has been assessed through the cystotomy or via cystoscopy, attention is turned to the repair. Although vesicovaginal fistula may develop even with early recognition and injury repair, the incidence is lower than if the injury remains undiagnosed.

Bladder Repair. The extent of an injury should be evaluated and adhesions lysed as needed to ensure a tension-free repair. The bladder is closed in two to three layers with 3-0 absorbable or delayed-absorbable suture (Fig. 40-40). The first layer is usually running. The second may be running or interrupted and should invert the first layer. In the area of the trigone, the ureters are typically stented, and the repair may be performed with interrupted sutures to avoid ureteral kinking (Popert, 2004). Bladder drainage should then be continuous and unobstructed typically for 7 to 10 days.

Alternatively, if injury involves errant sutures placed through the bladder mucosa, sutures should be cut. Persistent sutures can lead to cystitis symptoms or stone formation or both.

Urethral Injury

The female urethra is rarely injured during gynecologic surgery. Procedures that may result in injury include urethral diverticulum repairs, sling procedures, and possibly anterior colporrhaphy. Repair is undertaken with 3-0 or 4-0 absorbable suture in an interrupted fashion, in two layers if possible. A Foley catheter should be placed for the postoperative period (Francis, 2002).

■ Ureteral Injury

This is a serious complication of gynecologic surgery as patients may suffer significant morbidity and long-term sequelae. These injuries are uncommon in benign gynecologic surgery, and incidences associated with all hysterectomy approaches range from 0.03 to 6.0 percent (Harkki-Siren, 1998; Ostrzenski, 2003; Visco, 2001). Generally, vaginal hysterectomy has the lowest rate of ureteral injury, whereas laparoscopic hysterectomy has the highest. In cases without routine intraoperative cystoscopy, ureteral injury rates per procedure have been identified as follows: (1) vaginal hysterectomy 0.2/1000, (2) supracervical abdominal hysterectomy 0.5/1000, (3) total abdominal hysterectomy 0.9/1000, and (4) laparoscopic hysterectomy 7/1000. The rates are significantly

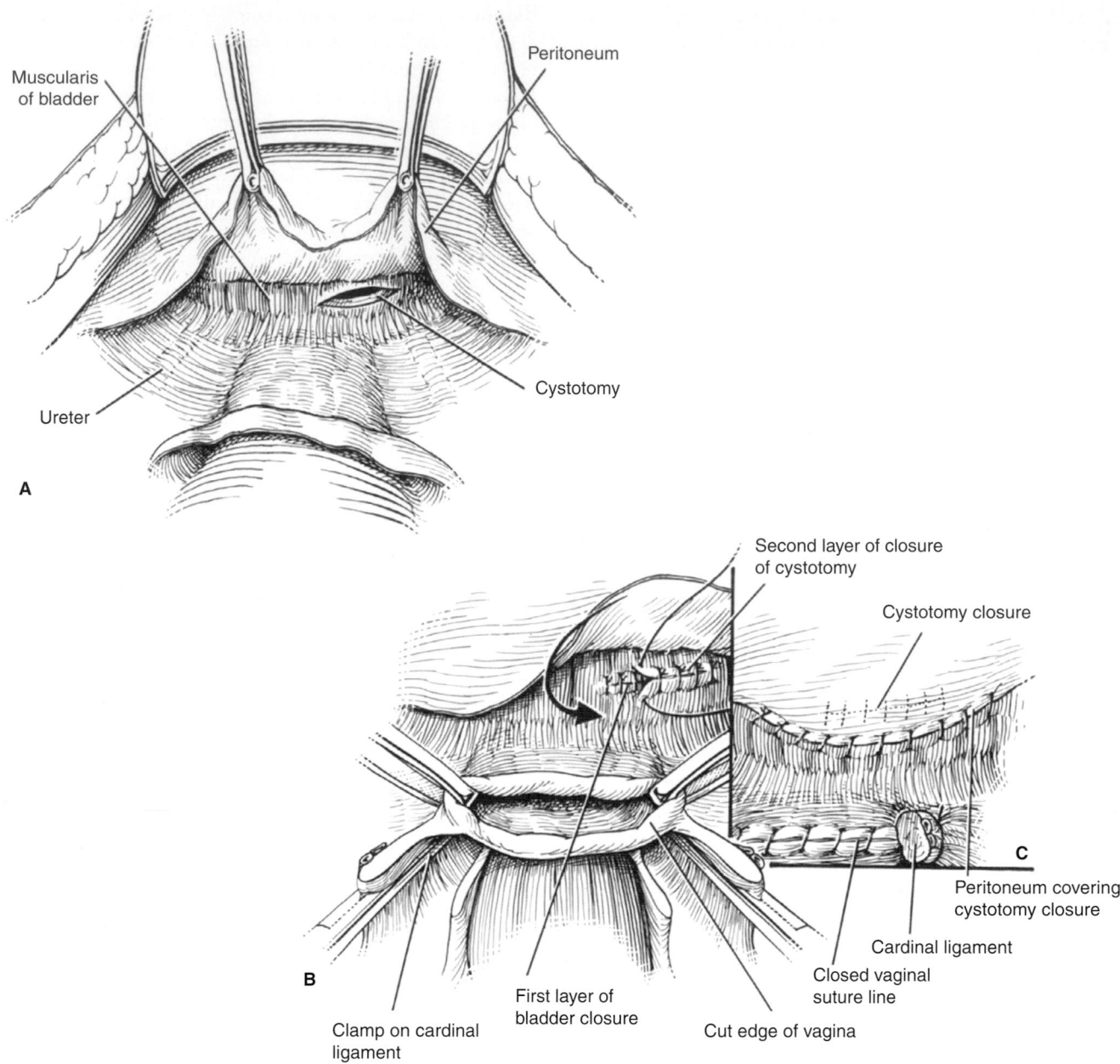

FIGURE 40-40 Cystotomy repair. **A.** Cystotomy occurring during hysterectomy. **B.** The primary layer inverts the bladder mucosa with running or interrupted sutures of 3-0 delayed-absorbable or absorbable suture. **C.** A second and possibly a third layer approximate the bladder muscularis to reinforce the incision closure. The bladder flap peritoneum is then reapproximated over the cystotomy repair. *(From Cunningham, 2010a, with permission.)*

higher if intraoperative cystoscopy is routinely performed, as this procedure identifies otherwise occult injuries (Gilmour, 2006).

The ureter is 25 to 30 cm long. It courses beneath the peritoneum and atop the psoas muscle until it enters the pelvis at the bifurcation of the common iliac artery and vein (Fig. 38-15, p. 931). The ureter then passes into the medial leaf of the broad ligament, anterior and medial to the internal iliac artery. It passes under the uterine artery approximately 1.5 cm lateral to the cervix (water under the bridge) and courses to reach the trigone. In the pelvis, its blood supply reaches the ureter from its lateral aspect. Accordingly, when necessary, the ureter should be mobilized in a direction medial to lateral to avoid devascularization.

The ureter may be injured at the pelvic brim (the level of the infundibulopelvic ligament), at the level of the uterine artery, at the vaginal fornices, and at the uterosacral ligaments. Obstruction may be the result of crushing with a clamp, ligating and transecting at the uterine arteries or the infundibulopelvic ligaments, or kinking. Delayed injuries may result in stricture or leak via thermal insult or devascularization.

Diagnosis

Intraoperative recognition during the initial surgery is associated with improved repair and lower patient morbidity (Neuman, 1991; Sakellariou, 2002). Approximately 75 percent of lower urinary tract injuries are unsuspected, thus many are not detected until the postoperative period (Ibeanu, 2009). Delayed diagnosis may result in more extensive complications such as fistula, urinoma, infection, and possible loss of the kidney. Renal damage may begin 24 hours after the obstruction and can be irreversible in 1 to 6 weeks (Walter, 2002). Signs and symptoms of injury postoperatively include flank pain, hematuria, anuria, vaginal urinary leakage, incontinence, ileus, fever, and elevated serum creatinine (Brandes, 2004). Interestingly, creatinine elevations greater than 0.2 mg/dL in the first 24 to 48 hours postoperatively may be helpful in early recognition of unilateral ureteral trauma (Walter, 2002). This increase is transient as the other kidney will begin compensating fairly quickly.

If ureteral injury is suspected postoperatively, a serum creatinine level and urinalysis should be obtained. If the serum creatinine level is elevated, additional calculation of the fractional excretion of sodium (FENa) or assessment of urine sodium levels may help clarify the source of renal injury as prerenal, intrarenal, or postrenal, as described in Chapter 39 (p. 965). Additionally, any fluid leaking from the vagina or obtained via drainage of an intraabdominal collection should be sent for a creatinine level. High creatinine levels confirm the presence of urine.

Imaging studies can be helpful in confirming the diagnosis. Intravenous pyelography is useful in localizing the injury. Computed tomography (CT) can demonstrate extravasation of contrast, ascites, urinoma, and hydronephrosis (Brandes, 2004; Francis, 2002). If delayed images are obtained, lack of contrast in the distal ureter on CT confirms a total obstruction (Armenakas, 1999). Retrograde pyelography is the most accurate modality in assessing location and extent of injury, and stents may also be placed at the time of the study.

Treatment

Management of ureteral injury will depend on the location and mode of injury. Additionally, the timing of the diagnosis, whether intraoperative or postoperative, will often influence treatment. If the ureter has been entrapped by suture and injury is identified early, often all that is needed is to release the suture and place a stent. Injuries to the distal third of the ureter are usually managed by ureteral reimplantation into the bladder (ureteroneocystotomy). If the injury occurs at a location that would create undue tension on the reimplantation site, then a psoas hitch is performed. With this, the bladder is dissected free on the side of the injury and sutured to the tendon of the psoas minor. This moves the bladder upward and relieves tension at the reimplantation site. Alternatives to the psoas hitch are an anterior bladder wall flap (Boari flap) or a ureteroureterostomy. With the Boari flap, the bladder ipsilateral to the injury is mobilized, and a pedicle of bladder wall is fashioned into a tube to bridge to the ureter. Transureteroureterostomy is rarely performed, but may be necessary with a more proximal injury or one in which the bladder cannot be mobilized. In this procedure, the injured ureter is tunneled across and connected to the healthy ureter (Brandes, 2004).

In the setting of delayed diagnosis, retrograde stenting is often attempted, although it may be unsuccessful. Typically, a percutaneous nephrostomy tube will be placed with a plan for a delayed definitive repair (Armenakas, 1999). Occasionally an antegrade stent can be placed, which will obviate the need for an open repair provided there is no leak or stricture.

Prevention of all ureteral injuries is not an attainable goal, however, gynecologic surgeons should be able to minimize their incidence and recognize them early. Proper exposure should be attained, with the ureter definitively identified and avoided. A surgeon should reidentify the ureter as necessary throughout a procedure. Preoperative stenting or intravenous pyelography have been advocated to assist in prevention, but they have not been found to be particularly effective or cost-efficient (Francis, 2002). Broad use of cystoscopy has also been advocated to assist in early detection (Ferro, 2003; Vakili, 2005).

Universal Cystoscopy

There is much ongoing discussion regarding adoption of universal cystoscopy to aid early detection of bladder and ureteral injuries. Up to 90 percent of unsuspected ureteral injuries and 85 percent of unsuspected bladder injuries may be identified with the use of cystoscopy (Gilmour, 1999, 2006; Gustilo-Ashby, 2006). Ibeanu and colleagues (2009) reported an approximately 97-percent intraoperative detection rate of urinary tract injury with universal cystoscopy. Of injuries, only 26 percent were noted intraoperatively and prior to cystoscopy.

Alternatively, many gynecologists selectively choose cystoscopy in those cases that pose greater risk for injury. These include cases in which an injury is actually suspected or cases with severe endometriosis, extensive adhesions, or broad ligament or cervical leiomyomas. Cost analysis indicates that if the ureteral injury rate exceeds 1.5 percent for abdominal hysterectomy, and 2 percent for vaginal or for laparoscopically assisted vaginal hysterectomy, then universal cystoscopy is cost effective (Visco, 2001). Other issues that play a role in this debate are credentialing problems for cystoscopy at some institutions for gynecologic surgeons and defining the appropriate resident training for performance of screening cystoscopy (Brubaker, 2009).

Bowel Injury

Injury to the bowel infrequently complicates gynecologic surgery, and rates in general lie below 1 percent (Harris, 1997; Hoffman, 1999; Makinen, 2001). Complications, however, may be more common in those with adhesions from prior surgery, infection, or endometriosis. Diagnosis may be obvious with gross fecal spill. However, subtle injury can occur. Thus, following extensive bowel adhesiolysis, examination of the bowel along the span involved with dissection is prudent. Moreover, diagnosis may be delayed in cases of thermal injury, in which tissues necrose, slough, and perforate only after time. Management of enterotomy varies considerably and typically is dictated by the size of the injury, skill and experience of the surgeon, and portion of the intestine entered. Short enterotomy wounds into the small intestine may be repaired with a layered closure using fine absorbable suture. The defect is closed perpendicular to the axis of the bowel rather than parallel to avoid narrowing the lumen. Multiple or long enterotomies may require resection and anastomosis to avoid narrowing the bowel lumen (Atkinson, 2004). During repair, rubber shod clamps are placed across the intestinal lumen on either side of the wound to prevent content spill. The large intestine carries a greater risk of contamination, but small enterotomies here may be managed like those of the small intestine. Injuries of the rectum below the peritoneal reflection can be managed by primary repair without significant sequelae. These are seen with procedures involving the posterior vaginal wall, such as posterior colpotomy during vaginal hysterectomy (Hoffman, 1999). For most general gynecologists, however, larger incisions of either the small or large bowel merit consultation with a general surgeon.

REFERENCES

Aletti GD, Dowdy SC, Podratz KC, et al: Surgical treatment of diaphragm disease correlates with improved survival in optimally debulked advanced stage ovarian cancer. Gynecol Oncol 100 (2):283, 2006

Amaral J: Electrosurgery and ultrasound for cutting and coagulating tissue in minimally invasive surgery. In Soper N, Swanstrom L, Eubanks W (eds): Mastery of Endoscopic and Laparoscopic Surgery. Philadelphia, Lippincott Williams & Wilkins, 2005, p 67

American Society for Reproductive Medicine, Society of Reproductive Surgeons: Pathogenesis, consequences, and control of peritoneal adhesions in gynecologic surgery. Fertil Steril 90(5 Suppl):S144, 2008

American Society of Anesthesiologists: Practice guidelines for blood component therapy: a report by the American Society of Anesthesiologists Task Force on Blood Component Therapy. Anesthesiology 84(3):732, 1996

Anderson RM, Romfh RF: Technique in the Use of Surgical Tools. New York, Appleton-Century-Crofts, 1980

Anderton J, Keen R, Neave R: The lithotomy position. In Positioning the Surgical Patient. London, Butterworths, 1988, p 20

Armenakas NA: Current methods of diagnosis and management of ureteral injuries. World J Urol 17:8, 1999

Aszmann OC, Dellon ES, Dellon AL: Anatomical course of the lateral femoral cutaneous nerve and its susceptibility to compression and injury. Plast Reconst Surg 100(3):600, 1997

Atkinson S: Techniques from the gastrointestinal surgeons. In Maxwell DJ (ed): Surgical Techniques in Obstetrics and Gynaecology. Edinburgh, Churchill Livingstone, 2004, p 182

Ayers JW, Morley GW: Surgical incision for cesarean section. Obstet Gynecol 70(5):706, 1987

Baskett PJ: ABC of major trauma. Management of hypovolaemic shock. BMJ 300(6737):1453, 1990

Batra EK, Franz DA, Towler MA, et al: Influence of surgeon's tying technique on knot security. J Appl Biomater 4:241, 1993

Baxter Healthcare: Floseal matrix hemostatic sealant: instructions for use. 2005. Available at: http://www.baxter.com/products/biopharmaceuticals/downloads/FloSeal_PI.pdf. Accessed January 13, 2011

Beckley ML, Ghafourpour KL, Indresano AT: The use of argon beam coagulation to control hemorrhage: a case report and review of the technology. J Oral Maxillofacial Surg 62:615, 2004

Bennett RG: Selection of wound closure materials. J Am Acad Dermatol l18(4 Pt 1):619, 1988

Benson AB, Moss M, Silliman CC: Transfusion-related acute lung injury (TRALI): a clinical review with emphasis on the critically ill. Br J Haematol 147(4):431, 2009

Bhende S, Rothenburger S, Spangler DJ, et al: In vitro assessment of microbial barrier properties of Dermabond topical skin adhesive. Surg Infect 3(3):251, 2002

Bleich AT, Rahn DD, Wieslander CK, et al: Posterior division of the internal iliac artery: anatomic variations and clinical applications. Am J Obstet Gynecol 197(6):658.e1, 2007

Blomstedt B, Osterberg B, Bergstrand A: Suture material and bacterial transport. An experimental study. Acta Chirurg Scand 143(2):71, 1977

Blondeel PNV, Murphy JW, Debrosse D, et al: Closure of long surgical incisions with a new formulation of 2-octylcyanoacrylate tissue adhesive versus commercially available methods. Am J Surg 188(3):307, 2004

Bose P, Regan F, Paterson-Brown S: Improving the accuracy of estimated blood loss at obstetric haemorrhage using clinical reconstructions. BJOG 113(8):919, 2006

Brandes S, Coburn M, Armenakas N, et al: Consensus on genitourinary trauma: diagnosis and management of ureteric injury: an evidence-based analysis. BJUI 94:277, 2004

Brecher ME, Goodnough LT: The rise and fall of preoperative autologous blood donation. Transfusion 42(12):1618, 2002

Brill AI, Nezhat F, Nezhat C, et al: The incidence of adhesions after prior laparotomy: a laparoscopic appraisal. Obstet Gynecol 85:269, 1995

Brubaker L: Is routine cystoscopy an essential intraoperative test at hysterectomy? Obstet Gynecol 113:2, 2009

Bucknall TE: Factors influencing wound complications: a clinical and experimental study. Ann R Coll Surg Engl 65(2):71, 1983

Burchell RC: Physiology of internal iliac artery ligation. J Obstet Gynaecol Br Commonwealth 75 (6):642, 1968

Burkhart SS, Wirth MA, Simonick M, et al: Loop security as a determinant of tissue fixation security. Arthroscopy 14:773, 1998

Campbell JA, Temple WJ, Frank CB, et al: A biomechanical study of suture pullout in linea alba. Surgery 106:888, 1989

Cardosi RJ, Cox CS, Hoffman MS: Postoperative neuropathies after major pelvic surgery. Obstet Gynecol 100(2):240, 2002

Carley ME, McIntire D, Carley JM, et al: Incidence, risk factors and morbidity of unintended bladder or ureter injury during hysterectomy. Int Urogynecol J 13:18, 2002

Carlson MA, Condon RE: Polyglyconate (Maxon) versus nylon suture in midline abdominal incision closure: a prospective randomized trial. Am Surgeon 61(11):980, 1995

Chanrachakul B, Likittanasombut P, Prasertsawat P, et al: Lidocaine versus plain saline for pain relief in fractional curettage: a randomized controlled trial. Obstet Gynecol 98(4):592, 2001

Chen SS, Lin AT, Chen KK, et al: Femoral neuropathy after pelvic surgery. Urol 46 (4):575, 1995

Cicinelli E, Didonna T, Ambrosi G, et al: Topical anaesthesia for diagnostic hysteroscopy and endometrial biopsy in postmenopausal women: a randomised placebo-controlled double-blind study. Br J Obstet Gynaecol 104(3):316, 1997

Cicinelli E, Didonna T, Schonauer LM, et al: Paracervical anesthesia for hysteroscopy and endometrial biopsy in postmenopausal women: a randomized, double-blind, placebo-controlled study. J Reprod Med Obstet Gynecol 43(12):1014, 1998

Colombo M, Maggioni A, Parma G, et al: A randomized comparison of continuous versus interrupted mass closure of midline incisions in patients with gynecologic cancer. Obstet Gynecol 89(5 Pt 1):684, 1997

C.R. Bard, Inc: Avitene Microfibrillar Collagen Hemostat Package Insert Information, 2002. Available at: http://www.davol.com/products/surgical-specialties/hemostasis/avitene-sheets/. Accessed September 19, 2011

Cunningham FG: Needles, sutures, and knots. In Gilstrap LC, Cunningham FG, Vandorsten JP (eds): Operative Obstetrics, 2nd ed. McGraw-Hill, New York, 2002, p 6

Cunningham FG, Leveno KJ, Bloom SL, et al: Cesarean delivery and peripartum hysterectomy. In Williams Obstetrics, 23rd ed. New York, McGraw-Hill, 2010a, p 560

Cunningham FG, Leveno KJ, Bloom SL, et al: Obstetrical hemorrhage. In Williams Obstetrics, 22nd ed. New York, McGraw-Hill, 2005, p 840

Cunningham FG, Leveno KJ, Bloom SL, et al: Obstetrical hemorrhage. In Williams Obstetrics, 23rd ed. New York, McGraw-Hill, 2010b, p 796

Deatrick KB, Doherty GM: Power sources in surgery. In Doherty GM (ed): Current Surgical Diagnosis and Treatment, 13th ed. New York, McGraw-Hill, 2010

Demirci F, Ozdemir I, Safak A, et al: Comparison of colour Doppler indices of pelvic arteries in women with bilateral hypogastric artery ligation and controls. J Obstet Gynaecol 25(3):273, 2005

Deppe G, Malviya VK, Malone JM Jr: Debulking surgery for ovarian cancer with the Cavitron Ultrasonic Surgical Aspirator (CUSA)—a preliminary report. Gynecol Oncol 31(1):223, 1988

Dinsmore RC: Understanding surgical knot security: a proposal to standardize the literature. J Am Coll Surg 180(6):689, 1995

Dodd R: Managing the microbiological safety of blood for transfusion: a US perspective. Future Microbiol 4(7):807, 2009

Dorian R: Anesthesia of the surgical patient. In Brunicardi F, Andersen D, Billiar T, et al (eds): Schwartz's Principles of Surgery. New York, McGraw-Hill, 2005, p 200

Ducic I, Dellon L, Larson EE: Treatment concepts for idiopathic and iatrogenic femoral nerve mononeuropathy. Ann Plast Surg 55(4):397, 2005

Ducic I, Moxley M, Al Attar A: Algorithm for treatment of postoperative incisional groin pain after cesarean delivery or hysterectomy. Obstet Gynecol 108(1):27, 2006

Dunn DL: Wound Closure Manual. Somerville, NJ, Ethicon, 2004, pp 49, 53

Dzieczkowski JS, Anderson KC: Transfusion biology and therapy. In Fauci AS, Braunwald E, Kasper DL, et al (eds): Harrison's Principles of Internal Medicine, 17th ed. New York, McGraw-Hill, 2008, p 709

Edlich RF, Panek PH, Rodeheaver GT, et al: Physical and chemical configuration of sutures in the development of surgical infection. Ann Surg 177(6):679, 1973

El-Gamal HM, Dufresne RG, Saddler K: Electrosurgery, pacemakers and ICDs: a survey of precautions and complications experienced by cutaneous surgeons. Dermatol Surg 27(4):385, 2001

Erber WN, Perry DJ: Plasma and plasma products in the treatment of massive haemorrhage. Best Pract Res Clin Haematol 19(1):97, 2006

Ferro A, Byck D, Gallup D: Intraoperative and postoperative morbidity associated with cystoscopy performed in patients undergoing gynecologic surgery. Am J Obstet Gynecol 189(2):354, 2003

Franchi M, Ghezzi F, Benedetti Panici PL, et al: A multicentre collaborative study on the use of cold scalpel and electrocautery for midline abdominal incision. Am J Surg 181(2):128, 2001

Franchi M, Ghezzi F, Zanaboni F, et al: Nonclosure of peritoneum at radical abdominal hysterectomy and pelvic node dissection: a randomized study. Obstet Gynecol 90(4 Pt 1):622, 1997

Francis, SL, Magrina JF, Novicki D, et al: Intraoperative injuries of the urinary tract. J Gynecol Oncol 7:65, 2002

Gallup DC, Gallup DG, Nolan TE, et al: Use of a subcutaneous closed drainage system and antibiotics in obese gynecologic patients. Am J Obstet Gynecol 175:358, 1996

Geiger D, Debus ES, Ziegler UE, et al: Capillary activity of surgical sutures and suture-dependent bacterial transport: a qualitative study. Surg Infect 6(4):377, 2005

Giacalone PL, Daures JP, Vignal J, et al: Pfannenstiel versus Maylard incision for cesarean delivery: a randomized controlled trial. Obstet Gynecol 99(5 Pt 1):745, 2002

Gilmour DT, Das S, Flowerdew G: Rates of urinary tract injury from gynecologic surgery and the role of intraoperative cystoscopy. Obstet Gynecol 107(6):1366, 2006

Gilmour DT, Dwyer PL, Carey MP: Lower urinary tract injury during gynecologic surgery and its detection by intraoperative cystoscopy. Obstet Gynecol 94(5 Pt 2):883, 1999

Gilstrap LC, Cunningham FG, Vandorsten JP: Operative Obstetrics, 2nd ed. New York, McGraw-Hill, 2002, p 412

Glantz JC, Shomento S: Comparison of paracervical block techniques during first trimester pregnancy termination. Int J Obstet Gynaecol 72(2):171, 2001

Goldman JA, Feldberg D, Dicker D, et al: Femoral neuropathy subsequent to abdominal hysterectomy. A comparative study. Eur J Obstet Gynecol Reprod Biol 20(6):385, 1985

Goodnough LT: Autologous blood donation. Anesthesiol Clin North Am 23(2):263, 2005

Gorgas D: Transfusion Therapy: Blood and blood products. In Roberts J, Hedges J, Chanmugam AS, et al (eds): Roberts Clinical Procedures in Emergency Medicine. Philadelphia, WB Saunders, 2004

Gostout BS, Cliby WA, Podratz KC: Prevention and management of acute intraoperative bleeding. Clin Obstet Gynecol 45(2):481, 2002

Grantcharov TP, Rosenberg J: Vertical compared with transverse incisions in abdominal surgery. Eur J Surg 167(4):260, 2001

Greenall MJ, Evans M, Pollock AV: Midline or transverse laparotomy? A random controlled clinical trial. Part I: influence on healing. Br J Surg 67(3):188, 1980

Greenberg CC, Regenbogen SE, Studdert DM, et al: Patterns of communication breakdowns resulting in injury to surgical patients. J Am Coll Surg 204:533, 2007

Gunderson PE: The half-hitch knot: a rational alternative to the square knot. Am J Surg 54:538, 1987

Gupta JK, Dinas K, Khan KS: To peritonealize or not to peritonealize? A randomized trial at abdominal hysterectomy. Am J Obstet Gynecol 178(4):796, 1998

Gustilo-Ashby AM, Jelovsek JE, Barber MD, et al: The incidence of ureteral obstruction and the value of intraoperative cystoscopy during vaginal surgery for pelvic organ prolapse. Am J Obstet Gynecol 194(5):1478, 2006

Guvenal T, Duran B, Kemirkoprulu N, et al: Prevention of superficial wound disruption in Pfannenstiel incisions by using a subcutaneous drain. Int J Gynecol Obstet 77:151, 2002

Gyr T, Ghezzi F, Arslanagic S, et al: Minimal invasive laparoscopic hysterectomy with ultrasonic scalpel. Am J Surg 181(6):516, 2001

Hambley R, Hebda PA, Abell E, et al: Wound healing of skin incisions produced by ultrasonically vibrating knife, scalpel, electrosurgery, and carbon dioxide laser. J Dermatol Surg Oncol 14(11):1213, 1988

Harkki-Siren P, Sjoberg J, Tiitinen A: Urinary tract injuries after hysterectomy. Obstet Gynecol 92(1):113, 1998

Harold KL, Pollinger H, Matthews BD, et al: Comparison of ultrasonic energy, bipolar thermal energy, and vascular clips for the hemostasis of small-, medium-, and large-sized arteries. Surg Endosc 17(8):1228, 2003

Harris WJ: Complications of hysterectomy. Clin Obstet Gynecol 40(4):928, 1997

Healey MA, Davis RE, Liu FC, et al: Lactated Ringer's is superior to normal saline in a model of massive hemorrhage and resuscitation. J Trauma Inj Inf Crit Care 45(5):894, 1998

Hébert PC, Wells G, Blajchman MA, et al: A multicenter, randomized, controlled clinical trial of transfusion requirements in critical care. Transfusion Requirements in Critical Care Investigators, Canadian Critical Care Trials Group. N Engl J Med 340(6):409, 1999

Heniford BT, Matthews BD, Sing RF, et al: Initial results with an electrothermal bipolar vessel sealer. Surg Endosc 15(8):799, 2001

Henry DA, Carless PA, Moxey AJ, et al: Pre-operative autologous donation for minimising perioperative allogeneic blood transfusion. Cochrane Database Syst Rev 2.CD003602, 2002

Hill SR, Carless PA, Henry DA, et al: Transfusion thresholds and other strategies for guiding allogeneic red blood cell transfusion. Cochrane Database Syst Rev 2:CD002042, 2002

Hoffman MS, Lynch C, Lockhart J, et al: Injury of the rectum during vaginal surgery. Am J Obstet Gynecol 181:274, 1999

Hong JY, Kim J: Use of paracervical analgesia for outpatient hysteroscopic surgery: a randomized, double-blind, placebo-controlled study. Amb Surg 12(4):181, 2006

Hsieh LF, Liaw ES, Cheng HY, et al: Bilateral femoral neuropathy after vaginal hysterectomy. Arch Phys Med Rehabil 79(8):1018, 1998

Hurt J, Unger JB, Ivy JJ, et al: Tying a loop-to-strand suture: is it safe? Am J Obstet Gynecol 192:1094, 2005

Ibeanu OA, Chesson RR, Echols KT, et al: Urinary tract injury during hysterectomy based on universal cystoscopy. Obstet Gynecol 113:6, 2009

Irvin W, Andersen W, Taylor P, et al: Minimizing the risk of neurologic injury in gynecologic surgery. Obstet Gynecol 103(2):374, 2004

Ivy JJ, Unger JB, Hurt J, et al: The effect of number of throws on knot security with non-identical sliding knots. Am J Obstet Gynecol 191:1618, 2004a

Ivy JJ, Unger JB, Mukherjee D: Knot integrity with nonidentical and parallel sliding knots. Am J Obstet Gynecol 190:83, 2004b

Jallo GI: CUSA EXcel ultrasonic aspiration system. Neurosurgery 48(3):695, 2001

Jenkins TR: It's time to challenge surgical dogma with evidence-based data. Am J Obstet Gynecol 189(2):423, 2003

Joint Commission: Universal protocol for preventing wrong site, wrong procedure, and wrong person surgery. Oakbrook Terrace (IL), Joint Commission, 2009. Available at: http://www.jointcommission.org/PatientSafety/UniversalProtocol. Accessed September 15, 2010

Kanter MH, van Maanen D, Anders KH, et al: A study of an educational intervention to decrease inappropriate preoperative autologous blood donation: its effectiveness and the effect on subsequent transfusion rates in elective hysterectomy. Transfusion 39(8):801, 1999

Kanter MH, van Maanen D, Anders KH, et al: Preoperative autologous blood donations before elective hysterectomy. JAMA 276(10):798, 1996

Karger R, Kretschmer V: Modern concepts of autologous haemotherapy. Transfus Apher Sci 32(2):185, 2005

Katz KH, Desciak EB, Maloney ME: The optimal application of surgical adhesive tape strips. Dermatol Surg 25(9):686, 1999

Kauko M: New techniques using the ultrasonic scalpel in laparoscopic hysterectomy. Cur Opin Obstet Gynecol 10(4):303, 1998

Ketchum L, Hess JR, Hiippala S: Indications for early fresh frozen plasma, cryoprecipitate, and platelet transfusion in trauma. J Trauma Inj Infect Crit Care 60(6 Suppl):S51, 2006

Khelifi A, Amamou K, Salem A, et al: [Therapeutic ligature of hypogastric arteries: color Doppler follow-up]. [French]. J Radiol 81(6):607, 2000

Kisielinski K, Conze J, Murken AH, et al: The Pfannenstiel or so called "bikini cut": still effective more than 100 years after first description. Hernia 8(3):177, 2004

Knockaert DC, Boonen AL, Bruyninckx FL, et al: Electromyographic findings in ilioinguinal-iliohypogastric nerve entrapment syndrome. Acta Clin Belg 51(3):156, 1996

Kolle D, Tamussino K, Hanzal E, et al: Bleeding complications with the tension-free vaginal tape operation. Am J Obstet Gynecol 193(6):2045, 2005

Kuuva N, Nilsson CG: A nationwide analysis of complications associated with the tension-free vaginal tape (TVT) procedure. Acta Obstet Gynecol Scand 81(1):72, 2002

Kvist-Poulsen H, Borel J: Iatrogenic femoral neuropathy subsequent to abdominal hysterectomy: incidence and prevention. Obstet Gynecol 60(4):516, 1982

Lacy PD, Burke PE, O'Regan M, et al: The comparison of type of incision for transperitoneal abdominal aortic surgery based on postoperative respiratory complications and morbidity. Eur J Vasc Surg 8(1):52, 1994

Lammers R, Trott A: Methods of wound closure. In Roberts J, Hedges J (eds): Clinical Procedures in Emergency Medicine. Philadelphia, WB Saunders, 2004, p 655

Lau WC, Lo WK, Tam WH, et al: Paracervical anaesthesia in outpatient hysteroscopy: a randomised double-blind placebo-controlled trial. Br J Obstet Gynaecol 106(4):356, 1999

Leaper DJ, Pollock AV, Evans M: Abdominal wound closure: a trial of nylon, polyglycolic acid and steel sutures. Br J Surg 64(8):603, 1977

Lichtenberg ES, Paul M, Jones H: First trimester surgical abortion practices: a survey of National Abortion Federation members. Contraception 64(6):345, 2001

Lin KY, Long WB: Scientific basis for the selection of surgical needles and sutures. 2006. Available at: http://www.woundclosures.com/article.cfm?id=6. Accessed November 15, 2006

Lipscomb GH, Ling FW: Wound healing, suture material, and surgical instrumentation. In Rock JA, Thompson JD (eds): Telinde's Operative Gynecology, 8th ed. Philadelphia, Lippincott Williams & Wilkins, 1997, p 278

Lipscomb GH, Ling FW, Stovall TG, et al: Peritoneal closure at vaginal hysterectomy: a reassessment. Obstet Gynecol 87(1):40, 1996

Lo IKY, Burkhart SS, Chan KC, et al: Arthroscopic knots: determining the optimal balance of loop security and knot security. Arthroscopy 20:489, 2004

Long JB, Elland RJ, Hentz JG, et al: Randomized trial of preemptive local analgesia in vaginal surgery. Int Urogynecol J Pelvic Floor Dysfunct 20(1):5, 2009

Luban NL: Transfusion safety: where are we today? Ann NY Acad Sci 1054:325, 2005

Luijendijk RW, Jeekel J, Storm RK, et al: The low transverse Pfannenstiel incision and the prevalence of incisional hernia and nerve entrapment. Ann Surg 225(4):365, 1997

Madjdpour C, Spahn DR, Weiskopf RB: Anemia and perioperative red blood cell transfusion: a matter of tolerance. Crit Care Med 34(5 Suppl):S102, 2006

Makinen J, Johansson J, Tomas C, et al: Morbidity of 10110 hysterectomies by type of approach. Hum Reprod 16(7):1473, 2001

Manning J: Fluid and blood resuscitation. In Tintinalli J, Gabor D, Stapczynski J, et al (eds): Tintinalli's Emergency Medicine. New York, McGraw-Hill, 2004

Masterson B: Intraoperative hemorrhage. In Nichols D, DeLancey J (eds): Clinical Problems, Injuries and Complications of Gynecologic and Obstetric Surgery. Baltimore, Williams & Wilkins, 1995, p 14

Mathevet P, Valencia P, Cousin C, et al: Operative injuries during vaginal hysterectomy. Eur J Obstet Gynecol Reprod Biol 97:71, 2001

McQuarrie HG, Harris JW, Ellsworth HS, et al: Sciatic neuropathy complicating vaginal hysterectomy. Am J Obstet Gynecol 113(2):223, 1972

Michelassi F, Hurst R: Electrocautery, argon beam coagulation, cryotherapy, and other hemostatic and tissue ablative instruments. In Nyhus L, Baker R, Fischer J (eds): Mastery of Surgery. Boston, Little, Brown, 1997, p 234

Moore FA, McKinley BA, Moore EE: The next generation in shock resuscitation. Lancet 363(9425):1988, 2004

Morris ML: Electrosurgery in the gastroenterology suite: principles, practice, and safety. Gastroenterol Nurs 29(2):126, 2006

Murovic JA, Kim DH, Tiel RL, et al: Surgical management of 10 genitofemoral neuralgias at the Louisiana State University Health Sciences Center. Neurosurg 56(2):298, 2005

Murphy MF, Wallington TB, Kelsey P, et al: Guidelines for the clinical use of red cell transfusions. Br J Haematol 113(1):24, 2001

Nagpal K, Vats A, Ahmed K, et al: A systematic quantitative assessment of risks associated with poor communication in surgical care. Arch Surg 145(6):582, 2010

Naguib M, Magboul MM, Samarkandi AH, et al: Adverse effects and drug interactions associated with local and regional anaesthesia. Drug Safety 18(4):221, 1998

Naumann RW, Hauth JC, Owen J, et al: Subcutaneous tissue approximation in relation to wound disruption after cesarean delivery in obese women. Obstet Gynecol 85:412, 1995

Neuman M, Eidelman A, Langer R, et al: Iatrogenic injuries to the ureter during gynecologic and obstetric operations. Surg Gynecol Obstet 173(4):268, 1991

Neumann G, Rasmussen KL, Lauszus FF: Perioperative bladder injury during hysterectomy for benign disorders. Acta Obstet Gynecol Scand 83(10):1001, 2004

Newton M: Intraoperative complications. In Newton M, Newton E (eds): Complications of Gynecologic and Obstetric Management. Philadelphia, WB Saunders, 1988, p 36

Nichols DH, Clarke-Pearson DL: Gynecologic, Obstetric, and Related Surgery, 2nd ed. Baltimore, Mosby, 2000, p 119

Nizard J, Barrinque L, Frydman R, et al: Fertility and pregnancy outcomes following hypogastric artery ligation for severe post-partum haemorrhage. Hum Reprod 18(4):844, 2003

Nygaard IE, Squatrito RC: Abdominal incisions from creation to closure. Obstet Gynecol Surv 51(7):429, 1996

Oderich GS, Panneton JM, Hofer J, et al: Iatrogenic operative injuries of abdominal and pelvic veins: a potentially lethal complication. J Vasc Surg 39(5):931, 2004

O'Neal MG, Beste T, Shackelford DP: Utility of preemptive local analgesia in vaginal hysterectomy. Am J Obstet Gynecol 189(6):1539, 2003

Orr JW Jr, Orr PF, Barrett JM, et al: Continuous or interrupted fascial closure: a prospective evaluation of No. 1 Maxon suture in 402 gynecologic procedures. Am J Obstet Gynecol 163(5 Pt 1):1485, 1990

Ostrzenski A, Radolinski B, Ostrzenska KM: A review of laparoscopic ureteral injury in pelvic surgery. Obstet Gynecol Surv 58(12):794, 2003

Penfield JA: Gynecologic surgery under local anesthesia. Baltimore, Urban and Schwarzenberg, 1986, p 48

Pfizer: Gelfoam Absorbable Gelatin Powder. Package Insert. 2008. Available at: www.pfizer.com/pfizer/download/uspi_gelfoam_powder.pdf. Accessed January 13, 2011

Phair N, Jensen JT, Nichols MD: Paracervical block and elective abortion: the effect on pain of waiting between injection and procedure. Am J Obstet Gynecol 186(6):1304, 2002

Philosophe R: Avoiding complications of laparoscopic surgery. Fertil Steril 80(Suppl 4):30, 2003

Pinski SL, Trohman RG: Interference in implanted cardiac devices, part II. Pacing Clin Electrophysiol 25(10):1496, 2002

Popert R: Techniques from the urologists. In Maxwell DJ (ed): Surgical Techniques in Obstetrics and Gynaecology. Edinburgh, Churchill Livingstone, 2004, pp 189, 195

Quinn J, Wells G, Sutcliffe T, et al: A randomized trial comparing octylcyanoacrylate tissue adhesive and sutures in the management of lacerations. JAMA 277(19):1527, 1997

Rahn DD, Phelan JN, Roshanravan SM, et al: Anterior abdominal wall nerve and vessel anatomy: clinical implications for gynecologic surgery. Am J Obstet Gynecol 202:234.e1, 2010

Roberts I, Alderson P, Bunn F, et al: Colloids versus crystalloids for fluid resuscitation in critically ill patients. Cochrane Database Syst Rev 4:CD000567, 2004

Robinson JB, Sun CC, Bodurka-Bevers D, et al: Cavitational ultrasonic surgical aspiration for the treatment of vaginal intraepithelial neoplasia. Gynecol Oncol 78(2):235, 2000

Rodeheaver GT, Halverson JM, Edlich RF: Mechanical performance of wound closure tapes. Ann Emerg Med 12(4):203, 1983

Rogers R Jr: Basic pelvic neuroanatomy. In Steege J, Metzger D, Levy B (eds): Chronic Pelvic Pain: an Integrated Approach. Philadelphia, WB Saunders, 1998, p 31

Rooney CM, Crawford AT, Vassallo BJ, et al: Is previous cesarean section a risk for incidental cystotomy at the time of hysterectomy? A case-controlled study. Am J Obstet Gynecol 193(6):2041, 2005

Sakellariou P, Protopapas AG, Voulgaris Z, et al: Management of ureteric injuries during gynecological operations: 10 years experience. Eur J Obstet Gynecol and Reprod Biol 101(2):179, 2002

Salom EM, Penalver M: Complications in gynecologic surgery. In Cohn SM, Barquist E, Byers PM, et al (eds): Complications in Surgery and Trauma. New York, Informa Healthcare USA, 2007, p 554

Santoso JT, Dinh TA, Omar S, et al: Surgical blood loss in abdominal hysterectomy. Gynecol Oncol 82(2):364, 2001

Schubert DC, Unger JB, Mukherjee D, et al: Mechanical performance of knots using braided and monofilament absorbable sutures. Am J Obstet Gynecol 187:1438, 2002

Schwartz D, Kaplan K, Schwartz S: Hemostasis, surgical bleeding, and transfusion. In Brunicardi F, Anersen D, Billiar T, et al (eds): Schwartz's Principles of Surgery. New York, McGraw-Hill, 2006

Sharp WV, Belden TA, King PH, et al: Suture resistance to infection. Surgery 91(1):61, 1982

Shepherd JH, Cavanagh D, Riggs D, et al: Abdominal wound closure using a nonabsorbable single-layer technique. Obstet Gynecol 61(2):248, 1983

Silliman CC, Ambruso DR, Boshkov LK: Transfusion-related acute lung injury. Blood 105(6):2266, 2005

Singer AJ, Hollander JE, Quinn JV: Evaluation and management of traumatic lacerations. N Engl J Med 337(16):1142, 1997

Singer AJ, Quinn JV, Clark RE, et al: Closure of lacerations and incisions with octylcyanoacrylate: a multicenter randomized controlled trial. Surgery 131(3):270, 2002a

Singer AJ, Quinn JV, Thode HC Jr, et al: Determinants of poor outcome after laceration and surgical incision repair. Plast Reconst Surg 110(2):429, 2002b

Singh S, Maxwell D: Tools of the trade. Best Pract Res Clin Obstet Gynaecol 20(1):41, 2006

Sinha UK, Gallagher LA: Effects of steel scalpel, ultrasonic scalpel, CO_2 laser, and monopolar and bipolar electrosurgery on wound healing in guinea pig oral mucosa. Laryngoscope 113(2):228, 2003

Soper DE, Bump RC, Hurt WG: Wound infection after abdominal hysterectomy: effect of the depth of subcutaneous tissue. Am J Obstet Gynecol 173(2):465, 1971

Stramer SL, Hollinger FB, Katz LM, et al: Emerging infectious disease agents and their potential threat to transfusion safety. Transfusion 49(Suppl 2):1S, 2009

Strumper-Groves D: Perioperative blood transfusion and outcome. Curr Opin Anaesthesiol 19(2):198, 2006

Swanson K, Dwyre DM, Krochmal J, et al: Transfusion-related acute lung injury (TRALI): current clinical and pathophysiologic considerations. Lung 184(3):177, 2006

Tikoo R, Jones W: Neurologic injury. In Orr J, Shingleton H (eds): Complications in Gynecologic Surgery: Prevention, Recognition, and Management. Philadelphia, JB Lippincott, 1994, p 221

Tomacruz RS, Bristow RE, Montz FJ: Management of pelvic hemorrhage. Surg Clin North Am 81(4):925, 2001

Toy P, Popovsky MA, Abraham E, et al: Transfusion-related acute lung injury: definition and review. Crit Care Med 33(4):721, 2005

Trimbos JB: Security of various knots commonly used in surgical practice. Obstet Gynecol 64:274, 1984

Trimbos JB, van Rijssel EJC, Klopper PJ: Performance of sliding knots in monofilament and multifilament suture material. Obstet Gynecol 68:425, 1986

Trolice MP, Fishburne C Jr, McGrady S: Anesthetic efficacy of intrauterine lidocaine for endometrial biopsy: a randomized double-masked trial. Obstet Gynecol 95(3):345, 2000

Tulandi T, Hum HS, Gelfand MM: Closure of laparotomy incisions with or without peritoneal suturing and second-look laparoscopy. Am J Obstet Gynecol 158(3 Pt 1):536, 1988

Vakili B, Chesson RR, Kyle BL, et al: The incidence of urinary tract injury during hysterectomy: a prospective analysis based on universal cystoscopy. Am J Obstet Gynecol 192(5):1599, 2005

Valleylab: Principles of electrosurgery. 2006. Available at: http://www.valleylab.com/education/poes/index.html. Accessed September 17, 2011

van Dam PA, Tjalma W, Weyler J, et al: Ultraradical debulking of epithelial ovarian cancer with the ultrasonic surgical aspirator: a prospective randomized trial. Am J Obstet Gynecol 174(3):943, 1996

van Rijssel EJC, Trimbos JB, Booster MH: Mechanical performance of square knots and sliding knots in surgery: a comparative study. Am J Obstet Gynecol 162:93, 1990

Vasilev SA: Obturator nerve injury: a review of management options. Gynecol Oncol 53(2):152, 1994

Vermillion ST, Lamoutte C, Soper DE, et al: Wound infection after cesarean: effect of subcutaneous tissue thickness. Obstet Gynecol 95(6 Pt 1):923, 2000

Visco AG, Taber KH, Weidner AC, et al: Cost-effectiveness of universal cystoscopy to identify ureteral injury at hysterectomy. Obstet Gynecol 97(5 Pt 1):685, 2001

Walter AJ, Magtibay PM, Morse AN, et al: Perioperative changes in serum creatinine after gynecologic surgery. Am J Obstet Gynecol 186.1315, 2002

Wang CJ, Yen CF, Lee CL, et al: Comparison the efficacy of laparosonic coagulating shears and electrosurgery in laparoscopically assisted vaginal hysterectomy: preliminary results. Int Surg 85(1):88, 2000

Warner MA: Perioperative neuropathies. Mayo Clin Proc 73(6):567, 1998

Warner MA, Warner DO, Harper CM, et al: Lower extremity neuropathies associated with lithotomy positions. Anesthesiology 93(4):938, 2000

Waters JH: Indications and contraindications of cell salvage. Transfusion 44(12 Suppl):40S, 2004

Waters JH: Red blood cell recovery and reinfusion. Anesthesiol Clin North Am 23(2):283, 2005

Whiteside JL, Barber MD, Walters MD, et al: Anatomy of ilioinguinal and iliohypogastric nerves in relation to trocar placement and low transverse incisions. Am J Obstet Gynecol 189(6):1574, 2003

Wiebe ER, Rawling M: Pain control in abortion. Int J Gynecol Obstet 50(1):41, 1995

Wind GG, Rich NM: Principles of Surgical Technique: The Art of Surgery, 2nd ed. Urban and Schwarzenberg, Baltimore, 1987, p 65

Winfree CJ: Peripheral nerve injury evaluation and management. Curr Surg 62(5):469, 2005

Wissing J, van Vroonhoven TJ, Schattenkerk ME, et al: Fascia closure after midline laparotomy: results of a randomized trial. Br J Surg 74(8):738, 1987

Zimmer CA, Thacker JG, Powell DM, et al: Influence of knot configuration and tying technique on the mechanical performance of sutures. J Emerg Med 9:107, 1991

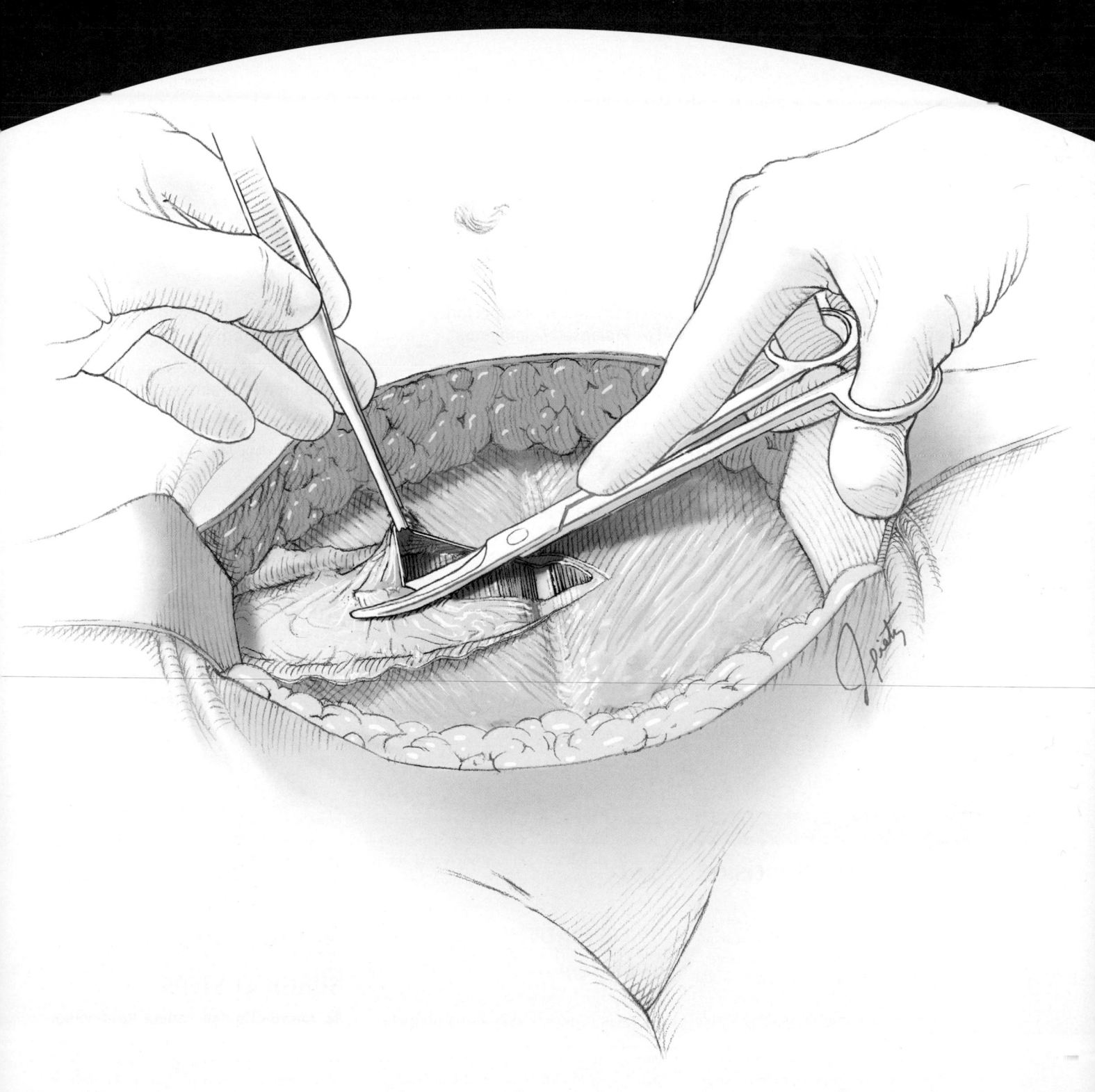

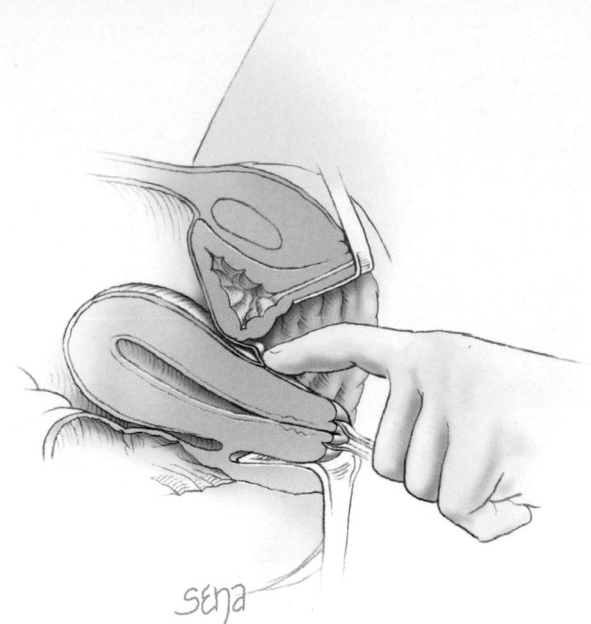

41-1

Midline Vertical Incision

Abdominal entry is the first step for many gynecologic surgeries. Either vertical or transverse incisions may be used to gain access, and each offers particular advantages. Vertical incisions may be midline or paramedian, but of the two, the midline is chosen more often. This incision offers quick entry, minimal blood loss, superior access to the upper abdomen, generous operating room, and the flexibility for easy wound extension if greater space or access is needed. No important neurovascular structures traverse this incision. Thus, this incision may be favored in the patient who is using anticoagulation agents.

PREOPERATIVE

Consent

Despite these advantages, midline incisions are more frequently associated with greater postoperative pain, poorer cosmetic results, and increased risk of incisional hernia compared with low transverse incisions. Risk of bowel injury is present with any abdominal entry, especially when extensive adhesions are present. Wound infection and venous thromboembolism may complicate abdominal surgery and are discussed in Chapter 39.

INTRAOPERATIVE

SURGICAL STEPS

❶ **Anesthesia and Patient Positioning.** After administration of adequate regional or general anesthesia, the patient is positioned supine. If needed, hair in the path of the planned incision is clipped; a Foley catheter is placed; and abdominal preparation is completed.

❷ **Skin and Subcutaneous Layer.** A midline vertical incision is made sharply beginning 2 to 3 cm above the symphysis pubis and is extended cephalad to within 2 cm of the umbilicus. In cases that require larger operating space or extensive access to the upper abdomen, the incision may arch around to the left of the umbilicus and continue cephalad as needed. The subcutaneous layers of Camper and Scarpa are incised to reach the fascia.

❸ **Fascia.** Tendinous fibers from the anterior abdominal wall aponeuroses merge in the midline of the abdomen to form the linea alba. This fascia layer is sharply entered near the midpoint of the incision to avoid potential injury to the bladder. This incision is extended cephalad and caudally to mirror the length of the skin incision. During this extension of the fascial incision, the linea alba may be elevated with finger tips or the ends of a Pean clamp to minimize injury to tissues below (Fig. 41-1.1).

❹ **Peritoneum.** The peritoneum is identified between the bellies of the rectus abdominis muscle, grasped with two fine forceps or hemostats, and sharply cut. Similarly, this incision is extended cephalad and caudally (Fig. 41-1.2). Fingers are placed underneath and elevate the peritoneum to prevent bowel injury. As the incision is extended caudally, the bladder dome can be identified by the increasing vascularity and thickness of the peritoneum.

Also, the urachus, which is the remnant of the allantois, may be seen as a white cord extending from the bladder dome toward the umbilicus in the midline.

During abdominal entry, prior surgery may blur clear tissue planes between the fascia, peritoneum, and viscera. In this situation, a gradual layered entry is required to avoid organ injury. One technique uses Metzenbaum scissors. Scissor tips are insinuated between tissue layers such that the tips are seen each time prior to cutting. This minimizes the risk that the thicker bowel or bladder wall will be cut.

❺ **Operative Field.** After the abdominal cavity is entered, a self-retaining retractor is commonly placed to retract the muscles of the abdominal wall, the bowel, and omentum. Moist laparotomy sponges are placed around the bulk of bowel, and it is gently directed cephalad. Adhesiolysis may be required to adequately free intestines for retraction. Upper blades of the retractor assist in holding these loops up and away from the pelvis and operating field. With the pelvic organs exposed, the planned abdominal surgery can proceed.

❻ **Wound Closure.** The fascia is closed from one end to the other using a continuous running suture with a 0-gauge delayed-absorbable suture. If the subcutaneous layer measures less than 2 cm, no closure is typically necessary. For deeper wounds, interrupted stitches of 4-0 delayed-absorbable suture are used to close this layer. The skin is closed with a subcuticular stitch using 4-0 delayed-absorbable suture, staples, or other suitable method (Chap. 40, p. 987).

POSTOPERATIVE

For most gynecologic surgeries, recovery from the abdominal incision constitutes the greatest portion of postsurgical healing. Midline incisions lead to significant pain with ambulation, coughing, and deep breathing. As a result, women undergoing laparotomy are at greater risk of postoperative thrombotic and pulmonary complications. For this reason, prevention of these complications is warranted, as described in Chapter 39 (p. 948). In addition, return of normal bowel function is commonly slowed, and signs of ileus should be monitored.

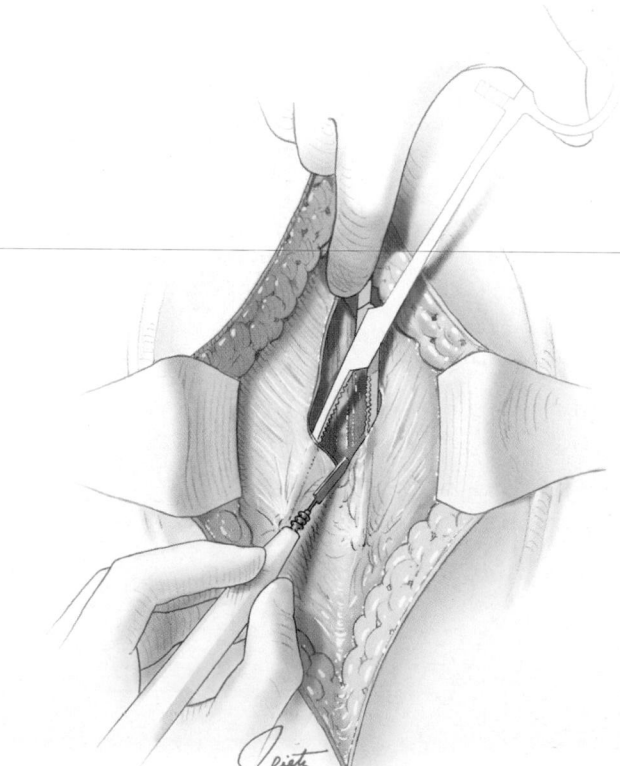

FIGURE 41-1.1 Fascial incision.

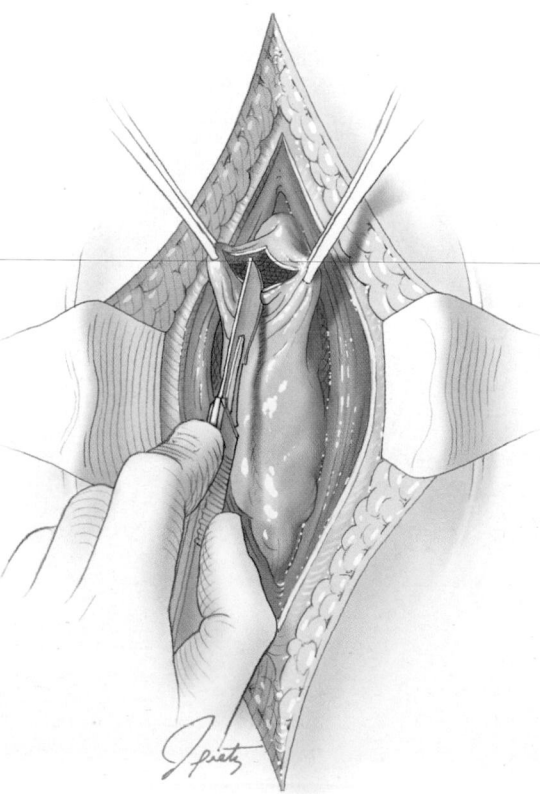

FIGURE 41-1.2 Peritoneal incision.

41-2

Pfannenstiel Incision

The Pfannenstiel, Cherney, and Maylard incisions are transverse abdominal incisions used for gynecologic procedures. Of these, the Pfannenstiel incision is the most commonly used incision for laparotomy in the United States. As discussed in Chapter 38 (p. 919), because the transverse incision follows Langer lines of skin tension, excellent cosmetic results can be achieved. Additionally, decreased rates of postoperative pain, fascial wound dehiscence, and incisional hernia are noted. Use of the Pfannenstiel incision, however, is often discouraged for cases in which a large operating space is essential or in which access to the upper abdomen may be needed. Lastly, because of the layers created by incision of the internal and external oblique aponeuroses, purulent fluid can collect between these. Therefore, most cases involving abscess or peritonitis favor use of a midline incision.

PREOPERATIVE

Consent

General risks associated with transverse laparotomy incisions are similar to those for vertical incisions (Section 41-1, p. 1020). These incisions, however, carry risk of injury to the iliohypogastric, ilioinguinal, and genitofemoral nerves (Chap. 40, p. 982). These injuries

more commonly involve sensory function and are typically transient. Wound infection and venous thromboembolism may complicate abdominal surgery and are discussed in Chapter 39.

INTRAOPERATIVE

SURGICAL STEPS

❶ **Anesthesia and Patient Positioning.** After administration of adequate regional or general anesthesia, the patient is positioned supine. If needed, hair in the path of the planned incision is clipped; a Foley catheter is placed; and abdominal preparation is completed.

❷ **Skin and Subcutaneous Layer.** Two to 3 cm above the symphysis pubis, an 8 to 10 cm transverse incision is made sharply with its lateral margins arching slightly cephalad. The incision is extended deeply with electrosurgical blade until the anterior rectus sheath fascia is reached.

❸ **Fascia.** The anterior rectus sheath is then incised transversely in the midline. At the level of the incision, the anterior rectus sheath is typically composed of two visible layers, the aponeuroses from the external oblique muscle and a fused layer containing aponeuroses of the internal oblique and transversus abdominis muscles (Fig. 38-2, p. 919). Therefore, lateral extension of the anterior rectus sheath incision requires transverse incision of each layer individually (Fig. 41-2.1).

Of note, the inferior epigastric artery and vein typically lie outside the lateral border of the rectus abdominis muscle and beneath the fused aponeuroses of the internal oblique and transversus abdominis muscles (Figs. 38-2 and 38-3, p. 919). Thus, lengthening the incision farther laterally may cut these vessels. If extension is required, these vessels are identified and cauterized or ligated. This prevents bleeding and vessel retraction with later hemorrhage. In addition, risk of injury to the iliohypogastric and ilioinguinal nerves increases as the incision is carried lateral to the borders of the rectus abdominis muscles (Rahn, 2010).

The superior edge of the fascial incision is grasped with a Kocher clamp on either side of the midline. Traction is directed cephalad and slightly upward.

In the area superior to the initial incision, the anterior rectus sheath is then bluntly or sharply separated from the underlying rectus abdominis muscle. The fascia separates easily from the bellies of the rectus muscle, but may be densely adhered along the midline. Several small perforating nerves and vessels traverse the space between the anterior rectus sheath and rectus muscle. Coagulation of these vessels, while avoiding injury to the nerves, should be undertaken during the separation. Upon completion of this dissection, a semicircular area with a radius of 6 to 8 cm has been created (Fig. 41-2.2). A similar separation is performed in the area inferior to the initial incision.

❹ **Rectus Abdominis Muscle.** The rectus abdominis muscle bellies are then separated

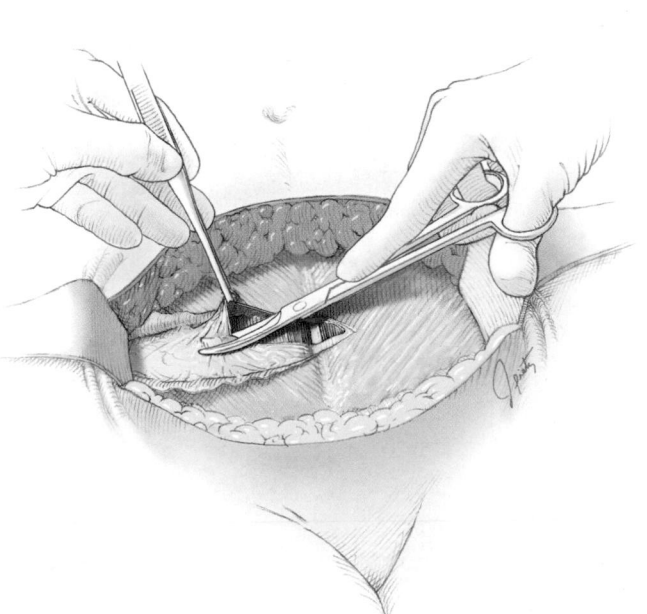

FIGURE 41-2.1 Incision of deeper fascial layer.

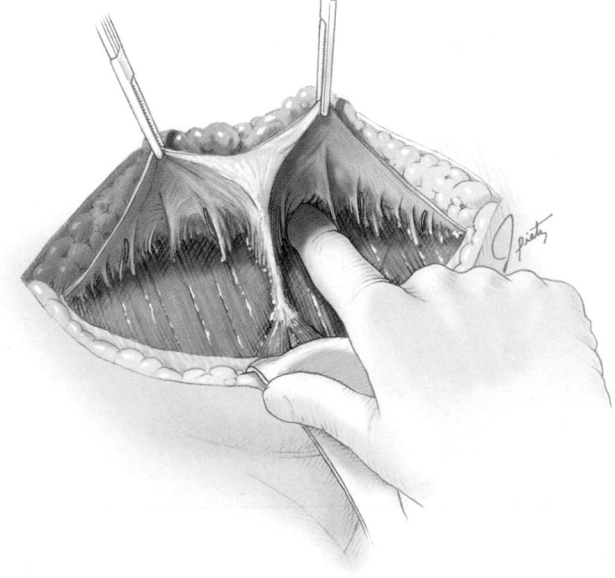

FIGURE 41-2.2 Anterior rectus sheath is separated from the underlying rectus abdominis muscle.

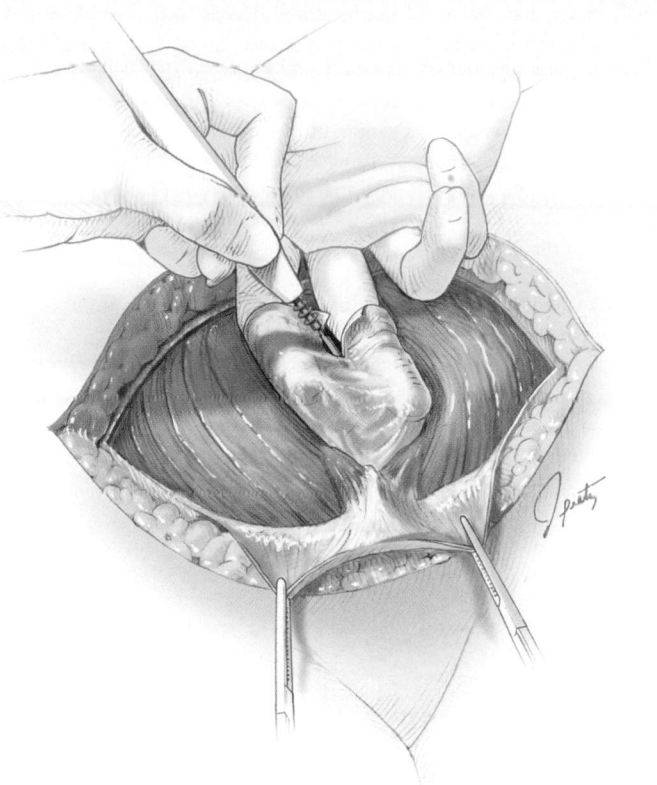

FIGURE 41-2.3 Peritoneal incision.

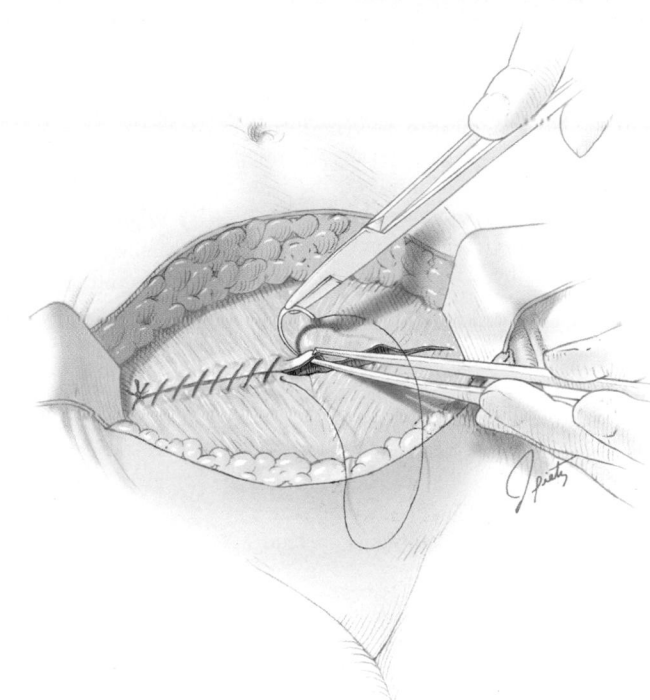

FIGURE 41-2.4 Fascial closure.

along the midline either bluntly or sharply. The pyramidalis muscles, located superficial to the rectus muscle, usually require sharp division at the midline.

❺ Peritoneum. Upon separation of the rectus muscle bellies, the thin, filmy peritoneum is identified, grasped with two hemostats, and sharply incised. The peritoneal incision is then extended superiorly and inferiorly (Fig. 41-2.3). Elevation of the peritoneum during its incision will minimize injury to bowel below. Similar to entry through a vertical incision, the bladder dome is identified during division of the peritoneum caudally to avert cystotomy. Once the abdominal cavity has been entered, the surgeon can proceed with the planned operation.

❻ Wound Closure. At completion of the intraabdominal portion of surgery, closure of the incision begins. Closure of the visceral or parietal peritoneum is not required (Chap. 40, p. 986). The fascial layer is closed with a running suture using 0-gauge delayed-absorbable suture (Fig. 41-2.4). In those patients with a greater than 2-cm layer, closure of the subcutaneous layer can decrease rates of wound infection and dehiscence. The skin may be closed with staples, a subcuticular stitch of 4-0 delayed-absorbable suture, or other suitable skin closure.

POSTOPERATIVE

The postoperative course for low transverse incisions follows that is described for midline incisions (Section 41-1, p. 1021).

Cherney Incision

The Cherney incision is a transverse abdominal incision that is similar to the Pfannenstiel incision in its early steps. After the anterior rectus sheath is opened, however, the tendons of the rectus abdominis and pyramidalis muscles are transected 1 to 2 cm above their insertion into the symphysis pubis. These muscles are then lifted cephalad to provide access to the peritoneum.

This incision offers greater operating space as well as access to the space of Retzius and, therefore, may be a primary choice in cases when these requirements are anticipated. Additionally, Pfannenstiel incisions may be converted to Cherney incisions when an unexpected need for additional operating space arises.

PREOPERATIVE

Preparation and consenting prior to Cherney incision are similar to that for Pfannenstiel incision (Section 41-2, p. 1022).

INTRAOPERATIVE

SURGICAL STEPS

❶ **Initial Steps.** The initial steps mirror that of the Pfannenstiel incision (Section 41-2, steps 1 through 3, p. 1022). Thus, the skin is incised transversely beginning 2 to 3 cm above the symphysis, the fascia is divided transversely in layers, and the rectus sheath is dissected off the rectus abdominis muscle bellies. After these steps, however, the techniques diverge.

❷ **Fascia.** The fascial opening reveals the rectus abdominis muscle and the smaller, triangular-shaped pyramidalis muscles, which lie more caudad and superficial. Cephalad to the symphysis pubis, fingers are insinuated underneath the rectus muscle tendons into the space of Retzius, also termed the prevesical or retropubic space. This blunt dissection begins laterally and extends toward the midline. The insinuated fingers exert pressure dorsally and against the bladder. As a result, the tendons are separated away from the underlying bladder to lessen the chance of accidental cystotomy during tendon transection. The tendons of both muscles are then transected 1 to 2 cm above the symphysis pubis (Fig. 41-3.1). The muscles are lifted cephalad. The peritoneum is grasped with two hemostats and sharply incised. This incision is extended laterally.

Once the abdominal cavity has been accessed, the planned surgery can proceed. It should be noted, however, that risk of nerve injury, particularly to the femoral nerve, is increased when self-retaining retractors are used within this generally wider incision. This is also true for the Maylard incision. Care should be taken to ensure that the lateral blades fit just under the edges of the incision.

❸ **Wound Closure.** During wound closure, the cut ends of the rectus muscle tendons are affixed with interrupted sutures of 0-gauge delayed absorbable sutures to the undersurface of the inferior fascia (Fig. 41-3.2). To avoid osteitis pubis or osteomyelitis, the tendons should not be affixed directly to the symphysis pubis. The fascia is then closed in a running fashion using 0-gauge delayed-absorbable suture. In those patients with a greater than 2-cm layer, closure of the subcutaneous layer can decrease rates of wound infection and dehiscence. The skin may be closed with staples, a subcuticular stitch of 4-0 delayed-absorbable suture, or other suitable skin closure.

POSTOPERATIVE

The postoperative course for low transverse incisions follows that described for midline incisions (Section 41-1, p. 1020).

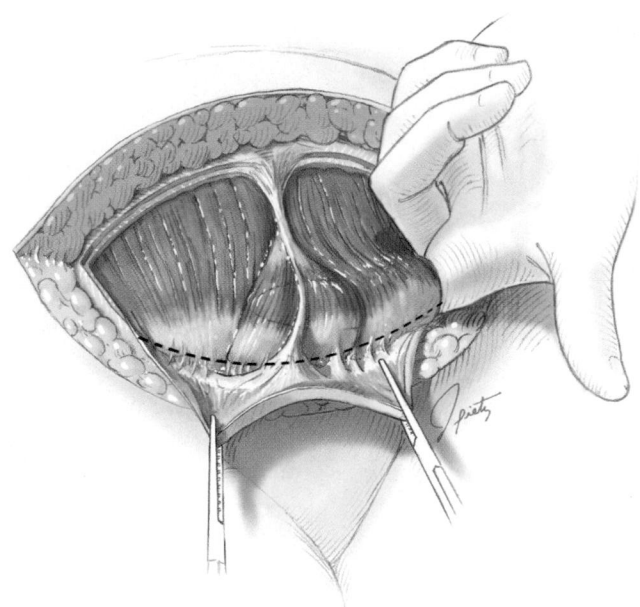

FIGURE 41-3.1 Tendon transection.

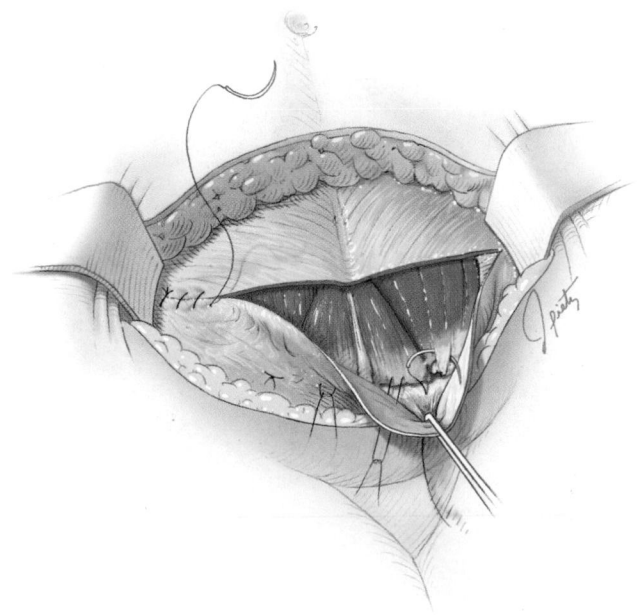

FIGURE 41-3.2 Wound closure.

41-4

Maylard Incision

The Maylard incision differs mainly from the Pfannenstiel and Cherney incisions in that the bellies of the rectus abdominis muscle are transected. The main advantage to this incision is the greater operating space it affords, and therefore it is often selected for cases in which extensive access to the pelvis is needed. Technically more difficult due to its required isolation and ligation of the inferior epigastric arteries, the Maylard incision has also been used infrequently because of concerns regarding greater postoperative pain, decreased abdominal wall strength, longer operating times, and increased febrile morbidity. Randomized studies, however, have not supported these concerns (Ayers, 1987; Giacalone, 2002). The Maylard incision should be avoided in those patients in whom the superior epigastric vessels have been interrupted, as this leaves the rectus abdominis muscles with inadequate blood supply. Also, patients with significant peripheral vascular disease may rely on the inferior epigastric arteries for collateral blood supply to their lower extremities. Ligation of this artery may lead to claudication (Salom, 2007).

PREOPERATIVE

Preparation and consenting prior to Maylard incision are similar to that for Pfannenstiel incision (Section 41-2, p. 1022).

INTRAOPERATIVE

SURGICAL STEPS

❶ **Initial Steps.** The initial steps mirror that of the Pfannenstiel incision (Section 41-2, steps 1 through 3, p. 1022). Thus, the skin is incised transversely beginning 2 to 3 cm above the symphysis, and the fascia is divided transversely in layers. After these steps, however, the techniques diverge.

The inferior epigastric artery and vein lie posterolateral to the bellies of the rectus abdominis muscle. Bilaterally, these vessels are identified, ligated, and transected. This step avoids their later laceration and hemorrhage when the rectus muscle is transected.

❷ **Rectus Abdominis Muscle.** The rectus abdominis muscle is bluntly dissected away from the underlying transversalis fascia and peritoneum. Of note, below the level of the arcuate line, the rectus sheath is absent posterior to the rectus abdominis muscle (Fig. 38-2, p. 919). The surgeon's fingers are slid behind the rectus muscle bellies, and this muscle is then transected using an electrosurgical blade (Fig. 41-4.1). Unlike the Pfannenstiel incision, the anterior rectus sheath should not be dissected away from the underlying rectus muscle. On the contrary, simple interrupted or mattress sutures using 0-gauge delayed-absorbable suture are placed 1 to 2 cm from the cut edge of the muscle and fascia to reinforce the anterior sheath

attachment to the rectus muscle. This reinforcement is performed on both the cephalad and caudad sections of the transected muscle and will improve muscle reapproximation during incision closure (Fig. 41-4.2).

❸ **Peritoneum.** The peritoneum is grasped with two hemostats and sharply incised, with extension of the incision laterally (see Fig. 41-4.2). After access is obtained to the abdominal cavity, the planned surgery can proceed. As mentioned in regard to the Cherney incision, careful placement of self-retaining retractors used in conjunction with a Maylard incision is necessary to lessen the risk of femoral or genitofemoral nerve compression injury.

❹ **Wound Closure.** At incision closure, the fascia is closed with a running stitch using 0-gauge delayed-absorbable suture. Closing the fascia adequately reapproximates the transected muscle fibers, and therefore the divided muscle bellies are not directly sutured together. In those patients with a greater than 2-cm layer, closure of the subcutaneous layer can decrease rates of wound infection and dehiscence. The skin may be closed with staples, a subcuticular stitch of 4-0 delayed-absorbable suture, or other suitable skin closure.

POSTOPERATIVE

The postoperative course for low transverse incisions follows that described for midline incisions (Section 41-1, p. 1021).

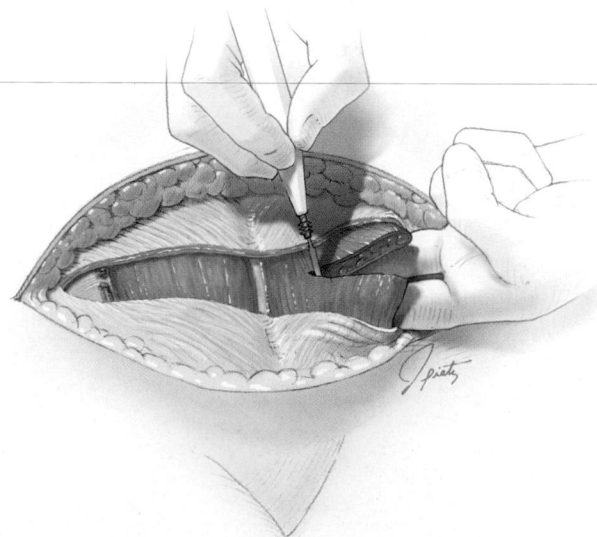

FIGURE 41-4.1 Rectus abdominis muscle transection.

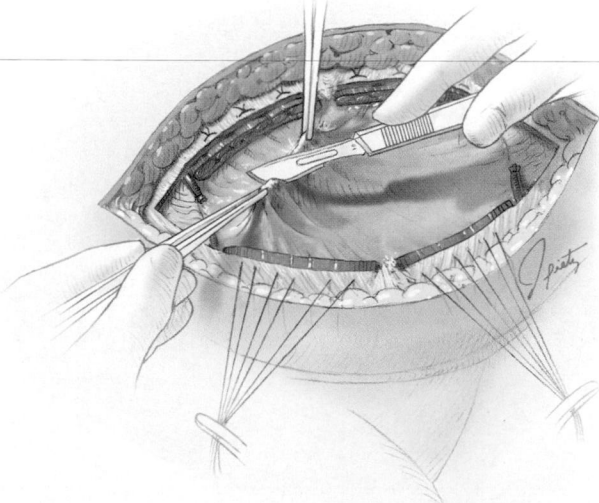

FIGURE 41-4.2 Placement of sutures through rectus abdominis muscle and fascia, and peritoneal incision.

41-5

Ovarian Cystectomy

The removal of ovarian cysts is usually prompted by patient symptoms or by concerns of ovarian malignancy. Rather than excision of the entire ovary, removal of the cyst alone can offer women with suspected benign ovarian pathology an opportunity to preserve hormonal function and reproductive capacity. For these reasons, goals of ovarian cystectomy include gentle handling of tissues to limit postoperative adhesion formation and reconstruction of normal ovarian anatomy to aid the transfer of ova to the fallopian tube.

In some patients, a cystectomy may be performed laparoscopically rather than through laparotomy (Section 42-6, p. 1133). Several studies support the safe and effective use of laparoscopy for this problem (Lin, 1995; Mais, 1995; Pittaway, 1991; Yuen, 1997). Although laparoscopy is often preferred, there are certain settings in which its role may be limited. In general, when the cyst is large, adhesive disease limits access and mobility, or the risk of malignancy is great, laparotomy is instead typically performed. As summarized in Chapter 9 (p. 262), malignancy is suspected when cysts exceed 10 cm, concurrent ascites is present, preoperative serum tumor markers are elevated, and cyst contents appear complex or borders appear irregular during imaging.

PREOPERATIVE

Consent

In addition to general surgical risks of laparotomy, the major risk of cystectomy is extensive bleeding from or injury to the ovary that necessitates removal of the entire ovary. Also, a variable degree of ovarian reserve may be lost with ovarian cystectomy. If ovarian cancer is suspected prior to surgery, patients should be educated regarding the possibility of surgical staging, including the need for hysterectomy, omentectomy, and removal of both ovaries (Chap. 35, p. 868).

Many patients undergoing cystectomy for ovarian pathology have associated pain. Although in most cases, cystectomy will be curative, in other instances, pain may persist despite cystectomy. This is especially true in those with coexistent endometriosis. Thus, patients are counseled that cystectomy may not relieve chronic pain in all cases.

Patient Preparation

Antibiotics are typically not required preoperatively. If hysterectomy is required during ovarian staging, antibiotics may be given intraoperatively.

INTRAOPERATIVE

SURGICAL STEPS

❶ Anesthesia and Patient Positioning. Because of the potential need for upper abdominal staging if malignancy is found, general anesthesia is typically indicated for this inpatient procedure. The patient is placed in a supine position, the abdomen is surgically prepared, and a Foley catheter is placed. Because of a possible need for hysterectomy if malignancy is found, the vagina is also surgically prepared.

❷ Abdominal Entry. Most ovarian cysts can be removed through a Pfannenstiel incision. Extremely large cysts or those in which a greater concern for malignancy is present may require a vertical incision. Vertical incisions allow adequate access to the upper abdomen if ovarian cancer staging is required and provide a large intraabdominal operating space.

Cell washings from the pelvis and upper abdomen are collected and are saved if a cancer is found. The upper abdomen and pelvis are explored and excrescences or suspicious areas are sampled and sent for intraoperative frozen-section analysis.

A self-retaining retractor is placed within the incision, and the bowel and omentum are packed from the operating field. The ovary is brought into view, and moist laparotomy sponges are placed in the cul-de-sac and underneath the ovary. This helps to minimize contamination of the pelvis if the cyst ruptures during excision.

❸ Ovarian Incision. The ovary is held between the surgeon's thumb and opposing fingers. The ovarian capsule that overlies the dome of the cyst is then incised with either scalpel or electrosurgical needle tip. This incision is ideally on the antimesenteric surface of the ovary to minimize dissection into extensive vascularity at the ovarian base. Care is taken to extend the incision into the ovarian stroma to the level of the cyst wall, but not to enter and rupture the cyst (Fig. 41-5.1). Allis clamps are placed on the incised edges of the ovarian capsule.

❹ Cyst Dissection. Blunt dissection with fingertip or knife handle is used to develop the cleavage plane between the cyst wall and the remaining ovarian stroma (Fig. 41-5.2). In certain cases, adhesions may obliterate the cleavage plane, and sharp dissection with scissor tips may be necessary. As an assistant

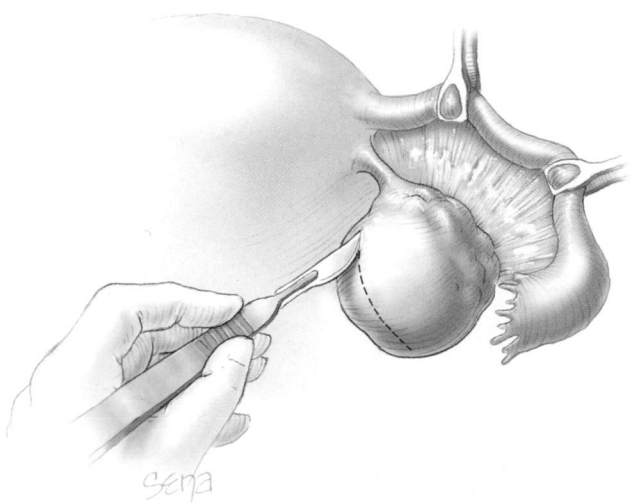

FIGURE 41-5.1 Ovarian incision.

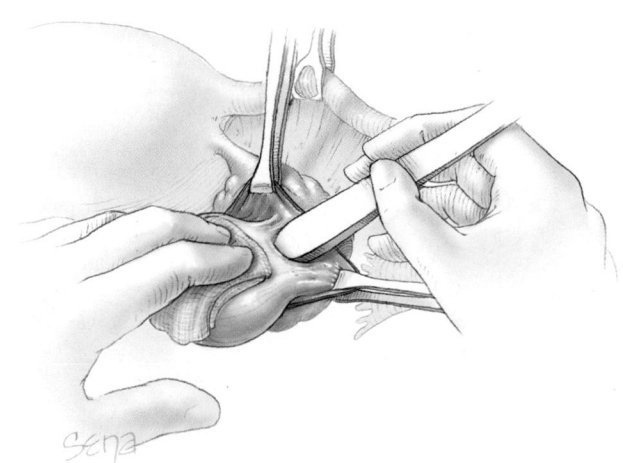

FIGURE 41-5.2 Cyst dissection.

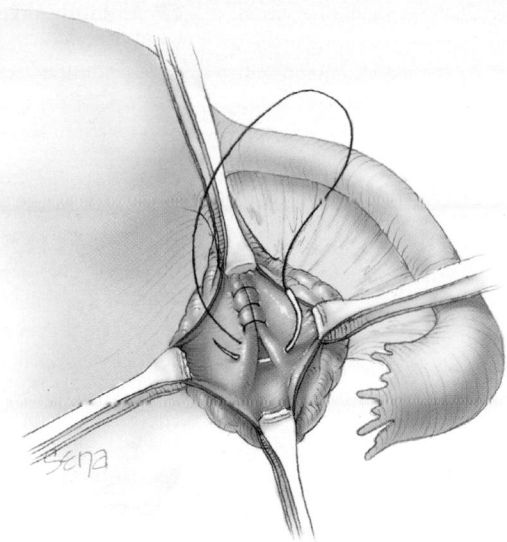

FIGURE 41-5.3 Ovarian closure.

gently retracts the Allis clamps in a direction away from the cyst wall, the surgeon places fingers near the advancing cleavage plane and retracts the cyst in the direction opposite the Allis clamps. Such traction and countertraction across the cleavage plane aids in dissection. Because the surface of the cyst wall may be smooth and slippery, the surgeon may place an unfolded thin gauze sponge between fingers and the cyst wall to afford a better grip.

❺ **Cyst Excision.** Once the cyst is removed, it may be sent to the pathology department for intraoperative frozen-section analysis. The ovarian bed is examined, and bleeding points are coagulated. In cases in which large cysts have stretched and thinned the ovarian surface, excess capsule can be sharply removed. This excision is performed to restore normal ovarian anatomy. But because ovarian follicles are contained within even extremely thinned capsules, this tissue is preserved whenever possible.

❻ **Ovarian Closure.** The ovarian bed is then closed in layers using 3-0 or 4-0 delayed-

absorbable suture. These sutures reapproximate the ovarian tissue that previously surrounded the cyst on both sides (Fig. 41-5.3). In cases where the ovarian surface has been thinned, the needle tip should not be driven through the capsule. The resulting exposed suture on the ovarian surface may increase adhesion formation.

The ovarian incision is closed with a running subcortical stitch (similar to subcuticular stitch) using 4-0 or 5-0 delayed-absorbable suture.

❼ **Incision Closure.** Laparotomy sponges are removed from the cul-de-sac, and the pelvis is copiously irrigated with an isotonic solution such as lactated Ringer solution. Irrigation assumes an even greater importance in the event of ovarian cyst rupture. For example, spill from a mature cystic teratoma (dermoid), if neglected, may induce a chemical peritonitis. Depending on the surgeon's preference and the patient's anatomy, an adhesion barrier may be placed around the ovary. The remaining packs and retractor are removed, and the abdominal incision is closed.

POSTOPERATIVE

After surgery, care may follow that described for laparotomy in general (Section 41-1, p. 1021).

Oophorectomy

Removal of an ovary is more commonly performed by laparoscopy. However, laparotomy is typically indicated if the potential for malignancy is great, if the ovary is larger than 8 to 10 cm, or if significant adhesions are anticipated. In many of these instances a salpingo-oophorectomy is performed as presented in Section 41-12 (p. 1047). However, if future fertility is desired, then the fallopian tube is preserved whenever possible.

PREOPERATIVE

Patient Evaluation

Oophorectomy is typically performed to remove ovarian pathology that has been identified using transvaginal or transabdominal sonography. In cases in which anatomy may be unclear, magnetic resonance imaging may add additional information. As described in Chapters 35 and 36 (pp. 861 and 879), blood levels of tumor markers may be measured prior to surgery if malignancy is suspected.

Consent

In general, serious complications with oophorectomy are low, are similar to those with other intraabdominal surgeries, and include organ injury, hemorrhage, wound infection, and anesthesia complications. In addition, the risk of injury to the adjacent fallopian tube or ureter is small but should be specifically discussed during the consenting process.

Ovarian cysts are the most common indication for oophorectomy. Because malignancy may be found, patients are informed of the steps of ovarian cancer surgical staging. Also, if a malignant cyst ruptures and spills its contents, patients should be aware of the possible negative effects on prognosis.

Lastly, many patients undergoing oophorectomy for ovarian pathology have associated pain. Although in most cases removal of the ovary will be curative, in other instances, pain may persist despite oophorectomy.

Patient Preparation

Unless an ovarian abscess is identified, antibiotic prophylaxis is generally not required. The American College of Obstetricians and Gynecologists (2009a) does not recommend antibiotic prophylaxis for women undergoing exploratory laparotomy. If hysterectomy is required during ovarian staging, antibiotics may be given intraoperatively (Table 39-6, p. 959).

INTRAOPERATIVE

SURGICAL STEPS

❶ Anesthesia and Patient Positioning. Oophorectomy performed via laparotomy typically requires general anesthesia to allow staging of the upper abdomen if malignancy is found. Following administration of anesthesia, the patient is positioned supine, a Foley catheter is placed, and the abdomen is surgically prepared.

❷ Abdominal Entry. Either transverse or vertical incision may be used for oophorectomy. Clinical factors such as ovarian size and risk of malignancy influence this selection (Section 41-1, p. 1020).

❸ Exposure. Following entry into the abdomen, a self-retaining retractor such as an O'Connor-O'Sullivan or Balfour retractor is placed. The pelvis and abdomen are visually and manually explored, and the bowel is packed from the operating field. The affected adnexa is grasped and elevated from the pelvis. If extensive adhesions are present, normal anatomic relationships are restored.

❹ Ureter Location. Because of the close proximity of the ureter to the infundibulopelvic ligament, the ureter is identified prior to any clamp placement. In many instances, the ureter can be seen beneath the posterior abdominal wall peritoneum. In other cases, the peritoneum may be opened directly to isolate the ureter.

❺ Mesovarium. The adnexa is lifted from the pelvis and inspected. If malignancy is suspected, pelvic washings are obtained and set aside until analysis of a frozen-section sample from the affected ovary is completed. Two Babcock clamps grasp the fallopian tube at points equidistant along its length. The clamps are then extended and retracted away from the ovary by an assistant. The ovary is elevated and placed on gentle tension in the opposite direction from the tube (Fig. 41-6.1). This effectively fans out the mesovarium.

Pean or other suitable clamps are placed in pairs, one close to the ovarian wall and the other across the distal mesovarium.

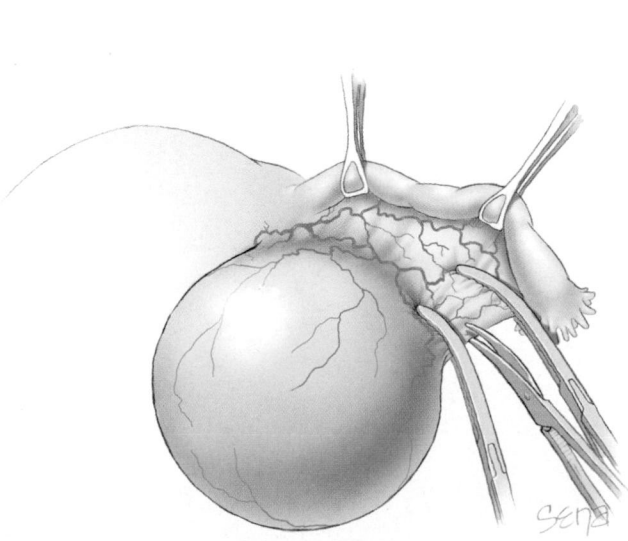

FIGURE 41-6.1 Clamping mesovarium.

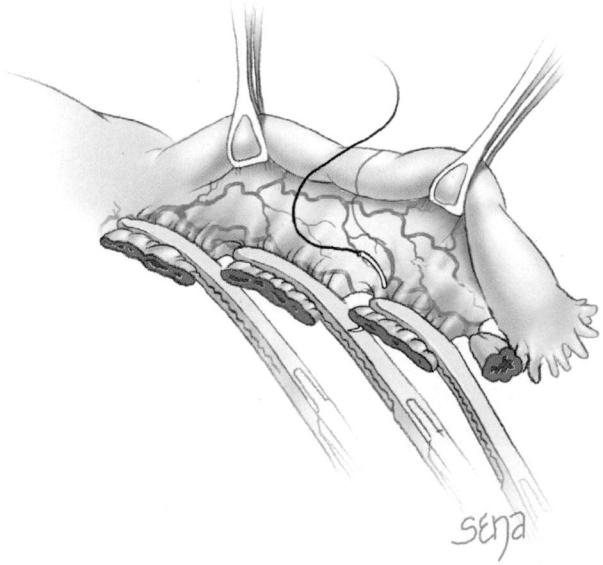

FIGURE 41-6.2 Ovary excision.

Tissue between the clamps is cut with scissors and ligated with 2-0 delayed-absorbable suture prior to placement of the next pair of clamps. Alternatively, especially with large cysts, serial clamps may be placed across the mesovarium in a line toward the uterus (Fig. 41 6.2). Small bites are taken to avoid kinking of the fallopian tube. Once the most medial clamp is placed across the ovarian ligament, curved Mayo scissors can be used to cut between the clamps and ovary. The freed ovary is removed from the operative site and sent to pathology for evaluation. All clamps on the mesovarium are then ligated. If malignancy is suspected, an intraoperative frozen section is requested.

❻ **Wound Closure.** The retractor and packing sponges are removed from the abdomen. The abdominal incision is then closed as described in Section 41-1 or 41-2 (p. 1021).

POSTOPERATIVE

Patient recovery is typically without complication and is similar to that described for laparotomy (Section 41-1, p. 1021). In reproductive-aged women, if only one ovary is removed, hormonal and reproductive function is preserved. However, if both are excised, then surgical menopause follows, and hormone replacement may be considered as described in Chapter 22 (p. 585).

41-7

Interval Partial Salpingectomy

Interval partial salpingectomy is similar to puerperal midsegment salpingectomy and differs mainly in procedure timing and the method of abdominal entry. In contrast to postpartum or postabortal sterilization, the term *interval* designates performance unrelated in time to pregnancy. Accordingly, for most women undergoing interval sterilization, the uterus is small and lies within the confines of the pelvis. Thus, fallopian tubes are reached either laparoscopically or through a low transverse incision.

In general with interval partial salpingectomy, a midtubal segment of fallopian tube is excised, and the severed ends seal by fibrosis and reperitonealization. Commonly used methods of interval sterilization include the Parkland, Pomeroy, and modified Pomeroy techniques (American College of Obstetricians and Gynecologists, 2003). Rarely, Irving and Uchida techniques are used. Increased dissection, operative time, and chance of mesosalpingeal injury are significant disadvantages with these latter two methods.

Of methods for tubal sterilization, interval partial salpingectomy is infrequently selected, and only approximately 4 percent of U.S. women who elect sterilization undergo this procedure (Peterson, 1996). More commonly, laparoscopic techniques are employed, mainly because of the postsurgical advantages linked with laparoscopy (Section 42-1, p. 1095). Accordingly, interval partial salpingectomy is typically selected for cases in which laparoscopy may not be indicated, such as those complicated by extensive adhesions, those in which other concurrent pelvic pathology dictates laparotomy, or those in which laparoscopic equipment or surgical skills are lacking.

PREOPERATIVE

Patient Evaluation

As with any sterilization procedure, pregnancy should be excluded prior to the procedure by means of either urine or serum β-human chorionic gonadotropin (hCG) testing. Similarly, to limit the possibility of an early, undetected luteal-phase conceptus, sterilization is ideally performed during the follicular phase of the menstrual cycle, and an effective contraceptive method should be used until surgery.

Consent

Women can be reassured that partial salpingectomy is an effective method of sterilization. Pregnancy rates of less than 2 percent are typical. Failures may result from tubal recanalization or technical errors, such as ligation of the wrong structure.

Tubal sterilization is a safe surgical procedure, and complication rates range below 2 percent (Pati, 2000). Of these, anesthesia complications, organ injury, and infection are the most frequent. In addition, although pregnancy is uncommon following sterilization, when pregnancy does occur, the risk of ectopic pregnancy is high and approximates 30 percent (Peterson, 1996; Ryder, 1999). However, because tubal sterilization is highly effective contraception, the overall risk of pregnancy is low, and therefore also the risk of ectopic pregnancy.

Aside from physical risks, a small percentage of women experience regret following sterilization (Chap. 5, p. 145). In studies, rates of regret approach 15 percent (Hillis, 1999; Trussell, 2003). For this reason, prior to surgery women are counseled regarding the risk of regret, the permanence of the procedure, and alternative effective long-term contraceptive methods.

INTRAOPERATIVE

SURGICAL STEPS

❶ Anesthesia and Patient Positioning. Interval partial salpingectomy is typically an outpatient procedure, performed under general or regional anesthesia. Following administration of anesthesia, the patient is placed supine or in low dorsal lithotomy position, the abdomen surgically prepared, and the bladder drained.

❷ Minilaparotomy. For most patients, a 3- to 5-cm transverse minilaparotomy incision at the level of the uterine fundus is suf-

ficient and should follow the steps outlined in Section 41-2 (p. 1022) for abdominal entry. Small Richardson or Army-Navy retractors provide adequate intraabdominal visualization in most cases. If the patient is in low dorsal lithotomy position, a uterine manipulator or vaginal sponge stick may be helpful in bringing the fallopian tubes into view.

❸ Tubal Identification. A common reason for sterilization failure is ligation of the wrong structure, typically the round ligament. Identification and isolation of the fallopian tubes prior to ligation and submission of both tubal segments for pathologic confirmation is therefore required. In some cases, especially those with associated tubal adhesions, this step may be challenging.

Initially, the uterine fundus is identified. At the cornu, insertion of the fallopian tube lies posterior to that of the round ligament, and this orientation can initially guide the surgeon to the correct structure. A primary Babcock clamp is used to elevate the fallopian tube proximally, while a second clamp grasps the tube more distally. The first clamp is then moved again and is placed distal to the second. The second is then removed and again placed distal to the first. In this manner, the surgeon "marches" down the length of the tube to reach the ampulla and identify the fimbria.

❹ Parkland Method of Tubal Ligation. At the midpoint of the fallopian tube, an avascular space in the mesosalpinx is identified, and a hemostat is placed directly beneath the tube. The selected site should allow excision of a 2-cm segment that does not incorporate the fimbrial portion of the tube. Ligation of the fimbrial portion leads to a greater risk of tubal recanalization and higher failure rates.

The hemostat is bluntly advanced through the mesosalpinx as counter pressure is applied with the index finger. Once advanced through the defect, the hemostat jaws are gently opened to expand the aperture (Fig. 41-7.1). The end

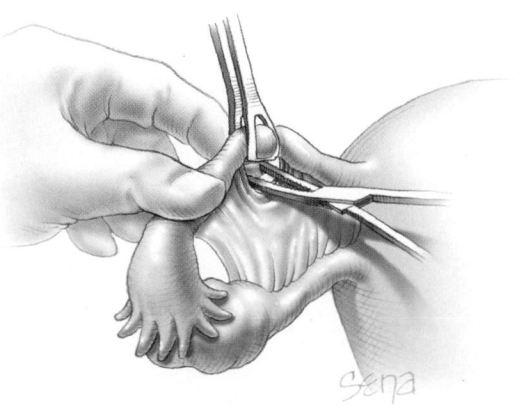

FIGURE 41-7.1 Parkland method: opening in mesosalpinx created.

of a 2-0 chromic free tie is placed in the tip of the hemostat and pulled through the opening. This is repeated, bringing another tie through the rent. The distal portion of the tubal mid-segment is lifted, and the distal suture tied. This elevation allows for a larger tubal segment to be obtained, which helps the cut ends to remain widely separated. The second tie is then secured around the proximal fallopian tube.

❺ Tubal Excision. The tip of Metzenbaum scissors is inserted through the mesosalpin-geal defect, and the proximal portion of the fallopian tube is cut. A 0.5-cm pedicle is left to ensure that the tube will not slip through its ligature (Fig. 41-7.2). The tube is sharply dissected from the mesosalpinx toward the distal ligature, thereby freeing the tube from the mesosalpinx. The distal end is excised to leave a 0.5-cm pedicle, and an adequate 2-cm segment of tube is obtained. The pedicles and mesosalpinx are inspected for hemosta-sis. The procedure is then repeated on the other side. Tubal segments are sent for histo-logic evaluation.

❻ Pomeroy Method. This technique in-volves grasping and elevating a 2-cm midseg-ment of tube, ligating the tubal loop with a 2-0 chromic or plain catgut suture, and then excising the distal portion of the loop (Fig. 41-7.3). Prompt absorption of the suture following surgery causes the ligated ends to fall away, with a resulting 2- to 3-cm gap.

❼ Modified Pomeroy Method. Many modifications of the Pomeroy technique have been described. One technique creates

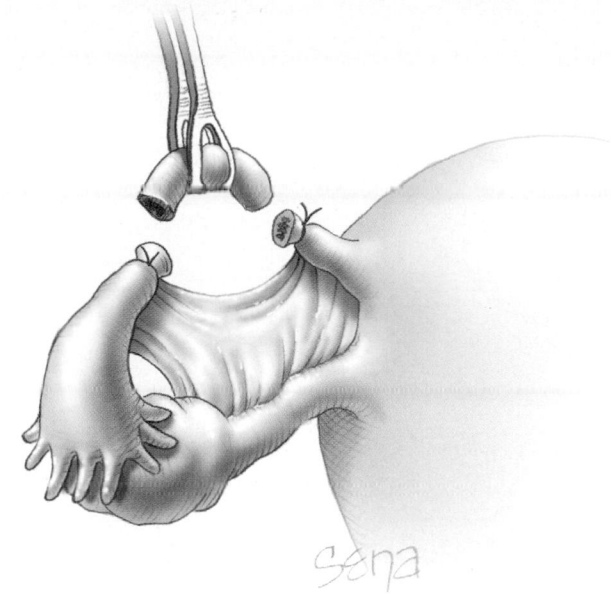

FIGURE 41-7.2 Parkland method: tubal excision.

an avascular window in the mesosalpinx at a midpoint along the tube. Through this window, suture similar to that used for the Pomeroy method is passed. The proxi-mal portion of fallopian tube is first ligated (Fig. 41-7.4). The long ends of this suture are then tied around the entire tubal loop, as in the Pomeroy method (see Fig. 41-7.3). The loop is then excised approximately 0.5 cm beyond the ligature.

❽ Uchida Method. Tubal serosa is first separated from the muscularis by a subsero-

sal injection of a dilute saline solution of epi-nephrine (1:100,000). A longitudinal incision is made in the ballooned serosa on its surface opposite the mesosalpinx. The serosal perito-neum is then grasped and dissected away from the underlying tubal muscularis. Following this dissection, a 5-cm midsegment of dissected fallopian tube is ligated proximally and dis-tally with 2-0 chromic or plain catgut suture and then resected. The raw serosal edges are reapproximated, burying the proximal cut tubal end and exteriorizing the distal end (Fig. 41-7.5) (Zurawin, 2011).

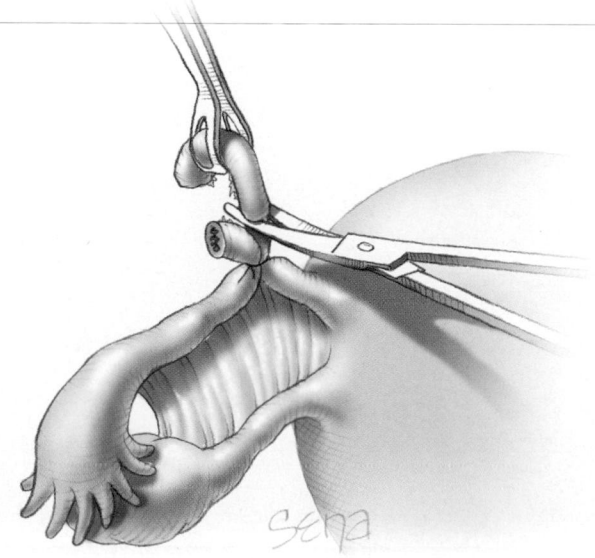

FIGURE 41-7.3 Pomeroy method.

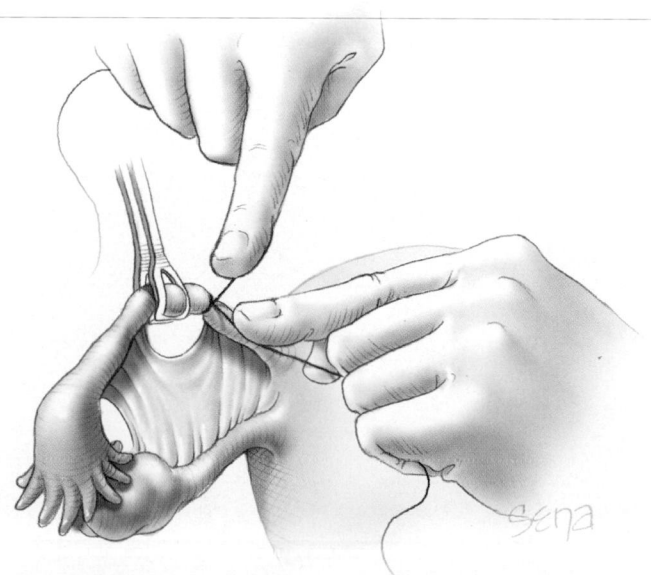

FIGURE 41-7.4 Modified Pomeroy method.

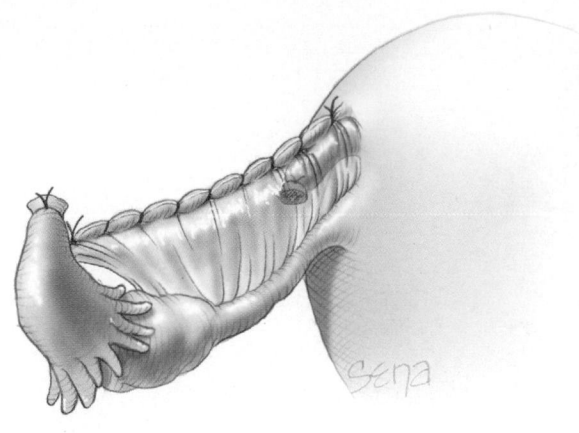

FIGURE 41-7.5 Uchida method.

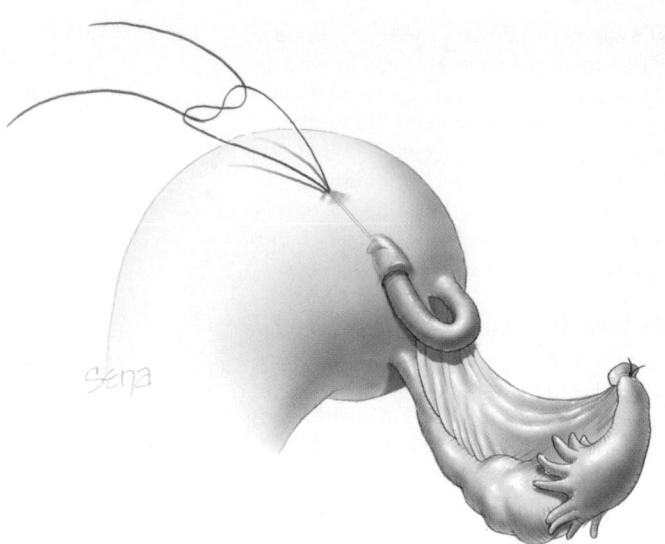

FIGURE 41-7.6 Irving method.

❾ **Irving Method.** The Irving method begins similarly to the Parkland method. However, after the knot on the proximal tubal segment is secured, the ties are left long. The distal segment is ligated and the intervening tubal segment excised as described previously. Near the cornu, a 1-cm incision is made into the uterine serosa on the posterior uterine wall (Fig. 41-7.6). From this incision, a hemostat is used to tunnel into the myometrium, creating a 1- to 2-cm pocket that lies deep but parallel to the serosa. The two free ends of the proximal stump ligature are then threaded onto a curved needle. The needle is driven deep into the myometrial tunnel and exits out onto the uterine serosa. The needle is removed, and traction on the sutures pulls the proximal tubal stump into the pocket. Sutures are then tied on the outside of the serosa. The opening of the tunnel is then closed around the tube with interrupted 2-0 absorbable sutures.

❿ **Wound Closure.** The wound is closed as for other transverse abdominal incisions (Section 41-2, p. 1023).

POSTOPERATIVE

The recovery following minilaparotomy is typically rapid and without complication, and women may resume their regular diet and activities as tolerated. Sterilization is immediate following surgery, and intercourse may resume at the patient's discretion. Aside from regret, the risk of long-term physical or psychologic sequelae is low.

41-8

Salpingectomy and Salpingostomy

Salpingectomy involves removal of the fallopian tube with sparing of the ovary, and its predominant use is in the treatment of ectopic pregnancy. This procedure, however, may be used as a method of sterilization or may also be employed to remove hydrosalpinges to improve in vitro fertilization success rates (Chap. 9, p. 273). Alternatively, *salpingostomy* describes a lengthwise linear incision of the fallopian tube and is typically used to remove intraluminal ectopic pregnancy contents.

Laparoscopic surgery offers patients the advantages of shorter hospitalizations, quicker recoveries, and less postoperative pain (Murphy, 1992; Vermesh, 1989). For these reasons, laparoscopic treatment of ectopic pregnancy is generally preferred. As a result, laparotomic approaches for salpingectomy and salpingostomy are now reserved typically for patients with ruptured ectopic pregnancies who are hemodynamically unstable or in those who have contraindications to laparoscopy. In these instances, laparotomy offers fast entry into the abdomen for control of bleeding.

PREOPERATIVE

Consent

Most complications associated with salpingectomy and salpingostomy occur in conjunction with ectopic pregnancies, and the risk of bleeding is prominent. Injury to the ipsilateral ovary, however, is an attendant risk regardless of the indication. In certain cases, if severe, this damage can demand concurrent oophorectomy. Additionally, involvement of the ovary with tubal pathology may necessitate ovarian removal.

Persistent Trophoblastic Tissue

Following any surgical treatment of ectopic pregnancy, trophoblastic tissue can persist. Remnant implants typically involve the fallopian tube, but extratubal trophoblastic implants have been found on the omentum and on pelvic and abdominal peritoneum. Peritoneal implants typically measure 0.3 to 2.0 cm and appear as red–black nodules (Doss, 1998).

The risk of persistent trophoblast tissue is lower with salpingectomy compared with salpingostomy. In addition, because morcellation of the tube during laparoscopic salpingectomy may leave trophoblastic tissue behind, the risk is lowest with laparotomic salpingectomy (Farquhar, 2005).

Preservation of Fertility

Most, but not all, studies show comparable subsequent fertility rates whether salpingectomy or salpingostomy is performed to treat ectopic pregnancy (Bangsgaard, 2003; Clausen, 1996; Mol, 1998; Tulandi, 1999). A further discussion of fertility and the long-term outcomes from these procedures can be found in Chapter 7 (p. 211). In the presence of a healthy contralateral tube, therefore, neither salpingostomy nor salpingectomy offers an advantage with respect to future fertility. However, salpingostomy should be considered as the primary treatment option for tubal pregnancy in the presence of disease in the contralateral tube and the desire for future fertility. Unfortunately, in some cases of rupture, the extent of tubal damage or bleeding may limit tubal salvage, and salpingectomy may be required.

Patient Preparation

If performed for ectopic pregnancy, either of these procedures may be associated with substantial bleeding. Baseline complete blood count (CBC) and β-human chorionic gonadotropin (β-hCG) level are obtained. The patient is typed and crossmatched for at least two units of packed red blood cells and other blood products as indicated. Salpingectomy and salpingostomy are associated with low rates of infection. Accordingly, preoperative antibiotics are usually not required.

INTRAOPERATIVE

SURGICAL STEPS

❶ Anesthesia and Patient Positioning. In most cases of ectopic pregnancy managed by laparotomy, surgery is an inpatient procedure and requires general anesthesia. The patient is positioned supine, a Foley catheter is placed, and the abdomen is surgically prepared.

❷ Abdominal Entry. Most laparotomic salpingectomy procedures can be managed using a Pfannenstiel incision (Section 41-2, p. 1022).

❸ Salpingectomy. Once access to the pelvic organs has been reached, the adnexa is elevated. A Babcock clamp is placed around the fallopian tube and directs the tube away from the uterus and ovary. This extends the mesosalpinx (Fig. 41-8.1).

Beginning at the distal, fimbriated end of the tube, one Kelly clamp is placed across a 2-cm long segment of the mesosalpinx, close to the fallopian tube. Another clamp is similarly placed, but lies closer to the ovary. These clamps occlude vessels that traverse the mesosalpinx. Scissors then cut the interposed mesosalpinx.

❹ Vessel Ligation. Each vascular tissue pedicle is tied with 2-0 or 3-0 delayed-absorbable suture. This step is repeated serially with each clamp incorporating approximately 2 cm of mesosalpinx. Progression is directed from the ampullary end of the fallopian tube toward the uterus.

The last clamp is placed across the proximal mesosalpinx and fallopian tube. Scissors then cut the mesosalpinx and free the tube from the uterus. This pedicle is similarly ligated with suture.

❺ Wound Closure. If the surgeon so desires, the exposed vascular pedicles may be covered by a running suture that approximates the peritoneum (Fig. 41-8.2). The

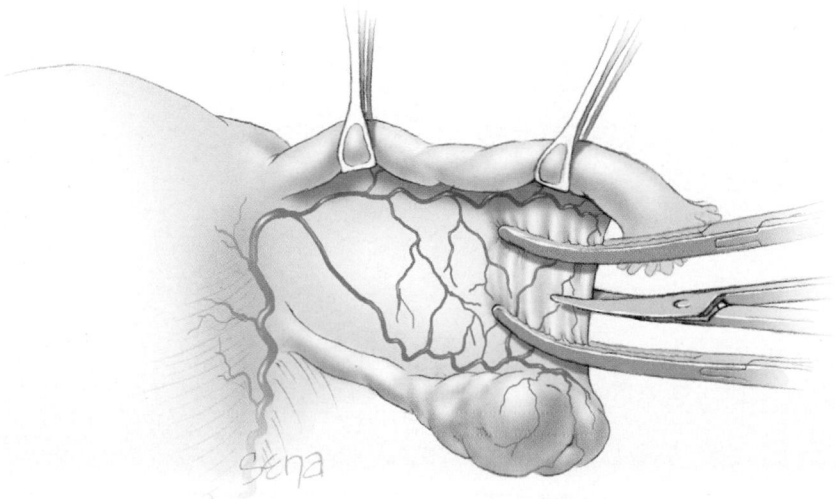

FIGURE 41-8.1 Salpingectomy.

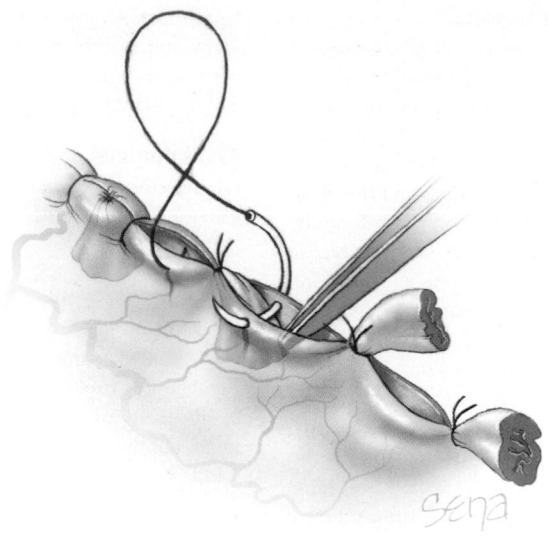

FIGURE 41-8.2 Peritoneal closure.

pelvis is irrigated and rid of blood and tissue debris. The abdominal incision is closed as previously described in Section 41-2 (p. 1023).

❻ Salpingostomy. Surgical steps for salpingostomy mirror those used in laparoscopic salpingostomy and can be reviewed in Section 42-5 (p. 1131). To summarize, the affected fallopian tube is elevated with Babcock clamps. The tube is then sharply incised along its length on its antimesenteric border at the ectopic pregnancy site. The incision, usually 1 to 2 cm long, varies based on pregnancy size. The products of conception are grasped and gently extracted. Bleeding sites are made hemostatic with electrosurgical coagulation, and the tubal incision is left to heal by secondary intention.

POSTOPERATIVE

In cases performed for ectopic pregnancy, salpingectomy or salpingostomy represents pregnancy termination. For this reason, the Rh status of the patient should be evaluated. Administration of 50 or 300 μg (1500 IU) Rh₀ (D) immune globulin intramuscularly within 72 hours after pregnancy termination in Rh-negative women can dramatically lower the risk of isoimmunization in future pregnancies.

Because of the increased risk of persistent trophoblastic tissue in patients undergoing salpingostomy, serial weekly serum β-hCG levels should be measured until undetectable levels are reached. During this time, contraception should be used to avoid confusion between persistent trophoblastic tissue and a new pregnancy.

Resumption of activity and diet may follow that of laparotomy in general, as discussed in Section 41-1 (p. 1021).

41-9

Cornuostomy and Cornual Wedge Resection

Interstitial pregnancy develops in a distensible portion of the tube surrounded by myometrium (Fig. 41-9.1). This location often permits pregnancies to attain greater size than ectopic pregnancy at other sites. Also, uterine rupture at the cornu, where uterine and ovarian arteries anastomose, can lead to significant hemorrhage. Fortunately, high-resolution sonography, β-hCG testing, and use of established diagnostic criteria have led to earlier diagnosis of interstitial pregnancy. This averts rupture in many cases, similar to the much more common tubal ectopic pregnancy.

In selected cases, this unusual type of ectopic pregnancy may be managed medically, but is more frequently managed by a variety of surgical techniques. *Cornuostomy* is analogous to linear salpingostomy for tubal ectopic pregnancies (Section 42-5, p. 1131), whereas *cornual wedge resection* removes the interstitial pregnancy with its surrounding myometrium. Cornual wedge resection, often performed via laparotomy, has remained a cornerstone of therapy. However, many cases of interstitial pregnancy are now managed laparoscopically, and some authors feel this may be the most appropriate treatment (Moawad, 2010).

Factors to consider in selecting surgical route and specific procedure include gestational age, presence of rupture, hemodynamic stability, patient's desire for future fertility, and surgeon's preference and skill.

In this discussion, a laparotomic approach is described. However, the principles and surgical steps presented here are applicable to laparoscopic management with only minor modifications.

PREOPERATIVE

Patient Evaluation

In some cases, particularly those in which the patient has undergone rupture of an interstitial pregnancy and is hemodynamically unstable, fluid resuscitation and blood transfusion are initiated preoperatively. Further, as risk exists for excessive bleeding intraoperatively, a patient is typed and crossmatched for at least two units of packed red blood cells and other blood products as indicated. Patients should be counseled regarding the possible need for blood products, which includes Rh_0 (D) immune globulin for those with Rh-negative blood. Baseline CBC and β-hCG levels are obtained.

Additional risks include removal of the ipsilateral tube and/or ovary and the possibility of hysterectomy for uncontrollable bleeding. In the event that the patient has completed her childbearing or has failed a prior sterilization procedure, bilateral tubal ligation or bilateral salpingectomy or even hysterectomy may be acceptable at the time of surgery.

Patient Preparation

Other than optimizing hemodynamic stability of the patient and ensuring blood availability, no special preparation is required. Prophylactic antibiotics are generally not required, unless hysterectomy is planned. For hysterectomy, antibiotics found in Table 39-6 (p. 959) are suitable options.

INTRAOPERATIVE

SURGICAL STEPS

❶ Anesthesia and Patient Positioning. Cornual wedge resection and cornuostomy are usually performed under general anesthesia, particularly if cornual rupture is suspected. The patient is positioned supine, and a Foley catheter is inserted if not done earlier. The abdomen is prepped and draped in the usual sterile fashion. The vaginal may also be surgically prepared if hysterectomy is anticipated.

❷ Abdominal Entry. Either a transverse or vertical incision may be used depending on the clinical situation as discussed in Section 41-1 (p. 1020).

❸ Exposure. In the absence of cornual rupture and active bleeding, the bowel is packed away to provide adequate exposure of the pelvis. A self-retaining retractor may then be placed. Should significant hemoperitoneum be encountered upon abdominal entry, the operator should attempt to remove obscuring blood with suction and laparotomy sponges. Failing this, the surgeon may consider manually elevating the uterus out of the pelvis where it may be visually inspected for rupture and bleeding. The uterus may be compressed between the operator's thumb anteriorly and fingers posteriorly in an effort to control bleeding. In addition, compression of the aorta may be helpful if bleeding is brisk.

❹ Inspection of the Pelvis. The location of the ectopic pregnancy is identified. Additional information including presence or absence of rupture, pregnancy size, amount of bleeding, and appearance of the contralateral (unaffected) adnexa is needed before deciding on the exact procedure to be performed.

❺ Injection of Vasopressin. For either cornuostomy or cornual wedge resection, dilute vasopressin (20 units in 30 to 100 mL of normal saline) may be injected into the myometrium surrounding the interstitial pregnancy to aid hemostasis. Needle aspiration prior to injection is imperative to avoid intravascular injection of this potent vasoconstrictor. The anesthesiologist should be informed of vasopressin injection, as a sudden increase in patient blood pressure may potentially occur following injection. Blanching at the injection site is common.

❻ Cornuostomy: Incision. A linear incision through the uterine serosa and myometrium overlying the interstitial pregnancy is made (Fig. 41-9.2). As the incision is carried downward, some products of conception may

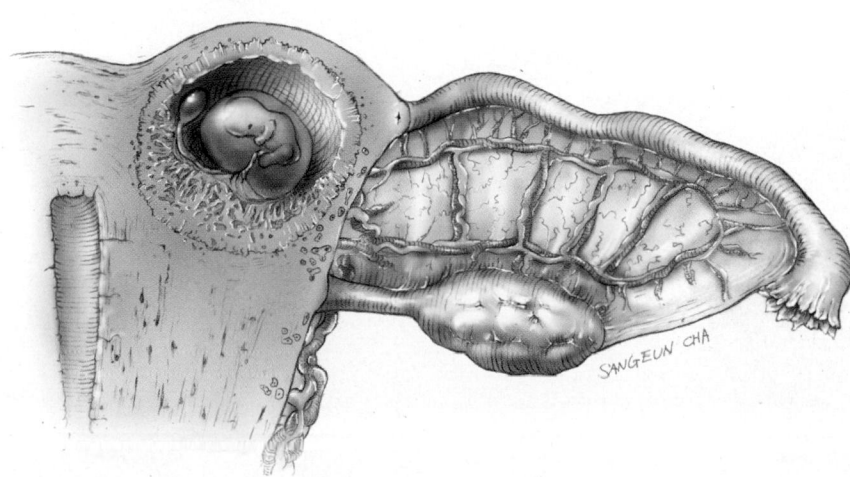

SANGEUN CHA

FIGURE 41-9.1 Interstitial pregnancy.

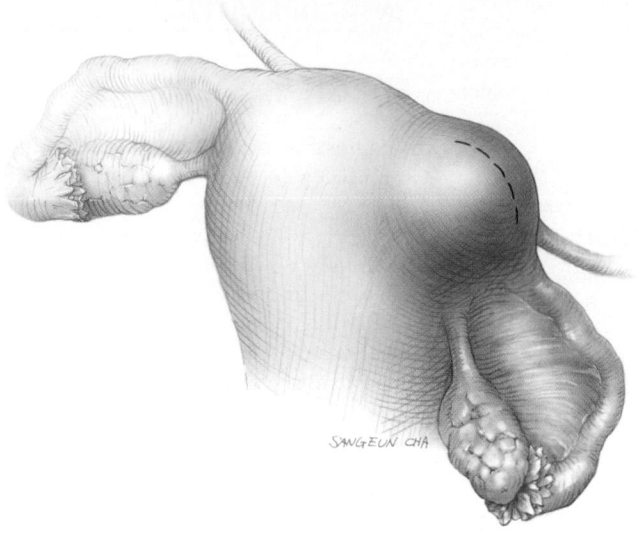

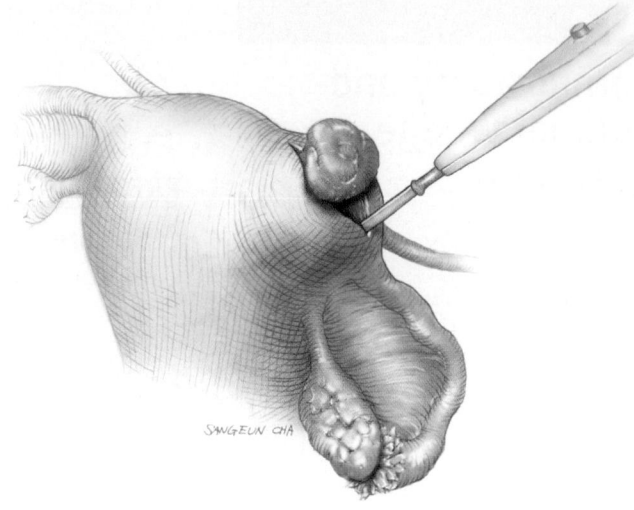

FIGURE 41-9.3 Cornuostomy with extrusion of products of conception.

FIGURE 41-9.2 Line of incision for cornuostomy.

be forced through the incision (Fig. 41-9.3). Products of conception may be removed by means of blunt or sharp dissection, by suction, or by hydrodissection (Fig. 41-9.4). Despite vasopressin, bleeding from the myometrium is common and is best managed with electrosurgical coagulation or figure-of-eight stitches with 2-0 absorbable or delayed-absorbable suture.

❼ Cornuostomy: Incision Closure. The myometrial incision is usually closed with absorbable or delayed-absorbable suture in an interrupted or continuous running fashion (Fig. 41-9.5) A gauge of sufficient strength

to prevent breakage during muscle approximation is selected, typically 2-0 or 0-gauge. Closure may be completed with one layer of sutures or may require two to three layers to aid hemostasis and reapproximate myometrium. Additionally, some prefer a subserosal closure, similar to a subcuticular running stitch, as a final layer. This theoretically minimizes the amount of exposed suture and thereby limits adhesion formation.

❽ Cornual Wedge Resection: Salpingectomy. With this approach, the pregnancy, surrounding myometrium, and ipsilateral fallopian tube are excised en bloc.

Initially, salpingectomy is completed as described in Section 41-8.1 (p. 1033). To summarize, the mesosalpinx is serially clamped and ligated across its length (Fig. 41-9.6). This separates the tube from its mesosalpinx and ipsilateral ovary (Fig. 41-9.7).

❾ Cornual Wedge Resection: Myometrial Incision. Following vasopressin injection, the cornu serosa surrounding the pregnancy is incised with an electrosurgical blade (Fig. 41-9.8). The incision is angled inward as it is deepened. This creates the characteristic wedge shape into the myometrium (Fig. 41-9.9). Hemostasis can be

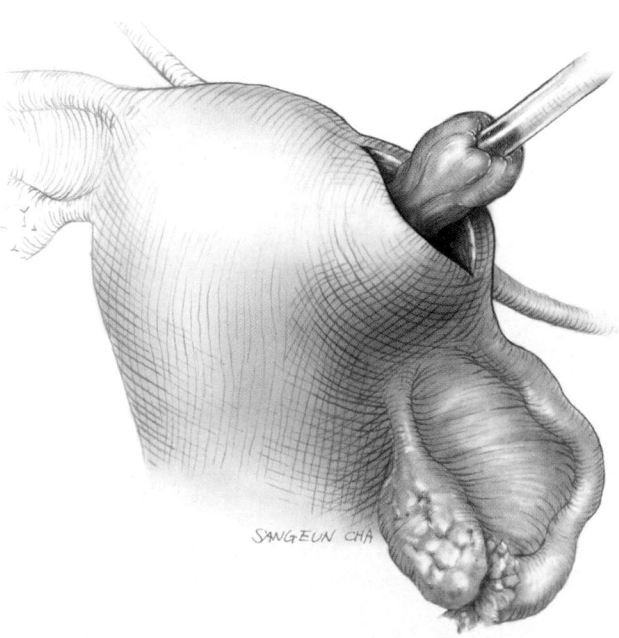

FIGURE 41-9.4 Suction removal of products of conception.

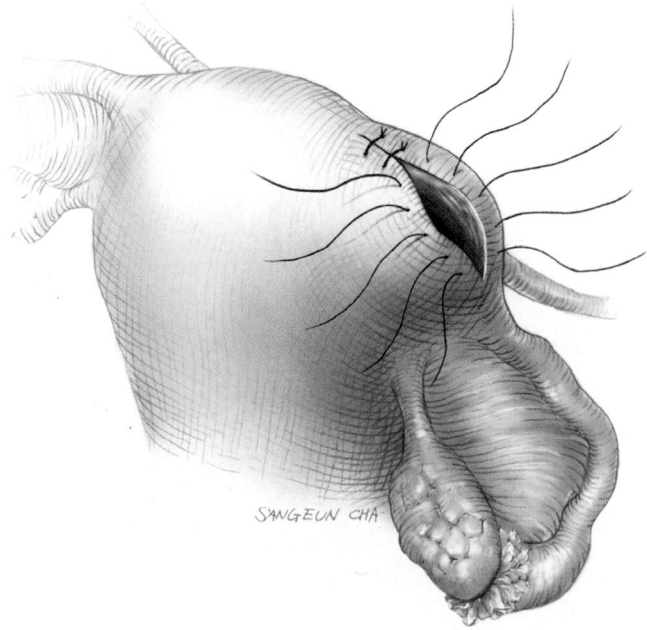

FIGURE 41-9.5 Myometrial incision closure.

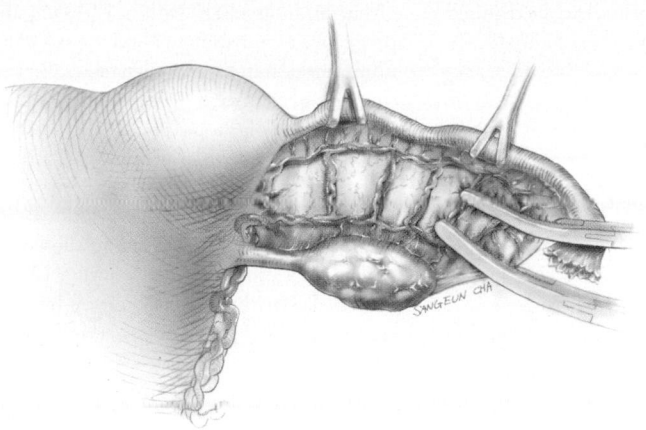

FIGURE 41-9.6 Mesosalpinx serially clamped and ligated.

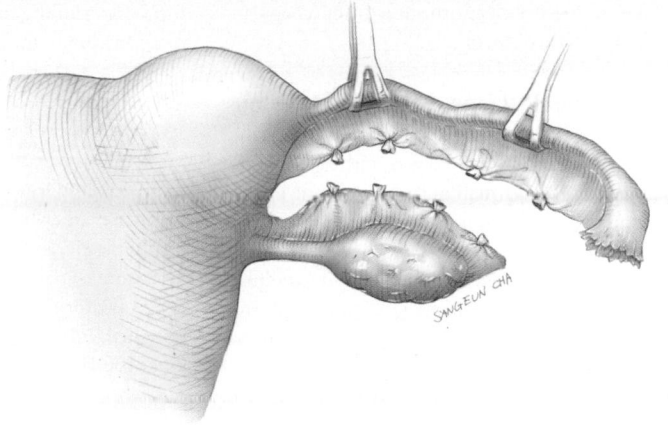

FIGURE 41-9.7 Salpingectomy completed.

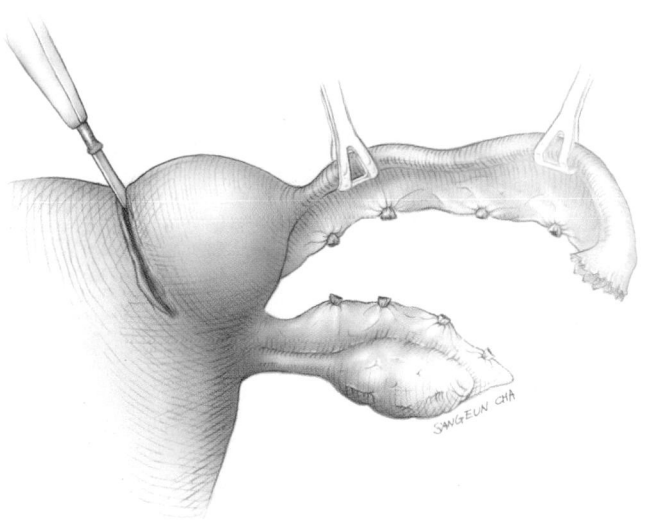

FIGURE 41-9.8 Myometrial incision.

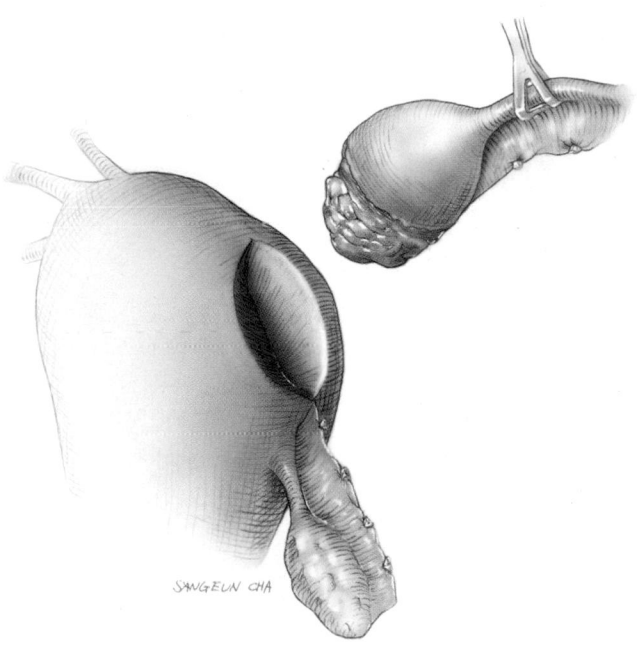

FIGURE 41-9.9 En bloc excision of interstitial pregnancy.

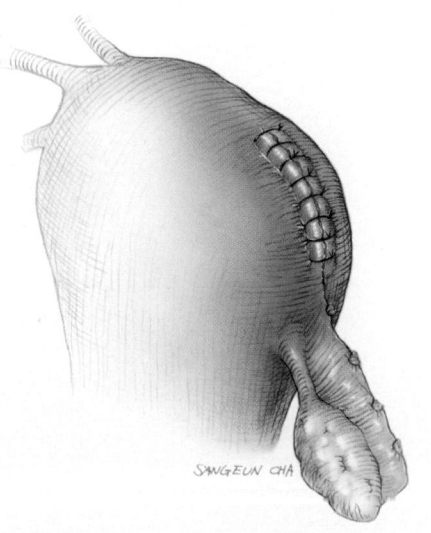

FIGURE 41-9.10 Incision closure.

achieved with electrosurgical blade coagulation or with sutures.

⑩ Cornual Wedge Resection: Incision Closure. The myometrial incision is usually closed in two to three layers with absorbable or delayed-absorbable suture in an interrupted or continuous running fashion. As with cornuostomy, some recommend a final subserosal layer closure. However, depending on the degree of wound tension created by the contracted myometrium, this suture may pull through the serosa, and a simple inter-

rupted or running suture line may be required to approximate the serosa (Fig. 41-9.10).

POSTOPERATIVE

As with salpingostomy for treatment of tubal pregnancy, there is increased risk of persistent trophoblastic tissue following cornuostomy. Therefore, serial β-hCG levels should be followed postoperatively until a negative test is obtained. For Rh-negative women, 50 or 300 μg (1500 IU) of Rh_0 (D) immune globulin is

given intramuscularly within 72 hours after pregnancy termination to lower the risk of isoimmunization in future pregnancies. Patients should be counseled that there is also an increased risk of ectopic pregnancy in general following an interstitial pregnancy. Lastly, as is the case with other types of uterine surgery such as classical cesarean delivery or myomectomy, the uterine rupture rate in subsequent pregnancies and particularly during labor is increased. For this reason, delivery by cesarean at term before labor onset is generally recommended.

41-10

Abdominal Myomectomy

Myomectomy involves surgical removal of leiomyomas from their surrounding myometrium. Indications can include abnormal uterine bleeding, pelvic pain, infertility, and recurrent miscarriage. For these problems, approximately 500,000 myomectomies were performed in the United States from 1979 to 2001. Although surgeons performed hysterectomies at nearly 12 times this frequency within the same time period, myomectomy rates still nearly doubled (Burrows, 2005). Suggested causes for this increased rate of organ preservation include desire to delay childbearing and concern about sexual dysfunction following hysterectomy (Section 41-12, p. 1045).

Myomectomy often requires laparotomy. However, laparoscopic excision may be performed by those with skills in laparoscopic suturing and suture ligation and is described in Section 42-9 (p. 1140).

PREOPERATIVE

Patient Evaluation

Because of their impact on preoperative and intraoperative planning, leiomyoma size, number, and location should be evaluated prior to surgery with sonography, magnetic resonance imaging, or hysteroscopy, as described in Chapter 9 (p. 252). For example, submucous tumors are more easily removed hysteroscopically (Section 42-16, p. 1166), whereas intramural and serosal types typically require laparotomy or laparoscopy. Leiomyomas may be small and buried within the myometrium. Therefore, accurate information as to leiomyoma number and location aids complete excision. Lastly, multiple large tumors or those that are located in the broad ligament, encroach upon the tubal ostia, or involve the cervix may increase the risk of conversion to hysterectomy. Patients should be so counseled.

Consent

Myomectomy has several risks including significant bleeding and transfusion. Moreover, uncontrolled hemorrhage or extensive myometrial injury during tumor removal may force hysterectomy. Fortunately, rates of conversion to hysterectomy during myomectomy are low and range from 0 to 2 percent (Iverson, 1996; LaMorte, 1993; Sawin, 2000).

Postoperatively, the risk of adhesion formation is significant, and leiomyomas can recur.

Patient Preparation
Hematologic Status

Abnormal uterine bleeding is a common indication for myomectomy. As a result, many women who elect to undergo this surgery are anemic. In addition, significant intraoperative blood loss during myomectomy is possible (Iverson, 1996, LaMorte, 1993; Sawin, 2000).

For these reasons, attempts to resolve anemia and bleeding prior to surgery should be pursued. Toward this goal, oral iron therapy and gonadotropin-releasing hormone (GnRH) agonists may have benefits (Chap. 9, p. 254). Benagiano and associates (1996) administered oral iron therapy alone or in combination with GnRH agonists and found the combination of the two to be significantly more effective in correcting preoperative anemia than either agonist use or iron therapy alone.

GnRH Agonists. In addition to preoperative control of abnormal uterine bleeding, these agents have been shown to significantly decrease uterine volume after several months of use (Benagiano, 1996; Friedman, 1991). As a result, decreased uterine size following treatment may allow a less invasive surgical procedure. For example, myomectomy may be completed through a smaller laparotomy incision or by laparoscopy or hysteroscopy (Crosignani, 1997; Lethaby, 2005; Mencaglia, 1993; Stovall, 1994). These agents have also been found to diminish leiomyoma vascularity and uterine blood flow (Matta, 1988; Reinsch, 1994). A final benefit may be adhesion prevention. Imai and associates (2003) noted lower rates of adhesion formation at second-look laparoscopy in women undergoing myomectomy who had received preoperative GnRH agonist therapy.

The use of preoperative GnRH agonists, however, may also have disadvantages. Within leiomyomas, GnRH agonists can incite hyaline or hydropic degeneration, which may obliterate the pseudocapsule connective tissue interface between the tumor and the myometrium. Such obliterated cleavage planes may lead to tedious and lengthy enucleation (Deligdish, 1997). Moreover, studies have shown higher rates of leiomyoma recurrence in women treated with GnRH agonists prior to myomectomy (Fedele, 1990; Vercellini, 2003). Leiomyomas treated with these agents may shrink in volume and be missed during surgical removal.

For these reasons, GnRH agonists are not used routinely in all patients undergoing myomectomy. They can be recommended

for preoperative use in women with greatly enlarged uteri or preoperative anemia or in cases in which a decrease in uterine volume would allow a less invasive approach to leiomyoma removal (Broekmans, 1996; Lethaby, 2002).

Autologous Blood Donation. The risk of blood transfusion varies among studies and ranges from less than 5 percent to nearly 40 percent (Darwish, 2005; LaMorte, 1993; Sawin, 2000; Smith, 1990). For this reason, in cases involving large uteri, especially those with multiple leiomyomas, autologous blood donation may be considered. Similarly, cell-saver blood scavenger and reuse techniques have been advocated (Yamada, 1997). Indication, benefits, and limitations to these forms of transfusion are discussed more fully in Chapter 40 (p. 1002).

Preoperative Uterine Artery Embolization. In select cases in which large leiomyomas are involved, administration of adequate volumes of vasopressin to control bleeding may pose risks of dangerous hypertension. Moreover, tourniquets may fail to adequately limit bleeding. In such cases, preoperative uterine artery embolization (UAE) on the morning of surgery may be an effective tool to limit blood loss. And, unlike GnRH agonist use, UAE allows tissue planes to be preserved (Chua, 2005; Ngeh, 2004; Ravina, 1995).

Several disadvantages have been noted with UAE, including collateral infarction of adjacent tissue and complications in subsequent pregnancies (Chap. 9, p. 256). For these reasons, preoperative UAE may best be limited to patients with large uteri in whom excessive blood loss is expected and in those not seeking future pregnancy.

Antibiotic Prophylaxis

There are few studies addressing the benefits of preoperative antibiotic use. Iverson and coworkers (1996), in their analysis of 101 myomectomy cases, found that although 54 percent of cases received prophylaxis, infectious morbidity was not lowered compared with cases in which antibiotics were not used.

In cases of myomectomy performed for infertility, because of the potential for tubal adhesions associated with pelvic infection, antibiotic prophylaxis has been advocated (Marquard, 2008). For those in whom prophylaxis is planned, 1 g of a first- or second-generation cephalosporin intravenously is appropriate (Iverson, 1996; Periti, 1988; Sawin, 2000).

Bowel Preparation

Because of the low risk of bowel injury with this procedure, bowel preparation is typically not required unless extensive adhesions are anticipated, and thereby the risk for bowel perforation is increased. In contrast, because the risk of conversion to hysterectomy is present, vaginal preparation immediately prior to surgical draping is warranted.

INTRAOPERATIVE

SURGICAL STEPS

❶ Anesthesia and Patient Positioning. Myomectomy performed through a laparotomy incision is typically an inpatient procedure performed under general or regional anesthesia. The patient is placed supine, the vagina and abdomen are surgically prepared, and a Foley catheter is inserted.

❷ Abdominal Entry. The choice of Pfannenstiel incision is typically appropriate for uteri 14 weeks' size or smaller (Section 41-2, p. 1022). Larger uteri usually require a midline vertical abdominal incision.

❸ Leiomyoma Identification. Following abdominal entry, the surgeon should inspect the serosal surface to identify leiomyomas to be removed. Additionally, firm squeezing palpation of the myometrium before and during the surgery will help identify buried intramural or submucous leiomyomas.

❹ Use of Uterine Tourniquet. Tourniquets have been used for years to temporarily occlude blood flow through the uterine arteries. Because the uterus receives collateral flow through the ovarian arteries, some tourniquet techniques include occlusion of both uterine and ovarian vessels. During these procedures, bilateral windows are created in the leaves of the broad ligament at the level of the internal cervical os. A Penrose drain or Foley catheter is threaded through the opening to encircle the uterine isthmus. Once in place, the Penrose drain is tied or the ends of the Foley catheter are clamped to compress the uterine vessels. In combination with this, occlusion of the uteroovarian ligaments or infundibulopelvic ligaments with rubber-shod clamps has been described to compress the ovarian arteries (Sapmaz, 2003; Taylor, 2005). Large, bulky uteri or those with leiomyomas in the broad ligament, however, may limit the use of tourniquets in some patients. In addition to temporary occlusion of the uterine arteries, permanent ligation of the uterine arteries has been described and shown to lower blood loss during myomectomy (Liu, 2004; Taylor, 2005).

❺ Use of Vasopressin. Pitressin (8-arginine vasopressin) is a sterile, aqueous solution of synthetic vasopressin. It is effective in limiting uterine blood loss during myomectomy because of its ability to cause vascular spasm and uterine muscle contraction. Compared with placebo, synthetic vasopressin injection has been shown to significantly decrease blood loss during myomectomy (Frederick, 1994). Compared with tourniquet techniques, vasopressin injection has also been associated with either comparable or less intraoperative blood loss and with equally low patient morbidity (Fletcher, 1996; Ginsburg, 1993). Moreover, Darwish and colleagues (2005) found lower rates of myometrial hematoma formation in those cases using vasopressin compared with those using tourniquet techniques.

Each vial of vasopressin is standardized to contain 20 pressor units/mL, and doses used for myomectomy range from 20 U diluted in 30 to 100 mL of saline (Bieber, 1998; Fletcher, 1996; Iverson, 1996). Vasopressin is typically injected along the planned serosal incision(s). The plasma half-life of this agent is 10 to 20 minutes. For this reason, injection of vasopressin is ideally discontinued 20 minutes prior to uterine repair to allow evaluation of bleeding from myometrial incisions (Hutchins, 1996).

The main risks associated with local vasopressin injection result from inadvertent intravascular infiltration and include transient increases in blood pressure, bradycardia, atrioventricular block, and pulmonary edema (Deschamps, 2005; Tulandi, 1996). For these reasons, patients with a medical history of angina, myocardial infarction, cardiomyopathy, congestive heart failure, uncontrolled hypertension, migraine, asthma, or severe chronic obstructive pulmonary disease may not be candidates for vasopressin use.

❻ Serosal Incision. Because of postoperative adhesion formation risks, surgeons ideally minimize the number of serosal incisions and attempt to place incisions on the anterior uterine wall. Tulandi and colleagues (1993) found that posterior wall incisions result in a 94-percent adhesion formation rate compared with a 55-percent rate for anterior incisions.

For most patients, a midline vertical uterine incision allows removal of the greatest number of leiomyomas through the fewest incisions. The length should accommodate the approximate diameter of the largest tumor. The incision depth should afford access to all leiomyomas (Fig. 41-10.1). To reach lateral tumors, a surgeon may create lateral myometrial incisions within the initial central incision. However, at times, a separate serosal incision may be required to excise tumors from these locations. In these instances, a horizontal serosal incision decreases the number of vessels transected.

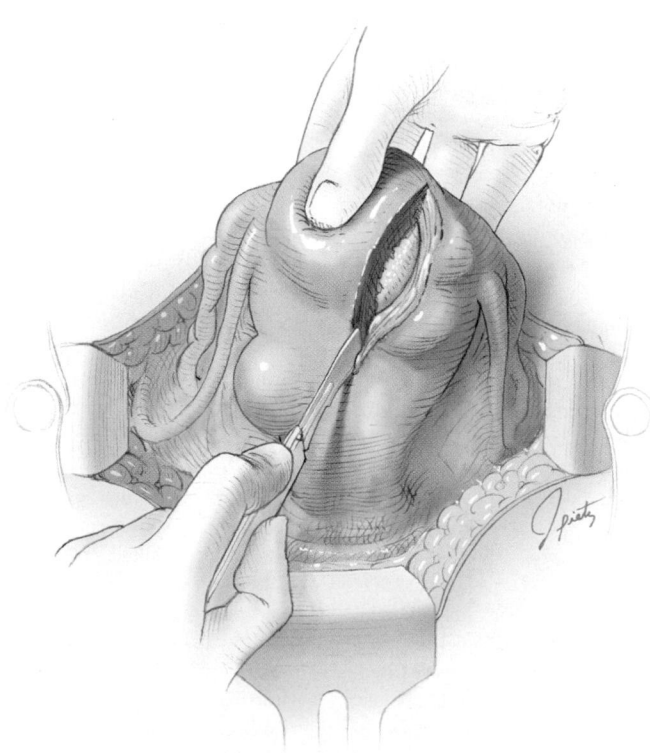

FIGURE 41-10.1 Uterine incision.

❼ Tumor Enucleation. The first leiomyoma is grasped with a Lahey or single-tooth tenaculum (Fig. 41-10.2). Applying traction on the leiomyoma aids in the development of a tissue plane between myometrium and leiomyoma. A leiomyoma screw can also be used for this same purpose. Sharp and blunt dissection of the pseudocapsule surrounding the leiomyoma frees the tumor from the adjacent myometrium.

❽ Bleeding. Hemorrhage during myomectomy primarily develops during tumor enucleation and is positively correlated with preoperative uterine size, total weight of leiomyomas removed, and operating time (Ginsburg, 1993). Approximately two to four main arteries feed each leiomyoma and enter the tumor at unpredictable sites. For this reason, surgeons should watch for these vessels, ligate them prior to transection when possible, and be ready to immediately grasp them with hemostats for ligation or fulguration if lacerated during tumor excision (Fig. 41-10.3).

❾ Myometrial Incision. Smaller, internal incisions into the myometrium may be required to excise all leiomyomas. If the endometrial cavity is entered, it should be closed with a running suture of 4-0 or 5-0 delayed-absorbable suture, as shown by the left needle in Figure 41-10.4.

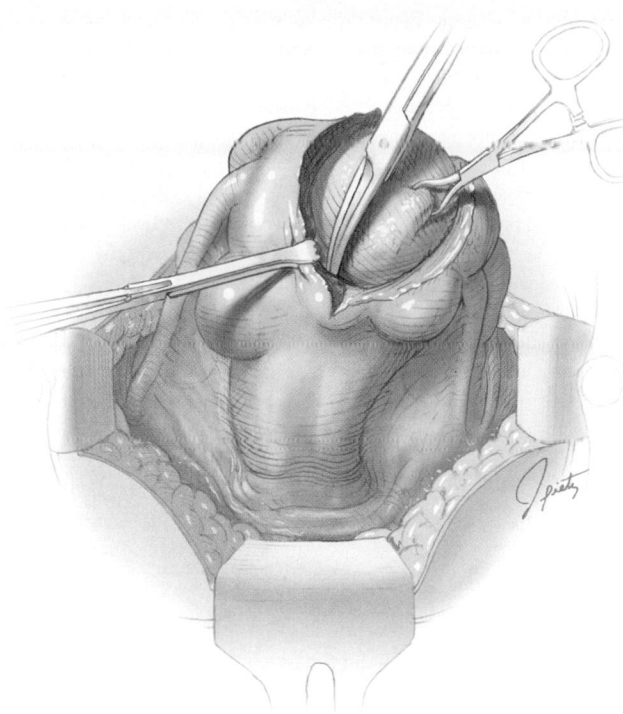

FIGURE 41-10.2 Tumor enucleation.

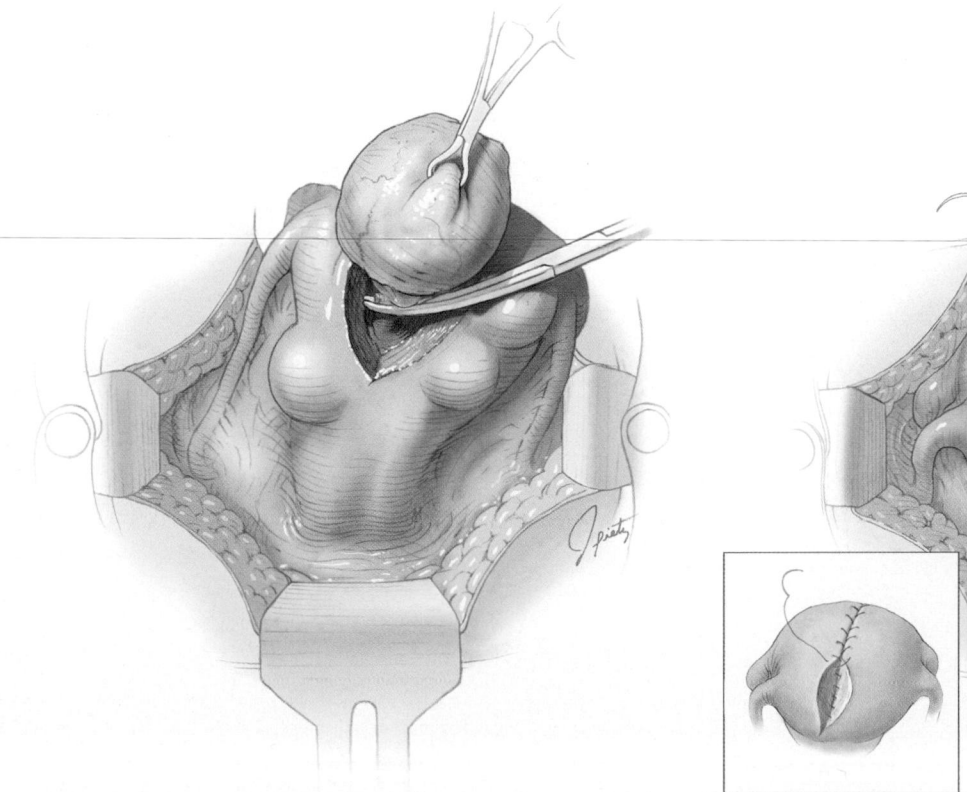

FIGURE 41-10.3 Vessel ligation.

FIGURE 41-10.4 Uterine incision closure.

⑩ Myometrial Closure. Following removal of all tumors, redundant serosa may be excised. As seen in the left uterine wall in Figure 41-10.4, smaller internal myometrial incisions are closed first with delayed-absorbable suture. The myometrium is then closed in several layers to improve hemostasis and prevent hematoma formation. A gauge of sufficient strength to prevent breakage during muscle approximation is selected, typically 2-0 or 0-gauge.

⑪ Serosal Closure. Closure of the serosal incision using a running baseball stitch or a subserosal running closure, similar to a running subcuticular closure, may help to limit adhesion formation. For this, 4-0 or 5-0 monofilament, delayed-absorbable suture may be selected. Moreover, absorbable adhesion barriers may help reduce the incidence of adhesion formation following myomectomy (Ahmad, 2008).

POSTOPERATIVE

Following abdominal myomectomy, postoperative care follows that for any major abdominal surgery (Chap. 39, p. 962). Hospitalization typically varies from 1 to 4 days, and return of normal bowel function and febrile morbidity usually dictates this course. Postoperative activity in general can be individualized, although vigorous exercise is usually delayed until 4 to 6 weeks after laparotomy.

Fever

Febrile morbidity of greater than 38.0°C is a common event following myomectomy (Iverson, 1995; LaMorte, 1993; Rybak, 2008). Purported causes include atelectasis, myometrial incisional hematomas, and factors released with myometrial destruction. Although fever is common following myo-

mectomy, pelvic infection is not. For example, LaMorte and colleagues (1993) noted only a 2-percent rate of pelvic infection in their analysis of 128 myomectomy cases.

Subsequent Pregnancy

There are no clear guidelines as to the timing of pregnancy attempts following myomectomy. Darwish and associates (2005) performed sonographic examinations on 169 patients following myomectomy. Following myometrial indicators, they concluded that wound healing is usually completed within 3 months. There are no clinical trials that address the issue of uterine rupture and therefore the route of delivery of pregnancies occurring after myomectomy (American College of Obstetricians and Gynecologists, 2008a). Management of these cases requires sound clinical judgment and individualization of care.

41-11

Vaginal Myomectomy for Prolapsed Leiomyoma

Prolapse of a pedunculated submucosal leiomyoma is an unusual occurrence but certainly not rare. Vaginal myomectomy is usually a relatively simple procedure and is frequently curative for the patient. In some cases, simply twisting the leiomyoma off its stalk may be sufficient for removal. Stalk diameter and patient discomfort typically dictate whether removal can be performed safely and comfortably in a clinic setting or in the operating room.

PREOPERATIVE

Patient Evaluation

In many cases, diagnosis of a prolapsed pedunculated submucosal leiomyoma will be obvious, as will the size of the prolapsed leiomyoma. However, as many of these patients present with abnormal uterine bleeding, evaluation for other less obvious causes of abnormal bleeding is appropriate. In other cases, partial prolapse of a leiomyoma through the cervix may preclude assessment of leiomyoma size, or the mass may be of unclear etiology. Accordingly, imaging studies, particularly transvaginal or transabdominal sonography or both, may yield additional information beyond pelvic examination. Specifically, uterine size, shape, and degree of involvement with leiomyomas or other pathology can be obtained. In addition, biopsy of any mass of uncertain etiology should always be considered. Tischler biopsy forceps may be selected for such biopsy (Fig. 29-15, p. 750). If required, Monsel solution can be applied to control bleeding from the biopsy site similar to that following colposcopic biopsy.

Consent

The risk of complications from vaginal myomectomy is low. Resection of the uterine wall can occur with possible concomitant injury to intraabdominal organs. Uncontrollable bleeding and procedural failure are other potential risks. Hysterectomy and its consequences should be discussed with the patient beforehand. Leiomyoma prolapse recurrence is uncommon but may occur if additional submucosal leiomyomas are present or develop within the uterus.

Patient Preparation

In an otherwise healthy woman, little preparation is needed for vaginal myomectomy.

However, in the event of moderately severe to severe anemia, improvement in the patient's hemodynamic status is initiated if the patient is symptomatic, is unstable, and/or is being taken to the operating room for the procedure. Anemia may be corrected with blood transfusion, oral iron therapy, or both. Resuscitative treatment varies with each individual and clinical situation and is discussed in detail in Chapter 40 (p. 1006). If fever is present and infection of the prolapsed leiomyoma or lower genital tract is suspected, treatment with broad-spectrum antibiotics should be initiated prior to vaginal myomectomy. Suitable options are found in Table 3-31 (p. 103).

INTRAOPERATIVE

SURGICAL STEPS

❶ **Anesthesia and Patient Positioning.** The patient is placed in dorsal lithotomy position. Vaginal myomectomy may be performed under general or regional anesthesia, intracervical or paracervical blockade, conscious sedation, or no anesthesia or analgesia. For those individuals who are taken to the operating room at our institution, we usually prefer general anesthesia for several reasons. First, hysteroscopy is often done following vaginal myomectomy to further evaluate the uterine cavity and status of the stalk. Secondly, many of the leiomyomas are bulky and require at least a moderate amount of manipulation and vaginal retraction for removal.

An examination is done once the patient is relaxed to assess the size of the prolapsed leiomyoma; location, length, and thickness of the stalk; and general pelvic anatomy. The vagina is then surgically prepared, and a Foley catheter inserted into the bladder.

❷ **Leiomyoma Ligation.** An Auvard weighted vaginal speculum is positioned to retract the posterior vaginal wall. Heaney retractors are used as needed for sidewall and anterior vaginal wall retraction. The prolapsed leiomyoma is grasped with a single-tooth tenaculum. Traction is applied on the leiomyoma to allow access to the stalk (Fig. 41-11.1). Excessive traction on the leiomyoma is avoided. This has the potential to create an inversion of the uterine wall at the site of stalk attachment and thereby expose the uterine wall to resection when the stalk is incised. In addition, undue traction may avulse the tumor prior to ligation of its muscular stalk and lead to bleeding.

The stalk is doubly ligated with delayed-absorbable suture. Preformed knotted loops with a knot pusher (as used in laparoscopy cases) work well in this setting, as manually tying a knot may be technically difficult given the size of the leiomyoma, the length

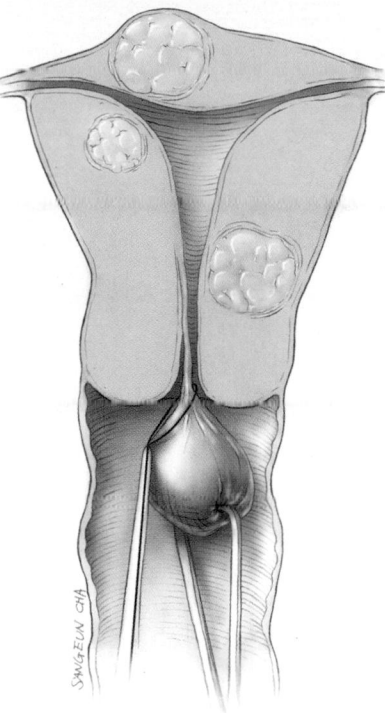

FIGURE 41-11.1 Exposure of prolapsed leiomyoma and ligation of stalk.

of the stalk (or lack thereof), and the limited amount of space in which to work.

❸ **Leiomyoma Removal.** The stalk is then sharply incised at an appropriate point distal to the ligature to prevent the ligature from slipping off (Fig. 41-11.2).

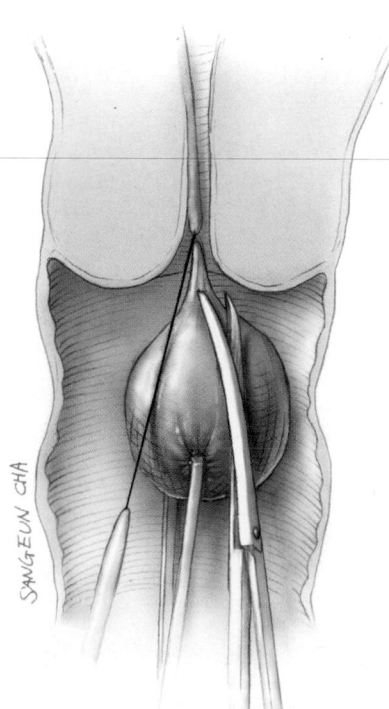

FIGURE 41-11.2 Suture loop cinched and tumor stalk transected.

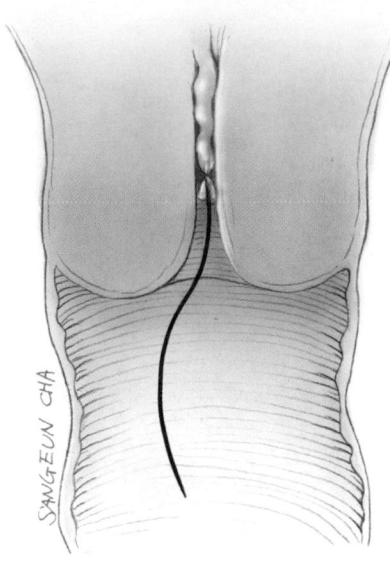

FIGURE 41-11.3 Leiomyoma excision completed.

With complete stalk transection, the prolapsed leiomyoma is freed for removal, and the stalk retracts into the uterine cavity (Fig. 41-11.3). Alternatively, the stalk may be incised electrosurgically without placement of ligatures, or the leiomyoma may be twisted from its stalk if the stalk is not excessively thick.

As mentioned previously, hysteroscopy is usually performed at our institution after leiomyoma removal to assess hemostasis and the uterine cavity. However, this step may be omitted.

POSTOPERATIVE

No special care beyond routine postoperative surveillance is necessary following vaginal myomectomy for a pedunculated prolapsed leiomyoma. Those patients who have the procedure performed in the operating room can be managed like any outpatient surgery patient.

41-12

Abdominal Hysterectomy

Hysterectomy is one of the most frequently performed gynecologic procedures, with approximately 600,000 women undergoing this procedure annually in the United States (Whiteman, 2008). The reasons for hysterectomy are varied and include both benign and malignant etiologies. Of benign indications, symptomatic leiomyomas and pelvic organ prolapse are the most frequent, although abnormal bleeding, endometriosis, chronic pain, and premalignant neoplasia are also relatively common.

PREOPERATIVE

Patient Evaluation

A spectrum of tests may be required to reach the preoperative diagnosis. These tests vary depending on the clinical setting and are discussed within the respective chapters covering those etiologies. Prior to hysterectomy, however, all patients require Pap smear screening, and abnormal findings require evaluation for cervical cancer prior to surgery (Chap. 29, p. 744). Similarly, women at risk for endometrial cancer and whose indication includes abnormal bleeding typically are also screened before surgery (Chap. 8, p. 223).

Hysterectomy Approach

Hysterectomy may be completed by a surgeon using an abdominal, vaginal, laparoscopic, or robotic approach, and selection is influenced by many factors. For example, physical properties of the uterus and pelvis, surgical indications, presence or absence of adnexal pathology, surgical risks, costs, hospitalization and recovery length, hospital resources, surgeon expertise, and anticipated postoperative quality of life are all weighed once hysterectomy is planned. Each of these approaches carries distinct advantages and disadvantages.

Abdominal Hysterectomy

Most uteri in the United States are removed through an abdominal incision (Farquhar, 2002). Either a transverse or vertical incision may be selected depending on the clinical setting (Sections 41-1 and 41-2, p. 1020). In general, if a uterus is large, a midline vertical incision is chosen to provide sufficient operating space.

Abdominal hysterectomy allows the greatest ability to manipulate pelvic organs and thus is preferred if large pelvic organs or extensive adhesions are anticipated. In addition, an abdominal approach affords access to the ovaries if oophorectomy is desired, to the space of Retzius or presacral space if concurrent urogynecologic procedures are planned, or to the upper abdomen for cancer staging. Abdominal hysterectomy typically requires less operating time than laparoscopic hysterectomy and requires no advanced laparoscopic instrumentation or expertise (Falcone, 1999).

However, abdominal hysterectomy is associated with longer patient recovery and hospital stays, increased incisional pain, and greater risk of postoperative fever and wound infection (Johns, 1995; Marana, 1999; Nieboer, 2009). Additionally, compared with a vaginal approach, abdominal hysterectomy is associated with greater risk of transfusion and ureteral injury, but lower rates of postoperative bleeding complications and bladder injury (Harris, 1996).

Vaginal Hysterectomy

This approach is usually chosen by surgeons if pelvic organs are small, extensive adhesions are not anticipated, no significant adnexal pathology is expected, and some degree of pelvic organ prolapse is present. When this procedure is compared with abdominal hysterectomy, patients more often benefit from faster recovery and from reduced hospital stays, costs, and postoperative pain.

Laparoscopic Hysterectomy

This approach is typically selected for patients if pelvic organs are small, extensive adhesions are not expected, uterine descent is poor, and surgeons are skilled in laparoscopic techniques. Although patient recovery, hospital stays, and postoperative pain scores are comparable with those for vaginal hysterectomy,

this approach allows greater visualization and access to the abdomen and pelvis. This may be advantageous if oophorectomy is planned or if adhesive disease or bleeding is encountered. However, laparoscopy typically requires longer operating times and more expensive equipment. In addition, it has been associated with greater rates of ureteral injury (as high as 14 percent) than either abdominal (0.4 percent) or vaginal hysterectomy (0.2 percent) (Harkki-Siren, 1997a,b). Laparoscopically assisted vaginal hysterectomy may be considered in those cases in which one or more factors are amenable to laparoscopic manipulation and thus, once corrected, allow hysterectomy to be completed vaginally.

Approach Selection

If all factors are equal, vaginal hysterectomy should be considered (American College of Obstetricians and Gynecologists, 2009b). However, when large pelvic organs, risk of associated malignancy, extensive adhesions, or poor uterine descent is present, either abdominal or laparoscopic hysterectomy may be required. Of note, surgical expertise is factored into the decision and heavily dictates the approach selected.

Total versus Supracervical Hysterectomy

Prior to hysterectomy, the decision to concurrently remove the cervix is typically discussed with the patient. Hysterectomy may include removal of the uterus and cervix, termed *total hysterectomy*, or may involve only the uterine corpus, called *supracervical hysterectomy* (Fig. 41-12.1). The term *subtotal hysterectomy* refers to the supracervical type but is not preferred usage.

During the latter half of the 20th century, most hysterectomies performed were total hysterectomies. The supracervical technique was reserved for cases in which excision of the

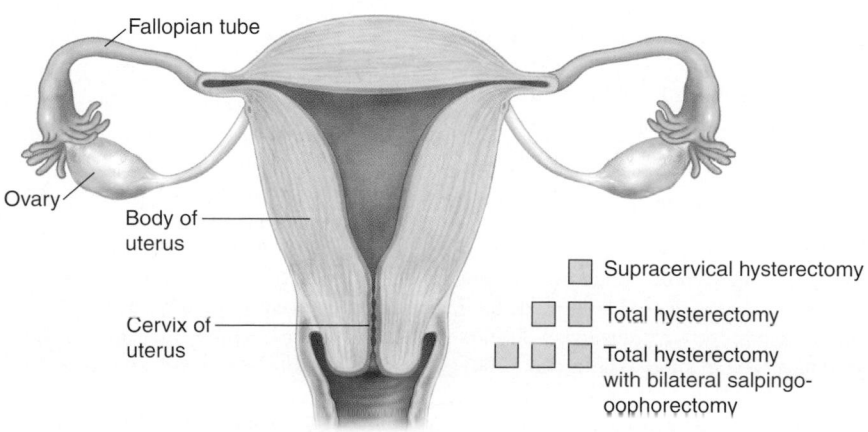

FIGURE 41-12.1 Hysterectomy classification.

Fallopian tube

Ovary

Body of uterus

Cervix of uterus

☐ Supracervical hysterectomy

☐☐ Total hysterectomy

☐☐☐ Total hysterectomy with bilateral salpingo-oophorectomy

cervix risked increased bleeding, surrounding organ damage, or increased operating time. However, suggested improvement in urinary symptoms and preservation of sexual function have been attributed to cervical conservation, and a trend began in the 1980s toward supra-cervical hysterectomy (Kilkku, 1983, 1985). Proponents suggest that the cervix provides an important stabilizing function for pelvic support and that the Frankenhäuser nerve plexus can be disrupted during total hysterectomy, causing bladder, bowel, or sexual dysfunction. Additionally, advocates argue that this approach decreases surrounding pelvic organ injury and operating times, especially during a laparoscopic approach to hysterectomy (Baggish, 2005).

However, randomized studies have failed to support differences in sexual or urinary function following total abdominal or supracervical hysterectomy (Gimbel, 2005a; Kuppermann, 2005; Roussis, 2004; Thakar, 2002). In addition, Learman and coworkers (2003) found no statistically significant differences between the two in surgical complications and clinical outcomes during 2 years of surveillance. Moreover, chronic bleeding may follow supracervical hysterectomy. Ten to 20 percent of women will still note vaginal bleeding, presumably from retained isthmic endometrium following hysterectomy. Most of these cases end in trachelectomy (Gimbel, 2005b; Okaro, 2001). Procedures that ablate or core out the endocervical canal may help prevent this complication (Jenkins, 2004; Schmidt, 2011).

Critics of supracervical hysterectomy have also noted the persistent risk for cancer in the conserved stump. However, the risk for cervical cancer in these women is comparable with those without hysterectomy, and the prognosis for cervical stump cancer mirrors that in those with a uterus (Hannoun-Levi, 1997; Hellstrom, 2001; Silva, 2004).

In sum, abdominal supracervical hysterectomy for benign diseases offers no distinct advantage compared with total abdominal hysterectomy (American College of Obstetricians and Gynecologists, 2007). The risks of persistent bleeding following surgery may deter many women and clinicians from its use.

Consent

Hysterectomy for most women is a safe and effective treatment that typically leads to an improved postoperative quality of life and psychological outcome (Hartmann, 2004; Thakar, 2004). However, pelvic organs may be injured during surgery, and vascular, bladder, and ureteral injury are most commonly cited. Accordingly, these and the risks of

blood loss and transfusion are discussed with the patient before surgery.

Concurrent Bilateral Oophorectomy

Hysterectomy is frequently performed with other surgical procedures. Pelvic reconstructive surgeries and bilateral salpingo-oophorectomy are among the most common.

Ovaries are prophylactically removed in approximately 40 percent of hysterectomy cases performed for benign indications in the United States (Asante, 2010). In women younger than 40 years, ovaries are typically conserved because the number of years of expected hormone production is great. In those older than 50 years, bilateral oophorectomy is common. However, for those in their 40s, the decision to prophylactically remove ovaries is controversial.

Proponents of prophylactic oophorectomy argue that the procedure eliminates future ovarian cancer risk and is estimated to prevent 1000 new cases of ovarian cancer each year (American College of Obstetricians and Gynecologists, 2008b). In addition, patients with retained ovaries may require future surgery for subsequent benign ovarian disease, and this risk ranges from 1 to 5 percent (Bukovsky, 1988; Zalel, 1997). Specifically, women with endometriosis, pelvic inflammatory disease, and chronic pelvic pain are at greater risk for reoperation. Lastly, the duration of significant ovarian estrogen production for many will be shortened following hysterectomy. For example, Siddle and coworkers (1987) noted the mean age of ovarian failure in a group undergoing hysterectomy was 45 years. This was significantly lower than the mean age of 49 years in a control group not receiving surgery.

Importantly, in women retaining their ovaries, the risk for ovarian cancer is still decreased by 40 to 50 percent by hysterectomy alone (Chiaffarino, 2005; Green, 1997). Additional disadvantages to oophorectomy include long-term effects of hypoestrogenism such as risks for osteoporosis and coronary artery disease. Parker and colleagues (2005) noted an increased rate of survival to 80 years in women after hysterectomy at ages 50 to 54 years with ovarian conservation (62 percent) compared with those electing oophorectomy without estrogen replacement therapy (ERT) (54 percent). Although these rates became nearly equal in those electing oophorectomy and then receiving postoperative ERT, concerns regarding ERT compliance have been noted. Castelo-Branco and coworkers (1999) found that after 5 years following hysterectomy and oophorectomy, only one third of patients still continued their ERT. Most stopped due to cancer concerns.

In addition to the loss of estrogen, ovarian androgen production is lost, and its importance in later life has not been entirely delineated (Olive, 2005). The American College of Obstetricians and Gynecologists (2008b) recommends strong consideration be given for retention of normal ovaries in premenopausal women not at increased genetic risk for ovarian cancer.

▨ Patient Preparation

Because of the risk of postoperative vaginal cuff cellulitis and urinary tract infection following hysterectomy, patients typically receive antibiotic prophylaxis with either a first- or second-generation cephalosporin. These and suitable alternative choices are found in Table 39-6 (p. 959). The risk of bowel injury with hysterectomy is low. Accordingly for most women, an enema administered prior to surgery to evacuate the rectum is sufficient. A more extensive preparation may be indicated if extensive pelvic adhesive disease is anticipated. Also, prophylaxis for venous thromboembolism is provided as outlined in Table 39-9 (p. 962).

INTRAOPERATIVE

SURGICAL STEPS

❶ Anesthesia and Patient Positioning. Abdominal hysterectomy is typically performed under general or regional anesthesia. The patient is positioned supine, a Foley catheter is placed, and the abdomen and vagina are prepared for surgery.

❷ Abdominal Entry. Either a transverse or a vertical incision may be used for hysterectomy, and clinical factors influence selection (Section 41-1, p. 1020).

❸ Exposure. Following entry into the abdomen, a self-retaining retractor such as an O'Connor-O'Sullivan or a Balfour retractor is placed. The pelvis and abdomen are visually and manually explored, and the bowel is packed from the operating field. The uterus is grasped and elevated from the pelvis. If extensive adhesions are present, normal anatomic relationships are restored to aid surgery. Hysterectomy may be performed by one surgeon, but commonly two surgeons are present with each typically operating on his or her side of the uterus.

❹ Round Ligament Transection. Curved Kelly clamps are placed bilaterally across each fallopian tube and uteroovarian ligament immediately lateral to the uterus (Fig. 41-12.2).

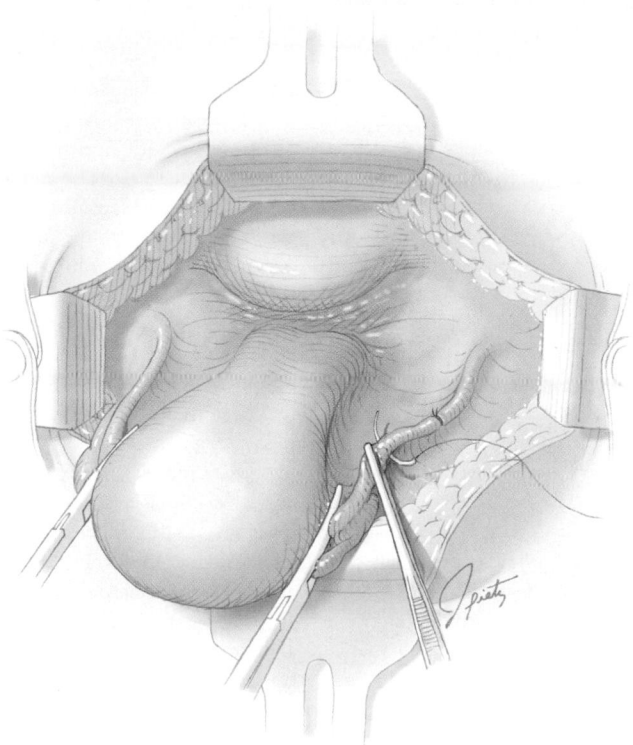

FIGURE 41-12.2 Round ligament transection.

Hysterectomy is begun with midsection division of one of the round ligaments. This provides entry into the retroperitoneum for identification of the ureter and also for access to the uterine artery and cardinal ligament for transection later in the procedure. A transfixing suture using 0-gauge delayed-absorbable suture is placed approximately 1 cm proximally and

another suture 1 cm distally to this planned division. These sutures are held by hemostats and directed upward and outward to create tension along the interposed segment of round ligament. The round ligament is divided, and the line of incision is directed inferiorly into the first 1 to 2 cm of the broad ligament.

❺ **Broad Ligament Leaves**. With this action, the broad ligament separates to create anterior and posterior leaves. Between them, gauzy areolar connective tissue is seen. The leading medial and lateral edges of the anterior leaf are grasped with smooth atraumatic forceps. Tension on these edges is directed upward and outward. The tented anterior leaf is then incised sharply with the line of incision curving inferiorly and medially to the level of the vesicouterine fold (Fig. 41-12.3). These last two steps are repeated on the contralateral side. At this point, it is advantageous to identify the ureters in the retroperitoneal space. Ideally this should be performed before any tissue clamps are placed. The posterior leaf of the broad ligament on either side can be opened once the ureters are identified. With the ureter safely out of the way, the posterior leaf of the broad ligament is sharply incised with extension inferomedially toward the uterosacral ligaments. Figure 41-12.4 shows the appearance of the broad ligament and adnexa following these steps.

❻ **Ovarian Conservation.** With the leaves of the broad ligament now open, if adnexa are to be preserved, the surgeon's index finger can be curved under the fallopian tube and uteroovarian ligament. One Kelly clamp was already placed at the beginning of surgery

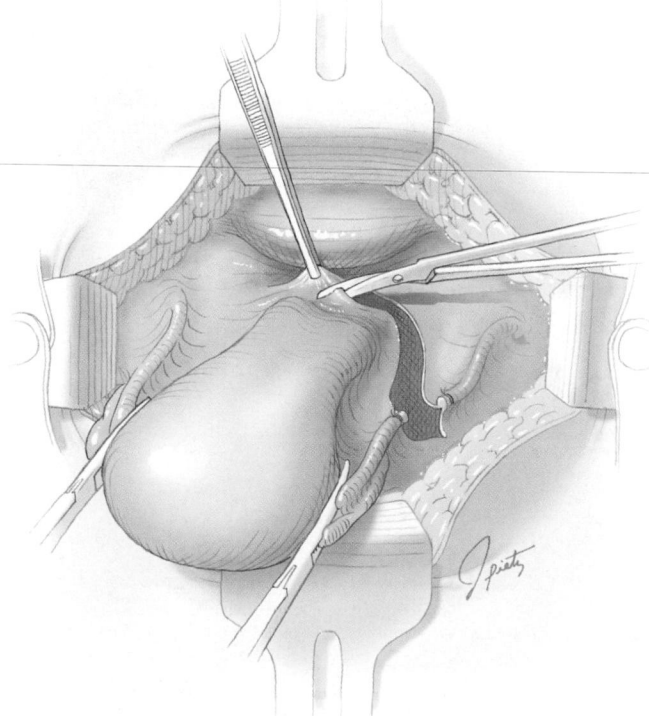

FIGURE 41-12.3 Anterior leaf of broad ligament opened.

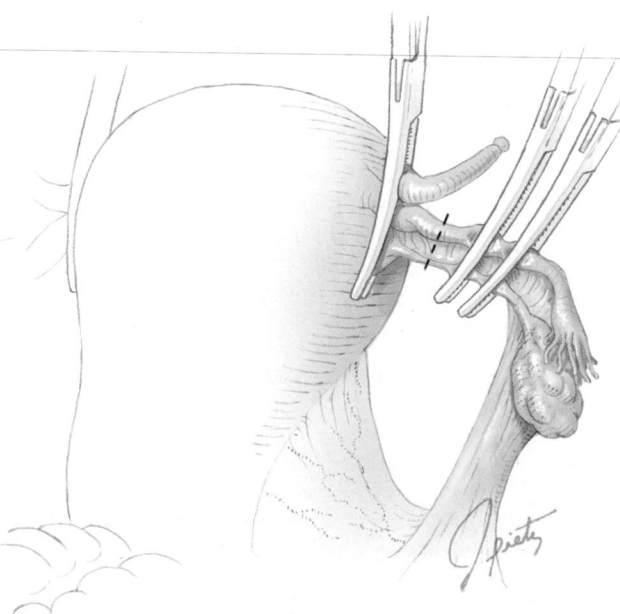

FIGURE 41-12.4 Ovarian conservation.

across the fallopian tube and uteroovarian ligament and lies medial to the surgeon's finger. Two Heaney or other appropriate clamps are then placed lateral to the finger, with each clamp's arc directed toward the uterus (see Fig. 41-12.4).

The surgeon's finger is removed, and the intervening segment of fallopian tube and uteroovarian ligament is incised between the medial Heaney clamp and Kelly clamp (dotted line). A free tie of 0-gauge delayed-absorbable suture is placed around the tissue pedicle held by the more lateral of the two Heaney clamps. As the knot of this suture is tied securely, the lateral of these two clamps is removed. A transfixing suture is then placed around the pedicle held by the remaining Heaney clamp (Fig. 40-38, p. 1004). This suture is placed above and distal to the first free tie. As the knot is cinched in place, the Heaney clamp is removed. The Kelly clamp is left in place. The adnexa is now freed from the uterus.

❼ Oophorectomy. If the adnexa are to be removed, the fallopian tube and ovary are grasped with a Babcock clamp and elevated away from the infundibulopelvic (IP) ligament (Fig. 41-12.5). The peritoneum lateral to this ligament is incised, and this incision is extended cephalad and laterally. The peritoneum medial to the IP ligament was earlier incised as part of the posterior leaf of the broad ligament.

With the IP ligament now isolated and the ureter visualized, curved Heaney clamps can be placed around this ligament. As with the uteroovarian ligaments, two clamps are placed lateral to the planned site of incision and one clamp is placed medially. All arcs of these curved clamps are directed toward the site of planned incision.

Once the clamps have been placed, the IP ligament is transected (dotted line). Ligation of the IP is carried out as in step 6. That is, a free tie 0-gauge delayed-absorbable suture is placed around the more proximal of the two Heaney clamps. As the knot of this suture is tied securely, the proximal clamp is removed. A transfixing suture is then placed around the tissue pedicle held by the remaining Heaney clamp. This suture is placed above and distal to the first free tie. As the knot is cinched in place, the remaining Heaney clamp is removed.

The adnexa is now freed from the pelvic sidewall, and its increased mobility may obstruct surgery. For this reason, the adnexa can be tied to the Kelly clamp still located on the uteroovarian ligament or is simply excised and removed.

❽ Bladder Flap. Attention is next turned to the bladder. The peritoneum that connects the superior edge of the bladder to the uterine isthmus is cut when the anterior leaf of the broad ligament is opened. Only loose areolar connective tissue joins the posterior surface of the bladder and anterior surface of the uterine isthmus and cervix. There are several techniques for mobilization of the bladder off the uterine isthmus and cervix. At our institution, sharp dissection is the preferred method of bladder mobilization. The vesicouterine fold is grasped and elevated to create tension between it and the underlying cervix. Concurrently, countertraction on the uterus is created by pulling upward on the Kelly clamps, previously placed at the fundus. Connective tissue bands within this vesicouterine space are then cut with fine Metzenbaum scissors. Incision of these bands is kept close to the cervix to avoid cystotomy. Sharp dissection is particularly useful for patients with prior cesarean deliveries who may have scar tissue connecting the posterior surface of the bladder to the anterior uterine surface.

Alternatively, to mobilize the bladder, a hand can be wrapped around the uterus, and a thumb used to exert gentle pressure under the bladder and against the cervix. Pressure is directed inferiorly toward the vagina. Similarly, a sponge stick can be used to create this pressure.

❾ Uterine Arteries. Next, the uterine arteries are identified along the lateral aspects of the uterus at the level of the isthmus. A variable amount of posterior peritoneum and loose areolar tissue remains from the broad ligament and surrounds the uterine vessels. Incising such tissue from around a vessel is termed *skeletonizing*. This ultimately creates a smaller volume of tissue contained in the vascular pedicle to be clamped. With a larger pedicle, cinching pressure produced by tying the knot may be wasted on surrounding tissue and may allow the uterine artery to retract before adequate ligation.

To skeletonize, the surgeon grasps the excess tissue with fine smooth forceps and gently retracts it laterally and away from the vessels. Curved Metzenbaum scissors incise this tissue close to the uterus, beginning superiorly and proceeding inferiorly toward the vessels.

Once skeletonization is completed, two curved Heaney clamps are placed on the uterine vessels inferiorly to the planned site of vessel transection. These clamp tips are placed horizontally across the vertical axis of the uterine vessels (Fig. 41-12.6). A third curved clamp is placed above the planned incision. Its tip crosses the vessels at an approximate 45-degree angle. The uterine vessels are then sharply transected.

A simple stitch of 0-gauge delayed-absorbable suture is placed below the lowest clamp's tip, and the suture ends are wrapped to the heel of the clamp. As the knot is cinched, the middle of the three clamps is opened and then immediately closed. The lowest of the three is then removed. A simple stitch is then placed above the first suture and below the middle clamp. As the knot is cinched, this clamp is removed. The upper clamp is left in place to prevent vessel bleeding due to the rich collateral uterine circulation.

❿ Fundal Amputation. After bilateral ligation of the uterine arteries, if the uterus is large and bulky, the uterine fundus may be sharply severed from the isthmus and cervix. After removal of the corpus, Kocher clamps can be placed on the anterior and posterior walls of the uterine isthmus to elevate the cervix.

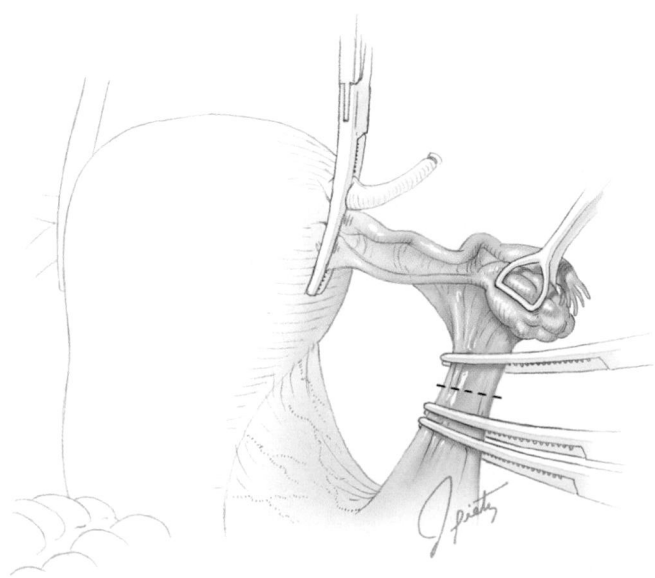

FIGURE 41-12.5 Oophorectomy.

the vertical axis of the uterus. A scalpel is used to transect the portion of the cardinal ligament held by the clamp. A simple or a transfixing suture of 0-gauge delayed-absorbable suture is placed below the clamp, the knot cinched, and clamp removed. A similar transection of the cardinal ligament is then performed on the opposite side.

Because of the vertical length and vascularity of the cardinal ligament, it may be necessary to repeat step 11 several times. In this manner, the cardinal ligament is ligated from its superior to inferior extent down the lateral aspect of the cervix.

⓬ **Uterosacral Ligament Transection.** At this point, the uterosacral ligaments are the last remaining support structures still attached to the uterus (Fig. 41-12.8). These ligaments are more easily felt and visualized by placing upward traction on the uterus. Each ligament is grasped with a straight Heaney clamp close to its uterine attachment. Importantly, because of the close proximity of the ureter, these clamps are placed as close to the uterus as possible. The ligament is severed medial to the clamp, a transfixing suture is placed, and the clamp is removed.

⓭ **Vaginal Entry.** The surgeon's hand palpates through the anterior and posterior vaginal walls to identify the most inferior level of the cervix. Here, curved Heaney clamps are

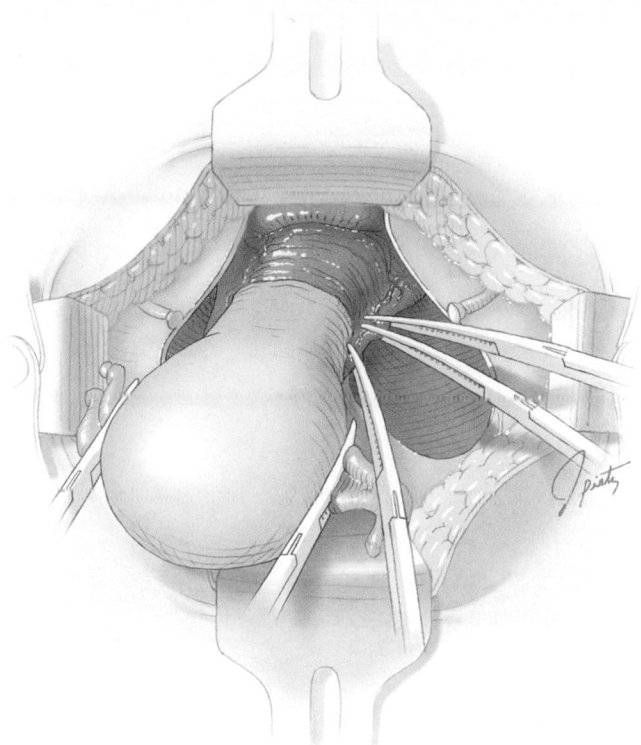

FIGURE 41-12.6 Uterine artery ligation.

⓫ **Cardinal Ligament Incision.** These ligaments lie lateral to the uterus and are inferior to the uterine vessels. A straight Heaney clamp is used to clamp the cardinal ligament

(Fig. 41-12.7). As the Heaney clamp initially grasps the ligament, it is oriented parallel to the lateral side of the uterus. As the clamp is slowly closed, it is angled slightly away from

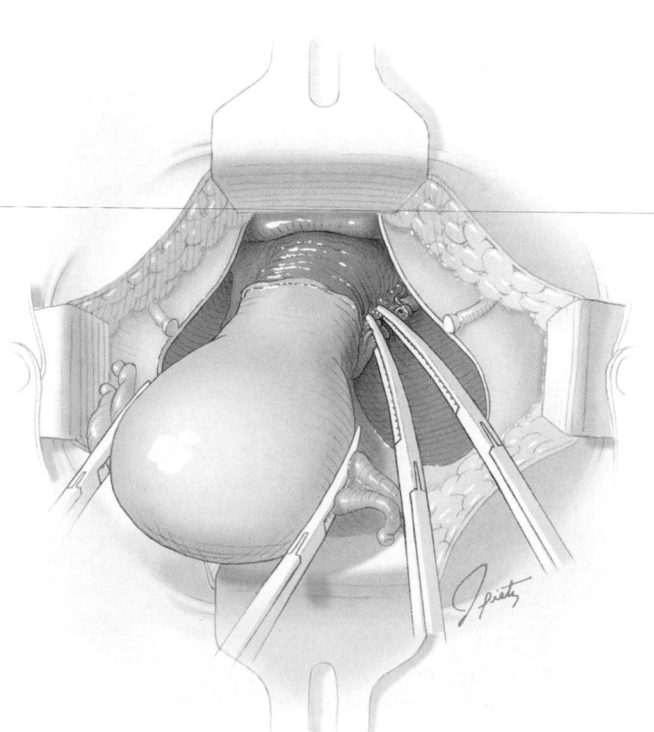

FIGURE 41-12.7 Cardinal ligament transection.

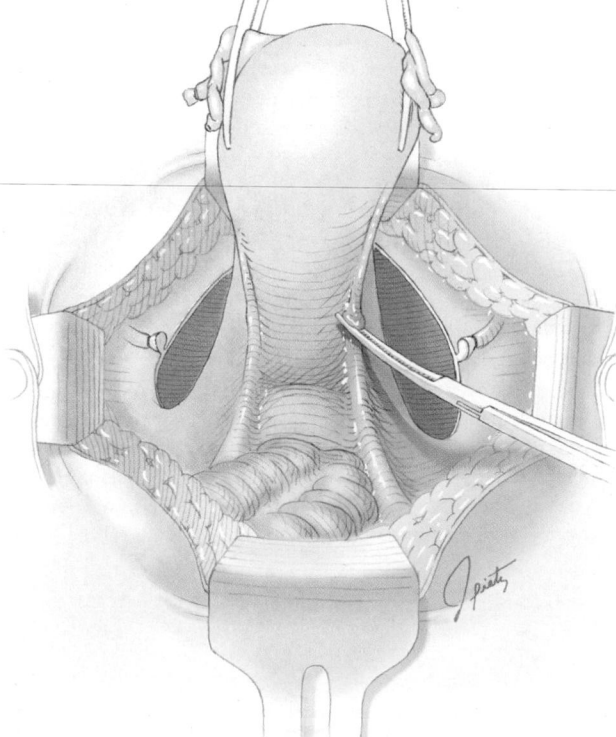

FIGURE 41-12.8 Uterosacral ligament transection.

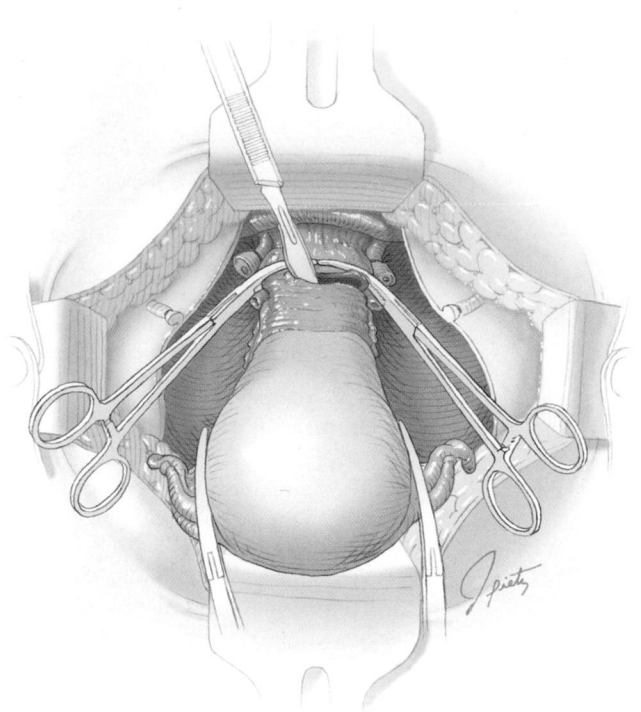

FIGURE 41-12.9 Uterine excision.

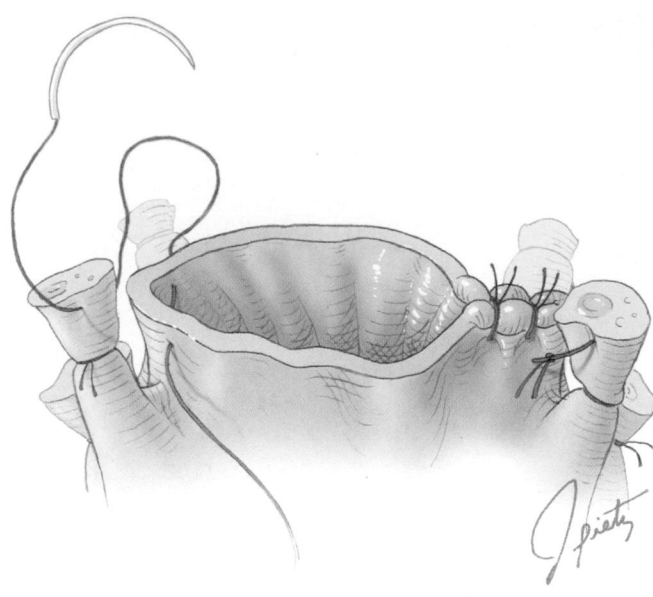

FIGURE 41-12.10 Vaginal cuff closure.

used to grasp and bring together the anterior and posterior vaginal walls at the point just below the cervix (Fig. 41-12.9).

⓮ Removal of the Uterus. The vaginal tissue above the level of these clamps is then incised. Either a scalpel or scissors may be used for incision. This procedure frees the uterus from the pelvis. Transfixing sutures are placed below the Heaney clamps, and the clamps are removed.

⓯ Vaginal Cuff Closure. A 0-gauge delayed-absorbable suture may be placed to suspend the vaginal apex to the utero-sacral ligament pedicle on either side (Fig. 41-12.10). This stitch incorporates the anterior and posterior vaginal walls with the distal portion of the uterosacral ligament and helps to prevent vaginal cuff prolapse following surgery.

These sutures are kept long and are grasped with hemostats. Upward and lateral traction with the hemostats elevates the vaginal cuff. The incised anterior and posterior vaginal edges are then reapproximated with several figure-of-eight sutures or with a running, locking suture line using 0-gauge delayed-absorbable suture. The peritoneum overlying the posterior vaginal margin should be included in this closure to lessen the risk of postoperative bleeding from the vaginal cuff. The pedicle line should be inspected on either side for bleeding. The lateral elevating sutures are then cut.

⓰ Wound Closure. The abdominal incision is closed as described in Section 41-1 or 41-2 (p. 1021).

POSTOPERATIVE

Following abdominal hysterectomy, postoperative care follows that for any major abdominal surgery (Chap. 39, p. 962). Hospitalization typically varies from 1 to 4 days, and return of normal bowel function and febrile morbidity usually dictate this course. Postoperative activity in general can be individualized, although intercourse is usually delayed until 4 to 6 weeks after surgery to allow time for vaginal cuff healing.

Febrile morbidity is common following abdominal hysterectomy and exceeds that seen with vaginal or laparoscopic approaches (Peipert, 2004). Frequently, fever is unexplained, but pelvic infections are common. Additionally, abdominal wound infection, urinary tract infection, and pneumonia should be considered and evaluated as described in Chapter 39 (p. 971). Because of the high rate of unexplained fever, which resolves spontaneously, observation for 24 to 48 hours for mild temperature elevations is reasonable. Alternatively, antibiotic treatment may be initiated. A second-generation cephalosporin may be selected, and other appropriate choices are found in Table 3-31 (p. 103). Additional testing, including transvaginal sonography or CT, may be indicated if a pelvic hematoma or abscess is suspected.

41-13

Vaginal Hysterectomy

In general, vaginal hysterectomy offers short patient recovery, operating times, and hospitalization as well as decreased surgical morbidity. Ideally, it is used when pelvic organs are small, some degree of uterine descent is present, and access to the upper abdomen is not required. This approach is typically not selected in those with a contracted pelvis or with significant pelvic adhesions.

PREOPERATIVE

Patient evaluation, consenting, and patient preparation are similar to that for abdominal hysterectomy (Section 41-12, p. 1045).

INTRAOPERATIVE

SURGICAL STEPS

❶ Anesthesia and Patient Positioning. After adequate general or regional anesthesia is administered, the patient is carefully placed in high dorsal lithotomy position to avoid injury to the sciatic, femoral, or common peroneal nerves (Fig. 40-6, p. 985). The vagina is surgically prepared, and the bladder

is drained. Some surgeons may prefer to wait until the case is completed before inserting a Foley catheter. A right-angle or other suitable retractor is placed along the anterior vaginal wall, and an Auvard weighted vaginal speculum is placed posteriorly.

❷ Vaginal Wall Incision. A Lahey-thyroid clamp is used to grasp both the anterior and posterior cervical lips and close them together. Ten to 15 mL of a dilute saline solution containing vasopressin (20 U diluted in 30 to 100 mL of saline) or 0.5-percent lidocaine and epinephrine (1:200,000 dilution) is injected circumferentially beneath the mucosa at a level above the cervicovaginal junction but below the inferior margin of the bladder. The margin of the bladder is identified as a crease in the overlying vaginal epithelium and can be accentuated by in-and-out displacement of the cervix (Sheth, 2005). This injection decreases bleeding during dissection and aids in defining tissue planes. The vaginal wall above the cervix is then circumcised. To avoid dissection into the cervix, this incision is kept at a depth superficial to the pubocervical fascia.

❸ Anterior Peritoneal Entry. The anterior vaginal wall is grasped and elevated with an Allis clamp. Tension is created by outward traction on the Lahey-thyroid clamp. This traction will reveal fibrous bands connecting the bladder and cervix. With surgical gauze covering the index finger, a surgeon

pushes downward and cephalad against the cervix to bluntly dissect through these fibers and move the bladder cephalad. This motion is continued until the vesicouterine fold is reached. Alternatively, and particularly for cases in which these cervicovesical fibrous bands are dense, sharp dissection is used to avoid blunt cystotomy by a surgeon's finger (Fig. 41-13.1).

The vesicouterine fold can be seen as a transverse white line across the anterior cervix. Palpation reveals two thin smooth layers of peritoneum slipping against one another (Fig. 41-13.2). The vesicouterine fold is grasped and elevated to place this peritoneal layer on tension. The peritoneum is then incised (Fig. 41-13.3). An index finger explores the opening to confirm peritoneal entry and palpate for any unanticipated pathology. The anterior retractor is then repositioned with its distal blade entering the peritoneal cavity and elevating the bladder.

❹ Posterior Entry. The Lahey-thyroid clamp and cervix are lifted anteriorly to expose the posterior vaginal vault. An Allis clamp is placed on the posterior vaginal wall and on the outer edge of the previously created circumferential incision. The Allis clamp is pulled downward to create tension across the exposed posterior peritoneum. The posterior vaginal vault may be grasped with forceps and is cut with curved Mayo scissors, and the cul-de-sac of Douglas is entered (Fig. 41-13.4). The posterior peritoneum is

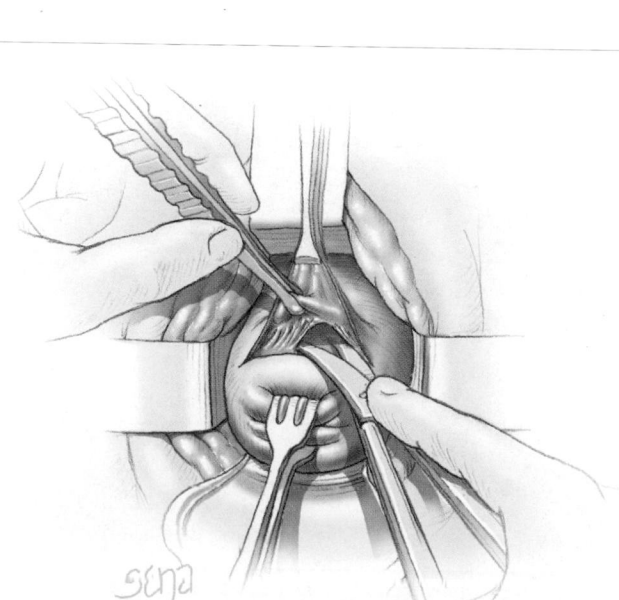

FIGURE 41-13.1 Sharp dissection of vaginal mucosa.

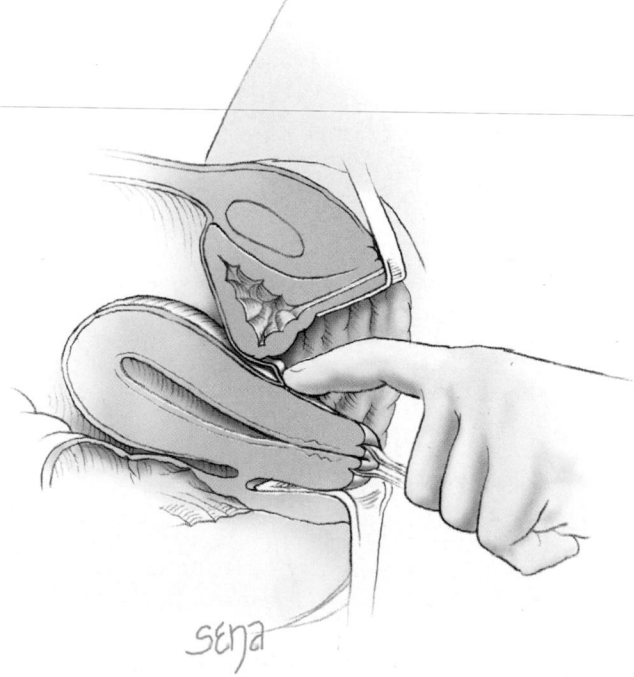

FIGURE 41-13.2 Vesicouterine fold identification.

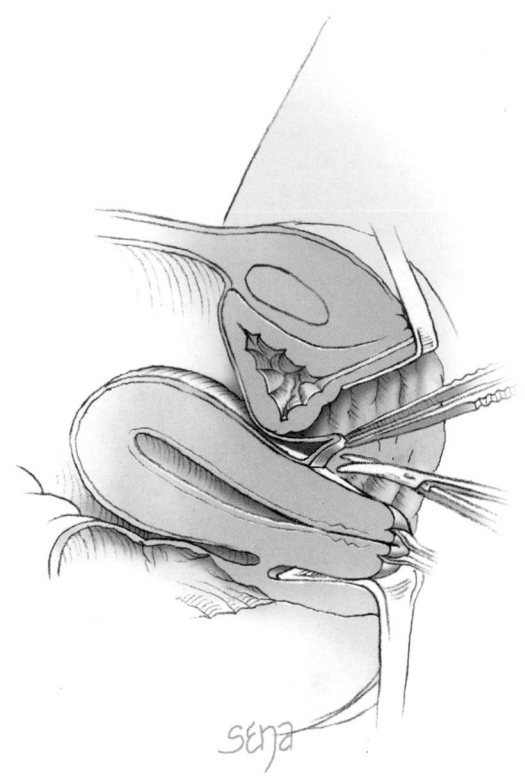

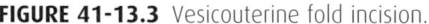

FIGURE 41-13.3 Vesicouterine fold incision.

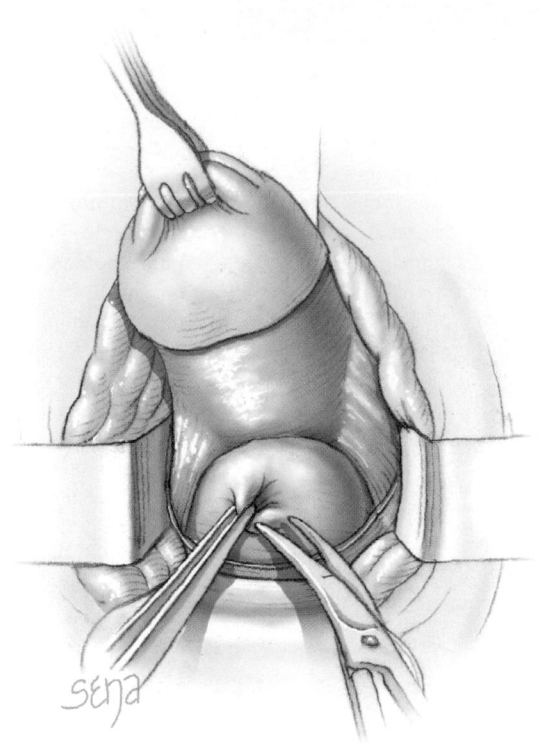

FIGURE 41-13.4 Entry into the cul-de-sac of Douglas.

then affixed centrally to the posterior vaginal wall incision with a single stitch of delayed-absorbable suture. This approximation will assist with closure of the peritoneum at the procedure's end. The short-weighted vaginal speculum is replaced by one with a longer blade, which enters the cul-de-sac.

❺ **Transection of Uterosacral and Cardinal Ligaments.** Outward traction on the Lahey-thyroid clamp pulls the supporting uterine ligaments into view. Such traction also aids in preventing ureteral injury. The uterosacral ligament is identified, clamped with a curved Heaney clamp, transected,

and ligated with 0-gauge delayed-absorbable suture using a transfixing stitch (Fig. 41-13.5). The opposite uterosacral ligament is then ligated.

After ligation of the uterosacral ligaments, the cardinal ligaments are similarly clamped, cut, and sutured (Fig. 41-13.6).

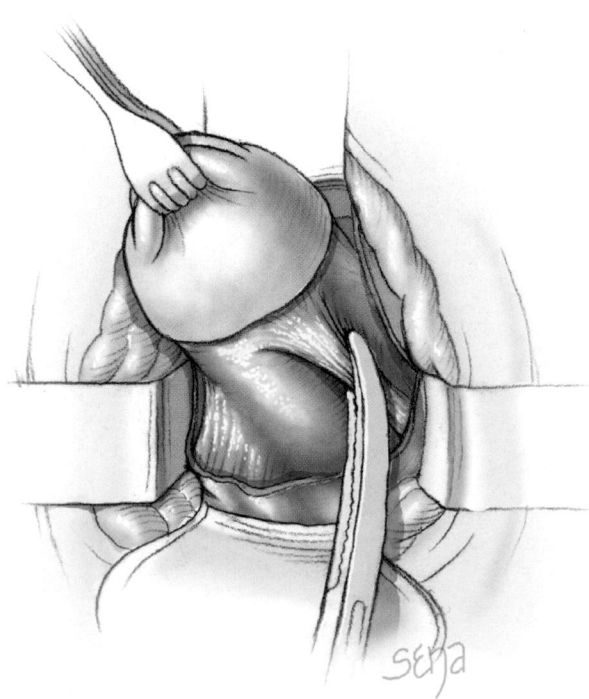

FIGURE 41-13.5 Uterosacral ligament transection.

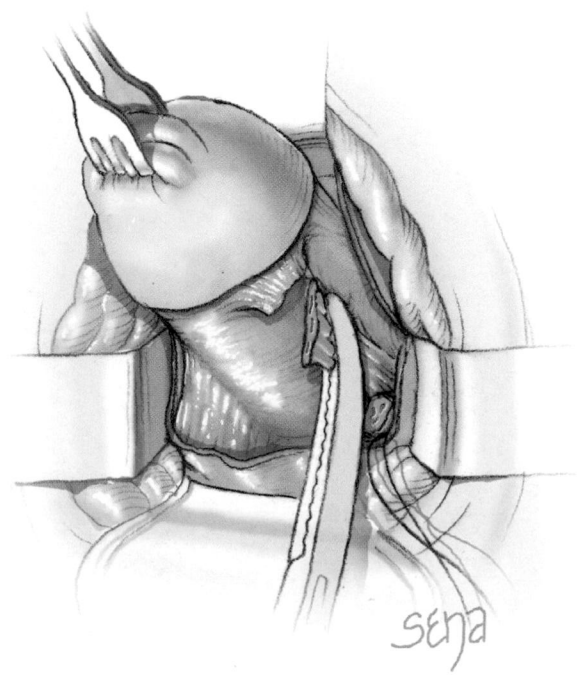

FIGURE 41-13.6 Cardinal ligament transection.

The uterosacral and cardinal ligaments may be isolated, clamped, and ligated individually or in combination depending on the size of each. Once the knots of these pedicles are secured, the suture ends are not cut but rather held by hemostats. These will be sutured to the vaginal cuff at a later time to aid in long-term vaginal support.

6 Uterine Arteries. The uterine artery is identified on one side and clamped with a curved Heaney clamp. A simple suture of 0-gauge delayed-absorbable suture is placed behind the clamp and is secured as this clamp is removed. The uterine artery on the opposite side is then similarly ligated.

7 Uteroovarian and Round Ligaments. If the uterus is small and descent is adequate, two curved Heaney clamps may be placed in tandem across the uteroovarian ligament, round ligament, and fallopian tubes. Each pedicle is doubly ligated, first with a simple suture placed proximally, and then with a transfixing stitch placed distally.

Alternatively, if the uterus is larger, the uterine corpus may be delivered through either the anterior or posterior colpotomy incision to expose the uteroovarian ligament, round ligament, and fallopian tubes (Fig. 41-13.7). To deliver the fundus, either fingers or a tenaculum can be used to gently pull the fundus into the vagina.

8 Morcellation. In some cases, a uterine fundus may be too large to deliver, and debulking of the uterus may be required prior to ligation of the cornual attachments. This can be done by enucleating individual large leiomyomas or by cervix-to-fundus central coring using scissors or scalpel. Once the bulk has been diminished, a Heaney clamp may be placed around the uteroovarian ligament, round ligament, and fallopian tube as described in step 7.

9 Oophorectomy. If removal of the ovaries is desired, the adnexa is grasped with a Babcock clamp and gently pulled toward the incision. An index finger is wrapped around the infundibulopelvic (IP) ligament to isolate it from surrounding structures. The IP ligament is clamped and ligated similarly to the uteroovarian pedicle (Fig. 41-13.8). The ends of its final transfixing suture are held by hemostat.

10 Evaluation of Hemostasis. Following removal of the uterus, the surgical pedicles are inspected for bleeding (Fig. 41-13.9). Electrosurgical coagulation or figure-of-eight sutures will typically control bleeding. If hemostasis is adequate, sutures to the IP ligament sutures are cut. If an enterocele repair is planned, it is performed at this time.

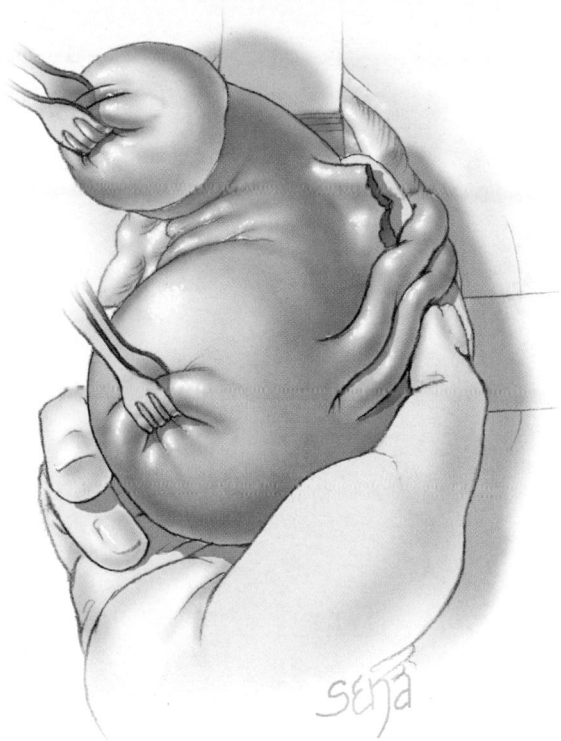

FIGURE 41-13.7 Uteroovarian and round ligament transection.

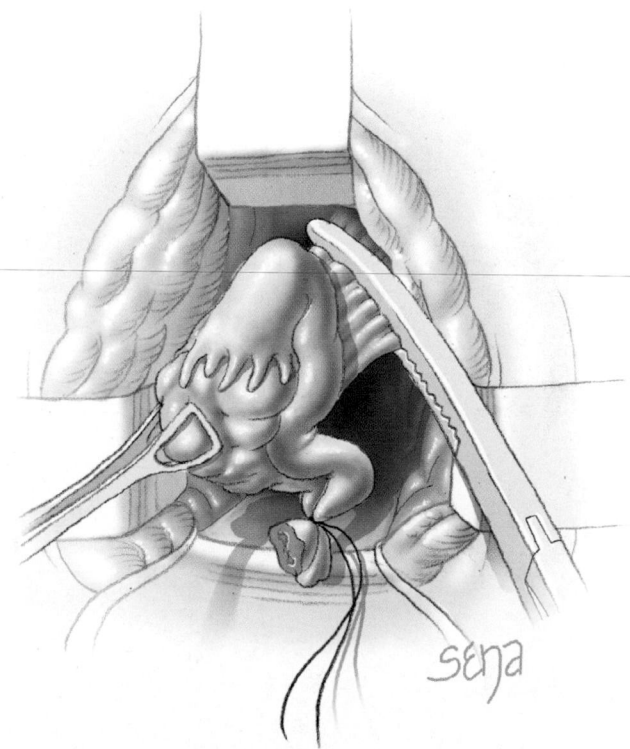

FIGURE 41-13.8 Oophorectomy.

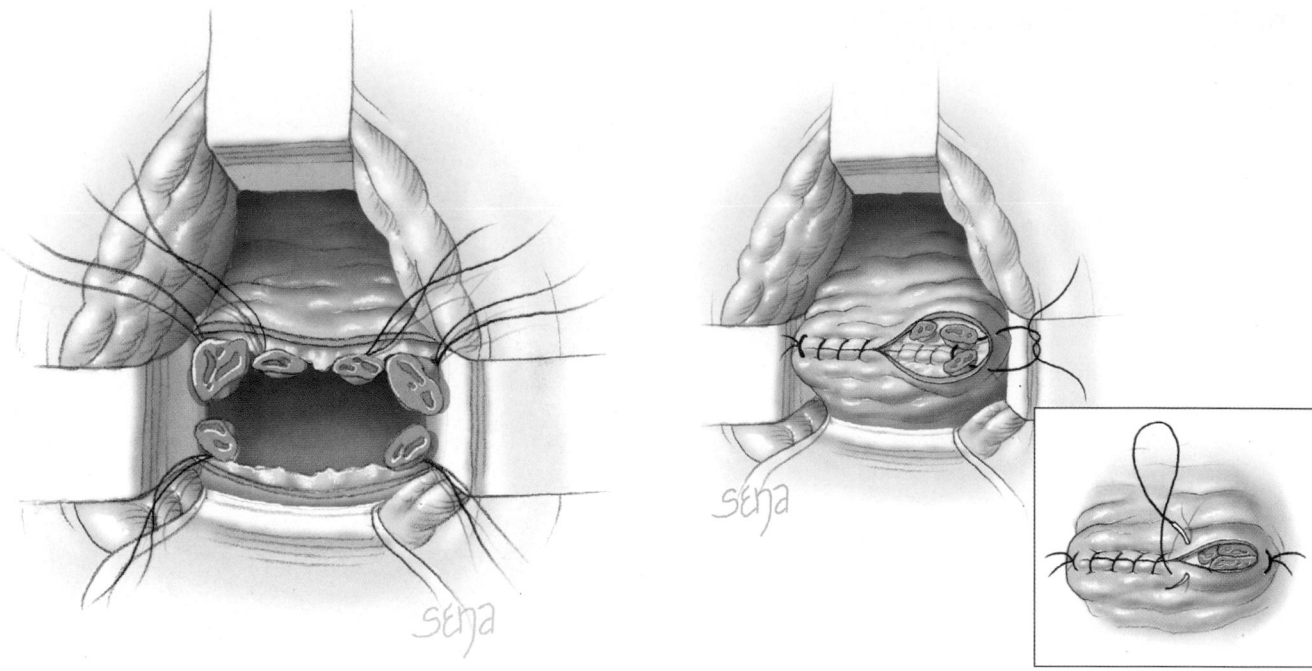

FIGURE 41-13.9 Inspection of surgical pedicles.

FIGURE 41-13.10 Vaginal cuff closure.

⓫ **Vaginal Cuff Closure.** As shown by the deep layer in Figure 41-13.10, peritoneum is closed in a purse-string manner using 2-0 gauge delayed-absorbable suture. A suspensory suture may be included in which the cardinal or uterosacral or both ligaments are sutured to the lateral vaginal cuff on each side to improve final suspension and support for the vaginal vault. Lastly, the vaginal wall incision is closed left to right with interrupted or continuous running sutures of 0-gauge delayed-absorbable material.

POSTOPERATIVE

In general, patients who undergo vaginal hysterectomy, as compared with abdominal hysterectomy, typically have faster return of normal bowel function, easier ambulation, and decreased analgesia requirements. Evaluation and treatment of postoperative complications mirrors that for abdominal hysterectomy.

41-14

Trachelectomy

During the 1920s through 1950s, most abdominal hysterectomies were supracervical due to the lack of adequate blood banking and antibiotic therapy. For many women who had supracervical hysterectomy, later surgical removal of the cervix, termed *trachelectomy*, was often indicated for complaints of vault prolapse, persistent cyclical bleeding, or preinvasive cervical lesions (Pasley, 1988).

The cervix may be removed either vaginally or abdominally, but for most women without concurrent pelvic pathology, vaginal trachelectomy is preferred (Pratt, 1976). With the resurgence of supracervical hysterectomy, now performed via laparoscopy, rates of trachelectomy for benign causes are expected to rise.

PREOPERATIVE

Patient Evaluation

As with hysterectomy, women require preoperative Pap smear screening to exclude cervical cancer.

Consent

As with vaginal hysterectomy, patients are at risk for urinary tract and bowel injury.

Similarly, postsurgical vaginal cuff complications may include hematoma, abscess, and cellulitis. Fortunately, complications are infrequent for most. Although Pratt and Jefferies (1976) noted complications in 91 of 262 patients, complication rates in several series range below 10 percent (Riva, 1961; Welch, 1959).

Patient Preparation

Entry into the peritoneal cavity is common during trachelectomy. Accordingly, as with vaginal hysterectomy, antibiotic prophylaxis is warranted, and appropriate choices are found in Table 39-6 (p. 959).

INTRAOPERATIVE

SURGICAL STEPS

❶ **Anesthesia and Patient Positioning.** For most women, trachelectomy is performed as an inpatient procedure under general or regional anesthesia. The patient is placed in a high dorsal lithotomy position, the vagina is surgically prepared, and a Foley catheter is placed.

❷ **Vaginal Wall Incision.** The beginning steps of trachelectomy mirror those for vaginal hysterectomy (Section 41-13, step 2, p. 1051).

❸ **Extraperitoneal Dissection.** However, unlike vaginal hysterectomy, because the cervical stump lies outside the peritoneum, entry into the peritoneal cavity is not required for trachelectomy. Accordingly, once circumcision of the vaginal wall around the cervix is completed, dissection proceeds to the vesicouterine fold, but without peritoneal entry.

In many cases, the bladder is more densely adhered to the anterior cervix, and the clear tissue planes often encountered during vaginal hysterectomy are absent. Moreover, if at completion of the original hysterectomy, the peritoneum was reapproximated to cover the cervical stump, then the bladder may be draped over and scarred to the apex of the stump as well. For this reason, dissection of the vaginal wall, bladder, and rectum from the surface of the cervix typically requires sharp rather than blunt dissection (Fig. 41-14.1). As with vaginal hysterectomy, outward traction on the cervix in combination with countertraction of the vaginal wall aids dissection. To avoid cystotomy and proctotomy, scissor blades and dissecting pressure are directed against the cervix.

❹ **Transection of Uterosacral and Cardinal Ligaments.** Once dissected free from the vaginal wall, the uterosacral and cardinal ligaments are clamped and ligated as with vaginal hysterectomy (Fig. 41-14.2). The cervical branches of the uterine artery are typically clamped and ligated with the cardinal ligament. Depending on cervical length,

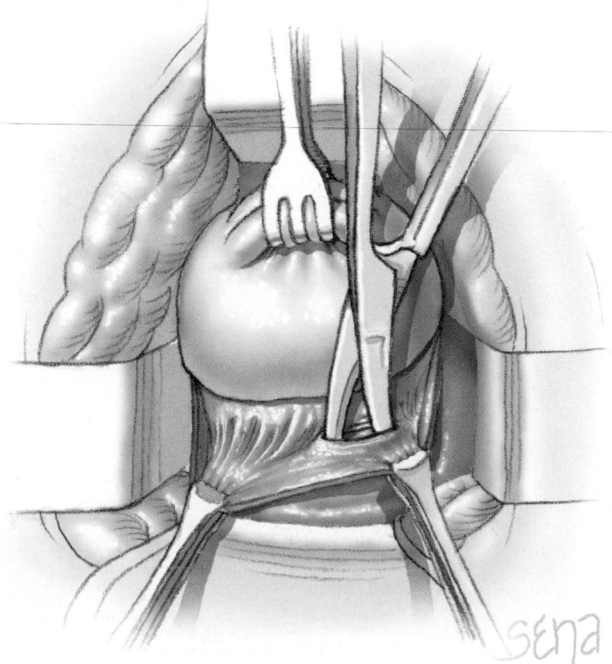

FIGURE 41-14.1 Extraperitoneal dissection.

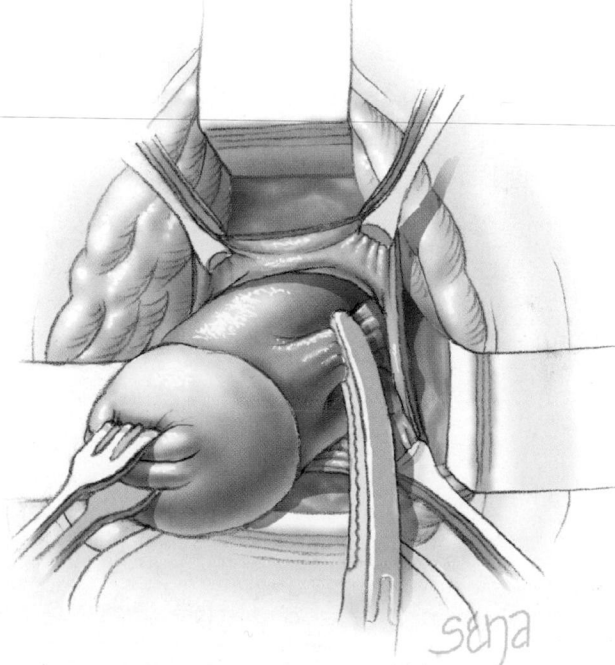

FIGURE 41-14.2 Uterosacral and cardinal ligament transection.

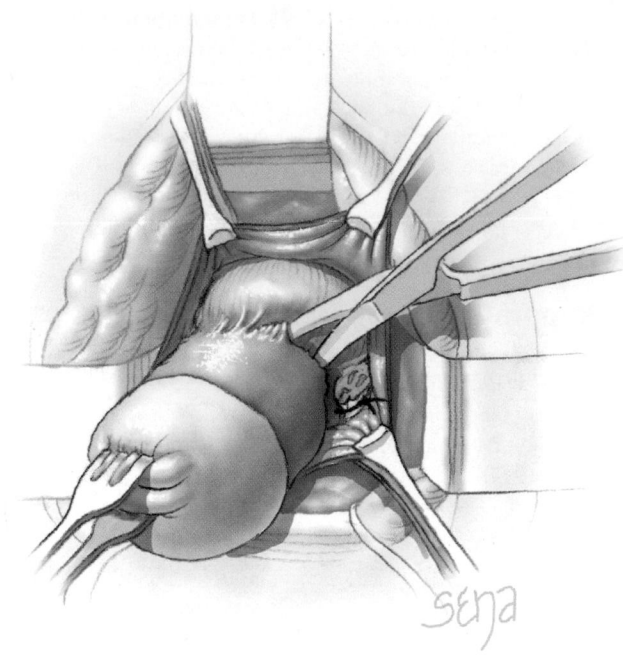

FIGURE 41-14.3 Stump excision.

serial transection and ligation of the cardinal ligament is continued until the stump apex is reached.

❺ Stump Excision. Once the apex is reached, sharp dissection across the top of the stump will free it from the vagina (Fig. 41-14.3).

❻ Incision Closure. Incorporation of the uterosacral and cardinal ligaments and reapproximation of the vaginal walls follows that for vaginal hysterectomy (p. 1054).

POSTOPERATIVE

As with hysterectomy, a significant number of women will have unexplained febrile morbidity following trachelectomy. Pasley (1988) in his series of 55 cases noted a rate of 9 percent. Similar to hysterectomy, patients with persistent or high-degree fevers require evaluation and possible antibiotic treatment (Chap. 39, p. 971).

41-15

Sharp Dilatation and Curettage

Although used for diagnostic evaluation and treatment of abnormal uterine bleeding during the past 150 years, the indications for dilatation and sharp curettage (D&C) have decreased with the development of less invasive methods (Chap. 8, p. 225). In the evaluation of abnormal uterine bleeding, sharp curettage may be used alone or more commonly in combination with hysteroscopy for those women with persistent bleeding despite normal findings with sonography and endometrial biopsy. Moreover, mechanical cervical dilatation may be required to gain access to the uterine cavity when a stenotic cervical os prohibits in-office endometrial sampling. In the treatment of severe acute menorrhagia, D&C may be used to remove hypertrophic endometrium if bleeding must be stopped promptly or if bleeding is refractory to medical management. Although suction curettage is used more commonly for removal of products of first-trimester pregnancy, sharp D&C may also be an option (Chap. 6, p. 189). Finally, in case of suspected ectopic pregnancy, D&C is sometimes used to document the absence of intrauterine trophoblastic tissue (Chap. 7, p. 208).

PREOPERATIVE

Consent

For most women, sharp dilatation and curettage poses only a small risk of complication, and rates typically fall below 1 percent (Radman, 1963; Tabata, 2001). Infection and uterine perforation are among the most common complications.

Patient Preparation

Because the indications for sharp D&C are diverse, diagnostic testing prior to evacuation will vary. Prophylactic antibiotic administration is typically not required when sharp D&C is performed for gynecologic indications. However, because pelvic infection may follow this procedure when performed in an obstetric setting, antibiotics are usually prescribed postoperatively, and doxycycline, 100 mg orally twice daily for 10 days, is commonly given (American College of Obstetricians and Gynecologists, 2009a). The risk of bowel injury with this procedure

is small, and thus preoperative enemas may or may not be completed.

INTRAOPERATIVE

SURGICAL STEPS

❶ Anesthesia and Patient Positioning. Dilatation and curettage is typically performed as an outpatient procedure under general or regional anesthesia or with local nerve blockade combined with intravenous sedation. The patient is placed in the dorsal lithotomy position, the vagina is surgically prepared, and the bladder drained.

A bimanual examination to determine uterine size and inclination is performed prior to introduction of uterine instruments. Information obtained from this examination aids the surgeon in avoiding uterine perforation. With insertion of instruments along the long axis of the uterus, there is less chance of injury.

❷ Uterine Sounding. Suitable vaginal exposure can be achieved with either a Graves speculum or individual vaginal retractors. The anterior lip of the cervix is grasped with a single-tooth tenaculum to stabilize the uterus during dilatation and curettage. A Sims uterine sound is then held as a pencil with the thumb and first two fingers (Fig. 41-15.1). The sound is slowly guided through the cervical os, into the uterine cavity, and to the fundus. Instruments should not be forced, as this increases the risk of perforation.

Once gentle resistance is met at the fundus, the distance from the fundus to the external os is measured by score marks along the length of the sound. Knowledge of the depth to which dilators and curettes can safely be inserted decreases the risk of uterine perforation.

At times, cervical stenosis may preclude easy access to the endocervical canal. In these cases, smaller caliber tools, such as a lacrimal duct probe, may be guided into the external cervical os to define the canal path. Sonography may be helpful when done simultaneously with D&C in these situations. Sonographic visualization of instruments as

they are being passed may help ensure proper placement (Christianson, 2008).

In addition, pretreatment with the prostaglandin E₁ analog misoprostol (Cytotec) may allow adequate cervical softening for instrument passage. Commonly used dosing options include 200 or 400 μg vaginally or 400 μg orally once at 12 or 24 hours prior to surgery. Common side effects include cramping, uterine bleeding, or nausea.

❸ Uterine Dilatation. After the uterus is sounded, dilators of sequentially increasing caliber are inserted to open the endocervical canal and internal cervical os as described in Section 41-16 (p. 1060). A Hegar, Hank, or Pratt dilator is held by the thumb and first two fingers, while the fourth and fifth fingers and heel of the hand rest on the perineum and buttock. Each dilator is gently and gradually advanced through the internal cervical os. Serial dilatation continues until the cervix will admit the selected curette (Fig. 41-15.2).

During sounding or dilatation, uterine perforation may occur and is suspected when the instrument travels deeper than previously measured by the uterine sound. Because of the blunt, narrow shape of these tools, risk of significant uterine or abdominal organ injury is low. In such cases, if significant bleeding is absent, reassessment of uterine inclination and completion of the D&C is reasonable. Alternatively, surgery may be terminated and repeated at a later date, thus allowing myometrial healing.

❹ Uterine Curettage. Prior to curettage, a sheet of nonadherent wound dressing material (Telfa pad) is spread out in the vagina beneath the cervix. The uterine curette is then inserted and advanced to the fundus, following the long axis of the corpus. On reaching the fundus, the sharp surface of the curette is positioned to contact the adjacent endometrium (Fig. 41-15.3). Pressure is exerted against the endometrium as the curette is pulled toward the internal cervical os.

After reaching the os, the curette is redirected to the fundus and positioned immediately lateral and adjacent to the path of the first curettage pass. After several passes,

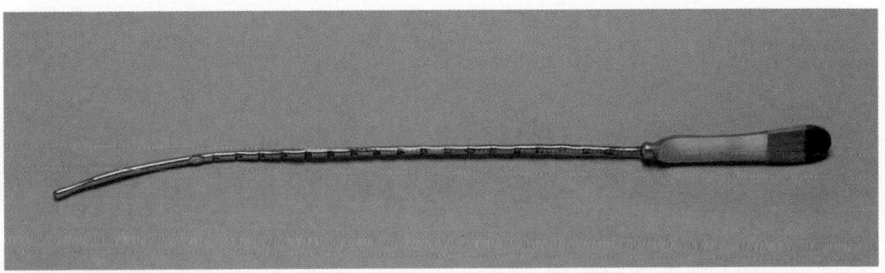

FIGURE 41-15.1 Sims uterine sound. *(Photograph contributed by Steven Willard.)*

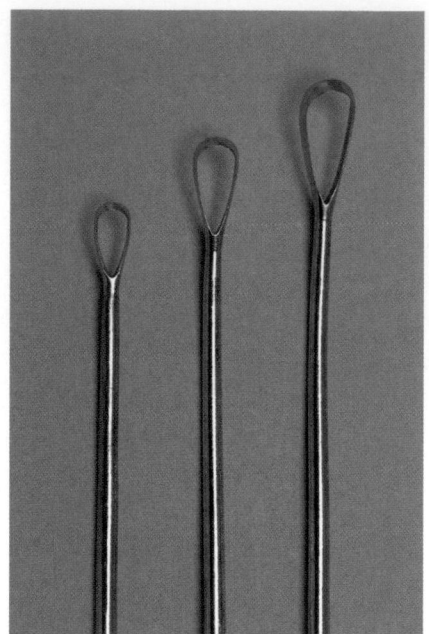

FIGURE 41-15.2 Uterine curette.

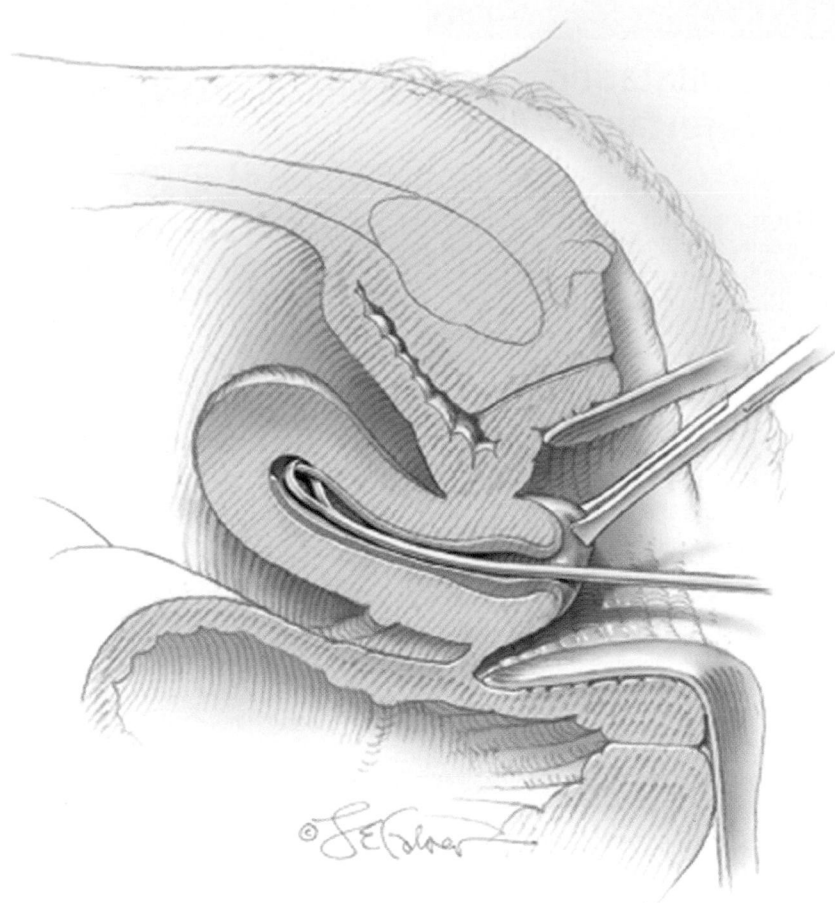

FIGURE 41-15.3 Uterine curettage.

tissues collected in the isthmic region are scraped out onto the Telfa pad. In this fashion, the entire uterine cavity is sequentially and circumferentially curetted. The collected tissue is sent for pathologic evaluation.

As with dilatation, the uterus may be perforated during curettage. However, the sharp curette has the potential to lacerate bowel, vessels, and other abdominal organs. Accordingly, diagnostic laparoscopy should be considered to evaluate for such injuries.

❺ **Uterine Exploration.** Because uterine polyps, both large and small, may be missed with sharp curettage, uterine exploration with Randall kidney stone forceps is advisable in women undergoing evaluation of abnormal bleeding. Closed forceps are inserted into the endometrial cavity. Upon reaching the fundus, forceps are opened against the uterine walls, closed, and then pulled away from

the endometrium. In this manner, anterior, posterior, proximal, and distal cavity surfaces are explored. With capture of a polyp within the jaws, a tug against the closed forceps is felt as they are pulled away from the uterine wall. Firm traction typically frees the polyp. Removed tissue is sent for pathologic evaluation.

Alternatively, hysteroscopy is a more accurate means than D&C alone to diagnose and remove focal lesions such as polyps.

Nonetheless, the techniques may be used together.

POSTOPERATIVE

Recovery from sharp D&C is typically fast and without complication. Light bleeding or spotting is expected, and patients may resume normal activities at their individual paces.

41-16

Suction Dilatation and Curettage

Suction dilatation and curettage (D&C) is the most common method used to remove first-trimester products of conception (Chap. 6, p. 189). Vacuum aspiration, the most common form of suction curettage, requires a rigid cannula attached to an electric-powered vacuum source. Alternatively, manual vacuum aspiration uses a similar cannula that attaches to a handheld syringe for its vacuum source (MacIsaac, 2000; Masch, 2005).

PREOPERATIVE

Patient Evaluation

For most women, dilatation and curettage is preceded by transvaginal sonography. This imaging modality aids in documenting pregnancy nonviability, location, and size. In addition to sonographic evaluation, blood typing is performed to assess Rh status. Administration of 50 or 300 µg (1500 IU) Rh_0 (D) immune globulin intramuscularly within 72 hours of first-trimester pregnancy termination in Rh-negative women can lower the risk of isoimmunization in future pregnancies (Chap. 6, p. 176).

Consent

Suction D&C is a safe and effective method of uterine evacuation (Tunçalp, 2010). Short-term complication rates are low and have been cited at 1 to 5 percent (Hakim-Elahi, 1990; Zhou, 2002). Complications include uterine perforation, retained products, infection, and hemorrhage, and rates increase after the first trimester. Accordingly, sharp or suction curettage should ideally be performed before 14 to 15 weeks' gestation.

The incidence of uterine perforation associated with elective abortion varies. Important determinants are the skill of the physician, uterine position, and uterine size. Rates of perforation increase with a retroverted or large uterus and with a less experienced surgeon. Accidental uterine perforation usually is recognized when the instrument passes without resistance deep into the pelvis. Observation may be sufficient if the uterine perforation is small, as when produced by a uterine sound or narrow blunt dilator. Considerable intraabdominal damage, however, can be caused by some instruments—especially suction cannulas and sharp curettes—passed through a uterine defect into the peritoneal cavity

(Keegan, 1982). Because unrecognized bowel injury can cause severe peritonitis and sepsis, laparoscopy or laparotomy to examine the abdominal contents is often the safest course of action in these cases (Kambiss, 2000).

Rarely, women may develop cervical incompetence or intrauterine adhesions following D&C. Those contemplating abortion should understand the potential for these rare but significant complications.

Patient Preparation

Suction D&C may be performed for cases of incomplete or inevitable abortion and require no cervical dilatation for procedure completion. However, other settings require physical dilatation of the cervical os with metal dilators, a procedural step closely associated with uterine perforation and patient discomfort. Therefore, to obviate this need, hygroscopic dilators may be placed in the endocervical canal to the level of the internal os to accomplish cervical dilatation.

Hygroscopic dilators draw water from cervical tissues and expand, which gradually dilates the cervix. One type of hygroscopic dilator originates from the stems of *Laminaria digitata* or *Laminaria japonica,* a brown seaweed. The stems are cut, peeled, shaped, dried, sterilized, and packaged according to their hydrated size—small, 3 to 5 mm diameter; medium, 6 to 8 mm; and large, 8 to 10 mm (Fig. 41-16.1). The strongly hygroscopic laminaria presumably act by drawing water from cervical proteoglycan complexes. The complexes dissociate, and thereby allow the cervix to soften and dilate.

An acrylic-based synthetic hygroscopic dilator, Dilapan-S, is also available. In 1995, Dilapan was removed from the U.S. market because of concerns over device fragmentation. It was reintroduced following Food and Drug Administration approval of a new device design (Food and Drug Administration, 2009).

For placement of a hygroscopic dilator, the cervix is cleansed with povidone-iodine solution and is grasped anteriorly with a tenaculum. A laminaria of appropriate size is then inserted using a uterine packing forceps so that the tip rests at the level of the internal os (Fig. 41-16.2). After 4 to 6 hours, the laminaria will have swollen to dilate the cervix sufficiently and allow easier mechanical D&C. Cramping frequently accompanies expansion of the laminaria.

In addition to hygroscopic dilators, various prostaglandin preparations have been investigated as cervical "ripening" agents for subsequent dilation. Misoprostol has been used effectively to induce uterine evacuation in properly selected patients. Studies investi-

gating its use preoperatively to ease or obviate cervical dilatation, however, have not found it consistently effective in this clinical setting (Bunnasathiansri, 2004; Sharma, 2005).

Antibiotic prophylaxis should be provided at the time of transcervical surgical abortion. Based on their review of 11 randomized trials, Sawaya and associates (1996) concluded that perioperative antibiotics decreased the risk of infection by 40 percent. Although no regimen appears superior to others, a convenient, inexpensive, and effective one is doxycycline, 100 mg orally twice daily for 10 days. Alternatives are found in Table 39-6 (p. 959).

INTRAOPERATIVE

Instruments

Suction D&C requires an electric suction unit; stiff, translucent, large-bore sterile suction tubing; and sterile Karman suction cannulas (Fig. 41-16.3). Plastic suction cannulas are available in varying diameters. Choosing the most appropriately sized cannula balances competing factors. Small cannulas risk retained intrauterine tissue postoperatively, whereas large cannulas risk cervical injury and greater discomfort. For most first-trimester evacuations, a No. 8 to 12 Karman cannula is sufficient.

SURGICAL STEPS

❶ Anesthesia and Patient Positioning. In the absence of maternal systemic disease, abortion procedures do not require hospitalization. When abortion is performed

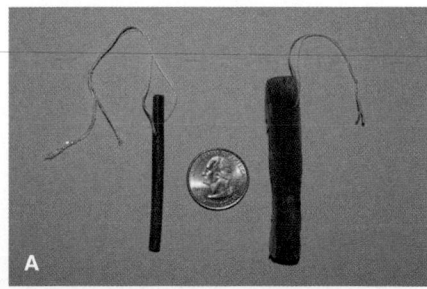

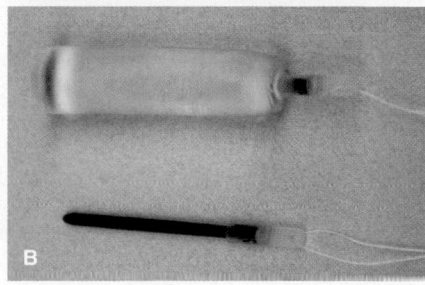

FIGURE 41-16.1 Hygroscopic dilators, dry and expanded. **A.** Laminaria. **B.** Dilapan-S.

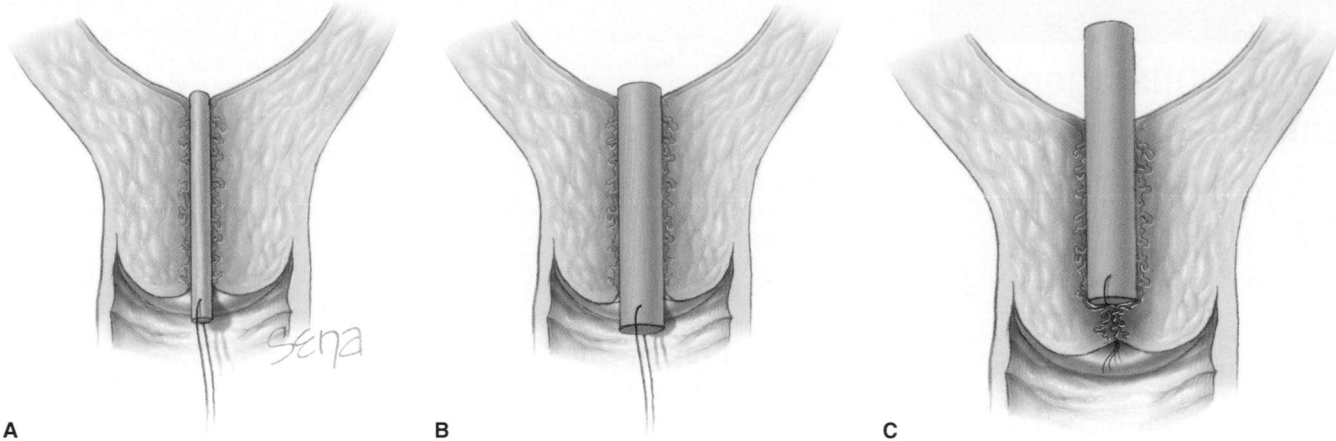

A   **B**   **C**

FIGURE 41-16.2 A. Correct placement of laminaria. **B.** Expanded laminaria. **C.** Laminaria inserted too deeply past the internal cervical os.

outside a hospital setting, capabilities for cardiopulmonary resuscitation and for immediate transfer to a hospital must be available. Anesthesia or analgesia used may vary and includes general anesthesia, paracervical block plus intravenous sedation, or intravenous sedation alone. After delivery of anesthesia or analgesia, the patient is placed in dorsal lithotomy position, the bladder is drained, and the vulva and vagina are surgically prepared.

❷ **Uterine Sounding.** A Sims uterine sound (see Fig. 41-15.1, p. 1057) is placed through the cervical os and into the uterine cavity to measure the depth and indicate the inclination of the uterine cavity prior to dilatation.

❸ **Cervical Dilatation.** A Graves speculum is placed in the vagina to allow access to the cervix. In cases of incomplete or inevitable abortion, the cervical os will already be dilated. Alternatively, metal Pratt, Hegar, or Hank dilators (Fig. 41-16.4) of sequentially

increasing diameter are placed through the external and internal os to gently dilate the cervix. The uterus is especially vulnerable to perforation during this step. For this reason, the metal dilator should be grasped as one would a pencil. The heel of the hand and fourth and fifth fingers rest on the perineum and buttock. Gentle pressure from only the thumb and first two fingers is used to push the dilator through the cervical os (Fig. 41-16.5).

❹ **Uterine Evacuation.** The cannula is inserted through the open cervix and into the endometrial cavity (Fig. 41-16.6). The suction unit is then turned on. The cannula is moved toward the fundus, then back toward the os, and is turned circumferentially to cover the entire surface of the uterine cavity (Fig. 41-16.7). Uterine contents are thereby removed (Fig. 41-16.8).

Tissue is collected in a container at the distal end of the tubing and is sent for pathologic evaluation. Occasionally, the Karman cannula may become obstructed with excess

tissue. The suction unit is turned off prior to cannula removal. Once the cannula opening is cleared of obstructing tissue, it may be reinserted, the suction unit restarted, and curettage completed.

❺ **Sharp Curettage.** Although no more tissue is aspirated, a gentle sharp curettage should follow to remove any remaining placental or fetal fragments as more fully described in Section 41-15 (p. 1057) (Fig. 41-16.9).

POSTOPERATIVE

Recovery from suction D&C is typically fast and without complication. Patients may resume normal activities as they desire, but abstinence from intercourse is usually encouraged during the first week following surgery.

Ovulation may resume as early as 2 weeks after an early pregnancy ends. Therefore, if contraception is desired, methods should be initiated soon after abortion.

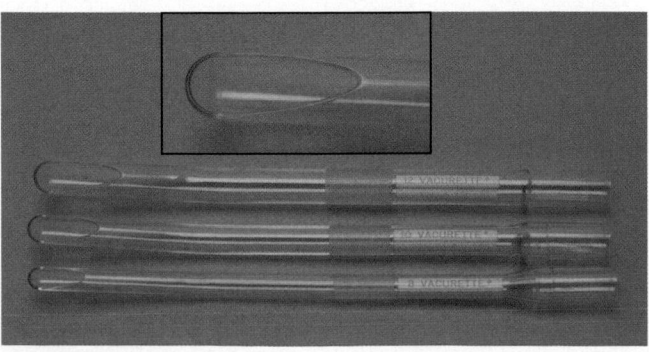

FIGURE 41-16.3 Karmen cannulas (sizes 8 mm to 12 mm). Inset: Cannula tip.

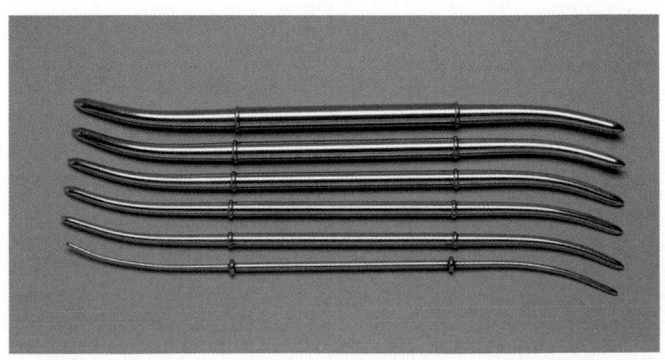

FIGURE 41-16.4 Hank dilators of serially increasing diameter.

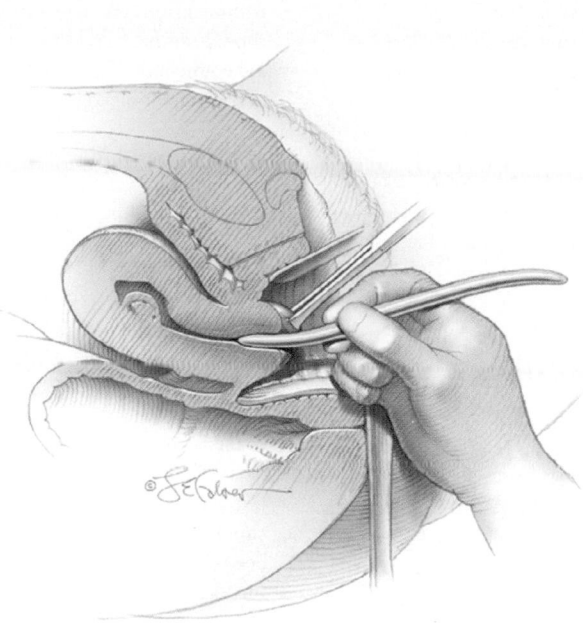

FIGURE 41-16.5 Uterine dilatation.

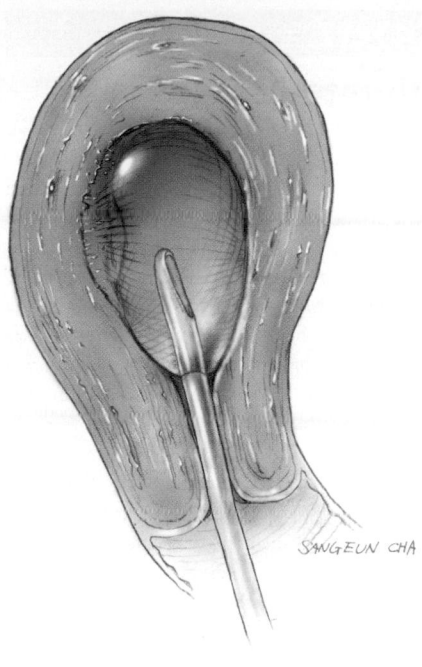

FIGURE 41-16.6 Suction cannula inserted into cavity and amnionic sac.

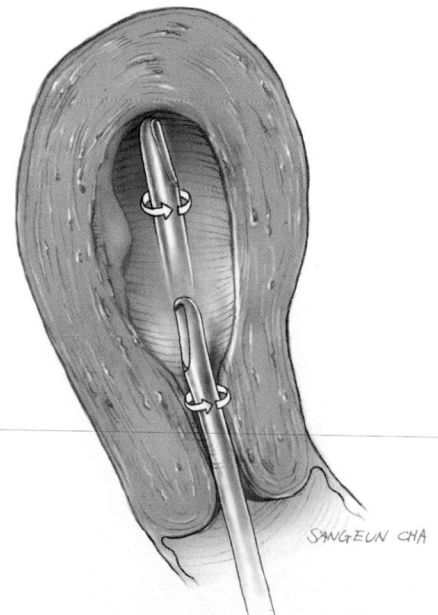

FIGURE 41-16.7 Movement of suction cannula during curettage.

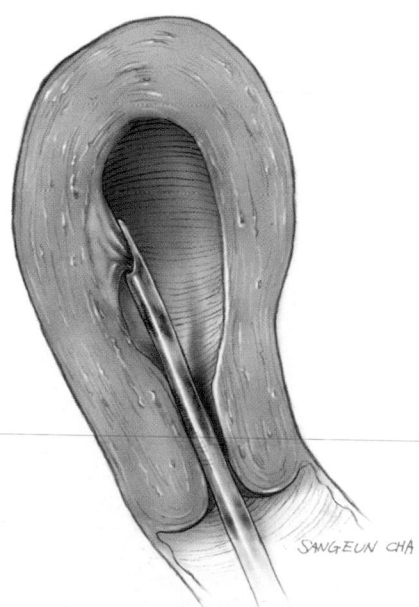

FIGURE 41-16.8 Removal of uterine contents.

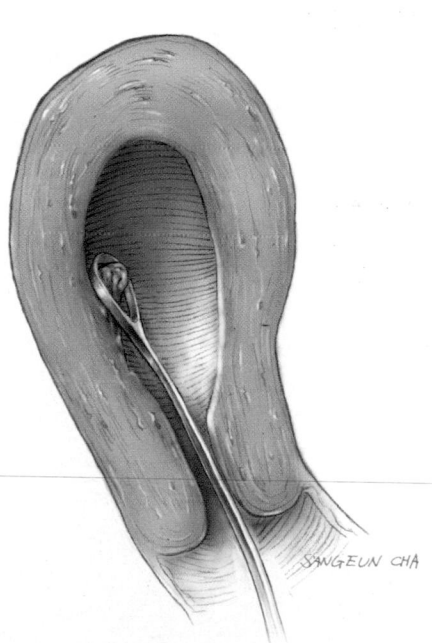

FIGURE 41-16.9 Sharp curettage following suction curettage.

41-17

Hymenectomy

Imperforate hymen results from failure of the hymen to canalize during the perinatal period. Many imperforate hymens are diagnosed after they have become symptomatic, usually during adolescence. Accordingly, the indications for hymenectomy may include complaints of amenorrhea, pain, abdominal mass, and urinary and defecation dysfunction (Chap. 18, p. 492).

An asymptomatic imperforate hymen may also be found early, during childhood. If there is no associated mucocele, these lesions can be managed expectantly. Elective hymenectomy can then be performed during puberty, when tissues are estrogenized, but prior to menarche to avoid the development of hematometra or hematocolpos. The presence of estrogen stimulation can aid surgical repair and healing.

PREOPERATIVE

Consent

Hymenectomy is a simple gynecologic procedure, and most patients recover with no short- or long-term complications. Uncommonly, the hymeneal edges may reepithelialize and a repeat procedure may be required (Joki-Erkkilä, 2003; Liang, 2003).

Patient Preparation

Conflicting opinions exist as to the need for prophylactic antibiotics, and little evidence exists to support either view (Adams-Hillard, 2010; Anania, 1994). If employed, intravenous antibiotics with polymicrobial coverage are given just prior to surgery.

INTRAOPERATIVE

SURGICAL STEPS

1 Anesthesia and Patient Positioning. Hymenectomy is typically performed as a day surgery procedure using general anesthesia. The patient is placed in the dorsal lithotomy position, the bladder is drained, and a sterile perineal prep is performed.

2 Hymen Incision. To avert injury to the urethra anteriorly and to the rectum posteriorly, the surgeon avoids creating pure vertical and horizontal incisions. Instead, a cruciate incision is made anteroposteriorly from 10 to 4 and from 2 to 8 o'clock into the hymeneal membrane (Fig. 41-17.1). Immediately, a stream of dark menstrual blood in the case of hematocolpos or mucoid fluid with mucocolpos will follow.

The hymeneal leaflets are then sharply trimmed from the hymeneal ring. The leaflets should not be excised too closely to the vaginal epithelium. This avoids increased scarring at the hymeneal ring.

3 Irrigation. The vagina is copiously irrigated using a sterile saline solution with either a red rubber catheter or bulb syringe.

4 Suturing. The cut edges of the leaflet bases are then oversewn with interrupted sutures using 3- or 4-0 delayed-absorbable suture, thus creating a ring of sutures (Fig. 41-17.2). A running interlocking suture line is avoided to minimize circumferential narrowing of the introitus (Adams-Hillard, 2010).

Intraoperative evaluation or manipulation of the upper vagina, cervix, and uterus is discouraged as the walls of these organs may have been thinned by hematocolpos or hematometra and may be at greater risk for perforation.

POSTOPERATIVE

Following surgery, the patient may use oral analgesics and topical anesthetics such as 2-percent lidocaine jelly. Local wound care includes twice-daily sitz baths. The patient is counseled that retained fluid may continue to drain from the uterus and vagina for several days following the procedure. The patient is seen 1 to 2 weeks following surgery, at which time the introitus is inspected for patency and assessment of healing.

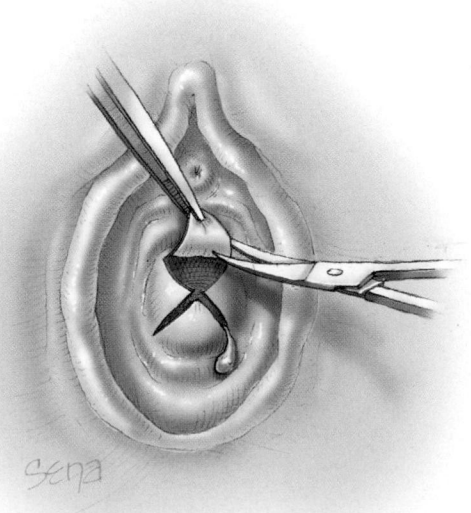

FIGURE 41-17.1 Trimming of hymenal leaflets.

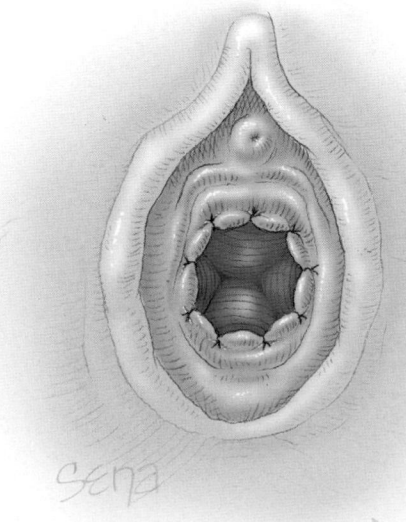

FIGURE 41-17.2 Suturing of leaflets' bases.

41-18

Bartholin Gland Duct Incision and Drainage

Bartholin gland duct cysts and abscesses are common vulvar masses encountered routinely in office gynecology (Chap. 4, p. 123). Bartholin duct cysts typically measure 1 to 4 cm in diameter and are frequently asymptomatic. Patients with larger cysts, however, may complain of vaginal pressure or dyspareunia. In contrast, patients with gland duct abscesses typically present with complaints of rapid unilateral vulvar enlargement and significant pain. Classically, a fluctuant mass is found on one side of the introitus, external to the hymenal ring, and at the lower aspects of the vulva.

Bartholin cysts or abscesses result from ductal opening obstruction followed by accumulation of mucus or pus within the duct. Bartholin abscesses are polymicrobial infections, and *Bacteroides* species, *Peptostreptococcus* species, *Escherichia coli,* and *Neisseria gonorrhoeae* are commonly found from culture of purulent drainage. Less typically, *Chlamydia trachomatis* may be involved (Bleker, 1990; Saul, 1988; Tanaka, 2005).

Incision and drainage (I&D) alone may give immediate but sometimes only temporary relief. Often, unless a new duct ostium is created, the incised edges following I&D will seal and mucus or pus will reaccumulate. Therefore, I&D with subsequent steps to create a new ostium are surgical goals.

Permanent resolution of the cyst or abscess is common following either marsupialization or I&D with Word catheter placement. However, if obstruction recurs, repeating either of these procedures is preferable to gland excision for most cases.

Bartholinectomy, as discussed later, carries significantly more morbidity than either of these less invasive procedures.

PREOPERATIVE

Consent

Repeated obstruction of the Bartholin gland duct following initial incision and drainage (I&D) is not uncommon during the weeks and months following drainage. Patients should be aware of the possible need to repeat the procedure should the duct obstruct again. Dyspareunia may be a long-term sequela, and patients are counseled accordingly.

INTRAOPERATIVE

Instruments

As noted, the goal of Bartholin gland I&D is to empty the cystic cavity and create a new epithelialized tract for gland drainage. For this purpose, a Word catheter is used. Named after Dr. Buford Word (1964), this catheter appears similar to a small, 10-French Foley catheter. Word catheters are constructed of a 1-inch latex tube stem that has an inflatable balloon at one end and a saline-injection hub at the other (Fig. 41-18.1). In place, pus drains around the tube rather than though the catheter.

SURGICAL STEPS

❶ **Analgesia and Patient Positioning.** Most procedures are performed as an outpatient procedure in the office or emergency room. Rarely, if the abscess is large or if adequate patient analgesia cannot be obtained, then I&D in the operative room

may be required. The patient is placed in dorsal lithotomy position, and the wound is cleaned with a povidone-iodine solution or other suitable antiseptic agent. Local analgesia is sufficient for most cases and can be obtained by infiltrating the skin overlying the planned incision with an aqueous 1-percent lidocaine solution.

❷ **Drainage.** A 1-cm incision is made using a scalpel with a No. 11 blade to pierce the skin and underlying cyst or abscess wall (Fig. 41-18.2) The incision should be made along the inner surface of the cyst or abscess and placed just outside and parallel to the hymen at 5 or 7 o'clock (depending on the side involved). This position mimics the normal anatomy of the gland duct opening and avoids creation of a fistulous tract to the outer surface of the labium majus (Hill, 1998). General anaerobic and aerobic cultures as well as samples for *Neisseria gonorrhoeae* and *Chlamydia trachomatis* identification can be obtained from spontaneously extruded pus. Mucus drained from a Bartholin cyst need not be cultured. Following drainage, some prefer to explore the cavity with the cotton tip of a small swab to open potential loculations of pus or mucus.

❸ **Word Catheter Placement.** The tip of a deflated Word catheter is placed within the empty cyst cavity. A syringe is used to inject 2 to 3 mL of sterile saline through the port of the catheter to inflate the catheter's balloon. The balloon is inflated to reach a diameter that will prohibit the catheter from falling out of the incision (Fig. 41-18.3).

The needle hub of the Word catheter can then be tucked inside the vagina to prevent it from being dislodged by traction from perineal movement. This positioning of the catheter hub allows for drainage while providing greater patient comfort.

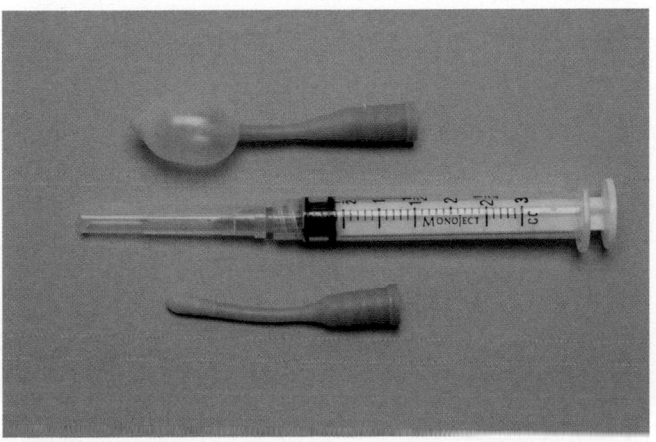

FIGURE 41-18.1 Word catheter. *(Photograph contributed by Steven Willard.)*

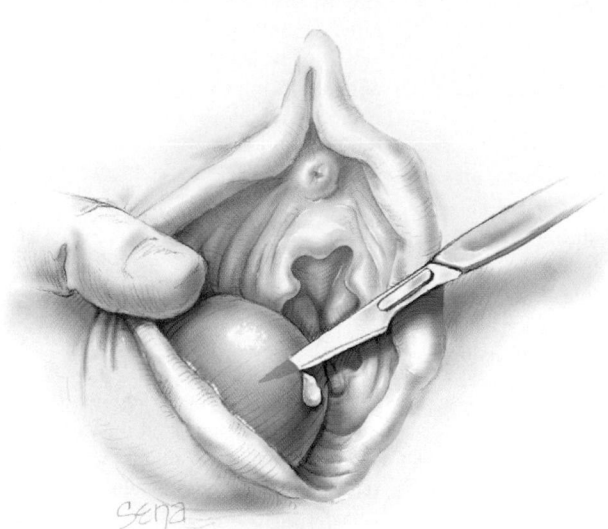

FIGURE 41-18.2 Abscess or cyst incision.

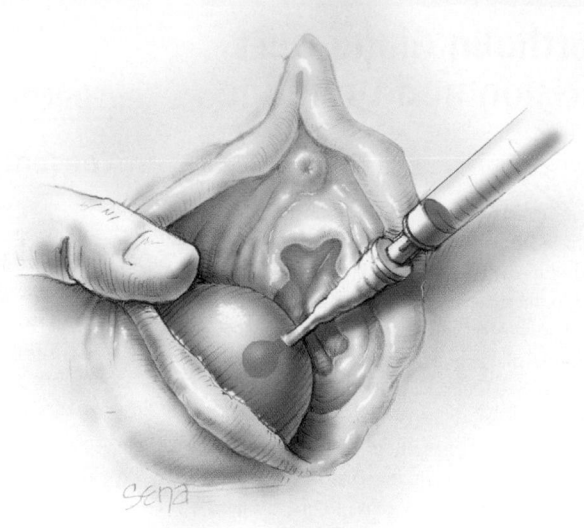

FIGURE 41-18.3 Word catheter in place.

POSTOPERATIVE

Abscesses are typically surrounded by significant cellulitis, and in such cases, antibiotics are warranted. Suitable oral choices include trimethoprim-sulfamethoxazole (Bactrim DS, Septra DS), doxycycline, or cephalexin (Keflex), prescribed for 7 to 10 days. Drainage of Bartholin gland duct cysts do not require antibiotic treatment.

Patients are encouraged to soak in warm tub baths twice daily. Coitus should be avoided for patient comfort and to prevent Word catheter displacement. Ideally, the catheter is left in place for 4 to 6 weeks. Often, however, a catheter will be dislodged before this time. There is no need to try and replace the catheter if displaced, and attempts to reinsert it are typically not possible due to cavity closure.

41-19

Bartholin Gland Duct Marsupialization

High recurrence rates follow simple I&D of a Bartholin duct cyst or abscess. As noted earlier, a new duct ostium must be created to prevent the incised edges from adhering and allowing mucus or pus to reaccumulate. For this reason, marsupialization was developed as a means to create a new accessory tract for gland drainage (Jacobson, 1950; Matthews, 1966).

With introduction of the Word catheter, however, use of marsupialization has declined. Word catheter placement following I&D offers several advantages over marsupialization, and recurrence rates are equal (Blakely, 1966; Jacobson, 1960). Marsupialization requires a greater degree of analgesia, a larger incision, placement of sutures, and longer procedure time. It may be preferred if Word catheters have been previously placed, yet cysts or abscesses repeatedly recur.

PREOPERATIVE

Consent

The consent for marsupialization mirrors that for Bartholin gland I&D. Accordingly, patients should be aware of the risk for repeated obstruction of the Bartholin gland duct following marsupialization. Patients should be aware of the possible need to repeat the procedure if ductal obstruction recurs. Dyspareunia may be a long-term sequela, and patients are counseled accordingly.

INTRAOPERATIVE

SURGICAL STEPS

❶ **Anesthesia and Patient Positioning.** Marsupialization is an outpatient procedure typically performed in an operating suite using a unilateral pudendal nerve block or general anesthesia. Some authors, however, have described performance of the procedure in an emergency room setting (Downs, 1989). The patient is placed in the dorsal lithotomy position, and the vagina and vulva are surgically prepared.

❷ **Skin Incision.** A vertical incision measuring 2 to 3 cm is made using a scalpel with either a No. 10 or 15 blade. The incision is made on the vestibule near the medial edge of the labia minora and approximately 1 cm lateral and parallel to the hymenal ring (Fig. 41-19.1). Care is taken to incise the skin, but not to puncture the underlying cyst wall.

❸ **Cyst Incision.** The cyst wall is then incised with a scalpel, and the incision is extended with scissors. Cultures of purulent material may be obtained as mentioned previously for I&D. Allis clamps are then placed on the superior, inferior, right, and left lateral edges. Each clamp should grasp and contain the skin and cyst wall edges. These clamps are then fanned out. Following drainage, some prefer to explore the cavity with the cotton tip of a small swab to open potential loculations of pus or mucus.

❹ **Wound Closure.** The edges of the cyst wall are sutured to adjacent skin edges with interrupted sutures using 2- or 3-0 delayed-absorbable suture (Fig. 41-19.2).

POSTOPERATIVE

Cool packs during the first 24 hours following surgery can minimize pain, swelling, and hematoma formation. After this time, warm sitz baths, one or two times each day, are suggested for pain relief and wound hygiene. Intercourse is postponed until after incision healing.

Patients may be seen within the first week following surgery to ensure that ostium edges have not adhered to each other (Novak, 1978). Within 2 to 3 weeks, the wound shrinks to create a duct opening typically 5 mm or less. Recurrence rates following marsupialization are low. Jacobson (1960) noted only 4 recurrences in his series of 152 cases.

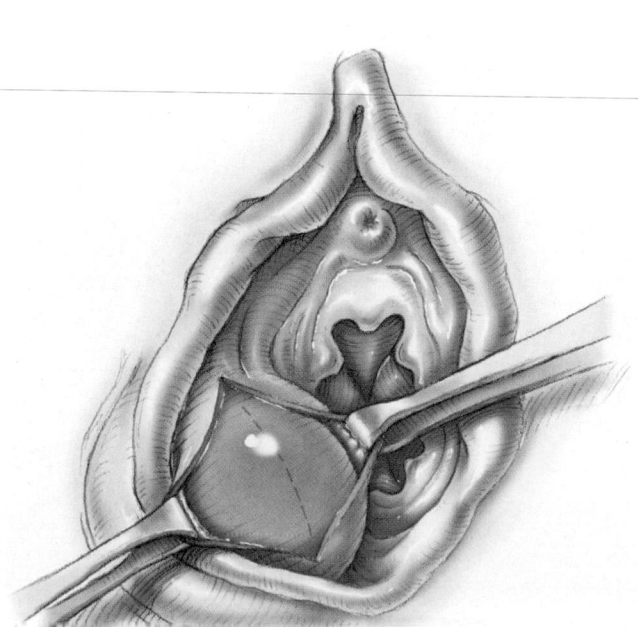

FIGURE 41-19.1 Skin incision.

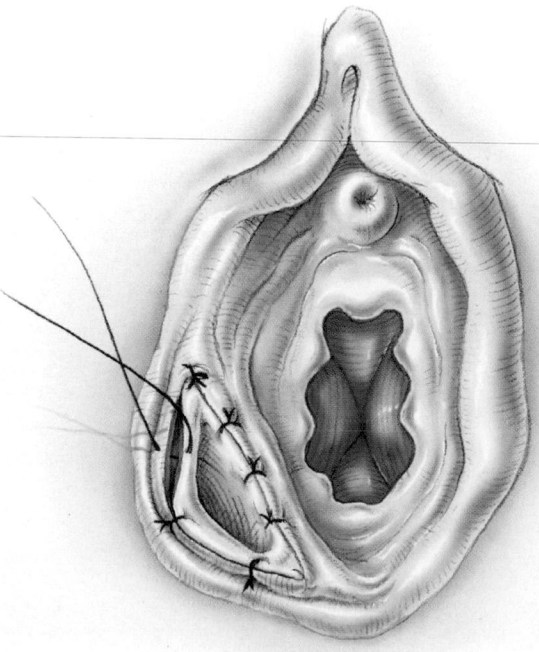

FIGURE 41-19.2 Cyst wall sutured open.

41-20

Bartholin Gland Duct Cystectomy

Most Bartholin gland duct cysts can be managed with incision and drainage (I&D) and Word catheter placement or with marsupialization. Symptomatic cysts, however, which repeatedly recur and refill following I&D or marsupialization are typical candidates for excision. Moreover, massive cysts, multilocular cysts, or those with solid components are best managed with excision. Bartholin gland duct abscesses are not suitable for excision and are instead incised and drained as described in Sections 41-18 and 41-19 (p. 1063).

Many had previously suggested excision of all Bartholin gland cysts in women older than 40 to exclude cancer. However, a study by Visco and Del Priore (1996) suggests that the morbidity of gland excision may not be justified for this rare cancer (Chap. 4, p. 123). Instead, they recommend cyst I&D and biopsy of the cyst wall for this age group.

PREOPERATIVE

Consent

Because of the rich venous plexus of the vestibular bulb, significant bleeding can be encountered during bartholinectomy (Fig. 38-26, p. 942). In addition, gland excision can be associated with other morbidities such postoperative wound cellulitis, hematoma formation, failure to remove the entire cyst wall with risk of recurrence, and pain or dyspareunia or both from postoperative scarring.

Patient Preparation

These cysts should only be excised in the absence of concurrent abscess or surrounding cellulitis. Therefore, antibiotic administration is typically not required.

INTRAOPERATIVE

SURGICAL STEPS

❶ Analgesia and Patient Positioning. Excision of most Bartholin cysts is performed as an outpatient procedure, in an operative suite, and under general or regional anesthesia. The patient is placed in the dorsal lithotomy position, and the vagina and perineum are surgically prepared.

❷ Skin Incision. A gauze sponge held by a ring forceps is placed inside the vagina by an assistant, and pressure is directed outward along the posterior aspect of the cyst. This pushes the full extent of the cyst forward. The surgeon's fingers retract the labia minora laterally to expose the medial surface of the cyst.

A linear incision that extends nearly the length of the cyst is made on the vestibule near and parallel to the medial edge of the labia minora. Care is taken to incise the skin, but not to puncture the underlying cyst wall. Allis clamps are placed on the medial skin edges and fanned out medially toward the contralateral labia.

❸ Cyst Dissection. The greatest vascular supply to these cysts is located at the posterosuperior aspect of these cysts. For this reason, dissection should begin at the lower cyst pole and be directed superiorly.

The inferomedial cyst wall is bluntly and sharply dissected away from the surrounding tissue. Dissection planes should be kept close to the cyst wall to avoid bleeding from the venous plexus of the vestibular bulb and to avoid injury to the rectum (Fig. 41-20.1). Because the lowermost pole of a Bartholin gland cyst may extend to lie adjacent to the rectum, the rectum can be entered accidentally during dissection. Placing a finger at times in the rectum can help orient the surgeon to the spatial relationship between the two. Bleeding from the venous plexus of the vestibular bulb can be troublesome. Most cases can be managed with ligation of individual vessels (if identified), placement of hemostatic sutures, closure of dead space, or a combination of these techniques.

Allis clamps are then placed along the lateral skin edge and fanned out laterally, and dissection is begun near the inferolateral cyst wall.

❹ Vessel Ligation. As dissection is completed superiorly, the main vascular bundle to the cyst is identified and clamped with a hemostat. The bundle is cut and ligated with 2-0 or 3-0 delayed-absorbable or chromic suture (Fig. 41-20.2).

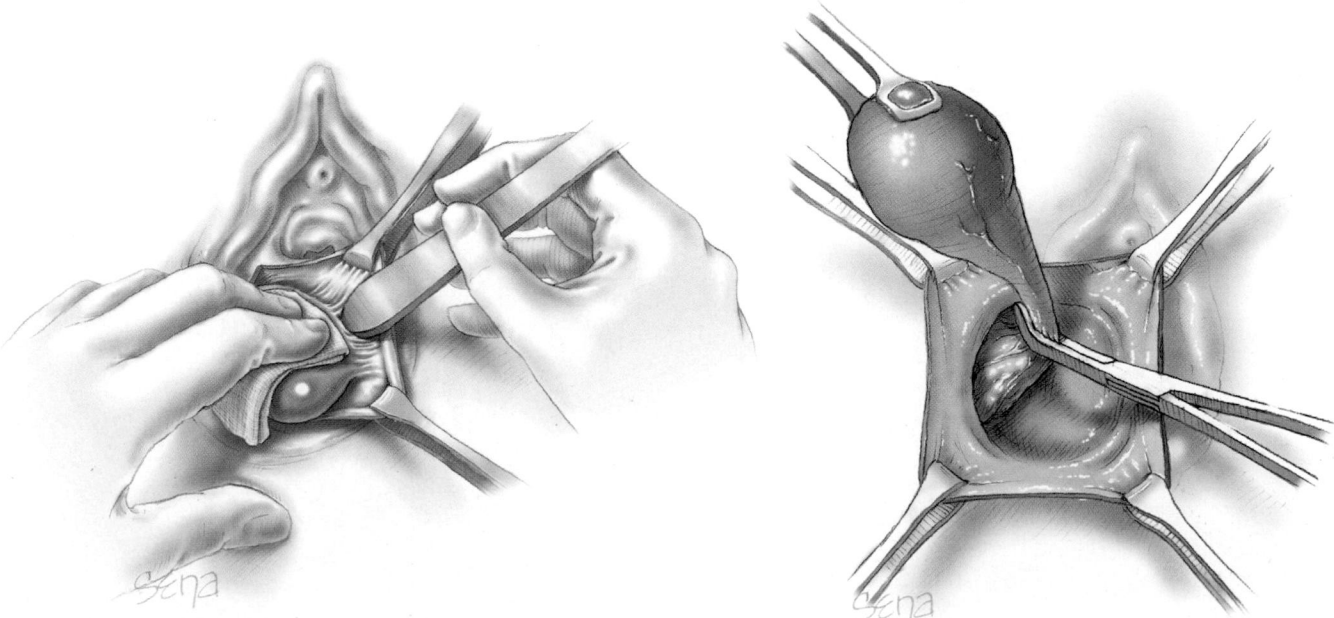

FIGURE 41-20.1 Cyst dissection.

FIGURE 41-20.2 Vessel clamping prior to ligation.

⑤ Wound Closure. The remaining cyst bed is closed in layers with running or interrupted sutures of 3-0 delayed-absorbable suture. Typically, two layers are required to close the space prior to skin closure, but in the case of large or vascular cyst beds, additional layers may be required. The skin is approximated with a running subcuticular suture of 4-0 delayed-absorbable suture.

POSTOPERATIVE

Cool packs during the first 24 hours following surgery can minimize pain, swelling, and hematoma formation. After this time, warm sitz baths, one or two times each day, are suggested for pain relief and wound hygiene. Intercourse is delayed for several weeks to permit wound healing, and then resumption is typically dictated by patient comfort.

41-21

Vulvar Abscess Incision and Drainage

A patient with a vulvar abscess may typically present with pain, vulvar edema and erythema, and a fluctuant mass that should be differentiated from the more common Bartholin gland duct abscess (Fig. 41-21.1). Little information exists in the literature regarding management of vulvar abscesses. In some cases, the abscess may be draining spontaneously, and treatment consists of antibiotics to resolve surrounding cellulitis. In other cases, small abscesses measuring approximately 1 cm or less may be treated with local warm compresses or baths and oral antibiotics. Larger abscesses typically require incision and drainage for clinical resolution of infection.

PREOPERATIVE

Patient Evaluation

Many patients with smaller abscesses can undergo incision and drainage in an ambulatory setting. In contrast, to attain adequate analgesia, larger abscesses may require drainage in the operating room. In addition, some women may require hospital admission for management of other medical comorbidities. Specifically, Kilpatrick and colleagues (2010) noted diabetes mellitus, immunosuppression, vulvar trauma, labial shaving, and pregnancy to be associated risk factors. These investigators found that coexistent diabetes was significantly related to hospitalization greater than 7 days, reoperation, and progression to necrotizing fasciitis.

Consent

Incomplete drainage and persistence of the abscess may follow initial incision and drainage, particularly if the abscess contains loculations. The abscess may also reform after drainage. Although uncommon, progression to or already coexisting necrotizing fasciitis may complicate the infection course.

Patient Preparation

Intravenous antibiotics are given preoperatively, and coverage for methicillin-resistant *Staphylococcus aureus* (MRSA) should be considered. Thurman (2008) and Kilpatrick (2010) and their coworkers found MRSA to be a common pathogen in vulvar abscesses (43 and 64 percent, respectively). Thurman and associates (2008) reported more frequent use of clindamycin or vancomycin for inpatient therapy at their institution and recommended use of trimethoprim-sulfamethoxazole (Bactrim, Septra) for first-line therapy if an oral antibiotic was prescribed.

INTRAOPERATIVE

SURGICAL STEPS

❶ Anesthesia and Patient Positioning. The patient is placed in dorsal lithotomy position, and the involved area of the vulva is cleaned with povidone-iodine solution or another acceptable antiseptic. If drainage is completed with local analgesia, the skin overlying the abscess is injected with a 1-percent lidocaine solution. However, regional or general anesthesia may be appropriate in some cases, such as those complicated by a large abscess or suspicion of necrotizing fasciitis.

❷ Drainage. A 1- to 2-cm incision is made with a No. 11 scalpel blade into the area of the abscess that is thought to be most likely pointing. The incision should penetrate into the abscess cavity with resultant drainage of pus. Aerobic and anaerobic cultures are obtained at this time. The abscess cavity is digitally explored to bluntly dissect any loculations within the cavity (Fig. 41-21.2). At our institution, digital exploration is preferred over that with a pointed surgical instrument, which may injure underlying vascular structures.

❸ Completion of Procedure. Depending upon surgeon preference, a drain may be placed in the abscess cavity and brought

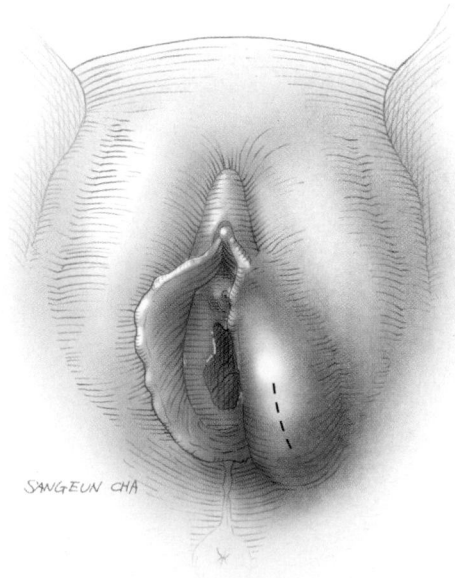
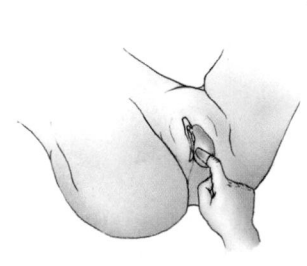

FIGURE 41-21.1 Vulvar abscess incision.

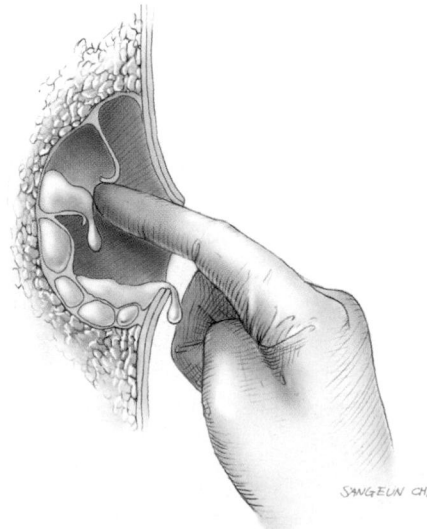

FIGURE 41-21.2 Digital exploration and blunt disruption of abscess loculations.

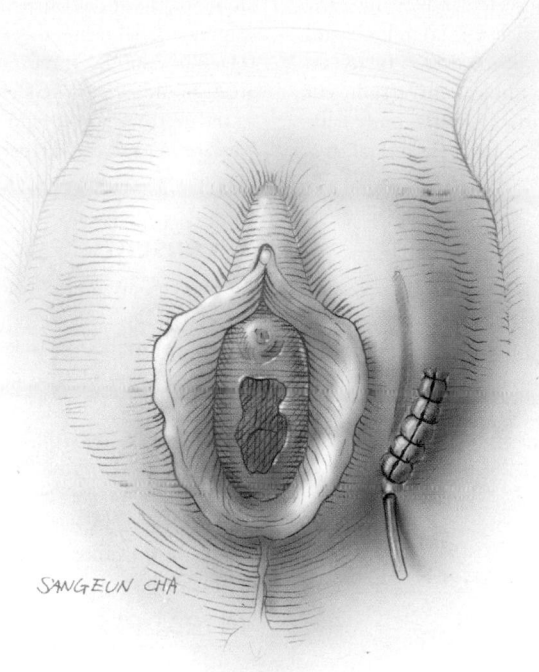

SANGEUN CHA

FIGURE 41-21.3 Drain placement and incision closure.

out through a separate incision. The edges of the primary incision are then reapproximated with delayed-absorbable suture (Fig. 41-21.3). Alternatively, the wound may be packed with iodoform gauze, or the incision may simply be left open to allow for spontaneous healing. Marsupialization of the abscess cavity may also be acceptable in some cases.

POSTOPERATIVE

As comorbidities such as diabetes and immunosuppression are often seen with women with vulvar abscesses, treatment of these associated conditions is important. Perineal hygiene and avoidance of labial shaving should be emphasized. Appropriate antibiotic coverage should be continued for several days. In those without gauze packing, warm sitz baths, one or two times each day, may aid pain relief and wound hygiene. Follow-up care is scheduled to ensure infection resolution.

41-22

Vestibulectomy

Anatomically, the vestibule extends along the inner labia minora, from the clitoris to the fourchette. Additional borders include the hymenal ring and Hart line, which lies along the inner labia minora and demarcates the boundary between skin and mucosa. For some women, inflammation in this region can lead to vulvodynia and dyspareunia.

Most cases of vulvodynia are managed conservatively, but for refractory cases, three surgeries have been employed: vestibuloplasty, vestibulectomy, and perineoplasty (Chap. 4, p. 126) (Edwards, 2003). Vestibuloplasty involves denervation of the vestibule by incision, undermining, and then closure of the mucosa, but without excision of the painful epithelium. It generally has been found to be ineffective (Bornstein, 1995).

Alternatively, vestibulectomy incorporates excision of vestibular tissue (Fig. 41-22.1). Incisions extend from the periurethral area down to the superior edge of the perineum and include the fourchette. The incisions laterally are carried along Hart line and medially should excise the hymen. In sum, mucous membrane, hymen, and minor vestibular glands are removed and Bartholin gland ducts are transected. Following excision, the vaginal mucosa is mobilized and pulled distally to cover the defect. In certain cases, a modified vestibulectomy is sufficient and only extends partially up the inner labia minora, well short of the periurethral area (Haefner, 2000; Lavy, 2005).

Perineoplasty is the most extensive of the three procedures and extends from just below the urethra to the perineal body, usually terminating above the anal orifice (see Fig. 41-22.1). Similarly, following tissue resection, the vaginal epithelium is advanced to cover the defect. Although most commonly used to treat vulvodynia, perineoplasty may also treat fissuring of the fourchette and its associated pain caused by lichen sclerosus (Kennedy, 2005; Rouzier, 2002).

PREOPERATIVE

Patient Evaluation

The most important factor for surgical success in treating vulvar pain is identifying the proper candidate (Chap. 4, p. 124). For example, vaginismus coexists in approximately half of patients with vulvodynia and when present, is associated with lower rates of postsurgical pain relief (Goldstein, 2005).

Prior to administration of anesthesia, the patient should undergo testing with a cotton swab to outline the areas of pain. These areas are marked with permanent marker prior to surgery to delineate the extent of excision (Haefner, 2005). Importantly, all sensitive areas should be removed, even those adjacent to the urethra. If not, tender foci that should have been resected as part of the primary operation may remain (Bornstein, 1999).

Consent

Vestibulectomy and perineoplasty are effective in treating vulvodynia, and in 80 to 90 percent of patients, pain either improves or resolves (Bornstein, 1999; McCormack, 1999; Schneider, 2001). Complications are infrequent but may include bleeding, infection, wound separation, Bartholin gland duct cyst formation, anal sphincter weakness, vaginismus, vaginal stenosis, and failure to alleviate pain (Haefner, 2000).

INTRAOPERATIVE

SURGICAL STEPS

❶ Anesthesia and Patient Positioning. Surgical marking of the sensitive areas to be excised precedes administration of anesthesia. In most cases, vestibulectomy is an outpatient procedure, conducted using general or regional anesthesia. The patient is placed in dorsal lithotomy position, and the vulvovaginal area is surgically prepared.

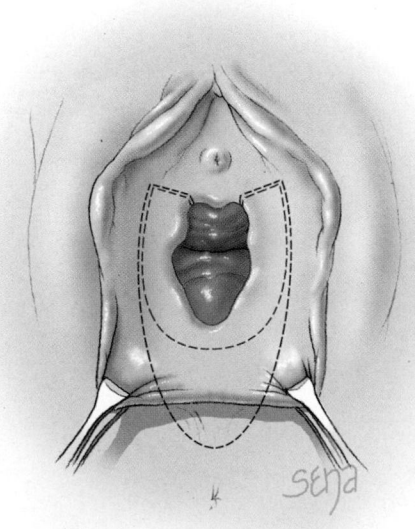

FIGURE 41-22.1 Incisions for vestibulectomy (*red line*) and for perineoplasty (*blue line*).

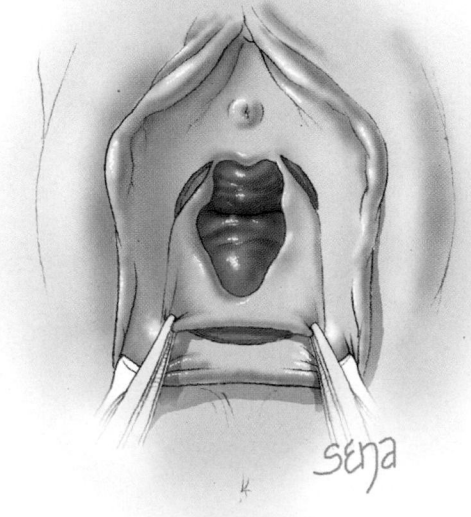

FIGURE 41-22.2 Vaginal mucosal advancement.

❷ Surgical Excision. The primary incision, which is the lateral border, is made to a depth of 2 to 4 mm along Hart line. It is extended inferiorly to the superior edge of the fourchette. The medial incision is placed just proximal to the hymenal ring. The amount of tissue removed anteroposteriorly varies according to sensitivity mapping, but traditionally it begins in the periurethral area and extends from the openings of the Skene ducts to the fourchette. Accordingly, care is taken to avoid urethral injury.

❸ Vaginal Mucosal Advancement. Following tissue excision, the incised edge of the vaginal mucosa is undermined 1 to 2 cm cephalad and then pulled distally to cover the defect (Fig. 41-22.2). To prevent hematoma and wound separation, hemostasis should be achieved prior to final suturing.

❹ Wound Closure. A deep closure layer using interrupted 3-0 gauge delayed-absorbable sutures approximates the vaginal wall to its new site covering the vestibular defect. The superficial incision between the skin and vaginal epithelium is closed in an interrupted fashion with 4-0 gauge delayed-absorbable suture.

POSTOPERATIVE

Cool packs are used to relieve immediate discomfort, and sitz baths are initiated after the first 24 hours. Recovery is typically fast and without complications, and wound healing takes 4 to 8 weeks. Patients usually meet with their surgeon during this time and are instructed to gradually resume intercourse 6 to 8 weeks following surgery (Bergeron, 2001).

41-23

Labia Minora Reduction

When outstretched, most labia minora span 5 cm or less from their base to lateral edge. In some women, this span may be greater and may cause aesthetic dissatisfaction, discomfort with tight clothing, pain with exercise, and insertional dyspareunia. As a result, some elect to have their labia minora surgically reduced.

Goals of surgery include reduction in labial size and maintenance of normal vulvar anatomy. Early reductive procedures involved anteroposterior excision along the base of the labia and reapproximation of the surgical edges. Drawbacks to this approach include a marked color contrast at the suture line, where the dark outer labial minoral surface abuts the lighter inner surface. Moreover, the labial edge is often replaced by a stiff suture line. To reduce these effects, alternate techniques have incorporated labial wedging or Z- or W-plasty incisions (Alter, 1998; Giraldo, 2004; Maas, 2000).

PREOPERATIVE

Consent

Labial minora reductive surgery is a safe and effective means to remove excess labial tissues. As with any aesthetic procedure, women who are seeking cosmetic correction should have realistic expectations as to the final size, shape, and color of the labia. Wound complications such as hematoma, cellulitis, or incisional dehiscence are rare but should be discussed during counseling. Similarly, postoperative dyspareunia is uncommon but should be noted in the consenting process.

Patient Preparation

Antibiotics are not required for infection prevention, and no special preoperative patient preparation is needed.

INTRAOPERATIVE

SURGICAL STEPS

❶ **Anesthesia and Patient Positioning.** Labial minora reduction may be performed as an outpatient procedure using general

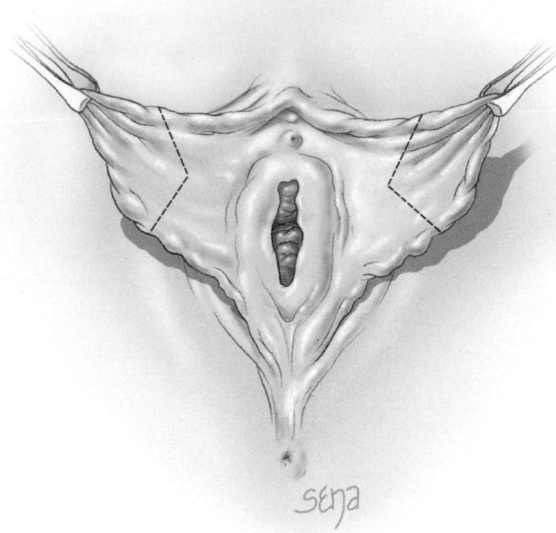

FIGURE 41-23.1 Incision lines.

or regional anesthesia. After anesthesia has been delivered, the patient is placed in dorsal lithotomy position, and the vulva is surgically prepared.

❷ **Labial Marking.** Excessive tissue removal should be avoided, as aggressive reduction may lead to anteroposterior narrowing and discomfort during subsequent intercourse. For this reason, during surgical marking, the surgeon may chose to place several fingers in the vagina to distend its caliber. The labia minora are then gently extended laterally.

The desired lateral span of the labia will vary between women, but most surgeons strive to create a span of 1 to 2 cm. Asymmetry between labia is common, and surgical marking helps to even this difference. With a surgical marker, the surgeon draws a V-shaped wedge on the ventral and dorsal surfaces of the labia minora demarcating the tissue for excision (Fig. 41-23.1).

❸ **Incision Infiltration.** The labia minora have a rich blood supply. To decrease bleeding, the incision may be infiltrated with a solution of 1-percent lidocaine and epinephrine in a 1:200,000 dilution.

❹ **Wedge Excision.** The tissue wedge is then sharply excised. Hemostasis may be achieved using electrosurgical coagulation

and is important in avoiding hematoma formation.

❺ **Incision Closure.** The subcutaneous layers of the labia are reapproximated beginning proximally at the tip of the wedge. Interrupted sutures of 4-0 delayed-absorbable suture are then added outward toward the base to close the remainder of the wound. The skin is reapproximated with 5-0 delayed-absorbable suture in a running subcuticular or interrupted fashion.

POSTOPERATIVE

Cool packs are used to relieve immediate discomfort, and sitz baths are initiated after the first 24 hours. Perineal hygiene is emphasized during the initial weeks following surgery. Exercise and intercourse may resume after wound healing.

41-24

Transverse Vaginal Septum Excision

Failure of the vaginal plate to completely regress during embryologic development can result in formation of a transverse septum at various levels of the vagina (Fig. 18-12, p. 494). Some septa may have small perforations that allow prolonged menstrual blood egress, whereas others have no openings. This latter situation may lead to accumulation of menstrual blood and distension in the upper reproductive tract. Some septa may be managed conservatively with observation, whereas those associated with pain, infertility, or hematometra require excision.

PREOPERATIVE

Patient Selection

Similar to the McIndoe procedure, this procedure is best performed in a mature adolescent or young adult rather than in a child. First, production of estrogen following puberty can improve healing. Moreover, excision of a transverse vaginal septum requires some degree of postoperative vaginal dilatation to avoid stricture, and regimen compliance may be limited in young girls. Unfortunately, not all cases can be delayed. Limitations include chronic pain or development of hematocolpos or hematometra, which is accompanied by an increased risk of endometriosis. A more complete discussion of conservative management and surgical indications is found in Chapter 18 (p. 493).

Consent

Risks of transverse septum excision mirror those associated with the McIndoe procedure. However, skin grafting and its attendant risks are usually avoided, except in cases in which the vaginal septum is long. Vaginal stricture following excision is a significant risk. In their small series, Joki-Erkkilä and Heinonen (2003) found that two of three adolescents required reexcision of scar tissue following initial septum removal.

INTRAOPERATIVE

SURGICAL STEPS

❶ **Anesthesia and Patient Positioning.** After administration of general anesthesia, a second-generation cephalosporin such as cefoxitin, 2 g intravenously, is given. The patient is placed in dorsal lithotomy position, and the perineum and vagina are surgically prepared. A Foley catheter serves as a guide to avoid urethral injury during septum excision.

❷ **Incision.** Retractors are placed to reveal the upper extent of the vagina. With higher-level septa, diagnostic needle aspiration of the suspected hematocolpos can help to locate the upper vagina to determine the direction of dissection (Fig. 41-24.1). The septum is then incised transversely to avoid laceration of the urethra, bladder, or rectum (Fig. 41-24.2).

❸ **Dissection.** Depending on septum thickness, both blunt and sharp dissection may be required to transect the septum. Blunt probing of septal tissue to identify the upper vagina may be necessary to direct dissection. Similarly, the Foley catheter or a finger in the rectum may assist with orientation.

❹ **Excision.** Once the septum is transected, the cervix is identified. The septum is widely excised to its base to minimize postoperative stricture (see Fig. 41-24.2, dotted line).

❺ **Wound Closure.** The vaginal mucosa is undermined and the cephalad mucosal edge is sutured to the opposite caudad edge. A circumferential ring of interrupted sutures

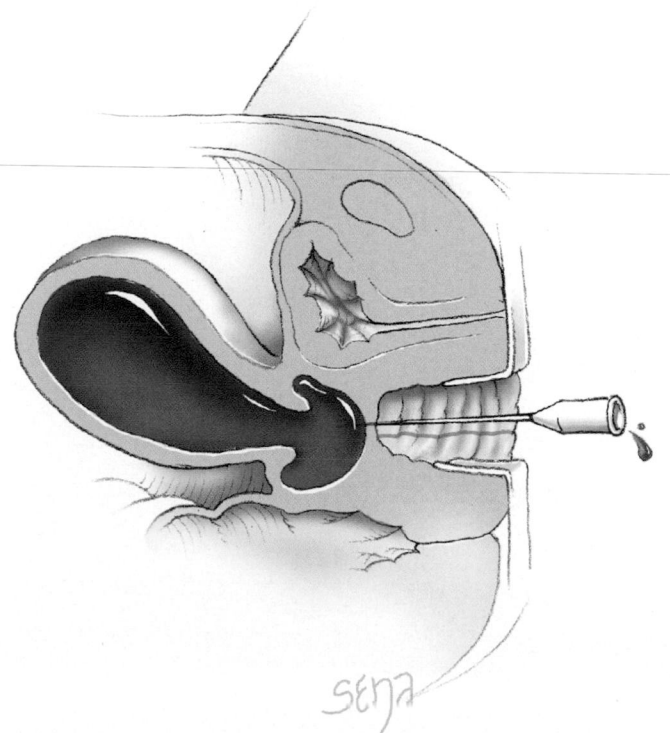
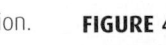

FIGURE 41-24.1 Diagnostic needle aspiration to direct dissection.

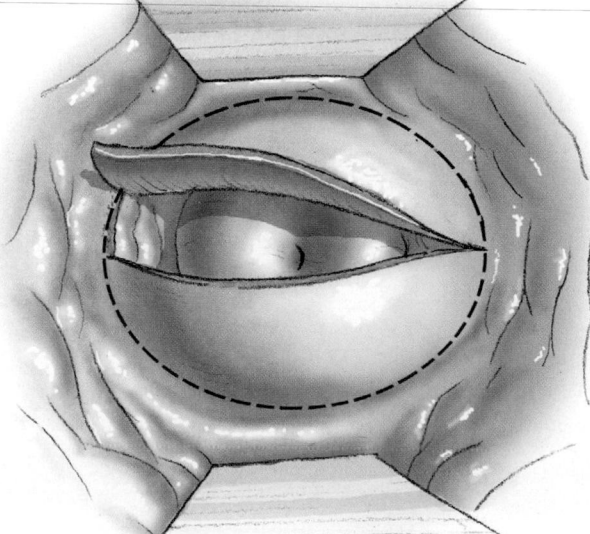

FIGURE 41-24.2 Septum incision.

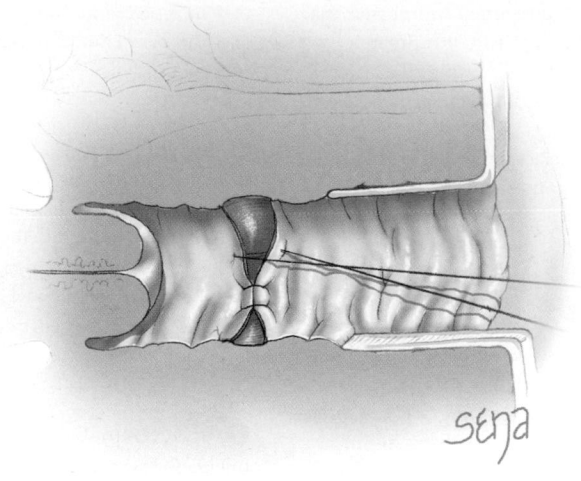

FIGURE 41-24.3 Vaginal mucosa reapproximation.

is thus constructed using 2-0 delayed-absorbable suture (Fig. 41-24.3). A soft cylindrical stent is placed into the vagina. If the vaginal septum is long and mucosal reapproximation is not possible, a skin graft can be taken and applied in a manner similar to the McIndoe procedure.

POSTOPERATIVE

The Foley catheter may be removed on the first postoperative day. The remaining postoperative care mirrors that for the McIndoe procedure.

41-25

McIndoe Procedure

Creation of a functional vagina is the treatment goal for many women with congenital agenesis of the vagina. Although several surgical and nonsurgical approaches have been used, the McIndoe procedure is the most commonly employed in the United States (Chap. 18, p. 497). With this technique, a canal is formed between the urethra and urinary bladder anteriorly and the rectum posteriorly (McIndoe, 1938). A skin graft obtained from the patient's buttock, thigh, or inguinal region is then wrapped around a soft mold and placed into the newly created vagina to allow epithelialization. Alternatively, other materials have been used to line the neovagina. These include amnionic membrane, cutaneous and myocutaneous flaps, buccal mucosa, and absorbable adhesion barrier (Ashworth, 1986; Lin, 2003; McCraw, 1976; Motoyama, 2003).

PREOPERATIVE

Patient Selection

Vaginal stricture can be a significant complication following the McIndoe procedure (Alessandrescu, 1996). Thus, adherence to a postoperative regimen of vaginal dilatation is mandatory. For this reason, surgery may be postponed until the patient has reached a level of maturity to comply (American College of Obstetricians and Gynecologists, 2002).

Consent

Prior to surgery, patients should be informed of overall success rates with this procedure. In a Mayo Clinic series of 225 patients, the McIndoe procedure provided a functional vagina to afford "satisfactory" intercourse in 85 percent of patients. In this review, the cumulative complication rate was 10 percent and included vaginal stricture, pelvic organ prolapse, graft failure, postcoital bleeding, and fistulas involving either the bladder or rectum (Klingele, 2003). Additionally, complications at the skin graft harvest site involved keloid formation, wound infection, and postoperative dysesthesias.

Patient Preparation

Intravenous administration of a second-generation cephalosporin such as cefoxitin 2 g in a single intravenous preoperative dose is recommended. Bowel preparation is completed the evening prior to surgery.

INTRAOPERATIVE

Instruments

Electrodermatome

The skin grafts used to line the neovagina are harvested from the donor site with the aid of an electrodermatome, which is able to shave grafts of varying size and depth. Both split-thickness and full-thickness skin grafts have been used in the McIndoe procedure, and the electrodermatome settings are adjusted to shave the desired depth.

Vaginal Mold

Following graft harvesting and neovagina formation, a stent is needed to apply the graft to the vaginal walls and hold it in place. Both soft and rigid forms have been used. Rigid mold materials have included balsa wood, Pyrex, plastic, and synthetic silicone-based materials (McIndoe, 1938; Ozek, 1999; Seccia, 2002; Yu, 2004). Unfortunately, rigid or semirigid stents have led to graft loss, fibrosis, contracture, and pressure-related bladder or rectal fistulas.

Use of soft stents has decreased the number of these complications. Inflatable rubber stents or condoms filled with foam rubber or other soft compressible materials are examples (Adamson, 2004; Barutcu, 1998; Concannon, 1993). The vagina graft produces abundant exudates, and poor drainage may lead to graft maceration, sloughing, and graft detachment. Accordingly, suction is attached to the soft stents to aid drainage of the neovagina (Yu, 2004).

SURGICAL STEPS

❶ Anesthesia and Patient Positioning. General anesthesia is administered, and the patient is initially positioned prone for skin graft harvesting from the buttock. Alternatively, skin may be obtained from the thigh, hip, or inguinal area. Choosing a location that has minimal hair growth and is cosmetically discreet is desired. The assistance of a plastic surgeon may be enlisted for skin graft procurement.

❷ Skin Graft. The surgeon first marks the outline of the wound on the skin of the donor site, enlarging it by 3 to 5 percent to allow for skin shrinkage immediately after excision. The surgeon uses the electrodermatome to remove a single strip of skin that is typically 0.018 inch thick, 8 to 9 cm wide, and 18 to 20 cm long (Fig. 41-25.1). Alternatively, two smaller strips of 5 cm × 10 cm can be obtained from each buttock.

Following excision, the graft is placed in a pan of sterile saline. The harvest sites on the buttocks are sprayed with a topical hemostatic agent and dressed with a clear occlusive dressing (Tegaderm).

❸ Perineal Incision. The patient is then placed in dorsal lithotomy position, perineal cleansing is performed, and a Foley catheter inserted.

The lower edge of each of the labia minora is grasped with Allis clamps and extended laterally. A third Allis clamp is placed on the vestibular skin below the urethra and is lifted superiorly. A dimple in the vestibule is typically identified below the urethra and a 2- to 3-cm transverse incision is made across it. Allis clamps are then placed on the superior and inferior edges of this incision and retracted.

❹ Neovaginal Dissection. In creation of the new vagina, the goal is to create a canal that is bounded anteriorly by the pubovesical fascia that supports the urethra and bladder,

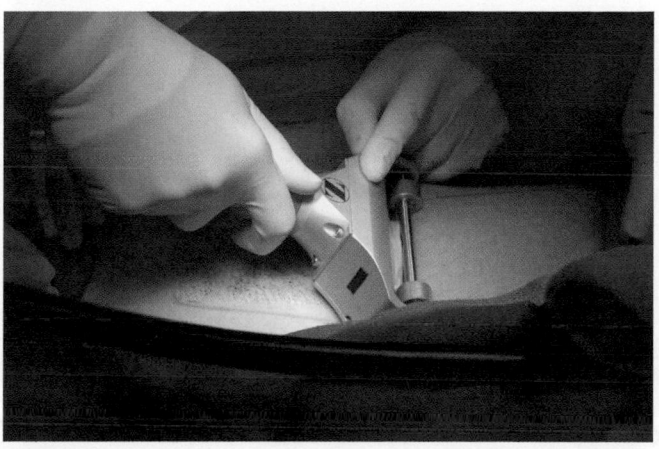

FIGURE 41-25.1 Skin graft harvest.

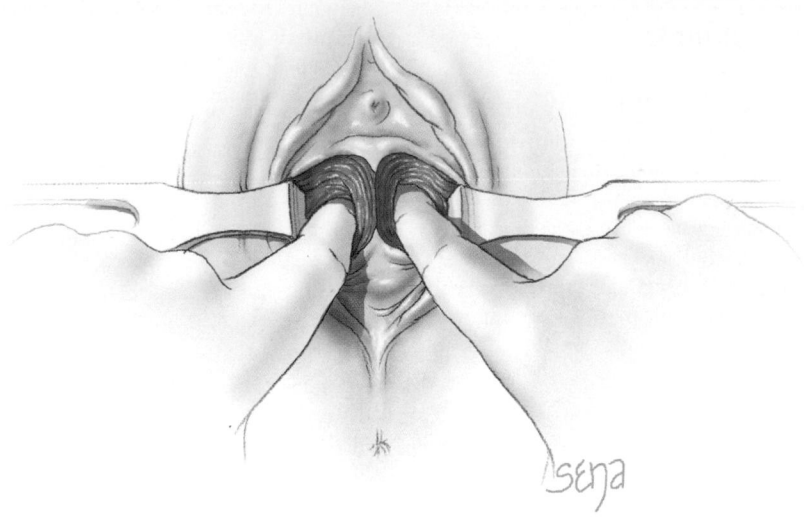

FIGURE 41-25.2 Neovaginal dissection.

posteriorly by the rectovaginal fascia and rectum, and laterally by the puborectalis muscles. Initially, two canals are created on either side of the median raphe, which is a midline collection of dense connective tissue bands that stretch between the urethra and bladder above and the rectum below (Fig. 41-25.2). These canals are initially formed using a spreading motion with blunt-tipped scissors. Fingers are then insinuated into the forming canals. Pressure is exerted cephalad to extend the canal depth. To widen the canals, finger pads are rolled outward, and lateral pressure is applied. Posterior pressure should be avoided to prevent entering the rectum. Each canal is created to reach a depth of 10 to 12 cm. Entering the cul-de-sac of Douglas should also be avoided.

During dissection, several points are noteworthy. First, with initial caudal dissection, the surgeon may meet greater resistance than with the tissues more cephalad. Second, remaining in the correct dissection plane can be difficult. Accordingly, the surgeon's finger may be placed into the rectum to identify its location and avert perforation. Similarly, the Foley catheter may serve as an orientation tool anteriorly.

To expand the space, retractors can be placed along the lateral walls of the forming canals and stretched outward. Moreover, incising the medial fibers of the puborectalis muscles can add further width. These muscles are cut along the lateral aspect of each canal and at a level midway along the anteroposterior length of the canals.

Cephalad, the canal is extended to within 2 cm of the cul-de-sac of Douglas. This leaves a layer of connective tissue affixed to the peritoneum. The skin graft will attach more effectively to this connective tissue than to a smooth peritoneal surface. Rates of subsequent enterocele formation are also lowered when this technique is employed.

❺ Cutting the Median Raphe. Once the formation of the two canals is completed, the median raphe is cut. The final single canal measures approximately 10 to 12 cm deep and three fingerbreadths wide.

❻ Hemostasis. As collections of blood can separate the skin graft from the canal bed, hemostasis is required prior to mold insertion.

❼ Mold Preparation. The vaginal mold may now be covered with the harvested skin. The graft is removed from the saline bath. One end of the graft is placed at the base of the mold with the keratinized surface of the skin facing the mold. The long axis of the graft is laid parallel to the long axis of the mold. The graft is then draped up and over the mold tip (Fig. 41-25.3). The lateral edges of the skin graft are then approximated on either side of the mold using interrupted stitches of 3-0 catgut.

❽ Mold Customizing. Customizing the mold to the size of the created neovaginal canal is essential. If the mold width is too large, pressure necrosis or inadequate drainage may result, which as noted earlier may lead to tissue maceration. Moreover, at the time of postoperative mold removal, a mold that is too large and snugly fitted into the neovagina may pull the graft loose. Once appropriately sized and constructed, the mold is then inserted (Fig. 41-25.4).

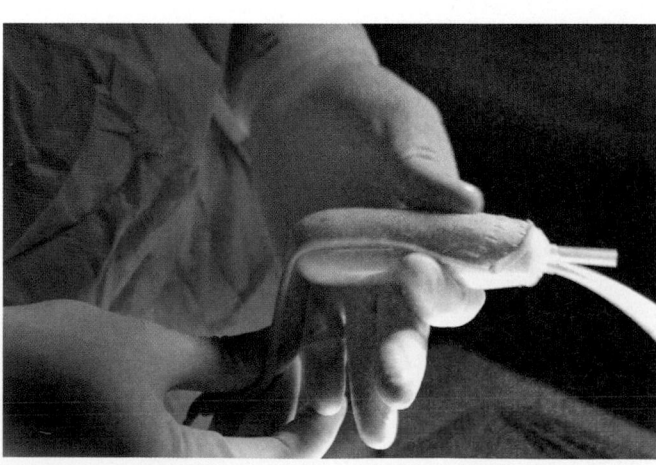

FIGURE 41-25.3 Mold creation.

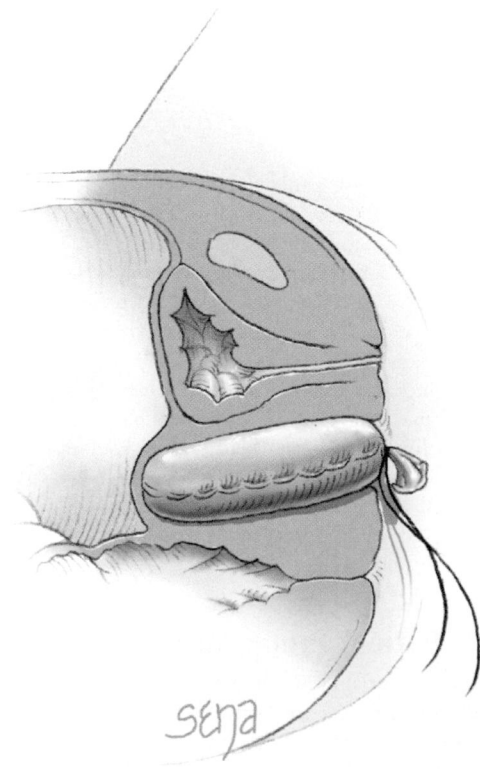

FIGURE 41-25.4 Skin graft and mold in place.

❾ **Perineal Sutures.** The edges of the skin graft at the distal end of the mold are then reapproximated to the distal opening of the neovagina using interrupted stitches of 4- or 5-0 delayed-absorbable suture.

The labia minora, if sufficiently long, can be sutured together along the midline with 2-0 silk sutures to help hold the mold in place for the first 7 postoperative days. An elastic compression dressing is placed on the perineum.

POSTOPERATIVE

The soft stent and Foley catheter are left in place for 7 days following surgery. To minimize dislodgement of the mold and wound contamination, a low-residue diet and loperamide, 2 mg orally twice daily, are used to limit defecation.

At the time of mold removal, an operating room, general anesthesia, and dorsal lithotomy position are employed. Stitches in the labia minora are cut, and the mold is removed. To lessen the risk of graft avulsion, irrigation is used to reduce adherence between graft and mold.

Several schedules for postoperative dilatation have been described. Commonly, the size of the mold placed at surgery is too large for maintenance use. Therefore, a smaller dilator may initially be used and then gradually replaced with larger ones as the vagina stretches.

For the first 6 weeks following surgery, the dilator is worn continuously except during defecation. During the subsequent 6 weeks, it is used only at night. Following these initial 3 months, patients are then instructed to either wear the dilator at night or engage in intercourse twice each week.

41-26

Treatment of Preinvasive Ectocervical Lesions

CERVICAL CRYOTHERAPY

Cryotherapy is an ablative method used to eliminate cervical intraepithelial lesions. This method uses compressed gas to create extremely cold temperatures that necrose cervical epithelium. In theory, as compressed gas expands, it draws heat away from its surroundings. In this case, heat is drawn from the cervical epithelium.

The *cryoprobe*, an interfacing tip made of silver or copper, allows contact with and conduction of extreme cold across the surface of the cervix. When nitric oxide gas is used, probe temperatures can reach –65°C. Cell death occurs at –20°C (Ferris, 1994; Gage, 1979).

As the cervical epithelium is cooled, an expanding layer of ice, called the *iceball*, forms beneath the center of the cryoprobe and grows circumferentially outward and past the margins of the probe. The portion of the iceball in which temperatures fall below –20°C is termed the *lethal zone*. This zone extends from the center of the cryoprobe to a point 2 mm inside the outer iceball edge. Outside this 2-mm point, tissue temperatures are warmer and necrosis may be incomplete.

The expanding iceball grows in depth as well as circumference during treatment. Although this dimension cannot be seen, iceball depth is estimated to equal the lateral spread of the iceball away from the cryoprobe margin. To treat the endocervical glandular crypt involvement of most lesions, a depth of 5 mm is sufficient (Anderson, 1980; Boonstra, 1990a). For this reason, when cryotherapy is performed, the iceball is allowed to enlarge until reaching a mark 7 mm distal to the probe margin. This will ensure creation of a freezing depth of 7 mm, that is, a 5-mm lethal zone and a 2-mm zone of indeterminate tissue death (Ferris, 1994).

Many surgeons use a double-freeze method for cryotherapy in which time rather than iceball dimensions define the process. Refrigerant gas is delivered for 3 minutes to create the iceball. After this, the iceball is allowed to thaw for 5 minutes, at which point a second 3-minute freeze is performed (Creasman, 1984). Studies show a single freezing period should be avoided due to high rates of dysplasia recurrence in the first year following treatment with this method (Creasman, 1984; Schantz, 1984).

The specific indications and long-term rates of success for cryotherapy are discussed in Chapter 29 (p. 752). In general, cryotherapy is appropriate for squamous cervical intraepithelial neoplasia (CIN) that does not extend deeper than 5 mm into the endocervical canal, does not span more than two quadrants of the ectocervix, and is not associated with unsatisfactory colposcopic examination or abnormal glandular cytology. Moreover, cryosurgery is generally not favored for the treatment of CIN 3 due to higher rates of disease persistence following treatment and lack of a histologic specimen to exclude occult invasive cancer (Martin-Hirsch, 2010). Lastly, cryosurgery and other ablative techniques are not favored for women with CIN and human immunodeficiency virus (HIV) infection due to high failure rates (Spitzer, 1999).

PREOPERATIVE

Patient Evaluation

In the United States, women receive colposcopic evaluation and histologic interpretation of cervical biopsies prior to cryotherapy. A "see and treat" approach is also an option. With this, immediate treatment rather than biopsy is initiated during colposcopy for abnormal cervical cytology (Dainty, 2005; Numnum, 2005). However, this type of approach, particularly in low-resource settings, is most successful when linked with excisional and not ablative procedures.

Consent

Although cryotherapy complications are uncommon, women should be counseled on expected postoperative changes and surgical risks. Watery vaginal discharge and vaginal spotting may persist for several weeks following treatment. Fortunately, severe hemorrhage is rare (Denny, 2005). Abdominal cramping is common but typically subsides within the first 24 hours. Infrequently, women may experience a vasovagal reaction during treatment, and care should be supportive.

Cryosurgery may have both short- and long-term effects. Risks include cervical stenosis, pelvic inflammatory disease (PID), and treatment failure. Rates for cervical stenosis and PID are very low. Treatment failures for CIN II have been cited at 6 to 10 percent (Benedet, 1981, 1987; Jacob, 2005; Ostergard, 1980). In addition, Jobson and Homesley (1984) reported retraction of the squamocolumnar junction into the endocervical canal in patients following cryotherapy. In their study, postoperative surveillance

revealed that this retraction resulted in a 47-percent rate of subsequent inadequate colposcopic examination, which often requires more invasive subsequent evaluation. Infertility and pregnancy complications have not been associated with this treatment modality (Weed, 1978).

Patient Preparation

Ideally, cryotherapy is performed after completion of menstruation. This decreases the chance of a coexistent early pregnancy and allows cervical healing prior to the next menses. If it is performed prior to menses, postsurgical swelling can block menstrual flow and intensify cramping. A normal bimanual examination should be confirmed before cryosurgery. If there is a possibility of pregnancy, β-hCG testing should precede treatment.

INTRAOPERATIVE

Instruments

Cryotherapy typically requires a tank of refrigerant gas plus a cryogun, connecting tubing, pressure gauge, and sterilizable cryoprobe. Nitric oxide is the most commonly used refrigerant gas, although carbon dioxide has also been employed. A 20-pound tank is sufficiently large to deliver gas under the 20 pounds of pressure needed to cool tissues adequately. In contrast, smaller tanks may fail to generate sustained pressures and hinder formation of a sufficiently large iceball. Gas moves through connecting tubing, into the barrel of the cryogun, and then to the cryoprobe tip. Circumferential grooves within the cryoprobe stem allow it to be screwed securely into position at the end of the cryogun.

Selection of an appropriate probe is individualized but should cover the transformation zone and lesion. For this reason, cryoprobes come in different sizes and shapes (Fig. 41-26.1). For example, flat-faced probes are used for lesions located on the cervical portio. Advantageously, this shape has a lower tendency to push the resulting squamocolumnar junction toward the endocervical canal and decreases the risk of unsatisfactory colposcopic examination following treatment (Stienstra, 1999). Use of smaller (19 mm) flat probes, however, has been discouraged following studies that indicated insufficient lethal zones and inadequate tissue destruction (Boonstra, 1990b; Ferris, 1994). Cone-shaped probes and those with nipple-shaped tips allow extension of the iceball into the endocervical canal. To minimize cervical stenosis, such nipple tips should not measure longer than 5 mm.

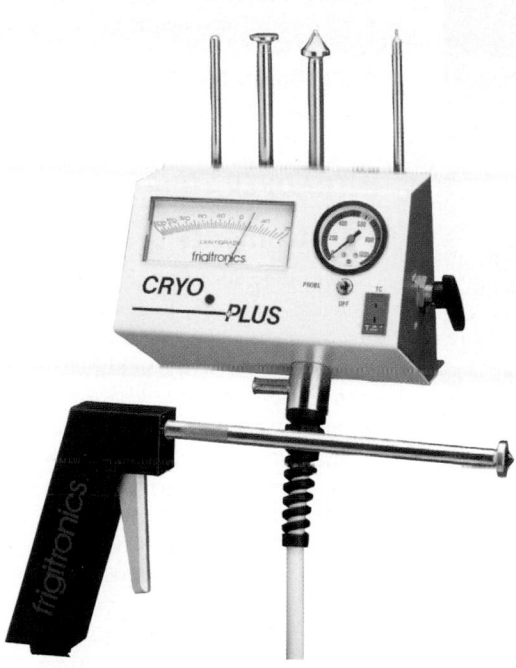

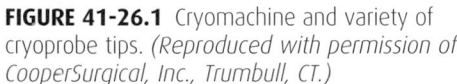

FIGURE 41-26.1 Cryomachine and variety of cryoprobe tips. *(Reproduced with permission of CooperSurgical, Inc., Trumbull, CT.)*

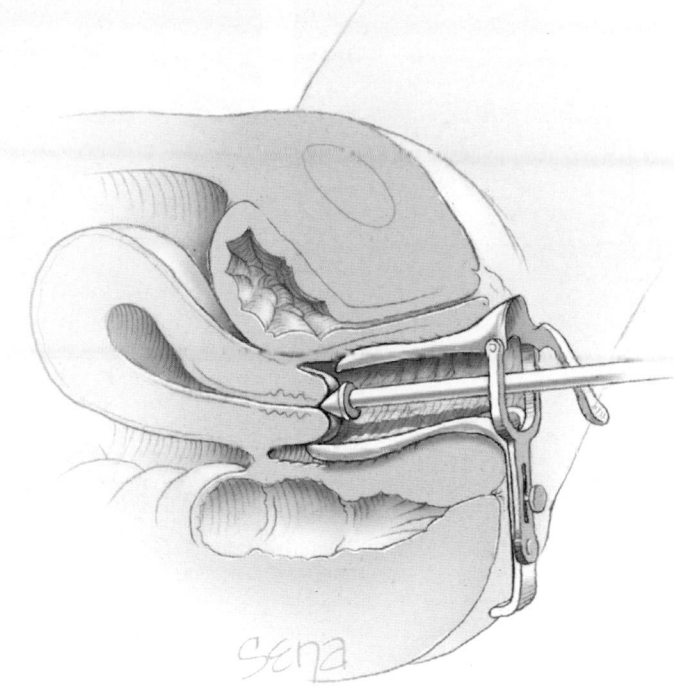

FIGURE 41-26.2 Cryoprobe placement.

Prior to treatment, the gas tank valve is opened, and the pressure gauge should indicate delivery of 20 pounds of pressure. The cryogun trigger is squeezed to confirm that the cryoprobe adequately cools and that no excess gas escapes at the junction of cryogun and cryoprobe. Soft hissing is expected, but loud hissing and gas escape indicate that the thin rubber O-ring that interfaces between the cryogun and cryoprobe should be replaced.

SURGICAL STEPS

❶ **Analgesia and Patient Positioning.** Cryotherapy may be performed in an office setting and requires no significant analgesia. However, to help attenuate associated uterine cramping, women are commonly given a nonsteroidal antiinflammatory drug (NSAID), such as naproxen sodium, 550 mg orally 30 to 60 minutes prior to therapy. Although not routinely used, paracervical blockade and cervical subepithelial injection of 1-percent lidocaine have been associated with decreased pain scores (Harper, 1997, 1998).

The patient is positioned in the dorsal lithotomy position, and a vaginal speculum is placed. No vaginal cleansing prep is required. The appropriate-sized cryoprobe is attached onto the end of the cryogun barrel.

A water-based lubricant jelly is smeared on the end of the cryoprobe to ensure even tissue contact.

❷ **Cryoprobe Placement.** The probe is then pressed firmly against the cervix (Figs. 41-26.2 and 41-26.3A). The cryogun trigger is squeezed, a light hissing sound is typically heard, and frost begins to cover the probe.

The cryoprobe should not contact the vaginal sidewalls. If this is identified, gas delivery is stopped to allow probe warming. The probe is then gently teased away from the wall, after which the procedure is continued.

❸ **Iceball Formation.** The trigger is held until the iceball extends 7 mm distal to the outer margin of the cryoprobe (Fig. 41-26.3B). Freezing typically requires 3 minutes. During the freezing process, ice may form that blocks the gas tubing. For this reason, many manufacturers recommend pushing the defrost button for less than 1 second every 20 seconds during freezing.

❹ **First Thaw.** At this point, the trigger is released. The probe quickly warms and can be removed from the cervix. Attempts to remove the probe prior to complete defrosting can cause patient discomfort and bleeding. The surface of the cervix is allowed to thaw during the following 5 minutes.

❺ **Second Cycle.** Subsequently, the freezing cycle is repeated for an additional 3 minutes. At completion of the second cycle, the cryoprobe and speculum are removed. Because vasovagal responses can be seen with this procedure, patients are assisted to a sitting position slowly.

POSTOPERATIVE

Copious watery vaginal discharge that develops after treatment usually requires sanitary pad use, but tampons are discouraged. Although some advocate debridement of the necrotic eschar to decrease the amount of discharge, Harper and colleagues (2000) reported no effect in the amount or duration of this discharge with this method. Vaginal spotting is expected and can persist for weeks. During the first few days following cryotherapy, patients may complain of diffuse mild lower abdominal pain or cramping for which NSAIDs typically provide relief. Infrequently, severe pain and cramping may result from necrotic tissue obstructing the endocervical canal and is termed *necrotic plug syndrome*. Removal of the obstructing tissue typically resolves symptoms.

Because a large area of the cervix is denuded after cryotherapy, there is an increased potential for infection. Accordingly, patients should abstain from intercourse during the

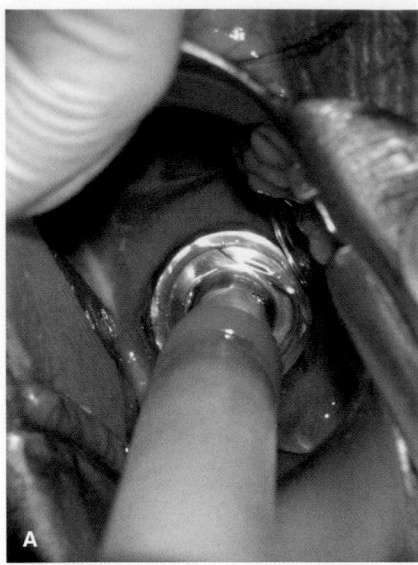 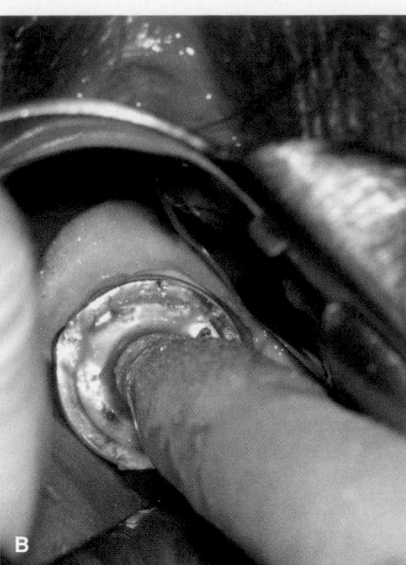

FIGURE 41-26.3 Photographs of cryotherapy. **A.** Cryotip applied to cervix. **B.** Creation of advancing iceball. *(Photographs contributed by Dr. Claudia Werner.)*

4 weeks following surgery. If abstinence is not feasible, then condom use is encouraged. Depending on patient symptoms, work and exercise may resume following treatment.

LOOP ELECTROSURGICAL EXCISION PROCEDURE (LEEP)

Loop electrosurgical excision procedure (LEEP), also known as *large loop excision of the transformation zone* (LLETZ), uses electric current to generate waveforms through a metal electrode that either cuts or coagulates cervical tissues. These thin, wire semicircular electrodes allow clinicians to excise cervical lesions in an office setting with minimal patient discomfort, cost, and complications. In addition, LEEP permits submission of a surgical specimen for additional evaluation. In the United States, electrosurgical treatment of cervical intraepithelial neoplasia is popular and often preferred over cryotherapy or laser ablation.

Although often performed in a clinic setting, several factors may dictate performance in the operating room. First, markedly relaxed vaginal sidewalls may require significant retraction for adequate visualization. Secondly, a lesion or transformation zone that lies near the cervix periphery may risk vaginal or bladder injury during completion of the electrode pass. Lastly, patient anxiety and an inability to remain relatively motionless with an office procedure may necessitate greater sedation.

PREOPERATIVE

Patient Evaluation

As with cryotherapy and laser ablation, women in the United States undergo colposcopy and histologic review of colposcopic biopsies prior to LEEP. Presurgical patient preparation mirrors that for cryotherapy (p. 1078).

Consent

This procedure is associated with low morbidity, and overall complication rates approximate 10 percent (Dunn, 2004). Major complications are rare (0.5 percent) and may include bowel or bladder injury and hemorrhage (Dunn, 2003; Kurata, 2003). Short-term complications such as abdominal pain, vaginal bleeding, vaginal discharge, and bladder spasm may be treated symptomatically.

Long-term complications include failure to completely treat the cervical lesion and cervical stenosis. Persistent disease is typically noted in the initial surveillance Pap smear or HPV testing following LEEP. However, such treatment failure rates are low (approximately 5 percent) and are positively correlated with initial excised lesion size (Alvarez, 1994; Gunasekera, 1990; Mitchell, 1998). Cervical stenosis is estimated to complicate less than 6 percent of cases. Risk factors include the presence of an endocervical lesion and excision of a large tissue volume (Baldauf, 1996; Suh-Burgmann, 2000).

The effects of LEEP with regard to obstetric outcomes are unclear. Several studies have shown that pregnancy does not appear to be

adversely affected by LEEP, whereas others have noted increased risks of premature labor and premature rupture of membranes (Crane, 2003; Ferenczy, 1995; Kyrgiou, 2006; Tan, 2004; Werner, 2010).

INTRAOPERATIVE

Instruments

Tissue excision during LEEP requires an electrosurgical unit, wire loop electrodes, insulated speculum, and smoke evacuation system. Electrosurgical units used in LEEP procedures generate high-frequency (350 to 1200 kHz), low-voltage (200 to 500 V) electric current. Because of the risk for electric burns to the patient from stray current, grounding pads should be placed on conductive tissue that is close to the operative site (Chap. 40, p. 999).

Similarly, an insulated speculum is used in LEEP procedures to limit the risk of stray current conductance to the patient. The insulated speculum should have a port for smoke evacuation tubing, which assists in clearing smoke from the operating field to improve visualization.

Surgical smoke plumes have contents including carbon monoxide, polyaromatic hydrocarbons, and a variety of trace toxic gases (National Institute for Occupational Safety and Health, 1999). Although there has been no documented transmission of infectious disease through surgical smoke, the potential for generating infectious viral fragments may exist. For these reasons, local smoke evacuation systems are recommended.

Electric current is directed to tissue via a 0.2-mm stainless steel or tungsten wire electrode. These are available in various sizes to customize treatment to lesion dimensions (Fig. 41-26.4). These instruments are disposable and discarded after each patient procedure.

SURGICAL STEPS

❶ Anesthesia and Patient Positioning. The patient is placed in the dorsal lithotomy position, and the electrosurgical grounding pad is placed on the upper thigh or buttock. The insulated speculum is inserted into the vagina, and smoke evacuation tubing is attached. The application of Lugol solution outlines lesion margins before starting the procedure (Chap. 29, p. 748).

For in-office anesthesia, vasoconstricting solutions of either vasopressin and 1-percent lidocaine solution (10 units Pitressin in 30 mL of lidocaine) or 1-percent lidocaine and epinephrine (1:100,000 dilution) may be used. A 25- to 27-gauge needle is used to circumferentially aspirate and then inject 5

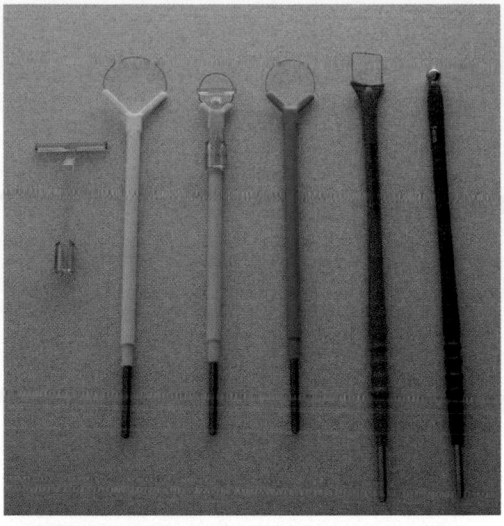

FIGURE 41-26.4 Variety of loop electrosurgical excision procedure (LEEP) electrodes.

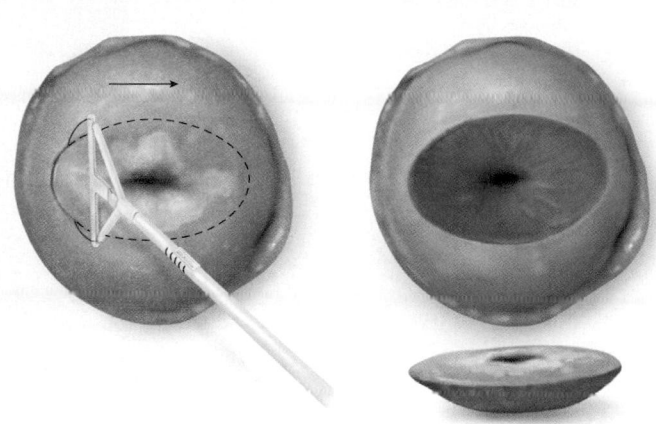

FIGURE 41-26.5 Single-pass loop electrosurgical excision.

to 10 mL of either solution 1 to 2 cm deep into the cervix outside the area to be excised. Cervical blanching is usually seen.

❷ **Single-Pass Excision.** Ideally, the lesion should be excised in one pass, and the appropriately sized loop is selected for this goal. If colposcopy is satisfactory, the correct loop diameter should incorporate the entire lesion diameter to a depth of 5 to 8 mm. The electrosurgical unit is set to cutting mode, and typically 30 to 50 W is used depending on the loop size. Larger loops require higher wattage.

To excise the lesion, a loop is positioned 3 to 5 mm outside the lateral perimeter of the lesion (Fig. 41-26.5). Current through the loop is activated prior to tissue contact, during which electric sparks at the loop tip may be seen. The loop is introduced to the cervix at a right angle to its surface. The loop is drawn parallel to the surface until a point 3 to 5 mm outside the opposite border of the lesion is reached. The loop is then withdrawn slowly, positioning it again at right angles to the surface. Current is stopped as soon as the loop exits the tissue. Following excision, the specimen is placed in formalin for pathologic evaluation.

❸ **Multiple-Pass Excision.** Less commonly, bulky lesions may require multiple passes using a combination of loop electrode sizes (Fig. 41-26.6).

❹ **Control of Bleeding Sites.** Despite use of vasoconstrictors, bleeding following LEEP is common. Sites of active bleeding may be controlled using a 3- or 5-mm ball electrode, and the electrosurgical unit

switched to coagulation mode. Alternatively, Monsel solution can be applied with direct pressure to bleeding sites.

POSTOPERATIVE

Following excision, patients typically will experience light spotting and cramping. Postoperative healing and patient care in general follows that for cryotherapy (p. 1079).

CARBON DIOXIDE LASER CERVICAL ABLATION

The carbon dioxide (CO_2) laser produces a beam of infrared light, with a wavelength of 10.6 μm. At its focal point, the laser energy produces heat sufficient to boil intracellular water and vaporize tissue.

Indications and success rates are discussed more fully in Chapter 29 (p. 752). In general, laser ablation may be used in cases in which

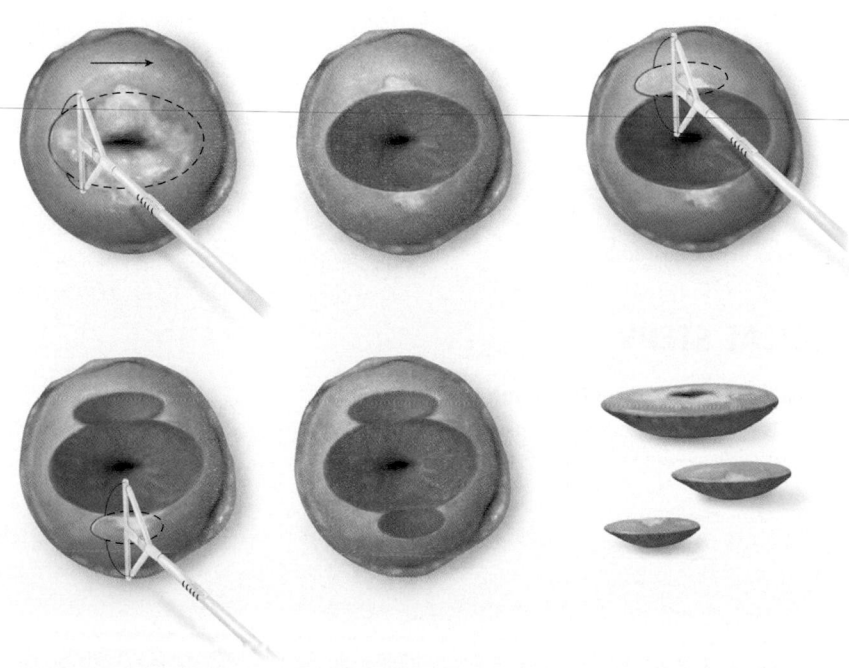

FIGURE 41-26.6 Multiple-pass excision.

the entire transformation zone can be seen with satisfactory colposcopy. There should be no evidence of microinvasive, invasive, or glandular disease, and cytology and histology should positively correlate.

Although research has shown laser ablation to be an effective tool in treating cervical intraepithelial neoplasia, its popularity is decreasing. Laser units are significantly more expensive than those used for cryotherapy and LEEP. In addition, lesions are destroyed with ablation, and unlike LEEP, the opportunity for additional pathologic evaluation of surgical margins is lost. Finally, physician and staff training and certification are typically required for safe, effective use of laser equipment.

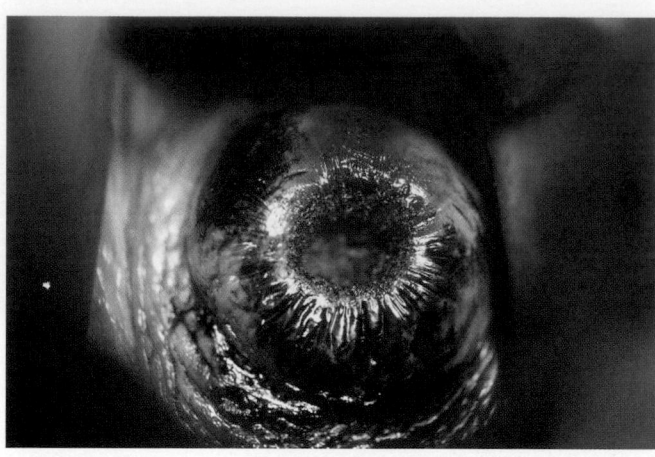

FIGURE 41-26.7 Cervical bed following laser ablation. *(Photograph contributed by Dr. Eddie McCord.)*

PREOPERATIVE

Consent

As with any treatment of cervical dysplasia, patients should be counseled on the risks of disease persistence and recurrence following treatment. These risks and surgical complications are low and comparable with LEEP (Alvarez, 1994; Nuovo, 2000).

INTRAOPERATIVE

Instruments

Carbon dioxide lasers suitable for cervical ablation are mobile, self-contained units. Tissue effects vary depending on the interval at which energy bursts are released. As a result, continuous waves (cutting) or pulsed energy (coagulation) can be released. Laser guidance is accomplished through attachment to a colposcopic sled device.

Because laser light is reflective, protective eyewear is required for the patient and all participants, and a sign is posted on the suite door warning that a laser procedure is in progress. For this same reason, a matte-surface speculum is necessary. As with LEEP, noxious smoke is generated, and a smoke evacuation system is required.

SURGICAL STEPS

❶ Anesthesia and Patient Positioning. Laser ablation for many women is an outpatient procedure and performed in either an operating suite or office depending on laser equipment location and patient characteristics. In most cases, local analgesia combined with a vasoconstrictor is sufficient, and administration mirrors that used for LEEP (p. 1080). The patient is placed in dorsal lithotomy position. A matte-surfaced speculum is inserted, and smoke evacuation tubing is attached to a port on the speculum. Misdirected laser energy can burn surrounding tissues and ignite paper drapes. Therefore, moistened cloth towels are draped outside the vulva to absorb misdirected energy. To delineate the area of excision, Lugol solution is applied to the cervix.

❷ Laser Settings. The colposcope-laser assembly is brought into position and focused on the ectocervix. The laser is set to achieve a power density (PD) of 600 to 1200 W/cm^2 in a continuous-wave mode. Calculation of power density is described in Section 41-28 (p. 1089).

❸ Ablation. Initially, four laser spots are placed at 12, 3, 6, and 9 o'clock positions on the perimeter of the cervix to surround the entire lesion. These spots serve as landmarks and are connected in an arching pattern to create a circle. Once encircled, the area is ablated to a depth of 5 to 7 mm (Fig. 41-26.7).

❹ Endocervical Eversion. To help prevent postoperative retraction of the squamocolumnar junction cephalad into the endocervical canal, the tissue immediately surrounding the endocervix is ablated less deeply. This allows an apparent eversion of the endocervical lining and retention of the squamocolumnar junction on the ectocervix.

❺ Hemostasis. Bleeding is common during CO_2 laser vaporization. A defocused laser beam and a lower power setting in a super pulse wave mode will coagulate vessels and aid hemostasis. Bleeding present at the end of surgery may also be controlled with an application of Monsel solution.

POSTOPERATIVE

Cramping is common following surgery, and light bleeding may persist for a week. Postoperative patient counseling is similar to that for cryotherapy.

41-27

Cervical Conization

Cervical conization removes ectocervical lesions and a portion of the endocervical canal by means of a cone-shaped tissue biopsy (Fig. 41-27.1). It is a safe, effective means to treat CIN, carcinoma in situ (CIS), and adenocarcinoma in situ (AIS). Moreover, cervical conization is a standard treatment for women with unsatisfactory colposcopy and biopsies suggestive of high-grade CIN, those with positive endocervical curettage, or those with discordant cytologic and histologic findings. Excision may be completed via scalpel, termed *cold-knife conization.* Alternatively, laser or LEEP conization may be performed. Success rates for these excisional methods in the treatment of CIN have been found equivalent. However, LEEP conization has gained popularity because of its ease of use and cost effectiveness. Indications for and differences among these modalities are discussed in Chapter 29 (p. 753).

PREOPERATIVE

Patient Evaluation

Prior to conization, patients will have undergone colposcopic examination and histologic evaluation of biopsies. β-hCG testing is warranted prior to conization if pregnancy is suspected. If pregnancy is confirmed and invasion is not suspected colposcopically, postpartum patient management is reasonable. Conization during pregnancy has great morbidity because of increased vascularity and bleeding.

Consent

Risks associated with conization mirror those for LEEP excision of ectocervical lesions. However, cold-knife conization has a greater risk of bleeding compared with that of laser and LEEP conization. Moreover, cold-knife and laser conizations carry higher risks of cervical stenosis compared with LEEP conization (Baldauf, 1996; Houlard, 2002). Increasing age and depth of endocervical excision are significant cervical stenosis risks. Penna and coworkers (2005) noted a lower risk of stenosis in postmenopausal women using estrogen replacement therapy compared with postmenopausal nonusers.

Conization of the cervix for the treatment of CIN has been associated with adverse outcomes in subsequent pregnancies including preterm delivery, low-birthweight infants, incompetent cervix, and cervical stenosis (Crane, 2003; Kristensen, 1993a,b; Raio, 1997;

Samson, 2005). Although there is no major difference in obstetric outcome among the three techniques, increased cone biopsy size has been shown to positively correlate with rates of preterm delivery and premature membrane rupture (Mathevet, 2003; Sadler, 2004). Cold-knife conization generally removes more cervical stroma than other excisional methods.

COLD-KNIFE CONIZATION

SURGICAL STEPS

❶ Anesthesia and Patient Positioning. For most women, cold-knife conization is a day-surgery procedure performed under general or regional anesthesia. Following administration of anesthesia, the patient is placed in the dorsal lithotomy position. The vagina is surgically prepared, the bladder drained, and vaginal sidewalls retracted to reveal the cervix. Areas of planned excision may be more easily identified with Lugol solution application and with preoperative colposcopic examination.

❷ Injection   of Vasoconstrictors. Bleeding during cold-knife conization can be brisk and obscure the operating field. Accordingly, preventative steps can be taken both during and before surgery. First, vasoconstrictors as described for LEEP are injected circumferentially into the cervix (Section 41-26, step 1, p. 1080). Additionally, descending cervical branches of the uterine arteries can be ligated with figure-of-eight sutures using a nonpermanent material placed along the lateral aspects of the cervix at 3 and 9 o'clock. After these knots are secured, the sutures are kept long and held by hemostats.

❸ Conization. A uterine sound or small-caliber uterine dilator is placed into the endocervical canal to orient the surgeon as to the depth and direction of the canal. Using a No. 11 blade, the surgeon initiates the incision on the lower lip of the cervix . Starting here limits blood from running downward and obscuring the operative field. Alternatively, a Beaver blade, which is a triangular-shaped knife blade with a 45-degree bend, may be used (Fig. 41-27.2). A circumscribing incision creates a 2- to 3-mm border around the entire lesion (Fig. 41-27.3). The 45-degree angle of the blade is directed centrally and cephalad to excise a conical specimen. Toothed forceps or tissue hooks may be used to retract the ectocervix during creation of the cone. Scalpel or Mayo scissors may be used to cut the tip of the cone and release the specimen. A suture is placed on the site of the specimen that corre-

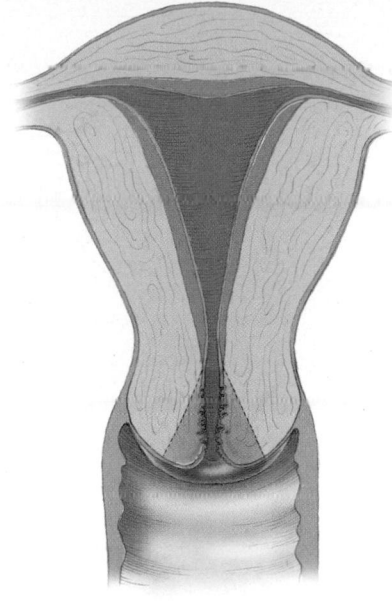

FIGURE 41-27.1 Cone-shaped tissue biopsies.

sponds to the 12 o'clock position in situ. The location of this suture aids the pathologist in orientation of the specimen and is noted on the pathology requisition form.

❹ Endocervical   Curettage. Following removal of the cone specimen, endocervical curettage is performed to evaluate for residual disease distal to the excised cone apex (Husseinzadeh, 1989; Kobak, 1995). This is sent as a separate specimen for evaluation.

❺ Hemostasis. With excision of the specimen, bleeding is common and can be controlled with individual suturing of isolated vessels, with electrosurgical coagulation, or

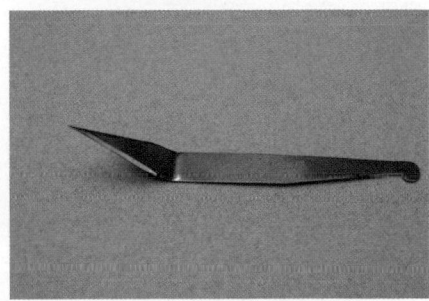

FIGURE 41-27.2 Beaver blade.

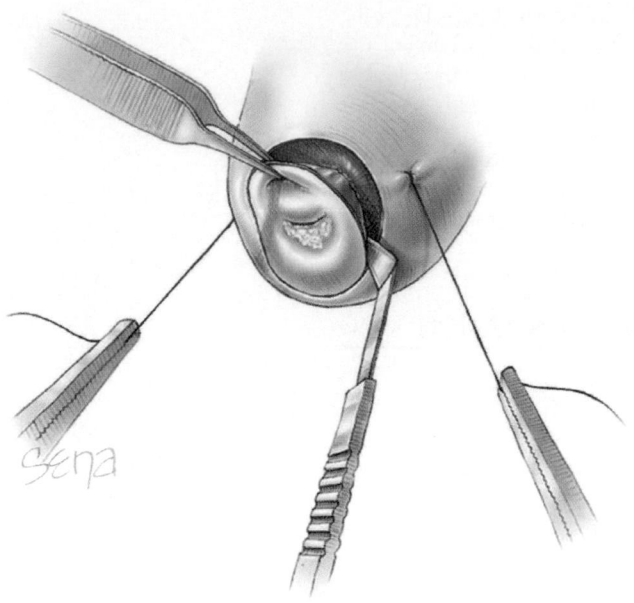

FIGURE 41-27.3 Conization incision.

with Sturmdorf sutures. In addition, a topical absorbable hemostat mesh (Surgicel) can be placed in the cone bed.

With placement of Sturmdorf sutures, a running locked suture line closes the cone bed by circumferentially folding the cut ectocervical edge inward toward the endocervix. This technique is less favored due to increased rates of postoperative dysmenorrhea, inadequate postoperative surveillance Pap smears, and concerns that the flap might conceal residual disease (Kristensen, 1990; Trimbos, 1983).

LOOP ELECTROSURGICAL EXCISION PROCEDURE (LEEP) CONIZATION

SURGICAL STEPS

The surgical steps for this more extensive LEEP mirror those used for excision of ectocervical lesions (p. 1080). However, to remove a portion of the endocervical canal, a deeper pass must be made through the cervical stroma. This may be accomplished with a single pass using a larger loop. Alternatively, in an effort to minimize the volume of tissue excised, a tiered or *top hat technique* can be used. With this method, an initial pass is made to remove ectocervical lesions as previously described (Fig. 41-26.5, p. 1081). To remove the endocervical canal, a second smaller loop is passed more deeply into the cervical stroma (Fig. 41-27.4). As a result, the tissue is excised in two pieces, and both are sent for evaluation. Similar to cold-knife conization, the specimen is marked with suture to note its 12 o'clock position in situ.

LASER CONIZATION

Excision of a laser cone biopsy specimen uses similar techniques as those described for laser

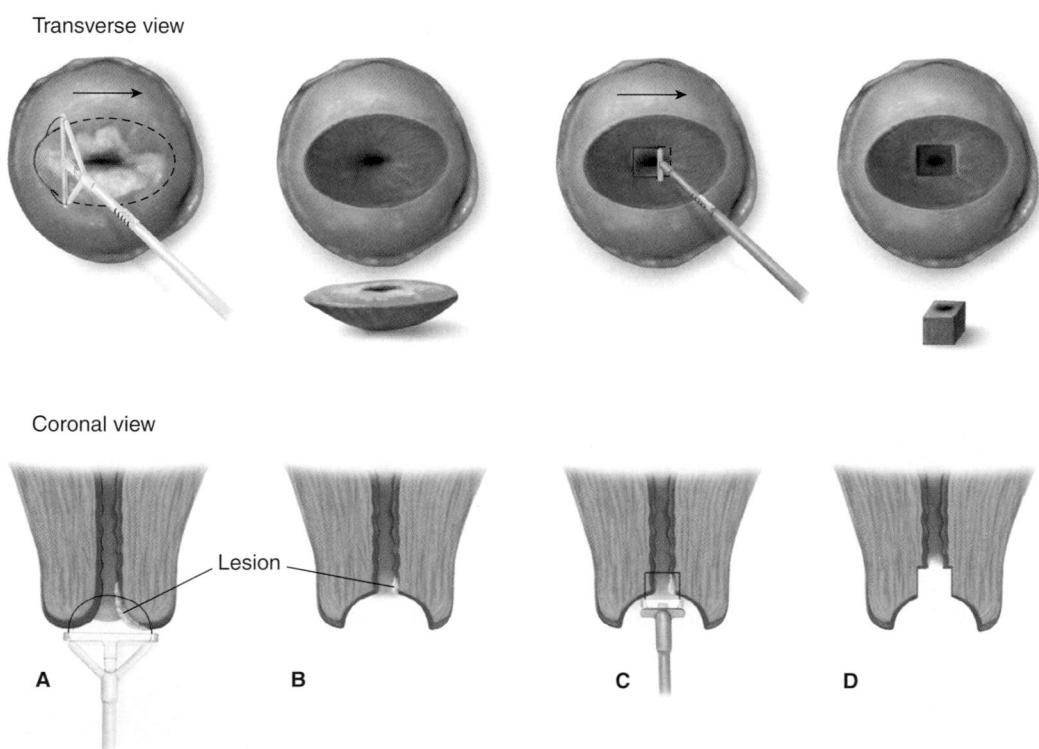

Transverse view

Coronal view

Lesion

A   B   C   D

FIGURE 41-27.4 Loop electrosurgical excision procedure (LEEP) "top hat" cervical conization procedure transverse (*upper row*) and coronal (*lower row*) views. **A.** Excision of ectocervical portion of lesion. **B.** Appearance of cervix following ectocervical excision. **C.** Excision of endocervical portion of lesion. **D.** Appearance of cervix upon completion of procedure.

ablation (Section 41-26, p. 1081). However, rather than ablating the involved tissue, laser energy is directed to cut and remove the cone-biopsy specimen. A higher power density is used to create a cutting effect, for example, 25 W with a 1-mm spot size (PD = 2500 W/cm^2). A cone-shaped specimen is then excised. During excision of the cone specimen, nonreflective tissue hooks may be needed to retract the ectocervical edge away from the laser beam path and to create tissue tension along the plane of incision.

POSTOPERATIVE

Recovery following all excisional methods is rapid and follows that for other surgeries of the cervix previously described (p. 1079). Patients require postoperative surveillance for identification of disease persistence or recurrence, and this is described in detail in Chapter 29 (p. 754).

41-28

Treatment of Vulvar Intraepithelial Neoplasia

WIDE LOCAL EXCISION

With high-grade vulvar intraepithelial neoplasia (VIN), treatment goals include prevention of invasive vulvar cancer and when possible, the preservation of normal vulvar anatomy and function. For more widespread VIN, simple vulvectomy may be appropriate treatment and is described in Section 44-26 (p. 1335). However, less extensive methods such as wide local excision of lesions, ablative modalities, and medical treatments have also been evaluated as alternative options (Chap. 29, p. 760) (Hillemanns, 2006).

Of these, wide local excision of lesions is favored by many. It removes the preinvasive lesion, offers a tissue specimen for exclusion of invasive disease and evaluation of surgical margins, and compared with simple vulvectomy, lowers patient morbidity. In cases where excision involves the clitoris, urethra, or anus, a combined surgical excision and laser ablation approach is sometimes helpful. This combined technique uses CO_2 laser vaporization at sites where excision might lead to dysfunction or poor cosmesis (Cardosi, 2001).

PREOPERATIVE

Patient Evaluation

Prior to excision, full evaluation of the lower reproductive tract for evidence of invasive disease should be completed as outlined in Chapter 29 (p. 747). Importantly, vulvar biopsies are obtained during this evaluation and should exclude invasive disease, which would warrant more extensive excision (Chap. 31, p. 799).

Consent

Wide local excision of high-grade VIN successfully treats disease, and progression to invasive vulvar cancer is low (3 to 5 percent) (Jones, 2005; Rodolakis, 2003). However, VIN recurrence is common, and even in those patients with tissue margins negative for disease, recurrence ranges from 15 to 40 percent (Kuppers, 1997; Modesitt, 1998).

In the immunocompetent, surgical and postoperative risks are few and typically include wound infection or separation, chronic vulvodynia, dyspareunia, and scar-

ring or altered vulvar appearance. Any vulvar operation requires thorough preoperative counseling regarding expectations for anatomic outcome and for sexual function.

INTRAOPERATIVE

SURGICAL STEPS

❶ **Anesthesia and Patient Positioning.** The choice of anesthesia or analgesia will vary depending upon the location and size of the lesion being treated. Whereas smaller labial or perineal lesions may easily be excised using local analgesia in an office setting, larger lesions or those involving the urethra and/or clitoris may require general or regional anesthesia. The patient is placed in dorsal lithotomy position, pubic hair at the surgical site is clipped, and the vulva is surgically prepared.

❷ **Lesion Identification.** The area of excision should be well demarcated. For this, colposcopic examination following application of 3- to 5-percent acetic acid to the vulva will aid identification of lesion margins. A 5-mm circumferential surgical margin surrounding the lesion is recommended by most (Joura, 2002). In the past, toluidine blue has been used to stain nuclear chromatin and enhance vulvar lesions. However, normal tissue can also absorb the stain and distort true disease margins and is therefore not recommended.

❸ **Incision.** A scalpel with a No. 15 surgical blade is used to incise the lesion (Fig. 41-28.1). An elliptical incision is preferred and aids wound reapproximation. Most VIN lesions fail to extend deeper than 2 mm on non-hair-bearing areas such as the labia minora. However, in hair-bearing areas of the vulva, VIN may extend to the deepest hair follicles. This is generally deeper than 2 mm, but not more than 4 mm. Thus, incision depth will vary depending on lesion location (Preti, 2005). Once the incision is created, Adson forceps or skin hooks can elevate and put traction along the incision line. Dissection beneath the lesion begins at the incision periphery and progresses toward the center and then to the opposite incision margin.

Disease recurrence is related to the presence or absence of disease-free surgical margins. Thus, frozen sections of the specimen margins can be evaluated intraoperatively (Friedrich, 1983).

❹ **Margin Undermining.** Reapproximation of the wound edges without tension will decrease the risk of postoperative superficial separation. For this reason, a surgeon may need to sharply undermine the wound margins with fine scissors to mobilize the skin and immediate underlying subcutaneous tissue.

❺ **Wound Closure.** The edges of the skin are then reapproximated with interrupted stitches using 3-0 or 4-0 delayed-absorbable sutures.

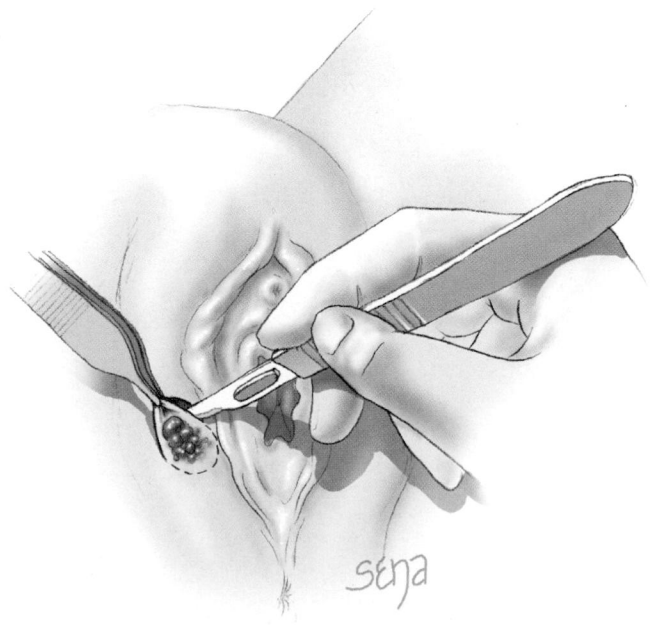

FIGURE 41-28.1 Vulvar incision.

POSTOPERATIVE

Without complication, recovery from wide local excision is typically rapid, and patients may resume normal activities as desired. Sitz baths and oral analgesics are usually recommended for the first week following surgery. Intercourse is delayed until wounds have fully healed, and this time will vary depending on wound site and size. Superficial wound separation is not uncommon, and sites of separation will heal by secondary intention.

There is significant risk for VIN recurrence. Accordingly, postprocedural surveillance is essential, with colposcopic vulvar examination every 6 months for 1 year and then annually thereafter.

CAVITATIONAL ULTRASONIC SURGICAL ASPIRATION (CUSA)

Indications for use and mechanism of action of cavitational ultrasonic surgical aspiration are discussed more fully in Chapter 40 (p. 1002). Briefly, cavitational changes are produced within tissue, causing fragmentation and disruption of the tissue, which is then aspirated and collected. Thus, the tissue, although fragmented, can be sent for histologic or cytologic evaluation.

Treatment of high-grade VIN with CUSA usually produces excellent cosmetic results, and complications such as scarring and dyspareunia are rare. However, the recurrence rate is high, as it is with other treatment modalities for VIN. It should generally be reserved for non-hair-bearing vulvar skin. Miller (2002) found higher rates of VIN recurrence if CUSA was used on these areas compared with its use on hair-bearing areas. Although the procedure allows for tissue evaluation, tissue disruption may preclude adequate examination of all parts of the specimen and their associated relationships. Cost is greater than for excisional therapy and is similar to the cost of laser therapy. Depending on lesion size, CUSA can be more time consuming compared with excision or laser ablation. However, compared with laser therapy, CUSA lacks a smoke plume, which may carry carcinogenic materials and avoids the risks associated with radiant energy, such as burns, eye injuries, and fires.

In addition to treatment for VIN, cavitational therapy works well for condyloma acuminata, particularly bulky or multifocal condyloma or condyloma that are refractory to topical treatment (Fig. 41-28.2). Information regarding cavitational therapy for condyloma acuminata is included in this section due to the similarity of treatment for VIN. Further, the underlying cause of condyloma and VIN is often similar, that is, human papillomavirus (HPV).

PREOPERATIVE

Patient Evaluation

The same principles apply as for excisional treatment of VIN. Specifically, a full evaluation of the lower genital tract is indicated to exclude an invasive process. Although condyloma acuminata are often diagnosed and treated on the basis of clinical appearance, a complete evaluation of the lower genital tract should likewise be undertaken preoperatively.

Consent

Risks of cavitational therapy for VIN or condyloma are few and are similar to wide local excision. Postoperative healing is by secondary intention and may take several weeks.

INTRAOPERATIVE

Instruments

The CUSA unit consists of a console, an operative handpiece, and a foot pedal, by which the system is activated (Fig. 41-28.3). The console allows control of amplitude or intensity, irrigation, and aspiration. Amplitude determines the relative amount of tissue fragmentation. A setting at 1 will produce cellular fragmentation to a depth of 30 μm, whereas a setting at 10 will produce cellular fragmentation to a depth of 300 μm. Fragmentation of a specific tissue is dependent on the water content of a given tissue. Therefore, less power is required for tissues with high water content

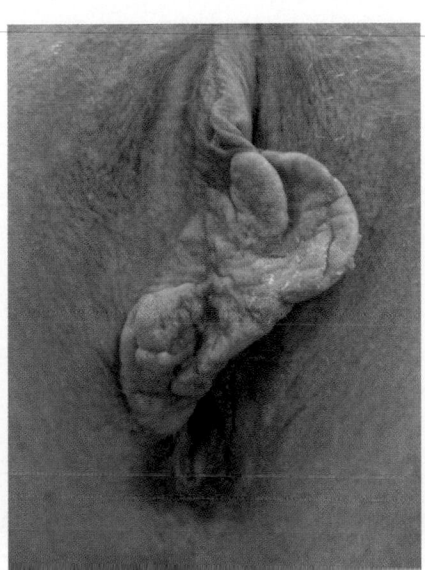

FIGURE 41-28.2 Bulky condyloma involving the right labium minorum.

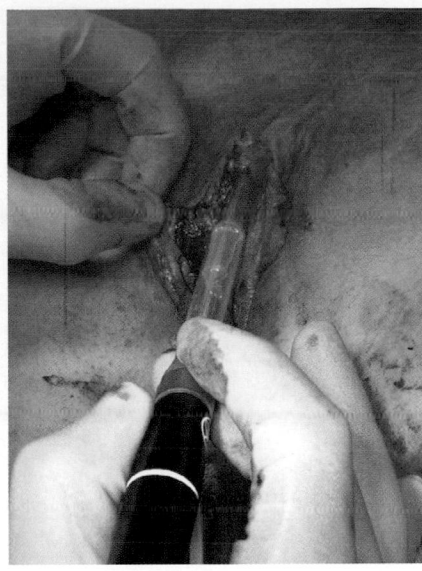

FIGURE 41-28.3 Operative handpiece of the CUSA unit.

such as skin and condyloma. Irrigation is used to control the considerable heat generated by the vibrating titanium tip of the handpiece and for suspension of the fragmented tissue. The tip has a hollow 2-mm diameter and will remove tissue within a 1- to 2-mm radius of the tip. Vaporized and fragmented tissue is aspirated through the hollow tip of the handpiece and collected in a tissue trap. Each console setting may be varied depending on the needs of the operator.

SURGICAL STEPS

❶ **Anesthesia and Patient Positioning.** Cavitational therapy is performed in the operating room under regional or general anesthesia. The patient is placed in the dorsal lithotomy position. The vulva and the perianal region, if involved with disease, are surgically prepped.

❷ **Lesion Identification.** The same colposcopic identification techniques used prior to wide local excision apply for CUSA (p. 1086). In Figure 41-28.4, two areas of VIN are evident even prior to application 3- to 5-percent acetic acid. The larger of the two is located in the midportion of the right labium minorum, and the smaller is more anterior and toward the clitoris.

❸ **Console Settings.** For treatment of VIN and condyloma acuminata, an amplitude setting at 5 to 6 produces cellular fragmentation to a tissue depth of 150 μm to 180 μm and should allow adequate removal of tissue without significant thermal injury.

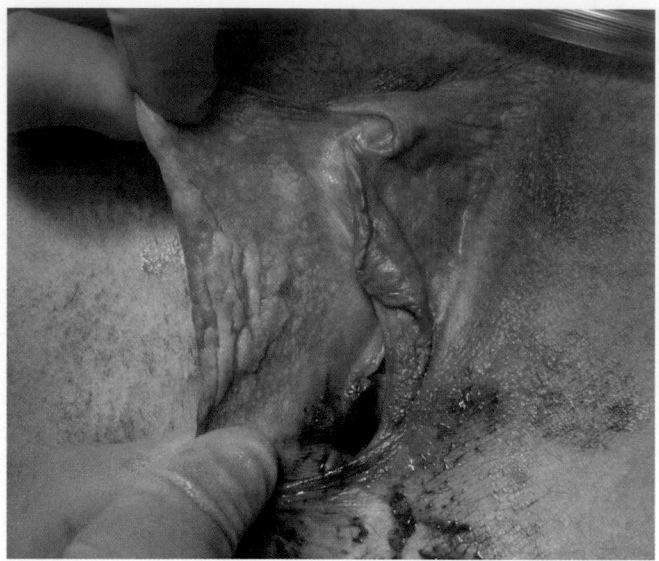

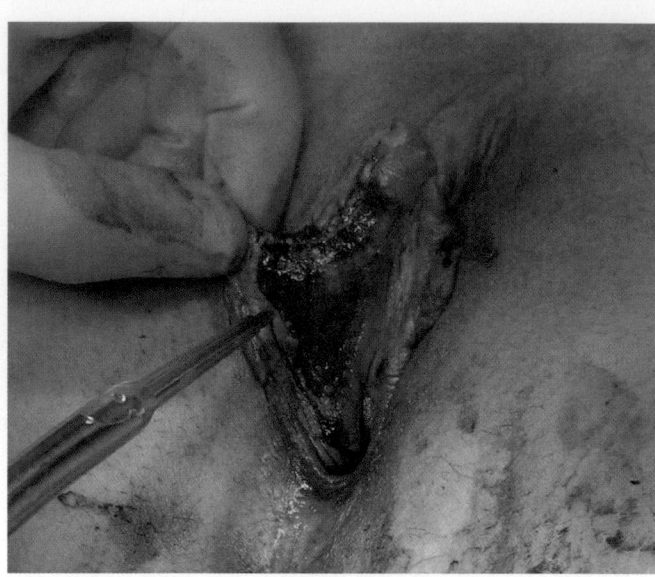

FIGURE 41-28.4 VIN involving the right labium minorum.

FIGURE 41-28.5 Treatment of VIN completed.

However, some studies have used amplitude settings at 6 to 8 for treatment of VIN (Miller, 2002). Irrigation and aspiration rates may be varied depending on the need of the operator. For example, if tissue fulguration is desired, a decrease in the irrigation rate will permit additional heat production at the handpiece tip. Aerosolization can be minimized with proper balance of irrigation and aspiration rates.

❹ **Ablation.** As with wide local excision, the area of treatment should extend at least 5 mm beyond the identified lesion(s). The tip of the handpiece is moved over the vulva in a back-and-forth movement. Only close contact with the skin of the vulva is required; no pressure is necessary. Repeat movements of the tip over the involved area dictate the depth of tissue removal. However, depth of destruction is often difficult to assess. Collagen bundles and elastic fibers become visible in the reticular dermis (Reid, 1985). Tissue destruction beyond this point increases the likelihood of scarring. For treatment of VIN, depth of treatment may vary between 1.5 and 2.5 mm (Miller, 2002; Rader, 1991). For condyloma acuminata, depth of treatment need not extend beyond the basement membrane (Ferenczy, 1983). Bleeding, if any, is usually minor and is controlled with pressure. Figure 41-28.5 shows the end result for the same patient shown in Figure 41-28.4.

POSTOPERATIVE

A 1-percent silver sulfadiazine cream may be applied to the vulva immediately following ablative therapy and continued once or twice daily for a short time. Oral analgesics and sitz baths are helpful in pain management following therapy. Patients may be seen for follow-up 2 to 4 weeks postoperatively.

CARBON DIOXIDE LASER VAPORIZATION OF VIN

In theory, the CO_2 laser is an ideal means to treat VIN. When used with the colposcope, the laser can accurately eradicate disease while preserving normal tissue structure and function. Associated bleeding is scant, healing is usually excellent, and scarring is minimal. Rates of significant complications are generally low. CO_2 laser vaporization may also be considered as an addition to an excisional procedure. One example is if there is multifocal disease involving both hair-bearing and non-hair-bearing areas, such as the clitoris, where excision may not be ideal.

As is the case with other destructive techniques, invasive disease must be excluded before laser vaporization is performed. Since VIN is often multifocal, a thorough examination of the vulva and the lower genital tract with biopsy of any abnormally appearing area is imperative. No tissue sample will be available for analysis following CO_2 laser vaporization.

Reid and colleagues (1985) recommend that only those surgeons experienced with CO_2 lasers should attempt VIN vaporization by this method. Indeed, there is literally a thin margin between the depth of therapy needed to eradicate disease and a depth that may produce delayed healing, scarring, and a poor cosmetic result.

PREOPERATIVE

Consent

As is true also with other methods for treatment of VIN, recurrence or persistence of VIN following CO_2 laser vaporization is possible. Factors such as length of patient surveillance, number of therapy courses, specific area of treatment, and total area of treated disease affect these rates. Patients should understand the need for postoperative surveillance.

Pain, infection, fever, skin depigmentation, alopecia, scarring, and dyspareunia may result from treatment. Healing is generally compete in 4 to 6 weeks, but may be delayed if treatment extends significantly into the dermis (Wright, 1987). Laser vaporization also carries a risk of inhalation of the plume and aerosolized HPV (Cardosi, 2001).

INTRAOPERATIVE

Instruments

A general description of the CO_2 laser is found in Section 41-26 (p. 1081). Recommendations regarding its use for cervical ablation of CIN are likewise appropriate for treatment of VIN.

SURGICAL STEPS

❶ **Anesthesia and Patient Positioning.** Laser ablation of VIN is nearly always performed as an outpatient procedure either in an office setting or in an operative suite depending on laser availability. The procedure may be performed under general, regional, or local anesthesia. Ferenczy and associates (1994) used disease greater than 6 cm^2 as a criterion for general anesthesia. The patient is placed in the dorsal lithotomy position. To lessen the risk of injury from misdirected laser energy to tissues beyond those being treated, wet towels are positioned around the operative field. Paper drapes are avoided due to risk of fire. A moistened sponge is placed inside the rectum to prevent possible ignition of flatal gas.

❷ Laser Settings. The laser is coupled to the colposcope, and the assembly is brought into focus on the vulva. A power density (PD) of 600 to 1200 W/cm^2 delivered in continuous mode is sufficient for therapy, although Reid and associates (1985) caution that PD >600 W/cm^2 may be difficult to control on the vulva. Average PD = 100 × W/D^2, where D = spot diameter in mm at 10 W at 0.1 s pulse. A power of 10 W with a spot diameter of 1 mm will yield a PD of 1000 W/cm^2.

❸ Examination of Treatment Area. After a soaking application of 3- to 5-percent acetic acid solution is applied to the vulva, the area to be treated is examined colposcopically to delineate the zone of vaporization. This may be marked with the laser beam, incorporating a margin of 5 mm or upward to 1 cm of normal appearing tissue (Helmerhorst, 1990; Hoffman, 1992).

❹ Ablation. The location of VIN will determine the needed depth of laser beam penetration for treatment. As hair root sheaths may harbor VIN up to a depth of 2.5 mm, involved hairy areas of the vulva will require laser penetration into the reticular dermis (Mene, 1985). Wright and Davies (1987) recommend a depth of 3 mm for hair-bearing areas and consider this depth to correspond well with destruction into the third surgical plane as described by Reid and coworkers (1985). Further, Cardosi and coworkers (2001) do not recommend laser treatment of VIN involving hair-bearing areas due to the chance of excessively deep tissue destruction and possible scarring and disfigurement. An important point to remember in this regard is that a zone of thermal necrosis will extend beyond the crater depth produced by the laser beam. Non-hair-bearing areas contain no adnexal structures and therefore, if laser is used, do not require deeper treatment. One millimeter or less of laser penetration is adequate for treatment of VIN in these areas, that is, no deeper than the basement membrane.

❺ Reexamination. Carbonized debris is removed, and 3- to 5-percent acetic acid solution applied to the vulva, which is again examined colposcopically to confirm no remaining areas of disease.

POSTOPERATIVE

Care should be taken to avert adhesion formation (labial coaptation) of treated areas. Avoidance of restricting clothing and separation of the labia at least daily are recommended. Salt water sitz bath two to three times per day is cleansing and frequently gives temporary relief of postoperative vulvar discomfort. Other measures that may be helpful include application of 1-percent silver sulfadiazine cream two to three times per day, oral analgesics, topical anesthetics, and cool blow drying of the vulva. The patient should refrain from sexual activity until healing is complete.

The first postoperative visit may be scheduled at 4 to 6 weeks following the laser vaporization procedure. An acceptable schedule for surveillance of persistent or recurrent VIN is examination every 6 months for 1 year and then yearly thereafter. This is identical to that for wide local excision or CUSA. However, more frequent visits, particularly in the first year after treatment, may be warranted depending on individual patient characteristics.

REFERENCES

Adams-Hillard PJ: Imperforate hymen. 2010. Available at: http://emedicine.medscape.com/article/269050-overview. Accessed March 13, 2011

Adamson CD, Naik BJ, Lynch DJ: The vacuum expandable condom mold: a simple vaginal stent for McIndoe-style vaginoplasty. Plast Reconstr Surg 113:664, 2004

Ahmad G, Duffy JM, Farquhar C, et al: Barrier agents for adhesion prevention after gynaecological surgery. Cochrane Database Syst Rev 2:CD000475, 2008

Alessandrescu D, Peltecu GC, Buhimschi CS, et al: Neocolpopoiesis with split-thickness skin graft as a surgical treatment of vaginal agenesis: retrospective review of 201 cases. Am J Obstet Gynecol 175:131, 1996

Alter GJ: A new technique for aesthetic labia minora reduction. Ann Plast Surg 40:287, 1998

Alvarez RD, Helm CW, Edwards RP, et al: Prospective randomized trial of LLETZ versus laser ablation in patients with cervical intraepithelial neoplasia. Gynecol Oncol 52:175, 1994

American College of Obstetricians and Gynecologists: Alternatives to hysterectomy in the management of leiomyomas. Practice Bulletin No. 96, August 2008a

American College of Obstetricians and Gynecologists: Antibiotic prophylaxis for gynecologic procedures. Practice Bulletin No. 104, May 2009a

American College of Obstetricians and Gynecologists: Benefits and risks of sterilization. Practice Bulletin No. 46, September 2003

American College of Obstetricians and Gynecologists: Choosing the route of hysterectomy for benign disease. Practice Bulletin No. 96, November 2009b

American College of Obstetricians and Gynecologists: Elective and risk-reducing salpingo-oophorectomy. Practice Bulletin No. 89, January 2008b

American College of Obstetricians and Gynecologists: Nonsurgical diagnosis and management of vaginal agenesis. Committee Opinion No. 274, July 2002

American College of Obstetricians and Gynecologists: Supracervical hysterectomy. Committee Opinion No. 388, November 2007

Anania C, Malinak L: Developmental anomalies of the vulva and vagina. In Kaufman RH, Faro S (eds): Benign Diseases of the Vulva and Vagina. St. Louis, MO, Mosby, 1994, p 28

Anderson MC, Hartley RB: Cervical crypt involvement by intraepithelial neoplasia. Obstet Gynecol 55:546, 1980

Asante A, Whiteman MK, Kulkarni A, et al: Elective oophorectomy in the United States: trends and in-hospital complications, 1998-2006. Obstet Gynecol 116(5):1088, 2010

Ashworth MF, Morton KE, Dewhurst J, et al: Vaginoplasty using amnion. Obstet Gynecol 67:443, 1986

Ayers JW, Morley GW: Surgical incision for cesarean section. Obstet Gynecol 70(5):706, 1987

Baggish MS: Total and subtotal abdominal hysterectomy. Best Pract Res Clin Obstet Gynaecol 19:333, 2005

Baldauf JJ, Dreyfus M, Ritter J, et al: Risk of cervical stenosis after large loop excision or laser conization. Obstet Gynecol 88:933, 1996

Bangsgaard N, Lund CO, Ottesen B, et al: Improved fertility following conservative surgi-cal treatment of ectopic pregnancy. Br J Obstet Gynaecol 110:765, 2003

Barutcu A, Akguner M: McIndoe vaginoplasty with the inflatable vaginal stent. Ann Plast Surg 41:568, 1998

Benagiano G, Kivinen ST, Fadini R, et al: Zoladex (goserelin acetate) and the anemic patient: results of a multicenter fibroid study. Fertil Steril 66:223, 1996

Benedet JL, Miller DM, Nickerson KG, et al: The results of cryosurgical treatment of cervical intraepithelial neoplasia at one, five, and ten years. Am J Obstet Gynecol 157:268, 1987

Benedet JL, Nickerson KG, Anderson GH: Cryotherapy in the treatment of cervical intraepithelial neoplasia. Obstet Gynecol 58:725, 1981

Bergeron S, Binik YM, Khalife S, et al: A randomized comparison of group cognitive-behavioral therapy, surface electromyographic biofeedback, and vestibulectomy in the treatment of dyspareunia resulting from vulvar vestibulitis. Pain 91:297, 2001

Bieber E: Myomectomy by laparotomy. In Bieber E, Maclin V (eds): Myomectomy. Malden, MA, Blackwell Science, 1998, p. 96

Blakely DH, Dewhurst CJ, Tipton RH: The long term results after marsupialization of Bartholin cysts and abscesses. J Obstet Gynaecol British Commonw 73:1008, 1966

Bleker OP, Smalbraak DJ, Schutte MF: Bartholin's abscess: the role of Chlamydia trachomatis. Genitourin Med 66:24, 1990

Boonstra H, Aalders JG, Koudstaal J, et al: Minimum extension and appropriate topographic position of tissue destruction for treatment of cervical intraepithelial neoplasia. Obstet Gynecol 75:227, 1990a

Boonstra H, Koudstaal J, Oosterhuis JW, et al: Analysis of cryolesions in the uterine cervix: application techniques, extension, and failures. Obstet Gynecol 75:232, 1990b

Bornstein J, Zarfati D, Goldik Z, et al: Perineoplasty compared with vestibuloplasty for severe vulvar vestibulitis. Br J Obstet Gynaecol 102:652, 1995

Bornstein J, Zarfati D, Goldik Z, et al: Vulvar vestibulitis: physical or psychosexual problem? Obstet Gynecol 93:876, 1999

Broekmans FJ: GnRH agonists and uterine leiomyomas. Hum Reprod 11:3, 1996

Bukovsky I, Liftshitz Y, Langer R, et al: Ovarian residual syndrome. Surg Gynecol Obstet 167:132, 1988

Bunnasathiansri S, Herabutya Y, Prasertsawat P: Vaginal misoprostol for cervical priming before dilatation and curettage in postmenopausal women: a randomized, controlled trial. J Obstet Gynaecol Res 30:221, 2004

Burrows LJ, Meyn LA, Weber AM: Rates of hysterectomy for uterine myomas and myomectomy in the United States, 1979–2001. J Pelvic Med Surg 2:84, 2005

Cardosi RJ, Bomalaski JJ, Hoffman MS: Diagnosis and management of vulvar and vaginal intraepithelial neoplasia. Obstet Gynecol Clin North Am 28:685, 2001

Castelo-Branco C, Figueras F, Sanjuan A, et al: Long-term compliance with estrogen replacement therapy in surgical postmenopausal women: benefits to bone and analysis of factors associated with discontinuation. Menopause 6:307, 1999

Chiaffarino F, Parazzini F, Decarli A, et al: Hysterectomy with or without unilateral oophorectomy and risk of ovarian cancer. Gynecol Oncol 97:318, 2005

Christianson MS, Barker MA, Lindheim SR: Overcoming the challenging cervix: techniques to access the uterine cavity. J Low Genit Tract Dis 12(1):24, 2008

Chua GC, Wilsher M, Young MPA, et al: Comparison of particle penetration with nonspherical polyvinyl alcohol versus trisacryl gelatin microspheres in women undergoing premyomectomy uterine artery embolization. Clin Radiol 60:116, 2005

Clausen I: Conservative versus radical surgery for tubal pregnancy: a review. Acta Obstet Gynecol Scand 75:8, 1996

Concannon MJ, Croll GH, Puckett CL: An intraoperative stent for McIndoe vaginal construction. Plast Reconstr Surg 91:367, 1993

Crane JM: Pregnancy outcome after loop electrosurgical excision procedure: a systematic review. Obstet Gynecol 102:1058, 2003

Creasman WT, Hinshaw WM, Clarke-Pearson DL: Cryosurgery in the management of cervical intraepithelial neoplasia. Obstet Gynecol 63:145, 1984

Crosignani PG, Vercellini P, Mosconi P, et al: Levonorgestrel-releasing intrauterine device versus hysteroscopic endometrial resection in the treatment of dysfunctional uterine bleeding. Obstet Gynecol 90:257, 1997

Dainty LA, Elkas JC, Rose GS, et al: Controversial topics in abnormal cervical cytology: "see and treat." Clin Obstet Gynecol 48:193, 2005

Darwish AM, Nasr AM, El Nashar DA: Evaluation of postmyomectomy uterine scar. J Clin Ultrasound 33:181, 2005

Deligdisch L, Hirschmann S, Altchek A: Pathologic changes in gonadotropin-releasing hormone agonist analogue treated uterine leiomyomata. Fertil Steril 67:837, 1997

Denny L, Kuhn L, De Souza M, et al: Screen-and-treat approaches for cervical cancer prevention in low-resource settings: a randomized, controlled trial. JAMA 294:2173, 2005

Deschamps A, Krishnamurthy S: Absence of pulse and blood pressure following vasopressin injection for myomectomy. Can J Anesth 52:552, 2005

Doss BJ, Jacques SM, Qureshi F, et al: Extratubal secondary trophoblastic implants: clinicopathologic correlation and review of the literature. Hum Pathol 29:184, 1998

Downs MC, Randall HW Jr: The ambulatory surgical management of Bartholin duct cysts. J Emerg Med 7:623, 1989

Dunn TS, Killoran K, Wolf D: Complications of outpatient LLETZ procedures. J Reprod Med 49:76, 2004

Dunn TS, Woods J, Burch J: Bowel injury occurring during an outpatient LLETZ procedure: a case report. J Reprod Med 48:49, 2003

Edwards L: New concepts in vulvodynia. Am J Obstet Gynecol 189:S24, 2003

Falcone T, Paraiso MF, Mascha E: Prospective, randomized clinical trial of laparoscopically assisted vaginal hysterectomy versus total abdominal hysterectomy. Am J Obstet Gynecol 180:955, 1999

Farquhar CM, Steiner CA: Hysterectomy rates in the United States, 1990–1997. Obstet Gynecol 99:229, 2002

Farquhar CM: Ectopic pregnancy. Lancet 366:583, 2005

Fedele L, Vercellini P, Bianchi S, et al: Treatment with GnRH agonists before myomectomy and the risk of short-term myoma recurrence. Br J Obstet Gynaecol 97:393, 1990

Ferenczy A: Using the laser to treat condyloma acuminata and intradermal neoplasia. Can Med Assoc J 128:135, 1983

Ferenczy A, Choukroun D, Falcone T, et al: The effect of cervical loop electrosurgical excision on subsequent pregnancy outcome: North American experience. Am J Obstet Gynecol 172:1246, 1995

Ferenczy A, Wright JR, Richart RM: Comparison of CO_2 laser surgery and loop electrosurgical excision/fulguration for the treatment of vulvar intraepithelial neoplasia (VIN). Int J Gynecol Cancer 4:22, 1994

Ferris DG: Lethal tissue temperature during cervical cryotherapy with a small flat cryoprobe. J Fam Pract 38:153, 1994

Fletcher H, Frederick J, Hardie M, et al: A randomized comparison of vasopressin and tourniquet as hemostatic agents during myomectomy. Obstet Gynecol 87:1014, 1996

Food and Drug Administration: October 2002 PMA approvals. 2009. Available at: http://www.fda.gov/MedicalDevices/ProductsandMedicalProcedures/DeviceApprovalsandClearances/PMAApprovals/ucm113094.htm. Accessed March 2, 2011

Frederick J, Fletcher H, Simeon D, et al: Intramyometrial vasopressin as a haemostatic agent during myomectomy. Br J Obstet Gynaecol 101:435, 1994

Friedman AJ, Hoffman DI, Comite F, et al: Treatment of leiomyomata uteri with leuprolide acetate depot: a double-blind, placebo-controlled, multicenter study. The Leuprolide Study Group. Obstet Gynecol 77:720, 1991

Friedrich EJ: Surgical procedures. In Vulvar Disease. Philadelphia, Saunders, 1983, p 61

Gage AA: What temperature is lethal for cells? J Dermatol Surg Oncol 5:459, 1979

Giacalone PL, Daures JP, Vignal J, et al: Pfannenstiel versus Maylard incision for cesarean delivery: a randomized controlled trial. Obstet Gynecol 99(5 Pt 1):745, 2002

Gimbel H, Zobbe V, Andersen BJ, et al: Lower urinary tract symptoms after total and subtotal hysterectomy: results of a randomized, controlled trial. Int Urogynecol J 16:257, 2005a

Gimbel H, Zobbe V, Andersen BM, et al: Total versus subtotal hysterectomy: an observational study with one-year follow-up. Aust N Z J Obstet Gynaecol 45:64, 2005b

Ginsburg ES, Benson CB, Garfield JM, et al: The effect of operative technique and uterine size on blood loss during myomectomy: a prospective, randomized study. Fertil Steril 60:956, 1993

Giraldo F, Gonzalez C, de Haro F: Central wedge nymphectomy with a 90-degree Z-plasty for aesthetic reduction of the labia minora. Plast Reconstr Surg 113:1820, 2004

Goldstein AT, Marinoff SC, Haefner HK: Vulvodynia: strategies for treatment. Clin Obstet Gynecol 48:769, 2005

Green A, Purdie D, Bain C, et al: Tubal sterilisation, hysterectomy and decreased risk of ovarian cancer: survey of Women's Health Study Group. Int J Ca 71:948, 1997

Gunasekera PC, Phipps JH, Lewis BV: Large loop excision of the transformation zone (LLETZ) compared to carbon dioxide laser in the treatment of CIN: a superior mode of treatment. Br J Obstet Gynaecol 97:995, 1990

Haefner HK: Critique of new gynecologic surgical procedures: surgery for vulvar vestibulitis. Clin Obstet Gynecol 43:689, 2000

Haefner HK, Collins ME, Davis GD, et al: The vulvodynia guideline. J Low Gen Tract Dis 9.40, 2005

Hakim-Elahi E, Tovell HM, Burnhill MS: Complications of first-trimester abortion: a report of 170,000 cases. Obstet Gynecol 76:129, 1990

Hannoun-Levi JM, Peiffert D, Hoffstetter S, et al: Carcinoma of the cervical stump: retrospective analysis of 77 cases. Radiother Oncol 43:147, 1997

Harkki-Siren P, Kurki T: A nationwide analysis of laparoscopic complications. Obstet Gynecol 89:108, 1997a

Harkki-Siren P, Sjoberg J, Makinen J, et al: Finnish national register of laparoscopic hysterectomies. a review and complications of 1165 operations. Am J Obstet Gynecol 176:118, 1997b

Harper DM: Paracervical block diminishes cramping associated with cryosurgery. J Fam Pract 44:71, 1997

Harper DM, Cobb JL: Cervical mucosal block effectively reduces the pain and cramping from cryosurgery. J Fam Pract 47:285, 1998

Harper DM, Mayeaux EJ, Daaleman TP, et al: The natural history of cervical cryosurgical healing: the minimal effect of debridement of the cervical eschar. J Fam Pract 49:694, 2000

Harris WJ, Daniell JF: Early complications of laparoscopic hysterectomy. Obstet Gynecol Surv 51:559, 1996

Hartmann KE, Ma C, Lamvu GM, et al: Quality of life and sexual function after hysterectomy in women with preoperative pain and depression. Obstet Gynecol 104:701, 2004

Hellstrom AC, Sigurjonson T, Pettersson F: Carcinoma of the cervical stump: the radium-hemmet series 1959–1987. Treatment and prognosis. Acta Obstet Gynaecol Scand 80:152, 2001

Helmerhorst TJM, van der Vaart CH, Dijkhuizen GH, et al: CO_2-laser therapy in patients with vulvar intraepithelial neoplasia. Eur J Obstet Gynecol Repro Biol 34(1-2):149, 1990

Hill DA, Lense JJ: Office management of Bartholin gland cysts and abscesses. Am Fam Physician 57:1611, 1998

Hillemanns P, Wang X, Staehle S, et al: Evaluation of different treatment modalities for vulvar intraepithelial neoplasia (VIN): CO2 laser vaporization, photodynamic therapy, excision and vulvectomy. Gynecol Oncol 100:271, 2006

Hillis SD, Marchbanks PA, Tylor LR, et al: Poststerilization regret: findings from the United States Collaborative Review of Sterilization. Obstet Gynecol 93:889, 1999

Hoffman MS, Pinelli DM, Finan M, et al: Laser vaporization for vulvar intraepithelial neoplasia. J Reprod Med 37(2):135, 1992

Houlard S, Perrotin F, Fourquet F, et al: Risk factors for cervical stenosis after laser cone biopsy. Eur J Obstet Gynaecol Reprod Biol 104:144, 2002

Husseinzadeh N, Shbaro I, Wesseler T: Predictive value of cone margins and post-cone endocervical curettage with residual disease in subsequent hysterectomy. Gynecol Oncol 33:198, 1989

Hutchins FL Jr: A randomized comparison of vasopressin and tourniquet as hemostatic agents during myomectomy. Obstet Gynecol 88:639, 1996

Imai A, Sugiyama M, Furui T, et al: Gonadotrophin-releasing hormones agonist therapy increases peritoneal fibrinolytic activity and prevents adhesion formation after myomectomy. J Obstet Gynaecol 23:660, 2003

Iverson RE Jr, Chelmow D, Strohbehn K, et al: Relative morbidity of abdominal hysterectomy and myomectomy for management of uterine leiomyomas. Obstet Gynecol 88:415, 1996

Jacob M, Broekhuizen FF, Castro W, et al: Experience using cryotherapy for treatment of cervical precancerous lesions in low-resource settings. Int J Gynaecol Obstet 89:S13, 2005

Jacobson P: Marsupialization of vulvovaginal (Bartholin) cysts. Am J Obstet Gynecol 79:73, 1960

Jacobson P: Vulvovaginal cyst (treatment by marsupialization). West J Surg 58:704, 1950

Jenkins TR: Laparoscopic supracervical hysterectomy. Am J Obstet Gynecol 191:1875, 2004

Jobson VW, Homesley HD: Comparison of cryo-surgery and carbon dioxide laser ablation for treatment of cervical intraepithelial neoplasia. Colposc Gynecol Laser Surg 11:73, 1984

Johns DA, Carrera B, Jones J, et al: The medical and economic impact of laparoscopically assisted vaginal hysterectomy in a large, metropolitan, not-for-profit hospital. Am J Obstet Gynecol 172:1709, 1995

Joki-Erkkilä MM, Heinonen PK: Presenting and long-term clinical implications and fecundity in females with obstructing vaginal malformations. J Pediatr Adolesc Gynecol 16:307, 2003

Jones RW, Rowan DM, Stewart AW: Vulvar intraepithelial neoplasia: aspects of the natural history and outcome in 405 women. Obstet Gynecol 106:1319, 2005

Joura EA: Epidemiology, diagnosis and treatment of vulvar intraepithelial neoplasia. Curr Opin Obstet Gynecol 14:39, 2002

Kambiss SM, Hibbert ML, Macedonia C, et al: Uterine perforation resulting in bowel infarction: sharp traumatic bowel and mesenteric injury at the time of pregnancy termination. Milit Med 165:81, 2000

Keegan GT, Forkowitz MJ: A case report: ureterouterine fistula as a complication of elective abortion. J Urol 123:137, 1982

Kennedy CM, Dewdney S, Galask RP: Vulvar granuloma fissuratum: a description of fissuring of the posterior fourchette and the repair. Obstet Gynecol 105:1018, 2005

Kilkku P: Supravaginal uterine amputation versus hysterectomy with reference to subjective bladder symptoms and incontinence. Acta Obstet Gynaecol Scand 64:375, 1985

Kilkku P, Gronroos M, Hirvonen T, et al: Supravaginal uterine amputation versus hysterectomy: effects on libido and orgasm. Acta Obstet Gynaecol Scand 62:147, 1983

Kilpatrick CC, Alagkiozidis I, Orejuela FJ, et al: factors complicating surgical management of the vulvar abscess. J Reprod Med 55:139, 2010

Klingele CJ, Gebhart JB, Croak AJ, et al: McIndoe procedure for vaginal agenesis: long-term outcome and effect on quality of life. Am J Obstet Gynecol 189:1569, 2003

Kobak WH, Roman LD, Felix JC, et al: The role of endocervical curettage at cervical conization for high-grade dysplasia. Obstet Gynecol 85:197, 1995

Kristensen GB, Jensen LK, Holund B: A randomized trial comparing two methods of cold knife conization with laser conization. Obstet Gynecol 76:1009, 1990

Kristensen J, Langhoff-Roos J, Kristensen FB: Increased risk of preterm birth in women with cervical conization. Obstet Gynecol 81:1005, 1993a

Kristensen J, Langhoff-Roos J, Wittrup M, et al: Cervical conization and preterm delivery/low birth weight: a systematic review of the literature. Acta Obstet Gynaecol Scand 72:640, 1993b

Kuppermann M, Summitt RL Jr, Varner RE, et al: Sexual functioning after total compared with supracervical hysterectomy: a randomized trial. Obstet Gynecol 105:1309, 2005

Kuppers V, Stiller M, Somville T, et al: Risk factors for recurrent VIN: role of multifocality and grade of disease. J Reprod Med 42:140, 1997

Kurata H, Aoki Y, Tanaka K: Delayed, massive bleeding as an unusual complication of laser conization: a case report. J Reprod Med 48:659, 2003

Kyrgiou M, Koliopoulos G, Martin-Hirsch P, et al: Obstetric outcomes after conservative treatment for intraepithelial or early invasive cervical lesions: systematic review and meta-analysis. Lancet 367:489, 2006

LaMorte AI, Lalwani S, Diamond MP: Morbidity associated with abdominal myomectomy. Obstet Gynecol 82:897, 1993

Lavy Y, Lev-Sagie A, Hamani Y, et al: Modified vulvar vestibulectomy: simple and effective surgery for the treatment of vulvar vestibulitis. Eur J Obstet Gynaecol Reprod Biol 120:91, 2005

Learman LA, Summitt RL Jr, Varner RE, et al: A randomized comparison of total or supracervical hysterectomy: surgical complications and clinical outcomes. Obstet Gynecol 102(3):453, 2003

Lethaby A, Vollenhoven B: Fibroids (uterine myomatosis, leiomyomas). Am Fam Physician 71:1753, 2005

Lethaby A, Vollenhoven B, Sowter M: Efficacy of pre-operative gonadotrophin hormone–releasing analogues for women with uterine fibroids undergoing hysterectomy or myomectomy: a systematic review. Br J Obstet Gynaecol 109:1097, 2002

Liang CC, Chang SD, Soong YK: Long-term follow-up of women who underwent surgical correction for imperforate hymen. Arch Gynecol Obstet 269:5, 2003

Lin P, Falcone T, Tulandi T: Excision of ovarian dermoid cyst by laparoscopy and by laparotomy. Am J Obstet Gynecol 173:769, 1995

Lin WC, Chang CY, Shen YY, et al: Use of autologous buccal mucosa for vaginoplasty: a study of eight cases. Hum Reprod 18:604, 2003

Liu WM, Tzeng CR, Yi-Jen C, et al: Combining the uterine depletion procedure and myomectomy may be useful for treating symptomatic fibroids. Fertil Steril 82:205, 2004

Maas SM, Hage JJ: Functional and aesthetic labia minora reduction. Plast Reconstr Surg 105:1453, 2000

MacIsaac L, Darney P: Early surgical abortion: an alternative to and backup for medical abortion. Am J Obstet Gynecol 183:S76, 2000

Mais V, Ajossa S, Piras B, et al: Treatment of nonendometriotic benign adnexal cysts: a randomized comparison of laparoscopy and laparotomy. Obstet Gynecol 86:770, 1995

Marana R, Busacca M, Zupi E, et al: Laparoscopically assisted vaginal hysterectomy versus total abdominal hysterectomy: a prospective, randomized, multicenter study. Am J Obstet Gynecol 180:270, 1999

Marquard KL, Chelmow D: Gynecologic myomectomy. 2008. Available at: http://emedicine.medscape.com/article/267677-overview. Accessed March 13, 2011

Martin-Hirsch PL, Paraskevaidis E, Kitchener H: Surgery for cervical intraepithelial neoplasia. Cochrane Database Syst Rev 6:CD001318, 2010

Masch RJ, Roman AS: Uterine evacuation in the office. Contemp Obstet Gynecol 51:66, 2005

Mathevet P, Chemali E, Roy M, et al: Long-term outcome of a randomized study comparing three techniques of conization: cold knife, laser, and LEEP. Eur J Obstet Gynaecol Reprod Biol 106:214, 2003

Matta WH, Stabile I, Shaw RW, et al: Doppler assessment of uterine blood flow changes in patients with fibroids receiving the gonadotropin-releasing hormone agonist Buserelin. Fertil Steril 49:1083, 1988

Matthews D: Marsupialization in the treatment of Bartholin cyst and abscesses. J Obstet Gynaec Br Commonw 73:1010, 1966

McCormack WM, Spence MR: Evaluation of the surgical treatment of vulvar vestibulitis. Eur J Obstet Gynaecol Reprod Biol 86:135, 1999

McCraw JB, Massey FM, Shanklin KD, et al: Vaginal reconstruction with gracilis myocutaneous flaps. Plast Reconstr Surg 58:176, 1976

McIndoe AH, Banister JB: An operation for the cure of congenital absence of the vagina. J Obstet Gynaecol Br Empire 45:490, 1938

Mencaglia L, Tantini C: GnRH agonist analogs and hysteroscopic resection of myomas. Int J Gynaecol Obstet 43:285, 1993

Mene A, Buckley CH: Involvement of the vulvar skin appendages by intraepithelial neoplasia. Br J Obstet Gynaecol 92:634, 1985

Miller BE: Vulvar intraepithelial neoplasia treated with cavitational ultrasonic surgical aspiration. Gynecol Oncol 85:114, 2002

Mitchell MF, Tortolero-Luna G, Cook E, et al: A randomized clinical trial of cryotherapy, laser vaporization, and loop electrosurgical excision for treatment of squamous intraepithelial lesions of the cervix. Obstet Gynecol 92:737, 1998

Moawad NS, Mahajan ST, Moniz MH, et al: Current diagnosis and treatment of interstitial pregnancy. Am J Obstet Gynecol 202:15, 2010

Modesitt SC, Waters AB, Walton L, et al: Vulvar intraepithelial neoplasia III: occult cancer and the impact of margin status on recurrence. Obstet Gynecol 92:962, 1998

Mol BW, Matthijsse HC, Tinga DJ, et al: Fertility after conservative and radical surgery for tubal pregnancy. Hum Reprod 13:1804, 1998

Motoyama S, Laoag-Fernandez JB, Mochizuki S, et al: Vaginoplasty with Interceed absorbable adhesion barrier for complete squamous epithelialization in vaginal agenesis. Am J Obstet Gynecol 188:1260, 2003

Murphy AA, Nager CW, Wujek JJ, et al: Operative laparoscopy versus laparotomy for the management of ectopic pregnancy: a prospective trial. Fertil Steril 57:1180, 1992

National Institute for Occupational Safety and Health: Control of smoke from laser/electric surgical procedures. Appl Occup Environ Hyg 14:71, 1999

Ngeh N, Belli AM, Morgan R, et al: Pre-myomectomy uterine artery embolisation minimises operative blood loss. Br J Obstet Gynaecol 111:1139, 2004

Nieboer TE, Johnson N, Lethaby A, et al: Surgical approach to hysterectomy for benign gynaecological disease. Cochrane Database Syst Rev 3:CD003677, 2009

Novak F: Marsupialization of Bartholin cysts and abscesses. In Novak F (ed): Surgical Gynecologic Techniques. New York, Wiley, 1978, p 191

Numnum TM, Kirby TO, Leath CA, III, et al: A prospective evaluation of "see and treat" in women with HSIL Pap smear results: is this an appropriate strategy? J Low Gen Tract Dis 9:2, 2005

Nuovo J, Melnikow J, Willan AR, et al: Treatment outcomes for squamous intraepithelial lesions. Int J Gynaecol Obstet 68:25, 2000

Okaro EO, Jones KD, Sutton C: Long term outcome following laparoscopic supracervical hysterectomy. Br J Obstet Gynaecol 108:1017, 2001

Olive DL: Dogma, skepsis, and the analytic method: the role of prophylactic oophorectomy at the time of hysterectomy. Obstet Gynecol 106:214, 2005

Omole F, Simmons BJ, Hacker Y: Management of Bartholin's duct cyst and gland abscess. Am Fam Physician 68:135, 2003

Ostergard DR: Cryosurgical treatment of cervical intraepithelial neoplasia. Obstet Gynecol 56:231, 1980

Ozek C, Gurler T, Alper M, et al: Modified McIndoe procedure for vaginal agenesis. Ann Plast Surg 43:393, 1999

Parker WH, Broder MS, Liu Z, et al: Ovarian conservation at the time of hysterectomy for benign disease. Obstet Gynecol 106:219, 2005

Pasley WW: Trachelectomy: a review of fifty-five cases. Am J Obstet Gynecol 159:728, 1988

Pati S, Cullins V: Female sterilization: evidence. Obstet Gynecol Clin North Am 27:859, 2000

Peipert JF, Weitzen S, Cruickshank C, et al: Risk factors for febrile morbidity after hysterectomy. Obstet Gynecol 103:86, 2004

Penna C, Fambrini M, Fallani MG, et al: Laser CO_2 conization in postmenopausal age: risk of cervical stenosis and unsatisfactory follow-up. Gynecol Oncol 96:771, 2005

Periti P, Mazzei T, Orlandini F, et al: Comparison of the antimicrobial prophylactic efficacy of cefotaxime and cephazolin in obstetric and gynaecological surgery: a randomised multi-centre study. Drugs 35:133, 1988

Peterson HB, Xia Z, Hughes JM, et al: The risk of pregnancy after tubal sterilization: findings from the U.S. Collaborative Review of Sterilization. Am J Obstet Gynecol 174:1161, 1996

Pittaway DE, Takacs P, Bauguess P: Laparoscopic adnexectomy: a comparison with laparotomy. Am J Obstet Gynecol 171:385, 1991

Pratt JH, Jefferies JA: The retained cervical stump: a 25-year experience. Obstet Gynecol 48:711, 1976

Preti M, Van Seters M, Sideri M, et al: Squamous vulvar intraepithelial neoplasia. Clin Obstet Gynecol 48:845, 2005

Rader JS, Leake JF, Dillon MB, et al: Ultrasonic surgical aspiration in the treatment of vulvar disease. Obstet Gynecol 77:573, 1991

Radman HM, Korman W: Uterine perforation during dilatation and curettage. Obstet Gynecol 21:210, 1963

Rahn DD, Phelan JN, Roshanravan SM, et al: Anterior abdominal wall nerve and vessel anatomy: clinical implications for gynecologic surgery. Am J Obstet Gynecol 202(3):234.e1, 2010

Raio L, Ghezzi F, Di Naro E, et al: Duration of pregnancy after carbon dioxide laser conization of the cervix: influence of cone height. Obstet Gynecol 90:978, 1997

Ravina JH, Bouret JM, Fried D, et al: Value of preoperative embolization of uterine fibroma: report of a multicenter series of 31 cases. Fertil Contracep Sex 23:45, 1995

Reid R, Elfont EA, Zirkin RM, et al: Superficial laser vulvectomy. II. The anatomic and biophysical principles permitting accurate control over the depth of dermal destruction with carbon dioxide laser. Am J Obstet Gynecol 152(3):261, 1985

Reinsch RC, Murphy AA, Morales AJ, et al: The effects of RU 486 and leuprolide acetate on uterine artery blood flow in the fibroid uterus:

a prospective, randomized study. Am J Obstet Gynecol 170:1623, 1994

Riva HL, Hefner JD, Marchetti AA, et al: Prophylactic trachelectomy of cervical stump: two hundred and twelve cases. South Med J 54:1082, 1961

Rodolakis A, Diakomanolis E, Vlachos G, et al: Vulvar intraepithelial neoplasia (VIN): diagnostic and therapeutic challenges. Eur J Gynaecol Oncol 24:317, 2003

Roussis NP, Waltrous L, Kerr A, et al: Sexual response in the patient after hysterectomy: total abdominal versus supracervical versus vaginal procedure. Am J Obstet Gynecol 190:1427, 2004

Rouzier R, Haddad B, Deyrolle C, et al: Perineoplasty for the treatment of introital stenosis related to vulvar lichen sclerosus. Am J Obstet Gynecol 186:49, 2002

Rybak EA, Polotsky AJ, Woreta T, et al: Explained compared with unexplained fever in postoperative myomectomy and hysterectomy patients. Obstet Gynecol 111(5):1137, 2008

Ryder RM, Vaughan MC: Laparoscopic tubal sterilization: methods, effectiveness, and sequelae. Obstet Gynecol Clin North Am 26:83, 1999

Sadler L, Saftlas A, Wang W, et al: Treatment for cervical intraepithelial neoplasia and risk of preterm delivery. JAMA 291:2100, 2004

Salom EM, Penalver M: Complications in gynecologic surgery. In Cohn SM, Barquist E, Byers PM, et al (eds): Complications in Surgery and Trauma. New York, Informa Healthcare USA, 2007, p 554

Samson SLA, Bentley JR, Fahey TJ, et al: The effect of loop electrosurgical excision procedure on future pregnancy outcome. Obstet Gynecol 105:325, 2005

Sapmaz E, Celik H, Altungul A: Bilateral ascending uterine artery ligation vs tourniquet use for hemostasis in cesarean myomectomy: a comparison. J Reprod Med 48:950, 2003

Saul HM, Grossman MB: The role of *Chlamydia trachomatis* in Bartholin's gland abscess. Am J Obstet Gynecol 158:76, 1988

Sawaya GF, Grady D, Kerlikowske K, et al: Antibiotics at the time of induced abortion: the case for universal prophylaxis based on a meta-analysis. Obstet Gynecol 87:884, 1996

Sawin SW, Pilevsky ND, Berlin JA, et al: Comparability of perioperative morbidity between abdominal myomectomy and hysterectomy for women with uterine leiomyomas. Am J Obstet Gynecol 183:1448, 2000

Schantz A, Thormann L: Cryosurgery for dysplasia of the uterine ectocervix: a randomized study of the efficacy of the single- and double-freeze techniques. Acta Obstet Gynaecol Scand 63:417, 1984

Schmidt T, Eren Y, Breidenbach M, et al: Modifications of laparoscopic supracervical hysterectomy technique significantly reduce postoperative spotting. J Minim Invasive Gynecol 18(1):81, 2011

Schneider D, Yaron M, Bukovsky I, et al: Outcome of surgical treatment for superficial dyspareunia from vulvar vestibulitis. J Reprod Med Obstet Gynecol 46:227, 2001

Seccia A, Salgarello M, Sturla M, et al: Neovaginal reconstruction with the modified McIndoe

technique: a review of 32 cases. Ann Plast Surg 49:379, 2002

Sharma S, Refaey H, Strafford M, et al: Oral versus vaginal misoprostol administered one hour before surgical termination of pregnancy: a randomised, controlled trial. Br J Obstet Gynaecol 112:456, 2005

Sheth SS: Vaginal hysterectomy. Best Pract Res Clin Obstet Gynaecol 19:307, 2005

Siddle N, Sarrel P, Whitehead M: The effect of hysterectomy on the age at ovarian failure: identification of a subgroup of women with premature loss of ovarian function and literature review. Fertil Steril 47:94, 1987

Silva CS, Cardoso CO, Menegaz RA, et al: Cervical stump cancer: a study of 14 cases. Arch Gynecol Obstet 270:126, 2004

Smith DC, Uhlir JK: Myomectomy as a reproductive procedure. Am J Obstet Gynecol 162:1476, 1990

Spitzer M: Lower genital tract intraepithelial neoplasia in HIV-infected women: guidelines for evaluation and management. Obstet Gynecol Surv 54(2):131, 1999

Stienstra KA, Brewer BE, Franklin LA: A comparison of flat and shallow conical tips for cervical cryotherapy. J Am Board Fam Pract 12:360, 1999

Stovall TG, Summit RL Jr, Washburn SA, et al: Gonadotropin-releasing hormone agonist use before hysterectomy. Am J Obstet Gynecol 170:1744, 1994

Suh-Burgmann EJ, Whall Strojwas D, Chang Y, et al: Risk factors for cervical stenosis after loop electrocautery excision procedure. Obstet Gynecol 96:657, 2000

Tabata T, Yamawaki T, Ida M, et al: Clinical value of dilatation and curettage for abnormal uterine bleeding. Arch Gynecol Obstet 264:174, 2001

Tan L, Pepra E, Haloob RK: The outcome of pregnancy after large loop excision of the transformation zone of the cervix. J Obstet Gynecol 24:25, 2004

Tanaka K, Mikamo H, Ninomiya M, et al: Microbiology of Bartholin's gland abscess in Japan. J Clin Microbiol 43:4258, 2005

Taylor A, Sharma M, Tsirkas P, et al: Reducing blood loss at open myomectomy using triple tourniquets: a randomised, controlled trial. Br J Obstet Gynaecol 112:340, 2005

Thakar R, Ayers S, Clarkson P, et al: Outcomes after total versus subtotal abdominal hysterectomy. N Engl J Med 347:1318, 2002

Thakar R, Ayers S, Georgakapolou A, et al: Hysterectomy improves quality of life and decreases psychiatric symptoms: a prospective and randomised comparison of total versus subtotal hysterectomy. Br J Obstet Gynaecol 111:1115, 2004

Thurman AR, Satterfield TM, Soper DE: Methicillin-resistant *Staphylococcus aureus* as a common cause of vulvar abscesses. Obstet Gynecol 112: 538, 2008

Trimbos JB, Heintz AP, van Hall EV: Reliability of cytological follow-up after conization of the cervix: a comparison of three surgical techniques. Br J Obstet Gynaecol 90:1141, 1983

Trussell J, Guilbert E, Hedley A: Sterilization failure, sterilization reversal, and pregnancy after

sterilization reversal in Quebec. Obstet Gynecol 101:677, 2003

Tulandi T, Beique F, Kimia M: Pulmonary edema: a complication of local injection of vasopressin at laparoscopy. Fertil Steril 66:478, 1996

Tulandi T, Murray C, Guralnick M: Adhesion formation and reproductive outcome after myomectomy and second-look laparoscopy. Obstet Gynecol 82:213, 1993

Tulandi T, Saleh A: Surgical management of ectopic pregnancy. Clin Obstet Gynecol Ectop Pregn 42:31, 1999

Tunçalp O, Gülmezoglu AM, Souza JP: Surgical procedures for evacuating incomplete miscarriage. Cochrane Database Syst Rev 9:CD001993, 2010

Vercellini P, Trespidi L, Zaina B, et al: Gonadotropin-releasing hormone agonist treatment before abdominal myomectomy: a controlled trial. Fertil Steril 79:1390, 2003

Vermesh M, Silva PD, Rosen GF, et al: Management of unruptured ectopic gestation by linear salpingostomy: a prospective, randomized clinical trial of laparoscopy versus laparotomy. Obstet Gynecol 73:400, 1989

Visco AG, Del Priore G: Postmenopausal Bartholin gland enlargement: a hospital-based cancer risk assessment. Obstet Gynecol 87:286, 1996

Weed JC Jr, Curry SL, Duncan ID, et al: Fertility after cryosurgery of the cervix. Obstet Gynecol 52:245, 1978

Welch JS, Cousellor VS, Malkasian GD Jr: The vaginal removal of the cervical stump. Surg Clin North Am 39:1073, 1959

Werner CL, Lo JY, Heffernan T, et al: Loop electrosurgical excision procedure and risk of preterm birth. Obstet Gynecol 115(3):605, 2010

Whiteman MK, Hillis SD, Jamieson DJ, et al: Inpatient hysterectomy surveillance in the United States, 2000-2004. Am J Obstet Gynecol 198(1):34.e1, 2008

Word B: New instrument for office treatment of cysts and abscesses of Bartholin's gland. JAMA 190:777, 1964

Wright VC, Davies E: Laser surgery for vulvar intraepithelial neoplasia: principles and results. Am J Obstet Gynecol 156(2):374, 1987

Yamada T, Yamashita Y, Terai Y, et al: Intraoperative blood salvage in abdominal uterine myomectomy. Int J Gynaecol Obstet 56:141, 1997

Yu KJ, Lin YS, Chao KC, et al: A detachable porous vaginal mold facilitates reconstruction of a modified McIndoe neovagina. Fertil Steril 81:435, 2004

Yuen PM, Yu KM, Yip SK, et al: A randomized, prospective study of laparoscopy and laparotomy in the management of benign ovarian masses. Am J Obstet Gynecol 177:109, 1997

Zalel Y, Lurie S, Beyth Y, et al: Is it necessary to perform a prophylactic oophorectomy during hysterectomy? Eur J Obstet Gynecol Reprod Biol 73:67, 1997

Zhou W, Nielsen GL, Moller M, et al: Short-term complications after surgically induced abortions: a register-based study of 56,117 abortions. Acta Obstet Gynaecol Scand 81:331, 2002

Zurawin RK, Sklar AJ: Tubal sterilization. 2011. Available at: http://emedicine.medscape.com/article/266799-overview. Accessed March 13, 2011

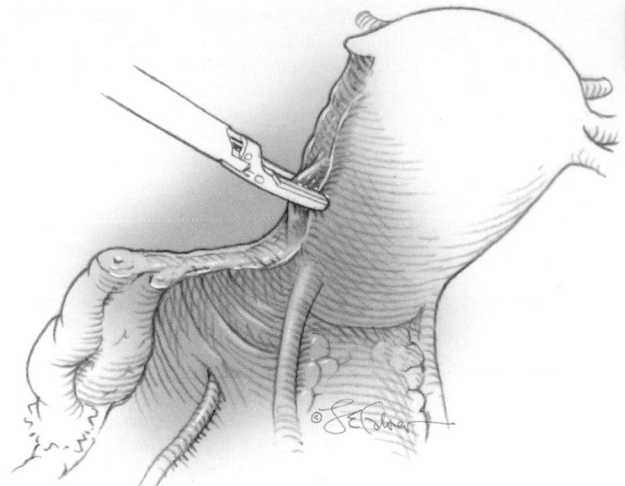

Minimally Invasive Surgery

Minimally invasive surgery (MIS) is characteristically performed through a small incision or no incision, and visualization is provided by endoscopes. Both laparoscopy and hysteroscopy are considered in this category. With laparoscopy, small abdominal incisions provide access to introduce an endoscope and surgical instruments into the abdomen. To increase operative space, a pneumoperitoneum is created through one of these incisions. As such, laparoscopy provides a minimally invasive option for women undergoing intraabdominal gyne-

cologic surgery. Initially used in diagnostic and sterilization procedures, laparoscopy and its improvements in technology, instrumentation, and surgical technique now allow almost all major intraabdominal gynecologic procedures to be performed in a minimally invasive manner. With advancements in robotic technology, options continue to expand and enable surgeons to perform more complex procedures.

Hysteroscopy uses an endoscope and uterine distending medium to provide an internal view of the endometrial cavity. This

tool permits both the diagnosis and operative treatment of intrauterine pathology. During the past two decades, the role of hysteroscopy has expanded rapidly with development of more effective instruments and smaller endoscopes. Indications for hysteroscopy vary and include evaluation as well as treatment of infertility, recurrent miscarriage, abnormal uterine bleeding, amenorrhea, and retained foreign bodies. Additionally, for those seeking sterilization, tubal occlusion devices can serve as an effective and safe method of contraception.

42-1

Laparoscopy Fundamentals

PREOPERATIVE CONSIDERATIONS

■ Decision for Laparoscopy versus Laparotomy

Theoretically, laparoscopic surgery differs from laparotomy only by its mode of access to the operative field. However, inherent qualities can make it more difficult to perform. These include counterintuitive motion, indirect palpation of tissue, finite number of ports for abdominal access, restricted tool movement, and replacement of normal three-dimensional vision by two-dimensional video images. The trade-off in appropriately selected patients, however, is a faster recovery, improved cosmesis, less postoperative pain, diminished adhesion formation, and at least equivalent surgical results (Ellström, 1998; Falcone, 1999; Lundorff, 1991; Mais, 1996; Nieboer, 2009). The decision to perform a laparoscopic procedure is based on several parameters. Primary among these are patient factors, availability of appropriate instrumentation, and surgeon skill.

■ Patient Factors

Laparoscopy using a pneumoperitoneum is contraindicated in very few clinical conditions, but these include acute glaucoma, increased intracranial pressure, and peritoneal shunts. Thus, laparoscopy is appropriate for many patients, although modifications may be warranted for certain clinical situations. Several are discussed subsequently.

Prior Surgeries

With laparoscopy, adhesive disease increases the risk of visceral injury during abdominal entry. Adhesions are also associated with higher conversion rates to laparotomy because long and tedious adhesiolysis may be completed by some surgeons more quickly with open surgical dissection techniques. Thus, during preoperative physical examination, a surgeon should note the location of previous surgical scars and ascertain the risk of possible intraabdominal adhesive disease (Table 42-1.1). Similarly, a history of endometriosis, pelvic inflammatory disease, or radiation treatment may predispose to adhesions. Predetermining this risk and the risk for associated anatomic distortion may help prevent vascular and visceral injury. In addition, abdominal wall hernias or hernia repairs and reparative mesh should be identified and avoided during trocar insertion.

If abnormal findings are found during this preoperative evaluation, plans for an alternative entry site should be considered (p. 1114). Risks of visceral and vascular injury and the possible need to convert to an open procedure should always be discussed with patients preoperatively.

Laparoscopic Physiology

Compared with traditional open laparotomy, laparoscopy produces several distinct cardiovascular and pulmonary physiologic changes. These result mainly from: (1) absorption across the peritoneum and into circulation of carbon dioxide used for insufflation, (2) increased intraabdominal pressure created by the pneumoperitoneum, and (3) head-down Trendelenburg positioning. These physiologic changes are typically tolerated by those in generally good health but may be less so in those with cardiovascular or pulmonary compromise. Thus, to improve patient safety and to appropriately select patients for laparoscopy, surgeons should be familiar with these physiologic changes.

Cardiovascular Changes. During laparoscopy, a pneumoperitoneum is created, in most cases, with carbon dioxide (CO_2). Absorption of this gas across the peritoneum can lead to systemic CO_2 accumulation and hypercarbia. In turn, hypercarbia produces sympathetic stimulation that raises systemic and pulmonary vascular resistance and increases blood pressure. If hypercarbia is not cleared by compensatory ventilation, then acidemia develops. From this, direct myocardial contractility depression and decreased cardiac output can follow (Ho, 1995; Reynolds, 2003; Sharma, 1996). Hypercarbia can also lead to tachycardia and arrhythmia. Although heart rate is typically increased during laparoscopy, less commonly, bradycardia from vagal stimulation can also occur. This may follow pelvic organ manipulation, cervical stretching during uterine manipulator placement, or peritoneal stretching during pneumoperitoneum creation.

Insufflation of any gas will increase intraabdominal pressure. This increased pressure decreases flow in the inferior vena cava, causes blood pooling in the legs, and increases venous

TABLE 42-1.1. Frequency of Umbilical Adhesions Found at Laparoscopy in Women Categorized by Their Prior Abdominal Surgery

		Prior Surgical History			
	Evaluated Patients	No Prior Surgery	Prior Laparoscopy	Prior LT	Prior VML
Agarwala (2005)	918 with prior surgery	—	16%	22%	62%
Audebert (2000)	814 undergoing laparoscopy	0.68%	1.6%	19.8%	51.7%
Brill (1995)	360 with prior laparotomy	—	—	27%	55% with VML below umbilicus 67% with VML above umbilicus
Sepilian (2007)	151 with prior laparoscopies only	—	21%	—	—

LT = low transverse incision; VML = vertical midline incision.

resistance. In sum, venous return to the heart is decreased, and thereby cardiac output is lowered. In addition to decreased cardiac output, increased intraabdominal pressure can also directly lower splanchnic blood flow.

Pulmonary Changes. Features of laparoscopy can also impair intraoperative pulmonary function. First, the diaphragm is displaced upward by intraabdominal pressure from the pneumoperitoneum. This can be accentuated by organs also being pushed cephalad against the diaphragm during Trendelenburg positioning. Moreover, insufflation pressures stiffen the diaphragm and chest wall. Together, these changes lead to higher required airway pressures to achieve adequate mechanical ventilation.

As the diaphragm moves up, lung volume and functional residual capacity are diminished, which in turn reduces the reserve volume for oxygenation. Moreover, this lung volume decline favors a tendency of the lung to collapse and create atelectasis. This can create ventilation and perfusion mismatching and an increased alveolar-arterial oxygen gradient. All of these factors can lead to poor oxygenation.

Renal Changes. Commonly, urinary output is decreased during laparoscopy. This may be the result of lowered cardiac output, decreased splanchnic blood flow, direct renal parenchymal compression, or the release of renin, aldosterone, or antidiuretic hormone (ADH). Together, these bring about decreased renal blood flow, reduced glomerular filtration rate, and diminished urine output. Importantly, renal function returns to normal following decompression of the pneumoperitoneum (Demyttenaere, 2007).

Health Conditions

Several coexistent medical disorders are particularly concerning for laparoscopy. These include cardiac and pulmonary disease, intestinal obstruction, hemoperitoneum with hemodynamic instability, and pregnancy. As just described, in those with severe cardiac or pulmonary disease, elevated intraabdominal pressures and steep Trendelenburg positioning may not be tolerated as they decrease venous return and pulmonary reserve. With laparoscopy, these techniques are often required for adequate visualization and instrument manipulation. In addition, CO_2 is used to distend the abdomen during laparoscopy. As noted, it is absorbed across the peritoneum into circulation, and hypercarbia may result. Accordingly, in those with pulmonary or cardiovascular limitations, lowering intraabdominal pressures and flattening the degree of Trendelenburg may be advantageous.

For a clinically stable patient with hemoperitoneum, laparoscopy is not contraindicated. Thus, ruptured ectopic pregnancies or ruptured bleeding ovarian cysts may be treated via this approach. Although an unstable patient was previously considered a contraindication to laparoscopic surgery, many skilled surgeons feel they can safely and quickly enter the abdomen laparoscopically.

Concurrent intestinal obstruction and its associated bowel distension may increase risks for bowel injury during abdominal entry. In these situations, open entry to gain initial abdominal access may be beneficial (p. 1113). Furthermore, assurance of gastric decompression is important.

Obesity

In the past, obesity had been considered a relative contraindication for gynecologic laparoscopy. It complicates adequate ventilation, hinders abdominal entry, and encumbers laparoscopic instrument manipulation. The fattier omentum also often obstructs the operative field (Gomel, 1995). Placement of an extra ancillary port for adequate manipulation of omentum and bowel out of the operative field can be helpful. In addition, coordination with the anesthesia team to find a comfortable degree of Trendelenburg for both the successful operative manipulations and adequate ventilation is essential.

Thus, with a skilled surgeon, obese patients may actually benefit from a minimally invasive approach. Specifically, research suggests that healthy obese patients experience less pain, quicker recovery, and fewer postoperative complications such as wound infections and postoperative ileus after laparoscopy compared with laparotomy (Eltabbakh, 1999, 2000; Scribner, 2002). Certain operative parameters may be adversely affected in obese patients undergoing laparoscopy compared with normal-weight patients. Some studies have noted higher conversion rates to laparotomy, longer operating times, and longer hospitalizations (Chopin, 2009; Heinberg, 2004; Hsu, 2004; Thomas, 2006). However, this has not been found by all investigators (Camanni, 2010b; O'Hanlan, 2003).

Pregnancy

Treatment of nonurgent conditions identified during pregnancy may often be delayed and addressed postpartum. However, laparoscopy may be performed during any trimester. Therefore, providers should be familiar with the superimposed physiologic changes of pregnancy and understand how these may be exacerbated during laparoscopy (O'Rourke, 2006; Reynolds, 2003).

To improve maternal and fetal safety during laparoscopy, several precautions can be instituted. Perioperatively, left uterine displacement with a wedge for second- or third-trimester pregnancies can minimize the decreased venous return that results from an enlarged uterus compressing pelvic veins and the inferior vena cava. Also, rates of venous thromboembolism are increased during pregnancy due to gestational hypercoagulability, and placing sequential compression stockings can lower this risk. Pre- and postoperative contraction and fetal monitoring should be implemented for more advanced pregnancies.

Intraoperatively, steps include avoiding placement of an intracervical uterine manipulator, limiting insufflation pressures to 10 to 15 mm Hg, maintaining end-tidal CO_2 levels between 32 and 34 mm Hg, moving trocar placement appropriately cephalad to avoid puncture of the gravid uterus, and limiting uterine manipulation (Society of American Gastrointestinal and Endoscopic Surgeons, 2008). Of note, the routine use of perioperative prophylactic tocolytics is not recommended in these cases.

Underlying Pathology

For adnexal masses, myomectomy, and supracervical hysterectomy, operative planning involves assessing appropriate specimen removal. As discussed later, options include endoscopic bags, morcellation, colpotomy, or minilaparotomy incisions. To guide this selection, specimen size and the risks for malignancy and abdominal tumor seeding are assessed. Importantly, for adnexal masses that are known or strongly suspected to be malignant, laparoscopy is avoided if patient outcome could be compromised by specimen rupture or morcellation or by incomplete resection or staging.

▣ Facility Factors

In addition to patient factors, a surgeon must also consider environmental factors. The availability of appropriate anesthesia care, surgical nursing, support staff, and proper instrumentation should influence procedure selection. Advanced operative laparoscopy is a coordinated team effort that requires multiple simultaneous activities, which should be overseen and directed by the surgeon. Together, accurate assessment of these patient and environmental factors leads to improved strategic planning and operative outcomes.

▣ Patient Preparation
Infection Prophylaxis

Randomized clinical trials have demonstrated that prophylactic antibiotics significantly reduce the risk of postoperative infectious morbidity following abdominal or vaginal hysterectomy. During laparoscopic hysterectomy, the vagina is similarly opened to remove the uterus. Therefore, preoperative antibiotics are recommended, and selection can be aided by guidelines from the American College of Obstetricians and Gynecologists (2009a) found in Table 39-6 (p. 959). Antibiotics are generally given at the induction of anesthesia. For other types of laparoscopic procedures, data do not support antibiotic prophylaxis for clean surgical cases, that is, those that do not enter the vagina, bowel, or urinary tract (Chap. 3, p. 99) (American College of Obstetricians and Gynecologists, 2009a; Kocak, 2005).

Preoperative Bowel Preparation

In general, the benefits from routine mechanical bowel preparation can be debated, and thus plans for bowel preparation are typically individualized (Chap. 39, p.958). If considered, bowel preparation prior to laparoscopy can effectively evacuate the rectosigmoid to permit improved colon manipulation and pelvic anatomy visualization. Moreover, if the risk of bowel injury and stool spillage is increased because of pelvic adhesions or endometriosis, then bowel preparation may limit fecal contamination at the surgical site.

Venous Thromboembolism (VTE) Prevention

The same principles used for thromboprophylaxis for other abdominal surgeries should be applied to laparoscopic cases (American College of Obstetricians and Gynecologists, 2007c). Specific to laparoscopy, pneumoperitoneum pressure may decrease venous return from the lower extremities (Caprini, 1994; Ido, 1995). Thus, for those in whom VTE prophylaxis is planned, preventative measures should be administered early and prior to anesthesia induction. A complete list of VTE prophylaxis and guidelines for their use can be found in Table 39-9 (p. 962).

Anesthesia Selection

Laparoscopy can be completed using regional or general anesthesia. In most cases, general anesthesia with endotracheal intubation is selected for several important reasons. These include requirements for: (1) adequate patient comfort, (2) controlled ventilation to correct hypercarbia, (3) muscle relaxation, (4) airway protection from regurgitation due to increased intraabdominal pressures, and (5) orogastric tube placement. Some studies have suggested that injection of local anesthesia at port sites prior to incision may diminish postoperative pain.

Consent

Laparoscopy is usually associated with few complications. Of major complications, the most common is organ injury caused by puncture or by electrosurgical tools and is described subsequently. If these occur or if surgery is hindered by bleeding or adhesions, conversion to laparotomy may be necessary. Overall, this risk of conversion is low, and logically, rates decline as surgeon experience accrues.

Minor complications of laparoscopy occur more frequently. These may include wound infection or hematoma, subcutaneous emphysema from CO_2 infiltration, vulvar edema, and postoperative peritoneal irritation from retained intraabdominal CO_2. Specifically, some CO_2, once instilled into the abdomen, is converted to carbonic acid, which can irritate the peritoneum.

Puncture Injuries

Because a sharp Veress needle and trocars may be used during laparoscopic entry, vessels and abdominal organs may be punctured. Risk factors have been identified and include intraabdominal adhesions, insufficient gastric emptying, full bladder, insufficient pneumoperitoneum, poor muscle relaxation, thin patient habitus, and inappropriate angle or force of trocar insertion. As discussed later, several authors have advocated use of the open entry method as a means to lower rates of puncture injury (Catarci, 2001; Hasson, 2000; Long, 2008).

Bowel Injury

The most common type of organ injury during laparoscopy is bowel injury. Its rate of occurrence has been cited as 0.6 and 1.6 per 1000 cases (Chapron, 1999; Harkki-Siren, 1997a). Women with previous laparotomy have a higher incidence of abdominal adhesions and are at greatest risk for this complication.

Unfortunately, bowel injury sustained during laparoscopy is often missed at the time of surgery. For example, in an observational study by Chandler and coworkers (2001), nearly 50 percent of both small and large bowel injuries were unrecognized for 24 hours or longer. Typically, these patients present with fever, abdominal pain, nausea, and vomiting within 48 hours of surgery (Li, 1997).

In laparoscopic cases, decompression of the stomach with an orogastric tube prior to Veress needle or primary trocar placement can assist in lowering the risk of stomach puncture. Moreover, in those with risks for abdominal adhesive disease, several preventative steps can help avoid bowel injury.

These include: (1) use of the open entry technique, (2) umbilical introduction of a microlaparoscope to scout for adhesions, (3) periumbilical sonography to exclude bowel adhered to the anterior abdominal wall, and (4) primary trocar entry in the left hypochondrium rather than at the umbilicus.

Vascular Injury

Major vascular injury associated with laparoscopy is rare and typically results during primary trocar insertion. Rates of injury have been cited as 0.09 to 5 per 1000 cases, and characteristically, the terminal aorta, inferior vena cava, and iliac vessels have been injured (Bergqvist, 1987; Catarci, 2001; Nordestgaard, 1995). Rarely, air embolism from gas insufflation following vessel puncture may occur.

Although infrequent, a significant number of deaths result from large vessel injury (Baadsgaard, 1989; Munro, 2002). Prevention may include use of the open entry technique or awareness of the angle and force of trocar entry. Despite these steps, if a large vessel is punctured, the Veress needle or trocar should not be removed because it may act as a vascular plug. In most cases, laparotomy, direct manual pressure on the vessel, steps for hemodynamic resuscitation, and notification of a vascular surgeon should follow.

In contrast, if the inferior epigastric artery is injured, several simple techniques can control hemorrhage. First, electrosurgical coagulation of the bleeding site may suffice in many cases. If this is unsuccessful in controlling bleeding, a 14F Foley catheter can be threaded through the cannula of the wounding trocar or through the defect created by this trocar. The Foley balloon then is inflated and pulled upward to create pressure against the posterior surface of the anterior abdominal wall. At the skin surface, a Kelly clamp is placed perpendicular across the Foley catheter and parallel to the skin to apply the balloon firmly in place. The balloon and catheter can be removed 12 hours later. Alternatively, Chatzipapas and Magos (1997) described a process that directs sutures from the skin surface through the abdominal wall and peritoneum to arch under the bleeding vessel to allow direct vessel ligation (Fig. 42-1.1).

Nerve Injury

During some procedures, patients may be placed for extended periods in the dorsal lithotomy position with arms abducted. From this, injury to the common peroneal, femoral, lateral femoral cutaneous, obturator, sciatic, and ulnar nerves and to the brachial plexus is possible (Barnett,

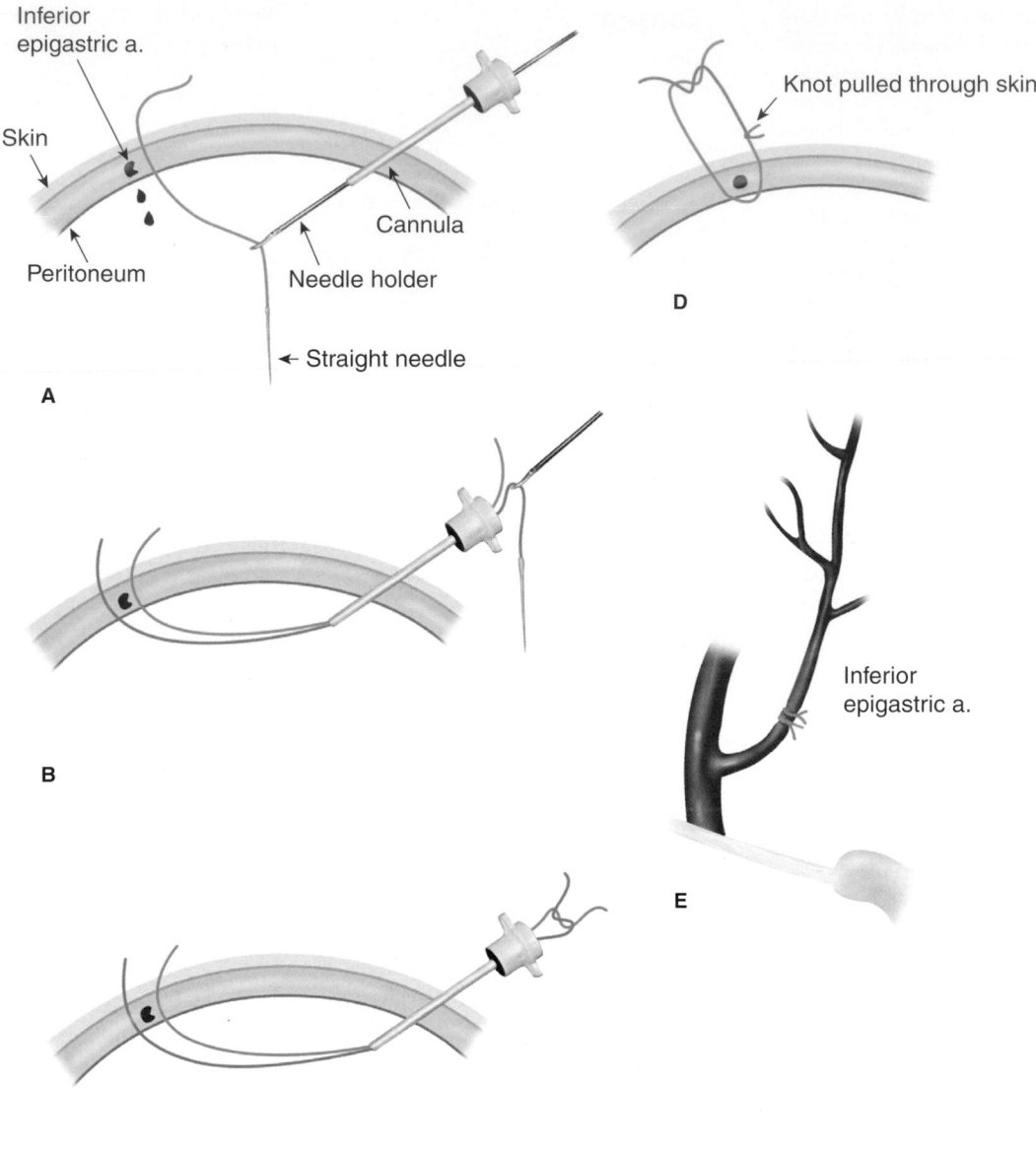

FIGURE 42-1.1 A. Suture with an attached straight Keith needle is driven through the anterior abdominal wall lateral and caudal to the bleeding vessel. This is performed using direct laparoscopic visualization to avoid organ injury. A laparoscopic needle driver or atraumatic grasping forceps grabs the suture. Both needle and driver are drawn up and out of a contralateral cannula. **B.** A similar procedure is repeated medial and caudal to the bleeding vessel as depicted here by the blue suture. **C.** The needles are cut from the two suture strands, and the strands are tied together outside the abdominal cavity. The knot is dragged back through the cannula. This creates a suture sling caudal to the point of vessel bleeding. **D.** Both suture strings then are tied again outside the abdomen over a pressure dressing to occlude the caudal portion of the inferior epigastric vessel. **E.** The entire process is repeated cephalad to the bleeding vessel. This places pressure sutures proximal and distal to the site of vessel laceration.

2007). Specific injuries and prevention are described in Chapter 40 (p. 982). Attention paid to patient position and surgery duration can prevent many of these complications.

Urinary Tract Injury

Bladder puncture is an uncommon risk of laparoscopy. Bladder decompression prior to and during surgery and careful placement of secondary trocars under direct visualization will prevent many cases of injury. However, with increased rates of laparoscopic hysterectomy, rates of bladder and ureteral injury have concurrently increased. These injuries occur at the same surgical steps associated with urinary tract injury during abdominal hysterectomy.

Thermal Injury

Electrosurgical complications may lead to accidental burns by direct contact of the instrument or by stray electric current. Fortunately, the risk of this complication is low. Steps to avoid these injuries include keeping instrument tips within the visual field when electric current is applied, strict instrument maintenance to identify insulation defects, employment of bipolar coagulation or harmonic energy for hemostasis when feasible, and use of lower-voltage (cutting) current whenever possible to reduce the applied voltage (Wu, 2000).

Incisional Hernia

Incisional hernias have been described as a potential long-term consequence of laparoscopy. The incidence approximates 1 percent but may rise in the future with the increasing use of larger trocars for operative laparoscopy and single-port umbilical techniques. Approximately one fourth of hernias are umbilical, and the remainder develops at secondary trocar sites (Lajer, 1997).

A major risk for this complication is the use of large trocars measuring 10 mm or greater in diameter. Accordingly, to reduce the frequency of these hernias, it is recommended to use smaller trocars when possible and to use a fascial suture closure at larger trocar wound sites. In addition, the use of conical tipped trocars as opposed to pyramidal trocars has been shown to lower this incidence (Leibl, 1999). Finally, care should be taken to ensure that peritoneal tissue is not drawn into the superficial layers of the wound when removing the cannulas (Boughey, 2003; Montz, 1994).

Trocar-Site Metastasis

Rates of trocar-site cancer metastasis are low and complicate the clinical course of approximately 1 percent of patients in whom gynecologic malignancy is identified. These metastases are more frequent with ovarian cancer than other malignancies, and higher rates are seen with more advanced disease (Abu-Rustum, 2004; Childers, 1994; Zivanovic, 2008). Although most trocar-site metastases are associated with advanced stages of disease, metastasis has followed surgery for tumors of low malignant potential. As a result, the steps of laparoscopy itself have been evaluated as a risk for tumor spread to the trocar sites (Ramirez, 2004). Currently, no evidence-based consensus addresses prevention of this complication.

INTRAOPERATIVE CONSIDERATIONS

■ Operating Room Organization

A well-organized operating room and operating fields are important aspects of a successful laparoscopic procedure. In laparoscopy, a surgeon has more limited movement compared with laparotomy, secondary to instrument angle restrictions and fixed ports (Berguer, 2001). Thus, thoughtful preparation of room organization is essential, with close attention to the positioning of equipment *before* the procedure is initiated. Also preoperatively, all instruments should be checked and tested to confirm proper functioning.

Although equipment positioning may vary based on surgeon preference, the following is suggested to optimize surgical efficiency and safety. The operating room table should be in the center of the room with the surgical lights directly above the operative field. Prior to surgery, the operating room bed should be checked to ensure that it moves up and down and into steep Trendelenburg position. Obese patients may require a larger bariatric operating bed.

Video monitors may be fixed to the ceiling with articulating arms or may be placed on portable stands. One monitor may suffice for simple procedures, however, we recommend at least two monitors for optimal surgeon and assistant viewing. When operating in the pelvis, the monitor should be placed directly in front of the surgeon. The surgeon, forearm-instrument axis, and video monitor should be aligned in a straight line. Thus, placement of the video monitor for most gynecologic surgeries should be near the patient's upper thigh (Fig. 42-1.2). For best surgeon ergonomics, the monitors should be 10 to 20 degrees below eye level to prevent neck strain (van

Det, 2009). The surgeons should also be standing at an appropriate distance and height such that their arms are slightly abducted, their shoulders are inwardly rotated, and their elbows are extended from 90 to 120 degrees. This positioning can minimize surgeon fatigue. The scrub technician and Mayo stand generally are positioned on the side of the primary surgeon near the patient's legs. Here, instruments can be easily passed to both surgeons. The Mayo stand is organized with frequently used handheld instruments.

A dedicated cabinet or "tower" houses the laparoscopic light source, gas insufflator, and image capture equipment. The tower is positioned on the side opposite the primary surgeon such that he or she has an unobstructed view of equipment display panels. Insufflation tubing, camera, and light cords should exit the operating field in the same direction and connect to the equipment tower. Electrosurgical equipment and pedals are organized so that all cords are aligned in one direction to reach a separate cart that houses these electrosurgical units. Pedals are oriented appropriately for the primary surgeon to comfortably reach

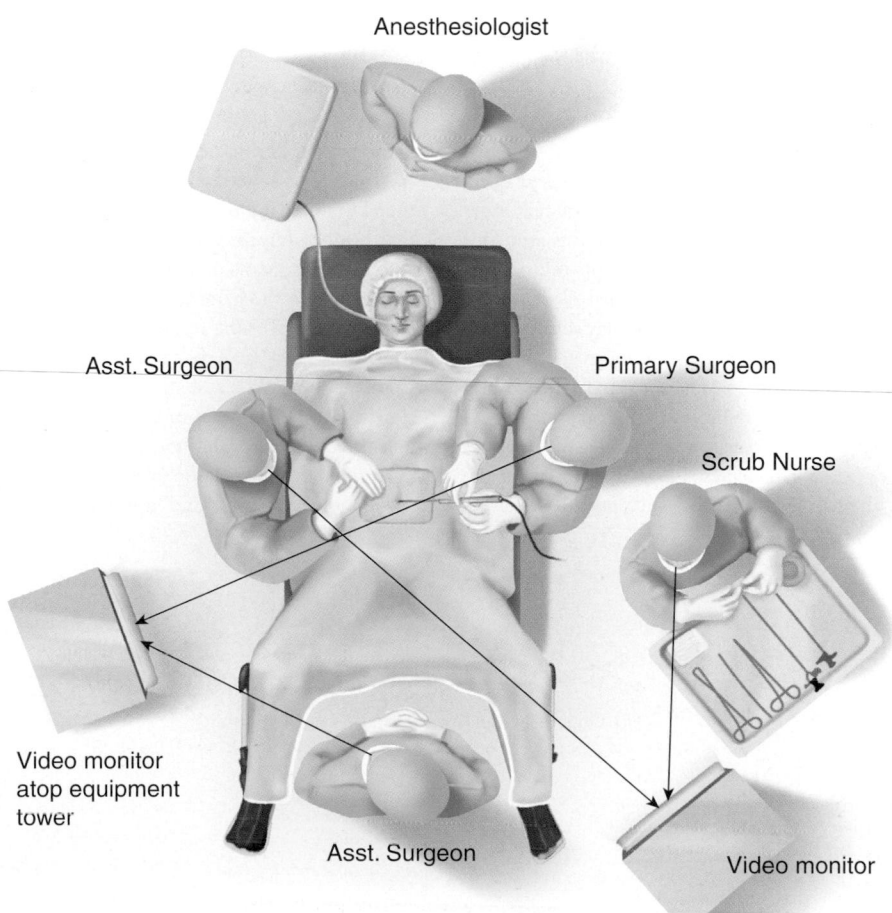

FIGURE 42-1.2 Operating room arrangement for laparoscopy.

without adjusting his body or moving his eyes from the monitor.

Patient Positioning

Preoperative attention to patient positioning is another essential component of safe laparoscopy. Following induction of anesthesia, a patient is placed in low dorsal lithotomy position with the legs in padded Allen stirrups (see Fig. 42-1.2). To aid proper positioning, the stirrup brackets, which holster the stirrups, are attached to the table at the level of the patient hips. To prevent femoral nerve injury, the hips should be positioned without sharp flexion, abduction, or external hip rotation. The knees should not be flexed more than 90 degrees to prevent excess stretch of the femoral nerve and are appropriately positioned and padded to avoid common peroneal nerve compression (Fig. 40-6, p. 985). To avert slipping when in steep Trendelenburg position and to minimize lower back pressure, a patient can be placed directly on an antiskid material such as egg-crate or gel pad with patient skin in direct contact with the padding (Klauschie, 2010; Lamvu, 2004). If uterine manipulation is needed, the buttocks should be placed slightly past the edge of the table.

Patient arms are tucked to the side in military position. This allows improved patient access and prevents hyperextension of the upper extremity, which can result in brachial plexus injury. The arms may be tucked using an extended draw sheet, which is placed under the gel pad. This relationship limits arm slippage during surgery and prevents injury from undue pressure on the brachial plexus. Even in obese patients, the use of antiskid material and arm tucking is useful in preventing slippage for long periods in steep Trendelenburg position (Klauschie, 2010). The arms should be padded to avert compression of the ulnar and median nerves. Fingertips are facing the thighs, well-padded, and positioned away

from the moving foot of the bed to prevent unintentional amputation. During arm positioning, finger oxygen monitors and intravenous access should not be dislodged.

Shoulder braces are padded brackets that are placed on the cephalic side of the operating room bed and positioned around the patient's acromion. Their goal is to brace the shoulder and prevent the head from slipping off the bed when in Trendelenburg. If shoulder braces are required, we recommend tucking the arms in addition to using well-padded braces. However, due to the risk of nerve injury, the use of shoulder braces in general should be limited. Specifically, brachial plexus injury complicates 0.16 percent of gynecologic laparoscopic procedures. When shoulder braces are used, compression over the acromion may apply pressure that stretches the plexus. Moreover, compression by braces laterally may compress the humerus against the plexus. Both predispose to brachial plexus injury (Romanowski, 1993).

Laparoscopic Instruments

The success of laparoscopic surgery depends greatly on the use of appropriate surgical instruments. Most surgeons are already aware of this in traditional surgery and have designated preferences for certain types of graspers, dissectors, and cutting instruments. Many of these have been adapted and subsequently improved for laparoscopic surgery. Moreover, newer models have been designed to further aid retraction and dissection, thereby increasing the number of procedures that can be performed laparoscopically.

The components of a laparoscopic instrument include the hand grip, shaft, jaw, and tip (Fig. 42-1.3). The tip defines instrument function. Jaws may be double action or single action. With a single-action jaw, one tip is fixed, lies in the same axis as the shaft, and offers greater stability during the action performed. Double-action jaws have tips that move synchronously, and this jaw offers a

wider angle in which to perform its function. The instrument tip's diameter is typically concordant with its shaft diameter, and standard sizes fit through 5-mm or 10-mm diameter cannulas. Additionally, 3-mm, 8-mm, and 15-mm instrument diameters are available for many tips.

Important instrument qualities are comfort and ease of use, which stem primarily from the hand grip shape, the instrument length, and its locking capability. Most laparoscopic instruments have a standard 33-cm length. More recently, extended instruments have been developed for procedures in obese patients. Specifically, long Veress needles and trocars and longer instrument shaft lengths offer improved manipulation through the thickened pannus. Although permitting better access, these longer instruments are often more difficult to manipulate due to altered operating angles caused by the extended length.

A locking feature in the hand grip allows a surgeon or assistant to hold tissue without maintaining constant pressure against the grip, and this decreases hand fatigue. Lastly, the ability to rotate an instrument tip 360 degrees is now preferred. This versatility allows access to additional anatomic spaces and decreases the need for uncomfortable surgeon wrist or arm positioning.

Disposable versus Reusable

Many laparoscopic instruments are available in both reusable and disposable forms, each having its own advantages. The main advantage to reusable instruments is lowered expense. Cost analyses have demonstrated that disposable instruments add significant cost compared with reusable ones (Campbell, 2003; Morrison, 2004). The main advantage to disposable instruments is the consistent sharpness of laparoscopic Veress needles, trocars, and scissors and the avoidance of lost instrument parts. For example, Corson and associates (1989) showed that reusable trocars, although sharpened at regular inter-

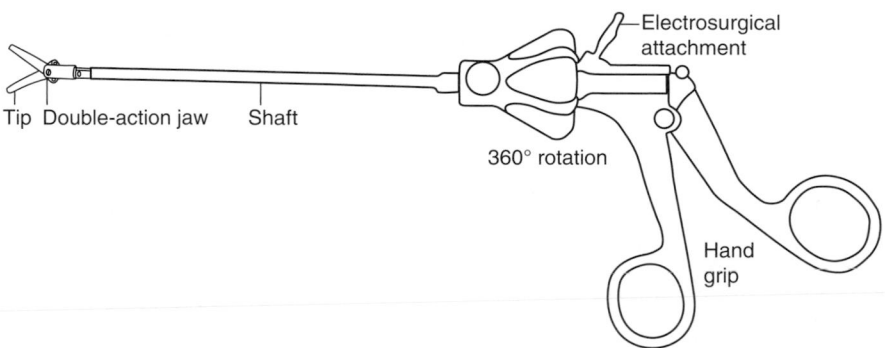

FIGURE 42-1.3 Parts of a typical laparoscopic instrument.

vals, still required twice the force for entry compared with disposable trocars. Dull scissors may lead to longer operating times and ineffectual surgical technique. As a result, these advantages and disadvantages must be balanced when selecting either a reusable or disposable tool.

Manipulators

During laparoscopic surgery, abdominopelvic organs may be elevated, retracted, or placed on tension (Fig. 42-1.4). Most current instrument designs have incorporated safety considerations to minimize organ trauma yet allow effective manipulation.

Atraumatic Manipulators. The *blunt probe* has an end that is modified to decrease

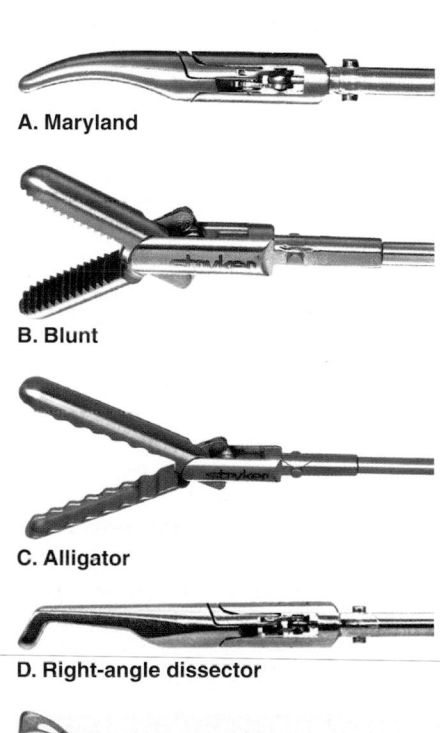

A. Maryland

B. Blunt

C. Alligator

D. Right-angle dissector

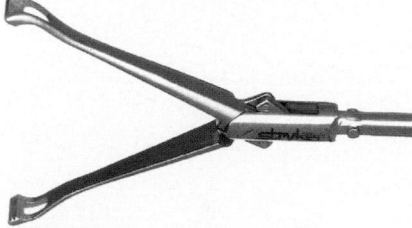

E. Babcock

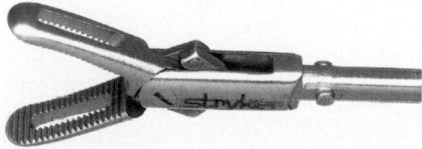

F. Fenestrated

FIGURE 42-1.4 Laparoscopic atraumatic graspers. (*Reproduced with permission of Stryker Endoscopy.*)

the perforation risk to retracted tissues. It is used for exploration and retraction and is a preferred tool during diagnostic laparoscopy. Most blunt probes are stainless steel and are conductive of electric current. However, disposable probes constructed of nonconductive materials are available.

Graspers are divided into two main categories, atraumatic and those with toothed or serrated tips. Atraumatic graspers are used for exploration, gentle traction, and delicate tissue handing. The 5-mm diameter is a popular size, although 3-mm and 10-mm sizes are available. Most of these graspers have a double-action jaw, and the hand grip is typically nonlocking. Their gradually tapering curved tip permits tissue separation and plane definition and is generally preferred for blunt dissection.

The Maryland clamp is an example of a curved blunt tip used for dissection and grasping. It compares to the peon, hemostat, or munion, which are used in open surgery. Additionally, it can double as a needle driver if one is unavailable. Although technically considered atraumatic, this clamp may crush delicate tissues such as the fallopian tube or bowel.

The Alligator clamp is a blunt grasper with a long, wide tip that handles delicate tissues with minimal risk of crushing. It is useful for manipulating bowel, larger vessels, or reproductive organs or for exploration of vascular compartments that may be easily injured. However, its ability to retract tissues under tension is limited due to its atraumatic characteristics.

The Babcock clamp is another atraumatic tip that handles delicate tissues with minimal crushing. The use of this instrument is similar to its use in open techniques. However, similar to the alligator clamp, its ability to retract or grasp on tension is poor due to slippage.

Ideally, all of these clamps are included in a general laparoscopic surgical tray for most laparoscopic surgical procedures. Figure 42-1.4 shows additional tips with similar characteristics. As seen, some tips have window openings and are described as *fenestrated*. These are useful for tissue elevation or retraction or for passing sutures during vessel ligation.

Traumatic Graspers. Graspers with tips that are serrated or toothed are used in procedures that involve tissue resection and tissue approximation (Fig. 42-1.5). Generally, such tissues are placed on tension, and a strong hold is required. In addition, a locking hand grip is typically preferred to keep grasped tissues secured. Most of these instruments have double-action jaws. However, in situations

where greater grip and tension strength is required, a tip with a single-action jaw and locking hand grip may be beneficial.

Toothed graspers have teeth at their tip's end. These are superior for tissue manipulation but function poorly as graspers for sutures or needles. One example is the laparoscopic tenaculum. Single-tooth tenaculums and double-tooth tenaculums are both available and effectively hold and retract dense, heavy tissue. The single-tooth tenaculum usually has a double-action jaw, whereas the double-tooth tenaculum is available with either a single- or double-action jaw. Both usually offer a locking hand grip. Tenaculums are very traumatic to tissue and thus are generally used only on tissue to be resected or repaired. One common use is to grasp and remove tissue during morcellation.

The cobra grasper is a toothed instrument with a double action jaw. It has short teeth on each side and is excellent for tissue retraction due to its strong grip strength. It is considered a traumatic grasper and should not be used on delicate tissues such as bowel or fallopian tubes.

Some of the toothed instruments are designed with less traumatic teeth and are selected when less tissue crushing is desired. For example, ovarian biopsy forceps provide adequate retraction with minimal tissue crushing. An appropriate setting for their use includes ovarian cyst resection and subsequent ovarian repair. An Allis grasper has

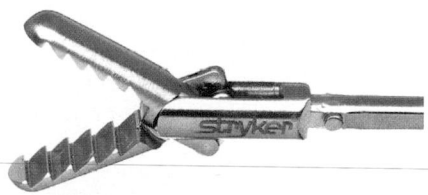

A. Serrated

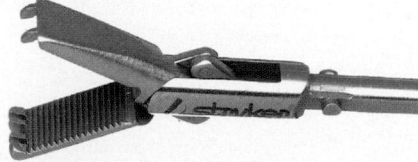

B. Cobra

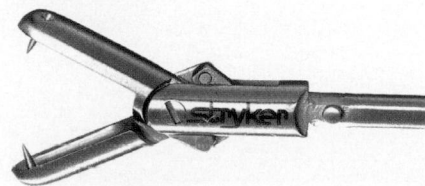

C. Biopsy forceps

FIGURE 42-1.5 Laparoscopic traumatic graspers. (*Reproduced with permission of Stryker Endoscopy.*)

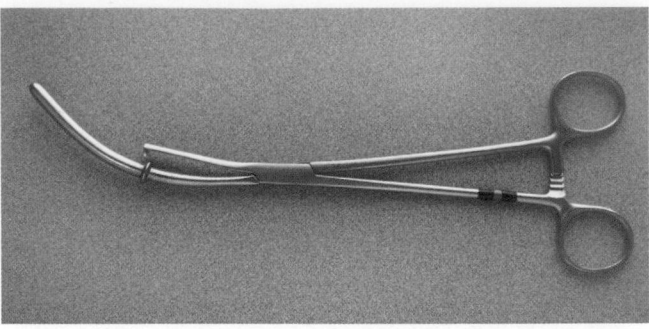

FIGURE 42-1.6 Hulka uterine manipulator.

blunter teeth for grasping and holding tissue during resection. However, it provides less gripping strength than the cobra.

Serrated graspers are considered traumatic but are less damaging than toothed graspers. They offer a secure grasp with minimal tissue damage and generally are used in repairs or tissue approximation. Because of their variety, a surgeon should be familiar with their grips and tissue effects to select the one that best fits the procedure planned. Serrated graspers may be fenestrated or nonfenestrated, may offer a locking hand grip, and may have single-action or double-action jaws.

A *corkscrew tip probe* is frequently used for retraction of more solid masses such as leiomyomas. It offers superior grip and strength, but is limited by the trauma created as it is screwed into the tissue to be held. Additionally, a surgeon should be mindful of the tip location when advancing it into tissue. Because of the downward force required to place the corkscrew tip, adjacent tissues can be perforated inadvertently. Despite this risk, this tool can be invaluable when manipulating solid, bulky leiomyomas or uteri.

Uterine Manipulators. These devices were originally designed to offer manipulation of the uterus to create tension, expand operating space, or improve access to specific parts of the pelvis. The Hulka and the Sargis uterine manipulators are reusable stainless steel instruments that contain the following: a stiff blunt tip for insertion into the endocervical canal, a toothed tip that affixes to the cervical lip for stabilization, and a handle for vaginal placement (Fig. 42-1.6). For these manipulators, the cervix should be patent to allow entry into the lower uterine cavity.

Uterine manipulators have become increasingly versatile and offer additional functions. The Cohen cannula manipulator has a hard-rubber conical tip with a patent cannula for dye injection into the uterus, such as with chromotubation (Fig. 42-1.7). For placement, a single-tooth tenaculum is placed on the anterior cervical lip. The manipulator's conical tip wedges firmly against the cervix and thereby minimizes retrograde dye egress back through the os. The distal end of the Cohen manipulator then articulates with the crossbar that extends between the tenaculum's finger rings. Although commonly used, its range of motion is hindered by its straight shaft. Thus, the ability to dramatically flex a uterus anteriorly or posteriorly may be limited. The Rubin cannula manipulator is similar, with the same disadvantages. Greater flexion may be offered by the Hayden and Valtchev uterine manipulators. These have tip options, either conical or longer blunt intrauterine probes, which attach to a wristed joint at the proximal end of the vaginal shaft. This wristed joint permits improved anteflexion and retroflexion. All of the manipulators just described affix to the cervical lip for stability. Thus, the risk of cervical trauma, although usually minimal, is disadvantageous.

Disposable uterine manipulators such as the Harris-Kronner Uterine Manipulator Injector (HUMI) or the Zinnati Uterine Manipulator Injector (ZUMI) also have a cannula for introducing dye to assess uterine and tubal patency (Fig. 42-1.8). Prior to threading the cannula through the cervical os and into the endometrial cavity, the surgeon sounds the uterus to determine the depth of safe insertion. Rather than affixing to the cervix, an intracavitary balloon at the manipulator's uterine end is expanded similar to a Foley balloon, once the manipulator is placed within the cavity. This prevents the device from dislodging. Due to the length and firmness of the material used, these devices are advantageous for oversized uteri.

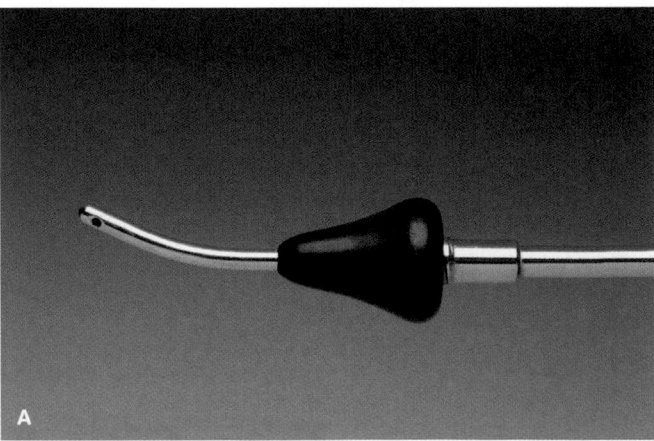
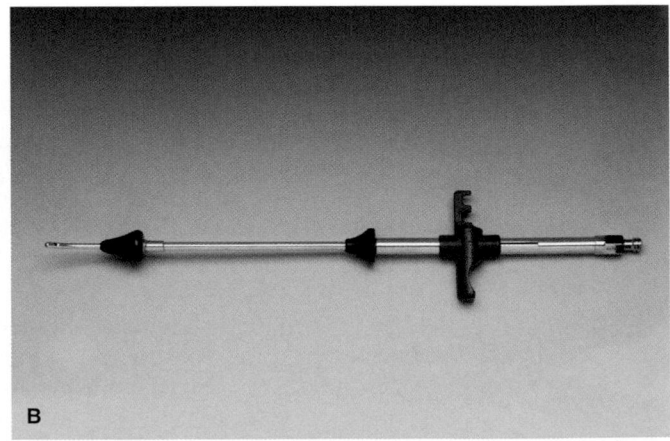

FIGURE 42-1.7 Cohen cannula. This device is used in conjunction with a separate tenaculum. The tenaculum is placed horizontally on the anterior cervical lip. **A.** The narrow cephalad tip of the cannula fits into the endocervical canal. The conical head abuts the external cervical os and limits insertion into the endometrial cavity. **B.** The caudad portion contains a crossbar into which the ratcheted handle of the cervical tenaculum fits. Caudally, the grooved end permits attachment of tubing for chromopertubation, if desired.

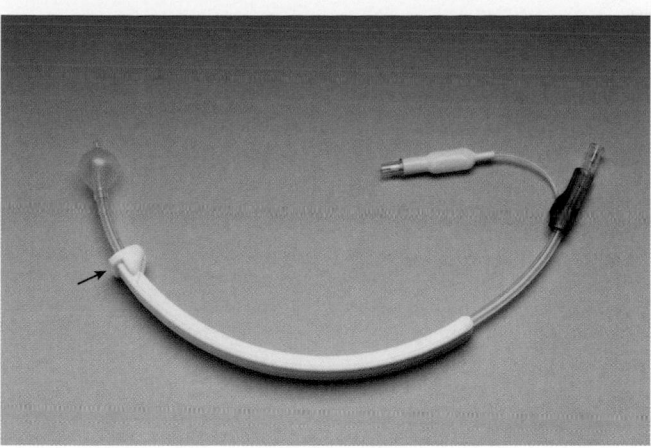

FIGURE 42-1.8 A balloon-type uterine manipulator. The deflated balloon tip is inserted into the endometrial cavity. The balloon is inflated to hold the stiff manipulator in place. The curved white plastic guard adds stiffness to the manipulator. Its head (*arrow*) abuts the external cervical os and limits insertion into the endometrial cavity. At the end opposite the balloon, the white port allows balloon insufflation, whereas the blue tip permits attachment of tubing for chromopertubation, if desired.

Suction and Irrigation Devices

Successful laparoscopy requires a clear visual field. Thus, an effective and efficient suction and irrigation system is integral to procedures that require fluid or smoke removal (Fig. 42-1.11). Older systems were extremely slow and thereby prolonged operative time or in the case of active bleeding, failed to adequately clear the field to permit procedure completion. Newer motorized systems provide faster irrigation and evacuation, and motors usually have two speeds, which can be manually adjusted. The suction tips are available in 3-, 5-, and 10-mm diameters, thereby tailoring instrument capability to the clinical setting. The latest generation systems also permit additional instruments to be placed through the hollow suction tip for concurrent electrosurgical techniques. Among others, there is a spatula, needle, hook, and blunt tips, which are attached to monopolar energy.

Tissue Retrievers

Morcellators. These tools cut excised tissues into smaller pieces, which can then be removed through a cannula. Available morcellators use either thin cutting blades or pulsatile kinetic energy. Bladed morcellators consist of a hollow large-bore shaft that contains razorlike blades to pare tissues into thin strips (p. 1151). One of these, the Storz

Newer manipulator designs have emerged to accommodate laparoscopic hysterectomy (Fig. 42-1.9). These permit adequate uterine manipulation but also contain an intravaginal cup. This cup serves as a guide during colpotomy with hysterectomy. Moreover, these guide cups are paired with an occlusive balloon or cup to decrease pneumoperitoneum loss during colpotomy.

At times, a vaginal sponge stick is a simple practical manipulator for elevation and identification of pelvic structures. This may selected by an advanced surgeon who wishes to eliminate the manipulator or chosen in cases in which the uterine fundus is absent.

Scissors

These are an important part of most laparoscopic procedures, and tips vary depending on the type of dissection or resection needed (Fig. 42-1.10). Scissors preferred for dissection commonly have a curved, somewhat blunted, tip that tapers similarly to Metzenbaum scissors. This shape allows a surgeon to use

standard techniques for tissue separation and resection with minimal trauma to the surrounding tissues (Fig. 40-12, p. 989). These curved blades may be smooth or slightly serrated. A serrated edge tends to hold tissue and minimize slippage prior to cutting. The smooth blade is preferred for strict dissection, such as with adhesiolysis.

Straight scissors also come with smooth or serrated blades. They are used more for cutting and are less desired for dissection. Many straight scissors are designed with a single-action jaw, and some surgeons feel this offers better control. However, many instrument choices are based on surgeon preference.

Hooked scissors have a rounded, blunt tip and arching hooked blades. When initially approximated, the blades close around the tissue without cutting and then cut from the tip toward the hinge. This offers a controlled transection and is useful for partial transection of tissues. Moreover, its design allows a surgeon to confirm optimum placement prior to the cutting. This type of scissors is commonly used for suture cutting.

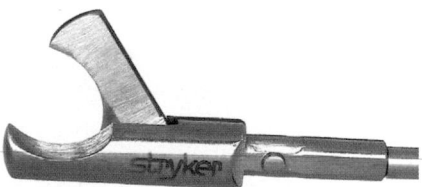

A. Hook

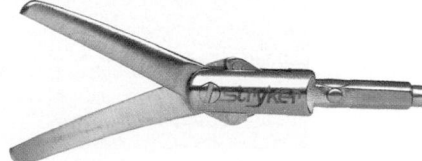

B. Curved

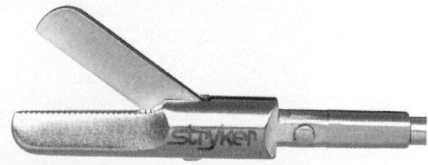

C. Straight

FIGURE 42-1.10 Laparoscopic scissors. (*Reproduced with permission of Stryker Endoscopy.*)

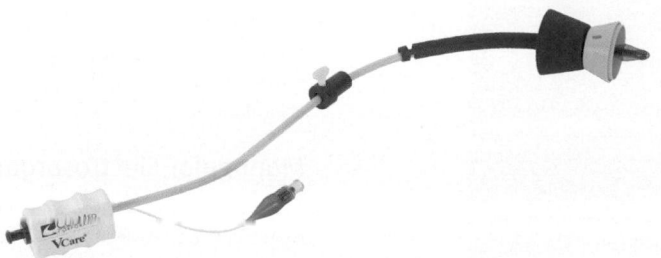

FIGURE 42-1.9 VCare uterine manipulator. (*Reproduced with permission of ConMed Corp.*)

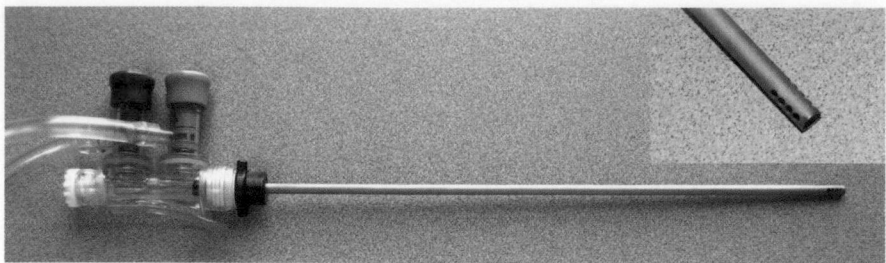

FIGURE 42-1.11 Suction-irrigator. Inset: Irrigator tip.

Rotocut, is nondisposable but houses disposable stainless steel blades that are efficient in cutting through tough smooth muscle or connective tissue masses. Although bulkier and heavier than others, it is among the fastest and most effective. Another mechanical, bladed instrument, the Gynecare Morcellex, is slower but more ergonomic and is disposable. Each mechanical morcellator provides advantages, and familiarity with both allows selection of the instrument most suited to the pathology to be removed.

A third morcellator, the PKS PlasmaSORD Bipolar Morcellator, is bladeless and uses plasma kinetic energy, which is a form of pulsatile bipolar energy. It works well for hysterectomy and myomectomy specimen morcellation. However, it produces a large smoke plume, which reduces visibility and thereby increases operative time. For this reason, cases with larger specimens to be excised may have extended operative times with this instrument compared with bladed

instruments. However, no randomized studies support the superiority of one morcellator over another.

Endoscopic Retrieval Pouches. Endoscopic bags for tissue retrieval are available currently from most instrument manufacturers and vary in sizes and vinyl strength. Some are free-standing sacs designed for manual introduction into the abdominal cavity through cannulas and are preferred for larger and dense masses. Other types are manufactured as pouches attached to support arms at the end of a laparoscopic shaft to create a self-contained unit. As shown in Figure 42-1.12, the support arms open the sac. Once the mass is bagged, the arms and pouch are retracted and removed through the cannula. The cannula is then removed, bringing the bag to the incision where it is extracted (p. 1135). If the specimen does not collapse or cannot be drained, the incision may require slight enlargement.

Self-Retaining Retractors

Designed to complement minimally invasive surgery, nonmetal and disposable self-retained retractors consist of two equal-sized plastic rings connected by a cylindrical plastic sheath. One ring collapses into a canoe shape that can be threaded through the incision and into the abdomen. Once inside the abdomen, it springs again to its circular form. The second ring remains exteriorized. Between these rings, the plastic sheath spans the thickness of the abdominal wall. To hold the retractor in place, a surgeon everts the exterior ring multiple times until the plastic sheath is tight against the skin and subcutaneous layers. This creates 360-degree retraction. These retractors maximize incision size because of their circular shape and by the elimination of thick metal retractors blades within the wound opening. Brands include the Alexis and Mobius retractors, and available sizes range from extra small to extra large. In addition, these retractors provide wound protection and subsequent lower rates of wound infection in some studies (Horiuchi, 2007; Reid, 2010).

For minimally invasive surgery, these devices have several functions. First, they provide retraction of minilaparotomy incisions to aid large specimen removal. Moreover, certain procedures, such as laparoscopic myomectomy, can also be completed through these incisions (Section 42-9, p. 1140).

Energy Systems in Minimally Invasive Surgery

Understanding principles and correct use of electrosurgical instruments is essential to the safe practice of laparoscopy. The same principles of electrosurgery in open surgery apply to laparoscopy (Chap. 40, p. 999). However, special considerations must also be made in a closed, minimally invasive environment. For example, the entire length of an instrument may extend past a surgeon's visual field, thus risking unintended electrosurgical burns. Fortunately, advances in instrumentation have enabled surgeons to mitigate many of the physical constraints inherent in minimally invasive surgery. Thus, electrosurgery can be used to cut with its desiccating properties and to achieve hemostasis through coagulation.

Monopolar Electrosurgery

Monopolar instruments may be useful for tissue cutting, dissection, vaporization, and desiccation. Delivery of this energy is usually through scissors or needle point tip. Other

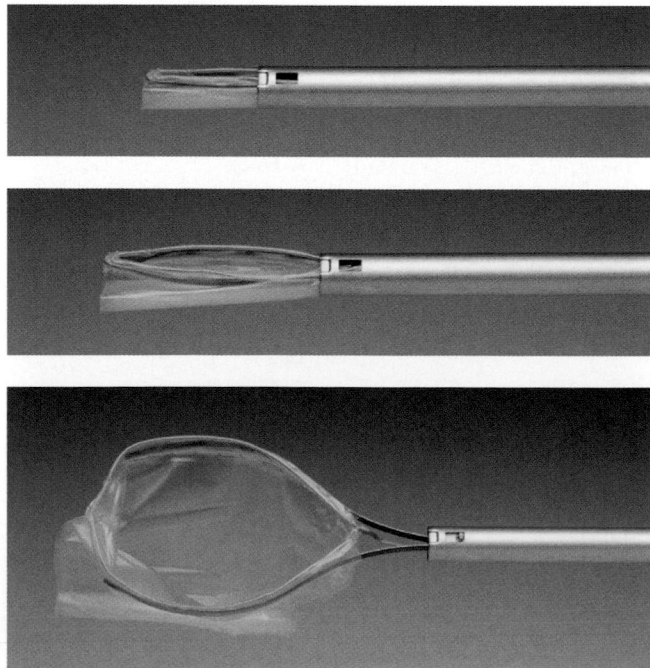

FIGURE 42-1.12 Endoscopic sac.

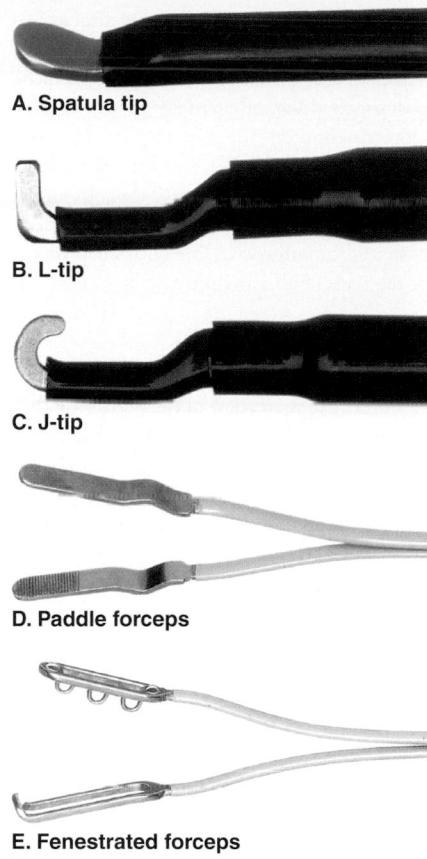

A. Spatula tip

B. L-tip

C. J-tip

D. Paddle forceps

E. Fenestrated forceps

FIGURE 42-1.13 Laparoscopic monopolar (**A-C**) and bipolar (**D**, **E**) tools. *(Reproduced with permission of Stryker Endoscopy.)*

tips, as shown in Figure 42-1.13, may be used for dissection or hemostasis. Monopolar scissors coagulate tissues within their jaws prior to incision. This is typically used for thin tissues and small vessels. Monopolar energy delivered though a needle point tip is used for functions varying from ovarian drilling to development of peritoneal planes during hydrodissection.

Unintended thermal injuries comprise the main risk with this energy type. With monopolar instruments, insulation failures, direct coupling, or capacitive coupling may each result in unintended, potentially serious electrosurgical burns. First, insulation failures are breaches in an instrument's insulation. This break provides an alternate pathway for current flow. When a monopolar instrument is activated, electric current may travel from the electrode through the insulation breach and discharge to any tissue in contact with this breach. This current flow may cause thermal damage to surrounding visceral and vascular structures without the surgeon ever being aware. For these reasons, before electrosurgical tool use, systematic inspection should exclude insulation cracks or aberrant or loose cord connections and should ensure that a grounding pad is correctly placed on the patient.

Another monopolar effect is direct coupling, which occurs when an activated electrode contacts another metal object—either intentionally or unintentionally. This technique is frequently used during open surgery to achieve hemostasis of small vessels, such as when the electrosurgical blade tip is touched to a hemostat around a small vessel. However, in laparoscopy, unintentional direct coupling may occur when a metal instrument or object (such as a metal cannula) contacts an active monopolar instrument and thus provides an alternate and undesired current flow to surrounding viscera.

Another hazard when using monopolar electrosurgical instruments is the risk of capacitive coupling. A capacitor is defined as two conductors separated by a nonconducting medium. During laparoscopy, an "inadvertent capacitor" can be created when a conductive active electrode (e.g., a monopolar scissor) is surrounded by a nonconducting medium (insulation around the scissors) and is placed through another conductive medium (a metal cannula). This capacitor creates an electrostatic field between the two conductors. When current is activated through one of the conductors, this in turn will induce a current in the second conductor. Capacitive coupling occurs when this system discharges current into other surrounding conductive material. In the case of an all-metal cannula, current can be dissipated throughout the abdominal wall. With hybrid cannula systems, in which a metal cannula is anchored by a plastic sleeve or collar, the capacitor that is created has no place to discharge. Stray current can then exit to adjacent tissue that is in contact with the metal portion of the cannula, thereby damaging nearby vascular or visceral structures. This risk can be reduced by avoiding hybrid cannulas and by selecting bipolar instruments. Moreover, the addition of an integrated shield on the electrode shaft of some monopolar instruments, which monitors for stray current, can prevent this complication.

Bipolar Energy

Bipolar energy is mainly used in laparoscopy for tissue desiccation and hemostasis. Many types of bipolar forceps are available for various uses (see Fig. 42-1.13). The 3-mm paddle forceps are used for tubal coagulation during sterilization procedures. Flat-tip forceps desiccate larger vessels and tissue pedicles. Fine-tip, "microbipolar" forceps aid hemostasis near or on vulnerable structures such as the ureter, bowel, and fallopian tubes. Burns are less of a concern with bipolar energy because the currents used are typically lower. In addition, currents, for the most part, stay confined between the two closely approximated electrodes.

Advanced Bipolar Devices. Various bipolar vessel sealing electrosurgical devices are currently commercially available. These devices were developed to produce a uniform mechanical compression while internally monitoring and adjusting the delivery of energy to tissues. Energy is delivered to denature collagen and elastin in vessel walls, thus sealing the vessel and creating hemostasis. When evaluating these devices, important considerations include thermal spread, ability to provide desired tissue effects, consistency of results, time required to achieve results, plume produced, and maximum vessel diameter that can be securely sealed (Lamberton, 2008; Newcomb, 2009).

Currently used advanced bipolar devices such as the Ligasure, Plasmakinetic (PK) Gyrus, and Enseal are multifunctional tools that can be used for both tissue desiccation and dissection. Each of these devices employs a low voltage to deliver energy to tissue and carry impedance feedback to the electrosurgical unit to locally regulate thermal tissue effects. These adaptations allow for reduced collateral injury from thermal spread, an improved tissue seal, less plume production, and diminished tissue sticking. Whereas the Ligasure delivers a continuous bipolar radiofrequency waveform, the PK delivers energy in a pulsed waveform. The Enseal system has a temperature controlled feedback mechanism at its tip, which "locally" modulates energy delivery.

Ultrasonic Energy

The harmonic scalpel, also known as an ultrasonic scalpel, uses ultrasonic energy, which is converted to mechanical energy at the active blade. Seen as the lower blade in Figure 42-1.14, the active blade vibrates to deliver high-frequency ultrasonically generated frictional force, whereas the inactive upper arm holds tissues in apposition against the active blade. Alternatively, the active blade may be used alone. Either tissue desiccation or separation effects can be achieved, and a balance between these two is created by controlling

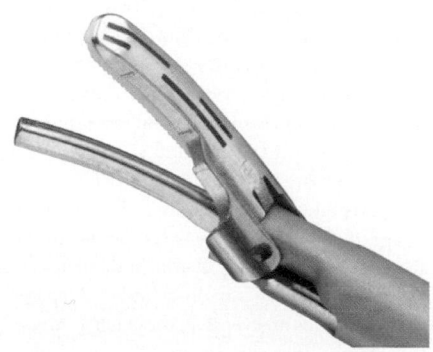

FIGURE 42-1.14 Laparoscopic harmonic scalpel. *(Reproduced with permission of Ethicon.)*

several factors: power levels, tissue tension, blade sharpness, and application time. A higher power level, greater tissue tension, and a sharp blade will lead to cutting. Lower power, decreased tissue tension, and a blunt blade will create slower cutting and greater hemostasis. Limitations of the harmonic scalpel include limited ability to coagulate vessels larger than 5 mm and the surgeon's ability to balance the factors just listed (Bubenik, 2005; Lamberton, 2008).

Laser Energy

Lasers were one of the most widely used types of energy in laparoscopy and served to popularize surgical laparoscopy in the 1980s through 1990s. The main types of lasers used for gynecologic laparoscopic surgery are the CO_2, argon, KTP (potassium titanyl phosphate), and Nd-YAG (neodymium:yttrium-aluminum-garnet) lasers. These are generally used through an operative channel on the laparoscope or via a suprapubic port. These lasers can cut, coagulate, and vaporize tissues and are commonly used for lysis of adhesions, tubal surgery, and endometriosis fulguration or resection. In the hands of skilled surgeons, advantages of the laser in laparoscopy are its precision and control with minimal effect on surrounding tissue. Thus, it may be used near or over sensitive structures such as bowel, bladder, ureters, and vessels. Disadvantages of the modality are its learning curve, expense, lack of portability, and smoke production.

Laparoscopic Optics

Laparoscope Construction

Successful minimally invasive surgery requires excellent visual acuity provided by high-intensity light sources and laparoscopes with focused lenses. Current rod lens systems contain a series of lenses that are the diameter of the laparoscope cylinder. At the periphery of each lens are small scalloped grooves that permit light-carrying fibers to reach the endoscope's end. This provides a well-lit image and minimal distortion. Uniquely, the space between lenses is filled with small, tightly packed glass rods. These rods are fitted exactly, which makes them self-aligning, requiring no other structural support. With the appropriate curvature and coatings to the rod ends and optimal choices of glass types, image quality is superb—even with laparoscope cylinders of only 1 mm in diameter.

In addition to its main cylinder, a laparoscope contains an eyepiece, to which a camera can attach. The cylinder also has an adapter on its exterior to attach the light source cable.

Laparoscope diameters range from 0.8 mm to 15 mm. In general, greater diameters offer superior optics, but require a larger incision. This trade-off typically dictates laparoscope selection for a given procedure.

In addition to typical straight-shaft endoscopes, operative laparoscopes are available and differ in shape. Operative endoscopes have an eye piece that comes off at a 45- or 90-degree angle from a straight operative channel. This permits tools to be placed through the operative channel, which are then visualized by the endoscope. Instruments used are generally longer than instruments that are typically placed in the accessory ports and approximate 45 cm, which is considered bariatric length. Lasers are also frequently placed through the operative port and can allow for precise application of energy. Although useful in single-port surgery, the lack of triangulation or articulation often limits the use of operative laparoscopes.

Angles of View

Similar to hysteroscopes and cystoscopes, laparoscopes vary in their angle of view. The most common are 0-, 30-, and 45-degree laparoscopes, and each offers a different view of the peritoneal cavity. A 0-degree endoscope offers a forward view and is preferred by most gynecologists (Fig. 42-13.1, p. 1158). This laparoscope is used in most diagnostic procedures or simple surgeries involving biopsies, simple adhesiolysis, and excision of small masses or organs such as the ovary or the appendix.

In contrast, angled-view endoscopes provide a larger field of view. For example, during difficult dissection in which multiple instruments are in action, an angled-view laparoscope offers a panoramic view at a distance. This provides a surgical field in which all instruments in use can be seen.

Angled-view endoscopes also allow a lateral view. This is useful during cases with more complicated pathology such as dense adhesions that obstruct the traditional forward view. For example, if an angled-view laparoscope is placed at one pelvic sidewall and is directed to the opposite sidewall, a surgeon is provided with a large lateral visual operating space. Angled views are also valuable along the sides of organs. With large myomatous uteri, it may be difficult to identify the uterine artery and cardinal ligaments. An angled-view laparoscope permits a surgeon to "slide" along the lateral border of the uterus to reach these. The advantage of this approach is also seen in small lateral or posterior spaces in the deep pelvis and in anterior spaces such as the space of Retzius.

Clearly, the 0-degree laparoscope is easier to master. However, the advantages in advanced procedures warrant the time needed to operate using an oblique view. Importantly, when orienting with an angled-view laparoscope, when the field of view is directed downward, the light cord attached to the endoscope is positioned up. Conversely, if the view is upward, the light cord will be positioned down. Regardless of the laparoscope orientation, the camera position is not changed by the surgeon, and the relationship of the light cord to the laparoscope should be manipulated. These steps will keep the orientation of the surgeon in line with the position of the patient and anatomy.

Flexible Laparoscopes

These special laparoscopes offer the advantage of a more extensive view of the peritoneal cavity due to their wide range of angled views. Usually the tip is able to bend to a greater degree than those of rigid endoscopes and can thereby travel into smaller spaces or around corners. Traditional fiberoptic laparoscopes are composed of fiber bundles that run the length of the endoscope. Alternatively, newer flexible endoscopes offer a camera chip at the end that transmits images in the form of an electrical signal. This technique offers less distortion and has opened the option of dual-camera technology for better optics and more advanced surgical procedures. Dual-camera technology involves placement of the camera at the end of the laparoscope. Instead of one chip, two are placed, resulting in superior optics. Some of the newer models provide a three-dimensional view and are used for single-port laparoscopic approaches, in which there is traditionally less maneuverability (p. 1115). Importantly, surgeons must choose the laparoscope that best suits their needs for the particular pathology or procedure.

Lighting

Light is transmitted through the laparoscope from a light source via a light cable. Originally, endoscopic light was provided by incandescent light bulbs, which produced little light and transmitted increased heat. Currently, a cold light source is used and provides a more intense beam. The term *cold light* describes the dissipation of heat along the length of the cable. Cold light sources use halogen, xenon, or halide modalities for the lamps. Despite heat dissipation, the light source still creates a hot tip at the end of the laparoscope. Thus, prolonged exposure of the tip to surgical drapes, patient skin, or internal organs should be avoided. Thermal injuries have resulted from such exposure.

Light cables connect the light source to the endoscope. Of these, two types are available: fiberoptic and fluid filled. The fiberoptic cable contains multiple coaxial quartz fibers that transmit light with relatively little heat conduction. However, these cables suffer from fiber breakage and need to be serviced often. In contrast, fluid-filled cables transmit more light and conduct more heat than the fiber cables. They are stiffer and have decreased maneuverability. This, coupled with difficulty in sterilization, may make this type less desired.

Most laparoscopes once attached to a camera and light source must be adjusted to a "true white." This will ensure that the colors in the field of vision are accurate. This is called *white balancing* and is performed at the procedure's beginning.

ROBOTIC SURGERY

A modern approach to minimally invasive surgery involves the use of robotic assistance, and most abdominal gynecologic

procedures can be completed with this technique. Similar to laparoscopy, robotic surgery uses abdominal ports to introduce instruments and a pneumoperitoneum to expand the operative field. However, one difference is the miniaturized and wristed articulating instrument tips that allow successful completion of complex procedures in tight operating spaces. Moreover, three-dimensional viewing, which is absent in traditional laparoscopy, permits a greater depth of field to dissect tissue in delicate areas with greater accuracy and fewer complications. This is accomplished by advanced video technology within an 8-mm laparoscope that provides a high-definition and magnified view.

Among the disadvantages, tactile feedback is lost with robotic surgery, forcing a surgeon to use visual cues. This is a learned skill that carries a significant learning curve. However, surgeons experienced in advanced laparoscopic techniques adapt more quickly. Other disadvantages include extended initial set-up time needed during each case, physician training costs, and robot and instrument expenses.

Robot

Currently, the only commercially available robot is the DaVinci system. As shown in Figure 42-1.15, one or two surgeon consoles are used to control robot arm movement. A

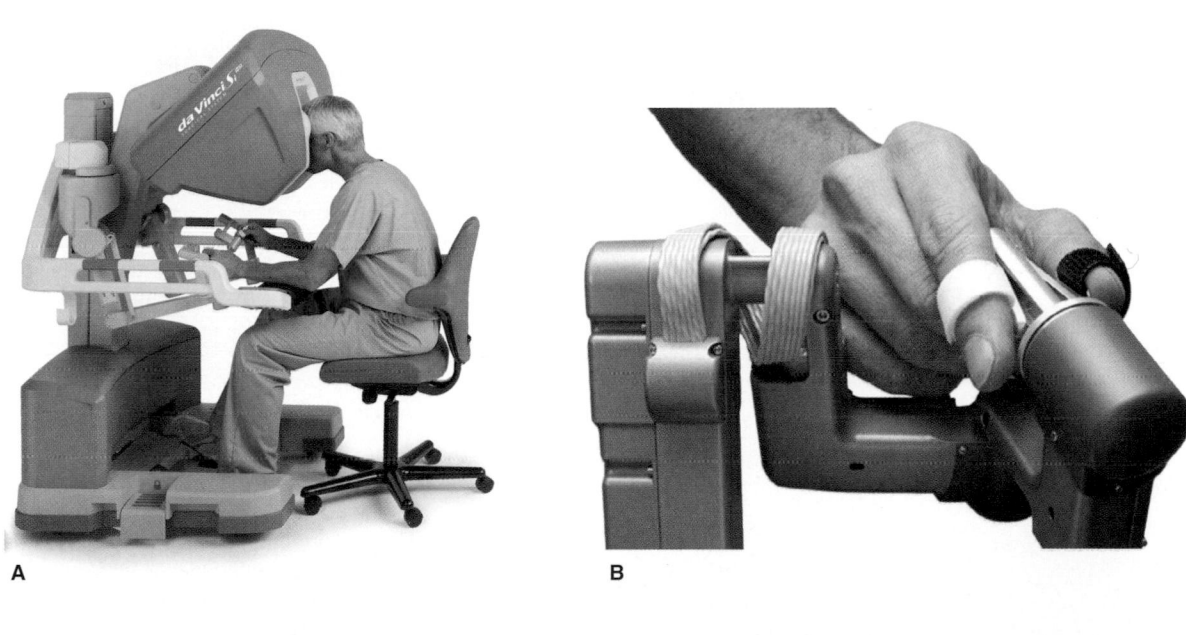

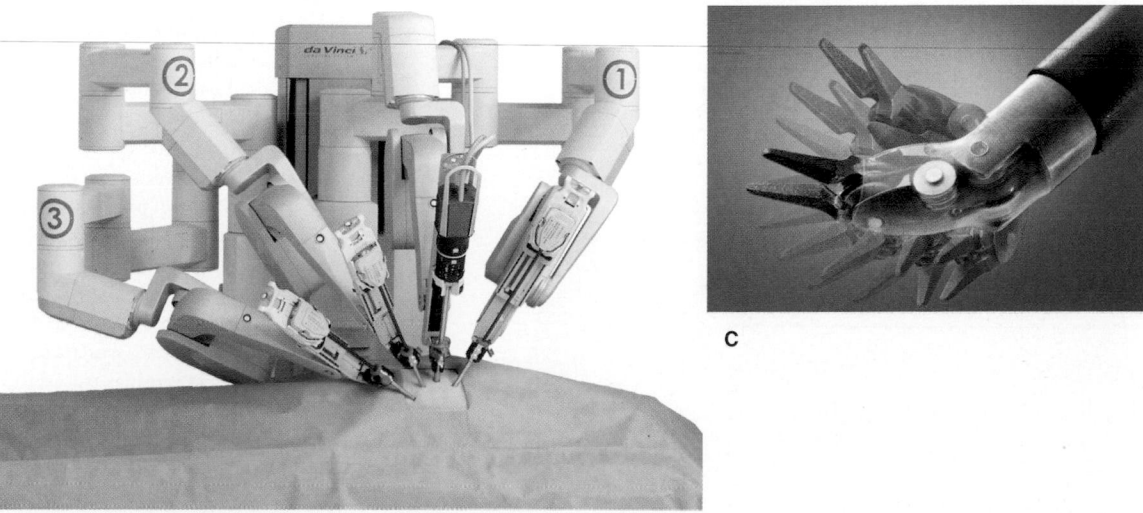

FIGURE 42-1.15 DaVinci Surgical System. **A.** Operator console. **B.** A surgeon's finger movements are translated into robotic instrument tip movement. **C.** Wristed instruments provide a wide range of motion. **D.** Robot at operative bedside. *(Reproduced with permission of Intuitive Surgical, Inc. © 2011.)*

separate cart stands at the surgical bedside and serves as the base for the four robotic arms. Of these arms, one controls the laparoscope, whereas the other arms hold robotic instruments. Procedures are performed using two or three of the instrument arms according to the procedure's needs and surgeon's preference. The second surgeon console is generally used for training. If additional ports are needed, an assistant surgeon works at the patient bedside through one or two traditional laparoscopic accessory ports, which are generally placed in the right or left upper quadrants. Typically, 5- to 15-mm trocars are used for the accessory port(s) depending upon instruments required for a given procedure. The instrument tips mimic those used in open surgery and in laparoscopy and include graspers, needle drivers, and cutting instruments.

Port placement for robotic surgery is unique in that ports must be placed with a minimum intervening distance of 8 cm. This avoids collision of the robot arms with each other and with the accessory ports. The level of the initial port placement depends on the procedure as well as the complexity of the pathology or previous surgery (Fig. 42-1.16).

Trocars are inserted to gain abdominal access similar to laparoscopy, described on page 1110. Importantly, a black ring around the cannula marks the depth to which a trocar is inserted. Insertion to this depth is essential to give the robot arms the correct fulcrum to function optimally and to minimize port-site tissue trauma.

■ Patient Selection for Robotic Surgery

When selecting a robotic approach, both patient and procedure characteristics should be considered. Patients chosen for this technique should be able to withstand conventional laparoscopic physiologic changes discussed earlier. As with laparoscopy, a high BMI may limit the robotic approach but is not a contraindication and must have the joint effort of the anesthesiologist. Procedures that are currently performed efficiently via conventional laparoscopy should not be replaced by robotic surgery. Rather, this modality should be an alternative to laparotomy and may offer the patient a more rapid recovery and decreased postoperative morbidity.

GASLESS LAPAROSCOPY

This variation of traditional laparoscopy was developed in response to the physiologic disadvantages of pneumoperitoneum with carbon dioxide insufflation described on page 1095. To counter these potential problems, gasless laparoscopy has been described. Additional advantages include the sustained visualization after colpotomy or with continuous suctioning. Despite advantages, drawbacks such as a "tent-shaped" operating space and the additional incisions and time needed for the abdominal wall lift device assembly currently limit its routine use. However, it may still have value in high-risk patients with cardiorespiratory diseases (Cravello, 1999; Goldberg, 1997; Negrin Perez, 1999).

LAPAROSCOPIC ANATOMY

An accurate knowledge of anatomy is the basis for sound surgical technique. However, the laparoscopic view of pelvic anatomy may differ slightly from laparotomy due to the effects of pneumoperitoneum, Trendelenburg positioning, and the translation of a three-dimensional reality into a two-dimensional image on the monitor.

■ Anterior Abdominal Wall

When planning abdominal entry, key structures of the anterior abdominal wall should be considered to avert neurovascular complications. Key landmarks are the umbilicus, anterior superior iliac spine, and pubic symphysis. Especially in the obese patient in whom a large pannus may alter anatomic relationships, bony landmarks should be used to plan safe port placement.

The umbilicus is generally located at the level of the L3-L4 vertebrae, although it may lie above or below depending on habitus. In most patients, the aorta bifurcates at the union of L4-L5 vertebrae (Nezhat, 1998). However, in obese patients, the umbilicus tends to be caudal to this aortic bifurcation. In normal weight individuals, the left common iliac vein crosses the midline approximately 3 to 6 cm inferior to the level of the umbilicus. These structures should be considered during initial trocar entry at the umbilicus as they lie approximately 6 cm deep to the base of the umbilicus in normal-sized supine patients (Hurd, 1992).

Accessory ports are placed with direct visualization of the trocar and of important anatomic structures including the bladder, bowel, and the inferior (deep) and superficial epigastric vessels. Of these, the inferior epigastric artery travels along the lateral third of

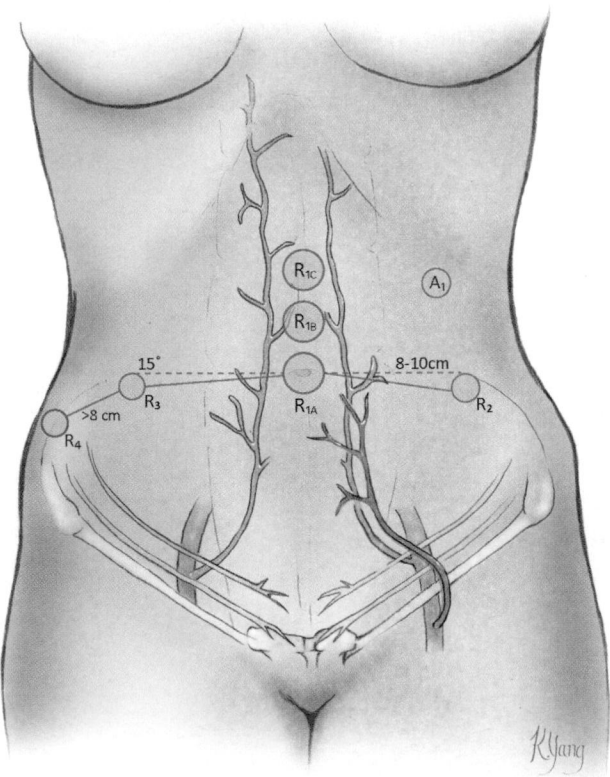

FIGURE 42-1.16 Typical port placements for robotic surgery. The R_1 port will house the laparoscope. Its site may be moved cephalad depending on the size of pelvic pathology as illustrated by R_{1A}–R_{1C}. Other robotic port sites are marked by R_2, R_3, and R_4. A_1 marks the assistant surgeon port site.

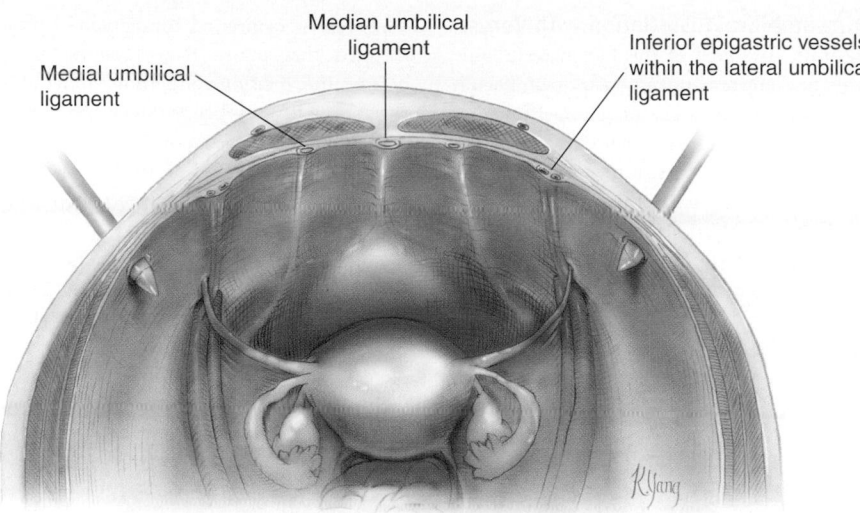

FIGURE 42-1.17 Umbilical ligaments relative to trocar placement.

the posterior surface of the rectus abdominis muscle. It can be easily visualized intraperitoneally, running lateral to the medial umbilical ligaments (Fig. 38-2, p. 919). The superficial epigastric artery, a branch of the femoral artery, travels in the subcutaneous tissue lateral to the rectus abdominis muscle in a similar path as the inferior epigastric vessels. The superficial epigastric artery may be identified by transillumination of the anterior abdominal wall with the laparoscope. Although not visualized, nerve supply to the anterior abdominal wall should also be considered to avoid injury from trocar placement. Both the ilioinguinal and iliohypogastric nerves can be injured during ancillary port placement (Fig. 38-3, p. 920). Steps to limit injury to these nerves and vessels are described later.

Superficial Landmarks to Retroperitoneal Structures

Five prominent anterior abdominal wall ligaments lie beneath peritoneal folds and can be easily visualized laparoscopically. These superficial intraperitoneal landmarks run cephalad to caudad and may be used to identify key anatomic structures in the retroperitoneum (Fig. 42-1.17). In the midline, the median umbilical ligament traverses from the bladder dome to the umbilicus and is the obliterated urachus.

Lateral to this lie the medial umbilical folds, which cover the obliterated umbilical arteries. Identification of the medial umbilical ligament is essential in the setting of a frozen pelvis and can lead to the internal iliac artery. In such cases, this ligament is followed underneath the round ligament, through the broad ligament, to the superior vesicle artery, and finally to the internal iliac artery.

Running laterally to the medial umbilical folds and the round ligaments are the lateral umbilical folds (Fig. 42-1.18). These folds are formed by peritoneum overlying the inferior epigastric vessels before they enter the rectus sheath. Direct intraperitoneal visualization of the lateral umbilical ligaments will prevent injury to these vessels during port placement.

Pelvic Anatomy

Knowledge of the anatomic location of the pelvic ureter and vessels of the pelvic sidewall is essential during laparoscopic surgery.

Often, the mobility and magnification provided by laparoscopy allows easy direct visualization of these structures. Moreover, the course of the pelvic ureter from the pelvic brim, along the pelvic sidewall, and to the cervix routinely should be appreciated with every laparoscopy to ensure normal peristalsis and caliber. Frequent identification and reidentification of the ureteric course is made when performing adnexal surgery, hysterectomy, and especially in cases of adhesive disease due to endometriosis or infection (Fig. 38-22, p. 938).

ABDOMINAL ACCESS

The optimal method of entry in the abdominal cavity has been debated since the advent of laparoscopy. The choice of entry site and entry method is influenced by factors including body habitus, prior surgery, risk of encountering adhesive disease, intended procedure, surgeon skill, and the site, size, and type of pathology. The most common and significant surgical complications during laparoscopy occur during abdominal entry. Specifically, nearly half of all laparoscopic complications occur while obtaining access, and nearly one quarter of these complications are undetected until the postoperative period (Bhoyrul, 2001; Chandler, 2001; Chapron, 1999; Jansen, 2004). Thus, the choice of entry should be made by careful consideration of the preceding variables. Each of the methods discussed next may be beneficial in different situations, but all have potential

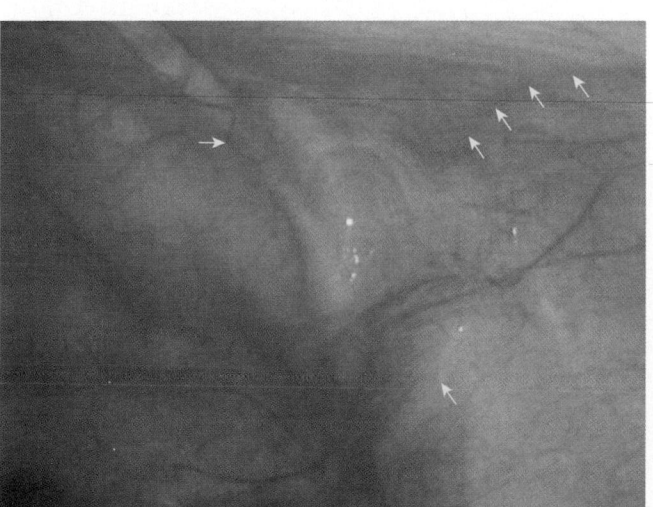

FIGURE 42-1.18 Laparoscopic photograph from the patient's right lower abdomen shows the round ligament (*single lower arrow*). The inferior epigastric vessels and the peritoneum that covers them comprise the lateral umbilical ligament, whose course is outlined by the four arrows on the upper left. The medial umbilical ligament (*single upper horizontal arrow*) is composed of the obliterated umbilical artery and its overlying peritoneum.

complications. It has not been established which entry method is safest.

Umbilical Entry

The umbilicus is the most frequent site of entry, although other sites include left upper quadrant or subxiphoid entry and less commonly, transuterine and transvaginal. The umbilicus is the preferred area of primary trocar placement because the subcutaneous and preperitoneal tissue layers are thinnest at the fused umbilical plate. Thus, the transumbilical approach is the shortest distance to the abdominal cavity, even in obese patients. From a cosmetic standpoint, the umbilical fossa also conceals the port-site scar.

Laparoscopic entry can be performed with an open or closed technique. With closed entry, either a 14-gauge Veress needle or laparoscopic trocar is used to pierce the fascia and peritoneum to gain abdominal entry. Closed entry techniques offer quick access to the abdominal cavity with a low risk of injury (Bonjer, 1997; Catarci, 2001).

With open entry, the fascia is grasped with Allis clamps or peans and surgically incised. The peritoneum is then grasped and opened. Some authors advocate an open entry method as means to lower rates of puncture injury. However, metaanalyses have not shown that any of the following techniques are superior to the others (Ahmad, 2008b; Vilos, 2007).

Closed Entry

Patient Preparation. During laparoscopic entry, surgeons should appropriately assess patient habitus and their physical relationship to the supine patient. To diminish the downward thrust when placing the Veress needle and trocars, a surgeon should adjust the table height and use a short step stool if necessary. The aorta and its bifurcation lie beneath the umbilicus. To maximize the distance between the puncturing instrument and these vessels and avert vascular injury, premature Trendelenburg positioning should be avoided, and the patient should lie flat. Moreover, to minimize visceral puncture during abdominal entry, the surgeon should empty the bladder and confirm with the anesthesiologist that an orogastric tube has been placed to empty the stomach. Palpation over these areas can confirm adequate decompression. The sacral promontory and aorta are also palpated, and a Veress needle with a length sufficient to reach the peritoneal cavity should be selected. Finally, once all equipment is checked and correctly connected, the surgeon should confirm with the anesthesiologist that the patient is fully paralyzed to prevent involuntary patient movement during abdominal entry.

Transumbilical Insufflation with Veress Needle. The goal of this closed technique is to first create a pneumoperitoneum with a 14-gauge needle. The pneumoperitoneum serves to tent the peritoneum and increases the distance of the viscera and retroperitoneal structures from the trocar entering the abdominal wall. This lowers the risk for puncture injury during trocar insertion. First, a Veress needle tip is placed through the fascia and peritoneum and into the intraabdominal cavity to allow abdominal cavity insufflation with CO_2. Once a pneumoperitoneum is created, the fascia and peritoneum are then secondarily punctured with a trocar.

With the closed method, a skin incision appropriate to the trocar size is created, usually at the umbilicus. The incision can be either horizontal or vertical, is placed centrally within the umbilicus, and can be made with a No. 11 or 15 blade. Skin hooks or Allis clamps can aid in everting the umbilicus.

During both Veress and trocar placement, many surgeons recommend abdominal wall elevation, either manually or with instruments such as towel clips (Fig. 42-1.19). A

study using computed tomography images revealed that up to 8 cm can be added between the incision and retroperitoneum by elevation with towel clips (Shamiyeh, 2009). Abdominal wall elevation also provides a controlled counter tension to the downward thrust of the Veress needle and subsequent trocar during insertion.

The Veress needle is a 14-gauge needle that has a spring-loaded obturator (Fig. 42-1.20). As the device contacts the fascia, the obturator is pushed back, and the needle pierces the fascia and peritoneum. As soon as the tip enters the abdominal cavity, the obturator springs back to prevent the needle from injuring abdominal viscera.

The Veress needle should be checked for patency by flushing saline through the needle and then withdrawing the fluid. It should also be checked to ensure that the spring mechanism is functioning appropriately. The patient and operating table are flat, and the anterior abdominal wall is elevated. The Veress needle is inserted at a 45- to 90-degree angle depending on patient habitus and abdominal wall thickness. In patients

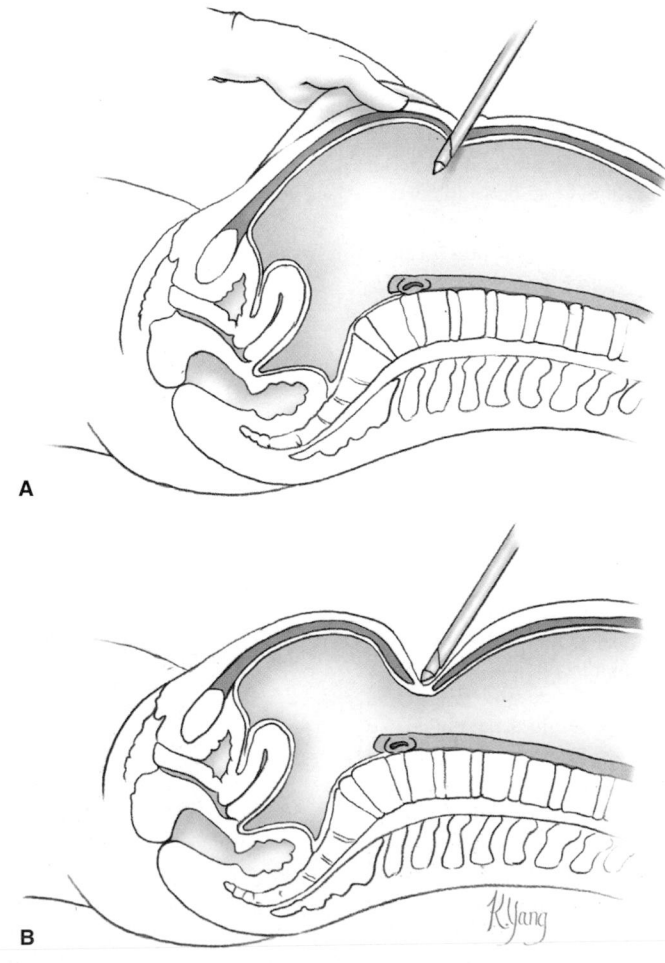

FIGURE 42-1.19 Primary trocar insertion. **A.** With anterior abdominal wall elevation. **B.** Without anterior abdominal wall elevation.

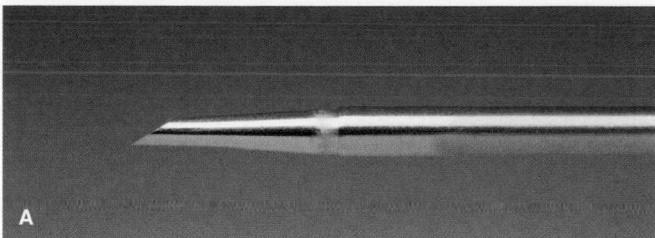 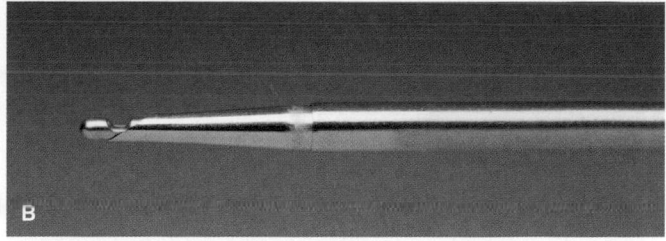

FIGURE 42-1.20 The Veress needle consists of a sharp outer needle **(A)**, which houses a blunt-tipped, spring-loaded inner stylet **(B)**.

with a normal BMI, angling the needle at a 45-degree angle permits abdominal entry yet minimizes the risk of great vessel injury (Fig. 42-1.21). With the Veress needle angled toward the hollow of the pelvis in the midline, it will give a sensation of two "pops" as the tip of the needle penetrates the fascia, and then the peritoneum. As shown in the figure, in overweight and obese individuals, smaller insertion angles are needed to successfully enter the abdomen.

Confirmation of Intraperitoneal Placement. Entry failures with this method usually stem from placement of the Veress needle tip into the preperitoneal space (Fig. 42-1.22). Flow of gas through the needle creates an extraperitoneal insufflation. This gaseous dissection of the peritoneum away from the anterior abdominal wall hinders the trocar in piercing the peritoneum. Instead, the trocar further stretches and pushes the peritoneum internally. Fortunately, this problem can often be overcome by a second attempt with the Veress needle above the umbilicus (Fig. 42-1.23).

Preperitoneal insertion of the Veress needle is a frequent complication of abdominal entry and can lead to abandonment of the laparoscopic procedure. Thus, confirmation

of correct needle placement in the peritoneal cavity is critical. For confirmation, a 10-mL syringe containing 5 mL of saline is attached to the hub of the inserted needle. With aspiration, air bubbles should be seen in the syringe. If blood or bowel contents are aspirated, concern for vascular or visceral injury should be high. In these cases, the needle should be left in place to help localize the puncture site and act as a vascular plug.

Normally after aspiration, saline should be easily injected with no resistance. The surgeon should be unable to reaspirate this saline, which has dispersed into the abdominal cavity. Similarly, a hanging drop test can be used. With this, a few drops of saline are placed on the external end of the Veress needle. If the needle tip is correctly inserted, the fluid should disappear into the negative pressure of the abdominal cavity. If incorrect entry is suspected, the needle should be withdrawn and checked for patency. Moving the Veress needle from side to side should be avoided at this stage. Such movement can create rents in the omentum or injure bowel.

Once correct placement is confirmed by these methods, the CO_2 insufflation tubing can be attached to the needle. A low-

volume flow of CO_2 is selected, and initial intraabdominal pressure recordings should be <8 mm Hg while the abdominal wall is manually lifted. If the pressure is elevated, the needle should immediately be removed. The initial pressure is the most sensitive measurement of correct intraperitoneal Veress needle placement (Vilos, 2007). With the needle correctly placed, pressure and gas flow may be increased. Simultaneously, the electronic insufflator parameters are closely monitored ensure a steady increase in the pressure and continued flow. If the intraperitoneal pressure rises rapidly prior to insufflation of 1.5 to 2 L of gas, one should be concerned for preperitoneal insufflation.

During insufflation, the abdomen should be observed for a uniform distension and dullness to percussion over the liver. The total volume required to appropriately insufflate an abdomen will vary depending on patient habitus. Thus, intraperitoneal pressure, rather than total volume of gas, should be used to determine adequate peritoneal insufflation. During normal insufflation, pressures should not be allowed to exceed 20 mm Hg. Such elevated pressure can lead to hemodynamic and pulmonary compromise. When an intraperitoneal pressure of 20 mm Hg is achieved, the Veress needle may

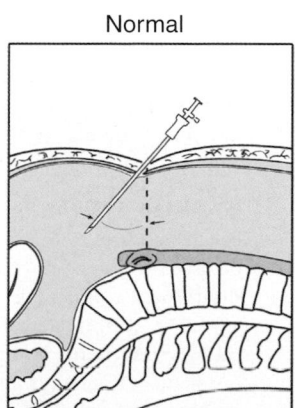 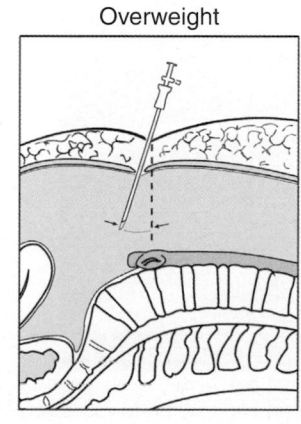 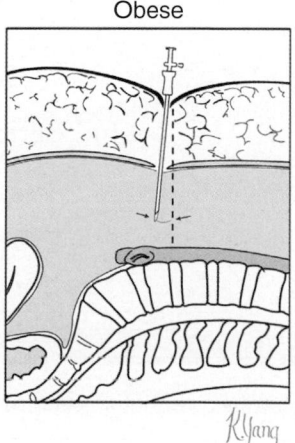

Normal   Overweight   Obese

FIGURE 42-1.21 The appropriate angle needed for the Veress needle to enter the abdomen without injury to the aorta varies with the degree of body fat.

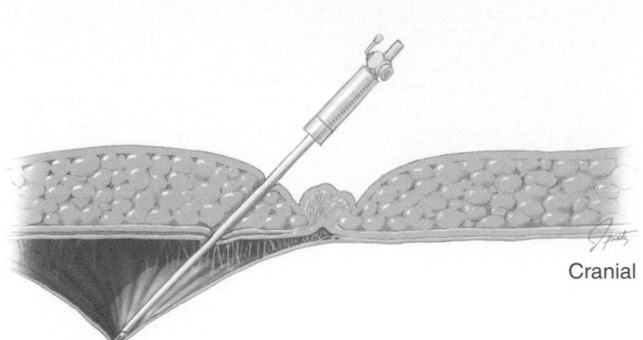

Cranial

FIGURE 42-1.22 Sagittal image showing a Veresss needle tenting the peritoneal layer.

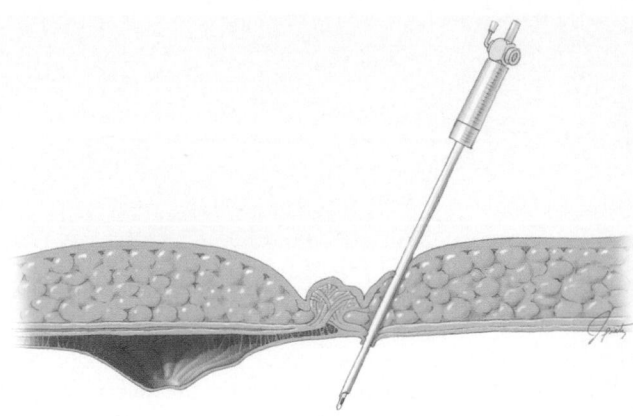

FIGURE 42-1.23 Veress needle replaced above the umbilicus.

be withdrawn, and the pneumoperitoneum should permit safe primary trocar insertion. This transient elevated intraabdominal pressure provides a volumetric counter tension for primary trocar insertion. However, once the primary trocar is placed, the insufflation pressure should be dropped to <15 mm Hg or to the lowest pressure to adequately visualize and safely perform the planned procedure.

Although data from multiple studies are conflicting, it has been proposed that the use of humidified CO_2 for insufflation may have several advantages. These include decreased postoperative pain, improved visualization from less lens fogging, and in animal studies, less de novo adhesion formation (Farley, 2004; Ott, 1998; Peng, 2009; Sammour, 2008).

Trocars. Once adequate insufflation is achieved, placement of the primary trocar may then be performed. Trocars are used to gain access to the abdominal cavity. First-generation trocars consist of a hollow, long, slender cannula that sheaths an inner obturator. Trocars typically range from 5 to 12 mm in diameter, and their tips may be pyramidal, conical, or blunt (Fig. 42-1.24).

Conical trocars are smooth except for their pointed tip and therefore have no cutting edges. They split the fascia rather than cut it and thus are preferred by some to lower risks of postoperative hernia formation and vessel injury (Hurd, 1995; Leibl, 1999). However, they require more penetration force to insert. In contrast, pyramidal trocars have sharp edges and tip and as result, cut the fascia as they are inserted into the abdomen.

In the 1980s, trocars with retractable shields were introduced. Similar to the concept used with the Veress needle, a hollow plastic retractable shield covers the trocar tip both before and after the trocar pierces the abdominal wall. In this manner, the cutting edge is exposed only during its passage through the fascia. Despite theoretical advantages to these shielded trocars in preventing organ injury, studies have failed to show superior results with their use (Fuller, 2003).

Primary Trocar Placement. Similar to Veress needle insertion, initial trocar entry is a blind procedure and thus associated with significant complications. It also is completed with the patient supine and flat. The Veress needle is removed, and a trocar is placed in the umbilical incision. The trocar head is cupped by the palm and the shaft of the cannula is grasped to add control and to splint the trocar from being inserted too deeply. The angle of trocar insertion should mirror that of the Veress needle. The anterior abdominal wall is elevated. With control and minimal downward force, the trocar punctures the fascia and underlying peritoneum and enters the abdominal cavity. After insertion, the trocar obturator is retracted, and the cannula may be advanced slightly to ensure adequate placement into the peritoneal cavity. At this point, the laparoscope may be inserted through the umbilical cannula to visually confirm safe and atraumatic entry.

Versastep System. Similar to the Veress needle method, the VersaStep system may be used. This consists of a stretchable nylon sheath over a disposable Veress needle (Fig. 42-1.25). The first step of insertion is identical to Veress needle insertion and peritoneal insufflation. Once insufflation is complete, the Veress needle is removed, leaving the nylon sheath in situ. A trocar with its blunt tipped obturator is inserted into the nylon sheath. Downward, gradual continuous pressure on the trocar causes the nylon sheath to

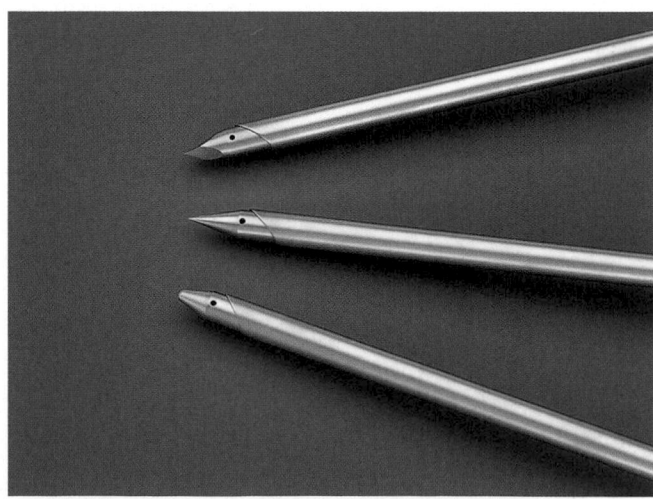

FIGURE 42-1.24 Trocars consist of an outer cannula and inner obturator. The trocar is used to gain access to the abdomen. The obturator then is removed, and the cannula serves as a conduit through which to introduce instruments. Obturators may have a pyramidal (*top*), conical (*middle*), or blunt tip (*bottom*). *(Reproduced with permission of Karl Storz America, Inc.)*

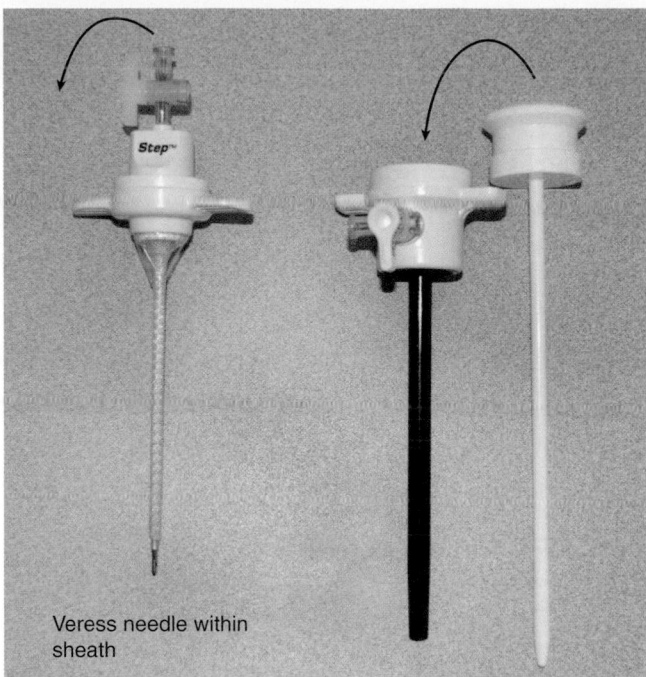

Veress needle within sheath

A

Cannula and obturator

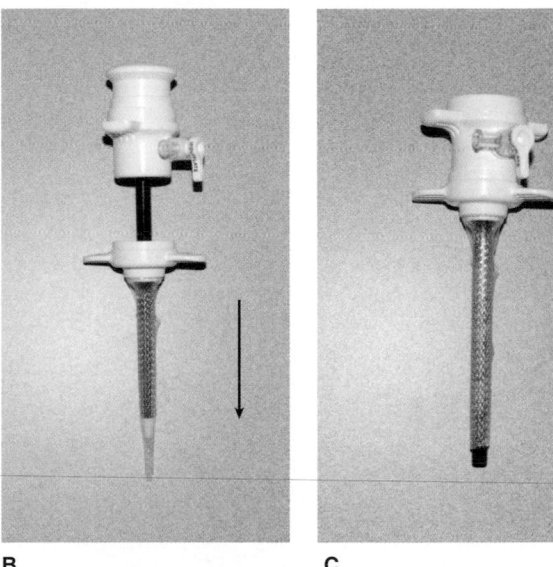

B   **C**

FIGURE 42-1.25 VersaStep system. **A.** The Veress needle housed within a nylon sheath is placed as a traditional Veress needle would be. Once inserted intraabdominally, the Veress needle is removed and the nylon sheath alone remains within the abdominal incision. Next, a white obturator is placed within the black cannula. **B.** Together, this assembled trocar is then threaded intraabdominally through the nylon sheath. **C.** Lastly, the obturator is removed. The black cannula is completely sheathed by the nylon sleeve and has gained access to the abdomen.

stretch and accommodate the trocar as the trocar is advanced. The conical obturator is then removed, leaving only the nylon sheath and cannula as the operative port. The benefit of this system is that a blunt trocar is used, thus potentially diminishing traumatic injuries from a cutting blade. Also, conical dilation may create a smaller fascial defect.

Optical Access Trocar Entry. To lower the risk of bowel injury at the time of primary trocar insertion, optical trocars were developed in the early 1990s. These devices, in essence, combine the laparoscope and trocar into one tool. Importantly, the laparoscope should be focused once it is housed within the trocar and prior to insertion. During use,

the optical trocar transmits images of the abdominal wall layers to the television monitor. These layers then are pierced under direct visualization by advancement of the trocar tip. If choosing a transumbilical entry, the layers visualized, in sequence, should be: the subcutaneous fat, the rectus sheath (fascia), preperitoneal fat, and peritoneum (Fig. 38-2, p. 919).

Despite the theoretical advantage to this type of trocar, major organ injury still has been reported with use of optical access trocars. Moreover, no large studies have been performed to establish its clinical superiority over other closed entry techniques (Sharp, 2002).

Direct Trocar Entry. Because of entry failures associated with preperitoneal insufflation, a direct trocar entry method was subsequently evaluated (Copeland, 1983; Dingfelder, 1978). The procedure involves elevating the abdominal wall and then directly piercing the anterior abdominal wall with a trocar without prior insufflation. Several comparative studies between Veress needle and direct trocar techniques have shown lower rates of entry failure with the direct method (Byron, 1993; Clayman, 2005; Gunenc, 2005). Moreover, these investigators found comparable or lower associated minor complication rates with the direct entry method.

Open Umbilical Entry

Because of associated risks of puncture injury with closed entry techniques, an open entry technique was described by Hasson (1971, 1974). This technique requires use of a trocar composed of a blunt-tipped obturator that is sheathed by an outer cannula. It is recommended by many surgeons for patients with prior abdominal surgery, for those following a closed technique entry failure, for those with a large cystic mass, and for pediatric or early-pregnant patients (Madeb, 2004).

In a retrospective review of more than 5000 open entry procedures, Hasson and associates (2000) noted that minor and medium-risk complications developed at a rate of 0.5 percent. Moreover, in studies comparing open and closed techniques, open methods showed lower rates of entry failure and organ injury (Bonjer, 1997; Merlin, 2003). This technique, however, is not foolproof, and organ injury, mainly bowel, has been described (Magrina, 2002). Typically, this method of entry takes longer than closed entry, and the pneumoperitoneum can be difficult to maintain in some cases due to air escape around the cannula.

Surgical Steps for Open Entry. A 1- to 2-cm transverse incision at the lower edge

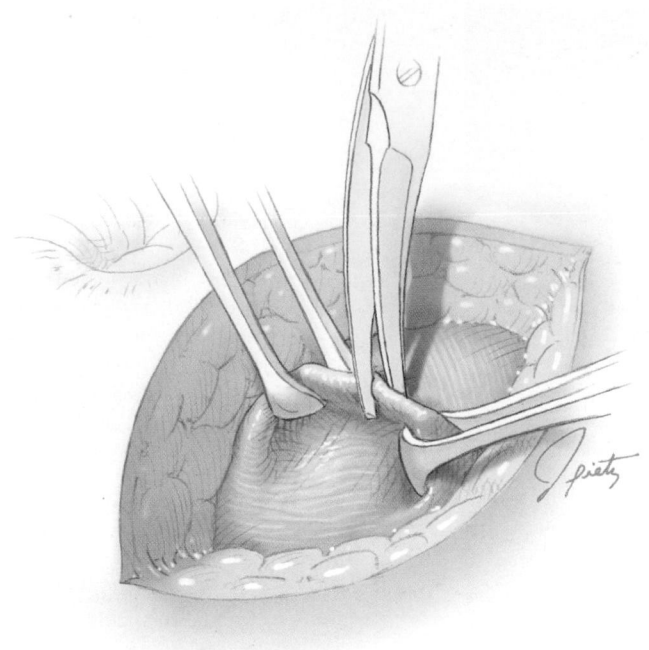

FIGURE 42-1.26 Infraumbilical fascial incision for open entry.

of the umbilicus is made while applying tension with fine-toothed forceps to its lateral borders. Skin edges are retracted laterally to expose the linea alba, and the fascia is dissected free of adhesions and adipose tissue.

The fascia is lifted and everted upward with two Allis clamps (Fig. 42-1.26). A 0.5- to 1-cm incision with scalpel or scissors then transects the fascia. The Allis clamps are repositioned, one on each free fascial edge.

A hemostat or finger is used to bluntly open the peritoneum, and the end of an S-retractor is placed into the abdomen. The abdominal portion of the retractor is used to elevate the abdominal wall and shield the underlying organs as a stitch of 0-gauge delayed-absorbable suture is place parallel on

one side of the fascial opening (Fig. 42-1.27). This suture is not tied. This suturing step is repeated on the opposite fascial edge.

The distal, blunt end of the trocar then is inserted into the incision. The fascial tag sutures are pulled firmly upward and threaded into the suture holders found on either side of the cannula's proximal end (Fig. 42-1.28). The blunt obturator is removed, and the laparoscope is threaded through the cannula.

Alternative Entry Sites

Anterior Abdominal Wall

In some situations, the umbilicus may be unsuitable for initial abdominal entry, and surgeons should develop comfort with entry at an alternative site. Specifically, if periumbilical anatomy is distorted or if umbilical entry may be challenging due to suspected adhesive disease, prior ventral hernia repair, large abdominal mass, advanced pregnancy, or BMI extremes, then other sites of entry are considered. Adhesive disease should be suspected in women with prior intraabdominal surgery, infection, endometriosis, or malignancy (see Table 42-1.1). Similarly, surgical mesh placed during umbilical herniorrhaphy is also linked with adhesive disease, and entry at this site may also disrupt the hernia repair. Nonumbilical entry can also be used to avoid inadvertently traumatizing or rupturing a large intraabdominal mass or gravid uterus.

Nonumbilical anterior abdominal wall entry has been described at various locations. The left upper quadrant is most common, but a subxiphoid approach can also be selected.

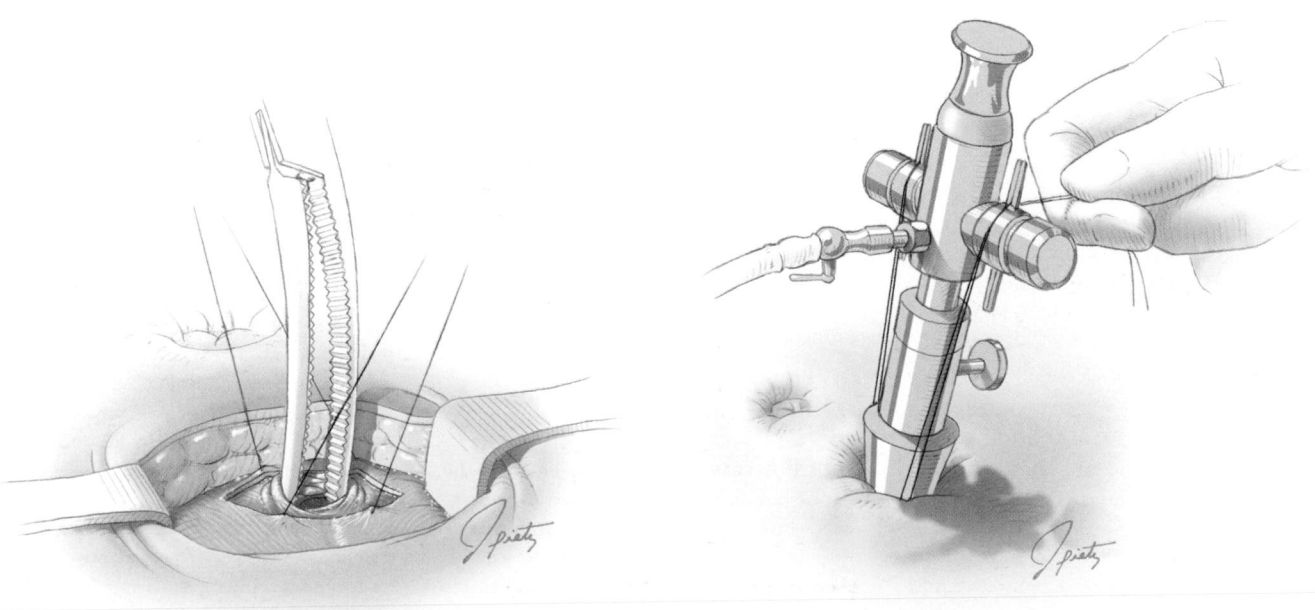

FIGURE 42-1.27 Peritoneal entry during open entry.

FIGURE 42-1.28 Primary trocar placement with open entry.

Left upper quadrant and subxiphoid entry have the advantage of providing working ports at these sites once safe entry is achieved.

Left upper quadrant entry is simple to perform, has a low risk of complications, and usually is free of adhesions (Agarwala, 2005; Howard, 1997; Palmer, 1974). Although left upper quadrant access may be obtained at either Palmer point or the ninth intercostal space, the easy accessibility of Palmer point makes this a favorable entry site. Palmer point is located 3 cm below the left costal margin in the midclavicular line. Organs in close proximity to this point are the stomach, left lobe of the liver, spleen, and retroperitoneal structures, which may be as close as 1.5 cm (Giannios, 2009; Tulikangas, 2000).

When performing laparoscopic entry at Palmer point, one should ensure that the stomach is emptied using suction with an orogastric or nasogastric tube. Palpation of the area will ensure adequate emptying as well as appreciation of incidental splenomegaly. A skin incision adequate for trocar insertion is made at Palmer point. With anterior abdominal wall elevation, the Veress needle is inserted in the skin incision at an angle slightly less than 90 degrees and is directed caudad to avoid liver injury. Initial intraabdominal pressure of <10 mm Hg indicates correct intraperitoneal placement. Once adequate insufflation is obtained, the Veress needle may be removed and a trocar inserted. Alternatively, direct trocar entry may be performed at Palmer point as well. We favor the use of an optical access trocar in this setting with visualization of each layer of the anterior abdominal wall as it is penetrated (Vellinga, 2009). Using an optical trocar, the anterior abdominal wall is elevated, and the trocar with laparoscope is placed into the skin incision. The trocar is directed toward the sacral promontory at a near 90-degree angle. During insertion, one should observe the following in sequence: subcutaneous fat, outer fascial layer, muscle layer, inner fascial layer, peritoneum, and finally, abdominal organs. This method allows for a controlled entry using both visual and tactile cues.

Natural Orifice Transluminal Endoscopic Surgery (NOTES)

This method uses existing natural orifices such as the vagina, stomach, bladder, and rectum to access the peritoneum. In addition, a transuterine approach has been described. Although infrequently used in current practice, there has been renewed interest in laparoscopic access through the posterior fornix. Proposed advantages of this method are improved access to organs, better cosmesis from elimination of an external scar, shorter hospitalizations, and possibly less postoperative pain and fewer postoperative complications.

In gynecologic surgery, large masses not amenable to morcellation or removal through an abdominal port may be removed transvaginally either through creation of a posterior colpotomy or at the time of hysterectomy. Additionally, the transvaginal route for appendectomy has been reported as a convenient method to perform incidental appendectomy during hysterectomy. Nezhat and associates (2009) described appendectomy performed with an endoscopic stapler introduced transvaginally for amputation and retrieval following total laparoscopic hysterectomy or laparoscopically assisted vaginal hysterectomy. This has also been a preferred route for appendectomy and cholecystectomy in the initial trials for NOTES procedures in nongynecologic patients (Palanivelu, 2008; Ramos, 2008; Zornig, 2008).

Single-Port Access Laparoscopy

Single-incision surgery, also known as single-incision laparoscopic surgery (SILS), laparo-endoscopic single-site surgery (LESS), and single-port access (SPA), is a laparoscopic approach in which only one 2- to 3-cm incision is used to place multiple instruments into the peritoneal cavity for surgery (Fig. 42-1.29). The proposed advantages of

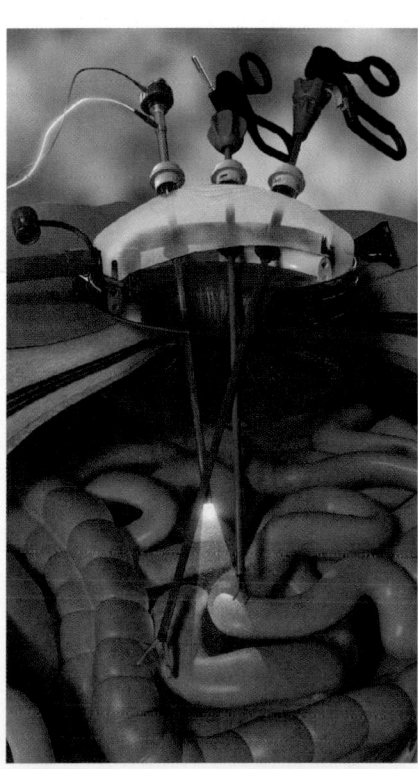

FIGURE 42-1.29 GelPOINT Advanced Access System. *(Reproduced with permission from Applied Medical Resources Corporation. ©2011. All rights reserved.)*

this method are improved cosmesis from a single port site, which is usually buried in the umbilicus, and possibly faster return to normal activity and fewer port-associated complications. Single-incision surgery is technically more challenging than conventional laparoscopy due to instrument crowding in a single port, loss of instrument triangulation, and limited visualization (Uppal, 2011). However, the technique has been popularized with advances in articulating instruments and flexible-tip endoscopes, which may aid these challenges of working from a single multichannel port. The use of single-incision surgery with robotic instrumentation is also being developed.

Ancillary Port Placement

During laparoscopy, once primary abdominal access is achieved, additional operative ports are needed to insert instruments. The number, location, and size of these cannulas will vary depending on the tools required for the laparoscopic procedure. For additional port placement, the patient is placed in Trendelenburg position to displace bowel from the pelvis and provide an unobstructed view of the pelvis. Ancillary trocars should always be placed under direct laparoscopic visualization to minimize the puncture risk to anterior abdominal wall vessels or abdominal viscera. The camera is generally driven by the first assistant or in some cases by the second assistant to free up two surgeons' hands for the actual operative tasks.

Site Selection

Appropriate ancillary port site selection is a key step in operative planning. Correct placement permits instruments to create opposing forces, termed triangulation, which is essential for effective tissue retraction, dissection, and resection. Poorly placed ports may create instrument angles that lead to ineffective movement, cause surgeon fatigue, and increase iatrogenic complications. As an ancillary site, the suprapubic midline site is most frequently used. Prior to trocar insertion, the bladder is emptied, and the trocar is placed after identification of both the bladder and the urachus.

For operative laparoscopy, placement of two lower quadrant ports, placed lateral to the inferior epigastric vessels, is also common. The height at which these are placed should be individualized and based on the patient's anatomy and pathology. Generally, the higher the port is placed, the easier it is to manipulate large masses such as large cysts or myomatous uteri.

Port Placement

Within the anterior abdominal wall, the superficial and inferior epigastric arteries course

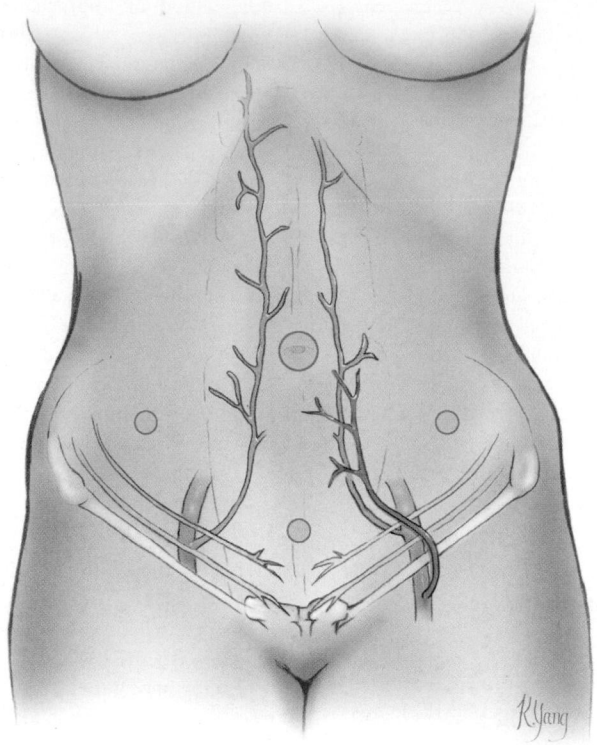

FIGURE 42-1.30 Abdominal access sites. The primary entry site is commonly placed at the umbilicus. Smaller blue circles mark other frequently used accessory trocar sites. As shown here, these are placed lateral to the inferior epigastric artery, which originates from the external iliac artery, and placed lateral to the superficial epigastric artery, which is a branch of the femoral artery.

parallel to the rectus abdominis muscles (Fig. 42-1.30). Specific to avoiding puncture of the superficial epigastric vessels, transillumination of the anterior abdominal wall is useful. During this process, the laparoscope, within the abdominal cavity, is placed directly against the peritoneal surface of the anterior wall. This light is seen externally as a red circular glow, and the superficial epigastric arteries are seen as dark vessels traversing it.

Unfortunately, the inferior epigastric arteries lie deep to the rectus abdominis muscle and are poorly seen with transillumination. These arteries, however, can be seen by direct laparoscopic visualization in most cases (Hurd, 2003). Anatomic landmarks also can be used to limit vessel puncture risks. For example, Epstein and coworkers (2004) noted that the main stem of the inferior epigastric artery can be avoided if trocars are inserted within the lateral third of the distance between the midline and anterior superior iliac spine. Rahn and colleagues (2010) noted that the inferior epigastric vessels were 3.7 cm from the midline at the level of the ASIS and were always lateral to the rectus abdominis muscle at a level 2 cm superior to the pubic symphysis.

Ideally, port placement will also minimize the risk of ilioinguinal and iliohypogastric nerve injury. Most injuries to these nerves and to the inferior epigastric vessels can be averted by placing the accessory ports superior to the anterior superior iliac spine and >6 cm from the abdomen's midline (Rahn, 2010).

Abdominal Entry Closure

Intraabdominal pressure produced by a pneumoperitoneum has an excellent hematostatic effect. Thus, at the end of cases, sites of potential bleeding are evaluated under a reduced pressure. A portion of the pneumoperitoneum is allowed to escape, and the intraabdominal pressure gauge is reset to 7 or 8 mm Hg. Vessels that need sealing will be seen and treated prior to procedure completion.

With surgery completed, CO_2 insufflation is halted, and the gas tubing is disconnected from the primary cannula. The gas ports on all cannulas are opened to deflate the abdominal cavity. To prevent diaphragmatic irritation from retained CO_2, manual pressure is placed on the abdomen to help expel remaining gas. During this process, cannulas are removed under laparoscopic

visualization. This allows evaluation for bleeding from punctured vessels that may have been tamponaded by the cannula or the pneumoperitoneum. These sites as well as other potential bleeding sites should be reinspected as the pneumoperitoneum is diminished. Additionally, visualization prevents herniation of bowel or omentum up through the cannula track and into the anterior abdominal wall. Once all secondary cannulas are out, the laparoscope and then the primary cannula are removed.

Many surgeons recommend reapproximation of fascial defects at port sites to prevent anterior abdominal wall hernia formation. Although closure of the fascial defect does not obviate the risk of hernia formation, in general, most surgeons close ancillary ports sites that are greater than 10 mm. Nonbladed trocars may decrease this risk (Liu, 2000). The fascia can be closed by direct visualization with the assistance of S-retractors. The fascia is grasped with Allis clamps and then reapproximated with interrupted stitches of 0-gauge delayed-absorbable suture. Also, several laparoscopic closure devices (Carter-Thomason system and EndoClose device) are available. With these, fascial defects are reapproximated under direct laparoscopic visualization.

Skin incisions are closed with a subcuticular stitch of 4-0 delayed-absorbable suture. Alternatively, the skin may be closed with cyanoacrylate tissue adhesive (Dermabond) or with skin tape (Steri-Strip Elastic) and benzoin tincture (Chap. 40, p. 987).

Open Entry Incision Closure

During removal of the Hasson trocar, sutures originally placed in the fascia are unthreaded from the cannula. Each of these sutures then is brought to the midline of the incision, and square knots are tied to close the fascial defect. The skin is reapproximated in a manner similar to that described with closed abdominal entry.

TISSUE APPROXIMATION

During many gynecologic surgeries, tissue reapproximation is required. Although basic principles are the same as with laparotomy, techniques to achieve tissue closure are modified to adapt to the constraints of laparoscopic surgery.

Suturing

Following tissue excision, reapproximation with suture is often needed. Subsequent knot tying may be performed, and either an

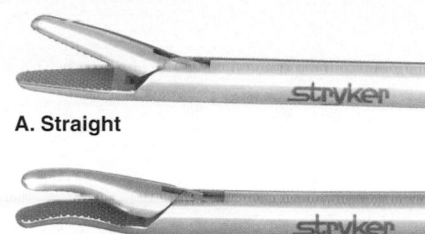

A. Straight

B. Curved

FIGURE 42-1.31 Laparoscopic needle drivers. *(Reproduced with permission of Stryker Endoscopy.)*

intracorporeal or extracorporeal technique can be used. With laparoscopic suturing and knot tying, a learning curve demands an investment of time, not only in the operating room, but also with box trainers or simulators to improve technique, operating time, and patient outcome. Many new devices make these essential steps of surgery less challenging. Thus, surgeons should be familiar and skilled with these techniques and devices to safely complete planned procedures. Typically, selection is based on the procedure planned, surgeon preference, and goals of reapproximation.

Needle Drivers

There are many styles of needle drivers, and preference is surgeon-driven based on ergonomics and the type of procedure performed. Available drivers are either curved or straight and have either a smooth or finely serrated inner surface (Fig. 42-1.31). Driver tips are tapered to limit tissue trauma. They also have a single-action jaw to provide a stable needle grasp, which avoids undesirable rotation or slippage. To assist with grasping and regrasping the needle during suturing, some needle driver tips are designed to guide the needle into a correct driving position. Termed *self-righting*, these needle drivers may be less desirable for suturing in difficult-to-reach anatomic spaces. Here, the needle may need to be grasped by the driver at an oblique angle to achieve correct suture placement. Other needle driver features include a coaxial (rotating) handle in combination with a locking grip. These are often desired because they hold the needle in place and decrease strain on the hand during suturing.

With suturing, the needle driver is held in the dominant hand, while the nondominant hand holds a tissue grasper. Alternatively, some surgeons prefer to use a second needle driver in the nondominant hand. This assists in grasping the tissue, retrieving the needle or sutures from the dominant hand, and providing counter traction when needed.

Sutures

Sutures are broadly categorized: (1) as absorbable, delayed-absorbable, and permanent, (2) as monofilament or braided, and (3) as natural or synthetic. As with traditional gynecologic surgery, the type of suture selected for laparoscopy depends primarily on the characteristics of tissues to be approximated and on the functional goals of reapproximation as discussed in Chapter 40 (p. 996). Importantly, compared with traditional surgery, laparoscopic knot tying creates increased friction and suture fraying, and time between knot throws is longer. Thus, greater tensile strength and increased memory become more valued suture traits. For example, synthetic delayed-absorbable suture offers high tensile strength, less tissue reactivity, knot reliability, and easy handling for either intracorporeal or extracorporeal knot tying. Of filament types, although monofilament suture passes more smoothly through tissues, braided suture ties more easily and breaks less frequently. Lastly, the most common absorbable suture is catgut. However, compared with delayed-absorbable suture, this material offers less tensile strength, and its knot security is less reliable. Accordingly, catgut is less popular for laparoscopic surgery. If used, intracorporeal knot tying is generally preferred due to the significant fraying that occurs with this suture during extracorporeal tying.

For many laparoscopic gynecologic procedures, narrow sutures in the 2-0 and 3-0 range are preferred. This diameter provides suitable tensile strength to prevent suture breakage. Yet, it is thin enough to limit scarring from foreign-body reaction and to harbor fewer bacteria compared with thicker suture. However, for some procedures, such as vaginal cuff closure, the greater tensile strength provided by a 0-gauge suture is required.

Newly designed barbed sutures offer the unique ability to maintain tensile pressure on a continuous suture line. With this synthetic suture, multiple barbs are evenly spaced around the suture's outer surface. These barbs flatten as they pass through the tissues to be approximated but flare out once through to the other side. These flared barbs prevent suture from slipping back through the approximated tissues. As a result, the tissues remain joined with evenly distributed tissue tension (Greenberg, 2008). By its design, this suture obviates the need for knot tying.

Available barbed-suture products include Quill and V-Loc sutures. For laparoscopy, these may be advantageous for myometrial reapproximation during myomectomy or for vaginal cuff closure during total laparoscopic hysterectomy. At completion of the running suture line, the suture is cut short. The use of the barbed suture on peritoneum is still under evaluation due to the theoretical risk of bowel injury from the terminal barbs. This needs additional study before more definitive recommendations can be made (Fig. 42-1.32) (Murtha, 2006).

Needles

For suturing, needles are passed through the ports, and thus, the needle type chosen will depend on the size of available cannulas. The ski needle offers the ability to

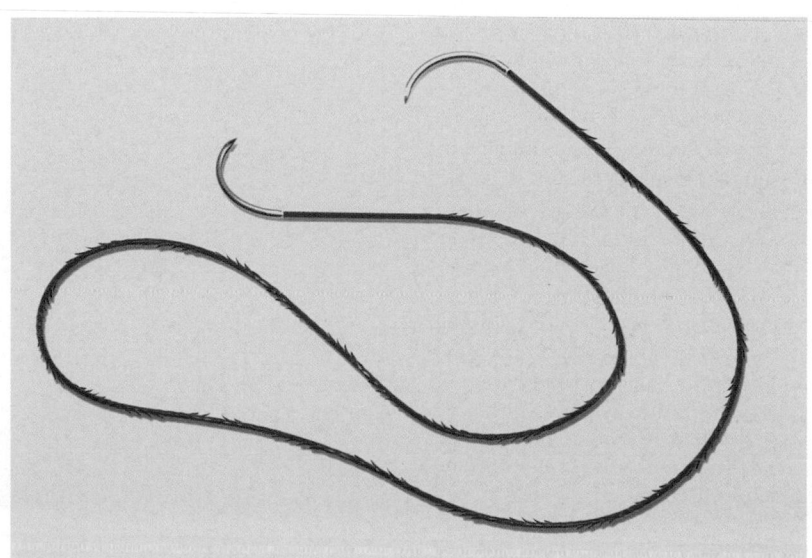

FIGURE 42-1.32 Barbed suture. *(Reprinted with permission of Angiotech Pharmaceuticals, Inc. © 2010.)*

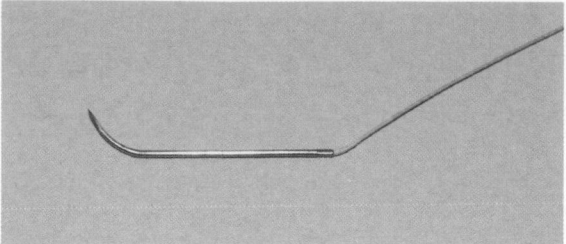

FIGURE 42-1.33 Ski needle.

introduce a needle through a narrow cannula (Fig. 42-1.33). However, its wide, flat arc prohibits its use in tight anatomic spaces, which require a needle with a smaller radius. Straight keith needles can also be easily passed through cannulas of any size. Placing higher-diameter ports in optimal locations allows the use of conventional needle shapes and sizes.

Technique

With suturing, the suture rather than the needle is grasped approximately 1 cm from the needle swage and passed through an appropriately sized cannula. The length of the suture will depend on the proposed suturing and knot-tying techniques and on the length of the tissue span to be reapproximated. In general, 6 to 8 cm is needed for intracorporeal knot tying, and 24 to 36 cm for extracorporeal tying. Longer lengths are needed for running stitches and for complicated knots compared with simple interrupted stitches. Once tissue approximation is completed, the needle is extracted, and the suture is knotted by either the intracorporeal or extracorporeal technique, and then trimmed.

Modern instrumentation has evolved to include disposable suturing devices that render needle drivers unnecessary to achieve tissue approximation. The EndoStitch is a 10-mm-diameter instrument with a double-action jaw. A short straight needle is attached to one tip at a right-angle. As the instrument tips are closed, the needle passes through the desired tissue. Then, with the tips still closed and with the flip of a toggle in the handle, the needle is released from the first tip and reanchors at a right angle to the opposite tip. Instruments containing either delayed-absorbable or nonabsorbable suture are available. Also, the LSI suturing device is a 5-mm instrument with a hooked tip that passes a straight needle through the tissue. Both suturing tools have benefits as well as limitations, and therefore, it is advisable to develop competency with both.

Knot Tying

At completion of stitch placement, a knot is placed to secure the suture. The throws for a

knot may be created inside the body, *intracorporeally*, or outside the body, *extracorporeally*. Of the two, intracorporeal tying has a steeper learning curve because the surgeon must use laparoscopic instruments rather than fingers to loop the suture (Fig. 42-1.34). Extracorporeal knot tying is simpler for most surgeons because the suture is looped with fingers as in traditional tying. Each formed knot throw is then guided through a laparoscopic cannula and cinched with a knot pusher to create the knot (Fig. 42-1.35). Of suture types, stronger braided suture is preferred if the knot pusher is used because suture fraying is a side effect of this technique. Another disadvantage of extracorporeal knot-tying techniques compared with intracorporeal knot tying is that it often causes more tissue tension and can cause tissue tearing when approximating or ligating delicate tissues.

As an alternative to manual knot tying, disposable clips can be placed at the end

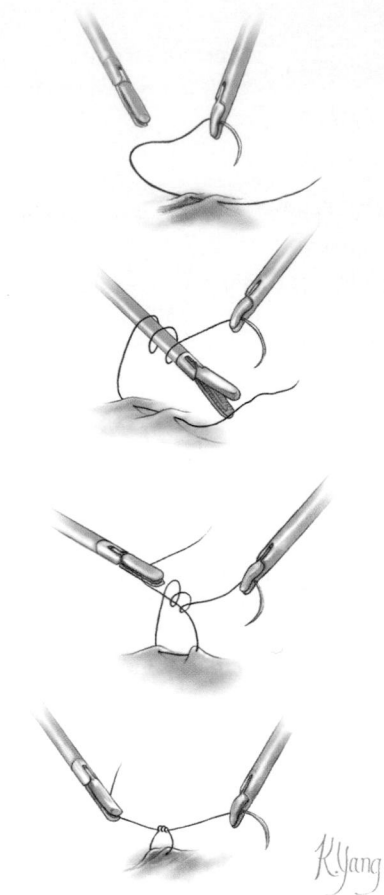

FIGURE 42-1.34 Intracorporeal knot tying.

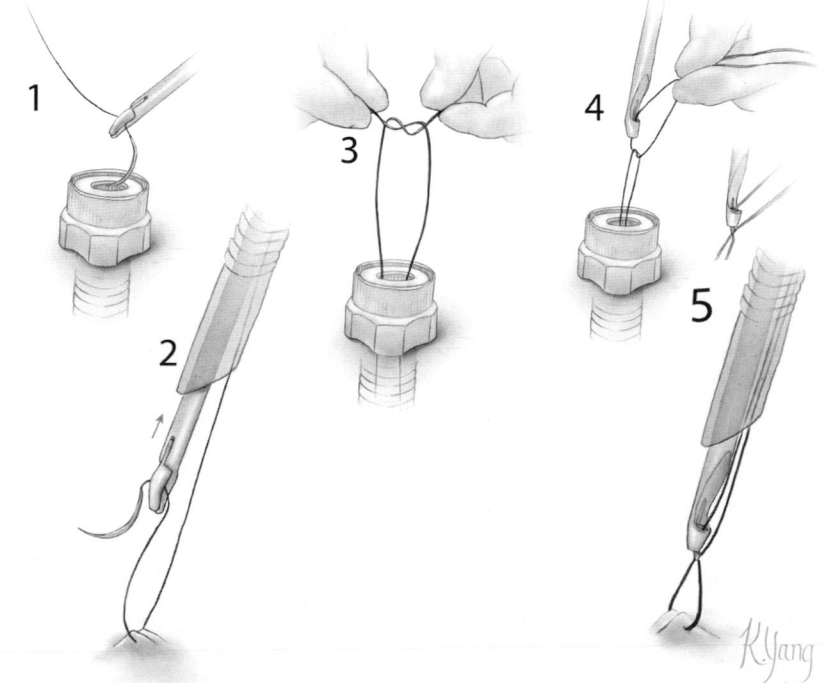

FIGURE 42-1.35 Extracorporeal knot typing.

of a suture line to keep stitches secure. Specifically, a hemoclip is a titanium V-shaped clip with arms that can be squeezed together during application. These clips were originally designed to compress vessels for hemostasis and are available in various sizes. At the end of a running suture line, hemoclips can also be placed across the suture tail to prevent stitch unraveling. If used for this purpose, two clips are advisable. More recent developments include the Lapra-Ty, which is a locking clip made of a delayed-absorbable material similar to Vicryl suture. Its ability to be absorbed and its lock are advantages, whereas its need for an 11- to 12-mm port may be a disadvantage in some settings. Also, these ties are only approved to anchor suture diameters greater than 4-0. Another option is the 5-mm Ti-KNOT instrument. With this disposable device, a special titanium clip may be placed around a single or a double strand of suture. With any of these alternatives to laparoscopic knot tying, the cost may be justified by the time saved in the operating room.

Stapling

In gynecologic surgery, vascular tissue is typically ligated first and then excised. Ligation may be achieved with electrosurgical tools described earlier, with stapling devices, or with suture loops. Linear staplers are mainly used for achieving anastomoses, as in bowel surgery, and are not frequently employed for gynecologic procedures. When selected in gynecologic laparoscopic surgery, they are chiefly used to ligate vascular pedicles, such as the infundibulopelvic ligament. Once fired, the stapler lays down three staggered double rows of staples while dividing tissue in between.

The staplers are available in 35-cm or 45-cm shaft lengths and contain an end called the "anvil," which houses the staple cartridges. *Vascular cartridges* apply staples that are 1 mm high when closed. *Tissue cartridges* apply those that are 1.5 mm when

closed and are suitable for thicker pedicles. Stapling provides hemostasis and gentle handling of tissue, which should lead to less necrosis and better healing.

Newer models have added articulating and rotating capabilities at the jaw. These attributes permit stapling at an angle and thereby increase access through operative laparoscopic ports. Although traditionally used for laparotomy or laparoscopy, newer models are also amenable for vaginal procedures, such as vaginal hysterectomy. Most staples are titanium. However, newer angled staplers for the vaginal cuff use delayed-absorbable material such as Polyglactin 910 for their staples. A main limitation to stapler use is generally the price of the device and cartridges, which can be costly compared with suture. However, if operating time is reduced, these costs can be negligible.

Suture Loops

Preformed suture loops, such as the Endoloop, may also be used to ligate tissue pedicles (Fig. 42-1.36). This instrument has a length of suture housed within a stiff, 5-mm-diameter rod and has a pre-tied loop at the end. The loop is guided around the pedicle by the stiff long rod and then is cinched similarly to a noose (p. 1130). The rod tip, similar to an index finger during manual knot tying, helps to add additional pressure to secure the knot in place. Loops of absorbable, delayed-absorbable, and permanent suture are available. Other types of knots that are pre-tied loops include the Roeder knot, Meltzer knot, and Tayside knot. These currently are not as popular as the square knot.

LAPAROSCOPIC DISSECTION TECHNIQUES

Sharp Dissection

Commonly during laparoscopy, pelvic adhesions will be encountered that require lysis to reestablish normal anatomy and

complete the planned surgery. Some situations require the use of sharp dissection, especially if adhesions are not amenable to blunt tissue separation. For cutting fine adhesions, the tissue band may be placed on gentle stretch using an atraumatic grasper or blunt probe. Curved scissors with a dissecting tip or an energy modality (monopolar, bipolar, or harmonic) are frequently used.

If denser adhesions are found, they are divided in layers to prevent injury to adjacent adhered organs. Traction and counter traction aid in tissue plane identification. As the surgeon begins to separate tissues with tension, the plane of attachment may be identified, and the scissor tips create a small incision. The tips are then eased between the tissue layers, creating an opening by spreading the blades outward (Fig. 40-12, p. 989). The initial incision carries the risk of injury to the underlying viscera or vessel and thus should be as short and shallow as possible. The use of energy sources in these situations is generally discouraged due to the type of injury that may result. Thermal injury may have a wider effect that may not be readily apparent. Conversely, a sharp cut is easier to identify and repair intraoperatively. The scissors used may be curved or straight, depending on the contour of the pelvic organs. Once a plane is developed, wider and deeper strokes are used to complete tissue dissection.

Hydrodissection

In addition to sharp dissection, hydrodissection is another technique often used in minimally invasive surgery. With this, normal saline or other irrigation fluid is injected under pressure to separate tissue planes. For example, peritoneal endometriosis can be lifted and excised with greater ease and less trauma to retroperitoneal structures. Other uses include resection of cysts from an ovary, removal of ectopic products from a fallopian tube, or separation of tissue planes that might be obscured or in close proximity to vascular spaces or bowel. As shown in Figure 42-1.37, an atraumatic grasper lifts the tissue, and a needle tip is inserted with the bevel away from the structure to be protected. Irrigation fluid is injected and creates a balloon effect. Depending on the location, 5 to 30 mL of fluid is instilled. A suction-irrigation system also is helpful for this technique. With this instrument, once the peritoneum is incised, the suction tip is insinuated into the opening. Fluid is forced to gently separate the tissue planes (pp. 1132 and 1134). Often, hydrodissection allows a surgeon to identify natural planes that might otherwise be obscured.

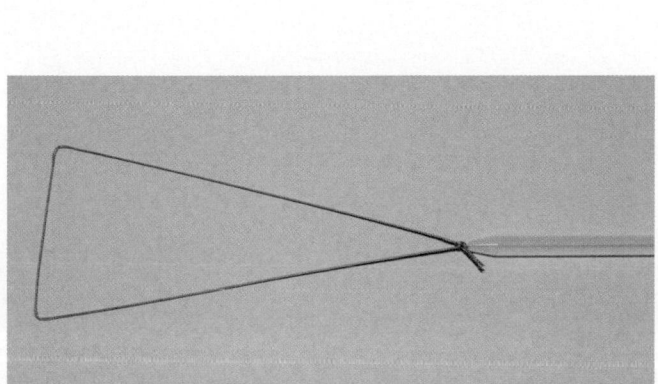

FIGURE 42-1.36 Laparoscopic suture loop.

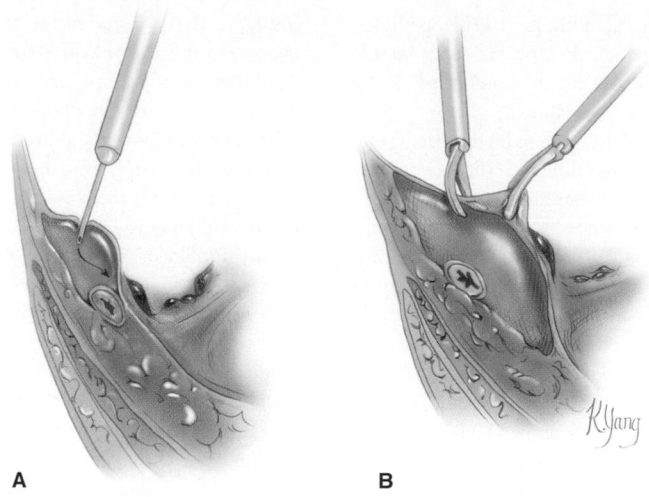

A   **B**

FIGURE 42-1.37 Hydrodissection. Needle insertion and fluid instillation (**A**) is followed by peritoneal excision of the endometriotic implant away from the ureter (**B**).

HEMOSTASIS

As tissue planes are developed, bleeding is invariably encountered. Requirements for vessel sealing are variable due to differing vessel diameters. For small vessels, spot coagulation is suitable, and a monopolar tool is satisfactory and mimics bovie use in open procedures. For larger vessels, the bipolar or harmonic technologies are preferred. Of these, the harmonic grasper coagulates or denatures the vessel tissue and can seal vessels up to 5 mm in diameter. Advanced bipolar technologies achieve vessel sealing by desiccation and can effectively seal vessels ranging from 5 to 7 mm in diameter. When choosing a modality, the thermal spread of a device should be considered. Lastly, microbipolar probes and needle-tip monopolar probes are useful for delicate tissues such as the fallopian tubes. The thermal spread is minimal, and the tip sizes are optimal for the small but friable vessels.

Liquid topical hemostatic agents have also gained popularity and have been adapted for laparoscopic use (Table 40-6, p. 1005). When using a laparoscopic adaptor, a portion of the matrix may remain in the applicator cannula. Thus, to avoid wasting retained sealant, a surgeon should flush the cannula following initial matrix application. Generally a plunger is included in many sealant kits. Alternatively, a syringe filled with air may be used to force matrix through the cannula and onto the desired tissue. Alternatively, an oxidized regenerated cellulose fabric sheet (Surgicel) can be used.

42-2

Diagnostic Laparoscopy

Diagnostic laparoscopy provides a minimally invasive option for thorough evaluation of the peritoneal cavity and pelvic organs. It is often performed to evaluate pelvic pain or causes of infertility, to diagnose endometriosis, or to ascertain the extent of adhesive disease or even the qualities of a pelvic mass. Importantly, systematic evaluation of the peritoneal cavity should be performed during every laparoscopy, either diagnostic or operative.

PREOPERATIVE

Consent

During the consenting process for diagnostic laparoscopy, a surgeon should review procedure goals, including diagnosis and possible treatment of identified pathology. This includes permission to perform procedures that may be required based on suspected pathology. Thus, consents for lysis of adhesions, peritoneal biopsy, and excision of endometriosis are commonly included. Importantly, a patient should be aware that diagnostic laparoscopy may not reveal any apparent pathology.

Laparoscopy is typically associated with few complications. Of these, organ injuries caused by puncture or by electrosurgery tools are the most common major complications, and these are summarized in Section 42-1 (p. 1097). Patients are also counseled regarding the possible need to complete the diagnostic evaluation via laparotomy. Reasons for conversion during diagnostic laparoscopy include failure to gain abdominal access, organ injury during entry, or extensive adhesions. Overall, the risk for conversion to laparotomy is low and approximates 5 percent.

Patient Preparation

In general, laparoscopy is associated with lower rates of postoperative infection and venous thromboembolism (VTE) compared with laparotomy. For diagnostic laparoscopy, antibiotics are typically not required, and VTE prophylaxis is implemented for those with risk factors (Table 39-8, p. 960). In addition, for most cases, bowel preparation is not administered. However, if extensive adhesiolysis is anticipated and the risk of bowel injury is thereby increased, bowel preparation may be indicated (Table 39-7, p. 960).

INTRAOPERATIVE

Instruments

Several instruments may prove especially helpful during diagnostic laparoscopy, and most are found in a standard laparoscopy instrument set. Of these, a blunt probe and atraumatic grasper are valuable to manipulate abdominal organs for complete inspection. A uterine manipulator that allows for chromopertubation may also be considered if performing diagnostic laparoscopy for infertility evaluation. If planned, indigo carmine dye is preferable to methylene blue, as methylene blue rarely may induce acute methemoglobinemia, particularly in patients with glucose-6-phosphate dehydrogenase deficiency. One 5-mL vial of indigo carmine is mixed with 50 to 100 mL of sterile saline for injection through the cervical cannula.

SURGICAL STEPS

❶ Anesthesia and Patient Positioning. Most laparoscopic surgery is performed in an operating room and requires general anesthesia. Some investigators, however, have described in-office microlaparoscopy using 2- to 3-mm microlaparoscopes for such diverse uses as second-look evaluation of cancer treatment, sterilization, and pelvic pain and infertility evaluation (Franchi, 2000; Kovacs, 1998; Mazdisnian, 2002; Palter, 1999).

In most cases, following anesthesia induction, the patient is placed in dorsal lithotomy position to permit manipulation of the uterus. The patient arms are tucked at the side. Correct patient positioning is critical to avoid nerve injury and is discussed in Section 42-1 (p. 1100). A bimanual examination is completed to determine uterine inclination. Inclination will direct positioning of the uterine manipulator, if used. The vagina and abdomen are surgically prepared, and the bladder is drained. If a longer procedure is anticipated, a Foley catheter may be required, as a full bladder can obstruct the operating view or increase the risk of bladder injury. The stomach is also decompressed. In many instances, a uterine manipulator is placed to provide uterine anteflexion or retroflexion during evaluation of the pelvis.

❷ Uterine Manipulator Placement. A surgeon is gowned and doubly gloved for placement of the uterine manipulator. A Graves speculum or vaginal retractors are used to display the cervix. To stabilize the cervix, a single-tooth tenaculum is placed on the anterior cervical lip. A Cohen or other uterine manipulator is then inserted

into the external os (Section 42-1, p. 1102). Alternatively, the balloon end of an endometrial cavity manipulator may be threaded into the endometrial cavity, and the balloon inflated. The outer pair of surgical gloves is removed, and the surgeon moves to either side of the patient.

❸ Primary Trocar Entry. Abdominal access may be attained by any of the four basic techniques described in Section 42-1 (p. 1110). These include Veress needle insertion, direct trocar insertion, optical-access insertion, and open entry methods. For diagnostic laparoscopy, one is not superior to the others. The umbilicus is usually chosen as the site of entry for diagnostic evaluation. However, if a patient's history suggests periumbilical adhesions, then entry at Palmer point may be preferred. A 5-mm or 10-mm umbilical port will house a suitable laparoscope for diagnostic examination. Generally, starting with a 5-mm incision and 5-mm laparoscope will allow for adequate visualization of the abdominopelvic cavity. Should improved optics be desired, this can be easily changed to a 10-mm size. Once safe initial entry is confirmed, the abdomen is insufflated to reach an intraabdominal pressure of 15 mm Hg.

❹ Additional Port Site Selection. During diagnostic laparoscopy, additional operative cannulas are needed. If minimal tissue manipulation is required, a suprapubic port may suffice. However, bilateral lower quadrant ports may be desired if lysis of adhesions or improved tissue manipulation is required. These are placed under direct laparoscopic visualization as described in Section 42-1 (p. 1115).

❺ Upper Abdomen Evaluation. All laparoscopic procedures begin with a systematic and thorough diagnostic evaluation of the entire peritoneal cavity, including the pelvis and upper abdomen. Once safe initial entry is confirmed, the area directly below the primary trocar entry site should be evaluated for bleeding or other signs of entry trauma. Prior to Trendelenburg positioning, the upper abdomen is evaluated. Specifically, the liver surface, gall bladder, falciform ligament, stomach, omentum, and right and left hemidiaphragms are inspected. The ascending, transverse, and descending colon are also examined. During inspection of the ascending portion, the appendix is identified. After Trendelenburg positioning, bowel and omentum fall toward the upper abdomen to expose the retroperitoneal structures. Now free of intestines, the area directly beneath the initial entry site is examined again. Previously unappreciated trauma to this area from initial abdominal entry may then be seen.

❻ Examination of Pelvis. Following evaluation of the upper abdomen, attention is turned to the pelvis. First, the uterus is retroflexed with the aid of the uterine manipulator to provide clear viewing of the anterior cul-de-sac. The manipulator then tilts the uterus up and to the right to permit left pelvic sidewall inspection. The uterus is then anteflexed to provide access to the posterior cul-de-sac. Lastly, the uterus is tilted to the left, and the right pelvic sidewall is viewed. Peritoneal surfaces are thereby sequentially and methodically inspected. During this, endometriotic implants, peritoneal defects or windows, studding concerning for malignancy, adhesions, or fibrosis are sought.

Next, both ureters are visualized coursing from the pelvic brim, along the pelvic sidewall, and to the cervix. Both peristalsis and caliber are evaluated. Uterine size, shape, and texture are also noted. To examine both fallopian tubes and ovaries, a surgeon may place a blunt probe into the cul-de-sac and sweep the probe forward and laterally. In doing so, the tubes and ovaries are lifted from the posterior cul-de-sac or ovarian fossa for inspection.

❼ Indicated Laparoscopic Procedures. After visual assessment of the pathology found, indicated procedures are then be performed. If adhesions are encountered, they may be divided as described in Section 42-1 (p. 1119).

❽ Abdomen Deflation and Port Removal. At laparoscopy completion, CO_2 insufflation is halted, and the gas tubing is disconnected from the primary cannula. The gas ports on all cannulas are opened to deflate the abdominal cavity. To prevent diaphragmatic irritation from retained CO_2, manual pressure is placed on the abdomen to help expel remaining gas. During this process, secondary cannulas are removed using laparoscopic visualization. This allows evaluation for bleeding from punctured vessels that may have been tamponaded by these cannulas. Additionally, it prevents herniation of bowel or omentum up through the cannula track and into the anterior abdominal wall. Of note, pneumoperitoneum can also act as an intraoperative tamponade. Accordingly, potential bleeding sites are reinspected as the pneumoperitoneum is released. Once all secondary cannulas are out, the primary cannula is removed while leaving the laparoscope in the abdomen. The laparoscope is then slowly removed to visualize the abdomen and entry site for any evidence of bleeding and to prevent viscera from being pulled into the port site.

❾ Incision Closure. Depending on their size, incisions may require deep fascial stitches. To prevent incisional hernia formation, fascial closure whenever trocars measuring 10 mm or greater are employed is often recommended (Lajer, 1997). Nonbladed trocars may decrease this risk (Liu, 2000). If open entry was used, then sutures originally placed in the fascia are unthreaded from the trocar. Each of these sutures then is brought to the midline of the incision, and square knots are tied to close the fascial defect.

Skin incisions are closed with a subcuticular stitch of 4-0 delayed absorbable suture. Alternatively, the skin may be closed with cyanoacrylate tissue adhesive (Dermabond Topical Skin Adhesive) or skin tape (Steri-Strips) (Chap. 40, p. 987).

POSTOPERATIVE

Depending on the procedure performed, most patients can be discharged home on the same day as surgery. For most, physical activities and diet can be resumed according to patient comfort.

42-3

Laparoscopic Sterilization

Approximately 700,000 tubal sterilization procedures are performed annually in the United States. Approximately half of these follow pregnancy delivery or termination, but the others are performed independent of pregnancy and are termed *interval sterilization* (Westhoff, 2000). Most interval procedures are performed laparoscopically, and most frequently involve tubal occlusion by electrosurgical coagulation, by mechanical clips, by Silastic bands, or by suture ligation (Pati, 2000).

PREOPERATIVE

Patient Evaluation
Concurrent Pregnancy

Several preventive steps can avoid sterilization of women with already early, undiagnosed pregnancies. Providing contraception well in advance of surgery, scheduling surgery in the follicular phase of the menstrual cycle, and preoperative serum β-human chorionic gonadotropin (β-hCG) level testing are effective methods to prevent or detect early pregnancy (American College of Obstetricians and Gynecologists, 2003).

Pap Smear Screening

Patients who require treatment of advanced cervical epithelial abnormalities and who desire sterilization may choose hysterectomy rather than tubal occlusion as a means to serve both needs.

For this reason, women should have current Pap smear screening results prior to surgery.

Consent

During the informed consent process, patients should be counseled regarding other reversible methods of contraception; other permanent methods, such as male sterilization; and the possibility of future regret (American College of Obstetricians and Gynecologists, 2007d). Tubal sterilization is effective and should be considered a permanent procedure by the patient. Tubal sterilization is safe and associated complications are few. In general, the risks of laparoscopic sterilization mirror those of laparoscopy as discussed in Section 42-1 (p. 1097).

Sterilizing clips and bands routinely fall from around the tube once occluded ends necrose and fibrose (Fig. 42-3.1). Most ectopic clips are incidental findings without untoward patient effects, but less commonly they can incite local foreign body reactions. Rarely, case reports of clip migration to sites such as the bladder, uterine cavity, and anterior abdominal wall have been noted in the literature (Gooden, 1993; Kesby, 1997; Tan, 2004).

In addition to surgical risks, contraceptive failure and pregnancy rates related to each procedure should be discussed with patients (Chap. 5, p. 145). Overall, these rates are low, and tubal sterilization is an effective method of contraception. For this reason, patients undergoing this procedure should be confident in their desires for permanent sterilization.

If pregnancy does occur, however, there is a greater risk of ectopic pregnancy. Bipolar

coagulation has the highest risk for this complication compared with that of clips or bands (Peterson, 1996). Accordingly, amenorrhea following any sterilization procedure should prompt serum β-hCG testing to aid in identifying ectopic pregnancies.

Patient Preparation

For sterilization procedures, antibiotics and bowel preparation are typically not administered. Venous thromboembolism prophylaxis is implemented for those at increased risk as listed in Table 39-8 (p. 960).

INTRAOPERATIVE

SURGICAL STEPS

❶ Anesthesia and Patient Positioning. Most laparoscopic tubal sterilization procedures are performed using general anesthesia, although a few investigators have described microlaparoscopic procedures using local or regional anesthesia (Siegle, 2005; Tiras, 2001).

In patients receiving general anesthesia, investigators have also evaluated the adjunctive use of several local analgesia techniques. Specific to sterilization procedures, 5 mL of a 0.25- or 0.5-percent bupivacaine solution from a needle and syringe may be dripped onto the serosal tubal surface prior to tubal occlusion (Brennan, 2004; Wrigley, 2000). Most studies comparing outcomes both with and without this topical analgesia have shown improvement in pain scores during the immediate postoperative period (30 minutes to 1 hour) but no overall differences in pain scores at later time intervals or in total pain medication consumption.

Alternatively, bupivacaine solutions have been delivered transcervically through balloon uterine manipulators into the fallopian tube lumen. In most evaluations, however, this method has proved ineffective in lessening postoperative pain (Ng, 2002; Schytte, 2003).

The patient is placed in the dorsal lithotomy position, and patient arms are tucked at the side as described in Section 42-1 (p. 1100). A bimanual examination is completed to determine uterine size and inclination. Uterine size will affect placement of the accessory trocar, and inclination will direct positioning of the uterine manipulator if used. The vagina and abdomen are surgically prepared, and the bladder is drained. Most sterilization procedures are brief, and a Foley catheter is seldom required. In many instances, a uterine manipulator or sponge stick is placed to provide uterine anteflexion or retroflexion

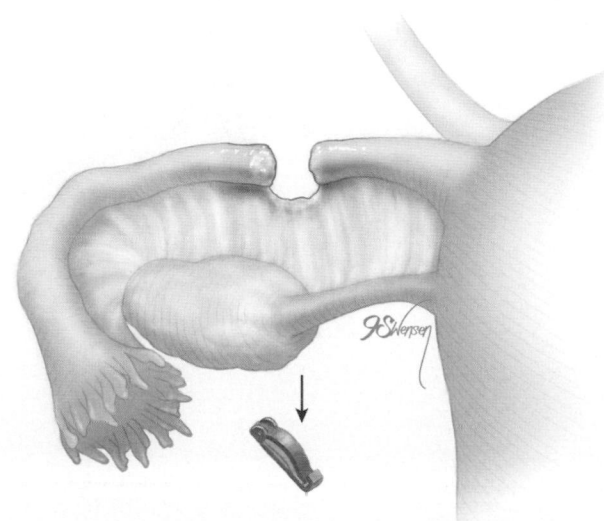

FIGURE 42-3.1 A Filshie clip may fall away following fibrosis of fallopian tube ends.

during evaluation of the pelvis (Section 42-1, p. 1102).

❷ Abdominal Entry and Accessory Ports. For all of the sterilization procedures described, the initial steps of laparoscopic abdominal entry are performed as described in Section 42-1 (p. 1110). In most instances, one accessory port is required and is placed suprapubically in the midline to provide an equal reach to both fallopian tubes. For a normal-sized uterus, this port is placed 2 to 3 cm above the symphysis pubis. However, for a larger uterus, this position is moved cephalad as needed to access both tubes. Once ports are in place, inspection of the abdomen and pelvis should be completed prior to the planned procedure.

❸ Filshie Clip. The titanium Filshie clip is applied with the aid of a customized metal applicator that houses the clip within its single-action jaw. As the jaw is closed, the shorter upper rim of the clip is forced beneath the longer lower clasp, and the clip is thereby locked into place around the fallopian tube.

❹ Fallopian Tube Manipulation. To begin, a blunt probe or atraumatic grasping forceps is placed through the accessory port. To aid clip positioning, the surgeon outstretches the fallopian tube horizontally and

laterally. Concurrently, a uterine manipulator can be used to tilt the uterus laterally and in the opposite direction. The blunt probe is then removed from the single port for insertion of the clip applicator.

❺ Applicator Insertion. At the beginning of clip application, a Filshie clip is held within its applicator and inserted through the accessory cannula into the abdomen. A surgeon half closes the applicator's upper jaw to insert it and the clip through the cannula. The handle of the applicator is not gripped tightly, as this may prematurely close and lock the clip (Penfield, 2000).

Once the Filshie clip emerges through the cannula, the applicator is opened slowly. The jaw of the applicator has the potential to spring open more quickly than the clip. This can result in the clip falling off the applicator and into the abdomen. Fallen clips are preferably retrieved, but if an open clip becomes lost and hidden by loops of bowel, laparotomy is typically not required for retrieval.

❻ Filshie Clip Placement. After the clip is completely open, the clip and applicator are positioned with one jaw above and one below the fallopian tube at a site along the isthmic portion of the tube and 2 to 3 cm from the uterine cornu (Fig. 42-3.2). The entire width of the tube should lie across the base of the clip. The distal hooked end of

the lower jaw should be visible through the mesosalpinx.

❼ Filshie Clip Application. Once satisfied that the clip is positioned correctly, a surgeon slowly squeezes the finger bar spring handle to its full limit, back toward the handle backstop. With this action, the upper ridge of the clip is slowly compressed and locked under the lower hooked end of the clip (Fig. 42-3.3). This flattens the entire tube within the clip (Fig. 42-3.4). As the applicator jaws are slowly opened, the clip releases automatically from the applicator as it has locked onto the tube. These steps are repeated on the opposite fallopian tube. If there is any doubt regarding proper clip placement, a second clip is applied correctly to the same tube.

Rarely, a fallopian tube may be transected by the clip. This is usually associated with a large fallopian tube, which has been clipped too quickly. For sterilization completion, a clip is applied to both ends of the transected tube.

❽ Bipolar Electrosurgical Coagulation. To begin, the fallopian tube is identified and grasped in the isthmic region at least 2 to 3 cm lateral to the cornu (Fig. 42-3.5). Placement here is important as pressure from retrograde menstrual flow against a coagulated stump that has been placed too close to the cornu can increase

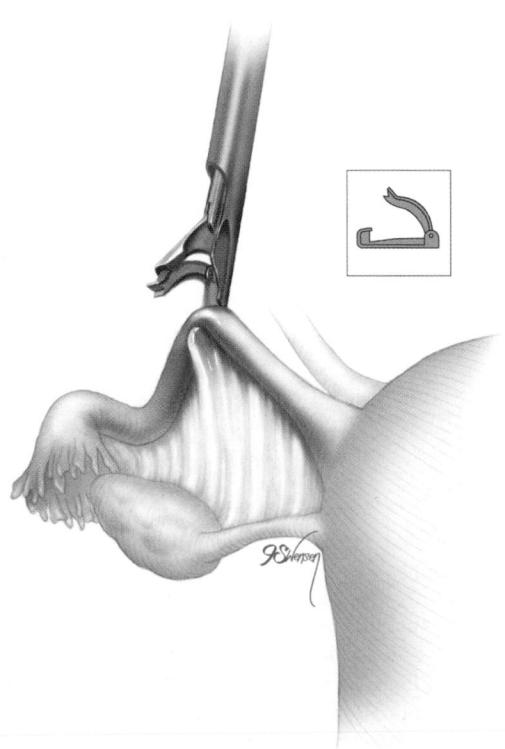

FIGURE 42-3.2 Open Filshie clip within applicator.

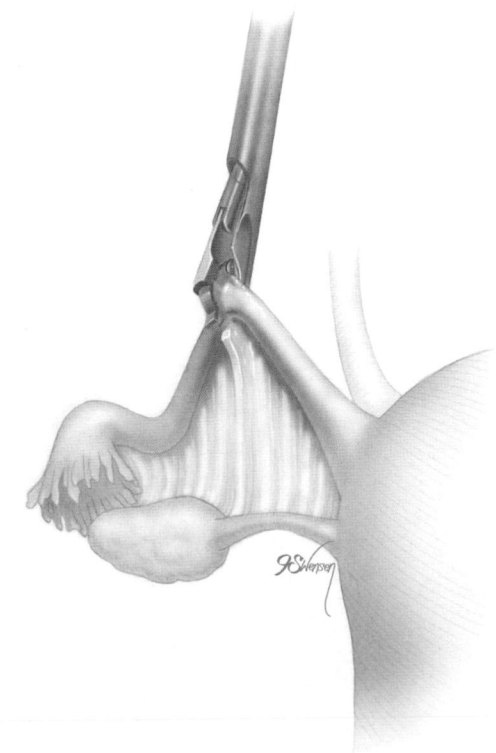

FIGURE 42-3.3 Clip application around fallopian tube.

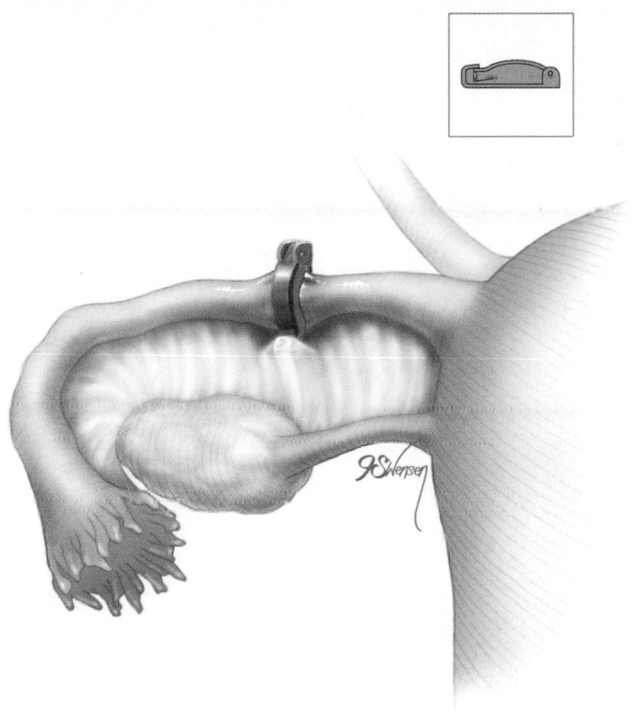

FIGURE 42-3.4 Closed clip around the tube.

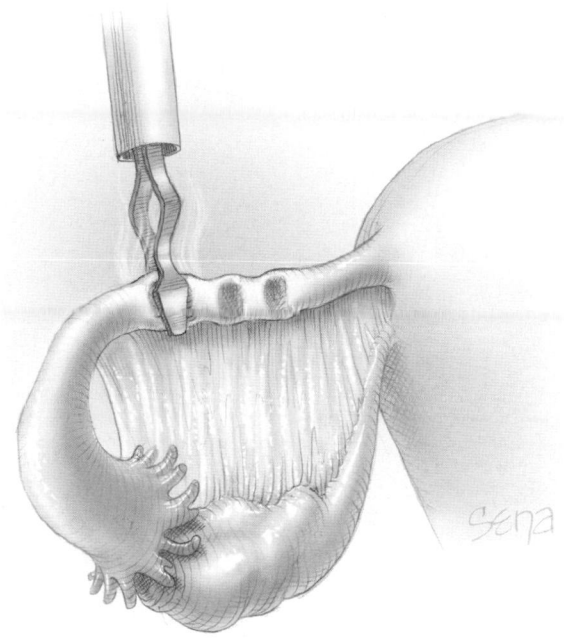

FIGURE 42-3.5 Bipolar electrosurgical coagulation.

the risk of stump recanalization and fistula formation. Leaving a 2- to 3-cm segment allows ample space for absorption of intrauterine fluid without creating excess pressure against the stump.

❾ Electrocoagulation. The coagulating paddles of the bipolar forceps should span the tube. Overextending their grasp may lead to partial coagulation of the mesosalpinx and incomplete coagulation of the entire tube width.

Before current is applied, the tube is slightly elevated and pulled away from other adjacent structures to prevent thermal injury to these structures. As current is applied, the tube swells and fluid often bubbles and pops from the tissue. Current is delivered until the tube is completely desiccated. Failure to reach this endpoint has been linked with increased contraceptive failures (Soderstrom, 1989). Because visual inspection of the tube is typically inadequate to assess complete desiccation, an ammeter is incorporated with most bipolar generators. Water conducts current through tissues. Thus, completely desiccated tissues are unable to conduct current. For this reason, current is maintained during coagulation until zero current flow across the tube is registered by the ammeter. The tube is then released.

A second site that is lateral but contiguous with the first coagulated segment is grasped and similarly coagulated. A total

of two to three contiguous sites are serially coagulated. This occludes a total span of 3 cm along the length of the tube (see Fig. 42-3.5). Coagulation of shorter distances along the tube can lead to recanalization and contraceptive failure (Peterson, 1999). These steps are then repeated on the opposite fallopian tube.

Occasionally, following coagulation the tube may stick to the bipolar paddles. To free the tube, a surgeon slowly opens the paddles and gently twist the forceps paddles to the right and then the left. Additionally, gentle fluid irrigation of the desiccated area may help release an adhered paddle.

❿ Falope Ring (Silastic Band). A Silastic Falope ring is applied with the aid of a custom metal applicator. To summarize the process, applicator tongs draw a portion of tube up into an inner sheath, and an outer sheath then pushes a Silastic band off the inner sheath and onto the loop of fallopian tube.

⓫ Ring Loading. Prior to its insertion into the abdomen, a Falope ring is stretched around the distal tip of the inner applicator sheath by means of a special ring loader and ring guide (Fig. 42-3.6).

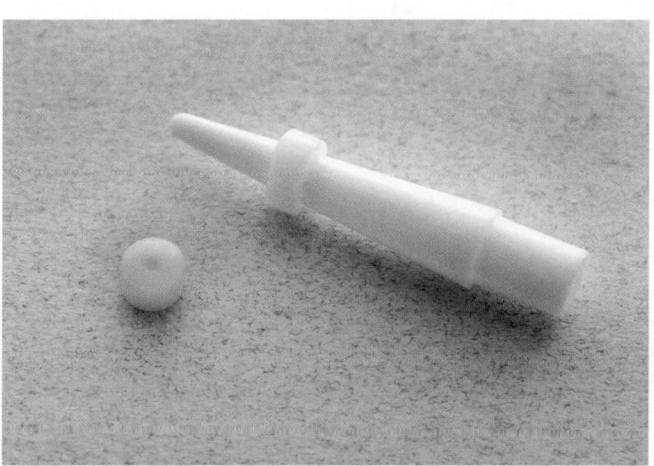

FIGURE 42-3.6 Falope ring (*left*) and ring stretched around ring loader (*right*).

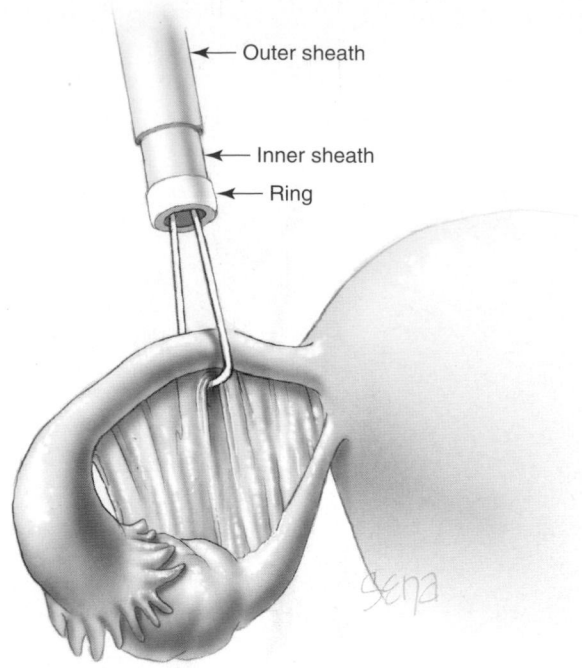

FIGURE 42-3.7 Falope ring applicator placement.

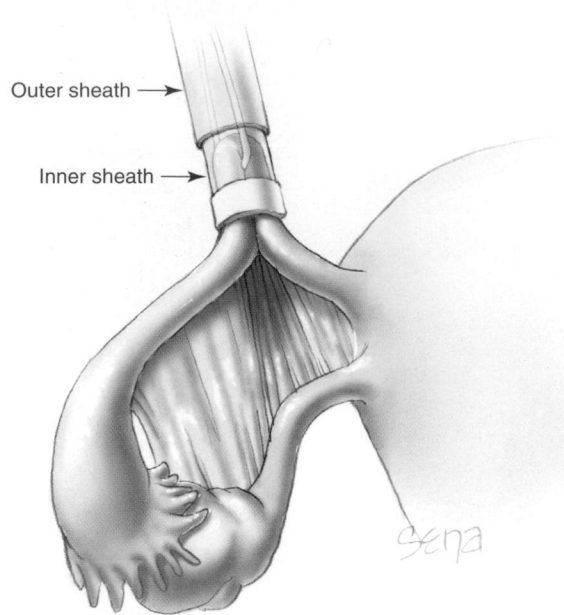

FIGURE 42-3.8 Tube drawn into inner sheath.

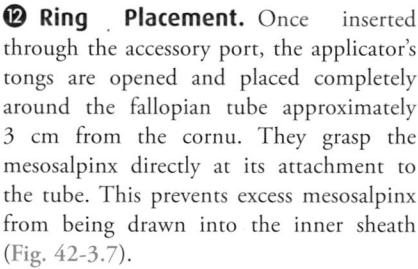

⑫ Ring Placement. Once inserted through the accessory port, the applicator's tongs are opened and placed completely around the fallopian tube approximately 3 cm from the cornu. They grasp the mesosalpinx directly at its attachment to the tube. This prevents excess mesosalpinx from being drawn into the inner sheath (Fig. 42-3.7).

⑬ Ring Application. A trigger on the applicator retracts the tongs and draws a loop of tube approximately 1.5 cm into the inner sheath. The total length of tube contained within the inner sheath is 3 cm (Fig. 42-3.8).

The outer sheath is then advanced toward the loop's base. This outer sheath pushes the Silastic band off the inner sheath and onto the loop base (Fig. 42-3.9). The loop base will blanch from ischemia following band placement (Fig. 42-3.10). These steps are repeated on the opposite fallopian tube.

⑭ Special Circumstances. Tubal transection is uncommon, and a Falope ring can be applied to each of the divided segments. Vessels of the mesosalpinx can occasionally tear and bleed as the tongs and tube are drawn into the inner sheath. The Silastic band, once applied to the loop base, will control bleeding in most instances. Thus, use of electrosurgical coagulation to achieve hemostasis is infrequently needed.

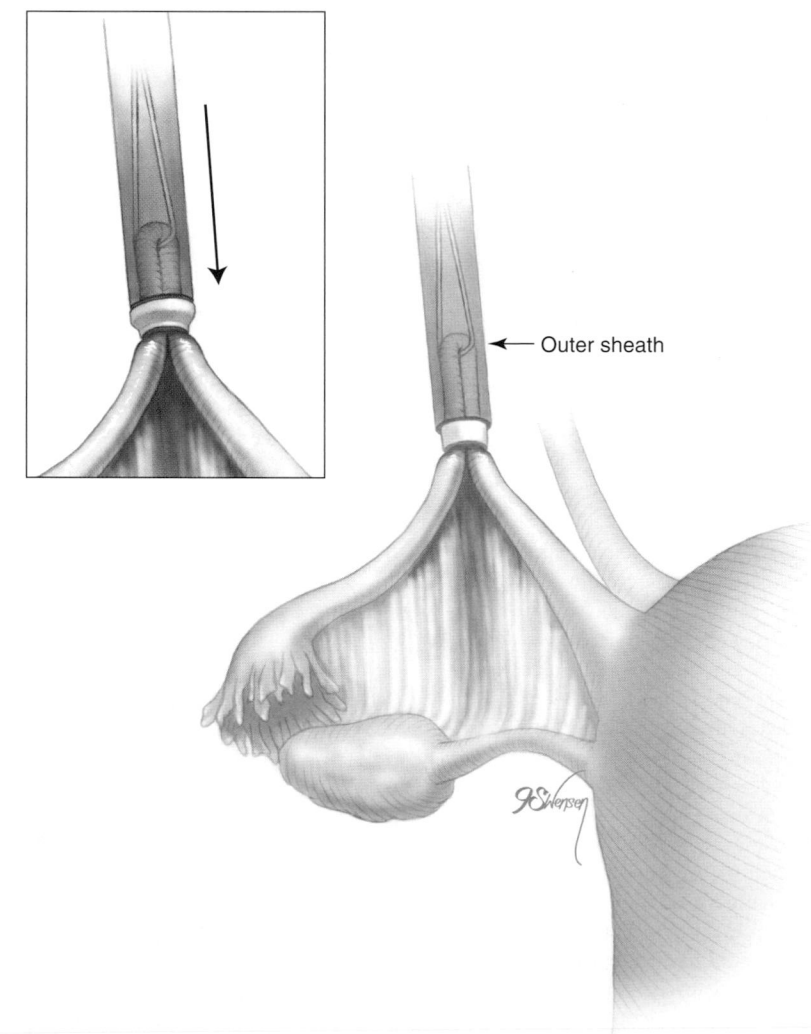

FIGURE 42-3.9 Outer sheath (*inset*) has slid over the inner sheath and forces the Falope ring off the inner sheath and onto the fallopian tube.

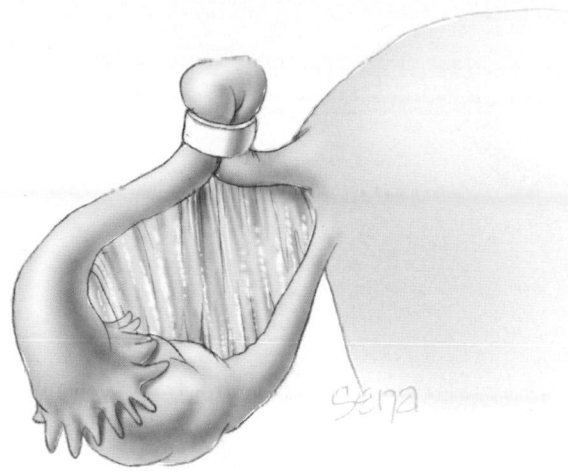

FIGURE 42-3.10 Falope ring in place.

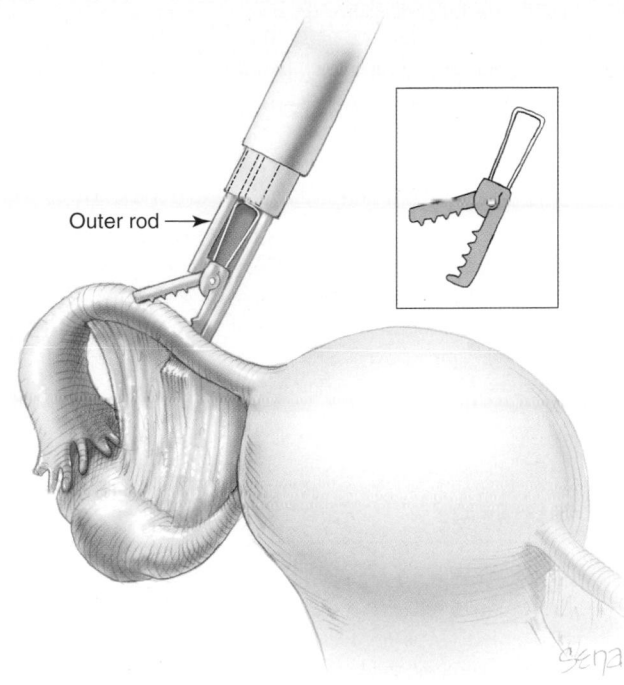

Outer rod →

FIGURE 42-3.11 Hulka clip application.

⑮ Hulka Clip Application. The plastic Hulka clip is also generically known as a spring clip because of the outer metal spring that locks the clip into place. Required equipment includes the clips themselves and a custom metal applicator, which holds the clip during application.

⑯ Fallopian Tube Manipulation. To begin, a blunt probe or atraumatic grasping forceps is placed through the accessory port. The fallopian tube is outstretched horizontally and laterally to aid clip application. Concurrently, a uterine manipulator can be used to tilt the uterus laterally and in the opposite direction.

⑰ Clip Loading. Prior to inserting the applicator and its clip through the accessory trocar, the trigger of the applicator is gently squeezed by the surgeon's thumb. This action advances the outer rod of the applicator down and over the top of the clip. This closes the jaws of the clip to within 1 mm of each other. This is an unlocked position yet allows the clip and applicator to be threaded down the accessory cannula.

⑱ Clip Application. Once inside the abdomen, the applicator trigger is drawn backward, the outer rod retracts, and the upper jaw of the clip reopens. Held within the applicator jaws, the open clip is positioned across the narrow isthmic portion of the fallopian tube, 2 to 3 cm from the cornu, and perpendicular to the long axis of the tube (Fig. 42-3.11). The jaws are positioned around the tube in a manner that directs the tube deeply into the crux of the clip jaws. This aids in total occlusion of the tube as it is flattened across the base of the closing clip. Additionally, positioning of the distal tip of the appli-

cator and clip should be such that when closed, the clip should incorporate a small portion of adjacent mesosalpinx.

⑲ Clip Closure. Once the applicator jaws are appropriately positioned, the thumb-action trigger is slowly squeezed to push

forward the outer rod of the applicator and close the clip around the tube (Fig. 42-3.12). The clip application is inspected to ensure that it has completely encompassed the tube.

If placement is deemed correct, the trigger is fully depressed. This forces the center

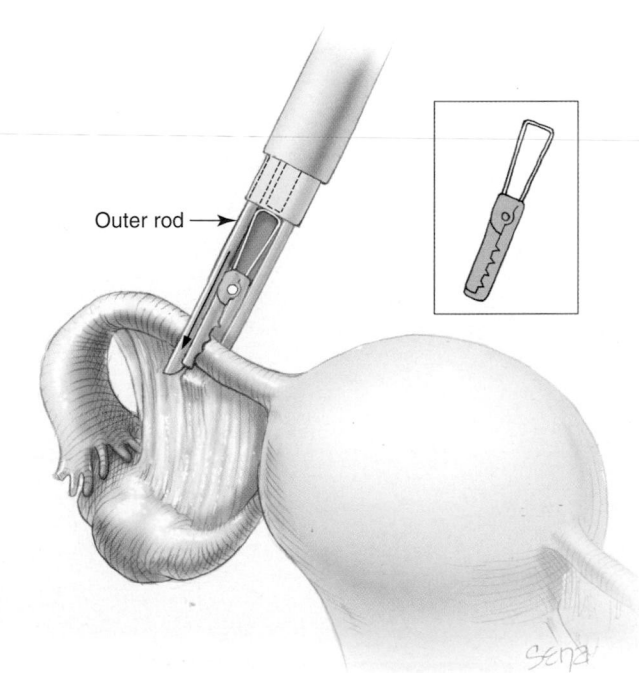

Outer rod →

FIGURE 42-3.12 Hulka clip closure.

rod of the applicator forward against the butt of the clip's metal spring (Fig. 42-3.13). The spring is pushed out and around the plastic frame of the clip to compress and lock the upper and lower clip jaws in place. One clip is placed on each tube. If a clip is misapplied, a second clip can be placed lateral to the first.

⑳ Pomeroy with Endoscopic Loop. This procedure can be used as a sterilization technique but is more commonly used to excise fallopian tube ectopic pregnancies. A description and figures can be found in Section 42-4 (p. 1130).

POSTOPERATIVE

Postoperatively, patients are given instructions similar to those following diagnostic laparoscopy. Sterilization is immediate, and intercourse may resume at the patient's discretion.

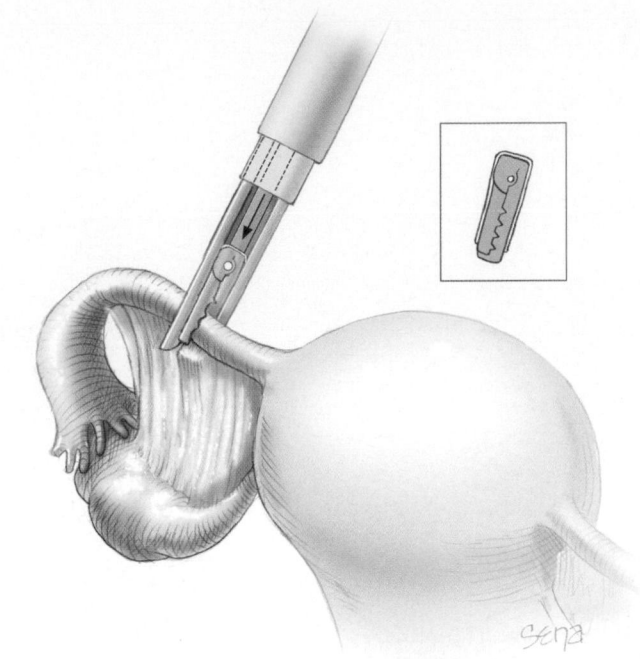

FIGURE 42-3.13 Hulka spring secured.

42-4

Laparoscopic Salpingectomy

For most women, laparoscopic management of ectopic pregnancy is the preferred surgical approach. It provides a safe and effective treatment of the affected fallopian tube while offering the patient-recovery advantages of laparoscopy. For some, laparoscopic salpingostomy is desired to treat the affected tube and preserve future fertility (Section 42-5, p. 1131). However, if fertility is not a consideration or if tubal damage or bleeding does not permit fallopian tube salvage, then laparoscopic salpingectomy is typically indicated.

In addition, salpingectomy may also be used to remove hydrosalpinges in women undergoing in vitro fertilization (IVF). Studies have shown improved pregnancy rates if such tubes are excised (Chap. 9, p. 273). Less commonly, total salpingectomy can be used as a method of sterilization. This may be especially attractive if a primary sterilization technique has failed.

PREOPERATIVE

Consent

The general risks of laparoscopic surgery are discussed in Section 42-1 (p. 1097). With salpingectomy, injury to the ipsilateral ovary is possible. Thus, the potential for oophorectomy, and its affects on fertility and hormone function, is discussed. Also, prior to surgery, a patient's desire for future fertility should be investigated. In the event that she has completed her childbearing or has failed a prior sterilization procedure, then contralateral tubal ligation or bilateral salpingectomy may be acceptable at the time of surgery.

Following any surgical treatment of ectopic pregnancy, trophoblastic tissue can persist. The risk of persistent trophoblastic tissue is lower with salpingectomy compared with salpingostomy and is discussed more fully in Section 42-5 (p. 1131).

Patient Preparation

Baseline complete blood count (CBC), β-hCG level, and Rh status are routinely assessed. If salpingectomy is performed in the setting of an ectopic pregnancy, substantial bleeding may be encountered. Thus, the patient is typed and crossmatched for packed red blood cells and other blood products as indicated. Salpingectomy is associated with low rates of infection. Accordingly, preoperative antibiotics are usually not administered. For those undergoing laparoscopic salpingectomy for ectopic pregnancy, venous thromboembolism (VTE) prophylaxis is typically indicated due to the hypercoagulability associated with pregnancy (Tables 39-8 and 39-9, p. 960). For VTE prophylaxis in those with active bleeding, intermittent pneumatic compression devices are preferred.

INTRAOPERATIVE

Instruments

Most instruments required for salpingectomy are found in a standard laparoscopy instrument set. However, a suction irrigation system is commonly needed during salpingectomy to remove blood from a ruptured ectopic pregnancy. Depending on the size of the ectopic or hydrosalpinges, an endoscopic retrieval bag may also be needed.

For salpingectomy, the fallopian tube and mesosalpinx require ligation and excision. This may be accomplished using bipolar instruments, harmonic scalpel, or laparoscopic suture loop (Endoloop). These may not be readily available in all operating suites, and desired tools should be requested prior to surgery.

SURGICAL STEPS

❶ Anesthesia and Patient Positioning. The patient is prepared and positioned for laparoscopic surgery (Section 42-1, p. 1100).

❷ Abdominal Entry. The abdomen is entered with laparoscopic techniques, and typically two or three accessory trocar sites are added (Section 42-1, p. 1110). Depending on the size of the ectopic, at least one 10-mm or larger accessory port may be necessary to allow specimen removal at surgery's end. Once ports are in place, inspection of the abdomen and pelvis should be completed prior to the planned procedure.

❸ Mesosalpingeal Incision. The affected fallopian tube is lifted and held with an atraumatic grasping forceps. Kleppinger bipolar electrode forceps are placed across a proximal portion of the fallopian tube. A cutting current at 25 W should suffice (Fig. 42-4.1). When zero amperage of flow is noted, scissors can then cut the desiccated, blanched tube.

Kleppinger forceps are then advanced across the most proximal portion of mesosalpinx. Again, current is applied, and the desiccated tissue cut. This process serially moves from the proximal mesosalpinx to its distal extent under the tubal ampulla (Fig. 42-4.2). Alternatively, monopolar scissors themselves may be attached to current. In this

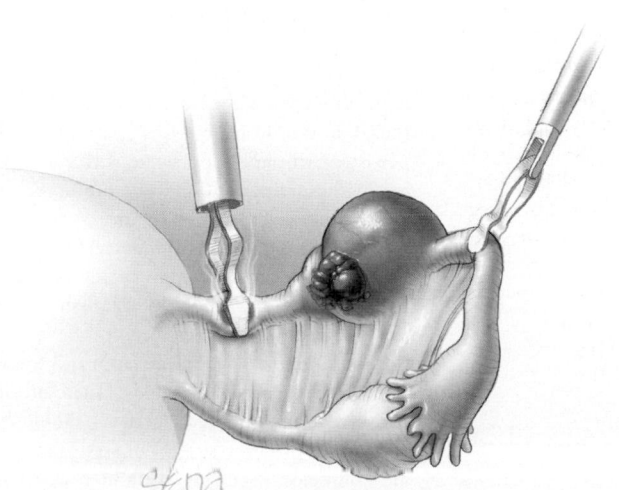

FIGURE 42-4.1 Fallopian tube desiccation.

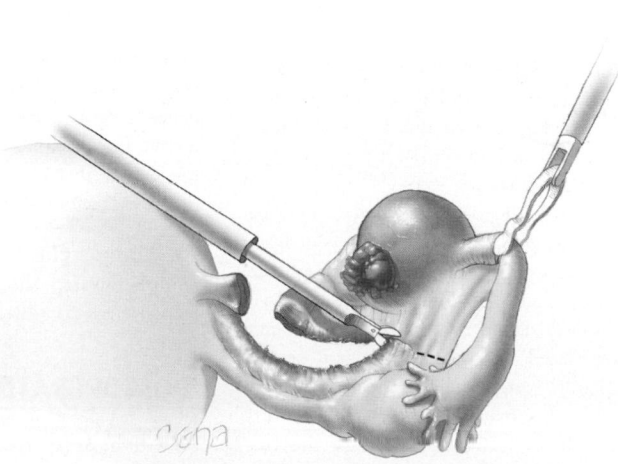

FIGURE 42-4.2 Mesosalpinx incision.

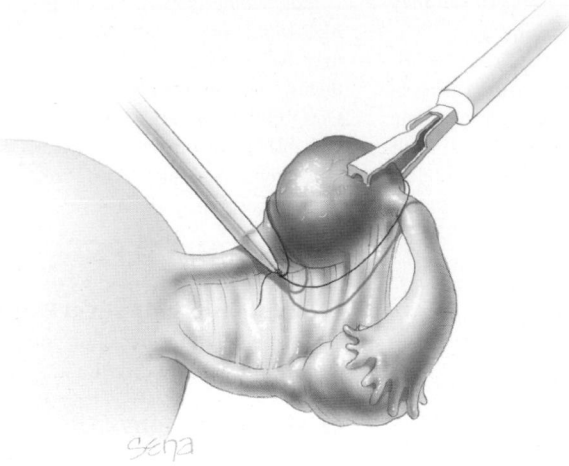

FIGURE 42-4.3 Endoscopic loop ligation.

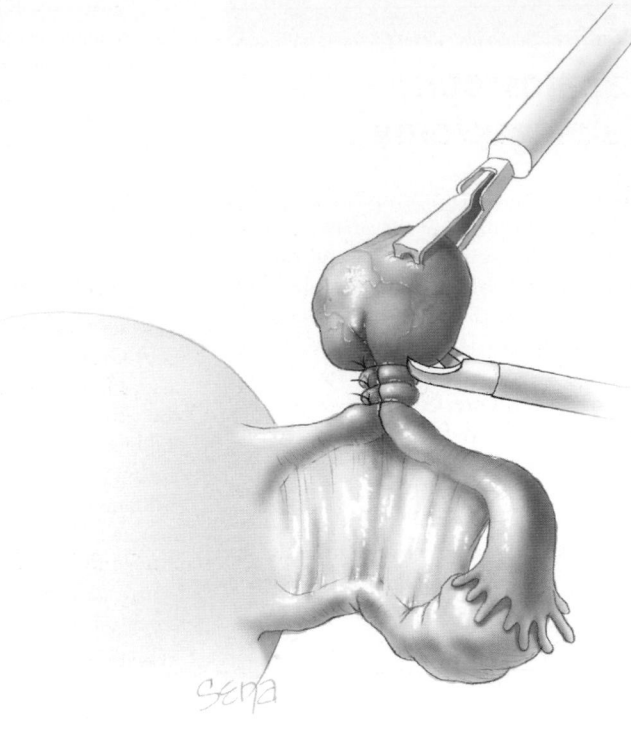

FIGURE 42-4.4 Looped portion of tube excised.

technique, vessels within the mesosalpinx are first electrosurgically coagulated and then cut. As the distal mesosalpinx is cut, the tube is freed.

Other energy sources are also available and work well. Advanced bipolar technologies (Ligasure, EnSeal), laser energy, and harmonic scalpel are suitable options. A surgeon's expertise with a particular modality dictates selection. One or more of these may be preferred based on the surrounding pelvic pathology or adhesions. The major concern with any of these tools is the amount of thermal spread to surrounding tissues.

❹ **Endoscopic Loop Ligation.** Alternatively, the vascular supply to the fallopian tube within the mesosalpinx can be ligated. Figure 42-4.3 shows an endoscopic suture loop encircling a loop of fallopian tube that contains an ectopic pregnancy. Absorbable and delayed-absorbable suture loops are available, and either is suitable for ligation. Two or three suture loops are sequentially placed, and the tube distal to these ligatures is then cut free with scissors (Fig. 42-4.4). Most tubal ectopic pregnancies are small and pliant. Accordingly, they can be held firmly by grasping forceps and drawn up into one of the accessory site cannulas. The cannula, grasping forceps, and ectopic tissue can then be removed together.

Larger tubal ectopic pregnancies may be placed in an endoscopic sac to prevent fragmentation as they are removed through the laparoscopic port site (Fig. 42-1.12, p. 1104). Alternatively, larger ectopic pregnancies can be morcellated with scissors or a laparoscopic morcellator, and the smaller fragments removed. This may be less desirable as this method theoretically may increase the risk for persistent trophoblast.

❺ **Irrigation.** To remove all trophoblastic tissue, the pelvis and abdomen should be irrigated and suctioned free of blood and tissue debris. This is especially true if morcellation was required for specimen removal. When using the suction irrigation system, the surgeon places all of the suction holes within the fluid pool to be suctioned. This avoids inadvertent removal of insufflation gas, which would collapse the visual and operative field. Additionally, the probe may cause damage to viscera, especially delicate structures such as tubal fimbria and bowel epiploica. To avoid damage, suction should be used when there is a safe distance from vulnerable structures and with the assistance of another instrument to move these structures away from the suction tip. Slow and systematic movement of the patient from Trendelenburg positioning to reverse Trendelenburg can also assist in dislodging stray tissue and fluid, which should be suctioned and removed from the peritoneal cavity.

❻ **Wound Closure.** Subsequent surgery completion steps should follow those of laparoscopy (Section 42-1, p. 1116).

POSTOPERATIVE

As with most laparoscopic surgeries, patients can resume presurgical diet and activity levels according to their comfort, typically within days.

Following Ectopic Pregnancy

If salpingectomy is performed for ectopic pregnancy, Rh-negative patients are given 50 or 300 µg (1500 IU) $Rh_0(D)$ immune globulin intramuscularly within 72 hours (Chap. 6, p. 176). To identify patients in whom trophoblastic tissue may persist, serial serum β-hCG levels should be monitored until undetectable (Seifer, 1997). Spandorfer and associates (1997) compared serum β-hCG levels 1 day postoperatively with those drawn prior to surgery. They found a significantly lower percentage of persistent trophoblastic tissue if the β-hCG level fell more than 50 percent and noted no cases if the level declined by greater than 77 percent. Until levels are undetectable, contraception should be used to avoid confusion between persistent trophoblastic tissue and a new pregnancy.

Ovulation may resume as early as 2 weeks after an early pregnancy ends. Therefore, if contraception is desired, methods should be initiated soon after surgery. Lastly, patients are counseled regarding their increased risk of future ectopic pregnancy.

42-5

Laparoscopic Salpingostomy

With surgical treatment of ectopic pregnancy, goals include hemodynamic support of the patient, removal of all trophoblastic tissue, repair or excision of the damaged tube, and preservation of fertility in those so desiring. For patients with ectopic pregnancy, laparoscopic linear salpingostomy offers the surgical advantages of laparoscopy and the opportunity to preserve fertility by preserving the involved fallopian tube (Chap. 7, p. 211). Accordingly, it is considered one of the first-line surgical treatments for women with an unruptured isthmic or ampullary ectopic pregnancy who desire future pregnancies. Success is mainly affected by the amount of bleeding, by the ability to control it, and by the degree of tubal damage.

Preoperative

Consent

Risks of laparoscopic salpingostomy mirror those for laparoscopic salpingectomy (Section 42-4, p. 1097). Importantly, with salpingostomy, a patient should be aware of the possible need for salpingectomy if the tube is irreparably damaged or bleeding from the tube cannot be controlled. Also, rates of persistent trophoblastic disease are higher with salpingostomy compared with removal of the entire affected tubal segment.

Bleeding

Because of the extreme vascularity of placental tissue, disruption of its vessels during ectopic pregnancy removal can lead to severe hemorrhage. The ability of tubal muscularis to contract is minimal, and thus bleeding during salpingostomy must be controlled with external modalities such as electrosurgical coagulation. Many devices are appropriate, and the microbipolar device is effective for achieving hemostasis while creating minimal thermal spread. At times, bleeding may be extensive and persistent and necessitate salpingectomy, partial or total.

In an effort to improve hemostasis, vasoconstrictive agents such as vasopressin have been evaluated. Dilutions of 20 U of vasopressin in 30 to 100 mL of saline are suitable. The mesosalpinx is then infiltrated with approximately 10 mL of solution. Because of the potential systemic vasoconstrictive effects of vasopressin, intravascular injection is avoided. Another approach is the injection of the solution into the portion of the tube to be incised. This is dictated by surgeon preference. Additional complications and contraindications to vasopressin use are discussed in Section 42-9 (p. 1141). Benefits to vasopressin use include less frequent use of electrosurgery, shorter operating time, and lower conversion rates to laparotomy for surgery completion.

In an attempt to avoid the cardiovascular complications of vasopressin, Fedele and colleagues (1998) diluted 20 U of oxytocin in 20 mL of saline and similarly injected the mesosalpinx. Oxytocin is purported to contract the smooth muscle fibers of the tube and cause vasoconstriction of mesosalpinx vessels. These researchers noted easier pregnancy enucleation, less bleeding, and less frequent use of electrosurgery.

Persistent Trophoblastic Tissue

During treatment of ectopic pregnancy, trophoblastic tissue can persist in as many as 3 to 20 percent of cases (Chap. 7, p. 212). Remnant implants typically involve the fallopian tube, but extratubal trophoblastic implants have been found on the omentum and on pelvic and abdominal peritoneal surfaces. Peritoneal implants typically measure 0.3 to 2.0 cm and appear as red-black nodules (Doss, 1998). Severe postoperative bleeding is the most serious complication of this persistent tissue (Giuliani, 1998).

The risk of persistent trophoblastic tissue is highest following laparoscopic salpingostomy, especially in those cases in which small, early pregnancies are removed. In these pregnancies, a less well-defined cleavage plane between the invading trophoblast and tubal implantation site develops. This may lead to a more difficult dissection and failure to completely remove all products of conception.

Preventive recommendations for this complication include irrigation and complete suctioning of the abdomen, limitation of Trendelenburg position to limit blood and tissue flow to the upper abdomen, and use of endoscopic bags for removal of larger ectopic pregnancies (Ben-Arie, 2001).

INTRAOPERATIVE

Instruments

Specific tools need for salpingostomy mirror those for salpingectomy and should be available in case salpingectomy is required (Section 42-4, p. 1129).

SURGICAL STEPS

❶ **Anesthesia and Patient Positioning.** The patient is prepared and positioned for laparoscopic surgery as described in Section 42-1 (p. 1100).

❷ **Abdominal Entry.** The abdomen is accessed with laparoscopic techniques, and typically two or three accessory port sites are used. Depending on the size of the ectopic pregnancy, at least one 10-mm or larger accessory port may be necessary to allow specimen removal at surgery's end. Once cannulas are in place, systematic inspection of the abdomen and pelvis should be completed prior to the planned procedure.

❸ **Salpingostomy.** The fallopian tube is lifted and held with atraumatic grasping forceps. By means of a 22-gauge needle through one of the accessory ports or through a separate abdominal wall needle puncture, a solution of vasopressin is injected into the mesosalpinx beneath the ectopic pregnancy. Prior to injection, aspiration should confirm that the needle is not within a vessel. If the serosal layer overlying the ectopic tissue is injected, then a smaller 25-gauge needle may be used.

A monopolar needle tip electrode is set at a cutting voltage and used to create a 1- to 2-cm longitudinal incision (Fig. 42-5.1). The incision should be positioned opposite the mesosalpinx and on the maximally distended portion of the tube that overlies the pregnancy. Laparoscopic scissors, CO_2 laser, bipolar needle, and harmonic scalpel have also been used.

❹ **Pregnancy Removal.** Atraumatic grasping forceps are used to hold one edge of the incision, while a suction-irrigation probe tip is insinuated into the tissue plane between the tubal wall and ectopic pregnancy (Fig. 42-5.2). Hydrodissection is performed on one side of the tube and then the other. A combination of high-pressure hydrodissection and gentle blunt dissection with the suction irrigator is used to remove the entire products of conception from the tube. Alternatively, the pregnancy or its fragments may require extraction with the assistance of smooth grasping forceps.

❺ **Hemostasis.** Bleeding points can be controlled with monopolar or bipolar electrosurgical coagulation (Fig. 42-5.3). The tubal incision is left open to heal by secondary intention. Tulandi and Guralnick (1991) found no differences in subsequent fertility and adhesion formation between salpingotomy with or without tubal suturing. Currently, fibrin products for hemostasis have been used in limited studies and warrant further investigation in regard to adhesion prevention and effects for future pregnancy (Mosesson, 1992).

❻ **Specimen Extraction.** Most ectopic pregnancies are small and pliant. Accordingly,

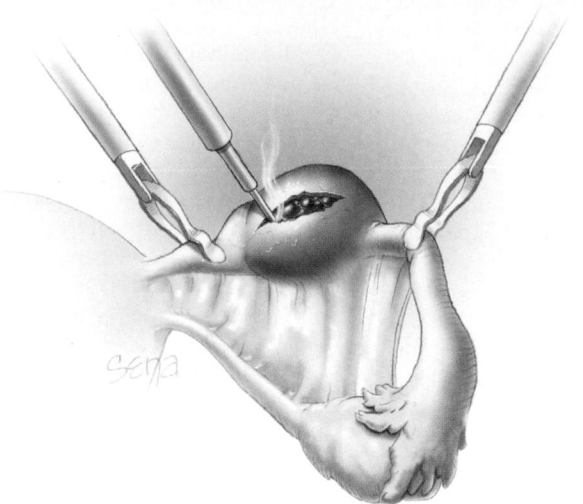

FIGURE 42-5.1 Salpingostomy.

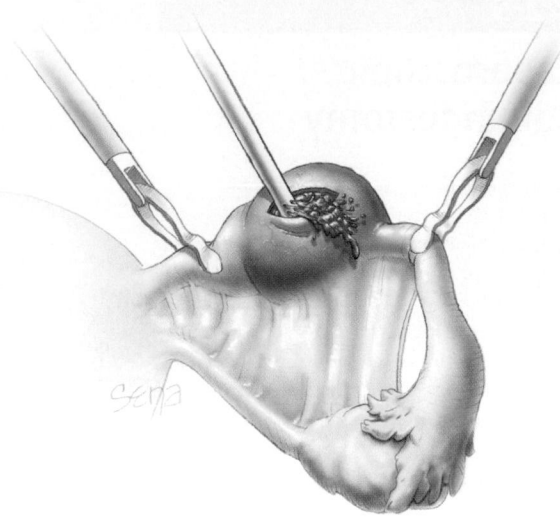

FIGURE 42-5.2 Hydrodissection.

they can be held firmly by grasping forceps and drawn up into one of the accessory cannulas. The cannula, grasping forceps, and ectopic tissue can then be removed together. Larger ectopic pregnancies may be placed in an endoscopic sac to prevent fragmentation as they are removed through the laparoscopic trocar site.

❼ Irrigation. To prevent persistent trophoblastic tissue postoperatively, the pelvis and abdomen should be irrigated and suctioned free of blood and tissue debris.

❽ Adhesion Prevention. There are adjuvants available and used for the prevention of postoperative adhesion formation. However, no substantial evidence documents that their use improves fertility, decreases pain, or prevents bowel obstruction (American Society for Reproductive Medicine, 2008).

❾ Wound Closure. Subsequent surgery completion steps follow those of laparoscopy (Section 42-1, p. 1116).

POSTOPERATIVE

As with most laparoscopic surgeries, patients can resume presurgical diet and activity levels according to their comfort, typically within days. As described more fully in Section 42-4 (p. 1130), postoperative topics specific to ectopic pregnancy include $Rh_0(D)$ immune globulin administration to Rh-negative women, surveillance for persistent trophoblastic disease, provision of contraception if desired, and counseling on future ectopic pregnancy risk.

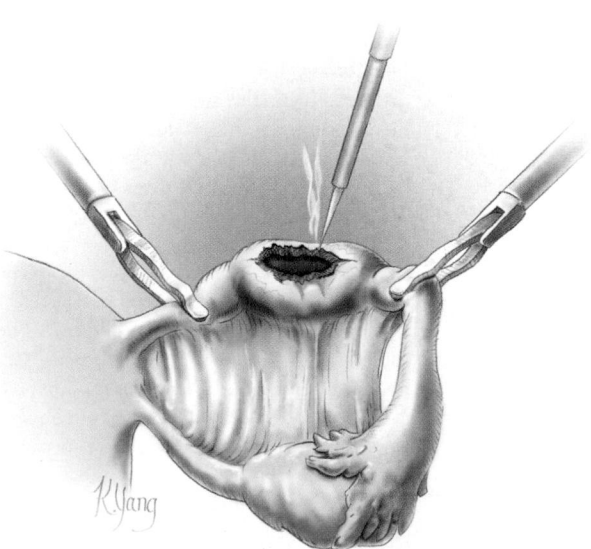

FIGURE 42-5.3 Coagulation of incision edges.

42-6

Laparoscopic Ovarian Cystectomy

Many studies have attested to the efficacy and safety of laparoscopic cystectomy for the management of ovarian cysts. Moreover, because of recovery-associated benefits, a laparoscopic technique is advocated by many as the preferred approach in women with ovarian cysts and a low risk of malignancy (Chap. 9, p. 263).

PREOPERATIVE

Patient Evaluation

Sonography

This is the primary tool used to diagnose ovarian pathology, and the sonographic characteristics of a cyst aid in determining preoperatively the malignant potential of a given lesion. Although uncommon, in those patients with indeterminate ovarian cysts following sonography, magnetic resonance imaging may enhance discrimination.

Tumor Markers

Serum cancer antigen 125 (CA125) levels are typically drawn preoperatively in postmenopausal patients and in any woman whose tumor displays other risk factors for ovarian epithelial cancer (Chap. 2, p. 41). Additionally, serum alpha-fetoprotein (AFP), lactate dehydrogenase (LDH), inhibin, and β-hCG levels may be measured to exclude germ cell or sex cord-stromal ovarian neoplasms, if these are suspected (Chap. 36, pp. 881 and 888).

Consent

Prior to surgery, patients should be informed of the unique complications associated with laparoscopy itself (Section 42-1, p. 1097). Specific to ovarian cystectomy, the risks of oophorectomy due to bleeding or extreme ovarian damage should be discussed. In many cases, cysts are investigated and removed due to concerns of potential malignancy. Accordingly, patients should be familiar with the steps involved in the surgical staging of ovarian cancer if malignancy is found.

Patient Preparation

Rates of pelvic and wound infection following ovarian cystectomy and laparoscopy are low, and antibiotic prophylaxis is typically not required. Bowel preparation is not usually required but may be considered if extensive adhesions are suspected. Venous thromboembolism (VTE) prophylaxis is typically not recommended for laparoscopic cystectomy. However, those with a greater risk of malignancy, with risks for VTE, or with an increased chance for conversion to laparotomy may benefit from these measures (Table 39-9, p. 962).

INTRAOPERATIVE

Instruments

Most instruments required for ovarian cystectomy are found in a standard laparoscopy instrument set. However, a suction irrigation system is commonly needed to remove cyst contents if rupture occurs. An endoscopic retrieval bag is also frequently used. Once contained in the sac, the cyst in some cases may be decompressed with a laparoscopic aspiration needle. If oophorectomy is required, the infundibulopelvic ligament is ligated. This may be accomplished using bipolar instruments, harmonic scalpel, laparoscopic suture loop, or stapler. These may not be readily available in all operating suites, and desired tools should be requested prior to surgery.

SURGICAL STEPS

❶ Anesthesia and Patient Positioning. The patient is prepared and positioned for laparoscopic surgery (Section 42-1, p. 1100). A bimanual examination is completed to determine ovarian size and position and uterine inclination. Ovarian information will affect placement of the accessory ports, and uterine inclination will direct positioning of the uterine manipulator if used. A uterine manipulator may assist with manipulation of the uterus and adnexa. In anticipation of possible hysterectomy as a part of ovarian cancer staging, the vagina and abdomen should be surgically prepared, and a Foley catheter is inserted. The patient is then draped to allow sterile access to the vagina and abdomen.

❷ Abdominal Entry. Primary and secondary trocars are placed as described in Section 42-1 (p. 1110). For insertion of most endoscopic sacs, at least one 10-mm or larger accessory trocar may be necessary to allow specimen removal at surgery's end. Typically, two or three accessory trocars are required.

Once the abdomen is entered, a diagnostic laparoscopy should be performed, inspecting the pelvis and upper abdomen for signs of malignancy such as ascites and peritoneal implants (Section 42-2, p. 1121). Cellular washings from these areas should be obtained and saved until frozen section analysis of the specimen has excluded malignancy. Similarly, identified peritoneal implants from suspicious areas should be biopsied and sent for intraoperative analysis. If pathology results indicate cancer, then cystectomy is aborted and intraoperative consultation with a gynecologic oncologist is preferred.

❸ Ovarian Incision. Prior to ovarian cystectomy, adhesions should be divided to restore proper anatomic relationships. A blunt probe is placed under the uteroovarian ligament and posterior ovarian surface to elevate the ovary. An atraumatic grasping forceps then steadies the ovary, and the blunt probe is removed (Fig. 42-6.1).

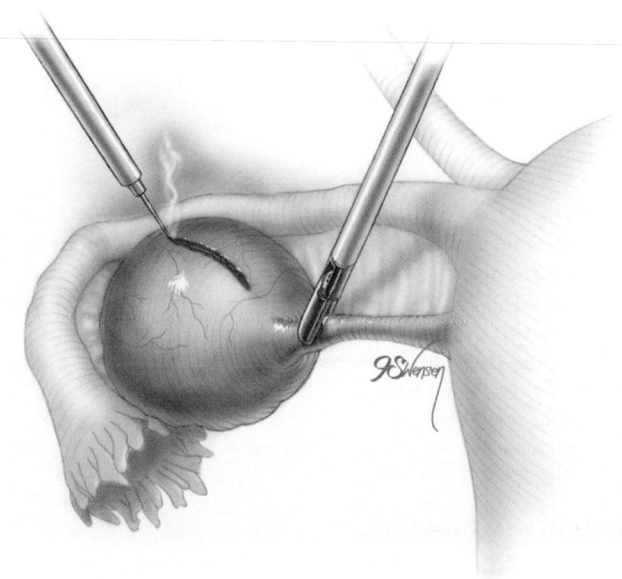

FIGURE 42-6.1 Ovarian incision.

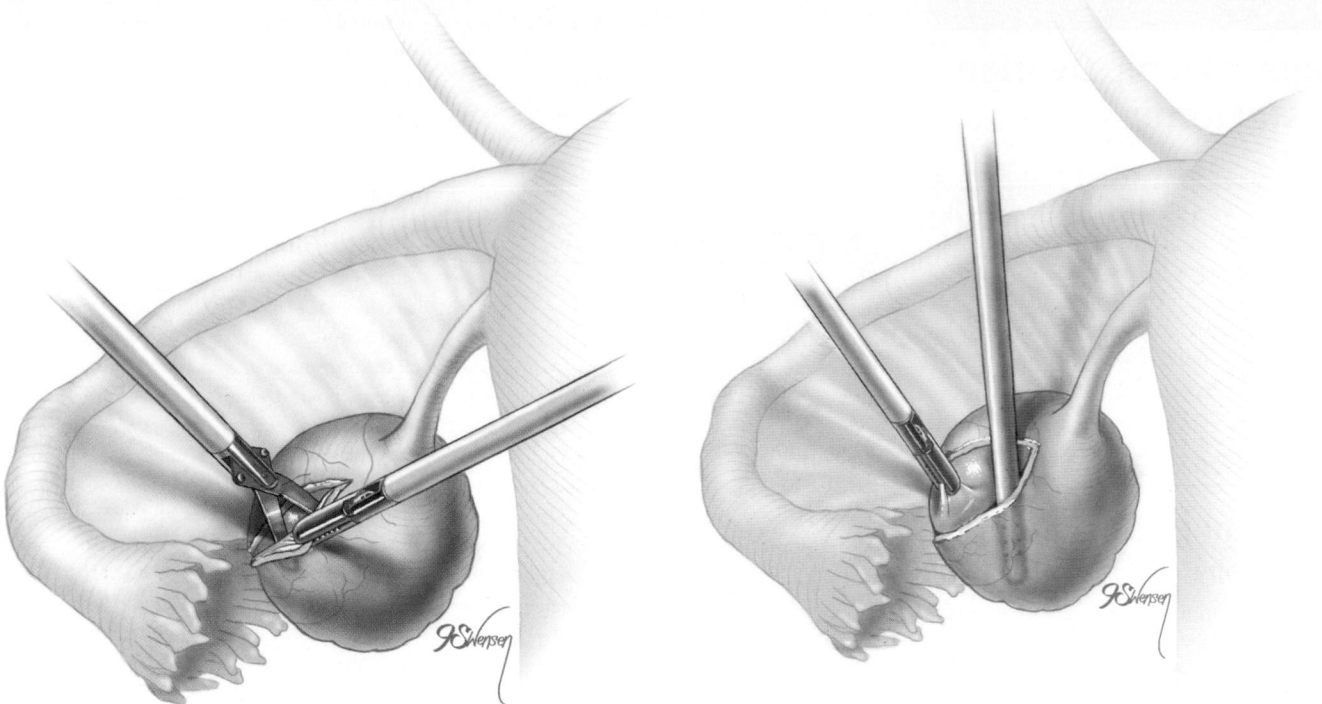

FIGURE 42-6.2 Dissection initiated.

FIGURE 42-6.3 Hydrodissection.

A monopolar needle tip electrode set at a cutting voltage is used to incise the ovarian capsule that overlies the cyst. Other suitable devices for incision include a monopolar scissor blade or harmonic scalpel. This incision is ideally on the antimesenteric surface of the ovary to minimize dissection into extensive vascularity at the ovarian base. The incision is extended into the ovarian stroma to the level of the cyst wall but should not rupture the cyst.

❹ **Cyst Dissection.** A space between the ovary and cyst wall is created using blunt forceps or dissecting scissors (Fig. 42-6.2). Atraumatic grasping forceps are used to hold one edge of the incision, while a blunt probe or suction-irrigation probe tip is insinuated into the tissue plane between the ovarian capsule and cyst wall (Fig. 42-6.3).

Blunt or hydrodissection is performed on one side of the cyst and then the other. Depending on the adherence of the cyst to its surrounding ovarian tissue, cystectomy may at times require sharp dissection with scissors. Following cyst enucleation, points of bleeding may be coagulated, or isolated vessels may be grasped and coagulated (Fig. 42-6.4).

❺ **Cyst Removal.** Following enucleation from the ovary, the cyst is placed into an endoscopic bag (Fig. 42-6.5). The opening of the sac is closed and brought up to the anterior abdominal wall (Fig. 42-6.6).

Depending on its size, the cyst and endoscopic bag may be removed in toto through one of the accessory incisions. In this setting, the laparoscopic cannula is removed first, followed by the cyst contained within the sac.

Alternatively, with larger cysts, the cannula is removed, and the entire pursed opening of the bag is drawn up through the trocar incision and fanned out onto the skin surface. The open edges of the bag are pulled upward to lift and

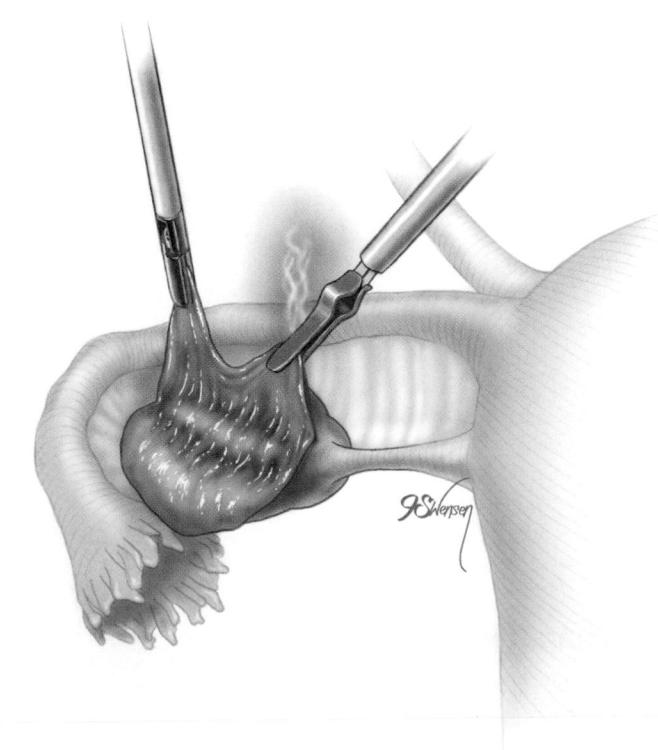

FIGURE 42-6.4 Following cyst enucleation, ovarian capsule edges are coagulated.

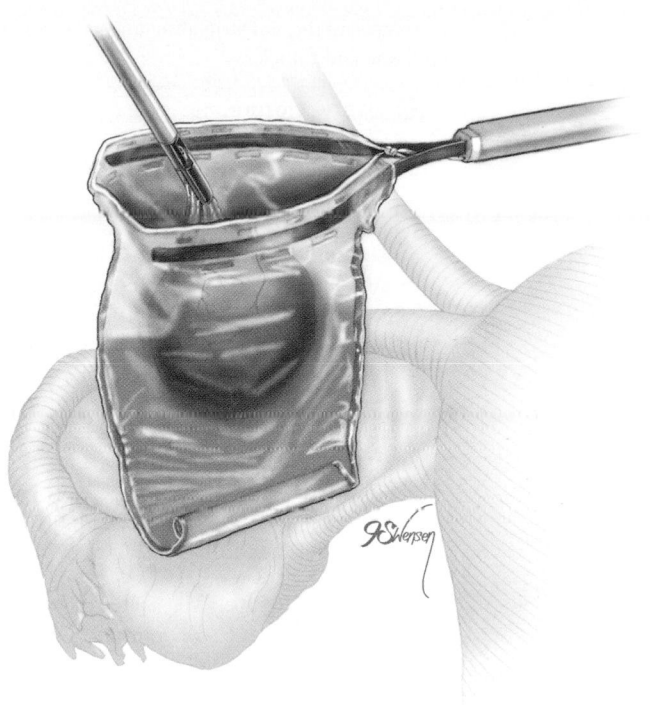

FIGURE 42-6.5 Cyst placed in endoscopic sac.

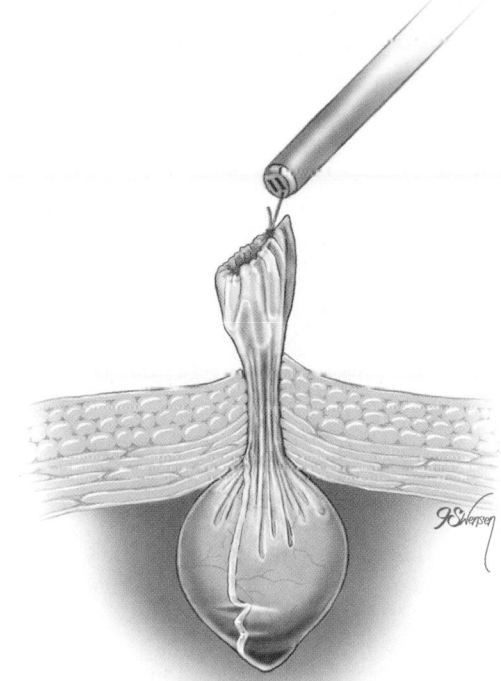

FIGURE 42-6.6 Endoscopic bag cinched and brought up to anterior abdominal wall.

press the cyst up against the incision. A needle tip is then directed into the incision and pierces the cyst contained within the endoscopic bag. An attached syringe is used to aspirate contents. Alternatively, the cyst may be ruptured by a toothed Kocher clamp placed through the skin incision and into the sac (Fig. 42-6.7). Thereby, cyst fluid is retained within the endoscopic sac. The endoscopic sac and decompressed cyst wall are then removed together through the incision (Fig. 42-6.8). During removal, care is taken to ensure that the endoscopic bag is not inadvertently punctured or torn, and all measures are used to prevent spill of cyst contents into the abdomen or port site.

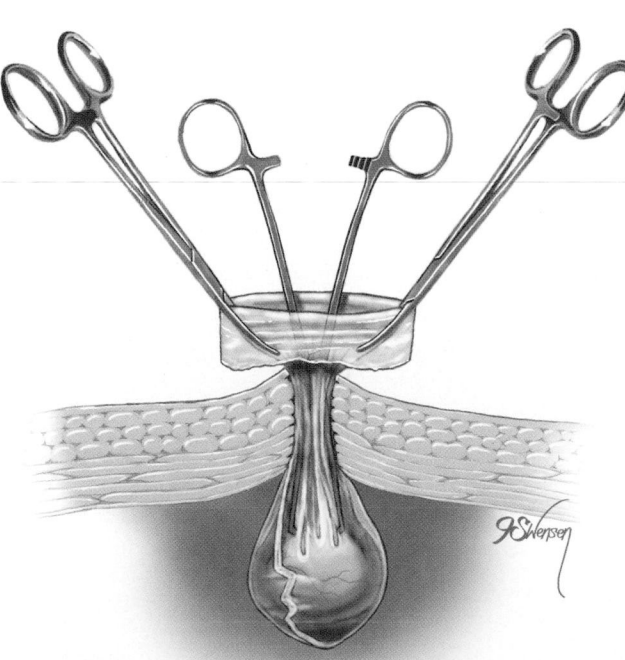

FIGURE 42-6.7 Cyst ruptured by toothed Kocher clamp within the endoscopic sac.

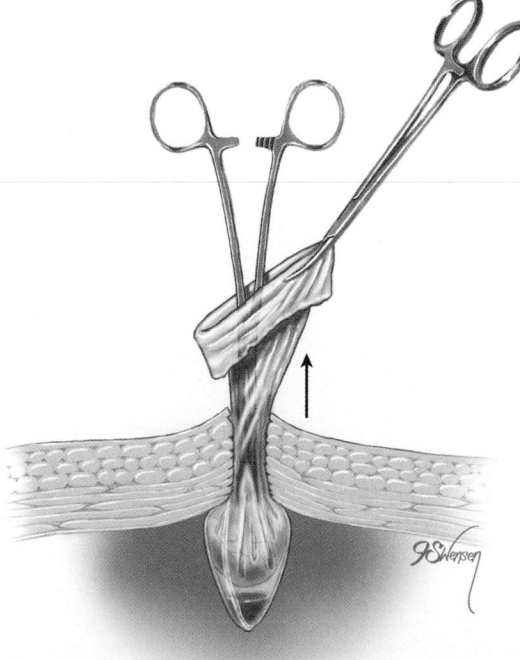

FIGURE 42-6.8 Sac and collapsed cyst are removed together.

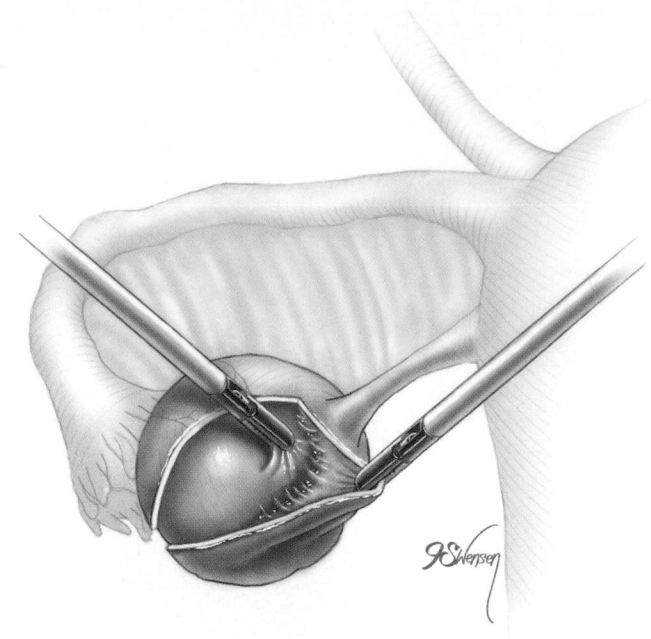

FIGURE 42-6.9 Stripping of collapsed cyst from ovarian capsule.

❻ **Cyst Rupture.** Not uncommonly during the dissection of the cyst away from the ovary, the cyst may rupture. The cyst wall is then removed using a "stripping" technique (Fig. 42-6.9). With this, both the cyst wall and cyst capsule can be grasped near the dissection plane by atraumatic forceps. Traction and counter traction can separate filmy connective tissue between these two to advance the dissection plane. As a result, the grasping forceps strip the cyst wall away from the underlying ovarian stroma (Mahdavi, 2004). To prevent damage to the underlying healthy ovary, the dissection plane between the cyst and stroma should be clearly delineated by traction on each side to prevent tearing. Injection of dilute vasopressin into this space may also help delineate the dissection plane and minimize bleeding. Histologically, Muzii and colleagues (2002) showed that this technique in nonendometriotic lesions spared ovarian tissue and did not strip away normal ovarian tissue and follicles.

❼ **Ovary Closure.** In general, the ovarian capsule is not sutured closed following cyst removal because of increased adhesion formation risk, technical difficulty, and time associated with laparoscopic suturing. Several studies have shown that leaving the capsule open does not lead to increased adhesion formation (Marana, 1991; Wiskind, 1990). Application of an adhesion barrier such as oxidized regenerated cellulose may be considered to prevent adhesion formation (Franklin, 1995; Wiseman 1999). However, no substantial evidence documents that their use improves fertility, decreases pain, or prevents bowel obstruction (American Society for Reproductive Medicine, 2008).

❽ **Wound Closure.** The specimen is submitted in most cases for immediate frozen section analysis. If benign findings are noted, then steps toward surgical closure begin. If malignancy is found, then surgical staging should ensue. Of note, if a large mass was removed and the port site was likely extended during the removal, one should consider fascial closure to prevent port site hernias. The finishing laparoscopic steps are found in Section 42-1 (p. 1116).

Postoperative

Following laparoscopic ovarian cystectomy, instructions similar to those after diagnostic laparoscopy are given (Section 42-2, p. 1122).

Laparoscopic Salpingo-Oophorectomy

Laparoscopy can be used to safely remove many adnexa and in most cases, offers a faster recovery and less postoperative pain compared with laparotomy. As discussed in Chapter 9 (p. 261), indications for adnexectomy vary but may include torsion, ovarian cyst rupture, suspicion of ovarian malignancy, and symptomatic ovarian remnant. In addition, prophylactic oophorectomy is often considered in women with or at risk for cancers involving the breast, ovary, and colon (Chap. 35, p. 857).

Laparoscopy is a preferred approach when possible and can be safely performed in pregnant women, preferably in the early second trimester. However, for all patients, there are clinical settings in which laparotomy may be preferred. These include a high suspicion of cancer, anticipation of extensive pelvic adhesions, and large ovarian mass size.

PREOPERATIVE

Patient Evaluation

Salpingo-oophorectomy is typically performed to remove ovarian pathology, and sonography is the primary tool used for diagnosis. In cases in which anatomy may be unclear, magnetic resonance imaging may add additional information. As discussed in Chapters 35 and 36, tumor markers may be drawn prior to surgery if malignancy is suspected.

Consent

Prior to surgery, patients should be informed of the unique complications associated with laparoscopy (Section 42-1, p. 1097). Specific to salpingo-oophorectomy, the risk of ureteral injury should be discussed. In addition, in some cases, unanticipated bilateral adnexectomy may be required, and patient's should be aware of its hormonal significance. Lastly, many adnexa are removed due to concerns of potential malignancy, and patients should be familiar with the steps involved in the surgical staging of ovarian cancer.

Patient Preparation

Unless an ovarian abscess is identified, antibiotic prophylaxis is administered according to the preference of the surgeon. In general, however, laparoscopic salpingo-oophorectomy does not require antibiotic prophylaxis (American College of Obstetricians and Gynecologists, 2009a). Bowel preparation is not usually

required, but may be considered if extensive adhesions are suspected. Venous thromboembolism prophylaxis is typically not recommended for laparoscopic cystectomy. However, those with a greater risk of malignancy, with VTE risks, or with an increased chance for conversion to laparotomy may benefit from these measures (Table 39-9, p. 962).

INTRAOPERATIVE

Instruments

Most instruments required for ovarian cystectomy are found in a standard laparoscopy instrument set. However, a suction irrigation system is commonly needed to remove cyst contents if rupture occurs. An endoscopic retrieval bag is also frequently used. During oophorectomy, the infundibulopelvic ligament is ligated. This may be accomplished using bipolar instruments, harmonic scalpel, laparoscopic suture loop, or stapler. These may not be readily available in all operating suites, and desired tools should be requested prior to surgery.

SURGICAL STEPS

1 Anesthesia and Patient Positioning. The patient is prepared and positioned for laparoscopic surgery as described in Section 42-1 (p. 1100). A bimanual examination is completed to determine ovarian size and position and uterine inclination. Ovarian information will affect placement of the accessory ports, and uterine inclination will direct positioning of the uterine manipulator if used. Because of possible hysterectomy as a part of ovarian cancer staging, the vagina and abdomen are surgically prepared. A Foley catheter is inserted. A uterine manipulator may also be placed to assist with manipulation of the uterus and adnexa.

2 Abdominal Access. Primary and secondary trocars are placed as described in Section 42-1 (p. 1110). Typically, two or three accessory ports are required. For insertion of most endoscopic sacs, at least one 10-mm or larger accessory port may be necessary to allow specimen removal at surgery's end.

3 Pelvic Inspection and Washings. Once the abdomen is entered, a diagnostic laparoscopy should be performed, inspecting the pelvis and upper abdomen for signs of malignancy such as ascites and peritoneal implants (Section 42-2, p. 1121). Cellular washings from these areas should be obtained and saved until frozen section analysis of the specimen has excluded malignancy. Similarly, identified peritoneal implants from these areas are biopsied and sent for intraoperative evaluation. If

intraoperative pathologic analysis reveals malignancy, operative consultation with a gynecologic oncologist is preferred for complete surgical cancer staging.

4 Ureter Location. Prior to adnexectomy, adhesions should be divided to restore proper anatomic relationships. The ureter lies close to the infundibulopelvic (IP) ligament, and its course should be noted. If the location of the ureter is not clear, the peritoneum is incised, and retroperitoneal isolation of the ureter is completed.

5 Infundibulopelvic Ligament Coagulation. Ligation of the ovarian vessels within the IP ligament can be completed with endoscopic loop ligatures, electrosurgical coagulating devices, harmonic scalpel, or stapler depending on surgeon preference (Fig. 42-7.1). Once these vessels are occluded, the IP is then severed distally.

6 Opening of the Broad Ligament. After transection of the IP, the fallopian tube and ovary are gently elevated with atraumatic forceps. Incision of the broad ligament's posterior leaf is then extended toward the uterus (Fig. 42-7.2).

7 Uteroovarian Ligament Coagulation. The uteroovarian ligament and proximal fallopian tube are identified posterior to the round ligament. Similarly to the IP, these may be coagulated, stapled, or ligated (Fig. 42-7.3). Distal to this occlusion, the uteroovarian ligament and fallopian tube are transected, and the adnexa is freed.

8 Adnexa Removal. A variety of endoscopic bags are available for tissue removal (Fig. 42-1.12, p. 1104). The specimen is dropped into the sac, which is closed and brought up to the anterior abdominal wall. Depending on its size, the adnexa and endoscopic bag may be removed in toto through one of the accessory port sites. In this setting, the laparoscopic cannula is removed first, followed by the specimen contained within the sac.

Alternatively, with larger cystic ovaries, the cannula is removed, and the entire pursed opening of the bag is drawn up through the incision and fanned out onto the skin surface. The open edges of the bag are pulled upward to lift and press the ovary against the incision. A needle tip is directed through the incision and into the sac. The ovary is pierced and aspiration drainage is completed by an attached syringe. Alternatively, the cyst may be ruptured by a toothed Kocher clamp placed through the skin incision and into the sac. Thereby, cyst fluid is retained in the endoscopic sac. The endoscopic sac and decompressed cyst wall are then removed together through the incision.

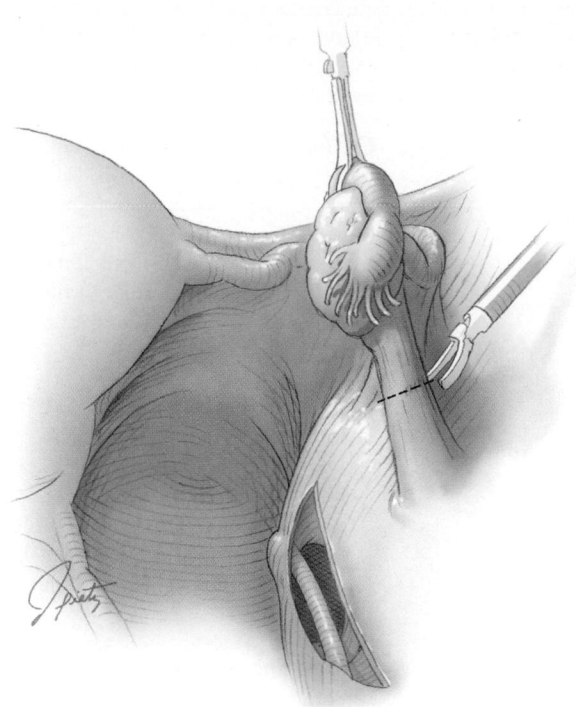

FIGURE 42-7.1 Infundibulopelvic ligament coagulation.

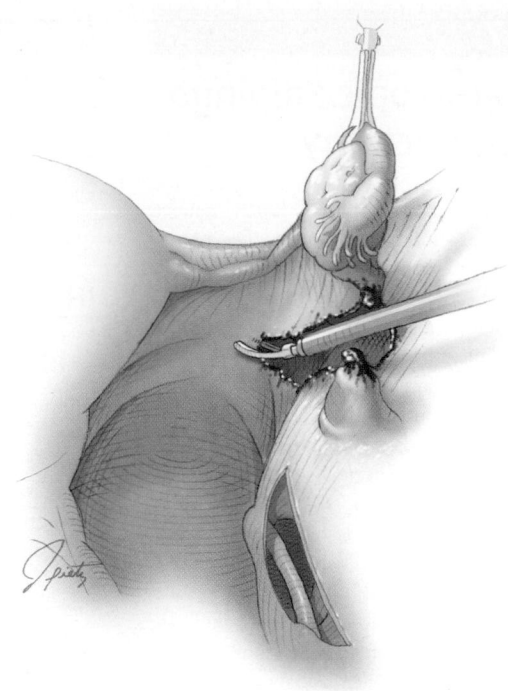

FIGURE 42-7.2 Opening of the broad ligament.

During removal, care is taken to ensure that the endoscopic bag is not inadvertently punctured or torn, and all measures are used to prevent spill of cyst contents into the abdomen or port site. Additionally, to prevent spill or in the case of large solid masses, one may remove the adnexa through a minilaparotomy incision or a colpotomy incision.

❾ **Colpotomy.** To enter the posterior cul-de-sac, attention is turned to the vagina, and handheld retractors are placed to expose the cervix and posterior fornix. The uterine manipulator is lifted anteriorly, and an Allis clamp is placed on the posterior vaginal wall 2 to 3 cm from the posterior cervicovaginal junction. The Allis clamp is pulled downward to create tension across the posterior vaginal wall. The posterior vaginal vault is then cut with curved Mayo scissors, and the cul-de-sac of Douglas is entered. Pneumoperitoneum is lost immediately. If a laparoscopic instrument is already holding the specimen, this can be passed through the colpotomy and removed vaginally. Following adnexa removal, the vaginal incision is closed with interrupted stitches or with a running suture line using 0-gauge delayed absorbable suture. If colpotomy is used for specimen removal, a single prophylactic dose of antibiotics is administered. Suitable agents are listed in Table 39-6 (p. 959).

❿ **Wound Closure.** If malignancy is suspected, the specimen is submitted for immediate frozen section analysis. If benign findings are noted, then steps toward surgical closure begin (Section 42-1, p. 1116). If malignancy is found, then surgical staging should ensue. Of note, if a large mass was removed and the port site was likely extended during the removal, one should consider fascial closure to prevent port site herniation.

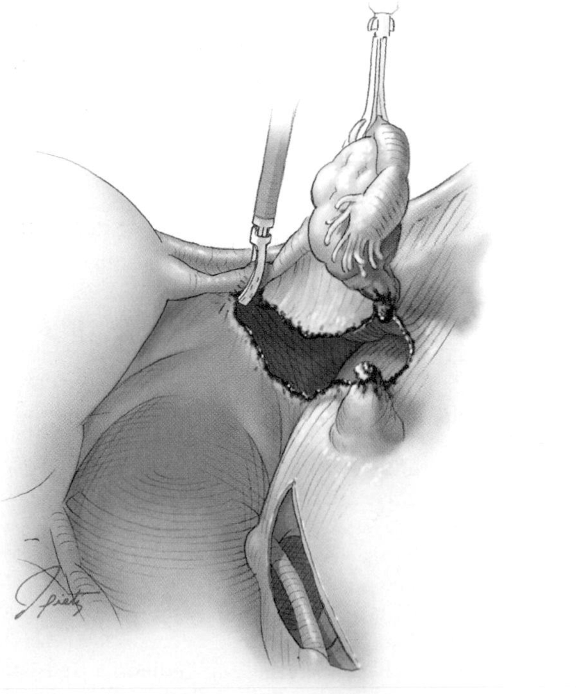

POSTOPERATIVE

Advantages to laparoscopy include a rapid return to normal diet and activities, and postoperative complication rates are low. If both adnexa are removed, then hormone replacement therapy is considered in appropriate candidates (Chap. 22, p. 585).

FIGURE 42-7.3 Fallopian tube and uteroovarian ligament coagulation and transection to free the specimen.

42-8

Ovarian Drilling

Ovarian drilling is a technique of puncturing the ovarian capsule with a laser beam or an electrosurgical needle using a laparoscopic approach. Similar to ovarian wedge resection, this procedure's end goal is to reduce the amount of androgen-producing tissue in women with polycystic ovarian syndrome (PCOS). However, in wedge resection, a long capsular incision is required for this degree of resection. As a result, infertility secondary to adhesions complicates many postoperative courses (Buttram, 1975; Toaff, 1976). To minimize this risk and avoid the need for laparotomy, ovarian drilling techniques using laparoscopy were developed in the early 1980s.

Compared with medical management, ovarian drilling has lower rates of ovarian hyperstimulation syndrome (OHSS) and of multifetal gestation (Farquhar, 2007). Disadvantages include the surgical risks of laparoscopy, risks of pelvic adhesion formation, and concerns regarding long-term effects on ovarian function (Donesky, 1995; Farquhar, 2007). For these reasons, ovarian drilling is viewed as a second-line therapy. It can be useful in patients who fail to ovulate with clomiphene citrate, who are at risk for OHSS, or who desire to minimize their risk for multifetal gestation. An additional discussion of this procedure's advantages, disadvantages, and indications can be found in Chapter 20 (p. 539).

PREOPERATIVE

Consent

There appear to be relatively few complications that arise immediately after ovarian drilling. Hemorrhage, infection, and thermal bowel injury are infrequent. Similarly, ovarian atrophy following drilling is rare but been reported (Dabirashrafi, 1989).

Adhesion formation following this procedure is common, however. Most of these adhesions at second-look laparoscopy have typically been graded as minimal or mild (Gürgan, 1991). Moreover, researchers have described only a minimal, if any, impact of these adhesions on fertility (Gürgan, 1992; Naether, 1993). The risk of infertility secondary to adhesive disease, however, should be discussed with the patient prior to surgery.

INTRAOPERATIVE

Instruments

Ovarian drilling has been described using monopolar or bipolar electrosurgical energy or using CO_2, argon, or Nd-YAG laser, all with the goal of causing focal damage to the ovarian stroma and cortex. Currently, no studies support the superiority of one modality (Strowitzki, 2005).

Number of Ovarian Punctures

Punctures into the ovarian capsule are typically 2 to 4 mm wide and 4 to 10 mm deep. Although techniques using as few as four or as many as 40 punctures per ovary have been described, there are a few studies that have investigated the optimum number of punctures (Farquhar, 2004). For example, Malkawi and Qublan (2005) showed that five punctures per ovary compared with 10 resulted in equally improved pregnancy rates and similarly low rates of postprocedural OHSS and multifetal gestation.

SURGICAL STEPS

❶ Anesthesia and Patient Positioning. Patient positioning and anesthesia mirror that for other laparoscopic procedures (Section 42-1, p. 1100).

❷ Abdominal Entry. Three incisions are used for this laparoscopic procedure. In addition to an umbilical incision, two bilateral lower abdominal incisions are made (Section 42-1, p. 1110). These incisions serve as entry sites for the electrosurgical needle tip and grasping forceps.

❸ Ovarian Drilling. The ovary is elevated with a blunt grasper. The electrosurgical current is set at 30 to 60 W cutting mode. A monopolar electrosurgery needle tip is used to puncture the ovary perpendicular to the capsular surface and to pierce the follicular cysts that are characteristic of PCOS. Four to five punctures are placed symmetrically on the antimesenteric surface of the ovary (Fig. 42-8.1). Drilling is avoided on the lateral surfaces of the ovaries to minimize adhesions to the pelvic sidewall and is avoided at the ovarian hilus to limit bleeding risks. The needle is inserted to a depth of 4 to 10 mm. Electrical current is applied for 3 to 4 seconds. The surface of the ovary can be irrigated with saline or lactated Ringer solution to cool the capsular surface (Strowitzki, 2005).

❹ Adhesion Barriers. Because of the risk for adhesion formation, some investigators have used adhesion barrier products following ovarian drilling. Greenblatt and Casper (1993), however, showed no improvement in adhesion prevention following this procedure using Interceed Adhesion Barrier. No other studies have addressed the efficacy of other adhesion prevention products.

POSTOPERATIVE

Postoperatively, patients are given instructions similar to those following diagnostic laparoscopy (Section 42-2, p. 1122).

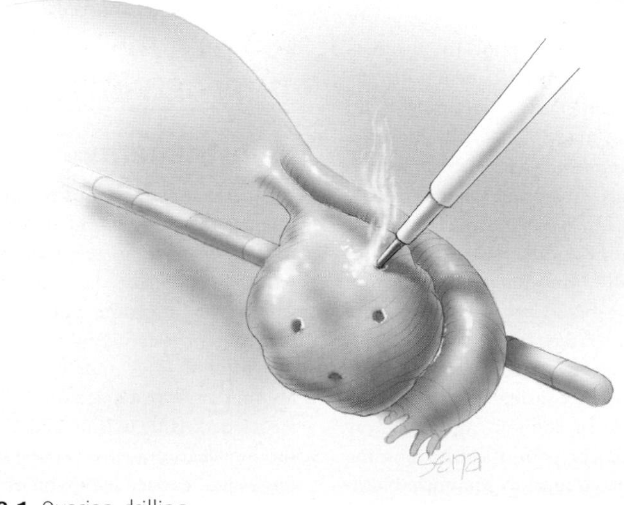

FIGURE 42-8.1 Ovarian drilling.

42-9

Laparoscopic Myomectomy

Myomectomy involves surgical removal of leiomyomas from their surrounding myometrium, and accepted indications include selected cases of abnormal uterine bleeding, pelvic pain, infertility, and recurrent miscarriage. Historically, removal of serosal and intramural tumors typically required laparotomy. However, laparoscopic excision may be performed by those with advanced skills in operative laparoscopy and laparoscopic suturing. Robotic myomectomy has also increased in popularity. For many, robotic technology permits easier leiomyoma dissection, enucleation, and multilayer suturing needed for hysterotomy closure (Visco, 2008).

In general, subserosal and intramural leiomyoma myomectomies are most appropriate for a laparoscopic approach. Submucous leiomyomas are best treated via hysteroscopic resection as discussed in Section 42-16 (p. 1166). The choice between abdominal myomectomy and laparoscopic myomectomy is based on various factors that include tumor number, size, and location. Surgical experience and comfort with laparoscopic dissection, morcellation, and suturing are also important. As a surgeon's laparoscopic experience accrues, many will complete a greater percentage of myomectomies with a minimally invasive approach.

PREOPERATIVE

Patient Evaluation

Because of their impact on preoperative and intraoperative planning, leiomyoma size, number, and location are evaluated prior to surgery with sonography, magnetic resonance (MR) imaging, or hysteroscopy, as described in Chapter 9 (p. 252). Specifically, leiomyomas may be small and buried within the myometrium. Therefore, accurate information as to tumor number and location ensures complete excision. Moreover, with a laparoscopic or robotic approach, the ability to palpate and appreciate smaller deep tumors may be compromised. In these cases, preoperative MR imaging may assist with leiomyoma location and surgical planning. Lastly, multiple large masses or those that are located in the broad ligament, are near the cornua, or involve the cervix may increase the risk of conversion to hysterectomy, and patients should be so counseled. Surgical expertise and comfort will vary and is the most important factor in determining the approach to myomectomy. However, studies have suggested that there is an increased risk of complications with the following: more than three leiomyomas, tumor size >5 cm, and intraligamentous location (Sizzi, 2007).

Consent

Myomectomy has several risks including significant bleeding and transfusion. Moreover, uncontrolled hemorrhage or extensive myometrial injury during tumor removal may necessitate hysterectomy. Patients should also be counseled regarding the risk of conversion to an open procedure, which ranges from 2 to 8 percent (American College of Obstetricians and Gynecologists, 2008).

Postoperatively, the risk of adhesion formation is significant, and leiomyomas can recur. In some series, the risk of leiomyoma recurrence after laparoscopic myomectomy compared with conventional myomectomy appears to be higher (Dubuisson, 2000; Fauconnier, 2000). As one explanation, with laparoscopic myomectomy, small, deep intramural leiomyomas may be missed because a surgeon's tactile sensation is diminished.

The use of electrosurgical energy on the uterus and challenges of laparoscopic multilayer hysterotomy closure also heighten concerns regarding uterine rupture during a subsequent pregnancy (Hurst, 2005; Parker, 2010; Sizzi, 2007). Women undergoing myomectomy who do plan to have future pregnancies should be counseled regarding the possible need for cesarean delivery based on the extent of myometrial disruption during the myomectomy.

PATIENT PREPARATION

Hematologic Status and Tumor Size

Many preparatory steps prior to myomectomy address associated patient anemia, anticipated intraoperative blood loss, and tumor size. First, many women who undergo this surgery are anemic secondary to associated menorrhagia. Correction prior to surgery may include oral iron therapy, gonadotropin-releasing hormone (GnRH) agonist administration, or both. In anticipation of blood loss, a complete blood count and type and crossmatch for packed red blood cells is obtained. Autologous blood donation or cell saver devices may be considered if great blood loss is expected. In addition, uterine artery embolization may be performed the morning of surgery for large uteri to minimize bleeding. However, this is most often used prior to laparotomy for significantly sized uteri.

GnRH agonists may be considered to decrease leiomyoma size, intraoperative blood loss, and adhesion rates. However, loss of pseudocapsule planes around the tumors and greater risk of recurrence due to missed smaller leiomyomas is the trade-off. A fuller evidence-based discussion of these same preoperative options is found in Section 41-10 (p. 1039).

Antibiotic Prophylaxis

There are few studies addressing the benefits of preoperative antibiotic use. Iverson and coworkers (1996), in their analysis of 101 open myomectomy cases, found that although 54 percent of cases received prophylaxis, infectious morbidity was not lowered compared with cases in which antibiotics were not used.

In cases of myomectomy performed for infertility, because of the potential for tubal adhesions associated with pelvic infection, antibiotic prophylaxis is commonly used. For those in whom prophylaxis is planned, 1 g of a first- or second-generation cephalosporin is appropriate (Iverson, 1996; Periti, 1988; Sawin, 2000).

Other Preparation

The risk of bowel injury with this procedure is low, and bowel preparation is typically not required unless extensive adhesions are anticipated. Because the risk of conversion to hysterectomy is present, vaginal preparation immediately prior to surgical draping is performed. With laparoscopic gynecologic surgery, the decision to provide or withhold prophylaxis should factor patient- and procedure-related risks for venous thromboembolism (VTE) (Geerts, 2008). Thus, if longer operating times or conversion to laparotomy are anticipated or preexisting VTE risks are present, then prophylaxis as outlined in Table 39-9 (p. 962) is reasonable.

INTRAOPERATIVE

Instruments

Many instruments required for laparoscopic myomectomy are found in a standard laparoscopy instrument set. However, a laparoscopic injection needle may be required for vasopressin injection, and a suction irrigation system is frequently needed to remove blood following tumor enucleation. A leiomyoma screw or tenaculum is helpful to create needed tissue tension and counter tension for enucleation. After enucleation and for removal of excised leiomyomas, electric morcellators are commonly used to pare down tumors (Section 42-1, p. 1103). These may not be readily available in all operating suites and should be requested prior to surgery.

SURGICAL STEPS

❶ Anesthesia and Patient Positioning. As with most laparoscopic procedures, the patient should be placed in dorsal lithotomy position after adequate general anesthesia has been delivered. This permits manipulation of a uterine manipulator, if desired, and access to the posterior fornix for colpotomy, if needed. A bimanual examination is completed to determine uterine size to aid port placement. Because of the risk of hysterectomy and because colpotomy may be used for tumor removal, both the vagina and abdomen are surgically prepared. A Foley catheter is inserted. A uterine manipulator may also be placed, including one that will allow chromotubation at the procedure's end (Section 42-1, p. 1102). If planned, one 5-mL vial of indigo carmine is mixed with 50 to 100 mL of sterile saline for injection through the cervical cannula.

❷ Trocar and Laparoscope Insertion. Primary and accessory trocars are placed as described in Section 42-1 (p. 1110). Port placement is customized to assist uterine manipulation, leiomyoma excision, and hysterotomy repair. Depending on uterine height, the primary port may need to be placed supraumbilically. In general, a distance 3 to 4 cm above the level of the fundus is helpful to provide a global view of the uterus. Typically, at least three accessory ports are required as depicted in Figure 42-1.30 (p. 1116). At minimum, one of the cannulas should be at least 12 mm to accommodate the electric morcellator if this will be employed.

After safe abdominal entry is obtained, a diagnostic laparoscopy is performed, and the serosal uterine surface should be inspected to identify leiomyomas to be removed (Section 42-2, p. 1121). Correlating with preoperative imaging, the surgeon selects the optimal uterine incision to minimize myometrial disruption and to remove the maximum number of tumors thorough one incision.

❸ Use of Vasopressin. Pitressin (8-arginine vasopressin) is a sterile, aqueous solution of synthetic vasopressin. It is effective in limiting uterine bleeding during myomectomy because of its ability to cause vascular spasm and uterine muscle contraction. Compared with placebo, vasopressin injection has been shown to significantly decrease blood loss during myomectomy (Frederick, 1994).

Each vial of Pitressin is standardized to contain 20 pressor units/mL, and doses used for myomectomy range from 20 U diluted in 30 to 100 mL of saline (Bieber, 1998; Fletcher, 1996, Iverson, 1996). Vasopressin is typically injected along the planned serosal incision(s), between the myometrium and leiomyoma

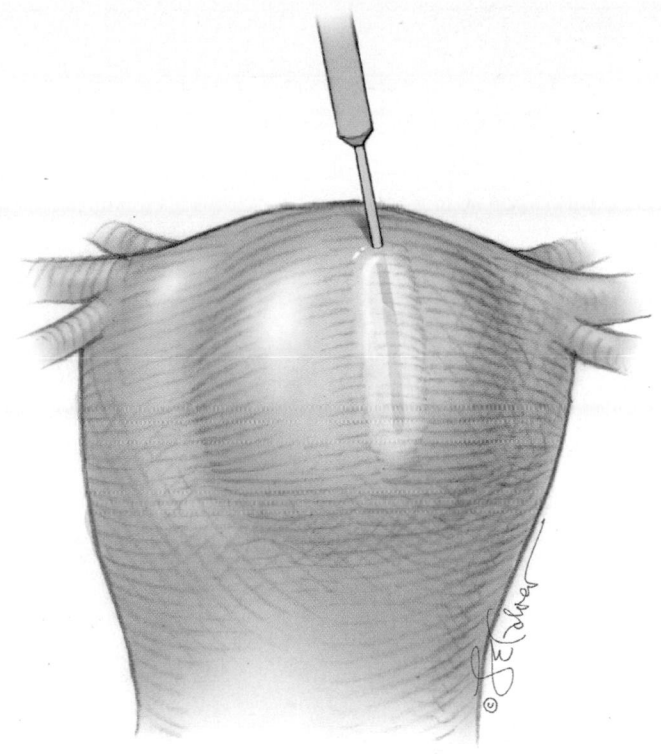

FIGURE 42-9.1 Vasopressin injection beneath serosa.

capsule (Fig. 42-9.1). A laparoscopic needle placed through one of the accessory ports or a 22-gauge spinal needle placed directly through the abdominal wall is suitable for injection. Needle aspiration prior to injection is imperative to avoid intravascular injection of this potent vasoconstrictor. The anesthesiologist should be informed of vasopressin injection, as a sudden increase in patient blood pressure may potentially occur following injection. Blanching at the injection site is common. The plasma half-life of this agent is 10 to 20 minutes. For this reason, injection of vasopressin should be discontinued 20 minutes prior to uterine repair to allow evaluation of bleeding from myometrial incisions (Hutchins, 1996).

The main risks associated with local vasopressin injection result from inadvertent intravascular infiltration and include transient increases in blood pressure, bradycardia, atrioventricular block, and pulmonary edema (Hobo, 2009; Tulandi, 1996). For these reasons, patients with a medical history of angina, myocardial infarction, cardiomyopathy, congestive heart failure, uncontrolled hypertension, migraine, asthma, or severe chronic obstructive pulmonary disease may not be candidates for vasopressin use.

❹ Serosal Incision. Because of postoperative adhesion formation risks, surgeons should minimize the number of serosal incisions and attempt to place incisions on the anterior

uterine wall. Tulandi and colleagues (1993) found that posterior wall incisions result in a 94-percent adhesion formation rate compared with a 55-percent rate for anterior incisions.

After instillation of vasopressin, hysterotomy may be performed using a harmonic scalpel, monopolar electrode, or laser. For most patients, an anterior midline vertical uterine incision allows removal of the greatest number of leiomyomas through the fewest incisions. The length should accommodate the approximate diameter of the largest tumor. The incision depth should afford access to all leiomyomas (Fig. 42-9.2).

❺ Tumor Enucleation. Once the hysterotomy is created, the myometrium will generally retract, and the first leiomyoma may be grasped with a laparoscopic single-toothed tenaculum. Alternatively, a leiomyoma screw can also be used to achieve tissue traction and create tissue tension between the myometrium and mass (Fig. 42-9.3). Using a blunt probe or suction-irrigator tip, blunt dissection of the pseudocapsule surrounding the leiomyoma frees the tumor from the adjacent myometrium. Areas requiring sharp dissection from the myometrium may be freed with any of the electrosurgical instruments that were used for the uterine incision.

❻ Bleeding. Hemorrhage during myomectomy primarily develops during tumor

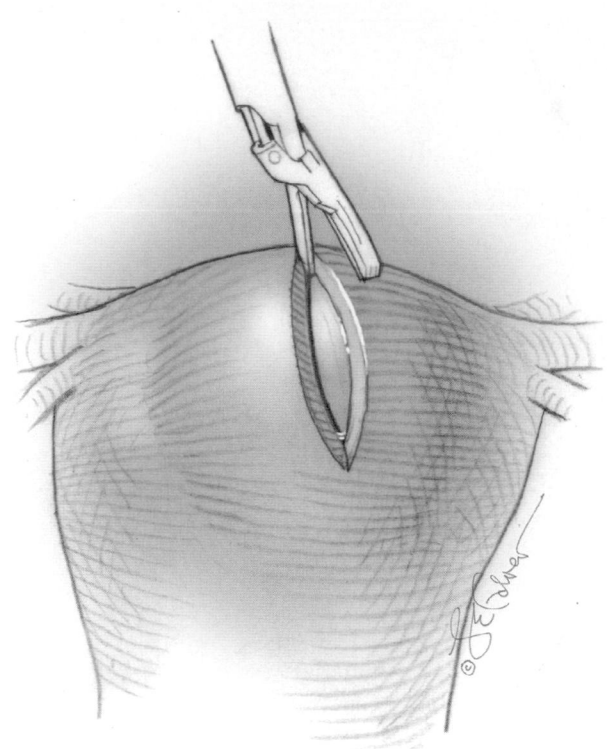

FIGURE 42-9.2 Serosal incision overlying leiomyoma.

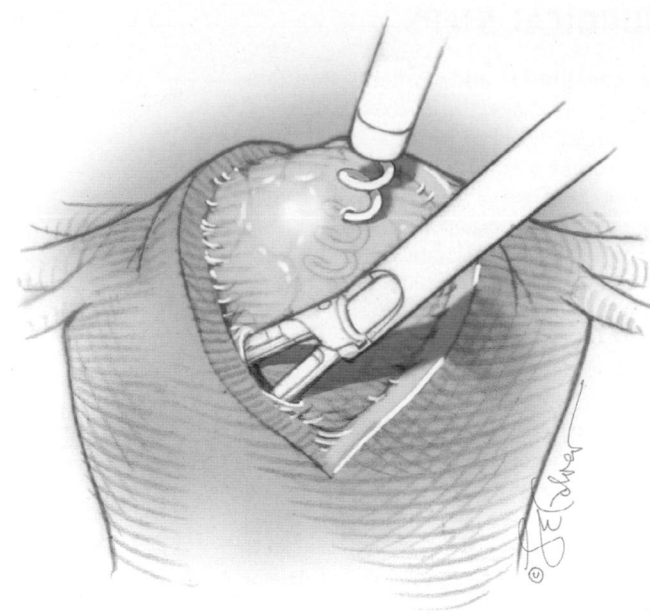

FIGURE 42-9.3 Tumor enucleation.

enucleation and is positively correlated with preoperative uterine size, total weight of leiomyomas removed, and operating time. Approximately two to four main arteries feed each leiomyoma and enter the tumor at unpredictable sites. For this reason, surgeons must watch for these vessels, coagulate them prior to transection when possible, and be ready to immediately fulgurate remaining bleeding vessels (Fig. 42-9.4). To avoid myometrial damage, the surgeon should apply electrosurgical energy only when necessary.

❼ Myometrial Closure. Following removal of all tumors, redundant serosa may be excised. Laparoscopic suturing techniques described in Section 42-1 (p. 1116) are used during incision reapproximation. The same general principles of myometrial closure for abdominal myomectomy are employed during laparoscopic myomectomy. This is true whether conventional laparoscopic needle drivers, a suturing device, or a surgical robot is used. In one method, for deep myometrial closure, a needle driver can be used with 0-gauge delayed-absorbable suture on a CT-2 needle in a continuous running fashion. Smaller internal myometrial incisions are closed first. The primary incision(s) is then closed in layers to improve hemostasis and prevent hematoma formation (Fig. 42-9.5). A gauge of sufficient strength to prevent breakage during muscle

approximation is selected, typically 0- or 2-0 gauge. Alternatively, barbed sutures (Quill or V-Loc) may aid closure of myometrial defects during laparoscopic myomectomy (p. 1117). These obviate the need for knot tying and yield consistent wound apposition (Einarsson, 2010; Greenberg, 2008).

❽ Serosal Closure. Closure of the serosal incision using a running baseball suture with 4-0 or 5-0 monofilament delayed-absorbable suture may help to limit adhesion formation (Fig. 42-9.6). Moreover, absorbable adhesion barriers have been shown to reduce the incidence of adhesion formation following myomectomy and may be introduced through laparoscopic ports (Ahmad, 2008a). However, no substantial evidence documents that adhesion barrier use improves fertility, decreases pain, or prevents bowel obstruction (American Society for Reproductive Medicine, 2008).

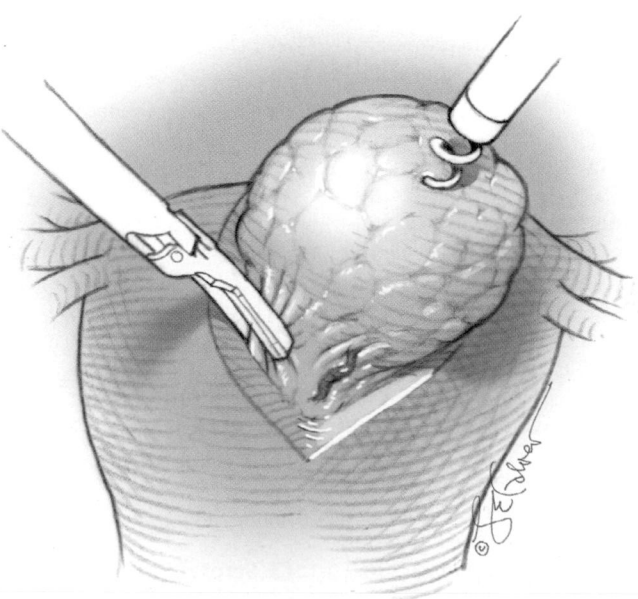

FIGURE 42-9.4 Coagulation of vascular attachments between the leiomyoma and the myometrium.

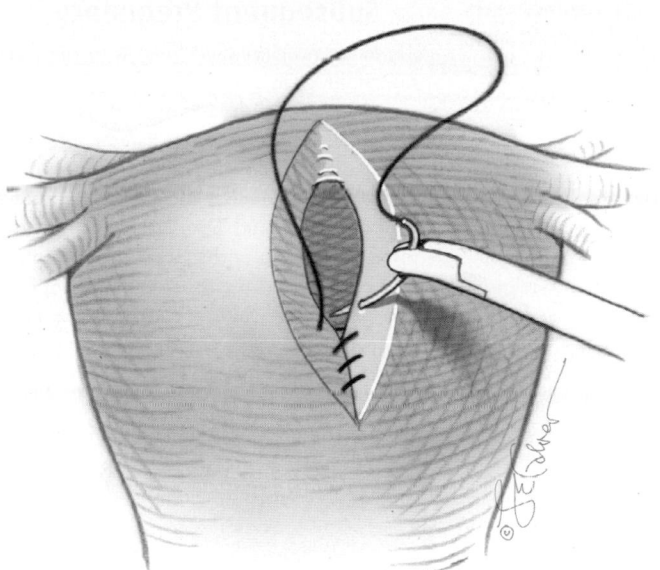

FIGURE 42-9.5 Myometrial closure.

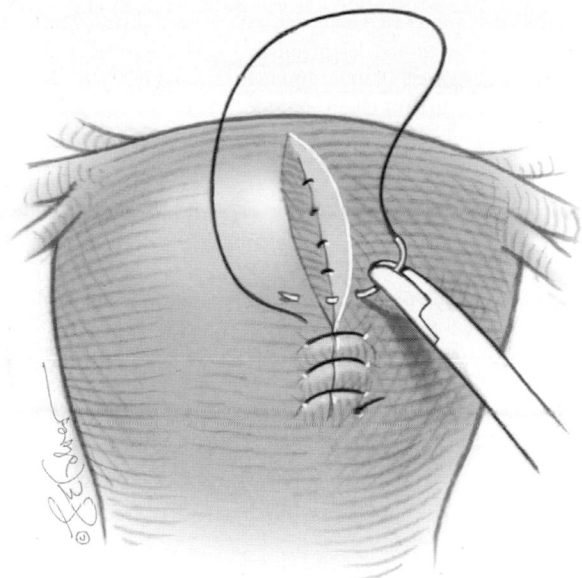

FIGURE 42-9.6 Serosal closure.

❾ Leiomyoma Removal. The task of tumor removal from the abdominal cavity may be as challenging as myometrial and serosal suturing. Electric morcellators allow for efficient leiomyoma removal from the abdomen by circumferentially paring the tumor into small strips that may be removed through a laparoscopic port. To prevent injury, the motorized morcellator blade should always be visible in the operative field and is placed away from vital structures. The morcellator remains immobile, and tissue is brought to the blade (p. 1151). A peeling, rather than a coring, technique should be used to debulk and remove the leiomyomas. Fragmentation of tissue is not uncommon during this process. Cases of iatrogenic seeding of the abdominal cavity with leiomyoma tissue, endometriosis, endometrial hyperplasia, and stromal

sarcomas have been reported (Della Badia, 2010; Kho, 2009; Kill, 2011; Nezhat, 2010; Sepilian, 2003). For this reason, removal of all tissue fragments is a priority.

Alternatively, as described in Section 42-7, step 9 (p. 1138), leiomyomas may be removed through a colpotomy incision. This is an attractive option for multiple large, calcified masses, which may be difficult or time-consuming to morcellate laparoscopically (Ou, 2002).

❿ Laparoscopically Assisted Myomectomy (LAM). Another minimally invasive technique that may allow for safe and efficient myomectomy is LAM. The procedure is initiated as described earlier, and abdominal cavity assessment, uterine inspection, and incision of the serosa and myometrium are performed laparoscopically. To aid the laparo

scopically challenging steps of myomectomy, LAM offers a hybrid approach. Specifically, tumor enucleation, morcellation, and uterine closure are completed through a 2- to 4-cm minilaparotomy incision placed suprapubically. With this, the pneumoperitoneum and visualization through the laparoscope are lost. Instead, application of a wound retraction system such as the Alexis or Mobius retractor provides visual access to the operative field (p. 1104). The uterus and leiomyoma are brought to the surface of the anterior abdominal wall and through the laparotomy incision. The tumors are then enucleated and morcellated through this incision (Fig. 42-9.7). This open incision also allows for conventional suturing techniques and aids suturing of large defects that require a multilayer closure (Fig. 42-9.8). Advantages include decreased operative time,

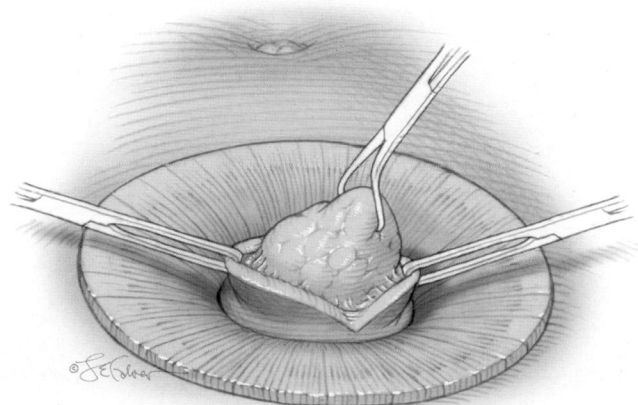

FIGURE 42-9.7 Tumor enucleation during laparoscopically assisted myomectomy.

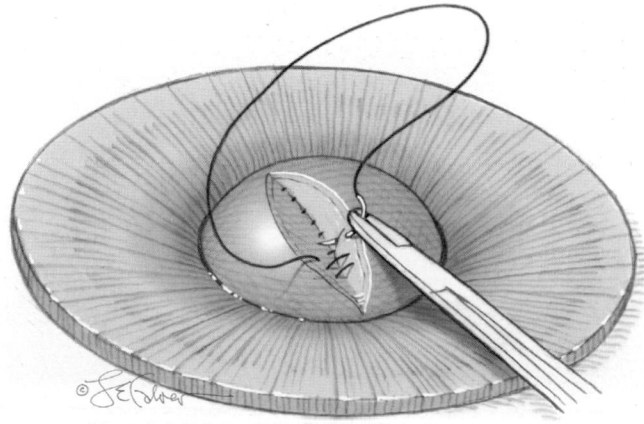

FIGURE 42-9.8 Myometrial closure during laparoscopically assisted myomectomy.

technical simplicity, improved tactile sensation to detect deep intramural leiomyomas, and easier removal of very large tumors (Prapas, 2009; Wen, 2010). Disadvantages stem mainly from the larger abdominal wall incision.

POSTOPERATIVE

Following abdominal myomectomy, postoperative care follows that for any major laparoscopic surgery. Hospitalization typically varies from 0 to 1 days, and return of normal bowel function and febrile morbidity usually dictates this course (Barakat, 2011). Postoperative activity in general can

be individualized, although vigorous exercise is usually delayed until 4 weeks after surgery.

Fever

Febrile morbidity of greater than 38.0°C is common following myomectomy (Iverson, 1996; LaMorte, 1993; Rybak, 2008). Purported causes include atelectasis, myometrial incisional hematomas, and factors released with myometrial destruction. Although fever is common following myomectomy, pelvic infection is not. For example, LaMorte and colleagues (1993) noted only a 2-percent rate of pelvic infection in their analysis of 128 open myomectomy cases.

Subsequent Pregnancy

There are no clear guidelines as to the timing of pregnancy attempts following myomectomy. Darwish and colleagues (2005) performed sonographic examinations on 169 patients following open myomectomy. Following myometrial indicators, they concluded that wound healing is usually completed within 3 months. There are no clinical trials that address the issue of uterine rupture and therefore the route of delivery of pregnancies occurring after myomectomy (American College of Obstetricians and Gynecologists, 2008). Management of these cases requires sound clinical judgment and individualization of care.

42-10

Laparoscopic Hysterectomy

With advancements in instrumentation and surgical skills, there has been a trend toward greater use of minimally invasive surgery for hysterectomy. Several laparoscopic techniques have been developed for hysterectomy and vary depending on the degree of laparoscopic dissection versus vaginal surgery required to remove the uterus (Garry, 1994). These include:

- Diagnostic laparoscopy prior to vaginal hysterectomy (VH)
- Vaginal hysterectomy assisted by laparoscopy, that is, lysis of adhesions and/or excision of endometriosis prior to VH
- Laparoscopically assisted vaginal hysterectomy (LAVH): laparoscopic dissection down to, but not including, uterine artery transection prior to VH
- Laparoscopic hysterectomy (LH): laparoscopic dissection, including uterine artery transection, but completion of hysterectomy vaginally
- Total laparoscopic hysterectomy (TLH): complete laparoscopic excision of the uterus

The laparoscopic approach offers advantages over traditional total abdominal hysterectomy (TAH). These include significant decreases in analgesic requirements, shorter hospital stays, rapid recovery, greater patient satisfaction, and lower rates of wound infection and wound hematoma formation (Kluivers, 2007; Schindlbeck, 2008). Disadvantageously, surgical time is lengthened, although the learning curve may be a factor. TLH offers fewer advantages compared with VH. Thus, in most cases, TLH should be an alternative to TAH (Johnson, 2009; Marana, 1999).

Poor candidates for a vaginal approach include poor uterine descent, extensive abdominal or pelvic adhesions, a large uterus not amenable to morcellation, adnexal pathology, a restricted vaginal vault due to scarring or radiation, or contracted pelvis. Patients with these findings are generally considered for TAH and are also considered for TLH (Schindlbeck, 2008).

PREOPERATIVE

Patient Evaluation

As described earlier, a thorough pelvic examination and history reveal factors that help determine the optimal surgical route for a patient. Uterine size and mobility are important. There is no agreed-upon size that precludes LH. However, a wide, bulky uterus with minimal mobility may make it difficult to visualize vital structures, to manipulate the uterus during surgery, and to remove it vaginally. Once a patient has been deemed eligible for a laparoscopic approach, the same preoperative evaluation as for abdominal hysterectomy applies (Section 41-12, p. 1045).

Consent

Similar to an open approach, possible risks of this procedure include increased blood loss and need for transfusion, unplanned adnexectomy, and injury to other pelvic organs, especially bladder, ureter, and bowel. The ureters are also at greater risk during LH compared with other hysterectomy approaches (Harkki-Siren, 1997b, 1998). Kuno and colleagues (1998) evaluated the use of ureteral catheterization to prevent such injury but found no benefit. Complications related specifically to laparoscopy include injury to the major vessels, bladder, and bowel during trocar placement (p. 1097).

The risk of conversion to an open procedure should also be discussed. In general, conversion to laparotomy may be necessary if exposure and organ manipulation is limited or if bleeding is encountered that cannot be controlled laparoscopically.

Patient Preparation

A blood sample is typed and crossed for potential transfusion. If considered, bowel preparation prior to laparoscopy may assist with colon manipulation and pelvic anatomy visualization by evacuating the rectosigmoid. Alternatively, enemas prior to surgery may be as effective for this goal. Antibiotic prophylaxis is administered within the hour prior to skin incision. Appropriate antibiotic options are listed in Table 39-6 (p. 960). With laparoscopic gynecologic surgery, the decision to provide or withhold prophylaxis should factor patient and procedure-related risks for venous thromboembolism (VTE) (Geerts, 2008). Thus, if longer operating times or conversion to laparotomy are anticipated or preexisting VTE risks are present, then prophylaxis as outlined in Table 39-9 (p. 962) is reasonable.

INTRAOPERATIVE

Instruments

A number of instruments have been developed to assist the laparoscopic surgeon and provide functions similar to those afforded by tools used in laparotomy. Vessel occlusion is an important component of any hysterectomy. For this, several different instruments have been used. These include monopolar or bipolar instruments, harmonic scalpel, stapling devices, traditional sutures, and suturing devices. Several instruments are multifunctional and can be used for dissection as well as hemostasis. The harmonic scalpel is frequently used for its ability to cut with minimal smoke plume and little surrounding thermal tissue damage, although it should only be used to seal vessels up to 5 mm. Several advanced bipolar devices also offer improved vessel sealing. With various instruments, vessels measuring up to 5 mm (Ligasure, Gyrus Plasma Kinetic) and up to 7 mm (Enseal) can be coagulated with minimal thermal spread (Lamberton, 2008; Landman, 2003; Smaldone, 2008).

SURGICAL STEPS

❶ Anesthesia and Patient Positioning. For most women, these procedures are performed as an inpatient procedure under general anesthesia. The patient is placed in a low dorsal lithotomy position, and a bimanual examination is completed to determine uterine size and shape to aid port placement. The abdomen and vagina are surgically prepared. To avoid stomach puncture by a trocar during primary abdominal entry, an orogastric or nasogastric tube should be placed to decompress the stomach. To avert similar bladder injury, a Foley catheter is placed. Uterine manipulators can assist with visualization. These should be considered in cases in which anatomic distortion is anticipated or in those with large uteri.

❷ Initial Steps. The introductory steps for LH mirror those for other laparoscopic procedures (Section 42-1, p. 1110). The number of ports and their caliber may vary, but in general, LH requires a 5- to 12-mm port placed at the level of the umbilicus, and two or three accessory ports placed through the lower abdominal wall. Specifically, two ports are positioned beyond the lateral borders of the rectus abdominis muscle, whereas a third may be positioned centrally and cephalad to the uterine fundus. Left upper quadrant or Palmer point entry is considered in cases of suspected periumbilical adhesions. For larger uteri, if the uterine fundus is close to or above the level of the umbilicus, the optical port should be placed approximately 3 to 4 cm above the fundus for optimal visualization.

❸ Pelvic Evaluation. With the ports and laparoscope inserted and the patient in Trendelenburg position, a blunt probe can aid organ manipulation. The pelvis and abdomen are inspected as described in Section 42-2 (p. 1122). At this point, the decision is made whether to continue with LH or convert to laparotomy. If needed, adhesions are lysed to restore normal anatomy. The bowel is displaced from the pelvis into the abdomen to expand available operating space and allow visualization of pelvic organs.

❹ Ureter Identification. Irrigating fluids and CO_2 used for insufflation can with time create edema of the peritoneum and hinder visualization of structures beneath it. For this reason, the ureters should be identified early. In many cases, the ureters can be visualized without difficulty beneath the pelvic peritoneum. However, it is sometimes necessary to open the peritoneum for identification. In such situations, the peritoneum medial to the infundibulopelvic (IP) ligament is grasped and tented using atraumatic forceps and incised with scissors. Hydrodissection techniques may be employed (Section 42-1, p. 1119). The opening in the peritoneum then is extended caudally and cephalad along the length of the ureter. Through this peritoneal window, the ureter is identified, and peristalsis

should be noted (Fig. 42-10.1) (Parker, 2004).

❺ Round Ligament Transection. The proximal round ligament is grasped and divided.

❻ Ovarian Conservation. If preservation of the ovaries is planned, proximal portions of the fallopian tube and uteroovarian ligament are also desiccated and transected (Figs. 42-10.1 and 42-10.2). With this, the tube and ovary are freed from the uterus and can be placed in the ovarian fossa.

❼ Oophorectomy. If removal of the ovaries is desired, the infundibulopelvic (IP) ligament is grasped and pulled up and away from retroperitoneal structures. The presence and path of the ureter is identified. The IP ligament is isolated and dissected away from the ureteral course. The pedicle is coagulated, desiccated, or stapled, and then is divided (Fig. 42-10.3).

❽ Broad Ligament Incision. Following transection of the round ligament, the leaves of the broad ligament fall open, and loose, gauzy connective tissue is found between these leaves. The anterior leaf is incised sharply. This incision is directed caudally and centrally to the midline above the vesicouterine fold (Fig. 42-10.4). The posterior

leaf requires incision caudally to the level of the uterosacral ligament. The loose areolar tissue separating the anterior and posterior leaves is dissected as well. Ultimately, opening the broad ligament provides access to lateral uterine anatomy, which is important for subsequent uterine artery ligation.

❾ Bladder Flap Development. After incision of the broad ligaments bilaterally, the vesicouterine fold is grasped with atraumatic forceps, elevated away from the underlying bladder, and incised (Fig. 42-10.5). This exposes connective tissue between the bladder and underlying uterus in the vesicouterine space. Loosely attached connections can be bluntly divided by gently pushing against the cervix and caudally to move the bladder caudad (Fig. 42-10.6). Denser tissue in the vesicouterine space is better divided sharply. With this, the tissue is elevated, and the scissors are kept close to the surface of the cervix to minimize inadvertent cystotomy risk. As this tissue is dissected, the vesicouterine space is opened. Electrosurgery may be needed to coagulate small bleeding vessels. Creating cephalad traction on the uterus with the uterine manipulator may also help with this dissection. Development of this space allows the bladder to be moved caudally and off the lower uterus and upper vagina. This mobilization of the bladder is necessary for final colpotomy and uterus

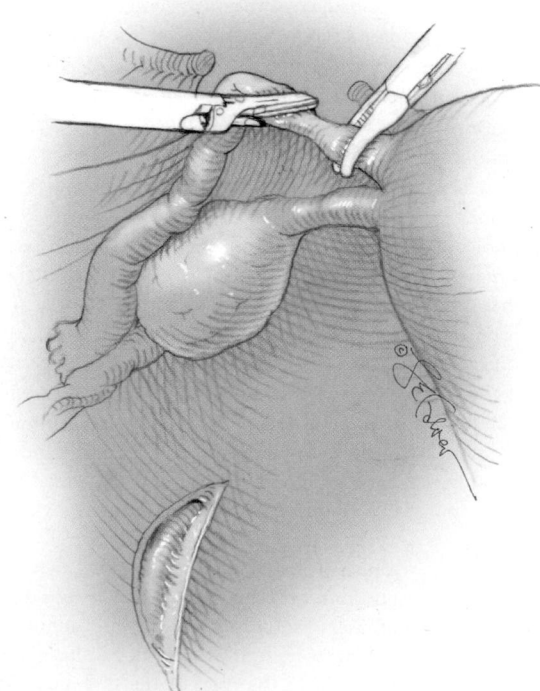

FIGURE 42-10.1 The ureter is first identified. With ovarian conservation, the round ligament is transected, and the fallopian tube is then grasped for transection.

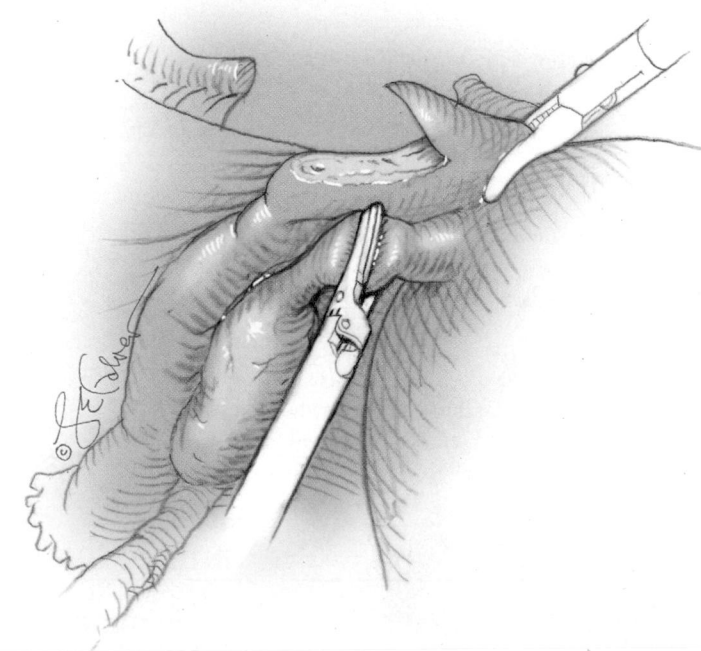

FIGURE 42-10.2 Uteroovarian ligament transection.

removal. Of the hysterectomy types, minimally invasive approaches have the highest risk of bladder injury, and injury occurs most frequently to the dome during this sharp or blunt dissection (Harkki, 2001). This risk is increased if scarring from prior cesarean delivery or from endometriosis is present.

❿ Uterine Artery Transection. After the uterine arteries are identified, the areolar connective tissue surrounding them is grasped, placed on tension, and incised. This skeletonizing of the vessels leads to superior occlusion of the uterine artery and vein. The arteries then are coagulated and transected (Fig. 42-10.7). Alternatively, surgeons may elect to terminate the laparoscopic portion prior to uterine artery transection and complete artery ligation from a vaginal approach (LAVH).

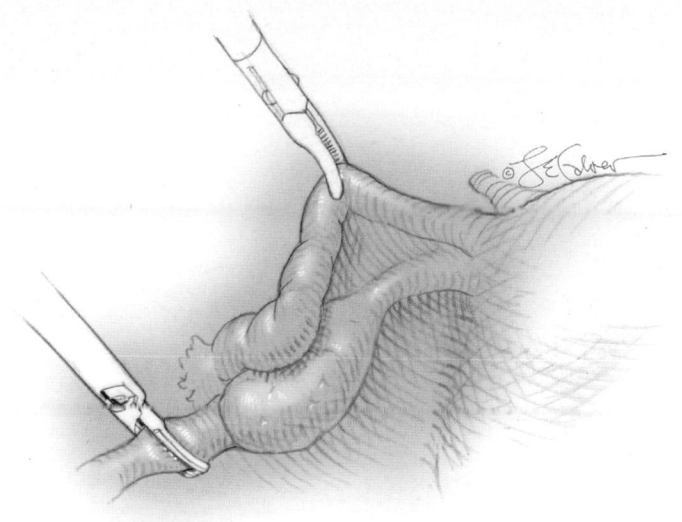

FIGURE 42-10.3 Infundibulopelvic ligament transection.

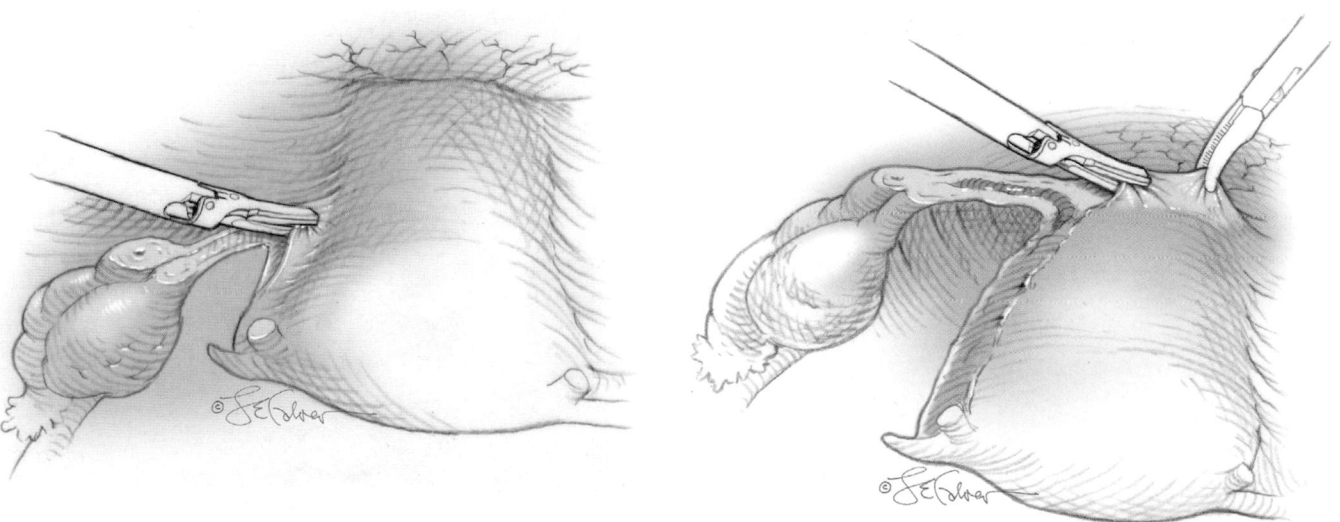

FIGURE 42-10.4 Anterior leaf of broad ligament incised caudally.

FIGURE 42-10.5 Vesicouterine fold incised.

⓫ Vaginal Hysterectomy. With LH, after the uterine arteries are transected, the surgical approach is converted to that for vaginal hysterectomy and is completed as outlined in Section 41-13 (p. 1051). In this transition, the patient is repositioned from low dorsal lithotomy to standard or high lithotomy positions.

⓬ Abdominal Inspection. After vaginal completion of the hysterectomy, attention is redirected to laparoscopic inspection of the pelvis for signs of bleeding. Prior to returning to the abdomen, surgeons will replace their surgical gloves. Copious irrigation of the abdominopelvic cavity and confirmation of hemostasis is performed.

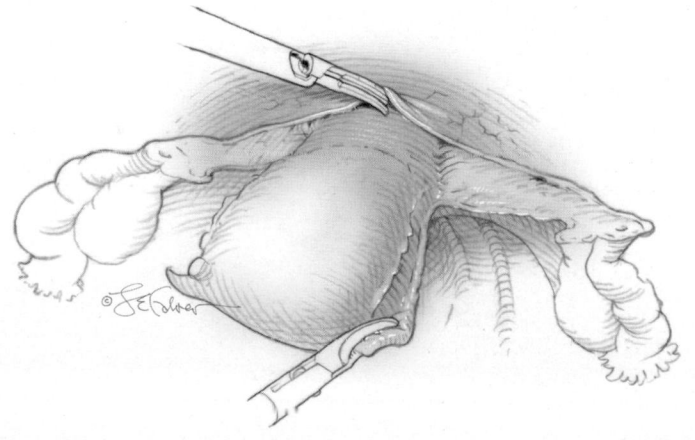

FIGURE 42-10.6 Bladder moved caudally.

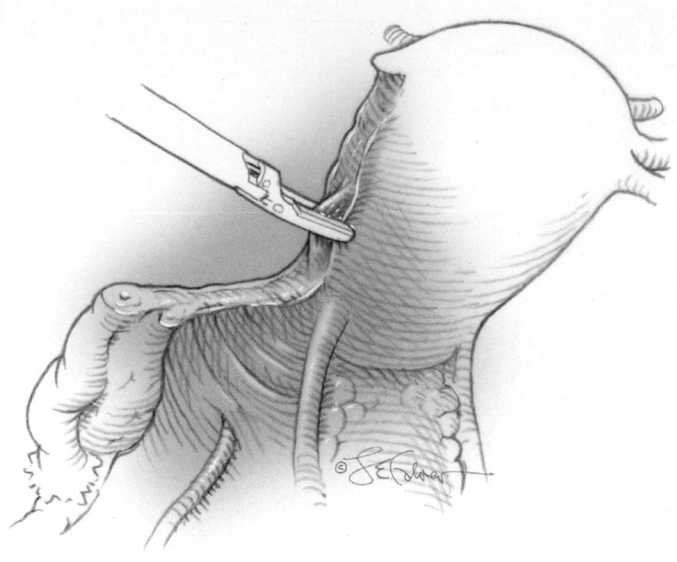

FIGURE 42-10.7 Uterine artery coagulation.

During this inspection, intraabdominal pressures are lowered to better identify sources of bleeding. The laparoscopic procedure is terminated as outlined in Section 42-1 (p. 1116).

POSTOPERATIVE

Following LH, patient recovery mirrors that for vaginal hysterectomy. In general, patients, compared with those undergoing abdominal hysterectomy, have faster return of normal bowel function, easier ambulation, and decreased analgesia requirements. A clear liquid diet can be initiated the day of surgery and advanced quickly as tolerated. Postoperative complications in general mirror those for abdominal hysterectomy, with the exception that superficial surgical site infection rates are lower.

42-11

Laparoscopic Supracervical Hysterectomy

Laparoscopic supracervical hysterectomy (LSH) differs from total laparoscopic hysterectomy (TLH) in that the uterine corpus is amputated, but the cervix remains. Once freed, the corpus either is delivered through a posterior colpotomy incision or more commonly, is morcellated and removed through laparoscopic ports. Advantageously, the uterosacral and cardinal ligaments, which are important to pelvic support, are retained. LSH is also an excellent alternative for cases complicated by extensive scarring. Specifically, adhesions between the bladder and the lower uterine segment in the vesico-uterine space or those in the cul-de-sac may make removal of the cervix difficult. Related to this, ureteral and bladder injury rates are decreased by avoiding difficult dissection.

Certain contraindications to preserving the cervix should be excluded prior to selecting supracervical hysterectomy. Examples include Pap smear findings of abnormal glandular cells or high-grade dysplasia suggesting endocervical neoplasia; endometrial hyperplasia with atypia or endometrial cancer; or a patient at risk for noncompliance with routine Pap smear screening.

PREOPERATIVE

Patient Evaluation

As described earlier, a thorough pelvic examination and history reveal factors that help determine the optimal surgical route for a patient (Section 42-1, p. 1095). Uterine size and mobility are important. There is no agreed-upon size that precludes LSH. However, a large, bulky uterus with minimal mobility may be difficult to adequately manipulate, may limit exposure during surgery, and may require significant time to morcellate. Once a patient has been deemed eligible for a laparoscopic approach, the same preoperative evaluation as for an abdominal hysterectomy applies (Section 41-12, p. 1045).

Consent

Similar to an open approach, possible risks of this procedure include blood loss and need for transfusion, unplanned adnexectomy, and injury to other pelvic organs, especially bladder, ureter, and bowel. Complications related specifically to laparoscopy include

injury to the major vessels, bladder, and bowel during trocar placement (p. 1097).

Postoperatively, with supracervical hysterectomy, endometrium within the lower uterine segment may be retained. As a result, the risk of cyclic long-term bleeding is a potential consequence of this approach. Rates quoted in early studies are as high as 24 percent but are lower in more recent investigations and range from 5 to 10 percent (Okaro, 2001; Sarmini, 2005; Schmidt, 2011; van der Stege, 1999). Techniques that resect more of the lower uterine and proximal endocervical tissue appear to lower these long-term bleeding risks (Schmidt, 2011; Wenger, 2006).

In some cases, secondary excision of the cervical stump may later be required. Termed trachelectomy, this excision may be indicated if refractory long-term bleeding or if significant subsequent cervical neoplasia develops postoperatively. Trachelectomy has the additional indication for residual persistent infection, although this is more anecdotal and not quoted with a consistent incidence. Overall rates of trachelectomy appear to mimic the bleeding rates just given and are on a downward trend.

The risk of conversion to an open procedure should also be discussed. In general, conversion to laparotomy may be necessary if exposure and organ manipulation are limited or if bleeding is encountered that cannot be controlled with laparoscopic tools and techniques.

Patient Preparation

A blood sample should be typed and crossmatched for potential transfusion. If considered, bowel preparation prior to laparoscopy may assist with colon manipulation and pelvic anatomy visualization by evacuating the rectosigmoid. Alternatively, enemas prior to surgery may be as effective for this goal. Antibiotic prophylaxis is administered within the hour prior to skin incision, and appropriate antibiotic options are listed in Table 39-6 (p. 959). With laparoscopic gynecologic surgery, the decision to provide or withhold venous thromboembolism (VTE) prophylaxis should factor patient- and procedure-related risks (Geerts, 2008). Thus, if longer operating times or conversion to laparotomy are anticipated or preexisting VTE risks are present, then prophylaxis as outlined in Table 39-9 (p. 962) is indicated.

INTRAOPERATIVE

Instruments

During cervical amputation, blunt scissors, harmonic scalpel, laser, monopolar needle,

or scissors may be used to excise the corpus. Vessel occlusion is an important component of any hysterectomy. For this, several different tools have been used and include monopolar or bipolar instruments, harmonic scalpel, stapling devices, traditional sutures, and suturing devices. Once the corpus has been freed, it must be removed from the abdomen. Previously, colpotomy was used. However, with the development of electric morcellating devices, vaginal removal of the specimen is less frequently required (Section 42-1, p. 1103). Many of these instruments may not be readily available in all operating suites, and desired tools should be requested prior to surgery.

SURGICAL STEPS

❶ Initial Steps. The initial surgical steps for LSH mirror those for LH, including coagulation of the uterine vessels as described in Section 42-10, steps 1 through 10 (p. 1145).

❷ Uterine Amputation. The corpus is amputated from the cervix at a point just below the internal cervical os and superior to the uterosacral ligaments (Fig. 42-11.1). To limit the possibility of residual endometrium, the incision is conical and extends down into the cervix (Figs. 42-11.2 through 42-11.4). Following amputation, adjunctive coring or ablation of the endocervical canal also may be performed to decrease the risk of long-term postoperative bleeding (Fig. 42-11.5).

❸ Morcellation. For morcellation, tissue is grasped securely with a toothed instrument such as a tenaculum. Because of the potential for surrounding organ injury, morcellators should not be moved toward the grasped tissue, but rather those tissues are brought to it (Fig. 42-11.6) (Milad, 2003). Importantly, the morcellator tip should always be kept in laparoscopic view. A peeling rather than coring technique is used to pare down the mass. During this, the tenaculum holding the corpus is drawn up into the morcellator cylinder and well past the edge of the morcellating blade. This avoids metal-to-metal contact, which dulls the blade. In cases of prolonged morcellation, such as with large leiomyomas, the blade may dull. For this, the generator allows a reverse in the blade's rotary direction. An improvement in cutting action is usually seen with this step and generally offers enough blade life to complete the procedure.

Feeding tissue to the morcellator may prevent excessive fragmentation of tissue. Following morcellation, any remnant uterine fragments should be removed entirely. To

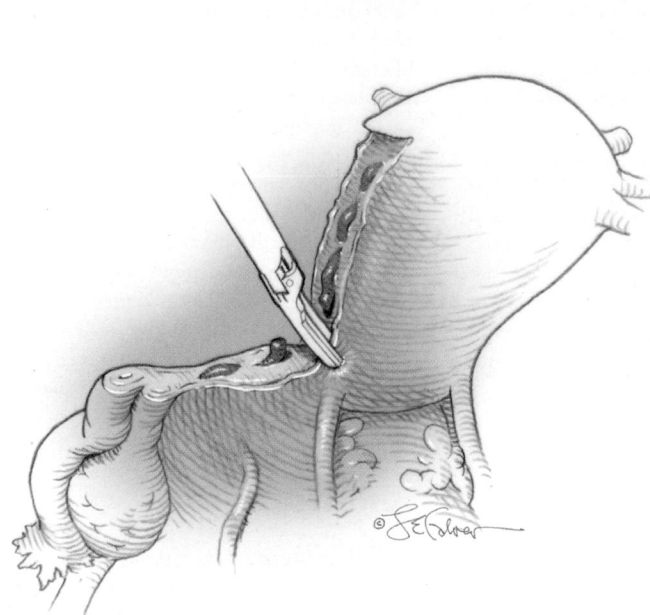

FIGURE 42-11.1 Incision initiated above uterosacral ligaments.

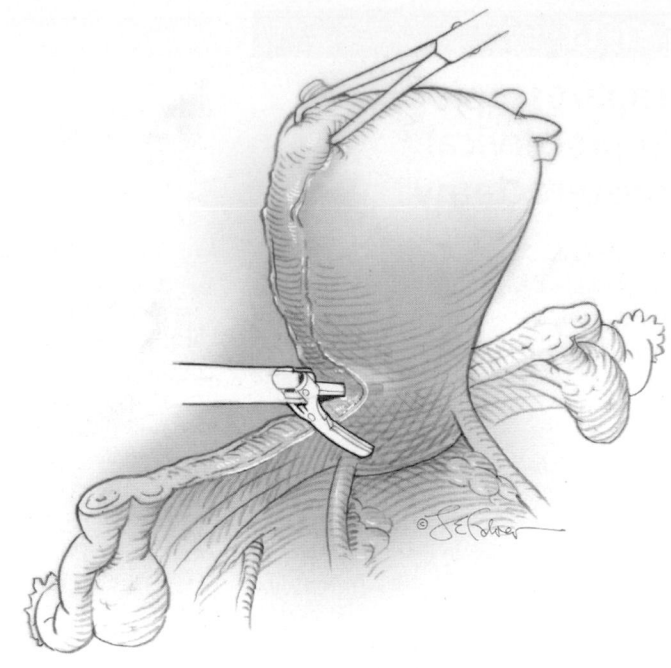

FIGURE 42-11.2 Incision extended posteriorly.

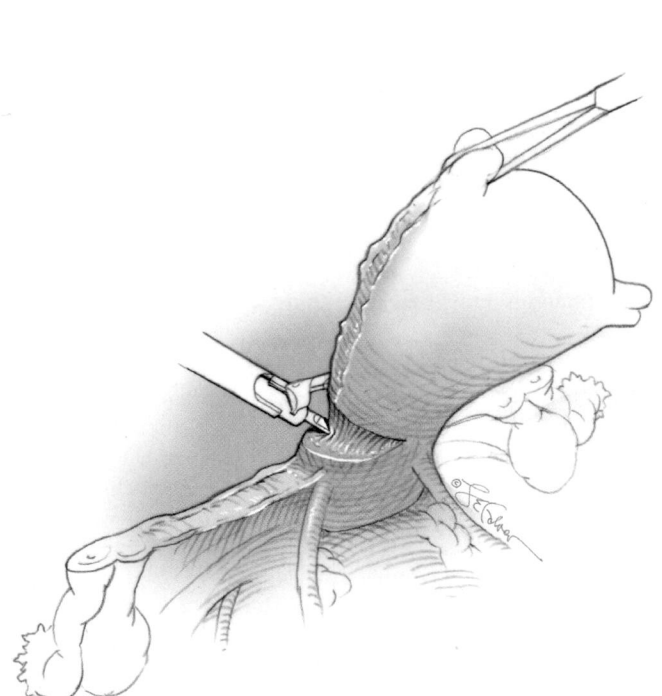

FIGURE 42-11.3 Cone-shape incision extended anteriorly.

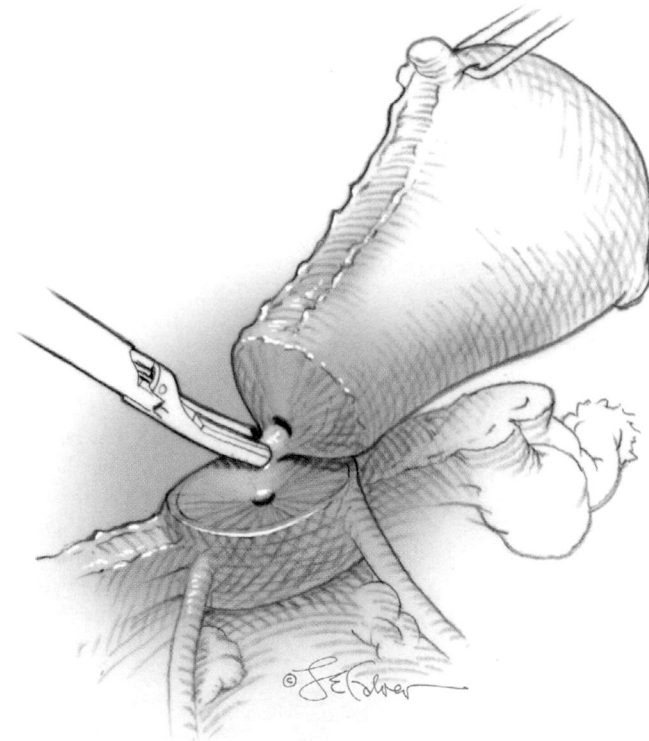

FIGURE 42-11.4 Excision completion.

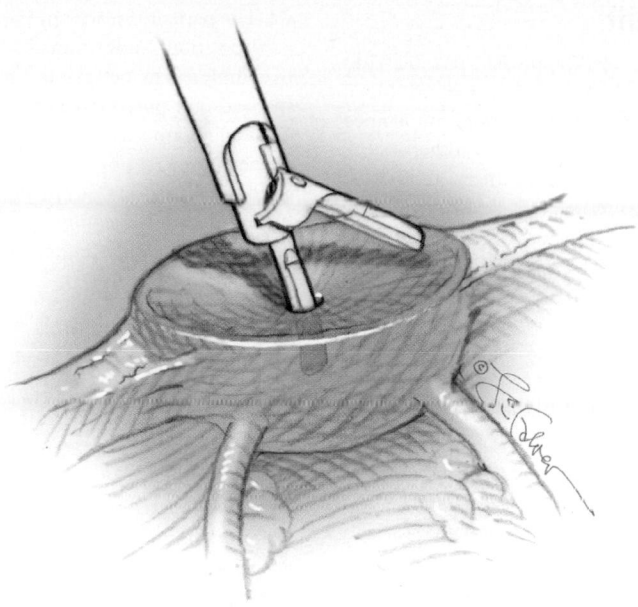

FIGURE 42-11.5 Endocervical canal coagulated.

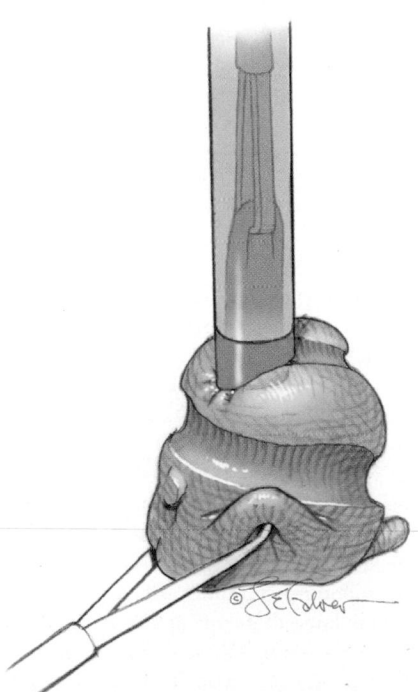

FIGURE 42-11.6 Uterine corpus morcellation.

myomatosis, and even development of endometriosis and endometrial stromal sarcoma following morcellation (Kho, 2009; Nezhat, 2010; Sinha, 2007; Takeda, 2007).

❹ **Hemostasis.** Points of bleeding are coagulated, and the surgeon may elect to reapproximate the anterior vesical and posterior cul-de-sac peritoneum to cover the cervical stump using 2-0 gauge delayed-absorbable suture. Alternatively, absorbable adhesion barriers (Interceed, Seprafilm) can be placed at the hemostatic surgical site.

❺ **Laparoscopy Final Steps.** Completion of the procedure follows that for general laparoscopic procedures (Section 42-1, p. 1116).

POSTOPERATIVE

Advantages to laparoscopy include a rapid return to normal diet and activities. With supracervical hysterectomy, there is no vaginal cuff that requires extended healing. Sexual intercourse, however, is typically delayed for 2 weeks following surgery to allow adequate internal healing.

aid this, copious irrigation of the abdominal cavity can dislodge and float these pieces for easier removal. Case reports have described peritoneal implantation of fragments, leio-

42-12

Total Laparoscopic Hysterectomy

Total laparoscopic hysterectomy (TLH) is similar to LAVH, LSH, and LH with the exception that the procedure is completed entirely from a laparoscopic approach. The procedure may be performed extrafascially (radical hysterectomy, type II or III) or intrafascially (simple hysterectomy, type I). After detachment, the specimen is removed vaginally or via morcellation if too large for vaginal delivery.

If all factors are equal, vaginal hysterectomy should be considered for women undergoing hysterectomy. Ideal candidates for TLH are those not suitable for vaginal hysterectomy (VH) (American College of Obstetricians and Gynecologists, 2009b). Specifically, successful vaginal hysterectomy may be limited by poor vaginal access, minimal vaginal descent, narrow pelvic angles, extensive pelvic adhesive disease, and significantly enlarged adnexa or uterus. TLH offers the added advantage of excellent visualization for performing uterosacral plication or McCall culdoplasty to guard against future prolapse.

TLH is viewed as a less invasive alternative to total abdominal hysterectomy (TAH). Compared with TAH, TLH benefits include rapid recovery, shorter hospitalizations, fewer wound or abdominal wall minor complications, and less blood loss (Johnson, 2009; Walsh, 2009). These benefits are dependent on a learning curve and may not be readily apparent (Schindlbeck, 2008). Moreover, longer operative times and higher rates of urinary tract injuries are negative balancing factors.

PREOPERATIVE

Patient Evaluation

As described earlier, a thorough pelvic examination and history reveal factors that help determine the optimal surgical route for a patient (Section 42-1, p. 1095). Uterine size and mobility are important. There is no agreed-upon size that precludes TLH. However, a wide, bulky uterus with minimal mobility may be difficult to adequately manipulate, may limit exposure during surgery, and may require significant time to morcellate. Once a patient has been deemed eligible for a laparoscopic approach, the same preoperative evaluation as for an abdominal hysterectomy applies (Section 41-12, p. 1045).

Consent

Similar to an open approach, possible risks of this procedure include increased blood loss and need for transfusion, unplanned adnexectomy, and injury to other pelvic organs, especially bladder, ureter, and bowel. Complications related to laparoscopy include entry injury to the major vessels, bladder, and bowel (Section 42-1, p. 1097). The ureters are also at greater risk during laparoscopic hysterectomies compared with other hysterectomy approaches (Harkki-Siren, 1998). Kuno and colleagues (1998) evaluated the use of ureteral catheterization to prevent such injury but found no benefit.

The risk of conversion to an open procedure should also be discussed. In general, conversion to laparotomy may be necessary if exposure and organ manipulation are limited or if bleeding is encountered that cannot be controlled with laparoscopic tools and techniques.

Patient Preparation

A blood sample should be typed and cross-matched for potential transfusion. If considered, bowel preparation prior to laparoscopy may assist with colon manipulation and pelvic anatomy visualization by evacuating the recto-sigmoid. Alternatively, enemas prior to surgery may be as effective for this goal. Antibiotic prophylaxis is administered within the hour prior to skin incision, and appropriate antibiotic options are listed in Table 39-6 (p. 959). With laparoscopic gynecologic surgery, the decision to provide or withhold prophylaxis should factor patient- and procedure-related risks for venous thromboembolism (VTE) (Geerts, 2008). Thus, if longer operating times or conversion to laparotomy are anticipated or preexisting VTE risks are present, then prophylaxis is indicated.

PREOPERATIVE

Instruments

The same instruments that are used for LH or LSH may be used for this procedure (p. 1145). In addition, a uterine manipulator that has a cupping device for the delineation of the cervicovaginal junction is helpful for colpotomy and also for final tissue extraction. If these are not available, a low-cost alternative is to use a right-angle retractor to delineate the anterior and posterior fornices for colpotomy.

SURGICAL STEPS

❶ Anesthesia and Patient Positioning. For most women, TLH is performed as an inpatient procedure under general anesthe-sia. The patient is placed in low dorsal lithotomy position, and a bimanual examination is completed to determine uterine size and shape to aid port placement. The abdomen and vagina are surgically prepared. To avoid stomach puncture by a trocar during primary abdominal entry, an orogastric or nasogastric tube is placed to decompress the stomach. To avert similar bladder injury, a Foley catheter is inserted.

❷ Uterine Manipulator. A uterine manipulator with its attached cervical cup (VCare or KOH Cup with RUMI manipulator) is placed vaginally to assist uterine manipulation and delineate the cervicovaginal junction for colpotomy. To accomplish placement, the cervical diameter and thickness are assessed. From this information, the manipulator colpotomy-cup size, which is small, medium, or large, is selected. To permit manipulator insertion, the cervical os is dilated to accept a No. 8 cervical dilator. The uterus is also sounded to determine cavity depth for correct manipulator placement. The surgeon tests the balloon at the manipulator's end for patency by filling it with air via a port at the opposite end. Once again deflated, it is passed through the cervical os to the fundus and then reinflated to hold the manipulator in place (Fig. 42-12.1A). Two stay sutures of 0-gauge delayed-absorbable suture are placed at 6 and 12 o'clock or at 3 and 9 o'clock, depending on surgeon preference. To securely anchor the colpotomy cup and cervix, stitches enter the ectocervix and exit just lateral to the endocervix. Each suture end is then passed through openings in the cup base (Fig. 42-12.1B). They are then tied firmly to the cervix on the outside face of the cup (Fig. 42-12.1C). Once in position, the proximal rim of this colpotomy cup will delineate the cervicovaginal junction. With the VCare, the blue vaginal cup is then advanced to join the colpotomy cup and is locked in place by a locking knob at the manipulator's distal end (Fig. 42-12.1D). This second cup will aid in maintaining the pneumoperitoneum during colpotomy. If the KOH Cup is used, then a pneumo-occluding balloon is positioned behind the colpotomy cup.

❸ Initial Laparoscopic Steps. The introductory steps for LH mirror that for other laparoscopic procedures (Section 42-1, p. 1110). The number of trocars and their caliber may vary, but in general, TLH requires a 5- to 12-mm optical port, usually at the umbilicus, and two or three accessory ports placed through the lower abdominal wall. Specifically, two trocars are placed beyond the lateral borders of the rectus abdominis muscle, whereas a third may be positioned centrally and cephalad to the uterine fundus

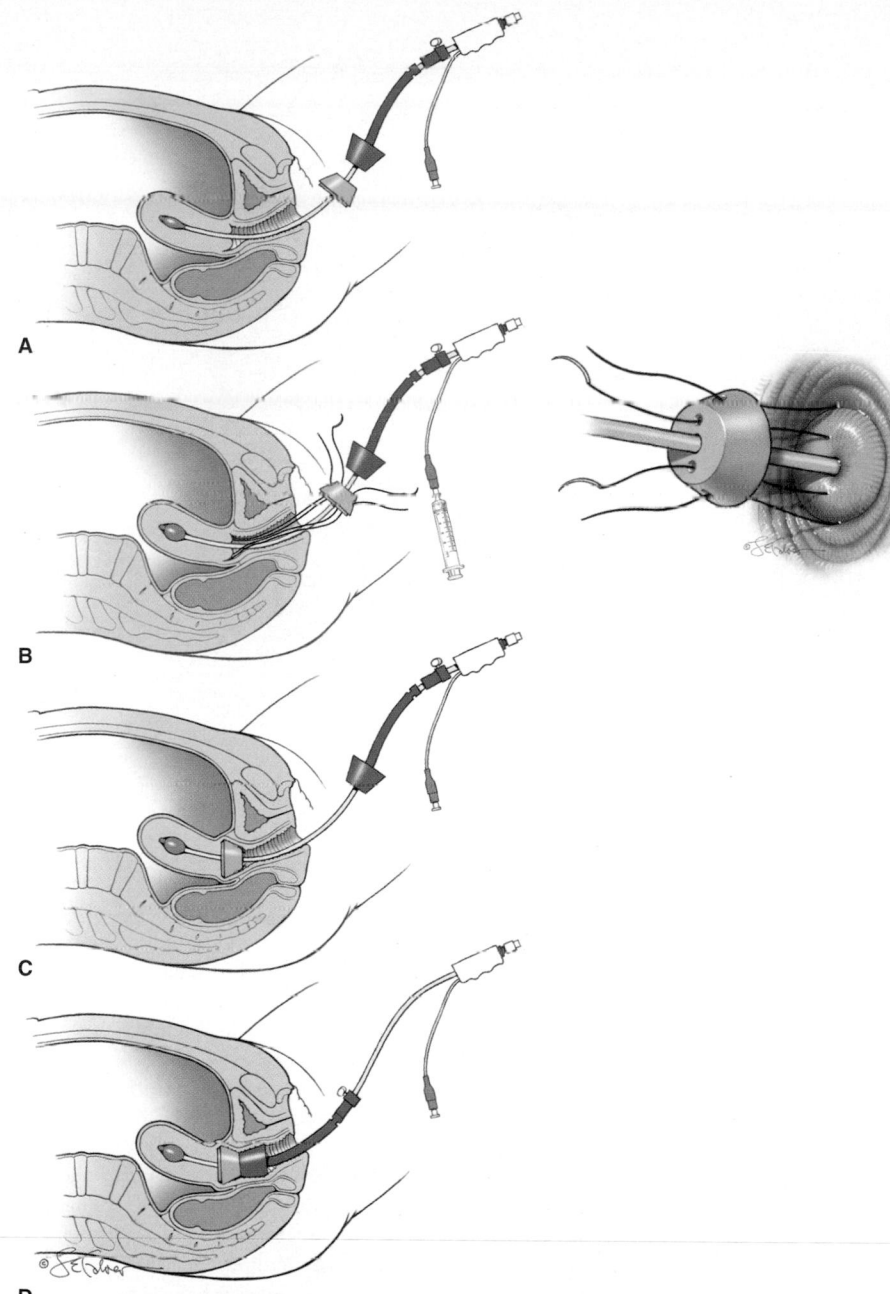

infundibulopelvic (IP) ligament is grasped and tented using atraumatic forceps and incised with scissors. An irrigating probe is used to force water beneath and elevate the peritoneum for easier incision. The opening in the peritoneum then is extended a short distance caudally and cephalad along the length of the ureter. Through this peritoneal window, the ureter is identified (Fig. 42-10.1) (Parker, 2004).

❻ Round Ligament Transection. The proximal round ligament is grasped and divided.

❼ Ovarian Conservation. If preservation of the ovaries is planned, proximal portions of the fallopian tube and uteroovarian ligament are then desiccated and transected (Figs. 42-10.1 and 42-10.2). With this, the tube and ovary are freed from the uterus and can be placed in the ovarian fossa.

❽ Oophorectomy. If removal of the ovaries is desired, the infundibulopelvic (IP) ligament is grasped and pulled up and away from retroperitoneal structures. The ureter's path is identified. The IP ligament is isolated and dissected away from the ureteral course. The pedicle is coagulated, desiccated, or stapled, and then is divided (Fig. 42-10.3).

❾ Broad Ligament Incision. Following round ligament transection, the leaves of the broad ligament fall open, and loose, gauzy connective tissue is found between these leaves. The anterior leaf is incised sharply. This incision is directed caudally and centrally to the midline above the vesicouterine fold (Fig. 42-10.4). The posterior leaf requires incision caudally to the uterosacral ligaments. The loose areolar tissue separating the anterior and posterior leaves is dissected as well. Opening the broad ligament provides access to lateral uterine anatomy, which is important for subsequent uterine artery ligation, cardinal ligament transection, and ureter identification.

❿ Bladder Flap Development. After incision of the broad ligaments bilaterally, the vesicouterine fold is grasped with atraumatic forceps, elevated away from the underlying bladder, and incised (Fig. 42-10.5). This exposes connective tissue between the bladder and underlying uterus within the vesicouterine space. Loosely attached connections can be bluntly divided by gently pushing against the cervix and caudally. This pushes the bladder caudad (Fig. 42-10.6). Denser tissue in the vesicouterine space is better divided sharply. For this, the tissue is elevated, and the scissors are kept close to the surface of the cervix to minimize inadvertent cystotomy. As

FIGURE 42-12.1 Uterine manipulator placement. **A.** Manipulator tip inserted into uterine cavity. **B.** Balloon tip inflated (*left*). Colpotomy cup sutured to cervix (*right*). **C.** Colpotomy cup sutured in place. **D.** Pneumo-occluding cup advanced and locked in place.

(Fig. 42-1.30, p. 1116). Left upper quadrant or Palmer point entry is considered in cases of suspected periumbilical adhesions.

❹ Pelvic Evaluation. With the cannulas and laparoscope inserted and the patient in Trendelenburg position, a blunt probe aids organ and bowel displacement. The pelvis and abdomen are inspected as described in Section 42-2 (p. 1121). At this point, the decision is made whether to continue with TLH or convert to laparotomy. If needed, adhesions are lysed to restore normal anatomy.

❺ Ureter Identification. The initial surgical steps for TLH mirror those for LH as described in Section 42-10, steps 1 through 10 (p. 1146). Irrigating fluids and CO_2 used for insufflation can with time create edema of the peritoneum and hinder visualization of structures beneath it. For this reason, the ureters should be identified early. In many cases, the ureters can be seen without difficulty beneath the pelvic peritoneum. However, it is sometimes necessary to open the peritoneum for identification. In such situations, the peritoneum medial to the

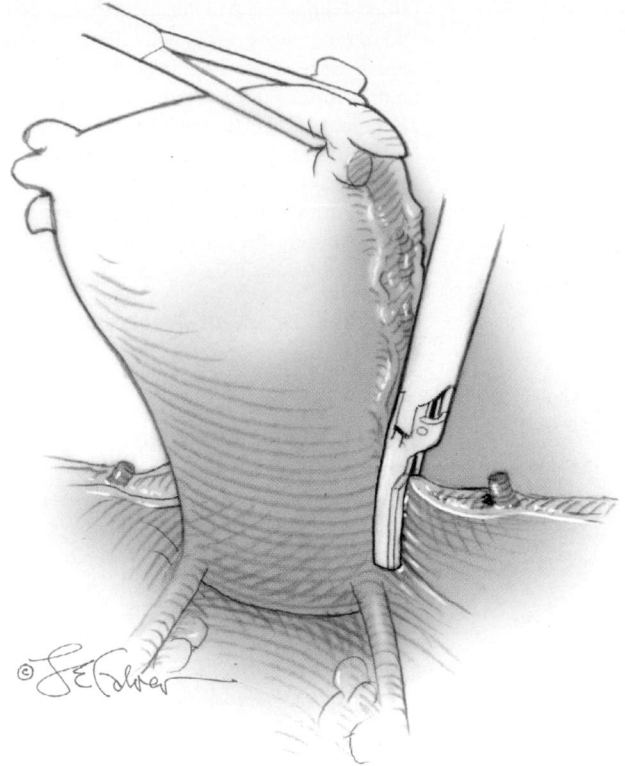

FIGURE 42-12.2 Cardinal ligament incised.

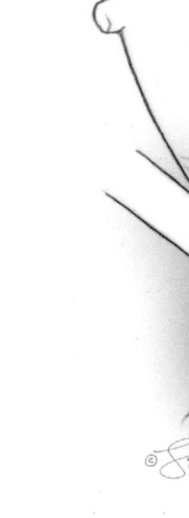

FIGURE 42-12.3 Posterior colpotomy.

this tissue is dissected, the vesicouterine space is opened. Electrosurgery may be needed to coagulate small bleeding vessels. Creating cephalad traction on the uterus with the uterine manipulator may also help with this dissection. Development of this space allows the bladder to be moved caudally and off the lower uterus and upper vagina. This mobilization is necessary for final colpotomy and uterus removal. Of the hysterectomy types, minimally invasive approaches have the highest risk of bladder injury, and injury occurs most frequently to the dome during this sharp or blunt dissection (Harkki, 2001). This risk is increased if scarring from prior cesarean delivery or from endometriosis is present.

⓫ **Uterine Artery Transection.** After the uterine arteries are identified, the areolar connective tissue surrounding them is grasped, placed on tension, and incised. This skeletonizing of the vessels permits superior occlusion of the uterine artery and vein. The arteries then are then coagulated and transected (Fig. 42-10.7).

⓬ **Cardinal Ligament Transection.** Transection of the cardinal ligaments to the level of the uterosacral attachments is performed bilaterally (Fig. 42-12.2).

⓭ **Colpotomy.** Incision at the cervicovaginal junction may be performed with

harmonic scalpel, monopolar scissors, monopolar hook, or plasma kinetic needle point. Prior to incision, the uterine manipulator is pushed cephalad to allow the colpotomy cup to displace the ureters laterally and expose the optimal location for colpotomy. Additionally, dissection within the vesicouterine space should be sufficient to mobilize the bladder caudad and away from the planned colpotomy site.

With these preparatory steps completed, colpotomy is begun by placing the incising tool at the posterior cervicovaginal junction, which is delineated by the cervical cup. If a colpotomy cup is not used, a simple tool such as right-angle retractor or sponge on a stick placed vaginally in the posterior fornix can also assist with delineation of the cervicovaginal junction. The posterior vaginal wall is opened first (Fig. 42-12.3). By extending this incision, the uterosacral ligament is next transected. The opposite uterosacral ligament is then divided close to the cervix (Fig. 42-12.4). Lastly, the anterior colpotomy incision is created (Fig. 42-12.5). To minimize twisting and disorientation of the specimen, the lateral vaginal cuff points are transected last (Fig. 42-12.6). Hemostasis is generally maintained using this technique. To prevent thermal damage to vaginal tissues and subsequent cuff dehiscence, surgeons should use the minimum amount of energy needed to incise tissues.

⓮ **Removal of Uterus.** The uterus is removed intact through the vaginal vault using the manipulator unless uterine size limits this (Fig. 42-12.7). In cases with a large uterus, the uterus is removed using the morcellator as described with the LSH procedure (Section 42-11, p. 1149). It can also be cored, bivalved, or morcellated vaginally.

⓯ **Repair of the Vaginal Cuff.** The cuff is closed laparoscopically with a running closure of absorbable suture, with interrupted figure-of-eight sutures, or with a suturing device. For this, delayed-absorbable material is preferred. To support the vaginal cuff long-term, the uterosacral ligament is incorporated into the closure (Fig. 42-12.8). If traditional suture is used, one must maintain tension to sufficiently close the space. If using barbed suture, the procedure is modified by manufacturer's recommendations to loosen stitch tension between the approximated cuff tissues. Moreover, if barbed suture is used, it is recommended to throw at least two bites at completion of cuff closure in the opposite direction to the original direction of closure to maintain tissue tension. For example, if closure is performed from right to left, the surgeon will reach the far left end and then will place two additional stitches in the left-to-right direction prior to final suture line cutting. It is advisable to cut the suture flush with the tissue to decrease risk of bowel damage from the barbed

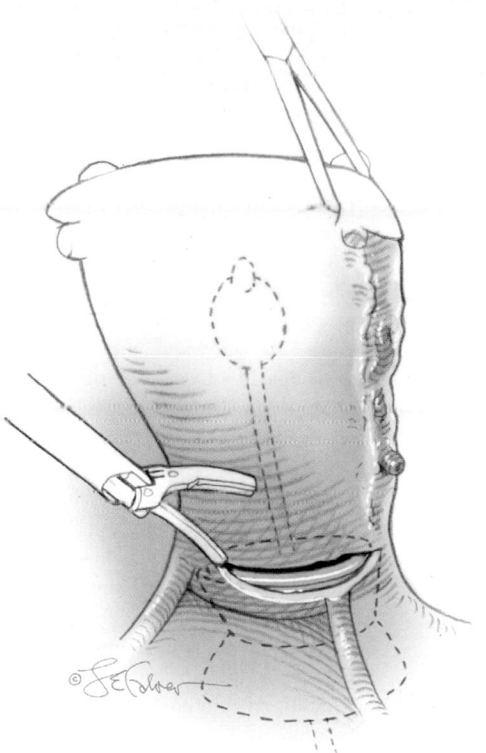

FIGURE 42-12.4 Right uterosacral ligament transected, and colpotomy extended toward the left.

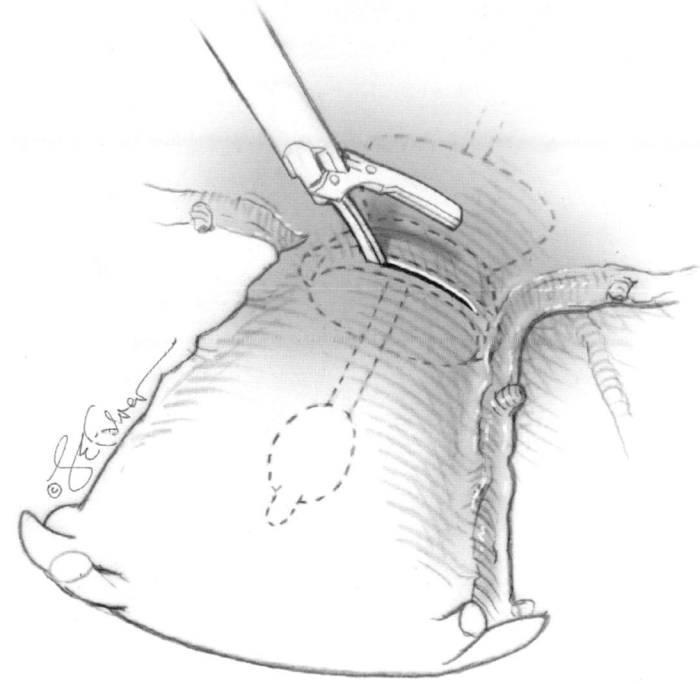

FIGURE 42-12.5 Anterior colpotomy.

end. Confirmation of full thickness closure is necessary to prevent later cuff dehiscence. Alternatively, for those less proficient with laparoscopic suturing, the cuff may be closed vaginally after removal of the uterus.

After cuff closure, irrigation and confirmation of hemostasis is performed. Intraabdominal pressures are lowered during this inspection to better identify sources of bleeding.

⓰ Laparoscopy Final Steps. Completion of this operation follows that for general laparoscopic procedures (Section 42-1, p. 1116).

Postoperative

The advantages of the laparoscopic approach include a rapid return to normal diet and activities. Generally, the evening of the surgery, the Foley catheter is removed, diet is advanced to a general diet, and the patient is allowed to ambulate early. Oral analgesics are quickly adopted in place of parenteral. The

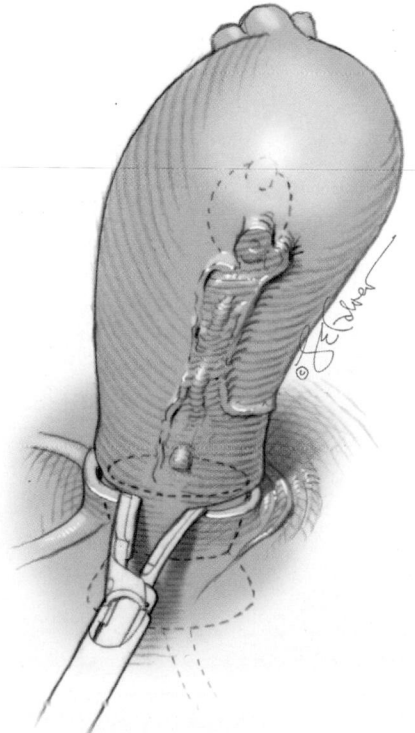
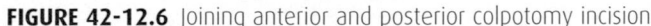

FIGURE 42-12.6 Joining anterior and posterior colpotomy incisions.

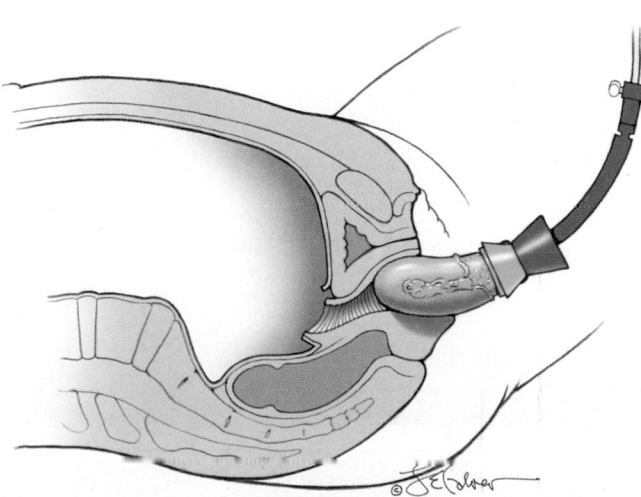

FIGURE 42-12.7 Uterus and manipulator removal.

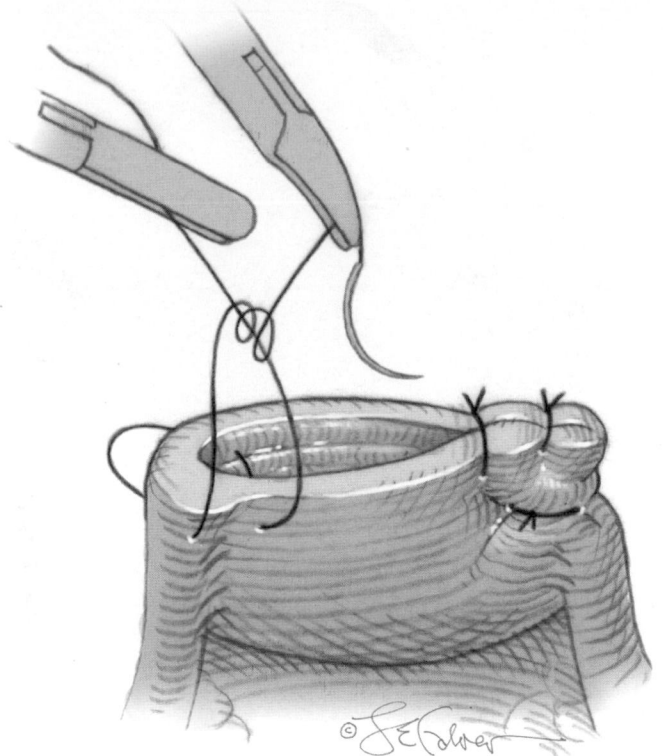

FIGURE 42-12.8 Vaginal cuff closure.

usual precautions for abdominal hysterectomy in regard to limitation of stress on the abdominal cavity by heavy lifting are followed. Delay of sexual activity mirrors that for abdominal hysterectomy, which is typically 6 weeks.

Vaginal cuff dehiscence is a serious postoperative complication that more frequently follows laparoscopic hysterectomy approaches compared with VH or TAH (Agdi, 2009; Walsh, 2007). In most cases, the precipitating event is sexual activity in premenopausal woman and increased intraabdominal pressure coupled with a weak, atrophic vagina in postmenopausal women (Lee, 2009). Patients present with vaginal bleeding or evisceration. Typical treatment includes debridement of vaginal cuff edges, reapproximation with delayed-absorbable suture, and administration of antibiotic prophylaxis. However, compromised bowel may require more extensive surgeries to repair.

Preventatively, sound initial surgical technique should strive to minimize thermal damage during colpotomy creation and limit undue desiccation of the vaginal cuff. Approximation of all tissue planes, particularly full thickness closure of the vaginal wall, should also be ensured. Reapproximation should include an adequate amount of viable tissue that is free of thermal effect. In addition, a two-layer closure may have an advantage over a single-layer figure-of-eight closure (Jeung, 2010).

42-13

Hysteroscopy Fundamentals

Hysteroscopy allows an endoscopic view of the endometrial cavity and tubal ostia for both the diagnosis and operative treatment of intrauterine pathology. During the past two decades, the role of hysteroscopy in modern gynecology has expanded rapidly with development of more effective hysteroscopic instruments and smaller endoscopes.

Indications for hysteroscopy vary and include evaluation and in some cases, treatment of infertility, recurrent miscarriage, abnormal uterine bleeding, amenorrhea, and retained foreign bodies. With hysteroscopic techniques, abnormal bleeding can be treated with endometrial ablation, polypectomy, or submucous myomectomy. Infertility may be improved with incision of intrauterine adhesions or septa. Additionally, obstructed tubal ostia may be unblocked or dilated. Alternatively, for those seeking sterilization, tubal occlusion devices can serve as an effective and safe method of contraception.

PREOPERATIVE CONSIDERATIONS

Patient Evaluation

Because the indications for hysteroscopy are varied, patient evaluations for specific disorders are discussed in their respective chapters. However, pregnancy is an absolute contraindication to hysteroscopy and should be excluded with serum or urine β-hCG testing prior to surgery. In addition, cervicitis or pelvic infection should be treated prior to hysteroscopy, and screening for *Neisseria gonorrhoeae* and *Chlamydia trachomatis* in those with risk factors is warranted (Table 1-2, p. 11). For those with abnormal bleeding and significant risks for endometrial cancer, preoperative endometrial Pipelle sampling is reasonable, as seeding of the peritoneal cavity with cancer cells has been noted following hysteroscopy (Chap. 8, p. 225).

If diagnostic hysteroscopy is planned to locate and remove a foreign body, preoperative imaging is recommended, usually with transvaginal sonography. For example, in some cases, an intrauterine device (IUD) or retained fetal bone may have perforated the uterine wall, lie predominantly outside the uterus, and thus be best removed by laparoscopy.

Consent

The risk of complications for women undergoing hysteroscopy is low and cited at less than 1 to 3 percent (Hulka, 1993; Jansen, 2000; Propst, 2000). Complications are similar to those associated with dilatation and curettage and include uterine perforation, inability to sufficiently dilate the cervix, hemorrhage, cervical laceration, and postoperative endometritis. In addition, because either gas or liquid media is required to distend the endometrial cavity during hysteroscopy, gas venous embolism and excessive intravascular fluid absorption are risks and are discussed later. In general, the risk of complication increases with the length and complexity of the procedure planned.

In the event of uterine perforation during hysteroscopy, diagnostic laparoscopy may be indicated for evaluation of the surrounding pelvic organs. Thus, patients should be additionally consented and aware of the possible need for laparoscopy.

Patient Preparation

Infectious and venous thromboembolic (VTE) complications following hysteroscopic surgery are rare. Accordingly, preoperative antibiotics or VTE prophylaxis is typically not required (American College of Obstetricians and Gynecologists, 2007c, 2009a).

Endometrial Thickness

In premenopausal women, hysteroscopy is ideally performed in the early proliferative phase of the menstrual cycle, when the endometrium is relatively thin. This allows small masses to be identified and easily removed. Alternatively, agents that induce endometrial atrophy such as progestins, combination oral contraceptives, danazol, and gonadotropin-releasing hormone (GnRH) agonists have been administered individually prior to an anticipated surgery. Although these effectively thin the endometrium, many of these agents have disadvantages including expense, adverse side effects, and surgical delay while atrophy ensues (Chap. 9, p. 254).

Cervical Dilatation

For operative hysteroscopy, dilatation of the cervix is typically required to insert an 8- to 10-mm hysteroscope or resectoscope. To minimize the risk of bleeding, which may obscure the operative view, and to lower the risk of uterine perforation, laminaria tents may be placed the day before surgery as described in Section 41-16 (p. 1059). Alternatively, misoprostol (Cytotec), a synthetic prostaglandin E_1 analog, may be administered orally the night before and if desired, again the morning of surgery to aid cervical softening. Commonly used dosing options include 200 or 400 μg vaginally or 400 μg orally once 12 to 24 hours prior to surgery. Common side effects include cramping, uterine bleeding, or nausea. Thus, the need for softening is balanced against these side effects, especially bleeding that might limit endoscopic visualization.

If cervical stenosis is encountered intraoperatively, the use of intracervical dilute vasopressin has also been demonstrated to diminish the force required for cervical dilation (Phillips, 1997). Because the onset of action is rapid, intracervical vasopressin is especially helpful if stenosis was not anticipated preoperatively. Also, smaller caliber tools, such as a lacrimal duct probe, may be guided into the external cervical os to define the canal path. In these situations, sonography may be helpful when done simultaneously with dilatation to help ensure proper placement (Christianson, 2008).

INTRAOPERATIVE

Instruments

Hysteroscopy requires a hysteroscope, light source, uterine distension medium, and in many cases, a video camera system.

Rigid Hysteroscope

Most hysteroscopes consists of a 3- to 4-mm diameter endoscope surrounded by an outer sheath. Smaller diameter hysteroscopes have been developed, although their use is limited by their decreased field of view and lower light intensity. Hysteroscopes may broadly be classified as diagnostic or operative. Diagnostic hysteroscopes offer a small diameter, which provides an adequate view of the endometrial cavity yet requires minimal if any cervical dilatation. Operative hysteroscopes with their added sheaths increase the overall diameter and necessitate cervical dilation in most cases. Thus, cases requiring operative hysteroscopes are best managed under general or regional anesthesia in the operating room for patient comfort and safety.

Hysteroscopic Lens. Individual endoscopes offer specific angles of view. Although 0- through 70-degree angles (0, 12, 25, 30, and 70 degrees) are available, 0- or 12-degree hysteroscopes allow the easiest orientation within the uterine cavity for most procedures (Fig. 42-13.1). The 12-, 25-, 30-, and 70-degree angles provide additional lateral views, which are often required for more

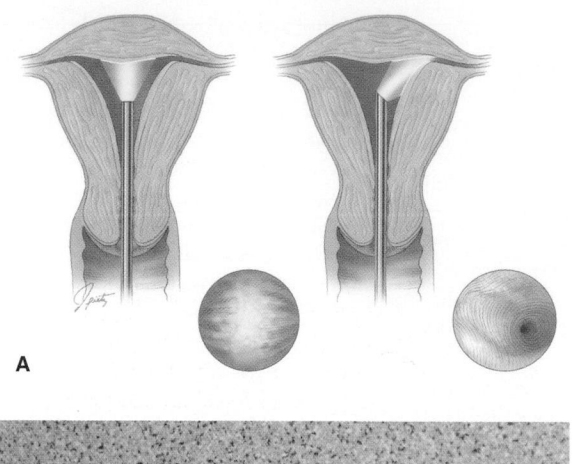

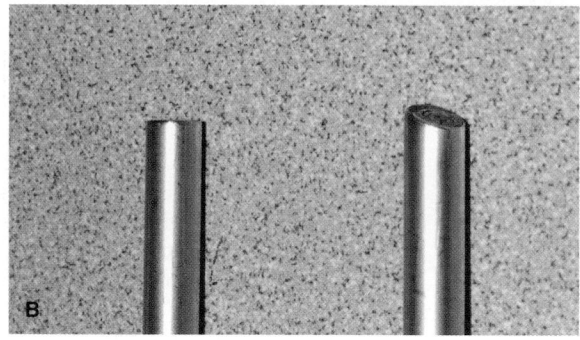

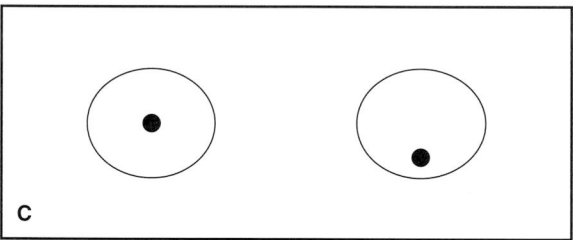

FIGURE 42-13.1 A. Differences between a 0-degree hysteroscope (*left*) and 30-degree hysteroscope (*right*). *Insert:* Intracavitary views. **B.** A 30-degree endoscope has an angled tip. **C.** Views of the endocervical canal (*black dot*) during hysteroscope insertion.

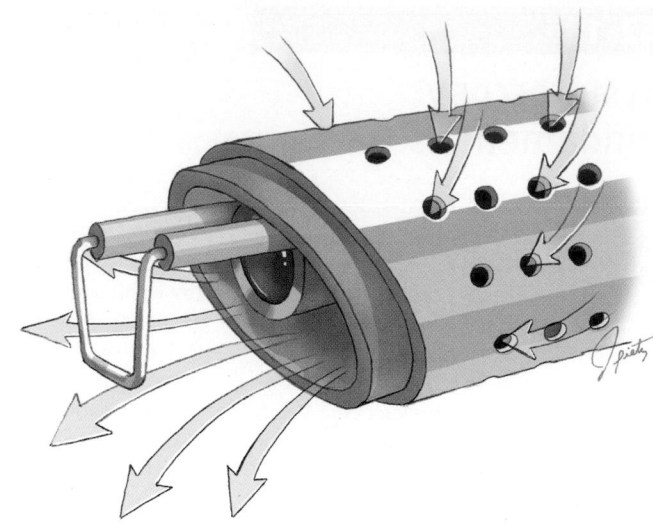

FIGURE 42-13.2 Distension medium flow through resectoscope.

complex operative procedures. There are also devices that have a 90- to 110-degree angle of view, although these are infrequently used.

Light Source. In general, the light source system used in hysteroscopy is the same type as for laparoscopy. However, the intensity is typically less than for most laparoscopic procedures. During assembly of the hysteroscope at the beginning of a procedure, the light source attaches directly to the endoscope.

Outer Sheath. The outer sheath surrounds the endoscope and directs fluid, and in some cases instruments, to the endometrial cavity. In directing fluid flow, sheaths are constructed to allow either unidirectional or bidirectional flow of distending media. Sheaths that allow continuous flow, that is, bidirectional inflow and outflow circulation of the distension medium, are most valuable in cases in which bleeding or large fluid

volume deficits are expected (Fig. 42-13.2). This circulation helps to clear blood from the operative field for better visualization and assists with fluid volume deficit calculation. The type of tubing attached to the hysteroscope sheath is dictated by the fluid management system. With diagnostic hysteroscopy, it may be as simple as intravenous tubing that provides solely inflow.

The operating sheath also allows the use of semirigid, rigid, and flexible instruments. The basic set that will suffice for most cases includes biopsy forceps, grasping forceps, and scissors. Of these, biopsy forceps are used for tissue sampling. They are somewhat sharp and cuplike. Grasping forceps permit removal of tissue or foreign bodies and may be toothed. Lastly, scissors can lyse adhesions, resect masses, or excise an intrauterine septum. Generally 5F in diameter and 34 to 40 cm long, these instruments are much smaller than the instruments used with the

resectoscope. None of these requires special distension media or energy. Flexible electrodes used to vaporize tissue may also be passed through this sheath.

Bettochi Hysteroscope

One of the smallest diameter operative hysteroscopes is the Bettochi hysteroscope. This 4-mm instrument has a 5F (1.67 mm) operating channel that provides both diagnostic and operative capability. Additionally, the shape of the hysteroscope is oblong rather than round, which conforms more naturally to the configuration of the cervical canal (Bradley, 2009). Biopsy forceps, monopolar and bipolar electrosurgical scissors, bipolar needle tip, or delivery devices for transcervical sterilization can easily pass through this hysteroscope's working channel. The 3.5-mm diagnostic continuous flow sheath has a small diameter yet permits sufficient flow to avoid a compromise in optical quality.

Flexible Hysteroscope

Flexible hysteroscopes are available whose tips can deflect over a range of 120 to 160 degrees. Although their optical view is less clear than that with rigid hysteroscopes, they offer surgeons the ease of maneuvering within irregularly shaped endometrial cavities and can be helpful when tubal access is required or during lysis of adhesions. Additionally, use of flexible hysteroscopes has been shown to cause less intraoperative pain than rigid ones (Unfried, 2001). This may be a consideration for patients undergoing in-office procedures.

Resectoscope

If resection of intrauterine tissues is planned, a resectoscope is often used (see Fig. 42-13.2).

This tool consists of inner and outer sheaths. The inner sheath houses a 3- to 4-mm endoscope and a channel for fluid inflow. The 8- to 10-mm outer sheath contains an electrosurgical resection loop and allows fluid egress from the uterus through a series of small holes near the sheath's distal end. By means of a spring mechanism, the resection loop can be extended and then retracted to shave off contacted tissues.

Larger instruments that are energy based for resection of intrauterine pathology are passed through the central cannula. These include the roller bar, roller ball, vaporizing electrodes (monopolar, bipolar, laser), hot scalpel, and motorized morcellators.

Hysteroscopic Morcellator

For resection of polyps or submucosal leiomyomas, a hysteroscopic morcellator may be used. The morcellator for hysteroscopic use offers different tips depending on the tissue type. For polyp resection, a rake-like tip is used. For resection of firmer tissue, such as a fibroid or septum, a cutting tip is selected. Both tips contain a mechanized rotary blade that fragments tissue. The tip is an extension of a hollow cannula that evacuates the tissue fragments using suction to a collection receptacle. The morcellator fits through the working channel of a 9-mm operative hysteroscopic cannula.

Distension Media

Because the anterior and posterior uterine walls lie in apposition, a distension medium is required to expand the endometrial cavity for viewing. Media include CO_2, saline, and low-viscous fluids, such as sorbitol, mannitol, and glycine solutions. Each group has distinct advantages and properties. To expand the cavity, intrauterine pressures of these media must reach 45 to 80 mm Hg (Tulandi, 1999). Rarely is more than 100 mm Hg required. Moreover, because for most women, mean arterial pressure approximates 100 mm Hg, higher pressures can result in increased intravasation of media into the patient's circulation and fluid volume overload (Fig. 42-13.3).

Carbon Dioxide

This commonly used distension medium, when used under pressure, tends to flatten the endometrium and provides excellent visibility. A continuous flow is necessary to replace any gas lost through the fallopian tubes, and typically flow rates of 40 to 50 mL/min are adequate. Rates higher than 100 mL/min are associated with increased risks for gas embolism and therefore are discouraged. Specialized hysteroscopic machines, which

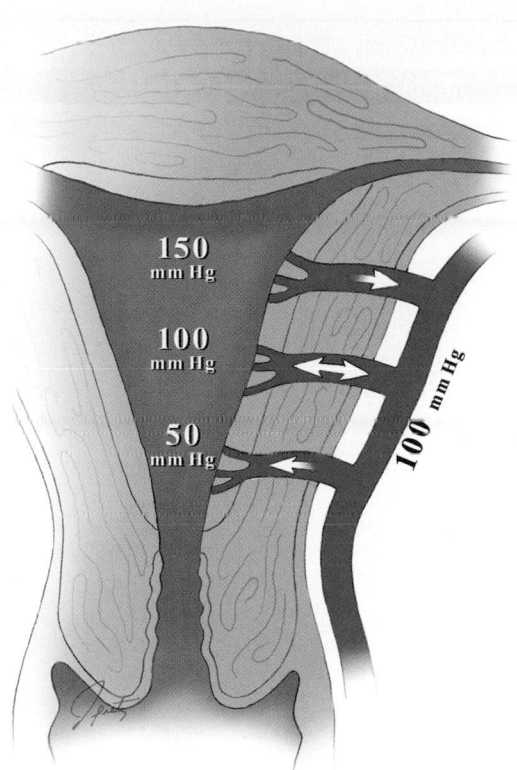

FIGURE 42-13.3 Distension medium flow varies depending on intrauterine pressure.

limit maximum flow rates, should be used. Importantly, because laparoscopic insufflating machines can permit flow rates greater than 1000 mL/min, these should not be used for hysteroscopy.

Disadvantages to CO_2 include its tendency, when mixed with blood or mucus, to form visually obstructive gas bubbles. Accordingly, prior to hysteroscope insertion, blood and mucus should be carefully removed from the cervical os with a dry swab (Sutton, 2006). Similarly, use of CO_2 with thermal energy sources is avoided, as smoke production prohibits adequate visualization. Because of these limitations, CO_2 is best used in cases in which minimal bleeding is anticipated, such as with diagnostic hysteroscopy or with simple operative excision (Bieber, 2003). The most serious complication associated with CO_2 use is venous gas embolism and is discussed on page 1161.

Fluid Media

Bleeding is common with operative hysteroscopy procedures, and fluid media are typically selected in these cases because of their optical clarity and ability to mix with blood.

The main risk of fluid distension media, however, involves increased fluid absorption and circulatory fluid volume overload. Volume overload may develop with any of the fluid media and results from a variety of mechanisms. For example, absorption across the endometrium, intravasation through surgically opened venous channels, and spill from the fallopian tubes with absorption by the peritoneum have all been suggested. Accordingly, clinical settings in which procedures are long, increased distension pressures are used, or large tissue areas are resected all carry a greater risk.

Fluid distension media can be divided according to their viscosity and electrolyte status. In general, low-viscosity fluids are used in modern hysteroscopy. An appropriate medium is selected based on its compatibility with electrosurgical instrumentation.

Low-Viscosity Electrolyte Fluids. Normal saline and lactated Ringer solutions are isotonic, electrolyte fluids. They are readily available in the operating room and are frequently used for diagnostic hysteroscopy. However, these fluids cannot be used with monopolar electrosurgery. Specifically, these solutions conduct current; thus, dissipate the energy; and thereby render the instrument useless.

Electrolyte-containing, isotonic fluids have lower associated risks of hyponatremia compared with hypoosmolar fluids, described in the next section. Still, rapid absorption can lead to pulmonary edema. In general, when using isotonic media in a healthy patient, a surgeon should consider terminating the procedure when the fluid deficit nears 2 L.

TABLE 42-13.1 Hysteroscopic Media

Class	Medium	Properties	Indications	Risks	Safety Measures
Gas	Carbon dioxide	Colorless gas	Diagnostic	Gas embolism	Avoid Trendelenburg Keep flow <100 mL/min Intrauterine pressure <100 mm Hg
Electrolyte fluid	0.9% saline	Isotonic, 380 mOsm/kg H_2O	Diagnostic Operative w/ bipolar tools	Volume overload	At 750 mL deficit, plan to complete procedure At 2.5 L deficit, stop procedure
	Lactated Ringer	Isotonic, 273 mOsm/kg H_2O	Diagnostic Operative w/ bipolar tools	Volume overload	Same as above
Electrolyte-poor fluid	Sorbitol 3%	Hypo-osmolar, 178 mOsm/kg H_2O	Operative w/ monopolar tools	Volume overload Hyponatremia Hypo-osmolality Hyperglycemia	At 750 mL deficit, plan to complete procedure At 1.5 L deficit, stop procedure
	Mannitol 5%	Iso-osmolar, 280 mOsm/kg H_2O	Operative w/ monopolar tools	Volume overload Hyponatremia	Same as above
	Glycine 1.5%	Hypo-osmolar, 200 mOsm/kg H_2O	Operative w/ monopolar tools	Volume overload Hyponatremia Hypo-osmolality Hyperammonemia	Same as above

Compiled from Cooper, 2000; Loffer, 2000.

Low-Viscosity, Electrolyte-Poor Fluids. Of other available media, 1.5-percent glycine, 3-percent sorbitol, and 5-percent mannitol are all low-viscosity, electrolyte-poor fluids. Because they are nonconducting, these media are used for electrosurgery involving monopolar instruments. Unfortunately, these fluids can create volume overload with concurrent development of hyponatremia and hypoosmolality and the potential for cerebral edema and death (American College of Obstetricians and Gynecologists, 2007b). Mechanistically, sorbitol is a six-carbon sugar and is metabolized following absorption. This effectively leaves free water in the intravascular space. Normal serum sodium levels are 135 to 145 mEq/L, and levels below this may lead to seizure followed by respiratory arrest. In addition, hypokalemia and hypocalcemia can often develop concurrently. Five-percent mannitol, also a six-carbon sugar, is isoosmolar and so has diuretic prop-

erties and does not lead to serum osmolality changes (Loffer, 2000).

In cases in which large fluid volume deficits are calculated, measurement of serum electrolyte levels is warranted. If a serum sodium level lower than 125 mEq/L is reached, postoperative care should be continued in a critical care setting. Treatment includes diuresis with furosemide (Lasix), 20 to 40 mg given intravenously, and correction of hyponatremia with 3-percent sodium chloride, administered 1 to 1.5 mEq/L/h. The goal of therapy is to reach a serum sodium level of 135 mEq/L within 24 hours. Overcorrection is avoided to prevent additional cerebral effects (Baggish, 2005).

To assist with fluid volume calculation, most operative hysteroscopes contain continuous flow systems that allow fluid deficits to be calculated. Calculation of deficits should be performed every 15 minutes during procedures. If a procedure has the

potential for larger deficits, a Foley catheter is also warranted for urine output monitoring. Moreover, an ongoing communication with participating anesthesia staff regarding large fluid deficits is prudent. The American Association of Gynecologic Laparoscopists recommends that if fluid discrepancy reaches 750 mL, a surgeon should plan for completion of the case. If fluid deficits reach 1500 mL of a nonelectrolyte solution or 2500 mL of normal saline, the procedure is immediately concluded, electrolytes measured, and diuretics given as indicated (Loffer, 2000). At the end of every hysteroscopic procedure, a final deficit is determined, and this value is recorded in the operative note.

Hysteroscopic Electrosurgery

Many widely used hysteroscopic tissue resection or desiccation techniques rely on monopolar current. Because current is dissipated and is thus ineffective in electrolyte solutions, these techniques have typically required nonelectrolyte solutions such as sorbitol, mannitol, and glycine. However, as discussed previously, these media can be associated with hyponatremia if fluid volume overload develops.

Alternatively, a bipolar electrosurgery system (Versapoint Bipolar Electrosurgery System) allows use of traditional hysteroscopic tools in a saline solution. The Versapoint system has attachments that include a loop resecting electrode, multiedged vaporizing electrodes, and ball, spring, and twizzle tips that can be employed for vaporization, desiccation, and cutting.

Surgical Complications

Uterine Perforation

In addition to fluid overload, uterine perforation or bleeding may complicate hysteroscopic procedures. The uterus may be perforated during uterine sounding, cervical dilatation, or hysteroscopic procedures (Cooper, 2000). Fundal perforations created by sounds, dilators, or hysteroscopes can be managed conservatively, as the myometrium will typically contract around these defects. In contrast, lateral perforation may perforate the broad ligament and injure larger pelvic vessels; posterior perforation may injure the rectum; and those caused by electrosurgical tools may cause organ laceration or burns. Diagnostic laparoscopy is indicated in these cases. Similarly, anterior perforations should prompt cystoscopy to evaluate associated bladder injury.

Gas Embolization

If vessels are opened during cervical dilation or endometrial disruption, gas under pressure can be forced into the vasculature. This can occur with gas or fluid media. Any undissolved portion can reach the lungs. CO_2 is many times more soluble in plasma than room air, and it typically dissolves sufficiently during transit from the pelvis (Corson, 1988). As a result, pulmonary embolism is rare. In a review of cases by Brandner and colleagues (1999), severe embolism complicated only 0.03 percent of nearly 4000 diagnostic hysteroscopic cases using CO_2.

Embolization can lead to rapid cardiovascular collapse. Signs and symptoms include chest pain, dyspnea, desaturation, hypotension, or a "mill wheel" heart murmur. To manage this emergency, the patient is placed in the left lateral decubitus position with the head tilted downward. This aids movement of the air from the right outflow tract to the apex of the right ventricle (American College of Obstetricians and Gynecologists, 2007b).

Surgeons can minimize the risk of gas embolism by avoiding Trendelenburg positioning of the patient during hysteroscopy, ensuring that air bubbles are removed from all tubing prior to introduction of the hysteroscope into the uterus, and maintaining intrauterine pressures at <100 mm Hg. Other preventions include minimizing the effort needed to dilate the cervix, avoiding deep myometrial resections, and limiting multiple removals and reinsertions of the hysteroscope in and out of the uterine cavity.

Hemorrhage

Heavy bleeding may develop during or following resection procedures. Although hysteroscopic electrosurgical electrodes may be used to contact and coagulate smaller vessels, these may be less effective for larger ones.

If heavy bleeding is encountered and is refractory to electrosurgical coagulation, termination of the procedure may be indicated. A Foley catheter balloon can be placed into the endometrial cavity and inflated incrementally with 5 to 10 mL of saline until moderate resistance to catheter tension is noted. An attached collection bag can be used to document blood loss and bleeding cessation, at which point the catheter may be removed.

42-14

Diagnostic Hysteroscopy

Hysteroscopy allows an endoscopic view of the endometrial cavity and tubal ostia. Indications are varied and include evaluation of abnormal uterine bleeding, infertility, or a sonographically identified uterine cavity mass.

PREOPERATIVE

Consent

Risks with diagnostic hysteroscopy are infrequent and include those described in Section 42-13 (p. 1157).

Patient Preparation

Infectious and venous thromboembolic (VTE) complications following hysteroscopic surgery are rare. Accordingly, preoperative antibiotics or VTE prophylaxis is typically not required (American College of Obstetricians and Gynecologists, 2007c, 2009a).

INTRAOPERATIVE

SURGICAL STEPS

❶ **Anesthesia and Patient Positioning.** Diagnostic hysteroscopy can be performed in an outpatient setting under local anesthesia with or without intravenous sedation. Alternatively, a day-surgery setting and general anesthesia may be selected.

The patient is placed in dorsal lithotomy position, the vagina is surgically prepared, and the bladder is drained. Because diagnostic hysteroscopy is a short procedure with little if any blood loss, CO_2 or saline is typically selected for uterine distension. Trendelenburg positioning should be avoided to prevent gas embolism.

❷ **Hysteroscope Assembly.** For assembly, the hysteroscope is placed within its outer sheath and locked into place. The light source is then attached to the endoscope. By convention, during hysteroscope insertion, the light source is kept pointing toward the floor. The distension media tubing port is attached to a port that typically lies 180 degrees away from the light source connection.

❸ **Hysteroscope Introduction.** For most diagnostic hysteroscopic procedures, cervical dilatation is not required to admit the 4- to 5-mm hysteroscope. Uterine sounding is not recommended by many because information regarding uterine depth and cavity inclination is provided by direct visualization during hysteroscope insertion. Moreover, the sound may disrupt the endometrium. This may alter endometrial anatomy prior to inspection and may cause obscuring bleeding.

For diagnostic purposes, a hysteroscope equipped with a 0-, 12-, or 30-degree forward oblique view lens is suitable. A single-toothed tenaculum is placed on the anterior cervical lip, the flow of distension medium is begun, and the hysteroscope is introduced into the endocervical canal. Pressure exerted by the medium opens the endocervical canal and allows entry of the hysteroscope. If using an angled lens, the surgeon should keep in mind that a panoramic image with a dark hole directly in the middle of the view is incorrect. The desired image would have the cervical canal at the bottom of the monitor if the light cord is directed downward, thus implying that the hysteroscope is in fact in the center of the cervical canal (Fig. 42-13.1, p. 1158).

❹ **Hysteroscopic Evaluation.** As the hysteroscope is inserted, the endocervical canal is examined for abnormalities. Upon entering the cavity, the hysteroscope is held at the distal portion of the cavity to allow a panoramic evaluation. Systematically, the hysteroscope is moved to the fundus and then to the left and right to permit inspection of the tubal ostia (Fig. 42-14.1). If an angled lens is employed, the hysteroscope may remain just beyond the internal cervical os and the light cord moved in a 180-degree rotational arc to obtain a global assessment of the endometrial cavity. Some surgeons also advocate keeping the hysteroscope in the cavity, evacuating it of distension medium, and evaluating the cavity in this decompressed stage. This helps identify lesions that may have been obliterated or flattened by the increased pressure of the distension medium.

❺ **Specific Procedures.** After complete cavity inspection, if specific lesions are identified, they are typically biopsied under direct visualization with hysteroscopic forceps. If IUD removal is planned, most are grasped by the string or stem with hysteroscopic grasping forceps and are easily extracted as the entire hysteroscope is removed (Fig. 42-14.2). However, embedded or fragmented devices may require removal in pieces. In these instances, a sturdy portion of the IUD is firmly grasped and traction on the forceps is exerted toward the vagina. For cases in which the IUD is deeply embedded, laparoscopy can assist in identifying uterine perforation and in determining whether the device is best removed hysteroscopically or laparoscopically.

❻ **Procedure Completion.** At the end of the procedure, the flow of distending medium is stopped, and hysteroscope and

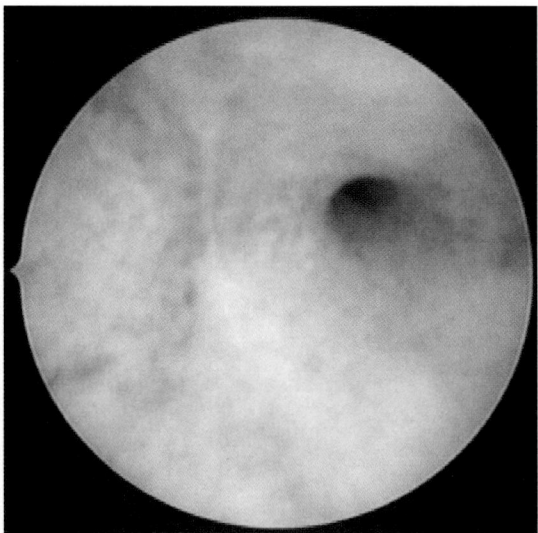

FIGURE 42-14.1 Hysteroscopic photograph of normal tubal ostia. (*Photograph contributed by Dr. Kevin Doody.*)

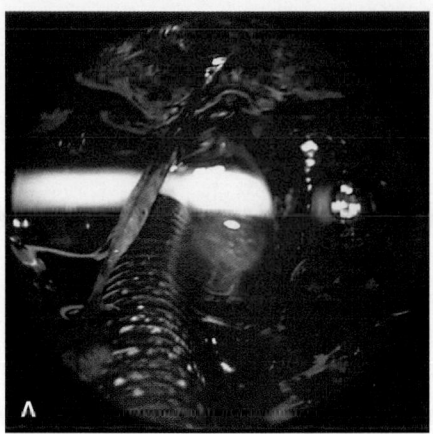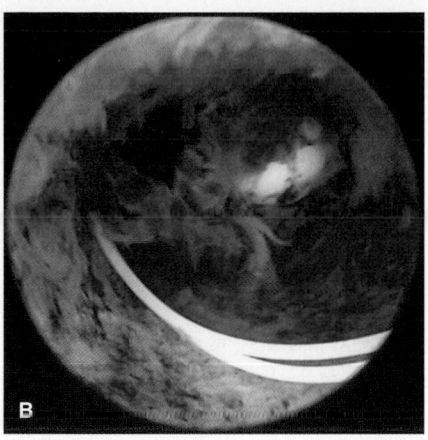

FIGURE 42-14.2 Hysteroscopic photograph of retained copper intrauterine device (IUD) prior to endoscopic removal. **A.** Copper coils around IUD body and white IUD crossbar are seen. **B.** In this view, two white IUD strings and white, ball-shaped distal end of IUD body are seen. *(Photographs contributed by Dr. Karen Bradshaw.)*

tenaculum are removed. A critical step at this point, and throughout the case, is to note the amount of distension fluid used and the amount retrieved. These values are used to calculate the final fluid deficit, which should be included in the operative report.

POSTOPERATIVE

Patient recovery is typically rapid and without complication and mirrors that following dilatation and curettage. Diet and activities may be resumed as desired by the patient. Spotting or light bleeding is not uncommon and typically stops within days.

42-15

Hysteroscopic Polypectomy

Indications for removal of endometrial polyps include abnormal uterine bleeding, infertility, and risk of malignant transformation (Chap. 8, p. 230). Hysteroscopic excision of these growths may be completed by incision of the polyp base with hysteroscopic scissors or resectoscope loop, avulsion of the polyp with hysteroscopic forceps, or morcellation. Of these, the resectoscope and morcellator offer the most versatility in managing lesions, both large and small.

PREOPERATIVE

Patient Evaluation

In many women undergoing polypectomy, preoperative transvaginal sonography or saline infusion sonography examinations have been completed. Information regarding the size, number, and location of polyps should be reviewed prior to surgery. In some instances, the use of magnetic resonance imaging may be indicated to fully distinguish a presumed polyp from a submucous leiomyoma. MR imaging often helps predict the success of this procedure if myomectomy is instead required (Section 42-16, p. 1166).

Consent

The complication rates for this procedure are low and mirror those for hysteroscopy in general (Section 42-13, p. 1157).

Patient Preparation

As with most hysteroscopic procedures, polypectomy is ideally performed during the follicular phase of the menstrual cycle, when the endometrial lining is thinnest and polyps would be most easily identified. Preoperative endometrial biopsy is optional but generally considered as part of the evaluation of abnormal uterine bleeding for those with risks for endometrial cancer (Chap. 8, p. 225). Preoperative antibiotics or VTE prophylaxis is typically not required (American College of Obstetricians and Gynecologists, 2007c, 2009a).

INTRAOPERATIVE

Instruments

As described in Section 42-13 (p. 1158), a resectoscope with a 90-degree loop electrode is ideal for polyp excision. Alternatively, an intrauterine morcellator with a hollow cannula that is attached to a suction mechanism can also quickly excise small to large growths. For smaller polyps, polyp forceps may also be used through the 5F channel of the operative port.

SURGICAL STEPS

❶ Anesthesia and Patient Positioning. Although simple polypectomy procedures under local analgesia in an office setting have been described, most cases are outpatient procedures performed under general or regional anesthesia. The complexity of fluid management, particularly with the use of hypotonic fluids as described in Section 42-13 (p. 1159), warrants a degree of safety that can be best provided in the operating suite. Following administration of adequate anesthesia, the patient is placed in dorsal lithotomy position, the vagina is surgically prepared, and a Foley catheter is inserted.

❷ Media Selection. Hysteroscopic morcellation may be performed with a physiologic saline solution. If a monopolar resectoscope is used, then a nonelectrolyte solution is required. Because of the risks for hyponatremia with sorbitol and glycine, 5-percent mannitol is preferred by many. Alternatively, selection of a bipolar resecting system (Versapoint) allows performance within an isotonic medium. As with any hysteroscopic procedure, fluid volume deficits are calculated and noted regularly during surgery.

❸ Cervical Dilatation. The larger diameter of an 8- or 10-mm resectoscope or morcellator typically requires dilatation up to 9 mm with Pratt or similar dilators (Section 41-16, p. 1060).

❹ Resection. Media flow is begun, and the resectoscope is inserted into the endocervical canal under hysteroscopic visualization. Upon entering the cavity, a panoramic inspection is completed to identify the location and number of polyps. The resectoscope loop is then extended to reach behind the polyp. Electrosurgical current is applied as the loop is retracted toward the cervix to cut the polyp base. The freed polyp is then grasped and delivered through the cervical os.

In cases in which the polyp is large, several passes with the loop electrode may be required for complete excision. Passes begin at the polyp tip and progress until the base is reached. To maintain visualization of the polyp and minimize the risks associated with multiple introductions and reintroductions of instruments into the cavity, the uterus is not emptied after each pass. Rather, resected segments are allowed to float within the cavity as resection continues. Once the entire polyp is excised, then the fragments are collected on a Telfa sheet as they flow out of the cavity along with the distending medium. For larger polyps, the number of floating fragments will accrue. Thus, the cavity may need to be emptied prior to complete resection to permit an unobstructed view during resection.

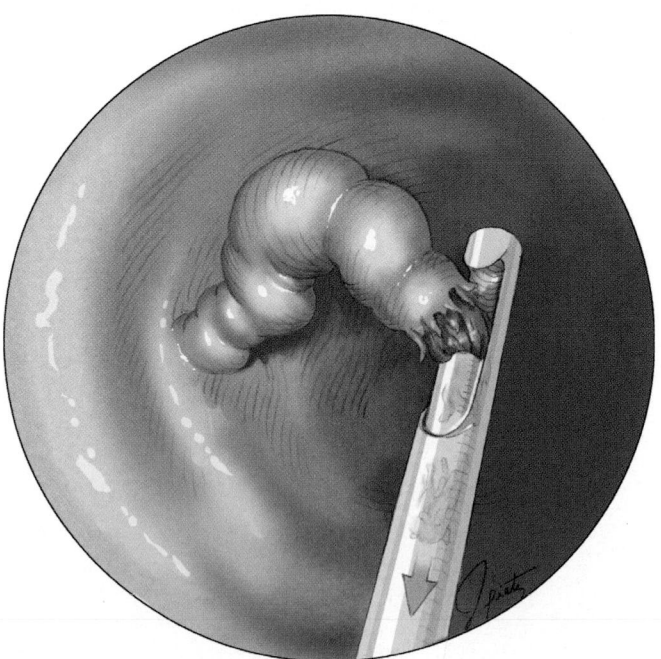

FIGURE 42-15.1 Hysteroscopic polypectomy.

❺ Morcellation. As with loop resection, distension medium flow is begun, and the morcellation unit is inserted. During morcellation, it is important to work from the polyp tip toward the base (Fig. 42-15.1). Moreover, the tumor should be kept between the morcellator opening and the optics of the camera.

The morcellator has suction action as well. This can be used apart from its cutting effects to clear blood, tissue debris, and clots during resection of large growths. Better visual acuity and the continuous retrieval of the tissue are two of the advantages to this approach.

❻ Control of Bleeding. Bleeding sites may be coagulated with the same resection loop using a coagulating current. Alternatively, for heavy bleeding, a Foley catheter balloon may be inflated as described in Section 42-13 (p. 1161).

❼ Instrument Removal. The resectoscope or morcellator is removed, and the surgical specimen is sent for pathologic evaluation. At the end of the procedure, the flow of distending medium is stopped, and hysteroscope and tenaculum are removed.

A critical step at this point, and throughout the case, is to note the amount of distension fluid used and retrieved to calculate the fluid deficit. This value is noted in the operative report.

POSTOPERATIVE

Recovery following polypectomy is rapid, is typically without complication, and follows that for other hysteroscopic procedures (Section 42-14, p. 1163).

42-16

Hysteroscopic Myomectomy

For symptomatic women with submucous leiomyomas, hysteroscopic resection of these tumors may provide relief of symptoms in most cases. Candidates may include those with abnormal uterine bleeding, those with dysmenorrhea, or those with infertility in which leiomyomas are suspected to be contributory. Tumors selected for resection should be either submucous or intramural with a prominent submucous component. During surgery, pedunculated submucous leiomyomas may be excised similarly to polyps as described in Section 42-15 (p. 1164). However, tumors with an intramural component require resection with a resectoscope, morcellator, or laser.

PREOPERATIVE

Patient Evaluation

Hysteroscopic myomectomy is a safe and effective option for most women. Contraindications to surgery, however, include pregnancy, potential endometrial cancer, current reproductive tract infection, and medical conditions sensitive to fluid volume overload.

Specific leiomyoma characteristics such as large size, great number, and degree of intramural penetration can raise the technical difficulty, complication rate, and clinical failure rate of this procedure (Di Spiezio Sardo, 2008). Thus, prior to resection, women should undergo transvaginal sonography, saline infusion sonography (SIS), or hysteroscopy to evaluate leiomyoma characteristics. Alternatively, magnetic resonance (MR) imaging can also accurately document uterine anatomy, but its high cost and lack of availability may limit its routine use.

During the evaluation by SIS or hysteroscopy, leiomyomas may be grouped according to criteria developed by Wamsteker and colleagues (1993) and adopted by the European Society of Gynaecological Endoscopy (ESGE):

Type 0: complete submucosal location

Type I: greater than 50-percent submucosal component

Type II: some submucosal involvement but greater than 50-percent myometrial component

These criteria help to predict which leiomyomas are suitable candidates for hysteroscopic resection based on tumor characteristics. A more recent classification has also been proposed by Lasmar and associates (2005, 2011). Similar to the ESGE system, their evaluation grades the degree of tumor penetration into the myometrium. But in addition, larger tumor size, wider tumor base, tumors in the upper portion of the cavity, or those found along the lateral wall receive higher scores. For higher scores, a nonhysteroscopic technique may be the safest and most successful.

Large or predominantly intramural tumors decrease clinical success rates, increase surgical risks, and increase the need for more than one surgical session to complete resection. For these reasons, many choose to resect only type 0 and I tumors and those measuring less than 3 cm (Vercellini, 1999; Wamsteker, 1993). More recent studies have reported resection of larger leiomyomas, although many need a two-step procedure and require a longer recovery (Camanni, 2010a).

Consent

Complications rates of this procedure mirror those for hysteroscopy in general. Rates of 2 to 3 percent have been reported (Section 42-13, p. 1157). Hysteroscopic myomectomy is associated with a greater risk of uterine perforation. This complication may follow cervical dilatation, but more frequently results during aggressive resection into the myometrium. Because of this risk, women should also give consent for laparoscopy to assess and treat this problem if it occurs.

Additionally, patients planning to seek pregnancy should be aware of possible intrauterine adhesion formation following resection and of rare uterine rupture during subsequent pregnancies (Batra, 2004; Howe, 1993).

During hysteroscopic myomectomy, distending medium is absorbed through open venous vasculature in the myometrium and also across the peritoneum as the fluid flows in a retrograde direction through the fallopian tubes. Thus, resection of type I or II tumors or of large leiomyomas may be halted due to advancing fluid volume deficits. Patients should be counseled that a second surgery may be required to finish resections in these cases. Fortunately, because of newer hysteroscopic morcellating tools, operating times and thus fluid deficits are decreased, even with large tumors. Additionally, although myomectomy is an effective treatment, 15 to 20 percent of patients will eventually require reoperation, either hysterectomy or repeat hysteroscopic resection, at a later time for either persistent or recurrent symptoms (Derman, 1991; Hart, 1999).

Patient Preparation

As discussed in Chapter 9 (p. 254), GnRH agonists can preoperatively shrink leiomyomas to enable resection of large tumors or allow patients to rebuild their red cell mass before surgery. However, disadvantages to their use include preoperative hot flashes, difficulty in cervical dilatation, increased risk of laceration or perforations, and reduced intracavitary volume, which limits instrument mobility. Thus, advantages and disadvantages of these drugs warrant individualization of their use.

To allow easier cervical dilatation and resectoscope insertion, laminaria tents may be placed the evening prior to surgery (Section 41-16, p. 1059). Alternatively, misoprostol (Cytotec) has also been shown to aid dilatation in some but not all studies, and postmenopausal women may benefit less from this pretreatment (Ngai, 1997, 2001; Oppegaard, 2008; Preutthipan, 2000). Commonly used dosing options include 200 or 400 µg vaginally or 400 µg orally once 12 to 24 hours prior to surgery. Common side effects include cramping, uterine bleeding, or nausea. Another alternative for cervical preparation prior to dilation is the use of dilute vasopressin (0.05 units/mL), 20 mL of which can be injected in divided doses intracervically at 4 and 8 o'clock. This method has the advantage of working rapidly at the time of surgery if the need for preoperative preparation was not anticipated (Phillips, 1997).

Although the risk of postoperative infection is low, because pelvic infections can have devastating effect on future fertility, most recommend antibiotic prophylaxis prior to extensive hysteroscopic resections, such as myomectomy. Suitable agents are found in Table 39-6 (p. 959).

Concurrent Ablation

In those women with menorrhagia and with no desire for future fertility, endometrial ablation may be concurrently performed (Section 42-17, p. 1169) (Loffer, 2005). However, because leiomyoma resection alone resolves abnormal bleeding in most women, we do not routinely perform concomitant endometrial ablation unless the patient desires hypomenorrhea.

INTRAOPERATIVE

Instruments

Hysteroscopic myomectomy can be performed using a resectoscope or hysteroscopic morcellator. Both procedures will be described.

SURGICAL STEPS

❶ **Anesthesia and Patient Positioning.** For most cases, hysteroscopic myomectomy is an outpatient procedure performed under general anesthesia. The patient is placed in dorsal lithotomy position, the

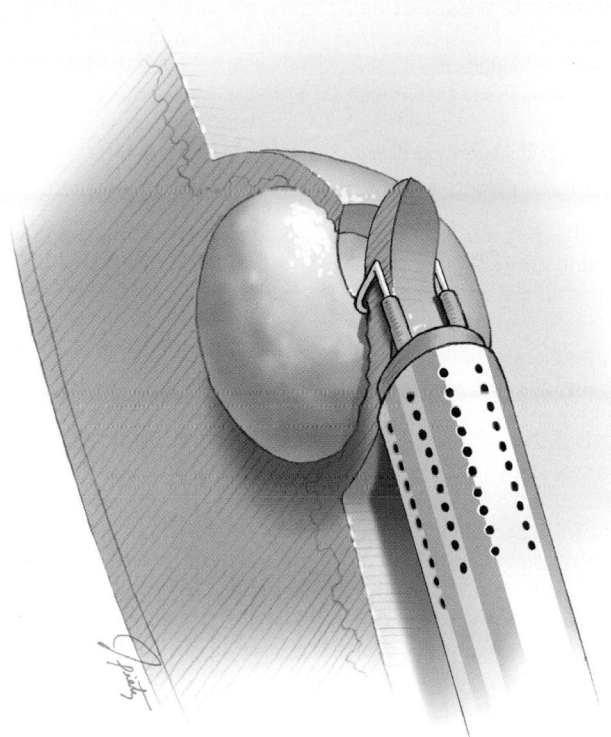

FIGURE 42-16.1 Hysteroscopic resection.

the resectoscope (Fig. 42-16.1). To ensure a clean cut and complete excision of the shaved strip, current is not stopped until the entire loop is retracted. The shaved strip of smooth muscle floats within the endometrial cavity.

This shaving process is repeated serially toward the leiomyoma's base until the tumor is removed. Although strips can be removed from the cavity after each pass, this results in a repetitive loss of uterine distension. Repeated removal and reinsertion of a resectoscope increases the risk of perforation, air embolism, and fluid intravasation. Thus in most cases, pushing removed strips to the fundus will help to adequately clear the operative field. However, if the view becomes obstructed, a pause in resection may be required to remove these strips.

❻ **Morcellation.** Morcellators currently available include Hologic's Myosure and Smith & Nephew's Truclear system. In general, sharp moving blades are contained within a hollow, rigid tube. By means of a vacuum source connected to the hollow tube, tissue is suctioned into the window opening at the device tip and is shaved off by the moving blade (Fig. 42-16.2).

vagina is surgically prepared, and a Foley catheter is inserted.

❷ **Medium Selection.** The choice of distending medium is dictated by the resecting tool used. Resection using a morcellator, bipolar electrosurgical loop, or laser can be performed in saline solution. Alternatively, cases using a monopolar electrosurgical loop require an electrolyte-free solution (Section 42-13, p. 1159).

❸ **Cervical Dilatation.** Using Pratt or other suitable dilators, the surgeon dilates the cervix as described in Section 41-16 (p. 1060).

❹ **Instrument Insertion.** The distending medium flow is begun, and the resectoscope or morcellator is inserted into the endocervical canal under direct visualization. Upon entering the endometrial cavity, a panoramic inspection is first performed to identify and assess leiomyomas.

❺ **Resection.** The electrosurgical unit is set to a continuous-wave mode (cutting). The resectoscope loop is advanced to lie behind the leiomyoma, and electric current is applied before the loop contacts the tissue. To minimize thermal injury and perforation, current should only be applied as the loop is retracted and not when it is being extended. Upon contact, the loop electrode is retracted toward

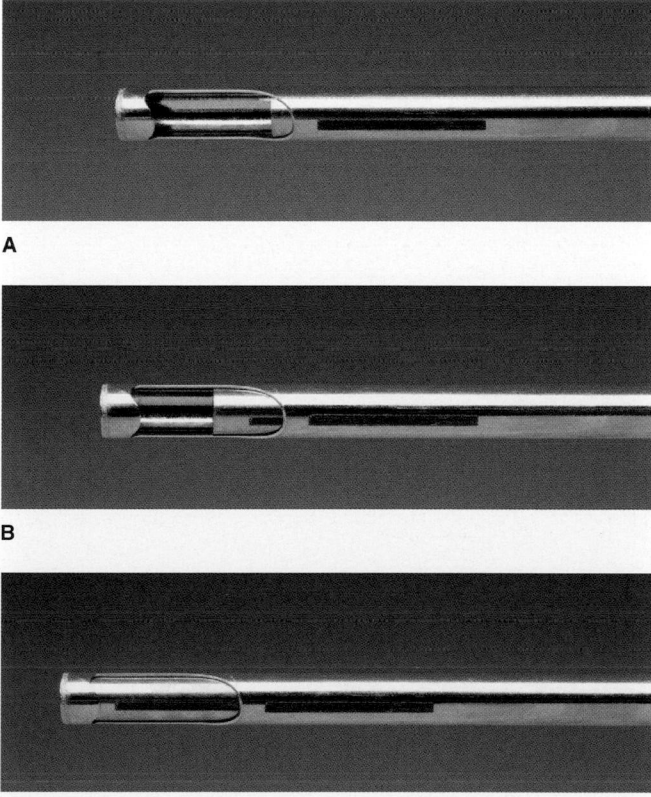

A

B

C

FIGURE 42-16.2 Hysteroscopic morcellator. **A.** Morcellator blade retracted. Suction draws tissue into the fluted opening. **B.** Blade partially advanced. The blade rapidly rotates as it is advanced and retracted. **C.** Blade is fully advanced and slices tissue drawn into the opening.

Suction also removes morcellated tissue fragments through the device cylinder and allows collection for pathologic analysis.

In retrospective comparisons, hysteroscopic morcellation is faster than resectoscopy and appears easier to perform. It is associated with fewer fluid-related complications and has a shorter learning curve compared with conventional resectoscopy (Emanuel, 2005).

❼ Intramural Leiomyomas. During removal of leiomyomas with an intramural component, uterine perforation risks are increased if resection extends below the level of the normal myometrium. Therefore, when resection reaches this level, the surgeon should pause and wait for the surrounding myometrium to contract around the now smaller tumor. This delivers deeper portions of the leiomyoma into the uterine cavity. Diminishing the intrauterine pressure, by decreasing the fluid inflow pressure, can also help to deliver the leiomyoma.

❽ Fluid Volume Deficit. Because of the hypervolemia risk during hysteroscopic myomectomy, fluid volume deficit should be carefully monitored throughout the procedure as discussed in Section 42-13 (p. 1159). The final fluid deficit is calculated and noted in the operative report.

❾ Hemostasis. Bleeding is common during myomectomy and will often cease as the myometrium fibers contract due to the reduction in intracavitary volume. Vessels that are actively bleeding may be coagulated with the edge of the resecting loop, and the electrosurgical unit set to a modulating (coagulating) current. At times, a ball electrode may be required to increase the surface area over which current is delivered. Global endometrial ablation offers a similar treatment in the case of multiple sites of bleeding. Rarely, hemorrhage may not be controlled with electrosurgical means. In such cases, mechanical pressure applied to bleeding vessels by a Foley balloon inflated with 5 to 10 mL of saline may be required (p. 1161).

POSTOPERATIVE

Recovery following myomectomy is quick and typically without complication. Patients may resume diet and activities as tolerated. Spotting or light bleeding may follow surgery for 1 to 2 weeks.

For patients desiring pregnancy, conception may be attempted in the menstrual cycle after the resection, unless the leiomyoma was broad-based or had a significant intramural component. In these patients, barrier contraception is advised for three cycles. For women who fail to conceive or continue to have abnormal bleeding following resection, postoperative hysterosalpingography or hysteroscopy is recommended to evaluate for synechiae.

42-17

Endometrial Ablation Procedures

Endometrial ablation broadly describes a group of hysteroscopic procedures that destroys or resects the endometrium and leads to eumenorrhea. For many women, ablation serves as a minimally invasive and effective treatment of abnormal uterine bleeding. Within the ablation group, techniques are defined as first or second generation depending on their temporal introduction into use and the need for hysteroscopic skills. First-generation tools require advanced hysteroscopic skills and longer operating times and can be associated with distension medium complications, such as volume overload. These techniques include endometrial vaporization with the neodymium:yttrium-aluminum-garnet (Nd-YAG) laser, rollerball electrosurgical desiccation, and endometrial resection by resectoscope.

It appears that all three first-generation methods produce similar outcomes in terms of bleeding and patient satisfaction. However, resection methods have been associated with more surgical complications, and thus desiccation methods may be preferred for women without intracavitary lesions (Lethaby, 2002; Overton, 1997).

To reduce risks and the specialized training required for use of these early ablative tools, second-generation nonresectoscopic methods have been introduced during the past 10 years. These tools use various modalities to ablate the endometrium but do not require direct hysteroscopic guidance. Modalities include thermal energy, cryosurgery, electrosurgery, and microwave energy.

PREOPERATIVE

Patient Evaluation

Prior to ablation, complete evaluation of abnormal uterine bleeding should be completed. Accordingly, the possibility of pregnancy, endometrial hyperplasia or endometrial cancer, and active pelvic infection should be excluded. During evaluation of bleeding, transvaginal sonography (TVS), saline infusion sonography (SIS), and hysteroscopy may be used solely or in combination (Chap. 8, p. 223). However, because many second-generation ablation techniques require a normal endometrial cavity and because endometrial pathology, if identified, can be treated concurrently by several of these ablative methods, SIS or hysteroscopy is preferred for preoperative evaluation. In addition, several

second-generation techniques are not appropriate for large endometrial cavities. Thus, uterine depth is also assessed preoperatively by uterine sounding or sonography.

Myometrial thinning from prior uterine surgery may increase the risk of damage to surrounding viscera during ablation. Thus, women with prior transmural uterine surgery should be evaluated for type and location of the uterine scar. A history of prior classical cesarean delivery or of abdominal or laparoscopic myomectomy may be considered a relative contraindication to ablation. Some experts advocate sonographic evaluation of myometrial thickness to determine if a patient is a candidate for ablation, although no specific thickness has been established (American College of Obstetrics and Gynecologists, 2007a).

Consent

Patients selecting ablation should be aware of success rates relative to other treatment options for abnormal bleeding as discussed in Chapter 8 (p. 237). In general, rates of decreased menstrual flow range from 70 to 80 percent and of amenorrhea, from 15 to 35 percent. Eumenorrhea, rather than amenorrhea, is considered the treatment goal. Therefore, a patient should not undergo ablation if guaranteed amenorrhea is desired. In addition, endometrial ablation effectively destroys the endometrium and is contraindicated in those who desire future fertility.

Endometrial tissue has tremendous regenerative capabilities. Therefore, premenopausal women should be counseled before surgery regarding the need for adequate postoperative contraception. If pregnancy does occur, complications after ablation may include miscarriage, prematurity, abnormal placentation, and perinatal morbidity. For this reason, many providers recommend concomitant tubal sterilization at the time of endometrial ablation (American College of Obstetricians and Gynecologists, 2007a).

Complications associated with ablation mirror those with operative hysteroscopy, although the risk of fluid volume overload is generally avoided with second-generation tools (Section 42-13, p. 1157).

Patient Preparation

During hysteroscopic surgeries, bacteria in the vagina may gain access to the upper reproductive tract and peritoneal cavity. However, postablation infection is rare, and preoperative prophylactic antibiotics are generally not indicated. Because the endometrium can thicken from only a few millimeters in the early proliferative phase to deeper than 10 mm in the secretory phase, all first-generation techniques and some

second-generation should be performed in the early proliferative phase. Otherwise, drugs that induce endometrial atrophy such as gonadotropin-releasing hormone (GnRH) agonists, combination oral contraceptives, or progestins may be used for 1 to 2 months prior to surgery. Alternatively, curettage may be performed immediately prior to surgery.

INTRAOPERATIVE

SURGICAL STEPS

❶ **Anesthesia and Patient Positioning.** Endometrial ablation is typically a day-surgery procedure, performed under general anesthesia. Some studies indicate that second-generation techniques may be satisfactorily completed in an outpatient setting with intravenous sedation, local anesthetic blockade, or both (Sambrook, 2010; Varma, 2010). The patient is placed in dorsal lithotomy position, and the perineum and vagina are surgically prepared.

❷ **Selection of Distending Medium.** With first-generation procedures, distending medium is required and selected based on the destructive energy used as described in Section 42-13 (p. 1159). In general, saline may be used for laser and bipolar electrical current, whereas monopolar tools require nonelectrolyte solutions.

❸ **Neodymium:Yttrium-Aluminum-Garnet (Nd-Yag) Laser.** Introduced in the 1980s, the Nd-YAG laser was the first ablative tool. Under direct hysteroscopic observation and uterine distension with saline, a Nd-YAG laser fiber touches the endometrium and is dragged across the endometrial surface. This creates furrows of photocoagulated tissue that are 5 to 6 mm deep (Garry, 1995; Goldrath, 1981).

❹ **Transcervical Resection of the Endometrium.** In attempts to lower cost from expensive laser equipment, transcervical resection of the endometrium (TCRE) was subsequently developed (DeCherney, 1983, 1987). In addition to less expense, because of the larger loop diameter, TCRE can be completed more quickly than laser fiber ablation and can thereby reduce the risk of excess media absorption due to long procedure duration.

This method uses a resectoscope with monopolar or bipolar electrical current to excise strips of endometrium. The resection technique is similar to that for hysteroscopic myomectomy as described in Section 42-16 (p. 1167). The excised tissue strips are sent for pathologic evaluation. In cases with concurrent intrauterine pathology such as endometrial polyps or submucous leiomyomas, TCRE can excise these lesions in addition to the endometrium.

However, TCRE has been associated with higher rates of perforation, especially at the cornual areas, where the myometrium is thinner. For this reason, many use a rollerball electrosurgical electrode in combination with TCRE, with the rollerball used in the cornua (Oehler, 2003).

❺ Rollerball. A 2- to 4-mm ball-shaped or barrel-shaped electrosurgical electrode can be rolled across the endometrium as an effective means of vaporizing the endometrium (Vancaillie, 1989). Advantages to rollerball ablation compared with TCRE include shorter operating time, less fluid absorption, and lower rate of perforation. Unfortunately, it is not effective in the treatment of intracavitary lesions, and pathology specimens are not obtained.

❻ Thermal Balloon Ablation. The first thermal balloon ablation system was initially used in the early 1990s. Several thermal balloon ablation systems are currently used worldwide (Fig. 42-17.1). Of these, only the ThermaChoice III Uterine Balloon Therapy System is approved for use in the United States. Other balloon systems available outside the United States include the Cavaterm Plus system and Thermablate Endometrial Ablation System.

The ThermaChoice III Uterine Balloon Therapy System is a software-controlled device designed to ablate endometrial tissue using thermal energy. After cervical dilation to 5.5 mm, the Thermachoice device is inserted into the uterine cavity. Once inside the cavity, a 5-percent dextrose and water solution is instilled into a disposable, clear silicone balloon at the tip and heated

to coagulate the endometrium. During the treatment, the fluid within the balloon is circulated to maintain a temperature of 87°C (186°F) for 8 minutes. The balloon can be introduced without hysteroscopic assistance into the uterine cavity and when inflated, conforms to the cavity contour.

All hot-liquid balloon devices require no advanced hysteroscopic skills, and complication rates are low (Gurtcheff, 2003; Vilos, 2004). Disadvantages include the requirement of an anatomically normal uterine cavity and of pharmacologic thinning prior to thermal ablation. Some studies, however, have demonstrated successful use in patients with small submucosal leiomyomas (Soysal, 2001). Alternatively, mechanical thinning can be accomplished with dilatation and curettage prior to ablation.

❼ Hysteroscopic Thermal Ablation. Several second-generation ablation procedures require a normal uterine cavity. However, the HydroThermAblator (HTA) (Boston Scientific) system allows treatment of the endometrium concurrent with submucous leiomyomas, polyps, or abnormal uterine anatomy. Another advantage of this system is that it is performed under direct hysteroscopic visualization, allowing the surgeon to observe the endometrium being destroyed. However, the risk of external burns from circulating hot water appears to be higher using

this method compared with other second-generation methods (Della Badia, 2007).

This tool is designed to ablate the endometrial lining of the uterus by heating an uncontained saline solution to a temperature of 90°C and recirculating it through the uterus for 10 minutes (Fig. 42-17.2). Spill through the fallopian tubes is avoided because hydrostatic pressure during the procedure remains below 55 mm Hg, which is well below pressures needed to open the tubes to the peritoneal cavity. Similarly, the water seal created between the hysteroscope and internal cervical os prevents leakage of fluid into the vagina. For this reason, care should be taken not to dilate the cervix to a diameter greater than 8 mm. Additionally, preoperative laminaria are not recommended.

Initially, a hysteroscope is inserted into the 7.8-mm diameter disposable HTA sheath. This combination is introduced into the endometrial cavity to enable visualization while room-temperature saline is instilled into the uterine cavity. The fluid is then gradually heated and circulated to treat the endometrium. At the completion of the treatment phase, cool saline replaces the heated fluid, and the instrument is then removed (Glasser, 2003).

❽ Impedance-controlled Electrocoagulation. The NovaSure endometrial ablation system was approved for marketing in the

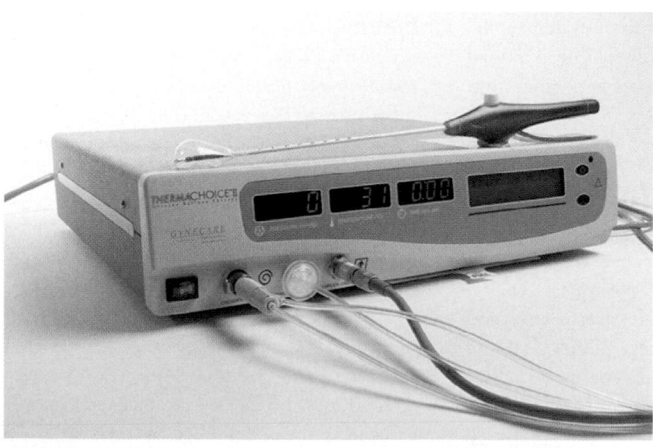

FIGURE 42-17.1 ThermaChoice III Uterine Balloon Therapy System. *(© Ethicon, Inc. Reproduced with permission.)*

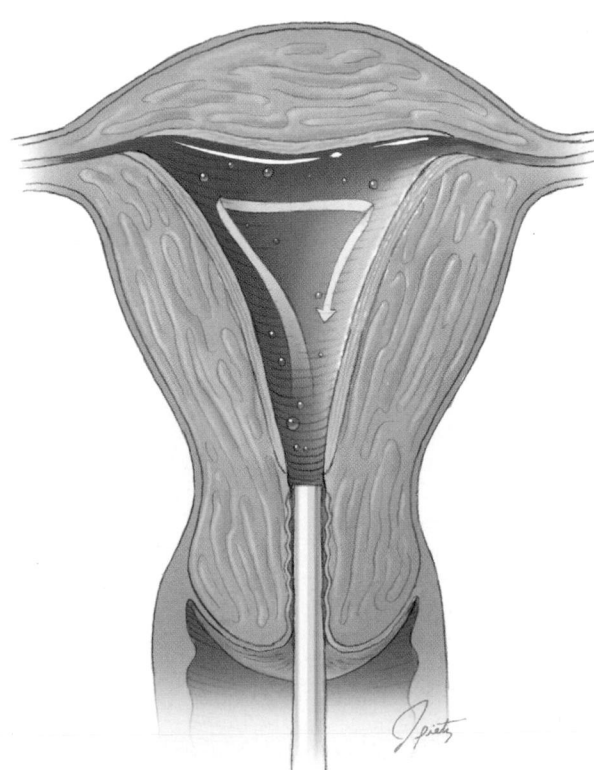

FIGURE 42-17.2 Hysteroscopic thermal ablation.

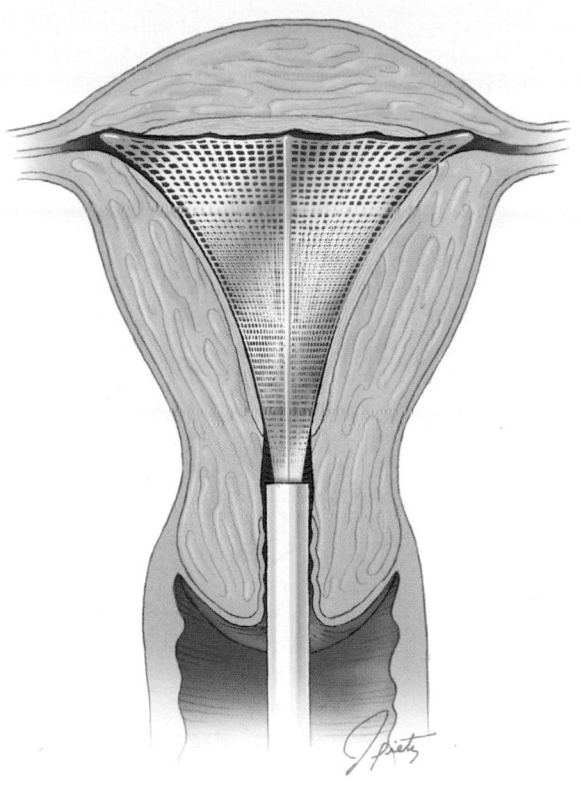

FIGURE 42-17.3 Impedance-controlled electrocoagulation.

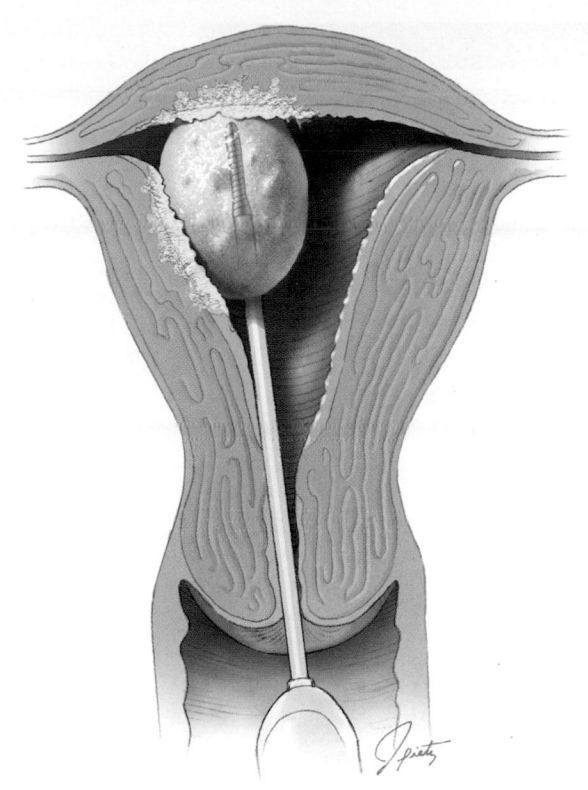

FIGURE 42-17.4 Cryoablation.

United States in 2001. The system consists of a high-frequency (radiofrequency) bipolar electrosurgical generator and a single-use, metal, fan-shaped device constructed of fabric-like mesh. The mesh fan is designed to contour to the shape of the endometrial cavity. During treatment, an attachment provides suction to draw the endometrium and myometrium up against the mesh electrode for improved contact and to remove generated vapor (Fig. 42-17.3). The treatment time of 2 minutes results in desiccation of the endometrium. An advantage of this system is that it does not require preoperative endometrial preparation. Although FDA-approval studies evaluated the system in normal uterine cavities, it has been used successfully in patients with small submucosal leiomyomas and polyps (Sabbah, 2006).

❾ Cryoablation. In addition to thermal damage, endometrial ablation can be achieved with extreme cold. The Her Option cryoablation system was approved for use in the United States in 2001. Similar to the physics of cervical cryotherapy, gases compressed under pressure with this unit can generate temperatures of −100° to −120°C at the cryoprobe tip to produce an iceball. As an iceball grows, its leading edge advances

through tissue, and cryonecrosis develops in those tissues reaching temperatures less than −20°C (Section 41-26, p. 1078).

The Her Option cryoablation system contains a metal probe, which is covered by a 5.5-mm disposable cryoprobe. After dilatation of the cervix, the cryoprobe's 1.4-inch cryotip is placed against one side of the endometrial cavity and advanced to one uterine cornu (Fig. 42-17.4). Concurrent transabdominal sonography is required to ensure accurate cryotip placement and surveillance of the increasing iceball diameter, which is seen as an enlarging hypoechoic area. The first freeze is terminated after 4 minutes or sooner, if the advancing iceball reaches to within 5 mm of the uterine serosa. The cryotip is allowed to warm, is removed from the cornu, and is redirected into the contralateral cornu. A second freeze is performed for 6 minutes or sooner, as with the initial freeze.

❿ Microwave Ablation. The Microwave Endometrial Ablation (MEA) technique uses microwave energy to destroy the endometrium. During the procedure, a microwave probe is inserted until the tip reaches the uterine fundus. Once inserted, the probe tip is maintained at 75° to 80°C and moved

slowly from side to side. Microwave energy is spread with a maximum penetration of 6 mm over the entire surface of the uterine cavity. Speed is an advantage, with the entire treatment completed in 2 to 3 minutes (Cooper, 1999). Due to complications of bowel burns in patients without evidence of uterine perforation, to obtain FDA approval, the manufacturers of the MEA system recommend preoperative assessment of myometrial thickness to document at least a 10-mm thickness throughout the uterus (Glasser, 2009; Iliodromiti, 2011). MEA was U.S. FDA approved in 2003. However, Microsulis discontinued worldwide sales of the MEA device in 2011 (McIntyre, 2011).

POSTOPERATIVE

Advantages to endometrial ablation include rapid patient recovery and low incidence of complications. Patients may resume normal diet and activities as tolerated. Patients may expect light bleeding or spotting during the first postoperative days as necrotic endometrial tissue is shed. A serosanguineous discharge follows for 1 week and is replaced by a profuse and watery discharge for another 1 to 2 weeks.

42-18

Transcervical Sterilization

Hysteroscopic sterilization is a minimally invasive, transcervical method to perform surgical sterilization. Currently, only two forms of transcervical sterilization are approved by the FDA (2009a,b). These are the *Essure Permanent Birth Control system* and *Adiana Permanent Contraception system* (Chap. 5, p. 147).

Essure employs a coil device, termed a *microinsert*, which is inserted hysteroscopically into the proximal section of each fallopian tube. Once in place and released from its delivery catheter, the microinsert expands to anchor itself within the fallopian tube (Fig. 42.18.1). Over time, synthetic fibers within the microinsert incite a chronic inflammatory response and a local tissue ingrowth from the surrounding tube. This ingrowth leads to complete tubal lumen occlusion, which is documented by hysterosalpingography (HSG) at 3 months following surgery.

The Adiana system was introduced in 2009 and employs a two-step process. A catheter is introduced hysteroscopically into the tubal ostium and delivers bipolar radiofrequency energy for 1 minute. This creates a superficial lesion within the proximal tubal lumen. Next, a 3.5-mm nonabsorbable silicone matrix is placed within the tube to create tubal occlusion similar to Essure (Fig. 42-18.2). As with the Essure system, a reliable form of contraception must be used until tubal occlusion is confirmed by HSG at 3 months.

As with any permanent birth control method, candidates should be confident in their decision for sterilization. Contraindications include pregnancy or pregnancy termination within the prior 6 weeks, recent pelvic infection, known tubal occlusion, and allergy to radiographic contrast media. Labeling for Essure regarding its use in those with nickel allergy has recently been relaxed by the FDA. Although prescribing information still notes that "patients who are allergic to nickel may have an allergic reaction to this device, especially those with a history of metal allergies," the risk of an allergic reaction to the nitinol alloy is extremely low (Yu, 2011; Zurawin, 2011).

PREOPERATIVE

Patient Evaluation

Pregnancy should be excluded prior to sterilization using a serum or urine β-hCG test.

Consent

For many women, hysteroscopic sterilization is a safe and effective method of birth control. Efficacy rates are comparable with current rates for laparoscopic sterilization, although long-term data are limited (Magos, 2004). Essure appears to have similar or superior contraceptive efficacy compared with other methods of sterilization (Levy, 2007). At 1 year, the Adiana system offers a contraceptive efficacy rate slightly higher than other methods, with the exception of spring clip sterilization (Vancaillie, 2008). However, an analysis of available data suggests a higher rate of subsequent pregnancy at 5-year follow-up (Basinski, 2010).

Effective bilateral tubal occlusion or insert placement may not be possible in all patients due to tubal ostium stenosis or spasm or an inability to visualize the ostia (Cooper, 2003; Gariepy, 2011). Rates of successful placement average 88 to 95 percent (Kerin, 2003; Ubeda, 2004).

In general, complications of transcervical sterilization are similar to those of hysteroscopy. However, rates of fluid volume overload are low because in most cases procedure lengths are short (15 to 30 minutes) and opening of endometrial vascular channels is minimal. Uterine or tubal perforation has been noted. Rates approximate 1 to 2 percent, and in most cases, the perforations are clinically insignificant (Cooper, 2003; Kerin, 2003). A perforated Essure insert may need to be removed from the peritoneal cavity to prevent complications. Insert erosion or migration may also occur.

Patient Preparation

Because menstrual bleeding and a thick endometrium can impair identification of tubal ostia, this procedure is typically performed during the early proliferative phase of the menstrual cycle. This also decreases the chance of an unidentified luteal-phase pregnancy. Preoperative analgesia may be considered and typically consists of a nonsteroidal antiinflammatory drug given 30 to 60 minutes before the procedure. Prophylactic antibiotics are not required for this operation.

INTRAOPERATIVE

Instruments

Both the Essure and Adiana Systems are disposable and come individually wrapped. Essure contains a handle, delivery catheter, release catheter, delivery wire, and microinserts. Each microinsert is attached to the end

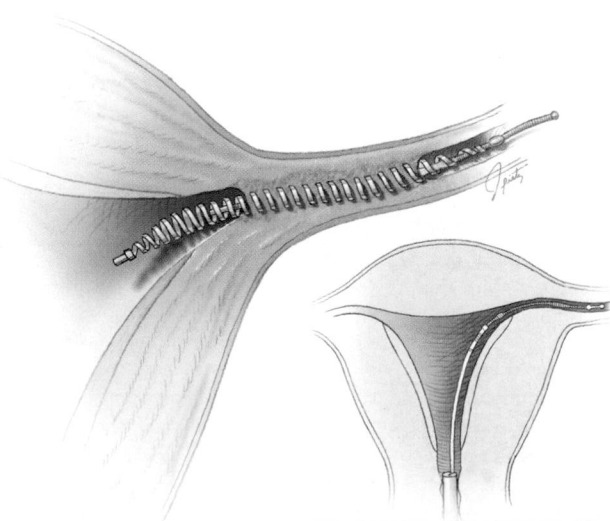

FIGURE 42-18.1 Essure microinsert placement and ingrowth of tissue.

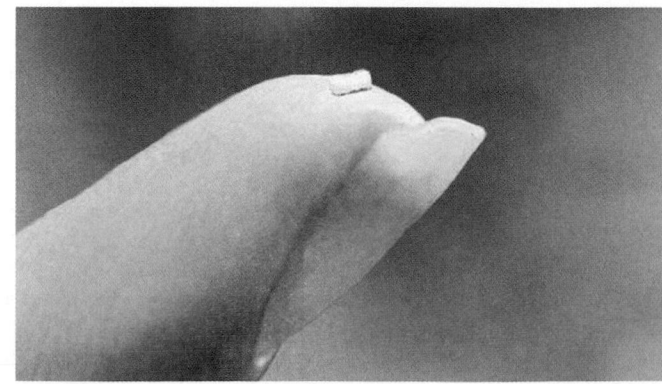

FIGURE 42-18.2 Adiana® matrix. *(Courtesy of Hologic, Inc. and affiliates.)*

of a delivery wire, which is housed within a release catheter. In turn, the release catheter is surrounded by a delivery catheter. The Adiana system consists of a delivery catheter with a bipolar array and implantable matrix at its tip, a split introducer sheath with obturator, and a radiofrequency (RF) generator.

SURGICAL STEPS

❶ Anesthesia and Patient Positioning. Transcervical sterilization can be performed in an outpatient setting under local analgesia with or without intravenous sedation. Alternatively, a day-surgery setting using general anesthesia may be selected. The patient is placed in the dorsal lithotomy position, and the vagina is surgically prepared.

❷ Medium Selection. For the Essure system, electrosurgery is not required, and therefore, 0.9-percent saline is commonly used to avoid the increased expense and risk of hyponatremia associated with nonelectrolyte solutions. For the Adiana system, nonionic hysteroscopic distension medium is recommended such as 1.5-percent glycine or 3-percent sorbitol. As with any hysteroscopic procedure, accurate calculation of fluid volume deficits during the procedure is essential (Section 42-13, p. 1159). The final deficit is recorded within the operative note.

❸ Hysteroscope Insertion. Vaginal retractors or speculum provides access to the cervix, and a tenaculum may be used for adequate cervical traction to insert the hysteroscope. Depending on the diameter of the operative hysteroscope, standard cervical dilatation may or may not be required as described in Section 41-16 (p. 1060). A 12- to 30-degree hysteroscope is preferred to provide easy

visualization of the cornua, and a 5F operating channel is required.

❹ Identification of Ostia. For completion of the procedure, both tubal ostia must be visualized.

❺ Essure Microinsert Delivery. The outermost catheter of the system, the *delivery catheter*, is threaded through the operating channel of the hysteroscope, and its tip is inserted into one tubal ostium. This delivers the tightly coiled, collapsed insert into the ostium. The delivery catheter is then retracted and coiled into the Essure device handle. With this, an inner cannula, which is the *release catheter*, is now seen. As the release catheter is retracted, the microinsert begins to uncoil. Ideally, if correctly placed, four to eight coils of the microinsert trail into the endometrial cavity (Fig. 42-18.3). As a final step, a guide wire that is attached to the distal end of the microinsert is detached and retracted. These steps are repeated at the opposite ostium.

❻ Adiana Matrix Implantation. With this system, the delivery catheter is threaded through the introducer sheath and then placed through the operating channel of the hysteroscope. Once it is threaded through the operating channel, the introducer sheath is removed. The catheter handle is used to guide the delivery catheter tip into the tubal ostium. The catheter tip is introduced until a black position mark is seen at the uterotubal junction. The RF generator will then automatically sense the position of the catheter in the fallopian tube. When all four detection arrays at the catheter tip are in contact with the tube, the RF energy may then be delivered for 60 seconds. At this point, the matrix release button on the catheter is pressed. This action deploys the matrix into the

tubal lumen. As a final step, the catheter is removed from the hysteroscope. These steps are repeated at the opposite ostium.

POSTOPERATIVE

Patients typically resume normal diet and activity within the first 24 hours following surgery. Cramping is common within the first few days, and light spotting or bleeding may be noted during the week following surgery.

To document complete tubal occlusion, HSG is performed at 3 months following insertion (Fig. 42-18.4). Until this time, an alternative method of contraception should be used. Rarely, in those with correct placement, tubal occlusion may not be complete at 3 months, and a second HSG at 6 months may be required to document sterilization. Of note, although Essure microinserts are radiopaque with fluoroscopy, the Adiana silicone implant is not visible. This has led to equivocal interpretations of HSGs and subsequent pregnancy in the Adiana pivotal trials (Basinski, 2010). Microinserts can be expelled. Thus, with Essure, if no device is identified during HSG or if 18 or more of its coils are seen trailing into the uterine cavity, then the microinsert should be replaced or an alternative method of contraception used (Magos, 2004).

Essure microinserts can conduct electric energy. Therefore, it is recommended that direct visualization of the inserts or the cornua be obtained hysteroscopically or laparoscopically prior to any subsequent electrosurgical procedures near the inserts. In contrast to Essure, after the Adiana silicone matrix is deployed, nothing remains in the endometrial cavity. This may be of importance to women who later choose to undergo a procedure such as endometrial ablation or in vitro fertilization (Di Spiezio Sardo, 2010).

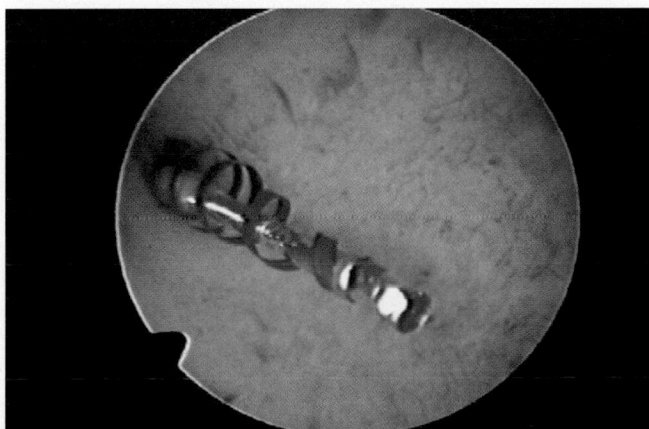

FIGURE 42-18.3 Hysteroscopic photograph of Essure microinsert coils within the tubal ostium. (© 2011 Conceptus, Inc. Reproduced with permission.)

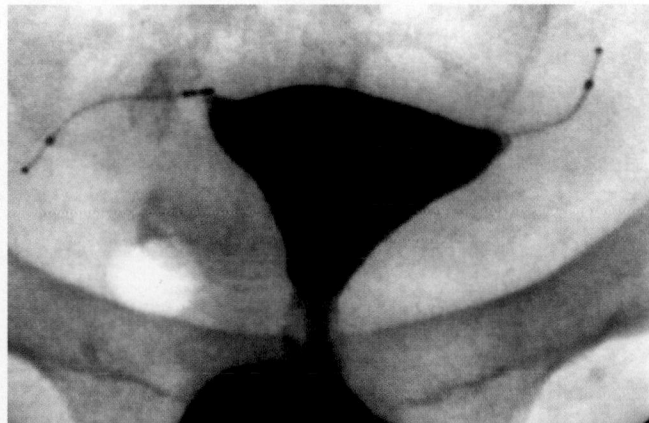

FIGURE 42-18.4 Hysterosalpingography displaying correct Essure microinsert placement. (© 2011 Conceptus, Inc. Reproduced with permission.)

42-19

Hysteroscopic Septoplasty

A uterine septum typically results from incomplete regression of the medial portion of the müllerian ducts during their fusion (Fig. 42-19.1) (Chap. 18, p. 500). These septa are associated with malpresentation and increased rates of first- and second-trimester spontaneous abortion. Recurrent pregnancy loss serves as the main indication for septoplasty.

Before the popularity of operative hysteroscopy, septoplasty was performed abdominally and with a hysterotomy incision. Fortunately, hysteroscopic septoplasty affords a minimally invasive procedure with decreased morbidity to the patient and uterus. *Septoplasty* refers to central division of the septum in a caudad-to-cephalad direction, generally with the use of hysteroscopic scissors. There is minimal bleeding due to the relative avascularity of the septum's fibroelastic tissue, which retracts upon incision. *Septum resection* is performed for broader, larger septa that have wider bases. The loop resectoscope or morcellator may be preferred for this approach.

PREOPERATIVE

Patient Evaluation

Diagnostic evaluation of a septate uterus follows guidelines outlined in Chapter 18 and commonly includes HSG, saline infusion sonography (SIS), and transvaginal sonography. Because of the frequent association between renal and müllerian anomalies, intravenous pyelography is also performed. Finally, although a septate uterus is associated with infertility and pregnancy loss, evaluation for other causes of these two conditions should be completed prior to septum excision. Contraindications to septoplasty include pregnancy and active pelvic infection, and these should be excluded.

Consent

Hysteroscopic septoplasty is a safe and effective treatment for recurrent pregnancy loss, and postoperative live birth rates approximate 85 percent (Fayez, 1987). In general, complications mirror those for operative hysteroscopy, although the risk of uterine perforation appears increased. For this reason, concurrent laparoscopy is recommended with septoplasty to help inform a surgeon as to the proximity of the uterine serosa. As the hysteroscope nears the fundal serosa, transillumination of the hysteroscopic light indicates the potential for uterine perforation. Accordingly, a patient should give consent for concurrent diagnostic laparoscopy as outlined in Section 42-1 (p. 1097).

Patient Preparation

Infectious and venous thromboembolic (VTE) complications following hysteroscopic surgery are rare. Accordingly, preoperative antibiotics or VTE prophylaxis is typically not required (American College of Obstetricians and Gynecologists, 2007c, 2009a). Laminaria tents or misoprostol may be used preoperatively to ease cervical dilatation (Section 42-13, p. 1157).

INTRAOPERATIVE

Instruments

Septum incision or resection may be completed using hysteroscopic scissors, resectoscope loop, neodymium: yttrium-aluminum-garnet (Nd-YAG) laser, or mechanical morcellators. Selection is according to surgeon preference and skill.

SURGICAL STEPS

❶ **Anesthesia and Patient Positioning.** Hysteroscopic septoplasty is typically a day-surgery procedure performed under general anesthesia. A woman is placed in dorsal lithotomy position. Because concurrent laparoscopy is recommended, the abdomen and vagina are surgically prepared. A Foley catheter is inserted.

❷ **Medium Selection.** The choice of distending medium is dictated by the incising tool used. Sharp incision with scissors, Nd:YAG laser, or bipolar instrument is commonly selected and can be performed in any liquid medium. Monopolar technology will require a hypotonic nonconductive medium (Section 42-13, p. 1159).

❸ **Concurrent Laparoscopy.** Because of the increased risk of uterine perforation, adjunctive laparoscopy is warranted. Placement of the laparoscope follows the steps described in Section 42-1 (p. 1110).

❹ **Cervical Dilatation.** A tenaculum is placed on the anterior cervical lip. Using Pratt or other suitable dilator, the surgeon

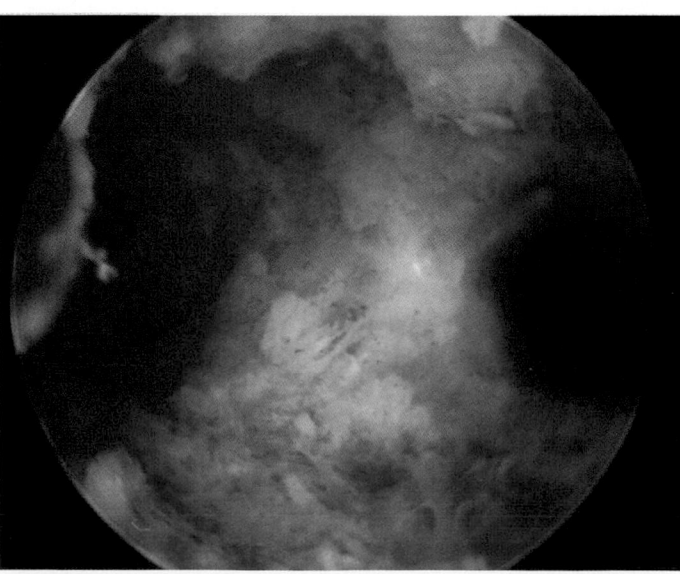

FIGURE 42-19.1 Hysteroscopic photograph of a uterine septum.

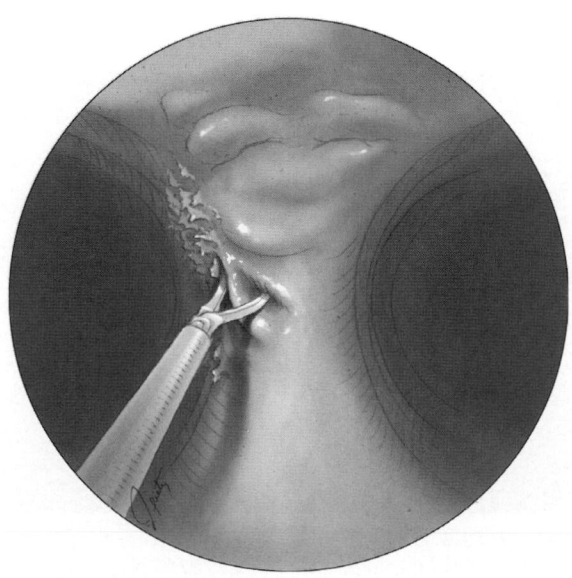

FIGURE 42-19.2 Septum incision.

dilates the cervix in the standard fashion as described in Section 41-16 (p. 1060).

❺ Instrument Insertion. The distending medium flow is begun, and the operative hysteroscope is inserted into the endocervical canal under direct visualization. Upon entering the endometrial cavity, a panoramic inspection is first performed to identify the septum.

❻ Septum Incision. When scissors are used, a surgeon should attempt to keep the line of incision in the anteroposterior midline. Transection begins caudally, at the septum apex, and continues cephalad toward the fundus. Bites with the scissors are taken bilaterally and are directed toward the horizontal midline (Fig. 42-19.2). During incision of the septum, drifting from the vertical midline is common. Incisions typically drift posteriorly in an anteverted uterus and anteriorly in a retroverted one. Thus, a surgeon may pause and reorient periodically.

During septoplasty, incision rather than complete resection of the septum is sufficient.

Septal stumps are retracted into the myometrium as the septum is transected. In most cases, the septum is relatively avascular, and cutting at its midpoint causes little bleeding. Signs that the transection is complete include increasing tissue vascularity, serosal transillumination of the hysteroscope at the uterine fundus, and reaching a level in line with the tubal ostia.

❼ Septum Resection. In some cases, the septum is broad, wide, and difficult to simply incise. Thus, to achieve the desired uterine cavity, a surgeon must completely excise or resect the septum. In general, scissors may be used, but in some instances, vaporizing electrodes, loop electrodes, or morcellators are more useful. Instruments are selected according to surgeon skill and preference.

❽ Procedure Completion. After incision, the hysteroscope and tenaculum are removed. The final fluid deficit should be calculated and noted in the operative report. Completion of laparoscopy follows the steps outlined in Section 42-1 (p. 1116).

POSTOPERATIVE

Recovery following septoplasty is rapid and typically without complication. Light bleeding or spotting may last 1 week or more. Patients may resume normal diet and activities as desired. Following resection, symptoms such as dysmenorrhea ultimately are greatly decreased.

To stimulate endometrial proliferation and prevent adhesion reformation, oral estrogen administration has proved effective. Although several regimens can be used, we prescribe 2 mg of estradiol orally for 30 days.

Attempts at conception should be delayed for 2 to 3 months following surgery. If septum resection appeared incomplete at the time of surgery or if recurrent miscarriage or amenorrhea develops, then postoperative HSG or a second hysteroscopy may be performed. Complete removal of the septum or adhesiolysis may be required (Section 42-21, p. 1178). With subsequent pregnancy, if the myometrium was not entered, cesarean delivery is required only for obstetric indications.

42-20

Hysteroscopic Proximal Fallopian Tube Cannulation

Proximal fallopian obstruction may results from pelvic inflammatory disease (PID), intratubal debris, congenital malformations, tubal spasm, endometriosis, tubal polyps, or salpingitis isthmica nodosa (SIN). It is generally diagnosed during evaluation of infertility when documentation of tubal patency is sought. Therefore, approaches to occlusion in this portion of the tube include tubal cannulation, surgical tubocornual anastomosis, and IVF (Kodaman, 2004). During cannulation, attempts are made to flush debris from within the tubes and perform chromotubation.

Proximal fallopian tube cannulation may be used to treat up to 85 percent of proximal tubal obstructions, but the occlusion may recur following the surgery. It may be performed as an outpatient radiologic procedure using fluoroscopy (Papaioannou, 2003). Alternatively, cannula placement may be completed with hysteroscopic guidance (Confino, 2003). If a hysteroscopic approach is selected, laparoscopy is typically used concurrently. This allows evaluation and treatment of both proximal and distal tubal disease as well as providing a view of tubal perforation by the cannulating guide wire if this occurs.

PREOPERATIVE

Patient Evaluation

Proximal tubal occlusion is typically identified with HSG during evaluation of female infertility. To avoid disruption of an early pregnancy, preoperative β-hCG testing is warranted prior to hysteroscopic tubal cannulation in most patients. Although this procedure may be performed at any time during the menstrual cycle, the early proliferative phase offers the advantage of a thinner endometrium to allow easy identification of tubal ostia and avoids disruption of an early luteal-phase pregnancy.

Consent

In addition to general complications associated with hysteroscopy and laparoscopy, patients undergoing proximal tubal cannulation should be informed of the small risk of tubal perforation. Fortunately, because the

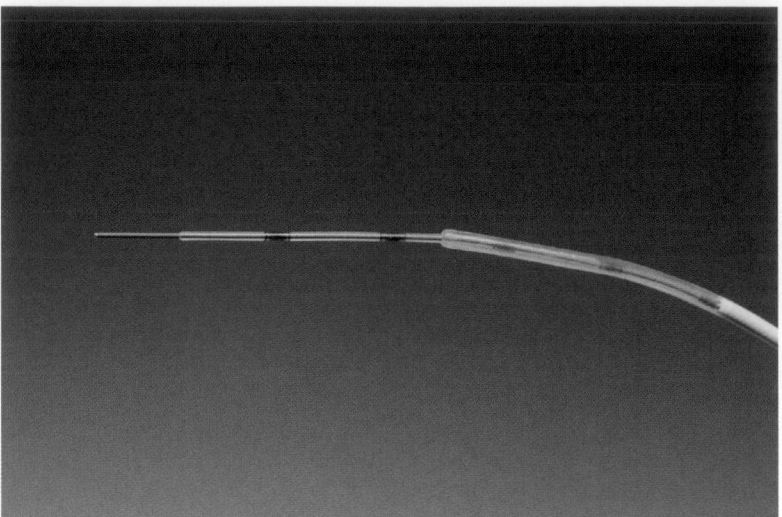

FIGURE 42-20.1 Photograph of hysteroscopic tubal cannulation catheter.

guide wire measures only 0.5 mm in diameter, tubal damage is rarely significant and can be assessed by concurrent laparoscopic examination of the perforated tube.

In most cases, patients with combined proximal and distal tubal disease are best managed with IVF. As discussed in Chapter 9 (p. 273), hydrosalpinges, when present, can lower IVF success rates and should be removed. Thus, consideration of and consent for salpingectomy should accompany plans for proximal tubal cannulation if concurrent laparoscopy is planned.

Patient Preparation

The risk of pelvic infection is low. However, because adhesions following such infection can have damaging effects on fallopian tube health, patients should receive either a first- or second-generation cephalosporin prior to surgery. In addition, laminaria tents or misoprostol may be used preoperatively to aid in hysteroscope insertion (Section 42-13, p. 1157).

INTRAOPERATIVE

Instruments

Fallopian tubes may be cannulated with a catheter system displayed in Figure 42-20.1. This system contains an outer cannula, inner cannula, and inner guide wire. The preset bend of the outer cannula aids placement of both the inner cannula and guide wire into the tubal ostium. Once the inner cannula has been threaded into the proximal fallopian tube, the guide wire is removed. The inner cannula, now emptied of the guide wire, can be use to flush debris from the fallopian tube and allow chromotubation, which is visualized laparoscopically (Fig. 19-10, p. 520).

SURGICAL STEPS

❶ Anesthesia and Patient Positioning.
Hysteroscopic tubal cannulation with con-

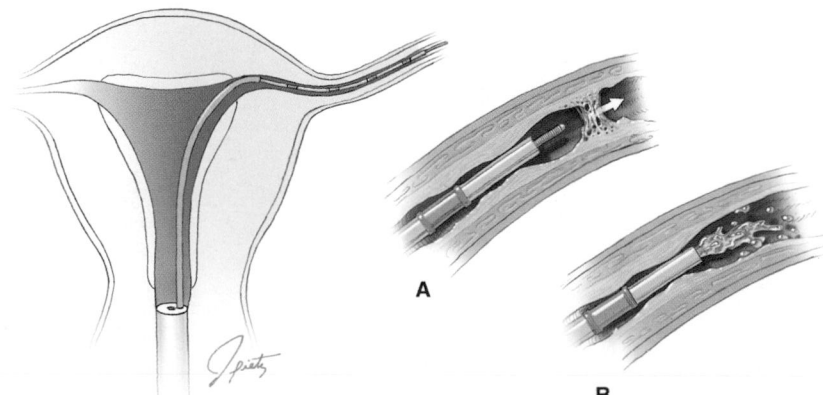

FIGURE 42-20.2 Tubal cannulation.

current laparoscopy is typically an outpatient procedure performed under general anesthesia. The patient is placed in dorsal lithotomy position, the abdomen and vagina are surgically prepared, and a Foley catheter is inserted.

❷ **Medium Selection.** No electrosurgery is required for tubal cannulation, thus saline is the preferred medium (Section 42-13, p. 1159).

❸ **Laparoscopy.** The laparoscope is inserted as described in Section 42-1 (p. 1110).

❹ **Cervical Dilatation.** Because a smaller diameter operative hysteroscope is required for tubal cannulation, cervical dilatation may not be required. If needed, it is performed as described in Section 41-16 (p. 1060).

❺ **Hysteroscope Insertion.** The flow of saline is begun, and a 0- or 30-degree hysteroscope is inserted. A panoramic inspection of the entire cavity is performed, and the tubal ostia are identified.

❻ **Tubal Cannulation.** The catheter system is threaded through an operating port of the hysteroscope. Under direct visual guidance, the outer catheter is advanced and placed at one of the tubal ostia. The inner catheter is then threaded approximately 2 cm into the proximal fallopian tube (Fig. 42-20.2). The guide wire is removed.

❼ **Tubal Flushing.** The inner catheter is flushed with water-soluble dye. Indigo carmine dye is preferable to methylene blue, as methylene blue rarely may induce acute methemoglobinemia, particularly in patients with glucose-6-phosphate dehydrogenase deficiency. One 5-mL vial of indigo carmine is mixed with 50 to 100 mL of sterile saline for injection. The laparoscope should be positioned to allow inspection of the distal tube to note the presence or absence of dye spill.

❽ **Concurrent Procedures.** If distal tubal adhesions are noted, laparoscopic lysis of adhesions may be concurrently performed.

❾ **Procedure Completion.** Following cannulation, the hysteroscope and cervical tenaculum are removed. Laparoscopy is completed as described in Section 42-1 (p. 1116).

POSTOPERATIVE

Recovery from hysteroscopic tubal cannulation and laparoscopy is typically quick and uncomplicated. Patients may resume diet, activity, and attempts at conception as desired.

42-21

Lysis of Intrauterine Adhesions

Intrauterine adhesions, also called *synechiae,* may develop following uterine curettage (Fig. 42-21.1). Less commonly, they may result from pelvic radiation, tuberculous endometritis, or endometrial ablation. The presence of these adhesions, also termed *Asherman syndrome,* may lead to hypo- or amenorrhea, pelvic pain, and infertility or pregnancy loss (Chap. 16, p. 444).

Treatment goals include surgical recreation of normal intrauterine anatomy and prevention of adhesion reformation. Surgery involves hysteroscopic transection rather than excision of adhesions. Thus, thin adhesions can usually be lysed using only gentle blunt force from the hysteroscopic sheath. However, dense adhesions usually require hysteroscopic division with scissors or laser.

Postsurgical pregnancy and live delivery rates are markers of surgical success, and these rates vary depending on the thickness of adhesions and degree of cavity obliteration. For this reason, various adhesion classification systems are useful to help predict the success of adhesiolysis for a given woman (Al-Inany, 2001).

PREOPERATIVE

Patient Evaluation

Although hysteroscopy and saline infusion sonography (SIS) can both accurately identify adhesions, HSG is preferred initially, because it allows concurrent assessment of tubal patency. However, after adhesions have been noted, diagnostic hysteroscopy is recommended to assess the thickness and density of these bands (Fayez, 1987). Additionally, completion of fertility assessment, including semen analysis and evaluation of ovulation, is recommended prior to surgery to help predict chances of conception following the procedure.

Consent

In general, hysteroscopic adhesiolysis is an effective tool to correct menstrual disorders and improve fertility in women with uterine adhesions (Valle, 2003). Although overall cumulative delivery rates in those with no other fertility factors range from 60 to 70 percent, lower rates generally are associated with more severe disease (Pabuccu, 1997; Zikopoulos, 2004). In addition, pregnancies following surgery may be complicated by placental implantation abnormalities or by preterm labor (Dmowski, 1969; Pabuccu, 2008).

The complications mirror those for operative hysteroscopy. However, the risk of uterine perforation may be increased. For this reason, patients smay also be consented for diagnostic laparoscopy.

Patient Preparation

Infectious and venous thromboembolic (VTE) complications following hysteroscopic surgery are rare. Accordingly, preoperative antibiotics or VTE prophylaxis is typically not required (American College of Obstetricians and Gynecologists, 2007c, 2009a). Additionally, laminaria tents, intracervical vasopressin, or misoprostol may be used preoperatively to ease cervical dilatation (Section 42-13, p. 1157).

INTRAOPERATIVE

SURGICAL STEPS

❶ Anesthesia and Patient Positioning. Hysteroscopic lysis of adhesions is typically a day-surgery procedure performed under general anesthesia. The patient is placed in dorsal lithotomy position, the vagina is surgically prepared, and a Foley catheter is inserted. If laparoscopy is concurrently planned, the abdomen is surgically prepared as well.

❷ Medium Selection. The choice of distending medium is dictated by the tool used. Sharp transection with scissors, neodymium: yttrium-aluminum-garnet (Nd:YAG) laser, or bipolar instrument can be performed in any liquid medium. However, thick adhesions often require resection rather than division, and they are severed close to the myometrium. Thus, the potential for creation of large denuded areas and fluid intravasation is great. Accordingly for many surgeons, 0.9-percent saline is preferred because hyponatremia is avoided if fluid overload does develop (Section 42-1, p. 1159).

❸ Concurrent Laparoscopy. Because of the increased risk of uterine perforation in those with more severe obliteration of the cavity, adjunctive laparoscopy may guide surgeons as to instrument proximity to the uterine serosa. The decision to use a laparoscope is individualized, and its placement follows the steps described in Section 42-1 (p. 1110).

❹ Cervical Dilatation. Using Pratt or other suitable dilators, the surgeon dilates the cervix in the standard fashion (Section 41-16, p. 1060).

❺ Instrument Insertion. The distending medium flow is begun, and the operative hysteroscope is inserted into the endocervical canal under direct visualization. Upon entering the endometrial cavity, a panoramic inspection is first performed to identify adhesions.

❻ Approach to Lysis. In general, a systematic approach to adhesiolysis begins with either blunt or sharp disruption of the most central adhesions and moves gradually to reach the most lateral. The size and qualities of adhesions may vary. Thin endometrial adhesions can usually be disrupted with gentle blunt force from the hysteroscopic sheath alone. More commonly, myofibrous and fibrous adhesions are denser and may require complete resection.

Adhesiolysis is continued until the endometrial cavity is restored to normal

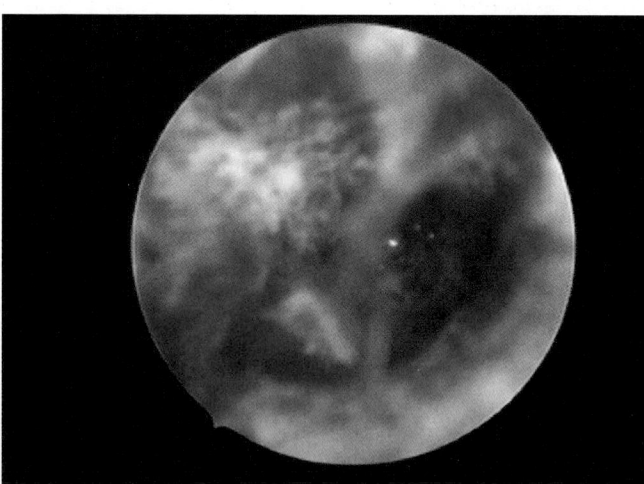

FIGURE 42-21.1 Hysteroscopic photograph of intrauterine adhesions. (*Photograph contributed by Dr. Kevin Doody.*)

and the tubal ostia are seen. Importantly, procedures may require termination before this, if significant fluid volume deficits are reached.

7 Chromotubation. At completion of adhesiolysis, transcervical chromotubation is performed to document tubal patency. Chromotubation may be performed by injecting dye into the uterine cavity through a uterine manipulator during simultaneous laparoscopy. Alternatively, tubal cannulation as described previously in Section 42-20 (p. 1176) may be performed to establish tubal patency.

8 Mechanical Uterine Distension. Mechanical endometrial cavity distension has been used to prevent treated areas from adhering following surgery. Either a copper IUD, placed for 3 months, or an 8F pediatric Foley catheter balloon, used for 10 days, may be chosen. In a comparison of the two, Orhue and colleagues (2003) noted fewer new adhesions and greater pregnancy rates in woman who had been treated with the balloon. If a Foley balloon is placed, antibiotic prophylaxis with either doxycycline 100 mg orally twice daily or other appropriate antibiotic is recommended.

POSTOPERATIVE

Recovery from hysteroscopic resection is rapid and typically without complication. Patients may resume normal activities and diet as tolerated.

To stimulate endometrial proliferation and prevent adhesion reformation, oral estrogen has proved effective. Although several regimens can be used, we prescribe 2 mg of estradiol orally for 30 days following adhesiolysis. Conjugated equine estrogen (Premarin) 1.25 may also be used. Following IUD insertion, 6 to 8 weeks of oral estrogen supplementation is given.

New adhesions can form following adhesiolysis. In their early stages, these bands are thinner and thus more amenable to successful resection. For this reason, another hysteroscopy or HSG is typically performed at 3 months following the initial resection. If significant new adhesions are found, a second surgical lysis of adhesions is planned. To allow adequate uterine healing, attempts at pregnancy by the patient should be delayed for 2 to 3 months.

REFERENCES

Abu-Rustum NR, Rhee EH, Chi DS, et al: Subcutaneous tumor implantation after laparoscopic procedures in women with malignant disease. Obstet Gynecol 103(3):480, 2004

Agarwala N, Liu CY: Safe entry techniques during laparoscopy: left upper quadrant entry using the ninth intercostal space—a review of 918 procedures. J Minim Invasive Gynecol 12(1):55, 2005

Agdi M, Al-Ghafri W, Antolin R, et al: Vaginal vault dehiscence after hysterectomy. J Minim Invasive Gynecol 16(3):313, 2009

Ahmad G, Duffy JM, Farquhar C, et al: Barrier agents for adhesion prevention after gynaecological surgery. Cochrane Database Syst Rev 2:CD000475, 2008a

Ahmad G, Duffy JM, Phillips K, et al: Laparoscopic entry techniques. Cochrane Database Syst Rev 2:CD006583, 2008b

Al-Inany H: Intrauterine adhesions: an update. Acta Obstet Gynaecol Scand 80:986, 2001

American College of Obstetricians and Gynecologists: Alternatives to hysterectomy in the management of leiomyomas. Practice Bulletin No. 96, August 2008

American College of Obstetricians and Gynecologists: Antibiotic prophylaxis for gynecologic procedures. Practice Bulletin No. 104, May 2009a

American College of Obstetricians and Gynecologists: Benefits and risks of sterilization. Practice Bulletin No. 46, September 2003

American College of Obstetricians and Gynecologists: Choosing the route of hysterectomy for benign disease. Practice Bulletin No. 96, November 2009b

American College of Obstetricians and Gynecologists: Endometrial ablation. Practice Bulletin No. 81, May 2007a

American College of Obstetricians and Gynecologists: Hysteroscopy. Technology Assessment No. 4, August 2005. Reaffirmed 2007b

American College of Obstetricians and Gynecologists: Prevention of deep vein thrombosis and pulmonary embolism. Practice Bulletin No. 84, August 2007c

American College of Obstetricians and Gynecologists: Sterilization of women, including those with mental disabilities. Committee Opinion No. 371, July 2007d

American Society for Reproductive Medicine, Society of Reproductive Surgeons: Pathogenesis, consequences, and control of peritoneal adhesions in gynecologic surgery. Fertil Steril 90(5 Suppl):S144, 2008

Audebert AJ, Gomel V: Role of microlaparoscopy in the diagnosis of peritoneal and visceral adhesions and in the prevention of bowel injury associated with blind trocar insertion. Fertil Steril 73(3):631, 2000

Baadsgaard SE, Bille S, Egeblad K: Major vascular injury during gynecologic laparoscopy: report of a case and review of published cases. Acta Obstet Gynaecol Scand 68:283, 1989

Baggish MS: Total and subtotal abdominal hysterectomy. Best Pract Res Clin Obstet Gynaecol 19:333, 2005

Barakat EE, Bedaiwy MA, Zimberg S, et al: Robotic-assisted, laparoscopic, and abdominal myomectomy: a comparison of surgical outcomes. Obstet Gynecol 117(2 Pt 1):256, 2011

Barnett JC, Hurd WW, Rogers RM Jr, et al: Laparoscopic positioning and nerve injuries. J Minim Invasive Gynecol 14(5):664, 2007

Basinski CM: A review of clinical data for currently approved hysteroscopic sterilization procedures. Rev Obstet Gynecol 3(3):101, 2010

Batra N, Khunda A, O'Donovan PJ: Hysteroscopic myomectomy. Obstet Gynecol Clin North Am 31:669, 2004

Ben-Arie A, Goldchmit R, Dgani R, et al: Trophoblastic peritoneal implants after laparoscopic treatment of ectopic pregnancy. Eur J Obstet Gynecol Reprod Biol 96(1):113, 2001

Bergqvist D, Bergqvist A: Vascular injuries during gynecologic surgery. Acta Obstet Gynaecol Scand 66:19, 1987

Berguer R, Forkey DL, Smith WD: The effect of laparoscopic instrument working angle on surgeons' upper extremity workload. Surg Endosc 15(9):1027, 2001

Bhoyrul S, Vierra MA, Nezhat CR, et al: Trocar injuries in laparoscopic surgery. J Am Coll Surg 192(6):677, 2001

Bieber E: Myomectomy by laparotomy. In Bieber E, Maclin V (eds): Myomectomy. Malden, MA, Blackwell Science, 1998, p 96

Bieber EJ: Distension media. In Bieber EJ, Loffer FD (eds): Hysteroscopy, Resectoscopy, and Endometrial Ablation. Boca Raton, FL, Parthenon, 2003, p 55

Bonjer HJ, Hazebroek EJ, Kazemier G, et al: Open versus closed establishment of pneumoperitoneum in laparoscopic surgery. Br J Surg 84:599, 1997

Boughey JC, Nottingham JM, Walls AC: Richter's hernia in the laparoscopic era: four case reports and review of the literature. Surg Laparosc Endosc Percutan Tech 13:55, 2003

Bradley LD, Falcone T: Hysteroscopy: Office Evaluation and Management of the Uterine Cavity, 1st ed. Philadelphia, Mosby Elsevier, 2009, p 4

Brandner P, Neis KJ, Ehmer C: The etiology, frequency, and prevention of gas embolism during CO_2 hysteroscopy. J Am Assoc Gynecol Laparosc 6:421, 1999

Brennan MC, Ogburn T, Hernandez CJ, et al: Effect of topical bupivacaine on postoperative pain after laparoscopic tubal sterilization with Filshie clips. Am J Obstet Gynecol 190:1411, 2004

Brill A, Nezhat F, Nezhat C, et al: The incidence of adhesions after prior laparotomy (a laparoscopic appraisal). Obstet Gynecol 85:269, 1995

Bubenik LJ, Hosgood G, Vasanjee SC: Bursting tension of medium and large canine arteries sealed with ultrasonic energy or suture ligation. Vet Surg (3):289, 2005

Buttram VC Jr, Vaquero C: Post-ovarian wedge resection adhesive disease. Fertil Steril 26:874, 1975

Byron JW, Markenson G, Miyazawa K: A randomized comparison of Veress needle and direct trocar insertion for laparoscopy. Surg Gynecol Obstet 177:259, 1993

Camanni M, Bonino L, Delpiano EM, et al: Hysteroscopic management of large symptomatic submucous uterine myomas. J Minim Invasive Gynecol 17(1):59, 2010a

Camanni M, Bonino L, Delpiano EM, et al: Laparoscopy and body mass index: feasibility and outcome in obese patients treated for gynecologic diseases. J Minim Invasive Gynecol 17(5):576, 2010b

Campbell ES, Xiao H, Smith MK: Types of hysterectomy: comparison of characteristics, hospital costs, utilization and outcomes. J Reprod Med 48:943, 2003

Caprini JA, Arcelus JI: Prevention of postoperative venous thromboembolism following laparo-

scopic cholecystectomy. Surg Endosc 8(7):741, 1994

Catarci M, Carlini M, Gentileschi P, et al: Major and minor injuries during the creation of pneumoperitoneum: a multicenter study on 12,919 cases. Surg Endosc 15:566, 2001

Chandler JG, Corson SL, Way LW: Three spectra of laparoscopic entry access injuries. J Am Coll Surg 192(4):478, 2001

Chapron C, Pierre F, Harchaoui Y, et al: Gastrointestinal injuries during gynaecological laparoscopy. Hum Reprod 14(2):333, 1999

Chatzipapas IK, Magos AL: A simple technique of securing inferior epigastric vessels and repairing the rectus sheath at laparoscopic surgery. Obstet Gynecol 90:304, 1997

Childers JM, Aqua KA, Surwit EA, et al: Abdominal-wall tumor implantation after laparoscopy for malignant conditions. Obstet Gynecol 84:765, 1994

Chopin N, Malaret JM, Lafay-Pillet MC, et al: Total laparoscopic hysterectomy for benign uterine pathologies: obesity does not increase the risk of complications. Hum Reprod (12):3057, 2009

Christianson MS, Barker MA, Lindheim SR: Overcoming the challenging cervix: techniques to access the uterine cavity. J Low Genit Tract Dis 12(1):24, 2008

Clayman RV: The safety and efficacy of direct trocar insertion with elevation of the rectus sheath instead of the skin for pneumoperitoneum. J Urol 174:1847, 2005

Confino E: Tubal catheterization and falloppioscopy. In Bieber EJ, Loffer FD (eds): Hysteroscopy, Resectoscopy, and Endometrial Ablation. Boca Raton, FL, Parthenon, 2003, p 113

Cooper JM, Brady RM: Intraoperative and early postoperative complications of operative hysteroscopy. Obstet Gynecol Clin North Am 27:347, 2000

Cooper JM, Carignan CS, Cher D, et al: Microinsert nonincisional hysteroscopic sterilization. Obstet Gynecol 102:59, 2003

Cooper KG, Bain C, Parkin DE: Comparison of microwave endometrial ablation and transcervical resection of the endometrium for treatment of heavy menstrual loss: a randomised trial. Lancet 354:1859, 1999

Copeland C, Wing R, Hulka JF: Direct trocar insertion at laparoscopy: an evaluation. Obstet Gynecol 62:655, 1983

Corson SL, Batzer FR, Gocial B, et al: Measurement of the force necessary for laparoscopic trocar entry. J Reprod Med 34:282, 1989

Corson SL, Hoffman JJ, Jackowski J, et al: Cardiopulmonary effects of direct venous CO_2 insufflation in ewes: a model for CO_2 hysteroscopy. J Reprod Med 33:440, 1988

Cravello L, D'Ercole C, Roger V, et al: Laparoscopic surgery in gynecology: randomized, prospective study comparing pneumoperitoneum and abdominal wall suspension. Eur J Obstet Gynaecol Reprod Biol 83:9, 1999

Dabirashrafi H: Complications of laparoscopic ovarian cauterization. Fertil Steril 52:878, 1989

Darwish AM, Nasr AM, El Nashar DA: Evaluation of postmyomectomy uterine scar. J Clin Ultrasound 33:181, 2005

DeCherney A, Polan ML: Hysteroscopic management of intrauterine lesions and intractable uterine bleeding. Obstet Gynecol 61:392, 1983

DeCherney AH, Diamond MP, Lavy G, et al: Endometrial ablation for intractable uterine bleeding: hysteroscopic resection. Obstet Gynecol 70:668, 1987

Della Badia C, Karini H: Endometrial stromal sarcoma diagnosed after uterine morcellation in laparoscopic supracervical hysterectomy. J Minim Invasive Gynecol 17(6):791, 2010

Della Badia C, Nyirjesy P, Atogho A: Endometrial ablation devices: review of a manufacturer and user facility device experience database. J Minim Invasive Gynecol 14:436, 2007

Demyttenaere S, Feldman LS, Fried GM: Effect of pneumoperitoneum on renal perfusion and function: a systematic review. Surg Endosc 21(2):152, 2007

Derman SG, Rehnstrom J, Neuwirth RS: The long-term effectiveness of hysteroscopic treatment of menorrhagia and leiomyomas. Obstet Gynecol 77:591, 1991

Dingfelder JR. Direct laparoscopic trocar insertion without prior pneumoperitoneum. J Reprod Med 21:45, 1978

Di Spiezio Sardo A, Bettocchi S, Spinelli M, et al: Review of new office-based hysteroscopic procedures 2003–2009. J Minim Invasive Gynecol 17(4):436, 2010

Dmowski WP, Greenblatt RB: Asherman's syndrome and risk of placenta accreta. Obstet Gynecol 34:288, 1969

Donesky BW, Adashi EY: Surgically induced ovulation in the polycystic ovary syndrome: wedge resection revisited in the age of laparoscopy. Fertil Steril 63:439, 1995

Doss BJ, Jacques SM, Qureshi F, et al: Extratubal secondary trophoblastic implants: clinicopathologic correlation and review of the literature. Hum Pathol 29:184, 1998

Dubuisson JB, Fauconnier A, Babaki-Fard K, et al: Laparoscopic myomectomy: a current view. Hum Reprod Update 6:588, 2000

Einarsson JI, Vellinga TT, Twijnstra AR, et al: Bidirectional barbed suture: an evaluation of safety and clinical outcomes. JSLS 14(3):381, 2010

Ellström M, Ferraz-Nunes J, Hahlin M, et al: A randomized trial with a cost-consequence analysis after laparoscopic and abdominal hysterectomy. Obstet Gynecol 91(1):30, 1998

Eltabbakh GH, Piver MS, Hempling RE, et al: Laparoscopic surgery in obese women. Obstet Gynecol 94(5 Pt 1):704, 1999

Eltabbakh GH, Shamonki MI, Moody JM, et al: Hysterectomy for obese women with endometrial cancer: laparoscopy or laparotomy? Gynecol Oncol 78(3 Pt 1):329, 2000

Emanuel MH, Wamsteker K: The Intra Uterine Morcellator: a new hysteroscopic operating technique to remove intrauterine polyps and myomas. J Minim Invas Gynecol 12:62, 2005

Epstein J, Arora A, Ellis H: Surface anatomy of the inferior epigastric artery in relation to laparoscopic injury. Clin Anat 17:400, 2004

Falcone T, Paraiso MF, Mascha E: Prospective, randomized clinical trial of laparoscopically assisted vaginal hysterectomy versus total abdominal hysterectomy. Am J Obstet Gynecol 180(4):955, 1999

Farley DR, Greenlee SM, Larson DR, et al: Double-blind, prospective, randomized study of warmed, humidified carbon dioxide insufflation vs standard carbon dioxide for patients undergoing laparoscopic cholecystectomy. Arch Surg 139(7):739, 2004

Farquhar C, Lilford RJ, Marjoribanks J, et al: Laparoscopic "drilling" by diathermy or laser for ovulation induction in anovulatory polycystic ovary syndrome. Cochrane Database Syst Rev 3:CD001122, 2007

Farquhar CM: The role of ovarian surgery in polycystic ovary syndrome. Best Pract Res Clin Obstet Gynaecol 18:789, 2004

Fauconnier A, Chapron C, Babaki-Fard, K, et al: Recurrence of leiomyomata after myomectomy. Hum Reprod Update 6:595, 2000

Fayez JA, Mutie G, Schneider PJ: The diagnostic value of hysterosalpingography and hysteroscopy in infertility investigation. Am J Obstet Gynecol 156:558, 1987

Fedele L, Bianchi S, Tozzi L, et al: Intramesosalpingeal injection of oxytocin in conservative laparoscopic treatment for tubal pregnancy: preliminary results. Hum Reprod 13:3042, 1998

Fletcher H, Frederick J, Hardie M, et al: A randomized comparison of vasopressin and tourniquet as hemostatic agents during myomectomy. Obstet Gynecol 87:1014, 1996

Food and Drug Administration: Adiana Permanent Contraception System—P070022 2009a. Available at: http://www.accessdata.fda.gov/scripts/cdrh/cfdocs/cfTopic/pma/pma.cfm?num=P070022. Accessed March 17, 2011

Food and Drug Administration: Essure™ System P020014. 2009b. Available at: http://www.fda.gov/medicaldevices/productsandmedicalprocedures/deviceapprovalsandclearances/recently-approveddevices/ucm083087.htm. Accessed March 17, 2011

Franchi M, Ghezzi F, Beretta P, et al: Microlaparoscopy: a new approach to the reassessment of ovarian cancer patients. Acta Obstet Gynaecol Scand 79:427, 2000

Franklin RR: Reduction of ovarian adhesions by the use of Interceed. Ovarian Adhesion Study Group. Obstet Gynecol 86(3):335, 1995

Frederick J, Fletcher H, Simeon D, et al: Intramyometrial vasopressin as a haemostatic agent during myomectomy. Br J Obstet Gynaecol 101:435, 1994

Fuller J, Scott W, Ashar B, et al: Laparoscopic trocar injuries: a report from a U.S. Food and Drug Administration (FDA) Center for Devices and Radiological Health (CDRH) Systematic Technology Assessment of Medical Products (STAMP) Committee. Finalized: November 7, 2003

Gariepy AM, Creinin MD, Schwarz EB, et al: Reliability of laparoscopic compared with hysteroscopic sterilization at 1 year: a decision analysis. Obstet Gynecol 118(2 Pt 1):273, 2011

Garry R, Reich H, Liu CY: Laparoscopic hysterectomy: definitions and indications. Gynaecol Endosc 3:1, 1994

Garry R, Shelley-Jones D, Mooney P, et al: Six hundred endometrial laser ablations. Obstet Gynecol 85:24, 1995

Geerts WH, Bergqvist D, Pineo GF, et al: Prevention of venous thromboembolism: American College of Chest Physicians Evidence-Based Clinical Practice Guidelines (8th ed). Chest 133(6 Suppl):381S, 2008

Giannios NM, Gulani V, Rohlck K, et al: Left upper quadrant laparoscopic placement: effects of insertion angle and body mass index on distance to posterior peritoneum by magnetic resonance imaging. Am J Obstet Gynecol 201(5):522.e1, 2009

Ginsburg ES, Benson CB, Garfield JM, et al: The effect of operative technique and uterine size on blood loss during myomectomy: a prospective, randomized study. Fertil Steril 60:956, 1993

Giuliani A, Panzitt T, Schoell W, et al: Severe bleeding from peritoneal implants of trophoblastic tissue after laparoscopic salpingostomy for ectopic pregnancy. Fertil Steril 70:369, 1998

Glasser MH: Practical tips for office hysteroscopy and second-generation "global" endometrial ablation. J Minim Invasive Gynecol 16(4):384, 2009

Glasser MH, Zimmerman JD: The HydroTherm-Ablator system for management of menorrhagia in women with submucous myomas: 12- to 20-month follow-up. J Am Assoc Gynecol Laparosc 10:521, 2003

Goldberg JM, Maurer WG: A randomized comparison of gasless laparoscopy and CO_2 pneumoperitoneum. Obstet Gynecol 90:416, 1997

Goldrath MH, Fuller TA, Segal S: Laser photovaporization of endometrium for the treatment of menorrhagia. Am J Obstet Gynecol 140:14, 1981

Gomel V, Taylor PJ: Indications and contraindications of diagnostic laparoscopy. In Diagnostic and Operative Gynecologic Laparoscopy, 1st ed. St. Louis, Mosby-Year Book, 1995, p 68

Gooden MD, Hulka JF, Christman GM: Spontaneous vaginal expulsion of Hulka clips. Obstet Gynecol 81:884, 1993

Greenberg JA, Einarsson JI: The use of bidirectional barbed suture in laparoscopic myomectomy and total laparoscopic hysterectomy. J Minim Invasive Gynecol 15(5):621, 2008

Greenblatt EM, Casper RF: Adhesion formation after laparoscopic ovarian cautery for polycystic ovarian syndrome: lack of correlation with pregnancy rate. Fertil Steril 60:766, 1993

Gunenc MZ, Yesildaglar N, Bingol B, et al: The safety and efficacy of direct trocar insertion with elevation of the rectus sheath instead of the skin for pneumoperitoneum. Surg Laparosc Endosc Percutan Tech 15:80, 2005

Gürgan T, Kisnisci H, Yarali H, et al: Evaluation of adhesion formation after laparoscopic treatment of polycystic ovarian disease. Fertil Steril 56(6):1176, 1991

Gürgan T, Urman B, Aksu T, et al: The effect of short-interval laparoscopic lysis of adhesions on pregnancy rates following Nd:YAG laser photo-coagulation of polycystic ovaries. Obstet Gynecol 80(1):45, 1992

Gurtcheff SE, Sharp HT: Complications associated with global endometrial ablation: the utility of the MAUDE database. Obstet Gynecol 102:1278, 2003

Harkki P, Kurki T, Sjoberg J, et al: Safety aspects of laparoscopic hysterectomy. Acta Obstet Gynaecol Scand 80:383, 2001

Harkki-Siren P, Kurki T: A nationwide analysis of laparoscopic complications. Obstet Gynecol 89:108, 1997a

Harkki-Siren P, Sjoberg J, Makinen J, et al: Finnish national register of laparoscopic hysterectomies: a review and complications of 1165 operations. Am J Obstet Gynecol 176:118, 1997b

Harkki-Siren P, Sjoberg J, Tiitinen A: Urinary tract injuries after hysterectomy. Obstet Gynecol 92:113, 1998

Hart R, Molnar BG, Magos A: Long-term follow-up of hysteroscopic myomectomy assessed by survival analysis. Br J Obstet Gynaecol 106:700, 1999

Hasson HM: A modified instrument and method for laparoscopy. Am J Obstet Gynecol 110:886, 1971

Hasson HM: Open laparoscopy: a report of 150 cases. J Reprod Med 12:234, 1974

Hasson HM, Rotman C, Rana N, et al: Open laparoscopy: 29-year experience. Obstet Gynecol 96:763, 2000

Heinberg EM, Crawford BL 3rd, Weitzen SH, et al: Total laparoscopic hysterectomy in obese versus nonobese patients. Obstet Gynecol 103(4):674, 2004

Ho HS, Saunders CJ, Gunther RA, et al: Effector of hemodynamics during laparoscopy: CO_2 absorption or intra-abdominal pressure? J Surg Res 59(4):497, 1995

Hobo R, Netsu S, Koyasu Y, et al: Bradycardia and cardiac arrest caused by intramyometrial injection of vasopressin during a laparoscopically assisted myomectomy. Obstet Gynecol 113(2 Pt 2):484, 2009

Horiuchi T, Tanishima H, Tamagawa K, et al: Randomized, controlled investigation of the anti-infective properties of the Alexis retractor/protector of incision sites. J Trauma 62(1)212, 2007

Howard FM, El-Minawi AM, DeLoach VE: Direct laparoscopic cannula insertion at the left upper quadrant. J Am Assoc Gynecol Laparosc 4(5):595, 1997

Howe RS: Third-trimester uterine rupture following hysteroscopic uterine perforation. Obstet Gynecol 81:827, 1993

Hsu S, Mitwally MF, Aly A, et al: Laparoscopic management of tubal ectopic pregnancy in obese women. Fertil Steril 81(1):198, 2004

Hulka JF, Peterson HB, Phillips JM, et al: Operative hysteroscopy: American Association of Gynecologic Laparoscopists 1991 membership survey. J Reprod Med 38:572, 1993

Hurd WW, Amesse LS, Gruber JS, et al: Visualization of the epigastric vessels and bladder before laparoscopic trocar placement. Fertil Steril 80:209, 2003

Hurd WW, Bude RO, DeLancey JO, et al: The relationship of the umbilicus to the aortic bifurcation: implications for laparoscopic technique. Obstet Gynecol 80(1):48, 1992

Hurd WW, Wang L, Schemmel MT: A comparison of the relative risk of vessel injury with conical versus pyramidal laparoscopic trocars in a rabbit model. Am J Obstet Gynecol 173:1731, 1995

Hurst BS, Matthews ML, Marshburn PB: Laparoscopic myomectomy for symptomatic uterine myomas. Fertil Steril 83:1, 2005

Hutchins FL Jr: A randomized comparison of vasopressin and tourniquet as hemostatic agents during myomectomy. Obstet Gynecol 88:639, 1996

Ido K, Suzuki T, Kimura K, et al: Lower-extremity venous stasis during laparoscopic cholecystectomy as assessed using color Doppler ultrasound. Surg Endosc 9(3):310, 1995

Iliodromiti S, Murage A: Multiple bowel perforations requiring extensive bowel resection and hysterectomy after microwave endometrial ablation. J Minim Invasive Gynecol 18(1):118, 2011

Iverson RE Jr, Chelmow D, Strohbehn K, et al: Relative morbidity of abdominal hysterectomy and myomectomy for management of uterine leiomyomas. Obstet Gynecol 88:415, 1996

Jansen FW, Kolkman W, Bakkum EA, et al: Complications of laparoscopy: an inquiry about closed- versus open-entry technique. Am J Obstet Gynecol 190(3):634, 2004

Jansen FW, Vredevoogd CB, van Ulzen K, et al: Complications of hysteroscopy: a prospective multicenter study. Obstet Gynecol 96:266, 2000

Jeung IC, Baek JM, Park EK, et al: A prospective comparison of vaginal stump suturing techniques during total laparoscopic hysterectomy. Arch Gynecol Obstet 282(6):631, 2010

Johnson N, Barlow D, Lethaby A, et al: Surgical approach to hysterectomy for benign gynaecological disease. Cochrane Database Syst Rev 3:CD003677, 2009

Kerin JF, Cooper JM, Price T, et al: Hysteroscopic sterilization using a micro-insert device: results of a multicentre phase II study. Hum Reprod 18:1223, 2003

Kesby GJ, Korda AR: Migration of a Filshie clip into the urinary bladder seven years after lapa-

roscopic sterilisation. Br J Obstet Gynaecol 104:379, 1997

Kho KA, Nezhat C: Parasitic myomas. Obstet Gynecol 114(3):611, 2009

Kill LM, Kapetanakis V, McCullough AE, et al: Progression of pelvic implants to complex atypical endometrial hyperplasia after uterine morcellation. Obstet Gynecol 117(2 Pt 2):447, 2011

Klauschie J, Wechter ME, Jacob K, et al: Use of anti-skid material and patient-positioning to prevent patient shifting during robotic-assisted gynecologic procedures. J Minim Invasive Gynecol 17(4):504, 2010

Kluivers KB, Hendriks JC, Mol BW, et al: Quality of life and surgical outcome after total laparoscopic hysterectomy versus total abdominal hysterectomy for benign disease: a randomized, controlled trial. J Minim Invasive Gynecol 14(2):145, 2007

Kocak I, Ustun C, Emre B, et al: Antibiotics prophylaxis in laparoscopy. Ceska Gynekol 70(4):269, 2005

Kodaman PH, Arici A, Seli E: Evidence-based diagnosis and management of tubal factor infertility. Curr Opin Obstet Gynecol 16:221, 2004

Kovacs GT, Baker G, Dillon M, et al: The microlaparoscope should be used routinely for diagnostic laparoscopy. Fertil Steril 70:698, 1998

Kuno K, Menzin A, Kauder HH, et al: Prophylactic ureteral catheterization in gynecologic surgery. Urology 52:1004, 1998

Lajer H, Widecrantz S, Heisterberg L: Hernias in trocar ports following abdominal laparoscopy: a review. Acta Obstet Gynaecol Scand 76:389, 1997

Lamberton GR, Hsi RS, Jin DH, et al: Prospective comparison of four laparoscopic vessel ligation devices. J Endourol 22(10):2307, 2008

LaMorte AI, Lalwani S, Diamond MP: Morbidity associated with abdominal myomectomy. Obstet Gynecol 82:897, 1993

Lamvu G, Zolnoun D, Boggess J, et al: Obesity: physiologic changes and challenges during laparoscopy. Am J Obstet Gynecol 191(2):669, 2004

Landman J, Kerbl K, Rehman J, et al: Evaluation of a vessel sealing system, bipolar electrosurgery, harmonic scalpel, titanium clips, endoscopic gastrointestinal anastomosis vascular staples and sutures for arterial and venous ligation in a porcine model. J Urol 169(2):697, 2003

Lasmar RB, Barrozo PR, Dias R, et al: Submucous myomas: a new presurgical classification to evaluate the viability of hysteroscopic surgical treatment—preliminary report. J Minim Invasive Gynecol 12(4):308, 2005

Lasmar RB, Xinmei Z, Indman PD, et al: Feasibility of a new system of classification of submucous myomas: a multicenter study. Fertil Steril 95(6):2073, 2011

Lee CK, Hansen SL: Management of acute wounds. Surg Clin North Am 89(3):659, 2009

Leibl BJ, Schmedt CG, Schwarz J, et al: Laparoscopic surgery complications associated with trocar tip design: review of literature and own results. J Laparoendosc Adv Surg Tech 9:135, 1999

Lethaby A, Hickey M: Endometrial destruction techniques for heavy menstrual bleeding: a Cochrane review. Hum Reprod 17:2795, 2002

Levy B, Levie MD, Childers ME: A summary of reported pregnancies after hysteroscopic sterilization. J Minim Invasive Gynecol 14(3):271, 2007

Li TC, Saravelos H, Richmond M, et al: Complications of laparoscopic pelvic surgery:

recognition, management and prevention. Hum Reprod Update 3:505, 1997

Liu CD, McFadden DW: Laparoscopic port sites do not require fascial closure when nonbladed trocars are used. Am Surg 66(9):853, 2000

Loffer FD: Improving results of hysteroscopic submucosal myomectomy for menorrhagia by concomitant endometrial ablation. J Minim Invasive Gynecol 12(3):254, 2005

Loffer FD, Bradley LD, Brill AI, et al: Hysteroscopic fluid monitoring guidelines: the Ad Hoc Committee on Hysteroscopic Training Guidelines of the American Association of Gynecologic Laparoscopists. J Am Assoc Gynecol Laparosc 7:167, 2000

Long JB, Giles DL, Cornella JL, et al: Open laparoscopic access technique: review of 2010 patients. JSLS 12(4):372, 2008

Lundorff P, Hahlin M, Källfelt B, et al: Adhesion formation after laparoscopic surgery in tubal pregnancy: a randomized trial versus laparotomy. Fertil Steril 55:911, 1991

Madeb R, Koniaris LG, Patel HR, et al: Complications of laparoscopic urologic surgery. J Laparoendosc Adv Surgical Tech [A] 14:287, 2004

Magos A, Chapman L: Hysteroscopic tubal sterilization. Obstet Gynecol Clin North Am 31:705, 2004

Magrina JF: Complications of laparoscopic surgery. Clin Obstet Gynecol 45:469, 2002

Mahdavi A, Berker B, Nezhat C, et al: Laparoscopic management of ovarian remnant. Obstet Gynecol Clin North Am 31:593, 2004

Mais V, Ajossa S, Guerriero S, et al: Laparoscopic versus abdominal myomectomy: a prospective, randomized trial to evaluate benefits in early outcome. Am J Obstet Gynecol 174(2):654, 1996

Malkawi HY, Qublan HS: Laparoscopic ovarian drilling in the treatment of polycystic ovary syndrome: how many punctures per ovary are needed to improve the reproductive outcome? J Obstet Gynaecol Res 31:115, 2005

Marana R, Busacca M, Zupi E, et al: Laparoscopically assisted vaginal hysterectomy versus total abdominal hysterectomy: a prospective, randomized, multicenter study. Am J Obstet Gynecol 180:270, 1999

Marana R, Luciano AA, Muzii L, et al: Reproductive outcome after ovarian surgery: suturing versus nonsuturing of the ovarian cortex. J Gynecol Surg 7:155, 1991

Mazdisnian F, Palmieri A, Hakakha B, et al: Office microlaparoscopy for female sterilization under local anesthesia: a cost and clinical analysis. J Reprod Med 47:97, 2002

McIntyre S: Specialists in microwave endometrial ablation. 2011. Available at: http://www.microsulis.com/index.php?c=Home. Accessed March 17, 2011

Merlin TL, Hiller JE, Maddern GJ, et al: Systematic review of the safety and effectiveness of methods used to establish pneumoperitoneum in laparoscopic surgery. Br J Surg 90:668, 2003

Milad MP, Sokol E: Laparoscopic morcellator-related injuries. J Am Assoc Gynecol Laparosc 10:383, 2003

Montz FJ, Holschneider CH, Munro MG: Incisional hernia following laparoscopy: a survey of the American Association of Gynecologic Laparoscopists. Obstet Gynecol 84:881, 1994

Morrison JE Jr, Jacobs VR: Replacement of expensive, disposable instruments with old-fashioned surgical techniques for improved cost-effectiveness in laparoscopic hysterectomy. J Soc Laparoendosc Surg 8:201, 2004

Mosesson MW: The roles of fibrinogen and fibrin in hemostasis and thrombosis. Semin Hematol 29(3):177, 1992

Munro MG: Laparoscopic access: complications, technologies, and techniques. Curr Opin Obstet Gynecol 14:365, 2002

Murtha AP, Kaplan AL, Paglia MJ: Evaluation of a novel technique for wound closure using a barbed suture. Plast Reconstr Surg 117(6):1769, 2006

Muzii L, Bianchi A, Croce C, et al: Laparoscopic excision of ovarian cysts: is the stripping technique a tissue-sparing procedure? Fertil Steril 77:609, 2002

Naether OG, Fischer R, Weise HC, et al: Laparoscopic electrocoagulation of the ovarian surface in infertile patients with polycystic ovarian disease. Fertil Steril 60:88, 1993

Negrin Perez MC, De La Torre FP, Ramirez A: Ureteral complications after gasless laparoscopic hysterectomy. Surg Laparosc Endosc Percutan Technol 9:300, 1999

Newcomb WL, Hope WW, Schmeltzer TM, et al: Comparison of blood vessel sealing among new electrosurgical and ultrasonic devices. Surg Endosc 23(1):90, 2009

Nezhat C, Datta MS, Defazio A, et al: Natural orifice-assisted laparoscopic appendectomy. JSLS 13(1):14, 2009

Nezhat C, Kho K: Iatrogenic myomas: new class of myomas? J Minim Invasive Gynecol 17(5):544, 2010

Nezhat F, Brill AI, Nezhat CH, et al: Laparoscopic appraisal of the anatomic relationship of the umbilicus to the aortic bifurcation. J Am Assoc Gynecol Laparosc 5:135, 1998

Ng A, Habib A, Swami A, et al: Randomized, controlled trial investigating the effect of transcervical papaverine and bupivacaine on postoperative analgesia following laparoscopic sterilization. Eur J Anaesth 19:803, 2002

Ngai SW, Chan YM, Ho PC: The use of misoprostol prior to hysteroscopy in postmenopausal women. Hum Reprod 16:1486, 2001

Ngai SW, Chan YM, Liu KL, et al: Oral misoprostol for cervical priming in non-pregnant women. Hum Reprod 12(11):2373, 1997

Nieboer TE, Johnson N, Lethaby A, et al: Surgical approach to hysterectomy for benign gynaecological disease. Cochrane Database Syst Rev 3:CD003677, 2009

Nordestgaard AG, Bodily KC, Osborne RW Jr, et al: Major vascular injuries during laparoscopic procedures. Am J Surg 169:543, 1995

Oehler MK, Rees MC: Menorrhagia: an update. Acta Obstet Gynaecol Scand 82:405, 2003

O'Hanlan KA, Lopez L, Dibble SL, et al: Total laparoscopic hysterectomy: body mass index and outcomes. Obstet Gynecol 102(6):1384, 2003

Okaro EO, Jones KD, Sutton C: Long term outcome following laparoscopic supracervical hysterectomy. Br J Obstet Gynaecol 108:1017, 2001

Oppegaard KS, Nesheim BI, Istre O, et al: Comparison of self-administered vaginal misoprostol versus placebo for cervical ripening prior to operative hysteroscopy using a sequential trial design. BJOG 115(5):663, 2008

Orhue AA, Aziken ME, Igbefoh JO: A comparison of two adjunctive treatments for intrauterine adhesions following lysis. Int J Gynaecol Obstet 82:49, 2003

O'Rourke N, Kodali BS: Laparoscopic surgery during pregnancy. Curr Opin Anaesthesiol 19(3):254, 2006

Ott DE, Reich H, Love B, et al: Reduction of laparoscopic-induced hypothermia, postopera-tive pain and recovery room length of stay by pre-conditioning gas with the Insuflow device: a prospective randomized controlled multi-center study. JSLS 2(4):321, 1998

Ou CS, Harper A, Liu YH, et al: Laparoscopic myomectomy technique. Use of colpotomy and the harmonic scalpel. J Reprod Med 47(10):849, 2002

Overton C, Hargreaves J, Maresh M: A national survey of the complications of endometrial destruction for menstrual disorders: the MISTLETOE study (Minimally Invasive Surgical Techniques—Laser, Endothermal or Endoresection). Br J Obstet Gynaecol 104:1351, 1997

Pabuccu R, Atay V, Orhon E, et al: Hysteroscopic treatment of intrauterine adhesions is safe and effective in the restoration of normal menstruation and fertility. Fertil Steril 68:1141, 1997

Pabuccu R, Onalan G, Kaya C, et al: Efficiency and pregnancy outcome of serial intrauterine device-guided hysteroscopic adhesiolysis of intrauterine synechiae. Fertil Steril 90(5):1973, 2008

Palanivelu C, Rajan PS, Rangarajan M, et al: Transvaginal endoscopic appendectomy in humans: a unique approach to NOTES—world's first report. Surg Endosc 22(5):1343, 2008

Palmer R: Safety in laparoscopy. J Reprod Med 13(1):1, 1974

Palter SF: Microlaparoscopy under local anesthesia and conscious pain mapping for the diagnosis and management of pelvic pain. Curr Opin Obstet Gynecol 11:387, 1999

Papaioannou S, Afnan M, Girling AJ, et al: Diagnostic and therapeutic value of selective salpingography and tubal catheterization in an unselected infertile population. Fertil Steril 79:613, 2003

Parker WH: Total laparoscopic hysterectomy and laparoscopic supracervical hysterectomy. Obstet Gynecol Clin North Am 31:523, 2004

Parker WH, Einarsson J, Istre O, et al: Risk factors for uterine rupture after laparoscopic myomectomy. J Minim Invasive Gynecol 17(5):551, 2010

Pati S, Cullins V: Female sterilization: evidence. Obstet Gynecol Clin North Am 27:859, 2000

Penfield AJ: The Filshie clip for female sterilization: a review of world experience. Am J Obstet Gynecol 182:485, 2000

Peng Y, Zheng M, Ye Q, et al: Heated and humidified CO_2 prevents hypothermia, peritoneal injury, and intra-abdominal adhesions during prolonged laparoscopic insufflations. J Surg Res 151(1):40, 2009

Periti P, Mazzei T, Orlandini F, et al: Comparison of the antimicrobial prophylactic efficacy of cefotaxime and cephazolin in obstetric and gynaecological surgery: a randomised multi-centre study. Drugs 35:133, 1988

Peterson HB, Xia Z, Hughes JM, et al: The risk of pregnancy after tubal sterilization: findings from the U.S. Collaborative Review of Sterilization. Am J Obstet Gynecol 174:1161, 1996

Peterson HB, Xia Z, Wilcox LS, et al: Pregnancy after tubal sterilization with bipolar electrocoagulation. U.S. Collaborative Review of Sterilization Working Group. Obstet Gynecol 94:163, 1999

Phillips DR, Nathanson HG, Milim SJ, et al: The effect of dilute vasopressin solution on the force needed for cervical dilatation: a randomized controlled trial. Obstet Gynecol 89(4):507, 1997

Prapas Y, Kalogiannidis I, Prapas N: Laparoscopy vs laparoscopically assisted myomectomy in the management of uterine myomas: a prospective study. Am J Obstet Gynecol 200(2):144.e1, 2009

Preutthipan S, Herabutya Y: Vaginal misoprostol for cervical priming before operative hysteroscopy: a randomized, controlled trial. Obstet Gynecol 96:890, 2000

Propst AM, Liberman RF, Harlow BL, et al: Complications of hysteroscopic surgery: predicting patients at risk. Obstet Gynecol 96:517, 2000

Rahn DD, Phelan JN, Roshanravan SM, et al: Anterior abdominal wall nerve and vessel anatomy: clinical implications for gynecologic surgery. Am J Obstet Gynecol 202(3):234.e1, 2010

Ramirez PT, Frumovitz M, Wolf JK, et al: Laparoscopic port-site metastases in patients with gynecological malignancies. Int J Gynecol Ca 14:1070, 2004

Ramos AC, Murakami A, Galvao Neto M, et al: NOTES transvaginal video-assisted cholecystectomy: first series. Endoscopy 40(7):572, 2008

Reid K, Pockney P, Draganic B, et al: Barrier wound protection decreases surgical site infection in open elective colorectal surgery: a randomized clinical trial. Dis Colon Rectum 53(10):1374, 2010

Reynolds JD, Booth JV, de la Fuente S, et al: A review of laparoscopy for non-obstetric-related surgery during pregnancy. Curr Surg 60(2):164, 2003

Romanowski L, Reich H, McGlynn F, et al: Brachial plexus neuropathies after advanced laparoscopic surgery. Fertil Steril 60:729, 1993

Rybak EA, Polotsky AJ, Woreta T, et al: Explained compared with unexplained fever in postoperative myomectomy and hysterectomy patients. Obstet Gynecol 111(5):1137, 2008

Sabbah R, Desaulniers G: Use of the NovaSure Impedance Controlled Endometrial Ablation System in patients with intracavitary disease: 12-month follow-up results of a prospective, single-arm clinical study. J Minim Invasive Gynecol 13:467, 2006

Sambrook AM, Jack SA, Cooper KG: Outpatient microwave endometrial ablation: 5-year follow-up of a randomised controlled trial without endometrial preparation versus standard day surgery with endometrial preparation. BJOG 117(4):493, 2010

Sammour T, Kahokehr A, Hill AG: Meta-analysis of the effect of warm humidified insufflation on pain after laparoscopy. Br J Surg 95(8):950, 2008

Sarmini OR, Lefholz K, Froeschke HP: A comparison of laparoscopic supracervical hysterectomy and total abdominal hysterectomy outcomes. J Minim Invasive Gynecol 12(2):121, 2005

Sawin SW, Pilevsky ND, Berlin JA, et al: Comparability of perioperative morbidity between abdominal myomectomy and hysterectomy for women with uterine leiomyomas. Am J Obstet Gynecol 183:1448, 2000

Schindlbeck C, Klauser K, Dian D, et al: Comparison of total laparoscopic, vaginal and abdominal hysterectomy. Arch Gynecol Obstet 277(4):331, 2008

Schmidt T, Eren Y, Breidenbach M: Modifications of laparoscopic supracervical hysterectomy technique significantly reduce postoperative spotting. J Minim Invasive Gynecol 18, 81, 2011

Schytte T, Soerensen JA, Hauge B, et al: Preoperative transcervical analgesia for laparoscopic sterilization with Filshie clips: a double blind, randomized trial. Acta Obstet Gynaecol Scand 82:57, 2003

Scribner DR Jr, Walker JL, Johnson GA, et al: Laparoscopic pelvic and paraaortic lymph node dissection in the obese. Gynecol Oncol 84(3):426, 2002

Seifer DB: Persistent ectopic pregnancy: an argument for heightened vigilance and patient compliance. Fertil Steril 68:402, 1997

Sepilian V, Della Badia C: Iatrogenic endometriosis caused by uterine morcellation during a supracervical hysterectomy. Obstet Gynecol 102(5 Pt 2):1125, 2003

Sepilian V, Ku L, Wong H, et al: Prevalence of infraumbilical adhesions in women with previous laparoscopy. JSLS 11(1):41, 2007

Shamiyeh A, Glaser K, Kratochwill H, et al: Lifting of the umbilicus for the installation of pneumoperitoneum with the Veress needle increases the distance to the retroperitoneal and intraperitoneal structures. Surg Endosc 23(2):313, 2009

Sharma KC, Brandstetter RD, Brensilver JM, et al: Cardiopulmonary physiology and pathophysiology as a consequence of laparoscopic surgery. Chest 110(3):810, 1996

Sharp HT, Dodson MK, Draper ML, et al: Complications associated with optical-access laparoscopic trocars. Obstet Gynecol 99:553, 2002

Siegle JC, Bishop LJ, Rayburn WF: Randomized comparison between two microlaparoscopic techniques for partial salpingectomy. JSLS 9(1):30, 2005

Sinha R, Sundaram M, Mahajan C, et al: Multiple leiomyomas after laparoscopic hysterectomy: report of two cases. J Minim Invasive Gynecol 14(1):123, 2007

Sizzi O, Rossetti A, Malzoni M, et al: Italian multicenter study on complications of laparoscopic myomectomy. J Minim Invasive Gynecol (4):453, 2007

Smaldone MC, Gibbons EP, Jackman SV: Laparoscopic nephrectomy using the EnSeal Tissue Sealing and Hemostasis System: successful therapeutic application of nanotechnology. JSLS 12(2):213, 2008

Society of American Gastrointestinal and Endoscopic Surgeons, Yumi H: Guidelines for diagnosis, treatment, and use of laparoscopy for surgical problems during pregnancy. Surg Endosc 22(4):849, 2008

Soderstrom RM, Levy BS, Engel T: Reducing bipolar sterilization failures. Obstet Gynecol 74:60, 1989

Soysal ME, Soysal SK, Vicdan K: Thermal balloon ablation in myoma-induced menorrhagia under local anesthesia. Gynecol Obstet Invest 51:128, 2001

Spandorfer SD, Sawin SW, Benjamin I, et al: Postoperative day 1 serum human chorionic gonadotropin level as a predictor of persistent ectopic pregnancy after conservative surgical management. Fertil Steril 68:430, 1997

Strowitzki T, von Wolff M: Laparoscopic ovarian drilling (LOD) in patients with polycystic ovary syndrome (PCOS): an alternative approach to medical treatment? Gynecol Surg 2:71, 2005

Sutton C: Hysteroscopic surgery. Best Pract Res Clin Obstet Gynaecol 20:105, 2006

Takeda A, Mori M, Sakai K, et al: Parasitic peritoneal leiomyomatosis diagnosed 6 years after laparoscopic myomectomy with electric tissue morcellation: report of a case and review of the literature. J Minim Invasive Gynecol 14(6):770, 2007

Tan BL, Chong HC, Tay EH: Migrating Filshie clip. Aust N Z J Obstet Gynaecol 44:583, 2004

Thomas D, Ikeda M, Deepika K, et al: Laparoscopic management of benign adnexal mass in obese women. J Minim Invasive Gynecol 13:311, 2006

Tiras MB, Gokce O, Noyan V, et al: Comparison of microlaparoscopy and conventional laparoscopy for tubal sterilization under local anesthesia with mild sedation. J Am Assoc Gynecol Laparosc 8:385, 2001

Toaff R, Toaff ME, Peyser MR: Infertility following wedge resection of the ovaries. Am J Obstet Gynecol 124:92, 1976

Tulandi T, Beique F, Kimia M: Pulmonary edema: a complication of local injection of vasopressin at laparoscopy. Fertil Steril 66:478, 1996

Tulandi T, Guralnick M: Treatment of tubal ectopic pregnancy by salpingotomy with or without tubal suturing and salpingectomy. Fertil Steril 55:53, 1991

Tulandi T, Murray C, Guralnick M: Adhesion formation and reproductive outcome after myomectomy and second-look laparoscopy. Obstet Gynecol 82:213, 1993

Tulandi T, Saleh A: Surgical management of ectopic pregnancy. Clin Obstet Gynecol Ectop Pregn 42:31, 1999

Tulikangas PK, Nicklas A, Falcone T, et al: Anatomy of the left upper quadrant for cannula insertion. J Am Assoc Gynecol Laparosc 7(2):211, 2000

Ubeda A, Labastida R, Dexeus S: Essure: A new device for hysteroscopic tubal sterilization in an outpatient setting. Fertil Steril 82:196, 2004

Unfried G, Wieser F, Albrecht A, et al: Flexible versus rigid endoscopes for outpatient hysteroscopy: a prospective randomized clinical trial. Hum Reprod 16:168, 2001

Uppal S, Frumovitz M, Escobar P, et al: Laparoendoscopic single-site surgery in gynecology: review of literature and available technology. J Minim Invasive Gynecol 18(1):12, 2011

Valle RF: Intrauterine adhesion. In Bieber EJ, Loffer FD (eds): Hysteroscopy, Resectoscopy, and Endometrial Ablation. Boca Raton, FL, Parthenon, 2003, p 93

Vancaillie TG: Electrocoagulation of the endometrium with the ball-end resectoscope. Obstet Gynecol 74:425, 1989

Vancaillie, TG, Anderson, TL, Johns, DA: A 12-month prospective evaluation of transcervical sterilization using implantable polymer matrices. Obstet Gynecol 112:1270, 2008

van der Stege JG, van Beek JJ: Problems related to the cervical stump at follow-up in laparoscopic supracervical hysterectomy. JSLS 3(1):5, 1999

van Det MJ, Meijerink WJ, Hoff C, et al: Optimal ergonomics for laparoscopic surgery in minimally invasive surgery suites: a review and guidelines. Surg Endosc 23(6):1279, 2009

Varma R, Soneja H, Samuel N, et al: Outpatient Thermachoice endometrial balloon ablation: long-term, prognostic and quality-of-life measures. Gynecol Obstet Invest 70(3):145, 2010

Vellinga TT, De Alwis S, Suzuki Y, et al: Laparoscopic entry: the modified Alwis method and more. Rev Obstet Gynecol 2(3):193, 2009

Vercellini P, Zaina B, Yaylayan L, et al: Hysteroscopic myomectomy: long-term effects on menstrual pattern and fertility. Obstet Gynecol 94:341, 1999

Vilos GA: Hysteroscopic and nonhysteroscopic endometrial ablation. Obstet Gynecol Clin North Am 31:687, 2004

Vilos GA, Ternamian A, Dempster J, et al: Laparoscopic entry: a review of techniques, technologies, and complications. J Obstet Gynaecol Can 29(5):433, 2007

Visco AG, Advincula AP: Robotic gynecologic surgery. Obstet Gynecol 112(6):1369, 2008

Walsh CA, Sherwin JR, Slack M: Vaginal evisceration following total laparoscopic hysterectomy: case report and review of the literature. Aust N Z J Obstet Gynaecol 47(6):516, 2007

Walsh CA, Walsh SR, Tang TY, et al: Total abdominal hysterectomy versus total laparoscopic hysterectomy for benign disease: a meta-analysis. Eur J Obstet Gynecol Reprod Biol 144(1):3, 2009

Wamsteker K, Emanuel MH, de Kruif JH: Transcervical hysteroscopic resection of submucous fibroids for abnormal uterine bleeding: results regarding the degree of intramural extension. Obstet Gynecol 82:736, 1993

Wen KC, Chen YJ, Sung PL, et al: Comparing uterine fibroids treated by myomectomy through traditional laparotomy and 2 modified approaches: ultraminilaparotomy and laparoscopically assisted ultraminilaparotomy. Am J Obstet Gynecol 202(2):144.e1, 2010

Wenger JM, Spinosa JP, Roche B, et al: An efficient and safe procedure for laparoscopic supracervical hysterectomy. J Gynecol Surg 21(4):155, 2006

Westhoff C, Davis A: Tubal sterilization: focus on the U.S. experience. Fertil Steril 73:913, 2000

Wiseman DM, Trout JR, Franklin RR, et al: Metaanalysis of the safety and efficacy of an adhesion barrier (Interceed TC7) in laparotomy. J Reprod Med 44(4):325, 1999

Wiskind AK, Toledo AA, Dudley AG, et al: Adhesion formation after ovarian wound repair in New Zealand White rabbits: a comparison of ovarian microsurgical closure with ovarian nonclosure. Am J Obstet Gynecol 163:1674, 1990

Wrigley LC, Howard FM, Gabel D: Transcervical or intraperitoneal analgesia for laparoscopic tubal sterilization: a randomized, controlled trial. Obstet Gynecol 96:895, 2000

Wu MP, Ou CS, Chen SL, et al: Complications and recommended practices for electrosurgery in laparoscopy. Am J Surg 179:67, 2000

Yu E: Important Essure® permanent birth control system labeling change FDA approval of the removal of the nickel contraindication for Essure. 7-22-11. email communication, August 5, 2011

Zikopoulos KA, Kolibianakis EM, Platteau P, et al: Live delivery rates in subfertile women with Asherman's syndrome after hysteroscopic adhesiolysis using the resectoscope or the VersaPoint system. Reprod Biomed Online 8:720, 2004

Zivanovic O, Sonoda Y, Diaz JP, et al: The rate of port-site metastases after 2251 laparoscopic procedures in women with underlying malignant disease. Gynecol Oncol 111(3):431, 2008

Zornig C, Mofid H, Emmermann A, et al: Scarless cholecystectomy with combined transvaginal and transumbilical approach in a series of 20 patients. Surg Endosc 22(6):1427, 2008

Zurawin RK, Zurawin JL: Adverse events due to suspected nickel hypersensitivity in patients with essure micro-inserts. J Minim Invasive Gynecol 18(4):475, 2011

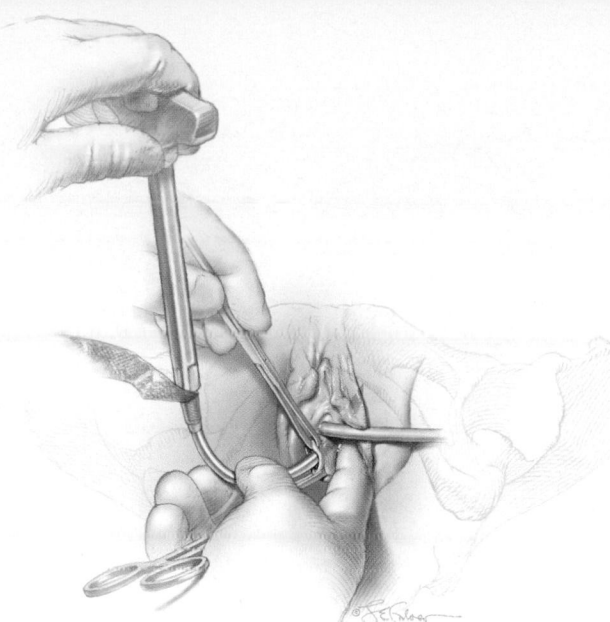

CHAPTER 43

Surgeries for Pelvic Floor Disorders

43-1

Diagnostic and Operative Cystoscopy and Urethroscopy

During gynecologic surgery, the lower urinary tract may be injured. Therefore, diagnostic cystoscopic evaluation is typically warranted following procedures in which the bladder and ureters have been placed at risk. Additionally, operative cystoscopy allows the passage of ureteral stents, lesion biopsy, and foreign-body removal. Of these, ureteral stenting may be indicated to assess ureteral patency following gynecologic surgery or to delineate the ureter's course in cases with abnormal pelvic anatomy.

Rigid and flexible cystoscopes are available, although in gynecology, a rigid scope is typically used. A cystoscope is composed of an outer sheath, a bridge, and an endoscope. The sheath contains one port for fluid infusion and a second port for fluid egress. For office cystoscopy, a sheath measuring 17 French affords greater comfort, whereas for operative cases, a 21 French or wider diameter cystoscope is preferred to allow rapid infusion of fluids. The sheath's end is sharp, and in cases in which the urethral meatus is narrow, an obturator can be placed inside the sheath to permit smooth introduction of the sheath and is then removed to insert the endoscope. The bridge attaches to the proximal portion of the sheath and allows coupling between the endoscope and sheath.

Several viewing angles are available and include 0-, 30-, and 70-degree optical views (Fig. 43-1.1). 0-degree endoscopes are used for urethroscopy. For cystoscopy, a 70-degree endoscope is superior in providing the most comprehensive view of the lateral, anterior, and posterior walls; trigone; and ureteral orifices. To achieve a comparable view, a 30-degree endoscope requires additional manipulation. However, a 30-degree endoscope does offer advantages and allows surgeons greater flexibility as it can be used for either urethroscopy or cystoscopy during a given case. For operative cystoscopic cases in which instruments are passed down the sheath, a 30-degree endoscope must be used because with 0- and 70-degree endoscopes, operative instruments lie outside the field of view.

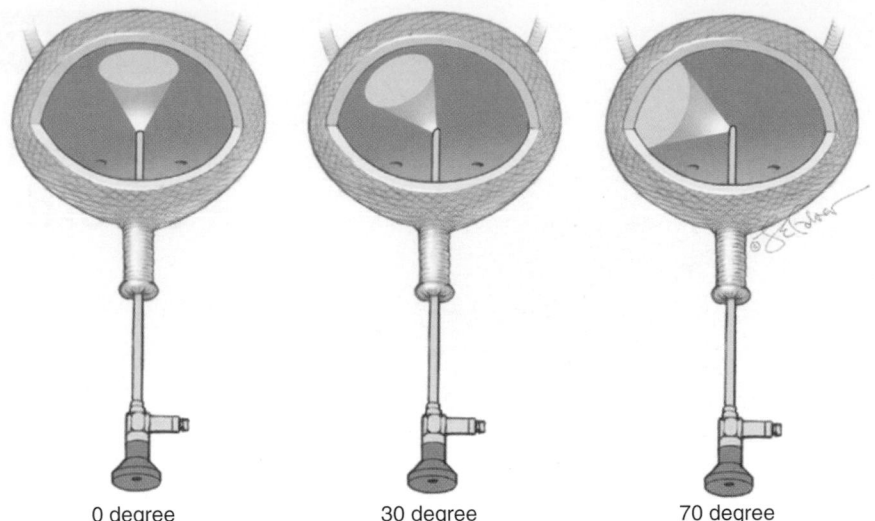

0 degree　　　30 degree　　　70 degree

FIGURE 43-1.1 Cystoscopic optical views.

PREOPERATIVE

Patient Evaluation

A significant incidence of bacteriuria follows cystoscopy. Thus, prior to office cystoscopy, urinary tract infection should be excluded.

Consent

If performed properly, complications of diagnostic cystoscopy are rare. Of these, infection is the most common.

Patient Preparation

Although evidence-based data are lacking for its use, oral antibiotic prophylaxis is commonly given postoperatively to cover common urinary tract pathogens.

INTRAOPERATIVE

SURGICAL STEPS

❶ Anesthesia and Patient Positioning. Cystoscopy may be performed in any lithotomy position with the legs positioned in stirrups. For office cystoscopy, 2-percent lidocaine jelly is instilled into the urethra 5 to 10 minutes prior to cystoscope insertion. For operative procedures, an additional 50 mL of 4-percent lidocaine solution is instilled into the bladder. The perineum and urethral meatus are surgically prepared.

❷ Distension Media. The bladder must be adequately distended to fully visualize all surfaces, and for diagnostic purposes, saline or sterile water may be used. To ensure adequate media flow, an infusion bag should be elevated significantly above the level of the

symphysis. The volume needed may vary, but is reached when bladder walls are not collapsing inward. Overdistending the bladder is avoided, as it may result in temporary urinary retention. If the bladder is distended beyond its capacity, excess fluid will leak out the urethra meatus and around the cystoscope rather than resulting in bladder rupture, which is rare.

❸ Indigo Carmine. If intraoperative cystoscopy is performed to document ureteral patency ½ to 1 ampule of indigo carmine is administered prior to the procedure.

❹ Cystoscopy. The anterior urethral wall is sensitive, and the sharp beveled sheath edge, if directed anteriorly, may cause increased discomfort. Therefore, a cystoscope is inserted into the urethral meatus with the bevel directed posteriorly. Immediately following insertion into the meatus, media flow is started. The cystoscope is advanced to the

bladder under direct visualization. During the procedure, the cystoscope may be steadied with one hand holding the sheath near the urethral meatus (Fig. 43-1.2).

❺ Bladder Inspection. Upon entry into the bladder, the cystoscope is slowly withdrawn until the bladder neck is identified. The cystoscope is then advanced and rotated 180 degrees. To maintain orientation during rotation, the camera is held in the same position while the light cord and cystoscope are rotated (Fig. 43-1.3). An air bubble is noted at the dome, which provides orientation for the remainder of the cystoscopic examination. The cystoscope is then withdrawn to the bladder neck and angled downward to provide a view of the trigone and both ureteral orifices. If ureteral patency is the topic of focus, brisk flow of indigo carmine should be seen from each orifice. Peristalsis of the ureteral orifice alone, without flow, is insufficient to document patency. Moreover, scant

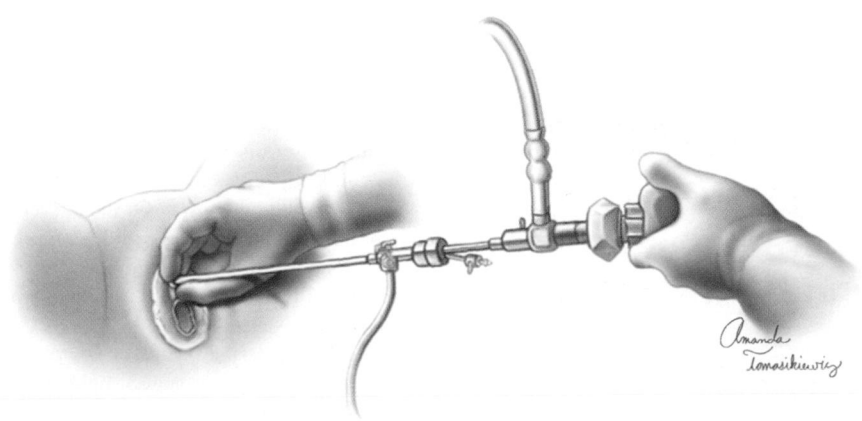

FIGURE 43-1.2 Cystoscope steadied during procedure.

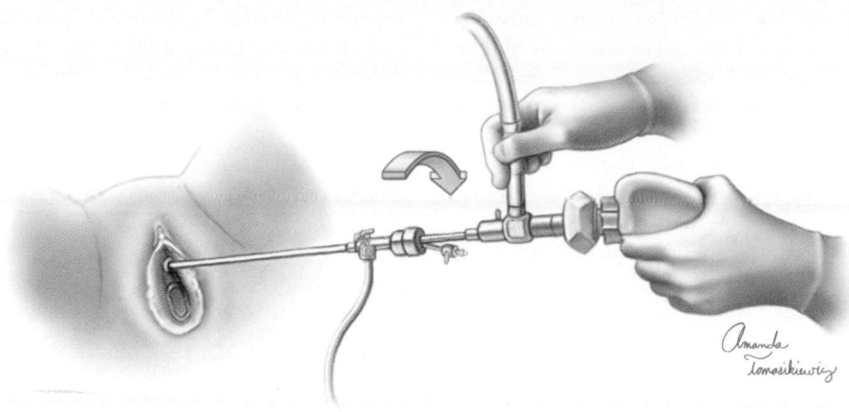

FIGURE 43-1.3 Orientation during cystoscopy is maintained by holding the camera steady while the light cord and cystoscope are rotated together.

flow may indicate partial ureteral obstruction. Bladder walls are inspected by rotating the cystoscope until all surfaces have been evaluated. During inspection, digital elevation of the anterior vaginal wall is beneficial if pelvic organ prolapse is present.

❻ **Operative Cystoscopy.** The operative instrument (biopsy or grasping forceps or scissors) is introduced through the operative port, until viewed at the end of the cystoscope. Prior to instrument insertion, a rubber adapter cap is positioned over the operative port to create a watertight seal with the operative instrument. Once in view, the instrument and cystoscope are moved together as a unit toward the area of interest.

❼ **Ureteral Stenting.** Ureteral stents may be placed at several junctures during surgery. They may be placed at the beginning of surgery and left through its duration to define anatomy in cases in which the ureter is at surgical risk of injury. Alternatively, they may be placed intraoperatively to document ureteral patency and exclude injury. Finally, ureteral stents may be positioned and left in place at the conclusion of surgery if ureteral injury is suspected or identified. Duration of postoperative stenting is variable and based on clinical indications.

Ureteral stents are available in a variety of sizes, and those ranging from 5 to 7F are commonly used. Stents vary in length from 12 to 30 cm, and a 24-cm length is appropriate for most adults. Generally, open-ended or whistle-tip stents are used to delineate anatomy in cases in which the ureter is at surgical risk or to exclude obstruction. Double- or single-pigtail stents are used in situations in which prolonged ureteral drainage is required.

❽ **To Exclude Ureteral Obstruction.** An open-ended or whistle-tip stent is threaded

through the operative channel of a 30-degree cystoscope and into the field of view. By advancing both the stent and cystoscope toward the orifice, the stent is passed into the ureteral orifice. After the stent has entered the orifice, it is manually threaded and advanced. Alternatively, an Albarrán bridge may be used. This specialized bridging sheath allows deflection and guidance of a stent into an orifice. Once a stent is placed within the orifice, it is advanced past the level of suspected obstruction. If a stent is easily advanced, obstruction is excluded. In most gynecologic surgery, this would not be higher than the pelvic brim. When passing a stent, undue pressure is avoided during advancement to avoid ureteral perforation.

❾ **To Delineate Anatomy.** For this purpose, the stent is advanced until resistance is

met, which indicates that the renal pelvis has been reached. The stent is tied securely to the transurethral catheter and drains into the Foley bag. At the conclusion of surgery, the stent is removed.

❿ **Ureteral Stenting.** In cases in which a ureteral stent is required postoperatively, a double-pigtail stent is used. The proximal coil of the stent prevents renal pelvis injury, and the distal coil secures placement in the bladder.

For placement, a guide wire is first threaded into the ureteral orifice and passed to the renal pelvis. The pigtail stent is then placed over the guide wire and advanced by a pusher device until the distal end enters the bladder. The guide wire is removed, allowing the ends to coil in the renal pelvis and bladder, respectively.

⓫ **Biopsy.** Mucosal lesions can be biopsied with a minimum amount of risk and discomfort to the patient. A biopsy instrument is introduced into the cystoscope's operative port and brought into the operative field. With the instrument directly in the field of view, the cystoscope is moved directly to the lesion. Biopsy is performed, and the cystoscope and instrument are withdrawn through the urethra together. In this way, a biopsy specimen is not pulled through the sheath and possibly lost. Bleeding is usually minor and will stop by itself. For brisk bleeding, electrosurgical coagulation can be used if a nonconducting solution was selected as the distension medium. As described in Section 42-13 (p. 1159), electrolyte solutions such as saline cannot be used with monopolar

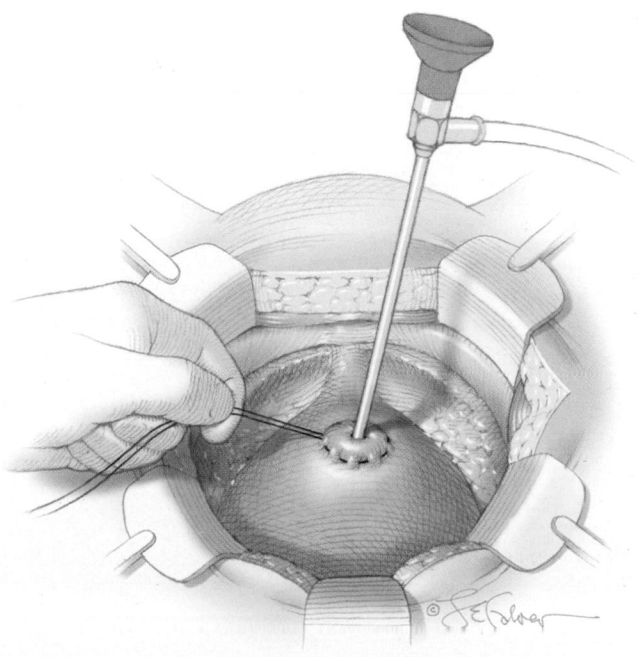

FIGURE 43-1.4 Suprapubic teloscopy.

electrosurgery. These solutions conduct current, thus dissipating the energy and thereby rendering the instrument useless.

⑫ **Removal of Foreign Bodies.** Foreign bodies, such as stones, are removed using the same technique as biopsy. The instrument is used to grasp the foreign body and then removed together with the cystoscope.

⑬ **Suprapubic Teloscopy.** Suprapubic teloscopy is a technique used to visualize the bladder through an abdominal approach. We have found this technique to be valuable when the ureters must be assessed during a difficult cesarean delivery or during a laparotomy in which a woman has not been positioned to allow easy cystoscopic access to the urethra. The bladder is distended using the transurethral Foley catheter until the bladder wall is tense. A wide purse-string using 2-0 absorbable suture is then placed at the bladder dome, taking deep bites into the bladder muscularis (Fig. 43-1.4). The two suture ends are elevated but held loosely. A small stab incision is then made in the purse-string's center, and a cystoscope is introduced into the bladder. For suprapubic teloscopy, a 30-degree cystoscope is most effective. The two suture ends are then pulled up and held tightly to prevent escape of the distending fluid. To allow visualization of the trigone and ureteral orifices, the Foley bulb is deflated but left in place. Indigo carmine is given if necessary to document ureteral efflux. If the ureteral orifices still cannot be visualized, the bladder incision is extended to allow direct visualization. At the conclusion of the teloscopy, the cystoscope is removed, and the purse-string suture is tied, closing the cystotomy.

POSTOPERATIVE

Office cystoscopy does not require specific postoperative management except for prophylactic antibiotics. With operative cystoscopy, hematuria may develop, generally clears within a few days, and is only considered significant if associated with symptomatic anemia. With long-term ureteral stenting, additional complications may include ureteral spasm, which typically presents as back pain.

43-2

Burch Colposuspension

Abdominal-approach antiincontinence procedures attempt to correct stress urinary incontinence (SUI) by stabilizing the anterior vaginal wall and urethrovesical junction in a retropubic location. Specifically, the Burch procedure, also known as *retropubic urethropexy*, uses the strength of the iliopectineal ligament (Cooper ligament) to stabilize the anterior vaginal wall and anchor the wall to the musculoskeletal framework of the pelvis (Fig. 38-24, p. 940).

The Burch colposuspension is usually performed through a Pfannenstiel or Cherney incision. More recently, however, some have introduced laparoscopic approaches that use suture or mesh to affix the paravaginal tissues to Cooper ligament (Ankardal, 2004; Zullo, 2004). However, compared with open Burch colposuspension, laparoscopic approaches appear to be less effective (el Toukhy, 2001; Moehrer, 2002).

PREOPERATIVE

Patient Evaluation

Prior to surgery, patients undergo complete urogynecologic evaluation. Urodynamic testing is recommended to differentiate stress and urge urinary incontinence as well as to assess bladder capacity and voiding patterns (Chap. 23, p. 621).

Many women with SUI may also have associated pelvic organ prolapse. For this reason, other indicated pelvic reconstructive surgeries commonly accompany Burch colposuspension. In women requiring hysterectomy, hysterectomy does not appear to improve or worsen success rates of Burch colposuspension (Bai, 2004; Meltomaa, 2001).

Consent

For most women with stress urinary incontinence, Burch colposuspension offers a safe, effective long-term treatment for incontinence. Success rates vary based on how "success" is defined, but it is generally believed that this operation provides symptomatic cure in approximately 85 percent of cases. Surgical risks compare similarly with other surgeries for SUI (Green, 2005; Lapitan, 2003). Intraoperative complications are rare and may include ureteral injury, bladder

perforation, and hemorrhage (Galloway, 1987; Ladwig, 2004).

Complications following surgery, however, are not uncommon and may include urinary tract or wound infection, voiding dysfunction, de novo urinary urgency, and pelvic organ prolapse, primarily enterocele formation (Alcalay, 1995; Demirci, 2000, 2001; Norton, 2006). Overcorrection of the urethrovesical angle has been suggested as a cause of these long-term urinary and prolapse complications.

Patient Preparation

The American College of Obstetricians and Gynecologists (2009) recommends antibiotic prophylaxis prior to urogynecologic surgery, and appropriate choices mirror those for hysterectomy as listed in Table 39-6 (p. 959). Bhatia (1989) showed significantly less febrile morbidity in women given 1-g doses of cefazolin intravenously before, during, and 8 hours after colposuspension compared with women receiving no prophylaxis. For all patients undergoing major gynecologic surgery, thromboprophylaxis is also recommended. Mechanical or heparin prophylaxis is appropriate as outlined in Table 39-9 (p. 962).

INTRAOPERATIVE

SURGICAL STEPS

❶ Anesthesia and Patient Positioning. The patient is placed supine with legs in Allen stirrups in low lithotomy position (Fig. 40-6, p. 985). The abdomen and vagina are surgically prepared, and a Foley catheter is inserted.

❷ Abdominal Incision. A low Pfannenstiel or Cherney incision is performed (Section 41-2, p. 1022). Surgery in the space of Retzius is easier to accomplish if the incision is placed low on the abdomen, approximately 1 cm above the upper border of the pubic symphysis. If hysterectomy, culdoplasty, or other intraperitoneal procedure is planned, the peritoneum is entered and concurrent surgery completed prior to beginning colposuspension.

❸ Entry into the Space of Retzius. Upon closure of the peritoneum, the avascular plane between the pubic bone and loose areolar tissue, that is, the space of Retzius, must be exposed. To enter this retropubic space, the fingers of one hand gently dissect along the cephalad surface of the pubic bone. Alternatively, gentle sponge dissection can be used to open this space (Fig. 43-2.1).

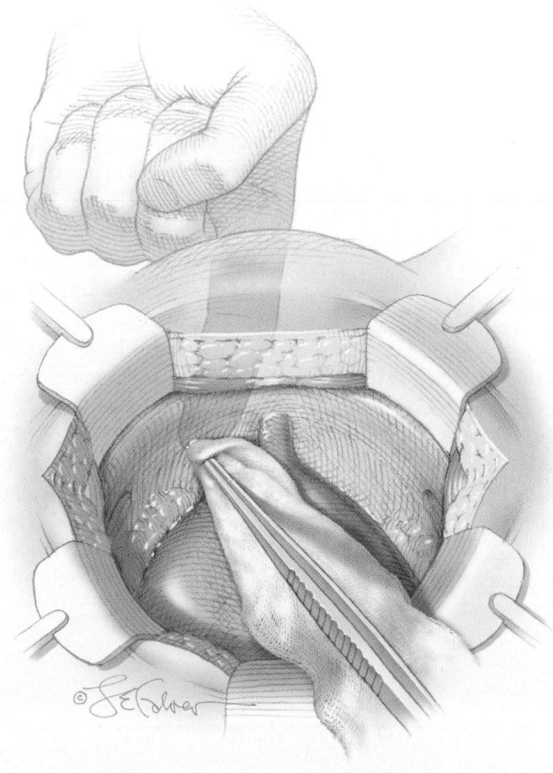

FIGURE 43-2.1 Entry into the space of Retzius.

The loose areolar tissue found behind the symphysis will easily separate from the bone. However, if the wrong plane is entered, bleeding can occur. Direct exposure of the back of the pubic bone ensures that the correct space has been entered. The bladder and urethra gently pull downward and away from the pubic bone, and the space of Retzius opens.

In those with prior surgery, sharp dissection may be required. Dissection begins with the curved tips of the Metzenbaum scissors directly on the pubic bone and progresses dorsally until the space is exposed. Clips and sutures can be used to control bleeding vessels.

During space of Retzius dissection, the obturator canal should be identified early to avoid neurovascular injury to the obturator vessels and nerves. The iliopectineal ligament (Cooper ligament) is identified as the space is opened.

❹ Exposing the Anterior Vaginal Wall. Following creation of this space, index and middle fingers of the surgeon's nondominant hand are placed in the vagina. With one on each side, the finger pads straddle the urethra and push the vagina ventrally. This maneuver alone will clear much of the fat off the anterior vaginal wall.

If necessary, a surgeon can use a Kitner (peanut) sponge or gauze sponge stick to wipe the fatty connective tissue laterally on either side of the urethra. Upward pressure by the vaginal fingers and downward, lateral pressure during this blunt separation removes this fatty tissue and reveals the white glistening anterior vaginal wall. Importantly, to protect the delicate urethral musculature, this dissection should remain lateral to the urethra.

Dissection may bring laceration of vessels within the Santorini plexus of paravaginal veins and a risk for significant bleeding (Fig. 38-24, p. 940). This is easily controlled with upward pressure from the vaginal fingers. Identified vessels can be sealed with electrosurgical coagulation, ligation, or placement of vascular clips.

❺ Identifying the Urethrovesical Junction. The urethrovesical junction is next identified to aid correct suture placement. This site can be found by using the surgeon's vaginal hand to position the Foley catheter balloon at the bladder neck. This should be done without pulling the Foley catheter. Tension may drag the bladder into the

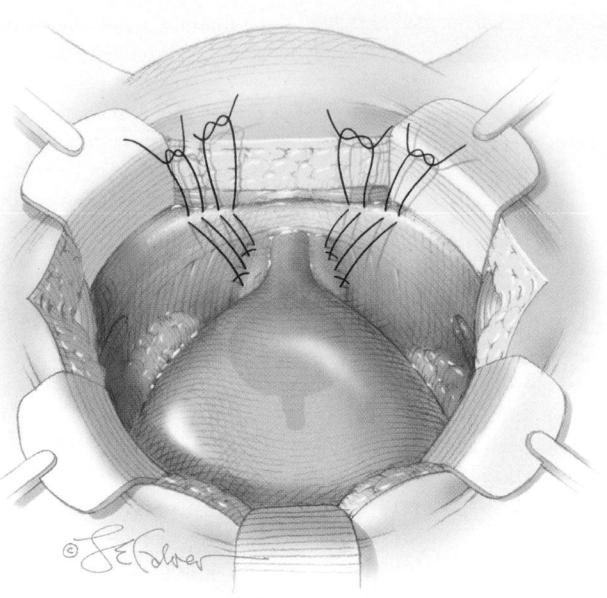

FIGURE 43-2.2 Suture placement.

operative field and increase the risk of suture entry into the bladder.

❻ Suture Placement. A double-armed suture of 2-0 nonabsorbable material is placed laterally on each side of the urethra. A surgeon's vaginal finger is pressed upward to expose the appropriate area, and the needle point is directed toward that finger. A thimble may be used to avoid needle-stick injury. A first suture is placed 2 cm lateral to the urethrovesical junction, and a second suture is placed 2 cm lateral to the proximal third of the urethra. For this suturing, a figure-of-eight stitch is used and incorporates a wedge of tissue for support (Fig. 43.2.2). Identical sutures are placed on the opposite side of the urethra.

Both ends of each suture are then placed through the nearest point of the ipsilateral iliopectineal ligament. Slack is removed from each suture, and knots are tied above the ligament. With knot securing, suture bridges are invariably formed, and these should stabilize but not elevate the anterior vaginal wall and urethrovesical junction.

❼ Cystoscopy. Following suture ligation, ½ or 1 ample of indigo carmine is given intravenously, and cystoscopy is performed. This allows identification and removal of any errant sutures that may traverse the bladder mucosa.

Moreover, it enables a surgeon to inspect the ureteral orifices and document flow as a means to exclude intraoperative ureteral injury.

❽ Catheterization. At the completion of colposuspension, the Foley catheter may remain and drain the bladder. Alternatively, a suprapubic catheter may be placed. Investigators comparing the two have found no differences in incontinence procedure success rates, length of hospitalization, or rates of infection. Urethral catheterization, however, was linked with a shorter duration of catheterization but also greater patient discomfort (Dunn, 2005; Theofrastous, 2002).

❾ Incision Closure. The abdominal wall fascia is then closed in a running fashion with 0-gauge delayed-absorbable suture. The skin is closed using a running subcuticular suture with 4-0 delayed-absorbable material or with another suitable skin-closure method (Chap. 40, p. 987).

POSTOPERATIVE

In general, recovery follows that associated with laparotomy, and it varies depending on concurrent surgeries and incision size. A voiding trial as described in Chapter 39 (p. 966) is performed prior to hospital discharge.

Tension-Free Vaginal Tape (TVT)

The tension-free vaginal tape procedure (TVT) is the most commonly performed operation worldwide for stress urinary incontinence. The procedure has been widely studied, and cure rates up to 10 years approximate 80 percent (Holmgren, 2005; Nilsson, 2008; Song, 2009). The TVT procedure has also become the prototype for a host of other antiincontinence operations, which include the TOT (transobturator tape), TVT-O (tension-free vaginal tape), and others. These are all based on the concept that midurethral support is vital to continence.

Tension-free vaginal tape placement is indicated for stress urinary incontinence (SUI) secondary to urethral hypermobility or to intrinsic sphincteric deficiency (Chap. 23, p. 615). It is used for primary cases as well as for those who have had prior antiincontinence procedures.

During TVT, a permanent sling material is placed underneath the midurethra, traverses behind the pubic bone, enters the space of Retzius, and is brought out through the anterior abdominal wall. Once positioned, tissue ingrowth ultimately holds the mesh in place. For placement, the TVT needle is placed blindly through the space of Retzius, and significant bleeding can occur. A modification of the TVT, the TOT (Section 43-4, p. 1194), was developed to avoid hemorrhage in this space. However, the TVT remains the primary operation for stress urinary incontinence.

The TVT device consists of a permanent polypropylene mesh covered with a plastic sheath that is removed after the mesh is placed. The plastic sheath is believed to prevent bacterial contamination of the mesh as it passes through the vagina and to protect the mesh from being damaged during passage. The mesh is attached to two metal disposable needles that are connected to a reusable metal introducer during placement. A metal catheter guide is used to displace the urethra away from the needle during the procedure.

PREOPERATIVE

Patient Evaluation

Prior to performing a TVT procedure, a diagnosis of SUI must be made. A woman should have bothersome symptoms of urine leakage with cough, sneeze, activity, exercise, or increased intraabdominal pressure. A urodynamic evaluation should be performed, and leakage with increases in intraabdominal pressure but in the absence of detrusor contractions should be documented (Chap. 23, p. 621). In some women, symptoms do not correlate with objective findings, and for these individuals, a surgical procedure should not be performed. In such cases, stress incontinence may not be present, and surgery may fail to improve or may aggravate symptoms. An exception might be a woman with pelvic organ prolapse that is obstructing the urethra. In these women, the prolapse should be replaced during urodynamic testing to attempt to document latent or potential stress incontinence.

Consent

The consenting process for TVT must include an honest discussion of outcomes. At best, the 5-year cure rate is 85 percent, with another 10 percent significantly improved. However, some patients will develop postoperative urge urinary incontinence, and others will develop bothersome voiding dysfunction. Additionally, with time and aging, incontinence may recur secondary to factors not related to urethral support.

The short-term complications of the procedure include incomplete bladder emptying requiring drainage with Foley catheter or intermittent self-catheterization for several days. A small percentage of patients will develop long-term urinary retention requiring reoperation for excision or removal of the tape (Section 43-8, p. 1202). In patients who require excision or removal of a piece of the tape, continence rates decrease. The TVT procedure is associated with a learning curve, and urinary retention rates decrease as the number of cases a physician performs accrues. Postoperatively, vaginal mesh erosion may develop as an early or late complication. This is managed by simple excision of the piece of eroding tape.

Intraoperative complications include hemorrhage, bladder perforation, and bowel injury. Major vessels are injured in less than 1 percent of cases.

Patient Preparation

The American College of Obstetricians and Gynecologists (2009) recommends antibiotic prophylaxis prior to urogynecologic procedures, and appropriate choices mirror those for hysterectomy as listed in Table 39-6 (p. 959). For all patients undergoing major gynecologic surgery, thromboprophylaxis is recommended. Mechanical or heparin prophylaxis is appropriate as outlined in Table 39-9 (p. 962). Bowel preparation is based on surgeon preference and on concurrent surgeries planned.

INTRAOPERATIVE

SURGICAL STEPS

❶ Anesthesia and Patient Positioning. The procedure was initially described as an ambulatory surgical procedure performed under local anesthesia. However, it can also be performed with regional or general anesthesia. The rationale for local anesthesia is that a cough stress test can be performed after placement of the tape to allow for proper tension setting of the tape. If performed without other procedures, TVT in most cases is a day-surgery operation. The procedure is performed in high lithotomy position (Fig. 40-6, p. 985). The vagina is surgically prepared, and an 18F Foley catheter is inserted to assist in deflection of the urethra during passage of the needle.

❷ Abdominal Incisions. Two ½-cm skin incisions are made 1 cm above the symphysis and 1 cm lateral to the midline. Although many surgeons incise the skin more laterally, we believe that near midline incisions decrease the risk of major vessel injury and do not increase the risk of bladder perforation.

❸ Vaginal Incisions. A midline incision is made sharply in the vaginal epithelium beginning 1 cm proximal to the urethral meatus and is extended 2 cm cephalad. Allis clamps are placed on the edges of the vaginal incision for traction. Using Metzenbaum scissors, bilateral submucosal tunnels are created beneath the vaginal epithelium on either side of the urethra. These tunnels extend several centimeters toward the pubic rami to allow placement of the TVT needle.

❹ Catheter-Guide Placement. A rigid guide is placed through the Foley catheter. During passage of the TVT needles, a surgical assistant uses this catheter guide to deflect the urethra to the contralateral side to prevent urethral injury.

❺ Mesh Placement. The TVT needle and mesh are attached to the introducer. The needle is placed through one of the submucosal tunnels so that its point touches the front surface of the ipsilateral pubic rami (Fig. 43-3.1). A hand placed in the vagina then carefully guides the needle around the back of the rami and then up toward the ipsilateral abdominal incision. The needle should always be directly behind the pubic bone. Pressure is applied to the introducer handle with the other hand, but the vaginal

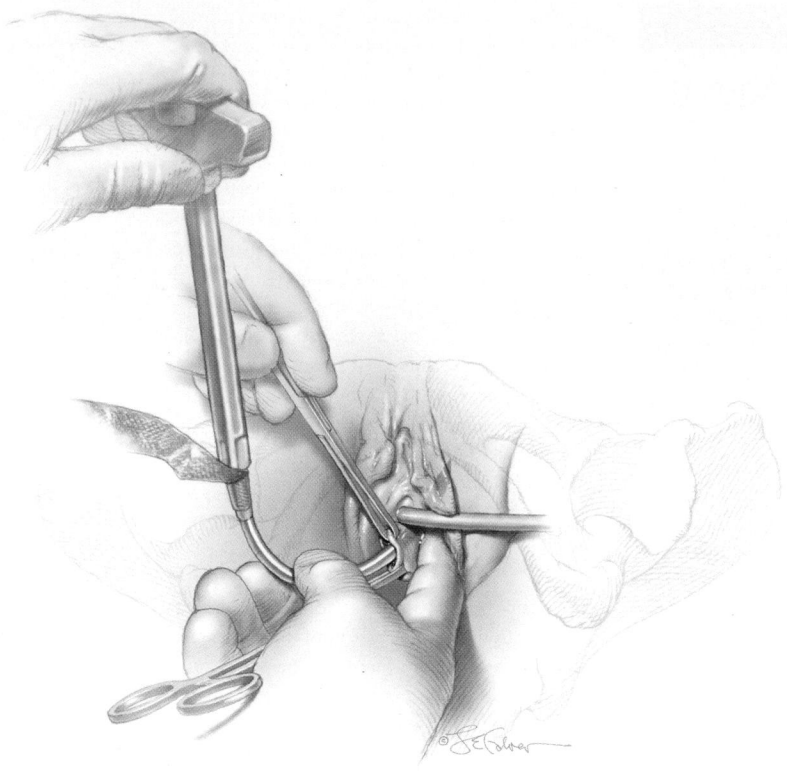

FIGURE 43-3.1 Needle placed through submucosal tunnel.

hand always controls the needle's direction. The handle of the introducer should always remain parallel to the ground to avoid lateral excursion into vessels (Fig. 43-3.2). Additionally, after the needle is passed around the pubic rami and behind the symphysis, its tip should always be directed toward the abdominal wall. The bladder may be perforated if excessive pressure is applied and if the needle is aimed cephalad rather than toward the abdominal wall (Fig. 43-3.3). Small changes in the position

of the hand applying pressure to the handle may lead to bladder perforation.

6 **Cystoscopy.** After the needle perforates the abdominal wall, the Foley and catheter guide are removed, and cystoscopy is performed with a 70-degree cystoscope. The bladder is distended with 200 to 300 mL of fluid. Inspection for perforation is completed. Generally, perforation will be obvious, and the TVT needle will be seen entering and exiting the bladder. In such cases,

the needle is removed and then correctly placed.

After cystoscopy, the introducer is unscrewed from the needle. The needle is brought through the abdominal wall. The needle is cut from the mesh, and the mesh is held by a hemostat. Next, the other TVT needle is attached to the introducer and is placed on the other side of the urethra, as in step 5. Cystoscopy is repeated. The second needle is then cut from the mesh.

7 **Setting Mesh Tension.** A hemostat is placed and opened between the urethra and mesh to act as a spacer and create distance between the mesh and urethra (Fig. 43-3.4). This spacing avoids excessive elevation of the urethra and lowers the risk for postoperative urinary retention.

8 **Sheath Removal.** An assistant surgeon then removes the plastic covering of the mesh, while the surgeon holds the mesh at the desired distance from the urethra using the hemostat. The plastic covering should be removed with a minimal amount of tension to avoid mesh stretching. The mesh is trimmed at the abdominal incisions (Fig. 43-3.5).

9 **Wound Closure.** The vaginal incision is closed in a running fashion with 2-0 delayed-absorbable suture. The abdominal skin incisions may be closed with Dermabond or with a single interrupted 4-0 delayed-absorbable skin suture.

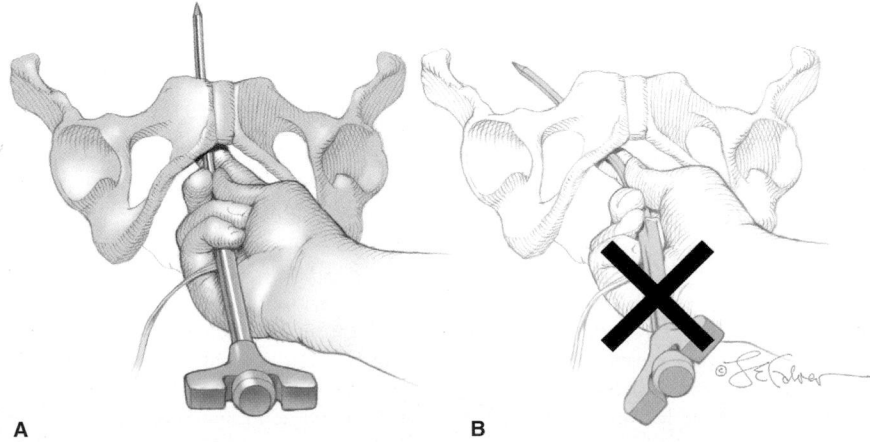

A   **B**

FIGURE 43-3.2 Correct and incorrect introducer positioning. **A.** Dark introducer, correct position. The tip is directed in the midline to a position behind the pubic bone. The handle is parallel to the ground. **B.** White introducer, incorrect position. The tip is directed laterally.

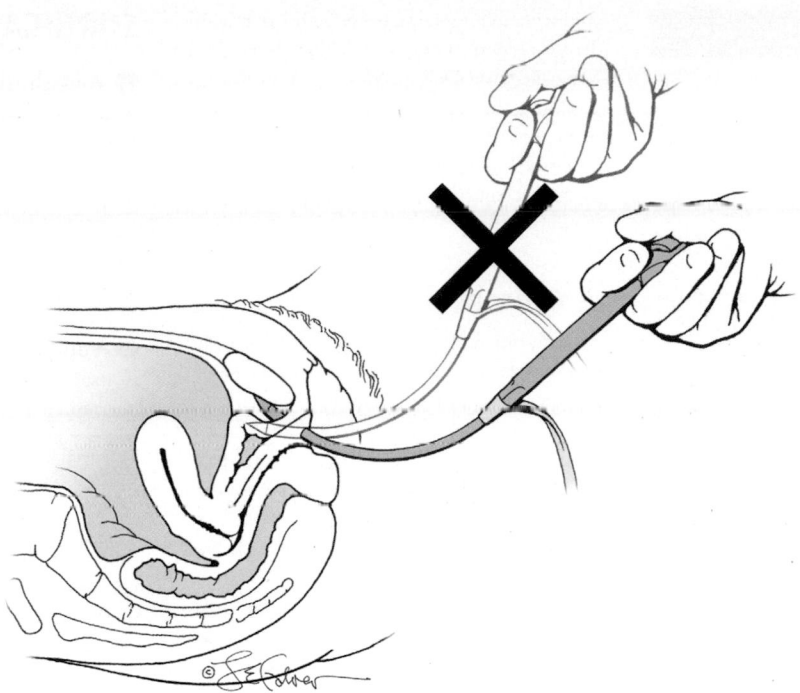

FIGURE 43-3.3 Correct (*dark introducer*) and incorrect (*light introducer*) hand and introducer positioning.

POSTOPERATIVE

Prior to discharge from a day-surgery unit, an active voiding trial is performed (Chap. 39, p. 966). If the patient fails this trial, a Foley catheter remains. A second voiding trial can be repeated in a few days or at the surgeon's discretion. Alternatively, a patient can be taught self-catheterization. This is continued until postvoid residuals fall below 100 mL.

Normal diet and activity can resume during the first postoperative days. Intercourse, however, should be postponed until the vaginal incision is healed. The time to resumption of exercise and strenuous physical activity is controversial. A standard recommendation has been to delay these at least 2 months, although there are no data to support this. However, logic would suggest that this is a reasonable amount of time to allow adequate healing.

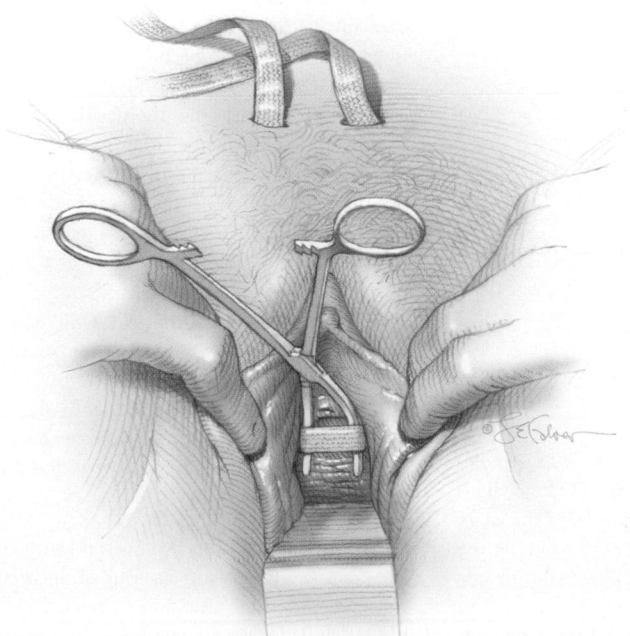

FIGURE 43-3.4 Setting mesh tension.

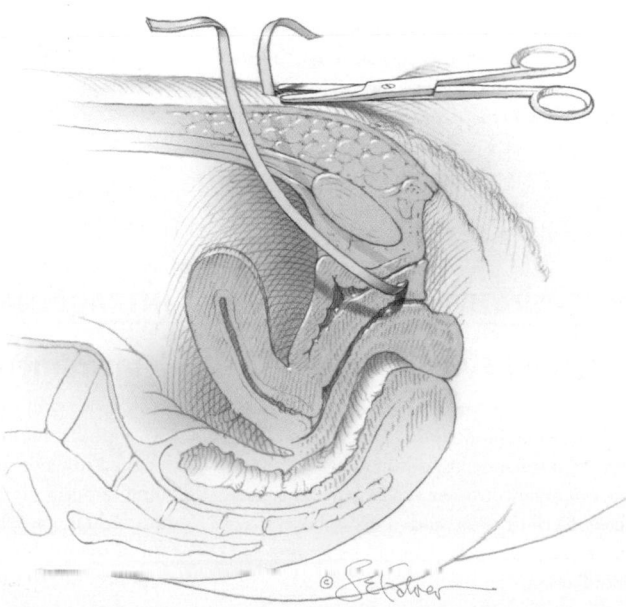

FIGURE 43-3.5 Sheath removal and tape trimming.

43-4

Transobturator Tape Sling

The transobturator tape (TOT) sling procedure is a variation of the midurethral sling procedures, which began with tension-free vaginal tape (TVT) (Section 43-3, p. 1191). The procedure is gaining popularity, although data regarding its long-term success are still not available. The procedure has several important differences from TVT, and there are also several modifications of the TOT procedure itself.

Generally, TOT is indicated for primary stress urinary incontinence (SUI) secondary to urethral hypermobility (Chap. 23, p. 615). It is currently not clear whether TOT will be of value in patients who have SUI secondary to intrinsic sphincteric deficiency.

During TOT procedures, a permanent sling material is placed bilaterally through the obturator fascia and extends underneath the midurethra. The entry point overlies the proximal tendon of the adductor longus muscle. Because of this entry approach, the space of Retzius is avoided. Bleeding in the space of Retzius is one of the primary complications of TVT, and avoidance of this space is an attractive TOT feature. Additionally, in patients who have had prior antiincontinence procedures and have scarring in the space of Retzius, bladder perforation may be averted by avoiding dissection in this space.

Kits containing required mesh and placement needles for TOT are produced by several companies, and each has its own modifications. The two major types of TOT procedures are defined by whether needle placement begins inside the vagina and is directed outward, termed an *in-to-out approach,* or starts outside the vagina and is directed inward, called an *out-to-in approach.* Currently, the out-to-in technique is more commonly performed and is described next.

PREOPERATIVE

Patient Evaluation

Prior to surgery, patients undergo complete urogynecologic evaluation. Urodynamic testing is recommended to differentiate stress and urge urinary incontinence. Many patients have mixed incontinence, and those whose stress symptoms predominate would be appropriate candidates.

Of note, caution must be exercised in patients who are Valsalva voiders. These women void with abdominal straining rather than with detrusor contraction and urethral relaxation. Most incontinence procedures prevent leakage by closing the urethra during cough or Valsalva maneuver. Therefore, these surgeries, when performed in women who rely on the Valsalva maneuver to urinate, will often results in voiding dysfunction.

Consent

As with other surgeries for incontinence, the major risks of this procedure are development of urge urinary incontinence, voiding dysfunction, urinary retention, and failure to correct stress incontinence. Groin pain appears to be another potential postoperative problem. Long-term complications may be associated with the supporting mesh and include mesh erosion.

Prior to surgery, patients should have realistic expectations and be informed of success rates in the literature as well as those of the individual surgeon. Moreover, the definition of "outcome success" varies from woman to woman. For example, in a patient with severe incontinence and 20 leakage episodes per day, improvement to one leakage episode every other day would be considered successful. However, in a woman with rare leakage, it may be more difficult to achieve an outcome considered satisfactory. Therefore, the patient's expectations should be discussed prior to surgery.

Intraoperatively, there is some risk of bladder perforation, although it is believed to be significantly less than that with TVT. There also may be risk of urethral perforation, and inappropriate TOT trocar placement can lead to significant hemorrhage if major pelvic vessels are lacerated.

Patient Preparation

Antibiotic and thromboprophylaxis are given as outlined in Tables 39-6 and 39-9 (p. 959). Bowel preparation is based on surgeon preference and on concurrent surgeries planned.

INTRAOPERATIVE

Instruments

A TOT kit will contain two TOT needles and synthetic mesh tape. The TOT needle is designed to navigate the path from the entry point, around the pubic rami, and to the midurethral epithelium. A plastic sheath surrounds the mesh tape and allows the mesh to be pulled into position smoothly. However, once these plastic sheaths are removed, the mesh remains fixed in position.

SURGICAL STEPS

❶ Anesthesia and Patient Positioning. If performed without other surgeries, a TOT procedure in most cases is a day-surgery procedure. It is performed in high lithotomy position under general, regional, or local anesthesia. The vagina is surgically prepared, and a Foley catheter is placed to assist in determination of urethral location.

❷ Vaginal Incisions. A midline incision is made sharply in the vaginal epithelium beginning 1 cm proximal to the urethral meatus and is extended 2 to 3 cm cephalad. Allis clamps are placed on the edges of the vaginal incision for traction. Using Metzenbaum scissors and blunt finger dissection, bilateral submucosal tunnels are created beneath the vaginal epithelium on either side of the urethra. These tunnels extend up to and behind the iliopubic rami.

❸ Thigh Incisions. A 0.5- to 1-cm entry incision is made bilaterally in the thigh-crease skin (genitocrural fold), 4 to 6 cm lateral to the clitoris, and at the point where the adductor longus insertion can be palpated.

❹ Mesh Placement. The TOT needle is grasped and the tip is placed in one of the thigh incisions (Fig. 43-4.1). The tip is directed cephalad until the obturator membrane is perforated, and a "popping" sensation is felt. A vaginal finger is placed in the ipsilateral vaginal tunnel and is positioned up to and behind the iliopubic rami. Using the curve of the TOT needle, the surgeon then directs the needle tip to the end of his finger and passes the needle into the vagina (Fig. 43-4.2). The TOT mesh is then attached to the end of the needle, the needle is withdrawn back through the thigh incision, and thereby, the covered mesh is threaded into position. The mesh is then removed from the needle. The procedure is repeated on the other side (Fig. 43-4.3).

❺ Setting Mesh Tension. A hemostat is placed and opened between the urethra and mesh to act as a spacer and create distance between the mesh and the urethra (Fig. 43-4.4). This spacing avoids excessive elevation of the urethra and lowers the risk for postoperative urinary retention.

❻ Sheath Removal. An assistant surgeon then removes the plastic covering of the mesh through the thigh incision. Concurrently, the surgeon holds the mesh at the desired distance from the urethra using the hemostat. The plastic covering should be removed

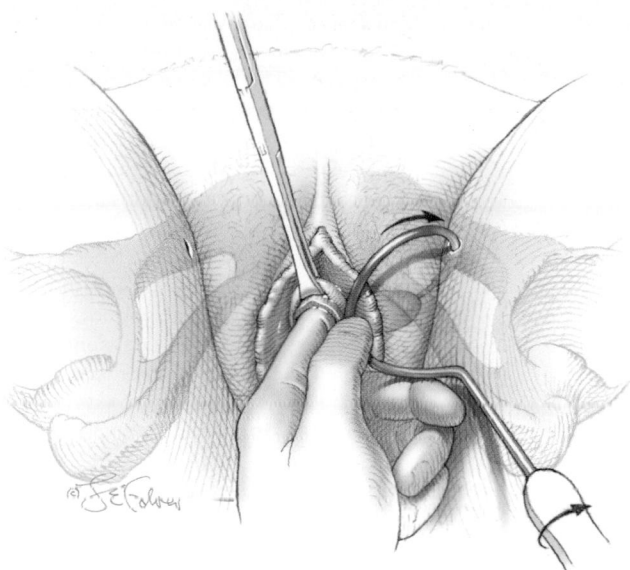

FIGURE 43-4.1 Needle introduction.

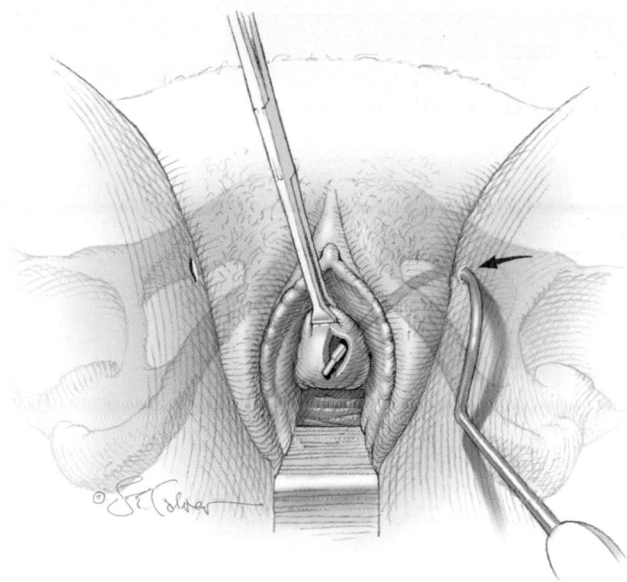

FIGURE 43-4.2 Needle passage.

with a minimal amount of tension to avoid mesh stretching. The mesh is trimmed at the thigh incisions.

❼ Wound Closure. The vaginal incision is closed in a running fashion with 2-0 delayed-absorbable suture. The thigh incisions may be closed with a single interrupted subcuticular stitch with 4-0 delayed-absorbable suture or with other suitable skin closure methods (Chap. 40, p. 987).

❽ Cystoscopy. The procedure is marketed as one in which cystoscopy is not necessary. However, because bladder and urethral injury can occur, we recommend postprocedural cystoscopy.

POSTOPERATIVE

Prior to discharge from a day-surgery unit, an active voiding trial is performed (Chap. 39, p. 966). If the patient fails this trial, a Foley catheter remains. A second voiding trial can be repeated in a few days or at the surgeon's discretion. Alternatively, a patient can be taught self-catheterization. This is continued until postvoid residuals fall below 100 mL.

Normal diet and activity can resume during the first postoperative days. Intercourse, however, should be delayed until the vaginal incision is healed. The time to resumption of exercise and strenuous physical activity is controversial. A standard recommendation has been to delay these at least 2 months, although there are no data to support this. However, logic would suggest that this is a reasonable amount of time to allow adequate healing.

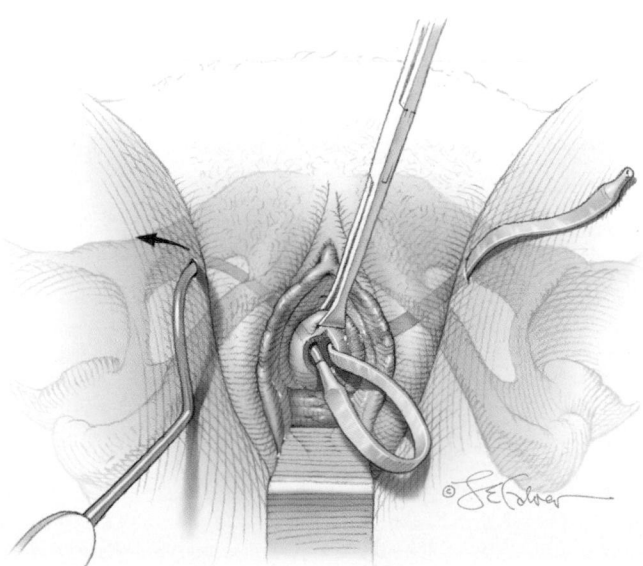

FIGURE 43-4.3 Tape placement.

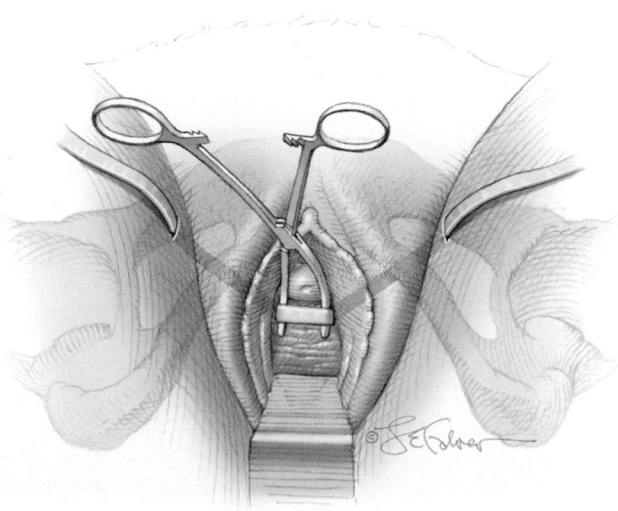

FIGURE 43-4.4 Setting mesh tension.

43-5

Pubovaginal Sling

Pubovaginal sling is a standard procedure for stress urinary incontinence (SUI). It has traditionally been used for SUI stemming from intrinsic sphincteric deficiency. This specific condition is characterized by a nonmobile urethra, a low maximum urethral closing pressure, or low Valsalva leak point pressure (Chap. 23, p. 616). In addition, pubovaginal sling may also be indicated for patients with prior failed antiincontinence operations. It is generally not employed in a woman having her first antiincontinence operation.

In the past, different materials have been used for the sling, however, autologous fascia is currently preferred. Generally, autologous fascia is obtained from the patient's rectus sheath, although fascia lata from the thigh may alternatively be used. With this surgery, a strip of fascia is placed at the bladder neck through the space of Retzius, and ends are secured above the rectus abdominis muscle.

PREOPERATIVE

Patient Evaluation

As with other antiincontinence procedures, patients require urogynecologic evaluation, including urodynamic testing to confirm SUI and intrinsic sphincteric deficiency.

Additionally, SUI often accompanies pelvic organ prolapse. Thus, the need for concurrent repair of associated prolapse should be assessed prior to surgery (Chap. 24, p. 641).

Consent

In addition to general surgical risks, patients should be counseled regarding the risk of recurrent incontinence and urinary retention following surgery.

Patient Preparation

Antibiotic and thromboprophylaxis are given as outlined in Tables 39-6 and 39-9 (p. 959). Bowel preparation is based on surgeon preference and on concurrent surgeries planned.

INTRAOPERATIVE

SURGICAL STEPS

❶ **Anesthesia and Patient Positioning.** Pubovaginal sling may be performed under general or regional anesthesia as an inpatient procedure. The patient is placed in high lithotomy position, and legs are held by candy-cane stirrups. The abdomen and vagina are surgically prepared, and a Foley catheter is placed.

❷ **Graft Harvest.** A transverse skin incision is made 2 to 4 cm above the symphysis

and should be large enough to allow removal of a fascial strip that measures, at minimum, 2 × 6 cm. The incision is carried down through subcutaneous tissue to the fascia.

The fascia to be harvested is outlined and then sharply dissected and removed. Following removal, the strip is cleaned of fat and adventitial tissue. A helical stitch using 0-gauge polypropylene suture is then placed against the grain of the fascia at each end of the strip. These sutures are not tied. The fascial incision is then closed in a running fashion with 0-gauge delayed-absorbable suture.

❸ **Vaginal Incision.** Two centimeters proximal to the urethral meatus, a 5- to 6-cm midline vertical incision is made sharply in the anterior vaginal wall. Sharp and blunt dissection is used to lift the vaginal epithelium off the underlying fibromuscular layer. The space of Retzius is entered bluntly or sharply bilaterally by penetrating the perineal membrane (Fig. 38-27, p. 943) (Fig. 43-5.1). The surgeon's finger should palpate the pubic bone in the space of Retzius (Fig. 43-5.2). Bleeding may be encountered, and this can be managed with compression or suturing.

❹ **Fascia Placement.** A long dressing or packing forceps or needle ligature carrier is used from above to perforate the rectus sheath caudad to the prior harvest incision. The instrument is placed against the back of the pubic bone and advanced toward the vagina. Concurrently, the surgeon guides the

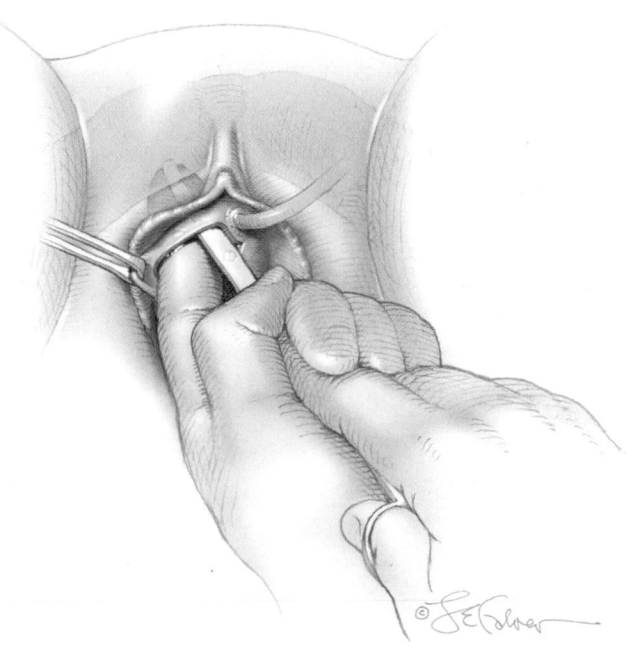

FIGURE 43-5.1 Entry into the space of Retzius.

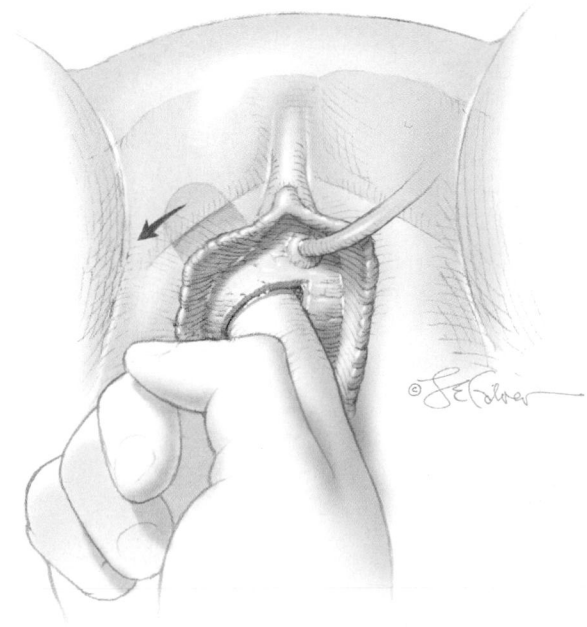

FIGURE 43-5.2 Palpation of pubic bone.

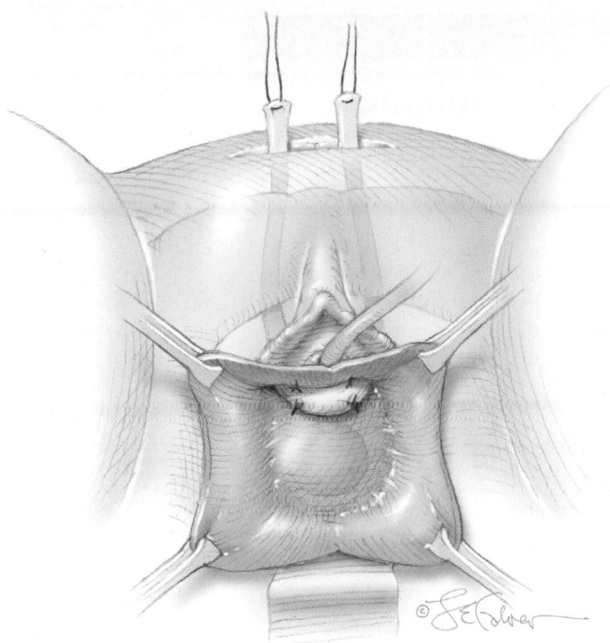

FIGURE 43-5.4 Fascial sling sutured in place.

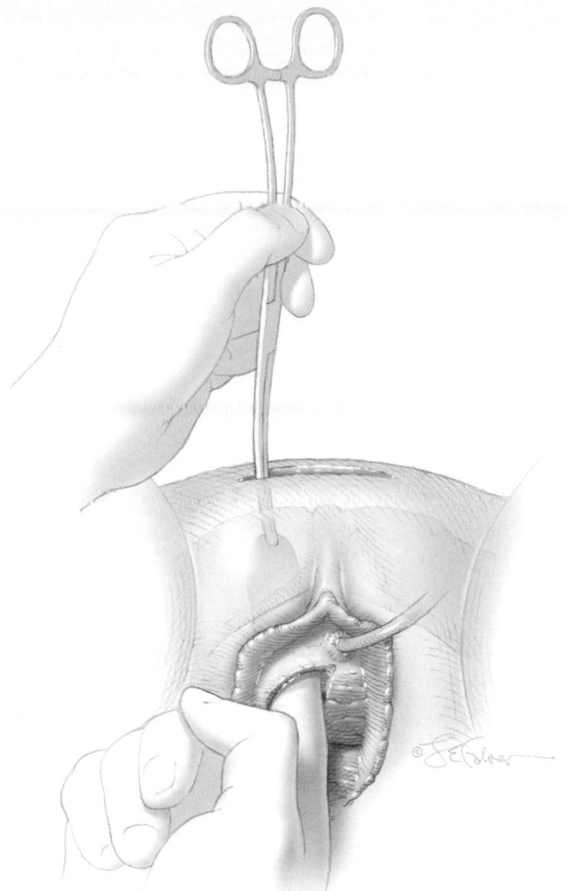

FIGURE 43-5.3 Fascial strip placement.

instrument to his finger within the space of Retzius (Fig. 43-5.3).

The suture at one end of the fascial strip is grasped with the perforating forceps and threaded up through the abdominal incision on one side of the urethra. A similar procedure is performed on the opposite side of the urethra with the other end of the sling. As a result, the fascial sling lies positioned beneath the bladder neck (Fig. 43-5.4). Three to four 2-0 delayed-absorbable sutures are used to fix the sling beneath the bladder neck to prevent movement.

❺ **Setting Sling Tension.** Sutures attached to the sling ends are then tied together above the rectus sheath. During knot tying,

a space of two to three fingerbreadths is left between the knot and fascia to prevent bladder neck obstruction and urinary retention. After the knot is secured, there should be no upward angulation of the urethra or bladder neck.

❻ **Cystoscopy.** Cystoscopy is performed to exclude bladder perforation and ureteral obstruction.

❼ **Vaginal Incision.** The vaginal incision is closed with 2-0 delayed-absorbable suture in a running fashion. A Foley catheter is left in place. In the past, it was common practice to insert a suprapubic tube. However, with a trend toward setting

tension loosely on the sling, the risk of prolonged urinary retention is lowered, and suprapubic drainage is therefore not typically required.

❽ **Abdominal Incision.** The remainder of the abdominal incision is closed as described in Section 41-2 (p. 1023).

POSTOPERATIVE

In general, recovery follows that associated with laparotomy and is heavily dependent on incision size. A voiding trial as described in Chapter 39 (p. 966) is performed prior to hospital discharge.

43-6

Urethral Bulking Injections

Injection of bulking agents into the urethral submucosa is one method available to treat stress urinary incontinence (SUI) resulting from intrinsic sphincter deficiency (ISD) (Chap. 23, p. 616). Although mechanisms are not completely clear, effectiveness may result from expansion of the urethral walls, which allows them to better approximate or *coapt* (Kershen, 2002). As a result, intraluminal resistance to flow is increased and continence is restored (Winters, 1995). Alternatively, injections may be effective by elongating the functional urethra. This may allow more even distribution of abdominal pressures across the proximal urethra to resist opening during stress (Monga, 1997).

Bulking agents are traditionally recommended for treatment of SUI solely due to ISD. However, some evidence suggests they can be used to treat SUI resulting from combined ISD and urethral hypermobility (Bent, 2001; Herschorn, 1997; Steele, 2000).

Urethral injection offers a cystoscopically assisted, minimally invasive treatment of SUI. It can be performed in an office setting under local anesthesia and is associated with a low risk of complications. For these reasons, it is often chosen for women who wish to avoid surgery or who are not surgical candidates due to other health reasons. Urethral injections can be performed both peri- and transurethrally. The transurethral approach is more commonly used and allows for more accurate placement of the bulking agent (Faerber, 1998; Schulz, 2004). Currently available agents approved for use in the United States include autologous fat and several synthetic agents. Until recently, a bovine collagen product was available in the United States and was a commonly used agent.

PREOPERATIVE

Patient Evaluation

Complex urodynamic testing with assessment of urethral structure and function should be completed. Maximum urethral closure pressure or leak point pressure are specifically evaluated (Chap. 23, p. 623). Additionally, urethral mobility should be assessed with Q-tip testing or similar evaluation (Fig. 23-13, p. 619).

Consent

Patients should be informed of the procedure's efficacy. Success rates in general are lower than those for surgery, although 1-year rates of curing or improving SUI range from 60 to 80 percent (Bent, 2001; Corcos, 2005; Lightner, 2002; Monga, 1995). Continence rates diminish with time, as would be intuitive with the breakdown of collagen and fat. However, Chrouser (2004) found similar rates of decline with time even when synthetic material was compared with collagen. Accordingly, these injections should be viewed as a nonpermanent treatment of SUI, and sustained continence is found in only 25 percent of patients at 5 years following injection (Gorton, 1999).

One major advantage to urethral injection is its low associated risk of complications. Side effects of injection are generally transient and may include vaginitis, acute cystitis, and voiding symptoms. Of these, urinary retention for a few days postprocedure is the most common. Long-term retention, however, is not a significant risk. A more serious complication is persistent de novo urgency, which may develop in as many as 10 percent of women following injection (Corcos, 1999, 2005).

Patient Preparation

Urinary tract infection can commonly follow urethral injection. Therefore, a suitable antibiotic is administered orally after the procedure is complete. Thromboprophylaxis is not typically required for this office procedure.

INTRAOPERATIVE

Choice of Bulking Agent

In the United States, several agents are currently available for urethral injection: autologous fat, carbon-coated synthetic microspheres (Durasphere), calcium hydroxylapatite particles (Coaptite), ethylene vinyl alcohol copolymer (Tegress), and polydimethylsiloxane (Macroplastique). Of these, autologous fat provides limited success in the treatment of SUI due to rapid degradation and reabsorption. Accordingly, it is not primarily employed for this use (Haab, 1997; Lee, 2001).

Synthetic agents are available and effective, but long-term comparative studies are currently lacking.

SURGICAL STEPS

❶ Anesthesia and Patient Positioning. Urethral injection for most patients can be performed in an office setting with cystoscopy capability. The patient is placed in the dorsal lithotomy position, the vulva is prepared and draped, and the bladder drained. Two-percent lidocaine jelly is instilled into the urethra 10 minutes prior to the procedure. If necessary, topical 20-percent benzocaine can be used as an analgesic on the vulva, and 4 mL of 1-percent lidocaine can be injected in divided doses at the 3 and 9 o'clock position of the external urethra.

❷ Transurethral Approach Needle Placement. A cystoscope is positioned within the distal urethra, so that the midurethra, proximal urethra, and bladder neck are viewed simultaneously. A 22-gauge spinal needle attached to a syringe carrying the bulking agent is introduced through the cystoscopic sheath. The needle is directed at a 45-degree angle to the urethral lumen and inserted through the urethral wall at the 9 o'clock position, at the level of the midurethra.

After the needle tip penetrates the urethral wall and the bevel is no longer seen, the needle is advanced parallel to the urethral lumen for 1 to 2 cm. This positions the needle at the level of the proximal urethra.

❸ Injection. The bulking agent is injected under constant pressure, and the submucosal lining begins to rise (Fig. 43-6.1). The needle is withdrawn slowly to bulk the proximal and midurethra. Bulking agent is administered until coaptation of the mucosa has developed (Fig. 43-6.2). In general, one to two syringes (2.5 to 5 mL) of agent is used per procedure. These steps are repeated then at the 3 o'clock position.

Ideally, the number of needle holes made into the urethral wall should be minimized to avoid leakage of bulking agent through these punctures. Thus, if a second syringe of agent is required to achieve coaptation, the originally positioned needle remains in place, and a second syringe of agent is attached.

❹ Cystoscope Removal. Once coaptation of the mucosa is achieved, as the cystoscope is

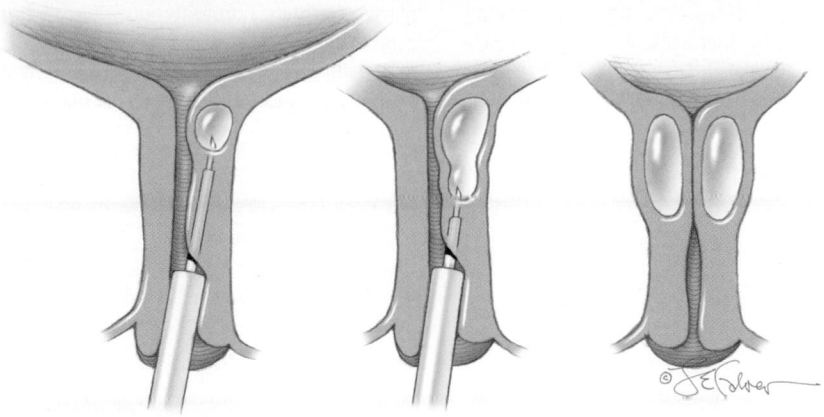

FIGURE 43-6.1 Injection of bulking agent.

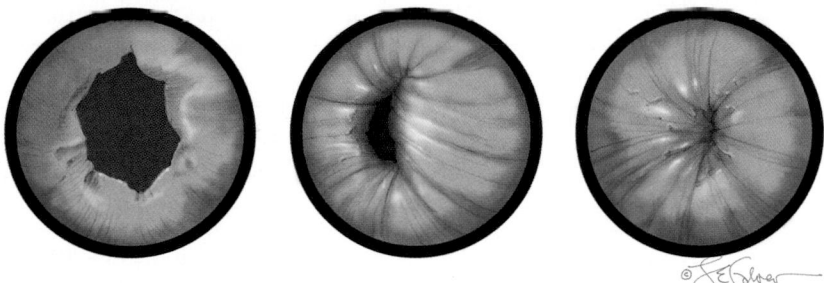

FIGURE 43-6.2 Corresponding cystoscopic views of urethral coaptation as bulking agent is injected, as shown in Figure 43-6.1.

removed, care should be taken not to advance it proximal to the injection site. This avoids forceful compression of the deposited agent and loss of coaptation.

POSTOPERATIVE

Women are discharged home following their first postinjection voiding, and oral antibiotic prophylaxis is recommended. Women should abstain from intercourse for 10 days following injection but may otherwise resume usual activities.

If urinary retention develops, then intermittent self-catheterization is begun and continued until retention resolves. If a woman is unable to perform self-catheterization, a temporary Foley catheter is placed. However, catheter placement can potentially compress deposited bulking agent collagen and diminish urethral coaptation.

Two weeks following injection, it is our practice to assess treatment success. If patients fail to achieve desired degrees of continence, additional injections are planned to improve urethral coaptation.

43-7

Urethrolysis

Urethrolysis is the loosening or release of a previous urethral suspension repair. This type of release is used in women with symptoms of urethral obstruction including urinary retention and voiding dysfunction following suspension. It can be performed either vaginally or abdominally. A vaginal approach is predominantly used and can successfully mobilize the urethra and bladder neck. An abdominal approach, however, may afford a better opportunity to mobilize the bladder from the pubic symphysis and may also be selected in instances in which the initial surgery was performed via laparotomy.

Debate exists as to the need of a concurrent antiincontinence procedure to compensate for urethral support lost with urethrolysis. However, in many cases, residual scarring prevents stress incontinence, and our belief is to avoid repeating a second potentially obstructing procedure. Accordingly, this decision should be individualized.

PREOPERATIVE

Patient Evaluation

In women with bladder neck obstruction, there is a temporal relationship between initial surgery and symptoms. Objective assessment with urodynamic testing is performed to determine the cause of voiding dysfunction and differentiate between a hypotonic bladder and obstruction. Obstruction may result from bladder neck obstruction or pelvic organ prolapse. Thus, a thorough examination for prolapse should be included.

Consent

In addition to the usual surgical risks, bleeding may be a significant complication due to vascularity in the space of Retzius. Additionally, dissection of dense scarring around the urethra and bladder may place these structures at risk of laceration.

Due to reformation of scar tissue, urethrolysis may fail to relieve symptoms. In contrast, postoperative incontinence may follow deconstruction of the prior antiincontinence support.

Patient Preparation

Bowel preparation prior to urethrolysis is individualized. Antibiotic prophylaxis is administered prior to surgery to decrease risks of postoperative wound and urinary tract infection (Table 39-6, p. 959). Thromboprophylaxis is given as outlined in Table 39-9 (p. 962).

INTRAOPERATIVE

SURGICAL STEPS—VAGINAL APPROACH

❶ **Anesthesia and Patient Positioning.** Urethrolyis may be performed under general or regional anesthesia. The patient is placed in high lithotomy position within candy-cane stirrups. The vagina is surgically prepared, and a Foley catheter containing a 30-mL balloon is inserted into the bladder.

❷ **Vaginal Incision.** Traction is placed on the Foley catheter to identify the bladder neck and assess the degree of scarring. Either a vertical midline or U-shaped incision is made in the anterior vaginal wall at the level of the proximal urethra and bladder (Fig. 43-7.1). Sharp dissection is used to separate the vaginal epithelium from underlying tissues and is extended bilaterally toward the inferior edge of each of the pubic rami.

Dissection frees the urethra by dividing scar tissue or prior sling material that lies between the urethra and pubic rami (Fig. 43-7.2). If prior sling material is identified, this may be incised or excised, if necessary. Bleeding is frequently encountered and can be controlled with direct pressure or vessel ligation.

After this lateral dissection, the perineal membrane is perforated, as described in Section 43-5, step 3 (p. 1196), and the space of Retzius is entered. Careful blunt dissection within this space and at the back of the symphysis pubis will additionally assist in mobilizing the proximal urethra.

❸ **Incision Closure.** Following adequate mobilization of the urethra, the vaginal incision is reapproximated with a running closure using 2-0 gauge delayed-absorbable suture.

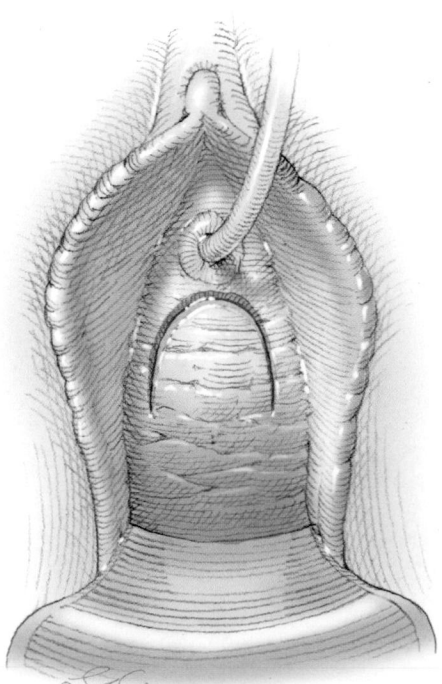
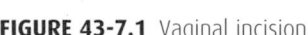

FIGURE 43-7.1 Vaginal incision.

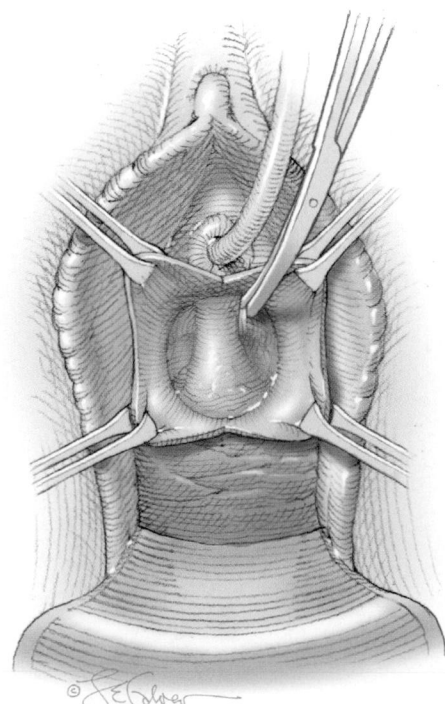

FIGURE 43-7.2 Urethral dissection.

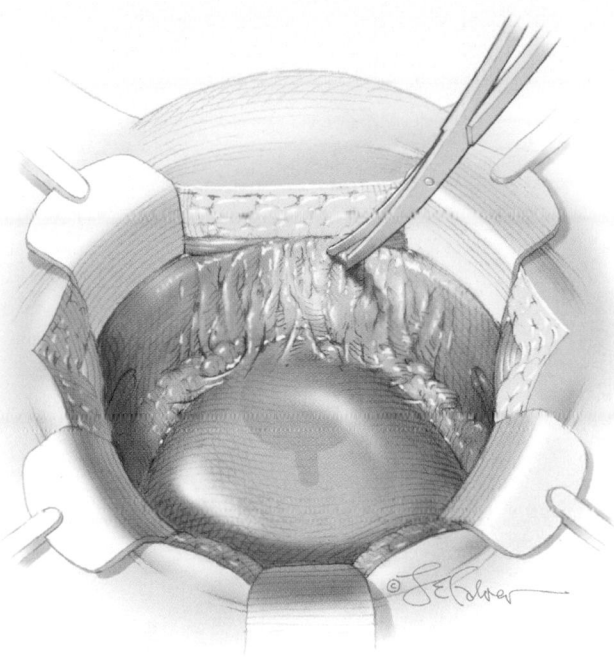

FIGURE 43-7.3 Dissection in the space of Retzius.

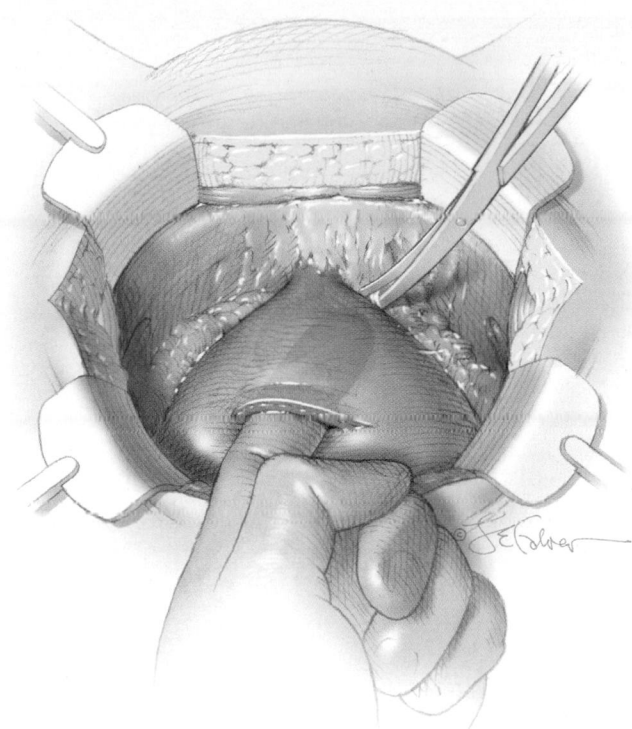

FIGURE 43-7.4 Intentional cystotomy to aid bladder and urethral dissection.

SURGICAL STEPS— ABDOMINAL APPROACH

❶ Anesthesia and Patient Positioning. As with a vaginal approach, urethrolysis may be completed under general or regional anesthesia. For an abdominal approach, Allen stirrups and standard lithotomy positioning are preferred. This positioning allows vaginal access for the surgeon's hand during dissection. The abdomen and vagina are surgically prepared, and a Foley catheter containing a 30-mL balloon is inserted within the bladder.

❷ Abdominal Incision. A low transverse incision is typically preferred for this procedure to permit easy access to the space of Retzius. Either Pfannenstiel or Cherney incisions are usually selected (Sections 41-2 and 41-3, p. 1022).

❸ Entry into the Space of Retzius. The correct plane of dissection to enter the space of Retzius lies directly behind the pubic

bone. Loose areolar tissue is gently dissected downward in a mediolateral fashion with fingers or sponge, beginning immediately behind the pubic bone. If the correct plane is entered, this potential space opens easily. However, women requiring urethrolysis have typically had prior surgery within this space. As a result, tissue may be densely adhered, and sharp downward dissection along the posterior surface of the symphysis may be needed to enter this space (Fig. 43-7.3).

❹ Bladder Dissection and Urethrolysis. The bladder is also typically densely adhered to the back of the symphysis. Sharp dissection with the curved surface of scissors facing the symphysis is directed against the symphysis to minimize the risk of bladder laceration. At times, however, an intentional cystotomy may be required so that a finger can be placed inside the bladder to aid dissection (Fig. 43-7.4).

Sharp dissection is continued inferiorly and laterally down the inner surface of the symphysis to free the bladder and eventually also the proximal urethra. Bleeding is

common during dissection and may be controlled with sutures or vascular clips.

❺ Abdominal Closure. The abdomen is closed in a standard fashion (Section 41-2, p. 1023).

POSTOPERATIVE

An active bladder test is performed following catheter removal. If large residual volumes are found, intermittent self-catheterization or replacement of the catheter is required. If cystotomy was performed, the duration of catheterization is dependent on cystotomy size and location. For example, small cystotomies in the bladder dome typically require drainage for 7 days or less. For larger cystotomies at the bladder base, however, drainage for several weeks may be needed. Antibiotic suppression is not required with this catheter use.

Normal diet and activity can resume during the first postoperative days. Intercourse, however, should be postponed until the vaginal incision is well healed.

43-8

Midurethral Sling Release

Symptoms of obstruction may develop following urethral sling procedures, specifically TVT and TOT procedures. This complication develops in 4 to 6 percent of patients after TVT and generally is identified days to weeks after surgery. When obstruction is diagnosed, surgical release is indicated and involves simple cutting of the sling material.

PREOPERATIVE

▊ Patient Evaluation

Inability to fully empty the bladder may be due to urethral obstruction or a hypotonic bladder. New-onset urinary retention after a midurethral sling procedure (TVT or TOT) is usually due to sling tightness. However, there may be other factors involved such as preexisting or de novo bladder hypotonia. Therefore, prior to TVT urethrolysis, urodynamic testing is often performed to prove that symptoms are due to obstruction rather than to bladder hypotonicity. Additionally, tape may erode into the bladder or urethra in cases of obstruction, and cystoscopy allows exclusion of this complication.

▊ Consent

Associated with midurethral sling release, the risks of incontinence recurrence, failure to adequately relieve retention, and intraoperative bladder or urethral injury should be presented in the consenting process.

▊ Patient Preparation

This is a minor surgical procedure, and no specific patient preparation is required.

INTRAOPERATIVE

SURGICAL STEPS

❶ Anesthesia and Patient Positioning. This surgery can be performed with local,

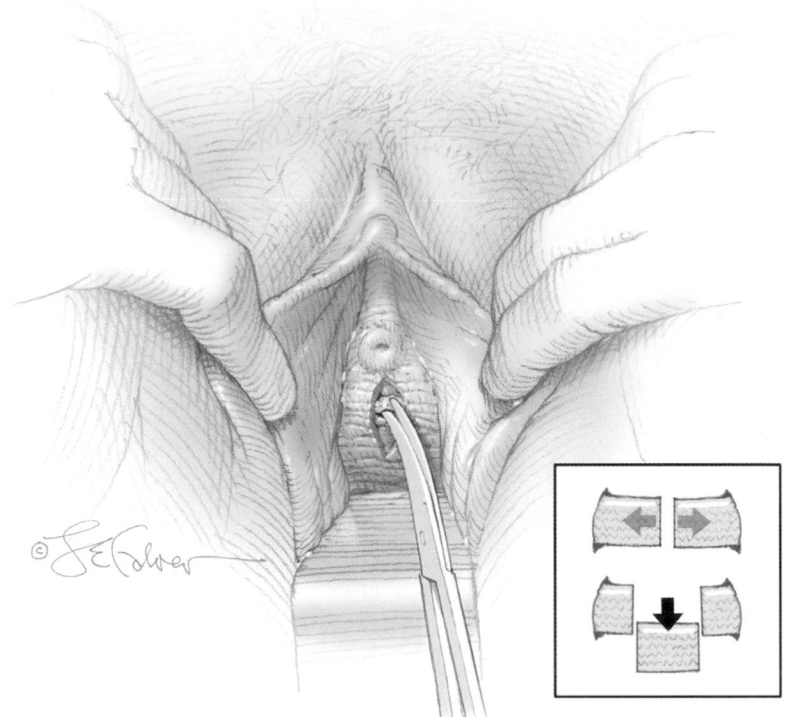

FIGURE 43-8.1 Mesh transection through vaginal incision. Inset top: Mesh incision and retraction. Inset bottom: Mesh excision.

regional, or general anesthesia as an outpatient procedure. A patient is placed in high lithotomy position within candy-cane or Allen stirrups. The vagina is surgically prepared, and a Foley catheter is inserted.

❷ Vaginal Incision and Tape Identification. A midline suburethral incision that follows the prior primary surgical incision is made sharply. Careful dissection is used to expose the sling material and to define the urethral borders.

Often because of increased sling tension, sling material is stretched and measures only one half of its expected width. Additionally, there is usually extensive tissue ingrowth into the sling material, and identification and mobilization can be difficult. Occasionally, a sling may migrate to the proximal urethra. In these instances, the vaginal incision may require cephalad extension.

❸ Incision of Sling Material. After mobilization of the material, a hemostat is opened between the sling and urethra.

Metzenbaum scissors are used to cut the sling material. In general, incision leads to immediate retraction of sling ends (Fig. 43-8.1, top inset). If retraction does not follow, a 1-cm segment of material should then be excised (see Fig. 43-8.1, bottom inset).

❹ Incision Closure. After vigorous irrigation, the vaginal epithelium is closed in a continuous running fashion using 2-0 delayed-absorbable suture.

POSTOPERATIVE

Prior to discharge, an active voiding trial is performed. If a Foley catheter remains, a second voiding trial can be repeated in a few days or at the surgeon's discretion. If a woman is performing self-catheterization, this is continued until postvoid residuals fall below 100 mL. Normal diet and activity can resume during the first postoperative days. Intercourse, however, should be postponed until the vaginal incision is healed.

43-9

Urethral Diverticulum Repair

The approach to urethral diverticulum repair varies and depends on the location, size, and configuration of the diverticular sac. For those that are near the bladder neck, partial ablation is often chosen to avoid damage to the bladder neck and continence mechanism. For midurethral diverticulum, simple diverticulectomy is typically indicated. For those located at the urethral meatus, the Spence procedure may be selected. With this technique, a distal diverticulum and urethral meatus are sharply opened together to form a large single meatus. Finally, for those with a complex diverticulum that may surround the urethra, a combination of techniques may be necessary.

PREOPERATIVE

Patient Evaluation

Accurate information regarding diverticular anatomy is essential to surgical planning

and patient counseling. Magnetic resonance (MR) imaging is a superior radiographic study to delineate diverticular configuration (Fig. 26-6, p. 685). Additionally, cystoscopy is valuable in locating sac openings along the urethral length (Fig. 26-7, p. 687).

Consent

With diverticular repair, damage to the urethral continence mechanism may lead to postoperative incontinence. Alternatively, urethral stricture or stenosis or urinary retention may develop depending on the extent and location of surgery. Additionally, urethrovaginal fistula and bladder injury may result. If a Spence procedure is selected, urethral meatus anatomy is typically altered, and a spraying pattern may result with urination.

Patient Preparation

Antibiotic and thromboprophylaxis are given as outlined in Tables 39-6 and 39-9 (p. 959).

At our institution, we recommend bowel preparation prior to diverticular repair to decompress the rectosigmoid, although this practice is not mandatory.

INTRAOPERATIVE

SURGICAL STEPS— DIVERTICULECTOMY

❶ **Anesthesia and Patient Positioning.** Diverticulum excision is typically performed as an inpatient procedure under general or regional anesthesia. A patient is placed in high lithotomy position within candy-cane stirrups to provide maximum surgical exposure. The vagina is surgically prepared, and a Foley catheter containing a 10-mL balloon is placed in the bladder to assist in identifying the bladder neck.

❷ **Cystourethroscopy.** This procedure is performed at the procedure's onset to locate the diverticular opening and exclude other abnormalities.

❸ **Vaginal Incision.** A midline incision is made on the anterior vaginal wall over the diverticulum, and the vaginal epithelium is dissected sharply off the fibromuscular layer of the vaginal wall (Fig. 43-9.1). Ample epithelium is freed to allow adequate exposure and to permit final tissue approximation without excess tension.

❹ **Diverticulum Exposure.** A longitudinal incision is then made through the

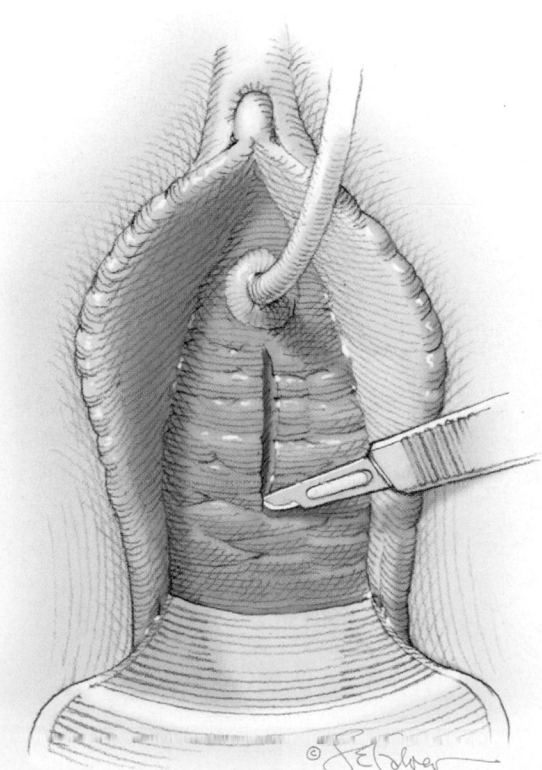

FIGURE 43-9.1 Vaginal incision.

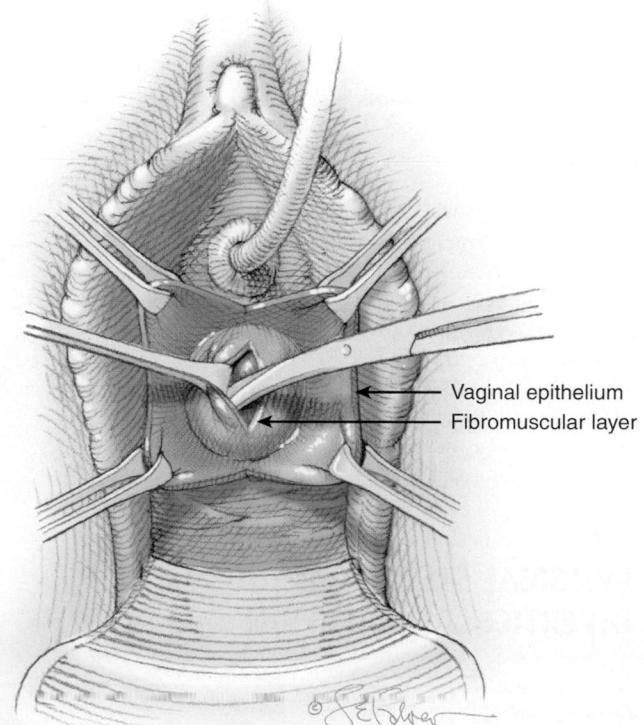

Vaginal epithelium
Fibromuscular layer

FIGURE 43-9.2 Diverticular sac dissection.

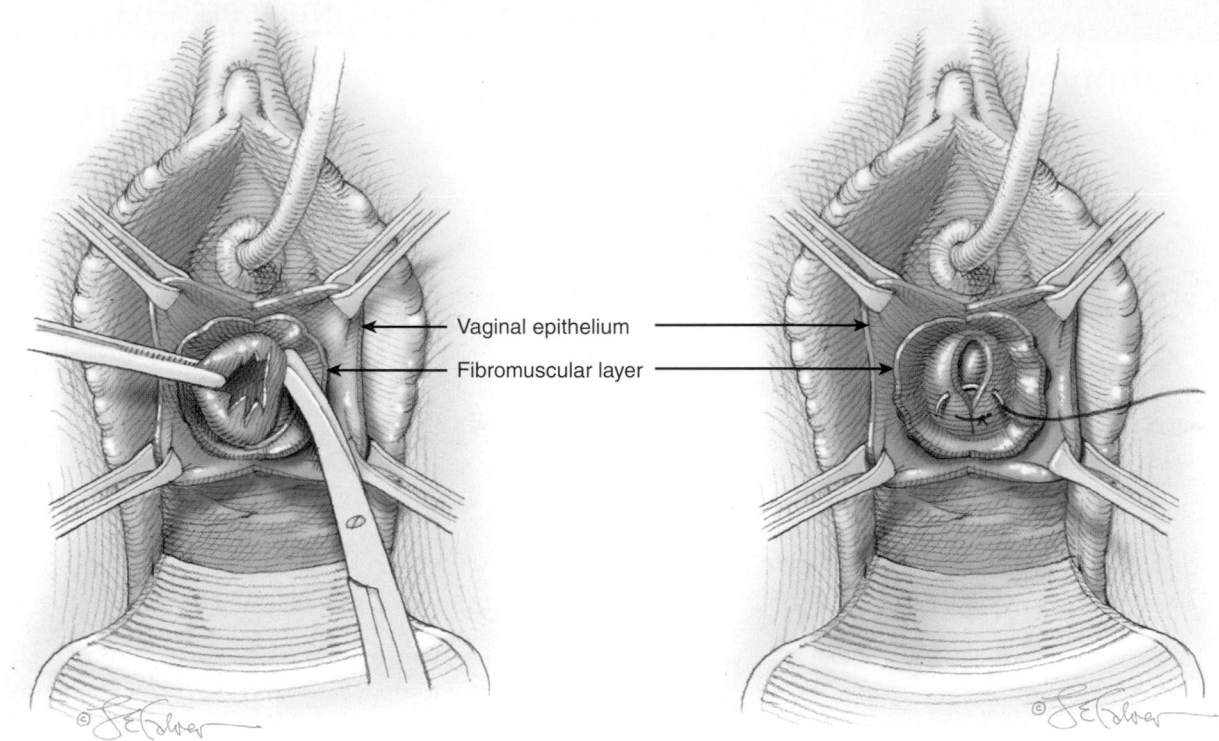

Vaginal epithelium

Fibromuscular layer

FIGURE 43-9.3 Diverticulum excision.

FIGURE 43-9.4 Urethral defect closure.

fibromuscular layer to reach the diverticular sac. Sharp dissection is used to completely mobilize and expose the diverticular sac and neck (Fig. 43-9.2). During dissection, the sac may be inadvertently or intentionally entered. If this happens, the diverticular walls are grasped with Allis clamps and dissection is continued. Caution and awareness of the location of the urethra are essential to avoid damage.

❺ **Diverticulum Excision.** At its neck, the diverticulum is excised from the urethra (Fig. 43-9.3).

❻ **Urethral Closure.** The urethral defect is closed with interrupted 4-0 delayed-absorbable sutures over the Foley catheter (Fig. 43-9.4). Fibromuscular layers are then reapproximated off tension in two or more layers in a vest-over-pants fashion with 2-0 delayed-absorbable suture (Fig. 43-9.5). Redundant vaginal epithelium is trimmed, and the epithelium is closed in a running fashion with 2-0 delayed-absorbable suture.

SURGICAL STEPS—PARTIAL DIVERTICULAR ABLATION

❶ **Vaginal Incision.** A midline incision is made on the anterior vaginal wall over the diverticulum, and the vaginal epithelium is dissected sharply off the fibromuscular layer

of the vaginal wall. Ample epithelium is freed to allow adequate exposure and permit later defect closure off tension. The Foley catheter and balloon can be placed on gentle tension to aid in identifying the bladder and bladder neck to avoid injury.

❷ **Diverticulum Exposure.** A longitudinal incision is made through the fibromuscular layer to the diverticular sac, and sharp dissection is used to completely mobilize and expose the sac. The diverticulum is open, and the communication with the urethra is identified. To avoid injury to the proximal urethra and bladder neck, the diverticular sac but not the neck of the diverticulum is sharply excised. As much of the sac that can be accessed is removed.

❸ **Sac Closure.** The base of the sac is then sutured side to side with 2-0 delayed-absorbable suture to cover the urethral

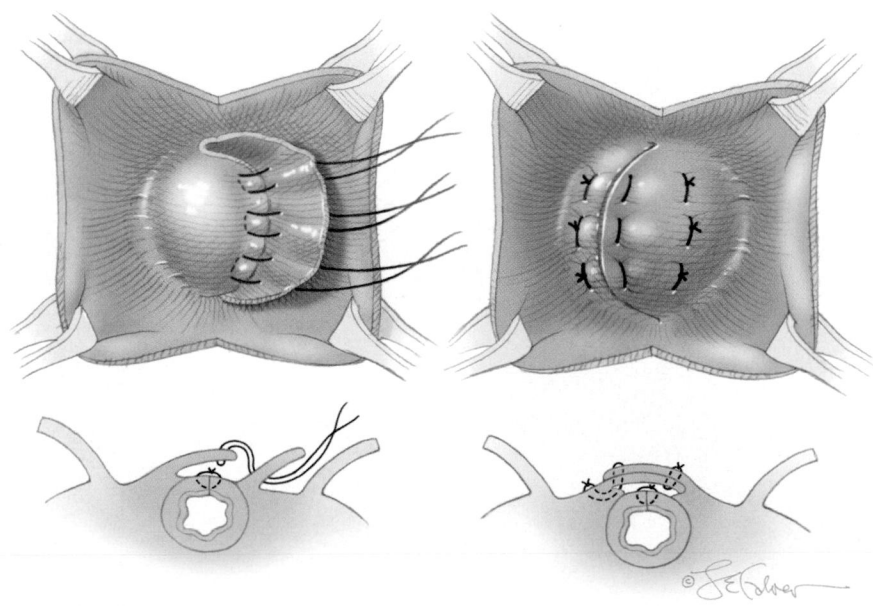

FIGURE 43-9.5 Fibromuscular layer reapproximation.

defect. A second, and possibly a third, imbricating layer using the vaginal muscularis is created with similar suture. Excess vaginal epithelium that had previously covered the diverticulum is excised. The vaginal epithelium is closed in a running fashion with a 2-0 delayed-absorbable suture.

SURGICAL STEPS—SPENCE MARSUPIALIZATION

❶ Meatal Incision. Tips of Metzenbaum scissors are inserted into the urethral meatus and vagina. An incision is made that incorporates and simultaneously incises the posterior urethral wall, entire thickness of the diverticulum, and distal anterior vaginal wall.

❷ Marsupialization. A running pattern using 4-0 delayed-absorbable suture is placed circumferentially around the enlarged meatus to approximate cut edges of the vaginal and urethral epithelia.

POSTOPERATIVE

Catheter management is an important aspect of postoperative care. Although no consensus guidelines exist, most experts recommend catheter placement for 5 to 7 days. Surgeries of increasing complexity may require longer duration. Antibiotic suppression is not required with this catheter use. Normal diet and activity can resume during the first postoperative days. Intercourse, however, should be postponed until the vaginal incision is well healed.

43-10

Vesicovaginal Fistula: Latzko Technique

Vesicovaginal fistulas may be repaired either vaginally or abdominally (Chap. 26, p. 682). A vaginal approach is preferred for most fistulas seen in the United States, which are posthysterectomy, apical fistulas. This approach is selected due to its comparable success rates, lower morbidity, and faster patient recovery. The most commonly performed vaginal procedure is the Latzko technique, which is a partial colpocleisis that obliterates the upper vagina for 2 to 3 cm around the fistula.

An abdominal approach may be necessary for cases in which a fistula cannot be accessed vaginally or in which prior vaginal repairs have been unsuccessful. With the abdominal approach, omentum or peritoneum can be mobilized and interposed as flaps between the bladder and vagina to prevent recurrence.

One principle of fistula repair dictates that a repair should be performed in noninfected and noninflamed tissues. A second principle states that tissues should be approximated without excess tension. If these guidelines are followed, success rates are typically good and range from 67 to 100 percent. In the United States, most fistulas follow hysterectomy for benign causes, and these fistulas are associated with high cure rates.

Fistulas associated with gynecologic cancer and radiation therapy, however, may require adjunctive surgical procedures such as vascular flaps. Such flaps provide supportive blood supply to these defects that develop in poorly vascularized or fibrotic tissue. Even with these measures, success rates are lower.

PREOPERATIVE

Patient Evaluation

Prior to repair, a fistula should be well characterized, and complex fistulas with multiple tracts or a ureterovaginal fistula should be identified. Proper evaluation should include intravenous pyelography (IVP) and cystoscopy (Fig. 26-1, p. 681). Ureterovaginal fistulas are usually associated with upper tract abnormalities such as hydroureter and hydronephrosis. Therefore, normal IVP findings should reassure a surgeon that ureteral involvement is absent. Additionally, this testing enables a surgeon to identify the proximity of ureters relative to a fistula for surgical planning. In general, routine posthysterectomy vesicovaginal fistulas develop at the vaginal

apex and well away from the ureters, which enter the bladder at the midvaginal level.

Whether or not surgery can be performed vaginally depends on the ability to obtain adequate exposure to a fistula. Therefore, during physical examination, a surgeon must assess if a fistula can be brought down into the surgical field and if a patient's pelvis affords adequate space for vaginal surgery. Some degree of vaginal apex prolapse is helpful for a vaginal approach to fistula repair.

Additionally, tissue infection or inflammation should be excluded. If these are identified, fistula repair should be delayed until resolution. If a fistula is recognized within a few days following hysterectomy, it may be repaired immediately, prior to a brisk inflammatory response. However, if surgical repair is not undertaken within a few days following the initial surgery, then a delay of 4 to 6 weeks is recommended to decrease tissue inflammation.

Consent

There is a significant recurrence rate with fistula repair, and patients should be aware that initial surgery may not be curative. With the Latzko procedure, the vagina is moderately shortened in most cases. Therefore, the risk of postoperative dyspareunia should be included in the consent.

Patient Preparation

Bowel preparation is administered the evening prior to surgery. This decompresses the rectosigmoid and minimizes fecal contamination of the surgical field. Immediately prior to surgery, intravenous antibiotic prophylaxis is commonly administered to decrease postoperative wound infection risks (Table 39-6, p. 959). Thromboprophylaxis is given as outlined in Table 39-9 (p. 960).

INTRAOPERATIVE

SURGICAL STEPS—LATZKO VAGINAL REPAIR

❶ Anesthesia and Patient Positioning. In most cases, repair is performed with general or regional anesthesia, and the need for postoperative hospitalization is individualized. A patient is placed in dorsal lithotomy position, and the vagina is surgically prepared. If ureters lie close to a fistula, ureteral stents should be placed (Section 43-1, p. 1187). Cystoscopy is required during the procedure to document ureteral patency and assess bladder integrity.

❷ Delineating a Fistulous Tract. The course of a fistulous tract must be identified.

If a tract is large enough to accept a pediatric catheter, the tube is threaded through the fistulous opening, and the balloon is inflated within the bladder. If a tract cannot be delineated in this manner, then lacrimal duct probes or other suitable narrow dilators should be used to trace the tract course and direction. Subsequently, attempts should be made to dilate the tract and place a pediatric catheter.

❸ Exposure. The fistula must be brought into the operative field. If catheterization of a fistulous tract is possible, tension on the tube will allow this. Alternatively, four sutures can be placed in the vaginal wall surrounding a fistula and used to pull the fistula into the operative field (Fig. 43-10.1). Some advocate performing a mediolateral episiotomy to gain exposure, although this is not our practice.

❹ Vaginal Incision. A vaginal incision is made circumferentially approximately 1 to 2 cm around the fistulous tract (Fig. 43-10.2). Vaginal mucosa surrounding the tract is then sharply mobilized and excised using Metzenbaum scissors.

❺ Tract Excision. The fistula tract may or may not be excised. If a tract is excised, surgeons should be aware that a larger defect for repair will result. However, in situations in which a tract is indurated, excision is warranted.

❻ Fistula Closure. If a tract is excised, the bladder mucosa is reapproximated with 3-0 delayed-absorbable sutures. Regardless of whether or not the tract is excised, subsequently, anterior and posterior vaginal fibromuscular layers are approximated over the fistula site. Interrupted stitches of 3-0 delayed-absorbable sutures are used (Fig. 43-10.3). After a first suture line is placed through the fibromuscular layer, a second and possibly a third line are created on top of the first (Fig. 43-10.4). Following this closure, the bladder should be filled with 100 mL of fluid to document a watertight repair. If not watertight, additional reinforcing sutures can be placed.

After fibromuscular layers of the vaginal wall are closed, the epithelium is closed in a continuous running fashion using 3-0 delayed-absorbable suture.

❼ Cystoscopy. Cystoscopy is performed to document ureteral patency and to inspect the incision site.

SURGICAL STEPS— ABDOMINAL REPAIR

❶ Anesthesia and Patient Positioning. In most cases, abdominal repair is performed under general anesthesia. The patient is placed

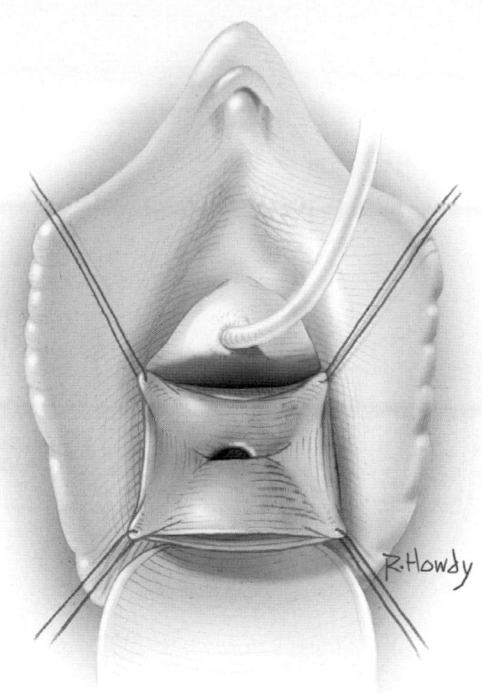

FIGURE 43-10.1 Stay sutures in the vaginal wall improve fistula access.

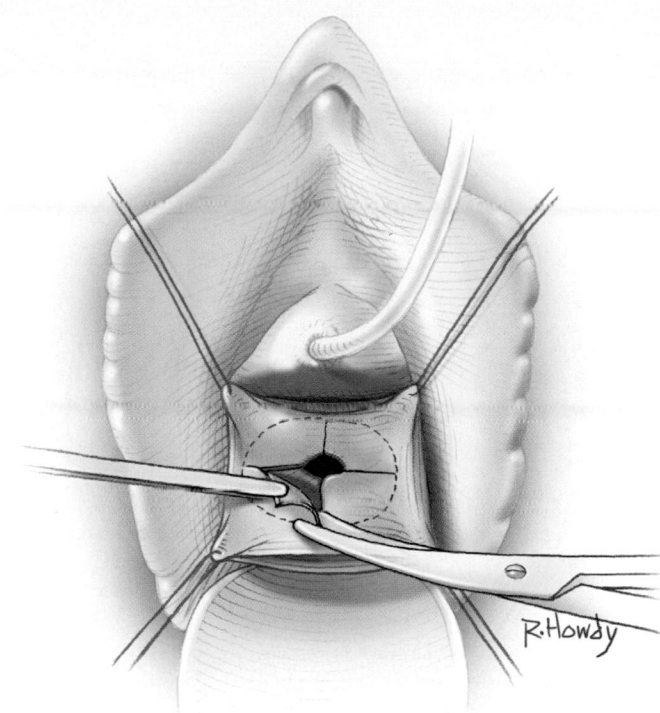

FIGURE 43-10.2 Vaginal epithelium incision.

in low lithotomy position with the use of Allen stirrups. With the patient's thighs parallel to the ground and the legs separated, access to the vagina is maximized. The abdomen and vagina are surgically prepared.

❷ **Abdominal Incision and Entry into the Bladder.** A Pfannenstiel or midline abdominal incision can be used. If mobilization of the omentum is anticipated, a midline incision may give easier access to the omentum.

Maylard or Cherney incisions may alternatively be selected (Sections 41-3 and 41-4, p. 1024). After the peritoneum is entered and the upper abdomen is explored, bowel is packed from the operating field, and a self-retaining abdominal

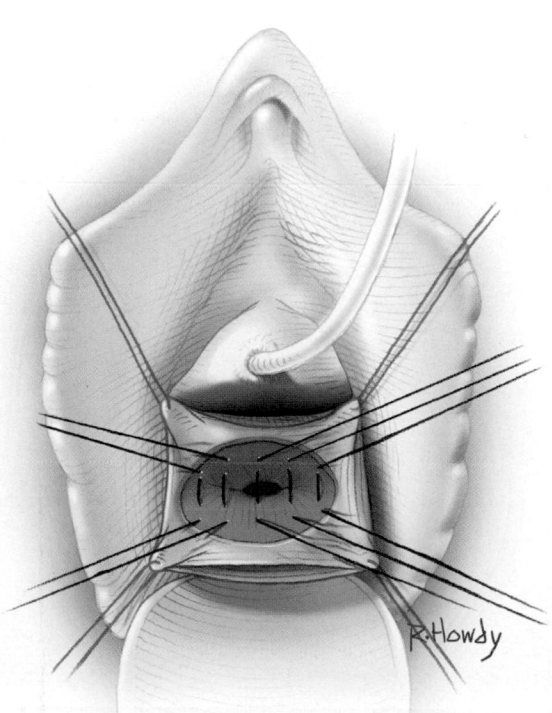

FIGURE 43-10.3 First-layer closure over fistula.

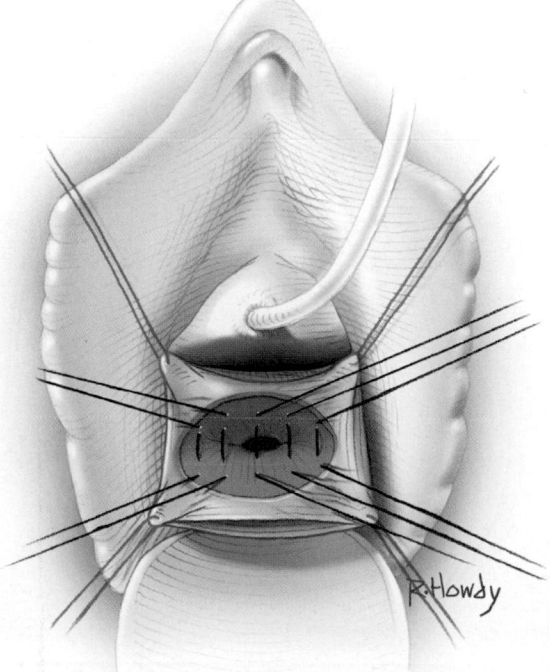

FIGURE 43-10.4 Second fibromuscular layer closure over fistula and vaginal epithelium reapproximation.

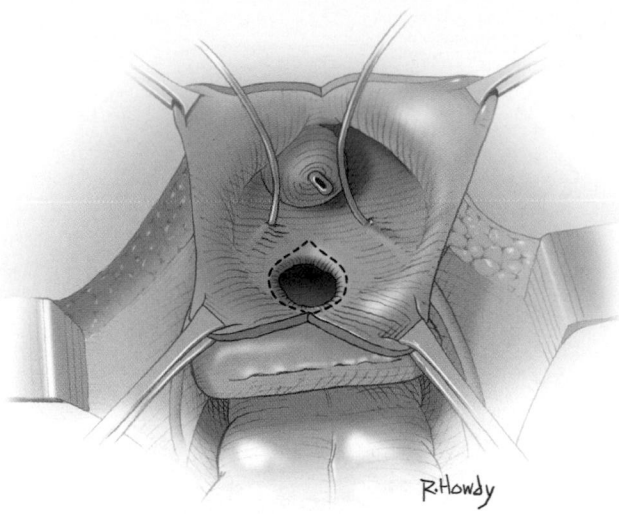

FIGURE 43-10.5 Bladder incision.

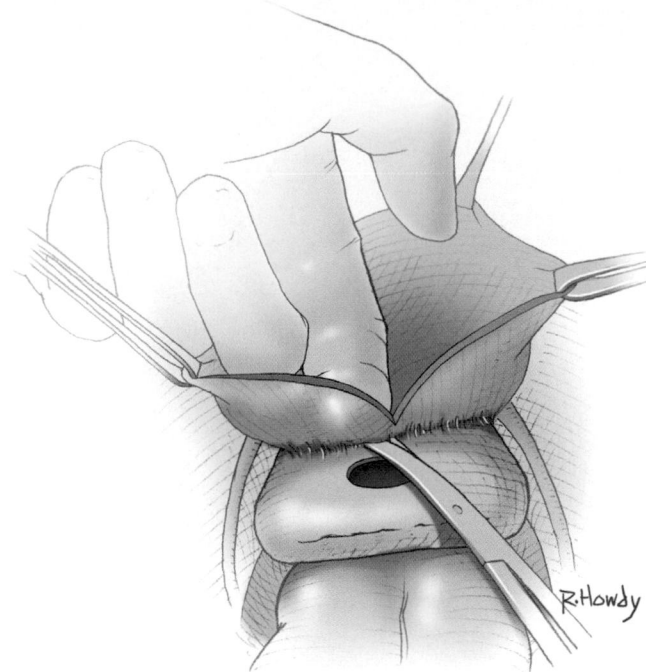

FIGURE 43-10.6 Separation of the bladder and vagina.

wall retractor is placed. The space of Retzius is opened using the technique described in Section 43-2, step 3 (p. 1189), and a vertical extraperitoneal incision is made in the bladder dome. Correct incision placement is aided by pulling the Foley balloon to the dome or by filling the bladder with fluid.

❸ **Delineation and Excision of the Fistulous Tract.** The fistula and ureteral orifices are visualized from within the bladder. If the fistula tract is near the orifices, ureteral stents are placed. The incision is then extended over the top and back of the bladder to reach the fistula tract (Fig. 43-10.5). A lacrimal probe or catheter may be placed into the fistula tract to delineate its course. The fistula tract is then excised.

❹ **Separation of the Bladder and Vagina.** Sharp dissection is used to dissect the vagina away from the bladder in the area of the fistula (Fig. 43-10.6). Scarring may be extensive, and sharp rather than blunt dissection should be used. To aid dissection, an EEA sizer may be placed in the vagina for manipulation (Fig. 43-17.5, p. 1228). The vagina should be widely separated from the bladder to allow omentum placement between the two.

❺ **Vaginal Closure.** The vagina is closed in two layers with 2-0 delayed-absorbable suture (Fig. 43-10.7). The EEA sizer or digital manipulation of the vagina will assist this closure.

❻ **Bladder Closure.** The bladder is closed in two layers using running sutures of 3-0 absorbable suture (Fig. 43-10.8). The second layer should be imbricated such that the first

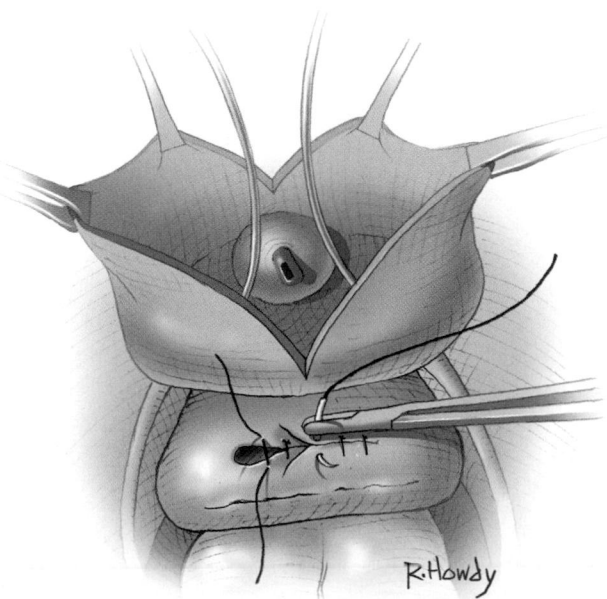

FIGURE 43-10.7 Vaginal closure.

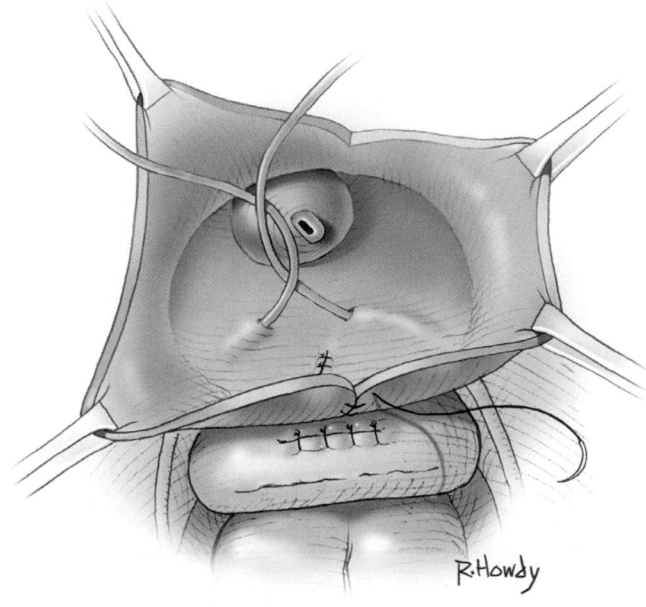

FIGURE 43-10.8 First-layer bladder closure.

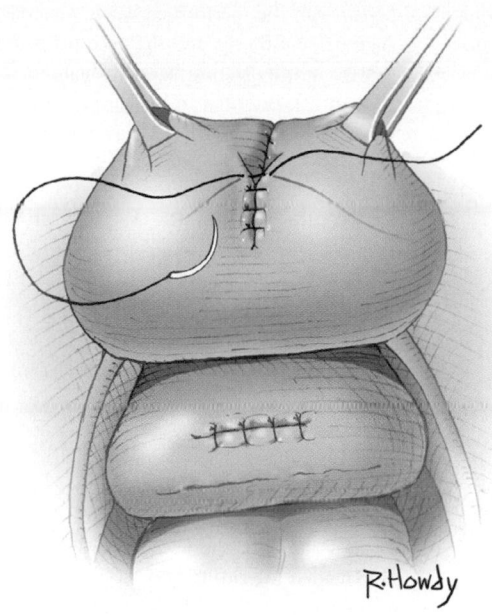

FIGURE 43-10.9 Second-layer bladder closure.

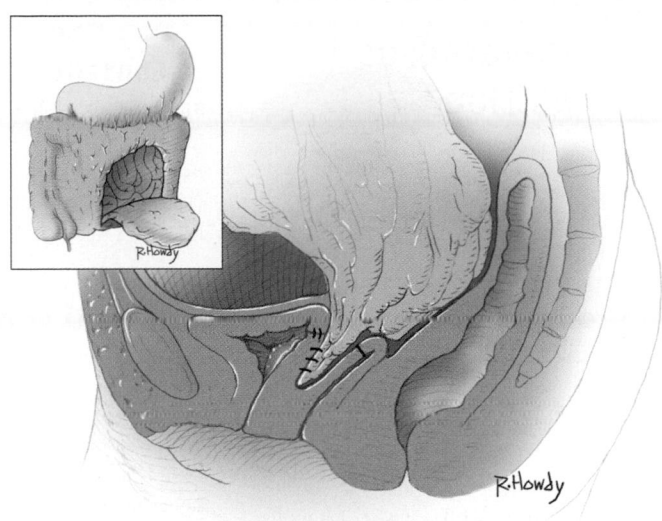

FIGURE 43-10.10 Omentum interposition.

suture line is covered and tension is released (Fig. 43-10.9).

❼ Omental or Peritoneal Interposition. As described in Section 44-16 (p. 1313), the omentum can be mobilized to create a J-flap. The omentum is then sutured to the anterior wall of the vagina to cover the incision line (Fig. 43-10.10). This provides a tissue layer between vagina and bladder, increases vascular flow to the area, and may improve tissue healing. Alternatively, if the omentum cannot be mobilized, peritoneum may be interposed between the bladder and vagina (Fig. 43-10.11).

❽ Cystoscopy. Cystoscopy is performed to document ureteral patency and to inspect the incision site.

❾ Incision Closure. The abdominal incision is closed as described in Sections 41-1 through 41-4 (p. 1020).

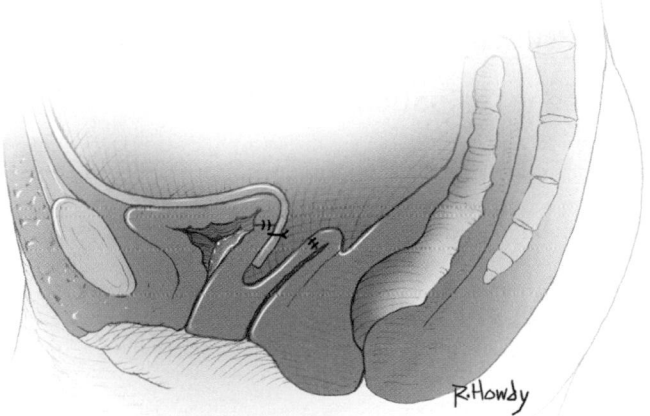

FIGURE 43-10.11 Peritoneum interposition.

POSTOPERATIVE

The bladder should be drained postoperatively to prevent overdistension and suture disruption. Placement of a transurethral or suprapubic catheter will ensure adequate drainage in the immediate postoperative period. At our institution, we generally continue catheterization for at least 3 weeks following vesicovaginal fistula repair. Antibiotic suppression is not required with this catheter use.

43-11

Martius Bulbocavernosus Fat Pad Flap

The Martius bulbocavernosus fat pad flap is a vascular graft that is commonly used in complex rectovaginal or vesicovaginal fistula repairs complicated by avascular or fibrotic tissue. Specifically, previously irradiated vaginal tissues often require this graft.

During graft placement, the fat pad overlying the bulbocavernosus muscle is first mobilized and subsequently brought to the fistula site through a vaginal incision. By means of this graft, fistula repair layers receive additional vascular support to increase rates of successful wound healing.

PREOPERATIVE

Patient Evaluation

In most instances, graft placement is anticipated for those with prior radiation or with fistula recurrence. Therefore, preoperative planning includes assessment of tissue vascularity, connective tissue strength, and ability to adequately mobilize vaginal tissues to create a multilayered fistula closure. To perform this procedure a woman must have adequate labial fat, and this should be assessed prior to surgery.

Consent

The consenting process for this procedure includes that for the primary fistula repair. Additionally, women are informed of the potential for postoperative vulvar numbness, pain, paresthesias, or hematoma.

Patient Preparation

Preoperative bowel preparation is indicated prior to use of a Martius flap to repair rectovaginal fistulas. Preparation protocols vary according to surgeon preference and may include administration of oral cathartic solutions, laxatives, or enemas (Table 39-7, p. 960). Because of the risk of poor wound healing in these complicated fistulas, antibiotic prophylaxis with a first- or second-generation cephalosporin or others listed in Table 39-6 (p. 959) is warranted. Thromboprophylaxis is given as outlined in Table 39-9 (p. 962).

INTRAOPERATIVE

SURGICAL STEPS

❶ Anesthesia and Patient Positioning. In most cases, a Martius flap graft and fistula repair can be performed with general or regional anesthesia, and the need for postoperative hospitalization is individualized. The patient is positioned in high lithotomy position, the vagina is surgically prepared, and a Foley catheter is placed.

❷ Fistula Repair. Rectovaginal or vesicovaginal fistulas are repaired as outlined in Sections 43-10 and 43-27 (pp. 1206 and 1255).

❸ Labial Incision. After completion of the fistula repair, the lateral margin of one labium majus is incised (Fig. 43-11.1). The length of the incision is tailored to specific labial anatomy and size of the graft needed. In many cases, a 6- to 8-cm incision is made beginning below the level of the clitoris and is extended inferiorly.

❹ Mobilization of the Fat Pad. Incision edges are retracted laterally, and sharp dissection is used to mobilize the bulbocavernosus fat pad (Fig. 43-11.2). This tissue is vascular, and vessels ideally are ligated prior to transection. A broad base is left inferiorly and the fat pad is detached superiorly.

❺ Graft Placement. After mobilization, a tunnel is created by bluntly dissecting with a hemostat from the vulvar incision underneath the vaginal epithelium to the fistula site. The tunnel must

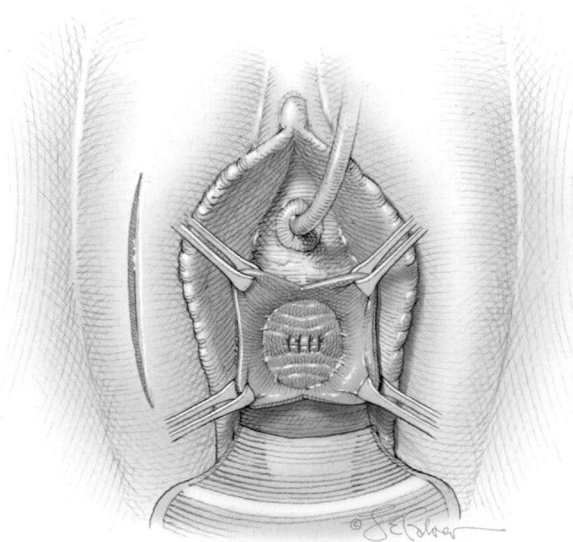

FIGURE 43-11.1 Labial incision.

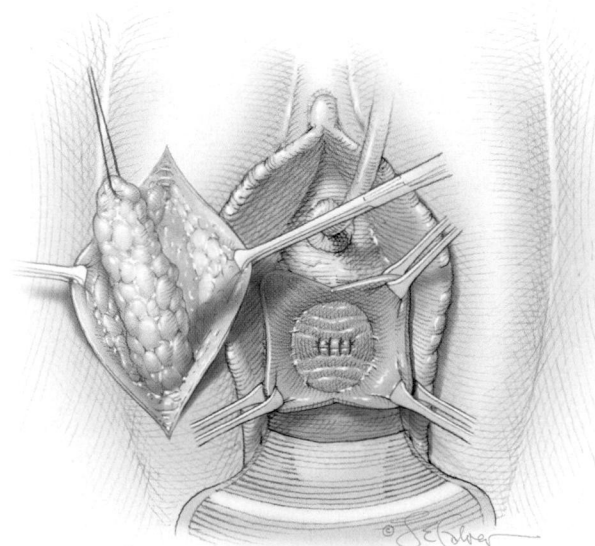

FIGURE 43-11.2 Mobilization of the fat pad.

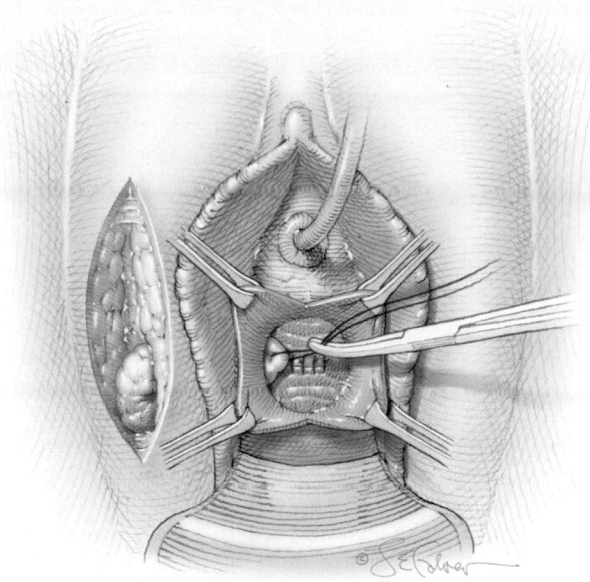

FIGURE 43-11.3 Graft placement.

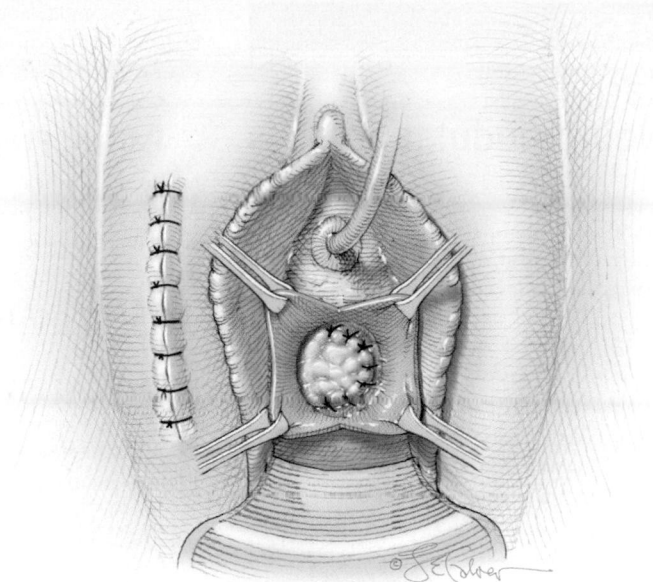

FIGURE 43-11.4 Graft fixation.

be of sufficient breadth to avoid vascular compression and graft necrosis. A suture is placed at the graft tip and used to pass the graft through the tunnel and into the vagina (Fig. 43-11.3).

❻ **Graft Fixation.** The graft is secured to the vaginal muscularis overlying the fistula repair with several interrupted stitches using 3-0 delayed-absorbable suture (Fig. 43-11.4).

❼ **Incision Closure.** The vulvar incision is closed along its length with interrupted 3-0 delayed-absorbable sutures. The vaginal mucosa overlying the fistula is closed with a continuous running technique using 3-0 delayed-absorbable suture.

POSTOPERATIVE

Care after surgery is predominantly dictated by the associated fistula repair. However, sitz baths twice daily are typically added to improve pain and healing of the vulvar incision.

43-12

Sacral Neuromodulation

Sacral neuromodulation is a technique that delivers electrical stimulation to the pelvic plexus and pudendal nerves. This device is a U.S. Food and Drug Administration (FDA)-approved treatment for selected cases of urinary urgency-frequency syndrome, urge urinary incontinence, nonobstructive urinary retention, and fecal incontinence. Although not FDA approved for pelvic pain and interstitial cystitis, it is sometimes used for these indications if they are associated with urgency, frequency, or retention. This surgery is typically performed on women who have failed to improve adequately with multiple other conservative therapies. The mechanism of action is unclear, but it is believed to modulate reflex pathways.

Sacral neuromodulation is generally completed in two steps. In the first stage, a lead is placed into the sacrum and connected to a temporary external stimulus generator via an extension device. A test stimulation period of approximately 2 weeks follows. If symptoms are decreased by 50 percent during the next several weeks, then a permanent implantable pulse generator (IPG) is placed in the superior buttock fat in a second surgical procedure.

PREOPERATIVE

Patient Evaluation

Prior to surgery, women should have completed full evaluation including urodynamic testing, voiding diary, cystoscopy, and other selected tests.

Consent

After the first stage, a 50-percent improvement in symptoms is considered a benchmark of success. Approximately 75 percent of patients achieve this level of improvement and are candidates for permanent IPG placement. Common complications following stage 1 include lack of clinical response or infection. For those who undergo second-stage implantation, approximately 80 percent reach the improvement benchmark and have greater than 50-percent improvement in symptoms.

Following the second stage, pain at the IPG site, infection, and lack of clinical response are common complications. After

sacral neuromodulation, magnetic resonance imaging and security wanding at airport security checkpoints are contraindications.

Patient Preparation

No specific patient preparation is needed. Antibiotic and thromboprophylaxis as well as bowel preparation are not required.

INTRAOPERATIVE

SURGICAL STEPS

❶ Anesthesia and Patient Positioning. General anesthesia is required to protect the airway, but neuromuscular blockade is contraindicated as this will prohibit neuromuscular stimulation evaluation. The patient is positioned prone on a Wilson frame or with a pillow under the abdomen and knees. The buttocks are separated to allow visualization of anus and perineum. The sacrum and perianal area are surgically prepared. A Foley catheter is typically not required due to the surgery's brevity.

❷ Identification of S3 Foramina. These landmarks are the site of lead placement and are located approximately 9 cm above the coccyx and 1 to 2 cm lateral to the midline. Foramina are outlined with a surgical marker. A foramina needle is placed horizontally at the suspected level of S3 and a confirmatory fluoroscopic image is obtained.

❸ Foramina Needle Insertion. The needle is inserted into the skin above the

foramina and is guided at a 60-degree-angle caudally into the opening (Fig. 43-12.1). If possible, the needle is placed concordant with patient handedness. Needle stimulation of S3 nerves causes contraction of the levator ani muscles, which appears as an inward bellows-like movement and causes great-toe dorsiflexion. Pelvic floor reflexes are checked, and when appropriate S3 reflexes are obtained (bellows and toe), lead placement is initiated.

❹ Lead Placement. A guide wire is placed down the foramina needle under fluoroscopic guidance. The needle is then removed, and a small stab incision is made at the point where the guide wire enters the skin. A sharp trocar is then passed over the guide wire into the foramina, again under fluoroscopic guidance. The guide wire is removed from the trocar. With continued fluoroscopy, a tined lead is then passed down the trocar into the appropriate position at the S3 foramina. All four electrodes on the lead are tested for S3 pelvic floor reflexes, and after the lead is correctly positioned, the trocar is removed. The tines lock into place when the trocar is removed. Thus, the lead cannot be repositioned after this point.

❺ Pulse Generator Incision and Lead Passage. A 4- to 6-cm incision is made over the lateral buttock. Sharp and blunt dissection is used to create a deep pocket that can house the extension device for the temporary external pulse generator and eventually can house the permanent IPG. The pocket should be deep enough into the subcutaneous tissue that it does not indent the skin, but it should not sit directly above the muscle.

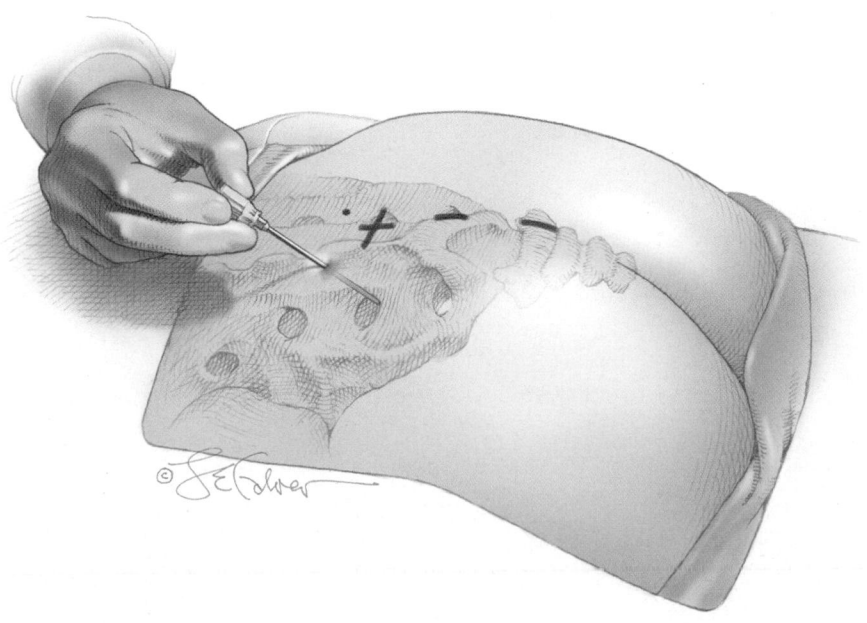

FIGURE 43-12.1 Foramen needle insertion.

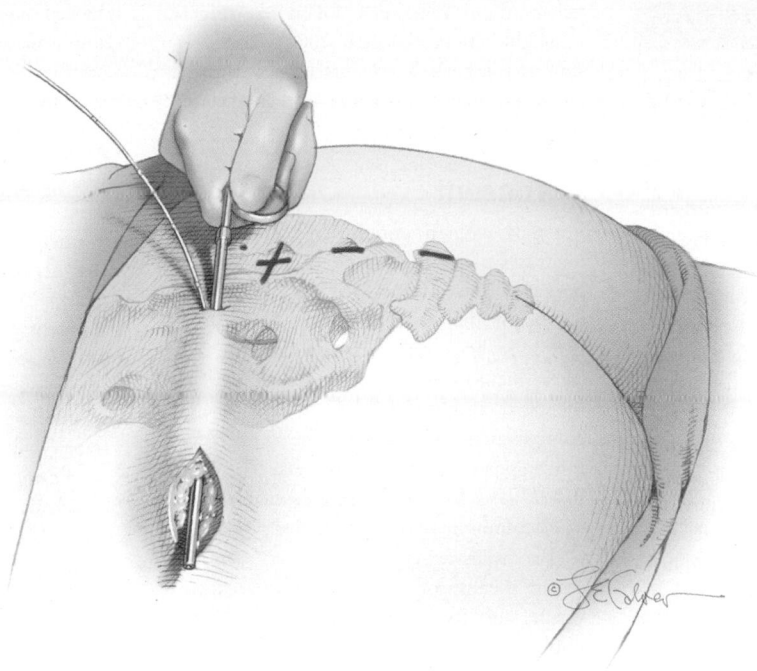

FIGURE 43-12.2 Pulse generator incision and lead passage.

After a pocket is created, a tunneling device is used to feed the lead laterally from the midline incision into the pocket (Fig. 43-12.2).

⑥ Placement of the Extension Device (First Stage). In the pocket, the lead is connected to an external extension wire. An additional stab incision is then created lateral to the pocket, and the tunneling device is used to guide the extension wire through the pocket and out this stab incision. The subcutaneous tissue is then closed with 2-0 delayed-absorbable suture in a running fashion. The skin is closed with a subcuticular stitch using 4-0 delayed-absorbable suture and Dermabond. The extension wire is connected to an external temporary pulse generator, which is used for 1 to 4 weeks to assess neuromodulation efficacy.

⑦ Implantable Pulse Generator Placement (Second Stage). If significant relief of symptoms is obtained, the permanent IPG is placed 1 to 4 weeks after the initial surgery. The procedure is performed with the patient prone and usually with general anesthesia for airway control. The buttock incision is opened down to the connection site between the lead and the external extension wire, and the previously created pocket is reopened. The external extender wire is removed, and the permanent IPG is connected to the lead (Fig. 43-12.3). The incision is closed as in step 6.

POSTOPERATIVE

Pain or erythema at the incision site suggests cellulitis, abscess, or seroma. These symptoms should be evaluated as soon as possible, and antibiotics are instituted if needed. Unusual pain should also be evaluated immediately as this could suggest lead malfunction. A woman can turn the device off by herself if necessary.

Symptoms are continually assessed postoperatively, and the IPG is reprogrammed as needed. Reprogramming the device or changing leads will often lead to symptom improvement.

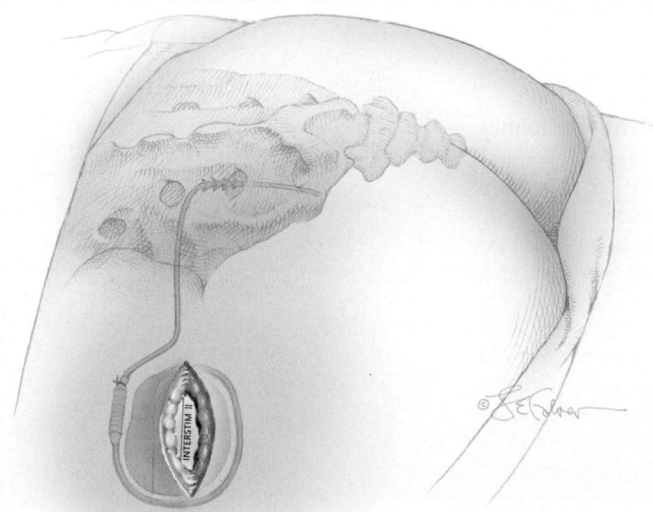

FIGURE 43-12.3 Implantable pulse generator placement.

43-13

Anterior Colporrhaphy

Anterior colporrhaphy is one of the more commonly performed gynecologic surgeries. Although it is still used as a primary choice for repair of anterior vaginal wall prolapse (cystocele), randomized trials suggest that anatomic cure is obtained in 50 percent or fewer patients (Weber, 2001). Therefore, several different techniques are used to augment traditional anterior colporrhaphy. These include vaginal paravaginal repair and reinforcement with synthetic or biologic mesh.

During the traditional anterior colporrhaphy procedure (midline plication), attenuated supporting fascia between the vagina and bladder is reapproximated and reinforced using plication sutures. This bolstering along the length of the vagina attempts to elevate the bladder and urethra to a more anterior and anatomically normal position. The vaginal paravaginal repair attempts to provide lateral support to the anterior vaginal wall, whereas mesh augmentation procedures may be used to add tissue strength and provide lateral and midline support.

In observational series, success rates for mesh augmentation range from 93 to 100 percent after 2 years (Julian, 1996; Mage, 1999; Migliari, 1999). However, in randomized studies, mesh repair compared with traditional colporrhaphy offered only a modest 15 to 23-percent greater improvement rate (Altman, 2011; Sand, 2001; Weber, 2001). Additionally, the associated risks of mesh erosion and infection should be factored into any decision to add reinforcing mesh (Cervigni, 2001). Cadaveric fascia has been similarly used. Gandhi and colleagues (2005), however, found no improved rates of surgical success using this material.

In women with cystocele, other points of pelvic support may also require concurrent repair. Accordingly, anterior colporrhaphy is frequently performed in combination with corrective surgeries for enterocele, rectocele, and vaginal apex prolapse.

PREOPERATIVE

Patient Evaluation

Women with anterior vaginal wall prolapse commonly have associated stress urinary incontinence (SUI) (Borstad, 1989). Even those who are continent, however, may have SUI unmasked following anterior vaginal wall prolapse correction. Thus, preoperative urodynamic evaluation is recommended. During this evaluation, the prolapse is reduced to its anticipated postoperative position to mimic

pelvic floor dynamics following surgery (Chaikin, 2000; Yamada, 2001). The decision to perform a concurrent prophylactic antiincontinence procedure is then dictated by individual urodynamic findings.

Consent

For most women, anterior colporrhaphy has low rates of complications. Of these, recurrence of the anterior vaginal wall defect is one of the most common. Several factors have been noted to increase this risk. These include a large original defect and an increased number of other prolapsed pelvic compartments. In addition to prolapse recurrence, postoperative dyspareunia has been noted. Less frequently, serious hemorrhage or cystotomy may complicate this procedure.

For transvaginal pelvic organ prolapse repair, the use of synthetic mesh is controversial, and recently, the U.S. FDA (2011) published a safety communication. They listed known risks, which include erosion, infection, chronic pain, dyspareunia, organ perforation, and urinary problems. Moreover, they noted that the consenting process should inform the patient of these risks, the possible need of additional surgery due to mesh-related complications, and the potential irreversibility of these complications in a small number of patients.

Patient Preparation

To decompress the rectum and thereby increase operating space within the vagina, bowel preparation is typically administered the evening prior to surgery. Suitable antibiotics for prophylaxis are found in Table 39-6 (p. 959). Thromboprophylaxis is given as outlined in Table 39-9 (p. 962).

INTRAOPERATIVE

SURGICAL STEPS

❶ Anesthesia and Patient Positioning. After adequate general or regional anesthesia is administered, a patient is placed in dorsal lithotomy position, the vagina is surgically prepared, and a Foley catheter is inserted. An Auvard weighted speculum is positioned to retract the posterior vaginal wall.

❷ Concurrent Surgery. If other reconstructive surgeries are required, they may precede or follow anterior colporrhaphy. Anterior colporrhaphy may be performed with the uterus in situ or alternatively, following hysterectomy.

❸ Vaginal Incision. One to 2 cm distal to the vaginal apex, two Allis clamps are placed on each side of the anterior vaginal wall (Fig. 43-13.1). These clamps are gently pulled laterally to create tension, and the vaginal wall between them

is incised transversely. Following incision, a third clamp is placed in the midline, 3 to 4 cm distal to this incision. All three clamps are held, creating gentle outward tension.

❹ Tissue Plane Dissection. The tips of curved Metzenbaum scissors are insinuated beneath the vaginal mucosa. Scissor blades are opened and closed, while the surgeon exerts gentle forward pressure that is parallel to and within the plane underlying the vaginal mucosa. This technique allows separation of the mucosa from the fibromuscular layer. This dissection continues caudad to reach the midline Allis clamp. The undermined vaginal wall is then incised longitudinally.

Additional Allis clamps are placed, one on each freed mucosal edge. The more distal central Allis clamp is moved 3 to 4 cm further distally. The steps of vaginal wall dissection are then repeated. This process continues until the wall has been bisected and dissected to within 2 to 3 cm of the urethral meatus (Fig. 43-13.2). This ending spot corresponds to a midpoint along the length of the urethra.

The lateral attachments of the vaginal wall to the underlying fibromuscular layer are next separated (Fig. 43-13.3). With one finger behind one of the incised vaginal walls, the scissors are held parallel to the wall, and the vaginal epithelial layer is sharply dissected from the fibromuscular layer. A combination of sharp and blunt dissection is used, and once the proper tissue plane is entered, the layers readily separate. This dissection is extended laterally and almost reaches the pubic rami.

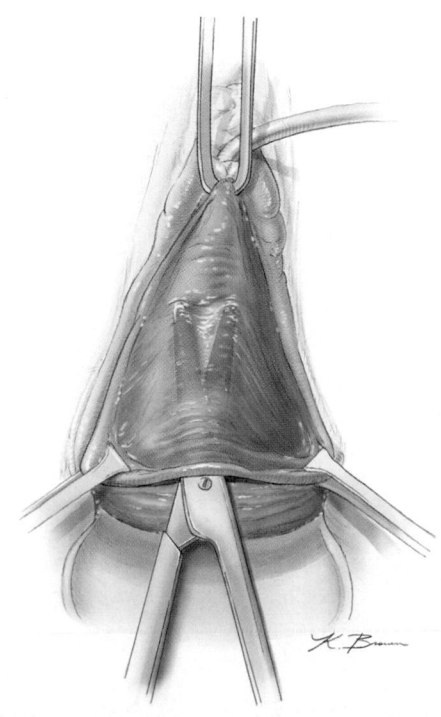

FIGURE 43-13.1 Tissue plane dissection.

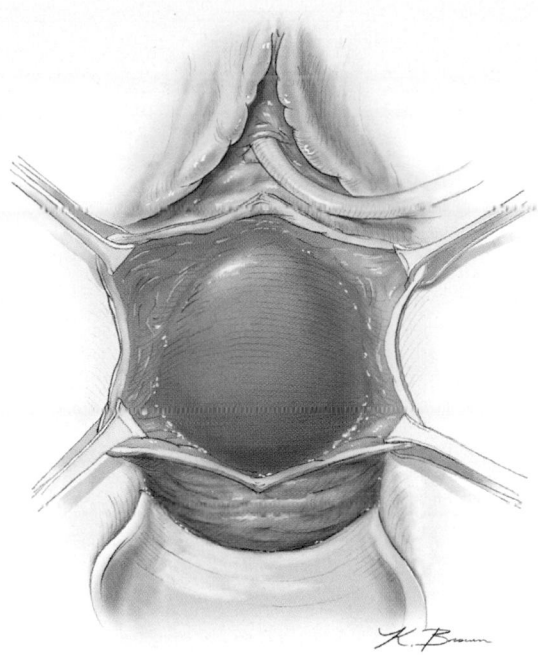

FIGURE 43-13.2 Vaginal incision.

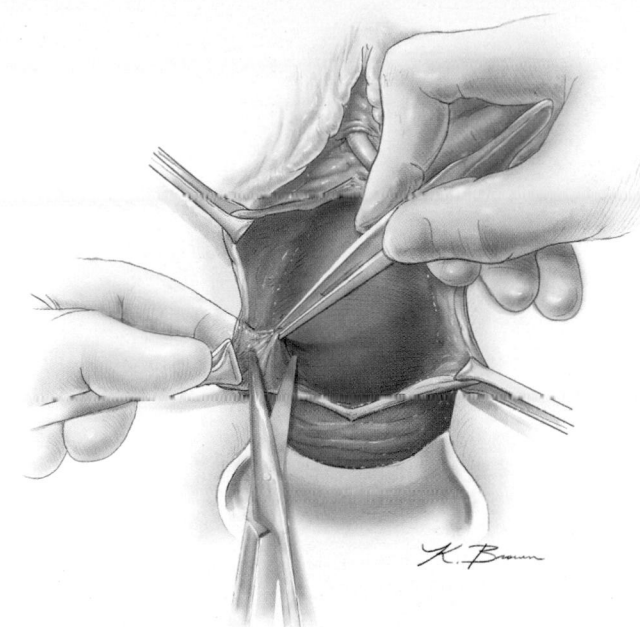

FIGURE 43-13.3 Separation of mucosa and fibromuscular layer.

❺ Traditional Anterior Colporrhaphy (Midline Plication). Plication of the fibromuscular layer is then begun. Interrupted sutures of 2-0 permanent or delayed-absorbable on an SH needle are placed in the midline along the length of the vaginal wall (Fig. 43-13.4). Plication of the fascia creates a double layer of fascia to support the bladder and urethra. Fascial tension should create a firm shelf overlying the bladder. Extreme tension is avoided to prevent sutures from pulling through the fascia or from excessively narrowing the vagina. As sutures are tied, the bladder is pushed by the surgeon gently upward and away from the incision line. A second layer of plication sutures is placed beginning lateral to the first if necessary (see Fig. 43-13.4).

❻ Vaginal Paravaginal Repair. If vaginal paravaginal repair is to be performed, lateral dissection proceeds along the ischiopubic rami from the pubic symphysis to the ischial spine. Blunt dissection is used to enter the space of Retzius. If a paravaginal defect is present, the space is easily entered. The arcus tendineus fascia pelvis is seen as a white line running from the ischial spine to the symphysis. Visualization is aided with the use of Breisky-Navratil and lighted retractors.

A series of four to six 0-gauge nonabsorbable sutures are placed in the arcus tendineus or obturator fascia and attached to the lateral edge of the vaginal fibromuscular layer (Fig. 43-13.5). This is then repeated on the other side. If necessary, a midline plication can be performed after the vaginal

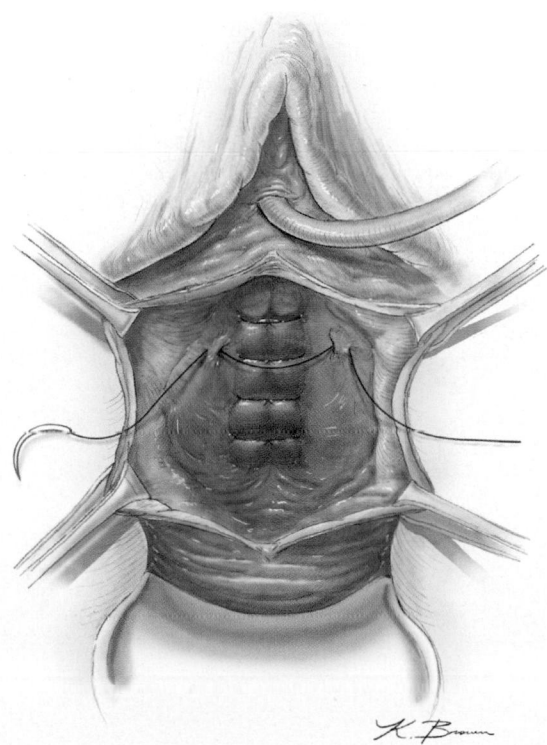

FIGURE 43-13.4 Midline plication.

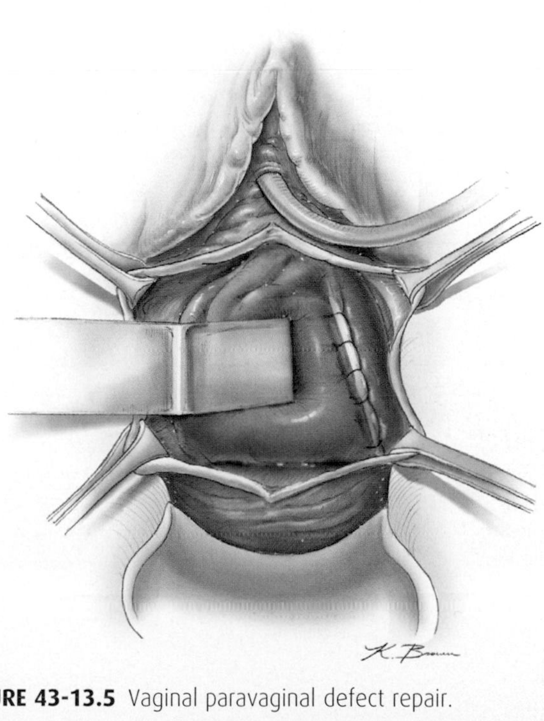

FIGURE 43-13.5 Vaginal paravaginal defect repair.

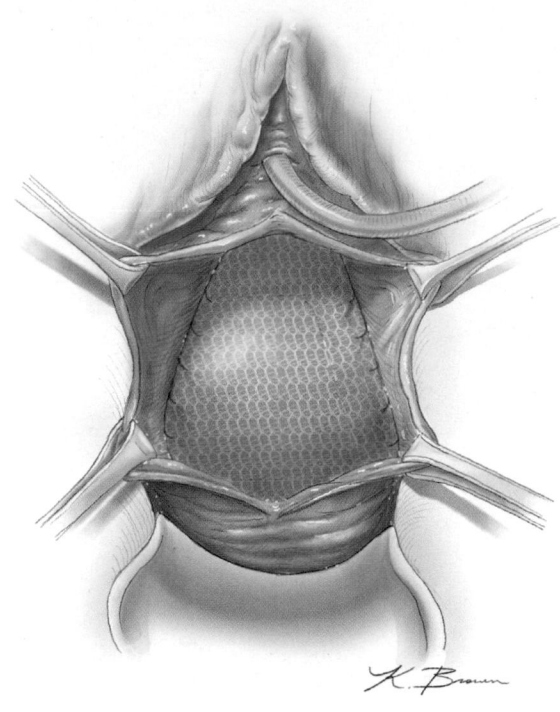

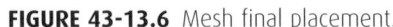

FIGURE 43-13.6 Mesh final placement.

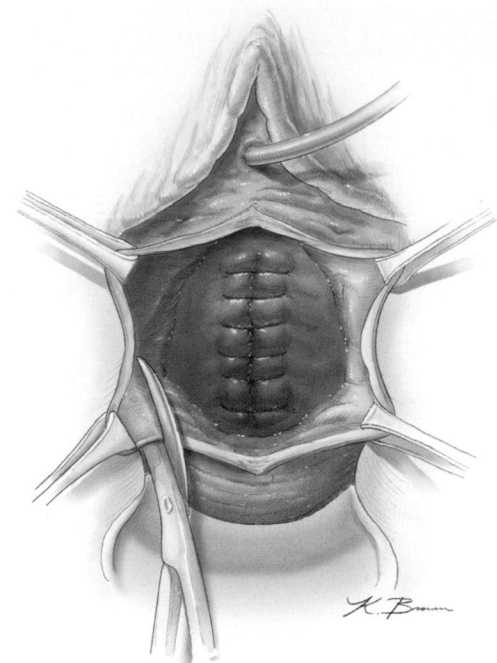

FIGURE 43-13.7 Second layer of plication and excess mucosa trimmed.

paravaginal sutures are tied. However, the vaginal wall should not be placed on tension.

❼ Mesh Augmentation. For the mesh augmentation procedure, the dissection proceeds similarly to that for the paravaginal repair. The mesh is cut in a trapezoidal shape and is attached to the arcus tendineus fascia pelvis with four 2-0 permanent sutures on each side (Fig. 43-13.6). Mesh augmentation may be used solely to reinforce an anterior wall defect or may be used after midline plication as described earlier in step 3.

❽ Incision Closure. Depending on the size of the original cystocele, some redundant vaginal wall will likely be present and require trimming (Fig. 43-13.7). Liberal trimming, however, can place the vaginal wall incision on excessive tension, affect wound healing, and narrow the vagina. Therefore, care should be taken to minimized tissue excision. The vaginal mucosa is reapproximated in a running fashion with 2-0 delayed-absorbable suture.

❾ Cystoscopy. Kwon and colleagues (2002) performed cystoscopy following 346 anterior colporrhaphy procedures and found unexpected injury in 2 percent of cases. These each required suture removal and replacement. Accordingly, cystoscopy may be warranted to document integrity of the ureteral orifices, bladder, and urethral lumen.

POSTOPERATIVE

Recovery following anterior colporrhaphy for most women is rapid and associated with few complications. Urinary retention or urinary tract infection, however, is common. In anticipation of retention, many advocate bladder drainage until urine residuals fall below 200 mL.

As with other vaginal surgery, diet and activity can be advanced as tolerated. Women, however, should abstain from intercourse until wound healing is complete, typically at 6 to 8 weeks following repair.

43-14

Abdominal Paravaginal Defect Repair

Paravaginal defect repair (PVDR) is a prolapse procedure that corrects lateral defects in the anterior vaginal wall. The procedure involves attachment of the lateral vaginal wall to the arcus tendineus fascia pelvis (Fig. 38-15, p. 931). Over the past 20 years, PVDR has become popular, as lateral defects in the anterior vaginal wall and their relationship to prolapse pathophysiology are more completely understood. Paravaginal defect repair is frequently performed in conjunction with the antiincontinence Burch procedure. Within this combination, paravaginal defect repair provides support to the mid- and upper vagina, whereas the Burch procedure provides mid- and distal support. PVDR is primarily a prolapse operation, and it has not been shown to be an effective treatment for stress urinary incontinence (SUI). This procedure can be performed alone or in combination with other prolapse procedures.

Paravaginal defect repair can also be performed laparoscopically by those with advanced laparoscopic skills. If sutures can be placed the same as in the abdominal approach, the results are expected to be equivalent.

PREOPERATIVE

Patient Evaluation

Demonstration of lateral vaginal wall defects on physical examination is required prior to surgery as outlined in Chapter 24 (p. 646). If significant anterior wall prolapse is identified, evaluation for SUI or potential SUI should be pursued. In women who have an isolated paravaginal defect, there is the risk that other pelvic support defects such as apical or posterior vaginal prolapse may develop. Thus, attempts to identify these potential defects should precede surgery. In some instances, prophylactic repair of potential defects is indicated.

Consent

Paravaginal defect repair provides effective support to the lateral vaginal walls, but as with other prolapse procedures, long-term success rates diminish with time. The procedure involves surgery in the space of Retzius, which has the potential for significant blood loss. In particular, those who have had prior surgery in this space are at increased risk of significant hemorrhage. Inaccurate suture placement can result in injury to the bladder and/or ureters, although this is uncommon. Additional complications include urinary incontinence or retention.

Patient Preparation

As with most abdominal urogynecologic surgeries, antibiotic prophylaxis is given to prevent wound infection (Table 39-6, p. 959). It is our practice to recommend bowel preparation prior to PVDR to decompress the bowel, although this practice is not mandatory (Table 39-7, p. 960). However, if this procedure is performed in combination with more extensive pelvic reconstructive surgeries, then thorough bowel evacuation is warranted. Thromboprophylaxis is given as outlined in Table 39-9 (p. 962).

INTRAOPERATIVE

SURGICAL STEPS

❶ Anesthesia and Patient Positioning. This surgery is typically performed as an inpatient procedure under general or regional anesthesia. Following administration of anesthesia, the patient should be positioned in Allen stirrups. Adequate exposure to the vagina is vital because a vaginal hand is used to elevate the paravaginal space to aid dissection. The abdomen and vagina are surgically prepared, and a Foley catheter with a 10-mL balloon is inserted.

❷ Abdominal Incision. A low transverse incision placed 1 cm superior to the symphysis pubis affords the best exposure to the space of Retzius (Section 41-2, p. 1022). Entry into the peritoneal cavity is not necessary. However, this may assist in placement of an abdominal self-retaining retractor.

❸ Entering the Space of Retzius. After incision of the fascia, the rectus muscles are separated in the midline and retractors are used to hold them in apposition. Careful dissection of this space decreases the risk of hemorrhage and creates accurate tissue planes for suture placement. The correct plane of dissection for opening the space of Retzius is directly behind the pubic bone. Loose areolar tissue is gently dissected in a mediolateral fashion with fingers or sponge beginning immediately behind the pubic bone (Fig. 43-14.1). If the correct plane is entered, this avascular potential space opens easily and without significant hemorrhage. If bleeding does occur, it is likely that the wrong tissue plane has been entered.

After the medial portion of the space of Retzius is opened, the obturator canal should be palpated bilaterally so that the vessels and nerve within this area can be avoided. The ischial spine is then palpated 4 to 5 cm directly below the obturator canal. The remainder of the paravaginal space is opened with gentle finger dissection or gentle insertion of 4 × 4-inch gauze sponges into the lateral paravaginal spaces. This is aided by a vaginal hand pushing up into the space.

Large paravaginal blood vessels are noted along the lateral vaginal wall. Bleeding from these vessels is easily controlled by upward pressure of the vaginal hand while hemostatic sutures are placed.

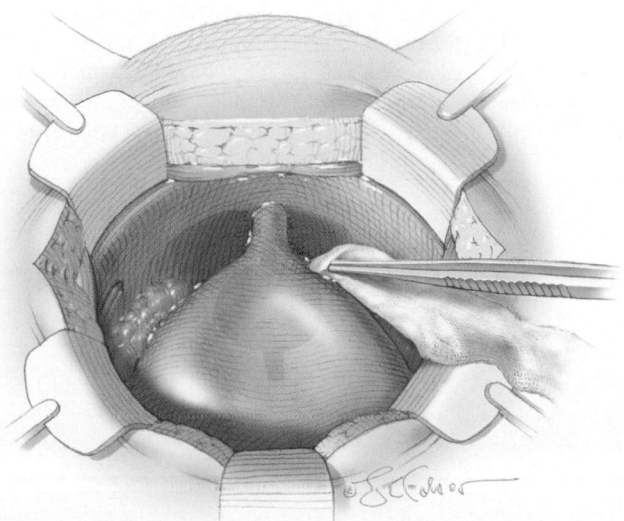

FIGURE 43-14.1 Dissection in the space of Retzius.

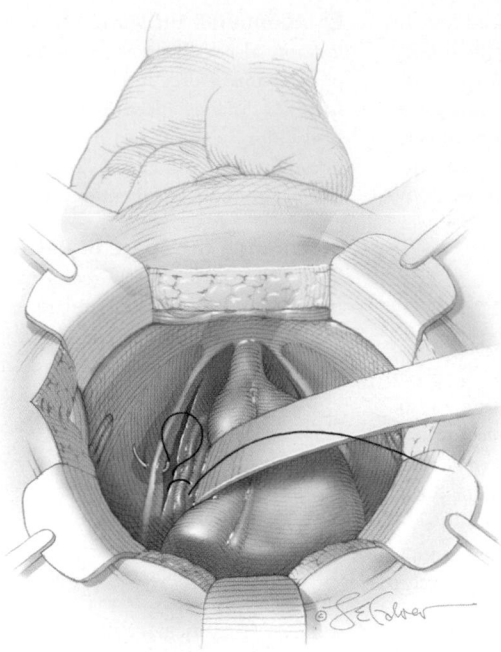

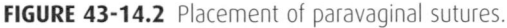

FIGURE 43-14.2 Placement of paravaginal sutures.

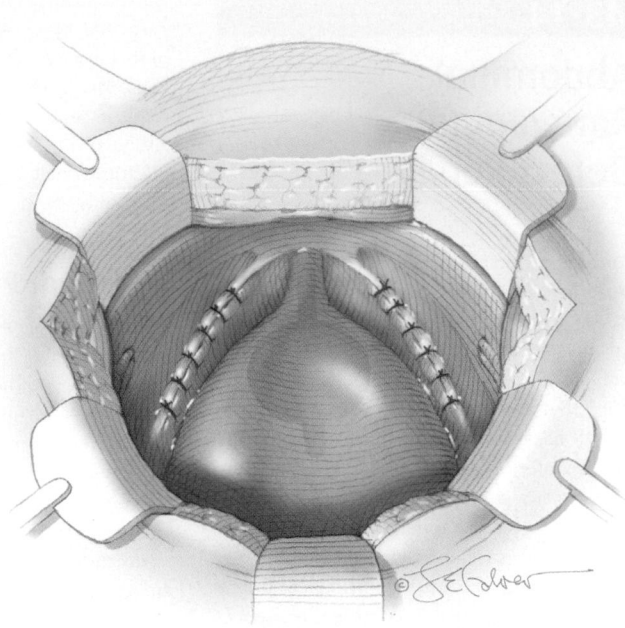

FIGURE 43-14.3 Final suture placement.

❹ Identification of the Arcus Tendineus Fascia Pelvis. The arcus tendineus fascia pelvis runs between the pubic symphysis and the ischial spine (Fig. 38-24, p. 940). It is observed in this location along the sidewall as a condensation of white connective tissue. In those with defects, it may be torn in the middle or completely avulsed from the sidewall.

❺ Placement of Paravaginal Sutures. With a hand in the vagina pressing upward into the paravaginal space, a medium-sized malleable retractor is used to reflect the bladder medially and protect it from inadvertent suture placement.

The most cephalad suture is the first one placed (Fig. 43-14.2). A thimble-covered vaginal finger presses upward, against the lateral vaginal wall, and a 2-0 permanent figure-of-eight suture is placed around the paravaginal vessels, taking care to avoid entry into the vaginal lumen. If bleeding follows,

the suture is tied to constrict involved vessels. The suture is then placed through the arcus tendineus fascia pelvis at a point 1 to 2 cm caudad to the ischial spine. Sutures are not tied until all paravaginal sutures have been placed. During suture placement, the obturator canal and neurovascular bundle should be visualized and avoided. Three to five more paravaginal stitches are then placed at 1-cm intervals until the level of the bladder neck is reached. After all sutures are placed, they are tied, and the procedure is repeated on the other side of the vagina (Fig. 43-14.3).

❻ Cystoscopy. One-half to one ampule of intravenous indigo carmine is administered, and cystoscopy is performed. Efflux from both ureteral orifices must be seen. In addition, the bladder surfaces should be inspected for sutures. A misplaced suture might be seen as a dimple in the bladder wall. If found, sutures entering the bladder should be removed and properly placed.

❼ Incision Closure. After vigorous irrigation of the space of Retzius, the abdomen is closed in a standard fashion (Section 41-2, p. 1023). If the peritoneum was opened, closure is recommended to prevent small bowel adhesions in the space of Retzius.

❽ Concurrent Procedures. In patients with stress urinary incontinence, a Burch procedure might be performed after placement of paravaginal sutures. In this case, cystoscopy is delayed until after the Burch procedure is completed.

POSTOPERATIVE

In general, recovery follows that associated with laparotomy and varies depending on concurrent surgeries and incision size. A voiding trial as described in Chapter 39 (p. 966) is performed prior to hospital discharge.

43-15

Posterior Colporrhaphy

Posterior colporrhaphy is traditionally used to repair prolapse of the posterior vaginal wall (rectocele). Specifically, posterior colporrhaphy techniques attempt to reinforce the fibromuscular layer of tissue between the vagina and rectum to prevent prolapse of the rectum into the vaginal lumen.

In many situations, the apex of the posterior vaginal wall must also be suspended to obtain successful repair. Thus, if care is not given to apical descent, recurrent prolapse may follow. Additionally, perineorrhaphy is often carried out in conjunction with posterior colporrhaphy.

Variations of posterior colporrhaphy have been developed to improve success rates. Current methods include midline plication, defect-directed repair, and placement of reinforcing materials. Evidence, however, does not indicate that one of these is more effective.

PREOPERATIVE

Patient Evaluation

A detailed discussion of symptoms should begin every patient evaluation prior to colporrhaphy. Often, patients may associate all of their bowel symptoms to the presence of a posterior wall bulge, but the two may not be related. Specifically, if constipation is a major complaint, then a trial of nonsurgical treatment may be indicated (Table 11-8, p. 323). Symptoms most likely to be to cured by this procedure include the need to digitally decompress the rectal vault and the sensation of vaginal bulge.

Posterior wall prolapse commonly accompanies other support defects, and patients should undergo a complete pelvic organ prolapse examination as described in Chapter 24 (p. 644). If concurrent anterior vaginal wall or vaginal apex prolapse is present, this should also be repaired.

Consent

In addition to standard surgical risks, this procedure may be associated with failure to correct symptoms or anatomy. Therefore, a patient and surgeon should identify treatment goals and discuss expectations. In the few randomized studies that have been done, current techniques give a less than optimal anatomic repair, and success rates approximate 70 percent. An additional common postoperative risk is dyspareunia. Injury to the rectum is rare.

For transvaginal pelvic organ prolapse repair, the use of synthetic mesh is controversial, and recently, the U.S. FDA (2011) published a safety communication. They listed known risks, which include erosion, infection, chronic pain, dyspareunia, organ perforation, and urinary problems. Moreover, they noted that the consenting process should inform the patient of these risks, the possible need of additional surgery due to mesh-related complications, and the potential irreversibility of these complications in a small number of patients.

Patient Preparation

A thorough bowel preparation is indicated to prevent fecal contamination during surgery (Table 39-7, p. 960). Additionally, delay of immediate postoperative defecation may be beneficial for patient comfort and can be achieved with a clear liquid or low-residue diet. Antibiotic and thromboprophylaxis are given as outlined in Tables 39-6 and 39-9 (p. 959).

INTRAOPERATIVE

SURGICAL STEPS

❶ **Anesthesia and Patient Positioning.** Posterior colporrhaphy is typically an inpatient procedure, performed under general or regional anesthesia. A patient is placed in high lithotomy position with stirrups of a surgeon's choosing, and the vagina is surgically prepared. A Foley catheter is not needed unless required by other concurrent surgeries.

❷ **Vaginal Incision and Dissection.** Corners of the introitus are grasped with Allis clamps. A third Allis clamp is placed in the vaginal midline at the proximal apex of the vaginal bulge. At the perineum, a horizontal incision is made and extended between the Allis clamps at the introitus.

Metzenbaum scissors are then used to develop the incision by undermining the vaginal mucosa (Fig. 43-15.1). Because of fusion

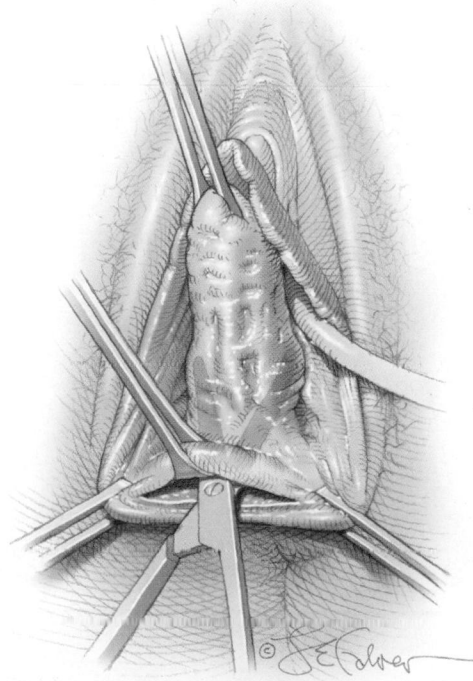

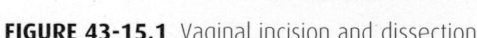

FIGURE 43-15.1 Vaginal incision and dissection.

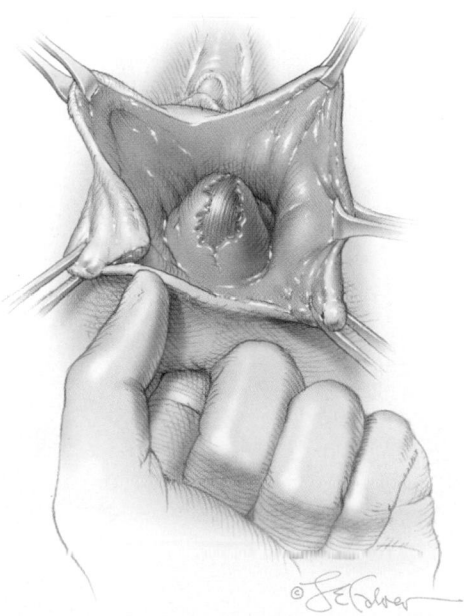

FIGURE 43-15.2 Rectal examination.

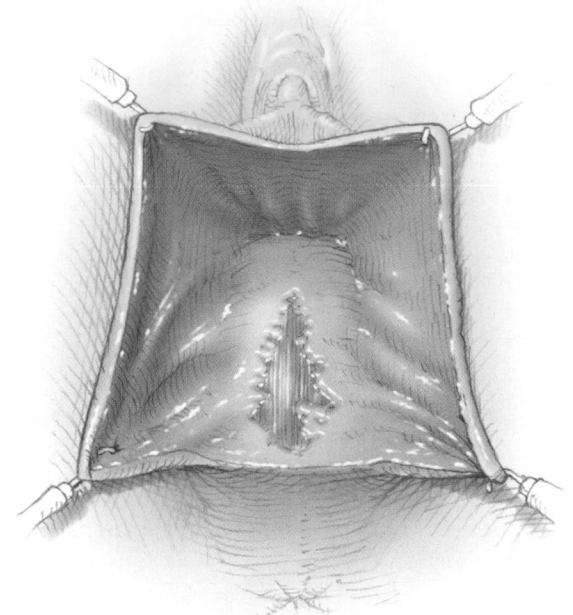

FIGURE 43-15.3 Midline defect.

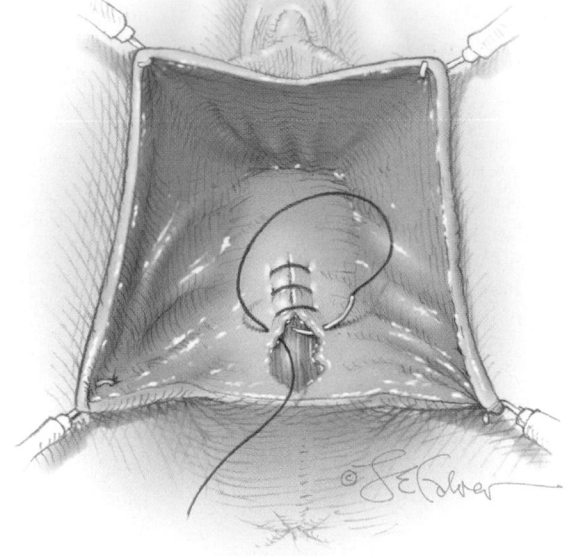

FIGURE 43-15.4 Midline plication.

of the fibromuscular layer within the perineal body, as well as possible scarring from prior episiotomy, clear tissue planes are not typically present. Thus, in the area immediately adjacent to the perineal body, sharp dissection is required. Once the vaginal mucosa is reached, however, clear tissue planes are typically encountered, and blunt dissection can be combined with sharp dissection.

During dissection, care should be taken to stay in the correct tissue plane. Scissor tips are positioned deep to and parallel to the vaginal mucosa. Deep dissection can lead to entry into the rectum, whereas superficial dissection can

create defects in the vaginal mucosa, often called "button holes." Dissection should extend cephalad to the level of the proximal Allis clamp previously placed at the apex.

A midline incision is then made from the perineal incision to the apex using Metzenbaum scissors. The edges of the midline incision are grasped with Allis clamps. Additional bilateral sharp and blunt dissection is typically necessary to further separate the fibromuscular layer from the vaginal epithelium laterally.

❸ **Rectal Examination.** Rectal examination is performed to identify the fibromuscular

layer as well as the rectal wall and the levator ani muscles (Fig. 43-15.2).

❹ **Midline Plication.** A series of interrupted 2-0 delayed-absorbable or permanent sutures are used to plicate the vaginal muscularis in the midline, and the line of plication sutures extends from the apex to the perineum (Figs. 43-15.3 and 43-15.4). A second layer of interrupted sutures then plicates muscularis that lies lateral to tissues approximated with the first layer. These sutures are secured in the midline over the first layer.

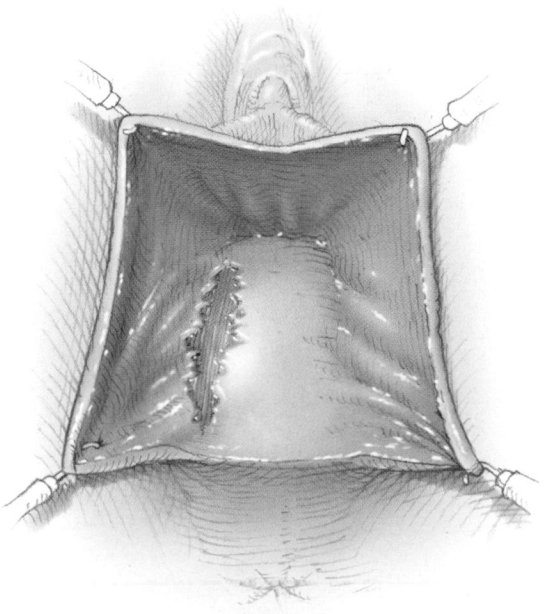

FIGURE 43-15.5 Lateral defect.

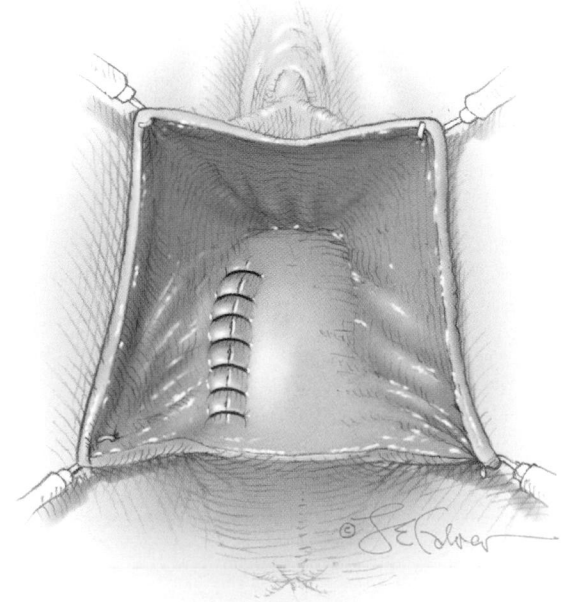

FIGURE 43-15.6 Defect-directed repair.

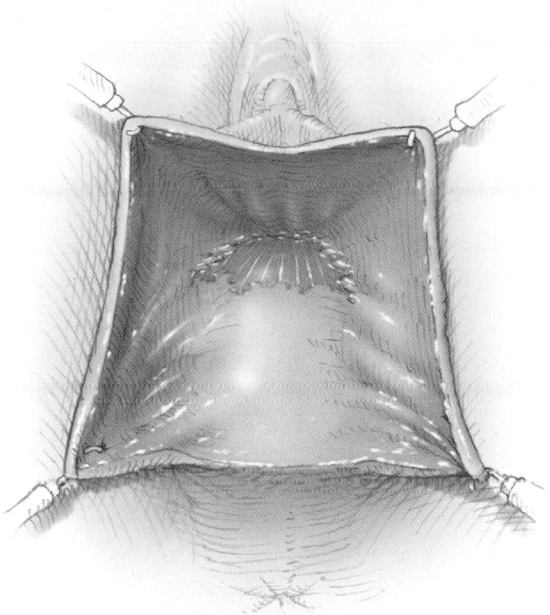

FIGURE 43-15.7 Proximal defect.

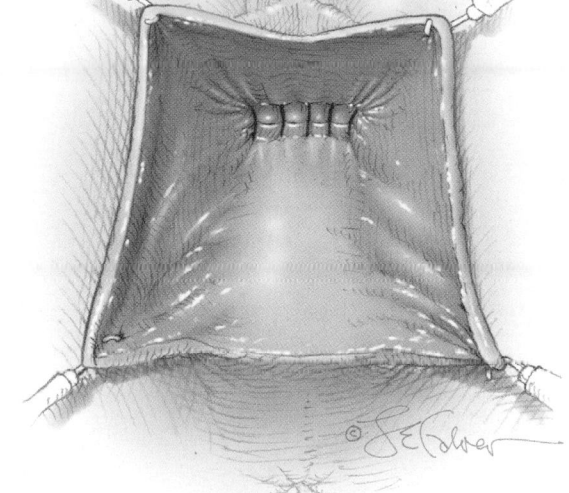

FIGURE 43-15.8 Defect-directed repair.

Care is taken to avoid placement of sutures too far laterally, as this will lead to a tissue bridge in the posterior vaginal wall and to potential resultant dyspareunia. Additionally, sutures should not be placed in the levator ani muscle, as this may also produce dyspareunia and chronic pain. Rectal examination should be performed after all sutures are placed to exclude inadvertent suture placement into the rectum.

Reinforcement of the apical aspect of the posterior vaginal wall is often beneficial. If the

uterosacral ligaments are identified at the lateral corners of the apex, interrupted sutures are used to connect these ligaments to the fibromuscular layer of the upper posterior wall.

❺ **Defect-Directed Repair.** In some instances, a discrete defect is identified in the posterior fibromuscular layer after the initial dissection. Defects may be lateral, midline, apical, or perineal (Figs. 43-15.5 through 43-15.10). In this situation, midline plication may not be effective, and a defect repair

should be performed. Interrupted stitches of 2-0 permanent or delayed-absorbable sutures are used to close the defect. This is generally a one-layered closure.

❻ **Mesh Augmentation.** In situations in which good fibromuscular tissue cannot be identified, synthetic or biologic material can be used for augmentation (Fig. 43-15.11). The initial epithelial dissection is continued laterally and to the apex. The material to be used is cut to size so that it lies flat. It

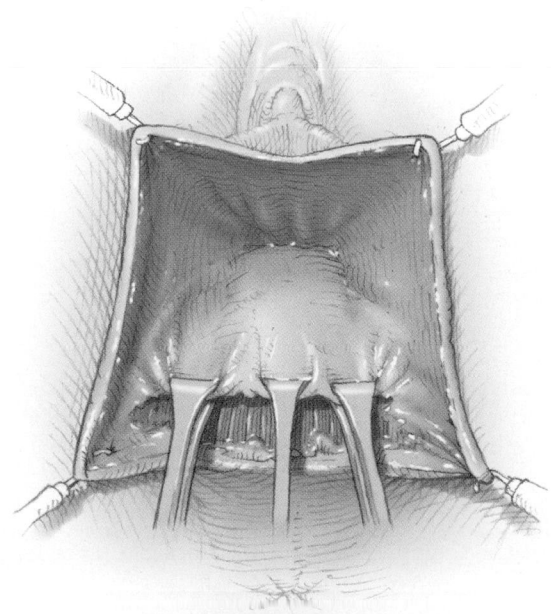

FIGURE 43-15.9 Distal defect.

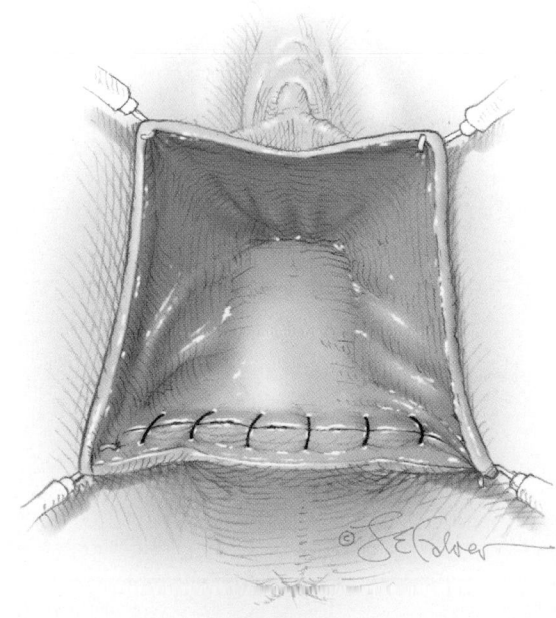

FIGURE 43-15.10 Defect-directed repair.

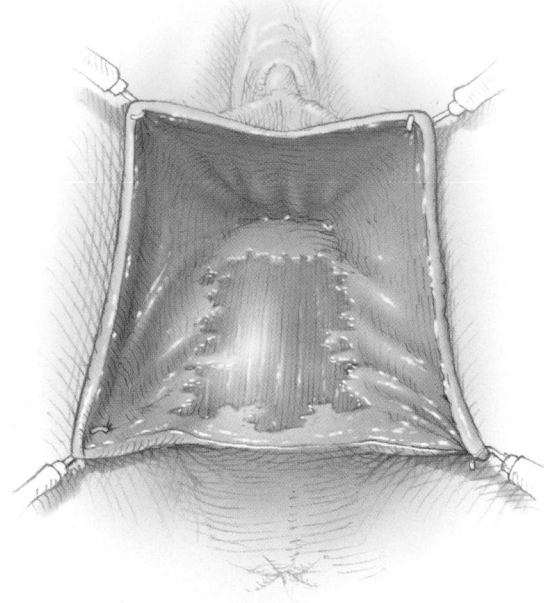

FIGURE 43-15.11 Large posterior wall defect.

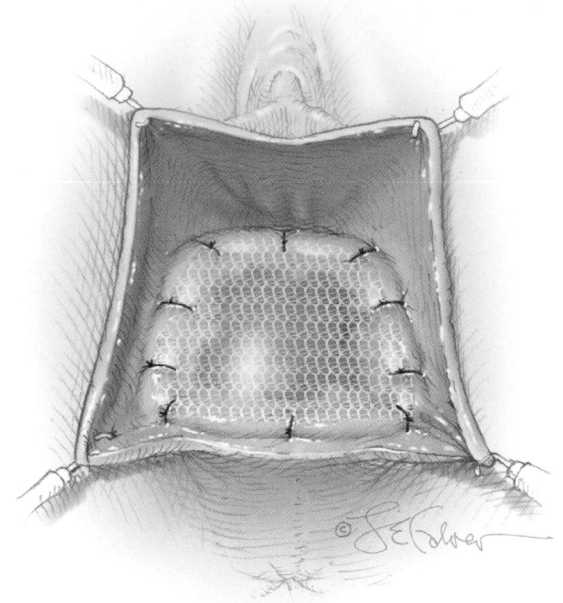

FIGURE 43-15.12 Mesh augmentation.

is then sutured with interrupted stitches of 2-0 delayed-absorbable suture to the vaginal apex as well as to the distal and lateral edges of the fibromuscular layer (Fig. 43-15.12). If permanent mesh is used, it should be kept at least 2 cm from the perineal body. The risk of mesh erosion increases as mesh is placed closer to the perineal body. Finally, if the need for mesh augmentation is anticipated, initial dissection is made in a deeper tissue plane to create greater distance between the mesh and vaginal lumen. This decreases the chance of mesh erosion into the vagina.

❼ Incision Closure. Following plication, redundant vaginal wall often remains and requires trimming. Liberal trimming, however, can narrow the vagina and can place the vaginal wall incision on excessive tension and impair wound healing.

The vaginal mucosa is reapproximated in a running fashion using a 2-0 delayed-absorbable suture. Care should be taken to avoid placement of suture bites too far apart. Widely positioned sutures can lead to accordion-type bunching of the vaginal epithelium and subsequent shortening of the vagina when the final suture is tied.

❽ Perineorrhaphy. Perineorrhaphy is often performed in conjunction with posterior repair (Section 43-16, p. 1223). If performed, it typically follows closure of the vaginal incision.

POSTOPERATIVE

Patients are instructed to use twice-daily sitz baths, stool softeners, and high-fiber diets. Constipation must be meticulously avoided. Intercourse is delayed until evaluation at 1 month postoperatively.

43-16

Perineorrhaphy

The perineal body serves as core support of the distal aspect of the vagina, rectum, and pelvic floor. Therefore, a damaged or weakened perineal body may contribute to distal prolapse. Reinforcement of this structure, that is, *perineorrhaphy*, is often performed in conjunction with other reconstructive procedures, such as posterior repair. As a result of perineorrhaphy, a shortened perineal body is lengthened, and the genital hiatus is concurrently shortened to reestablish distal support.

The degree to which the perineal body is lengthened can be tailored according to surgical goals. With high perineorrhaphy, incisions are placed to create a longer perineal body and narrower genital hiatus. This may be an advantageous adjunct to colpocleisis procedures (Sections 43-24 and 43-25, p. 1246). With low perineorrhaphy, the degree to which the perineal body is lengthened is minimized in an effort to create a genital hiatus wide enough to preserve comfortable coitus.

PREOPERATIVE

Patient Evaluation

The length of the genital hiatus is measured in centimeters both at rest and with Valsalva maneuver from the urethral meatus at 12 o'clock to the hymeneal ring at 6 o'clock. The perineal body is measured from the hymeneal ring at 6 o'clock to the anus. Normative data for these lengths do not exist. Therefore, the decision for perineorrhaphy must include an overall assessment of patient symptoms, clinical findings, and anatomy.

Perineorrhaphy is also sometimes performed for laxity of the introitus with the goal of narrowing the genital hiatus. However, care is taken to not decrease the caliber to the extent that dyspareunia results. Moreover, in sexually active postmenopausal women whose partners have decreased erectile tone, entry into the vagina may be difficult if the introitus is too small.

Consent

A patient preparing for perineorrhaphy should be counseled regarding risks of postoperative dyspareunia, prolapse recurrence, or wound complications, such as a stitch abscess.

Patient Preparation

Because of the surgical site's close proximity to the anus and also because bowel injury is possible, bowel preparation and antibiotic prophylaxis are administered prior to surgery to minimize the risks of fecal contamination and wound infection (Tables 39-6 and 39-7, p. 959). Thromboprophylaxis is given as outlined in Table 39-9 (p. 962).

INTRAOPERATIVE

SURGICAL STEPS

❶ Anesthesia and Patient Positioning. Perineorrhaphy is typically performed under general or regional anesthesia, and this choice is often dictated by concurrent surgeries planned. The patient is placed in dorsal lithotomy position. A vaginal and rectal examination under anesthesia is first performed to assess the size of the perineal body and defects of the posterior vaginal wall, which may also require repair. The vagina is surgically prepared, and a Foley catheter is inserted.

❷ Concurrent Surgery. If concurrent surgeries have been included, perineorrhaphy is the final procedure in most cases.

❸ Incision. To determine the approximate appearance of the final repair, Allis clamps are placed at the corners of the introitus at 3 and 9 o'clock. These are brought together in the midline. With this technique, a surgeon can judge the final size of the introitus and perineal body anticipated at the procedure's conclusion. Because scarring and retraction can occur, it is prudent to err on the side of leaving the genital hiatus larger rather than smaller. Although each case is individualized, in general, the introitus should admit three fingers at the end of surgery. A diamond-shape incision is made with its cephalad tip extending 2 to 3 cm into the vagina and the caudad tip extending to a point approximately 2 cm above the anus.

❹ Removal of Skin and Mucosa. For traction, an Allis clamp is placed at the lowermost tip of the diamond. Metzenbaum scissors are use to excise the perineal skin and vaginal mucosa within the diamond from the underlying tissue. During dissection, the scissor tips are held parallel to the perineal and vaginal tissues, respectively.

Sharp dissection must be performed over the perineal body. This area contains a normal condensation of tissue, and additionally scarring may be present. As a result, development of good tissue planes may not always be possible. Accordingly, frequent rectal examination during dissection may be required to prevent entry into the rectum.

❺ Suture Placement. One centimeter below the hymeneal ring, a 0-gauge delayed-absorbable suture on a CT-1 needle is used to approximate the perineal muscles. In suturing these muscles, a wide lateral bite is taken, and suture is directed first in an inward-to-outward and then outward-to-inward sequence (Fig. 43-16.1). This suture technique effectively buries knots below the

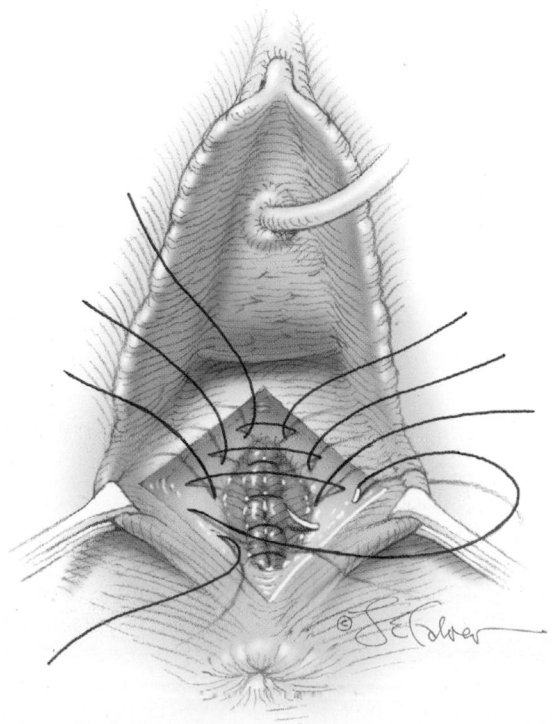

FIGURE 43-16.1 Suture placement.

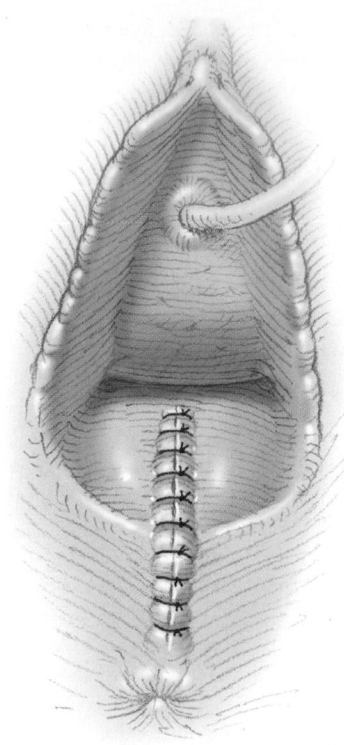

FIGURE 43-16.2 Wound closure.

plicated muscles. However, initially, the first suture is held and not tied.

Downward traction is placed, and a second suture is positioned approximately 1 cm cephalad. As with the first, this suture is not tied. A third suture can be placed 1 cm further cephalad to this, if necessary. In a similar fashion, one to two stitches are placed 1 cm apart and caudad to the primary suture. The sutures are then progressively tied beginning with the lowermost. In some cases, a second running layer is placed in the superficial perineal muscles for additional support.

❻ Vaginal and Perineal Closure. Starting at the vaginal apex, the vaginal mucosa is closed in a running fashion using 2-0 delayed-absorbable suture (Fig. 43-16.2). A surgeon should be mindful that sutures, when creating a running suture line in the vagina, should be placed close together. If suture bites are placed far apart during mucosal closure, the vagina can be shortened.

The running suture reapproximates the hymeneal ring and then is brought into the perineal area. The same suture is then used in a running mattress method to reapproximate the subcutaneous tissue to the end of the incision, near the anus. Interrupted stitches of 3-0 delayed-absorbable suture are used to close the skin.

POSTOPERATIVE

Patients are instructed to use twice-daily sitz baths, stool softeners, and high-fiber diets. Constipation must be meticulously avoided. Intercourse is delayed until evaluation at 1 month postoperatively. We have found that perineorrhaphy and posterior repair may be associated with short-term urinary retention. This is believed to result from spasm of the levator ani muscles. Therefore, a voiding trial is recommended postoperatively, with assessment of post-void residuals.

43-17

Abdominal Sacrocolpopexy

Since its introduction the early 1960s, abdominal sacrocolpopexy has become a widely accepted transabdominal procedure that suspends the vaginal vault to the sacrum using natural or synthetic grafts (Lane, 1962). This procedure is primarily performed to resuspend a prolapsed vaginal apex. Secondary indications include repair of apical segment descent of the anterior vaginal wall (cystocele) and posterior vaginal wall apical segment descent (enterocele and rectocele). A modification of the procedure, sacrocolpoperineopexy, is used to repair perineal descent (Weidner, 1997).

Sacrocolpopexy is one of several primary operations chosen for vaginal apex resuspension because of its ability to maintain normal vaginal anatomy and its durability. Long-term success rates range near 90 percent. It may be used as a primary procedure or alternatively, as a second surgery for patients with recurrences after failure of other prolapse repairs. In addition, it is ideal for those believed to be at high risk for recurrence. Examples include those with chronically increased intraabdominal pressure such as chronic obstructive pulmonary disease or chronic constipation; connective tissue disease; history of recurrent hernia; or obesity. In these patients, mesh provides augmentation to the patient's own tissues.

Although the vaginal apex can also be successfully suspended with vaginal approach procedures such as sacrospinous ligament fixation and uterosacral ligament suspension, sacrocolpopexy offers distinct advantages. Sacrocolpopexy maintains or lengthens the vagina, in contrast to vaginal approaches, which tend to shorten it. Secondly, the use of permanent mesh with multiple attachment sites to the vagina has a very low risk of failure. Finally, unlike vaginal approaches, the vaginal apex typically remains mobile, thus possibly lowering the risk for dyspareunia.

Sacrocolpopexy provides durable support by attaching the vaginal apex and the anterior and posterior vaginal walls to the anterior longitudinal ligament of the spine at the level of the sacrum. Although grafts of autologous, cadaveric, or synthetic materials may be used, permanent (synthetic) mesh has the best success rate and should be used unless otherwise contraindicated (Culligan, 2005).

Minimally invasive sacrocolpopexy may be performed laparoscopically or robotically by skilled minimally invasive surgeons

(Section 43-18, p. 1230). If the minimally invasive operation is performed in the same manner as the open operation, similar results can be expected.

PREOPERATIVE

▉ Patient Evaluation

Prior to sacrocolpopexy, patients with symptoms of urinary incontinence should undergo simple or complex urodynamic testing to determine the need for an antiincontinence procedure (Chap. 23, p. 621). Similarly, women without incontinence should also undergo testing with reduction of the prolapse to assess whether repair will unmask incontinence.

Prolapse of the vaginal apex often coexists with other sites of prolapse along the vaginal vault. For this reason, a careful preoperative assessment should be performed and concurrent prolapse of the anterior or posterior vaginal walls identified as described in Chapter 24 (p. 644). If necessary, sacrocolpopexy can be performed concurrently with paravaginal defect repair, posterior repair, or other prolapse procedures. In addition, a modification of the procedure known as sacrocolpoperineopexy may be performed to correct perineal descent. Beer and Kuhn (2005) found that approximately 70 percent of abdominal sacrocolpopexy procedures were performed with other pelvic reconstructive operations. With the technique we describe, a concurrent enterocele will be repaired by the colpopexy, and thus Halban or Moschcowitz-type enterocele repairs are unnecessary. These repairs close the cul-de-sac of Douglas but have not been proven to decrease prolapse recurrence and may worsen defecatory dysfunction.

In patients with real or potential stress urinary incontinence, a concurrent antiincontinence operation is performed. The CARE (Colpopexy After Reduction Efforts) trial found that patients without urinary incontinence symptoms undergoing sacrocolpopexy for prolapse of the anterior vaginal wall to within 1 cm of the hymen developed bothersome urinary incontinence in 24 percent of cases. Only 6 percent of those that had a concurrent Burch procedure developed bothersome incontinence (Brubaker, 2006).

▉ Consent

As with any prolapse repair, the most important long-term risk is recurrent prolapse. The individual surgeon should be aware of the recurrence rates quoted in the literature of 10 to 15 percent as well as his or her own personal recurrence rates. Although vaginal apex

prolapse recurrence is infrequent, subsequent prolapse of the anterior and posterior vaginal walls is common.

Mesh erosion is another frequent complication, developing in 2 to 5 percent of cases. This may develop soon after surgery or years later. Mesh erosion is generally found at the apex and is more common if sacrocolpopexy is performed concurrently with hysterectomy.

▉ Patient Preparation

Because of the risk of bowel injury during dissection of the sigmoid colon and rectum, a cleansing evacuation is recommended the evening prior to surgery (Table 39-7, p. 960). Antibiotic and thromboprophylaxis are given as outlined in Tables 39-6 and 39-9 (p. 959).

Vaginal estrogen cream use during the 6 to 8 weeks prior to surgery has been routinely recommended. It is believed that estrogen treatment enhances vascularity to promote healing and increase tissue strength. Although this is common practice and seems logical, there are no data to suggest that preoperative vaginal estrogen cream is beneficial.

INTRAOPERATIVE

▉ Instruments and Materials

The upper vagina and vaginal apex must be elevated and distended by a vaginal stent to allow adequate dissection and delineation of the fibromuscular layers of the vaginal wall and to aid mesh placement. The vaginal stent may be a large EEA (end-to-end anastomosis) sizer, which is present in most operating rooms, or a cylindrical Lucite rod.

The ideal bridging material for this procedure is permanent, nonantigenic, easily cut or customized, and readily available. Although autologous and cadaveric materials have been used, they are not as effective as synthetic mesh, and their use is discouraged. The ideal mesh has a large pore size to allow host tissue ingrowth, is monofilament to decrease bacterial adherence, and is easily manipulated.

SURGICAL STEPS

❶ Anesthesia and Patient Positioning. Following administration of general anesthesia, the patient is positioned supine in Allen stirrups. Correct positioning, with no pressure on the calf or thigh and with the thigh parallel to the ground, will decrease the risk of nerve injury. Moreover, this positioning allows excellent access to the vagina and proper placement of the abdominal self-retaining retractor. The buttocks are positioned at the edge of the table or slightly distal to allow full range of vaginal stent manipulation. The vagina and abdomen are surgically prepared, and a Foley catheter is inserted.

❷ Incision. A vertical or transverse abdominal incision as described in Sections 41-1 and 41-2 (p. 1020) may be used. Incision selection is directed by a woman's body habitus and by planned concurrent procedures. A Pfannenstiel incision generally provides adequate access to the sacrum and deep pelvis.

Prior to skin incision, the sacral promontory should be palpated through the abdominal wall deep to the umbilicus. The incision is then placed at a level that allows access to both vaginal apex and promontory. If a Burch colposuspension, paravaginal defect repair, or other surgery in the space of Retzius is planned, then a Pfannenstiel incision that is positioned closer to the symphysis is preferred.

❸ Bowel Packing. A self-retaining retractor, preferably a Balfour or Bookwalter type, is placed, and the bowel is packed up and out of the pelvis with laparotomy sponges (Chap. 40, p. 991). Bowel packing should attempt to shift the sigmoid colon farther to the patient's left, thereby allowing access to the sacrum.

❹ Identification of Anatomic Structures. The aortic bifurcation and iliac vessels are identified, and the middle sacral vessels are palpated ventral to the sacral promontory in the midline. In addition, tracing the course of both ureters aids in minimizing their injury. Specifically, the right ureter is at greater risk than the left during suture placement at the sacrum.

❺ Peritoneal Incision. The peritoneum overlying the sacral promontory in the midline is elevated with forceps and incised sharply. The incision is extended caudally into the Douglas cul-de-sac. This creates the peritoneal tunnel that will house the mesh. Closure of this incision at the end of surgery allows the mesh to lie beneath the peritoneum, and this may decrease the risk of future adhesion of bowel to mesh.

❻ Selection of Sacral Suture Site. To anchor the mesh proximally, sutures may be placed through the anterior longitudinal ligament at higher or lower sacral vertebrae. Suture placement at S3 or S4 vertebral bodies increases the risk of injury to the presacral venous plexus, whereas placement of sutures at S1 or the sacral promontory risks laceration of the middle sacral vessels or the left common iliac vein (Wieslander, 2006). However, at S1 the middle sacral vessels are readily visible and can be easily isolated and avoided. Additionally, at S1 the anterior longitudinal ligament is thicker and stronger. Affixing sutures into this thicker portion of the ligament minimizes the risk of suture avulsion. Many surgeons currently choose to place sutures at S1 or at the level of the sacral promontory (Nygaard, 2004). There have been a few reported cases of discitis related to suture placement at the sacral promontory. If sutures are placed here, care is taken to suture only the anterior longitudinal ligament and thereby avoid suture placement deep and into the disk.

❼ Bleeding Complications. Significant hemorrhage can develop during dissection and suture placement at the anterior longitudinal ligament. A thorough knowledge of pelvic anatomy is essential to prevent and manage such hemorrhage. The most common vessels lacerated during sacrocolpopexy are the presacral venous plexus and the middle sacral vessels (Fig. 38-23, p. 939).

With hemorrhage, several steps may be critical toward its control. First, pressure is applied immediately and held for several minutes. This may be particularly effective for venous bleeding. Sutures and clips may be useful, but injury of small veins frequently worsens with suturing. Additionally, as vessels retract into the bone, isolation and ligation become difficult. Sterile thumbtacks directed through the lacerated vessels and pushed into the sacrum can effectively compress such vessels. Unfortunately, these tacks are not routinely found in many operating rooms.

Alternatively, various local hemostatic agents have been used to control bleeding refractory to these initial steps (Table 40-6, p. 1005). Although no studies have compared these agents in urogynecologic procedures, animal and vascular studies have shown FloSeal Matrix to be very effective (Kheirabadi, 2002; Oz, 2000; Weaver, 2002). Moreover, the granular nature of FloSeal Matrix allows conformation to irregular wounds, which is a distinct advantage in managing the hemorrhage typical of sacrocolpopexy.

❽ Placement of Sacral Sutures. A Kitner sponge is used to gently dissect and remove fat and areolar tissue from the sacrum. Beneath these tissues, the shiny white anterior longitudinal ligament is seen to overlie the bone in the midline. As stated previously, sutures may be placed at S1 through S4. Three sutures of 2-0 gauge permanent material, each double armed with SH needles, are used (Fig. 43-17.1). The needle is driven either horizontally or vertically through the anterior longitudinal ligament. Suture placement is determined by each patient's anatomy and ease of placement. There is no evidence to suggest that horizontal placement is superior to vertical placement or vice versa. In some situations, damage to the middle sacral vessels may be avoided by horizontal placement of the sutures around the vessels. Ideally, the sutures lie approximately ½ cm apart. These sutures, with needles attached, are then held by a hemostat until later in the case.

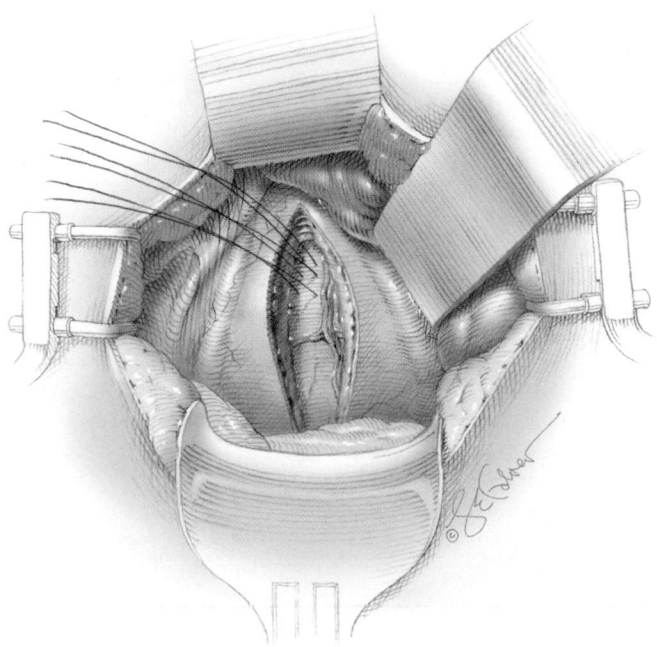

FIGURE 43-17.1 Placement of sacral sutures.

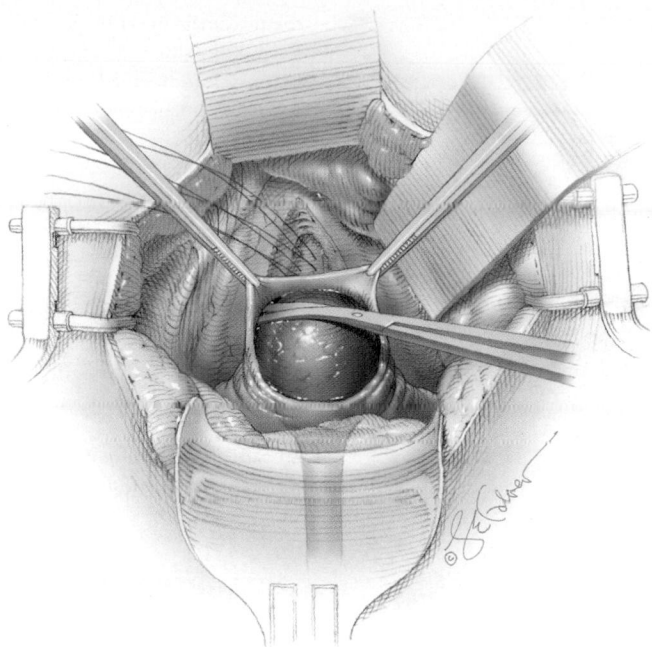

FIGURE 43-17.2 Dissection of the anterior vaginal wall.

⑨ Dissection of the Anterior Vaginal Wall. A vaginal stent is placed to elevate the vaginal apex, and the peritoneum covering it is incised transversely. Sharp and blunt dissection is used to separate the peritoneum and bladder from the anterior vaginal wall (Fig. 43-17.2). This anterior dissection extends approximately 5 to 6 cm caudally to create an extensive surface for mesh fixation. Dissection should progress at a depth above the fibromuscular layer of the vaginal wall. Entry into the proper plane above the fibromuscular layer will decrease the risk of

incidental entry into the vagina. Accidental opening of the vaginal wall increases the risk of future mesh erosion secondary to bacterial exposure. If the vaginal wall is opened, it should be irrigated copiously and followed by a two-layered imbricating closure with 2-0 or 3-0 delayed-absorbable suture.

⑩ Dissection of the Posterior Vaginal Wall. The vaginal apex is grasped with Allis clamps, pressure is released on the EEA sizer, and the peritoneum covering the posterior vaginal wall is then opened. The rectovaginal

space is identified and entered. Blunt dissection further opens this space to the level of the rectal reflection. If sacrocolpoperineopexy is planned, dissection continues beyond the rectal reflection to the level of the perineal body.

⑪ Posterior Mesh Placement. Two rectangular pieces of mesh are then cut to the width of the dissected anterior and posterior vaginal wall surfaces. They are left long to allow fixation to the sacrum later in the procedure. For mesh attachment, 2-0 nonabsorbable suture is recommended. The vaginal EEA sizer is once again pushed upward, and six sutures are used at the edges of the mesh to secure the mesh to the posterior vaginal wall's fibromuscular layer (Fig. 43-17.3). We prefer two rows of three sutures each, with the bottom row placed at the distal edge of the mesh. Care is taken to avoid placing sutures at the vaginal apex, as this is the least vascular region and therefore susceptible to suture and mesh erosion. Attempts are made to avoid penetration of the vaginal epithelium with these sutures. However, if the fibromuscular layer is thin, this will not be possible, and the epithelium is incorporated. These vaginal sutures will generally be epithelialized postoperatively.

⑫ Anterior Mesh Placement. With the vaginal stent serving as a support, mesh is sutured to the anterior vaginal wall in exactly the same fashion as was performed on the posterior vaginal wall (Fig. 43-17.4). In general, the length of the mesh used on the anterior vaginal wall is shorter than on the posterior vaginal wall.

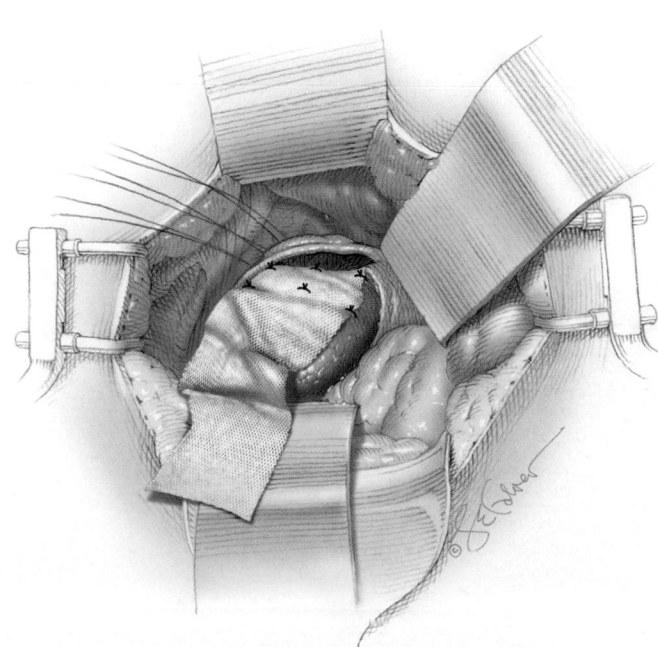

FIGURE 43-17.3 Posterior mesh secured and draped forward. Initially placed sacral sutures are seen in the background.

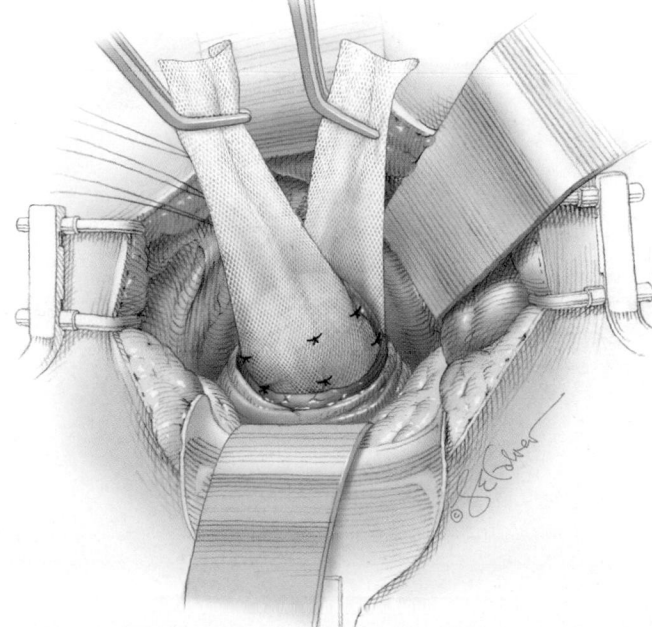

FIGURE 43-17.4 Anterior and posterior mesh in place.

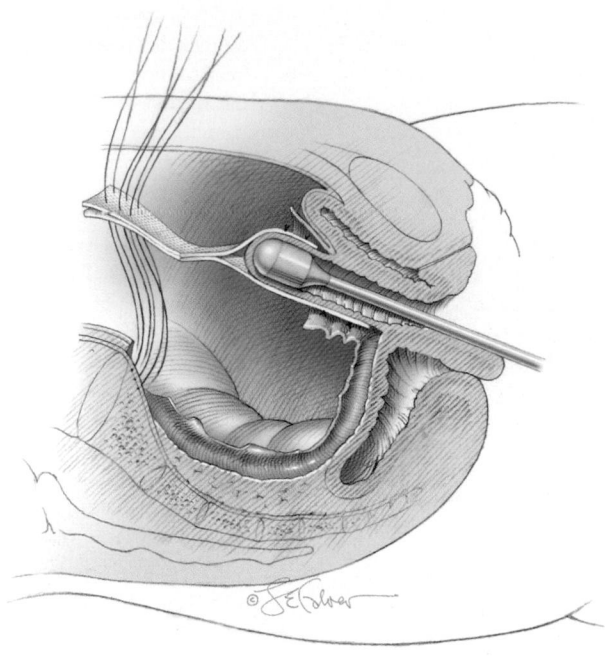

FIGURE 43-17.5 Mesh attachment to the sacrum.

⓭ Passage of Mesh into Peritoneal Tunnel. After the anterior and posterior meshes are secured, both are passed through the peritoneal tunnel to the sacral sutures.

⓮ Vaginal Peritoneal Closure. The peritoneum is closed over the vaginal apex with 2-0 delayed-absorbable suture in a running fashion.

⓯ Mesh Sizing and Attachment to the Sacrum. The vaginal stent is removed, and digital examination of the vagina is performed. The length of mesh necessary for adequate support is estimated by holding the mesh to the sacrum with the abdominal hand while palpating prolapse improvement vaginally. Apical suspension should reduce prolapse of the apex as well as the apical segments of the anterior and posterior vaginal walls. If possible, the mesh should not be placed on tension and is then cut to the appropriate length. The six needles of the three double-armed sacral sutures are then passed through

the proximal end of the mesh (Fig. 43-17.5). Each of the three paired sutures is then knotted to secure the mesh to the anterior longitudinal ligament (Fig. 43-17.6).

⓰ Peritoneal Closure. The peritoneum is then closed over the mesh to the level of the sacral promontory, thereby completely burying the mesh retroperitoneally (Fig. 43-17.7).

⓱ Cystoscopy. Cystoscopy is performed to insure ureteral integrity (Section 43-1, p. 1185).

⓲ Abdominal Closure. The abdomen is closed in a standard fashion (Section 41-1 or 41-2, p. 1021).

POSTOPERATIVE

Patient Care

Postoperative in-hospital management is similar to other intraabdominal surgeries. Foley catheter management depends on whether a concurrent antiincontinence procedure was performed. In the absence of such procedures, the catheter can be routinely removed on the first postoperative day. A stool softener should be prescribed as soon as a regular diet is tolerated, and care should be taken to avoid constipation after discharge from the hospital.

At routine postoperative visits, evaluation for prolapse recurrence and mesh or suture erosion should be performed. Symptoms of pelvic floor dysfunction should also be

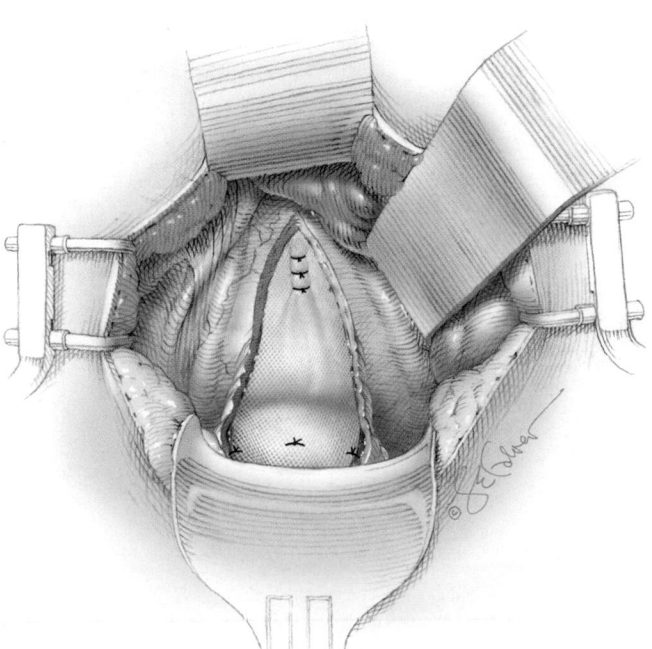

FIGURE 43-17.6 Final mesh placement.

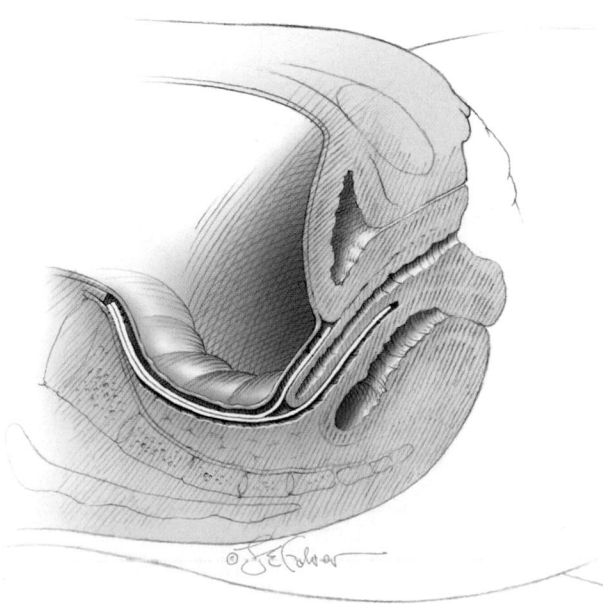

FIGURE 43-17.7 Peritoneal closure.

elicited at all postoperative visits. Anatomic success does not always correlate with functional success, and vice versa. Therefore, it is important to continually evaluate the results of surgery based on anatomy as well as symptoms such as urinary incontinence, defecatory dysfunction, pelvic pain, and sexual dysfunction.

Complications

Following sacrocolpopexy, the graft material or its attaching sutures can erode through the vaginal muscularis and then the mucosa. This is a frequently cited complication of the procedure, but fortunately is uncommon and develops in 2 to 5 percent of cases (Beer, 2005; Nygaard, 2004). On average, symptoms develop 14 months following surgery and classically consist of vaginal bleeding and discharge (Kohli, 1998). The diagnosis is straightforward, as mesh or sutures can be seen directly on speculum examination.

Mesh erosion through the vaginal mucosa may initially be treated with a 6-week course of intravaginal estrogen cream. For those in whom epithelium fails to cover the mesh, surgical removal is performed vaginally. The mesh is grasped, placed on tension, and as much mesh as can be identified is resected. The mucosal edges bordering the erosion site are dissected away from the mesh, undermined, and reapproximated. Failure of these wounds to heal should be interpreted as a sign of graft infection, and the graft material should be completely removed either vaginally or abdominally (Mattox, 2004). *Suture erosion* may be managed by removal in the office. Of note, recurrent bouts of granulation tissue without visible erosion most likely represent an invisible mesh or suture erosion. Fortunately, removal of sutures and eroding mesh does not compromise the prolapse repair, as in most cases, postoperative scarring continues to hold the vaginal apex suspended.

43-18

Minimally Invasive Sacrocolpopexy

Sacrocolpopexy may be performed with a minimally invasive technique using laparoscopy or robotic surgery. The basic steps of the procedure are the same and differ mainly by the method of abdominal entry. Although not as extensively studied as abdominal sacrocolpopexy, minimally invasive sacrocolpopexy is presumed to have similar results. In general, studies show that the minimally invasive procedures are associated with shorter hospitalization, but with longer operating times and greater cost (Judd, 2010).

PREOPERATIVE

Patient Evaluation

Candidates for minimally invasive sacrocolpopexy undergo the same prolapse and incontinence evaluation as that for abdominal sacrocolpopexy (Section 43-17, p. 1225). As discussed in Chapter 42 (p. 1095), factors that influence the decision regarding approach include patient overall health, body habitus, presence of intraabdominal adhesions, and surgeon skill.

Consent

Consent considerations mirror those with abdominal sacrocolpopexy. Additionally, with the minimally invasive approach, patients are counseled and consented for laparotomy if surgery cannot be completed laparoscopically. Complications more common to laparoscopy should also be discussed (Section 42-1, p. 1097). These include puncture injury to organs and vessels during abdominal entry and organ burns from electrosurgical tools.

Patient Preparation

Because of bowel injury risk during dissection of the sigmoid colon and rectum, a cleansing evacuation is recommended the evening prior to surgery. Additionally, some surgeons believe that a full bowel prep with Golytely decompresses the bowel, decreases risk of injury with laparoscopic instruments, and allows easier displacement of bowel out of the pelvis (Table 39-7, p. 960). Antibiotic and thromboprophylaxis are given as outlined in Tables 39-6 and 39-9 (p. 959).

Vaginal estrogen cream use during the 6 to 8 weeks prior to surgery has been routinely recommended. Estrogen treatment is believed to enhance vascularity to promote healing and increase tissue strength. Although this is common practice and seems logical, there are no data to suggest that preoperative vaginal estrogen cream is beneficial.

INTRAOPERATIVE

Instruments and Materials

The upper vagina and vaginal apex must be elevated and distended by a vaginal stent. This permits adequate dissection and delineation of the fibromuscular layers of the vaginal wall and aids mesh placement. The vaginal stent may be a large EEA (end-to-end anastomosis) sizer, which is present in most operating rooms, or a cylindrical Lucite rod.

The ideal bridging material for this procedure is permanent, nonantigenic, easily cut or customized, and readily available. Although autologous and cadaveric materials have been used, they are not as effective as synthetic mesh, and their use is discouraged. The ideal mesh has a large pore size to allow host tissue ingrowth, is monofilament to decrease bacterial adherence, and is easily manipulated.

SURGICAL STEPS

❶ **Anesthesia and Patient Positioning.** Following administration of general anesthesia, the patient is positioned supine in Allen stirrups in low lithotomy position. Correct positioning will decrease the risk of nerve injury. Moreover, this positioning allows excellent access to the vagina and full rotation of laparoscopic instruments. The buttocks are positioned at the edge of the table or slightly distal to permit full range of vaginal stent manipulation. The vagina and abdomen are surgically prepared, and a Foley catheter is inserted.

❷ **Incision and Trocar Placement.** A 10-mm incision is made in the base of the umbilicus, and a 10-mm trocar is placed to gain abdominal access as described in Section 42-1 (p. 1110). After safe abdominal entry, a diagnostic laparoscopy is performed (Section 42-2, p. 1121). Three accessory ports are then usually placed under direct laparoscopic visualization. We typically place a 5-mm port in the upper abdomen and two 10-mm ports in the right and left lower abdomen (Fig. 43-18.1).

❸ **Identification of Anatomic Structures.** The bed is moved into Trendelenburg position, and the bowel is gently swept out of the pelvis and above the pelvic brim. The aortic bifurcation and iliac vessels are identified, and the sacral promontory is visualized and palpated in the midline. In addition, tracing the course of both ureters aids in minimizing their injury. Specifically, the right ureter is at greater risk than the left during suture placement at the sacrum.

❹ **Peritoneal Incision.** The peritoneum overlying the sacral promontory in the midline is elevated with forceps and incised sharply (Fig. 43-18.2). The incision is extended caudally into the Douglas cul-de-sac (Fig. 43-18.3). This creates the peritoneal tunnel that will house the mesh. Closure of this incision at the end of surgery allows the mesh to lie beneath the peritoneum, and this may decrease the risk of future adhesion of bowel to mesh.

❺ **Dissection of the Anterior Vaginal Wall.** A vaginal stent is placed to elevate the vaginal apex, and the peritoneum covering it is incised transversely. Sharp and blunt dissection is used to separate the peritoneum and bladder from the anterior vaginal wall (Fig. 43-18.4). This anterior dissection extends approximately 5 to 6 cm caudally to create an extensive surface for mesh fixation. Dissection should progress at a depth above the fibromuscular layer of the vaginal wall. Entry into the proper plane above the fibromuscular layer will decrease the risk of incidental entry into the vagina. Accidental opening of the vaginal wall increases the risk of future mesh erosion secondary to bacterial exposure. If the vaginal wall is opened, it should be irrigated copiously followed by a two-layered closure with 2-0 or 3-0 delayed-absorbable suture.

❻ **Dissection of the Posterior Vaginal Wall.** The vaginal apex is next directed toward the anterior abdominal wall, and the peritoneum covering the posterior vaginal wall is opened (Fig. 43-18.5). With

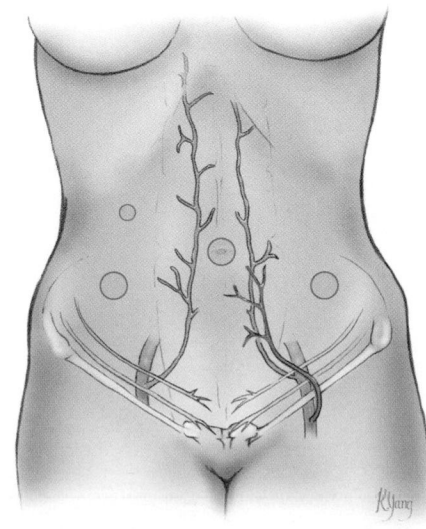

FIGURE 43-18.1 Port placement.

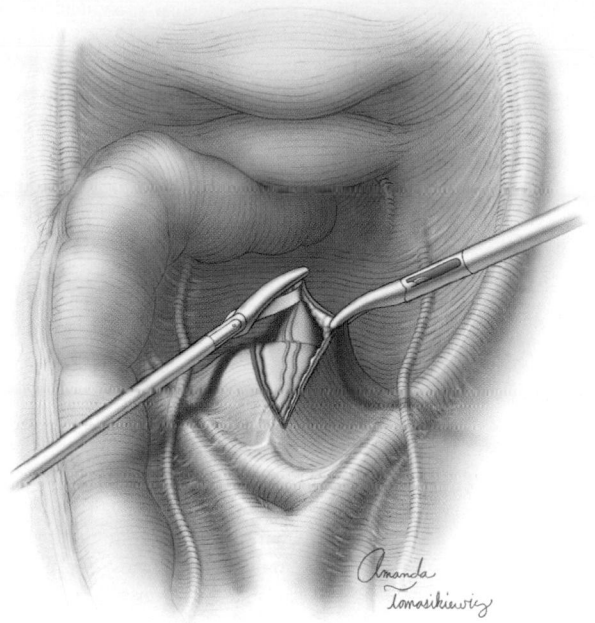

FIGURE 43-18.2 Peritoneal incision overlying the sacrum.

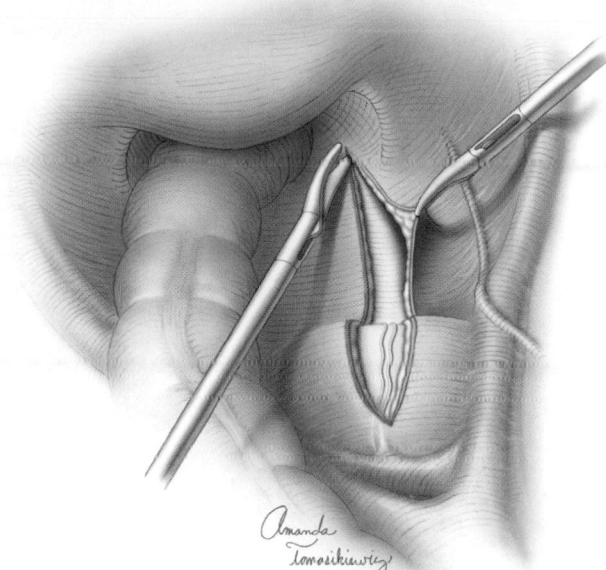

FIGURE 43-18.3 Peritoneal incision extended caudad.

dissection, the rectovaginal space is identified and entered. Blunt dissection further opens this space to the level of the rectal reflection. If sacrocolpoperineopexy is planned, dissection continues beyond the rectal reflection to the level of the perineal body.

❼ Posterior Mesh Placement. Two rectangular pieces of mesh are then cut to the

width of the dissected anterior and posterior vaginal wall surfaces. They are left long to allow fixation to the sacrum later in the procedure. Alternatively, a prefashioned Y-shaped mesh may be used. The mesh is placed into the peritoneal cavity through the lower right 10-mm cannula and guided into place with graspers in the accessory port. For mesh attachment, 2-0 permanent suture is recommended. With

upward pressure on the EEA sizer, six sutures are used at the edges of the mesh to secure it to the posterior vaginal wall's fibromuscular layer (Fig. 43-18.6). We prefer two rows of three sutures each with the bottom row placed at the distal edge of the mesh. Care is taken to avoid placing sutures at the vaginal apex, as this is the least vascular region and therefore is susceptible to suture and mesh erosion. During

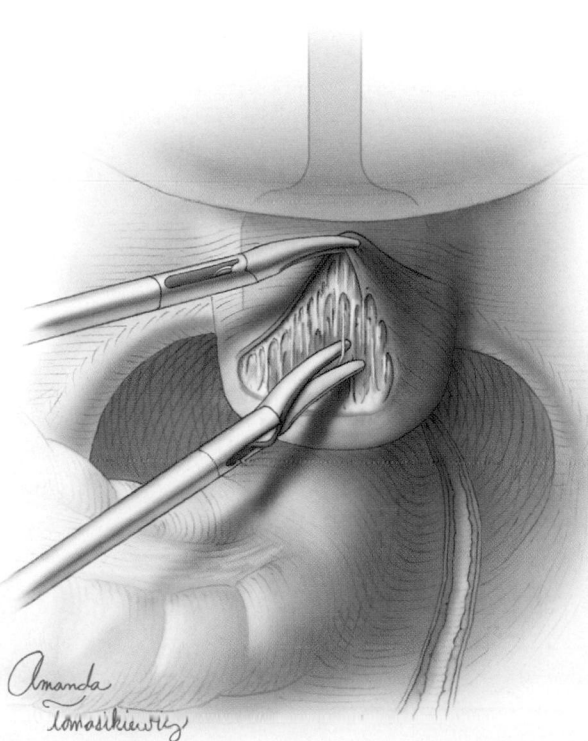

FIGURE 43-18.4 Dissection of the anterior vaginal wall.

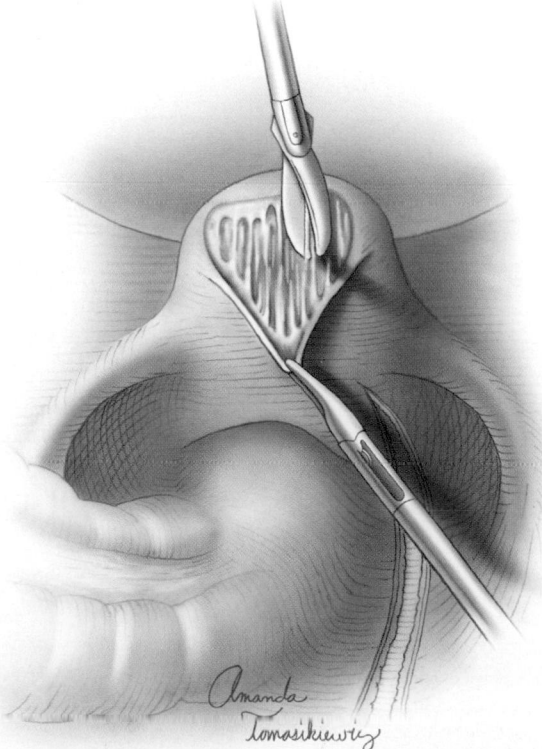

FIGURE 43-18.5 Dissection of the posterior vaginal wall.

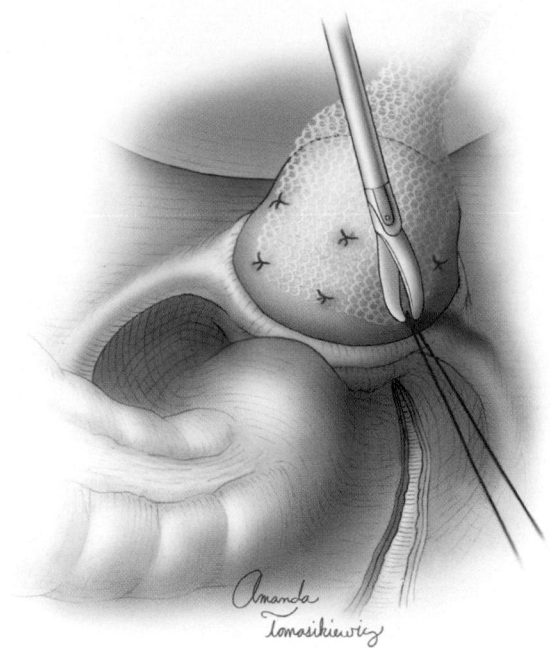

FIGURE 43-18.6 Posterior mesh placement.

suturing, penetration of the vaginal epithelium with these stitches is avoided. However, if the fibromuscular layer is thin, this will not be possible and the epithelium is incorporated. These vaginal sutures will generally be epithelialized postoperatively. Laparoscopic knot tying is used and illustrated in Figures 42-1.34 and 35 (p. 1118).

❽ Anterior Mesh Placement. With the vaginal stent serving as a support, mesh is sutured to the anterior vaginal wall in exactly the same fashion as was performed on the posterior vaginal wall (Figs. 43-18.7 and 43-18.8). In general, the length of the mesh used on the anterior vaginal wall is shorter than that on the posterior vaginal wall.

❾ Selection of Sacral Suture Site. To anchor the mesh proximally, sutures may be placed through the anterior longitudinal ligament at higher or lower sacral vertebrae. Suture placement at S3 or S4 vertebral bodies increases the risk of injury to the presacral

venous plexus, whereas placement of sutures at S1 or the sacral promontory risks laceration of the middle sacral vessels or the left common iliac vein (Wieslander, 2006). However, at S1 the middle sacral vessels are readily visible and can be easily isolated and avoided. Additionally, at S1 the anterior longitudinal ligament is thicker and stronger. Affixing sutures into this thicker portion of the ligament minimizes the risk of suture avulsion. For these reasons, many surgeons currently choose to place sutures at S1 or at the level of the sacral promontory (Nygaard, 2004).

❿ Bleeding Complications. Significant hemorrhage can develop during dissection and suture placement at the anterior longitudinal ligament. A thorough knowledge of pelvic anatomy is essential to prevent and manage such hemorrhage. The most common vessels lacerated during sacrocolpopexy are the presacral venous plexus and the middle sacral vessels (Fig. 38-23, p. 939).

With hemorrhage, several steps may be critical toward its control. First, pressure is applied immediately and held for several minutes. This may be particularly effective for venous bleeding. Sutures and clips may be useful, but injury of small veins frequently worsens with suturing. Additionally, as vessels retract into the bone, isolation and ligation become difficult.

Alternatively, various local hemostatic agents have been used to control bleeding refractory to these initial steps (Table 40-6, p. 1005). Although no studies have compared these agents in urogynecologic procedures,

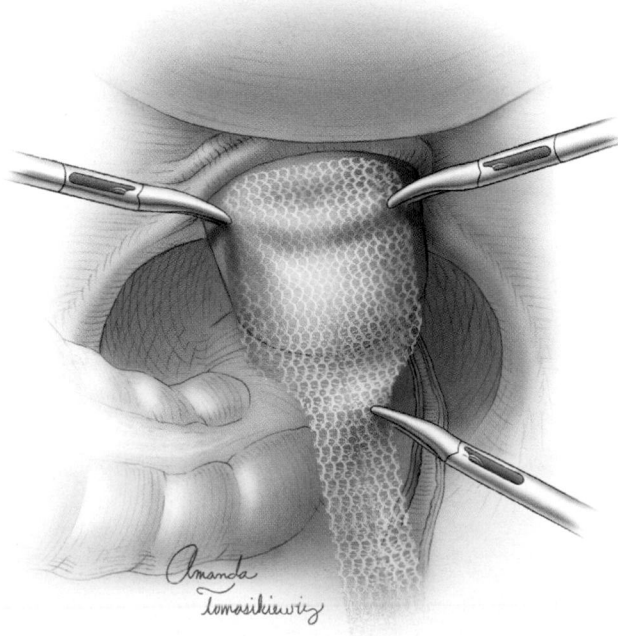

FIGURE 43-18.7 Anterior mesh placement.

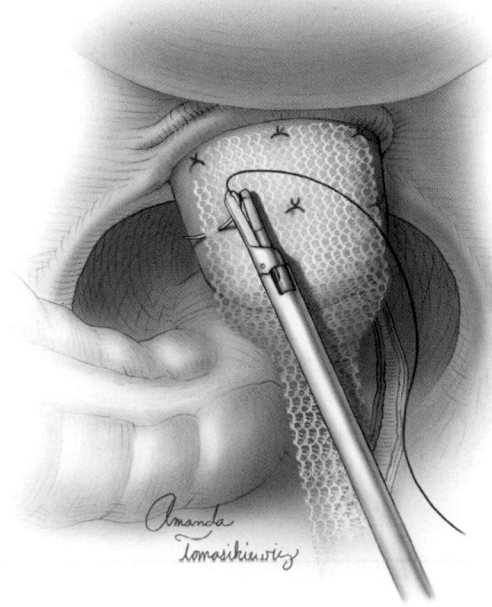

FIGURE 43-18.8 Anterior mesh sutured.

animal and vascular studies have shown FloSeal Matrix to be very effective (Kheirabadi, 2002; Oz, 2000; Weaver, 2002). Moreover, the granular nature of FloSeal Matrix allows conformation to irregular wounds, which is a distinct advantage in the managing hemorrhage typical of sacrocolpopexy.

⓫ Placement of Sacral Sutures. Gentle dissection with graspers and blunt instruments is used to remove fat and areolar tissue from the sacrum. Beneath these tissues, the shiny white anterior longitudinal ligament is seen to overlie the bone in the midline. As stated previously, sutures may be placed at S1 through S4. Three sutures of 2-0 gauge permanent material, each double-armed with SH needles, are used. The needle is driven either horizontally or vertically through the anterior longitudinal ligament. Suture placement is determined by each patient's anatomy and ease of placement. There is no evidence to suggest that horizontal placement is superior to vertical placement or vice versa. In some situations, damage to the middle sacral vessels may be avoided by horizontal placement of the sutures around the vessels. Ideally, the sutures lie approximately ½ cm apart.

⓬ Mesh Sizing and Attachment to the Sacrum. The vaginal stent is removed, and digital examination of the vagina is performed. The length of mesh necessary for adequate support is estimated by holding the mesh to the sacrum with a grasper and palpating prolapse improvement vaginally. Apical suspension should reduce prolapse

of the apex as well as the apical segments of the anterior and posterior vaginal walls. If possible, the mesh should not be placed on tension and is then cut to the appropriate length. The six needles of the three double-armed sacral sutures are then passed through the proximal end of the mesh. Each of the three paired sutures is then tied down with laparoscopic knot tying techniques (Fig. 43-18.9).

⓭ Vaginal Peritoneal Closure. The peritoneum is closed over the vaginal apex with 2-0 delayed-absorbable suture in a running fashion (Fig. 43-18.10).

⓮ Peritoneal Closure. The peritoneum is then closed over the mesh to the level of the sacral promontory, completely burying the mesh retroperitoneally (see Fig. 43-18.10).

⓯ Cystoscopy. Cystoscopy is performed to ensure ureteral integrity (Section 43-1, p. 1185).

⓰ Wound Closure. Subsequent surgery completion steps follow those of laparoscopy (Section 42-1, p. 1116).

POSTOPERATIVE

Patient Care

Patients are usually discharged from the hospital on postoperative day 1. Postoperative in-hospital management is similar to other laparoscopic surgeries. Management of the

Foley catheter depends on whether a concurrent antiincontinence procedure was performed. In the absence of such procedures, the catheter can routinely be removed on the first postoperative day. A stool softener should be prescribed as soon as a regular diet is tolerated, and constipation is avoided after discharge from the hospital.

At routine postoperative visits, evaluation for prolapse recurrence and mesh or suture erosion should be performed. Symptoms of pelvic floor dysfunction should also be elicited at all postoperative visits. Anatomic success does not always correlate with functional success, and vice versa. Therefore, it is important to continually evaluate the results of surgery based on anatomy as well as symptoms such as urinary incontinence, defecatory dysfunction, pelvic pain, and sexual dysfunction.

Complications

Following sacrocolpopexy, the graft material or its attaching sutures can erode through the vaginal muscularis and then the mucosa. This is a frequently cited complication of the procedure, but fortunately is uncommon and develops in 2 to 5 percent of cases (Beer, 2005; Nygaard, 2004). Symptoms develop on average 14 months following surgery and classically consist of vaginal bleeding and discharge (Kohli, 1998). The diagnosis is straightforward, as mesh or sutures can be seen directly during speculum examination. As discussed more fully in Section 43-17 (p. 1229), treatment options include intravaginal estrogen cream or partial or complete graft material excision.

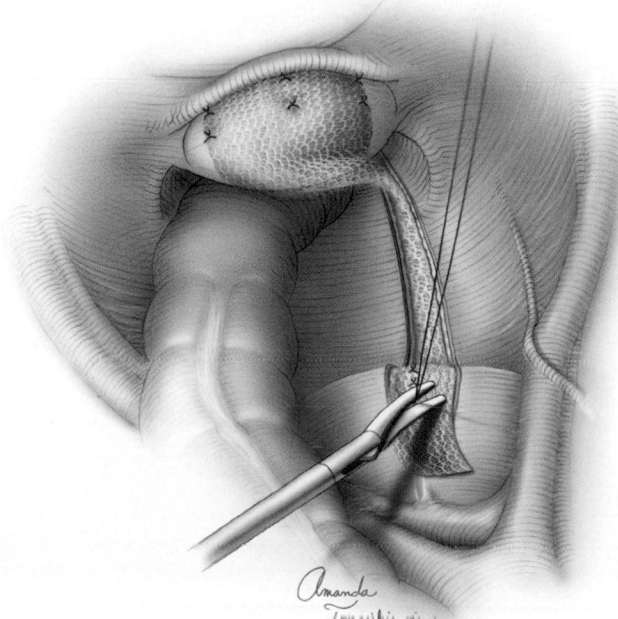

FIGURE 43-18.9 Mesh attachment to the sacrum.

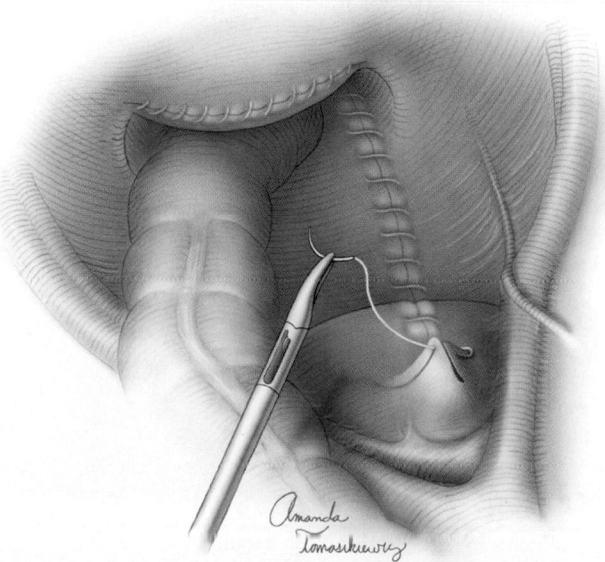

FIGURE 43-18.10 Peritoneal closure.

43-19

Abdominal Uterosacral Ligament Suspension

Suspension of the vaginal apex can be effectively performed with a variety of vaginal or abdominal surgeries, and success rates approximate 90 percent. Selection of procedure approach is based on a comprehensive assessment of a woman's symptoms and anatomy as well as surgeon preference. For patients undergoing abdominal surgery, there are two choices—abdominal uterosacral ligament suspension (USLS) or abdominal sacrocolpopexy (ASC) (Section 43-17, p. 1225). Uterosacral ligament suspension may be performed in patients with well-defined uterosacral ligaments. In addition, abdominal USLS is often preferred for those undergoing hysterectomy, because ASC carries an increased risk of mesh erosion if performed concurrently with hysterectomy.

During abdominal USLS, the uterosacral ligaments are sutured to the anterior and posterior vaginal walls at the vaginal apex. Because of this suspension, enteroceles are effectively closed. Thus, adjunctive Halban or Moschcowitz culdoplasty enterocele repairs are not required.

PREOPERATIVE

Patient Evaluation

Prior to USLS, patients with symptoms of urinary incontinence should undergo simple or complex urodynamic testing to determine the need for an antiincontinence procedure (Chap. 23, p. 621). Patients without incontinence should also undergo testing with reduction of their prolapse to assess whether repair will unmask incontinence.

Prolapse of the vaginal apex often coexists with other sites of prolapse along the vaginal vault. For this reason, a careful preoperative assessment should be performed, and concurrent prolapse of the anterior or posterior vaginal walls is sought as described in Chapter 24 (p. 644). If necessary, abdominal USLS can be performed with paravaginal defect repair, posterior repair, or other prolapse procedures. In patients with real or potential stress urinary incontinence, a concurrent antiincontinence operation is performed.

Consent

The consent process for USLS should include discussion of general risks associated with abdominal surgery and of specific risks associated with the procedure. As with any prolapse repair, the most important long-term risk is recurrence. Thus, surgeons should be aware of recurrence rates quoted in the literature of 10 to 15 percent as well as their own personal recurrence rates. Although recurrence of vaginal apex prolapse is infrequent, later prolapse of the anterior and posterior vaginal walls is common.

Urinary incontinence may also develop after USLS if an antiincontinence procedure is not performed. Therefore, preoperative discussion of bladder function after surgery is essential. Uterosacral ligament suspension does have a potential to shorten and fix the upper vagina. Thus, dyspareunia is a postoperative risk and should be discussed. Additionally, sacral plexus nerve injury with subsequent neuropathy has been reported.

Patient Preparation

During USLS, an end-to-end anastomosis (EEA) sizer may be placed for rectosigmoid colon manipulation. For this reason and because of the small, but potential, risk of bowel injury, bowel preparation is recommended (Table 39-7, p. 960). Additionally, antibiotic and thromboprophylaxis are given as outlined in Tables 39-6 and 39-9 (p. 959).

INTRAOPERATIVE

SURGICAL STEPS

① **Anesthesia and Patient Positioning.** This inpatient procedure is performed under general or regional anesthesia. A patient's legs are placed into Allen stirrups and positioned in low lithotomy with patient thighs parallel to the ground (Fig. 40-6, p. 985). The vagina and abdomen are surgically prepared, and a Foley catheter is inserted.

② **Incision.** The surgery can be performed through a vertical or Pfannenstiel incision. After the abdomen is opened, a self-retaining retractor is placed, and bowel is packed from the operative field. In most cases, USLS is performed at the completion of abdominal hysterectomy.

③ **Identification of the Ureters.** The ureters are identified bilaterally because of an increased risk of ureteral injury during suturing of the uterosacral ligaments.

④ **Identification of Uterosacral Ligaments.** Prior to beginning a hysterectomy, a surgeon should identify the uterosacral ligaments by applying contralateral upward traction to the uterine fundus. With this technique, the uterosacral ligaments are placed on stretch and can be identified. As their name implies, these ligaments originate from the lower and posterior uterine surface and extend to the sacrum. They also lie medial and posterior to the ischial spines.

Three double-armed sutures of 2-0 permanent suture are placed 1 cm apart in each uterosacral ligament and held (Fig. 43-19.1). This is the step of greatest risk to the ureters. However, it should be emphasized that if sutures are placed medial and posterior to the ischial spines, the ureters will not be in

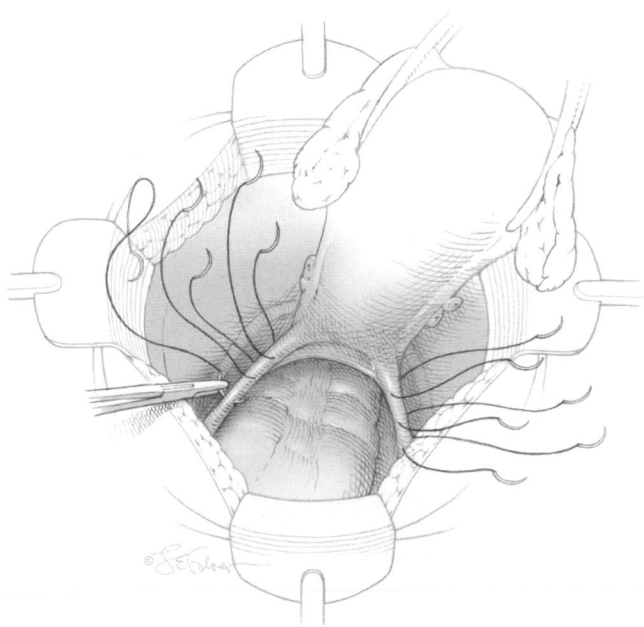

FIGURE 43-19.1 Uterosacral ligament suture placement.

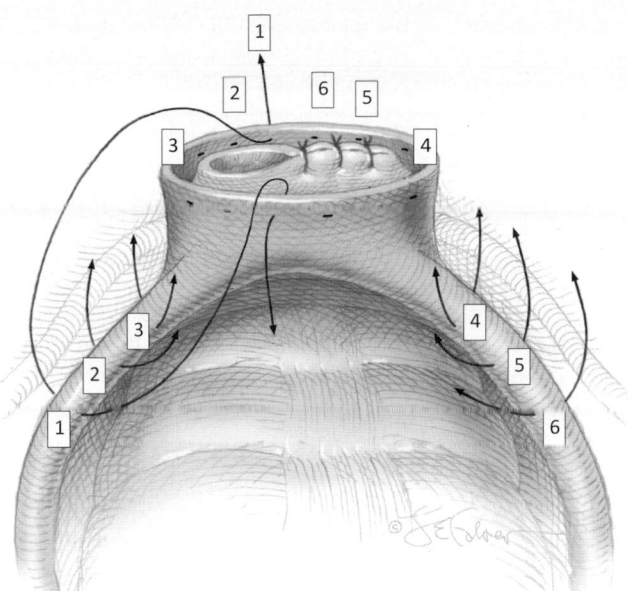

FIGURE 43-19.2 Vaginal cuff suture placement.

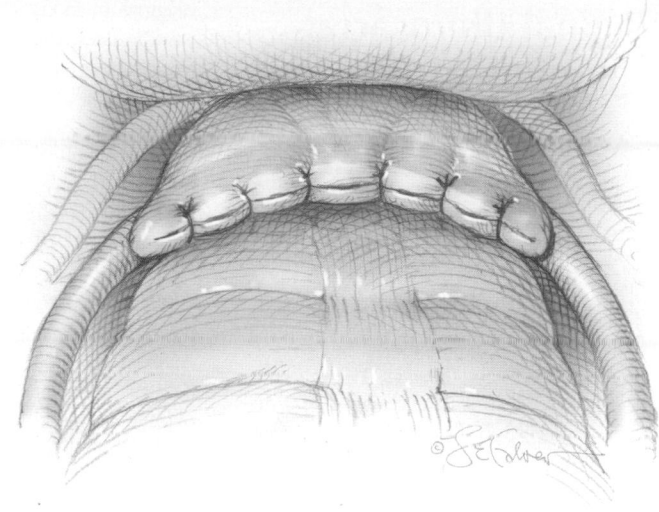

FIGURE 43-19.3 All sutures secured.

jeopardy. For this reason, an EES sizer may be placed rectally to identify the lateral rectal wall. This allows sutures to be placed as medial as possible to avoid the ureter, while also being placed lateral enough to avoid the rectal wall.

❺ Hysterectomy. If hysterectomy is planned, it is now completed, but the cuff is left open. A purse-string suture of 2-0 delayed-absorbable suture is placed 1.5 cm from the edge of the cuff in the vaginal epithelium to close the vaginal apex. This step will prevent many cases of erosion of permanent USLS sutures through the vaginal epithelium.

❻ Suture Placement. Six sutures are placed equidistant along the horizontal length of the vaginal cuff. These sutures are placed through the fibromuscular layer above the prior purse-string (Fig. 43-19.2). From both sides, the most cephalad sutures are placed through the horizontal midpoint of the vaginal cuff (sutures 1 and 2). One arm of the each suture is placed through the posterior fibromuscular layer of the vaginal wall, whereas the other arm sutures the anterior wall. The middle sutures (sutures 3 and 4)

are placed next in a similar fashion. Lastly, the angle sutures (sutures 5 and 6) are placed at the cuff angles through the fibromuscular layers of the anterior and posterior vaginal walls.

At this point, knots are secured starting with most medial sutures (sutures 1 and 2) and ending with the most lateral (sutures 5 and 6). This suturing order may prevent suture bridges in the lateral sutures. Care is taken to firmly secure all knots and to confirm that vaginal wall is directly approximated to the uterosacral ligaments (Fig. 43-19.3).

❼ Cystoscopy. Cystoscopy is performed following intravenous administration of indigo carmine to document ureteral patency. After cystoscopy, vaginal examination may be performed to assess the need for additional prolapse repair of the anterior and posterior vaginal walls.

❽ Incision Closure. The abdomen is closed in a standard fashion (Section 41-1 or 41-2, p. 1021).

❾ Concurrent Procedures. If necessary, prior to incision closure a paravaginal defect repair (Section 43-14, p. 1217) or

abdominal antiincontinence procedure may be performed. If posterior repair or vaginal antiincontinence surgery is required, these will follow incision closure.

POSTOPERATIVE

Following USLS, postoperative care follows that for any major abdominal surgery. Hospitalization typically varies from 2 to 4 days, and return of normal bowel function and febrile morbidity usually dictate this course. Postoperative activity in general can be individualized, although intercourse is usually delayed until after assessment of the vaginal cuff at 4 to 6 weeks following surgery. Catheter maintenance will vary and depend on whether or not antiincontinence procedures were performed.

Suture erosion with granulation tissue can be a short- or long-term complication. As discussed in Section 43-17 (p. 1229), patients will present with either an asymptomatic permanent suture seen at the vaginal apex or granulation tissue. Generally, these sutures can be removed in the office. However, if sutures are asymptomatic and difficult to remove, they may remain.

43-20

Vaginal Uterosacral Ligament Suspension

Vaginal uterosacral ligament suspension (USLS), also called high uterosacral ligament vault suspension, is a popular approach to vaginal apex suspension for women with symptomatic prolapse. In addition, this procedure is effective for repair of apical enteroceles.

During vaginal USLS, anterior and posterior aspects of the vaginal apex are attached to the uterosacral ligaments. As a result, continuity of the posterior and anterior vaginal walls is reestablished and the apex is resuspended.

Apical prolapse commonly develops concurrently with anterior and posterior compartment prolapse. Accordingly, vaginal USLS is often performed in conjunction with other surgeries to correct these defects, such as vaginal hysterectomy, anterior and posterior colporrhaphy, antiincontinence procedures, and perineorrhaphy.

PREOPERATIVE

Patient Evaluation

Prior to this procedure, patients with symptoms of urinary incontinence should undergo simple or complex urodynamic testing to determine the need for an antiincontinence procedure (Chap. 23, p. 621). Patients without incontinence should also undergo testing with reduction of the prolapse to assess whether suspension of the apex will unmask incontinence. In patients with real or potential stress urinary incontinence, a concurrent antiincontinence operation is performed.

Prolapse of the vaginal apex often coexists with other sites of prolapse along the vaginal vault. For this reason, a careful preoperative assessment should be performed as described in Chapter 24 (p. 644). If identified, prolapse of the anterior or posterior vaginal walls can be repaired as needed concurrently with USLS.

Consent

The consenting process for vaginal USLS should include discussion of general risks associated with major vaginal surgeries and of specific risks associated with the procedure. As with any prolapse repair, the most important long-term risk is recurrent prolapse. Although recurrence of vaginal apex prolapse is infrequent, prolapse of the anterior and posterior vaginal walls is common.

Urinary incontinence may also develop after USLS, if an antiincontinence procedure

is not performed. Therefore, preoperative discussion of bladder function after surgery is essential. In addition, uterosacral ligament suspension does have a potential to shorten and fix the upper vagina. Therefore, women should be aware of the potential for postoperative dyspareunia. Additionally, sacral plexus nerve injury and subsequent neuropathy have been reported after USLS and should be discussed.

The ureters are at risk during placement of uterosacral ligament suspension sutures. In the literature, the risk varies, and in some series, ureteral injury has been reported in up to 25 percent of cases. This complication appears to be related to surgeon experience. Knowledge of anatomy and correct suture placement should minimize this risk.

Permanent sutures are recommended for apical suspension. As a result, suture erosion and nonhealing granulation tissue can frequently develop. Therefore, efforts should be made to avoid suturing through the vagina epithelium.

Patient Preparation

Bowel preparation and evacuation of the rectum is recommended and is administered the evening prior to surgery (Table 39-7, p. 960). Antibiotic and thromboprophylaxis are given as outlined in Tables 39-6 and 39-9 (p. 959).

INTRAOPERATIVE

SURGICAL STEPS

1 Anesthesia and Patient Positioning. Vaginal USLS is typically performed under general or regional anesthesia. The patient is placed in dorsal lithotomy position using candy-cane stirrups. Examination under anesthesia is performed to assess degree of prolapse and confirm the need for surgeries planned. The vagina and abdomen are surgically prepared, and a Foley catheter is inserted.

2 Incision. The initial incision can be made in various ways. If in the context of vaginal hysterectomy, the vaginal cuff is already open and uterosacral ligaments are simply identified. However, if the procedure is performed in a woman who has previously undergone hysterectomy, then a vaginal incision can be created in one of two ways. A midline incision may be made in the posterior vaginal wall beginning at the perineum, and dissection proceeds cephalad to the vaginal apex. With this technique, vaginal epithelium is dissected off the vaginal wall. An enterocele sac is identified and entered.

Alternatively, an elliptical incision can be made directly over the enterocele sac at

the vaginal apex. The vaginal epithelium is excised in this region, and the enterocele sac is identified and entered.

3 Packing and Retraction. A key step of this procedure requires that bowel must be adequately packed away so that high uterosacral sutures can be placed without bowel injury. Several moist laparotomy sponges are placed in the Douglas cul-de-sac and hollow of the sacrum to elevate bowel from the operative field. Additionally, two Breisky-Navratil retractors are positioned. One reflects the rectum to the contralateral side, and a second is used to reflect remaining bowel. At times, a third may be necessary to adequately clear the field.

4 Identification of Uterosacral Ligaments. Initially, the ischial spines are palpated. The uterosacral ligaments are found medial and posterior to the spines and lateral to the rectum. Additionally, Allis clamps may be placed on the posterior vaginal wall at the apex. If traction is applied, uterosacral ligaments become taut and are more easily identified by their cordlike texture.

5 Placement of Sutures in the Uterosacral Ligament. Beginning at the level of the ischial spines and progressing cephalad, a surgeon places two or three double-armed 2-0 gauge permanent sutures approximately 1 cm apart in each uterosacral ligament (Figs. 43-20.1 and 43-20.2). Following the normal path of these ligaments, the most caudad sutures will be most medially. To avoid ureteral injury, it is critical that sutures be placed medial and posterior to the ischial spines. In addition, ureteral injury is averted by directing needles medially during suturing. Although this will place sutures near the lateral border of the rectum, bowel injury is avoided by retraction with a Breisky-Navratil retractor.

In some instances, uterosacral ligaments are attenuated and difficult to identify distinctly. In these circumstances, suturing may proceed by placing stitches in the expected anatomic area for these ligaments.

Hematomas may form occasionally following inadvertent laceration of the lateral rectal veins. Should this occur, application of pressure with a sponge stick will typically control bleeding.

6 Cystoscopy. After all six stitches are placed and tied, indigo carmine is administered intravenously. Cystoscopy is performed to exclude ureteral injury prior to proceeding with the remaining surgical steps.

7 Placement of Sutures in the Vaginal Wall. With the use of the double-armed suture, the most distal suspensory suture on

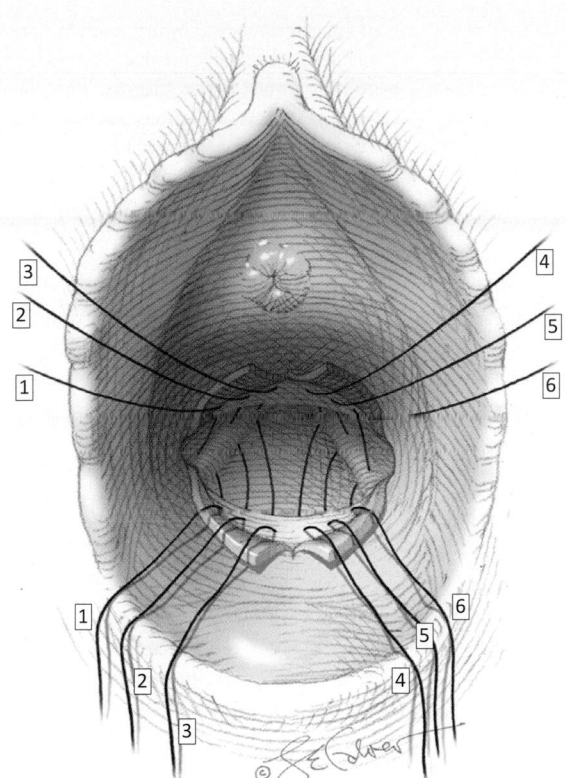

FIGURE 43-20.1 Vaginal view of sutures placed into uterosacral ligaments.

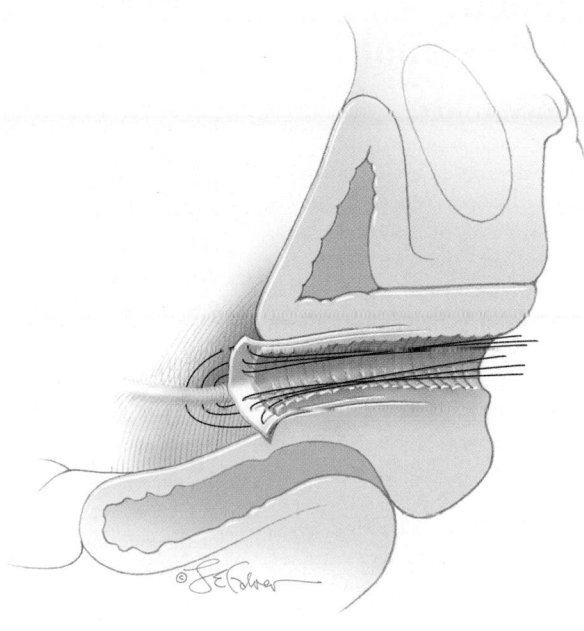

FIGURE 43-20.2 Lateral view of sutures placed into the left uterosacral ligament.

each side (sutures 1 and 6) is sewn to the most lateral portion of the anterior and posterior fibromuscular layers at the corner of the vaginal apices. The sutures (sutures 2 and 5) immediately cephalad to these most caudal ones are placed more medially. Finally, the most cephalad sutures (sutures 3 and 4) are placed in the midline of the anterior and posterior fibromuscular layers. Tangling of sutures is common. Thus, sutures may be tagged, numbered, and attached to surgical drapes.

Vaginal packing is removed, and sutures are tied beginning with the most cephalad (sutures 3 and 4). As knots are secured, the vaginal walls should be brought into immediate contact with the uterosacral ligaments to avoid "bow-stringing," which can lead to bowel obstruction.

❽ **Closure of the Vaginal Cuff.** The vaginal cuff is reapproximated in a running fashion with 2-0 gauge delayed-absorbable suture.

POSTOPERATIVE

Following USLS, postoperative care follows that for any vaginal surgery. Postoperative activity in general can be individualized, although intercourse is usually delayed until after assessment of the vaginal cuff at 4 to 6 weeks following surgery. Catheter maintenance will be dependent on whether or not antiincontinence procedures were performed concurrently.

43-21

Sacrospinous Ligament Fixation

Prolapse of the vaginal apex may be corrected by several procedures. One vaginal approach, termed *sacrospinous ligament fixation*, uses the strength of the sacrospinous ligament to resuspend the apex. Stretching from the ischial spine to the lateral surface of the sacrum's inner hollow, this ligament is a tough fibrous aponeurosis that lies within the body of the coccygeus muscle (Fig. 43-21.1). The great size and tensile strength of this ligament allow it to serve as an excellent support during suspensory surgery.

Although effective in correcting apical prolapse, sacrospinous ligament fixation compares less favorably with abdominal sacrocolpopexy (Benson, 1996; Maher, 2004). However, sacrospinous ligament fixation averts abdominal surgery and is associated with shorter operating times and quicker recovery. For these reasons, it often provides a superior choice for women with other significant health problems. Additionally, the vaginal approach allows other concurrent support defects to be repaired vaginally at the same time as fixation. Success rates are comparable to those of other vaginal approaches for vault suspension (Maher, 2001).

PREOPERATIVE

Patient Evaluation

Prior to sacrospinous ligament fixation, patients with symptoms of urinary incontinence should undergo urodynamic testing to determine the need for an adjunctive antiincontinence procedure (Chap. 23, p. 621). Patients without incontinence should also undergo testing with reduction of the prolapse to assess whether suspension of the apex will unmask incontinence. In patients with real or potential stress urinary incontinence, a concurrent antiincontinence operation is indicated.

Prolapse of the vaginal apex often develops with prolapse at other sites along the vaginal vault. Accordingly, careful preoperative assessment should be performed as described in Chapter 24 (p. 644). If identified, prolapse of the anterior or posterior vaginal walls can be repaired as needed concurrently with sacrospinous ligament fixation.

Consent

For most women, sacrospinous ligament fixation is effective in preventing recurrent apical prolapse, and success rates range from 70 to nearly 100 percent (Cruikshank, 2003; Lantzsch, 2001; Maher, 2004). The procedure is safe and associated with low rates of serious complications. Significant hemorrhage requiring transfusion is uncommon and typically results from injury to the pudendal, inferior gluteal, or inferior rectal vessels. Rates

of long-term nerve injury similarly are low, and injury typically involves the pudendal or inferior gluteal nerves (Sagsoz, 2002). Rarely, life-threatening infections such as necrotizing fasciitis and ischiorectal fossa abscess may develop (Hibner, 2005; Silva-Filho, 2005).

As with other pelvic reconstructive surgeries, new pelvic support defects may follow sacrospinous fixation, and rates for development of any support defect range from 15 to 40 percent (Paraiso, 1996; Shull, 1992). During fixation, the vagina's long axis is redirected posteriorly. As this axis is lowered, the anterior compartment of the pelvis widens and lies vulnerable to increased intraabdominal pressures. Accordingly, cystoceles develop postoperatively in 10 to 40 percent of cases (Lantzsch, 2001; Paraiso, 1996). As a result, increased rates of stress urinary incontinence may also be noted.

Concern is often expressed regarding shortening of the functional vaginal length by this procedure, and postoperative lengths approximate 8 cm (Given, 1993). Despite a resulting shorter vaginal length compared with an abdominal approach for suspension, de novo dyspareunia is infrequent. Indeed, for many women, replacement of the vagina to a more anatomic location leads to improved satisfaction with intercourse following surgery (Maher, 2004).

Patient Preparation

The risk of intraoperative rectal injury is not uncommon with sacrospinous ligament

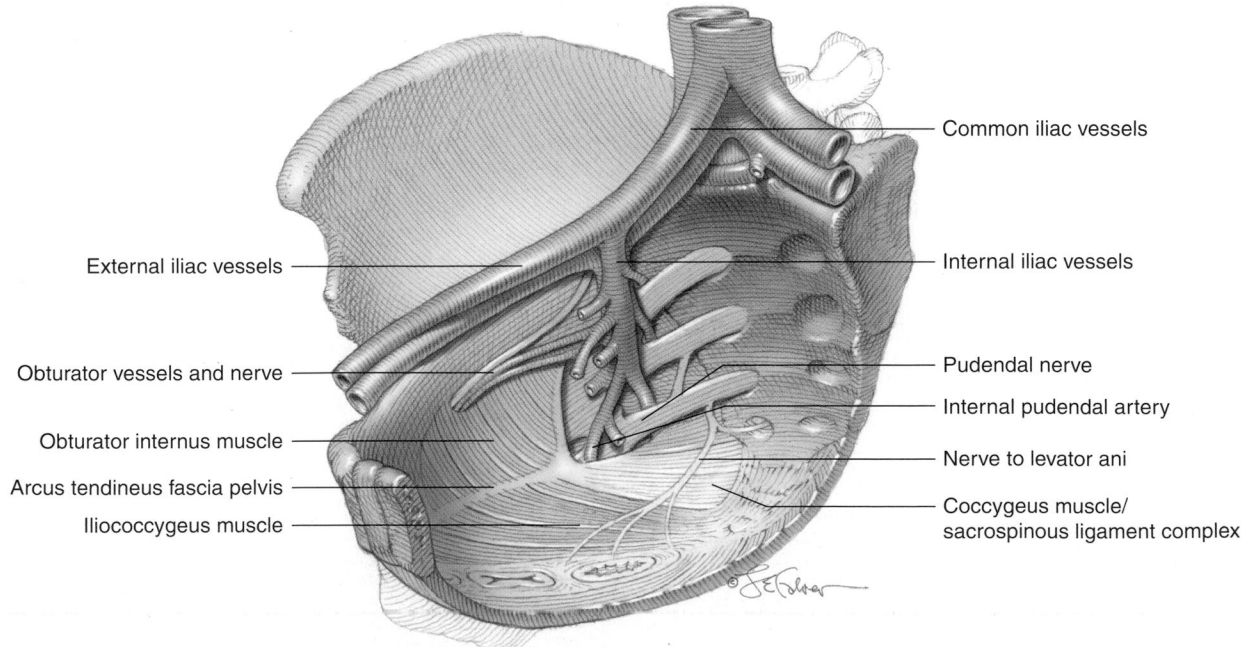

FIGURE 43-21.1 Sacrospinous ligament complex and surrounding pelvic anatomy.

fixation. For this reason, bowel preparation is performed the evening prior to surgery (Table 39-7, p. 960). As with most vaginal surgery, because of the risk posed by the normal vaginal flora for postoperative wound cellulitis and abscess, preoperative antibiotics are warranted. Typical agents are found in Table 39-6 (p. 959). Additionally, thromboprophylaxis is provided as outlined in Table 39-9 (p. 962).

INTRAOPERATIVE

Surgical Instruments

Placement of sutures into the sacrospinous ligament can be performed with various ligature carriers, which include the Deschamps ligature carrier, Miya hook, Capio ligature carrier, and EndoStitch. Using the Deschamps ligature carrier, a surgeon threads the suture through an eye at the needle-shaped tip of the carrier. Arcs and curves constructed into the instrument aid ease of suture placement into the ligament. Disadvantages to this device, however, include the relative thickness of the needle tip, which can add difficulty in perforating the ligament. Alternatively, Miyazaki (1987) described 74 cases using the Miya hook. This device aids in passage through the ligament. However, there is less control of the needle and suture because the device has moving parts. These first two carriers offer additional cost advantages because they are reusable. With adequate exposure, a long needle driver is another reusable device that can be used easily. Alternatively, disposable devices have become popular, in particular the Capio ligature carrier. This device is easier to manipulate than the Miya hook, and the needle is well controlled at all times.

SURGICAL STEPS

❶ Anesthesia and Patient Positioning.
After general anesthesia has been administered, a woman is placed in dorsal lithotomy position, the vagina is surgically prepared, and a Foley catheter is inserted. Initially, vaginal vault prolapse is reduced to place the vagina in a normal anatomic position. Enterocele or cystocele repairs, if planned, should precede sacrospinous ligament fixation.

❷ Unilateral or Bilateral Fixation.
A surgeon may choose to suture the vaginal apex to either one or both sacrospinous ligaments. In most instances unilateral fixation gives sufficient support. The right ligament is preferred because most surgeons are right handed. Additionally, fixation to the right side avoids anatomic difficulties posed by the rectum.

Alternatively, bilateral fixation has been advocated as a method to maintain the vaginal apex in a midline plane and to provide superior durability because of additional support given by two ligaments (Cespedes, 2000). Clear benefits between bilateral fixation and unilateral fixation have not, however, been evaluated in clinical trials. Moreover, greater rates of postoperative anterior compartment prolapse have been noted following bilateral fixation (Pohl, 1997).

❸ Access to the Sacrospinous Ligament.
The sacrospinous ligament is accessed through the pararectal space. Entering this space permits close proximity to the ligament with minimal dissection.

❹ Entry into Pararectal Space.
During a pararectal approach, the surgeon sharply incises the posterior vaginal wall and separates it from the underlying rectum as described in Section 43-15 (p. 1219). These steps reveal the perirectal fascia, and the rectal pillars are seen on either side of the rectum. The right rectal pillar is entered sharply by placing and opening a hemostat at the level of the ischial spine (Fig. 43-21.2). This blunt dissection permits entry into the pararectal space (Fig. 38-18, p. 934).

❺ Retractor Positioning.
Breisky-Navratil retractors are positioned within the pararectal space. The first, positioned anteriorly, lifts pelvic contents away from the surgical site. The second is placed to the patient's left and retracts the rectum. The last is held inferiorly and parallel to the sacrospinous ligament.

❻ Ligament Dissection.
After entering the right pararectal space, the ischial spine is located digitally, and the path of the sacrospinous ligament is traced medially. Blunt dissection with fingertips removes loose adventitial tissue overlying the midportion of the ligament.

During dissection within the pararectal space or retraction of the rectum, vessels in the area may be lacerated, most commonly including branches of the inferior rectal vessels. Hemorrhage in this area is often best managed with packing a sponge into the area and holding pressure.

❼ Ligature Placement.
Following dissection, the ligament may be grasped with a Babcock clamp at a spot approximately 2.5 cm medial to the ischial spine. This transforms the flat ligament into a thicker, more rounded structure and often allows the third, inferior retractor to be removed for greater visualization and mobility of the ligature carrier.

A ligature carrier is loaded with 0-gauge permanent suture. Although erosion of sutures through the vaginal apex postoperatively has been noted, use of permanent sutures increases repair durability (Chapin, 1997). In addition, use of monofilament sutures to lower infection risks in this procedure has been advocated (Hibner, 2005). The suture is threaded through the needle eye to its midpoint. As a result, the suture tails on either side of the eye are of equal length.

The pudendal and inferior gluteal vessels and nerves lie behind the sacrospinous ligament and may be injured during sacrospinous ligament fixation. For this

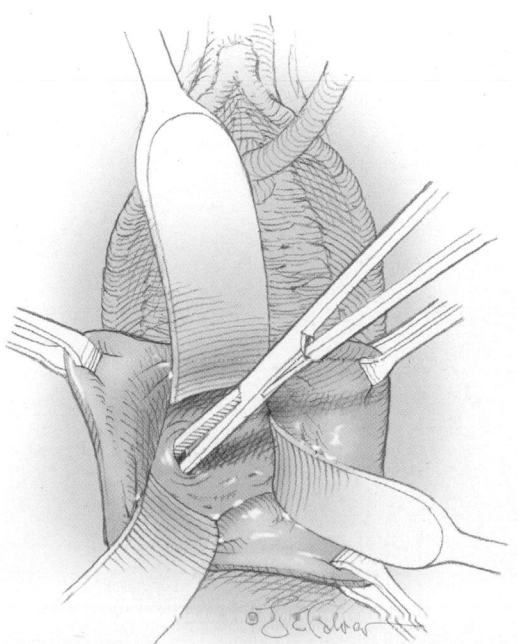

FIGURE 43-21.2 Entry into pararectal space.

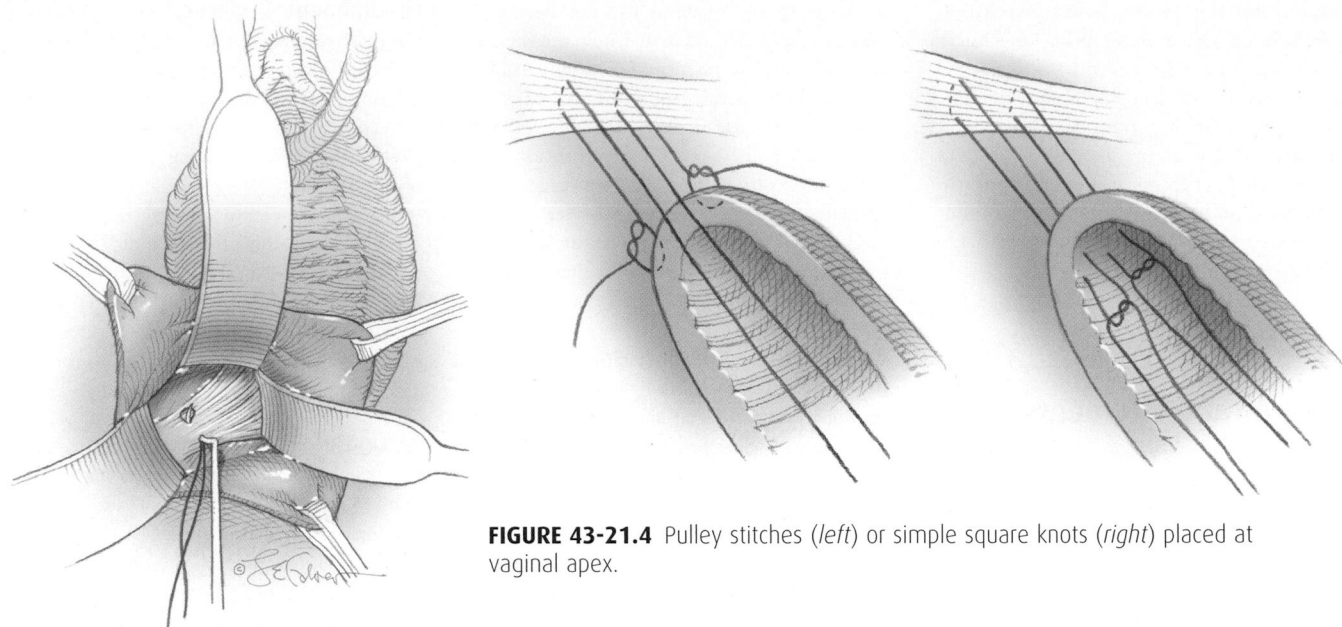

FIGURE 43-21.3 Ligature placement.

FIGURE 43-21.4 Pulley stitches (*left*) or simple square knots (*right*) placed at vaginal apex.

reason, sutures should be placed 2.5 to 3 cm medial to the ischial spine and are not placed completely through the entire thickness of the ligament (Sagsoz, 2002; Verdeja, 1995).

If a vessel is lacerated and immediate isolation and ligation is not possible, the area of hemorrhage may be packed with laparotomy sponges and pressure held for several minutes. As sponges are then gradually removed, a site of laceration can be identified and clipped with a vascular clip or ligated.

A ligature carrier is held in the surgeon's right hand, and the tip of the driver is placed toward the inferior edge of the ligament (Fig. 43-21.3). The tip then pierces the ligament with a clockwise motion of the carrier.

❽ **Vaginal Apex Suturing.** The suture loop is snagged with a nerve hook and pulled into the vagina. The loop is cut, thereby leaving two separate equal-length sutures within the ligament. This allows placement of two sutures with only one carrier pass and thus

minimizes adjacent tissue injury. The two sutures are used to create two pulley stitches (one stitch per suture) in the vaginal apex (Fig. 43-21.4, left). As shown at right in this image, simple square knots may be use to affix the vaginal apex to the sacrospinous ligament.

With the Michigan modification of this procedure, two suture passes are made through the ligament. This provides four sutures with two ligament passes (Fig. 43-21.5). Sutures are then used to attach the anterior and posterior vaginal walls to the sacrospinous ligament (Fig. 43-21.6).

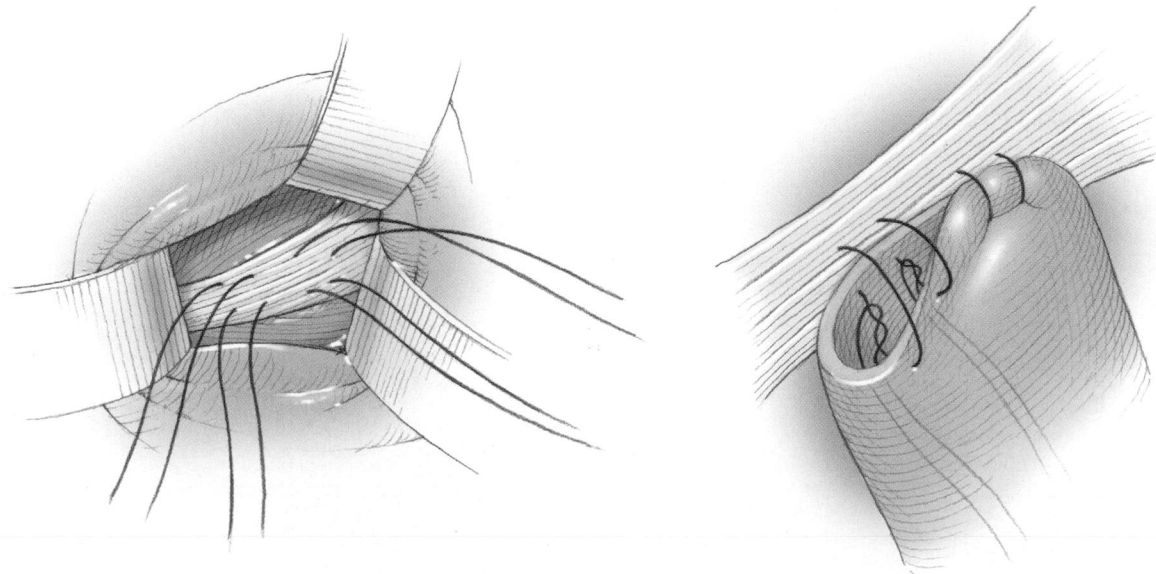

FIGURE 43-21.5 Michigan modification.

FIGURE 43-21.6 Vaginal apex approximated to ligament.

❾ Closure of Posterior Vaginal Wall and Pararectal Space. The proximal posterior vaginal wall is reapproximated with a running closure using 2-0 delayed-absorbable suture.

❿ Vault Resuspension. The pulley stitches are tightened, bringing the vaginal apex directly to the ligament. The remainder of the vaginal wall is then closed in a running fashion using 2-0 delayed-absorbable suture.

POSTOPERATIVE

Following surgery, patients may ambulate on the first postoperative day, and diet may be advanced as tolerated. Mild buttock pain may follow surgery and resolves typically in days to months. Such neuralgia is common following surgery. Lantzsch and associates (2001) found a rate of 8 percent in their series. Nonsteroidal antiinflammatory drugs in this setting may be helpful.

Occasionally, a patient may complain of severe pain and display sensory or motor neurologic symptoms or both. If motor symptoms are present, the chance for nerve entrapment of sciatic nerve branches is great. These women should undergo exploration of the pararectal space and removal of entrapping sutures.

Postoperative activity in general can be individualized, although intercourse is usually delayed until after assessment of the vaginal cuff at 4 to 6 weeks following surgery. Catheter maintenance will be dependent on whether or not antiincontinence procedures were performed concurrently.

43-22

McCall Culdoplasty

McCall culdoplasty is performed at the time of vaginal hysterectomy to close the cul-de-sac, add support to the posterior vaginal apex, and possibly prevent enterocele formation. With McCall culdoplasty, horizontal rows of sutures are placed. Each row begins with suturing into one uterosacral ligament, then incorporating colonic serosa with intervening suture bites, and ending at the opposite uterosacral ligament. The initial rows begin caudad, and sequential rows are added cephalad. This process essentially closes the posterior vaginal wall against the colon serosa and uterosacral ligament. This adds apical support to the vaginal cuff and obliterates a potential site for small bowel herniation into the vagina, that is, enterocele.

The main difference between McCall culdoplasty and the Halban and Moschcowitz methods lies in its vaginal approach. No data support the superior efficacy of one when these three are compared. Thus, the choice of procedure should be based on the approach planned for hysterectomy and on other concurrent surgeries.

Culdoplasty is suggested to prevent enterocele formation and vaginal vault prolapse. However, if significant vaginal apex prolapse or enterocele is already present, then either sacrospinous ligament fixation or vaginal uterosacral ligament suspension of the vaginal vault is preferred.

PREOPERATIVE

▢ Patient Evaluation

McCall culdoplasty is generally performed following vaginal hysterectomy in patients with enterocele or preventively in those without. Because the degree of pelvic organ prolapse will dictate the reconstructive surgeries planned, a thorough prolapse evaluation should be performed as described in Chapter 24 (p. 644).

▢ Consent

As with any pelvic reconstructive surgery to correct prolapse, the risk of enterocele formation or recurrence should be discussed. Risks of ureteral and bowel injury, although low, should be included in the consenting process.

▢ Patient Preparation

Postoperative vaginal cuff cellulitis and urinary tract infection may follow hysterectomy, and patients typically receive

antibiotic prophylaxis with a first-generation cephalosporin. Suitable options are found in Table 39-6 (p. 959). Additionally, thromboprophylaxis is provided as outlined in Table 39-9 (p. 962). Although the risk of bowel injury is low, bowel preparation is recommended prior to surgery to evacuate the rectum and thus decrease contamination should proctotomy occur (Table 39-7, p. 960).

INTRAOPERATIVE

SURGICAL STEPS

❶ Anesthesia and Patient Positioning. McCall culdoplasty is typically performed under general anesthesia, although epidural or spinal regional methods may also be appropriate. A patient is placed in high lithotomy position in candy-cane stirrups. The vagina is surgically prepared, and a Foley catheter is inserted. Vaginal hysterectomy is completed as described in Section 41-13 (p. 1051), but the vaginal cuff is left open for culdoplasty completion.

❷ Packing. After vaginal hysterectomy, a moist pack is placed into the posterior cul-de-sac to prevent descent of bowel or omentum into the operative field.

❸ Identification of Uterosacral Ligaments, Rectum, and Ureters. The uterosacral ligaments, which were previously tagged during vaginal hysterectomy, are placed on lateral traction to define the

course of the ligaments to the sacrum. The ureter always lies laterally to the uterosacral ligament, and although it may not be visualized per se, placement of sutures medial to the ligament will avoid ureteral injury. Additionally, rectal examination should delineate the lateral borders of the rectum to avoid needle-stick injury to the bowel.

❹ Suture Placement. The first suture row is placed caudad. Traction on these most caudad sutures helps to identify the ligaments. Each subsequent row is then placed progressively cephalad. With suturing, the first internal 2-0 permanent suture is placed into one uterosacral ligament. With placement, the needle is directed toward the midline to avoid ureteral injury. Subsequent serial bites are placed 1 cm apart across the rectosigmoid colon's serosa to reach and penetrate the opposite uterosacral ligament. This suture is left untied. More cephalad rows of sutures are similarly added, and 1 cm between rows is appropriate spacing. Thus, depending on the size and depth of the cul-de-sac, the number of rows will vary.

Following completion of the internal suture rows, one external suture row is placed using 2–0 delayed-absorbable suture and incorporates the posterior vaginal wall. As shown in Figure 43-22.1, this suture is initially placed through the full thickness of the posterior vaginal wall and into the uterosacral ligament. Progressive bites are then taken serially through the rectosigmoid serosa to reach the opposite uterosacral ligament. Finally, the suture enters the opposite uterosacral ligament

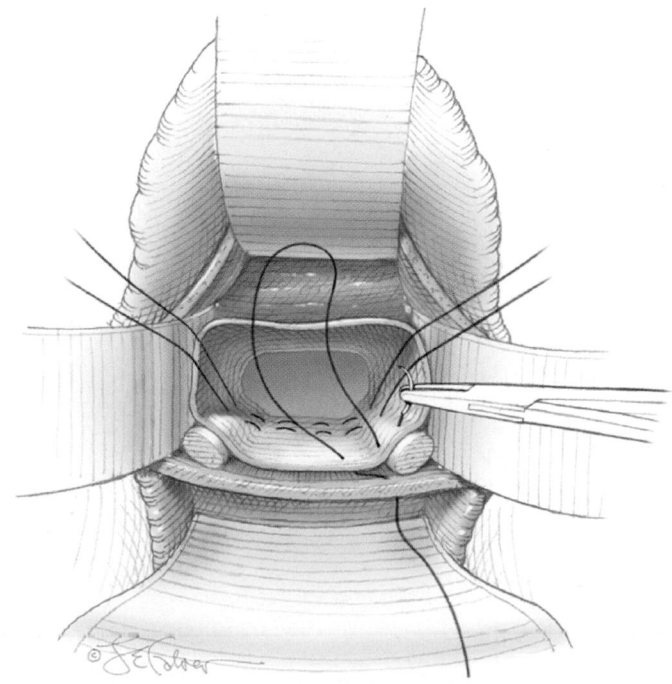

FIGURE 43-22.1 Uterosacral ligament suture placement.

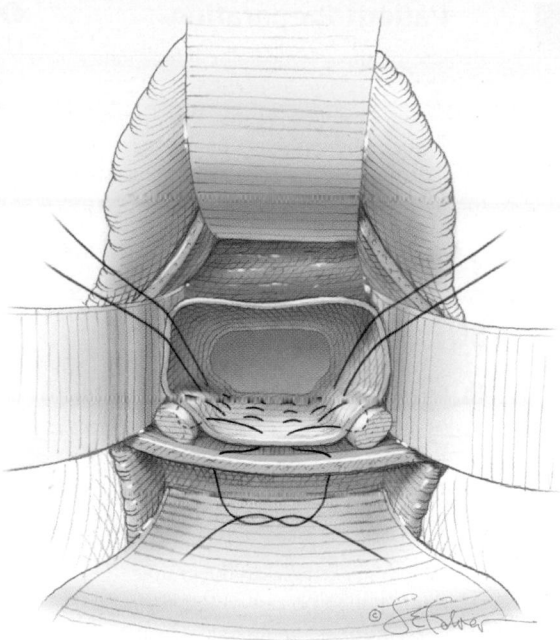

FIGURE 43-22.2 Suture reenters the vagina prior to securing.

and exits through the full vaginal wall thickness to reenter the vagina (Fig. 43-22.2).

⑤ Suture Tying. The sutures are sequentially tied beginning with the most proximal sutures and progressing caudad.

⑥ Cystoscopy. Because of the proximity of suture placement to the ureters, cystoscopy should be considered to document ureteral patency.

⑦ Vaginal Cuff Closure. Upon completion of McCall culdoplasty, the remaining steps of vaginal hysterectomy will follow as described in Section 41-13 (p. 1054).

POSTOPERATIVE

Following vaginal hysterectomy and McCall culdoplasty, postoperative care follows that for most vaginal surgeries. Hospitalization typically varies from 1 to 3 days, and return of normal bowel and bladder function usually dictates this course. Postoperative activity in general can be individualized. Intercourse is usually delayed for 4 to 6 weeks and after the first postoperative visit to allow inspection of vaginal cuff healing.

43-23

Abdominal Culdoplasty Procedures

Culdoplasty techniques are used to obliterate the cul-de-sac of Douglas and prevent herniation of small bowel into the vaginal wall. Thus, these procedures have traditionally been thought of as appropriate for repair and prevention of enteroceles. However, evidence-based studies have not born out these benefits, and current concepts of specific pelvic-support defect repair have decreased the popularity of culdoplasty. Nevertheless, this procedure is still performed and may have value when completed in conjunction with other prolapse procedures.

Included in this group are the Moschcowitz and Halban operations. In general, permanent sutures are used to close the cul-de-sac, and procedures vary based on the orientation of suture placement. Either the Halban or Moschcowitz procedure may be selected, and the decision is based on surgeon's preference and concurrent abdominal or vaginal pathology. No evidence exists that compares these techniques.

PREOPERATIVE

Patient Evaluation

Culdoplasty procedures are typically performed with other prolapse surgeries. Thus, thorough pelvic organ prolapse evaluation should be performed as described in Chapter 24 (p. 644). All sites of prolapse should be considered when planning surgical correction. Depending on the type of prolapse present, urodynamic testing may also be indicated to exclude potential stress urinary incontinence that may develop once prolapse has been corrected.

Consent

As with any pelvic reconstructive surgery to correct prolapse, the risk of enterocele recurrence following abdominal culdoplasty should be discussed. Additionally, risks of ureteral and bowel injury should be included in the consenting process. During Halban and Moschcowitz culdoplasty, the rectosigmoid is plicated to the posterior vaginal wall. Accordingly, defecatory dysfunction and technical difficulty in performing subsequent colonoscopy have been reported following these culdoplasty procedures.

Patient Preparation

Because of the potential for bowel injury, bowel preparation is performed the evening prior to surgery (Table 39-7, p. 960). Antibiotic and thromboprophylaxis are given as outlined in Tables 39-6 and 39-9 (p. 959).

INTRAOPERATIVE

SURGICAL STEPS

❶ **Anesthesia and Patient Positioning.** Abdominal culdoplasty is typically performed under general anesthesia, although regional techniques may also be used. The patient is positioned in low lithotomy position with the legs in Allen stirrups and with the thighs parallel to the ground. This positioning allows access to the vagina and provides normal abdominal laparotomy exposure. A Foley catheter is placed, and the abdomen and vagina are prepared for surgery.

❷ **Surgical Incision.** Either transverse or vertical incision may be used for culdoplasty. Incision choice is dependent on concurrent surgeries planned (Section 41-1 or 41-2, p. 1020). A self-retaining retractor such as an O'Connor-O'Sullivan or Balfour retractor is placed, and concurrent surgeries such as hysterectomy are performed.

❸ **Special Considerations.** Following completion of initial procedures, the cul-de-sac is exposed and evaluated for suture placement. Additionally, an end-to-end anastomosis (EEA) sizer may be placed within the vagina or rectum to identify borders and allow correct suture placement. Prior to culdoplasty, both ureters should be identified again.

In the past, these procedures have focused on suturing peritoneal and serosal surfaces. However, a more effective approach incorporates deep bites into the muscularis of the vagina and sigmoid, while taking care to avoid both bowel and vaginal lumens. During placement of rectosigmoid sutures, attempts are made to avoid adjacent rectosigmoid veins, as hematomas commonly form. If bleeding develops, direct vascular compression provides effective control in most instances.

❹ **Halban Culdoplasty.** Several rows of 2-0 gauge permanent sutures are placed longitudinally through the serosa and muscularis of the sigmoid (Fig. 43-23.1). Rows are placed 1 to 2 cm apart, and attention is given to avoiding entry into the lumen. The same sutures are then advanced through the peritoneum of the deep cul-de-sac and up toward the apex of the posterior vaginal wall. As much of the cul-de-sac as possible should be obliterated, but to avoid ureteral injury, sutures are not placed lateral to the uterosacral ligaments.

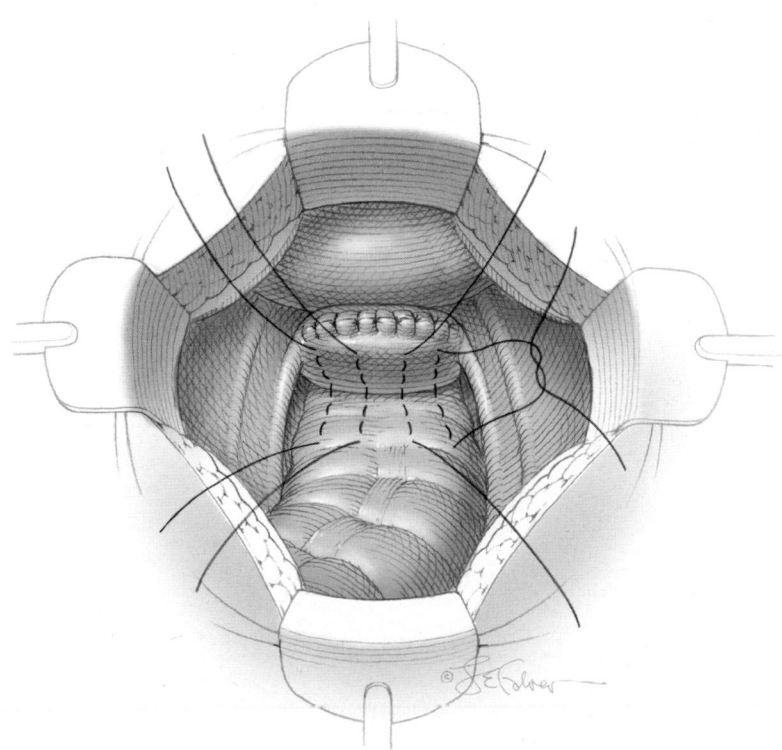

FIGURE 43-23.1 Halban culdoplasty.

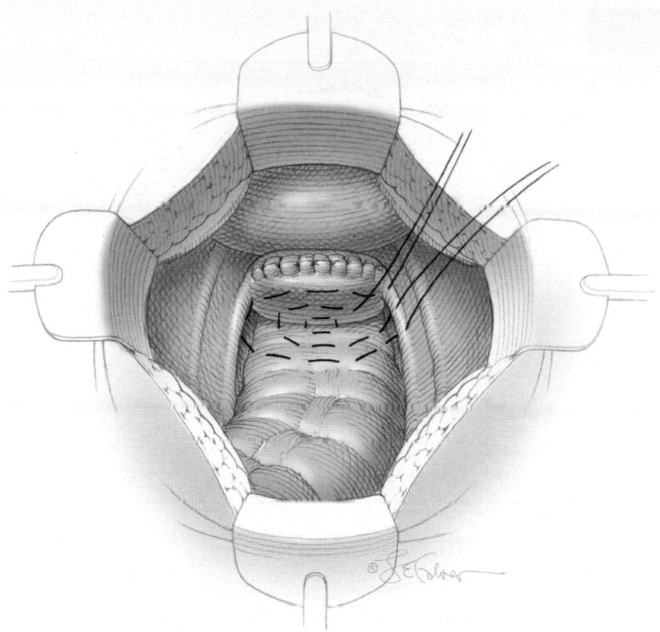

FIGURE 43-23.2 Moschcowitz culdoplasty.

❺ **Moschcowitz Culdoplasty.** Concentric 2-0 gauge permanent sutures are placed in the cul-de-sac beginning at the base and are directed upward almost to the level of the vaginal apex (Fig. 43-23.2). During placement, sutures are placed through the posterior vaginal wall and then advanced through the right uterosacral ligament, the sigmoid colon muscularis, and finally the left uterosacral ligament. The number of concentric rings required depends on the depth of the cul-de-sac, and usually three to four rings is sufficient. Rings are positioned 1 to 2 cm apart. With this procedure, ureteral kinking should be avoided during suture tying.

❻ **Cystoscopy.** Consideration should be given to performing cystoscopy after sutures are tied because of the potential risk of ureteral injury with culdoplasty procedures.

❼ **Incision Closure.** The abdominal incision is closed as described in Section 41-1 or 41-2 (p. 1021).

POSTOPERATIVE

Following culdoplasty, postoperative care follows that for any major abdominal surgery. Hospitalization typically varies from 2 to 4 days, and return of normal bowel function usually dictates this course. Stool softeners should be administered because defecatory dysfunction can develop due to a change in the rectosigmoid angle. These may be continued as needed to maintain normal bowel function.

43-24

LeFort Partial Colpocleisis

There are two basic approaches to the repair of vaginal vault prolapse: obliterative and reconstructive. Although reconstructive approaches recreate a functional vagina, obliterative procedures reach nearly 100-percent success rates in curing prolapse.

The LeFort partial colpocleisis is an obliterative vaginal procedure that approximates the anterior and posterior vaginal walls. This surgery effectively replaces the prolapsed vaginal vault into the abdominal cavity in women with or without a uterus (Fig. 43-24.1). The procedure is performed in women with significant prolapse beyond the hymen of the uterus, vagina, and anterior and posterior vaginal walls.

As opposed to complete colpocleisis, with LeFort partial colpocleisis, the vaginal mucosa is not excised in its entirely. Rather, rectangular sections of vaginal mucosa are dissected from the anterior and posterior vaginal walls, and the denuded fibromuscular layers are sewn together to close the vaginal vault. The remaining lateral tracts of vaginal epithelium create drainage tunnels on either side of the closed vagina.

This operation may be performed quickly with general, regional, or local anesthesia. Blood loss is minimal, and success rates are high. The procedure is only indicated in elderly women who have no future desire for sexual intercourse. Because of the high incidence of stress urinary incontinence (SUI) following LeFort partial colpocleisis, concurrent antiincontinence surgery should be considered. Additionally, high perineorrhaphy is recommended to decrease the risk of recurrent prolapse (Section 43-16, p. 1223).

PREOPERATIVE

Patient Evaluation

Because access to the cervix and endometrial cavity is not possible following this procedure, preinvasive lesions should be excluded. Specifically, a normal Pap smear should be documented prior to surgery, and evaluation of the endometrium with either endometrial biopsy or sonography is recommended.

Prolapse of the anterior, posterior, and apical compartments should be documented prior to surgery (Chap. 24, p. 644). Additionally, urodynamic testing is performed prior to surgery to evaluate for potential SUI (Chap. 23, p. 621). Even without documented SUI, an adjunctive antiincontinence procedure should be considered to prevent postoperative incontinence. Additionally, in those patients undergoing LeFort partial colpocleisis who have large, global prolapse, intravenous pyelography or cystoscopy is warranted to assess for ureteral obstruction preoperatively. Known obstruction will help with interpretation of findings during cystoscopy performed at the procedure's end.

Consent

Women considering this procedure must be fully aware that future vaginal intercourse will not be possible. Therefore, the decision to undergo this procedure should include a woman's partner. Patients expressing hesitation or doubt should be excluded as candidates.

Risks of the procedure include urinary incontinence, urinary retention, ureteral obstruction, and recurrent prolapse. Additionally, in the unlikely situation that malignancy of the cervix or endometrium develops after LeFort partial colpocleisis, the diagnosis may be potentially delayed.

Patient Preparation

Bowel preparation is administered the evening prior to surgery to effectively empty and decompress the rectum (Table 39-7, p. 960). This minimizes fecal contamination of the surgical field. Antibiotic prophylaxis is routinely administered to lower rates of postoperative wound infection (Table 39-6, p. 959). Additionally, thromboprophylaxis is provided as outlined in Table 39-9 (p. 962).

INTRAOPERATIVE

SURGICAL STEPS

❶ Anesthesia and Patient Positioning. General or regional anesthesia is preferred, although LeFort partial colpocleisis can be performed under local anesthesia. A patient is placed in high lithotomy position, the vagina is surgically prepared, and a Foley catheter is inserted. Although LeFort partial colpocleisis may be performed in women with or without a uterus, the following description outlines the steps in women without previous hysterectomy.

❷ Vaginal Marking. The rectangular areas of vaginal mucosa on the anterior and posterior vaginal walls are outlined with a surgical marker or electrosurgical blade. The size of the rectangular sections to be removed is determined by the length of vaginal wall.

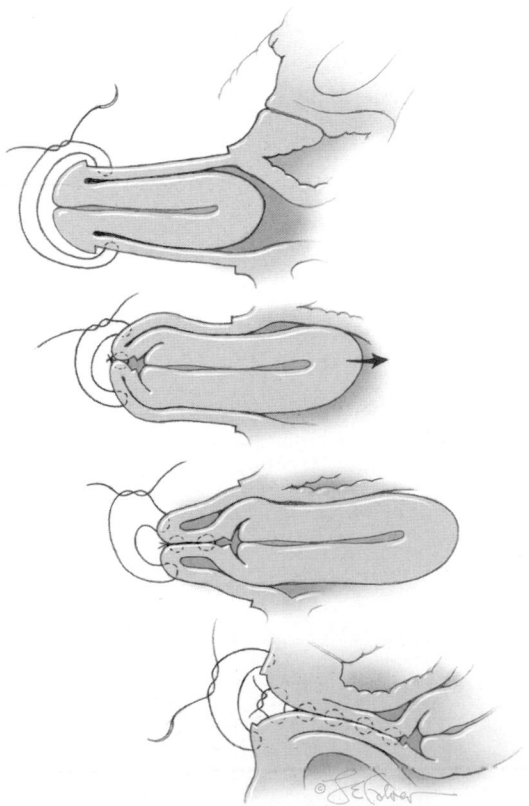

FIGURE 43-24.1 Prolapse correction following placement of serial sutures.

vasopressin in 60 mL of saline). Without infiltration, significant bleeding can result from disruption of multiple small vessels during dissection. This infiltration should extend beyond the anticipated incision boundaries.

Needle aspiration prior to injection is imperative to avoid intravascular injection of this potent vasoconstrictor. The anesthesiologist should also be informed of vasopressin injection, as a sudden increase in patient blood pressure may potentially occur following injection. Blanching at the injection site is common.

Due to its vasoconstrictive effects, patients with certain comorbidities may not be suitable candidates for vasopressin use. These can include a medical history of angina, myocardial infarction, cardiomyopathy, congestive heart failure, uncontrolled hypertension, migraine, asthma, or severe chronic obstructive pulmonary disease.

❹ **Vaginal Incision.** Previously outlined areas are sharply incised down to the fibromuscular layer.

❺ **Vaginal Dissection.** A combination of sharp and blunt dissection is used to lift the mucosa away from the fibromuscular layer (Figs. 43-24.2 and 43-24.3). Dissection in the correct plane will prevent inadvertent entry into the bladder or bowel. The technique for dissection involves a finger behind the vaginal wall and dissection with Merzenbaum scissors parallel to the vaginal wall. After entry into the correct plane, blunt dissection with a sponge may allow rapid and wide development of this avascular space.

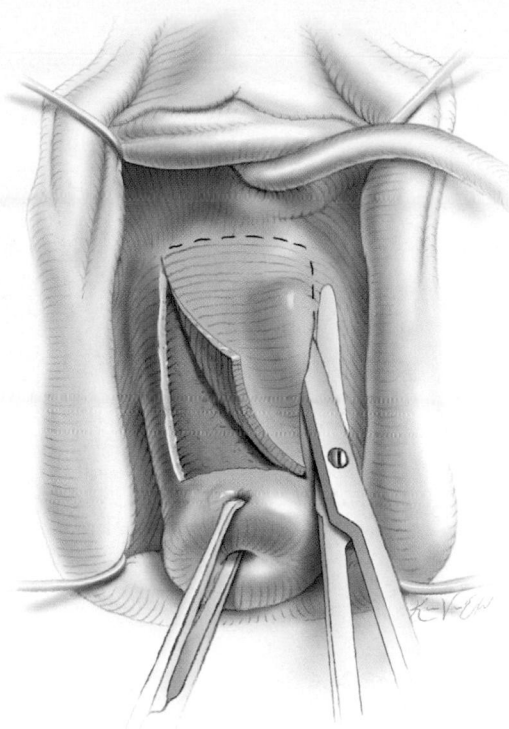

FIGURE 43-24.2 Anterior vaginal wall incision.

The distal transverse incision should be placed 1 to 2 cm above the cervical os. The proximal transverse incision should lie 2 to 3 cm below the urethral meatus. The width of the incision will be determined by the size of the uterus, cervix, and vaginal walls and should be almost as wide as the prolapsed bulge. This allows multiple sutures to be placed during closure.

❸ **Vaginal Infiltration.** The rectangular areas of the vaginal wall to be removed are thoroughly infiltrated with 50 mL of a dilute hemostatic solution (20 units of synthetic

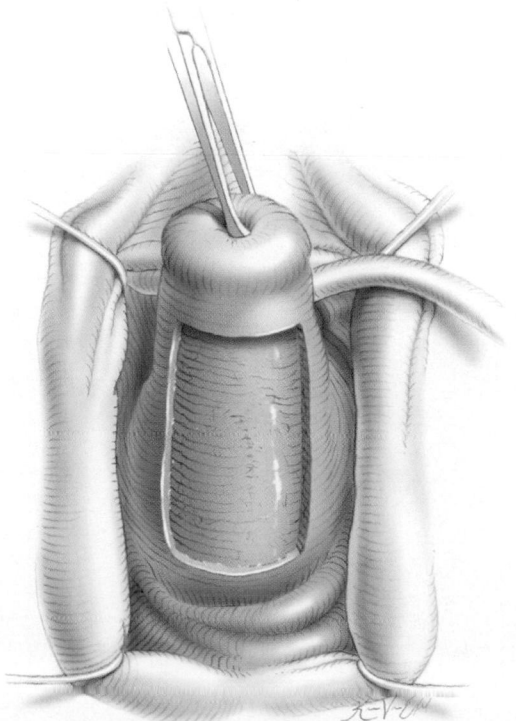

FIGURE 43-24.3 Posterior vaginal wall incision.

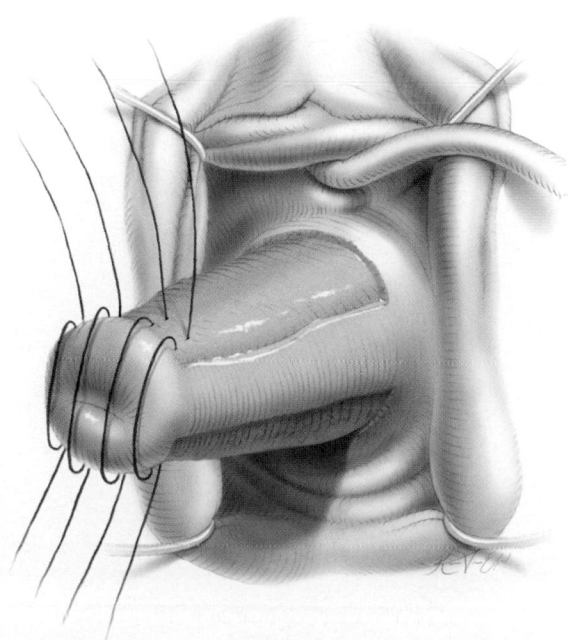

FIGURE 43-24.4 Initial suture placement.

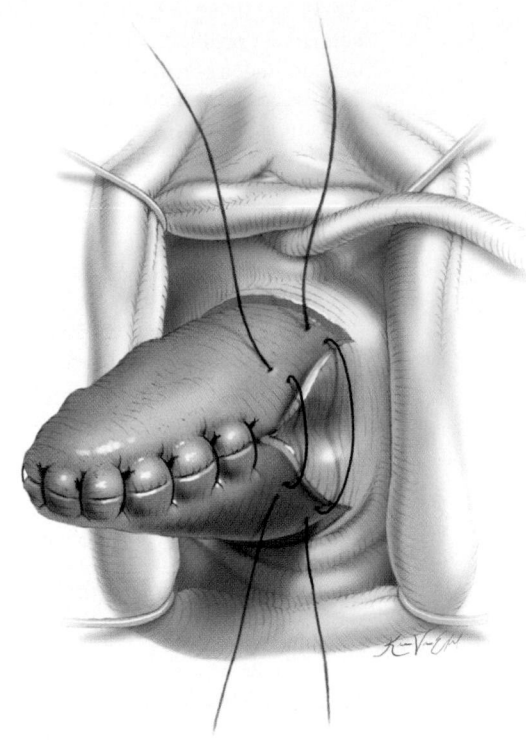

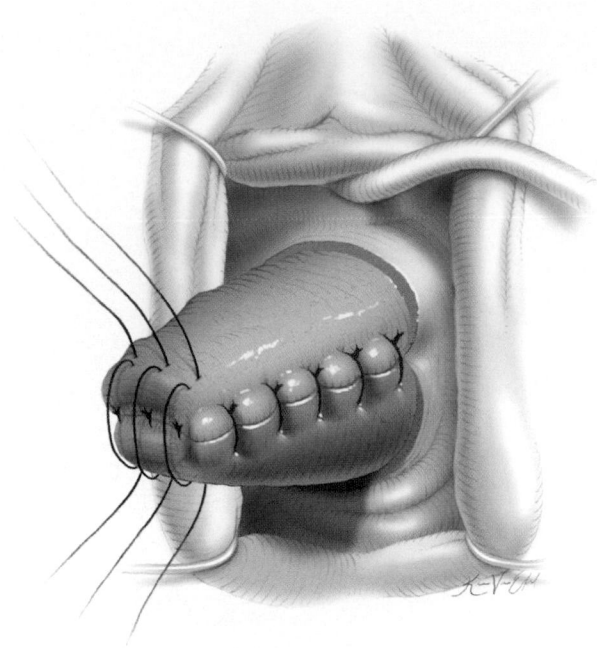

FIGURE 43-24.6 Second row of sutures.

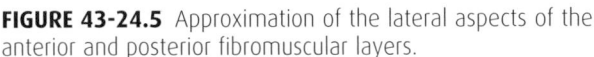

FIGURE 43-24.5 Approximation of the lateral aspects of the anterior and posterior fibromuscular layers.

❻ **Suture Placement.** After rectangles are removed, a row of interrupted stitches using 2-0 permanent suture is placed from the anterior to the posterior distal transverse edges (Fig. 43-24.4). These will effectively close the fibromuscular layer over the cervix.

Next, lateral vaginal drainage canals are created along both the right and left sides of the incision. These allow drainage of physiologic endometrial and cervical discharge into the vagina. On the first side, sutures approximate the superior and inferior edges of the rectangles. This lateral row of sutures begins distally and progresses proximally to the original proximal transverse incision (Fig. 43-24.5). A drainage canal is created on the opposite side in a similar fashion.

To elevate and replace the uterus into the pelvic cavity, a surgeon places progressively more caudal rows of interrupted sutures that approximate the anterior and posterior fibromuscular layers along the width of the incision (Fig. 43-24.6). Successive

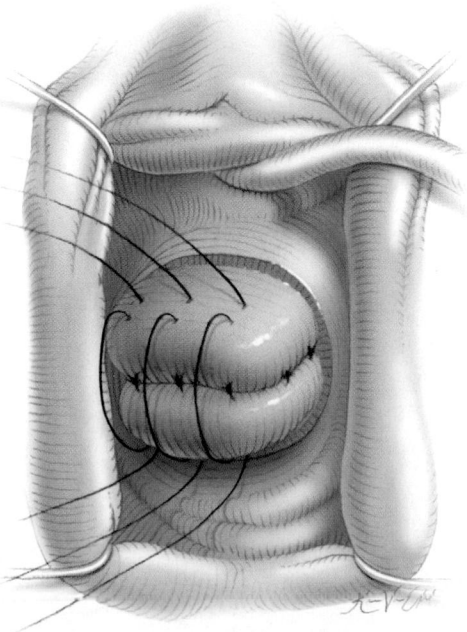

FIGURE 43-24.7 Subsequent row of sutures.

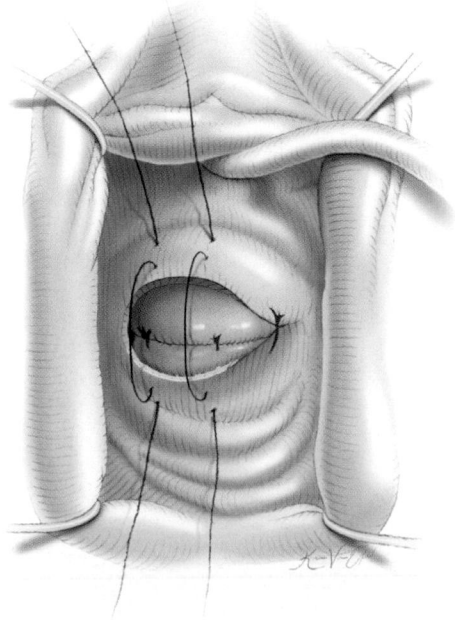

FIGURE 43-24.8 Vaginal mucosa closure.

transverse tiers of sutures are placed until the proximal transverse incision is reached (Fig. 43-24.7). These rows create a tissue septum that elevates and supports the uterus (see Fig. 43-24.1).

❼ Antiincontinence Surgery. At this point, an antiincontinence procedure may be performed.

❽ Closure of the Vaginal Mucosa. The vaginal mucosa is then closed in a running fashion with 2-0 delayed-absorbable suture, taking wide bites through the vaginal epithelium (Fig. 43-24.8).

❾ Perineorrhaphy. Following closure of the vaginal mucosa, perineorrhaphy is performed as described in Section 43-16 (p. 1223).

❿ Cystoscopy. Cystoscopy should be performed at the end of the procedure to exclude urinary tract injury and document ureteral patency (Section 43-1, p. 1185).

POSTOPERATIVE

Postoperative bladder function will depend on whether antiincontinence surgery is performed. In general, recovery with LeFort partial colpocleisis is quick and typically without complication. Postoperative drainage should not be anticipated save for mild spotting. As with any prolapse procedure, constipation should be avoided, and administration of stool softeners is recommended. Resumption of normal activities is encouraged with the exception of heavy lifting for several months.

CHAPTER 43

43-25

Complete Colpocleisis

Complete colpocleisis, also termed colpectomy, is an obliterative procedure used for those with posthysterectomy global prolapse who do not desire future sexual activity. If the uterus is present, concurrent total vaginal hysterectomy and closure of the peritoneum is performed prior to colpocleisis.

In contrast to LeFort partial colpocleisis, with complete colpocleisis, the vaginal wall is excised in its entirety. During complete colpocleisis, the epithelial and lamina proprial layers are removed down to the fibromuscular layer. The operation attaches the anterior fibromuscular layer to the posterior fibromuscular layer, effectively closing the vaginal tube and replacing it back into the abdominal cavity.

The operation obliterates the vagina and removes any potential for sexual intercourse. Thus, the operation is generally performed in elderly women. It may also be considered in those with high surgical risks because it can be performed quickly, under local or regional anesthesia, and with minimal blood loss. Complete colpocleisis should be performed in conjunction with high perineorrhaphy to decrease the risk of recurrence. Consideration should also be given to performing a prophylactic antiincontinence procedure, even in those without incontinence symptoms, as the risk of postoperative stress urinary incontinence is high.

PREOPERATIVE

Patient Evaluation

This procedure is used in patients who have complete eversion of the apical, anterior, and posterior vaginal walls. Patients with this severe degree of prolapse often do not have stress urinary incontinence (SUI) because the urethra is kinked by prolapsing organs. However, with replacement of the prolapse, many patients do develop postoperative SUI. Therefore, urodynamic testing has traditionally been performed prior to this procedure, and antiincontinence surgery is recommended for those who demonstrate latent SUI.

Frequently women with global prolapse have some degree of ureteral obstruction. Accordingly, consideration should be given to obtaining a preoperative intravenous pyelogram (IVP) or performing cystoscopy to document ureteral patency. If ureteral patency is not confirmed, then preoperative stent placement should be considered (Section 43-1, p. 1187).

Consent

Women must have absolutely no intention or desire for future intercourse. If there is a partner involved, they should be included in the decision and consenting process. Women who express any hesitancy or doubt should be excluded as candidates. Subsequent stress urinary incontinence is a definite risk with this surgery. If patients decline antiincontinence operations, they should be aware of the significant risk of postoperative urinary incontinence.

As with any prolapse surgery, the consenting process should include a discussion of prolapse recurrence risk, although this risk is low with complete colpocleisis. Additionally, ureteral injury has also been described with this procedure, and it should be included on consenting documents.

Patient Preparation

Bowel preparation is administered the evening prior to surgery to effectively empty and decompress the rectum (Table 39-7, p. 960). This minimizes fecal contamination of the surgical field. Antibiotic prophylaxis is routinely administered to lower rates of postoperative wound infection (Table 39-6, p. 959). Additionally, thromboprophylaxis is provided as outlined in Table 39-9 (p. 962).

INTRAOPERATIVE

SURGICAL STEPS

❶ Anesthesia and Patient Positioning. General or regional anesthesia is preferred, although complete colpocleisis can be performed with local anesthesia. Following anesthesia administration, a woman is placed in high lithotomy position, the vagina is surgically prepared, and a Foley catheter is inserted.

❷ Vaginal Infiltration. With the prolapsed vaginal tube replaced, Allis clamps are place laterally at 3 and 9 o'clock inside the hymenal ring and pulled to the midline without tension. This maneuver allows the surgeon to assess the amount of vaginal wall to be removed. With the vaginal tube prolapsed, the vaginal wall is then thoroughly infiltrated with 50 mL of a dilute hemostatic solution (20 units of synthetic vasopressin in 60 mL of saline). Without infiltration, significant blood loss can occur from disruption of multiple small vessels during dissection. Careful use of vasopressin is outlined in Section 43-24 (p. 1247).

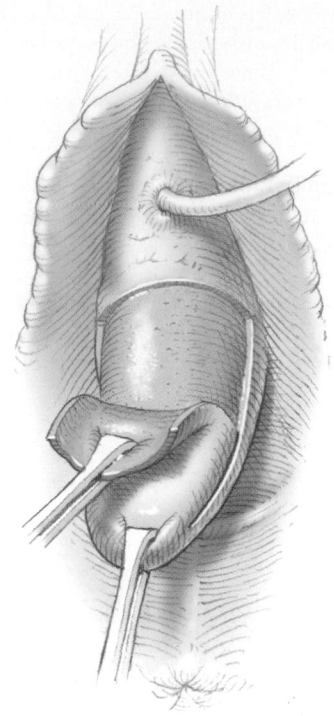

FIGURE 43-25.1 Anterior vaginal wall incision.

❸ Vaginal Incision. A circumferential incision is made 1 cm inside the hymenal ring around the base of the prolapsed vaginal tube. The incision should begin approximately 3 cm below the urethral meatus to allow concurrent antiincontinence procedures.

❹ Vaginal Dissection. A combination of sharp and blunt dissection is used to lift the vaginal epithelium and lamina propria off the fibromuscular layer (Figs. 43-25.1 and 43-25.2). Dissection in this correct plane will prevent inadvertent entry into the bladder or bowel. The technique for dissection involves positioning a finger behind the vaginal wall and dissecting with Metzenbaum scissors parallel to the vaginal wall. After entry into the correct plane, blunt dissection with a sponge may allow rapid and wide development of this avascular space. There are areas where dissection may be difficult. For example, upon reaching the prolapsed vaginal apex and remnants of the uterosacral ligaments, extensive scarring may be present that requires sharp dissection. The entire vaginal epithelium is removed from the prolapsed vaginal tube.

❺ Suture Placement. To plicate the anterior and posterior vaginal walls together and replace the vaginal tube into the abdominal cavity, a surgeon places a series of circumferential purse-string sutures around the

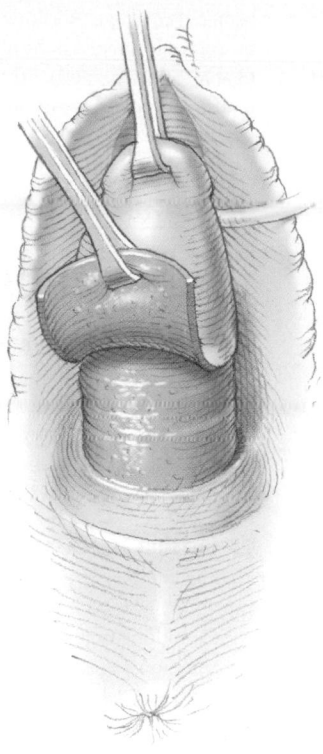

FIGURE 43-25.2 Posterior vaginal wall incision.

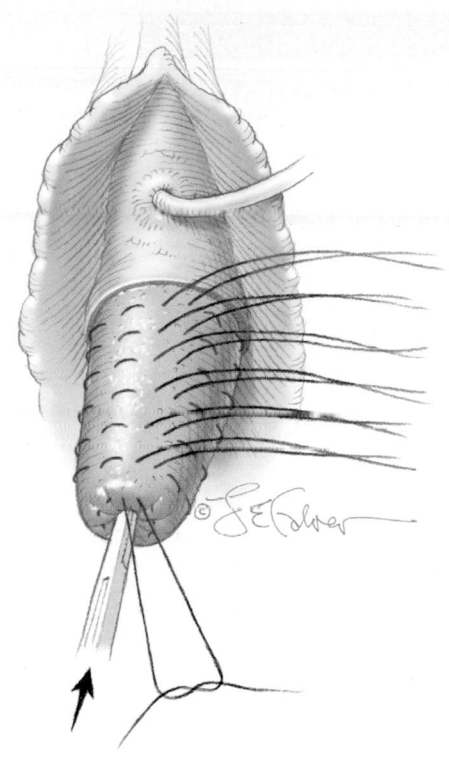

FIGURE 43-25.3 Circumferential suturing.

vaginal tube within the fibromuscular layer using 2-0 permanent suture (Fig. 43-25.3).

The first bite is taken at 12 o'clock at the distal end of the prolapsed tube. Bites are taken circumferentially around the vaginal tube, and the knot is secured at 12 o'clock. A hemostat is placed 1 cm above the knot, and the suture ends are cut. The next circumferential suture is then place 1 cm proximal to the first suture. Prior to securing the knot on this second suture, the surgeon presses the hemostat into the apex of the vaginal tube. This telescopes the tube cephalad and toward the abdominal cavity (Fig. 43-25.4A). The knot is then secured over the hemostat, effectively reducing this section of prolapsed vaginal tube. The hemostat is then removed and placed on the second suture above the knot, and the process is repeated. Depending on the size of the prolapse, approximately 6 to 8 suture rings are needed to completely invert the prolapsed vaginal tube (Fig. 43-25.4B).

❻ Antiincontinence Surgery. At this point, an antiincontinence procedure may be performed.

❼ Closure of Vaginal Mucosa. The vaginal mucosa is then closed with a running technique using 2-0 delayed-absorbable suture, taking wide bites through the vaginal epithelium. The completed incision lies approximately 2 to 3 cm above the hymenal ring.

❽ Perineorrhaphy. At this point, perineorrhaphy is performed as described in Section 43-16 (p. 1223).

❾ Cystoscopy. Cystoscopy should be performed at the procedure's completion, and ureteral patency documented (Section 43-1, p. 1185).

POSTOPERATIVE

Postoperative bladder function will depend on whether antiincontinence surgery is performed. In general, recovery with colpocleisis is quick and typically without complication. Postoperative drainage should not be anticipated save for mild spotting. As with any prolapse procedure, constipation should be avoided, and administration of stool softeners is recommended. Resumption of normal activities is encouraged with the exception of heavy lifting for several months.

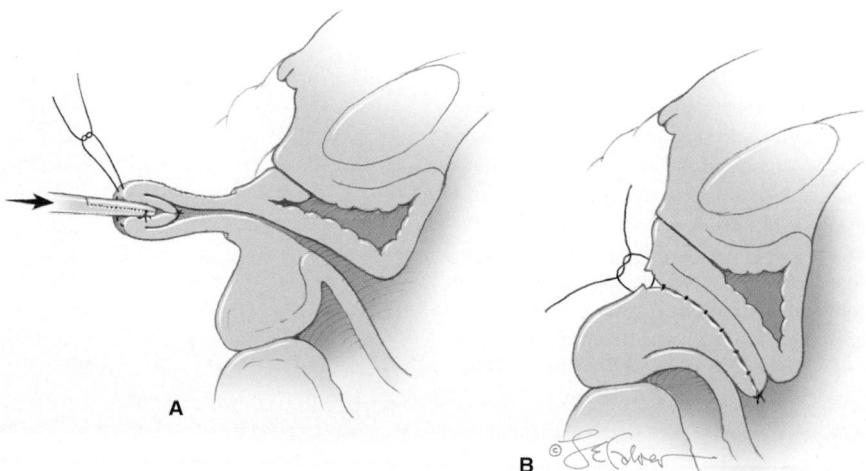

FIGURE 43-25.4 Cephalad pressure against telescoping vaginal tube as serial sutures are secured (*left*). Completely inverted vaginal tube (*right*).

43-26

Anal Sphincteroplasty

Anal sphincteroplasty reapproximates disrupted skeletal muscle fibers of the external anal sphincter (EAS) and disrupted smooth muscle fibers of the internal anal sphincter (IAS). Reapproximation may be accomplished by joining the ends of disrupted fibers, termed an *end-to-end sphincteroplasty*. Alternatively, disrupted ends may be overlapped and then sutured, called an *overlapping sphincteroplasty*.

Both techniques can be used to repair a third- or fourth-degree laceration immediately following a delivery or may be used in a nonobstetric setting to treat anal incontinence. Although incontinence secondary to sphincter disruption stands as a clear indication, surgical correction may also benefit those with incontinence from other etiologies, including pudendal neuropathy. A full discussion of anal incontinence is found in Chapter 25 (p. 659).

PREOPERATIVE

Patient Evaluation

Because some causes of anal incontinence are more amenable to surgical correction than others, careful preoperative evaluation should attempt to distinguish underlying sources. Evaluation for structural gastrointestinal (GI) tract pathology typically involves colonoscopy and/or barium enema. Additionally, radiographic bowel transit studies can be used to diagnose slow transit time, which may be related to symptoms of defecatory dysfunction.

Specific to the anorectum, endoanal sonography can accurately define structural disruption of the EAS and IAS (Fig. 25-7, p. 667). Anal manometry and pudendal nerve conduction studies may identify physiologic dysfunction such as neuropathy (Martinez Hernandez, 2003).

Clinicians have attempted to improve success rates by selecting only those women who may benefit most from surgery. Investigations have evaluated patient age, preoperative anal manometry readings, and pudendal nerve motor function as possible predictors of outcome. However, research findings have been conflicting, and none of these predictors has proved to be a consistent indicator of success (Bravo Gutierrez, 2004; Buie, 2001; Gearhart, 2005; Gilliland, 1998).

Consent

Although a significant number of women may have improved incontinence immediately following anal sphincteroplasty, the durability of this repair is poor. For example, 3 to 5 years following repair, only approximately 10 percent of women are fully continent of solid and liquid stool (Halverson, 2002; Malouf, 2000). The causes of long-term deterioration in function remain uncertain, but the effects of aging, postoperative scarring, and progressing pudendal neuropathy have been suggested (Madoff, 2004). In addition, it is believed that skeletal muscle repair has poor success because the resting tone of muscle places incision lines on constant tension. Therefore, preoperative counseling should inform that although most individuals will improve after the procedure, continence is rarely perfect, and deterioration of continence typically progresses with time.

In addition to persistent incontinence, sphincteroplasty is associated with other surgical risks. More common serious complications include wound dehiscence and fistula formation. For example, Ha and coworkers (2001) noted wound complication in 12 percent and fistula formation in 4 percent.

Patient Preparation

Because of the high associated risk of wound complications, antibiotic prophylaxis is warrant to minimize wound infection following surgical contamination from vaginal and rectal flora. We use a combination of ciprofloxacin and metronidazole to obtain broad bacterial coverage. Additionally, bowel preparation is administered the night before surgery (Table 39-7, p. 960). Thromboprophylaxis is also provided as outlined in Table 39-9 (p. 962).

INTRAOPERATIVE

SURGICAL STEPS

❶ Anesthesia and Patient Positioning. After administration of either general or regional anesthesia, a woman is placed in dorsal lithotomy position, the vagina and perineum are surgically prepared and draped, and a Foley catheter is inserted into the bladder.

❷ Incision and Dissection. A downward-arching curvilinear incision is placed between the fourchette and anus, and this connects with a midline vaginal incision (Fig. 43-26.1). The incision edges are placed on tension with Allis clamps. Metzenbaum scissors are used to dissect disrupted ends of the EAS from surrounding and intervening scar tissue. Because of the extensive scarring frequently found surrounding these muscles, fibers may be difficult to isolate. A nerve stimulator or a needle-tip electrosurgical blade can assist in delineating these fibers. Scar tissue in the midline may be cut but should not be excised, as this tissue is used in the sphincteroplasty repair to add strength to the muscle closure.

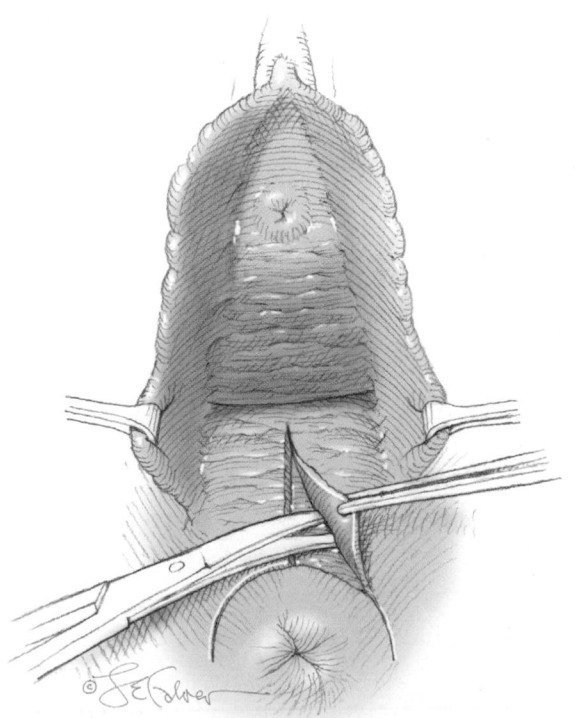

FIGURE 43-26.1 Vaginal dissection.

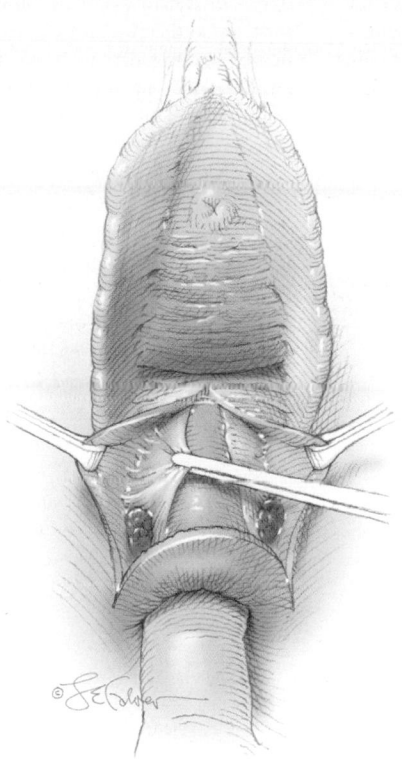

FIGURE 43-26.2 Internal anal sphincter identification.

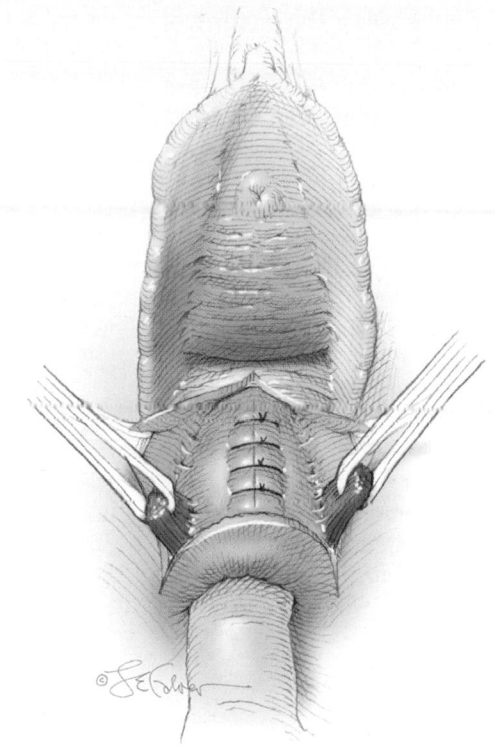

FIGURE 43-26.3 Following internal anal sphincter reapproximation, the external anal sphincter is identified and grasped.

The internal anal sphincter contributes significantly to the resting tone of the anal canal, and closure of this muscle should be included in the repair. Grasped in Figure 43-26.2, the IAS is identified as a smooth white sheet of tissue deep to the external sphincter and superficial to the rectal wall.

❸ **Suture Placement within the Internal Anal Sphincter.** Interrupted stitches of 3-0 delayed-absorbable suture are used to bring the edges of the internal anal sphincter together in the midline (Fig. 43-26.3). Sutures are spaced approximately 0.5 cm apart, and a second overlying row of sutures may be placed after the first is completed. Suture placement and exposure of the IAS is aided by a finger in the rectum.

❹ **Levator Ani Muscle Plication.** For additional support, the levator ani muscle can be plicated with interrupted stitches using 2-0

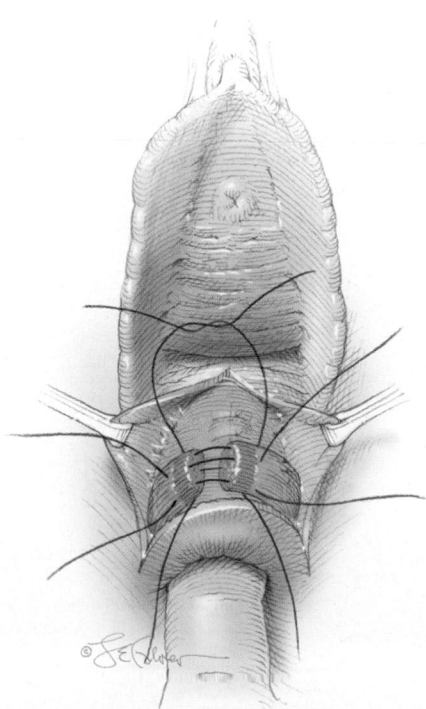

FIGURE 43-26.4 End-to-end sphincteroplasty.

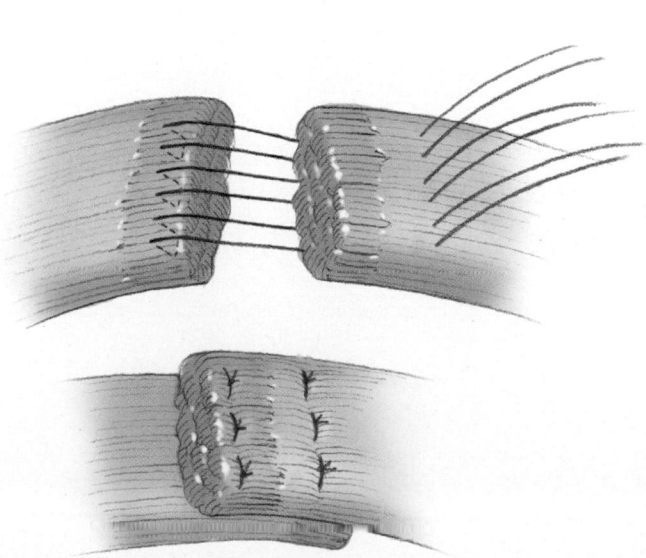

FIGURE 43-26.5 Overlapping sphincteroplasty.

delayed-absorbable suture. This is performed after IAS closure but prior to EAS closure.

❺ Suture Placement for End-to-End External Anal Sphincteroplasty. Each end of the disrupted EAS is identified and grasped with an Allis clamp (see Fig. 43-26.3). The ends of the EAS are brought to the midline, and a row of interrupted reapproximating stitches are placed (Fig. 43-26.4). Although many surgeons prefer the durability of permanent sutures for most pelvic reconstructive procedures, use of permanent sutures for sphincteroplasty has been associated with high rates of suture erosion and wound dehiscence (Luck, 2005). For this reason, 2-0 delayed-absorbable suture is used.

❻ Suture Placement for Overlapping External Anal Sphincteroplasty. With overlapping sphincteroplasty, at least 1 cm of the EAS is mobilized on each side. The ends are grasped with Allis clamps and brought to the midline, where they are overlapped. The overlapped ends are then sewn together with interrupted stitches of 2-0 delayed-absorbable suture placed in two rows, each containing two to three stitches (Fig. 43-26.5).

❼ Incision Closure. Excision of excess perineal skin may be required prior to closing the incision. Vaginal mucosa and perineal skin are then closed in a running fashion using 2-0 delayed-absorbable suture.

POSTOPERATIVE

Pain varies postoperatively, and some women can be discharged home on day 1, whereas others require longer hospitalization. The Foley catheter is removed on postoperative day 1 or 2. An active voiding trial is performed, and some women may have difficulty voiding due to pain, inflammation, and levator ani muscle spasm. To limit trauma to the healing repair, we try to delay defecation for several days. Patients do not eat or drink on day 1 and are subsequently advanced to clear liquids for 3 or 4 days. Stool softeners are given when a solid diet is begun and continued for at least 6 weeks. Because of the high risk of wound dehiscence and infection, oral ciprofloxacin and metronidazole are given for 10 days postprocedure. Local wound care involves sitz baths twice daily and perineal cleansing with a plastic water bottle following urination or defecation. Ambulation is encouraged, but physical exercise and sexual intercourse are delayed for 8 weeks. The first postoperative visit is typically 4 weeks following surgery.

Rectovaginal Fistula Repair

In general, rectovaginal fistulas that are encountered by gynecologists include those complicating fourth-degree obstetric lacerations. Less commonly, fistulas may result from gynecologic surgery or radiation therapy.

If a fistula is identified at the time or shortly after injury, then immediate repair may be undertaken. However, fistulas should not be repaired in the setting of inflammation, induration, or infection. In addition, fistulas that are associated with radiation therapy and recurrent fistula often require interposition of a vascular flap, such as a Martius bulbocavernosus fad pad graft, due to poor tissue vascularity (Section 43-11, p. 1210).

Approaches to fistula repair include perineoproctotomy or transvaginal, transperineal, or transrectal techniques. The approach favored by gynecologists is the transvaginal approach and is described here. Perineoproctotomy is not recommended unless fistulas involve the anal sphincter. This technique involves disruption of the sphincter to access a fistula and as a result, increases the risk of anal incontinence postoperatively.

PREOPERATIVE

Patient Evaluation

A thorough evaluation is necessary to delineate the full extent of a fistula. If there are questions regarding the complexity or number of fistulas, then testing as discussed in Chapter 25 (p. 674) may be needed. At times, pinpoint fistulas are difficult to identify and may be require examination under anesthesia with lacrimal duct probing.

Consent

In addition to general surgical risks, specific risks following rectovaginal fistula repair include fistula recurrence, dyspareunia, and vaginal narrowing or shortening. Fecal incontinence may follow some cases if the anal sphincter is disrupted during surgery, as with perineoproctotomy.

Patient Preparation

A rigorous bowel preparation is required to clear all stool from the rectal vault. Accordingly, a clear liquid diet and 1 gallon

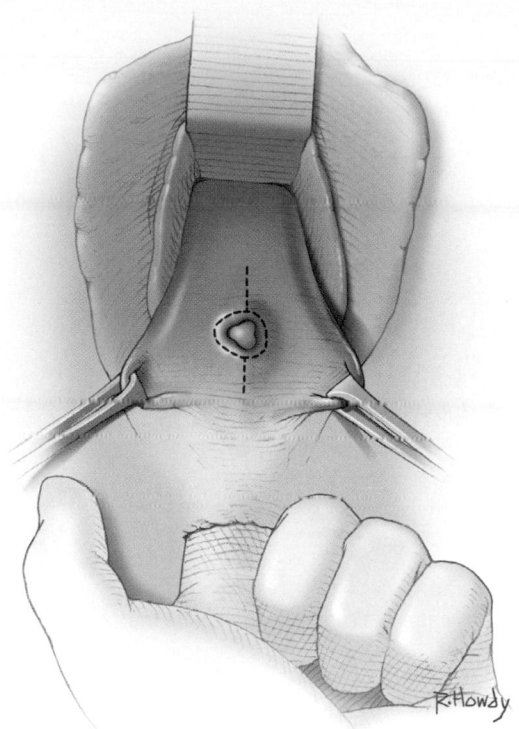

FIGURE 43-27.1 Vaginal incision.

of an orally administered polyethylene glycol and electrolyte solution (Golytely) is advised the day prior to surgery. If stool is still present in the rectum at the beginning of surgery, then a povidone-iodine (Betadine) flush with a Malecot drain may be needed. Antibiotic prophylaxis is given concurrent with surgery, however, additional doses during the days before surgery are not indicated. We use a combination of ciprofloxacin and metronidazole to obtain broad bacterial coverage. Additionally, thromboprophylaxis is provided as outlined in Table 39-9 (p. 962).

INTRAOPERATIVE

SURGICAL STEPS

❶ **Anesthesia and Patient Position.** Rectovaginal fistula repair is typically an inpatient procedure, performed under general or regional anesthesia. A patient is placed in high lithotomy position with stirrups of a surgeon's choosing. The vagina is surgically prepared, and a Foley catheter is inserted.

❷ **Fistula Identification.** The fistula is identified and its course is traced with the use of a probe or dilator. Small fistulas may be dilated to improve identification of the tract.

❸ **Vaginal Incision.** A circular incision is made in the vaginal epithelium surrounding the fistula (Fig. 43-27.1). The incision must be wide enough to allow excision of the tract and permit sufficient mobilization of surrounding tissues to close the defect without excess tissue tension (Fig. 43-27.2). The entire fistula tract is then excised (Fig. 43-27.3).

❹ **Closure of the Rectal Wall.** Using 3-0 delayed-absorbable suture, a purse string suture is placed around the defect a few millimeters from the mucosal edge. This suture is tied and inverts the defect's edges into the bowel lumen. One or two additional purse-string sutures may be placed in the rectal wall muscularis to reinforce the closure. Alternatively, the defect may be closed with serial interrupted sutures placed within the rectal wall muscularis (Fig. 43-27.4).

❺ **Closure of the Fibromuscular Layer.** The fibromuscular layer between the vagina and rectum is then reapproximated with interrupted stitches of 2-0 delayed-absorbable sutures (Fig. 43-27.5). If possible, two layers of closure are completed to minimize incision tension and reinforce the repair.

❻ **Martius Bulbocavernosus Fat Pad Graft.** In cases in which avascular or fibrotic

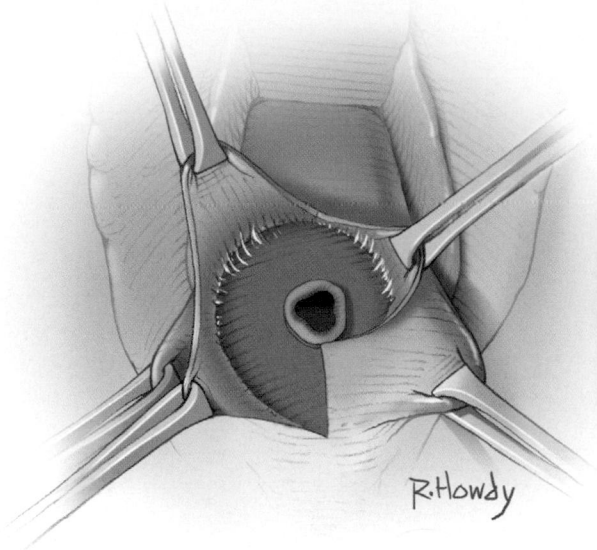

FIGURE 43-27.2 Mobilization of surrounding vaginal mucosa.

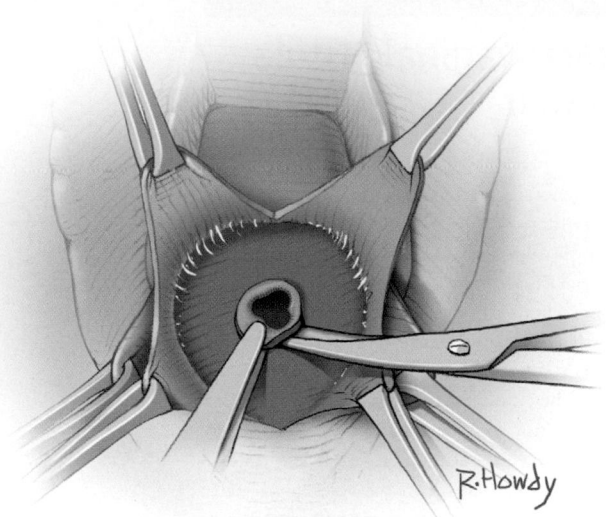

FIGURE 43-27.3 Fistulous tract excision.

tissue is extensive, a Martius graft may be placed between the fibromuscular layer and vaginal epithelium.

❼ **Vaginal Wall Closure.** Excess vaginal mucosa is trimmed, and the vaginal mucosa is closed in a continuous running fashion using 3-0 absorbable or delayed-absorbable suture.

POSTOPERATIVE

Normal activity can resume during the first postoperative days. Intercourse, however, should be delayed at least 1 month or until the vaginal incision is healed.

To limit trauma to the healing repair, we try to delay defecation for several days. Patients do not eat or drink on the first postoperative day and are subsequently advanced to clear liquids for 3 or 4 days. Stool softeners are given when a solid diet is begun and continued for at least 6 weeks. Constipation should be avoided. Local wound care involves sitz baths twice daily and perineal cleansing with a squeeze plastic water bottle following urination or defecation.

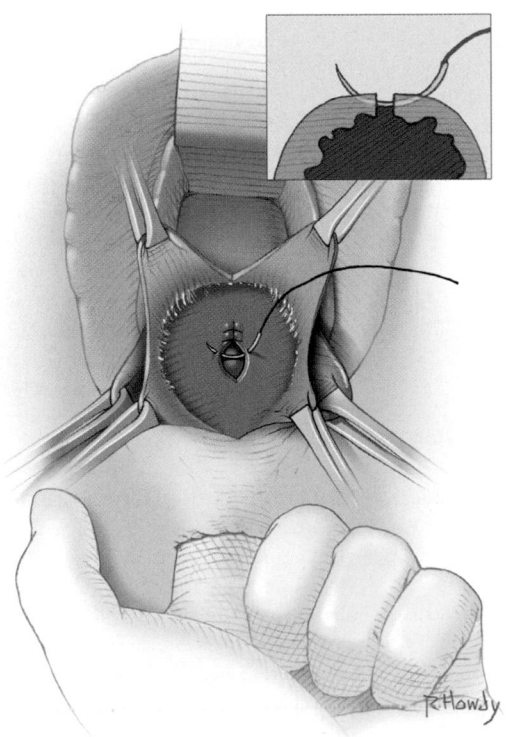

FIGURE 43-27.4 Closure of the rectal wall.

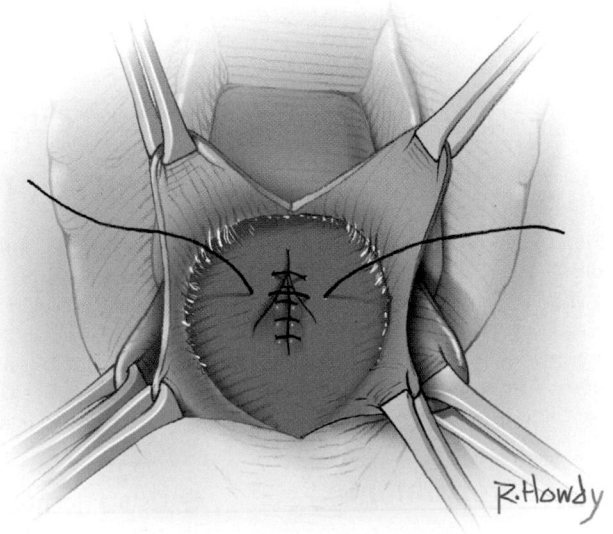

FIGURE 43-27.5 Closure of the fibromuscular layer.

REFERENCES

Alcalay M, Monga A, Stanton SL: Burch colposuspension: a 10-20 year follow up. Br J Obstet Gynaecol 102:740, 1995

Altman D, Väyrynen T, Engh ME, et al: Anterior colporrhaphy versus transvaginal mesh for pelvic organ prolapse. N Engl J Med 364(19):1826, 2011

American College of Obstetricians and Gynecologists: Antibiotic prophylaxis for gynecologic procedures. Practice Bulletin No. 104, May 2009

Ankardal M, Ekerydh A, Crafoord K, et al: A randomised trial comparing open Burch colposuspension using sutures with laparoscopic colposuspension using mesh and staples in women with stress urinary incontinence. Br J Obstet Gynaecol 111:974, 2004

Bai SW, Kim BJ, Kim SK, et al: Comparison of outcomes between Burch colposuspension with and without concomitant abdominal hysterectomy. Yonsei Med J 45:665, 2004

Beer M, Kuhn A: Surgical techniques for vault prolapse: a review of the literature. Eur J Obstet Gynecol Reprod Biol 119:144, 2005

Benson JT, Lucente V, McClellan E: Vaginal versus abdominal reconstructive surgery for the treatment of pelvic support defects: a prospective, randomized study with long-term outcome evaluation. Am J Obstet Gynecol 175:1418, 1996

Bent AE, Foote J, Siegel S, et al: Collagen implant for treating stress urinary incontinence in women with urethral hypermobility. J Urol 166:1354, 2001

Bhatia NN, Karram MM, Bergman A: Role of antibiotic prophylaxis in retropubic surgery for stress urinary incontinence. Obstet Gynecol 74:637, 1989

Borstad E, Rud T: The risk of developing urinary stress-incontinence after vaginal repair in continent women: a clinical and urodynamic follow-up study. Acta Obstet Gynaecol Scand 68:545, 1989

Bravo Gutierrez A, Madoff RD, Lowry AC, et al: Long-term results of anterior sphincteroplasty. Dis Colon Rectum 47:727, 2004

Brubaker L, Cundiff GW, Fine P, et al: Abdominal sacrocolpopexy with Burch colposuspension to reduce urinary stress incontinence. N Engl J Med 354:1557, 2006

Buie WD, Lowry AC, Rothenberger DA, et al: Clinical rather than laboratory assessment predicts continence after anterior sphincteroplasty. Dis Colon Rectum 44:1255, 2001

Cervigni M, Natale F: The use of synthetics in the treatment of pelvic organ prolapse. Curr Opin Urol 11:429, 2001

Cespedes RD: Anterior approach bilateral sacrospinous ligament fixation for vaginal vault prolapse. Urology 56:70, 2000

Chaikin DC, Groutz A, Blaivas JG: Predicting the need for anti-incontinence surgery in continent women undergoing repair of severe urogenital prolapse. J Urol 163:531, 2000

Chapin DS: Teaching sacrospinous colpopexy. Am J Obstet Gynecol 177:1330, 1997

Chrouser KL, Fick F, Goel A, et al: Carbon coated zirconium beads in β-glucan gel and bovine glutaraldehyde cross-linked collagen injections for intrinsic sphincter deficiency: continence and satisfaction after extended follow-up. J Urol 171:1152, 2004

Corcos J, Collet JP, Shapiro S, et al: Multicenter randomized clinical trial comparing surgery and collagen injections for treatment of female stress urinary incontinence. Urology 65:898, 2005

Corcos J, Fournier C: Periurethral collagen injection for the treatment of female stress urinary incontinence: 4-year follow-up results. Urology 54:815, 1999

Cruikshank SH, Muniz M: Outcomes study: a comparison of cure rates in 695 patients undergoing sacrospinous ligament fixation alone and with other site-specific procedures—a 16-year study. Am J Obstet Gynecol 188:1509, 2003

Culligan PJ, Blackwell L, Goldsmith LJ, et al: A randomized controlled trial comparing fascia lata and synthetic mesh for sacral colpopexy. Obstet Gynecol 106:29, 2005

Demirci F, Petri E: Perioperative complications of Burch colposuspension. Int Urogynecol J 11:170, 2000

Demirci F, Yucel O, Eren S, et al: Long-term results of Burch colposuspension. Gynecol Obstet Invest 51:243, 2001

Dunn TS, Figge J, Wolf D: A comparison of outcomes of transurethral versus suprapubic catheterization after Burch cystourethropexy. Int Urogynecol J 16:60, 2005

el Toukhy TA, Davies AE: The efficacy of laparoscopic mesh colposuspension: results of a prospective, controlled study. Br J Urol Int 88:361, 2001

Faerber GJ, Belville WD, Ohl DA, et al: Comparison of transurethral versus periurethral collagen injection in women with intrinsic sphincter deficiency. Tech Urol 4:124, 1998

Galloway NT, Davies N, Stephenson TP: The complications of colposuspension. Br J Urol 60:122, 1987

Gandhi S, Goldberg RP, Kwon C, et al: A prospective, randomized trial using solvent dehydrated fascia lata for the prevention of recurrent anterior vaginal wall prolapse. Am J Obstet Gynecol 192:1649, 2005

Gearhart S, Hull T, Floruta C, et al: Anal manometric parameters: predictors of outcome following anal sphincter repair? J Gastrointest Surg 9:115, 2005

Gilliland R, Altomare DF, Moreira H Jr, et al: Pudendal neuropathy is predictive of failure following anterior overlapping sphincteroplasty. Dis Colon Rectum 41:1516, 1998

Given FT Jr, Muhlendorf IK, Browning GM: Vaginal length and sexual function after colpopexy for complete uterovaginal eversion. Am J Obstet Gynecol 169:284, 1993

Gorton E, Stanton S, Monga A, et al: Periurethral collagen injection: a long-term follow-up study. Br J Urol Int 84:966, 1999

Green J, Herschorn S: The contemporary role of Burch colposuspension. Curr Opin Urol 15:250, 2005

Ha HT, Fleshman JW, Smith M, et al: Manometric squeeze pressure difference parallels functional outcome after overlapping sphincter reconstruction. Dis Colon Rectum 44:655, 2001

Haab F, Zimmern PE, Leach GE: Urinary stress incontinence due to intrinsic sphincteric deficiency: experience with fat and collagen periurethral injections. J Urol 157:1283, 1997

Halverson AL, Hull TL: Long-term outcome of overlapping anal sphincter repair. Dis Colon Rectum 45:345, 2002

Herschorn S, Radomski SB: Collagen injections for genuine stress urinary incontinence: patient selection and durability. Int Urogynecol J 8:18, 1997

Hibner M, Cornella JL, Magrina JF, et al: Ischiorectal abscess after sacrospinous ligament suspension. Am J Obstet Gynecol 193:1740, 2005

Holmgren C, Nilsson S, Lanner L, et al: Long-term results with tension-free vaginal tape on mixed and stress urinary incontinence. Obstet Gynecol 106(1):38, 2005

Judd JP, Siddiqui NY, Barnett JC, et al: Cost-minimization analysis of robotic-assisted, laparoscopic, and abdominal sacrocolpopexy. J Minim Invasive Gynecol 17(4):493, 2010

Julian TM: The efficacy of Marlex mesh in the repair of severe, recurrent vaginal prolapse of the anterior midvaginal wall. Am J Obstet Gynecol 175:1472, 1996

Kershen RT, Dmochowski RR, Appell RA: Beyond collagen: injectable therapies for the treatment of female stress urinary incontinence in the new millennium. Urol Clin North Am 29:559, 2002

Kheirabadi BS, Field-Ridley A, Pearson R, et al: Comparative study of the efficacy of the common topical hemostatic agents with fibrin sealant in a rabbit aortic anastomosis model. J Surg Res 106:99, 2002

Kohli N, Walsh PM, Roat TW, et al: Mesh erosion after abdominal sacrocolpopexy. Obstet Gynecol 92:999, 1998

Kwon CH, Goldberg RP, Koduri S, et al: The use of intraoperative cystoscopy in major vaginal and urogynecologic surgeries. Am J Obstet Gynecol 187:1466, 2002

Ladwig D, Miljkovic-Petkovic L, Hewson AD: Simplified colposuspension: a 15-year follow-up. Aus N Z J Obstet Gynaecol 44:39, 2004

Lane FE: Repair of posthysterectomy vaginal-vault prolapse. Obstet Gynecol 20:72, 1962

Lantzsch T, Goepel C, Wolters M, et al: Sacrospinous ligament fixation for vaginal vault prolapse. Arch Gynecol Obstet 265:21, 2001

Lapitan MC, Cody DJ, Grant AM: Open retropubic colposuspension for urinary incontinence in women. Cochrane Database Syst Rev 1:CD002912, 2003

Lee PE, Kung RC, Drutz HP: Periurethral autologous fat injection as treatment for female stress urinary incontinence: a randomized, double-blind controlled trial. J Urol 165:153, 2001

Lightner DJ, Itano NB, Sweat SD, et al: Injectable agents: present and future. Curr Urol Rep 3:408, 2002

Luck AM, Galvin SL, Theofrastous JP: Suture erosion and wound dehiscence with permanent versus absorbable suture in reconstructive posterior vaginal surgery. Am J Obstet Gynecol 192:1626, 2005

Madoff RD, Parker SC, Varma MG, et al: Faecal incontinence in adults. Lancet 364(9434):621, 2004

Mage P: [Interposition of a synthetic mesh by vaginal approach in the cure of genital prolapse]. [French]. J Gynecol Obstet Biol Reprod 28:825, 1999

Maher CF, Murray CJ, Carey MP, et al: Iliococcygeus or sacrospinous fixation for vaginal vault prolapse. Obstet Gynecol 98:40, 2001

Maher CF, Qatawneh AM, Dwyer PL, et al: Abdominal sacral colpopexy or vaginal sacrospinous colpopexy for vaginal vault prolapse: a prospective, randomized study. Am J Obstet Gynecol 190:20, 2004

Malouf AJ, Norton CS, Engel AF, et al: Long-term results of overlapping anterior anal-sphincter repair for obstetric trauma. Lancet 355:260, 2000

Martinez Hernandez MP, Villanueva SE, Jaime ZM, et al: Endoanal sonography in assessment of fecal incontinence following obstetric trauma. Ultrasound Obstet Gynecol 22:616, 2003

Mattox TF, Stanford EJ, Varner E: Infected abdominal sacrocolpopexies: diagnosis and treatment. Int Urogynecol J 15:319, 2004

Meltomaa SS, Haarala MA, Taalikka MO, et al: Outcome of Burch retropubic urethropexy and the effect of concomitant abdominal hysterectomy: a prospective long-term follow-up study. Int Urogynecol J 12:3, 2001

Migliari R, Usai E: Treatment results using a mixed fiber mesh in patients with grade IV cystocele. J Urol 161:1255, 1999

Miyazaki FS: Miya hook ligature carrier for sacrospinous ligament suspension. Obstet Gynecol 70:286, 1987

Moehrer B, Ellis G, Carey M, et al: Laparoscopic colposuspension for urinary incontinence in women. Cochrane Database Syst Rev 1:CD002239, 2002

Monga AK, Robinson D, Stanton SL: Periurethral collagen injections for genuine stress incontinence: a 2-year follow-up. Br J Urol 76:156, 1995

Monga AK, Stanton SL: Urodynamics: prediction, outcome and analysis of mechanism for cure of stress incontinence by periurethral collagen. Br J Obstet Gynaecol 104:158, 1997

Nilsson CG, Palva K, Rezapour M, et al: Eleven years prospective follow-up of the tension-free vaginal tape procedure for treatment of stress urinary incontinence. Int Urogynecol J Pelvic Floor Dysfunct 19(8):1043, 2008

Norton P, Brubaker L: Urinary incontinence in women. Lancet 367:57, 2006

Nygaard IE, McCreery R, Brubaker L, et al: Abdominal sacrocolpopexy: a comprehensive review. Obstet Gynecol 104:805, 2004

Oz MC, Cosgrove DM III, Badduke BR, et al: Controlled clinical trial of a novel hemostatic agent in cardiac surgery. The Fusion Matrix Study Group. Ann Thorac Surg 69:1376, 2000

Paraiso MF, Ballard LA, Walters MD, et al: Pelvic support defects and visceral and sexual function in women treated with sacrospinous ligament suspension and pelvic reconstruction. Am J Obstet Gynecol 175:1423, 1996

Pohl JF, Frattarelli JL: Bilateral transvaginal sacrospinous colpopexy: preliminary experience. Am J Obstet Gynecol 177:1356, 1997

Sagsoz N, Ersoy M, Kamaci M, et al: Anatomical landmarks regarding sacrospinous colpopexy operations performed for vaginal vault prolapse. Eur J Obstet Gynaecol Reprod Biol 101:74, 2002

Sand PK, Koduri S, Lobel RW, et al: Prospective randomized trial of polyglactin 910 mesh to prevent recurrence of cystoceles and rectoceles. Am J Obstet Gynecol 184:1357, 2001

Schulz JA, Stanton SL, Baessler K, et al: Bulking agents for stress urinary incontinence: short-term results and complications in a randomized comparison of periurethral and transurethral injections. Int Urogynecol J Pelvic Floor Dys 15:261, 2004

Shull BL, Capen CV, Riggs MW, et al: Preoperative and postoperative analysis of site-specific pelvic support defects in 81 women treated with sacrospinous ligament suspension and pelvic reconstruction. Am J Obstet Gynecol 166:1764, 1992

Silva-Filho AL, Santos-Filho AS, Figueiredo-Netto O, et al: Uncommon complications of sacrospinous fixation for treatment of vaginal vault prolapse. Arch Gynecol Obstet 271:358, 2005

Song PH, Kim YD, Kim HT, et al: The 7-year outcome of the tension-free vaginal tape procedure for treating female stress urinary incontinence. BJU Int 104(8):1113, 2009

Steele AC, Kohli N, Karram MM: Periurethral collagen injection for stress incontinence with and without urethral hypermobility. Obstet Gynecol 95:327, 2000

Theofrastous, Cobb DL, Van Dyke AH, et al: A randomized trial of suprapubic versus transurethral bladder drainage after open Burch urethropexy. J Pelvic Surg 872, 2002

U.S. Food and Drug Administration: FDA safety communication: UPDATE on serious complications associated with transvaginal placement of surgical mesh for pelvic organ prolapse. Available at: http://www.fda.gov/MedicalDevices/Safety/AlertsandNotices/ucm262435.htm. Accessed October 14, 2011

Verdeja AM, Elkins TE, Odoi A, et al: Transvaginal sacrospinous colpopexy: anatomic landmarks to be aware of to minimize complications. Am J Obstet Gynecol 173:1468, 1995

Weaver FA, Hood DB, Zatina M, et al: Gelatin-thrombin-based hemostatic sealant for intraoperative bleeding in vascular surgery. Ann Vasc Surg 16:286, 2002

Weber AM, Walters MD, Piedmonte MR, et al: Anterior colporrhaphy: a randomized trial of three surgical techniques. Am J Obstet Gynecol 185:1299, 2001

Weidner AC, Cundiff GW, Harris RL, et al: Sacral osteomyelitis: an unusual complication of abdominal sacral colpopexy. Obstet Gynecol 90:689, 1997

Wieslander CK, Rahn DD, McIntire DD, et al: Vascular anatomy of the presacral space in unembalmed female cadavers. Am J Obstet Gynecol 195:1736, 2006

Winters JC, Appell R: Periurethral injection of collagen in the treatment of intrinsic sphincteric deficiency in the female patient. Urol Clin North Am 22:673, 1995

Yamada T, Ichiyanagi N, Kamata S, et al: Need for sling surgery in patients with large cystoceles and masked stress urinary incontinence. Int J Urol 8:599, 2001

Zullo F, Palomba S, Russo T, et al: Laparoscopic colposuspension using sutures or Prolene meshes: a 3-year follow-up. Eur J Obstet Gynaecol Reprod Biol 117:201, 2004

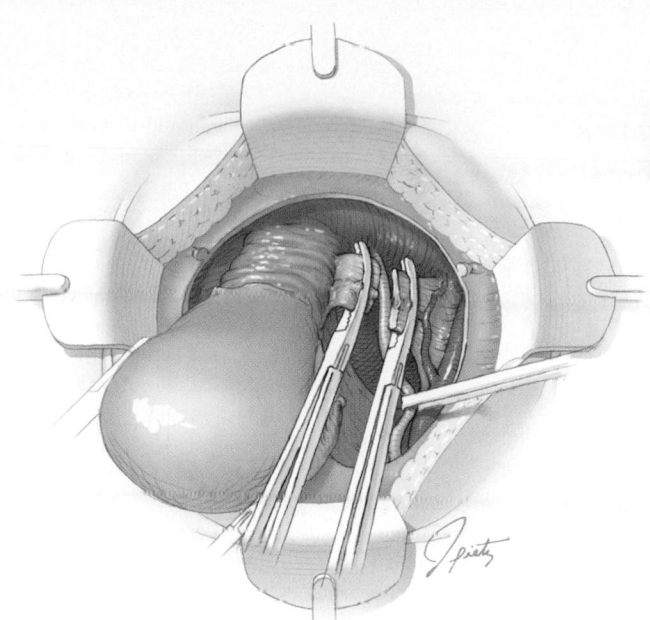

CHAPTER 44

Surgeries for Gynecologic Malignancies

44-1

Radical Abdominal Hysterectomy (Type III)

Radical hysterectomy differs from simple hysterectomy in that additional surrounding soft tissue is resected to achieve negative tumor margins. The operation involves wide radical excision of the parametrial and paravaginal tissues in addition to removal of intervening pelvic lymphatics.

The five "types" of extended hysterectomy are discussed in Chapter 30 (p. 783). Of these, type III (radical) hysterectomy is chiefly indicated for stage IB1 to IIA cervical cancer or small central recurrences following radiation therapy, or for clinical stage II endometrial cancer when tumor has extended to the cervix (Greer, 2011a,b).

Type III radical hysterectomy is increasingly being performed by a minimally invasive approach (Sections 44-3 and 44-4, p. 1267). With these approaches, the principles of the abdominal operation are still applied. Radical hysterectomy is a dynamic operation that always requires significant intraoperative decision making. Every step requires a focused, consistent surgical approach. In many ways, radical abdominal hysterectomy initially defined the field of gynecologic oncology. Familiarity with its concepts continues to be critically important in developing expertise in complex pelvic surgery.

PREOPERATIVE

Patient Evaluation

Radical hysterectomy is not appropriate for women with higher-stage cancers. Thus, accurate clinical staging is critical prior to selection of this surgery. Pelvic examination under anesthesia with cystoscopy and proctoscopy is not mandatory for smaller cervical cancer lesions, but the clinical staging described in Chapter 30 (p. 777) should be completed before proceeding surgically. For most patients with grossly visible cervical tumors, an abdominopelvic computed-tomography (CT), magnetic resonance (MR) imaging, or positron emission tomography (PET) scan is indicated to identify clinically obvious metastases or undetected local tumor extension (Greer, 2011a). Unfortunately, there are limitations in what can be reliably detected preoperatively (Chou, 2006).

Consent

Radical abdominal hysterectomy can result in significant morbidity and potentially unforeseen short- and long-term complications. These complications may develop more frequently in women with obesity, prior pelvic infections, and prior abdominal surgery, which may add difficulty to safely performing radical hysterectomy (Cohn, 2000). In addition, differences in patient morbidity rates among surgeons do exist and may be of significant magnitude (Covens, 1993).

Of potential intraoperative complications, the most common is acute hemorrhage. Blood loss averages 500 to 1000 mL, and transfusion rates are variable, but high (Estape, 2009; Naik, 2010). Subacute postoperative complications may include ureterovaginal or vesicovaginal fistula (1 to 2 percent), symptomatic lymphocyst formation (3 to 5 percent), and significant postoperative bladder or bowel dysfunction (20 percent) (Franchi, 2007; Hazewinkel, 2010; Likic, 2008). Additionally, long-term effects on sexual function, loss of fertility, and other body functions should be candidly reviewed (Jensen, 2004; Serati, 2009).

The tone of the consenting process should reflect the extent of the operation required to ideally cure or at least begin treatment of the malignancy. In addition, a patient must be advised that the procedure may be aborted if metastatic disease or pelvic tumor extension is found (Leath, 2004).

Patient Preparation

A blood sample should be typed and cross-matched for potential transfusion. Pneumatic compression devices or subcutaneous heparin or both are particularly important due to the long-anticipated length of the operation and longer duration of postoperative recovery (Table 39-9, p. 962) (Martino, 2006).

Bowel preparation with a polyethylene glycol-electrolyte solution (GoLytely) is no longer commonly used. Inadvertent bowel injury should be rare unless extenuating circumstances are identified. However, it may be helpful to empty the colon to limit fecal spill if extensive pelvic adhesive disease is anticipated due to prior infection, endometriosis, or radiation therapy.

Two doses of perioperative antibiotic prophylaxis with a third-generation cephalosporin such as cefoxitin are given at spaced intervals. This is sufficient to prevent most postoperative surgical site infections. High-volume blood loss is largely responsible for rapid clearance of antibiotics from the operative site during radical hysterectomy compared with extrafascial hysterectomy and necessitates the additional dose (Bouma, 1993; Sevin, 1991).

Concurrent Surgery

Early-stage cervical cancer most frequently spreads via the lymphatics. Accordingly, adjunctive removal of nodes is required to address this potential. Pelvic lymphadenectomy is typically completed just before or immediately after radical hysterectomy, and paraaortic lymphadenectomy may also be indicated in some circumstances (Sections 44-11 and 44-12, p. 1296) (Angioli, 1999).

Spread to the adnexa is much less common than via the lymphatics. Thus, removal of the adnexa should depend on a woman's age and potential for metastases (Shimada, 2006). In candidates for ovarian preservation, transposition of ovaries out of the pelvis may be considered in young women if postoperative radiation is anticipated. However, in transposed ovaries, symptomatic periadnexal cysts are commonplace, and sustained ovarian function may not result (Buekers, 2001).

INTRAOPERATIVE

SURGICAL STEPS

❶ Anesthesia and Patient Positioning. General anesthesia is mandatory, but epidural placement may aid effective postoperative pain control and decrease duration of postoperative ileus (Leon-Casasola, 1996).

Bimanual examination should be performed in the operating room before scrubbing. This reorients a surgeon to the patient's individual anatomy. Supine positioning is appropriate in most cases.

❷ Abdominal Entry. A midline vertical abdominal incision provides excellent exposure, but typically prolongs hospital stays and increases postoperative pain. Alternatively, Cherney or Maylard incisions offer postoperative advantages found with transverse incisions and allow access to the lateral pelvis (Sections 41-3 and 41-4, p. 1024). However, upper paraaortic nodes are not readily accessible through these transverse incisions. Pfannenstiel incisions offer limited exposure and should be reserved for selected patients only (Orr, 1995).

❸ Exploration. Following abdominal entry, a surgeon first thoroughly explores the abdomen for obvious metastatic disease. Suspicious lymph nodes and any other lesions should be removed or biopsied. Confirmation of metastatic disease or pelvic tumor extension should prompt a surgeon to decide whether to proceed or abort an operation based on overall intraoperative findings and clinical situation (Leath, 2004).

❹ Entering the Retroperitoneal Space. The uterus is placed on traction with curved Kelly clamps at the cornua. The round ligament is sutured with 0-gauge delayed-absorbable suture as laterally as possible, and the tie is held on tension to aid entry into the retroperitoneal space. Transection of the round ligament more laterally along its length aids later excision of the parametrium out to the pelvic sidewall. The round ligament is divided, and the broad ligament beneath separates into thin anterior and posterior leaves that contain loose areolar connective tissue between.

The anterior leaf of the broad ligament is placed on traction and is sharply dissected to the vesicouterine fold. The posterior leaf of the broad ligament is then placed on traction and sharply dissected along the pelvic sidewall parallel to the infundibulopelvic (IP) ligament.

❺ Ureter Isolation. Loose areolar connective tissue of the retroperitoneal space is bluntly dissected in the area lateral to the IP until the external iliac artery is palpated just medial to the psoas major muscle. The index and middle fingers are then placed on either side of the artery, and the areolar connective tissue is bluntly dissected by a "walking" motion toward the patient's head.

The medial portion of the posterior peritoneal leaf of the broad ligament is elevated

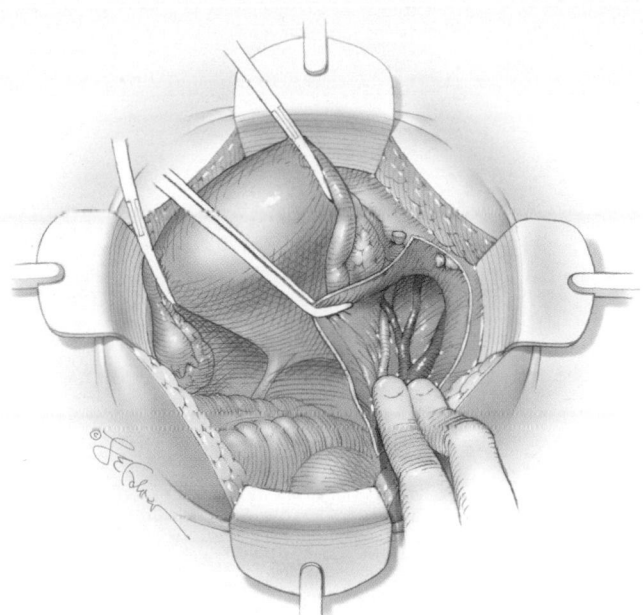

FIGURE 44-1.1 Finding the ureter.

and placed on traction to permit direct identification of the common iliac artery bifurcation and origins of the external and internal iliac arteries (Fig. 44-1.1). Blunt dissection with a finger or suction tip is used in a sweeping motion from top to bottom along the medial peritoneal leaf to identify and sufficiently mobilize the lateral surface of the ureter at this site. Here, the ureter crosses above the common iliac bifurcation.

A Babcock clamp is used to grasp the ureter, and a Mixter right-angle clamp is used to "pop" through an underlying avascular space where the ureter is still attached medially to the peritoneum. A quarter-inch-wide Penrose drain is then pulled through this space to isolate the ureter and assist in identifying its location throughout the remainder of surgery.

❻ Creating Spaces. The parametrium that will be removed with the hysterectomy specimens lies between the paravesical and pararectal spaces (Fig. 38-18, p. 934). Thus, creation of these spaces is needed to isolate the parametrium for transection. The pararectal space is developed by gently placing the right index finger between the internal iliac artery and the ureter and tracking in a gentle swirling motion at a 45-degree angle downward toward the midline and aiming for the coccyx (Fig. 44-1.2).

Subsequently, the paravesical space is formed by holding the lateral tie of the round ligament and bluntly following the external iliac artery to the pelvic bone. The index, middle, and ring finger of the right hand are then swept horizontally toward the midline.

❼ Uterine Artery Ligation. Reflection of the lateral peritoneal fold of the anterior broad ligament leaf just distal to the round ligament should reveal the superior vesical artery. This vessel is bluntly dissected to better define its location and then is grasped with a Babcock clamp and placed on traction. A right-angle clamp is "popped" through and beneath to create a space large enough to accommodate a narrow curved Deaver retractor (Fig. 44-1.3). This maneuver places the superior vesical artery on traction, prevents its inadvertent ligation, and aids location of the uterine artery.

A surgeon's left hand is inserted into the pelvis with the middle finger placed in the paravesical space, the index finger in the pararectal space, and the uterus with attached Kelly clamps cupped in the palm. The uterus is held on firm medial traction to expose the lateral pelvic sidewall. To visualize the uterine artery, a surgeon sharply dissects parametrial attachments and intervening areolar connective tissue beginning at the internal iliac artery and continuing caudad to the superior vesical artery.

Tissues immediately proximal and distal to the uterine artery are bluntly dissected, and a right-angle clamp is placed beneath this artery to retrieve a 2-0 silk suture. The uterine artery tie is placed as close as possible to its origin from the internal iliac artery. The process is repeated to place a separate silk suture far enough medial to enable vessel transection (see Fig. 44-1.3). Silk ties help identify the proximal and distal portions of the uterine artery throughout the remainder of the operation. A small vascular clip (Hemoclip) can also be placed lateral to the silk tie on the proximal uterine artery for additional security of hemostasis. The uterine artery is then cut. The underlying uterine vein may also then be isolated, clipped or tied, and cut.

❽ Uniting Paravesical and Pararectal Spaces. The parametrial tissues have been pressed together by development of the paravesical and pararectal spaces. Parametrial resection to unite the spaces can be performed by several methods: (1) clamping, cutting, and suturing (Fig. 44-1.4), (2) stapling with gastrointestinal anastomosis stapler (GIA stapler), (3) electrosurgical blade dissection to the pelvic sidewall using a right-angle clamp to elevate and isolate parametrial tissue, or

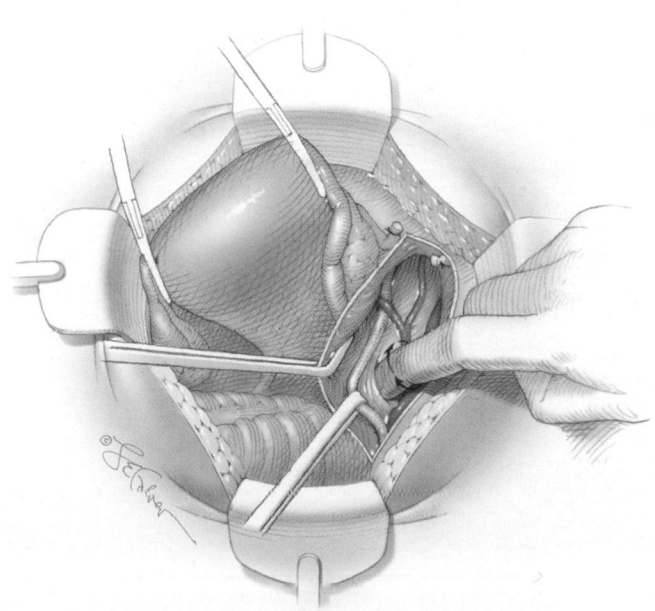

FIGURE 44-1.2 Making the pararectal space.

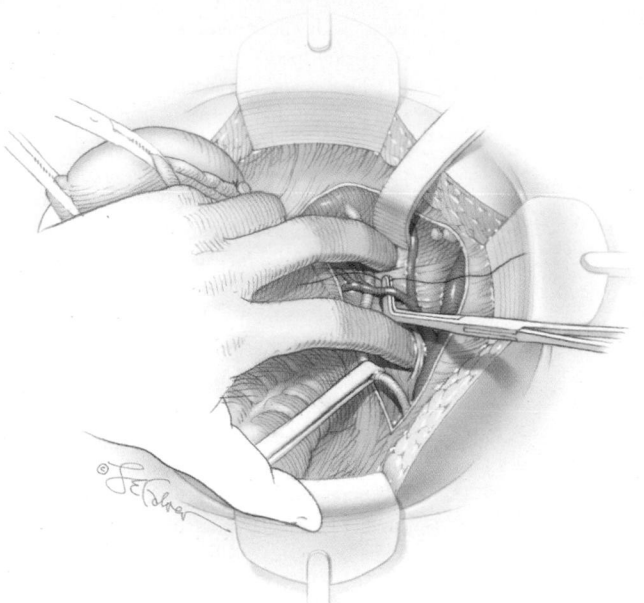

FIGURE 44-1.3 Ligating the uterine artery.

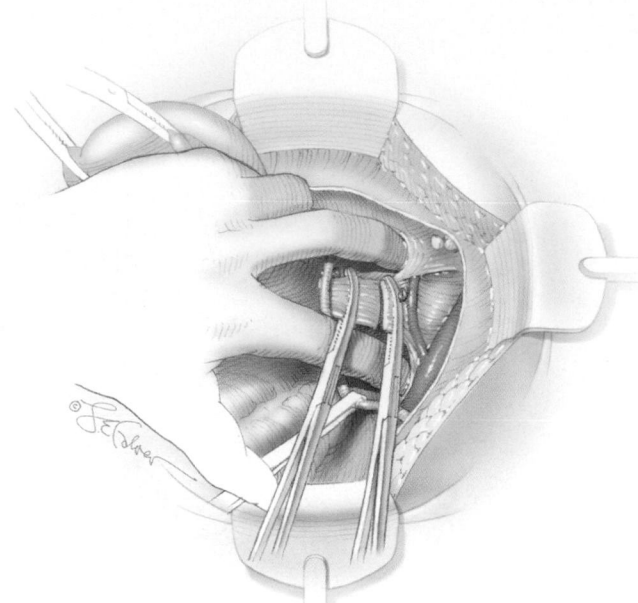

FIGURE 44-1.4 Uniting the spaces by parametrial resection.

(4) use of an electrothermal bipolar coagulator (LigaSure). Dissection is continued until the parametrium overlying the ureter is mobile.

❾ Ureter Mobilization. In this same area of the pelvis, tips of a right-angle clamp are positioned perpendicular to and just above the ureter to detach it from the medial leaf of the peritoneum. Opening the tips parallel to the ureter creates a plane that permits it to be bluntly dissected away from the peritoneum. The ureter is placed on gentle traction by grasping the previously placed Penrose drain with the left hand. The right index finger carefully sweeps the ureter downward and laterally until a "tunnel" through the

paracervical tissue can be palpated ventromedially as the ureter enters this tissue (Fig. 44-1.5). Additional parametrial dissection is often required to ensure that the uterine artery and surrounding soft tissue has been lifted medially over the ureter.

❿ Bladder Dissection. Electrosurgical dissection is performed to free the bladder distally from the cervix and onto the upper vagina. This may need to be repeated several times as the tunnel is progressively unroofed and the ureter is more directly visible. The bladder will eventually need to be dissected so that it lies several centimeters distal to the cervical portio and onto the upper vagina.

⓫ Unroofing the Ureteral Tunnel. The uterus is placed on lateral traction, and the proximal ureter is held on traction to straighten it by gently pulling on the Penrose drain. The tunnel opening should be palpated. Concurrently, a right-angle clamp is inserted with its tips directed upward, while direct visualization of the underlying ureter is confirmed. The tips are directed medially toward the cervix and "popped" through the paracervical tissue. A second clamp is placed through the opening. The ureter can be bluntly dissected and pushed posteriorly toward the tunnel floor. It should be visible below before cutting the overlying paracervical tissue (Fig. 44-1.6). Delayed-absorbable

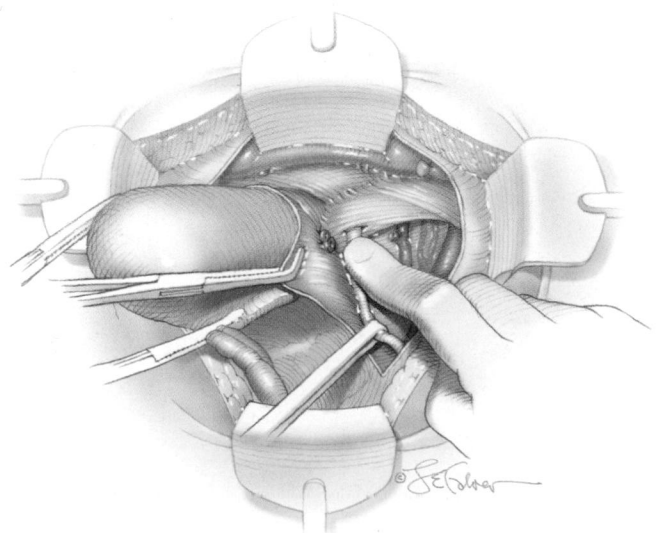

FIGURE 44-1.5 Mobilizing the ureter.

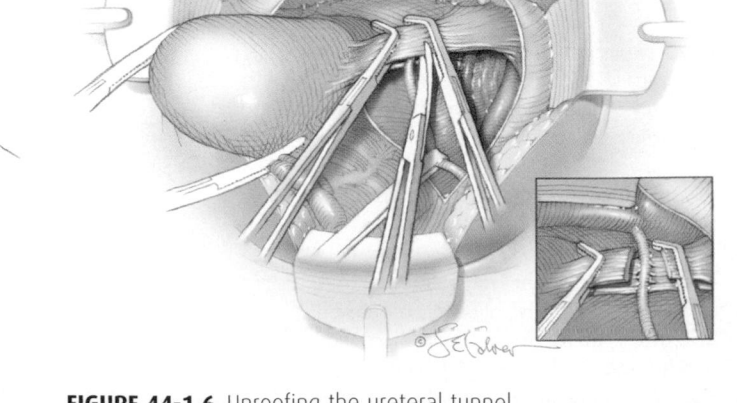

FIGURE 44-1.6 Unroofing the ureteral tunnel.

3-0 suture ties are used to secure the para-cervical tissue pedicles that are held by the right-angle clamps, but significant bleeding is commonplace during these steps. The same procedure may be repeated several times to completely unroof the tunnel and expose the ureter. The dissection should proceed in a proximal to distal fashion with direct visualization of the ureter at all times to prevent injury. Increasingly, the use of new technologies, such as the Harmonic scalpel, can decrease operating time and blood loss. After unroofing the ureter, it is retracted upward, and filmy attachments between the ureter and tunnel bed are sharply divided.

12 Uterosacral Resection. Posterior radical dissection is often best performed near the operation's end because exposed retroperitoneal tissues typically ooze until the vaginal cuff is closed. The cervical external os is palpated, and the electrosurgical blade is used to superficially incise or "score" the peritoneum between the uterosacral ligaments.

A plane is developed by gently pressing a finger toward the vaginal wall without poking through and into the vault. This rectovaginal plane should be developed by gentle pressure toward the sacrum and enlarged laterally until three fingers can be comfortably inserted. This maneuver frees the rectosigmoid away from the uterosacral ligaments and prevents inadvertent bowel injury. Remaining peritoneal attachments are sharply dissected to fully expose the rectovaginal space. The exposed uterosacral ligaments

can be visualized, palpated, clamped at the sacrum near the level of the rectum, then cut, and ligated with 0-gauge delayed-absorbable suture (Fig. 44-1.7). This procedure may need to be repeated to complete transection of the uterosacral ligament and adjacent supportive tissues.

13 Vaginal Resection. At this point in the operation, the radical hysterectomy specimen should be held in place only by the paracolpium and vagina. The bladder and ureters are further bluntly and sharply dissected free until at least 3 cm of upper vagina will be included with the resected specimen. Curved clamps are placed on the lateral paracolpium. The ureter should be lateral and directly visible. Tissue is then cut and suture ligated with 0-gauge delayed-absorbable suture. The upper vagina can then be: (1) clamped, cut, and suture ligated, (2) stapled, or (3) sharply transected with electrosurgical blade and suture ligated (Fig. 44-1.8). The specimen should be carefully examined to ensure an adequate upper vaginal segment and grossly negative margins.

14 Suprapubic Catheter Placement. Placement of a suprapubic catheter may aid postoperative voiding trials in carefully selected, motivated patients (Pikaart, 2007). The tip of a second Foley catheter is brought through a stab incision in the lateral anterior abdominal wall. The Foley catheter already within the bladder is held firmly and anteriorly in a distal extraperitoneal location. A 5-mm transverse incision is made through

the bladder mucosa using an electrosurgical blade set to a blended cutting mode. The Foley bulb should be directly visible to confirm bladder entry. After being incised, the bladder mucosal edges are held with two Allis clamps. The tip of a second Foley catheter is inserted into the bladder, and the balloon is inflated. A snug, but not tight, purse-string 3-0 chromic suture is placed around the bladder defect and tied. Delayed-absorbable suture in a running fashion is used to "bury" the visible Foley catheter tubing in a tunnel of overlying peritoneum to its exit at the lateral anterior abdominal wall. The Foley catheter should be fixed at the skin with a permanent suture that does not occlude the tubing. The original urethral Foley catheter can be discontinued postoperatively when urine is seen to be draining from the suprapubic catheter.

Alternatively, a sole urethral Foley catheter may be placed. Drainage is continued until postvoid residual volumes measure less than 100 mL.

15 Ovarian Transposition. Optionally, for those in whom ovarian function preservation is desired, adnexa may be transposed out of the anticipated pelvic radiation field. A distal portion of the adnexa is grasped with a Babcock clamp. Using traction, dissection is performed to mobilize the IP ligament so that the adnexa can be lifted into the upper abdomen. A large vascular clip is placed on the ovary at the residual uteroovarian ligament stump to allow postoperative visualization

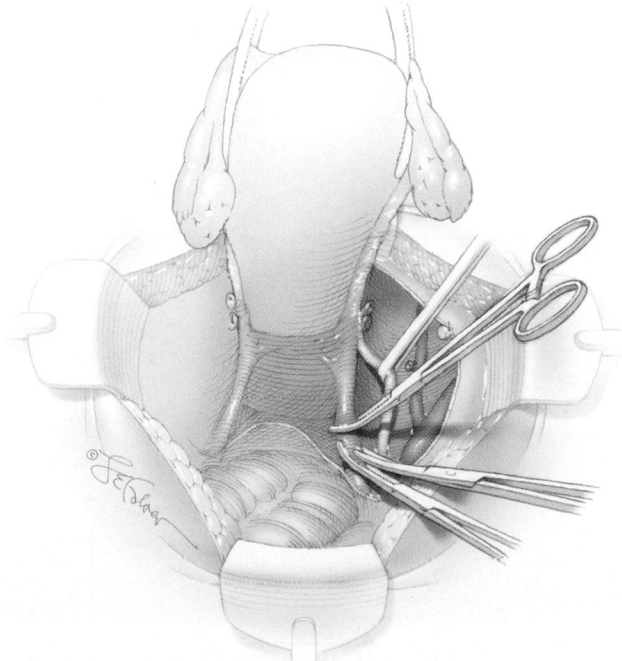

FIGURE 44-1.7 Uterosacral resection.

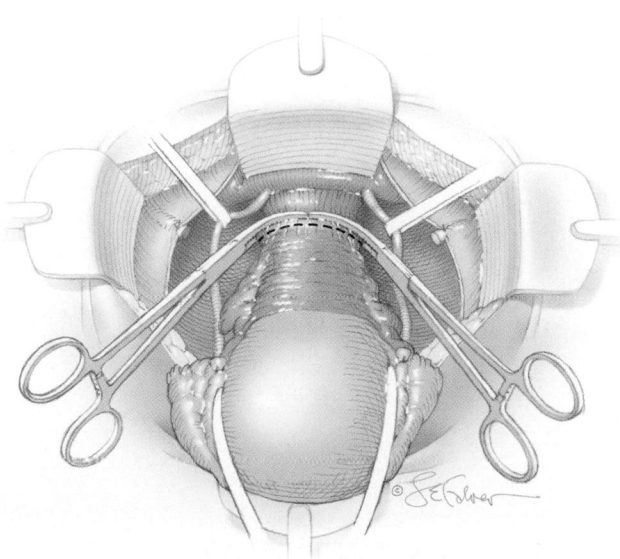

FIGURE 44-1.8 Vaginal resection.

of ovarian location by radiography or CT. Additionally, a 0-gauge silk suture is placed at this stump site and tied. Its needle is left in place.

A handheld abdominal retractor is then used to expose an area of the lateral posterior peritoneum as high as possible in the abdomen. The silk suture needle is then placed through the peritoneum, the adnexa is elevated by this "pulley-stitch," and tied. The lateral pelvic defect is closed with a continuous running stitch using 0-gauge delayed-absorbable suture to prevent internal herniation. The ovaries should be inspected before abdominal closure to exclude vascular compromise by transposition.

⑯ Final Steps. Active bleeding should be immediately controlled when the radical hysterectomy specimen has been removed. A dry laparotomy sponge may then be held firmly deep in the pelvis for several minutes to tamponade raw surfaces. With bleeding controlled, a surgeon should assess the vascular support to the ureter and other sidewall structures. To structures that appear particularly devascularized, an omental J-flap may provide additional blood supply (Section 44-16, p. 1314) (Fujiwara, 2003; Patsner, 1997). Routine pelvic suction drainage and closure of the peritoneum are not necessary (Charoenkwan, 2010; Franchi, 2007).

POSTOPERATIVE

Immediate postoperative care following radical hysterectomy in general follows that for laparotomy. Early ambulation after radical hysterectomy is especially important to prevent thromboembolic complications (Stentella, 1997). Early feeding, including rapid initiation of a clear liquid diet, may also shorten the hospital stay (Kraus, 2000). Tenesmus, constipation, and incontinence are common immediate symptoms that should improve significantly months or years later (Butler-Manuel, 1999; Sood, 2002).

Bladder tone returns slowly, and a major cause is thought to be partial sympathetic and parasympathetic denervation during radical dissection (Chen, 2002). Thus, Foley catheter drainage is commonly continued until a patient is passing flatus, as improving bowel function typically accompanies resolving bladder hypotonia. Removal of the catheter or clamping of the suprapubic tube should be followed by a successful voiding trial (Chap. 39, p. 966). A voiding trial may be attempted prior to hospital discharge or at the first postoperative visit. Patients with adequate voiding should be instructed to press gently on the suprapubic area for several days afterward to help completely empty the bladder and prevent retention. Successful voiding may take several weeks to achieve.

Nerve-sparing radical hysterectomy is a new method demonstrating an improvement in postoperative bladder function (Raspagliesi, 2006). However, many patients have preexisting abnormal urodynamic findings that are simply exacerbated by radical hysterectomy (Lin, 1998, 2004). In the 3 percent of women who develop long-term bladder hypotonia or atony, intermittent self-catheterization is preferred to indwelling urinary catheterization (Chamberlain, 1991; Naik, 2005).

Cervical cancer survivors treated with radical hysterectomy have much better sexual functioning than those who receive radiation therapy. Despite this, more than half of surgical patients postoperatively report a worse sex life (Butler-Manuel, 1999). Severe orgasmic problems, uncomfortable intercourse due to a reduced vaginal length, and severe dyspareunia may develop but often resolve within 6 to 12 months. However, a persistent lack of sexual interest and lubrication may be long-term or permanent changes (Jensen, 2004). Disturbances of vaginal blood flow response during sexual arousal may account for much of the reported constellation of symptoms (Maas, 2004). Eventually, patients treated by surgery alone can expect a quality of life and overall sexual function similar to peers without a history of cancer (Frumovitz, 2005).

44-2

Modified Radical Abdominal Hysterectomy (Type II)

Four procedural differences distinguish a modified radical hysterectomy (type II) hysterectomy from the more radical type III procedure (Section 44-1, p. 1259). First, the uterine artery is transected where it crosses the ureter (rather than at its origin from the internal iliac artery). Second, only the medial half of the cardinal ligament is resected (instead of division at the sidewall). Additionally, the uterosacral ligament is divided halfway between the uterus and sacrum (rather than at the sacrum near the level of the rectum). And lastly, a smaller margin of upper vagina is removed. These modifications serve to reduce surgical time and associated morbidity, while still enabling complete resection of smaller cervical tumors (Cai, 2009; Landoni, 2001).

Clear indications for modified radical hysterectomy are few and controversial (Rose, 2001). Stage IA2 cervical cancer is the most common presenting diagnosis (Orlandi, 1995). Type II hysterectomy is also performed on occasion for: (1) preinvasive or microinvasive disease when a more invasive lesion cannot be excluded, (2) selected stage IB1 disease with <2-cm lesions, and (3) small

central postirradiation recurrences (Cai, 2009; Coleman, 1994; Eisenkop, 2005). In addition, a variation of this operation may be performed if more extensive dissection is required for known benign disease. Anatomic landmarks that distinguish a type II hysterectomy are somewhat vague, and thereby allow a surgeon to sculpt the procedure to a patient's specific situation (Fedele, 2005). Similar to the type III radical procedure, modified radical hysterectomy is increasingly being performed using a minimally invasive approach.

PREOPERATIVE

Preparation for surgery should proceed with the same care and discretion that is essential for the success of radical (type III) abdominal hysterectomy.

INTRAOPERATIVE

SURGICAL STEPS

❶ Anesthesia and Patient Positioning. Modified radical hysterectomy is performed under general anesthesia with the patient supine. Bimanual examination is performed in the operating room before scrubbing to reorient a surgeon to a patient's individual anatomy. The abdomen is surgically prepared, and a Foley catheter is placed.

❷ Abdominal Entry. Modified radical hysterectomy may be safely performed through a midline vertical or transverse incision (Fagotti, 2004).

❸ Retroperitoneal Dissection. The initial steps of modified radical (type II) hysterectomy mirror those of the type III procedure. The retroperitoneum is opened to identify structures, the ureter is mobilized, and the paravesical and pararectal spaces are developed to exclude the possibility of parametrial tumor extension before proceeding with this less radical operation (Section 44-1, steps 3 through 6, p. 1260) (Scambia, 2001).

❹ Uterine Artery Ligation. At this point, type II hysterectomy begins to differ from the radical type III procedure. The superior vesical artery does not have to be identified, nor does the entire extent of the internal iliac artery need to be dissected free of adventitial tissue. The ureteral tunnel opening should be palpated, and the uterine vessels are divided at that location (Fig. 44-2.1). Ligation of the uterine artery as it crosses the ureter allows preservation of distal ureteral blood supply.

❺ Cardinal Ligament Resection. The bladder is mobilized distally off the cervix and onto the upper vagina. Parametrial tissue at the sidewall does not require mobilization over the ureter (as in a type III hysterectomy). Posterior attachments of the ureter remain intact, and only the medial half of the cardinal ligaments are resected by successive clamping, cutting, and suture ligation of the paracervical tissue medial to the ureter. In contrast to the type III hysterectomy, the ureter is not dissected out of the tunnel bed, but is rolled laterally to expose the medial cardinal ligament (Fig. 44-2.2).

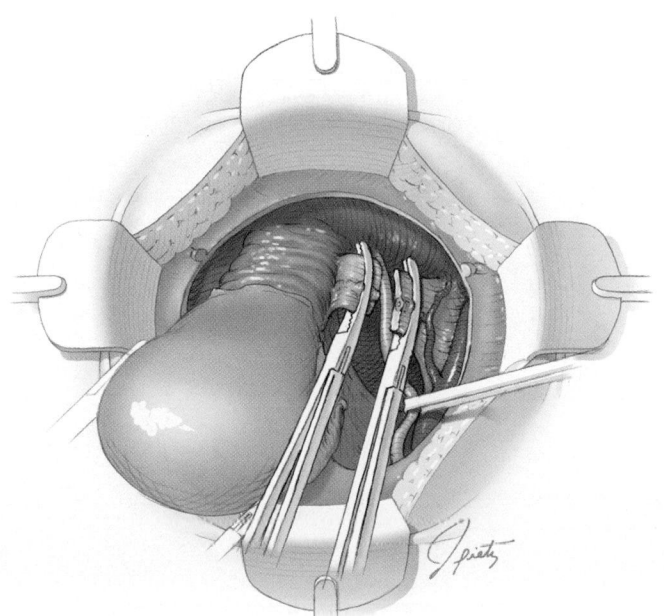

FIGURE 44-2.1 Uterine artery ligation.

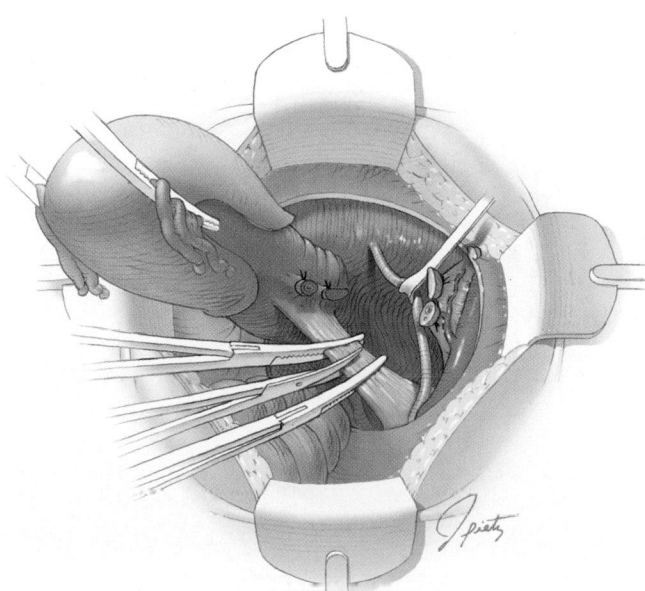

FIGURE 44-2.2 Cardinal ligament resection.

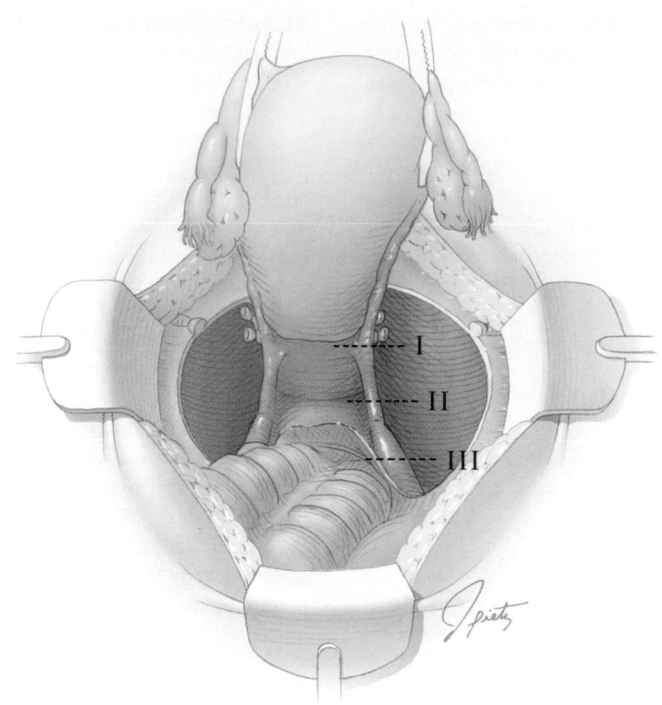

FIGURE 44-2.3 Uterosacral resection.

❻ **Uterosacral Resection.** Posterior dissection is also modified. Uterosacral ligaments are only clamped halfway to the sacrum (instead of "at" the sacrum near the level of the rectum) and are transected (Fig. 44-2.3). The uterus and adjacent parametrium can then be lifted well out of the pelvis, and any additional tissues are also clamped, cut, and ligated.

❼ **Vaginal Resection.** At this point in surgery, the modified radical hysterectomy specimen should be held in place only by the paracolpium and vagina. The bladder and ureters are further bluntly and sharply dissected free until at least 2 cm of upper vagina will be included in the specimen (instead of 3 to 4 cm). Curved clamps are placed on the lateral paracolpium, cut, and suture ligated. The upper vagina can then be closed with a continuous running method using 0-gauge delayed-absorbable suture. The specimen should be carefully examined to ensure an adequate upper vaginal segment and grossly negative margins.

POSTOPERATIVE

In general, postoperative care follows that for radical hysterectomy, but the incidence of complications is lower (Cai, 2009). Partial sympathetic and parasympathetic denervation should be much less extensive with a modified radical hysterectomy. Thus, bladder dysfunction is much less likely than following a type III radical hysterectomy, and successful voiding begins much earlier (Landoni, 2001; Yang, 1999). Foley catheter drainage may be discontinued on the second postoperative day and is followed by a voiding trial (Chap. 39, p. 966). In addition, bowel and sexual dysfunction should also be less pronounced.

44-3

Laparoscopic Radical Hysterectomy

The first laparoscopic radical hysterectomy was described in 1992 by Nezhat and colleagues. Since then, multiple series have reported favorable surgical outcomes and results that do not compromise oncologic outcome (Abu-Rustum, 2003; Ramirez, 2006; Spirtos, 1996, 2002; Yan, 2011). In addition, case series indicate distinct advantages to laparoscopic radical hysterectomy compared with an open approach. These include less intraoperative blood loss and shorter hospital stays. However, operative times are usually increased (Frumovitz, 2007a; Malzoni, 2009).

Whether completed by a laparoscopic or open approach, the indications for radical hysterectomy with pelvic lymphadenectomy are the same. Thus, patients with stage IB1 to IIA cervical cancer, or small central recurrences following radiation therapy, or with clinical stage II endometrial cancer when tumor has extended to the cervix are suitable candidates. Similarly, women who are candidates for modified (type II) radical hysterectomy can also benefit from a minimally invasive approach.

Selecting appropriate candidates is critical to successful laparoscopy. Potentially negative factors include a high body mass index (BMI), history of prior surgeries, extensive or bulky disease, and coexistent cardiopulmonary disease. Of these, obesity can hinder adequate ventilation and can limit instrument movement. However, laparoscopy can be a successful option for many obese patients and offers lower rates of postoperative wound infection, which is often a major complication after laparotomy in these patients (Eltabbakh, 2000; Obermair, 2005).

In addition, extensive prior abdominal surgeries with subsequent dense adhesions that limit exposure and visualization can require conversion to laparotomy. In such cases, inadequate adhesiolysis may limit access to the spaces needed for radical hysterectomy, and extensive adhesiolysis may significantly lengthen operative times.

Uterine and tumor size can also affect surgical approach. Specifically, a large bulky uterus may be difficult to manipulate, may block visualization, and may be too large for vaginal removal. Importantly, morcellation should be avoided when dealing with any gynecologic malignancy. At the same time, the extent of disease and spread of cancer to other organs should be determined before proceeding with laparoscopy.

Lastly, as described in Chapter 42 (p. 1095), laparoscopy creates unique physiologic cardiopulmonary changes that stem mainly from hypercarbia and pulmonary compliance changes. Thus, those with significant cardiac or pulmonary disease may not tolerate a laparoscopic approach.

In sum, these factors may prove laparoscopy to be a poor choice for some patients. However, in those who are suitable candidates, benefits include a shorter hospital stay, shorter recovery time, less postoperative pain, and lower surgical site infection rates.

In Section 44-1 (p. 1259), the steps of an open radical hysterectomy (type III) were outlined, and the surgical principles of laparoscopic radical hysterectomy are the same. Although the steps are quite similar to a simple laparoscopic hysterectomy (type I), dissection is more extensive and includes opening of the paravesical and pararectal spaces, unroofing and complete dissection of the ureter, and lateral transection of the uterine artery to allow removal of all parametrial tissue, which extends to the pelvic sidewall (Ramirez, 2006).

PREOPERATIVE

Patient Evaluation

As described earlier, a thorough pelvic examination and history reveal factors that help determine the optimal surgical route for a patient. Uterine size and mobility are important. There is no agreed-upon size that precludes total laparoscopic hysterectomy (TLH). However, a wide bulky uterus (width greater than 8 cm) with minimal mobility may be difficult to remove vaginally. Once a patient has been deemed eligible for a laparoscopic approach, the same preoperative evaluation as for an open procedure applies (Section 44-1, p. 1260).

Consent

Similar to an open approach, possible risks of this procedure include increased blood loss, need for transfusion, and bladder and bowel dysfunction. Vesicovaginal or ureterovaginal fistula is a known complication of radical hysterectomy, and postoperative rates appear comparable between open and laparoscopic approaches (Likic, 2008; Pikaart, 2007; Uccella, 2007; Xu, 2007; Yan, 2009). The rate of complication with laparoscopy is not increased compared with that of open procedures. Chi and associates (2004) reviewed more than 1400 laparoscopic procedures performed by a gynecologic oncology service during a 10-year period and reported an overall complication rate of 9 percent. Risk factors that contributed to all complications included older age, previous abdominal surgery, and prior radiation.

Complications related specifically to laparoscopy are discussed in Chapter 42 (p. 1097) and include entry injury to the major vessels, bladder, ureters, and bowel. In addition, the risk of conversion to an open procedure should be discussed. In general, conversion to laparotomy may be necessary if exposure and organ manipulation is limited.

Port-site metastasis or recurrence is another potential complication described with minimally invasive procedures. Potential causes include intraperitoneal spread of tumor cells by the pneumoperitoneum or contamination of the incision during specimen removal (Wang, 1999). The overall incidence varies in the literature but is low. Moreover, cases of recurrence within laparotomy incisions have also been reported. Therefore, the risk of surgical incisional recurrence is not unique to laparoscopy or robotic procedures.

Patient Preparation

A blood sample should be typed and crossmatched for potential transfusion. Pneumatic compression devices or subcutaneous heparin or both to prevent a venous thrombotic event are particularly important due to the long-anticipated length of the operation and venous stasis created by increased intraabdominal pressures from pneumoperitoneum and positioning. Antibiotic prophylaxis follows that for simple hysterectomy, and appropriate antibiotic options are listed in Table 39-6 (p. 959). The benefits from routine mechanical bowel preparation can be debated, and thus plans for bowel preparation are typically individualized (Chap. 39, p. 958). If considered, bowel preparation prior to laparoscopy can effectively evacuate the rectosigmoid to permit improved colon manipulation and pelvic anatomy visualization.

Concurrent Surgery

Pelvic lymphadenectomy is typically completed just before or immediately after radical hysterectomy, and paraaortic lymphadenectomy may also be indicated in some circumstances. A laparoscopic approach to lymphadenectomy in these areas is described in Section 44-13 (p. 1302).

Spread to the adnexa is much less common than via the lymphatics. Thus, removal of the adnexa should depend on a woman's age and potential for metastases (Shimada, 2006). If preservation of the ovaries is chosen, then based on the clinical picture, the adnexa can be transposed laparoscopically.

INTRAOPERATIVE

■ Instruments

Successful laparoscopy begins with adequate positioning of video monitors. Next, the cart or tower containing the laparoscopic light source and insufflation device should be positioned to permit easy viewing of these instruments' monitors and to avoid obstruction of the video screens.

Important laparoscopic instruments include 5- and 12-mm trocars, a monopolar electrosurgical instrument, a coagulation or vessel sealing device, a vaginal probe, laparoscopic suturing devices, and an irrigation and suction tool. There are a number of suitable electrosurgical and ultrasonic energy-based vessel sealing devices. These include the argon beam coagulator (ABC), the Harmonic scalpel, and the electrothermal bipolar coagulator (LigaSure, Enseal) device (Frumovitz, 2007b).

SURGICAL STEPS

❶ Anesthesia and Patient Positioning.
The patient is initially placed in the supine position for induction of anesthesia. Prior to induction, lower extremity compression devices are placed on the patient for venous thrombosis prophylaxis. General endotracheal anesthesia is administered. To avoid stomach puncture by a trocar during primary abdominal entry, an orogastric or nasogastric tube should be placed to decompress the stomach. To avert similar bladder injury, a Foley catheter should be placed.

Legs are then positioned in low lithotomy in Allen stirrups to permit adequate perineal access. The patient is positioned on the table so that a transvaginal uterine manipulator, if needed, can be moved in all directions. As described in Chapter 42 (p. 1100), appropriate positioning of the legs within the stirrups and arms at the side is especially crucial to reduce the risk of nerve injury due to the potential for lengthy operative time.

Bimanual examination is performed in the operating room before scrubbing to reorient a surgeon to the patient's individual anatomy. The abdomen, perineum, and vagina are then surgically prepared, and a Foley catheter is inserted.

Typically, effective uterine manipulation is critical when performing laparoscopic radical hysterectomy due to the delicate dissection required. Moreover, care should be taken to place a device that will help facilitate

an adequate vaginal margin. One very effective method is to first dilate the cervix and attach the 10-mm tip to the RUMI manipulator (CooperSurgical). The largest KOH ring is placed, followed by placement of the medium-size KOH ring onto the tip and within the large ring. The two KOH rings are tied together, and the tip is inserted into the uterus. With this technique, adequate uterine manipulation and the ability to obtain a broad vaginal margin is achieved. Alternatively, a VCare device can be used as described in Section 42-12, step 2 (p. 1152). However, in cervical cancer cases, if a bulky cervical lesion is present, a blunt vaginal probe in the vaginal fornix may be all that can be inserted.

For pelvic procedures, the primary surgeon stands on the patient's left side, the first assistant is on the right side, and the second assistant stands between the patient's legs. Ideally, each surgeon should have a video screen directly in front of him or her (Fig. 42-1, p. 1099).

Anatomical landmarks that help guide laparoscopic port placement should be assessed. As described in Chapter 42 (p. 1108), an understanding of the relationship between landmarks and the large vessels helps avert vascular puncture injuries during initial abdominal entry.

❷ Port Placement.
The abdominal cavity can be entered by several methods, which include the open technique, direct trocar insertion, or transumbilical insertion of a Veress needle (Chap. 42, p. 1110). An umbilical or supraumbilical site is preferred for primary entry. For gynecologic oncology cases, the open technique is often used, as it results in the fewest vascular and intestinal complications.

A 1- to 2-cm skin incision is made above the umbilicus. Alternatively, this incision can be made inside the umbilicus. If supraumbilical, S-shaped retractors can be used to dissect bluntly through subcutaneous tissue down to the fascia. The fascia is grasped with Allis clamps, elevated, and entered sharply with knife or scissors. To keep bowel away from the area of active cutting, the surgeon should continue to elevate the abdominal wall while making incisions. Once the fascia is entered, the peritoneum is grasped with hemostats and incised sharply. The fascial edges are tagged with 0-gauge delayed-absorbable sutures. A 10- or 12-mm trocar with a blunt obturator is then placed into the abdominal cavity and is secured in place with the fascial-anchoring sutures.

Insufflation of the abdomen can begin through this umbilical port by connecting the carbon dioxide (CO_2) tubing to the

trocar. High flow is appropriate for insufflation, and the intraabdominal pressure should be maintained at 15 mm Hg. The 10-mm laparoscope is then placed through the trocar. The abdomen and pelvis are thoroughly inspected to assess the extent of disease and adhesions. At this point, confirmation of metastatic disease or pelvic tumor extension should prompt a surgeon to decide whether to proceed or abort the operation based on overall intraoperative findings and clinical situation. In addition, the decision is made to proceed laparoscopically or convert to laparotomy.

The other ports are placed under direct laparoscopic visualization. For complex laparoscopic gynecologic procedures, four port sites are preferred. The initial trocar is placed at or above the umbilicus, and this port most often holds the laparoscope. Two 5-mm lateral ports and one 12-mm suprapubic port are used to introduce surgical instruments (Fig. 44-3.1). Additional ports can be placed according to surgeon preference.

❸ Entering the Retroperitoneum and Opening the Spaces.
Entering the retroperitoneum is the initial step to opening the paravesical and pararectal spaces bilaterally. Opening and developing these spaces allows the parametrial tissue to be isolated and therefore more easily resected (Fig. 38-18, p. 934).

First, the uterus is mobilized to one side by movement of the uterine manipulator and/or by an intraperitoneal blunt grasper holding one cornu. As shown on the left

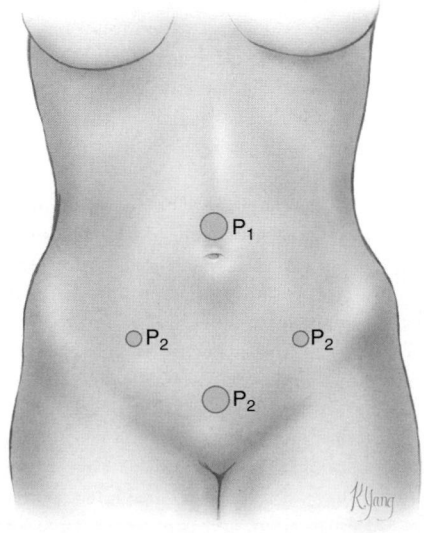

FIGURE 44-3.1 One example of port placement for laparoscopic radical hysterectomy.

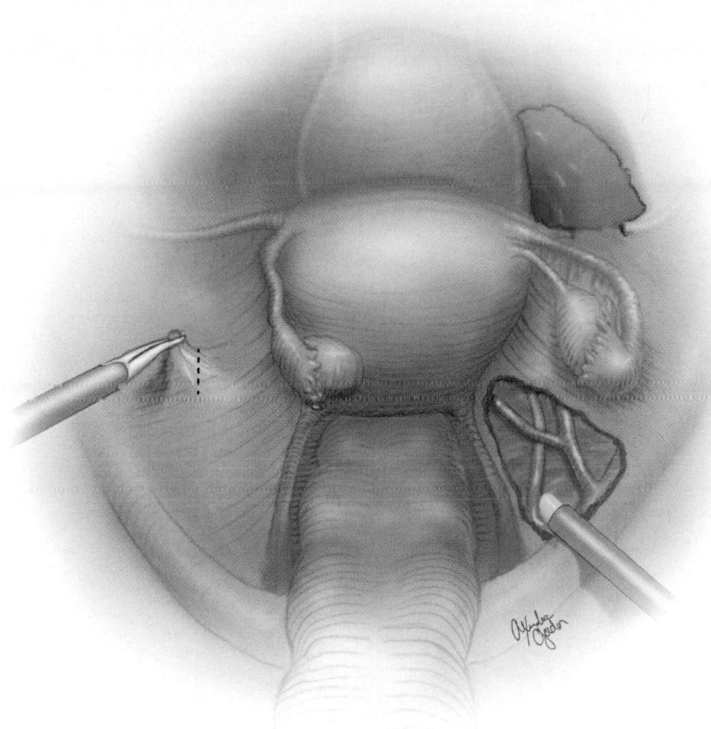

FIGURE 44-3.2 Peritoneal incision for retroperitoneal entry (*left*) and opened paravesical and pararectal spaces (*right*).

in Figure 44-3.2, the pelvic peritoneum above the psoas major muscle is tented upward and incised to open the retroperitoneum. Parallel to the infundibulopelvic (IP) ligament, the peritoneal incision is then extended both superiorly toward the pelvic brim and inferiorly to the round ligament. As shown on the lower right by the ABC tool, this exposes the iliac vessels and provides access to the ureter.

The round ligament is divided close to the pelvic sidewall. This ligament can be transected with the ABC, Harmonic scalpel, monopolar scissors, bipolar coagulation device, or clips and scissors. When using the ABC, it is set at 70 W of energy with a gas flow of 2 to 4 L/min and must be placed through a 12-mm port. Although the ABC serves as a coagulator, because of its blunt tip, it can be also used for gentle blunt dissection and retraction.

The peritoneum lateral to the medial umbilical ligament is also sharply incised and extended inferiorly parallel to the medial umbilical ligament. This allows entrance into the paravesical space. With blunt dissection using two instruments (coagulation device and a blunt grasper), the space is opened (see Fig. 44-3.2, upper right). This dissection mobilizes the bladder

and further exposes the external iliac vessels. With proper dissection of this avascular space, the pubic ramus is also exposed. The boundaries of the paravesical space include: the bladder and obliterated umbilical ligament medially, the external iliac vessels laterally, the pubic symphysis anteriorly, and the cardinal ligament posteriorly.

Next, the pararectal space is opened by dissecting bluntly below the IP ligament and bluntly entering the avascular plane between the ureter and the internal iliac vessels. The boundaries of the pararectal space are the following: the rectum and ureter medially, internal iliac artery laterally, cardinal ligament anteriorly, and the sacrum posteriorly. Once the paravesical and pararectal spaces are opened, the parametrium is now isolated between these two spaces and can be evaluated for disease.

❹ **Ureteral Isolation.** The ureters are located on the medial aspect of the broad ligament bilaterally. During a radical procedure, the ureters are unroofed in stages to the point of their insertion into the bladder. This allows parametrial tissue to be elevated off the ureter, which is necessary for the wide parametrial excision characteristic of radical hysterectomy. The ureters are isolated by dividing the tissue encasing them by blunt

dissection and preferably by bipolar coagulation. Mobilization of the bladder, next described, also helps to move the ureters laterally and away from the parametrium.

❺ **Bladder Mobilization.** To expose the vagina for transection, the bladder is dissected and moved downward off the anterior vagina. Initially, the bladder flap is created by grasping and elevating the vesicouterine fold with a blunt grasper. This peritoneum is incised, permitting entry into the vesicouterine space. Further dissection is performed in this plane between the posterior bladder and the uterus/anterior vagina using both sharp and blunt dissection. As the bladder is pushed inferiorly, the anterior vagina is exposed. It is crucial to adequately mobilize the bladder because up to a 3-cm vaginal margin may be resected with the specimen depending on the type of radical hysterectomy being performed.

❻ **Adnexectomy or Ovarian Preservation.** The infundibulopelvic (IP) ligament or the uteroovarian ligament will be transected, depending on whether adnexa will be removed or retained. For this, a window is made in the posterior broad ligament below the IP ligament. The ureter should be clearly identified to avoid its injury. The window can be made bluntly or with an electrosurgical tool, and the window is then enlarged. At this point, the IP ligament or the uteroovarian ligament is transected with an electrothermal bipolar coagulator, Harmonic scalpel, or endoscopic stapler.

The ovaries can be transposed laparoscopically if ovarian preservation is chosen. For this, the IP ligament is further dissected cephalad by extending the peritoneal incision on both the medial and lateral sides of the IP ligament. This mobilizes the adnexa, whose uteroovarian ligament stump is then sutured to the lateral peritoneum in the upper abdomen. Importantly, following transposition, the fallopian tube and ovary should be inspected to confirm adequate blood supply. A clip can be placed at the new site of the ovary so that it can be delineated on future imaging studies.

❼ **Uterine Artery Ligation and Parametrial Dissection.** Following development of the paravesical and pararectal spaces, the pelvic vessels are exposed. By moving down the common iliac artery to its bifurcation, a surgeon will identify the internal iliac artery and its spatial relationship to the ureter. The uterine artery branches medially from the internal iliac artery and crosses over the ureter. With blunt dissection, the uterine artery is isolated and ligated as close to its origin from the internal iliac artery as possible

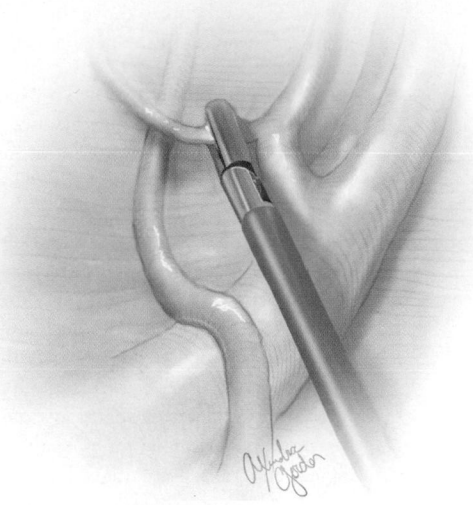

FIGURE 44-3.3 Uterine artery coagulation and transection.

using an electrothermal bipolar coagulator (Fig. 44-3.3). Alternatively, endoscopic vascular clips can also be placed across the uterine artery, which is then cut between the clips. Once the uterine artery has been ligated, further dissection and complete unroofing of the ureter can be then performed. Typically, the ureter is held on traction while a grasper is used to open the tunnel (Fig. 44-3.4). The tissue is held anteriorly away from the underlying ureter and divided in small increments. The uterine artery and parametrial tissue are pulled medially as they are dissected off the sidewall to be reflected over the ureter. Eventually, the ureteral insertion into the bladder is identified. The bladder pillars are isolated and transected with an electrothermal bipolar coagulator to complete parametrial tissue resection.

❽ Uterosacral Transection. After the ureter has been dissected and moved laterally and following further creation of the pararectal space, the uterosacral ligaments can be isolated. First, the uterus is retracted anteriorly, and the peritoneum between the isolated uterosacral ligaments is incised with an electrothermal bipolar coagulator at the level of the external os. The rectovaginal space is developed with a blunt dissector to further isolate the uterosacral ligaments and mobilize the rectum downward. The ureter should be retracted laterally before transecting the uterosacral ligament. The uterosacral ligaments, which are now isolated, can then be ligated close to the sacrum near the level of the rectum with an electrothermal bipolar coagulator (Fig. 44-3.5). An endoscopic stapler or a Harmonic scalpel can also be used to transect these ligaments.

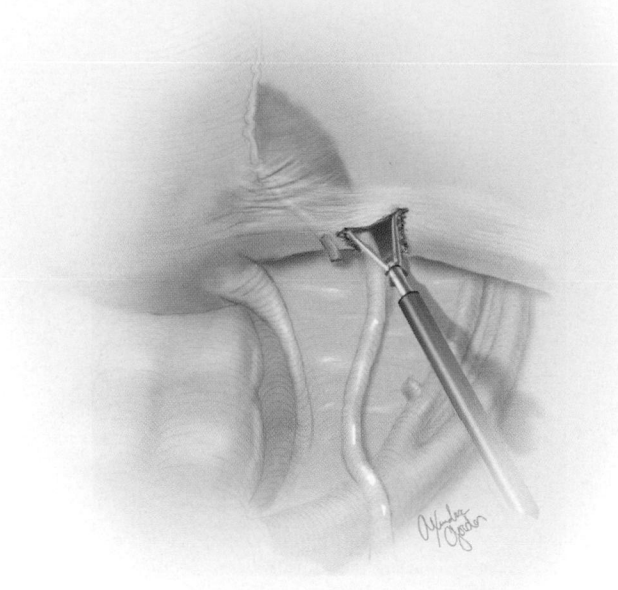

FIGURE 44-3.4 Unroofing the ureter.

❾ Vaginal Resection. With complete mobilization of the bladder and rectum, the anterior and posterior vagina should be easily identified. The radical hysterectomy specimen is now held in place only by the paracolpium and vagina. The upper vagina is incised distally on the vaginal wall to allow resection of a portion of proximal vagina (Fig. 44-3.6). The goal of radical hysterectomy resection is to remove approximately 3 cm of the upper vagina. An anterior colpotomy is made, and the incision is extended circumferentially around the cervix to its posterior aspect. An alternative

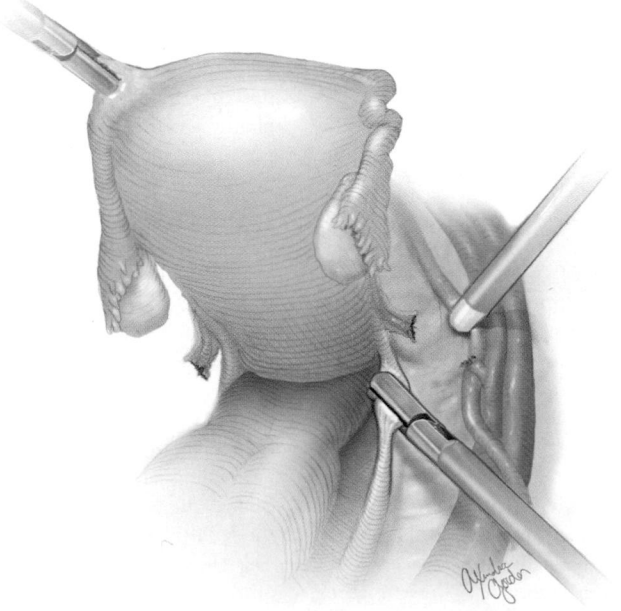

FIGURE 44-3.5 Uterosacral ligament coagulation and transection.

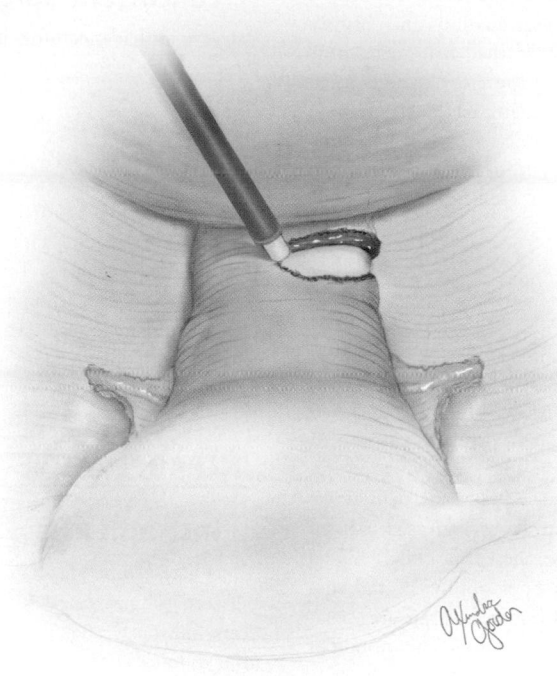

FIGURE 44-3.6 Anterior colpotomy.

step is to make the posterior cul-de-sac incision prior to the anterior colpotomy to help develop the rectovaginal septum. It is useful to have a vaginal delineator in the vagina to help direct colpotomy. As described earlier, a uterine manipulator with a cervical cup, such as a VCare Uterine Manipulator or KOH Colpotomizer, can be used if the cervical tumor is small (Fig. 42-12.1, p. 1152). The uterus, cervix, vaginal margin and parametrial tissue are then freed. This specimen is grasped with an instrument and removed

intact through the vagina. The final specimen is labeled "radical hysterectomy specimen" and includes cervix, uterus, vaginal margin, and parametrial tissue.

⑩ Vaginal Cuff Closure. Laparoscopic closure of the vaginal cuff can be performed by multiple methods. These are described and detailed in Section 42-12 (p. 1154). Another option to consider is cuff closure from a vaginal approach as done during simple vaginal hysterectomy (Section 41-13, p. 1054). Following

cuff closure, lymphadenectomy is begun and is described in Section 44-13 (p. 1302).

⑪ Port Removal and Fascial Closure. Once procedures have been completed, an inspection for hemostasis is performed. Ports are then removed under direct visualization. All fascial defects greater than 10 mm should be closed with 0-gauge delayed-absorbable suture to avoid hernia development at the site. Various methods of skin closure are available and include subcuticular suturing, skin adhesive (Dermabond), or surgical tape strips (Steristrips) plus tincture of benzoin.

POSTOPERATIVE

Immediate postoperative care following laparoscopic radical hysterectomy in general mirrors that for other minimally invasive procedures. Diet can be advanced more quickly than with open procedures, and most patients will tolerate a regular diet early on postoperative day 1. Patients are often discharged home on postoperative day 1 or 2 since their pain is well controlled. The same principles for retaining a Foley catheter do apply for open radical procedures. Therefore, many patients will be sent home with the Foley catheter and will return to clinic for a voiding trial.

Following radical hysterectomy, patients may be at increased risk for vaginal cuff dehiscence. In one series of 417 patients, the rate was 1.7 percent, and this rate was similar whether surgery was completed laparoscopically or robotically (Nick, 2011). This rate is higher than that with an open approach, and operative thermal damage during colpotomy or vaginal closure technique are suggested causes for this increased rate (Kho, 2009).

44-4

Robotic Radical Hysterectomy

Minimally invasive approaches to radical surgery offer specific recovery advantages. However, laparoscopic radical hysterectomy, described in Section 44-3 (p. 1267), is associated with long operative times and a steep learning curve, since meticulous dissection is required. In contrast, robotic radical hysterectomy is generally associated with faster skill acquisition compared with laparoscopy.

Moreover, compared with an open approach to radical hysterectomy, a robotic approach offers shorter hospital stays and equal or higher numbers of lymph nodes sampled during lymphadenectomy (Estape, 2009; Ko, 2008; Lowe, 2009). In addition, a recent study showed equal progression-free and overall-survival rates after 3 years following robotic radical hysterectomy compared with open radical hysterectomy (Cantrell, 2010). However, more long-term data on oncologic outcomes are needed. Thus, this approach has become an option for many gynecologic oncology surgeons, and the use of robotic surgery has become commonplace, particularly for surgical treatment of endometrial and cervical cancers.

Indications for a robotic approach to radical hysterectomy mirror those for laparoscopic and laparotomic approaches. Type III (radical) hysterectomy is chiefly indicated for stage IB1 to IIA cervical cancer or small central recurrences following radiation therapy, or for clinical stage II endometrial cancer when tumor has extended to the cervix. Similarly, for those women who are candidates for modified radical hysterectomy (type II), surgery can also be completed by a robotic approach.

PREOPERATIVE

Patient Evaluation

The same principles apply when choosing a patient for robotic surgery or for laparoscopy. As discussed in Section 44-3 (p. 1267), patients with significant cardiopulmonary disease, those with suspected extensive adhesive disease, or those with a large bulky uterus may be poor candidates for a minimally invasive approach. Specifically, a wide bulky uterus (width greater than 8 cm) with minimal mobility may be difficult to remove vaginally. Importantly, morcellation should be avoided when dealing with uterine or adnexal malignancy. For these reasons, a thorough pelvic examination and history should reveal factors that help determine the optimal surgical route for an individual patient. Once a patient has been deemed eligible for the robotic approach, the same preoperative evaluation as for an open radical hysterectomy applies (Section 44-1, p. 1267).

Consent

Inherent in the procedure, regardless of approach, possible risks include increased blood loss, need for transfusion, bladder and bowel dysfunction, and fistula formation. As described in Section 44-3, following a minimally invasive approach to radical hysterectomy, patients may be at increased risk for vaginal cuff dehiscence. This rate is higher than that with an open approach, and suggested causes for this increased rate are operative thermal damage during colpotomy or vaginal closure technique (Kho, 2009; Nick, 2011).

Complications related to robotic surgery are discussed in Chapter 42 (p. 1097) and include entry injury to the major vessels, bladder, ureters, and bowel. In addition, the risk of conversion to an open procedure should be discussed. Conversion to laparotomy may be necessary if exposure and organ manipulation are limited. Finally, port-site metastasis is an uncommon but possible complication, as described in Section 42-1 (p. 1099).

Patient Preparation

A blood sample should be typed and crossmatched for potential transfusion. Pneumatic compression devices or subcutaneous heparin or both to prevent venous thrombotic events are particularly important due to the long-anticipated length of the operation and venous stasis created by increased intraabdominal pressures from pneumoperitoneum (Chap. 39, p. 962). Due to lower associated blood loss with robotic radical hysterectomy, single-dose antibiotic prophylaxis is used and follows that for simple hysterectomy. Appropriate antibiotic options are listed in Table 39-6 (p. 959). The benefits from routine mechanical bowel preparation can be debated, and thus plans for bowel preparation are typically individualized (Chap. 39, p. 958). If considered, bowel preparation prior to surgery can effectively evacuate the rectosigmoid to permit improved colon manipulation and pelvic anatomy visualization.

Concurrent Surgery

Pelvic lymphadenectomy is typically completed just before or immediately after radical hysterectomy, and paraaortic lymphadenectomy may also be indicated in some circumstances. A robotic approach to lymphadenectomy in these areas is described in Section 44-14 (p. 1306).

Spread to the adnexa is much less common than via the lymphatics. Thus, removal of the adnexa should depend on a woman's age and potential for metastases (Shimada, 2006). As with laparoscopy, ovarian transposition can be performed with a robotic approach.

INTRAOPERATIVE

Instruments

There are some fundamental differences between robot-assisted surgery and laparoscopy. Currently, the only commercially available robotic system is the daVinci Surgical system. The specifics of this system and fundamentals of robot surgery are described in detail in Chapter 42 (p. 1107).

Important robotic instruments for radical hysterectomy include the EndoWrist monopolar scissors and the EndoWrist bipolar Maryland grasper. The PK dissecting forceps is an alternative bipolar cautery source for the robot. There are different additional graspers and retractors that can be used in the fourth robotic arm, as indicated for the procedure. The surgical assistant uses traditional laparoscopic instruments through the 12-mm assistant port. A suction irrigator is set up at the start of the procedure and can be used by the assistant if needed.

SURGICAL STEPS

❶ Anesthesia and Patient Positioning. The patient is initially placed supine for induction of general anesthesia. Prior to induction, lower extremity compression devices are placed for venous thrombosis prophylaxis. To avoid stomach puncture by a trocar during primary abdominal entry, an orogastric or a nasogastric tube should be placed to decompress the stomach. To avert similar bladder injury, a Foley catheter is placed.

Legs should be positioned in low lithotomy in Allen stirrups to permit adequate perineal access. The patient should be positioned on the table so that a transvaginal uterine manipulator, if needed, can be moved in all directions. As described in Section 42-1 (p. 1100), appropriate positioning of the legs within the stirrups is crucial to reduce the risk of nerve injury. The patient's arms are then tucked alongside her body to provide the surgeon with an increased area to move and operate. When tucking the patient's arms, a surgeon should be careful not to dislodge intravenous access lines and oxygen saturation finger monitors.

The patient should be secure on the table, as steep Trendelenburg position will be used. Robot arms do not move independently and remain locked in position. Thus, patient sliding can lead to muscle tears by the trocars and undesirable bleeding. In addition, sliding leads to limited uterine manipulator mobility and difficult vaginal specimen removal. Thus, after positioning in dorsal lithotomy and before the patient is prepped and draped, the patient should be placed in steep Trendelenburg to confirm secure positioning on the table. A bean bag on the bed or padding with securing adhesive can assist in keeping the patient in an appropriate position.

Bimanual examination is performed in the operating room before scrubbing to reorient a surgeon to the patient's individual anatomy. The abdomen, perineum, and vagina are then surgically prepared, and a Foley catheter is inserted.

A uterine manipulator, the same as used for laparoscopy, can be placed for the robotic procedure to aid uterine movement (Section 44-3, step 1, p. 1168). If a large cervical mass is present, a blunt probe can alternatively be used in the vagina.

❷ Abdominal Exploration. The abdomen and pelvis are thoroughly inspected to assess the extent of disease and adhesions. At this point, confirmation of metastatic disease or pelvic tumor extension should prompt a surgeon to decide whether to proceed or abort an operation based on overall intraoperative findings and clinical situation. In addition, the decision is made to proceed robotically or convert to laparotomy.

❸ Port Placement. Placement of the abdominal ports is different from that used in laparoscopy. In robotic surgery, the initial port, which is the laparoscope port, is placed above the umbilicus. The desired site is approximately 20 to 25 cm above the pubic symphysis either in the midline or just slightly off the midline, depending on the planned procedure. This is placed with the open abdominal entry technique described in Section 44-3, step 2 (p. 1268). Once the supraumbilical port is in place, other ports can be placed with direct laparoscopic visualization. The two main 8-mm robotic ports are placed 8 to 10 cm lateral to the midline

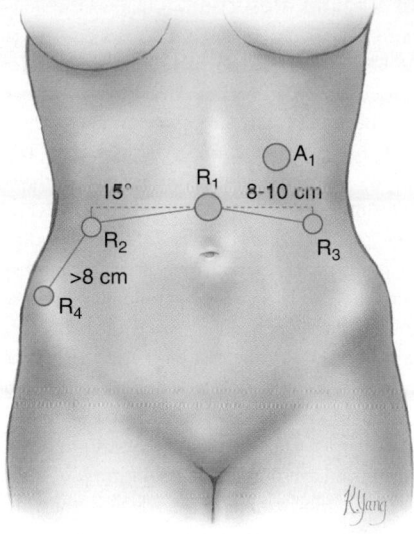

FIGURE 44-4.1 Port placement for robotic radical hysterectomy.

laparoscope port and 15 degrees downward (Fig. 44-4.1). Importantly, all robotic ports should have a minimum of 8 cm between them to allow appropriate robot arm range of motion and avoid arm collisions. If the robotic system has a fourth arm, it is usually placed in the lower quadrant approximately 2 cm above the anterior superior iliac spine and at least 8 cm from the other ports. It can be placed in either the right or left lower quadrant depending on where the bedside assistant will be standing. A fifth site, the assistant port, is placed in the upper abdomen and on the opposite side of the fourth arm. This port will house instruments that are manipulated by the assistant surgeon rather than the robot. Often, a 12-mm port is used as the assistant port and is placed between the laparoscope port and one of the main robotic arms. All of these trocars are placed under direct laparoscopic visualization before the robot arms are docked. The trocars are inserted to the level of the thick, black line on the cannula. This line is the fulcrum of the trocar cannula and permits optimal robot arm range of motion.

Once the ports are placed, the patient is then placed in steep Trendelenburg to help shift bowel out of the pelvis. The robot is then brought into position between the patient's legs, and the robotic arms are docked onto the trocars.

❹ Instrument Positioning. The surgeon is scrubbed at the bedside to place the trocars and to dock the robotic arms to these ports. A 0-degree laparoscope can be used while operating in the pelvis, although a laparoscope with a 30-degree lens system is

also available. Importantly, the robotic camera light source is hotter than the laparoscope used in traditional laparoscopy. Therefore, adjacent organs such as the bowel should not touch this laparoscope tip.

Several combinations of robotic arm instruments can be used. We recommend placing monopolar scissors in the right arm and a bipolar Maryland grasping forceps in the left arm. Another suitable bipolar option for the robot is the PK radiofrequency dissecting forceps. A blunt grasper can be placed in the fourth arm to assist with retraction. At the end of the case, these instruments will be changed to needle drivers for vaginal cuff closure. Once the robot is docked and the instruments placed, the surgeon leaves the sterile operative field and moves to the robot console to begin the procedure.

❺ Entering the Retroperitoneum and Opening the Spaces. The steps of robotic radical hysterectomy are the same as those of open and laparoscopic procedures. The procedure begins with opening of the paravesical and pararectal spaces to allow isolation and assessment of the parametrial tissue.

Initially, the uterus is manipulated to one side. This can be performed with the help of a grasper in the fourth robotic arm. The contralateral pelvic peritoneum above the psoas major muscle is grasped and incised with monopolar scissors in a blended mode. This peritoneum is opened both superiorly toward the pelvic brim and inferiorly toward the round ligament. This exposes the external iliac vessels and provides access to the ureter. The round ligament can be divided at this time using a combination of bipolar graspers to coagulate the ligament and monopolar scissors to transect it.

The peritoneum is further opened lateral to the medial umbilical ligament to open the paravesical space. Moving the laparoscope inward and using the right and left arm instruments, the surgeon bluntly opens the paravesical space down the levator muscles. Next, the pararectal space is opened by bluntly dissecting the avascular space between the ureter and the internal iliac vessels down toward the sacrum. The parametrium is now isolated between these two opened avascular spaces.

❻ Ureteral Isolation. The ureter, which lies on the medial aspect of the broad ligament, can be dissected using a bipolar forceps. The tissue encasing the ureter is dissected to allow the ureter to be moved medially and away from the iliac vessels. The ureter is unroofed to the point of its insertion into the bladder. This also allows parametrial tissue to be dissected off the ureters and away from the pelvic sidewall and to be removed with the final specimen. This dissection is made easier by the 360-degree articulation of the wristed robotic instruments.

❼ Bladder Mobilization. To expose the anterior vagina wall for resection, the bladder is mobilized inferiorly. First, the vesicouterine fold is grasped and incised, the bladder flap is then extended laterally with monopolar scissors, and the vesicouterine space is entered. The bladder is then mobilized by caudad dissection within this space. As with laparoscopy, dissection is performed using a combination of sharp and blunt dissection to push the bladder inferiorly off the anterior vagina.

❽ Adnexectomy or Ovarian Preservation. The infundibulopelvic (IP) ligament or the uteroovarian ligament will be transected depen-ding on whether adnexa will be removed or retained. A window is made in the posterior broad ligament below the IP ligament with monopolar scissors. The ureter should be clearly identified to avoid its injury. At this point, the IP ligament or the uteroovarian ligament is transected with the bipolar coagulation and cut with monopolar scissors.

❾ Uterine Artery Ligation and Parametrial Dissection. Following opening of the paravesical and pararectal spaces and dissection of the ureter, the uterine artery is isolated close to its origin from the internal iliac artery. The uterine artery is then coagulated with the bipolar instrument near its origin and is transected with the monopolar scissors. The parametrial tissue can be further dissected off the ureter and mobilized medially. Dissection of the bladder pillars is done with bipolar electrosurgery, and finally, the parametrial tissue dissection is complete.

❿ Uterosacral Transection. The uterosacral ligaments are next isolated. With the uterus retracted anteriorly, the posterior broad ligament incision is continued toward the uterosacral ligament with the help of monopolar scissors. This incision is made low on the uterosacral ligaments to permit an adequate vaginal margin to be obtained. The rectovaginal peritoneum is incised with monopolar scissor set on a blended mode. The rectovaginal space is then developed with blunt dissection. The isolated uterosacral ligaments are coagulated near the sacrum at the level of the rectum with the bipolar Maryland forceps. The ligaments are cut with monopolar scissors.

⓫ Vaginal Resection. Finally, the colpotomy can be made in the upper vagina with monopolar scissors and a blended mode. Different types of uterine manipulators can be used for laparoscopic hysterectomy. The KOH Colpotomizer system and the VCare Uterine Manipulator are two options (Section 42-12, p. 1152). These tools delineate the vagina and make colpotomy easier to perform. If a large cervical lesion is present, the uterus can be manipulated by the fourth arm and by the assistant's instrument, and a vaginal probe can be placed. In either case, a pneumooccluder balloon is placed in the vagina and inflated to help maintain the pneumoperitoneum during colpotomy. If a colpotomizer is used, the colpotomy incision is made approximately 3 cm below the ring and continued circumferentially with the monopolar scissors.

The entire specimen is then removed through the vagina either with traction on the uterine manipulator or by extraction with ring forceps. After the specimen is removed, the pneumooccluder balloon is replaced into the vagina. This allows sufficient insufflation for vaginal cuff closure. The final specimen is labeled "radical hysterectomy specimen" and includes cervix, uterus, proximal vagina, and parametrial tissue (Fig. 44-4.2).

⓬ Vaginal Cuff Closure. The robotic instruments are changed by the surgical assistant to perform the vaginal cuff closure. A Mega needle driver and a second needle driver are placed in the right and left arms. These are used for reapproximation of the vaginal walls with intracorporeal suturing and knot tying. A 0-gauge delayed-absorbable suture is passed through the 12-mm assistant port and handed to one of the needle drivers. The cuff

can be closed in a running, locking fashion or can be closed with interrupted figure-of-eight stitches. To begin closure, the needle is driven through the anterior vaginal wall and then through the posterior wall. The articulation of robotic instruments makes suturing and knot tying easier than in traditional laparoscopy. However, tactile feedback is absent with robotic surgery, and therefore, one must be cautious to cinch each knot throw snuggly yet avoid breaking the suture.

Once the vaginal cuff is closed, the needle is removed through the 12-mm assistant port. Generally, the suture adjacent to the needle rather than the needle itself is grasped by a needle driver in the assistant port. This permits safe needle removal without losing it within the peritoneal cavity. At this point, the needle drivers are removed from the robot arms. The original instruments are replaced into the arms by the assistant for completion of lymphadenectomy and other additional procedures.

⓭ Port Removal and Fascial Closure. Once procedures are completed, instruments are removed from the robotic arms, and the arms are undocked from the trocars. Once all of the arms are disengaged, the robot can be moved away from the patient. The laparoscope is handheld at this point, and the trocars are removed under direct laparoscopic visualization. All fascial defects greater than 10 mm should be closed with 0-gauge delayed-absorbable suture to avoid hernia development at those sites (Section 42-1, p. 1116). Various methods of skin closure are available and include subcuticular suturing, skin adhesive (Dermabond), or surgical tape strips (Steristrips) plus tincture of benzoin.

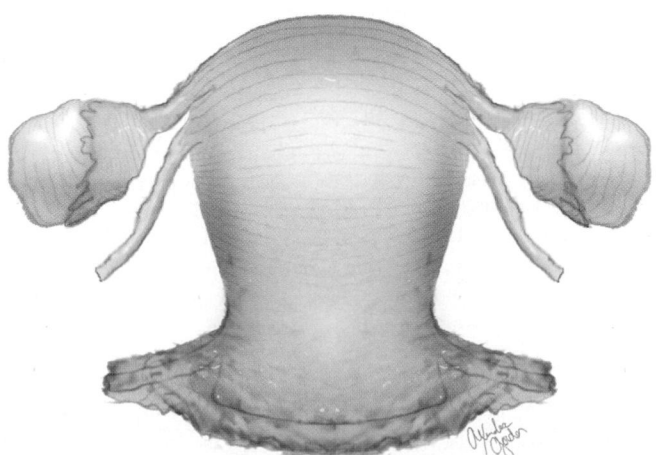

FIGURE 44-4.2 Anterior view of a radical hysterectomy specimen including uterus, cervix, portion of vagina, and parametria.

POSTOPERATIVE

Immediate postoperative care following robotic radical hysterectomy in general follows that for laparoscopic radical hysterectomy. The patient's diet can be advanced to a regular diet either on the day of the procedure or on postoperative day 1. Often pain is adequately controlled with oral medications, and intravenous narcotics are not needed. Patients are usually discharged home on postoperative day 1 or 2, once they are tolerating a regular diet and have adequate pain control. Patients are usually sent home with a Foley catheter and are seen in clinic 5 to 7 days after surgery for a voiding trial.

44-5

Total Pelvic Exenteration

Removal of the bladder, rectum, uterus (if present), and surrounding tissues is the most technically challenging single procedure in gynecologic oncology. Total pelvic exenteration is most commonly indicated for centrally persistent or recurrent cervical cancer after radiation therapy. Less common indications include some instances of recurrent endometrial adenocarcinoma, uterine sarcoma, or vulvar cancer; locally advanced carcinoma of the cervix, vagina, or endometrium when radiation is contraindicated, such as previous radiotherapy or malignant fistula; and melanoma of the vagina or urethra (Berek, 2005; Goldberg, 2006; Maggioni, 2009).

Total pelvic exenteration is generally indicated for curative situations when less radical surgery, chemotherapy, or radiation options have been exhausted. In some instances, intraoperative radiation therapy may be useful as an adjunct to the procedure due to an obviously positive or clinically suspicious resection margin (Greer, 2011a; Sharma, 2005). Palliative exenterations may be of benefit on rare occasions when selected patients have severe, unrelenting symptoms (Guimarães, 2011). Because exenteration commonly follows radiation therapy, the uterus and cervix usually have lost their distinct tissue architecture and boundaries. As a result, traditional hysterectomy steps and anatomical landmark identification are typically not possible. Minimally invasive exenterative procedures have been reported and may rarely be indicated in highly selected patients (Martinez, 2011; Puntambekar, 2006).

Total pelvic exenterations are subclassified based on the extent of pelvic floor muscle and vulvar resection (Table 44-5.1) (Magrina, 1997). Supralevator (type I) exenteration may be indicated when a lesion is relatively small and does not involve the lower half of the vagina. Most total pelvic exenterations will be infralevator (type II). This type is selected if vaginal contracture, prior hysterectomy, or the inability to otherwise achieve adequate margins is present. Rarely, tumor extension warrants an infralevator exenteration with vulvectomy (type III).

PREOPERATIVE

Patient Evaluation

Initially, biopsy confirmation of recurrent invasive disease should be performed. With confirmation, the single most impor-

TABLE 44-5.1 Differences among Type I (Supralevator), Type II (Infralevator), and Type III (with Vulvectomy) Pelvic Exenterations

Pelvic Structure	Degree of Resection		
	Type I	Type II	Type III
Viscera	Above levator	Below levator	Below levator
Levator ani muscles	None	Limited	Complete
Urogenital diaphragm	None	Limited	Complete
Vulvoperineal tissues	None	None	Complete

From Magrina, 1997, with permission.

tant preoperative challenge is to search for metastatic disease that would abort plans for surgery. Chest radiography is mandatory. Abdominopelvic computed tomography (CT) is also routinely indicated, but a positron emission tomography (PET) scan may be particularly helpful (Chung, 2006; Husain, 2007). Hydroureter and hydronephrosis are not absolute contraindications unless they are due to obvious pelvic sidewall disease.

Patients often initially reject the entire concept of this operation even when faced with the knowledge that it represents their only chance for cure. Counseling is essential. Overcoming denial may take several visits. Regardless, not all eligible women will wish to proceed.

Preexisting medical problems, morbid obesity, and malnutrition increase the potential morbidity of total pelvic exenteration. Thus, a surgeon should take all factors into consideration and candidly explore all possible alternatives before proceeding with surgical planning.

Consent

The consenting process is the ideal time to finalize plans for the type and location of urinary conduit, plans for colostomy or low rectal anastomoses, and need for vaginal reconstruction or other ancillary procedures. A patient should also be advised that the procedure may need to be aborted based on intraoperative findings.

For those who undergo exenteration, the perioperative mortality rate approaches 5 percent (Marnitz, 2006; Sharma, 2005). However, the mortality rate from progressive cancer would otherwise be 100 percent. Patients should be prepared for admission to an intensive care unit (ICU) postoperatively. Febrile morbidity, wound breakdown, bowel obstruction, and venous thromboembolic events are common short-term com-

plications. Additionally, intestinal fistulas or anastomotic leaks or strictures may develop. Most women will experience significant morbidity and unforeseen complications (Berek, 2005; Goldberg, 2006; Maggioni, 2009; Marnitz, 2006). Reoperation may be required.

Long-term effects on sexual function and other body functions should be candidly reviewed. Patients with two ostomies have a lower quality of life and poorer body image. However, in those who retain vaginal capacity, quality of life and sexual function is reportedly improved. Thus, counseling regarding vaginal reconstruction should be part of the preoperative dialogue (Section 44-10, p. 1292). A detailed approach to the consent process can help resolve many of these dilemmas and achieve the ideal balance for an individual patient (Hawighorst, 2004; Roos, 2004). In general, a woman's postoperative quality of life is most affected by her worries regarding tumor progression (Hawighorst-Knapstein, 1997). Therefore, patients should be aware that more than half will develop recurrent disease despite exenterative surgery (Berek, 2005; Goldberg, 2006; Sharma, 2005).

Patient Preparation

Patients require thorough preoperative counseling and preparation, occasionally necessitating admission the day before surgery. Stoma sites are marked, the consent form is reviewed, and final questions are answered.

To minimize fecal contamination during bowel excision, aggressive bowel preparation such as with a polyethylene glycol with electrolyte solution (GoLytely) is mandatory. Ileus is common following exenteration and nutritional demands are increased. Thus, total parenteral nutrition is often initiated as early as possible. In addition, routine antibiotic prophylaxis has been shown to decrease infectious complications (Goldberg, 1998). Pneumatic compression devices or subcutaneous heparin is particularly important due to the anticipated length of the operation and longer duration of postoperative recovery. Patients should be typed and crossmatched for potential packed red blood cell replacement. Critical care team consultation may be indicated, and an ICU bed should be requested.

INTRAOPERATIVE

Instruments

To prepare for complicated resections, a surgeon should have access to all types and sizes of bowel staplers. These include end-to-end anastomosis (EEA), gastrointestinal anastomosis (GIA), and transverse anastomosis (TA) staplers. Additionally, an electrothermal bipolar coagulator (LigaSure) may speed pedicle ligation while decreasing blood loss (Slomovitz, 2006).

SURGICAL STEPS

❶ Anesthesia and Patient Positioning.
General anesthesia with or without epidural placement for postoperative pain management is mandatory. Invasive monitoring is typically added as a necessary precaution. Bimanual examination is performed to reorient a surgeon to a patient's individual anatomy. The abdomen, perineum, and vagina are surgically prepared, and a Foley catheter is inserted. Legs should be positioned in low lithotomy in Allen stirrups to permit adequate perineal access.

❷ Abdominal Entry.
The type of abdominal entry may be dictated by an intended rectus abdominis flap, but otherwise a midline vertical incision is ideal. A less commonly employed option is to initially assess patients by laparoscopy. This minimally invasive approach may avoid unnecessary laparotomy in up to half of candidate patients (Kohler, 2002; Plante, 1998).

❸ Exploration.
The most common reason that exenterations are aborted is the presence of metastatic peritoneal disease (Miller, 1993). Thus, following positioning of an abdominal self-retaining retractor, a surgeon should thoroughly explore for disseminated disease that may not have been suspected preoperatively. Typically, numerous adhesions must also be lysed to inspect and palpate abdominal contents. Suspicious lesions should be removed or biopsied.

❹ Lymph Node Dissection.
A significant number of exenterations will be aborted intraoperatively due to identification of lymph node metastases (Miller, 1993). For this reason, pelvic and paraaortic node sampling is performed to exclude metastatic disease before proceeding (Sections 44-11 and 44-12, p. 1296). Additionally, retroperitoneal dissection provides a surgeon with a sense of the degree of pelvic sidewall fibrosis, which may render the vessels, ureters, and other important structures virtually indistinguishable from the surrounding soft tissue.

❺ Pelvic Sidewall Exploration.
As described in Section 44-1, steps 4 through 6 (p. 1269), the retroperitoneum is entered and the external iliac and internal iliac artery bifurcation is bluntly dissected free of overlying areolar connective tissue. The ureter is placed on a Penrose drain for identification. The paravesical and pararectal spaces are developed.

Parametrial tumor extension is the third most common reason for aborting exenteration (Miller, 1993). Thus, the pelvic sidewall should be verified to be clinically free of disease by inserting one finger into the paravesical space, another into the pararectal space, and palpating the intervening tissue down to the levator plane. There must be a grossly negative margin at the pelvic sidewall to proceed. Tissues may be biopsied to confirm this impression. Often, it is difficult to know with absolute certainty whether the margins are clear due to the varying extent of retroperitoneal fibrosis encountered.

❻ Bladder Mobilization.
The bladder blade is removed from the self-retaining retractor to permit entry into the space of Retzius and to bluntly reflect the bladder from the back of the pubic symphysis. Downward traction on the bladder and urethra will expose filmy attachments that may be electrosurgically incised (Fig. 44-5.1). Laterally positioned false ligaments of the bladder are divided between clamps or transected with an electrothermal bipolar coagulator. This joins the retropubic and paravesical spaces (Fig. 38-18, p. 934). The bladder should be floppy in the pelvis from loss of its supporting pelvic attachments and is completely freed anteriorly. However, the urethra is still attached to the bladder.

❼ Rectal Mobilization.
Following mobilization of the bladder, the ureters are held laterally, and the overlying peritoneum at the pelvic brim is divided in a medial direction up to the sigmoid mesentery. By inserting a finger into the pararectal space and sweeping medially, it should be possible to develop the avascular plane between the rectosigmoid and the sacrum (retrorectal space).

Surgeons should be confident that there is no sacral tumor invasion and that they will be able to lift the rectosigmoid out of the pelvis to achieve a posterior margin that is free of tumor. This is the last decision to be made before dividing the bowel and beginning steps of the operation that are irreversible.

Once the entire circumference of the tumor has been assessed, exenteration proceeds by dividing the sigmoid with a gastrointestinal

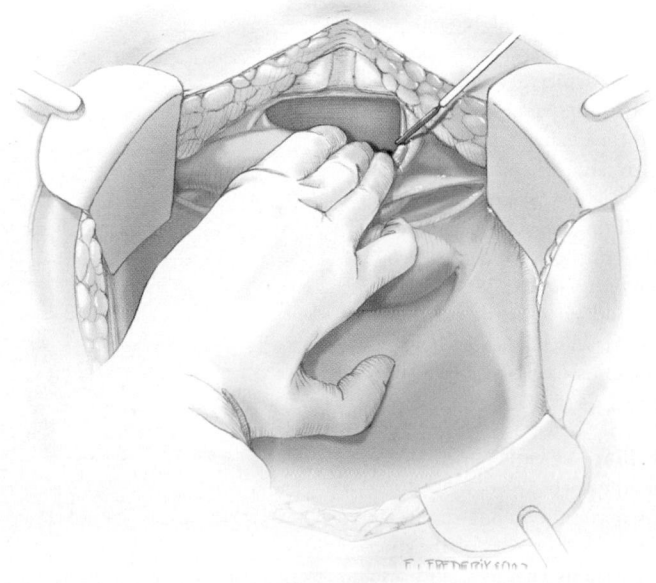

FIGURE 44-5.1 Mobilizing the bladder.

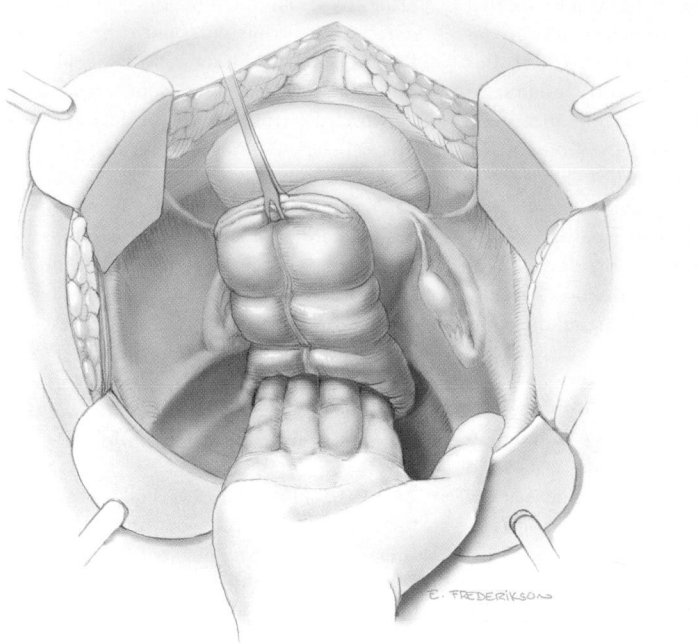

FIGURE 44-5.2 Mobilizing the rectum.

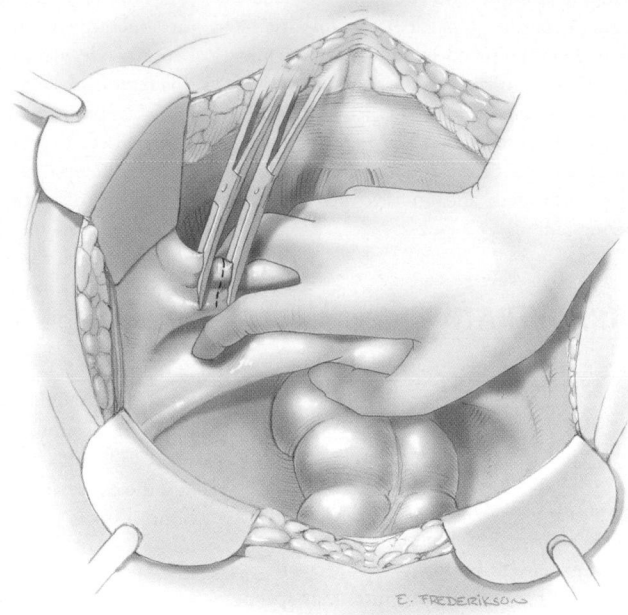

FIGURE 44-5.3 Dividing the cardinal ligaments.

anastomotic (GIA) stapler and dividing the intervening mesenteric tissue (Section 44-23, steps 5 and 6, p. 1327). The proximal sigmoid is then packed into the upper abdomen. The distal rectosigmoid is held ventrally and cephalad while a hand is inserted posteriorly to bluntly dissect the adventitial tissue between the rectum and sacrum in the midline (Fig. 44-5.2). This maneuver is continued distally to the coccyx to develop the retrorectal space and isolate the laterally located rectal pillars.

❽ **Cardinal Ligament Division.** The mobilized bladder and distal rectum with uterus (if present) are held together on contralateral traction, while a hand is placed with one finger in the paravesical space and the other in the pararectal space to isolate the lateral pelvic attachments. The cardinal ligaments, internal iliac vessels, and ureter are often not distinguishable in a typically radiated field, but lie within this tissue. Beginning anteriorly, these fibrous attachments are serially divided at the pelvic sidewall (Fig. 44-5.3). Vascular clips should be available in case of tissue slippage or inadvertent bleeding.

❾ **Internal Iliac Vessels and Ureter Division.** As the pelvic sidewall dissection continues posteriorly along the levator muscles, the anterior branches of the internal iliac artery, venous channels, and distal ureter ideally are individually located and ligated to optimize hemostasis (Fig. 44-5.4).

However, blood vessels and ureters frequently will lie within fibrous tissue and may be relatively indistinguishable. Thus, clamps or the electrothermal bipolar coagulator should be placed around smaller pedicles to minimize the possibility of inadvertent blood loss. At minimum, the ureter should be located, isolated, and divided as distally as possible to provide extra length for reaching the conduit. Later, any damage at the distal tip can be trimmed as needed to ensure healthy tissue for urinary conduit creation. A large vascular clip is placed on the proximal end of the ureter to distend the lumen and aid later anastomosis into the planned conduit. Dissection is then repeated on the contralateral side, and any remaining lateral attachments along the levator ani muscles are divided as the pelvic floor curves toward the perineum.

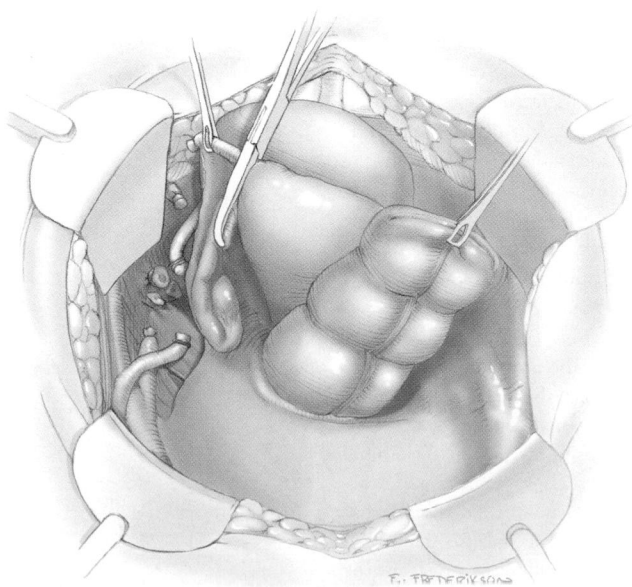

FIGURE 44-5.4 Dividing the hypogastric vessels and ureter.

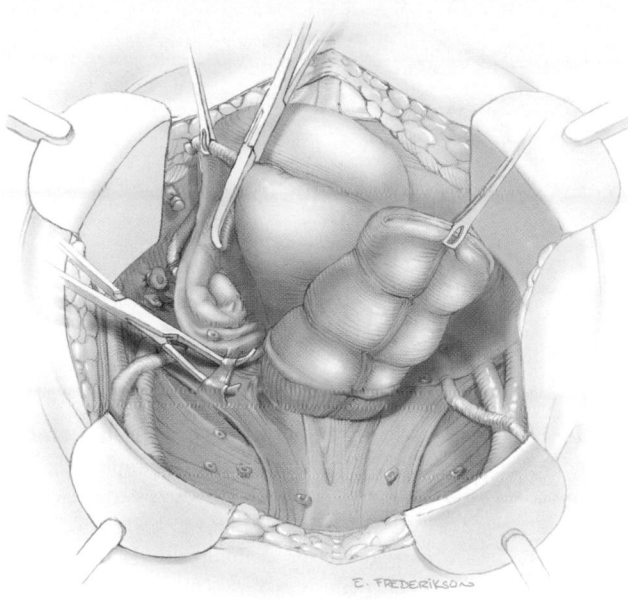

FIGURE 44-5.5 Dividing the rectal pillars.

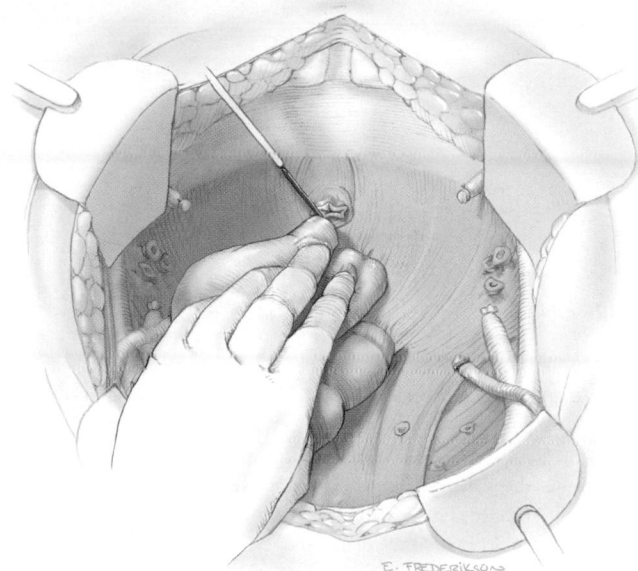

FIGURE 44-5.6 Supralevator exenteration: dividing the urethra.

❿ Rectal Pillar Division. The exenteration specimen is now chiefly tethered by the rectal stalks and distal mesenteric attachments posteriorly. These can be skeletonized with a right-angle clamp and divided along the pelvic floor (Fig. 44-5.5). This maneuver is continued distally to expose the entire posterior pelvic floor. The exenteration specimen is then circumferentially inspected and additional dissection is performed to completely release it from all attachments leading through the levator ani muscles.

⓫ Supralevator Exenteration: Final Steps. Removal of the specimen above the levator muscles begins by posterior traction on the bladder. The Foley catheter should be palpable within the urethra, and all surrounding tissue should already be dissected away. An electrosurgical blade is used to transect the distal urethra (Fig. 44-5.6). The distal opening does not require closure and may function as a natural orifice drain postoperatively. The vagina is then transected and closed with 0-gauge delayed-absorbable

suture in a running fashion. The transverse anastomosis (TA) or curved cutter stapler (Contour) is placed across the distal rectum and fired (Fig. 44-5.7). This completes detachment of the specimen, which includes bladder, uterus, rectum, and surrounding tissue. The pelvic floor is then carefully assessed to identify bleeding points (Fig. 44-5.8). A laparotomy pad is packed firmly into the pelvis to tamponade any surface oozing, while the exenteration specimen is inspected to confirm grossly negative margins.

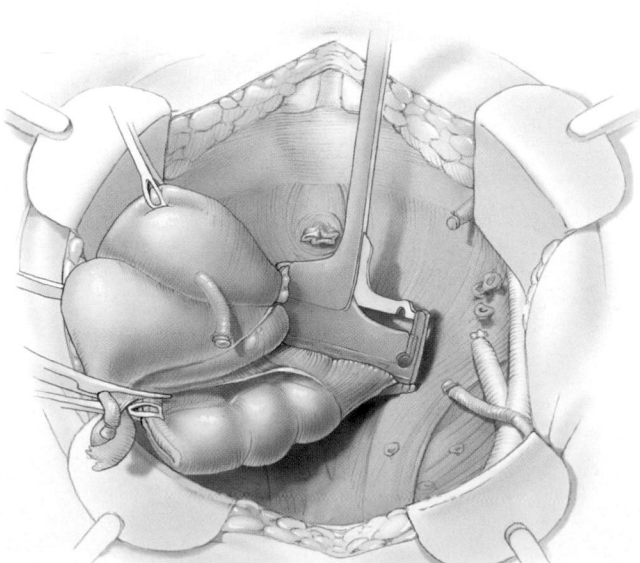

FIGURE 44-5.7 Supralevator exenteration: dividing the rectum.

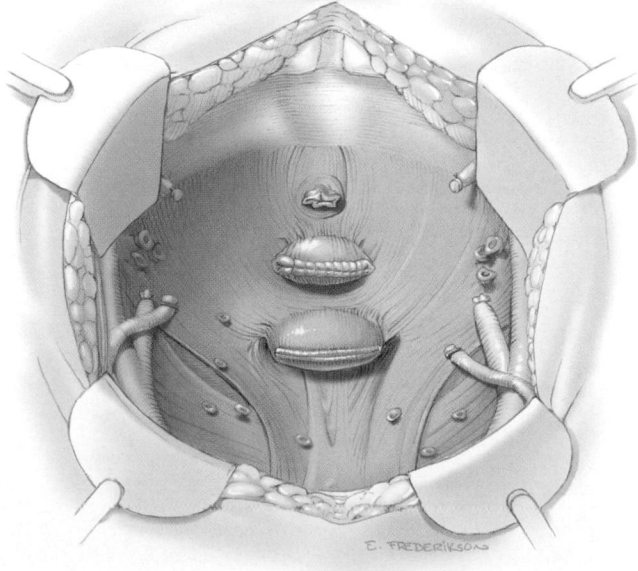

FIGURE 44-5.8 Supralevator exenteration: appearance of the pelvic floor.

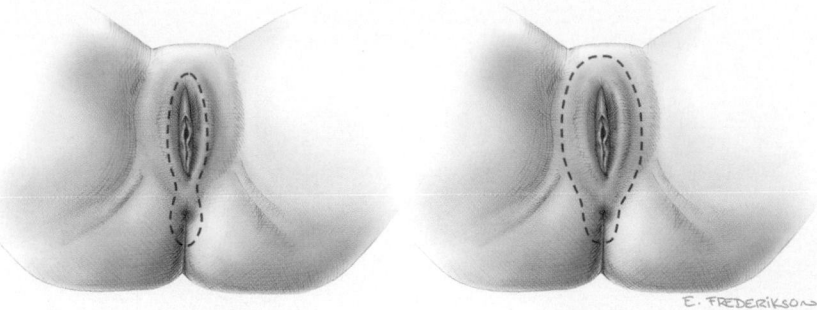

FIGURE 44-5.9 Infralevator exenteration: perineal phase incisions without vulvectomy (*left*) and with vulvectomy (*right*).

⑫ Infralevator Exenteration: Perineal Phase. When the abdominal dissection reaches the levator muscles, a second surgical team begins the perineal phase. The use of two teams typically shortens operative time and reduces bleeding. The planned perineal resection is outlined to encompass the tumor. As shown in Figure 44-5.9, resection may require infralevator exenteration without or with vulvectomy.

The perineal incision ideally begins concomitantly with division of the levator muscles by the abdominal team. At the perineum, a skin incision is first performed, followed by use of an electrosurgical blade to dissect through the subcutaneous tissues surrounding the urethra, vaginal opening, and anus.

⑬ Infralevator Exenteration: Partial Resection of the Levator Muscles. Within the abdomen, the primary surgical team places the specimen on traction. Electrosurgical blade dissection is used to

circumferentially incise the levator muscles lateral to the area of tumor extension (Fig. 44-5.10). The dissection proceeds distally toward the perineum.

⑭ Infralevator Exenteration: Connecting the Perineal and Abdominal Spaces. After the perineal incision has reached the fascial plane, four spaces are developed: subpubic space, left and right vaginal spaces, and retrorectal space. It is helpful to have the abdominal surgeon place a hand deep into the pelvis and guide the electrosurgical dissection by the perineal team (Fig. 44-5.11). Five pedicles should be identified that separate these avascular spaces: two pubourethral pedicles, two rectal pillar pedicles, and the midline posterior anococcygeal pedicle. Electrosurgical dissection that is directed by the abdominal surgeon's finger is performed to open the intervening spaces. From below, the five vascular pedicles are divided and ligated using the electrothermal bipolar coagulator.

⑮ Infralevator Exenteration: Removal of the Specimen. Circumferential dissection will result in complete detachment of the specimen that can be removed either vaginally or abdominally (Fig. 44-5.12). Hemostasis is then achieved with a series of sutures, vascular clips, or clamps and ties. Finally, the pelvic floor and pedicle sites are carefully reinspected (Fig. 44-5.13).

⑯ Infralevator Exenteration: Simple Closure. The most straightforward and quickest way to close the perineum is for the second team to perform a layered closure of the deep tissues with 0-gauge delayed-absorbable suture (Fig. 44-5.14). The perineal skin is closed with the same type of delayed-absorbable suture in a running fashion.

⑰ Final Steps. A dry laparotomy pad may be held firmly deep in the pelvis to tamponade surface oozing, while the urinary conduit, colostomy or bowel anastomosis, other

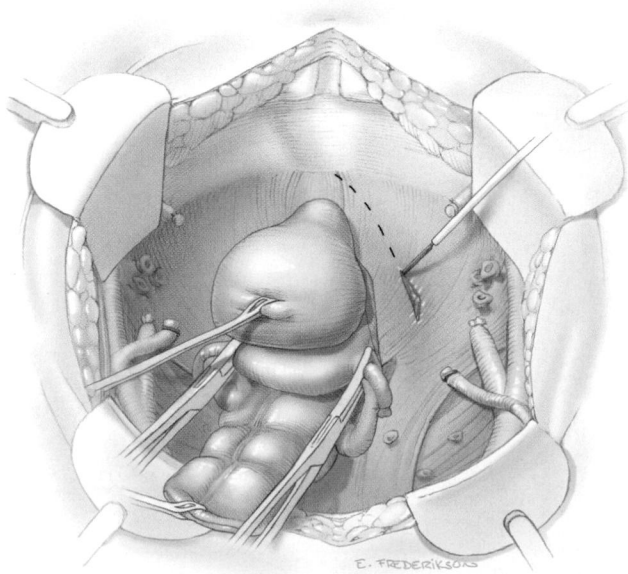

FIGURE 44-5.10 Infralevator exenteration: partial resection of the levator muscles.

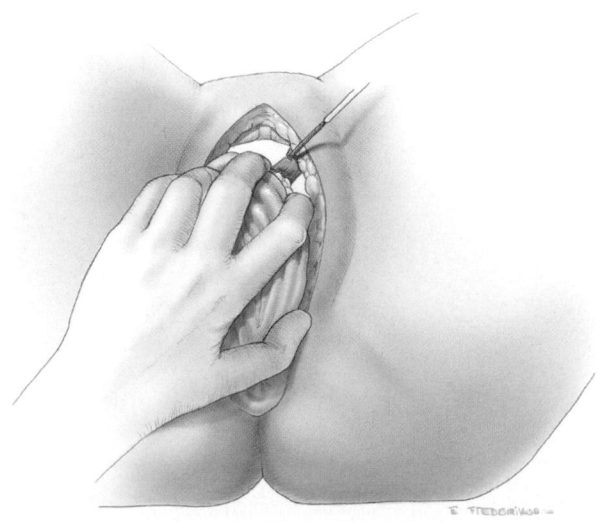

FIGURE 44-5.11 Infralevator exenteration: connecting the perineal and abdominal spaces.

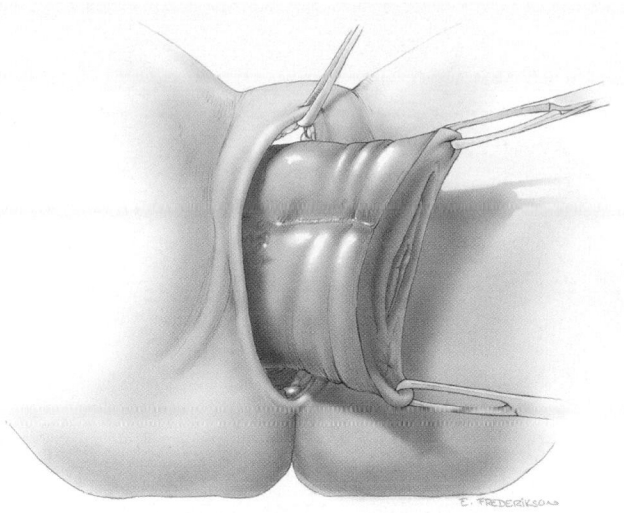

FIGURE 44-5.12 Infralevator exenteration: removal of the specimen.

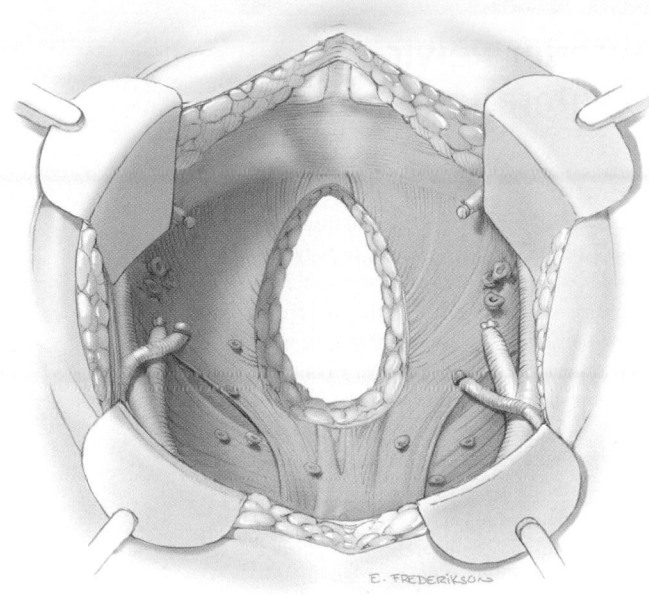

FIGURE 44-5.13 Infralevator exenteration: pelvic floor.

surgical procedures, vaginal reconstruction, or intraoperative radiation therapy are performed. An omental J-flap may provide additional blood supply to the irradiated, denuded pelvic floor (Section 44-16, p. 1314). The type of postoperative suction drainage may be dictated by these ancillary procedures, but should be judiciously used (Goldberg, 2006).

POSTOPERATIVE

The morbidity of total pelvic exenteration depends on various factors. These include preoperative health of the patient, intraoperative events, extent of the procedure, ancillary procedures, and postoperative vigilance. Hospitals that treat a relatively high volume of such patients report lower surgical in-hospital mortality rates (Maggioni, 2009). However, unlike a few decades ago, few institutions perform this operation on a regular basis.

The immediate life-threatening concerns are massive bleeding, adult respiratory distress syndrome, pulmonary embolism, and myocardial infarction (Fotopoulou, 2010). Every effort should be made to encourage early ambulation as soon as the patient is stable.

A prolonged ileus or small bowel obstruction will typically respond to expectant management, but may require total parenteral nutrition for weeks. Intestinal fistulas and leaks are more common when using mesh to cover the pelvic floor or when performing low rectal anastomoses. Omental pedicle grafts and rectus abdominis or gracilis myocutaneous flaps may prevent such complications (Section 44-10, p. 1293). Pelvic abscess and septicemia are additional subacute complications that occur commonly (Berek, 2005; Goldberg, 2006; Maggioni, 2009; Marnitz, 2006; Sharma, 2005).

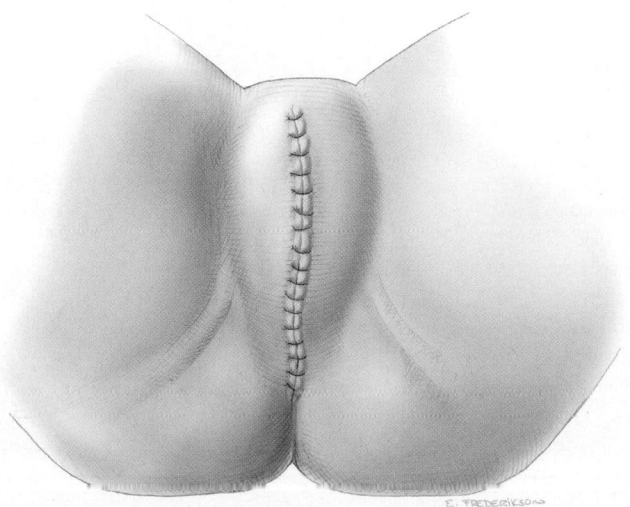

FIGURE 44-5.14 Infralevator exenteration: simple perineal closure.

44-6

Anterior Pelvic Exenteration

Removal of the uterus, vagina, bladder, urethra, distal ureters, and parametrial tissues with preservation of the rectum is meant to be a less morbid operation than total pelvic exenteration (Section 44-5, p. 1276). Patients are carefully selected for this more limited procedure to still achieve negative surgical margins. For this reason, women who have previously had a hysterectomy are not usually good candidates. The most common indications include small recurrences confined to the cervix or anterior vagina after pelvic radiation. In gynecologic oncology, up to half of all exenterations performed are anterior (Berek, 2005; Maggioni, 2009).

PREOPERATIVE

The preoperative evaluation is similar to that described for total pelvic exenteration. Although preservation of the rectum is planned, patients should be advised during the consenting process that potentially unforeseen clinical circumstances may dictate bowel resection and colostomy or low rectal anastomosis. Accordingly, a complete bowel preparation is still mandatory.

INTRAOPERATIVE

SURGICAL STEPS

❶ Initial Steps. Anterior exenteration is technically similar to total pelvic exenteration, described earlier. Patients are positioned in Allen stirrups, the appropriate skin incision is made, the abdomen is explored, lymph nodes are removed, and spaces are developed to exclude metastatic or unresectable disease. The procedure begins to differ after the bladder has been mobilized. A surgeon then makes the final decision to leave the rectum intact and proceed with anterior pelvic exenteration.

❷ Developing the Rectovaginal Space. Instead of mobilizing the rectum and dividing the sigmoid, the rectovaginal space is developed much as in a type III radical hysterectomy. The uterosacral ligament and the entire length of the rectal pillars are divided to free the exenteration specimen posteriorly (see Fig. 44-1.7, p. 1263).

❸ Lateral Pelvic Attachments. The mobilized bladder and uterus are held medially to aid isolation of the cardinal ligaments, internal iliac vessels, and ureter. These structures are

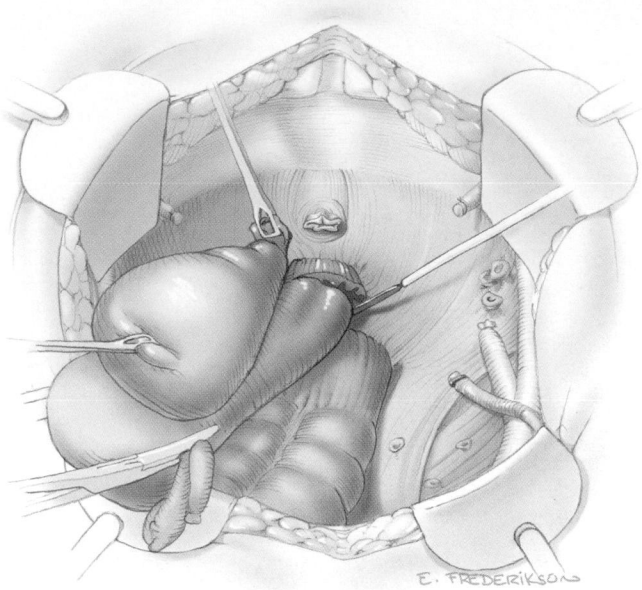

FIGURE 44-6.1 Removal of the specimen.

successively divided with an electrothermal bipolar coagulator (LigaSure) or clamped, cut, and individually ligated.

❹ Removal of the Specimen. After the anterior pelvic exenteration specimen has been completely mobilized, the urethra and vagina are divided (Fig. 44-6.1). The urethra is left open, and the vaginal cuff is closed with 0-gauge delayed-absorbable suture in a running fashion (Fig. 44-6.2).

❺ Final Steps. Typically, the lesion is small and lies above the levators, thus a perineal phase is not required. For this reason, placement of a

myocutaneous flap for vaginal reconstruction may be more problematic in these patients due to limited space in the pelvis.

POSTOPERATIVE

Morbidity of anterior pelvic exenteration is comparable with that of total pelvic exenteration (Sharma, 2005). Ideally, the operation is shorter in duration and restoration of bowel function is more rapid. Some patients will experience tenesmus or long-term rectal symptoms that likely stem from interruption of the autonomic nervous system in surrounding tissue.

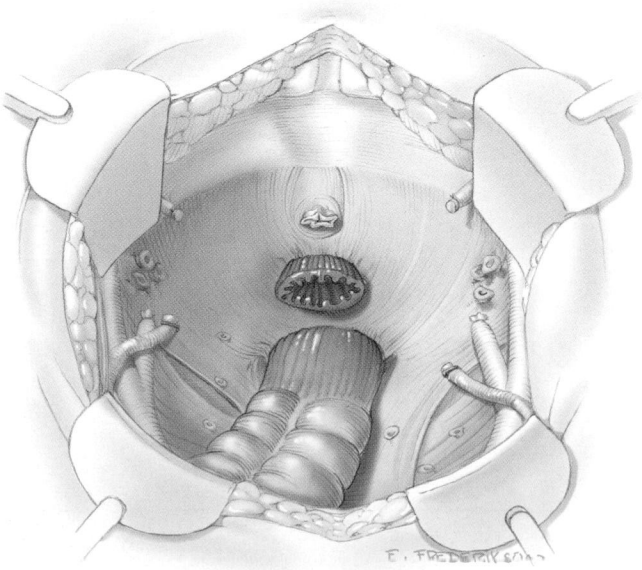

FIGURE 44-6.2 Appearance of the pelvic floor before vaginal cuff closure.

44-7

Posterior Pelvic Exenteration

Removal of the uterus, vagina, rectum, and parametrial tissues with preservation of the ureters and bladder is meant to be a less morbid operation than total pelvic exenteration (Section 44-5, p. 1276). Patients should be carefully selected for this more limited procedure to still achieve negative surgical margins. For this reason, women who have previously had a hysterectomy are not usually good candidates. The most common indications include small postirradiation recurrences primarily involving the posterior vaginal wall or coexisting with a rectovaginal fistula. In gynecologic oncology, fewer than 10 percent of exenterations are posterior (Berek, 2005; Maggioni, 2009).

PREOPERATIVE

Preoperative evaluation is largely identical to that described for total pelvic exenteration. A surgeon's judgment and experience are critical in deciding to proceed with a more limited operation. Although preservation of the bladder is planned, patients should be advised during the consenting process that potentially unforeseen clinical circumstances may dictate resection of the ureters and bladder with formation of a urinary conduit.

INTRAOPERATIVE

SURGICAL STEPS

❶ Initial Steps. Posterior pelvic exenteration is technically similar to a type III radical hysterectomy but with the addition of a more extended vaginectomy and rectosigmoid resection (Section 44-1, p. 1259). The operation begins as a total pelvic exenteration. Patients are positioned in Allen stirrups, the appropriate skin incision is made, the abdomen is explored, lymph nodes are removed, and spaces are developed to exclude metastatic or unresectable disease. A surgeon then

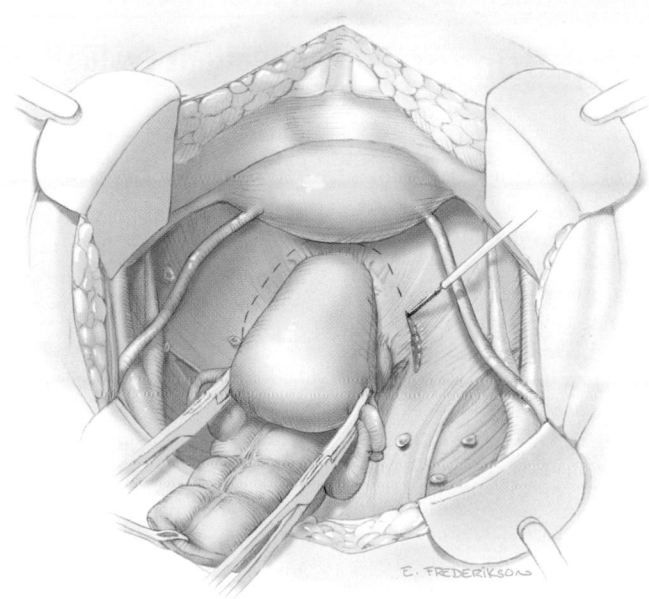

FIGURE 44-7.1 Incising the levator muscles.

makes the final decision to leave the bladder intact and proceed with posterior exenteration.

❷ Ureteral Dissection. As with type III radical hysterectomy, the retroperitoneum is entered, ureters are mobilized, uterine arteries are ligated at their internal iliac artery origin, and parametrial tissue is divided at the pelvic sidewall. The bladder is then dissected distally to aid in unroofing the ureters from the paracervical tunnels. The lateral attachments have been divided all the way to the levator ani muscles (Fig. 44-7.1). However, typically these steps are much more tedious in a previously irradiated field because of tissue fibrosis and scarring.

❸ Mobilizing the Rectum. The sigmoid is divided with the mesentery and peritoneal attachments, as earlier described for a total pelvic exenteration (Section 44-5, step 7 p. 1277). The retrorectal space is bluntly dissected to mobilize the rectum and enable transection of the rectal pillars.

❹ Removal of the Specimen. The dissection is continued circumferentially to (or through) the levator ani muscles to encom-

pass the tumor. The distal vagina is transected and sewn closed in a running fashion with 0-gauge delayed absorbable suture. The entire specimen may then be placed on traction to aid placement of the transverse anastomosis (TA) or curved cutter stapler (Contour) and division of the rectum. The rectum is divided below the tumor to leave grossly negative margins, and the specimen is removed.

❺ Final Steps. Typically, the lesion is small and lies above the levator ani muscles, and thus a perineal phase is not required. As a result, placement of a myocutaneous flap for vaginal reconstruction may be more problematic in such patients due to limited space in the pelvis.

POSTOPERATIVE

Morbidity of posterior pelvic exenteration is comparable with that of total pelvic exenteration (Section 44-5, p. 1281) (Sharma, 2005). Ideally, the operation is shorter in duration, and urinary complications are much less frequent. However, posterior exenteration in a previously irradiated patient frequently results in a contracted bladder and intractable urinary incontinence.

44-8

Incontinent Urinary Conduit

Removal of the bladder during total or anterior exenteration is the main indication for an incontinent urinary conduit. Less commonly, an otherwise irreparable postirradiation vesicovaginal fistula may warrant urinary diversion. Following cystectomy, an isolated resected segment of bowel that maintains its mesenteric connection and vascular supply is used as the new reservoir. A stoma is crafted using one end of the bowel segment and an opening in the anterior abdominal wall. Ureters are reimplanted into the opposite end of this isolated bowel segment.

Various diversion techniques are available to create such urinary conduits, and these are categorized as *incontinent diversions* or *continent diversions*. Incontinent diversion is the simplest to create, but postoperatively a patient must continuously wear an ostomy bag. These conduits are often preferable for medically compromised patients, the elderly, and anyone with a short life expectancy. Alternatively, a continent urinary reservoir can be created that is emptied by intermittent patient self-catheterization of the bowel stoma.

Of incontinent diversions, an *ileal conduit* has historically been the most common urinary diversion used in gynecologic oncology (Goldberg, 2006). However, this bowel segment and distal ureters invariably lie within a prior radiated field. Conduit construction with radiation-damaged bowel may lead to higher rates of stenosis or leakage at the ureteral anastomotic sites (Pycha, 2008). More recently, the *transverse colon conduit* has proven to be a very successful alternative for previously irradiated patients (Segreti, 1996b; Soper, 1989). *Sigmoid conduits* are generally less desirable due to preexisting radiation damage and proximity to a concurrent colostomy site. The *jejunal conduit* is another rarely used option that typically lies outside the radiation field.

The basic principles of constructing an incontinent urinary conduit are the same—regardless of the intestinal segment used. First, healthy-appearing bowel with a good blood supply should be selected. Second, wide ureterointestinal anastomoses and stenting are essential to minimize the risk of anastomosis stenosis. Third, sufficient mobility of the ureters and bowel segment is important to prevent tension that might lead to anastomotic leaks. Fourth, creation of a straight tunnel through the abdominal wall will prevent obstruction.

PREOPERATIVE

Patient Evaluation

The preoperative evaluation is usually dictated by the preceding exenterative procedure. The specific decision is whether to plan for an incontinent or continent urinary conduit. Patients should be extensively counseled regarding the differences. The type of conduit selected should be considered permanent, although later conversions are possible (Benezra, 2004).

Consent

Patients should be advised that intraoperative findings may dictate revision of an original surgical plan. Postoperatively, urinary infections with or without pyelonephritis are very common with any type of conduit. Anastomotic leaks are less frequent with routine ureteral stent placement, but can contribute to a prolonged ileus, the need for computed tomography-guided drainage, or potentially, surgical reexploration with revision. Episodes of small bowel obstruction are possible and often develop at the site where the bowel segment was harvested and the remaining bowel ends were reanastomosed. In the long term, strictures and ureteral stenosis may cause renal compromise. Infrequently, reoperation is necessary for complications that do not respond to conservative management (Houvenaeghel, 2004).

Patient Preparation

Bowel preparation is obviously mandatory, but preparation is typically dictated by the preceding exenterative surgery (Section 44-5, p. 1276). Ideally, an enterostomal therapist is available to mark a conduit stoma site, typically on the patient's right side, that is unobstructed in the supine, sitting, and standing positions.

INTRAOPERATIVE

SURGICAL STEPS

❶ **Initial Steps.** The incontinent urinary conduit is constructed as the last major intraabdominal procedure during exenterative surgery to avoid unnecessary traction on its anastomoses. Hemostasis should be achieved before beginning the conduit. Anesthesia, patient positioning, and skin incisions are typically dictated by the preceding operation.

❷ **Exploration.** The bowel segment for the planned conduit is carefully inspected. It must be healthy appearing, not tethered, and lie within range of the distal ureters. The final decision is now made regarding which type of incontinent conduit is best for the circumstances. If the distal ileum has the typical leathery, pale, mottled appearance of radiation injury, a conduit should be prepared from the transverse colon. Overlooking the importance of this decision can lead to a variety of otherwise preventable complications intraoperatively and postoperatively.

❸ **Ileal Conduit: Preparing the Bowel Segment.** The ileocecal junction is located, and the ileum is elevated to identify a bowel segment with the most mobility to reach the right side of the anterior abdominal wall where the stoma will be located. Ideally, the proximal point of the conduit lies 25 to 30 cm from the ileocecal valve. At the selected site, the mesentery is scored on each side with an electrosurgical blade to aid insertion of a hemostat directly beneath the ileal serosa. A Penrose drain is pulled through to mark this proximal site along the ileum that will eventually become the distal part of the conduit and will form the abdominal wall stoma.

The conduit length depends on subcutaneous tissue depth and ileum mobility but should measure approximately 15 cm. The conduit's butt end will house the ureteral anastomoses and is selected by measuring the ileum that lies distal to the Penrose drain, and again the mesentery is scored. The gastrointestinal anastomosis (GIA) stapler is then inserted to divide the distal bowel segment (Fig. 44-8.1). The point of division should ideally be at least 12 cm from the ileocecal valve. The conduit is remeasured prior to dividing the proximal ileum, to account for possible shrinkage of the intervening segment and to again ensure sufficient length.

The conduit mesentery is carefully divided on each side. This dividing of tissue is angled inward and toward the base of the mesentery at its insertion to the posterior abdominal wall. This provides adequate mobility. The vasculature may be compromised if too much mesentery is divided, whereas too little will result in tension on the conduit. A perfect balance is required. When convenient, intestinal continuity, minus the excised segment, is reestablished anterior to the conduit with a functional end-to-end anastomosis using the GIA and TA staplers (Fig. 44-22.2, p. 1326).

❹ **Ileal Conduit: Preparing the Ureters.** The staple line is excised from the stomal end of the conduit, and the conduit is irrigated. The ureters should now be engorged from the vascular clips placed earlier during exenteration. The distal end of the ureters should have a stay suture for traction and are never directly grasped with forceps or roughly

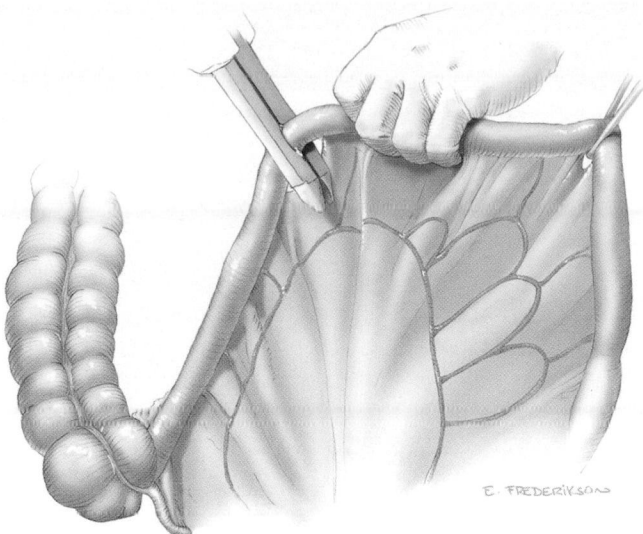

FIGURE 44-8.1 Ileal conduit: preparing the bowel segment.

handled to prevent focal necrosis that may impede successful anastomosis. They are freed from their retroperitoneal attachments so that they easily reach past the point of their planned anastomosis into the conduit. The left ureter is brought *under* the inferior mesenteric artery (IMA) to prevent acute angulation. The ureter ultimately exits from beneath the base of the sigmoid mesentery to reach the conduit.

❺ Ileal Conduit: Ureteral Anastomoses.
Adson forceps are used to grasp a small section of the ileal serosa to which the left ureter will reach. This site is ideally approximately 2 cm from the proximal end of the conduit on the anterior side of the antimesenteric surface. Metzenbaum scissors remove a small, full-thickness section of bowel wall (Fig. 44-8.2). The ileal mucosa should be easily visible.

The distal tip of the left ureter is cut at a 45-degree angle just behind the vascular clip placed during exenteration. If the distal ends of the ureters exhibit fibrosis, they are trimmed to reach healthy-appearing tissue. Urine will drain into the abdomen while a 4-0 delayed-absorbable stay suture is placed from outside-to-in through the ureter's distal tip. The needle is left on this traction stitch, since it will be the final suture in the anastomosis. Fine-tip scissors are used to spatulate the ureter for approximately 1 cm, but the length is customized depending on the caliber of the ureteral lumen (Fig. 44-8.3). This maneuver helps reduce the possibility of future stenosis.

The first suture is placed at the apex of the spatulation with a full-thickness bite through the ureteral wall and bowel mucosa (Fig. 44-8.4). Two or three adjoin-ing mucosa-to-mucosa sutures are placed. A 7-French ureteral stent is then placed through the stomal end of the conduit and advanced through the anastomosis into the left renal pelvis. This is held against the wall of the midsection of the conduit with one hand and secured with a 3-0 or 4-0 chromic catgut suture through the entire bowel wall around the stent to hold it in place. This left ureteral anastomosis is completed with additional circumferential sutures to achieve a water-tight closure.

The anastomotic site for the right ureter is selected at least 2 to 3 cm distal to that of the left along the length of the conduit. The entire procedure is then repeated. Saline with methylene blue dye is used to fill the conduit and observe for water-tight integrity. Any anastomotic leaks must be reinforced with additional suture and retested. If leakage persists or if there is concern about the mucosa-to-mucosa apposition, then the entire anastomosis should be redone.

This proximal or butt end of the conduit is next secured to the sacral promontory, iliopsoas muscle, or posterior peritoneum with two or three delayed-absorbable sutures through the seromuscular layer of the conduit. Stabilizing the conduit in this way will prevent undue tension on the ureteral anastomoses when the patient is upright and gravity allows the intestines to slide into the pelvis.

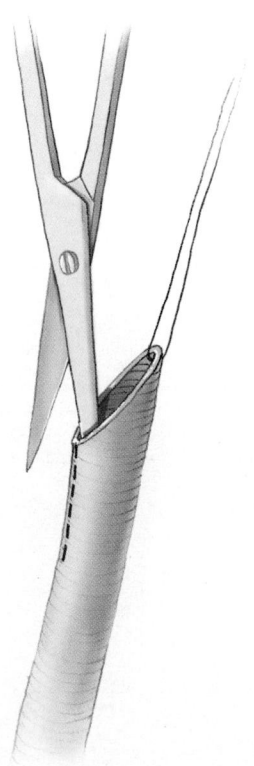

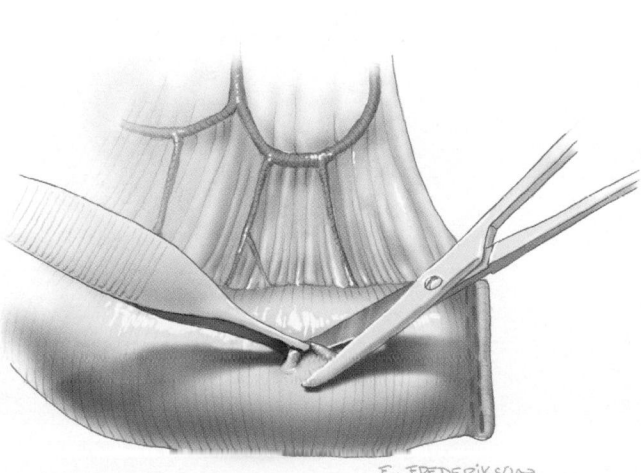

FIGURE 44-8.2 Ileal conduit: ileal incision.

FIGURE 44-8.3 Ileal conduit: spatulating the ureter.

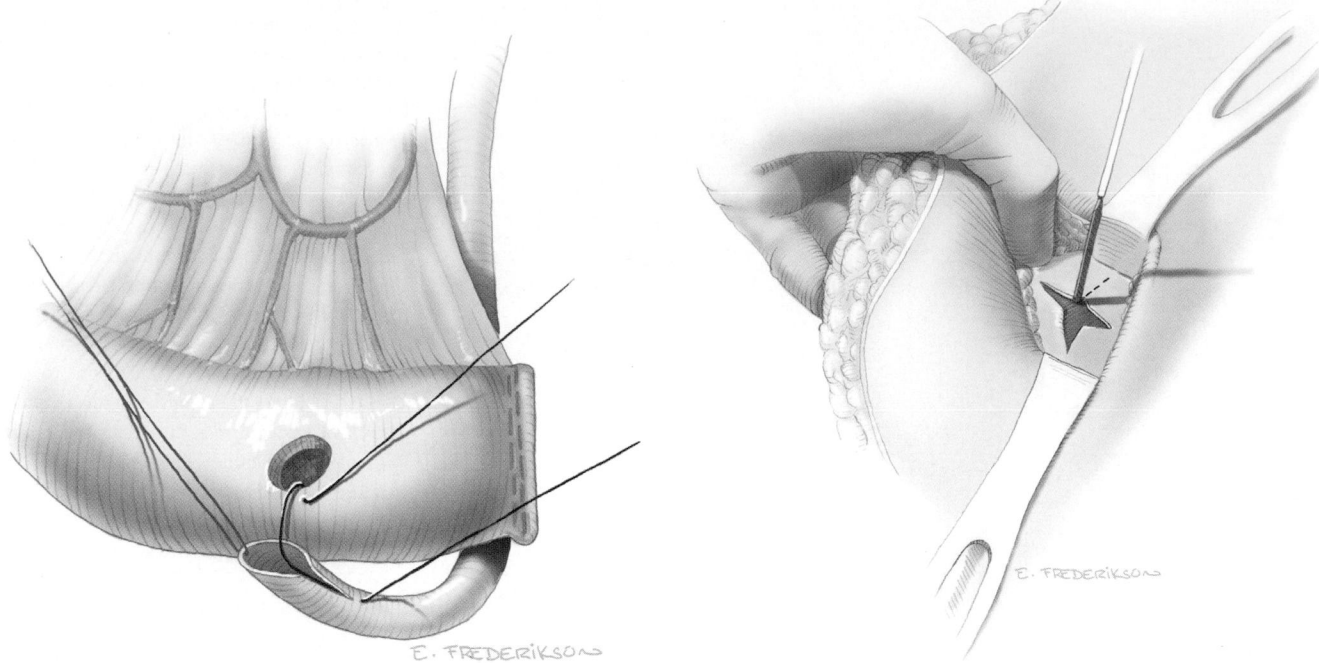

FIGURE 44-8.4 Ileal conduit: suturing ureter and ileal segment.

FIGURE 44-8.5 Ileal conduit: making the stoma.

❻ Ileal Conduit: Stoma Creation. The skin at the proposed stoma site is elevated with a Kocher clamp. An electrosurgical blade, set on cutting mode, is used to excise a small circle of skin. The subcutaneous fat is separated by blunt dissection until the fascia is visible. A cruciate incision is made with electrosurgical blade (Fig. 44-8.5). The rectus abdominis muscle is split longitudinally and another cruciate incision is created in the peritoneum. The opening is bluntly expanded until it easily accommodates two fingers.

The stoma and stents are carefully pulled through the incision until at least 2 cm of ileum protrudes through the skin (Fig. 44-8.6). The mesentery may need to be trimmed or the abdominal wall opening further dissected to accommodate the conduit. The mucosal edge of the bowel is everted. The stoma is completed with 3-0 delayed-absorbable "rosebud" stitches that include the ileal mucosa, intervening bowel serosa, and skin dermis (Fig. 44-8.7). Circumferential sutures are placed. Both stents are trimmed to fit in the stoma bag. To enable correct

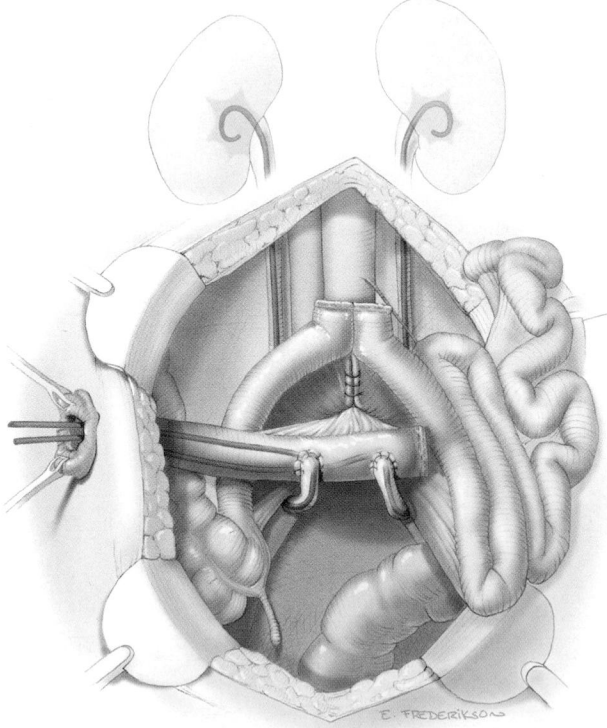

FIGURE 44-8.6 Ileal conduit: stoma with stents is carefully pulled through the incision.

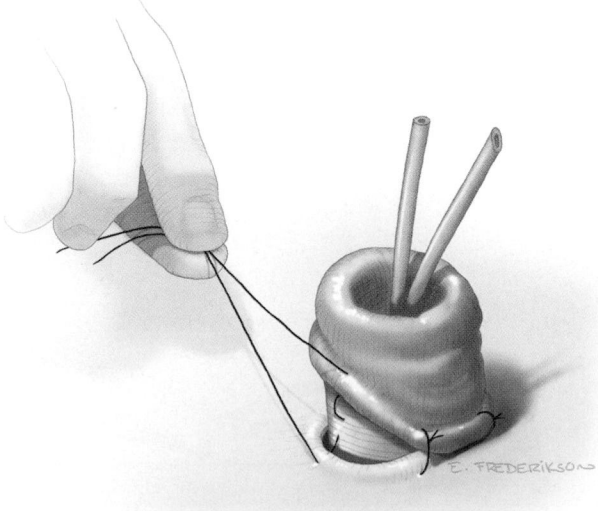

FIGURE 44-8.7 Ileal conduit: suturing the stoma.

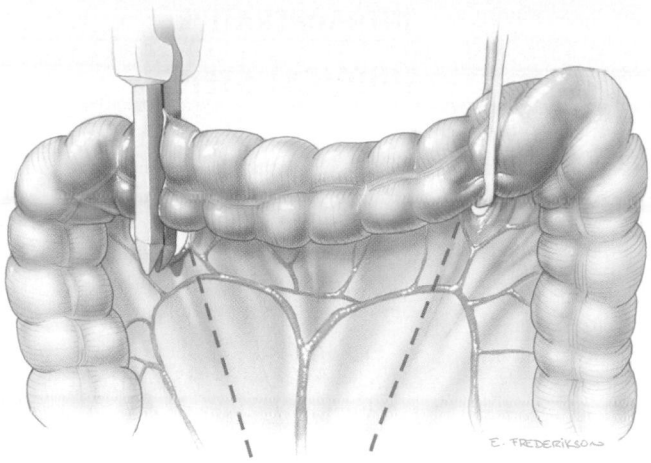

FIGURE 44-8.8 Transverse colon conduit: preparing the bowel segment.

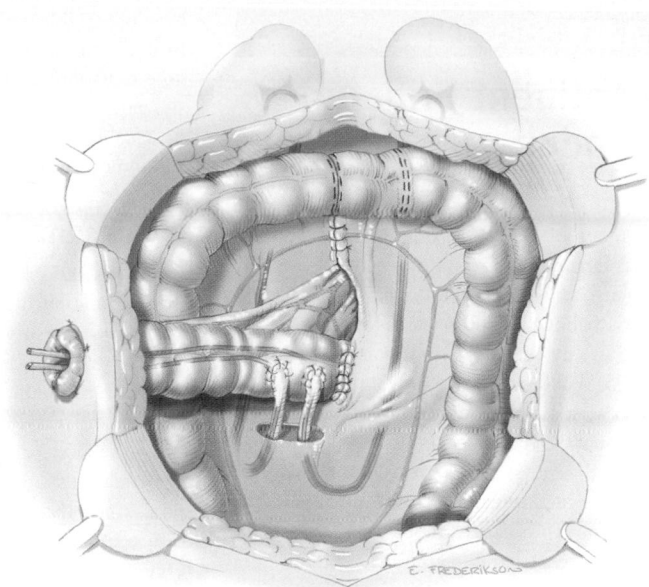

FIGURE 44-8.9 Transverse colon conduit: final appearance.

identification postoperatively, the right ureteral stent is cut at a "right" angle. Individual silk sutures placed through each stent may be secured at the skin to prevent stent dislodgement over the first few postoperative days.

❼ Transverse Colon Conduit. For this type of conduit, the hepatic and splenic flexures of the transverse colon are fully mobilized. In addition, the omentum is detached. Division points are marked with Penrose drains and transected (Fig. 44-8.8). The transverse mesocolon is then divided, as shown by the dotted lines, to provide sufficient mobility while preserving the middle colic artery. When performed in the usual setting of an exenteration with left lower quadrant colostomy, the bowel segment must measure approximately 20 cm to reach the right lower quadrant. Often, this requires incorporation of the hepatic flexure into the conduit and an antiperistaltic orientation. Thus, the proximal bowel segment (nearest the cecum) will be the end of the conduit that eventually is brought through the abdominal wall.

Ureters are sufficiently mobilized in the retroperitoneal space, and both are brought out through a commodious peritoneal opening to reach the conduit. The left ureter will need to be brought across the aorta *proximal* to the IMA (unlike the ileal conduit). The

ureteral anastomoses are then completed, ideally at the taenia coli, over stents. To prevent postoperative sliding and tension on the anastomoses, the conduit's butt end is secured to the sacrum, iliopsoas muscle, or posterior peritoneum with interrupted delayed-absorbable suture. Intestinal continuity is reestablished anterior to the conduit by a functional end-to-end anastomosis using EEA and TA staplers. The stoma can be made at the preselected site, but it can be repositioned almost anywhere that the conduit will comfortably reach. The stomal end of the conduit is brought through the anterior abdominal wall and secured (Fig. 44-8.9).

❽ Final Steps. Mesenteric defects require closure to prevent internal hernias, but not so tightly as to compromise blood supply. A suction drain may be placed if there is concern about the integrity of the anastomoses. If the stoma appears dusky, the abdominal wall tunnel may be too tight, the mesentery may be twisted or placed on too much tension, or the blood supply may not be sufficient. The worst circumstance is the last, which generally requires trimming of the distal end of the bowel or occasionally redoing the entire conduit. Either is preferable to avoid problematic retraction, stricture, or necrosis.

POSTOPERATIVE

The stoma should regularly be checked for viability during the immediate postoperative recovery period. Both stents should be functioning. A dry stent that does not respond to irrigation should prompt an imaging study to exclude obstruction. Urinary fistulas and obstruction are uncommon, but are potentially life threatening if not addressed with percutaneous drainage or reoperation. Prolonged bowel dysfunction may indicate an anastomotic urine leak or small bowel obstruction.

Patients often are readmitted within a few weeks of surgery due to partial small bowel obstruction, urinary infection, wound separation, or other relatively minor complications of exenteration. These typically resolve with targeted supportive care. Long-term complications include ureteral stenosis and renal loss. Renal function may deteriorate due to chronic infection and reflux. When patients cannot be otherwise managed, they may require long-term percutaneous nephrostomy tubes, indwelling stents, or reoperation and conduit or stoma revision. Predictably, the overall morbidity of creating an incontinent conduit is much higher in previously irradiated patients (Houvenaeghel, 2004). Tissue quality and mobility are especially important in these patients.

44-9

Continent Urinary Conduit

Removal of the bladder during total or anterior exenteration is the main indication for a continent urinary conduit. Vesicovaginal fistulas and disabling incontinence following radiation therapy are other less common reasons (Lentz, 1995). Following cystectomy, urine is diverted into a reservoir created from a resected bowel segment. Depending on their construction, these diversions may render a woman continent or incontinent. An incontinent conduit reservoir chronically drains into an ostomy bag, whereas that of a continent conduit does not leak urine. Patients empty the reservoir by intermittent self-catheterization.

Continent conduits, however, may not be appropriate for all patients. The operation is more complex than an incontinent diversion procedure and may lead to more postoperative complications (Karsenty, 2005). They also require a highly motivated patient who is capable of long-term self-catheterization. An ideal candidate for a continent conduit is a young, otherwise healthy woman without a colostomy.

There are several continent diversion methods. In gynecologic oncology, the continent ileocolonic urinary reservoir (Miami pouch) has become the most popular choice (Salom, 2004). This pouch is technically straightforward to construct and uses tissues that characteristically lie in nonirradiated areas (Penalver, 1998).

A Miami pouch includes a distal ileum segment, the ascending colon, and a portion of transverse colon. The basic steps involve opening the colon segment along the length of the taenia and folding it onto itself. The walls of the ascending and transverse colon are then sewn together to achieve a reservoir with low intraluminal pressure. The ileum segment is tapered, and purse-string sutures are placed at the level of the ileocecal valve to achieve continence. The ileal segment is then exteriorized as a stoma to allow catheterization (Penalver, 1989).

PREOPERATIVE

Patient Evaluation

Preoperative evaluation is usually dictated by the preceding exenterative procedure. The specific decision is whether to plan for an incontinent or continent urinary conduit. Patients should be extensively counseled regarding the differences. The presence of a permanent colostomy removes the apparent advantage of a continent conduit and an abdominal wall without draining stomas. Catheterization may

be more problematic in very obese women. In addition, some patients with prior high-dose radiation or chronic bowel disease may also not be good candidates due to poor tissue quality and increased associated risks of anastomotic leaks, ureteral stricture, or fistula.

Consent

Patients should be advised that intraoperative findings such as poor bowel appearance and dense adhesions may dictate a change in original surgical plans. In addition, complications are common and should be reviewed. Even in experienced centers, half of patients will have one or more early pouch-related complications: ureteral stricture with obstruction, anastomotic leak, fistula, difficulty in catheterization, pyelonephritis, or sepsis. One third will develop late complications beyond 6 weeks. Ten percent of patients will ultimately require reoperation to revise the Miami pouch (Penalver, 1998). As a result, many patients would not choose the continent urinary conduit again (Goldberg, 2006).

Patient Preparation

Bowel preparation is obviously mandatory, but generally is dictated by the preceding exenterative surgery. Ideally, an enterostomal therapist is available to mark a conduit stoma site in the right lower abdomen that is unobstructed in the supine, sitting, and standing positions.

INTRAOPERATIVE

SURGICAL STEPS

The continent urinary conduit is constructed as the last major intraabdominal procedure during exenterative surgery to avoid unnecessary traction on anastomoses. Before beginning the conduit, hemostasis should be achieved. Anesthesia, patient positioning, and skin incisions are typically dictated by the preceding operation.

❶ **Exploration.** The bowel segment is carefully inspected at the planned conduit site. It must be healthy appearing and without severe radiation injury. At this point, the final decision to proceed with creation of a Miami pouch is made.

❷ **Preparing the Bowel Segment.** The right colon is freed along the white line of Toldt from the cecum, around the hepatic flexure, to the proximal transverse colon. The conduit will require approximately 25 to 30 cm of colon and at least 10 cm of ileum. With these measurements in mind, a surgeon selects sites to divide the bowel.

The mesentery is scored with an electrosurgical blade, and a Penrose drain is placed around the sections to be divided. Within the mesentery, the underlying vasculature is reviewed to ensure sufficient conduit blood supply. A gastrointestinal anastomosis (GIA) stapler is used to divide the bowel at both sites marked with the Penrose drains (Fig. 44-9.1).

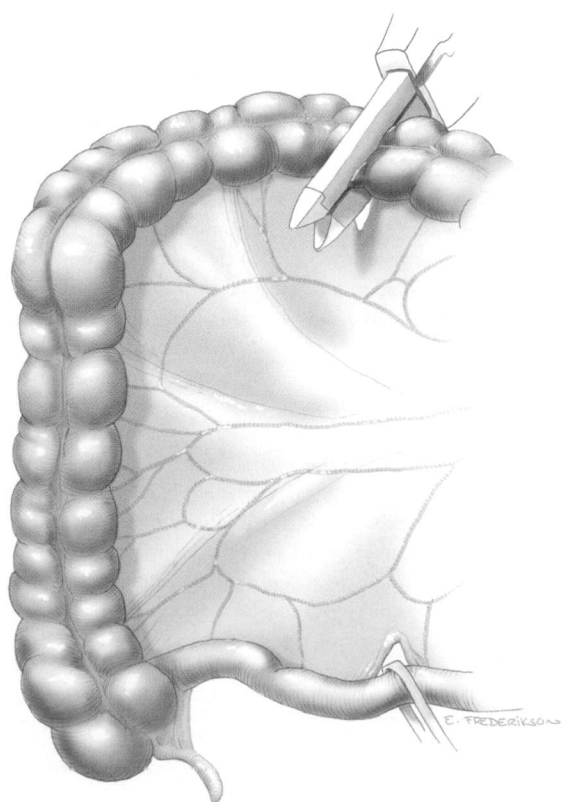

FIGURE 44-9.1 Preparing the bowel segment.

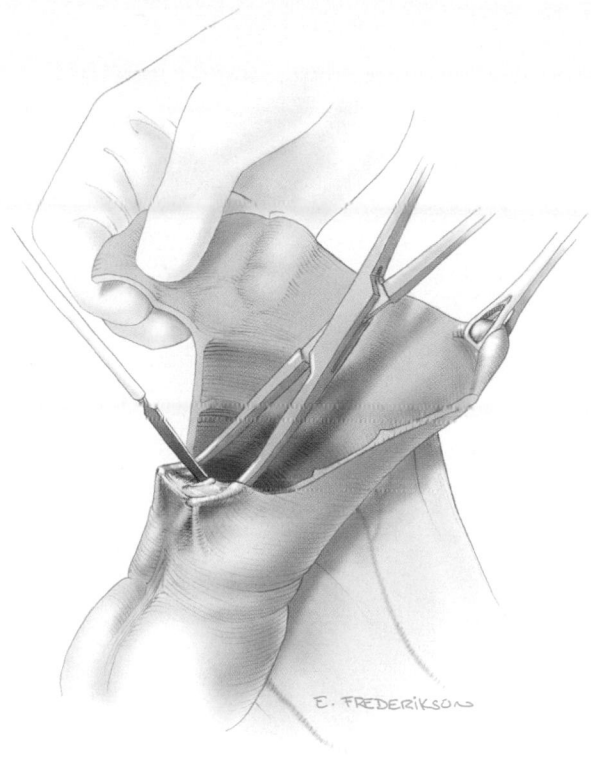

FIGURE 44-9.2 Detubularizing the bowel.

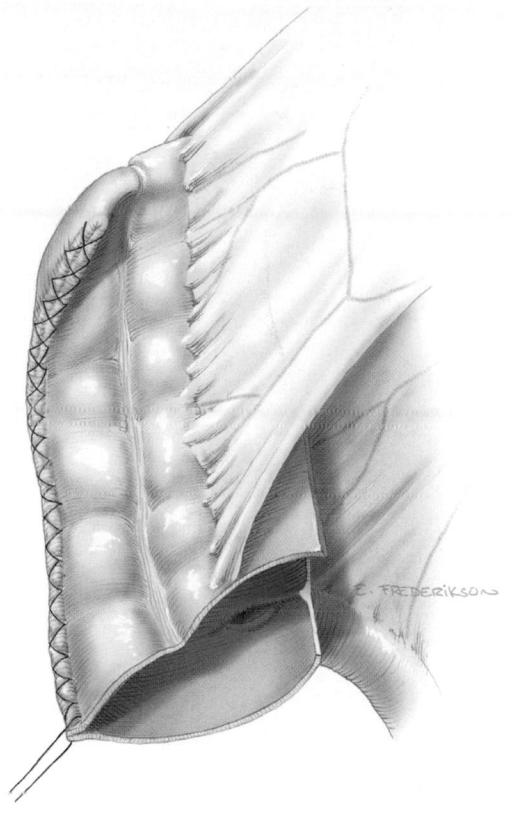

FIGURE 44-9.3 Creating the reservoir.

The mesenteries are incised down through the avascular areas to the posterior peritoneum. At this point, intestinal continuity is reestablished by a functional end-to-end stapled ileo-transverse enterocolostomy using the GIA and transverse anastomosis (TA) staplers. The mesenteric defect is closed with 0-gauge delayed-absorbable suture in a running fashion.

❸ **Detubularizing the Bowel.** The conduit staple lines on both ends of the bowel segment are removed with Metzenbaum scissors, and the bowel is irrigated into a basin. Of this bowel segment, the entire colon portion is opened with an electrosurgical blade along the taenia of the antimesenteric border to "detubularize" the bowel (Fig. 44-9.2). Distally, this is extended to remove the appendix.

❹ **Creating the Pouch.** The colon segment is folded in half, and four delayed-absorbable stay sutures are placed at the corners to begin creation of the pouch. The lateral edge is closed in two layers with 2-0 and 3-0 gauge delayed-absorbable suture in a running fashion (Fig. 44-9.3).

❺ **Tapering the Ileum.** A 14-French red rubber catheter is inserted through the terminal ileum segment into the pouch. Two purse-string, 0-gauge delayed-absorbable sutures are placed 1 cm apart at the ileocecal junction. The ileum is elevated with Babcock clamps, and a GIA stapler is used to taper the terminal ileum on its antimesenteric border over the catheter (Fig. 44-9.4). An anterior abdominal wall opening is made in the right lower quadrant so that the ileal segment of the conduit can be pulled through to approximate its final position (Fig. 44-8.5, p. 1286).

❻ **Ureteral Anastomoses.** Both ureters are further mobilized from their retroperitoneal attachments and brought into position under the ascending mesocolon using a 4-0 delayed absorbable stay suture at the tip to avoid crush injury and subsequent necrosis. As in the transverse colon conduit, the left ureter will need to be brought over the aorta and *above* the origin of the internal mesenteric artery (IMA). The ureteral anastomotic sites within the pouch are selected based on ureter length and their ability to have a straight course to the pouch.

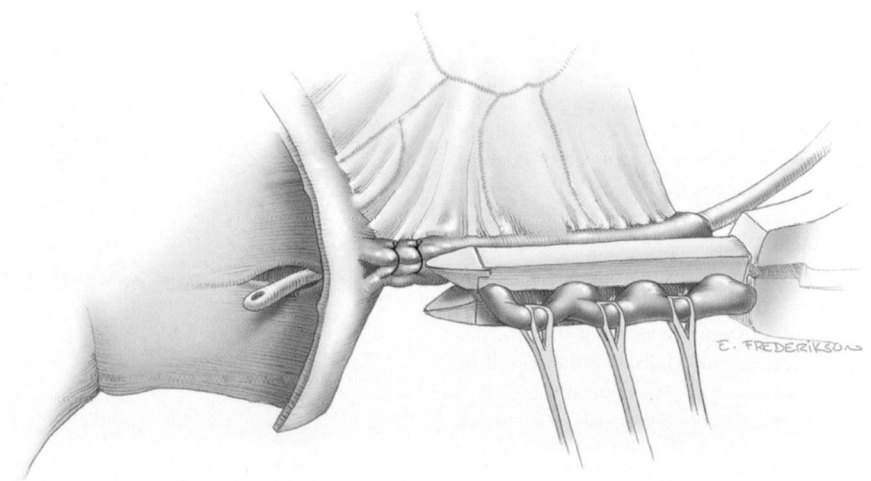

FIGURE 44-9.4 Tapering the ileum.

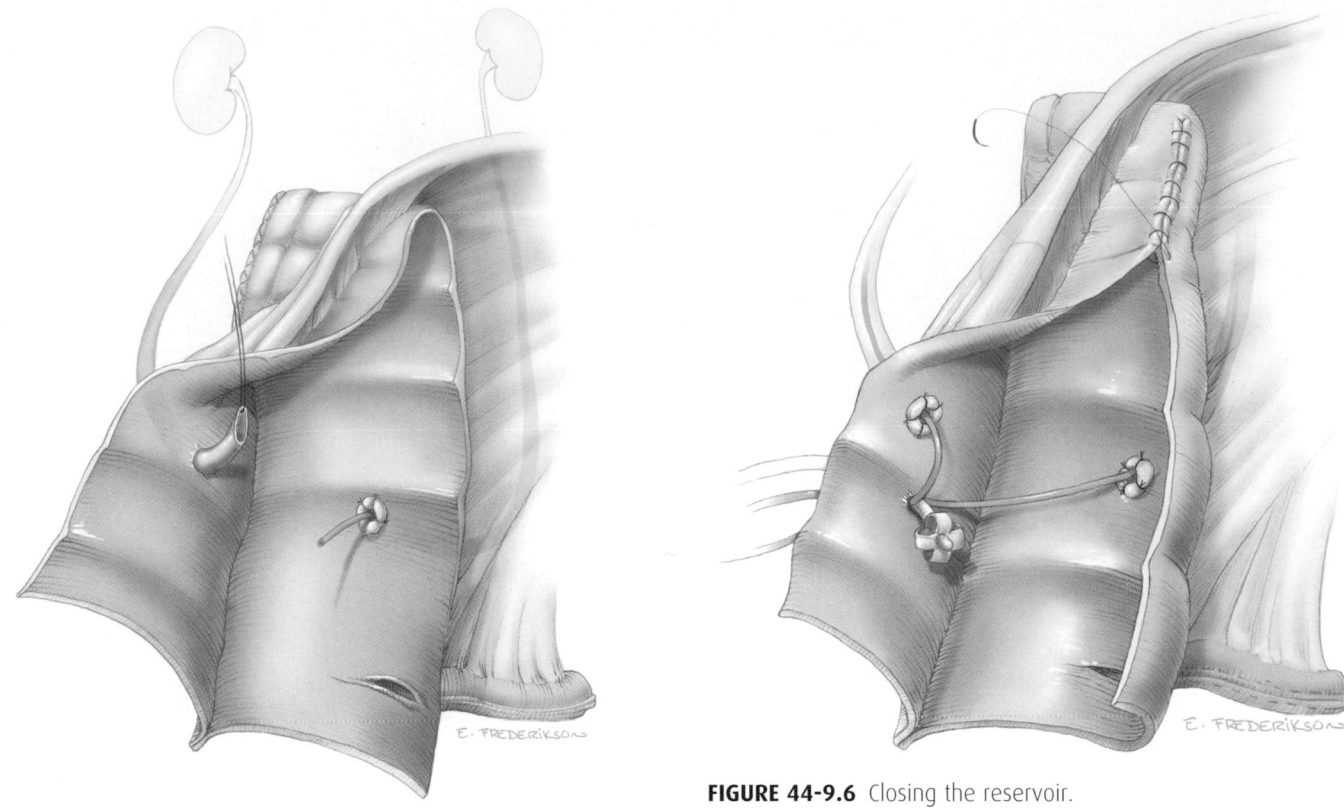

FIGURE 44-9.5 Ureteral anastomoses.

FIGURE 44-9.6 Closing the reservoir.

One ureter is usually brought through on either side of the pouch suture line. The ureters are trimmed and spatulated (Fig. 44-8.3, p. 1285). In creating the openings for the ureters, the bowel mucosa is incised away from the suture line, and a hemostat is poked through the bowel wall to bring 2 cm of each ureter into the pouch by pulling on the traction suture (Fig. 44-8.4, p 1286).

Each ureter is secured to the bowel mucosa with interrupted stitches of 4-0 delayed-absorbable suture (Fig. 44-9.5). Single-J ureteral stents (7 French) are inserted and sutured to the bowel wall with 3-0 chromic to stabilize their placement. To enable correct identification postoperatively, the right ureteral stent is cut at a "right" angle.

❼ Closing the Pouch. A large Malecot catheter is brought into the pouch through an incision made away from the ileocecal valve. The ureteral stents are brought out through the pouch next to the Malecot (Fig. 44-9.6). A watertight purse-string using 3-0 plain catgut suture is placed where the catheters exit the pouch. Absorbable suture is used for this purse-string as the Malecot catheter will be removed 2 to 3 weeks postoperatively.

The remaining edges of the pouch are closed with two layers of 2-0 and 3-0 delayed-absorbable suture in a running fashion. Continence may be tested by inserting a red rubber catheter through the plicated ileum, filling the pouch with 250 to 300 mL of saline, removing the red rubber catheter, and gently squeezing the pouch. Additional purse-string sutures may be placed at the ileocecal valve if incontinence is demonstrated. The completed pouch (Fig. 44-9.7) is now ready to be brought to the abdominal wall.

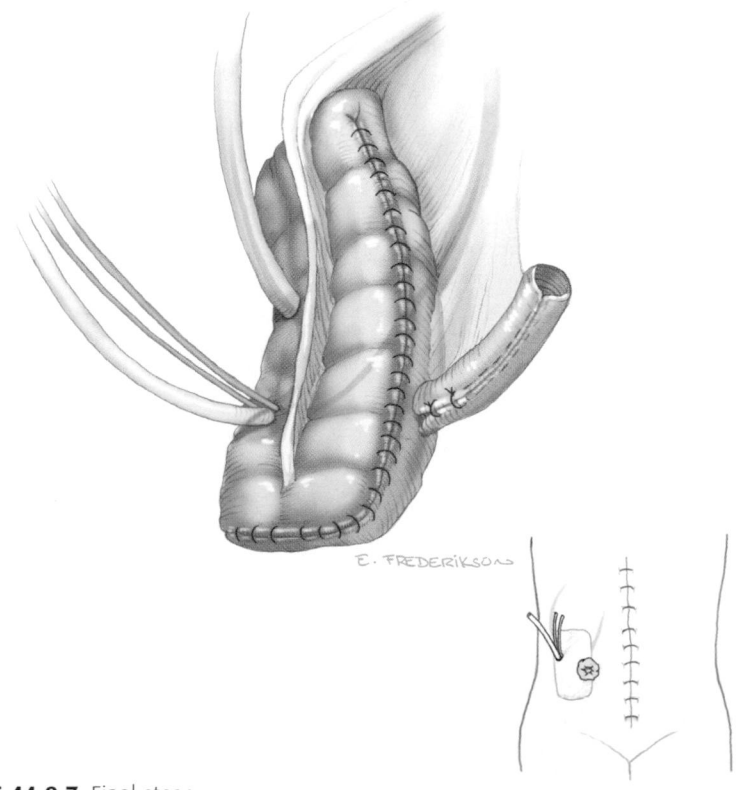

FIGURE 44-9.7 Final steps.

8 Final Steps. The two stents and Malecot drain are brought out through a separate stab wound away from the stoma site. The Malecot drain is individually fixed to the skin with nylon sutures. Stoma formation mirrors that for the incontinent conduit (Section 44-8, step 6, p. 1286). First, the abdominal wall is incised for the stoma. The ileal segment is pulled through the abdominal wall and may require trimming to sit flush. The pouch is stabilized by suturing it to the undersurface of the abdominal wall, and the stoma is created by placing interrupted stitches of 3-0 delayed-absorbable suture between the dermis and ileal mucosa. With a continent conduit, a red rubber catheter should be inserted and withdrawn to make sure that the pouch can be easily accessed. A Jackson-Pratt (JP) drain is then placed near the pouch and brought out through a separate stab wound away from the stoma.

POSTOPERATIVE

The Miami pouch initially requires more care than an incontinent urinary conduit. Mucus will be produced by the colonic bowel segment. Therefore, the Malecot catheter should be irrigated every few hours to permit urine drainage. In contrast, the ureteral stents are irrigated only if one of the catheters becomes obstructed. Two to 3 weeks postoperatively, an intravenous pyelogram (IVP) and gravity pouchogram should be performed. If these tests are normal, the ureteral stents, Malecot catheter, and JP suction drainage tube may all be removed. The hole in the conduit that housed these tubes will heal secondarily.

A patient may be taught self-catheterization using an 18- to 22-French red rubber catheter and antiseptic technique. The time between catheterizations may be progressively increased over weeks to reach 6 hours during the day and none at night. In addition, the pouch requires periodic irrigation to remove mucus. An IVP, pouchogram, and serum electrolytes and creatinine levels are obtained at 3 months postoperatively and then every 6 months to evaluate the pouch, renal function, and upper urinary tracts.

More than half of patients will have a conduit-related complication postoperatively. Fortunately, most may be successfully managed conservatively without the need for reoperation (Ramirez, 2002). The most common urinary complications are ureteral stricture or obstruction, difficult catheterization, and pyelonephritis (Angioli, 1998; Goldberg, 2006). The gastrointestinal complication rate attributed to Miami pouch is less than 10 percent and includes fistulas (Mirhashemi, 2004).

CHAPTER 44

44-10

Vaginal Reconstruction

Patients undergoing exenterative surgery are typical candidates for creation of a new vagina. Other less common indications include congenital absence of the vagina, postirradiation stenosis, and total vaginectomy. There are innumerable ways to perform the procedure, and the type of reconstruction is typically determined by both the surgeon's personal experience and the patient's clinical circumstances (Fowler, 2009).

Vaginal reconstruction at the time of exenteration is a very personal choice. Not every woman will desire a new vagina, and others will be unhappy with the functional result (Gleeson, 1994b). Moreover, reconstruction may significantly prolong an already lengthy operation and lead to additional perioperative morbidity (Mirhashemi, 2002). However, proponents suggest that filling the large pelvic defect and bringing in a new source of blood supply may actually prevent postoperative fistula or abscess formation (Goldberg, 2006; Jurado, 2000).

To create a functional neovagina, one of the following is performed: (1) surrounding skin and subcutaneous tissue is mobilized and positioned into the defect (skin flap), (2) skin from another part of the body is harvested and transferred to replace the vaginal mucosa (split-thickness skin graft), or (3) skin and underlying tissue outside the radiated field are mobilized on an attached section of muscle with its dominant blood supply (myocutaneous flap). Of the three choices for vaginal reconstruction, skin flaps, such as *rhomboid flaps, pudendal thigh fasciocutaneous flaps,* and *advancement* or *rotational flaps,* are technically the easiest to perform (Burke, 1994; Gleeson, 1994a; Lee, 2006). *Split-thickness skin grafts (STSG)* provide the ability to cover large surfaces if primary closure is not possible. However, these require that most of the native subcutaneous tissue has been retained at the neovagina site, and months of stenting with a vaginal mold are needed to prevent stricture (Kusiak, 1996). *Rectus abdominis myocutaneous (RAM) flaps* and *gracilis myocutaneous flaps* are technically more challenging and take longer to perform, but demonstrate the most satisfying functional results (Lacey, 1988; Smith, 1998). Importantly, RAM flaps may be inappropriate in those with a prior Maylard incision or any other procedure that resulted in ligation of the inferior epigastric artery, which is the dominant blood supply to this type of flap.

Regardless of reconstruction technique, sexual function is often significantly impaired in women after pelvic exenteration (Hockel, 2008; Ratliff, 1996). Other techniques are used less commonly and will not be covered in this section.

PREOPERATIVE

Patient Evaluation

The surgeon should have an open discussion with the patient regarding the risks and benefits of vaginal reconstruction. Some women may have unrealistic expectations that are important to address preoperatively. Others may not wish to incur additional morbidity. The patient should also be aware that intraoperative complications may dictate a change of plans and the need to abort reconstruction.

Consent

Patients who are motivated to undergo creation of a new vagina must be carefully counseled. Postoperative patient concerns are expected and include self-consciousness about being seen in the nude by their partner, vaginal dryness, and vaginal discharge (Ratliff, 1996). The potential morbidity of the neovagina depends on the type of reconstruction. Flap necrosis, prolapse, wound separation, or other complications may require reoperation and/or lead to an unsatisfying end result.

Patient Preparation

The preceding exenterative surgery typically dictates preoperative preparation. Modifications may be required, depending on the type of neovaginal reconstruction. For example, the legs may need to be surgically prepped beyond the knees for a gracilis flap or a suitable donor site identified for STSG.

INTRAOPERATIVE

SURGICAL STEPS

❶ **Pudendal Thigh Fasciocutaneous Flap.** From a perineal approach, the planned incisions are marked along the skin from the non-hair-bearing areas just lateral to the labia majora. Flaps should be roughly 15 × 6 cm. The most inferior skin margin should be level with the lower part of the gaping perineal defect. The skin incision is begun at the superior flap margin and dissected to include the underlying subcutaneous tissue and fascia lata (Fig. 44-10.1). The posterior labial artery, a branch of the internal pudendal artery, provides blood supply (Fig. 38-28, p. 944).

The flap's edges are approximated in a running, subcuticular suture line with 4-0 delayed-absorbable suture, and the neovagina is inserted into the perineal defect. The incision sites are closed with interrupted stitches of 3-0 delayed-absorbable suture, and bilateral Jackson Pratt (JP) drains are placed beneath these suture lines. The perineal defect requires resculpting of tissue folds and suturing to form a functional end result (Fig. 44-10.2). The apex of the neovagina may then be abdominally sutured to the hollow of the sacrum and covered with an omental J-flap to provide additional neovascularization.

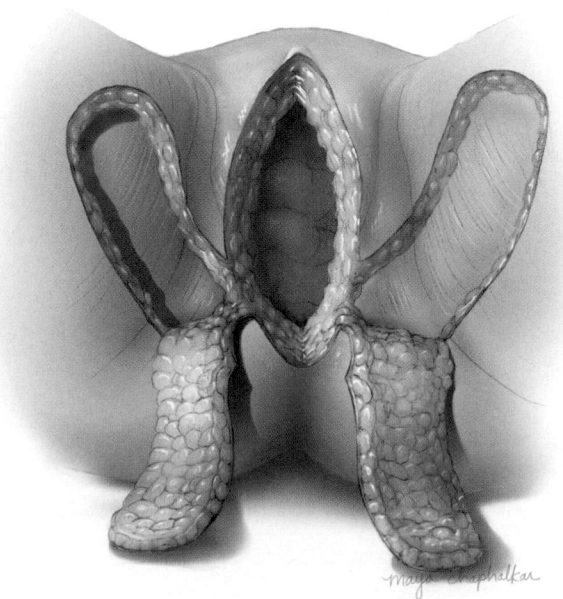

FIGURE 44-10.1 Raising the perineal flaps.

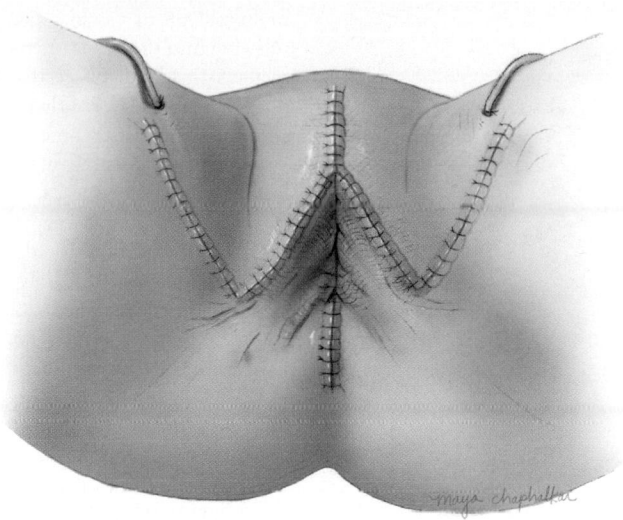

FIGURE 44-10.2 Perineal flap closure.

❷ **Split-Thickness Skin Graft with Omental J flap.** Modification of the omental flap, which is normally used to close off the pelvic inlet after exenteration, can create a cylinder providing anterior, posterior, and lateral walls for a new vagina. In thin patients with an attenuated omentum, a thin and poorly vascularized omentum may not be the best option for neovagina creation because there may not be enough tissue to form a cylinder and cover the mold.

From an abdominal approach, the omentum is detached from the stomach with a ligate-divide-staple (LDS) device or electrothermal bipolar coagulator (LigaSure). Resection is usually from right to left, until it will comfortably reach the pelvis as a J-flap (Section 44-16, p. 1313). Only three quarters of the omentum is divided, so as to preserve the left gastroepiploic artery. The distal omentum is rolled into a cylinder and sutured together with interrupted stitches of 3-0 gauge delayed-absorbable suture (Fig. 44-10.3).

The proximal end can be closed abdominally with interrupted sutures or the transverse anastomosis (TA) stapler without dividing it entirely. From the perineal side, the omental cylinder is then sutured to the vaginal introitus.

Next, the STSG is harvested from the donor site and sutured over a vaginal mold with 4-0 delayed-absorbable suture similar to the McIndoe procedure described in Section 41-25 (p. 1075). The mold is placed into the neovaginal space and sutured into place at the introitus (Fig. 44-10.4).

❸ **Gracilis Myocutaneous Flap.** From a perineal approach, a reference line is drawn on the medial thigh from the pubic tubercle to the medial tibial plateau following the adductor longus muscle. Posterior to this line, an island of skin, its associated subcutaneous tissue, and the gracilis muscle will serve as the flap. The planned elliptic incision is marked, and a full-thickness skin incision through the reference line is continued through the subcutaneous fat and the fascia lata. The belly of the gracilis muscle is isolated at its distal margin and divided. The remainder of the incision is completed around the marked skin island margin. The gracilis muscle is fully mobilized with blunt and sharp dissection from distal to proximal. This preserves the dominant vascular pedicle—a branch of the medial femoral circumflex artery—as it

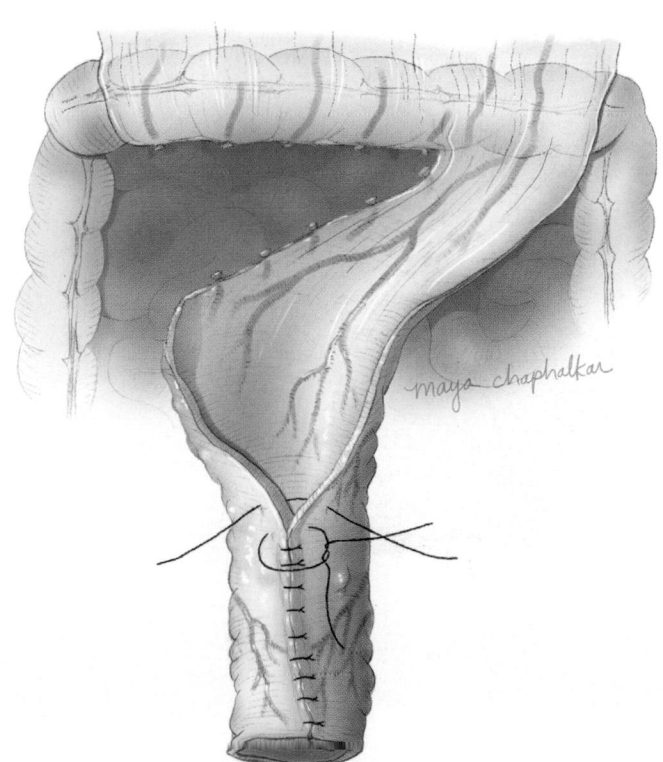

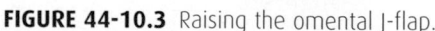

FIGURE 44-10.3 Raising the omental J-flap.

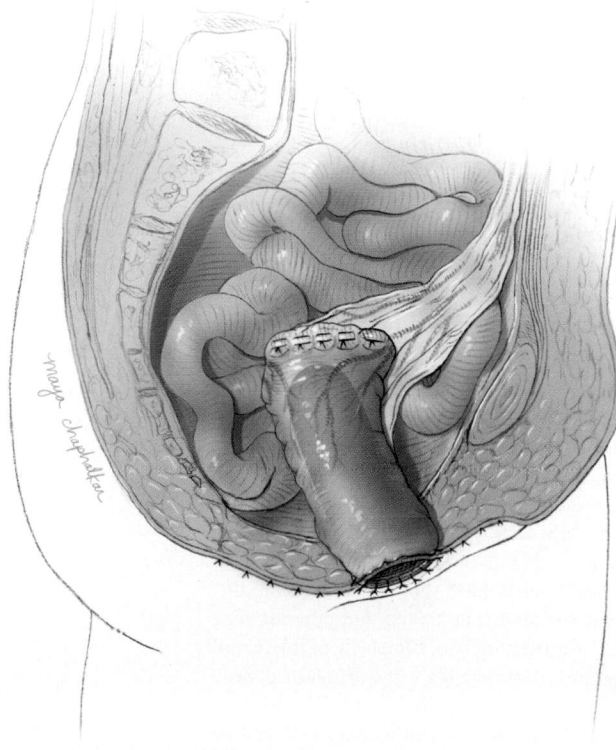

FIGURE 44-10.4 Insertion of the split-thickness skin graft.

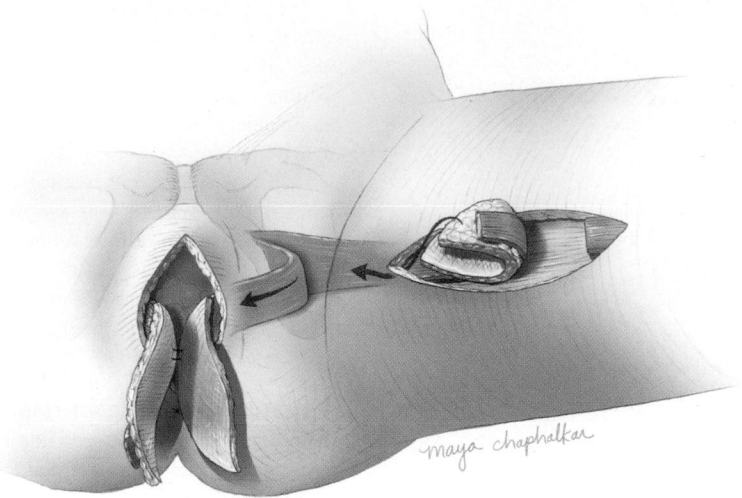

FIGURE 44-10.5 Gracilis myocutaneous flap.

enters the deep anterior belly of the muscle 6 to 8 cm from the pubic tubercle.

Through the operative site on the thigh, a subfascial tunnel is bluntly developed medially to the open perineal defect. The left gracilis muscle flap is rotated *clockwise* against the thigh, that is, rotated first posteriorly and then medially. It is placed through the tunnels and allowed to hang freely between the patient's legs. The right flap is rotated *counterclockwise* and similarly positioned (Fig. 44-10.5).

Beginning at the distal tip, the tubular gracilis neovagina is constructed by suturing the skin edges of the right and left skin islands together with interrupted stitches using 4-0 delayed-absorbable suture. The proximal opening should accommodate two or three fingers. The neovagina is rotated cephalad into the pelvis and posteriorly anchored to the levator plate abdominally with interrupted stitches of 0-gauge delayed-absorbable suture to prevent vaginal prolapse. Redundant flap skin is trimmed, and the proximal skin is sutured to the introitus with interrupted stitches of 3-0 gauge delayed-absorbable suture.

❹ Rectus Abdominis Muscle (RAM) Flap. A skin island can be harvested from any location on the abdominal wall as long as the base of its shape is at the umbilicus. Typically, a 10 × 15 cm skin island is marked. At the superior border of the island, which will ultimately form the vaginal opening, the skin, subcutaneous tissue, and anterior rectus sheath are incised. One belly of the rectus abdominis muscle is freed with blunt dissection from the posterior sheath. The belly is divided proximally, and anastomotic vessels connecting to the superior epigastric system are ligated.

The remaining borders of the skin island are incised through the anterior rectus sheath to the arcuate line. The subcutaneous fat is mobilized along the lateral and medial margins of the rectus muscle belly. The rectus muscle is then bluntly dissected from the posterior sheath until reaching the arcuate line. Next, the posterior peritoneum is cut inferiorly along the full length of the midline incision well beyond the flap. The RAM flap is now fully detached, but needs to be further

mobilized on its vascular pedicle to be able to swing into the pelvis. At the distal portion of the skin island, the rectus muscle is then bluntly dissected inferiorly from the anterior sheath to its insertion onto the pubic bone.

The flap, consisting of skin, subcutaneous tissue, anterior sheath, and rectus belly, is coiled around a syringe to form a tube (Fig. 44-10.6). The skin edges are approximated with 4-0 delayed-absorbable suture. The syringe is removed, and the tube is placed into the pelvis. The pelvic end is closed. The RAM flap must be put into the pelvis without tension to prevent occlusion of its dominant vascular supply from the inferior epigastric artery.

The open end of the neovagina is brought out under the pubic symphysis to the perineum where it is attached to the vulvar defect using interrupted vertical mattress stitches using 0-gauge delayed-absorbable suture. An omental J-flap may also be prepared to provide additional blood supply.

POSTOPERATIVE

For many women, the presence of a vagina significantly improves a woman's quality of life and reduces sexual problems after exenteration (Hawighorst-Knapstein, 1997). Reconstruction may be beneficial to a patient's self-image, and the knowledge that intercourse

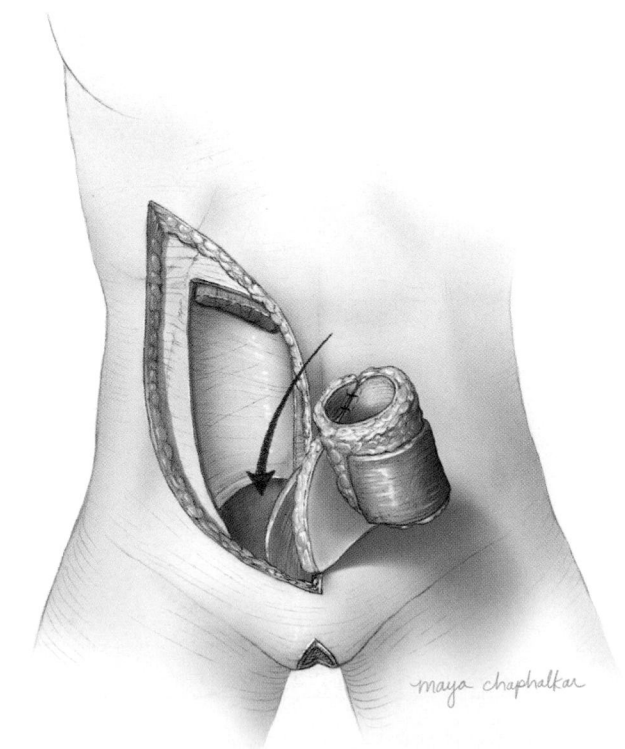

FIGURE 44-10.6 Rectus abdominis myocutaneous flap.

is possible may be reassuring even if she chooses not be sexually active postoperatively. Morbidity from the procedure largely depends on the type of neovagina.

Pudendal thigh flaps are reliable and easy to harvest, but perhaps are the most likely to be nonfunctional. Long-term sequelae may include vulvar pain, chronic vaginal discharge, hair growth, and protrusion of the flaps. These symptoms may discourage patients and their partners from attempting sexual activity (Gleeson, 1994a).

STSG neovaginas may become infected at the donor or recipient site. Sloughing due to vascular compromise or development of a seroma are other common complications.

Postoperatively, patients must initially be immobilized to aid healing, and stenting with a vaginal mold is required for months to prevent vaginal stenosis or contracture (Fowler, 2009).

Gracilis myocutaneous flaps may be difficult to pass into the pelvis during the procedure and have the potential for partial or complete tissue loss due to necrosis from an inherently tenuous blood supply (Cain, 1989). Flap loss is significantly more common if rectosigmoid anastomosis is performed concurrently during exenteration (Soper, 1995). Long-term prolapse is another relatively common problem. Residual scarring on the legs is a frequent, albeit relatively minor, complaint postoperatively.

Rectus abdominis muscle flaps are perhaps the best choice for vaginal reconstruction at the time of pelvic exenteration (Jurado, 2009). Ideally, they fill pelvic dead space, reduce the risk of fistulas, and provide fulfilling sexual activity (Goldberg, 2006). However, the donor site may be difficult to close primarily or lead to a postoperative hernia or dehiscence. The operating time is also increased because, unlike a gracilis flap where the abdominal team can be proceeding with exenteration while the perineal team is beginning the reconstruction, two surgical teams are not possible when performing a RAM flap. Flap necrosis, fistula, and vaginal stenosis are other frequent complications (Soper, 2005).

44-11

Pelvic Lymphadenectomy

Pelvic lymph node removal is one of the hallmarks of surgical staging and is commonly indicated for patients with uterine, ovarian, and cervical cancer. Pelvic lymphadenectomy implies a *complete* removal of all nodal tissue within an area bordered by well-defined anatomic landmarks: midportion of the common iliac artery (proximally), deep circumflex iliac vein (distally), midportion of the psoas major muscle (laterally), ureter (medially), and obturator nerve (posteriorly) (Whitney, 2010). The main indication of pelvic lymphadenectomy is its role as part of cancer staging surgery. However, in those with grossly involved nodes, this procedure may serve to optimally debulk tumor burden.

Additional definitions are commonly used in association with lymphadenectomy. For example, pelvic lymph node "sampling" is a more limited procedure within the same anatomic boundaries and is particularly intended to remove any enlarged or suspicious nodes (Whitney, 2010). Sampling is limited to easily accessible pelvic regions and does not address all nodal groups (Cibula, 2010). Pelvic lymph node "dissection" is a vague term that may range from sampling to lymphadenectomy.

The aim of lymphadenectomy is to remove all fatty lymphatic tissue from the predicted areas that carry a high incidence of nodal metastasis (Cibula, 2010). Ideally, the procedure should yield numerous pelvic nodes from multiple sites within the boundaries described earlier (Huang, 2010). However, removal of more lymph nodes increases the risk of postoperative complications (Franchi, 2001). Removal of at least four lymph nodes from each side (right and left) is a minimum requirement to validate that an "adequate" lymphadenectomy has been performed (Whitney, 2010). In general, the extent of pelvic lymphadenectomy will depend on the clinical circumstances and will vary by clinician. Moreover, lymphadenectomy completeness is also dependent on the diagnostic skills of the interpreting pathologist.

As noted, removal of enlarged pelvic nodes may be required to achieve optimal debulking of ovarian cancer. In addition, debulking of grossly involved pelvic lymph nodes may also confer a survival benefit in selected endometrial and cervical cancer patients (Havrilesky, 2005; Kupets, 2002). However, there is controversy whether systematic removal of pelvic nodes confers a true survival benefit or solely provides more accurate staging information in otherwise "understaged" patients (Panici, 2005).

Pelvic lymphadenectomy can be performed during laparotomy or via a minimally invasive approach (Sections 44-13 and 44-14, p. 1302). Extraperitoneal pelvic lymphadenectomy is not commonly performed (Larciprete, 2006). Additionally, preoperative identification of suspicious pelvic nodes by lymphatic mapping and sentinel node identification is not universally available.

PREOPERATIVE

Patient Evaluation

Depending on the situation, imaging studies such as computed tomography, magnetic resonance imaging, or positron emission tomography (PET) may suggest the presence of pelvic lymphadenopathy and help guide a surgeon to the most suspicious areas. However, the ability to preoperatively detect less obvious nodal metastases is limited.

Consent

Pelvic lymphadenectomy should be a straightforward procedure with few complications, but acute hemorrhage, postoperative lymphocyst, lymphedema, and obturator nerve injury are possible. Obesity, previous radiation therapy, prior pelvic infections, prior abdominal surgery, and other factors causing retroperitoneal fibrosis can add difficulty to dissection. These destroy tissue planes and can lead to an increased risk of complications.

Patient Preparation

Routine bowel preparation and antibiotic prophylaxis are not required for lymphadenectomy but may be indicated for other concurrent surgeries. Thromboprophylaxis is administered as outlined in Table 39-9 (p. 962).

INTRAOPERATIVE

SURGICAL STEPS

❶ Anesthesia and Patient Positioning. Lymphadenectomy may be performed under general or regional anesthesia with a patient in supine position. A Foley catheter is placed, and the abdomen is surgically prepared. The vaginal is also surgically prepared if concurrent hysterectomy is planned.

❷ Abdominal Entry. A midline vertical or transverse abdominal incision that allows adequate visualization is appropriate for this procedure. Self-retaining retractors should be adjusted to provide exposure of the external iliac artery in its entirety.

❸ Abdominal Exploration. Pelvic lymph nodes should be routinely palpated during initial abdominal exploration. Unexpected grossly positive nodes may indicate that a proposed operative plan should be abandoned (for example, radical hysterectomy for cervical cancer) or revised (Whitney, 2000).

❹ Retroperitoneal Exploration. The retroperitoneal space has typically already been entered through the round ligament during preceding surgical procedures. However, to improve visibility, surgeons may further extend dissection of the anterior and posterior leaves of the broad ligament.

Palpation of the external iliac artery pulsation just medial to the psoas major muscle should be the starting point. Its identification permits surgeons to locate relevant anatomy. Blunt dissection is then performed to visualize the bifurcation of the common iliac artery into the external and internal iliac arteries. The ureter is isolated as previously described (Section 44-1, step 5, p. 1260). The remaining pelvic sidewall structures are covered with fatty-lymphoid tissue and are not yet easily visible. To remove an en bloc specimen, the dissection will begin along the external iliac artery, proceed distally to reach the inguinal ring, reflect medially over the external iliac vein into the obturator space, and end at the internal iliac artery. Separately, nodes along the distal common iliac artery can be included.

❺ Lateral Dissection. An index finger is placed lateral to the common iliac bifurcation and is used to bluntly dissect parallel to the external iliac artery caudally along the psoas major muscle (Fig. 44-11.1). The general lack of arterial and venous branches along the external iliac vessels enables aggressive blunt dissection to be performed unless there is significant fibrosis. This maneuver separates the lateral preperitoneal fat from the fatty-lymphoid tissue covering the vessels.

Nodal tissue is next reflected medially to reveal the entire external iliac artery. Forceps traction and electrosurgical cutting are typically required to lift all adventitial tissue above the artery and maintain the correct plane of dissection. The deep circumflex iliac vein originates from the distal external iliac vein and serves as the caudal boundary for this node group. The deep circumflex iliac vein should be visible crossing laterally over the distal external iliac artery before proceeding. The genitofemoral nerve, which is visible parallel to the artery and overlying the psoas major muscle, should be kept intact whenever possible.

Bleeding is a common problem with pelvic lymphadenectomy and may be exacerbated by retroperitoneal fibrosis. Usually venous

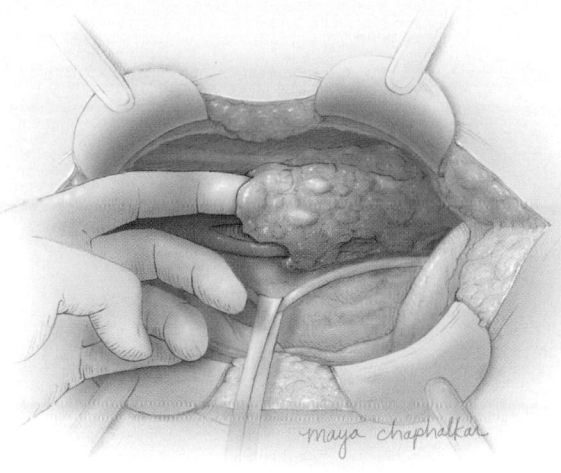

FIGURE 44-11.1 Mobilizing the lateral nodal tissue.

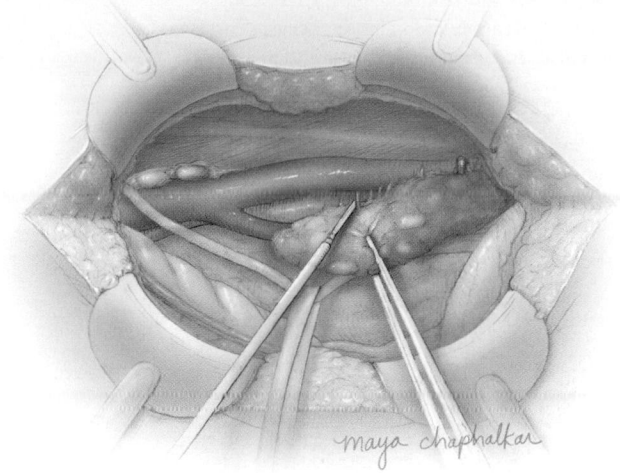

FIGURE 44-11.2 Medial dissection over the vein.

bleeding or avulsion of small vessel branches can be quickly controlled with vascular clips. Vascular anomalies are regularly encountered and may cause inadvertent hemorrhage if not properly identified in advance.

❻ Removal of Distal Nodes. A distal self-retaining retractor blade may need to be temporarily removed to resect all pelvic nodes heading toward the inguinal canal. The distal round ligament tie is elevated with one hand. The thumb of the other hand should be advanced directly beneath the round ligament and followed to the inguinal ring. Apposition of the tip of the thumb with the middle and adjoining fingertips will enable palpation, distal pinching, and removal of nodal tissue at the inguinal ring without cutting, clamping, or meaningful blood loss. The retractor blade may then be replaced.

❼ Dissection over the External Iliac Vein. The ureter can be held medially by a Penrose drain to promote visualization of the pelvic sidewall. Forceps are used to place the nodal tissue bundle overlying the external iliac vein on medial traction. Alternating electrosurgical and blunt dissections are performed to reflect the nodal tissue medially until the external iliac vein is visualized (Fig. 44-11.2). The dissection is continued from proximal to distal above the internal iliac vessels. Nodal tissue may be transected with blunt and electrosurgical blade dissection along the inferiomedial wall of the external iliac vein. The distal end of the bundle is usually tethered to the sidewall. Nodal tissue may be removed by placing a vascular clip and dividing the tethered attachment. Additional fatty-lymphoid tissue is typically seen within the anatomic boundaries. These nodes may be more adhered to vessels and can be separately removed and added to the specimen.

❽ Obturator Fossa Nodes. The index finger is gently inserted between the psoas major muscle and external iliac artery, and blunt dissection progresses downward to the obturator fossa. Lateral arterial or venous branches may need to be clipped and cut. Nodal tissue may be identified behind the external iliac vessels and added to the specimen.

A vein retractor is then used to elevate the external iliac vein and expose the obturator fossa (Fig. 44-11.3). Forcep tips can be used to mobilize nodal tissue inferiorly from the bottom of the vein. Accessory venous branches may be identified and clipped. The vein retractor is then removed and a hand inserted with the thumb directly beneath the vein. The tip of the thumb is advanced laterally and the nodal bundle is scooped over the fingertips. This nodal packet may be removed by gently pinching along the pelvic sidewall.

The obturator nerve will be palpable, and dissection should purposely remain superior. Firm fibrotic attachments may be electrosurgically dissected under direct visualization. The vein retractor is then reinserted, and the obturator nerve should be readily visible. Additional areas of fatty-lymphoid tissue can be visualized. Further blunt dissection is continued until the entire portion of the obturator fossa that lies anterior to the nerve is empty. Nodal tissue below the obturator nerve is not routinely removed since the obturator artery and vein traverse this area. Laceration of either of these vessels can result in vessel retraction and catastrophic hemorrhage that is difficult to control.

❾ Distal Common Iliac Lymph Node Dissection. The upper retractor blade is readjusted to allow increased visibility of the

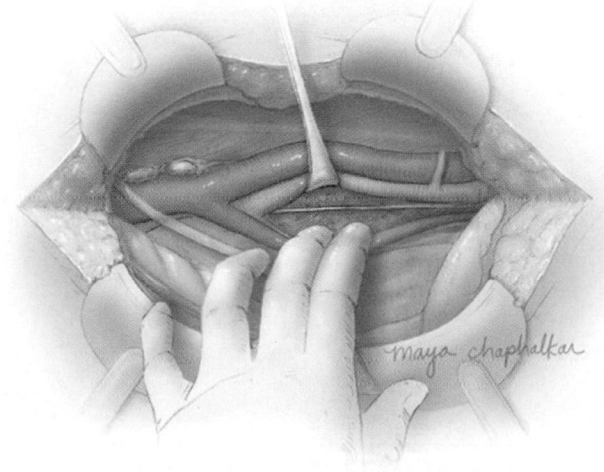

FIGURE 44-11.3 Obturator fossa dissection.

distal half of the common iliac artery. The colon may require mobilization using electrosurgical dissection along the white line of Toldt. Bowel can then be retracted sufficiently to allow access to the common iliac nodes.

The lateral fatty-lymphoid tissue may be removed by first grasping with DeBakey forceps and using electrosurgical dissection to establish a plane. Blunt dissection may then be performed in a proximal direction to further separate the nodal tissue from the artery. Electrosurgical coagulation or clips may then be used to detach the nodes (Fig. 44-11.4). Caution should be used on the right side due to the presence of the underlying external iliac and common iliac veins and inferior vena cava.

❿ **Final Steps.** Gauze sponges may be opened and tightly placed into the obturator fossa and medial to the external iliac vein to tamponade any surface oozing while additional procedures are performed. There is no benefit to closing the retroperitoneal space or routinely using pelvic suction drainage (Charoenkwan, 2010).

POSTOPERATIVE

Surgical blunt dissection techniques decrease the risk of inadvertent vessel or nerve injury, but may increase the chance of postoperative

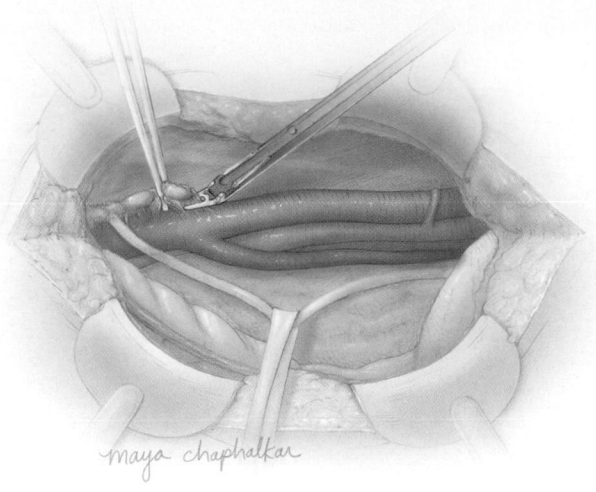

FIGURE 44-11.4 Distal common iliac dissection.

lymphocyst formation. Also known as lymphoceles, these cysts are usually asymptomatic, transient collections of lymph. Symptomatic or large lymphocysts will usually respond to percutaneous aspiration with or without drainage catheter placement. Sclerosis is uncommonly required, and laparotomy with marsupialization should be considered a last option (Karcaaltincaba, 2005; Liu, 2005).

Neurologic injuries involving the obturator, ilioinguinal, iliohypogastric, genitofemoral, or femoral nerves may result from direct surgical trauma, stretch injury, suture entrapment, or retractor placement (Cardosi, 2002). However, transection of the obturator nerve should ideally be immediately noted intraoperatively and an epineural repair performed (Vasilev, 1994). Motor deficits are best managed by physical therapy and typically resolve with time. Sensory changes, such as pain, may require long-term pharmacologic management or surgical intervention (Cardosi, 2002).

44-12

Paraaortic Lymphadenectomy

Paraaortic lymphadenectomy implies a complete removal of all nodal tissue from within an area with well-defined anatomic boundaries: inferior mesenteric artery (proximally), mid-common iliac artery (distally), ureter (laterally), and aorta (medial). The completeness of the procedure will vary by clinician, but an adequate dissection requires that lymphatic tissue at least be demonstrated pathologically from both the right and left sides (Whitney, 2010).

Removal of paraaortic lymph nodes is routinely indicated to surgically stage women with uterine and ovarian cancer because of these cancers' unpredictable patterns of lymphatic dissemination (Burke, 1996; Negishi, 2004). Moreover, removal of enlarged paraaortic nodes may be required to achieve optimal debulking of ovarian cancer and may also confer a survival benefit in selected endometrial and cervical cancer patients (Cosin, 1998; Havrilesky, 2005).

Paraaortic lymphadenectomy may be performed during laparotomy or using a minimally invasive technique (Sections 44-13 and 44-14, p. 1302). Regardless, the proximal dissection is usually only extended to the inferior mesenteric artery (IMA), unless there are indications for a "high" lymphadenectomy up to the renal vein (Whitney, 2010).

PREOPERATIVE

Patient Evaluation

As described in Section 44-11 (p. 1296), imaging studies may help guide the surgeon to the most suspicious areas but are not entirely reliable in identifying nodal metastases.

Consent

Paraaortic lymphadenectomy is not routinely performed worldwide due to the heightened technical difficulty of the procedure and potential for complications (Fujita, 2005). Of these, acute hemorrhage and postoperative ileus are most commonly associated. Other complications should be infrequent. In the obese patient, visibility in the area of dissection is decreased, and thus the complexity of performing this delicate procedure is increased. The operative time is also lengthened considerably in these women.

Patient Preparation

Routine bowel preparation and antibiotic prophylaxis is not typically required.

However, other concurrent surgeries may dictate their use. Thromboprophylaxis is provided as outlined in Table 39-9 (p. 962).

INTRAOPERATIVE

SURGICAL STEPS

❶ **Anesthesia and Patient Positioning.** Lymphadenectomy may be performed under general or regional anesthesia with a patient in supine position. A Foley catheter is placed, and the abdomen is surgically prepared. The vaginal is also surgically prepared if concurrent hysterectomy is planned.

❷ **Abdominal Entry.** A midline vertical abdominal incision that extends around and above the umbilicus provides optimal exposure. Alternatively, paraaortic lymphadenectomy can also be performed via Cherney or Maylard incisions (Sections 41-3 and 41-4, p. 1024) (Helmkamp, 1990). A Pfannenstiel incision, in contrast, provides limited exposure and may not allow sufficient abdominal access if bleeding develops (Horowitz, 2003).

❸ **Abdominal Exploration.** Paraaortic lymph nodes should be routinely palpated during initial abdominal exploration. A hand is placed beneath the small bowel mesentery to palpate the aorta. The index and middle fingers are then used to straddle the aorta and palpate for lymphadenopathy. Suspicious or

grossly positive paraaortic nodes should typically be removed as one of the initial steps in an abdominal operation. Unexpected positive nodes may indicate that the proposed operative plan should be abandoned or revised (Whitney, 2000). For most instances, in which no adenopathy is present, the dissection should usually be performed last due to the possibility of triggering catastrophic bleeding that might otherwise limit further surgery.

❹ **Visualization.** Exposure and proper retractor positioning is perhaps the most important part of the procedure. Thus, a self-retaining retractor is positioned to allow access to the aorta. The sigmoid colon should be gently retracted in a lower left direction, whereas small bowel and transverse colon are packed with laparotomy sponges into the upper abdomen. Modified Trendelenburg patient positioning is also helpful to shift bowel from the operative field. Additional sharp dissection along the right paracolic gutter may be necessary to sufficiently mobilize and move the cecum from the dissection plane. Once bowel has been cleared from the field, the peritoneum overlying the aorta and right common iliac artery should be visible. Both vessels should be palpated before proceeding.

❺ **Opening the Retroperitoneal Space.** As described in Section 44-1, step 5 (p. 1260), the ureter is isolated and held laterally on a Penrose drain. A right-angle

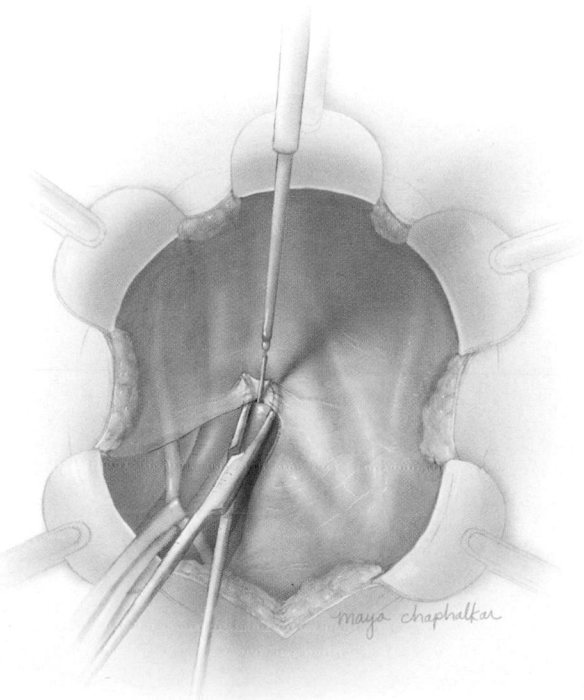

FIGURE 44-12.1 Opening the retroperitoneal spaces.

clamp is used to guide electrosurgical blade dissection of the posterior peritoneum in a medial and cephalad direction over the right common iliac artery and aorta (Fig. 44-12.1). Staying directly above these arteries is a safe location since no vital structures cross these vessels medial to the ureter. A surgeon intermittently stops to palpate the course of the artery before continuing dissection in a cephalad direction to the inferior duodenal fold. Blunt dissection is performed to mobilize the duodenum, and the cephalad self-retaining retractor blade is repositioned to retract this bowel.

❻ Exposing the Aorta and Inferior Vena Cava.
A surgeon returns to the area near the right ureter where the posterior peritoneal dissection began. Electrosurgical cutting is used to incise the areolar sheath on top of the right common iliac artery, and dissection is continued proximally past the aortic bifurcation to at least the IMA. Small perforating vessels may be encountered and coagulated.

❼ Removal of Right Paraaortic Nodes.
Lymphadenectomy begins lateral to the midportion of the right common iliac artery. The ureter is held medially by traction on the Penrose drain while the nodal bundle is elevated with forceps and blunt dissection is performed to better visualize its fibrinous attachments to the distal artery.

A right-angle clamp is placed under these fibers, and electrosurgical cutting is used to divide them and free the distal tip of the bundle. Blunt dissection will demonstrate the right common iliac vein as it crosses beneath the artery. The adventitial sheath surrounding the common iliac vein is incised and extended upward by electrosurgical cutting following the arterial direction to the level of the IMA to free the bundle medially. The lateral border is established by again holding the ureter laterally and bluntly dissecting along the iliopsoas muscle in a cephalad direction to separate the right lateral side of the inferior vena cava (IVC) from the retroperitoneal fat. The upper right abdominal retractor blade may need to be repositioned to improve visibility.

At this point, the right paraaortic node bundle has been largely detached medially, distally, and laterally. Lymph nodes are grasped distally with DeBakey forceps and elevated as gentle blunt dissection is performed in a proximal direction. Delicate perforating veins along the IVC warrant meticulous dissection to reduce bleeding. The "fellow's vein" is routinely encountered near the level of the aortic bifurcation and should be occluded with a vascular clip for hemostasis (Fig. 44-12.2). Upon reaching the level of the IMA, the nodal bundle can be removed by placing large vascular clips across the proximal end and transecting it.

❽ Repair of Venous Bleeding.
A surgeon should prepare for causing small lacerations in the wall of the IVC or common iliac veins by inadvertently avulsing perforating venous tributaries. Hemorrhage may be copious and immediate. Initially, pressure is applied with a sponge-stick or finger. Secondly, exposure is assessed. Blood is suctioned from the abdominal cavity, retractors are repositioned, and incisions are extended if necessary. Lastly, proper vascular instruments are obtained. Lacerated veins can usually be simply repaired with vascular clips (Fig. 44-12.3).

❾ Removal of Left Paraaortic Nodes.
The upper left abdominal retractor blade is repositioned under the posterior peritoneal edge to access the left side of the aorta. Electrosurgical dissection is performed to incise the adventitial sheath of the aorta distally to the midportion of the left common iliac artery. Lateral blunt dissection at the level of the bifurcation should demonstrate the left ureter and establish this lateral boundary. Blunt posterior dissection is performed directly adjacent to the left side of the aorta to develop the medial plane between the nodal bundle and aorta. This dissection is continued to the vertebral bodies and then extended distally to the midportion of the left common iliac artery.

The nodal bundle is held on traction to aid vascular clip placement and is distally transected unless already freed by proximal dissection during a preceding pelvic lymphadenectomy. Nodal tissue is elevated and progressively lifted proximally. Alternating blunt and electrosurgical dissection are performed to divide any remaining posterior attachments (Fig. 44-12.4). The dissection is

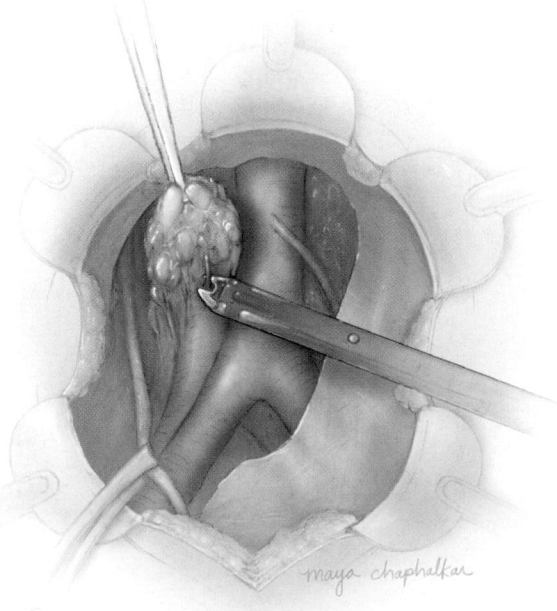

FIGURE 44-12.2 Removal of right paraaortic nodes.

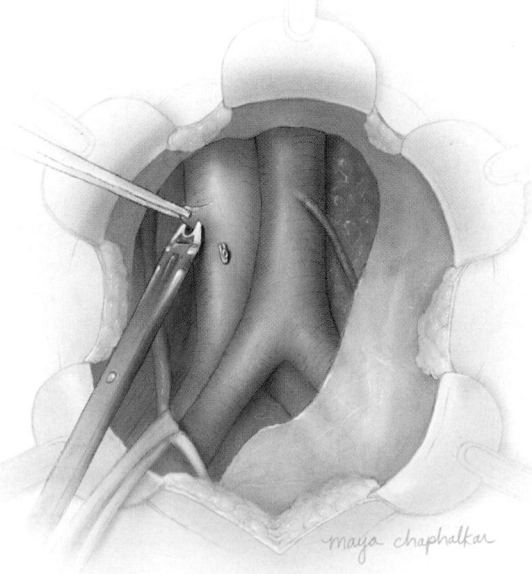

FIGURE 44-12.3 Repair of venous bleeding.

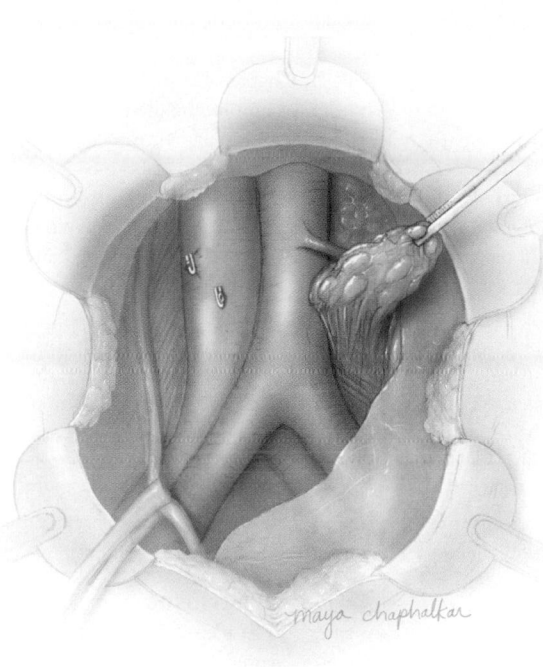

FIGURE 44-12.4 Removal of left paraaortic nodes.

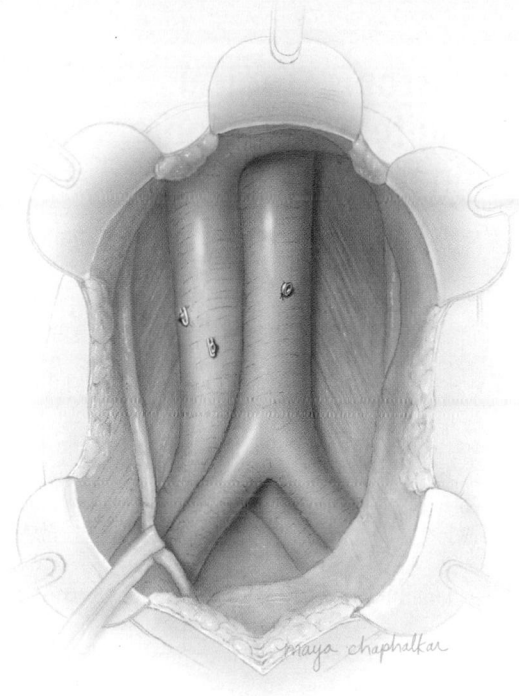

FIGURE 44-12.5 High paraaortic lymphadenectomy.

continued cephalad to the IMA where the nodal bundle is clipped and transected.

❿ Removal of Interiliac Nodes. Optionally, several additional lymph nodes may be removed by excising the fatty interiliac tissue between the common iliac vessels. The posterior peritoneum at the aortic bifurcation is grasped, and electrosurgical dissection is performed along the inner side of both common iliac arteries. The crossing left common iliac vein is visible directly beneath. Once the peritoneum is reflected, the fatty tissue beneath is grasped and placed on tension. Blunt dissection is performed along the surface of the common iliac vein because there are typically few small perforating vessels. Electrosurgical dissection can be performed from right to left to free the triangle-shaped area of fatty-lymphoid tissue after it has been mobilized between the common iliac arteries.

⓫ High Paraaortic Lymphadenectomy. A surgeon may elect an extended dissection to reach the renal veins. Most often, this is performed during ovarian cancer staging or in high-risk endometrial cancer cases (Mariani, 2008; Morice, 2003). The anatomic boundaries begin distally at the IMA and reach proximally to the entry level of the right ovarian vein and left renal vein (Whitney, 2010).

The midline peritoneal incision is incised more cephalad, and the duodenal loop is bluntly dissected off the aorta and IVC. Repositioning of the retractor blade to retract this loop aids exposure. The right-sided paraaortic nodal bundle is regrasped with DeBakey forceps, and dissection is continued in a cephalad direction until the right ovarian vein can be clipped, divided, and incorporated within the specimen. When the level of the left renal vein is reached, the bundle is clipped and transected.

Dissection of the left side begins with identification, clipping, and cutting of the IMA between ties. The mesenteric circulation has an extensive collateralization network that permits IMA ligation without subsequent bowel ischemia. Dividing the IMA allows access to upper nodal tissue. The proximal boundary is established by blunt dissection to visualize the left renal vein. Removal of the left paraaortic nodes includes elevation of the distal nodal bundle, blunt dissection to isolate and electrosurgically coagulate lymphatic attachments, and progression toward the left renal vein. Here, the bundle is clipped and transected (Fig. 44-12.5).

⓬ Retroaortic Lymphadenectomy. This more extended dissection is optional and begins after left-sided paraaortic lymphadenectomy has been completed. The left-sided lumbar arteries can be visualized branching directly from the aorta. These vessels may be clipped and cut to allow manual rolling of the aorta from left to right and allow access to the retroaortic nodal chain. Typically, this procedure is performed when imaging studies have demonstrated suspicious nodes in the region.

⓭ Final Steps. Gauze sponges may be opened and gently placed in areas of nodal dissection to tamponade any surface oozing. There is no benefit to closing the retroperitoneal space or routinely using suction drainage (Morice, 2001).

POSTOPERATIVE

The postoperative course following paraaortic lymphadenectomy in general follows that after laparotomy. However, the incidence of postoperative ileus is increased due to longer operative time, increased bowel manipulation, extension of the incision, and additional blood loss. Most episodes will be mild, but longer hospital stays may be expected (Fujita, 2005).

44-13

Laparoscopic Surgical Staging for Gynecologic Malignancies

Laparoscopic staging can be performed in selected patients with presumed early-stage gynecologic malignancies. Staging includes pelvic and paraaortic lymph node dissection and sometimes omentectomy and peritoneal biopsy. These procedures may also be completed laparoscopically in selected patients who did not undergo comprehensive surgical staging at the time of their initial operation.

Paraaortic lymphadenectomy implies a complete removal of all nodal tissue from within an area with well-defined anatomic boundaries: inferior mesenteric artery (proximally), mid-common iliac artery (distally), ureter (laterally), and aorta (medial). Within these boundaries, paraaortic lymph nodes are removed from the right and the left. Specific indications for paraaortic lymphadenectomy include surgical staging of women with uterine and ovarian cancer. In addition, removal of enlarged paraaortic nodes may be required to achieve optimal debulking of ovarian cancer and may also confer a survival benefit by aiding targeted radiotherapy in selected endometrial and cervical cancer patients.

Pelvic lymphadenectomy implies a complete removal of all nodal tissue within an area bordered by well-defined anatomic landmarks: midportion of the common iliac artery (proximally), deep circumflex iliac vein (distally), midportion of the psoas major muscle (laterally), ureter (medially), and obturator nerve (posteriorly). Within these boundaries, pelvic lymph nodes are removed near the external iliac, internal iliac, and obturator vessels. The main indication of pelvic lymphadenectomy is its role in cancer staging surgery. However, in those with grossly involved nodes, this procedure may serve to optimally debulk tumor burden.

PREOPERATIVE

Patient Evaluation

A thorough pelvic examination and history reveal factors that help determine the optimal surgical route for an individual patient. When considering a minimally invasive route, patients with suspected extensive adhesive disease or those with significant cardiopulmonary disease may be poor candidates. Regardless of approach, preoperative imaging studies prior to lymphadenectomy may help guide the surgeon to suspicious areas of lymph node involvement.

Consent

General complications related to laparoscopic surgery are discussed in Chapter 42 (p. 1097) and include entry injury to the major vessels, bladder, ureters, and bowel. Specific to laparoscopic pelvic and paraaortic lymphadenectomy, acute hemorrhage is the most commonly associated complication. Moreover, ureteral injury, postoperative lymphocyst, and nerve injuries, particularly to the obturator and genitofemoral nerve, can also occur. Preventatively, careful dissection and identification of retroperitoneal anatomy is mandatory before proceeding with any resection. For both lymphadenectomy procedures, obesity, previous radiation therapy, prior pelvic infections, and prior abdominal surgery may hinder dissection and lead to incomplete or limited lymph node sampling.

The risk of conversion to an open procedure should also always be discussed. Conversion to laparotomy may be necessary if exposure and organ manipulation are limited or if acute hemorrhage cannot be controlled laparoscopically. Finally, port-site metastasis is an uncommon but possible complication, as described in Section 42-1 (p. 1099).

Patient Preparation

Routine bowel preparation and antibiotic prophylaxis are not typically required. However, other concurrent surgeries may dictate their use. Thromboprophylaxis is administered as outlined in Table 39-9 (p. 962).

INTRAOPERATIVE

Instruments

For laparoscopic surgical staging, some type of energy-based device such as the argon beam coagulator (ABC), Harmonic scalpel, or monopolar scissors is required. Additionally, blunt graspers are needed, and Maryland forceps are useful for more fine dissection. Lymph nodes can be removed in a variety of ways, including use of an endoscopic specimen bag or by laparoscopic spoon graspers. Since bleeding may be encountered, a suction irrigator should be ready for use, and laparoscopic vascular clips should be available.

SURGICAL STEPS

❶ Anesthesia and Patient Positioning. Laparoscopic lymphadenectomy is performed under general anesthesia. Typically, dorsal lithotomy position is selected due to concurrent hysterectomy, although supine may be appropriate for a restaging procedure. As described fully in Chapter 42 (p. 1100), positioning is crucial for any minimally invasive procedure. Accordingly, the patient is secured to the bed by means of a gel pad or bean bag with appropriate protective padding. This avoids patient sliding when placed in steep Trendelenburg position. Patient arms are padded and tucked at her side to allow a broad range of surgeon movement during the procedure.

To avoid stomach puncture by a trocar during primary abdominal entry, an orogastric or nasogastric tube should be placed to decompress the stomach. To avert similar bladder injury, a Foley catheter is placed. The abdomen is then surgically prepared. The vaginal is also surgically prepared if concurrent hysterectomy is planned.

❷ Port Placement. As described in Section 44-3, step 2 (p. 1268), the 10- to 12-mm primary trocar is placed approximately 1 to 2 cm above the umbilicus using an open abdominal entry method. The 10-mm zero-degree laparoscope provides improved visualization compared with a 5-mm diameter and should be utilized. Accessory ports include two 5-mm trocars in the right and left lower quadrants and a 12-mm trocar placed midline above the pubic symphysis.

Lymph nodes should be evaluated during initial abdominal exploration. Unexpected positive nodes may alter a proposed operative plan and may require conversion to an open procedure.

❸ Paraaortic Lymphadenectomy: Positioning. Transperitoneal paraaortic lymphadenectomy is usually performed first as it is the most challenging part of the procedure. Exposure and proper positioning are essential for successful dissection. One technique is to move the video monitors toward the patient's shoulders. Each video monitor should be placed at a position comfortable for surgeon viewing. The primary surgeon stands on the patient's right at the level of the hips and faces the patient's head. The laparoscope is placed into the suprapubic port and is directed toward the upper abdomen for visualization of the aorta and inferior vena cava (IVC).

❹ Paraaortic Lymphadenectomy: Opening the Retroperitoneal Space. With the patient in steep Trendelenburg position, the small bowel is gently elevated into the right and left upper quadrants. The first landmark to identify is the bifurcation of the aorta and the right common iliac artery. The peritoneum above the right common iliac artery is grasped, elevated, and incised with the ABC, which has been placed in the 12-mm supraumbilical port, or with another type of energy-based device or scissors. This peritoneal incision is extended superiorly over the lateral aspect of the aorta and is continued to the level of the duodenum. Following entry into the retroperitoneal space, the peritoneum is held anteriorly and cephalad by the assistant surgeon using a grasper through the right lower quadrant trocar. Blunt and sharp dissection is performed by the surgeon to mobilize the duodenum cephalad and expose the aorta until reaching the inferior mesenteric artery (IMA) as it exits on the left. The peritoneal fold is regrasped by the assistant above the right common iliac artery, and the surgeon dissects laterally until the right ureter is located. The assistant surgeon releases the peritoneum to lift the ureter anterior and lateral with gentle blunt traction. The surgeon continues the dissection laterally along the common iliac artery, under the ureter, until identifying the psoas major muscle. A plane is bluntly developed between the lateral portion of the IVC and psoas muscle and extended cephalad to a level parallel to the IMA. With the anatomical boundaries having been identified, removal of the nodal bundle can be performed.

❺ Paraaortic Lymphadenectomy: Node Removal over the Inferior Vena Cava. The surgeon begins the dissection at the far right portion of the common iliac artery where it meets the psoas major muscle. The grasper is used to bluntly open small spaces to create fibrous pedicles that can be lysed or coagulated and divided. This is continued until the tip of the nodal bundle can be elevated and brought in a cephalad direction. The dissection continues medially until crossing the IVC and reaching the lower aorta. The lymph nodes overlying the IVC are grasped with a blunt grasper and gently elevated (Fig 44-13.1). This nodal tissue is then separated from the underlying vein with blunt dissection in a proximal direction, creating small pedicles that often contain small vessels. The multiple perforating vessels are sequentially isolated, clipped or coagulated, and then divided. Typically, this is the most difficult part of the dissection since when these vessels are inadvertently torn, significant bleeding may follow. Preventatively, laparoscopic hemostatic clips or coagulation can be used on the larger vascular pedicles. Moreover, a small sponge can be prophylactically placed through the periumbilical trocar into the abdomen in case quick tamponade is required to control bleeding. Dissection proceeds proximally along the IVC to reach the level of the IMA. Lymph nodes are removed intact using an endoscopic bag or spoon instrument though the 12-mm supraumbilical port.

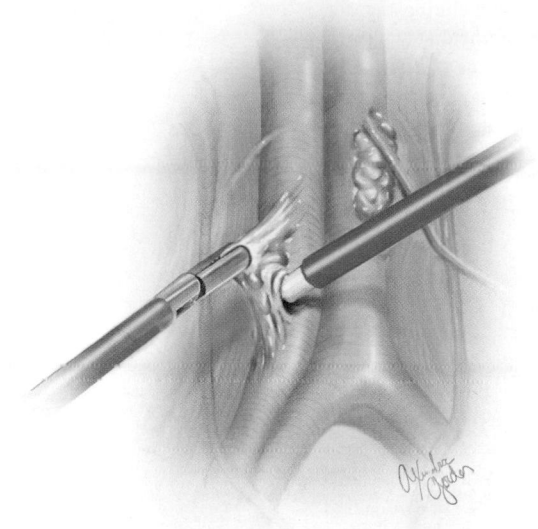

FIGURE 44-13.1 Dissection of right paraaortic lymph nodes.

❻ Paraaortic Lymphadenectomy: Removal of Left Paraaortic Nodes. Left paraaortic dissection is performed next, and the surgeon and assistant switch places. The mesentery of the sigmoid is retracted anteriorly and laterally by the assistant by grasping and retracting the left peritoneal edge through the left lower quadrant trocar. Alternatively, a 0-gauge delayed-absorbable suture can be placed laparoscopically to tack a portion of the sigmoid epiploica to the left lateral abdominal wall. The IMA is again identified as it exits the aorta. With blunt dissection under the IMA and lateral to the aorta, the left psoas major muscle is identified. The left ureter, which runs deep and lateral to the aorta, is also exposed. Once identified, it can be retracted anteriorly and laterally by the assistant after releasing the peritoneum. A plane is bluntly developed by gentle dissection medial to the ureter, from the IMA to the left common iliac artery. Lymph nodes adjacent to the aorta are detached by grasping with laparoscopic forceps and dissecting laterally. Fibrous pedicles and perforating vessels are isolated, coagulated, and divided. With the anatomic boundaries identified, the inferior tip of the nodal bundle is dissected and divided at the midportion of the left common iliac artery after rechecking the location of the ureter. The grasper is used to elevate the bundle as the dissection proceeds proximally until reaching the IMA. The bundle is then detached and removed.

❼ High Paraaortic Lymphadenectomy. In some instances, a surgeon may elect an extended laparoscopic dissection (Section 44-12, step 11, p. 1301). The anatomic boundaries of a high paraaortic lymphadenectomy begin distally at the IMA and reach proximally to the entry level of the right ovarian vein and left renal vein (Whitney, 2010). Typically, this transperitoneal procedure is only possible in selected patients with favorable anatomy, such as thin body habitus, since exposure is otherwise often problematic. Other helpful maneuvers include having a second surgical assistant and placing additional right and left mid-quadrant 5-mm trocars.

The peritoneum overlying the aorta at the level of the IMA is grasped and elevated anteriorly to displace small intestine into the upper abdomen while providing exposure to the aorta. If one grasper is not sufficient, then both right-sided ports are used by the assistant, while a second assistant holds the laparoscope. The surgeon performs retroperitoneal dissection proximally along the aorta to further mobilize the duodenum. Often a laparoscopic fan retractor will need to be inserted by the assistant through the periumbilical port and positioned in the retroperitoneal space to provide exposure of the upper aorta. Gentle dissection continues until the left renal vein is visualized as it crosses the aorta.

The right ureter is identified and again elevated by the assistant through the right-sided port. Then the nodal bundle overlying the IVC is regrasped by the surgeon and held on lateral traction to dissect and divide the fibrous attachments from the aorta. The lateral portion of the nodal bundle is bluntly separated from the psoas major muscle in a proximal direction. The gonadal vein will be encountered by the surgeon during the dissection and should be individually ligated using a bipolar coagulating device. The proximal border of the nodal bundle is then detached at the level of the renal vein and removed as described earlier.

Dissection of the left side begins by the surgeon and assistant switching places. This is followed by placement of laparoscopic clips on the IMA and dividing in between using a bipolar coagulating device. The left ureter is again identified and held laterally by the assistant through a left-sided port. Using both right-sided trocars, the surgeon performs blunt dissection with intermittent coagulation and division of fibrous or vascular pedicles to detach the nodal bundle in a proximal direction. The gonadal vein will be visualized at some point, and dissection continues parallel to it until reaching the left renal vein, where the bundle is divided and removed.

❽ Pelvic Lymphadenectomy: Positioning.
Once paraaortic dissection is completed, pelvic lymphadenectomy can be performed. The surgeons now turn to face the pelvis, and the video screens are moved to approximate the level of the patient's thighs. The laparoscope is replaced into the supraumbilical port. The primary surgeon now operates at the left side using the lateral and suprapubic ports, while the assistant stands on the right side and holds the laparoscope and the instrument in the right lower port.

❾ Pelvic Lymphadenectomy: Retroperitoneal Entry.
Preferably, the retroperitoneal spaces will have been opened if hysterectomy was performed first. Otherwise, the round ligament is transected and the posterior peritoneum is grasped, elevated, and dissected parallel to the infundibulopelvic ligament. Then, gentle anterior traction is applied to the transected round ligament to open the broad ligament. Medial traction on the obliterated medial umbilical ligament allows for exposure of the paravesical space and subsequently the obturator space and lymph nodes. The goal prior to pelvic lymph node removal is to open and to develop completely the pararectal and paravesical spaces, which is described in Section 44-3, step 3 (p. 1268). In the retroperitoneum, important structures to identify include the ureter, the psoas muscle, the genitofemoral and obturator nerves, and the external and internal iliac vessels (Fig. 38-16, p. 932).

❿ Pelvic Lymphadenectomy: Node Removal over the External Iliac Vessels.
Removal of lymphatic tissue begins over the common iliac artery and extends adjacent to the external iliac artery by creating a plane

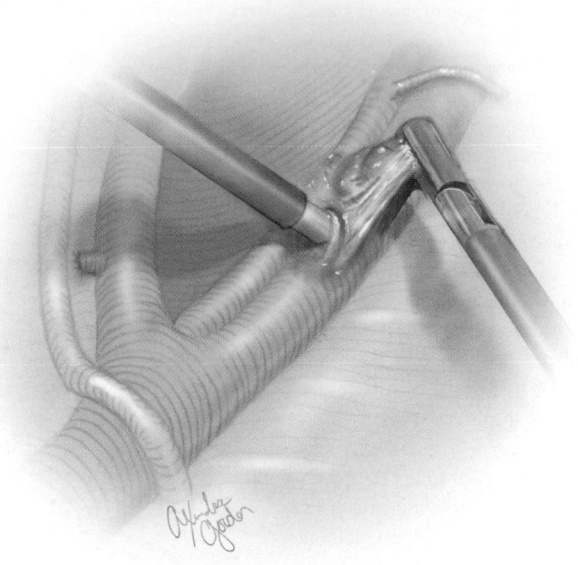

FIGURE 44-13.2 Pelvic lymph node dissection over the external iliac vessels.

between medially located lymphoid tissue and lateral preperitoneal fat above the psoas major muscle. The lymph node group is grasped with the blunt instrument and elevated. A blunt dissector can help create pedicles, which can then be coagulated. Electrosurgery can be used to obtain hemostasis as the lymph node packet is dissected bluntly (Fig. 44-13.2). Specifically, the ABC can be used both for coagulation and dissection. With small taps of energy, hemostasis can be achieved with minimal thermal energy spread. Then, the instrument can be used as a blunt probe to continue dissection until reaching the deep circumflex iliac vein as it crosses the external iliac artery (see Fig. 44-13.2). Alternatively, the Harmonic scalpel can serve the same function. The genitofemoral nerve running atop the psoas major muscle is identified and protected during this dissection.

As the dissection proceeds medially over the artery, the external iliac vein is visualized. Unlike performing open surgery, the pneumoperitoneum and Trendelenburg position used during laparoscopy result in collapse of the vein. As a result, this vein is harder to distinguish and can be easily injured. The nodal bundle is reflected medially, with traction applied as blunt dissection is performed with division of fibrous pedicles. The landmarks and extent of dissection are the same as those used for the open technique.

⓫ Pelvic Lymphadenectomy: Obturator Node Group Removal.
Next, the obturator lymph nodes and the internal iliac (or hypo-

gastric) lymph nodes, which are located near the origin of the uterine artery, are resected. With the assistant surgeon holding medial traction on the superior vesical artery, the obturator fossa can be exposed. The obturator space dissection may begin medial to the external iliac artery and the psoas major muscle. Thereafter, the external iliac vessels are retracted laterally, and the obturator space can be entered.

The obturator nerve is identified by blunt dissection and should be found before dividing any tissue pedicles. The obturator vessels run below this nerve. Gentle blunt dissection will expose the obturator internus muscle. The nerve is bluntly moved laterally as the nodes are grasped and elevated. The lymph nodes between the external iliac vein and the obturator nerve are removed using the same cautious technique of tissue dissection described earlier. That is, nodes are gently grasped with a blunt instrument, and the ABC or Harmonic scalpel is used for dissection and coagulation to free the nodal bundle (Fig. 44-13.3).

The lymph nodes located at the bifurcation of the internal and external iliac vessels are termed the internal iliac or hypogastric lymph nodes. Typically, these are the most difficult to remove as the final step. The anatomy, including ureteral location, should be confirmed before gentle medial blunt movements and electrosurgical dissection allow the entire pelvic lymph node bundle to be safely detached en bloc. Nodes are then removed via endoscopic bag or laparoscopic

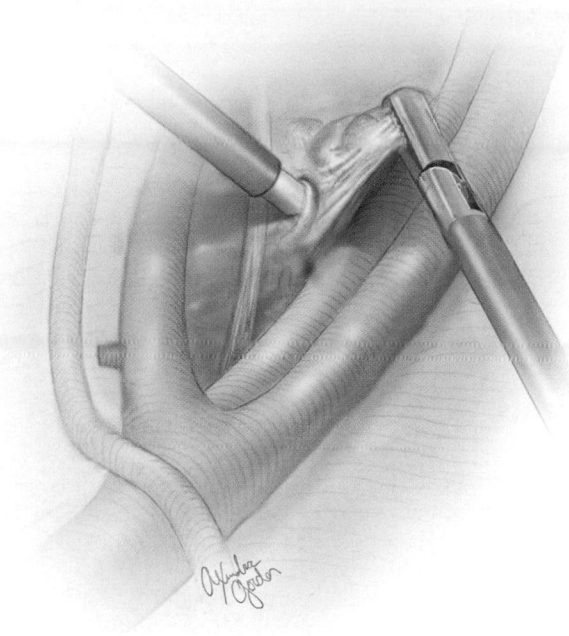

FIGURE 44-13.3 Obturator lymph node removal.

Chapter 40 (p. 1013). Ureteral repair may require laparotomy, depending on the laparoscopic expertise of the surgeon.

Small bladder injuries can be treated with continuous drainage with a Foley catheter, whereas larger defects require repair. Bladder injuries at the dome of the bladder or above the trigone can be closed primarily laparoscopically in layers with delayed-absorbable suture.

⓮ Port Removal and Fascial Closure.
Once laparoscopic procedures have been completed, an inspection for bleeding is performed. Topical hemostats may be used and are listed in Table 40-6 (p. 1005). If hemostasis is achieved, trocars are removed and port sites closed. Fascial defects larger than 10 mm are sutured to decrease the risk of herniation at those sites. Interrupted stitches of 0-gauge delayed-absorbable suture are used to reapproximate this fascia. Alternatively, a dedicated trocar-site closure device can be used. Regardless of technique, palpation of the defect should be performed to confirm adequate closure. Skin incisions are closed as described in Chapter 40 (p. 987).

POSTOPERATIVE

The postoperative course following laparoscopic staging lymphadenectomy in general follows that after other major laparoscopic surgery. In general, patients are able to tolerate clear liquids quickly, followed by a regular diet and discharge on postoperative day 1. With their pain typically controlled with oral pain medication, patients ambulate early.

Postoperative complications may include pelvic lymphocyst formation, neurologic injuries, or trocar-site herniation. One long-term potential complication of pelvic lymphadenectomy is lymphedema. The exact incidence is unknown, but the risk increases if a higher number of lymph nodes are removed or if pelvic radiation is administered after surgery. Treatments, which may or may not be successful, often include compression stockings, lower extremity wrapping, and massage therapy to manipulate lymph channels. Although generally not associated with an adverse outcome, this complication can significantly lower a patient's quality of life postoperatively.

spoon forceps. The identical procedure is performed on the contralateral side.

⓬ Completion of Laparoscopic Staging and Omentectomy. The staging procedure for ovarian cancer includes obtaining multiple peritoneal biopsies from the cul-de-sac, pelvic sidewalls, and pelvic gutters, and from the diaphragm bilaterally. This can be performed with a blunt grasper and laparoscopic scissors, with or without electrosurgical coagulation. The surgical staging for ovarian cancer and for certain histologic subtypes of endometrial cancer (papillary serous and clear cell carcinoma) also includes omental removal.

A laparoscopic omentectomy is performed by identifying and elevating the omentum off the transverse colon. Avascular windows are created within the proximal omentum. The intervening vascular attachments are then ligated with one of the following instruments: electrothermal bipolar coagulator (LigaSure), Harmonic scalpel, or endoscopic stapler. Once completely dissected, the

omentum is placed in an endoscopic bag and removed through a transabdominal 12-mm port. However, the omentum generally is too large and therefore is brought through the vagina if a laparoscopic hysterectomy is performed. All specimens should be minimally manipulated and should be removed through an endoscopic bag or an enclosed instrument, such as the laparoscopic spoon forceps, to help decrease the risk of port-site tumor implantation.

⓭ Cystoscopy. Both the ureters and bladder can be injured during these procedures. To decrease the occult injury rate, ureters are identified and traced from above the pelvic brim to the bladder. If injury is suspected, cystoscopy at the end of the procedure can aid injury recognition. Indigo carmine or methylene blue is administered intravenously. During cystoscopy, jets of blue dye effluxing from the ureteral orifices confirm ureteral patency. Options for repair of diagnosed ureteral injury are discussed in

44-14

Robotic Surgical Staging for Gynecologic Malignancies

The wrist-like articulation of robotic instruments allows meticulous, fine dissection. Accordingly, robotic surgery for lymph node dissection has become popular. The robot has been used to perform simple and radical hysterectomies with pelvic and paraaortic lymph node dissection to treat endometrial, ovarian, and cervical cancers. As described in Section 44-13 (p. 1302), the same principles for patient selection and preparation apply to robotic surgery as for laparoscopic surgery. Procedure steps are also the same in terms of landmarks and fields of dissection.

PREOPERATIVE

Patient Evaluation

A thorough pelvic examination and history reveal factors that help determine the optimal surgical route for a patient. When considering a minimally invasive route, patients with suspected extensive adhesive disease or those with significant cardiopulmonary disease may be poor candidates. Regardless of approach, preoperative imaging studies prior to lymphadenectomy may help guide the surgeon to suspicious areas of lymph node involvement.

Consent

With paraaortic lymphadenectomy, acute hemorrhage and possible postoperative ileus are the most commonly associated complications. With pelvic lymphadenectomy, hemorrhage, postoperative lymphocyst, and obturator nerve injury are possible. Ureteral injury is also a potential complication during both paraaortic and pelvic lymph node dissection. Therefore, the ureters should always be recognized and retracted out of the field of dissection. For both of these lymphadenectomy procedures, obesity, previous radiation therapy, prior pelvic infections, and prior abdominal surgery may hinder dissection and lead to incomplete or limited lymph node sampling.

General complications related to laparoscopic surgery are discussed in Chapter 42 (p. 1097) and include entry injury to the major vessels, bladder, ureters, and bowel. In addition, the risk of conversion to an open procedure should be discussed. Conversion to laparotomy may be necessary if exposure and

organ manipulation are limited. Finally, port-site metastasis is an uncommon but possible complication, as described in Section 42-1 (p. 1099).

Patient Preparation

Routine bowel preparation and antibiotic prophylaxis are not typically required. However, other concurrent surgeries may dictate their use. Thromboprophylaxis is administered as outlined in Table 39-9 (p. 962).

INTRAOPERATIVE

Instruments

Important robotic energy-source instruments for radical hysterectomy include the EndoWrist monopolar scissors and the EndoWrist bipolar Maryland grasper. The PK dissecting forceps is an alternative bipolar electrosurgical source for the robot. Additional blunt graspers and retractors are available that can be used in the fourth robotic arm depending on the procedure planned. The surgical assistant can operate with traditional laparoscopic instruments through an added 12-mm assistant port. Instruments used by the assistant include laparoscopic blunt graspers, spoon forceps, and suction irrigator.

SURGICAL STEPS

❶ Anesthesia and Patient Positioning. Robotic lymphadenectomy is performed under general anesthesia with the patient in low dorsal lithotomy position. As described in Section 44-4, step 1 (p. 1272), patient positioning should avoid patient sliding when placed in steep Trendelenburg position. The patient's arms are tucked at her side with padding to prevent injury.

To avoid stomach puncture by a trocar during primary abdominal entry, an orogastric or nasogastric tube should be placed to decompress the stomach. To avert similar bladder injury, a Foley catheter is placed. The abdomen is then surgically prepared. The vaginal is also surgically prepared if concurrent hysterectomy is planned.

❷ Port Placement. Port placement is as described in detail in Section 44-4 (p. 1273). Robotic staging surgery typically uses five port sites. One supraumbilical, two lateral, and one trocar above the left anterior superior iliac spine will be docked to the robot arms. The fifth site, an assistant surgeon's port, is often placed in the right upper quadrant. Importantly, robotic ports should be no closer than 8 cm apart to avoid robotic arm collision. Moreover, the port for the laparo-

scope must be placed proximal enough above the umbilicus to permit visualization of the lower aorta.

Paraaortic dissection is most easily performed with the 30-degree down laparoscope placed in the midline supraumbilical port. Here, the laparoscope is close to the paraaortic region, and the 30-degree down lens system allows for direct inspection of the lymph nodes and vessels. Monopolar scissors are placed in one robotic arm, and bipolar Maryland forceps or a PK dissecting forceps is placed in the other arm for dissection. The fourth robotic arm can hold a blunt grasper, which can assist in retraction.

Lymph nodes should be evaluated during initial abdominal exploration. Unexpected positive nodes may alter a proposed operative plan in certain cases, particularly in cervical cancer. In addition, the decision is made to proceed robotically or convert to laparotomy.

❸ Robotic Paraaortic Lymphadenectomy: Opening the Retroperitoneal Space. With the patient in steep Trendelenburg position, the small bowel is elevated into the right and left upper quadrants. The directional approach with robotic surgery is unique for paraaortic node dissection because the laparoscope remains in the supraumbilical port. As a result, the surgeon looks directly down on the aorta and inferior vena cava. This differs from laparoscopic paraaortic dissection, in which the laparoscope is housed in the suprapubic port.

As with all paraaortic lymph node dissections, the first step, whether performed open or by a minimally invasive approach, is to open the peritoneum above the right common iliac artery. This artery and its origin from the aorta are identified. The peritoneum above the right common iliac artery is grasped, elevated, and incised with the monopolar scissors. This incision is then extended upward over the aorta until the duodenum is exposed and mobilized. The inferior mesenteric artery (IMA) should be visible as it exits to the left, which is the cephalad border of the planned lymphadenectomy. A sponge may be prophylactically inserted through the assistant port to tamponade surface oozing or hold pressure on any sites of brisk bleeding that may be encountered.

❹ Paraaortic Lymphadenectomy: Removal of Right Paraaortic Nodes. The peritoneal dissection continues along the right common iliac artery laterally. Once the right ureter is identified, a blunt grasper in the fourth robotic arm can gently retract the peritoneum, which will lateralize the ureter (Fig. 44-14.1). The assistant surgeon holds the cephalad portion of the peritoneum to aid exposure and prevent loops of small intestine from obstructing the view. The psoas major

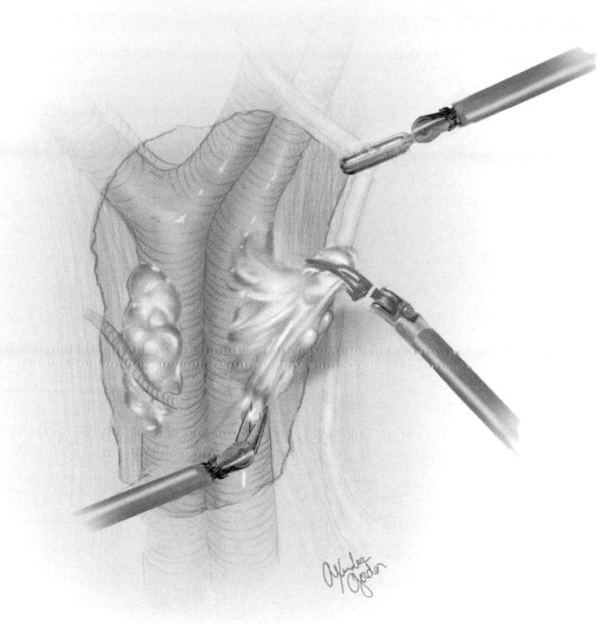

FIGURE 44-14.1 Robotic right paraaortic lymph node dissection.

muscle is identified laterally, and a plane is developed at the lateral border of the inferior vena cava (IVC). The distal tip of the nodal bundle is isolated at the convergence of the common iliac artery and psoas major muscle using blunt and electrosurgical dissection. At this point, the right paraaortic lymph nodes are grasped by the forceps and elevated upward to begin dissection. The monopolar scissors can create pedicles and coagulate them to further mobilize the nodes in a step-by-step fashion starting at the aorta and working laterally over the IVC (see Fig. 44-14.1). Once completely dissected to the proximal border of the IMA, the nodal bundle can be placed either in an endoscopic bag or in spoon forceps and removed through the assistant port.

❺ Paraaortic Lymphadenectomy: Removal of Left Paraaortic Nodes. The left paraaortic lymph node dissection is usually technically more challenging. The fourth arm is used to grasp the left side of the opened peritoneum above the aortic bifurcation and elevate it laterally to retract the left colon. The IMA and distal aorta are visualized, and exposure is aided by the assistant surgeon using suction, a fan retractor, or a blunt probe. The ureter, which is deep and lateral to the aorta and located adjacent to the psoas major muscle, is identified by blunt dissection and retracted laterally with a blunt probe held by the assistant. A plane is bluntly developed between the psoas major muscle and medial nodal bundle. The lymph nodes located

lateral to the aorta and below the IMA are grasped and elevated upward. The monopolar scissors can create pedicles and coagulate them to mobilize the nodal bundle medially from the aorta. Bipolar coagulation is used for small perforating vessels. Importantly, the lumbar vessels should be avoided if possible. The distal tip of the nodal bundle is isolated at the midportion of the left common iliac artery, transected, and mobilized cephalad to the IMA. Again, once completely resected, the

lymph nodes can be placed either in an endoscopic bag or in spoon forceps and then are removed through the assistant port.

Typically, robotic paraaortic lymphadenectomy stops at the level of the IMA. High paraaortic dissection to the level of the renal vein is technically difficult and infrequently performed due to poor visualization, limitations in spanning the distance with the robotic arms, and inability to turn the patient around without undocking and placing additional ports.

❻ Robotic Pelvic Lymphadenectomy. After the paraaortic nodal dissection is completed, the laparoscope can be changed to a 0-degree straight laparoscope to proceed with pelvic lymph node dissection. The 0-degree can provide a wider normal anatomic view of the pelvis. The anatomic landmarks for this dissection are as follows: midportion of the psoas major muscle and genitofemoral nerve (laterally), the ureter (medially), the deep circumflex iliac vein (distally), and the midportion of common iliac artery (proximally). The same steps apply for resection of the pelvic lymph nodes as described using the laparoscopic approach (Section 44-13, steps 9 through 11, p. 1304). However, with 360-degree movement, robotic instruments aid resection while avoiding nerves and vessels, thus preventing injury and bleeding. At the same time, the three-dimensional images provide clear delineation of small vessels and nerves, which can then be spared during the dissection.

In overview, dissection begins over the external iliac artery distally and moves cephalad. Alternatively, some surgeons will begin at the common iliac artery bifurcation and proceed caudad as shown in Figure 44-14.2.

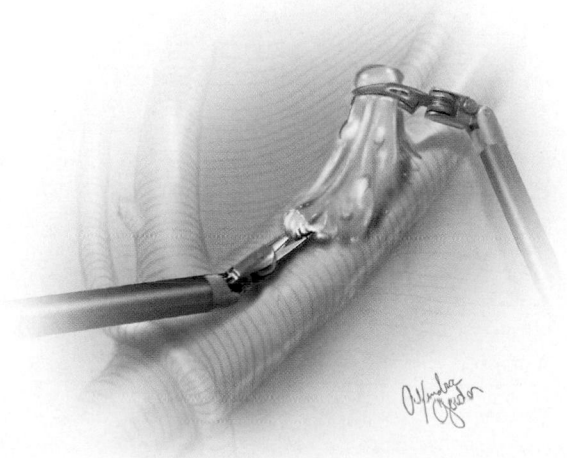

FIGURE 44-14.2 Robotic pelvic lymph node dissection over the external iliac vessels.

In either case, nodes are separated from the external iliac vessels. As described previously in Section 44-13, step 11 (p. 1304), dissection then continues deep to the external iliac vein to remove obturator and hypogastric (internal iliac) nodes. During this dissection, the external iliac vessels can be retracted either medially or laterally depending on the individual patient so that lymph nodes behind these vessels, in the obturator space, can be resected. While performing the pelvic lymph node dissection, the surgeon isolates the obturator nerve and keeps it in view to avoid injury. The obturator nerve will be completely exposed at the completion of the lymph node resection. The ureter runs medially to the dissection in the obturator space and should also be kept in view while being retracted medially to avoid injury. Due to the lack of tactile sensation using robotics, great caution is required when retracting retroperitoneal structures to provide exposure. Once completely resected, the nodes are placed either in an endoscopic bag or in spoon forceps and then are removed through the assistant port.

❼ Completion of Robotic Staging and Omentectomy. The staging procedure for ovarian cancer includes obtaining multiple peritoneal biopsies from the cul-de-sac, pelvic sidewalls, and pelvic gutters, and from the diaphragm bilaterally. This can be performed with a blunt grasper, scissors, and electro-surgical coagulation. The surgical staging for ovarian cancer and for certain histologic subtypes of endometrial cancer (papillary serous and clear cell carcinoma) also includes omental removal.

Omentectomy using a robotic approach employs the same fundamental steps as with laparoscopy (Section 44-13, step 12 p. 1305). The distal omentum can be held with blunt graspers, usually by instruments in the fourth arm and the assistant port. This allows for the omentum to be laid out across the field of vision. Then, the omentum can be separated from the transverse colon by creating avascular windows. The intervening vascular attachments are ligated with bipolar coagulation device and cut with the scissors. Once completely dissected, the omentum is placed in an endoscopic bag and removed through a transabdominal 12-mm port. However, the omentum generally is too large and therefore is brought through the vagina if a laparoscopic hysterectomy is performed. All specimens should be minimally manipulated and should be removed in an endoscopic bag or in an enclosed instrument, such as spoon forceps, to decrease the risk of port-site tumor implantation.

❽ Port Removal and Fascial Closure. Once procedures are completed, instruments are removed from the robotic arms, and the arms are undocked from the trocars. Once all of the arms are disengaged, the robot can be moved away from the patient by surgical nursing staff. The laparoscope is handheld at this point, and the trocars are removed under direct laparoscopic visualization. All fascial defects greater than 10 mm should be closed with 0-gauge delayed-absorbable suture to avoid hernia development at those sites. Various methods of skin closure are available and include subcuticular suturing, skin adhesive (Dermabond), or surgical tape strips (Steristrips) plus tincture of benzoin.

POSTOPERATIVE

The postoperative course following para-aortic lymphadenectomy in general follows that after other major laparoscopic surgery. Again, the benefit of minimally invasive surgery is mild postoperative pain. Therefore, only oral medication for pain control is usually necessary, and the patient is able to ambulate without difficulty. Patients are able to tolerate clear liquids quickly and may advance to a regular diet usually on postoperative day 1. With postoperative goals met, most patients are discharged home on postoperative day 2.

Some of the complications following pelvic lymphadenectomy may include lymphedema, lymphocyst formation, and neurologic injuries, as described in Section 44-11 (p. 1298).

44-15

En Bloc Pelvic Resection

Ovarian cancer with contiguous encasement of the reproductive organs, pelvic peritoneum, cul-de-sac, and sigmoid colon is the main indication for en bloc pelvic resection. Also known as radical oophorectomy, this effective technique aids a maximal cytoreductive surgical effort. As a result of removing all microscopic and infiltrative peritoneal tumor in the pelvis, improved survival in patients with advanced epithelial ovarian cancer may be anticipated (Aletti, 2006b). Moreover, pelvic recurrence rates are very low and reflect the completeness of pelvic tumor eradication (Hertel, 2001). Many of the principles of en bloc pelvic resection mirror those of other procedures in gynecologic oncology.

PREOPERATIVE

Patient Evaluation

Pelvic examination may reveal a relatively immobile mass, and abdominopelvic computed tomography (CT) images typically demonstrates a pelvic mass and ascites. With the presumed diagnosis of advanced ovarian cancer, patients are prepared preoperatively for anticipated cytoreductive surgery. However, the need for en bloc resection is usually dictated by intraoperative findings rather than preoperative testing.

Consent

In general, women with advanced ovarian cancer undergoing cytoreductive surgery are at significant risk for complications, and they should be counseled accordingly. Minor postoperative complications such as incisional cellulitis, superficial wound dehiscence, urinary tract infection, or ileus are common. Major postoperative complications of en bloc resection that should be discussed include anastomotic leaks and fistulas (Bristow, 2003; Park, 2006).

Patient Preparation

Primary anastomosis without colostomy is typical for most patients. Thus, bowel preparation is commonplace for any type of cytoreductive ovarian cancer surgery, but particularly if en bloc pelvic resection is a possibility. One or more bowel resections may be required to achieve optimal debulking, and often, preoperative determination of the exact location of tumor infiltration is not entirely accurate. The combination of pneumatic compression devices and subcutaneous heparin is particularly important due to the anticipated longer operation length, hypercoagulable features of ovarian malignancy, and possibility of extended postoperative recovery. Moreover, patients should routinely be typed and crossmatched for packed red blood cell replacement, as transfusions are frequently indicated (Bristow, 2003).

INTRAOPERATIVE

Instruments

En bloc pelvic resection requires access to multiple sizes of bowel staplers, including gastrointestinal anastomosis (GIA), transverse anastomosis (TA), and end-to-end anastomosis (EEA) staplers. Additionally, a ligate-divide-staple (LDS) device or electrothermal bipolar coagulator (LigaSure) may be used to divide vascular tissue pedicles.

SURGICAL STEPS

❶ Anesthesia and Patient Positioning. Bimanual examination under general anesthesia is especially important to confirm the necessity of leg positioning in Allen stirrups. Access to the perineum is crucial any time the EEA device may need to be placed in the rectum. The patient is properly positioned to avoid nerve injury while in stirrups (Chap. 40, p. 984). Sterile preparation of the abdomen, perineum, and vagina is performed, and a Foley catheter is placed.

❷ Abdominal Entry. Typically, a vertical incision is selected for ovarian cancer debulking surgery since the extent of disease cannot be precisely known beforehand and may extend up to the diaphragms. At first, the incision extends up to the umbilicus. After exploration and determination of tumor resectability, it can be extended as needed.

❸ Exploration. The abdomen is thoroughly explored to first determine whether all gross disease can be safely removed. For example, unresectable upper abdominal tumor makes the prospect of a radical pelvic operation less attractive.

Frequently during exploration, it is difficult to distinguish uterus, adnexa, and adjacent tumor. As demonstrated in Figure 44-15.1, both ovaries may be grossly enlarged with tumor and densely fixed into the posterior cul-de-sac with contiguous involvement of the uterus, rectosigmoid, and lateral sidewalls. Moreover, superficial implants often coat the fallopian tubes, the vesicouterine fold, and much of the surrounding pelvic peritoneum. En bloc pelvic resection will allow removal of all this gross disease.

❹ Lateral Pelvic Dissection. The lateral peritoneum is grasped with an Allis clamp, and an electrosurgical blade is used to enter the retroperitoneal space if the round

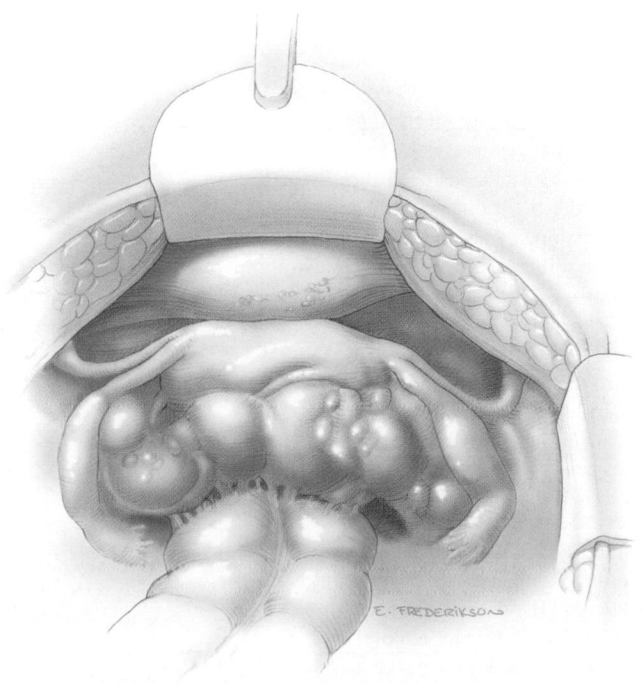

FIGURE 44-15.1 Extensive ovarian cancer.

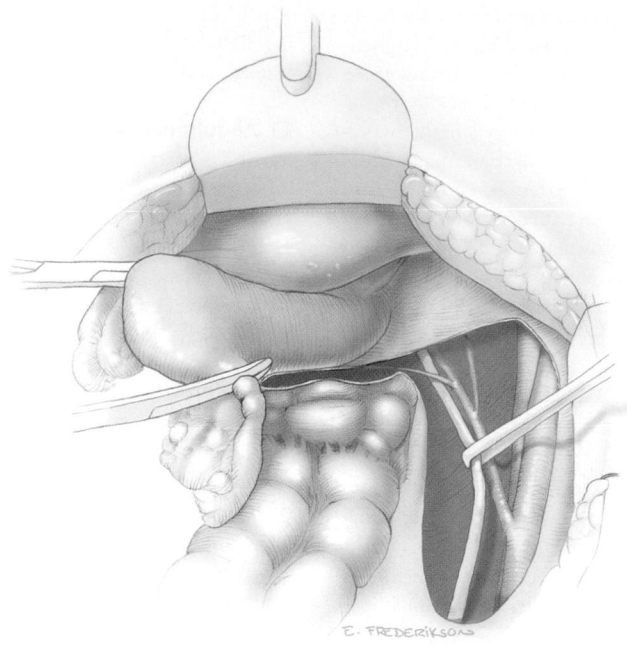

FIGURE 44-15.2 Lateral pelvic dissection.

ligaments cannot be located with certainty. The loose areolar connective tissue of this space is bluntly dissected and the overlying peritoneum is sharply incised to create an opening in which the external iliac artery can be palpated. This artery is bluntly followed to the bifurcation with the internal iliac artery. The medial peritoneal leaf of the broad ligament is elevated to identify the ureter, around which a one-quarter inch Penrose drain is looped (Fig. 44-15.2).

The infundibulopelvic (IP) ligament will typically not be entirely distinguishable due to induration and anatomical distortion by tumor. A window is bluntly opened just superior to the ureter as it crosses above the pelvic brim to isolate a tissue pedicle that will include the IP ligament. The ligament is isolated, clamped, cut, and tied with 0-gauge delayed-absorbable suture. The entire sequence is repeated on the contralateral side. The ureter may then be mobilized distally, and the anterior leaf of the broad ligament is incised toward the vesicouterine fold using an electrosurgical blade. The round ligament will be identified during this dissection and separately divided.

❺ Vesicouterine Dissection. The anterior broad ligament dissection is continued with a right-angle clamp guiding the electrosurgical blade (Fig. 44-15.3). The peritoneum is typically edematous and thick. En bloc removal of tumor implants within the vesicouterine fold will require a wide excision of the peritoneum over the dome of the bladder. Thus, the proxi-

mal end of the vesicouterine fold may be held on traction, and an electrosurgical blade used to sharply dissect in a caudal direction toward the cervix while encompassing the tumor. The bladder mucosa is typically not entered, but it may be simply repaired if an inadvertent cystotomy occurs (Chap. 40, p. 1011). After incorporating the peritoneal vesicouterine

tumor into the specimen, the bladder may then be advanced distally in the usual manner as for simple hysterectomy. The ureters are held laterally while the uterine vessels are freed of surrounding connective tissue (skeletonized), clamped, cut, and ligated.

❻ Dividing the Sigmoid. The ureters are held laterally while a right-angle clamp guides electrosurgical blade dissection of the posterior peritoneum to the sigmoid mesentery. The sigmoid segment that lies proximal to the tumor is selected, and the underlying mesentery is superficially incised on each side with the electrosurgical blade. A GIA stapler is inserted to divide the bowel. The remaining mesentery is scored superficially with the electrosurgical blade and divided with the LDS (small pedicles) or electrothermal bipolar coagulator. Larger pedicles, such as those including the inferior mesenteric vessels, will need to be clamped, cut, and ligated separately. As during total pelvic exenteration, the avascular retrorectal space between the rectum and the sacrum may then be bluntly dissected to completely mobilize the rectosigmoid down to the cervix (Fig. 44-15.4).

❼ Retrograde Hysterectomy. The bladder is advanced distally onto the upper vagina with sharp electrosurgical blade dissection. The distal anterior vaginal wall is grasped with a Kocher clamp. The anterior vaginal wall is then incised at 12 o'clock with the electrosurgical blade, and the incision is extended

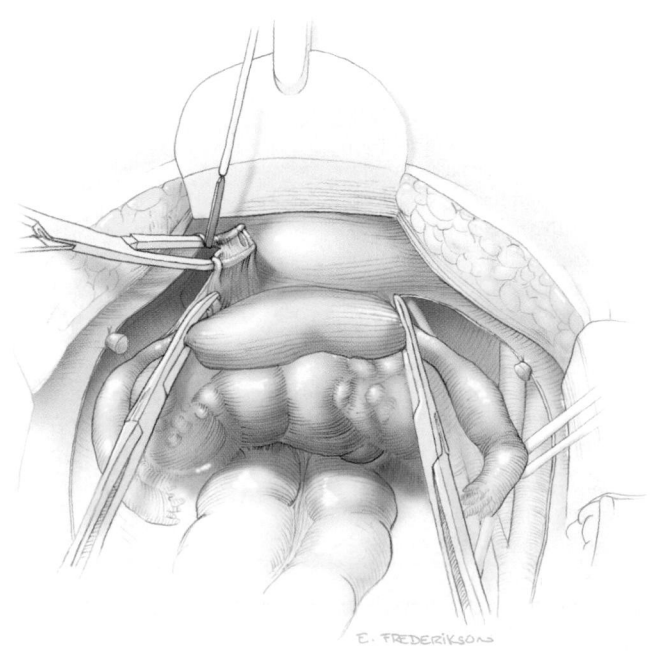

FIGURE 44-15.3 Vesicouterine dissection.

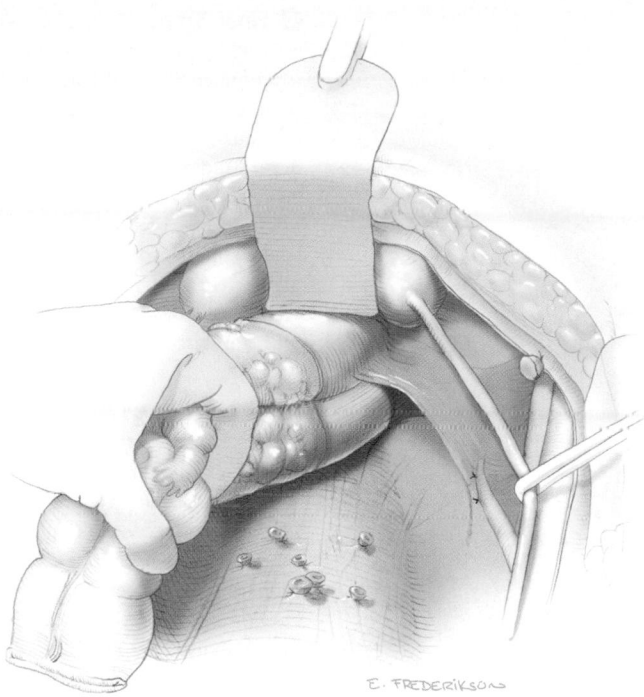

FIGURE 44-15.4 Rectosigmoid divided and mobilized.

laterally to the right and left. The cervix is grasped with a Kocher clamp and retracted to expose the posterior vaginal wall. An electrosurgical blade is used to incise this wall transversely and enter the rectovaginal space. An Allis clamp is used to grasp the en bloc specimen side of the upper vagina to apply caudad traction and aid further dissection. A retrorectal hand is placed to assess whether the tumor extends into the rectovaginal septum beyond the cervix. With large masses, distal dissection may be required into the rectovaginal septum to reach a point distal to the tumor's leading edge. Alternatively, smaller tumors may allow proximal dissection in the rectovaginal septum. This gains additional rectal length distal to the tumor and allows for creation of a higher colon reanastomosis. Finally, the remaining uterosacral and cardinal ligaments are clamped, analogous to a radical hysterectomy (Section 44-1, p. 1259), but in a retrograde fashion while confirming lateral ureteral positioning (Fig. 44-15.5).

❽ **Distal Rectal Division.** The mucosa of the rectal segment distal to the tumor is circumferentially dissected free of mesenteric attachments and rectal pillars by constant traction on the en bloc specimen (Fig. 44-15.6). The TA or contour cutting (Contour) stapler is inserted into the pelvis and fired to transect the rectum. The specimen, which contains the uterus, adnexa, rectosigmoid, and surrounding peritoneum, is then lifted out of the pelvis. The vaginal opening is closed in a running fashion with 0-gauge delayed-absorbable suture. The final appearance Figure 44-15.7 is shown with completed rectosigmoid anastomosis, which is described in Section 44-23 (p. 1327).

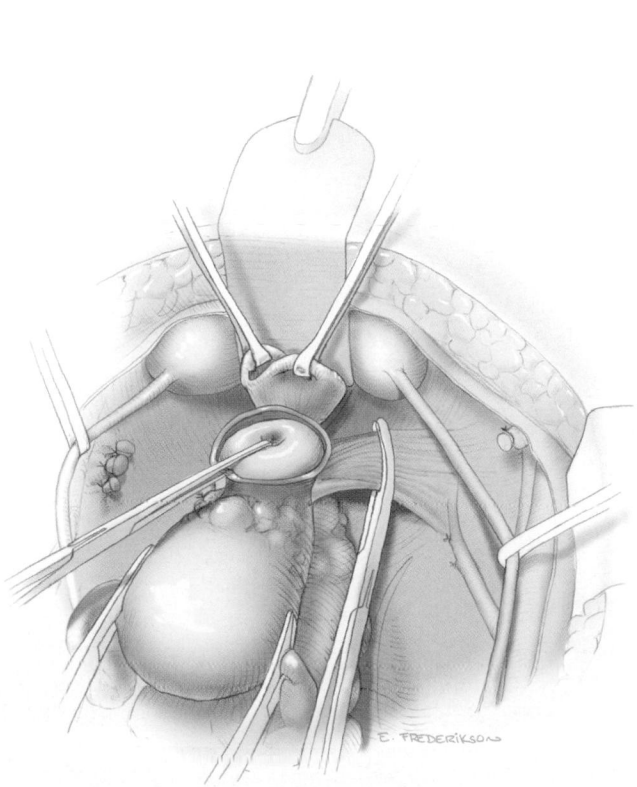

FIGURE 44-15.5 Retrograde hysterectomy.

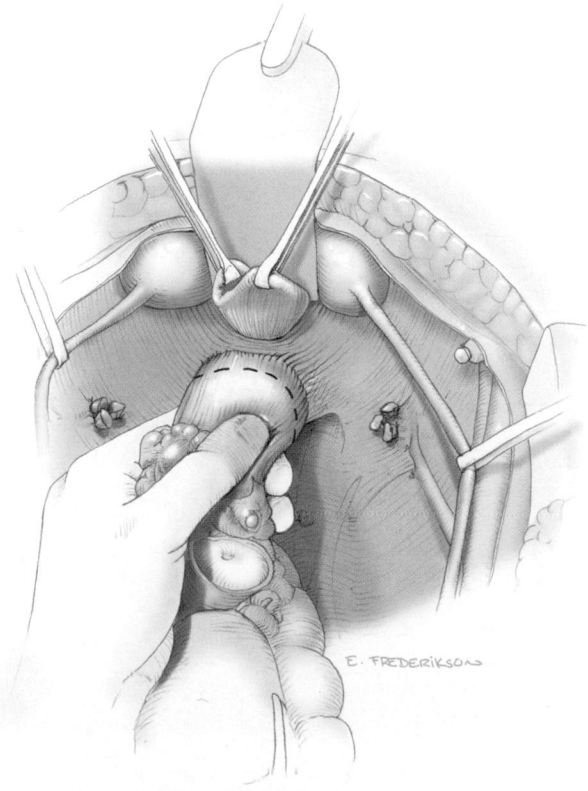

FIGURE 44-15.6 Rectosigmoid resection.

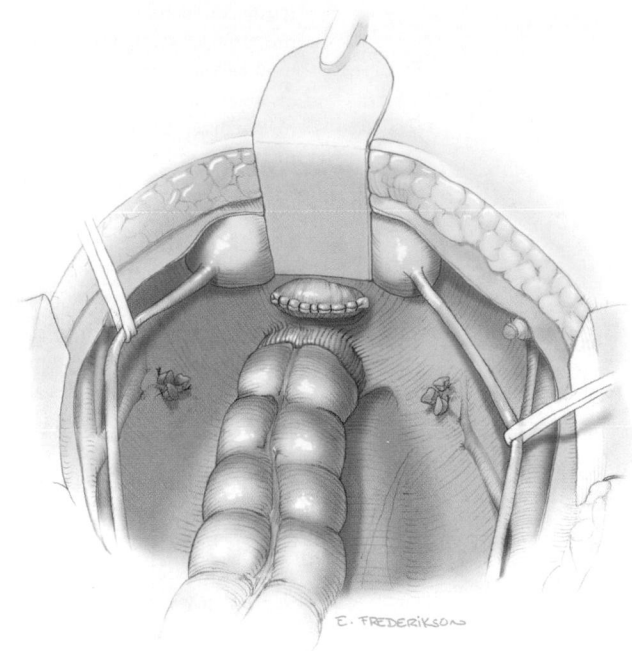

FIGURE 44-15.7 Final appearance.

❾ Final Steps. A surgeon will then proceed with additional procedures if necessary to complete the ovarian cancer debulking surgery. A colostomy or rectosigmoid anastomosis may require mobilization of the splenic flexure and is performed near the end of surgery. Postoperative drains may be placed at the surgeon's discretion. Occasionally, the bladder may also require testing to exclude inadvertent injury during vesicouterine dissection. All pedicle sites should be reexamined for hemostasis.

POSTOPERATIVE

En bloc pelvic resection of primary and recurrent ovarian cancer permits a high rate of complete debulking with acceptable morbidity and mortality rates (Park, 2006). Urinary tract infection, pneumonia, deep-vein thrombosis, wound cellulitis, and postoperative ileus are relatively common events following major abdominal surgery for ovarian cancer. Reoperation for anastomotic breakdown or postoperative hemorrhage specific to en bloc pelvic resection is uncommon (Bristow, 2003; Clayton, 2002).

44-16

Omentectomy

The omentum is typically removed for two reasons: tumor debulking or cancer staging. Patients who present with advanced ovarian cancer almost invariably have metastases to the omentum. The extent of this "omental cake" is often difficult to appreciate on imaging studies, and a tumor may be massive and involve the upper gastrocolic ligament, anterior abdominal wall, splenic hilum, and transverse colon (Fig. 35-16, p. 868). Thus, a surgeon should be prepared to encompass the entire tumor with an adequate resection.

Omentectomy is also routinely indicated for staging patients with ovarian cancer or with uterine papillary serous carcinoma who do not have obvious metastatic disease (Boruta, 2009; Greer, 2011b; Whitney, 2010). Infracolic (below the transverse colon) omentectomy is sufficient for most clinical circumstances. However, supracolic (total) omentectomy may be indicated for a large omental cake.

PREOPERATIVE

Patient Evaluation

Imaging studies may suggest the presence of an omental cake, but the extent is difficult to ascertain until exploration in the operating room.

Consent

Although bleeding may follow inadequate vessel ligation, complications from omentectomy are rare. Obesity and intraabdominal adhesive disease, however, may increase these risks. Obesity results in a much thicker omentum that has thicker vascular pedicles, which may slip from clamps or ligatures. Additionally, prior upper abdominal surgery—particularly gastric bypass—may cause adhesions and a more difficult resection. In addition to these risks, women with an omental cake should be informed of a possible need for bowel resection, splenectomy, or other radical debulking procedures to remove the entire tumor.

Patient Preparation

Bowel preparation should be performed when an omental cake is present due to the possibility of colon resection. The risk of infection following omentectomy is low, however, this surgery is typically performed with other gynecologic procedures that warrant antibiotic prophylaxis. Thromboprophylaxis is administered as outlined in Table 39-9 (p. 962).

INTRAOPERATIVE

SURGICAL STEPS

❶ Anesthesia and Patient Positioning. Omentectomy is typically performed as an inpatient procedure under general anesthesia. A patient is positioned supine, a Foley catheter is placed, and the abdomen is surgically prepared. The vaginal is also surgically prepared if concurrent hysterectomy is planned.

❷ Abdominal Entry. Infracolic omentectomy may be performed through any type of incision. However, because of the uncertain extent of disease that accompanies these cases, a midline vertical incision is most commonly selected. If only a portion of the omentum needs to be removed for staging purposes, the incision does not necessarily need to be extended above the umbilicus since the omentum is often accessible. In all other situations, the incision should be extended upward to provide sufficient exposure.

❸ Exploration. Palpation of the omentum is often the first step in exploring the abdomen. This organ is directly beneath a midline vertical incision and should be readily visible. Omentectomy is typically the first procedure performed in women with an omental cake and presumed ovarian cancer. The omentum can usually be quickly removed and sent for frozen section analysis while a surgeon places a self-retaining retractor and proceeds with the remainder of the planned operation.

❹ Visualization. A surgeon gently grasps the infracolic omentum and pulls it out of the abdomen through the incision. The borders of any omental cake can be seen directly or palpated. The extent of resection can then be determined, and the abdominal wall incision extended if necessary.

❺ Entrance into the Lesser Sac. The posterior leaf of the omentum is attached to the transverse colon primarily by filmy adventitial tissue with some intervening small vessel tributaries. The filmy attachments can be electrosurgically cut and vessels divided by the ligate-divide-staple (LDS) device or an electrothermal bipolar coagulator (LigaSure) to enter the lesser sac (Fig. 44-16.1). Dissection generally begins as far to the right as possible and continues as far to the left as possible. A right-angle clamp is opened beneath the omentum to guide the direction of the electrosurgical blade.

Entrance into the lesser sac mobilizes the colon and provides access to the tumor free proximal gastrocolic ligament. The omentum is then flipped over and held on distal traction.

❻ Gastrocolic Ligament Division. Dissection generally again begins on the far right. Numerous vertically coursing vessels can be

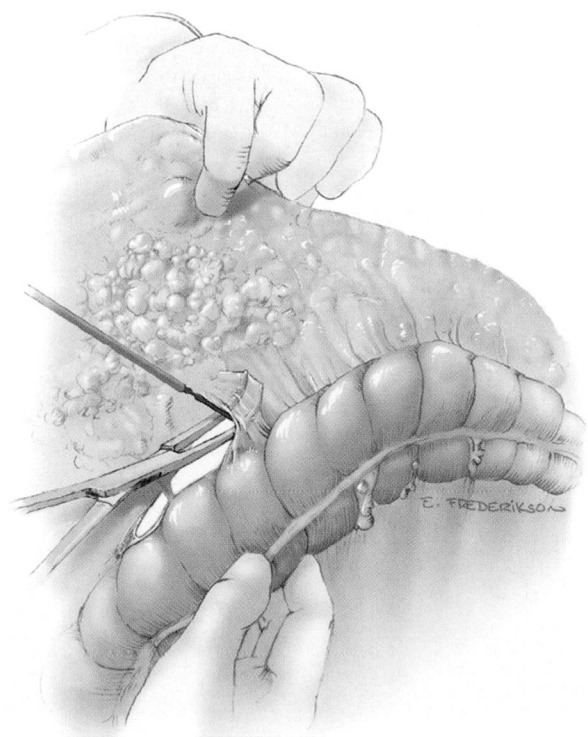

FIGURE 44-16.1 Posterior dissection to enter the lesser sac.

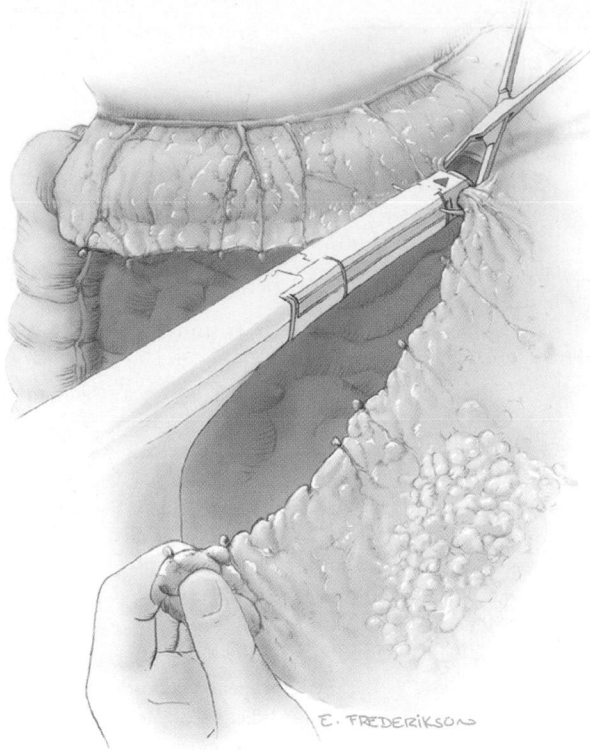

E. FREDERIKSON

FIGURE 44-16.2 Anterior ligation of gastrocolic ligament.

seen, but others are covered by fatty tissue and difficult to appreciate. A right-angle clamp is used by the surgeon to "pop" through an avascular portion of the gastrocolic ligament that is near, but safely distal to the colon. The clamp is then opened in a vertical direction (parallel to the vessels) and held in place to guide the LDS or electrothermal bipolar coagulator in safely and quickly dividing the tissue (Fig. 44-16.2).

This procedure is continued across the entire gastrocolic ligament, and the omental specimen is handed off. However, if a J-flap is being constructed instead of complete omentum resection, then only three-quarters

of the omentum is divided from right to left, to preserve the left gastroepiploic artery. The distal tip of the flap is brought into the pelvis and tacked to adjoining peritoneum with 2-0 or 3-0 gauge delayed-absorbable suture to provide additional blood supply wherever desired. Regardless of whether removing the infracolic omentum or fashioning a J-flap, it will need to be rotated back and forth intermittently to make certain that dissection remains away from the colon.

❼ Total Omentectomy. In cases in which an omental cake has extended proximally,

supracolic (total) omentectomy is indicated. This procedure requires a midline vertical incision to provide better exposure to the upper abdomen. Resection may simply involve transecting the omentum at a higher level in the gastrocolic ligament. Alternatively, anatomic boundaries of resection may need to be extended to the hepatic flexure, the stomach, and the splenic flexure to encompass the entire tumor.

Dissection again proceeds from right to left. Mobilization of the ascending colon around the hepatic flexure may be necessary. The right gastroepiploic artery is ligated, and the dissection is continued to the left by dividing the short gastric vessels until the lateralmost portion of the tumor is reached. Mobilization of the descending colon and takedown of the splenic flexure may be required if tumor extends that far laterally. The omentum is then detached from the transverse colon across the remaining gastrocolic ligament.

❽ Incision Closure. The remaining omentum should be reexamined at the completion of surgery before closing the abdomen. Occasionally, small bleeding vessels or a hematoma will need to be addressed with additional ligation. The abdominal entry incision is then closed as described in Section 41-1 (p. 1021).

POSTOPERATIVE

Nasogastric tube placement is only required if a total omentectomy has been performed. Decompression of the stomach for 48 hours protects the ligated gastric vessels from postoperative dislodgement due to gastric dilation. The remaining postoperative course follows that for laparotomy or for other specific concurrent surgeries performed.

44-17

Splenectomy

In gynecologic oncology, removal of the spleen is occasionally required to achieve optimal surgical cytoreduction of metastatic ovarian cancer (Magtibay, 2006). Most commonly, tumor is found directly extending from the omentum into the splenic hilum during primary debulking surgery. Splenectomy and other extensive upper abdominal resection techniques have been shown to improve survival with acceptable morbidity (Chi, 2010; Eisenhauer, 2006). However, the number of patients who will actually have their spleen removed during their initial operation ranges from 1 to 14 percent (Eisenkop, 2006; Goff, 2006). Splenectomy is also indicated for selected patients with isolated parenchymal recurrences to assist optimal secondary surgical cytoreduction of ovarian cancer (Manci, 2006). In some instances, a laparoscopic or hand-assisted approach may be possible (Chi, 2006). Lastly, intraoperative splenic trauma is the least common indication and often is unanticipated (Magtibay, 2006).

PREOPERATIVE

Patient Evaluation

Preoperative diagnosis of splenic involvement is often difficult to predict with certainty prior to primary cytoreduction. Typically, in such cases, an omental cake is seen on CT scan, but its proximity to the spleen is difficult to ascertain. Splenic involvement is more commonly distinguishable at the time of secondary cytoreduction. Ideally, relapsed patients have isolated disease and have had an extended progression-free survival of at least 12 months before they are considered for splenectomy.

Consent

Patients with presumed advanced ovarian cancer should provide consent for possible splenectomy, although the decision to perform the procedure will only be finalized intraoperatively. Removal of the spleen results in a longer operative time, greater blood loss, and longer hospital stay, but may ultimately determine whether tumor is optimally debulked or not (Eisenkop, 2006). Possible serious complications include hemorrhage, infection, and pancreatitis.

INTRAOPERATIVE

SURGICAL STEPS

❶ Anesthesia and Patient Positioning. Splenectomy is performed under general anesthesia and with the patient supine. As with other major intraabdominal surgery, the abdomen is surgically prepared, and a Foley catheter is inserted. The vaginal is also surgically prepared if concurrent hysterectomy is planned.

❷ Abdominal Entry and Exploration. During laparotomy, splenectomy requires a vertical incision for adequate exposure. Following entry, a surgeon should carefully assess the entire abdomen and pelvis to confirm the ability to resect all gross disease. Ideally, splenectomy is only performed if optimal tumor debulking can thereby be achieved. The spleen is grasped to assess its mobility, degree of tumor involvement, and potential difficulty in removal.

❸ Entrance into the Lesser Sac. The gastrocolic ligament is opened to the left of midline by dividing vascular pedicles as described in Section 44-16 (p. 1313). Dissection is continued in two directions: (1) along the superior transverse colon with mobilization of the entire splenic flexure to reach the splenocolic ligament and (2) upward to the greater curvature of the stomach toward the gastrosplenic ligament (Fig. 44-17.1). The intervening portion of omentum is often involved with tumor.

❹ Mobilization of the Spleen. The spleen is grasped, elevated, and pulled medially to expose the splenophrenic ligament. A surgeon uses alternating electrosurgical blade and blunt finger dissection to further mobilize the spleen. Additional blunt and sharp dissection is then performed circumferentially to free the spleen from the gastrosplenic and splenocolic ligaments. To avoid pancreatic injury, it is important to continually review the anatomy.

❺ Ligating the Splenic Vessels. The spleen is elevated into the incision, and the peritoneum overlying the splenic hilum is carefully incised. To aid this approach, a left index finger is held against the spleen. The pancreatic tail, which lies close to the splenic hilum (often within 1 cm), is displaced medially with the left thumb.

Blunt dissection parallel to the expected course of the splenic artery and vein aids identification of these vessels. The artery, vein, and vascular tributaries should be individually ligated. The artery is first isolated to prevent splenic engorgement (Fig. 44-17.2). A right-angle clamp is placed beneath the artery, and a 2-0 silk suture is pulled through and tied. A second silk tie is placed more distally, directly at the hilum. The proximal end of the artery is again tied or occluded with a vascular clip. The artery is then divided, and the procedure is repeated for the splenic vein. Vascular tributaries should be similarly divided. The remaining peritoneal attachments

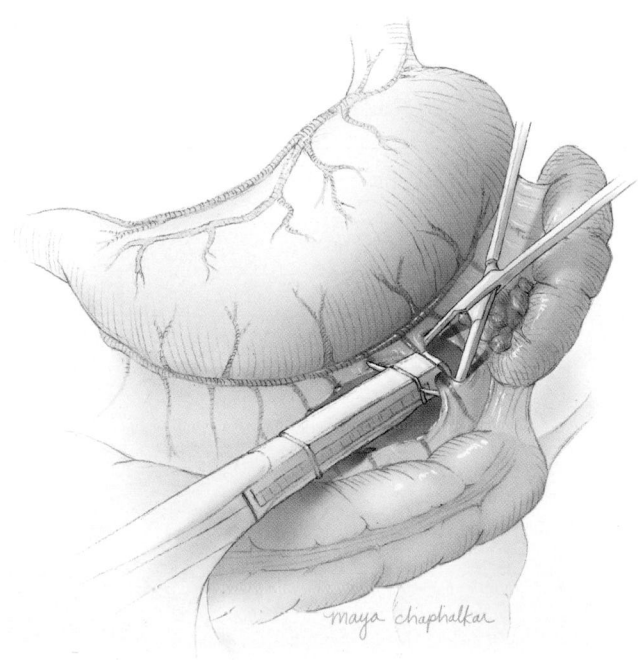

FIGURE 44-17.1 Mobilizing the spleen.

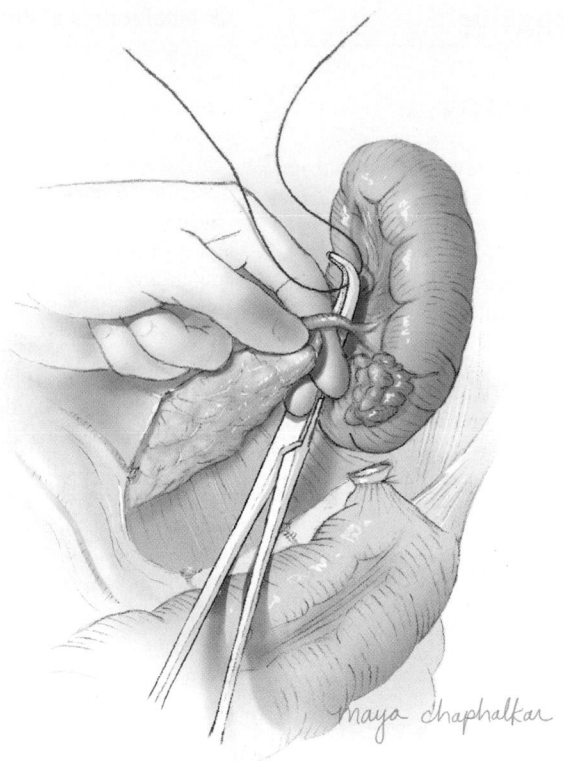

FIGURE 44-17.2 Vessel ligation.

are incised with the electrosurgical blade to remove the spleen.

❻ Final Steps. The distal pancreas should be carefully inspected to exclude injury. The splenic vessels should also be reexamined prior to abdominal closure. Suspicion of pancreatic trauma or bleeding should prompt placement of a suction drain in the splenic bed. Otherwise, drainage is not routinely required.

A nasogastric tube is placed to decompress the stomach and prevent displacement of gastric vessel staples.

POSTOPERATIVE

Hemorrhage is the most serious immediate complication and typically originates from the short gastric or splenic vessels. Bleeding from either site can be profuse and potentially catastrophic. Thus, the initial 12 to 24 postoperative hours require particular vigilance (Magtibay, 2006).

The most common postoperative "complication" is left lower lobe lung atelectasis. This will typically resolve with ambulation, pulmonary therapy, and time. Development of a postoperative intraabdominal abscess usually results from inadvertent injury to the stomach, splenic flexure, or distal pancreas.

Excessive pancreatic manipulation or laceration may lead to pancreatitis or leaking. When a distal pancreatectomy is required due to tumor adherence or injury, approximately one quarter of patients will develop a pancreatic leak. According to one set of criteria, this leak is defined by a left upper quadrant collection of fluid seen on imaging after postoperative day 3, and this fluid contains an amylase level >3 times that of serum amylase. If a drain has been placed, fluid may be sent to the laboratory if this complication is suspected. Pancreatic leak usually presents early in the postoperative period and can be managed conservatively with percutaneous drainage (Kehoe, 2009).

Patients undergoing splenectomy will be at lifelong risk for episodes of overwhelming sepsis. Accordingly, the pneumococcal and meningococcal vaccines are recommended, and the *Haemophilus influenzae* type b vaccine should be considered postoperatively (Centers for Disease Control and Prevention, 2010). Importantly, these vaccines may be given together but should not be administered earlier than 14 days following splenectomy. In addition, patients should be instructed to seek immediate medical attention for fevers that may rapidly progress to serious illness.

44-18

Diaphragmatic Surgery

Patients with advanced ovarian cancer will often have tumor implants or confluent plaques involving the diaphragm. The right hemidiaphragm is most frequently affected. Implants are typically superficial, but invasive disease can extend through the peritoneum to the underlying muscle. Accordingly, gynecologic oncologists should be prepared to perform diaphragmatic ablation, stripping (peritonectomy), or full-thickness resection. These surgical procedures increase the rate of optimal tumor debulking and correlate with improved survival (Aletti, 2006a; Tsolakidis, 2010).

PREOPERATIVE

Patient Evaluation

Imaging studies may suggest diaphragmatic nodularity, but the extent is difficult to ascertain until exploration in the operating room.

Consent

Patients with presumed advanced ovarian cancer should be informed of the possible need for extensive upper abdominal surgery to achieve optimal cytoreduction. Pulmonary complications after diaphragmatic surgical techniques most commonly include atelectasis and/or pleural effusion. However, empyema, subphrenic abscess, and pneumothorax are also possible (Chereau, 2011; Cliby, 2004).

INTRAOPERATIVE

Instruments

It is generally advisable to have a cavitational ultrasonic surgical aspiration (CUSA) system and/or argon beam coagulator (ABC) available for ovarian cancer debulking procedures, since one or both can be useful in eradicating diaphragmatic disease. These tools are discussed further in Chapter 40 (p. 1001).

SURGICAL STEPS

❶ Anesthesia and Patient Positioning. As with other major intraabdominal surgeries, diaphragmatic surgery requires general anesthesia. The patient is positioned supine, the abdomen is surgically prepared to accommodate an incision to the sternum,

and a Foley catheter is inserted. The vagina is also surgically prepared if concurrent hysterectomy is planned.

❷ Abdominal Entry. Diaphragmatic surgery requires a vertical midline incision that has been extended to the sternum, passing to the right side of xiphoid process, for maximum exposure. Following abdominal entry, a surgeon should carefully assess the entire abdomen and pelvis to confirm the ability to resect all gross disease. Ideally, diaphragmatic surgery is only performed if optimal tumor debulking can thereby be achieved.

❸ Diaphragmatic Ablation. A few scattered, small tumor implants on the surface of the right or left hemidiaphragm can usually be easily ablated with the CUSA or ABC. This simple technique may be all that is required.

❹ Diaphragmatic Stripping. Confluent plaques of tumor or extensive implants indicate the need for resection of the peritoneum. For this, the right side of the anterior rib cage is retracted sharply upward. The liver is manually retracted downward and medially to aid division of the falciform ligament with electrosurgical blade, ligate-divide-staple device (LDS), and/or electrothermal bipolar coagulator (LigaSure). This maneuver significantly mobilizes the liver and allows it to be held medially away from the diaphragm.

Allis clamps are used to grasp the peritoneum above the tumor plaque and place it on tension. The peritoneal incision is created transversely above the tumor with an electrosurgical blade, and a plane is developed with blunt dissection to separate the peritoneum

from the underlying muscle fibers of the diaphragm. The free peritoneal edge is placed on tension with Allis clamps to maintain traction. The incision is then extended medially and laterally to encompass the implants (Fig. 44-18.1). The specimen eventually becomes large enough to grasp with a left hand to aid "stripping" of the peritoneum off the diaphragm. Electrosurgical blade dissection proceeds dorsally until all implants are contained within the peritoneal specimen. At this point, it can be detached.

❺ Diaphragmatic Resection. Occasionally, tumor has penetrated through the peritoneum, and a plane cannot be developed to strip the diaphragm. In these circumstances, full-thickness diaphragmatic resection is required. A self-retaining retractor is placed, and the liver mobilized. A transverse peritoneal incision is made above the tumor plaque, and at this point, the inadequacy of stripping is determined.

The ventilator is temporarily turned off to avoid lung parenchymal injury, and an electrosurgical blade is used to cut through the diaphragmatic muscle into the pleural cavity above the tumor. Ventilation may then be resumed while Allis clamps are placed to retract the specimen into the peritoneal cavity. Both pleural and peritoneal surfaces should be visible to aid complete resection of the disease. Primary mass closure of the diaphragmatic defect is then performed with a running stitch using 0-gauge PDS suture or interrupted stitches of silk suture.

To evacuate the pneumothorax, a red rubber catheter is placed through the defect into the pleural space prior to securing the final

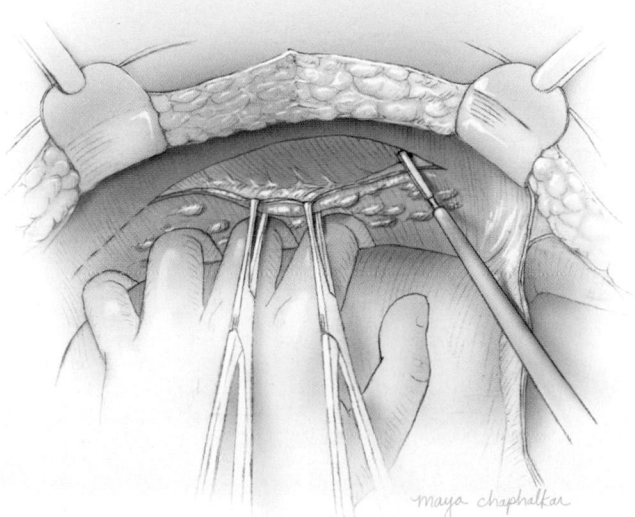

FIGURE 44-18.1 Diaphragm stripping.

knot. The ventilator is turned off at the end of inspiration to maximally inflate the lungs while the catheter is placed on suction. The catheter is removed concomitantly with tying the knot, and mechanical ventilation is resumed (Bashir, 2010). Grafts are not typically needed, even for large defects (Silver, 2004).

❻ Final Steps. The patient should be placed in Trendelenburg position at the completion of stripping or resection to check the integrity of the diaphragmatic closure. The upper abdomen is filled with saline and observed for air leaks as the patient is ventilated. The presence of air bubbles indicates the need to reintroduce the red rubber catheter through the hole, resuture the defect, and retest the closure. Chest tubes are not routinely required.

POSTOPERATIVE

Atelectasis is common with any diaphragmatic surgery, and routine postoperative respiratory expansion techniques are appropriate (Chap. 39, p. 950). Diaphragmatic stripping is associated with an increased incidence of pleural effusion, especially when the pleural space is entered. Fortunately, most will self-resolve, and only a few will require postoperative thoracentesis (Dowdy, 2008). Patients having full-thickness diaphragmatic resection should be carefully monitored with chest radiographs for evidence of a pneumo- or hemothorax. Those few who do not resolve with supportive care measures may require chest tube drainage to aid lung reexpansion (Bashir, 2010).

44-19

Colostomy

A colostomy is a surgical anastomosis between created openings in the colon and anterior abdominal wall to divert bowel contents into an external collection bag. Colostomies serve several purposes and may be used: (1) to protect distal bowel repair from disruption or contamination by feces, (2) to decompress an obstructed colon, and (3) to evacuate feces if the distal colon or rectum is excised. In gynecologic oncology, there are innumerable specific indications for performing a colostomy. Some of the more common reasons include rectovaginal fistula, severe radiation proctosigmoiditis, bowel perforation, and rectosigmoid resection in which reanastomosis is not feasible.

A colostomy may be temporary or permanent, and its duration is dictated by clinical circumstances. For instance, recurrent end-stage cervical cancer with obstruction may warrant a permanent colostomy. In contrast, only temporary diversion is needed to allow healing of an intraoperative bowel injury that occurred during benign gynecologic surgery.

In addition, the location of the stoma and the decision to perform an end or loop colostomy are also clinically based. A loop colostomy is constructed by creating an opening in a loop of colon and bringing both ends through the stoma. Alternatively, an end colostomy stoma contains only the proximal end of the transected colon. The distal end is stapled and left intraabdominally.

Regardless of the circumstances, the same surgical principles apply during colostomy: adequate bowel mobilization, sufficient blood supply, and a tension-free tunnel through the abdominal wall without bowel constriction. Strict attention to these seemingly straightforward steps will ensure the best possible outcome. In some circumstances, a laparoscopic colostomy may be possible (Jandial, 2008).

PREOPERATIVE

Patient Evaluation

The colostomy site, typically on the patient's left, is ideally marked preoperatively by an enterostomal therapist to ensure that the postoperative stoma will be located in an easily accessible area when sitting and standing.

Consent

Concerns regarding postoperative quality-of-life changes are common with this procedure. Accordingly, a surgeon should carefully describe a colostomy's medical purpose and its expected temporary or permanent duration. Much of the fear regarding "wearing a bag" can be assuaged with compassionate preoperative counseling and education. Many times, postoperative results are actually superior to a patient's current symptoms and quality of life.

Perioperative complications may include fecal leakage into the abdomen or retraction of the stoma. Long-term complications involve parastomal hernia, stricture, and the potential need for surgical revision.

Patient Preparation

To minimize fecal contamination during bowel incision, aggressive bowel preparation such as with a polyethylene glycol with electrolyte solution (GoLytely) may be performed the day prior to surgery unless contraindicated, such as with bowel obstruction or perforation. Broad spectrum antibiotics are given perioperatively due to the possibility of stool contamination of the operative site. Also, thromboprophylaxis is administered as outlined in Table 39-9 (p. 962).

INTRAOPERATIVE

SURGICAL STEPS

❶ **Anesthesia and Patient Positioning.** Colostomy is performed under general anesthesia with the patient positioned supine. Prior to surgery, the abdomen is surgically prepared, and a Foley catheter is inserted. The vaginal is also surgically prepared if concurrent hysterectomy is planned.

❷ **Abdominal Entry and Exploration.** Although concurrent surgery may dictate the approach, a midline vertical incision, due to its superior exposure, is generally preferred when colostomy is a possibility. The bowel segment is selected as distally as possible. Dissection and adhesiolysis are performed as necessary to mobilize the bowel to obtain sufficient length before creating the abdominal wall stoma opening. The colon is elevated to ensure that it will reach the selected stoma site without tension. If the bowel fails to reach the selected site without tension despite maximal mobilization, then the proposed stoma site is moved to accommodate the available bowel length.

❸ **End Colostomy.** This type of diversion is commonly used for rectovaginal fistulas and severe proctosigmoiditis after radiation. Ideally, a more distal colon site is used since bowel content becomes progressively more solid and less voluminous as it moves from the cecum to the rectum. As a result, the ostomy bag does not need to be changed as often, and the risk of dehydration or electrolyte abnormalities is reduced. If performing an end sigmoid colostomy, the distal bowel may simply be stapled closed and left in the pelvis (Hartmann pouch). In contrast, a more proximal end colostomy will require that the distal bowel also be brought to the abdominal wall and opened, either at the same site or as a second ostomy that serves as a "mucus fistula" to prevent a closed loop obstruction and subsequent colonic perforation.

The stoma site for a sigmoid colostomy is selected based on an imaginary line drawn from the umbilicus to the left-sided anterior superior iliac spine. The site should be lateral enough from the midline to allow application of the ostomy appliance. A Kocher clamp is used to elevate the skin and an electrosurgical blade, set to a cutting mode, is used to remove a 3-cm circle of skin. The fascia is exposed by blunt dissection. In obese patients, a cone of subcutaneous fat may need to be removed to prevent bowel constriction. A cruciate incision is made on the anterior rectus sheath. The fibers of the rectus abdominis muscle are bluntly separated, and another cruciate incision is cut on the posterior rectus sheath. The opening is bluntly expanded to accommodate two to three fingers.

After the colon is divided as described in Section 44-23, step 5 (p. 1327), the proximal bowel should be mobilized by incising the peritoneum toward the splenic flexure along the white line of Toldt, which is the reflection of posterior abdominal parietal peritoneum over the mesentery of the descending colon. A Babcock clamp is then placed through the skin opening to grasp the stapled end of the bowel and lift it through the abdominal opening (Fig. 44-19.1). The bowel should appear pink, and its mesentery must not be twisted. The primary vertical abdominal incision is then closed.

The stoma is "matured" by first tilting the table to the left to minimize bowel spillage and fecal contamination of the incision site and then excising the intestinal staple line. Circumferential interrupted 3-0 and 4-0 gauge delayed-absorbable sutures are placed through the bowel mucosa and skin dermis (Fig. 44-19.2). The ostomy bag appliance may then be attached.

❹ **Loop Colostomy.** The usual indications for this type of procedure include protection of a distal anastomosis, relief of colonic obstruction, and colonic perforation. Accordingly, loop colostomy can be performed at any site along the colon where indicated. A loop colostomy in general is intended to be a temporary or palliative procedure. It is easier to take down, often simpler to perform, and does not necessarily require

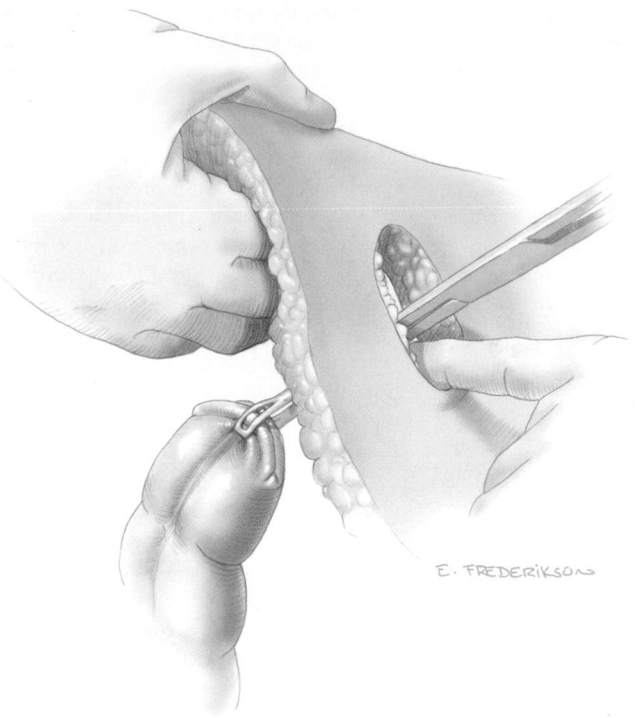

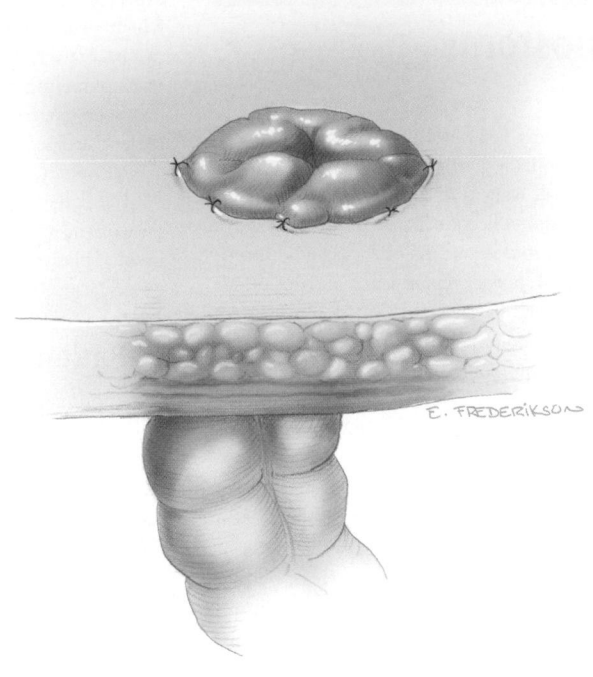

FIGURE 44-19.1 End-sigmoid colostomy: bowel pulled through abdominal wall incision.

FIGURE 44-19.2 End-sigmoid colostomy: bowel mucosa sutured to skin.

designation of loops as distal or proximal. However, fecal matter will eventually pass through to the distal segment. As a result, this type of colostomy is not a permanent solution to a fistula or proctosigmoiditis.

❺ Transverse Loop Colostomy. This colostomy is performed in the left upper quadrant by creating a 5-cm transverse incision over the rectus abdominis muscle midway between the costal margin and the umbilicus. The anterior and posterior fascia, rectus abdominis muscle, and peritoneum are opened longitudinally by sharp and blunt dissection. The omentum is separated from the underlying transverse colon for enough length that the bowel segment can be pulled up through the incision without it. Next, a one-quarter inch Penrose drain is placed through the mesocolon for traction, and the bowel loop is brought through the incision (Fig. 44-19.3). A Hollister bridge or similar device is passed through the mesenterotomy in place of the Penrose drain. The incision is then closed around the bowel loop without constricting it.

The bowel is then "matured" by opening the antimesenteric half of the bowel along the taenia with an electrosurgical blade and leaving a 1-cm margin on each end (Fig. 44-19.4). The colostomy edges are

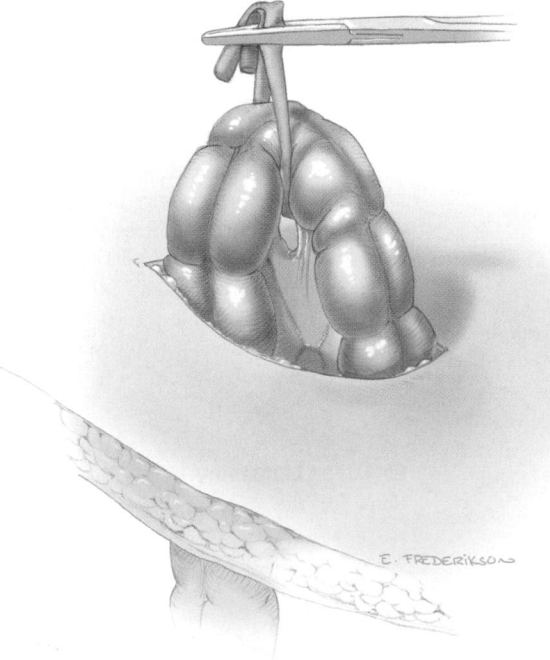

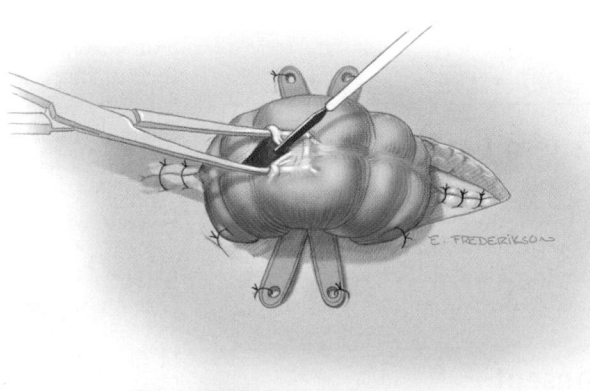

FIGURE 44-19.3 Transverse loop colostomy: elevation of bowel segment.

FIGURE 44-19.4 Transverse loop colostomy: opening of the bowel.

sutured to the skin with interrupted stitches of 3-0 gauge delayed-absorbable suture.

❻ Final Steps. The stoma should be carefully inspected. Ideally, a stoma is pink and comfortably positioned. A dusky color may indicate bowel ischemia, which can lead to sloughing, necrosis, and retraction. Tension on the bowel may be improved with additional mobilization. Constriction of a loop colostomy within the abdominal wall opening can be improved by broadening the fascial incision or removing additional subcutaneous fat. With end colostomy, on occasion, the tip may need to be transected further distally to reach a viable bowel segment. All of these steps are cumbersome but are much easier to perform during the operation rather than postoperatively after complications have become obvious.

POSTOPERATIVE

Morbidity is comparable for end and loop colostomies (Segreti, 1996a). Complications may be immediate or not evident for several months. Common complications with colostomy creation may include wound infection, necrosis, bowel obstruction, hematoma, retraction, fistula, fecal leakage, sepsis, stricture, and parastomal herniation (Hoffman, 1992). Many of these complications are manageable with supportive care and local measures. Dramatic symptoms are infrequent, but may require operative revision. Careful attention during initial surgery will prevent most of these morbidities.

44-20

Large Bowel Resection

Partial colectomy is most often performed as part of cytoreductive surgery for ovarian cancer, although other indications include radiation injury and colonic fistulas. Surgical principles are similar, whether a bowel segment to be removed is from the ascending, transverse, or descending colon. Rectosigmoid (low anterior) resection is somewhat more complex and is reviewed in Section 44-23 (p. 1327). Ideally during colectomy, a surgeon will achieve meticulous hemostasis, remove the smallest required length of colon, avoid fecal spill, and confirm bowel continuity by excluding possible sites of proximal or distal intestinal obstruction. In addition, bowel must be sufficiently mobilized to create a tension-free anastomosis that is watertight, large caliber, and supported by adequate blood supply.

A general familiarity with colonic blood supply is important for partial colectomy. The ascending and transverse colon are supplied by the superior mesenteric artery via the middle colic, right colic, and ileocolic branches. The descending and sigmoid colon are supplied by the left colic and sigmoid branches of the inferior mesenteric artery. As a result, these vessels form an effective anastomotic vascular network that allows large bowel resection at virtually any segment of the colon.

PREOPERATIVE

Patient Evaluation

The need for partial colectomy during ovarian cancer cytoreductive surgery is usually decided intraoperatively and is based on clinical circumstances. For example, although preoperative computed tomography (CT) images may suggest tumor at multiple sites near the colon, these lesions are often superficial and may be removed without colectomy. Typically, the need for colectomy is more obvious preoperatively for those with radiation damage or fistula. However, the extent of the resection will still generally be unclear until the operation is underway.

Consent

Patients should be fully informed of the potential for colostomy, anastomotic leak, and abscess formation. A postoperative ileus should also be anticipated.

Patient Preparation

To minimize fecal contamination during bowel incision, most surgeons still recommend aggressive bowel preparation. One choice, a polyethylene glycol with electrolyte solution (GoLytely) is given the day prior to surgery unless contraindicated, such as with bowel obstruction or perforation. However, there is no evidence that patients benefit from this practice, and bowel preparation may not lower the risk of postoperative complications (Guenaga, 2009; Zhu, 2010). If a bowel obstruction is present, then cleansing only the distal colon with enemas is a secondary option. The patient should also be marked for a colostomy if that is a possibility. Moreover, if a complicated resection or prolonged recovery is anticipated, postoperative total parental nutrition (TPN) administration should be considered. Antibiotic prophylaxis may be initiated prior to creating the abdominal incision. Also, thromboprophylaxis is administered as outlined in Table 39-9 (p. 962).

INTRAOPERATIVE

Instruments

To prepare for complicated resections, a surgeon should have access to all types and sizes of bowel staplers. These include end-to-end anastomosis (EEA), gastrointestinal anastomosis (GIA), and transverse anastomosis (TA) staplers. Additionally, a ligate-divide-staple (LDS) device or electrothermal bipolar coagulator (LigaSure) may aid vessel ligation.

SURGICAL STEPS

❶ **Anesthesia and Patient Positioning.** Rectovaginal examination under anesthesia is mandatory before positioning any patient for abdominal gynecologic cancer surgery. A palpable mass with compression of the rectum or rectovaginal septum indicates the need for dorsal lithotomy with legs comfortably positioned in Allen stirrups to prepare for possible low anterior resection and anastomosis. Supine positioning is otherwise appropriate. Sterile preparation of the abdomen, perineum, and vagina is completed, and a Foley catheter is placed.

❷ **Abdominal Entry.** A midline vertical incision is preferable if partial colectomy is anticipated, as this incision provides access to the entire abdomen. Required dissection, adhesiolysis, or other unanticipated findings may render exposure from a transverse incision inadequate.

❸ **Exploration.** A surgeon should first explore the entire abdomen to lyse adhesions, to "run" the bowel and evaluate its appearance from duodenum to rectum, to exclude other potential sites of obstruction proximally or distally, and to determine the extent of the bowel resection. Blood supply at the splenic flexure, hepatic flexure, and ileocecal valve can be tenuous. As a result, resection boundaries should lie beyond these areas if possible. For example, in Figure 44-20.1, because of the known tenuous blood supply at the hepatic flexure, the proximal line of transection includes several centimeters of transverse

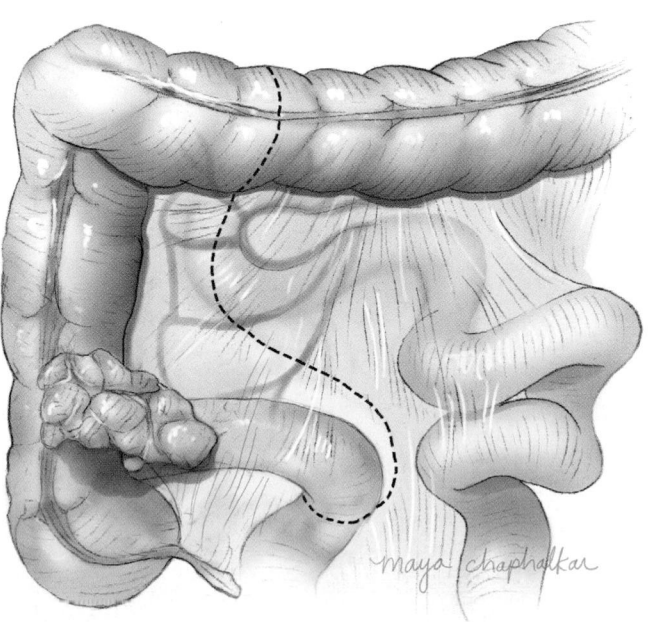

FIGURE 44-20.1 Area of resection is shown to encompass the tumor.

colon. Similarly, the distal line of transection includes 8 to 10 cm of the terminal ileum because the ileocecal artery is sacrificed.

A window is made in the mesocolon proximal and distal to the lesion. A one-quarter inch Penrose drain is pulled through each location's opening to provide traction.

❹ **Mobilization of the Colon.** The bowel is next mobilized by incising peritoneum along the white line of Toldt and/or along the hepatic or splenic flexures—depending on the resection site. The left or right retroperitoneal space is entered at a site beyond the distal Penrose drain. The entry opening is created with an electrosurgical blade just lateral to the colon. This space is bluntly expanded and electrosurgical dissection is guided cephalad past the proximal Penrose drain while providing countertraction on the colon. The bowel segment may be bluntly mobilized medially as necessary. Omentectomy may be required for resections involving the transverse colon.

❺ **Resection.** A GIA stapler is inserted to replace one Penrose drain, is positioned around the entire colon diameter, and is fired. This stapler lays two rows of staples and transects interposed bowel. A second stapling and transection is then repeated at the other Penrose drain site. The bowel segment may then be detached from the underlying mesentery using an LDS device, electrothermal bipolar coagulator, or individual clamps and 0-gauge delayed-absorbable suture ligation. During this process, as much of the mesentery as possible should be preserved to provide adequate blood supply to the anastomosis. The specimen is then removed.

❻ **"Side-to-Side" Anastomosis.** The proximal and distal bowel ends are held parallel against each other to estimate their position following anastomosis. Typically, additional mobilization of the bowel by incising adhesions and peritoneum is required using a combination of electrosurgical blade and blunt dissection. The two segments must comfortably approximate antimesenteric borders without tension. For larger resections, the mesentery of each segment may need to also be dissected to achieve sufficient mobility. The proximal and distal stapled bowel ends are skeletonized of fatty tissue to create an anastomosis with maximal mucosa-to-mucosa contact. To accomplish this, the proximal staple line is elevated with two Allis clamps at its lateral edges. DeBakey forceps grasp surrounding fatty tissue and place it on traction, while an electrosurgical blade is used to dissect this tissue away from the bowel serosa. The dissection is then performed on the distal segment in similar fashion.

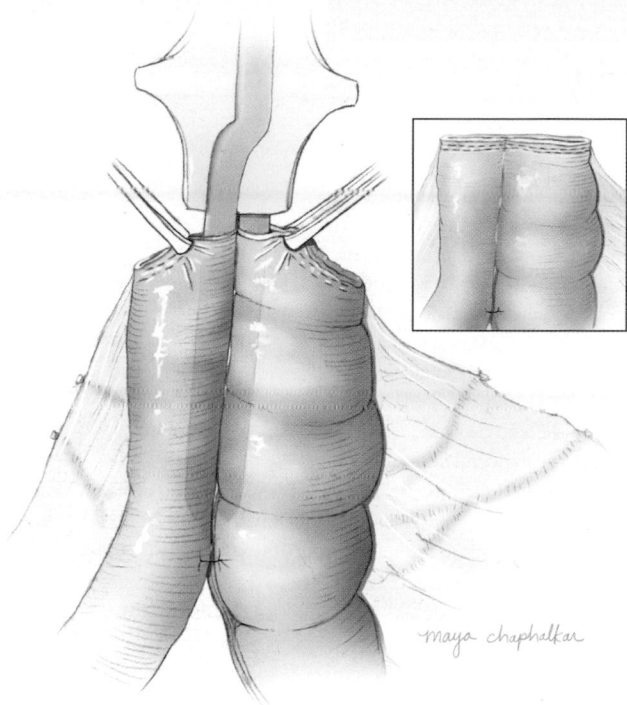

FIGURE 44-20.2 GIA stapler connects a side-to-side anastomosis of the ileum and transverse colon. **Inset:** TA stapler line closes the distal end of the anastomosis.

The antimesenteric tip of each staple line is excised with scissors, and the bowel is held vertically by Allis clamps to prevent fecal spill. One or two seromuscular silk stay sutures may be placed distally on each bowel end to help align the correct position and prevent slippage. One fork of the GIA stapler is then inserted as deeply as possible into each of the bowel lumens (Fig. 44-20.2). The bowel segments are evenly positioned, and the device is then fired along the antimesenteric surfaces and removed. This stapler places two staggered rows of titanium staples and simultaneously transects tissue between these rows.

The bowel interior should be examined for bleeding sites, which may be electrosurgically coagulated. The remaining opening may then be stapled across with a TA stapler, and residual bowel tissue above the TA staple line is excised. The mesenteric defect is reapproximated with interrupted or running 0-gauge delayed-absorbable suture to prevent an internal hernia.

❼ **Final Steps.** The abdomen is irrigated with copious warmed saline at the conclusion of any bowel resection, especially if feces have spilled during the procedure. Drains are not routinely required and may impair healing.

POSTOPERATIVE

Morbidity after large bowel resection is significantly increased by a variety of factors, but especially by preexisting obstruction, malignancy, obesity, radiation damage, and sepsis. Moreover, patients undergoing multiple bowel resections have a higher blood loss and longer hospital stay (Salani, 2007). Anastomotic leaks are the most specific complication and typically present as an abscess or fistula, or as peritonitis within days or weeks of surgery. Some localized leaks can be managed with initiation of TPN, CT-guided drainage, antibiotic administration, and bowel rest for a couple of weeks. However, urgent reoperation is indicated for nonlocalized intraperitoneal perforation and its resulting peritonitis. This will usually require temporary colostomy (Kingham, 2009).

Pelvic abscesses may also result from intraoperative fecal spillage or hematoma superinfection. Usually these will resolve with CT-guided drainage and antibiotics. Gastrointestinal hemorrhage should be rare with stapled procedures. In addition, symptomatic anastomotic strictures are infrequent and often present as colonic obstruction. Some strictures can be managed with endoscopic stents, but often they require reoperation. Small or large bowel obstructions may also result from postoperative adhesions or tumor progression. Lastly, a prolonged ileus can develop and be very slow to resolve. Most of these complications will depend primarily on the patient's underlying nutrition and the clinical circumstances prompting the primary surgery.

44-21

Ileostomy

Relatively few patients will require ileostomy for management of a gynecologic malignancy. For those who do, loop ileostomy is usually a temporary procedure that is performed to protect a distal anastomosis (Nunoo-Mensah, 2004). In addition, palliation of a large bowel obstruction or diversion of a colonic fistula may be other indications (Tsai, 2006). On occasion, ovarian cancer will involve the entire colon, requiring colectomy with a permanent end ileostomy and formation of a Hartmann pouch (Song, 2009).

PREOPERATIVE

■ Patient Evaluation

Stoma placement is particularly important for an ileostomy since the effluent will be more corrosive than that of a colostomy. Ideally, the site should be marked by an enterostomal therapist preoperatively.

■ Consent

In general, many of the complications from this procedure mirror those of colostomy: retraction, stricture, obstruction, and herniation. Patients should be informed that temporary loop ileostomies can be later taken down without a laparotomy.

■ Patient Preparation

Bowel preparation is preferred whenever there is a potential for more extensive bowel resection. However, ileostomy can safely be performed in virtually all circumstances without cleansing.

INTRAOPERATIVE

SURGICAL STEPS

❶ Anesthesia and Patient Positioning.
Ileostomy is performed under general anesthesia. Patients are generally supine, but dorsal lithotomy or other positioning with access to the abdominal wall is acceptable. Sterile preparation of the abdomen is completed, and a Foley catheter is placed. The vaginal is also surgically prepared if concurrent hysterectomy is planned.

❷ Abdominal Entry.
A midline vertical incision is preferable for most situations in which an ileostomy is considered.

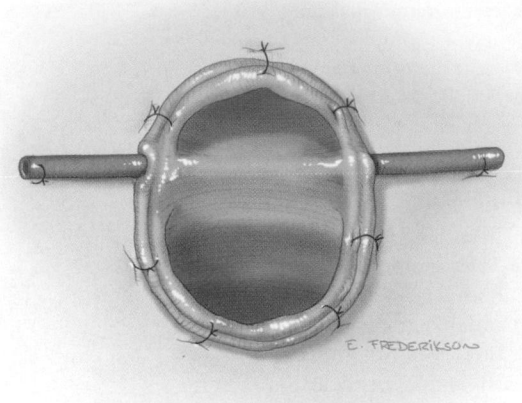

FIGURE 44-21.1 Ileal loop has been pulled through the abdominal wall and opened with an electrosurgical blade.

❸ Exploration.
After abdominal entry, a surgeon first explores the abdomen, lyses adhesions, "runs" the bowel length to identify obstructive sites, and determines the need for ileostomy. An ileum loop is selected that will reach several centimeters above the skin. Additionally, to reduce the effluent volume, the selected loop should be located as distally along the bowel length as possible. On occasion, tethering of small bowel by carcinomatosis or radiation injury will significantly reduce mobility and will require a more proximal diversion.

❹ Loop Ileostomy.
A one-quarter inch Penrose drain is placed through a mesenterotomy at the selected loop's apex. The loop can then be approximated to the stoma site, which is created to accommodate two fingers as described for an ileal conduit (Section 44-8, step 6, p. 1286). The loop is pulled through the abdominal wall opening so that several centimeters protrude above the skin surface. The Penrose drain is removed and replaced with either the cut end of a red rubber catheter or other device that can be sewn to the skin to elevate the loop. The loop should be tension-free and patent. The proximal end of the loop is placed in the lower position to reduce fecal flow into the distal bowel. The abdominal wall is then closed around the stoma.

The ileostomy is "matured" by longitudinally incising the bowel loop and everting its walls with Allis clamps. Circumferential interrupted stitches of 3-0 and 4-0 delayed-absorbable sutures are placed through the dermis and bowel mucosa (Fig. 44-21.1). An ostomy bag may then be applied.

❺ End Ileostomy.
If a total colectomy is performed or if the bowel is too tethered or the patient too obese for a loop to reach the abdominal wall, the distal ileum may need to

be divided instead of brought out as a loop. The segment is selected, a mesenterotomy is made, and the GIA stapler is fired. An appropriate stoma site is identified, and with a few modifications, the end ileostomy is matured similarly to colostomy (Section 44-19, p. 1319). Typically, the abdominal wall opening will be smaller in diameter. Unless there is a distal colon obstruction necessitating creation of a mucus fistula, the distal bowel segment can be left in the peritoneal cavity or just under the fascia. An attempt should be made to evert the single stoma by turning the bowel wall over on itself using Allis clamps. In each quadrant of the stoma, stitches of 3-0 delayed absorbable suture are placed through the dermis, the seromuscular layer of the bowel at the skin level, and a full-thickness bite at the cut edge of the everted bowel.

POSTOPERATIVE

The stoma should be carefully examined postoperatively for its appearance and function. The loop supporting rod may be removed in 1 to 2 weeks, but potentially earlier if the stoma becomes dusky or the loops seem constricted or are obstructed.

Ileostomy may be associated with significant postoperative complications. High-output effluent may result in electrolyte abnormalities that are difficult to correct. In addition, approximately 10 percent of patients will require early reoperation for small bowel obstruction or intraabdominal abscess (Hallbook, 2002). Specifically, if loop ileostomy is indicated to protect a low anterior anastomosis, it is more commonly associated with bowel obstruction and ileus than loop colostomy (Law, 2002). Long-term complications such as a peristomal hernia or retraction are also possible.

44-22

Small Bowel Resection

There are numerous indications for small bowel resection in gynecologic oncology, including obstruction, involvement with cancer, perforation, intraoperative injury, fistulas, and radiation damage. Unlike the large bowel, where greater attention is required to ensure an adequate blood supply to the anastomotic site, the small intestine has a consistent cascade of vessels that all arise from the superior mesenteric artery. However, unique situations such as radiation damage, obstructive dilatation, and edema can compromise this vasculature dramatically. In these situations, meticulous dissection is especially crucial to prevent inadvertent removal of the bowel serosa, enterotomy, and bowel damage that will impair anastomotic healing. In general, surgical principles with this procedure are much the same as those for large bowel resection (Section 44-20, p. 1322).

PREOPERATIVE

Patient Evaluation

Small bowel obstructions (SBO) that do not resolve with nasogastric suction decompression and bowel rest may result from postoperative adhesions or tumor progression. Patients with recurrent gynecologic malignancy, particularly those with ovarian cancer, should be evaluated with an upper gastrointestinal series and small bowel follow-through radiographic studies preoperatively. With these, numerous sites of obstruction may be identified that would indicate a woman with end-stage disease who might be better served by placement of a palliative percutaneous draining gastrostomy tube. Patients with an SBO following pelvic radiation almost invariably have stenosis at the terminal ileum.

Consent

Depending on circumstances, patients should be counseled regarding the intraoperative decision-making process for performing an anastomosis, bypass, or ileostomy. Leaking, obstruction, and/or fistula formation are possible complications. Less common outcomes include short-bowel syndrome and vitamin B_{12} deficiency.

Patient Preparation

Aggressive bowel preparation is often contraindicated, particularly in patients with obstruction. Antibiotic prophylaxis should be initiated. Also, thromboprophylaxis is administered as outlined in Table 39-9 (p. 962). If a complex fistula is present or an extensive resection for radiation damage is anticipated, then postoperative total parental nutrition (TPN) may be advisable.

INTRAOPERATIVE

Instruments

The surgeon should have access to all types and sizes of bowel staplers, such as end-to-end anastomotic (EEA), gastrointestinal anastomotic (GIA), and transverse anastomotic (TA) staplers, to prepare for complicated resections.

SURGICAL STEPS

❶ Anesthesia and Patient Positioning. Small bowel resection is performed under general anesthesia. Patients are generally supine, but dorsal lithotomy or other positioning with access to the anterior abdominal wall is acceptable. Sterile preparation of the abdomen is completed, and a Foley catheter is placed. The vaginal is also surgically prepared if concurrent hysterectomy is planned.

❷ Abdominal Entry. A midline vertical incision is preferable for most situations in which a small bowel resection is considered.

❸ Exploration. The surgeon explores the entire abdomen first to identify the obstruction. Infrequently, an adhesion may be located and lysed to quickly relieve an obstruction, thereby avoiding small bowel resection. More often, an area is discovered that warrants removal. Importantly, the remainder of the bowel must be examined to exclude other obstructive sites.

Peritoneum and adhesions attached to the involved portion of small bowel are dissected to mobilize the bowel. The small intestine can be damaged easily by rough handling and extensive blunt dissection—particularly if the bowel is edematous, densely adhered, or previously radiated. Trauma should be kept to an absolute minimum to reduce spillage of intestinal contents by inadvertent enterotomy. Ideally, healthy-appearing serosa for anastomosis is identified at sites both proximal and distal to the lesion while preserving a maximum amount of intestine.

❹ Dividing Small Bowel. The involved bowel is brought through the abdominal incision. A one-quarter inch Penrose drain is pulled through a mesenterotomy at the proximal and distal sites to be approximated. A GIA stapler is inserted to replace the Penrose drain and is fired (Fig. 44-22.1). This is repeated at the other bowel site. These staple lines minimize contamination of the abdomen with bowel contents.

A wedge of mesentery then is "scored" by superficially creating a V shape with an electrosurgical blade. The mesentery is divided by a ligate-divide-staple (LDS) device, electrothermal bipolar coagulator (LigaSure), or clamps and 0-gauge delayed-absorbable

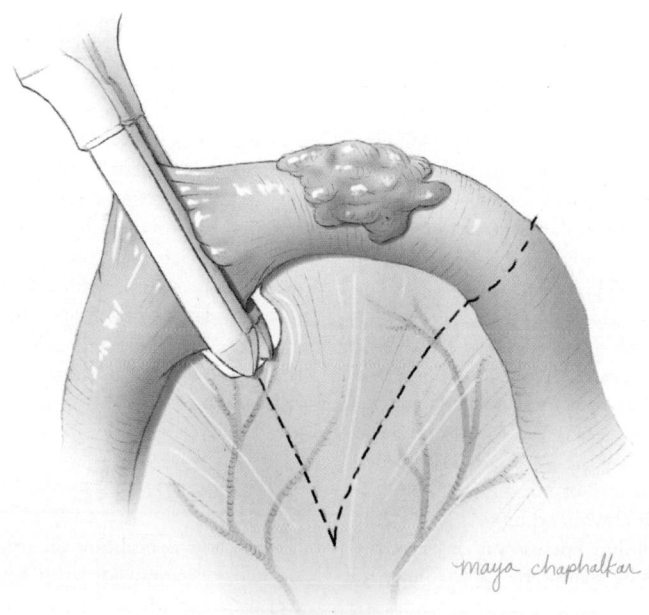

maya chaphalkar

FIGURE 44-22.1 Identifying the proximal and distal sites.

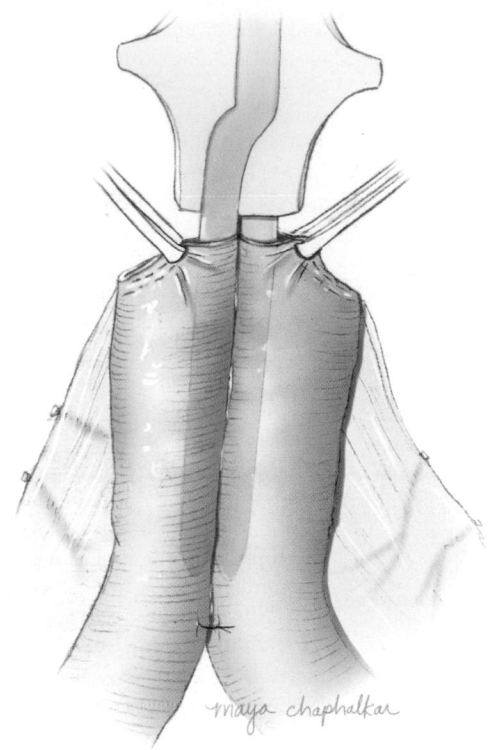

FIGURE 44-22.2 Side-to-side anastomosis.

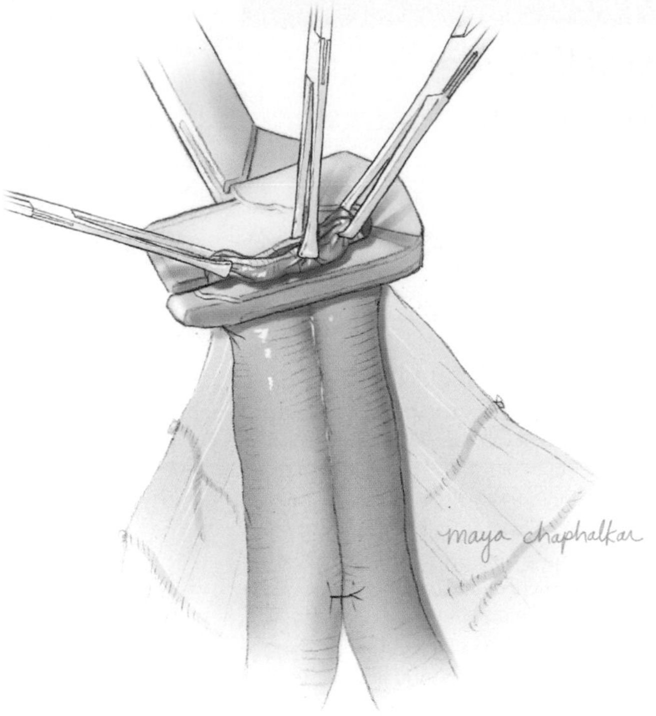

FIGURE 44-22.3 Closing the enterotomy.

suture ligatures. Hemostasis will be more difficult with edematous or inflamed tissue, and thus, smaller mesentery pedicles should be sequentially divided. The bowel specimen is then removed.

⑤ Performing Side-to-Side Anastomosis. The proximal and distal bowel segments are elevated with Allis clamps and matched parallel along their antimesenteric borders. One or two silk stay sutures are placed through the antimesenteric border of each segment beyond the tip of where the GIA stapler fork will reach. The antimesenteric corner of each segment is excised at the staple line just deeply enough to enter the lumen and sufficiently widely to permit passage of one GIA stapler fork. Massively distended bowel from an obstruction may be decompressed by inserting a pool suction tip into the proximal bowel end.

Allis clamps are replaced on the bowel at the edge of each opening. These clamps and silk stay sutures assist insertion of one fork of the GIA stapler into each segment and aid bowel positioning (Fig. 44-22.2). The bowel is rotated to bring the antimesenteric borders together, Allis clamps are removed, and the GIA stapler is closed and fired.

The remaining enterotomy is regrasped with three Allis clamps to approximate for closure. The TA stapler is placed around the bowel beneath the Allis clamps and is closed (Fig. 44-22.3). The Allis clamps elevate the enterotomy and assist correct positioning of

the TA stapler. The stapler is fired, excess tissue above the stapler is trimmed sharply, and the stapler is opened and removed. The mesenteric defect may be closed next with running 0-gauge delayed-absorbable suture to prevent internal herniation, that is, herniation of bowel or omentum through the mesenteric defect.

⑥ Final Steps. Copious irrigation with warmed saline should be performed at the conclusion of any bowel resection, but particularly if spillage is noted during the procedure. Drains are not required routinely and may impair healing. In general, placement of a nasogastric tube to decompress the stomach postoperatively until bowel function has resumed is prudent. Palpation of the stomach will confirm correct placement, or the anesthesiologist can be directed to advance or pull back the tube if necessary. If overlooked, correct location can only be reliably confirmed postoperatively by chest radiography.

POSTOPERATIVE

The underlying health of the patient, diagnosis, and indications for small bowel resection will dictate much of the potential postoperative morbidity. Common minor complications include wound infection and ileus. Fistula formation, anastomotic leakage, and obstruction

are more serious problems that may require reoperation. Two specific complications are unique to extensive small bowel surgery.

First, short-bowel syndrome may develop. More than half the small intestine can be removed without impairing nutritional absorption as long as the remaining bowel is functional. Accordingly, this syndrome is more likely to develop from extensive radiation damage than from resection. Symptoms include diarrhea and dehydration. Maldigestion, malabsorption, nutritional deficiencies, and electrolyte imbalance are noted commonly. As a result, home TPN may be required in some patients (King, 1993).

A second complication, vitamin B_{12} deficiency, results from inadequate absorption and depletion of available stores. Vitamin B_{12} and bile salts are only absorbed in the distal 100 cm of the ileum. Malabsorption in this segment may result from radiotherapy or extensive intestinal resection (Bandy, 1984). If vitamin B_{12} deficiency is suspected, a complete blood count (CBC), peripheral blood smear, and serum cobalamin (B_{12}) level are collected as part of an initial laboratory assessment. Accepted lower limits of serum vitamin B_{12} levels in adults range between 170 and 250 ng/L, but deficiency is considered levels <75 ng/L. One option for replacement is 1 mg intramuscularly weekly for 8 weeks, followed by long-term monthly injections (Centers for Disease Control and Prevention, 2009).

44-23

Low Anterior Resection

Rectosigmoid resection, also known as low anterior resection, is mainly used in gynecologic oncology to achieve optimal cytoreduction of primary or recurrent ovarian cancer (Mourton, 2005). This procedure is distinguished from other types of large bowel resection in that it requires mobilization and transection of the rectum distally, below the peritoneal reflection. Following resection of the involved rectosigmoid segment, proximal and distal bowel ends are usually anastomosed.

Low anterior resection is the most common bowel operation for primary tumor debulking (Hoffman, 2005). For example, en bloc pelvic resection combines low anterior resection with hysterectomy, bilateral salpingo-oophorectomy, and removal of surrounding peritoneum (Section 44-15, p. 1309) (Aletti, 2006b). In addition, total and posterior pelvic exenterations incorporate many of the same principles of tissue dissection to remove centrally recurrent cervical cancer with widely negative soft tissue margins. Other less common indications for low anterior resection are radiation proctosigmoiditis and intestinal endometriosis (Urbach, 1998). Occasionally, additional large or small bowel resections will be performed concomitantly with low anterior resection (Salani, 2007).

PREOPERATIVE

Patient Evaluation

Bowel symptoms may or may not be present in women with rectosigmoid involvement of ovarian cancer. However, a surgeon should have a high suspicion if patients describe rectal bleeding or progressive constipation, and a rectovaginal examination may help predict a need for low anterior resection. Additionally, computed tomography (CT) scanning may suggest rectosigmoid invasion of tumor. However, prior to surgery, prediction is difficult. Many ovarian cancers intraoperatively may be easily lifted away from the bowel or surface tumors may be removed without resection.

Consent

Patients should be prepared for the possibility of low anterior resection any time ovarian cytoreductive surgery is discussed. The survival benefit of achieving minimal residual disease warrants the risks of this procedure. However, low anterior resection significantly extends operative time, and hemorrhage may contribute to a need for blood transfusion (Tebes, 2006).

In general, progressively higher complication rates and poorer long-term bowel function follow anastomoses that are more distal and approach the anal verge. However, the operation is designed to encompass the tumor. Thus, an end sigmoid colostomy with Hartmann pouch is another, albeit less attractive, option for very low resections.

In general, a protective loop colostomy or ileostomy is not required, but patients should be counseled for that possibility. Anastomotic leaks should develop in fewer than 5 percent of procedures (Mourton, 2005).

Patient Preparation

To minimize fecal contamination during resection, bowel preparation such as with a polyethylene glycol with electrolyte solution (GoLytely) is generally recommended prior to surgery. Antibiotic prophylaxis may be initiated in the operating room, and suitable options are found in Table 39-6 (p. 959). Also, thromboprophylaxis is administered as outlined in Table 39-9 (p. 962).

INTRAOPERATIVE

Instruments

All types and sizes of bowel staplers such as end-to-end anastomosis (EEA), gastrointestinal anastomosis (GIA), and transverse anastomosis (TA) staplers should be available. Additionally, a ligate-divide-staple (LDS) device or electrothermal bipolar coagulator (LigaSure) may be used for vessel ligation.

SURGICAL STEPS

1 Anesthesia and Patient Positioning. Low anterior resection requires general anesthesia. Rectovaginal examination under anesthesia is mandatory before positioning any patient for abdominal gynecologic cancer surgery. A palpable mass with compression of the rectum or rectovaginal septum warrants patient positioning in dorsal lithotomy with legs safely placed in Allen stirrups. This allows access to the rectum in cases requiring EEA stapler insertion for anastomosis. Alternatively, supine positioning may be appropriate if no mass is palpable by rectovaginal examination. In such cases, if a mass is more proximally located, low rectal anastomosis can be performed entirely within the pelvis. After positioning, sterile preparation of the abdomen is completed, and a Foley catheter is placed. The vaginal is also surgically prepared if concurrent hysterectomy is planned.

2 Abdominal Entry. A midline vertical incision provides generous operating space and upper abdominal access. This is preferable if low rectal anastomosis is anticipated because the descending colon may need to be mobilized around and beyond the splenic flexure. In contrast, transverse incisions often fail to provide sufficient exposure.

3 Exploration. A surgeon should first explore the entire abdomen to determine if disease is resectable. If not, then the procedure's benefit should be reevaluated. On occasion, imminent bowel obstruction, infection, or other clinical circumstances may dictate resection regardless of residual tumor. The pelvis and rectosigmoid should be palpated to mentally plan for the resection and determine whether en bloc pelvic resection or an exenterative procedure is indicated.

4 Visualization. The bowel is packed into the upper abdomen, and retractor blades are positioned to allow access to the deep pelvis and the entire rectosigmoid colon. Ureters are identified at the pelvic brim and are held laterally on Penrose drains to expose the peritoneum and mesentery that can next be safely dissected.

5 Dividing the Proximal Sigmoid. The sigmoid colon is held on traction proximal to the tumor and in the approximate area where it will be divided. The ureter is located, and a right-angle clamp is used to guide superficial electrosurgical blade dissection of the peritoneum and mesentery up to the bowel serosa. A similar dissection is repeated on the other side. Blunt dissection may then be performed to define the entire circumference of the sigmoid. Epiploica and adjacent fatty tissue are held with DeBakey forceps and dissected away with an electrosurgical blade from the proposed area of transection. The GIA stapler is placed across the sigmoid, fired, and removed (Fig. 44-23.1).

6 Dividing the Mesentery. Occasionally, the tumor is small and superficially located, requiring only a wedge resection of underlying mesentery to remove it with the bowel segment. More frequently, the entire mesentery needs to be divided to provide access to the avascular plane between the rectosigmoid and the sacrum (retrorectal space). Gentle blunt dissection is performed inferior to the divided sigmoid to better characterize the underlying fatty tissue and small vessels. A right-angle clamp is placed through sections of the mesentery, and an LDS device or electrothermal bipolar coagulator divides this tissue. Dissection is continued anteroposteriorly through approximately two thirds of the mesentery (Fig. 44-23.2). Typically, one or more pedicles will have a blood vessel that slips out and requires clamping with a

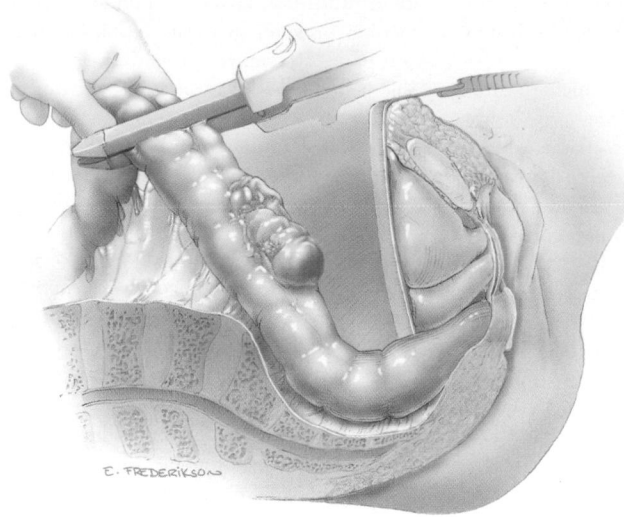

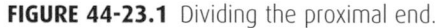

FIGURE 44-23.1 Dividing the proximal end.

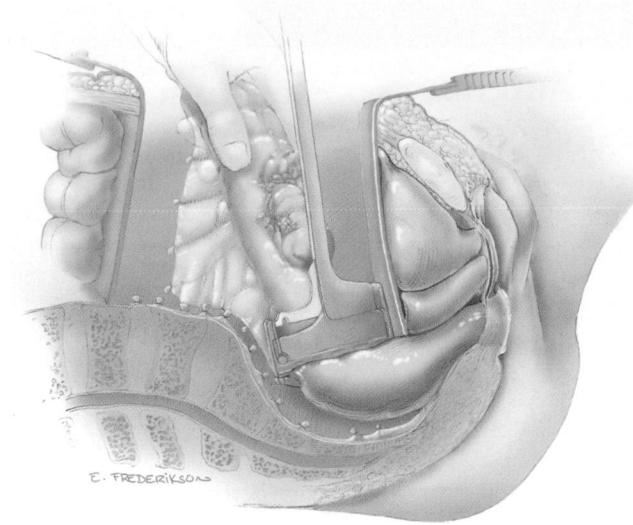

FIGURE 44-23.2 Dividing the distal end.

right-angle clamp and ligation with 0-gauge delayed-absorbable suture.

Blunt dissection is performed in the pelvic midline to identify the large superior rectal vessels, which are branches of the inferior mesenteric artery (IMA). This artery and vein are large and should be separately doubly clamped, cut, and ligated with 0-gauge delayed-absorbable suture. Dissection is continued to the other side of the pelvis until there is no tissue visible between the ureters. The common iliac artery bifurcation and sacrum should be entirely visible.

❼ **Dividing the Rectum.** The proximal sigmoid and attached mesentery is repacked into the upper abdomen to improve pelvic exposure. The rectosigmoid is held superiorly, and blunt dissection is performed posteriorly in the retrorectal space to mobilize the distal bowel beyond the tumor to define the location of planned resection. The ureters are traced along the pelvic sidewall. Lateral blunt dissection is performed to further mobilize the rectosigmoid. Lateral mesenteric attachments are isolated and divided with an LDS device or electrothermal bipolar coagulator, or are grasped between Pean clamps, cut, and ligated. Self-retaining retractor blades may require repositioning as dissection proceeds more distally.

The anterior bowel serosa is generally visible throughout its course beyond the peritoneal reflection and into the levator muscles. Lateral and posterior bowel margins are surrounded by fatty tissue, mesentery, and rectal pillars. The distal rectum beyond the tumor is grasped and rotated to aid exposure of these attachments. Attachments are divided using alternating electrosurgical blade dissection and vascular pedicle division and/or right-angle clamping and transection. Division continues circumferentially until the rectal serosa is entirely visible. The curved cutter stapler (Contour) is often a good

choice for the limited space of the deep pelvis. The rectosigmoid is held on traction, while the stapler is gently inserted into the pelvis around the rectal segment (see Fig. 44-23.2). The ureters and any lateral tissue are pushed safely away, the stapler is fired, and the low anterior resection specimen is removed. The pelvis is irrigated, and a laparotomy sponge is left in place to tamponade any surface oozing.

❽ **Mobilization.** The final decision is now made to perform an anastomosis instead of an end sigmoid colostomy. The upper

abdominal retractors are removed, and the proximal sigmoid colon is mobilized by incising peritoneum along the white line of Toldt toward the splenic flexure. A combination of electrosurgical blade and blunt dissection is typically used. The proximal sigmoid colon is intermittently placed into the deep pelvis to assess the extent of further dissection needed to achieve a tension-free anastomosis. Ideally, the proximal sigmoid colon sits comfortably on top of the distal rectum. To achieve this, mobilization may encompass the entire splenic flexure (Fig. 44-23.3).

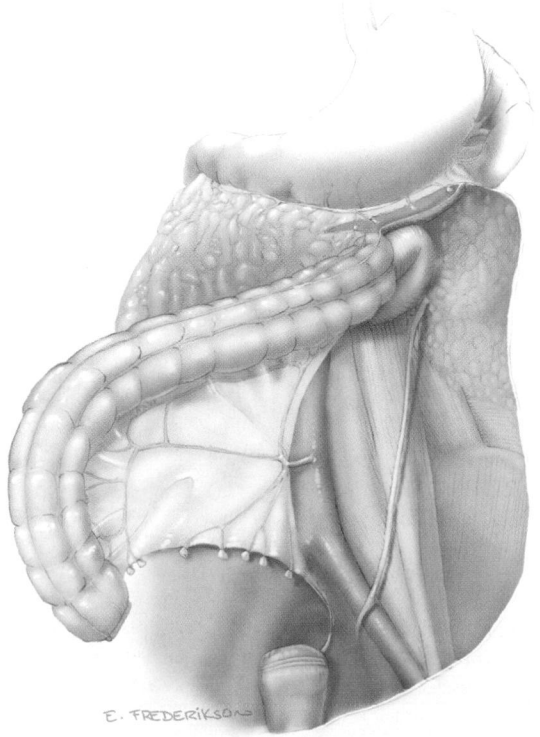

FIGURE 44-23.3 Mobilizing the descending colon.

Occasionally, the hepatic flexure may need to be mobilized also. Sufficient mobilization is critical to ensure a tension-free anastomosis.

❾ Preparing the Anastomotic Sites.

The proximal and distal stapled bowel ends now must be cleared of any fatty tissue or epiploica to allow sufficient mucosa-to-mucosa contact during anastomosis. The staple line of the proximal sigmoid is grasped with two Allis clamps at the lateral edges and elevated. Adson forceps are used to delicately place any surrounding fatty tissue on traction, and an electrosurgical blade is used to dissect these away from the bowel serosa. This can be particularly difficult in patients with prominent diverticulosis. A similar dissection may also be required on the distal rectal segment.

❿ Placing the Anvil.

The largest possible EEA circular stapler that will fit the bowel segments, typically 31- or 34-mm size, should be used. This provides a commodious anastomosis that will lessen the chances of symptomatic rectal stenosis. The proximal sigmoid colon is again held with Allis clamps, and scissors are used to remove the entire staple line. The Allis clamps are replaced to grasp the mucosa/serosa and hold open the proximal sigmoid. Sizing instruments may be used if necessary to decide which EEA instrument is best. The EEA device contains an anvil that will be placed in the proximal bowel and a stapler that is placed in the distal bowel. Articulation of the anvil and stapler head allows firing of a staple ring at this articulation site to form the anastomosis.

First, the anvil is detached from the stapler, lubricated, and gently inserted by rotating it into the proximal sigmoid. Its concave surface faces proximally, away from the anticipated anastomotic site (Fig. 44-23.4, inset). The surgeon adds sequential stitches that pierce through bowel serosa, muscularis, and mucosa to create a purse string around the anvil. These "through-and-through" stitches using 2-0 Prolene suture are placed 5 to 7 mm from the mucosal edge. The purse string begins and ends on the outside of the bowel serosa around the anvil spike and is then tied securely. Allis clamps are removed. A quicker alternative is to use a stapler purse-string suture device. Irrigation may be performed if bowel contents have spilled.

⓫ Placing the Stapler.

The distal rectal stump is reexamined to ensure that all surrounding fatty tissue has been dissected free. The surgical team then reviews the details of using an EEA instrument. A phantom application is helpful. After this, the shaft of the stapler is extended and its spike is attached. The shaft and spike are then retracted into the instrument. The EEA is lubricated and gently inserted into the anus until the circular outline is visible and seen to be gently pressing on the rectal staple line. A wing nut located on the device handle is gently rotated, and this extends the shaft and its spike. This is guided by the abdominal surgeon so that the spike is brought out just posterior to the staple midline. With a hand in the abdomen, gentle countertraction held against the bowel may be helpful as the sharp spike tip pops through the entire bowel thickness. The shaft subsequently becomes visible, and the spike is removed.

⓬ Stapling.

The abdominal surgeon lowers the proximal sigmoid to the distal rectum and connects the hollow tip of the anvil into the metal shaft of the EEA. An audible "click" should be heard to confirm articulation. The tip of the EEA is held perfectly still, while the wing nut is again rotated to retract the shaft back into the EEA until the handle indicator is in the correct position (Fig. 44-23.4). This draws the anvil into apposition with the stapler head. The safety is released, and the instrument is fired by squeezing and depressing the handles completely. Incomplete squeezing can result in partial stapling. The wing nut is then turned to the specified position to release the staple line. The EEA with its attached anvil is then gently rotated and slowly removed from the rectum. The anastomosis should be visualized by the abdominal surgeon throughout the process. Distal retraction of the anastomosis or inability to remove the EEA suggests that the stapler was not completely fired. This situation may be salvaged by gently pulling the EEA through the anus and cutting inside the staple line to release the anastomosis. The anvil is removed from the EEA instrument and inspected to confirm that two completely intact circular "donuts" of rectal tissue are present.

⓭ Rectal Insufflation.

Warmed saline is irrigated into the pelvis. The integrity of the anastomosis may now be checked by gently inserting a proctoscope or red rubber catheter into the anus, but distal to the anastomosis. Air is then insufflated into the bowel. The abdominal surgeon should gently palpate the sigmoid to make certain that air is entering the sigmoid proximal to the anastomotic site. No air bubbles should be visible if the connection is watertight (Fig. 44-23.5). The appearance of bubbles suggests a leak, but this should be double-checked for authenticity. Occasionally, air is being erroneously pumped into the vagina rather than the rectum due to incorrect placement of the red rubber catheter.

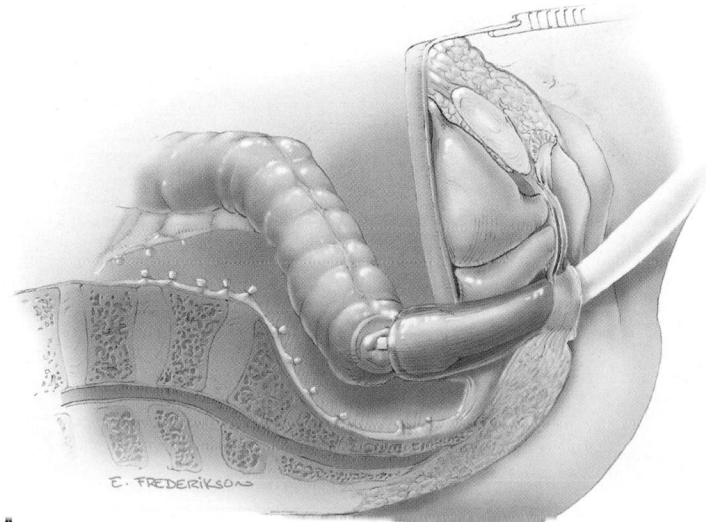

A

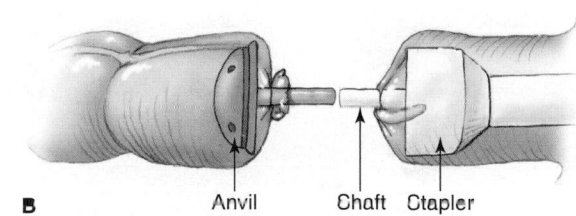

B

Anvil   Shaft   Stapler

FIGURE 44-23.4 Performing the end-to-end anastomosis. **Inset:** The EEA stapler device head.

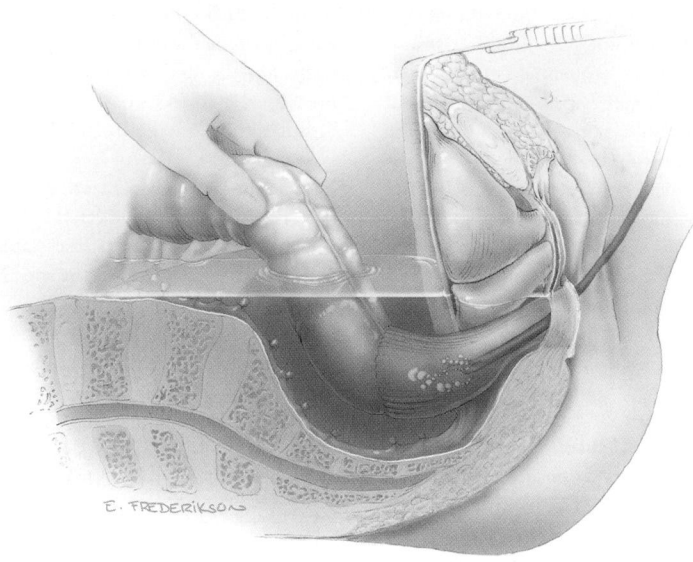

E. FREDERIKSON

FIGURE 44-23.5 Testing the anastomosis.

If there is any valid suspicion for a leak, the distal rectum should be divided again and the anastomosis redone. Reinforcing interrupted suture to close the air leak may be attempted in select situations, but this is riskier. Diverting colostomy may also be considered if the problem cannot otherwise be managed.

14 Final Steps. All pedicle sites should be rechecked for hemostasis and the pelvis irri-gated. Nasogastric suction is not routinely required. In addition, prophylactic suction drainage of the pelvis does not improve outcome or influence the severity of complications (Merad, 1999).

POSTOPERATIVE

The most common early postoperative complications are similar to other major abdominal operations and include fever, self-limiting ileus, wound separation, and anemia requiring transfusion. Serious events such as bowel obstruction and fistula should develop infrequently (Gillette-Cloven, 2001). Long-term, some patients will have a poor functional result, including fecal incontinence or chronic constipation (Rasmussen, 2003).

Low rectal anastomoses have much higher leak rates than intraperitoneal large bowel anastomoses. Leakage of stool leads to fever, leukocytosis, lower abdominal pain, and ileus. Any suspicious constellation of these signs and symptoms should prompt an abdominopelvic computed tomography (CT) scan with oral contrast. When a leak is present, it may appear as a pelvic abscess, or at times, contrast extravasation can be demonstrated into the fluid collection. Occasionally, this complication can be successfully managed with percutaneous drainage of the abscess, bowel rest, and broad-spectrum antibiotics. Otherwise, a temporary diverting loop ileostomy or colostomy may be required (Mourton, 2005). Risk factors for postoperative leakage include previous pelvic irradiation, diabetes mellitus, low preoperative serum albumin, long surgical duration, and a low anastomosis (≤6 cm from the anal verge) (Matthiessen, 2004; Mirhashemi, 2000; Richardson, 2006).

44-24

Intestinal Bypass

This bowel anastomotic procedure typically connects a section of the ileum to the ascending or transverse colon and thereby "bypasses" a portion of diseased bowel. Following anastomosis, the closed, bypassed small-bowel segment remains.

There are relatively few indications for intestinal bypass in gynecologic oncology, and this procedure accounts for only approximately 5 percent of all bowel operations performed for these cancers (Barnhill, 1991; Winter, 2003). In all circumstances, removal of diseased bowel and end-to-end anastomosis is preferable. However, some patients will have unresectable tumor, dense adhesions, extensive radiation injury, or other prohibitive factors. In these cases, a poor decision to proceed with an aggressive dissection can result in numerous enterotomies, hemorrhage, or other intraoperative catastrophes with major postoperative sequelae. Instead, an intestinal bypass can often quickly be performed with minimal morbidity. Many times a bypass is selected because it is the easiest palliative maneuver for a terminally ill patient. The main purpose is to relieve an obstruction, to reestablish an adequate bowel communication, and to regain the ability to take oral nourishment.

PREOPERATIVE

Patient Evaluation

The intestinal tract should be carefully evaluated by an upper gastrointestinal (GI) series with small bowel follow-through and/or computed tomography (CT) scanning. Invariably, pelvic radiation injuries are located at the terminal ileum, but there may be complex fistulas or multiple sites of obstruction to be addressed. In most circumstances in which a bypass is considered, a surgeon should anticipate limitations in adequately exploring the abdomen intraoperatively. Careful analysis of preoperative findings will help ensure that bypass encompasses the entire lesion and does not leave a distal obstruction.

Consent

Patients usually have a miserable quality of life when bypass is considered, and the operation's goal is mainly to improve patient symptoms. The counseling process should emphasize that intraoperative judgment will dictate whether a small bowel resection, ileostomy, large bowel resection, colostomy, or bypass is indicated. Many risks are similar to those of other intestinal surgical procedures and include anastomotic leaks, obstruction, abscess formation, and fistula. Blind loop syndrome, discussed later, is one long-term complication that is characteristic to the bypass procedure.

Patient Preparation

Aggressive bowel preparation with oral agents is usually contraindicated due to bowel obstruction or other dire circumstances. Broad-spectrum antibiotics are given perioperatively due to the possibility of stool contamination. Also, thromboprophylaxis is administered as outlined in Table 39-9 (p. 962). If a prolonged recovery is anticipated, postoperative total parenteral nutrition should be considered.

INTRAOPERATIVE

Instruments

To prepare for complicated resections, bowel staplers such as an end-to-end anastomosis (EEA), gastrointestinal anastomosis (GIA), and transverse anastomosis (TA) staplers should be available.

SURGICAL STEPS

❶ **Anesthesia and Patient Positioning.** Bypass is performed under general anesthesia with the patient positioned supine. Prior to surgery, the abdomen is surgically prepared, and a Foley catheter is inserted.

❷ **Abdominal Entry and Exploration.** Intestinal bypass generally requires a midline vertical incision for adequate exposure. A surgeon should first explore the entire abdomen to identify bowel lesions. In addition, the remaining bowel should be examined to exclude other obstructive sites. Healthy-appearing bowel proximal and distal to the lesion is selected with the intent of preserving the maximal amount of intestine. Typically, the bypass will entail connecting a section of the ileum to the ascending or transverse colon.

❸ **Aligning the Bowel.** The two bowel segments selected for the anastomosis are aligned side-to-side without tension or twisting. The hepatic or splenic flexure of the transverse colon may require mobilization from its peritoneal attachments to achieve a tension-free connection. The antimesenteric borders of the bowel segments are held in position by 2-0 silk stay sutures that are placed approximately 6 cm apart along the length of the aligned bowel segments. Two Adson forceps hold up the small bowel serosa laterally and transversely on traction. An electrosurgical blade is then used to enter the small bowel lumen on its antimesenteric surface (Fig. 44-24.1). The same maneuver is performed on the taenia coli to enter the colon.

❹ **Performing the Side-to-Side Anastomosis.** One fork of the GIA stapler is inserted into each bowel segment lumen. The bowel is adjusted, if necessary, to position the antimesenteric surfaces between the stapler forks. The stapler is then closed and

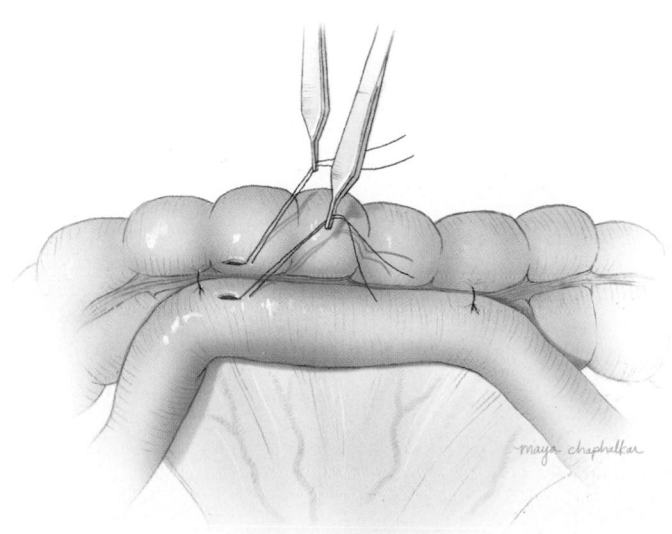

FIGURE 44-24.1 Aligning the bowel.

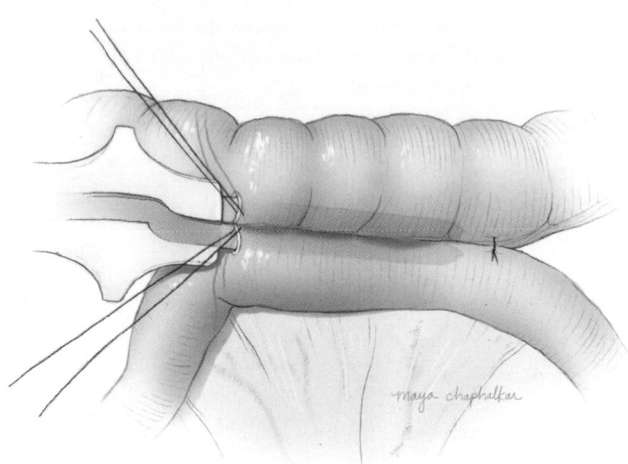

FIGURE 44-24.2 Performing the side-to-side anastomosis.

fired (Fig. 44-24.2). With stapling, the initial bowel openings that were cut to slip the stapler forks into are fused into one open defect. This opening can be closed with the TA stapler and the excess bowel trimmed.

❺ Final Steps. Occasionally, small bleeding sites will be electrosurgically coagulated on the staple line. The anastomosis should also be palpated to verify an adequate lumen. The bowel should be reexamined to make certain that the connection is watertight and that there is no tension on the anastomosis.

POSTOPERATIVE

Recovery after bypass surgery should be rapid compared with that following a large resection with anastomosis. In general, a postoperative ileus will resolve in several days, and patients may begin oral alimentation. The underlying clinical situation prompting the need for bypass surgery will dictate most of the clinical course. Relatively minor complications such as febrile morbidity and wound infection or wound separation occur commonly. Fistulas, obstruction, anastomotic leaks, abscesses, peritonitis, and perforation are more difficult to manage and often lead to a prolonged postoperative course or death.

Blind loop syndrome is a condition of vitamin B_{12} malabsorption, steatorrhea, and bacterial overgrowth of the small intestine. The usual scenario is a bypass procedure that leaves a segment of nonfunctional, severely irradiated bowel behind. Stasis of the intestinal contents leads to dilatation and mucosal inflammation. Symptoms resemble a partial small bowel obstruction and include nausea, vomiting, diarrhea, bloating, abdominal distension, and pain. Bowel perforation is possible. Antibiotics will often alleviate the condition, but recolonization and resumption of the blind loop syndrome is common (Swan, 1974). The only definitive therapy for recurrent episodes is exploration with resection of the bypassed segment. To avoid this syndrome, a surgeon may intraoperatively divide the bowel proximal and distal to the lesion and perform a side-to-side anastomosis. The closed loop can be relieved by creation of a mucus fistula at the abdominal wall.

44-25

Appendectomy

Removal of the appendix may be indicated during gynecologic surgery for a variety of reasons. The need, however, is commonly not recognized until an operation is already underway as signs and symptoms of benign gynecologic conditions can mimic appendicitis (Bowling, 2006; Fayez, 1995; Stefanidis, 1999).

In addition, malignancies may involve the appendix. Ovarian cancer frequently metastasizes to the appendix and thereby often warrants removal (Ayhan, 2005). Primary tumors of the appendix are rare, but commonly metastasize to the ovaries. Thus, the initial surgical intervention is often performed by a gynecologic oncologist (Dietrich, 2007). Pseudomyxoma peritonei is the classic type of mucinous tumor of appendiceal origin that spreads to the ovaries and may implant throughout the abdomen (Prayson, 1994).

Elective coincidental appendectomy is defined as the removal of an appendix at the time of another surgical procedure unrelated to appreciable appendiceal pathology. Possible benefits include preventing a future emergency appendectomy and excluding appendicitis in patients with chronic pelvic pain or endometriosis. Other groups that may benefit include women in whom pelvic or abdominal radiation or chemotherapy is anticipated, women undergoing extensive pelvic or abdominal surgery in which major adhesions are anticipated postoperatively, and patients such as the developmentally disabled in whom making the diagnosis of appendicitis may be difficult because of diminished ability to perceive or communicate symptoms (American College of Obstetricians and Gynecologists, 2009).

PREOPERATIVE

Specific preoperative tests or preparations are not required prior to appendectomy. In general, the consenting process for gynecologic surgery should include a discussion of possible "other indicated procedures" such as appendectomy when anticipated intraoperative findings and the potential for performing an appendectomy are uncertain.

Most studies suggest that there is at most, a small increased risk of nonfatal complications associated with elective coincidental appendectomy at the time of gynecologic surgery, whether performed during laparotomy or during laparoscopy (American College of Obstetricians and Gynecologists, 2009; Salom, 2003). Hematoma formation at the mesoappendix may cause an ileus or partial small bowel obstruction. Perforation of the stump is rare and typically follows insecure suture placement.

INTRAOPERATIVE

SURGICAL STEPS

❶ Anesthesia and Patient Positioning. Appendectomy is performed under general anesthesia in a supine position. Postoperative hospitalization is individualized and is dependent on concurrent surgeries and associated clinical symptoms.

❷ Abdominal Entry. Appendectomy can be performed through almost any incision. A laparoscopic approach or an oblique McBurney incision in the right lower quadrant of the abdomen is traditionally selected for appendectomy. However, in gynecologic cases, the needs of planned concurrent procedures will commonly dictate incision choice.

❸ Locating the Appendix. The appendix is located by first grasping the cecum and gently elevating it upward into the incision. Insertion of the terminal ileum should be visible, and the appendix is typically obvious at this point. Infrequently, an appendix is retrocecal or otherwise difficult to identify. In this situation, the convergence of the three teniae coli can be followed to locate the appendiceal base.

❹ Mesoappendix Division. The appendix tip is elevated with a Babcock clamp, and the cecum is held laterally to place the mesoappendix on gentle traction. The appendiceal artery is usually very difficult to distinguish reliably due to abundant surrounding fatty tissue. Thus, curved hemostats are used to successively clamp the mesoappendix and its vessels to reach the appendiceal base (Fig. 44-25.1).

The first hemostat is placed horizontally—aiming directly toward the base of the appendix. The second hemostat is placed at a 30-degree angle so that the tips meet, but Metzenbaum scissors have room to cut between the two clamps. The mesoappendix pedicle is ligated with 3-0 delayed-absorbable suture. This step is typically repeated once or twice to comfortably reach the base of the appendix. An alternative is to use an electrothermal bipolar coagulator (LigaSure) to divide the mesoappendix.

❺ Appendix Ligation. At this point, the appendix has been completely isolated from the mesoappendix and is still held vertically by a Babcock clamp. A first hemostat is placed at the appendiceal base, and a second is positioned directly above (Fig. 44-25.2). A third hemostat is closed with a few millimeters of intervening tissue to allow for passage of a knife blade. The knife then cuts between the second and third clamps, and the appendix is removed. The "contaminated" knife and appendix are then handed off the field.

A 2-0 silk suture is placed beneath the first hemostat with removal of that clamp. A separate suture is placed underneath the second hemostat for added security of the appendiceal stump. Gentle electrosurgical coagulation at the stump surface may also be performed.

❻ Final Steps. There is no need to invert the stump or to place a purse-string suture around it. The cecum may be returned to the abdomen, and remaining concurrent surgeries completed.

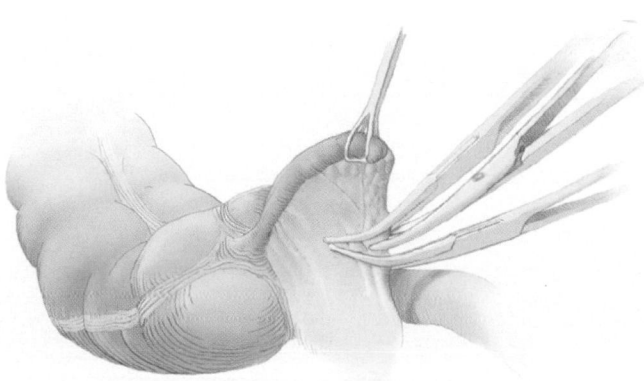

FIGURE 44-25.1 Clamping the mesoappendix.

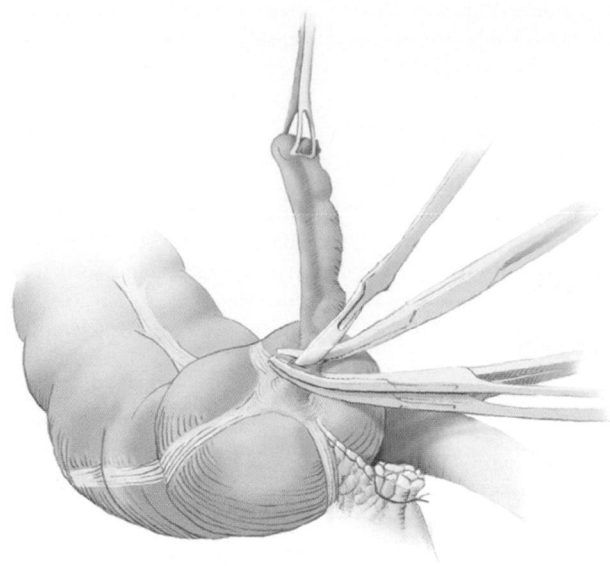

FIGURE 44-25.2 Ligation of the appendix.

POSTOPERATIVE

Patient care postoperatively is dictated by other surgeries performed. Delayed initiation of oral intake or administration of additional antibiotics is not required for appendectomy alone.

44-26

Skinning Vulvectomy

The term *skinning vulvectomy* implies a wide, superficial resection that encompasses both sides of the vulva, that is, a complete simple vulvectomy. A less extensive, unilateral procedure is better referred to as a *wide local excision* or *partial simple vulvectomy* (Section 41-28, p. 1086). The usual indication for skinning vulvectomy is a woman with confluent, bilateral vulvar intraepithelial neoplasia (VIN) 2 to 3 who is not a candidate for directed ablation with carbon dioxide (CO_2) laser or Cavitron Ultrasonic Surgical Aspirator (CUSA). Fortunately, patients with such extensive VIN are infrequently encountered. Paget disease without underlying adenocarcinoma and vulvar dystrophies refractory to standard therapy are other rare indications (Ayhan, 1998; Curtin, 1990; Rettenmaier, 1985).

The surgical procedure is straightforward and removes the entire lesion with negative margins. It is distinguished from a radical complete vulvectomy in that skinning vulvectomy removes only the skin surface and preserves the subcutaneous fat and deeper tissues. Despite this, the disfiguring result can still be psychologically devastating. In addition, the defect is often large and cannot be closed primarily without a split-thickness skin graft (STSG) or other type of flap (Section 44-30, p. 1346).

PREOPERATIVE

Patient Evaluation

Colposcopy with directed diagnostic biopsy is required to exclude a squamous lesion with invasion, which would warrant a more radical procedure. Familiarity with an array of possible STSGs or flaps is crucial to planning the operation in the event primary closure is not possible.

Consent

Patients should be informed that other more limited treatment options either have been exhausted or are inappropriate. The surgery may result in significant sexual changes, which may be permanent. Accordingly, surgeons should emphasize that all efforts will be made to restore a functional, normal-appearing vulva. Fortunately, most physical complications will be minor, such as cellulitis or partial wound dehiscence.

Patient Preparation

Complete bowel preparation is only indicated if perianal skin is to be excised. In these cases, bowel preparation will minimize fecal soiling and will also permit initial wound healing prior to the first stool. Otherwise, enemas are sufficient. Prophylactic antibiotics are typically given. Also, thromboprophylaxis is administered as outlined in Table 39-9 (p. 962). Grafts are typically taken from the upper thigh, and selection of the donor site for STSG is described in Section 44-30.

INTRAOPERATIVE

SURGICAL STEPS

❶ **Anesthesia and Patient Positioning.** Regional or general anesthesia is generally required. The patient is placed in dorsal lithotomy position, and adjustments provide access to the entire lesion. Vulvar hair should be clipped, and the vulva is surgically prepared. Intraoperative colposcopy may be needed to better delineate VIN lesion margins.

❷ **Skin Incision.** The inner and outer incision lines are drawn to encompass the disease with margins of at least a few millimeters (Fig. 44-26.1). As an overview, once final markings are placed, the skin is dissected from one side of the vulva. The skin on the opposite side of the vulva is then dissected, and the bridging skin overlying the perineal body is excised last. In performing this, the clitoris may be spared in many cases by making a horseshoe-shaped incision (as shown).

To begin, if preserving the clitoris, the outer incision is started on one side of the vulva at the anterolateral margin of the clitoris and is continued inferiorly along the length of the labia majora at least halfway to the perineal body. The inner incision on that same side of the vulva is then also taken through the full skin thickness to the same inferior halfway point. Incising the skin in stages reduces blood loss.

❸ **Beginning the Dissection.** The specimen edge may then be reflected with an Allis clamp to provide traction as the avascular plane underneath the skin is dissected from the subcutaneous fatty tissue (Fig. 44-26.2). When the anterior skin edge is large enough, a hand is placed underneath to reflect the specimen more firmly and guide dissection inferiorly. The outer and inner skin incision is then extended on that same side downward toward the perineal body. Electrosurgical coagulation is used to achieve hemostasis before repeating the process on the contralateral side.

❹ **Removal of the Specimen.** The left and right outer skin incisions are joined in the midline superficial to the perineal body. The posterior vulvar tissue is held with an Allis clamp to provide traction for upward dissection toward the inner incision. This portion of the skinning vulvectomy is typically performed last because an avascular tissue plane superficial to the subcutaneous tissue is absent, and bleeding can be brisk. The specimen can be removed

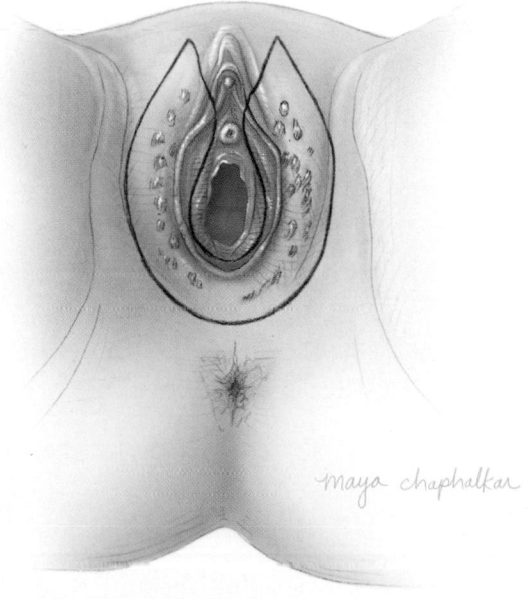

FIGURE 44-26.1 Marking the incisions.

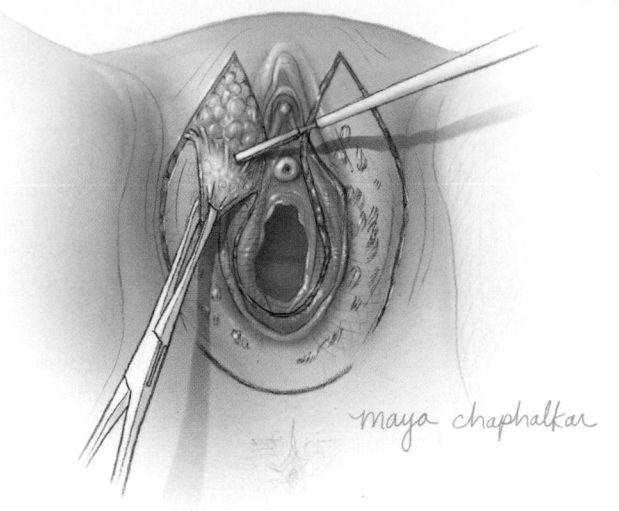

FIGURE 44-26.2 Performing the dissection.

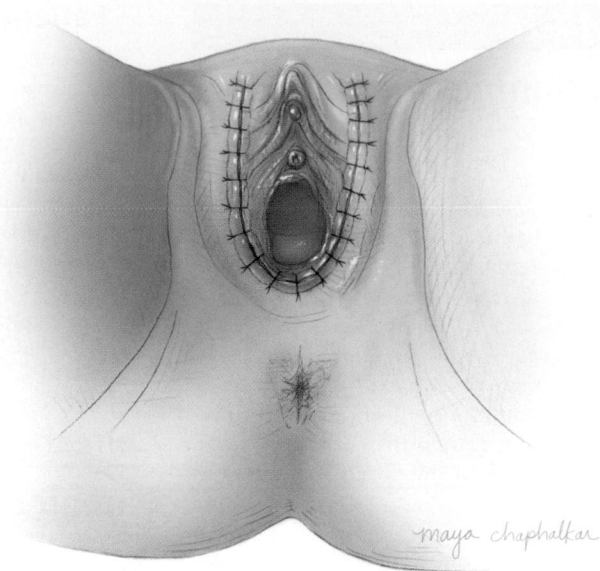

FIGURE 44-26.3 Primary closure.

following detachment from the inner posterior incision.

The skinning vulvectomy should be carefully examined to grossly determine the margins. A frozen section may be warranted if close VIN margins are suspected, to determine if more tissue requires excision. However, the margins of vulvar Paget disease cannot reliably be judged visually or by frozen-section analysis (Fishman, 1995). A stitch should be placed on the specimen to orient the pathologist.

❺ Closure of the Defect. A dry laparotomy pad is held against the vulvar defect and slowly rolled downward to halt surface bleeding and aid meticulous electrosurgical coagulation of vessels. The operative site is irrigated and assessed.

If the width of the defect is sufficiently narrow to permit primary closure, the surrounding tissue is mobilized. Lateral undermining may be particularly useful to create a tension-free closure. Typically, 0-gauge or 2-0 delayed-absorbable vertical mattress sutures are then placed circumferentially with the knots laterally positioned (Fig. 44-26.3). However, if a split-thickness skin graft is required, the graft is now harvested and placed as described in Section 44-30, p. 1346).

❻ Final Steps. A CO_2 laser may be used to vaporize multifocal lesions outside the operative field. This is described in Section 41-28 (p. 1088).

POSTOPERATIVE

If a primary closure is performed, postoperative care is essentially the same as described for patients undergoing radical partial vulvectomy (Section 44-27). Long-term surveillance is mandatory regardless of margin status to identify recurrent or de novo sites of preinvasive disease. The Foley catheter can be removed without regard to urine spill unless a graft is placed or the patient is otherwise immobilized.

44-27

Radical Partial Vulvectomy

For vulvar cancer, to reduce the high morbidity associated with radical complete vulvectomy yet without sacrificing cure, a less extensive resection may be used. Patients with well-localized, unifocal, clinical stage I invasive lesions are ideal candidates (Stehman, 1992). Radical partial vulvectomy is a somewhat ambiguously defined operation that generally refers to complete removal of the tumor-containing portion of the vulva, wherever it is located, with 1- to 2-cm skin margins and excision to the perineal membrane (Fig. 38-26, p. 942) (Whitney, 2010). Radical hemivulvectomy refers to a larger resection that may be anterior, posterior, right, or left. Vulvectomy is typically performed concurrently with inguinal lymphadenectomy to add prognostic information. However, in those with microinvasive disease undergoing wide local excision or skinning vulvectomy, lymphadenectomy is not required.

The chief concern in performing a less extensive operation for vulvar cancer is the possibility of an increased risk of local recurrence due to multifocal disease. However, survival after partial or complete radical vulvectomy is comparable if negative margins are obtained (Chan, 2007; Landrum, 2007; Scheistroen, 2002; Tantipalakorn, 2009). Following less aggressive surgical resection, 10 percent of patients will develop a recurrence at the ipsilateral vulva, and this may be treated by reexcision (Desimone, 2007).

PREOPERATIVE

Patient Evaluation

Biopsy confirmation of invasive cancer is an obvious necessity. An isolated squamous lesion with less than 1 mm of invasion, that is, microinvasion, may be adequately managed with only wide local excision (Section 41-28, p. 1086). Multiple microinvasive lesions may require skinning vulvectomy (Section 44-26, p. 1335). In general, patients undergoing radical partial vulvectomy do not require reconstructive grafts or flaps to cover operative defects.

Consent

Morbidity after radical vulvar surgery is common. Wound separation or cellulitis develops frequently. Long-term changes may include displacement of the urine stream, dyspareunia, vulvar pain, and sexual dysfunction. Surgeons should be sensitive to these possible sequelae and counsel the patient appropriately, emphasizing the curative intent and limited scope of the operation.

Patient Preparation

Bowel preparation may be indicated with posteriorly located resections. In such instances, bowel preparation will minimize fecal soiling and will also permit initial wound healing prior to the first stool. Prophylactic antibiotics, such as a single dose of cefazolin, are typically given prior to the initial incision. Thromboprophylaxis is administered as outlined in Table 39-9 (p. 962).

INTRAOPERATIVE

SURGICAL STEPS

❶ Anesthesia and Patient Positioning. Radical partial vulvectomy has been performed under local anesthesia combined with sedation in medically compromised patients (Manahan, 1997). However, regional or general anesthesia is typically required.

Inguinal lymphadenectomy (Section 44-29, p. 1343) is typically performed before vulvar resection. Patients may then be repositioned to provide full exposure to the vulva, and the vulva is surgically prepared.

❷ Radical Partial Vulvectomy: Variations. The area of tissue to be removed when radically excising a small cancer depends on the size and location of the tumor (Fig. 44-27.1). The dotted line indicates a planned skin incision for a 1-cm right labia majora tumor with 2-cm margins (left image), a 2.5-cm periclitoral tumor necessitating anterior hemivulvectomy (middle), and (a 2.5-cm midline posterior fourchette tumor requiring posterior hemivulvectomy (right).

❸ Right Hemivulvectomy: Making the Lateral Incision. The planned excision is drawn on the vulva with a surgical marking pen to provide 2-cm margins (Fig. 44-27.2). Tapering the incision anteriorly and posteriorly will aid a tension-free closure. The lateral skin incision is made with a knife (No. 15 blade) into the subcutaneous fat. Forceps are used to place the skin edges on traction and aid electrosurgical dissection downward and lateral until reaching the perineal membrane (Fig. 44-27.3). An index finger can then be

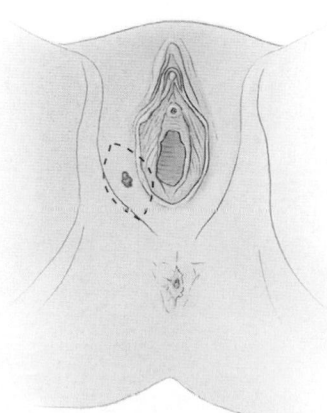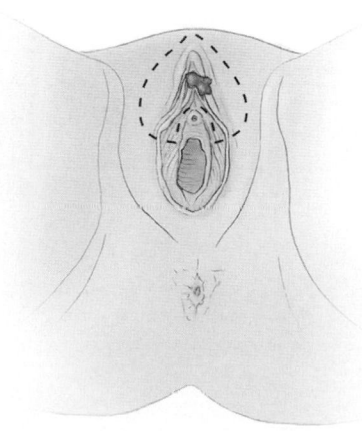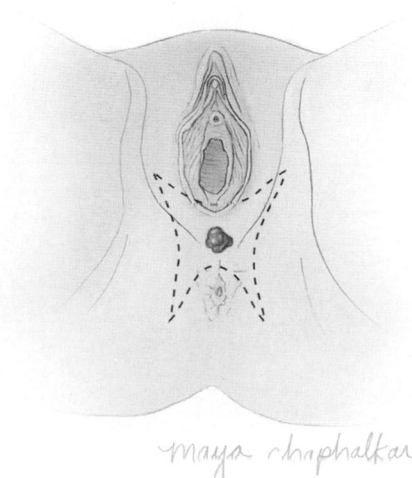

FIGURE 44-27.1 Partial radical vulvectomy: variations.

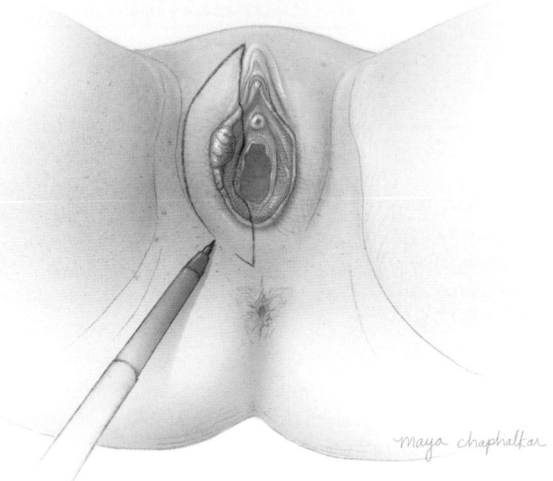

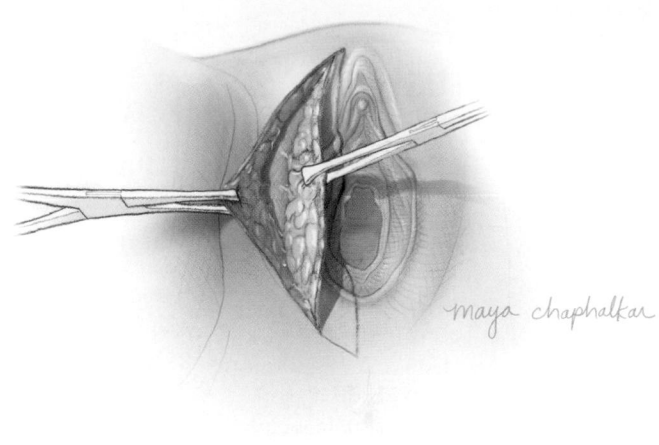

FIGURE 44-27.2 Right hemivulvectomy: outlining the skin incision.

FIGURE 44-27.3 Right hemivulvectomy: lateral dissection to the fascia lata.

used to develop the plane between the fat pad of the labia majora and the subcutaneous tissue of the lateral thigh.

❹ Right Hemivulvectomy: Completing the Resection. The lateral plane that has been developed is mobilized medially by blunt and electrosurgical dissection along the perineal membrane. The skin edge of the specimen is then placed on lateral traction, and the medial (vaginal mucosa) incision is incised from anterior to posterior. The labial fat pad is transected anteriorly, and the entire radical right hemivulvectomy specimen is placed on downward traction to aid final

dissection along the mucosal incision in an anterior to posterior direction (Fig. 44-27.4). The specimen is marked at 12 o'clock and examined to ensure adequate margins.

❺ Right Hemivulvectomy: Closing the Defect. A gauze sponge may be held firmly in the cavity and rolled downward to guide the electrosurgical blade in achieving hemostasis. The defect can then be irrigated and evaluated to determine requirement for a tension-free closure while minimizing anatomic distortion (Fig. 44-27.5). Several pedicles are visible, particularly at the vaginal margin, where vessels were clamped and tied.

In general, lateral undermining of the subcutaneous tissue will provide sufficient mobility to allow primary closure. Interrupted 0-gauge delayed-absorbable suture is used to create a layered reapproximation of deeper tissues. Interrupted vertical mattress sutures, often alternating 0-gauge and 2-0 suture, with knots placed laterally are used to close the skin (Fig. 44-27.6).

❻ Anterior Hemivulvectomy. This variation requires removal of the clitoris and partial resection of the labia minora, labia majora, and mons pubis. The most anterior portion of the incision is first created on the

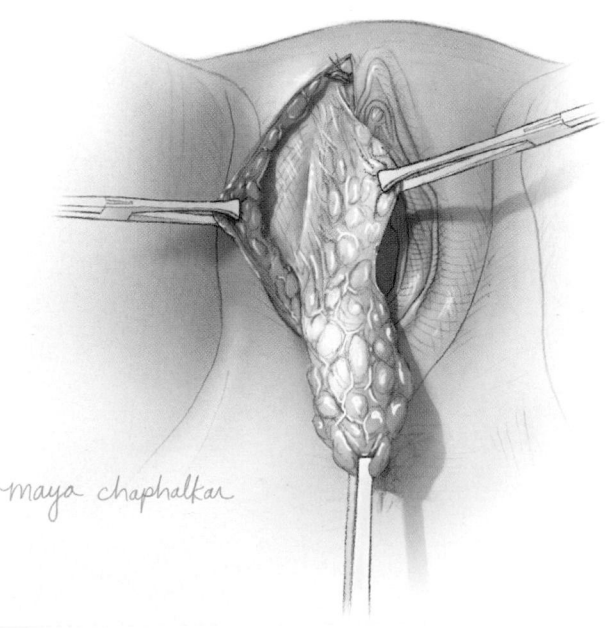

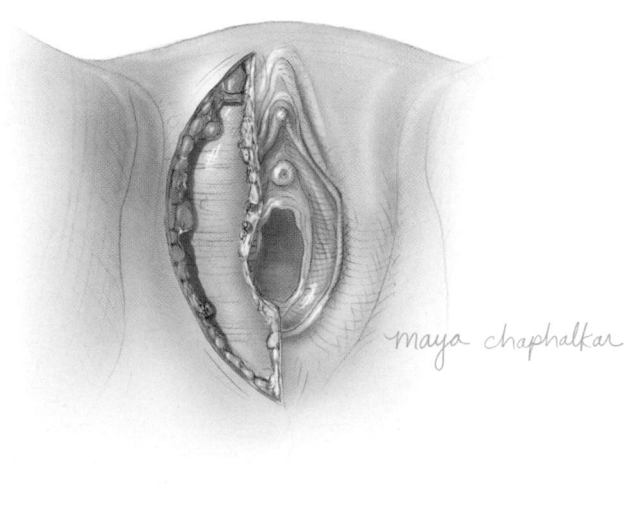

FIGURE 44-27.4 Right hemivulvectomy: removal of the specimen.

FIGURE 44-27.5 Right hemivulvectomy: evaluation of the surgical defect.

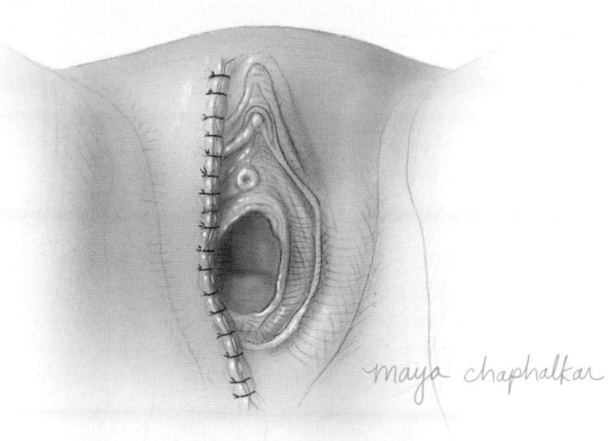

FIGURE 44-27.6 Right hemivulvectomy: closure of the surgical defect.

mons and carried down to the aponeurosis over the pubic symphysis. The specimen is reflected posteriorly to guide dissection. In the midline, the clitoral vessels are separately clamped, divided, and ligated with 0-gauge suture. The posterior incision is made above the urethral meatus, and careful attention to Foley catheter location should avoid urethral injury. Layers of interrupted 0-gauge delayed-absorbable sutures are used to close the defect. Usually, the area surrounding the urethral meatus is left to granulate secondarily.

❼ Posterior Hemivulvectomy. This variation entails removal of a portion of the labia majora, Bartholin glands, and upper perineal body. It is generally necessary to compromise the deep margin in this resection because of anal sphincter and rectum proximity. The skin is first incised posteriorly and a finger is placed into the rectum to guide proximal dissection. The specimen is gradually retracted upward off the sphincter. Dissection proceeds laterally until the anterior margin at the introitus can be incised to complete the resection. The perineal body will need to be reinforced with interrupted sutures of 0-gauge delayed-absorbable material to provide bulk and to allow reapproximation of skin edges for a tension-free closure. Rectal examination should be performed at the end of surgery to confirm the absence of palpable stitches or stenosis. Incontinence of flatus or stool may develop postoperatively despite efforts to preserve the sphincter.

❽ Partial Urethral Resection (Optional). If an anterior lesion encroaches on the urethral meatus, then a distal urethrectomy may be required to achieve a negative margin. Radical partial vulvectomy should otherwise be almost entirely completed. The urethra may be transected anywhere distal to the pubic arch. The length of resection is first measured against the Foley catheter. The meatus is held with an Allis clamp and the specimen placed on traction. The posterior urethra is incised with a knife, and the underlying mucosa is sewn to the adjacent wall with 4-0 delayed-absorbable suture at the 6 o'clock position. The urethral incision is extended laterally with additional sutures at 3 and 9 o'clock, and the Foley balloon is deflated with removal from the bladder. The transection is completed and a final stitch is placed at 12 o'clock. The Foley catheter is then replaced. Alternatively, the surgeon may forgo stitch placement altogether and allow the meatus to heal by secondary intent. Although urethral plication may be indicated in selected cases, resection of 1 to 1.5 cm of the distal urethra does not result in a significant increase in urinary incontinence (de Mooij, 2007).

❾ Final Steps. Suction drains are not typically required but should be at least considered in some circumstances. Copious irrigation is indicated at various times during closure of the defect to minimize infection postoperatively. No formal dressing is applied at the end of surgery. However, fluffed-out gauze

may be placed at the perineum and held in place with mesh underwear to tamponade any subcutaneous bleeding and to promote a clean and dry operative site in the immediate postoperative period.

POSTOPERATIVE

Meticulous care of the vulvar wound is mandatory to prevent morbidity. The vulva should be kept dry by use of a blow dryer or fan. Within a few days, brief sitz baths or bedside irrigation followed by air drying will help keep the incision clean. Patients should be instructed not to wear tight-fitting underwear upon discharge from the hospital. Moreover, instructions should encourage loose-fitting gowns to aid healing and efforts to minimize wound tension. For posteriorly located defects near the anus, a low-residue diet and stool softeners will prevent straining and potential disruption of the perineal incisions.

Typically, the Foley catheter is removed on postoperative day 1 unless a distal urethrectomy was performed or extensive periurethral dissection was required. In these circumstances, the catheter is removed within a few days, after tissue swelling has resolved and obstructive urinary retention is no longer a concern. Early removal prevents ascending urinary infection. When the patient is purposely immobilized to aid healing of a reconstructive graft or flap, the timing of catheter removal is individualized. Moreover, urine that comes in contact with the vulvar incision during normal voiding is not of great clinical concern.

Incision separation is the most common postoperative complication and often will only involve a portion of the incision (Burke, 1995). The wound should be debrided and stitches removed if necessary, while efforts to keep the site clean and dry are continued. Granulation tissue will eventually allow healing by secondary intention, but recovery time will be significantly extended. Although negative-pressure wound therapy (wound vacuum-assisted closure) may be practical in rare instances, the location of most defects precludes effective device placement.

Sexual dysfunction may relate to a sense of disfigurement. Scarring may also result in discomfort or altered sensation that affects a woman's sexual satisfaction. Sensitivity to these concerns will enable a dialogue to develop that can lead to possible management options (Janda, 2004).

44-28

Radical Complete Vulvectomy

If cancers are so extensive that no meaningful portion of the vulva can be preserved, radical complete vulvectomy is indicated over the more limited procedure—radical partial vulvectomy (Section 44-27, p. 1337). The operation is typically performed concurrently with bilateral inguinal lymphadenectomy (Section 44-29, p. 1343). With currently used radical complete vulvectomy technique, intact skin bridges remain between these three incisions (vulvectomy incision and two lymphadenectomy incisions) to aid wound healing. Traditionally, the en bloc incision, colloquially termed the *butterfly* or *longhorn* incision, was used to remove these skin bridges and the underlying lymphatic channels that potentially harbored "in transit" tumor emboli (Fig. 31-7A, p. 800) (Gleeson, 1994c). However, such recurrences are rare, and the en bloc technique has been largely abandoned (Rose, 1999). Thus, the three-incision procedure is preferred because survival rates are equivalent, and major morbidity is dramatically reduced (Helm, 1992).

Removal of an extensive vulvar lesion with an adequate margin and with resection down to the perineal membrane usually creates a large surgical defect. In some cases, wound margins may be primarily closed without tension by undermining and mobilizing adjacent tissues. On other occasions, a split-thickness skin graft, lateral skin transposition, rhomboid flap, or other reconstructive procedure will be indicated to reduce the chances of wound separation.

PREOPERATIVE

Patient Evaluation

Biopsy confirmation of invasive cancer should precede surgery. Depending on the location of the tumor, the clitoral-sparing modification of radical complete vulvectomy is also an option (Chan, 2004). Frequently, patients are elderly, obese, or have significant coexisting medical problems that must be considered.

Consent

Major morbidity is common soon after radical complete vulvectomy, and partial wound separation or cellulitis occurs frequently. Complete wound breakdown is more problematic, and weeks of aggressive hospital care may be required to promote secondary healing. Premature hospital discharge may result in poor home wound care, and resulting tissue necrosis often requires readmission and surgical debridement. Thus, meticulous attention to the wound site while the patient is hospitalized and frequent office visits thereafter are critically important.

Long-term changes may include displacement of the urine stream, dyspareunia, vulvodynia, and sexual dysfunction. Accordingly, surgeons should be aware of possible sequelae and counsel appropriately. Emphasis is placed on the curative intent of the operation and the need for adequate tumor-free margins to lessen local recurrence risks.

Patient Preparation

Bowel preparation may be indicated with posteriorly located lesions. In addition, evaluation of potential graft donor sites is completed. Prophylactic antibiotics, such as a single dose of cefazolin, are typically given prior to making the initial incision. Also, thromboprophylaxis is administered as outlined in Table 39-9 (p. 962).

INTRAOPERATIVE

SURGICAL STEPS

❶ Anesthesia and Patient Positioning. Regional or general anesthesia is required, and inguinal lymphadenectomy is performed first. A patient is then placed in dorsal lithotomy position. Exposure and surgical preparation of the operative field should be planned to accommodate resection and reconstruction. Sites of potential donor graft harvest are also prepared as described in Section 44-30 (p. 1346).

❷ Planning the Skin Incision. The medial and lateral incisions are drawn to encompass the tumor and provide a 1 to 2 cm margin around the tumor. The clitoris is included if necessary. Tapering the incision anteriorly and posteriorly will also aid a tension-free closure (Fig. 44-28.1).

❸ Anterior Dissection. The skin incision begins anteriorly with the knife (No. 15 blade) cutting into the subcutaneous fat. The incision is extended downward approximately three quarters of its length. The remainder of the posterior skin incision is completed later to decrease bleeding. Much of the anterior dissection is described in the preceding section on partial radical vulvectomy (Section 44-27, step 6, p. 1338). However, use of the Harmonic scalpel in this more extensive resection may decrease operative time and blood loss compared with a conventional electrosurgical blade (Pellegrino, 2008). Briefly, the incision is carried down to the pubic aponeurosis. The specimen is reflected downward on traction to guide dissection. The vascular base of the clitoris is clamped in the midline, transected, and suture ligated with 0-gauge delayed-absorbable suture (Fig. 44-28.2). Electrosurgical or Harmonic scalpel dissection then proceeds dorsally off the pubic bone until the medial incision line is reached anteriorly. The medial incision is made above the urethral meatus to avoid injury to the urethra unless a distal urethrectomy is required (Section 44-27, step 8, p. 1339).

❹ Lateral Dissection. Blunt finger dissection is performed to establish a plane lateral to the labial fat pads and at a depth to reach the perineal membrane. The vulvectomy specimen is placed on traction to guide dissection medially to reach the vaginal walls. Vascular vestibular tissue along the sides of the vagina will need to be divided

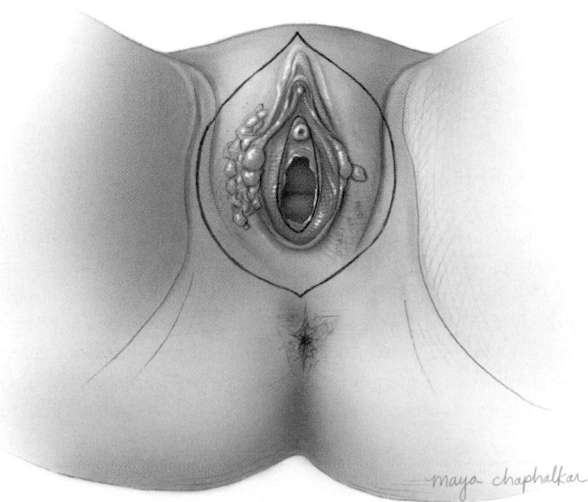

FIGURE 44-28.1 Incisions.

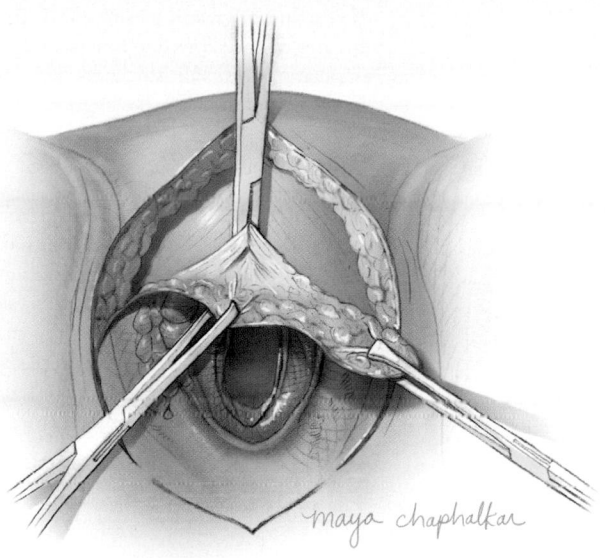

FIGURE 44-28.2 Anterior dissection.

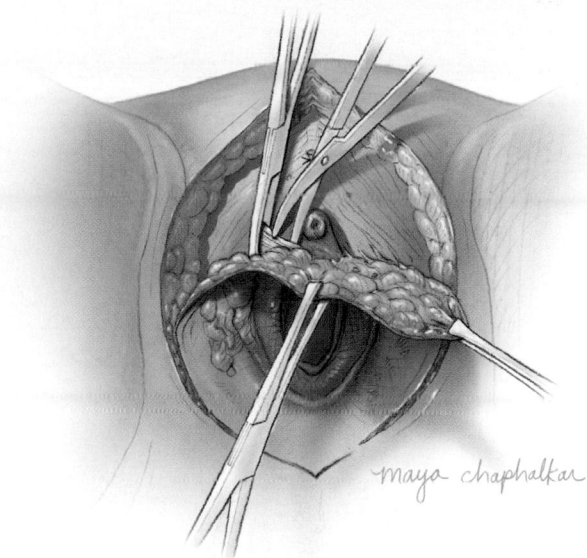

FIGURE 44-28.3 Medial dissection.

with the Harmonic scalpel or clamped, cut, and ligated with 0-gauge delayed-absorbable suture to reduce bleeding (Fig. 44-28.3).

❺ Posterior Dissection. The outer skin incision is completed inferiorly with a knife as the vulvectomy proceeds posteriorly toward the perineal body. A finger is then placed into the rectum to prevent inadvertent injury, and the specimen is now held upward on traction. Electrosurgical dissection along the deep fascia plane extends the outer incisions

toward the midline. The dissection continues anteriorly away from the anus until the medial incision can be made. This completes detachment of the entire complete radical vulvectomy specimen (Fig. 44-28.4).

❻ Evaluating the Specimen. A stitch is placed at 12 o'clock on the specimen to orient the pathologist, and this is noted on the pathology requisition. Skin retraction of the specimen will make it appear narrower and smaller than the defect. However, it

should be carefully inspected to assess its margins. Additional lateral or medial tissue margins can be separately sent if necessary. Alternatively, a frozen section can be requested to evaluate an equivocal margin.

❼ Closing the Defect. The wound is copiously irrigated, and hemostasis is achieved with a combination of electrosurgical coagulation, clamping, and suturing. The defect is then evaluated to determine the best method of closure (Fig. 44-28.5). Undermining

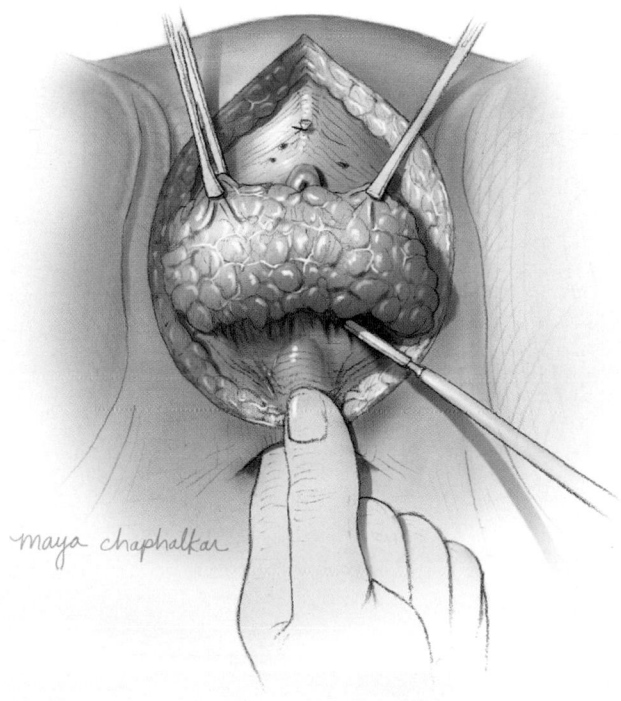

FIGURE 44-28.4 Posterior dissection.

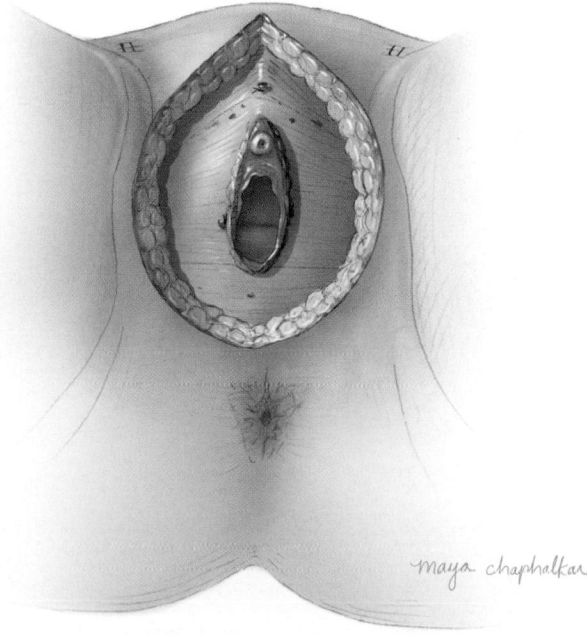

FIGURE 44-28.5 Surgical defect.

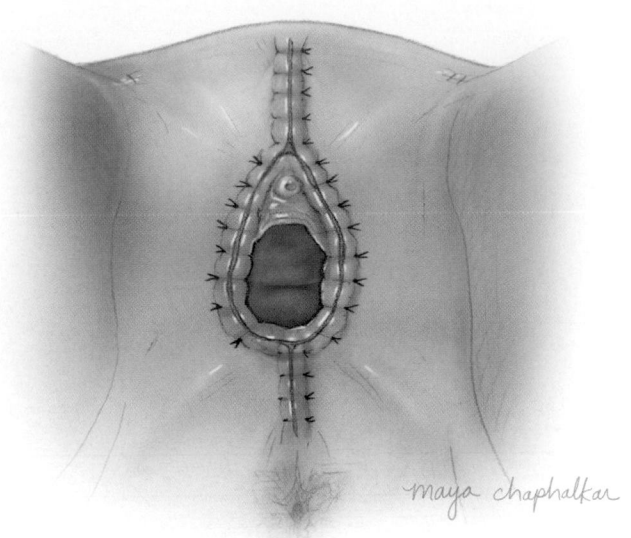

FIGURE 44-28.6 Simple closure.

lateral tissues will aid a tension-free primary closure. Deeper tissues are first reapproximated with 0-gauge interrupted delayed-absorbable suture. The vulvar skin is then closed with 0-gauge, or alternating with 2-0, delayed-absorbable vertical mattress sutures (Fig. 44-28.6). No stitches are placed between the skin and urethra if this displaces the urethra or creates tension on it. Instead, this area can be allowed to heal secondarily by granulation. If a split-thickness skin graft or flap is required to close the incision, the graft is now harvested and placed as described in Section 44-30, p. 1346)

❽ **Final Steps.** Suction drains do not prevent wound infection or breakdown but may be considered in some cases if there is a large defect (Hopkins, 1993). If primary closure is performed, then fluffed-out gauze may be placed at the perineum and held in place with mesh underwear to keep the operative site clean and dry in the immediate postoperative period.

POSTOPERATIVE

If a primary closure is performed, postoperative care is essentially the same as described for patients undergoing radical partial vulvectomy (Section 44-27, p. 1339). Because of a larger operative defect, the likelihood of morbidity is correspondingly increased. Management of reconstructive grafts and flaps is reviewed in Section 44-30 (p. 1347).

44-29

Inguinofemoral Lymphadenectomy

The main indication for removal of groin nodes is staging surgery for vulvar cancer. Inguinal metastases are the most significant prognostic factor in vulvar squamous cancer, and their detection will necessitate additional therapy (Chap. 31, p. 801) (Homesley, 1991). However, the utility of this dissection is more controversial in the management of malignant melanoma, where the presence of positive nodes is generally only of prognostic value. Occasionally, suspicion of inguinal metastases will prompt removal in patients with ovarian or uterine cancer.

The proper extent of an inguinal lymphadenectomy for vulvar cancer is controversial and varies widely. The terminology is also inconsistent. Based on a survey of gynecologic oncologists, the most common procedure is a superficial (above the cribriform fascia) inguinal lymphadenectomy with (40 percent) or without (34 percent) additional removal of some deeper nodes medial to the femoral vein. Fewer practitioners (22 percent) routinely resect all of the deep nodes below the cribriform fascia (Levenback, 1996).

In general, lymphatic drainage from the vulva rarely bypasses the superficial nodes. Therefore, a superficial node dissection with or without selective removal of deep nodes within the fossa ovalis is generally advisable (DeSimone, 2007; Kirby, 2005). Unroofing the cribriform fascia to remove the deep nodes is best avoided due to the unacceptable risks of major morbidity, such as postoperative erosion into the skeletonized femoral vessels by breakdown of the overlying skin flap (Bell, 2000). Moreover, ipsilateral lymphadenectomy is sufficient for patients with unilateral lesions distant from the midline (Gonzalez Bosquet, 2007).

Described in Chapter 31 (p. 800), sentinel lymph node mapping is a promising modality that has demonstrated vast potential in reducing the radicality of detecting inguinal metastases (Van der Zee, 2008). Implementation of this minimally invasive strategy is emerging as the future standard of care for staging vulvar cancer. Currently, it remains under investigation, largely as an experimental option.

PREOPERATIVE

Patient Evaluation

Clinical palpation is not an accurate means to evaluate the groin nodes (Homesley, 1993). Magnetic resonance (MR) imaging and posi-

tron emission tomography (PET) scanning are also relatively insensitive (Bipat, 2006; Cohn, 2002; Gaarenstroom, 2003). Fixed, large, clinically obvious groin metastases that appear unresectable should be treated preoperatively with radiation before attempting removal.

Consent

Patients should understand the need for unilateral or bilateral groin dissection and its relationship to their cancer treatment. They should be prepared for a potentially several-week recovery in which postoperative complications are common and may include cellulitis, wound breakdown, chronic lymphedema, and lymphocyst formation. These events may develop within a few days, several months, or even years later. In contrast, intraoperative complications are less common, and hemorrhage from the femoral vessels is rarely encountered.

Patient Preparation

When both groins are dissected, a two-team approach is ideal to reduce operative time. Prophylactic antibiotics may be administered but have not been shown to prevent complications (Gould, 2001). Thromboprophylaxis is administered as outlined in Table 39-9 (p. 962).

INTRAOPERATIVE

SURGICAL STEPS

❶ Anesthesia and Patient Positioning. General or regional anesthesia may be used. Inguinal lymphadenectomy is performed prior to partial or complete radical vulvectomy (Sections 44-27 and 44-28, p. 1337). Legs are placed in Allen stirrups in low lithotomy position, are abducted approximately 30 degrees,

and flexed minimally at the hip to flatten the groin. Rotation of the thigh a few degrees outward will open the femoral triangle.

❷ Skin Incision. The groin is incised 2 cm below and parallel to the inguinal ligament starting 3 cm distal and medial to the anterior superior iliac spine—aiming toward the adductor longus tendon (Fig. 44-29.1). The incision is 8 to 10 cm long and is taken through full skin thickness and 3 to 4 mm into the fat.

❸ Developing the Upper Flap. Adson forceps elevate and provide traction to the dermal surface of the upper skin edge while a hemostat is opened underneath to begin dissection down through the subcutaneous fat and Scarpa fascia—aiming for a position in the midline of the incision and 3 cm above the inguinal ligament. Dissection proceeds downward until the glistening white aponeurosis of the external oblique muscle is identified. Adson forceps are then replaced with skin hooks to provide better traction.

A semicircle of fatty tissue is rolled inferiorly and laterally along the aponeurosis using electrosurgical dissection and intermittent blunt dissection. During dissection, the superficial circumflex iliac vessels are divided with a Harmonic scalpel or clamped and ligated (Fig. 38-29, p. 945). Additionally, superficial epigastric and superficial external pudendal vessels are divided as they are encountered. Dissection proceeds until the lower margin of the inguinal ligament is exposed (Fig. 44-29.2).

❹ Developing the Lower Flap. The posterior skin flap is now raised in a similar manner to the upper flap. Dissection progresses through the subcutaneous fat to the deep fascia of the thigh—aiming approximately 6 cm from the inguinal ligament toward the

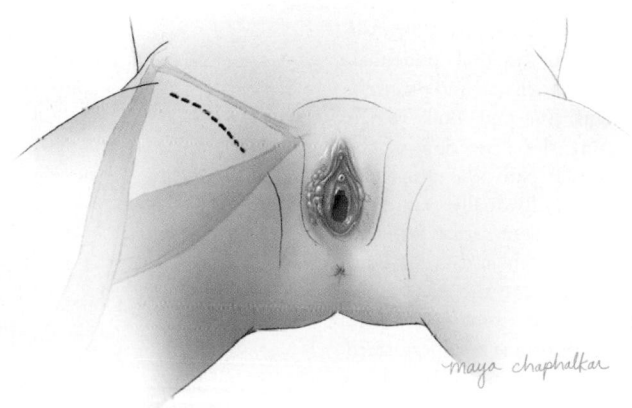

FIGURE 44-29.1 Incisions.

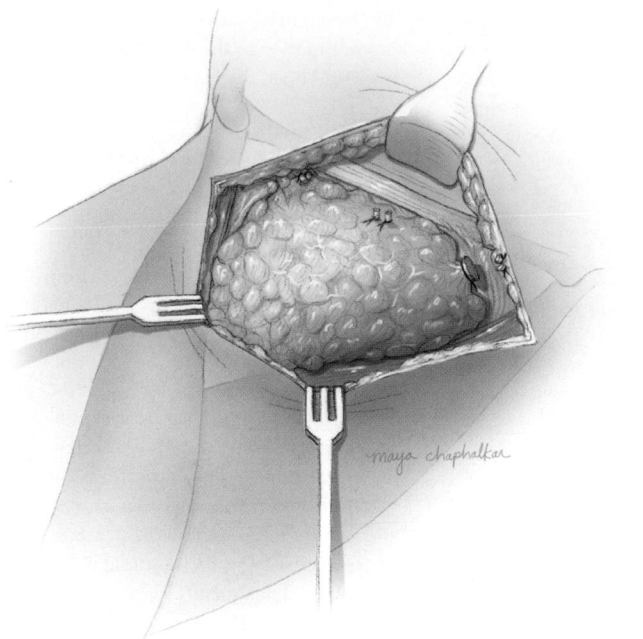

FIGURE 44-29.2 Dissection of the upper flap.

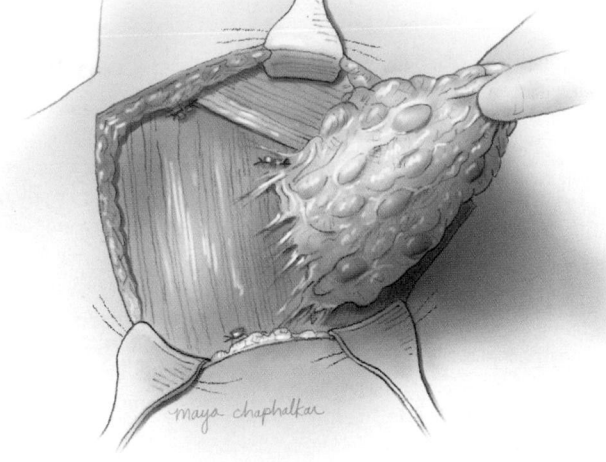

FIGURE 44-29.3 Dissection of the lower flap and removal of the superficial nodes.

apex of the femoral triangle. As shown in Figure 44-29.1, the femoral triangle is bordered by the inguinal ligament superiorly, by the sartorius muscle laterally, and by the adductor longus muscle medially. Blunt finger dissection along the inner portion of the sartorius and adductor longus muscles aids development of the lower flap boundaries. The dissection progressively becomes deeper into the subcutaneous tissue of the thigh, but remains superficial to the fascia lata. The tissue exiting at the apex of the femoral triangle is divided. Dissection is continued circumferentially toward the fossa ovalis (Fig. 38-29, p. 945). Node-bearing tissue is held on traction to aid its dissection. Venous tributaries are ligated as they are encountered.

❺ Removal of the Superficial Nodes. The superficial lymph nodes lie within the fatty tissue at various locations along the saphenous, superficial external pudendal, superficial circumflex iliac, and superficial epigastric veins. The saphenous vein is encountered during the dissection of the medial side of the fat pad. The distal end this vein should be individually transected and ligated with permanent suture for identification. If desired, saphenous vein transection can be avoided, and the vein can be salvaged by dissecting it from the fat pad. Circumferential dissection is next performed to isolate and remove the nodal bundle as it exits the fossa ovalis (Fig. 44-29.3). The proximal end of the saphenous vein should be separately ligated, unless the vessel has

been preserved and can be dissected away from the nodal bundle. Remaining attachments are dissected from the cribriform fascia or clamped and cut to remove the specimen.

❺ Removal of the Deep Nodes. The femoral vein should be visible within the fossa ovalis. The deep groin nodes are consistently located just medial and parallel to this vessel. Of these, Cloquet node is the uppermost. The residual deep femoral

nodal tissue is excised by removing any fatty tissue along the anterior and medial surfaces of the femoral vein above the lower limit of the fossa ovalis. The femoral sheath and cribriform fascia should remain intact if possible.

If a clinically positive deep node cannot otherwise be reached, the cribriform fascia may be unroofed by making a longitudinal incision distally along the overlying femoral sheath (Fig. 44-29.4). Seven or eight underlying deep inguinal nodes are revealed, and

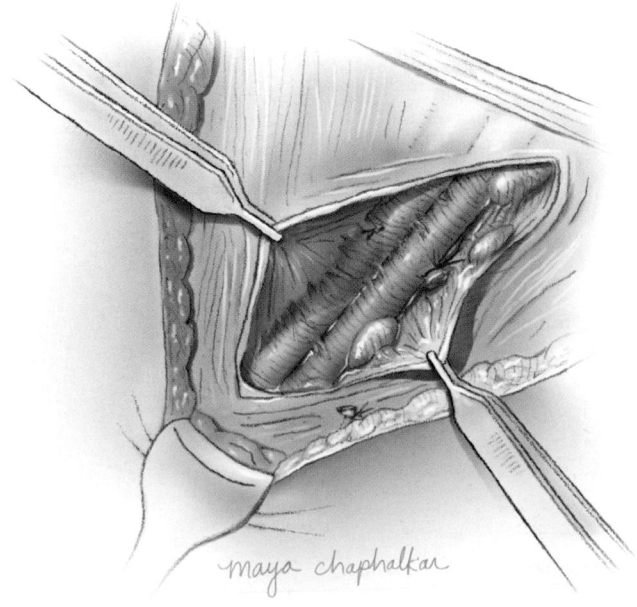

FIGURE 44-29.4 Unroofing the cribiform fascia to remove the deep nodes.

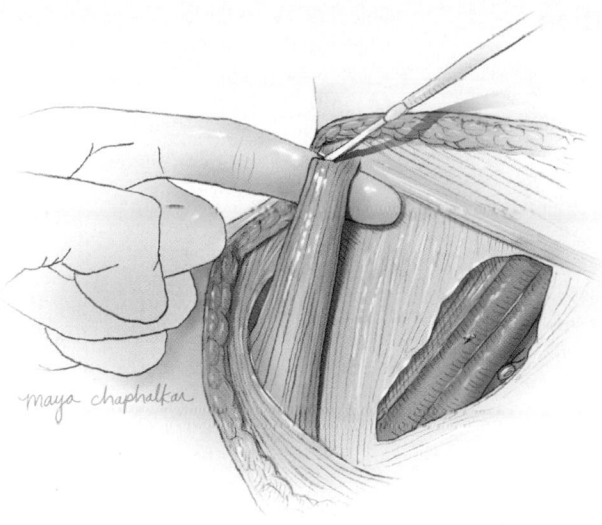

FIGURE 44-29.5 Sartorius muscle transposition.

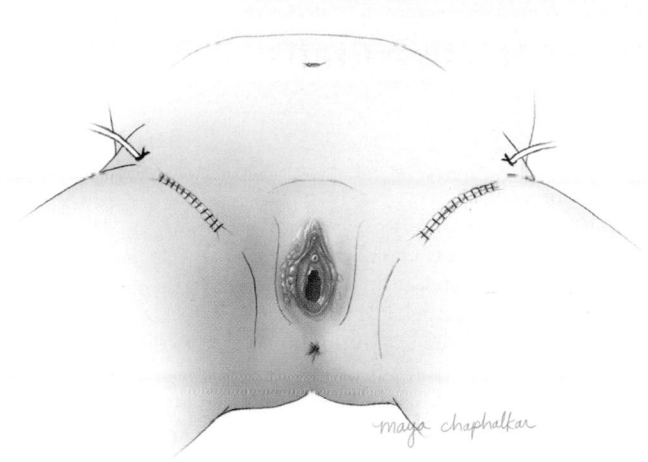

FIGURE 44-29.6 Wound closure.

these deep nodes are typically located in a more orderly fashion than the superficial nodes. Fatty-lymphoid tissue is then dissected from the anterior and medial surfaces of the femoral vein. Following node removal, the femoral sheath edges may then be reapproximated using 3-0 delayed-absorbable suture and/or covered with the sartorius muscle.

❻ Sartorius Muscle Transposition (Optional). The fascia lata is incised to allow blunt dissection of the sartorius muscle (Fig. 44-29.5). The proximal sartorius muscle is then transected at its insertion to the anterior superior iliac spine. A finger is wrapped around the upper part of the muscle to aid electrosurgical blade transection directly off the spine. Transection should be as high as possible with care taken to avoid the lateral femoral cutaneous nerve. The muscle is then further mobilized to cover the femoral vessels and sutured to the inguinal ligament with 2-0 delayed-absorbable suture.

❼ Wound Closure. The surgical defect should be carefully examined, made hemostatic, and irrigated. The groin is closed with layers of delayed-absorbable suture, and a Blake or Jackson-Pratt drain is brought out superolaterally and tied in place with permanent suture (Fig. 44-29.6). Staples are placed to reapproximate skin edges.

POSTOPERATIVE

Suction drainage enables the incision to heal and the underlying space to be obliterated. Drain tubing should be manually milked or stripped regularly with index finger and thumb toward the suction device to prevent blockage. Drains may be removed when output declines to 20 to 25 mL per day. Typically, this requires approximately 2 weeks (Gould, 2001). Premature removal may result in a symptomatic lymphocyst that requires drain reinsertion or outpatient needle aspiration.

The groin incision should be left uncovered and regularly examined. Postoperative complications are very common, particularly wound cellulitis and breakdown. Preoperative radiation and removal of bulky, fixed nodes increase the risk of these complications. Unroofing the deep fascia can also unnecessarily expose the femoral vessels to erosion or sudden hemorrhage. A protective sartorius muscle transposition may be especially indicated in these selected situations to prevent morbidity (Judson, 2004; Paley, 1997).

Chronic lymphedema is another frequent complication of inguinal lymphadenectomy. In most reports, preservation of the saphenous vein has been shown to reduce the incidence (Dardarian, 2006; Gaarenstroom, 2003). Regardless, this condition is typically much more problematic with the addition of groin radiation. Supportive management is meant to minimize the edema and prevent symptomatic progression. Foot elevation, compression stockings, and on occasion, diuretic therapy may be helpful.

44-30

Reconstructive Grafts and Flaps

Primary closure of a vulvar wound is typically not advised if closure of a large defect would create excessive incision tension or if other untoward factors are present. In these cases, a reconstructive skin graft or flap is preferable to a defect healing by secondary intent. In general, the simplest procedure that will achieve the best functional result should be selected.

The decision to perform a split-thickness skin graft (STSG), lateral skin transposition, or rhomboid skin flap depends on clinical circumstances and surgeon experience. Variations of these techniques are occasionally used in gynecologic oncology (Burke, 1994; Dainty, 2005; Saito, 2009). Typical candidates for a skin graft or flap have undergone a large wide local excision, skinning vulvectomy, or partial or complete radical vulvectomy. Myocutaneous flaps, most commonly using the rectus abdominis and gracilis muscles, are used primarily in patients with prior radiation, very large defects, or a need for vaginal reconstruction (Section 44-10, p. 1292). However, a full description of the innumerable types of local flaps is beyond the scope of this section.

PREOPERATIVE

Patient Evaluation

Fortunately, a broad range of operative procedures are available—each with its advantages and disadvantages (Weikel, 2005). The size of the lesion and the anticipated postsurgical defect will largely dictate reconstructive options. In some complicated cases, plastic surgery consultation may be indicated.

Consent

A woman's body image may be significantly altered following extensive vulvar surgery, and sexual dysfunction may be problematic (Green, 2000). When discussing these effects, patient responses vary widely. Some express minimal concern, whereas others are devastated by the thought of a disfiguring result. Accordingly, counseling is individualized, specifically addressing patient concerns.

In addition, wound separation, infection, and wound healing by secondary intention are common complications. Moreover, patients should also be advised that recurrences of their underlying disease may recur within the graft or flap (DiSaia, 1995).

Patient Preparation

Complete bowel preparation is generally indicated for most reconstructions. Because a patient may be relatively immobile postoperatively and the need to prevent wound contamination is absolute, enemas are usually insufficient. In addition, prophylactic antibiotics are typically given. Early ambulation may be detrimental to graft or flap healing. Therefore, to prevent deep-vein thrombosis, use of pneumatic compression devices or subcutaneous heparin is especially warranted (Table 39-9, p. 962).

For patients undergoing STSG, the hip, buttock, and inner thigh should be carefully examined. The selected donor sites should contain healthy skin, be hidden by a patient's clothing postoperatively, and accessible in the operating room. Typically, a graft is taken from the upper thigh.

INTRAOPERATIVE

SURGICAL STEPS

❶ Anesthesia and Patient Positioning. General or regional anesthesia is required. The patient will need to be positioned in dorsal lithotomy with complete access to the vulva, upper thighs, and mons pubis. Sterile preparation of the lower abdomen, perineum, thighs, and vagina is performed, and a Foley catheter is placed. Infrequently, the buttock or hip will be selected as the STSG donor site—this will require additional repositioning.

❷ Evaluating the Surgical Defect. After the vulvar resection has been completed and hemostasis is achieved, the wound is examined to confirm that primary closure is impossible (Fig. 44-30.1). The best graft or flap that will adequately cover a defect is determined.

❸ Split-Thickness Skin Graft (STSG). A dermatome is required to harvest the graft from the donor site when performing an STSG. At a setting of 18/1000ths to 22/1000ths, normal epithelium is harvested from the donor site (Fig. 41-25.1, p. 1075). The STSG is placed in a basin and moistened with saline. The donor site is then sprayed with thrombin (Table 40-6, p. 1005). It is covered with a transparent film dressing (Tegaderm) and wrapped firmly with gauze.

The recipient site is irrigated with antibiotic solution, and hemostasis must be absolute. The graft is then held over the defect and cut to fit so that there is some overlap. Meticulous care is required to smooth graft wrinkles and avoid graft tension. Edges are then sutured to the skin with interrupted 3-0 nylon suture (Fig. 44-30.2). Moistened gauze or cotton balls are placed over the graft and covered with opened and fluffed gauze squares to provide light pressure. To create a stable dressing, a few ties are usually placed through the covering dressing and lateral to the graft site. Alternatively, fibrin tissue adhesives and/or vacuum-assisted closure devices may further augment graft adherence and viability (Dainty, 2005).

❹ Lateral Skin Transposition. In some cases, the skin lateral to the surgical defect is extensively undermined but still may not be able to cover a large defect and reach the medial skin margin. To perform a lateral skin transposition, a surgeon makes separate curvilinear relaxing skin incisions in the upper thigh bilaterally. The relaxing incisions are each undermined laterally out to the dotted line as

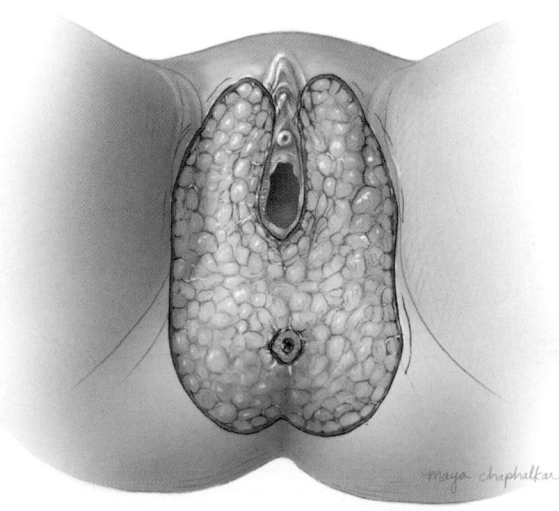

FIGURE 44-30.1 Large vulvar surgical defect.

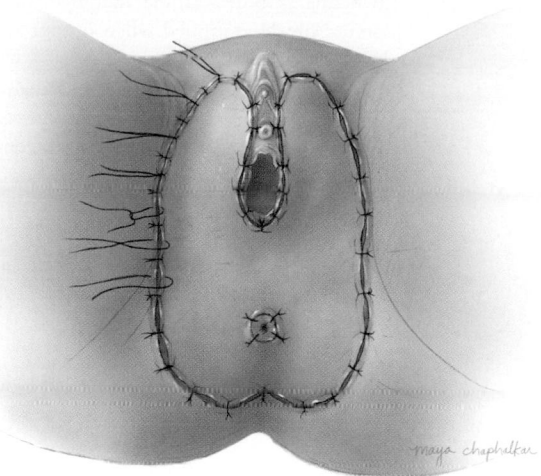

FIGURE 44-30.2 Split-thickness skin graft.

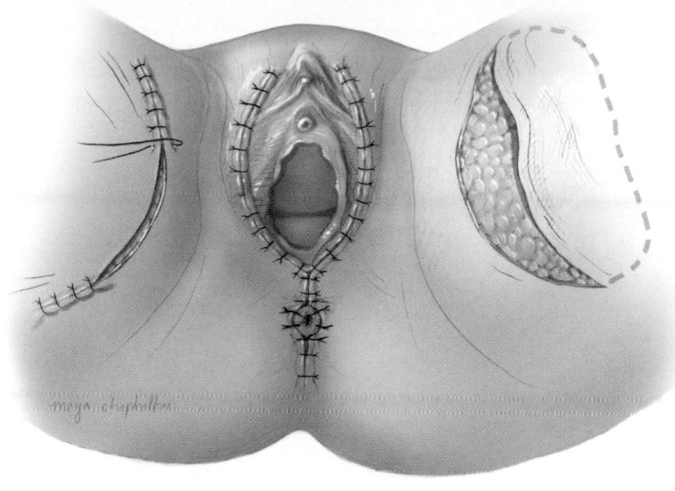

FIGURE 44-30.3 Lateral skin transposition.

shown in Figure 44-30.3. The resulting mobility of the intervening vulvar skin bridge should allow for a tension-free primary closure using interrupted vertical mattress sutures. Lastly, the relaxing incisions are closed with interrupted 0-gauge delayed-absorbable suture.

❺ **Rhomboid Flaps.** A rhomboid is a four-sided parallelogram with unequal angles at its corners. When creating a rhomboid flap from adjacent tissue, a marking pen is used to draw all sides the same length as the short axis of the defect (Fig. 44-30.4, A–C). This minimizes wound tension and prevents necrosis. The diagonal A-C is continued in a straight line onto the adjacent vulvar skin lateral to the defect, and marked so that the

length of AC = CE. The remaining rhomboid sides are drawn in parallel.

Incisions are made through the skin and into the subcutaneous fat. A flap is developed to include underlying fatty tissue and is mobilized medially to cover the surgical defect (Fig. 44-30.5). In repositioning the flap, (as shown by the arrow), line CE is swung medially to appose line AB and secured with stay sutures at the corners CA and EB. Flap edges are reapproximated with vertical mattress stitches using 0-gauge delayed-absorbable suture (Fig. 44-30.6). Typically, excess tissue folding at the corners requires significant trimming or undermining to provide a reasonably smooth contour and is needed to aid closure of the remaining

defects above and below the flap. Finally, a suction drain is placed at the donor site to prevent seromas caused by extensive tissue dissection and which could otherwise result in wound dehiscence.

POSTOPERATIVE

Patients should be kept relatively immobile for the first 5 to 7 postoperative days to prevent tension on the reconstruction. Foley catheter drainage is also continued during these initial postoperative days. A low-residue diet, diphenoxylate hydrochloride (Lomotil), or loperamide hydrochloride (Imodium) tablets will aid healing by delaying defecation and prevent straining (Table 25-6, p. 669).

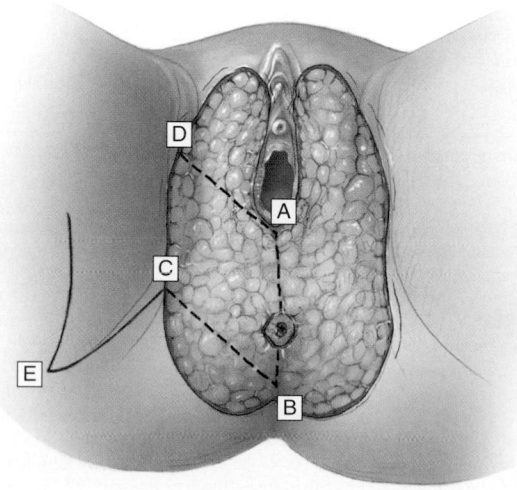

FIGURE 44-30.4 Rhomboid flap: incisions.

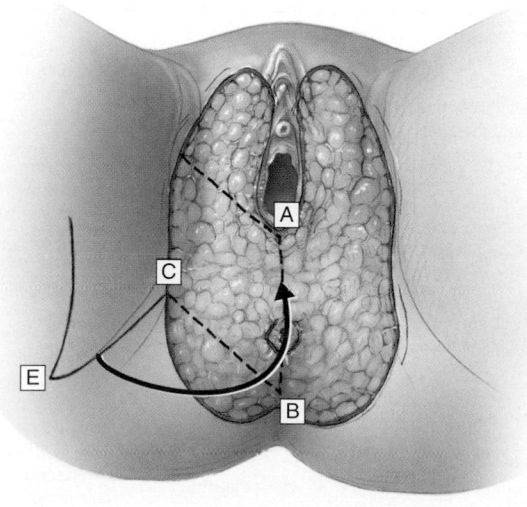

FIGURE 44-30.5 Rhomboid flap: flap positioning.

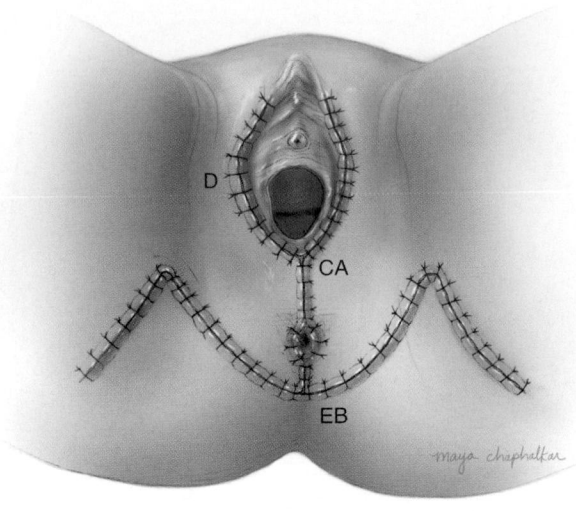

FIGURE 44-30.6 Rhomboid flap: closure.

ischemia is noted at the margins. Suction drains are discontinued when output is less than 30 mL per 24 hours.

Women experience significant sexual dysfunction after vulvectomy. However, the extent of the surgery and need for reconstruction is less important than preexisting depression and hypoactive sexual dysfunction. Accordingly, postoperative psychological counseling and treatment of depression may be particularly helpful (Green, 2000; Weijmar Schultz, 1990).

Thromboembolic prophylaxis should be continued until the patient is ambulatory.

During the first few days postoperatively, the wound should be examined frequently to identify signs of hematoma or infection.

For STSGs, the transparent dressing may be removed from the donor site after approximately 7 days and an antibiotic ointment applied. For skin flaps, positioning changes or release of some sutures may be helpful if

REFERENCES

Abu-Rustum NR, Gemignani M, Moore K, et al: Total laparoscopic radical hysterectomy with pelvic lymphadenectomy using the argon-beam coagulator: pilot data and comparison to laparotomy. Gynecol Oncol 91:402, 2003

Abu-Rustum NR, Rhee EH, Chi DS, et al: Subcutaneous tumor implantation after laparoscopic procedures in women with malignant disease. Obstet Gynecol 103:480, 2004

Aletti GD, Dowdy SC, Podratz KC, et al: Surgical treatment of diaphragm disease correlates with improved survival in optimally debulked advanced stage ovarian cancer. Gynecol Oncol 100:283, 2006a

Aletti GD, Podratz KC, Jones MB, et al: Role of rectosigmoidectomy and stripping of pelvic peritoneum in outcomes of patients with advanced ovarian cancer. J Am Coll Surg 203:521, 2006b

American College of Obstetricians and Gynecologists: Elective coincidental appendectomy. Committee Opinion No. 323, November 2005, Reaffirmed 2009

Angioli R, Estape R, Cantuaria G, et al: Urinary complications of Miami pouch: trend of conservative management. Am J Obstet Gynecol 179:343, 1998

Angioli R, Estape R, Salom E, et al: Radical hysterectomy for cervical cancer: hysterectomy before pelvic lymphadenectomy or vice versa? Int J Gynecol Cancer 9:307, 1999

Ayhan A, Gultekin M, Taskiran C, et al: Routine appendectomy in epithelial ovarian carcinoma: is it necessary? Obstet Gynecol 105:719, 2005

Ayhan A, Tuncer ZS, Dogan L, et al: Skinning vulvectomy for the treatment of vulvar intraepi-thelial neoplasia 2–3: a study of 21 cases. Eur J Gynaecol Oncol 19:508, 1998

Bandy LC, Clarke-Pearson DL, Creasman WT: Vitamin-B12 deficiency following therapy in gynecologic oncology. Gynecol Oncol 17:370, 1984

Barnhill D, Doering D, Remmenga S, et al: Intestinal surgery performed on gynecologic cancer patients. Gynecol Oncol 40:38, 1991

Bashir S, Gerardi MA, Giuntoli RL 2nd, et al: Surgical technique of diaphragm full-thickness resection and trans-diaphragmatic decompression of pneumothorax during cytoreductive surgery for ovarian cancer. Gynecol Oncol 119:255, 2010

Bell JG, Lea JS, Reid GC: Complete groin lymphadenectomy with preservation of the fascia lata in the treatment of vulvar carcinoma. Gynecol Oncol 77:314, 2000

Benezra V, Lambrou NC, Salom EM, et al: Conversion of an incontinent urinary conduit to a continent urinary reservoir (Miami pouch). Gynecol Oncol 94:814, 2004

Berek JS, Howe C, Lagasse LD, et al: Pelvic exenteration for recurrent gynecologic malignancy: survival and morbidity analysis of the 45-year experience at UCLA. Gynecol Oncol 99:153, 2005

Bipat S, Fransen GA, Spijkerboer AM, et al: Is there a role for magnetic resonance imaging in the evaluation of inguinal lymph node metastases in patients with vulva carcinoma? Gynecol Oncol 103(3):1001, 2006

Boruta DM 2nd, Gehrig PA, Fader AN, et al: Management of women with uterine papillary serous cancer: a Society of Gynecologic Oncology (SGO) review. Gynecol Oncol 115:142, 2009

Bouma J, Dankert J: Infection after radical abdominal hysterectomy and pelvic lymphad-enectomy: prevention of infection with a two-dose peri-operative antibiotic prophylaxis. Int J Gynaecol Cancer 3:94, 1993

Bowling CB, Lipscomb GH: Torsion of the appendix mimicking ovarian torsion. Obstet Gynecol 107:466, 2006

Bristow RE, del Carmen MG, Kaufman HS, et al: Radical oophorectomy with primary stapled colorectal anastomosis for resection of locally advanced epithelial ovarian cancer. J Am Coll Surg 197:565, 2003

Buekers TE, Anderson B, Sorosky JI, et al: Ovarian function after surgical treatment for cervical cancer. Gynecol Oncol 80:85, 2001

Burke TW, Levenback C, Coleman RL, et al: Surgical therapy of T1 and T2 vulvar carcinoma: further experience with radical wide excision and selective inguinal lymphadenectomy. Gynecol Oncol 57:215, 1995

Burke TW, Levenback C, Tornos C, et al: Intraabdominal lymphatic mapping to direct selective pelvic and paraaortic lymphadenectomy in women with high-risk endometrial cancer: results of a pilot study. Gynecol Oncol 62:169, 1996

Burke TW, Morris M, Levenback C, et al: Closure of complex vulvar defects using local rhomboid flaps. Obstet Gynecol 84:1043, 1994

Butler-Manuel SA, Summerville K, Ford A, et al: Self-assessment of morbidity following radical hysterectomy for cervical cancer. J Obstet Gynaecol 19:180, 1999

Cai HB, Chen HZ, Zhou YF, et al: Class II radical hysterectomy in low-risk IB squamous cell carcinoma of cervix: a safe and effective option. Int J Gynecol Cancer 19:46, 2009

Cain JM, Diamond A, Tamimi HK, et al: The morbidity and benefits of concurrent gracilis myocutaneous graft with pelvic exenteration. Obstet Gynecol 74:185, 1989

Cantrell LA, Mendivil A, Gehrig PA, et al: Survival outcomes for women undergoing type III robotic radical hysterectomy for cervical cancer: a 3-year experience. Gynecol Oncol 260, 2010

Cardosi RJ, Cox CS, Hoffman MS: Postoperative neuropathies after major pelvic surgery. Obstet Gynecol 100:240, 2002

Centers for Disease Control and Prevention: Recommended adult immunization schedule—United States, 2010. MMWR 59(1):1, 2010

Centers for Disease Control and Prevention: Vitamin B12 deficiency. 2009. Available at: http://www.cdc.gov/ncbddd/b12/index.html. Accessed February 2, 2011

Chamberlain DH, Hopkins MP, Roberts JA, et al: The effects of early removal of indwelling urinary catheter after radical hysterectomy. Gynecol Oncol 43:98, 1991

Chan JK, Sugiyama V, Pham H, et al: Margin distance and other clinico-pathologic prognostic factors in vulvar carcinoma: a multivariate analysis. Gynecol Oncol 104:636, 2007

Chan JK, Sugiyama V, Tajalli TR, et al: Conservative clitoral preservation surgery in the treatment of vulvar squamous cell carcinoma. Gynecol Oncol 95:152, 2004

Charoenkwan K, Kietpeerakool C: Retroperitoneal drainage versus no drainage after pelvic lymphadenectomy for the prevention of lymphocyst formation in patients with gynaecological malignancies. Cochrane Database Syst Rev 1:CD007387, 2010

Chen GD, Lin LY, Wang PH, et al: Urinary tract dysfunction after radical hysterectomy for cervical cancer. Gynecol Oncol 85:292, 2002

Chereau E, Rouzier R, Gouy S, et al: Morbidity of diaphragmatic surgery for advanced ovarian cancer: retrospective study of 148 cases. Eur J Surg Oncol 37(2):175, 2011

Chi DS, Abu-Rustum NR, Sonoda Y, et al: Laparoscopic and hand-assisted laparoscopic splenectomy for recurrent and persistent ovarian cancer. Gynecol Oncol 101:224, 2006

Chi DS, Abu-Rustum NR, Sonoda Y, et al: Ten-year experience with laparoscopy on a gynecologic oncology service: analysis of risk factors for complications and conversion to laparotomy. Am J Obstet Gynecol 191:1138, 2004

Chi DS, Zivanovic O, Levinson KL, et al: The incidence of major complications after the performance of extensive upper abdominal surgical procedures during primary cytoreduction of advanced ovarian, tubal, and peritoneal carcinomas. Gynecol Oncol 119:38, 2010

Chou HH, Chang TC, Yen TC, et al: Low value of [^{18}F]-fluoro-2-deoxy-d-glucose positron emission tomography in primary staging of early-stage cervical cancer before radical hysterectomy. J Clin Oncol 24:123, 2006

Chung HH, Kim SK, Kim TH, et al: Clinical impact of FDG-PET imaging in post-therapy surveillance of uterine cervical cancer: from diagnosis to prognosis. Gynecol Oncol 103(1):165, 2006

Cibula D, Abu-Rustum NR: Pelvic lymphadenectomy in cervical cancer—surgical anatomy and proposal for a new classification system. Gynecol Oncol 116:33, 2010

Clayton RD, Obermair A, Hammond IG, et al: The Western Australian experience of the use of en bloc resection of ovarian cancer with concomitant rectosigmoid colectomy. Gynecol Oncol 84:53, 2002

Cliby W, Dowdy S, Feitoza SS, et al: Diaphragm resection for ovarian cancer: technique and short-term complications. Gynecol Oncol 94:655, 2004

Cohn DE, Dehdashti F, Gibb RK, et al: Prospective evaluation of positron emission tomography for the detection of groin node metastases from vulvar cancer. Gynecol Oncol 85:179, 2002

Cohn DE, Swisher EM, Herzog TJ, et al: Radical hysterectomy for cervical cancer in obese women. Obstet Gynecol 96:727, 2000

Coleman RL, Keeney ED, Freedman RS, et al: Radical hysterectomy for recurrent carcinoma of the uterine cervix after radiotherapy. Gynecol Oncol 55:29, 1994

Cosin JA, Fowler JM, Chen MD, et al: Pretreatment surgical staging of patients with cervical carcinoma: the case for lymph node debulking. Cancer 82:2241, 1998

Covens A, Rosen B, Gibbons A, et al: Differences in the morbidity of radical hysterectomy between gynecological oncologists. Gynecol Oncol 51:39, 1993

Curtin JP, Rubin SC, Jones WB, et al: Paget's disease of the vulva. Gynecol Oncol 39:374, 1990

Dainty LA, Bosco JJ, McBroom JW, et al: Novel techniques to improve split-thickness skin graft viability during vulvo-vaginal reconstruction. Gynecol Oncol 97:949, 2005

Dardarian TS, Gray HJ, Morgan MA, et al: Saphenous vein sparing during inguinal lymphadenectomy to reduce morbidity in patients with vulvar carcinoma. Gynecol Oncol 101:140, 2006

de Mooij Y, Burger MP, Schilthuis MS, et al: Partial urethral resection in the surgical treatment of vulvar cancer does not have a significant impact on urinary incontinence. A confirmation of an authority-based opinion. Int J Gynecol Cancer 17:294, 2007

Desimone CP, Van Ness JS, Cooper AL, et al: The treatment of lateral T1 and T2 squamous cell carcinomas of the vulva confined to the labium majus or minus. Gynecol Oncol 104(2):390, 2007

Dietrich CS 3rd, Desimone CP, Modesitt SC, et al: Primary appendiceal cancer: gynecologic manifestations and treatment options. Gynecol Oncol 104:602, 2007

DiSaia PJ, Dorion GE, Cappuccini F, et al: A report of two cases of recurrent Paget's disease of the vulva in a split-thickness graft and its possible pathogenesis-labeled "retrodissemination." Gynecol Oncol 57:109, 1995

Dowdy SC, Loewen RT, Aletti G, et al: Assessment of outcomes and morbidity following diaphragmatic peritonectomy for women with ovarian carcinoma. Gynecol Oncol 109:303, 2008

Eisenhauer EL, Abu-Rustum NR, Sonoda Y, et al: The addition of extensive upper abdominal surgery to achieve optimal cytoreduction improves survival in patients with stages III-IV epithelial ovarian cancer. Gynecol Oncol 103(3):1083, 2006

Eisenkop SM, Spirtos NM, Lin WC: Splenectomy in the context of primary cytoreductive operations for advanced epithelial ovarian cancer. Gynecol Oncol 100:344, 2006

Eisenkop SM, Spirtos NM, Lin WM, et al: Laparoscopic modified radical hysterectomy: a strategy for a clinical dilemma. Gynecol Oncol 96:484, 2005

Eltabbakh GH, Shamonki MI, Moody JM, et al: Hysterectomy for obese women with endometrial cancer: laparoscopy or laparotomy? Gynecol Oncol 78:329, 2000

Estape R, Lambrou N, Diaz R, et al: A case matched analysis of robotic radical hysterectomy with lymphadenectomy compared with laparoscopy and laparotomy. Gynecol Oncol 113:357, 2009

Fagotti A, Fanfani F, Ercoli A, et al: Minilaparotomy for type II and III radical hysterectomy: technique, feasibility, and complications. Int J Gynaecol Cancer 14:852, 2004

Fayez JA, Toy NJ, Flanagan TM: The appendix as the cause of chronic lower abdominal pain. Am J Obstet Gynecol 172:122, 1995

Fedele L, Bianchi S, Zanconato G, et al: Tailoring radicality in demolitive surgery for deeply infiltrating endometriosis. Am J Obstet Gynecol 193:114, 2005

Fishman DA, Chambers SK, Schwartz PE, et al: Extramammary Paget's disease of the vulva. Gynecol Oncol 56:266, 1995

Fotopoulou C, Neumann U, Kraetschell R, et al: Long-term clinical outcome of pelvic exenteration in patients with advanced gynecological malignancies. J Surg Oncol 101:507, 2010

Fowler JM: Incorporating pelvic/vaginal reconstruction into radical pelvic surgery. Gynecol Oncol 115:154, 2009

Franchi M, Ghezzi F, Riva C, et al: Postoperative complications after pelvic lymphadenectomy for the surgical staging of endometrial cancer. J Surg Oncol 78:232, 2001

Franchi M, Trimbos JB, Zanaboni F, et al: Randomised trial of drains versus no drains following radical hysterectomy and pelvic lymph node dissection: a European Organisation for Research and Treatment of Cancer-Gynaecological Cancer Group (EORTC-GCG) study of 234 patients. Eur J Cancer 43:1265, 2007

Frumovitz M, dos Reis R, Sun CC, et al: Comparison of total laparoscopic and abdominal radical hysterectomy for patients with early-stage cervical cancer. Obstet Gynecol 110(1):96, 2007a

Frumovitz M, Ramirez PT: Total laparoscopic radical hysterectomy: surgical technique and instrumentation. Gynecol Oncol 104: S13, 2007b

Frumovitz M, Sun CC, Schover LR, et al: Quality of life and sexual functioning in cervical cancer survivors. J Clin Oncol 23:7428, 2005

Fujita K, Nagano T, Suzuki A, et al: Incidence of postoperative ileus after paraaortic lymph node dissection in patients with malignant gynecologic tumors. Int J Clin Oncol 10:187, 2005

Fujiwara K, Kigawa J, Hasegawa K, et al: Effect of simple omentoplasty and omentopexy in the prevention of complications after pelvic lymphadenectomy. Int J Gynaecol Cancer 13:61, 2003

Gaarenstroom KN, Kenter GG, Trimbos JB, et al: Postoperative complications after vulvectomy and inguinofemoral lymphadenectomy using separate groin incisions. Int J Gynaecol Cancer 13:522, 2003

Gillette-Cloven N, Burger RA, Monk BJ, et al: Bowel resection at the time of primary cytoreduction for epithelial ovarian cancer. J Am Coll Surg 193:626, 2001

Gleeson NC, Baile W, Roberts WS, et al: Pudendal thigh fasciocutaneous flaps for vaginal reconstruction in gynecologic oncology. Gynecol Oncol 54:269, 1994a

Gleeson N, Baile W, Roberts WS, et al: Surgical and psychosexual outcome following vaginal reconstruction with pelvic exenteration. Eur J Gynaecol Oncol 15:89, 1994b

Gleeson NC, Hoffman MS, Cavanagh D: Isolated skin bridge metastasis following modified radical vulvectomy and bilateral inguinofemoral lymphadenectomy. Int J Gynaecol Cancer 4(5):356, 1994c

Goff BA, Matthews BJ, Wynn M, et al: Ovarian cancer: patterns of surgical care across the United States. Gynecol Oncol 103(2):383, 2006

Goldberg GL, Sukumvanich P, Einstein MH, et al: Total pelvic exenteration: the Albert Einstein College of Medicine/Montefiore Medical Center Experience (1987–2003). Gynecol Oncol 101:261, 2006

Goldberg JM, Piver MS, Hempling RE, et al: Improvements in pelvic exenteration: factors responsible for reducing morbidity and mortality. Ann Surg Oncol 5:399, 1998

Gonzalez Bosquet J, Magrina JF, Magtibay PM, et al: Patterns of inguinal groin metastases in squamous cell carcinoma of the vulva. Gynecol Oncol 105(3):742, 2007

Gould N, Kamelle S, Tillmanns T, et al: Predictors of complications after inguinal lymphadenectomy. Gynecol Oncol 82:329, 2001

Green MS, Naumann RW, Elliot M, et al: Sexual dysfunction following vulvectomy. Gynecol Oncol 77:73, 2000

Greer BE, Koh WJ, Abu-Rustum N, et al: Cervical cancer, version 1.2011. 2011a. National Comprehensive Cancer Network Clinical Practice Guidelines in Oncology. Available at: http//www.nccn.org/professionals/physician-gls/PDF/uterine.pdf. Accessed January 19, 2011

Greer BE, Koh WJ, Abu-Rustum N, et al: Uterine neoplasms, version 1.2011. 2011b. National Comprehensive Cancer Network Clinical Practice Guidelines in Oncology. Available at: http//www.nccn.org/professionals/physician-gls/PDF/uterine.pdf. Accessed January 19, 2011.

Guenaga KK, Matos D, Wille-Jorgensen P: Mechanical bowel preparation for elective colorectal surgery. Cochrane Database Syst Rev 1:CD001544, 2009

Guimarães GC, Baiocchi G, Ferreira FO, et al: Palliative pelvic exenteration for patients with gynecological malignancies. Arch Gynecol Obstet 283(5):1107, 2011

Hallbook O, Matthiessen P, Leinskold T, et al: Safety of the temporary loop ileostomy. Colorectal Dis 4:361, 2002

Havrilesky LJ, Cragun JM, Calingaert B, et al: Resection of lymph node metastases influences survival in stage IIIC endometrial cancer. Gynecol Oncol 99:689, 2005

Hawighorst S, Schoenefuss G, Fusshoeller C, et al: The physician-patient relationship before cancer treatment: a prospective longitudinal study. Gynecol Oncol 94:93, 2004

Hawighorst-Knapstein S, Schönefussrs G, Hoffmann SO, et al: Pelvic exenteration: effects of surgery on quality of life and body image—a prospective longitudinal study. Gynecol Oncol 66:495, 1997

Hazewinkel MH, Sprangers MA, van der Velden J, et al: Long-term cervical cancer survivors suffer from pelvic floor symptoms: a cross-sectional matched cohort study. Gynecol Oncol 117:281, 2010

Helm CW, Hatch K, Austin JM, et al: A matched comparison of single and triple incision techniques for the surgical treatment of carcinoma of the vulva. Gynecol Oncol 46:150, 1992

Helmkamp BF, Krebs HB: The Maylard incision in gynecologic surgery. Am J Obstet Gynecol 163:1554, 1990

Hertel H, Diebolder H, Herrmann J, et al: Is the decision for colorectal resection justified by histopathologic findings: a prospective study of 100 patients with advanced ovarian cancer. Gynecol Oncol 83:481, 2001

Hockel M, Dornhofer N: Vulvovaginal reconstruction for neoplastic disease. Lancet Oncol 9:559, 2008

Hoffman MS, Barton DP, Gates J, et al: Complications of colostomy performed on gynecologic cancer patients. Gynecol Oncol 44:231, 1992

Hoffman MS, Griffin D, Tebes S, et al: Sites of bowel resected to achieve optimal ovarian cancer cytoreduction: implications regarding surgical management. Am J Obstet Gynecol 193:582, 2005

Homesley HD, Bundy BN, Sedlis A, et al: Assessment of current International Federation of Gynecology and Obstetrics staging of vulvar carcinoma relative to prognostic factors for survival (a Gynecologic Oncology Group study). Am J Obstet Gynecol 164:997, 1991

Homesley HD, Bundy BN, Sedlis A, et al: Prognostic factors for groin node metastasis in squamous cell carcinoma of the vulva (a Gynecologic Oncology Group study). Gynecol Oncol 49:279, 1993

Hopkins MP, Reid GC, Morley GW: Radical vulvectomy: the decision for the incision. Cancer 72:799, 1993

Horowitz NS, Powell MA, Drescher CW, et al: Adequate staging for uterine cancer can be performed through Pfannenstiel incisions. Gynecol Oncol 88:404, 2003

Houvenaeghel G, Moutardier V, Karsenty G, et al: Major complications of urinary diversion after pelvic exenteration for gynecologic malignancies: a 23-year mono-institutional experience in 124 patients. Gynecol Oncol 92:680, 2004

Huang M, Chadha M, Musa F, et al: Lymph nodes: is total number or station number a better predictor of lymph node metastasis in endometrial cancer? Gynecol Oncol 119:295, 2010

Husain A, Akhurst T, Larson S, et al: A prospective study of the accuracy of ^{18}fluorodeoxyglucose positron emission tomography (18FDG PET) in identifying sites of metastasis prior to pelvic exenteration. Gynecol Oncol 106:177, 2007

Janda M, Obermair A, Cella D, et al: Vulvar cancer patients' quality of life: a qualitative assessment. Int J Gynecol Cancer 14:875, 2004

Jandial DD, Soliman PT, Slomovitz BM, et al: Laparoscopic colostomy in gynecologic cancer. J Minim Invasive Gynecol 15:723, 2008

Jensen PT, Groenvold M, Klee MC, et al: Early-stage cervical carcinoma, radical hysterectomy, and sexual function: a longitudinal study. Cancer 100:97, 2004

Judson PL, Jonson AL, Paley PJ, et al: A prospective, randomized study analyzing sartorius transposition following inguinal-femoral lymphadenectomy. Gynecol Oncol 95:226, 2004

Jurado M, Bazan A, Alcazar JL, et al: Primary vaginal reconstruction at the time of pelvic exenteration for gynecologic cancer: morbidity revisited. Ann Surg Oncol 16:121, 2009

Jurado M, Bazan A, Elejabeitia J, et al: Primary vaginal and pelvic floor reconstruction at the time of pelvic exenteration: a study of morbidity. Gynecol Oncol 77:293, 2000

Karcaaltincaba M, Akhan O: Radiologic imaging and percutaneous treatment of pelvic lymphocele. Eur J Radiol 55:340, 2005

Karsenty G, Moutardier V, Lelong B, et al: Long-term follow-up of continent urinary diversion after pelvic exenteration for gynecologic malignancies. Gynecol Oncol 97:524, 2005

Kehoe SM, Eisenhauer EL, Abu-Rustum NR, et al: Incidence and management of pancreatic leaks after splenectomy with distal pancreatectomy performed during primary cytoreductive surgery for advanced ovarian, peritoneal and fallopian tube cancer. Gynecol Oncol 112:496, 2009

King LA, Carson LF, Konstantinides N, et al: Outcome assessment of home parenteral nutrition in patients with gynecologic malignancies: what have we learned in a decade of experience? Gynecol Oncol 51:377, 1993

Kingham TP, Pachter HL: Colonic anastomotic leak: risk factors, diagnosis, and treatment. J Am Coll Surg 208:269, 2009

Kirby TO, Rocconi RP, Numnum TM, et al: Outcomes of stage I/II vulvar cancer patients after negative superficial inguinal lymphadenectomy. Gynecol Oncol 98:309, 2005

Kho RM, Akl MN, Cornella JL, et al: Incidence and characteristics of patients with vaginal cuff dehiscence after robotic procedures. Obstet Gynecol 114(2 Pt 1):231, 2009

Ko EM, Muto MG, Berkowitz RS, et al: Robotic versus open radical hysterectomy: a comparative study at a single institution. Gynecol Oncol 111(3):425, 2008

Kohler C, Tozzi R, Possover M, et al: Explorative laparoscopy prior to exenterative surgery. Gynecol Oncol 86:311, 2002

Kraus K, Fanning J: Prospective trial of early feeding and bowel stimulation after radical hysterectomy. Am J Obstet Gynecol 182:996, 2000

Kupets R, Thomas GM, Covens A: Is there a role for pelvic lymph node debulking in advanced cervical cancer? Gynecol Oncol 87:163, 2002

Kusiak JF, Rosenblum NG: Neovaginal reconstruction after exenteration using an omental flap and split-thickness skin graft. Plast Reconstr Surg 97:775, 1996

Lacey CG, Stern JL, Feigenbaum S, et al: Vaginal reconstruction after exenteration with use of gracilis myocutaneous flaps: the University of California, San Francisco, experience. Am J Obstet Gynecol 158:1278, 1988

Landoni F, Maneo A, Cormio G, et al: Class II versus class III radical hysterectomy in stage IBIIA cervical cancer: a prospective, randomized study. Gynecol Oncol 80:3, 2001

Landrum LM, Lanneau GS, Skaggs VJ, et al: Gynecologic Oncology Group risk groups for vulvar carcinoma: improvement in survival in the modern era. Gynecol Oncol 106:521, 2007

Larciprete G, Casalino B, Segatore MF, et al: Pelvic lymphadenectomy for cervical cancer: extraperitoneal versus laparoscopic approach. Eur J Obstet Gynaecol Reprod Biol 126:259, 2006

Law WL, Chu KW, Choi HK: Randomized clinical trial comparing loop ileostomy and loop transverse colostomy for faecal diversion following total mesorectal excision. Br J Surg 89:704, 2002

Leath CA III, Straughn JM Jr, Estes JM, et al: The impact of aborted radical hysterectomy in patients with cervical carcinoma. Gynecol Oncol 95:204, 2004

Lee PK, Choi MS, Ahn ST, et al: Gluteal fold V-Y advancement flap for vulvar and vaginal reconstruction: a new flap. Plast Reconstr Surg 118:401, 2006

Lentz SS, Homesley HD: Radiation-induced vesicosacral fistula: treatment with continent urinary diversion. Gynecol Oncol 58:278, 1995

Lentz SS, Shelton BJ, Toy NJ: Effects of perioperative blood transfusion on prognosis in early-stage cervical cancer. Ann Surg Oncol 5:216, 1998

Leon-Casasola OA, Karabella D, Lema MJ: Bowel function recovery after radical hysterectomies: thoracic epidural bupivacaine-morphine versus intravenous patient-controlled analgesia with morphine: a pilot study. J Clin Anesth 8:87, 1996

Levenback C, Morris M, Burke TW, et al: Groin dissection practices among gynecologic oncologists treating early vulvar cancer. Gynecol Oncol 62:73, 1996

Likic IS, Kadija S, Ladjevic NG, et al: Analysis of urologic complications after radical hysterectomy. Am J Obstet Gynecol 199:644.e1, 2008

Lin HH, Sheu BC, Lo MC, et al: Abnormal urodynamic findings after radical hysterectomy or pelvic irradiation for cervical cancer. Int J Gynaecol Obstet 63:169, 1998

Lin LY, Wu JH, Yang CW, et al: Impact of radical hysterectomy for cervical cancer on urodynamic findings. Int Urogynecol J Pelvic Floor Dysfunct 15:418, 2004

Liu FS, Hung MJ, Hwang SF, et al: Management of pelvic lymphocysts by ultrasound-guided aspiration and minocycline sclerotherapy. Gynecol Obstet Invest 59:130, 2005

Lowe MP, Chamberlain DH, Kamelle SA, et al: A multi-institutional experience with robotic-assisted radical hysterectomy for early stage cervical cancer. Gynecol Oncol 113(2):191, 2009

Maas CP, ter Kuile MM, Laan E, et al: Objective assessment of sexual arousal in women with a history of hysterectomy. Br J Obstet Gynaecol 111:456, 2004

Maggioni A, Roviglione G, Landoni F, et al: Pelvic exenteration: ten-year experience at the European Institute of Oncology in Milan. Gynecol Oncol 114:64, 2009

Magrina JF, Stanhope CR, Weaver AL: Pelvic exenterations: supralevator, infralevator, and with vulvectomy. Gynecol Oncol 64:130, 1997

Magtibay PM, Adams PB, Silverman MB, et al: Splenectomy as part of cytoreductive surgery in ovarian cancer. Gynecol Oncol 102:369, 2006

Malzoni M, Tinelli R, Cosentino F, et al: Total laparoscopic radical hysterectomy versus abdominal radical hysterectomy with lymphadenectomy in patients with early cervical cancer: our experience. Ann Surg Oncol 16(5):1316, 2009

Manahan KJ, Hudec J, Fanning J: Modified radical vulvectomy without lymphadenectomy under local anesthesia in medically compromised patients. Gynecol Oncol 67:166, 1997

Manci N, Bellati F, Muzii L, et al: Splenectomy during secondary cytoreduction for ovarian cancer disease recurrence: surgical and survival data. Ann Surg Oncol 13:1717, 2006

Mariani A, Dowdy SC, Cliby WA, et al: Prospective assessment of lymphatic dissemination in endometrial cancer: a paradigm shift in surgical staging. Gynecol Oncol 109:11, 2008

Marnitz S, Kohler C, Muller M, et al: Indications for primary and secondary exenterations in patients with cervical cancer. Gynecol Oncol 103:1023, 2006

Martinez A, Filleron T, Vitse L, et al: Laparoscopic pelvic exenteration for gynaecological malignancy: is there any advantage? Gynecol Oncol 120(3):374, 2011

Martino MA, Borges E, Williamson E, et al: Pulmonary embolism after major abdominal surgery in gynecologic oncology. Obstet Gynecol 107:666, 2006

Matthiessen P, Hallbook O, Andersson M, et al: Risk factors for anastomotic leakage after anterior resection of the rectum. Colorectal Dis 6:462, 2004

Merad F, Hay JM, Fingerhut A, et al: Is prophylactic pelvic drainage useful after elective rectal or anal anastomosis? A multicenter controlled randomized trial. French Association for Surgical Research. Surgery 125:529, 1999

Miller B, Morris M, Rutledge F, et al: Aborted exenterative procedures in recurrent cervical cancer. Gynecol Oncol 50:94, 1993

Mirhashemi R, Averette HE, Estape R, et al: Low colorectal anastomosis after radical pelvic surgery: a risk factor analysis. Am J Obstet Gynecol 183:1375, 2000

Mirhashemi R, Averette HE, Lambrou N, et al: Vaginal reconstruction at the time of pelvic exenteration: a surgical and psychosexual analysis of techniques. Gynecol Oncol 87:39, 2002

Mirhashemi R, Lambrou N, Hus N, et al: The gastrointestinal complications of the Miami pouch: a review of 77 cases. Gynecol Oncol 92:220, 2004

Morice P, Joulie F, Camatte S, et al: Lymph node involvement in epithelial ovarian cancer: analysis of 276 pelvic and paraaortic lymphadenectomies and surgical implications. J Am Coll Surg 197:198, 2003

Morice P, Lassau N, Pautier P, et al: Retroperitoneal drainage after complete para-aortic lymphadenectomy for gynecologic cancer: a randomized trial. Obstet Gynecol 97:243, 2001

Mourton SM, Temple LK, Abu-Rustum NR, et al: Morbidity of rectosigmoid resection and primary anastomosis in patients undergoing primary cytoreductive surgery for advanced epithelial ovarian cancer. Gynecol Oncol 99:608, 2005

Naik R, Jackson KS, Lopes A, et al: Laparoscopic assisted radical vaginal hysterectomy versus radical abdominal hysterectomy—a randomized phase II trial: perioperative outcomes and surgicopathological measurements. BJOG 117:746, 2010

Naik R, Maughan K, Nordin A, et al: A prospective, randomised, controlled trial of intermittent self-catheterisation vs supra-pubic catheterisation for post-operative bladder care following radical hysterectomy. Gynecol Oncol 99:437, 2005

Negishi H, Takeda M, Fujimoto T, et al: Lymphatic mapping and sentinel node identification as related to the primary sites of lymph node metastasis in early stage ovarian cancer. Gynecol Oncol 94:161, 2004

Nezhat CR, Burrell MO, Nezhat FR: Laparoscopic radical hysterectomy with paraaortic and pelvic node dissection. Am J Obstet Gynecol 166(3):864,1992

Nick AM, Lange J, Frumovitz M, et al: Rate of vaginal cuff separation following laparoscopic or robotic hysterectomy. Gynecol Oncol 120(1):47, 2011

Nunoo-Mensah JW, Chatterjee A, Khanwalkar D, et al: Loop ileostomy: modification of technique. Surgeon 2:287, 2004

Obermair A, Manolitsas TP, Leung Y, et al: Total laparoscopic hysterectomy versus total abdominal hysterectomy for obese women with endometrial cancer. Int J Gynecol Cancer 15:319, 2005

Orlandi C, Costa S, Terzano P, et al: Presurgical assessment and therapy of microinvasive carcinoma of the cervix. Gynecol Oncol 59:255, 1995

Orr JW Jr, Orr PJ, Bolen DD, et al: Radical hysterectomy: does the type of incision matter? Am J Obstet Gynecol 173:399, 1995

Paley PJ, Johnson PR, Adcock LL, et al: The effect of sartorius transposition on wound morbidity following inguinal-femoral lymphadenectomy. Gynecol Oncol 64:237, 1997

Panici PB, Maggioni A, Hacker N, et al: Systematic aortic and pelvic lymphadenectomy versus resection of bulky nodes only in optimally debulked advanced ovarian cancer: a randomized clinical trial. J Natl Cancer Inst 97:560, 2005

Park JY, Seo SS, Kang S, et al: The benefits of low anterior en bloc resection as part of cytoreductive surgery for advanced primary and recurrent epithelial ovarian cancer patients outweigh morbidity concerns. Gynecol Oncol 103(3):977, 2006

Patsner B, Hackett TE: Use of the omental J-flap for prevention of postoperative complications following radical abdominal hysterectomy: report of 140 cases and literature review. Gynecol Oncol 65:405, 1997

Pellegrino A, Fruscio R, Maneo A, et al: Harmonic scalpel versus conventional electrosurgery in the treatment of vulvar cancer. Int J Gynaecol Obstet 103:185, 2008

Penalver MA, Angioli R, Mirhashemi R, et al: Management of early and late complications of ileocolonic continent urinary reservoir (Miami pouch). Gynecol Oncol 69:185, 1998

Penalver MA, Bejany DE, Averette HE, et al: Continent urinary diversion in gynecologic oncology. Gynecol Oncol 34:274, 1989

Pikaart DP, Holloway RW, Ahmad S, et al: Clinical-pathologic and morbidity analyses of types 2 and 3 abdominal radical hysterectomy for cervical cancer. Gynecol Oncol 107:205, 2007

Plante M, Roy M: Operative laparoscopy prior to a pelvic exenteration in patients with recurrent cervical cancer. Gynecol Oncol 69:94, 1998

Prayson RA, Hart WR, Petras RE: Pseudomyxoma peritonei: a clinicopathologic study of 19 cases with emphasis on site of origin and nature of associated ovarian tumors. Am J Surg Pathol 18:591, 1994

Puntambekar S, Kudchadkar RJ, Gurjar AM, et al: Laparoscopic pelvic exenteration for advanced pelvic cancers: a review of 16 cases. Gynecol Oncol 102(3):513, 2006

Pycha A, Comploj E, Martini T, et al: Comparison of complications in three incontinent urinary diversions. Eur Urol 54:825, 2008

Ramirez PT, Modesitt SC, Morris M, et al: Functional outcomes and complications of continent urinary diversions in patients with gynecologic malignancies. Gynecol Oncol 85:285, 2002

Ramirez PT, Slomovitz BM, Soliman PT, et al: Total laparoscopic radical hysterectomy and lymphadenectomy: the M.D. Anderson Cancer Center experience. Gynecol Oncol 102:252, 2006

Rasmussen OO, Petersen IK, Christiansen J: Anorectal function following low anterior resection. Colorectal Dis 5:258, 2003

Raspagliesi F, Ditto A, Fontanelli R, et al: Type II versus type III nerve-sparing radical hysterectomy: comparison of lower urinary tract dysfunctions. Gynecol Oncol 102(2):256, 2006

Ratliff CR, Gershenson DM, Morris M, et al: Sexual adjustment of patients undergoing gracilis myocutaneous flap vaginal reconstruction in conjunction with pelvic exenteration. Cancer 78:2229, 1996

Rettenmaier MA, Braly PS, Roberts WS, et al: Treatment of cutaneous vulvar lesions with skinning vulvectomy. J Reprod Med 30:478, 1985

Richardson DL, Mariani A, Cliby WA: Risk factors for anastomotic leak after recto-sigmoid resection for ovarian cancer. Gynecol Oncol 103(2):667, 2006

Roos EJ, de Graeff A, van Eijkeren MA, et al: Quality of life after pelvic exenteration. Gynecol Oncol 93:610, 2004

Rose PG: Skin bridge recurrences in vulvar cancer: frequency and management. Int J Gynaecol Cancer 9:508, 1999

Rose PG: Type II radical hysterectomy: evaluating its role in cervical cancer. Gynecol Oncol 80:1, 2001

Saito A, Sawaizumi M, Matsumoto S, et al: Stepladder V-Y advancement medial thigh flap for the reconstruction of vulvoperineal region. J Plast Reconstr Aesthet Surg 62:e196, 2009

Salani R, Zahurak ML, Santillan A, et al: Survival impact of multiple bowel resections in patients undergoing primary cytoreductive surgery for advanced ovarian cancer: a case-control study. Gynecol Oncol 107:495, 2007

Salom EM, Mendez LE, Schey D, et al: Continent ileocolonic urinary reservoir (Miami pouch): the University of Miami experience over 15 years. Am J Obstet Gynecol 190:994, 2004

Salom EM, Schey D, Penalver M, et al: The safety of incidental appendectomy at the time of abdominal hysterectomy. Am J Obstet Gynecol 189:1563, 2003

Scambia G, Ferrandina G, Distefano M, et al: Is there a place for a less extensive radical surgery in locally advanced cervical cancer patients? Gynecol Oncol 83:319, 2001

Scheistroen M, Nesland JM, Trope C: Have patients with early squamous carcinoma of the vulva been overtreated in the past? The Norwegian experience 1977–1991. Eur J Gynaecol Oncol 23:93, 2002

Segreti EM, Levenback C, Morris M, et al: A comparison of end and loop colostomy for fecal diversion in gynecologic patients with colonic fistulas. Gynecol Oncol 60:49, 1996a

Segreti EM, Morris M, Levenback C, et al: Transverse colon urinary diversion in gynecologic oncology. Gynecol Oncol 63:66, 1996b

Serati M, Salvatore S, Uccella S, et al: Sexual function after radical hysterectomy for early-stage cervical cancer: is there a difference between laparoscopy and laparotomy? J Sex Med 6:2516, 2009

Sevin BU, Ramos R, Gerhardt RT, et al: Comparative efficacy of short-term versus long-term cefoxitin prophylaxis against postoperative infection after radical hysterectomy: a prospective study. Obstet Gynecol 77:729, 1991

Sharma S, Odunsi K, Driscoll D, et al: Pelvic exenterations for gynecological malignancies: twenty-year experience at Roswell Park Cancer Institute. Int J Gynaecol Cancer 15:475, 2005

Shimada M, Kigawa J, Nishimura R, et al: Ovarian metastasis in carcinoma of the uterine cervix. Gynecol Oncol 101(6):234, 2006

Silver DF: Full-thickness diaphragmatic resection with simple and secure closure to accomplish complete cytoreductive surgery for patients with ovarian cancer. Gynecol Oncol 95:384, 2004

Slomovitz BM, Ramirez PT, Frumovitz M, et al: Electrothermal bipolar coagulation for pelvic exenterations. Gynecol Oncol 102:534, 2006

Smith HO, Genesen MC, Runowicz CD, et al: The rectus abdominis myocutaneous flap: modifications, complications, and sexual function. Cancer 83:510, 1998

Song YJ, Lim MC, Kang S, et al: Total colectomy as part of primary cytoreductive surgery in advanced Mullerian cancer. Gynecol Oncol 114:183, 2009

Sood AK, Nygaard I, Shahin MS, et al: Anorectal dysfunction after surgical treatment for cervical cancer. J Am Coll Surg 195:513, 2002

Soper JT, Berchuck A, Creasman WT, et al: Pelvic exenteration: factors associated with major surgical morbidity. Gynecol Oncol 35:93, 1989

Soper JT, Havrilesky LJ, Secord AA, et al: Rectus abdominis myocutaneous flaps for neovaginal reconstruction after radical pelvic surgery. Int J Gynaecol Cancer 15:542, 2005

Soper JT, Rodriguez G, Berchuck A, et al: Long and short gracilis myocutaneous flaps for vulvovaginal reconstruction after radical pelvic surgery: comparison of flap-specific complications. Gynecol Oncol 56:271, 1995

Spirtos NM, Eisenkop SM, Schlaerth JB, et al: Laparoscopic radical hysterectomy (type III) with aortic and pelvic lymphadenectomy: surgical morbidity and intermediate-term follow up. Am J Obstet Gynecol 187:340, 2002

Spirtos NM, Schlaerth JB, Kimball RE, et al: Laparoscopic radical hysterectomy (type III) with aortic and pelvic lymphadenectomy. Am J Obstet Gynecol 174:1763, 1996

Stefanidis K, Kontostolis S, Pappa L, et al: Endometriosis of the appendix with symptoms of acute appendicitis in pregnancy. Obstet Gynecol 93:850, 1999

Stehman FB, Bundy BN, Dvoretsky PM, et al: Early stage I carcinoma of the vulva treated with ipsilateral superficial inguinal lymphadenectomy and modified radical hemivulvectomy: a prospective study of the Gynecologic Oncology Group. Obstet Gynecol 79:490, 1992

Stentella P, Frega A, Cipriano L, et al: Prevention of thromboembolic complications in women undergoing gynecologic surgery. Clin Exp Obstet Gynecol 24:58, 1997

Swan RW: Stagnant loop syndrome resulting from small-bowel irradiation injury and intestinal bypass. Gynecol Oncol 2:441, 1974

Tantipalakorn C, Robertson G, Marsden DE, et al: Outcome and patterns of recurrence for International Federation of Gynecology and Obstetrics (FIGO) stages I and II squamous cell vulvar cancer. Obstet Gynecol 113:895, 2009

Tebes SJ, Cardosi R, Hoffman MS: Colorectal resection in patients with ovarian and primary peritoneal carcinoma. Am J Obstet Gynecol 195:585, 2006

Tsai MS, Liang JT: Surgery is justified in patients with bowel obstruction due to radiation therapy. J Gastrointest Surg 10:575, 2006

Tsolakidis D, Amant F, Van Gorp T, et al: Diaphragmatic surgery during primary debulking in 89 patients with stage IIIB-IV epithelial ovarian cancer. Gynecol Oncol 116:489, 2010

Uccella S, Laterza R, Ciravolo G, et al: A comparison of urinary complications following total laparoscopic radical hysterectomy and laparoscopic pelvic lymphadenectomy to open abdominal surgery. Gynecol Oncol 107(1 Suppl 1):S147, 2007

Urbach DR, Reedijk M, Richard CS, et al: Bowel resection for intestinal endometriosis. Dis Colon Rectum 41:1158, 1998

Van der Zee AG, Oonk MH, De Hullu JA, et al: Sentinel node dissection is safe in the treatment of early-stage vulvar cancer. J Clin Oncol 26:884, 2008

Vasilev SA: Obturator nerve injury: a review of management options. Gynecol Oncol 53:152, 1994

Wang P, Yuan C, Lin G, et al: Risk factors contributing to early occurrence of port-site metastases of laparoscopic surgery for malignancy. Gynecol Oncol 72:38, 1999

Weijmar Schultz WC, van de Wiel HB, Bouma J, et al: Psychosexual functioning after the treatment of cancer of the vulva: a longitudinal study. Cancer 66:402, 1990

Weikel W, Hofmann M, Steiner E, et al: Reconstructive surgery following resection of primary vulvar cancers. Gynecol Oncol 99:92, 2005

Whitney CW: GOG Surgical Procedures Manual. Gynecologic Oncology Group, 2010. Available at: https://gogmember.gog.org/manuals/pdf/surgman.pdf. Accessed January 23, 2011

Whitney CW, Stehman FB: The abandoned radical hysterectomy: a Gynecologic Oncology Group study. Gynecol Oncol 79:350, 2000

Winter WE, McBroom JW, Carlson JW, et al: The utility of gastrojejunostomy in secondary cytoreduction and palliation of proximal intestinal obstruction in recurrent ovarian cancer. Gynecol Oncol 91:261, 2003

Xu H, Chen Y, Li Y, Zhang Q, et al: Complications of laparoscopic radical hysterectomy and lymphadenectomy for invasive cervical cancer: experience based on 317 procedures. Surg Endosc 21(6):960, 2007

Yan X, Li G, Shang H, et al: Complications of laparoscopic radical hysterectomy and pelvic lymphadenectomy—experience of 117 patients. Int J Gynecol Cancer 19(5):963, 2009

Yan X, Li G, Shang H, et al: Twelve-year experience with laparoscopic radical hysterectomy and pelvic lymphadenectomy in cervical cancer. Gynecol Oncol 120(3):362, 2011

Yang YC, Chang CL: Modified radical hysterectomy for early Ib cervical cancer. Gynecol Oncol 74:241, 1999

Zhu QD, Zhang QY, Zeng QQ, et al: Efficacy of mechanical bowel preparation with polyethylene glycol in prevention of postoperative complications in elective colorectal surgery: a meta-analysis. Int J Colorectal Dis 25:267, 2010

INDEX